PRINCIPLES OF ORTHOPAEDIC PRACTICE

With the editorial assistance of

Steven P. Sampson, M.D.
Assistant Professor of Clinical Orthopaedics
    and Chief of Foot and Ankle Service
Department of Orthopaedics
State University of New York at Stony Brook
    Health Sciences Center
Stony Brook, New York

The Foot and Ankle Section

Lawrence G. Lenke, M.D.
Assistant Professor of Orthopaedic Spinal Surgery
Washington University School of Medicine
Director of Spinal Deformity Surgery
St. Louis Shriners Hospital
Barnes–Jewish Hospital
St. Louis, Missouri

The Spine Section

Keith Bridwell, M.D.
Professor of Orthopaedic Surgery
Department of Orthopaedic Surgery
Barnes–Jewish Hospital
Washington University School of Medicine
Director of Spinal Surgery
St. Louis Shriners Hospital
St. Louis, Missouri

The Spine Section

SECOND EDITION

PRINCIPLES OF ORTHOPAEDIC PRACTICE

Roger Dee, M.D., Ph.D., F.R.C.S. (ENG.)
Chairman of Orthopaedics
Winthrop-University Hospital
Professor of Orthopaedics
Department of Orthopaedics
State University of New York at Stony Brook
 Health Sciences Center
Stony Brook, New York

Lawrence C. Hurst, M.D.
Chairman and Professor
Chief, Division of Hand Surgery
Department of Orthopaedics
State University of New York at Stony Brook
 Health Sciences Center
Stony Brook, New York

Martin A. Gruber, M.D.
Professor of Clinical Orthopaedics and Chief
Division of Pediatric Orthopaedics
Department of Orthopaedics
State University of New York at Stony Brook
 Health Sciences Center
Stony Brook, New York

Stephen A. Kottmeier, M.D.
Chief, Division of Orthopaedic Trauma
Assistant Professor of Orthopaedics
Department of Orthopaedics
State University of New York at Stony Brook
 Health Sciences Center
Stony Brook, New York

McGRAW-HILL

HEALTH PROFESSIONS DIVISION

New York St. Louis San Francisco Auckland Bogotá Caracas Lisbon London Madrid
Mexico City Milan Montreal New Delhi San Juan Singapore Sydney Tokyo Toronto

McGraw-Hill

A Division of The McGraw·Hill Companies

PRINCIPLES OF ORTHOPAEDIC PRACTICE

Copyright © 1997, 1988 by *The McGraw-Hill Companies, Inc.* All rights reserved.
Printed in the United States of America. Except as permitted under the United States
Copyright Act of 1976, no part of this publication may be reproduced or distributed
in any form or by any means, or stored in a data base or retrieval system, without
the prior written permission of the publisher.

345678910   QPKQPK   076543210

ISBN 0-07-016356-1

This book was set in Cheltenham Book by York Graphic Services, Inc.
The editors were Martin J. Wonsiewicz and Muza Navrozov.
The production supervisor was Richard Ruzycka.
The cover was designed by Robert Freese.
The index was prepared by Alan Shaw.
Quebecor Printing/Kingsport was printer and binder.

This book is printed on recycled, acid-free paper.

Library of Congress Cataloging-in-Publication Data

Principles of orthopaedic practice/Roger Dee...[et al.].—2nd ed.
    p.   cm.
    Includes bibliographical references and index.
    ISBN 0-07-016356-1
    1. Orthopedics.   I. Dee, Roger, date–
    [DNLM: 1. Orthopedics.   WE 168 P957 1997]
RD731.P92   1997
617.3—dc20
DNLM/DLC
   for Library of Congress

CONTENTS

PART II   GENERAL ORTHOPAEDICS

PART III   ORTHOPAEDIC TRAUMA

Section 1   General Complications and Principles of Treatment

Section 2   Fractures and Dislocations of the Upper Limb and Shoulder Girdle

PART V   REGIONAL ORTHOPAEDICS

Section 1   The Hip

Section 2   The Knee

PART VI   THE SPINE

Index   1483

CONTRIBUTORS*

Edward Akelman, M.D. [24]
Vice Chairman, Department of Orthopaedics
Chief, Division of Hand, Upper Extremity,
  and Microvascular Surgery
Rhode Island Hospital
University Orthopaedics
Providence, Rhode Island

Hormozan Aprin, M.D. [17]
Associate Clinical Professor of Orthopaedics
State University of New York at Stony Brook
Pediatric Orthopaedic Sugeon
Great Neck, New York

Douglas G. Avella, M.D. [40]
Pediatric Orthopaedic Surgeon
Ridgewood, New Jersey

Marie A. Badalamente, Ph.D. [59, 67]
Professor, Department of Orthopaedics
State University of New York at Stony Brook
  Health Sciences Center
Stony Brook, New York

Louis U. Bigliani, M.D. [55]
Professor of Orthopaedic Surgery
Chief, The Shoulder Service
New York Orthopaedic Hospital
Columbia-Presbyterian Medical Center
New York, New York

Shawn J. Bird, M.D. [13]
Assistant Professor of Neurology
Department of Neurology
University of Pennsylvania School of Medicine
Philadelphia, Pennsylvania

David A. Boone, C.P. [18]
Clinical Instructor
Department of Orthopaedics and Rehabilitation Medicine
University of Washington
Director, Prosthetics Research Study
Seattle, Washington

Christopher T. Born, M.D. [22, 23]
Adjunct Assistant Professor of Orthopaedic Surgery
University of Pennsylvania School of Medicine
Adjunct Clinical Professor of Orthopaedic Surgery
Jefferson Medical College
Associate Professor of Clinical Surgery (Orthopaedics)
UMDNJ/Robert Wood Johnson Medical School
Cooper Hospital/University Medical Center
Camden, New Jersey

J. Richard Bowen, M.D. [42]
Professor of Orthopaedics
Alfred I. duPont Institute
Thomas Jefferson University
Wilmington, Delaware

R. Jay Bradley, Jr., M.D. [14]
Orthopaedic Research Laboratory
Department of Orthopaedic Surgery
Medical University of South Carolina
Charleston, South Carolina

Mark J. Brown, M.D. [13]
Professor of Neurology
Department of Neurology
University of Pennsylvania School of Medicine
Philadelphia, Pennsylvania

Ernest M. Burgess, M.D. [18]
Professor of Orthopaedic Surgery
Department of Orthopaedics
University of Washington
Seattle, Washington

Donald K. Bynum, Jr., M.D. [69]
Associate Professor of Orthopaedic Surgery
University of North Carolina
Chapel Hill, North Carolina

Wesley Carrion, M.D. [32]
Assistant Professor
Department of Orthopaedics
State University of New York at Stony Brook
  Health Sciences Center
Stony Brook, New York

Norris C. Carroll, M.D. [48]
Professor of Orthopaedic Surgery
Northwestern University Medical School
Head, Division of Pediatric Orthopaedic Surgery
Department of Orthopaedic Surgery
The Children's Memorial Hospital
Chicago, Illinois

*The numbers in parentheses following each contributor's name
refer to the chapter(s) written or co-written by that contributor.

Edmund Y. S. Chao, Ph.D. [14]
Professor of Orthopaedic Surgery
Orthopaedic Biomechanics Laboratory
Department of Orthopaedic Surgery
The Johns Hopkins University Medical School
Baltimore, Maryland

Michael P. Chapman, M.D. [72]
Attending Orthopaedic Spine Surgeon
Mercy Hospital of Dubuque
Finley Hospital of Dubuque
Musculoskeletal Center
Dubuque, Iowa

Stuart Cherney, M.D. [51]
Assistant Clinical Professor
Department of Orthopaedics
State University of New York at Stony Brook
Stony Brook, New York

Stephen F. Conti, M.D. [53, 54]
Assistant Professor and Chief
Division of Foot and Ankle Surgery
Department of Orthopaedics
University of Pittsburgh School of Medicine
Pittsburgh, Pennsylvania

Michael P. Coyle, Jr., M.D. [68]
Clinical Professor of Surgery
Co-Director, Hand Surgical Service
University Orthopaedic Associates, P.A.
New Brunswick, New Jersey

Burke A. Cunha, M.D. [17]
Professor of Medicine
State University of New York at Stony Brook
   School of Medicine
Stony Brook, New York
Chief, Infectious Disease Division
Vice Chairman, Department of Medicine
Winthrop-University Hospital
Mineola, New York

David A. Cutcliffe, M.D. [65]
Hand Fellow in Orthopaedic Surgery
Department of Orthopaedics
State University of New York at Stony Brook
Stony Brook, New York

Alexander Bee Dagum, M.D., F.R.C.S. (C) [64, 67]
Lecturer, Department of Surgery
University of Toronto
Co-Director of Research, The Toronto Hand Program
Attending Plastic Surgeon
St. Michael's Hospital
Attending Hand and Microsurgeon
The Toronto Hospital
Toronto, Ontario, Canada

Christian H. Dee, M.D. [56]
Clinical Instructor of Orthopaedic Surgery
Department of Orthopaedic Surgery
University of California Medical Center
San Francisco, California

Roger Dee, M.D., Ph.D., F.R.C.S. (Eng.) [3, 17, 32, 38, 39, 41, 49, 56]
Chairman of Orthopaedics
Winthrop-University Hospital
Professor of Orthopaedics
Department of Orthopaedic Surgery
State University of New York at Stony Brook
   Health Sciences Center
Stony Brook, New York

William G. DeLong, Jr., M.D. [21, 22]
Associate Professor of Surgery
Robert Wood Johnson Medical School
Chief, Division of Orthopaedic Surgery
Cooper Hospital/University Medical Center
Camden, New Jersey

Gina C. Del Savio, M.D. [57]
Robert E. Carroll Hand Fellow
New York Orthopaedic Hospital
Columbia-Presbyterian Medical Center
New York, New York

Harold M. Dick, M.D. [62]
Attending in Orthopaedic Surgery
Professor and Chairman
Department of Orthopaedic Surgery
Columbia-Presbyterian Medical Center
New York, New York

Frank DiMaio, M.D. [49]
Orthopaedic Surgeon
Garden City Medical Center
Garden City, New York

James C. Drennan, M.D. [47]
Professor of Orthopaedics and Pediatrics
University of New Mexico School of Medicine
Medical Director/CEO
Carrie Tingley Hospital
University of New Mexico Health Sciences Center
Albuquerque, New Mexico

Kenneth A. Egol, M.D. [26]
Resident, Department of Orthopaedic Surgery
Hospital for Joint Diseases
New York, New York

Robert E. Eilert, M.D. [46]
Professor of Orthopaedic Surgery
University of Colorado Health Sciences Center
Chairman, Department of Orthopaedic Surgery
The Children's Hospital
Denver, Colorado

Thomas A. Einhorn, M.D. [7]
Professor of Orthopaedics
Director, Orthopaedic Research
Mount Sinai Medical Center
New York, New York

Jerry L. Ellstein, M.D., F.A.C.S. [58]
Clinical Professor of Orthopaedic Surgery
Department of Orthopaedics
State University of New York at Stony Brook
Attending Staff
Huntington Hospital
Huntington, New York

Christopher H. Evans, Ph.D. [10]
Henry J. Mankin Professor of Orthopaedic Surgery
Professor of Molecular Genetics and Biochemistry
Department of Orthopaedic Surgery
University of Pittsburgh Medical Center
Musculoskeletal Research Center
Pittsburgh, Pennsylvania

Kathleen Finzel, M.D. [15]
Co-Director, Musculoskeletal Radiology
Assistant Professor of Radiology
State University of New York at Stony Brook
    Health Sciences Center
Stony Brook, New York

Cyril B. Frank, M.D., F.R.C.S.(C) [11]
Professor, Department of Surgery
University of Calgary
Calgary, Alberta, Canada

Gary E. Friedlaender, M.D. [8]
Professor and Chairman
Department of Orthopaedics and Rehabilitation
Yale University School of Medicine
Chief, Orthopaedics and Rehabilitation
Yale–New Haven Hospital
New Haven, Connecticut

Richard J. Friedman, M.D., F.R.C.S. (C) [14]
Professor of Orthopaedic Surgery
Attending in Orthopaedic Surgery
Department of Orthopaedic Surgery
Medical University of South Carolina
Charleston, South Carolina

Freddie H. Fu, M.D. [50]
Blue Cross Professor of Orthopaedic Surgery
Executive Vice Chairman and Professor
Department of Orthopaedic Surgery
University of Pittsburgh
Medical Director
Center for Sports Medicine
University of Pittsburgh Medical Center
Pittsburgh, Pennsylvania

Abraham Ganel, M.D. [37]
Sheba Medical Center
Tel Hashomer
Sackler School of Medicine
Tel Aviv University
Tel Aviv, Israel

Timothy M. Ganey, Ph.D. [45]
Director for Orthopaedic Research
Georgia Baptist Medical Center
Atlanta, Georgia

Francis H. Gannon, M.D. [4]
Attending, Surgical Pathology
Assistant Professor of Pathology
Department of Pathology
Hospital of the University of Pennsylvania
Philadelphia, Pennsylvania

William E. Garrett, Jr., M.D., Ph.D. [12]
Professor of Orthopaedic Surgery
Assistant Professor of Cell Biology
Duke University Medical Center
Durham, North Carolina

Robert Y. Garroway, M.D. [66]
Assistant Professor of Clinical Orthopaedics
State University of New York at Stony Brook
Stony Brook, New York
Assistant Chief of Orthopaedics
South Nassau Communities Hospital
Oceanside, New York

Daniel E. Gelb, M.D. [71]
Department of Orthopaedics and Rehabilitation
The Milton S. Hershey Medical Center
Hershey, Pennsylvania

Evan R. Geller, M.D., F.A.C.S. [19]
Associate Professor of Surgery
Chief of Trauma
St. Charles Hospital
Port Jefferson, New York

Joan T. Gold, M.D. [18]
Clinical Director of Children's Rehabilitation Services
Associate Clinical Professor of Rehabilitation Medicine
The Howard A. Rusk Institute of Rehabilitation Medicine
New York University Medical Center
New York, New York

Antoni B. Goral, M.D. [5]
Montgomery Orthopaedics, PA
Rockville, Maryland

Dennis P. Grogan, M.D. [36, 37]
Chief of Staff
Associate Clinical Professor
Department of Orthopaedics
Shriners Hospital for Children
Tampa, Florida

Martin A. Gruber, M.D. [39, 40, 41]
Professor of Clinical Orthopaedics and Chief
Division of Pediatric Orthopaedics
Department of Orthopaedics
State University of New York at Stony Brook
    Health Sciences Center
Stony Brook, New York

Kenneth J. Guidera, M.D. [45]
Associate Clinical Professor
University of South Florida
Assistant Chief of Staff
Shriners Hospital for Children
Tampa, Florida

James T. Guille, M.D. [42]
Resident in Orthopaedic Surgery
Department of Orthopaedic Surgery
Allegheny University Hospitals–Center City
Philadelphia, Pennsylvania

Matthew F. Halsey, M.D. [2, 32]
Clinical Instructor
Department of Orthopaedics
State University of New York at Stony Brook
   Health Sciences Center
Stony Brook, New York

Christopher L. Hamill, M.D. [73, 74]
Orthopaedic Surgeon
Simmons Orthopaedic Spine Associates
Buffalo, New York

Robert M. Henshaw, M.D. [16]
Consultant, Surgical Branch
National Institutes of Health
Bethesda, Maryland
Junior Faculty, Orthopaedic Oncology
Department of Orthopaedic Oncology
The Washington Cancer Institute
   at Washington Hospital Center
Washington, D.C.

Kevin A. Hildebrand, M.D., F.R.C.S. (C) [11]
Post Doctoral Research Fellow
Alberta Heritage Clinical Fellow
Musculoskeletal Research Center
University of Pittsburgh Medical Center
Pittsburgh, Pennsylvania

M. Mark Hoffer, M.D. [33]
Lowman Professor
Orthopaedic Hospital
University of Southern California
Los Angeles, California

John D. Hsu, M.D. [35]
Chairman, Department of Surgery
Chief of Orthopaedics
Clinical Professor of Orthopaedics
University of Southern California School of Medicine
Downey, California

Gregory L. Hung, M.D. [53, 54]
Clinical Instructor in Orthopaedic Surgery
University Orthopaedics
University of Pittsburgh Medical Center
Pittsburgh, Pennsylvania

Lawrence C. Hurst, M.D. [59, 65, 67]
Chairman and Professor
Chief, Division of Hand Surgery
Department of Orthopaedics
State University of New York at Stony Brook
   Health Sciences Center
Stony Brook, New York

Eric T. Johnson, M.D. [21]
White Clay Creek Medical Center
Newark, Delaware

Frederick S. Kaplan, M.D. [4]
Associate Professor of Orthopaedic Surgery and Medicine
Chief of Metabolic Bone Disease Service
Department of Orthopaedic Surgery
Hospital of the University of Pennsylvania
Philadelphia, Pennsylvania

Donald M. Kastenbaum, M.D. [40]
Orthopaedic Surgeon
Private office
New York, New York

Kenneth Keller, M.D. [44]
Clinical Instructor
Department of Orthopaedics
State University of New York at Stony Brook
Stony Brook, New York

Donald T. Kirkendall, Ph.D. [12]
Assistant Clinical Professor
Department of Physical and Occupational Therapy
Duke University Medical Center
Durham, North Carolina

Natalie C. Klein, M.D., Ph.D. [17]
Assistant Professor of Medicine
State University of New York at Stony Brook
   School of Medicine
Stony Brook, New York
Associate Director, Infectious Disease Division
Winthrop-University Hospital
Mineola, New York

Stephen A. Kottmeier, M.D. [27, 28]
Chief, Division of Orthopaedic Trauma
Assistant Professor of Orthopaedics
Department of Orthopaedics
State University of New York at Stony Brook
   Health Sciences Center
Stony Brook, New York

Kenneth J. Koval, M.D. [26]
Assistant Professor
New York University Medical School
Chief, Fracture Service
Hospital for Joint Diseases
New York, New York

Klaus E. Kuettner, Ph.D. [9]
Professor and Chairman
Department of Biochemistry
Associate Dean of Basic Sciences and Research
Rush Medical College
Chicago, Illinois

Peter Larcom, M.D. [52]
Fellow on Joint Reconstruction Service
University of Pennsylvania Medical Center
Philadelphia, Pennsylvania

Joseph P. Leddy, M.D. [60]
Clinical Professor and Chief
Section of Hand Surgery
Division of Orthopaedics
Department of Surgery
University of Medicine and Dentistry of New Jersey
Robert Wood Johnson Medical School
New Brunswick, New Jersey

Timothy P. Leddy, M.D. [60]
Orthopaedic Surgery Resident
Division of Orthopaedic Surgery
Robert Wood Johnson Medical School
University of Medicine and Dentistry of New Jersey
New Brunswick, New Jersey

Steven J. Lee, M.D. [65]
Assistant Clinical Instructor of Orthopaedic Surgery
Department of Orthopaedics
State University of New York at Stony Brook
Stony Brook, New York

Wallace B. Lehman, M.D. [40]
Chief, Pediatric Orthopaedic Surgeon
Hospital for Joint Diseases
New York, New York

Lawrence G. Lenke, M.D. [70, 75]
Assistant Professor of Orthopaedic Spinal Surgery
Washington University School of Medicine
Director of Spinal Deformity Surgery
St. Louis Shriners Hospital
Barnes–Jewish Hospital
St. Louis, Missouri

John J. Leppard, M.D. [61]
Assistant Clinical Professor
Department of Orthopaedics
State University of New York at Stony Brook
Stony Brook, New York
Chief, Division of Orthopaedics
North Shore University at Plainview
Woodbury, New York

Merv Letts, M.D., F.R.C.S.(C) [43]
Professor and Head, Division of Orthopaedics
University of Ottawa
Head, Department of Surgery
Children's Hospital of Eastern Ontario
Ottawa, Ontario, Canada

Roger N. Levy, M.D. [6]
Chief of Arthritis Surgery
Clinical Professor of Orthopaedic Surgery
Mount Sinai Medical Center
New York, New York

Paul A. Lotke, M.D. [52]
Professor of Orthopaedic Surgery
Department of Orthopaedic Surgery
University of Pennsylvania Medical Center
Philadelphia, Pennsylvania

Martin M. Malawer, M.D. [16]
Professor of Orthopaedic Surgery
George Washington University
Consultant, Surgery Branch
National Cancer Institute
National Institutes of Health
Director, Orthopaedic Oncology
Washington Cancer Institute
  at the Washington Hospital Center
Washington, D.C.

Fred C. McCue III, M.D. [66]
Alfred R. Shands Professor of Orthopaedic Surgery
  and Plastic Surgery of the Hand
Director, Division of Sports Medicine and Hand Surgery
University of Virginia
Charlottesville, Virginia

Kenneth McLeod, Ph.D. [2]
Associate Professor of Orthopaedics and Physiology
Musculoskeletal Research Laboratory
Department of Orthopaedics
State University of New York at Stony Brook
  Health Sciences Center
Stony Brook, New York

Theodore T. Miller, M.D. [15]
Assistant Professor of Radiology
New York University School of Medicine
Attending Radiologist and Director
North Shore Radiology at the Musculoskeletal Institute
North Shore University Hospital
Great Neck, New York

M. Ather Mirza, M.D. [64]
Assistant Clinical Professor of Orthopaedics
State University of New York at Stony Brook
Stony Brook, New York
Hand Surgery Service
  at St. John's Hospital
Smithtown, New York

Juergen Mollenhauer, Ph.D., D.Sc.(Med.) [9]
Associate Professor
Department of Biochemistry
Rush Medical College
Chicago, Illinois

Michael F. O'Brien, M.D. [70]
Assistant Clinical Professor
University of Colorado
Lutheran Medical Center
St. Anthony's Hospital North
North Suburban Medical Center
Denver Orthopaedic Specialists
Wheat Ridge, Colorado

John A. Ogden, M.D. [45]
Clinical Professor of Orthopaedics
Emory University
Director of Orthopaedics
Georgia Baptist Medical Center
Atlanta, Georgia

Robert Pae, M.D. [49]
Clinical Instructor
Department of Orthopaedics
State University of New York at Stony Brook
   Health Sciences Center
Stony Brook, New York

Wayne T. Pan, M.D. [22]
Orthopaedic Resident
University of Pennsylvania School of Medicine
Cooper Hospital University Medical Center
Camden, New Jersey

Gregory M. Pastores, M.D. [6]
Assistant Professor of Human Genetics
Director, Comprehensive Gaucher Disease Program
Mt. Sinai School of Medicine
New York, New York

Stuart Polisner, M.D. [32]
Assistant Clinical Professor of Orthopaedics
Department of Orthopaedics
State University of New York at Stony Brook
Stony Brook, New York
Pediatric Orthopaedic Surgeon
Comack, New York

Thomas M. Reilly, M.D. [23]
Hospital of the University of Pennsylvania
University of Medicine and Dentistry of New Jersey
Robert Wood Johnson Medical School
Camden, New Jersey

Michael D. Ries, M.D. [56]
Orthopaedic Surgeon
Bassett Hospital
Bassett Healthcare
Cooperstown, New York

Mark W. Rodosky, M.D. [20, 55]
Assistant Professor of Orthopaedic Surgery
The Shoulder Service
Minneapolis Sports Medicine Center
University of Minnesota
Minneapolis, Minnesota

Samuel R. Rosenfeld, M.D. [34]
Assistant Clinical Professor
University of California, Irvine
Director, Spina Bifida Clinic
Rancho Los Amigos Medical Center
Orange, California

Melvin P. Rosenwasser, M.D. [57]
Associate Professor of Orthopaedic Surgery
Columbia University College of Physicians and Surgeons
Attending Orthopaedic Surgeon
Columbia-Presbyterian Medical Center
New York, New York

M. L. Chip Routt, Jr., M.D. [25]
Associate Professor
Department of Orthopaedics
Harborview Medical Center
Seattle, Washington

Clinton T. Rubin, Ph.D. [2]
Professor and Director
Program in Biomedical Engineering
Musculoskeletal Research Laboratory
Department of Orthopaedics
State University of New York at Stony Brook
Stony Brook, New York

Steven P. Sampson, M.D. [24, 53]
Assistant Professor of Clinical Orthopaedics
   and Chief of Foot and Ankle Service
Department of Orthopaedics
State University of New York at Stony Brook
   Health Sciences Center
Stony Brook, New York

Alan J. Schefer, M.D. [66]
Assistant Clinical Instructor of Orthopaedic Surgery
State University of New York at Stony Brook
   Health Sciences Center
Lake Worth, Florida

Barry M. Shmookler, M.D. [16]
Director, Surgical Pathology
Department of Pathology
Washington Hospital Center
Washington, D.C.

Peter T. Simonian, M.D. [25]
Fellow, Department of Orthopaedic Surgery
Hospital for Special Surgery
New York, New York

Jeffrey D. Stone, M.D. [50]
Orthopaedic Resident
Department of Orthopaedic Surgery
University of Pittsburgh Medical Center
Pittsburgh, Pennsylvania

Robert J. Strauch, M.D. [62]
Assistant Professor of Orthopaedic Surgery
Columbia University
Assistant Professor of Orthopaedic Surgery
Columbia-Presbyterian Medical Center
New York, New York

James W. Strickland, M.D. [58, 63]
Clinical Professor
Department of Orthopaedic Surgery
Indiana University School of Medicine
Chairman, Department of Hand Surgery
St. Vincent Hospitals
The Indiana Hand Center
Indianapolis, Indiana

Stuart T. Styles, M.D. [7]
Resident, Orthopaedic Surgery
Maimonides Medical Center
Brooklyn, New York

Paul Tornetta III, M.D. [29, 30]
Associate Professor
State University of New York
    Health Sciences Center at Brooklyn
Director of Orthopaedic Trauma
Kings County Hospital
Brooklyn, New York

Ronald J. Turker, M.D. [47]
Assistant Professor of Orthopaedics and Pediatrics
University of New Mexico School of Medicine
Director of Residency Education
University of New Mexico Health Sciences Center
Carrie Tingley Hospital
Albuquerque, New Mexico

Ashok Vaswani, M.D. [3]
Associate Director
Department of Endocrinology
Winthrop-University Hospital
Mineola, New York

Oksana Volshteyn, M.D. [76]
Assistant Professor, Division of Rehabilitation
Department of Neurology
Jewish Hospital of St. Louis
    at Washington University Medical Center
St. Louis, Missouri

Douglas Wisch, M.D. [24]
Orthopaedic Surgeon
Orthopaedic Associates
Torrington, Connecticut

T. Scott Woll, M.D. [31]
Adjunct Assistant Professor
Division of Orthopaedics and Rehabilitation
Oregon Health Sciences University
Northwest Surgical Specialists
Southwest Washington Medical Center
Vancouver, Washington

David J. Zaleske, M.D. [1]
Associate Professor of Orthopaedics
Harvard Medical School
Chief, Pediatric Orthopaedics
Wang Ambulatory Care Center
Massachusetts General Hospital
Boston, Massachusetts

Joseph D. Zuckerman, M.D. [26]
Professor and Chairman
Department of Orthopaedics
Hospital for Joint Diseases
New York, New York

PREFACE

Now is an exciting time to be practicing orthopaedic surgery as our specialty is renewed by the introduction of new technologies and clinical methods.

The rapid pace of change has necessitated a complete revision of our text. This is a completely new book. The scientific foundations of the discipline are presented here by a stellar international group of scientists newly recruited for this edition. The clinical sections have been expanded in key areas, particularly fractures and dislocations, spinal disorders, sports medicine, and reconstructive orthopaedics.

We are grateful for the kind letters we have received from orthopaedic students throughout the world and for their many suggestions concerning our text. Many of their ideas have been incorporated into this new edition, but we have not lost sight of the goals which we set ourselves in the first edition and which we believe were responsible for that volume being so well received.

Once again, we have endeavored to produce a well-referenced, comprehensive single source text. Our book should enable the student of orthopaedics to rapidly acquire a knowledge base that will form a foundation and preparation for a future study of the large volume of orthopaedic literature.

On a personal note, I would like to acknowledge with gratitude the work of the collaborative editors, without whose effort a book of this size could not have been completed. I would also like to acknowledge the indispensable contributions of Mr. M. Wonsiewicz, Editorial Director, and Muza Navrozov, Senior Editing Supervisor, at McGraw-Hill, without whose labors we would certainly still be struggling in the wilderness.

Roger Dee, M.D.

PART I

Scientific Foundations
of Orthopaedics

Development of Components of the Skeletal System (Bone, Cartilage, Synovial Joints, Growth Plate)

David J. Zaleske

CYTODIFFERENTIATION AND MORPHOGENESIS

The development of multicellular organisms can be divided into three fundamental processes: cytodifferentiation, morphogenesis, and growth.[1] In cytodifferentiation, pluripotential cells express individual characteristics. In morphogenesis or organogenesis, cells collectively migrate, condense, or change shape in establishing tissues, organs, and body plan. Cytodifferentiation and morphogenesis are generally the two processes occurring during the embryonic period of vertebrate development. The general body plan has been established by the end of the embryonic period, and the fetal period is largely devoted to rapid growth.

Bone tissue forms during development; it is the one tissue that normally regenerates in response to injury throughout postnatal life. The term *bone growth* used in the sense of bone tissue formation and maintenance includes biological and physical phenomena frequently studied in various fracture and remodeling models. Bone growth may also imply morphogenesis of entire structures (organs), such as the femur, and their subsequent growth, collectively producing the growth of the organism in the fetal and postnatal periods. Mammals generally have relatively limited regenerative capacity of entire musculoskeletal structures postnatally. Thus a structure that has not formed appropriately during the embryonic period or that is lost postnatally will not usually reform. The first part of this chapter is concerned with bone growth in this second sense.

INTRAMEMBRANOUS AND ENDOCHONDRAL BONE

During development, bone tissue may be formed by two pathways: intramembranous bone and endochondral bone.[2] The bone tissue so formed appears to be identical or at least extremely similar by most biochemical assays. Yet various clinical phenomena suggest that some regulatory mechanisms must be different. For example, the cranial vault is formed as intramembranous bone and the vertebrae and appendicular skeleton as endochondral bone. The cranial vault is not affected by senile osteoporosis, as are the vertebrae and long bones.

Intramembranous bone is formed directly from mesenchymal condensations (*blastema;* pl., *blastemata*) without going through a cartilage intermediate. Toward the end of the embryonic period and at the beginning of the fetal period, the mesenchymal condensations destined to form intramembranous bone begin to transform. The mesenchymal cells differentiate into osteoblasts. These cells elaborate the matrix termed *osteoid,* a complex of collagen and proteoglycans, which calcifies and forms bone. As the osteoblasts elaborate more osteoid, some become encased in this matrix and become osteocytes. The bones of the cranial vault, the facial bones, and part of the clavicle form by the process of intramembranous ossification.

Endochondral bone is formed through a cartilage intermediate. It goes through a mesenchymal or blastemal condensation, subsequently changing into a cartilaginous miniature precursor (*anlage;* pl., *anlagen*). Toward the end of the embryonic period, mesenchymal condensations destined to form endochondral bone first transform into cartilage. The mesenchymal cells differentiate into chondrocytes, which also produce a matrix, but a matrix richer in proteoglycans and a collagen (type II) different from bone collagen (type I). The cartilaginous structure so formed is a miniature of the bone structure. These cartilaginous anlagen will direct the formation of osseous tissue in very specific ways. The cartilaginous anlagen of long bones will form bone tissue at the midshaft or diaphysis, termed the *primary center of ossification,* in the early fetal period. The cartilaginous ends or chondroepiphyses will grow away from the advancing ossification front of the primary center of ossification.

It is this process of interstitial cartilage growth linked to replacement with advancing ossification that is the basis for the growth of bone as an organ. In the long bones, secondary centers of ossification will form within the chondroepiphyses at specified postnatal times, the one exception being the secondary center of ossification of the distal femur, which forms at 36 weeks of gestation. The small bones, such as the carpus and tarsus, also form what constitute primary centers of ossification, some prenatally and some postnatally. These bones have spherical proliferating cartilage at the surface but never form secondary centers of ossification. The appearance and evolution of the primary centers of ossification of the wrist and the secondary centers of ossification of the hand can be used as a measure of biological age.[3] Proliferating cartilage is also present in the sutures and base of the skull, at the edges of flat bones such as the scapula and iliac crest (apophyses), at either end of the vertebrae (vertebral end plates), and in special arrangements such as the triradiate cartilage of the acetabulum in specialized anatomic configurations.

DEVELOPMENT OF BODY PLAN AND ITS SIGNIFICANCE FOR BONE

High Degree of Phylogenetic Conservation of Developmental Mechanisms

In the past, embryology was to a large degree a descriptive science.[2,4] By contrast, embryology has become an experimental discipline. Molecular biology is revealing, startlingly, that the mechanisms underlying development have been highly conserved phylogenetically. Indeed, mechanisms in existence prior to the vertebrates have continued to be employed in structuring body plans with quite different components. *Drosophila* has a well-described genetics and an embryology that may easily be observed. This fortuitous combination led to the description of homeobox genes that are ordered on the chromosome corresponding to the order of body segments. By using probes developed with *Drosophila* ("fly genes"), investigators have found a similar conservation of such genes throughout phylogeny. Experimental work has also been done on the chick, exploiting the ability to remove the shell, operate on the developing embryo, observe further development, and make inferences about tissue interactions directing morphogenesis. This has been especially important in formulating models of vertebrate limb development.[5,6] Such models can now be reexamined at the molecular level.

The mouse has been the favored model of general mammalian development. It has well-described genetics, and transgenic and "knockout" (of a particular gene) mice can be made experimentally, although actual development is less observable. While experimental work is not possible with *Homo sapiens,* kindreds of naturally occurring congenital musculoskeletal differences can be used to map the gene to the human chromosome, to regions with known analogies to lower species.[7] The enormous importance of this family of genes in explaining development was recognized in the 1995 Nobel Prizes in Medicine and Physiology, the first time in 60 years that developmental biology was so recognized.[8]

Truncal Development

In *Homo sapiens,* the notochord forms at 15 days of development. It is a rod of cells running the length of the craniocaudad axis, embedded in mesoderm. The ectoderm overlying the dorsal side of the notochord will form the neural tube, from which will develop the central nervous system. The endoderm underlying the ventral side of the notochord will form the gut.

Shortly after the formation of the notochord, the mesoderm dorsal to and on either side of the notochord con-

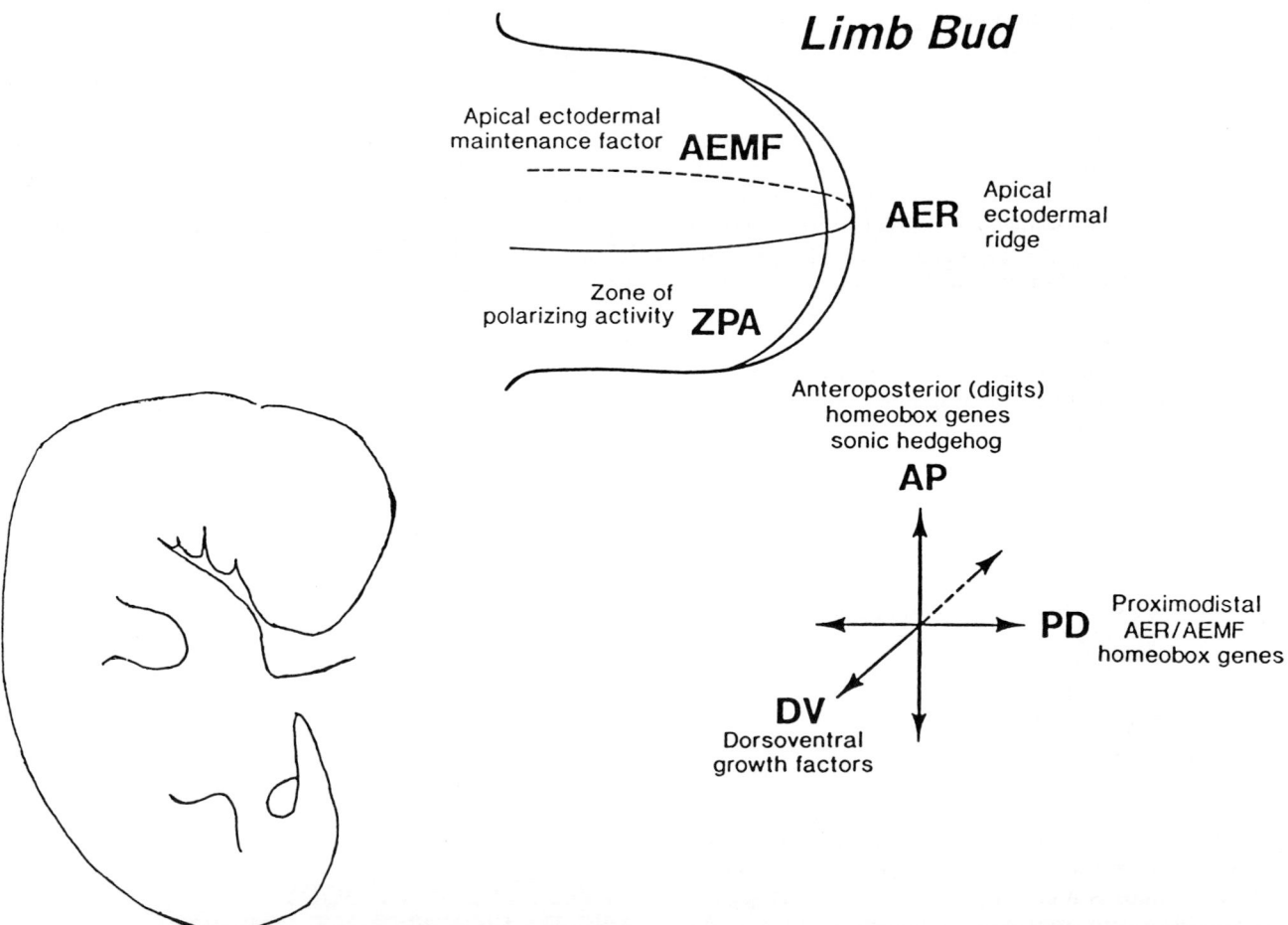

Figure 1-1 Diagram of a 4-week-old human embryo at lower left corner, side view, and enlargement of limb bud. The limb bud is mesoderm covered by ectoderm. A thickening of the ectoderm forms at the apex of the limb bud, the apical ectodermal ridge (AER). An information network is established along the three axes: proximodistal (PD), anteroposterior (AP), and dorsoventral (DV). Outgrowth along the PD axis is mediated by the AER. The digits are specified along the AP axis, which is under the control of the zone of polarizing activity (ZPA). Growth factors are important in signaling along the DV axis.

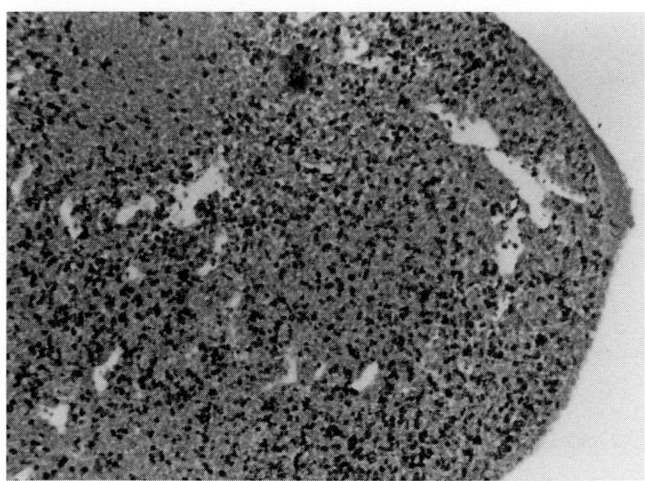

Figure 1-2 Autoradiograph of a hindlimb bud from a 3-day-old chick embryo (×100). No mesenchymal condensations are present; the label is distributed homogeneously throughout the mesenchyme.

denses and forms somites. These paired somites reflect the primarily segmental nature of the trunk. Their total numbers generally correspond (but not on a strict one-to-one basis) to the various postnatal truncal regions (8 cervical, 12 thoracic, 5 lumbar, 5 sacral). Each somite further divides into a dermatome, from which will form the dermis of the truncal skin, a myotome from which will form the truncal musculature, and a sclerotome from which will form the vertebrae and ribs. The sclerotome from a somite on either side of the notochord migrates ventrally and medially to surround the notochord. The superior halves of one pair of somites and the inferior halves of another pair form the blastemal condensations of the vertebrae. The costal processes in the thoracic region form the blastemal condensations of the ribs. Toward the end of the embryonic period (6 to 8 weeks of development), the blastemal condensations of the ribs and vertebrae separate and become cartilaginous anlagen, parts of which will subsequently be replaced by (endochondral) bone in the early fetal period.

The regions between the vertebrae form the intervertebral disks. The somitic mesoderm in this region, which came to surround the notochord, develops into the fibrocartilaginous annulus fibrosus. The notochordal tissue persists as the nucleus pulposus of the disks.

Limb Development

Limb development in *Homo sapiens* begins as an outpouching at the lateral body wall at 4 weeks of gestation (Fig. 1-1).[2,9] There is a craniocaudad time gradient, with the upper limb bud appearing and developing slightly ahead of the lower limb bud. The limb bud begins as mesenchyme, undifferentiated at the light microscopic level and covered by a jacket of ectoderm (Fig. 1-2). A genetic and epigenetic information network is established along the three axes of the limb bud.[10–13] While the molecular

events underlying this network are presently being elucidated and will be discussed further in the next section, the events at the level of histogenesis have been established by surgical experiments on the chick embryo. A thickening of the distal ectoderm covering the limb bud, the apical ectodermal ridge (AER), forms soon after limb bud formation. The AER is essential in directing the longitudinal growth of the limb bud along the proximodistal (PD) axis. There is also a time gradient along this axis, with proximal structures being formed before distal structures. Along the anteroposterior (AP) axis, the digits are specified, representing an example of unique variations of a morphogenetic theme at each digit. The dorsoventral (DV) axis appears to be mediated by messengers between the ectoderm and the underlying mesoderm. The combined signals along the three axes interact to specify the blastemal condensations of the skeleton (Fig. 1-3).[14,15] As indicated, such condensations form in a PD sequence. Much developmental time is devoted to the cytodifferentiation and morphogenesis of the blastemata, with further modifications, such as joint cavitation and growth, to occur later. This means that elements such as the terminal appendages, the carpus, and the tarsus will initially constitute a large percentage of

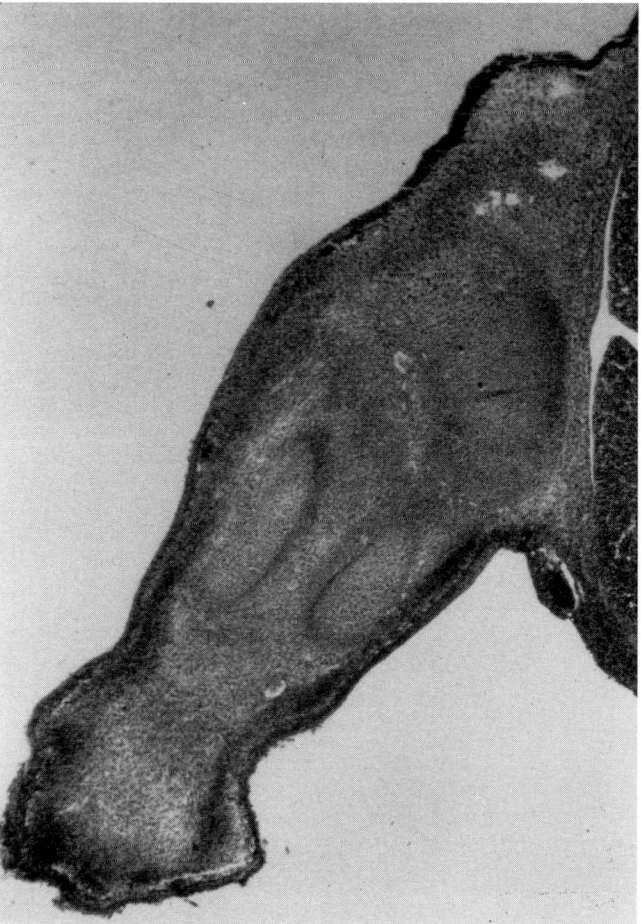

Figure 1-3 Longitudinal section of the developing hindlimb from a 13-day mouse embryo (H&E, ×40). Mesenchymal condensations are forming.

the length of the limb, with changes in proportion occurring with growth.

During the sixth week of gestation in the human embryo, the mesenchymal condensations of the limb bones begin to chondrify (Fig. 1-4). The regions between the continuous condensations start to break down in the process of joint cavitation, which will also be discussed in greater detail in a later section. The cartilage attains some of the cytodifferentiation, which persists in fetal and postnatal articular and physeal or growth regions. The growth regions may be considered as hydraulic jacks continually moving away from each other in the case of the ends of a long bone or growing more or less spherically in the case of the bones of the carpus and tarsus. The rate of growth is programmed differently at different anatomic locations, with the distal femoral growth area being the most active in the body.

The end of the embryonic and beginning of the fetal period in the human occurs at 8 weeks of gestation. The vascular invasion at the midshaft of the cartilaginous anlage of the humerus is the event that marks this transition. A similar sequence soon follows at all the long bone anlagen, forming the primary centers of ossification throughout the skeleton (Fig. 1-5). The cartilaginous ends, the chondroepiphyses, continue to grow away from the advancing primary center of ossification. The chondrocyte proliferation is now well ordered into zones within the chondroepiphysis.[16–20] In the immature skeleton, there is a population of chondrocytes dividing to increase the size of the articular surface. There is a population of chondrocytes devoted to increasing the size of the chondroepiphysis and also the secondary center of ossification when it appears within the chondroepiphysis. Finally, there is the proliferative zone of the physeal growth region, which becomes a "plate" or "physis" contributing to longitudinal growth (Figs. 1-6 and 1-7).

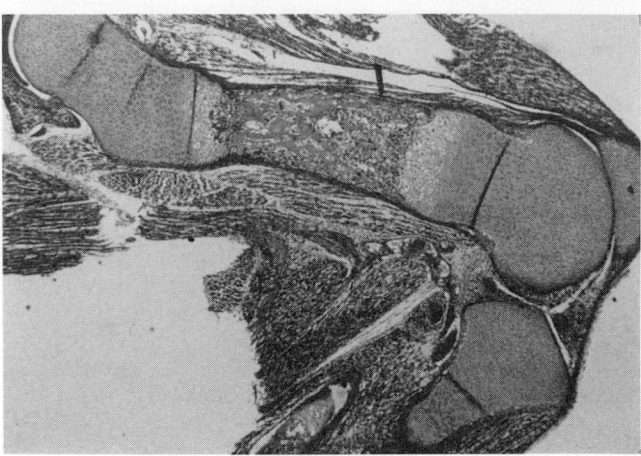

Figure 1-5 Longitudinal section of the hindlimb from an 18-day mouse fetus (H&E, ×40). The primary center of ossification has formed in the midshaft of the femur.

Formation of secondary centers of ossification usually occurs at predictable postnatal stages of development. The secondary center of ossification of the distal femur, however, begins to form at 36 weeks of gestation in the human fetus. At times, the terms *secondary center of ossification* and *epiphysis* are used synonymously. The bone age of a child may be judged radiologically by interpreting from tables those "epiphyses" present. At other times, the terms *epiphysis* and *chondroepiphysis* may be used to refer to the entire cartilaginous end of a long bone, whether or not the secondary ossification centers have appeared.[12] The crucial point to appreciate is that osseous tissue is really following the lead of the cartilaginous tissue in forming endochondral bone. Cartilage transformation is seen in the formation of the primary and secondary centers of ossification and in the continual function of the growth plate. Cartilage transformation is a change from a tissue with small, round chondrocytes embedded in an abundant matrix to one with large, hypertrophic chondrocytes and a relatively scant matrix that calcifies and elicits vascular invasion.[21,22]

The perichondrial groove of Ranvier, part of which forms a bony ring, and the adjacent fibrous perichondrial ring of LaCroix should also be noted (Fig. 1-7). These structures are circumferential restraints to the growth plate, add to its latitudinal growth, and anchor the growth plate to the metaphysis.[23–25] The ring also demarcates that portion of the metaphysis which is not yet remodeled and consists of circumferential collagen fibers.

Genes and Messengers Mediating the Morphogenesis of Skeletal Anlagen

The three-dimensional informational network within the limb bud was discussed previously at the level of tissue interactions (Fig. 1-1). The basic model of vertebrate limb development was established with extensive surgical experiments (ablations, transplantations) on the chick limb

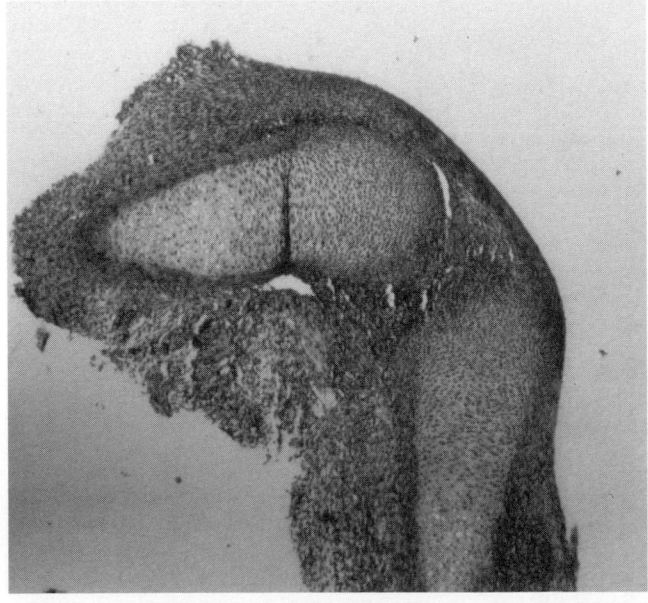

Figure 1-4 Longitudinal section of the knee region from a 15-day mouse embryo (H&E, ×40). Joint cavitation is occurring.

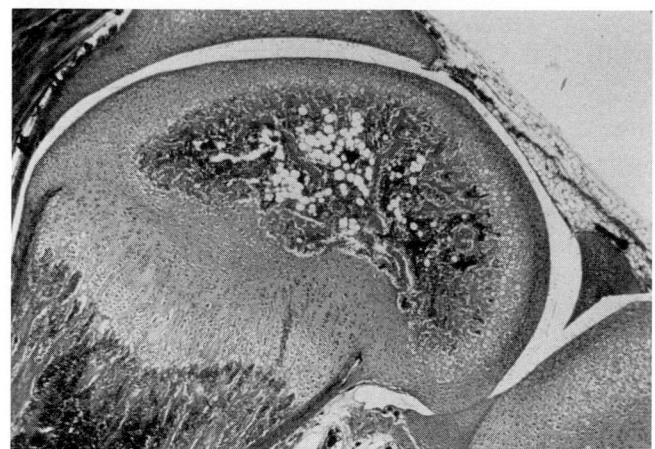

Figure 1-6 Longitudinal section of the distal femur from a 10-day postnatal mouse (H&E, ×40). With the presence of the secondary center of ossification, the growth plate or physis is clearly defined.

group of homeobox genes. In humans, the HOX D genes are then important in specifying digits.[10,11] In the DV axis, the polypeptide growth factors are attractive candidates for communication between the ectoderm and mesoderm. Bone morphogenetic protein (BMP) was originally described for its activity in mediating bone formation.[33] It is really a collection of several molecules that are part of the transforming growth factor-beta (TGF-β) superfamily, which generally upregulates cellular functions important in healing.[34–37] Interestingly, in the mouse AER FGF-4 stimulates proliferation of the underlying mesenchyme but BMP-2 inhibits limb growth; a combination of these molecules may be important in regulating growth along the PD axis.[28] Related TGF-β growth factors are responsible for the mutation *brachypodism* (bp), which alters the length and number in limb bones in the mouse.[38] It may be appreciated from this that it is the appropriate combination of many factors which leads to normal histogenesis. An effect of a given growth factor documented in vitro may be difficult to extrapolate to the very complicated and dynamic situation of development, with interacting factors and responsive cells.

bud.[5,6,26,27] This model is now being restudied at the level of genes and molecular messengers. The outgrowth along the PD axis was noted earlier to be under the control of the apical ectodermal ridge (AER) and the underlying mesoderm. It has now been established that this activity can be replicated by the fibroblast growth factors (FGFs).[28–31] A zone of tissue at the posterior aspect of the limb bud, the zone of polarizing activity (ZPA), was demonstrated by tissue interactions to be important in specifying the number of digits along the anteroposterior (AP) axis. This activity seems to be mediated by the gene *sonic hedgehog*, which is being shown to have far-reaching implications in development.[32] *Sonic* seems to activate a

VASCULOGENESIS

Limb

The development of the vascular tree during development (vasculogenesis) proceeds simultaneously with the events specifying the skeletal elements. Soon after formation of the limb bud, there is a diffuse capillary invasion into it from the flank. The capillary invasion fills the mesoderm except for a thin zone of mesoderm under the surface ectoderm, from which it is apparently excluded by a high

Figure 1-7 Diagram of the end of a growing long bone.

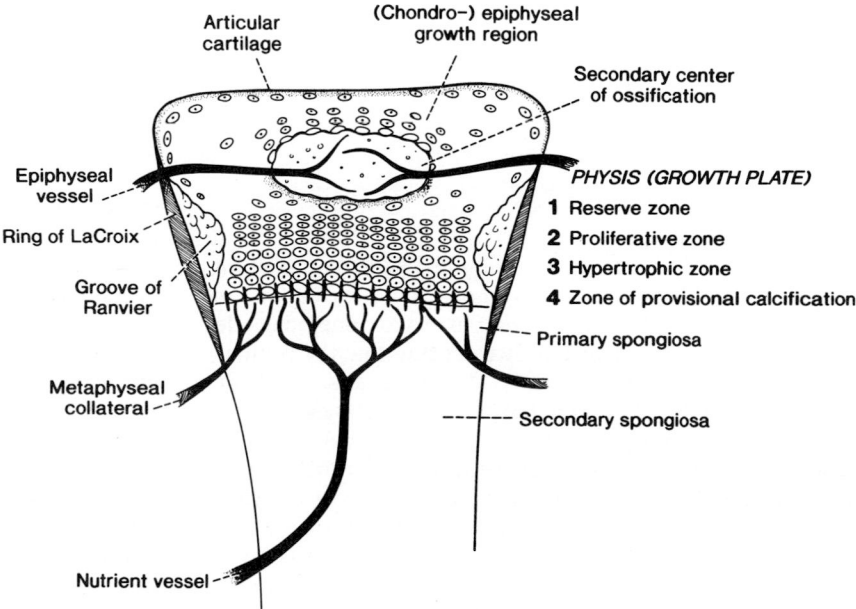

content of hyaluronate.[39,40] As the mesenchymal condensations form, these regions also become avascular, again apparently related to a high hyaluronate content.[41] As the mesenchymal condensations turn into cartilage, they remain avascular. The surrounding myogenic precursor tissue remains highly vascular. With limb growth, the capillary system condenses and rearranges to form the large vascular tree. With the transformation of the cartilage at the midshaft of the anlage of a long bone, the chondrocytes become hypertrophic, apparently releasing angiogenic or angiotropic substances; the matrix calcifies; and vascular invasion occurs at the midshaft to form the primary center of ossification.[22,42–46]

It can be seen that the processes of skeletal anlagen generation and vasculogenesis of the limb are closely linked. Abnormal limb vascularity has been reported in a number of congenital limb differences for both humans[47] and experimental animals.[48] There can, of course, be variability in cause versus effect. Thalidomide has recently been demonstrated to be an inhibitor of angiogenesis, which may explain its role in limb teratogenicity.[49]

Cartilage and Growth Plate

The growth plate has a dual blood supply (Fig. 1-7), the origins of which may be traced back to development. The epiphyseal (proliferative) side of the plate is supplied by epiphyseal vessels.[43,50,51] Prior to the formation of the secondary center of ossification within the chondroepiphysis, large species (including humans) have a network of canals permeated by nutrients. These cartilage canals are also the conduits along which the definite epiphyseal vessels grow as the secondary center of ossification forms.[43,52,53] The metaphyseal side of the growth plate is supplied by metaphyseal vessels, which are largely derived from the nutrient artery that formed the primary center of ossification. Metaphyseal collaterals also exist. In general, injury or inhibition of the metaphyseal supply is an insult from which recovery is possible. Injury to the epiphyseal vasculature and therefore the proliferative side of the growth plate may result in permanent damage to the physis.[51] The ring of LaCroix also has a blood supply from its peripheral tissues.

Bone

The blood supply of bone is a complex topic[43] of great importance in the biology of osseous tissue formation, remodeling, and repair. The nutrient artery of long bones develops from the vascular ingrowth at the time the primary center of ossification is formed, and this artery remains the main supply of the diaphysis and metaphysis of long bones. Cortical bone at the diaphysis is largely supplied from the endosteal side, with the inner two-thirds dependent ultimately on the nutrient artery. The outer one-third can derive its supply from periosteal collaterals. Under conditions such as injury and intramedullary nailing of fractures, there can be reversal of this ratio, with relatively more supply coming from the periosteum.[54]

Special Anatomic Considerations of the Proximal Femur

The blood supply to the proximal femur deserves special mention because of its unique anatomic features. In order to allow ball-and-socket configuration and motion, the proximal femoral epiphysis cannot be relatively tightly tethered to the surrounding soft tissues, as it is in other anatomic configurations. The hip capsule originates on the pelvis and inserts into the base of the femoral neck. At this attachment vessels leave the protection of the capsule becoming closely applied to the femoral neck and traveling to the proximal femur to form the epiphyseal circulation.[55,56] An understanding of these anatomic features is important in appreciating the vulnerability of these vessels to direct injury in fractures or dislocations of the hip or to occlusion by increased intracapsular pressure resulting from hematoma, purulence, or synovitis. These features also have relevance in the etiology and treatment of such clinical conditions as Legg-Perthes disease, slipped capital femoral epiphysis, and femoral head osteonecrosis.

JOINT DEVELOPMENT

Interzone Formation, Cavitation, Intraarticular Structures

Joint development is customarily divided into three phases. In the first phase, the blastemal condensations of the skeletal elements are formed, juxtaposed against each other as continuous masses of tissues (Fig. 1-3). In the second, joint cavitation occurs (Fig. 1-4). In the third and final phase, the synovium and intraarticular structures are formed, producing a diarthrodial joint (Fig. 1-5). While there are some variations depending upon the individual joint, the three stages, merging into each other, may be seen underlying joint development.

Centers of chondrification begin within each blastema and spread peripherally. As chondrification proceeds, turning the blastemata into cartilaginous anlagen, arcs of flattened cells develop in the regions between adjacent anlagen. This tissue is termed the *interzone*. The interzone itself forms three layers. The middle layer consists of rather loosely packed, randomly arranged cells. The layers subjacent to each chondroepiphyseal region consist of more densely packed, flattened cells parallel to the chondroepiphysis. The middle layer forms hyaluronate.[57] This tissue merges with the surrounding matrix, from which the synovium will form. A still more peripheral layer of the mesenchyme surrounding the joint condenses into the fibrous capsule. The middle layer of the interzone gives way completely to the joint cavity. The layers adjacent to the epiphyseal cartilages form the articular cartilage.[58]

The precise mechanism underlying joint cavitation is unknown. It would appear to be either programmed cell death (apoptosis) or enzyme-mediated degradation. Recent work with mice with a defect in apoptosis in thymocytes did not demonstrate other disruptions in development.[59] It has been demonstrated that motion is required for cavitation to proceed normally.[60] Chicks paralyzed with curare at the crucial stage of cavitation proceed to joint ankylosis.

Soon after joint cavitation, synovial cells form a smooth surface, one or two cells thick, overlying a richly vascularized mesenchyme. Remaining intracapsular structures such as tendons, ligaments, and menisci form from this mesenchyme.

Heterogeneity of Articular and Anlagen Cartilage

The development of joints emphasizes the differences between articular and anlagen or epiphyseal cartilage. Articular cartilage arises from the interzone. It will remain avascular, aneural, and alymphatic throughout its life, deriving its nutrition primarily from the synovial cavity.[61] (In the immature skeleton, prior to formation of the tide mark or calcified basal layer of the articular cartilage, it is possible for nutrition to diffuse in retrograde fashion from the underlying epiphysis. This becomes an important pathway only in states such as prolonged immobilization.) The anlagen cartilage or the chondroepiphysis will get its nutrition through the cartilage canals[52,53] prior to the formation of the secondary centers of ossification and from the epiphyseal vasculature thereafter (Fig. 1-7).[50]

Motion and Physical Factors

As discussed under joint development, motion is a crucial element in the normal formation of diarthrodial joints. It is also important in the repair of articular cartilage postnatally.[62,63] Articular cartilage in the mature skeleton is absolutely dependent upon nutrition from the synovial cavity, and motion is important in propelling nutrients through the pores of the matrix.[64] Compressive loads can either increase or decrease the synthetic response of articular cartilage explants in culture, depending on specific parameters.[65] Generally, intermittent compressive load in the physiologic range (5 to 10 MPa, or megapascals) appears to enhance the synthetic response of articular cartilage.[65-68] The secondary center of ossification within the chondroepiphysis is aligned to support the cartilaginous structures.[69] Loads exceeding physiologic range lead to premature degeneration of articular cartilage.[70,71]

ZONE OF THE GROWTH PLATE

The growth plate of a long bone provides an exceptional correlation between histology, ordered cytodifferentiation, molecular biology, and physical function (Figs. 1-5 through 1-8). Several zones may be distinguished in moving from the secondary center of ossification to the metaphysis.[72,73]

Reserve Zone—Metabolic Storage

Adjacent to the secondary center of ossification is the reserve zone. Chondrocytes here are round, embedded in an abundant matrix, and not clearly ordered in columns. At one point, it was felt that this was the germinal zone of the growth plate. It is not very active in cell division. The precise role of this zone remains somewhat unclear. One function may be to provide a physical barrier between the advancing ossification of the secondary center and the rest of the growth plate. Epiphyseal vessels pass through this region but do not form terminal capillaries. The oxygen tension of this region is therefore relatively low. The chondrocytes of this region do participate in the synthesis and storage of glycogen, lipids, and protein, which may be used by other zones of the physis.

Proliferative Zone—Chondrocyte Division and Matrix Synthesis

Past the reserve zone, the chondrocytes are highly ordered in columns directed along the axis of growth of the long bone. The chondrocytes are relatively small and flattened. Kember demonstrated with tritiated thymidine that this is the kinetically active zone of the growth plate.[17-19] Mitosis occurs exclusively in this zone, with the cells so formed marching down the column in line and progressing through ordered cytodifferentiation. Finally, at the metaphysis, the terminal chondrocyte dies. In normal growth, chondrocyte removal at the metaphyseal side is precisely matched by chondrocyte generation from the proliferative zone on the epiphyseal side. The growth plate therefore

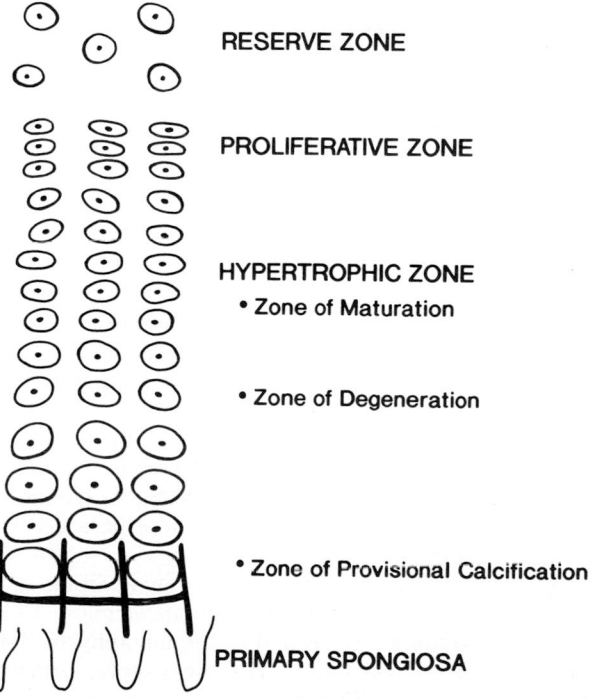

RESERVE ZONE

PROLIFERATIVE ZONE

HYPERTROPHIC ZONE
• Zone of Maturation

• Zone of Degeneration

• Zone of Provisional Calcification

PRIMARY SPONGIOSA

Figure 1-8 Diagram of the zones of the growth plate.

remains relatively constant as it moves continually away from the advancing ossification front at the metaphysis. It is really continuing the function which began with the formation of the primary center of ossification (Fig. 1-5) and will continue until growth plate closure and growth cessation in adolescence. The proliferative zone is also engaged in matrix synthesis. The proteoglycans in this region are large aggregates (aggrecans) made up of glycosaminoglycans attached to core proteins. Many such proteoglycan subunits (PGS) are linked to a hyaluronic acid backbone, forming a structure likened to the bristle region of a test-tube brush.[74] Aggrecans in their large form inhibit calcification of the cartilage matrix. Oxygen tension in the proliferative zone is high, as the epiphyseal vessels arborize in a capillary network at the top of the zone.

Hypertrophic Zone—Chondrocyte and Matrix Changes

The hypertrophic zone can be divided into upper and lower zones. In the upper hypertrophic zone, also termed the *zone of maturation,* the chondrocytes begin to swell. The size of the aggrecans begins to diminish as a result of enzymatic degradation.[75,76] By moving down the cell column, the chondrocytes move away from the epiphyseal vessels and into increasingly lower oxygen tension. The mitochondria of the chondrocytes switch their activity from generating adenosine triphosphate (ATP) in the proliferative zone to accumulating calcium in the upper hypertrophic zone.[72]

In the lower hypertrophic zone, the chondrocytes swell still further. The mitochondria now begin to discharge the calcium accumulated in the upper hypertrophic zone. The calcium is packaged in vesicles and deposited into the surrounding matrix.[77–81] The precise role of such vesicles in calcification is unclear.[82] Concomitantly, the aggrecan of the matrix is further degraded, removing its inhibitory role in calcification.[83] While the entire growth plate synthesizes type II collagen, only the lower hypertrophic zone synthesizes type X collagen, a unique type associated with endochondral ossification.[84,85] The sudden appearance of type X collagen in the lower hypertrophic zone is another example of the very highly ordered cytodifferentiation in correlation with chondrocyte progression down the cellular columns. Similarly, the cartilage that had resisted vascular invasion in the upper part of the growth plate now actively attracts it.[39,42,86,87] Earlier textbooks of histology suggested that all of this was a rather passive process as the chondrocytes become senescent. It is now clear that these changes leading to chondrocyte death at the last intact transverse septum are very active.[21,22,88–91] Since the longitudinal septa begin to calcify in this region, the end of the lower hypertrophic zone is also called the *zone of provisional calcification.* The last transverse septa are degraded at the metaphysis. Bone is laid down on the calcified longitudinal septa, forming the primary spongiosa. With normal osteoclast function, the primary spongiosa is soon removed and replaced by the secondary spongiosa. The metaphyseal flare regions or "cut-back zones" are active sites of remodeling, normally keeping the flare sharp and close to the growth plate.

The pertinent biochemical events in moving from the reserve zone to the metaphysis can now be summarized. Glycogen is stored in the reserve and proliferative zones and then consumed in the hypertrophic zone. All the zones of the growth plate are relatively inefficient, lacking glycerol phosphate dehydrogenase and a shuttle for glycerol phosphate into the mitochondria.[92] Even when sufficient oxygen is present, cartilage metabolizes glucose to lactate. In the lower hypertrophic zone, changes occur to calcify the matrix. Alkaline phosphatase activity is pronounced.[93] Type II or cartilage collagen is synthesized throughout the growth plate. Type X collagen appears in the lower hypertrophic zone. Type I or bone collagen appears in the metaphysis. Proteoglycans are progressively degraded down the growth plate.[94,95] The enzymatic degradation is mediated by metalloproteinases such as collagenase, stromelysin, and neutral growth plate proteases,[75,76,83] rendering the matrix calcifiable at the zone of provisional calcification. Cytokines such as interleukin-1 (IL-1) and plasmin also have a role in regulating matrix calcification and endochondral bone formation.[94,96,97]

GROWTH AND ITS CONTROL

Growth results from the coordination of all the molecular, cellular, and tissue functions described. Disruptions in any one may result in abnormal growth. Various short stature syndromes are manifestations of such disruptions.[98,99] Longitudinal growth is the rate of production of cells in the proliferative zones multiplied by the size of the hypertrophic cells being lost at the metaphysis.[18] The contribution to proportionate growth from a given growth plate is normally quite predictable, implying that the pool of cells available for cell division, the rate at which they enter mitosis, and the duration over which they do so are all regulated. Matrix swelling and cellular hypertrophy must be maintained in columns oriented along the axis of growth by septa. The entire physeal structure must be kept contained latitudinally by the groove of Ranvier and the ring of LaCroix. Dissociation between longitudinal endochondral and perichondrial growth has been demonstrated as the basis of metatropic dwarfism.[100]

Physical force is an important regulator of the interstitial growth of cartilage, which is the distracting force underlying longitudinal endochondral bone growth. This clinical observation is the Hueter-Volkmann law of growth plates,[71,101] stating that increased pressure causes decreased growth and decreased pressure causes increased growth. (The Hueter-Volkmann law of growth plates is therefore somewhat opposite to Wolff's law of internal bone remodeling, which states that bone is laid down according to the stress upon it.[102]) The Hueter-Volkmann law implies that when a deformation of a growth plate occurs that does not correct, yet further inhibition of growth may result. One example of this is infantile tibia vara or Blount's disease. The cellular basis underlying the Hueter-Volkmann law is just beginning to be elucidated.[69,103,104]

Hormones—Endocrine Control

Various hormones—agents synthesized at a distance and released into the systemic circulation—have regulatory effects upon growth plates. It should be appreciated that in vivo regulation of growth plates is complex. Generally, a hormone or other agent is isolated and studied in vitro. However, in the body, it is the combination of factors working in a given physical environment on a group of cells with special responsiveness that produces clinical growth.

The thyroid hormones are important regulators of proliferating cartilage. Triiodothyronine (T3) stimulates cartilage proliferation and maturation by different mechanisms[105]: it stimulates increased chondrocyte division by interacting with somatomedin and it regulates transformation independently from somatomedin.

Growth hormone, secreted by the pituitary, is the prototypical agent regulating growth.[106] Its absence will lead to pituitary dwarfism, which, in turn, can be circumvented by the provision of exogenous growth hormone. Yet the stimulation of the growth plates is not primarily a direct one. Growth hormone is either converted in the liver or causes the liver to produce somatomedin or insulinlike growth factor (IGF), which is the potent direct stimulator of chondrocyte proliferation.[107] Insulinlike growth factor is the postnatal hormone; IGF-II is fetal somatomedin. Insulin cross-reacts with the IGF receptor. This would appear to be a mechanism whereby nutrition can influence growth.[108,109]

Parathyroid hormone (PTH) and parathyroid-related peptide (PTHrp) also regulate the growth plate.[110] Parathyroid hormone stimulates growth plate chondrocytes to produce inositol triphosphate (IP3) from phosphoinositol bis-phosphate, and IP3 mediates the release of intracellular calcium. By another mechanism, PTH works through membrane G (guanine nucleotide-binding) proteins to activate cyclic AMP (cAMP) and calcium release.[111,112] Parathyroid hormone also mediates an increase in proteoglycan synthesis through the activation of protein kinase C (PKC).

Glucocorticoids inhibit growth and may do this by interfering with glucose utilization and energy production.[113] Androgens and estrogens increase chondrocyte division but also interact with the other regulators of the growth plate. They promote growth plate closure by an incompletely understood mechanism.[114–116]

Several vitamins have effects on the growth plate, in essence making them hormones.[117] Vitamin D and its metabolites are required for calcification of the matrix. Vitamin D deficiency causes rickets, which at the histologic level is a failure of calcification of the matrix with marked elongation of the hypertrophic zone. Vitamin C is a necessary cofactor for the synthesis of collagen. Deficiency of vitamin C causes scurvy. Collagen fibers of poor quality are produced. Blood vessels rupture easily, and bone formed with such collagen is weakened. The histology of the growth plate in scurvy is particularly abnormal at the physeal-metaphyseal junction, with persistence of calcified cartilage and sparse bony trabeculae. This produces the white line of

Fraenkel seen radiologically. The similar phenomenon at the proliferating cartilage of the chondroepiphysis produces ringed epiphyses or Wimberger's sign. Vitamin A is required for appropriate chondrocyte maturation. Deficiency disrupts this process; excess leads to bone fragility.

Growth Factors—Autocrine and Paracrine Control

In addition to the systemic circulating hormones, small polypeptide regulators, the growth factors or cytokines, are employed in more local control of growth. These factors are important in the embryogenesis of the growth plate. Such factors can both be synthesized by and have an effect upon the same cell (autocrine regulation). Alternatively, these factors can influence other cells in proximity to the signaling cell (paracrine regulation).

The fibroblast growth factors are divided into acidic and basic (aFGF, bFGF). The various FGFs upregulate endothelial cell division, neovascularization, and chondrocyte proliferation.[118] Both FGF and IGF-I work synergistically to upregulate mitosis in the physeal proliferative zone.[36,119] The transforming growth factor-beta (TGF-β) superfamily consists of several different factors (including the bone morphogenetic proteins, or BMPs) that generally upregulate cartilage and bone molecules as well as other components of repair and healing.[34] The effects of this family of growth factors can be dramatically altered by their interactions with other factors.[36] While TGF-β can inhibit cartilage transformation to the full hypertrophic phenotype, thyroid hormones can overcome this inhibition.[120] Interleukin-1 is an inflammatory cytokine that promotes matrix degradation through the metalloproteinases, while TGF-β inhibits IL-1 mediated matrix degradation. Prostaglandins have variable effects on connective tissues.[121] In the physis, prostaglandins increase proteoglycan synthesis but decrease collagen synthesis and alkaline phosphatase activity.

THE MOLECULAR BIOLOGY OF SOME CLINICAL CONDITIONS AND THE GROWTH PLATE

Advances in molecular biology are rapidly establishing genetic linkage and, in some cases, the mechanism for many short-stature conditions.[122] Reports come so frequently that a text cannot be truly current. Yet it is fitting to conclude this chapter with several correlations between molecular biology and short-stature conditions.

Achondroplasia

Achondroplasia is the prototypical short-limb/short-stature condition. Endochondral growth is affected throughout the body, with the most severe inhibition occurring at what would otherwise have been the most rapidly growing regions of the skeleton. It has recently been mapped to a region coding for the receptor for fibroblast growth factor 3

(FGFR-3).[123,124] Mutations in other receptors for FGFs have been demonstrated to be responsible for syndromes that include abnormalities in other areas of endochondral bone. In the Crouzon syndrome, there are abnormal cranial sutures; the underlying mutation is in the receptor for FGF2.[125] In the Jackson-Weiss and Pfeiffer syndromes, there are abnormal cranial sutures and limb defects; mutations exist in both FGF1 and FGF2 receptors.[126,127] Coordination of the various FGFs and their receptors seems to be a crucial part of the regulation of proportionate growth.[128]

Type II Collagen Abnormalities

Since type II collagen is an important component of cartilage, including the growth plate, it would be logical that mutations in this collagen produce problems in articulation and growth. Further, as collagen is a large molecule, there can be room for heterogeneity. Mutations at different positions in the molecule can produce different clinical syndromes. This is indeed the case with mutations in type II collagen underlying spondyloepiphyseal dysplasia congenita, Stickler syndrome, and Kniest dysplasia.[129,130]

Diastrophic Dwarfism

Diastrophic dwarfism is notable for short limbs with deformities that are particularly recalcitrant to treatment. The associated equinovarus feet are very inflexible. Auricular cartilages can sustain hemorrhages and become hypertrophic. A unique sulfate transporter with an abnormality has been established as the basis for this short-stature condition.[131] It leads to undersulfated proteoglycans. As discussed under "Zones of the Growth Plate," proteoglycan swelling is part of the mechanism producing growth. The proteoglycan abnormality in diastrophic dysplasia probably leads to the abnormal growth throughout the skeleton.

Jansen Metaphyseal Chondrodysplasia

Metaphyseal chondrodysplasias can be mistaken for rickets. In the Jansen type, there is a constitutively active mutant in the parathyroid hormone–parathyroid hormone–related peptide receptor. Therefore, even in the presence of a normal serum calcium and parathyroid hormone, the growth cartilage behaves as if these parameters were abnormal.[128]

The examples cited here represent the fundamental link between the basic science of the growth plate and clinical conditions.[132] The future should bring capabilities for molecular repair of the growth plate, which will be of benefit to many pediatric orthopaedic patients.

REFERENCES

1. Trinkaus JP: *Cells into Organs.* Englewood Cliffs, NJ, Prentice-Hall, 1984, pp 1–5.
2. Netter FH: *The Ciba Collection of Medical Illustrations:* Vol 8. *Musculoskeletal System.* Summit, NJ, Ciba-Geigy Corporation, 1987, pp 125–136.
3. Greulich WW, Pyle SI: *Radiographic Atlas of Skeletal Development of the Hand and Wrist,* 2d ed. Stanford, CA, Stanford University Press, 1959.
4. Crelin ES: Development of the musculoskeletal system. *CIBA Clin Symp* 33(1):1–36, 1981.
5. Saunders JW Jr: The experimental analysis of chick limb bud development, in Ede DA, Hinchliffe JR, Balls M (eds): *Vertebrate Limb and Somite Morphogenesis.* Cambridge, England, Cambridge University Press, 1977, pp 1–24.
6. Zwilling E, Saunders JW Jr, Gasseling MT: Involvement of the apical ectodermal ridge in chick limb development. *Anat Rec* 136:307, 1960.
7. Tsukurov O, Boehmer A, Flynn J, et al: A complex bilateral polysyndactyly disease locus maps to chromosome 7q36. *Nature Genet* 6:282–286, 1994.
8. Rousch W: Nine make the Nobel grade: Fly development works bears prize-winning fruit. *Science* 270:380–381, 1995.
9. Sledge CB, Zaleske DJ: Developmental anatomy of joints, in Resnick D, Niwayama G (eds): *Diagnosis of Bone and Joint Disorders,* 2d ed. Philadelphia, Saunders, 1988, pp 604–624.
10. Scott MP: Vertebrate homeobox gene nomenclature. *Cell* 71:551–553, 1992.
11. Tabin CJ: Retinoids, homeoboxes, and growth factors: Toward molecular models for limb development. *Cell* 66:199–217, 1991.
12. Hinchliffe JR, Johnson DR: *The Development of the Vertebrate Limb.* Oxford, England, Clarendon Press, 1980, pp 85–90.
13. Yokouchi Y, Sasaki H, Kuroiwa A: Homeobox gene expression correlated with the bifurcation process of limb cartilage development. *Nature* 353:443–445, 1991.
14. Newman SA, Frisch HL: Dynamics of skeletal pattern formation in developing chick limb. *Science* 205:662, 1979.
15. Duboule D: How to make a limb? *Science* 266:575–576, 1994.
16. Diao E, Zaleske DJ, Avella D, et al: Kinetic and biochemical heterogeneity in vertebrate chondroepiphyseal regions during development. *J Orthop Res* 7:502–510, 1989.
17. Kember NF: Cell kinetics and the control of growth in long bones. *Cell Tissue Kinet* 11:477–485, 1978.
18. Kember NF: Cell divisions in endochondral ossification: A study of cell proliferation in rat bones by the method of tritiated thymidine. *J Bone Joint Surg [Br]* 42:824–839, 1960.
19. Kember NF: Cell population kinetics of bone growth: The first ten years of autoradiographic studies with tritiated thymidine. *Clin Orthop* 76:213–230, 1971.
20. Mankin HJ: Localization of tritiated thymidine in articular cartilage of rabbits. *J Bone Joint Surg [Am]* 44:682–688, 1962.
21. Cowell HR, Hunziker EB, Rosenberg L: The role of hypertrophic chondrocytes in endochondral ossification and in the development of secondary centers of ossification. *J Bone Joint Surg [Am]* 69:159–161, 1987.
22. Floyd WE III, Zaleske DJ, Schiller AL, et al: Vascular events associated with the appearance of the secondary center of ossification in the murine distal femoral epiphysis. *J Bone Joint Surg [Am]* 69A:185–190, 1987.
23. Langenskiold A, Elima K, Vuorio E: Specific collagen mRNAs eluciate the histogenetic relationship between the growth plate, the tissue in the ossification groove of Ranvier, and the cambium layer of the adjacent periosteum. *Clin Orthop* 297:51–54, 1993.
24. Langenskiold A, Videman T, Nevalainen T: Vital staining indicating cell migration towards the periphery in the growth plate. *Acta Orthop Scand* 64:683–687, 1993.
25. Shapiro F, Holtrop ME, Glimcher MJ: Organization and cellular biology of the perichondrial ossification groove of Ranvier. *J Bone Joint Surg [Am]* 59:703–723, 1977.
26. Saunders JW Jr, Gasseling MT, Gfeller MD: Interaction of ectoderm and mesoderm in the origin of axial relationships in the wing of the fowl. *J Exp Zool* 137:39, 1958.

27. Saunders JW Jr, Gasseling MT, Saunders LC: Cellular death in morphogenesis of the avian wing. *Dev Biol* 5:147, 1962.
28. Niswander L, Martin GR: FGF-4 and BMP-2 have opposite effects on limb growth. *Nature* 361:68–71, 1993.
29. Niswander L, Martin GR: FGF-4 expression during gastrulation, myogenesis, limb and tooth development in the mouse. *Development* 114:755–768, 1992.
30. Tabin C: The initiation of the limb bud: Growth factors, *Hox* genes, and retinoids. *Cell* 80:671–674, 1995.
31. Cohn MJ, Izpisua-Belmonte JC, Abud H, et al: Fibroblast growth factors induce additional limb development from the flank of chick embryos. *Cell* 80:739–746, 1995.
32. Riddle RD, Johnson RL, Laufer E, Tabin C: Sonic hedgehog mediates the polarizing activity of the ZPA. *Cell* 75:1401–1416, 1993.
33. Urist MR, DeLange RJ, Finerman GAM: Bone cell differentiation and growth factors. *Science* 220:680–686, 1983.
34. Centrella M, McCarthy TL, Canalis E: Transforming growth factor-beta and remodeling of bone. *J Bone Joint Surg [Am]* 73:1418–1428, 1991.
35. Sporn M, Roberts AB, Wakefield LM, Assoian RK: Transforming growth factor-beta: Biological function and chemical structure. *Science* 233:532–534, 1986.
36. O'Keefe RJ, Crabb ID, Puzas JE, Rosier RN: Effects of transforming growth factor-beta₁ and fibroblast growth factor on DNA synthesis in growth plate chondrocytes are enhanced by insulin-like growth factor-1. *J Orthop Res* 12:299–310, 1994.
37. Border WA, Noble NA: Transforming growth factor beta in tissue fibrosis. *N Engl J Med* 331:1286–1292, 1994.
38. Storm EE, Huynh TV, Copeland NG: Limb alterations in *brachypodism* mice due to mutations in a new member of the TGFb-superfamily. *Nature* 368:639–643, 1994.
39. West DC, Hampson IN, Arnold F, Kumar S: Angiogenesis induced by degradation products of hyaluronic acid. *Science* 228:1324–1326, 1985.
40. Feinberg RN, Beebe DC: Hyaluronate in vasculogenesis. *Science* 220:1177–1179, 1983.
41. Toole BP: Proteoglycans and hyaluronan in morphogenesis and differentiation, in Hay ED (ed): *Cell Biology of Extracellular Matrix*, 2d ed. New York, Plenum Press, 1991, pp 305–341.
42. Howell DS, Carreno MR, Ryan U: Evidence for an angiotrophic factor in growth plate hypertrophic cell cartilage. *Trans Orthop Res Soc* 11:50, 1986.
43. Brookes M: *The Blood Supply of Bone: An Approach to Bone Biology.* London: Butterworths, 1971, pp 123–132.
44. Sorgente N, Kuettner KE, Soble LW, Eisenstein R: The resistance of certain tissues to invasion: II. Evidence for extractable factors in cartilage which inhibit invasion by vascularized mesenchyme. *Lab Invest* 32:217–222, 1975.
45. Bright RW: Further canine studies with medical elastomer X7-2370 after osseous bridge resection for partial physeal plate closure. *Trans Orthop Res Soc* 6:108, 1981.
46. Brem H, Folkman J: Inhibition of tumor angiogenesis mediated by cartilage. *J Exp Med* 141:427–439, 1975.
47. Hootnick DR, Levinsohn EM, Randall PA, Packard DS Jr: Vascular dysgenesis associated with skeletal dysplasia of the lower limb. *J Bone Joint Surg [Am]* 62:1123, 1980.
48. Zaleske DJ, Holmes LB: Vascular patterns in the malformed hindlimb of Dh/+ mice, in Fallon JF, Caplan AI (eds): *Limb Development and Regeneration: Progress in Clinical Biological Research 110A.* New York, Liss, 1983, pp 317–326.
49. D'Amato RJ, Loughnan MS, Flynn E, Folkman J: Thalidomide is an inhibitor of angiogenesis. *Proc Natl Acad Sci USA* 91:4082–4085, 1994.
50. McKibbin B: The structure of the epiphysis, in Owen R, Goodfellow J, Bullough P (eds): *Scientific Foundations of Orthopaedics and Traumatology.* Philadelphia, Saunders, 1980, pp 169–175.
51. Trueta J, Morgan JD: The vascular contribution to osteogenesis: I. Studies by the injection method. *J Bone Joint Surg [Br]* 42:98–109, 1960.
52. Chappard D, Alexandre C, Riffat G: Uncalcified cartilage resorption in human fetal cartilage canals. *Tissue Cell* 18:701–707, 1986.
53. Ganey TM, Love SM, Ogden JA: Development of vascularization in the chondroepiphysis of the rabbit. *J Orthop Res* 10:496–510, 1992.
54. Rhinelander FW: Tibial blood supply in relation to fracture healing. *Clin Orthop* 105:34–81, 1974.
55. Chung S: The arterial supply of the developing proximal end of the human femur. *J Bone Joint Surg [Am]* 58:961, 1976.
56. Shapiro F: Epiphyseal disorders. *N Engl J Med* 317:1702–1710, 1987.
57. Pitsillides AA, Archer CW, Prehm P, et al: Alterations in hyaluronan synthesis during developing joint cavitation. *J Histochem Cytochem* 43:263–273, 1995.
58. McKibbin B, Holdsworth FW: The dual nature of epiphyseal cartilage. *J Bone Joint Surg [Br]* 49:351, 1967.
59. Kuida K, Lippke JA, Ku G, et al: Altered cytokine export and apoptosis in mice deficient in interleukin-1b converting enzyme. *Science* 267:2000–2003, 1995.
60. Drachman DB, Sokoloff L: The role of movement in embryonic joint development. *Dev Biol* 14:401, 1966.
61. Mankin HJ: The reaction of articular cartilage to injury and osteoarthritis. *N Engl J Med* 291:1285–1292, 1974.
62. Salter RB, Simmonds DF, Malcolm BW, et al: The biological effect of continuous passive motion on the healing of full-thickness defects in articular cartilage. *J Bone Joint Surg [Am]* 62:1232–1251, 1980.
63. O'Driscoll SW, Keeley FW, Salter RB: The chondrogenic potential of free autogenous periosteal grafts for biological resurfacing of major full-thickness defects in joint surfaces under the influence of continuous passive motion. *J Bone Joint Surg [Am]* 68:1017, 1986.
64. Maroudas A, Bullough P, Swanson SAV, Freeman MAR: The permeability of articular cartilage. *J Bone Joint Surg [Br]* 50:166–177, 1968.
65. Sah RL-Y, Kim Y-J, Doong J-YH, et al: Biosynthetic response of cartilage explants to dynamic compression. *J Orthop Res* 7:619–636, 1989.
66. Hall AC, Urban JPG, Gehl KA: The effects of hydrostatic pressure on matrix synthesis in articular cartilage. *J Orthop Res* 9:1–10, 1991.
67. Parkkinen JJ, Lammi MJ, Helminen HJ, Tammi M: Local stimulation of proteoglycan synthesis in articular cartilage explants by dynamic compression in vitro. *J Orthop Res* 10:610–620, 1992.
68. Freeman PM, Natarajan RN, Kimura JH, Andriacchi TP: Chondrocyte cells respond mechanically to compressive loads. *J Orthop Res* 12:311–320, 1994.
69. Carter DR, Wong M: Mechanical stresses and endochondral ossification in the chondroepiphysis. *J Orthop Res* 6:148–154, 1988.
70. Murphy SB, Ganz R, Muller ME: The prognosis in untreated dysplasia of the hip. *J Bone Joint Surg [Am]* 77:985–989, 1995.
71. Hueter C: Anatomische Studien an den Extremitatengelenken Neugebornener und Erwachsener. *Virchows Archiv* 25:572–599, 1862.
72. Brighton CT: Longitudinal bone growth: The growth plate and its dysfunctions, in Griffin PP (ed): *Instructional Course Lectures: XXXVI.* Park Ridge, IL: American Academy of Orthopaedic Surgeons, 1987, pp 3–25.
73. Robertson WW Jr: Newest knowledge of the growth plate. *Clin Orthop* 253:270–278, 1990.
74. Buckwalter JA: Proteoglycan structure in calcifying cartilage. *Clin Orthop* 172:207, 1982.

75. Ehrlich MG, Armstrong AL, Mankin HJ: Partial purification and characterization of a proteoglycan-degrading neutral protease from bovine epiphyseal cartilage. *J Orthop Res* 2:126–133, 1984.

76. Ehrlich MG, Armstrong AL, Neuman RG, et al: Patterns of proteoglycan degradation by a neutral protease from human growth-plate epiphyseal cartilage. *J Bone Joint Surg [Am]* 64:1350–1354, 1982.

77. Ali SY: Analysis of matrix vesicles and their role in calcification of epiphyseal cartilage. *Fed Proc* 35:135–142, 1976.

78. Felix R, Felisch H: Role of matrix vesicles of calcification. *Fed Proc* 35:169–171, 1976.

79. Anderson HC: Vesicles associated with calcification in the matrix of epiphyseal cartilage. *J Cell Biol* 41:59–72, 1969.

80. Anderson HC: Molecular biology of matrix vesicles. *Clin Orthop* 314:266–280, 1995.

81. Iannotti JP, Naidu S, Noguchi Y, et al: Growth plate matrix vesicle biogenesis. *Clin Orthop* 306:222–229, 1994.

82. Landis WJ, Glimcher MJ: Electron optical and analytical observations of rat growth plate cartilage prepared by ultracryomicrotomy: The failure to detect a mineral phase in matrix vesicles and the identification of heterodispersed particles as the initial solid phase of calcium phosphate deposited in the extracellular matrix. *J Ultrastruct Res* 78:227–268, 1982.

83. Boskey AL, Maresca M, Armstrong A, Ehrlich MG: Treatment of proteoglycan aggregates with physeal enzymes reduces their ability to inhibit hydroxyapatite proliferation in a gelatin gel. *J Orthop Res* 10:313–319, 1992.

84. Burgeson RE, Nimni ME: Collagen types: Molecular structure and tissue distribution. *Clin Orthop* 282:250–272, 1992.

85. Sandell LJ, Sugai JV, Trippel SB: Expression of collagens I, II, X, and XI and aggrecan mRNAs by bovine growth plate chondrocytes in situ. *J Orthop Res* 12:1–14, 1994.

86. Brooks PC, Clark RAF, Cheresh DA: Requirement of vascular integrin alpha(v)beta(3) for angiogenesis. *Science* 264:569–571, 1994.

87. Langer R, Brem H, Falterman K, et al: Isolation of a cartilage factor that inhibits tumor neovascularization. *Science* 193:70–72, 1976.

88. Hunziker EB, Schenk RK, Cruz-Orive L-M: Quantitation of chondrocyte performance in growth-plate cartilage during longitudinal bone growth. *J Bone Joint Surg [Am]* 69:162–173, 1987.

89. Breur GJ, VanEnkevort BA, Farnum CE, Wilsman NJ: Linear relationship between the volume of hypertrophic chondrocytes and the rate of longitudinal bone growth in growth plates. *J Orthop Res* 9:348–359, 1991.

90. Farnum CE, Wilsman NJ: Condensation of hypertrophic chondrocytes at the chondro-osseous junction of growth plate cartilage in Yucatan swine: Relationship to kinetics of long bone growth. *Am J Anat* 188:346–358, 1989.

91. Farnum CE, Turgai JA, Wilsman NJ: Visualization of living terminal hypertrophic chondrocytes of growth plate cartilage in situ by rectified interference contrast microscopy and time lapse cinematography. *J Orthop Res* 8:750–763, 1990.

92. Brighton CT, Lackman RD, Cuckler JM: Absence of the glycerol phosphate shuttle in the various zones of the growth plate. *J Bone Joint Surg [Am]* 65:663–666, 1983.

93. Kuhlman RE: Phosphatases in epiphyseal cartilage: Their possible role in tissue synthesis. *J Bone Joint Surg [Am]* 47:545–550, 1965.

94. Iannotti JP, Goldstein S, Kuhn J, et al: Growth plate and bone development, in Simon SR (ed): *Orthopaedic Basic Science*. Rosemont, IL: American Academy of Orthopaedic Surgeons, 1994, pp 185–217.

95. Poole AR: Review article: Proteoglycans in health and disease: Structures and functions. *Biochem J* 236:1–14, 1986.

96. DeSimone DP, Reddi AH: Vascularization and endochondral bone development: Changes in plasminogen activator activity. *J Orthop Res* 10:320–324, 1992.

97. Appleton I, Tomlinson A, Colvill-Nash PR, Willoughby DA: Temporal and spatial immunolocalization of cytokines in murine chronic granulomatous tissue. *Lab Invest* 69:405–414, 1993.

98. Armstrong PF: Cell kinetics and control of physeal growth, in Uhthoff HK, Wiley JJ (eds): *Behavior of the Growth Plate*. New York: Raven Press, 1988, pp 233–236.

99. Hinchliffe JR, Johnson DR: Growth of cartilage, in Hall BK (ed): *Cartilage:* Vol 2. New York, Academic Press, 1983, pp 255–295.

100. Boden SD, Kaplan FS, Fallon MD, et al: Metatropic dwarfism: Uncoupling of endochondral and periochondrial growth. *J Bone Joint Surg [Am]* 69:174–184, 1987.

101. Moss ML: The design of bones, in Owen R, Goodfellow J, Bullough P (eds): *Scientific Foundations of Orthopaedics and Traumatology*. Philadelphia, Saunders, 1980, pp 59–66.

102. Wolff J: *Das Gesetz der Transformation dem Knochen*. Berlin, Hirschwald, 1892.

103. Elmer EB, Ehrlich MG, Zaleske DJ, et al: Chondrodiatasis in rabbits: A study of the effect of transphyseal bone lengthening on cell division, synthetic function, and microcirculation in the growth plate. *J Pediatr Orthop* 12:181–190, 1992.

104. Greco F, DePalma L, Speddia N, Mannarini M: Growth plate cartilage metabolic response to mechanical stress. *J Pediatr Orthop* 9:520–524, 1989.

105. Burch WM, Van Wyk JJ: Triidothryronine stimulates cartilage growth and maturation by different mechanisms. *Am J Physiol* 252:E176–E182, 1987.

106. Trippel SB: Basic science of the growth plate. *Curr Opin Orthop* 1:279–288, 1990.

107. Trippel SB, Corvol MT, Dumontier MF, et al: Effect of somatomedin-C/insulin-like growth factor I and growth hormone on cultured growth plate and articular chondrocytes. *Pediatr Res* 25:76–82, 1989.

108. Crawford JD: Meat, potatoes, and growth hormone. *N Engl J Med* 305:163, 1981.

109. Macey LR, Kana SM, Jinguishi S, et al: Defects of early fracture-healing in experimental diabetes. *J Bone Joint Surg [Am]* 71:722–733, 1989.

110. Iannotti JP, Brighton CT, Iannotti V, Ohishi T: Mechanism of action of parathyroid hormone-induced proteoglycan synthesis in the growth plate chondrocyte. *J Orthop Res* 8:136–145, 1990.

111. Lefkowitz RJ: G proteins in medicine. *N Engl J Med* 332:186–187, 1995.

112. Loveys LS, Gelb D, Hurwitz SR, et al: Effect of parathyroid hormone-related peptide on chick growth plate chondrocytes. *J Orthop Res* 11:884–891, 1993.

113. Balogh K, Kunin AS: The effect of cortisone on the metabolism of epiphyseal cartilage. *Clin Orthop* 80:208–215, 1971.

114. Silbermann M: Hormones and cartilage, in Hall BK (ed): *Cartilage*. New York, Academic Press, 1983, pp 327–368.

115. Corvol MT, Carrascosa A, Tsagris L, et al: Evidence for a direct in vitro action of sex steroids on rabbit cartilage cells during skeletal growth: Influence of age and sex. *Endocrinology* 120:1422–1429, 1987.

116. Carrascosa A, Audi L, Ferrandez MA, Ballabriga A: Biological effects of androgens and identification of specific dihydrotestosterone-binding sites in cultured human fetal epiphyseal chondrocytes. *J Clin Endocrinol Metab* 70:134–140, 1990.

117. Mankin HJ: Metabolic bone disease. *J Bone Joint Surg [Am]* 76:760–788, 1994.

118. Kato Y: Roles of fibroblast growth factor and transforming growth factor-b families in cartilage formation, in Adolphe M (ed): *Biological Regulation of the Chondrocytes.* Boca Raton, FL: CRC Press, 1992, pp 141–160.

119. Trippel SB, Wroblewski J, Makower A-M, et al: Regulation of growth-plate chondrocytes by insulin-like growth-factor I and basic fibroblast growth factor. *J Bone Joint Surg [Am]* 75:177–189, 1993.

120. Alini M, Kofsky Y, Poole AR: Thyroid hormone, T3, negates the inhibitory effect of TGF-b1 on growth plate chondrocytes hypertrophy (abstr). *Trans Orthop Res Soc* 20:471, 1995.

121. Bennett A, Harvey W: Prostaglandins in orthopaedics. *J Bone Joint Surg [Br]* 63:152–154, 1981.

122. Francomano CA: Clinical implications of basic research: The genetic basis of dwarfism. *N Engl J Med* 332:58–59, 1995.

123. Shiang R, Thompson LM, Zhu Y-Z, et al: Mutations in the transmembrane domain of FGFR3 cause the most common genetic form of dwarfism achondroplasia. *Cell* 78:335–342, 1994.

124. LeMerrer M, Rousseau F, Legeai-Mallet L, et al: A gene for achondroplasia-hydrochondroplasia maps to chromosome 4p. *Nature Genet* 6:318–321, 1994.

125. Reardon W, Winter RM, Rutland P, et al: Mutations in the fibroblast growth factor receptor 2 gene cause Crouzon syndrome. *Nature Genet* 8:98–103, 1994.

126. Jabs EW, Li X, Scott AF, et al: Jackson-Weiss and Crouzon syndromes are allelic with mutations in fibroblast growth factor receptor 2. *Nature Genet* 8:275–279, 1994.

127. Muenke M, Schell U, Hehr A, et al: A common mutation in the fibroblast growth factor receptor 1 gene in Pfeiffer syndrome. *Nature Genet* 8:269–274, 1994.

128. Erlebacher A, Filvaroff EH, Gitelman SE, Derynck R: Toward a molecular understanding of skeletal development. *Cell* 80:371–378, 1995.

129. Prockop DJ: Mutations in collagen genes as a cause of connective-tissue diseases. *N Engl J Med* 326:540–546, 1992.

130. Kuivaniemi H, Tromp G, Prockop DJ: Mutations in collagen genes: Causes of rare and some common diseases in humans. *FASEB J* 2052–2060, 1991.

131. Hastbacka J, de la Chapelle A, Mahtani MM, et al: The diastrophic dysplasia gene encodes a novel sulfate transporter: Positional cloning by fine-structure linkage disequilibrium mapping. *Cell* 78:1073, 1994.

132. Rosenberg LC: The physis as an interface between basic research and clinical knowledge. *J Bone Joint Surg [Am]* 66A:815–816, 1984.

CHAPTER 2

The Biology of Bone

Matthew F. Halsey, Kenneth McLeod, and Clinton Rubin

An understanding of the complex and heterogenous nature of bone is an essential prerequisite for the knowledgeable treatment of musculoskeletal anomalies, diseases, and injuries. Advances in our understanding of the basic biology of bone continue to promote the development of innovative clinical applications. It is important that the surgeon appreciate the many responsibilities of the skeletal organ and the numerous biochemical and biophysical factors to which the bone tissue is sensitive.

The skeleton fulfills several indispensable functions. These include facilitation of effective and efficient locomotion and the protection of vital organs, including the brain, heart, and lungs. Bone tissue is also the principal reservoir for mineral metabolism, specifically calcium, phosphate, and magnesium. A key component to the success of the skeleton is its plasticity; bone is a dynamic tissue that can rapidly adapt to the structural and metabolic demands placed upon it. This is achieved by an intricate balance between the formation and resorption of bone tissue, orchestrated by the complex interaction of osteoblasts, osteoclasts and osteocytes.

It is important to understand how, at the cellular level, the body regulates matrix formation and removal, mineralization, and bone structure. This chapter also presents an overview of those regulatory messages, both chemical and physical, that define the bone's mass and morphology.

BONE ARCHITECTURE

The remarkable structural capabilities of bone, in both time and space, are derived from the advantageous utilization and placement of its constituent materials on the gross and microscopic levels. In comparison to common building materials, bone has nearly the same ultimate tensile strength as cast iron and twice the energy absorption capacity of oak. The most interesting aspect of bone, though, is its capacity to remodel, adapt, and repair itself in response to a variety of stimuli, whether physiologic, traumatic, or pathologic. At the gross level, each bone has a distinct morphology comprising both cortical bone, found in the outer shell, and cancellous bone, found within the epiphyseal and metaphyseal regions of long bones as well as throughout the interior of short bones. At the microscopic level, two types of bone are identified: the disorganized, hypercellular woven bone and the highly organized, relatively hypocellular lamellar bone. Essentially, all bone tissue can be described by either of these two morphologies, whether mature, growing, pathologic, or healing.

Woven bone is a product of rapid bone formation, which is characterized by an irregular, disorganized pattern of collagen orientation and osteocyte distribution. While it is characteristic of embryonic and fetal development, woven bone is also found in the healthy adult skeleton at ligament and tendon insertions. More importantly, woven bone is elaborated in response to bony injury, whether metabolic or traumatic, as well as dramatic changes in mechanical stimulation.[1,2] Because woven bone can be produced so quickly in comparison to lamellar bone, it is utilized as a temporary mechanical adjunct that allows the bone to maintain or to return quickly to its role as a structural support. While many consider woven bone to represent an aberrant response, it appears that it in fact represents a wise use of metabolic energies in accommodating new, intense structural challenges.

Lamellar, or mature, bone can be packed tightly to form the dense cortex of a bone or organized as the trabecular struts in cancellous bone. In contrast to the random and disorganized structure of woven bone, the lamellar appearance of this mature bone is the product of highly organized, mineralized plates. In cancellous bone, the lamellae run parallel to the trabeculae. In cortical bone, several patterns occur. The predominant one is that found in osteons, which are made up of small, concentric, lamellar cylinders surrounding a central vascular channel, not unlike the rings in a tree trunk. Osteons are typically 200 to 300 μm in diameter, consisting of up to six or seven concentric osteocyte rings comprising up to 20 lamellar plates[3] (Fig. 2-1). Canaliculi in lamellar bone are consistent in diameter and orientation and in toto contain fewer osteocytes per unit volume than woven bone (20,000 cells versus 80,000 cells per cubic millimeter).

The birefringent pattern of both circumferential lamellae and single osteons is believed to be produced by the altering of direction of collagen bundles from one layer to the next, therefore maximizing strength in a number of different planes (Fig. 2-2). Although the collagen bundles within each of these lamellar plates are highly oriented, individual fibers will often traverse interlamellar spaces. Such a composite integration will increase both the individual osteon's resistance to external loads and the effective strength of the bone structure.[4] An alternative theory for the polarized light birefringence of an osteon is based on alternating fiber-rich and fiber-poor lamellar rings, in which the thinner (1- to 2-μm) plates contain a greater degree of glycosaminoglycans (ground substance) than the adjacent 5- to 7-μm collagen-rich layers.[5] These glycosaminoglycans are thought to be continuous from the "thin" lamellar plate, through the cement line, to interdigitate with the ground substance of the "thick" plate. This architecture, with a true continuity between plates, would produce an increase in the stiffness of each osteon or each circumferential plate. Perhaps the morphology of lamellar bone will prove to be some combination of these two postulations, thus maximizing both the stiffness of the material (continuity of ground substance) and its toughness (integration of collagen layers).

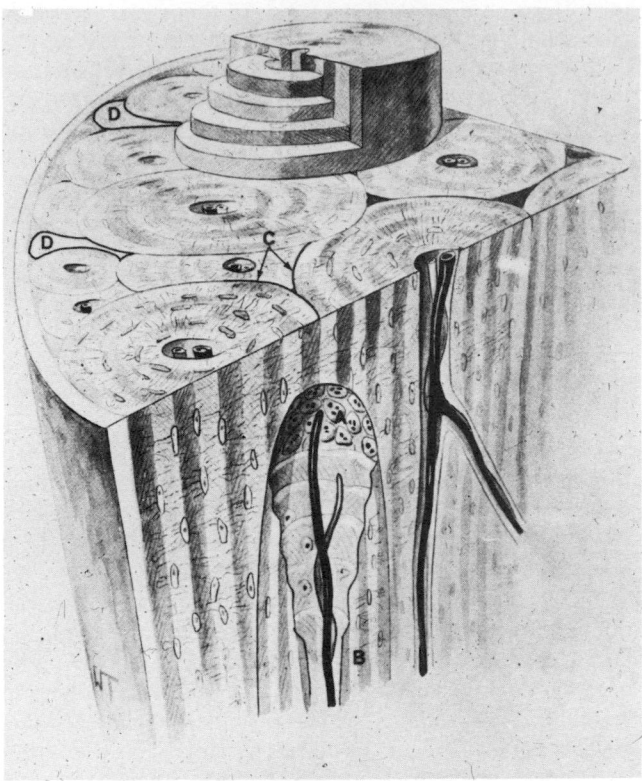

Figure 2-1 Schematic reconstruction of a segment of cortical bone. A, The cutting cone where osteoclasts are actively creating a tunnel along which new bone is laid; B, creation of a new osteon; C, cement lines; D, interstitial lamellae. [From Bullough PG, in Wren R, Goodfellow J, Bullough P (eds): *Scientific Foundations of Orthopaedics and Traumatology.* Philadelphia, Saunders, 1980. With permission.]

THE CELLS OF BONE

The success with which bone meets its principal responsibilities is largely a result of an active cell population derived from two distinct cellular lineages. Multipotential primitive mesenchymal cells form the pool from which osteoblasts, bone lining cells, and osteocytes arise. Osteoclasts, on the other hand, originate in the hematopoietic monocyte-macrophage series. Despite their separate beginnings, these cells are coupled to provide essential physiologic functions, including bone modeling and remodeling, fracture healing, and mineral homeostasis.[6]

Osteoblasts

The primary role of osteoblasts is to synthesize osteoid, the nonmineralized portion of the bone matrix. Differentiation of mesenchymal progenitor cells into preosteoblasts and osteoblasts marks the first stage of formation of new bone rather than other phenotypes such as muscle, fat, or cartilage.[7] The progenitor cells, in turn, most likely originate from vessel endothelial cells, pericytes, or reticular cells.[8] The progression from progenitor cell to preosteoblast is marked by migration, proliferation, and differentiation of the cells, with a concomitant change in appearance from thin and flat to plump, eosinophilic, and cuboidal[9,10] (Fig 2-3). These events are inducible by cytokines.[11]

Differentiation into a full-fledged osteoblast is immediately preceded by an intermediate, or preosteoblast, stage, which lasts 2 to 3 days and is highlighted by formation of a contiguous layer of cells and increased alkaline phosphatase levels.[12] The most notable product of early

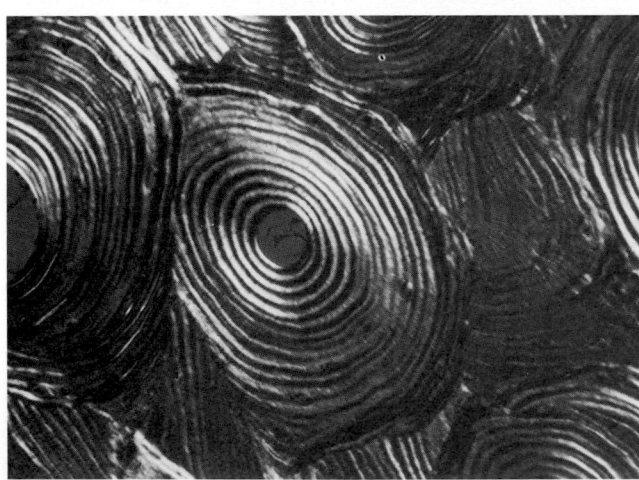

Figure 2-2 Lamellar bone viewed with polarized light. The collagen-rich bundles are arranged in concentric rings approximately 7 μm thick about the haversian canal. Straight, rather than circular, bundles are interstitial lamellae. ($\times$350). [From Sokoloff L, Bland JH (eds): *The Musculoskeletal System.* Baltimore, Williams & Wilkins, 1975. With permission.]

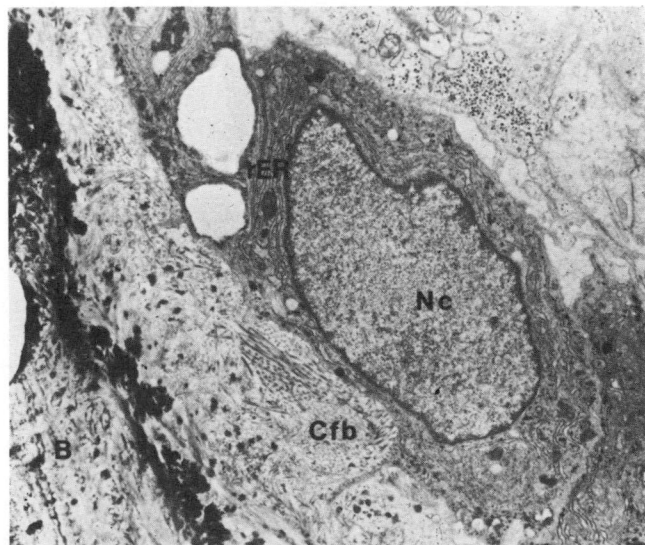

Figure 2-3 Electron micrograph of an osteoblast. There is a well-developed rough endoplasmic reticulum (rER) close to the nucleus (Nc); along the bone (B) surface are disposed several collagen fibers (Cfb). (Decalcified bone, $\times$7200.)[From Marie PG, in Cruess R (ed): *The Musculoskeletal System.* New York: Churchill Livingstone, 1982. With permission.]

osteoblast activity is pro-α1 collagen, which constitutes the majority of osteoid.[6] Osteocalcin and bone morphogenetic proteins are other notable products.[13] Mineralization of the osteoid material is also initiated by osteoblasts, which appear to modulate electrolyte fluxes between the extracellular fluid (ECF) volume and osseous fluid.[10,12,14] An individual osteoblast can produce 0.5 to 1.5 μm/day of an osteoid seam for approximately 8 weeks.[15,16] Osteoblast histology is notable for its extensive endoplasmic reticulum with multiple cisternae, well-developed Golgi bodies, and numerous ribosomes, which all point to its massive synthetic efforts. Interestingly, it has been noted that osteoblasts are connected by numerous gap junctions, 9 nm in size, which facilitate communication between cells via chemical or electrical signals.[17] Osteoblasts follow one of three fates: cell death (apoptosis), differentiation into a bone lining cell, or differentiation into an osteocyte surrounded by matrix.

Bone Lining Cells

Quiescent bone surfaces, including endosteal, periosteal, and intracortical surfaces, are lined with osteocytelike cells. These cells are differentiated from osteoblasts and, like osteocytes, maintain cytoplasmic extensions into the bone to contact osteocytes.[14,18] They maintain a flattened appearance and have fewer active organelles than osteoblasts. Their main function is to isolate the bone surface and to moderate site-specific mineralization or resorption.[19] Parfitt[20] has described the bone lining cell as a "gatekeeper: which mediates bone resorption activity after activation by PTH [parathyroid hormone]." Gatekeeper-mediated functions include resorption, site activation and preparation, mononuclear recruitment, capillary budding, and attraction of preosteoclasts.[21] Martin and Rodan[21] have also postulated that initiation of resorption by PTH, 1,25-dihydroxycholecalciferol (vitamin D), or prostaglandins leads to decreased synthesis of collagen and alkaline phosphatase. It also increases production of cyclic adenosine monophospate (cAMP), which causes the cell to become more rounded, exposing the bone surface to osteoclastic activity. Collagenase secretion dissolves the endosteal membrane, contributing to the exposure of the bone surface. Indirectly, the bone lining cell also activates osteoclasts and inhibits osteoblastic anabolic activity.

Osteocytes

Osteocytes are the main cellular component of bony tissue, making up 90 percent of all bone cells. These cells originate from osteoblasts that are trapped by osteoid produced by surrounding osteoblasts, forming a lacuna.[22] Histologically, osteocytes possess a single nucleus and, compared to osteoblasts, are smaller in size and have a decreased number of organelles (Fig. 2-4). Collagen synthesis is essentially halted. Osteocytes continue to maintain the cytoplasmic extensions that characterized the osteoblasts, forming a large canalicular system. This system essentially constitutes a three-dimensional array or "syncytium," ex-

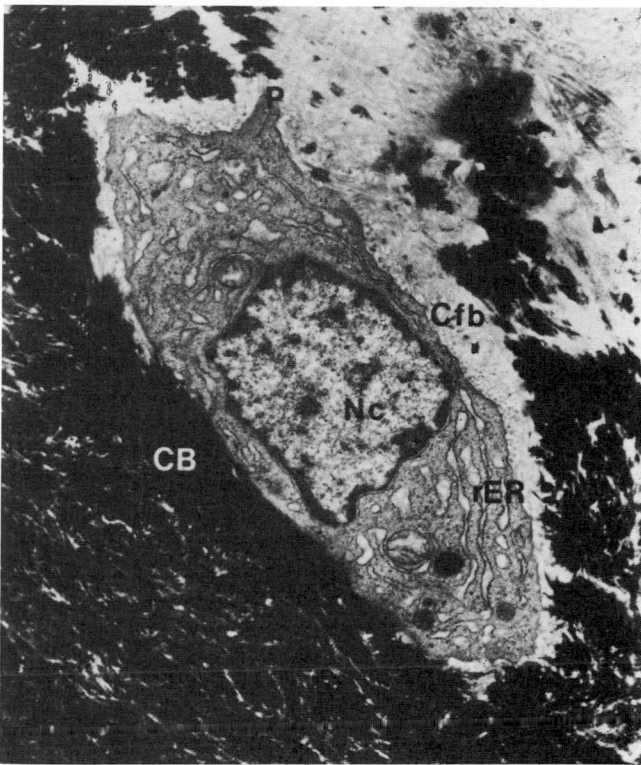

Figure 2-4 Electron micrograph of a young osteocyte within its lacuna. It is surrounded by collagen fibers (Cfb). It possesses a large nucleus (Nc) and has well-developed rough endoplasmic reticulum (rER). A process from the osteocyte (P) extends into the calcified bone (CB). (Undecalcified bone, $\times$6600.) [From Marie PG, in Cruess R (ed): *The Musculoskeletal System.* New York, Churchill Livingstone, 1982. With permission.]

tending beyond osteonal limits, which is ideal for chemical, electrical, and stress-generated fluid communication[23] (Fig. 2-5). Osteocytes communicate with osteoblasts and bone lining cells, as well as other osteocytes.[24] The connections are made up of gap junctions formed by six identical membrane-protein subunits termed *connexins.*[25] Besides the obvious role of metabolic support, it has been proposed that this vast, interconnected system moves biophysical data to cells within and at the surface of the bone. This is supported by the fact that the osteocytes' surface area exceeds that of the lining cells by two orders of magnitude.[26] It is postulated that this array can either sense mechanical deformations directly and/or pick up the electric potentials produced by the flow of ions across the negatively charged bone surface. Also, Weinbaum et al.[27] have modeled the ability of osteocyte processes to detect small shear stresses produced by the flow of the surrounding fluid. Of interest is the fact that the extent of the osteocyte syncytium slowly diminishes with age,[28] decreasing its sensitivity to biophysical signals.

Osteoclasts

Osteoclasts are the cells responsible for bone resorption and as such constitute the counterweight to osteoblasts. In fact, the lack of properly functioning osteoclasts leads to

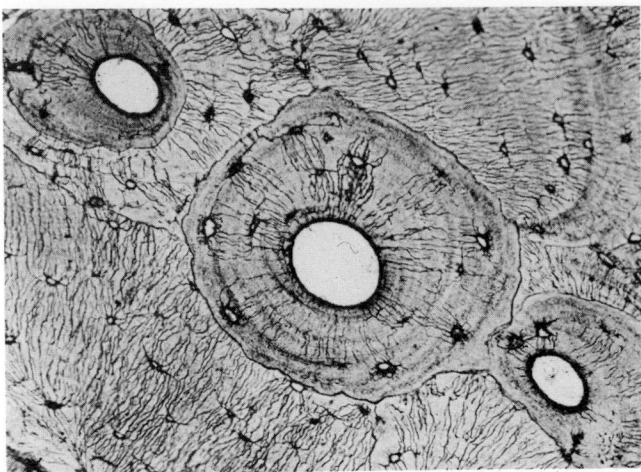

Figure 2-5 Nutritional and communication pathways through bone. The cement line encircles the osteon with its Haversian canal and circumferentially arranged lamellae. The fine filaments extending radially from the lacunae are canaliculi. (Bodian, ×250.) [From Sokoloff L, Bland JH (eds): *The Musculoskeletal System.* Baltimore, Williams & Wilkins, 1975. With permission.]

the development of osteopetrosis, or marble bone disease. This potentially fatal disorder is characterized by inadequate bone resorption, which eventually results in an altered hematopoietic homeostasis. In contrast to osteoblasts, osteoclasts are multinucleated and motile, capable of traveling 100 μm in a day. As it moves, the osteoclast will resorb bone in a 300-μm-diameter tunnel, excavating up to 200,000 μm^3 each day.

Like the osteoblast, the osteoclast has been the focus of intense study in attempts to discern its origins, development, structure, and function. Early microscopic studies appeared to indicate that the osteoclast, rather than arising from mesenchymal progenitors, arose instead from the hematopoietic cell lines based on its multinuclear appearance.[29] Using a model of osteopetrosis, Walker[30] was able to demonstrate that bone resorption activity could be reestablished with hematopoietic stem cell transplants. Other studies focusing on the osteoclast found strong evidence to support the hypothesis that macrophages and osteoclasts shared a common origin.[31,32] Regulation of osteoclastic proliferation and differentiation appears to be coincident with the macrophage/monocyte lineage. Both interleukin-3 (IL-3) and granulocyte-macrophage colony stimulating factor (GM-CSF) are needed to form the original colony forming unit. Loss of GM-CSF action engenders deficiencies of both osteoclasts and macrophages: the osteopetrotic op/op mouse, which secretes an ineffective GM-CSF, is cured by infusions of recombinant GM-CSF.[33] Beyond this point the signals required for differentiation are less well delineated, though there is strong evidence to suggest that further development and activation of osteoclasts is mediated by osteoblast cell products.[34,35]

The primary signals for osteoclast activation include 1,25(OH)$_2$D$_3$, PTH, and tumor necrosis factor (TNF); these hormones, in the presence of bone stromal elements, induce the production of calcitonin receptors, the expression of carbonic anhydrase, and intense tartrate-resistant alkaline phosphatase (TRAP) activity. Interestingly, though, osteoclast precursors do not possess receptors to any of these chemical signals, while osteoblasts do.[6] The activation of osteoclasts by insulin-like growth factors is also mediated by osteoblasts.[36] The association of IL-6 with osteoporosis[37] and of IL-11 with Paget disease[38] has highlighted a potential role for these cytokines in the appropriate development of osteoclasts.

Osteoclast functionality is made possible by several ultrastructural modifications that enable the cell to isolate a bone surface, dissolve the mineral component, and then lyse the remaining organic matrix. Before the process of bone resorption can occur, the osteoclast must recognize and adhere to the bone surface in question, forming a resorption compartment. This is mediated via *integrin,* a cell surface glycoprotein, which binds the arginyl-glysyl-aspartyl (RGD) ligand found in vitronectin, a bone matrix molecule (blocking the integrin activity prevents osteoclastic bone resorption).[39] An apical clear zone and ruffled border form, guided by intracellular contractile proteins attached to the integrins[40] (Fig. 2-6). Numerous vacuolar proton-ATPase pumps then localize to the ruffled border and, in concert with the intracellular carbonic anydrase II, lower the pH of the extracellular bone compartment, which forms a resorption pit.[41] This metabolic activity is supported by numerous pleiomorphic mitochondria[30] (Fig. 2-6). At physiologic pH (7.4), hydroxyapatite is essentially insoluble; lowering the pH allows the pericellular concentration of Ca^{2+} to increase 10- to 20-fold up to 40 mM.[42] Lysosomal enzymes—for example, cathepsin B[43] and acid proteases[12]—then digest the exposed organic matrix, completing the dissolution of the bone.

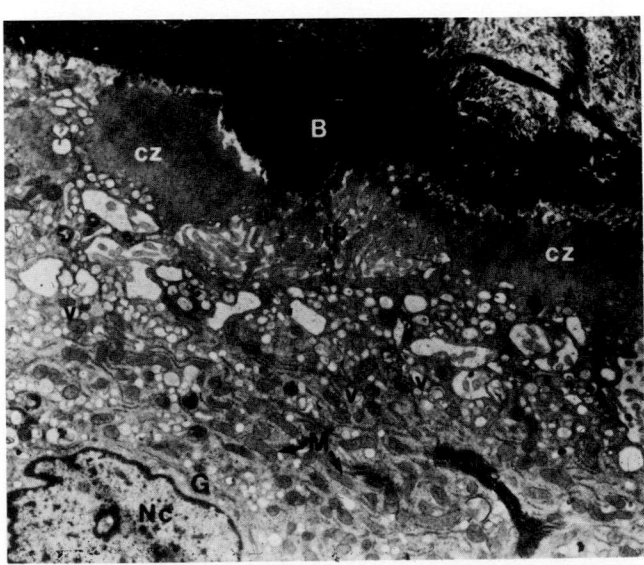

Figure 2-6 Electron micrograph of an osteoclast showing one nucleus (Nc), a large number of mitochondria (M), Golgi apparatus (G), and numerous vacuoles (V). The ruffled border (rb) is surrounded by a clear zone (cz) and applied to the bone matrix (B). (Undecalcified bone, ×5400.) [From Marie PG, in Cruess RL (ed): *The Musculoskeletal System.* New York, Churchill Livingstone, 1982. With permission.]

THE COMPOSITION OF BONE MATRIX

Bone cells lie on and in a matrix which consists of both organic and inorganic components. By wet weight, bone tissue is 70 percent mineralized matrix, 25 percent organic matrix and cells, and 5 percent water. Collagen constitutes 94 percent of the organic component, while the rest is made up of noncollagenous proteins, proteoglycans, osteonectin,[44] sialoproteins,[45] osteocalcin,[46] and bone morphogenic proteins (BMPs),[47] which influence matrix organization, mineralization, and bone cell behavior. Structurally, the organic matrix is responsible for resisting deformation in tension: bone that possesses inadequate or abnormal collagen, as with osteogenesis imperfecta, is especially brittle and easily fractured. The organic matrix also contains enzymes, hormones, and growth factors that most likely play a part in bone cell regulation.[48] The inorganic phase consists of hydroxyapatite and maintains, in solid form, 99 percent of the body's calcium, 85 percent of the phosphorus, and 66 percent of the magnesium. The mineral phase is also responsible for resisting mechanical deformation in compression, while collagen provides tensile properties.[49] Together, the organic and inorganic matrix of bone form a material that is both very durable and stable.

Collagen

The collagen found in bone is primarily type I, though trace amounts of types III, V, and XI, usually attributed to blood vessel walls found in the bone, have been found as well.[50] Type I collagen is a heterotrimer, formed by two $\alpha 1$(I)chains, or tropocollagen molecules, and one $\alpha 2$(I) chain.[51] Tropocollagen is notable for the long central portion formed by the repeating amino acid sequence Gly-X-Y, where X and Y are usually lysine and hydroxylysine, respectively. This attribute is essential for the quaternary structure of type I collagen, which is characterized by its 300-nm linear triple helix.[52] Bone collagen molecules align themselves head-to-tail longitudinally and with a one-quarter stagger laterally, resulting in a well-defined microscopic periodicity of 640 nm.[53] The resultant collagen fibril possesses gaps within its structure that are postulated to be where mineralization is initiated.[48] Type I collagen found in bone is very similar to type I collagen found in skin and tendons except for a few notable differences. Bone collagen forms significantly fewer covalent allysine and hydroxyallysine cross links[54] and has higher levels of glycosylated hydroxylysyl residues, as opposed to the glucosyl-galactosyl hydroxylysine residues characterizing the soft tissue type I collagen.[55]

Proteoglycans

The proteoglycans biglycan (PG-I) and decorin (PG-II) constitute an early and substantial portion of noncollagenous proteins in the bone matrix. These molecules are formed by a thin protein core (5 percent by weight) and multiple covalently bound disaccharide units (95 percent by weight).[56] Different types of disaccharide units, or glycosaminoglycans, can be attached, including dermatan sulfate, heparan sulfate, keratan sulfate, and chondroitan sulfate.[57] The latter is the most common in bone matrix. Both types of proteoglycans are localized to matrix and cells, but biglycan alone is detected in the canaliculi and osteonal walls of osteocytes.[58] The function of proteoglycans has not yet been clearly defined, but evidence suggests several important roles with respect to the reservation of space for bone development,[59] the initiation of mineralization,[60,61] the deposition and structuring of collagen fibrils,[62] and the binding and availability of local growth factors.[59] Skerry et al.,[63] noting that physiologic strains lead to proteoglycan deformation (which resolves slowly over 48 h), have suggested that these molecules, through direct interactions with the osteocyte membrane and cytoskeleton, act as mediators in the transfer of mechanical strain information from tissue to cell.

Osteonectin

Osteonectin is an acidic 38-kDa glycoprotein,[64] constituting 15 percent of the noncollagenous protein in developing bone.[61] Both osteoblasts and osteocytes produce this moiety constitutively. Chemically, this molecule is notable for multiple acid phosphate groups and a tertiary structure similar to the Ca^{2+} binding region of calmodulin. Functionally, osteonectin appears to play a role in mineralization,[65] as it binds collagen, has a high affinity for both Ca^{2+} and hydroxyapatite,[66] and localizes to crystal-producing matrix vesicles.[67]

RGD-Containing Proteins

Another family of noncollagenous bone matrix proteins is characterized by the Arg-Gly-Asp (RGD) amino acid sequence, which is preferentially recognized by cell surface integrin molecules. This protein family is represented by fibronectin, thrombospondin, and the bone sialoproteins, including osteopontin. Fibronectin, which is produced by osteoblasts, mediates osteoblast interaction with bone matrix via cell attachment and dispersion.[68] Bone sialoprotein is produced by osteoblasts and osteocytes as well as uterine trophoblasts and represents 15 percent of noncollagenous bone matrix proteins. Osteopontin, or bone sialoprotein-I (BSP-I), is an 80-kDa protein composed of 3 percent sialic acid and appears in multiple forms depending on the amount of sulfonation.[69] Like fibronectin, osteopontin mediates the attachment of cells to bone matrix.

Osteocalcin

The last major noncollagenous matrix protein, osteocalcin, is small, 5.3-kDa, with three to five gamma-carboxylated glutamic acid residues.[51] Osteocalcin is specific for mineralized tissues and represents 2 percent of total bone protein. Increased osteocalcin synthesis is induced by $1,25(OH)_2D_3$,[70] while vitamin K mediates glutamic acid carboxylation.[71] As with several other noncollagenous matrix proteins, osteocalcin function is not clearly delineated, but it is associated with bone remodeling—i.e., osteoclast recruitment and bone formation.[72] Indirectly, serum levels of osteocalcin are used to discern bone formation activity.[73] Furthermore, bone deficient in osteocalcin does not undergo resorption in vivo[74] and is associated with premature closure of epiphyseal growth plates.[75]

Hydroxyapatite

The inorganic matrix is composed chiefly of hydroxyapatite, a calcium crystal which is also found in geologic formations. The chemical composition of hydroxyapatite is represented by the formula $Ca_{10}(PO_4)_6(OH)_2$, and its structural dimensions are approximately 80 nm by 20 nm by 3 nm.[76] The biological version is smaller (100 versus 400 nm^2) and has numerous molecular impurities, including sodium, fluoride, strontium, lead, and radium as well as carbonate and acid phosphate groups, which are particular to biological crystals.[77] These "characteristics" combine to make this molecular species more reactive,[78] which may facilitate resorption and repair by the bone cell population. It is generally agreed that the inorganic matrix, like the organic matrix, undergoes change as it ages. Specifically, the crystalline structure of hydroxyapatite becomes less impure, with fewer carbonate and acid phosphate groups attached, which results in a smaller surface-to-volume ratio and a less reactive molecule.[79]

MINERALIZATION

The process of tissue mineralization is not completely understood but is a critical aspect of bone physiology that has significant clinical applications. Stated simply, mineralization is the transformation of hydroxyapatite from a soluble form into a solid form, starting at multiple nucleation sites and then spreading by accretion. Mineralization in organic tissues represents a complex, dynamic, and site-specific process that integrates the actions of multiple cells, enzymes, and other proteins to create a structurally and biologically competent tissue.[49]

The mineralization of osteoid begins 10 to 15 days after its formation.[80] Yet within hours of the beginning of the process, 70 percent of the ultimate mineral contents is deposited.[81] Initiation of mineralization occurs at multiple independent nucleation sites, separated by 640 nm, that coincide with the collagen hole zones.[49] Glimcher[82] demonstrated not only that nucleation sites appeared at 640-nm intervals but also that without the collagen hole zones, calcium phosphate crystals would not form. The formation of nucleation sites within the hole zones is most likely mediated by a number of organic components found within the hole zones, including osteonectin,[48] fibronectin,[83] and phosphoproteins.[49] Continued mineralization is driven by the decreasing free energy associated with increasing mineral accretion.[49] As the crystals expand, the collagen fibrils help to direct their alignment and orientation so that, in their final form, the crystals are aligned parallel with the collagen.[84]

Formation of calcium phosphate particles does not occur exclusively in the collagen hole zones; microscopic studies have also revealed these particles in osteoblastic mitochondria[85,86] and matrix vesicles.[87,88] *Matrix vesicles* develop as buds from hypertrophic chondrocytes or osteoblastic plasma membranes undergoing apoptosis. Nucleation within the vesicles occurs at the internal membrane and is mediated by membrane-bound acidic phospholipids (which in vitro are efficient apatite nucleators)[89] and a membrane-bound calcium pump. Both direct and indirect roles for vesicles and mitochondria in bone mineralization have been proposed, but none have been clearly established.[49]

The necessity of limiting the calcification of biological tissues to appropriate sites points to the importance of the agents inhibiting mineralization. Proteoglycans appear to play a large part in this process. The molecules bind calcium ions, inhibit their diffusion, and exclude the inorganic phosphate necessary for continued mineralization.[82] The high concentration of proteoglycans in ligaments, tendons, and skin may be what prevents mineralization in these tissues.[90] During the process of endochondral ossification, proteoglycan moieties gradually decrease in amount and size, thus decreasing the number of bound calcium ions.[91,92] Some authors postulate a possible role for matrix vesicles, suggesting that they release enzymes that degrade proteoglycans, allowing mineralization to proceed.[93] Collagen structure may also play a role in resisting mineralization if collagen fibrils are packed so tightly that ion diffusion is severely hindered.[94]

Clinically, the importance of mineralization is evident in a number of clinical states. "Greenstick" fractures and plastic deformation of bone are possible only because immature bone is less mineralized. As the bone matures, these fracture patterns become less common. Rickets and osteomalacia represent pathologic states characterized by adequate production of osteoblastic osteoid but insufficient mineralization. As the percentage of unmineralized matrix increases, the skeleton becomes subject to deformity and pathologic fracture.

BONE MINERAL METABOLISM

Calcium, magnesium, and phosphorus ions all play an integral role in numerous organ functions throughout the body, including muscle contraction, neural activity, and cardiac rhythm. Because of the relationship of these ions with normal body function, the concentration of these species in the ECF compartments, both intra- and extravascular, is fairly rigidly controlled. Mineral homeostasis is performed through the actions of several different systemic hormones—PTH, $1,25(OH)_2D_3$, and calcitonin—that monitor the entry and release of ions from bone, kidney, and intestine.

Parathyroid Hormone

The organ responsible for sensing and responding to changing levels of calcium in the plasma, normally 8 to 10 mg/dL, is the parathyroid. The parathyroid controls ECF Ca^{2+} levels via its hormone product, PTH. This is a single-chain polypeptide secreted by the parathyroid chief cells.[26] The target organs of PTH include the kidneys and bone: in the former, it inhibits tubular reabsorption of phosphate, improves Ca^{2+} resorption, and indirectly stimulates the production of $1,25(OH)_2D_3$ by 1-hydroxylase, while in the latter, PTH mobilizes Ca^{2+} from the bone mineral.[95] Parathyroid hormone acts indirectly, via $1,25(OH)_2D_3$, on the small intestine to increase Ca^{2+} ion absorption and on bone to stimulate differentiation of osteoclast precursors.[96,97]

Parathyroid hormone stimulation in bone tissue elicits a biphasic response: initially PTH activates osteoclasts, starts bone resorption, and inhibits collagen synthesis; 2 to 5 days later, PTH increases collagen synthesis and bone formation.[3,98] As osteoclasts do not possess receptors for PTH, they are activated indirectly via osteoblasts.[99] Once activated, the osteoclasts undergo profound morphologic and metabolic changes, including an increase in overall size and in the volume of the ruffled border.[98,100] Bone lining cells undergo retraction from the bone surface to allow access to the osteoclasts. It appears that these changes are mediated via increased intracellular concentrations of cAMP and Ca^{2+}.[101]

Vitamin D

Vitamin D is intimately involved with a number of metabolic activities, including intestinal absorption of Ca^{2+}, bone resorption, and bone mineralization.[102] The active metabolites of vitamin D, most of which is in the D_3 form, act as systemic asteroid hormones.[103] Cholecalciferol, vitamin D_3, is first hydroxylated in the liver to 25-hydroxy D_3 by microsomal 25-hydroxylase.[104] The most active form is 1,25-dihydroxy D_3 [$1,25(OH)_2D_3$, or calcitriol], which is formed in the kidney by 1-hydroxylase.[3] The primary action of $1,25(OH)_2D_3$ is to increase the absorption of Ca^{2+} by increasing the production of a transport protein.[3] Acting as a hormone, calcitrol localizes to the cell nucleus, where it induces the biosynthesis of new mRNA molecules.[3] In bone, $1,25(OH)_2D_3$ stimulates the differentiation of osteoclast precursors to increase bone resorption.[96] Its precise relationship to the process of bone mineralization is unclear, although insufficient levels of $1,25(OH)_2D_3$ are associated with osteomalacia and rickets.

Calcitonin

Calcitonin is a polypeptide, elaborated by thyroid parafollicular C cells, which modulates serum calcium and phosphate ion concentrations.[105,106] Secretion of calcitonin is regulated by serum Ca^{2+} levels.[107] Specifically, calcitonin acts on osteoclasts directly via calcitonin receptors[108] to inhibit their activation and to promote division into mononuclear cells.[109,110] It appears that the effects of calcitonin are mediated by increasing levels of cAMP and Ca^{2+}.[111] Because of its effects on osteoclastic activity, calcitonin has been suggested as a possible therapeutic agent for hypercalcemia, Paget disease, and hyperresorptive osteoporosis.[112]

HORMONE, GROWTH FACTOR, AND CYTOKINE REGULATION OF BONE METABOLISM

Sex Hormones

Estrogen is a systemic hormone, largely synthesized by the ovaries, that has potent if unclear effects on bone tissue metabolism. Postmenopausal osteoporosis is associated with the concomitant decrease in estrogen levels; bone loss increases dramatically for approximately a decade, affecting both cortical and trabecular bone, especially the latter.[113] The principal benefit of estrogen appears to be a decrease in the rate of bone turnover by inhibition of osteoclastic bone resorption, but some anabolic potential is also evident.[26] Research into estrogenic effects on bone resorption are hampered by the fact that estrogen has no effect upon in vitro resorption systems. It appears that some estrogenic effects are mediated by other systemic hormones. Estrogen increases calcitonin synthesis and secretion[114,115] and decreases the secretion and peripheral effects of PTH.[116,117]

A major breakthrough in estrogen research occurred when it was discovered that bone tissue, specifically osteoblasts, synthesized estrogen receptors.[118,119] Interestingly, osteoblasts in males possess androgen receptors,[120] which mediate the same effects as estrogen receptors.[121] Oursler et al.[122] demonstrated that osteoclasts also express estrogen receptor proteins. Elevated levels of estrogen increase osteoblast proliferation,[123] decrease osteoblast sensitivity to PTH,[99] increase collagen gene expression,[123] and increase the synthesis of insulin-like growth factor-1 (IGF-1), insulin-like growth factor-2 (IGF-2),[124] and transforming growth factor-beta (TGF-β). Estrogen also inhibits the production of IL-6, TNF, and lymphokine inhibiting factor (LIF).[118,119,124,125] More important, decreased levels of estrogen are associated with an increased concentration of bone resorption factors—including prostaglandins, IL-1, and IL-6,[126,127]—which is reversed with estrogen therapy.[128] Girasole et al.[125] suggested that it is the increased levels of IL-6, secondary to decreasing concentrations of estrogen, that drives the development of postmenopausal osteoporosis.

Thyroid

Thyroxine (T4) and triiodothyronine (T3) are systemic hormones that have effects on numerous tissues including bone. Increased levels of T4 and T3 are associated with enhanced osteoclastic bone resorption and premature loss of bone density.[129] Hyperthyroidism can occasionally lead to hypercalcemia; histologic sections from patients with this condition demonstrate findings similar to those of primary hyperparathyroidism or osteitis fibrosa cystica.[130] It has also been demonstrated that hypothyroidism decreases the rate of bone turnover.[131]

Glucocorticoids

The glucocorticoids also have clinically important effects on bone and mineral metabolism. Specifically, cortisol inhibits intestinal Ca^{2+} absorption via direct effects on the endothelium and indirect effects on vitamin D and PTH. In fact, cortisol has been suggested as a treatment for intestinally mediated hypercalcemia, as seen in sarcoid and vitamin D toxicity.[132] Dietrich et al.,[98] using fetal rat bone, showed that elevated concentrations of glucocorticoids increase collagen synthesis and that lower concentrations inhibit it.[98] Other in vitro studies have shown that glucocorticoids inhibit osteoclast formation and differentiation.[133,134] More importantly, glucocorticoid therapy, administered for extended periods, is associated with bone resorption and osteopenia.[135–137]

Transforming Growth Factor-Beta

TGF-β is a 25-kDa polypeptide and one of the most prevalent growth factors found in bone matrix.[138,139] Its activity is regulated by its conversion into an active peptide, which, in turn, is controlled by PTH.[140] After it is released during bone resorption,[141] TGF-β enhances osteoblast activity; via increased collagen synthesis,[142,143] it increases the bone apposition rate and inhibits the differentiation of osteoclasts.[144,145] Oursler[146] hypothesized that TGF-β may be the coupling agent in the bone remodeling unit, linking bone resorption to bone formation. Clinically, TGF-β is associated with wound and fracture repair and has been studied as an adjuvant to induce bone ingrowth in porous implant models.[147] Also, it appears that glucocorticoids oppose TGF-β effects in vitro, suggesting a possible pathogenetic mechanism for steroid-induced osteoporosis.[148]

Insulin-like Growth Factors

Insulin-like growth factors 1 and 2 (IGF-1 and IGF-2) are closely related 7.5-kDa polypeptides that are found in the systemic circulation; they are produced in the liver under the control of growth hormone and in local tissues.[149,150] In bone tissue, IGF-1 and IGF-2 are among the most common growth factors produced locally by fibroblasts and osteoblasts.[151] The synthesis of IGF is under hormonal control; PTH and prostaglandin E2 enhance IGF-1 synthesis,[151,152] while cortisol diminishes its production.[153] Insulinlike growth factor 1 increases bone apposition rates by increasing preosteoblast cell replication and osteoblastic collagen synthesis and decreasing bone resorption.[145] Centrella et al.[154] demonstrated that 2-microglobulin potentiates the effects of IGF via increased IGF binding to target cells. Overall, IGF appears to help maintain normal bone mass.

Platelet-Derived Growth Factor

In bone tissue, platelet-derived growth factor (PDGF) is a 30-kDa polypeptide dimer that most likely serves as a local cytokine regulator.[155] In rat calvarial cultures, it has been demonstrated to increase cell replication rates as well as collagen synthesis.[156] Pfeilschifter et al.[157] revealed that PDGF will increase matrix apposition rates. The effects of PDGF are regulated at the receptor level: IL-1 increases the number of binding sites, while TGF-β decreases its binding affinity.[148]

Heparin-Binding Growth Factors

Bone matrix also contains two osteoblast-synthesized[158] heparin-binding growth factors (HBGFs) that are significantly homologous and are 16 to 17 kDa in mass: acidic fibroblast growth factor (aFGF) and basic fibroblast growth factor (bFGF).[159] Both of them enhance mitogenesis and increase protein synthesis of collagen and noncollagen proteins.[160,161] A specific role for these local growth factors is unclear, but Montesano et al.[162] have hypothesized that they play a role in wound repair and fracture healing.

Colony-Stimulating Factors

Generally, colony-stimulating factors (CSFs) are responsible for the proliferation of osteoclast precursors as well as other cells of the hematopoietic system.[163] Specifically, Yoshida et al.[164] described an osteopetrosis mouse model, the op/op mouse, which possessed a bioinert version of CSF-M. When this model was treated with CSF-M, bone resorption was restored and the marrow cavity was allowed to progress.[165,166] The effects of CSF-M appear to be mediated by a receptor of tyrosine kinase, the c-*fms* protooncogene,[167] which in turn may stimulate IL-1 and prostaglandin synthesis.[168,169]

Interleukin-1

Interleukin-1 is a powerful stimulant of bone resorption,[170] capable of acting through either a prostaglandin-dependent or prostaglandin-independent mechanism.[167] It is mitogenic for osteoclast precursors and promotes the proliferation and differentiation of committed precursors.[141,170,171] The bone-resorptive effects of IL-1 are potentiated by tumor necrosis factor alpha (TNF-α).[172] Interleukin-1 also acts synergistically with PTH[173] and with PTH-related peptide.[174] Surprisingly, IL-1 has also been demonstrated to stimulate proliferation of osteoblast precursors while inhibiting differentiated osteoblast function.[175,176] Clinically, IL-1 may be associated with the hypercalcemia of malignant disease as well as the bone destruction in chronic inflammatory processes and osteoporosis.[125,167,174,177]

Interleukin-6

Interleukin-6 is primarily responsible for acute-phase protein response and plays a major role as a paracrine growth factor in myeloma.[178,179] It also potentiates the bone-resorbing effects of IL-1 and TNF-α by stimulating early osteoclast lineage mitogenesis; its role in differentiated osteoclast function is unclear.[167] The synthesis of IL-6 is regulated by PTH, IL-1, and 1,25$(OH)_2D_3$ and is performed by osteoblasts.[167] Girasole et al.[125] have shown that estrogen regulates IL-6 by limiting its production and have suggested that the ability of estrogen to prevent osteoporosis is related to this regulatory relationship. Interleukin-6 may also be associated with Paget disease of bone: Kurihara et al.[180] demonstrated that pagetoid osteoclasts produce increased amounts of IL-6.

Tumor Necrosis Factor-Alpha

In bone tissue, TNF-α, which is synthesized by activated lymphocytes, activated monocytes, and macrophages, stimulates osteoclastic bone resorption.[167,181] These effects, while similar to those of IL-1, are more dependent on prostaglandin synthesis.[167] Also like IL-1, TNF-α stimulates osteoblast precursor proliferation but inhibits differentiated osteoblast function.[176] In vivo, TNF-α has been demonstrated to produce increased bone resorption and hypercalcemia;[182,183] it is associated clinically with myeloma and chorionic inflammatory disease and their concomitant bone destruction.[167]

Prostaglandins

Prostaglandins (PGs) are found throughout the circulation and are potent effector molecules for a variety of organs, including the vascular, cardiac, and intestinal systems. In bone, PGs act as local modulators of bone-cell activity, such as local inflammatory responses, blood flow, and ion transport.[10,12,184] Of all the biologically active products of arachidonic acid metabolism seen in bone, which include PGI (prostacyclin) and PGF_2, PGE_2 is the most abundant[185,186] and most potent with respect to bone resorption.[187,188] Prostaglandins help to increase bone resorption by increasing the production of osteoclastlike multinuclear cells. Surprisingly, it appears that PGs can stimulate both osteoblastic as well as osteoclastic cell lines in vitro.[189] Prostaglandin activity is mediated by increased intracellular concentrations of Ca^{2+} and cAMP as well as activation of the phosphatidyl inositol pathway[190] and protein kinase C.[191] Prostaglandin synthesis in vitro is regulated by a number of systemic and local signals: production is stimulated by PTH[192] and IL-1[193] via increased arachondonic acid release and increased cyclooxygenase activity,[192,194] while production is inhibited by glucocorticoids and sex hormones.[195] More interestingly, biophysical stimuli, such as bone cell stretching[196] or fluid shear stress,[197] enhance PG synthesis. Clinically, PGs are associated with the hypercalcemia of malignancy, inflammatory bone loss in periodontal disease, and rheumatoid arthritis as well as with loosening of joint replacements.[198–200]

Leukotrienes

Other eicosanoids include the leukotrienes, which also play a role in bone tissue turnover. In rat calvaria models, leukotrienes were discovered to stimulate osteoclasts to increase TRAP production and to increase the formation of resorption pits.[201] Indeed, Gallwitz et al.[201] have suggested that leukotrienes act as the message from osteoblasts to osteoclasts to begin resorption. Finally, leukotrienes are clinically associated with the bone destruction found in giant cell tumors.[202]

Bone Morphogenetic Protein

A number of studies over the last 65 years have demonstrated that certain tumor cells, epithelial cells, and demineralized bone can produce ectopic bone formation.[203–207] The molecular moiety discovered to be responsible for this osteoinductive response is a member of the TGF-β superfamily of growth factors and is termed *bone morphogenetic protein* (BMP). This factor is a dimeric polypeptide, where each subunit has a mass of 16 to 18 kDa and is found in only small amounts (1 μg/kg).[208–210] Since its initial characterization, six related human proteins (BMP-2 through BMP-7) have been identified.[211–213] The BMPs act on progenitor cells to induce differentiation into osteoblasts and chondroblasts. In fact, BMP may be the main signal that regulates skeletal formation and skeletal repair; it induces de novo bone formation, following the same pathways as endochondral ossification.[214] The amount and rate of bone formation depends on the dose of BMP implanted.[215] As with TGF-α, it appears that BMP is stored with the bone matrix and released with the resorptive activity that often follows injury.[214] In animal trials, rhBMP-2 is capable of inducing bone growth in a 2.5-cm cortical defect, a defect that usually heals with fibrotic tissue, restoring functional strength to the bone within 3 months.[216] Clinically, BMP is being studied to determine its potential action as an osteoinductive agent indicated for catastrophic bone loss, complex fracture sites, spinal fusions, and repair of fracture nonunions.

BONE MODELING AND REMODELING

As initially emphasized, bone is a dynamic tissue, which, under the influence of chemical, matrix, biophysical, and cellular constituents, undergoes constant turnover. Modeling is strictly a process that increases the amount of bone tissue in the absence of resorption (e.g., periosteal surface apposition). Remodeling, on the other hand, changes bone morphology by the coordinated processes of bone formation and resorption (e.g., drilling and refilling of an osteon or cortical drift). The rate of bone turnover varies dramatically throughout life, from nearly 100 percent turnover at infancy to less than 10 percent turnover during adulthood.[217] Frost developed a cellular model for physiologic remodeling that he called the *basic multicellular unit* (BMU),[218] which comprises both osteoclasts and osteoblasts. He emphasized the different phases that occur during remodeling. These are activation of the site, bone resorption, and subsequent new bone formation within the resorption pocket.[218,219] Knowledge of this process has served as the basis for clinically relevant studies of bone adaptation and osteoporosis, providing many insights into their underlying mechanisms.

Physiologic Remodeling

Physiologic remodeling is a continuous process, mediated by the BMU.[218] This process occurs within cortical bone as well as on trabecular, endosteal, and periosteal surfaces. Each BMU is a distinct entity comprising osteoclasts and osteoblasts. Remodeling begins with activation of osteoclasts, which subsequently create a cutting cone[220] (Fig 2-7). In cortical bone, the resorption process drills a tunnel as large as 2.5 mm in length and 100 μm in diameter, while on bone surfaces it forms a 50-μm-deep saucer-shaped crater[221] (Fig 2-8). Cement lines are formed where the BMU ceases resorption and starts to form new bone. Factors that mediate the reversal phase are not well characterized, though possible candidates include osteoclast cytokines and bone matrix proteins such as TGF-β or BMP-3.[222] Bone formation occurs via layers of osteoblasts forming successive lamellae of new-bone matrix. After a 20-day period, the matrix begins mineralization, which proceeds rapidly at first; 75 percent of final mineral content is achieved in the first few days, but the process takes up to a year to reach completion.[223]

As elaborate as this process is, ironically neither the factors that control physiologic remodeling nor its purpose are clear. Currey[224] has suggested that random remodeling plays a role in fracture prevention, removing potentially dangerous fatigue cracks. Remodeling may also have a role in mineral homeostasis. Selective remodeling, though, suggests the presence of a local signal that mediates the initiation of remodeling. Indeed, research into the adaptive response of bone has elucidated several candidate signal mechanisms.

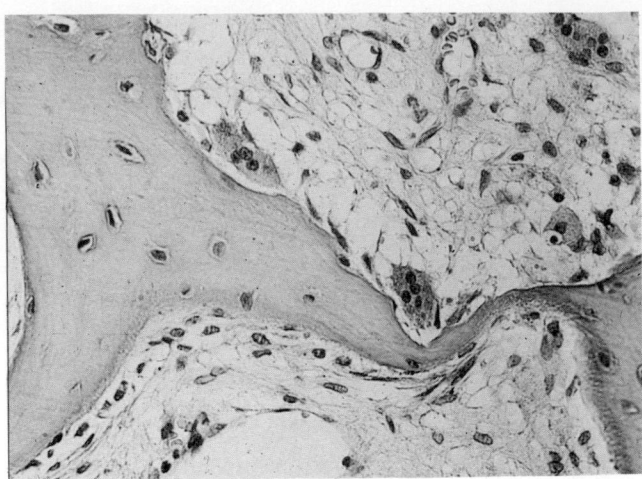

Figure 2-8 An osteoclast in Howship's lacuna absorbing bone on the surface of a trabecula. The patient has secondary hyperparathyroidism, and the adjacent marrow is fibrous (osteitis fibrosa). (H&E, ×350.) [From Sokoloff L, Bland JH (eds): *The Musculoskeletal System.* Baltimore, Williams & Wilkins, 1975.]

Bone Adaptation

The ability of bone to modify its morphology in the face of an altered biomechanical environment has long been recognized. Wolff, in the nineteenth century, demonstrated the intimate relationship between bone morphology and mechanical function. Furthermore, he developed a mathematical model, now called *Wolff's law,* that attempted to predict bone adaptation in the face of an altered loading environment.[225] One striking example of the skeleton's capacity to adapt to its functional environment was demonstrated in professional tennis players.[226] By comparing the cortical thickness in the humerus of the racquet arm to that of the contralateral arm, they observed a significant increase in the cortical thickness of the more active humerus, 35 percent in men and 28 percent in women. Conversely, decreased loading diminishes both bone strength and mass.[227,228] Donaldson et al.[229] demonstrated, after 36 weeks of bed rest, a 4.2 percent total body calcium loss and, more impressively, a 34 percent decrease in calcaneal bone mineral content.

These observations only raise further questions. What component of the functional environment is regulatory, and what is the structural objective of bone morphology? The simplest model states that bone attempts to minimize both mass and strain. There is mounting evidence suggesting that the relationship of bone morphology to the biomechanical environment is much more complex. For example, the curvature of long bones is directed away from the neutralization of bending loads, which accounts for over 80 percent of the total measured strain;[230] in fact, some long bones are oriented so that bending is increased.[231] This suggests that, rather than minimizing

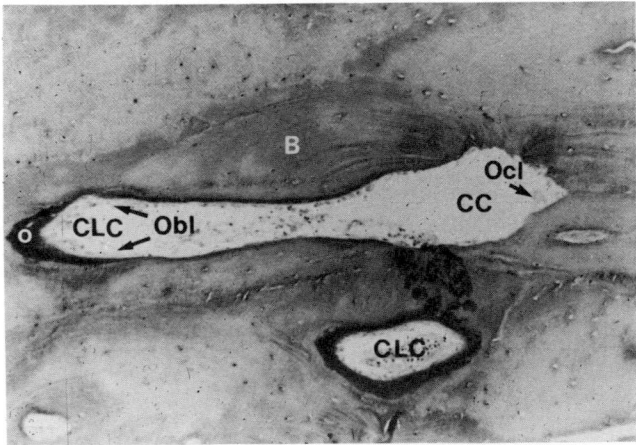

Figure 2-7 Events in cortical bone remodeling, shown in this longitudinal section of an osteon. Bone (B) is being reabsorbed by osteoclasts (Ocl), eroding a cutting cone (CC). The canal is being progressively filled by the deposition of osteoid (o) laid down by osteoblasts (Obl), forming a closing cone (CLC), which also appears circular in transverse section in the lower part of the slide. (Undecalcified, Goldner stain; 5-μm section of human cortical bone, ×100.) [From Marie PG, in Cruess RL (ed): *The Musculoskeletal System.* New York, Churchill Livingstone, 1982. With permission.]

strain, bending could be a means of regulating strain and strain distribution.

The Functional Strain Environment

Peak strain magnitudes measured in adult species—including horse, human, lizard, sheep, goat, goose, pig, macaque, turkey, sunfish, and dog—are remarkably similar, ranging from 2000 to 3500 microstrain (1000 microstrain is a 1-mm change in length over an original length of 1000 mm). This relationship has been called *dynamic strain similarity* and suggests that skeletal morphology and locomotion character combine to elicit a very specific and perhaps beneficial level of strain.[232] The interspecies similarities in peak strain magnitudes are strong evidence for the existence of a common strain-sensitive cellular population within the skeletal tissues of each of these animals. Further, it suggests that a generic cellular mechanism exists that strives toward a common, strain-determined structural goal.

Attempts to identify those aspects of the skeleton's functional milieu that are responsible for generating and controlling this adaptive response have demonstrated that alterations in bone mass, turnover, and internal replacement are sensitive to changes in the magnitude,[233] distribution,[234] and the rate of strain[235] generated within the bone tissue. A loading regimen must be dynamic in nature, as static loads do not influence bone morphology,[236] yet its full osteogenic potential is achieved following only an extremely short exposure to this stimulus.[237] The potency of the stimulus is proportional to the magnitude of the strain.[233] As strain levels that are acceptable in one location induce adaptive remodeling in others, it would suggest that each region of each bone is genetically programmed to accept a particular amount and pattern of intermittent strain as normal. Deviation from this optimal strain environment will stimulate changes in the bone's remodeling balance, resulting in adaptive increases or decreases in its mass.

Isolating specific components of the physical milieu that actually regulate skeletal morphology has been difficult; no single parameter of the mechanical environment has been shown to reliably predict bone remodeling in all naturally observed or experimentally created conditions.[238] Perhaps the engineering perspective that strain is harmful to bone and that remodeling is a repair-driven process needs to be reconsidered. Instead, there may be some byproduct of strain—such as stress-generated potentials, piezoelectric currents, or increased perfusion—that enhances the cell population's vitality.

Extremely low-intensity electric fields (below 1 mV/cm),[239] as well as low-magnitude strains (less than 100 microstrain),[240] when induced within a specific, hyperphysiologic frequency (10 to 50 Hz) band, influence bone mass as effectively as stimuli of greater intensity induced at more "physiologic" frequencies. Importantly, strains at this frequency and magnitude are induced as byproducts of muscle contractions, which resonate between 20 and 50 Hz.[241]

Transducing a Physical Signal to a Cellular Response

While these data demonstrate some relationship of function to form, they do not suggest the means by which the physical signal is transduced by the cell and extracellular matrix into the adaptive process. A potential mechanism for the coupling of mechanical deformation and control of cellular metabolic activity may be the stress-generated electrical potential (SGP). A change in the bone's level or type of activity will, in turn, alter the magnitude of this potential charge at the bone/fluid interface. Vascular channels within haversian systems, combined with the lacunae and canaliculi occupied by cells and the microporosity of the matrix, may consume as much as 10 percent of the bone tissue's volume and are filled with fluids and/or cellular components. The deformation or straining of the skeleton caused by functional activity will prompt this fluid to flow, like water flowing through a sponge that is stretched or compressed. While at one level this fluid behavior may contribute to increased perfusion and nutrient delivery, the ionic constituents of the fluid will interact with the charged nature of the mineral to generate electrokinetic potentials.[242] In 1962, Bassett and Becker hypothesized that a primary step in translating functional load bearing to an adaptive cellular response was linked to the electrical potential generated by the mechanical deformation of the bone tissue.[243] This postulation has been strongly supported by many subsequent investigators showing the relationship between electrical potential and regulation of bone cell activity.[244,245]

As fluid pressure gradients and the resultant streaming potentials would affect primarily those cells confined within the cortices of the extracellular matrix (osteocytes), and changes in the "normal" electrokinetic signal would be generated by alterations in the type and/or amplitude of function, this intracortical syncytium could be a key regulator of osteoblast or osteoclast activity. This potential, in turn, may act to effect proliferation of osteoprogenitor cells[246] or to catalyze the production[247] or mineralization[248] of the extracellular matrix. Indeed, extremely low-magnitude electrical fields can affect both differentiation of osteoblasts[249] and recruitment of osteoclasts.[250]

Whatever the signal transduction pathway of transforming physical information to something the cell population can perceive and respond to, it is clear that the capacity of bone tissue to adapt to its functional demands is critical to the skeleton's structural success. Indeed, as we attempt to evaluate the cellular mechanisms responsible for the positive control of bone mass, the osteogenic potential of physical stimuli cannot be ignored.

MECHANICAL PROPERTIES OF BONE

There is little argument that the intricate balance of bone formation and resorption, the tightly controlled, multifaceted aspects of bone cell kinetics, bone's ability to heal itself without scar and adapt its morphology to changes in the functional milieu, reflect a sophisticated and elegant tissue. Ultimately, however, the success of bone as a structure is, in large part, a product of its mechanical properties: how stiff it is, how resilient to fatigue, and how effectively it withstands the extremes of physical activity.[251] For normal tensile or compressive loading, the stiffness of the material, or elastic modulus, shows human haversian bone to be about 17.0 GPa (gigapascals) in the longitudinal direction, 11.5 GPa in the transverse direction, and 3.3 GPa in shear. The degree of mineralization (young bone) or porosity (old bone) will compromise the stiffness of the bone and thereby lower the elastic modulus. The "effective" modulus of the bone can compensate for decreased stiffness by changes in morphology (e.g., periosteal expansion).

The strength of bone is derived by two distinct strategies. The first and most obvious is the composite nature of the material. The tensile properties of the collagen, combined with the compressive behavior of the mineral, result in an extremely strong material, not unlike the reinforcing of brittle concrete with steel. A second, less obvious means of contributing to the strength of bone is by the composite nature of the bone structure—haversian, circumferential, and interstitial lamellae working synergistically to avoid yield or ultimate strain.

The yield strain of bone, or that degree of deformation reached where the bone will not elastically recover, is approximately 7000 microstrain—i.e., a 0.7 percent change in length will cause irreversible damage to the tissue. Ultimate strain in bone, or that degree of deformation where the material actually fractures, is 15,000 microstrain.[252] From the material viewpoint, a metabolic bone disease resulting in a disorganized or low level of collagen will produce a bone material with inferior tensile and compressive behavior. The collagen not only contributes to the tensile strength of the bone but also governs the orderly deposition of the material. The converse is also true; a metabolic disease that produces inadequate or inappropriate mineral will also have poor material properties, with dangerously low yield and ultimate strain.

The ability of the bone to resist load also comes from the architecture, or organization, of the bone tissue. Consider an analogy of a bundle of straws versus a solid stick as an illustration of how a composite structure such as bone can prove more successful in resisting loads by avoiding yield and ultimate strain of the material. The solid stick breaks with relatively little bending, because relatively high strains are generated within the periphery of the material. However, the bundle of straws made up of the same mass and subjected to the same bending conditions will continue to deform (strain) rather than break, as each independent element slips relative to adjacent bundles. By dissipating the strains generated by identical forces, the chance of exceeding yield strains or ultimate failure is greatly diminished. Dissipating energy and minimizing strain levels within the material allows the entire system to react in a more elastic manner rather than sustaining brittle failure or ultimate fracture.

Bone, as an organ, has a requirement to be both stiff (to resist deformation) and tough (to prevent crack propagation). Again, the composite material, both architec-

turally and ultrastructurally, helps in both circumstances, and the relative proportions of collagen and mineral are tuned to optimize the structure to accommodate the functional demand. The resiliency to crack propagation is provided by both the tensile component of collagen and the haversian system (i.e., working as a strain relief to the growth of fractures), and the resiliency to deformation is provided by mineral. Comparatively small changes in the mineral content of bone tissue can have substantial effects on its properties as a material, as demonstrated by Curry in his determination of the mechanical properties of divers types of bone.[253] By comparing the bovine femur, the deer antler, and the whale tympanic bulla, he illustrated that as the morphologic responsibility of the skeletal element changed, so did its mineral content. In the extreme, the mineral content ranged from 86 percent in the bulla, which requires a high acoustic impedance, to 59 percent in the antler, which must be resilient to high-impact loads. The consequence of this high mineral content is revealed by comparing the relative work to fracture of these bones; that required to fracture the bulla is only 3 percent of that needed to do the same to the antler.

The material properties of the appendicular skeleton, however, remain remarkably consistent through a wide range of animals.[254] Examining an animal mass range of 0.09 to 700.0 kg, the bending strength of those bones relegated to traditional load-bearing responsibilities is approximately 200 to 250 MPa (megapascals), with an elastic modulus around 20 GPa. To adapt to changes in the physical demands placed upon it, it appears that the appendicular skeleton responds not by changing its material properties but by altering its shape and morphology.[255] This is achieved via functionally regulated alterations in bone mass and architecture.

Compatibility of Bone with Biomaterials

Orthopaedic surgery, more than any other surgical subspecialty, relies on implantating foreign materials, usually metals and/or hardened plastics, as therapeutic adjuncts to strengthen or replace diseased or damaged musculoskeletal tissues. The field of biomaterials is expanding rapidly and has made major inroads into the medical sphere, as exemplified by vascular grafts, heart valves, insulin pumps, and breast reconstruction. As always, the major concern with implant material is how the adjacent tissues will react. Total hip arthroplasty utilizing porous-coated components provides a good starting point to explore the relationship of bone to the mechanical, biological, and biophysical properties of implant materials.

The biochemical environment at the bone-implant interface affords researchers multiple opportunities to actively alter the response of bone to the porous implant. Techniques for bone ingrowth enhancement have included the use of bioactive materials such as bone autograft and allograft,[256,257] bone chips and powder,[258,259] hydroxyapatite,[260,261] calcium phosphate,[262] and polysulfone beads.[263,264] These materials act as osteoconductive materials, guiding the ingrowth of bone into the porous surface via alterations (i.e., increased local calcium concentrations) in the local biochemical environment; they have demonstrated the ability to increase bony ingrowth even in the face of gaps[261] and micromotion.[265] Other researchers have focused on the local hormonal environment and have studied the effects of growth hormones and basic fibroblast growth factor (bFGF).[266] The application of bone morphogenetic protein (BMP)[267,268] presents an especially intriguing alternative because of its osteoinductive capabilities: it can induce the formation of bone de novo.[214] Obviously, considering the anabolic potential of these growth factors, extensive in vitro and in vivo work must still be done to minimize any aberrant responses.

Surface chemistry characteristics also appear to play a role at the bone-implant interface. Hazan et al.[269] have demonstrated a differential growth of bone into heat-treated intramedullary screws, both titanium and stainless steel, using a rat femur model. They characterized the changes at the implant surface using Auger electron spectroscopy, noting that there was a twofold increase in the titanium oxide layer in the former and a conversion from chromium oxide to ferrous oxide in the latter. They did not elucidate a mechanism whereby bony ingrowth was increased but raised the possibility that it could be associated with changes in the surface electrical properties. With continued research into the relationship between biomaterials and musculoskeletal tissues, the development of more durable and compatible implants is increasingly possible.

REFERENCES

1. Jones BH, Harris J McA, Vinh TN, Rubin CT: Exercise-induced stress fractures and stress reactions of bone: Epidemiology, etiology, and classification. *Exerc Sport Sci Rev* 17:379–422, 1989.
2. Rubin CT, Gross T, McLeod K, Bain SD: Morphologic stages in lamellar bone formation stimulated by a potent mechanical stimulus. *J Bone & Min Res* 10:488–493, 1995.
3. Albright JA, Skinner HCW: Structural organization and remodeling dynamics, in Albright JA, Brand RA (eds): *The Scientific Basis of Orthopaedics,* 2d ed. East Norwalk, CT, Appleton & Lange, 1987, pp 161–198.
4. Ascenzi A, Benvenuti A: Orientation of collagen fibers at the boundary between two successive osteonic lamellae and its mechanical interpretation. *J Biomech* 19:455–463, 1986.
5. Schaffler MB, Burr DB, Frederickson RG: Morphology of the osteonal cement line in human bone. *Anat Rec* 217:223–228, 1987.
6. Martin TJ, Ng KW: Mechanisms by which cells of the osteoblast lineage control osteoclast formation and activity: A review. *J Cell Biochem* 56:357–366, 1994.
7. Grigoriadis AE, Heersche JN, Aubin JE: Differentiation of muscle, fat, cartilage, and bone from progenitor cells present in a bone-derived clonal cell population: Effect of dexamethasone. *J Cell Biol* 106:2139–2151, 1988.
8. Brighton CT, Lorich DG, Kupcha R, et al: The pericyte as a possible osteoblast progenitor cell. *Clin Orthop* 275:287–299, 1992.
9. Wozney JM: Bone morphogenetic proteins and their gene expression. *Cellular Molecular Biology of Bone.* New York, Academic Press, 1993, pp 131–167.
10. Raisz LG, Kream BE: Regulation of bone formation. *N Engl J Med* 309:29–35, 1983.
11. Urist MR, Mikulski A, Lietze A: Solubilized and insolubilized bone morphogenetic protein. *Proc Natl Acad Sci USA* 76:1828–1832, 1979.
12. Raisz LG, Rodan GA: Cellular basis of bone turnover, in Avioli LV, Krane SM (eds): *Metabolic Bone Disease and Clinically Related Disorders,* 2d ed. Philadelphia, Saunders, 1990, pp 1–41.
13. Mundy GR: Local control of bone formation by osteoblast: A Review. *Clin Orthop* 313:19–26, 1995.
14. Matthews JL: Bone structure and ultrastructure, in Urist MR (ed): *Fundamental and Clinical Bone Physiology.* Philadelphia, Lippincott, 1980, pp 4–44.
15. Jaworski ZF: Lamellar bone turnover system and its effector organ. *Calcif Tiss Int* 36(suppl 1):S46–S55, 1984.
16. Jowsey J: *Metabolic Diseases of Bone.* Philadelphia, Saunders, 1977, p 61.
17. Doty SB: Morphological evidence of gap junctions between bone cells. *Calcif Tiss Int* 33:509–512, 1981.
18. Recker RR: Embryology, anatomy, and microstructure of bone, in Coe FL, Favus MJ (eds): *Disorders of Bone and Mineral Metabolism.* New York, Raven Press, 1992, pp 219–240.
19. Rodan GA, Martin TJ: Role of osteoblasts in hormonal control of bone resorption—A hypothesis. *Calcif Tiss Int* 33:349–351, 1981.
20. Parfitt AM: Osteonal and hemi-osteonal remodeling: The spatial and temporal framework for signal traffic in adult human bone. A review. *J Cell Biochem* 55:273–286, 1994.
21. Martin TJ, Rodan GA: Role of osteoblasts in hormonal control of bone resorption: A hypothesis. *Calcif Tiss Int* 33:349–351, 1981.
22. Menton DN, Simmons DJ, Chang SL, Orr BY: From bone lining cell to osteocyte: An SEM study. *Anat Rec* 209:29–39, 1984.
23. Curtis TA, Ashrafi SH, Weber DF: Canalicular communication in the cortices of human long bones. *Anat Rec* 212:336–344, 1985.
24. Palumbo C, Palazzini S, Marotti G: Morphological study of intercellular junctions during osteocyte differentiation. *Bone* 11:401–406, 1990.
25. VanderMolen M, Rubin C, Donahue H: Decreased hormonal responsiveness in gap junction deficient osteoblasts. *Trans 41st Orthop Res Soc* 20(2):295, 1996.
26. Buckwalter JA, Glimcher MJ, Cooper RR, Recker R: Bone biology: I. Structure, blood supply, cells, matrix and mineralization. *J Bone Joint Surg* 77A:1256–1275, 1995.
27. Weinbaum S, Cowin SC, Zeng Y: A model for the excitation of osteocytes by mechanical loading-induced bone fluid shear stresses. *J Biomech* 27:339–360, 1994.
28. Atkinson PJ, Hallsworth B: The changing pore structure of aging human mandibular bone. *Gerontology* 2:57–63, 1983.
29. Hancox NM: The osteoclast. *Biol Rev* 24:448–467, 1949.
30. Walker DG: Enzymatic and electron microscopic analysis of isolated osteoclasts. *Calcif Tiss Res* 9:296–309, 1975.
31. Gothlin G, Ericsson JLE: The osteoclast, review of ultrastructure, origin and structure-function relationship. *Clin Orthop* 120:201–231, 1975.
32. Kahn AJ, Simmons DJ: Investigation of cell lineage in bone using a chimera of chick and quail embryonic tissue. *Nature* 258:325–327, 1975.
33. Felix R, Cecchini M, Fleisch H: Macrophage colony stimulating factor restores *in vivo* bone resorption in the op/op osteopetrotic mouse. *Endocrinology* 127:2592–2594, 1990.
34. Rodan GA, Martin TJ: Role of osteoblasts in hormonal control of bone resorption—A hypothesis. *Calcif Tiss Int* 33:349–351, 1981.

35. Chambers TJ: Osteoblasts release osteoclasts from calcitonin-induced quiescence. *J Cell Sci* 57:247–260, 1982.

36. Hill PA, Reynolds JJ, Meikle MC: Osteoblasts mediate insulin-like growth factor-1 and -11 stimulation of osteoclast formation and function. *Endocrinology* 136:124–131, 1995.

37. Jilka RL, Hangoc G, Girasole G, et al: Increased osteoclast development after estrogen loss: Mediation by interleukin-6. *Science* 257:88–91, 1992.

38. Roodman G, Kurihara N, Ohsaki Y, et al: Interleukin-6: A potential autocrine/paracrine factor in Paget's disease of bone. *J Clin Invest* 89:46–52, 1992.

39. Dresner-Pollak R, Rosenblatt M: Blockade of osteoclast-mediated bone resorption through occupancy of the integrin receptor: A potential approach to the therapy of osteoporosis. *J Cell Biochem* 56:323–330, 1994.

40. Baron R: Polarity and membrane transport in osteoclasts: A review. *Connect Tiss Res* 29:109–120, 1989.

41. Blair HC, Teitelbaum SLO, Ghiselli R, Gluck S: Osteoclastic bone resorption by a polarized vacuolar proton pump. *Science* 245:855–857, 1989.

42. Silver JA, Murrills RJ, Etherington DJ: Microelectrode studies on the acid microenvironment beneath adherent macrophages and osteoclasts. *Exp Cell Res* 175:266–276, 1988.

43. Jones SJ, Boyde A, Ali NN, Maconnachie E: A review of bone cell substratum interactions: An illustration of the role of scanning electron microscopy. *Scanning* 7:5–24, 1985.

44. Fisher LW, Gehron RP, Tuross N, et al: The mr 24,000 phosphoprotein from developing bone is the NH 2-terminal propeptide of the alpha chain of type 1 collagen. *J Biol Chem* 161:13457, 1987.

45. Noda M, Yoon K, Prince CW, et al: Transcriptional regulation of osteopontin production in rat osteosarcoma cells by type B transforming growth factor. *J Biol Chem* 263:13916, 1988.

46. Price PA, Otsuka AS, Poser JW, et al: Characterization of 8-carboxyglutamic acid containing protein from bone. *Proc Natl Acad Sci USA* 73:1447, 1976.

47. Urist MR, Juo YK, Brownell AD, et al: Purification of bovine bone morphogenetic protein by hydrosyapatie chromatography. *Proc Natl Acad Sci USA* 81:371, 1984.

48. Termine JC, Belcourt AB, Conn KM: Mineral and collagen-binding proteins of fetal calf bone. *J Biol Chem* 256:10403, 1981.

49. Glimcher MJ: The nature of the mineral component of bone and the mechanisms of calcification, in Coe FL, Favus MJ (eds): *Disorders of Bone and Mineral Metabolism.* New York, Raven Press, 1992, pp 265–286.

50. Niyibizi C, Eyre DR: Identification of cartilage α1(XI) chain in type V collagen from bovine bone. *FEBS Lett* 242:314–418, 1989.

51. Robey PG. The biochemistry of bone. *Endocrinal Metab Clin North Am* 18:859–902, 1989.

52. Glimcher MJ: Studies of the structure, organization and reactivity of bone collagen, in Gibson T (ed): *Proceedings of the International Symposium on Wound Healing, Montreaux.* Foundation of International Cooperative Medical Science, 1975, p 253.

53. Piez KA: Structure and assembly of the native collagen fibril. *Connect Tiss Res* 10:25, 1982.

54. Eyre DR: Collagen: Molecular diversity in the body's protein scaffold. *Science* 207:1315, 1980.

55. Pinnell SR, Fox R, Krane SM: Human collagens: Differences in glycosylated hydroxylysines in skin and bone. *Biochem Biophys Acta* 229:119, 1971.

56. Herring GM: The chemical structure of tendon cartilage, dentin, and bone matrix. *Clin Orthop* 60:261, 1968.

57. Herring GM: The organix matrix of bone, in Browne GH (ed): *The Biochemistry and Physiology of Bone,* 2d ed. New York, Academic Press, 1972, p 127.

58. Bianco P, Fisher LW, Young MF, et al: Expression of bone sialoprotein in human developing bone as revealed by immunostaining and in situ hybridization. *J Bone Min Res* 4(suppl):S321, 1989.

59. Robey, PG: The biochemistry of bone. *Endocrinal Metab Clin North Am* 18:859–902, 1989.

60. Blumenthal NC, Posner AS, Silverman LC, et al: The effects of proteoglycans on in vitro hydroxyapatite formation. *Calcif Tiss Int* 27:75, 1979.

61. Fisher LW: in *The Chemistry and Biology of Mineralized Tissues.* Birmingham, AL, LBSCO Media, 1985, p 188.

62. Johannson S, Hadman K, Kjellen L: Structure and interactions of proteoglycans in the extracellular matrix produced by cultured human fibroblasts. *Biochem J* 232:161, 1985.

63. Skerry TM, Suswillo R, Lanyon LE: Loading-related reorientation of bone proteoglycans in vivo and in vitro: A possible signal to control adaptive remodeling. *Calcif Tiss Int* 44:599, 1989.

64. Young MF, Bolander ME, Day AA, et al: Osteonectin mRNA: Distribution in normal and transformed cells. *Nucleic Acids Res* 14:4483, 1986.

65. Termine JD, Kleinman HK, Whitson SW, et al: Osteonectin: A bone-specific protein linking mineral to collagen. *Cell* 26:99, 1981.

66. Romberg RW, Werness PG, Lollar P, et al: Isolation and characterization of native adult osteonectin. *J Biol Chem* 260:2728, 1985.

67. Termine JD, Eaves ED, Conn KM: Phosphoprotein modulation of apatite crystallization. *Calcif Tiss Int* 31:247–251, 1980.

68. Weiss RE, Reddi AH: Synthesis and localization of fibronectin during collagenous matrix-mesenchymal cell interaction and differentiation of cartilage and bone in vivo. *Proc Natl Acad Sci USA* 77:2074–2078, 1980.

69. Oldberg A, Franzen A, Heinegard D: Cloning and sequence analysis of rat bone sialoprotein (osteopontin) cDNA reveals an Arg-Gly-Asp cell-binding sequence. *Proc Natl Acad Sci USA* 83:8819, 1986.

70. Lian JB, Coutts M, Canalis E: Studies of hormonal regulation of osteocalcin synthesis in cultured fetal rat calvariae. *J Biol Chem* 260:8706–8710, 1985.

71. Hauschka PV, Lian JB, Cole DEC, Gundberg CM: Osteocalcin and matrix Gla protein: Vitamin K-dependent protein in bone. *Phys Rev* 69:990–1047, 1988.

72. Canalis E, McCarthy T, Centrella M: Growth factors and the regulation of bone remodeling. *J Clin Invest* 81:277–281, 1988.

73. Lian JB, Gundberg CM: Osteocalcin: Biochemical considerations and clinical applications. *Clin Orthop* 262:267–291, 1988.

74. Lian JB, Tassihari M, Glowecki J: Resorption of implanted bone prepared from normal and warfarin-treated rats. *J Clin Invest* 73:1223, 1984.

75. Price PA, Williamson MK: Effects of warfarin on the vitamin K-dependent protein in rat bone. *J Biol Chem* 256:127–154, 1981.

76. Moradien-Oldak J, Weiner S, Addadi L, et al: Electron imaging and diffraction study of individual crystals of bone mineralized tendon and synthetics carbonate apatite. *Connect Tiss Res* 25:219–228, 1991.

77. Skinner HCW: Studies in the basic mineralizing system CaO-P_2O_5-H_2O. *Calcif Tiss Res* 14:3, 1974.

78. Weiner S, Traub W: Bone structure: From angstroms to microns. *FASEB J* 6:879–885, 1992.

79. Bonar LC, Roufosse AH, Sabine WK, et al: X-ray diffraction studies of the crystallinity of bone mineral in newly synthesized and density fractionated bone. *Calcif Tiss Int* 35:202–209, 1983.

80. Christoffersen J, Landis WJ: A contribution with review to the description of bone and other calcified tissues in vivo. *Anat Rec* 230:435–450, 1991.

81. Jowsey J: *Microradiography: A Morphologic Approach to Quantitating Bone Turnover.* Excerpta Medical Intl Congress Series No. 270. Amsterdam, Excerpta Medica Foundation, 1972, p 114.

82. Glimcher MJ, Krane SM: The organization and structure of bone, and the mechanism of calcification, in Ramachandran GN, Gould BS (eds): *Treatise on Collagen.* New York, Academic Press, 1968, pp 67–251.

83. Hynes RD: The molecular biology of fibronectin. *Annu Rev Cell Biol* 1:67, 1985.

84. Veis A, Sharkey M, Dickson I: Non-collagenous proteins of bone and dentin extracellular matrix and their role in organized mineral deposition, in Wasserman RH (ed): *Calcium Binding Proteins and Calcium Function.* New York, Elsevier, 1977, p 409–418.

85. Shapiro IM, Greenspan JS: Are mitochondria directly involved in biological mineralization? *Calcif Tiss Res* 3:100–102, 1969.

86. Lehninger AL: Mitochondria in calcium ion transport. *Biochem J* 119:129–138, 1970.

87. Anderson HC: Vesicles associated with calcification in the matrix of epiphyseal cartilage. *J Cell Biol* 41:59–72, 1969.

88. Bonucci F: The locus of initial calcification in cartilage and bone. *Clin Orthop* 78:108–139, 1971.

89. Odutuga AA, Prout RES, Hoare J: Hydroxyapatite precipitator in vitro by lipids extracted from mammalian hard and soft tissues. *Arch Oral Biol* 20:311–316, 1976.

90. Baylink D, Wengedal J, Thompson E: Loss of protein polysaccharides at sites where bone mineralization is initiated. *J Histochem Cytochem* 20:279, 1972.

91. Pita JC, Muller F, Howell DS: Disaggregation of proteoglycan aggregates during endochondrial calcification: Physiological role of cartilage lysozyme, in Burleigh M, Poole R (eds): *Dynamics of Connective Tissue Macromolecules.* Amsterdam, North Holland, 1975, pp 247–258.

92. Chen CC, Boskey AL: Mechanisms of proteoglycan inhibition of hydroxyapatite growth. *Calcif Tiss Int* 36:285–290, 1985.

93. Thyberg J, Friberg U: Ultrastructure and acid phosphatase of matrix vesicles and cytoplasmic dense bodies in the epiphyseal plate. *J Ultrastruct Res* 33:554–573, 1970.

94. Katz EP, Li S-T: Structure and function of bone collagen fibrils. *J Mol Biol* 80:1–15, 1973.

95. Albright JA, Skinner HCW: Bone: Structural organization and remodeling dynamics, in Albright JA, Brand RA (eds): *The Scientific Basis of Orthopaedics,* 2d ed. East Norwalk, CT, Appleton & Lange, 1986, pp 161–198.

96. Pharoah MJ, Heersche JNM. 1,25 dihydroxyvitamin D3 causes an increase in the number of osteoclast-like cells in cat bone marrow cultures. *Calcif Tiss Int* 37:276–281, 1985.

97. Suda T, Takahashi N, Martin TJ: Modulation of osteoclast differentiation: A review. *Endocr Rev* 13(1):66–80, 1992.

98. Dietrich JW, Mundy GR, Raisz LG: Inhibition of bone resorption in tissue culture by membrane-stabilizing drugs. *Endocrinology* 104:1644–1648, 1979.

99. Rouleau MF, Warshawsky H, Goltzman D: Parathyroid hormone binding in vivo to renal, hepatic and skeletal tissues of the rat using a radioautographic approach. *Endocrinology* 118:919–931, 1986.

100. McSheehy PMJ, Chambers TJ: Osteoblast-like cells in the presence of parathyroid hormone release soluble factor that stimulates osteoclastic bone resorption. *Endocrinology* 119:1654–1659, 1986.

101. Donahue HJ, Fryer MJ, Eriksen EF, Heath H III: Differential effects of parathyroid hormone and its analogues on cytosolic calcium ion and cAMP levels in cultured rat osteoblast-like cells. *J Biol Chem* 263:13522–13527, 1988.

102. Stern PH. Vitamin D and bone. *Kidney Int* 38:S17–S21, 1990.

103. Haddad JG, Hahn TJ: Natural and synthetic sources of circulating 25-hydroxyvitamin D in man. *Nature* 244:515–517, 1973.

104. Henry HL, Neuman AW. Vitamin D: Metabolism and biological actions. *Annu Rev Nutr* 4:493, 1984.

105. Austin LA, Heath H III: Calcitonin: Physiology and pathophysiology, *N Engl J Med* 304:269–278, 1981.

106. Friedman J, Raisz LG: Thyrocalcitonin: Inhibitor of bone resorption in tissue culture. *Science* 150:1465–1467, 1967.

107. Arnaud CD, Kolb FO. The calciotropic hormones and metabolic bone disease, in Greenspan FS, Forsham PH (eds.): *Basic & Clinical Endocrinology.* Los Altos, CA, Lange Medical Publications, 1983, pp 187–250.

108. Nicholson GC, Moseley JM, Sexton PM, et al: Abundant calcitonin receptors in isolated rat osteoclasts—Biochemical and autoradiographic characterization. *J Clin Invest* 78:355–360, 1986.

109. Chambers TJ, Athanasou NA, Fuller K: Effects of parathyroid hormone and calcitonin on the cytoplasmic spreading of isolated osteoclasts. *J Endocrinol* 102:281, 1984.

110. Murrills RJ, Dempster DW: The effects of stimulators of intracellular cyclic AMP on rat and chick osteoclasts *in vitro:* Validation of a simplified light microscope assay of bone resorption. *Bone* 11:333–344, 1990.

111. Deftos LJ, Roos B. Medullary thyroid carcinoma and calcitonin gene expression, in Peck WA (ed): *Bone and Mineral Research.* Amsterdam, Excerpta Medica, 1989, pp 267–316.

112. Martin TJ, Moseley JM: Calcitonin, in Avioli LV, Krane SM (eds): *Metabolic Bone Disease and Clinically Related Disorders,* 2d ed. Philadelphia, Saunders, 1990, pp 131–154.

113. Mundy GR: Hormonal factors which regulate bone resorption, in Mundy GR, Martin TJ (eds): *Handbook of Experimental Pharmacology:* Vol 107. *Physiology and Pharmacology of Bone.* New York, Springer-Verlag, 1992, pp 215–247.

114. Stevenson JC, Abeyasekera G, Hillyard CJ, et al: Regulation of calcium-regulating hormones by exogenous sex steroids in early postmenopause. *Eur J Clin Invest* 13:481–487, 1983.

115. Greenberg C, Kirkreja SC, Bowser EN, et al: Effect of estradiol and progesterone on calcium secretion. *Endocrinology* 118:2594–2598, 1990.

116. Heaney RP: A unified concept of osteoporosis. *Am J Med* 39:377–380, 1965.

117. Riggs BL, Melton LJ III: Clinical review 8: Clinical heterogenity of involutional osteoporosis: Implications for preventative therapy. *J Clin Endocrinol Metab* 70:1229–1232, 1990.

118. Erikssen EF, Colvard DS, Berg NJ, et al: Evidence of estrogen receptors in normal human osteoblast-like cells. *Science* 241:84–86, 1988.

119. Komm BS, Terpening CM, Benz DJ, et al: Estrogen binding, receptor mRNA, and biologic response in osteoblast-like osteosarcoma cells. *Science* 24:81–84, 1988.

120. Colvard DS, Eriksen EF, Keeting PE, et al: Identification of androgen receptors in normal human osteoblast-like cells. *Proc Natl Acad Sci USA* 86:854–857, 1989.

121. Fukayama S, Tashjian AH: Direct modulation by androgens of the response of human bone cells (SaOS-2) to human parathyroid hormone (PTH) and PTH-related protein. *Endocrinology* 125:1789–1790, 1989.

122. Oursler MJ, Pyfferoen J, Osdoby P, et al: Osteoclasts express mRNA for estrogen receptor. *J Bone Min Res* 5(suppl 2):S203, 1990.

123. Ernst M, Heath JK, Rodan GA: Estradiol effects on proliferation, messenger ribonucleic acid for collagen and insulin-like growth factor-1 and parathyroid hormone-stimulated adenylate cyclase activity in osteoblastic cells from calvariae and long bones. *Endocrinology* 125:825–833, 1988.

124. Gray TK, Mohan S, Linkhart TA, Baylink DJ: Estradiol stimulates in vitro the secretion of insulin-like growth factors by

the clonal osteoblastic cell line, UMR-106. *Biochem Biophys Res Commun* 158:407–412, 1989.

125. Girasole G, Sakagami J, Hustmyer FG, et al: 17-β estradiol inhibits cytokine induced IL-6 production by bone marrow stromal cells and osteoblasts. *J Bone Min Res* 5(suppl 2):S273, 1990.

126. Pacifici R, Rifas L, Teitelbaum S, et al: Spontaneous release of interleukin-1 from human blood monocytes reflects bone formation in idiopathic osteoporosis. *Proc Natl Acad Sci USA* 84:4616–4620, 1987.

127. Feyen JHM, Raisz LG: Prostaglandin production by calvariae from sham operated and oopherectomized rats: Effects of 17β-estradiol in vivo. *Endocrinology* 121:819–821, 1987.

128. Pacifici R, Rifas L, Vered I, et al: Interleukin-1 secretion from human blood monocytes in normal and osteoporotic women: Effect of menopause and estrogen/progesterone treatment. *J Bone Min Res* 3(suppl 1):S204, 1988.

129. Mundy GR, Shapiro JL, Bandelin JG, et al: Direct stimulation of bone resorption by thyroid hormones. *J Clin Invest* 58:529–534, 1976.

130. Follis RH: Skeletal changes associated with hyperthyroidism. *Bull Johns Hopkins Hosp* 92:405–421, 1953.

131. Mosekilde L, Melsen F: Morphometric and dynamic studies of bone changes in hypothyroidism. *Acta Pathol Microbiol Scand* 86:56–62, 1978.

132. Kimberg DV, Baerg RD, Gershon E, Graudusius RT: Effect of cortisone treatment on the active transport of calcium by the small intestine. *J Clin Invest* 50:1309–1321, 1971.

133. Raisz LG, Trummel CL, Simmons H: Induction of bone resorption in tissue culture: Prolonged response after brief exposure to parathyroid hormone or 25-hydroxycholecalciferol. *Endocrinology* 90:744–751, 1972.

134. Suda T, Testa NG, Allen TD, et al: Effects of hydrocortisone on osteoclasts generated in cat bone marrow cultures. *Calcif Tiss Int* 35:82–86, 1983.

135. Bockman RS, Weinerman SA: Steroid-induced osteoporosis. *Orthop Clin North Am* 21:97–107, 1990.

136. LoCascio V, Bonucci E, Imbimbo B, et al: Bone loss in response to long-term glucocorticord therapy. *Bone Min* 8:39–51, 1990.

137. Lukert BP, Raisz LG: Glucocorticoid-induced osteoporosis: Pathogenesis and management. *Ann Intern Med* 112:352–364, 1990.

138. Centrella M, Canalis E: Transforming and non-transforming growth factors are present in medium conditioned by fetal rat calvariae. *Proc Natl Acad Sci USA* 82:7335–7339, 1985.

139. Seyedin SM, Thompson AY, Bentz H, et al: Cartilage-inducing factor-A: Apparent identity to transforming growth factor-beta. *J Biol Chem* 261:5693–5696, 1986.

140. Pfeilschifter J, Erdmann J, Schmidt W, et al: Differential regulation of plasminogen activator and plasminogen activator inhibitor by osteotropic factors in primary cultures of mature osteoblasts and osteoblast precursors. *Endocrinology* 126:703–711, 1990.

141. Pfeilschifter J, Chenu C, Bird A, et al: Interleukin-1 and tumor necrosis factor stimulate the formation of human osteoclast-like cells in vitro. *J Bone Min Res* 4:113–118, 1989.

142. Centrella M, McCarthy TL, Canalis E: Transforming growth factor beta is a bifunctional regulator of replication and collagen synthesis in osteoblast enriched cell cultures from fetal rat bone. *J Biol Chem* 262:2869–2874, 1987.

143. Noda M, Camilliere JJ: *In vivo* stimulation of bone formation by transforming growth factor-beta. *Endocrinology* 124:2991–2994, 1989.

144. Chenu C, Pfeilschifter J, Mundy GR, Roodman GD: Transforming growth factor B inhibits formation of osteoclast-like cells in long-term human marrow cultures. *Proc Natl Acad Sci USA* 85:5683–5687, 1988.

145. Canalis E, McCarthy T, Centrella M: Isolation and characterization of insulin-like growth factor I (somatomedin C) from cultures of fetal rat calvariae. *Endocrinology* 122:22–27, 1988.

146. Oursler MJ: Osteoclast synthesis and secretion and activation of latent transforming growth factor beta. *J Bone Min Res* 9:443–452, 1994.

147. Joyce ME, Roberts AB, Sporn MB, Bolander ME: Transforming growth factor-β and the initiation of chondrogenesis and osteogenesis in the rat femur. *J Cell Biol* 110:2195–2207, 1990.

148. Centrella M, McCarthy TL, Canalis E: Glucocorticoid control of transforming growth factor β (TGF-β) binding and effects on osteoblast-enriched cultures from fetal rat bone. *J Bone Min Res* 5(suppl 2):S211, 1990.

149. Daughaday WH, Rotwein P: Insulin-like growth factors I and II: Peptide, messenger ribonucleic acid and gene structures, serum, and tissue concentrations. A review. *Endocrinol Rev* 19:68–91, 1989.

150. Mathews LS, Hammer RE, Brinster RL, Palmiter RD: Expression of insulin-like growth factor I in transgenic mice with elevated levels of growth hormone is correlated with growth. *Endocrinolgy* 124:1247–1253, 1989.

151. Canalis E, McCarthy TL, Centrella M: Differential effects of continuous and transient treatment with parathyroid hormone related peptide (PTHrp) on bone collagen synthesis. *Endocrinology* 126:1806–1812, 1990.

152. McCarthy TL, Centrella M, Raisz LG, Canalis E: Prostaglandin E2 stimulates insulin-like growth factor I synthesis in osteoblast-enriched culture from fetal rat bone. *J Bone Min Res* 5(suppl 2):S86, 1990.

153. McCarthy TL, Centrella M, Canalis E: Cortisol inhibits the synthesis of insulin-like growth factor I in skeletal cells. *Endocrinology* 126:1569–1575, 1990.

154. Centrella M, McCarthy TL, Canalis E: Platelet-derived growth factor enhances deoxyribonucleic acid and collagen synthesis in osteoblast-enriched cultures from fetal rat bone. *J Bone Min Res* 5(suppl 2):S211, 1989.

155. Graves DT, Valentin-Opran A, Delgado R, et al: The potential role of platelet-derived growth factor as an autocrine or paracrine factor for human bone cells. *Connect Tiss Res* 23:209–218, 1989.

156. Centrella M, McCarthy TL, Canalis E: Platelet-derived growth factor enhances deoxyribonucleic acid and collagen synthesis in osteoblast-enriched cultures from fetal rat parietal bone. *Endocrinology* 125:13–19, 1989.

157. Pfeilschifter J, Oechsner M, Naumann A, et al: Stimulation of bone matrix apposition in vitro by local growth factors: A comparison between insulin-like growth factor I, platelet-derived growth factor, and transforming growth factor. *Endocrinology* 127:69–75, 1990.

158. Globus RK, Plouet J, Gospodarowicz D: Cultured bovine bone cells synthesize basic fibroblast growth factor and store it in their extracellular matrix. *Endocrinology* 124:1539–1547, 1989.

159. Burgess WH, Mehlman T, Friesel R, et al: Multiple forms of endothelial cell growth factor: Rapid isolation and biological and clinical characterization. *J Biol Chem* 260:11389–11392, 1985.

160. Canalis E, Lorenzo J, Burgess WH, Maciag T: Effects of endothelial cell growth factor on bone remodeling in vitro. *J Clin Invest* 79:52–58, 1987.

161. McCarthy TL, Centrella M, Raisz LG, Canalis E: Prostaglandin E2 stimulates insulin-like growth factor I synthesis in osteoblast-enriched culture from fetal rat bone. *J Bone Min Res* 5(suppl 2):S86, 1986.

162. Montesano R, Vassalli JD, Baird A, et al: Basic fibroblast growth factor induces angiogenesis in vitro. *Proc Natl Acad Sci USA* 83:7297–7301, 1986.

163. Metcalf D: The molecular biology and functions of the granulocyte-macrophage colony-stimulating factors. A review. *Blood* 67:257–267, 1986.

164. Yoshida H, Hayashi SI, Kunisada T, et al: The murine mutation osteopetrosis is in the coding region of the macrophage colony stimulating factor gene. *Nature* 345:442–444, 1990.

165. Felix R, Cecchini MG, Fleisch H: Macrophage colony stimulating factor restores in vivo bone resorption in the *op/op* osteopetrotic mouse. *Endocrinology* 127:2592–2594, 1990.

166. Kodama H, Yamasaki A, Nose M, et al: Congenital osteoclast deficiency in osteopetrotic (*op/op*) mice is cured by injections of macrophage colony-stimulating factor. *J Exp Med* 173:269–272, 1991.

167. Mundy GR: Cytokines and growth factors in the regulation of bone remodeling: A review. *J Bone Min Res* 8(suppl 2)S505–S510, 1993.

168. Moore RN, Oppenheim JJ, Farrar JJ, et al: Production of lymphocyte-activating factor (interleukin-1) by macrophages activated with colony-stimulating factors. *J Immunol* 125:1302–1305, 1980.

169. Kurland JI, Pelus LM, Ralph P, et al: Induction of prostaglandin E synthesis in normal and neoplastic macrophages: Role for colony-stimulating factors distinct from effects on myeloid progenitor cell proliferation. *Proc Natl Acad Sci USA* 76:2326–2330, 1979.

170. Gowen M, Meikle MC, Reynolds JJ: Stimulation of bone resorption in vitro by a non-prostanoid factor released by human monocytes in culture. *Biochim Biophys Acta* 762:471–474, 1983.

171. Thomson BM, Saklatvala J, Chambers TJ: Osteoblasts mediate interleukin-1 stimulation of bone resorption by rat osteoclasts. *J Exp Med* 164:104–112, 1986.

172. Sabatini M, Garrett IR, Mundy GR: TNF potentiates the effects of interleukin-1 on bone resorption in vitro. *J Bone Min Res* 2(suppl 1):34, 1987.

173. Stashenko P, Dewhirst FE, Peros WJ, et al: Synergistic interactions between interleukin-1, tumor necrosis factor, and lymphotoxin in bone resorption. *J Immunol* 138:1464–1468, 1987.

174. Sato K, Fujii Y, Kasano K, Ozawa M, et al: Parathyroid hormone-related protein and interleukin-1 synergistically stimulate bone resorption in vitro and increase the serum calcium concentration in mice in vivo. *Endocrinology* 124:2172–2178, 1989.

175. Canalis E: Interleukin-1 has independent effects on deoxyribonucleic acid and collagen synthesis in cultures of rat calvariae. *Endocrinology* 118:74–81, 1986.

176. Smith DD, Gowen M, Mundy GR: Effects of interferon gamma and other cytokines on collagen synthesis in fetal rat bone cultures. *Endocrinology* 120:2494–2499, 1987.

177. Fried RM, Voelkel EF, Rice RH, et al: Two squamous cell carcinomas not associated with humoral hypercalcemia produce a potent bone resorption-stimulating factor which is interleukin-1 alpha. *Endocrinology* 125:742–751, 1989.

178. Klein B, Zhang XG, et al: Cytokines involved in human multiple myeloma. *Monoclonal Gammopathies II* 12:55–59, 1989.

179. Bataille R, Jourdan M, Zhang XG, Klein B: Serum levels of interleukin-6, a potent myeloma cell growth factor, as a reflect of disease severity in plasma cell dyscrasias. *J Clin Invest* 84:2008–2011, 1989.

180. Kurihara N, Chenu C, Miller M, et al: Identification of committed mononuclear precursors for osteoclast-like cells formed in long term human marrow cultures. *Endocrinology* 126:2733–2741, 1990.

181. Bertolini DR, Nedwin GE, Bringman TS, et al: Stimulation of bone resorption and inhibition of bone formation in vitro by human tumor necrosis factor. *Nature* 319:516–518, 1986.

182. Tashjian AH Jr, Voelkel EF, Lazzaro M, et al: Tumor necrosis factor α (cachectin) stimulates bone resorption in mouse calvaria via a prostaglandin-mediated mechanism. *Endocrinology* 120:2029–2036, 1987.

183. Garrett, IR, Durie BG, Nedwin GE, et al: Production of lymphotoxin, the bone resorbing cytokine, by cultured human myeloma cells. *N Engl J Med* 317:526–532, 1987.

184. Klein DC, Raisz LG: Prostaglandins: Stimulation of bone resorption in tissue culture. *Endocrinology* 86:1436–1440, 1970.

185. Raisz LG, Vanderhoek JY, Simmons HA: Prostaglandin synthesis by fetal rat bone in vitro: Evidence for a role of prostacyclin. *Prostaglandin* 17:905–914, 1979.

186. Voelkel EF, Tashjian AH Jr, Levine L: Cyclo-oxygenase products of arachindonic acid metabolism by mouse bone in organ culture. *Biochim Biophys Acta* 620:418–428, 1980.

187. Raisz LG, Alander CB, Simmons HA: Effects of prostaglandin E3 and eicosapentaenoic acid on rat bone in organ culture. *Prostaglandins* 37:615–625, 1989.

188. Raisz LG, Woodiel FN: Effects of alteration in the cyclopentane ring on bone resorptive activity of prostaglandin. *Prostaglandins* 37:229–235, 1989.

189. Raisz LG, Niemann I: Effect of phosphate, calcium and magnesium on bone resorption and hormonal responses in tissue culture. *Endocrinology* 85:446–452, 1969.

190. Yamaguchi DT, Hahn TJ, Beeker TG, et al: Relationship of cAMP and calcium messenger systems in prostaglandin-stimulated UMR-106 cells. *J Biol Chem* 263:10745–10753, 1988.

191. Hakeda Y, Hotta T, Kurihara N, et al: Prostaglandin E and F2α stimulate differentiation and proliferation, respectively, of clonal osteoblastic MC3T3-E1 cells by different second messengers in vitro. *Endocrinology* 121:1966–1974, 1987.

192. Klein-Nulend J, Pilbeam CC, Harrison JR, et al: Mechanism of regulation of prostaglandin production by parathyroid hormone, interleukin-1, and cortisol in cultured mouse parietal bone. *Endocrinology* 128:2503–2510, 1991.

193. Harrison JR, Lorenzo JA, Kawaguchi H, Raisz LG, Pilbeam CC: Stimulation of prostaglandin E2 production by interleukin-1α and transforming growth factor α in osteoblastic MC3T3-E1 cells. *J Bone Min Res* 9:817–823, 1994.

194. Kawaguchi H, Raisz LG, Voznesensky OS, et al: Regulations of the two prostaglandin G/H synthases by parathyroid hormone, interleukin-1, cortisol and prostaglandin E2 in cultured neonatal mouse calvariae. *Endocrinology* 135:1157–1164, 1994.

195. Pilbeam CC, Kawaguchi H, Hakeda Y, et al: Differential regulation of inducible and constitutive prostaglandin endoperoxide synthase in osteoblastic MC3T3-E1 cells. *J Biol Chem* 268:25643–25649, 1993.

196. Harell A, Dekel S, Binderman I: Biochemical effect of mechanical stress on cultured bone cells. *Calcif Tiss Res* 22(suppl):202–207, 1979.

197. Reich KM, Frangos JA: Protein kinase-C mediates flow-induced prostaglandin E2 production in osteoblasts. *Calcif Tiss Int* 52:62–66, 1993.

198. Minkin C, Fredericks RS, Pikress S, et al: Bone resorption and humeral hypercalcemia of malignancy: Stimulation of bone resorption in vitro by tumor extracts is inhibited by prostaglandin synthesis inhibitors. *J Clin Endocrinal Metab* 53:941–947, 1981.

199. Harris M, Jenkins MV, Bennett A, Wills MR: Prostaglandin production and bone resorption by dental cysts. *Nature* 245:213–215, 1973.

200. Robinson DR, Tashjian AH Jr, Levine L: Prostaglandin-stimulated bone resorption by rheumatoid synovia: A possible mechanism for bone destruction in rheumatoid arthritis. *J Clin Invest* 56:1181–1187, 1975.

201. Gallwitz WE, Mundy GR, Lee CH, et al: 5-lipoxygenase metabolites of arachidonic acid stimulate isolated osteoclasts to resorb calcified matrices. *J Biol Chem* 268:10087–10094, 1993.

202. Oreffo RO, Marshall GJ, Kirchen M, et al: Characterization of a cell line derived from a giant cell tumor that stimulates osteoclastic bone resorption. *Clin Orthop* 296:229–241, 1993.

203. Huggins CB. The formation of bone under the influence of epithelium of the urinary tract. *Arch Surg* 22:377–408, 1931.

204. Wlodarski K: The inductive properties of epithelial established cell lines. *Exp Cell Res* 57:446–448, 1969.

205. Urist MR: Bone formation by autoinduction. *Science* 150:883–889, 1965.

206. Wlodarski K, Poltorak A, Koziorowska J: Species specificity of osteogenesis induced by WISH cell line and bone induction by vaccinia virus transformed human fibroblasts. *Calcif Tiss Res* 7:345–352, 1971.

207. Hall BK, Van Exan RJ: Induction of bone by epithelial cell products. *J Embryol Exp Morphol* 69:37–46, 1982.

208. Wang EA, Rosen V, Cordes P, et al: Purification and characterization of other distinct bone-inducing factors. *Proc Natl Acad Sci USA* 85:9484–9488, 1988.

209. Luyten FP, Cunningham NS, Ma S, et al: Purification and partial amino acid sequence of osteogenin, a protein initiating bone differentiation. *J Biol Chem* 264:13377–13380, 1989.

210. Sampath TK, Coughlin JE, Whitsone RM, et al: Bovine osteogenic protein is composed of dimers of OP-1 and BMP-2A, two members of the transforming growth factor β superfamily. *J Biol Chem* 265:13198–13205, 1990.

211. Wozney JM, Rosen V, Celest AJ, et al: Novel regulators of bone formation: Molecular clones and activities. *Science* 242:1528–1534, 1988.

212. Wozney JM: Bone morphogenetic proteins: A review. *Prog Growth Factor Res* 1:267–280, 1989.

213. Celeste AJ, Iannazzi JA, Taylor RC, et al: Identification of transforming growth factor β family members present in bone-inductive protein purified from bovine bone. *Proc Natl Acad Sci USA* 87:9843–9847, 1990.

214. Wozney JM, Rosen V: Bone morphogenetic proteins, in Mundy GR, Martin TJ (eds): *Handbook of Experimental Pharmacology: Vol 107. Physiology and Pharmacology of Bone.* New York, Springer-Verlag, 1995, pp 725–748.

215. Wang EA, Rosen V, D'Allesandro JS, et al: Recombinant human bone morphogenetic protein induces bone formation. *Proc Natl Acad Sci USA* 87:2220–2224, 1990.

216. Gerhart TN, Kirker-Head CA, Kriz MJ, et al: Healing of large mid-femoral segmental defects in sheep using recombinant human bone morphogenetic protein (BMP-2). *Trans Orthop Res Soc* 16:172, 1991.

217. Avioli LV, Lindsay R: The female osteoporotic syndrome(s), in Avioli LV, Krane SM (eds): *Metabolic Bone Disease and Clinically Related Disorders.* Philadelphia, Saunders, 1990, pp 397–451.

218. Frost HM: *Bone Remodeling and Its Relationship to Metabolic Bone Disease.* Springfield, IL, Charles C Thomas, 1973.

219. Frost HM: *Intermediate Organization of the Skeleton:* Vol 1. Boca Raton, FL, CRC Press, 1986.

220. Tran VP, Vignery A, Baron R: An electron microscope study of the bone-remodeling sequence in the rat. *Cell Tiss Res* 225:283–289, 1982.

221. Dempster DW: Bone remodeling, in Coe FL, Favus MJ (eds): *Disorders of Bone and Mineral Metabolism.* New York, Raven Press, 1992, pp 344–380.

222. Mundy GR, Roodman GD: Osteoclast ontogeny and function, in Peck WA (ed): *Bone and Mineral Research.* New York, Elsevier, 1987, pp 209–280.

223. Amprino R, Engstrom A: Studies on x-ray absorption and diffraction of bone tissue. *Acta Anat* 15:1–22, 1952.

224. Currey J: *The Mechanical Adaptations of Bones.* Princeton, NJ, Princeton University Press, 1984.

225. Wolff J: *The Law of Remodeling.* Maquet P, Furlong R, (trans). Berlin, Springer-Verlag, 1986 (1892).

226. Jones HH, Priest JD, Hayes WC, et al: Humeral hypertrophy in response to exercise. *J Bone Joint Surg* 59A:204–208, 1977.

227. Buckwalter JA, Woo SL-Y: Effects of repetitive loading and motion on the musculoskeletal tissues, in DeLee JC, Drez D Jr (eds): *Orthopaedic Sports Medicine, Principles and Practice.* Philadelphia, Saunders, 1994, pp 60–72.

228. Carter DR: Mechanical loading histories and cortical bone remodeling. *Calcif Tiss Int* 36(suppl 1):S19–S24, 1984.

229. Donaldson CL, Hulley SB, Vogel JM, et al: Effect of prolonged bedrest on bone mineral. *Metabolism* 19:1071–1084, 1970.

230. Rubin CT, Lanyon LE: Limb mechanics as a function of speed and gait: A study of functional strains in the radius and tibia of horse and dog. *J Exp Biol* 101:187–211, 1982.

231. Rubin CT: Skeletal strain and functional strain significance of bone architecture. *Calcif Tiss Int* 6(suppl 1):S11–S18, 1984.

232. Rubin CT, Lanyon LE: Dynamic strain similarity in vertebrates: An alternative to allometric limb bone scaling. *J Theor Biol* 107:321–327, 1984.

233. Rubin CT, Lanyon LE: Regulation of bone mass by mechanical loading: Ether effect of peak strain magnitude. *Calcif Tiss Int* 37:411–417, 1985.

234. Lanyon LE, Goodship AE, Pye C, MacFie H: Mechanically adaptive bone remodeling *J Biomech* 15:141–154, 1982.

235. O'Connor JA, Lanyon LE, MacFie H: The influence of strain rate on adaptive bone remodeling. *J Biomech* 15:767–781, 1982.

236. Lanyon LE, Rubin CT: Static vs dynamic loads as an influence on bone remodeling. *J Biomech* 17:897–905, 1984.

237. Rubin CT, Lanyon LE: Regulation of bone formation by applied dynamic loads. *J Bone Joint Surg* 66A:397–402, 1984.

238. Brown TD, Pederson DR, Gray ML, et al: Toward an identification of mechanical parameters initiating periosteal remodeling: A combined experimental and analytic approach. *J Biomech* 23:893–905, 1990.

239. McLeod KJ, Rubin CT: The effect of low frequency electric fields on osteogenesis. *J Bone Joint Surg* 74A:920–929, 1992.

240. Rubin CT, McLeod KJ: Promotion of bony ingrowth by frequency-specific, low-amplitude mechanical strain. *Clin Orthop* 298:165–174, 1994.

241. McLeod KJ, Rubin CT: Strain frequency spectra in the appendicular skeleton during normal activity. *J Biomech* 1995. In press.

242. Berretta DA, Pollack SR: Ion concentration effects on the zeta potential of bone. *J Orthop Res* 4:337–345, 1986.

243. Bassett CA: Biophysical principles affecting bone structure, in Bourne GH (ed): *The Biochemistry and Physiology of Bone.* New York, New Academic Press, 1971, pp 1–76.

244. Brighton CT, McCluskey WP: Cellular response and mechanism of action of electrically induced osteogenesis, in Peck WA (ed): *Bone and Mineral Research 4.* New York, Elsevier, 1986, pp 213–254.

245. Bassett CA: Fundamental and practical aspects of therapeutic uses of pulsed electromagnetic fields (PEMFs): A review. *Crit Rev Biomed Eng* 17:451–529, 1989.

246. Ashihara T, Kagawa K, Kimiih M, et al: 3H-Thymidine autoradiographic studies of the cell proliferation and differentiation in electrically stimulated osteogenesis, in Brighton CT, Black J, Pollack SR (eds): *Electrical Properties of Bone and Cartilage.* New York, Grune & Stratton, 1979, pp 401–426.

247. McLeod KJ, Lee RC, Ehrlich HP: Frequency dependence of electic field modulation of fibroblast protein synthesis. *Science* 236:1465–1469, 1987.

248. Bassett CA, Chokshi HR, Hernandez E, et al: The effect of pulsing electromagnetic fields on cellular calcium and calcification of nonunions, in Brighton CT, Black J, Pollack SR (eds): *Electrical Properties of Bone and Cartilage.* New York, Grune & Stratton, 1979, pp 427–442.

249. McLeod KJ, Donahue HJ, Fontaine MA, et al: Electric fields modulate bone cell function in a density dependent manner. *J Bone Min Res* 8:977–984, 1993.

250. Rubin J, McLeod KJ, Titus L, et al: Formation of osteoclast-like cells is suppressed by low frequency, low intensity electric fields. *J Orthop Res* 14:7–15, 1996.

251. Cowin SC: *Bone Mechanics.* Boca Raton, FL, CRC Press, 1989, p 313.

252. Carter DR, Harris WH, Caler WE: The mechanical and biological response of cortical bone to in vivo strain histories, in Cowin SC (eds): *Mechanical Properties of Bone.* AMD-ASME Publ 45. American Society of Mechanical Engineers, 1981, pp 81–92.

253. Curry JD: Mechanical properties of bone with greatly differing functions. *J Biomech* 12:313, 1979.

254. Lanyon LE, Rubin CT: Functional adaptation in skeletal structures, in Hildebrand M, Bramble DM, Leim KF, Wake DB (eds): *Functional Vertebrate Morphology.* Cambridge, MA: Harvard University Press, 1985, pp 1–25.

255. Woo SLY: The relationships of changes in stress levels on long bone remodeling, in Cowen S (ed): *Mechanical Properties of Bone.* AMD-ASME Publ 45. American Society of Mechanical Engineers, 1981, p 107.

256. Lewis GC, Jones LC, Connor KM, et al: An evaluation of grafting materials in cementless arthroplasty. *Trans Orthop Res Soc* 12:319, 1987.

257. Soballe K, Hansen ES, B-Rasmussen H, et al: Early fixation of allogenic bone graft in titanium and hydroxyapatite coated implants. *Trans Orthop Res Soc* 14:385, 1989.

258. Dai KR, Liu YK, Park JB, et al: Bone-particle impregnated bone cement: An in vivo weight bearing study. *J Biomed Mater Res* 25:141, 1991.

259. Kotani S, Yamamuro T, Nakamura T, et al: Enhancement of bone bonding to bioactive ceramics by demineralized bone powder. *Clin Orthop* 278:226, 1992.

260. Cook SD, Thomas KA, Haddad RJ: Histologic analysis of retrieved porous-coated total joint components. *Clin Orthop* 232:90, 1988.

261. Soballe K, Gotfredsen K, B-Rasmussen H, et al: Histologic analysis of a retrieved hydroxyapatite-coated femoral prosthesis. *Clin Orthop* 272:255–258, 1991.

262. Jasty M, Rubash HE, Paiement GD, et al: Porous-coated uncemented components in experimental total hip arthroplasty in dogs: Effect of plasma-sprayed calcium phosphate coating on bone ingrowth. *Clin Orthop* 280:300, 1992.

263. Shen WJ, Chung KC, Wand GJ, McLaughlin RE: Mechanical failure of hydroxyapatite- and polysulfone-coated titanium rods in a weight-bearing canine model. *J Arthropl* 7:43–49, 1992.

264. Spector M, Davis RJ, Lunceford EM, Harmon SL: Porous polysulfone coatings for fixation of femoral stems by bony ingrowth. *Clin Orthop* 1786:34, 1983.

265. Goodman S, Aspenberg P, Song Y, et al: Effects of intermittent micromotion versus polymer particles on tissue ingrowth: Experiment using a micromotion chamber implanted in rabbits. *J Appl Biomat* 5117–123, 1994.

266. Aspenberg P, Wang JS, Choong P, Thorngren KG: No effect of growth hormone on bone graft incorporation: Titanium chamber study in the normal rat. *Acta Orthop Scand* 65:456–461, 1991.

267. Aspenberg P, Goodman S, Toksvig-Larsen S, et al: Intermittent micromotion inhibits bone ingrowth: Titanium implants in rabbits. *Acta Orthop Scand* 63:141–145, 1992.

268. Yasko AW, Lane JM, Fellinger EJ, et al: The healing of segmental bone defects induced by recombinant human bone morphogenetic protein (rhBMP-2). *J Bone Joint Surg* 74A:659, 1992.

269. Hazan R, Brener R, Oron U: Bone growth to metal implants is regulated by their surface chemical properties. *Biomaterials* 14:570–574, 1993.

CHAPTER 3

Generalized Metabolic Disorders of the Skeleton

Ashok Vaswani
and Roger Dee

BONE METABOLISM

Calcium

Bone is the reservoir for 99 percent of the body's calcium. Of this, 1 percent may be considered as a readily exchangeable reservoir; access to the rest is initiated by some combination of cellular (e.g., osteoclast), paracrine (e.g., osteoclast-stimulating factor), or endocrine—e.g., parathyroid hormone (PTH)—factors (Table 3-1, Fig. 3-1).

Control of extracellular calcium concentration is important. The excitability of the muscle cell membrane is proportional to the ratio

$$\frac{[HCO_3^-][HPO_4]}{[Ca^{2+}Mg^{2+}][H^+]}$$

According to the formula, a fall in the level of the calcium in the extracellular fluid can promote tetany. This is the basis of the well-known Chvostek sign, when tapping the masseter muscle often induces spasm in that muscle. There may be associated carpopedal spasm. The treatment of hypocalcemia is described later in this chapter.

Excessive administration of vitamin D preparations together with oral calcium supplements can result in hypercalcemia, which, in excess of 40 mg/dL, can be rapidly fatal. Serum levels greater than 15 mg/dL require prompt treatment. The treatment of hypercalcemia is described later in this chapter. The symptoms of hypercalcemia may vary from mental depression and lethargy to psychosis. The effect on the muscles is to induce hypotonia and weakness, and there may be cardiac arrhythmias. Alterations may be seen on the electroencephalogram (EEG) as well as the electrocardiogram (ECG).[1] The differential diagnosis includes malignancy with bone involvement, primary hyperparathyroidism, vitamin D intoxication, and sarcoidosis. There are also rare inherited forms of hypercalcemia.

Plasma calcium exists in three forms: 48 percent of it is present in the free ionized form; 46 percent is ionized but bound to serum proteins, mainly albumin; and the remainder is complexed with citrate and phosphates.[2] Consequently, changes in serum protein may affect serum calcium. In order to exclude factitious hypercalcemia due to hyperproteinemia or prolonged venous stasis during blood collection, a correction factor may be necessary. A general guideline is to adjust the observed serum calcium level by 0.8 mg/dL for each increase or decrease of 1 g of albumin outside the normal range. It will be seen from the above equation that even in the presence of normal serum

calcium, an alkaline pH, such as one induced by hyperventilation, may cause the physiologic effects of hypocalcemia. Other causes include surgically produced hypoparathyroidism, pseudohypoparathyroidism, malabsorption syndromes, and vitamin D deficiencies.

Calcium is absorbed from the gut by means of active transport in the brush border of certain lining epithelial cells. This process is regulated by 1,25-dihydroxyvitamin D_3 [1,25(OH)$_2$D$_3$]. At the luminal surface of the mucosal cell, the absorption of calcium into the cell is mediated by a 1,25(OH)$_2$D$_3$–dependent calcium carrier in the brush border. Calcium transport *from* the mucosal cell into the blood is enhanced by stimulation of alpha-adrenergic receptors (e.g., by epinephrine).[3]

The rate of production of 1,25(OH)$_2$D$_3$ at the kidney is increased when the plasma calcium level is decreased, and it is reduced when the plasma calcium is elevated (Fig. 3-2). Calcium absorption is thus adjusted to body needs. Calcium is also possibly secreted into the gut, but by cells different from those that reabsorb it, by means of a calmodulin-dependent calcium-transporting ATPase.[3] Some calcium is absorbed by passive diffusion and by certain substances that form insoluble compounds with calcium—for example, oxylates. Phosphates may therefore have some effect on decreasing absorption of calcium, which produces defective skeletal mineralization (osteomalacia). Calcium ingestion varies greatly and is often subnormal in the elderly.

Reabsorption of almost all filtered calcium is accomplished by the kidney. Some 60 percent of the reabsorption occurs in the proximal tubule; the remainder takes place in the distal tubule and is regulated by parathyroid hormone.

Phosphate

Plasma levels of phosphate vary from 2.4 to 4.4 mg/dL. Most of this is in a diffusible form, only 12 percent being bound to protein. Apart from its role in key cellular enzyme systems and molecular interactions, phosphate is a component of bone mineral. It is not surprising, therefore, that of the total body phosphorus of 500 to 800 g, some 85 to 90 percent is found in the skeleton.

The movement of calcium and phosphate ions is often linked (Fig. 3-1). Phosphate is the normal accompanying anion in the calcium transport system during absorption from the gut, but an independent phosphate absorption system that shows vitamin D dependence has been postulated. The absorption of phosphate from the gut seems to be linearly proportionate to dietary intake.[4]

Only 10 percent of the phosphate passing through the glomerulus is excreted in the urine, the rest being reabsorbed. There are two mechanisms for reabsorption. Active reabsorption in the proximal tubule of the nephron is by active transport, a process that, when inhibited by PTH, is responsible for the phosphaturic action of that hormone. A second mechanism seems to be independent of parathyroid gland functions, so that as the serum level of inorganic phosphate rises and renal tubular reabsorption of phosphate diminishes, this can be shown to occur

TABLE 3-1   Some Agents Affecting Bone Metabolism and Their Actions at Different Target Sites

Agent	Gut	Kidney	Bone
PTH	Increases Ca^{2+} absorption via effect on $1,25(OH)_2D_3$ production.	Increases renal reabsorption of Ca^{2+}. Inhibits active reabsorption of phosphate: phosphaturia (via cyclic AMP). Stimulates $1,25(OH)_2D_3$ production by renal 1α hydroxylase.	Acts on osteoblasts (via cyclic AMP and Ca^{2+} second messengers). Indirect stimulation of osteoclasts.
$1,25(OH)_2D_3$	Promotes binding and absorption of Ca^{2+} from lumen.	Inhibits activity of renal 1α hydroxylase Promotes $24,25(OH)_2D_3$ pathway.	$\downarrow$Bone matrix synthesis. $\uparrow$Osteocalcin synthesis. $\uparrow Ca^{2+}$ in ECF (active transport across bone cells).
Calcitonin		Increases excretion of sodium and phosphate.	Induces quiescence in osteoclasts. Phosphate enters BF and bone cells; probably Ca^{2+} also.

Key: PTH, parathyroid hormone; AMP, adenosine monophosphate; ECF, extracellular fluid; BF, bone fluid.

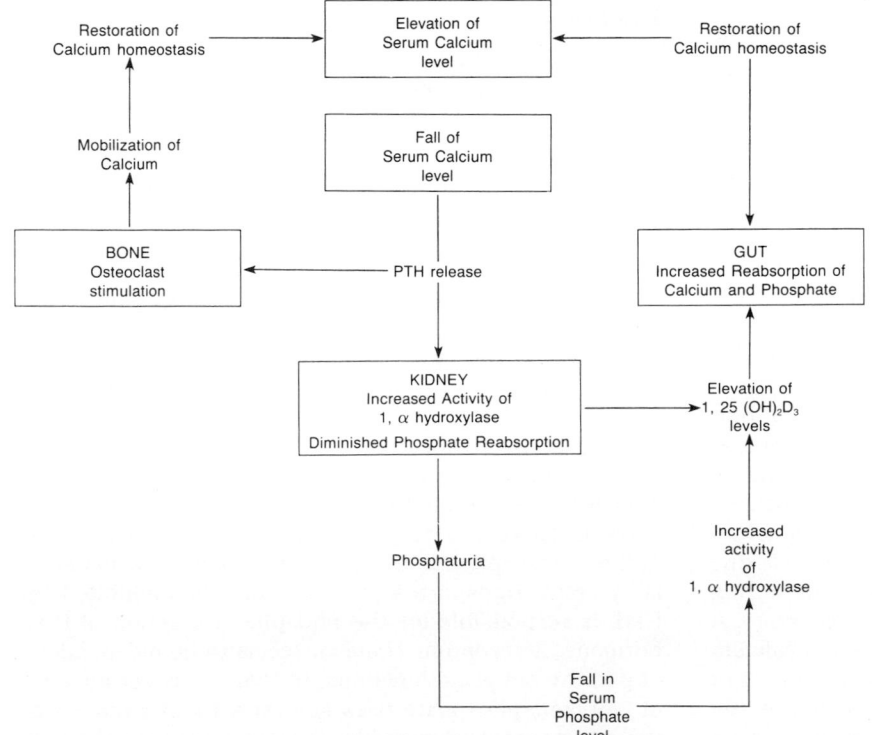

Figure 3-1 Feedback mechanisms affecting kidney, bone, and gut that maintain calcium homeostasis.

in isolated tubular segments. It is not simply dependent upon variations in the amount of phosphate filtered at the glomerulus.

A feedback mechanism exists between the level of plasma phosphate and the activity of the renal 1α-hydroxylase enzyme responsible for converting 25-OH-D_3 to the more active form $1,25(OH)_2D_3$ (Fig. 3-2). High plasma phosphate levels inhibit this enzyme, thus reducing production of the active metabolite. Plasma phosphate levels seem to have no effect upon parathyroid gland production of PTH.

A decrease in blood calcium level is caused by hyperphosphatemia (such as that which may occur with the low filtration rates of chronic renal disease), related to diminished production of calcitriol. The low calcium stimulates increased parathyroid activity, which will increase the renal clearance of phosphate as well as blood calcium levels to restore homeostasis (Fig. 3-2). If the kidney cannot respond with increased phosphate loads, since PTH is also mobilizing phosphate from the bone, phosphate levels will remain high. Eventually, however, the low levels of $1,25(OH)_2D_3$ will affect the ability to maintain adequate calcium balance. There may be undiminished stimulation of the parathyroids, resulting in renal osteodystrophy. Inadequate levels of $1,25(OH)_2D_3$ lead to osteomalacia; the secondary hyperparathyroidism may cause changes of osteitis fibrosis cystica.

In renal tubular diseases, there may similarly be low levels of $1,25(OH)_2D_3$, associated, however, with abnormally high levels of phosphate excretion by the kidney.[5]

Parathyroid Hormone

The stimulus for the release of stored PTH from the production site—the chief cells in the parathyroid glands—is a diminution in the level of ionized calcium in the extracellular fluid (Fig. 3-2). When serum calcium levels are elevated, secretion is inhibited. According to Rosenblatt,[1] the relationship of calcium to parathyroid hormone is linear within a narrow physiologic range; but below 8 mg/dL, hormone secretion decreases dramatically. The hormone mobilizes calcium from bone by action upon cells lining the bone surfaces, and it also mobilizes phosphate from bone. At the kidney, it has a phosphaturic action and also influences vitamin D metabolism.

There are data suggesting that cyclic adenosine monophosphate (AMP) and, perhaps, ionic calcium (Ca^{2+}) function as second intracellular messengers in response to PTH.[6,7] This certainly seems to be true in bone, where the osteoblast is the target cell for PTH. In bone, PTH interacts with receptors on the osteoblast cell membrane, promoting the activity of adenylate cyclase located on the membrane and the entry of calcium into the cell. The changes in levels of calcium and cyclic AMP inside the cell produce the desired cellular result. At the kidney, cyclic AMP can be detected in the urine after exposure to PTH, and such a finding can be used clinically as an indicator of hormone activity.

At the kidney, the phosphaturic effect of PTH occurs rapidly. The half-life of the polypeptide hormone is less than 20 min, and it is quickly metabolized by liver Kupffer cells.[4]

Figure 3-2 The metabolic pathways for vitamin D_3 and factors that affect them. Vitamin D_3 is the naturally occurring animal form, but synthetically produced D_2 is the usual supplement in the diet. Vitamin D_2 produces metabolic analogues similar to the D_3 compounds shown in the figure.

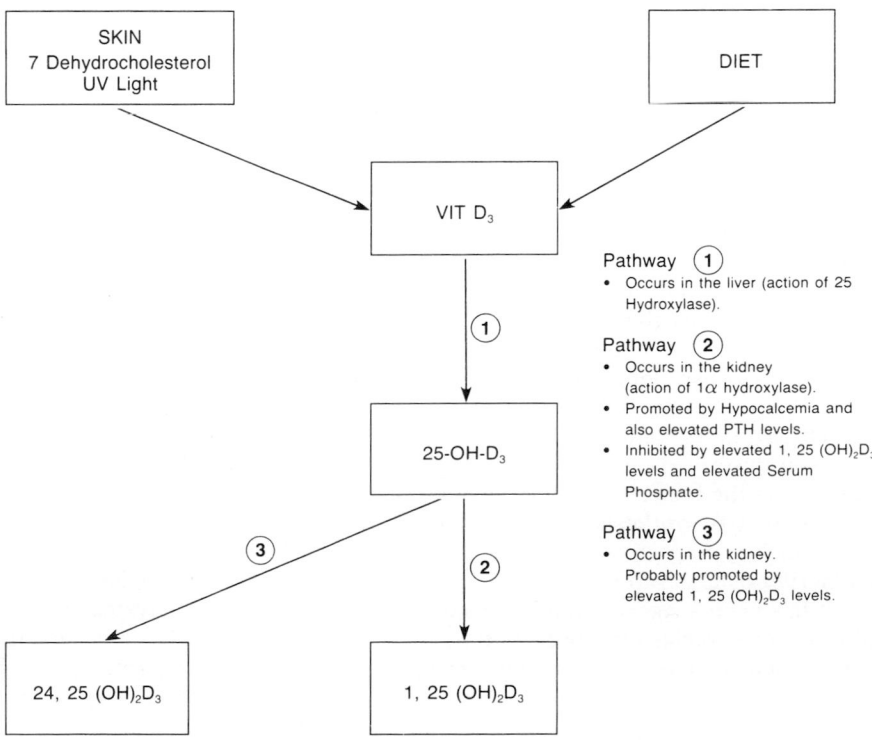

SKIN
7 Dehydrocholesterol
UV Light

DIET

VIT D_3

25-OH-D_3

24, 25 $(OH)_2D_3$

1, 25 $(OH)_2D_3$

Pathway ①
• Occurs in the liver (action of 25 Hydroxylase).

Pathway ②
• Occurs in the kidney (action of 1α hydroxylase).
• Promoted by Hypocalcemia and also elevated PTH levels.
• Inhibited by elevated 1, 25 $(OH)_2D_3$ levels and elevated Serum Phosphate.

Pathway ③
• Occurs in the kidney. Probably promoted by elevated 1, 25 $(OH)_2D_3$ levels.

Parathyroid hormone provides an appropriate physiologic response to low ionic calcium by stimulating the production of $1,25(OH)_2D_3$ by 1α-hydroxylase in the kidney. The hormone acts directly on bone to increase bone resorption and mobilize calcium, which contributes to restoration of appropriate blood levels (Fig. 3-1).

Since the resorption of bone is associated with osteoclastic simulation and yet the osteoblast is the *primary* target cell of this hormone, it is now evident that both in bone morphogenesis and in response to hormonal stimulation, many of the functions of the osteoclasts seem to be mediated via the osteoblast[8] (Table 3-1).

There is evidence that hormones such as PTH $1,25(OH)_2D_3$ and PGE_2 (one of the prostaglandin E series) stimulate osteoclasts indirectly following a primary hormonal interaction with osteoblasts.[8,9] In addition to inducing changes in the osteoblasts on the bone surface, which then assume a spindlelike shape, PTH inhibits bone collagen synthesis by altering the activity of procollagen messenger RNA.[10]

Vitamin D

The naturally occurring animal form of vitamin D is termed D_3 and has minor chemical differences from the synthetic form (D_2). The precursor 7-dihydrocholesterol is restored in the skin and may be converted to cholecalciferol (vitamin D_3) by the effect of ultraviolet irradiation in sunlight.

At the liver, vitamin D_3 is converted to 25-hydroxycholecalciferol (25-OH-D_3). Like all vitamin D derivatives, this metabolite is transported bound in the plasma to a specific globulin (vitamin D–binding protein). Within the mitochondria of cells of the proximal renal tubules, 25-OH-D_3 is converted by the action of the enzyme renal 1α hydroxylase to 1,25-dihydroxycholecalciferol [$1,25(OH)_2D_3$] (Fig. 3-1). The activity of renal 1α hydroxylase in the production of $1,25(OH)_2D_3$ is inhibited both when the plasma phosphate level is high and when the level of PTH is low. This provides a mechanism for controlling extracellular fluid calcium levels. Further specific hydroxylation in the kidney of 25-OH-D_3 also produces another metabolite, 24,25-dihydroxycholecalciferol [$24,25(OH)_2D_3$], this pathway being facilitated by elevated $1,25(OH)_2D_3$ levels (Fig. 3-2).

It follows from this description of the production of active metabolites that vitamin D is more appropriately thought of as a hormone—one with critical roles within the body—whose depletion or absence induces severe bone disease. The action of the active metabolite $1,25(OH)_2D_3$ in regulating calcium absorption from the gut has been described, but it also has important actions directly upon the bone. It can have similar reactions to PTH on bone matrix synthesis, which it may diminish in vitro by as much as 50 percent.[11] It also increases the synthesis and serum concentration of osteocalcin (Table 3-1).

It has been suggested that the role of vitamin D in inhibiting bone collagen synthesis (studied in tissue culture) is a useful mechanism when calcium and phosphate are in short supply.

Recent work has shown that $1,25(OH)_2D_3$ inhibits the proliferation of first-generation mesenchymal cells in the bone induction promoted by intramuscular implants of demineralized bone graft. There is a delay in the proliferation of mesenchymal tissue and the beginning of chondrogenesis. However, at a later stage in the induction of bone, when capillary sprouts are prominent, the hormone stimulates the differentiation of the cells associated with the vascular ingrowth. These cells differentiate into osteoblasts, with an increase in alkaline phosphatase levels that can be measured.[11] The evidence suggests also that a receptor for $1,25(OH)_2D_3$ is present in osteoblasts. Its effect upon osteoblasts lining bone surfaces may be similar to that upon gut mucosal cells, where it modulates calcium transport across the cells.

It has been observed that serum levels of $1,25(OH)_2D_3$ do not increase in the summer months. There are, however, seasonal trends for the incidence of such conditions as osteomalacia and certain fractures, which tend to increase in the winter months, and for renal nephrolithiasis, which seems to increase in the summer months. The data would seem to suggest that metabolites of vitamin D other than $1,25(OH)_2D_3$ may have an important physiologic role.[12] The metabolite $24,25(OH)_2D_3$ was thought to represent a shunting of hormone that might act as a storage mechanism when high levels of calcitriol were not required. However, it is now believed that this metabolite has a role of its own, since it seems to be necessary together with $1,25(OH)_2D_3$ for adequate healing in experimental rickets and also has a potent influence on chondrogenesis and mineralization during endochondral bone development and in fracture repair.[13]

Calcitonin

Calcitonin is a polypeptide hormone synthesized and secreted by parafollicular cells derived from the ultimobranchial body. These cells are identified in humans as clear cells (C cells) primarily in the thyroid gland. In fish, where calcitonin is probably more important metabolically, the ultimobranchial body is distinct from the thyroid. The exact role of the hormone is uncertain (Table 3-1), but it is secreted when the thyroid gland is perfused with solutions containing high calcium concentrations, and it seems to have a half-life of only about 10 min.[4] Calcitonin seems to induce quiescence in osteoclasts and consequently lowers serum calcium. Thyroidectomy does not affect plasma calcium levels if the parathyroid glands are preserved.

Osteoclasts have membrane receptors for calcitonin; the hormone causes loss of ruffled borders on these cells, associated with a rise and intracellular cyclic AMP levels. Prostaglandin (PGI_2) has a similar effect, increasing intracellular levels of cyclic AMP in osteoclasts and inducing cytoplasmic quiescence. Quiescent osteoblasts can be reactivated and stimulated by PGE_2, PTH, and $1,25(OH)_2D_3$ in vivo; however, these cells are not directly affected in vitro, suggesting that their stimulants act indirectly by means of a primary interaction with osteoblasts.[8]

Other Hormones

Mineral homeostasis is normally maintained primarily by the mechanisms described, and these mechanisms function smoothly during growth and normal bone remodeling.

Although changes in levels of other hormones do not cause such dramatic skeletal manifestations, nevertheless gross changes will lead to bone disease. With thyroid hormone excess, for example, there is a generalized increase in bone turnover, with a balance tipped toward bone reabsorption and the development of osteoporosis.

Patients chronically treated with glucocorticoids demonstrate a decrease in bone formation associated with inhibition of collagen synthesis. Increase in bone reabsorption is also observed and is thought to be due in part to increased PTH activity.[14] Certainly an increase in the blood levels of parathyroid hormone and alkaline phosphatase coupled with an increase in calcium excretion was observed after the administration of prednisone in human subjects.[14] There is an increase in urinary cyclic AMP levels as a response to the raised PTH. It seems that in the gut, gluocorticoids stimulate active calcium secretion by mucosal cells, resulting in a decrease of net calcium absorption in that portion of the gut concerned with the active transport of calcium. However, some increase in the passive diffusion of calcium in the duodenum is mediated by glucocorticoid, which seems to cancel out the effect on active transport.

The mechanism by which postmenopausal bone loss is associated with diminished estrogen levels is presently unknown. Estrogens may moderate the action of other hormones, such as PTH.[15] On the other hand, some evidence is now accumulating that specific estrogen receptors are present in bone cells.[16]

Insulin seems to participate in the regulation of bone growth; in particular, it is necessary for the anabolic effect of growth hormone.[17]

Growth hormone increases calcium excretion in urine but also increases intestinal absorption of calcium, with a resulting positive calcium balance.[4] Normal thyroid hormone levels are also necessary for normal maturation and growth. Some of the effects of growth hormone on epiphyseal cartilage are mediated by the somatomedins. The latter are a group of five separate peptides released in the liver by the effect of growth hormone.[4]

METABOLIC AND ENDOCRINE SYNDROMES AFFECTING BONE

Primary Hyperparathyroidism

The incidence of hyperparathyroidism in the general population is approximately 1 in 1000 subjects. More cases are now detected due to the increased availability of automated laboratory techniques that detect hypercalcemia, a diagnostic feature of hyperparathyroidism.[18] Since PTH fragments can circulate in the blood, it is important to emphasize that intact PTH should be measured in the blood simultaneously with the serum calcium levels. Thus, if serum calcium and PTH are elevated, hyperparathyroidism is most likely the cause of hypercalcemia. If PTH is suppressed and the serum calcium is elevated, then other causes of hypercalcemia should be sought (Table 3-2).

Pathogenesis

Under physiologic conditions, ionized calcium is the most important regulator of parathyroid hormone secretion. Other substances that affect plasma calcium levels—such as calcitonin, 1,25-dihydroxyvitamin D_3, and beta-adrenergic catecholamines—also play a role in the secretory control of PTH. In primary hyperparathyroidism, there is overproduction of hormone, leading to elevated and nonsuppressible levels of PTH. Excessive production of

TABLE 3-2   Differential Diagnosis of Hypercalcemia

Etiology	Differentiating features
Factitious	High serum proteins
Primary hyperparathyroidism	High PTH, low phosphate; mild metabolic acidosis
Familial hypercalcemia:	
Multiple endocrine neoplasia type I	Pituitary and pancreatic endocrine hyperfunction
Multiple endocrine neoplasia type II	Catecholamine and calcitonin excess
Hypocalciuric hypercalcemia	Low urinary calcium excretion, elevated serum magnesium
Malignant diseases:	
Multiple myeloma	Proteinuria, anemia, plasma cells in bone marrow
Lymphomas	Lymph node biopsy
Other causes:	
Thyrotoxicosis	Symptoms, elevated T_4, low PTH
Addison disease	Low cortisol, high ACTH, hyponatremia, hyperkalemia
Sarcoidosis	Chest x-ray; usually negative PPD, increased ACE levels
Tuberculosis	Chest x-ray; usually positive PPD
Paget's disease (during immobilization)	High alkaline phosphatase
Drugs:	
Vitamin D intoxication	Serum 25-hydroxyvitamin D
Vitamin A intoxication	Serum levels of vitamin D
Thiazide diuretics	History of drug use
Antacids	Excessive use of milk or calcium-containing antacids

Key: T_4, thyroid function tests; ACE, angiotensin converting enzyme; ACTH, adrenocorticotropic hormone; PPD, purified protein derivative tuberculin tests.

parathyroid hormone may be due to the presence of an adenoma (80 percent), hyperplasia (19 percent), or parathyroid carcinoma (1 percent). Certain nonparathyroid tumors may produce excessive PTH or PTH-related peptides. These peptides can be measured in the serum and, if the PTH is normal and the serum calcium is elevated, should be included in the workup of the patient.

Excessive parathyroid hormone enhances the urinary loss of phosphate and bicarbonate, leading to hypophosphatemia and mild hyperchloremic metabolic acidosis. The hypercalcemia may be associated with hypercalciuria, which occurs due to increased filtration of calcium. Bone resorption is enhanced by osteoclastic stimulation, raising serum calcium and increasing calcium excretion. Parathyroid hormone increases the synthesis of 1,25-dihydroxy vitamin D_3, which enhances intestinal absorption of calcium and may contribute to hypercalcemia. Thus, the overall effect of PTH excess is to resorb bone calcium and enhance excretion of urinary calcium, with a net loss of total body calcium.

Clinical Features

In its mildest form, primary hyperparathyroidism may be entirely asymptomatic and may be detected incidentally during routine laboratory screening tests. Symptomatic hyperparathyroidism may present as renal colic if hypercaliuria predominates. Hyperparathyroidism may also occur rapidly, presenting with weight loss, bone pain, compression fractures, and hypercalcemia. Other symptoms may include depression, emotional lability, and proximal muscle weakness.[19]

Although there are no classic physical findings, there may be fasciculations of the tongue and proximal muscle weakness. Other causes of hypercalcemia must be excluded before the diagnosis of primary hyperparathyroidism can be established (Table 3-2).

Laboratory and Radiologic Findings

Hypercalcemia is a hallmark of hyperparathyroidism, although in the early stages it may be intermittent. Hypophosphatemia in the presence of hyperphosphaturia is an important clue to the excessive production of PTH. Since the effect of parathyroid hormone is mediated by activation of the adenylate cyclase system, elevated levels of urinary cyclic AMP are commonly encountered in primary hyperparathyroidism. The finding of an elevated blood level of either the intact PTH or N-terminal PTH is required to establish the diagnosis of primary hyperparathyroidism in the presence of hypercalcemia. Since PTH activates the renal 1α-hydroxylase, elevated blood levels of 1,25-dihydroxyvitamin D_3 are often seen in hyperparathyroid patients with renal stones or colic.[20]

In long-standing hyperparathyroidism, bone changes of osteitis fibrosa cystica may be readily apparent radiographically. There may also be generalized osteopenia or localized bone resorption at the terminal phalanges (Fig. 3-3) or distal clavicles, or changes in the skull (Fig. 3-4). Subcortical bone resorption in the jaw may produce characteristic "brown tumor," which may resolve spontaneously after correction of the hyperparathyroidism. Chondrocalcinosis may be seen in primary hyperparathyroidism. Osteoclastic bone resorption, reactive osteoblastic activity, and peritrabecular fibrosis are commonly seen histologically.

The differential diagnosis of hyperparathyroidism includes all the causes of hypercalcemia (Table 3-2). Primary hyperparathyroidism must be distinguished from familial hypercalcemic syndromes and hypercalcemia of non-PTH causes (Fig. 3-5).

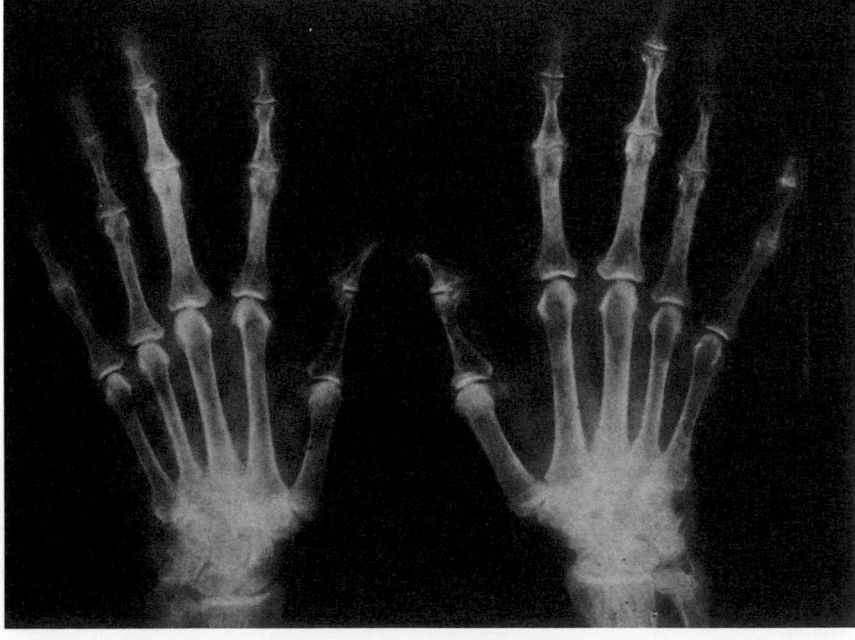

Figure 3-3 Extensive bone resorption in hyperparathyroidism. Note the cystic appearance of the proximal phalanges. [Reproduced with permission from Greenfield GB (ed): *Radiology of Bone Disease,* 3d ed. Philadelphia, Lippincott, 1979.]

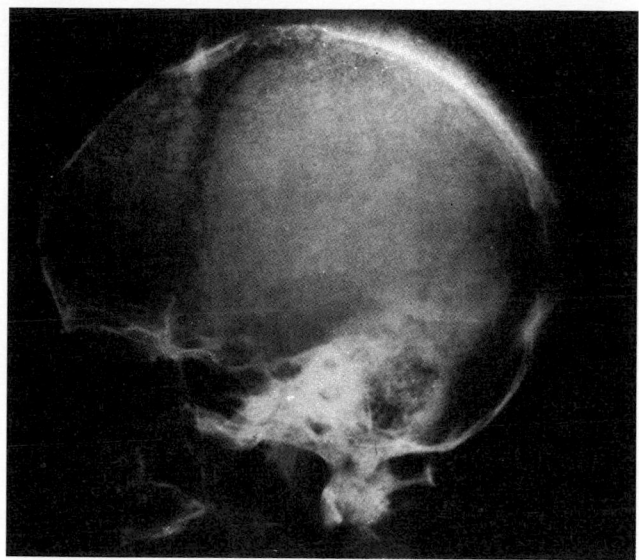

Figure 3-4 Characteristic "hair on end" appearance of the skull in primary hyperparathyroidism. [Reproduced with permission from Greenfield GB (ed): *Radiology of Bone Diseases,* 3d ed. Philadelphia, Lippincott, 1975.]

Familial Syndrome

Hypercalcemia may occur as a distinct entity in three familial syndromes. In multiple endocrine neoplasia type I (MEN-I), there may be associated pituitary of pancreatic adenomas. Serum gastric levels may be elevated. In MEN type II, increased levels of calcitonin or catecholamines along with the hypercalcemia are usually encountered. The patients may present with a thyroid nodule (reflecting the calcitonin-producing tumor) and/or hypertension (due to the excess catecholamines). Familial hypocalciuric hypercalcemia (FHH) is a distinct syndrome that can be diagnosed by a low calcium/creatinine clearance (< .01) in the urine and a high serum magnesium level. In FHH, there may be hyperplasia of the parathyroid glands, and the response to surgery is usually poor. In the MEN syndromes, it is imperative to diagnose the pheochromocytoma (catecholamine excess) first. Thus, the syndromes of familial hypercalcemia must be carefully excluded before exploration of the neck (Table 3-2).

Non-PTH–Related Hypercalcemia

Although there are a number of causes within this group, malignant disease is by far the most important in the differential diagnosis of non-PTH–related hypercalcemia. Weight loss, anorexia, constipation, and depression, although nonspecific, should heighten the suspicion of malignant disease. If malignant disease is suspected, a search for bony metastases or myelomatosis must be instituted with appropriate diagnostic procedures.

A thorough history and physical examination is usually sufficient to diagnose hyperthyroidism, which can be confirmed by thyroid function tests (T_4, T_3 uptake, and free thyroxine index or equivalent test) and a radioisotope scan. Hypercalcemia is often an associated electrolyte abnormality in Addison's disease. The presence of hyperpigmentation and hypotension along with other electrolyte abnormalities—such as hyperkalemia and hyponatremia—and the finding of a low serum cortisol will confirm the diagnosis of Addison's disease. Drugs, such as thiazides and absorbable antacids as well as excessive ingestion of vitamins A and D, taken individually or in combination, may precipitate hypercalcemia.

Hypercalcemia is frequently reported in patients with granulomatous diseases, particularly sarcoidosis.[21] An increased synthesis of vitamin D (1,25-dihydroxyvitamin D_3) is believed to cause the hypercalcemia. Similar alterations in vitamin D metabolism have been reported in patients with tuberculosis.[22] Destruction of the adrenal gland by tuberculosis should be considered if clinical symptoms are suggestive of Addison's disease.

Immobilization from any cause, particularly inpatients with active bone turnover, may be an important cause of hypercalcemia.[23] There is typically increased bone reabsorption, presumably unrelated to PTH, which leads to hypercalciuria. If renal function is impaired, rapid hypercalcemia may ensue.

Treatment of Hypercalcemia

No treatment may be necessary in asymptomatic subjects with minimal (less than 11.2 mg/dL) elevations in serum calcium. Mild symptomatic hypercalcemia can be treated in an outpatient setting with increased hydration and nonthiazide diuretics as needed. Bony involvement or abnormalities of renal function must be carefully sought and followed up at 6- to 12-month intervals. In addition, a detailed family history must be obtained to exclude familial or multiple endocrine neoplasia before contemplating surgery. Surgery may be indicated in case of primary hyperparathyroidism with symptomatic disease or in any asymptomatic individual with renal involvement and/or bone densitometry changes suggestive of osteoporosis.

During hypercalcemic crisis, intravenous therapy will be necessary to correct the dehydration. As much as 4 to 6 L of fluid may be given intravenously, depending on the age of the patient and on the severity of the hypercalcemia or coexisting diseases. Calcium excretion may be more effectively accomplished by the addition of a nonthiazide or loop diuretic. Since sodium and calcium are transported in the proximal tubule, a brisk diuresis with normal or half-normal saline should be instituted.

Salmon calcitonin (Calcimar) may be used in doses of 50 to 100 U every 6 h to control hypercalcemia. Its effect may be transient. It may also acutely induce facial flushing and nausea. Pamidronate (Aredia) in doses of 60 to 90 mg given over 24 h will reduce serum calcium for approximately 1 week. However, the drug needs 1 to 2 days to be effective and is, therefore, used in combination with the above therapies. Mithramycin, an inhibitor of RNA synthesis, may be used as a single dose (25 μg/kg per IV bolus). The effect of a single dose usually lasts between 24 and 48 h. The use of intravenous phosphates is not recommended, since soft tissue calcifications may occur. Oral

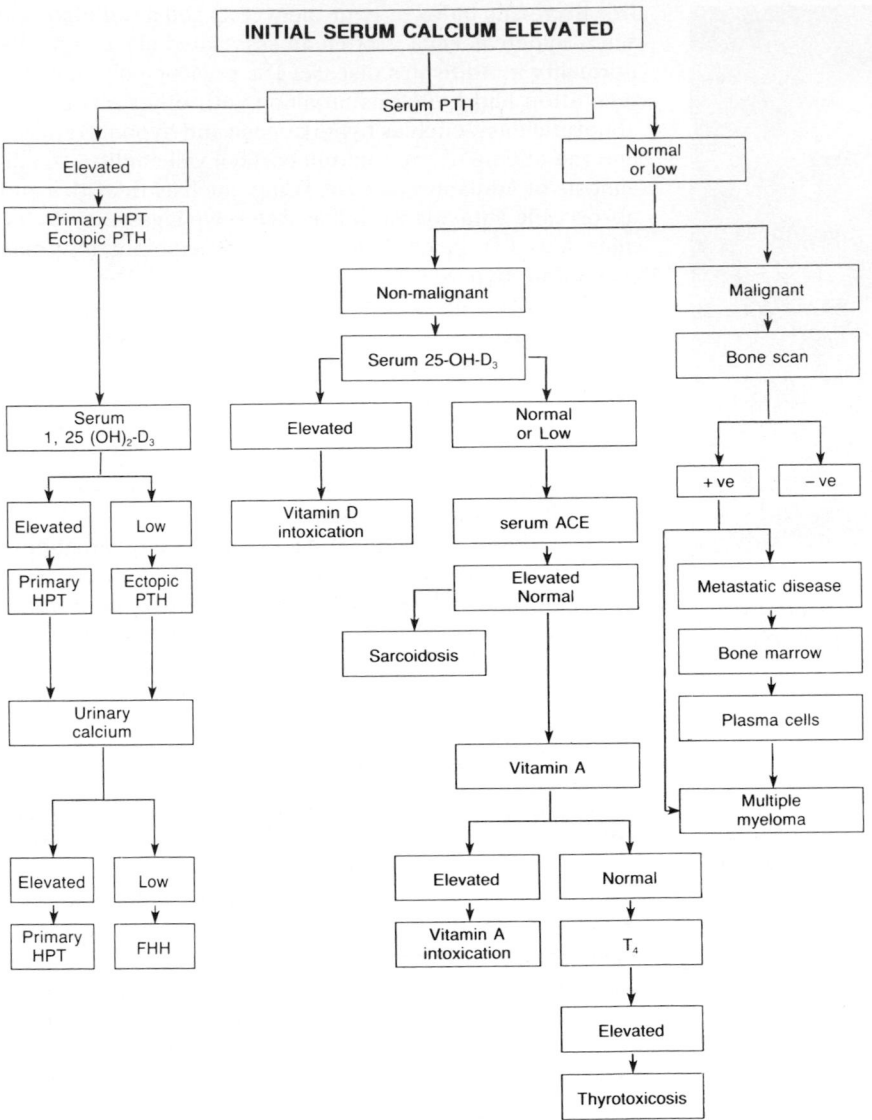

Figure 3-5 An algorithm that may be used for the diagnosis of hypercalcemic disorders.

phosphate may be less toxic and can be used in doses of 2 to 3 g of elemental phosphate daily. Serum calcium and phosphate must be monitored closely during therapy with phosphates. Serum electrolytes must also be monitored at periodic intervals during the saline infusion.

Specific therapy for hypercalcemia is directed toward the known or established cause of the disease. Discontinuation of excess vitamin D may not immediately lower the serum calcium, since the drug is fat-soluble. The use of steroids may be useful, since glucocorticoids antagonize the gastrointestinal absorption of calcium. In addition, glucocorticoid therapy will be lifesaving in patients with hypercalcemia of Addison's disease. Patients with hypercalcemia due to sarcoidosis, multiple myeloma, and certain lymphomas may also benefit from glucocorticoid therapy. Glucocorticoids should not be used in untreated tuberculosis.

Hypoparathyroidism and Other Hypocalcemic States

Hypocalcemia occurs as a result of deficiency or inadequate function of parathyroid hormone or vitamin D. It is not caused by dietary deficiency of calcium alone, because this is corrected by the secondary hyperparathyroidism, which increases bone resorption and corrects the hypocalcemia. Increased synthesis of $1,25(OH)_2D_3$ also helps correct low calcium levels.

Clinical Features

The symptoms of hypocalcemia include neuromuscular irritability, seizures, and tetany. Patients may have a positive Chvostek or Trousseau signs. In the former, there is irritability of the masseter muscle to percussion; in the latter, the characteristic position of the hand occurs, with flexion of the thumb and wrist and extension of the fingers. Physical examination may reveal lenticular cataracts or fungal infections of the nails, or there may be the obvious phenotypic features of pseudohypoparathyroidism described below. In this condition, x-ray films will reveal a short fourth metacarpal and metatarsal. Routine radiographs of the abdomen may reveal pancreatic calcification, indicating a malabsorption syndrome as an etiologic factor in the hypocalcemia. The ECG may show a prolonged Q interval.

Hypoparathyroid Syndromes

Hypoparathyroidism may be defined as an absolute or relative deficiency or inadequacy of PTH function. Hypocalcemia and hyperphosphatemia is associated with the diminished action of PTH. Since PTH mediates its action by the adenylate cyclase system, any receptor abnormalities or lack of cofactors (particularly magnesium) at the target cell can render the hormone ineffective.[24] Consequently, in these syndromes there may be normal or even markedly elevated levels of PTH. There may also be diminution in $1,25(OH)_2D_3$ production, which, in turn, affects calcium balance. Severe magnesium deficiency, which may be seen in chronic alcoholism, may mimic hypoparathyroidism. Hypoparathyroidism may be idiopathic, or it may occur as part of an autoimmune syndrome of polyglandular dysfunction. Hypoparathyroidism may also occur as a complication of thyroid or parathyroid surgery.

Clinical Features

The decrease in ionized serum calcium leads to neuromuscular irritability and tetany. Symptoms range from mild circumoral tingling to paresthesia or tetany. Chronic hypocalcemia leads to elevated cerebrospinal fluid (CSF) pressure, papilledema, and occasionally seizures. Lenticular cataract is an important feature of long-standing hypoparathyroidism.[25]

When the condition occurs as part of the pluriglandular syndrome, there may be associated thyroid and gonadal hypofunction with occasional pernicious anemia. When hypoparathyroidism occurs early in life, there may be delayed dentition or dental hypoplasia. Hypoparathyroidism may be associated with mucocutaneous candidiasis.

Hypoparathyroidism Associated with Parathyroid Hormone Resistance

Some patients with the typical biochemical features of hypoparathyroidism present with a characteristic physical appearance, indicating a syndrome of PTH resistance, sometimes termed *pseudohypoparathyroidism (PHP)*, or Albright's hereditary osteodystrophy.

In PHP, PTH levels are elevated in the presence of hypocalcemia and hyperphosphatemia, this being consis-

tent with hormone resistance. Recent evidence suggests that the guanine nucleotide regulatory components of the membrane-bound adenylate cyclase system may be defective, accounting for the deficiency in PTH function.[26] Thus, after injection of PTH, there may be no increase in cyclic AMP. However, in some affected family members, cyclic AMP response to an injection of PTH is normal. These subjects also have the characteristic familial type of PHP, however, and are classified as a separate subtype of hormone resistance known as *pseudopseudohypoparathyroidism (PPHP)*.

Clinical Features

The symptoms of PTH resistance are indistinguishable from those of idiopathic hypoparathyroidism. The characteristic familial type of short stature and bony abnormalities helps to distinguish the two. Bony abnormalities include shortening of the metacarpals and metatarsals (particularly the fourth metacarpal), brachydactyly, and exostoses. The patients are obese, with a round face, and usually have diminished intelligence. Patients with PHPP may have coexistent hypothyroidism and subcutaneous or basal ganglia calcification.

Differential Diagnosis

The history, physical examination, and laboratory tests usually permit an appropriate diagnosis. The presence of a neck scar is suggestive of postsurgical hypoparathyroidism, whereas monilial infection of the nails, alopecia, or vitiligo is more commonly associated with autoimmune or idiopathic hypoparathyroidism. Detectable or low levels of serum PTH will usually confirm the diagnosis of hypoparathyroidism, whereas higher levels suggest a PTH resistance syndrome. A history of alcoholism may suggest hypomagnesemia, which may cause impaired secretion of PTH from the gland and may decrease the effect of PTH at its target cells in the bone and kidney. A history of chronic diarrhea, abdominal pain, or chronic alcohol abuse should heighten the suspicion of pancreatitis or other malabsorption syndromes, particularly if there is pancreatic calcification. Reabsorption of vitamin D and calcium can be affected by malabsorption, thus worsening the problem of hypocalcemia.

The phenotype of PHP is characteristic, and there is no history of neck surgery. The bony exostoses of PHP are typical and do not occur in idiopathic hypoparathyroidism. Brachydactyly may also be seen in PHP. Factitious hypocalcemia can easily be excluded by correcting for abnormal serum albumin levels; serum phosphate is usually normal. All the causes of hypoparathyroid dysfunction should be considered in the differential diagnosis of hypocalcemia. Hypocalcemia with hyperophosphatemia and a markedly elevated level of PTH usually indicates the secondary hyperparathyroidism of chronic renal failure. Abnormal renal function tests will confirm the diagnosis of renal disease.

Serum calcium levels must be determined in any newborn infant with a seizure disorder. Neonatal hypocalcemia is often seen in premature infants as well as infants of diabetic mothers. Massive blood transfusion in premature infants or adults with hepatic insufficiency may induce hypocalcemia due to the chelating effect of citrate on calcium. Intravenous phosphate therapy for hypercalcemic crises also carries a risk of inducing acute hypocalcemia and should never be used to correct hypercalcemia. Calcitonin, used for the treatment of hypercalcemia, rarely produces hypocalcemia. Hypocalcemia can occasionally occur following surgical treatment of long-standing hyperparathyroidism. Chronic suppression of the normal remaining parathyroid tissue and a delayed release of PTH may be the cause of the transient hypocalcemia.

Treatment of Hypocalcemia and Hypoparathyroidism

Acute tetany requires immediate correction with intravenous calcium. A 10% solution of calcium gluconate (10 to 20 mL) can be given slowly over a period of several hours. Vitamin D therapy is required, with supplemental calcium, in the management of hypoparathyroidism of all types discussed. If the condition is due to magnesium deficiency, replacement of magnesium either orally or intravenously is sufficient to correct the biochemical abnormality; 1 to 2 g of elemental calcium will correct the hypocalcemia. The goal of therapy is to maintain serum calcium in the normal range so that the patient is free of symptoms of hypoparathyroidism and does not develop significant hypercalciuria or hypercalcemia.

Renal Osteodystrophy

Renal osteodystrophy is a complex bone disorder in patients with chronic renal failure. The renal impairment leads to an inability to excrete phosphate, with a compensatory reduction in serum calcium.[27]

Clinical Features

The hallmark of this syndrome is hyperphosphatemia, hypocalcemia, and markedly elevated blood levels of PTH. Bone histomorphometry reveals a mixture of both osteoporosis and osteomalacia. Radiographically, the changes may resemble hyperparathyroidism. X-ray films of the spine may reveal the typical "rugger jersey" appearance, associated with sclerosis, in the region immediately beneath the vertebral end plates. Slipped capital femoral epiphysis is a common orthopedic problem in children with renal osteodystrophy.

Rickets

Rickets includes several diseases of different etiologies, all of which severely affect normal skeletal development (Table 3-3).

Vitamin D–Deficiency Rickets

At the turn of the century, dietary deficiency of vitamin D was by far the commonest cause of rickets in this country.

TABLE 3-3   Differential Diagnosis of Hypocalcemia

Etiology	Differentiating features
Factitious	Low serum protein (albumin)
Primary hypoparathyroidism	Low to absent PTH, calcified basal ganglia
Pseudohypoparathyroidism (PHP)	Normal to high PTH, shortened metacarpals
Pseudopseudohypoparathyroidism (PPHP)	Phenotype of PHP, usually normal serum calcium
Magnesium deficiency	Low PTH, low serum Mg^{2+}
Chronic renal failure	Markedly elevated PTH, renal function abnormal
Vitamin D deficiency	Low phosphate, high PTH, low 25-hydroxyvitamin D
Pancreatitis	Diarrhea, malabsorption
Neonatal hypocalcemia	Maternal diabetes mellitus

Drugs:
  Intravenous phosphates
  Citrate
	Ectopic calcification during blood transfusions

This public health problem has been eliminated by the fortification of dairy products with vitamin D. Dietary sources of vitamin D include fish oils and vitamin D_2 ergocalciferol, present in plants. Vitamin D is also synthesized in the skin from 7-dehydrocholesterol by ultraviolet irradiation. In countries such as the United Kingdom, where vitamin D is not added to dairy products, rickets is occasionally seen, particularly in the children of Asian immigrants. Lack of exposure to sunlight can pose an additional health hazard in the perpetuation of rickets. Premature infants receiving prolonged therapy with total parenteral nutrition may exhibit radiographic changes of rickets.[28]

A reduction in the absorption of calcium and phosphorus occurs in the vitamin D–deficient state. There is a compensatory increase in parathyroid hormone when the serum calcium levels decline. Increased bone resorption is initially able to maintain serum calcium levels in the normal range. Continued unavailability of vitamin D intensifies in the secondary hyperparathyroidism, leading to a loss of phosphorus and decreased ability to maintain a normal serum calcium. At the skeletal level, deficient mineralization may be most evident in the regions of rapid bone turnover.

Clinical Features

In the first year of life, there may be delayed closure of the fontanelles, leading to widened cranial sutures. Flattening of the occiput (craniotabes) and thickening of the skull (frontal bossing) are also common. In the thorax, bulging and enlargement of the costochondral junction (rachitic rosary) may be an early indication of vitamin D deficiency. Other thoracic abnormalities include a posterior displacement of the sternum and the appearance of Harrison's groove, which manifests itself as an indentation of the lower ribs at the site of diaphragmatic insertion.

The rachitic bone lacks strength and is prone to stress fracture. The lower extremity bones bend and deformities appear as soon as the child is able to stand or walk. Long-standing disease may lead to coxa vara, saber shin, or lordosis of the spine. In addition to the skeletal deformities, there is a peculiar waddling gait. If the hypotonia of muscles is profound, it may lead to a delay in standing or walking. Dental enamel may be hypoplastic, and there may be delayed eruption of teeth.

In older children, vitamin D deficiency may manifest as short stature or an increased tendency to pathologic fractures of the long bones. In premature infants, symptoms of vitamin deficiency may occur in the first few months of life, due to delayed maturation of the hepatic enzyme systems.

Laboratory Findings

Since serum calcium levels are usually in the low normal range, tetany is uncommon. However, serum calcium is maintained in the low-normal range by an increase in the circulating level of PTH, leading to the classic manifestations of secondary hyperparathyroidism—i.e., increased phosphaturia, low serum phosphate, and mild hyperchloremic acidosis. The plasma level of alkaline phosphatase is usually elevated. The plasma concentration of the metabolites of vitamin D is low, in particular 25-OH-D$_3$. Inability to absorb sufficient calcium in the absence of vitamin D usually leads to a decrease in urinary calcium excretion. There may be a tendency to aminoaciduria.

Radiology

Radiographically, the poorly mineralized but abundant cartilage creates cupped metaphyses. The physis appears enlarged with increased height and width. The bone appears demineralized, with a thin cortex and few trabeculae. Features of secondary hyperparathyroidism, such as subperiosteal erosion of metaphyses of long bones, may be present. Radiography of the rachitic bone depends to some extent on the severity of the metabolic defect. Histologically, the growth plate in a rachitic child shows irregular widening, disrupted maturation, and delayed endochrondral ossification. There is irregularity of calcification and vascular invasion in the zone of provisional calcification; the osteoid in the primary spongiosa remains uncalcified.[29] There is peripheral splaying of cartilage cells, and the physis herniates into microfractures in the primary spongiosa, causing the cupped appearance of the metaphysis. The mineralization front may be absent or decreased. There is deficient mineralization of osteoid in cortical and trabecular bone. In some areas of the bone, osteoclastic activity may be increased if secondary hyperparathyroidism supervenes.

Differential Diagnosis

In addition to dietary deficiency of vitamin D to account for low levels of circulating 25(OH)D$_3$ found in nutritional rickets, malabsorption syndromes and renal and hepatic diseases must be considered as possibilities.

Treatment

Correction of bony abnormalities must be attempted only after the vitamin deficiency has been adequately treated. This can be satisfactorily achieved by giving 5000 U of vitamin D (as ergocalciferol) daily. In the early stages of treatment, since bone mineralization may be rapid, the serum calcium level may decrease, giving rise to hypocalcemia. Supplemental calcium, up to 3 g daily, may be required to avoid symptoms of hypocalcemia. In an emergency, 15 mg/kg of calcium chloride may be infused intravenously, slowly, over a few hours, in order to maintain serum calcium in the normal range.

Calcification in the unmineralized osteoid may begin after 1 week of treatment with vitamin D and calcium supplements. Serum alkaline phosphatase may increase above the baseline levels. As the vitamin and mineral deficits are corrected, mild to moderate bony abnormalities may resolve spontaneously. If a severe deformity persists after growth is complete, an osteotomy may be indicated.

Hereditary Vitamin D–Dependent Rickets

This condition has been called *pseudo–vitamin D deficiency*. As the name implies, this variety of rickets is unresponsive to the usual physiologic replacement doses of vitamin D. Hereditary vitamin D dependency, which is inherited as an autosomal recessive trait, can be categorized into two groups, distinguished only by low (type I) or normal (type II) levels of 1,25-dihydroxyvitamin D$_3$.

Pathogenesis

Vitamin D dependency may represent a defect in the renal 1α hydroxylation of 25-dihydroxyvitamin D$_3$. The resultant decrease in the synthesis of 1,25(OH)$_2$D$_3$ will impair calcium absorption, leading to the typical features of low serum calcium, secondary hyperparathyroidism, and clinical manifestations of vitamin D deficiency.[30]

Clinical Features

The clinical characteristics of this syndrome are identical to those of nutritional vitamin D deficiency, although the disease may be more florid. Occasionally, the child may present with tetany or convulsions as the initial manifestation of this disease. Alopecia totalis, which is a distinctive feature of the type II syndrome, has been reported in several kindreds with this disorder. In the adult, pseudo–vitamin D deficiency may present as osteomalacia.

Laboratory Findings

Serum calcium may be low, owing to the relatively low levels of 1,25-dihydroxyvitamin D_3. Serum phosphate may be decreased and the urinary phosphate increased as a result of the secondary hyperparathyroidism. The plasma level of alkaline phosphatase is usually elevated. The plasma concentration of 1,25-dihydroxyvitamin D_3 is low in the type I syndrome and normal or elevated in type II vitamin D–dependent rickets. The radiographic abnormalities are similar to those seen in vitamin D–deficiency rickets.

Differential Diagnosis

Nutritional vitamin D rickets is characterized by extremely low levels of circulating 25-OH-D_3 and can be readily distinguished from the pseudodeficiency syndromes by the therapeutic response to lower levels of vitamin D therapy. The presence of alopecia totalis can be helpful in diagnosing the type II syndrome. Moreover, patients with alopecia are often the most resistant to treatment with vitamin D.

Treatment

High doses of vitamin D (ergocalciferol) are required to correct the metabolic abnormalities. The usual doses for therapy of this disorder range from 20,000 to 100,000 U of vitamin D daily. Normalization of serum calcium can be achieved by physiologic doses of an analogue of $1,25(OH)_2D_3$ (Rocaltrol), thereby suggesting a defect in the 1α-hydroxylase system as the potential pathogenic mechanism for this syndrome.[31] Therapy with these potent compounds should be carefully monitored in order to prevent hypercalcemia. Frequent (weekly) serum and urine calcium determinations may be necessary in the initial phase of therapy. If surgical correction of the skeletal deformities is necessary and prolonged immobilization is anticipated, appropriate reductions in the vitamin D dosage are required to prevent hypercalcemia and hypercalciuria. Normalization of the biochemical parameters can be expected in 1 to 6 months. The maintenance dosage of Rocaltrol may vary from 0.25 to 2.0 μg daily.

Familial Hypophosphatemic Rickets (Vitamin D–Resistant Rickets)

This familial disease is transmitted via an abnormal gene on the X chromosome. Accordingly, an affected male will transmit this disease to all of his daughters but to none of his sons, and half the children of an affected female will be normal.

Pathogenesis

This most characteristic abnormality present in all the affected individuals is hypophosphatemia and decreased renal tubular reabsorption of phosphate. There may be an associated abnormality in the intestinal absorption of phosphate. Physiologically, low phosphate should stimulate the synthesis of $1,25(OH)_2D_3$, which is inappropriate

for the circulating level of phosphate.[30] Hereditary hypophosphatemic rickets has recently been reported in one kindred with normal serum calcium, marked hypercaliuria, and elevated levels of 1,25-dihydroxyvitamin D_3.[32]

Clinical Features

Short stature in childhood and osteomalacia in adulthood are the commonest manifestations of this disorder. Tetany and myotonia are typically absent. If there is a family history of this disease, recognition of the characteristic features in childhood is not difficult. Within the families, female members have a lower incidence of the bone disease. Calcification of joint capsules, ligaments, and tendons without inflammatory or degenerative disease has been reported.[33]

Laboratory Findings

In the typical syndrome, hypophosphatemia may be the only manifestation in some family members; these individuals may be entirely asymptomatic. Serum calcium is usually normal. The alkaline phosphatase may be elevated. Urinary phosphate excretion is high, whereas calcium excretion is low in untreated individuals. The serum PTH may be slightly elevated.

Radiographically, the features of familial hypophosphatemic rickets may be indistinguishable from those of vitamin D deficiency. There may be bowing of the lower extremities and occasionally genu varum or genu valgum. Calcium deposits in the hand and sacroiliac joints were observed in 50 to 60 percent of the patients in one kindred. Histomorphometry of bone in hypophosphatemic rickets indicates a marked decrease in the calcification rate and a reduction in the bone formation rate.[34]

Differential Diagnosis

Absence of tetany or seizures and normal muscle strength and tone are features of hypophosphatemic rickets, which are uniquely different from symptoms of vitamin D–deficient or –dependent rickets. Hypophosphatemia with only minimal elevation of PTH can also serve to distinguish this disease from the marked secondary hyperparathyroidism seen in vitamin D–deficient rickets.

Treatment

Large doses of vitamin D usually result in incomplete healing of bone, with little or no effect on the hypophosphatemia. Satisfactory treatment of this disease requires the addition of phosphate to correct the specific biochemical abnormality of low serum phosphate. The usual dose for phosphate replacement is 1 to 4 g of neutral phosphate daily, in divided doses, given orally. It should be recalled that phosphate therapy alone—i.e., without vitamin D—can initiate bone mineralization. The process of remineralization, however, may be patchy or incomplete with phosphate alone. Therefore, a combination of phosphate with vitamin D, such as 1,25-dihydroxyvitamin

D_3, is most beneficial and can prevent some of the complications encountered with high-dose phosphate therapy.[35,36] These include the development of secondary hyperparathyroidism, since increasing serum phosphate is a stimulus for the release of PTH. Once the doses of vitamin D and oral phosphate have been finely titrated, accelerated growth can be achieved in children, with remission of the rachitic changes in bone (radiographic and histologic). Genu valgum deformity may be corrected surgically.[37] If a new proband has been identified, skeletal and biochemical abnormalities should be sought in other members of the family. Genetic counseling may be necessary.

Hypophosphatasia

Hypophosphatasia is probably an autosomal recessive disorder, which may present in its more severe form as childhood rickets and is less severe in adults.

Pathogenesis

Alkaline phosphatase is required for bone mineralization, in addition to the vitamin D, calcium, and phosphate. The enzyme alkaline phosphatase is present in vesicles in the matrix; it hydrolyzes pyrophosphate to yield inorganic phosphate. This step is believed to be necessary to initiate apatite formation in the matrix. Hypophosphatasia is characterized by a low alkaline phosphatase, the lack of which gives rise to the typical features of rickets.[38]

Clinical Features

In infancy, the disease is invariably severe and may present with rickets and hypercalcemia. A less severe variety of this disorder in childhood and in adults is characterized by premature loss of deciduous teeth and a tendency to bone fracture.

Laboratory Findings

A low serum alkaline phosphatase is the hallmark of this disease. Substrates from the enzyme, such as phosphorylethanolamine, are typically excreted in increased quantities in the urine. Serum calcium and urinary calcium may be elevated in the severe form of the disease. Radiographically, the epiphyses appear irregular and notched. Other features of rickets may be common.

Differential Diagnosis

The laboratory finding of a low alkaline phosphatase in the presence of rickets is an important consideration for differentiating this disease from the other types of rickets discussed above. Hypercalcemia or hypercalciuria are unusual in untreated rickets.

Treatment

There is no satisfactory treatment for this disorder, although phosphate therapy has been tried with some success. Surgical correction of pathologic fractures may be difficult to achieve.[39]

Hyperphosphatasia

In this uncommon disease (also called *juvenile Paget's disease*), there is elevation of alkaline phosphatase and also acid phosphatase of bone origin. The disease is autosomal recessive in hereditary transmission and resembles Paget's disease in children.

Osteomalacia

Clinically and histologically, osteomalacia may be considered an adult counterpart of rickets. Many of the hereditary or familial disorders discussed under the heading of rickets are equally applicable in this section and may be considered in the differential diagnosis of osteomalacia.

The primary underlying defect seen in osteomalacia in adults is a disproportionately large amount of unmineralized osteoid associated with a failure of mineralization. This can be quantified using the technique of histomorphometry.

Etiology

A low 25-hydroxyvitamin D_3 level causing osteomalacia is commonly seen in patients with malabsorption or with hepatic or pancreatic disease. Impaired fat absorption, as occurs in steatorrhea, reduces calcium and vitamin D absorption. Gastric bypass surgery also has this effect. Celiac disease will occasionally induce osteomalacia. Phosphate-binding antacids (aluminum hydroxide), if used in excess, may also induce osteomalacia. Levels of PTH will typically be increased in an attempt to maintain the serum calcium in the normal range. Anticonvulsant drugs (e.g., phenobarbital, phenytoin) may induce the hepatic microsomal dihydroxylase enzyme systems, which enhance 25-hydroxyvitamin D_3 degradation. The clinical and biochemical profile will be identical to that of hepatic disease.

Renal tubular acidosis (which may have multiple causes) should be suspected if there is hypophosphatemia and phosphaturia accompanied by glycosuria, aminoaciduria, or bicarbonate excretion. In patients with chronic renal failure, there is hyperphosphatemia along with low or undetectable levels of 1,25-dihydroxyvitamin D_3. Aluminum toxicity may present as osteomalacia in patients with chronic renal failure undergoing hemodialysis. Bone morphometry in these patients suggests that the aluminum may inhibit mineralization directly.[40]

Tumor-induced osteomalacia should be considered if rickets or hypophosphatemia is not responsive to treatment, since surgical correction of benign tumor may reverse the osteomalacia.[41]

Diagnosis

Laboratory Studies Serum calcium may be low or normal, whereas the phosphate is usually low. Serum alkaline phosphate is generally elevated in all types of osteomalacia. Indices of renal and hepatic function are necessary.

Bone Biopsy Histologically, osteomalacia is characterized by an increased width of unmineralized bone as well as blurred or discontinuous mineralization.

An increase in the osteoid width is demonstrated using double tetracycline labeling, but it may also be seen in other diseases associated with an accelerated synthesis of matrix, such as Paget's disease and thyrotoxicosis. The rate of mineralization, however, is normal in these disorders.[42] Thyrotoxicosis is readily recognized by its specific symptoms and is confirmed if the results of thyroid function tests are elevated. Serum PTH in both these conditions is low or normal unless primary hyperparathyroidism coexists.

Radiologic Diagnosis Radiology in osteomalacia may be normal, but Looser's zones, also known as *pseudofractures,* may be seen and confirmed by bone scan. These radiolucencies occur as bands at right angles to the cortex. They occur at points of stress on the cortex of long bones, are often symmetrical, and tend to occur on concave surfaces of long bones as well as on flat bones. They may become complete fractures and are also seen in Paget's disease and osteogenesis imperfecta.[43]

Treatment Initially the primary cause of the osteomalacia must be treated. Anticonvulsant osteomalacia can be treated with vitamin D in doses sufficient to overcome the biochemical abnormalities. Patients with chronic renal failure usually respond to treatment with 1,25-dihydroxyvitamin D_3 or other synthetic analogues of vitamin D. Hypophosphatemic syndromes may require supplemental phosphate in addition to the vitamin D.

In treating osteomalacia, serum calcium and phosphate should be monitored frequently, particularly if the more potent forms of vitamin D are used. During treatment, serum calcium may decrease at first due to rapid remineralization of bone. Supplemental calcium should be provided.

Vitamin C–Deficiency (Scurvy)

Ascorbic acid, which is a low-molecular-weight water-soluble vitamin, is an essential nutrient, since it cannot be synthesized by humans. Ascorbic acid is required for normal repair and growth of collagen as well as for the absorption of iron. It is derived from rapidly growing fresh fruits and vegetables. The recommended allowance of this vitamin is about 60 mg daily—an amount readily available in the average American diet. When ascorbic acid is consumed in large quantities, the percent of ascorbic acid absorbed is reduced. Moreover, excretion of ascorbic acid is enhanced above a certain renal threshold. If an individual is fed a diet deficient in vitamin C, symptoms or signs of scurvy may not appear for at least 2 months.[44]

Clinical Features

Deficiency of vitamin C may manifest itself as generalized fatigue, bleeding gums, perifollicular hemorrhage, or ecchymoses. There may be pain in the joints and occasional joint effusions. Bone pain and deformities at the costochondral junction may mimic rickets.

Diagnosis

Iron deficiency anemia may occur, but this is a nonspecific finding. Serum ascorbic acid determinations may not be helpful, since depletion of vitamin C may take 2 or 3 months. Radiographically, the cortices may be thin and the trabeculae poorly defined. As the disease progresses, spurs and zones of rarefaction may develop. Metaphyseal clefts are characteristic of scurvy. There may be generalized subperiosteal hemorrhage.

The typical clinical presentation, normal serum calcium, and PTH will readily distinguish scurvy from vitamin D deficiency.

Treatment

Initially, vitamin C should be given in doses of 100 mg three times daily. This is usually sufficient to replenish tissue stores within a week, with marked improvement of symptoms. Massive doses of vitamin C are unnecessary.

Pituitary, Thyroid, and Steroid Hormone Dysfunction: Their Effect on Bone

Pituitary, thyroid, and gonadal hormones are required for somatic growth at the time of puberty. The effect of each of these hormones is varied; however, under physiologic conditions, they are required for accelerating the linear growth spurt. Overproduction of any of these hormones will disrupt normal growth and produce abnormalities specific to each hormone.

Pathophysiology

Growth hormone exerts its effect on somatic growth indirectly by increasing synthesis of insulinlike growth factors (IGF-1), or somatomedins. Chromophobe or eosinophilic adenoma of the pituitary, which produces excessive growth hormone, present in a child as gigantism and in an adult as acromegaly. Thyroid hormone enhances bone resorption, and thyroid hormone production—e.g., in Graves' disease—leads to demineralization of bone rather than alterations in height. Glucocorticoids directly inhibit bone growth and affect collagen synthesis.[45]

Clinical Features

Headache, changes in visual field (hemianopsia), and excessive somatic growth are symptoms and signs of growth hormone excess. If the disorder develops before puberty, tall stature is the rule. There is laxity of ligaments and joints. Arthritis, enlargement of the hands and feet, and carpal tunnel syndrome also occur in acromegaly. Encroachment of the tumor onto the normal pituitary gland may cause hypofunction of other pituitary hormones.

A history of weight loss, tremors, nervousness, and heat intolerance is highly suggestive of thyroid hyperfunction. The gland is usually palpable and enlarged in Graves' disease, whereas symptoms of thyroid hormone excess and no glandular enlargement are compatible with factitious thyrotoxicosis. There may be proximal muscle weakness on physical examination. Bone pain, fracture, and osteoporosis occur in hyperthyroidism, with significant bone loss in the axial and appendicular skeleton.[46] There may be intracortical striations in the phalangeal hands and feet.

Glucocorticoid excess—e.g., Cushing's syndrome—is highlighted by truncal obesity, "moon facies," supraclavicular fat pad, hypertension, and occasionally glucose intolerance or overt diabetes mellitus. Short stature is a hallmark of excess glucocorticoid production in childhood. Glucocorticoid excess may also present as osteoporosis, and diminished bone density may be seen with photon absorptiometry.

Diagnosis

Growth hormone and somatomedin C levels are elevated in acromegaly and gigantism. Serum phosphate is usually elevated, whereas the serum calcium and PTH are normal unless hyperparathyroidism is associated, as in multiple endocrine neoplasia. Thyroid function tests are diagnostic in thyrotoxicosis of any cause, and 24-h urine collection for cortisol is the best test to diagnose Cushing's syndrome. Dexamethasone suppression tests may be necessary to further define the exact cause of the excess cortisol production (adrenal versus pituitary tumor).

Radiography of the hands may reveal cortical thickening or tufting of the distal phalanges in acromegaly. On skull x-ray films, the sinuses may be enlarged, and there may be a thickened mandible, with its characteristic underbite. Computed tomography of the sella turcica should be done in patients suspected of having growth hormone excess. Cushing's syndrome and thyrotoxicosis may present as osteoporosis or demineralization of bone. The characteristic features of the various hormonal excess syndromes should not pose any difficulty in the diagnosis of specific disorders.

Treatment

Growth hormone excess can be treated by transsphenoidal hypophysectomy or the drug bromocriptine (Parlodel). Thyrotoxicosis can be managed by the use of antithyroid drugs or ablation with radioactive iodine. Adrenal or pituitary adenomas as a cause of Cushing's syndrome should be treated surgically. Patients receiving prednisone in high doses may not improve bone mass even with supplements of calcium and vitamin D.

Endocrine Hypofunction

Hypofunction of growth hormone or thyroid hormone usually manifests itself as short stature in a child.[47] In an adult, disorder or hypofunction of endocrine glands may appear insidiously over a number of years. The presentation is usually less dramatic and therefore more often missed.

Pathogenesis

Surgical ablation of endocrine glands to treat hormonal excess may lead to an endocrine hypofunction syndrome. Pituitary gonadal deposits of excess iron may occur in patients receiving chronic blood transfusion and may impair the release of any of the pituitary or gonadal hormones. Eating disorders, such as anorexia nervosa, produce changes in the hypothalamic-pituitary axis and present as hypofunction of gonadal hormones.

Clinical Features

Symptoms of hypofunction of any hormone may occur insidiously, depending upon the severity of the inciting events. In disorders such as thalassemia, which require repeated blood transfusions, symptoms of iron overload may occur before those of hormonal inadequacy. Patients with hemochromatosis may exhibit diabetes mellitus, a bronze discoloration of the skin, and hepatic or cardiac abnormalities. Pain and stiffness of the metacarpophalangeal (MCP) joints are not uncommon.[48]

There may be no musculoskeletal manifestation in early anorexia nervosa. Chronic deficiency of estrogen, due to the impaired pituitary gonadal axis, eventually leads to osteopenia. Fatigue is a common symptom of many of these disorders, and hypofunctioning thyroid or adrenal function should be suspected. There may be no history of weight loss or salt craving in primary hypopituitary disease. Amenorrhea and diminished bone mass may be seen in athletes.[49]

Diagnosis

In general, hypofunction of endocrine glands is not easily diagnosed by single measurements of the hormones believed to be deficient. Repeat testing or dynamic testing is often necessary (see "Differential Diagnosis," below). A complete blood count, hepatic function tests, serum iron, and ferritin assays are also required to distinguish the disorders of iron overload.

A low-normal thyroid test may be due to primary thyroid or primary pituitary hypofunction. A TRH [hypothalamic thyroid-stimulating hormone (TSH)–releasing hormone] test may be required to establish the diagnosis of hypopituitary disease. In primary hypothyroidism, the TSH level is markedly elevated. Low levels of luteinizing hormone (LH) and follicle-stimulating hormone (FSH) may be seen in hypopituitary disease or anorexia nervosa. The history and physical findings are usually sufficient to distinguish the two disorders. Growth hormone is typically elevated in anorexia nervosa, whereas it may be deficient in hypofunction of the pituitary.

The radiographic features of hemochromatosis are characteristic. The initial swelling of the MCP joints should not be confused with rheumatoid arthritis, since the characteristic ulnar deviation is not present. Chondrocalcinosis is a characteristic finding on x-ray examination in hemochromatosis. There is irregularity of the articular surfaces and loss of joint space with sclerosis, typically affecting the second and third MCP joints. Osteopenia may be the only manifestation of disorders of the hypothalamic-pituitary axis.

Treatment

Treatment must be directed to the primary cause of endocrine hypofunction.

Osteoporosis

Osteoporosis is characterized by diminution in bone mass. There is a tendency for the bone to fracture. An estimated 15 to 20 million persons in the United States may be afflicted with osteoporosis, accounting in 1993 for over 275,000 hip fractures annually, at an estimated cost of more than $8 billion.[50] Osteoporotic fractures commonly occur at sites of a large volume of trabecular bone, such as the proximal femur, the distal radius, and the vertebral body.

Classification

Osteoporosis may be either primary or secondary.

Primary osteoporosis has additionally been subclassified into types I and II, but there is overlap between them.[51–53] Type I is characterized by excessive loss of cancellous bone and relative sparing of cortical bone. It occurs six times more commonly in women than men, within 15 to 20 years following the menopause, and is believed to be associated with estrogen deficiency in women and testosterone deficiency in men.

Type II osteoporosis affects elderly individuals beyond the seventh or eighth decade and is probably associated with an aggregate deficit of bone remodeling occurring over many years (*low-turnover osteoporosis*). There may be a long history of calcium dietary deficiency. Another possibility is an age-related decline in renal production of 1,25-dihydroxyvitamin $D_3[1,25(OH)_2D_3]$, with subsequent secondary hyperparathyroidism. In type II osteoporosis, there is a simultaneous loss of both cortical and cancellous bone, and it is the hyperparathyroidism that is largely responsible for the cortical bone loss. Hip fractures (mainly femoral neck) are the common fractures seen in this group.[53] By contrast, in type I osteoporosis, there is excessive loss of cancellous bone with relative sparing of cortical bone. This produces an environment suitable for the occurrence of distal radius or vertebral body compression fractures, which typically occur in type I disease. If these patients get hip fractures, they tend to be mainly intertrochanteric.[53] As well as having a different age distribution, type II osteoporosis has less of an imbalance between the sexes than type I disease. Nevertheless,

women are twice as likely as men to suffer from the condition.[51]

The excessive bone loss that occurs in osteoporosis results from abnormalities in bone remodeling. As old bone is resorbed and replaced by newly deposited bone, there is a marginal deficit in bone formation and a net loss of bone in these patients. Because osteoblast recruitment becomes more inefficient with normal aging, the deficit between new bone formation and bone resorption increases progressively with each remodeling cycle, and the accumulated bone loss increases even when skeletal remodeling rates are diminished. This, again, is low-turnover osteoporosis, as is seen in type II primary osteoporosis.

By contrast, any conditions that increase the rate of bone remodeling or increase the amount of bone being remodeled will increase the rate of bone loss. This is thought to be the mechanism in so-called secondary osteoporosis. It is sometimes termed *high-turnover osteoporosis.*

A number of hormonal diseases—such as hyperparathyroidism, hyperthyroidism, diabetes, and hypercortisolism—have been associated with the development of secondary osteoporosis (Table 3-4). Infiltrative disorders—such as thalassemia, multiple myeloma, and leukemia—may also produce localized areas of osteoporosis as they expand the marrow cavity at the expense of the trabecular bone.[55] Localized osteoporosis at the site of metastic bone disease may be associated with the production of osteoclast-activating factors in neoplasia.

Risk Factors

The multifactorial nature of osteoporosis has led to the risk-factor approach (Table 3-5). Men have a greater bone mass than women at maturity, and blacks have a greater bone mass than whites. Clinical osteoporosis, which is rare in black women, is common in fair-complexioned whites with blonde or reddish hair, freckles, and a northwest European background. Other risk factors are an early menopause, chronic smoking, and use of alcohol.[2,51,53–55]

Clinical Presentation

The presence of kyphosis, giving rise to the typical dowager's hump, may be the only finding on physical examination. This deformity may occur rapidly or following surgically induced menopause without estrogen replacement. The commonest presentation, however, is a vertebral body compression fracture or hip fracture. Although kyphoscoliosis and blue sclera in the child or young adult suggest osteogenesis imperfecta, the tarda II variety of this condition may present undiagnosed in an adult with no deformity of the lower extremities and with normal height and appearance. This disease, characterized by abnormal collagen production, may be diagnosed by bone biopsy.

Laboratory Findings

Initial laboratory tests should include serum and urine calcium, serum protein, inorganic phosphorus, alkaline phosphatase, and a complete blood count. Renal function tests, 24-h urinary calcium, creatinine, and hydroxyproline will

TABLE 3-4   Factors Commonly Associated with Osteopenic and/or Osteoporotic Syndrome(s)

Genetic
  White or Asiatic ethnicity
  Positive family history
  Small body frame (<127 lb)
Lifestyle
  Smoking
  Inactivity
  Nulliparity
  Excessive exercise (producing amenorrhea)
  Early natural menopause
  Late menarche
Nutritional factors
  Milk intolerance
  Lifelong low dietary calcium intake
  Vegetarian dieting
  Excessive alcohol intake
  Consistently high protein intake
Medical disorders
  Anorexia nervosa
  Thyrotoxicosis
  Parathyroid overactivity
  Cushing's syndrome
  Type I diabetes
  Alterations in gastrointestinal and hepatobiliary function
  Occult osteogenesis imperfecta
  Mastocytosis
  Rheumatoid arthritis
  "Transient" osteoporosis
  Prolonged parenteral nutrition
  Prolactinoma
  Hemolytic anemia
Drugs
  Thyroid replacement therapy
  Glucocorticoid drugs
  Anticoagulants
  Chronic lithium therapy
  Chemotherapy (breast cancer or lymphoma)
  Gonadotropin-releasing hormone agonist or antagonist
    therapy
  Anticonvulsants
  Chronic phosphate binding antacid use
  Extended tetracycline use[a]
  Diuretics producing calciuria[a]
  Phenothiazine derivatives[a]
  Cyclosporin A[a]

[a]Not yet associated with decreased bone mass in humans, although identified as either toxic to bone in animals or as inducing calciuria and/or calcium malabsorption in humans.
Source: Reproduced with permission from Kleerekoper M, Avioli LV: Evaluation and treatment of postmenopausal osteoporosis, in Favus MJ (ed): *Primer on the Metabolic Diseases and Disorders of Mineral Metabolism.* New York, Raven Press, 1993, pp 223–229.

TABLE 3-5   Osteoporosis Risk Factors

Genetic and biological
  Family history
  Fair skin and hair
  Northern European background
  Scoliosis
  Osteogenesis imperfecta
  Early menopause
  Slender body build

Behavioral and environmental
  Excessive alcohol use
  Cigarette smoking
  Inactivity
  Malnutrition
  Low calcium intake
  Exercise-induced amenorrhea
  High-fiber diet
  High-phosphate diet
  High-protein diet

Source: From Lucas TS, Einhorn TA: Osteoporosis: The role of the orthopedist. © 1993, American Academy of Orthopaedic Surgeons. Reprinted from the *Journal of the American Academy of Orthopaedic Surgeons* 1:49–50, 1993, with permission.

min D_3, the level of $1,25(OH)_2D_3$, as well as PTH and thyroid levels are recommended in all cases where there is appropriate clinical suspicion.

Evaluation of Vertebral Fracture

Investigation of a vertebral crush fracture should take into account whether there was a significant injury. In osteoporosis, spontaneous collapse will often follow no trauma or the mildest stress to the dorsal spine. A convenient algorithm has been developed by Lane.[51] A modified version of this is shown in Fig. 3-6. Nuclear bone scans may be helpful in differentiating crush fractures due to osteoporosis from the multiple foci of metastatic disease. Tumor exclusion may require imaging studies such as computed tomography (CT) and MRI. The typical anteriorly wedged vertebral body fracture may be seen together with typical osteopenic changes in other vertebrae. It should be recalled that at least 30 percent of the bone mass from the vertebrae must be removed before there is significant radiologic abnormality. In the spine, since the small horizontal trabeculae disappear first, there is a characteristic prominence of the vertically oriented trabeculae, which appear as vertical striation. In addition, the vertebral end plates become more prominent due to the resorption of the trabeculae. There is biconcavity of vertebral bodies due to the intervertebral pressure against the weakened vertebral end plates. Compression fractures occur most frequently at T12, followed by T11 and then L1. Vertebrae above T3 are rarely involved, and neither is the cervical spine. Destruction of the pedicles will indicate other pathologic processes.

give information about mineral and collagen turnover disorders. More recently, cross-linked telopeptides (NTx) have been measured in the urine to determine the bone turnover rate. Studies of plasma cortisol, 25-hydroxyvita-

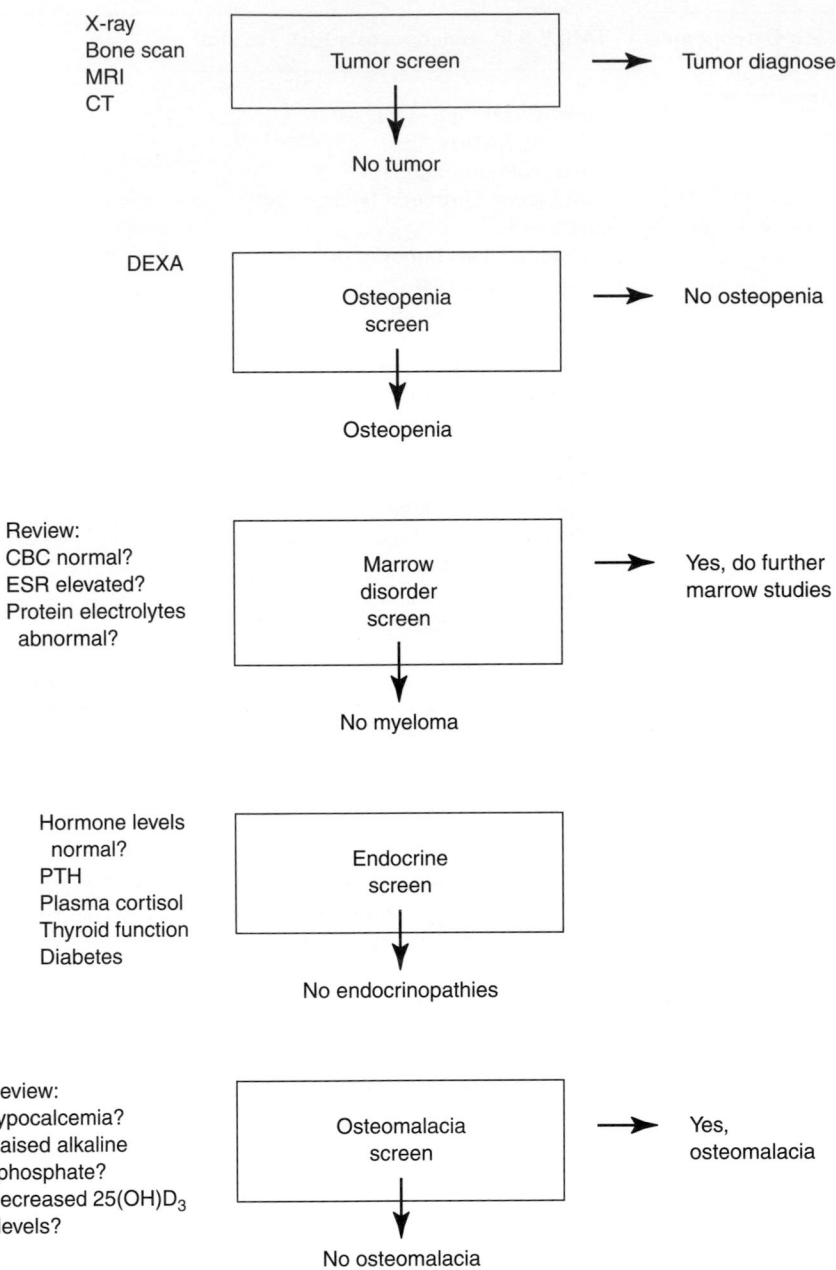

Figure 3-6 Diagnostic algorithm for low-energy vertebral compression fracture. (Modified and reproduced with permission from Lane ML: Osteoporosis: etiology, diagnosis, prevention, and treatment. *Orthopedic Special Edition,* Vol. 2, No. 1. New York, McMahon, 1996, pp 27–29.)

Measurement of Bone Mass

When local malignancy or tumor has been excluded, evaluation of bone density using dual-energy x-ray absorptiometry (DEXA) is the logical next step in the diagnosis and confirmation of the presence of osteopenia. In this technique, the use of two photons of different energies allows measurement of bone where there may be prominent soft tissue cover, as at the hip and spine. Quantitative CT of the vertebrae has also been used to determine bone mass, but it exposes the patient to more radiation.[56] DEXA is by far the most readily available and well-established technique for the determination of bone mass. It is highly reproducible and is accomplished in less than 10 min with most modern scanning devices. The results are based on the bone mineral density (BMD) of the spine or hip for women between the ages of 20 and 40 years. A T score is reported along with a Z score, which permits the comparison of the patient's BMD with that of an age-matched counterpart. The response to treatment for osteoporosis can also be conveniently followed sequentially, with the measurement of BMD at periodic intervals.

Differential Diagnosis

The generalized osteoporosis of hyperthyroidism, primary hyperparathyroidism, and Cushing's syndrome should be detected in the endocrine screen. Cushing's syndrome has characteristic stigmata. A history of weight loss, anorexia, and anemia is suggestive of malignant disease, and diagnosis of multiple myeloma can be established by the finding of Bence Jones protein in the urine, increased plasma cells in the bone marrow, and appropriate plasma protein electrophoretic patterns. Often there is associated hypercalcemia, which responds to a course of steroid therapy. It can be seen that the diagnosis of postmenopausal osteoporosis is primarily made by exclusion (Fig. 3-6).

Treatment

Treatment is directed to the specific etiology. A period of analgesia and bed rest should be prescribed for the patient with compression fracture of the spine, and surgery for the hip fracture, as needed. Bracing should be provided only for minimal periods, since physical activity is recommended as soon as possible to prevent further bone loss.

Drug Treatment

The treatment of osteoporosis with a combination of calcium supplements and sodium fluoride has been shown to increase bone mass and to decrease the fracture rate in postmenopausal osteoporosis.[57] Treatment with fluoride increases trabecular thickness and volume. Sodium fluoride promotes transformation of lining cells to osteoblasts, bypassing the normal remodeling mechanism. Additional osteoid is produced, which has to be mineralized; hence, there is a need for calcium supplements. Adverse reactions reported with the use of fluoride have included gastrointestinal upset and arthritic-type symptoms. Radiographic changes resembling fluorosis have also been reported, including increased bone density and trabeculation and partial obliteration of the medullary cavity.[58] Skeletal scintigraphy has been used to evaluate the skeletal response to fluoride treatment.[59] Lane and coworkers, in their study, found that 66 percent of patients suffered no fractures following the onset of this treatment, and in over 90 percent no more fractures developed in the spine after 18 months of treatment. Hip fracture rates were not influenced during the first 2 years of treatment, but then they seemed to diminish somewhat, although these changes were not statistically significant.[60]

Calicimar (salmon calcitonin) has been used with some success in preventing bone loss in postmenopausal osteoporosis.[61] The drug can be given intramuscularly or subcutaneously, 25 U three times a week. Side effects are minimal and include nausea, flushing, and a mild diuretic effect. These effects may be transient. The drug is now available as a nasal spray (Miacalcin, Sandoz) delivering a metered dose of 200 U per spray daily. Hypocalcemia or tachyphylaxis do not develop with Calcimar therapy. Calcitonin induces osteoclast quiescence, and attempts are now being made to stimulate bone remodeling with other agents such as PTH. These experimental regimens are termed ADFR (activation-depression free release), a protocol during which there is alternate activation and depression of bone cells to promote maximal bone growth.

One of the bisphosphonates (Alendronate) has recently been approved by the FDA. This drug is to be given by mouth 10 mg daily, intermittently. It inhibits bone resorption via activity on the osteoclasts. In a 2-year study, the drug showed an improvement in spinal bone density of approximately 6 to 9 percent. The fracture reduction was less dramatic.[62]

Preventive Therapy

Women at risk for the development of osteoporosis should consider preventive measures. Recommended preventive therapy includes increased physical activity (weight bearing), a calcium intake of 1000 to 1500 mg of elemental calcium daily, and, in some cases, judicious use of estrogens.[63] Estrogen use has been clearly shown to improve bone mineral density in the early postmenopausal years and currently is highly recommended in those subjects who are not at risk for any side effects or complications of estrogen. In a long-term study involving several thousand women, the beneficial effects of estrogen therapy were evident for approximately 5 years without adverse effects.[64] Treatment should commence as soon as possible after the menopause. If the uterus is still in situ, cycling estrogen with progestin probably diminishes the risk of endometrial (but not breast) cancer.[53]

Therapy in Endocrine Disorders

The osteoporosis associated with hormonal diseases, such as thyrotoxicosis, does not improve once the thyroid disease has been treated. Similarly, bone mineral content does not improve in patients on long-term steroid therapy, even when a combination of fluoride, calcium, and vitamin D is used.[65]

REFERENCES

1. Rosenblatt M: Hormonal regulation of calcium metabolism, in Smith LH, Their SO (eds): *Pathophysiology: The Biological Principles of Disease.* Philadelphia, Saunders, 1985.
2. Lingarde F: Potentiometric determination of serum ionized calcium in the normal human population. *Clin Chem Acta* 40:477–484, 1972.
3. Hyun CS, Cragoe JE Jr, Field M: Adrenergic receptor mediated regulation of internal calcium transport. *Am J Physiol* 249:117–123, 1985.
4. Ganong WP: *Review of Medical Physiology,* 11th ed. Los Altos, CA, Lange, 1983.
5. Krane SM, Near RM: Connective tissue, in Smith LH, Thier SO (eds): *Pathophysiology: The Biological Principles of Disease.* Philadelphia, Saunders, 1985.
6. Gennari C, Imbimbo B, Montagnani M, et al: Effects of prednisone and deflazacort on mineral metabolism and parathyroid hormone activity in humans. *Calcif Tissue Int* 36:245–252, 1984.
7. Kohler G, Schen U, Peck WA: Adriamycin inhibits PTH-mediated but not PGE2-mediated stimulation of cyclic AMP formation in isolated bone cells. *Calcif Tissue Int* 36:279–284, 1984.

8. Chambers TJ, Dunne CJ: Prostacyclin inhibits the cytoplasmic activity of isolated osteoclases, in Silbermann M, Slavkin HC (ed): *Current Advances in Skeletogenesis*. Exerpta Medica. Amsterdam, Elsevier, 1982, pp 149–153.

9. Chambers TJ, Dunne CJ: Osteoclast activities determined by intracellular AMP levels, in Silbermann M, Slavkin HC (eds): *Current Advances in Skeletogenesis*. Excerpta Medica. Amsterdam, Elsevier, 1982, pp 154–157.

10. Raisz LG, Kream BE: Regulation of bone formation. *N Engl J Med* 309:29–35, 1983.

11. Vukicevoc S, et al: One alpha dihydroxy vitamin D_3 stimulates alkaline phosphatase activity and inhibits soft tissue proliferation in implants of bone matrix. *Clin Orthop* 196:285–291, 1985.

12. Clayton J, Clayton J, Guilland-Cumming DF, et al: Seasonal trends in vitamin D metabolism, in Silbermann M, Slavkin HC (eds): *Current Advances in Skeletogenesis*. Exerpta Medica. Elsevier, Amsterdam, 1982, pp 224–229.

13. Norman AW, Edelstein S: Overview of vitamin D sessions, in Silbermann M, Slavkin HC (eds): *Current Advances in Skeletogenesis*. Exerpta Medica. Amsterdam, Elsevier, 1982, pp 230–232.

14. Gennari C, Imbimbo B, Montagnani M, et al: Effects of prednisone and deflazacort on mineral metabolism and parathyroid hormone activity in humans. *Calcif Tissue Int* 36:245–252, 1984.

15. Langeland N: The in vitro effect of oestradiol on collagen metabolism in metaphyseal rat bone. *Acta Orthop Scand* 48:226–272, 1977.

16. Erisken EF, Colvard DS, Berg NJ, et al: Evidence of oestrogen receptors in normal human osteoblast-like cells. *Science* 241:84–86, 1988.

17. Vaughan J: *The Physiology of Bone,* 2d ed. Oxford, England, Clarendon Press, 1975.

18. Scholz DA, Purnell DC: Asymptomatic primary hyperparathyroidism: Ten-year prospective study. *Mayo Clin Proc* 56:473–478, 1981.

19. Mallette LE, Bilezikian JP, Heath DA, Aurbach GD: Primary hyperparathyroidism: Clinical and biochemical features. *Medicine* 53:127–146, 1974.

20. Broadus AE, Horst RL, Lang R, et al: The importance of circulating 1,25 dihydroxy vitamin D in the pathogenesis of hypercalcuria and renal stone disease in primary hyperparathyroidism. *N Engl J Med* 302:421, 1980.

21. Sharma OP: Hypercalcemia in sarcoidosis. The puzzle finally solved [editorial]. *Arch Intern Med* 145:626–627, 1985.

22. Gnokos PJ, London R, Hendler ED: Hypercalcemia and elevated 1,25 dihydroxy vitamin D levels in a patient with end-stage renal disease and active tuberculosis. *N Engl J Med* 311:1683–1685, 1984.

23. Stewart AF, Adler M, et al: Calcium homeostasis in immobilization. *N Engl J Med* 306:1136, 1982.

24. Rude RK, Oldham SB, Sharp CF Jr, et al: Parathyroid hormone secretion in magnesium deficiency. *J Clin Endocrinol Metab* 48:800–806, 1978.

25. Breslau NA, Pak CYC: Hypoparathyroidism. *Metabolism* 28:1261–1276, 1979.

26. Farfel Z, Brickman AS, Kasslow HR, et al: Defect of receptor cyclase coupling protein in psueodhypoparathyroidism. *N Engl J Med* 303:237–242, 1980.

27. Klein KL, Maxwell MH: Renal osteodystrophy. *Orthop Clin North Am* 15:687–695, 1984.

28. Toomey F, Hoag R, Batton D, et al: Rickets associated with cholestasis and parenteral nutrition in premature infants. *Radiology* 142:85–86, 1982.

29. Doppelt SH: Vitamin D, rickets and osteomalacia: Symposium on metabolic bone disease. *Orthop Clin North Am* 15:671–686, 1984.

30. Scriver CR, Frazer D, Koch SW: Hereditary rickets, in Heath DA, Marx SJ (eds): *Calcium Disorders*. Boston, Butterworth, 1982, pp 1–46.

31. Liberman UA, Eil C, Marx SJ: Resistance to 1,25 dihydroxy vitamin D: Association with heterogenous defects in skin fibroblasts. *J Clin Invest* 71:192–200, 1982.

32. Tieder M, Modai D, Samuel R, et al: Hereditary hypophosphatemic rickets with hypercalciuria. *N Engl J Med* 312:611–617, 1985.

33. Pollison RP, Martinez S, Khoury M, et al: Calcification of entheses associated with X-linked hypophosphatemic osteomalacia. *N Engl J Med* 313:1–7, 1985.

34. Marie PJ, Glorieux FH: Histomorphometric study of bone remodeling and hypophosphatemic vitamin D–resistant rickets. *Metab Bone Dis Rel Res* 3:31–38, 1981.

35. Chesny RW, Mazess RB, Rose P, et al: Long-term influence of calcitriol (1,25 dihydroxy vitamin D) and supplemental phosphate in X-linked hypophosphatemic rickets. *Pediatrics* 71:559–567, 1983.

36. Rasmussen H, Pechet M, Anast C, et al: Long-term treatment of familial hypophosphatemic rickets with oral phosphate and 1-alpha-hydroxy vitamin D. *J Pediatr* 99:16–25, 1981.

37. Evans GA, Arulanantham K, Gage JR: Primary hypophosphatemic rickets: Effects of oral phosphate and vitamin D on growth and surgical treatment. *J Bone Joint Surg* 62A:1130–1137, 1980.

38. Rasmussen H: Hypophosphatasia, in Stanbury JB, Fredrickson DS, et al (eds): *The Metabolic Basis of Inherited Disease,* 5th ed. New York, McGraw-Hill, 1983, pp 1497–1507.

39. Anderton JM: Orthopedic problems in adult hypophosphatasia: A report of two cases. *J Bone Joint Surg* 61B:82–84, 1979.

40. Dunstan CR, Evans RA, Hills E, et al: Effect of aluminum and parathyroid hormone on osteoblasts and bone mineralization in chronic renal failure. *Calcif Tissue Int* 36:133–138, 1984.

41. Parker MS, Klein I, Haussler MR, et al: Tumor-induced osteomalacia: Evidence of a surgically correctable alteration in vitamin D metabolism. *JAMA* 245:492–493, 1981.

42. Meunier PJ: Bone biopsy in diagnosis of metabolic bone disease, in Cohn DV, Talmage RV, Matthews JL (eds): *Hormonal Control of Calcium Metabolism: Proceedings of the Seventh International Conference on Calcium Regulating Hormones*. Exerpta Medica, 1980.

43. Schneider R: Radiologic methods of evaluating generalized osteopenia. *Orthop Clin North Am* 15:631–651, 1984.

44. Hodges R: Ascorbic acid, in Goodhartt RS, Shilis ME (eds): *Modern Nutrition in Health and Disease,* 6th ed. Philadelphia, Lea & Febiger, 1980, pp 259–273.

45. Thompson JS, Palmieri GMA, Crawford RL: The effect of porcine calcitonin on osteoporosis induced by adrenal cortical steroids. *J Bone Joint Surg* 54A:1490–1496, 1972.

46. Stulberg BN, et al. Hyperparathyroidism, hyperthyroidism and Cushing's disease. *Orthop Clin North Am* 15:697–710, 1984.

47. Rimoin DL, Horton WA: Short stature, Part I. *J Pediatr* 95:523, 1978.

48. Bellamy RE: The orthopedic surgeon and hemochromatosis. *Orthopedics* 3:419–423, 1980.

49. Drinkwater BL, Nilson K, Chestnut CH, et al: Bone mineral content of amenorrheic and eumenorrheic athletes. *N Engl J Med* 311:277–280, 1984.

50. Kleerekoper M, Avioli LV: Evaluation and treatment of postmenopausal osteoporosis, in Favus MJ (ed): *Primer on the Metabolic Bone Diseases and Disorders of Mineral Metabolism.* New York, Raven Press, 1993, pp 223–229.

51. Lane ML: *Osteoporosis: Etiology, Diagnosis, Prevention and Treatment.* Orthopedic Special Edition, Vol. 2, No. 1, pp 27–29. New York, McMahon, 1996, pp 27–29.

52. Riggs BL, Wahner HW, Dunn RB, et al: Differential changes in bone density of the appendicular and axial skeleton with aging. *J Clin Invest* 67:328–335, 1981.

53. Lucas TS, Einhorn TA: Osteoporosis: The role of the orthopedist. *J Am Acad Orthop Surg* 1:49–56, 1993.

54. Lane JM, Vigorita VJ: Osteoporosis: Symposium on Metabolic Bone Disease. *Orthop Clin North Am* 15:711–727, 1984.

55. Lane JM, Vigorita VJ: Current concepts review: Osteoporosis. *J Bone Joint Surg* 65A:274–278, 1983.

56. Genant HK, Cann CE, Ettinger MB, et al: Quantitative computed tomography of vertebral spongiosa: A sensitive method for detecting early bone loss after oophorectomy. *Ann Intern Med* 97:699–7055, 1982.

57. Riggs BL, Seeman E, Hodgson SF, et al: Effect of the fluoride calcium regimen on vertebral fracture occurrence in postmenopausal osteoporosis. *N Engl J Med* 306:446–460, 1982.

58. El-Khoury GY, Moore TE, Albright JP, et al: Sodium fluoride treatment of osteoporosis: Radiologic findings. *AJR* 139:39–43, 1982.

59. Schulz EE, Libanti CR, Farley SM, et al: Skeletal scintigraphic changes in osteoporosis treated with sodium fluoride: Concise communication. *J Nucl Med* 25:651–655, 1984.

60. Lane JM, Healey JH, Schwartz E, et al: Treatment of osteoporosis with sodium fluoride and calcium: Effects on vertebral fracture incidence and bone histomorphometry. *Orthop Clin North Am* 15:729–745, 1984.

61. Aloia JF, Cohn SH, Vaswani AN, et al: Risk factors for postmenopausal osteoporosis. *Am J Med* 78:95–100, 1985.

62. Riggs BL: A new option for treating osteoporosis. *N Engl J Med* 323:124–125, 1990.

63. Aloia JF, Cohn SH, Vaswani AN, et al: Risk factors for postmenopausal osteoporosis. *Am J Med* 78:95–100, 1985.

64. Doran M, Reuther G, Minnie HW, Schneider HPG: Superior compliance and efficacy of continuous combined oral estrogen-progestogen replacement therapy in post-menopausal women. *Am J Obstet Gynec* 173:1446–1451, 1995.

65. Rickers H, Deding A, Christiansen C, et al: Mineral loss in cortical and trabecular bone during high-dose prednisone treatment. *Calcif Tissue Int* 36:269–273, 1984.

CHAPTER 4

Paget's Disease of Bone: Pathophysiology and Medical Management

Frederick S. Kaplan
and Francis H. Gannon

EPIDEMIOLOGY

Paget's disease of bone, or osteitis deformans, was described in 1876 by Sir James Paget.[1] The disorder occurs rarely before age 40, in 3 to 4 percent of the population over 50 years of age,[2] and in as many as 10 to 15 percent of the population by the ninth decade of life. The disease is slightly more common in men.[3]

As many as 25 percent of patients have one or more family members afflicted with the disorder.[4]

Paget's disease is most prevalent in England, western Europe, the United States, Australia, and New Zealand. The disease is uncommon in Scandinavia, the Orient, and India.[5]

PATHOLOGY

The primary cellular abnormality in Paget's disease is a focal increase in osteoclastic bone resorption with a compensatory increase in bone formation (Fig. 4-1). The focal rate of bone remodeling is accelerated, resulting in bone that is highly vascular, structurally weak, and prone to deformities or pathologic fractures.[2,3,5,6]

Pagetic osteoclasts are numerous, large, and active. These bone-resorbing cells contain nuclear and cytoplasmic inclusions of the Paramyxoviridae family of viruses.[7]

Paget's disease may be divided into lytic and sclerotic phases. Intense osteoclastic bone resorption prevails early in the lytic phase. Later, compensatory bone formation is apparent (mixed phase), followed by intense osteoblastic bone formation (sclerotic phase). Pagetic bone exhibits a mosaic pattern with irregularly shaped areas of lamellar bone and an erratic pattern of cement lines. This mosaic pattern is a consequence of dramatically accelerated bone remodeling.[6] Immature woven bone may predominate in active lesions or in regions of poorly mineralized osteoid.

ETIOLOGY

Studies of pagetic osteoclasts have revealed the mRNA and antigens of the paramyxoviruses (particularly measles and respiratory syncytial virus). Infectious virus has not been isolated from long-term cultures of pagetic bone cells. This may not be achieved if the putative virus is highly defective.[5,7]

While current data are by no means conclusive, they suggest that Paget's disease may be caused by hematogenous infection with one of several paramyxoviruses.[7] Following an acute viremia, osteoclasts or their precursors become chronically infected with a virus that mutates rapidly and loses infectivity but is able to stimulate osteoclast proliferation and cytokine production, with dramatic local osseous effects.[8,9] Familial or genetic factors may provoke susceptibility and may influence the clinical expression of disease.[4,6,7,10]

CLINICAL MANIFESTATIONS AND COMPLICATIONS

Any bone may be affected with Paget's disease. The condition is most often asymptomatic and may not require treatment. Clinical features vary depending on the site and severity of lesions. Paget's disease may be detected incidentally on roentgenograms obtained for other purposes or may be suspected following unexpected elevation of serum alkaline phosphatase on a routine blood test.[2,3,5]

Patients with symptomatic Paget's disease often have bone pain unrelated to physical activity. Acute pain may develop as a consequence of pathologic fractures.

Bone enlargement occurs with Paget's disease and may cause spinal stenosis or a cauda equina syndrome. Increased blood flow through the highly vascular pagetic bone may provoke the "steal" syndrome, a condition of high-flow shunting away blood from the neural elements, thus exacerbating the neurologic signs.[11]

Cranial nerves may be impinged as a result of pagetic involvement of the skull. Temporal bone involvement is a common cause of conductive hearing loss in this condition. Extreme thickening and enlargement of the skull may result in platybasia and, in rare instances, impaired flow of cerebrospinal fluid and resultant hydrocephalus.[10]

Pseudofractures and completed pathologic fractures may occur in areas of high stress, particularly in the weight-bearing bones of the lower limbs. Fracture healing may be impaired, resulting in delayed union or nonunion.[2,5,6]

Degenerative arthritis is a common feature of Paget's disease.[12,13] Pagetic bone remodeling results in juxtaarticular bony enlargement, abnormal joint biomechanics, and altered subchondral support. Gout may result from hyperuricemia often due to accelerated nucleic acid turnover.[12,13]

Metabolic complications of Paget's disease are uncommon but include hypercalciuria and hypercalcemia.[2,5] These complications are seen in only the most severely affected and immobilized patients. The association of mild hyperparathyroidism and Paget's disease may be coincidental.[2,5]

Malignant bone tumors[14] are exceedingly rare. Osteosarcomas, chondrosarcomas, fibrosarcomas, or tumors of mixed histology may develop in a preexisting pagetic lesion. Primary giant cell tumors and secondary metastatic carcinoma are also common.

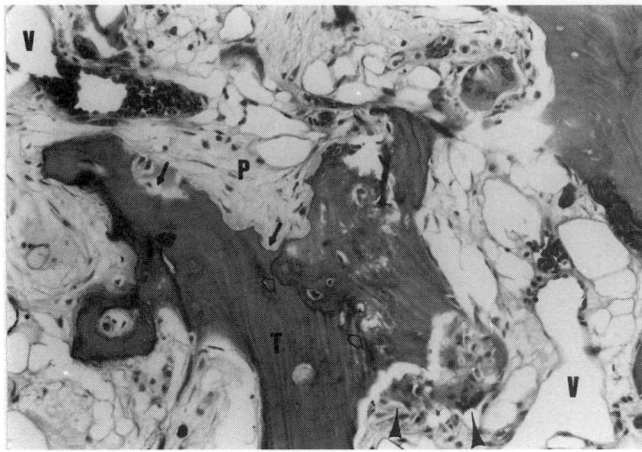

Figure 4-1 Photomicrograph reveals characteristic features of Paget's disease. These include irregularly shaped and remodeled islands of trabecular bone (T), peritrabecular fibrous tissue (P), and multiple blood vessels (V). The remodeling is evidenced by the osteoclasts (*arrowheads*), which have multiple nuclei, and Howship's lacunae (*arrows*), which are scalloped defects in the trabecular surface. The multiple cement lines (*open arrows*) give a mosaic appearance to the bone. (Original magnification, H&E, ×125.)

Paget's sarcoma occurs in less than 1 percent of cases and seldom before 70 years of age.[14] A marked and sustained increase in pain in an area of long-standing Paget's disease suggests this serious complication. Night pain and radiographic evidence of bone destruction may also suggest the diagnosis. Serum alkaline phosphatase activity may be normal or elevated. Rapid worsening of bone pain or deformity indicates the need for radiologic evaluation, followed by bone biopsy if suspicion of a tumor remains. Magnetic resonance imaging and computed tomography are particularly helpful in delineating the presence of bone tumors. Despite recent advances in the therapy of malignant bone tumors, the prognosis for patients who have Paget's disease remains dismal.[14]

DIAGNOSTIC EVALUATION

Radiology

Skeletal involvement can be adequately assessed by a radionuclide bone scan. Complete roentgenographic examination should be obtained of all skeletal sites that demonstrate an increase in radionuclide uptake.[3,5]

The earliest pagetic lesions are osteolytic. In the skull, discrete oval or round areas of osteolysis are termed *osteoporosis circumscripta*. In the limbs, the disease begins as a localized metaphyseal involvement. The osteolytic lesion usually has a V or arrowhead shape at its advancing edge.[3,5] Over time, the bone become chaotic in structure, thickened, and sclerotic. Bone size may increase remarkably (Fig. 4-2).

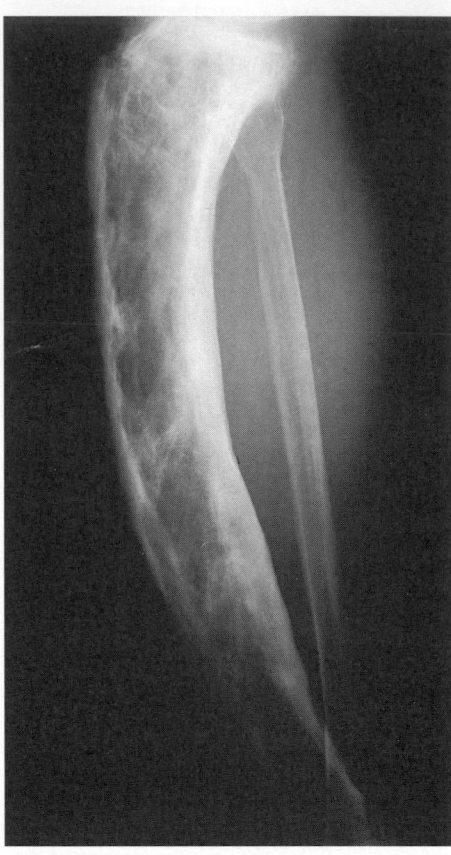

Figure 4-2 Lateral roentgenogram of leg in a 68-year-old woman with monostotic Paget's disease of the tibia. Note the metaphyseal and diaphyseal involvement, with bowing of the tibia, and lack of fibular involvement.

In the lower limbs, bowing, pseudofractures, and complete transverse pathologic fractures are common. These transverse or "chalk-stick" pathologic fractures can also be seen in osteomalacia or fibrous dysplasia (Fig. 4-3). Asymmetrical metaphyseal involvement may lead to joint incongruity and subsequent arthritis.[2,3,5]

With symptomatic pagetic involvement of the spine, MRI and computed tomography have been useful in defining the extent of degenerative arthritis, spinal stenosis, or nerve root impingement.[11] Enlargement of a vertebral body is a radiographic hallmark of Paget's disease of the spine (Fig. 4-4) and can distinguish an osteosclerotic pagetic vertebra from one affected with lymphoma or metastatic carcinoma.

Biochemistry

Serum alkaline phosphatase is a useful biochemical marker of pagetic activity. Alkaline phosphatase levels correlate roughly with the extent of skeletal involvement as established by radionuclide bone scans. Serial alkaline phosphatase determinations provide a simple and inexpensive biochemical index of disease activity.

Urinary excretion of pyridinoline cross links is a biochemical index of bone matrix collagen resorption and is

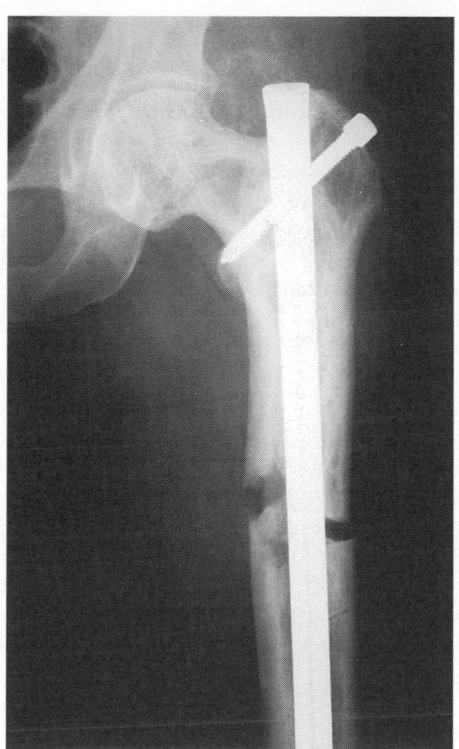

Figure 4 3 Anteroposterior view of the proximal femur in a 67-year-old woman with Paget's disease of the femur following an intramedullary rodding of a pathologic "chalk-stick" fracture of the femoral shaft.

measured over 24 h. Like serum alkaline phosphatase activity, urinary excretion of pyridinoline cross links correlates well with the extent of pagetic involvement.[15] This test is expensive and is usually not considered to be a routine test in the assessment or follow-up of a patient with Paget's disease.[2,3,5]

Due to tight metabolic coupling between bone resorption and bone formation, calcium levels in serum and urine are usually normal except when there is concurrent immobilization, hyperthyroidism, hyperparathyroidism, or malignancy.[2,3,5]

MANAGEMENT

Evaluation of symptoms, physical findings, roentgenograms, and alkaline phosphatase levels will allow the clinician to determine whether treatment of Paget's disease is indicated. Not everyone who has Paget's disease requires treatment. In evaluating a symptomatic patient, it is critical to determine whether the complaints are, in fact, due to Paget's disease. The symptoms that cause the patient to seek care are often due to an associated disorder.

Aspirin and other nonsteroidal anti-inflammatory medications play an important role in treating the symptomatic arthritis of Paget's disease. Patients with end-stage Paget's disease commonly have low alkaline phosphatase

levels, limited disease activity, but moderate joint degeneration that can be controlled symptomatically with nonsteroidal anti-inflammatory agents. The analgesic effects of these medications are important and are commonly overlooked in practice. A cane may be helpful for patients with Paget's disease of the lower limbs. The increased stability, prevention of falls, and load-sharing ability provided by a cane make good sense and should be standard treatment in the elderly.

The most important indications for treatment of Paget's disease are bone pain, neurologic involvement, congestive heart failure, or preparation for orthopaedic surgery.[5,16]

A thorough explanation of the disease should be offered to the patient prior to considering the use of specific therapy for Paget's disease. Relief of pain and restoration of function should be emphasized in all discussions. Long-term follow-up should be stressed. All patients should be reexamined annually and a repeat alkaline phosphatase level determined. Roentgenograms may be performed periodically, as dictated by symptoms, but repeat bone scans are generally not necessary. The patient's home environ-

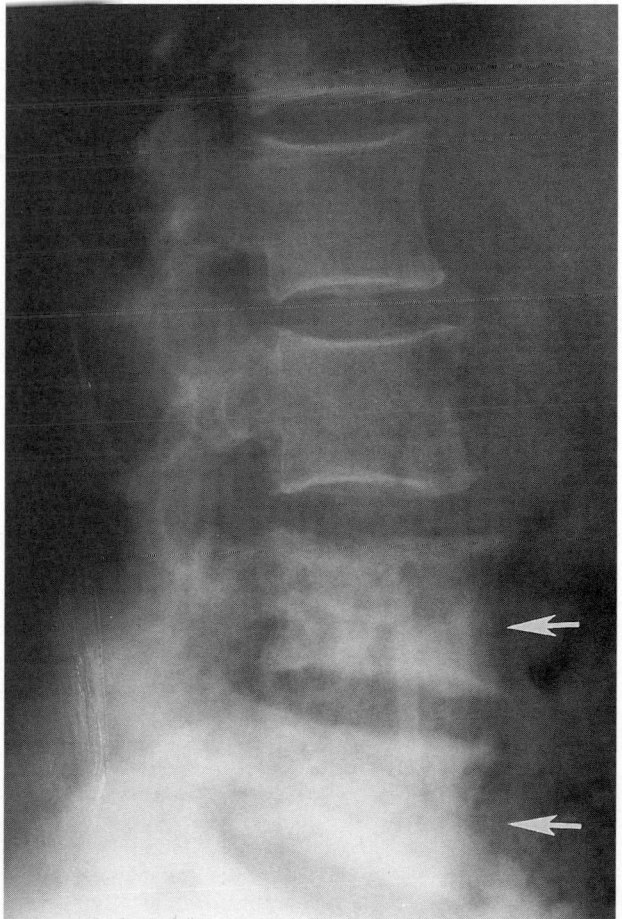

Figure 4-4 Lateral roentgenogram of lumbar spine in a 73-year-old man with severe pagetic spinal stenosis. Note pagetic involvement with enlargement of lower lumbar vertebrae (*arrows*).

ment should be discussed, with the goal of offering advice on the prevention of accidents that could lead to pathologic fractures. Patients who have maxillary or mandibular involvement should be referred for dental evaluation, and those who have auditory deficits should be referred for medical treatment and hearing aids.[10] Finally, The Paget Foundation may be helpful in providing patient information on the disease. (Their address is The Paget Foundation, 200 Varick Street, New York, NY 10014.)

DRUG THERAPY

Calcitonin and bisphosphonates are the two major therapeutic agents used in the treatment of symptomatic Paget's disease.[2,16] The treatment schedules and special characteristics of each agent are indicated in Table 4-1. The observed benefits of therapy include relief of bone pain, a reduction of increased cardiac output, reversal of certain neurologic deficits, stabilization of hearing loss, healing of osteolytic lesions, and reduction in bone bleeding during orthopaedic surgery.

Calcitonin is a remarkably safe and effective agent for the treatment of Paget's disease and is self-administered subcutaneously with daily injections. Minor side effects occur in 20 percent of patients treated with either salmon or human calcitonin; these include nausea, facial flushing, and polyuria. Resistance to salmon calcitonin therapy develops in more than 20 percent of patients after a successful initial treatment period.[16]

Bisphosphonates are another class of drugs useful in the treatment of Paget's disease. These long-acting pyrophosphate analogues, potent inhibitors of bone resorption, bind and stabilize hydroxyapatite crystals in bone.[16]

Disodium etidronate, a bisphosphonate, is administered orally. After absorption, the drug localizes to bone or is excreted unchanged in the urine. The recommended dose of disodium etidronate (5 mg/kg of body weight daily for 6 months) produces suppression of disease activity and symptoms in a time course similar to that of calcitonin. The medication is taken daily on an empty stomach at least 2 h away from meals, as absorption with food is poor. Disodium etidronate should not be used in the treatment of patients who have osteolytic pagetic lesions of weight-bearing bones. Side effects with disodium etidronate appear to be less common than with calcitonin; loose bowel movements and nausea occur but are infrequent. High doses or long-term uninterrupted use can also lead to a mineralization defect and predispose to pathologic fractures.[2,3,16] After a 6-month course of treatment, biochemical and symptomatic remissions may persist for months or years.

Second-generation bisphosphonates are more potent than etidronate and do not impair mineralization. The most widely evaluated of these is pamidronate,[17] which has been approved by the U.S. Food and Drug Administration for use in the treatment of Paget's disease. Medication is administered intravenously, due to its poor absorption otherwise. The approved treatment regimen is 30 mg by slow (3 1/2 to 4 h) intravenous infusion daily for 3 consecutive days; this is repeated as needed. The drug

Table 4-1 Drug Treatment of Paget's Disease

Drug	Dosage	Special Characteristics
Salmon calcitonin	50–100 IU subcutaneously daily. After symptomatic improvement, dosage may be reduced to 3 times weekly.	Anti–salmon calcitonin antibodies develop in 60%; clinical resistance appears in > 20%.
Human calcitonin	0.5 mg subcutaneously daily. After symptomatic improvement, dosage may be reduced to 3 times weekly.	Effective in salmon calcitonin–resistant patients with high antibody titers.
Disodium etidronate	5 mg/kg of body weight orally for 6 months. May repeat after recurrence of symptoms or biochemical exacerbation, but not sooner than 6 months.	A remission of years may occur after 6 months of therapy. Some patients experience transient increased bone pain. Osteolytic lesions rarely heal. Osteomalacia occurs at high doses
Disodium pamidronate	30–60 mg intravenously, slowly, over 3 1/2 to 4 h. Repeat three times daily. Repeat course as needed. Patients with more severe disease may need 60 mg weekly, monthly, or quarterly for variable periods.	Potent new bisphosphonate; potent antiresorption effects. Transient fever is a common side effect.
Alendronate sodium	40 mg orally daily for 6 months. May repeat after recurrence of symptoms or biochemical exacerbation, but not sooner than 6 months.	Potent new oral bisphosphonate; potent antiresorption effects. Esophageal irritation is a common side effect.

has also been administered in a 60-mg single dose or weekly, monthly, or quarterly, depending on the severity of the disease and the patient's response. A brief postinfusion fever or acute flare of pain may occur. Short courses of treatment with pamidronate can produce long-term remissions of the disease. New-generation oral bisphosphonates will likely become the most commonly used and effective therapy of Paget's disease.[17] Alendronate has recently been approved for oral administration at a dose of 40 mg daily for no longer than 6 months continuous duration. The medication must be taken on an empty stomach with water only, due to its poor gastrointestinal absorption. Esophageal irritation is the most common side effect and has been reported in as many as 15 percent of patients taking the medication.

REFERENCES

1. Paget J: On a form of chronic inflammation of bones (osteitis deformans). *Med-Chir Trans* 60:37–64, 1877.
2. Kaplan FS, Singer FR: Paget's disease, in Morley JE, Korenman SG (eds): *Endocrinology and Metabolism in the Elderly.* Cambridge, MA, Blackwell, 1992, pp 230–240.
3. Merkow RL, Lane JM: Paget's disease of bone. *Orthop Clin North Am* 21:171–189, 1990.
4. Siris ES, Ottman R, Flaster E, Kelsey JL: Familial aggregation of Paget's disease of bone. *J Bone Min Res* 6:495–500, 1991.
5. Kaplan FS, Singer FR: Paget's disease of bone: Pathophysiology and diagnosis. *Instr Course Lect* 42:417–424, 1993.
6. Teitelbaum SL: The pathology of Paget's disease, in Singer FR, Wallach S (eds): *Paget's Disease of Bone: Clinical Assessment, Present & Future Therapy.* New York, Elsevier, 1991, p 313.
7. Mills, BG, Singer FR: Critical evaluation of viral antigen data in Paget's disease in bone. *Clin Orthop Rel Res* 217:16–25, 1987.
8. Hoyland JA, Freemont AJ, Sharpe PT: Interleukin-6, IL-6 receptor, and IL-6 nuclear factor gene expression in Paget's disease. *J Bone Min Res* 9:75–80, 1994.
9. Ralston SH, Hoey SA, Gallacher SJ, et al: Cytokine and growth factor expression in Paget's disease: Analysis by reverse-transcription/polymerase chain reaction: *Br J Rheum* 33:620–625, 1994.
10. Kaplan FS, Haddad JG, Singer FR: Paget's disease: Complications and controversies. *Calcif Tissue Int* 55:75–78, 1994.
11. Hadjipavlou A, Lander P: Paget disease of the spine. *J Bone Joint Surg* 73A:1376–1381, 1991.
12. Krane SM, Kroop SF: Arthritis and Paget's disease of bone, in Singer FR, Wallach S (eds): *Paget's Disease of Bone: Clinical Assessment, Present and Future Therapy.* New York, Elsevier, 1991, pp 191–199.
13. Franck WA, Bress NM, Singer FR, Krane SM: Rheumatic manifestations of Paget's disease of bone. *Am J Med* 56:592–603, 1974.
14. Huvos AG, Butler A, Bretsky SS: Osteogenic sarcoma associated with Paget's disease of bone: A clinicopathologic study of 65 patients. *Cancer* 52:1489–1495, 1983.
15. Delmas PD, Gineyts E, Bertholin A, et al: Immunoassay of pyridinoline crosslink excretion in normal adults and in Paget's disease. *J Bone Min Res* 8:643–648, 1993.
16. Bockman RS, Weinerman SA: Medical treatment for Paget's disease of bone. *Instr Course Lect* 42:425–433, 1993.
17. Siris ES: Perspectives: A practical guide to the use of pamidronate in the treatment of Paget's disease. *J Bone Min Res* 9:303–304, 1994.
18. Meyers MH, Singer FR: Osteotomy for tibia vara in Paget's disease under cover of calcitonin. *J Bone Joint Surg* 60A:810–814, 1978.

CHAPTER 5

Paget's Disease: Surgical Management

Antoni B. Goral

Orthopedic complications related to Paget's disease are common, with upwards of one-third of patients having deformities of the tubular bone, and 20 percent having joint damage associated with their disease.[1] Medical management of active Paget's disease through the use of calcitonin, pamidronate, or other bisphosphonates perioperatively has been described as having varying effect on perioperative hypercalcemia and blood loss at surgery.[2,3] Surgical intervention is indicated in situations of severe skeletal deformity of the long bones or joints, pathologic fracture, malignant transformation, or spinal stenosis.

FRACTURES IN PAGET'S DISEASE

A pathologic fracture through pagetoid bone may be the initial presenting sign of the disease in as many as two-thirds of patients.[4] The most common site for fracture is the femur; this often occurs with relatively minor trauma through an area of typical lateral bowing. Fractures are generally transverse, with disruption of the periosteal tissue and comminution. Hypercalcemia associated with immobilization often requires medical management. Intramedullary fixation in combination with internal or external osteoclasis/osteotomy has a high success rate, achieving union and correction of deformity in select cases.[5,6] Subtrochanteric and intertrochanteric fractures usually go on to union after internal fixation, whether with compression plates/screws or intramedullary rod fixation. Newer-generation "reconstruction"-type intramedullary nails offer the benefits of improved fixation into the proximal femur/neck.[5] On the other hand, although only 7 percent of femoral fractures in Paget's disease involve the femoral neck, nonunion rates after internal fixation may approach 100 percent in some series.[7] Treatment with hemiarthroplasty may also have a poor outcome due to early loss of implant fixation.[8,9]

Fractures of the tibia will commonly show stress fractures on the convex aspect of the typically anteriorly bowed bone (by contrast with Looser's zones, seen on the concave aspect in osteomalacia). Complete fractures are treated by the same principles and techniques as femoral fractures, with the need for internal fixation either intramedullary with metadiaphyseal osteotomy or plating.[10] Avulsion of the tibial tubercle and disruption of the extensor mechanism through pagetoid bone with successful surgical repair have been described.[11] The few reported cases of metacarpal fractures through pagetoid bone have been of traumatic origin and generally achieve union by conservative means.[12]

CORRECTIVE OSTEOTOMY

The surgical correction of long bone deformity may be indicated for limb dysfunction associated with intractable joint (coxa vara), bone pain (femoral and tibial vara), or impending pathologic fracture. Corrective diaphyseal osteotomy may take a longer time to heal, while metaphyseal osteotomy generally achieves union satisfactorily. Plate fixation of the osteotomy offers a lower complication rate as compared with the use of external fixation.[3]

Coxarthropathy is seen in upwards of 10 percent of patients with Paget's disease. Radiographic findings of acetabular protrusio, medial joint or concentric joint space narrowing, and coxa vara deformity suggest both a metaphyseal as well as subchondral bone abnormality.[13] Surgical treatment is most frequently performed as total hip replacement. However, intertrochanteric osteotomy with bone grafting may be the procedure of choice if the joint space is well preserved.[14] Roper reported an improved postoperative range of motion in Paget's disease patients as compared with primary osteoarthritis after osteotomy.[15] Surprisingly, union is achieved in virtually all such patients treated with osteotomy.[16]

TOTAL HIP ARTHROPLASTY

The indications for total hip arthroplasty are similar to those for nonpagetoid degenerative hip disease. Care must be taken to be certain that the pain is in the joint and not related to bony changes remote from the joint surface. Arthroplasty may be indicated in the setting of intracapsular fracture with associated acetabular disease.

The technical difficulties of hip arthroplasty are compounded by coexistent proximal femoral deformity of coxa vara. Medical management to avoid hypercalcemia, acidosis, and excessive bleeding through the use of calcitonin and bisphosphonates is commonly cited.[4,17] Merkow, however, found that in two-thirds of patients undergoing arthroplasty, the disease was already quiescent. Intraoperative bleeding does not seem to be excessive,[4,18,19] whether calcitonin or bisphosphonates are used preoperatively. Heterotopic ossification occurs in as many as 52 percent of patients undergoing hip arthroplasty for Paget's disease, compared to under 5 percent for routine hip arthroplasty.[4,20,21] The concern that the underlying bone disease may predispose to early prosthetic loosening has not been statistically proven in all studies.[17,18,19] MacDonald described in 91 hips a slight statistically significant increase in the revision rate for Paget's patients, although commenting that the overall success rate of 74 percent was good to excellent for cemented total hip replacement in this population.[22] Modular reconstruction with diaphyseal osteotomy utilizing noncemented press-fit components has also been described.[23]

TOTAL KNEE ARTHROPLASTY

Painful malalignment at the knees with degenerative changes not amenable to proximal metaphyseal osteotomy may be an indication for total knee arthroplasty. Although concern exists that in pagetoid bone subchondral hyperemia may lead to subsequent remodeling and loosening of the implants, results with total knee arthroplasty are satisfactory at follow-up of 12 years.[24] Successful use of both cemented and noncemented components has been cited.[13,24]

MALIGNANT DEGENERATION

Malignant degeneration in Paget's disease has been reported in 6½ percent of documented cases.[20,25] The most frequent sites of malignant change include the femur, humerus, pelvis, and tibia, in order of frequency. Vertebral tumors do occur, but rarely. Tumors take the form of osteogenic sarcoma, giant cell sarcoma, and fibrosarcoma as well as reticulum cell sarcoma and a mixed anaplastic type. The occurrence of tumor at a site of previous fracture through pagetoid bone has been reported, but there is no direct correlation.[26] Sarcomatous degeneration is generally seen in patients with the polyostotic form of the disease. Treatment consists of palliative resection or amputation. Surgery may be combined with chemotherapy but is generally not well tolerated in these patients, who are often elderly. Survival beyond 2 years from diagnosis is a rarity.[25,26]

REFERENCES

1. Zollinger H, Goldmann A: Indikation und Möglichkeiten operativer Therapie bei der Osteodystrophia deformans Paget. *Orthopadie* 17:397–403, 1988.
2. Brumsen C, Bloem RM, Papapoulos SE: Paget's disease with osteolytic lesions: combining medical and surgical treatments. *Netherlands J Med* 40:292–298, 1992.
3. Frankle M, Tiegs RD, Sim FH: A review of corrective osteotomies for deformity in Paget's disease. *Semin Arthritis Rheum* 23:253, 1994.
4. Merkow RL, Pellicci PM, Help DP, Salvati E: Total hip replacement for Paget's disease of the hip. *J Bone Joint Surg* 66A:752–757, 1984.
5. Barlow IW, Thomas NP: Reconstruction nailing for subtrochanteric fractures in the pagetic femur. *Injury* 25:426–428, 1994.
6. Haddad JGJ: Paget's disease of bone: Problems and management. *Orthop Clin North Am* 3:775–780, 1972.
7. Barry HC: Fractures of the femur in Paget's disease of bone in Australia. *J Bone Joint Surg* 49A:1359–1370, 1967.
8. Grundy M: Fractures of the femur in Paget's disease of bone: Their etiology and treatment. *J Bone Joint Surg* 52B:252–263, 1970.
9. Nicholas JA, Hilloram P: Fracture of the femur in Paget's disease: Results of treatment in 23 cases. *J Bone Joint Surg* 47A:450–461, 1965.
10. Berruex P: Traitement par plague des fractures et deformations axicles des membres dans la maladie de Paget. *Rev Chir Orthop* 64:123–129, 1978.
11. Lapinsky AS, Padgett DE, Hall FW: Disruption of the extensor mechanism in Paget's disease. *Am J Orthop* 24:165–167, 1995.
12. Oglivie-Harris DJ, Formasier VL: Pathologic fractures of the hand. *Clin Orthop* 143:168–170, 1979.
13. Cameron HU: Total knee replacement in Paget's disease. *Orthop Rev* 18:206–208, 1989.
14. Turek SI: *Orthopedics,* 4th ed. Philadelphia, Lippincott, 1984, pp 734–743.
15. Roper BA: Paget's disease involving the hip joint: A classification. *Clin Orthop* 80:33–38, 1971.
16. Roper BA: Paget's disease at the hip with osteoarthrosis: Results of intertrochanteric osteotomy. *J Bone Joint Surg* 53B:660–662, 1971.
17. Stauffer RN, Sim FH: Total hip arthroplasty in Paget's disease of the hip. *J Bone Joint Surg* 58A:476–478, 1976.
18. Ludkowski P, Wilson-MacDonald J: Total arthroplasty in Paget's disease of the hip: A clinical review and review of the literature. *Clin Orthop Rel Res* 255:160–167, 1990.
19. Nerubay J, Caspi I: Total hip replacement in two patients with Paget's disease. *Orthop Rev* 15:605–607, 1986.
20. Kaplan FS: Paget's disease of bone: Orthopedic complications. *Semin Arthritis Rheum* 23:250–252, 1994.
21. *Mercer's Orthopedic Surgery,* 8th ed. Baltimore, University Press, 1983, pp 279–290.
22. McDonald DJ, Sim FH: Total hip arthroplasty in Paget's disease. *J Bone Joint Surg* 69A:766–772, 1987.
23. Brodner W, Eyb R, Engel A: Paget-Coaxarthrose. Implantation eines modularen Tumor-Reckonstruktionssystems. Fallbericht. *Zeitschr Orthop Grenzgebiete* 132:295–299, 1994.
24. Broberg MA, Cass JR: Total knee arthroplasty in Paget's disease of the knee. *J Arthrop* 1:139–142, 1986.
25. Schajawicz F: *Tumours and Tumourlike Lesions of Bone and Joint.* New York: Springer-Verlag, 1981, pp 399–407.
26. Brice CHG, Goldie W: Paget's sarcoma of bone. *J Bone Joint Surg* 51B:205–224, 1969.

CHAPTER 6

Gaucher's Disease

Gregory M. Pastores
and Roger N. Levy

THE NATURE OF THE DISEASE

Gaucher's disease, the most common lysosomal storage disease, results from an inborn error of glycosphingolipid metabolism.[1] The accumulation of the undegraded substrate glucosylceramide in cells of the monocyte/macrophage system leads to a multisystemic disease characterized by involvement of the bone marrow, liver, spleen, and bone.[2] It is inherited as an autosomal recessive trait and affects people of all ethnic backgrounds, although it is most prevalent among individuals of Ashkenazi (central and eastern European) Jewish descent.

General Clinical Features

A broad spectrum of clinical problems may be encountered in patients with Gaucher's disease. Three clinical subtypes have been delineated on the basis of the absence (type 1) or presence and severity (acute type 2 and subacute type 3) of neurologic involvement. Bone disease is usually seen as a problem only for types 1 and 3 disease, because patients with type 2 disease rarely live beyond 2 years of age.

Common presentations include anemia, thrombocytopenia, and hepatosplenomegaly. Other hematologic problems reported in patients with Gaucher's disease include in vitro monocyte dysfunction following glucosylceramide incubation, with resultant suppressed superoxide generation and decreased (NBT) reduction, staphylococcal killing, and phagocytosis.[3] This may be the basis for increased infections in some patients. Although major bleeding episodes are infrequently observed among patients with Gaucher's disease, an abnormal coagulation profile is usually noted. This is presumably due to reduced clotting factors in the presence of severe liver dysfunction and the inactivation of clotting factors by and nonspecific adsorption to retained sphingolipids. In some patients of Jewish ancestry, factor XI deficiency may also be encountered due to independent segregation of this trait, which also happens to be prevalent among the Ashkenazim. Interestingly, neoplastic disorders, notably lymphoproliferative diseases, have been reported to be more common in patients with Gaucher's disease.[4]

Serum angiotensin converting enzyme and tartrate-resistant acid phosphatase levels are often found to be elevated in these patients.

Orthopedic Aspects of Gaucher's Disease

Although the majority of patients with Gaucher's disease are diagnosed because of hematologic problems and/or splenomegaly, skeletal disease often coexists and can be a source of debility. The pattern of bone involvement does not always reflect the extent of visceral disease and, in fact, the relationship may even be discordant. As the bone disease can be insidious, all diagnosed patients should have a careful skeletal assessment even in the absence of bone complaints.

The pathogenesis of observed bone changes in Gaucher's disease is incompletely understood. Although, presumably, the progressive marrow infiltration triggers the primary reactions that result in the loss of trabecular bone, the mechanisms that lead to the development of lytic lesions and "bone crises" most likely have a multifactorial basis. Gaucher cells are believed not to be directly involved with bone resorption; however, it is possible that they create a "toxic milieu" for bone and chronically secrete or stimulate the secretion of inflammatory enzymes (including the release of interleukin-1, which is known to stimulate osteoclasts).[5] Studies in our laboratory have suggested high collagenase levels in tissues obtained from the proximal femur at the time of surgery.[6] Medullary expansion and increased intraosseous pressure—with resultant extravascular compression and ischemia—are believed to play a contributory role.

Virtually any bone can be involved. However, major disability usually results from osteonecrosis of the femoral or humeral heads. Severely affected type 1 Gaucher's disease patients may develop neurologic complications secondary to vertebral compression fractures.

Radiologic Changes

A variety of radiologic modalities, including plain radiography,[7] computed tomography (CT),[8,9] MRI,[7,10] and nuclear bone[11] and marrow[10] scans using technetium-99m (^{99m}Tc) methylene-diphosphonate (MDP) and ^{99m}Tc sulfur colloid (SC), respectively, have been utilized to define the pattern and extent of bone involvement. More recently, studies using dual-energy x-ray absorptiometry (DEXA),[12] MRI of the spine with quantitative chemical shift imaging (QCSI),[13] and xenon-133 (^{133}Xe) scintigraphy[14] have been undertaken to evaluate Gaucher's bone disease and its progression. A classification scheme based on x-ray findings enumerates the most important bone changes, as outlined in Table 6-1.

Osteopenia

A diffuse osteopenia is often present. Although frequently asymptomatic, it may increase the risk of pathologic fractures in certain patients. Routine radiographs or CT scans show cortical thinning, endosteal scalloping, and coarsened, decreased, or absent trabecular markings.[7] It is well known that conventional radiographs are relatively insen-

TABLE 6-1   Radiographic Staging of Skeletal Lesions in Gaucher's Disease

Stage	Description	Findings
1	Osteopenia	Decreased bone density, which may be localized or diffuse, and is associated with a coarse trabecular pattern
2	Medullary expansion	Loss of normal contour above femoral condyles (Erlenmeyer-flask deformity)
3	Localized destruction (osteolysis)	Small, well-defined, or moth-eaten erosions in bone associated with endosteal notching gives a "ground-glass" appearance
4	Osteonecrosis	Patchy densities and erosions usually observed in the femoral and humeral heads
5	Diffuse destruction; epiphyseal collapse; osteoarthrosis	Flattening or irregular destruction of femoral heads with mixed lytic and sclerotic foci gives a "soap bubble" appearance

Source: Reproduced with permission from Hermann G, Goldblatt J, Levy RN, et al: Gaucher's disease type 1: Assessment of bone involvement by CT and scintigraphy. *Am J Radiol* 147: 943–948, 1986.

sitive in quantifying rates of bone loss, with estimates of radiographically detectable minimal bone losses ranging between 25 and 60 percent. Our studies show that a significant proportion of patients with Gaucher's disease have bone densities less than one standard deviation below the age- and sex-matched norm, which correlates with increased risk for pathologic fractures and/or osteonecrosis of the femoral heads.[12]

Localized Areas of Bone Erosion

In some patients, an extraosseous extension of Gaucher cell deposits, often associated with an apparent soft tissue mass, occurs secondary to destruction of the overlying cortex. In patients with vertebral involvement who develop masses in the epidural space, there is often compromise of the thecal sac, with neurologic deficits arising as a result of spinal cord compression. Biopsies confirm the diagnosis of conglomerate Gaucher cells (Fig. 6-1). These localized areas of bone loss create stress risers within bone and can lead to pathologic fracture.

Osteosclerosis

Osteosclerosis, which is noted primarily among patients with more severe bone disease, is considered to be the sequela of localized or diffuse medullary osteonecrosis.[15] Sclerotic areas are often noted as serpiginous streaks touching the endosteal surface or isolated from it. Osteosclerosis can cause significant pain when the subchondral bone attains an abnormally high stiffness and is no longer resilient with respect to its support of articular cartilage.

Medullary Expansion

Failure of remodeling, characterized by Erlenmeyer-flask deformity of the distal femurs with widening of the metaphyseal-diaphyseal regions, is a common skeletal finding in Gaucher's disease. These changes probably result from a defect in osteoclastic activity during the remodeling phase of skeletal growth, when, in the area of primary spongiosa, normal resorption and funnelization of calcified cartilage fail to take place. It is not pathognomonic of Gaucher's disease and can be associated with a number of skeletal disorders, including Pyle's disease, craniometaphyseal dysplasia, osteopetrosis, and some of the hemoglobinopathies.[15]

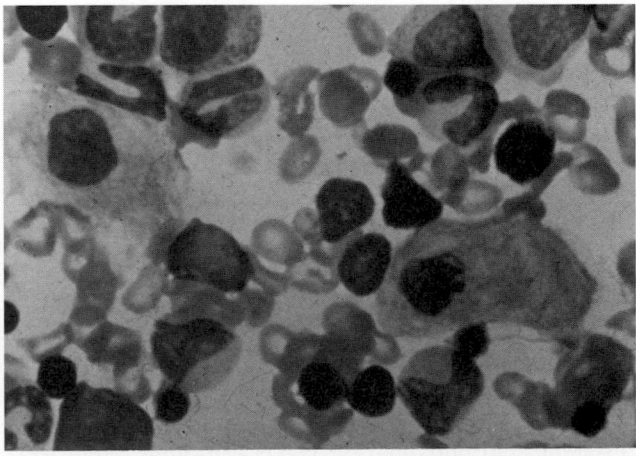

Figure 6-1 Lipid-laden "foamy" macrophages; the typical Gaucher cell.

Complications

Osteonecrosis

Osteonecrosis is the most debilitating skeletal complication in Gaucher's disease.[1,16] It may affect articular areas of bone, such as the femoral (Fig. 6-2) or humeral head or a condyle of the knee. Alternatively, it may present as an infarct involving the shaft of a long bone. Osteonecrosis is probably due to chronic infarction, possibly from occlusion of arterioles or of even larger vessels as a consequence of the progressive marrow infiltration and vasospastic or thrombotic episodes. Clinically, patients experience pain, which is most likely due to increased intraosseous pressure and, in some cases, alteration of joint contours. Children may present with a limp or show a silent course, mimicking a case of Perthes' disease. Weight bearing is extremely painful, as is any movement of the limb. [99m]Tc MDP scans performed very early have revealed avascularity of the femoral heads, while MRI often shows evidence of extensive marrow infiltration (by Gaucher cells) and edema, with osteonecrosis of the femoral head manifest by the double-line sign (i.e., parallel black and white lines). In many cases, there is a slow and steady progression in symptomatology leading to chronic pain, diminished range of motion, pathologic fracture, and joint collapse. Progressive fragmentation and flattening of the capital segment results in deformity of the femoral head and accounts for the leg-length discrepancies and gait abnormalities.

Gaucher "Bone Crises"

Bone crises are acute episodes of excruciating pain, similar to those seen in sickle cell anemia, which occur most often in the first two decades of life.[17] Radiologically, scintigraphic scans may show a localized area of transient photopenia with or without evidence of periosteal elevation on x-rays.[18,19] In the absence of cortical interruption, the presumed mechanism for the periosteal elevation is fluid accumulation secondary to microscopic egress through the

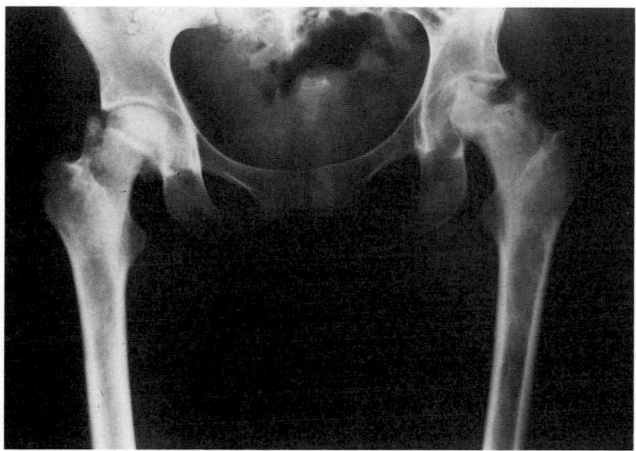

Figure 6-2 Pathologic fracture of femoral neck following bilateral ischemic necrosis due to Gaucher's bone disease.

haversian systems and Volkmann canals persisting in the devitalized cortex.[20] Nonspecific laboratory abnormalities include a mildly elevated erythrocyte sedimentation rate (equal to or greater than 50/h) and leukocytosis of up to 30,000 cells/mm[3]. In contrast to osteomyelitis, with which Gaucher's disease is frequently confused, blood cultures in patients with Gaucher's disease and bone crises are consistently negative and signs of toxemia are not observed.[19]

Treatment

Prior to the introduction of enzyme replacement therapy, treatment of symptomatic patients was supportive, with blood product infusions, total or partial splenectomy, and the use of analgesics. In selected patients with rapidly progressing disease, "cure" was achievable—but at high risk—through bone marrow transplantation. As splenectomy leads to redistribution of the undegraded substrate to other end organs (e.g., liver, bone), there were concerns regarding development of progressive bone complications in splenectomized patients. However, other studies show that bone disease remained stable in some patients and that the incidence of bone disease at autopsy was similar between splenectomized and nonsplenectomized patients. Bone crises are managed with rest, analgesics, and external support. Acute episodes of osteonecrosis may be managed surgically or conservatively. A few patients treated with a specific bisphosphonate, aminohydroxy-propylidene, have shown relief from bone pain and improvements in relevant laboratory parameters such as serum alkaline phosphatase, calcium, and urinary hydroxyproline levels. Our experience with core decompression in the early acute phase has been successful, but numbers are limited. Late problems of secondary degenerative joint disease, especially at the hip, can be managed by joint replacement. Such an endeavor requires care and considerable experience, since the bone anatomy is often atypical and the patients are young. Bleeding and infection hover as threats to success. The treatment of pathologic fractures can be challenging. Because of the paucity of bone cells, delay or failure of union may occur. Internal fixation devices must be selected carefully if surgical treatment is elected. Pathologic fracture in the spine can lead to neurologic compression syndromes and may require vertebrectomy and stabilization with spinal rods. With considerable attention to detail, results can be encouraging.

Enzyme replacement therapy has led to hematopoietic reconstitution and significant reduction of the visceromegaly in patients who received regular intravenous infusions of the placenta-derived (alglucerase) or recombinant (imiglucerase) product.[21] There is also increasing evidence of skeletal regeneration, particularly when treatment is initiate early in the disease.[22,23] With 42 months of high-dose treatment, marked improvement in marrow composition and bone mass was observed in both children and adults initiated.[24] The skeletal response may be dependent on degree of bone involvement at the time that therapy is initiated and may signify the limitations of enzyme therapy when administration is delayed beyond a point of irreversible bone changes.

REFERENCES

1. Beighton P, Beighton G: *The Man Behind the Syndrome.* Berlin, Springer-Verlag, 1986.
2. Beutler E, Grabowski GA: *Gaucher Disease,* 7th ed. New York, McGraw-Hill, 1995.
3. Liel Y, Rudich A, Nagauker-Shriker O, et al: Monocyte dysfunction in patients with Gaucher disease: Evidence for interference of glucocerebroside with superoxide generation. *Blood* 83:2646–2653, 1994.
4. Shiran A, Brenner B, Laor A, Tatarsky I: Increased risk of cancer in patients with Gaucher disease. *Cancer* 72:219–224, 1993.
5. Stowens DW, Teitelbaum SL, Kahn AJ, Barranger JA: Skeletal complications of Gaucher disease. *Medicine (Baltimore)* 64:310–322, 1985.
6. Levy RN, Oronsky AL, Guzman NA, et al: *Collagen Biosynthesis and Degradation in Gaucher's Disease.* New York, Petrie Arthritis Research Laboratory, Department of Orthopedics, Mount Sinai School of Medicine, 1984.
7. Rosenthal DI, Barton NW, McKusick KA, et al: Quantitative imaging of Gaucher disease. *Radiology* 185:841–845, 1992.
8. Hermann G, Goldblatt J, Levy RN, et al: Gaucher's disease type 1: Assessment of bone involvement by CT and scintigraphy. *Am J Radiol* 147:943–948, 1986.
9. Rosenthal DI, Mayo-Smith W, Goodsitt MM, et al: Bone and bone marrow changes in Gaucher disease: Evaluation with quantitative CT. *Radiology* 170:143–146, 1989.
10. Hermann G, Shapiro RS, Abdelwahab IF, Grabowski G: MR imaging in adults with Gaucher disease type 1: Evaluation of marrow involvement and disease activity. *Skel Radiol* 22:247–251, 1993.
11. Katz K, Mechlis-Frish S, Cohen IJ, et al: Bone scans in the diagnosis of bone crisis in patients who have Gaucher disease (published erratum appears in *J Bone Joint Surg Am* 73:791, 1991.) *J Bone Joint Surg Am* 73:513–517, 1991.
12. Pastores GM, Wallenstein S, Desnick RJ, Luckey M: Bone density in type 1 Gaucher disease. *J Bone Miner Res,* 1997 (in press).
13. Johnson LA, Hoppel BE, Gerard EL, et al: Quantitative chemical shift imaging of vertebral bone marrow in patients with Gaucher disease. *Radiology* 182:451–455, 1992.
14. Castronovo FP Jr, McKusick KA, Doppelt SH, Barton NW: Radiopharmacology of inhaled ^{133}Xe in skeletal sites containing deposits of Gaucher cells. *Nucl Med Biol* 20:707–714, 1993.
15. Mankin HJ, Doppelt SH, Rosenberg AE, Barranger JA: Metabolic bone disease in patients with Gaucher disease, in Avioli LV, Krane SM (eds): *Metabolic Bone Disease,* 2d ed. Philadelphia: Saunders, 1990, pp 730–752.
16. Katz K, Cohen IJ, Ziv N, et al: Fractures in children who have Gaucher disease. *J Bone Joint Surg* 69A:1361–1370, 1987.
17. Yosipovitch Z, Katz K: Bone crisis in Gaucher disease—An update. *Isr J Med Sci* 26:593–595, 1990.
18. Bilchik TR, Heyman S: Skeletal scintigraphy of pseudo-osteomyelitis in Gaucher's disease: Two case reports and a review of the literature. *Clin Nucl Med* 17:279–282, 1992.
19. Noyes FR, Smith WS: Bone crises and chronic osteomyelitis in Gaucher's disease. *Clin Orthop* 79:132–140, 1971.
20. Jaffe H (ed): *Metabolic Degenerative and Inflammatory Diseases of Bone and Joints.* Philadelphia, Lea & Febiger, 1972.
21. Pastores GM, Sibille AR, Grabowski GA: Enzyme therapy in Gaucher disease type 1: Dosage efficacy and adverse effects in 33 patients treated for 6 to 24 months. *Blood* 82:408–416, 1993.
22. Pastores GM, Hermann G, Norton K, Desnick RJ: Resolution of a proximal defect in type 1 Gaucher disease by enzyme replacement therapy. *Pediatr Radiol* 25:486–487, 1995.
23. Pastores GM, Hermann G, Norton K, et al: Skeletal regeneration in a patient with Gaucher disease on enzyme replacement therapy. *Skeletal Radiol* 25:485–488, 1996.
24. Rosenthal DI, Doppelt SH, Mankin HJ, et al: Enzyme replacement therapy for Gaucher disease: Skeletal responses to macrophage-targeted glucocerebrosidase. *Pediatrics* 96:629–637, 1995.

CHAPTER 7

Fracture Healing and Responses to Skeletal Injury

Stuart T. Styles
and Thomas A. Einhorn

The sequence of events that leads to the restoration of skeletal integrity after a fracture can be divided into distinct stages that are identifiable both histologically and clinically.

Molecular techniques have recently identified many of the mediators of the healing response. The mechanisms for intercellular communication and the modulation of cellular signaling within the healing fracture have also recently begun to be elucidated. There is promise that we will eventually be able to manipulate the variables associated with reparative osteogenesis and improve clinical fracture care.

THE SEQUENCE OF FRACTURE HEALING

This complex series of events should be viewed as a continuum of overlapping biological processes. Initially, there is bleeding from the bone ends and the associated soft tissue injury, resulting in the formation of local hematoma. Devascularization of the bone ends may occur due to the local interruption of vascular supply and stripping or rupture of the periosteum. The degree of soft tissue injury and bone comminution is related to the amount of energy absorbed before failure occurs. This, in turn, is greater in a bone of large volume and also where the modulus of the bone is reduced. The amount of energy absorbed by the bone is also directly related to the rate of force application to the bone.

The Inflammatory Response

Immediately after a fracture, the inflammatory response is initiated; it corresponds with the pain, swelling, erythema, and increased tissue temperature observed clinically. Injured tissues and platelets release potent vasoactive mediators, growth factors, and other cytokines, such as the immunomodulatory agents interleukin-1 and interleukin-6. Another factor produced is platelet-derived growth factor (PDGF). In addition, the polypeptides transforming growth factor beta (TGF-β) and fibroblast growth factor (FGF) are present at the site of the fracture, and these can influence cell migration, proliferation, differentiation, and matrix synthesis (Table 7-1).[1-7] Polymorphonuclear leukocytes, histiocytes, and mast cells soon make their appearance, and the

process of removing tissue debris begins.[8] Macrophages are the first cells to arrive at the fracture site,[3] and mast cells are present within 48 h.[10,11] Mast cells that stain positively for heparin[12] play a role in altering the local vascularity and thus influence the migration of cells to the fracture site. In addition to these cells, a loose connection of reticulin fibers and collagen fibrils forms in the hematoma, and cell fragments lie scattered within the fibrin scaffold.[13,14] Within the bone ends adjacent to the fracture, lacunae are seen extending a variable distance from the fracture.[15]

The Reparative Response and Callus Formation

The inflammatory response persists for 24 to 72 h.[16-19] As inflammation abates, the initial events of repair commence. Undifferentiated mesenchymal cells migrate to the site of the injury. These migrating cells have the capacity to form

TABLE 7-1 The Transforming Growth Factor Beta Superfamily of Genes[a]

Transforming growth factor beta (TGF-β) subfamily
  TGF-β_1
  TGF-β_2
  TGF-β_3
  TGF-β_4 (chicken)
  TGF-β_5 (*Xenopus*)
Bone morphogenetic protein subfamily
  Bone morphogenetic protein 2
  Bone morphogenetic protein 3
  Bone morphogenetic protein 4
  Bone morphogenetic protein 5
  Bone morphogenetic protein 6
  Bone morphogenetic protein 7
  (also known as osteogenic protein 1)
  Bone morphogenetic protein 8
  (also known as osteogenic protein 2)
  Bone morphogenetic protein 9
  Bone morphogenetic protein 10
  Decapentophegic gene (*Drosophila*)
  Growth and differentiation factor 1
  Vegetal pole-derived gene (*Xenopus*)
  Drosophila 60A
Inhibin-activin subfamily
  Inhibin-α
  Inhibin-βA
  Inhibin-βB
  Mullerian inhibiting substance

[a]Members of each subfamily show close genetic-sequence identity among themselves (50 to 90 percent sequence homology) and lesser identity with members of the other subfamilies (30 to 40 percent sequence homology).

Bone morphogenetic protein 1 is not a member of the TGF-β superfamily.

Source: Derived in part from Einhorn TA: Current concepts review: Enhancement of fracture healing. *J Bone Joint Surg* 77A:940–956, 1995. With permission.

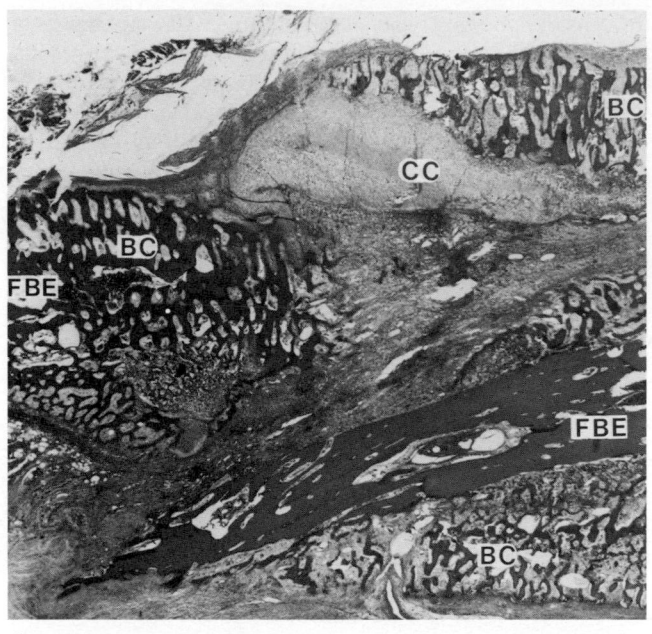

A

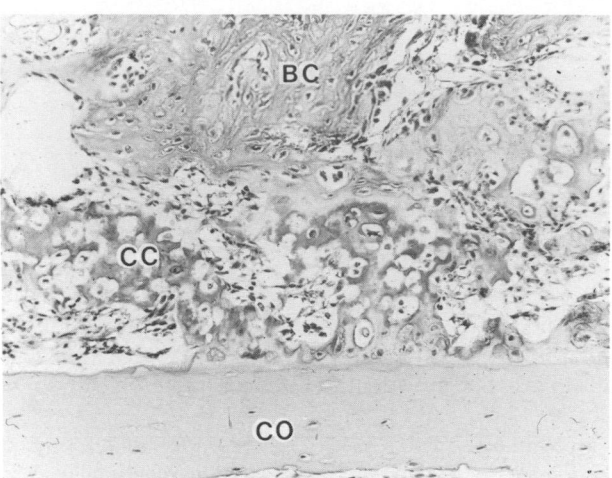

B

Figure 7-1 Bone formation in early external callus. *A.* Fracture in a child aged 2 years showing proliferative bone and cartilage formation (H&E, ×9.6.) *B.* Same fracture as in *A.* BC, bony callus; CC, chondroid callus; CO, cortex; FBE, fracture bone ends. (H&E, ×193.) (Courtesy of Dr. L. Sokoloff.)

bone, cartilage, or fibrous tissue.[17] Removal and replacement of necrotic and damaged tissue is occurring concurrently. Cellular proliferation and differentiation results in the formation of an extracellular matrix. These events are stimulated by growth factors and biophysical modulating signals. They require a microenvironment with appropriate pH, oxygen tension, and nutrition. The invading mantle of capillaries demonstrates ATPase activity, which can be identified by histochemical studies and mirrors the great increase in vascularity at the repair site. Periosteal cells stain positively for alkaline phosphatase, indicating osteoblastic activity. Osteoclasts responsible for removing debris can be identified, since they stain intensely for acid phosphatase. As a result of this increased cellularity, vascularity, and metabolic activity, the hematoma becomes organized and fibroblasts and chondroblasts appear between the bone ends. The presence of cartilage is accompanied by the appearance of type 2 collagen. Cartilage is later replaced by woven bone by the process of enchondral ossification, and then type 1 collagen is seen to predominate.

The subperiosteal woven bone that forms external callus (Fig. 7-1) originates directly from osteoprogenitor cells of the inner periosteal cell layer (the cambial layer). This bone forms by intramembranous ossification. Simultaneously, endochondral bone formation occurs elsewhere in the healing fracture.

Remodeling of the Healing Fracture

There are regional differences in bone remodeling. In cortical bone, remodeling occurs by the mechanism of invasion by a resorption "cutting cone," with osteoclasts re-

moving bone and osteoblasts depositing new bone in organized lamellae. It may take a few years before all the dead bone is removed and replaced by new bone. In cancellous bone, on the other hand, the process of remodeling occurs on the surface of the individual trabeculae. Cancellous bone is rich in osteoprogenitor cells that differentiate into osteoblasts after they have invaded dead bone. There is therefore an increase in the thickness of the trabecular bone mass after a fracture of cancellous bone.[18]

The remodeling of newly deposited woven bone during fracture healing is also affected by the mechanical forces imposed upon the fracture. The primary external callus is relatively uninfluenced by mechanical factors until it becomes bridging callus.[22] When bridging has occurred, inductive mechanisms come into play that speed up or, alternatively, delay the mineralization of the chondroosteoid, depending upon the mechanical environment.

Under a rigid plate, stress shielding will cause cortical thinning and osteoporosis, but there is likely to be little if any external callus produced in this situation. The fracture may heal by a mechanism resembling normal bone remodeling if the interosseous gap at the fracture is completely eliminated (which is rarely the case microscopically). Where the bone is in such close apposition, it is possible for a remodeling cutting cone of osteoclasts to traverse the fracture followed by a mantle of osteoblasts. This produces a haversian system (osteon) traversing the fracture (Fig. 7-2). It is unlikely that such direct "osteonal" union occurs without some initial callus being formed, even beneath a compression plate. Even with the most rigid plate, there is sufficient micromotion between the bone ends that stresses exceeding the failure point of this type of haversian osteon are generated.[19]

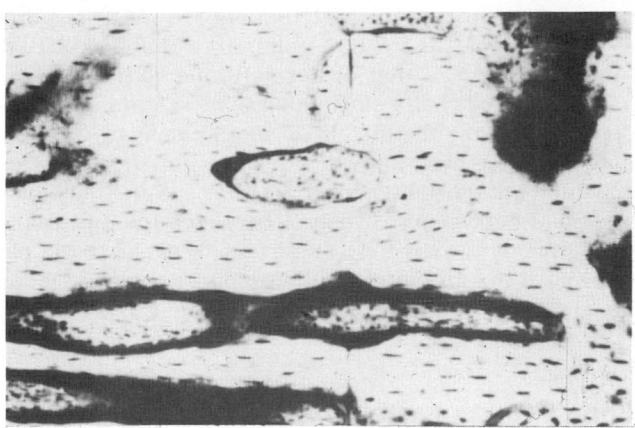

A

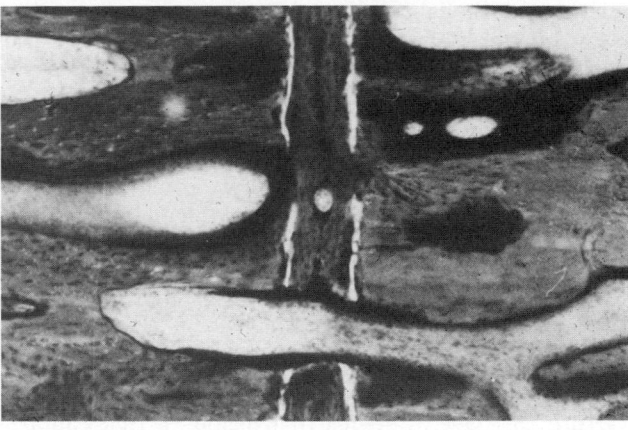

B

Figure 7-2 *A.* Histology of the cortex of the sheep tibia beneath a rigid plate, 12 weeks after operation. Primary fracture healing is seen in spite of full weight bearing. No specific resorption of the compressed surfaces is visible. *B.* Histology of the opposite side of the same tibia shown in *A.* The gap between the fragments is first filled by lamellar bone ("transverse osteon"), which, in turn, will be remodeled later in an axial direction. Fluorescent label given 3 weeks after the operation is found in such a transverse osteon. This animal was sacrificed at 12 weeks. (Reproduced with permission from Perren SM, Russenberger M, Steinemann S, et al.: A dynamic compression plate. *Acta Orthop Scand* (Suppl) 125:31–41, 1969.*)*

Woo and coworkers have considered the theoretical requirements for fixation plates to maximize the environmental conditions necessary for fracture union (Fig. 7-3). They have concluded that during the early stage of fracture management, a plate should be stiff enough in bending in torsional directions to prevent bone angulation or implant failure; thus they caution against using very flexible materials that may not fulfill these requirements. They point out that in the late phase of callus or bone remodeling, the plate must be stiff enough under axial loading to ensure that the underlying bone shares a higher proportion of the physiologic stresses needed to facilitate its normal remodeling and avoid osteoporosis.[19]

Fractures treated with intramedullary (IM) rods show more periosteal callus than fractures treated with rigid compression plates because the mechanical situation is different at the fracture. The bone porosity is less with a rigid IM rod than with a loosely fitted rod.[20] However, the IM rod, particularly if reamed, may delay union by damaging the formation of endosteal callus and injuring the endosteal blood supply.

BIOLOGICAL CONSIDERATIONS IN FRACTURE HEALING

Many systemic and local factors have been reported as either impeding or preventing fracture healing.[3] The vascular response seems to be particularly critical. Normally the cortex is supplied primarily through a centrifugal medullary vascular system and most of the blood supply to the fracture is derived from this source. The periosteum contributes little to the blood supply of the fracture. An extraosseous blood supply to the injured area arises

PRE-UNION

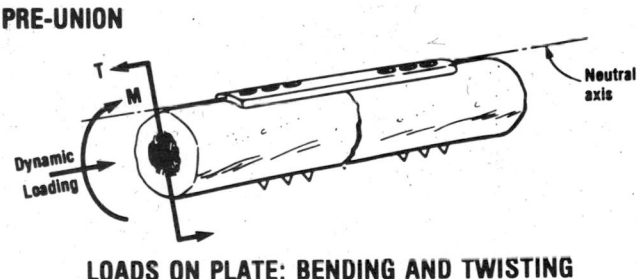

LOADS ON PLATE: BENDING AND TWISTING

POST-UNION

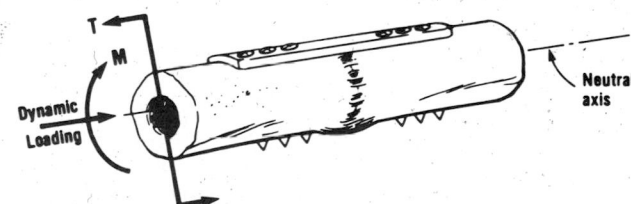

LOADS ON PLATE: TENSION OR COMPRESSION

Figure 7-3 Diagram demonstrating the changes in the loading conditions on the internal fixation plates between the pre- and postunion stages of a long bone fracture. Under identical dynamic in vivo loads, the plate is subjected to bending and torsional loads in the early healing phase because of the discontinuity of bone. However, as healing progresses, the neutral axis of the plate-bone structure shifts toward the bone and the plate is subjected to tensile or compressive loads. (Reproduced with permission from Woo SLY, Lothringer KS, Akeson WH, et al: Less rigid internal fixation plates: Historical perspectives and new concepts: *J Orthop Res* 1:431–449, 1984.)

quickly. Endothelial cells from blood vessels in the soft tissues near the injury proliferate and form new capillaries that extend into the injury.[18,21,22] This response peaks at 10 days postfracture. Once the medullary system has been disrupted, this extraosseous blood supply may supply some blood to the necrotic bone cortex, but its main focus appears to be development of external callus. When the fracture is completely healed and the medullary blood supply has been restored, the extraosseous blood supply regresses.

Brighton[23] has drawn attention to the paradox between the increased local blood flow, which can be measured with radioisotopes, and the finding of diminished oxygen tension in fracture hematomas and newly formed fracture cartilage. It seems that despite a rich capillary bed in the fracture callus, hypoxia does exist at the cellular level. During mineralization of osteoid in fracture callus, cellular hypoxia may trigger the release of accumulated calcium by chondrocyte mitochondria into the matrix by exocytosis in the same way that this process occurs in the hypertrophic zone in the physis. The devascularization associated with soft tissue stripping in high-velocity injuries to the limbs clearly affects the potential for healing of the fracture negatively because of the extent of the vascular injury to the bone ends. The vascular response to a fracture is responsible for the ultimate oxygen gradient. An optimal vascular reparative response must occur to ensure osteogenesis. Where the local anatomy of the supply to the bone is specifically disrupted by the fracture, thus creating avascularity (for example, in the scaphoid and the talus and femoral neck), the fracture can still heal, but the rate and incidence of healing is reduced.[24,25]

Failure to develop an adequate vascular response in high-velocity injuries may be responsible for the so-called atrophic nonunion, where all cellular activities seem to be suppressed. No callus is produced, the bone ends are sclerotic, and the medullary cavities are closed over at the fracture site, indicating that no further biological activity will occur without intervention. Eventually there may be a fully developed pseudarthrosis. This condition should be differentiated from delayed union, when union does not occur within an expected time frame. In delayed union, no irreversible biological changes have occurred. One cannot rule out the possibility that union in the fracture may still occur.

Another type of identifiable nonunion seen radiologically is the so-called hypertrophic nonunion, where there is an abundant proliferative radiopaque callus but none of it bridges the fracture, which is still visible as a lucent line. Intervention to create a more favorable mechanical environment is necessary (e.g., by IM rodding) if union is to be achieved.

Other factors that may contribute to nonunion include infection and ischemia. Skeletally immature patients have the greatest healing potential and heal most rapidly.[26] The elderly often heal more slowly and less effectively due to a combination of factors. Comorbid medical conditions and nutritional status are important in surgical decision making. Nutritional demands in fracture healing can exceed caloric intake.[27,28] Leung and coauthors[29] re-

ported that the adenosine triphosphate (ATP) requirement of 2-week-old fracture callus in a rabbit was 1000 times greater than that of normal bone. Other authors have suggested that a single long bone fracture can temporarily increase the metabolic requirement by 22 to 25 percent.[30] It is well known that poor nutritional status may increase mortality, infection rate, and the incidence of wound dehiscence. It can also reduce fracture callus strength.[31] It is extremely important to evaluate the nutritional status of injured patients and to provide nutritional support if needed.[32-35]

Bone Growth Factors in Fracture Repair

Studies have demonstrated changes in collagen gene expression corresponding to the development of the healing fracture. During the initial stages of healing in mechanically stable fractures, type 3 and 5 collagen is laid down first.[36,37] By week 2, the cartilaginous stage has appeared, with some type 2 and type 9 collagen. This is followed by a brief period of expression of type 10 collagen by hypertrophic chondrocytes, which may correspond with cartilage calcification and associated bone formation. Type 1 collagen then appears in mechanically stable fractures. In unstable fractures, however, type 2 and type 9 collagen predominate in the cartilage and little of type 1 appears.[36] Extracellular matrix protein genes vary in activity and expression during different stages of fracture healing and within different areas of the callus. When rat femur fracture callus was examined, mRNA for osteonectin, alkaline phosphatase, and type 1 procollagen varied in peak expression in hard and soft callus.[38] Soft callus corresponds to the stage in which the developing matrix is composed primarily of fibrocartilage, which corresponds clinically to decreasing pain, swelling, and motion at the fracture site. Hard callus develops as a result of woven bone formation. Osteonectin mRNA is detected in hard and soft callus throughout repair. Osteonectin expression has been localized in preosteoblasts and early osteoblasts and is an early marker of bone formation.[39] Osteocalcin gene expression is detected in hard callus only, but circulating levels have been shown to be increased in the serum after local skeletal injuries or bone marrow stimulation.[38] It seems that osteocalcin and osteonectin are extracellular matrix components whose presence is required to increase osteogenic activity. The information available suggests that genetic regulation is influenced by signals within the developing callus and that local regulatory factors are required for the orderly genetic activation of the required polypeptide sequences during fracture healing.

The TGF-β superfamily of growth-regulatory peptides (Table 7-1) may be essential in the regulation of fracture healing.[39] These factors appear to be potent inducers of collagen expression as well as inhibitors of osteoclast activity.[40-42] Almost all cells make TGF-β in one of its forms, although the most prolific producers are bone cells and platelets. There are at least five types of TGF-β, two of which are found in humans. All show similarity in the amino acid sequence.[43] These agents have a broad range of cellular activities, including control of the proliferation of the mesenchymal precursor cells for chondrocytes, osteoblasts, and osteoclasts.[44,45] They stimulate the differentiation of periosteally derived cells. Fibroblast growth factor has also been shown to exhibit the same effect,[45] and TGF-β has been shown to be a chemotactic factor attracting macrophages to the sites of injury and also increasing the production of other extracellular matrix components, such as collagen, fibronectin, and proteoglycan.[42] It has powerful osteoinductive potential. (Osteoinduction is the process that leads to the production of osteoprogenitor cells with a capacity to form new bone even in extraskeletal sites.) Recombinant TGF-β can stimulate the formation of bone even in the cartilage of the rabbit ear.[46] Injected subperiosteally into the rat femur, TGF-β will produce local bone; when it is combined with bFGF (basic FGF), even more bone formation will occur.[47]

Other members of the TGF-β superfamily, called the bone morphogenetic proteins (BMPs), have been cloned, allowing for the investigation of their activities. These agents were the first growth factors to be identified as a result of Urist's pioneering work on the implantation of demineralized bone at extraskeletal sites.[48] When recombinant BMP is linked to a carrier and subcutaneously implanted into rats, complete endochondral ossification is seen with a normal event sequence.[49] Other studies have shown varying amounts of cartilage and bone formation depending on the type of BMP used.[50]

The clinical use of recombinant human BMP has recently been investigated in gap healing of fractures in long bones.[51] A segmental defect in the femur of the sheep was stabilized with a plate and screws, and those animals who received recombinant human BMP-2 with a carrier achieved radiographic healing 1 month after implantation. Mechanical testing has shown that these femora subsequently exhibited mechanical properties comparable to those on the contralateral side.[52]

Osteoconductive Materials and Their Role in Fracture Repair

Osteoconductive substances cannot induce the formation of bone at extraskeletal sites. In many cases they act as scaffolding and are used to augment the supply of autogenous bone for grafting, which is available from the patient only in limited quantities. These substances support vascular ingrowth and bone formation by their physical and chemical composition. Those in common clinical use include a hydroxyapatite matrix obtained from marine coral calcium phosphate. This material is commonly used to augment fusion masses and fill some defects in bone that may occur in severe fractures.[53] Other materials available include mixtures of calcium phosphate and collagen.[54] Much publicity has attended the announcement of the development of an inorganic calcium phosphate material that can form a paste, can be injected into a fracture site, and will then harden, forming the mineral structure "dahllite." Unlike some of the materials previously mentioned, this material appears to be remodeled after being incorporated in vivo.[55]

BIOPHYSICAL ENHANCEMENT OF BONE REPAIR

The ability of bone to adapt to mechanical stimuli has been recognized for well over a century and is known as *Wolff's law*. The consequences of this relationship for fracture healing are readily apparent. Bone loss associated with the rigid fixation of a plate is often a concern, yet excessive motion may lead to hypertrophic nonunion. The beneficial effects of controlled weight bearing have been demonstrated by Sarmiento et al. to have important clinical applications.[56] There is striking evidence of the potential for biophysical influences on fracture healing in the work of Kenwright and coworkers. They compared the effects of controlled axial micromotion with static external fixation alone on tibial diaphysial fractures. The beneficial effect of cycling the load was shown by shortened healing times in these experiments. Similar animal studies have investigated the influence of the number of cycles, the degree of displacement, and the rate at which the bone is loaded.[57]

In 1953, Yasuda demonstrated new bone formation in the region of the negative electrode after electric current had been continuously applied to a rabbit femur.[58] He also demonstrated that electric currents are generated when dry bone is loaded. The discovery of load-induced piezoelectric potentials in bone suggested a means by which stress or strain could intrinsically alter the cellular environment in the bone and thus influence proliferation and function. This hypothesis became even more attractive when it was demonstrated that in wet bone, two sources of electric current coexisted. The piezoelectric currents arise from deformation of collagen. The relatively large electrokinetic (streaming) potentials are produced by the strain-induced interaction of charged constituents of extracellular fluids flowing past the mineral phase of the matrix.[59]

Friedenberg[60-62] and Bassett[63-67] and their colleagues were pioneers in the use of electromagnetic stimulation in the treatment of nonunions. The noninvasive methods utilizing these principles are still in clinical use, while the earlier invasive procedures have been abandoned. The efficacy of a pulsed electromagnetic field (PEMF) in stimulating ununited fractures has been shown in several double-blinded clinical trials. Sharrard showed, in a double-blind trial, that PEMF significantly influenced healing in tibial fractures with delayed union.[68] Similar results have followed the application of PEMF to open tibial osteotomy, revealing that this treatment doubles the number of patients who are 50 to 100 percent healed within the first 60 days of treatment.[69]

An additional approach to the use of biophysical stimulation of fracture healing has recently been demonstrated using acoustic power. Heckman and coworkers, in a prospective randomized double-blind trial, demonstrated the efficacy of ultrasound in 67 closed or grade 1 open fractures of the tibia and showed a significant decrease in the time for both clinical healing and radiologic union.[70] Kristiansen reported similar benefits in the treatment of fractures of the distal radius.[71] Cook and coworkers recently showed this type of stimulation to be particularly beneficial in smokers, who are notoriously slow to heal their fractures.[72] The FDA had approved the marketing of devices delivering acoustic power to enhance fracture union.

SYSTEMIC AGENTS INFLUENCING FRACTURE HEALING

Einhorn et al. examined distant skeletal sites after the insertion of an IM into rat femora.[73] By thus mimicking closed rodding of the femur, rates of mineral apposition were measured in both tibias and an increase of as much as 350 percent over controls was seen in both. These results suggest that marrow injury alone can lead to the production of a circulating growth factor that can enhance osteogenic potential in healing fractures. Simply stimulating bone marrow even by simple aspiration can also evoke a systemic osteogenic response, producing an agent known as *osteogenic growth peptide*.[74-76] The role of circulating growth factors in the well-observed phenomenon of ectopic bone formation in comatose patients (after head injury) is unknown, but these patients' fractures heal more quickly and with more callus than those in patients without head injury.[77-80]

CONCLUSION

Recent advances in the ability to produce individual bone-growth factors coupled with the ongoing development of suitable carriers to deliver the active molecules to the healing fracture promises a revolution in fracture care. Stimulation of tardy healing and reactivation of active biological healing processes in established nonunion seem to be techniques soon to be within our grasp. At the same time, the availability of new devices to produce these effects by biophysical stimulation will hopefully reduce the number of surgical interventions and the associated morbidity.

REFERENCES

1. Joyce ME, Jingushi S, Bolander, MA: Transforming growth factor beta in the regulation of fracture repair. *Orthop Clin North Am* 21:199–209, 1990.
2. Brown GL, Curtsinger LJ, White M, et al: Acceleration of tensile strength of incisions treated with EGF and TGF-beta. *Ann Surg* 208:788–794, 1988.
3. Canalis E: Effects of growth factors on bone cell replication. *Clin Orthop* 193:246–263, 1985.
4. Canalis E, McCarthy T, Centrella M: Growth factors and the regulation of bone remodeling. *J Chem Invest* 81:277–288, 1988.
5. Joyce ME, Jingushi S, Skully SP, Bolander MA: Role of growth factors in fracture healing. *Prog Clin Biol Res* 365:391–416, 1991.
6. Lucas PA: Chemotactic response of osteoblast-like cells to TGF-beta (abstr). *Trans Orthop Res Soc* 14:86, 1989.
7. Noda M, Camillier JJ: In vivo stimulation of bone formation by transforming growth factor beta. *Endocrinology* 124:2991–2994, 1989.
8. Lindholm R, Lindholm S, Liukko P, et al: The mast cell as a component of callus in fracture healing. *J Bone Joint Surg* 51B:148–155, 1969.
9. Benfu C, Xueming T: Ultrastructural investigation of experimental fracture healing: I. Electron microscopic observation of cellular activity. *Chin Med J* 92:530, 1979.
10. Duthie RB, Barker AM: An autoradiographic study of mucopolysaccharide and phosphate complexes in bone growth and repair. *J Bone Joint Surg* 37B:304, 1955.
11. Duthie RB, Barker AM: The histochemistry of the preosseous stage of bone repair studied by autoradiography. *J Bone Joint Surg* 37B:691, 1955.
12. Rebecca RO, Bassett CO, Bachman CH: *Bone Biodynamics.* Boston, Little, Brown, 1964, p 209.
13. Aho AJ: Electron microscopic and histological evaluations on fracture repair in young and old rats. *Acta Pathol Microbiol Scand Suppl* 184:25, 1966.
14. Benfu C, Xueming T: Ultrastructural investigation of experimental fracture healing: II. Electron microscopic observation on fibrillogenesis. *Chin Med J* 92:600, 1979.
15. Hamm AW: A histological study of the early phase of bone repair. *J Bone Joint Surg* 12:825–844, 1930.
16. Benfu C, Xueming T: Ultrastructural investigation of experimental fracture healing: I. Electron microscopic observation of cellular activity. *Chin Med J* 92:530, 1979.
17. Buckwalter JA, Cooper RR: The cells and matrices of skeletal connective tissue, in Albright JA, Brand RA (eds): *The Scientific Basis of Orthopedics,* Norwalk, CT: Appleton & Lange, 1987, pp 1–25.
18. McKibbins B: The biology of fracture healing in long bones. *J Bone Joint Surg* 60B:150–161, 1978.
19. Woo SLY, Lothringer KS, Akeson WH, et al: Rigid internal fixation plates: Historical perspectives and new concepts. *J Orthop Res* 1:431–449, 1984.
20. Rand JA, An KN, Chao EYS, Kelly PJ: A comparison of the effect of open intramedullary nailing and compression plate fixation on fracture site blood flow and fracture union. *J Bone Joint Surg* 63A:427–442, 1981.
21. Brighton CT, Hunt RM: Early histological and ultrasound changes in medullary fracture callus. *J Bone Joint Surg* 73A:832–847, 1991.
22. Books M: *The Blood Supply of Bone: An Approach to Bone Biology.* London, Butterworths, 1971.
23. Brighton CT: The biology of fracture repair. *AAOS Instr Lect* 33:60–82, 1984.
24. Blade HB, Salvitor JE: Acute fractures of the femoral neck: Internal fixation or prosthesis? *J Bone Joint Surg* 46A:1066–1068, 1964.
25. Marsh JL, Buckwalter JA, Evarts CM: Non union, delayed union, malunion and avascular necrosis, in Epps CH (ed): *Complications in Orthopedic Surgery.* Philadelphia, Lippincott, 1994, pp 183–211.
26. Bak B, Jorgenson PH, Andreassen TT: The stimulating effect of growth hormone on fracture healing is dependent on onset and duration of administration. *Clin Orthop* 264:295–301, 1991.
27. Cuthbertson DB: Further observation of a disturbance of metabolism caused by injury, with particular reference to the dietary requirements of fracture cases. *Br J Surg* 23:505–520, 1936.

28. Jenson JE, Jenson TG, Smith TK, et al: Nutrition in orthopedic surgery. *J Bone Joint Surg* 64A:1236–1272, 1982.

29. Leung KS, Sher AH, Lamb TSW, Leung PC: Energy metabolism in fracture healing. *J Bone Joint Surg* 71B:567–660, 1989.

30. Cuthbertson DB: Further observation of a disturbance of metabolism caused by injury, with particular reference to the dietary requirements of fracture cases. *Br J Surg* 23:505–520, 1936.

31. Einhorn TA, Bonnarens F, Burstein AH: The contributions of dietary protein and mineral to the healing of experimental fractures: A biomechanical study. *J Bone Joint Surg* 68A:1389–1395, 1986.

32. Braun RM, Schorr R: Surgical nutrition in patients with multiple injuries: Report of a case. *J Bone Joint Surg* 65A:123–127, 1983.

33. Herbsman H, Powers JC, Herschman A, Schafton GW: Retardation of fracture healing in experimental diabetes. *J Surg Res* 8:424–431, 1968.

34. Jacobs SJ, Gilbert MS, Einhorn TA: The treatment of fractures in uremic bone disease: Causes of failure and optimization of healing. *Contemp Orthop* 18:23–25, 1989.

35. Mikelson CG, Askinazi J: Current concepts review: The metabolic response to injury: Mechanisms and clinical implications. *J Bone Joint Surg* 68A:782–787, 1986.

36. Page M, Hog J, Asherst DE: The effects of mechanical stability on the macromolecules of the connective tissue matrices produced during fracture healing: No. 1. The collagens. *Histochem J* 18:251–265, 1986.

37. Sandberg M, Aro H, Mokamake T, Aho AJ: In situ localization of collagen production by chondrocytes and osteoblasts in fracture callus. *J Bone Joint Surg* 71A:69–77, 1989.

38. Jingushi S, Joyce ME, Bolander ME: Genetic expression of extracellular matrix proteins correlates with histologic changes during fracture repair. *J Bone Min Res* 7:1045–1055, 1992.

39. Massague J: The transforming growth factor beta family. *Annu Rev Cell Biol* 6:597, 1990.

40. Pfeilschifter J, Suiden SM, Munde GR: Transforming growth factor beta inhibits bone reabsorption in fetal rat long bone cultures. *J Clin Invest* 82:680, 1988.

41. Centrella M, McCarthy TL, Canalis E: Current concepts review: Transforming growth factor beta and remodeling of bone. *J Bone Joint Surg* 73A:1418–1428, 1991.

42. Sporn MB, Roberts AB: Transforming growth factor beta: Multiple actions and potential clinical applications. *JAMA* 262:938–941, 1989.

43. Glowacki J, Kaban LB, Murray JE, et al: Application of the biological principle of induced osteogenesis for craniofacial defects. *Lancet* 1:959–962, 1981.

44. Sporn MB, Roberts AB: Transforming growth factor beta: Multiple actions and potential clinical applications. *JAMA* 262:938–941, 1989.

45. Iwasaki M, Haruhiko N, Nakase T, et al: Regulation of proliferation and osteochondrogenic differentiation of periosteum derived cells by transforming growth factor beta and basic fibroblast growth factor. *J Bone Joint Surg* 77A:543–553, 1995.

46. Beck LS, Amman AJ, Aufdemorte TB, et al: In vivo induction of bone by recombinant human transforming growth factor beta. *J Bone Min Res* 6:961–968, 1991.

47. Pierce T, Kuz J, Deheer D, Swanson A: Stimulation of osteogenesis by transforming growth factor beta and fibroblastic growth factor in mature rat bone. *Contemp Orthop* 30:331–335, 1995.

48. Urist MR: Bone formation by autoinduction. *Science* 150:893–899, 1965.

49. Wang EA, Rosen V, Allesandro JS, et al: Recombinant human bone morphogenetic protein induces bone formation. *Proc Natl Acad Sci USA* 87:2220–2224, 1990.

50. Wozney JM, Rosen V: Bone morphogenetic proteins and their gene expression, in Noda M (ed): *Cellular and Molecular Biology of Bone*. San Diego, CA, Academic Press, 1993, pp 131–167.

51. Crook SD, Baffes GC, Wolf MW, et al: The effect of recombinant human osteogenic protein-1 on healing of large segmental bone defects. *J Bone Joint Surg* 76:827–838, 1994.

52. Gerhart TN, Kerkerdashead CA, Vett MA, et al: Healing segmental femoral defects in sheep using recombinant human bone morphogenetic protein. *Clin Orthop* 293:317–326, 1993.

53. Bucholz RW, Carlton RPT, Holmes R: Interporous hydroxyapatite as a bone graft substitute in tibial plateau fractures. *Clin Orthop* 240:53–62, 1989.

54. Cornell CN: Initial clinical experience with use of Collagraft as a bone graft substitute. *Tech Orthop* 7:55–63, 1992.

55. Constantz BR, Ison IC, Fulner MT, et al: Skeletal repair by in-site formation of the mineral phase of bone. *Science* 267:1796–1799, 1995.

56. Sarmiento A, Schaeffer JF, Beckerman L, et al: Fracture healing in rat femora is affected by functional weight bearing. *J Bone Joint Surg* 59A:369–375, 1977.

57. Kenwright J, Richardson JB, Cunningham JL, et al: Axial movement and tibial fractures: A controlled randomized trial of treatment. *J Bone Joint Surg* 73B:654–659, 1991.

58. Yasudua I: Fundamental aspects of fracture treatment. *J Kyoto Med Soc* 4:395–406, 1953.

59. Hastings GW, Mahmud FA: *J Biomed Eng* 10:515–521, 1988.

60. Friedenberg ZB, Andrews ET, Smolenski BI, et al: Bone reaction to varying amounts of direct current. *Surg Gynecol Obstet* 131:894, 1970.

61. Friedenberg ZB, Zemsky LM, Pollis RP, Brighton CT: The response of non-traumatized bone to direct current. *J Bone Joint Surg* 56A:1023, 1974.

62. Friedenberg ZB, Brighton CT: Biophysical induction of fracture repair, in Lang JM (ed): *Fracture Healing*. New York, Churchill Livingstone, 1987, pp 75–80.

63. Bassett CAL, Becker RO: Generation of electrical potentials by bone in response to mechanical stress. *Science* 137:1063–1064, 1962.

64. Bassett CAL: Biophysical principles affecting bone structure, in Bourne GA (ed): *The Biochemistry and Physiology of Bone*, 2d ed. Vol 3. New York, Academic Press, 1971, pp 1–76.

65. Brighton CT: The semi-invasive method of treating non union with direct current. *Orthop Clin North Am* 15:33–45, 1984.

66. Brighton CT, Hozach WJ, Brager MD: Fracture healing in the rabbit fibula when subjected to various capacitively coupled electrical fields. *J Orthop Res* 3:331–340, 1985.

67. Brighton CT, Pollack SL: Treatment of recalcitrant non union with a capacitively coupled electrical field: A preliminary report. *J Bone Joint Surg* 67A:577–585, 1985.

68. Sharrard WJW: A double blind trial of pulsed electromagnetic fields for delayed union of tibial fractures. *J Bone Joint Surg* 72B:347–355, 1990.

69. Mammie GI, Rocchi R, Cadossi R, et al: The electrical stimulation of tibial osteotomies. *Clin Orthop* 288:246–253, 1993.

70. Heckman JB, Ryaby JP, McCabe J, et al: Acceleration of tibial fracture healing by non invasive low intensity pulsed ultrasound. *J Bone Joint Surg* 76A:26–34, 1994.

71. Kristiansen TK: The effect of low power specifically programmed ultrasound on the healing time of fresh fractures using a Colles model. *J Orthop Trauma* 4:227–228, 1990.

72. Cook D, Heckman JD, McCabe J, Ryaby JP: Low intensity pulsed ultrasound accelerates tibia fracture healing in smokers. AAOS Meeting, February 1996.

73. Einhorn TA, Simon G, Devlin VJ, et al: The osteogenic response to distant skeletal injury. *J Bone Joint Surg* 72A:1374–1378, 1990.

74. Bab I, Gazit D, Chorev M, et al: Histone H4-related osteogenic growth peptide (OGP): A novel circulating stimulator of osteoblastic activity. *EMBO J* 11:1867, 1992.

75. Foldes J, Naparstek E, Statter M, et al: Osteogenic response to marrow aspiration: Increased serum osteocalcin and alkaline phosphatase in human bone marrow donors. *J Bone Min Res* 4:643, 1989.

76. Bab I, Gazit D, Muhlrad A, Shteyer A: Regenerating bone marrow produces a potent growth factor activity to osteogenic cells. *Endocrinology* 123:345, 1988.

77. Perkins R, Skaving AP: Callus formation and the rate of healing of femoral fractures in patients with head injuries. *J Bone Joint Surg* 69B:521–524, 1987.

78. Smith R: Head injury fracture healing and callus (editorial). *J Bone Joint Surg* 69B:518–520, 1987.

79. Spencer RF: The effect of head injury on fracture healing. *J Bone Joint Surg* 69B:525–528, 1987.

80. Garland DE, Toder L: Fractures of the tibial diaphysis in adults with head injuries. *Clin Orthop* 150:198–202, 1980.

CHAPTER 8

Bone Grafting

Gary E. Friedlaender

Bone possesses the unusual biological capacity to regenerate and does so routinely in the course of normal skeletal homeostasis as well as fracture repair. These same physiologic mechanisms are associated with bone grafts. Consequently, osseous grafts are frequently and successfully used to repair or replace skeletal deficits associated with a wide variety of bony disorders spanning congenital, traumatic, degenerative, and neoplastic etiologies. Specific applications include the filling of cystic defects, repair of nonunions, supplementation of arthrodeses, and provision of segmental replacements.[19]

In one form or another, bone grafts have been used for centuries, as documented by numerous biblical, ecclesiastic, and medical records of varying credibility.[4] The modern science associated with bone grafts began in the nineteenth century with contributions by Ollier[39] and Macewen[34]; practical applications were further developed in the early twentieth century by Albee,[1] Lexer,[33] and Phemister,[42] to name only a few.

BIOLOGICAL CONSIDERATIONS

Today, the armamentarium of alternative bone graft sources and bone graft substitutes is extensive. Cortical and cancellous autograft can be transplanted alone or as composites with musculoskeletal soft tissues, and the procedures may be accomplished with or without an intact or immediately reestablished blood supply. Similarly, a variety of allogeneic and even xenogeneic preparations treated and preserved by a wide spectrum of approaches are available. Indeed, the choice of appropriate bone graft material is now as complex as the diversity of disorders for which these transplants are employed. Nonetheless, autografts remain the standard by which all other approaches must be measured and of which our knowledge, although incomplete, is most comprehensive.

Autografts

Autografts are tissues removed from one place in the body and returned to another site in the *same individual* (whether within an animal or a human). By definition, these tissues are histocompatible, and transfer of disease from donor to recipient is not an issue. Consequently, the biological potential of autogenous tissues is considered to represent the maximum achievable. Much of the physiologic control over bone graft incorporation remains unknown or a matter of

speculation, but considerable new information is evolving in terms of characterizing the molecular messengers—e.g., the transforming growth factor β (TGF-β) superfamily—responsible for bone remodeling activities.[23,38] The histologic sequence of events, however, has been well described and serves as a basis for discussing rational clinical applications of these tissues.[8,9,24,47]

Bone graft incorporation is an interactive process between the graft and the host bed, with contributions from each source that can either enhance or detract from success of the overall process. In general, grafts must be invaded by blood vessels. The blood vessels emanate from the recipient site and carry with them multipotential cells that differentiate into populations specialized in bone formation or resorption. The graft itself serves as a passive scaffold or template for this influx of activity (osteoconduction) and may also provide active signals to the host response capable of influencing, if not regulating, the process of incorporation (osteoinduction).[57]

Fresh autogenous bone is replete with the many growth factors and osteoinductive agents, which play important roles in the local regulation of bone formation, including bone morphogenetic proteins (BMPs).[3] These are a family of low-molecular-weight, noncollagenous proteins, most of which are related through amino acid homology to the supergene family of TGF-β.[11] These BMPs—1 through 7—have been isolated from bone matrix[54–56]; BMP-2 and BMP-7 (OP-1) are now available through recombinant DNA synthesis and are being evaluated in clinical trials.[46,60] These molecules stimulate bone formation by inducing undifferentiated cells to proliferate and to differentiate into osteoblasts.[12,30] Local factors, systemic hormones, and mechanical stresses may all play a role in the initiation and regulation of new bone formation intrinsic to the process of osteoinduction and bone graft incorporation.[3] Once formed, this new bone enters into the normal homeostatic routine of remodeling, a process that responds to physiologic stresses, be they mechanical or biological.

Nonvascularized Grafts

The histologic pattern observed with nonvascularized bone graft incorporation—that is, a graft transferred without an intact blood supply or without immediate reestablishment of blood flow by vascular reanastomosis—begins with hematoma formation (similar to fracture repair), followed by a gradual transformation to a fibrovascular response. The graft itself undergoes substantial cell necrosis except for those cells within approximately 0.1 to 0.3 mm of the surface, which can survive by diffusion.[25] The necrosis causes an inflammatory response within the contiguous fibrovascular stroma, the tissue that is also responsible for ingrowth of new blood vessels into the bony architecture.

Up to this point, cortical and cancellous grafts behave in a similar fashion, but significant differences can be identified both qualitatively and quantitatively in a now-ongoing repair process. Cancellous grafts are rapidly vascularized by virtue of their porous structure. Osteoblastic activity then follows, with the deposition of osteoid on surfaces of acellular trabeculae, and mineralization proceeds to engulf the initially surface-oriented osteogenic cell population. This new bone activity causes cancellous grafts at first to appear increased in radiographic density. Osteoclastic activity begins later in this sequence, and eventually the preexisting acellular graft is resorbed and replaced as remodeling ensues. The incorporation process of cancellous bone is relatively rapid and relatively complete as compared with that of cortical grafts.

Cortical bone revascularizes more slowly, with an initial ingrowth of blood vessels occurring peripherally and through preexisting haversian canals. Revascularization is aided by and, in part, is dependent upon a vigorous osteoclastic response, which causes increased porosity (decreased radiographic density) and reduced mechanical strength during the early stages of cortical graft incorporation. Resorption is followed by osteoblastic activity, resulting in "creeping substitution" of the original cortex, along with an increased mechanical strength; this phase of repair is followed by an ongoing remodeling mode. Cortical bone graft incorporation is slower and less complete than that seen with cancellous tissue, but the end result is substantial and is both biologically and biomechanically effective.

Revascularized Grafts

Revascularized grafts—those tissues transferred along with their vascular pedicles, which are reanastomosed at their site of implantation, and those grafts transferred limited distances such that their usual blood supply remains intact—do not undergo the incorporation process described for nonvascularized grafts. Instead, they unite to the recipient-site skeleton by a process analogous to fracture repair.[59] Theoretically, these grafts remain in a remodeling mode and do not sustain the initial cell necrosis, matrix resorption, and transient loss of mechanical strength characteristic of nonvascularized tissues.

Allografts

Allografts are tissues transferred between members of the *same species* (human to human, rabbit to rabbit, etc.). Unlike autografts, they do not require sacrifice of a normal structure when recovered from cadavers or when removed incidentally from a living donor in the course of an unrelated operative procedure. Furthermore, the potential morbidity associated with a second operative site, which is required to obtain autograft, is avoided; also, the limits in size, shape, and quantity of autogenous tissues are circumvented by allogeneic sources. On the other hand, allografts raise issues relevant to their biological potential, possible transfer of disease from donor to recipient, and immune responses to clearly foreign tissues.

At the present time, allografts in humans cannot be transferred successfully with an intact blood supply because of the effects of acute immunologic rejection on vascular endothelium. Results with immediately revascularized bone allografts in animals subjected to immunosuppressive regimens have, however, been encouraging.[47,58] Instead, al-

logeneic bone used clinically is usually subjected to some form of long-term preservation, especially freezing or lyophilization. In any case, cell viability within the graft is lost. This cellular activity is not prerequisite to the biological efficacy of bone grafts, but the relatively few cells that remain viable in fresh autografts undoubtedly contribute to the biological momentum observed during the initial stages of bone graft incorporation. Allografts, therefore, incorporate more slowly and, perhaps, less completely, but they are otherwise qualitatively similar to autografts. Various preservation techniques can, however, influence subsequent allograft repair.[8,9,24,31] For example, demineralization of allogeneic bone appears to enhance the osteoblastic response but reduces the initial strength of the graft. Lyophilization and high-dose irradiation contribute to long-term storage but also sacrifice mechanical characteristics.[19,41]

Xenografts

Xenografts are tissues transferred *between species* (cow to human, etc.), and although they are used clinically in some countries, past experience in the United States has been unsatisfactory. Lack of reliable bone graft incorporation, in particular, has detracted from the clinical application of these tissues. Efforts to combine xenografts with autogenous marrow and osteogenic factors are being explored and may stimulate renewed interest and reconsideration of the role of xenogeneic bone grafts in the future.[45]

Synthetic Bone Graft Materials

Despite their efficiency, the limited availability and potential donor site morbidity associated with autografts and the possibility of disease transmission intrinsic to allografts[18,19] have stimulated the use of synthetic bone graft materials. In general, these products have only osteoconductive properties and serve well as adjuncts to the repair of defects requiring limited biomechanical strength or as supplementation of fusion masses.[7] Similarly, these materials may be useful when combined with autologous bone marrow or bone grafts or as carriers for osteogenic proteins.[50,53]

A variety of synthetic hydroxyapatite (HA) and tricalcium phosphate (TCP) preparations, or combinations of these ceramics, have been manufactured for use as bone graft substitutes or supplements. Hydroxyapatite is not bioresorbable,[7,26] while TCP is slowly resorbed, accommodating increased new bone formation, but it is brittle.[29] By varying the ratio of HA to TCP as well as their pore sizes, composites with a range of osteoconductive, bioresorbable, and biomechanical properties have been developed. A nonceramic, bioresorbable, osteoconductive "cement" is also being evaluated.[14]

Collagen has been used in conjunction with HA and bone marrow[13] and as a carrier for osteoinductive proteins (BMPs),[40,43] as have biodegradable polymers of polylactic and/or polyglycolic acid.[37]

CLINICAL APPLICATIONS

The choice of appropriate graft material should be based upon knowledge of the biological and biomechanical advantages and disadvantages of specific types of bone as well as a clear understanding of the clinical circumstances and goals of the reparative procedure. As such, there may be more than one satisfactory solution for specific problems, but there are also relative inadequacies inherent to some alternatives. As already described, bone graft incorporation is a partnership between the graft and its host bed. The graft's primary contributions are its structural and osteoconductive nature, with the limited presence of osteogenic cells or proteins (depending upon its source and manner of preparation). On the other hand, virtually all of the cells and neovascularization required to incorporate the graft are derived from the host bed. An understanding of these principles will help guide the surgeon to utilize graft materials in the most efficacious manner and to recognize those circumstances that have the potential to interfere with graft success.[15]

General Considerations

Local host factors that interfere with host contributions to graft incorporation include the interposition of an inert material, such as polymethylmethacrylate, between the host bed and graft (thereby blocking the ingress of cells and blood supply); infection; incomplete removal of diseased or neoplastic tissue at the graft site (leading to tumor recurrence); the irradiation of bone and soft tissue at the host bed sufficient to interfere with vascularity; or inadequate coverage of the graft by well-vascularized soft tissue. Incorporation cannot occur if the graft's only contiguous support is metal or polyethylene. Systemic host factors that detract from bone graft incorporation are exemplified by chemotherapy, whereby required osteoprogenitor cells are adversely affected by these antimetabolic drugs, and the use of other drugs that interfere with the remodeling cycle. Doxorubicin (Adriamycin) and methotrexate, for example, are toxic to both osteoblastic and osteoclastic cells, in addition to their adverse influence on neoplastic tissues.[22]

Graft-related factors of importance to successful incorporation include both mechanical loading and stability for structural grafts, the nature of graft pretreatment or preservation, and the biological consequences of immunologic events (discussed in more detail below).

Autografts (Nonvascularized)

In general, the biological potential of autografts is maximal if not superior as compared with all other bone graft preparations.[8,9,24] Autografts must be highly considered for all circumstances requiring bone graft and especially where previous failure of biological potential has occurred (e.g., fracture nonunion) or where rapid incorporation, especially across relatively large gaps between bone ends, is crucial to success (e.g., arthrodesis of major joints).

Decisions regarding the choice of cortical or cancellous bone reflect the specific expectations of the graft material. It may have to act as a structural element, characteristic of cortex (struts, wafers, blocks, plates, etc.), or it may be used in filling cystic defects or in some other intrinsically stable circumstances ideally addressed by cancellous bone graft.

Autografts (Revascularized)

Revascularized autografts do not depend upon the host bed for their success, and their potential applications reflect this uniqueness.[59] They can therefore function in locations compromised by irradiation-induced changes (characterized by fibrosis and obliteration of small blood vessels). In addition, these grafts can be used in circumstances that may involve infection, generally a contraindication to the use of nonvascularized autografts or allografts. They also function in a superior fashion, as compared with alternatives, when the host bed has been compromised by irradiation, when there has been loss of adequate soft tissue coverage (e.g., due to trauma or after tumor resection), or when the patient is more generally (systemically) impaired (e.g., by chemotherapy). Vascularized bone autografts also offer the opportunity to bridge substantial distances of segmental loss with a tissue that rapidly unites at each osteosynthesis site and remains viable rather than undergoing necrosis followed by creeping substitution.

Potential disadvantages to this approach include its technically demanding and time-consuming nature and the limitations imposed by available donor sites, currently confined to the fibula, rib, or iliac crest. The shape and quantity of vascularized autograft is also, obviously, limited, as is the scope of mechanical properties; e.g., the fibula alone may be structurally inadequate to compensate properly for femoral or tibial bone stock.

Allografts

Allografts avoid the need for a donor site (characterized by postoperative discomfort, sacrifice of normal structures, etc.) and are available in virtually unlimited supply and any anatomic shape. At the present time, only nonvascularized allografts are feasible, but these can be preserved for elective reconstructive approaches, making them particularly well suited for the treatment of traumatic injuries and for limb-sparing tumor resections. Available clinical information suggests that 70 to 80 percent of massive frozen osteochondral allografts are associated with successful resolution of the problem for which they are employed.[36] Unsuccessful circumstances usually involve infection, failure to unite at the osteosynthesis site, or graft fracture.[35] The use of systemic chemotherapy also appears to have an adverse effect on bone graft repair.[22] Animal studies suggest that the biological capacity of allografts, especially those that have been deep-frozen or closely matched with respect to histocompatibility antigens, is qualitatively similar to that of autografts but temporally prolonged in terms of repair.[9,31]

Allografts should be highly considered where massive segmental loss is incurred provided that adequate soft tissue coverage and an aseptic environment can be anticipated. Allografts have also been used for filling cystic defects, in joint arthrodeses, and in fracture repair; clinical observations support their efficacy in these circumstances as well.[19]

IMMUNOLOGIC CONSIDERATIONS

Foreign tissues evoke immune responses, the nature and scope of which are influenced by a variety of factors. The degree of genetic disparity between donor and recipient, the route of immunization, as well as dose and time of exposure to antigen and the general immunocompetence of the recipient—all influence the expression of transplantation immunity. In addition, immune responses are manifest by both cellular and humoral components that are interrelated, often apparently reciprocal in intensity, and, in the case of bone, rarely of straightforward significance. Immunologic rejection is usually defined as an adverse influence on biological function resulting from a specific immune response. It is difficult to quantitate bone graft biology or function in vivo and by noninvasive techniques. Therefore, most approaches to assessing bone graft immunology and its significance have relied upon animal models.[17]

Animal Studies

Numerous approaches have been used to define bone allograft antigenicity in animals over the past 40 years. Virtually all these studies suggested that fresh allografts were strongly immunogenic, that deep-freezing prior to implantation significantly reduced the intensity of response, and that lyophilization decreased immunogenicity to negligible levels.[5,6,10,17,20] The most potent sources of bone graft–related antigens are associated with cells, particularly of the marrow. Nonetheless, recent studies by Horowitz and associates[27,28] have demonstrated that even bone depleted of marrow elements remains highly immunogenic in in vitro assays. Cell-surface antigens of the major histocompatibility complex (MHC) specifically activate T cells of the killer/suppressor phenotype. These cells are then presumed to act both as direct effectors of immune responses and as sources of cytokines (e.g., interleukin-1, tumor necrosis factor α) capable of activating osteoblasts. Osteoblasts, in turn, through secretion of soluble mediators, may cause osteoclast activation and bone graft resorption. Studies by Stevenson and colleagues[48] have demonstrated that allografts exchanged between closely matched dogs were more successfully incorporated than grafts transplanted across a strong MHC barrier. These observations suggest a relationship in animals between a graft's immunogenicity and its biological fate.

Experience in Humans

The evaluation of bone graft immunogenicity in humans has been relatively limited; however, available information parallels that obtained in animals.[16] Human recipients of fresh bone allografts usually develop humoral antibodies following transplantation.[32] The response seen after implantation of massive frozen allograft appears to be reduced modestly in both frequency and intensity, and even more so if the bone has been freeze-dried.[21,44] In a multi-institutional study, immunologic responses were monitored in 84 patients receiving massive frozen osteochondral allografts.[49] Sixty-seven percent of patients were sensitized to class I, class II, or classes I and II human leukocyte antigens (HLA). Attempts to correlate these responses with the biological fate of bone grafts have, to date, been inconclusive.

BONE BANKING

The goals of bone banking are to provide adequate quantities of biologically useful tissues at times dictated by clinical circumstance and without concern for transferring disease from donor to recipient. Guidelines and standards that address these requirements have been developed by the American Association of Tissue Banks.[2,18,51]

Donor Selection Criteria

Bone grafts can be recovered from living donors "incidentally" in the course of operative procedures necessitating the removal of bone (e.g., femoral heads during joint replacement) or from cadaveric sources. In either event, appropriate authorization from the individual or next of kin is required, and the history of the potential donor is carefully reviewed. The basic principle in screening donors is to avoid the use of bone as a vector for transmission of a potentially serious illness to the recipient and to avoid the use of bone whose biological or physical properties may be compromised or may be viewed as unpredictable. Contraindications to tissue donation, therefore, include evidence of sepsis or infection of the bone to be recovered; malignancies, particularly those with a propensity to metastasize to the skeleton; viral diseases, including hepatitis, rabies, Creutzfeld-Jakob disease (and other slow-virus disorders), and acquired immunodeficiency syndrome (AIDS); venereal diseases; the presence of toxic substances in toxic amounts; systemic collagen disorders; and diseases of unknown etiology.

Tissue Recovery, Preservation, and Storage

Bone may be recovered in a sterile fashion using an operating room environment and customary technique, or tissues may be removed under clean conditions that require secondary sterilization. High-dose irradiation and chemicals (e.g., ethylene oxide or concentrated acids) have been used widely to render tissues free from pathogens, but these may, in turn, influence the mechanical properties of bone.[41]

Once removed, tissues may be preserved for later application by a wide variety of approaches, including deep-freezing, lyophilization, or combinations of chemical extractions and chemosterilization. Again, manipulation of the graft may cause changes in its biological or biomechanical properties,[41] but the importance of these changes will vary with intended clinical applications. For example, lyophilization causes gross structural cracks that render bone less capable of withstanding loads. Such tissue may not be suitable for segmental replacements unless methods of internal fixation compensate for this weakness; however, loss of mechanical strength will be of no significance when such tissue is used to fill cystic defects. The author's preferred method of tissue acquisition and long-term preservation is sterile recovery and frozen storage at −70 to −80°C.

Unlike that of bone, the preservation of cartilage requires retention of cell viability. For this purpose, the articular surface is exposed to either glycerol or dimethyl sulfoxide (DMSO) prior to freezing. This results in viability of no more than 40 percent of chondrocytes but appears to be compatible with matrix homeostasis.[52]

Record Keeping

Record keeping should document the donor's medical history as well as results of laboratory tests, including those for hepatitis and venereal diseases. Records also provide an opportunity to identify donor-recipient combinations in the event of adverse reactions that may be related to bone graft.

SUMMARY

In summary, the future will undoubtedly provide opportunities to use fresh vascularized allografts, but their applications and logistics will remain complex and limited. Other forms of providing reliable osteogenic potential, either by treatment of allogeneic or xenogeneic bone or by using factors and cells of skeletal tissue origin, will emerge and decrease reliance upon autografts. In addition, methods to enhance the body's own osteogenic activity, either by systemic drugs or physical signals, will continue to be pursued. At this time, it is important to understand the biological aspects of bone graft repair, including the contributions of the graft and of the recipient site. Only then can one appreciate the biomechanical consequences of graft incorporation biology and use this knowledge to make an appropriate choice of graft material and of surgical methodology. Further, one can then also recognize and utilize responsible ways to bank allografts for later clinical applications. The surgeon must clearly understand the goals of the operative procedure in which bone graft will play a

role and must match these circumstances (including changes anticipated over time) with the graft material appropriate for such intended use.

REFERENCES

1. Albee FH: *Bone-Graft Surgery.* Philadelphia, Saunders, 1915.
2. American Association of Tissue Banks: *Standards for Tissue Banking.* Arlington, VA, American Association of Tissue Banks, 1993.
3. Baylink DJ, Finkelman RD, Mohan S: Growth factors to stimulate bone formation. *J Bone Min Res* 8:5565–5572, 1993.
4. Bick EM: *Source of Orthopaedics.* New York, Hafner, 1968.
5. Bonfiglio M, Jeter WS, Smith CL: The immune concept: Its relation to bone transplantation. *Ann NY Acad Sci* 59:417–432, 1955.
6. Brooks DB, Heiple KG, Herndon CH, Powell AE: Immunological factors in homogeneous bone transplantation. IV: The effect of various methods of preparation and irradiation on antigenicity. *J Bone Joint Surg* 45A:1617–1626, 1963.
7. Bucholz RW, Carlton A, Holmes RE: Hydroxyapatite and tricalcium phosphate bone graft substitutes. *Orthop Clin North Am* 18:323–334, 1987.
8. Burchardt H: The biology of bone graft repair. *Clin Orthop* 174:28–42, 1983.
9. Burwell RG: The fate of bone grafts, in Apley AG (ed): *Recent Advances in Orthopaedics.* Baltimore, Williams & Wilkins, 1963, pp 115–207.
10. Burwell RG, Gowland G: Studies in the transplantation of bone. III: The immune response of lymph nodes draining components of fresh homogeneous bone treated by different methods. *J Bone Joint Surg* 44B:131–148, 1963.
11. Centrella M, McCarthy TL, Canalis E: Current concepts review: Transforming growth factor-beta and remodeling of bone. *J Bone Joint Surg* 73A:1418–1428, 1991.
12. Chen TL, Bates RL, Dulley A, et al: Bone morphogenetic protein-2B stimulation of growth and osteogenic phenotypes in rat osteoblast-like cells: Comparison with TGF-alpha 1. *J Bone Min Res* 6:1387–1393, 1991.
13. Cornell C, Lane J, Chapman M, et al: Multicenter trial of collograft as bone graft substitute. *J Orthop Trauma* 5:1–8, 1991.
14. Costantino PD, Friedman CD, Jones K, et al: Experimental hydroxyapatite cement. *Cranioplasty Plastic Reconstr Surg* 90:174–185, 1992.
15. Friedlaender GE: Bone grafts: The basic science rationale for clinical applications. *J Bone Joint Surg* 69A:786–790, 1987.
16. Friedlaender GE: Immune responses to preserved bone allografts in humans, in Friedlaender GE, Mankin HJ, Sell KW (eds): *Osteochondral Allografts: Biology, Banking and Clinical Applications.* Boston, Little, Brown, 1983, pp 159–164.
17. Friedlaender GE: Immune responses to osteochondral allografts: Current knowledge and future directions. *Clin Orthop* 174:58–68, 1983.
18. Friedlaender GE, Mankin HJ: Bone banking: Current methods and suggested guidelines. *Instr Course Lect* 30:36–55, 1981.
19. Friedlaender GE, Mankin HJ, Sell KW: *Osteochondral Allografts: Biology, Banking and Clinical Applications.* Boston, Little, Brown, 1983.
20. Friedlaender GE, Strong DM, Sell KW: Studies on the antigenicity of bone. I: Freeze-dried and deep-frozen bone allografts in rabbits. *J Bone Joint Surg* 58A:854–858, 1976.
21. Friedlaender GE, Strong DM, Sell KW: Studies on the antigenicity of bone. II: Donor-specific anti-HLA antibodies in human recipients of freeze-dried bone allografts. *J Bone Joint Surg* 66A:107–112, 1984.

22. Friedlaender GE, Tross RB, Doganis AC, et al: Effects of chemotherapeutic agents on bone. I: Short-term methotrexate and doxorubicin (Adriamycin) treatment in a rat model. *J Bone Joint Surg* 66A:602–607, 1984.

23. Goldring SR, Goldring MB: Cytokines and skeletal physiology. *Clin Orthop* 323:13–23, 1996.

24. Heiple KG, Chase SW, Herndon CH: A comparative study of the healing process following different types of bone transplantation. *J Bone Joint Surg* 45A:1593–1616, 1963.

25. Heslop BF, Zeiss IM, Nisbet MW: Studies on transference of bone. I: A comparison of autologous and homologous bone implants with reference to osteocyte survival, osteogenesis and host reaction. *Br J Exp Pathol* 41:269–287, 1960.

26. Hoogendoorn HA, Renooij W, Akkermans LM, et al: Long-term study of large ceramic implants (porous hydroxyapatite) in dog femora. *Clin Orthop* 187:281–288, 1984.

27. Horowitz MC, Friedlaender GE: Induction of specific T-cell responsiveness to allogeneic bone. *J Bone Joint Surg* 73A: 1157–1168, 1991.

28. Horowitz MC, Friedlaender GE, Qian H-Y: The immune response: The efferent arm. *Clin Orthop* 326:25–34, 1996.

29. Jarcho M: Calcium phosphate ceramics as hard tissue prosthetics. *Clin Orthop* 157:259–278, 1981.

30. Knutsen R, Mohan S, Wergedad J, et al: Osteogenic protein-1 stimulates proliferation and differentiation of human bone cells in vitro. *J Bone Min Res* 6:231, 1991.

31. Kreuz FP, Hyatt GW, Turner TC, Bassett AL: The preservation and clinical use of freeze-dried bone. *J Bone Joint Surg* 33A:863–872, 1951.

32. Langer F, Gross AE, West M, Urovitz EP: The immunogenicity of allograft knee joint transplants. *Clin Orthop* 132:155–162, 1978.

33. Lexer E: Joint transplantation and arthroplasty. *Surg Gynecol Obstet* 40:782, 1925.

34. Macewen W: Observations concerning transplantation of bone: Illustrated by a case of interhuman osseous transplantation, whereby over two-thirds of the shaft of a humerus was restored. *Proc R Soc Lond* 32:232, 1881.

35. Mankin HJ: Complications of allograft surgery, in Friedlaender GE, Mankin HJ, Sell KW (eds): *Osteochondral Allografts: Biology, Banking and Clinical Applications.* Boston, Little, Brown, 1983, pp 259–274.

36. Mankin HJ, Doppelt SH, Sullivan TR, Tomford WW: Osteoarticular and intercalary allograft transplantation in the management of malignant tumors of bone. *Cancer* 50:613–630, 1982.

37. Miyamoto S, Takaoka K, Okada T, et al: Evaluation of polylactic acid homopolymers as carriers for bone morphogenetic protein. *Clin Orthop* 272:274–285, 1992.

38. Mundy GR: Regulation of bone formation by bone morphogenetic proteins and other growth factors. *Clin Orthop* 323:24–28, 1996.

39. Ollier L: *Traite experimental et clinque de la regeneration des os.* Paris, Masson, 1867.

40. Ono I, Ohura T, Murata, et al: A study on bone induction in hydroxyapatite combined with bone morphogenetic protein. *Plast Reconstr Surg* 40:870–879, 1992.

41. Pelker RR, Friedlaender GE, Markham TC: Biomechanical properties of bone allografts. *Clin Orthop* 174:54–57, 1983.

42. Phemister DB: The fate of transplanted bone and regenerative power of its various constituents. *Surg Gynecol Obstet* 19:33–39, 1914.

43. Ripamonti U, Ma S, Van den Heever B, Reddi H: Osteogenins: A bone morphogenetic protein, absorbed in porous hydroxyapatite substrata, induces rapid bone differentiation in calvarial defects of adult primates. *Plast Reconstr Surg* 90:382–393, 1992.

44. Rodrigo JJ, Fuller TC, Mankin HJ: Cytotoxic HLA antibodies in patients with bone and cartilage allografts. *Trans Orthop Res Soc* 1:131, 1976.

45. Salama R: Xenogeneic bone grafting in humans. *Clin Orthop* 174:113–121, 1983.

46. Sampath TK, Maliakal JC, Hacischka PV, et al: Recombinant human osteogenic protein induces new bone formation in vivo with specific activity comparable to natural bovine OP and stimulates osteoblast proliferation and differentiation in vitro. *J Biol Chem* 267:20352–20362, 1992.

47. Stevenson S, Emery SE, Goldberg VM: Factors affecting bone graft incorporation. *Clin Orthop* 323:66–74, 1996.

48. Stevenson S, Li XQ, Martin B: The fate of cancellous and cortical bone after transplantation of fresh and frozen tissue-antigen-matched and mismatched osteochondral allografts in dogs. *J Bone Joint Surg* 73A:1143–1156, 1991.

49. Strong DM, Friedlaender GE, Tomford WW, et al: Immunological responses in human recipients of osseous and osteochondral allografts. *Clin Orthop* 326:107–114, 1996.

50. Takaoka K, Nakahara H, Yosmikawa H, et al: Ectopic bone induction on and in porous hydroxyapatite combined with collagen and bone morphogenetic protein. *Clin Orthop* 234: 250–254, 1988.

51. Tomford WW, Friedlaender GE: 1983 bone banking procedures. *Clin Orthop* 174:15–21, 1983.

52. Tomford WW, Mankin HJ: Investigational approaches to articular cartilage preservation. *Clin Orthop* 174:22–27, 1983.

53. Uchida A, Nade S, McCartney E, Ching W: Bone ingrowth into three different porous ceramics implanted into the tibia of rats and rabbits. *J Orthop Res* 3:65–77, 1985.

54. Urist MR: Bone formation by autoinduction. *Science* 150: 893–899, 1965.

55. Urist MR, Delange RJ, Finerman GAM: Bone cell differentiation and growth factors. *Science* 220:680–686, 1983.

56. Urist MR, Sato K, Brownell AG, et al: Human bone morphogenetic protein (hBMP). *Proc Soc Exp Biol Med* 173:194–199, 1983.

57. Urist MR, Silverman BG, Buring K, et al: The bone induction principle. *Clin Orthop* 53:243, 1967.

58. Weiland AJ: Current concepts review: Vascularized free bone transplants. *J Bone Joint Surg* 63A:166–169, 1981.

59. Weiland AJ, Moore JR, Daniel RK: Vascularized bone autografts: Experience with 41 cases. *Clin Orthop* 174:87–95, 1983.

60. Yasko A, Lane J, Fellinger E, et al: The healing of segmental bone defects induced by recombinant human bone morphogenetic protein (rhBMP-2): A radiographic histological and biomechanical study in rats. *J Bone Joint Surg* 74A:659–670, 1992.

CHAPTER 9

Articular Cartilage

Juergen Mollenhauer
and Klaus E. Kuettner

The chondrocyte, the resident cell of the cartilage tissue, is embedded in its very own specific environment. This "universe" is filled with the extracellular hydrated cartilage matrix and, in the absence of vascular elements, penetrated only by small biomolecules that provide nutrition and by regulatory biomolecules—i.e., tissue hormones. Cartilage is an aneural, bradytrophic, and immunologically privileged tissue.

Typically, each chondrocyte is separated from the neighboring cells by an extracellular matrix. In the absence of direct cellular communication, the chondrocyte receives all essential information for the control and maintenance of its extracellular matrix and for its intracellular activities from the biophysical (biomechanical) modulation of the tissue. This biophysical behavior is governed by the physical properties of the extracellular matrix molecules and by ion fluxes. During mechanical loading, both the matrix molecules and the ion fluxes undergo alterations in very characteristic patterns. Hence, a chondrocyte is in a cross point between the physical and the chemical aspects of life. Superimposed on these normal functions are events that require significantly different capabilities of a chondrocyte: repair of damaged tissue and response to infections, wherein the chondrocyte acts as an autonomous repair and self-defense unit.

TISSUE ARCHITECTURE

The structure of articular cartilage, as revealed by histologic techniques, is described elsewhere in this book but is briefly summarized here in order to familiarize the reader with the terms in the following segments.

Adult articular cartilage, an avascular and noninnervated tissue, can be grossly subdivided into four horizontal layers with different cell types and molecular compositions: (1) the superficial zone, (2) the middle and deep zones, (3) the tidemark, and (4) the calcified zone at the subchondral bone interface (Fig. 9-1).[1]

The Superficial Zone

The superficial zone consists of one to three layers of flattened cells. These cells, less than 10 percent of all the cells in articular cartilage, are distinctly different from the other cells of the articular cartilage. They produce their own particular subset of extracellular matrix proteins,[2,3] including a very special proteoglycan.[4] Joints are not surrounded by a basement membrane; the superficial zone itself probably serves as a "basement membrane" equivalent, with the function to separate cartilage from the peripheral tissue and body fluid. In addition, the superficial cells are very sensitive to irritation, respond strongly to interleukin-1,[5,6] exhibit stimulated phagocytosis[7] and Ia antigen presentation,[8] and can be triggered to release reactive oxygen species and eicosanoids, making them very similar in their capacities to macrophages.[9–11]

The Middle and Deep Zones

The deeper layers of chondrocytes are made up of articular chondrocytes of spherical shape, surrounded by a distinct halo of "territorial" or "pericellular" matrix that has different properties and compositions than the "interterritorial" or "further removed" matrix.[1] These cells are the major providers for the function of the articular cartilage and represent and control most (over 80 percent) of the tissue. The chondrocytes of the deeper layers produce all the extracellular matrix components found in the articular cartilage: collagens, proteoglycans, glycoproteins, hyaluronan, and degradative enzymes (mostly metalloproteinases) needed for tissue turnover.[12]

Depending upon the joint and the location within a joint, they appear either as single cells or grouped together in "chondrons" of two to several cells, most likely representing a clonal colony.[1] The chondrons can be seen as a functional subcompartment within the cartilage matrix designed to host the chondrocytes.[13,14] A chondron's matrix is both structurally and functionally different from the interterritorial matrix and may represent the equivalent of the territorial matrix of single chondrocytes.[14] The extracellular matrix in a chondron has a higher turnover rate than in the interterritorial matrix. Its quantitative composition is not well known. However, even in a chondron, no cellular junctions exist between adjacent chondrocytes.

The Calcified Zone and the Tidemark

The deepest layers of chondrocytes in articular cartilage are situated within a calcified extracellular matrix and form a transitional tissue to the underlying bone.[15] However, differing from bone, the calcification is sparse. The calcified zone prevents the diffusion of nutrients from the bone tissue into the cartilage. The tidemark is a cell-free line of about 10-μm thickness made visible by histologic staining at the border between the uncalcified and the calcified cartilage. Its molecular composition is unknown except for some accumulated calcium-containing mineral deposits. The staining behavior toward certain dyes indicates increased concentrations of glycoproteins and extracellular lipids. The tidemark may mark the line of the most recent turnover of the calcified tissue, or a "sink" for metabolic (end) products, since it tends to migrate upward with age.[16]

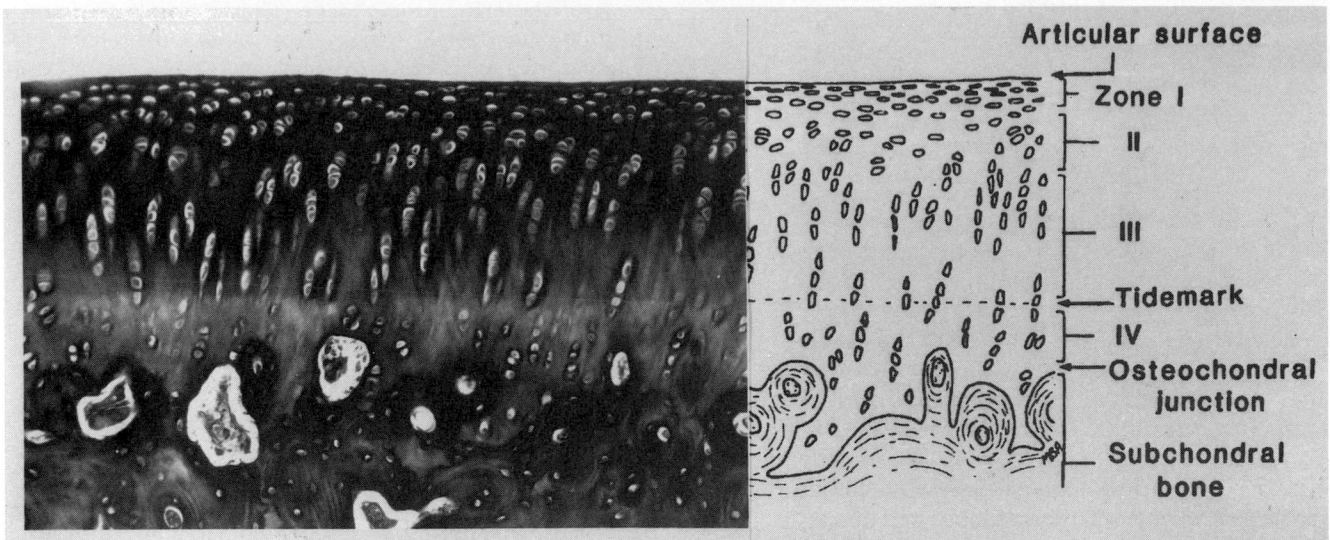

Figure 9-1 Vertical section through the articular cartilage and subchondral bone of canine femural condyle, showing the superficial zone (zone I), the middle and deep zones (zones II and III), the tidemark, the calcified zone (zone IV), and the subchondral bone, with a diagrammatic representation on the right (stained Mallroy-Heidenhain, ×170). (Courtesy of M. B. Aydelotte.)

MOLECULAR FINE STRUCTURE

The articular cartilage of the adult is dominated by the extracellular matrix, since cells age-dependently occupy only 5 percent or less of the tissue mass. The importance of the extracellular matrix is also apparent in the function: the biomechanical properties are governed by the extracellular matrix,[17,18] in contrast to, for example, striated muscle, where the myotubes determine the biomechanical behavior.

Cartilage matrix is a compound structure. Its major elements are water, fibers (collagen), hydrophilic aggregates (proteoglycans, hyaluronan, glycoproteins), and ions. The collagen fiber bundles with a diameter of about 60 nm and a length of several micrometers are grossly arranged in patterns like those found in the pillars of gothic cathedrals: extending vertically from their basis in the calcified zone and forming a cross-vault underneath the superficial zone (which itself has horizontal layers of diagonally arranged fibers). It is believed that the vertical fibers help to guide load vertically through the cartilage into the bone, whereas the horizontal fibers of the articular surface might guide lateral shear forces during joint motion into the adjacent connective tissue of the synovium. The diameter of the collagen fiber increases in the deeper zones.[1]

This gross orientation is supported by a network of "random"-oriented short and very fine fibrils. Within collagen fibers, about 0.8 g of water is bound per gram of collagen. At a collagen content of about 20 percent wet weight, the 200-mg collagen fibers in 1 g of cartilage bind approximately 160 mg water.[17] Interdispersed within this meshwork and attached to it are aggregates of proteoglycans, hyaluronan, and glycoproteins. The ability of these macromolecules to bind large quantities of water builds up the hydrostatic pressure of the tissue. It is the proteoglycan content that is mostly responsible for the water content of cartilage tissue: 50 mg of proteoglycans correspond to about 400 mg of cartilage water.[17] The collagen meshwork allows expansion of the hydrated aggregates to about only 40 percent of maximum hydration. Thus, there is a permanent tendency of cartilage to take up water. The swelling of the tissue is counteracted by the loading forces during motion, which can exceed 1 metric ton per joint. This enormous pressure releases the water molecules from the matrix molecules into the joint space, where it contributes to joint lubrication.[19–22] The constant movement of water and ions during the cyclic loading and unloading of the joint cartilage is the pump mechanism that provides nutrients for the chondrocytes[23] and eliminates metabolic waste products into the synovial fluid through pores (about 2 nm in size) within the extracellular matrix.[17] Larger pores (greater than 3 nm) allow for the movement of regulatory peptides and hormones into the cartilage and the release of degraded extracellular matrix fragments into the synovial fluid during cyclic loading.[17]

MACROMOLECULAR COMPONENTS

Three components dominate the quantitative picture of cartilage matrix molecules: cartilage-specific type II collagen, the large proteoglycan aggrecan, and the polysaccharide hyaluronan. Together, they make up approximately 90 percent of the tissue dry mass.[12] These three major elements are accompanied by a number of minor but functionally important collagens, small proteoglycans, and other glycoproteins.[12] Their molecular properties are listed in Table 9-1. Most of the matrix proteins are able not only

TABLE 9-1   Structural Macromolecules of the Extracellular Cartilage Matrix

Macromolecule	Location in cartilage	Molecular properties—molecular weight, subunits or core protein
Collagens in normal cartilage		
II	Fibers, ubiquitous	300,000; homotrimer
XI	Fiber cores	450,000; heterotrimer
IX	Fiber periphery	500,000; heterotrimer, 1 chondroitin sulfate chain
VI	Independent meshwork	570,000; heterotrimer
X	Hypertrophic portion of growth plate	180,000; heterotrimer
Collagens in osteoarthritic cartilage		
I	Fibers, ubiquitous	300,000; heterotrimer
III	Pericellular (?) fibers	300,000; homotrimer
X	Pericellular meshwork	180,000; heterotrimer
Proteoglycans		
Aggrecan	Ubiquitous	240,000
Decorin	Preferentially superficial layer	35,000
Byglycan	Codistributed with aggrecan	36,000
Fibromodulin	Codistributed with aggrecan	37,000
Syndecan	Cell surface-intercalated	30,000
Lumican	Codistributed with aggrecan	38,000
SZP (superficial zone protein)	Joint surface and synovial fluid	345,000
Glycosaminoglycans		
Hyaluronan = hyaluronic acid (HA)	Ubiquitous, complexed with aggrecan via → link protein	>1,000,000
Chondroitin sulfate (CS)	Aggrecan, syndecan, collagen type IX	2,000–20,000
	Biglycan, decorin, SZP	20,000–50,000
Keratan sulfate (KS)	Aggrecan, fibromodulin, SZP	1,000–12,000
Heparan sulfate (HS)	Syndecan	1,000–10,000
Glycoproteins		
Fibronectin	Pericellular (?) fibers	440,000; homodimer
Cartilage oligomeric protein (COMP) = thrombospondin 3	Ubiquitous, independent meshwork?	524,000; homopentamer
Tenascin	Perichondrial network	1,900,000; heterohexamer
Chondroadherin	Pericellular	38,400
Cartilage matrix protein (CMP)	Ubiquitous, binding-dependent on divalent cations	148,000; homotrimer
58-kDa matrix protein	Interstitial	41,600
Lubricin	Joint surface	227,500
Laminin	Perichondrium	900,000; heterotrimer
Chondrocyte matrix glycoprotein (CMGP)	Cell surface, membrane–associated (oxidase activity)	550,000
Chondronectin	Cell surface–associated	175,800; homotrimer

to assemble into a defined extracellular matrix element and bind to other matrix molecules but also to bind to receptors and binding proteins on the chondrocyte surface. This feature may anchor the chondrocyte in the matrix and provide metabolic information on the status of each matrix molecule within the tissue.

Collagens

The major collagen type in cartilage is collagen type II, representing about 90 percent of all collagens.[24] The collagen fibers of articular cartilage are composed of a core of types XI and II collagen, surrounded by multiple layers of type II collagen molecules and finally some type IX collagen attached to the fiber surface (Fig. 9-2).[25,26] The quantitative balance of the different collagen types in a fiber determines the size and shape of one individual collagen fiber bundle.[26,27] Type IX collagen has one chondroitin sulfate side chain that makes it a transitional molecule between the collagens and the proteoglycans. This feature might link both macromolecular elements together to form one functional [collagen fiber:proteoglycan aggregate] complex.[28] Other minor collagens are dispersed within this major fiber network. Type VI collagen, a collagen that forms a three-dimensional meshwork but not fibers,[29] is found in particular in the chondrons.[30] Since type VI collagen is found in all tissues with high tensile stresses (trabecular meshwork of the eye, synovial tissue), its function might be in carrying part of the shear stress in joints. Type X

collagen is found primarily in the hypertrophic zone of fetal growth plate cartilage.[31] As type VI, it forms a meshwork but not fibers.[28] Type X collagen is not processed from procollagen to a mature triple-helical collagen but maintains its procollagen peptides, through which it is cross-linked with other collagen molecules. Functionally, it seems to be related to the calcification process of the fetal cartilage. In adult articular cartilage, it can be detected only in (early) osteoarthritis.[32,33]

Proteoglycans

The major proteoglycan in cartilage is aggrecan (Fig. 9-3).[34] Aggrecan consists of five different domains: three globular (G) and two extended domains. The N-terminal protein portion starts with the G1 domain, which carries the binding site for link protein. The G1 domain possesses oligosaccharide side chains and highly susceptible cleavage sites for metalloproteinases. The extended domains carry the polysulfated polysaccharide side chains keratan sulfate and chondroitin sulfate. The C-terminal G3 domain is unglycosylated and, as the G1 domain, is readily cleaved off by metalloproteinases during catabolism. The large carbohydrate side chains of the extended domains guarantee the strongly hydrophilic nature of the molecule and allow for the maintenance of a large hydration radius of each aggrecan molecule in solution. However, as mentioned before, the hydration of the proteoglycans in the tissue is restricted by the collagen meshwork. Thus, both types of

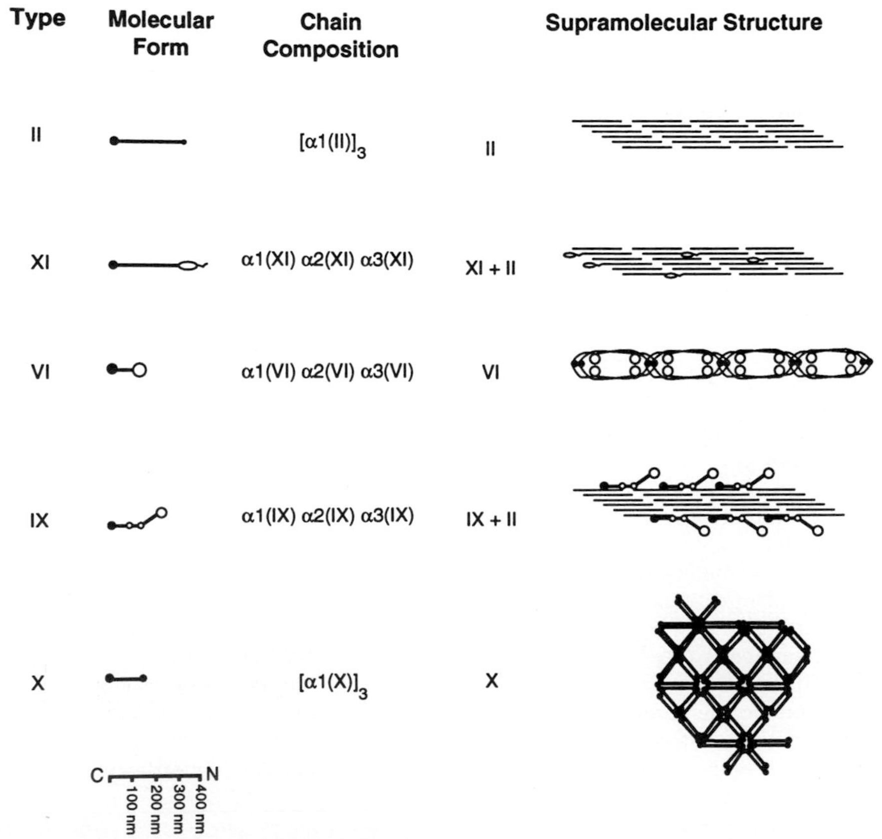

Type	Molecular Form	Chain Composition	Supramolecular Structure
II		$[\alpha1(II)]_3$	II
XI		$\alpha1(XI)\ \alpha2(XI)\ \alpha3(XI)$	XI + II
VI		$\alpha1(VI)\ \alpha2(VI)\ \alpha3(VI)$	VI
IX		$\alpha1(IX)\ \alpha2(IX)\ \alpha3(IX)$	IX + II
X		$[\alpha1(X)]_3$	X

Figure 9-2 Diagrammatic representation of the collagen types found in cartilage. *Left panel:* individual collagen molecules, drawn to scale. *Right panel:* schematic representation of possible supramolecular fiber and network assemblies.

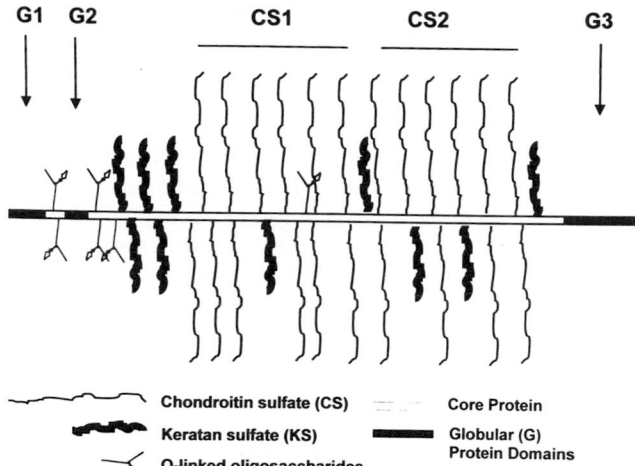

Chondroitin sulfate (CS)
Keratan sulfate (KS)
O-linked oligosaccharides
Core Protein
Globular (G)
Protein Domains

Figure 9-3 Diagrammatic representation of aggrecan, the large cartilage proteoglycan. The globular domains of the core protein are drawn in black boxes, the extended domains in white boxes. The presentation is not to scale and does not depict the correct number of glycosylation sites and polysaccharide side chains.

molecules together lay the foundation for the hydromechanical properties of cartilage tissue described above. As to the collagens, the so-called minor proteoglycans—decorin, lumican, fibromodulin, and biglycan (Table 9-1)—complete the functional pattern and fine-tune the structural properties of the cartilage proteoglycan matrix.[34–36] For example, lumican is found in many connective tissues as a glycoprotein. However, in cartilage, it is substituted with a keratan sulfate side chain and therefore a transitional molecule to proteoglycans. The keratan sulfate–bearing variant is predominantly found in juvenile articular cartilage, whereas adult cartilage contains more of the keratan sulfate–free modification.[36]

A distinct proteoglycan, superficial zone protein (SZP), is secreted from the superficial cell layer. It has similarities in amino acid composition to the large mucoproteins secreted by the epithelial layers of the gastrointestinal tract, but it also carries a keratan sulfate side chain that makes it unique for cartilage.[4] Since the protein is found only in the superficial zone of the articular cartilage—in the synovial lining cells and the synovial fluid—it may be involved in joint lubrication.

The major protein-free polysaccharide in cartilage is hyaluronan.[37] Along its chain of several 10,000 disaccharide units of [glucose–glucuronic acid], it binds proteoglycans stabilized by a link protein.[38,39] Cartilage link protein is a very hydrophobic protein with the unique property to bind simultaneously to hyaluronan and the G1 domain of aggrecan.[38,39] This results in the formation of molecular aggregates of several million daltons, the size of an average virus particle. These aggregates are too large to escape from the collagen network and are therefore not found in body fluids outside the cartilage tissue.[34,35] The appearance of fragments of the proteoglycan aggregates in body fluids is therefore a very sensitive indicator of the normal turnover and of pathologic conditions in cartilage.[40,41] Hyaluronan is also involved in joint lubrication,

first by its high water-binding capacity and also because of its "rheodynamic" behavior.[19–22,42,43] Without mechanical load, hyaluronan is a three-dimensional globular polymer. Under sudden pressure, it contributes to high viscosity of the pressurized solution in the joint space. Under shear stress, the molecule forms linear filaments that permit smooth gliding along the longitudinal axis, thus allowing for smooth, dampened gliding of the joint surfaces.

Glycoproteins

Although minor in abundance, the glycoproteins in the extracellular matrix of articular cartilage carry a significant portion of the functional properties of the tissue. They may represent a "tissue cement," but at the same time they may be involved in the regulation of the chondrocyte phenotype. A major glycoprotein of cartilage is cartilage oligomeric protein (COMP),[44] composed of five monomers assembled in a spiderlike configuration.[45] The oligomer is able to bind to other matrix proteins as well as to the chondrocyte surface. Fibronectin, the dominant glycoprotein of the noncartilagenous matrix, is present only in relatively small amounts in normal cartilage.[46] The detection of significant quantities is an indicator of pathologic changes.[47] However, since fibronectin also binds to the chondrocyte surface via integrins, its small quantity might not reflect its importance in the metabolic regulation of the tissue. Chondrocalcin is a calcium-binding glycoprotein exclusively found in cartilage.[48,49] It is the N-terminal propeptide of collagen type II and therefore synchronized with type II collagen metabolism.[48] However, unlike other procollagen peptides that are released and quickly degraded during the processing of the collagen fiber, chondrocalcin resides in the tissue as an independent structural element.[49,50] Laminin has been detected in the pericellular matrix of articular chondrocytes.[50,51] In other tissues, laminin is a major component of basement membranes. As there is no basement membrane in cartilage, the function of laminin in cartilage is still unclear. Lubricin has been described as a component of the synovial fluid and obtained its name because of its postulated function as a joint lubricant.[52,53] Tenascin is a glycoprotein found in many connective tissues in several isoforms.[54] Its extended three-dimensionality as a six-armed spiderlike molecule indicates a particular role in tissue cross-linking. Normal articular cartilage contains some pericellular tenascin; osteoarthritic conditions cause a significant upregulation and deposition throughout the extracellular matrix.[55] Chondroadherin has been described first as a glycoprotein that promotes adhesion of chondrocytes to solid substrates. It has a high content of leucine and an unusually high isoelectrical point of 9.5 to 9.8,[56] features shared by several novel cartilage glycoproteins.[57,58] Cartilage matrix protein (CMP) is anchored in the cartilage matrix by complexation with divalent (possibly calcium) cations.[59] As part of the chondrocyte surface and anchored on the plasma membrane, cartilage matrix glycoprotein (CMGP) forms a connection from the class of extracellular matrix proteins to the class of molecules that helps to anchor the chondrocyte in the extracellular matrix.[60] It is closely related to ceruloplasmin and might be involved in metal ion transport. Another member of such cell surface–associated glycoproteins is chondronectin.[61] Like chondroadherin, it promotes chondrocyte adhesion.

Matrix Metalloproteinases and Their Inhibitors

Matrix metalloproteinases are intrinsic components of the cartilage matrix (Table 9-2).[62–65] The classic definition is "members of a family of zinc metalloproteinases of animal origin that act outside the cell on components of the extracellular matrix and that are homologous to interstitial collagenase."[62] They can be classified into stromelysins, gelatinases, collagenases, and membrane-associated metalloproteinases. Collagenases are endoproteinases that cleave intact collagen triple helices, including those in the supramolecular fiber structures. The resulting cleavage products are thermally unstable and denature from the typical triple helix into a random coil. Gelatinases are able to degrade only already precleaved and denatured single collagen polypeptide chains. Both types are not restricted to collagen as a substrate but also degrade other matrix proteins as well. Stromelysins are metalloproteinases with a broad spectrum of substrates, including proteoglycans and other matrix (glyco-) proteins. Typical proteoglycan cleavage products lose their ability to bind to hyaluronan and other matrix components and therefore are lost from cartilage. A new class of cell surface membrane-intercalated metalloproteinases are called ADAMs.[66] It is the transmembrane domain that makes them unique among the metalloproteinases, although they are closely related to the other metalloproteinases from their proteinase domains. Metalloproteinases are involved in the normal turnover of matrix molecules by cleaving the macrostructures of collagen fibers and proteoglycan aggregates into defined and, for the chondrocyte, accessible fragments. It is currently not clear how many of the known metalloproteinases are expressed in normal cartilage. If excessively upregulated, they might contribute significantly to the development and progression of osteoarthritis.[65]

The natural counterparts of the metalloproteinases are proteinase inhibitors such as tissue-induced metalloproteinase inhibitors (TIMP).[67,68] Four isoforms have been characterized: TIMP-1, -2, -3 and cartilage-derived inhibitor (CDI); the last of these has a unique status in cartilage, as it is most likely not produced by chondrocytes.[69] Its acquisition from the lymphatic fluid and accumulation in cartilage is passive. The TIMPs are acidic polypeptides that bind readily to the basic elements of matrix proteins—i.e., collagen. Thus they may prevent excessive degradation of the cartilage matrix by metalloproteinases. Inhibitors such as TIMP are also responsible for the "antiangiogenic" property of cartilage, which results in the avascularity of the tissue (even in chondrosarcomas!). Angiogenesis depends strongly on the degradation of the tissue by proteinases released by the migrating vascular endothelium and is impossible in the presence of large tissue concentrations of TIMPs and related molecules. The specificity of TIMPs for matrix metalloproteinases makes them interesting models for xenobiotic drugs to act as specific metalloproteinase inhibitors.

Extracellular Ions

The cation composition of cartilage is different from that of the plasma and lymphoid fluids.[70,71] Cartilage is characterized by a high content of sodium and potassium ions. These ions act as counterions for the sulfate anion residues on proteoglycans. Calcium ions are unevenly distributed in articular cartilage. The superficial and deeper zones have lower calcium concentrations than blood plasma, whereas the calcified zone has significantly elevated levels of extracellular calcium.[72,73] However, the sulfate anions of proteoglycans have a tendency to complex calcium ions and shift the equilibrium toward tissue-bound calcium.[18] For example, tracheal cartilage has been shown to serve as an ion buffer and calcium reservoir for the tracheal tissues. Tracheal tissue depleted of cartilage has lower smooth muscle cell contractility and a reduced reaction of smooth muscle to histamine than tissue preparations with cartilage.[74]

It is known that compression of cartilage results in deformation of cells and matrix, hydrostatic pressure gradients, interstitial fluid flow, and electrical fields called "streaming potentials."[75–77] These mechanical, chemical, and electrical phenomena can regulate cell behavior. Thus (in vitro) static loading decreases proteoglycan and collagen synthesis, while dynamic loads at walking frequency can stimulate synthesis (as in vivo). These electromagnetic effects have been mimicked and used to treat osteoarthritis.[78] It is not known which cellular structures are able to recognize the alterations in electromagnetic fields, since no molecular element is known that reacts to capacity changes in the range observed in cartilage. Classic voltage-dependent channels of the neuromuscular tissues depend on much stronger (orders of magnitude) electrical fluxes.

TABLE 9-2   Matrix Metalloproteinases and Their Extracellular Substrates

Metalloproteinase	Substrate
Neutral collagenase	Native collagens
Stromelysin-1	Native collagen types II and IX
Stromelysin-2	Proteoglycans
Gelatinase A (72 kDa)	Denatured collagens, native collagen type X
Gelatinase B (92 kDa)	Denatured collagens, native collagen type XI
Aggrecanase	Aggrecan (and other proteoglycans?)
Membrane-associated metalloproteinases	?

Source: Adapted from Werb Z, Huttenlocher A: Proteinases and their inhibitors, in Schumacher HR, Klippel JH, Koopman WJ (eds): *Primer on Rheumatic Diseases,* 10th ed. Chicago, IL, Arthritis Foundation, 1991, pp 52–56.

THE CHONDROCYTE

The chondrocyte is derived from the mesenchymal cell lineage.[79–81] During embryogenesis, chondroblasts are rapidly generated by zonal proliferation in the presumptive cartilage and bone tissue and are the structural basis for the majority of the skeletal bone formed by endochondral ossification.[82] Fetal growth cartilage is characterized by a terminal differentiation process via the development of a hypertrophic chondrocyte phenotype. The hypertrophic chondrocyte is irreversibly postmitotic, undergoes apoptosis (controlled cell death), and is ultimately replaced by bone cells.[83,84] A very characteristic product of the hypertrophic chondrocyte is type X collagen.[85,86]

During development, during fracture healing, and when brought into tissue culture after enzymatic depletion of the extracellular matrix, chondrocytes are metabolically very active and produce vast amounts of extracellular matrix molecules. In general, these highly activated populations are unstable. They either undergo terminal differentiation, as in the growth plate and in fracture healing, or are modulated or "dedifferentiated" into an unspecific "fibroblastoid" phenotype that is unable to produce cartilage matrix components.[87] However, they do release collagen type I and other components of the interstitial connective tissue.[87]

Basic Metabolism

Chondrocytes maintain a very low metabolic rate in the resting cartilage of an adult organism.[88] Cell proliferation cannot be observed and could be totally absent throughout the entire adult life. The basic turnover rate of the extracellular matrix proteins is very low.[89,90] Proteoglycans have a half-life in the range of weeks to months; collagen half-life is estimated at several years, at least. Some data suggest a lifelong persistence of the individual collagen molecules in the fiber network once it has been established at adolescence. The exceptions are the territorial matrix surrounding each single chondrocyte and the chondrons. Here the turnover rate may be higher, resulting in the previously mentioned different organization of the extracellular matrix characterized by very fine collagen fibers. The role of this differential matrix turnover is still unclear. Taken together, chondrocytes are "bradytrophic."

The bradytrophic metabolism is supported by particular features of the energy metabolism in chondrocytes. Chondrocytes are able to cover a significant portion of their energy consumption via the lactic acid pathway, even in the presence of saturation concentrations of oxygen and glucose.[91,92] Chondrocytes consume about one-tenth of the oxygen per time unit as compared to metabolically very active cells such as muscle and liver cells.[93] This led to the assumption that chondrocytes may prefer slightly anaerobic conditions. However, in vivo, the availability of oxygen in the different zones of articular cartilage from the superficial zone down to the calcified zone is similar.[94] It is the presence of glucose concentrations typical for synovial fluid (about 5 mM) that suppresses oxygen consumption ("Crabtree effect") in the upper zones.[94] This situation causes a "facultative" anaerobic metabolism. The Crabtree effect allows diffusion of sufficient oxygen for aerobic glycolysis into the deeper zones. The deeper zones have at the same time a reduced glucose availability because of the limited diffusion of glucose through the extracellular matrix. In consequence, cells of the upper zones produce more lactate per unit glucose consumed, and cells from the deeper zones consume more oxygen per unit glucose burned in order to produce equal amounts of chemical energy. An excess of glucose is stored as glycogen granules and utilized upon glucose shortages.[94] Only in the case of acute oxygen deprivation in pathologic situations (inflammation) or in vitro with artificial oxygen depletion do all the cells completely rely on anaerobic glycolysis.[95] Diabetic conditions immediately destroy the balanced glucose and oxygen utilization in the different zones of articular cartilage, since the Crabtree effect depends upon the regulated uptake of glucose into the chondrocyte.[94]

The Cell Surface

The exclusion of cell-to-cell communication of chondrocytes with cells from other tissues places very specific demands on the chondrocyte's ability to sense its environment by specific subsets of plasma membrane proteins. The unique ion distribution of the extracellular matrix imposes additional tasks on ion channels in the chondrocyte membrane. The extracellular matrix molecules can be recognized by specific receptors. Tissue hormone signals have to be recognized and processed, even under the restrictions imposed by the solid extracellular matrix. Finally, the chondrocyte should be able to react to acute events, such as inflammation and trauma, by expressing receptors to cytokines, for example. Although much work has been done on these structures in many tissues, only relatively few attempts have been made to characterize the corresponding elements in cartilage.

Cartilage Lipids

The lipid composition in cartilage is in part distinct from that in other tissues.[96–104] Chondrocytes from different cartilage tissues vary considerably in their relative contents of cholesterol, phosphatidylserine, and phosphatidylcholine, especially in plasma membranes. The lowest cholesterol content is found in proliferating chondrocytes (about 19 percent of all nonpolar lipids); chondrocytes from adult joint tissue have somewhat higher values, with the highest in plasma membranes of hypertrophic chondrocytes. Matrix vesicles from growth plates have up to 32 percent cholesterol. The lipids of the matrix vesicles may be involved in the calcification process. The triacylglycerol content in nonpolar lipids is reduced from 44 percent in proliferative chondrocytes to 22 percent in hypertrophic chondrocytes.

Similar significant changes are found for polar phospholipids. Phosphatidylserine in plasma membranes of young, proliferating chondrocytes makes up about 3 percent of all phospholipids, increased to 5 percent in hypertrophic chondrocytes and 9 percent in matrix vesicles. The phosphatidylethanolamine content drops from 19 percent in fetal proliferating chondrocytes to 9 percent in hypertrophic cells. Dipalmytoyl phosphatidylcholine, as the major lipid found in synovial fluid, may also contribute to joint lubrication, since it behaves as a boundary lubricant between two surfaces under loading.[105]

Ion Channels

Two types of voltage-gated channels have been identified by electrophysiologic measurements: potassium channels and calcium channels.[106–113] Their electrophysiologic properties correspond to those reported in other tissues but exclude participation in the recognition of ion fluxes during loading. However, the potassium and the calcium channels have not been further characterized as to their molecular properties. It has been shown, however, that articular chondrocytes respond to mechanical loading with ion fluxes typical for calcium-dependent potassium channels.[109] Cartilage annexin V (Anchorin CII)[111,112] is another candidate for a calcium channel, having been described as a slow, voltage-dependent channel in artificial lipid bilayers.[113] However, although the molecule has been analyzed in more detail as to its collagen-binding properties, its role as a functional calcium channel unit in chondrocytes has not as yet been investigated.

Integrins

Integrins comprise a large family of cell surface proteins involved in both cell-cell and cell-matrix interaction.[114] An alpha and a beta subunit must be combined for ligand specificity and signal transmission capacities.[115] Both units reach through the plasma membrane and bind to the cytoskeleton. Signal transduction is achieved by intracellular protein phosphorylation induced by binding of the extracellular ligand. The ligand structures exist on many proteins. For example, the ligand sequence argine-glycine-aspartic acid is typically recognized by β1-integrins and is present in many matrix proteins; however, it may be a hidden domain in the normal protein conformation, to be exposed upon proteolytic cleavage of the proteins in trauma or inflammation. Articular chondrocytes express mainly α3β1 and αVβ3 combinations, the latter predominantly in the superficial zone.[116] The ligand molecules for these combinations are collagens, fibronectin, COMP, and decorin (i.e., in fetal and adult articular cartilage, α6β1 integrin expression with a specificity for laminin has been described).[116] The level of integrin expression in resting cartilage is low. However, metabolically activated chondrocytes express much higher integrin levels that include the expression of additional integrin subtypes.[117,118]

Hyaluronan Receptors

The hyaluronan receptors appear to play a major role in chondrocyte matrix assembly at the cell surface[119] as well as in matrix metabolism.[120] Proteoglycans bound to fila-

ments of hyaluronan become anchored to the chondrocyte cell surface via interactions with these hyaluronan receptors. It has been suggested that hyaluronan receptors are related to the lymphocyte homing receptor, CD44.[119,120]

Hormones and Their Receptors

The chondrocyte has been shown to respond to a wide variety of tissue hormones and growth factors: acidic and basic fibroblast growth factor (FGF), insulin-like growth factor (IGF), parathyroid hormone (PTH), and several members of the transforming growth factor-beta (TGF-β) superfamily [i.e., TGF-β itself and some bone morphogenic factors such as BMP-2 and BMP-7 (OP-1)].[121–133] Although not all receptors have been structurally characterized, the specific responses of chondrocytes to these growth factors imply a specific ligand-receptor interaction and receptor constellation. These hormone-receptor pairs are important during cartilage differentiation during development and in balancing the steady-state metabolism of adult cartilage. They provide anabolic activation for macromolecule synthesis, although sometimes in context with the induction of dedifferentiation of chondrocytes into a fibroblastic phenotype (FGF, TGF-β). Steroid receptors, in particular for vitamin D, play a key role in cartilage differentiation in the growth plate and transition to calcified tissues.[134,135] It is not known to what extent they also control adult chondrocyte metabolism. Thyroxin has been identified recently as a potent stimulus for matrix protein synthesis in chondrocytes in vitro.[136] However, little is known about its potential role in vivo.

Catabolic Mediators

A number of inflammatory mediators (i.e., interleukin-1, histamine, serotonin, beta-endorphin, and eicosanoids) also affect chondrocyte metabolism.[5,6,125–127,137–142] Of the cytokines, IL-1 has been best characterized in its actions on chondrocytes via the IL-1 receptor. More recently, variations in IL-1 response and receptor configuration among different cartilages have been shown, a finding that might be important in context with arthritis pathology. The action of histamine and histamine binding to chondrocytes also has been shown in pharmacologic approaches.[125,127]

Chondrocytes also produce small quantities of prostaglandins (E2 and F2α) during normal metabolism. As in other tissues, they may contribute to the control of steady-state metabolism. Prostaglandin output is about 10-fold increased upon stimulation with IL-1 and might then serve as a cofactor for an intense stimulation of repair and inflammation pathways.[10,127,137] Chondrocytes have receptors for interferon-gamma.[8] Chondrocytes express receptors for immunoglobulins (Fc receptors) and are able to activate the complement system after the Fc receptors have bound immunoglobulins.[7,9,10] In inflammatory activated joints and triggered by interferon gamma, chondrocytes express Ia-antigen, a histocompatibility antigen subtype that allows an interaction of the chondrocyte with immune-competent cells.[8] Chondrocytes, in particular the superficial zone cells, are able to perform activated phagocytosis, possibly via scavenger receptors,[7] and release reactive oxygen species in an oxidative burst otherwise typical for macrophages.[6,11] This unique equipment of the chondrocyte's surface enables these cells to respond autonomously to viral or bacterial infections.

Intracellular Elements

Intermediate Filaments

The chondrocyte possesses a distinct intermediate filament network. In addition to actin, it contains cytokeratin and vimentin filaments that may be specific subtypes of the intermediate filaments found in other tissues.[143–145] The fine structural analysis of the intracellular filament architecture of chondrocytes has not been undertaken thus far. In particular, little is known about the architecture and even the existence of a transition site from the extra- to the intracellular fiber network in cartilage.

Mitochondria

Despite their bradytrophic metabolism, chondrocytes possess well-developed mitochondria.[1] In in vitro studies, it has been shown that chondrocytes are able to adapt the number and size of their mitochondria to the amount of oxygen available and to the metabolic demands on energy production.[146,147] Chondrocytes utilize their mitochondria to control the calcium metabolism, a feature that is particularly obvious in growth-plate cartilage. Here, calcium is accumulated in the mitochondria, starting in the proliferative zone, released from the cell, and incorporated into the mineralizing vesicles.[147] It is possible to connect such processes to pathologic calcification patterns in osteoarthritis.

The Golgi Apparatus and Matrix Protein Synthesis

Although chondrocytes are a "resting" tissue, they possess a well-developed Golgi system and are therefore able to generate a significant output of matrix proteins per time unit via Golgi export.[148,149] The dominating posttranslational modification is the addition of the sulfated glycosaminoglycan side chains to the proteoglycan core proteins. The best known cartilage-specific modification is the introduction of keratan sulfate side chains to keratan sulfate–bearing proteoglycans. For proper sulfation, high levels of specific glycosyl-sulfotransferase activities are necessary. Sulfate enters chondrocytes most likely via a sulfate transporter and is not a limiting step in proteoglycan synthesis.[150] Limiting, however, is the production of the polyglycosyl chain itself, depending upon the activity and capacity of the UDP-transferase system. Since this system is highly energy-dependent, a redirection of the energy consumption into catabolic processes leads to an immediate interruption and downregulation of proteoglycan production, even without regulation on transcription or translation of the core protein. Therefore, proteoglycan synthesis is one of the most sensitive parameters available for measuring anabolic or catabolic activities in cartilage.

Heat Shock Proteins

Heat shock proteins are important functional components of the protein folding and transport system of cells under metabolically normal conditions[151] and are expressed in normal cartilage.[152] Their particular acute protective function during cellular stress situations is well established. Expression of heat shock proteins can be very prominent in chondrocytes, as shown in in vitro activated chondrocytes[152–154] and during chronic inflammation in rheumatoid arthritis.[155]

PATHOPHYSIOLOGIC EVENTS

Repair Following Mechanical Trauma

Superficial injuries and laceration of articular cartilage do not heal. Chondrocyte proliferation and cell migration into the lesion does not occur sufficiently actively (nor does cartilage-specific matrix synthesis), and such activity ceases early.

Injuries that penetrate to subchondral bone produce hematoma and a fibrin clot that serves as a scaffold for some repair. A modified form of hyaline cartilage is formed but without any layered zonal organization. Also, this repair cartilage is subsequently transformed to a tissue containing matrix components that are untypical for articular cartilage, such as collagen type I fiber bundles (similar to fibrocartilage), a tissue unsuitable for repetitive load bearing.[156]

Osteoarthritis

The analysis of pathophysiological developments in cartilage is hampered by the fact that most patients visit their physician after osteoarthritis has reached its clinically overt phase. Although the diseased joint may be classified as mildly affected in clinical terms, the alterations of the molecular and biophysical properties of cartilage tissue might already have a long history of unnoticed degeneration and repair and may be beyond the stage where spontaneous repair could occur. Much available biochemical data are from such cases and signify terminal alterations rather than onset or intermediate events (the cell biological and biochemical basis for the pathophysiologic alterations has been presented in the preceding sections and is not detailed below).

However, some insights into early stages of arthritis can be deduced from cell and tissue culture experiments with normal cartilage and linked to the data from the more advanced stages obtained from surgical biopsy specimens.

Repair Mechanisms

Chondrocytes have a significant metabolic capacity enabling them to repair damaged cartilage tissue. In vitro, under optimal culture conditions, they produce and deposit large quantities of extracellular matrix.[12] These quantities can be increased if the cells are treated with tissue hormones such as bone morphogenic proteins.[132,133] In three-dimensional suspension cultures embedded in agarose or alginate, the cells produce a newly formed matrix that resembles closely in morphology (fiber size) and composition that from normal cartilage.[2,3] These data suggest that a significant amount of repair takes place in joint cartilage before irreversible negative changes occur.

Acute Pathophysiologic Events

The activation of chondrocytes can be induced by physical damage to cartilage, joint irritation and damage by bacterial or viral infection, and autoimmune processes. *Minor physical damage* (microtraumata) will activate molecular repair processes immediately. Infection will cause inflammatory activation first and subsequently lead to repair. In these cases, activation may start by the diffusion of external inflammatory agents into the joint, i.e., IL-1, tumor necrosis factor-alpha (TNF-α), prostaglandins, and histamine.[6,11,125,126,139,141] Immune complexes may bind to Fc receptors and activate phagocytosis.[7] Immune complexes are thought to play a role in chronic immunologic responses in joints since they induce phagocytosis in cultured chondrocytes and cause damage of the superficial zone in a rabbit model.[7] Bleeding into the joint could therefore cause an activation of these metabolic processes and might be one of the reasons for the negative prognosis in cases of joint injuries without direct initial affliction of the cartilage tissue.

The impact of inflammatory mediators on cartilage and their induction in a joint also can be seen in vitro. The administration of IL-1, for example, leads to (1) downregulation of matrix protein (especially proteoglycan) synthesis; (2) release of prostaglandins; (3) production, release, and activation of matrix metalloproteinases; (4) and degradation of the pericellular matrix.[65] Once IL-1 is removed from the system, the repair processes with the production of new matrix occur. Protease-generated fragments of fibronectin have been shown to induce articular cartilage breakdown.[157] This is of particular interest, since the induction of degradation by fibronectin fragments is independent of the appearance of cytokines. It is not known, however, how many cycles of activation of repair can occur and how long an activated state can be perpetuated until a chondrocyte can no longer respond properly.

Chronic Pathophysiologic Events

The transition into permanent changes in cartilage is marked by several changes in the extracellular matrix, and the irreversible loss of proteoglycans is the most prominent feature.[12] It can be visualized by a lack of Safranin O staining or Alcian blue staining in sections from osteoarthritic cartilage. More detailed analysis revealed a specific loss of aggrecan.[40,41] Since the large proteoglycans are mainly responsible for the biomechanical properties of cartilage, many alterations typical for arthritic cartilage may be related to this, i.e., loss of water, leading to softening and fibrillation of the tissue, followed by cessation of collagen type II production. However, the long half-life and the stability of collagen fibers prevent losses of collagen as prominent as losses of proteoglycans. The action of metalloproteinases causes cleavage of the collagen cross links and thus destabilizes the fiber network, making it, in turn, further vulnerable to mechanical destruction. The metabolic fragments of the degraded extracellular matrix components are released into (peripheral) body fluids and can be used as markers for cartilage turnover.[40,41,158]

The chondrocytes start to proliferate. The mitotic activation in late osteoarthritis has two additional features: the remittance of the embryonic phenotype and the dedifferentiation into an atypical cell type. The embryonic phenotype includes the expression of type X collagen[32,33,159] and the development of the hypertrophic growth plate chondrocyte, possibly leading into apoptosis (controlled cell death) and eventual calcification of the remaining tissue.[160,161] This may also be responsible for the observed age-related migration of the tidemark, for the formation of secondary ossification centers, and for the ingrowth of osteophytes into the cartilage.[15,32]

Phenotypic modulation into a fibroblastoid cell type causes the production and deposition of type I collagen, type III collagen, and fibronectin in large quantities and, ultimately, the formation of a callus tissue.[162] Since type I collagen and fibronectin form an entirely different fiber network with very prominent thick fiber bundles and a relatively low water content, the biomechanical properties of this replacement tissue are quite different from those of the original cartilage and not suited to replace the missing cartilage matrix functionally.

CONCLUSIONS

Articular cartilage is an aneural bradytrophic tissue with the biomechanical task to function as a shock-absorbing structure. This task is achieved mainly by the tissue water and the tissue-specific extracellular matrix, which together make up approximately 95 percent of the tissue volume. Although they represent only 5 percent of the tissue mass, the chondrocytes tightly control the tissue properties. Nutrients and soluble metabolic mediators are provided via the synovial fluid and help to maintain the metabolic status of the cartilage. Early events in osteoarthritis are characterized by a possibly reversible loss of proteoglycans and an activation of repair mechanisms in chondrocytes. Late, clinically overt osteoarthritic modifications include the modulation of the extracellular matrix into a variant with inferior biomechanical properties and an irreversible switch in the chondrocyte phenotype. A major task for future research in the biochemistry and cell biology of osteoarthritis is the development of diagnostic markers for the very early stages of osteoarthritis and of support for the natural repair mechanisms, based upon cartilage-specific drug development.

ACKNOWLEDGMENTS The authors wish to thank Jennifer Thonar for her help in preparing the manuscript. Select research components reported in this chapter were supported in part by a chapter grant from the Arthritis Foundation and by the NIH/NI-AMS SCOR grant 1-P50-AR39239.

REFERENCES

1. Schenk RK, Eggli PS, Hunzicker EB: Articular cartilage morphology, in Kuettner KE, Schleyerbach R, Hascall VC (eds): *Articular Cartilage Biochemistry.* New York, Raven Press, 1986, pp 3–22.

2. Aydelotte MB, Kuettner KE: Differences between sub-populations of cultured bovine articular chondrocytes: I. Morphology and cartilage matrix production. *Connect Tissue Res* 18:205, 1988.

3. Aydelotte MB, Greenhill RR, Kuettner KE: Difference between sub-populations of cultured bovine articular chondrocytes: II. Proteoglycan metabolism. *Connect Tissue Res* 18:223, 1988.

4. Schumacher BL, Block JA, Schmid TM, et al: A novel proteoglycan synthesized and secreted by chondrocytes of the superficial zone of articular cartilage. *Arch Biochem Biophys* 311:144, 1994.

5. Aydelotte MB, Raiss RX, Caterson B, Kuettner KE: Influence of interleukin-1 on the morphology and proteoglycan metabolism of cultured bovine articular chondrocytes. *Connect Tissue Res* 28:142, 1992.

6. Häuselmann HJ, Flechtenmacher J, Michal L, et al: The superficial layer of human articular cartilage is more susceptible to interleukin-1 induced damage than the deeper layers. *Arthritis Rheum* 39:478, 1996.

7. Cooke TDV, Sumia M, Elliott S, Maeda M: Immune complex mediated destruction of cartilage in antigen induced arthritis in rabbits. *J Rheumatol Suppl* 11:103, 1983.

8. Jahn B, Burmester, GR, Schmid HJ, et al: Changes in cell surface antigen expression on human articular chondrocytes induced by γ-interferon. *Arthritis Rheum* 29:1, 1986.

9. Takagi T, Jasin H: Interactions of synovial fluid immunoglobulins with chondrocytes. *Arthritis Rheum* 35:1502, 1992.

10. Jasin HE: Structure and function of the articular cartilage surface. *Scand J Rheumatol Suppl* 101:51, 1995.

11. Häuselmann HJ, Oppliger L, Michel BA, et al: Nitric oxide and proteoglycan synthesis by human articular chondrocytes. *FEBS Lett* 352:361, 1994.

12. Kuettner KE: Biochemistry of articular cartilage in health and disease. *Clin Biochem* 25:155, 1992.

13. Poole CA, Flint MH, Beaumont BW: Chondrons in cartilage: Ultrastructural analysis of the pericellular microenvironment in adult human articular cartilages. *J Orthop Res* 5:509, 1987.

14. Poole CA, Matsuoka A, Schofield JR: Chondrons from articular cartilage: III. Morphologic changes in the cellular microenvironment of chondrons isolated from osteoarthritic cartilage. *Arthritis Rheum* 34:22, 1991.

15. Oegema TR, Thompson R: Cartilage-bone interface (tidemark), in Brandt K (ed): *Cartilage Changes in Osteoarthritis.* Indianapolis: Indiana School of Medicine Publishers, 1990, pp 43–52.

16. Oegema TR Jr, Thompson RC Jr: Metabolism of chondrocytes derived from normal and osteoarthritic human cartilage, in Kuettner KE, Schleyerbach R, Hascall VC (eds): *Articular Cartilage Biochemistry.* New York, Raven Press, 1986, pp 257–272.

17. Maroudas A, Katz EP, Wachtel EJ, et al: Physicochemical properties and functional behavior of normal and osteoarthritic human cartilage, in Kuettner KE, Schleyerbach R, Hascall VC (eds): *Articular Cartilage Biochemistry.* New York, Raven Press, 1986, pp 311–330.

18. Comper WD: Extracellular matrix interactions: Sulfation of connective tissue polysaccharides creates macroion binding templates and conditions for dissipative structure formation. *J Theor Biol* 145:497, 1990.

19. Radin EL, Paul IL: A consolidated concept of joint lubrication. *J Bone Joint Surg Am* 54:607, 1972.

20. Wright V, Dowson D: Lubrication and cartilage. *J Anat* 121:107, 1976.

21. Mow VC, Ateshian GA, Spilker RL: Biomechanics of diarthrodial joints: A review of twenty years of progress. *J Biomech Eng* 115:460, 1993.

22. Hou JS, Mow VC, Lai WM, Holmes MH: An analysis of the squeeze-film lubrication mechanism for articular cartilage. *J Biomech* 25:247, 1992.

23. Mansour JM, Mow VC: The permeability of articular cartilage under compressive strain and at high pressures. *J Bone Joint Surg Am* 58:509, 1976.

24. Miller EJ: Structural studies on cartilage collagen employing limited cleavage and solubilization with pepsin. *Biochemistry* 11:4903, 1972.

25. Bruckner P, van der Rest M: Structure and function of cartilage collagens. *Microsc Res Tech* 28:378, 1994.

26. Müller-Glauser W, Humbel B, Glatt M, et al: On the role of type IX collagen in the extracellular matrix of cartilage. Type IX collagen is localized to intersections of collagen fibrils. *J Cell Biol* 102:1931, 1986.

27. Wu J-J, Woods PE, Eyre DR: Identification of cross-linking sites in bovine cartilage type IX collagen reveals an antiparalell type II–type IX molecular relationship and type IX to type IX bonding. *J Biol Chem* 267:23007, 1992.

28. Thomas JD, Ayad S, Grant ME: Cartilage collagens: Strategies for the study of their organisation and expression in the extracellular matrix. *Ann Rheum Dis* 53:488, 1994.

29. Timpl R, Engel J: Type VI collagen, in Mayne R, Burgeson RE (eds): *Structure and Function of Collagen Types.* Orlando, FL, Academic Press, 1987, pp 223–259.

30. Poole CA, Ayad S, Schofield JR: Chondrons extracted from articular cartilage: I. Immunolocalisation of type VI collagen in the pericellular capsule of isolated canine chondrons. *J Cell Sci* 90:635, 1988.

31. Schmid TM, Linsenmayer TF: Type X collagen, in Mayne R, Burgeson RE (eds): *Structure and Function of Collagen Types.* Orlando, FL, Academic Press, 1987, pp 223–259.

32. Aigner T, Dietz U, Stöss H, von der Mark K: Differential expression of collagen types I, II, III, and X in human osteophytes. *Lab Invest* 73:236, 1995.

33. Aigner T, Reichenberger E, Bertling W, et al: Type X collagen expression in osteoarthritic and rheumatoid articular cartilage. *Virchows Arch B Cell Pathol Incl Mol Pathol* 63:205, 1993.

34. Hardingham TE, Fosang AJ, Dudhia J: The structure, function and turnover of aggrecan, the large aggregating proteoglycan from cartilage. *Eur J Clin Chem Clin Biochem* 32:249, 1994.

35. Paulsson M: The cartilage proteoglycan aggregate: Assembly through combined protein-carbohydrate and protein-protein interactions. *Biophys Chem* 50:113, 1994.

36. Roughley PE, Lee ER: Cartilage proteoglycans: Structure and potential functions. *Microsc Res Tech* 28:385, 1994.

37. Laurent TC, Fraser JRE: Hyaluronan. *FASEB J* 6:2397, 1992.

38. Sandy JD, Plaas AHK: Studies on the hyaluronate binding affinity of newly synthesized proteoglycans in chondrocyte cultures. *Arch Biochem Biophys* 271:300, 1989.

39. Neame PJ, Barry FP: The link proteins. *EXS* 70:53, 1994.

40. Thonar EJ-MA, Lenz ME, Klintworth GK, et al: Quantification of keratan sulfate in blood as a marker of cartilage catabolism. *Arthritis Rheum* 28:1367, 1985.

41. Thonar EJ-MA, Glant T: Serum keratan sulfate—A marker of predisposition to polyarticular osteoarthritis. *Clin Biochem* 25:175, 1992.

42. Hlavacek M: The role of synovial fluid filtration by cartilage in lubrication of synovial joints: I. Mixture model of synovial fluid. *J Biomech* 26:1145, 1993.

43. Hlavacek M: The role of synovial fluid filtration by cartilage in lubrication of synovial joints: II. Squeeze-film lubrication: Homogeneous filtration. *J Biomech* 26:1151, 1993.

44. Oldberg A, Antonsson P, Lindblom K, Heinegard D: COMP (cartilage oligomeric matrix protein) is structurally related to the thrombospondins. *J Biol Chem* 267:22346, 1992.

45. Efimov VP, Lustig A, Engel J: The thrombospondin-like chains of cartilage oligomeric matrix protein are assembled by a five-stranded alpha-helical bundle between residues 20 and 83. *FEBS Lett* 341:54, 1994.

46. Burton-Wurster N, Butler M, Harter S, et al: Presence of fibronectin in articular cartilage in two animal models of osteoarthritis. *J Rheumatol* 13:175, 1986.

47. Chevalier X, Groult N, Labat-Robert J: Biosynthesis and distribution of fibronectin in normal and osteoarthritic human cartilage. *Clin Physiol Biochem* 9:1, 1992.

48. Van der Rest M, Rosenberg LC, Oslen BR, Poole AR: Chondrocalcin is identical with the C-propeptide of type II procollagen. *Biochem J* 237:923, 1986.

49. Poole AR, Rosenberg LC: Chondrocalcin and the calcification of cartilage: A review. *Clin Orthop* 208:114, 1986.

50. Silbermann M, von der Mark K, Heinegard D: An immunohistochemical study of the distribution of matrical proteins in the mandibular condyle of neonatal mice: II. Non-collagenous proteins. *J Anat* 170:23, 1990.

51. Lawlor P, Archer CW: Expression of laminin and laminin receptor in mature articular cartilage. *Orthop Res Soc Trans* 20:273, 1995.

52. Swann DA, Radin EL: The molecular basis of articular lubrication: I. Purification and properties of a lubricating fraction from bovine synovial fluid. *J Biol Chem* 247:8069, 1972.

53. Swann DA, et al: The molecular structure of lubricating glycoprotein I, the boundary lubricant for articular cartilage. *J Biol Chem* 256:5921, 1981.

54. Hofer U, Chiquet-Ehrismann R: Tenascin variants: Ligands and expression. *Prog Clin Biol Res* 383B:455, 1993.

55. Chevalier X, Groult N, Larget-Piet B, et al: Tenascin distribution in articular cartilage from normal subjects and from patients with osteoarthritis and rheumatoid arthritis. *Arthritis Rheum* 37:1013, 1994.

56. Neame PJ, Sommarin Y, Boynton RE, Heinegard D: The structure of a 38-kDa leucine-rich protein (chondroadherin) isolated from bovine cartilage. *J Biol Chem* 269:21547, 1994.

57. Sommarin Y, Neame PJ, Wendel M, et al: Three novel extracellular matrix proteins from cartilage or bone with similar structure. *Trans 2nd Comb Orthop Res Soc* 1, 1995.

58. Grover J, Chen XN, Korenberg JR, Roughley PJ: The human lumican gene: Organization, chromosomal location, and expression in articular cartilage. *J Biol Chem* 270:21942, 1995.

59. Hauser N, Paulsson M: Native cartilage matrix protein (CMP): A compact trimer of subunits assembled via a coiled-coil alpha-helix. *J Biol Chem* 269:25747, 1994.

60. Fife RS, Kluve-Beckerman B, Houser DS, et al: Evidence that a 550,000-dalton cartilage matrix glycoprotein is a chondrocyte membrane-associated protein closely related to ceruloplasmin. *J Biol Chem* 268:4407, 1993.

61. Varner HH, Furthmayr H, Nilsson B, et al: Chondronectin: Physical and chemical properties. *Arch Biochem Biophys* 243:579, 1985.

62. Nagase H, Barrett AJ, Woessner JF Jr: Nomenclature and glossary of the matrix metalloproteinases, in Birkedal-Hansen H, Werb Z, Welgus H, Van Wart H (eds): *Matrix Metalloproteinases*

and Inhibitors. Gustav-Fischer-Verlag, New York, 1992, pp 421–424.

63. Werb Z, Huttenlocher A: Proteinases and their inhibitors, in Schumacher HR, Klippel JH, Koopman WJ (eds): *Primer on Rheumatic Diseases*, 10th ed. Chicago, IL, Arthritis Foundation, 1991, pp 52–56.

64. Nagase H, Woessner JF Jr: Role of endogenous proteinases in the degradation of cartilage, in Woessner JF, Howell DS (eds): *Joint Cartilage Degradation.* New York, Marcel Dekker, 1993, pp 159–186.

65. Woessner JF Jr, Gunja-Smith Z: Role of metalloproteinases in human osteoarthritis. *J Rheumatol Suppl* 27:99, 1991.

66. Wolfsberg TG, Straight PD, Gerena RL, et al: ADAM, a widely distributed and developmentally regulated gene family encoding membrane proteins with a disintegrin and metalloproteinase domain. *Dev Biol* 169:378, 1995.

67. Denhardt DT, Feng B, Edwards DR, et al: Tissue inhibitor of metalloproteinases (TIMP, aka EPA): Structure, control of expression and biological functions. *Pharmacol Ther* 59:329, 1993.

68. Gunja-Smith Z, Woessner JF Jr: Activation of cartilage stromelysin-1 at acid pH and its relation to enzyme pH optimum and osteoarthritis. *Agents Actions* 40:228, 1993.

69. Böhm B, Aigner T, Kinne R, Burkhardt H: The serine-protease inhibitor of cartilage matrix is not a chondrocyte gene product. *Eur J Biochem* 207:773, 1992.

70. Urban JPG, Hall AC, Gehl KA: Regulation of matrix synthesis rates by the ionic and osmotic environment of articular chondrocytes. *J Cell Physiol* 154:262, 1993.

71. Urban JPG: The chondrocyte: A cell under pressure. *Br J Rheumatol* 33:901, 1994.

72. Shitama, K: Calcification of aging articular cartilage in man. *Acta Orthop Scand* 50:613, 1979.

73. Benderly H, Maroudas A: Equilibria of calcium and phosphate ions in human articular cartilage. *Ann Rheum Dis* 34(suppl 2):46, 1975.

74. Reaburn D, Hay DWP, Framer SG, Fedan JS: Influence of cartilage on reactivity and on the effectiveness of verapamil in guinea pig isolated airway smooth muscle. *J Pharm Exp Ther* 242:450, 1987.

75. Frank EH, Grodzinsky AJ: Cartilage electromechanics: I. Electrokinetic transduction and the effects of electrolyte pH and ionic strength. *J Biomech* 6:615, 1987.

76. Gu WY, Lai WM, Mow VC: Transport of fluid and ions through a porous-permeable charged-hydrated tissue, and streaming potential data on normal bovine articular cartilage. *J Biomech* 26:709, 1993.

77. Sah RL-Y, Kim Y-J, Doogn J-YH, et al: Biosynthetic response of cartilage explants to dynamic compression. *J Orthop Res* 7:619, 1989.

78. Trock DH, Bollett AJ, Dyer RH Jr, et al: A double-blind trial of the clinical effects of pulsed electromagnetic fields in osteoarthritis. *J Rheumatol* 20:456, 1993.

79. Ahrens PB, Solursh M, Reiter RS: Stage-related capacity for limb chondrogenesis in cell culture. *Dev Biol* 60:69, 1977.

80. Ahrens PB, Solursh M, Reiter RS, Singley CT: Position-related capacity for differentiation of limb mesenchyme in cell culture. *Dev Biol* 69:436, 1979.

81. Tickle C, Eichele G: Vertebrate limb development. *Annu Rev Cell Biol* 10:121, 1994.

82. Caplan AI, Peshak DG: The cellular and molecular embryology of bone formation. *Bone Min Res* 5:117, 1987.

83. Roach HI, Shearer JR: Cartilage resorption and endochondral bone formation during the development of long bones in chick embryos. *Bone Miner* 6:289, 1989.

84. Roach HI, Erenpreisa J, Aigner T: Osteogenic differentiation of hypertrophic chondrocytes involves asymmetric cell divisions and apoptosis. *J Cell Biol* 131:483, 1995.

85. Bonen DK, Schmid TM: Elevated extracellular calcium concentrations induce type X collagen synthesis in chondrocyte cultures. *J Cell Biol* 115:1171, 1991.

86. Stephens M, Kwan APL, Bayliss MT, Archer CW: Human articular surface chondrocytes initiate alkaline phosphatase and type X collagen synthesis in suspension culture. *J Cell Sci* 103:1111, 1992.

87. Mayne R, Vail MS, Mayne PM, Miller EJ: Change in type of collagen synthesized as clones of chick chondrocytes grow and eventually lose division capacity. *Proc Natl Acad Sci USA* 73:1674, 1976.

88. Handley CJ, McQuillan DJ, Campbell MA, Bolis S: Steady-state metabolism in cartilage explants, in Kuettner KE, Schleyerbach S, Hascall VC (eds): *Articular Cartilage Biochemistry.* New York, Raven Press, 1986, pp 163–179.

89. Mok SS, Masuda K, Häuselmann HJ, et al: Aggrecan synthesized by mature bovine chondrocytes suspended in alginate. *J Biol Chem* 269:33021, 1994.

90. Petit B, Masuda K, D'Souza A, et al: Comparative studies of the rate of formation, compartmentalization and crosslinking of the collagenous network formed by fetal and adult articular chondrocytes in vitro. *Trans Orthop Res Soc* 20:405, 1995.

91. Lane JM, Brighton CT, Menkwitz BJ: Anaerobic and aerobic metabolism in articular cartilage. *J Rheumatol* 4:4, 1977.

92. Vittur F, Grandolfo M, Fragonas E, et al: Energy metabolism replicative ability, intracellular calcium concentration, and ionic channels of horse articular chondrocytes. *Exp Cell Res* 210:130, 1994.

93. Holm S, Maroudas A, Urban JPG, et al: Nutrition of the invertebral disc: Solute transport and metabolism. *Conn Tissue Res* 8:101, 1981.

94. Otte P: Basic metabolism of articular cartilage. *Z Rheumatol* 50:304, 1991.

95. Marcus RE: The effect of low oxygen concentration on growth, glycolysis, and sulfate incorporation by articular chondrocytes in monolayer culture. *Arthritis Rheum* 16:646, 1973.

96. Mandi B, Hadhazy C, Rethy A, et al: Studies on cartilage formation: XVI. Chemical and histochemical assay of lipids in the regenerating articular cartilage. *Acta Biol Acad Sci Hung* 26:115, 1975.

97. Stockwell RA: Lipid content of human costal and articular cartilage. *Ann Rheum Dis* 26:481, 1967.

98. Stockwell RA: Lipid in the matrix of ageing articular cartilage. *Nature* 207:427, 1965.

99. Bonner WM, Jonsson H, Malanos C, Bryant M: Changes in the lipids of human articular cartilage with age. *Arthritis Rheum* 18:461, 1975.

100. Rabinowitz JL, Gregg JR, Nixon JE, Schumacher HR: Lipid composition of the tissues of human knee joints: I. Observations in normal joints (articular cartilage, meniscus, ligaments, synovial fluid, synovium, intra-articular fat pad and bone marrow). *Clin Orthop* 260–265, 1979.

101. Wuthier RE: Lipid composition of isolated epiphyseal cartilage cells, membranes and matrix vesicles. *Biochim Biophys Acta* 409:128, 1975.

102. Wuthier RE: Lipids of matrix vesicles. *Fed Proc* 35:117, 1976.

103. Boyan BD, Schwartz Z, Swain LD, Khare A: Role of lipids in calcification of cartilage. *Anat Rec* 224:211, 1989.

104. Watkins EL, Stillo JV, Wuthier RE: Subcellular fractionation of epiphyseal cartilage: Isolation of matrix vesicles and profiles of enzymes, phospholipids, calcium and phosphate. *Biochim Biophys Acta* 631:289, 1980.

105. Williams PF, Powell GL, LaBerge M: Sliding friction analysis of phosphatidylcholine as a boundary lubricant for articular cartilage. *Proc Inst Mech Eng [H]* 207:59, 1993.

106. Middleton JF, Hunt S: Cation movement in rat articular and non-articular cartilage and in isolated chondrocytes: Calcium influx and efflux. *Comp Biochem Physiol* A 91:837, 1988.

107. Grandolfo MD, d'Andrea P, Martina M, et al: Calcium-activated potassium channels in chondrocytes. *Biochem Biophys Res Commun* 182:1429, 1992.

108. Kirsch T, Wuthier RE: Stimulation of calcification of growth plate cartilage matrix vesicles by binding to type II and X collagen. *J Biol Chem* 269:11462, 1994.

109. Wright MO, Stockwell RA, Nuki G: Response of plasma membrane to applied hydrostatic pressure in chondrocytes and fibroblasts. *Connect Tiss Res* 28:49, 1991.

110. Walsh KB, Cannon SD, Wuthier RE: Characterization of a delayed rectifier potassium current in chicken growth plate cartilage. *Am J Physiol* 262:C1335, 1992.

111. von der Mark K, Pfäffle M, Hofmann C, et al: Anchorin CII, a collagen-binding protein of the calpactin-lipocortin family, in McDonald JA, Mecham R (eds): *Receptors for ECM.* New York, Academic Press, 1991, pp 301–322.

112. Böhm BB, Wilbrink B, Kuettner KE, Mollenhauer J: Structural and functional comparison of anchorin CII (cartilage annexin V) and muscle annexin V. *Arch Biochem Biophys* 314:64, 1994.

113. Huber R, Schneider M, Mayr I, et al: The calcium binding sites in human annexin V by crystal structure analysis at 2.0 Å resolution. *FEBS Lett* 275:15, 1990.

114. Ruoslahti E: Integrins. *J Clin Invest* 87:1, 1991.

115. Juliano RL, Haskill S: Signal transduction from the extracellular matrix. *J Cell Biol* 120:577, 1993.

116. Woods VL, Schreck PJ, Gesink DS, et al: Integrin expression by human articular chondrocytes. *Arthritis Rheum* 37:537, 1994.

117. Dürr J, Goodman S, Potocnik A, et al: Localization of beta$_1$-integrins in human cartilage and their role in chondrocyte adhesion to collagen and fibronectin. *Exp Cell Res* 207:235, 1993.

118. Loeser RF: Modulation of integrin-mediated attachment of chondrocytes to extracellular matrix proteins by cations, retinoic acid, and transforming growth factor beta. *Exp Cell Res* 211:17, 1994.

119. Knudson CB: Hyaluronan receptor-directed assembly of chondrocyte pericellular matrix. *J Cell Biol* 120:825–834, 1993.

120. Hua Q, Knudson CB, Knudson W: The role of hyaluronan receptors in the internalization of hyaluronan and proteoglycans by chondrocytes. *Ortho Trans* 17:29, 1992.

121. Morales TI, Roberts AB: Transforming growth factor β regulates the metabolism of proteoglycans in bovine cartilage organ cultures. *J Biol Chem* 263:12828, 1988.

122. Lewinson D, Silbermann M: Parathyroid hormone stimulates proliferation of chondroprogenitor cells in vitro. *Calcif Tissue Int* 38:155, 1986.

123. Deshmukh K, Kline WG, Sawyer BD: Effects of calcitonin and parathyroid hormone on the metabolism of chondrocytes in culture. *Biochim Biophys Acta* 499:28, 1977.

124. Livne E, Weiss A, Silbermann M: Articular chondrocytes lose their proliferative activity with aging yet can be restimulated by PTH-(1-84), PGE1, and dexamethasone. *J Bone Miner Res* 4:539, 1989.

125. Fukuda K, Matsumura F, Tanaka S: Histamine H2 receptor mediates keratan sulfate secretion in rabbit chondrocytes: Role of cAMP. *Am J Physiol* 265:C1653, 1993.

126. Taylor DJ, Woolley DE: Evidence for both histamine H1 and H2 receptors on human articular chondrocytes. *Ann Rheum Dis* 46:431, 1987.

127. Taylor DJ, Yoffe JR, Brown DM, Woolley DE: Histamine stimulates prostaglandin E production by rheumatoid synovial cells and human articular chondrocytes in culture. *Arthritis Rheum* 29:160, 1986.

128. Guerne PA, Blanco F, Kaelin A, et al: Growth factor responsiveness of human articular chondrocytes in aging and development. *Arthritis Rheum* 38:960, 1995.

129. Chai Y, Mah A, Crohin C, et al: Specific transforming growth factor-beta subtypes regulate embryonic mouse Meckel's cartilage and tooth development. *Dev Biol* 162:85, 1994.

130. Wu LNY, Genge BR, Ishikawa Y, Wuthier RE: Modulation of cultured chicken growth plate chondrocytes by transforming growth factor-$\beta 1$ and basic fibroblast growth factor. *J Cell Biochem* 49:181, 1992.

131. Watanabe N, Rosenfeld RG, Hintz RL, et al: Characterization of a specific insulin-like growth factor-I/somatomedin-C receptor on high-density, primary monolayer cultures of bovine articular chondrocytes: Regulation of receptor concentration by somatomedin, insulin and growth hormone. *J Endocrinol* 107:275, 1985.

132. Reddi AH: Bone morphogenetic proteins, bone marrow stroma cells, and mesenchymal cells: Maureen Owen revisited. *Clin Orthop* 313:115, 1995.

133. Chen P, Vukicevic S, Sampath TK, Luyten FP: Bovine articular chondrocytes do not undergo hypertrophy when cultured in the presence of serum and osteogenic protein-1. *Biochem Biophys Res Commun* 197:1253, 1993.

134. Langston GG, Swain LD, Schwartz Z, et al: Effect of 1,25(OH)$_2$D$_3$ and 24,25(OH)$_2$D$_3$ on calcium fluxes in costochondral chondrocyte cultures. *Calcif Tissue Int* 47:230, 1990.

135. Dayani N, Corvol MT, Robel P, et al: Estrogen receptors in cultured rabbit articular chondrocytes: Influence of age. *J Steroid Biochem* 31:351, 1988.

136. Ballock RT, Reddi AH: Thyroxine is the serum factor that regulates morphogenesis of columnar cartilage from isolated chondrocytes in chemically defined medium. *J Cell Biol* 126:1311, 1994.

137. Richard M, Vignon E, Peschard MJ, et al: Serotonin-stimulated phospholipase A2 and collagenase activation in chondrocytes from human osteoarthritic articular cartilage. *FEBS Lett* 278:38, 1991.

138. Morales TI, Hascall VC: Factors involved in the regulation of proteoglycan metabolism in articular cartilage. *Arthritis Rheum* 32:1197, 1989.

139. Loyau G, Pujol JP: The role of cytokines in the development of osteoarthritis. *Scand J Rheumatol Suppl* 81:8, 1990.

140. Lefebvre V, Peeters-Joris C, Vaes G: Modulation by interleukin 1 and tumor necrosis factor α of production of collagenase, tissue inhibitor of metalloproteinases and collagen types in differentiated and dedifferentiated articular chondrocytes. *Biochem Biophys Acta* 1052:366, 1990.

141. Wilbrink B, Nietfeld JJ, den Otter W, et al: Role of TNF-α, in relation to IL-1 and IL-6 in the proteoglycan turnover of human articular cartilage. *Br J Rheumatol* 30:265, 1991.

142. Castano MT, Freire-Garabal M, Giraldez M, et al: Autoradiographic evidence of 125-I-β-endorphin binding sites in the articular cartilage of the rat. *Life Sci* 49:PL-103, 1991.

143. Bang H, Mollenhauer J, Schulmeister A, et al: Isolation and characterization of a cartilage-specific membrane antigen (CH65): Comparison with cytokeratins and heat-shock proteins. *Immunology* 81:322, 1994.

144. Casey R, Wilbrink B, Mollenhauer J: CH65, an arthritis autoantigen from chondrocytes, is related to intermediate filament proteins. *Trans Orthop Res Soc* 20:311, 1995.

145. Ralphs BM Jr, Archer CW, Mason RM, et al: Cytoskeletal changes in articular fibrocartilage are an early indicator of osteoarthritis in STR/ort mice. *Trans Orthop Res Soc* 20:246, 1995.

146. Shapiro LM, Burke A, Lee NH: Heterogeneity of chondrocyte mitochondria: A study of the Ca^{2+} concentration and density banding characteristics of normal and rachitic cartilage. *Biochim Biophys Acta* 451:583, 1976.

147. Appleton J, Lyon R, Swindin KJ, Chesters J: Ultrastructure and energy-dispersive X-ray microanalysis of cartilage after rapid freezing, low temperature freeze drying, and embedding in Spurr's resin. *J Histochem Cytochem* 33:1073, 1985.

148. Vertel BM, Walters LM, Mills D: Subcompartments of the endoplasmic reticulum. *Semin Cell Biol* 3:325, 1992.

149. Kearns AE, Vertel BM, Schwartz NB: Topography of glycosylation and UDP-xylose production. *J Biol Chem* 268:11097, 1993.

150. Morcuende JA, Kimura JH, Plaas AHK: Identification of the sulfate transport channel SAT-1 in chondrocytes. *Trans 2nd Comb Orthop Res Soc* 1995, p 50.

151. Morimoto RI: Cells in stress: Transcritional activation of heat shock genes. *Science* 259:1409, 1993.

152. Zafarullah M, Su S, Gedamu L: Basal and inducible expression of metallothionine and heat shock protein 70 genes in bovine articular chondrocytes. *Exp Cell Res* 208:371, 1993.

153. Cruz TF, Kandel RA, Brown IR: Interleukin 1 induces the expression of a heat-shock gene in chondrocytes. *Biochem J* 277:327, 1991.

154. MacGinitie LA, Gluzband YA, Grodzinsky AJ: Electric field stimulation can increase protein synthesis in articular cartilage explants. *J Orthop Res* 12:151, 1994.

155. Karlsson-Parra A, Söderström K, Ferm M, et al: Presence of human 65 kD heat shock protein (hsp) in inflamed joints and subcutaneous nodules of RA patients. *Scand J Immunol* 31:283, 1990.

156. Dee R, Goral A, Blyznak N: Articular cartilage, in Dee R, Mango E, Hurst L (eds): *Principles of Orthopaedic Practice.* New York, McGraw-Hill, 1989.

157. Homandberg GA, Meyers R, Xie DL: Fibronectin fragments cause chondrolysis of bovine articular cartilage slices in culture. *J Biol Chem* 267:3597, 1992.

158. Lohmander LS, Saxne T, Heinegard DK: Release of cartilage oligomeric matrix protein (COMP) into joint fluid after knee injury and in osteoarthritis. *Ann Rheum Dis* 53:8, 1994.

159. von der Mark K, Kirsch T, Nerlich A, et al: Type X collagen synthesis in human osteoarthritic cartilage. *Arthritis Rheum* 35:806, 1992.

160. Hulth A: Does osteoarthritis depend on growth of the mineralized layer of cartilage? *Clin Orthop* 287:19, 1990.

161. Derfus BA, Rachow JW, Mandel NS, et al: Articular cartilage vesicles generate calcium phosphate dihydrate-like crystals in vitro. *Arthritis Rheum* 35:231, 1992.

162. Aigner T, Bertling W, Stöss H, et al: Independent expression of fibril-forming collagens I, II, and III in chondrocytes of human osteoarthritic cartilage. *J Clin Invest* 91:829, 1993.

CHAPTER 10

Synovial Membrane

Christopher H. Evans

Noncartilaginous intraarticular surfaces are covered by a tissue known as the *synovium*. All other body cavities are lined by a highly structured basement membrane, but synovium is a loose connective tissue continuous with the subsynovium that lies beneath.

Synovium plays an important role in the nutrition of the joint and in maintaining intraarticular biochemical homeostasis. These roles reflect the fact that intraarticular tissues, particularly ligaments and the medial aspects of the knee menisci, receive a very limited blood supply, and articular cartilage is completely avascular. Thus, to a very considerable extent, these tissues rely upon the rich subsynovial capillary network for nutrition and removal of waste products. The biochemical environment of the joint is also modified by products secreted by synoviocytes. Synovium also has a role in regulating the volume and composition of the synovial fluid and, indirectly, intraarticular pressure.

Given the influence of the synovium over the intraarticular environment, it is not surprising that synovial pathology leads to disturbances in the other tissues of the joint. This is seen at its fullest extent in rheumatoid arthritis, where the inflammation of the synovium leads to destruction of bone, cartilage, and ligaments; changes in the volume and composition of synovial fluid; and joint instability.

This chapter summarizes the structure and function of the normal synovium and indicates some of the more salient changes it undergoes in disease. Previous reviews are to be found in Refs. 1 through 6.

STRUCTURE OF THE NORMAL SYNOVIUM

Strictly speaking, the normal synovium is a thin structure, less than 30 μm in depth, that lines the joint cavity. It is sometimes referred to as the *intima*. It lacks blood vessels or nerves. Immediately beneath this intimal layer lies a subsynovial zone which, depending upon its anatomic location, can be fibrous, areolar, or adipose. It is far less cellular than the synovium proper but, unlike the intimal layer, is innervated, is richly perfused with blood capillaries, and contains lymphatics. Most of the nerve endings are associated with the vasculature, with some free endings in the matrix.[41] Beneath the subsynovium is the thick, fibrous capsule of the joint.

Like all connective tissues, synovium comprises a population of cells, in this case synoviocytes, contained within an extensive extracellular matrix. The precise nature of the synoviocytes has been difficult to determine, particu-

larly with regard to how many different types exist and what their defining characteristics are. Early studies using electron microscopy of normal human synovium identified two morphologically and functionally distinct types of synoviocytes—type A and type B.[7] Subsequent investigators have attempted to modify this classification in various ways. Some have postulated the existence of a third type of synoviocyte, variously called the type III, type C, or type AB cell, with a morphology intermediate between that of types A and B (see, for example, Refs. 8 through 10). Others have denied the existence of distinct types of synoviocytes, claiming instead the presence of a single cell type capable of changing its morphology to reflect the ambient physiologic environment.[11] Nevertheless, most commentators now agree that the normal synovium indeed contains two types of synoviocytes and the original nomenclature (types A and B) of Barland et al.[7] has been retained (Fig. 10-1).

The resemblance of type A cells to macrophages, originally postulated on morphologic grounds, has been further supported by biochemical and immunologic evidence, such as the presence of nonspecific esterase, receptors for the F_c component of immunoglobulin and the C_3 component of complement,[12] and a variety of other macrophage markers.[13] Like macrophages, these cells are phagocytic and derived from the bone marrow.[14]

Type B cells, in contrast, remain less well characterized and their origin is unknown. Although these cells have a standard fibroblastic morphology, there is increasing evidence that type B synoviocytes constitute a distinct cell type and are not merely those capsular cells that happen to be nearest to the joint space. For instance, they are unusual in possessing an epitope recognized by a monoclonal antibody known as Mab67,[15] and they contain high amounts of the enzyme uridine diphosphoglucose dehydrogenase,[16] the rate-limiting enzyme in the production of UDP-glucouronate, a molecule essential for the biosynthesis of hyaluronan (hyaluronic acid). This presumably reflects the large amounts of hyaluronan that these cells synthesize. Unlike type A cells, type B synoviocytes also express prolyl hydroxylase, a key enzyme in collagen biosynthesis, at high levels.[17] Type B synoviocytes are also unusual in expressing constitutively vascular cell adhesion molecule 1 (VCAM-1), the significance of which is unclear.[18]

Estimates of the relative proportions of type A and type B cells in synovia vary. There may be species differences, as type B cells have been reported to predominate in pigs[19] and rabbits,[20] whereas most studies of human synovium (see, for example, Refs. 7 and 21) have reached the opposite conclusion. Jilani and Ghadially[22] have evidence that the proportion of type A to type B synoviocytes increases with age. There is no information on how this proportion may vary between different joints of the same individual or between different anatomic locations within the same joint.

It is often stated that the synovium is two to three cell layers in depth (Fig. 10-2), and some authors describe a structured cellular arrangement in which type A cells are at the limit of the joint space, with type B cells forming a slightly deeper layer of cells behind them. This may, however, give

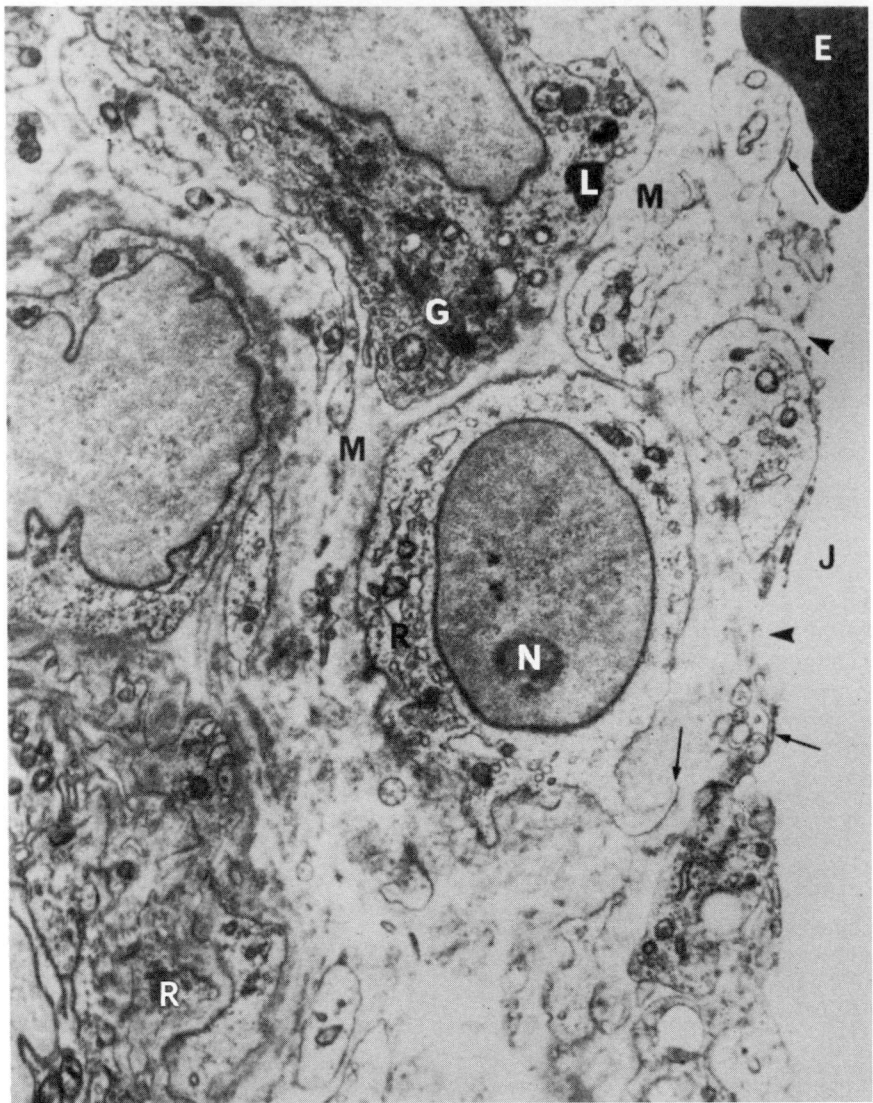

Figure 10-1 Synovial intima from a normal human knee joint. The synovial cells are set loosely in a matrix (M) which is exposed (*arrowheads*) to the joint space (J) in places. A type A cell with prominent Golgi complex (G) and lysosome (L) is easily distinguished from a type B cell with some rough endoplasmic reticulum (R) even at this low magnification. Note nucleus containing a nucleolus (N), cell process (*arrow*), and an erythrocyte (E) lying in the adjoining space. Original × 9250. (Reproduced with permission from Ghadially FN: *Fine Structure of Synovial Joints.* London, Butterworth, 1983.)

a false sense of structure of a tissue in which the distribution of cells is less regimented. Although fibroblastic cells are to be seen on the synovial surface, large areas of this surface are acellular, instead presenting naked interstitium to the joint space. It has been calculated that approximately 20 percent of the internal surface of the unstretched rabbit's knee joint is naked interstitium.[23] Within this joint, approximately 84 percent of the synovium lies above an areolar subsynovium, with adipose and fibrous subsynovium making up 8 and 7 percent, respectively, of the total.[24]

There has been some disagreement as to the surface morphology of the synovial intima. This is probably due in

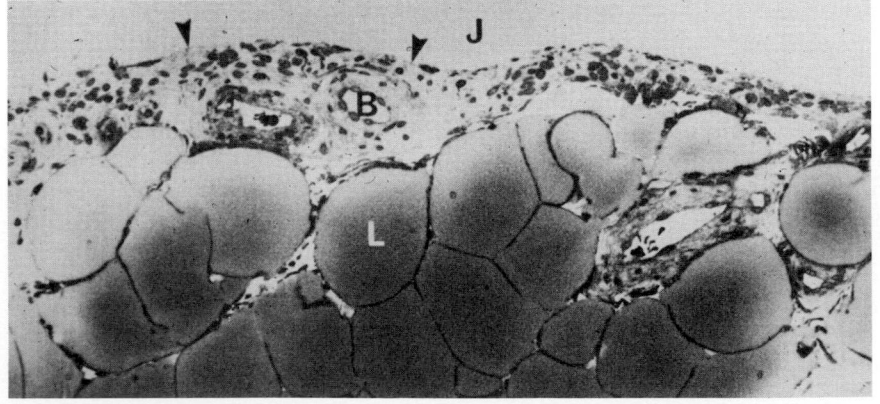

Figure 10-2 Adipose synovial membrane from a normal human knee joint. The synovial intima presents as a layer of cells (three or four cells deep) lying in a matrix that in some places is exposed (*arrowheads*) to the joint space (J). Blood vessels (B) and lipocytes containing large lipid (L) droplets are seen in the subintimal tissue. Original × 216. (Reproduced with permission from Ghadially FN: *Fine Structure of Synovial Joints.* London, Butterworth, 1983.)

large part to artifacts generated by the various fixation techniques used. A detailed examination of this matter by McDonald and Levick[23] concluded that the synovial surface in situ is smooth, with a cobblestone appearance in those parts underlain by adipose tissue. Each of the "cobblestones" appears to reflect the presence of an underlying fat cell. Although long cytoplasmic processes are present on the synovial surface, intercellular junctions are rare. Microarthroscopic examination conducted in conjunction with in vivo methylene blue staining confirms that normal human synovium also has a smooth surface in vivo.[25]

The turnover kinetics of synoviocytes are poorly understood. It has been estimated that both the type A and B cells are replaced in approximately 20 weeks,[2] but there is little hard, detailed information. It is assumed that the type A cells, being macrophages, do not divide but are replaced as necessary from precursors within the hematopoietic progenitors in the bone marrow. Type B synoviocytes divide readily in culture, but it has been extremely difficult to detect evidence of cell division in normal synovium in vivo. Henderson et al.,[26] for example, noted labeling indices of 0 to 0.3 percent following a 1- to 2-h pulse with radiolabeled thymidine injected intraarticularly into the knee joints of young adult rabbits. Similarly low labeling indices were noted for cells in the subsynovium. En vivo incubation of normal human synovium provided equally low values.[27] These low indices are not an artifact of the thymidine labeling technique, as measurements based upon Feulgen cytophotometry[28] and immunostaining for an epitope present only in dividing cells[29] gave equivalent results. This may indicate that there is little cell turnover or, alternatively, that when type B cells are lost they are replaced by cells migrating from elsewhere. The latter implies an extrasynovial source of type B progenitor cells, but its location is unknown.

The extracellular matrix of the synovium is predominantly collagenous, with collagens type I, III, IV, V, and VI all identified within the intimal and subintimal layers,[30–35] although the presence of type IV collagen is controversial.[31,34,35] Biochemical analysis[30] suggests that at least half the total collagen is type III. According to Okada et al.,[31] the normal, human synovium contains only types III and VI collagen, with type I being restricted to the subsynovium and type IV to the blood vessels. Similar investigations of rabbit synovium, in contrast, identified types I, III, V, and VI collagens throughout the synovium and subsynovium.[33]

Other proteinaceous components of the synovial matrix include fibronectin[36,37] and tenascin,[38] but elastin is absent. Laminin has also been detected, but in normal synovium this may be restricted to the walls of blood vessels.[35]

Little analysis has been made of the glycosaminoglycans and proteoglycans present in normal synovium. Type B synoviocytes synthesize large amounts of hyaluronan, and this has been localized to the intimal, pericellular environment, with little present in the subsynovium except within the walls of blood vessels.[39] Perlecan, a large heparan sulfate proteoglycan, has recently been immunolocalized to the intimal and subintimal layers of normal human synovium. Cultures of type B synoviocytes were shown to synthesize perlecan in culture, and approximately 25 percent of the proteoglycan synthesized by these cells was shown to contain heparan sulfate.[40]

The presence of perlecan within synovium is as interesting as it is unexpected. This proteoglycan is normally found as a characteristic component of basement membrane, a structure that is not found in synovium. Nevertheless, there is evidence that two other components of basement membrane, type IV collagen and laminin, may also present in synovium, although their expression may be limited to rheumatoid conditions.[31,34,35] The significance of this is unknown.

NORMAL SYNOVIAL PHYSIOLOGY

Study of the synovial vasculature goes back at least 250 years, with William Hunter in 1743[42] observing vessels within the synovium, which he named the *circulus articuli vasculosus*. Knight and Levick[43] found that in normal rabbit knee synovium, the majority of the capillaries occur within 25 μm of the joint space, being at their most concentrated 6.2 to 11.5 μm below the synovial surface.[43] The tissue is richly vascularized, with 670 to 830 capillaries per square millimeter, irrespective of whether the subsynovium is areolar or adipose. This exceeds the density of 289 capillaries per square millimeter reported for the adjacent gastrocnemius muscle.[44]

About half of the synovial capillaries contain fenestrations, which are oriented toward the joint space.[47] This reinforces the importance of the synovial blood vessels in providing for the poorly perfused intraarticular structures of the joint.

In diffusing from the synovial capillaries into the joint space, fluid and dissolved species have to diffuse through the capillary endothelium and the matrix of the synovium.[48] Neither of these barriers is freely permeable under normal conditions. Large proteins, in particular, are subjected to a sieving effect, which lowers their concentration in the synovial fluid as compared with plasma.[49,50] Examples of proteins excluded from synovial fluid by this process are α_2-macroglobulin, a large proteinase inhibitor, and fibrinogen. The absence of the latter from synovial fluid contributes to the observation that normal synovial fluid does not clot. Although proteins enter the joint space by diffusion from the synovial capillaries, they leave the joint via the lymphatics present within the subsynovium. Unlike the former process, the rate at which proteins are removed from the joint is independent of molecular weight. The capillary endothelium of the normal synovium also presents a barrier to the extravasation of leukocytes, which are poorly represented in both synovium and synovial fluid.

Although synovial fluid is depleted in certain plasma proteins, it is enriched by a number of other substances synthesized locally by the synovium and cartilage. The type B synoviocytes synthesize prodigious quantities of hyaluronic acid (hyaluronan), which accumulates to a concentration of approximately 3 mg/mL in normal joints. Hyaluronan is commonly but incorrectly held responsible for the impressive lubricating properties of synovial fluids. This function is actually performed by lubricin, a large glycoprotein that is also a product of synoviocytes.[51,52] Both synoviocytes and chondrocytes[53,54] are highly glycolytic cells; therefore they produce large amounts of lactic acid. Although the buffering capacity of normal synovial fluid is sufficient to maintain a pH of 7.3 to 7.6,[55] it can become considerably acidotic in chronic inflammation.

SYNOVIUM AND JOINT STABILITY

Although the most obvious function of synovium is to regulate the intracellular biochemical environment in the manner described above, it also plays an indirect and less appreciated role in the maintenance of joint stability. The ligaments, capsule, and surrounding musculature make the most obvious contributions to the mechanical stability of joints, but there is evidence that synovium, a mechanically weak tissue, plays an indirect stabilizing role. There are two aspects to this.

The first involves the manner in which fluid enters and leaves the joint. As stated above, fluid enters the joint space by diffusing through both the endothelial lining of the synovial capillaries and the matrix of the synovium. Fluid egress from the joint, in contrast, occurs largely via the lymphatics and is more efficient, possibly because joint movement repeatedly compresses and decompresses the lymphatic vessels, leading to a "sucking" effect. When joints are immobilized, therefore, intraarticular pressures rise. Because egress is more efficient than ingress, the joint space pressure is normally subatmospheric. In the normal human knee, this negative pressure difference is approximately 4 mmHg,[56,57] although it is not clear whether this is true for all joints.[57,58] The negative pressure is thought to make an important contribution to the stability of joints.

A second stabilizing mechanism involves the adhesive properties of synovial fluid. As pointed out by Simkin,[5] although synovial fluid has an important lubricating function and facilitates the smooth, lateral motion of cartilage moving against cartilage, it has a stickiness that resists the distraction of two surfaces in contact. For the reasons given above, the volume of synovial fluid is normally low and is limited to a thin coating over the articulating surfaces. When two cartilaginous surfaces come into contact, the thin layer of synovial fluid that is trapped between them resists their distraction, thus contributing to stability.

Both of these stabilizing mechanisms are compromised under conditions where there is a joint effusion.

SYNOVIAL PATHOPHYSIOLOGY

The most obvious change to the synovium occurs during inflammation. Regardless of the cause of the inflammation, the early response is the ingress of polymorphonuclear leukocytes (PMNs) into the joint. In a more chronic situation, the population of infiltrating leukocytes shifts from one dominated by PMNs to one dominated by macrophages. Lymphocytes also accumulate in chronic inflammation, especially if the inflammation is driven by immune mechanisms. The presence of large numbers of mast cells in these conditions is increasingly recognized.[59]

The earliest synovial changes leading to the influx of leukocytes occur in the endothelial cells of the subsynovial capillaries. A class of adhesion molecules known as *selectins* is present in increased amounts on the endothelial surface. These bind to carbohydrate moieties on the leukocyte surface, leading to a weak interaction between the two cells and a characteristic rolling of the leukocyte along the inner surface of the vessel. This is followed by upregulation of leukocyte selectins and then the expression of different classes of adhesion molecules on the surfaces of both the leukocyte and endothelium. The former now express adhesion molecules known as *integrins* on their cell surface, and these bind strongly to adhesion molecules of the immunoglobulin superfamily, such as the intercellular adhesion molecule 1 (ICAM-1), on the endothelial surface. When these two types of adhesion molecules engage each other, strong intercellular interaction occurs, and the rolling motion of the leukocytes is supplanted by firm binding which immobilizes the leukocytes as a prelude to diapadesis and extravasation out of the capillary and into the synovium and synovial fluid. These matters are reviewed by Springer.[60] Human synovial tissue expresses a number of selectins, integrins, and ICAMs as well as the hyaluronan receptor CD44.[61–65]

The distribution of leukocytes within the inflamed joint is not uniform: PMNs are not highly abundant in the synovium but tend to congregate in the synovial fluid. The opposite is true for macrophages and lymphocytes. The reasons for this are not known but are thought to reside within the different adhesion molecules present upon the surfaces of the various leukocytes.[63]

Synoviocyte hyperplasia also contributes to the increased cellularity of the inflamed synovium. This involves largely type B synoviocytes. In the knee joints of rabbits, for example, the mitotic index of synoviocytes rose from 0 to 0.3 percent in normal knee joints to 15.3 ± 2.6 percent 3 days after the onset of antigen-induced arthritis.[26] This proliferative potential is presumably also realized during the regrowth of synovium after synovectomy. The increase in synovial cell mass is seen at its most exuberant in the rheumatoid pannus. Despite this impressive increase in cellularity, it has proved very difficult to identify mitotic cells in human rheumatoid pannus.[27,29] This may mean that most of the increase in cell mass occurred early in the disease, before biopsy was performed, that cell number increased through migration rather than through mitosis, or that there is a decreased rate of cell death rather than an increased rate of cell division. The last of these possibilities is interesting in view of recent evidence that synoviocytes in rheumatoid joints have a defect in their ability to undergo programmed cell death.[66]

Much interest has been generated by the detection within rheumatoid synovium of an unusual synovial cell with a distinct stellate morphology.[67,68] After much debate about its nature and origins, the present consensus is that this represents a type B synoviocyte that has undergone morphologic and functional modification in response to the local inflammatory environment.[69]

Another type of cell found in the synovium of diseased but not normal joints is the giant cell.[70,71] In certain cases, these accumulate in response to large wear particles of bone and cartilage that occur in osteoarthritis. Synovial responses to such particles are likely to be involved in the pathophysiology of such joints.[72]

The cells of the diseased synovium are abnormal not only in number and type but also in function. In particular, many of the cells are in an activated state, where they secrete mediators of inflammation and tissue destruction. Such mediators include cytokines, eicosanoids, free radicals, and proteinases.

In addition to the increase in cell mass and the presence of an increased variety of cell types, the rheumatoid synovium exhibits a hypertrophy resulting from increased deposition of matrix. The organization of the matrix is also disturbed in rheumatoid synovium. For example, type VI collagen is no longer restricted to the intimal layer but occurs throughout the both the synovium and subsynovium.[31] A similar extension in the synovial distribution of hyaluronan[39] and tenascin[38] has been noted in rheumatoid tissue. The type III collagen of rheumatoid synovium is more than normally susceptible to pepsin solubilization,[30] which may reflect less cross-linking, possibly because of more recent biosynthetic origin or the actions of synovial proteinases.

Early rheumatoid synovium also shows evidence of neovascularization, presumably in response to the increased cellularity and size of the tissue. There is evidence that in late rheumatoid disease, the rate of matrix deposition exceeds the rate of neovascularization, leading to a decreased synovial density of capillaries below the joint surface.[45]

Many of these pathologic changes occur in response to locally produced cytokines and other such mediators. Discussion of these lies outside the scope of this chapter, but they include interleukins 1, 6, 8, and 10; tumor necrosis factor α; basic fibroblast growth factor (bFGF); transforming growth factor-β (TGF-β); various colony stimulating factors; free radicals; and eicosanoids.

The synovia of osteoarthritic joints often show changes that are qualitatively similar to those of rheumatoid synovia but which are quantitatively reduced. Pannus, of course, is absent, but discrete areas of synovium are sometimes microscopically indistinguishable from the rheumatoid appearance.[73]

In addition to the structural and cellular changes described above, the inflamed synovium is physiologically altered. The synovial capillaries are far more permeable to fluid egress, resulting in large increases in the volume of synovial fluid.[45,48] These vessels also permit freer passage of macromolecules, thus increasing the protein concentration of the synovial fluid and enhancing the representation within it of large proteins.[42,44] The concentration of hyaluronan is, however, lower, and the fluid is consequently less viscous.[74] It is unclear whether the decrease in hyaluronan concentration reflects reduced synthesis or increased breakdown of this macromolecule. As noted earlier in this chapter, the capillaries of the inflamed synovium are also more permeable to cells, and the cellularity of synovial fluid is consequently much higher (Tables 10-1 and 10-2). Most of the cells recovered from the synovial fluids of inflamed joints are PMNs.

These changes have several important consequences. One is that the synovial fluid becomes anoxic and acidotic. The anoxia presumably reflects the higher oxygen demand imposed by the increased cellularity of the inflamed joints. In chronic rheumatoid disease, anoxia may additionally be engendered by the reduced capillary perfusion of the synovium.[45] The acidosis of inflammatory synovial fluid is primarily a lactate acidosis reflecting increased glycolytic ac-

TABLE 10-1 Classification of Synovial Effusions

	Normal	Noninflammatory, group 1	Inflammatory, group 2	Septic, group 3	Hemorrhagic
Viscosity	High	High	Low	Variable	Variable
Color	Pale yellow	Pale to dark yellow	Yellow to green	Variable	Bloody
Clarity	Transparent	Transparent	Translucent	Opaque	Opaque
WBC, mm^3	200	200–100	2000–75,000	Often 100,000	Same as blood
PMNs, %	25	25	50 (often)	75	Same as blood
Culture	Negative	Negative	Negative	Often positive	Negative
Mucin clot	Firm	Firm	Friable	Friable	Friable
Glucose	Nearly equal to blood	Nearly equal to blood	25 mg per 100 mL, lower than blood	25 mg per 100 mL, lower than blood	Same as blood

Source: Reproduced with permission from Morrey BF: *The Elbow and Its Disorders.* Philadelphia, Saunders, 1985.

TABLE 10-2 Conditions Associated with Types of Synovial Fluid

Group 1	Group 2	Group 3	Hemorrhagic
Acromegaly	Acute rheumatic fever	Acute tuberculosis	Anticoagulant therapy
Acute rheumatic fever	Ankylosing spongylitis	Bacterial infections	Hemophilia and other bleeding disorders
Aseptic necrosis	Arthritis of inflammatory bowel disease		Neuropathic joint disorders
Degenerative joint disease	Chronic infectious tuberculosis		Pigmented villonodular synovitis
Hypertrophic osteo-arthropathy	Crystal-induced synovitis		Synovioma
Neuropathic arthropathy	Fungous arthritis		Thrombocytopenia
Osteochondritis dissecans	Psoriatic arthritis		Thrombocytosis
Osteochondromatosis	Reiter syndrome		Trauma
Systemic lupus erythematosus	Rheumatoid arthritis		
Trauma	Systemic lupus erythematosus		
	Viral arthritis		

Source: Reproduced with permission from Morregy BF: *The Elbow and Its Disorders.* Philadelphia, Saunders, 1985.

tivity assumed to result from lowered ambient oxygen tensions.[75–78] These further lead to increased glucose consumption and elevated CO_2 production (Table 10-1). Recent studies have shown that cytokines such as IL-1 can increase lactate production under conditions of stable oxygen tension,[54] suggesting a mechanism of intraarticular acidosis that does not require reduced pO_2 values. The pH of synovial fluid can fall as low as 6.6 in rheumatoid arthritis.

The increased volume of synovial fluid reduces the stability of the joint when an effusion is present; intraarticular pressures exceed atmospheric pressure, and external air pressure no longer exerts its stabilizing influence. This effect increases quantitatively with the volume of the fluid.[79,80] Rheumatoid joints develop higher pressures than normal joints, probably because the thickened fibrotic tissue present in the former is less compliant.[79]

Another destabilizing influence of effusions results from the way in which the synovial fluid no longer forms a thin adhesive bond between the opposed cartilaginous surfaces. Instead, the cartilages are held apart by a comparatively thick layer of fluid, which fails to resist distraction of these surfaces.[4,5] As well as destabilizing the joint, chronically increased intraarticular pressures are thought to contribute to the development of popliteal cysts.

The magnitude of the intraarticular pressure varies with the degree of flexion of the joint, and increases with contracture of the surrounding musculature. Pressures in the knee joint are minimal at a flexion angle of 30°, which is why afflicted individuals tend to maintain the joint at this angle. Muscle contracture can generate enormous intraarticular pressures. Jayson and Dixon have recorded a peak pressure of over 500 mmHg is response to quadriceps contraction following the injection of 40 mL of saline into a rheumatoid knee.[80] In this instance, rupture of the joint capsule resulted. Such pressures are sufficient to interrupt the flow of blood through the synovial capillaries. It has been suggested that the motion of joints with large effusions leads to repetitive interruptions of the synovial blood supply and consequent ischemia-reperfusion injury.[58,81]

SYNOVIUM AND PARTICLES

Particles are generated within joints by biological, chemical, and physical processes. The most obvious example from the first category is the intraarticular accumulation of erythrocytes that occurs as a result of bleeding into the joint. Chemical mechanisms lead to the intraarticular deposition of crystals, particularly urate in gout, pyrophosphate in pseudogout, and hydroxyapatite in osteoarthritis. In addition, the articulating surfaces of joints undergo the physical process of wear. When these surfaces are cartilaginous, they release particles of cartilage. When prosthetic surfaces are involved, they generate particles of the prosthetic material which, in the case of most total joint replacements, are made up of metal, polyethylene, and, often, bone cement.

Irrespective of the origin or chemical nature of the particles, they initially engage the synovium. Once the particles have been engaged by the synovium, they can undergo one of three fates—retention in the synovium, intracellular degradation, or transport out of the joint and to the regional lymph nodes. Size and composition are key determining factors. Transfer to lymph nodes has been observed in humans for particles of polyethylene,[86,87] carbon,[87] and metal.[88] These types of particles are all small and indigestible; they were presumably transported to the lymph nodes following phagocytosis by synovial leukocytes. Larger particles of this type (larger than 20 μm), in contrast, may remain embedded within the extracellular matrix of the synovium for considerable periods of time.

Crystals are much more soluble within the acidic endosomes of synovial cells. McCarty et al.[89] injected radioactive crystals of calcium pyrophosphate into normal knee joints of rabbits and knee joints with hemosiderosis[90] as well as into the knee joints of four patients with arthritis.[89] Clearance rates were inversely related to the sizes of the crystals. Half-lives for the clearance of 10- to 20-μm crystals were 9.5 days in the knees of normal rabbits but 30 to 90 days in human knees. Hemosiderosis decreased the rate of clearance from the knees of rabbits. The mechanism of clearance was by intracellular crystal dissolution, and 99 percent of the radioactivity cleared from the joint appeared in the urine within 72 h.

Less is known of the fate of biological wear particles. Particles of bone and cartilage have been found within synovial fluid[91,92] and both intracellularly and extracellularly, depending upon their size, within human synovium.[93-95] The fate of these particles is unknown, although data with rabbits[96] would suggest a prolonged dwell time in the synovium.

Synoviocytes readily phagocytose erythrocytes. Although most components of the erythrocyte are readily digestible within synovial lysosomes, there often remains an iron-rich residue known as a siderosome.[82] In many cases there is a chronic inflammatory reaction to the intrasynovial presence of erythrocytes.[83,84] The addition of iron complexes to cultures of synovial fibroblasts leads to increased collagenase expression,[85] suggesting a mechanism for increased cartilage breakdown. Reactions of this nature explain the severe destructive arthropathies seen in hemarthrosis.[82-84]

Crystals are usually highly inflammatory in joints. This may reflect their small sizes, which permit ready phagocytosis. The cellular capture of various types of crystal found in joints has been associated with the release of a number of inflammatory mediators, including prostaglandins,[97] collagenase,[98] and interleukin-1[99] as well as the activation of complement.[100] Certain crystals may also be mitogenic for synoviocytes.[101] In view of these properties, it is not surprising that the synovia of joints in which crystals are deposited show a rampant, acute inflammatory reaction, with a heavy leukocytic infiltration and evidence of synovial hyperplasia.

Wear particles can trigger many of the same responses. Injection of cartilaginous particles into the knees of rabbits leads to synovial inflammation and loss of articular cartilage.[96] There is evidence that similar reactions occur in human joints and that this may partly explain the benefits of articular lavage[102] in certain patients with arthritis (reviewed in Ref. 103).

Tissue reactions to wear debris released from prosthetic joints are presently the subject of considerable study, as these may be responsible for the process of aseptic loosening.[104] Of particular interest is a membrane with many of the histologic features of synovium that forms at the interface of the prosthesis with the surrounding bone.[105] This membrane contains particles of metal, polyethylene, and—for cemented prostheses—bone cement. Many of these particles are small, intracellular, and associated with the production of modulators of bone metabolism including prostaglandins,[105] collagenase,[105] interleukins,[106] and nitric oxide.[107]

SYNOVIUM AND INFECTION

Microorganisms enter the synovium hematogenously or following injury. It appears that certain bacteria preferentially localize in joints. The presence of microbial agents within joints triggers a massive influx of leukocytes, particularly polymorphonuclear leukocytes, which phagocytose and attempt to kill the invading organisms. In the process they release very large amounts of a wide variety of inflammatory mediators, including prostaglandins, cytokines, and free radicals as well as proteolytic enzymes. Under these conditions a purulent synovitis occurs, with rapid destruction of articular cartilage. The speed with which the cartilage is lost may be explained by the production of bacterial factors that induce very rapid chondrolysis.[108]

GENE TRANSFER TO SYNOVIUM

It has been proposed that the transfer of certain genes to the synovial lining of joints could be a useful therapeutic strategy for the treatment of arthritis[109] and other joint disorders.[110] The original idea[109] was to introduce into the cells of the synovial lining genes that encode secreted, antiarthritic proteins.

Gene transfer may be accomplished by direct injection of the gene, in association with an appropriate vector (in vivo gene delivery), or by removing synoviocytes and manipulating them genetically outside the body and reimplanting them (ex vivo gene delivery). In vivo gene delivery to synovium may be achieved with a number of vectors,[111,112] but none is yet suitable for human use. Ex vivo gene delivery is more laborious, but it can make use of vectors based on murine retroviruses, which are very well developed. Also, because all genetic manipulations occur outside the body and no infectious agents are introduced into the patient, it is presently safer.

Ex vivo delivery of a gene encoding a blocker of interleukin-1, known as the interleukin-1 receptor antagonist (IL-1Ra or IRAP), has been successfully transferred to the synovial lining of rabbits' knee joints, where it exerts an antiarthritic effect.[113-116]

Based on these findings a human trial was proposed and approved by the FDA.[117] The first patient was treated on July 17, 1996, thus initiating the world's first human gene therapy for arthritis or any other chronic nonfatal condition.

REFERENCES

1. Davies DV: Synovial membrane and synovial fluid of joints. *Lancet* 7:815–819, 1946.
2. Henderson B, Pettipher ER: The synovial lining cell: Biology and pathobiology. *Arthritis Rheum* 15:1–32, 1985.
3. Henderson B, Edwards JCW: *The Synovial Lining in Health and Disease.* London, Chapman and Hall, 1987.
4. Simkin PA: Physiology of normal and abnormal synovium. *Semin Arthritis Rheum* 21:179–183, 1991.
5. Simkin PA: Biology and function of synovium, in Finerman G, Noyes FR (eds): *Biology and Biomechanics of the Traumatized Synovial Joint: The Knee as a Model.* American Academy of Orthopaedic Surgeons, Park Ridge, Illinois. 1994, pp 5–15.
6. Hung GL, Evans CH: Synovium, in: Fu FH, Harner C, Vince KG (eds): *Knee Surgery.* Baltimore, Williams & Wilkins, 1994, pp 141–154.
7. Barland P, Novikoff AB, Hammerman D: Electron microscopy of the human synovial membrane. *J Cell Biol* 14:207–220, 1962.
8. Burmester GR, Dimitriu-Bona A, Waters SJ, Winchester RJ: Identification of three major synovial lining cell populations by monoclonal antibodies directed to Ia antigens and antigens associated with monocytes/macrophages and fibroblasts. *Scand J Immunol* 17:69–82, 1983.
9. Kinsella TD, Baum J, Ziff M: Studies of isolated synovial lining cells of rheumatoid and non-rheumatoid synovial membranes. *Arthritis Rheum* 13:734, 1970.
10. Ghadially FN: *Fine Structure of Synovial Joints.* London, Butterworths, 1983.
11. Ghadially FN: The articular territory of the reticuloendothelial system. *Ultrastruct Pathol* 1:249–264, 1980.
12. Theofilopoulos AN, Carson DA, Tavassoli M, et al: Evidence for the presence of receptors for C_3 and $IgGF_c$ of human synovial cells. *Arthritis Rheum* 23:1–19, 1980.
13. Athanasou NA, Quinn J: Immunocytochemical analysis of human synovial lining cells: Phenotypic relation to other marrow derived cells. *Ann Rheum Dis* 50:311–315, 1991.
14. Edwards JCW, Willoughby DA: Demonstration of bone marrow derived cells in synovial lining by means of giant intracellular granules as genetic markers. *Ann Rheum Dis* 41:177–182, 1982.
15. Stevens CR, Mapp PI, Revell PA: A monoclonal antibody (Mab67) marks type B synoviocytes. *Rheumatol Int* 10:103–106, 1990.
16. Pitsillides AA, Wilkinson LS, Mehdizadeh S, et al: Uridine diphosphoglucose dehydrogenase activity in normal and rheumatoid synovium: The description of a specialized synovial lining cell. *Int J Exp Pathol* 74:27–34, 1993.
17. Wilkinson LS, Pitsillides AA, Worrall JG, Edwards JCW: Light microscopic characterization of the fibroblast-like synovial intimal cell (synoviocyte). *Arthritis Rheum* 35:1179–1184, 1992.
18. Wilkinson LS, Edwards JCW, Ponston RN, Haskard DO: Expression of vascular cell adhesion molecule-1 in normal and inflamed synovium. *Lab Invest* 68:82–88, 1993.
19. Fell HB, Glauert AM, Barratt MEJ, Greer R: The pig synovium. I: The intact synovium *in vivo* and in organ culture. *J Anat* 122:663–680, 1976.
20. Krey PR, Cohen AS: Fine structural analysis of rabbit synovial cells. The normal synovium and changes in organ cultures. *Arthritis Rheum* 16:324–340, 1973.
21. Castor CW: The microscopic structure of human synovial tissue. *Arthritis Rheum* 3:140–151, 1960.
22. Jilani M, Ghadially FN: An ultrastructural study of age-associated changes in the rabbit synovial membrane. *J Anat* 146:201–215, 1986.
23. McDonald JN, Levick JR: Morphology of surface synoviocytes *in situ* at normal and raised joint pressure, studied by scanning electron microscopy. *Ann Rheum Dis* 47:232–240, 1988.
24. Knight AD, Levick JR: Morphometry of the ultrastructure of the blood-joint barrier in the rabbit knee. *Q J Exp Physiol* 69:271–288, 1984.
25. Frizziero L, Georgountzos A, Zizzi F, Focherini MC: Microarthroscopic study of the morphological features of normal and pathological synovial membrane. *Arthroscopy* 8:504–509, 1992.
26. Henderson B, Glynn LE, Chayen J: Cell division in the synovial lining in experimental allergic arthritis: Proliferation of cells during the development of chronic arthritis. *Ann Rheum Dis* 41:275–281, 1982.
27. Mohr W, Beneke G, Mohing W: Proliferation of synovial lining cells and fibroblasts. *Ann Rheum Dis* 34:219–224, 1975.
28. Coulton LA, Henderson B, Bitensky L, Chayen J: DNA synthesis in human rheumatoid and non-rheumatoid synovial lining. *Ann Rheum Dis* 39:241–247, 1980.
29. Lalor PA, Mapp PI, Hall PA, Revell PA: Proliferative activity of cells in the synovium as demonstrated by a monoclonal antibody, Ki67. *Rheumatol Int* 7:183–186, 1987.
30. Eyre DR, Muir H: Type III collagen: A major constituent of rheumatoid and normal human synovial membrane. *Connect Tissue Res* 4:11–16, 1975.
31. Okada Y, Naka K, Minamoto T, et al: Localization of type VI collagen in the lining cell layer of normal and rheumatoid synovium. *Lab Invest* 63:647–656, 1990.
32. Ashhurst DE, Bland YS, Levick JR: An immunohistochemical study of the collagens of rabbit synovial interstitium. *J Rheumatol* 18:1669–1672, 1991.
33. Wolf J, Carsons SE: Distribution of type VI collagen expression in synovial tissue and cultured synoviocytes: Relation to fibronectin expression. *Ann Rheum Dis* 50:493–496, 1991.
34. Pollock LE, Lalor O, Revell PA: Type IV collagen and laminin in the synovial intimal layer: An immunohistochemical study. *Rheumatol Int* 9:277–280, 1990.
35. Schneider M, Voss B, Rauterberg J, et al: Basement membrane proteins in synovial membrane: Distribution in rheumatoid arthritis and synthesis by fibroblast-like cells. *Clin Rheumatol* 13:90–97, 1994.
36. Linck G, Stocker S, Grimauld JA, Porte A: Distribution of immunoreactive fibronectin and collagen (types I, III, IV) in mouse joints. *Histochemistry* 70:323–328, 1983.
37. Mapp PI, Revell PA: Fibronectin production by synovial intimal cells. *Rheumatol Int* 5:229–237, 1985.
38. McCachren SP, Lightner VA: Expression of human tenascin in synovitis and its regulation by interleukin-1. *Arthritis Rheum* 35:1185–1196, 1992.
39. Worrall JG, Bayliss MT, Edwards JCS: Morphological localization of hyaluronan in normal and diseased synovium. *J Rheumatol* 18:1466–1472, 1991.
40. Dodge GR, Boesler EW, Jimenez SA: Expression of the basement membrane heparan sulfate proteoglycan (perlecan) in human synovium and in cultured human synovial cells. *Lab Invest* 73:649–657, 1995.
41. Freeman M: The innervation of the knee joint: An anatomical and histological study in the cat. *J Anat* 101:502–532, 1967.

42. Hunter W: Of the structure and diseases of articulating cartilages. *Phil Trans R Soc Lond* 42:514–421, 1743.

43. Knight AD, Levick JR: The density and distribution of capillaries around a synovial cavity. *Q J Exp Physiol* 68:629–644, 1983.

44. Perry MA: Capillary filtration and permeability coefficients calculated from measurement of interendothelial cell functions in rabbit lung and skeletal muscle. *Microvasc Res* 19:142–157, 1980.

45. Stevens CR, Blake DR, Merry P, et al: A comparative study by morphometry of the microvasculature in normal and rheumatoid synovium. *Arthritis Rheum* 34:1508–1513, 1991.

46. Wilkinson LS, Edwards JCW: Microvascular distribution in normal human synovium. *J Anat* 167:129–136, 1989.

47. Suter ER, Majno G: Ultrastructure of the joint capsule in the rat: Presence of two kinds of capillaries. *Nature* 102:920–921, 1964.

48. Levick JR: Synovial fluid exchange—A case of flow through fibrous mats. *News Physiol Soc* 4:198–202, 1989.

49. Simkin PA, Pizzorno JE: Transynovial exchange of small molecules in normal human subjects. *J Appl Physiol* 36:581–587, 1974.

50. Levick JR: Permeability of rheumatoid and normal human synovium to specific plasma proteins. *Arthritis Rheum* 24:1550–1560, 1981.

51. Swann DA, Slayter HS, Silver FH: The molecular structure of lubricating glycoprotein-1, the boundary lubricant for articular cartilage. *J Biol Chem* 256:5921–5925, 1981.

52. Swann DA, Silver FH, Slayter HS, et al: The molecular structure and lubricating activity of lubricin isolated from bovine and human synovial fluids. *Biochem J* 225:195–201, 1985.

53. Bywaters EGL: The metabolism of joint tissues. *J Pathol Bacteriol* 44:247–268, 1937.

54. Stefanovic-Racic M, Stadler J, Georgescu HI, Evans CH: Nitric oxide and energy production in articular chondrocytes. *J Cell Physiol* 159:274–280, 1994.

55. Cummings NA, Nordby GL: Measurement of synovial fluid pH in normal and arthritic knees. *Arthritis Rheum* 9:47–56, 1966.

56. Levick JR Jr: Point pressure-volume studies: Their importance, design and interpretation. *J Rheumatol* 10:353–357, 1983.

57. Simkin P, Benedict R: Hydrostatic and oncotic determinants of microvascular fluid balance in normal canine joints. *Arthritis Rheum* 33:80–86, 1990.

58. Gaffney K, Williams RB, Jolliffe VA, Blake DR: Intraarticular pressure changes in rheumatoid and normal peripheral joints. *Ann Rheum Dis* 54:670–673, 1995.

59. Gruber B, Poznansky M, Boss E, et al: Characterization and functional studies of rheumatoid synovial mast cells. *Arthritis Rheum* 29:944–955, 1986.

60. Springer TA: Traffic signals for lymphocyte recirculation and leukocyte emigration: The multistep paradigm. *Cell* 76:301–314, 1994.

61. Johnson BA, Haines GK, Harlow LA, Koch AE: Adhesion molecule expression in human synovial tissue. *Arthritis Rheum* 36:137, 1993.

62. Haynes BF, Hale LP, Patton KL, et al: Measurement of an adhesion molecule as an indicator of inflammatory disease activity: Up-regulation of the receptor for hyaluronate (CD44) in rheumatoid arthritis. *Arthritis Rheum* 34:1434–1443, 1991.

63. Morales-Ducret J, Wayner E, Elices MJ, et al: α_4/β_1 integrin (VLA-4) ligand in arthritis: Vascular cell adhesion molecule-1 expression in synovium and on fibroblast-like synoviocytes. *J Immunol* 149:1424–1431, 1992.

64. Abbot SE, Kaul A, Stevens CR, Blake DR: Isolation and culture of synovial microvascular endothelial cells: Characterization and assessment of adhesion molecule expression. *Arthritis Rheum* 35:401–406, 1992.

65. Nikkari L, Aho H, Yli-Jama T, et al: Expression of integrin family of cell adhesion receptors in rheumatoid synovium: α_6 Integrin subunit in normal and hyperplastic synovial lining cell layer. *Am J Pathol* 142:1019–1027, 1993.

66. Firestein GS: Invasive fibroblastlike synoviocytes in rheumatoid arthritis: passive responders or transformed aggressors? *Arthritis Rheum.* In press, 1996.

67. Winchester RJ, Brumester GM: Demonstration of Ia antigens on certain dendritic cells and on a novel elongate cell found in human synovial tissue. *Scand J Immunol* 14:439–444, 1981.

68. Gadher SJ, Woolley DE: Comparative studies of adherent rheumatoid synovial cells in primary culture: Characterization of the dendritic (stellate) cell. *Rheumatol Int* 7:13–22, 1987.

69. Clarris BJ, Leizer T, Fraser JRE, Hamilton JA: Diverse morphological responses of normal human synovial fibroblasts to mononuclear leukocyte products: Relationship to prostaglandin production and plasminogen activator activities and comparison to the effects of purified interleukin-1. *Rheumatol Int* 7:35, 1987.

70. Soren A, Waugh TR: The giant cells in the synovial membrane. *Ann Rheum Dis* 40:496–500, 1981.

71. Donald HF, Kerr JFR: Giant cells in the synovium in rheumatoid arthritis. *Med J Aust* 1:761–762, 1950.

72. Evans CH, Brown TD: Role of physical and mechanical agents in degrading the matrix, in Wossner JF, Howell DS (eds): *Joint Cartilage Degradation. Basic and Clinical Aspects.* New York, Marcel Dekker, 1993, pp 187–208.

73. Lindblad S, Hedors E: Arthroscopic and immunohistologic characterization of knee joint synovitis in osteoarthritis. *Arthritis Rheum* 30:1081–1088, 1987.

74. Dahl LB, Dahl IMS, Engstrom-Laurent A, Granath K: Concentration and molecular weight of sodium hyaluronate in synovial fluid from patients with rheumatoid arthritis and other arthropathies. *Ann Rheum Dis* 44:817–822, 1985.

75. Levick JR: Hypoxia and acidosis in chronic inflammatory arthritis: Relation to vascular supply and dynamic effusion pressure. *J Rheumatol* 17:579–582, 1990.

76. Simkin PA, Bassett JE: Lactate in synovial effusions. *J Rheumatol* 19:1017–1019, 1992.

77. Richman AI, Su EY, Ho G: Reciprocal relationship of synovial fluid volume and oxygen tension. *Arthritis Rheum* 24:701–705, 1981.

78. Lund-Oleson K: Oxygen tension in synovial fluids. *Arthritis Rheum* 13:769–776, 1970.

79. Jayson MIV, Dixon A St J: Intraarticular pressure in rheumatoid arthritis of the knee: I. Pressure changes during passive joint distention. *Ann Rheum Dis* 29:261–265, 1970.

80. Jayson MIV, Dixon A St J: Intraarticular pressure in rheumatoid arthritis of the knee: III. Pressure changes during joint use. *Ann Rheum Dis* 29:401–408, 1970.

81. Blake DR, Merry P, Unsworth J, et al: Hypoxic-reperfusion injury in the inflamed human joint. *Lancet* 1:289–293, 1989.

82. Roy S, Ghadially FN: Ultrastructure of the synovial membrane in human hemarthrosis. *J Bone Joint Surg* 49(A):1636–1646, 1967.

83. Roy S, Ghadially FN: Synovial membrane in experimentally produced chronic haemarthrosis. *Ann Rheum Dis* 28:402–413, 1969.

84. Mainardi CL: Proliferative synovitis in hemophilia. *Arthritis Rheum* 21:137–144, 1978.

85. Okazaki I, Brinckerhoff CE, Sinclair JF, et al: Iron increases collagenase production by rabbit synovial fibroblasts. *J Lab Clin Med* 97:396–402, 1981.

86. Morawski DR, Coutts RD, Handal EG, et al: Polyethylene debris in lymph nodes after a total hip arthroplasty. *J Bone Joint Surg* 77A:772–776, 1995.

87. Bauer TW, Saltarelli M, McMahon JT, Wilde AH: Regional dissemination of wear debris from a total knee prosthesis: A case report. *J Bone Joint Surg* 75A:106–111, 1993.

88. Shinto Y, Uchida A, Yoshikawa H, et al: Inguinal lymphadenopathy due to a metal release from a prosthesis: A case report. *J Bone Joint Surg* 75B:266–269, 1993.

89. McCarty DJ, Palmer DW, Halverson PB: Clearance of calcium pyrophosphate dihydrate crystals *in vivo:* I. Studies using ^{169}Yb labeled triclinic crystals. *Arthritis Rheum* 22:718–727, 1979.

90. McCarty DJ, Palmer DW, Garancis JC: Clearance of calcium pyrophosphate dihydrate crystals *in vivo:* III. Effects of synovial hemosiderosis. *Arthritis Rheum* 24:706–710, 1981.

91. Evans CH, Mears DC, McKnight JL: A preliminary ferrographic survey of the wear particles in human synovial fluid. *Arthritis Rheum* 24:912–918, 1981.

92. Evans CH, Mears DC, Stanitski CL: Ferrographic analysis of wear in human joints: Evaluation by comparison with arthroscopic examination of symptomatic knees. *J Bone Joint Surg* 64B:572–578, 1982.

93. Muirden KD: Giant cells, cartilage and bone fragments within rheumatoid synovial membrane: Clinico-pathological correlations. *Aust Ann Med* 2:105–110, 1970.

94. Gordon GV, Villamiera T, Schumacher HR, Gohel V: Autopsy study correlating degree of osteoarthritis, synovitis and evidence of articular calcification. *J Rheumatol* 11:681–686, 1984.

95. Revell PA, Mayston V, Lalor P, Mapp PP: The synovial membrane in osteoarthritis: A histological study including the characterization of the cellular infiltrate present in inflammatory osteoarthritis using monoclonal antibodies. *Ann Rheum Dis* 47:300–307, 1988.

96. Evans CH, Mazzocchi RA, Nelson DD, Rubash HE: Experimental arthritis induced by the intraarticular injection of allogeneic cartilaginous particles into rabbit knees. *Arthritis Rheum* 27:200–207, 1984.

97. McCarty DJ, Cheung HS: Prostaglandin (PG) E$_2$ generation by cultured canine synovial fibroblasts exposed to microcrystals containing calcium. *Ann Rheum Dis* 44:316–320, 1985.

98. Hasselbacher P, McMillan RM, Vater CA, et al: Stimulation of secretion of collagenase and prostaglandin E$_2$ by synovial fibroblasts in response to crystals of monosodium urate monohydrate: A model for joint destruction in gout. *Trans Assoc Am Physiol* 94:243–252, 1981.

99. Alwan WH, Dieppe PA, Elson CJ, Bradfield JWB: Hydroxyapatite and urate crystal induced cytokine release by macrophages. *Ann Rheum Dis* 48:476–482, 1989.

100. Hasselbacher P: C3 activation by monosodium urate monohydrate and other crystalline material. *Arthritis Rheum* 22:571–578, 1979.

101. McCarthy GM, Mitchell PG, Cheung HS: The mitogenic response to stimulation with basic calcium phosphate crystals is accompanied by induction and secretion of collagenase in human fibroblasts. *Arthritis Rheum* 34:1021, 1991.

102. Chang RW, Falconer J, Stulberg SD, et al: A randomized, controlled trial of arthroscopic surgery versus closed-needle joint lavage for patients with osteoarthritis of the knee. *Arthritis Rheum* 36:289, 1993.

103. Evans CH, Brown TD: Role of physical and mechanical agents in degrading the matrix, in Woessner JF and Howell DS (eds): in: *Joint Cartilage Degradation: Basic and Clinical Aspects.* New York, Marcel Dekker, 1993, pp 187–208.

104. Galante JO, Lemons J, Spector M, et al: The biologic effect of implant materials. *J Orthop Res* 9:760–775, 1991.

105. Goldring SR, Schillar AR, Ruelke MS, et al: The synovial-like membrane at the bone cement interface in loose total hip arthroplasty and its proposed role in bone lysis. *J Bone Joint Surg* 65A:575–584, 1983.

106. Kim KJ, Chiba J, Rubash HE: *In vivo* and *in vitro* analysis of membranes from hip prostheses inserted without cement. *J Bone Joint Surg* 76A:172–180, 1994.

107. Watkins SC, Macaulay W, Turner D, et al: Identification of nitric oxide synthase in human macrophages surrounding loosened hip prostheses. *Am J Pathol.* In press.

108. Smith RL, Kajiyama GK, Schurman DJ: Staphylococcal septic arthritis: Staph factor induces cartilage degradation but does not inhibit GAG synthesis *in vitro. Trans Orthop Res Soc* 21:220, 1996.

109. Bandara G, Robbins PD, Georgescu HI, et al: Gene transfer to synoviocytes: Prospects for gene treatment for arthritis. *DNA Cell Biol* 11:227–231, 1992.

110. Evans CH, Robbins PD: Possible orthopaedic applications of gene therapy. *J Bone Joint Surg* 77A:1103–1114, 1995.

111. Roessler BJ, Alloen ED, Wilson JM, et al: Adenoviral mediated gene transfer to rabbit synovium *in vivo. J Clin Invest* 92:1085–1092, 1993.

112. Nita I, Ghivizzani SC, Galea-Lauri J, et al: Direct gene delivery to synovium: An evaluation of potential vectors *in vitro* and *in vivo. Arthritis Rheum* 39:820–828, 1996.

113. Bandara G, Mueller GM, Galea-Lauri J, et al: Intraarticular expression of biologically active interleukin-1 receptor antagonist protein by *ex vivo* gene transfer. *Proc Natl Acad Sci USA* 90:10764–10768, 1993.

114. Hung GL, Galea-Lauri J, Mueller GM, et al: Suppression of intraarticular responses to interleukin-1 by transfer of the interleukin-1 receptor antagonist gene to synovium. *Gene Ther* 11:64–69, 1994.

115. Otani K, Nita I, Macaulay W, et al: Suppression of antigen-induced arthritis in rabbits *ex vivo* gene therapy. *J Immunol* 156:3558–3562, 1996.

116. Makarov SS, Olsen JC, Johnston WN, et al: Suppression of experimental arthritis by gene transfer of interleukin-1 receptor antagonist cDNA. *Proc Natl Acad Sci USA* 93:402–406, 1996.

117. Evans CH, Robbins PD, et al: Clinical trial to assess the safety, feasibility, and efficacy of transferring a potentially antiarthritic cytokine gene to human joints with rheumatoid arthritis. *Human Gene Ther* 7:1261–1280, 1996.

CHAPTER 11

Ligaments: Structure, Function, and Response to Injury and Repair

Kevin A. Hildebrand
and Cyril B. Frank

Ligament injuries occur virtually any time a joint is "sprained"[1-3]; therefore the treatment of ligament injuries is an important part of orthopaedic surgery. The clinical management of ligament injuries requires the clinician to understand normal ligament structure and function as well as the response of ligaments to injury and treatment. With this knowledge, treatment can be instituted to optimize ligament healing.

This chapter begins with a brief description of normal ligament structure and function and soft tissue biomechanics. Subsequently, injury mechanisms, responses to clinically relevant conditions, and surgical interventions are discussed. Finally, ligament reconstruction is reviewed, with consideration given to the future direction of ligament research clinically and in the laboratory. The treatment of ligament injuries is a growing area of orthopaedic surgery, as evidenced by the many excellent reviews available to the interested reader.[4-8]

NORMAL LIGAMENT STRUCTURE AND FUNCTION

Anatomy

Skeletal ligaments are fibrous bands of dense connective tissue that connect bones across joints. In combination with bone geometry, muscle action, and other soft tissues, ligaments stabilize and help to guide the motion of joints.[7,8] There is also evidence to support the existence of a proprioceptive "ligamentomuscular reflex loop,"[9,10] but the exact role and relative importance of this neuromuscular mechanism in joint function remains to be determined.[6]

Macroscopically, ligaments are strong white bands of tissue (Fig. 11-1). Some ligaments have well-defined edges, while others blend into adjacent tissues (e.g., joint capsules).[7] Ligaments vary in size, shape, orientation, and location; however, all ligaments attach to bones via some very specialized insertions.[11]

Microscopically, ligaments are composed of cells and matrix. Most of the cells are called *fibroblasts,* which appear as elongated structures parallel to the matrix fibers. Since ligaments contain relatively few cells, however, fibroblasts represent a small portion of the total ligament volume.[5,12] While fibroblasts create the surrounding solid matrix, recent evidence suggests that constituents of the matrix can affect fibroblast function.[6,13,14]

The term *matrix* refers to the material that surrounds ligament cells. Water constitutes the largest component, at approximately 70 percent of ligament wet weight (Fig. 11-2). The role of water in ligaments is poorly defined, but possible functions include the transportation of nutrients and ions and an incompressible spacer.[15] In addition, water definitely contributes to the viscoelastic behavior of ligaments.[16] The most abundant solid constituent of ligaments is collagen, which represents 65 to 90 percent of their dry weight.[6,7] Collagen, a complex protein, is the primary tensile load-bearing substance in ligaments.[6,8] Three polypeptide chains (each a left-handed helix) come together in a right-handed triple helix to form a tropocollagen molecule. The tropocollagen units aggregate into smaller (fibrils) and larger (fibers) components (Fig. 11-3). Collagen fibers are characterized by their "crimped" or undulating appearance when the ligament is viewed unloaded (Fig. 11-4). Recent evidence suggests that there are at least three types of fibrillar collagen in any quantity (types I, III, and VI) in normal ligaments,[17] with other minor collagens also likely to be present; type I collagen, however, represents approximately 90 percent of all the collagen in ligaments.[4] Matrix components present in smaller proportions include proteoglycans, elastin, fibronectin, laminin, and others. Their roles are poorly understood, but it is evident that they are involved with the interaction between cells and matrix and the organization of the matrix.[4,6,13,14]

Compared to other organ systems, ligaments are relatively avascular.[18] Some vessels penetrate ligament surfaces and course between fibrils.[19,20] These vessels come mostly from adjacent soft tissues, with little or no contribution from the ligament-bone insertion sites.[6] Nerves in ligaments appear to follow a similar path, with both sensory endings and some proprioceptive-type nerve receptors having been identified on and in ligaments.[7,10] A surface tissue known as the *epiligament* envelops certain ligaments (e.g., the medial collateral ligament, or MCL, in the rabbit) and is characterized by a fibroblast population unique in appearance, some blood vessels, and nerves.[12]

Biomechanics

Standardized testing protocols[21-24] have been developed to test the knee joints of various species. Tests have been conducted on the anterior cruciate ligament (ACL) and the MCL. Data obtained have to be interpreted in the context of the testing conditions, since many variables can affect the results, including animal model, test protocols, tissue tested, manipulations of the tissues, and other factors.[8]

Ligaments take up the tensile loads applied to joints. Both laboratory tests and the clinical examination of joints attempt to apply tensile loads to ligaments. Therefore some comparisons between clinical and laboratory tests can be made. When a tensile load is applied to a ligament in a laboratory setting, a curve describing the load-deformation behavior of that structure can be plotted (Fig. 11-5).[25] Three regions are recognized: a toe region, a linear region, and a failure region. The toe region is the first nonlinear

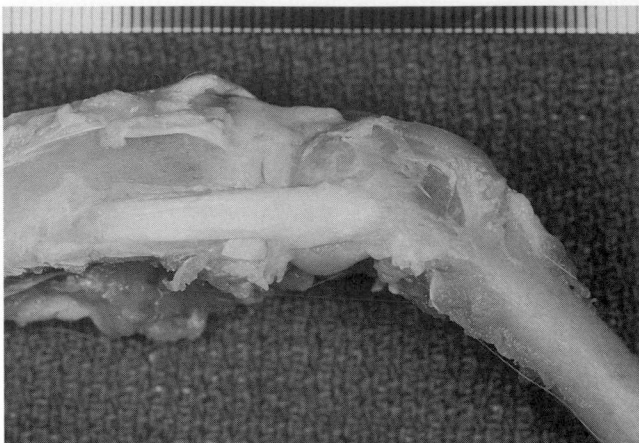

Figure 11-1 Photograph of the medial collateral ligament of a skeletally mature (12-month-old) New Zealand white rabbit. (Reproduced with permission from Frank CB, Bray RC, Hart DA, et al: Soft tissue healing, in Fu FH, Harner CD, Vince KG (eds): *Knee Surgery*. Baltimore, Williams & Wilkins, 1994, pp 189–229.)

that fibers in the anterior cruciate ligament (ACL) are being recruited to resist that load.[6] This phenomenon would be viewed microscopically as the straightening of the crimp in the collagen fibers as well as the aligning of the collagen fibers to the direction of loading.[7]

The second region of the load-deformation curve shows increased load with increased deformation, more linear in appearance. This region describes ligament stiffness experimentally. Clinically, *stiffness* refers to the load required to displace two bones, attached by a ligament, relative to one another.[6] Microscopically, individual fibers become taut and progressively more fibers are recruited to resist load. The more fibers recruited, the greater the load required to deform the ligament. Damage to fibers decreases ligament stiffness and consequently allows a greater translation of the bone than would normally be expected with specific loads. This concept can be observed in the clinic when the end point of a ligament test is "softer" or absent (e.g., the positive Lachman test). The third region of the load-deformation curve shows a slower rise in load toward a peak as individual fibers begin to fail, followed by a precipitous decrease in load, representing total ligament failure. Microscopically, collagen fibers fail in a progressive, sequential fashion until enough fibers have failed to cause the whole ligament to rupture. The peak or ultimate load is referred to as the *structural strength* of the ligament.

The load-deformation curve defines the structural properties of the ligament. Structural properties (stiffness, ultimate load) represent those of the entire bone-ligament-

portion of the curve, characterized by larger deformations with only small increases in load. This region of low load displacement could be tested in the clinical setting by a maneuver such as the Lachman test. When the test is negative, the tibia is drawn anteriorly relative to the femur, with little resistance until an "end point" is felt, signaling

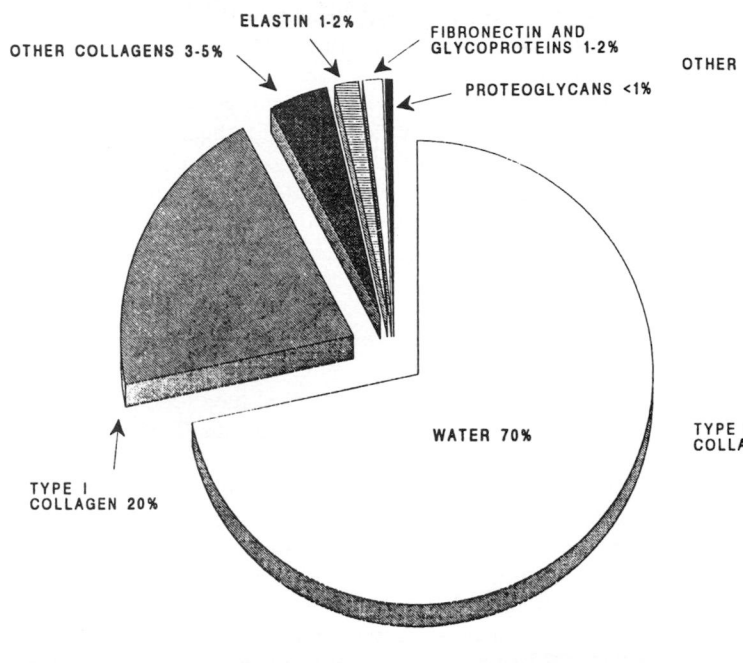

NORMAL LIGAMENT

A

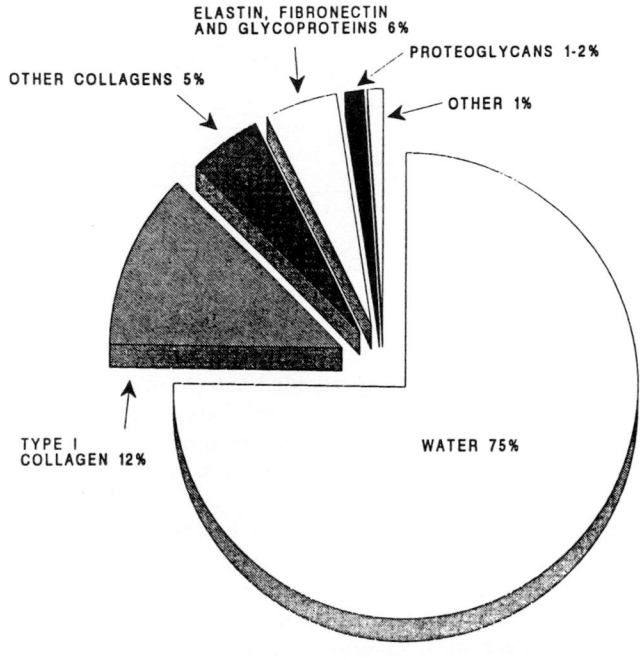

LIGAMENT SCAR

B

Figure 11-2 Pie charts showing approximate proportions of important biochemical components: *A,* in normal medial collateral ligament; *B,* in rabbit medial collateral scar. (Reproduced with permission from Frank CB, Bray RC, Hart DA, et al: Soft tissue healing, in Fu FH, Harner CD, Vince KG (eds): *Knee Surgery*. Baltimore, Williams & Wilkins, 1994, pp 189–229.)

Figure 11-3 Ligament architecture. (Reproduced with permission from Kastelic J, Galeski A, Baer E: The multicomposite ultrastructure of tendons. *Connect Tissue Res* 6:11–23, 1978.)

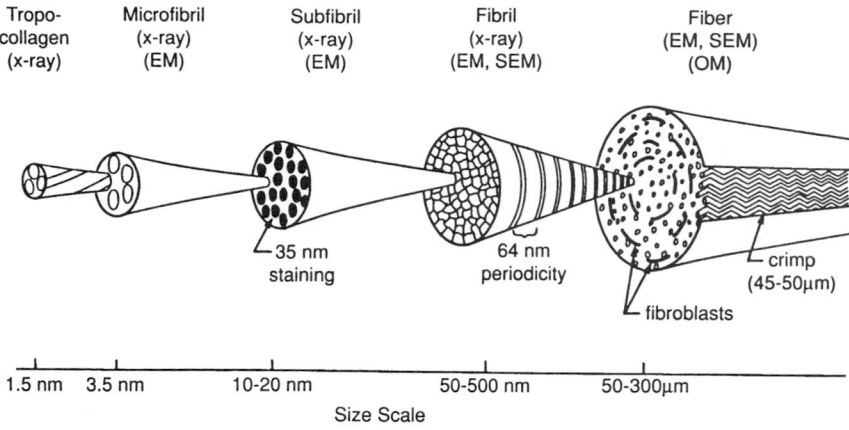

Tropo-collagen (x-ray)	Microfibril (x-ray) (EM)	Subfibril (x-ray) (EM)	Fibril (x-ray) (EM, SEM)	Fiber (EM, SEM) (OM)

35 nm staining

64 nm periodicity

crimp (45-50µm)

fibroblasts

| 1.5 nm | 3.5 nm | 10-20 nm | 50-500 nm | 50-300µm |

Size Scale

bone complex. These values are size-dependent. However, by normalizing the data to the cross-sectional area of the ligament, the effect of size is taken into account. *Material* or *mechanical properties,* as these normalized values are known, describe the ligament substance only and represent the quality of the ligament tissue. Stress (force/area) and strain (change in length/resting length) values can be determined, as well as the modulus of elasticity (the slope of the stress-strain relationship) for the ligament substance.

Both the structural and mechanical properties of ligaments are a function of the three-dimensional orientation of the loads applied, since fiber recruitment is related to the collagen fiber organization. Collagen fibers in ligaments are generally oriented with the long axis of the tissue, but they are not completely parallel and there also appear to be some connections between fibers.[5] On a gross scale, fibers run in a spiral fashion, with that spiral being a function of insertion sites, ligament shape, and joint position.[26] As a result, ligament fibers become recruited in different fashions, depending on how load is applied, thus accounting for the dependence of ligament structural and mechanical properties on the direction of load. The three-dimensional dependence of structural and mechanical properties is speculated to be more unique to ligaments than to tendons, since the collagen fibers found in tendons are more likely to be parallel.[5,27]

Ligaments are also viscoelastic materials, since they have both time- and history-dependent loading behaviors.[8] A ligament exposed to a constant stress, for example, will lengthen over time, or "creep." A ligament elongated to a certain length and held at this length experiences a decrease in stress with time, known as *stress relaxation.* Both the increase in length (creep) and decrease in the stress (stress relaxation) become smaller over time and eventually become negligible. Viscoelasticity contributes to the perceived stiffness and laxity of ligaments in a minor way; these properties are difficult to appreciate clinically. However, the viscoelastic properties of ligaments are important in that they probably represent a very interesting fine-tuning mechanism for both ligament lengths and loads over time.

The tensile loading behavior of ligaments can be considered in two broad categories: low load and high load.[6] As illustrated in Fig. 11-5, most daily activities appear to involve only low loads[25,28]; however, much clinical prac-

tice and laboratory experiments have focused on high-load behaviors. To characterize a normal ligament fully or to evaluate the healing of a ligament, both low- and high-load parameters should be considered.

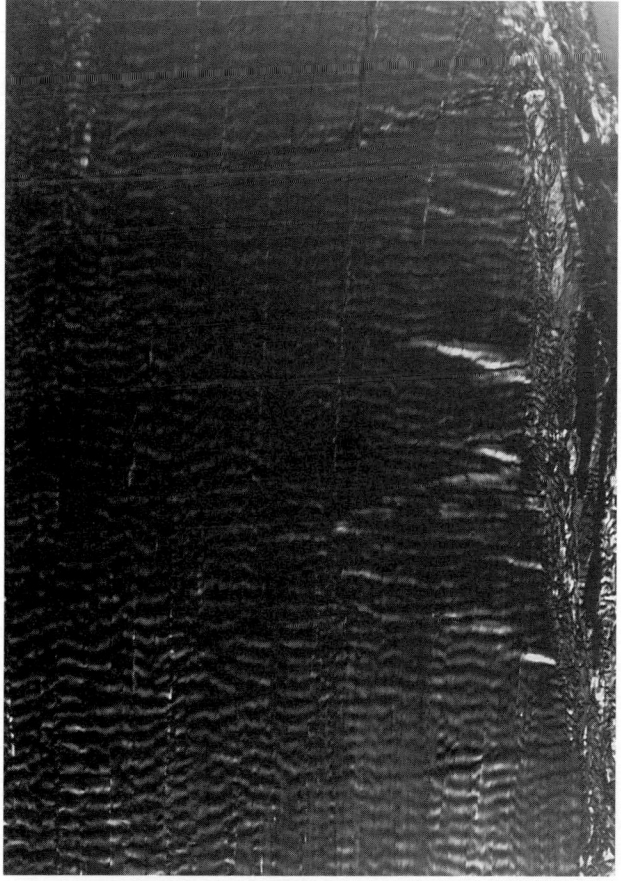

Figure 11-4 Low-power polarized photomicrograph of the rabbit medial collateral ligament cut parallel to its long axis. Note the density of the tissue and the periodic banding pattern of crimp throughout. The delicate surface tissue of the medial collateral ligament, the epiligament, which can be seen on the right side of this photograph, has a finer crimp. (Photograph courtesy of Dr. J. R. Matyas, University of Calgary, Calgary, Alberta, Canada.)

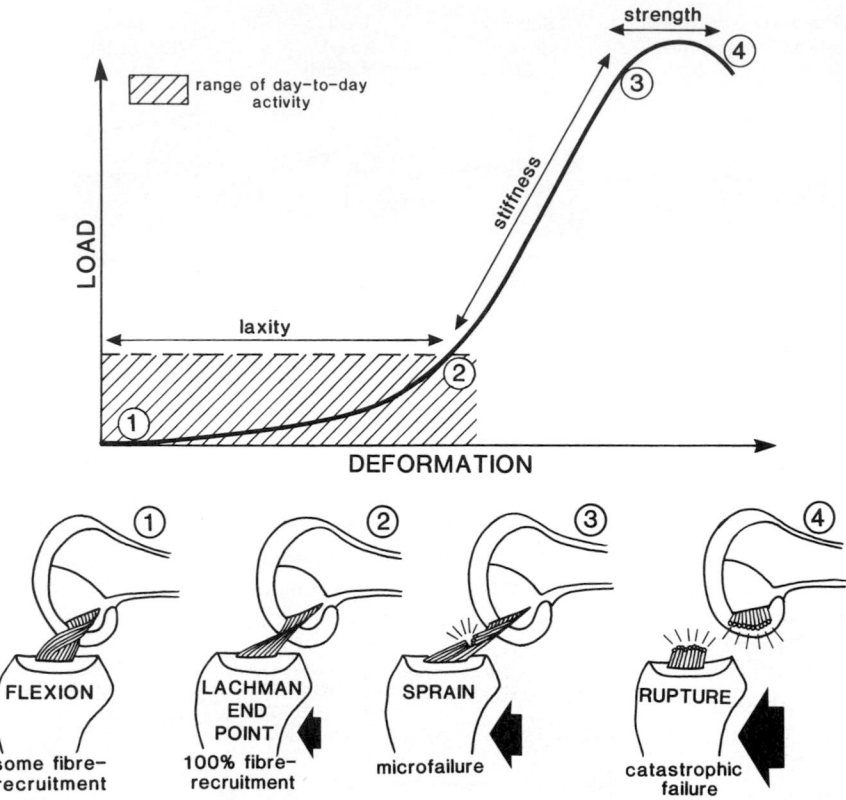

Figure 11-5 Schematic diagram to illustrate ligament structural properties from a clinical perspective. Diagrams are intended to be illustrative rather than comprehensive. (Reproduced with permission from Frank CB: Ligament healing: Current knowledge and clinical applications. *J Am Acad Orthop Surg* 4:74–83, 1996.)

Changes with Maturation and Aging

Maturation and aging affect both the structural and mechanical properties of ligaments.[29,30] In rabbits with open physes, the structural properties of the femur-MCL-tibia complex and the mechanical properties of the MCL substance increase rapidly. With maturity, these properties stabilize. It has been hypothesized that an asynchronous rate of maturity exists between the ligament substance and the ligament insertions to bone[29]: the ligament substance matures faster than the insertions, but eventually the insertion sites get stronger, as witnessed by the change in failure locations with maturity from the tibial insertion to the ligament midsubstance. Some of the effects of aging on ligaments were demonstrated in a study on human cadavers in which ACLs showed decreased stiffness, energy absorbed, and ultimate strength with increasing age.[30] In the young specimens, the ultimate load was 2160 ± 157 N; in the elderly human specimens, it was 658 ± 129 N.[30] Amiel and coworkers have also shown changes in cell metabolism and matrix quality with age.[31] Thus it is apparent that ligament properties change throughout life, making the definition of normal ligament behavior a moving target.

TRAUMATIC INJURY TO LIGAMENTS

Mechanisms of ligament failure vary. Ligaments can fail within their substance, at their bony interfaces, or pull away some bone with their attachments (avulsion). Ligaments can be damaged in more than one location,[32,33] and with complete disruptions of a ligament, there quite often occur concomitant injuries of varying degrees to other joint structures, including bone, cartilage, and other ligaments.[32] Ligaments fail by a progressive, sequential mechanism of microfiber failure. In most cases, structural failure is signaled by physical disruption of the ligament, but there is clinical evidence of functional failure of ligaments that remain in continuity morphologically.[34] This is almost certainly due to "partial" or microscopic disruption of functional components.

OTHER CAUSES OF LIGAMENT DETERIORATION

Immobilization

Immobilization causes the deterioration of both the mechanical and structural properties of ligaments. Woo et al.[35] demonstrated a rapid decrease in the mechanical properties of otherwise uninjured rabbit MCLs and also a decrease in structural properties of the femur-MCL-tibia complexes of rabbits with 9 to 12 weeks of immobilization. The MCL-tibia junction was reported to be especially sensitive, with osteoclastic resorption associated with failure occurring by ligament insertional failure at this interface. Longer periods of immobilization were found to increase deterioration. Remobilization was found to restore the mechanical and structural properties to normal levels, but the rate of return was different. The ligament substances recovered within 9 to 12 weeks, but it took up to 1 year for the MCL-tibia insertions to return to normal. In other words, there appears to be a very long term requirement for ligament recovery from a few months of immobilization.

Cortisone Injection

Corticosteroids have been shown to have detrimental effects on normal and healing ligaments. Noyes et al.[36] gave intraarticular methylprednisolone (10 times human-equivalent doses) to primate knees and demonstrated structural and mechanical compromise in ACLs up to 15 weeks later. Wiggins et al.[37] found that human-equivalent doses of betamethasone implanted on top of rabbit MCLs impaired healing. After 10 days of healing, one-third of the steroid group failed to form healing tissue when all of the controls had, and after 3 weeks of healing, the peak load for the steroid group was 50 percent of non-steroid-treated MCL injury controls. The study was not extended beyond 3 weeks, so long-term effects were not determined; however, it appears that cortisone injections have the potential to weaken the biomechanical qualities of both normal and healing ligaments.

Joint Inflammation

Inflammatory processes of synovial joints, such as rheumatoid arthritis, are well known for their effects on articular cartilage, but it is likely that such processes also affect the other soft tissues of joints. Neurath[38] used electron microscopy to show that collagen fiber diameters were much smaller, their courses were irregular, and atypical thick collagenous structures (Luse bodies) were present in cruciate ligament specimens from rheumatoid arthritis patients undergoing total knee replacements. In a rabbit model of immune synovitis, Goldberg et al.[39] found the strength of the femur-ACL-tibia complex to be one-third that of controls; however, the effects of pain and disuse, caused by the inflammation, on the structural properties were not accounted for in this model. Nevertheless, it appears that joint inflammation can directly or indirectly alter and weaken ligaments.

LIGAMENT HEALING

A synovial joint consists of various elements, some of which are subject to tensile stresses while others experience compressive forces.[25] The joint functions through a dynamic equilibrium between these elements (Fig. 11-6). If one particular element (e.g., a ligament) is damaged, the balance is disturbed and the remaining structures try to establish a new equilibrium to maintain joint function. Three points arise from this adaptation. First, a lack of symptoms does not necessarily mean that an individual ligament has healed, since other structures may simply compensate for it. Second, if the other stabilizers are not able to establish a new equilibrium to protect a healing ligament, the load this ligament experiences may be too much

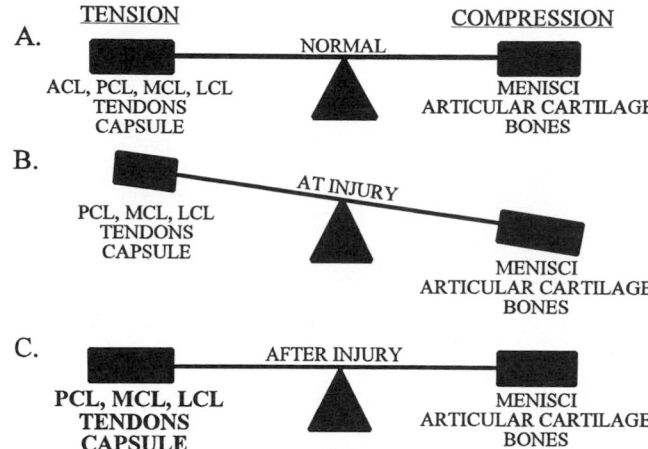

Figure 11-6 Schematic diagram to illustrate the balance between the tension-bearing elements and the compression-bearing elements in a knee joint. In the uninjured knee joint, the tensile and compressive elements are in equilibrium (*A*), but immediately following the failure of one or more of those structures, there is imbalance (*B*). To restore joint function, the same forces become redistributed among the remaining structures (indicated here with bold, large lettering), predisposing some of them to subsequent failure (*C*). (Reproduced with permission from Frank CB. Ligament healing: Current knowledge and clinical applications. *J Am Acad Orthop Surg* 4:74–83, 1996.)

and it may heal poorly or not at all. A lack of healing in this sense is related not to the intrinsic inability of the ligament to heal but to the excessive load it experiences while healing. Third, it can be surmised that with time, certain structures or elements could fail if the increased load they accept exceeds their ability to adapt.

Descriptions of ligament healing have most commonly been defined from animal investigations of the MCL of the knee. The MCL is an extraarticular ligament and is typical of most ligaments in the body in that it appears to heal well in a functional sense. However, some ligaments, such as the intraarticular ACL, have different (poorer) healing in a functional sense. A description of general ligament healing, using the MCL model, is followed by a closer look at what is known about the specific differences between MCL and ACL healing.

Healing Response—General

Once a collateral ligament is damaged, a biological response is mounted to repair the injury. Ligament repair follows a process qualitatively similar to wound healing to produce a scar to fill the gap.[6] There are three main phases of healing that overlap (Fig. 11-7). The first, or hemorrhagic, phase occurs within minutes to hours of an injury, with hemorrhage and the formation of a blood clot within the damaged region. This induces an inflammatory response, bringing in polymorphonuclear cells and monocytes/macrophages to remove damage and attract reparative cells to the area. The inflammatory stage initiates the

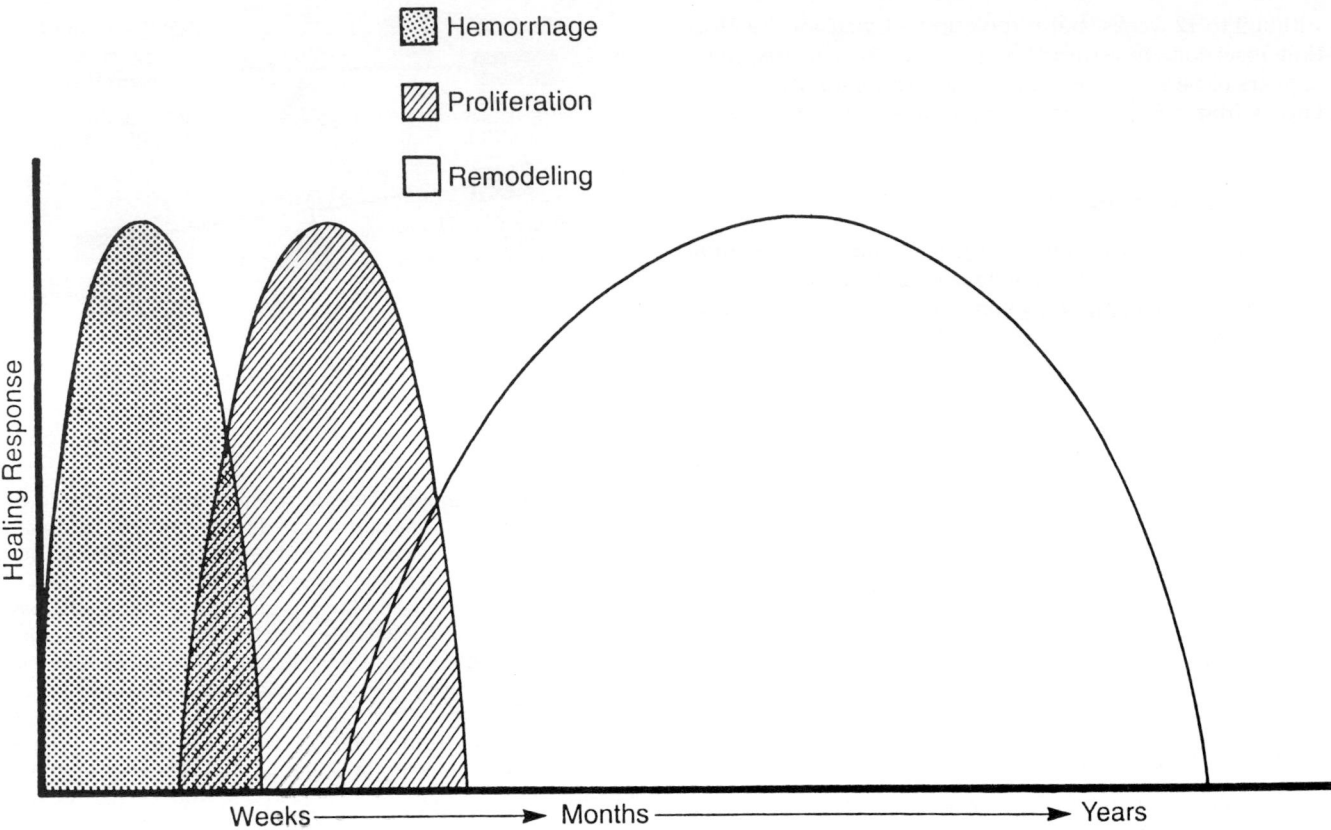

Figure 11-7 A theoretical representation of ligament healing showing relative durations and overlap of stages. (Reproduced with permission from Frank CB, Bray RC, Hart DA, et al: Soft tissue healing, in Fu FH, Harner CD, Vince KG (eds): *Knee Surgery.* Baltimore, Williams & Wilkins, 1994, pp 189–229.)

formation of granulation tissue. The second phase is the proliferative phase. It begins within days of the injury and lasts several weeks. New blood vessels are formed while fibroblasts are recruited from the local environment or circulation to produce and excrete new matrix material. The third, or remodeling, phase starts within weeks of the injury, overlaps with the proliferative phase, and continues for several years. Elements within the tissue reorganize the material produced by the fibroblasts to improve the properties of the healing ligament scar over time.

The biological and some of the biomechanical properties of all healed ligaments remain abnormal for long periods of time (if not permanently).[15,22,24,40] In animal models, ligament scars contain slightly more water, cells, and blood vessels as well as collagen fibrils with smaller diameters.[41] High-load structural properties (ultimate load, stiffness, energy absorbed to failure) and material properties also remain inferior.[23,24,40,42] In contrast, low-load behaviors return toward normal levels considerably sooner (6 to 14 weeks postinjury).[6,22]

Healing Response—Specific Ligaments

As mentioned above, different ligaments respond in a tissue-specific manner to various injuries and treatments. The best clinical and laboratory examples are the ACL and MCL of the knee. Clinical studies support the favorable functional healing response of the MCL[43,44] in contrast to the ACL.[45,46] Laboratory studies also show a superior healing potential for the MCL[22,24] compared to the ACL.[40,47] Many reviews imply that the ACL "lacks a healing response," but at least from a biological perspective, this is not entirely true. Healing occurs with partial ACL transections in rabbits.[48] In humans, ACLs often "heal" to the posterior cruciate ligament.[25] In most cases, though, this healing does not provide substantial stability over time,[45,46] suggesting that it is not "functional healing." On the other hand, it does show some healing response, perhaps limited by the sites of attachment of the healing ACL rather than by a total failure of new tissue to form.

The reasons for the differences in the functional healing responses of MCLs and ACLs are unknown, but many factors have been suggested. Most obvious is the location of these ligaments in the joint; the MCL is an extraarticular ligament, while the ACL is an intraarticular ligament. With injury, the ACL may be exposed to a "hostile" synovial environment; however, some studies have shown positive effects of synovial fluid on ligament fibroblasts.[49,50] Other differences noted between the ACL and MCL include cell morphology,[51] cell adhesion and migration,[13,14,52] cellular response to growth factors,[53,54] biomechanical properties,[8] and biochemical factors.[4] The role and importance of these differences in the healing potential of these two ligaments remain to be determined.

Differences in location may also lead to different load histories for each healing ligament. According to the dynamic equilibrium theory (Fig. 11-6),[25] after an MCL injury, the other tensile stabilizers (e.g., ligaments) may be better able to take up the load to allow the MCL to heal. Conversely, after an ACL injury, the remaining tensile stabilizers may be unable to take up sufficient load to allow ACL healing in a functional sense. Evidence suggests that joint motion improves healing for isolated MCL injuries,[55] but in a combined ACL-MCL injury model, MCL healing is impaired.[56] The implied difference in these two forms of MCL healing is that the load environment for the healing MCL is altered, although this remains to be proven experimentally. For the ACL, clinical strategies to lessen the load on ACL grafts have been developed.[57,58] Very little is known of the in vivo loads experienced by ligaments,[28,59] and the optimal load for ligament healing is unknown.

Ligament Repair

Some potential to enhance ligament healing is in the surgeon's control. Three factors have been investigated to date: suture repair, mobilization, and joint instability. Suturing of a ligament has produced modest improvements in healing.[25] In a rabbit model comparing the healing of a 4-mm gap to transection and end-to-end repair of an MCL injury, only modest increases (10 to 30 percent) in structural strength occurred with suture repair, while mechanical properties did not improve.[22]

Motion after injury definitely affects the healing ligament. Motion in a stable joint produces larger scars and improves scar stiffness and strength.[60,61] Immobilization leads to scars that are smaller, weaker, and not as stiff.[23,62] Combined ligament injuries also affect the quality of ligament healing. With combined ACL and MCL injuries in rabbits,[42] MCL scars regain less strength, are less stiff, and are made of inferior tissue compared to MCL scars from an isolated MCL injury equivalent. These data imply that too much load to a healing ligament—for example, in an unstable joint caused by multiple ligament injuries—is detrimental. Unfortunately, it is hard to define stable and unstable joints precisely in terms of each injured ligament. Nevertheless, it is clear clinically that in some combined injury cases, surgical joint stabilization may be required to protect other healing ligaments from excessive stress.

Ligament Reconstruction

Clinical experience[63] and laboratory studies on primary ACL repairs[40,47] reveal substantial functional failure rates. Therefore, in patients requiring surgery for instability due to ACL deficiency, substitute tissues are typically used to reconstruct the ligament. Replacements include human tissue (autograft or allograft) and synthetic material (biological or nonbiological). There are to date no grafts to mimic all the structural and mechanical properties of the normal ACL.[40,64]

Studies have been performed on the incorporation and maturation of graft materials for the ACL. The most common sources of replacement tissue are the tendons around the knee, specifically the patellar tendon and the medial hamstring tendons. Biomechanical, histologic, ultrastructural, and biochemical changes with time have been studied in these grafts. Biomechanically, a variety of animal models and various autograft and allograft tissues have shown a drop in high-load structural properties that have not recovered[18,40] or have recovered slowly with time.[65] Some 1 to 2 years after grafting, autograft and allograft ultimate loads have been shown to range from 11 to 52 percent and stiffness ranged from 13 to 45 percent of control ACLs.[18,40,65]

Concomitant with the biomechanical changes over time, ACL grafts undergo histologic modification. Necrosis occurs with cell death in the first week of healing. Blood vessels are reestablished within the first 6 to 8 weeks, together with cells and matrix production. Similar steps to those discussed above for ligament healing take place in the grafts, with remodeling continuing to the longest time periods studied (up to 2 years).[18,66] Biochemical changes include early increases in water content with a return closer to control levels. Total proteoglycan content, collagen distributions, and reducible collagen cross links approach normal ACL qualities with remodeling.[18] In contrast, ultrastructural studies of patellar tendon and hamstring autografts have not revealed normal ACL architectural reconstitution.[67,68] Thus, while many grafts appear to "do the job" clinically in terms of improving the functional stability of the knee, they do not reconstruct normal ACLs.

FUTURE DIRECTIONS

Investigations over the last 20 to 25 years have increased our knowledge of normal ligament structure and function, thus helping us appreciate the ligament as a dynamic structure that responds to its environment. Work continues to improve our understanding of normal ligament structure and function, while information concerning the basic processes of ligament healing and the effects of some of the more common orthopaedic treatment methods is ongoing. Growth factors, modifying joint stability, applying loads to healing ligaments, and other modalities to improve healing are new areas of research. Further work is necessary to understand the effects of maturation and aging on normal tissue and the healing differences between intraarticular (e.g., ACL) and extraarticular (e.g., MCL) ligaments. Until we have this information, we will not fully understand normal ligaments and will be unable to optimize their healing, replacement, or both.

REFERENCES

1. Miyasaka KC, Daniel DM, Stone ML, Hirshman P: The incidence of knee ligament injuries in the general population. *Am J Knee Surg* 4:3–8, 1991.
2. Praemer A, Furner S, Rice D: *Musculoskeletal Conditions in the United States.* Rosemont, Illinois, American Academy of Orthopaedic Surgeons, 1992.

3. Warme WJ, Feagin JA Jr, King P, et al: Ski injury statistics, 1982 to 1993, Jackson Hole ski resort. *Am J Sports Med* 23:597–600, 1995.

4. Amiel D, Billings E, Akeson WH: Ligament structure, chemistry, and physiology, in Daniel DM, Akeson WH, O'Connor JJ (eds): *Knee Ligaments: Structure, Function, Injury, and Repair.* New York, Raven Press, 1990, pp 77–91.

5. Carlstedt CA, Nordin M: Biomechanics of tendons and ligaments, in Nordin M, Frankel VH (eds): *Basic Biomechanics of the Musculoskeletal System,* 2d ed. Philadelphia, Lea & Febiger, 1989, pp 59–74.

6. Frank CB, Bray RC, Hart DA, et al: Soft tissue healing, in Fu FH, Harner CD, Vince KG (eds): *Knee Surgery.* Baltimore, Williams & Wilkins, 1994, pp 189–229.

7. Loitz BJ, Frank CB: Biology and mechanics of ligament and ligament healing. *Exerc Sport Sci Rev* 21:33–64, 1993.

8. Woo SL-Y, Smith BA, Johnson GA: Biomechanics of knee ligaments, in Fu FH, Harner CD, Vince KG (eds): *Knee Surgery.* Baltimore, Williams & Wilkins, 1994, pp 155–172.

9. Solomonow M, Baratta R, Zhou BH, et al: The synergistic action of the anterior cruciate ligament and thigh muscles in maintaining joint stability. *Am J Sports Med* 15:207–213, 1987.

10. Madey SM, Cole KJ, Brand RA: The sensory role of the anterior cruciate ligament, in Jackson DW (ed): *The Anterior Cruciate Ligament: Current and Future Concepts.* New York, Raven Press, 1993, pp 23–33.

11. Maytas JR, Bodie D, Andersen M, Frank CB: The developmental morphology of a "periosteal" ligament insertion: Growth and maturation of the tibial insertion of the rabbit medial collateral ligament. *J Orthop Res* 8:412–424, 1990.

12. Chowdhury P, Maytas JR, Frank CB: The "epiligament" of the rabbit medial collateral ligament: A quantitative morphological study. *Connect Tissue Res* 27:33–50, 1991.

13. Sung K-LP, Kwan MK, Maldonado F, Akeson WH: Adhesion strength of human ligament fibroblasts. *J Biomech Eng* 116:237–242, 1994.

14. Sung K-LP, Steele LL, Whittermore D, et al: Adhesiveness of human ligament fibroblasts to laminin. *J Orthop Res* 13:166–173, 1995.

15. Frank CB, Loitz B, Bray R, et al: Abnormality of the contralateral ligament after injuries of the medial collateral ligament. *J Bone Joint Surg Am* 76:403–412, 1994.

16. Wilson AN, Frank CB, Shrive NG: The behaviour of water in the rabbit medial collateral ligament, in *Second World Congress of Biomechanics,* vol 2. Amsterdam: Stichting World Biomechanics, 1994, p 226.

17. Bray DF, Bray RC, Frank CB: Ultrasound immunolocalization of type-VI collagen and chondroitin sulphate in ligament. *J Orthop Res* 11:677–685, 1993.

18. McFarland EG: The biology of anterior cruciate ligament reconstructions. *Orthopedics* 16:403–410, 1993.

19. Arnoczky SP, Maytas JR, Buckwalter JA, Amiel D: Anatomy of the anterior cruciate ligament, in Jackson DW (ed): *The Anterior Cruciate Ligament: Current Concepts and Future Concepts.* New York, Raven Press, 1993, pp 5–22.

20. Bray R, Rangayyan R, Eng K: A study of vascular behavior in normal and healing medial collateral ligaments. *Trans Orthop Res Soc* 18:57, 1993.

21. Amiel D, Kleiner JB, Roux RD, et al: The phenomenon of "ligamentization": Anterior cruciate ligament reconstruction with autogenous patellar tendon. *J Orthop Res* 4:162–172, 1986.

22. Chimich D, Frank C, Shrive N, et al: The effects of initial end contact on medial collateral ligament healing: A morphological and biomechanical study in a rabbit model. *J Orthop Res* 9:37–47, 1991.

23. Lechner CT, Dahners LE: Healing of the medial collateral ligament in unstable rat knees. *Am J Sports Med* 19:508–512, 1991.

24. Weiss JA, Woo SL-Y, Ohland KJ, et al: Evaluation of a new injury model to study medial collateral ligament healing: Primary repair vs nonoperative treatment. *J Orthop Res* 9:516–528, 1991.

25. Frank CB: Ligament healing: Current knowledge and clinical application. *J Am Acad Orthop Surg* 4:74–83, 1996.

26. Woo SL-Y, Adams DJ, Takai S: The human anterior cruciate ligament and its replacement: Biomechanical considerations, in Niwa S, Perron SM, Hattori T (eds): *Biomechanics in Orthopedics.* Tokyo, Springer-Verlag, 1992, pp 13–30.

27. Woo SL-Y, Young EP: Structure and function of tendons and ligaments, in Mow VC, Hayes WC (eds): *Basic Orthopaedic Biomechanics.* New York, Raven Press, 1991, pp 199–243.

28. Holden JP, Grood ES, Korvick DL, et al: In vivo forces in the anterior cruciate ligament: Direct measurements during walking and trotting in a quadruped. *J Biomech* 27:517–526, 1994.

29. Woo SL-Y, Ohland KJ, Weiss JA: Aging and sex-related changes in the biomechanical properties of the rabbit medial collateral ligament. *Mech Ageing Dev* 56:129–142, 1990.

30. Woo SL-Y, Hollis JM, Adams DJ, et al: Tensile properties of the human femur-anterior cruciate ligament-tibia complex: The effect of specimen age and orientation. *Am J Sports Med* 19:217–225, 1991.

31. Amiel D, Kuiper SD, Wallace CD, et al: Age-related properties of medial collateral ligament and anterior cruciate ligament: A morphologic and collagen maturation study in the rabbit. *J Gerontol* 46:B159–B165, 1991.

32. Garvin GJ, Munk PL, Vellet AD: Tears of the medial collateral ligament: Magnetic resonance imaging findings and associated injuries. *Can Assoc Radiol J* 44:199–204, 1993.

33. O'Donoghue DH: Surgical treatment of fresh injuries to the major ligaments of the knee. *J Bone Joint Surg (Am)* 32:721–738, 1950.

34. Noyes FR, Bassett RW, Grood ES, Butler DL: Arthroscopy in acute traumatic hemarthrosis of the knee: Incidence of anterior cruciate tears and other injuries. *J Bone Joint Surg (Am)* 62:687–695, 1980.

35. Woo SL-Y, Gomez MA, Sites TJ, et al: The biomechanical and morphological changes in the medial collateral ligament of the rabbit after immobilization and remobilization. *J Bone Joint Surg (Am)* 69:1200–1211, 1987.

36. Noyes FR, Grood ES, Nussbaum NS, Cooper SM: Effect of intraarticular corticosteroids on ligament properties. *Clin Orthop* 123:197–209, 1977.

37. Wiggins ME, Fadale PD, Barrach H, et al: Healing characteristics of a type I collagenous structure treated with corticosteroids. *Am J Sports Med* 22:279–288, 1994.

38. Neurath MF: Detection of luse bodies, spiralled collagen, dysplastic collagen, and intracellular collagen in rheumatoid connective tissues: An electron microscope study. *Ann Rheum Dis* 52:278–284, 1993.

39. Goldberg VM, Burnstein A, Dawson M: The influence of an experimental immune synovitis on the failure mode and strength of the rabbit anterior cruciate ligament. *J Bone Joint Surg (Am)* 64:900–906, 1982.

40. Newton PO, Horibe S, Woo SL-Y: Experimental studies on anterior cruciate ligament autografts and allografts, in Daniel DM, Akeson WH, O'Connor JJ (eds): *Knee Ligaments: Structure, Function, Injury and Repair.* New York, Raven Press, 1990, pp 389–399.

41. Shrive NG, Chimich DD, Marchuk L, et al: "Flaws" in scar matrix correlate with material properties of ligament scars. *Trans Orthop Res Soc* 19:630, 1994.

42. Anderson DR, Weiss JA, Takai S, et al: Healing of the medial collateral ligament following a triad injury: A biomechanical and histological study of the knee in rabbits. *J Orthop Res* 10:485–495, 1992.

43. Indelicato PA: Isolated medial collateral ligament injuries in the knee. *J Am Acad Orthop Surg* 3(1):9–14, 1995.

44. Petermann J, von Garrel T, Gotzen L: Non-operative treatment of acute medial collateral ligament lesions of the knee joint. *Knee Surg Sports Trauma Arthrosc* 1:93–96, 1993.

45. Johnson RJ, Beynnon BD, Nichols CE, Renstrom PAFH: The treatment of injuries of the anterior cruciate ligament. *J Bone Joint Surg (Am)* 74:140–151, 1992.

46. O'Donoghue DH: An analysis of end results of surgical treatment of major injuries to the ligaments of the knee. *J Bone Joint Surg (Am)* 37:1–13, 1955.

47. O'Donoghue DH, Rockwood CC, Frank GR: Repair of the anterior cruciate ligament in dogs. *J Bone Joint Surg (Am)* 48:503–519, 1966.

48. Hefti FL, Kress A, Fasel J, Morscher EW: Healing of the transected anterior cruciate ligament in the rabbit. *J Bone Joint Surg Am* 73:373–383, 1991.

49. Dahlin LB, Hanff G, Myrhage R: Healing of ligaments in synovial fluid: An experimental study in rabbits. *Scand J Plast Reconstr Surg Hand Surg* 25:97–102, 1991.

50. Nickerson DA, Joshi R, Williams S, et al: Synovial fluid stimulates the proliferation of rabbit ligament fibroblasts in vitro. *Clin Orthop* 274:294–299, 1992.

51. Lyon RM, Akeson WH, Amiel D, et al: Ultrastructural differences between the cells of the medial collateral and the anterior cruciate ligaments. *Clin Orthop* 272:279–286, 1991.

52. Schreck PJ, Kitabayashi LR, Amiel D, et al: Integrin display increases in the wounded rabbit medial collateral ligament but not the wounded anterior cruciate ligament. *J Orthop Res* 13:174–183, 1995.

53. Lee J, Green MH, Amiel D: Synergistic effect of growth factors on cell outgrowth from explants of rabbit anterior cruciate and medial collateral ligaments. *J Orthop Res* 13:435–441, 1995.

54. Schmidt CC, Georgescu HI, Kwoh CK, et al: Effect of growth factors on the proliferation of fibroblasts from the medial collateral and anterior cruciate ligaments. *J Orthop Res* 13:184–190, 1995.

55. Woo SL-Y, Weiss JA, Gomez MA, Hawkins DA: Measurement of changes in ligament tension with knee motion and skeletal maturation. *J Biomech Eng* 112:46–51, 1990.

56. Woo SL-Y, Young EP, Ohland KJ, et al: The effects of transection of the anterior cruciate ligament on healing of the medial collateral ligament: A biomechanical study of the knee in dogs. *J Bone Joint Surg (Am)* 72:382–392, 1990.

57. Fowler PJ: Synthetic augmentation, in Jackson DW (ed): *The Anterior Cruciate Ligament: Current and Future Concepts.* New York, Raven Press, 1993, pp 339–341.

58. Lewis JL, Poff BC, Smith JJ, et al: Method for establishing and measuring in vivo forces in an anterior cruciate ligament composite graft: Response to differing levels of load sharing in a goat model. *J Orthop Res* 12:780–788, 1994.

59. Beynnon BD, Johnson RJ, Fleming BC, et al: The measurement of elongation of anterior cruciate-ligament grafts in vivo. *J Bone Joint Surg (Am)* 76:520–531, 1994.

60. Gomez MA, Woo SL-Y, Inoue M, et al: Medial collateral ligament healing subsequent to different treatment regimens. *J Appl Physiol* 66:245–252, 1989.

61. Hart DP, Dahners LE: Healing of the medial collateral ligament in rats: The effects of repair, motion, and secondary stabilizing ligaments. *J Bone Joint Surg (Am)* 69:1194–1199, 1987.

62. Inoue M, Woo SL-Y, Gomez MA, et al: Effects of surgical treatment and immobilization on the healing of the medial collateral ligament: A long-term multidisciplinary study. *Connect Tissue Res* 25:13–26, 1990.

63. Engebretsen L: The acute repair of anterior cruciate tears, in Jackson DW (ed): *The Anterior Cruciate Ligament: Current and Future Concepts.* New York, Raven Press, 1993, pp 273–279.

64. Jackson DW, Grood ES, Goldstein JD, et al: A comparison of patellar tendon autograft and allograft used for anterior cruciate ligament reconstruction in the goat model. *Am J Sports Med* 21:176–185, 1993.

65. Ng GY, Oakes BW, Deacon OW, et al: Biomechanics of patellar tendon autograft for reconstruction of the anterior cruciate ligament in the goat: Three year study. *J Orthop Res* 13:602–608, 1995.

66. Boynton MD, Fadale PD: The basic science of anterior cruciate ligament surgery. *Orthop Rev* 22:673–679, 1993.

67. Frogameni AD, Jackson DW, Simon TM: Collagen remodeling in ACL reconstruction (goat model), in Jackson DW (ed): *The Anterior Cruciate Ligament: Current and Future Concepts.* New York, Raven Press, 1993, pp 219–226.

68. Oakes BW: Collagen ultrastructure in the normal ACL and in ACL graft, in Jackson DW (ed): *The Anterior Cruciate Ligament: Current and Future Concepts.* New York, Raven Press, 1993, pp 209–218.

CHAPTER 12

The Structure and Function of Skeletal Muscle

William E. Garrett, Jr.,
and Donald T. Kirkendall

Skeletal muscle is uniquely constructed to adapt its contractile response to the functional requirements of varying loading conditions.

MUSCLE DEVELOPMENT

The four major characteristics of skeletal muscle—contractility, excitability, extensibility, and elasticity—are all related to its anatomic structure, derived during embryonic development. Skeletal muscle develops in four distinct phases: axonal outgrowth, myogenesis, synaptogenesis, and synapse elimination.[1]

Motor neurons from the anterior horn of the spinal cord project into the muscle mass[2] "searching for their appropriate muscle fiber." This is not a random procedure but rather a coordinated series of events that will eventually link a motor neuron with its correct muscle fiber. At the same time, mononuclear muscle fiber precursors (myoblasts) begin to congregate into clusters that fuse, resulting in multinucleated myotubes. The fiber increases in length by the addition of myoblasts at the end of the tubes. The first myoblasts (myoblast I) form only small myotubes. Larger secondary myotubes with more nuclei are formed by myoblast II fibers. Myoblast III fibers with recognizably adult muscle protein finally appear in a nerve-dependent event sequence. Secondary myotubes form next to primary tubes under a development basal lamina. Unfused myoblasts settle under the basal lamina as satellite cells. As maturation proceeds, the myotubes begin to take on the characteristic appearance of skeletal muscle (Fig. 12-1). Along the surface of the developing myotube, receptors for acetylcholine (Ach) are widely dispersed over the maturing membrane. As the projecting axon nears its fiber, the Ach receptors migrate to the neuron. The attraction appears to be a result of end-plate potentials.

Multiple axons innervate the developing muscle, but the hyperinnervation is subsequently corrected, establishing the definitive innervation ratio for each motor neuron. The mechanisms behind the process and elimination of synapses is still unclear. The major factor is believed to be elimination of collateral axonal sprouts.[3,4]

The heterogeneity of muscle fibers is also established during this developmental process. The influence of the motor neuron on muscle fiber characteristics is well es-

tablished. However, three distinct clonal fiber types are already evident during the myoblast stage.[5]

THE SKELETAL MUSCLE CELL

The muscle cell is termed a *myofiber* (muscle fiber). Each fiber contains thousands of contractile elements called *myofibrils,* which extend throughout its length. Individual myofibers are wrapped in connective tissue endomysium. Bundles of myofibers encased in the perimysium form a *fasciculus.* Bundles of fasciculi, in turn, are bound by the epimysium within the fascia that surrounds the entire muscle. Beneath the connective tissue basal lamina surrounding the muscle fibers are satellite cells that do not contribute to the development of tension. These cells can differentiate into myoblasts, but regeneration potential after injury is poor in the adult.

Each myofiber is limited by a cell membrane called the *sarcolemma.* This is a typical cell membrane except that there are periodic invaginations, the transverse tubules or T tubules, that project deep inside the fiber. Each myofiber has many nuclei located peripherally beneath the sarcolemma. Within the cytoplasm are found typical cell organelles, including mitochondrial lysosomes, ribosomes, glycogen, and lipid droplets. The myofiber also contains a system of membrane-bound sacs (outer vesicles or cisterns) termed the *sarcoplasmic reticulum* (Fig. 12-1). The vesicles accumulate calcium ions available for release into the myofiber cytoplasm to initiate contraction.

Contractile Components

The distinctive contractile machinery (Figs. 12-2 and 12-3) is arranged in an orderly manner. The distinguishing feature of the myofiber's structure is its appearance of alternately wide and then narrow dark bands, giving a striated appearance on light microscopy. The electron microscopy of the myofibrils within each fiber shows a regular pattern of repeating contractile units called *sarcomeres,* arranged in series. Repeating wide bands known as A (anisotropic) bands are seen; they are composed of thick myosin filaments. Primarily alternating with these bands is a thin dark line called the Z line (the German *zwischen* means between). The functioning sarcomere extends from one Z line to another. Within the A band is a lighter H zone (the German *helle* means bright). In the center of the A band is the dense M line. A narrow light band on either side of the Z line is the I (isotropic) band composed of thin actin filaments.

Contractile Proteins

The arrangements of the contractile proteins define the bands. The Z lines extend perpendicular to the contractile elements of the sarcomere and serve as an anchor for the thin actin filaments (Fig. 12-2). Actin is a double-stranded helix made up of g-actin monomers. These fibers reach to-

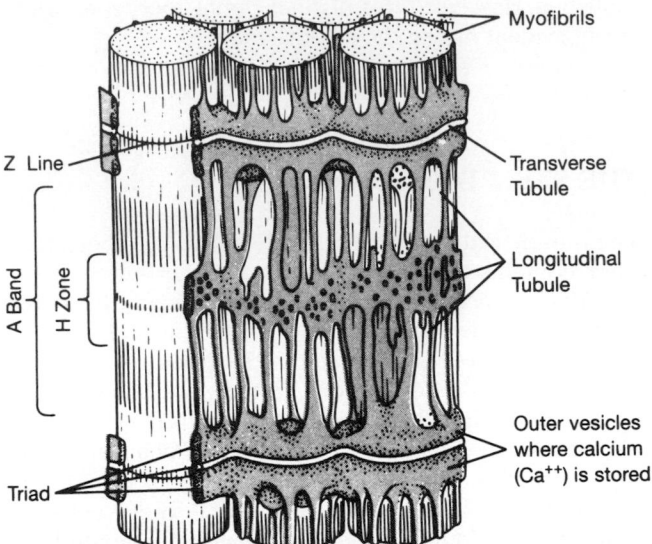

Figure 12-1 The sarcoplasmic reticulum and transverse tubules form a netlike system of tubules and vesicles surrounding the myofibrils. The outer vesicles store large quantities of calcium ions (Ca^{2+}), one of the ingredients required for the contractile process. The transverse tubules are concerned with conduction of the nervous impulses deep into the myofibrils. The two outer vesicles and the transverse tubule separating them are known as a triad. There are two triads per sarcomere. (From Fox EL et al: *The Physiological Basis for Exercise and Sport,* 5th ed. Dubuque, IA, Brown and Benchmark, 1988. Reproduced by permission.)

ward the center of the sarcomere and, on cross section, are arranged in a hexagonal array. The actin filament contains the *active site* where the two contractile proteins will interact.

In the middle of the sarcomere are the thick myosin filaments, one within each hexagonal array of actin filaments (Fig. 12-2). The myosin filament is composed primarily of a single protein, which can be enzymatically

cleaved into smaller moieties, the light meromyosin (LMM) backbone of the filament, and the globular heavy meromyosin (HMM), which makes up the cross-bridge. These are arranged in an antiparallel (tail-to-tail) pattern, so that the cross-bridges extend away from the center of the sarcomere in a feathered appearance. The heavy subunit is made up of two subunits—referred to as the S_1 and S_2 units—that make up the cross-bridge. These proteins are systematically spaced so that the heads of the cross-bridges make a complete circle around the myosin at the predictable distances of separation (Fig. 12-2).

Regulatory Proteins

While the interaction of the actin and myosin filaments is what generates tension, this interaction is regulated by two proteins that are a part of the actin filament. Along the grooves of the actin filament are the tropomyosin molecules. Covering the active sites and connected to tropomyosin is the troponin molecule. This molecule is made up of three units. The I unit inhibits the active site on the actin filament, the C unit has a high affinity for calcium, and the T unit joins the whole molecule to tropomyosin. In the absence of calcium, the troponin-tropomyosin complex inhibits the active site from interacting with the myosin cross-bridge. When calcium binds the troponin C, the tropomyosin molecule "rolls away," exposing the active site to the myosin cross-bridges (Fig. 12-3).

Architecture of Skeletal Muscle

The orderly arrangement of muscle elements also extends from the microscopic to the macroscopic level. Architecture is defined as the arrangement of fibers relative to the axis of the generation of force.[1] Parallel muscles have fibers that extend parallel to the axis of force generation. If the fibers are arranged in a single angle to the axis of force generation, the muscle is termed *unipennate.* Fibers in bipennate muscles have two such angles, and

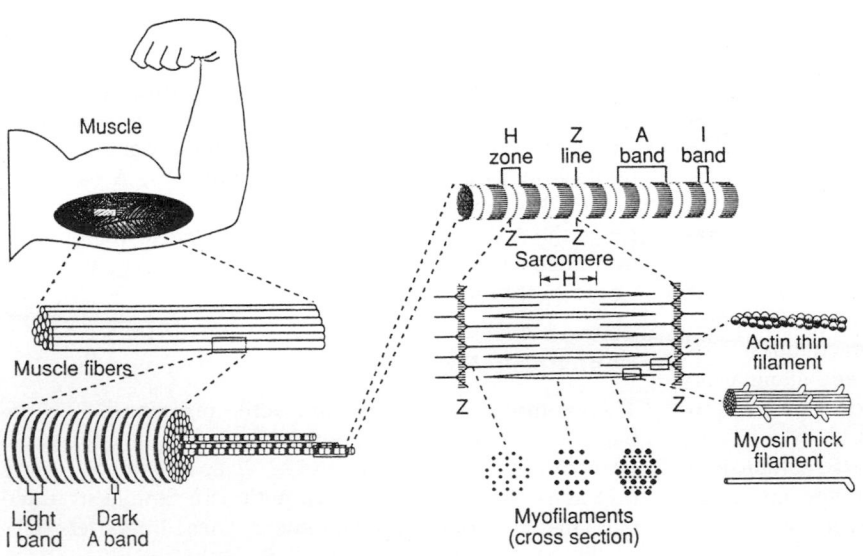

Figure 12-2 Microscopic organization of skeletal muscle. The whole muscle is composed of fibers; these in turn are made up of myofibrils, of which the actin and myosin protein filaments are a part. If viewed under a microscope, magnification would be approximately × 205,000. (From McArdle WD et al: *Exercise Physiology: Energy, Nutrition and Human Performance,* 3d ed. Malvern, PA, Lea & Febiger, 1991. Reproduced with permission.)

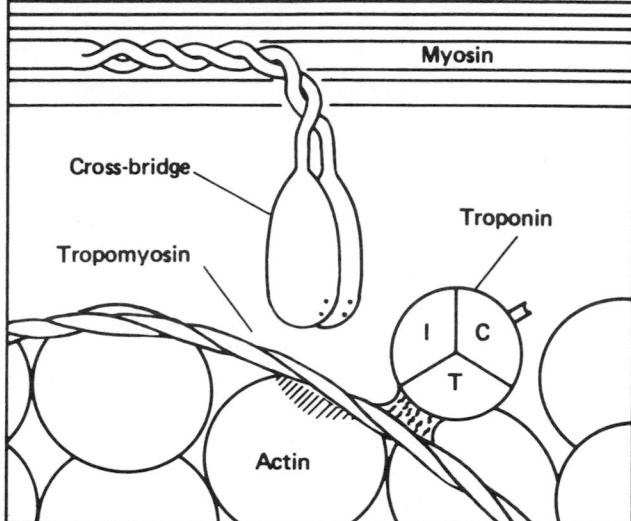

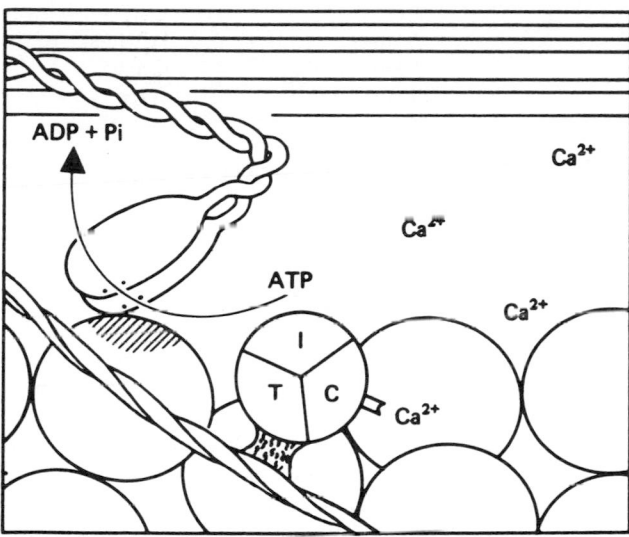

Figure 12-3 Initiation of muscle contraction by calcium (Ca^{2+}). The cross-bridges (heads of myosin molecules) attach to binding sites on actin (*striped areas*) and swivel when tropomyosin is displaced laterally by binding of Ca^{2+} to troponin C. [From Ganong WF (ed): *Review of Medical Physiology*. Los Altos, Lange Medical, 1983. Reproduced with permission.]

multipennate muscle fibers are aligned at multiple angles to the axis of force generation. Muscle fiber length also can influence rate of force production; not all fibers within a muscle are of the same length. Details of pennation and fiber length, critical values for calculating force production, are published.[1]

THE CONTRACTILE PROCESS

Contraction is made up of three conceptual steps: membrane excitation, excitation-contraction coupling, and contraction.

Membrane Excitation

The spinal motor neuron's action potential travels down the axon to the neuromuscular junction. In a calcium-mediated mechanism, acetylcholine (Ach) is released into the synaptic cleft and diffuses to the sarcolemmal receptors, resulting in local depolarization of the muscle cell. This area of local depolarization initiates an action potential in the muscle membrane similar to that in a neuron membrane. The impulse travels, via local current flow, away from the junction and along the membrane to the T tubules.

Excitation-Contraction Coupling

The action potential follows the membrane into the T tubules. These invaginations of the membrane carry the action potential deep into the muscle fiber. At the base of the T tubules, the action potential triggers the release of calcium from the terminal cisternae of the sarcoplasmic reticulum (SR). Calcium diffuses out of the SR and is drawn toward troponin C. Once calcium is bound with troponin C, the tropomyosin "rolls away," exposing the active site on the actin molecule for interaction with the myosin cross-bridges.

When the active site opens, the cross-bridge heads reach out and attach to the site. Energy from the breakdown of adenosine triphosphate (ATP) is needed for the cross-bridges to fold toward the center of the sarcomere, pulling the actin filaments which are attached to the Z lines. The repeated cross-bridge cycling shortens the sarcomere and develops tension. This mechanism, multiplied over thousands of sarcomeres, myofibrils, and fibers, achieves overall shortening of the whole muscle. The process of cross-bridge movement is energy-dependent. For the cross-bridge to detach one active site and attach to the next active site, ATP is required.

For relaxation to occur, the calcium is actively transported back into the terminal cisternae, causing the active site to be inhibited by the troponin-tropomyosin complex.

Muscle Fiber Type

Not all myofibers are identical, and relatively different types occur with varying physiologic, biochemical, and structural properties. Although the variability may be continuous, the fibers are considered to belong to two major categories: type I, the so-called slow-twitch type, and type II, the fast-twitch fiber (Table 12-1). Type I fibers have slow contraction and relaxation times and good resistance to fatigue. Type IIB fibers have the fastest contraction times and poor resistance to fatigue. Type IIA fibers are intermediate. They have fast contraction times and good fatigue resistance.

Energy Production in Muscle

Aerobic metabolism utilizes the Krebs cycle to regenerate ATP molecules by consuming pyruvate (from glucose)

TABLE 12-1   Fiber Type Summary

	Type I	Type IIA	Type IIB
Mechanical aspects			
Time to peak tension	Slow	Faster	Fastest
Twitch tension	Low	Higher	Highest
Fatigue resistance	High	Lower	Lowest
Elasticity	Low	High	High
Structural aspects			
Motor neuron size	Small	Large	Large
Motor neuron conduction velocity	Slow	Fast	Fast
Motor neuron recruitment threshold	Low	High	High
Fiber diameter	Small	Larger	Largest
Sarcoplasmic reticulum development	Least	More	Most
Mitochondrial density	Highest	Less	Least
Capillary density	Very dense	Less	Poor
Myoglobin content	High	Moderate	Low
Metabolic aspects			
Phosphocreatine	Low	Higher	Highest
Glycogen	Low	High	High
Triglyceride	High	Moderate	Low
ATPase activity	Low	High	High
Glycolytic enzyme activity	Low	High	High
Oxidative enzyme activity	High	High	Low

within muscle mitochondria. Fibers utilizing primarily this pathway are rich in mitochondria and oxidative enzymes (type I fiber type).

The glycolytic (anaerobic) pathway generates ATP by the metabolism of glucose to lactic acid. By this mechanism, only two molecules of ATP are produced (compared with 38 molecules by oxidative phosphorylation) per glucose molecule. Type IIB fibers have fewer mitochondria and are rich in anaerobic enzyme systems. Another occasional source of high-energy phosphate bonds is contained in the muscle's creatine phosphate.

REGULATION OF TENSION

The basic response of muscle to a single stimulus (either a nerve stimulus or direct stimulation of the fiber membrane) is the twitch (Fig. 12-4). When stimulated, the fiber develops tension rapidly to a peak (twitch tension) prior to relaxing. Tension can be increased by more rapid stimulation provided that these stimuli reach the fiber prior to full relaxation. The twitch tensions for each higher stimulation rate also increase in a steplike manner until tetanus—the full and complete contraction of the muscle.

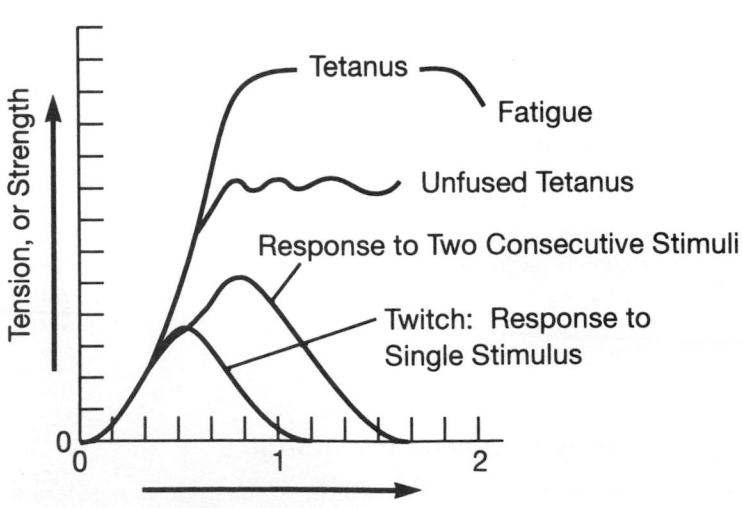

Figure 12-4 Wave summation. A motor unit responds to a single stimulus (nerve impulse) by giving a twitch (i.e., a brief period of contraction followed by relaxation). When a second stimulus is applied to the motor unit before it completely relaxes from the previous twitch, the two twitches summate so that the tension developed is greater than that produced by a single twitch alone. If the stimuli are repeated, summation continues until the individual twitches are completely fused (tetanus). Eventually fatigue occurs and tension is reduced. (From Fox EL et al: *The Physiological Basis for Exercise and Sport,* 5th ed. Dubuque, IA, Brown and Benchmark, 1988. Reproduced with permission.)

A single motor neuron and all the muscle fibers it innervates is called a *motor unit*. The number of fibers per neuron is termed the *innervation ratio;* it may be as low as 10 in muscles where fine gradation of force is required, such as extraocular muscles. Innervation ratios as high as 2000 may occur in the gastrocnemius muscle.

In addition to changing the rate of stimulation to alter muscle tension, the force of muscle contraction can also be increased by incremental recruitment of additional motor units by the central nervous system. Both these mechanisms may act together. As additional motor units are recruited by the central nervous system, the various muscle fiber types are recruited in an orderly manner. For low-force output activity, the slow-twitch type I fibers are recruited first. Increasing the force output requires the addition of the intermediate fibers. Highly intense contractions then add the fastest type IIB fibers.[6]

Length-Tension Relationship

The prestimulation length of an isometric muscle preparation dictates the eventual tension produced by the muscle (Fig. 12-5). The muscle's resting or optimal length offers the ideal possibility for maximum twitch tension, since there is the opportunity for optimal cross bridge and active site interaction. If the muscle is shortened prior to contraction, the expanded diameter of the sarcomere separates the actin and myosin filaments. Thus, less tension is produced. If the fiber is lengthened prior to stimulation, cross-bridges may be reaching for active sites that are not accessible, because the actin filaments have been pulled from the center of the sarcomere. With fewer cross-bridges interacting with actin, less tension is produced.

Some resting tension is produced within the muscle, in the absence of any contraction, at lengths beyond the optimal. This passive tension is believed to be exerted by the connective tissue sheaths around fibers, fasciculi, and the muscle bundles.

Force-Velocity Relationship

The tension that a muscle can exert is also related to its velocity of shortening or lengthening.[7] The fastest velocity of shortening will occur during concentric (shortening) contraction of the muscle in an unloaded condition, and the muscle tension falls as the shortening velocity increases (Fig. 12-6). When the load exceeds that which the muscle can maintain, the muscle is lengthened. The velocity of lengthening is less than the velocity of shortening for a given increment of force. Notice that tension maintained during a lengthening ("eccentric") contraction is very much higher relative to that produced during a shortening contraction. The level of force production has a hyperbolic relationship with the velocity of shortening or lengthening.

NEUROLOGIC CONTROL OF MUSCLE FORCE

Control in the Spinal Cord

The nerve supply to myofibers stems from fibers originating from alpha motor neurons in the anterior horn of the spinal cord. The summation of all facilitatory and inhibitory influences upon its cell membrane determines whether an individual alpha motor neuron will fire. An alpha motor neuron provides a single axon, which supplies numerous neuromuscular junctions on adjacent myofibers. Central control over the alpha motor neurons is achieved by means of descending axons in the principal efferent tracts of the spinal cord (cortico- and vestibulospinal). These enable a

Figure 12-5 The sarcomere length-tension curve for frog skeletal muscle obtained using sequential isometric contractions in single muscle fibers. Insets show schematic arrangement of myofilaments in different regions of the length-tension curve. Dotted line represents passive muscle tension. (From Lieber RL: *Skeletal Muscle Structure and Function: Implications for Rehabilitation and Sports Medicine.* Media, PA, Williams & Wilkins, 1992. Reproduced by permission.)

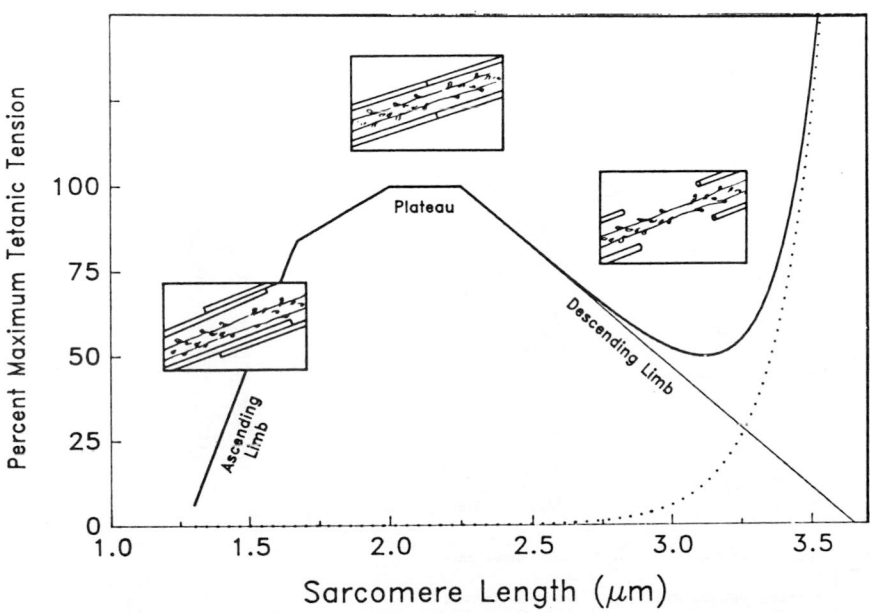

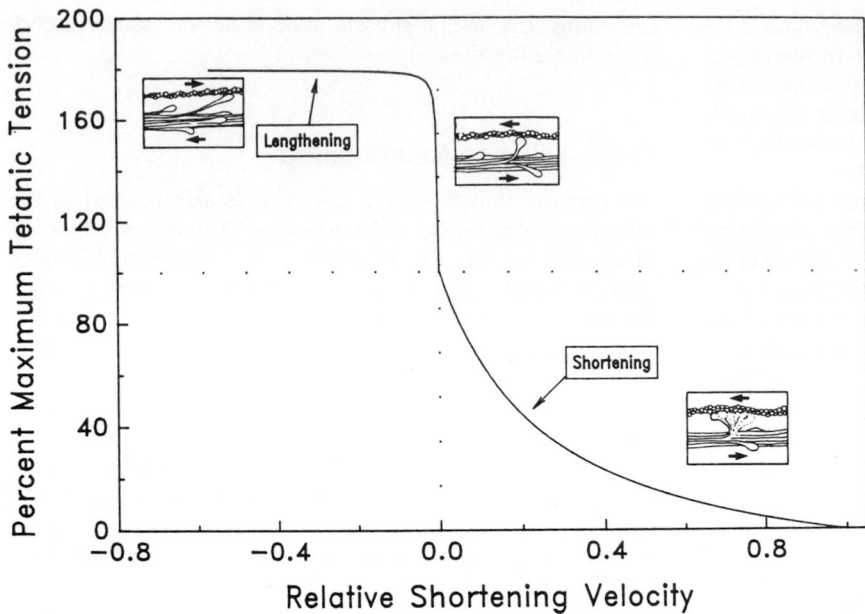

Figure 12-6 The muscle force-velocity curve for skeletal muscle obtained using sequential isotonic contractions in single fibers. *Insets* show schematic representation of cross-bridges. Note that force increases dramatically upon forced muscle lengthening (concentric contraction). (From Lieber RL: *Skeletal Muscle Structure and Function: Implications for Rehabilitation and Sports Medicine.* Media, PA, Williams & Wilkins, 1992. Reproduced by permission.)

programmed pattern of movement to occur. At the spinal level, afferent fibers with their endings in the muscle spindles exert facilitatory influences monosynaptically on alpha motor neurons. They are responsible for the well-known stretch reflex so useful in clinical practice.

Peripheral Mechanisms: Muscle Spindles

Other important influences impinging upon motor neurons are the afferent fibers from joint and muscle receptors as well as those from skin, tendon, and fascia. Until recently, it was thought that the afferent input from muscle spindles was not represented in the cortex. Thus, muscle sense was thought to be limited to joint receptors. However, it is now known that muscle spindles indeed contribute to joint-position sense and that their afferent discharge is represented in the cortex. Figure 12-7 shows the structure of the muscle spindle. It consists of 8 to 10 myofibers called *intrafusal fibers,* which run within a capsule in parallel with normal myofibers (sometimes called *extrafusal fibers*). In the equatorial region of each intrafusal fiber is a large ag-

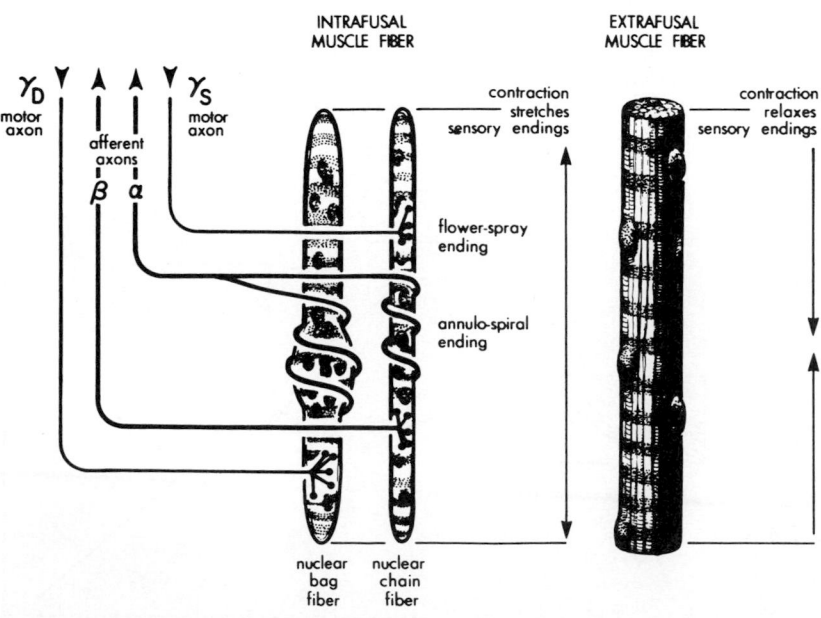

Figure 12-7 The mammalian muscle spindle consists of intrafusal and extrafusal fibers. Contraction responses of both fibers are schematically represented.

gregation of nuclei. One may differentiate, primarily according to appearance of the nuclei, two kinds of fibers, the so-called nuclear-bag and nuclear-chain fibers. The primary afferent endings consist of annulospiral terminals and large alpha afferent axons (with a diameter of 12 to 20 mm), which supply the central parts of both bag and chain fibers. Somewhat smaller beta afferent axons (4 to 12 mm) form secondary, flow-spray endings, which supply the less central regions of the fibers, primarily the chain fibers. The two types of endings respond differently. The primary endings are sensitive mainly to the rate of change of stretch, so their frequency of discharge is maximal while the stretch is applied but subsides to a resting level while the stretch is maintained (dynamic response). The secondary endings, on the other hand, are relatively unaffected by the rate of stretch but are sensitive to a particular steady level of tension (static response).

The intrafusal fibers are separately innervated from gamma motor neurons in the spinal cord, ensuring a sophisticated servomechanism.[8] The gamma fibers control the contraction of the intrafusal fibers and thereby adjust the level of sensitivity of the muscle spindle and its afferent range of discharge during muscle stretch. The gamma motor neurons themselves are influenced by polysynaptic peripheral reflexes and also central control mechanisms. The balance of these is normally inhibitory. When gamma motor neurons are released from central control (which may occur, for example, in spinal cord transection), there are changes in the level at which the muscle spindle is set. This accounts for the spasticity that then develops. Changes in the higher centers are known to exert influence upon the alpha and gamma motor neurons, particularly the reticular formation and the cerebellum. This explains the various changes in muscle tone accompanying brain damage.

There is more than one kind of termination from fusimotor axons. They vary from a structure that closely resembles a motor end plate to another kind of termination described as a trail ending, in which the axon seems to be distributed on the fiber through diffuse branching. To further complicate the matter, intrafusal myofibers may each be innervated by several motor axons. There may be more than one type of gamma motor neuron, each responding differently to dynamic and static parameters.

Control at the Level of Muscle Fiber

When motor units are recruited, the motor goal is achieved by increasing the firing rate of motor neurons.[9] Although in the laboratory repetitive stimulation of a myofiber within its relative refractory period (but not within its even shorter absolute refractory period) produces tetanic contraction, this probably rarely occurs in vivo. It should be emphasized that depolarization, both at the neuromuscular junction and at the myofibril membrane, is an all-or-none phenomenon.

Pathologic contractions of muscle fibers can occur if there are gross changes in the environment. Changes in the pH in the level of critical ions (particularly magnesium and calcium) affect the myofiber. Tetany is caused by levels of calcium in the extracellular fluid when they are sufficiently low to cause membrane depolarization. Rigor oc-

curs when muscles are depleted of ATP and phosphocreatine—for example, postmortem. This is accompanied by fixed bonding of actin and myosin.

ADAPTATION TO TRAINING

Muscle responds specifically to a wide variety of functional requirements, and its functional adaptability forms the basis of differing training regimens.

Endurance Training

Prolonged low intensity exercise requires aerobic energy production. Under these conditions all myofiber types increase their rates of synthesis of mitochondria. These sites for oxidative ATP generation increase in number and volume. Endurance exercise training also induces an increase in a muscle's capacity to oxidize fatty acids through the aerobic mechanism. This change favors the utilization of fat and spares muscle glycogen. Overall, the oxidative capacity of the cells, particularly types I and IIA, increases.

There is also an increase in the number of capillary blood vessels and the level of muscle myoglobin. Both these changes facilitate more efficient oxygen transport to the mitochondria.

Resistance Training

High intensity, short duration exercises such as weight lifting produce an increase in the contractile proteins in muscle with few metabolic changes. Regular resistance training results at first in a rapid improvement in strength in the absence of hypertrophy. This is due to increased recruitment of additional fibers as well as an increased activation frequency of recruited fibers. However, after a period of such training, which varies according to the individual, fiber hypertrophy begins with an increase in protein synthesis leading to increased contractile proteins (for increased force output) and sarcomeres in series (for increased shortening velocity). Fiber hypertrophy is primarily of the fast fiber population and consequently accompanied by little mitochondrial adaptation. There is an adaptation by the central nervous system improving the synchronicity of muscular recruitment.

Exercises that are very high resistance and short duration ("high weight, low reps") stress contractile aspects. With less weight and more repetitions, there is a move toward increases in local muscle endurance. This indicates that local improvements in oxygen use occur even when lifting weights. Table 12-2 summarizes training adaptations.

Anabolic Steroids

In male body builders no difference was observed in muscle fiber cross section after 8 weeks administration of either anabolic steroids or placebo during strength training.[10]

TABLE 12-2 Summary of Muscle Fiber Adaptations to Training

	Slow-twitch fibers		Fast-twitch fibers	
	Resistance training	Endurance training	Resistance training	Endurance training
Fiber type	⇔ or ?	⇔ or ?	⇔ or ?	⇔ or ?
Fiber size	⇑	⇔ or ⇑	⇑⇑⇑	⇔
Contractile properties	⇔	⇔	⇔	⇔
Anaerobic capacity	⇑ or ?	⇔	⇑ or ?	⇔
Aerobic capacity	⇔	⇑⇑⇑	⇔	⇑
Glycogen	⇔	⇑⇑⇑	⇔	⇑⇑⇑
Oxidation of fats	⇔	⇑⇑⇑	⇔	⇔
Density of capillaries	?	⇑	?	⇑ or ?
Exercising muscle blood flow	?	⇑ or ?	?	?

Key: ⇑ = increase; ⇔ = no change; ? = unknown.

Source: Modified with permission from McArdle WD, Katch FI, Katch FL: *Exercise Physiology: Energy, Nutrition and Human Performance.* Philadelphia, Lea & Febiger, 1991, p 351.

However, the American College of Sports Medicine believes small but significant increases in strength can occur in some individuals.[11] Fiber type transformation in favor of a preponderance of slow type I fibers is seen in experimental animals.[12,13] There is also a transitory reduction of collagen biosynthesis which may predispose to tendon rupture.[14]

Many of the performance effects may be due to generalized action on the body, including the central nervous system. Some of these, such as cardiomyopathy, are highly undesirable.[15]

ADAPTATIONS TO DETRAINING

Detraining can be a result of exercise cessation or restriction. Similar changes will follow central nervous system injury, limb immobilization, or bed rest. Detraining will mostly affect those fibers previously involved in training. Fibers that are minimally recruited prior to immobilization are going to suffer the least. The number of type I fibers and the aerobic profile regress, leading to reductions in the oxidative capacity of the muscle.[16]

The most visible adaptation of detraining is a loss of muscle mass due to atrophy. Those fibers that have the greatest change in their use as a result of immobilization lose the greatest mass. For example, the quadriceps femoris group will atrophy following knee immobilization. However, the vastus muscle atrophies to a greater extent than the rectus femoris, which is a two-joint muscle and still involved in hip flexion during walking. Furthermore, the vastus medialis, in its role as a patellar stabilizer, is probably recruited more often than the vastus lateralis. Thus, its change in recruitment is greater than that for the vastus lateralis, and its atrophy is also greater.

Both fast and slow fibers lose mass. This may be selective, depending on the muscle studied. For example, in the immobilized knee of the dog, the fast fibers of the vastus medialis and lateralis lose more protein than the fast fibers of the rectus femoris. The slow fibers of the medialis lose more protein than those of the lateralis, and the slow fibers of the rectus femoris lose the least.[1]

Immobilization also affects the metabolic aspects of muscle. The muscle is not required to be as active, so the adaptations favoring oxygen transport and utilization will reverse. Fewer capillaries around the fibers will result, and there will be less myoglobin, fewer mitochondria, and less active aerobic enzymes.[1,17]

INJURIES TO SKELETAL MUSCLE

Myofibers have a very limited ability to regenerate following injury.[16] In newborn muscle, satellite cells possess some capacity to regenerate new myofibers up to 3 weeks postinjury. However, the nuclei of mature myoblasts do not divide and regenerate. Fibroblasts lay down collagen fibrils at right angles to the axis of a surgical incision in muscle, whether the line of incision is parallel to the direction of existing muscle fibers or perpendicular to it.[18]

Few if any myofibers penetrate the scar. Active joint and muscle movement seems to provide the ideal tissue environment for repair of muscles in the injured limb provided that reinjury is prevented.[19,20] This is further discussed below, under "Contusion Injury."

Delayed-Onset Muscle Soreness

Muscle soreness develops over the 1- to 3-day period following the performance of unaccustomed exercise.[13] This predictable occurrence seems to be a result of eccentric contractions, during which the muscle is lengthened. The number of fibers necessary to move a load during a concentric contraction is much greater than the number of fibers needed to move the same load eccentrically.[21] As a result, the force per unit of active fiber is greater during an eccentric contraction. This appears to damage the Z lines as well as some of the connective tissue. Most of the damage seems to be isolated to the muscle-tendon junction. During the period of soreness, the muscle is weaker[21,22] and the range of motion is less.[23] The soreness then disappears within a few days as the muscle adapts to the prior activity. The adaptation is obvious because a repeat bout of the same exercise does not result in similar soreness. An inflammatory response contributes to the immediate discomfort and subsequent repair.[22,24]

Muscle Strain Injury

Strain injuries are not due to impact. Instead, strains are a result of excessive stretch or tension on the muscle, resulting in either partial muscle tears or complete rupture of the muscle.[16,25]

When a muscle is forcibly stretched passively or during a contraction, a muscle tear is possible. The susceptible muscles are two-joint muscles that may already be lengthened at time of injury. Another characteristic of frequently strained muscles is that they are used in the control of regulation of motion promoted by other muscle groups—e.g., during sprinting, the hamstrings function eccentrically to limit the amount of knee extension. In sports, strain injuries occur in activities that demand speed, acceleration/deceleration, and changes of direction, as in sprinting and team ball sports.

The patient with a strained limb muscle may show asymmetry or swelling due to hemorrhage by comparison with the contralateral side, especially when the muscle is contracted. The specific location of the injury appears to be at the muscle-tendon junction (a few sarcomeres into the muscle).[26,27] However, lesions can extend well into the muscle belly, because fibers within any given muscle are often of considerably different lengths. The locations of any associated hemorrhage can be demonstrated with imaging methods such as computed tomography or magnetic resonance imaging.[28] The bleeding may take several days to be detectable as ecchymosis.

Rest, ice, and compression constitute the recommended treatment. Physical therapy goals include improving functional strength and range of motion.

Nonsteroidal anti-inflammatory drugs can be started as soon as possible. However, they are administered only for a short period (5 to 7 days), because they can interfere with repair and remodeling of the tissue.

With improvement in strength and range of motion, light activity can be resumed. Comfort will dictate when exercise intensity can be increased. Resumption of competition prior to full recovery frequently leads to reinjury. Prophylactic stretching programs and warmup appear to be acceptable preventive measures.

Laceration Injury

Skeletal muscle laceration is a common injury seen by trauma surgeons. The recovery of muscle from a laceration injury varies depending upon whether the injury was a partial or a complete laceration of the tissue. In an incomplete laceration injury, the muscle will recover and then be able to generate only about 60 percent of its tension, but it will regain the normal ability to shorten. Following a complete laceration, the muscle may recover up to 50 percent of its ability to generate tension but will be able to shorten only to 80 percent of normal. Necrosis of fibers in the proximal or distal segment is not seen. The distal segment may exhibit signs of denervation atrophy: fiber area variability, fibrosis, and centralization of the nuclei. A dense scar forms between the two tissue fragments. Normal function does not return after the injury, and the distal segment then functions as a soft tissue bridge connecting the innervated segment with the tendon.[29]

Contusion Injury

Muscle contusions are a result of nonpenetrating blunt trauma that acutely crushes muscle fibers, leading to bleeding and hematomas. Contusions may be either intramuscular (within the epimysium) or intermuscular (spread outside of muscle facia). The former may be quite painful and disabling, leading to surgery. The latter, less serious injury can lead to ecchymosis or effusion just below the area of impact within 2 to 3 days.[30]

The severity of the injury is dictated by the impact energy per unit area, the contused tissue's material properties, and the underlying tissue (e.g., bone). A high-energy impact to a discrete area can lead to fiber disruption, while the same impact to a larger area may result only in a large hematoma. Edema and other components of the inflammatory response will occur. Some regeneration and repair of the crushed muscle cells may occur within the scar formation.[30] Occasionally the damaged muscle will ossify (myositis ossificans).

The inflammatory response is necessary for vascular and connective tissue ingrowth; therefore the use of nonsteroidal anti-inflammatory agents is probably questionable.[31] A short period of immobilization (5 days or less) promotes the beneficial granulation of the tissue matrix. If the immobilization is extended, the scar is contracted and functional muscle recovery is poor. Stretching the muscle promotes lymphatic and venous drainage and lowers tissue pressure.[30] Any suggestion of ossification, however, prohibits continuation of the exercise program.

Muscle Cramps

Cramps are a unique aspect of muscle contraction. Their appearance immediately reduces the ability to perform activities. These are somewhat difficult to define because disruption of any step in the sequence of events leading to contraction—motor neuron activity, membrane excitability, contraction coupling—can be a logical culprit for cramps and spasms.

Electrodiagnostic evidence indicates cramps are usually due to abnormal motor neuron excitability rather than abnormalities within the muscle fibers. Why this occurs is unknown. Spontaneous muscle fiber activity does not appear to be the mechanism. A frequent variable in muscle cramps is dehydration or rapid changes in sodium levels. Similar changes in muscle can occur in dialysis patients, who can exhibit electrolytic changes similar to those triggered by intense physical activities.

Muscle spasms, which originate from the central nervous system nociceptive protective reflexes, should be differentiated from cramps. In spasms, the pain of the injury triggers the central nervous system to contract selected motor units in an attempt to protect the area.

REFERENCES

1. Lieber RL: *Skeletal Muscle Structure and Function: Implications for Rehabilitation and Sports Medicine.* Baltimore, Williams & Wilkins, 1992.
2. Landmesser LT: The generation of neuromuscular specificity. *Annu Rev Neurosci* 3:279, 1980.
3. Thompson WJ, Sutton LA, Riley DA: Fiber type composition of single motor units during synapse elimination of neonatal rat soleus muscle. *Nature* 309:709, 1984.
4. Engel AG: The neuromuscular junction, in Engel AG, Banker BQ (eds): *Myology:* Vol 1. New York, McGraw-Hill, 1986.
5. Miller JB, Stockdale FE: Developmental origins of skeletal muscle fibers: Clonal analysis of myogenic cell lineages based on expression of fast and slow myosin heavy chains. *Proc Natl Acad Sci USA* 83:3860, 1986.
6. Henneman E, Somjen G, Carpenter DO: Functional significance of cell size in spinal motoneurons. *J Neurophysiol* 28:560, 1965.
7. Perrine JJ, Edgerton VR: Muscle force-velocity and power-velocity relationships under isokinetic loading. *Med Sci Sports* 10:159–166, 1978.
8. Granit R: *Muscle Afferents and Motor Control.* New York, Wiley, 1966.
9. Milner Brown HS, Stein RB, Yemor R: The orderly recruitment of human motor units during voluntary isometric contraction. *J Physiol* 230:359–370, 1973.
10. Kuipers H, Peeze Binkhorst FM, Hartgens F: Muscle ultrastructure after strength training with placebo or anabolic steroid, *Can J Physiol* 18(2):189–196, 1993.
11. American College of Sports Medicine position stand on the use of anabolid androgenic steroids in sports medicine. *Sci Sports Exerc* 19:534–539, 1987.
12. Salmon S: Myotrophic effects of an anabolic steroid in rabbit limb muscles. *Muscle Nerve* 15:806–812, 1992.
13. Fritzsche D, Krakos R, Asmussen E, et al: Effect of an anabolic steroid (metenolon) on contractile performance of the chronically stimulated latissimus dorsi in sheep. *Eur J Cardiothorac Surg* 8:214–219, 1993.
14. Karpakka JA, Pesola MK, Takala TES: The effects of anabolic steroids on collagen synthesis in rat skeletal muscle and tendon. *Am J Sports Med* 20:262–267, 1992.
15. Celotti F, Negri C: Anabolic steroids: A review of their effects on the muscles of their possible mechanisms of action and of their use in athletics. *J Steroid Biochem Molec Biol* 43:469–477, 1992.
16. Caplan A, Carlson B, Faulkner J, et al: Skeletal muscle, in Savio LY, Buckwalter JA (eds): *Injury and Repair of the Musculoskeletal Soft Tissues.* Rosemont, IL, American Academy of Orthopaedic Surgeons, 1988.
17. Gollnick PD, Saltin B: Skeletal muscle adaptability: Significance for metabolism and performance, in Peachy LD (ed): *Handbook of Physiology:* Sec 10. *Skeletal Muscle.* Bethesda, MD, American Physiological Society, 1983.
18. Rizk NN: SEM of the structural reconstruction of the abdominal wall after experimental paramedian incision. *J Surg Res* 35:354–364, 1983.
19. Allbrook DB, Baker N de C, Kirkaldy-Willis WH: Muscle regeneration in experimental animals and man. *J Bone Joint Surg* 48B:153–169, 1966.
20. Cooper RR: Alterations during immobilization and regeneration of skeletal muscle in rats. *J Bone Joint Surg* 54B:919–925, 1972.
21. Stauber WT: Eccentric action of muscle: Physiology, injury and adaptation. *Exerc Sports Sci Rev* 17:157, 1989.
22. Evans J, Cannan JG: The metabolic effects of exercise-induced muscle damage. *Exerc Sports Sci Rev* 19:99, 1991.
23. Howell JN, Chila JG, Ford G, et al: An electromyographic study of elbow motion during post exercise soreness. *J Appl Physiol* 58:1713, 1985.
24. Smith LL: Acute inflammation: The underlying mechanism in delayed onset muscle soreness? *Med Sci Sports Exerc* 23:542, 1991.
25. Garrett WE Jr: Muscle strain injuries: Clinical and basic science aspects. *Med Sci Sports Exerc* 22:436, 1990.
26. Almekinders LC, Garrett WE Jr, Seaber AV: Histopathology of muscle tears in stretching injuries. *Trans Orthop Res* 9:306, 1984.
27. Almekinders LC, Garrett WE Jr, Seaber AV: Pathophysiologic response to muscle tears in stretching injuries. *Trans Orthop Res* 9:307, 1984.
28. Garrett WE Jr, Rich FR, Nikolaou PK, Vogler JB III: Computed tomography of hamstring strains. *Med Sci Sports Exerc* 21:506, 1989.
29. Garrett WE Jr, Seaber AV, Boswick J, et al: Recovery of skeletal muscle after laceration and repair. *J Hand Surg* 9A:683, 1984.
30. Crisco JJ, Jokl P, Heinen GT, et al: A muscle contusion injury model: Biomechanics, physiology and histology. *Am J Sports Med* 22:702, 1994.
31. Mishara DK, Smitz MC, Giangreco C, et al: Anti-inflammatory medication after muscle injury provides short-term improvement but long-term loss of muscle function. *Trans Orthop Res Soc* 161:689, 1994.

Lieber RL, McKee-Woodburn T, Frieden J, Gershuni DH: Recovery of the dog quadriceps after ten weeks of immobilization followed by four weeks of remobilization. *J Orthop Res* 7:408, 1989.

Armstrong RB: Mechanisms of exercise induced delayed onset muscle soreness. *Med Sci Sports Exerc* 16:529, 1984.

CHAPTER 13

Peripheral Nerve

Shawn J. Bird
and Mark J. Brown

STRUCTURE OF PERIPHERAL NERVE

Gross Anatomy of Peripheral Nerve

The peripheral nervous system includes all the neural structures that lie outside the brain, spinal cord, and brainstem. The somatic peripheral nerves consist of efferent motor fibers to cranial, trunk, and limb muscles; afferent sensory fibers from cutaneous and deep sensory receptors; and receptors in muscles and tendons. The peripheral autonomic nervous system includes both sympathetic and parasympathetic components.

The motor limb of the somatic peripheral nervous system begins with nerve cell bodies in the spinal cord or brainstem. In the spinal cord these are located in the anterior or ventral horns of the central gray matter. Each cell body gives rise to an axon that accompanies others to form rootlets, which, in turn, combine to form the ventral or motor roots. The ventral roots join with dorsal roots to form the spinal nerves, or spinal roots. The spinal nerves leave the vertebral canal through neural foramina and split into dorsal and ventral rami. Motor axons from dorsal rami innervate paraspinal muscles. Motor axons in the ventral rami continue directly or through a plexus and then along nerves to supply individual muscles. The sensory (afferent) limb of the somatic nervous system begins in receptors in skin, muscle, or tendon. The sensory axons ascend rostrally through nerve, plexus, and then ventral rami to join the spinal nerve. The sensory cell bodies are clustered in dorsal root ganglia in intervertebral foramina, located just proximal to the union of the ventral root and distal to the end of the dural sleeve. The central projections of sensory neurons enter the spinal cord through the dorsal roots and then synapse within the central nervous system.

Individual muscles are supplied by specific nerves but also have a segmental relation to ventral nerve roots. All muscles supplied by an individual ventral nerve root are called *myotomes*. Most muscles are supplied by one nerve but receive innervation from two or more other roots. For example, the deltoid muscle is supplied by the axillary nerve and receives motor fibers from the C5 and C6 myotomes. The myotomal pattern of innervation may vary among individuals. For example, the anterior tibialis muscle is always supplied by the peroneal nerve. It most often receives components from both the L4 and L5 myotomes but may be innervated solely by L4- or L5-derived motor fibers. Cutaneous sensory receptors project centrally through specific peripheral nerves, such as the median nerve, and also have a segmental relation to spinal nerve roots. The region of skin supplied by an individual dorsal nerve root is a dermatome. The sensory borders of skin supplied by a nerve are relatively sharply demarcated, whereas dermatomal areas are less distinct and partially overlap.

The peripheral autonomic nervous system is divided into craniosacral (parasympathetic) and thoracolumbar (sympathetic) divisions. Unlike the somatic system, where a single neuron precisely connects the central nervous system with the peripheral receptor or muscle, there are two neurons, preganglionic and postganglionic, in the autonomic peripheral system. The cranial portion of parasympathetic division arises from preganglionic special visceral nuclei in the brainstem. It supplies, through cranial nerves III, VII, and IX, the pupil sphincter muscles and lacrimal and salivary glands, after synapsing in ganglia close to its target. The vagus nerve carries parasympathetic fibers to the heart and other thoracoabdominal organs. The sacral portion of the parasympathetic divisions arises from preganglionic cell bodies in the lateral horn of the S2 to S4 levels of the spinal cord. These fibers travel with the S2 to S4 spinal nerves and pelvic nerves to synapse with pelvic ganglia that lie on effector organs in the genitourinary and lower gastrointestinal tracts.

The sympathetic division originates from preganglionic neurons in the anteromedial cell column of the thoracolumbar (C8 to L2) spinal cord. Axons travel with spinal nerves and then myelinated white rami to a chain of paravertebral ganglia. Some pass through to synapse in the celiac, superior, or inferior mesenteric ganglia to regulate splanchnic blood flow. Others synapse in the paravertebral ganglia. There are 3 cervical, 11 thoracic, and 4 to 6 lumbar sympathetic ganglia. These fibers then rejoin the ventral rami in somatic nerves to innervate the sympathetic components of the head and limbs. They function to regulate peripheral blood vessels (vasomotor), sweat glands (sudomotor), and muscles of the hair follicle (pilomotor). The sympathetic vasomotor, sudomotor, and pilomotor nerve fibers approximate the distribution of somatosensory fibers with which they travel. For example, the cutaneous radial sensory distribution is also supplied by sympathetic fibers that control sweating and vasomotor changes over the dorsum of the hand.

Microscopic Anatomy of Peripheral Nerve

Peripheral neurons consist of cell bodies (the soma or perikaryon) and long axonal processes. Like other cells, the soma contains the nucleus, mitochondria, rough endoplasmic reticulum, and ribosomes. It is the endoplasmic reticulum that forms the floccular-appearing Nissl substance in stained histologic sections. Peripheral nerve cells are unique in that the soma must maintain a cytoplasmic extension, the axon, that is more than 200 times its size. This places unique metabolic and structural demands on these cells. There are two principal mechanisms for moving molecules to and from the soma, anterograde (centrifugal) and retrograde (centripetal) axonal transport. Neurotransmitter molecules and axonal membrane components, used to renew axonal and synaptic terminal membranes, are transported by a fast anterograde transport

TABLE 13-1   General Properties of Axons in Peripheral Nerves

	Myelinated	Unmyelinated
Axonal size	1–18 μm	0.2–2 μm
Population	Bimodal (small and large)	Unimodal
Conduction velocity	12–70 m/s	0.5–2.0 m/s
Mode of conduction	Saltatory	Continuous
Axons per Schwann cell	1	>1
Functions	Somatic motor	Some sensory
	Some sensory	Most autonomic
	Muscle afferents	
	Some preganglionic autonomic	

Source: Modified with permission from Stewart JD: *Focal Peripheral Neuropathies,* 2d ed. New York, Raven Press, 1993, p 5.

system with a speed of about 400 mm per day. A fast retrograde transport system moves material from the periphery to the cell body at about 250 mm per day. This recycles metabolic and structural breakdown products and allows the soma to interact with the periphery by delivering to it products taken up by peripheral endocytosis. A slow transport system, about 1 mm per day, carries axonal cytoskeletal elements from the cell body down the axon.

Dendrites are short cytoplasmic extensions from the cell body with complex branches. They and the soma provide a membrane surface to integrate synaptic input from other nerve cells. The axon, the long nerve fiber extension from the cytoplasm, is a complex specialized structure. It originates from a thickened extension of the cell body, the axon hillock. The axonal membrane (axolemma) is a double phospholipid membrane. It contains ion channels that maintain a transmembrane ionic and electrical gradient and also voltage-dependent channels, which underlie the propagation of nerve action potentials. The axolemma encloses the axoplasm; it is filled with microtubules and neurofilaments that serve as the axonal cytoskeleton as part of the transport system.

Peripheral axons are either myelinated or unmyelinated (Table 13-1).[1] Both types are associated with supporting glial cells, the Schwann cells. The proportion of myelinated to unmyelinated axons in a nerve varies depending on its function; but in general, unmyelinated fibers predominate. Unmyelinated axons are enveloped in groups by Schwann cell cytoplasm. In contrast, myelinated fibers are surrounded individually by a sequence of single Schwann cells along their lengths. Myelinated fibers occur in a bimodal size distribution (Fig. 13-1). The myelin sheath is made up of compacted layers of Schwann cell plasma membrane. Each segment of myelin or internode is adjacent to another; the gap of exposed axolemma between them is the node of Ranvier. The myelinated internodes have increased transmembrane resistance and reduced capacitance compared to the nodes of Ranvier. This allows conduction to skip rapidly from node to node (saltatory conduction). The conduction velocities of myelinated axons range from 40 to 70 m/s. This compares to 0.5 to 2.0 m/s for unmyelinated fibers, which rely on continuous conduction along bare axolemmae membrane.

The thickness of the myelin sheath is related to axonal diameter, increasing with larger-diameter axons.[2] Internodal length also increases with diameter and is typically about 200 to 2000 μm long. Increased axonal diameter, myelin sheath thickness, and internodal length lead to a greater conduction velocity and allow faster transmission of electrical impulses. Functions that require intense information demands, such as efferent motor impulse and proprioceptive feedback from muscle stretch and joint position receptors, are mediated by larger, faster-conducting myelinated axons (40 to 70 m/s). Autonomic and some sensory functions are conveyed by slowly conducting, unmyelinated axons (0.5 to 2.0 m/s).

The compound nerve action potential elicited by electrical stimulation consists of discrete peaks, each corresponding to populations of nerve fibers with characteristic conduction velocities (Table 13-2).[3,4] These populations, designated A, B, and C, can be differentiated by their physiologic and histologic properties. The A fibers, myelinated somatic efferent or afferent axons, are the largest and conduct the fastest (20 to 70 m/s). The A fibers may be further separated by their function, size, and conduction velocity. For example, cutaneous nerves are commonly divided into two peaks, A-alpha and A-delta. The B fibers are the small, myelinated, efferent preganglionic axons of the autonomic nerves. The C fibers are unmyelinated and conduct the slowest (0.5 to 2.0 m/s). These make up the smallest afferent sensory and postganglionic autonomic axons.

Myelinated and unmyelinated axons are bundled together as fascicles surrounded by a thin connective tissue layer, the perineurium (Fig. 13-1). Within the perineurium is the endoneurium, a space that includes axons, connective tissue elements, small capillaries, and extracellular fluid. An outer layer of connective tissue and vessels, the epineurium, loosely joins the fascicles together as a nerve. The longitudinally oriented endoneurial collagen and the circumferential perineurial and epineurial collagen protect the nerve from compression and trauma and give it tensile strength. The vascular supply of peripheral nerve is provided by abundant segmental branches from adjacent arteries. These enter the epineurium as the vasa nervorum, branch into arterioles, and pierce the perineurium to form an anastomotic network of endoneurial capillaries. These

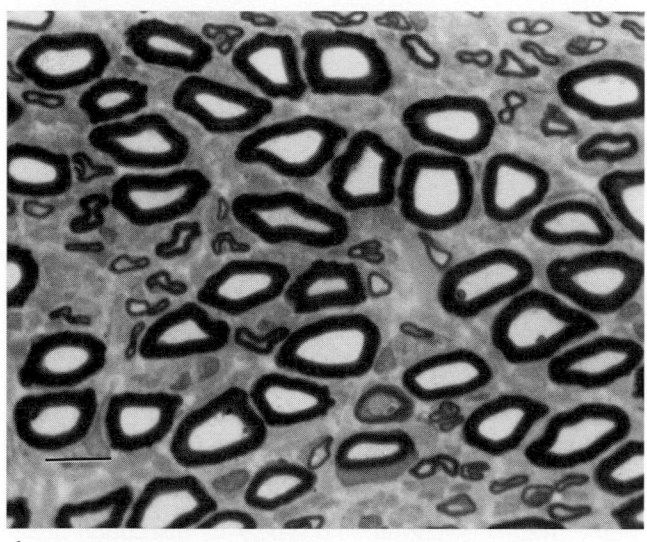

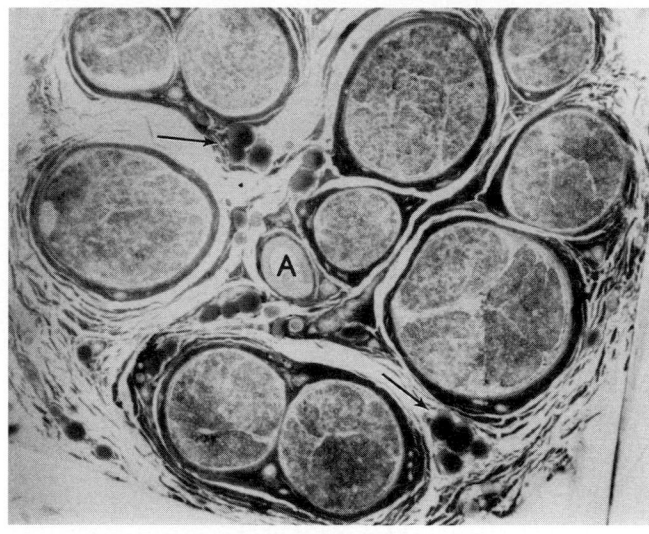

A
B

Figure 13-1 *A.* High-magnification cross-section light micrograph of a normal human sural nerve. There are both large-diameter myelinated fibers with thick sheaths and smaller myelinated fibers with thin sheaths. Epoxy-embedded. Bar = 10 μm. *B.* Very low magnification cross-section light micrograph of a normal sural nerve, obtained at biopsy from the lateral ankle. There are 10 fascicles, each enclosed by darker-staining perineurium. The fascicles are surrounded by epineurium, a matrix of collagen, blood vessels (A) and lipid (*arrows*). Epoxy-embedded.

capillaries have tight junctions, and, with the perineurium, form a barrier that isolates the endoneurial compartment from blood, analogous to the blood-brain barrier. Trauma, toxins, inflammation, ischemia, or immune-mediated mechanisms may damage this barrier, leading to destructive changes within the endoneurium.

Fascicular Arrangements within Peripheral Nerve

Sunderland demonstrated that there is intermingling of axons among fascicles, leading to the branching and formation of new fascicles (Fig. 13-2).[5] After reconstructing multiple serial cross sections of nerve, he concluded that more proximal nerve contained fascicles that held axons destined for diverse locations, whereas axons in more distal locations were more likely to have common destinations. The more proximal the site in the nerve, the more intermixing of axons would be expected. With characterization of a motor and sensory deficit and knowledge of the nerve anatomy, a lesion site could be accurately identified.

Recent observations indicate that Sunderland's concept of fascicular anatomy is an oversimplification. For example, the relative sparing of ulnar forearm muscles with ulnar neuropathy at the elbow [6] suggests that the motor fascicle to those muscles is distinct and separate at the elbow and less susceptible to compression. Similarly, studies of radial nerve compression at the spiral groove[7] and peroneal nerve at the fibular head[8] have shown sparing of

---

TABLE 13-2 Classification of Peripheral Nerve Fibers by Size and Function

---

A fibers   Somatic nerve (myelinated fibers)
          Muscle nerve
             Afferent: group I (12–21 μm), II (6–12 μm), III (1–6 μm), IV (C fiber)
             Efferent: alpha motor neuron
                 gamma motor neuron
          Cutaneous nerve
             Afferent: alpha (6–17 μm)
                 delta (1–6 μm)

B fibers   Autonomic preganglionic myelinated nerve (<3 μm)

C fibers   Somatic or autonomic unmyelinated nerve (<1.3 μm)

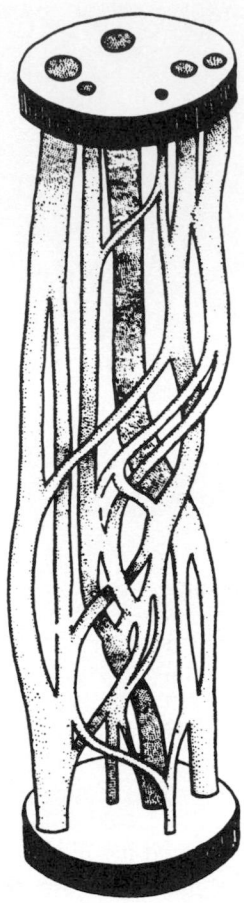

Figure 13-2 Drawing of the fascicular rearrangement along a nerve, constructed from serial cross sections. (Reproduced with permission from Sunderland S: *Nerves and Nerve Injuries,* 2d ed. Edinburgh, Churchill Livingstone, 1978, p 32.)

distal sensory branches or of individual muscles. This sparing is best explained by selective involvement of fascicles going to these distal motor or sensory branches. In addition, evidence from dissection studies of human nerve indicate less fascicular rearrangement than expected from Sunderland's work.[9] Lesion experiments in dogs,[10] anatomic studies after specific nerve fiber labeling,[11] and microneurographic studies[12,13] have shown relatively modest fascicular rearrangement. Although Sunderland's theory of fascicular intermixing explains many clinical observations, the concept should not cause one to overlook the unique fascicular anatomy of some nerves.

RESPONSE TO INJURY

Classification of Nerve Injuries

Peripheral nerves have a limited repertoire of responses to injury (Fig. 13-3). The axons, myelin sheaths, and the supporting connective tissue elements may be involved in a predictable, stereotypical way. Most lesions of peripheral nerve have some degree of involvement of all of these

structures, but it is critical to determine clinically and electrophysiologically how much of each is contributing.

Seddon first subdivided nerve injuries into three basic categories. This classification remains useful today.[14] He used the term *neurapraxia* to describe nerve fibers whose axons are intact but are unable to conduct an action potential. Focal demyelination from compression is the usual cause. *Axonotmesis* and *neurotmesis* indicate the loss of axonal continuity, but with the latter there is also loss of integrity of supporting Schwann cell tubes and connective tissue elements. Sunderland subsequently proposed a more detailed classification system (Table 13-3).[15] His type 1 injury corresponds to neurapraxia, whereas his type 5 is neurotmesis. Sunderland further subdivided axonotmesis into three types. Type 2 has preservation of all other nerve elements and is most often seen with severe chronic compression. Type 3 is characterized by disruption of the endoneurium and type 4 by disruption of the perineurium. Types 3 and 4 are most often seen after acute blunt trauma or incomplete nerve transection. Most closed traumatic injuries, including crush or stretch, and nerve ischemia cause loss of axonal continuity or axonotmesis. Laceration, or severe stretch, crush, and percussion injuries, may result in neurotmesis.

Clinically, nerve injuries result in both negative neurologic manifestations, or loss of functions, and positive manifestations. Loss of axonal function, due to either conduction block or axonal loss, results in weakness and sensory loss. Positive manifestations, such as paresthesias and pain, may result from the injury, ischemia, or wound-site neuromas.[16] The mechanism of pain in nerve lesions remains incompletely understood, however.

Neurapraxia and Acute Compression

There are three levels of injury when nerve is subject to a compression. The mildest, physiologic conduction block, is usually quickly and completely reversible if the compression is relieved. This is the process that occurs after brief leg crossing and is due to transient nerve ischemia.[17]

With more severe compression, there may be persistent conduction block (neuropraxia) or Wallerian degeneration (axonotmesis). Acute compressive nerve injuries are a combination of demyelination-induced conduction block and axonal degeneration, but one process may predominate. A region of persisting conduction block will result in loss of function distal to those blocked axons. This kind of lesion occurs after prolonged peroneal nerve compression at the fibular head. Recovery occurs by remyelination of the involved segments.[18,19] Electrophysiologically, regions of conduction block (neurapraxia) can be identified using conventional nerve conduction tests. Renewed conduction across the segment is followed by functional recovery.

In studies of acute experimental nerve compression, Gilliatt and colleagues, using tourniquet-induced pressure in a limb of the baboon, demonstrated the importance of mechanical factors under the compressed region.[20–24] Mild compression results in paranodal demyelination, but moderate compression causes myelin displacement away from the site of compression. The displaced myelin invaginates

Figure 13-3 Drawing of a normal motor neuron and muscle (*left*) and the basic responses to injury (Wallerian degeneration and segmental demyelination). (Reproduced with permission from Asbury AK, Johnson PC: *Pathology of Peripheral Nerve.* Philadelphia, Saunders, 1978, p 51.)

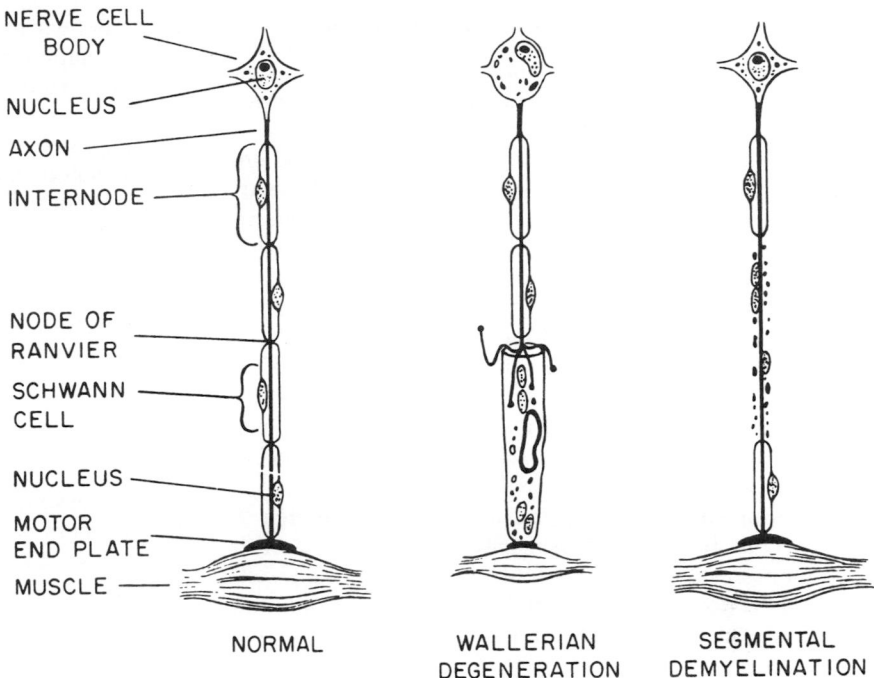

NERVE CELL BODY

NUCLEUS

AXON

INTERNODE

NODE OF RANVIER

SCHWANN CELL

NUCLEUS

MOTOR END PLATE

MUSCLE

NORMAL   WALLERIAN DEGENERATION   SEGMENTAL DEMYELINATION

the adjacent paranodes and produces segmental demyelination, with conduction block. Recovery occurs coincident with remyelination. The histologic changes observed strongly support a direct mechanical effect due to pressure gradient at the edge of the region of compression as the principal pathogenetic factor.

The hypothesis that ischemia plays a major role in acute compressive lesions[25,26] has not been supported by subsequent studies. Pressures just above systolic do not produce conduction block.[27] Also, ischemia produced by a proximal tourniquet does not potentiate the effects of mild experimental distal compression.[28] Experimentally produced acute nerve ischemia results in Wallerian degeneration, not focal demyelination.[29,30] Regardless of the

mechanism that produces neurapraxia with acute compression, the larger motor and sensor myelinated nerves are preferentially susceptible to the pressure effect. There is relative sparing of small myelinated and unmyelinated fibers unless compression is severe enough to result in Wallerian degeneration.[27,31]

The third level of injury, axonal degeneration (axonotmesis), occurs with more intense and prolonged compression. Percussion injuries, occasionally studied as a model of acute crush injuries,[19,32] cause additional axonal injury through intraneural hemorrhage, endoneurial edema, and disruption of the supporting structures (perineurium). The final result, Wallerian degeneration, is common to severe acute compressive and percussive injuries.

TABLE 13-3   Methods of Classifying Traumatic Nerve Lesions[a]

Seddon	Sunderland	Pathophysiology
Neurapraxia	1	Temporary block of nerve conduction without axonal degeneration (conduction block)
Axonotmesis	2	Axonal degeneration (loss of continuity) with intact endoneurium
	3	Endoneurial disruption with intact perineurium; axonal degeneration
	4	Perineurium and endoneurium disrupted with intact epineurium; axonal degeneration
Neurotmesis	5	Complete nerve disruption; axonal degeneration

[a]Based on data from Seddon HJ: Three types of nerve injury. *Brain* 66:236, 1943; and Sunderland S: A classification of peripheral nerve injuries producing loss of function. *Brain* 74:491, 1951.

Chronic Nerve Compression and Entrapment

Chronic nerve compression, such as carpal tunnel syndrome or ulnar neuropathy at the elbow, is characterized by clinical and electrophysiologic signs of focal neurapraxia. The basis of this is thought to be segmental demyelination. Experimental models have supported the argument that histologic and electrophysiologic changes after chronic compression are similar to those seen with acute tourniquet compression. Gilliatt and colleagues showed that the guinea pig spontaneously develops compressive neuropathy in the hindfoot that histologically shows prominent segmental demyelination and electrophysiologic hallmarks of slowing and conduction block.[33] With more severe compression, there is also axonotmesis (axonal loss) with endoneurial and perineurial thickening.[34]

Early myelin changes occur under the entire area of chronic compression, not primarily at the edges as with acute compression.[35,36] After chronic compression, each internode is distorted, with myelin heaped up at one end, away from the center, and thinned at the other end. This is followed by demyelination of the internode. Aguayo and coworkers made similar observations in studies of experimental entrapment of rabbit sciatic nerve by using a siliconized rubber tube.[37] Studies of chronic nerve compression in rats and monkeys showed that the earliest changes were thickening of the epineurium and perineurium, followed by thinning of myelin and focal conduction abnormalities.[38,39] Histologic studies of human nerves from sites of entrapment have demonstrated focal demyelination.[23,40] Postmortem studies of severe compressive neuropathy in humans have confirmed a similar increase in endoneurial and perineurial connective tissue under the site of compression.[41]

Some have advocated a prominent role for ischemia, like acute compression, in chronic nerve compression.[42] Severe, long-standing ischemia produces nerve infarction with axonal loss and connective tissue reaction.[43,44] Pressure may also restrict venous outflow and increase endoneurial pressure, which could alter the nerve microcirculation. Interruption of axonal transport may also occur even at relatively low compressive pressures.[45–47] These perturbations may produce axonal loss, added to the direct effects of compression. However, ischemia cannot account for the earliest pathologic changes and the persistent conduction block seen at sites of compression. Conduction block may occur with acute nerve ischemia, but it is transient.[48]

Axonotmesis and Wallerian Degeneration

Axonotmesis is the loss of axonal continuity with an intact endoneurium and is followed by Wallerian degeneration distal to the lesion. When the axon is interrupted, regardless of the cause, changes occur distal and proximal to the lesion.[49] Proximal to the lesion the cell body undergoes central chromatolysis, with an enlarged eccentric nucleus, enlarged nucleolus, Nissl granules displaced into dendrites from the soma, and reduced membrane excitability.[50] If the lesion is near the cell body, some proportion of cells will die, precluding any recovery.

Distal to the site of axonal interruption, granular fragmentation of the axonal cytoskeleton occurs along the entire length of the distal axon.[49] The structural breakdown is associated with a loss of electrical excitability of the axonal membrane, and the ability to conduct action potentials is lost. The axonal and myelin debris, seen as myelin ovoids on histologic sections, is taken up by macrophages. Remaining Schwann cells proliferate and create an environment for remyelination after axonal regeneration.

The timing of these changes depends on several factors, including species and distal stump length. Axonal disintegration is considerably slower in larger animals than in rats or mice.[51,52] Most data on Wallerian degeneration in humans come from serial electrophysiologic studies following nerve transection. Motor responsiveness is lost after an injury when stimulating across the lesion site due to the loss of axonal continuity through that region. A motor response can be recorded distal to the lesion for 4 to 5 days. The amplitude of the motor response falls steadily and is unmeasurable after 6 to 8 days.[53,54] The sensory response is more persistent, remaining normal for 5 to 8 days. It then declines and disappears by 10 to 12 days after injury. The length of the distal nerve stump influences the response; the larger the stump, the greater the delay in conduction failure.[54,55] This may alter the time of conduction failure by up to 3 days. These studies have practical implications in the timing of electrophysiologic studies following nerve injury.

The influence of stump length on axonal survival has been demonstrated in a number of species and has suggested that fast axonal transport plays a pivotal role in maintaining distal stump integrity.[56–58] Fast transport can continue after nerve transection and therefore maintain distal nerve terminals and neuromuscular transmission. Slow axonal transport may play a similar role in nonmammalian nerve.[49] The structural breakdown of the axon may be initiated by an increase in axoplasmic calcium concentration. This disintegration is likely mediated by calcium-sensitive proteases present in the axon in many species.[59–61] The axoplasmic concentration of calcium is ordinarily kept low by an energy-dependent calcium pump and organelles that also sequester the ion. Transection of nerve results in a rise in axoplasmic calcium concentration,[62] and chelation of calcium can delay the granular fragmentation of the axon.[63]

Compression Neuropathy in Association with Polyneuropathy

Nerve may be more susceptible to compression in the setting of a generalized peripheral neuropathy. Compressive plantar neuropathies occur more readily in rats with experimental diabetic neuropathy.[64] Humans with uremic or diabetic polyneuropathy appear to have increased susceptibility to compressive neuropathy. Although the evidence is best for carpal tunnel syndrome (CTS), focal neuropathy appears more frequent at other conventional sites of compression, including the ulnar nerve at the elbow and the peroneal nerve at the knee. Retrospective studies of diabetics have suggested an increased incidence of CTS.[65,66] Prospective population studies of diabetics have unequivocally demonstrated an increased incidence of CTS.[67,68] The overall prevalence of median neuropathy at the wrist is about 30 percent, but only about 9 percent are symptomatic. The occurrence of median neuropathy at the wrist increases with longer duration of diabetes.[67,68]

Carpal tunnel syndrome also occurs in greater frequency in those with neuropathy from chronic renal failure. This is especially true after long-standing dialysis and with secondary generalized amyloidosis.[69] Dialysis shunts placed in the forearm may cause ischemic neuropathy in all nerves distally in the arm (ischemic monomelic neuropathy),[70–72] but it may also produce CTS.[73] Management of CTS in these circumstances includes surgical decompression, with biopsy of the flexor reticulum for amyloid, or closure of the fistula.

Ulnar neuropathy may occur at greater frequency in diabetics.[66,67] Peroneal and other focal neuropathies are infrequent enough that they may be a coincidental occurrence with generalized polyneuropathy.[65,74] Patients with focal compression neuropathy associated with polyneuropathy should be managed like any others.[75,76] However, they must understand that the portion of the symptoms from the polyneuropathy will not be relieved by decompressive surgery.

The Double-Crush Syndrome

The double-crush hypothesis, first proposed by Upton and McComas, postulated additive effects of two lesions along a common nerve component.[77] This hypothesis remains an uncertain one to date. It is supported by experimental studies but not convincingly by clinical data.

Clinical studies have reported the coincident presence of CTS and cervical radiculopathy,[77–80] using this as evidence in favor of the double-crush hypothesis. Osterman reported that 18 percent of patients with electrodiagnostically confirmed CTS had electromyographic (EMG) evidence of upper cervical radiculopathy. These patients appeared to be symptomatic with less severe electrophysiologic abnormalities than those with CTS alone.[81] Frith and Litchy reported 18 similar patients and found bilateral CTS in 10 with unilateral radiculopathy; they found contralateral CTS in 2.[82] Frith and Litchy used this as evidence against a double-crush mechanism. Several papers have suggested that thoracic outlet syndrome (TOS) may predispose to CTS through a double-crush mechanism.[83,84] However, these studies base the diagnosis of TOS on clinical grounds. Given the controversy about the validity of clinically diagnosed TOS,[85] such data should be regarded suspiciously. Additionally, Carroll and Hurst have shown that the coexistence of TOS and CTS is rare.[86] There have been no clinical studies with the statistical power to prove that the coexistence of CTS and another lesion is not the result of chance alone.

More convincing data on the double-crush hypothesis have been provided by experimental studies. Gilliatt and coworkers demonstrated axonal atrophy distal to an experimental constriction in rabbit sciatic nerve and also impaired recovery from a distal crush injury.[87,88] They also showed that plantar compressive neuropathies developed more readily distal to the site of a unilaterally placed ligature constricting the sciatic nerve, suggesting an increased susceptibility to the effects of chronic compression.[89] Nemoto and coworkers produced a compressive lesion with distal axonal atrophy by clamping canine sciatic nerves.[90] A second distal compression lesion resulted in conduction block and distal axonal degeneration. The investigators demonstrated that the effect of removing the distal clamp was more beneficial than removing the proximal one. This experiment supports the current clinical view that the distalmost should be approached surgically first.[81]

A double-crush effect could result from alterations in axonal transport, with increased vulnerability to distal nerve segments. Evidence for this was provided by Rydevik and colleagues, who showed reversible block of rapid axonal transport at the site of compression in rabbit vagus nerve.[91] Others have demonstrated effects of compression on retrograde axonal transport[92] and have speculated that this could render the entire proximal axon more susceptible as well.

Recovery from Nerve Injury

There are three basic mechanisms by which nerve recovers from injury. These include remyelination through areas of focal neurapraxia, collateral sprouting from surviving motor axon terminals to denervated muscle, and nerve regeneration from the site of injury (Table 13-4). The timing and ultimate extent and success of recovery depend on the contribution of each of these processes.

Focal block of conduction (neurapraxia) from demyelination can recover rapidly through remyelination. Schwann cells proliferate and form new myelin, restoring more normal electrical properties to the axon. If the lesion is predominantly one of focal conduction block (neurapraxia), then function may be fully restored within several weeks following the injury. If several adjacent segments had been demyelinated, remyelinated internodal lengths will be abnormally short. This process of remyelination typically takes 2 to 6 weeks, with recovery of function following shortly thereafter. With extensive demyelination, conduction velocity along the remyelinated nerve may be slowed without any apparent deficit in function.[93]

With axonotmesis (axonal degeneration), recovery requires reinnervation, which can result from collateral sprouting or nerve regeneration. The role of each is dictated by the extent of axonal loss and the distance of the injury from the target muscle. Recovery through collateral sprouting is faster than nerve regeneration. Nerve regeneration is less effective and may produce aberrant patterns of regeneration that limit functional recovery.

TABLE 13-4   Methods for Recovery from Peripheral Nerve Injury

Type of injury	Mode of recovery
Conduction block (neurapraxia)	Remyelination Clinical improvement over 2 to 12 weeks
Limited[a] axonal loss (axonotmesis)	Collateral sprouting from surviving motor axons Clinical improvement over 2 to 6 months
Intermediate[b] axonal loss	Both collateral sprouting from surviving motor axons and regeneration from the site of injury Two phases of recovery: early, as with collateral sprouting, and late, from regeneration
Severe[c] axonal loss	Regeneration from the site of nerve injury Rate and success of recovery dependent on the distance to be traversed Clinical improvement over 2 to 18 months

[a]Less than 70 percent axonal loss.
[b]About 70 to 90 percent axonal loss.
[c]More than 90 percent axonal loss.

Recovery through collateral sprouting is effective if no more than 70 to 80 percent of the motor axons have been injured. This process of reinnervation by collateral sprouting occurs over a 3- to 6-month period following the injury, with return of the full contractile force of the muscle. When the degree of partial nerve injury exceeds this, the surviving axons are insufficient to supply the denervated muscle fibers. Only partial return of contractile force in the muscle will occur, and further recovery will require nerve regeneration from the site of injury. There are two phases of recovery, collateral sprouting from remaining motor axons and nerve regeneration. When nerve injuries result in more than 90 percent motor axon loss, regeneration is the predominant mode of recovery. Electrophysiologic studies can predict the mode and degree of recovery with a useful degree of accuracy.[19]

After a nerve injury and Wallerian degeneration, Schwann cells line up and proliferate along the nerve.[49] Axonal sprouts develop from the proximal tip of the axon and, if still intact, grow along the distal Schwann cell tubes. Recovery by this mechanism is slower than with collateral sprouting. After crush or stretch injuries that produce axonotmesis, proximal regeneration is approximately 6 to 8 mm/day, with distal regeneration 1 to 2 mm/day.[5] With knowledge of the site of injury, an approximate estimate of the time for regenerating axons to reach the target muscle can be determined. For example, a severe lesion that produces axonotmesis in the peroneal nerve at the fibular head will also produce foot drop, which can be expected to recover through axonal regeneration within 6 to 10 months. Alternatively, when there is a partial sciatic (peroneal division) injury with foot drop at the level of the sciatic notch, as may occur often with a hip injury, it may take longer than a year for nerve regeneration to occur, and recovery may be incomplete. This is a major limitations of nerve regeneration. Schwann cell basal lamina tubes remain viable for nerve regeneration for only about 18 to 24 months.

Therefore, when the target muscles are distant from the injury, much reinnervation may not occur. This is a feature of severe brachial plexus injuries, where proximal muscles recover more fully than distal hand muscles despite equally severe axonal injury across the plexus.

With severe disruption of the endoneurium (Sunderland grades 3 and 4) or nerve transection (neurotmesis), the orderly matrix of Schwann cells and basal lamina is not available and axonal sprouts are not able to regenerate in a useful way down the distal nerve. The axonal sprouts may terminate blindly, sometimes forming a mass of painful neuroma tissue.

Severe injuries that must recover through axonal regeneration face several obstacles. The distance from the injury to the target muscle may be too great for effective regeneration. This is especially so when a distance of more than 18 must be traversed. There may be misguided or aberrant regeneration to an inappropriate target.[94] Sensory axons may run the course of motor fibers, and the reverse may occur. Aberrant regeneration is especially prominent after proximal injuries, or where there is extensive fascicular rearrangement. This is the case after severe traumatic brachial and lumbosacral plexopathies. A common example is facial synkinesis after a facial nerve injury. Another common example is that seen after a phrenic nerve injury. Motor unit responses in C5-supplied muscles such as the deltoid may be activated rhythmically with phrenic nerve activation with respiration. Some axons originally destined for the diaphragm instead supply proximal arm muscles. Thomas and coworkers found aberrantly directed motor axons in intrinsic hand muscles following median and ulnar injuries at the wrist.[95] Although strength was recovered through nerve regeneration, dexterity remained limited because of aberrant regeneration. This process may not be apparent when one is testing full contractile force, but more refined movements such as playing a musical instrument may be impaired.

DIAGNOSTIC ELECTROPHYSIOLOGIC PROCEDURES

Nerve Conduction Studies and Needle Electromyography

Nerve conduction studies and the needle EMG examination are complementary techniques that are together called *EMG*. These studies are an essential part of the evaluation of a patient with a nerve or muscle disorder.[96–98] The test is objective and is especially helpful when the clinical evaluation is limited by the patient's pain or incomplete cooperation. Electromyography allows the localization of disorders of roots or peripheral nerves, measures the type and severity of injury, and provides prognostic information. Unsuspected causes of weakness may be identified, including neuromuscular junction disorders or myopathy and the presence of a polyneuropathy.

Electrophysiologic testing may be technically challenging and is dependent on the skills of the examiner. In an individual patient, the approach is designed to extend the physical examination and frequently must be redirected during its course by the initial electrodiagnostic findings. Therefore, these studies are best performed by those trained in both EMG and neuromuscular disorders. The EMG study is mildly uncomfortable, but it poses few risks. Patients with altered hemostasis may develop a hematoma at the site of the EMG needle entry. Patients with external cardiac pacemakers or implantable cardiac defibrillators should not have nerve conduction studies performed except in special circumstances with appropriate safeguards. A description of the electrodes, equipment, filter settings, and other technical aspects of EMG are reviewed in standard tests.[99,100]

Nerve Conduction Studies

The nerve conduction study (NCS) portion of the examination is divided into recordings from sensory, motor, and mixed nerves. The individual nerve of interest is stimulated through the skin with a surface electrical stimulator. The evoked motor or sensory response is recorded either directly from the sensory or mixed nerve or, in the case of motor conduction studies, indirectly from a muscle supplied by that nerve. Stimulation begins at a low intensity (5 to 10 mA) and with a short duration (approximately 0.1 ms). The intensity is slowly increased until the amplitude of the response no longer rises. This supramaximal stimulation ensures that all nerve fibers have been stimulated, giving the maximal response possible from that nerve. The relative threshold to stimulation of A delta and C fibers, both of smaller diameter, are 10 and 20 times greater, respectively, than those of the larger-diameter A alpha fibers. Therefore, nerve conduction studies generally reflect conduction in the larger-diameter somatic sensory and motor axons.

For motor nerve conduction studies, recording electrodes are placed over one of the muscles supplied by the nerve under study, and the evoked compound motor action potential (CMAP) is recorded. The motor nerve is stimulated percutaneously at two points along the nerve,

the time difference is determined, the distance between the stimulation sites is measured, and the conduction velocity is calculated. Other values measured include the distal motor latency (DML) and distal and proximal CMAP amplitudes (Fig. 13-4). The DML is the time delay to the onset of the motor response, determined at the initial electronegative or upward deflection following stimulation at the distal site. This distal site is at the wrist for the median and ulnar nerves and at the ankle for peroneal and posterior tibial nerves. The DML is a reflection of the conduction time in the distal motor nerves and also neuromuscular transmission. The CMAP amplitude is proportional to the number of motor nerve axons stimulated in the nerve and is conventionally recorded from the baseline to the onset of the negative (upward) peak. Other features of the CMAP may be recorded, including the duration and area under the negative peak. The CMAP duration is the time interval from the onset to the end of the initial large negative CMAP waveform. The area may be calculated automatically on many current machines, but measuring the amplitude is easier and is currently the standard technique.

For sensory nerve conduction studies, only one point is stimulated (Fig. 13-4). The time to the response is measured from the shock artifact to the peak of the sensory nerve action potential (SNAP). Alternatively, the conduction velocity can be calculated using the recorded distance between stimulation and recording electrodes and the time from the shock artifact to the onset of the response. The parameters recorded include the SNAP amplitude and either the latency to peak or the conduction velocity. Sensory potentials may be elicited in two ways. The orthodromic method involves distal stimulation with proximal recording, whereby impulses propagate in the physiologic direction. Antidromic methods stimulate proximally with recording distally, and the impulse propagates opposite to the afferent direction. There are differences in the normal values for these two techniques. Mixed sensory and motor nerve conduction studies (MNAP) are similar to sensory studies in that the nerve is stimulated along one point of its course and recording is made from the nerve at another point. The amplitude of the response and the conduction velocity are measured. Sensory and mixed nerve conduction studies produce responses that are much smaller than those of motor studies. Typically these responses are in the order of 5 to 20 μm, compared to CMAP values of 5 to 10 mV. Averaging techniques are frequently necessary to eliminate baseline noise and define the sensory potentials, especially if they are abnormally low. Even with averaging, it may be difficult to detect the responses of some smaller nerves of healthy individuals. These include the saphenous, lateral cutaneous nerve of the thigh, and medial and lateral plantar sensory responses.

Nerve Conduction Studies: Basic Abnormalities

The hallmark of disorders that produce motor axonal loss (axonotmesis) is a generalized reduction in the CMAP amplitudes after stimulation at any point along the motor nerve (Fig. 13-5). This reflects the loss of axons distal to the

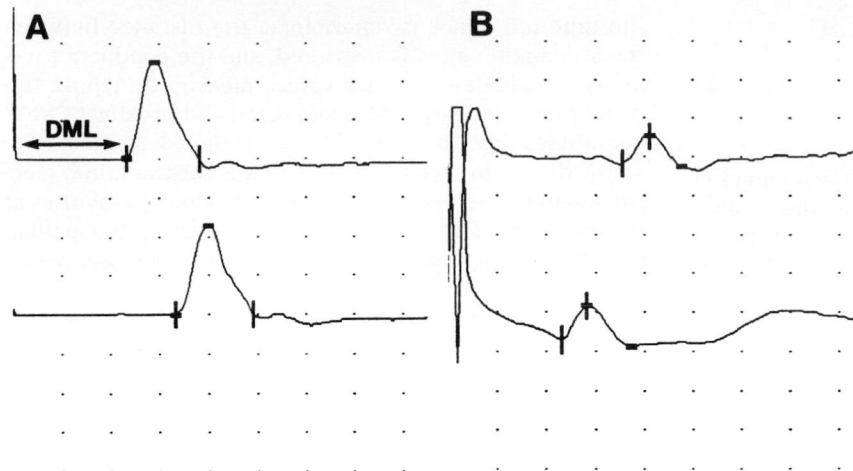

Figure 13-4 Motor and sensory nerve conduction studies of a median neuropathy at the wrist (carpal tunnel syndrome). *A. Top:* median compound muscle action potential (CMAP) recorded from the abductor pollicis brevis muscle after stimulation at the wrist. The distal motor latency (DML) is prolonged to 7.5 ms (normal < 4.6 ms), reflecting the slow conduction across the wrist. *Bottom:* CMAP after stimulation at the elbow. Median conduction in the forearm is normal. (Vertical sensitivity = 5 mV/div; horizontal sweep = 5 ms/div.) *B. Top:* median sensory nerve action potential (SNAP), recorded from the wrist after stimulation of the median digital branches in the index finger. *Bottom:* median palmar study with stimulation in the palm and the same recording site. The latencies from the stimulus to peak (marked by vertical dash) are prolonged, reflecting slow conduction across the wrist. The amplitude of the responses is also reduced. (Sensitivity = 5 μV/div; sweep = 1 ms/div.)

site of injury. Conduction velocity may be mildly reduced due to the loss of the fastest-conducting motor fibers but will not fall below 70 percent of the lower limit of normal values for that nerve.[101,102] Similarly, the amplitude of the SNAP is proportional to the number of functioning myelinated sensory fibers in that nerve, and a reduction in amplitude reflects axonal loss.

A focal compressive neuropathy or demyelinating process produces localized conduction abnormalities at the site of injury. In this circumstance, the CMAP amplitude after proximal stimulation will be smaller than that of the distal CMAP (Fig. 13-5). This reflects conduction block and temporal dispersion between the proximal and distal sites, physiologic hallmarks of focal segmental demyelination (neuropraxia).[103] Segmental demyelination may also

produce significant slowing of conduction velocity, greater than that which can be produced by axonal loss alone. These physiologic features allow one to assess the relative degree of axonal loss and demyelination.

F- and H-Wave Studies

F waves are often recorded as part of the motor nerve conduction studies and have a much longer latency than the direct CMAP.[104] The F wave is the surface recorded response of a late motor unit discharge due to the antidromic activation and backfiring of a motor neuron. These recorded responses reflect antidromic motor discharges that travel centrally to the anterior horn cells, a small proportion of which fire orthodromically back down the

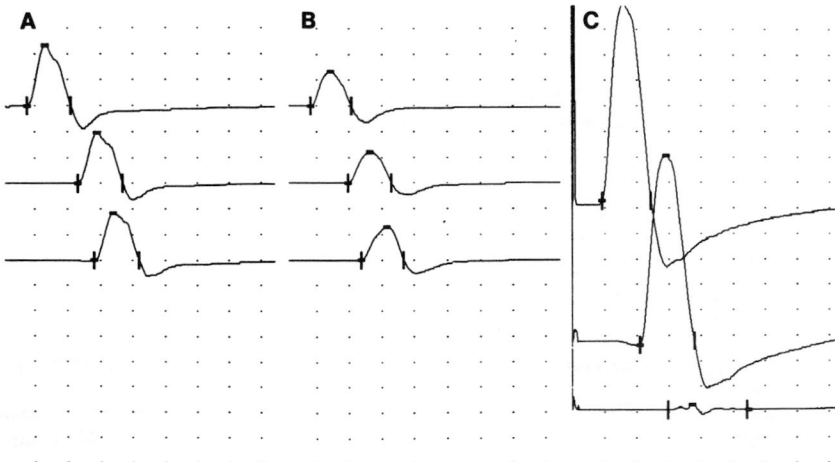

Figure 13-5 Peroneal motor conduction studies. *A.* Normal. A CMAP recorded from the extensor digitorum brevis muscle after stimulation at the ankle (*top trace*), below fibular head (*middle*), and above fibular head (*bottom*). The amplitude is the same with all sites of stimulation. *B.* After axonal loss (axonotmesis). The amplitude of the CMAP is reduced, following distal and proximal stimulation (displayed at a different sensitivity than *A*). *C.* With conduction block (neurapraxia) at the fibular head. The responses after stimulation at the ankle and below the fibular head are normal. The response after stimulation above the fibular head is markedly reduced, reflecting conduction block. (*A,* sensitivity = 2 mV/div; *B* and *C,* 0.5 mV/div; in each sweep = 5 ms/div.)

course of the motor axon. Each motor stimulation produces different motor axon discharges back down the nerve, so the F waves vary in latency and morphology. The latency reflects the time after the stimulus that is necessary for the action potential to reach the motor neuron antidromically and then to travel orthodromically back down the motor axon to the muscle. Consequently, F-wave measurements involve conduction through the proximal portions of the motor axon—nerve segments that are not directly accessible by other means. F waves are often absent or occur with a delayed latency in disorders that produce involvement of proximal motor axons— e.g., demyelinating disorders like the Guillain-Barré syndrome or proximal motor root lesions. F waves are less helpful in the evaluation of radiculopathies and plexopathies than they are in the diagnosis of acute demyelinating polyneuropathies.[105,106]

H reflexes, or H waves, are recorded with surface electrodes over the soleus muscle after stimulation of the posterior tibial nerve in the popliteal fossa. This monosynaptic reflex is the electrical equivalent of the ankle jerk reflex, provoked by electrical stimulation of afferents in the mixed nerve instead of mechanical muscle stretch. The H reflex latency, unlike F-wave latencies, does not vary. The H reflex in adults is normally obtained only from the gastrocnemius-soleus muscle complex. The H reflex is lost or latency delayed in processes that affect the S1 root, such as radiculopathy or proximal demyelination.

Needle Electromyography

Needle EMG studies are essential in separating neurogenic causes (nerve, root, or anterior horn cell) from myopathic ones. They help differentiate the pattern of involvement that allows localization to a particular nerve, plexus, or root and quantifies the extent of involvement. The studies are performed with placement of a fine needle electrode into the muscle; the electrical activity is then evaluated with the muscle initially at rest and then during voluntary contraction.[107,108]

A healthy muscle at rest is electrically silent. Spontaneous electrical discharges at rest, fibrillation potentials, and positive sharp waves (Fig. 13-6) appear after muscle denervation. Fibrillations develop in muscle 2 to 6 weeks after the axonal loss. Fibrillations may also be seen in muscle disorders. Fibrillation potentials and positive sharp waves are the action potentials of single muscle fibers that discharge spontaneously. They fire at a regular rate, most often 1 to 15 Hz. Other abnormal spontaneous

discharges at rest include myotonic discharges, myokymia, and fasciculation potentials.

During the voluntary portion of the needle EMG examination, the state of the motor unit (the motor axon and the muscle fibers it innervates) and the recruitment of motor units are assessed. An EMG needle records from an area of muscle that contains multiple overlapping motor units (Fig. 13-7). The needle records the nearly synchronous muscle fiber action potentials from all of the activated muscle fibers in the recording area. This summated electrical waveform is the motor unit potential (MUP). The amplitude, duration, and number of phases of the MUP are determined by the number and distribution of muscle fibers of the motor unit in that recording area. In normal muscle, the amplitude is determined by the few fibers closest to the needle and the duration by the number and location of more distant ones. In neurogenic disorders, with loss of motor axons to other motor units in that recording area, there is collateral spouting from surviving axons that innervate some of those muscle fibers. There are more muscle fibers close to the needle, and they are more widely distributed. This larger, longer, and more complex MUP is the hallmark of chronic neurogenic injury and repair. The extra components may result in greater complexity of the waveform, producing a polyphasic (greater than four phases) appearance. With muscle disorders, there is loss of muscle fibers in the motor unit. There are a few muscle fibers close to the needle and in the recording area, so that the recorded MUP is both small in amplitude and short in duration. These changes occur over time in a fairly predictable fashion (Fig. 13-7). Immediately after acute partial denervation, there is no change in the MUP amplitude or duration, since sprouting from surviving motor axons has not had time to occur. With early collateral sprouting, where the poorly myelinated small sprouts reach denervated muscle fibers, long-duration, complex MUPs of relatively normal amplitude are seen. Over time, the collateral sprouts mature and the MUP enlarges in amplitude.

Recruitment is the manner in which the MUPs increase their firing rates and new MUPs begin to fire as the muscle contraction is increased in a graded fashion. In normal muscle, recruitment of new units occurs with relatively little effort, and there is only modest increase in the firing rates of those already recruited. In neurogenic disorders with loss of motor axons, the MUPs are recruited abnormally, with increased firing rates of individual motor units after only mild muscle contraction. Myopathic disorders, in contrast, recruit with the appearance of numerous MUPs despite very low contractile forces.

Figure 13-6 Needle EMG appearance of abnormal spontaneous activity at rest. Fibrillation potentials (*closed arrow*) and positive sharp waves (*open arrow*) are the action potentials of single muscle fibers that spontaneously discharge after loss of nerve innervation. (Sensitivity = 50 μV/div; sweep = 10 ms/div.)

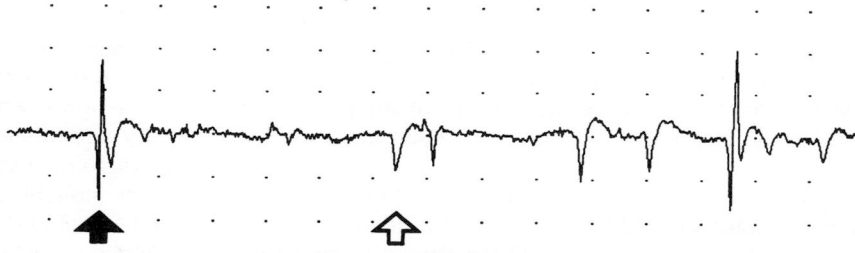

Motor Unit Territory **MUP Morphology** **Needle EMG**

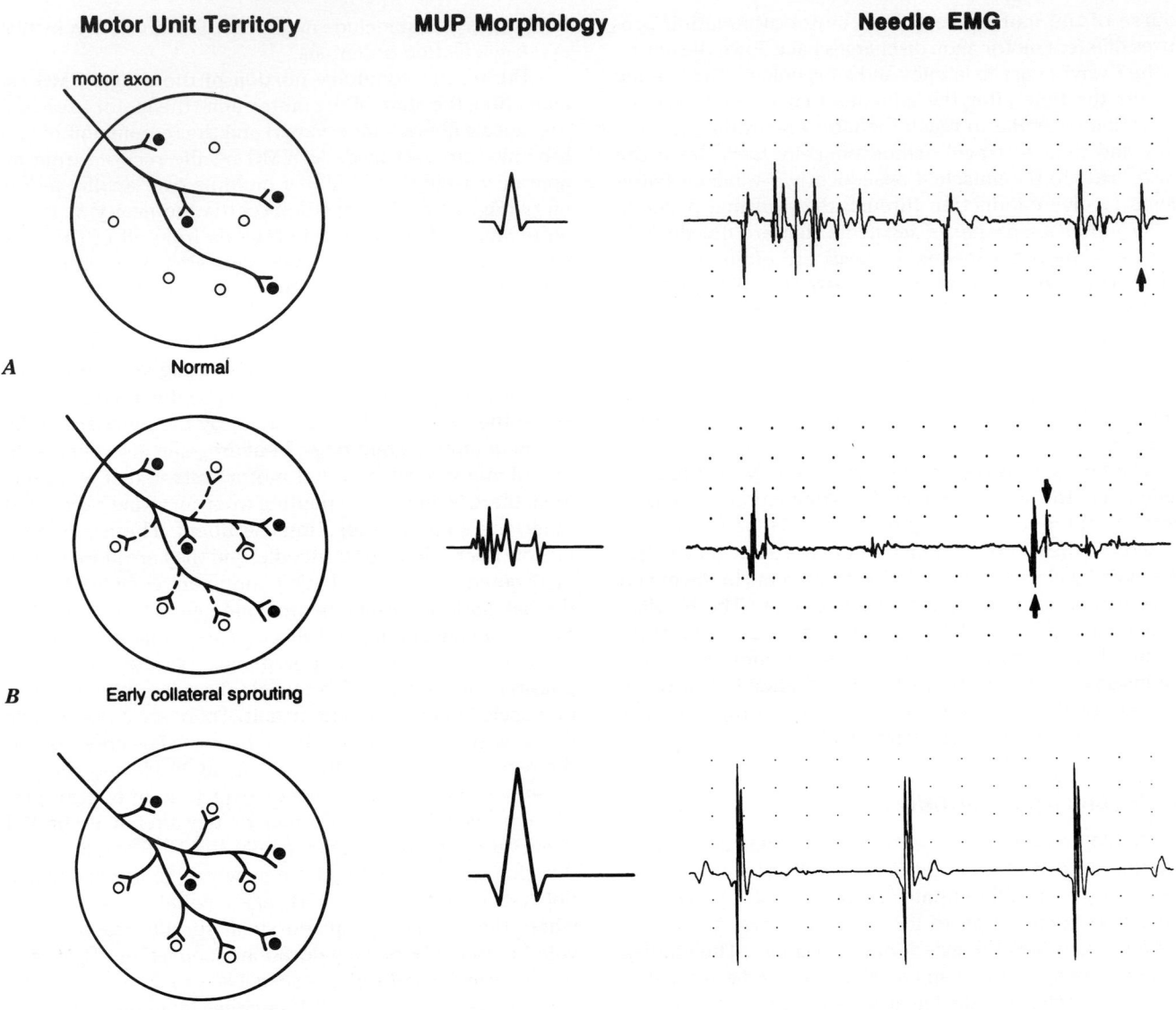

Figure 13-7 The motor unit and its relation to motor unit potential (MUP) morphology. *A.* The motor unit territory within the recording area of the EMG needle is schematized by the large circle. The small dark circles represent the muscle fibers innervated by a motor axon in that territory. In a recording area, there are overlapping motor units. A normal MUP is shown (*middle column*), with a corresponding example of the needle EMG appearance (*arrow*). *B.* Early after a partial lesion, with loss of the axon to an adjacent motor unit represented by the open circle, there is collateral sprouting with immature nerve twigs. This produces a longer, more complex MUP. Needle EMG shows a complex MUP (*upward arrow*) with a late component (*downward arrow*). *C.* With maturation of the sprouts, the MUPs are longer and larger. (Needle EMG: *A* and *B,* sensitivity = 200 μV/div; *C,* 1000 μV/div; sweep = 10 ms/div.)

Principles of Electrodiagnostic Localization

In addition to the clinical examination, electrodiagnostic studies play and important role in defining the localization of a disorder in the peripheral nervous system, including anterior horn cells, nerve roots, brachial and lumbosacral plexus, individual nerves, muscle, or neuromuscular junction.

In certain nerve disorders, focal abnormalities on nerve conduction studies are critical in identifying localization. These include nerve conduction slowing or conduction block in the median nerve across the wrist in CTS, in the ulnar nerve across the elbow, and across the fibular head with peroneal neuropathy.

Sensory potentials are spared in lesions that are proximal to the dorsal root ganglia (preganglionic). Unlike motor neurons, whose cell bodies are in the spinal cord, sensory neurons have cell bodies in the dorsal root ganglia, distal to the usual site of compression in radiculopathy. As such, radiculopathy produces sensory losses due to involvement of the sensory axon proximal to the dorsal root ganglion. The sensory axon's continuity is preserved distal to the ganglia, and the sensory response is normal despite clinical sensory loss. Lesions distal to the dorsal root ganglion result in Wallerian degeneration from that level and are reflected in a fall in amplitude of the sensory response. Therefore, sensory potentials are spared in root lesions but are reduced in more distal lesions of the plexus or individual peripheral nerve.[106,109] For example, the loss of a superficial peroneal sensory response with a significant foot drop may reflect peroneal neuropathy, whereas sparing of that response would be expected in an L5 radiculopathy. Sensory responses are segmentally represented, and recording the appropriate SNAP may help differentiate nerve or plexus versus root involvement (Table 13-5).

The detection of muscle involvement by needle EMG is critical in identifying the localization to a root, plexus, or nerve level. The pattern of needle EMG abnormalities is matched with that expected from a nerve, plexus, or root distribution.[106,110] For example, a patient with intrinsic hand muscle weakness with mild medial hand numbness could have a lesion of the ulnar nerve, the lower trunk of the brachial plexus, or the C8 root. With ulnar neuropathy, the ulnar hand muscles would be involved by needle EMG, with sparing of the C8/median and radial-innervated muscles. A lower trunk lesion would involve all of the latter muscles with a reduced or absent ulnar sensory potential, since it is a lesion distal to the dorsal root ganglia. In a C8 root lesion all of the C8/ulnar, median, and radial-innervated muscles would be abnormal, with a preserved ulnar sensory nerve action potential. Thus, a combination of the nerve conduction study and needle EMG abnormalities allows localization along the neuraxis.

Limitations

Electrodiagnostic studies have limitations. Unavoidable limitations include the inherent limits on the sensitivity of the studies and the inability to measure the smallest nerve fibers. Avoidable limitations include improper timing of the studies and overinterpretation of minor abnormalities by an inexperienced examiner.

The ideal eletrodiagnostic test would identify all patients with an abnormality as abnormal and all normal in-

dividuals as normal. Unfortunately there is overlap between normal and abnormal values in virtually any test, including EMG. The normal limits for a value are set after statistical examination of a normal population.[111,112] Abnormalities two standard deviations from the mean value will identify 95 percent of the normal population as normal. Using two standard deviations from the mean as a criterion, 5 percent of the normal population will have abnormal values, half of which (2.5 percent) will be abnormal at one end of the distribution. Thus 2.5 percent of the normal population will be incorrectly identified as abnormal, a false-positive result. For most clinical situations, this 2.5 percent false-positive rate is an acceptable compromise, since this usually allows a reasonable proportion of abnormal patients to be identified. Additional studies are often added to increase the diagnostic sensitivity, although each test introduces a 2.5 percent probability of a false-positive result. Typically the studies are not truly independent and the false-positive rates are not additive, but additional tests do increase the number of false-positive studies and degrade the predictive value of the test. The standard methods of nerve conduction studies and electrodiagnostic testing are interpreted such that the sensitivity is maximized with an acceptable degree of false-positive results.

"More sensitive" techniques introduce an unacceptable number of false-positive studies. This is more fully discussed under CTS. Using that example, "more sensitive" techniques such as short segment inching studies and conductions with stress maneuvers at the wrist slightly increase the sensitivity of the technique and identify most patients with CTS. However, they also introduce an extraordinarily high false-positive rate,[113] reducing the predictive value of the study to unacceptably low levels.

The corollary is that there will also be false-negative studies. To maximize the predictive value of the study, there will be some proportion of false-negative studies as an inherent limitation of the test. This not preventable, regardless of the experience of thoroughness of the examiner. A negative study does not exclude a particular diagnosis. False-negative studies may be as small as 8 percent in the investigation of CTS or as high as 50 percent when

---

TABLE 13-5 Segmental Relation of Sensory Responses to Peripheral Sensory Distributions

SNAP[a] from cutaneous nerve	Plexus (trunk/cord)	Nerve root
Musculocutaneous	Upper/lateral	C5
Radial or median[b]	Upper/posterior	C6
Median[c]	Middle/lateral	C7
Ulnar[d]	Lower/medial	C8
Saphenous	—	L4
Superficial peroneal	—	L5
Sural	—	S1

[a]SNAP = sensory nerve action potential.
[b]D1(thumb) or D2.
[c]D3.
[d]D5.

patients have acute radiculopathy with only pain and sensory symptoms.

The EMG is insensitive to abnormalities of the smallest fibers.[114] Small-diameter fibers, such as those that mediate pain and temperature sensation, as well as autonomic fibers, cannot be studied using routine EMG techniques. Consequently, disorders that preferentially affect small-diameter fibers must be investigated using other techniques. These include quantitative sensory testing (QST) and specialized autonomic studies.

From the referring physician's standpoint, an avoidable limitation is improper timing of the study. For traumatic nerve injury, the desired information regarding the nature of the pathologic lesion (neurapraxia or axonotmesis) will not be apparent for at least 7 to 10 days following the injury. A study performed only several days after the injury will give false information regarding the nature and prognosis of the injury. In addition, after acute radiculopathy, many of the needle EMG findings do not develop for 4 weeks or more.

Electrodiagnosis in Peripheral Nerve Injury

Electrodiagnostic studies provide the clinician with critical information regarding the localization, severity, and the pathologic nature of the injury as well as evidence of nerve continuity.[115] They also provide important information regarding prognosis, with estimates of the timing and the extent of recovery, and are particularly helpful for localization when the clinical examination is limited by pain or poor cooperation on the part of the patient. They allow an assessment of improvement by following recovery during conservative treatment or following surgical repair.

The pathologic nature of the lesion, neuropraxia (conduction block), or axonotmesis (axonal loss), can be directly determined with nerve conduction studies. Electrodiagnostic studies provide information that directly relates to the underlying pathophysiologic state of nerve if sufficient time has elapsed between the injury and the test. After nerve sectioning or injury, focal conduction block (neurapraxia) or distal Wallerian degeneration may occur. However, when a peripheral nerve is injured, the eletrophysiologic hallmarks that provide information regarding the underlying pathologic state of nerve are not expressed immediately. Axons that will undergo Wallerian degeneration (axonotmesis) continue to conduct electrically for a number of days following the injury as the distal degeneration occurs. Stimulation of the nerve proximal to the axonal discontinuity will not result in recordable responses distally. This is the case despite the fact that stimulation distally beyond the site of injury will elicit an evoked electrical response for some days. This may give the false impression of conduction block across that nerve segment and underestimate the severity of the lesion. After experimental nerve transection[53,116] or following sequential nerve injuries in humans,[54,55] the motor responses (CMAP) fall in amplitude over a period of 5 to 7 days. Sensory responses (SNAP) fall in amplitude over 7 to 10 days. The motor responses fail earlier due to the loss of neuromuscular transmission that occurs prior to the inability of the axon to conduct electrical impulses.[117]

For these reasons the optimal time to perform the nerve conduction studies is 10 days to 2 weeks following an injury. At that time the pathologic nature of the underlying injury can be inferred. The examiner can usually determine whether focal demyelination (neurapraxia) is an important part of the neurologic deficit produced by the injury. This provides important prognostic information, since conduction block (neurapraxia) recovers quickly and fully, despite the presence of even marked weakness. When there is significant axonal loss (axonotmesis), as reflected in the reduction of the CMAP and SNAP amplitudes, recovery will be slower and will occur by the methods of collateral sprouting from surviving axons or nerve regeneration (see "Recovery from Nerve Injury," above).

The physical examination does not allow the distinction of conduction block (neurapraxia) from axonal loss. A profoundly weak muscle may occur as a result of proximal conduction block, and yet there may be full and complete recovery within several weeks. Electrodiagnostic studies play an important role in the assessment of the severity of the injury. The principal factor determining recovery from an injury is the degree of axonal degeneration, as may be estimated by the reduction in the CMAP and SNAP amplitudes. These studies provide the best objective way of measuring the degree of axonal loss, especially so if a side-to-side comparison can be performed. In addition, in markedly weak muscles, evidence of nerve continuity may be obtained. The demonstration of sensory or motor responses on the nerve conduction studies or the presence of any voluntarily recruited MUPs on the needle EMG portion of the examination prove nerve continuity.

Recovery from nerve injury occurs in several phases.[115] The earliest phase occurs within 2 to 12 weeks as conduction block (neurapraxia) resolves after remyelination of the focal lesion. The focal conduction abnormalities resolve coincident with the clinical recovery. With axonal loss, recovery occurs either by collateral sprouting from surviving axons or by nerve regeneration from the point of injury. A partial nerve injury with mild or moderate axonal loss can be expected to recover substantially by collateral sprouting within 2 to 6 months. As reinnervation by collateral sprouting occurs, the needle EMG examination shows evidence of the incorporation of more muscle fibers into the territory of each surviving motor unit. This is reflected by longer-duration polyphasic MUPs (Fig. 13-8). The process of reinnervation by collateral sprouting occurs over 2 to 6 months from the time of injury and is accompanied by a progressive increase in muscle strength. If the nerve injury is more severe, recovery must occur at least in part by nerve regeneration—a slower and generally less successful mode of recovery. Electromyographic evidence of reinnervation by regeneration may be found in muscles long before there is any clinical evidence of return of muscle function. Therefore, when a patient has severe axonal loss it may be helpful performing a needle EMG examination to look for early nerve regeneration. The early reinnervation MUPs are of very low amplitude and long duration. They progressively mature as more sprouting occurs and strength slowly recovers coincident with those electrophysiologic changes.

Figure 13-8 The EMG appearance of an abnormal polyphasic MUP with effort. The MUP is extremely complex, of long duration, and with normal to low amplitude. This reflects early reinnervation by regeneration. (Sensitivity = 200 μV/div; sweep = 10 ms/div.)

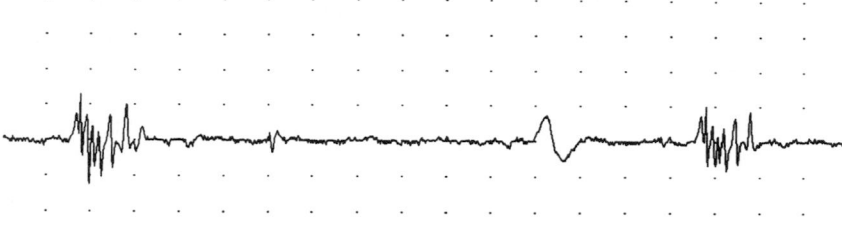

A suggested protocol for the timing EMG studies after nerve injury is shown in Table 13-6.

Electrodiagnosis in Compression/ Entrapment Neuropathy

Median Neuropathy

Compressive median neuropathy at the wrist, the carpal tunnel syndrome, is the most common focal neuropathy. Although CTS is a clinical diagnosis, the best way to confirm the diagnosis of median neuropathy at the wrist is with EMG studies. Compression leads to focal demyelination, resulting in slowed conduction across the wrist. In time there is axonal loss, with a reduction of motor and sensory evoked responses. This results in prolonged median distal motor latencies with stimulation at the wrist[118] and slowed sensory latencies across the wrist, stimulating the index finger (Fig. 13-4).[119] These simple motor and sensory conduction studies can provide convincing evidence of CTS in about 85 percent of patients with symptoms suggesting this disorder.[120,121] Techniques like comparison of median to radial sensory latency differences or palmar sensory studies increase the diagnostic sensitivity to about

92 percent.[121–125] Palmar studies (stimulation in the palm, recording at the wrist) add to the diagnostic sensitivity because of the shorter length of nerve studied, since a focal area of slowing is more evident over a shorter segment. Using all of the currently recommended techniques,[126] the sensitivity of EMG for CTS is in the low 90 percent range, with false positives less than 5 percent. Those patients with falsely negative studies are those with the mildest neuropathy. The severity of the CTS can be estimated by considering the degree of median sensory and motor slowing, the reduction in the SNAP and CMAP amplitudes, and the amount of denervation by needle EMG examination of median-innervated hand muscles. Needle EMG is also helpful in identifying a coexisting radiculopathy or other second lesions (double-crush). A generalized polyneuropathy can produce similar clinical symptoms to CTS, so sensory and motor conduction studies of other nerves are tested when CTS is suspected.

Multiple studies have attempted to increase the diagnostic yield for suspected CTS.[124] However, any increase in the yield of positive studies degrades the predictive value of the test by introducing a larger number of false-positive studies. Inching techniques, multiple nerve comparisons,[127] and changes in the definition of "normal" cri-

TABLE 13-6 Optimal Timing for Electrodiagnostic Studies after Peripheral Nerve Injury

Timing of study	Information obtained
Baseline study, in the first week after injury	Usually unnecessary[a] Baseline NCS/EMG for later comparison at initial study Presence of voluntary MUPs on EMG[b]
Initial study at 10 days to 3 weeks after injury	SNAP amplitude (pre- versus postganglionic)[b] Distal CMAP amplitude[b] Examine for conduction block (neurapraxia) Voluntary MUP recruitment in weak muscles[b]
Follow-up study at 3 to 6 months	Examine for reinnervation in markedly weak muscles before surgical intervention/intraoperative studies
Follow-up study at 6 to 12 months	As above, for injuries at a greater distance from the weak muscle to be examined

[a]Do test if there is a preexisting condition and baseline study is likely to be abnormal.
[b]Presence indicates nerve continuity
Key: NCS = nerve conduction studies; EMG = needle electromyography; SNAP = sensory nerve action potential; CMAP = compound muscle action potential; MUP = motor unit potential.

teria for abnormality have resulted in false-positive rates as high as 46 percent.[111,113] More recent studies have attempted to use multiple electrodiagnostic tests in a more systematic way to allow the assignment of a probability of having CTS.[128] Provocative "stress" tests have not been useful to differentiate normals from those with CTS. Comparison before and after wrist flexion or other maneuvers does change conduction across the wrist, but this has not allowed differentiation between patients or control subjects.[129,130] Claims that new techniques provide more sensitive diagnosis in early or mild CTS should be regarded with caution. If there is a high clinical suspicion of CTS and the disorder worsens, nerve conduction studies will become abnormal in time.[131]

Ulnar Neuropathy

Ulnar nerve compression may occur at the elbow or the wrist. Electrophysiologic studies allow localization of the entrapment site and provide information about the severity of the injury. Localization is based on evidence of focal demyelination.[132,133] Slowing of motor conduction may localize the lesion to the elbow in more than half of patients with ulnar neuropathy.[134] The yield is increased to more than two-thirds by studying sensory or mixed nerve conduction across the elbow.[135] Investigators have used short segments of stimulation across the elbow, the "inching technique," to more precisely localize elbow lesions to the postcondylar groove or the cubital tunnel. This is possible in 80 percent of those with focal conduction abnormalities.[136] With ulnar axon loss, there may be a reduction in the sensory nerve action potential amplitude. This is a very sensitive indicator of ulnar nerve injury, but it has no localizing value.

Ulnar neuropathy at the wrist (ulnar tunnel syndrome) leads to prolongation of the ulnar distal motor latency. The dorsal ulnar cutaneous sensory response may distinguish lesions at the elbow from those at the wrist. This cutaneous sensory nerve does not cross the wrist with the remainder of the ulnar nerve, so it is spared with wrist lesions.[137] Needle EMG of ulnar-innervated hand and forearm muscles may distinguish elbow from wrist lesions. When ulnar-innervated forearm muscles are abnormal, the lesion must be at or proximal to the elbow. These muscles may be normal, however, in up to half of patients with ulnar neuropathy at the elbow.[6,138]

Other Upper Extremity Mononeuropathies

Electrodiagnostic studies are important in the localization of other mononeuropathies and of plexopathies.[1,139] Needle EMG is especially helpful when the nerve of interest is deep and cannot be stimulated directly, such as the long thoracic nerve.

With compressive radial neuropathy at the spiral groove, testing may show primarily motor conduction block (neurapraxia) across the compressed segment.[140] More significant axonal loss (axonotmesis), which has a more guarded prognosis, occurs with humeral fracture or other trauma.[141]

Conduction studies of the posterior interosseous nerve are insensitive for entrapment of this nerve.[139] This neuropathy is best demonstrated by needle EMG abnormalities in the appropriate muscles. Studies of the "radial tunnel syndrome," in which there is pain but no definite neurologic deficit, may be misleading. The demonstration of increased motor latencies, with without forced supination, does not have proven clinical significance. Most electrophysiologic studies have not demonstrated convincing electrophysiologic abnormalities of the posterior interosseous nerve in this syndrome.[142,143] The wide range of diagnostic yields of these various studies ranges from 9 to 80 percent, emphasizing the uncertain sensitivity and specificity.[144]

Other mononeuropathies include isolated lesions of the radial sensory, anterior interosseus, musculocutaneous, axillary, suprascapular, long thoracic, spinal accessory, medial and lateral pectoral, dorsal scapular, and medial cutaneous nerves as well as the brachial plexus itself.[139]

The thoracic outlet syndrome (TOS) occurs in three forms, but only in neurogenic TOS are electrodiagnostic studies clearly abnormal. The other two are the symptomatic, or disputed, form and vascular TOS. The neurogenic form of TOS, often associated with a cervical rib or band, is a real but very uncommon disorder. Electrophysiologic features are reduced or absent ulnar sensory potentials, reduced median and ulnar motor amplitudes, and denervation evident on needle EMG in the lower plexus-innervated muscles in the arm and hand.[145,146]

Unlike the neurogenic TOS, symptomatic TOS, or disputed TOS, is much more difficult to define. It is characterized by a variable constellation of upper extremity pains, sensory symptoms, and provocative maneuvers. It is as amorphous as the neurogenic form is concise, and the neurologic examination and conventional electrophysiologic studies are normal.[85,147,148] Various techniques have been described to increase the diagnostic sensitivity in symptomatic TOS. Early data on slowing of ulnar and motor conduction across the brachial plexus suggested that plexus conduction may be helpful.[149] However, the value of plexus conduction has been challenged[150] and has not been duplicated by many others.[151] Other techniques including positional brachial plexus conduction studies,[152] needle stimulation of the C8 nerve root,[153] and somatosensory evoked potentials,[154] and positional somatosensory evoked potentials[155] have been advocated. However, the claimed high sensitivity of these studies has not been duplicated, and many have found great variability in normal populations using these techniques, thus greatly limiting their diagnostic value. One feature arguing against the involvement of neural structures in this controversial disorder is the lack of a spectrum of disease. Other compression neuropathies have a range of severity extending from the mildest symptoms, with little in the way of clinical and electrophysiologic findings, to the more severe, where there are substantial neurologic and electrophysiologic abnormalities. This is not the case in the symptomatic, or disputed, form of TOS. There also has not been documentation of cases that begin symptomatically, with normal physical and EMG findings, and progress without treatment to neurologic deficits and abnormal conventional electrophysiologic findings.

Lower Extremity Mononeuropathies

Peroneal neuropathy at the fibular head is the most common mononeuropathy in the lower extremity, and is usually the result of compression. Focal abnormalities of conduction across the fibular head, in the form of conduction block or focal slowing, occurs in up two-thirds of patients studied electrophysiologically.[8,156] The superficial peroneal sensory response amplitudes are usually reduced. The needle EMG examination demonstrates denervation in the distribution of the peroneal nerve, with sparing of the short head of the biceps femoris, which is the only muscle above the knee supplied by the peroneal division of the sciatic nerve.

Nerve conduction studies with needle EMG will localize the peroneal lesions to the level of the knee in most patients. This is particularly helpful when the examination may be misleading, particularly from sciatic nerve lesions.[157] Many injuries to the sciatic nerve especially affect the lateral or peroneal division and appear clinically to represent a peroneal neuropathy. Other nerve lesions that may be localized electrophysiologically include focal tibial neuropathy at the ankle (tarsal tunnel syndrome),[158] sciatic neuropathy, femoral neuropathy, meralgia paresthetica (lateral cutaneous nerve of the thigh), and lesions of the lumbosacral plexus itself.[159]

Electrodiagnosis in Radiculopathy

The diagnosis of cervical and lumbosacral radiculopathy is primarily a clinical one, but radiographic and electrodiagnostic studies provide important information in most patients. The electrodiagnostic studies in particular provide information not often obtainable by the clinical examination or radiographic studies. Standard sensory and motor nerve conduction studies are most often normal. Because root lesions are proximal to the dorsal root ganglion in radiculopathy, the SNAP amplitude is preserved. Motor nerve conduction studies are most often normal unless multiple roots are involved. The CMAP amplitude is preserved in acute radiculopathy, since most muscles have multiple root innervation, and in chronic radiculopathy, where collateral sprouting compensates for any lost motor nerve supply to that muscle. As a result, the sensory and motor nerve conduction studies are most helpful for excluding other disorders that may mimic a radiculopathy. Focal compressive neuropathies, plexopathies, and other peripheral nerve lesions may simulate radiculopathy.[106] Attempts to stimulate the nerve roots proximal to the lesion, either electrically or with magnetic stimulation, have provided inconsistent results. The techniques are limited because of the difficulty in demonstrating short segments of focal conduction abnormality over a long length of nerve. Also, stimulation with these techniques still occurs distal to the root foramina and thus distal to the lesion.[160] F waves may occasionally be delayed or absent but are

generally insensitive and not specific for focal root lesions.[104,106] H-reflex studies are a sensitive measure of S1 radiculopathy. However, they are limited to this particular nerve root and do not add more information than an absent ankle jerk reflex.

Other studies have been advocated to increase the diagnostic yield with radiculopathy. Somatosensory evoked potentials can be performed by stimulating a peripheral nerve, a sensory cutaneous nerve of one dermatome (such as the radial sensory nerve), or a dermatomal portion of skin. Somatosensory evoked responses from major peripheral nerves have little diagnostic yield because of the mixed root supply to major nerves. Although segmental cutaneous or dermatomal evoked potentials may demonstrate abnormalities with radiculopathy, the yield is less than with EMG studies.[105,161,162] Some have found dermatomal somatosensory evoked potentials to be more sensitive in patients with radiculopathy than standard EMG studies, but by the same criteria, abnormalities were also noted in multiple adjacent asymptomatic dermatomes.[163] This suggests that the criteria for abnormality may be too sensitive and degrade the positive predictive value of the study. Thermography has also been studied in patients with radiculopathy and is of little or no value in this setting.[164]

Following an acute radiculopathy, the role of EMG is primarily in the differential diagnosis. This is particularly helpful when the patient is in pain and the clinical examination is limited. The strength examination is the best way to asses the severity of the root injury after an acute radiculopathy. This is because the degree of motor axon loss is directly reflected in the extent of weakness. Collateral sprouting from the remaining motor axons to that muscle has not had time to occur to compensate for this partial denervation.

Needle EMG examination is most helpful in evaluating a chronic radiculopathy and is superior to the clinical examination. Collateral sprouting will have occurred in previously denervated muscle fibers. This repair process will mask clinically detectable axonal loss from the injury, since contractile force will largely have been restored. Only after 70 to 80 percent of motor axons are lost will weakness be clinically evident. Needle EMG will detect a much milder degree of denervation.

The diagnostic yield in radiculopathy depends on a number of factors, including whether the problem is acute or chronic. These studies should not be used to exclude radiculopathy. False-negative studies can occur with predominantly pain and sensory root symptoms, presumably as a result of selective dorsal root compression. This is an important limitation in these studies, in that motor, not sensory, axons are studies. Also, mild abnormalities on EMG may be incidental and unrelated to the patient's symptoms, as may radiographic ones. A coexistent disease, like polyneuropathy, may also limit the yield of EMG by masking more modest changes that occur at the root level. Considering these factors, the needle EMG examination has a diagnostic yield of 50 to 75 percent for all patients with radiculopathy.[105,106,163,165,166] The yield increases when there is weakness and the disorder is chronic.

REFERENCES

1. Stewart JD: *Focal Peripheral Neuropathies,* 2d ed. New York, Raven Press, 1993.
2. Smith KJ, Blakemore WF, Murray JA, Patterson RC: Internodal myelin volume and axon surface area: A relationship determining myelin thickness? *J Neurol Sci* 55:231, 1982.
3. Dyck PJ, Lambert EH: Compound nerve action potentials and morphometry. *Electroencephalogr Clin Neurophysiol* 36:573,1974.
4. Lambert EH, Dyck PJ: Compound nerve action potentials of sural nerve in vitro in peripheral neuropathy, in Duck PJ, Thomas PK, Lambert EH, Bunge R (eds): *Peripheral Neuropathy,* 2d ed. Philadelphia, Saunders, 1984, pp 1030–1044.
5. Sunderland S: *Nerve and Nerve Injuries,* 2d ed. Edinburgh, Churchill Livingstone, 1978.
6. Stewart JD: The variable clinical manifestations of ulnar neuropathy at the elbow. *J Neurol Neurosurg Psychiatry* 50:252, 1987.
7. Trojaborg W: Rate of recovery in motor and sensory fibers of the radial nerve: Clinical and electrophysiologic aspects. *J Neurol Neurosurg Psychiatry* 33:625, 1970.
8. Soukes M, Stewart JD: Common peroneal neuropathy: A study of selective motor and sensory involvement. *Neurology* 41:1117, 1991.
9. Jabaley ME, Wallace WH, Heckler FR: Internal topography of major nerves of the forearm and hand: A current view. *J Hand Surg* 5:1, 1980.
10. Ueyama T: The topography of root fibers within the sciatic nerve trunk of the dog. *J Anat* 127:277, 1978.
11. Brushart TME: Central course of digital axons within the median nerve of *Macaca mulatta. J Comp Neurol* 311:197, 1991.
12. Schady W, Ochoa JL, Torebjork HE, Chen LS: Peripheral projections of fascicles in the human median nerve. *Brain* 106:745, 1983.
13. Hallin RG: Microneurography in relation to intraneural topography: Somatotopic organization of median nerve fascicles in humans. *J Neurol Neurosurg Psychiatry* 53:736, 1990.
14. Seddon HJ: Three types of nerve injury. *Brain* 66:236, 1943.
15. Sunderland S: A classification of peripheral nerve injured producing loss of function. *Brain* 74:491, 1951.
16. Sivak M, Ochoa J, Fernandez JM: Positive manifestations of nerve fiber dysfunction: Clinical, electrophysiologic, and pathologic correlates, in Brown WF, Bolton CF (eds): *Clinical Electromyography,* 2d ed. Boston, Butterworth-Heinemann, 1993, pp 117–148.
17. Lewis T, Pickering GW, Rothschild P: Centripetal paralysis arising out of arrested blood flow to the limb, including notes on a form of tingling. *Heart* 16:1, 1931.
18. Miller RG: Acute versus chronic compressive neuropathy. *Muscle Nerve* 7:427, 1984.
19. Miller RG: Injury to peripheral motor nerves. *Muscle Nerve* 10:698, 1987.
20. Ochoa J, Danta G, Fowler TJ, Gilliatt RW: Nature of the nerve lesion caused by a pneumatic tourniquet. *Nature* 233:265, 1971.
21. Ochoa J, Fowler TJ, Gilliatt RW: Anatomic changes in peripheral nerves compressed by a pneumatic tourniquet. *J Anat* 113:433, 1972.
22. Rudge P, Ochoa J, Gilliatt RW: Acute peripheral nerve compression in the baboon. *J Neurol Sci* 23:403, 1974.
23. Neary D, Ochoa J, Gilliatt RW: Subclinical entrapment neuropathy in man. *J Neurol Sci* 24:283, 1975.
24. Bolton CF, McFarlane RM: Human pneumatic tourniquet paralysis. *Neurology* 28:787, 1978.
25. Denny-Brown D, Brenner C: Paralysis of nerve induced by direct pressure and by tourniquet. *Arch Neurol Psychiatry* 51:1, 1944.
26. Lundborg G: Ischemic nerve injury: Experimental studies on intraneural microvascular pathophysiology and nerve function in a limb subjected to temporary circulatory arrest. *Scand J Plast Reconstr Surg* 6:1, 1970.
27. Fowler TJ, Danta G, Gilliatt RW: Recovery of nerve conduction after a pneumatic tourniquet: Observations on the hind limb of the baboon. *J Neurol Neurosurg Psychiatry* 35:638, 1972.
28. Williams IR, Jefferson D, Gilliatt RW: Acute nerve compression during limb ischemia: An experimental study. *J Neurol Sci* 46:199, 1980.
29. Hess K, Eames RA, Darveniza P, Gilliatt RW: Acute ischemic neuropathy in the rabbit. *J Neurol Sci* 44:19, 1979.
30. Parry GP, Brown MJ: Arachidonate-induced experimental nerve infarction. *J Neurol Sci* 50:123, 1981.
31. Fowler TJ, Ochoa J: Unmyelinated fibers in normal and compressed peripheral nerves of the baboon: A quantitative electron microscopic study. *Neuropathol Appl Neurobiol* 1:247, 1975.
32. Richardson PM, Thomas PK: Percussive injury to peripheral nerve in rats. *J Neurosurg* 51:178, 1979.
33. Fullerton PM, Gilliatt RW: Pressure neuropathy in the hind foot of the guinea-pig. *J Neurol Neurosurg Psychiatry* 30:18, 1967.
34. Anderson MH, Fullerton PM, Gilliatt RW, Hern JEC: Changes in the forearm associated with median nerve compression at the wrist in guinea-pig. *J Neurol Neurosurg Psychiatry* 33:70, 1970.
35. Ochoa J, Marcotte LR: The nature of the nerve lesion caused by chronic entrapment in the guinea-pig. *J Neurol Sci* 19:492, 1973.
36. Marcotte LR: An electron microscope study of chronic median nerve compression in the guinea-pig. *Acta Neuropathol* 27:69, 1971.
37. Aguayo A, Nair CPU, Midgley R: Experimental progressive compression neuropathy in the rabbit: Histologic and electrophysiologic studies. *Arch Neurol* 24:358, 1971.
38. MacKinnon SE, Dellon AL, Hudson AR, Hunter DA: Chronic nerve compression in an experimental model in the rat. *Ann Plast Surg* 13:113, 1984.
39. MacKinnon SE, Dellon AL, Hudson AR, Hunter DA: Chronic human nerve compression: A histological assessment. *Neuropathol Appl Neurobiol* 12:547, 1986.
40. Jefferson D, Eames RA: Subclinical entrapment of the lateral femoral cutaneous nerve: An autopsy study. *Muscle Nerve* 2:145, 1978.
41. Thomas PK, Fullerton PM: Nerve fiber size in the carpal tunnel syndrome. *J Neurol Neurosurg Psychiatry* 26:520, 1963.
42. Lundborg G, Dahlin L: The pathophysiology of nerve compression. *Hand Clin* 4:215, 1992.
43. Lundborg G: Ischemic nerve injury: Experimental studies on intraneural microvascular pathophysiology and nerve function in a limb subjected to temporary circulatory arrest. *Scand J Plast Reconstr Surg* 6(suppl):1, 1970.
44. Sunderland S: Nerve lesion in the carpal tunnel syndrome. *J Neurol Neurosurg Psychiatry* 39:615, 1976.
45. Rydevik B, Lundborg G: Permeability of intraneural microvessels and perineurium following acute, graded experimental nerve compression. *Scand J Plast Reconstr Surg* 11:179, 1977.
46. Dahlin LB, McLeon WG: Effects of graded experimental compression on slow and fast axonal transport in rabbit vagus nerve. *J Neurol Sci* 72:19, 1986.
47. Gelbermann RH, Szabo RM, Williamson RU: Tissue pressure

threshold for peripheral nerve viability. *Clin Orthop* 178:285, 1983.

48. Parry GJ, Cornblath DR, Brown MJ: Transient conduction block following acute peripheral nerve ischemia. *Muscle Nerve* 8:409, 1985.

49. Griffin JW, Hoffman PN: Degeneration and regeneration in the peripheral nervous system, in Dyck PJ, Thomas PK, Griffin JW, Low PA, Poduslo JF (eds): *Peripheral Neuropathy,* 3d ed. Philadelphia, Saunders, 1993, pp 361–376.

50. Selzer ME: Regeneration of peripheral nerve, in Sumner AJ (ed): *The Physiology of Peripheral Nerve Disease.* Philadelphia, Saunders, 1980, pp 358–431.

51. Pellegrino RG, Politis MJ, Ritchie JM, Spencer PS: Events in degenerating cat peripheral nerve: Induction of Schwann cell S phase and its relation to nerve fiber degeneration. *J Neurocytol* 15:17, 1986.

52. Ramon Y Cajal: *Study on Degeneration and Regeneration of the Nervous System.* London, Oxford University Press, 1928.

53. Gilliatt RW, Taylor JC: Electrical changes following section of the facial nerve. *Proc R Soc Med* 52:1080, 1959.

54. Chaudry V, Cornblath DR: Wallerian degeneration in human nerves: A serial electrophysiologic study. *Muscle Nerve* 15:687, 1992.

55. Pilling JB: Nerve conduction study during Wallerian degeneration in man. *Muscle Nerve* 1:81, 1978.

56. Birks R, Katz B, Miledi R: Physiological and structural changes at the amphibian myoneural junction, in the course of nerve degeneration. *J Physiol* 150:145, 1960.

57. Davidovich A, Luco JV: The synaptic transmission of sympathetic ganglia during Wallerian degeneration: Effect of length of degenerating nerve fibers. *Acta Physiol Lat Am* 6:49, 1956.

58. Vial JD: the influence of axon length on the course of Wallerian degeneration of the motor end-plates. *Acta Physiol Lat Am* 5:94, 1955.

59. Schlaeper WW: Calcium-induced degeneration of axoplasm in isolated segments of rat phrenic nerve. *Brain Res* 69:203, 1974.

60. Schlaepfer WW: Structural alterations in peripheral nerve induced by the calcium ionophore A223187. *Brain Res* 136:1, 1977.

61. Johnson GVW, Greenwood JA, Costello AC, Troncoso JC: The regulatory role of calmodulin in the proteolysis of individual neurofilament proteins by calpain. *Neurochem Res* 16:869, 1991.

62. Lopachin RM, Lopachin VR, Saubermann AJ: Effects of axotomy on distribution and concentration of elements in rat sciatic nerve. *J Neruochem* 54:320, 1990.

63. Schlaepfer WW, Bunge RP: The effects of calcium ion concentration on the degradation of amputated axons in tissue culture. *J Cell Biol* 59:456, 1973.

64. Brown MJ, Sumner AJ, Greene DA, et al: Distal neuropathy in experimental diabetes mellitus. *Ann Neurol* 8:168, 1980.

65. Mulder DW, Lambert EH, Bastron JA: The neuropathies associated with diabetes mellitus. *Neurology* 11:275–284, 1961.

66. Fraser DM, Campbell IW, Ewing DJ: Mononeuropathy in diabetes mellitus. *Diabetes* 28:96–101, 1979.

67. Dyck PJ, Kratz KM, Karnes JL, et al: The prevalence by staged severity of various types of diabetic neuropathy, retinopathy, and nephropathy in a population-based cohort: The Rochester Diabetic Neuropathy Study. *Neurology* 43:817, 1993.

68. Albers JW, Brown MB, Sima AAF, Greene DA: Frequency of median mononeuropathy in patients with mild diabetic neuropathy in the early diabetes intervention trial (EDIT). *Muscle Nerve* 19:140–146, 1996.

69. Asbury AK: Neuropathies with renal failure, hepatic disorders, chronic respiratory insufficiency, and critical illness, in Dyck PJ, Thomas PK, Griffin JW, et al (eds): *Peripheral Neuropathy,* 3d ed. Philadelphia, Saunders, 1993, pp 1251–1265.

70. Bolton CF, Driedger AA, Lindsay RM: Ischaemic neuropathy in uremic patients due to a bovine arteriovenous shunt. *J Neurol Neurosurg Psychiatry* 42:810, 1979.

71. Wilbourn AJ, Furlan AJ, Hulley W, Ruschaupt W: Ischemic monomelic neuropathy. *Neurology* 33:447, 1983.

72. Wyrtzes L, Markley HG, Fisher M, Alfred HJ: Brachial neuropathy after brachial artery-antecubital vein shunts for chronic hemodialysis. *Neurology* 37:1398, 1987.

73. Harding AE, Le Fanu J: Carpal tunnel syndrome related to antebrachial fistula. *J Beurol Neurosurg Psychiatry* 40:511, 1977.

74. Shahani B, Spalding DMK: Diabetes mellitus presenting with bilateral foot-drop. *Lancet* 2:930–931, 1969.

75. Brown MJ, Asbury AK: Diabetic neuropathy. *Ann Neurol* 15:2, 1984.

76. Clayburgh RH, Beckenbough RD, Dobyns JH: Carpal tunnel release in patients with diffuse peripheral neuropathy. *J Hand Surg* 12A:380, 1987.

77. Upton AR, McComas AJ: The double crush in nerve entrapment syndromes. *Lancet* 2:359, 1973.

78. Yu J, Bendler EM, Mentori A: Neurologic disorders associated with carpal tunnel syndrom. *Electromyogr Clin Neurophysiol* 19:27, 1979.

79. Massey EW, Riler TL, Pleet AB: Coexistent carpal tunnel syndrome and cervical radiculopathy. *South Med J* 74:957, 1981.

80. Hurst LC, Weissberg D, Carrol RE: The relationship of the double crush to carpal tunnel syndrome: An analysis of 1,000 cases of carpal tunnel syndrome. *J Hand Surg* 108:202, 1985.

81. Osterman AL: The double crush syndrome. *Orthop Clin North Am* 19:147, 1988.

82. Frith RW, Litchy WJ: Electrophysiologic abnormalities of peripheral nerves in patients with cervical radiculopathy. *Muscle Nerve* 8:613, 1985.

83. Narakas AO: The role of thoracic outlet syndrome in the double crush syndrome. *Ann Hand Surg* 9:331, 1990.

84. Wood UE, Biondi J: Double crush nerve compression in thoracic outlet syndrome. *J Bone Joint Surg* 72A;85, 1990.

85. Wilbourn AJ: The thoracic outlet syndrome is overdiagnosed. *Arch Neurol* 47:328, 1990.

86. Carroll RE, Hurst LC: The relationship of thoracic outlet syndrome and carpal tunnel syndrome. *Clin Orthop* 164:149, 1982.

87. Baba M, Fowler CJ, Jacobs JM, Gilliatt RW: Changes in peripheral nerve fibers distal to a constriction. *J Neurol Sci* 54:197, 1982.

88. Reiners K, Gilliatt RW, Harding AE, O'Neill JH: Regeneration following tibial nerve crush in the rabbit: The effect of proximal constriction. *J Neurol Neurosurg Psychiatry* 50:6, 1987.

89. Shimpo T, Gilliatt RW, Kennett RP, Allen PJ: Susceptibility to pressure neuropathy distal to a constricting ligature in the guinea pig. *J Neurol Neurosurg Psychiatry* 50:1625, 1987.

90. Nemoto K, Matsumoto N, Tazaki K: An experimental study on the "double crush" hypothesis. *J Hand Surg* 12A:542, 1987.

91. Rydevik B, McLean WG, Sjostrand J, Lundborg G: Blockage of axonal transport induced by graded compression of the rabbit vagus nerve. *J Neurol Neurosurg Psychiatry* 43:690, 1980.

92. Dahlin LB, Lundborg G: The neurone and its response to peripheral nerve compression. *J Hand Surg* 158:5, 1990.

93. Cragg BG, Thomas PK: The conduction velocity of regenerating peripheral nerve fibres. *J Physiol* 171:164, 1964.

94. Sumner AJ: Aberrant reinnervation. *Muscle Nerve* 13:801, 1990.

95. Thomas PK, Stein RB, Gordon RB: Patterns of reinnervation and motor unit recruitment in human hand muscles after complete ulnar and median nerve section and resuture. *J Neurol Neurosurg Psychiatry* 50:259, 1987.

96. Asbury AK: The clinical view of neuromuscular electrophysiology, in Sumner AJ (ed): *The Physiology of Peripheral Nerve Disease.* Philadelphia, Saunders, 1980, pp 484–491.

97. Wilbourn AJ: Electrodiagnostic testing of neurologic injuries in athletes. *Clin Sports Med* 9:229, 1990.

98. Kimura J: Nerve conduction studies and electromyography, in Dyck PJ, Thomas PK, Griffin JW, Low PA, Poduslo JF (eds): *Peripheral Neuropathy,* 3d ed. Philadelphia, Saunders, 1993, pp 598–644.

99. Kimura J: *Electrodiagnosis in Diseases of Nerve and Muscle: Principles and Practice,* 2d ed. Philadelphia, Davis, 1989.

100. Dumitru D: *Electrodiagnostic Medicine.* Philadelphia, Hanley & Belfus, 1995.

101. Albers JW, Kelly JJ: Acquired inflammatory demyelinating polyneuropathies: Clinical and electrodiagnostic features. *Muscle Nerve* 12:435, 1985.

102. Cornblath DR: Electrophysiology in Guillian-Barré syndrome. *Ann Neurol* 27(suppl):S17, 1990.

103. Cornblath DR, Sumner AJ, Daube J, et al: Conduction block in clinical practice. *Muscle Nerve* 14:869, 1991.

104. Fisher MA: H reflexes and F waves: Physiology and clinical application. *Muscle Nerve* 15:1223, 1992.

105. Aminoff MJ, Gooden DS, Parry GJ, et al: Electrophysiologic evaluation of lumbosacral radiculopathy: Electromyography, late responses, and somatonsensory evoked potentials. *Neurology* 35:1514, 1985.

106. Wilbourn AJ, Aminoff MJ: The electrophysiologic examination in patients with radiculopathies. *Muscle Nerve* 11:1099, 1988.

107. Daube JR: Needle examination in clinical electromyography. *Muscle Nerve* 14:645, 1991.

108. Dumitru D: Needle electromyography, in Dumitru D (ed): *Electrodiagnostic Medicine.* Philadelphia, Handley & Belfus, 1995, pp 211–248.

109. Branstader ME, Fullerton M: Sensory nerve conduction studies in cervical root lesions. *Can J Neurol Sci* 10:152, 1983.

110. Levin KH, Maggiano HJ, Wilbourn AJ: Cervical rediculopathy: Comparison of surgical and EMG localization of single root lesions. *Neurology* 46:1022, 1996.

111. Rivner MH: Statistical errors and their effects on electrodiagnostic medicine. *Muscle Nerve* 17:811, 1994.

112. Schulzer M: Diagnostic tests: A statistical review. *Muscle Nerve* 17:815, 1994.

113. Redmond MD, Rivner MH: False positive tests in carpal tunnel syndrome. *Muscle Nerve* 11:511, 1988.

114. Dyck PJ: Limitations in predicting pathologic abnormalities of nerve from the EMG examination. *Muscle Nerve* 13:371, 1990.

115. Parry GP: Electrodiagnostic studies in the evaluation of peripheral nerve and brachial plexus injuries. *Neurol Clin* 10:921, 1992.

116. Gilliatt RW, Hjorth RJ: Nerve conduction during Wallerian degeneration in the baboon. *J Neurol Neurosurg Psychiatry* 35:335, 1972.

117. Miledi R, Slater CR: On the degenration of rat neuromuscular junctions after nerve section. *J Physiol* 207:507, 1970.

118. Simpson JA: Electrical signs in the diagnosis of carpal tunnel and related syndromes. *J Neurol Neurosurg Psychiatry* 19:275, 1956.

119. Gilliatt RW, Sears TA: Sensory nerve action potentials in patients with peripheral nerve lesions. *J Neurol Neurosurg Psychiatry* 21:108, 1958.

120. Thomas JE, Lambert EH, Cseuz KA: Electrodiagnostic aspects of the carpal tunnel syndrome. *Arch Neurol* 16:635, 1967.

121. Stevens JC: The electrodiagnosis of carpal tunnel syndrome. *Muscle Nerve* 2:99, 1987.

122. Pease WS, Cannell CD, Johnson EW: Median to radial latency difference test in mild carpal tunnel syndrome. *Muscle Nerve* 12:905, 1989.

123. Jackson DA, Clifford JC: Electrodiagnosis of mild carpal tunnel syndrome. *Arch Phys Med Rehabil* 70:199, 1989.

124. American Association of Electordiagnostic Medicine Quality Assurance Committee: Literature review of the usefulness of nerve conduction studies and electromyography for the evaluation of patients with carpal tunnel syndrome. *Muscle Nerve* 16:1392, 1993.

125. Ross MA, Kimura J: The carpal tunnel syndrome. *Muscle Nerve* 18:567, 1995.

126. American Academy of Neurology: Practice parameters for electrodiagnostic studies in carpal tunnel syndrome. *Neurology* 43:2404, 1993.

127. Seror P: Sensitivity of the various tests for the diagnosis of carpal tunnel syndrome. *J Hand Surg* 19B:725, 1994.

128. Eisen A, Schilzer M, Pant B, et al: Receiver operating characteristic curve analysis in the prediction of carpal tunnel syndrome: A model for reporting electrophysiologic data. *Muscle Nerve* 16:787, 1993.

129. Dunnon JB, Waylonis GW: Wrist flexion as an adjunct to the diagnosis of carpal tunnel syndrome. *Arch Phys Med Rehabil* 72:211, 1991.

130. Novak CB, MacKinnon SE, Brownlee R, Kelly L: Provocative testing in carpal tunnel syndrome. *J Hand Surg* 17B:204, 1992.

131. Rivner MH, Kumar J, Crout BO: Long-term outlook in patients with mild carpal tunnel syndrome. *Muscle Nerve* 12:764, 1989.

132. Miller RG: The cubital tunnel syndrome: Diagnosis and precise localization. *Ann Neurol* 6:56, 1979.

133. Miller RG: Ulnar neuropathy at the elbow. *Muscle Nerve* 14:97, 1991.

134. Kincaid JC: The electrodiagnosis of ulnar neuropathy at the elbow. *Muscle Nerve* 11:1005, 1988.

135. Raynor EM, Shefner JM, Prestion DC, Logigian EL: Sensory and mixed nerve conduction studies in the evaluation of ulnar neuropathy at the elbow. *Muscle Nerve* 17:785, 1994.

136. Campbell WW, Pridgeon RM, Sahni KS: Short segment incremental studies in the evaluation of ulnar neuropathy at the elbow. *Muscle Nerve* 15:1050, 1992.

137. Jabre JF: Ulnar nerve lesions at the wrist: New technique for recording from the sensory dorsal branch of the ulnar nerve. *Neurology* 30:873, 1980.

138. Campbell WW, Pridgeon RM, Riaz G, et al: Sparing of the flexor carpi ulnaris in ulnar neuropathy at the elbow. *Muscle Nerve* 12:965, 1989.

139. Fisher MA: Other mononeuropathies of the upper extremities, in Brown WF, Bolton CF (eds): *Clinical Electromyography,* 2d ed. Boston, Butterworth-Heinemann, 1993, pp 271–304.

140. Trojaborg W: Rater of recovery in motor and sensory fibers of the radial nerve: Clinical and electrophysiologic aspects *J Neurol Neurosurg Psychiatry* 32:354, 1969.

141. Culp RW, Osterman AL, Davidson RS, et al: Neural injuries associated with supracondylar fractures of the humerus in children. *J Bone Joint Surg* 72A:1211, 1990.

142. Van Rossum J, Buruma OJ, Kamphuisen HA: Tennis elbow—A radial tunnel syndrome. *J Bone Joint Surg* 60B:197, 1978.

143. Verhaar J, Spaans F: Radial tunnel syndrome: An investigation of compression as a possible cause. *J Bone Joint Surg* 73A:539, 1991.

144. Roles NC, Maudsley RH; Radial tunnel syndrome: Resistant tennis elbow as a nerve entrapment. *J Bone Joint Surg* 54B:499, 1972.

145. Gilliatt RW, LeQuesne PM, Logue V, Sumner AJ: Wasting of the hand associated with a cervical rib or band. *J Neurol Neurosurg Psychiatry* 33:615, 1970.

146. Wilbourn AJ: Brachial plexus disorders, in Dyck PJ, Thomas PK, Griffin JW, et al (eds): *Peripheral Neuropathy,* 3d ed. Philadelphia, Saunders, 1993, pp 911—950.

147. Cuetter AC, Barostek DM: The thoracic outlet syndrome: Controversies, overdiagnosis, overtreatment, and recommendations for management. *Muscle Nerve* 12:410, 1989.

148. Cherington M: A conservative view of the thoracic outlet syndrome. *Am J Surg* 158:394, 1989.

149. Urschel HC, Razzuk MA: Management of the thoracic outlet syndrome. *N Engl J Med* 286:1140, 1972.

150. Wilbourn AJ, Lederman RJ: Evidence of conduction delay in thoracic-outlet is challenged. *N Engl J Med* 310:1052, 1984.

151. Daube JR: Nerve conduction studies in the thoracic outlet syndrome. *Neurology* 25:347, 1975.

152. Stanton PE, Vo NM, Haley T, et al: Thoracic outlet syndrome: A comprehensive evaluation. *Am Surg* 54:129, 1988.

153. Pavot AP, Ignucis DR, Gargom GW: Assessment of conduction from C8 nerve root exit to supraclavicular fossa—Its value in the diagnosis of thoracic outlet syndrome. *Electromyogr Clin Neurophysiol* 29:445, 1989.

154. Yiannikas C, Walsh JC: Somatosensory evoked responses in the diagnosis of thoracic outlet syndrome. *J Neurol Neurosurg Psychiatr* 46:234, 1983.

155. Chodoroff G, Lee DW, Honet JC: Dynamic approach in the diagnosis of thoracic outlet syndrome using somatosensory evoked responses. *Arch Phys Med Rehabil* 65:4, 1985.

156. Katriji B, Wilbourn AJ: Common peroneal mononeuropathy: A clinical and electrophysiologic study of 116 lesions. *Neurology* 38:1723, 1988.

157. Katriji B, Wilbourn AJ: High sciatic lesion mimicking peroneal neuropathy at the fibular head. *J Neurol Sci* 121:172, 1994.

158. Oh SJ, Sarala PK, Kuba T: Tarsal tunnel syndrome: Electrophysiologic study. *Ann Neurol* 5:327, 1979.

159. Stewart JD: Mononeuropathies of the lower extremities, in Brown WF, Bolton CF (eds): *Clinical Electromyography,* 2d ed. Boston, Butterworth-Heinemann, 1993, pp 305–322.

160. Schmid VD, Walker G, Hess CW, Schmid J: Magnetic and electrical stimulation of cervical motor roots: Technique, site, and mechanisms of excitation. *J Neurol Neurosurg Psychiatry* 53:770, 1990.

161. Walk P, Fisher MA, Poundoulakis SH, Hemmati M: Somatosensory evoked potentials in the evaluation of lumbosacral radiculopathy. *Neurology* 42:1197, 1992.

162. Dumitru D, Dreyfuss P: Dermatiomal/segmental SEP evaluation of L5/S1 unilateral/unilevel radiculopathies. *Muscle Nerve* 19:442, 1996.

163. Leblhuber F, Reisecker F, Boehm-Jurkovic H, et al: Diagnostic value of different electrophysiologic tests in cervical disk prolapse. *Neurology* 38:1879, 1988.

164. So YT, Olney RK, Aminoff MJ: A comparison of thermography and electromyography in the diagnosis of cervical radiculopathy. *Muscle Nerve* 13:1032, 1990.

165. Tonzola RF, Ackil AA, Shahani BT, Young RR: Usefulness of electrophysiologic studies in the diagnosis of lumbosacral root disease. *Ann Neurol* 9:305, 1981.

166. Hall S, Bartleson JD, Onofrio et al: Lumbar spinal stenosis: Clinical features, diagnostic procedures, and results of surgical treatment in 68 patients. *Ann Intern Med* 103:271, 1985.

CHAPTER 14

Biomechanics and Biomaterials

R. Jay Bradley, Jr., Edmund Y. S. Chao, and Richard J. Friedman

BIOMECHANICS

Basic Concept of Force and Moment in Static Analysis

Definition of Statics

The study of the relationship between the *external applied forces* and *internal reactive forces* of a *rigid body system* in *static equilibrium.*

Concept of Force

Force is a *vector quantity,* with *magnitude* and *direction,* which will cause a rigid body to *accelerate* in the direction of application. Different forces acting on a body cannot be added or subtracted algebraically unless they are all in the same direction.

Units of Force

dyne: A force magnitude capable of producing an acceleration of 1 cm/s^2 to a rigid body with 1 g of mass.
newton (N): A force magnitude capable of producing an acceleration of 1 m/s^2 to a rigid body with 1 kg of mass.
kgf: A force magnitude causing an acceleration of 1 g (9.8 m/s^2) to a mass of 1 kg; 1 kgf = 9.8 N.
lbf: A force magnitude causing an acceleration of 1 g (32.2 ft/s^2) to a mass of 1 lb; 1 kgf = 2.2 lbf.

Force Vector and Components

Force is a *vector quantity* that has both magnitude and direction. Vector quantities cannot be added or subtracted algebraically unless they have identical direction. Any force can be decomposed into two *orthogonal components* (two-dimensional problem) along the *x* and *y* directions of a *Cartesian coordinate system* (Fig. 14-1).

After forces are decomposed into orthogonal components, they can be added and subtracted algebraically along both the *x* and *y* directions separately.

Types of Forces in Joint Biomechanics

1. *External forces:* Ground reaction force, gravitational force, and applied force through contact.
2. *Internal forces:* Muscle contracting force, joint contact and shear forces, and capsuloligamentous constraint force.

Muscles, tendons, and ligaments can carry only *tensile forces,* while joint articulating surfaces can transmit only *compression forces.* Normally, joint *shear force* (parallel to the joint surface) is very small due to the extremely low frictional coefficient of the cartilage, synovial fluid, and prosthetic materials.

Moment of a Force

The moment of a force acting on a rigid body with respect to a point is equal to the force times the *perpendicular distance* from the point to the line of force action (moment arm). The direction of the moment is always perpendicular to the plane of forces in a two-dimensional case. The units of moment are kg-cm or lb-in. A moment of force will cause the rigid body to *rotate* as well as to *translate.* In the case of holding a ball with the arm in the horizontal position, as shown in Fig. 14-2, the moments of the weight of the ball with respect to the wrist joint center (O″), the elbow joint center (O′), and the shoulder joint center (O) can easily be determined.

Moment about the wrist:

$$M_w = 5 \times 3 = 15 \text{ lb-in.}$$

Moment about the elbow:

$$M_e = 5 \times 12 = 60 \text{ lb-in.}$$

Moment about the shoulder:

$$M_s = 5 \times 23 = 115 \text{ lb-in.}$$

Torque of a Couple

A couple is a pair of two equal and opposite forces parallel to each other at a distance *d*. The product of one of the forces and the distance *d* is defined as the torque of a couple, which has the same unit as moment. A couple only causes the rigid body to *rotate.*

Bending Couple (Moment) in a Beam

When a beamlike member is loaded laterally, every transverse cross section carries an internal *bending* couple, commonly defined as *bending moment.* This bending moment is the result of an infinite number of couples acting in the longitudinal direction along the fibers of the beam. The main function of the bending couple is to *bend the beam* in the direction of load application.

Frictional Force

If a rigid body is in contact with another surface, the resistive force to sliding motion along the contact surface is defined as the *frictional force.* The maximum frictional force before sliding motion occurs is equal to the product of the normal compressive force between the body and the surface and the *frictional coefficient μ* (Fig. 14-3).

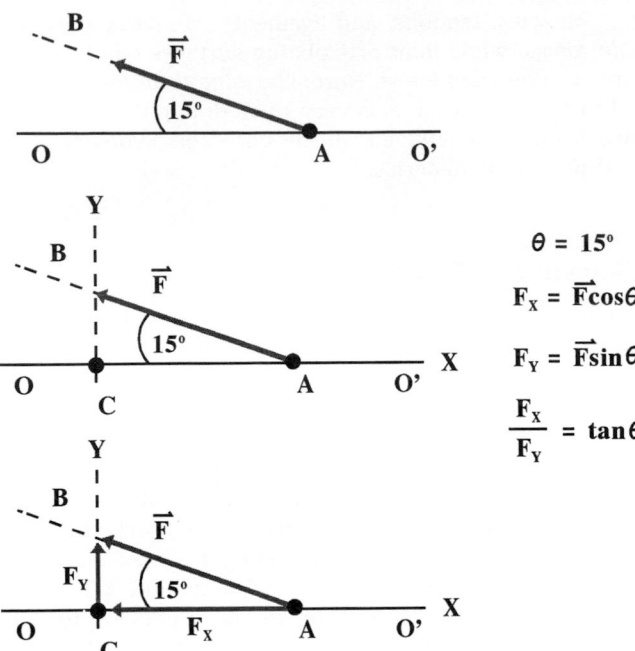

$$\theta = 15°$$

$$F_X = \vec{F}\cos\theta$$

$$F_Y = \vec{F}\sin\theta$$

$$\frac{F_X}{F_Y} = \tan\theta$$

Figure 14-1 Force vector and components.

Two-Dimensional Static Force Analysis in Joint Biomechanics

Newton's Law of Static Equilibrium

When a rigid body system is in *static equilibrium* (no motion is involved), then (1) the summation of all the external forces acting on the body will be zero and (2) the summation of all the moments of all the forces with respect to a point will be zero. Since not all the forces will be in the same direction, each force has to be decomposed into *x* and *y* components before summation. As a result, the static equilibrium condition implies that Eq. 5 in Fig. 14-4 must be satisfied (Fig. 14-4).

These are the three basic equations required to relate unknown internal muscle and joint forces with the known external forces. Three equations can be used only to solve

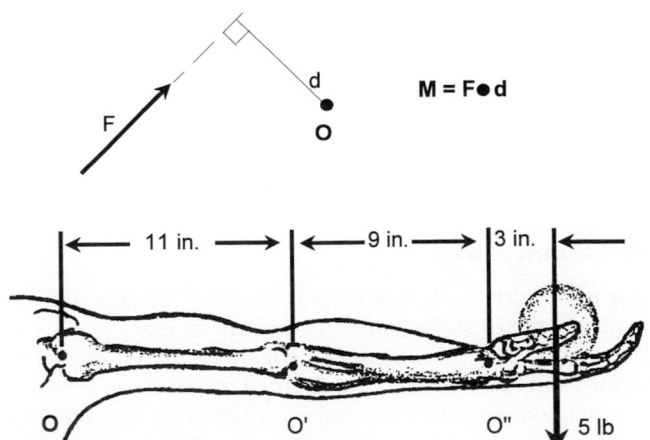

Figure 14-2 Force moments about the upper extremity.

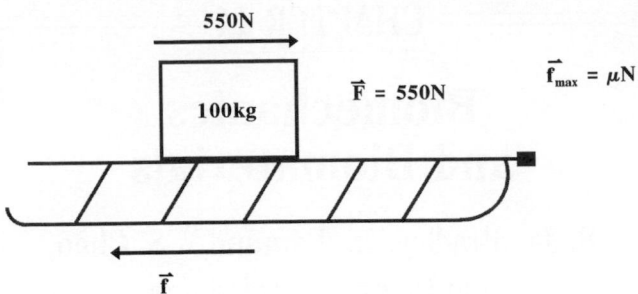

Figure 14-3 Frictional force.

three unknown muscle or joint constraint forces. If the unknown forces are more than three in two-dimensional cases, the problem is defined as *statically indeterminate,* where there is *no unique solution.* All joint mechanic problems are of this type because of the *redundant nature* of muscle action. Special methods and assumptions must be used in order to solve these problems.

Free-Body Diagram

A free-body diagram (FBD) represents the entire rigid body system or a portion of it isolated from all its physical contacts with the environment in which all the externally applied forces and the joint constraint forces and moments are clearly identified. If the FBD is isolated from a *point contact* without friction, then there is only one joint force that must be normal to the contact surface. When a *hinge joint* is isolated from the FBD, there will be two forces perpendicular to each other acting through the center of the hinge joint. Note that these two forces are *resultant* in nature, representing the combined resistance of the joint articulating surface and the ligamentous constraints. When an FBD is taken from a *rigid joint* (does not allow free rotation in the plane of motion), there will be two forces and one moment occurring at the isolated site of the imaginary joint. If muscles or tendons are active across the joint being isolated in the FBD, their forces have to be included in the system, with their directions along the fiber of the muscle or tendon. A few examples of the free-body diagram isolated at various joints are shown in Fig. 14-5.

If the entire rigid body system is in equilibrium, any portion of it must also be in equilibrium. Therefore, the FBD of a rigid body system in static equilibrium must satisfy the *three equilibrium equations:*

$$\sum F_x = 0, \qquad \sum F_y = 0, \qquad \sum M_o = 0$$

All the forces acting on the FBD and the internal force at the joints isolated will appear in these equations as either the known quantities or the unknown forces to be determined.

Static Force Analysis by Graphical Method

If a rigid body is in static equilibrium, all the force vectors acting on the rigid free body must form a *closed polygon* when these forces are joined from *head to tail in any sequence.* Based on this principle, the unknown force can be determined by closing the open polygon formed by all known forces or known force directions acting on the sys-

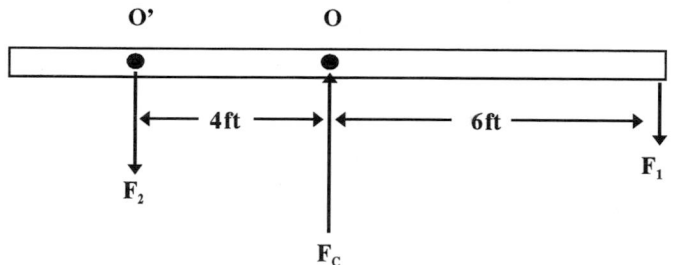

$$\begin{cases} \vec{F_c} = \vec{F_1} + \vec{F_2} \\ 4\vec{F_2} = 6\vec{F_1} \end{cases}$$

$$\sum F_X = 0$$
$$\sum F_Y = 0$$
$$\sum M_O = 0$$

Figure 14-4 Static equilibrium.

tem. Consider the following pulley traction device in equilibrium: $W = 10$ N, the cable force is along the line OA, and the traction force is along OB. If the FBD is taken around the point O, ignoring the gravity force of the foot and leg, the three forces must form a closed triangle, which allows us to determine T_A and T_B graphically. In this case, $T_A = 12.5$ N, and $T_B = 7.5$ N (Fig. 14-6).

Graphical methods can be used only to solve a rigid body subjected to *concurrent force systems* (all forces intersect at one point).

Static Force Analysis by the Algebraic Method

If all forces acting on an FBD in equilibrium are decomposed into x and y components, these forces must satisfy the following equilibrium equations:

$$\sum F_x = 0, \qquad \sum F_y = 0, \qquad \sum M_o = 0$$

Basic Concepts of Kinematics and Kinetics
Definitions

Kinematics: The study of rigid body motion without concern for the cause.
Kinetics: The study of the relationship between rigid body motion *and the* forces *causing the motion.*

Degrees of Freedom of Joint Motion

The number of *independent* modes of motion in a joint are called the *degrees of freedom* (DOF). In two-dimensional cases, a joint can have three independent modes of motion (three DOF): translation in x direction, translation in y direction, and rotation in z direction (defined by the *right-hand rule*) (Fig. 14-7).

However, in a *closely packed* hinge joint, there is only one DOF in rotation, since the joint is constrained not to

Figure 14-5 Free-body diagrams for various joints.

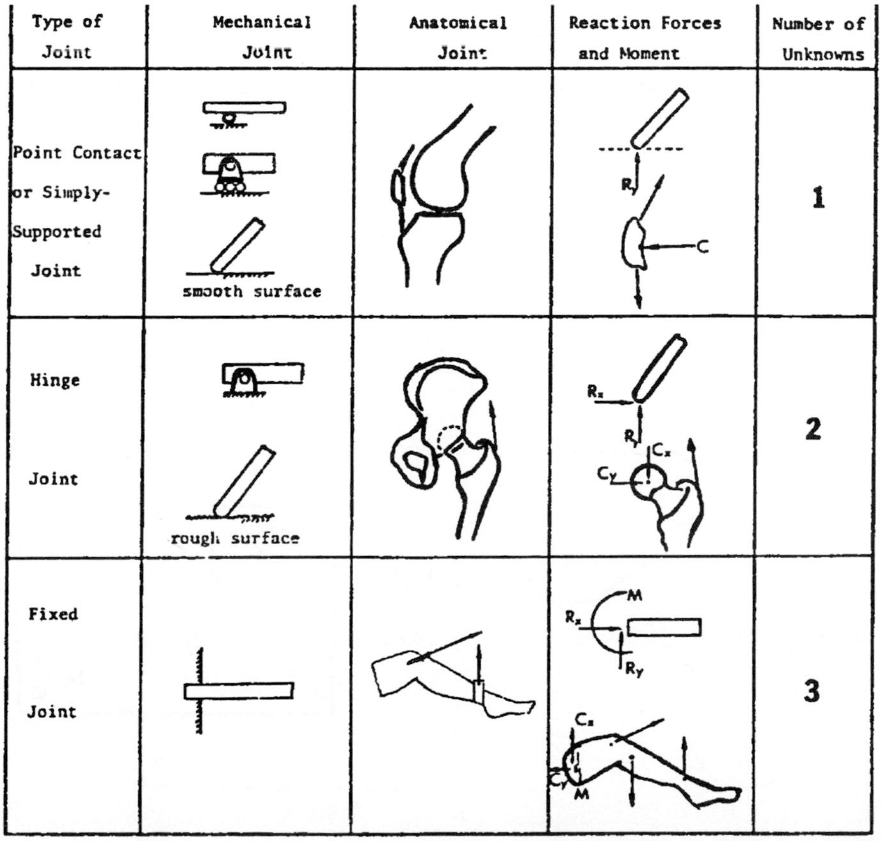

Type of Joint	Mechanical Joint	Anatomical Joint	Reaction Forces and Moment	Number of Unknowns
Point Contact or Simply-Supported Joint	smooth surface			1
Hinge Joint	rough surface			2
Fixed Joint				3

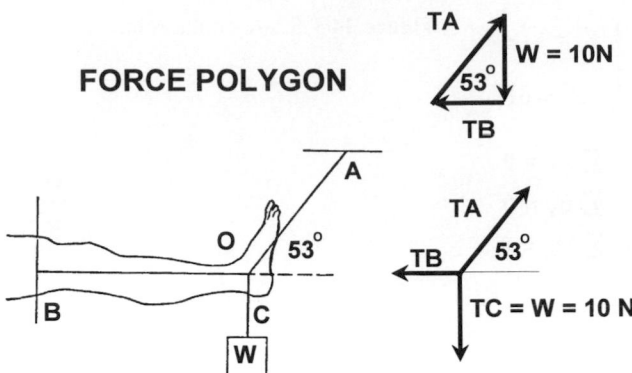

Figure 14-6 Force polygon.

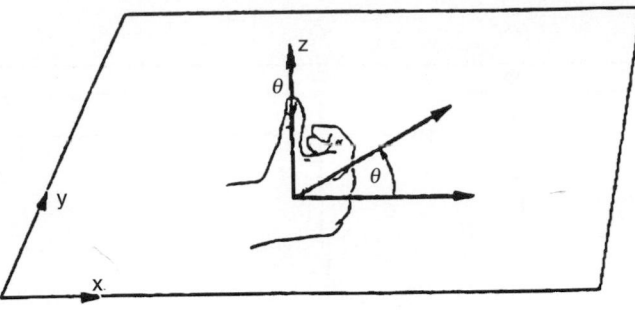

Figure 14-7 Degrees of freedom of joint motion.

allow translation in any direction. The ulnohumeral joint can be considered as an example of this type. A *universal joint* has two DOF and a *ball-and-socket* joint contains three DOF, all in rotation. In three-dimensional cases, a free joint would have a total of six DOF: three in rotation and three in translation along three mutually perpendicular directions (*x, y,* and *z* axes of a Cartesian coordinate system). A hip joint possesses three DOF in rotation: flexion-extension, abduction-adduction, and axial rotation with respect to three perpendicular axes.

The DOF and joint constraint forces and moment are directly related. If there is a degree of freedom in motion along a specific direction, then the constraint force or moment in that direction will be zero. In two-dimensional cases, the total number of DOF plus the constraint force and moment should be three; while in three-dimensional cases, the sum becomes six. For example, when the proximal interphalangeal (PIP) joint of a finger is analyzed only in the sagittal plane (two-dimensional case), it has one DOF in flexion-extension and two constraint forces of axial compression and volar-dorsal shear. If the wrist joint is considered in three-dimensional motion, it has two DOF (flexion-extension and ulnar-radial deviation). Consequently, the wrist joint should have a total of four constraint forces and moment ($6 - 2 = 4$). These constraint forces and moment are (1) axial compressive force, (2) medial-lateral shear force, (3) volar-dor-

sal shear force, and (4) axial rotational torque. The concept of DOF and joint constraints is very important in joint motion and force analysis in biomechanics.

Basic Types of Motion

Translation: All particles of a rigid body move along parallel paths (Fig. 14-8).
Rotation: Particles of a rigid body move in parallel planes along circles centered on the same axis (axis of rotation) (Fig. 14-9).

In two-dimensional motion, the rotation is with respect to an axis perpendicular to the plane of motion. The intersection of this axis with the plane is a point defined as the *center of rotation*. Any *general motion* of a rigid body can always be decomposed into a *translation plus a rotation*.

Linear Motion

A rigid body under pure translation along a *straight path* is said to have *linear motion*. If the position of the rigid body can be identified at two time instances, then the *average velocity V* can be calculated as shown in Fig. 14-10.

If the rigid body is undergoing nonuniform linear motion (changing velocity), the *average acceleration a* can be determined as shown in Fig. 14-11.

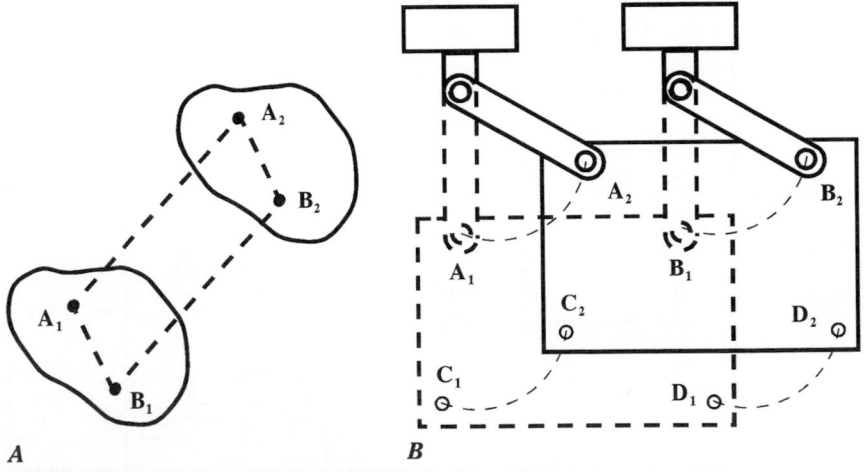

Figure 14-8 Translation. *A.* Linear translation. *B.* Curvilinear translation.

Figure 14-9 *A* and *B.* Rotation.

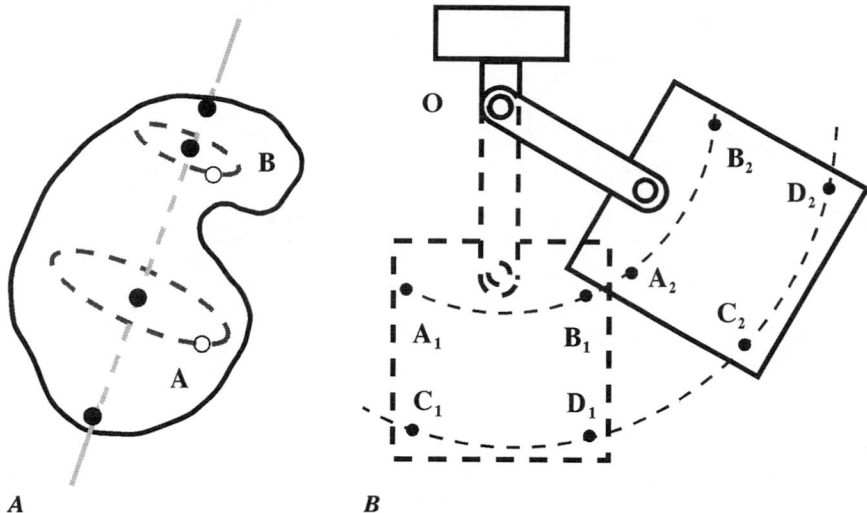

A	*B*

Uniform Circular Motion

If a plane rigid body is rotating about a fixed point (center of rotation) in the plane of the body, it is said that the body is undergoing circular motion. The *angular velocity ω* is measured in units of rads per second or revolutions per minute. Under uniform circular motion, the angular velocity will be constant. Under constant circular motion, the velocity of any point on the plane rigid body is always perpendicular to the line (radius of rotation *r*) joining the

point and the center of rotation. The magnitude of such velocity is $V = r\omega$ (Fig. 14-12).

Under such motion, the rotating point has an acceleration pointing towards the center of rotation defined as *centripetal acceleration* (or *normal acceleration*) a_n with a magnitude

$$a_n = r\omega^2$$

When the angular velocity is not uniform, there will be an angular acceleration α measured in units of rads per sec-

Figure 14-10 Instantaneous velocity.

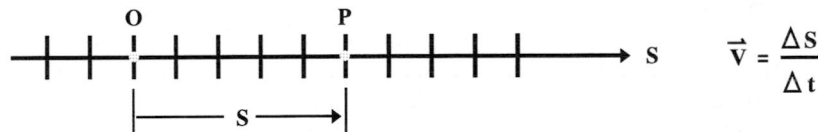

$$\vec{V} = \frac{\Delta s}{\Delta t}$$

The **instantaneous velocity**, v, is defined as

$$\vec{V} = \lim_{\Delta t \to 0} \frac{\Delta s}{\Delta t}$$

Figure 14-11 Instantaneous acceleration.

$$\vec{v} > 0$$

$$\vec{a} = \frac{\Delta s}{\Delta t}$$

The **instantaneous acceleration**, $\vec{a}$, is defined as

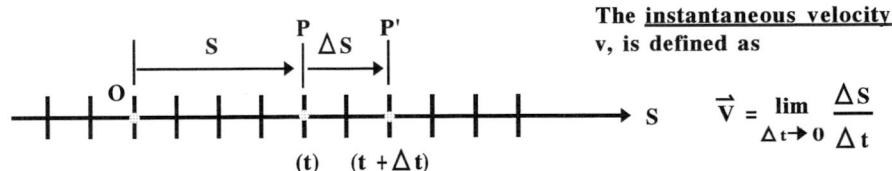

$$\vec{a} = \lim_{\Delta t \to 0} \frac{\Delta v}{\Delta t}$$

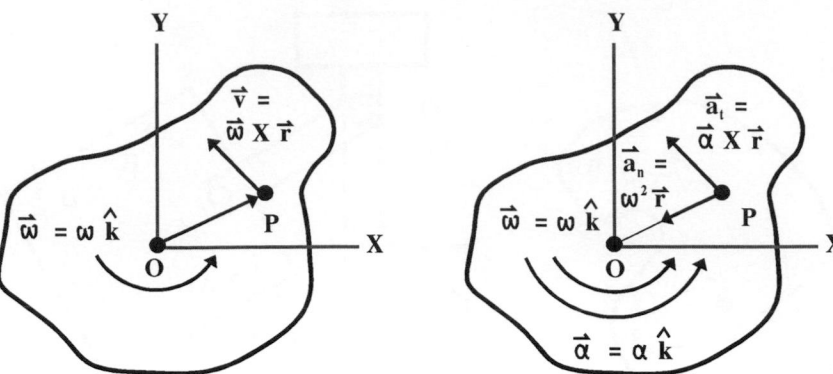

Figure 14-12 Angular velocity.

ond squared. In this case, the rotating point will have an additional acceleration in the tangential direction of the circular path of motion, defined as the tangential acceleration a_t with the magnitude:

$$a_t = r\alpha$$

Instantaneous Center of Rotation in Two-Dimensional Motion

When a two-dimensional rigid body is moving freely in a plane, it can have both translation and rotation. Because of the translational component of motion, the center of rotation for the body will change throughout the course of motion. At any instance of time, an approximate center of rotation can be determined which is defined as the *instantaneous center of rotation* (ICR). Since the velocity of a point on a rigid body experiencing rotation during a short period of time must be perpendicular to a line joining the point and the center of rotation, one can use this specific property to determine the ICR. If the velocities of two separate points on the body are known, then the ICR at that instant can be determined graphically, as shown in Fig. 14-13. In experimental measurements, it will be nearly impossible to determine the velocity of different points on

the body in motion. A different method will be used to determine the approximate ICR. This method was first described by Franz Reuleaux, a German engineer, in 1876. If the instantaneous location of two points, A and B, on a plane rigid body can be identified from two consecutive positions (A_1,B_1 and A_1',B_1') within a short period of time, then the *intersection of the bisectors* of the lines joining the same points (A_1,A_1' and B_1,B_1') at the two positions defines the ICR, as illustrated in Fig. 14-14. Note that the instantaneous center determined in this manner is *averaged* in nature, which describes the *mean center of rotation* between the unprimed and primed positions during the short period of motion. Although the *method of Reuleaux* has been widely applied in the field of biomechanics, one must recognize three potential drawbacks of this technique: (1) The motion must occur in a two-dimensional plane; (2) this method is graphical in nature, and therefore it is tedious and cannot utilize the advantage of computer manipulation; and (3) it is an approximate method and very sensitive to error.

In order to use this method, pure two-dimensional motion must be ensured and the time interval between positions should be kept as short as possible. In true three-dimensional motion, ICR does not exist and the concept of *instantaneous axis of rotation (screw axis)* must be applied.

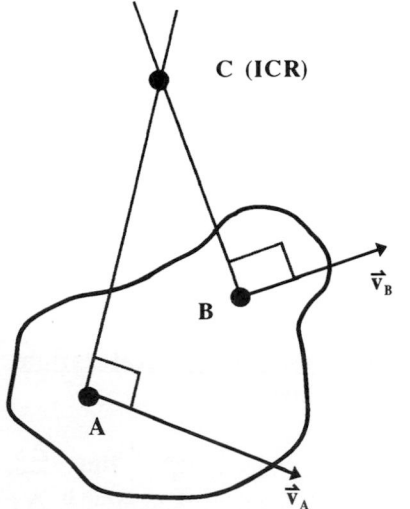

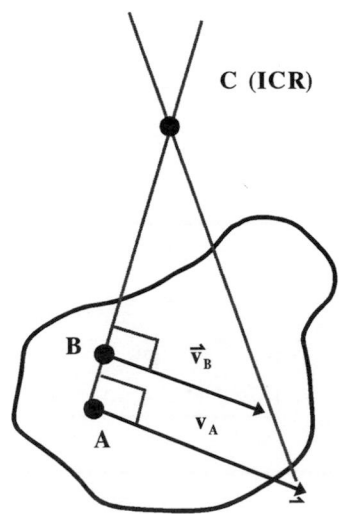

Figure 14-13 Instantaneous center of rotation.

Figure 14-14 Mean center of rotation.

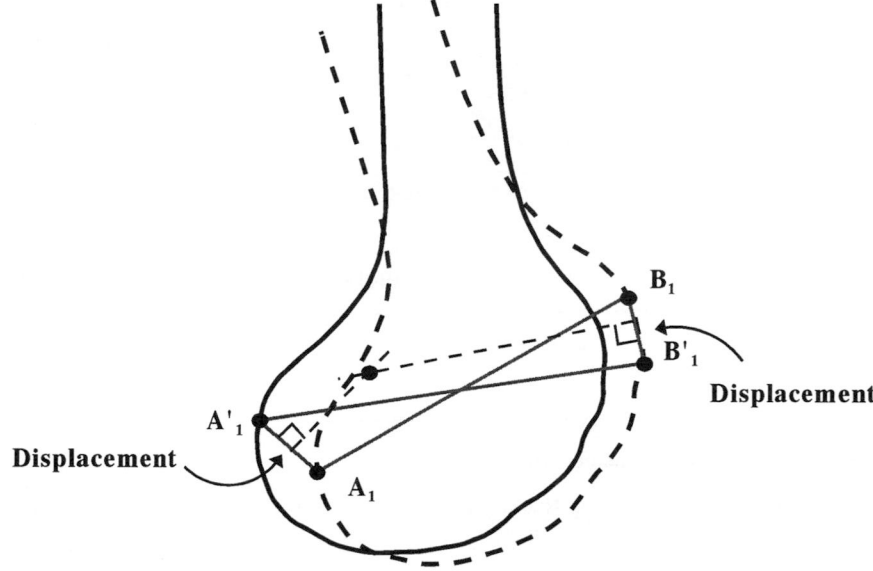

Basic Types of Joint-Articulating Surface Motion

In studying joint kinematics, two types of motion are involved: (1) the *gross joint motion* and (2) the *joint-articulating surface motion*. The gross motion is important in evaluating joint function and calculating the resultant force and moment passing through the joint center under dynamic conditions. The articulating surface motion of a joint can help to describe the precise joint function in terms of relative surface motion, surface contact forces, and the effects of friction and wear on the joint surface materials. There are three basic types of articulating surface motion in anatomic and prosthetic joints:

1. *Sliding motion:* The relative motion between the contact surfaces is a pure translation. If one surface is flat, then the ICR is located at infinity. The contact point on the circular body does not change, while its mating flat surface has a constantly changing contact point.

2. *Spinning motion:* This motion is an exact reverse of the sliding motion; the circular body is rotating and the contact point on the flat surface is unchanged. The ICR in this case is located at the center of the spinning circular body, which is undergoing pure rotation.

3. *Rocking motion (rolling without slip):* In this case, the points of contact on the circular and flat surfaces are constantly changing. The arc length of the circle matches the linear path on the flat surface so that the two surfaces have point-to-point contact without any slip (relative motion). The relative motion of the circle with respect to the flat surface is a combination of translation and rotation. The ICR in this case is located at the contact point of the two surfaces.

These three types of articulating surface motion in human joints are illustrated in Fig. 14-15.

A pure hinge type of joint will exhibit a spinning motion, while most of the anatomic joints are moving according to certain combinations of the three basic types of motion described above. In this case, the ICR will change depending upon the amount of sliding and rocking motion involved. From the friction and wear point of view, the rocking motion is ideal, while the other two types of mo-

Figure 14-15 Articulating surface motion.

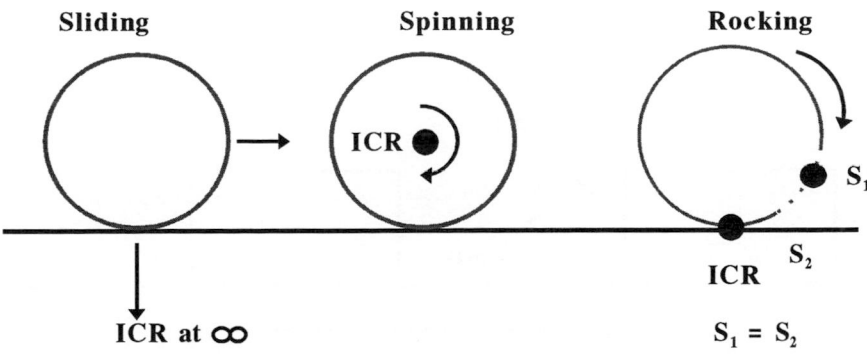

FEMOROTIBIAL ARTICULATING CONTACT

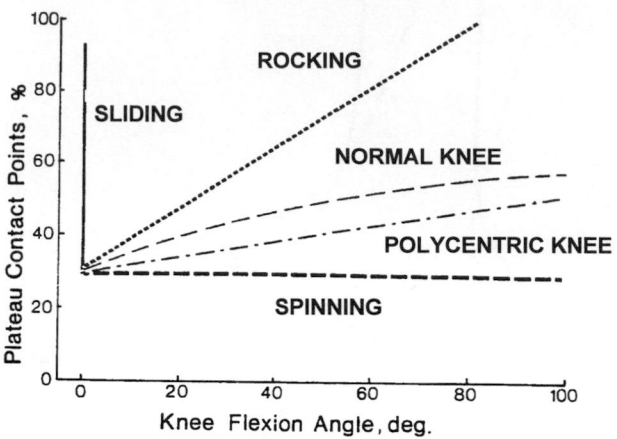

Figure 14-16 Femoral-tibial articulating contact.

tion will cause excessive wear to one or the other articulating surfaces. Using the knee joint as an example, Fig. 14-16 shows different types of motion in terms of plateau contact point change and the knee joint angle.

Basic Concepts in Kinetics

1. Work (W): Product of force along the direction of displacement and the displacement of a rigid body in motion. The unit of work is N-m or lb-in. In the following example, $W = (F \cos \theta) \cdot s$ (Fig. 14-17).
2. Potential energy (E_p): The potential of doing work due to the *position* or *configuration* of the rigid body. If the rigid body is elevated to a height of h from the ground or a spring is stretched x length beyond its neutral position, then the potential energies for both systems are expressed as seen in Fig. 14-18.
3. Kinetic energy (E_k): The amount of work required to stop a moving body at velocity v or to move a body from rest to velocity v is defined as the E_k. If a rigid body has mass of m and velocity of v, its E_k is

$$E_k = \frac{1}{2} mv^2$$

The work done from point 1 to point 2 is equal to the change of E_k provided that no energy is being dissipated through friction (conservative system). This is described as the *work-energy principle*. In a conservative system, the total energy ($E_p + E_k$) of a

body at position 1 is equal to that at position 2. This is described as the *law of conservation of energy*.
4. Power (P): The work done per unit time is called *power*.
5. Momentum (L): The momentum of a body is equal to the product of its mass and velocity: $L = mv$.
6. Impulsive force and impulse: A large force applied to a rigid body through a small period of time is defined as *impulsive force*. The product of impulsive force and the time period is called *impulse*. This concept is useful in studying *impact problems* in biomechanics.
7. Mass moment of inertia (I): An *inertial resistance to rotation* is defined as the mass moment of inertia as opposed to the pure mass, which is a measurement of *resistance to translation*. Mass moment of inertia depends on the *magnitude of the mass* as well as its *geometric distribution*. If mass is distributed far away from the center of rotation, it will have larger I.

Two-Dimensional Kinetic Analysis of Plane Rigid Body

Following Newton's law of motion, an FBD must satisfy the following *equations of motion* (Fig. 14-19):

$$\Sigma F_x = ma_x, \quad \Sigma F_y = ma_y, \quad \Sigma M_G = I\alpha$$

where a_x, a_y = accelerations of the center of mass G along x and y directions
     m = mass of the rigid body
     I_G = mass moment of inertia of the rigid body with respect to the mass center
     α = angular acceleration of the body

The above three equations can be used to calculate the unknown variables (forces or motion) based on the known quantities (forces or motion), similar to the equation of equilibrium in static analysis.

Direct Dynamic Problem and Inverse Dynamic Problem

In the equation of motion, if one knows all the forces and proceeds to determine the resulting rigid body motion, such a process is defined as the direct dynamic problem (DDP). On the other hand, if motion of the rigid body is known through experimental measurements and the objective is to determine the forces causing such motion, this type of problem is defined as the inverse dynamic

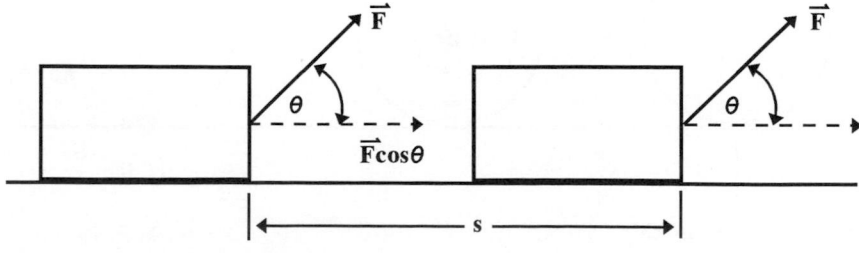

Figure 14-17 Work.

Figure 14-18 Potential energy.

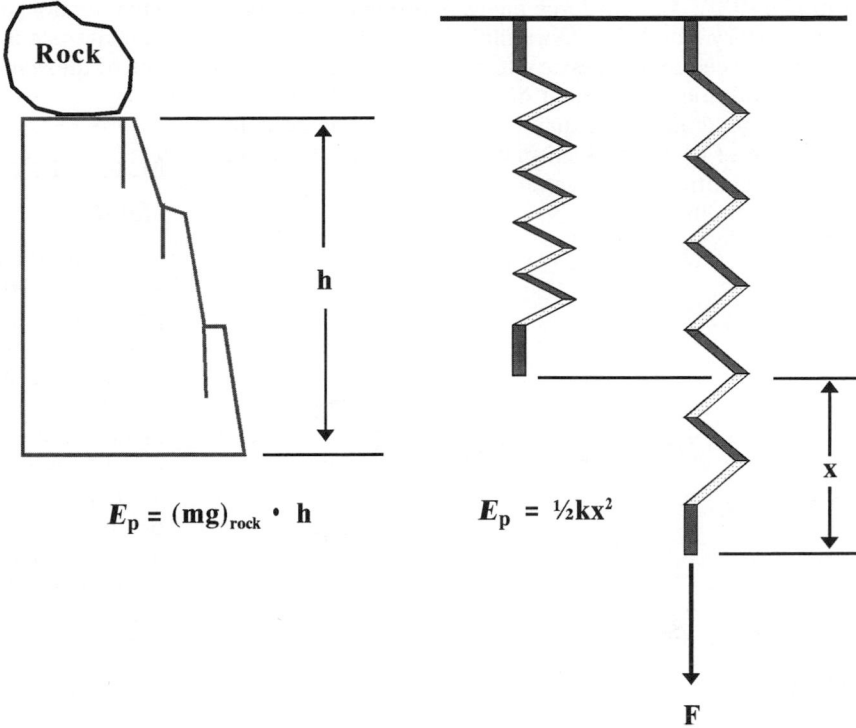

$$E_p = (mg)_{rock} \cdot h \qquad\qquad E_p = \tfrac{1}{2}kx^2$$

Figure 14-19 Kinetic analysis.

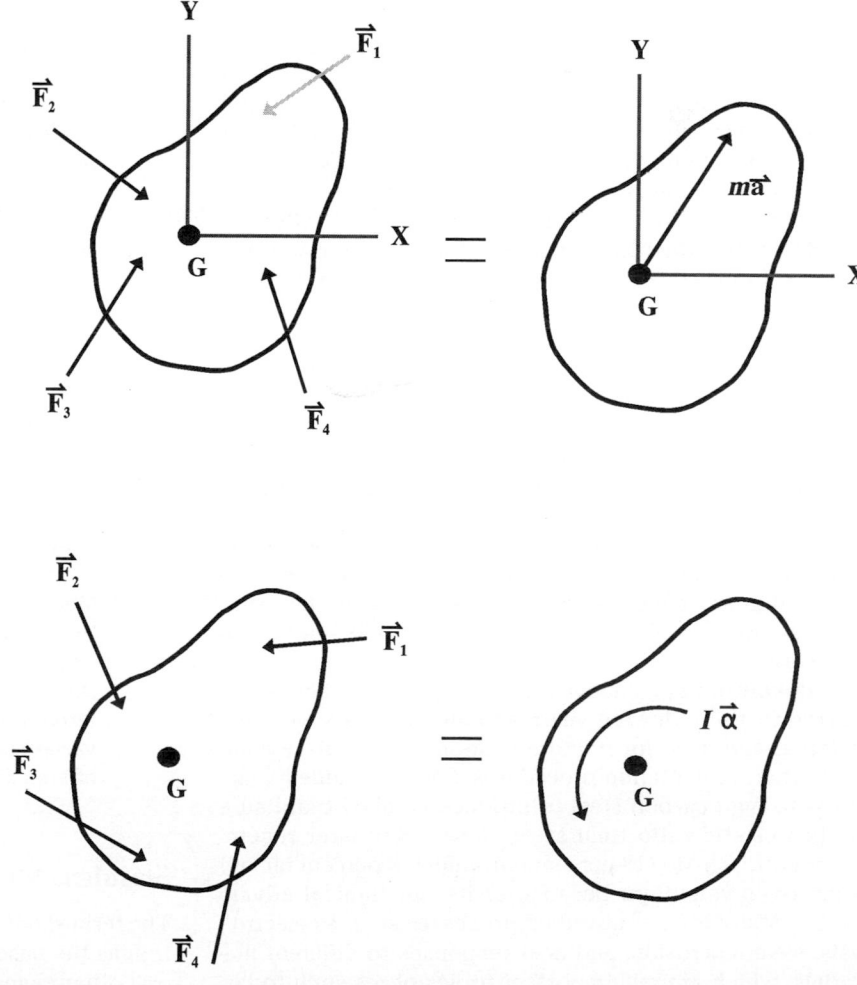

problem (IDP). All joint force analysis problems belong to this category. The IDP is more difficult to solve due to the tedious procedures necessary to measure the system motion. In addition, the number of unknown muscle and joint forces is generally more than the number of the available equations of motion, which makes the system indeterminate. Assumptions and simplifications must be applied in order to obtain solutions.

$$\Sigma F_x = ma_x \qquad \Sigma F_x = ma_x$$
$$\rightarrow \qquad\qquad \leftarrow$$
$$\Sigma F_y = ma_y \qquad \Sigma F_y = ma_y$$
$$\rightarrow \qquad\qquad \leftarrow$$
$$\Sigma M_G = I_G m\alpha \qquad \Sigma M_G = I_G m\alpha$$
$$\rightarrow \qquad\qquad \leftarrow$$
$$\text{DDP} \qquad\qquad \text{IDP}$$

BIOMATERIALS

History

Choosing the best biomaterials for varied clinical situations has long been an important aspect of orthopaedic practice. Even as early as the 1700s, physicians were using biomaterials for the internal fixation of fractures.[1] Icart wrote in 1775 accusing Lapuyade and Sicre, his two colleagues, of causing the death of a patient after fixating a fracture internally with iron wire.[2] Both Levert and Lister made subsequent discoveries about biomechanics and host responses regarding other metals such as silver, gold, platinum, and lead. Levert did tolerance studies with dogs in 1889, from which he concluded that platinum was the least irritating of all the buried sutures he tested.

By the early 1900s, Lane and Lambotte were each having success with the use of metal plates screwed to bone, and this established a new method of internal fracture fixation.[3] Sepsis was a major problem at the time, and Lane began to use an aseptic "no touch" technique, where the surgeon never directly touched the tissues. Instead, he used forceps, clamps, and other instruments.[1] He also believed that the less metal placed into the tissue, the lower the chances of infection. Lambotte made observations regarding the use of different metals and finally recommended gold or nickel-plated soft steel, since the other metals—such as aluminum, silver, and copper—were too malleable.

Revolutionary changes in orthopaedic practice occurred in the following years as new materials were developed and used for fracture fixation, joint replacement, and other implantation procedures. Sherman added vanadium to high carbon steel to produce an alloy that had a higher elastic ratio than steel alone.[1] Key later recommended 18-8 S-Mo (18 percent chromium, 8 percent nickel) steel over vanadium because of its mechanical advantages.[1] Many others described processes such as electrolysis, wear, corrosion, and host responses to different materials, which are still important topics of research today.

This section discusses the properties of contemporary biomaterials and current issues regarding the design and use of these materials in orthopaedic practice.

Material Properties

Metals

Metals are the most widely used orthopaedic biomaterials and are employed in fracture fixation, joint replacement, prosthetics, braces, and other areas of structural need.[4] The most commonly used metals in orthopaedic practice are stainless steel, cobalt-chromium (CoCr), commercially pure (cp) titanium, and titanium alloy. Several of the basic mechanical properties of these and other materials are listed in Table 14-1. The rheological properties of a metal are dependent on its elemental composition and the various processing techniques used in its production. Before discussing specific metals and alloys, it is important to understand the meaning of certain mechanical properties as well as why they are desirable for orthopaedic use. Several of these properties are as follows:

1. The relatively high yield point (when plastic deformation occurs without an increase in the load) of metals allows them to bear relatively high loads without any plastic deformation. The term *plastic deformation* refers to a permanent change in dimension that is unrecoverable with a reduction in load.
2. *Ductility* refers to the ability of a material to be "drawn out" by forces acting parallel to the plane of the material (i.e., tensile force). If a material is relatively ductile, then it will undergo considerable plastic deformation or "necking-down" before breaking.[5] In contrast, brittle materials rupture soon after the elastic limit with little plastic deformation. *Elasticity* is the ability to fully recover from deformation; it denotes a linear relationship between the degree of deformity and the amount of force. The elastic limit is the maximum stress that a metal can sustain before permanent deformation occurs.[1] Metals are ductile enough that stresses exceeding the yield point will produce plastic deformation as opposed to brittle fracture.
3. The plastic nature of metals is such as to allow them to withstand a high number of load/unload cycles, which occur physiologically as materials are used for structural or load-bearing devices.
4. Metals are often affordable and in good supply, and they can be fashioned into many different parts for orthopaedic use. Different techniques of processing (i.e., annealing, cold working, forging, etc.) and different combinations of metals (alloys) provide for a variety of mechanical properties suitable for a range of specific clinical and surgical needs.

Stainless Steel

The term *stainless steel* denotes numerous alloys including iron as the base element, with various proportions of several other elements such as chromium, nickel, and molyb-

TABLE 14-1 Representative Values in MPa (psi) of Biological and Biomaterial Properties

Material	Ultimate strength		Yield strength (0.2% offset) (tension)	Fatigue strength (10^8 cycles)	Modulus of elasticity [b] (Young's—E)	Modulus of rigidity (Shear—G)	Poisson's ratio	Maximum elongation
	Tensile	Compressive						
Muscle	0.2 (30)	NA	NA.	NA	NA	NA	0.49	60%
Skin	8 (1,000)	NA	NA	NA	50 (7,000)	NA	0.49	100%
Cartilage (hyaline)	4 (600)	10 (1,500)	<3 (400)	NA	20 (3,000)	NA	NA	25%
Fascia	10 (1,500)	NA	NA	NA	NA	NA	NA	15%
Tendon [c]	70 (10,000)	NA	NA	NA	400 (60,000)	NA	0.4	10%
Bone, cortical [d]	100 (15,000)	175 (25,000)	80 (12,000)	30 (4,000)	15,000 (2×10^6)	350 (50,000)	0.4	2%
Bone, cancellous (without marrow)	2 (300)	3 (400)	NA	NA	1,000 (150,000)	NA	NA	10%
Plaster of paris	70 (10,000)	75 (11,000)	20 (3,000)	NA	NA	NA	NA	NA
Polyethylene (UHMW—HDP)	40 (6,000)	20 (3,000)	20 (3,000)	NA	1,000 (150,000)	150 (20,000)	0.45	500%
Polytetrafluoroethylene (PTFE—Teflon)	25 (3,500)	NA	NA	NA	500 (70,000)	200 (30,000)	0.4	400%
Acrylic bone cement (PMMA: F-451)	40 (6,000)	80 (12,000)	NA	<15 (2,000)	2,000 (300,000)	1,000 (150,000)	0.4	5%
Polyamide (nylon)	80 (12,000)	NA	NA	NA	3,000 (400,000)	1,000 (150,000)	0.4	50%
Aluminum (annealed, pure)	70 (10,000)	NA	30 (4,000)	NA	70,000 (10×10^6)	25,000 (4×10^6)	0.33	60%
Titanium [e] (cold worked) (pure, F-67)	500 (70,000)	NA	400 (60,000)	250 (35,000)	100,000 (15×10^6)	45,000 (6×10^6)	0.35	15%
Titanium 6A1-4V (alloy: F-136)	900 (130,000)	NA	800 (120,000)	400 (60,000)	100,000 (15×10^6)	NA	NA	10%
Stainless steel (316, 316L) Wrought, annealed (F-55, 56, 138, 139)	>500 (75,000)	NA	>200 (30,000)	250 (35,000)	200,000 (30×10^6)	80,000 (12×10^6)	0.28	40%
Wrought, cold worked (F-55, 56, 138, 139)	>850 (125,000)	NA	>700 (100,000)	300 (40,000)	200,000 (30×10^6)	80,000 (12×10^6)	0.28	15%
Cobalt-chromium alloys Cast (F-75) (Co, Cr, Mo)	>450 (95,000)	NA	>50 (65,000)	300 (40,000)	200,000 (30×10^6)	NA	NA	8%
Wrought, annealed (F-90) (Co, Cr, W, Ni)	>300 (125,000)	NA	>300 (45,000)	NA	230,000 (33×10^6)	NA	NA	50%
Wrought, cold worked (F-90) (Co, Cr, W, Ni)	1,500 (200,000)	NA	1,000 (150,000)	500 (70,000)	230,000 (33×10^6)	NA	NA	10%
"Super alloys" (F562) (wrought, special heat treated, cold working, etc.) (Co, Ni, Cr, Mo, etc.)	1,800 (260,000)	NA	1,600 (230,000)	600 (90,000)	230,000 (33×10^6)	NA	NA	10%

This table gives a composite of values from a variety of sources. Data represent *typical* values rounded to facilitate recall. All materials listed have a wide range of values due to biologic, compositional, or manufacturing process variations. NA indicates that a representative single value is not readily available. For soft tissues, modulus of elasticity represents tangent to the relatively linear portion of the stress-strain curve.

[a] MPa, megapascals = mega (10^6) N/m^2, psi, lbs/in^2. 1 MPa = 145 psi. To convert to psi, multiply MPa value by 145, but values given have been rounded and are *not* exact conversions.

[b] This modulus is more conveniently quoted in gigapascals (10^9) (GPa): 1000 MPa = 1 GPa. Thus E for steel = 200 GPa.

[c] Individual collagen fibers have a much higher tensile strength (3000 MPa).

[d] Like other tissues, bone is anisotropic: values would be *higher* if bone were tested parallel to bone axis (with the grain), lower when tested perpendicular to bone axis (across the grain). Ultimate shear strength of bone is roughly 60 MPa (9000 psi).

[e] For metals, F refers to applicable ASTM standard. Properties of all these alloys depend heavily on the finishing process—annealing, cold working, etc. In metals, maximum elongation usually is determined for a 50.8 mm (2 inch) sample.

denum.[1] Chromium and molybdenum both impart strength and corrosion resistance to the iron-based alloy, while molybdenum also increases the resistance of stainless steel to pitting corrosion and attack by chlorides. It is the chromium that reacts with oxygen to form a protective, stable, passive oxide layer on the surface of the implant.[6] Nickel allows the addition of more chromium and molybdenum, and it serves to lower the tendency of the alloy to harden with cold work.

The three basic classes of stainless steel include *ferritic*, *martensitic*, and *austenitic* steel, and each class is dependent on the appearance of its characteristic phase at room temperature.[4] Ferritic steels have the lowest nickel content and are magnetic. The ferrite state is characterized by the *body-centered* cubic crystalline structure.[5] These permanently ferritic steels have excellent corrosion resistance but poor strength; hence, they are not often employed as surgical steels.[1] Martensitic steels have a transitional strained structure due to a failure to convert completely back to ferrite from austenite on cooling. As opposed to ferrite, martensitic steels are very strong but have little corrosion resistance. Therefore, martensite such as AISI (American Iron and Steel Institute) 420 is favored for use in the production of surgical instruments such as scalpel blades, where strength and hardness are essential.[4] Iron in the austenitic state has a *face-centered* cubic structure that is stabilized at room temperature with the addition of nickel.[5] The austenitic alloys have superior corrosion resistance and good strength, and the addition of molybdenum allows these steels to resist attack within the sea of chloride ions present in the human body.[1]

The stainless steel most commonly used for orthopaedic biomaterials is AISI 316L, which contains 16 to 20 percent chromium, 8 to 17 percent nickel, 2 to 4 percent molybdenum, 60 to 70 percent iron, less than 1 percent carbon, and the remainder a small percentage of manganese, silicon, and other elements.[5] The development of this austenitic steel from earlier alloys such as EV85J, 18-8 S-Mo, and AISI 316 is characterized by progressive improvements in their corrosion-resistant properties.[4] The "L" designation refers to a carbon content below 0.03 percent. A low carbon content allows the formation of strength-enhancing carbides, but these are limited because they are more corrosive in vivo than the alloy matrix itself.

Due to the addition of chromium and molybdenum, stainless steel is generally highly resistant to corrosion. However, stainless steels are very susceptible to cracking from stress corrosion if the exposed surface is under tension for long periods of time while in a corrosive medium such as the chloride solution of the human body.[1] Pitting corrosion is also likely to be due to differential oxygenation between different metal surfaces that touch (i.e., a screw and the implant itself).

The AISI 316L stainless steel (annealed) has a tensile strength of 280 MPa, while cold working yields a tensile strength of 1000 MPa and a fatigue strength of 300 MPa.[7] Although cold working increases strength, ductility drops significantly.

Type 316L stainless steel (annealed) is highly ductile and can be worked to improve strength while sacrificing ductility. It is a highly economical material and is easily fabricated for orthopaedic use. The highly ductile version is a good choice for use in fracture fixation devices due to its ability to remain ductile after large amounts of cold work, while stronger wrought and forged alloys are commonly used in joint replacement components.[4,8] Porous, coated stainless steel components in cementless arthroplasties are not used because of their relatively poor corrosion characteristics.[9]

Cobalt Chrome Alloys

Cobalt-chromium alloys have been used for medical purposes since the 1930s and make up a considerable portion of the orthopaedic implants used today.[8] The original cobalt-chromium alloy was named *stellite,* being a star among metals, and uses a mixture of 25 percent chromium and 75 percent cobalt.[1] *Stellite* is now a generic term for many cobalt-based alloys. These alloys basically have the austenitic phase structure (face-centered cubic), and can undergo a strength-enhancing partial conversion to the martensitic phase.[4]

Two basic types of cobalt-chromium alloys exist: cast and wrought. Casting is the process whereby molten material is poured into molds and allowed to solidify. Cast cobalt-chromium is composed of approximately 60 percent cobalt, 30 percent chromium, 5 percent molybdenum, and 2.5 percent nickel.[5] The ASTM (American Society for Testing and Materials) F-75 is the traditional cast cobalt-chromium alloy and was originally called vitallium.[4] It was strong, relatively brittle, and nearly impossible to machine.[5] Improvements in manufacturing, however, have eliminated many of the problems associated with the cast alloys.

Wrought cobalt-chromium has been worked or work-hardened to change its mechanical properties before fabrication of a component.[4] F-90 is a wrought cobalt-chromium superalloy and is quite strong. It is composed of approximately 50 percent cobalt, 20 percent chromium, 10 percent nickel, and 15 percent tungsten.[5] The addition of tungsten decreases the brittle qualities, while work-hardening imparts strength to the alloy. Like steel, the variable manufacturing of wrought cobalt-chromium makes it available in a wide range of yield strengths, ultimate strengths, and strain to failure. F-562 is another cobalt-chromium alloy and is referred to as MP35N (multiphase, 35 percent Ni). Like wrought cobalt-chromium, MP35N is a superalloy, but it contains approximately 35 percent nickel and no tungsten. It is characterized by strength properties similar to those of other cobalt-based alloys but possesses higher than typical ductility.

Carbon imparts strength in the cobalt-chromium alloys, much as it does in stainless steel, and implants use low carbon alloys.[1] These are strong alloys with high moduli, but their ductility is usually less than that of stainless steel. Cobalt-chromium alloys are more susceptible to work-hardening than AISI 316L, and this intrinsic hardness makes them difficult to machine. Stainless steel is also cheaper, because of the relatively high cost of cobalt and tungsten. However, cast cobalt-chromium is valued for its resistance to corrosion cracking, and it is significantly more resistant to wear than the other metal alloys currently used in total hip replacements.[9] Corrosion resistance, as with stainless steel, is obtained from the passive chromium oxide film on the surface of the implant.[6] It appears that cobalt-chromium alloys are the most corrosion- and fatigue-resistant of all implant alloys; only titanium is more resistant to corrosion.

CP Titanium and Titanium Alloys

Titanium is a readily available element that makes up 0.6 to 0.7 percent of the earth's crust.[1] It is used both in the pure form and as an alloy and is a more recent development in orthopaedic materials science relative to the stainless steel and cobalt-chromium alloys. One of the primary advantages of using titanium for orthopaedic devices is its superior biocompatibility and lack of known immunogenicity.[10–14] It also has superior resistance to corrosive forces as compared to either stainless steel or cobalt-chrome alloys.[7] The corrosion resistance seen in titanium and titanium alloys is once again due to the passive oxide film that is chemically formed on the surface of the implant after exposure to oxygen.[5] The protective oxide coatings on stainless steel and cobalt-chromium alloys are generated as oxygen reacts with the added chromium to form chromium oxides. In contrast, it is the titanium that reacts with oxygen to form stable titanium dioxides on the surface of the implants in clinical use.[9] Thus, the tissue around the implant is exposed to the inert ceramic titanium dioxide surface rather than directly to the titanium metal. This allows titanium and its alloys to be especially resistant to crevice corrosion and stress corrosion cracking.[1]

Commercially pure titanium, also known as ASTM F-67, is composed of approximately 0.03 percent carbon, 0.06 percent oxygen, 0.04 percent nitrogen, and 0.25 percent iron, with the balance (more than 99 percent) being titanium.[1] Commercially pure titanium is manufactured in several grades, and those used primarily for orthopaedic devices have the highest oxygen content.[4] Although considerably weaker than the titanium alloys, cp titanium is remarkably corrosion-resistant and provides excellent osseointegration.[10,15,16] Thus, it seems to have potential for use as a surface coating in some orthopaedic devices.[4] Commercially pure titanium is generally weaker than 316L and cobalt-chromium alloys, but it is easily weldable and machineable, and it can be cold worked to increase strength and hardness.[1]

Titanium alloy Ti-6Al-4V (ASTM F-136) was developed in part because of the inferior qualities of cp titanium.[9] Titanium alloy is composed of approximately 6 percent aluminum, 4 percent vanadium, 0.25 percent iron, 0.03 percent nitrogen, and 0.0125 percent hydrogen, with the balance being titanium.[7] F-136 is stronger than cp titanium, with a higher yield strength; it has been used extensively in other industries such as aerospace design and manufacturing.[4] It is considered a superalloy in view of its tensile strength and corrosion resistance. Titanium alloy is considered a combined α and β alloy because of the presence of an α phase that is stable at high temperatures and a β or martensitic phase that occurs at lower tempera-

tures. The α phase is stabilized by the addition of the aluminum, while vanadium stabilizes the β phase. The relationship of these elements to these phases allows for microstructural manipulation through chemical and heat treatments that provide a range of resultant mechanical properties.

Another advantage with the use of titanium is its lower modulus of elasticity, which is approximately one-third to one-half that of stainless steel and cobalt-chromium.[4,5,7] Low moduli combined with low ductility and relatively high strength make this a relatively brittle alloy. Although the elastic modulus of titanium is still significantly greater than that of cortical bone, stress shielding of the surrounding tissue is less than with the stainless steel and cobalt-chromium alloys.

The significance of this lower elastic modulus is understood after a brief explanation of Wolff's law. It states that bone, whether normal or abnormal, develops the structure most suited to resist the forces acting upon it. Simply put, bone formation occurs along the lines of stress. The arthroplasty-induced reconstruction of diaphyseal bone produces a composite load-sharing system, the result of which is a decrease in the load share or stress transmitted through the bone.[17] When the stress or load on bone is reduced, periprosthetic bone mass is resorbed, leading to lower bone density and decreased stiffness. This process may ultimately contribute to the failure of total joint arthroplasty.

The lower modulus may help to reduce the cortical bone remodeling and osteogenic stress shielding.[9] In comparison to cp titanium, Ti-6Al-4V has superior strength and mechanical properties, with similar resistance to corrosion, and the elastic modulus is essentially unchanged.[18] Concern about the host's biological response to vanadium led to the development of more recent titanium alloys. Ti-5Al-2.5Fe is composed of approximately 5 percent aluminum, 2.5 percent iron, 0.8 percent carbon, 0.2 percent oxygen, and the balance titanium.[4,5] It has increased ductility, which makes this suitable for a wide range of applications because of the ease in fabrication.

Ti-13Nb-13Zr is a more recent, lower-modulus alloy that possesses strength and toughness properties comparable to those of the existing Ti-6Al-4V.[19] However, it does not contain any elements associated with adverse cell responses (i.e., Co, Cr, Mo, Ni, Fe, Al, V). This biocompatible alloy seems well suited for press-fit hip replacement applications, but it is also easier to forge into more complex stem designs.

Ceramics

The Greek root of the word ceramic is *keramo*, which means "burnt stuff," referring generally to pottery.[4] Ceramics represent a poorly defined class of composite substances that are basically made up of dense, randomly oriented masses of crystal.[5] They are nonmetallic materials that can be characterized as either *bioactive* or *inorganic*. Bioactive materials, according to a 1986 Consensus Conference held at the European Society of Biomaterials, are materials which have been designed to induce specific biological activity.[9,20–23] Bioactive ceramics include bioactive glasses such as silicon dioxide (SiO_2) and calcium phosphate ceramics (i.e., hydroxyapatite, tricalcium phosphate, and fluorapatite).[9,20] Alumina (Al_2O_3) and zirconia (ZrO_2) are examples of inorganic oxide ceramics. Both are used as components of implantable orthopaedic devices. Ceramics include very few class-characteristic qualities, but as a whole they are stiff, hard, brittle, and water-insoluble; they lack ductility and are highly resistant to compressive forces.

The use of hydroxyapatite (HA) in orthopaedic applications has grown dramatically over the last decade. As a bioactive ceramic, HA has been used as a coating to enhance bony ingrowth into prosthetic devices, resulting in osseointegration and direct bonding to bone without any unmineralized tissue layer at the HA-bone interface.[9,20,24–31] It is predominantly used at this time in cementless total hip arthroplasty as a coating on the surface of the implant.[6,9,24–30] This serves to enhance bone tissue formation around and into the prosthetic surface and to establish a mechanical anchoring of the implant.[28]

Hydroxyapatite has been shown in numerous studies to be nontoxic, noninflammatory, and biocompatible because it is considered to be a physiologic component of bone closely associated with collagen.[4,9,32–46] *Apatite* is a term that generally refers to a family of structurally related compounds including HA, fluorapatite, chlorapatite, and others.[47] The "deception" and confusion surrounding the early investigation of HA is evidenced by the Greek derivation of the term *apatite*, which means "to deceive."[48]

Calcium phosphate ceramics are also utilized as bulk material or granules to promote osteoconduction into gaps and deficiencies between bone.[32,48] The brittle nature of bioactive ceramics dictates that they be used in applications such as granular bone filler (e.g., ear, nose, and throat implants, replacement of hearing ossicles, etc.), where loads are limited to purely compressive forces.[49,50]

As calcium hydroxyapatite, HA has the chemical formula $Ca_{10}(PO_4)_6(OH)_2$.[9,32] The Ca/P ratio is 1.67, but the ratio of HA-type materials may be as low as 1.5.[4,9] Tricalcium phosphate (TCP) is formed by the precipitation of HA, and contact with water autocatalytically transforms it back to HA.[48,51] Tricalcium phosphate appears to have less osteogenic potential than HA, and it is less stable.[52,53] It is thought that the presence of TCP in the HA coating contributes to increased resorption.[9] Fluorapatite (FA) [$Ca_5(PO_4)_3F$] has been used experimentally and is able to bond directly with bone.[20] However, FA-coated titanium implants have been found to have less bone contact than those with HA coatings, resulting in lower tensile strength values for the FA-coated implants.[20] At this time, HA is the preferred choice to provide an osteoconductive coating on metal implants.

The plasma spray technique for HA that was first described by de Groot et al.[38] in the 1980s made it possible for HA to be utilized as a coating for implants, with the high mechanical requirements needed for total joint arthroplasty.[9] Hydroxyapatite plasma spray occurs as HA particles are injected into a high-temperature (15,000°C) plasma tail flame and solidify on impact with the metal substrate. The quality of the HA coating is dependent on many factors, such as Ca/P ratio, purity, crystallinity, and variables in the velocity and heat content of the plasma flame.[24,54] The behavior of the coating is dependent on its quality, microstructure, adhesive strength relative to the implant, porosity, and thickness.[9]

The probability of finding defects is reduced with decreasing thickness of the coating.[24] Thus, the mechanical properties of the coating are inversely proportional to its thickness. Thicker HA coatings have inferior properties regarding toughness and fatigue resistance. Approximately 15 μm of the HA coating is lost within the first year, prior to the stabilization that occurs as bone covers the surface of the implant.[55] Although coatings as thin as 1 μm have been made, 50 to 75 μm coatings are most widely used due to the relatively low risk of HA fracture and preservation of the porosity of the implant surface.[24,38,56,41] The porous surface must not be "filled in" by too thick a coating, since it is believed that the prosthesis bears the body weight primarily through the porous layer.[25]

The osteoconductive properties of the calcium-phosphate ceramics are used in applications beyond that of coating implant surfaces. Bulk supplies of HA available in porous or dense forms are used to fill gaps between the bone and prosthesis[57] and serve to fill bone defects.[32] Maruyama has recently used granulated HA and sodium alginate to develop HA clay that is easily handled and able to fill any irregular gap.[32,54]

The use of HA-coated porous implants has allowed the maximum interface shear strength to be reached in half the time compared to porous implants without HA coating.[37,58,59] Other factors governing the osteoconductive potential of these implants include the ability to achieve a static fit with minimal movement at the HA-bone interface and the gap size between the bone and the prosthesis.[32,60–63] Although ingrowth may be achieved under conditions of micromotion, bone apposition and initial implant fixation occur more rapidly when the implant is well fixed with little or no gap at the HA-bone interface.[32,63,64] It is possible to achieve surface ongrowth of 60 to 80 percent of the available surface of femoral stems when these conditions are met.[24]

Aluminum oxide and zirconium oxide are inorganic materials known as oxide ceramics. These bioinert compounds are fully stable,[65–68] and their use in orthopaedics is rising due to their great strength and superior hardness.[6] They are primarily used as femoral heads in total hip arthroplasty, and a ceramic ball on the stem combined with a conventional polyethylene socket is now available in most hip systems.[9,69] This combination is used due to the reduced friction and favorable wear behavior of ceramic-polyethylene surfaces in comparison to those of metal-polyethylene combinations.[70] Oxide ceramics have not been widely used in the knee, partly because of the high cost of manufacturing the ceramic-knee femoral component.[69] As late as 1988, only one clinical series reported routine use of ceramic components in total knee arthroplasty.[71] However, recent developments in ceramic materials and the formation of hard ceramic surfaces on metals have increased the use of ceramic-knee femoral components.[72]

It is well known that the rate of polyethylene debris production in total hip arthroplasty can be reduced by using more wettable materials (better able to maintain lubricant on the surface) for the articular surface of the femoral component.[6,69,70,73–77] The intrinsic hardness of these materials makes them abrasion-resistant and allows them to maintain their polished surface finish in the presence of polymethylmethacrylate (PMMA) or bone debris.[78–80] Ceramic surfaces also have less than half the friction relative to metals in articulation with ultrahigh-molecular-weight polyethylene (UHMWPE).[73,81] This decreases the levels of torque on the acetabular cup and may decrease the incidence of loosening.[6]

Another aspect of wear reduction with oxide ceramics is the reduced amount of adhesive wear compared to the alloys.[82] The metals and alloys previously discussed have a protective, passive, oxide film on the implant surface that is formed as chromium or titanium reacts with oxygen.[6] Although these surface films form extremely quickly (nanoseconds), they can be sheared off, adhering to the opposing UHMWPE surface and resulting in transfer of the passivated layer to the polymer.[81] This loss of the protective film to the opposing surface leaves the metal surface temporarily exposed to the environment and allows metal ions to be released locally. The constant loss and reforming of the passive film that occurs with hip motion provides a continuous source of "polishing powder" that accelerates the roughening process of the articular surfaces. The end result is the development of three-body wear, with the oxide film as the third body, and increased surface roughness as metal is consumed from oxidative wear. Oxide ceramics do not have this passive, oxide type of film and thus can be expected to have less long-term wear than metal surfaces.

Zirconia and alumina are presently available as the bore (female portion) of the Morse taper in modular components.[81] This eliminates the electrochemical corrosion that occurs with the use of a cobalt-chrome bore in contact with a trunion (male portion) made of titanium alloy. However, the metal trunion may still undergo corrosion due to differential oxygen concentrations at the trunion-bone interface as compared with the outside of the prosthesis. The superior strength of zirconia (versus alumina) does not negate the great importance of correctly matching the bores to the trunions when either of the oxide ceramics is used. This can be especially difficult at the time of revision, and it is necessary that products from different manufacturers not be mixed, as dissociation may occur. Friedman et al.[81] have discussed the need to standardize Morse tapers within the orthopaedic industry. They also report that the FDA has suggested standard dimensions for these components in order to prevent excessive hoop stresses, which may cause catastrophic failure.

Polymers

Synthetic polymers and polymer-based composites are among the most rapidly expanding areas of modern materials science.[4] These ubiquitous materials are as well known as plastics, but they may be more generally defined as chemical compounds formed by the joining of smaller, repeating structural units known as monomers. Polymer molecules are named according to their monomeric derivatives, and most monomers exist as gases or low-viscosity liquids. Polymethylmethacrylate is used in bone cement, and UHMWPE is predominantly employed as a bearing surface in total joint arthroplasty, and these are the most widely used in clinical practice (Table 14-2).

A polymer chain is not unlike a string of pearls. Polymerization is the process whereby each monomer, or "pearl," is added to the growing chain. This occurs by two different mechanisms, *addition* and *condensation* polymerization. Addition polymers are formed as monomers combine, without the formation of any other products. Addition polymerization is primarily used to produce linear or simply branched molecules.[4] Polymers formed by addition include polyethylene, PMMA, polystyrene, and polyvinyl chloride. Condensation polymerization produces interlocking networks formed by the reaction of smaller, dissimilar molecules. As the polymer forms, simple compounds such as water are eliminated (condensation). These materials (e.g., nylon, Dacron) are relatively unaffected by temperature change and may be referred to as *thermoset* polymers. The physical properties of *thermoplastic* (addition) polymers, however, are greatly dependent on temperature. Thermoplastic materials are more widely used in clinical orthopaedics.

TABLE 14-2 Monomers and Polymers

Monomer	Polymer	Application
Ethylene	Polyethylene	Bearing of surface components in joint arthroplasty
Vinyl chloride	Polyvinyl chloride	Tubing for blood and infusion sets
Methyl methacrylate	Polymethylmethacrylate	Bone cement
Dichlorodiphenyl sulfone	Polysulfone	Fabrication of composites
Dimethylsiloxane	Polydimethylsiloxane	"Silicone rubber," fabrication of PIP and MCP joint prostheses

Key: PIP = proximal interphalangeal; MCP = metacarpophalangeal.

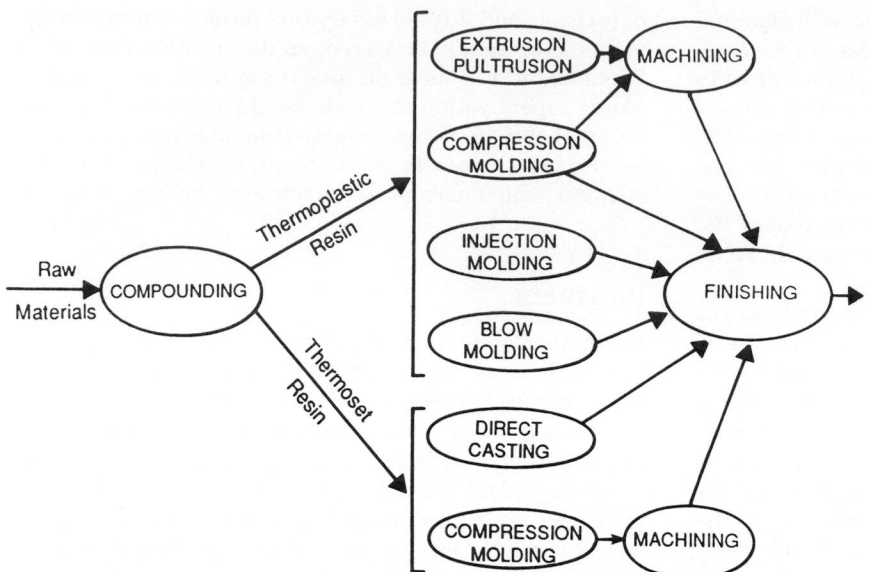

Figure 14-20 Manufacture and processing of polymers.

Polymer fabrication begins with formation of the basic polymer compound, resulting in a *resin* material. Different types of molding procedures (i.e., injection, compression, and blow molding) are used preferentially to machining, and direct casting is additionally used for thermoset resins (Fig. 14-20). Before finishing the polymer, cross-linking may be necessary to enhance the wear-resistant properties of the material surface.

The behavioral characteristics of polymers may be described as *glassy, leathery, rubbery,* and *viscous* (Fig. 14-21). Below the glass transition temperature (T_G), even amorphous polymers are brittle and behave much like ceramics or metals. Leathery polymers exhibit slowly recoverable deformations, and these exist at temperatures just above the T_G. More rapid recovery defines the elastic or rubbery behavior of polymers. The melting point (T_M) is the temperature at which the polymer creeps irreversibly under the force of gravity. A second, rapid drop in the

modulus occurs near the T_M, and the polymer then behaves as a viscous fluid.

Creep is related to the viscous behavior of polymers and is defined as slow, continuous deformation over time.[5] Unlike plastic deformations, which recover, viscous deformation remains when the load is removed. Thus, creep is a continuous wear process, and it contributes significantly to the loss of polyethylene thickness in acetabular components. *Crazing* refers to the production of fine networks of cracks on a material surface. This fatigue or stress cracking may cause material failure. Polymers such as UHMWPE are particularly prone to creep and crazing, and this must be considered in the design and fabrication of orthopaedic devices using these materials.

Polymethylmethacrylate

Primarily used as a bone cement in orthopaedic applications, PMMA provides mechanical fixation and load distribution between host tissues and prosthetic devices. The fixative mechanism of PMMA rests in the ability of this polymer to form an interlocking network between irregularities in the bone and implant surface.[5] The term *cement* refers to this mechanical anchoring between the two substrates and should not imply any adhesive character. In fact, PMMA adheres poorly to most surfaces, including old bone cement.[4]

The first significant use of PMMA bone cement for orthopaedic implant fixation is credited to Sir John Charnley in the early 1960s.[83] Charnley described the ability of the cement to produce gradual load transmission to the femoral shaft, which resulted in greatly increased load-bearing capacity of the femoral prosthesis.[84] This revolutionary development led to dramatic improvements in the short-term relief of pain and disability but increased the long-term rate of mechanical loosening in young patients and those with rheumatoid arthritis.[85–91]

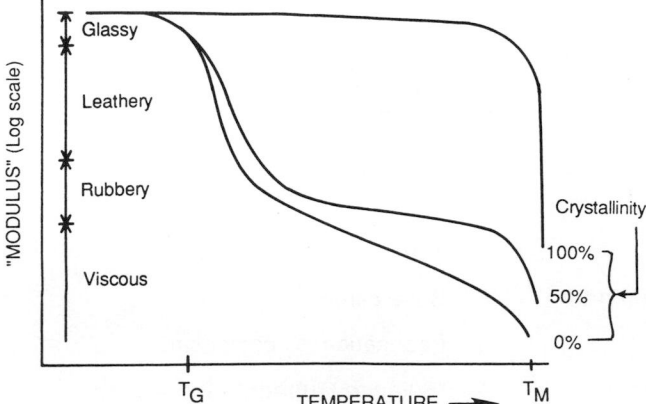

Figure 14-21 Temperature dependence of polymer modulus.

The typical PMMA bone cement used in orthopaedic procedures is produced by mixing a dry and a liquid component. The liquid usually contains an initiator and one or more stabilizers to prevent premature polymerization; the balance is methylmethacrylate monomer. The dry component is usually 10 weight percent barium sulfate ($BaSO_4$), with the remainder consisting of microspherical PMMA powder and a small amount of free radical source. The addition of $BaSO_4$ makes this a radiopaque material. A more recent development is the addition of antibiotics to the dry component in order to prevent and treat infection after total joint arthroplasty.

Curing is the polymerization process that occurs when the dry and liquid components are combined. This forms long-chain polymers that are essentially linear and relatively free of cross linking. The mixing process affects the absolute porosity of the material and may lead to variations in the mechanical properties of a certain "batch" of cement. Whereas the introduction of air that occurs with rapid mixing increases porosity, treatments such as centrifugation and vacuum mixing of the powder greatly decrease porosity and may improve the fatigue life of the bone cement. The curing process may be characterized by the following time periods:

1. *Dough time* begins at the point when the bone cement mixture will not stick to unpowdered surgical gloves. This occurs approximately 2 to 3 min after the beginning of mixing for most PMMA cements.

2. The polymerization process is an exothermic chemical reaction that liberates 12 to 14 kcal/100 g of typical bone cement. *Setting time* is the period measured from the beginning of mixture until the surface temperature of the dough mass is one-half its maximum value. This is typically 8 to 10 min.

3. The *working time* represents the difference between the setting and dough times, and it roughly estimates the period during which a specific batch of cement may be used.

Although PMMA provides significant initial implant fixation, long-term loosening remains a major concern.[92,93] Thermal damage to surrounding bone during polymerization may ultimately contribute to loosening and subsequent implant failure.[94,95] Newer cements with a lower curing temperature may increase the long-term survival of these implants.[96–99] Recently developed hydroxyapatite composite resin shows promise for future improvements in bone cement materials.[100] This new material possesses superior mechanical and biological properties to PMMA cement and allows bone ingrowth comparable to that of hydroxyapatite.[100]

Despite recent advances, PMMA-based cements remain the gold standard for fixation of prostheses used in cemented total joint arthroplasty. No substitute exists for good operative technique, and controllable factors may be the most important for long-term joint stability (Table 14-3).

TABLE 14-3   Factors in Optimizing Bone Cement (BC) Strength

Factors	Outcome
Uncontrollable factors	
Aging	Gradual 10% loss of strength resulting from postcuring chemical changes
Environmental temperature	10% weaker at body temperature than at room temperature
Fatigue	Fatigue strength (10^6 cycles) 20–25% of single-cycle strength
Moisture content	Loss of 3–10% strength due to water absorption
Strain rate	Significant increase in strength with increasing strain rate
Partially controllable factors	
Cement thickness	Important; "intermediate" BC thicknesses minimize both fatigue stresses and shrinkage effects
Constraint	Significant; BCs far stronger in compression than in tension
Inclusion of blood or tissue	Considerable effect; up to 70% loss of strength, depending on amount
Stress risers (bony bed, prosthesis)	Significant; BCs are quite notch sensitive
Fully controllable factors	
Antibiotic inclusion	5–10% loss of strength
Centrifugation/vacuum degassing	10–25% increase in strength, possible increase in fatigue strength
Insertion	Delay may produce up to 40% loss of strength, whereas pressurization increases strength by up to 20% by reduction of porosity
Mixing speed	Up to 21% loss of strength due to too slow or too rapid mixing
Radiopaque fillers	5% weaker than unfilled

Note: "strength," "fatigue strength" are in tension; behavior in compression is different and less sensitive to external conditions.

(Adapted from Lee AJC, Ling RSM, Vangala SS: Some clinically relevant variables affecting the mechanical behavior of bone cement. *Arch Orthop Traumat Surg* 92:1–18, 1978.)

Ultrahigh-Molecular-Weight Polyethylene (UHMWPE)

Low-friction arthroplasty was the term Charnley first used to describe his original total hip arthroplasty utilizing a metal-polymer interface.[84] The polymer was poly(fluoroethylene), and it was soon replaced by UHMWPE after failure due to relatively rapid wear and exuberant foreign-body response.[4] As a newer, linear polymer, UHMWPE has widespread uses as a bearing surface in joint replacement. Most commonly employed in total hip replacement as an all-polyethylene or metal-backed modular component for the acetabulum, it is also used in total knee, total shoulder, and total elbow arthroplasty. The ultrahigh molecular weight of this polymer is obtained by polymerization with metallic catalysts at low pressure until molecular weights of 1×10^7 are reached.

Very ductile relative to metals, UHMWPE has a modulus of elasticity less than one-tenth that of bone.[5] Although it is presently the best polymer for load-bearing surfaces in metal-polymer pairs, there is need for significant improvement in the biomechanical properties pertaining to its wear.

Mention was previously made of the relatively high susceptibility of polyethylene materials to creep and fatigue cracking (crazing). These components are highly prone to abrasive wear also, and a great deal of literature has been devoted to polyethylene wear, wear debris, and the host response to this debris. Surface wear is commonly seen in polyethylene components retrieved at autopsy and revision arthroplasty.[101-103] The many factors that contribute to polyethylene failure include articular geometry, joint alignment, femoral component bearing-surface material, manufacturing processes, modularity, material quality and thickness, third-body wear debris, patient weight and activity level, and surgical technique, to name a few. One of the most important of these factors pertaining to design criteria for minimizing applied stresses is UHMWPE thickness—the thicker the better.[104]

Polyethylene wear debris is associated with destructive inflammatory processes, bursitis and bursal distension,[105-111] osteolysis,[81,109,112-115] bone resorption,[116,117] loosening,[116-121] and arthroplasty failure.[104] Debris production occurs primarily from direct, abrasive articulation with the opposing metal bearing surface, third-body wear, and adhesive wear. The PMMA cement, bone fragments, and metallic debris[69] act as a *third body,* which concentrates stress and secondarily increases the wear rate.[81] *Abrasive wear* is related to the hardness and roughness of opposing surfaces and is dependent on the contact stress between them. The roughness R may be expressed as the average roughness R_a, peak roughness R_{max}, or root mean square roughness R_{rms},[122] but controversy exists as to which measurement best predicts minimum wear.

Hardness enables a surface to remain smooth,[123] and treatments such as ion implantation and nitriding are available to increase the hardness of metal surfaces. Thus, maintenance of a smooth, hard metal surface will logically reduce the rate of wear in the opposing polyethylene surface.

Adhesive wear also affects UHMWPE surfaces and acts by two primary mechanisms. As polyethylene articulates with the opposing surface, it is transferred to the metal, with subsequent shearing of this layer into the joint space. Also, the previously mentioned passive oxide layer on the opposing metal surface may adhere to the UHMWPE. This adhesion eventually results in free metal oxide third bodies that subsequently roughen the metal surface.

The biomechanical properties of UHMWPE make it an excellent choice for an articulating surface in total joint arthroplasty. This has been the material of choice for acetabular bearing surfaces in total hip arthroplasty and tibial bearing surfaces in total knee arthroplasty. However, polyethylene appears to be the weakest link of the implantable materials in these joint arthroplasties. Although newer femoral head components such as alumina and zirconia reduce the wear associated with polyethylene, improvement in the polymer material is essential to make more significant gains in the in vivo survival of these prostheses.

Bioabsorbable Materials

Bioabsorbable materials for bone repair were employed in the late 1960s for mandibular and maxillofacial surgery as implantable rods and pins.[124,125] Screws and plates became available in the next decade, but these were not strong enough for orthopaedic use.[126] Subsequent advances in polymer chemistry yielded materials that are currently used for the internal fixation of many fractures and osteotomies.

The terminology surrounding the use of these materials can be misleading. Terms such as *bioabsorption, bioresorption,* and *biodegradation* are often used to refer to these resorbable polymers. *Biodegradation* should be reserved for the description of cell-mediated effects that would not occur in the same conditions in the absence of cellular activity (i.e., enzymatic degradation). *Bioresorption* and *bioabsorption* usually refer to the physiochemical processes that direct the dissolution of these materials.

A number of bioabsorbable polymers are currently used; they are chemically known as alpha polyesters.[126] The most common polyesters in orthopaedic use are poly-glycolic acid (PGA), polyparadioxanone (PDS), polylactic acid (PLA), and a copolymer of PGA/PLA. Both PGA and PLA are discussed further in order to introduce the properties of bioabsorbable materials used in orthopaedic practice.

Bioabsorbable implants are designed to maintain proximity between tissues (soft tissue/bone or bone/bone) while facilitating their long-term stability through regrowth and attachment.[127] Speer and Warren suggest the following basic criteria for the development of bioabsorbable implants:

1. The implant must have adequate strength of initial fixation to coapt the tissues together.
2. The bioabsorption profile of the material must allow it to maintain satisfactory strength while the healing tissues are regaining mechanical stability.
3. Bioabsorption must not proceed too slowly or the implant may perform as its metal counterpart, with fracture and migration.

4. The materials must be completely safe—not toxic, immunogenic, pyrogenic, or carcinogenic.

The most widely used bioabsorbable material in orthopaedic applications is PGA. The polygluconate copolymer tack used in one study was composed of approximately 67.5 percent glycolide (CH_2COOCH_2COO) and 32.5 percent trimethylene carbonate ($CH_2CH_2CH_2OCOO$).[127] This substance has not been found to be antigenic, pyrogenic, carcinogenic, teratogenic, or systemically toxic. It is degraded by hydrolysis of the ester bonds, without any need of passive or active degradation from host tissues. The absorption profile of PGA is such that most of its strength is lost on the order of weeks. This may be a benefit over the longer-acting copolymers such as PLA, since PGA implants are less likely to act as loose bodies if breakage occurs.

Both PLA and its stereoisomer, poly-levo lactic acid (PLLA), have the longest half lives, at 6 months. The former is also degraded by hydrolytic depolymerization,[128] and the lactic acid metabolite then enters the Cori cycle, where it is converted to a more usable carbohydrate.

Although PGA is more widely used as a bioabsorbable material in orthopaedics, its use is associated with sterile sinus formation in up to 25 percent of patients receiving implants.[129] This complication is unique to bioabsorbable implants and occurs as the partially degraded polymer is extruded through the skin after the surgical site has healed.[130] The metabolites cannot be cleared before they trigger a foreign-body reaction.[17] Hence, a sterile sinus forms.

In comparison to metals and other materials, bioabsorbable implants are relatively new to the field of orthopaedics. These materials are finding use in the fixation of soft tissue to bone and for internal fixation of fractures and osteotomies. The lack of initial fixation strength compared to metal components requires stricter immobilization until the tissues regain stability.[127] Future developments should aim to provide stronger materials, reduced local toxicity, and bioabsorption profiles compatible with the rate of tissue healing.

Processes Affecting Orthopaedic Materials

Nitriding and Ion Implantation

Nitriding and *ion implantation* are two processes used to enhance the surface hardness of several alloys employed in orthopaedic materials. Nitriding is the general process whereby the surface of materials is modified by reaction with nitrogen to form nitrides on the surface of the metal. This occurs specifically as steel or titanium alloys have a portion of their surface (iron or titanium, respectively) converted to nitrides by reaction with gaseous ammonia or molten potassium cyanate at elevated temperatures. The resultant implantation of nitrogen ions approximately 0.1 μm into the surface of the metal causes local atomic strain, which hardens the surface.[81]

Nitriding produces remarkable increases in surface hardness, as evidenced by the greater than twofold increase in the surface hardness of Ti-6Al-4V (Table 14-4).[81,122] This process also imparts a golden color to titanium. The bene-

TABLE 14-4 Hardness of Different Surfaces Which Articulate Against UHMWPE in Joint Replacement

Material	Surface hardness
Ti-6Al-4V	330
Cobalt-chromium alloy	400
Nitrogen ion-implanted Ti-6Al-4V	770
Zirconia	1430

fits of surface hardening are primarily related to the decrease in abrasive wear, as the treated material maintains its smooth, polished surface for a longer period of time.[131]

Ion implantation also increases the durability of metal surfaces.[9] This process is a result of the direct implantation of ionized species from the gaseous phase, which occurs as the surface of the metal is bombarded with ions at high velocity that penetrate and rest in the lattice of the metal itself. Ion implantation of the articulating surfaces of implants has been shown to reduce the wear rate[132] and corrosion wear[133] of these surfaces.

Corrosion

Corrosion is the metal-releasing reaction that results in solution equilibrium concentrations of metal-bearing ions greater than 10^{-6} M. *Immunity* is the resistance to corrosion that occurs when the surface of the metal does not have enough free energy to initiate significant reaction with an electrolyte. The concentration of metal ions in solution around immune metals will by definition be less than 10^{-6} M. As previously discussed with metals, *passivation* is the process in which an oxide or hydroxide layer forms on the surface of the implant as chromium or titanium reacts with oxygen. Passivation is actually a brief period of corrosion where metal is consumed. This thin oxide film mechanically separates the metal from the surrounding environment.

Uniform attack is the most common type of corrosion and occurs with all metals in electrolyte solution. Galvanic current is not required because the solution itself corrodes the metal. Thus, all metals experience a finite rate of corrosion in vivo.

Galvanic or *bimetallic corrosion* continues to be a factor in orthopaedic practice, especially with the advent of modular components and other applications where dissimilar metals are used in close proximity to each other. This process requires the following physical conditions:

1. Two different metals or two areas on the same metal that exist at different energy levels
2. Electronic conduction between the two metals, either through the metal or through a connecting wire
3. Ionic conduction through a bathing solution of free ions

TABLE 14-5   Effects of Mixed Metals on Corrosion Rates

Pair	Result
Stainless steel/carbon	Increased stainless steel corrosion
Stainless steel/cobalt-base	Increased stainless steel corrosion
Cobalt-base (cast)/cobalt-base (forged)	No effect
Cobalt-base/titanium-base	No significant effect
Cobalt-base/carbon	No significant effect
Titanium-base/carbon	No effect

Oxidation occurs at the anode (metal with higher free energy) and is corrosive. The cathode is considered immune. Although it is good policy to avoid using dissimilar metals together, the only absolute contraindication is the use of a stainless steel component with other metals (Table 14-5).

Crevice corrosion occurs in a crevice or crack and is characterized by oxygen depletion. This sets up an oxygen gradient and a resultant difference in free energy. These areas are in the crevices between implanted parts, such as a screw head and an acetabular cup, or in the microcracks that form from incomplete fatigue failure. The presence of chloride ions accelerates this process. Thus, certain materials in vivo undergo a significant amount of crevice corrosion due to the presence of chloride ions in the body. Stainless steel is the most susceptible, and cobalt-based alloys are only mildly prone to this corrosive process. Titanium-based alloys are relatively protected from crevice corrosion.

Pitting corrosion is similar to crevice corrosion, but the attack is more isolated and symmetrical. The presence of chlorides accelerates the process, but the oxygen depletion and static conditions associated with crevice corrosion seem less important. Pitting may be initiated by inclusions or scratches, and the pits may occur in large numbers along a defect or damaged area. As with crevice corrosion, the presence of molybdenum in an alloy increases its resistance to attack by chlorides. Pitting is especially detrimental to highly stressed implants, as the pits serve as points of stress concentration, which may lead to fatigue failure. The once common pitting of stainless steel implants has been greatly reduced with the use of more advanced manufacturing processes such as vacuum melting and remelting. Again, the cobalt-chrome alloys are moderately resistant, and this process is rare in titanium-based implants.

The increase in the chemical activity of metals that results from tensile stress may lead to *stress corrosion* and *cracking*. For example, electrochemical potential is generated between the convex and concave surfaces of a fracture plate that is flexed. The convex surface behaves as the anode, and the rate of corrosion is accelerated in this area. The continued stress may cause rapid growth of the cracks, and they extend between the grains. This process could lead to rapid failure of the implant.

Fretting results from fine, abrasive movements between components that serve to physically remove the passivating layer and then metal ions. This may occur be-tween a screw head and a poorly fixed acetabular cup or fracture fixation plate. Fretting corrosion may progress rapidly as the passivated layer forms and reforms. Although less symmetrical, the physical damage from fretting resembles that of pitting corrosion. The serum proteins that increase the rate of uniform attack appear to reduce the rate of fretting corrosion.

Another corrosive process is galvanic in nature and is related to the granular structure of the metal or alloy. Grains are regions of continuous structure, and the disordered areas between them are the grain boundaries. These two regions are often composed of different materials, resulting in the formation of a galvanic cell. The cathodic behavior of the grain boundaries renders them immune, while the grain surface becomes corroded. Hence, *intergranular corrosion* refers to this process, which occurs because of the differing free energies along the crystal planes within the material. This may be enhanced by stresses that serve to accentuate the differing zones of activity within a material. Alloys are infinitely more susceptible than metals to intergranular corrosion, but any level of impurity predisposes a metal to this process.

The last two types of corrosion also contain a galvanic element. They include *leaching* and *inclusion corrosion*. Leaching is similar to intergranular corrosion, but is the result of electrochemical differences within, rather than between, the grains themselves. This may also be considered an *intra*granular corrosive process, and it has increased activity in the multiphase alloys. Although few of these alloys are used in orthopaedic practice, MP35N is an exception. This cobalt-chrome superalloy has proven to be quite corrosion resistant in vivo. However, the relatively high rate of nickel release has limited its clinical use.

Inclusion corrosion occurs when impurities are left in the surface of cast materials. The inclusion acts as a cathode and allows galvanic corrosion at the interface surface of the implant. Pitting may occur if the inclusion is released from the metal surface. As with pitting corrosion, these pits may concentrate stress and initiate fatigue failure of the implant. Cold welding and metallic transfer also cause inclusion corrosion (i.e., a screwdriver may leave bits of metal cold welded to a screw). Thus, instruments are now produced from the same alloys as the implants.

Technological advances in materials science continue to provide more effective methods of producing orthopaedic devices. Improved manufacturing processes and new alloys have contributed to increased material purity, better implant fabrication, and improved corrosion resistance. It is hoped that further study will serve to increase the corrosion resistance and durability of orthopaedic materials in vivo.

Host Response to Biomaterials

Orthopaedic biomaterials must interact with host tissues under specific circumstances in order to produce adverse host responses. When this happens, inflammation, infection, and osteolysis may lead to loosening and subsequent failure of the implanted device. These interactions may be understood as processes of coupling between the implant material and the human body, and they often define the limiting factor for the in vivo use of a specific biomaterial.[81] Whereas the intact form of the implant material may induce little or no host response, the particulate debris of certain materials may couple with the host tissues with devastating results. Host responses may occur locally, systemically, or at sites remote from the implant. Metabolic, bacteriologic, immunologic, and neoplastic processes broadly characterize these reactions to biomaterials, and "local response" may also refer to the osteolytic and resorptive (structural) mechanisms of bone loss.[81,134,135]

The classic foreign-body response results from the body's attempt to degrade all non-self material. What cannot be degraded is generally encapsulated. Hence, the typical orthopaedic biomaterial in bulk form is surrounded in vivo by a fibrous capsule. Bioactive ceramics (i.e., hydroxyapatite), however, chemically resemble host tissues and are free from capsule formation. This is advantageous in the uncemented prosthesis, where fibrous tissue may intervene between the bone and the implant surface. This weakens the interface and may predispose the implant to loosening and failure. Prostheses coated with HA allow for improved bony ingrowth, direct bonding of bone to the implant, and stronger fixation of the prosthetic device.[9,31]

More severe responses are seen when the implant serves as a source of particulate debris.[136] Loosening is a common cause of clinical failure and is often associated with osteolysis.[137] The macrophage response to particulate wear debris was first implicated in causing osteolysis and eventual loosening by Willert and Semlitch in 1977.[138] In the same year, this was associated with PMMA[138,139] and

came to be known as cement disease.[140] More recent clinical studies have shown similar phenomena occurring around cementless prostheses, which suggests a role for UHMWPE and metal debris.[141,142]

Osteolysis

Periprosthetic bone loss resulting from osteolysis may pose clinical problems for joint replacement through implant fixation failure, host bone fracture, disability, and pain.[135] When infectious causes are eliminated, bone loss is attributable to one of two mechanisms: periprosthetic bone remodeling and focal osteolysis.[81] The structural remodeling of bone was discussed previously in regard to Wolff's law and periprosthetic stress shielding. While stress-induced remodeling may lead to significant complications, focal osteolysis has the greatest potential for periprosthetic bone destruction with aseptic loosening and eventual failure.

Focal osteolysis is roentgenographically visualized as diffuse cortical thinning, and is also recognized by the more problematic focal cystic lesion.[135] Peri- and retroacetabular lesions are seen as well and are localized in the peripheral and central areas of the acetabulum, respectively.[81] Bone loss has been associated with both cemented and uncemented implants and is known to occur in all prosthetic systems and all biomaterials used to date.

The factors that lead to osteolytic bone resorption basically involve the production of particulate debris and implant loosening. A loose, uncemented implant can be as damaging to the periprosthetic bone and surrounding tissues as a loose, cemented implant.[81] Although the presence of either of these exacerbates the clinical complications produced by the other, particle generation seems to be the most common pathogenic mechanism.[143–146] Particle-induced aseptic loosening is thought to be due to the excessive release of wear-associated debris that overwhelms the capacity of lymphatic clearance from the synovial cavity.[136] The local particle accumulation produces an intense foreign-body reaction due to the migration and proliferation of macrophages in the synovial cavity and periprosthetic space.[81,138] Subsequent release of inflammatory mediators from activated macrophages stimulates osteoclastic activity and bone resorption (Fig. 14-22).[81,147] Despite the complex cascade of cytokine-mediator interactions involved in bone resorption, *prostaglandin E₂* and *interleukin-1* have emerged as central

Figure 14-22 Diagram representing a hypothesis of wear particle–induced bone resorption.

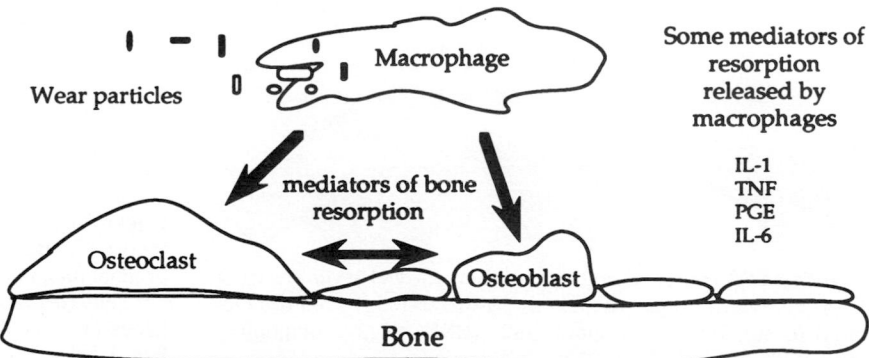

components in this process.[148,149] This pathogenic effect of particulate debris is a function of its size, concentration, surface properties, and composition.[150,151]

One of the more difficult tasks involving the characterization of the osteolytic response to debris is to determine the nature and type of particulate matter most likely to precipitate this reaction. Wear debris results predominantly in microscopic and submicroscopic particles of metals, UHMWPE, and PMMA cement. Metallic debris is generated from the articular surface, porous coating, metal backing of the acetabular component, Morse taper junctions, contaminants from surgical instruments, acetabular fixation screws, and fretting, whether implant-implant or femoral stem-bone fretting. It is most common in loose implants.[135] Debris due to UHMWPE originates from the back of the modular insert and the articular surface. Articular surface wear may be abrasive or adhesive, and both decrease polyethylene thickness. Last, PMMA cement may be generated from fracture, fretting, or fragmentation, resulting in particulate debris that easily migrates into the joint space.

Studies have demonstrated that the in vitro response of macrophages and fibroblasts to particulate debris is dependent on particle size, composition, and dose.[152] For the macrophage response to develop, particles must be internalized into the cell through phagocytosis. Fragments larger than 7 μm are generally too large to be phagocytosed.[153] Thus, macrophage-induced bone resorption is due to very fine particles (less than 7 μm), which may be seen in phagocytic cytoplasms and necrotic tissues.[141,142,154,155]

Particle composition is a factor in that the type and severity of host response is dependent on which material the particle is from. La Budde et al. have quantitatively described some of the inflammatory host responses to various types of debris, including metal (cobalt-chrome and titanium alloy), polyethylene, and PMMA cement particles (Figs. 14-23 through 14-26).[136] Chronic inflammatory cells represented by leukocytes and plasma cells were seen in variable amounts among all the tissue samples, with no statistical difference between the response to cobalt-chrome

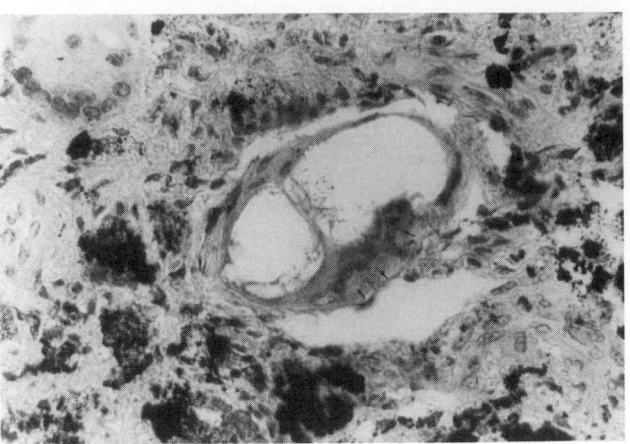

Figure 14-24 Photomicrograph showing a large space resulting from dissolution of methylmethacrylate from tissue sections by standard processing procedures and surrounded by spindly giant cells (*arrows*). (H&E, magnification ×200.)

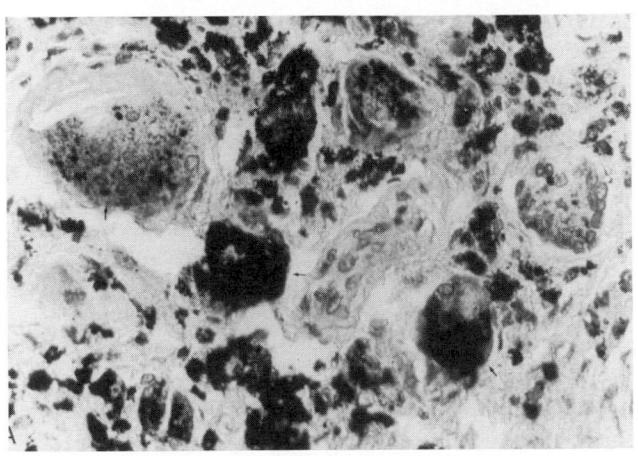

A

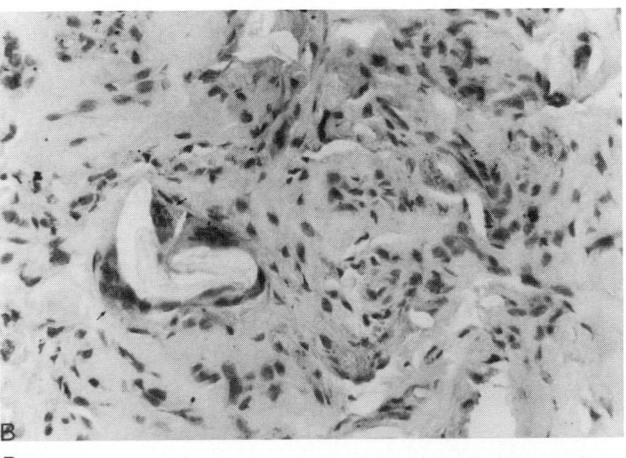

B

Figure 14-25 *A.* Photomicrograph showing giant cells associated with titanium alloy particulate debris (*arrows.*) (H&E, original magnification ×200.) *B.* Photomicrograph showing giant cells (*arrows*) associated with polyethylene in Co-Cr alloy knees but not directly associated with metallic Co-Cr particulate debris. (H&E, original magnification ×200.)

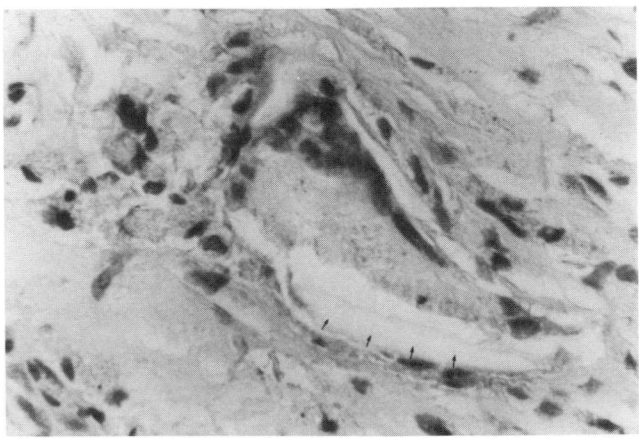

Figure 14-23 Photomicrograph of the synovial layer showing a polyethylene fragment (*arrows*) surrounded by multinucleated foreign-body–type giant cells. (H&E, original magnification ×400.)

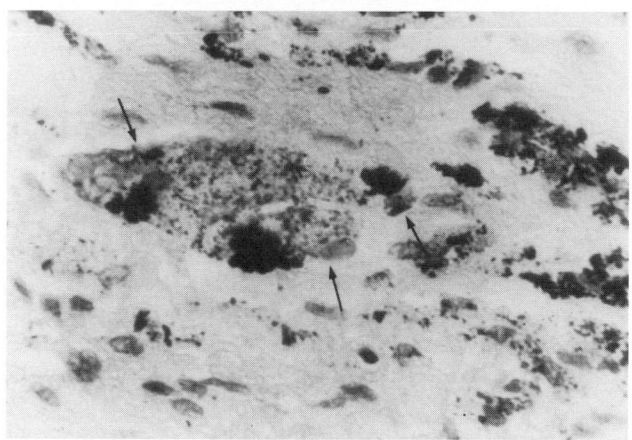

Figure 14-26 Photomicrograph showing black metallic titanium debris within histiocytes (*arrows*). (H&E, original magnification ×400.)

versus titanium alloys. Multinucleated giant cells (histiocytes) were also seen among all the samples and were consistently associated with particulate debris. Metal debris examined histologically appeared as 1- to 4-μm spheres for both types, and also as 10- to 20-μm flakes of titanium. Titanium alloy was associated with giant cell formation, whereas cobalt-chromium was not. Although significant giant cell counts were present in cobalt-chrome–containing sections, histologic examination demonstrated the proximity of the giant cells to the polyethylene debris rather than metallic particles. Cobalt-chrome alloy particles were more often associated with a *mononuclear* histiocytic response compared to the *multi-nucleated* histiocyte response seen with titanium alloy. The significance of polyethylene debris and cement disease has previously been mentioned, and both of these factors have been linked to the multinucleated giant cell inflammatory response.[136]

The obvious solution would be to eliminate the corrosion and wear-liberated debris from any implantable orthopaedic biomaterial. Current methods include nitriding and ion implantation, surface polishing, development and use of potentially superior materials (e.g., alumina, zirconium), implant surface coating, improvements in modular tapers, and other factors regarding the design and fabrication of implants previously discussed.

Systemic and Remote Site Effects

Systemic and remote site effects have been characterized as metabolic, bacteriologic, immunologic, and neoplastic.[134] *Metabolic* consideration is given to the elemental components of the nonphysiologic metals (other than Na^+, K^+, Ca^+, and Fe^+) used as biomaterials. Except for titanium, all metallic elements in orthopaedic implants serve in a toxic or essential role in body metabolic functions.[156] Unfortunately, toxic effects may even occur with high enough doses of essential elements.[157,158]

Bacteriologic effects include deep sepsis, osteomyelitis, implant corrosion, and so on. Deep wound sepsis following

arthroplasty was historically a major complication; now it is a smaller but potentially serious concern.[159] Foreign materials promote infectious complications of the musculoskeletal system by providing a neutral surface for the colonization of microorganisms. The protective surface of the material combined with formation of a virulent biofilm may serve to sequester bacterial colonies from host defenses. Thus, the minimum titer of organisms required to cause an infection is significantly reduced. While contamination during the implant procedure may cause early infection, late infection is associated with activation of a previously existing, latent source or hematogenous seeding from a remote site. Further predisposition to local infection occurs with ionic suppression of chemotaxis and particulate suppression of the respiratory burst in leukocytes.[160–162] Concern about systemic infection arises from the possibility of leukocyte suppression at remote sites, which is suggested by the dose-response increase of lung infections in rats with remotely placed large-area cobalt-alloy implants.[163]

Type IV delayed hypersensitivity reactions in previously sensitized individuals are characteristic of the host's *immune* response to many metallic ions such as cobalt, chromium, and nickel.[164] Also, high release rates of metallic debris may sensitize previously unsensitized individuals.[165] Dermatitis, urticaria, and eczematous reactions result from type IV reactions, but a clearly defined association of these and other, more subtle immune phenomena with implants and their debris has not been produced.

The association of implantable biomaterial with *neoplastic* effects seems rather distant, but the carcinogenic potential of implant-generated metallic debris such as chromium, cobalt, and nickel is well established.[166,167] Although the procedure is still considered low risk, the number of reported tumors in association with joint replacement is increasing.[168] Further epidemiologic evidence suggests an elevated risk of leukemia and lymphoma in patients after total hip arthroplasty.[169,170] As the life spans of patients and in vivo prosthetic devices continue to increase, concerns about the toxic and carcinogenic potential of orthopaedic biomaterials may well become extremely important.

CHOICES OF BIOMATERIALS

The orthopaedic surgeon has historically been required to make knowledgeable choices from a growing list of biomaterials available for use in prosthetic applications. The essence of clinically applied materials science is to help provide information suggesting which of the biomaterials are more appropriate for particular applications. As mentioned, some of the desirable properties of orthopaedic biomaterials include strength, hardness, ductility, modulus, biological response, and use with or without cement. Each material possesses a different biomechanical profile, and some general conclusions may be made as to the choices of biomaterials in specific situations. The remainder of this section discusses current thinking regarding the most appropriate choices of biomaterials in total hip and total knee arthroplasty.

The particular applications of certain biomaterials may generally be grouped according to anatomic location. Total hip arthroplasty requires an acetabular component, femoral head, and femoral stem component, while total knee arthroplasty uses femoral and tibial implants along with a prosthetic patella. These implants may also be used in applications with and without cement. Friedman et al. have suggested the following choices of biomaterials[81]:

1. For a cemented femoral component to be used in total hip or total knee arthroplasty, cobalt-chromium alloys are preferred at present due to the clinical data supporting their superior ability as bearing surfaces. Forged cobalt-chromium alloy is optimal in that the remote chance of fatigue failure is further lessened. The lack of difference regarding bony ingrowth into the commercially available prostheses of differing metal materials and surface morphologies suggests that selection of the cemented femoral component should be based on the properties of the bearing surface.[171] Titanium alloy has been shown to generate excessive amounts of particulate metallic debris,[172–174] but the advent of treatments such as nitriding and ion implantation may help decrease this wear by increasing surface hardness. The decrease in stress shielding is an obvious benefit to using this material for the reduction of stress shielding and subsequent bone remodeling. However, the widespread use of titanium in cemented joint replacement must be precluded by a lack of clinical evidence supporting the long-term in vivo stability of these surface treatments. Newer ceramic materials such as alumina and zirconia have been shown to decrease the rate of wear and debris production compared even to cobalt-chromium femoral heads. The use of these materials as modular components is increasing rapidly, and these ceramic devices may be the "gold standard" in the near future.

2. Flexibility is much more important in the uncemented femoral component due to the absolute necessity for osseointegration that results in a strong bone-implant interface. The low modulus of titanium alloy provides for decreased stress shielding and a reduction in the periprosthetic bone remodeling as compared to cobalt-chromium alloys. Since implant flexibility has been inversely related to thigh pain[175,176] and stress shielding,[177] a titanium-alloy femoral implant should be used to minimize these complications.

3. Acetabular and tibial components are typically metal-backed UHMWPE or may be composed of all UHMWPE. Use of metal-backed components introduces the possibility of material fracture and the additional component of fretting corrosion between the UHMWPE and the metal. The metal-backed components may be fine-tuned more precisely regarding the ligamentous tension and load distribution in total knee arthroplasty by varying the UHMWPE insert after implantation.[178] However, the clinical superiority of these implants over all-polyethylene components has not been demonstrated. The use of a metal-backed implant may also increase the cost more than twofold. Thus, the UHMWPE prosthesis must be considered an adequate alternative to the metal-backed prosthesis in cemented acetabular and tibial components.

4. Uncemented acetabular and tibial components should be composed of cobalt-chromium or titanium alloy as the osseointegrative surface and UHMWPE as the bearing surface. Material properties should have little bearing on the selection due to the compressive loading of these prostheses. Both cobalt-chromium and titanium alloy may be produced with sufficient strength so that bony ingrowth and other design considerations become more important.

5. The choice of material for the patellar component in total knee arthroplasty is relatively uncontroversial.[179–182] An all-UHMWPE component is generally preferred at this time.

REFERENCES

1. Bechtol CO, Ferguson AB, Laing PG: *Metals and Engineering in Bone and Joint Surgery.* Baltimore, Waverly Press, 1959.
2. Icart: Letter in response to the memorandum of Mr. Rujol. *J Med Chir Pharm,* Roux, 44:169, 1775.
3. Bick EM: *Sourcebook of Orthopaedics,* 2d ed. Baltimore, Williams & Wilkins, 1948.
4. Black J: *Orthopaedic Biomaterials in Research and Practice.* New York, Churchill Livingstone, 1988.
5. Cochran GVB: *A Primer of Orthopaedic Biomechanics.* New York, Churchill Livingstone, 1982.
6. Davidson JA: Characteristics of metal and ceramic total hip bearing surfaces and their effect on long-term ultra-high molecular weight polyethylene wear. *Clin Orthop Rel Res* 294:361–378, 1993.
7. Pugh J, Dee R: Properties of musculoskeletal tissues and biomaterials, in Dee R, Mango E, Hurst LC (eds): *Principles of Orthopaedic Practice:* Vol 1. New York, McGraw-Hill, 1988, pp 134–146.
8. Crowninshield R: An overview of prosthetic materials for fixation. *Clin Orthop* 235:166–172, 1988.
9. Søballe K: Hydroxyapatite-ceramic coating for bone-implant fixation: Mechanical and histological studies in dogs. *Acta Orthop Scand* 64(suppl 255):1–58, 1993.
10. Black J: Requirements for successful total knee replacement: Material considerations. *Orthop Clin North Am* 20:1, 1989.
11. Black J: Systemic effects of biomaterials. *Biomaterials* 5:11, 1984.
12. Rae T: The toxicity of metals used in orthopaedic prosthesis: An experimental study using cultured human synovial fibroblasts. *J Bone Joint Surg* 63B:435, 1981.
13. Agins HJ, Alcock NW, Bansal M, et al: Metallic wear in failed titanium-alloy total hip replacements: A histological and quantitative analysis. *J Bone Joint Surg* 70A:347, 1988.
14. Williams DF: Titanium as a metal for implantation. *J Med Eng Technol* 1:266, 1977.
15. Albrektsson T, Branemark PI, Hansson HA, Lindstrom J: Osteo integrated titanium implants. *Acta Orthop Scand* 52:155, 1981.

16. Hofmann AA, Bloebaum RD: Bone chip incorporation in porous coated total knee replacement. *Trans Orthop Res Soc* 14:533, 1989.
17. Burstein AH, Wright TM: *Fundamentals of Orthopaedic Biomechanics.* Baltimore, Williams & Wilkins, 1994.
18. Keller JC, Lautenschlager EP: Metals and alloys, in von Recum AF (ed): *Handbook of Biomaterials Evaluation: Scientific, Technical, and Clinical Testing of Implant Materials.* New York, Macmillan, 1986, pp 3–23.
19. Davidson JA, Mishra AK, Kovacs P, Poggie RA: New surface-hardened, low-modulus, corrosion-resistant Ti-13Nb-13Zr alloy for total hip arthroplasty. *Biomed Mater Eng* 4:231–243, 1994.
20. Kangasniemi IMO, Verheyen CCPM, van der Velde EA, de Groot K: In vivo tensile testing of fluorapatite and hydroxy-lapatite plasma-sprayed coatings. *J Biomed Mater Res* 28:563–572, 1994.
21. Williams DF (ed): *Proceeding of a Consensus Conference of the European Society for Biomaterials, Hester, England, 1986.* Amsterdam, Elsevier, 1987.
22. Williams DF: *Definitions in Biomaterials: Progress in Biomedical Engineering,* 4th ed. New York, Elsevier, 1987.
23. Williams DF: Consensus and definitions in biomaterials, in de Putter C, de Lange GL, de Groot K, Lee AJC (eds): *Advances in Biomaterials.* Amsterdam, Elsevier, 1988, pp 11–16.
24. Geesnick RGT, Hoefnagels NHM: Six year results of hydrox-yapatite-coated total hip replacement. *J Bone Joint Surg (Br)* 77B:534–547, 1995.
25. Kazuhiro I, Yasutaka M, Takao Y, et al: Cementless total hip replacement: Bio-active glass ceramic coating studied in dogs. *Acta Orthop Scand* 64:607–610, 1993.
26. Jarcho M: Calcium phosphate ceramics as hard tissue prosthetics. *Clin Orthop* 157:259–278, 1981.
27. Bauer TW, Geesink RC, Zimmerman R, McMahon JT: Hydroxyapatite-coated femoral stems: Histological analysis of components retrieved at autopsy. *J Bone Joint Surg (Am)* 73:1439–1452, 1991.
28. Ducheyne P, Cuckler JM: Bioactive ceramic prosthetic coatings. *Clin Orthop* 276:102–114, 1992.
29. Furlong RJ, Osborn JF: Fixation of hip prosthesis by hydroxya-patite ceramic coatings. *J Bone Joint Surg (Br)* 73:741–745, 1991.
30. Hardy DC, Frayssinet P, Guilhem A, et al: Bonding of hydrox-yapatite-coated femoral prosthesis: Histopathology of specimens from four cases. *J Bone Joint Surg (Br)* 73:732–740, 1991.
31. Tracy BM, Doremus RH: Direct electron microscopy studies of the bone hydroxyapatite interface. *J Biomed Mater Res* 18:719–726, 1984.
32. Maruyama M: Hydroxyapatite clay used to fill the gap between implant and bone. *J Bone Joint Surg* 77B:213–218, 1995.
33. Jarcho M: Calcium phosphate ceramics as hard tissue prosthetics. *Clin Orthop* 157:259–278, 1981.
34. Kamegaya M, Shinohara Y, Shinada Y, et al: The use of a hydroxyapatite block for innominate osteotomy. *J Bone Joint Surg (Br)* 76B:123–126, 1994.
35. Uchida A, Araki N, Shinto Y, et al: The use of calcium hydroxyapatite ceramic in bone tumour surgery. *J Bone Joint Surg (Br)* 72B:298–302, 1990.
36. Bauer TW, Geesink RGT, Zimmerman R, McMahon JT: Hydroxyapatite-coated femoral stems: Histological analysis of components retrieved at autopsy. *J Bone Joint Surg (Am)* 73:1439–1452, 1991.
37. Cook SD, Thomas KA, Kay JF, Jarcho M: Hydroxyapatite-coated titanium for orthopaedic implant application. *Clin Orthop* 232:225–243, 1988.
38. de Groot K, Geesink RGT, Klein CPAT, Serekian P: Plasma sprayed coatings of hydroxylapatite. *J Biomed Mater Res* 21:1375–1381, 1987.
39. Denissen HW, de Groot K, Makkes PC, et al: Tissue response to dense apatite implants in rats. *J Biomed Mater Res* 14:713–721, 1980.
40. Geesink RGT: Hydroxyl-apatite coated hip implants. Thesis, The Netherlands, University of Maastricht, 1987.
41. Geesink RGT, de Groot K, Klein CPAT: Chemical implant fixation using hydroxyl-apatite coatings. *Clin Orthop* 225:147–170, 1987.
42. Geesink RGT, de Groot K, Klein CPAT: Bonding of bone to apatite-coated implants. *J Bone Joint Surg (Br)* 70:17–23, 1988.
43. Jarcho M, Kay JF, Gumaer KI, et al: Tissue, cellular and subcellular events at a bone-ceramic hydroxyapatite interface. *J Bioeng* 1:79–92, 1977.
44. Klein CPAT: Calcium phosphate implant materials and biodegradation. Thesis, Amsterdam, Free University, 1983.
45. Thomas KA, Cook SD, Haddad RJ, et al: Biological response to hydroxyapatite-coated titanium hips. *J Arthroplasty* 4:43–53, 1989.
46. Thomas KA, Kay JF, Cook SD, Jarcho M: The effect of surface macrotexture and hydroxyapatite coating on the mechanical strengths and histological profiles of titanium implant materials. *J Biomed Mater Res* 21:1395–1414, 1987.
47. Posner AS: The structure of bone mineral. *Clin Orthop* 9:5–14, 1957.
48. Patka P: *Bone Replacement by Calcium Phosphate Ceramics.* Amsterdam, Free University Press, 1984.
49. Heimke G: Ceramics, in von Recum AF (ed): *Handbook of Biomaterials Evaluation: Scientific, Technical, and Clinical Testing of Implant Materials:* New York, Macmillan, 1986, pp 38–54.
50. Osborn JF: Preservation and reconstruction of the alveolar bone using hydroxyapatite ceramic, in Hjorting-Hansen E (ed): *Oral and Maxillofacial Surgery: Proceedings from the 8th International Conference on Oral and Maxillofacial Surgery.* Chicago, Quintessence Publishing, 1985, pp 552–556.
51. Blumenthal NC, Posner AS: Hydroxyapatite: Mechanism of formation and properties. *Calc Tiss Res* 13:235–243, 1975.
52. Klein CPAT, Patka P, van der Lubbe HBM, et al: Plasma-sprayed coatings of tetracalciumphosphate, hydroxylapatite, and alpha-TCP on titanium alloy: An interface study. *J Biomed Mater Res* 25:53–65, 1991.
53. Klein CPAT, Driessen AA, de Groot K: Biodegradation behavior of various calcium phosphate material in bone tissue. *J Biomed Res* 12:769–784, 1983.
54. Herman H: Plasma-sprayed coatings: *Sci Am* 259:78–83, 1988.
55. van Blitterswijk CA, Grote JJ, Kuijpers W, et al: Macropore tissue ingrowth: A quantitative study on hydroxyapatite ceramic. *Biomaterials* 7:137–143, 1986.
56. Berndt CC, Haddad GN, Gross KA: Thermal spraying for bioceramics application, in Heimke G (ed): *Bioceramics: Proceedings of the 2nd International Symposium on Ceramics in Medicine.* Heidelberg, 1989, p 201.
57. Maruyama M, Terayama K, Ito M, et al: Hydroxyapatite clay for gap filling and adequate bone ingrowth. *J Biomed Mater Res* 29:329–336, 1995.
58. Anderson RC, Cook SD, Weinstein Am, Haddad RJ: An evaluation of skeletal attachment to LT1 purolytic carbon, porous titanium and carbon-coated porous titanium implants. *Clin Orthop* 182:242–257, 1984.
59. Cook SD, Walsh KA, Haddad RJ: Interface mechanics and bone growth onto porous Co-Cr-Mo alloy implants. *Clin Orthop* 193:271–280, 1985.
60. Geesink RGT, de Groot K, Klein CPAT: Bonding of bone to apatite-coated implants. *J Bone Joint Surg (Br)* 70B:17–22, 1988.
61. Schulte KR, Callaghan JJ, Kelley SS, Johnston RC: The outcome of Charnley total hip arthroplasty with cement after a minimum twenty-year follow-up: The results of one surgeon. *J Bone Joint Surg (Am)* 75A:961–975, 1993.

62. Schen WJ, Chung KC, Wang GJ, McLaughlin RE: Mechanical failure of hydroxyapatite- and polysulfone-coated titanium rods in a weight-bearing canine model. *J Arthroplasty* 7:43–49, 1992.

63. Soballe K, Hansen ES, Brockstedt-Rasmussen H, Bunger C: Hydroxyapatite coating converts fibrous tissue to bone around loaded implants. *J Bone Joint Surg (Br)* 75B:270–278, 1993.

64. Søballe K, Hansen ES, Brockstedt-Rasmussen H, et al: Gap healing enhanced by hydroxyapatite coating in dogs. *Clin Orthop* 272:300–307, 1991.

65. Cooke FW: Ceramics in orthopedic surgery. *Clin Orthop* 276:135, 1992.

66. Drummond JL, Lenke JW: In vivo and in vitro aging of dense alumina. *Adv Ceram Mater* 3:159, 1988.

67. Pourbaix M: *Atlas of Electrochemical Equilibria in Aqueous Solutions.* Houston, TX, National Association of Corrosion Engineers, 1974.

68. Rhodes G: Stability of medical grade yttria stabilized zirconia. 4th International Symposium on Ceramics in Medicine, London, England, Sept. 11–13, 1991.

69. White SE, Whiteside LA, McCarthy DS, et al: Simulated knee wear with cobalt chromium and oxidized zirconium knee femoral components. *Clin Orthop Rel Res* 309:176–184, 1994.

70. Schwartz GL: Wear and strength of zirconia and alumina ceramic materials. Trans 36th Annual Meeting. *Orthop Res Soc* 15:483, 1990.

71. Yammamuro T: Total knee replacement with ceramics. Presentation at the 6th DePaul International Joint Replacement Symposium. St Louis, 1988.

72. Davidson JA: Characteristics of metal and ceramic total hip bearing surfaces and their effect on long-term ultra high molecular weight polyethylene wear. *Clin Orthop* 294:361–378, 1993.

73. Kumar P, Masanori O, Ikeuchi K, et al: Low wear rate of UHMWPE against zirconia ceramic (Y-PSZ) in comparison to alumina ceramic and SUS 316L alloy. *J Biomed Mater Res* 25:813, 1991.

74. Oonishi H, Igaki H, Takayama Y: Comparisons of wear of UHMWPE sliding against metal and alumina in total hip prosthesis. *Bioceramics* 1:272, 1989.

75. Poggie RA, Wert JJ, Mishra AK, Davidson JA: Friction and wear characterization in reciprocating sliding contact with Co-Cr, Ti-6Al-4V and zirconia implant bearing surfaces, in Denton R, Keshavan M (eds): *Wear and Friction of Elastomers,* ASTM STP 1145. Philadelphia, American Society for Testing and Materials, 1992.

76. Schuller H, Marti R.: Ten-year socket wear in 66 hip arthroplasties—Ceramic versus metal heads. *Acta Orthop Scand* 61:240, 1990.

77. Weber BG: Total hip replacement: Rotating versus fixed and metal versus ceramic heads, in *The Hip.* St. Louis, Mosby, 1981, pp 264–275.

78. Caravia L, Dowson D, Fisher J, Jobbins B: The influence of bone and bone cement debris on counterface roughness in sliding wear tests of UHMWPE on stainless steel. *Proc Inst Mech Eng* 204:65, 1990.

79. Cooper JR, Dowson D, Fisher J, Jobbins B: Ceramic bearing surfaces in total artificial joints: Resistance to third body wear damage from bone cement particles. *J Med Eng Technol* 15:63, 1991.

80. Mishra AK, Davidson JA: Abrasion resistance of candidate coatings for orthopaedic articulating surfaces. *Proceedings of the 9th European Conference on Biomaterials,* Chester, UK, Sept 9–11, 1991.

81. Friedman RJ, Black J, Galante JO, et al: Current concepts in orthopaedic biomaterials and implant fixation, in Heckman JD (ed): *Instr Course Lect:* Vol 43. Rosemont, IL, The American Academy of Orthopaedic Surgeons, 1994.

82. Davidson JA, Mishra AK: Surface modification issues for orthopaedic implant bearing surfaces, in *Surface Modification Technologies,* 5th ed. Torrington, CT, Torrington, 1992.

83. Charnley J, Kettlewell L: The elimination of slip between prosthesis and femur. *J Bone Joint Surg* 47B:56–60, 1965.

84. Charnley J: *Acrylic Cement in Orthopaedic Surgery.* Baltimore, Williams & Wilkins, 1970.

85. Ahlfelt L, Herberts P, Malchau H, Anderson GBJ: Prognosis of total hip replacement: A swedish multicenter study of 4664 revisions. *Acta Orthop Scand* 61(suppl 238):1–26, 1990.

86. Almby B, Hierton T: Total hip replacement: 10 year follow-up of an early series. *Acta Orthop Scand* 53:397–406, 1982.

87. Callaghan JJ, Salvati EA, Pellicci PM, et al: Results of revision for mechanical failure after cemented total hip replacement, 1979–1982. *J Bone Joint Surg* 67:1074–1085, 1985.

88. Charnley J, Cubic Z: The nine and ten year results of the low friction arthroplasty of the hip. *Clin Orthop* 95:9–25, 1973.

89. Gruen TA, McNeice GM, Amstutz HC: "Modes of failure" of cemented stem type femoral components: A radiographic analysis of loosening. *Clin Orthop* 141:17–27, 1979.

90. Søballe K, Boll KL, Kofod S, et al: Total hip replacement after medial-displacement osteotomy of the proximal part of the femur. *J Bone Joint Surg* 71:692–697, 1989.

91. Tew M, Waugh W: Estimation of the survival time of knee replacements. *J Bone Joint Surg (Br)* 64:579–582, 1982.

92. Stauffer RN: Ten-year follow-up study of total hip replacement, with particular reference to roentgenographic loosening of the components. *J Bone Joint Surg* 64A:983–990, 1982.

93. Sutherland CJ, Wilde AH, Borden LS, Marks KE: A ten-year follow-up of one hundred Müller curved-stem total hip replacement arthroplasties. *J Bone Joint Surg* 64A:970–982, 1982.

94. Goldring SR, Schiller AL, Roelke M, et al: The synovial-like membrane at the bone-cement interface in loose total hip replacements and its proposed role in bone lysis. *J Bone Joint Surg* 65A:575–584, 1983.

95. King JW: Some physiological aspects of prosthesis stabilization with acrylic polymer. *Clin Orthop* 83:317–328, 1972.

96. Harving S, Søballe K, Bünger C: A method for bone-cement interface thermometry. An in vitro comparison between low temperature curing cement Palavit and Surgical Simplex P. *Acta Orthop Scand* 62:546–548, 1991.

97. Harving S, Søballe K, Hoy K, et al: Interface bone repair enhanced by low temp curing cement. *Trans 37th Annual Meeting Orthop Res Soc* 16:496, 1991.

98. Mjöberg B: Loosening of the cemented hip prosthesis: The importance of heat injury. *Acta Orthop Scand Suppl* 221:57, 1986.

99. Nimb L, Stürup J, Jensen JS: Improved cortical histology after cementation with a new MMA-DMA-IBMA bone cement: An animal study. *J Biomed Mater Res* 27:565–574, 1993.

100. Masanobu S, Akira M, Toshikazu M, et al: Experimental studies on a new bioactive bone cement: Hydroxyapatite composite resin. *Biomaterials* 15:156–160, 1994.

101. Landy MM, Walker PS: Wear of ultra-high molecular weight polyethylene components of 90 retrieved knee prosthesis. *J Arthroplasty* 3:S73–S85, 1988.

102. Weightman B, Swanson SAV, Isaac GH, et al: Polyethylene wear from retrieved acetabular cups. *J Bone Joint Surg* 73B:806–810, 1991.

103. Wright TM, Burnstein AH, Bartel DL: Retrieval analysis of total joint replacement components: A six-year experience, in Fraker AC, Griffin CD (eds): *Corrosion and Degradation of Implant Materials: Second Symposium.* Philadelphia, American Society for Testing and Materials, 1985, pp 415–428.

104. Spector M: Biomaterial failure. *Orthop Clin N Am* 23:211–217, 1992.

105. Berquist TH, Bender CE, Maus TP, et al: Pseudobursae: A useful finding in patients with painful hip arthroplasty. *Am J Roentgenol* 148:103, 1987.

106. Binek R, Levinsohn EM: Enlarged iliopsoas bursae: An unusual case of thigh mass and hip pain. *Clin Orthop* 224:158, 1987.

107. Griffiths HJ, Burke J, Bonfiglio TA: Granulomatous pseudotumors in total joint replacement. *Ske Radiol* 16:146, 1987.

108. Howie DW, Cain CMJ, Cornish BL: Pseudo-abscess of the psoas bursae in failed double-cup arthroplasty of the hip. *J Bone Joint Surg* 73B:29, 1991.

109. Kilgus DJ, Funahashi TT, Campbell PA: Massive femoral osteolysis and early disintegration of a polyethylene-bearing surface of a total knee replacement: A case report. *J Bone Joint Surg* 74A:770, 1992.

110. Kolmert L, Persson BM, Herrlin K, Ekelund L: Iliopectineal bursitis following total hip replacement. *Acta Orthop Scand* 55:63, 1984.

111. Matsumoto K, Hukuda S, Nishioka J, Fujita T: Iliopsoas bursal distension caused by acetabular loosening after total hip arthroplasty: A rare complication of total hip arthroplasty. *Clin Orthop* 279:144, 1992.

112. Howie DW, Vernon-Roberts B, Oakeshott R, Manthey B: A rat model of resorption of bone at the cement-bone interface in the presence of polyethylene wear particles. *J Bone Joint Surg* 70A:257, 1988.

113. Peters PC, Engh GA, Dwyer KA, Vinh TN: Osteolysis after total knee arthroplasty without cement. *J Bone Joint Surg* 74A:864, 1992.

114. Ranawat CS, Johanson NA, Rimnac CM, et al: Retrieval analysis of porous-coated components for total knee arthroplasty: A report of two cases. *Clin Orthop* 209:244, 1986.

115. Wright TM, Bartel DL: The problem of surface damage in polyethylene total knee components. *Clin Orthop* 205:67, 1986.

116. Howie DW, Vernon-Roberts B, Oakeshott R, Manthey B: A rat model of resorption of bone at the cement-bone interface in the presence of polyethylene wear particles. *J Bone Joint Surg* 70A:257, 1988.

117. Harris WH, Schiller AL, Scholler JM, et al: Extensive localized bone absorption in the femur following total hip replacement. *J Bone Joint Surg* 58A:612, 1976.

118. Charnley J: The reaction of bone to self-curing acrylic cement. *J Bone Joint Surg* 52B:340, 1970.

119. Goldring SR, Schiller AL, Roelke M, et al: The synovial-like membrane at the bone-cement interface in loose total hip replacements and its proposed role in bone lysis. *J Bone Joint Surg* 65A:575–584, 1983.

120. Howie DW, Cornish BL, Vernon-Roberts B: Resurfacing hip arthroplasty classification of loosening and the role of prosthesis wear particles. *Clin Orthop* 255:144, 1990.

121. Howie DW, Vernon-Roberts B, Oakeshott R, Manthey B: A rat model of resorption of bone at the cement-bone interface in the presence of polyethylene wear particles. *J Bone Joint Surg* 70A:257, 1988.

122. Davidson JA: Characteristics of metal and ceramic total hip bearing surfaces and their effect on long-term ultra-high molecular weight polyethylene wear. *Clin Orthop Rel Res* 294:361–378, 1993.

123. McKellop HA, Rostlund TV: The wear behavior of ion-implanted Ti-6Al-4V against UHMW polyethylene. *J Biomed Mater Res* 24:1413–1425, 1990.

124. Beiser I, Kanat I: Biodegradable internal fixation: A literature review. *J Am Podiatr Med Assoc* 80:70–75, 1990.

125. Bostman O: Current concepts review of bioabsorbable implants for fixation of fractures. *J Bone Joint Surg* 73A:148–152, 1991.

126. Strycker ML: Biodegradable internal fixation. *J Foot Ankle Surg* 34:82–88, 1995.

127. Speer KP, Warren RF: Arthroscopic shoulder stabilization. *Clin Orthop Rel Res* 291:67–74, 1993.

128. Bucholz RW, Henry S, Henley MB: Fixation with bioabsorbable screws for the treatment of fractures of the ankle. *J Bone Joint Surg* 76A:319–324, 1994.

129. Bostman O: Osteolytic changes accompanying degradation of absorbable fracture fixation implants. *J Bone Joint Surg* 73B:679–682, 1991.

130. Wetter L, Dineen M, Levitt M, Motson R: Controlled trial of polyglycolic acid versus catgut and nylon for appendectomy wound closure. *Br J Surg* 78:985–987, 1991.

131. McKellop HA, Rostlund TV: The wear behavior of ion-implanted Ti-6Al-4V against UHMW polyethylene. *J Biomed Mater Res* 24:1413–1425, 1990.

132. Röstlund TV: On the development of a new arthroplasty, with special emphasis on the gliding elements in the knee. Thesis. Göteborg, Sweden, University of Göteborg, 1990.

133. Williams DF, Buchanan RA: Ion implantation of surgical Ti-6Al-4V alloy. *Mater Sci Eng* 69:237, 1985.

134. Black J: Systemic effects of biomaterials. *Biomaterials* 5:11–18, 1984.

135. Jacobs JJ, Sumner DR, Galante GO: Mechanisms of bone loss associated with total hip replacement. *Orthop Clin North Am* 24:583–590, 1993.

136. La Budde JK, Orosz JF, Bonfiglio TA, Pellegrini VD: Particulate titanium and cobalt-chrome metallic debris in failed total knee arthroplasty. *J Arthroplasty* 9:291–305, 1994.

137. Shanbhag AS, Jacobs JJ, Glant TT, et al: Composition and morphology of wear debris in failed uncemented total hip replacement. *J Bone Joint Surg* 76B(1):60–77, 1994.

138. Willert HG, Semlitch M: Reactions of the articular capsule to wear products of artificial joint prostheses. *J Biomed Mater Res* 11:157–164, 1977.

139. Vernon-Roberts D, Freeman MAR: The tissue response to total joint replacement prosthesis, in Swanson SAV, Freeman MAR (eds): *The Scientific Basis of Joint Replacement.* Tunbridge Wells, England: Pitman Medical, 1977, pp 86–129.

140. Jones LC, Hungerford DS: Cement disease. *Clin Orthop* 225:192–206, 1987.

141. Jacobs J, Urban RM, Schajowicz F, et al: Particulate associated endosteal osteolysis in titanium-based alloy cementless total hip replacement, in St John KR (ed): *Particulate Debris from Metal Implants: Mechanisms of Formation and Biological Consequences,* ASTM STP 1144. Philadelphia, American Society for Testing and Materials, 1992, pp 52–60.

142. Maloney WJ, Jasty M, Harris WH, et al: Endosteal erosion in association with stable uncemented femoral components. *J Bone Joint Surg* 72A:1025–1034, 1990.

143. Dannenmaier WC, Haynes DW, Nelson CL: Granulomatous reaction and cystic bony destruction associated with high wear rate in a total knee prosthesis. *Clin Orthop* 198:224, 1985.

144. Mirra JM, Marder RA, Amstutz HC: The pathology of failed total joint arthroplasty. *Clin Orthop* 170:175, 1982.

145. Willert HG, Semlitch M: Reactions of the articular capsule to wear products of artificial joint prostheses. *J Biomed Mater Res* 11:157–164, 1977.

146. Winter GD: Tissue reactions to metallic wear and corrosion products in human patients. *J Biomed Mater Res* 5:11, 1974.

147. Howie DW, Haynes DR, Rogers SD, et al: The response to particulate debris. *Orthop Clin North Am* 24:571–581, 1993.

148. Glant TT, Jacobs JJ, Tabith K, Galante JO: Particulate titanium induced bone resorption in organ culture. *Orthop Trans* 15:540, 1991.

149. Shanbhag AS, Jacobs JJ, Black J, Glant TT: Pro- and anti-inflammatory mediators secreted by cells of interfacial membranes from revision total hip replacements. *Trans Orthop Res Soc* 18:517, 1993.

150. Glant TT, Jacobs JJ, Molnar G, et al: Bone resorption activity of particle-stimulated macrophages. *J Bone Min Res* 8:1071–1079, 1993.

151. Shanbhag AS, Glant TT, Jacobs JJ, Black J: Macrophage stimulation of fibroblastic proliferation is affected by size, composition and surface area of the particulates. *Trans Orthop Res Soc* 17:342, 1992.

152. Shanbhag AS, Glant TT, Jacobs JJ, Black J: Macrophage stimulation of fibroblastic proliferation is affected by size, composition and surface area of the particulates. *Trans Orthop Res Soc* 17:342, 1992.

153. Robert J, Quastel JH: Particle uptake by polymorphonuclear leucocytes and Ehrlich ascites–carcinoma cells. *Biochem J* 89:150–156, 1963.

154. Glant TT, Jacobs JJ, Molnar G, et al: Bone resorption activity of particle-stimulated macrophages. *J Bone Min Res* 8:1071–1079, 1993.

155. Glant TT, Jacobs JJ: Particulate-induced bone resorption in organ cultures: A comparison of the stimulatory effects of three different macrophage populations. *J Orthop Res* 12:720–731, 1994.

156. Mertz W: *Trace Elements in Human and Animal Nutrition,* 5th ed. Orlando, FL, Academic Press, 1986.

157. Friberg L, Nordberg GF, Vouk VB: *Handbook on the Toxicology of Metals.* Amsterdam, Elsevier, 1986.

158. Luckey TD, Venugopal B: *Metal Toxicity in Mammals:* Vol 1. New York, Plenum Press, 1977.

159. Esterhai JL, Gristina AG, Poss R: *Musculoskeletal Infection.* Park Ridge, IL, American Academy of Orthopaedic Surgeons, 1992.

160. Pascual A, Tsukayama DT, Wicklund BH, et al: The effect of stainless steel, cobalt-chromium, titanium alloy and titanium on respiratory burst activity of human polymorphonuclear leukocytes. *Clin Orthop* 280:281–288, 1992.

161. Rae T: Cell biochemistry in relation to the inflammatory response to foreign materials, in Williams DF (ed): *Fundamental Aspects of Biocompatibility:* vol 1. Boca Raton, FL, CRC Press, 1981, pp 159–181.

162. Shanbhag A, Yang J, Lilien J, Black J: Decreased neutrophil respiratory burst on exposure to cobalt-chrome alloy and polystyrene in vitro. *J Biomed Mater Res* 26:185–195, 1992.

163. Wapner KL, Morris DM, Black J: Release of corrosion products by F-75 cobalt base alloy in the rat: II. Morbidity apparently associated with chromium release in vivo: A 120-day rat study. *J Biomed Mater Res* 20:219–233, 1986.

164. Hildebrand HF, Champy M: *Biocompatibility of Co-Cr-Ni Alloys.* New York, Plenum Press, 1988.

165. Elves MW: Immunological aspects of biomaterials, in Williams DF (ed): *Fundamental Aspects of Biocompatibility:* vol 2. Boca Raton, FL, CRC Press, 1981, pp 159–173.

166. Black J: Metallic ion release and its relationship to oncogenesis, in *The Hip: Proceedings of the Thirteenth Open Scientific Meeting of The Hip Society.* St. Louis, Mosby, 1986, pp 199–213.

167. Sugano N, Nishii T, Nakata K, et al: Polyethylene sockets and alumina ceramic heads in cemented total hip arthroplasty. *J Bone Joint Surg* 77B:548–556, 1995.

168. Jacobs JJ, Rosenbaum DH, Hay RM, et al: Early sarcomatous degeneration near a cementless hip replacement: A case report and review. *J Bone Joint Surg* 74B:740–744, 1992.

169. Gillespie WJ, Frampton CM, Henderson RJ, Ryan PM: The incidence of cancer following total hip replacement. *J Bone Joint Surg* 70B:539–542, 1988.

170. Visuri T, Koskenvuo M: Cancer risk after McKee-Farrar total hip replacement. *Orthopaedics* 14:137–142, 1991.

171. Hulbert SF, Cooke FW, Klawitter JJ, et al: Attachment of prostheses to the musculoskeletal system by tissue ingrowth and mechanical interlocking. *J Biomed Mater Res* 7:1–23, 1973.

172. Agins HJ, Alcock NW, Bansal M, et al: Metallic wear in failed titanium-alloy total hip replacements: A histological and quantitative analysis. *J Bone Joint Surg* 70A:347–356, 1988.

173. Black J, Sherk H, Bonini J, et al: Metallosis associated with a stable titanium-alloy femoral component in total hip replacement: A case report. *J Bone Joint Surg* 72A:126–130, 1990.

174. McKellop HA, Sarmiento A, Schwinn CP, Ebramzadeh E: In vivo wear of titanium-alloy hip prostheses. *J Bone Joint Surg* 72A:512–517, 1990.

175. Franks E, Mont MA, Maar DC, et al: Thigh pain as related to bending rigidity of the femoral prosthesis and bone. *Trans Orthop Res Soc* 17:296, 1992.

176. Skinner HB, Curlin FJ: Decreased pain with lower flexural rigidity of uncemented femoral prostheses. *Orthopedics* 13:1223–1228, 1990.

177. Bobyn JD, Glassman AH, Goto H, et al: The effect of stem stiffness on femoral bone resorption after canine porous-coated total hip arthroplasty. *Clin Orthop* 261:196–213, 1990.

178. Hsu HP, Garg A, Walker PS, et al: Effect of knee component alignment on tibial load distribution with clinical correlation. *Clin Orthop* 248:135–144, 1989.

179. Bayley JC, Scott RD, Ewald FC, Holmes GB: Failure of the metal-backed patellar component after total hip replacement. *J Bone Joint Surg* 70A:668–674, 1988.

180. Lombardi AV, Engh GA, Volz RG, et al: Fracture/dissociation of the polyethylene in metal-backed patellar components in total knee arthroplasty. *J Bone Joint Surg* 70A:675–679, 1988.

181. Stulberg BN, De Swart RJ, Reger S, Gaisser DM: Factors influencing wear of all-polyethylene patellar components: A retrieval study. Read at the American Society for Testing and Materials Symposium on Biocompatibility of Particulate Implant Materials, San Antonio, Texas, Oct 31, 1990.

182. Sutherland CJ: Patellar component dissociation in total knee arthroplasty: A report of two cases. *Clin Orthop* 228:178–181, 1988.

PART II

General Orthopaedics

CHAPTER 15

Imaging of the Musculoskeletal System

Kathleen Finzel
and Theodore T. Miller

The first radiograph ever made was of a hand of the wife of Wilhelm Conrad Roentgen, the discoverer of x-rays, in 1895. It did not take long for the clinical applicability of "Roentgen's ray" to be appreciated, especially in cases of trauma and skeletal disease. How appropriate that, over 100 years later, radiographs are still the most common imaging procedure for musculoskeletal disease and indeed are the sine qua non of any radiologic workup. The basic principle of radiographic evaluation is the taking of two views orthogonal to each other. Only in this manner can true spatial relationships be appreciated. Similarly, there is no substitute for a properly exposed film, and the reader is cautioned not to attempt interpretation of underexposed (too light), overexposed (too dark), or blurry films. A description of radiographic appearances of individual diseases is beyond the scope of this chapter, and the reader is referred to any of several bone radiology texts.[1–5]

While radiography will suffice in many instances, other imaging modalities in the radiologist's armamentarium include nuclear medicine, computed tomography (CT), ultrasound, and magnetic resonance imaging. In this chapter, the role and contributions of each of these modalities to musculoskeletal imaging are discussed. In addition, the radiologic workup and appearances of avascular necrosis, infection, and bony and soft tissue tumors are reviewed.

MODALITIES

Nuclear Medicine

Radionuclide imaging has evolved since the days of crude rectilinear scanning, with its coarse images, to sophisticated single photon emission computed tomography (SPECT) imaging, which can provide tomographic sections in sagittal, coronal, and axial planes. The mainstay of musculoskeletal radionuclide imaging is the bone scan. In this technique, intravenously administered technetium 99m (^{99m}Tc) methylene diphosphonate (MDP) is incorporated into bone by adsorption onto hydroxyapatite. Tracer uptake is a reflection of bone turnover (osteoblastic activity) and is greatly influenced by regional blood flow. The study can be performed either in a single static phase, in which images of the skeleton are obtained 2 to 4 h after injection, or in three phases, in which the first phase is a radionuclide angiogram consisting of sequential images every 2 to 5 s for 30 to 60 s, immediately followed by the static blood pool second phase, which is a reflection of soft tissue distribution, and concludes with the 2- to 4-h delayed views of the skeleton. The four major areas of utility are infection, trauma, avascular necrosis, and neoplasia.

Scintigraphy is frequently called upon to evaluate infection in cases of normal radiographs but high clinical suspicion of osteomyelitis. Radiographs may not demonstrate any osseous abnormality in the first 2 to 3 weeks of infection. Moreover, interpretation of radiographs in cases complicated by previous trauma or degenerative/neuropathic changes can be difficult. Single-phase bone scanning is sensitive but has a low specificity due to update of ^{99m}Tc-MDP by any process that has increased osteoblastic activity (e.g., infection, trauma, avascular necrosis, degenerative change). Specificity can be increased by doing a three-phase study to evaluate for inflammatory hyperemia in the angiographic and blood pool phases. Osteomyelitis, which displays increased uptake on all three phases, can be distinguished from soft tissue infection by the latter's lack of focal increased uptake on the delayed skeletal images. Reported sensitivity and specificity for a three-phase study are 94 and 95 percent, respectively, for cases of uncomplicated osteomyelitis.[6]

Due to the nonspecific uptake of ^{99m}Tc-MDP and the myriad clinical settings of infection, specificity drops to 33 percent when underlying bony pathology is present, even though sensitivity remains high.[6] For this reason, other agents such as gallium-67 (Ga^{67}) citrate and indium-111 (^{111}In), leukocytes, both alone and in various combinations, are also used. There is uptake at infectious sites of ^{67}G citrate for two reasons: (1) it is incorporated into the hydroxyapatite matrix of bone, like ^{99m}Tc-MDP, making it a weak bone-scanning agent for reflecting areas of bony activity, and (2) it is an iron analog and is bound to serum transferrin, bacterial siderophores, and leukocyte lactoferrins, thus accumulating as a result of hyperemia and chemotaxis.[7] Sensitivity ranges from 62 to 100 percent and specificity from 0 to 100 percent.[6] Borman et al. report 91 percent accuracy in a pediatric population,[8] a group for which bone scanning has had disappointing results. Some investigators have tried combining bone scanning and gallium imaging, with osteomyelitis suggested when uptake is incongruent or when focal uptake of gallium exceeds that of technetium.[6,9] One study using this combination reported a 38 percent sensitivity and 86 percent specificity, with an overall accuracy of 57 percent,[10] while Palestro cites a 60 to 80 percent accuracy with this technique.[9] Most authors conclude that leukocyte imaging is superior to gallium imaging for cases of complicated osteomyelitis, making it the procedure of choice.[6,9]

Leukocyte imaging uses neutrophils labeled with ^{111}In or, less commonly, ^{99m}Tc to diagnose infection. Since uptake of ^{111}In-labeled white blood cells (WBC) is not related to bone turnover, it is more specific for infection than bone scanning or gallium imaging. Wegener and Alavi cite sensitivities of 80 to 100 percent and specificities of 50 to 100 percent,[7] while Schauwecker combined the results of 16 studies and obtained an overall sensitivity and specificity of 88 and 85 percent, respectively.[6] Normally, ^{111}In-labeled WBC are distributed in areas of red marrow (e.g., axial skeleton). Palestro et al. believe that the wide range of results is in large part due to variable red marrow distribution, particularly in the axial skeleton, which makes it difficult to choose a normal marrow reference point on the scan. They advocate combining a ^{99m}Tc–sulfur colloid marrow scan with the leukocyte study, with osteomyelitis suggested when there is increased ^{111}In-labeled WBC uptake but decreased sulfur colloid uptake. Using this combination, they achieved a sensitivity, specificity, and accuracy of 100, 94, and 96 percent, respectively.[11] Achong and Oates achieved nearly similar results.[12]

Leukocyte scanning does have several weaknesses: (1) Nonbacterial infections, in which neutrophils are not the major responders, may not be well demonstrated. Similarly, chronic bacterial infections in which the neutrophilic response has diminished may not have intense focal uptake,[6,7,9] although Datz disagrees.[13] (2) Leukocyte imaging of vertebral osteomyelitis has a reported accuracy of only 66 percent.[9] Spinal infection may manifest as a cold defect rather than focal "hot spot," a situation occurring in 10 to 60 percent of studies.[6,13] Cold spots are difficult to detect and are not specific for infection.[6] Whalen et al.[14] found a correlation between cold spots and prior antibiotic treatment,[14] but Wegener and Alavi claim that antibiotic treatment and steroids do not alter the efficacy of leukocyte scanning as long as the clinical setting is still suggestive of infection.[7] Palestro et al. reported that cold spots represented a more chronic stage of infection.[15] In contrast to ^{111}In-labeled WBC, Modic reported 94 percent accuracy of bone scan–gallium imaging for vertebral osteomyelitis.[16] (3) Indium is cyclotron-produced, making it less available than technetium, and the process of labeling the WBC takes approximately 2 h[7] and is labor-intensive.[9] (4) Neutropenic patients may not be well labeled.[7,9]

Attention is recent years has focused on an array of newer agents such as polyclonal and monoclonal immunoglobulins,[6,7] Fab fragments of IgG,[6,7,17] ^{111}In-labeled chloride,[7] and ^{99m}Tc-labeled citrate.[18] The immunoglobulins and Fab fragments can be labeled with either ^{111}In or ^{99m}Tc. Sensitivity and specificity for ^{111}In-labeled polyclonal IgG ranges from 91 to 100 percent and 56 to 100 percent, respectively,[6,7] whereas Ang et al. report 95 percent sensitivity and 100 percent specificity for ^{99m}Tc-labeled polyclonal IgG.[19]

In the realm of trauma, the patient with a clinically suspected hip fracture but normal or equivocal radiographs poses a therapeutic dilemma. Patients with hip fractures will be managed surgically, patients with pelvic fractures but without hip fractures may be allowed protected weight bearing, and patients without any osseous injury can be ambulated immediately. The two imaging options for resolving the problem of occult fracture are scintigraphy and MRI. On the three-phase bone scan, acute fracture is characterized by increased perfusion on the angiographic phase and intense, ill-defined uptake on both the blood pool and delayed images.[20] Holder et al.[20] report a 98 percent sensitivity for this technique in 145 patients with radiographically occult hip fracture; in a subset of patients older than 70 years and imaged within 72 h of injury, sensitivity and specificity were 86 and 95 percent, respectively. Those authors concluded that bone scan should be the imaging modality of choice for occult hip fractures, even in elderly patients soon after injury, and that a repeat

study be performed 2 to 3 days later if the initial study is negative. Rizzo et al. disagree, however, choosing MRI as the preferred modality.[21] In their study of 62 patients, MRI was more sensitive than bone scan, and the MRI exams could be performed in 15 min or less. They, as well as Quinn et al., advocate an abbreviated MRI scan, consisting of only a coronal T1-weighted sequence, to screen for suspected hip fracture, thus reducing the cost of the MRI and eliminating the cost of an initial and sometimes repeat bone scan[22] (Fig. 15-1). Moreover, Rubin et al.[23] found that using MRI instead of bone scanning reduced the frequency of hospital admission for the workup of hip fracture and decreased the time interval between hospital admission and surgery. A similar conclusion regarding the cost-effectiveness of immediate MRI examination was reached by

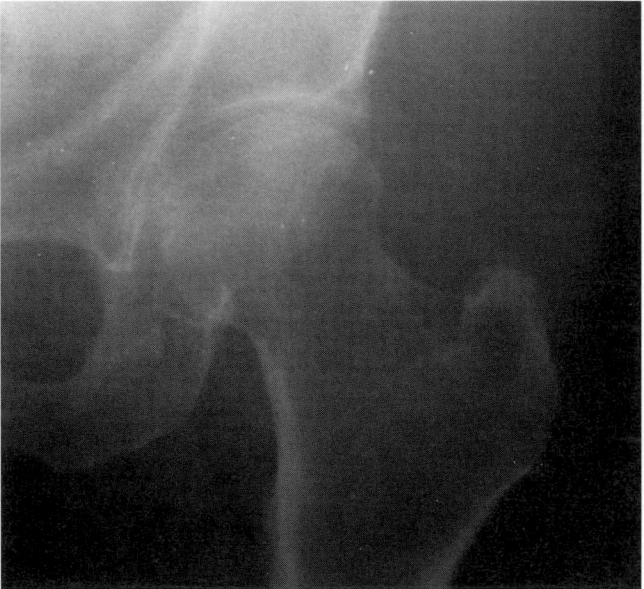

A

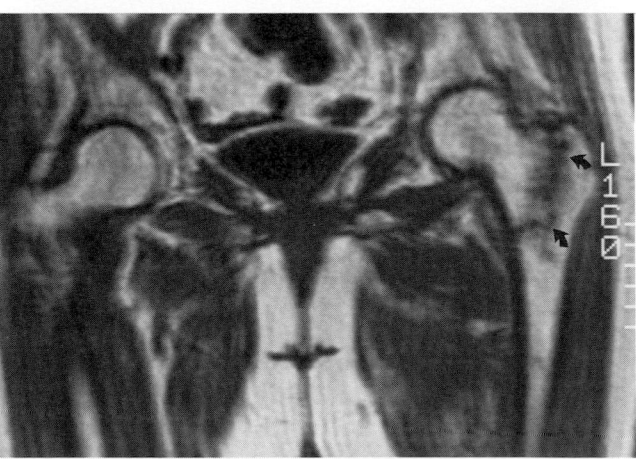

B

Figure 15-1 Ninety-one-year-old woman with left hip pain after a fall. *A.* Anteroposterior radiograph of the hip shows no osseous injury. *B.* Coronal T1-weighted image (TR/TE 550/20) of an abbreviated MRI examination shows an intertrochanteric fracture (*arrows*) of the left hip.

Guanche et al.[24] We prefer MRI because of its unparalleled anatomic resolution (and resultant increased specificity) and demonstration of associated soft tissue injury.

Stress fractures and shin splints may also be evaluated with bone scan,[20,25] and bone scan can also provide a whole-body screening survey in cases of suspected child abuse.[26] Mesgarzadeh et al.[27] recommend three-phase bone scan as the procedure of choice for the evaluation of mechanical stability of osteochondritis dessicans, reserving MRI for instances of indeterminate bone scans; however, we prefer MRI as the initial imaging modality.

The most common use of bone scanning in our department is the search for metastatic disease. Radiographs are insensitive for the demonstration of metastases, requiring 30 to 50 percent loss of mineralization before being radiographically visible. Bone scan is sensitive for most metastatic tumors, but some tumors—such as myeloma, lymphoma, highly anaplastic carcinomas, and renal cell and papillary thyroid carcinomas—are not well demonstrated by bone scan because of their highly aggressive and lytic nature, which causes little osteoblastic response.[26] Bone scan may have a 40 percent false-negative rate for these tumors.[28] In these instances, evaluation is best performed with radiographs, followed by MRI if the radiographs are normal but clinical suspicion remains high. Moreover, uptake is not specific and sites of trauma and bone infarct can be mistaken for metastatic disease. Certain patterns of uptake are helpful, however, such as focal uptake in adjacent sites in several ribs, which is suggestive of previous fracture rather than metastatic disease. Areas of increased uptake, particularly if single, should be further evaluated by radiographs; a normal radiograph without an obvious benign reason for the uptake, such as callus, is suggestive of metastasis, and further imaging with CT or MRI may need to be performed.[29] We have also used bone scanning to evaluate, preoperatively, the long bones of patients who are going to have prophylactic nailing of a destructive lesion seen on radiographs, to make sure there are no radiographically occult lesions that might act as stress risers at the planned tip of the intramedullary rod.

The role of scintigraphy in the evaluation of suspected primary bone tumors is severely limited due to the poor specificity of the exam and the poor anatomic resolution in determining a lesion's boundaries and extent.[30] Moreover, benign and malignant lesions cannot be distinguished by either bone scan or gallium imaging, with uptake of both by osteosarcoma, Ewing's sarcoma, metastases, healing fracture, Paget's disease, fibrous dysplasia, and other benign processes.[26,30]

Imaging with thallium 201 (^{201}Th) is also being used in the evaluation of both primary bone tumors and bony metastases.[31] Thallium has sensitivity for osteosarcoma equal to that of bone scan, but its importance may not lie so much of its diagnostic as in its prognostic capability. Unlike MDP, which is incorporated into new bone formation, thallium is taken up by the osteosarcoma itself and thus may be able to assess tumor viability after chemotherapy, thereby distinguishing which tumors are good responders to preoperative chemotherapy and which are not.[31] (See discussion of tumors, further on). Unfortunately, thallium is plagued by the same problems of speci-

ficity as bone scan and gallium imaging, showing increased activity in benign processes such as eosinophilic granuloma, Paget's disease, fibrous dysplasia, stress fracture, fracture, and inflammatory processes as well as in other malignancies such as Ewing's sarcoma.[31] Nonetheless, there are reports using thallium chloride to differentiate benign from malignant processes. Van der Wal et al.[32] reported uptake in 7 of 8 malignant tumors but in only 1 of 17 benign processes. In contrast, Caluser et al.[33] described 88 percent sensitivity but only 69 percent specificity and 83 percent accuracy of thallium for diagnosing sarcomas. They concluded that the ratio of thallium uptake in the tumor to that in normal tissue could not differentiate benign and malignant processes, but that this ratio, combined with a ratio of ^{99m}Tc-MDP blood pool uptake in abnormal and normal tissue, had 100 percent sensitivity and 100 percent positive predictive value for malignancy if the thallium ratio was greater than the blood pool ratio. It is recommended that thallium ratios be calculated from SPECT rather than planar images.[34]

A discussion of various modalities available to image osteonecrosis, particularly avascular necrosis (AVN) of the femoral head, is found elsewhere in this chapter, but a brief mention of scintigraphic ability is worthwhile. Acute AVN of the femoral head manifests on bone scan as a photopenic defect. Reported sensitivities and specificities for planar imaging range from 55 to 89 percent and 50 to 100 percent, respectively.[35–38] Imaging with SPECT has been advocated to increase the sensitivity, the rational being that overlying activity from the pelvis would be eliminated by the tomographic technique. While isolated case reports have confirmed the helpfulness of SPECT in equivocal planar imaging cases,[39] reported sensitivities and specificities are 58 to 85 percent and 78 to 100 percent, respectively, for single-head SPECT cameras.[38,40] Using a triple-head SPECT unit does not substantially increase the sensitivity (88.5 percent).[41] In addition, bone scan had not proved useful in predicting collapse of the avascular femoral head, either in children[42] or in adults.[43]

Computed Tomography

Computed tomography (CT) uses a tightly collimated, fan-like beam of x-rays to produce tomographic images. The x-ray tube is mounted on the inside of a ring, with detectors placed on the ring across from the tube. The tube rotates 360° during each exposure, and an image is created by the process of "back-transformation," using a Fourier transform algorithm. The ring of a conventional CT scanner needs to be "unwound" back to the zero position between exposures, and the tabletop (carrying the patient) moves a discrete incremental amount between exposures but does not move during the exposure. In contrast, spiral (also called *helical*) CT units have slip-ring technology, allowing the x-ray tube and detectors to rotate continuously as the tabletop is fed nonstop through the ring. This allows rapid exams (on the order of 30 to 90 s) and the acquisition of a volume of raw data that can then be displayed in any two- or three-dimensional plane; while there is a minimal loss of resolution caused by scanning a moving object, this is offset by the large advantage of obviating patient motion. Spiral scanners can be operated in a conventional mode if desired. With the emergence of MRI, CT is no longer the "workhorse" of musculoskeletal imaging, and its role in the evaluation of trauma, neoplasia, and infection is being redefined.

In the evaluation of complex or comminuted fractures, CT is better than MRI because of its superior spatial resolution and its ability to demonstrate small cortical fragments. Although MRI is exquisitely sensitive to the presence of fracture, fracture detail itself may be masked by the accompanying marrow and soft tissue edema (Fig. 15-2). Fracture evaluation is greatly enhanced by the reconstruction of axial data into either two-dimensional coronal and sagittal planes or into three-dimensional images, and these reconstructions may be more informative than the plain radiographs.[44,45] This is particularly true for horizontal fractures that are in the plane of the axial CT image and for sites of complex anatomy such as the acetabulum[46,47] and the ankle.[44–48] Even sagittal and coronal reconstruction of less complex sites such as the tibial plateau may yield information not well appreciated on radiographs.[49] Similarly, Nakamura et al.[50] reported that three-dimensional reconstruction of scaphoid fractures demonstrated fracture displacement better than radiographs. Rosenberg et al. found that routine radiographs underestimated the amount of posterior articular facet depression in their study of CT of calcaneal fractures,[51] and Johnston et al. reported that CT changed management of distal radius injury by demonstrating both fractures and intraarticular extension, which were not seen on radiographs.[52] In instances of shoulder fracture, in which it may be difficult to assess the humeral head radiographically due to its spherical shape and limitation of patient positioning, we use CT to assess displacement of the tuberosities and to evaluate for "head split." Computed tomography is also excellent for evaluation of the sternoclavicular joint, an area notoriously hard to assess radiographically.[53] In the wrist, we prefer directly acquired coronal and sagittal images instead of reconstructed images if the patient is able to cooperate with positioning.

Although CT is inferior to MRI for depiction of soft tissue detail, associated soft tissue injury can be identified on CT. Twenty-two instances of peroneal tendon injury were found in 24 cases of calcaneal fracture assessed by CT, the most common injury being lateral displacement.[54] In contrast, a comparison of MRI and CT for the evaluation of tibial plateau fractures found MRI far superior for diagnosing concomitant soft tissue injuries such as meniscal and ligamentous tears.[55] These authors also found MRI equal to or better than CT in evaluating routine plateau fractures, whereas CT was better in complex or severely comminuted cases. At our institution, we use CT with sagittal and coronal reconstructions, rather than MRI, to evaluate plateau fractures.

Other uses of CT after trauma include assessment of fracture nonunion. Kuhlman et al. studied 19 patients with clinically suspected nonunion using CT with two-dimensional reconstruction.[56] Radiographs in these cases were indeterminate because of metallic hardware, prior operations, or presence of bone graft. Lack of osseous bridging across the fracture was identified in 13 cases, and variable amounts of bony bridging were identified in 6. The presence of orthopedic hardware was not detrimental to the reconstructed images. We too have found CT useful in this clinical situation (Fig. 15-3).

By scanning through a joint after intraarticular injection of contrast and air, one can use CT to evaluate the cartilage and other articular structures. The most common use of CT arthrography in the shoulder is the evaluation of the glenoid labrum. Sensitivity for labral abnormalities in patients with glenoid instability range from 73 to 95 percent[57,58] and 94 percent for detection of superior labrum anterior and posterior (SLAP) lesions.[59] Recurrent instability after repair has also been successfully assessed with this technique.[60] In the knee, chondromalacia patellae,[61] synovial plicae,[62] and the cruciate ligaments[63] can be well visualized by CT arthrography. Although MRI is the preferred method of evaluating articular cartilage, osteo-

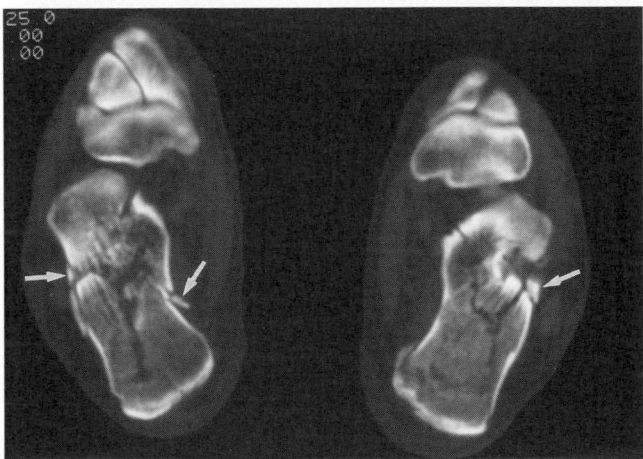

A

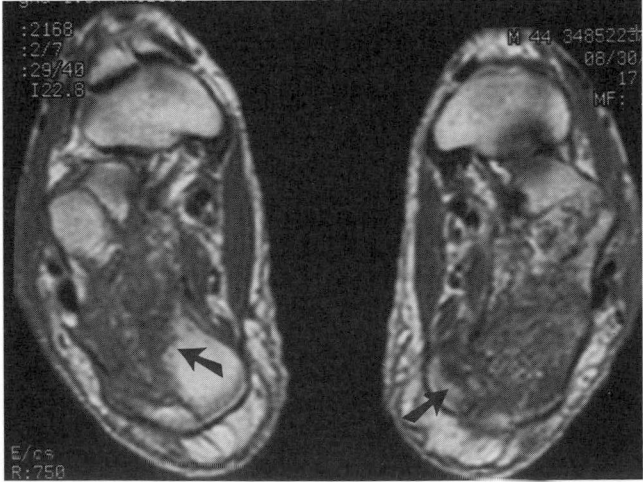

B

Figure 15-2 Forty-four-year-old man who sustained bilateral calcaneal fractures after an attempted suicide jump. *A.* Axial CT scan through both calcanei shows numerous fracture lines and small cortical fragments (*arrows*). *B.* Axial T1-weighted image at same level as the CT shows diffuse marrow edema (*arrows*) that obscures the fracture lines.

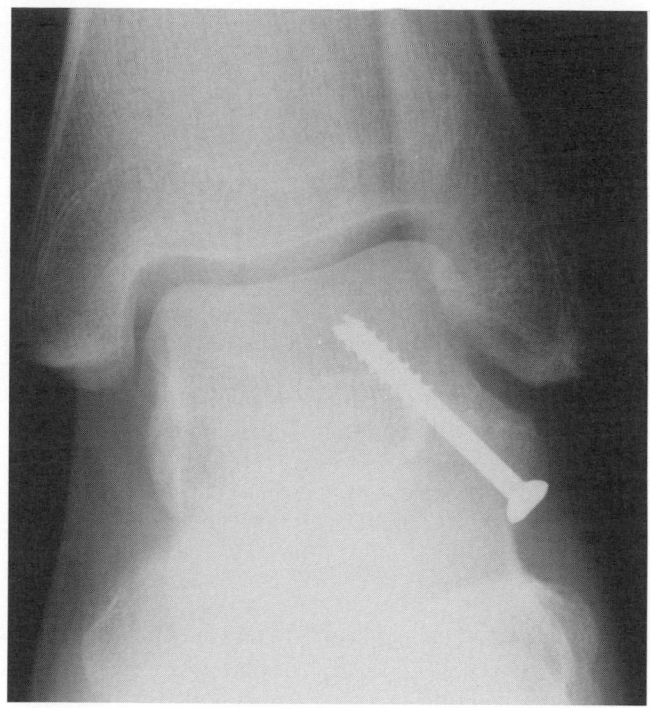

A

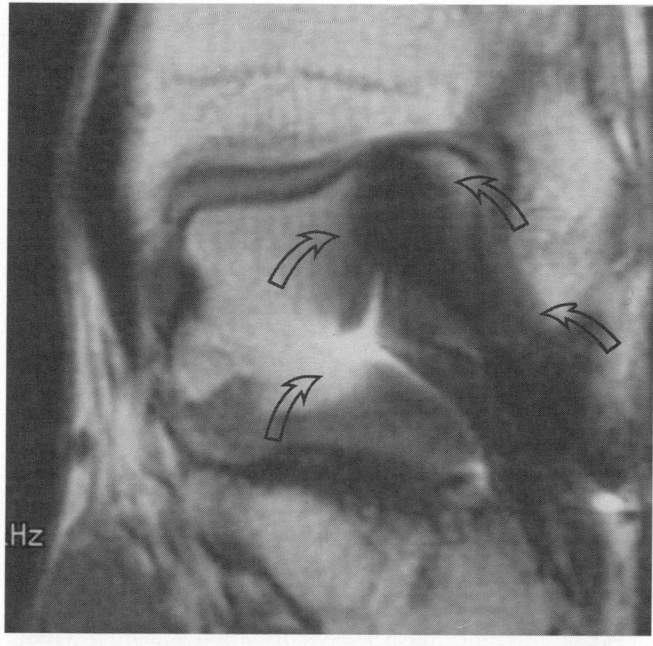

B

C

Figure 15-3 Twenty-three-year-old man with persistent pain 9 months after screw fixation of a fracture of the inferior aspect of the talus. *A.* Anteroposterior radiograph demonstrates the lag screw. The fracture site could not be visualized on this or any other radiograph. *B.* Coronal T1-weighted image (500/20) MRI performed to evaluate for a possible osteochondral injury of the dome of the talus as a source of the persistent pain. The screw causes dephasing artifact (*arrows*), which distorts the talar dome and subtalar region. *C.* Coronal CT-arthrogram of the ankle performed to better evaluate for osteochondral injury of the talar dome shows a normal cartilage surface. Instead, a delayed union of the original fracture was identified (*arrow*). The screw causes mild artifact.

chondritis dessicans is well evaluated by CT arthrography. We also use this technique to look for suspected, but radiographically occult intraarticular loose bodies, as has been described by others.[60] A major disadvantage of CT arthrography is that it is an invasive procedure.

Imaging of infection and tumors is discussed elsewhere in this chapter, and so only brief mention will be made here. We prefer MRI to CT for the evaluation of osteomyelitis and soft tissue infection because of the superb soft tissue contrast of the former. Some patients, however, cannot be scanned with MRI (e.g., those with pacemakers, ICU patients with non-MRI-compatible monitoring devices), and in these situations CT is an acceptable alternative. Beauchamp et al. have recently reviewed the CT appear-

ances of cellulitis, lymphedema, necrotizing fasciitis, myonecrosis, and abscess.[64] Findings range from swelling and change in attenuation of the involved tissue to frank air and walled-off collections. They advocate the use of intravenous contrast to enhance inflammatory tissue. Subtle early changes of osteomyelitis—such as demineralization, periosteal reaction, and soft tissue edema—are better seen with CT than radiographs. More advanced acute changes include replacement of the normal low-attenuation fatty marrow by intermediate-attenuation edema, and chronic cases may show medullary sclerosis. Computed tomography is superior to MRI for demonstrating subtle cortical destruction and evaluation of sequestra.[65] Similarly, bone tumor characteristics—such as margination, periosteal reaction, and matrix mineralization—can be well appreciated on CT even when at an early stage that might not be as well visualized on radiographs.[66] In the evaluation of subtle cortical destruction and matrix and soft tissue mineralization, CT is better than MRI.[67] Magid advocates two-dimensional reconstruction in the sagittal and coronal planes in order to fully appreciate the extent and characteristics of the tumor.[66]

Ultrasound

Although in the mainstream of abdominal imaging since its invention, ultrasound is quickly becoming appreciated for its musculoskeletal applications as well. The modality is based on the transmission of sound waves through tissue and the time it takes for the waves to be reflected back to the transducing probe. Since different tissues transmit sound waves at different velocities and the waves are reflected at tissue interfaces, sound waves that originate from the transducer at the same time will return to the transducer at different times. This information is used to create an image. Ultrasound is readily available and inexpensive; on the other hand, it is operator-dependent and has a long learning curve. Orthopedic applications include trauma, sports injuries, soft tissue tumor evaluation, infection, congenital and acquired pediatric disorders, bone mineral density, arthropathies, and several other miscellaneous topics.

In the setting of trauma, ultrasound has been used to detect acute bony and soft tissue injury and to assess the quality of callus formation. The cortex of bone is a highly reflective sonographic surface, appearing as a bright ("echogenic") line. Any discontinuity or step-off of that cortical surface may represent a fracture. In this regard, sonography's role is not to replace radiography but to complement it in the instance of a clinically suspected fracture and negative plain films. The ability of ultrasound to detect radiographically occult fractures is not good, however. Christiansen et al.[68] reported only 37 percent sensitivity and 61 percent specificity for occult scaphoid fractures. Sonographic techniques other than imaging of the fracture itself have been tried in attempts to diagnose scaphoid fractures. Hodgkinson et al. measured displacement of the radial artery from the injured scaphoid and compared it to the patient's uninjured side;[69] using a ratio of the two distances, they found 100 percent sensitivity but 74 percent specificity. Finkenberg et al. used vibratory sound waves and achieved 100 percent sensitivity and 95 percent specificity for scaphoid fractures.[70] Since the management of true and suspected scaphoid fractures is the same, sonographic diagnosis may be a moot point, since radiography can be repeated 1 to 2 weeks later, more quickly and less expensively, albeit with ionizing radiation. Ultrasound may be helpful in fractures in children because of its ability to depict the radiolucent cartilaginous growth centers, thus demonstrating the extent of fracture lines not appreciated on radiographs.[71]

Degree and quality of fracture healing can also be assessed sonographically, with callus demonstrated earlier than on radiographs[72] and nonunion demonstrated by a disorganized echo pattern.[73] However, comparison of this technique with CT and MRI has not been made. Moreover, despite the demonstration of callus formation, ultrasound may not be able to quantitatively evaluate the mechanical status of the callus.[74]

Sports-related soft tissue injuries, as of the rotator cuff and Achilles tendon, can be evaluated sonographically (see below), as can posttraumatic injury such as rupture of the interosseous membrane in Weber B and C ankle fractures[75] and injury to the lateral ligament complex of the ankle.[76]

Ultrasound is an appealing modality for the detection of osteomyelitis, particularly in children, since it does not use ionizing radiation. The earliest ultrasound finding in osteomyelitis is deep soft tissue swelling, followed by periosteal elevation and subperiosteal fluid or abscess, and, last, cortical destruction.[77] The first two stages can be demonstrated before any radiographic manifestations of infection,[78–80] thus allowing prompt diagnosis and treatment. Most reported results are excellent, with sensitivities and specificities ranging from 86 to 100 percent and 91 to 100 percent, respectively[79–82] Larcos et al.,[83] however, reported only 63 percent sensitivity and 58 percent accuracy. Ultrasound can distinguish osteomyelitis, manifest as a subperiosteal collection, from a soft tissue abscess, manifest as a collection not near bone, and from cellulitis, demonstrated as ill-defined soft tissue thickening,[79,80] and it can be used to guide the aspiration and/or drainage of subperiosteal abscesses. As with all aspects of ultrasound, experience is necessary for accuracy in both scanning and interpretation.

Ultrasound is becoming popular in the evaluation of sports injuries, because it is inexpensive and readily available compared to MRI and is noninvasive compared to arthrography and arthroscopy. In the knee, the utility of MRI for diagnosing meniscal tears ranges from 82 to 94 percent sensitivity and 78 to 88 percent specificity.[84–86] In Gerngross and Sohn's subset of patients who received both ultrasound and arthrography, sensitivity of the former for meniscal tear was 100 percent, while that of arthrography was only 91 percent.[84] Friedl and Glaser, reporting a series of 84 patients studied with ultrasound, found 70 and 98 percent sensitivity and specificity, respectively, for rupture of the anterior cruciate ligament, and 87 percent sensitivity and 96 percent specificity for rupture of the medial collateral ligament.[85] In Maffulli et al.'s series of 52 athletes, however, the cruciate ligaments could not be visualized well enough to be evaluated.[87] We do not believe that knee sonography is a reasonable alternative to MRI for the general evaluation of the injured knee.

In the shoulder, however, ultrasound may be a reasonable alternative to MRI. Sonographic findings of supraspinatus tendon tear include nonvisualization, focal thinning, and focal defect.[88] Experiences of different investigators for detecting full-thickness cuff tears are fairly similar, with sensitivity and specificity ranging from 74 to 95 percent and 91 to 95 percent, respectively.[88–93] Sensitivity of detecting partial-thickness tears is less well agreed upon, however, with results ranging from 41 to 93 percent.[88,89,94] Newman et al.[95] described the use of power Doppler sonography as a helpful adjunct to conventional gray-scale ultrasound to show the hyperemia associated with cuff injuries. Several authors advocate ultrasound as a screening tool or initial imaging modality for assessment of rotator cuff tears because of its high sensitivity, low cost, and widespread availability.[90,93,96] Van Moppes et al. caution, however, that the technique has a long learning curve,[92] which has been our experience, also.

Calcific tendinitis of the supraspinatus tendon can also be demonstrated by ultrasonography,[97] and Farin et al. have described ultrasonically guided treatment with aspiration and lavage of the calcific deposits.[98] In Farin's and Jaroma's review of 951 patients, radiographs were only slightly better at detecting cuff calcification than ultrasound.[97] However, the authors of that study urge, and we agree, that radiographs *must* be performed prior to *any* musculoskeletal sonography to give a general overview of the region and to rule out any abnormality of the underlying bone.

Diseases of tendons other than the supraspinatus have also been investigated with ultrasound. The Achilles tendon, being large and superficially located, is well suited to sonographic evaluation. Sensitivity for Achilles tendon abnormality other than acute complete rupture is 72 to 96 percent, with 83 to 100 percent specificity.[99,100] Neuhold et al. found MRI more sensitive than ultrasound for detection of partial Achilles tear but recommended sonography as the initial imaging modality, reserving MRI for sonographically indeterminate cases.[101] After repair of Achilles rupture, ultrasound can demonstrate the morphologic changes of healing,[102,103] but it may not be able to predict functional results.[102] Other uses of ultrasound related to tendons include detection of early thickening in the fingers in rheumatoid arthritis,[104] evaluation of spondyloarthropic enthesopathy,[105] and assessment of tendon thickening as marker of dialysis-related amyloid infiltration.[106]

Although radiographs should be obtained in every case of suspected soft tissue mass (see discussion of tumors, further on), most soft tissue tumors cannot be characterized on plain films. Because of its ubiquity, low cost, and lack of ionizing radiation, ultrasound has been advocated as the next imaging modality after radiography.[107] While excellent for confirming the nature of cystic masses, like ganglia and Baker's cysts[108,109] (Fig. 15-4), gray-scale sonography cannot accurately diagnose solid or mixed masses.[108] Latifi and Siegel used color Doppler ultrasound to examine 50 pediatric soft tissue masses and reported that the pattern of blood flow could not reliably diagnose lesions or make a distinction between benign and malignant with the exception that abscesses tended to have a peripheral rim of flow.[110] Ozbek et al. measured the resistive indices of soft tissue tumors in 86 patients with color Doppler ultrasound and found a lower index in acute inflammatory processes.[111] Except in locations where a mass is likely to be a cyst (e.g., wrist, popliteal fossa of knee) and therefore diagnosable by ultrasound, we prefer MRI evaluation because of the greater soft tissue characterizability of MRI and the clearer overall depiction of the mass relative to the surrounding structures. For follow-up of soft tissue sarcomas after therapy, Pino et al. found a 77 percent sensitivity of recurrence with sonography and only 62 percent with CT,[112] whereas Choi et al. reported 83 percent sensitivity and 93 percent specificity of MRI and 100 percent sensitivity and 79 percent specificity of ultrasound.[113] Fornage recommends follow-up with ultrasound,

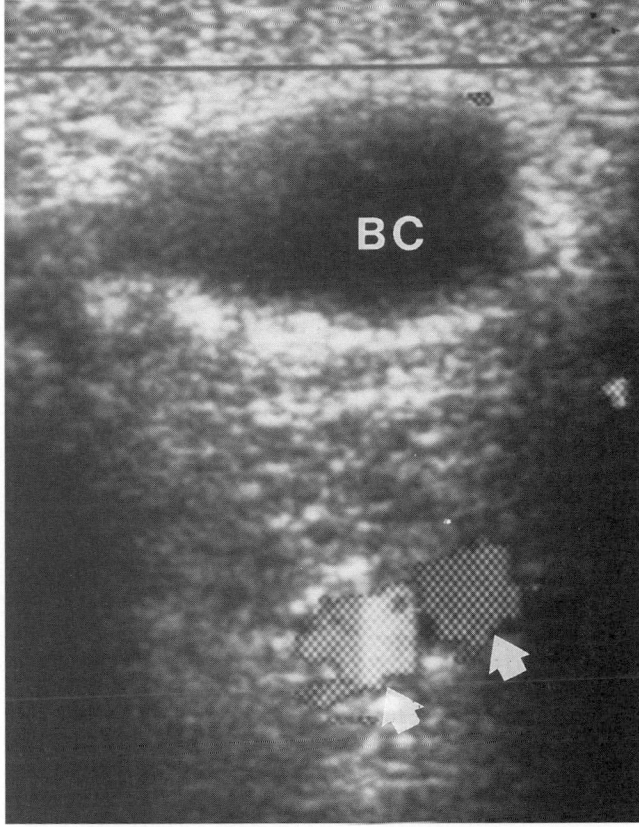

Figure 15-4 Transverse sonographic image of the popliteal fossa of the knee in a woman with a palpable mass demonstrates an anechoic mass consistent with a Baker's cyst (BC). The popliteal artery and vein are deep to this mass (*arrows*).

reserving MRI for inconclusive cases,[114] but we prefer MRI as the surveillance modality (see discussion of tumors, further on).

Several other uses of ultrasound have been described. For example, in patients with carpal tunnel syndrome, ultrasound demonstrates a swollen median nerve in the proximal tunnel and flattened nerve distally, as well as increased palmer bowing of the transverse ligament.[115,116] Synovitis in patients with rheumatoid arthritis and secondary carpal tunnel syndrome can also be well depicted.[117] Ultrasound can be used to determine the presence of the plantaris muscle and tendon of the calf prior to tendon harvesting, to avoid unnecessary surgical exploration if the tendon is congenitally absent[118]; Simpson et al. reported 95 percent sensitivity for detecting a tendon suitable for grafting and 100 percent specificity.[119] While most types of glass foreign bodies are radiopaque and thus visible on radiographs, most wood and plastic foreign bodies are not.[120] On ultrasound all foreign bodies, regardless of composition, are echogenic and thus likely to be visualized on a targeted exam. However, shape and size often cannot be determined because the reflective surface of the object causes acoustic shadowing, which obscures the remainder of the object.[121] Sensitivity and specificity for detection of foreign bodies is 89 percent and 93 percent, respectively.[122]

Ultrasound may also be able to provide a quantitative assessment of bone quality without the radiation of photon or x-ray absorptiometry and CT methods. There are two types of measurement, both of which are typically performed through the calcaneus: (1) ultrasound transmission velocity (UTV) and (2) attenuation of ultrasound signal, called broadband ultrasound attenuation (BUA). These parameters are not mere reflections of bone mineral density but rather are also affected by bone elasticity and bone microarchitecture, respectively.[123] As such, they provide an estimation of bone quality, not bone density; indeed, correlation between these techniques and bone mineral density is only 0.56 to 0.75.[123] A recent study of almost 4700 women found no significant difference in assessment of fracture risk between quantitative ultrasound techniques and absorptiometrically derived bone mineral density; the investigators concluded that the former technique may complement the latter.[124]

Ultrasound is particularly suited to pediatric disorders because of its ability to depict unossified cartilaginous growth centers and its lack of ionizing radiation. This is especially true in infants, in whom radiographic assessment of clubfoot and developmental hip dysplasia may be difficult. Several recent articles suggest the utility and helpfulness of ultrasound for assessing clubfoot.[125–128] While the ability of ultrasound to depict the neonatal cartilaginous femoral head is undisputed, criteria for sonographic determination of hip dislocation and appropriate timing and use of ultrasound are still debated. The two most common methods of determining dislocation are those of Graf,[129] which is based on measurements of the osseous and cartilaginous convexity of the acetabulum relative to the ilium, thus assessing acetabular development, and of Harcke,[130] which dynamically assesses femoral head position in stress, thus evaluating position and stability of the femoral head. A compromise technique, called the *dynamic standard minimum examination,* incorporates features of both methods.[131,132] Other methods include measurement of femoral head coverage by the bony acetabulum[133] and measurements of acetabular cartilage thickness.[134] Harcke and Grissom advocate clinical screening, reserving ultrasound for cases with risk factors for hip dysplasia or with physical findings of instability or hip click.[132] It must be stressed that hip ultrasound is labor-intensive and requires extensive training and practice in order to achieve accurate and reliable results.[132,135,136] A limited CT scan, consisting of only a few slices, is also an excellent way to evaluate alignment of the congenitally dislocatable hip that has been placed in a plaster cast.[137]

Hip disease in older children may also benefit from sonographic evaluation. Wirth et al.[138] compared ultrasound and radiography in 23 children with Legg-Perthes disease and found that sonography was able to demonstrate both healing and lateral extrusion of the femoral head earlier than radiographs; these authors suggest that ultrasound may thus influence the timing of containment treatment and obviate the need to perform arthrography for evaluation of extrusion. Similarly, in a study of 21 patients with 26 instances of slipped capital femoral epiphyses, Kallio et al. found sonographic detection of slippage slightly more sensitive than radiography and free of the projectional errors that plague radiographs.[139] However, they caution that knowledge of the normal appearance of the hip as well as comparison with the asymptomatic side are essential to avoid false-positive diagnoses; examination of both hips in their study took less than 20 min.

Magnetic Resonance Imaging

The advent of MRI has had a profound effect on the evaluation of musculoskeletal disease. Foremost among the numerous advantages of this imaging technique is its reliance upon the principles of magnetism rather than ionizing radiation.

Magnetic resonance imaging has great sensitivity to physical differences among tissues and fluids and has the ability to display these differences as image contrast. It shares with CT the ability to produce high-quality cross-sectional images of the human body, but MRI can do so in any imaging plane with greater contrast resolution and equal or greater spatial resolution. It shares with nuclear medicine the capability of providing physiologic data, but it does so without the need for radiation-emitting pharmaceutical agents. It can provide information about blood vessel anatomy and blood flow similar to that defined with angiography, but it does so without the need for iodinated contrast material. With particular relevance to the musculoskeletal system, MRI can define intra- and periarticular anatomy with results similar or superior to those of arthrography. Magnetic resonance imaging accomplishes these goals without significant biological ill effects.[140]

In order to harness the tremendous strengths of this imaging modality, an understanding of the physical principles upon which MRI is based is necessary.[141–147] After a review of these physical principles, a discussion of the methodology of generating an MR image as well as the specific parameters that affect image contrast is provided. Subsequently, specific applications of MRI in the evaluation of musculoskeletal disease are discussed.

Physical Principles

Nuclear spin is the underlying principle of MRI. Only those nuclei with an odd number of protons or neutrons possess nuclear spin. These nuclei can be thought of as spinning charged particles that behave like tiny magnets. The hydrogen nucleus (proton), due to its natural abundance in the human body and its favorable magnetic properties, is utilized in medical MRI.

The normal situation within the human body is for the hydrogen nuclei (protons) to be randomly oriented, with their tiny magnetic fields canceling each other; thus there is no net magnetization. With the application of an external magnetic field, the protons align parallel and antiparallel to the field (Fig. 15-5). Since the lower-energy state is to be aligned parallel to the field, a very small excess of protons are aligned parallel to the field, creating a net magnetization. It has been calculated that at a magnetic field strength of 1.5T (used in many clinical scanners), this excess of protons aligned with the magnetic field is only about 8 per 2 million protons. It is the signal from this tiny excess of protons that is utilized in MRI.

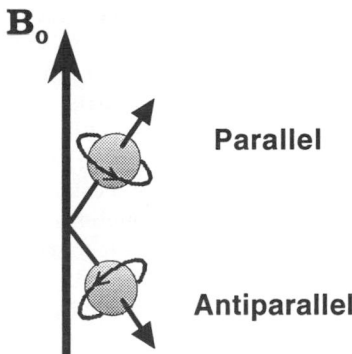

Figure 15-5 Spinning protons align parallel and antiparallel to an applied magnetic field.

The concept of precession is central to understanding MRI. Common examples of precession are the movement of the earth and planets about the sun or the rotation of a spinning top. In these examples the precession results from the effect of an orienting gravitational field on the motion of the object. Similarly, when a patient is placed in a strong magnetic field, alignment of the magnetic moments of the protons in water and fat creates a net magnetization in the tissue. The aligned magnetic moments also precess about the main magnetic field (Fig. 15-6). This precession is a cyclic process with a characteristic frequency.

The relationship between the magnetic field's strength and the characteristic precessional frequency is governed by the Larmor equation $v = \gamma \cdot B_0$, where v is the Larmor, or precessional, frequency; γ is the gyromagnetic ratio (which equals 42.58 MHz/T for the proton); and B_0 is the strength (in teslas) of the external magnetic field.

Next we must define the term *resonance.* This refers to the change in energy states of the nucleus, caused by absorption of a specific radiofrequency. The small net magnetism produced by precessing protons in tissue in a strong external magnetic field cannot be measured directly with any accuracy. Instead it is detected indirectly with a second perturbing magnetic field (B_1) perpendicular to the main magnetic field (B_0). This perturbing magnetic field (B_1) is applied through a short pulse of a radio-frequency (RF) wave at the Larmor frequency. The synchronization of the RF pulse with the precessing (Larmor) frequency of the spinning protons causes energy to be transmitted efficiently to the protons, which then resonate and begin to precess around the perturbing magnetic field (B_1) (Fig. 15-7). After excitation, the net magnetization of the protons in the tissue generates a transverse magnetic field. This can induce a voltage in a receiver coil, which can be detected and translated into an MR signal. This transverse magnetization does not persist after the exciting RF pulse is turned off and the perturbing magnetic field removed. This transverse magnetization decays to zero through a process called *free induction decay* with a characteristic time constant. The amplitude of the voltage detected in the receiver coil as a result of the transverse magnetization also decays to zero. The initial signal amplitude is proportional to the net transverse magnetization, which is itself proportional to the number of protons excited in a particular volume element (voxel) of tissue. Thus differences in proton density become discernible in the MR image.

Generation of the MR Image

The generation of an MR image can be thought of as a four-dimensional problem. The spatial origin of the MR signal must be defined with suitable resolution in three orthogonal planes or three dimensions. The fourth dimension to be resolved is that of contrast and is reflected by the intensity of the signal within each volume element of tissue.

How is the spatial origin of the MR signal identified? In a perfectly homogeneous static magnetic field, all of the water and fat protons would precess at the same Larmor frequency. However, the strength of the magnetic field can be made to vary in a linear, predictable fashion in each of three dimensions through the use of magnetic-field gradient coils. Every MR scanner makes use of such gradient coils to induce a linear change in the magnetic field B_0 in each of three dimensions. Since the precessional frequency of a proton in a particular voxel of tissue is dependent upon the effective magnetic field strength as governed by the Larmor equation, the precessional frequency can be made to vary as a function of spatial location by the use

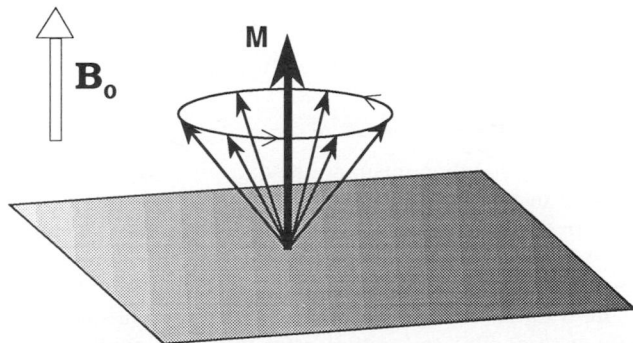

Figure 15-6 The aligned magnetic moments of the protons precess (*horizontal circular arrowed path*) about the magnetic field B_0, creating net magnetization M.

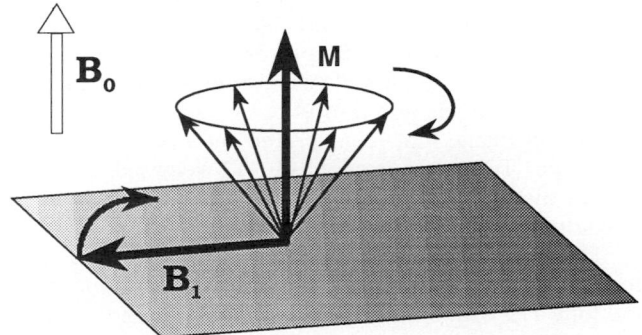

Figure 15-7 Transverse magnetization is induced by a perturbing magnetic field B_1, which is perpendicular to B_0.

of gradient coils. In this way, the three-dimensional origin of the MR signal is identified. It is the gradient coils that cause the loud clanging noise familiar to any patient who has undergone an MR examination.

An MR image is created by a particular schedule or sequence of radiofrequency pulses. After a particular slice or volume of tissue is excited, the MR signal can be detected for only a short time. The decay of the signal is a result of two different types of relaxation processes.

When a perturbing magnetic field or RF pulse is applied for a time sufficient to deflect the magnetic moment to a plane perpendicular to the main magnetic field (B_0), this is called a 90° pulse. After a 90° excitation pulse, the nuclei are in phase with one another and precess as a unit. In a very short time, however, due to interactions with neighboring nuclei, the nuclei spin out of phase with one another thus causing decay of the transverse magnetization. The time required for 63 percent of the signal to disappear irreversibly is called the T2 relaxation time. The T2 relaxation time of a tissue is an intrinsic property with a fixed value. The T2 relaxation time is also known as the transverse or spin-spin relaxation time.

The second type of relaxation involves the transfer of energy from the excited magnetic moments in a slice of tissue to the surrounding lattice of magnetic moments in other molecules. This spin-lattice relaxation time is also known as the longitudinal or T1 relaxation time. Just as the T2 relaxation time is an exponential function, so is the T1 relaxation time. It is defined as the time required to restore 63 percent of the equilibrium population of magnetic moments to be aligned with the external magnetic field (B_0) after being deflected by a 90° pulse. The T1 relaxation time for any tissue is always greater than or equal to the T2 relaxation time. For most soft tissues, the range of T1 relaxation time varies from 220 to 3000 ms. T2 relaxation times vary from 55 to 200 ms.

Pulse Sequences

There is an ever-increasing array of pulse sequences that can be utilized to generate an MR image. The most commonly used is called *spin echo*. In a spin echo sequence, a 90° pulse produces transverse magnetization. The maximal transverse magnetization immediately begins to decay through T1 and T2 relaxation. However, if a second RF pulse is applied (a 180° pulse), the dephasing of the magnetization is reversed and the magnetic moments are refocused, forming an echo or MR signal. TR is the repetition time or the time between RF pulses. TE, or echo time, is the time between the initial perturbing RF pulse and the center of the acquisition period of the echo.

An MR image that is generated by a pulse sequence using short TR and TE is said to be T1-weighted. The contrast in the image primarily reflects any differences in T1 relaxation between adjacent tissues.

Fluids and edema can be accentuated on T2-weighted images. A T2-weighted image is generated with a long TR and long TE. With a long TE, the attenuation of the signal from fluid or edema occurs more slowly than signal from fat, muscle, or connective tissue. Thus fluid and edema appear bright on T2-weighted images.

Many other pulse sequences besides standard spin-echo sequences are currently used in musculoskeletal imaging. Small-flip-angle gradient-echo sequences may produce T2-weighted images in a shorter acquisition time than standard spin-echo sequences. Other sequences have been devised to suppress the signal from fat. In many cases, detection of a pathologic process is hindered by the presence of a large signal from neighboring adipose tissue. Fat suppression can be effectively accomplished and thus increase the conspicuity of a lesion. Other sequences have been devised to assess blood flow, either arterial or venous, in a particular tissue.

The appearance of an MR image is determined by many parameters. Intrinsic parameters have a fixed value governed by the physics of MR. Intrinsic parameters are tissue-dependent. They include the density of water and fat within tissue, blood flow, and the relaxation rate (T1 and T2) of the magnetic moments after excitation. These intrinsic parameters cannot be altered.

Extrinsic parameters are under operator control. They include the series of pulse sequences utilized; the thickness, spacing, and plane of the slices; the matrix size (voxel size); and the number of signal averages from which the image is derived. The choice of these parameters is complex but critical to the success of the examination.

The radiologist must strive for a balance, with the overall general goal of achieving optimal signal-to-noise ratio and therefore the best resolution and tissue contrast in the shortest possible imaging time.

For example, if the MR image is generated by a single signal average, the signal-to-noise ratio will not be as great as when the image is generated by two or more signal averages. An increased number of signal averages, however, requires longer imaging time. Similarly, the slice thickness can be made smaller to improve resolution, but this decreases the signal-to-noise ratio, and a longer imaging time is required to cover the same distance. When the length of the MR examination becomes excessive, patients have difficulty remaining motionless. This can then cause image degradation due to motion artifacts.

It is through a thorough understanding of the fundamental principles by which the MR image is generated that the radiologist can design an MR examination that will be diagnostic for the particular clinical problem to be addressed. Since the design of the examination should be tailored to the specific question of the referring orthopedist, open communication between the orthopedist and radiologist is essential.

Applications

Magnetic resonance imaging has extremely diverse applications in the evaluation of musculoskeletal disorders. The spectrum of conditions that can be evaluated includes disorders of cartilage, muscle, tendons, ligaments, and bone marrow. Imaging may take place in the setting of acute trauma, or the condition may be more chronic in nature, with some intervention being contemplated.

Cartilage A great deal of research in recent years has focused upon optimizing pulse sequences for evaluation of articular cartilage abnormalities.[148–152] Pulse sequences that optimize contrast differences between articular cartilage and the subjacent subchondral bone are necessary to measure cartilage thickness. Sufficient contrast between articular cartilage and adjacent joint effusion is required to identify focal cartilage defects.[151–154] From an orthopedic perspective, both acute and chronic cartilage abnormalities are common. Acute osteochondral or purely chondral injuries are detectable with MRI.[155–156] In patients with osteochondritis dessicans, knowledge of fragment stability and the presence of an articular cartilage defect is useful for determining treatment. DeSmet et al.[157] used a high signal interface between the osteochondral lesion and the parent bone on T2-weighted sequences, as evidence for fragment instability. With this criterion, they correctly identified 14 of 15 lesions, with the final lesion questionably stable at surgery. Six additional patients with displaced fragments and large articular cartilage defects were also correctly identified.

The term *chondromalacia patellae* has been used to describe pathologic softening of the patellar cartilage. Most authors who have correlated MRI of the patellar cartilage with the arthroscopic grading system of chondromalacia established by Shahriaree[158] agree that detection of low-grade disease by MRI is only fair,[159–162] whereas moderate and advanced chondromalacia (stages III and IV) can be reliably identified.[161,162] Yulish and colleagues report an overall accuracy of 89 percent for detection of chondromalacia patellae using standard spin-echo techniques. Quinn and coworkers utilized fast spin-echo and fat-suppression techniques, which improved their ability to detect early disease but did not change their overall accuracy of 79 percent when all stages of chondromalacia were combined.

Chronic or progressive cartilage changes such as those from osteoarthritis may require evaluation to assess for extent and severity of cartilage loss when therapeutic intervention such as partial or complete joint replacement is being considered. In patients with inflammatory arthritides that cause focal cartilage thinning or focal erosions, MRI may play a role in assessing efficacy of different treatment plans.

Muscle Magnetic resonance imaging has proven to be an effective tool in demonstrating normal and diseased muscle. Skeletal muscle has signal intensity intermediate between that of fat and that of cortical bone on most commonly used pulse sequences. Because the difference in signal intensity between fat and muscle is so distinct, intermuscular fat planes are normally readily identified and thus individual muscle groups are well delineated. Magnetic resonance imaging is capable of documenting focal muscle abnormalities or quantifying extent of involvement in more generalized conditions.[163,164]

Polymyositis is a noninfectious inflammatory disorder of muscle that is difficult to diagnose. Because the prognosis for these patients is poor without treatment, a biopsy is commonly required to confirm the diagnosis.[165] The MRI findings in this entity are not specific (diffusely increased signal intensity within the involved musculature on T2-weighted images); but when MRI is used as a method of

guidance to improve biopsy yield, costs of patient care can be decreased.[166] The false-negative rate with non-guided biopsies in polymyositis approaches 25 percent.[166]

Pyomyositis is a well-recognized, serious infection affecting children and young adults in tropical regions. In the United States, the vast majority of cases occur in children and are related to *Staphylococcus aureus* infection. Skeletal muscle is generally highly resistant to metastatic infection, and the pathogenesis of staphylococcal localization in muscle with the development of abscesses is not clear, although it is suggested that an initial muscular insult is required to allow such localization.[167] Magnetic resonance imaging is a useful modality in identifying extent of muscle involvement and in localizing abscess collections (Fig. 15-8). Surgical myotomy and abscess drainage when combined with antimicrobial therapy usually ensure complete resolution.

Regional Magnetic Resonance Imaging

Magnetic Resonance Imaging of the Knee In 1985, Reicher et al.[168,169] proposed that MRI might be a clinically useful tool in evaluating meniscal pathology. Since that time, imaging of the knee has become the most commonly performed nonneurologic MRI examination.[170,171] This modality has virtually replaced arthrography, which is now utilized only in very limited settings,[169,171] such as evaluation of loosening of a joint prosthesis, documentation of communication between the joint and a popliteal mass believed to be an atypical popliteal cyst when the communication is not identified on MRI examination, and in the evaluation of suspected re-tear of the meniscus in a patient with prior meniscal repair or partial meniscectomy.

Magnetic resonance imaging of the knee has also changed the role of arthroscopy since it, unlike arthroscopy, is noninvasive, painless, requires no anaesthesia, results in no postprocedural disability, and is capable of simultaneously assessing both intra- and extraarticular structures. These advantages over arthroscopy have shifted its role from a diagnostic tool to one of therapeutic intervention.

Significant advances have been made in MRI of the knee since its initial application to the evaluation of the meniscus, and routine examinations now encompass a wide spectrum of internal knee derangements and articular disorders.[172,173] Initial MRI of the knee was performed with planar surface coils, which resulted in anterior to posterior signal drop-off. Circumferential extremity coils are now widely available; these provide uniform signal across the knee. The availability of these dedicated wrap-around extremity coils has had the single greatest impact on image quality, speed of examination, and the ability to obtain high-resolution coronal images.[172]

Meniscal Degeneration and Tears The normal fibrocartilaginous menisci have few mobile protons and demonstrate uniformly low signal intensity on all pulse sequences. They are triangular in cross section, with an outer convex curve, and the apex is directed toward the intercondylar notch. Degeneration and tears of the meniscus demonstrate increased signal intensity, which is attributed to imbibed synovial fluid.[172] An MRI grading system for intra-

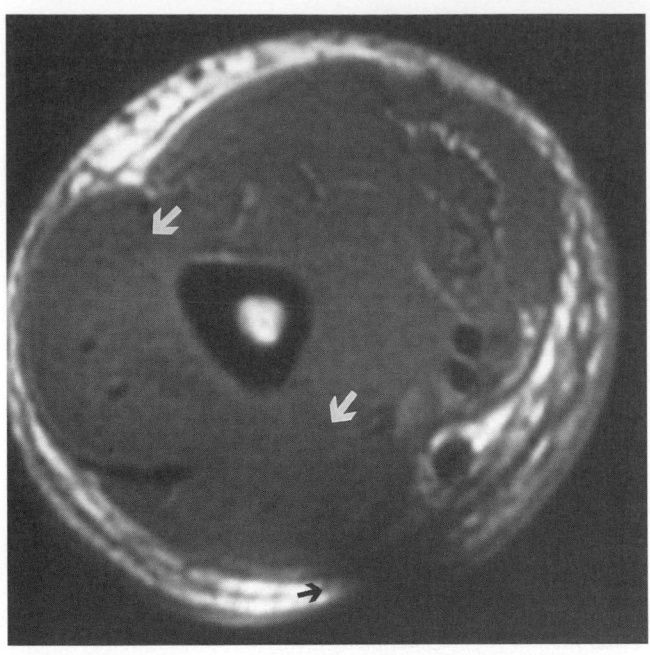

A

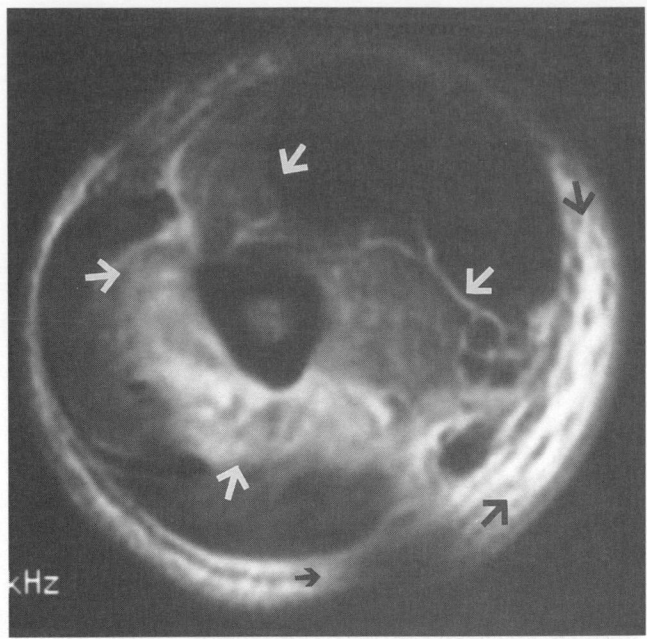

B

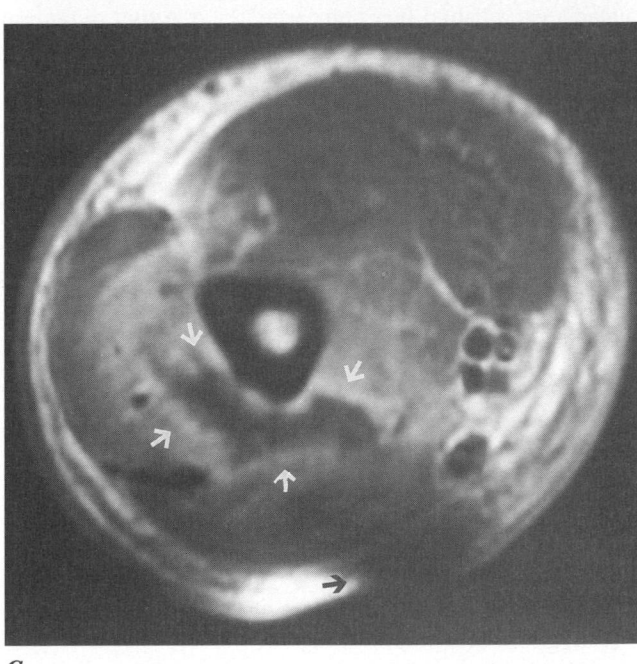

C

Figure 15-8 Pyomyositis. This 25-year-old neutropenic patient had local nonpenetrating trauma to the elbow. Increasing induration and decreasing range of motion occurred despite antibiotic therapy. *A.* T1-weighted axial image (TR/TE 700/18) at level of distal humeral shaft shows enlargement of the medial and lateral heads of the triceps (*white arrows*). *B.* T2-weighted axial image (TR/TE 5000/100) shows edematous/inflammatory changes of the brachialis, brachioradialis, and triceps muscles (*white arrows*) with relative sparing of the biceps brachii. Extensive subcutaneous edema is also present (*large black arrows*). *C.* T1-weighted postcontrast image (TR/TE 700/18) depicts extent of muscular involvement but also outlines a focal intramuscular abscess (*white arrows*). Patient did well after surgical myotomy, debridement, and abscess drainage. Cultures were positive for *Staphylococcus aureus.* (*Small black arrows point to coil artifact.*)

meniscal signal has been developed and correlated with a histologic model.[174] Grade 1 signal is an irregularly marginated or globular increased intrasubstance signal. Grade 2 is a horizontal, linear intrasubstance increased signal that usually extends from the capsular periphery of the meniscus but does not involve an articular margin. An articular margin is the superior or inferior surface of the meniscus directly facing the articular cartilage of the femoral condyle or tibial plateau. The meniscocapsular junction is not considered an articular margin. Grade 3 (Fig. 15-9) is increased signal intensity communicating with at least one articular margin. Histologically, grade 1 and grade 2 signals represent areas of mucinous degeneration.[175] Only those menisci with grade 3 signal represent frank meniscal tears. The prevalence of grades 1 and 2 signals approaches 23 percent in asymptomatic volunteers[176] and can be seen as early as the second decade. Thus differentiation between grade 2 degenerative signal, which is found incidentally, and grade 3 signal, representing a true tear, is important.

Equally important in the assessment of meniscal pathology is evaluation of meniscal morphology (size and shape). The anterior and posterior horns of the lateral meniscus are roughly equivalent in size, while the poste-

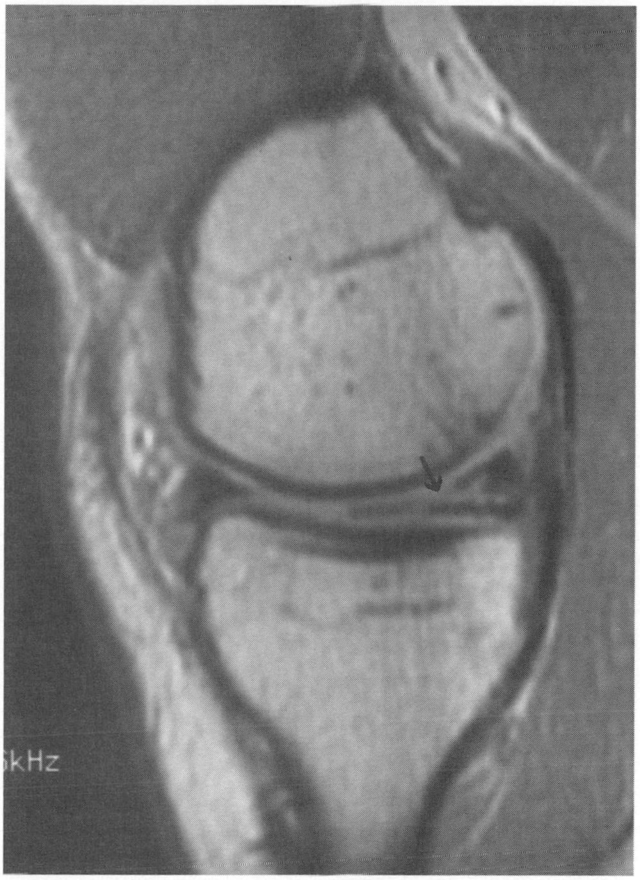

Figure 15-9 Grade 3–signal posterior horn medial meniscus. Tear of the posterior horn identified on sagittal balanced MR image (TR/TE 2000/12) has both oblique and horizontal components with communication to the superior articular surface (*arrow*).

rior horn of the medial meniscus is larger than the anterior horn. Truncation of the sharp apex of a meniscal horn is abnormal in the absence of a history of partial meniscectomy.

Using arthroscopy as the gold standard of measurement, the sensitivity of MRI for detecting meniscal tears has been reported to be between 83 and 98 percent.[173,175,177–184] In one large series by Mink and colleagues, 600 menisci were studied with an accuracy rate of 92 percent.[184] Of perhaps the greatest significance is MRI's high negative predictive value. The chance of failing to detect a clinically significant meniscal tear on MRI is certainly low, with the negative predictive value of MRI approaching 100 percent.[173,186] This very high negative predictive value has greatly diminished the number of purely diagnostic, nontherapeutic, and retrospectively unnecessary arthroscopies.[187] Ruwe et al.[188] showed that the use of MRI could preclude the need for diagnostic arthroscopy in 51 percent of patients, with resulting significant monetary savings.

Magnetic resonance imaging has had less success in identifying tears in meniscal remnants after partial meniscectomy or in identifying retears after primary meniscal

repair. Each of these subsets may demonstrate persistent grade 3 signal. Applegate et al.,[189] increased their overall accuracy for diagnosing recurrent tears in the postoperative meniscus with the administration of intraarticular gadolinium. This increased their accuracy from 66 percent with MRI alone to 88 percent when MR arthrography was used.

Cruciate Ligaments The cruciate ligaments are directly visualized with MRI. Tears of the anterior cruciate ligament (ACL) are a common component of knee injuries. In one large series, 69 percent of all knee injuries requiring surgery had such tears.[190] Although acute ACL injuries can occur in isolation, approximately 65 percent have associated intraarticular injuries, most commonly medial meniscal tears.[185,191]

The normal ACL is composed of two major fiber bundles that course obliquely from their origin on the lateral femoral condyle to their insertion on the tibial plateau anterior to the tibial spines. It is best seen on sagittal T2-weighted images paralleling the intercondylar roof as a continuous low-signal band, with separate fiber striations visible near attachment points (Fig. 15-10). Coronal images may be a helpful adjunct to differentiate between abnormal signal due to partial volume averaging and abnormal signal due to a true tear.

The accuracy of MRI for detecting complete ACL tears is 94 to 95 percent.[173,192] This compares favorably with the best arthrographic results reported[193] and was more sensitive than the commonly applied clinical tests of ACL in-

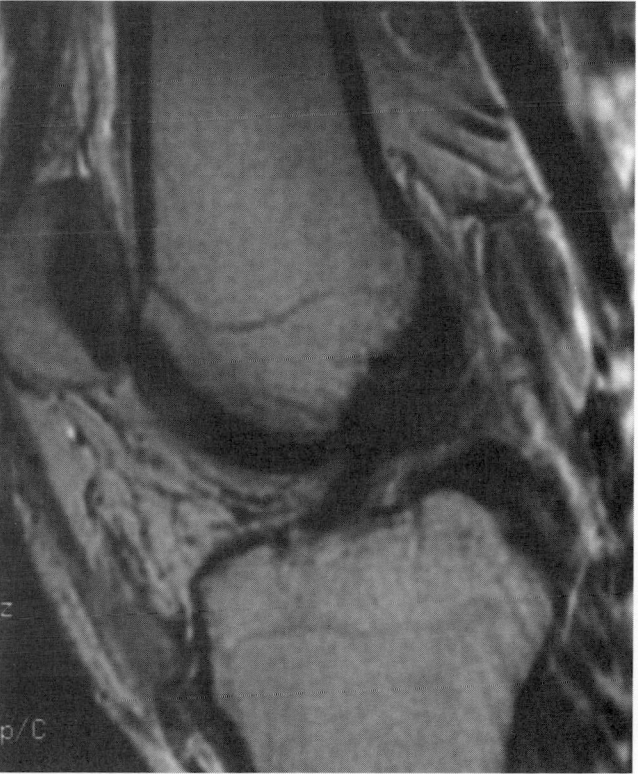

Figure 15-10 Normal appearance of anterior cruciate ligament.

stability, the Lachman test and the anterior drawer test.[192] The criteria for diagnosing complete ACL tear on MRI include discontinuity of the low-signal band on sagittal images, (Fig. 15-11), an irregular wavy contour to the anterior margin of the ACL, or high signal intensity within the substance of the ACL on T2-weighted images (Fig. 15-12).

In addition to the direct signs of ACL injury, Murphy and colleagues have reported an additional, specific, associated sign of complete ACL tear. In their study of 32 adult patients, 92 percent had bone contusions known as *bone bruises* in the posterolateral tibial plateau and the lateral femoral condyle (Fig. 15-13). These bone abnormalities are manifest as poorly marginated areas of low signal on T1-weighted images and high signal intensity on T2-weighted images in comparison to the signal intensity of normal marrow. These bone changes are presumed to occur during injury when the lateral femoral condyle impacts the posterior tibia.[194]

Interestingly, although Murphy found this pattern of bone bruises in the lateral compartment to be a reliable specific sign of complete ACL disruption, Snearly and colleagues[195] showed that this was not true in the pediatric population. In their study of 53 adolescent patients, 28 percent had this same pattern of bone contusions, but with intact ACLs, presumably due to ligamentous laxity in this age group.

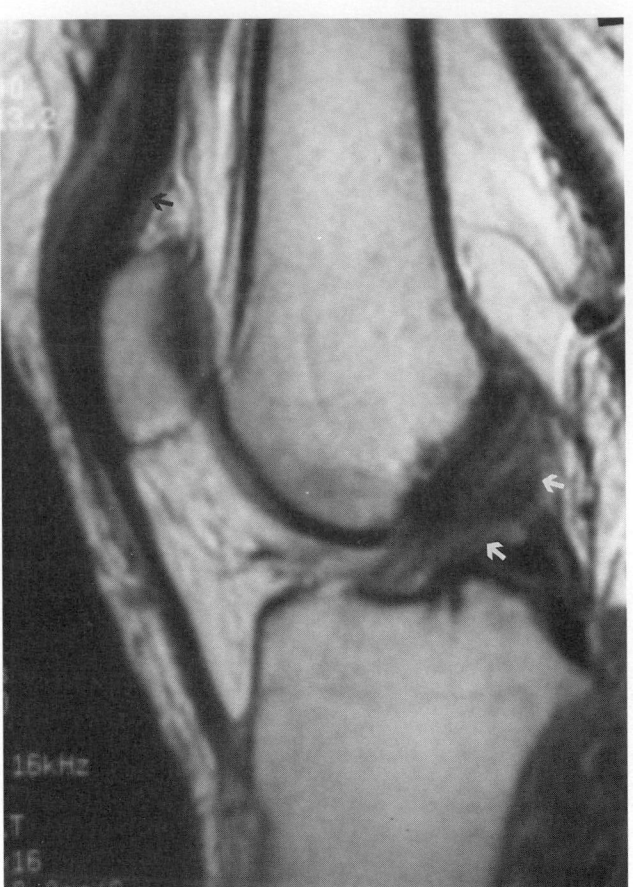

Figure 15-12 Tear of the anterior cruciate ligament. T2-weighted image (TR/TE 2000/12/80) shows complete tear of ACL near its femoral origin (*white arrow*) as well as partial tear of quadriceps tendon (*black arrow*).

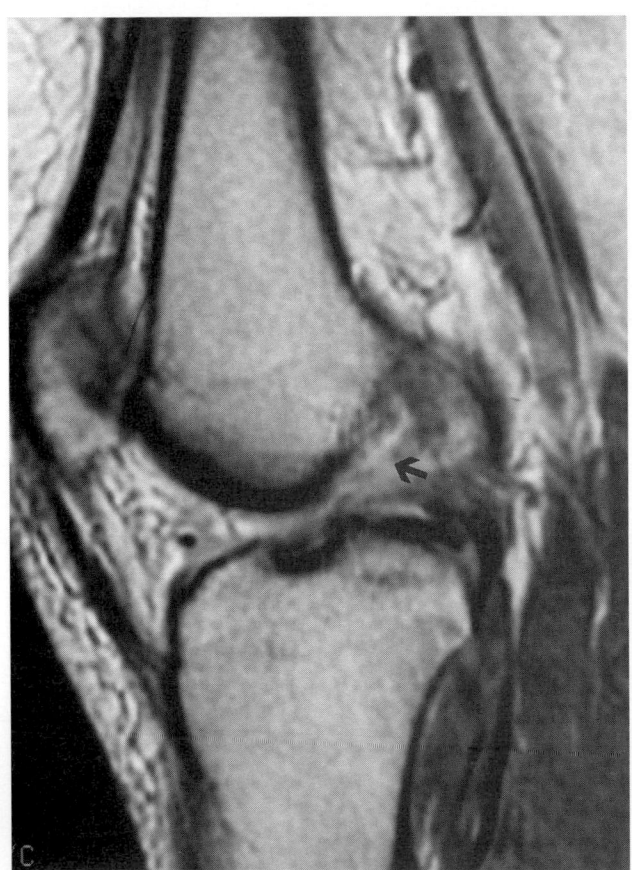

Figure 15-11 A complete midsubstance tear of the anterior cruciate ligament.

In chronic tears of the ACL, the ligament may not be visualized at all; it may be focally angulated or more horizontal in orientation than normal, or it may be scarred down upon the posterior cruciate ligament (PCL).[196]

Magnetic resonance imaging has also proved to be a reliable method for detecting injury to the PCL. It is rare for the PCL to be injured in isolation; such injury is usually associated with tears of the ACL, the meniscus, or the collateral ligaments.[197,198] In the sagittal plane, the normal PCL is seen as a broad band of low signal with an arcuate shape, with the entire length of the ligament normally visualized on a single sagittal image. Because the PCL is thicker than the ACL, it is less affected by knee rotation and volume averaging in the intercondylar notch. Any increase in signal on either T1- or T2-weighted images within the ligament should be regarded as abnormal (Fig. 15-14). Grover et al.[199] reported a 100 percent sensitivity for detection of PCL injury in 202 patients who underwent arthroscopy or surgery. All of the 11 injuries were detected including 4 not detected on clinical exam. None of the 202 patients had an abnormal PCL identified at surgery in the presence of a normal MRI examination.

Occult Bone Injuries Various traumatic bone abnormalities may not be detectable with conventional radiography

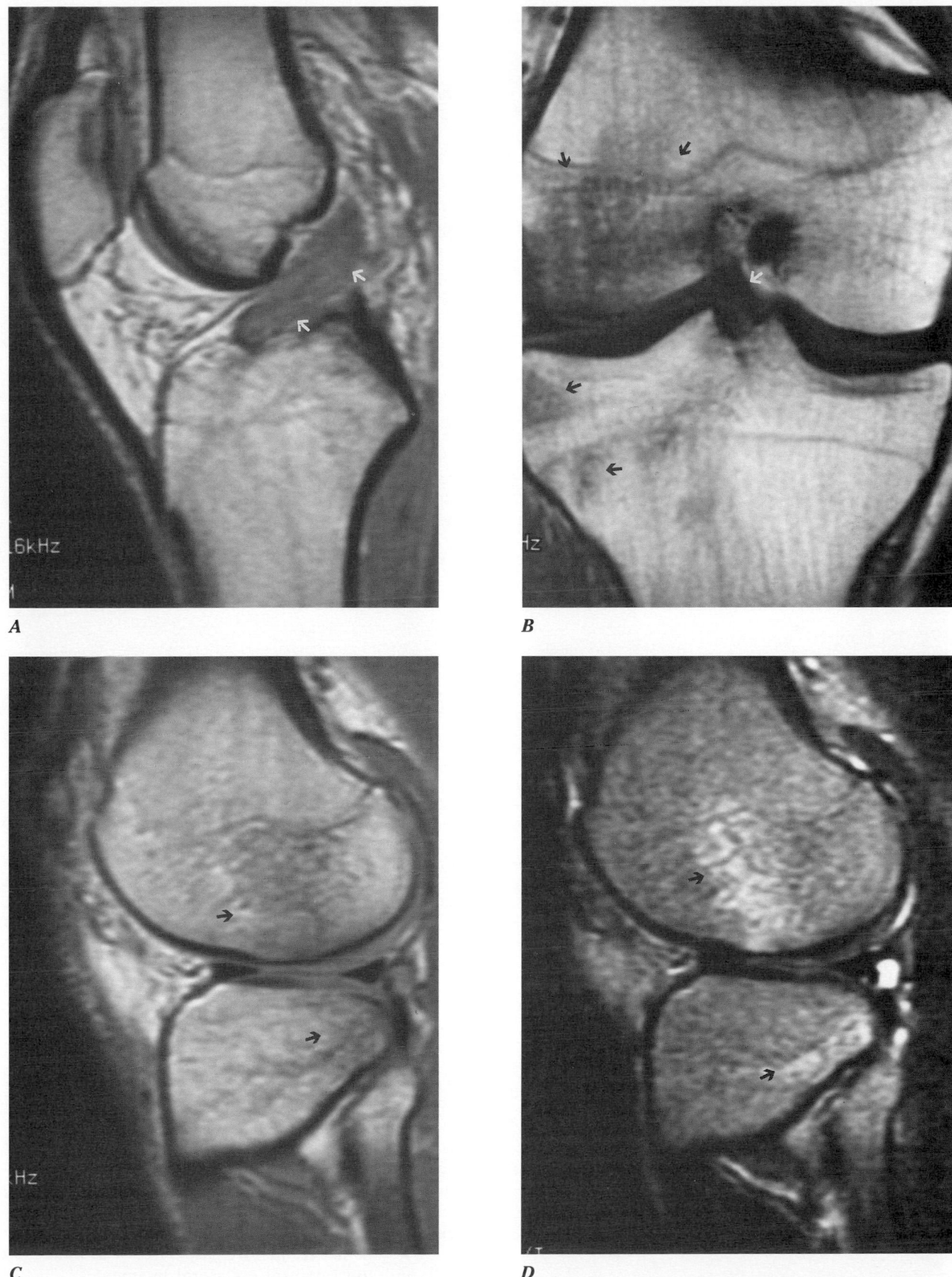

A

B

C

D

Figure 15-13 Tear of the anterior cruciate ligament with associated bone contusions. *A.* Proton-density-weighted sagittal MR image (TR/TE 2000/12). *B.* T1-weighted coronal MR image (TR/TE 500/15). *C.* Sagittal T1-weighted (TR/TE 2200/30) MR image. *D.* Sagittal T2-weighted (TR/TE 2200/80) MR image. Torn and edematous anterior cruciate ligament (*white arrows*) with blurring of the ligamentous fibers. The marrow edema pattern, low signal intensity with T1 weighting, and high signal intensity with T2 weighting in the lateral femoral condyle and posterolateral tibial plateau reflect associated bone contusions (*black arrows*).

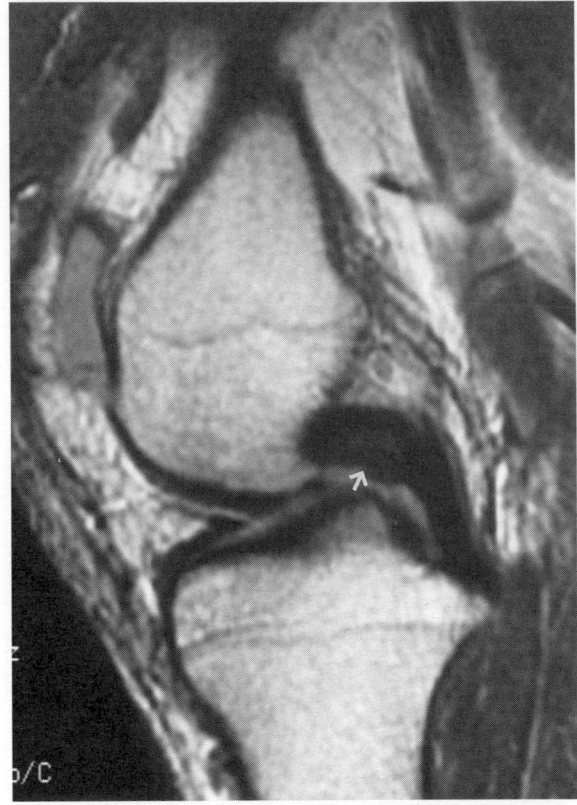

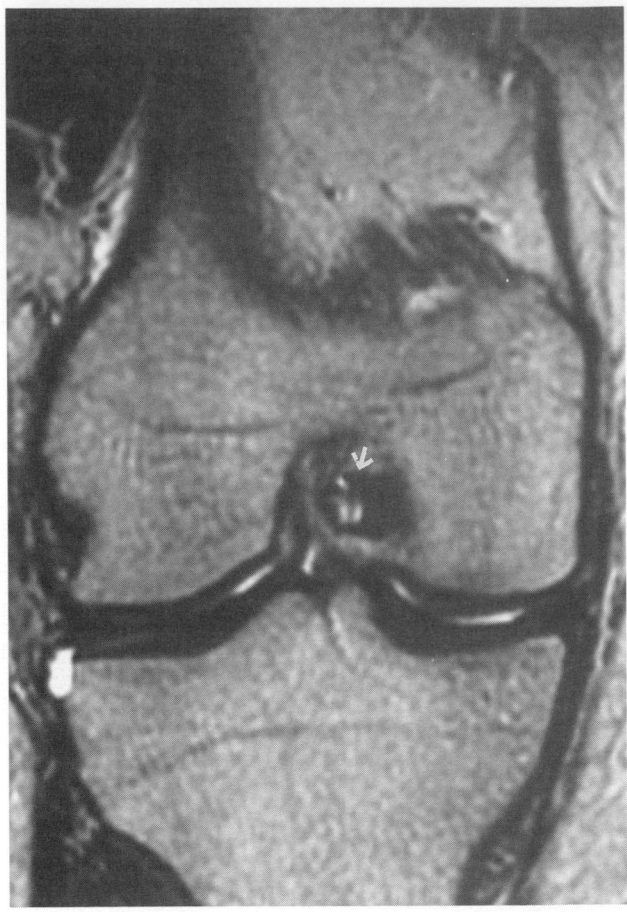

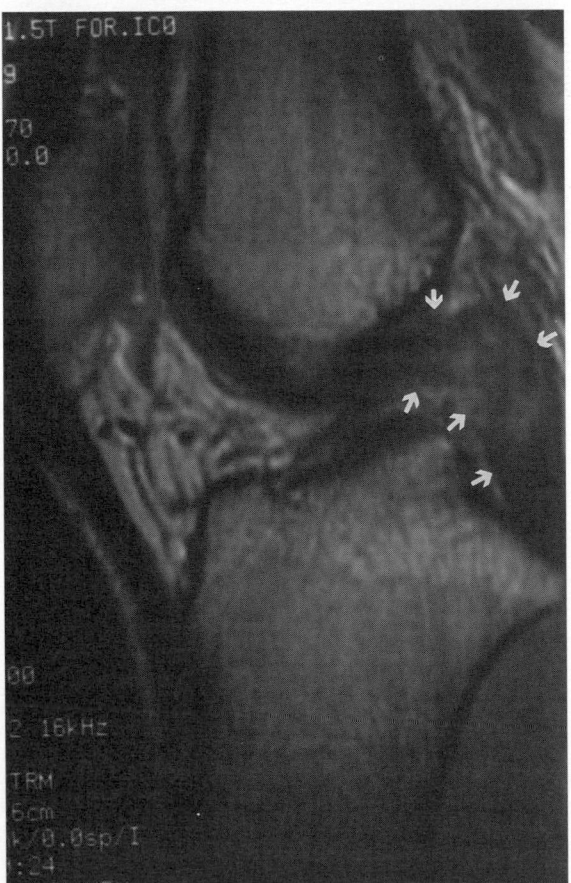

Figure 15-14 Injuries to the posterior cruciate ligament. *A.* Sagittal proton-density (TR/TE 2200/30) MR image shows enlargement and heterogeneous signal in PCL near femoral origin (*white arrow*). *B.* T2-weighted coronal (TR/TE 4000/100) MR image demonstrates high signal intensity within horizontal portion of PCL due to partial tear (*white arrow*). *C.* In this patient with complete rupture of the PCL, the sagittal proton-density-weighted (TR/TE 2000/16) image shows an ill-defined intermediate-signal-intensity mass roughly conforming to the shape of the posterior cruciate ligament (*white arrows*).

(Fig. 15-1). Mink and Deutsch[155] identified four types of occult fracture in their review of 66 patients with the most common injury, classified as a bone bruise. A bone bruise is defined as either a diffuse or localized area of decreased signal on T1-weighted images involving the subcortical bone, with signal brightening on T2-weighted images, representing a combination of edema, hyperemia, hemorrhage, and trabecular microfracture.[155,200] These bone lesions are frequently associated with injury of the ACL and contralateral collateral ligament.[201–203] In the study by Mink and Deutsch,[155] if the mechanism of injury included twisting or rotation, 100 percent of patients with bone bruises also had a severe ligament tear. Lynch and coworkers advocate a delay in full weight bearing in patients with bone contusions. They feel that these regions of bone are at increased risk for the subsequent devel-

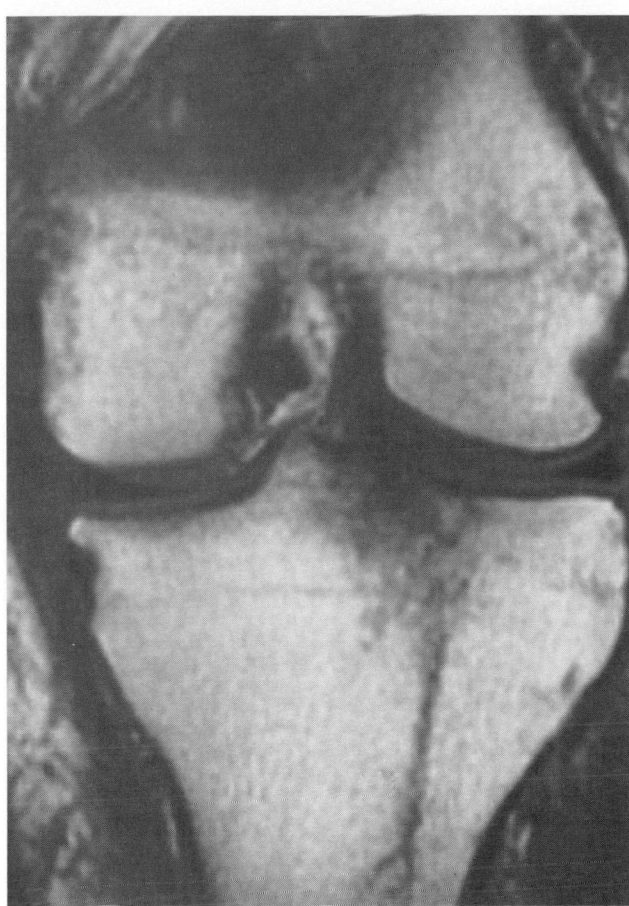

Figure 15-15 Occult tibial plateau fracture. T1-weighted (TR/TE 500/12) coronal MR image shows a tibial plateau fracture with vertical extension into the metaphysis not detected on plain film examination.

opment of insufficiency fractures if the bone is not adequately protected during trabecular healing.[201]

Vellet and coworkers[156] have recently proposed modifications to the original classification of occult fractures, suggesting that these lesions should not be collectively described as bone bruises, which implies that they resolve with little sequelae. Their study group consisted of 120 consecutive patients with acute hemarthrosis. The prevalence of occult subcortical femoral and tibial fractures in this population was 72 percent, which is similar to the prevalence in the study of Mink and Deutsch[155] (Fig. 15-15). They identified a subset of patients, described as having occult geographic subcortical fractures, who demonstrated a remarkably high incidence (67 percent) of osteochondral sequelae. All of these patients had no evidence of cartilaginous injury at initial arthroscopy, but, upon follow-up MRI 6 to 12 months after their trauma, 14 percent showed apparent cartilage thinning, 48 percent showed overt cartilaginous loss or defect, and 14 percent showed an osteochondral defect.

Thus the relevance of occult fractures is not in their presence but rather in the osteochondral and chondral sequelae. Modifications in immediate and rehabilitative management of patients with these injuries should ensure the best possible outcome.

Magnetic Resonance Imaging of the Shoulder Magnetic resonance imaging of the shoulder is technically more difficult than that of the knee. It is not possible to place the shoulder joint in the isocenter of the magnetic field and thus requires imaging offset capabilities. The optimal imaging planes for the shoulder are not conventional, necessitating the use of oblique planes. As with knee imaging, the development of surface coils that conform to the surface anatomy of the joint has markedly improved image quality.

The glenohumeral joint is the most mobile joint within the body, allowing a wide range of motion. Since it is also an essentially unstable joint with only one-third of the humeral head articular surface in contact with the shallow glenoid fossa, joint stability is achieved by surrounding osseous and soft tissue structures. The rotator cuff muscles and their tendinous insertions are best demonstrated on coronal oblique and sagittal oblique images (Fig. 15-16). The anatomy of the distal acromion and acromioclavicular (AC) joint and any pathologic changes that may contribute to impingement syndrome are best assessed on oblique sagittal images. Transaxial images are the most useful in evaluation of the glenoid labrum, the capsular mechanism, and the tendon of the long head of the biceps.

Impingement Syndrome Shoulder impingement is a relatively common clinical condition in which the soft tissues of the subacromial space—specifically the subacromial/subdeltoid bursa, the supraspinatus tendon, and the biceps tendon—become anatomically confined and compressed between the coracoacromial arch and the humeral head. This places the supraspinatus tendon at risk for acute injury and chronic wear. The impingement syndrome is considered a continuous pathologic process in which bursal inflammation and tendinitis can lead to tendon degeneration and can progress to complete disruption of the rotator cuff. The typical location of injury is a zone of relative hypovascularity in the distal supraspinatus tendon. Various proposed etiologies for the painful shoulder impingement syndrome include mechanical trauma, sudden macrotrauma, or repetitive microtrauma from overuse, as from throwing sports or work activities that emphasize overhead motions.[204]

Magnetic resonance imaging is useful for documenting anatomic findings that can be associated with the clinical syndrome of impingement.[205] Factors that could contribute to mechanical trauma to the supraspinatus tendon include inferior acromial spurs, hypertrophic bone or callus formation around the AC joint, and acromial shape.[206] The shape of the acromion as seen on radiographs of the supraspinatus outlet have been divided into three types. The type 1 acromion is flat; type 2 is smoothly curved in shape; and there is anteroinferior hooking of the acromion in type 3, which is correlated with a greater predisposition to and association with rotator cuff tears.[206,207]

The accuracy of MRI in demonstrating the full spectrum of rotator cuff pathology has been evaluated.[208–212] Seeger and colleagues[205] have proposed a classification of impingement based upon oblique coronal images. Zlatkin[213] has also devised a grading system for characterization of the rotator cuff tendons, attempting to correlate these grades with the three types of impingement identified by arthroscopic surgery. In both systems, increased signal in-

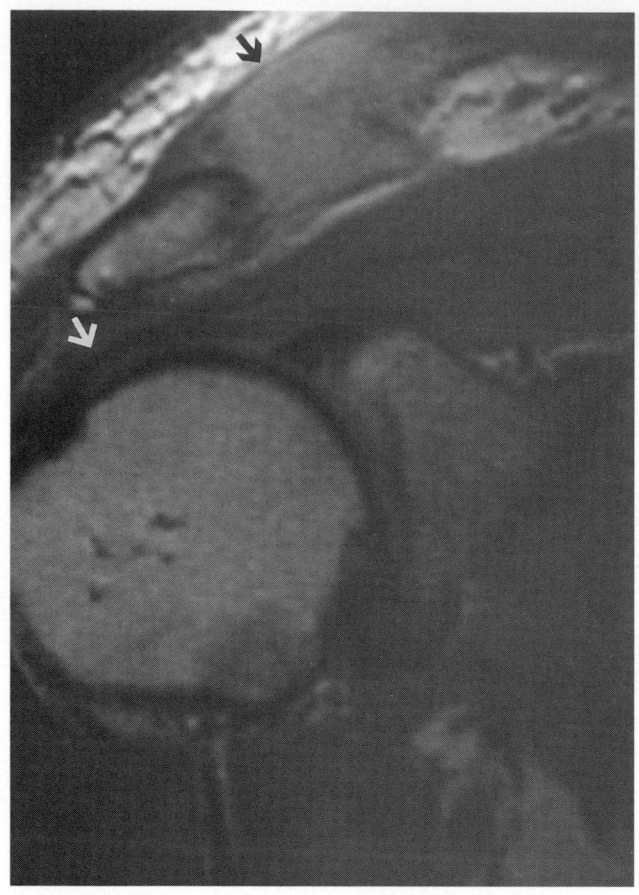

A

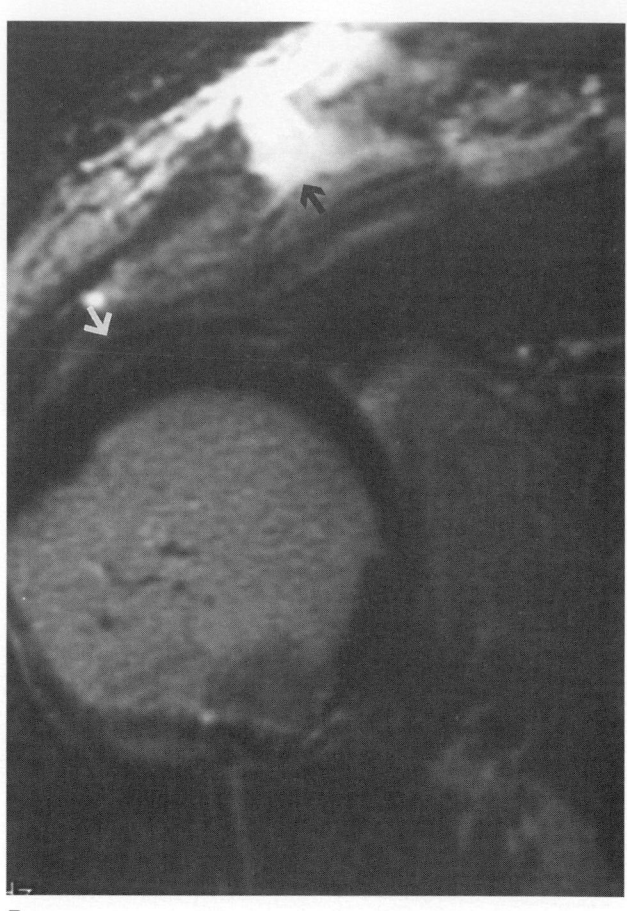

B

Figure 15-16 Young male patient with continued pain after shoulder trauma. *A.* Oblique coronal proton-density-weighted MR image (TR/TE 2500/30) demonstrates intermediate-signal-intensity fluid collection in separated acromioclavicular (AC) joint (*black arrow*). *B.* T2-weighted (TR/TE 2500/80) oblique coronal image shows high-signal-intensity fluid (hematoma) of AC joint (*black arrow*) with intact supraspinatus tendon (*white arrows*).

tensity within the supraspinatus tendon can be seen on T1-weighted and balanced images, with relative preservation of articular and bursal tendon surface outlines in early impingement. Biopsy specimens show inflammation and mucoid degeneration, which may account for this increased signal intensity on short-TR/TE images.[214] Rafii and coworkers,[215] however, feel that this increased signal intensity is due to degeneration (eosinophilic, fibrillar, or mucoid) and scarring rather than active inflammation. This is further supported by observations of increased signal intensity within the supraspinatus tendon on short-TR/TE images in asymptomatic volunteers.[208]

With continued entrapment of the tendon, changes in tendon morphology are identified as tendon thinning or irregularity. Further damage to the tendon results in a partial- or full-thickness tear. Zlatkin and coworkers[213] report 91 percent sensitivity for MRI in detecting rotator cuff tears. In their group of 32 patients, arthroscopy was utilized as the standard of reference. No attempt was made to differentiate partial from complete tears. Similarly, Rafii and colleagues[215] report an MRI accuracy of 95 percent for detection of full-thickness cuff tears. In the study of Burk and coworkers,[216] MRI and arthrography showed identical

sensitivities of 92 percent in the detection of cuff tears. Criteria used for diagnosing rotator cuff tears included increased signal intensity on T2-weighted images, with abnormal morphology or discontinuity.[205,213,215] Proximal retraction of the muscle-tendon junction is an indication of a significant tear but is not specific for irreparable tear[217] (Fig. 15-17). While Rafii and coworkers[215] report that, less commonly, the torn region is manifest as an extremely degenerated or attenuated tendon with only moderate signal intensity on T2-weighted images, Stoller feels that without demonstration of a defined defect, retraction of the muscle belly, or extension of fluid across the supraspinatus tendon into the subacromial-subdeltoid bursa, a complete tear cannot be diagnosed unequivocally.[218]

Reinus and coworkers[219] reported improved sensitivity for detection of rotator cuff tears using fat-saturated T2-weighted images. With standard spin-echo imaging, they had 80 percent sensitivity for full-thickness tears, which improved to 100 percent with fat saturation. Detection of partial-thickness tears also improved but remained poor with both techniques. Magnetic resonance arthrography is an additional alternative for increasing sensitivity in detecting partial-thickness tears (Fig. 15-18).

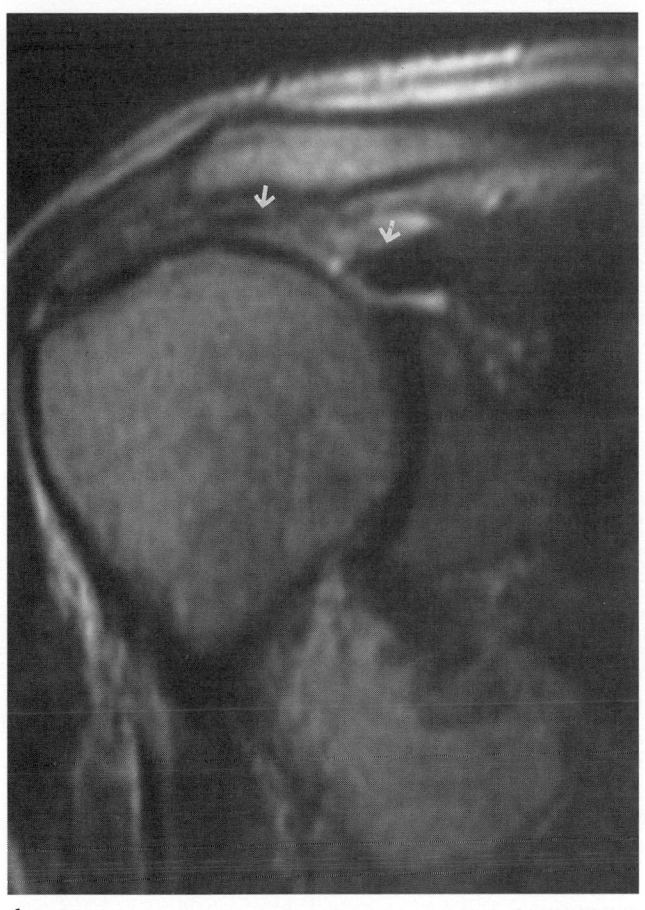

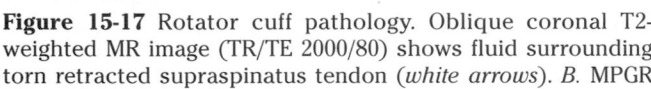

A

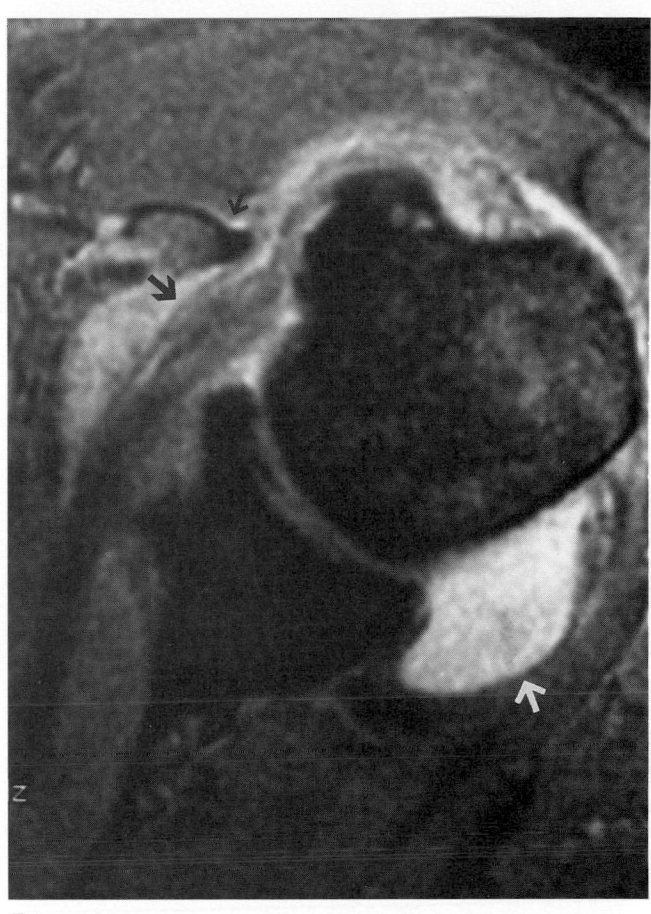

B

Figure 15-17 Rotator cuff pathology. Oblique coronal T2-weighted MR image (TR/TE 2000/80) shows fluid surrounding torn retracted supraspinatus tendon (*white arrows*). B. MPGR axial image (350/20/20) shows additional tear of subscapularis tendon (*large black arrow*), displaced bicipital tendon (*small black arrow*), and large joint effusion (*white arrow*).

Shoulder Instability In addition to evaluating the patient with clinical symptoms of impingement/rotator cuff pathology, the other major area in which the role of MRI has been studied is in the patient with instability.[220]

One definition of instability is simply the slipping of the humeral head out of the glenoid socket during activities.[221] In the past, instability was considered evident in a patient only if previous dislocation had occurred. Other authors contend, however, that an earlier dislocation does not necessarily make a shoulder unstable.[222] Different degrees of instability are now being recognized, including subluxations. Instability can be classified according to antecedent trauma (acute versus recurrent), degree (subluxation versus dislocation), or direction (unidirectional versus multidirectional).

Four anatomic areas should be evaluated in imaging the patient with symptoms of instability. These areas are the humeral head, joint capsule, glenohumeral ligaments, and glenoid labrum.[221]

Defects in the posterolateral humeral head, or Hill-Sachs lesions, are readily and perhaps most accurately identified with MRI.[223] Feller and colleagues[221] caution against mistaking the normal anatomic indentation of the posterior aspect of the humeral head, seen on axial images below the level of the coracoid, for a Hill-Sachs lesion. The presence of a Hill-Sachs lesion is, however, only a marker for previous dislocation. Its presence does not change most orthopedists' management, nor does it indicate an increased risk for recurrent dislocation. [223–225]

Three types of joint capsule have been described based upon their anterior insertion site upon the glenoid.[226,227] Type 1 capsules are attached on or at the base of the labrum. Type 2 capsules insert within 1 cm of the base of the labrum. Type 3 capsules insert upon the scapular neck at least 1 cm medial to the labrum. The laxity of type 3 capsules is believed to be a predisposing factor in the development of shoulder instability.[228,229]

The glenohumeral ligaments are three congenitally variable focal thickenings in the anterior capsule. The presence, normal anatomic features, and relative functional contributions of each of the glenohumeral ligaments in the maintenance of shoulder stability has been debated ex-

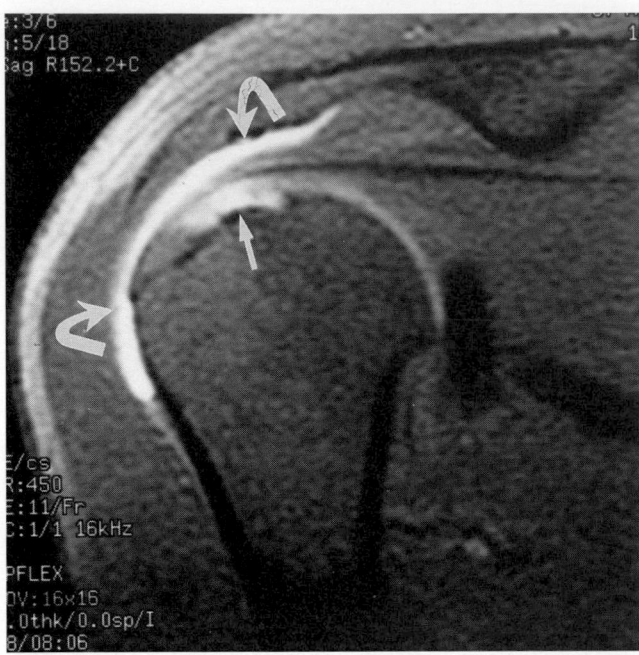

Figure 15-18 Oblique coronal fat-suppressed T1-weighted image (TR/TE 450/11) of the right shoulder after intraarticular injection of dilute gadolinium in a 57-year-old male. The gadolinium fills a large tear in the undersurface of the supraspinatus tendon (*white arrow*). A full-thickness perforation elsewhere in the tendon (not shown) allowed gadolinium to flow into the subacromial-subdeltoid bursa (*curved arrows*).

tensively.[230–232] It is now fairly well accepted that the inferior glenohumeral ligament–labral complex is the major structure stabilizing the shoulder and limiting anterior subluxation and dislocation.[222] The glenohumeral ligaments are best seen with MR arthrography[233] (Fig. 15-19). It should be noted, at this juncture, that the technique of MR arthrography is not without its critics. They argue that MR arthrography negates one of the main advantages of MRI, namely, its noninvasiveness. Additionally, the use of gadopentate dimeglumine for intraarticular injection is not as yet approved by the Food and Drug Administration for routine use. Thus, its use remains investigational, as an unapproved indication for an approved drug.

Using MR arthrography, Chadnani and coworkers report identification of the superior glenohumeral ligament in 85 percent, middle glenohumeral ligament in 85 percent, and inferior glenohumeral ligament in 91 percent of their 46-patient study population. They also report sensitivities of 100, 89, and 88 percent for diagnosing tears of the superior, middle, and inferior glenohumeral ligaments respectively, with surgical correlation for all patients.[229] Other researchers advocate MR arthrography as well as special patient positioning. By imaging the patient with the patient's palm underneath his or her head, the so-called dislocation position of abduction and external rotation is achieved. Stoller[234] describes enhanced detection of tears of the inferior glenohumeral ligament–labral complex with this positioning.

The final structure requiring evaluation in the instability patient is the glenoid labrum. Studies performed using conventional MRI for the detection of labral tears have produced mixed results, with reported sensitivities ranging from 44 to 90 percent.[235–238] A number of factors contribute

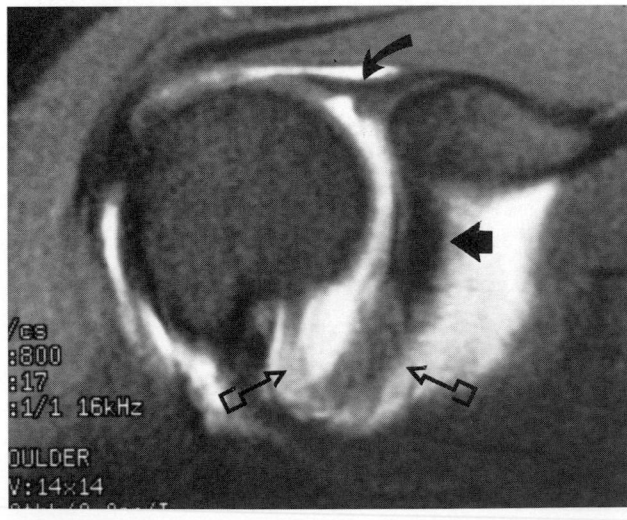

A

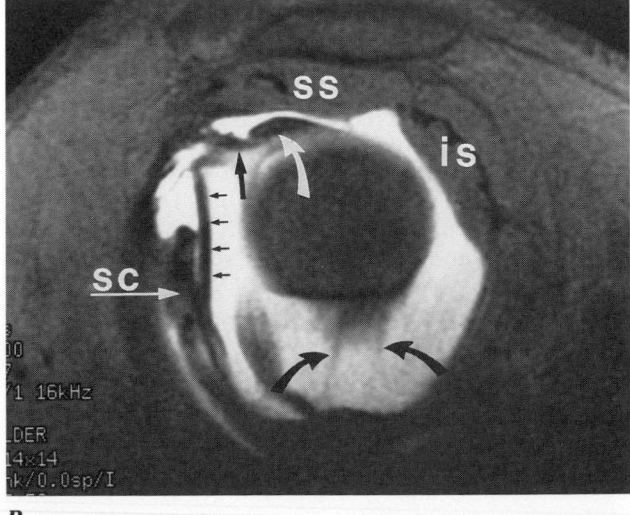

B

Figure 15-19 Normal MR arthrogram of the shoulder. *A.* Oblique coronal fat-suppressed T1-weighted image (TR/TE 800/17). The biceps-labral complex (*curved black arrow*) and anterior rim of the glenoid labrum (*short black arrow*) are demonstrated. The anterior band of the inferior glenohumeral ligament (*blocked black arrows*) forms the axillary recess. *B.* Oblique sagittal fat-suppressed T1-weighted image (TR/TE 800/17). Subscapularis muscle (*sc, arrow*), supraspinatus muscle (*ss*), infraspinatus muscle (*is*), biceps-labral complex (*white arrow*), superior glenohumeral ligament (*large black arrow*), middle glenohumeral ligament (*small black arrows*), inferior glenohumeral ligament (*curved black arrows*).

to the difficulty in accurately assessing the labrum. First, there is considerable variation in the normal shape of the anterior labrum. The labrum may appear triangular, round, or crescentic, or it may be absent.[239–241] Second, the middle and inferior glenohumeral ligaments lie closely apposed to the anterior labrum in the absence of a joint effusion. The cleavage plane between these ligaments and the anterior labrum can mimic a labral tear.[240,242]

To enhance the detection of labral abnormalities, MR arthrography can be used. Flannigan and coworkers studied 23 patients, all of whom had surgical correlation. They detected all of the 9 labral tears using MR arthrography, but only 3 of 9 were detected with conventional MRI.[243] Chadnani and coworkers compared CT arthrography, conventional MRI and MR arthrography for the detection of labral tears, detached labral fragments, and labral degeneration. They found MR arthrography to be the most sensitive technique, with 96 percent sensitivity for labral tears and 96 percent sensitivity for detached labral fragments. This compared favorably to conventional MRI, with sensitivities of 93 and 46 percent respectively, as well as CT arthrography, with sensitivities of 73 and 52 percent respectively.[244]

Magnetic Resonance Imaging of the Spine Magnetic resonance imaging of the spine has utility in a variety of clinical settings, including evaluation of degenerative disk disease, the postoperative spine, infection, trauma, and neoplasia.

Degenerative Disk Disease In the evaluation of degenerative disk disease, the availability of MRI has sharply reduced the number of myelograms performed at many centers. Unlike myelography, which is an invasive procedure and provides only indirect evaluation of the disk by its effect upon the contour of the thecal sac and nerve root sleeves, MRI is capable of directly demonstrating the separate components of the disk: the nucleus pulposus, the annulus fibrosus, and the cartilaginous end plate. On conventional T1-weighted sequences, the yellow fatty marrow of the vertebral bodies demonstrates bright signal intensity, the disks are intermediate in signal intensity, and cerebrospinal fluid (CSF) is of low signal intensity, contrasting with the higher signal intensity of the cord (Fig. 15-20). A myelographic effect is obtained on conventional T2-weighted sequences, in which the bright CSF creates excellent cord-CSF contrast (Fig. 15-21). True myelogramlike images of the thecal sac can also be generated by MRI. Krudy[245] first reported a new method for generating myelogramlike images using a heavily T2-weighted fast spin-echo pulse sequence and obliterating fat signal by presaturation. El Gammal et al. reported further refinements in technique and illustrated the usefulness of MR myelography not only in the thoracic and lumbar regions but also in the cervical region.[246,247] As these techniques become more widely utilized, the need for intrathecal contrast myelography may be completely averted.

The cause of disk degeneration is as yet unknown. Multiple factors—autoimmune, genetic, and biomechanical—may precipitate degeneration.[248] A variety of biochemical and structural changes take place during the processes of aging and degeneration.[249–252] Early degenerative disk disease may be identified on conventional T2-

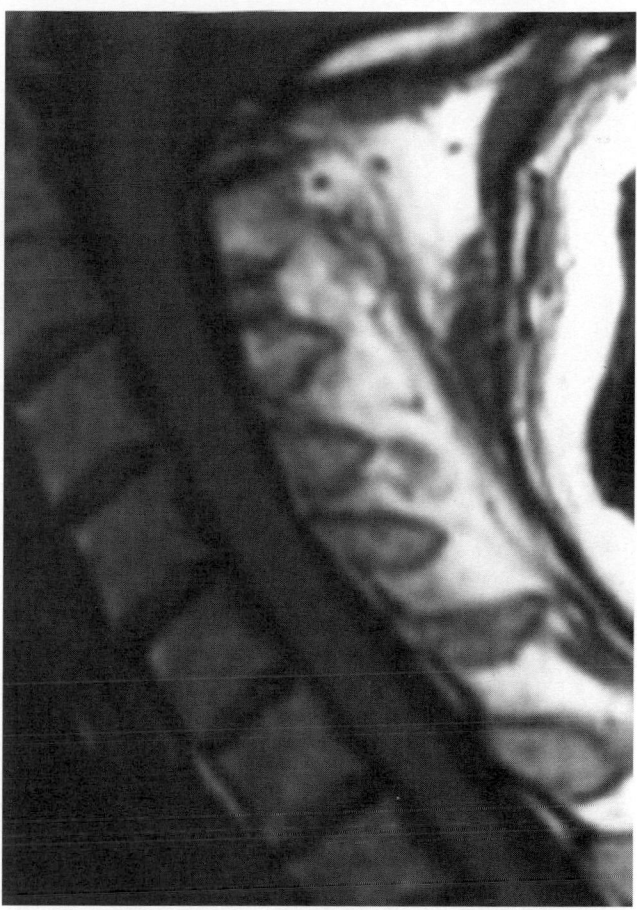

Figure 15-20 Normal cervical spine. This normal T1-weighted sagittal MR image (TR/TE 600/20) shows the intervertebral disks, which are of intermediate signal intensity. The low-signal-intensity CSF contrasts with the homogeneous higher signal intensity of the spinal cord.

weighted sagittal images and is characterized by loss of signal intensity, which is presumed to be due to disk dessication.[248,253,254] However, correlation is not straightforward, as differences in signal intensity appear to be somewhat exaggerated for the degree of water loss noted with degeneration (e.g., 15 percent).[255]

Changes in signal intensity are commonly observed on MR images in vertebral marrow adjacent to end plates of degenerative disks. Modic has classified these end-plate changes into three types.[248] In type I end plates, signal is decreased on T1-weighted images and increased on T2-weighted images, with corresponding histopathologic specimens demonstrating disruption and fissuring of the end plate and vascularized fibrous tissue in the adjacent marrow. Type II end plates demonstrate hyperintense signal on T1-weighted images with iso- or slightly hyperintense signal on T2-weighted images, which corresponded histopathologically to end-plate disruption with fatty marrow replacement in the adjacent vertebral body. In type III end plates, there is decreased signal on both T1- and T2-weighted images correlating with extensive bone sclerosis on plain radiographs (Fig. 15-22).

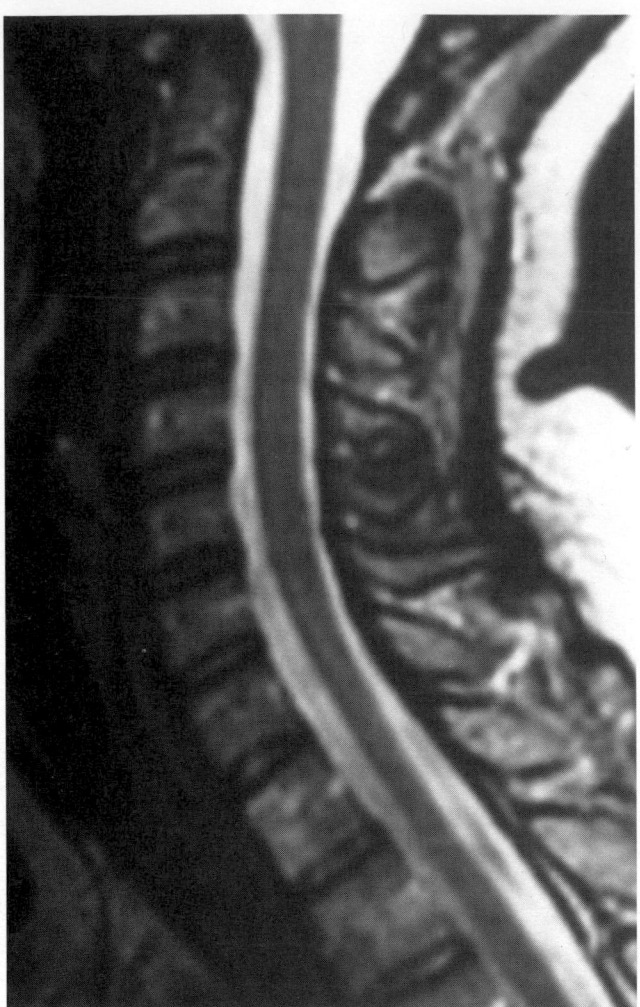

Figure 15-21 Normal cervical spine. On this normal FSE T2-weighted sagittal MR image (TR/TE 4000/102), a myelographic effect is obtained with the bright CSF contrasting with the intermediate signal intensity of the cord and the very low signal intensity of the annulus fibrosus/posterior longitudinal ligament complex.

The accuracy of MRI in the assessment of thoracic and lumbar disk herniations is equivalent to that of CT and myelography.[253,256–259] Sagittal images are sensitive in identifying the posterior disk margin, the annular complex, and the interface with the ventral aspect of the thecal sac. Axial images provide more accurate assessment of the degree of secondary central canal or neural foraminal stenoses and nerve root impingement. Other factors that contribute to central canal stenosis—including facet joint arthrosis and hypertrophy of the ligamentum flavum—are also best assessed on axial images. The criteria for the diagnosis of a herniated disk on MRI are similar to those on CT scans. Disk herniations are characterized by a focal extension of the disk beyond the margins of the adjacent vertebral end plates. Most disk herniations demonstrate low signal intensity on T1- and T2-weighted images.[260] Large extrusions or sequestered disk fragments, however, may

have high signal intensity on T2-weighted images, while the disk of origin shows the typical decreased signal intensity associated with degenerative disk disease.[248] Thornbury and coworkers studied 95 patients with acute low back and radicular pain with MRI and either plain CT or CT myelography for diagnosis of herniated nucleus pulposus–caused nerve root compression. They found MRI to have a sensitivity of 91.9 percent and the overall sensitivity of both CT techniques to be 89.2 percent.[261]

Modic and coworkers studied 25 patients with symptoms of acute lumbar radiculopathy. The patients underwent physical examination and MRI at presentation, 6 weeks, and 6 months. Initial symptoms were correlated with type, size, location, and enhancement of disk herniations. The investigators found excellent agreement between clinical and MRI findings for level and side of herniated nucleus pulposus and radicular symptoms[262] (Fig. 15-23).

Imaging of cervical disk disease poses special requirements.[263] Early reports including that of Modic et al.[264] demonstrated a slight deficiency of MRI compared with CT myelography for the detection of cervical radicular compression and noted a relative lack of specificity of MRI for separating soft disk protrusion from osteophytic spur. These early studies, using standard spin-echo imaging, were limited by section thickness and artifacts created by CSF pulsation. These pulsation artifacts, which are especially prevalent in the cervical region, can be minimized by the use of flow compensation, which is currently performed routinely.[265] Gating signal acquisition to the cardiac cycle also minimizes CSF pulsation artifact.[266,267] Gradient recalled echo (GRE) sequences with small flip angles are effective in demonstrating low-signal-intensity osteophytic spurs and higher-signal-intensity herniated disk[268,269] (Fig. 15-24). With the use of three-dimensional volume-acquisition imaging, very thin sections can be acquired (1.5 to 2 mm). These thin sections are critical for accurate evaluation of the cervical intervertebral foramina.[270,271] Since the prevalence of cervical degenerative disk disease is so high (by some estimates over 80 percent in patients over 55 years of age),[272] the necessity of correlating imaging findings with patient symptomatology before any surgical intervention is contemplated cannot be overemphasized.

Imaging of the Postoperative Spine The syndrome of failed back surgery is characterized by intractable pain and varying degrees of disability after spine surgery. Common etiologies include misdirected surgery (wrong level, wrong diagnosis, unrelated incidental disk herniation), bony stenosis, either central or lateral recess, instability, arachnoiditis, recurrent disk herniation, and postoperative epidural fibrosis or scar.[273]

Three MRI categories for arachnoiditis have been described. Group 1 consists of a central conglomeration of nerve roots within the thecal sac (Fig. 15-25). In group 2, the nerve roots are adherent peripherally to the meninges, giving rise to an "empty sac" appearance. In group 3, a soft tissue signal-intensity mass occupies the thecal sac with no discrimination of nerve roots. T2-weighted axial images are often required to display the distortion of the thecal sac and nerve roots.[274] Enhancement of a decompressed nerve root extending proximally toward the conus

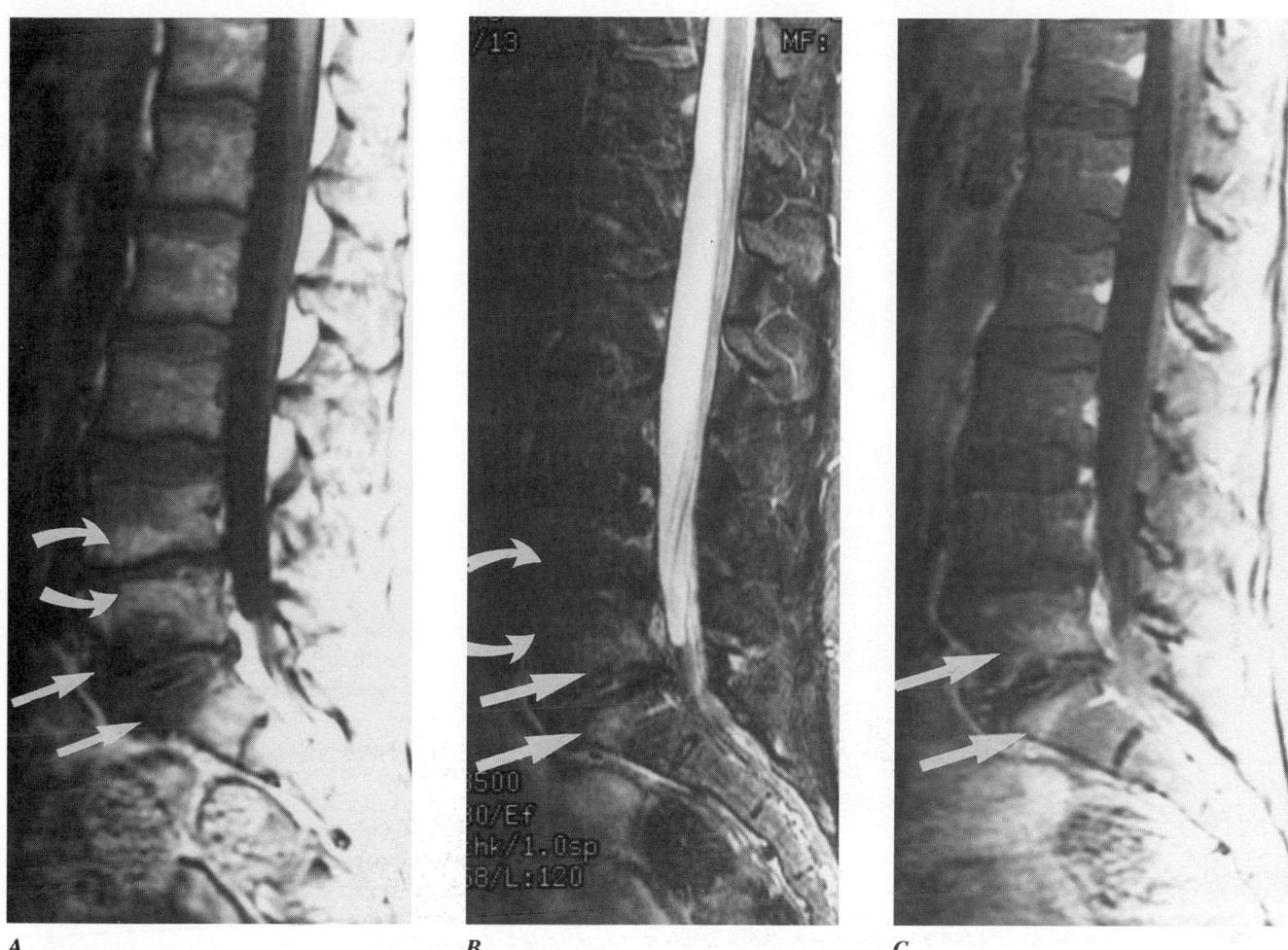

A   *B*   *C*

Figure 15-22 MRI of the lumbar spine in a 42-year-old woman with low back pain. *A.* Sagittal T1-weighted image (TR/TE 550/11) demonstrates fatty high signal intensity at the inferior end plate of L4 and superior end plate of L5 (*curved arrows*), consistent with fibrofatty change (Modic type II). Low signal intensity is present in the inferior end plate of L5 and superior end plate of S1 (*straight arrows*), consistent with granulation-type changes (Modic type I). *B.* Sagittal fat-suppressed fast T1-weighted image (TR/TE 3500/80) shows suppression of the fatty end plates (*curved arrows*) and increased signal intensity of the granulation-type end plates (*straight arrows*). *C.* Sagittal fat-suppressed T1-weighted image (TR/TE 600/11) after intravenous gadolinium administration shows enhancement of the granulation-type end-plate changes (*arrows*).

medullaris occurred in 62 percent of asymptomatic patients when imaged in the first 6 months after successful lumbar disk surgery[275,276] and should not be mistaken as evidence for arachnoiditis.

The distinction between epidural fibrosis/scar and recurrent disk herniation is important, since reoperation on scar unaccompanied by disk material generally leads to a poor surgical result.[277] Myelography and CT have not proven very reliable in making this distinction.[278,279] With MRI, the most useful criteria for separating disk from scar has been the lack of enhancement of disk on early contrast-enhanced T1-weighted images. The recurrent or residual disk fragment remains low in signal on T1-weighted images obtained shortly after contrast administration (Fig. 15-26). Conversely, epidural fibrosis or scar will enhance after Gd-DTPA administration (Fig. 15-27). Ross and coworkers[280] found maximal enhancement of epidural fibrosis to occur at 5 min after contrast injection. Glickstein and Sussman[281] caution

that this distinction may not hold true in patients examined long after surgery. They found that the degree of enhancement of epidural fibrosis was related to the postoperative interval and was greatest in those patients examined no later than 9 months after surgery. In their study, patients examined long after surgery showed less intense or even nonexistent enhancement of epidural fibrosis. Hueftle et al.[282] demonstrated 100 percent sensitivity, 71 percent specificity, and 89 percent accuracy in differentiating postoperative fibrosis from recurrent disk herniation in 17 patients at 19 disk levels. None of their 12 surgically proven cases of recurrent disk herniation showed early contrast enhancement. Ross and coworkers reported similar results with MRI, demonstrating 96 percent accuracy in differentiating scar from disk in 44 patients at 50 reoperated levels.[283]

Infection Magnetic resonance imaging for the detection of infectious spondylitis (discitis, vertebral osteomyelitis, epidural abscess) has been proved to be an extremely sen-

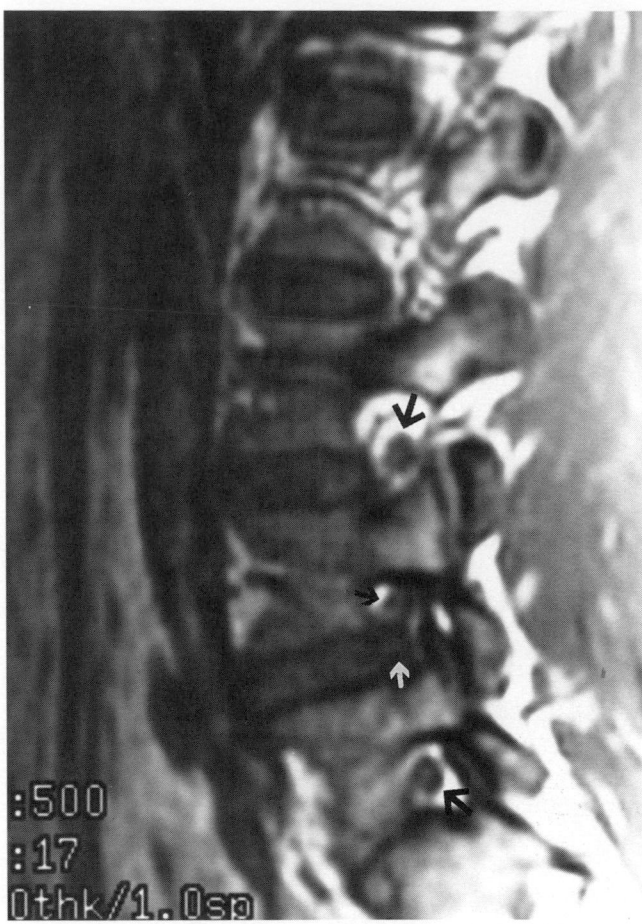

Figure 15-23 Lateral herniated nucleus pulposus (HNP). This very lateral L4/5 HNP (*white arrow*) compresses the right L4 nerve root (*small black arrow*). On the sagittal T1-weighted image (TR/TE 500/17), note the right L3 and L5 nerve roots exiting beneath their respective pedicles, surrounded by fat (*large black arrows*).

sitive modality. Modic and coworkers[284] studied 23 patients with microbiological and histologic diagnosis of spinal osteomyelitis and found MRI to have a 96 percent sensitivity, 92 percent specificity, and 94 percent accuracy.

Friedman and Hills[285] studied 18 patients with cervical discitis/osteomyelitis as well as inflammation in the epidural space. They found that multilevel involvement was the rule, with the C5 and C6 levels affected most frequently. Involvement of the epidural space was usually anterior, with frequent abscess formation. Cord compression was present in 74 percent of their patients, making prompt diagnosis and treatment mandatory.

The most characteristic MRI findings are as follows.[286,287] On T1-weighted sagittal images, there is low signal intensity in the marrow of at least two adjacent vertebrae, the disk space is narrowed, subligamentous or epidural soft tissue masses are present, and there is erosion of cortical bone. On T2-weighted images, the major findings are a narrowed disk space with variable signal changes, abnormal high signal in the marrow of two adjacent vertebrae bodies, high-signal subligamentous or

epidural masses, and cortical bone erosion. Gadolinium-enhanced images can be especially helpful for delineating the epidural extent of disease and in characterizing the epidural abscess.[288,289] Homogeneous enhancement of the epidural abscess correlates with the phlegmonous stage of infection, with granulomatous, thickened tissue and no significant drainable pus collection. A peripheral enhancement pattern corresponds to a liquid abscess core surrounded by inflammatory tissue (Fig. 15-28).

Gillams and coworkers[290] reviewed 25 patients retrospectively to assess the temporal evolution and resolution of infectious spondylitis. They found the first sign of response to treatment was reduction in the inflammatory soft tissue mass. A second definitive sign of healing was a peripheral rim of high T1 signal in bone. Gadolinium enhancement can persist or even increase after symptom resolution and should not be mistaken for evidence of treatment failure.

Trauma After initial plain-film examination, MRI has become the study of choice in the evaluation of patients presenting with neurologic deficit.[291,292] Most trauma centers have halo vests made of MRI-compatible material as well as MRI-compatible ventilators, so that patients requiring such stabilization or respiratory support are not excluded from MRI examination.

Magnetic resonance imaging plays a complementary role to CT in evaluating vertebral fracture patterns. It alone has the capability of directly visualizing associated ligamentous injury, traumatic disk herniations, and the spinal cord itself. Until recently, clinical evaluation was the only method available to predict the outcome in patients with injury to the spinal cord. Clinical assessment, however, does not allow distinction between edema, hemorrhage, and transection of the spinal cord. Several recent studies have focused upon the MRI appearance of the spinal cord in the acute stages following trauma and the prediction of neurologic outcome[293–296] (Fig. 15-29).

Spinal cord edema, which is manifest as low signal intensity on T1-weighted images and bright signal intensity on T2-weighted images, is associated with a more favorable outcome than is hemorrhage, especially when limited to one spinal segment.[291,295] In the study by Silberstein and coworkers,[293] 73 percent of patients with cord edema at presentation had useful motor function at outcome. All of these patients had complete motor paralysis at presentation.

Acute hematoma in the spinal cord is seen as an area of decreased signal intensity on T2-weighted images and as an isointense or hypointense area on T1-weighted images (Fig. 15-30). Patients with acute hematoma typically have no neurologic function below the level of the hemorrhage, and recovery is not likely.[291,294,295]

Neoplasia This subject is covered more extensively further on in this chapter. However, a few words covering neoplastic disease of the vertebral column are indicated.

Radionuclide bone scanning, the standard method for screening the skeleton for metastatic disease, is relatively insensitive to certain marrow neoplasms such as leukemia, lymphoma, and myeloma. Aggressive metastatic tumors may be falsely negative on radionuclide scans. Magnetic resonance imaging has the major benefit of visualizing bone marrow directly. The majority of malignant marrow

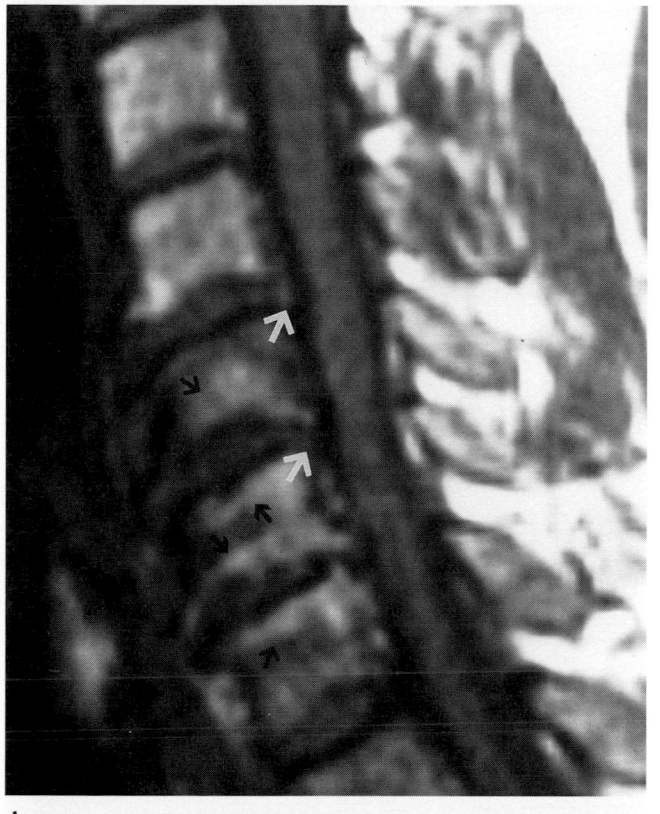

A

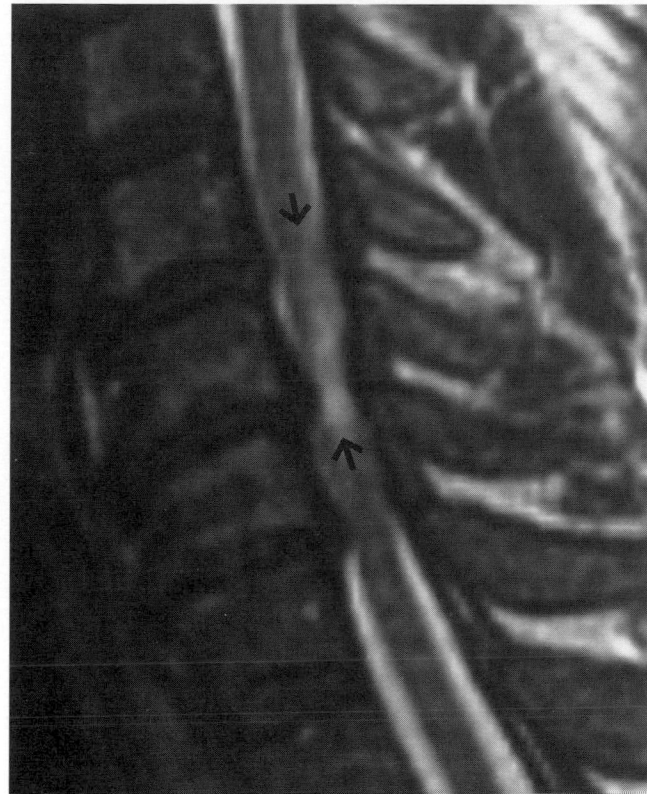

B

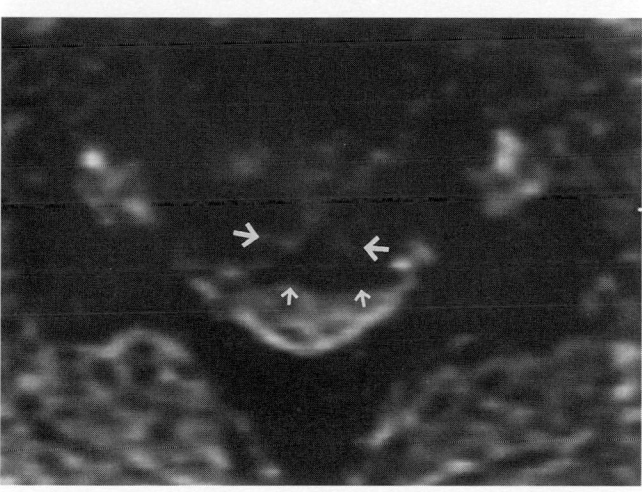

C

Figure 15-24 Cervical stenosis. *A*. Sagittal T1-weighted MR image (TR/TE 600/20). *B*. Sagittal T2-weighted image (TR/TE 4000/102). *C*. Axial gradient recalled echo (GRE) image (52/15/5). Disk herniation (*large white arrows*) and associated posterior bony ridge formation (*small white arrows*) is causing cervical stenosis. The cord compression is evident. Associated edema is designated by the bright signal seen on the sagittal T2-weighted image (*B*) (*large black arrows*). Modic type 2 degenerative end-plate changes are present at both the C5-6 and C6-7 disk levels (*small black arrows*).

disorders have long T1 and T2 values. Thus, on T1-weighted images, areas of marrow infiltration will often demonstrate decreased signal intensity in relation to normal yellow (fatty) marrow. Short T1 inversion recovery (STIR) sequences have proved extremely valuable in increasing the conspicuity of lesions. On STIR images, fat is black, combinations of red and yellow marrow are light gray, and most marrow tumors are bright white.[297]

In our department, a relatively common clinical situation is the patient with no known malignancy and with back pain. Radionuclide imaging may show foci of abnor-mal tracer uptake in the spine, but it sometimes remains unclear if this is related to metastatic disease or degenerative disk disease. Magnetic resonance imaging is a useful problem solver in this situation and can often clarify the cause of the increased radiotracer uptake.

Another common clinical scenario is the elderly patient presenting with back pain due to a compression fracture of the spine. Plain films and radionuclide bone scans may not be reliable in distinguishing benign osteoporotic compression fractures from malignant ones, but MRI has proved to be of value in making this distinction.[298–301]

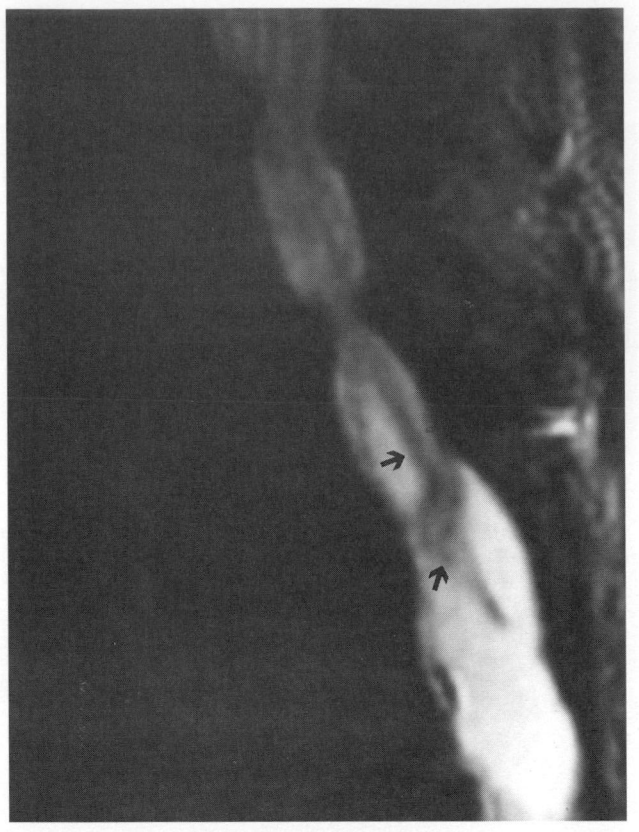

A

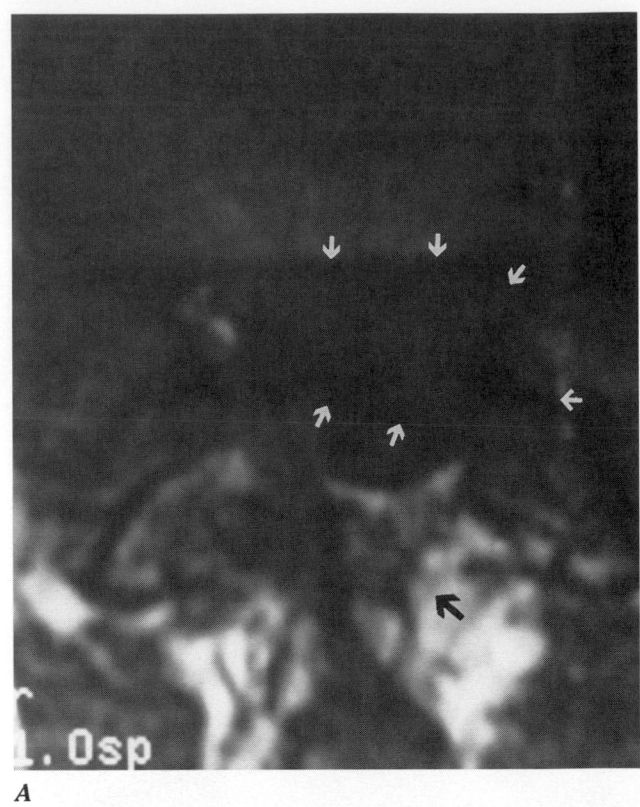

A

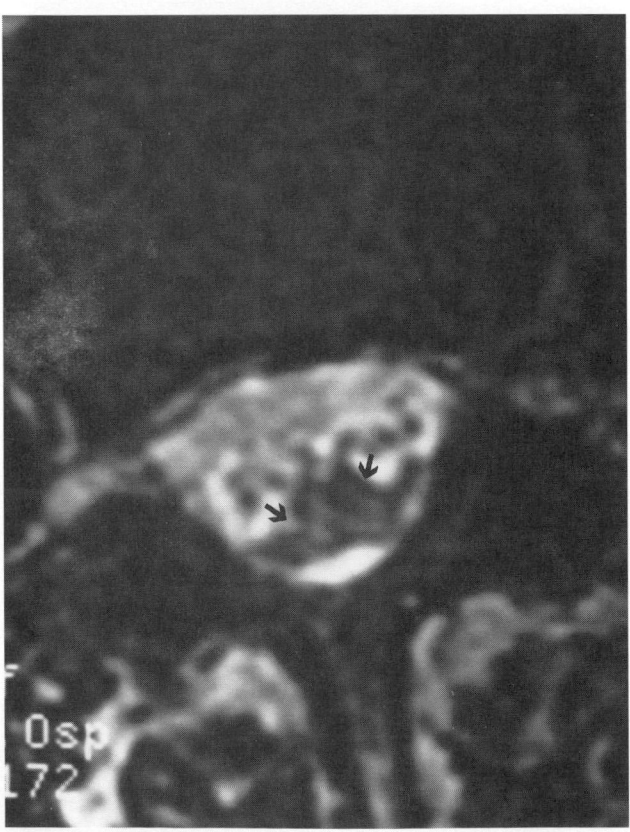

B

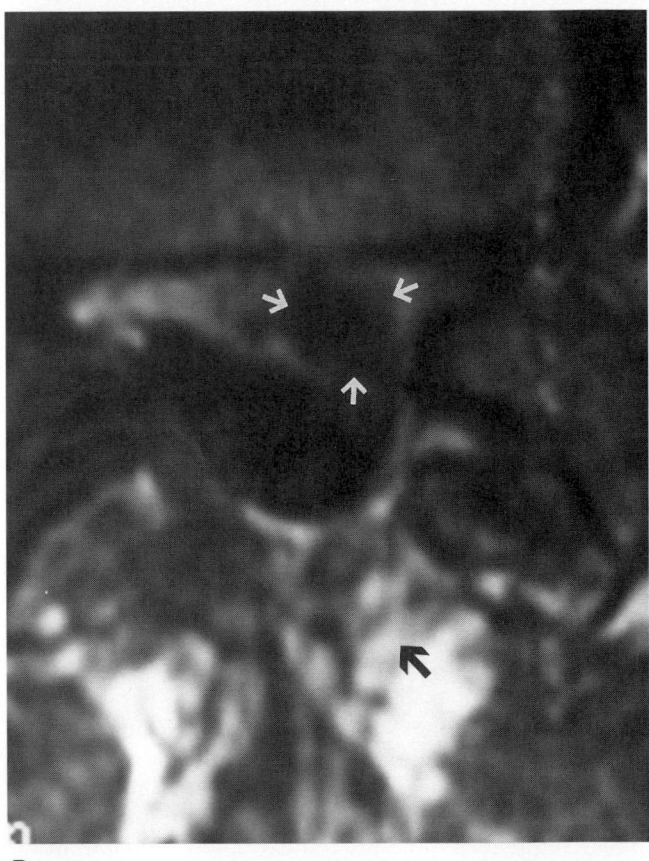

B

Figure 15-25 Arachnoiditis. T2-weighted sagittal (*A*) and T2-weighted axial (*B*) images (TR/TE 3400/95). Irregularly clumped nerve roots are present (*arrows*).

Figure 15-26 Axial T1-weighted (TR/TE 600/10) images obtained before (*A*) and after (*B*) contrast administration demonstrate enhancing granulation tissue surrounding a large nonenhancing recurrent disk fragment (*white arrows*) deforming the thecal sac. Note the left laminectomy defect (*black arrows*).

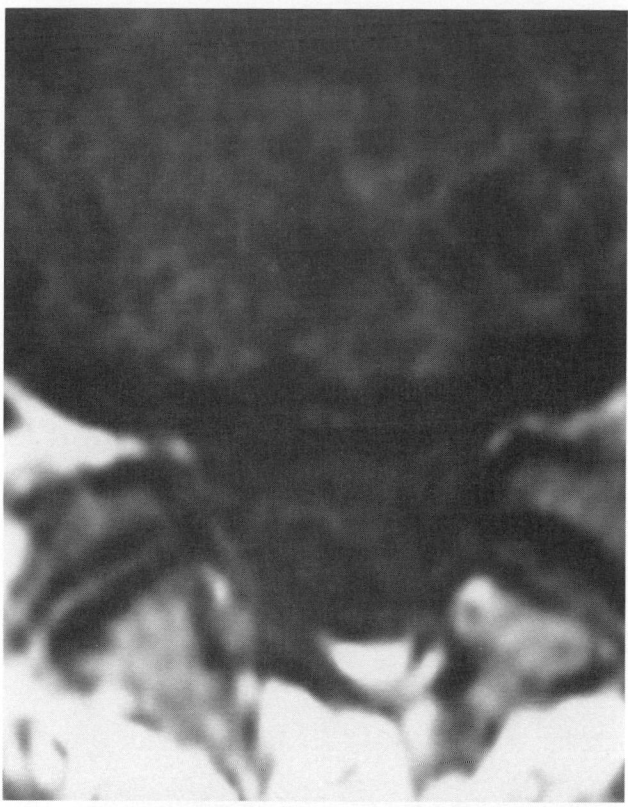

A

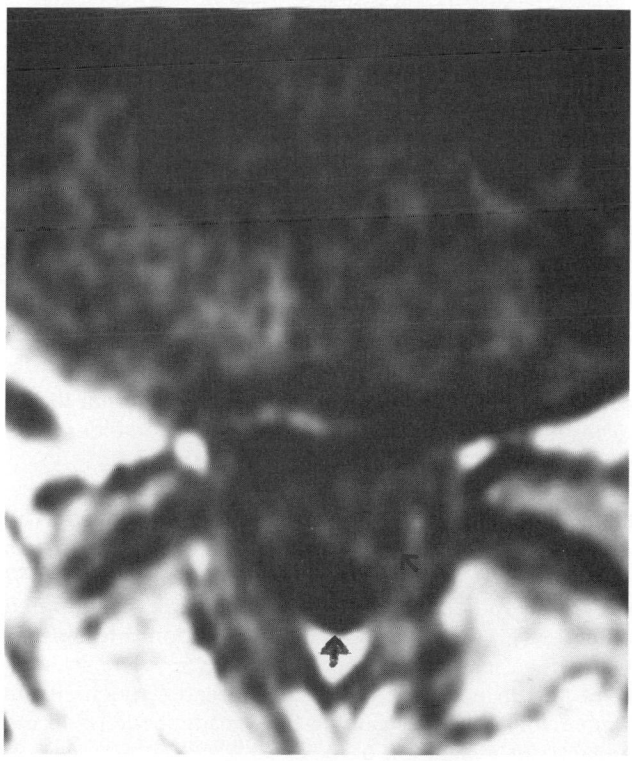

B

Figure 15-27 Epidural fibrosis. Enhancing epidural fibrosis deforming the thecal sac (*large black arrow*) and encasing the left L5 nerve root (*small black arrow*) is seen on these T1-weighted (TR/TE 600/11) axial MR images before (*A*) and after (*B*) Gd-DTPA.

SELECTED TOPICS

Osteonecrosis

Osteonecrosis is a relatively common disease entity in which there is death of the cellular elements of bone and marrow. *Avascular necrosis* (AVN) is the term most often used when this process involves the epiphysis or subarticular bone. *Bone infarct* is the term commonly applied to sites of metaphyseal or diaphyseal involvement.[302]

The femoral heads are the most commonly affected sites for clinically significant AVN. Important predisposing causes include corticosteroid use, previous trauma—including femoral neck fractures or prior dislocation—alcohol abuse, collagen vascular diseases, and hemoglobinopathies. This potentially disabling disorder often affects young or middle-aged adults. The condition can lead to early osteoarthritis through epiphyseal collapse and joint incongruity. Disabling hip pain may thus result in the need for total joint replacement in early adulthood.

Currently, core decompression of the avascular femoral head has been utilized as a method to reduce the likelihood of subsequent femoral head collapse. In all published series, the indication for core decompression has been based on the plain film radiographic stage of AVN, with the majority of authors agreeing that core decompression should be performed before the development of subchondral fracture. This technique has shown good results in some series but not in others, with the frequency of progression to collapse varying from 20 to 80 percent.[303–307] Other treatment options include free bone grafts, vascularized bone grafts, electrical stimulation; and rotational osteotomy to reposition the necrotic portion of the femoral head away from the weight-bearing surface.[303,308] Since there are no specific laboratory tests or physical findings to establish the diagnosis, clinically suspected AVN is confirmed with diagnostic imaging or biopsy. The goals of imaging include accurate diagnosis as well as staging. Staging of AVN is important in assessing prognosis and guiding treatment. Staging of AVN will also be essential in evaluating the efficacy of any treatment devised in the future. The imaging modalities utilized for detection of AVN include plain films, radionuclide bone scans, CT, and MRI.

Plain films should be obtained as the initial study in any patient with suspected AVN. Most authors recommend both anteroposterior and frog-leg lateral views, because a subchondral fracture or segmental collapse of the femoral head may be seen on only one of the two views. The plain-film classification of staging AVN developed by Ficat[303] is as follows: Stage 0 is preclinical and preradiographic. The diagnosis is suspected in a patient with known predisposition and with definite disease in the contralateral hip. Stage I involves a symptomatic patient with a normal radiograph, while in stage II there are changes in the trabecular pattern of the femoral head with sclerosis. The sclerosis may be diffuse, localized, or in a linear arc concave superiorly. At stage III, there is subchondral fracture with segmental collapse, while stage IV involves progressive collapse and deformity of the femoral head, loss of joint space, and osteophyte formation due to secondary osteoarthritis. Since plain films lack sensitivity for the de-

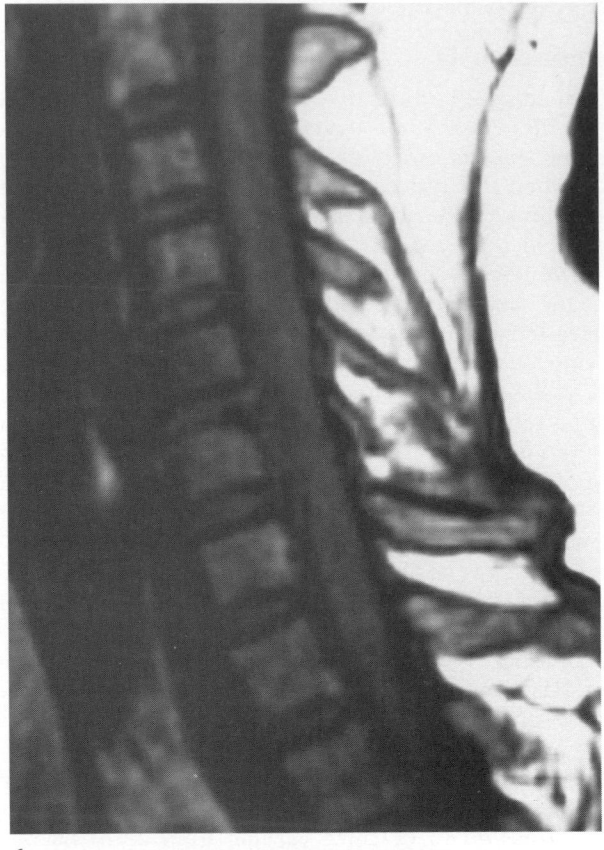

A

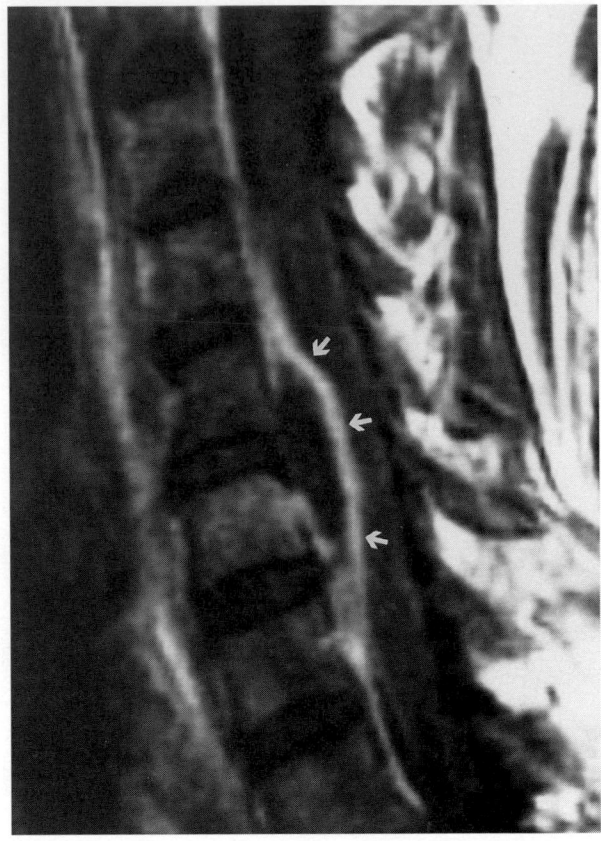

B

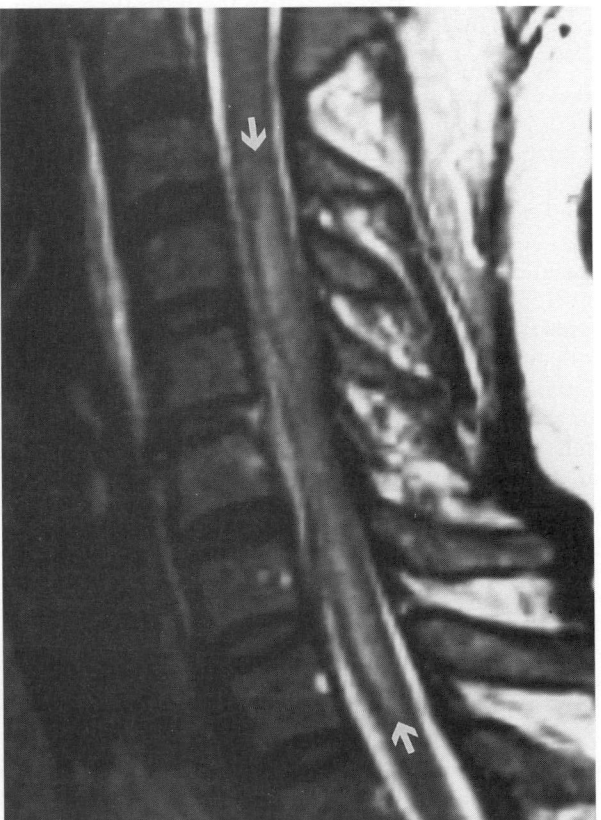

C

Figure 15-28 Discovertebral osteomyelitis with epidural abscess. T1-weighted (TR/TE 600/10) MRI before (*A*) and after (*B*) gadolinium enhancement and T2-weighted (TR/TE 4000/100) sagittal images. The epidural abscess extending from C4 to T1 causes cord edema/compression (*large white arrows*). The peripheral enhancement pattern with central low signal intensity corresponds to a liquid abscess core, with surrounding inflammatory tissue (*small white arrows*).

tection of AVN[304,309,310] and in fact remain normal in the earliest stages of the disorder, alternative modalities were explored.

For the detection of radiographically occult AVN, radionuclide bone scanning and MRI have both proved to be sensitive methods. Sensitivity for detection of AVN has ranged from 89 to 100 percent on MRI and from 72 to 87 percent on radionuclide bone scanning.[308–314] Computed tomography with multiplanar reconstruction is less sensitive than either of these modalities.[308,312,315] The sensitivity of MRI in conjunction with its greater specificity in comparison to bone scanning have made it the preferred modality for evaluation of AVN.[308,312,314,316,317]

Criteria for diagnosing AVN by MRI include a segmental pattern with the abnormal segment of the femoral head marginated by a line of very low signal or signal void seen on both T1- and T2-weighted sequences (Fig. 15-31). This segmental defect most commonly involves the anterosuperior aspect of the femoral head initially.[35] The line of sig-

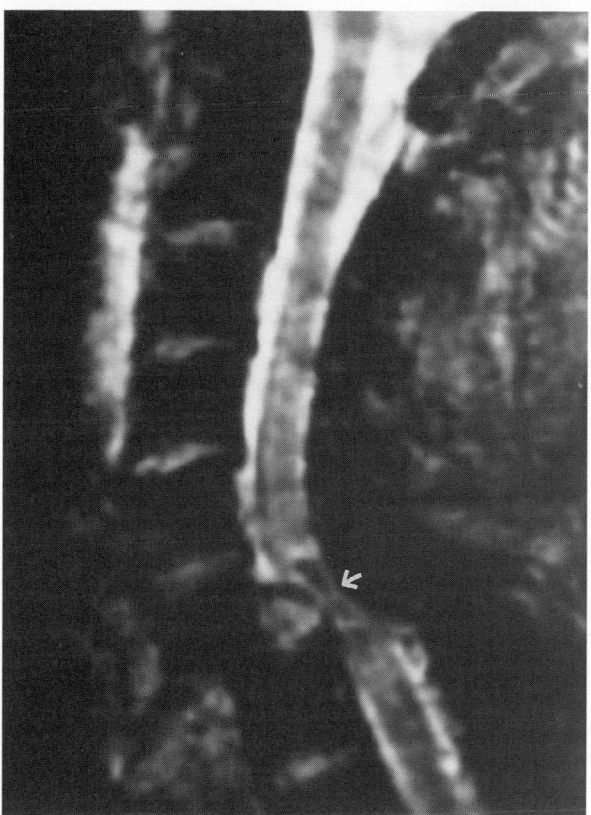

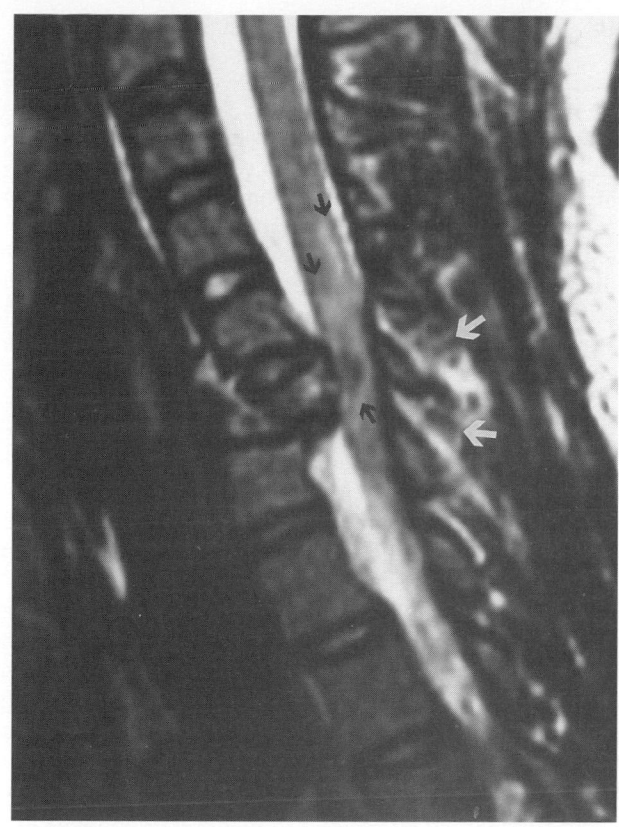

Figure 15-29 Cord contusion/partial transection. GRE (550/25/20) sagittal image shows C6-7 subluxation with associated disk herniation and partial cord transection. The low signal within the cord (*white arrow*) on this T2-weighted image represents contusion. The patient did not regain any neurologic function below the level of injury.

Figure 15-30 Fracture and cord contusion. A C6 burst fracture is present. Associated cord contusion is hypointense relative to the remainder of the cord, with surrounding high-signal-intensity rim (*black arrows*). Sagittal T2-weighted MR image (TR/TE 3400/102). Posterior ligamentous injury is also present (*white arrows*).

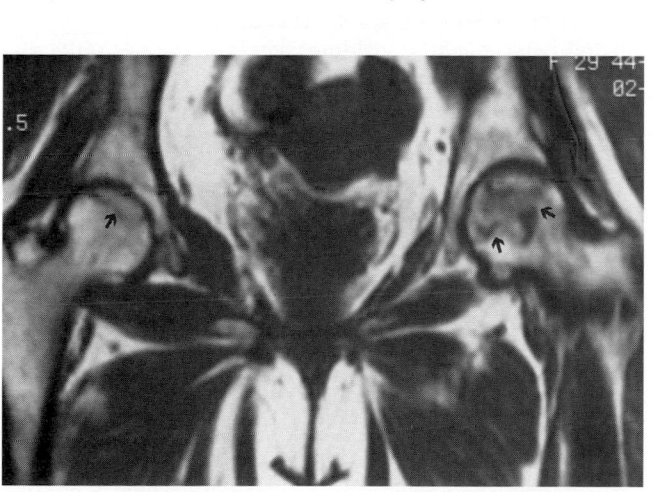

A

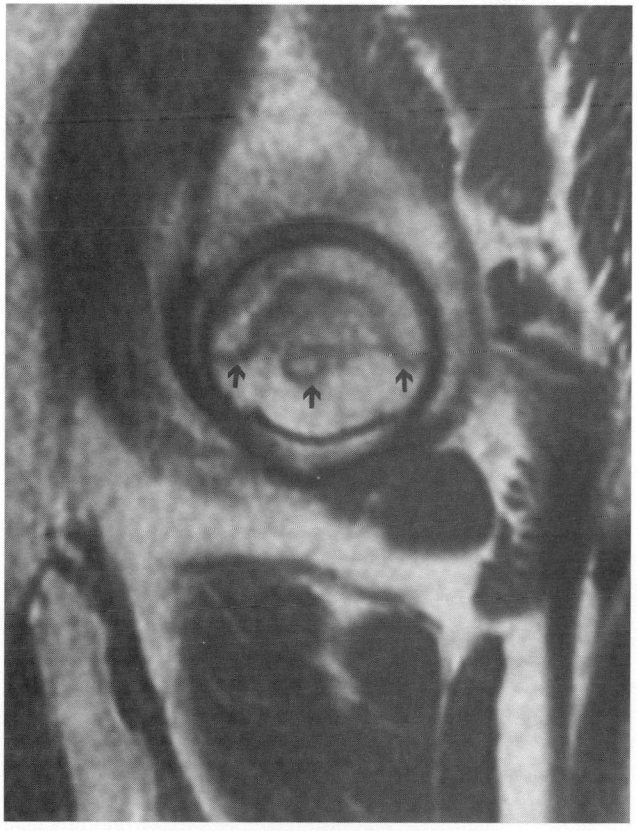

B

Figure 15-31 Avascular necrosis. This 29-year-old lupus patient, treated with steroids, developed bilateral hip pain. Coronal (*A*) T1-weighted (TR/TE 600/15) and (*B*) sagittal T1-weighted (TR/TE 600/15) MR images of the left femoral head. The serpiginous low-signal line (*black arrows*) delineates the extent of involvement of the femoral heads. Note the involvement of 100 percent of the weight-bearing cortex of the left femoral head, best seen on the sagittal image.

nal void marginating the segmental defect is felt to represent the interface between necrotic and viable bone. Mitchell et al. described a hyperintense rim of granulation tissue abutting this line of signal void, creating the "double-line sign," which is considered pathognomic for AVN but is identified in only 80 percent of patients.[316] The subchondral fracture associated with AVN may be difficult to see on T1-weighted images, but fluid within the fracture cleft can be readily identified as a high-signal-intensity line on T2-weighted images.[318]

In addition to its high sensitivity and specificity for detection of AVN, MRI also has an additional role. Other imaging modalities had never been successful in predicting which patients would proceed to collapse of the femoral head. With the extremely high spatial resolution afforded by MRI, it was possible to test the hypothesis that the development of collapse is closely related to the extent and location of the avascular necrosis rather than to the radiographic stage. One recent study quantitatively assessed the percentage of weight-bearing cortex of the femoral head involved by avascular necrosis and found consistently poor outcome in those patients with more than 45 percent involvement.[319] Magnetic resonance imaging may thus prove accurate in the prediction of long-term outcome. The efficacy of treatment modalities such as core decompression could then be reevaluated.

Infection

Infection, either of soft tissue and/or bone, can range from a mild nuisance to a major headache for the clinician. Its diagnosis runs a similar gamut for the radiologist. In a straightforward case, radiographs may show periosteal reaction, trabecular and cortical destruction, soft tissue swelling, and blurring of adjacent fat planes. The bony changes are relatively late, however, not being radiographically evident until approximately 10 to 12 days.[320] The soft tissue changes can be seen earlier, but they may be subtle.

Other modalities can be used in this early period, however. Nuclear medicine offers an array of various radiopharmaceuticals, such as ^{99m}Tc-MDP bone scan, ^{67}Ga citrate, leukocyte imaging with either ^{111}In or ^{99m}Tc, and newer agents like polyclonal immunoglobulins, with sensitivities and specificities for various techniques as high as 100 and 100 percent, respectively (see discussion of nuclear medicine, above). General disadvantages of scintigraphy are the need to label cells or pharmaceuticals with radionuclides, delays in imaging of 4 to 48 h after the intravenous administration of the agent, and lack of anatomic resolution, particularly with respect to soft tissue infection.

Magnetic resonance imaging, with its exquisite sensitivity to changes in the water content of marrow and soft tissue, is excellent for demonstrating the inflammatory edema of early infection. Acute osteomyelitis and cellulitis are suggested when there is replacement of normal fatty marrow signal intensity by low signal intensity on T1-weighted images and high signal intensity on T2-weighted images and similar signal intensity changes in the soft tissues, respectively[321,322] (Fig. 15-32). Early investigations of MRI in infection compared this modality to scintigraphy and CT. Unger et al. reported equal sensitivity but better specificity of MRI versus ^{99m}Tc-MDP bone scan for diagnosing osteomyelitis, yielding overall accuracy of 94 and 71 percent, respectively.[322] Beltran et al., in two different

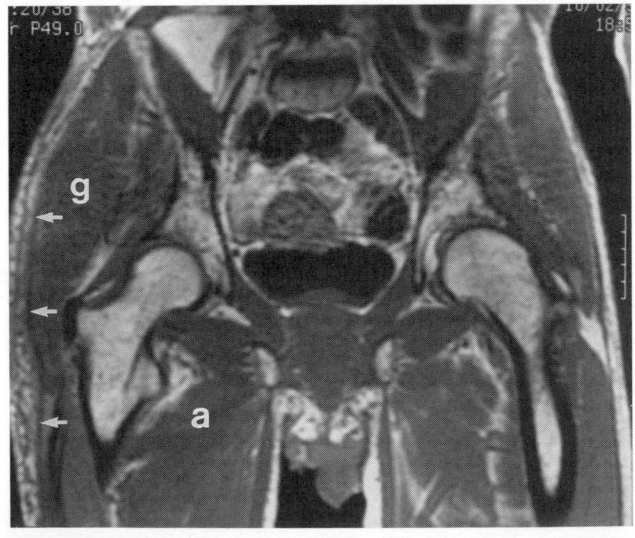

A

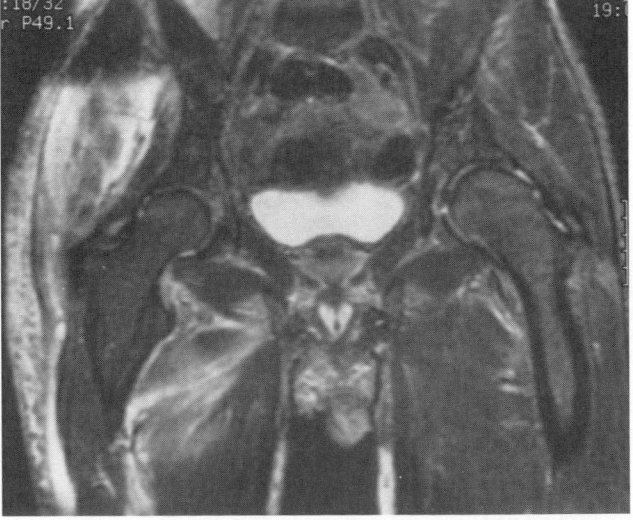

B

Figure 15-32 MRI of a 47-year-old man with cellulitis, ordered to assess extent of the process and rule out bony involvement. *A.* Coronal T1-weighted (TR/TE 600/20) MRI. The subcutaneous fat is infiltrated with inflammatory edema (*white arrows*), and the gluteus medius (g) and adductors (a) are swollen by a similar process (compare to the opposite side). The femur retains its normal fatty marrow (high signal intensity), thus ruling out osteomyelitis. *B.* Coronal fat-suppressed fast T2-weighted (TR/TE 6000/80) MRI demonstrates the high-signal-intensity soft tissue inflammatory edema and the normal low signal intensity of the suppressed fatty marrow.

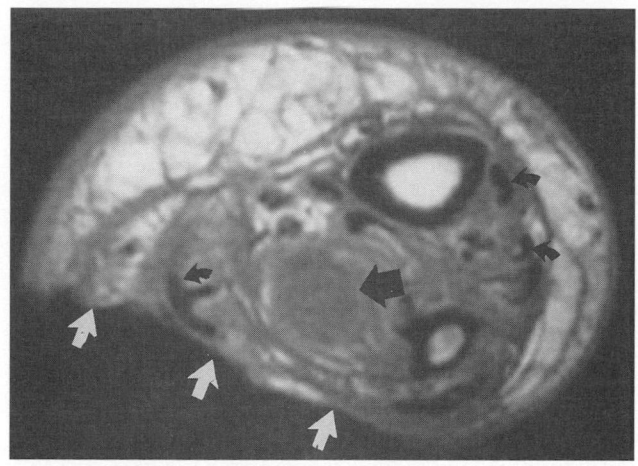

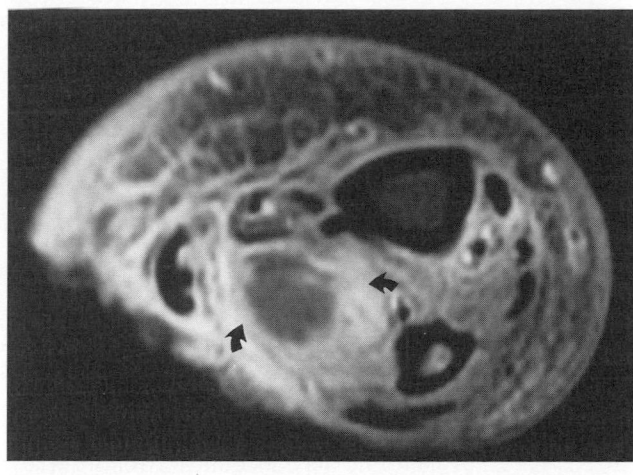

A

B

Figure 15-33 Forty-two-year-old diabetic woman after debridement of soft tissue abscesses in the thigh. Patient continued to have spiking fevers, and MRI was ordered to evaluate for residual collections. *A.* Axial T1-weighted (TR/TE 700/20) MRI of the thigh shows a large surgical defect posteriorly (*white arrows*), residual postoperative air (*small black arrows*), and a deep space-occupying process (*large black arrow*) with edematous infiltration of the surrounding deep fat. *B.* Axial fat-suppressed T1-weighted (TR/TE 800/17) MRI after intravenous gadolinium administration shows enhancement of the wall of the collection (*small black arrows*) but not of the contents, consistent with abscess.

studies, reported equal sensitivity of MRI and bone scan for osteomyelitis but superior sensitivity of MRI for soft tissue infection, with the added ability to distinguish cellulitis from abscess.[323,324] In a series of experimentally produced musculoskeletal infections in rabbits, MRI was more sensitive than CT for detecting osteomyelitis and abscess (94 versus 66 percent and 97 versus 52 percent, respectively).[325] Similarly, Beltran et al. reported better definition of abscesses on MRI than CT.[324] In vertebral osteomyelitis, MRI and combined gallium–bone scan both had 94 percent accuracy, whereas bone scan alone had 86 percent accuracy,[16] and MRI was superior to CT in evaluating epidural spread of infection.[326]

The utility of gadolinium enhancement has also been investigated. In cases of infection not complicated by underlying pathology, Miller et al. found no difference in extent and conspicuity of inflammatory change in bone and soft tissue between fat-suppressed T1-weighted images with gadolinium enhancement versus fat-suppressed fast spin-echo T2-weighted images, but they did find the fat-suppressed T1-weighted images with gadolinium helpful for identifying abscesses[327] (Fig. 15-33). Similar conclusions have been reached by others.[328,329] In complicating osteomyelitis, (i.e., osteomyelitis complicating a fracture or neuropathic joint), the addition of a fat-suppressed gadolinium-enhanced T1-weighted sequence increased the sensitivity and specificity of the study to 88 and 93 percent, respectively, up from 79 and 53 percent, respectively, for the unenhanced study, whereas three-phase bone scan in this study demonstrated 61 percent sensitivity and 33 percent specificity.[330]

Evaluation of chronic osteomyelitis can also be challenging. Radiographs may show mixed lucency and sclerosis, sequestra, cloacae, and involucrum (cloaking periosteal reaction). Activity is difficult to assess, however.

Magnetic resonance imaging will display active areas as high signal intensity on T2-weighted images. It has been shown to have 100 percent sensitivity, while ^{111}In-WBC had 45 percent.[331] Moreover, while CT can demonstrate sequestra and sinus tracts well, studies have shown MRI to be superior to CT because of MRI's ability to demonstrate areas of active infection in addition to the demonstration of sequestra and sinus tracts [321,332] (Fig. 15-34).

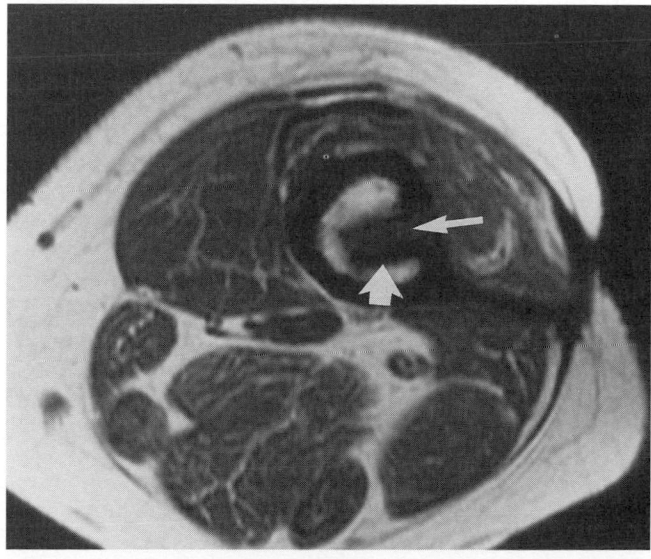

Figure 15-34 Chronic osteomyelitis in the midshaft of the femur in a 51-year-old woman. Axial T1-weighted (TR/TE 600/30) MRI demonstrates a sequestrum (*thick arrow*) and sinus tract (*thin arrow*). The marrow signal around the sinus tract is normal, suggesting that there is no active osteomyelitis.

Some clinical situations are particularly challenging and require special mention, such as infection in children, around prostheses, and in diabetic feet. The diagnosis of acute osteomyelitis in children can be difficult; symptomatology may be misleading due to referred pain, and laboratory tests may be falsely normal or only mildly elevated.[333,334] Radiographs of the immature skeleton can be hard to interpret because of lucent open growth plates and unossified growth centers. Moreover, radiographic bony changes are late findings. Investigations of bone scan and gallium scintigraphy have reported mixed results. Unlike uptake of MDP in adults, which is increased in the case of osteomyelitis, uptake in children may be decreased due to decreased blood flow resulting from the compression of vessels by subperiosteal pus. "Cold" spots may be hard to recognize, and this may account for reported low sensitivities. Nonetheless, Bressler et al. have reported 100 percent sensitivity for ^{99m}Tc-MDP bone scan, but they stressed the need for meticulous imaging technique using a high-resolution collimator and magnification.[335] On the other hand, ^{67}Ga-citrate, which is less dependent on blood flow, has been reported to have 91 percent sensitivity and accuracy.[8] An advantage of scintigraphy is the ability to image the entire body—an important consideration, since osteomyelitis can be multifocal in 19 percent of children overall, with 31 percent incidence in neonates and 44 percent in children 9 to 12 years old.[336]

A recent comparison of MRI and bone scan revealed 97 percent sensitivity and 92 percent specificity for MRI versus 64 percent sensitivity and 71 percent specificity for bone scan.[337] Disadvantages of MRI are the cost, the need to sedate young children, and the ability to image only a focal anatomic region, while an advantage is its use of magnetic radiation instead of ionizing radiation. It is recommended that scintigraphy be the next modality performed, if needed, after radiographs, reserving MRI for suspected infection of the pelvis and spine, infections not responding to antibiotic treatment, and for preoperative evaluation of suspected abscess prior to drainage and debridement.[333,334] For suspected pediatric hip infection, ultrasound has excellent negative predictive value for septic arthritis if an effusion is absent, but it cannot distinguish a sterile effusion from an infected one, and it cannot exclude osteomyelitis.[337]

The diagnosis of infection around a prosthesis is mostly the domain of nuclear medicine, since the presence of the metallic prosthesis causes artifacts on CT and MRI that degrade or distort the image. Radiographs should be obtained in all cases of painful prostheses, and while investigations show that streak artifact due to metal prostheses can be markedly diminished on reconstructed images,[338,339] neither radiographs nor CT can distinguish between the changes of noninfectious mechanical loosening versus those of septic loosening. Bone scan with ^{99m}Tc-MDP has been extensively investigated; in a cemented total hip replacement, focal uptake at the tip of the femoral stem is suggestive of mechanical loosening, whereas diffuse uptake around the entire stem is suggestive of infection.[340] Unfortunately, there are problems with this technique:[7,341] (1) there may be diffuse or variable uptake within the first year after implantation, which makes in-

terpretation impossible; (2) approximately 10 percent of asymptomatic people will still have some degree of uptake even after the first postoperative year; and (3) noncemented ingrowth components may normally demonstrate variable uptake for several years after implantation. Consequently, other techniques have been tried. Some authors have reported near perfect sensitivity and specificity of ^{67}Ga-citrate,[9] but this nuclide is a weak bone agent that is plagued by the same problems as ^{99m}Tc-MDP. Others have combined gallium imaging and bone scan, with infection suggested when uptake is spatially incongruent, or congruent but more intense for gallium, with accuracies of 60 to 80 percent.[341] Leukocyte imaging sounded promising because of its theoretical specificity for infection, but sensitivities and specificities have ranged from 73 to 100 percent and 50 to 93 percent, respectively.[7] Leukocytes normally accumulate in sites of red marrow, which is variable from person to person, making interpretation of uptake difficult. This difficulty can be ameliorated by the addition of a ^{99m}Tc–sulfur colloid scan, which demonstrates normal marrow distribution.[11] Currently, this combined leukocyte-marrow imaging technique is the study of choice to evaluate suspected infected prostheses, with infection suggested when uptake is spatially incongruent. Palestro et al. reported 95 and 98 percent accuracies for this combination in evaluating total knee replacements[342] and total hip replacements,[345] respectively. Some investigators have even reported the use of ultrasound to evaluate suspected infected hip prostheses, with infection suggested when joint effusion caused displacement of the pseudocapsule more than 3.2 mm from the anterior femoral cortex.[344]

The most challenging situation is the diagnosis of infection complicating a diabetic foot. Radiographs can be hard to interpret secondary to the neuropathic changes of joint destruction, bony fragmentation, and soft tissue swelling. Results of different studies vary because of different clinical and laboratory criteria used to diagnose infection and the severity of the underlying neuropathic disease. One study reported sensitivity and specificity for radiographs of 75 percent,[345] while another reported 83 percent sensitivity and 43 percent specificity.[82] Bone scan with ^{99m}Tc-MDP is sensitive but lacks specificity due to uptake by the bone turnover of the neuropathic foot itself.[83,345] Gallium citrate has also been tried, but combined leukocyte–bone scan imaging is the currently preferred scintigraphic technique. Sensitivity and specificity ranges from 73 to 100 percent and 78 to 91 percent, respectively,[82] and Schauwecker cites 89 percent accuracy.[346] However, these scintigraphic methods are hindered by their lack of anatomic resolution, which makes preoperative planning difficult. This point is particularly important, since accurate surgical debridement is necessary to eradicate infection, and surgical attention is now directed toward foot-sparing procedures. Because of its superb anatomic resolution and multiplanar capability, MRI is excellent for delineating the extent of disease in both bone and soft tissue. Studies have reported high sensitivities and specificities for MRI,[345,347] and Horowitz et al. praised its utility in preoperative planning.[348] Morrison et al. reported 89 percent accuracy for gadolinium-enhanced MRI and concluded that, the accuracy of leukocyte imaging and MRI being equal, MRI was superior to scintigraphy for two reasons: (1) its ability to accurately delineate the extent of infection and (2) its better cost-effectiveness than scintigraphy because of the decreased preoperative hospital stay resulting from its more rapid performance.[349] In a recent study of 16 diabetic feet with clinically suspected infection, ^{111}In-WBC imaging was 78 percent sensitive and 86 percent specific, while MRI using gadolinium-enhanced fat-suppressed T1-weighted images was 89 percent sensitive and 86 percent specific.[350]

Tumors

The subject of tumors is broad, encompassing both bony tumors (primary, metastatic, and infiltrative marrow disorders) and soft tissue tumors. A description of individual tumors is beyond the scope of this chapter; therefore we will concentrate instead on the principles of radiologic evaluation. The radiologic workup of any suspected tumor must begin with plain radiographs. In the case of bony tumors, radiographic features such as pattern (permeative, moth-eaten, geographic), margin definition, matrix, location (long/flat bone, end-of-bone/shaft, medulla/cortex), and periosteal reaction are important clues to the lesion's identity. If the age and sex of the patient are also known, a correct diagnosis can be made from radiographs in most cases.

The role of other imaging modalities in the workup of bony tumors, therefore, is to stage rather than diagnose the lesions. Magnetic resonance imaging is the favored modality for staging the solitary bone tumor, having been shown superior to both CT and bone scan for evaluating intra- and extramedullary extent.[66,351–357] It is this superiority that has led to a staging system for bone tumors based on the MRI demonstration of extent of bony involvement and breakthrough into the surrounding soft tissues.[357] The addition of gadolinium does not further the evaluation of tumor margin or of extent of the lesion.[358]

Certain benign lesions, however—like fractures, infections, eosinophilic granuloma, and chondroblastoma—can have a deceptively aggressive appearance on MRI, mimicking malignant lesions[359–361] (Fig. 15-35). Interpretation of a bone lesion on MRI without the corresponding radiograph is analogous to driving a car with one's eyes closed; both are inviting disaster. In addition, there are situations in which CT and scintigraphy are better approaches. Computed tomography is the modality of choice for the evaluation of flat bones such as the scapula and iliac wing and for visualizing matrix mineralization, cortical destruction, and subtle soft tissue calcifications.[352,355,356] Osteoid osteoma is also best imaged with CT.[362] Bone scan is the modality of choice for screening suspected multifocal disease.[363]

Patients with primary bony malignancies, such as osteosarcoma and Ewing's sarcoma, should undergo chest CT as part of the preoperative staging workup. If limb-salvage surgery is planned, current levels of technology make MR angiography an acceptable alternative to conventional angiography, thus allowing noninvasive preoperative assessment of tumor vascularity and providing a vascular "road map" for the surgeon.[363]

Radiographs of soft tissue tumors may also provide a clue as to their identity by demonstrating such features as phleboliths in a hemangioma or low density in a lipoma. Most soft tissue masses are not characterizable on radiographs, however, and additional imaging must be performed. Both CT and MRI have been used, and while CT is superior for the evaluation of subtle calcification, MRI, due to its excellent soft tissue contrast and multiplanar capability, is superior for demonstrating size and extent of the

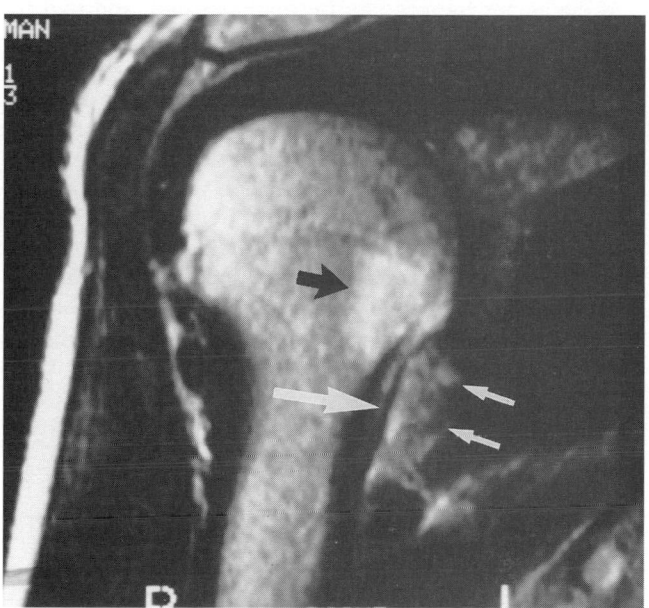

A

B

Figure 15-35 Nineteen-year-old male with right shoulder pain. *A.* Coronal oblique T2-weighted MRI of the right shoulder shows focal marrow edema (*black arrow*), periosteal reaction (*large white arrow*), and soft tissue edema (*small white arrows*), which suggest an aggressive, possibly malignant process. *B.* Frontal radiograph of the right shoulder demonstrates the lucent nidus of an osteoid osteoma (*short arrows*) with a small central calcification (*long arrow*).

mass, margin definition, and surrounding edema as well as for defining its relationship to adjacent structures.[365,366] Numerous articles have addressed the issue of MRI's ability to distinguish benign and malignant soft tissue tumors, with conflicting conclusions. Features that have been investigated as potential discriminators of benignancy and malignancy have included tumor size, margin definition, presence and amount of peritumoral edema, signal intensity and homogeneity, and involvement of neurovascular or other adjacent structures.[367–370] Studies of soft tissue tumors of the hands and wrists,[371,372] foot,[373] and the body in general[375] have suggested that in most instances benign and malignant tumors can be distinguished, and that for many masses a specific diagnosis can be made. There are two reasons for these results. First, some benign soft tissue tumors have characteristic appearances. For example, lipomas are homogeneous masses with signal intensity paralleling that of subcutaneous fat, desmoids are low in signal intensity on all sequences due to their hypocellularity and collagenous stroma, and hemangiomas have a lacelike pattern of alternating low and high signal intensity due to their mixed fatty and vascular components. Second, there are tendencies which, although not 100 percent accurate, do suggest the lesion's nature.[366] For example, a small well-circumscribed, homogeneous mass without peritumoral edema is most likely benign. Most masses, however, have a nonspecific pattern of low signal intensity on T1-weighted images and high signal intensity on T2-weighted images as well as a mixture of features; when benign masses with typical appearances are excluded from analysis or do not make up a large percentage of the sample population, the ability of MRI to differentiate benign and malignant soft tissue lesions is nullified.[367,368]

Other techniques have attempted to succeed where conventional MRI has failed. Erlemann et al.[375] and Verstraete et al.[376] both achieved 80 percent accuracy by measuring the rate of enhancement on dynamically enhanced MRI studies, with malignant tumors having steeper slopes, but these results are no better than the unenhanced MRI results of Moulton et al.[367] Despite a statistically significant difference in rates of enhancement, there is enough overlap of malignant lesions of low vascularity and highly vascular benign lesions to make completely accurate separation of the two impossible. For example, by choosing a higher slope value as the threshold for malignancy, specificity can be increased to 100 percent, but sensitivity will drop to 55 percent.[376] Li et al. approached the problem by using magnetization-transfer contrast MRI, but they found no significant difference in the magnetization transfer ratios between benign and malignant processes.[377] Scintigraphic techniques have also been described, such as assessing uptake of ^{99m}Tc(V) dimercaptosuccinic acid (DMSA).[378] This tracer has been shown to accumulate in all cases of malignant and many cases of recurrent/aggressive benign processes; Kobayashi et al. therefore suggest that lack of uptake of this material by a tumor excludes malignancy.[378] Other investigators have used ^{201}Th chloride to distinguish benign and malignant processes (see elsewhere).

The role of MRI in the workup of soft tissue tumors is not to provide a histologic diagnosis but to aid surgical planning. It is necessary to assess features such as margin definition, location, involvement of adjacent tissue planes or compartments, and encasement of neurovascular bundles prior to operation in order to avoid surprises in the operating room and to ensure the greatest chance of complete resection.

Arguably more important than the pretherapy imaging evaluation of osseous and soft tissue tumors is the determination of tumor response to preoperative chemo- or radiotherapy and the reliability of posttherapy imaging surveillance. The goal of preoperative chemo- or radiotherapy is to necrose as much of the tumor as possible. Greater than 90 percent necrosis is considered a good response and an implication of good prognosis. The assessment of tumor response has been made with MRI, MR angiography, MR spectroscopy, color Doppler sonography, and scintigraphy.

Post chemotherapy appearances of osteosarcoma[379] and Ewing's sarcoma[380] suggestive of good response have been described, including decrease in size of the extraosseous soft tissue component and change in the MRI signal intensity or pattern of the tumor. These descriptions are limited, however, by the overlap in appearance and signal intensity of residual tumor and tumor necrosis and/or hemorrhage, such that other investigators concluded that these and other characteristics were not useful for predicting which patients would have a good histologic response or clinical outcome.[381–383]

The difficulty in distinguishing residual tumor from tumor necrosis on unenhanced MRI had led some workers to investigate the use of gadolinium. Hanna et al.[384] found that static gadolinium-enhanced T1-weighted images overestimated the amount of residual tumor because of the nonspecific uptake of gadolinium by both tumor and posttherapy inflammation/granulation tissue.[384] They and others, however, describe 100 percent accuracy for this distinction using dynamically enhanced MRI based on differential rates of enhancement between residual tumor and necrosis/granulation tissue.[384,385] Erlemann et al.[386] reported 86 percent accuracy with the dynamic technique, compared to 74 percent for three-phase bone scan and 71 percent for static-enhanced MRI. De Baere et al. cite excellent results using a subtraction technique of pre- and postdynamically enhanced images to predict response to chemotherapy.[387]

Similar to assessing the differential uptake of gadolinium between tumor and granulation tissue, which is a reflection of differences in vascularity, other investigators have studied the vascularity itself. Carrasco and colleagues had mixed results differentiating responders from nonresponders using conventional angiography,[388] but a recent study by Lang et al. using MR angiography reported excellent results, with responders showing a decrease both in tumor neovascular density and in the number and caliber of feeder vessels.[389] Changes in the blood supply as an indication of tumor response have also been assessed with color Doppler sonography. Van der Woude et al.[390] compared color Doppler sonography, contrast-enhanced MRI, and three-phase bone scan in the evaluation of tumor perfusion after chemotherapy and found color Doppler most accurate. This same group of authors[391] recently reported another series of patients assessed with color Doppler sonography after chemotherapy, again with excellent results, concluding that an increased resistive index is indicative of a good response.

Scintigraphy with [201]Th chloride is also being used to assess response to chemotherapy. Two groups of investigators[392,393] noted decreased uptake of thallium in tumors that showed a good histologic response and no change in uptake in poor responders. Lin et al.[396] advocate a quantitative assessment of thallium uptake by measuring a ratio of tumor uptake to contralateral normal tissue uptake. They, too, noted that a decrease in the ratio correlated well with good response.

Investigation of other modalities, such as positron emission tomography (PET) and MR spectroscopy, is also being performed in the pre- and posttherapy evaluation of musculoskeletal sarcomas. Zlatkin et al. noticed a correlation between an increased ratio of phosphomonoester to β-nucleotide triphosphate with high-grade tumors and suggested using MRI to select the site of the spectroscopic interrogation.[395] Kern et al. correlated a high glucose utilization rate on PET with high-grade tumors,[398] and Sostman et al. suggest that a long T2 relaxation time and alkaline pH of a soft tissue sarcoma before treatment predicts a good response to therapy.[397] In their study of osteosarcoma, Redmond et al. found that the postchemotherapy T2 values of the intramedullary component of the tumor did not correlate with the percentage of tumor necrosis, but that those of the extraosseous component did.[398] Moreover, these authors noted changes in the phosphorus-31 spectra of the tumors, which may have implications for assessing tumor necrosis. Clearly, though much investigation is under way, no single modality has yet emerged as the clear and unequivocal technique for evaluating tumor response.

For the follow-up surveillance of tumors after definitive treatment, Reuther and Mutschler reported sensitivities for recurrence of 82.5 and 57.5 percent for MRI and CT, respectively.[399] Vanel and colleagues, reporting two different studies of the MRI follow-up of treated lesions, noted that low signal intensity on T2-weighted images correlated well with lack of recurrence; high signal intensity, however, was nonspecific, representing either recurrence, hygroma, or postradiation change. They recommended gadolinium enhancement in these cases.[400,401] Similarly, posttherapy seroma, hematoma, fat necrosis, and even herniated bowel and bladder have been described as other, nonrecurrence causes of high signal intensity on T2-weighted images.[402] A comparison of MRI and sonography for the detection of recurrent soft tissue tumors showed no statistical difference in sensitivity and specificity between the two modalities (MRI, 83 percent sensitive, 93 percent specific; sonography, 100 percent sensitive, 79 percent specific); the authors suggest that sonography be used for follow-up, since it is inexpensive and can guide needle biopsies of suspicious sites.[113] We prefer MRI because sonography is highly operator-dependent, and comparison with previous sonographic examinations can be difficult if imaging is not done the same way each time.

The MRI appearance of allografts has also been reported. Levin et al. described low signal intensity on T1-weighted images and high signal intensity on T2-weighted images in allografts of three pediatric patients.[403] This pattern is nonspecific and could be seen with recurrence, but their patients had no clinical evidence of recurrent disease. The authors surmised that water content within the marrow cavity of the sterilized allograft accounted for the signal intensities. This observation has been confirmed subsequently by Hoefner et al. and has been shown to represent "gelatinous transformation" or "serous atrophy" of the allograft marrow cavity.[404] A study of the MRI appearance of bone lesions after cryotherapy has also been reported; the authors describe a marginal zone of variable thickness—showing low signal intensity on T1-weighted images and high signal intensity on T2-weighted images—surrounding the frozen site; the authors believe that this zone represents osteonecrosis.[405]

REFERENCES

1. Resnick D, Niwayama G: *Diagnosis of Bone and Joint Disorders.* Philadelphia, Saunders, 1988.
2. Edeiken J, Dalinka M, Karasick D: *Roentgen Diagnosis of Diseases of Bone,* 4th ed. Baltimore, Williams & Wilkins, 1990.
3. Greenfield GB: *Radiology of Bone Diseases,* 5th ed. Philadelphia, Lippincott, 1990.
4. Greenspan A: *Orthopedic Radiology,* 2d ed. New York, Raven Press, 1992.
5. Chew F: *Skeletal Radiology: The Bare Bones.* Rockville, MD, Aspen, 1989.
6. Schauwecker DS: The scintigraphic diagnosis of osteomyelitis. *AJR* 158:9–18, 1992.
7. Wegener WA, Alavi A: Diagnostic imaging of musculoskeletal infection: Roentgenology; gallium, indium-labeled white blood cell, gammaglobulin, bone scintigraphy; and MRI. *Orthop Clin North Am* 22:401, 1991.
8. Borman TR, Johnson RA, Sherman FC: Gallium scintigraphy for diagnosis of septic arthritis and osteomyelitis in children. *J Pediatr Orthop* 6:317–325, 1986.
9. Palestro CJ: The current role of gallium imaging in infection. *Semin Nucl Med* 24:128, 1994.
10. Merkel KD, Brown ML, Dewanjee MK, et al: Comparison of indium-labeled-leukocyte imaging with sequential technetium-gallium scanning in the diagnosis of low-grade musculoskeletal sepsis. *J Bone Joint Surg* 67A:465, 1985.
11. Palestro CJ, Roumanas P, Swyer AJ, et al: Diagnosis of musculoskeletal infection using combined In-111 labeled leukocyte and Tc-99m SC marrow imaging. *Clin Nucl Med* 17:269, 1992.
12. Achong DM, Oates E: The computer-generated bone marrow subtraction image: A valuable adjunct to combined In-111 WBC/Tc-99m sulfur colloid scintigraphy for musculoskeletal infection. *Clin Nucl Med* 19:188, 1994.
13. Datz FL: Indium-111–labeled leukocytes for the detection of infection: Current status. *Semin Nucl Med* 24:92, 1994.
14. Whalen JL, Brown ML, McLeod R, Fitzgerald RH Jr: Limitations of indium leukocyte imaging for the diagnosis of spine infections. *Spine* 16:193, 1991.
15. Palestro CJ, Kim CK, Swyer AJ, et al: Radionuclide diagnosis of vertebral osteomyelitis: Indium-111-leukocyte and technetium-99m-methylene diphosphonate bone scintigraphy. *J Nucl Med* 32:1861, 1991.
16. Modic MT, Feiglin DH, Piraino DW, et al: Vertebral osteomyelitis: Assessment using MR. *Radiology* 157:157, 1985.

17. Harwood SJ, Camblin JG, Hakki S, et al: Use of technetium antigranulocyte monoclonal antibody fab' fragments for the detection of osteomyelitis. *Cell Biophys* 99:24–25, 1994.

18. Caglar M, Tokgozoglu AM, Ercan MT, et al: The value of Tc-99m citrate scintigraphy in chronic osteomyelitis: An indicator of the involved bone. *Clin Nucl Med* 20:712, 1995.

19. Ang ES, Sundram FX, Goh AS, Aw SE: 99Tcm-Polyclonal IgG and 99Tcm nanocolloid scans in orthopaedics: A comparison with conventional bone scan. *Nucl Med Commun* 14:419, 1993.

20. Holder LE: Bone scintigraphy in skeletal trauma. *Radiol Clin North Am* 31:739, 1993.

21. Rizzo PF, Gould ES, Lyden JP, Asnis SE: Diagnosis of occult fractures about the hip: Magnetic resonance imaging compared with bone-scanning. *J Bone Joint Surg* 75A:395 1993.

22. Quinn SF, McCarthy JL: Prospective evaluation of patients with suspected hip fracture and indeterminate radiographs: Use of T1-weighted MR images. *Radiology* 187:469, 1993.

23. Rubin SJ, Marquardt J, Meyers SP, et al: Magnetic resonance imaging compared to bone scanning in the evaluation of patients with suspected hip fractures. *AJR* 166(suppl):117, 1996.

24. Guanche CA, Kozin SH, Levy AS, Brody LA: The use of MRI in the diagnosis of occult hip fractures in the elderly: A preliminary review. *Orthopedics* 17:327, 1994.

25. Nussbaum AR, Treves ST, Micheli L: Bone stress lesions in ballet dancers: Scintigraphic assessment. *AJR* 150:851, 1988.

26. Mettler FA, Guiberteau MJ: *Essentials of Nuclear Medicine Imaging,* 2d ed. Philadelphia, Saunders, 1985.

27. Mesgarzadeh M, Sapega AA, Bonakdarpour A, et al: Osteochondritis dessicans: Analysis of mechanical stability with radiography, scintigraphy and MR imaging. *Radiology* 165:775, 1987.

28. Woolfenden JM, Pitt MJ, Durie BGM, Moon TE: Comparison of bone scintigraphy and radiology in multiple myeloma. *Radiology* 134:723, 1980.

29. Jacobson AF, Harley JD, Lipsky BA, et al: Diagnosis of osteomyelitis in the presence of soft-tissue infection and radiologic evidence of osseous abnormalities: Value of leukocyte scintigraphy. *AJR* 157:807–812, 1991.

30. Vande Streek PR, Carretta RF, Weiland FL: Nuclear medicine approaches to musculoskeletal disease: Current status. *Radiol Clin North Am* 32:227, 1994.

31. Nadel HR: Thallium-201 for oncological imaging in children. *Semin Nucl Med* 23:243, 1993.

32. Van der Wal H, Murray IP, Huckstep RL, Philips RL:The role of thallium scintigraphy in excluding malignancy in bone. *Clin Nucl Med* 18:551, 1993.

33. Caluser CI, Abdel-Dayem HM, Macapinlac HA, et al: The value of thallium and three-phase bone scans in the evaluation of bone and soft tissue sarcomas. *Eur J Nucl Med* 21:1198, 1994.

34. Abdel-Dayem H: 201Tl-Chloride uptake ratios in differentiating benign from malignant lesions: Recommendations for ratio calculations and interpretation. *Nucl Med Commun* 16:145, 1995.

35. Markisz JA, Knowles RJR, Altchek DW, et al: Segmental patterns of avascular necrosis of the femoral heads: Early detection with MR imaging. *Radiology* 162:717, 1987.

36. Conklin JJ, Alderson PO, Zizic TM, et al: Comparison of bone scan and radiographic sensitivity in the detection of steroid-induced ischemic necrosis of bone. *Radiology* 147:221, 1983.

37. Beltran J, Herman LJ, Burk JM, et al: Femoral head avascular necrosis: MR imaging with clinical-pathologic and radionuclide correlation. *Radiology* 166:215, 1988.

38. Collier BD, Carrera GF, Johnson RP, et al: Detection of femoral head avascular necrosis in adults by SPECT. *J Nucl Med* 26:979, 1985.

39. Sadeleer C, Audiens H, De Boeck H, Piepsz A: Legg-Perthes disease: Partial or total loss of femoral head? Contribution of SPECT images. *Clin Nucl Med* 19:830, 1994.

40. Miller IL, Savory CG, Polly DW Jr, et al: Femoral head osteonecrosis: Detection by magnetic resonance imaging versus single-photon emission computed tomography. *Clin Orthop Rel Res* 247:152, 1989.

41. Kim KY, Lee SH, Moon DH, Nah HY: The diagnostic value of triple head single photon emission computed tomography (3H-SPECT) in avascular necrosis of the femoral head. *Int Orthop* 17:132, 1993.

42. Mortensson W, Rosenborg M, Gretzer H: The role of bone scintigraphy in predicting femoral head collapse following cervical fractures in children. *Acta Radiol* 31:291, 1990.

43. Kokubo T, Takatori Y, Ninomiya S, et al: Magnetic resonance imaging and scintigraphy of avascular necrosis of the femoral head: Prediction of subsequent segmental collapse. *Clin Orthop Rel Res* 277:54, 1992.

44. Magid D, Michelson JD, Ney DR, et al: Adult ankle fractures: Comparison of plain films and interactive two- and three-dimensional CT scans. *AJR* 154:1017–1023, 1990.

45. Fishman EK, Ney DR, Scott WW, Robertson DD: The role of CT with multiplanar reconstruction. *Appl Radiol* 36–40, 1992.

46. Magid D, Fishman EK, Mandelbaum BM, et al: Computed tomography with multiplanar reconstructions in the assessment and management of acetabular fractures. *J Comput Assist Tomogr* 10:778–783, 1996.

47. Scott WW Jr, Fishman EK, Magid D: Acetabular fractures: Optimal imaging. *Radiology* 165:537–539, 1987.

48. Feldman F, Singson R, Rosenberg ZS, et al: Distal tibial triplane fractures: Diagnosis with CT. *Radiology* 164:429–435, 1987.

49. Rafii M, Firooznia H, Golimbu C, et al: Computed tomography of tibial plateau fractures. *AJR* 142:1181–1185, 1984.

50. Nakamura R, Imaeda T, Horii E, et al: Analysis of scaphoid fracture displacement by three-dimensional computed tomography. *J Hand Surg* 16A:485–492, 1991.

51. Rosenberg ZS, Feldman F, Singson RD: Intra-articular calcaneal fractures: Computed tomographic analysis. *Skel Radiol* 16:105–113, 1987.

52. Johnston GH, Friedman L, Kriegler JC: Computerized tomographic evaluation of acute distal radial fractures. *J Hand Surg* 17A:738–744, 1992.

53. Dalinka MK, Boorstein JM, Zlatkin MB: Computed tomography of musculoskeletal trauma. *Radiol Clin North Am* 27:933, 1989.

54. Rosenberg ZS, Feldman F, Singson RD, et al: Peroneal tendon injury associated with calcaneal fractures: CT findings. *AJR* 149:125–129, 1987.

55. Kode L, Lieberman JM, Motta AO, et al: Evaluation of tibial plateau fractures: Efficacy of MR imaging compared with CT. *AJR* 163:141–147, 1994.

56. Kuhlman JE, Fishman EK, Magid D, et al: Fracture nonunion: CT assessment with multiplanar reconstruction. *Radiology* 167:483–488, 1988.

57. Chandnani VP, Yeager TD, DeBerardino T, et al: Glenoid labral tears: Prospective evaluation with MRI, MR arthrography, and CT arthrography. *AJR* 161:1229–1235, 1993.

58. Rafii M, Minkoff J, Bonamo J, et al: Computed tomography (CT) arthrography of shoulder instabilities in athletes. *Am J Sports Med* 16:352–361, 1988.

59. Hunter JC, Blatz DJ, Escobedo EM: SLAP lesions of the glenoid labrum: CT arthrographic and arthroscopic correlation. *Radiology* 184:513–518, 1992.

60. Singson RD, Feldman F, Bigliani LU, et al: Recurrent shoulder dislocation after surgical repair: Double-contrast CT arthrography. Work in progress. *Radiology* 164:425–428, 1987.

61. Gagliardi JA, Chung EM, Chandnani VP, et al: Detection and staging of chondromalacia patellae: Relative efficacies of conventional MR imaging, MR arthrography, and CT arthrography. *AJR* 163:629–636, 1994.

62. Hodge JC, Ghelman B, O'Brien SJ, et al: Synovial plicae and chondromalacia patellae: Correlation of results of CT arthrography with results of arthroscopy. *Radiology* 186:827–831, 1993.

63. Ihara H: Double-contrast CT arthrography of the cruciate ligaments. *Nippon Seikeigeka Gakkai-Zasshi* 65:477–487, 1991.

64. Beauchamp NJ, Scott WW, Gottlieb LM, et al: CT evaluation of soft tissue and muscle infection and inflammation: A systematic compartmental approach. *Skel Radiol* 244:317–324, 1995.

65. Magid D: Computed tomographic imaging of the musculoskeletal system: Current status. *Radiol Clin North Am* 32:255, 1994.

66. Magid D: Two-dimensional and three-dimensional computed tomographic imaging in musculoskeletal tumors. *Radiol Clin North Am* 31:425, 1993.

67. Pettersson H, Gillespy T, Hamlin DJ, et al: Primary musculoskeletal tumors: Examination with MR imaging compared with conventional modalities. *Radiology* 164:237–241, 1987.

68. Christiansen TG, Rude C, Lauridsen KK, Christensen OM: Diagnostic value of ultrasound in scaphoid fractures. *Injury* 22:397, 1991.

69. Hodgkinson DW, Nicholson DA, Stewart G, et al: Scaphoid fracture: A new method of assessment. *Clin Radiol* 48:398, 1993.

70. Finkenberg JG, Hoffer E, Kelly C, Zinar DM: Diagnosis of occult scaphoid fractures by intrasound vibration. *J Hand Surg* 18A:4, 1993.

71. Davidson RS, Markowitz RI, Dormans J, Drummond DS: Ultrasonographic evaluation of the elbow in infants and young children after suspected trauma. *J Bone Joint Surg* 76A:1804, 1994.

72. Young JWR, Kostrubiak IS, Resnick CS, Paley D: Sonographic evaluation of bone production at the distraction site in Ilizarov limb-lengthening procedures. *AJR* 154:125, 1990.

73. Maffulli N, Thorton A: Ultrasonographic appearance of external callus in long-bone fractures. *Injury* 26:5, 1995.

74. Ricciardi L, Perissinotto A, Dabala M: Mechanical monitoring of fracture healing using ultrasound imaging. *Clin Orthop Rel Res* 293:71, 1993.

75. Christodoulou G, Korovessis P, Giarmenitis S, et al: The use of sonography for evaluation of the integrity and healing process of the tibiofibular interosseous membrane in ankle fractures. *J Orthop Trauma* 9:98, 1995.

76. Singh AK, Malpass TS, Walker G: Ultrasonic assessment of injuries to the lateral complex of the ankle. *Arch Emerg Med* 7:90, 1990.

77. Mah ET, LeQuesne GW, Gent RJ, et al: Ultrasonic features of acute osteomyelitis in children. *J Bone Joint Surg (Br)* 76:969–974, 1994.

78. Riebel TW, Nasir R, Nazarenko O: The value of sonography in the detection of osteomyelitis. *Pediatr Radiol* 26:291, 1996.

79. Taneja K, Mittal SK, Marya SK, et al: Acute osteomyelitis: Early diagnosis by ultrasonography. *Australas Radiol* 36:77–79, 1992.

80. Nath AK, Sethu AU: Use of ultrasound in osteomyelitis. *Br J Radiol* 65:649–652, 1992.

81. Mah ET, LeQuesne GW, Gent RJ, et al: Ultrasonic signs of pelvic osteomyelitis in children. *Pediatr Radiol* 24:484–487, 1994.

82. Howard CB, Einhorn M, Dagan R, et al: Ultrasound in diagnosis and management of acute haematogenous osteomyelitis in children. *J Bone Joint Surg (Br)* 75:79–82, 1993.

83. Larcos G, Antico VF, Cormick W, et al: How useful is ultrasonography in suspected acute osteomyelitis? *J Ultrasound Med* 13:707–709, 1994.

84. Gerngross H, Sohn C: Ultrasound scanning for the diagnosis of meniscal lesions of the knee joint. *Arthroscopy* 8:105–110, 1992.

85. Friedl W, Glaser F: Dynamic sonography in the diagnosis of ligament and meniscal injuries of the knee. *Arch Orthop Trauma Surg* 110:132–138, 1991.

86. Casser HR, Sohn C, Kiekenbeck A: Current evaluation of sonography of the meniscus: Results of a comparative study of sonographic and arthroscopic findings. *Arch Orthop Trauma Surg* 109:150–154, 1990.

87. Maffulli N, Regine R, Carrillo F, et al: Ultrasonographic scan in knee pain in athletes. *Br J Sports Med* 26:93–96, 1992.

88. Farin PU, Jaroma H: Acute traumatic tears of the rotator cuff: Value of sonography. *Radiology* 197:269–273, 1995.

89. Brenneke SL, Morgan CJ: Evaluation of ultrasonography as a diagnostic technique in the assessment of rotator cuff tendon tears. *Am J Sports Med* 20:287–289, 1992.

90. Olive RJ Jr, Marsh HO: Ultrasonography of rotator cuff tears. *Clin Orthop Rel Res* 282:110–113, 1992.

91. Wiener SN, Seitz WH Jr: Sonography of the shoulder in patients with tears of the rotator cuff: Accuracy and value for selecting surgical options. *AJR* 160:103–107; discussion, 109–110, 1993.

92. Paavolainen P, Ahovuo J: Ultrasonography and arthrography in the diagnosis of tears of the rotator cuff. *J Bone Joint Surg (Am)* 76:335–340, 1994.

93. van Moppes FI, Veldkamp O, Roorda J: Role of shoulder ultrasonography in the evaluation of the painful shoulder. *Europ J Radiol* 19:142–146, 1995.

94. van Holsbeeck MT, Kolowich PA, Eyler WR, et al: US depiction of partial-thickness tear of the rotator cuff. *Radiology* 197:443–446, 1995.

95. Newman JS, Adler RS, Bude RO, Rubin JM: Detection of soft-tissue hyperemia: Value of power Doppler sonography. *AJR* 163:385–389, 1994.

96. Middleton WD: Ultrasonography of rotator cuff pathology: *Topics in magnetic resonance imaging* 6:133–138, 1994.

97. Farin PU, Jaroma H: Sonographic findings of rotator cuff calcifications. *J Ultrasound Med* 14:7–14, 1995.

98. Farin PU, Jaroma H, Soimakallio S: Rotator cuff calcification: Treatment with US-guided technique. *Radiology* 195:841–843, 1995.

99. Lehtinen A, Peltokallio P, Taavitsainen M: Sonography of Achilles tendon correlated to operative findings. *Ann Chir Gynaecol* 83:322–327, 1994.

100. Kalebo P, Allenmark C, Peterson L, et al: Diagnostic value of ultrasonography in partial ruptures of the Achilles tendon. *Am J Sports Med* 20:378–381, 1992.

101. Neuhold A, Stiskal M, Kainberger F, et al: Degenerative Achilles tendon disease: Assessment by magnetic resonance and ultrasonography. *Eur J Radiol* 14:213–220, 1992.

102. Rupp S, Tempelhof S, Fritsch E: Ultrasound of Achilles tendon after surgical repair: Morphology and function. *Br J Radiology* 68:454–458, 1995.

103. Massari L, Cinotti A, Mannella P, et al: Clinical and ultrasound follow-up of 62 patients submitted to the surgical treatment of subcutaneous rupture of the Achilles tendon. *Chir Organi Mov* 79:213–218, 1994.

104. Grassi W, Tittarelli E, Blasetti P, et al: Finger tendon involvement in rheumatoid arthritis: Evaluation with high-frequency sonography. *Arthritis Rheum* 38:786–794, 1995.

105. Lehtinen A, Taavitsainen M, Leirisalo-Repo M: Sonographic analysis of enthesopathy in the lower extremities of patients with spondylarthropathy. *Clin Exp Rheumatol* 12:143–148, 1994.

106. Jadoul M, Malghem J, Van de Berg B, et al: Ultrasonographic detection of thickened joint capsules and tendons as marker of dialysis-related amyloidosis: A cross-sectional and longitudinal study. *Nephrol Dial Transplant* 8:1104–1109, 1993.

107. Sintzoff SA Jr, Gilard I, Van Gansbeke D, et al: Ultrasound evaluation of soft tissue tumors. *J Belge Radiol* 75:276–280, 1992.

108. Cardinal E, Buckwalter KA, Braunstein EM, Mih AD: Occult dorsal carpal ganglion: Comparison of US and MR imaging. *Radiology* 193:259, 1994.

109. Abiezzi SS, Miller LS: The use of ultrasound for the diagnosis of soft-tissue masses in children. *J Pediatr Orthop* 15:566–573, 1995.

110. Latifi HR, Siegel MJ: Color Doppler flow imaging of pediatric soft tissue masses. *J Ultrasound Med* 13:165–169, 1994.

111. Ozbek SS, Arkun R, Killi R, et al: Image-directed color Doppler ultrasonography in the evaluation of superficial solid tumors. *J Clin Ultrasound* 23:233–238, 1995.

112. Pino G, Conzi GF, Murolo C, et al: Sonographic evaluation of local recurrences of soft tissue sarcomas. *J Ultrasound Med* 12:23–26, 1993.

113. Choi H, Varma DGK, Fornage BD, et al: Soft-tissue sarcoma: MR imaging vs sonography for detection of local recurrence after surgery. *AJR* 157:353, 1991.

114. Fornage BD: Soft-tissue masses. *Clin Diagn Ultrasound* 30:21, 1995.

115. Buchberger W, Judmaier W, Berbamer G, et al: Carpal tunnel syndrome: Diagnosis with high-resolution sonography. *AJR* 159:793, 1992.

116. Buchberger W, Schon G, Strasser K, Jungwirth W: High-resolution ultrasonography of the carpal tunnel. *J Ultrasound Med* 10:531, 1991.

117. Nakamichi K, Tachibana S: The use of ultrasonography in detection of synovitis in carpal tunnel syndrome. *J Hand Surg* 18B:176, 1993.

118. Mackay IR, McCulloch AS: Imaging the plantaris tendon with ultrasound. *Br J Plast Surg* 43:689–691, 1990.

119. Simpson SL, Hertzog MS, Barja RH: The plantaris tendon graft: An ultrasound study. *J Hand Surg (Am)* 16:708–711, 1991.

120. Friedberg EB, Miller TT, Staron R, Feldman F: Imaging techniques for evaluation of foreign bodies. Presented at the annual meeting of the Association of University Radiologists, 1996.

121. Kaplan PA, Anderson JC, Norris MA, Matamoros A Jr: Ultrasonography of post-traumatic soft-tissue lesions. *Radiol Clin North Am* 27:973, 1989.

122. Gooding GAW: Foreign bodies. *Clin Diagn Ultrasound* 30:99, 1995.

123. Fuerst T, Gluer CC, Genant HK: Quantitative ultrasound. *Eur J Radiol* 20:188, 1995.

124. Gluer CC, Cummings SR, Bauer DC, et al: Osteoporosis: Association of recent fractures with quantitative US findings. *Radiology* 199:725, 1996.

125. Chami M, Daoud A, Maestro M, et al: Ultrasound contribution in the analysis of the newborn and infant normal and clubfoot: A preliminary study. *Pediatr Radiol* 26:298, 1996.

126. Maiza D, Themar-Noel C, Legrand I, et al: Ultrasonographic approach to the neonatal foot: Preliminary study. *J Pediatr Orthop Part B* 4:123, 1995.

127. Tolat V, Boothroyd A, Carty H, Klenerman L: Ultrasound: A helpful guide in the treatment of congenital talipes equinovarus. *J Pediatr Orthop Part B* 4:65, 1995.

128. Napiontek M: Intraoperative ultrasound for evaluation of reduction in congenital talipes equinovarus. *J Pediatr Orthop Part B* 4:55, 1995.

129. Graf R: Fundamentals of sonographic diagnosis of infant hip dysplasia. *J Pediatr Orthop* 4:735–740, 1984.

130. Harcke HT, Grissom LE: Performing dynamic sonography of the infant hip. *AJR* 155:837–844, 1990.

131. Harcke HT: Hip in infants and children. *Clin Diagn Ultrasound* 30:179, 1995.

132. Harcke HT: Screening newborns for developmental dysplasia of the hip: The role of sonography. *AJR* 162:395–397, 1994.

133. Holen KJ, Terjesen T, Tegnander A, et al: Ultrasound screening for hip dysplasia in newborns. *J Pediatr Orthop* 5:667–673, 1994.

134. Soboleski DA, Babyn P: Sonographic diagnosis of developmental dysplasia of the hip: Importance of increased thickness of acetabular cartilage. *AJR* 161:839–842, 1993.

135. Rosendahl K, Aslaksen A, Lie RT, Markestad T: Reliability of ultrasound in the early diagnosis of developmental dysplasia of the hip. *Pediatr Radiol* 25:219–224, 1995.

136. Jomha NM, McIvor J, Sterling G: Ultrasonography in developmental hip dysplasia. *J Pediatr Orthop* 15:101–104, 1995.

137. MacDonald J, Barrow S, Carty HM, Taylor JF: Imaging strategies in the first 12 months after reduction of developmental dislocation of the hip. *J Pediatr Orthop Part B* 4:95–99, 1995.

138. Wirth T, LeQuesne GW, Paterson DC: Ultrasonography in Legg-Calvé-Perthes disease. *Pediatr Radiol* 22:498–504, 1992.

139. Kallio P, LeQuesne GW, Paterson DC, et al: Ultrasonography in slipped capital femoral epiphysis. *J Bone Joint Surg (Br)* 73B:884–889, 1991.

140. Heiken JP, Glazer HS, Lee JKT, et al: *Manual of Clinical Magnetic Resonance Imaging.* New York, Raven Press, 1986.

141. Berquist TH: *MRI of the Musculoskeletal System,* 2d ed. New York, Raven Press, 1990, pp 1–25.

142. Stoller DW: *Magnetic Resonance Imaging in Orthopaedics and Sports Medicine.* Philadelphia, Lippincott, 1993, pp 1–22.

143. Resnick D, Niwayama G: *Diagnosis of Bone and Joint Disorders,* 2d ed. Philadelphia, Saunders, 1988, pp 203–212.

144. Curry TS, DowHdey JE, Murry RC: *Christensen's Physics of Diagnostic Radiology*, 4th ed. Philadelphia, Lea & Febiger, 1990, pp 432–469.

145. NMR A perspective on imaging. General Electric Manual, 1983.

146. Scott JA, Rosenthal DI, Brdy TJ: The evaluation of musculoskeletal disease with magnetic resonance imaging. *Radiol Clin North Am* 22:917, 1984.

147. Bradley WG, Newton TH, Crooks LE: Physical principles of nuclear magnetic resonance, in TH Newton, DG Potts (eds): *Modern Neuroradiology: Advanced imaging techniques.* San Anselmo, California, Clavadel Press, 1983.

148. Chadnani VP, Ho C, Chu P, et al: Knee hyaline cartilage evaluated with MR imaging: A cadaveric study involving multiple imaging sequences and intraarticular injection of gadolinium and saline solution. *Radiology* 178:557–561, 1991.

149. Recht MP, Kramer J, Marcelis S, et al: Abnormalities of articular cartilage in the knee: Analysis of available MR techniques. *Radiology* 187:473–478, 1993.

150. Reiser MF, Bongartz G, Erlemann R, et al: Magnetic resonance in cartilaginous lesions of the knee joint with three-dimensional gradient-echo imaging. *Skel Radiol* 17:465–471, 1988.

151. Konig H, Sauter R, Deimling M, et al: Cartilage disorders: Comparison of spin echo. CHESS. and flash sequence MR images. *Radiology* 164:753–758, 1987.

152. Hodler J, Berthiaume MJ: Knee joint hyaline cartilage defects: A comparative study of MR and anatomic sections. *J Comput Assist Tomogr* 16:597–603, 1992.

153. Glys-Morin VM, Hajek PC, Sartoris DJ, et al: Articular cartilage defects: Detectability in cadaver knees with MR. *AJR* 148:1153–1157, 1987.

154. Winalski CS, Aliabadi P, Wright RJ, et al: Enhancement of joint fluid with intravenously administered gadopentate dimeglumine: Technique, rationale, and implications. *Radiology* 187:179–185, 1993.

155. Mink JH, Deutsch AL: Occult cartilage and bone injuries of the knee: Detection, classification and assessment with MR imaging. *Radiology* 170:823–829, 1989.

156. Vellet AD, Marks PH, Fowler PJ, et al: Occult posttraumatic osteochondral lesions of the knee: Prevalence, classification,

and short-term sequelae evaluated with MR imaging. *Radiology* 178:271–276, 1991.

157. DeSmet AA, Fisher DR, Graf BK, Lange RH: Osteochondritis dessicans of the knee: Value of MR imaging in determining lesion stability and the presence of articular cartilage defects. *AJR* 155:549–553, 1990.

158. Shahriaree H: Chondromalacia. *Contemp Orthop* 11:27–39, 1985.

159. Hayes CW, Conway WF: Evaluation of articular cartilage: Radiographic and cross-sectional imaging techniques. *Radiographics* 12:409–428, 1992.

160. Hayes CW, Sawyer RS, Conway WF: Patellar cartilage lesions: In vitro detection and staging with MR imaging and pathologic correlation. *Radiology* 176:479–483, 1990.

161. Yulish BS, Montanez J, Goodfellow DB, et al: Chondromalacia patellae: Assessment with MR imaging. *Radiology* 164: 763–766, 1987.

162. Quinn SF, Rose PM, Brown TR, Demlow TA: MR imaging of the patellofemoral compartment. *MRI Clin North Am* 2:425–440, 1994.

163. Murphy WA, Totty WG, Carroll JE: MRI of normal and pathological skeletal muscle. *AJR* 146:565–574, 1986.

164. Hernandez RJ, Keim DR, Chenevert TL, et al: Fat-suppressed MR imaging of myositis. *Radiology* 182:217–219, 1992.

165. Bohan A, Peter JB: Polymyositis and dermatomyositis (first of two parts). *N Engl J Med* 292:344–347, 1975.

166. Schweitzer ME, Fort J: Cost effectiveness of MR imaging in evaluating polymyositis. *AJR* 165:1469–1471, 1995.

167. Resnick D, Niwayama G: *Diagnosis of Bone and Joint Disorders*. Philadelphia, Saunders, 1988, p 2595.

168. Reicher MA, Basset LW, Gold RH: High resolution magnetic resonance imaging of the knee joint: Pathologic correlations. *AJR* 145:903–909, 1985.

169. Reicher MA, Rauschning W, Gold RH, et al: High resolution magnetic resonance imaging of the knee joint: Normal anatomy. *AJR* 145:895–902, 1985.

170. Langer JE, Meyer SJ, Dalinka MK: Imaging of the knee. *Radiol Clin North Am* 28:975–990, 1990.

171. Resnick D, Niwayama G: *Diagnosis of Bone and Joint Disorders*, 2d ed. Vol 1. Philadelphia, Saunders, 1988, p 239.

172. Stoller DW: *Magnetic Resonance Imaging in Orthopaedics and Sports Medicine: The Knee*. Philadelphia, Lippincott, 1993, pp 139–369.

173. Mink JH, Levy T, Crues JV: Tears of the anterior cruciate ligament and menisci of the knee: MR imaging evaluation. *Radiology* 167:769–774, 1988.

174. Stoller DW: *Magnetic Resonance Imaging in Orthopaedics and Sports Medicine*. Philadelphia, Lippincott, 1993, p 178.

175. Polly DW Jr, Callaghan JJ, Sikes RA, et al: The accuracy of selective magnetic resonance imaging compared with the findings of arthroscopy of the knee. *J Bone Joint Surg (Am)* 70:192, 1988.

176. Kornick J, Trefelner E, McCarthy S, et al: Meniscal abnormalities in the asymptomatic population at MR imaging. *Radiology* 177:463–465, 1990.

177. Crues JV III, Mink J, Levy TL, et al: Meniscal tears of the knee: Accuracy of MR imaging. *Radiology* 164:445, 1987.

178. Glashow JL, Katz R, Schneider M, Scott W: Double-blind assessment of the value of magnetic resonance imaging in the diagnosis of anterior cruciate and meniscal lesions. *J Bone Joint Surg (Am)* 71:113, 1989.

179. Crues JV, Ryu R, Morgan FW: Meniscal pathology: the expanding role of magnetic resonance imaging. *Clin Orthop Rel Res* 252:80–87, 1990.

180. Fischer SP, Fox JM, DelPizzo W, et al: Accuracy of diagnosis from magnetic resonance imaging of the knee. *J Bone Joint Surg (Am)* 73:2, 1991.

181. Justice WW, Quinn SF: Error patterns in the MR imaging evaluation of menisci of the knee. *Radiology* 196:617–621, 1995.

182. Firooznia H, Golimbu C, Rafii M: MR imaging of the menisci. *MRI Clin North Am* 2:325–347, 1994.

183. DeSmet AA, Norris MA, Yandow DR, et al: Diagnosis of meniscal tears of the knee with MR imaging. *AJR* 160:555–559, 1993.

184. Reicher MA: MR imaging of the knee: Part 1, traumatic disorder. *Radiology* 162:547–551, 1987.

185. Mink JH, Reicher MA, Crues JV: *Magnetic Resonance Imaging of the Knee*. New York, Raven Press, 1987.

186. Stoller DW: *Magnetic Resonance Imaging in Orthopaedics and Sports Medicine*. Philadelphia, Lippincott, 1993, p 177.

187. Bonamo JT, Saperstein AL: Contemporary magnetic resonance imaging of the knee: The orthopedic surgeon's perspective. *MRI Clin North Am* 2:481–495, 1994.

188. Ruwe PA, Wright J, Randall RL, et al: Can MR imaging effectively replace diagnostic arthroscopy? *Radiology* 183:335–339, 1992.

189. Applegate GR, Flannigan BD, Tolin BS, et al: MR diagnosis of recurrent tears in the knee: Value of intraarticular contrast material. *AJR* 161:821–825, 1993.

190. Torg JS, Conrad W, Kalen V: Clinical diagnosis of anterior cruciate ligament instability in the athlete. *Am J Sports Med* 4:84–93, 1976.

191. Indelicato PA, Bittar ES, et al: A perspective of lesions associated with ACL insufficiency of the knee: A review of 100 cases. *Clin Orthop* 198:77, 1985.

192. Lee JK, Yao L, Phelps CT, et al: Anterior cruciate ligament tears: MR imaging compared with arthroscopy and clinical test. *Radiology* 166:861–864, 1988.

193. Pavlov H, Warren RF, Sherman MF, Cayea PD: The accuracy of double-contrast arthrographic evaluation of the anterior cruciate ligament. *J Bone Joint Surg (Am)* 65:175–183, 1983.

194. Murphy BJ, Smith RL, Uribe JW, et al: Bone signal abnormalities in the posterolateral tibia and lateral femoral condyle in complete tears of the anterior cruciate ligament: A specific sign? *Radiology* 182:221–224, 1992.

195. Snearly WN, Kaplan PA, Dussault RG: Lateral compartment bone contusions in adolescents with intact anterior cruciate ligaments. *Radiology* 198:205–208, 1996.

196. Vahey TN, Broome DR, Kayes KJ, et al: Acute and chronic tears of the anterior cruciate ligament: Differential features at MR imaging. *Radiology* 181:251, 1991.

197. Clancy WG, Shelbourne KD, Zoellner GB, et al: Treatment of knee joint instability secondary to rupture of the posterior cruciate ligament: Report of a new procedure. *J Bone Joint Surg (Am)* 65:310, 1983.

198. Sonin AH, Fitzgerald SW, Hoff FL, et al: MR imaging of the posterior cruciate ligament: Normal, abnormal, and associated injury patterns. *Radiographics* 15:551–561, 1995.

199. Grover JS, Bassett LW, Gross ML, et al: Posterior cruciate ligament: MR imaging. *Radiology* 174:527–530, 1990.

200. Stoller DW: *Magnetic Resonance Imaging in Orthopaedics and Sports Medicine*. Philadelphia, Lippincott, 1993, p 339.

201. Lynch TCP, Crues JV II, Morgan FW, et al: Bone abnormalities of the knee: Prevalence and significance at MR imaging. *Radiology* 171:761–766, 1989.

202. Yao L, Lee JK: Occult intraosseous fracture: Detection with MR imaging. *Radiology* 167:749–751, 1988.

203. Vellet D: Magnetic resonance imaging of bone marrow and osteochondral injury. *MRI Clin North Am* 2:413–423, 1994.

204. Bigliani LU, Morrison DS: Subacromial impingement syndrome, in Dee R (ed): *Principles of Orthopaedic Practice*. New York, McGraw-Hill, 1989, p 627.

205. Seeger LL, Gold RH, Bassett LW, et al: Shoulder impingement syndrome: MR findings in 53 shoulders. *AJR* 150:343–347, 1988.

206. Bigliani LU, Morrison DS, April EW, et al: The morphology of the acromion and its relationship to rotator cuff tears. *Orthop Trans* 10:228, 1986.

207. Ozaki J, Fujimoto S, Nakagawa Y, et al: Tears of the rotator cuff of the shoulder associated with pathologic changes in the acromion. *J Bone Surg (Am)* 70:1224, 1988.

208. Mirowitz SA: Normal rotator cuff: MR imaging with conventional and fat-suppression techniques. *Radiology* 180:735–740, 1991.

209. Seeger LL, Ruszkowski JT, Bassett LW, et al: MR imaging of the normal shoulder: Anatomic correlation. *AJR* 148:83–91, 1987.

210. Middeton WD, Kneeland JB, Carrera GF, et al: High-resolution MR imaging of the normal rotator cuff. *AJR* 148:559–564, 1987.

211. Evancho AM, Stiles RG, Fajman WA, et al: MR imaging diagnosis of rotator cuff tears. *AJR* 151:751–754, 1988.

212. Kneeland JB, Middleton WD, Carrera GF, et al: MR imaging of the shoulder: Diagnosis of rotator cuff tears. *AJR* 149:333–337, 1987.

213. Zlatkin MB, Iannotti JP, Roberts MC, et al: Rotator cuff tears: Diagnostic performance of MR imaging. *Radiology* 172:223–229, 1989.

214. Kieft GJ, Bloem JL, Rozing PM, et al: Rotator cuff impingement syndrome: MR imaging. *Radiology* 166:211–214, 1988.

215. Rafii M, Firooznia H, Sherman O, et al: Rotator cuff lesions: Signal patterns of MR imaging. *Radiology* 177:817–823, 1990.

216. Burk DL, Karasick D, Kurtz AB, et al: Prospective comparison of MR imaging with arthrography, sonography, and surgery. *AJR* 153:87–92, 1989.

217. Stoller DW: *Magnetic Resonance Imaging in Orthopaedics and Sports Medicine.* Philadelphia, Lippincott, 1993, p 576.

218. Stoller DW: *Magnetic Resonance Imaging in Orthopaedics and Sports Medicine.* Philadelphia, Lippincott, 1993, p 568.

219. Reinus WR, Shady KL, Mirowitz SA, Totty WG: MR diagnosis of rotator cuff tears of the shoulder: Value of using T2-weighted fat-saturated images. *AJR* 164:1451–1455, 1995.

220. Seeger LL, Gold RH, Bassett LW, et al: Shoulder instability: Evaluation with MR imaging. *Radiology* 168:695–697, 1988.

221. Feller JF, Tirman PF, Steinbach LS, Zucconi F: Magnetic resonance imaging of the shoulder: Review. *Semin Roentgenol* 30:224–240, 1995.

222. Mohtadi NGH: Advances in the understanding of anterior instability of the shoulder. *Clin Sports Med* 10:863–885, 1991.

223. Workman TL, Burkhard TK, Resnick D, et al: Hill-Sachs lesion: Comparison of detection with MR imaging, radiography, and arthroscopy. *Radiology* 185:847–852, 1992.

224. Schweitzer ME: MR arthrography of the labral-ligamentous complex of the shoulder. *Radiology* 190:641–643, 1994.

225. Thomas SC, Matsen FA: An approach to the repair of avulsion of the glenohumeral ligaments in the management of traumatic anterior glenohumeral instability. *J Bone Joint Surg (Am)* 71:506–513, 1989.

226. Zlatkin MB, Bjorkengren AG, Glys-Morin V, et al: Cross sectional imaging of the capsular mechanism of the glenohumeral joint. *AJR* 150:151–158, 1988.

227. Rafii M, Firooznia H, Golimbu C, et al: CT arthrography of capsular structures of the shoulder. *AJR* 146:361–367, 1986.

228. Moseley HF, Overgaard B: The anterior capsular mechanism in recurrent anterior dislocation of the shoulder. *J Bone Joint Surg (Br)* 44:913–927, 1962.

229. Chandnani VP, Gagliardi JA, Murnane TG, et al: Glenohumeral ligaments and shoulder capsular mechanism: Evaluation with MR arthrography. *Radiology* 196:27–32, 1995.

230. Matsen FA, Harryman DT, Sidles JA: Mechanics of glenohumeral instability. *Clin Sports Med* 10:783–788, 1991.

231. Turkel SJ, Panio MW: Stabilizing mechanisms preventing anterior dislocation of the glenohumeral joint. *J Bone Joint Surg (Am)* 63:1208–1217, 1981.

232. O'Brien SJ, Neves SC, Arnoczsky SP, et al: The anatomy and histology of the glenohumeral ligament complex of the shoulder. *Am J Sports Med* 18:449–456, 1990.

233. Palmer WE, Brown JH, Rosenthal DI: Labral-ligamentous complex of the shoulder: Evaluation with MR arthrography. *Radiology* 190:645–651, 1994.

234. Stoller DW: *Magnetic Resonance Imaging in Orthopaedics and Sports Medicine.* Philadelphia, Lippincott, 1993, p 512.

235. Coumas JM, Waite RJ, Goss TP, et al: CT and MR evaluation of the labral capsular ligamentous complex of the shoulder. *AJR* 158:591–597, 1992.

236. Garneau RA, Renfrew DL, Moore TC, et al: Glenoid labrum: Evaluation with MR imaging. *Radiology* 179:519–522, 1991.

237. Legan JM, Burkhard TK, Goff WB II, et al: Tears of the glenoid labrum: MR imaging of 88 arthroscopically confirmed cases. *Radiology* 179:241–246, 1991.

238. Gross ML, et al: Magnetic resonance imaging of the labrum. *Am J Sports Med* 18:229, 1990.

239. Loredo R, Longo C, Salonen D, et al: Glenoid labrum: MR imaging with histologic correlation. *Radiology* 196:33–41, 1995.

240. Liou JTS, Wilson AJ, Totty WG, Brown JJ: The normal shoulder: Common variations that simulate pathologic conditions at MR imaging. *Radiology* 186:435–441, 1993.

241. Neumann CH, Peterson SA, Jahnke AH: MR imaging of the lobral-capsular complex: Normal variations. *AJR* 157:1015–1021, 1991.

242. Kaplan PA, Bryans KC, Davick JP, et al: MR imaging of the normal shoulder: Variants and pitfalls. *Radiology* 184:519–524, 1992.

243. Flannigan B, Kursunog LU-Grahme S, Snyder S, et al: MR arthrography of the shoulder. *AJR* 155:829–832, 1990.

244. Chadnani VP, Yaeger TD, DeBerardino T, et al: Glenoid labral tears: Prospective evaluation with MR imaging, MR arthrography and CT arthrography. *AJR* 161:1229–1235, 1993.

245. Krudy AG: MR myelography using heavily T2-weighted fast spin-echo pulse sequences with fat saturation. *AJR* 159:1315–1320, 1992.

246. El Gammal TA, Brooks BS, Freedy RM, Crews CE: MR myelography: Imaging findings. *AJR* 164:173–177, 1995.

247. El Gammal TA, Crews CE: MR myelography of the cervical spine. *Radiographics* 16:77–88, 1996.

248. Modic MT, Masaryk TJ, Ross JS, Carter JR: Imaging of degenerative disk disease. *Radiology* 168:177–186, 1988.

249. Adams P, Eyre DR, Muir H: Biochemical aspects of development and aging of human lumbar intervertebral discs. *Rheumatol Rehabil* 16:22–29, 1977.

250. Coventry MB, Ghormley RK, Kernohan JW: The intervertebral disc: Its microscopic anatomy and pathology. Part I. anatomy, development and physiology. *J Bone Joint Surg* 27:105–112, 1945.

251. Coventry MB, Ghormley RK, Kernohan JW: The intervertebral disk: Its microscopic anatomy and pathology. Part II. changes in the intervertebral disc concomitant with age. *J Bone Joint Surg* 27:233–247, 1945.

252. Coventry MB, Ghormley RK, Kernohan JW: The intervertebral disc: Its microscopic anatomy and pathology. Part III. pathologic changes in the intervertebral disc. *J Bone Joint Surg* 27:460–474, 1945.

253. Stoller DW: *Magnetic Resonance Imaging in Orthopaedics and Sports Medicine.* Philadelphia, Lippincott, 1993, p 892.

254. Haughton VM: MR imaging of the spine. *Radiology* 166:297–301, 1988.

255. Modic MT, Pavlicek W, Weinstein MA, et al: Magnetic resonance imaging of intervertebral disc disease: Clinical and pulse sequence considerations. *Radiology* 152:103–111, 1984.

256. Berger PE, Atkinson D, Wilson WJ, et al: High resolution surface coil magnetic resonance imaging of the spine: Normal and pathologic anatomy. *Radiographics* 6:573, 1986.

257. Modic MT, Masaryk T, Boumphrey F, et al: Lumbar herniated disc disease and canal stenosis: Prospective evaluation by surface coil MR, CT, and myelography. *AJNR* 7:709–717, 1986.

258. Ross JS, Perez-Reyes N, Masaryk TJ, et al: Thoracic disc herniation: MR imaging. *Radiology* 165:511–515, 1987.

259. Edelman RR, Shoukimas GM, Stark DD, et al: High-resolution surface-coil imaging of lumbar disk disease. AJNR 6:479–485, 1985.

260. Stoller DW: *Magnetic Resonance Imaging in Orthopaedics and Sports Medicine.* Philadelphia, Lippincott, 1993, p 893.

261. Thornbury JR, Fryback DG, Turski PA, et al: Disk caused nerve compression in patients with acute low-back pain: Diagnosis with MR, CT myelography, and plain CT. *Radiology* 186:731–738, 1993.

262. Modic MT, Ross JS, Obuchowski NA, et al: Contrast enhanced MR imaging in acute lumbar radiculopathy: A pilot study of the natural history. *Radiology* 195:429–435, 1995.

263. Russell EJ: Cervical disc disease. *Radiology* 177:313–325, 1990.

264. Modic MT, Masaryk TJ, Mulopulos GP, et al: Cervical radiculopathy: Prospective evaluation with surface coil MR imaging, CT with metrizamide, and metrizamide myelography. *Radiography* 161:753–759, 1986.

265. Enzmann DR, Rubin JB, Wright A: Use of cerebiospinal fluid gating to improve T2 weighted images: I. Spinal cord. *Radiology* 162:763–767, 1987.

266. Rubin JB, Enzmann DR, Wright A: CSF-gated MR imaging of the spine: Theory and clinical implementation. *Radiology* 163:784–792, 1987.

267. Hedberg MC, Drayer BP, Flom RA, et al: Gradient echo (GRASS) MR imaging in cervical radiculopathy. *AJNR* 9:145–151, 1988.

268. Enzmann DR, Rubin JB: Cervical spine: MR imaging with a partial flip angle, gradient-refocused pulse sequence. *Radiology* 166:467–472, 1988.

269. Kulkarni MV, Narayna PA, McArelle CB, et al: Cervical spine MR imaging using multislice gradient echo imaging: Comparison with cardiac gated spin echo. *Magn Reson Imaging* 6:517–525, 1988.

270. Czervionke LF, Daniels DL, Ho PSP, et al: Cervical neural foramina: Correlative anatomic and MR imaging study. *Radiology* 169:753–759, 1988.

271. Tsuruda JS, Norman D, Dillon W, et al: Three-dimensional gradient recalled MR imaging as a screening tool for the diagnosis of cervical radiculopathy. *AJNR* 10:1263–1271, 1990.

272. Brain WR: Some unresolved problems of cervical spondylosis. *Br Med J* 1:771–777, 1963.

273. Burton CV, Kirkaldy-Willis WH, Yong-Hing K, et al: Causes of failure of surgery on the lumbar spine. *Clin Orthop* 157:191–199, 1981.

274. Ross JS, Masaryk TJ, Modic MT, et al: MR imaging of the lumbar arachnoiditis. *AJR* 149:1025–1032, 1987.

275. Boden SD, Davis DO, Dina TS, et al: Contrast-enhanced MR imaging performed after successful lumbar disc surgery: Prospective study. *Radiology* 182:59–64, 1992.

276. Dina TS, Boden SD, Davis DO: Lumbar spine after surgery for herniated disk: Imaging findings in the early postoperative period. *AJR* 164:665–671, 1995.

277. Finnegan WJ, Fenlin JM, Marvel JP, et al: Results of surgical intervention in the symptomatic multiply-operated back patient. *J Bone Joint Surg (Am)* 61:1077–1081, 1979.

278. Teplick JG, Haskin ME: Computed tomography of the postoperative lumbar spine. *AJR* 141:865–884, 1983.

279. Sotiropoulos S, Chafetz NI, Lang P, et al: Differentiation between postoperative scar and recurrent disc herniation: Prospective comparison of MR, CT, and contrast-enhanced CT. *AJNR* 10:639–643, 1989.

280. Ross JS, Delamarter R, Hueftle MG: Gadolinium-DTPA–enhanced MR imaging of the postoperative lumbar spine: Time course and mechanism of enhancement. *AJNR* 10:37–46, 1989.

281. Glickstein MF, Sussman SK: Time dependent scar enhancement in magnetic resonance imaging of the postoperative lumbar spine. *Skel Radiol* 20:333–337, 1991.

282. Hueftle MG, Modic MT, Ross JS, et al: Lumbar spine: Postoperative MR imaging with Gd-DTPA. *Radiology* 167:817–824, 1988.

283. Ross JS, Masaryk TJ, Schrader M, et al: MR imaging of the postoperative lumbar spine: Assessment with gadopentetate dimeglumine. *AJNR* 11:771–776, 1990.

284. Modic MT, Feiglin DH, Piraino DW, et al: Vertebral osteomyelitis: Assessment using MR. *Radiology* 157:157–166, 1985.

285. Friedman DP, Hills JR: Cervical epidural spinal infection: MR imaging characteristics. *AJR* 163:699–704, 1994.

286. Thrush A, Enzmann D: MR imaging of infectious spondylitis. *AJNR* 11:1171–1180, 1990.

287. Smith AS, Weinstein MA, Mizushima A, et al: MR imaging characteristics of tuberculous spondylitis vs vertebral osteomyelitis. *AJR* 153:399–405, 1989.

288. Sandhu FS, Dillon WP: Spinal epidural abscess: Evaluation with contrast-enhanced MR imaging. *AJNR* 12:1087–1093, 1991.

289. Numaguchi Y, Rigamonti D, Rothman MI, et al: Spinal epidural abscess: Evaluation with gadolinium-enhanced MR imaging. *Radiographics* 13:545–559, 1993.

290. Gillams AR, Chaddha B, Carter AP: MR appearances of the temporal evolution and resolution of infectious spondylitis. *AJR* 166:903–907, 1996.

291. Mirvis SE, Geisler FH, Jelinek JJ, et al: Acute cervical spine trauma: Evaluation with 1.5T MR imaging. *Radiology* 166:807–816, 1988.

292. El-Khoury GY, Kathol MH, Daniel WW: Imaging of fracture injuries of the cervical spine: Value of plain radiography, CT, and MR imaging. *AJR* 164:43–50, 1995.

293. Silberstein M, Tress BM, Hennessy O: Prediction of neurologic outcome in acute spinal cord injury: The role of CT and MR. *AJNR* 13:1597–1608, 1992.

294. Kulkarni MV, McArdle CB, Kopanicky D, et al: Acute spinal cord injury: MR imaging at 1.5T. *Radiology* 164:837–843, 1987.

295. Flanders AE, Schaefer DM, Doan HT, et al: Acute cervical spine trauma: Correlation of MR imaging findings with degree of neurologic deficit. *Radiology* 177:25–33, 1990.

296. Kulkarni MV, Bondurant FJ, Rose SL, Narayana PA: 1.5 tesla magnetic resonance imaging of acute spine trauma. *Radiographics* 8:1059–1082, 1988.

297. Stoller DW: *Magnetic Resonance Imaging in Orthopaedics and Sports Medicine.* Philadelphia, Lippincott, 1993, p 968.

298. Cuenod CA, Laredo JD, Chevret S, et al: Acute vertebral collapse due to osteoporosis or malignancy: Appearance on unenhanced and gadolinium-enhanced MR images. *Radiology* 199:541–549, 1996.

299. Yuh WT, Zachar CK, Barloon TJ, et al: Vertebral compression fractures: Distinction between benign and malignant causes with MR imaging. *Radiology* 172:215–218, 1989.

300. Baker LL, Goodman SB, Perkash I, et al: Benign versus pathologic compression fractures of vertebral bodies: Assessment with conventional spin-echo, chemical-shift, and STIR MR imaging. *Radiology* 174:495–502, 1990.

301. Frager D, Elkin C, Swerdlow M, Bloch S: Subacute osteoporotic compression fracture: Misleading magnetic resonance appearance. *Skel Radiol* 17:123–126, 1988.

302. Resnick D, Niwayama G: Osteonecrosis: Diagnostic techniques, specific situations, and complications, in Resnick D, Niwayama G (eds): *Diagnosis of Bone and Joint Disorders.* Philadelphia, Saunders, 1988, pp 3238–3287.

303. Ficat RP: Idiopathic bone necrosis of the femoral head. *J Bone Joint Surg* 67(B):3–9, 1985.

304. Coleman BG, Kressel HY, Dalinka MK, et al: Radiographically negative avascular necrosis: Detection with MR imaging. *Radiology* 168:525–528, 1988.

305. Camp JF, Colwell CW: Core decompression of the femoral head for osteonecrosis. *J Bone Joint Surg* 68(A):1313–1319, 1986.

306. Tooke SMT, Nugent PJ, Bassett LW, et al: Results of core decompression for femoral head osteonecrosis. *Clin Orthop* 288:99–104, 1988.

307. Seiler JG, Cristie MJ, Homra L: Correlation of the findings of magnetic resonance imaging with those of bone biopsy in patients who have stage-I or II ischemic necrosis of the femoral head. *J Bone Joint Surg* 71(A):28, 1989.

308. Thickman D, Axel L, Kressel HY, et al: Magnetic resonance imaging of avascular necrosis of the femoral head. *Skel Radiol* 15:133–140, 1986.

309. Kokubo T, Takatori Y, Ninomiya S, et al: Magnetic resonance imaging and scintigraphy of avascular necrosis of the femoral head: Prediction of subsequent segmental collapse. *Clin Orthop* 277:54, 1992.

310. Glickstein MF, Burk DL, Schiebler ML, et al: Avascular necrosis versus other diseases of the hip: Sensitivity of MR imaging. *Radiology* 169:213, 1988.

311. Robinson HJ, Hartleben PD, Lund G, Schreiman J: Evaluation of magnetic resonance imaging in the diagnosis of osteonecrosis of the femoral head. *J Bone Joint Surg* 71(A):650, 1989.

312. Hauzeur JP, Pateels JI, Schoutens A, et al: The diagnostic value of magnetic resonance imaging in nontraumatic osteonecrosis of the femoral head. *J Bone Joint Surg* 71(A):641, 1989.

313. Conklin JJ, Alderson PO, Zizic TM, et al: Comparison of bone scan and radiograph sensitivity in the detection of steroid-induced ischemic necrosis of bone. *Radiology* 147:221–226, 1983.

314. Beltran J, Herman LJ, Burk JM, et al: Femoral head avascular necrosis: MR imaging with clinical-pathologic and radionuclide correlation. *Radiology* 166:215–220, 1988.

315. Lee MJ, Corrigan J, Stack JP, Ennis JT: A comparison of modern imaging modalities in osteonecrosis of the femoral head. *Clin Radiol* 42:427, 1990.

316. Michell DG, Rao VM, Dalinka MK, et al: Femoral head avascular necrosis: Correlation of MR imaging, radiographic staging, radionuclide imaging, and clinical findings. *Radiology* 162:709–715, 1987.

317. Mitchell M, Kundel H, Steinberg M, Kressel H, et al: Avascular necrosis of the hip: Comparison of MR, CT, and scintigraphy. *AJR* 147:67–71, 1985.

318. Mitchell DG, Kressel HY, Arger PG, et al: Avascular necrosis of the femoral head: Morphologic assessment by MR imaging, with CT correlation. *Radiology* 161:739–742, 1986.

319. Laffargue P, Dahan E, Chagnaud C, et al: Early stage avascular necrosis of the femoral head: MR imaging for prognosis in 31 cases with at least 2 years follow-up. *Radiology* 187:199, 1993.

320. Capitanio MA, Kirkpatric JA: Early roentgen observations in acute osteomyelitis. *Radiology* 108:488–496, 1970.

321. Tang JS, Gold RH, Bassett LW, et al: Musculoskeletal infection of the extremities: Evaluation with MR imaging. *Radiology* 166:205–209, 1988.

322. Unger E, Moldofsky P, Gatenby R, et al: Diagnosis of osteomyelitis by MR imaging. *AJR* 150:605–610, 1988.

323. Beltran J, McGhee RB, Shaffer PB, et al: Experimental infections of the musculoskeletal system: Evaluation with MR imaging and Tc-99m MDP and Ga-67 scintigraphy. *Radiology* 167:167–172, 1988.

324. Beltran J, Noto AM, McGhee RB, et al: Infections of the musculoskeletal system: High-field-strength MR imaging. *Radiology* 164:449–454, 1987.

325. Chandnani VP, Beltran J, Morris CS: Acute experimental osteomyelitis and abscesses: Detection with MR imaging versus CT. *Radiology* 174:233–236, 1990.

326. Angtuaco EJ, McConnell JR, Chadduck WM, et al: MR imaging of spinal epidural sepsis. *AJNR* 8:879–883, 1987.

327. Miller TT, Randolph DA Jr, Staron RB, et al: Evaluation of musculoskeletal infection using gadolinium-enhanced fat-suppressed T1 weighted sequences vs fat-suppressed fast T2 weighted techniques. *AJR* 166(suppl):51, 1996.

328. Hopkins KL, King MD, Li CP, et al: Gadolinium-DTPA-enhanced magnetic resonance imaging of musculoskeletal infectious processes. *Skel Radiol* 24:325–330, 1995.

329. Dangman BC, Hoffer FA, Rand FF, et al: Osteomyelitis in children: Gadolinium-enhanced MR imaging. *Radiology* 182:743–747, 1992.

330. Morrison WB, Schweitzer ME, Bock GW, et al: Diagnosis of osteomyelitis: Utility of fat-suppressed contrast-enhanced MR imaging. *Radiology* 189:251–257, 1993.

331. Mason MD, Zlatkin MB, Esterhai JL: Chronic complicated osteomyelitis of the lower extremity: Evaluation with MR imaging. *Radiology* 173:355–359, 1989.

332. Quinn SF, Murray W, Clark RA, et al: MR imaging of chronic osteomyelitis. *J Comput Assist Tomogr* 12:113–117, 1988.

333. Jaramillo D, Treves ST, Kasser JR, et al: Osteomyelitis and septic arthritis in children: Appropriate use of imaging to guide treatment. *AJR* 165:399–403, 1995.

334. Mazur JM, Ross G, Cummings RJ, et al: Usefulness of magnetic resonance imaging for the diagnosis of acute musculoskeletal infections in children. *J Pediatr Orthop* 15:144–147, 1995.

335. Bressler EL, Conway JJ, Weiss SC, et al: Neonatal osteomyelitis examined by bone scintigraphy. *Radiology* 152:685–688, 1984.

336. Howman-Giles R, Uren R: Multifocal osteomyelitis in childhood: Review by radionuclide bone scan. *Clin Nucl Med* 17:274–278, 1992.

337. Zawin JK, Hoffer FA, Rand FF, et al: Joint effusion in children with an irritable hip: US diagnosis and aspiration. *Radiology* 187:459–463, 1993.

338. Robertson DD, Magid D, Poss R, et al: Enhanced computed tomographic techniques for the evaluation of total hip arthroplasty. *J Arthrop* 4:271–276, 1989.

339. Fishman EK, Magid D, Robertson DD, et al: Metallic hip implants: CT with multiplanar reconstruction. *Radiology* 160:675–681, 1986.

340. Williamson BRJ, McLaughlin RE, Wang GJ, et al: Radionuclide bone imaging as a means of differentiating loosening and infection in patients with a painful total hip prosthesis. *Radiology* 133:723, 1979.

341. Palestro CJ: Radionuclide imaging after skeletal interventional procedures. *Semin Nucl Med* 25:3–14, 1995.

342. Palestro CJ, Swyer AJ, Kim CK, et al: Infected knee prosthesis: Diagnosis with In-111 leukocyte, Tc-99m sulfur colloid, and Tc-99m MDP imaging. *Radiology* 179:645–646, 1991.

343. Palestro CJ, Kim CK, Swyer AJ, et al: Total-hip arthroplasty: Periprosthetic indium-111–labeled leukocyte activity and complementary technetium-99m-sulfur colloid imaging in suspected infection. *J Nucl Med* 31:1950–1955, 1990.

344. van Holsbeeck MT, Eyler, WR, Sherman LS, et al: Detection of infection in loosened hip prostheses: Efficacy of sonography. *AJR* 163:381–384, 1994.

345. Yuh WT, Corson JD, Baraniewski HM, et al: Osteomyelitis of the foot in diabetic patients: Evaluation with plain film, 99mTc-MDP bone scintigraphy, and MR imaging. *AJR* 152:795–800, 1989.

346. Schauwecker DS, Park HM, Burt RW, et al: Combined bone scintigraphy and indium-111 leukocyte scans in neuropathic foot disease. *J Nucl Med* 29:1651–1655, 1988.

347. Beltran J, Campanini DS, Knight C, et al: The diabetic foot: Magnetic resonance imaging evaluation. *Skel Radiol* 19:37–41, 1990.

348. Horowitz JD, Durham JR, Nease DB, et al: Prospective evaluation of magnetic resonance imaging in the management of acute diabetic foot infections. *Ann Vasc Surg* 7:44–50, 1993.

349. Morrison WB, Schweitzer ME, Wapner KL, et al: Osteomyelitis in feet of diabetics: Clinical accuracy, surgical utility, and cost-effectiveness of MR imaging. *Radiology* 196:557–564, 1995.

350. Colon E, Judkewicz A, Jelinek J, et al: Osteomyelitis in the diabetic foot: MRI vs indium scan, prospective double blind study with pathologic correlation. *AJR* 166(suppl):49, 1996.

351. Aisen AM, Martel W, Braunstein EM, et al: MRI and CT evaluation of primary bone and soft-tissue tumors. *AJR* 146:749–756, 1986.

352. Zimmer WD, Berquist TH, McLeod RA, et al: Bone tumors: Magnetic resonance imaging versus computed tomography. *Radiology* 155:709–718, 1985.

353. Bohndorf K, Reiser M, Lochner B, et al: Magnetic resonance imaging of primary tumours and tumour-like lesions of bone. *Skel Radiol* 15:511–517, 1986.

354. Bloem JL, Taminiau HM, Eulderink F, et al: Radiologic staging of primary bone sarcoma: MR imaging, scintigraphy, angiography, and CT correlated with pathologic examination. *Radiology* 169:805–810, 1988.

355. Tehranzadeh J, Mnaymneh W, Ghavam C, et al: Comparison of CT and MR imaging in musculoskeletal neoplasms. *J Comput Assist Tomogr* 13:466–472, 1989.

356. Beltran J, Noto AM, Chakeres DW, et al: Tumors of the osseous spine: Staging with MR imaging versus CT. *Radiology* 162:565–569, 1987.

357. Berquist TH: Magnetic resonance imaging of primary skeletal neoplasms. *Radiol Clin North Am* 31:411, 1993.

358. Seeger LL, Widoff BE, Bassett LW, et al: Preoperative evaluation of osteosarcoma: Value of gadopentetate dimeglumine-enhanced MR imaging. *AJR* 157:347–351, 1991.

359. Ma LD, Frassica FJ, Scott WW, et al: Differentiation of benign and malignant musculoskeletal tumors: Potential pitfalls with MR imaging. *RadioGraphics* 15:349–366, 1995.

360. Hayes CW, Conway WF, Sundaram M: Misleading aggressive MR imaging appearance of some benign musculoskeletal lesions. *RadioGraphics* 12:1119–1134, 1992.

361. Seeger LL, Dungan DH, Eckardt JJ, et al: Nonspecific findings on MR imaging. *Clin Orthop Rel Res* 270:306–312, 1991.

362. Assoun J, Richardi G, Railhac J-J, et al: Osteoid osteoma: MR imaging versus CT. *Radiology* 191:217–223, 1994.

363. Frank JA, Ling A, Patronas NJ, et al: Detection of malignant bone tumors: MR imaging vs scintigraphy. *AJR* 155:1043–1048, 1990.

364. Swan JS, Grist TM, Sproat IA, et al: Musculoskeletal neoplasms: Preoperative evaluation with MR angiography. *Radiology* 194:519–524, 1995.

365. Petasnick JP, Turner DA, Charters JR, et al: Soft-tissue masses of the locomotor system: Comparison of MR imaging with CT. *Radiology* 160:125–133, 1986.

366. Totty WG, Murphy WA, Lee JK: Soft-tissue tumors: MR imaging. *Radiology* 160:135–141, 1986.

367. Moulton JS, Blebea JS, Dunco DM, et al: MR imaging of soft-tissue masses: Diagnostic efficacy and value of distinguishing between benign and malignant lesions. *AJR* 164:1191–1199, 1995.

368. Crim JR, Seeger LL, Yao L, et al: Diagnosis of soft-tissue masses with MR imaging: Can benign masses be differentiated from malignant ones? *Radiology* 185:581–586, 1992.

369. Kransdorf MJ, Jelinek JS, Moser RP, et al: Soft-tissue masses: Diagnosis using MR imaging. *AJR* 153:541–547, 1989.

370. Hermann G, Abdelwahab IF, Miller TT, et al: Tumour and tumour-like conditions of the soft tissue: Magnetic resonance imaging features differentiating benign from malignant masses. *Br J Radiol* 65:14–20, 1992.

371. Miller TT, Potter HG, McCormack RR, et al: Benign soft tissue masses of the wrist and hand: MRI appearances. *Skel Radiol* 23:327–332, 1994.

372. Binkovitz LA, Berquist TH, McLeod RA: Masses of the hand and wrist: Detection and characterization with MR imaging. *AJR* 154:323–326, 1990.

373. Wetzel LH, Levine E: Soft-tissue tumors of the foot: Value of MR imaging for specific diagnosis. *AJR* 155:1025–1030, 1990.

374. Berquist TH, Ehman RL, King BF, et al: Value of MR imaging in differentiating benign from malignant soft-tissue masses: Study of 95 lesions. *AJR* 155:1251–1255, 1990.

375. Erlemann R, Reiser MF, Peters PE, et al: Musculoskeletal neoplasms: Static and dynamic Gd-DTPA-enhanced MR imaging. *Radiology* 171:767–773, 1989.

376. Verstraete KL, Vanzieleghem B, De Deene Y, et al: Static dynamic and first-pass MR imaging of musculoskeletal lesions using gadodiamide injection. *Acta Radiol* 36:27–36, 1995.

377. Li KC, Hopkins KL, Moore SG, et al: Magnetization transfer contrast MRI of musculoskeletal neoplasms. *Skel Radiol* 24:21–25, 1995.

378. Kobayashi H, Sakahara H, Hosono M, et al: Soft-tissue tumors: Diagnosis with Tc-99m(V) dimercaptosuccinic acid scintigraphy. *Radiology* 190:277–280, 1994.

379. Pan G, Raymond AK, Carrasco CH, et al: Osteosarcoma: MR imaging after preoperative chemotherapy. *Radiology* 174:517–526, 1990.

380. MacVicar AD, Olliff JF, Pringle J, et al: Ewing sarcoma: MR imaging of chemotherapy-induced changes with histologic correlation. *Radiology* 184:859–864, 1992.

381. Lawrence JA, Babyn PS, Chan HS, et al: Extremity osteosarcoma in childhood: Prognostic value of radiologic imaging. *Radiology* 189:43–47, 1993.

382. Holscher HC, Bloem JL, Vanel D, et al: Osteosarcoma: Chemotherapy-induced changes at MR imaging. *Radiology* 182:839–844, 1992.

383. Sanchez RB, Quinn SF, Walling A, et al: Musculoskeletal neoplasms after intraarterial chemotherapy: Correlation of MR images with pathologic specimens. *Radiology* 174:237–240, 1990.

384. Hanna S, Parham DM, Fairclough DL, et al: Assessment of osteosarcoma response to preoperative chemotherapy using dynamic flash gadolinium-DTPA-enhanced magnetic resonance mapping. *Invest Radiol* 27:367–373, 1992.

385. Fletcher BD, Hanna SL, Fairclough DL, et al: Pediatric musculoskeletal tumors: Use of dynamic, contrast-enhanced MR imaging to monitor response to chemotherapy. *Radiology* 184:243–248, 1992.

386. Erlemann R, Sciuk J, Bosse A, et al: Response of osteosarcoma and Ewing sarcoma to preoperative chemotherapy: Assessment with dynamic and static MR imaging and skeletal scintigraphy. *Radiology* 175:791–796, 1990.

387. de Baere T, Vanel D, Shapeero LG, et al: Osteosarcoma after chemotherapy: Evaluation with contrast material-enhanced subtraction MR imaging. *Radiology* 185:587–592, 1992.

388. Carrasco CH, Charnsangavej CC, Raymond AK, et al: Osteosarcoma: angiographic assessment of response to preoperative chemotherapy. *Radiology* 170:839–842, 1989.

389. Lang P, Grampp S, Vahlensieck M, et al: Primary bone tumors: value of MR angiography for preoperative planning and monitoring response to chemotherapy. *AJR* 165:135–142, 1995.

390. van der Woude H-J, Bloem JL, Schipper J, et al: Changes in tumor perfusion induced by chemotherapy in bone sarcomas: Color Doppler flow imaging compared with contrast-enhanced MR imaging and three-phase bone scintigraphy. *Radiology* 191:421–431, 1994.

391. van der Woude HJ, Bloem JL, van Oostayen JA, et al: Treatment of high-grade bone sarcomas with neoadjuvant chemotherapy: The utility of sequential color Doppler sonography in predicting histopathologic response. *AJR* 165:125–133, 1995.

392. Rosen G, Loren GJ, Brien EW, et al: Serial thallium-201 scintigraphy in osteosarcoma: Correlation with tumor necrosis after preoperative chemotherapy. *Clin Orthop Rel Res* 293:302–306, 1993.

393. Menendez LR, Fideler BM, Mirra J: Thallium-201 scanning for the evaluation of osteosarcoma and soft-tissue sarcoma. A study of the evaluation and predictability of the histological response to chemotherapy. *J Bone Joint Surg (Am)* 75:526–531, 1993.

394. Lin J, Leung WT, Ho SK, et al: Quantitative evaluation of thallium-201 uptake in predicting chemotherapeutic response of osteosarcoma. *Eur J Nucl Med* 22:5533–5535, 1995.

395. Zlatkin MB, Lenkinski RE, Shinkwin M, et al: Combined MR imaging and spectroscopy of bone and soft tissue tumors. *J Comput Assist Tomogr* 4:1–10, 1990.

396. Kern KA, Brunetti A, Norton JA, et al: Metabolic imaging of human extremity musculoskeletal tumors by PET. *J Nucl Med* 29:181–186, 1988.

397. Sostman HD, Prescott DM, Dewhirst MW, et al: MR imaging and spectroscopy for prognostic evaluation in soft-tissue sarcomas. *Radiology* 190:269–275, 1994.

398. Redmond OM, Stack JP, Dervan PA, et al: Osteosarcoma: Use of MR imaging and MR spectroscopy in clinical decision making. *Radiology* 172:811–815, 1989.

399. Reuther G, Mutschler W: Detection of local recurrent disease in musculoskeletal tumors: Magnetic resonance imaging versus computed tomography. *Skel Radiol* 19:85–90, 1990.

400. Vanel D, Lacombe M-J, Couanet D, et al: Musculoskeletal tumors: Follow-up with MR imaging after treatment with surgery and radiation therapy. *Radiology* 164:243–245, 1987.

401. Vanel D, Shapeero LG, DeBaere T, et al: MR imaging in the follow-up of malignant and aggressive soft-tissue tumors: Results of 511 examinations. *Radiology* 190:263–268, 1994.

402. Panicek DM, Schwartz LH, Heelan RT, et al: Non-neoplastic causes of high signal intensity at T2-weighted MR imaging after treatment for musculoskeletal neoplasm. *Skel Radiol* 24:185–190, 1995.

403. Levin TL, Miller TT, Panicek DM, et al: MR signal characteristics of cadaveric bone allografts in three children with primary bone tumors treated with limb salvage therapy. *Pediatr Radiol* 24:488–490, 1994.

404. Hoeffner EG, Ryan JR, Qureshi F, et al: Magnetic resonance imaging of massive bone allografts with histologic correlation. *Skel Radiol* 25:165–170, 1996.

405. Richardson ML, Loough LR, Shuman WP: MR appearance of skeletal neoplasms following cryotherapy. *Skel Radiol* 23:121–125, 1994.

CHAPTER 16

Principles of Orthopaedic Oncology

Martin M. Malawer, Robert M. Henshaw,
and Barry M. Shmookler

I. Musculoskeletal Oncology

Martin M. Malawer, Robert M. Henshaw, and Barry M. Shmookler

Neoplasms of the musculoskeletal system still rank among the least common diagnoses made by orthopaedists: only 8000 new cases (6000 soft tissue and 2000 bone) of sarcoma are estimated to have been seen in 1995 by the American Cancer Society. A high degree of clinical suspicion, necessary for early diagnosis, is ever more important as fundamental changes in health care delivery alter patient access to both specialists and expensive imaging studies. Early detection combined with proper techniques of diagnosis and treatment can dramatically improve the chances of achieving functional limb salvage. Continued progress in radiographic imaging, chemotherapy, radiation therapy, and biotechnology—coupled with a better understanding of the biological behavior of mesenchymal neoplasms—has led to a rational basis for diagnosis, staging, and surgical treatment.[1-11]

NATURAL HISTORY OF BONE AND SOFT TISSUE TUMORS

Mesenchymal neoplasms have characteristic patterns of behavior and growth that distinguish them from other malignancies.[8,12] These patterns form the underlying basis of a staging system and provide a focus for current treatment strategies.[12]

Biology and Growth

Spindle cell sarcomas form solid lesions through circumferential growth, in which the periphery of each lesion is composed of the least mature cells. In contradistinction to benign lesions, which are surrounded by a true capsule composed of compressed normal cells, the malignant tumor is generally enclosed by a pseudocapsule consisting of viable tumor cells and a fibrovascular zone of reactive tissue with a variable inflammatory component that interdigitates with the normal tissue adjacent to and beyond the lesion. The thickness of the reactive zone varies with the degree of malignancy and histogenetic type.

High-grade sarcomas characteristically have a poorly defined reactive zone that may be locally invaded and destroyed by the tumor. In addition, tumor nodules not in continuity with the main tumor may be present in tissue that appears to be normal (see "Skip Metastasis," below). Low-grade sarcomas rarely form tumor nodules beyond the reactive zone.

Local anatomy influences the growth of sarcomas by setting natural barriers to extension.[13] In general, bone sarcomas take the path of least resistance. The three mechanisms of growth and extension of bone tumors are compression of normal tissue, resorption of bone by reactive osteoclasts, and direct destruction of normal tissue. Benign tumors grow and expand by the first two mechanisms, whereas direct tissue destruction is characteristic of malignant bone tumors. Most benign bone tumors are unicompartmental; they remain confined and may expand the bone in which they arise. Most malignant bone tumors are bicompartmental; they destroy the overlying cortex and push directly into the adjacent soft tissue. Soft tissue tumors may start in one compartment (intracompartmental) or between compartments (extracompartmental).[14] The determination of anatomic compartment involvement has become more important with the advent of limb preservation surgery.

Advances in molecular biology and cytogenetics have led to the discovery that many neoplasms have characteristic chromosomal abnormalities.[15] Specific families of oncogenes have been identified in a number of sarcomas, including the RB1 gene, seen in both retinoblastoma and osteosarcoma[16]; the p53 tumor suppressor gene, which is mutated in almost 50 percent of human tumors and nearly all types of sarcomas, including osteosarcoma, rhabdomyosarcoma, and neurofibrosarcoma[17]; the NF1 gene, associated with neurofibromatosis, malignant nerve sheath tumors, and neurofibrosarcomas[18]; and the EWS split gene product, produced by a specific chromosomal translocation t(11;22) or t(21;22), seen in Ewing's sarcoma and peripheral neuroectodermal tumors (PNETs). Recently, a variety of benign tumors have also been shown to have specific chromosomal alterations.[19] Ongoing research in this field may lead to more precise diagnostic techniques and novel treatment alternatives in the near future.

Patterns of Behavior

Based on biological considerations and natural history, all bone and soft tissue tumors, benign and malignant, may be classified into five categories; tumors within each of these share certain clinical characteristics and radiographic patterns and require similar surgical procedures. The five general patterns of behavior are as follows[12]:

1. *Benign/latent* Lesions whose natural history is to grow slowly during normal growth of the individual and then to stop, with a tendency to heal sponta-

neously. They never become malignant and heal rapidly if treated by simple curettage.

2. *Benign/active*   Lesions whose natural history is progressive growth: excision leaves a reactive zone with some tumors.

3. *Benign/aggressive*   Lesions that are locally aggressive but do not metastasize. Pathologically, there is tumor extension through the capsule into the reactive zone. Local control can be obtained only by removing the lesion with a margin of normal tissue beyond the reactive zone.

4. *Malignant, low-grade*   Lesions that have a low potential to metastasize. Histologically there is no true capsule but a pseudocapsule. Tumor nodules exist within the reactive zone but rarely beyond. Local control can be accomplished only by removal of all tumor and reactive tissue with a margin of normal bone or muscle. These lesions can be treated successfully by surgery alone; systemic therapy is not required.

5. *Malignant, high-grade*   Lesions whose natural history is to grow rapidly and to metastasize early. Tumor nodules are usually found within and beyond the reactive zone and at some distance in the normal tissue. Surgery is necessary for local control, and systemic therapy is warranted to prevent metastasis.

Examples of bone and soft tissue tumors in each of these categories are shown in Table 16-1.

Tumor Spread

Unlike carcinomas, bone and soft tissue sarcomas disseminate almost exclusively through the blood. Soft tissue tumors occasionally (5 to 10 percent) spread through the lymphatic system to regional nodes.[20] Hematogenous spread is manifest by pulmonary involvement in the early stages and by bony involvement in later stages.[1,2,21,22] Bone metastasis occasionally is the first sign of dissemination.

Skip Metastasis

The histologic hallmark of malignant sarcomas is their potential to break through the pseudocapsule to form satellite lesions called *skip metastases*. A skip metastasis is a tumor nodule that is located within the same bone as the main tumor but is not contiguous to it. Transarticular skip metastases are located in the joint adjacent to the main tumor (Fig. 16-1).[14] Although relatively uncommon, skip metastases occur most frequently with high-grade sarcomas. Skip lesions develop via embolization of tumor cells within the marrow sinusoids; they are, in effect, local micrometastases that have not passed through the circulation. Soft tissue sarcomas, similarly, may be associated with noncontinuous tumor nodules away from the main tumor mass. These nodules are responsible for local recurrences that develop in spite of apparently negative margins after a resection.

Local Recurrence

Local recurrence following surgery results from incomplete removal and subsequent regrowth of either benign or malignant cells. Adequacy of surgical removal is the main determinant of local control. The aggressiveness of the lesion determines the choice of surgical procedure. Some 95 percent of all local recurrences, regardless of the histologic findings, develop within 24 months of surgery.[12,14]

STAGING SYSTEM OF MUSCULOSKELETAL TUMORS

Selection and use of a prognostically significant staging system is fundamental both for the rational selection of treatment protocols and for the development of tumor registries necessary for basic research analysis. In 1980, the Musculoskeletal Tumor Society adopted a surgical staging system (SSS) for both bone and soft tissue sarcomas.[8] This system is based upon the fact that mesenchymal sarcomas of bone and soft tissue behave alike, irrespective of histogenetic type. The SSS encompasses the GTM classification: grade (G), location (T), and lymph node involvement and metastases (M).

1. *Surgical grade (G)*   The letter *G* represents both the histologic grade of a lesion and clinical factors related to aggressiveness, such as growth rate. A

TABLE 16-1   Behavioral Classification of Bone and Soft Tissue Tumors

	Typical example	
Classification	**Bone**	**Soft tissue**
Benign/latent	Nonossifying fibroma	Lipoma
Benign/active	Aneurysmal bone cyst	Angiolipoma
Benign/aggressive	Giant-cell tumor	Aggressive fibromatosis
Malignant/low-grade	Parosteal osteosarcoma	Myxoid liposarcoma
Malignant/high-grade	Classic osteosarcoma	Malignant fibrous histiocytoma

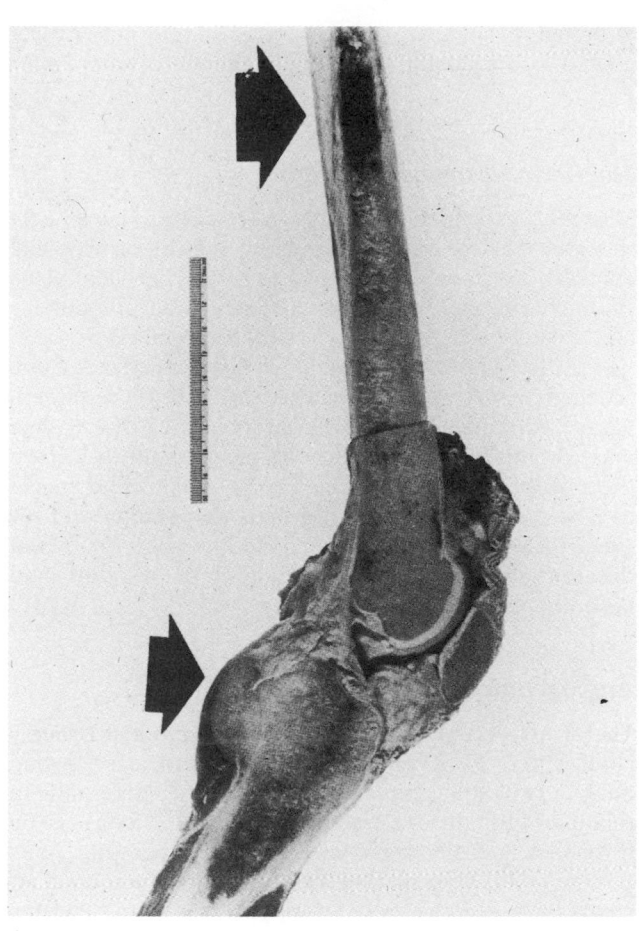

A

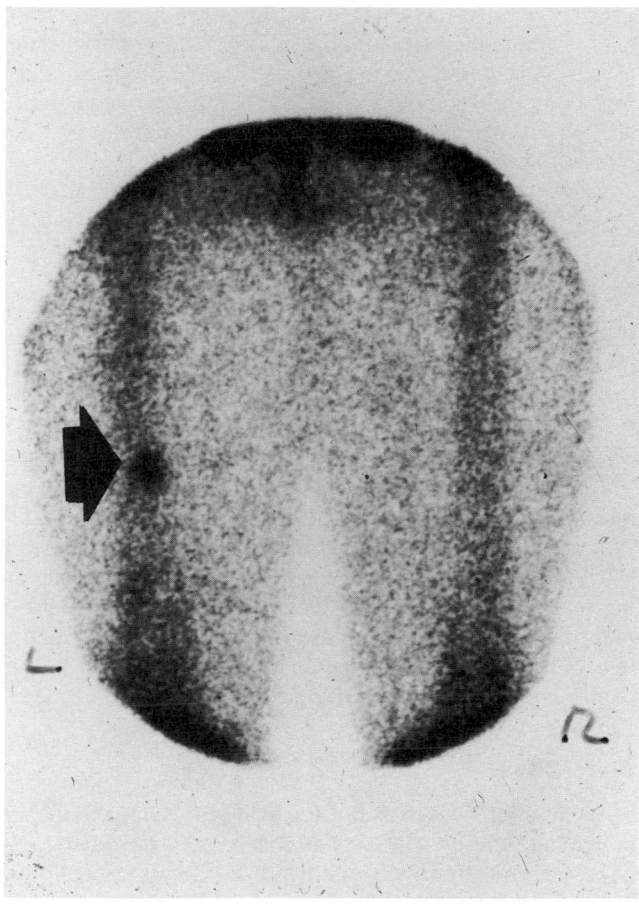

B

Figure 16-1 A skip metastasis from an osteosarcoma of the proximal tibia to the ipsilateral femur. Satellite nodules that occur from a bony sarcoma are termed *skip metastases*. These may occur within the same bone as the primary lesion or across the adjacent joint, termed a *transarticular skip metas-* *tasis. A.* Gross specimen following an above-knee amputation, showing the primary tumor (*lower arrow*) and the skip metastasis (*upper arrow*). *B.* Bone scan of the same lesion (*solid arrow*), demonstrating a small well-defined area of uptake of the skip lesion.

low-grade tumor is rated G1, while a high-grade tumor is rated G2. Low-grade lesions represent malignancies with little potential to metastasize.

2. *Surgical site (T)*   The letter *T* represents anatomic site, either intracompartmental (T1) or extracompartmental (T2). *Compartment* is defined as "an anatomic structure or space bounded by natural barriers of tumor extension." T1 lesions are easier to delineate clinically, surgically, and radiographically than T2 lesions and have a correspondingly better chance of adequate removal without amputative procedures.

3. *Lymph nodes and metastases (M)*   Local disease without evidence of metastasis is designated M0. When a bone or soft tissue sarcoma has metastasized (M1), the prognosis is extremely poor. Lymphatic spread is a sign of extensive dissemination. Regional lymphatic involvement is equated with distal metastases.

The SSS developed for surgical planning and assessment of bone sarcomas is summarized as follows[8]:

Stage IA (G1, T1, M0) Low-grade intracompartmental lesion without metastasis

Stage IB (G1, T2, M0) Low-grade extracompartmental lesion without metastasis

Stage IIA (G2, T1, M0) High-grade intracompartmental lesion without metastasis

Stage IIB (G2, T2, M0) High-grade extracompartmental lesion without metastasis

Stage IIIA (G1 or G2, M1) Intracompartmental lesion, any grade, with metastasis

Stage IIIB (G1 or G2, T1 or T2, M1) Extracompartmental lesion, any grade, with metastasis

PREOPERATIVE EVALUATION, STAGING, AND BIOPSY

If the clinical examination and/or plain radiographs suggest an aggressive or malignant tumor, staging studies should be performed before biopsy. All radiographic studies are influenced by surgical manipulation of the lesion, making interpretation more difficult.[12,23] Bone scintigraphy, computed tomography (CT) or MRI, and angiography are required to delineate local tumor extent, vascular displacement, and compartmental localization.[7,14,24–36]

Radiographic Evaluation
X-rays

Plain radiographs taken in perpendicular planes—anteroposterior (AP) and lateral—remain essential to the characterization and diagnosis of lesions involving the skeleton. Selection and interpretation of other imaging techniques is often guided by the radiographic properties of the lesion. Proper interpretation of a lesion seen on a radiograph can be summarized by answering Enneking's "four questions"[37]: What is the anatomic location and extent of the lesion? What is the lesion doing to the bone? What is the bone doing to the lesion? Are there any radiographic peculiarities of the lesion that give a hint as to its tissue type? Distinction between benign, aggressive, and frankly malignant lesions can be made based upon this analysis.

Bone Scans

Bone scintigraphy is useful for evaluating both bony and soft tissue tumors. It assists in detecting metastatic disease, polyostotic involvement, intraosseous extension of tumor, and the state of the bone underlying a primary soft tissue sarcoma.[27,38–40] Malignant bone tumors may present with skeletal metastasis (1.6 percent).[24] The initial flow phase correlates to the vascularity of the tumor. Recent studies utilizing quantitative techniques and the isotope thallium 201 have shown that the histologic tumor response to chemotherapy can be predicted based upon comparison of pre- and posttreatment studies.[41–44]

Computed Tomography

Computed tomography scanning allows accurate determination of intra- and extraosseous extension of skeletal neoplasms.[7,38,39,45,46] It accurately depicts the transverse anatomic relationship of a tumor to the surrounding structures. By varying window settings, one can study cortical bone, intramedullary space, adjacent muscles, and extraosseous soft tissue extension. The anatomic compartmental involvement by soft tissue sarcomas is easily determined.[14] High-resolution CT scans (1-mm cuts) and two- or three-dimensional (2D or 3D) reconstruction can be extremely valuable in preoperative planning, particularly in the pelvis or spine. Evaluation by CT must be individualized to obtain the maximum benefit of image reconstruction: close interaction between the surgeon and the radiologist facilitates accurate and effective imaging.

Core needle biopsies guided by CT have proved to be effective in obtaining tissue for diagnosis from difficult to reach or clinically occult sites. Proper utilization of this technique requires a skilled radiologist working in concert with a tissue pathologist to ensure that adequate tissue is obtained. A negative needle biopsy should never be accepted as diagnostic, given the likelihood of sampling error.

Magnetic Resonance Imaging

Magnetic resonance imaging is now accepted as an accurate and valuable imaging technique and can provide high-contrast images in multiple planes.[36,47–49] Excellent visualization of anatomic compartments, neurovascular bundles, and areas of reactive tissue allows for detailed preoperative planning of resection margins. Skip metastases can be strikingly apparent and readily identifiable on sagittal images.[50] Although the signal characteristics of any given mass on the traditional T1- or T2-weighted images (or on the more recent fat-suppressed and gradient-echo images) can be diagnostic, distinction between benign and low-grade malignant lesions (such as lipomas versus well-differentiated liposarcomas) cannot be reliably made based upon the MRI images alone.

Angiography

The arteriographic technique for bone and soft tissue lesions differs from that used for arterial disease. A minimum of two views (biplane) is necessary to determine the relation of the major vessels to the tumor.[32] Extraosseous extension is easily demonstrated by angiography. As experience with limb-sparing procedures has increased, surgeons have become more aware of the need to determine the individual vascular patterns prior to resection. This is especially crucial for tumors of the proximal tibia, where vascular anomalies are common.[51] The increasing use of preoperative intraarterial chemotherapy has also increased the need for accurate angiography. Reduction of vascularity following chemotherapy can be correlated to the overall histologic response of the tumor.[52,53] Preoperative embolization of highly vascular tumors prior to surgical resection can significantly reduce blood loss and intraoperative morbidity.

The combination of plain radiographs, bone scintigraphy, cross-sectional anatomic imaging (via CT or MRI scans), and longitudinal imaging of vascular supply (angiography) allows the surgeon to develop a 3D construct of the local tumor area prior to resection and to formulate a detailed surgical approach for limb salvage.

Biopsy Considerations

A biopsy should be performed after the staging studies are obtained. If a resection is to be performed, it is crucial that the location of the biopsy be in line with the anticipated incision for the definitive procedure. Extreme care should be taken before biopsy not to contaminate potential tissue planes or flaps, thus compromising the management of the lesion. Improper biopsy technique often eliminates the opportunity for limb salvage. Mankin[54] documented that 60 percent of referred patients had a major error in diagnosis, and 18 percent had less than optimal treatment secondary to problems related to the biopsy. A repeat study 10 years after publication of this study revealed no improvement in overall management of referred patients.[55] The Musculoskeletal Tumor Society has adopted the policy that biopsies should be performed only by the surgeon who will ultimately perform the final tumor resection.

To minimize contamination and reduce patient morbidity, needle biopsy of soft tissue masses or of extraosseous components should be attempted prior to an incisional biopsy whenever possible. Needle or core biopsy of bone tumors often provides an adequate specimen for diagnosis.[56,57] Cooperation between the radiologist and pathologist is vital to ensure that adequate tissue is obtained. Radiographs should be obtained to document the position of the trocar. Core biopsy is preferable if a limb-sparing option exists, since it entails less local contamination than an open biopsy does. In addition, core needle biopsy has been shown to be as accurate as and more cost-effective than open biopsies.[58–61] Core biopsy is especially helpful in difficult areas such as the spine, pelvis, and hips. If a core biopsy proves to be inadequate, a small incisional biopsy is performed.

Proper techniques for open biopsies are necessary to minimize contamination.[60] A tourniquet is used, if feasible, to facilitate visualization of the tumor. Transverse incisions are to be avoided at all costs; consideration of subsequent surgery for limb salvage should guide positioning of the biopsy incision. Since sarcomas are characteristically surrounded by the most immature cells, biopsy of the lesion's peripheral tissue is recommended. If a soft tissue component is present, there is no need to biopsy the underlying bone. If it is necessary to biopsy the underlying bone, a small, rounded, cortical window should be used. This is especially true for a tumor that requires primary radiotherapy. Large segments will not reossify, leading to fracture and subsequent amputation. To decrease postoperative hemorrhage and minimize the risk of pathologic fracture, polymethylmethacrylate is used to plug any cortical windows. Gelfoam and the electrocautery are useful for hemostasis in the soft tissue. The overlying pseudocapsule is carefully closed for maximum hemostasis. Closed suction drainage, while useful in preventing extensive hematoma formation, increases the area of tumor contamination. When used, the drain should always be brought out of the wound in line with the biopsy incision. Regardless of the technique utilized, tumor cells will contaminate all tissue planes and compartments traversed. All open biopsy and drain sites must therefore be removed en bloc when the tumor is resected.

Frozen section analyses are performed on all biopsy specimens prior to closure of the wound.[12,62] Many bone tumors can be adequately sectioned with a microtome: touch preps allow for collection of cells for examination. The purpose of the frozen section is not to make the diagnosis; rather, it is to demonstrate that adequate viable tumor has been obtained for diagnostic evaluation. If not, additional specimens must be obtained. Frozen section studies may also suggest that additional material should be obtained for electron microscopy and/or immunohisto-

chemical staining techniques to ensure an accurate histologic diagnosis.

CLASSIFICATION OF SURGICAL PROCEDURES

Surgical removal—including curettage, resection, and amputation—is the traditional method of managing skeletal neoplasms. The advent of advanced imaging techniques, improved understanding of the biological behavior of sarcomas, and adoption of effective adjuvant therapy has led to widespread acceptance of limb-sparing techniques.[4,22,23,34,62–69] Retrospective analysis of disease-free survival and overall survival has shown no difference between limb salvage and amputation for osteosarcoma of the distal femur.[70]

A classification scheme of surgical procedures based on the surgical plane of dissection in relation to the tumor and the method of accomplishing the removal has recently been developed. This system, summarized below, permits meaningful comparison of various operative procedures and gives surgeons a common language.[8,14]

1. *Intralesional* An intralesional procedure passes through the pseudocapsule and directly into the lesion. Macroscopic tumor is left, and the entire operative field is potentially contaminated. Biopsies are by definition intralesional.
2. *Marginal* A marginal procedure is one in which the entire lesion is removed in one piece. The plane of dissection passes through the pseudocapsule or reactive zone around the lesion. When performed for a sarcoma, it leaves macroscopic disease because of tumor involvement of the pseudocapsule.
3. *Wide (intracompartmental)* This is commonly termed *en bloc resection*. A wide excision includes the entire tumor, the reactive zone, and a marginal cuff of normal tissue. The entire structure of origin of the tumor is not removed. In patients with high-grade sarcomas, this procedure may leave skip nodules.
4. *Radical (extracompartmental)* The entire tumor and the structure of origin of the lesion are removed. The plane of dissection is beyond the limiting fascial or bony borders.

It is important to note that any of these procedures may be accomplished *either* by a local (i.e., limb-sparing) procedure or by amputation. An amputation may entail a marginal, wide, or radical excision, depending upon the plane through which it passes in relation to the tumor. Therefore, an amputation is not automatically an adequate cancer operation, and careful consideration to the desired final margin is required prior to selection of the amputation level. The local anatomy dictates how a specific margin can be obtained surgically, and proper preoperative staging (as discussed above) is necessary to assess both local tumor extent and relevant local anatomy. In general, benign bone tumors can be adequately treated with either an intralesional procedure (curettage) or a marginal excision. Malignant tumors require a minimum of wide (intracompartmental) excision or a radical (extracompartmental) resection. This can be accomplished by amputation, or by an en bloc procedure (limb salvage). Similarly, benign soft tissue tumors are treated by marginal excision, aggressive tumors by wide excision, and malignant tumors by wide or radical resection.

SOFT TISSUE SARCOMAS

Soft tissue sarcomas (STSs) are a heterogeneous group of tumors arising from the supporting extraskeletal mesenchymal tissues of the body—i.e., muscle, fascia, connective tissues, fibrous tissues, and fat. They are rare lesions, constituting less than 1 percent of all cancers. There are wide morphologic differences among these tumors, probably resulting from the different cells of origin. All STSs, like bone sarcomas, however, share certain biological and behavioral characteristics.

The clinical, radiographic, and surgical management of most STSs is identical, regardless of histogenesis. The surgical grading system developed by the Musculoskeletal Tumor Society applies to both bone sarcomas and soft tissue sarcomas.

Clinical Findings

Soft tissue sarcomas are a disease of adulthood, occurring in persons between 30 and 60 years of age. The sole exception is rhabdomyosarcoma, which occurs in young children. Approximately one-half of STSs are found in the extremities; the remainder arise in the head/neck and trunk. The lower extremity is the most common anatomic site; 40 percent of all STSs occur in this location.[71] The anterior thigh (quadriceps) is the most common compartment, followed by the adductors and hamstrings.[13,14]

Most STSs present as a painless mass. Systemic signs such as fever, weight loss, or anemia are rare. There are no useful laboratory screening examinations. Clinical suspicion is therefore crucial to diagnosis. Any adult presenting with an extremity mass must be presumed to have a sarcoma until proved otherwise and should be further evaluated. History of coincident trauma can often be especially misleading. Unfortunately, a presumptive diagnosis of lipoma, ganglion, hematoma, or muscle tear is often made, thereby delaying definitive evaluation and treatment. Local examination reveals a well-localized, nontender mass that may be movable. The lesion may be firm or cystic. (The latter indicates that necrosis has occurred and is a sign of high-grade sarcoma.)

Biological Behavior and Natural History

The pattern of growth, metastasis, and recurrence of STSs is similar to that of spindle cell sarcomas arising in bone. The major distinctions are (1) the tendency of STSs to remain intracompartmental and (2) a significant incidence of lymphatic involvement in a few of the less common entities such as the epithelioid, synovial, and alveolar soft-part sarcomas. The prognosis of an STS is most closely related to its histologic grade and the presence or absence of metastases.[8,14] Historically, high-grade STS had an overall survival rate of 40 to 60 percent.[8,13,30,72,73] In half of all cases, wide local excision was followed by local recurrence within 12 to 24 months, followed by pulmonary metastases resulting from hematogenous dissemination to the lungs. Enneking has noted that if a local recurrence develops, the risk of pulmonary metastases doubles.[14,30] Visceral and lymphatic involvement was rare. Pulmonary metastasis and/or local recurrence are the most common sites of relapse. Aggressive surgical resection of local recurrences should be considered if distant metastasis has not occurred: a 5-year salvage rate of 50 to 80 percent can be achieved.[74]

Pathology and Staging

The STSs are classified based upon the histologic cell of origin, as listed in Table 16-2. Individual grading is often difficult; in general, however, the extent of pleomorphism, atypia, mitosis, and necrosis correlates with the degree of malignancy. Notable exceptions are synovial sarcomas, which tend to behave like high-grade lesions even in the absence of these findings. The exact histogenesis of some soft tissue sarcomas often cannot be accurately defined, although grading can still be adequately performed. The surgical stage is determined by grade, location, and the presence or absence of pulmonary or lymphatic metastases.[8] Staging studies must be done prior to treatment.

Because of its better visual contrast and ability to image in coronal and sagittal planes, MRI has surpassed CT as the most useful study for evaluating STS of the extremities[36]; while CT scanning remains valuable for retroperitoneal tumors and for the assessment of lung metastases. Either imaging method can delineate the cross-sectional anatomic extent and compartmentalization of the lesion. Unique features of modern MRI—including use of gadolinium contrast, mixed spin-echo images, and fat-suppression images—appear to facilitate visualization of tumor extent and may prove crucial to longitudinal study of postoperative patients to allow for early detection of local recurrences.

Biplane angiography remains the standard technique for demonstrating the position of the major vessels. Although MRI and contrast-enhanced CT often show the vessels, angiography is helpful in planning an operative approach, especially if displacement is noted on the CT scan. Bone scintigraphy is used to determine the relation of adjacent bony structures to the tumor. Increased uptake of the tracers by a bone in close proximity to an STS usually indicates a reactive rim of tumor near the periosteum, rather than direct intraosseous tumor extension. Such findings indicate that surgical resection of the underlying bony cortex or periosteum may be required.

TABLE 16-2 Histologic Types and Grades of Soft Tissue Sarcomas

Histological Type	Grade[a] 1	2	3
Well-differentiated liposarcoma	X	—	—
Myxoid liposarcoma	X	—	—
Round cell liposarcoma	—	X	X
Pleomorphic liposarcoma	—	—	X
Fibrosarcoma	—	X	X
Malignant fibrous histiocytoma	—	X	X
Inflammatory malignant fibrous histiocytoma	—	X	X
Myxoid malignant fibrous histiocytoma	—	X	—
Dermatofibrosarcoma protuberans	X	—	—
Malignant giant-cell tumor	—	X	X
Leiomyosarcoma	X	X	X
Malignant hemangiopericytoma	X	X	X
Embryonal rhabdomyosarcoma	—	—	X
Alveolar rhabdomyosarcoma	—	—	X
Pleomorphic rhabdomyosarcoma	—	—	X
Combined rhabdomyosarcoma	—	—	X
Chondrosarcoma	X	X	X
Mesenchymal chondrosarcoma	—	—	X
Myxoid chondrosarcoma	X	X	—
Osteosarcoma	—	—	X
Soft tissue sarcoma resembling Ewing's sarcoma	—	—	X
Synovial sarcoma	—	—	X
Epithelioid sarcoma	—	X	X
Clear cell sarcoma	—	X	X
Malignant superficial schwannoma	—	X	—
Neurofibrosarcoma	X	X	X
Epithelioid schwannoma	—	X	X
Malignant Triton tumor	—	—	X
Angiosarcoma	—	X	X
Alveolar soft part sarcoma	—	—	X
Malignant granular cell tumor	—	X	X
Kaposi's sarcoma	—	X	X

[a]The usual variation in grade is indicated for each recognized common histologic type.
Source: Reproduced with permission from Costa J, Wesley RA, Glatstein E, et al: The grading of soft tissue sarcoma. Results of a clinicopathologic correlation in a series of 163 cases. *Cancer* 53:530–541, 1984.

Treatment

The treatment of high-grade STS has undergone fundamental changes within the past decade. Successful management requires cooperation of the surgeon, chemotherapist, and radiation oncologist. The appropriate role of each modality is continuously changing, but it can be described in general as follows.

Chemotherapy

Combination chemotherapy has been shown to be more effective in preventing pulmonary dissemination from high-grade sarcomas than single-agent therapy.[71] However, significant toxicity can occur and doses must be reduced when compared to single-agent therapy. The most effective drugs in use today are doxorubicin hydrochloride (Adriamycin) and ifosfamide.[75] Dacarbazine (DTIC), methotrexate, and cisplatin also have activity and are included in many current protocols. The various combinations are traditionally given in an adjuvant (postoperative) setting and are presumed effective against clinically undetectable micrometastases.[76] Neoadjuvant (preoperative) chemotherapy is presently being evaluated in several institutions.[77–81] Early results indicate that significant reduction in tumor size can occur, thereby facilitating attempts at limb salvage.[82–84] Intraarterial administration of chemotherapy has been shown to increase local control in several studies.

Radiation Therapy

Radiation in the range of 5000 to 6500 cGy is effective in an adjuvant setting in decreasing local recurrence following nonablative resection.[73,85] The degree to which the initial surgical volume should be decreased in these circumstances is controversial, although local recurrence following a wide excision and postoperative radiotherapy is less than 51 percent. The technique of radiation therapy includes irradiating all the tissues at risk, shrinking fields, preserving a strip of unirradiated skin, and using filters and radiosensitizers. The local morbidity has been greatly decreased within the past decade. Preoperative radiation is effective in reducing tumor volume but is associated with increased morbidity resulting from significant wound healing complications.[86] Brachytherapy, or implantation of catheters for delivery of local radiation during the postoperative period, can reduce the time of treatment substantially.[87]

Surgery

Removal of the tumor is necessary to achieve local control. This may be accomplished by either a nonablative resection (limb salvage) or an amputation. The procedure chosen depends on results of the preoperative staging studies. A prospective randomized National Cancer Institute (NCI) trial established that a multimodality approach employing limb salvage surgery combined with adjuvant radiation and chemotherapy offered local control and survival rates comparable to amputation plus chemotherapy while simultaneously preserving a functional extremity.[88,89]

Surgical Management

The use of adjuvant therapy (chemotherapy or radiation) permits limb-sparing procedures for the majority of extremity STSs.[88,90] Enneking has shown that a radical resection for an STS has about a 5 percent local recurrence rate with surgery alone.[8,14] Wide excision (without adjuvant radiation or chemotherapy) has a 50 percent rate of local failure. Results from the NCI showed that the rate of local recurrence decreased to 5 percent following local excision (either a marginal or wide excision) when combined with postoperative radiation therapy and chemotherapy.[88] Others have reported similar good results from preoperative radiation, with or without preoperative chemotherapy. Contraindications to limb-sparing surgery are similar to those for the bony sarcomas. In general, nerve or major vascular involvement is a contraindication. Most stage IIA lesions can be treated by a limb-sparing procedure, whereas stage IIB lesions often require amputation to achieve negative margins. Introduction of neoadjuvant chemotherapy appears to improve the chances of limb salvage dramatically, with one study showing a 92 percent rate of limb salvage in stage IIB extremity STSs.[84]

Studies of referred patients show that approximately 50 percent of all patients with STSs treated with attempted excisional biopsy by the referring surgeon will have microscopic or gross tumor remaining.[91,92] As a result, referred patients undergo routine re-resection of the surgical site to ensure adequate local control prior to the institution of adjuvant treatment.

Surgical Technique

The technique of resection for specific anatomic compartments is discussed in their respective sections. The general surgical and oncologic principles are summarized as follows:

1. All tissue at risk should be removed with a wide en bloc excision. This includes the tumor, a cuff of normal muscle, and all potentially contaminated tissues. The entire muscle group need not be removed. The biopsy site should be removed along with 3 cm of normal skin and subcutaneous tissue en bloc with the tumor.
2. The tumor and/or pseudocapsule should never be visualized during the procedure. Contamination of the wound with tumor greatly increases the risk of local recurrence.
3. Distant flaps should not be developed at the time of resection. This may contaminate an uninvolved area.
4. The margin surrounding the surgical wound should be marked with metallic staples. This helps the radiotherapist determine the high-risk area, should radiation treatment be decided upon at a later date.
5. Reconstruction of the defect should include local muscle transfers to protect exposed neurovascular bundles and bone cortex.
6. All dead space should be closed, and there should be adequate drainage to prevent hematoma.
7. Perioperative antibiotics should be given. These procedures are associated with a low but significant rate of postoperative infection, especially following preoperative adjuvant therapy.

Characteristics of Specific Soft Tissue Sarcomas

Malignant Fibrous Histiocytoma

Malignant fibrous histiocytoma (MFH), first described as a specific entity in 1963, is the most common STS in older adults.[93–95] It occurs primarily in adults and is most prevalent in the lower extremity, followed in frequency by the upper extremity and the retroperitoneum. The histologic grade, usually intermediate to high, is a good prognosticator of metastatic potential. The myxoid variant, particularly when located in the superficial soft tissues, tends to have a more favorable prognosis than the other subtypes.[95] In fact, pure myxoid tumors with bland spindle cells are considered to be low-grade neoplasms with minimal metastatic potential.[96] It has been suggested that high-grade pleomorphic MFHs are a heterogeneous collection of poorly differentiated sarcomas, many of which can be specifically classified with the application of immunohistochemical and electron microscopic techniques.[97]

Gross Characteristics The lesions may be solitary or multinodular with well-circumscribed or ill-defined infiltrative borders. The size at the time of diagnosis is often directly related to the ease of clinical detection; superficial variants may be but a few centimeters in diameter, whereas those arising in the retroperitoneum often attain a diameter of 15 cm or more. Color and consistency vary considerably and relate to the proportion of stromal and cellular elements. The myxoid variant contains a predominance of white-gray, soft, mucoid tumor lobules, reflecting the high content of myxoid ground substance. Red-brown areas of hemorrhage and necrosis are not uncommon. Approximately 5 percent of MFHs undergo extensive hemorrhagic cystification, often leading to a clinical diagnosis of hematoma.[94]

Microscopic Characteristics The broad histologic spectrum encompasses many variants that were formerly considered to be distinct clinicopathologic entities. These variants had been named according to the predominant cell type and included fibroxanthosarcoma, malignant fibroxanthoma, inflammatory malignant fibrous histiocytoma, and malignant giant cell tumor of soft parts. The basic cellular constituents of all fibrohistiocytic tumors include fibroblasts, histiocyte-like cells, and mesenchymal cells. The proportion of these cellular elements and their degree of maturation account for the wide variety of histologic patterns. The storiform type, which is the most common variant, is so named because the spindle and histocytic cells form a storiform, that is, a cartwheel, pattern. There can be a considerable degree of pleomorphism, with the appearance of atypical and bizarre giant cells, often containing abnormal mitotic figures. Chronic inflammatory cells along with xanthoma cells often permeate the stroma. In the myxoid variant, the tumor cells are dispersed in a richly myxoid matrix. Diagnosis depends on the recognition of the cytologic atypia and presence of mitotic figures. The less common giant-cell type (malignant giant-cell tumor of soft parts) is characterized by abundant osteoclast-like giant cells diffusely distributed among the fibrohistiocytic elements. Finally, inflammatory MFH contains a rich component of acute and/or chronic inflammatory cells. It can be confused with inflammatory pseudotumor or lymphoma, particularly Hodgkin's disease.

Fibrosaroma

Fibrosarcoma used to be considered the most common STS. Following the identification of MFH as a distinct entity and the establishment of reproducible criteria for the recognition of other definitive spindle cell sarcomas, fibrosarcoma is less commonly diagnosed. Clinical and histologic difficulty occasionally arises in differentiating low-grade fibrosarcoma from fibromatosis and its variants. The anatomic site, age, and histologic findings must be carefully evaluated. This is a neoplasm of midadulthood and most commonly affects the lower extremity.

Gross Characteristics This neoplasm usually arises from the fascial and aponeurotic structures of the deep soft tissues; superficial variants are rare. The smaller tumors present as partially to completely circumscribed masses. As the lesions enlarge, a more diffusely infiltrative pattern predominates.

Microscopic Characteristics The fundamental cell of this neoplasm is the fibroblast, a spindle cell capable of producing collagen fiber. The collagen matrix can be easily identified in the better differentiated fibrosarcomas; moreover, its presence can be confirmed with the application of Masson's trichrome stain. Well-differentiated fibrosarcoma is characterized by intersecting fascicles of relatively uniform spindle cells showing minimal atypical features and sparse mitotic figures. The fascicles often intersect at acute angles and form the typical herringbone pattern (Fig. 16-2). In contrast, poorly differentiated fibrosarcoma often has a barely discernible fascicular arrangement. Furthermore, the cells show increased pleomorphism and nuclear atypia and often have a brisk mitotic rate. In the latter presentation, distinction from MFH may be exceedingly difficult and arbitrary, since both behave as high-grade sarcomas.

Liposarcoma

Liposarcoma is a common STS. It has a wide range of malignant potential, depending upon the grade of the individual tumor. Determination of subtype and grade is essential to appropriate management. Well-differentiated (grade I) liposarcomas rarely metastasize. Unlike other sarcomas, liposarcomas may be multiple and occur in unusual sites within the same individual. Careful evaluation of other masses in a patient with a liposarcoma is mandatory. Occasionally, these lesions occur in children.[98]

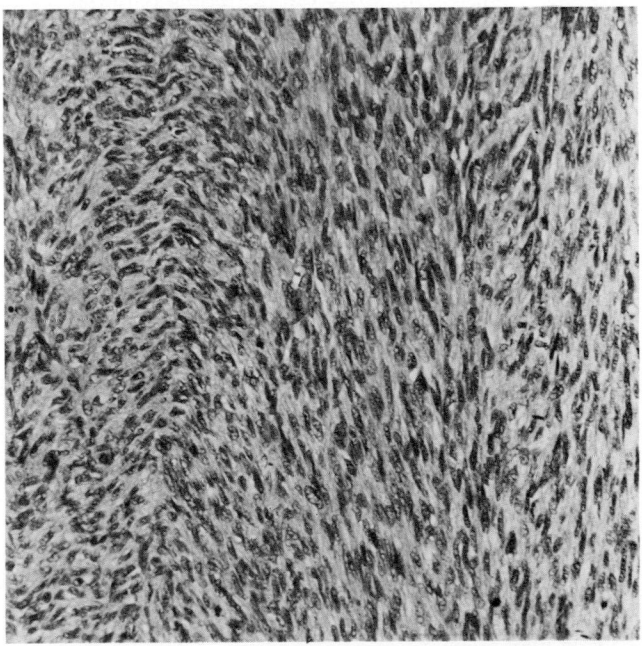

Figure 16-2 Elongated spindle cell fascicles intersecting at acute angles form the characteristic "herringbone" pattern of fibrosarcoma.

Liposarcomas very rarely arise from preexisting benign lipomas.

Gross Characteristics Liposarcomas, particularly those arising in the retroperitoneum, can become quite large; examples measuring 10 to 15 cm in diameter are not unusual. The tumors tend to be well circumscribed and multilobulated. The color and consistency observed on cut section usually correlate with the histologic type. Well-differentiated liposarcomas, containing variable proportions of relatively mature fat and fibrocollagenous tissue, vary from yellow to white-gray and can be soft, firm, or rubbery. A tumor that is soft and pink-tan and reveals a mucinous surface is typical of myxoid liposarcoma. The high-grade liposarcomas (round cell and pleomorphic) vary from pink-tan to brown and may disclose hemorrhagic and necrotic foci.

Microscopic Characteristics A current histologic classification of liposarcoma recognizes four distinct types (Table 16-3). Regardless of the histologic type, the identification of typical lipoblasts is mandatory to establish the diagnosis of liposarcoma. The lipoblast contains one, several, or multiple round, cytoplasmic fat droplets that form sharp, scalloped indentations on the central or peripheral nucleus.

Well-differentiated liposarcomas often contain a predominance of mature fat cells with a few widely scattered lipoblasts. In the sclerosing subtype, delicate collagen fibrils that encircle fat cells and lipoblasts constitute a prominent part of the matrix (Fig. 16-3). Spindle cell liposarcoma has recently been added to the subtypes of well-differentiated liposarcoma.[99] It is often subcutaneous, with a predilection for the upper extremity and shoulder girdle. A diagnosis of myxoid liposarcoma is based on the presence of a delicate, plexiform capillary network associated with both primitive mesenchymal-type cells and a variable number of lipoblasts. The stroma contains a high proportion of myxoid ground substance (hyaluronic acid), which, in areas, may form microcyst-like collections. In round cell liposarcoma, the lipoblasts are interspersed within sheets of poorly differentiated round cells. Pleomorphic liposarcoma is characterized by an admixture of bizarre, often multivacuolated lipoblasts and atyp-

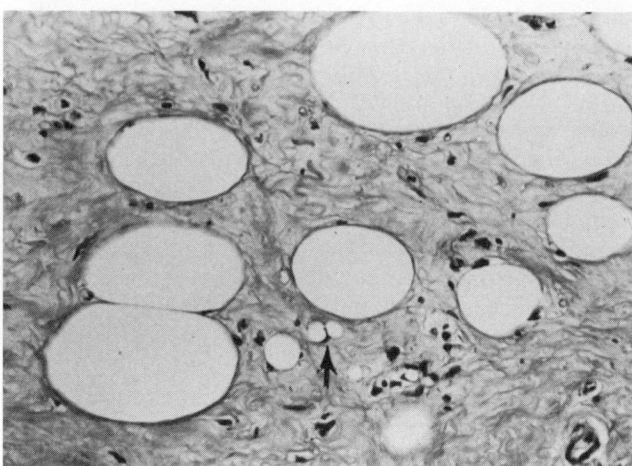

Figure 16-3 In the sclerosing type of well-differentiated liposarcoma, delicate collagen fibrils constitute a prominent part of the matrix. Note the bivacuolated lipoblast (*arrow*).

ical stromal cells, many of which contain highly abnormal mitotic figures. Areas of hemorrhage and necrosis are common. *Dedifferentiated liposarcoma* refers to a neoplasm that contains both a well-differentiated liposarcomatous component and elements of undifferentiated spindle cell sarcoma, often resembling MFH. This tumor arises most frequently in the retroperitoneum, but it may affect the groin or the extremity.[100,101]

Synovial Sarcoma

Synovial sarcomas are the fourth most common STS. They characteristically have a biphasic pattern that gives the impression of glandular formation, which was originally thought to be indicative of synovial origin. These tumors, however, rarely arise within a joint but rather have distributions similar to those of other STSs. Uncommon primary sites include retropharynx, orofacial area, and retroperitoneum. Synovial sarcomas occur in a younger age group than other sarcomas; 72 percent of patients in one large study were below the age of 40 years.[102] There is a propensity for the distal portions of extremities; hand (5 percent), ankle (9 percent), or foot (13 percent). The plain radiograph often shows small calcifications within a soft tissue mass; this should alert the physician to the diagnosis. Occasionally lymphatic spread occurs (5 to 7 percent). Virtually all synovial sarcomas are high grade.

Gross Characteristics Typically the tumor presents as a deep-seated, well-circumscribed, firm multinodular mass. Actual contiguity with a synovium-lined space is rare. It is common to find solitary or multiple cysts on sectioning the lesion. The poorly differentiated variety is likely to present as an ill-defined, infiltrative lesion with a soft, somewhat gelatinous consistency.

Microscopic Characteristics The classic form of this tumor has a biphasic pattern (Fig. 16-4). This implies the presence of two distinct cell populations: spindle cells and epithelioid cells. The plump spindle cells, usually the

---

TABLE 16-3   Histological Classification of Liposarcoma

Well-differentiated liposarcoma
  Lipoma-like
  Sclerosing
  Inflammatory
  Dedifferentiated

Myxoid liposarcoma

Round cell liposarcoma

Pleomorphic liposarcoma

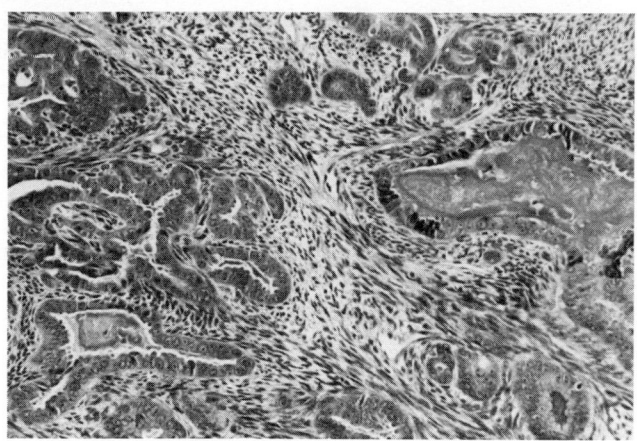

Figure 16-4 Typical synovial sarcoma in its biphasic form, characterized by glandlike structures lined by cuboidal cells intimately associated with a spindle cell sarcomatous component.

predominant component, form an interlacing fascicular pattern. The epithelioid cells form either solid nests or glandlike structures. When constituting glandular spaces, the cells range from cuboidal to tall columnar and rarely undergo squamous metaplasia. The application of special stains demonstrates that the lumina of these glandular spaces often contain epithelial-type mucins. The neoplasm may contain extensive areas of dense stromal hyalinization, and focal calcification is common. The presence of extensive areas of calcification, sometimes with modulation to benign osteoid, deserves recognition, as this rare, calcifying variant imparts a significantly more favorable prognosis.[103] Within the spindle cell portion of the tumor, areas resembling the branching vascular pattern of hemangiopericytoma commonly occur. The existence of a monophasic spindle cell sarcoma is recognized, although distinction from fibrosarcoma can be exceedingly difficult.

Epithelioid Sarcoma

Epithelioid sarcoma was first described in 1970.[102] It is an unusually small tumor that is often misdiagnosed as a benign lesion. It occurs in the forearm and wrist one-half the time and is the most common sarcoma of the hand. This lesion has a propensity for eventual lymph node involvement. Rarely, it presents as a metastasis to the epitrochlear lymph node. Unlike other sarcomas, it occurs predominantly in adolescents and young adults (average age, 26 years). When it arises in the dermis, where it presents as a nodular or ulcerative process, it often clinically simulates benign cutaneous diseases, such as granulomatous dermatitis.

Gross Characteristics The tumor usually arises in the deep soft tissues, particularly in relation to tendons, fascia, and aponeuroses, and presents as a firm, often multinodular mass. Central nodular hemorrhage and/or necrosis is occasionally encountered.

Microscopic Characteristics The typical low-power picture is that of nodules or granuloma-like collections of epithelioid cells. These are large cells with deeply eosinophilic cytoplasm and nuclei that tend to be angulated and hyperchromatic. Mitotic figures are occasionally seen. The predominant epithelioid cells often transform to plump spindle cells. A characteristic feature of this tumor is the propensity for diffuse infiltration of tendinous and fascial structures by small, elongated nests of tumor cells.

Clear Cell Sarcoma (Malignant Melanoma of Soft Parts)

Clear cell sarcoma is a small, unusual neoplasm that arises in conjunction with tendons or aponeuroses. It occurs most often around the foot and ankle (46 percent) and in persons between 20 and 40 years of age.[102] The histogenesis is unknown but is considered by some to be related to melanoma; 50 percent of these lesions contain melanin. Appropriate diagnosis depends on special histologic stains: Fontana preparation for melanin, periodic acid–Schiff (PAS) for intracellular glycogen, and reticulin stains to demonstrate a nesting pattern. Lymphatic as well as hematogenous spread occurs. One must examine the regional lymph nodes carefully. If there is any suggestion of enlargement, a lymph node dissection is recommended.

Gross Characteristics The neoplasm presents as a solitary or multinodular firm mass, frequently attached to tendons or aponeuroses. The tumor infrequently exceeds 6 cm in diameter and varies from white to brown on cut surface.

Microscopic Characteristics The characteristic feature of this neoplasm is the formation of distinct fascicles and nests of spindle cells that are separated by well-defined collagenous trabeculae. The uniform spindle cells are often plump and contain pale to faintly eosinophilic cytoplasm. In addition, the cells contain a vesicular nucleus with a prominent solitary nucleolus. Frequently, bland-appearing multinucleated giant cells are found within the spindle cell fascicles. Application of special stains discloses that the clear spindle cells contain glycogen (PAS-positive) and that melanin pigment is present in half of the tumors.

Malignant Peripheral Nerve Sheath Tumor (Malignant Schwannoma)

Malignant peripheral nerve sheath tumors (MPNSTs) are malignant tumors that arise from the various cellular constituents of peripheral nerves. They represent about 10 percent of all sarcomas. A large percentage (25 to 67 percent) are associated with von Recklinghausen's disease.[102] This subset of patients is at high risk (3 to 13 percent) for developing sarcomas, and the risk increases with each decade of life. Unlike other sarcomas, the MPNST often presents with neurologic symptoms (pain, paresthesia, and weakness), reflecting its relation to major peripheral nerves. Those tumors not associated with neurofibromatosis tend to occur in an older age group. An extremity mass associated with neurologic symptoms must be considered malignant and should be evaluated with the appropriate staging studies.

Gross Characteristics This neoplasm presents as a fusiform or bulbous enlargement of a large nerve, usually within the deep soft tissues. When associated with von Recklinghausen's disease, MPNST can often be demonstrated to arise in a preexisting neurofibroma. As the tumor enlarges and infiltrates the adjacent soft tissues, its origin from and relation to the nerve structure is frequently obscured. On section, the gray-to-white neoplasm varies from firm to soft, with areas of necrosis and hemorrhage.

Microscopic Characteristics The basic pattern consists of intersecting spindle cell fascicles, not unlike that observed with fibrosarcoma or leiomyosarcoma. However, the presence of certain differential features supports the diagnosis of a malignant peripheral nerve sheath tumor. The slender nuclei of the spindle cells tend to be wavy or buckled. A palisading pattern, although not pathognomonic, typifies this entity. In areas, the spindle cells may form whorled, tactoid, or plexiform arrangements. The rarely encountered epithelioid variant may closely resemble malignant melanoma or even carcinoma. Infrequently, heterologous elements such as osteoid, chondroid, skeletal muscle, or glandular structures arise within the spindle cell background. The MPNST combined with rhabdomyosarcomatous elements, a rare variant often presenting in the context of von Recklinghausen's disease, has been called a malignant Triton tumor.

BENIGN SOFT TISSUE TUMORS

All mesenchymal tissue can give rise to benign lesions. Occasionally these can be confused with malignant lesions, or they may become symptomatic due to their size, anatomic location, or both. Although these tumors are benign, local recurrence or difficult anatomic location can cause significant morbidity. Some, such as lipomas, are easily cured by simple removal, while others, most notably fibromatoses, require extensive resection. Thus, it is important to differentiate these lesions from their malignant counterparts, establish a correct diagnosis, and remove them surgically.

There are a large number of benign lesions. The more common lesions and their unique characteristics are described.

Benign Adipose Tumors

Simple Lipoma

Lipomas, the most common mesenchymal neoplasms, arise from normal fat and appear during adulthood. They may be single or multiple; the latter occur in only 5 percent of all patients. They are found either subcutaneously or deeply embedded. Eighty percent of all lipomas are of

the subcutaneous type.[102] The shoulder girdle and proximal thigh are the two most common sites. Simple surgical excision is curative.

Gross Characteristics Superficial lipomas, arising within the subcutaneous layer, present as well-circumscribed, movable, round to ovoid masses. The lesions reveal, on cut section, a homogeneous pale- to bright-yellow tissue. Deep lipomas, which are much rarer than the superficial variety, may occur in an intermuscular space. The gross appearance of these lipomas is indistinguishable from that of the superficial type.

Microscopic Characteristics Both types of lipoma consist of monotonous sheets of mature fat cells that are ovoid to round and usually contain a single fat droplet, which compresses the nucleus along the cell membrane. Capillary-like vessels occasionally appear between the fat lobules. Areas of myxoid change or dense fibrous trabeculae are sometimes encountered.

Spindle Cell Lipoma

This is a variant of lipoma, consisting of benign spindle cells in addition to mature fat. The tumor has a predilection for males (90 percent) and most commonly occurs in the neck and shoulder. Spindle cell lipomas are encapsulated and are easily removed by simple excision. It is essential to distinguish this lesion clinically from a well-differentiated liposarcoma.

Gross Characteristics Both these benign lipomatous tumors are similar to and usually indistinguishable from the ordinary lipoma. They invariably arise within the subcutis and are encapsulated with a delicate fibrous membrane. On sectioning, they vary from diffuse yellow to having foci of white, firm, fibrous tissue or even gray myxoid areas.

Microscopic Characteristics Spindle cell lipoma reveals a component of mature adipose tissue with rare to abundant clusters of spindle cells dispersed throughout the fat. The spindle cells are uniform and in parallel arrangement. Mitotic figures are rarely noted.

Pleomorphic lipomas also consist of mature fat cells, but they are more variable in size. Instead of spindle cells, both pleomorphic and distinctive multinucleated giant cells are found. These giant cells contain multiple peripheral overlapping nuclei. Occasionally, lipoblast-like cells occur.

Intramuscular and Intermuscular Lipoma

Lipomas occurring within (intramuscular) and between (intermuscular) muscle groups often become large, produce few symptoms, and present as a mass mimicking an STS. Clinical evaluation and staging are similar to those of any suspected sarcoma. The pathologist must be aware of the clinical setting, and an adequate sample must be obtained in order to differentiate a low-grade liposarcoma from a true benign lipoma. Unlike superficial lipomas, these lesions often do not have a capsule and tend to infiltrate the surrounding muscle. A marginal or wide resection is required to obtain local control. These lesions never become malignant.

Gross Characteristics This tumor presents either as a relatively well delineated yellow mass clearly distinguishable from the surrounding skeletal muscle or as an ill-defined infiltrative lesion that gradually blends into the adjacent muscle tissue, imparting a marbled appearance.

Microscopic Characteristics The lesion is characterized by sheets and nests of mature adipose tissue insinuating themselves between bundles and individual fibers of viable skeletal muscle. The fat cells lack features of cytologic atypia, and lipoblasts never occur.

Benign Tumors of Peripheral Nerves

The two most common nerve tumors are neurilemmoma (schwannoma) and neurofibroma.

Neurilemmoma

These benign growths arise within a nerve and are surrounded by a true capsule composed of the epineurium. They are composed of Antoni A (cellular) and Antoni B (loose myxoid) components. These lesions generally are not associated with von Recklinghausen's disease. Surgical treatment entails opening the capsule and enucleating the growth from the nerve. "Ancient" neurilemmoma refers to a cystic degeneration of a neurilemmoma. These lesions clinically present as a large mass with some cellular atypia. They must be differentiated from malignant lesions. Simple excision, done for diagnostic purposes or if the lesion is symptomatic, is curative.

Gross Characteristics These tumors are invariably encapsulated and range from fusiform to ovoid. It is usually possible to demonstrate the nerve of origin. The tissue varies from white to yellow. As the lesion increases in size, there is a greater likelihood of cystic degeneration and focal hemorrhage.

Microscopic Characteristics Reliable diagnosis depends on the identification of the two basic cell patterns, the so-called Antoni A and Antoni B areas. The Antoni A pattern, the more cellular of the two, is characterized by plump spindle cells arranged in fascicles, palisaded rows, or whorls (Fig. 16-5). The parallel alignment of two rows of nuclei has been called a *Verocay body.* An Antoni B area discloses an unpatterned distribution of spindle cells in a loose, somewhat myxoid matrix (Fig. 16-6). There may be a sprinkling of chronic inflammatory cells and clusters of xanthoma cells.

Neurofibroma

Neurofibromas may be solitary or multiple. Unlike the neurilemmomas, they are not encapsulated, often enlarge the nerves, and may undergo malignant degeneration.

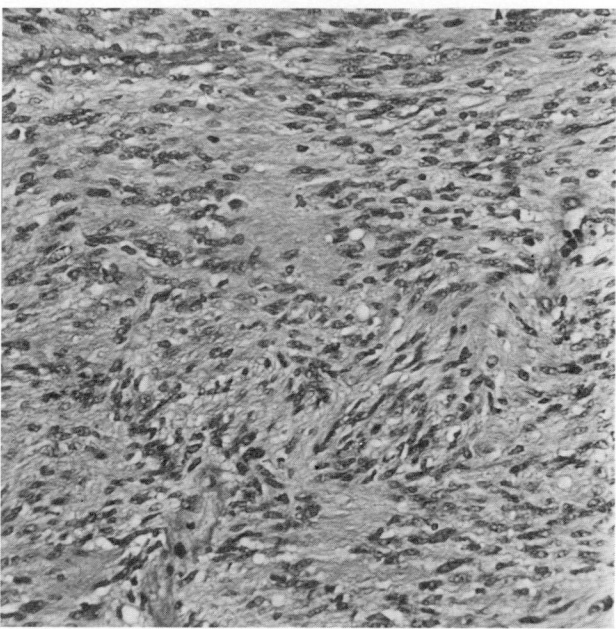

Figure 16-5 The solid, or Antoni A, portion of a neurilemmoma with an area of nuclear palisading.

Histologically they consist of Schwann cells associated with collagen fibrils and myxoid material. Multiple neurofibromas are found in patients with von Recklinghausen's disease (multiple neurofibromatosis). These lesions cannot be surgically detached from the underlying nerve. Surgery is indicated only if malignant degeneration is suspected. Between 20 and 65 percent of patients with neurofibromatosis ultimately develop a sarcoma.

Gross Characteristics These lesions may be encapsulated, although they usually infiltrate into adjacent soft tissues.

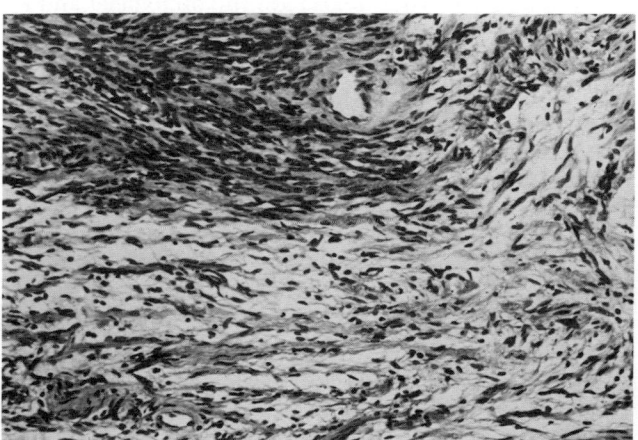

Figure 16-6 In contrast to the Antoni A pattern, the Antoni B region reveals a less organized cellularity dispersed in a loose myxoid matrix.

Microscopic Characteristics The tumor is characterized by individual or slender bundles of elongated wavy spindle cells closely opposed to dense fibers of mature collagen. Groups of these spindle cell–collagen units randomly intersect at variable angles. The matrix, which is rich in hyaluronic acid, can be sparse or may present as a highly myxoid background; in the latter case, it may often obscure the nerve sheath origin of the lesion. The spindle cell nuclei occasionally appear hyperchromatic or pleomorphic, yet mitotic figures are exceedingly rare.

Benign Fibrous Tumors

There is a large variety of benign fibrous tumors.[102] Most are treated by simple excision. Aggressive fibromatosis is a benign but locally aggressive lesion deserving special consideration.

Aggressive Fibromatosis

This tumor, which appears bland microscopically, is the most serious of all the benign soft tissue tumors. It does not have a capsule and tends to infiltrate far beyond its clinically recognized boundaries. This lesion does not respect fascial borders and, if untreated, can attain a large size involving multiple anatomic compartments. The most common locations are the neck, shoulder, and pelvic girdle. Death results from intrathoracic or retroperitoneal extension. The clinical history often reveals multiple recurrences despite "adequate" surgical removal. The appropriate surgical procedure is wide excision. Local recurrence uniformly follows excision with positive margins. Surgical staging studies should be performed prior to resection. Amputation is occasionally required. Radiation and chemotherapy have recently been utilized for unresectable fibromatosis.

Gross Characteristics The general category of fibromatosis can be split into two subtypes. The superficial fibromatoses encompass, among others, the palmar (Dupuytren's contracture) and plantar types. Among the deep fibromatoses (desmoids) are the abdominal and extraabdominal varieties. Palmar and plantar fibromatoses appear identical and range from foci of thickened fascia to individual or coalescent firm nodules. In contrast, the abdominal and extraabdominal fibromatoses present as firm, often multinodular masses, which arise from fascial planes and infiltrate, to some extent, the adjacent skeletal muscle. These lesions can attain a rather large size. They tend to be firm, and the cut surface reveals a white-gray tissue.

Microscopic Characteristics The hallmark of both the superficial and the deep varieties is the uniformity of the spindle cells and the regularity of the pattern. The cellularity can be focally increased, particularly in the superficial types, yet the arrangement of uniform spindle cells in a typical nodular or fascicular pattern is maintained. Mitoses are infrequent and abnormal forms are never present. The matrix consists of a variable quantity of mature, dense collagen bundles. At the periphery of the deep fibromatoses, infiltration of adjacent skeletal muscle is characteristic and does not by itself serve as a valid basis for a diagnosis of fibrosarcoma.

Benign Vascular Tumors

Hemangioma

Benign tumors of the blood vessels consist of a variety of hemangiomas. It is not certain if these are true neoplasms, hamartomas, or vascular malformations. In general there are two types of hemangiomas—generalized and localized; localized are more common. Hemangiomas are classified based upon their pathologic appearance—capillary, cavernous, venous, or arteriovenous. Capillary hemangiomas are the most common type. Most hemangiomas occur during childhood. Venous hemangiomas occur during adulthood and are often deeply situated. Intramuscular hemangiomas are rare and are occasionally difficult to differentiate from angiosarcomas. Evaluation requires angiography and venography. Surgery is indicated if symptoms develop. Hemangiomas rarely become malignant.

Gross Characteristics The gross characteristics depend in large part on the histological variety and anatomic distribution of the hemangioma (Table 16-4). The localized types tend to appear as a well-circumscribed, red-to-purple mass, although examples with poorly defined, infiltrative borders, particularly in the deep-seated hemangiomas, are not uncommon. Intramuscular hemangioma (infiltrating angiolipoma) can present as a red, highly vascular lesion or as a yellow-to-gray firm mass, depending on the proportion of the vascular component to the amount of accompanying adipose tissue and fibrous stroma.

TABLE 16-4 Classification of Soft Tissue Vascular Tumors

I. Benign
  Localized hemangioma
    Capillary hemangioma
    Cavernous hemangioma
    Venous hemangioma
    Arteriovenous hemangioma
    Epithelioid hemangioma
    Deep soft tissue hemangiomas (synovial, intramuscular, neural)
  Diffuse hemangioma
    Angiomatosis

II. Borderline malignancy
  Epithelioid hemangioendothelioma

III. Malignant
  Angiosarcoma
  Kaposi's sarcoma

Source: Reproduced with permission from Enzinger FM, Weiss SW: *Soft Tissue Tumors,* 3d ed. St Louis, Mosby, 1995, p 757.

Angiomatosis indicates a benign condition in which multiple types of mesenchymal tissues are involved. Large anatomic regions, even an entire limb, may be affected. These extensive vascular lesions, which are probably hamartomatous, can involve the skin, subcutaneous fat, skeletal muscle, fascia, and bone. Involvement of an entire extremity can cause hypertrophy of the limb.

Microscopic Characteristics Pure types of vascular tumors are uncommon; there tends to be some degree of admixture of small and large vessels. Capillary hemangioma consists of myriad small vascular channels lined by a flattened endothelial layer. Particularly in some juvenile types of capillary hemangioma, the vascular channels may be miniature, and a highly cellular stroma predominates. Cavernous hemangioma, in contrast, is characterized by large, engorged vascular channels separated by fibrocollagenous septa.

The diagnosis of intramuscular hemangioma or angiomatosis usually requires clinical and gross pathologic correlation. At the microscopic level, these entities are nonspecific except that the identification of adjacent skeletal muscle or other soft tissue elements indicates the extensive involvement of the lesion. The vessels, as in the circumscribed hemangiomas, are well formed and vary from capillary to venous size. There is a single flat endothelial layer. The extravascular stroma contains adipose tissue and sometimes fibromuscular fascicles.

Other Benign Tumors

Pigmented Villonodular Synovitis

Pigmented villonodular synovitis (PVNS) is a rare primary disease of the synovium characterized by exuberant proliferation with the formation of villi and nodules. It presents with localized pain, joint swelling, a thickened synovium, and an effusion that, on aspiration, shows either a brownish or a serosanguineous discoloration. This tumor commonly occurs between the second and the fifth decade of life. The knee is most commonly involved (75 to 90 percent), followed by the hip and the ankle joint. Treatment is often delayed because PVNS is not considered in the differential diagnosis. Clinical suspicion is the key to early diagnosis. Pigmented villonodular synovitis should always be considered in the differential diagnosis of a monoarticular arthritis of the knee or hip joint. Simple aspiration is often suggestive, and a synovial biopsy is definitive. Plain radiographs demonstrate juxtacortical erosions of both sides of an affected joint and may show marked joint and/or bone destruction if the disease has been present for a long time. Arthrography and/or arthroscopy are helpful in establishing the correct diagnosis. Arthrography shows diffuse nodular masses, while arthroscopy shows a brownish, discolored synovium with large, flattened nodules and villous proliferation. Rarely, PVNS may present as a primary bony or soft tissue tumor due to marked proliferation of the synovium with destruction of the adjacent joint and/or a soft tissue mass. The histologic findings in this clinical situation may incorrectly suggest an MFH.

This lesion is best treated by surgical excision. Localized lesions require simple excision, while extensive involvement requires a synovectomy. The anterior and/or posterior compartments of the knee may be extensively involved. This necessitates a staged approach. The anterior joint is treated through a standard midline incision and arthrotomy. The posterior knee is best approached by a popliteal incision with complete exposure of the posterior capsule. In general, it is the author's preference to first proceed with the anterior synovectomy and regain knee motion, and secondarily to perform a posterior synovectomy. Joint manipulation is often required at 10 days. Recurrent disease should be retreated by surgical excision. If there is extensive bony destruction, arthrodesis or prosthetic replacement, combined with an extraarticular joint resection, is required. Low-dose radiation treatment may be beneficial in improving local control, particularly in high-risk patients.

Gross Characteristics The thick synovium is variegated tan-brown to yellow and ranges from villous to nodular.

Microscopic Characteristics The typical lesion consists of a heterogeneous population of cells. The villi are lined by several layers of plump synovial cells (Fig. 16-7). Beneath the synovium are found sheets of histiocytes, xanthoma cells, hemosiderin-laden macrophages, and multinucleated giant cells, all in variable proportion. Occasionally, slitlike spaces are present within the more cellular areas.

Ganglion

Ganglia are among the most common soft tissue lesions treated by the orthopaedic surgeon. The wrist is the most common location; other sites include the metatarsophalangeal joints and the ankle and knee joints. When the lesions are located in unusual sites, the diagnosis is often less obvious. Ganglia represent benign myxoid degeneration. It must be emphasized that not all masses are ganglia

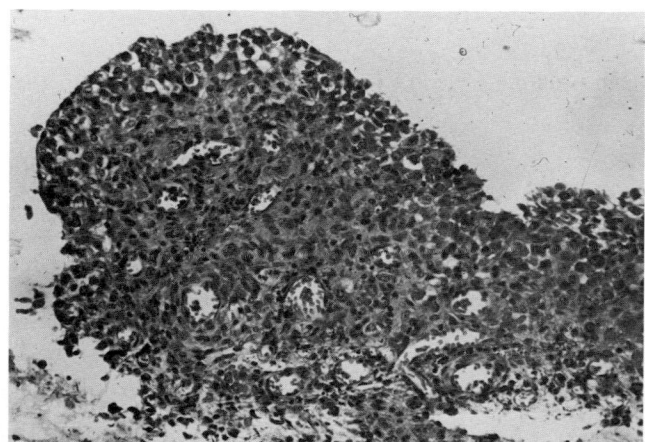

Figure 16-7 In pigmented villonodular synovitis, there is hyperplasia of the surface synovial cells and the stroma is filled with inflammatory cells, histiocytes, and hemosiderin-laden macrophages.

and therefore all should be critically evaluated. All too often a sarcoma of the hand or ankle is assumed to be a ganglion. Excision is undertaken, and the correct diagnosis is made only after extensive soft tissue contamination has occurred. This unfortunate circumstance leads to many lost limbs. Treatment of ganglia is simple excision or aspiration.

Gross Characteristics Ganglia are uniloculated or multiloculated cystic lesions arising in dense ligamentous tissue. The cysts contain a translucent gelatinous material, the expression of which results in the partial collapse of the thin-walled cysts.

Microscopic Characteristics The cyst walls consist of a dense paucicellular fibrocollagenous tissue lacking an epithelial or synovial lining. The intercystic connective tissue often contains small foci of myxoid stroma with scattered spindle cells. The cyst(s) may contain a pale-blue, acellular myxoid ground substance.

MALIGNANT BONE TUMORS

Primary malignancies of bone arise from mesenchymal cells (sarcomas) and bone marrow cells (myeloma and lymphoma). Bone is also a common site of metastasis from a variety of carcinomas. Osteosarcoma and Ewing's sarcoma, the most common malignant mesenchymal bone tumors, usually occur during childhood and adolescence. Other mesenchymal tumors (MFH, fibrosarcoma, chondrosarcoma), while occasionally seen in childhood, are more common in adults. Multiple myeloma and metastatic carcinoma typically increase in frequency with increasing patient age. This section describes the clinical, radiographic, and pathologic characteristics and treatment of the primary bone sarcomas. Table 16-5 presents a general classification of the benign and malignant bone tumors as described by Dahlin.[21] Their characteristic locations within a bone are shown schematically in Fig. 16-8.

Osteosarcoma provides the model on which treatment of all other sarcomas is based. The effectiveness of multiagent chemotherapy regimens has been proved by increasing overall survival rates from the bleak 15 to 20 percent with surgery alone in the 1970s to 55 to 80 percent by the 1980s.[104–108] In parallel with improved survival, dramatic advances in reconstructive surgery have resulted in limb salvage supplanting amputation as the standard method of treatment.[10,22,63,64,67,69,109] Techniques of reconstruction include resection-arthrodesis, massive allograft or prosthetic-allograft composite replacement, custom endoprosthetic replacement, or, more recently, modular endoprosthetic replacement (Fig. 16-9).

TABLE 16-5 General Classification of Bone Tumors[a]

Histological type	Distribution, %[b]	Benign	Malignant
Hematopoietic	41.4		Myeloma Reticulum cell sarcoma
Chondrogenic	20.9	Osteochondroma Chondroma Chondroblastoma Chondromyxoid fibroma	Primary chondrosarcoma Secondary chondrosarcoma Dedifferentiated chondrosarcoma Mesenchymal chondrosarcoma
Osteogenic	19.3	Osteoid osteoma Benign osteoblastoma	Osteosarcoma Parosteal osteogenic sarcoma
Unknown origin	9.8	Giant cell tumor (Fibrous) histiocytoma	Ewing's tumor Malignant giant cell tumor Adamantinoma (Fibrous) histiocytoma
Fibrogenic	3.8	Fibroma Desmoplastic fibroma	Fibrosarcoma
Notochordal	3.1		Chordoma
Vascular	1.6	Hemangioma	Hemangioendothelioma Hemangiopericytoma
Lipogenic	<0.5	Lipoma	
Neurogenic	<0.5	Neurilemmoma	

[a]Classification based on Lichtenstein: *Cancer* 4:335–351, 1951.
[b]Distribution based on Mayo Clinic experience.
Source: Adapted with permission from Dahlin DC: *Bone Tumors: General Aspects and Data on 6,221 Cases,* 3d ed. Springfield, IL, Charles C Thomas, 1978.

Figure 16-8 Common anatomic location of benign and malignant bone tumors with respect to the diaphysis, metaphysis, and epiphysis of the bone. (Modified and reproduced with permission from Madewell JE, Ragsdale BD, Sweet DE: Radiographic and pathologic analysis of solitary bone lesions: parts I, II, and III. *Radiol Clin North Am* 19:715–814, 1981).

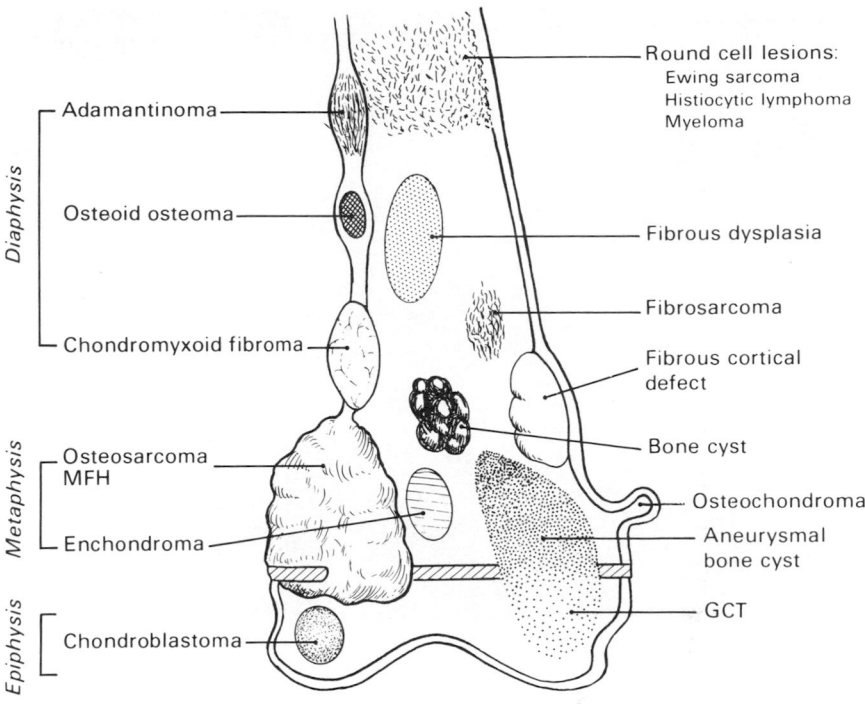

Classic Osteosarcoma

Osteosarcoma (OS) is a high-grade malignant spindle cell tumor arising within a bone. Its distinguishing characteristic is the production of "tumor" osteoid, or immature bone, directly from a malignant spindle cell stroma.[21,46,110,111]

Clinical Characteristics

Osteosarcoma typically occurs during childhood and adolescence. In patients over the age of 40, it is usually associated with a preexistent disease such as Paget's disease, irradiated bones, multiple hereditary exostosis, or polyostotic fibrous dysplasia.[21,110] The most common sites are bones of the knee joint (50 percent) and the proximal humerus (25 percent). While 80 to 90 percent of OS occurs in the long tubular bones,[21,24,110,112,113] the axial skeleton is rarely affected.

With the exception of the level of serum alkaline phosphatase, which is elevated in 45 to 50 percent of patients, laboratory findings are usually not helpful.[114] Furthermore, an elevated alkaline phosphatase level per se is not diagnostic, since it is also found in association with other skeletal diseases such as hyperparathyroidism (brown tumor), fibrous dysplasia, and Paget's disease. Pain is the most common complaint on presentation, with a firm, soft-tissue mass fixed to the underlying bone found on physical examination. Systemic symptoms are rare. The incidence of pathologic fracture is less than 1 percent.[114]

Radiographic Characteristics

Typical radiographic findings include increased intramedullary sclerosis (due to tumor bone or calcified cartilage), an area of radiolucency (due to nonossified tu-

mor), a pattern of permeative destruction with poorly defined borders, cortical destruction, periosteal elevation, and extraosseous extension with soft tissue ossification.[113,115] This combination of characteristics is not seen with any other lesions. Wilner classified 600 radiographs of OS seen at New York's Memorial Sloan-Kettering into three broad categories[113]: sclerotic OS (32 percent), osteolytic OS (22 percent), and mixed OS (46 percent) (Fig. 16-10). Although there was no statistically significant difference in overall survival rates among these types, it is important to recognize the patterns. The sclerotic and mixed types offer few diagnostic problems. Errors of diagnosis most often occur with pure osteolytic tumors. The differential diagnosis of osteolytic OS includes giant cell tumors, aneurysmal bone cyst, fibrosarcoma, and MFH.[25]

Gross Characteristics

This tumor is central in origin, but at the time of diagnosis there is often already substantial cortical destruction. Continued growth of the lesion results in bulky involvement of the adjacent soft tissues. As the neoplasm extends through the cortex, the periosteum may be elevated; this stimulates reactive bone formation and accounts for the radiologic features of the so-called Codman's triangle. Longitudinal sectioning of the involved bone often reveals wide extension within the marrow cavity. Rarely, skip areas can be demonstrated.[112] The consistency of the tumor varies greatly and generally reflects the predominant histologic composition. There may be soft, necrotic and hemorrhagic foci. Sclerotic and bony regions reflect a preponderance of fibrotic or osteoblastic elements, respectively. Occasionally, a lobulated cartilaginous appearance is observed.

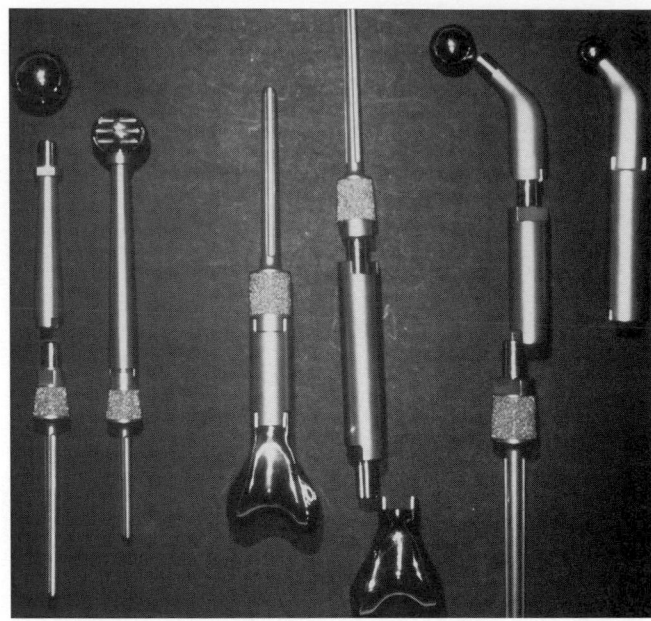

A

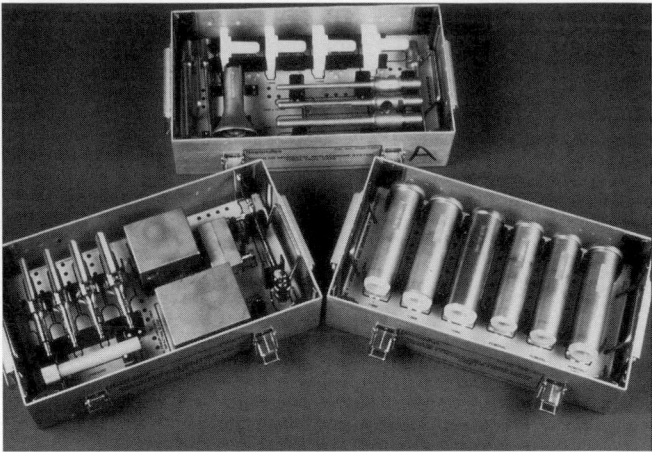

B

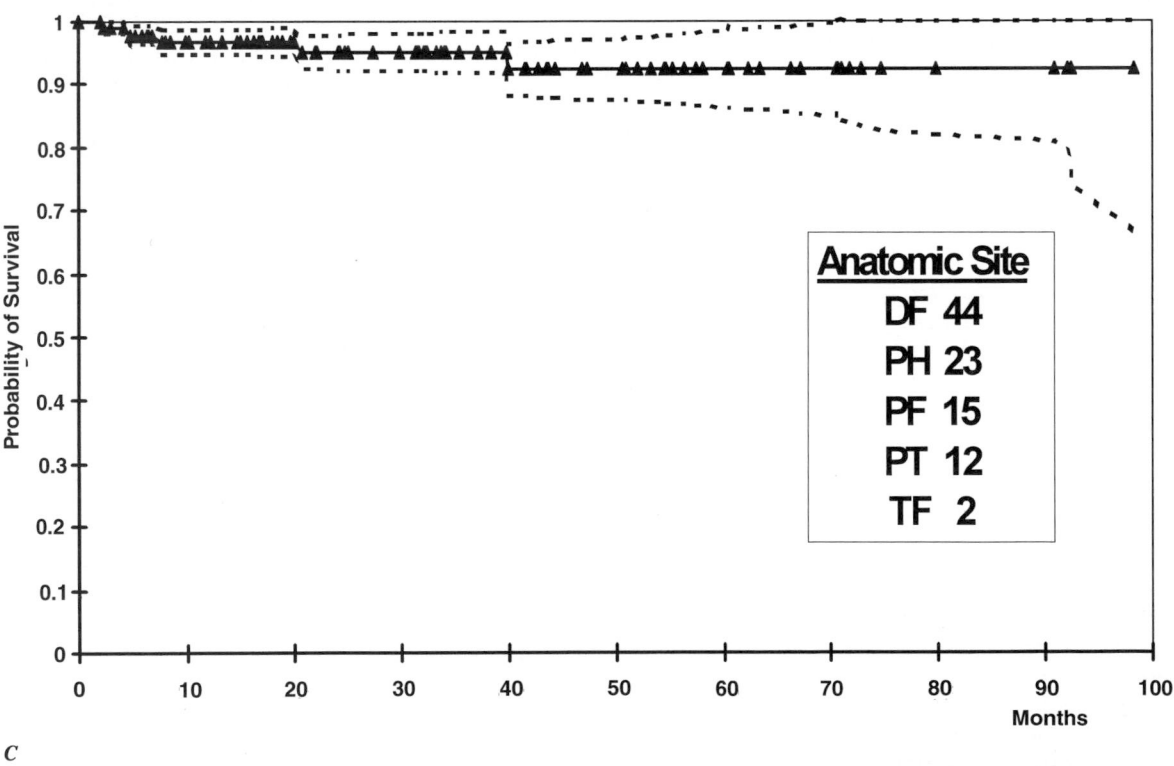

C

Figure 16-9 The modular segmental replacement system (MSRS) permits intraoperative selection and assembly of endoprostheses, allowing replacement of the proximal humerus, proximal femur, distal femur, proximal tibia, and total femur. *A.* Modular components are assembled using interlocking Morse tapers. *B.* Universal instrumentation for prosthetic assembly and preparation of bone for cemented insertion of the selected stem. *C.* Kaplan-Meier survival analysis of 96 consecutive MSRS replacements demonstrating 92.3% overall survival at all sites after a median follow-up of 32.2 months. (Adapted from Henshaw RM, Jones V, Malawer MM: Skeletal reconstruction with noncustom modular endoprostheses. Results of the first 96 consecutive MSRS prosthetic replacements. Presented at the Ninth Annual Symposium of the International Society of Technology in Arthroplasty, Amsterdam, The Netherlands, August 1996.)

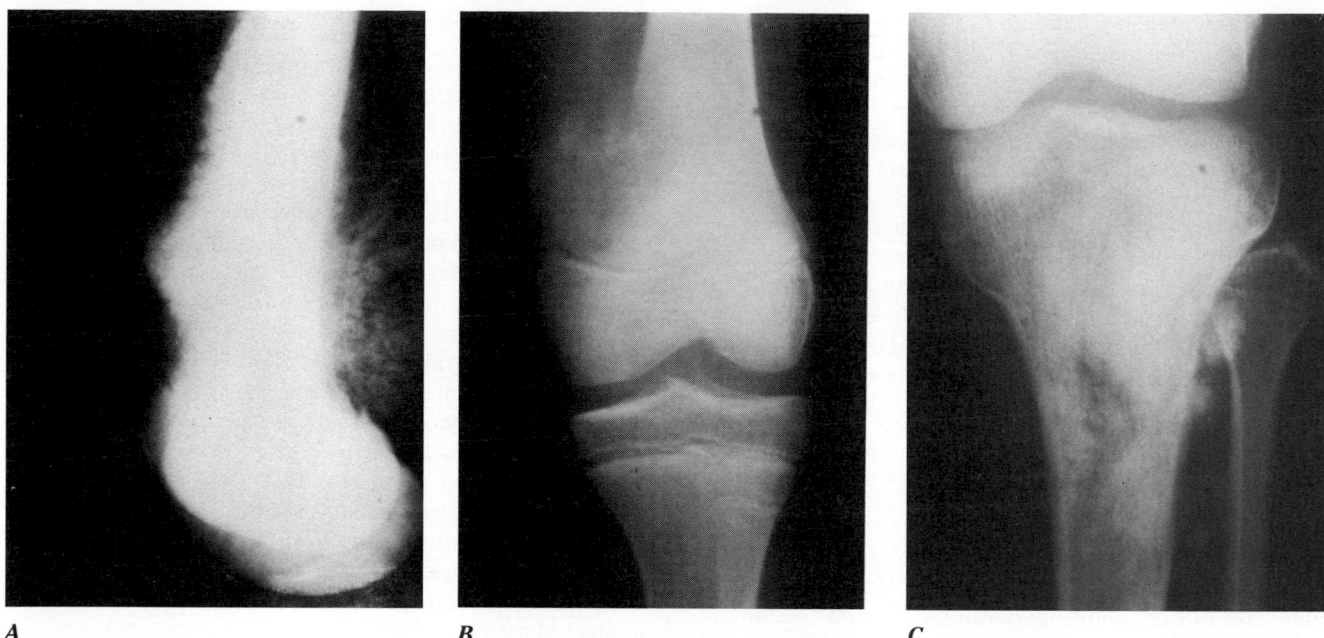

A   *B*   *C*

Figure 16-10 The three radiographic patterns of osteosarcoma. *A.* Sclerosing. *B.* Osteolytic. *C.* Mixed (osteolytic and osteoblastic). Mixed is the most common. There is no correlation between radiographic type and survival. All three show extraosseous new bone formation. This is pathognomonic of a bone-forming neoplasm. (Reproduced with permission from Malawer MM, Abelson HT, Suit HD: Sarcomas of bone, in DeVita VT, Hellman S, Rosenberg SA (eds): *Cancer: Principles and Practice of Oncology,* 2d ed. Philadelphia, Lippincott, 1985, pp 1293–1343.)

Microscopic Characteristics

The diagnosis of OS is based on the identification of a malignant stroma that produces unequivocal osteoid matrix. The stroma consists of a haphazard arrangement of highly atypical cells. The pleomorphic cells contain hyperchromatic, irregular nuclei. Mitotic figures, often atypical, are usually easy to identify. Between these cells is a delicate, lacelike eosinophilic matrix, assumed to be malignant osteoid. Both malignant and benign osteoblast-like giant cells can be found in the stroma. An abundance of the latter type can create confusion with giant-cell tumor of bone. A predominance of one tissue type has resulted in a histologic subclassification of OS.[116] The term *osteoblastic osteosarcoma* is utilized for those tumors in which the production of malignant osteoid prevails. The pattern is usually that of a delicate meshwork of osteoid, as noted above, although broader confluent areas can be present (Fig. 16-11). Calcification of the matrix is variable. Some tumors reveal a predominance of malignant cartilage production; hence the term *chondroblastic osteosarcoma.* Even though the malignant cartilaginous elements may be overwhelming, the presence of a malignant osteoid matrix warrants the diagnosis of OS. Yet another variant is characterized by large areas of proliferating fibroblasts, arranged in intersecting fascicles. Such areas are indistinguishable from fibrosarcoma, and thorough sampling may be necessary to identify the malignant osteoid component. The so-called *telangiectatic* type of OS contains multiple blood-filled cystic and sinusoidal spaces of variable size. There

may be minimal osteoid production; benign giant cells are invariably present. However, identification of marked cytologic atypia in the septa and in more solid areas rules out the possibility of aneurysmal bone cyst or giant-cell tumor. A rare low-grade central osteosarcoma has been de-

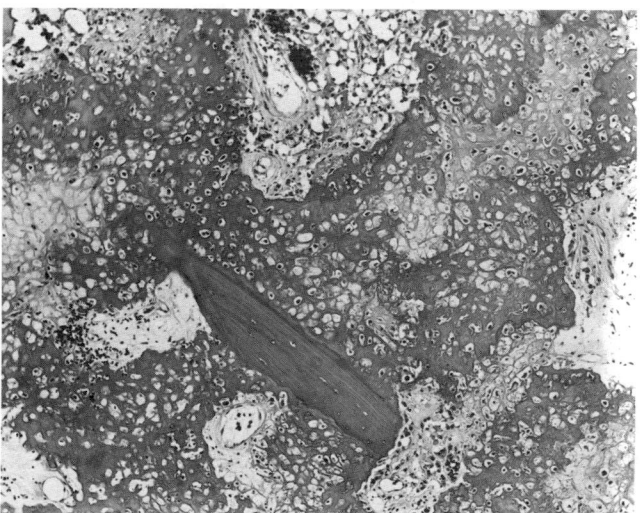

Figure 16-11 Broad coalescent sheets of malignant osteoid typify this osteoblastic osteosarcoma. The spicule of lamellar bone is a remnant of the normal medullary bone.

scribed that may be difficult to diagnose, since it can closely resemble desmoplastic fibroma or fibrous dysplasia.[117] It is important to recognize this variant, for while it has an excellent prognosis, metastasis may occur.

The advent of several successful chemotherapeutic regimens for OS has permitted the examination of multiple posttherapy radical resection specimens.[118] The degree of tumor necrosis is variable and ranges between 0 and 100 percent. The osteoid or osseous matrix remains, without its accompanying cellular component. There may be growth of a reparative type of connective tissue with fibroblastic proliferation and clusters of small vessels. The spindle cells may reveal a degree of cytologic atypia.

Prognosis

Prior to adjuvant chemotherapy, effective treatment was limited to radical margin amputation. Metastasis to the lungs and other bones generally occurred within 24 months. Overall survival ranged from 5 to 20 percent at 2 years.[1,119,120] No significant correlation between overall survival and histologic subtypes, tumor size, patient age, or degree of malignancy was seen. The most significant clinical variable discovered was anatomic site: pelvic and axial lesions have a lower survival rate than extremity tumors, while tibial lesions have a better survival rate than femoral lesions.

The dismal outcome associated with osteosarcoma has been dramatically altered by adjuvant chemotherapy as well as by aggressive thoracotomy for pulmonary disease.[6,121–123] A recent update[124] of the Musculoskeletal Tumor Society's combined tumor registry of 227 patients showed that 48 percent remained alive at an average 11 years after surgery. Of critical importance was that no difference in local recurrence or overall survival was seen between patients undergoing amputation versus limb-sparing surgery. Recently described prognostic indicators include tumor necrosis in response to neoadjuvant chemotherapy and the surgical margins achieved at the time of resection.[125,126]

Chemotherapy protocols have typically included various combinations and dosage schedules of high-dose methotrexate (HDMTX), doxorubicin hydrochloride (Adriamycin), and cisplatin. Recently, ifosfamide, which is as effective as Adriamycin in single-agent studies, has supplanted methotrexate in many ongoing protocols.[127,128] Multiagent chemotherapy, using various dosing schedules, is now considered standard treatment for osteosarcoma.[104,105,129,130] Success with adjuvant chemotherapy led to investigation of treatment in the neoadjuvant (preoperative) setting. When chemotherapy is used in the neoadjuvant setting, tumor response results in shrinkage of the soft tissue components, facilitating surgical excision and subsequent limb salvage.[131]

The unique features of evaluation, management, and surgical resection of tumors of the most common anatomic areas are discussed further on in this chapter. Guidelines and principles discussed in the following section are applicable to all bone sarcomas except round cell tumors.

Limb-Sparing Resection

Limb salvage surgery is a safe operation in approximately 85 percent of individuals.[22,34,62–65,67,68] This technique may be utilized for all spindle cell sarcomas, regardless of histogenesis. When combined with effective adjuvant treatments, the majority of OSs can be treated safely by a limb-sparing resection. The successful management of localized OS and other sarcomas requires careful coordination and timing of staging studies, biopsy, surgery, and preoperative and postoperative chemotherapy and/or radiation therapy. The site of the lesion is evaluated as previously described. Preoperative studies allow the surgeon to conceptualize the local anatomy and the volume of tissue to be resected and reconstructed. All patients should be considered candidates for limb-sparing procedures unless a surgical oncologist familiar with these procedures feels that a nonamputative option has little chance of success. Contaminated tissue planes from misplaced biopsy sites remain a major impediment to successful limb salvage.

Successful limb-sparing procedures consist of three surgical phases.[9]

1. *Resection of tumor* Resection strictly follows the principles of oncologic surgery. Avoiding local recurrence is the criterion of success and the main determinant of the amount of bone and soft tissue to be removed.
2. *Skeletal reconstruction* The average skeletal defect following adequate bone tumor resection measures 15 to 20 cm. Techniques of reconstruction (prosthetic replacement, arthrodesis, allograft, or combination) vary and are independent of the resection, although the degree of resection may favor one technique over the others.
3. *Soft tissue and muscle transfers* Muscle transfers are performed to cover and close the resection site and to restore lost motor power. Adequate skin and muscle coverage is mandatory to decrease postoperative morbidity. Distal tissue transfers are not used because of the possibility of contamination.

Based on the above, the surgical guidelines and techniques of limb-sparing surgery utilized by the authors are summarized as follows[9]:

1. The major neurovascular bundle must be free of tumor.
2. Wide resection of the affected bone with a normal muscle cuff in all directions should be performed.
3. All previous biopsy sites and all potentially contaminated tissues should be removed en bloc.
4. Bone should be resected 3 to 4 cm beyond abnormal uptake as determined by bone scan. This is a safe margin to avoid intraosseous tumor extension. Magnetic resonance imaging is extremely useful in delineating the zone of involvement and allows for accurate resection above the tumor.
5. The adjacent joint and joint capsule should be resected. Extraarticular resection is preferred; it is mandatory in the presence of effusion.
6. A tourniquet should be placed proximal to the lesion if possible. This allows amputation to proceed

proximal to the tourniquet without iatrogenic contamination of the amputation site if the tumor is found to be unresectable at the time of surgery.

7. Adequate motor reconstruction must be accomplished by regional muscle transfers. The type of transfer depends upon the anatomic site and the patient's functional requirements.

8. Adequate soft tissue coverage is needed to decrease the risk of skin flap necrosis and secondary infection.

Contraindications to Limb-Sparing Surgery

The relative contraindications to limb-sparing surgery are as follows[9]:

1. *Major neurovascular involvement*   Though vascular grafts may be utilized, the adjacent nerves are usually at risk, making a successful resection less likely. In addition, the magnitude of resection in combination with vascular reconstruction is often prohibitive.

2. *Pathologic fractures*   A fracture through a bone affected by a tumor spreads tumor cells via the hematoma beyond accurately determined limits. The risk of local recurrence is increased following a pathologic fracture. Neoadjuvant chemotherapy can lead to healing of pathologic fractures, thus permitting a limb-sparing procedure in some individuals.

3. *Inappropriate biopsy sites*   An inappropriate or poorly planned biopsy jeopardizes local tumor control by inadvertently contaminating normal tissue planes and compartments.

4. *Infection*   Implantation of a metallic device or allograft in an infected area is contraindicated. Sepsis jeopardizes the ability to give effective doses of adjuvant chemotherapy.

5. *Immature skeletal age*   In the lower extremity, the predicted leg-length discrepancy should not be greater than 6 to 8 cm. Upper extremity reconstruction is independent of skeletal maturity.

6. *Extensive muscle involvement*   There must be enough muscle remaining for a functional extremity to be reconstructed.

Treatment Considerations

Four clinical scenarios may be encountered in the treatment of patients with classic OS. These and the general considerations are discussed below.

Localized Extremity Disease without Demonstrable Metastases

The patient with a primary tumor of the extremity without evidence of metastases requires surgery to control the primary tumor and chemotherapy to control micrometastatic disease. Surgery alone results in a 15 to 20 percent cure rate at best, according to Marcove.[120] The choice between amputation and limb-sparing resection must be made by an experienced orthopaedic oncologist, taking into account several interrelated factors, including tumor loca-

tion, size or extramedullary extent, the presence or absence of distant metastatic disease, and patient factors such as age, skeletal development, and lifestyle preference that might dictate the suitability of limb salvage or amputation. Routine amputations are no longer performed; all patients should be evaluated for limb-sparing options. Intensive, multiagent chemotherapeutic regimens have provided the best results to date (see Tables 16-6 and 16-7). Patients who are judged unsuitable for limb-sparing options may be candidates for presurgical chemotherapy; those with a good response may then become suitable candidates for limb-sparing operations. The management of these patients mandates close cooperation between the chemotherapist and the surgeon.

Localized Extremity Disease with Synchronous Pulmonary Metastases

Metastatic pulmonary disease detected at initial diagnosis (approximately 10 percent of patients) does not preclude a curative treatment strategy, although the presence of extrathoracic metastases makes cure extremely unlikely. Newly diagnosed patients have not been exposed to chemotherapy and are thus less likely to have drug-resistant tumors. For the patient presenting with resectable disease (i.e., usually fewer than 15 pulmonary nodules and a primary tumor of the extremity), the traditional approach has been resection of all macroscopic disease by median sternotomy and limb amputation or resection, followed by intensive adjuvant chemotherapy. The tumor burden is thereby reduced to a minimum before adjuvant therapy begins. Although the timing of surgery for the primary tumor and metastatic sites has been variable, most modern approaches entail alternating chemotherapy and surgery. Treatment usually begins with a course of chemotherapy, followed by resection of the primary tumor, followed by a second course of chemotherapy, surgical ablation of metastatic sites, and the remaining courses of chemotherapy. In patients with inoperable metastases, primary treatment with chemotherapy is probably appropriate; metastases may respond sufficiently to allow complete resection. Because these patients usually require surgery for the primary tumor as a palliative procedure, early surgery may be recommended, despite the presence of unresectable pulmonary disease. Although improving, the outlook for patients presenting with metastatic disease remains poor.[6,132]

Pelvic Tumors and Unresectable Disease

Most pelvic osteosarcomas (occurring in about 5 percent of patients) can be treated by hemipelvectomy; however, more centrally located pelvic tumors, especially those involving the sacrum, are unresectable. Only a few pelvic osteosarcomas can be treated by limb-sparing resection (internal hemipelvectomy). Contraindications to resection are unusually large extraosseous extensions with sacral plexus or major vascular involvement. Patients with primary tumors of the axial skeleton have traditionally had poor outcomes because local control was rare. Patients whose tumors can be completely resected should be approached with curative intent; radiotherapy provides sig-

TABLE 16-6 Results of Adjuvant Therapy for Osteosarcoma

Institution[a]/Year	Chemotherapy[b]	Percent relapse-free/Number of patients
NCI 1979	HDMTX, VCR ± BCG	38% of 39 patients
SWOG 1980	CTX, VCR, ADRIA, PAM, HDMTX CONPADRI III	38% of 84 patients
CALGB 1981	ADRIA ± HDMTX	50% of 88 patients
DFCI 1986	ADRIA + VCR + HDMTX (weekly)	60% of 46 patients
CCG 1987	ADRIA + VDR + (HDMTX vs IDMTX) (study III)	38% of 166 patients
UCLA 1987	BCD + HDMTX + ADRIA + CDDP (+IA ADRIA + XRT) versus no adjuvant therapy	55% of 59 patients 20% of "no chemo" patients
St. Jude 1990	ADRIA + HDMTX + CTX (OSTEO)77)	56% of 50 patients
MIOS 1996 (in press)	BCD + HDMTX + ADRIA + CDDP versus no adjuvant therapy	63% of 201 patients 12% of "no chemo" patients

[a]NCI = National Cancer Institute; SWOG = Southwest Oncology Group; CALGB = Cancer and Acute Leukemia Group B; DFCI = Dana-Farber Cancer Institute; CCG = Children's Cancer Group; UCLA = University of California, Los Angeles; MIOS = Multi-Institutional Osteosarcoma Study.
[b]HDMTX = high-dose methotrexate (5 g/m^2 or more) + leucovorin rescue; VCR = vincristine; BCG = bacillus Calmette-Guérin; ADRIA = Adriamycin; IDMTX = intermediate-dose methotrexate (750 mg/m^2) + leucovorin rescue; CTX = cyclophosphamide; PAM = phenylalanine mustard; CDDP = cisplatin; BCD = bleomycin, cyclophosphamide, actinomycin D combination; IA = intraarterial administration; XRT = radiotherapy.

TABLE 16-7 Results of Neoadjuvant Chemotherapy for Osteosarcoma

Institution[a]/Year	Chemotherapy[b]	Percent relapse-free/Number of patients
MSKCC 1983	HDMTX + VCR + ADRIA + BCD ± CDDP (T-10 protocol)	76% of 79 patients
GPO 1988	HDMTX + ADRIA + CDDP + IFOS (COSS-82)	58% of 125 patients
Mt. Sinai 1989	HDMTX + ADRIA + CDDP	77% of 25 patients
Rizzoli 1990	IA CDDP + (HDMTX versus IDMTX) + ADRIA ± BCD	51% of 127 patients (58% with HDMTX)
MD And. 1990	(IA CDDP versus HDMTX) + ADRIA (TIOS I)	60% of 43 patients
POG 1995	HDMTX + ADRIA + CDDP + BCD (POG 8651)	70% of 100 patients
CCSG 1996 (in press)	HDMTX + VCR + ADRIA + BCD ± CDDP (CCG-782)	56% of 231 patients

[a]MSKCC = Memorial Sloan-Kettering Cancer Center; GPO = German Society for Pediatric Oncology; Rizzoli = Instituto Ortopedico Rizzoli; MD And. = MD Anderson Cancer Center; POG = Pediatric Oncology Group; CCG = Children's Cancer Study Group.
[b]HDMTX = high-dose methotrexate (5 g/m^2 or more) + leucovorin rescue; VCR = vincristine; BCG = bacillus Calmette-Guérin; ADRIA = Adriamycin; IDMTX = intermediate-dose methotrexate (750 mg/m^2) + leucovorin rescue; CDDP = cisplatin; BCD = bleomycin, cyclophosphamide, actinomycin D combination; IFOS = ifosfamide; IA = intraarterial administration.

nificant palliation in patients with unresectable primary tumors. Palliative decompression of the spine is often required to avoid neurologic damage. There is growing interest in using regional chemotherapy plus concurrent radiation therapy, in addition to systemic chemotherapy, for patients with nonresectable pelvic osteosarcoma.[133,134]

Management of Patients with Recurrent Disease

Historically, patients who developed recurrent disease had a poor prognosis and were treated palliatively; most died within a year of the development of metastases. With the advent of thoracic CT, metastatic nodules can be detected when they are quite small and more easily resectable. Complete surgical resection of all overt metastatic disease is a prerequisite for long-term salvage after relapse.[135,136] Patients not treated by thoracotomy have little hope for cure, because complete responses of macroscopic metastases to chemotherapy are rare.[137,138] The discovery of unresectable extrathoracic metastases or unresectable pulmonary disease is a contraindication to aggressive thoracotomy, and the patient should be treated palliatively. Radiotherapy may be particularly useful.

There is no doubt that survival after relapse has been enhanced by approaches that incorporate repeated aggressive surgery to remove overt disease. With such treatment, 30 to 40 percent of patients have been reported to survive beyond 5 years after relapse.[139,140] Not all of these patients, however, will ultimately be cured. Such considerations emphasize the value of close follow-up, and frequent chest radiographs and thoracic CT scans to detect recurrent disease when it is still resectable.

Variants of Osteosarcoma

There are 11 recognizable variants of classic OS.[111] Osteosarcoma arising in the jawbones is the most common of all variants. Parosteal and periosteal OS are the most common variants of classic OS occurring in the extremities. In contrast to classic (intramedullary) OS, which arises within a bone, parosteal and periosteal (juxtacortical) OS arise on the surface of the bone.

Parosteal Osteosarcoma

Parosteal osteosarcoma (POS) is a distinct variant of conventional osteosarcoma, accounting for 4 percent of all OS.[112] It arises from the cortex of a bone and generally occurs in older individuals. It has a better prognosis than classic osteosarcoma.

Clinical Characteristics There is a slight predominance of POS in women. The distal posterior femur is involved in 72 percent of all cases; the proximal humerus and proximal tibia are the next most frequent sites. Parosteal osteosarcoma metastasizes slowly and has an overall survival rate of 75 to 85 percent.[112,141] Unni and colleagues noted that all patients who died of tumor lived more than 5 years.[141] The natural history of POS involves progressive enlargement and late metastasis. This condition presents primarily with a mass and is occasionally associated with pain. In contrast with conventional OS, the duration of symptoms varies from months to years. Tumor size, location, and duration of symptoms did not correlate with survival.[112] Table 16-8 summarizes the radiographic and clinical differential of classic, parosteal, and periosteal OS.

Radiographic Findings Roentgenograms characteristically show a large, dense, lobulated mass broadly attached to the underlying bone without involvement of the medullary canal (Fig. 16-12). If old enough, the tumor may encircle the entire bone. The periphery of the lesion is characteristically less mature than the base. Ahuja et al. emphasized that intramedullary extension is difficult to determine from plain radiographs.[112] Unni et al. empha-

TABLE 16-8   Radiographic and Clinical Differential of Classic, Parosteal, and Periosteal Osteosaroma

Type of tumor	Common anatomic site	Location	Radiographic appearance	Histology	Metastases
Classic	Distal femur Proximal tibia	Intramedullary	Destructive, osteoblastic/ osteolytic	High-grade (fibroblastic, chondroblastic, and osteoblastic)	Early
Parosteal	Posterior distal femur	Cortical	Dense, homogeneous new bone	"Mature" bone and fibroblastic stroma, low-grade	Late
Periosteal	Proximal tibia and humerus	Cortical	"Scooped-out" lesion with calcification	Chondroblastic high-grade	Intermediate

Source: Reproduced with permission from Malawer MM, Abelson HT, Suit HD, in DeVita V, Hellman S, Rosenberg SA (eds): *Cancer: Principles and Practice of Oncology*, 2d ed. Philadelphia, Lippincott, 1985, pp 1293–1343.

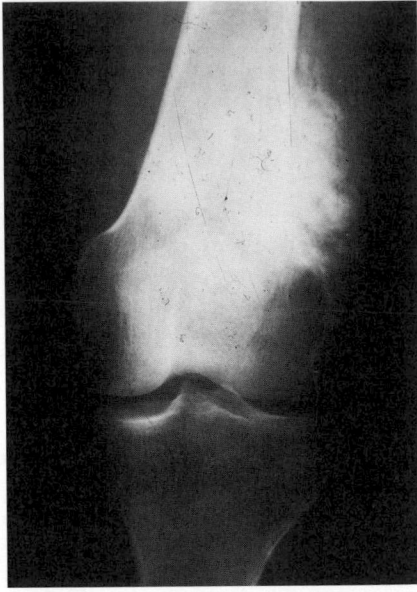
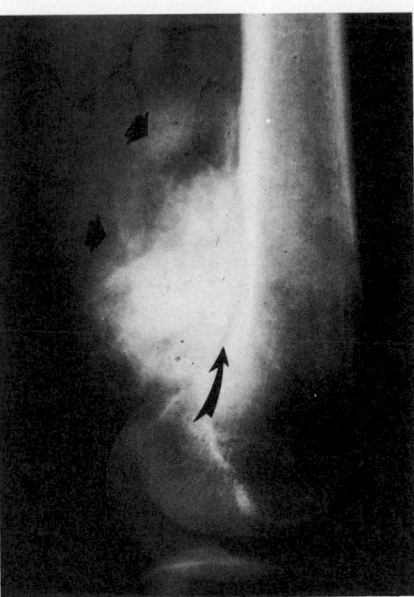

A   *B*

Figure 16-12 Parosteal osteosarcoma. *A* and *B.* Anteroposterior and lateral radiographs of a typical parosteal osteosarcoma. There is a dense, lobulated broad-based mass attached to the posterior aspect of the distal femur. Note that the periphery (*arrowheads*) is less mature than the center. There is a characteristic radiolucent line (*curved arrow*) at the base denoting an attempt of the tumor to surround the bone along the cortex. A large intramedullary extension found at surgery was not well seen on these plain radiographs.

sized that high-grade foci did not usually alter the roentgenographic appearance of these tumors.[141]

Diagnosis and Grading The diagnosis is difficult and must include evaluation of the radiographs, age of the patient, and location of tumor. The differential diagnosis includes osteochondroma, myositis ossificans, and conventional OS. Cortical tumors of the posterior femur should always be suspected of malignancy; this is a rare location for a benign osteochondroma. In contrast to sarcoma, myositis ossificans is rarely attached to the underlying bone. In addition, the periphery is more mature, both radiographically and histologically, than in sarcoma.

Parosteal sarcomas are graded from low to high grade: grade I (low grade), grade II (intermediate), and grade III (high grade).[112] The majority (85 percent) are grade I. It is important to evaluate the fibroblastic, cartilaginous, and osseous components independently. The survival rate of patients with grade III tumors is similar to that of patients with conventional OS. Intramedullary involvement does not imply a worse prognosis unless it is also a high-grade lesion.

Gross Characteristics The tumor arises from the periosteal surface and presents as a protuberant, multinodular, firm mass. The surface may be covered in part by a cartilaginous cap, whereas the tumor in other areas may infiltrate into adjacent soft tissue. The tumor usually encircles, partially or even completely, the shaft of the underlying bone. Unlike the osteochondroma, in POS the medullary canal of the bone is not contiguous with that of the neoplasm.

Microscopic Characteristics This neoplasm is generally low grade. Irregularly formed osteoid trabeculae are surrounded by a spindle cell stroma containing widely spaced,

bland-appearing spindle cells. There may be foci of atypical chondroid differentiation. (Infrequently, more cellular foci with appreciable atypia and mitotic activity are present). A four-step grading system based on features of the fibrous and chondroid components has been proposed.[3] With the higher grades, the likelihood of intramedullary involvement increases. This, in turn, correlates well with the occurrence of distant metastasis.

Treatment Wide excision of the tumor is the treatment of choice. This may be accomplished by an amputation or a limb-sparing procedure. No experience has been reported with preoperative chemotherapy or radiotherapy. Parosteal osteosarcomas are often amenable to limb preservation due to their distal location, low grade, and lack of local invasiveness. Vascular displacement is not a contraindication for resection; if the adjacent neurovascular bundle is free of tumor, resection is feasible. The major surgical decision is usually whether to remove the entire end of the bone and the adjacent joint or to preserve the joint. If the lesion is small, the joint can be preserved. If the medullary canal is involved or if extensive cortical involvement is present, then the joint usually cannot be preserved. Techniques of resection and reconstruction are similar to those described for conventional osteosarcoma. The major difference is that only a small amount of soft tissue usually needs to be resected; consequently, a good functional result is obtained. Grade III parosteal lesions warrant systemic therapy because of the risk of metastasis.

Periosteal Osteosarcoma

Periosteal OS is a rare cortical variant of OS that arises superficially on the cortex, most often on the tibial shaft.[142] Radiographically, it is a small, radiolucent lesion with some evidence of bone spiculation. The cortex is

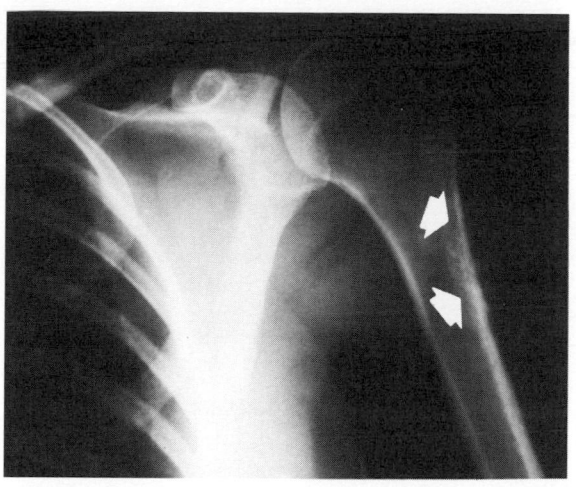
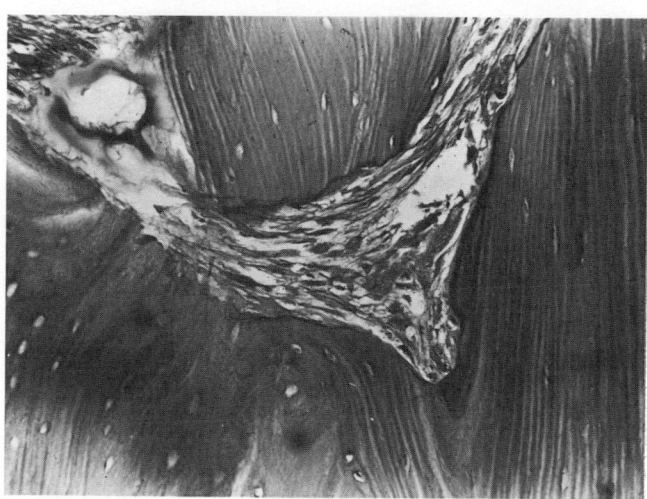

A   *B*

Figure 16-13 Periosteal osteosarcoma. *A.* Typical radiograph of a periosteal osteosarcoma of the humerus. Note the cortical location *(arrowheads)* with a scooped-out defect on the lateral shaft and the diaphyseal location. *B.* High-power photomicrograph of the underlying cortex demonstrating early extension of tumor within the cortex. Periosteal osteosarcomas most commonly involve the humerus and tibia and are diaphyseal, in contrast to parosteal osteosarcomas, which arise from the posterior aspect of the distal femur. (Reproduced with permission from Hall RB, Robinson LH, Malawer MM, et al: Periosteal osteosarcoma. *Cancer* 55:165–171, 1985.)

characteristically intact, with a scooped-out appearance and a Codman's triangle (Fig. 16-13). By contrast, POSs are large, broad-based, and radiodense. Periosteal OSs are relatively high-grade chondroblastic OSs composed of malignant cartilage with areas of anaplastic spindle cells and osteoid production. Periosteal OSs are one-third as frequent as the parosteal variant.[142] Treatment is similar to that of other high-grade lesions. En bloc resection should be performed when feasible; otherwise, amputation is indicated.

Gross Characteristics Like POS, this lesion arises from the periosteal surface. It projects as a well-circumscribed mass into the overlying soft tissues. On section, the tumor often reveals a chondroid consistency (Fig. 16-12*A*).

Microscopic Characteristics The features are essentially those of a chondroblastic OS. The cartilagenous lobules can contain markedly atypical chondrocytes. At the periphery of the lobule a cellular spindle cell component is situated, wherein a fine intercellular osteoid matrix is produced. Areas of malignant osteoid and chondroid can infiltrate into the cortical bone at the base of the neoplasm (Fig. 16-12*B*).

Small Cell Osteosarcoma

Small cell OS is a rare variant of OS. The cells are round, rather than spindle-shaped. There is definite evidence of osteoid production; thus the inclusion of this entity as an OS. Because of the presence of small cells, this entity is often classified as an "atypical" Ewing's sarcoma.[143,144] The

recommendations for treatment vary; radiation and chemotherapy are used at some institutions, while others choose primary surgical ablation with pre- and/or postoperative chemotherapy. Too few cases have been reported to make definitive recommendations.

Microscopic Characteristics The tumor consists of nests and sheets of small round cells separated by fibrous septa, a pattern reminiscent of Ewing's sarcomas. Occasionally, transition to spindle cells is noted. The cells have well-defined borders and a distinct rim of cytoplasm. The round nuclei disclose a delicate chromatin pattern. The presence of a characteristic, delicate, lacelike osteoid matrix, often surrounding individual or small nests of cells, confirms the diagnosis of OS.

Chondrosarcoma

Chondrosarcoma, the second most common primary malignant spindle cell tumor of bone,[21] is a heterogeneous group of tumors whose basic neoplastic tissue is cartilaginous without evidence of direct osteoid formation. Bone formation occasionally results from differentiation of cartilage. If there is evidence of direct osteoid or bone production, the lesion is classified as an OS. There are five types of chondrosarcoma: central, peripheral, mesenchymal, dedifferentiated, and clear cell.[21,116,145,146] The classic chondrosarcomas are central (arising within a bone) or peripheral (arising from the surface of a bone). The other three are variants and have distinct histologic and clinical characteristics. Their characteristics are summarized in Table 16-9.

TABLE 16-9   Classification and General Characteristics of Chondrosarcomas

Type	Size, location, grade	Primary[a] or secondary[b]
Central	Intramedullary Moderate to high-grade Small extraosseous component Little calcification	Usually primary
Peripheral	Cortical Usually low-grade, myxomatous Large soft tissue component Heavily calcified	Usually secondary
Mesenchymal	Intramedullary High-grade, may respond to radiotherapy Small round cells	Primary
Dedifferentiated	High-grade anaplastic (osteosarcoma, MFH) in association with recognizable low-grade chondrosarcoma	Primary
Clear cell chondrosarcoma	Low-grade Appears as a chondroblastoma Locally recurrent	Primary

[a]76% of primary chondrosarcomas are central.
[b]Usually from benign cartilage tumors, e.g., osteochondromas.

Both central and peripheral chondrosarcomas can arise as primary tumors or secondary to underlying neoplasm. Seventy-six percent of primary chondrosarcomas arise centrally.[21,146–148] Secondary chondrosarcomas most often arise from benign cartilage tumors. The multiple forms of the benign osteochondromas or enchondromas have a higher rate of malignant transformation than do the corresponding solitary lesions.[46,148–150]

Central and Peripheral Chondrosarcomas

Clinical Characteristics Half of all chondrosarcomas occur in persons above the age of 40.[21,151] The most common sites are the pelvis, femur, and shoulder girdle.[147,151] The clinical presentation varies. Peripheral chondrosarcomas may become quite large without causing pain, and local symptoms develop only because of mechanical irritation. Pelvic chondrosarcomas are often large and present with referred pain to the back or thigh, sciatica secondary to sacral plexus irritation, urinary symptoms from bladder neck involvement, unilateral edema due to iliac vein obstruction, or as a painless abdominal mass. Conversely, central chondrosarcomas present with dull pain. A mass is rarely present. Pain, which indicates active growth, is an ominous sign of a central cartilage lesion. This cannot be overemphasized. An adult with a plain radiograph suggestive of a "benign" cartilage tumor but associated with pain most likely has a chondrosarcoma.

Radiographic Findings Central chondrosarcomas have two distinct radiologic patterns.[152] One is a small, well-de-fined lytic lesion with a narrow zone of transition and surrounding sclerosis with faint calcification. This is the most common malignant bone tumor that may appear radiographically benign. The second type has no sclerotic border and is difficult to localize. The key sign of malignancy is endosteal scalloping. This type is difficult to diagnose on plain radiographs and may go undetected for a long period of time. In contrast, peripheral chondrosarcoma is easily recognized as a large mass of characteristic calcification protruding from a bone. Its differential diagnosis includes large benign osteochondroma, POS, and juxtacortical myositis ossificans. Correlation of the clinical, radiographic, and histologic data is essential for accurate diagnosis and evaluation of the aggressiveness of cartilage tumor. In general, proximal or axial location, skeletal maturity, and pain point toward malignancy, even though the cartilage may appear benign.

Grading and Prognosis Chondrosarcomas are graded I, II, and III; the majority are either grade I or grade II.[21,46,147,151] The metastatic rate of moderate-grade versus high-grade is 15 to 40 percent versus 75 percent.[21,46,146,148,153–155] Grade III lesions have the same metastatic potential as osteosarcomas (Fig. 16-14).[147,150]

In general, peripheral chondrosarcomas are lower in grade then central lesions. Forty-three percent of the peripheral lesions are grade I, compared with 13 percent of the central lesions.[155] The 10-year survival rate among those with peripheral lesions is 77 percent, compared with 32 percent among those with central lesions. Secondary chondrosarcomas arising from osteochondromas also

Figure 16-14 High-grade chondrosarcoma associated with enchondromatosis. *A.* Plain radiograph of a radiolucent lesion of the proximal humerus with little calcification. *B.* The gross specimen. The incidence of malignant degeneration associated with multiple enchondromas increases with each decade of life, with an overall risk of 15 to 25 percent. Chondrosarcomas arising centrally tend to be high grade.

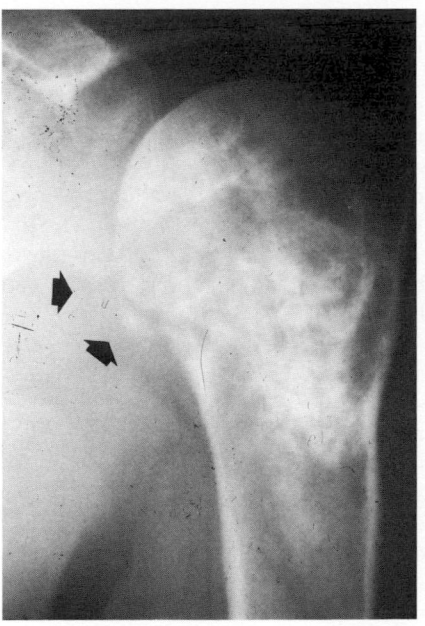

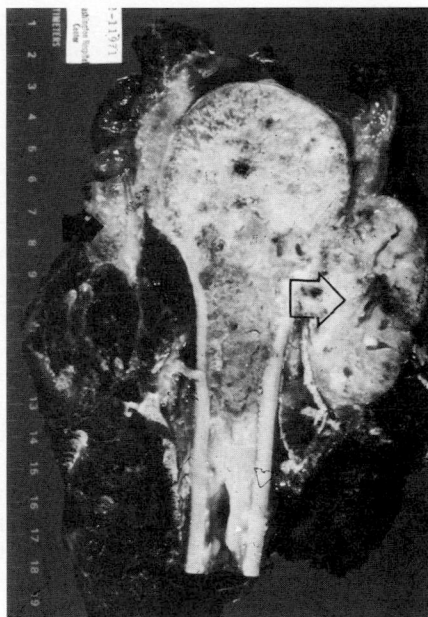

A

B

have a low malignant potential; 85 percent are grade I. The multiple forms of benign osteochondromas or enchondromas have a higher rate of malignant transformation than the corresponding solitary lesions.[148–150]

Gross Characteristics Primary intraosseous (central) chondrosarcoma is an expansile lesion that eventuates in cortical destruction. Subsequent extension into soft tissue often occurs. Chondrosarcoma arising from a rib or from the pelvis may protrude, as a smooth-surfaced multinodular mass, into the pleural cavity or pelvic retroperitoneum, respectively.

Typically, the tumor consists of fused, variably sized nodules, which on cut section are composed of a white-gray hyaline tissue. Areas of calcification and even ossification are common. There may be focal myxoid areas. The nodules occasionally contain degenerative cysts of various sizes.

Microscopic Characteristics The histologic spectrum of this neoplasm varies tremendously: high-grade examples can easily be identified, whereas certain low-grade tumors are exceedingly difficult to distinguish from chondromas. Correlation of the histologic features with both the clinical setting and the radiographic changes is therefore of utmost importance in avoiding serious diagnostic error. The grade of malignant cartilagenous tumors correlates with clinical behavior. Grade I tumors are characterized by an increased number of condrocytes set in a matrix that is chondroid to focally myxoid. The cells contain hyperchromatic nuclei and occasionally binucleate forms; they show minimal variation in size (Fig. 16-15).

Areas of increased cellularity with more marked variation in cell size, significant nuclear atypia, and frequent pleomorphic forms define a grade II lesion. Binuclear forms are more common in this group.

Grade III chondrosarcomas, which are relatively uncommon, disclose still greater cellularity, often with spin-dle cell areas, and reveal prominent mitotic activity. Chondrocytes may contain large, bizarre nuclei. Areas of myxoid change are common.

Areas of calcification and enchondral ossification can be observed in tumors of all grades. However, the presence of unequivocal malignant osteoid production, even in the face of chondrosarcomatous areas, dictates that the tumor be classified as OS.

Treatment The treatment of chondrosarcoma is surgical removal.[146–148,157,158] Guidelines of resection for high-grade chondrosarcomas are similar to those for OSs. The sites of origin and the fact that chondrosarcomas tend to be low grade make them amenable to limb-sparing procedures.

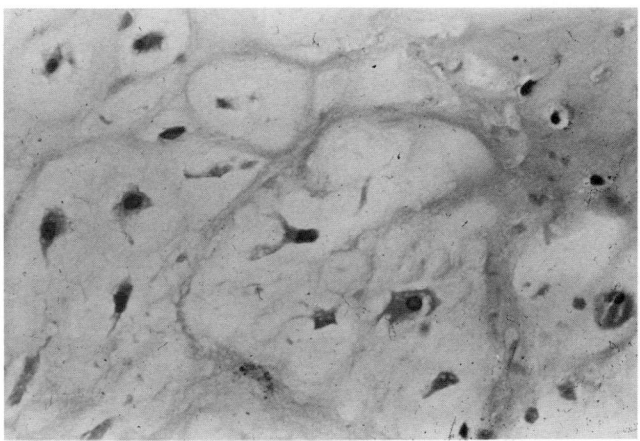

Figure 16-15 The presence of chondrocytes with central hyperchromatic nuclei is typical of chondrosarcoma, grade I. Binucleate forms are not uncommon. The matrix may vary from chondroid to myxoid.

The four most common sites are the pelvis, proximal femur, shoulder girdle, and diaphyseal portions of long bones.

Effective adjuvant treatment is limited: there are no reports of effective adjuvant chemotherapy and few reports of effective radiation therapy.[159] High-grade chondrosarcomas warrant consideration of adjuvant chemotherapy, given risk of metastatic potential. Chondrosarcomas have generally been considered to be radio-resistant; however, radical radiotherapy is useful for local control in unresectable or inoperable lesions.

Cryosurgery, as pioneered by Marcove,[154,155] is advocated as an effective adjuvant for obtaining local control. Cryosurgery involves thorough curettage followed by freezing of the resulting cavity with liquid nitrogen.[154,155,160] This technique allows for preservation of bone stock and avoidance of resection. Use of polymethylmethacrylate cement and internal fixation to reconstruct the cavity reduces the risk of subsequent pathologic fracture. Cryosurgery has recently been used for central, low-grade chondrosarcomas.[154,155] With increasing experience, Marcove has expanded the cryosurgery indications to low-grade intramedullary cartilage tumors as well as a few high-grade lesions. With these indications, he has treated 30 chondrosarcomas with only one local recurrence.

Variants of Chondrosarcoma

Clear Cell Chondrosarcoma

Clear cell chondrosarcoma, the rarest form of chondrosarcoma, is a slow-growing, locally recurrent tumor resembling a chondroblastoma but with some malignant potential typically occurring in adults.[23,161] The most difficult clinical problem is early recognition; it is often confused with chondroblastoma. Metastases occur only after multiple local recurrences. Primary treatment is wide excision. Systemic therapy is not required.

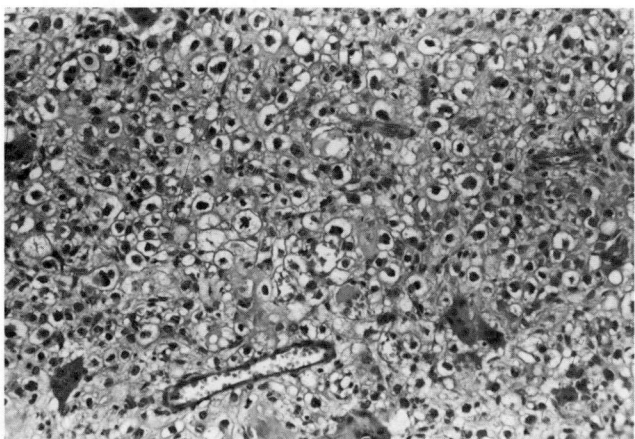

Figure 16-16 Sheets of round cells with clear cytoplasm and central nuclei point to a diagnosis of clear cell chondrosarcoma. Multinucleated giant cells, very rare in the usual chondrosarcoma, are common in this entity.

Gross Characteristics The neoplasm commonly presents as a solid expansile mass with focal cystic changes.

Microscopic Characteristics The diagnostic features consist of sheets or vague lobules composed of round clear cells (Fig. 16-16). Variably perichromatic nuclei is typical of chondrosarcoma grade I. Binucleate forms are not uncommon. The matrix may vary from chondroid to myxoid. In addition, areas indistinguishable from other primary bone lesions can obscure the underlying clear cell neoplasm. Foci resembling aneurysmal bone cyst, OS, osteoblastoma, chondroblastoma, and giant-cell tumor have been identified.[162]

Mesenchymal Chondrosarcoma

Mesenchymal chondrosarcoma is a rare, aggressive variant of chondrosarcoma, characterized by a biphasic histologic pattern; i.e., small compact cells intermixed with islands of cartilaginous matrix.[31,163] This tumor has a predilection for flat bones; long tubular bones are rarely affected. It tends to occur in the younger age group and has a high metastatic potential. The 10-year survival rate is 28 percent.[163] This entity responds favorably to radiotherapy. Treatment is surgical removal combined with adjuvant chemotherapy. Radiotherapy is recommended if the tumor cannot be completely removed.[31]

Gross Characteristics The firm white-gray tumor usually contains hard calcified or ossified areas. Prominent cartilaginous features are unusual.

Microscopic Characteristics The hallmark of this neoplasm is the juxtaposition of foci of poorly differentiated round cells with islands of relatively mature chondroid tissue. The small, round to slightly spindled cells are arranged in broad sheets and typically form a hemangiopericytoma-like pattern. Scattered islands of chondroid, which can be focally calcified or ossified, arise abruptly among the sheets of round cells.

Dedifferentiated Chondrosarcoma

Around 10 percent of chondrosarcomas may dedifferentiate into either a fibrosarcoma or an OS.[21,146,150] They occur in older individuals and are often fatal. Surgical treatment is similar to that described for other high-grade sarcomas. Adjuvant therapy is warranted.

Gross Characteristics The central region of the tumor is comparable to that of ordinary chondrosarcoma and is characterized by distinctly lobulated gray-white translucent tissue. Calcified foci are commonly found within this zone. Peripheral to this chondroid portion, but contiguous to it, is a firm to soft, often focally necrotic component which, after eroding the cortical bone, often extends into the adjacent soft tissue.

Microscopic Characteristics Two distinct components are identified. The central portion shows features of a low-grade chondrosarcoma (grade I or II), identical to that described elsewhere in this chapter. At the periphery of the lobules arises an anaplastic high-grade infiltrative sarcoma that can present features of MFH, OS, or fibrosarcoma.

Giant-Cell Tumor of Bone

Giant-cell tumor of bone (GCT) is an aggressive, locally recurrent tumor with a low metastatic potential.[26,151,164–168] *Giant-cell sarcoma of bone* refers to a de novo, malignant GCT, not to the tumor that arises from the transformation of a GCT previously thought to be benign. These two lesions are separate clinical entities.

Clinical Characteristics

GCTs occur slightly more often in females than in males. Eighty percent of GCTs in the long bones occur after skeletal maturity; 75 percent of these develop around the knee joint.[21,26,116] A joint effusion or pathologic fracture, uncommon with other sarcomas, is common with GCTs. Occasionally, GCTs occur in the vertebrae (2 to 5 percent) and the sacrum (10 percent).[21,145]

Natural History Although GCTs are rarely malignant de novo (2 to 8 percent), they may undergo transformation and demonstrate malignant potential histologically and clinically after multiple local recurrences. Between 8 and 22 percent of known GCTs become malignant following local recurrence.[151,164–166,169] This rate decreases to less than 10 percent if patients who have undergone radiotherapy are excluded. Approximately 40 percent of malignant GCTs became malignant at the first recurrence.[165] The remainder become malignant by the second and third recurrences; thus, each recurrence increases the risk of malignant transformation. A recurrence after 5 years is

extremely suspicious for a malignancy. Primary malignant GCT generally has a better prognosis than secondary malignant transformation of typical GCT, especially if the transformation occurs after radiation therapy. Local recurrence of a GCT is determined by the adequacy of surgical removal rather than histologic grade.

Radiographic and Clinical Evaluation Giant-cell tumors are eccentric lytic lesions without matrix production (Fig. 16-17). They have poorly defined borders with a wide area of transition. They are juxtaepiphyseal with a metaphyseal component. Although the cortex is expanded and appears destroyed, at surgery it is usually found to be attenuated but intact. Periosteal elevation is rare; soft tissue extension is common. In the skeletally immature patient, aneurysmal bone cyst must be differentiated, although both lesions are closely related.

Pathology

Gross Characteristics The typical lesion presents as a large expansile mass in the region of the epiphysis. Cortical destruction of the adjacent bone is not uncommon. The periphery of the tumor is often partially surrounded by a thin, delicate rim of reactive bone. The soft, somewhat gelatinous tumor tissue varies from gray-tan to red-brown. (Areas of hemorrhage with hemosiderin deposition account for the color of the latter.) Small, cystlike foci frequently occur; however, occasionally the cystic degeneration can become so extensive that the tumor resembles an aneurysmal bone cyst. Firm fibrous or osteoid tissue can be associated with a site of pathologic fracture.

Microscopic Characteristics Two basic cell types constitute the typical GCT. The stroma is characterized by polygonal to somewhat spindled cells containing central round

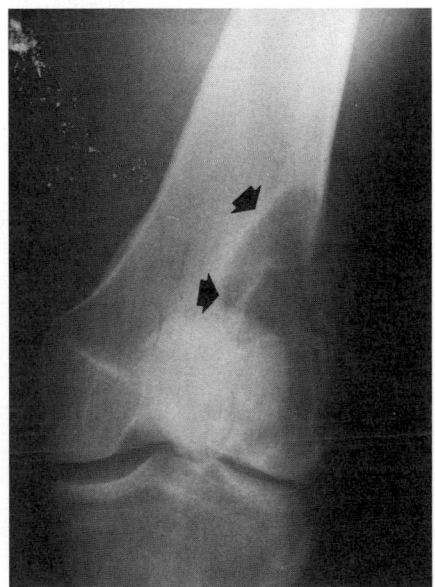 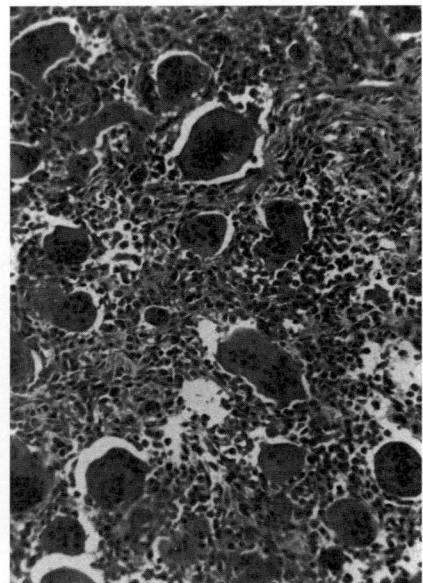

Figure 16-17 Aggressive giant-cell tumor. *A.* Typical GCT of bone. GCTs are eccentric, without matrix formation, and metaphyseal. They often have poorly defined margins with some sclerosis (*arrows*). Pathologic fracture is common. Cortical expansion and poorly defined margins are signs of aggressivity. *B.* Low-power photomicrograph showing a uniform distribution of giant cells in a benign stroma. The stroma cells tend to be ovoid. No mitoses are seen, but they are occasionally present. (Reproduced with permission from Malawer MM, Abelson HT, Suit HD, in DeVita VT, Hellman S, Rosenberg SA (eds): *Cancer: Principles and Practice of Oncology,* 2d ed. Philadelphia, Lippincott, 1985.)

A

B

nuclei. Mitotic figures, sometimes numerous, are often noted, but they are not atypical and do not warrant a malignant interpretation.

Scattered diffusely throughout the stroma are benign multinucleated giant cells. Small foci of osteoid matrix, produced by the benign stroma cells, can be observed; however, chondroid matrix never occurs. Extensive hemorrhage, pathologic fracture, or previous surgery can significantly alter the usual histologic picture of GCT. These events must be recognized at the time of histologic interpretation in order to prevent diagnostic errors. Cystic areas with surrounding hemosiderin pigment and xanthoma cells correspond to the grossly observed cysts.

Grading The grading of GCTs into three groups in order to predict clinical behavior, as originally proposed by Jaffe,[145] has been generally abandoned. Recognition of the overtly malignant type (grade III), as described below, is valid; however, lesions rated as histologically benign (grade I or II) have been shown to metastasize.[116,170] Malignant GCT contains areas of unequivocal sarcomatous transformation, usually typical fibrosarcoma or OS. The sarcomatous component is devoid of GCT features; thus, it is only by the recognition of foci of residual benign GCT or by the confirmation of preexisting benign GCT that an accurate diagnosis of malignant GCT can be established.

Treatment

Treatment of GCT of bone is surgical removal. En bloc resection is curative in 90 percent of these cases.[26,33,164–166] In contrast, curettage, with or without bone grafts, has a recurrence rate of 40 to 75 percent.[26,164,165] Johnson and Dahlin reported a recurrence rate of 29 percent within 1 year of curettage and of 54 percent within 5 years.[166] Figure 16-18 summarizes the results of treatment by the various techniques. Though en bloc excision offers reliable results, routine resection is not recommended because of the morbidity associated with resection of a joint.[2,171] Primary resection is recommended for GCT of the proximal radius and fibula, distal ulna, tubular bones of hand and foot, coccyx, sacrum, and pelvic bones. In general, curettage does not rule out a later curative resection.

Today, curettage is supplemented with extensive use of a high-speed burr through a large cortical window equal to the length of the bony defect, referred to as *curettage/resection*.[172] Bone graft and/or polymethylmethacrylate is used to reconstruct the defect. This technique has reduced recurrence rates to 8 percent within 2 years initially,[173] but longer-term follow-up reveals a 25 percent recurrence rate.[174] Recently, curettage with polymethylmethacrylate augmentation of the bony defect has been performed with the intent of inducing thermal necrosis of regional tumor cells utilizing the heat of polymerization. This technique does not provide better local control than curettage alone.

Amputation is reserved for massive recurrence, malignant transformation, or infection. Because of the risk of malignant transformation and pathologic fracture, as well as lack of effectiveness, radiation is used only for surgically inaccessible sites.[26,164,175] Treatment of GCTs of the vertebrae and sacrum is difficult and must be individualized. A combination of surgical excision, cryosurgery, and/or radiotherapy is required for tumor eradication and the prevention of neurologic impairment.[176–178]

Cryosurgical Treatment Cryosurgery has been utilized more successfully for GCTs than for any other type of bone tumor.[33,154,155,160,179] Cryosurgery was developed by Marcove in an attempt to overcome the high recurrence rates after curettage and the significant risk of sarcomatous degeneration in GCTs treated by irradiation. Figure 16-19*A* shows the technique of cryosurgery. Marcove found cryosurgery effective in eradicating the tumor while preserving joint motion and avoiding resection or amputation. Recently he reported a 17-year experience of 100 GCTs treated by thorough curettage and cryosurgery.[154] He noted a recurrence rate of 16 percent in the first 50 cases and 2 percent in the following 50 cases. The major complications of cryosurgery are necrosis of the adjacent bone (Fig. 16-19*B*), which is liable to develop a late pathologic fracture, and delayed union. The rate of secondary pathologic fracture has been decreased by a combination of polymethylmethacrylate augmentation, bone graft, and internal fixation of the cavity.[180] Malawer et al.[181] reported on 102 patients with GCTs treated with wide curettage and

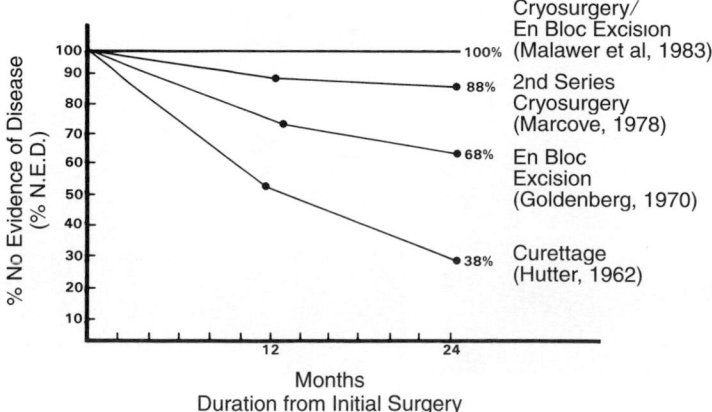

Figure 16-18 Reported cure rates of GCTs of bone treated by various modalities.

Figure 16-19 Cryosurgery. *A.* Intraoperative photograph demonstrating the direct-pour method of cryosurgery. After thorough curettage of the lesion, liquid nitrogen is poured directly into the cavity through a funnel. This ensures complete contact of the liquid nitrogen with the wall of the cavity in order to kill any remaining tumor cells. The temperature of the freeze is monitored by thermocouples (*solid arrow*); −20 to −40°C is necessary for cryonecrosis. The base of the funnel is packed with Gelfoam to prevent leakage. *B.* GCT of the distal tibia treated by curettage and cryosurgery. Radiograph at 18 months demonstrates the typical "cryonecrotic" rim (*arrows*), an area of necrotic and reparative bone at the limit of the original freeze. Presumably any tumor cells remaining within the cavity or the bony interstices following curettage were killed by the liquid nitrogen. A radiograph at 2 years shows no evidence of recurrence, incorporation of the graft with a normal appearing joint space, and some persistence of the cryonecrotic rim.

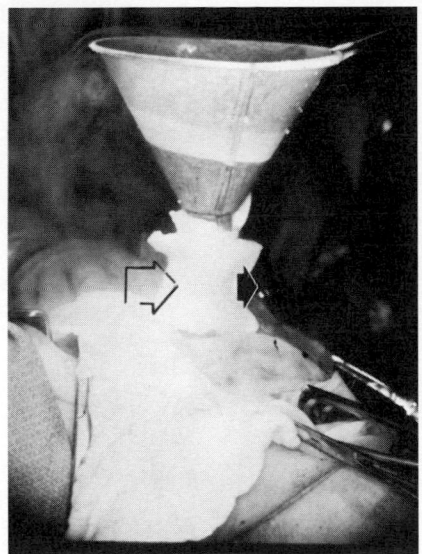

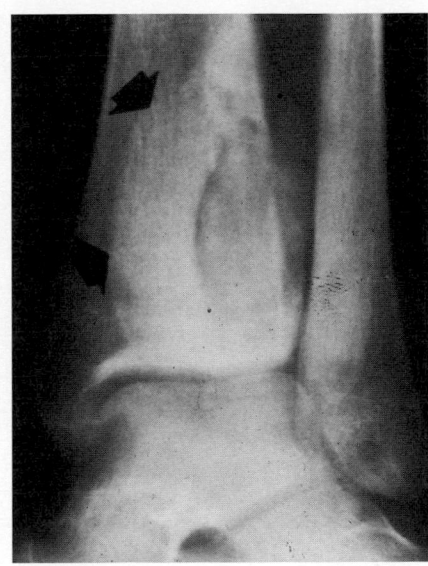

A

B

cryosurgery followed by reconstruction with polymethylmethacrylate and/or bone graft. Local recurrence was less than 8 percent and the incidence of pathologic fracture was only 5 percent. Liquid nitrogen is a very effective physical adjuvant and is recommended following curettage resection. Curettage alone is not recommended because of the associated high rate of local recurrence.

Radiation Therapy Radiation is considered when surgical excision is not technically feasible. Most often this is the case when the tumor occurs in the vertebrae. Dahlin[164] reported a significant risk of radiation-induced sarcoma following radiation alone or in conjunction with surgery for the treatment of GCT of bone. However, malignant degeneration also occurs independent of radiation, suggesting that this may simply be the natural history of the disease. Recent series have demonstrated that GCT is not radioresistant, as once believed: local control rates of 75 to 85 percent have been achieved.[182–184] As a result, local curettage followed by megavoltage radiation appears to be a suitable alternative to complex and difficult surgery, particularly for the medically inoperable.

Malignant Fibrous Histiocytoma

Clinical Characteristics

Malignant fibrous histiocytoma (MFH) is a high-grade bone tumor histologically similar to its soft tissue counterpart.[185–187] Osteoid production is absent. It is a disease of adulthood. The most common sites are the metaphyseal ends of long bones, especially around the knee. Alkaline phosphatase values are normal, helping to rule out an osteosarcoma or fibrosarcoma.[185] Pathologic fracture is common, as MFH disseminates rapidly. Lymphatic involvement, although rare for other bone sarcomas, has been reported.

Radiographic Characteristics

This is an osteolytic lesion associated with marked cortical disruption, minimal cortical or periosteal reaction, and no evidence of matrix formation. The extent of the tumor routinely exceeds plain radiographic signs. It may be multicentric (10 percent) and associated with bone infarcts (10 percent).[186]

Pathology

Gross Characteristics The features are nonspecific and vary greatly. Firm, fibrous areas can alternate with soft, necrotic foci. Some lesions are relatively homogeneous white-gray, whereas others are more variegated, with ill-defined brown-red and yellow regions.

Microscopic Characteristics As in its soft tissue counterpart, primary MFH of bone reveals a remarkably broad histologic spectrum. Plump histiocyte-like cells and spindled fibroblastic cells, in variable proportion, are the main elements. Characteristic is the storiform or pinwheel pattern, in which the fibroblasts radiate from a central focus. The histiocyte-like cells can form sheets or transform into markedly bizarre, often multinucleated forms with atypical mitotic figures (Fig. 16-20). The spindle cell component may predominate, forming areas resembling fibrosarcoma. Chronic inflammatory cells and occasional osteoblast-like giant cells are usually scattered throughout the stroma. Occasionally small foci of osteoid matrix production by

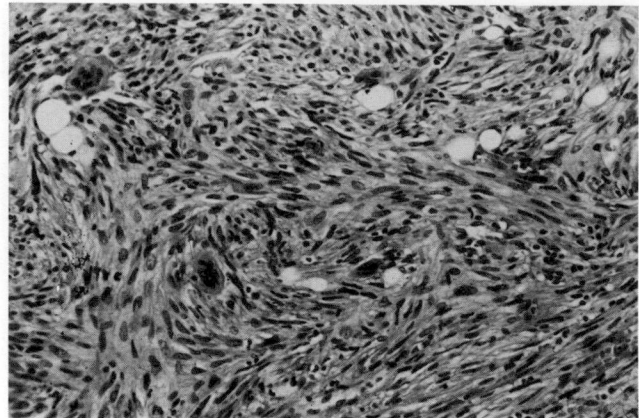

Figure 16-20 This example of malignant fibrous histiocytoma of bone demonstrates pleomorphic and bizarre tumor cells admixed with spindle cells and inflammatory cell infiltrates.

tumor cells can be observed. Metastatic pleomorphic carcinoma, particularly from the kidney, can closely mimic MFH; such a possibility must be excluded in the differential diagnosis. Application of immunohistochemical tests for cytokeratins can be very helpful in this dilemma, since sarcomas rarely contain abundant keratin-positive cells.

Treatment

Treatment is similar to that of other high-grade sarcomas. Several studies suggest that adjuvant chemotherapy has similar results to those seen in the treatment of osteosarcoma.[188,189]

Fibrosarcoma of Bone

Clinical Characteristics

Fibrosarcoma of bone is a rare entity characterized by interlacing bundles of collagen fibers (herringbone pattern) without any evidence of tumorous bone or osteoid formation.[190] Fibrosarcoma occurs in middle age. The long bones are most affected. Fibrosarcomas occasionally arise secondarily in conjunction with an underlying disease such as fibrous dysplasia, Paget's disease, bone infarcts, osteomyelitis, postirradiation bone, and GCT.[190] Fibrosarcoma may be either central or cortical (termed *periosteal*). The histologic grade is a good prognosticator of metastatic potential. The overall survival rate is 27 percent and 52 percent for central and peripheral lesions, respectively.[190] Late metastases do occur, and 10- and 15-year survival rates vary. In general, periosteal tumors have a better prognosis than central lesions do.

Radiographic Features

Fibrosarcoma is a radiolucent lesion that shows minimal periosteal and cortical reaction. The radiographic appearance closely correlates with the histologic grade of the tumor.[190] Low-grade tumors are well defined, whereas high-grade lesions demonstrate indistinct margins and bone destruction similar to those seen in osteolytic OS. Plain radiographs often underestimate the extent of the lesion. Pathologic fracture is common (30 percent) because of the lack of matrix formation.[191] Differential diagnosis includes GCT, aneurysmal bone cyst, MFH, and osteolytic OS.

Pathology

Gross Characteristics The presentation correlates reasonably well with the histologic grade. Low-grade lesions tend to be firm and white-gray and may appear encapsulated. With the higher-grade tumors, the tissue becomes soft, somewhat myxoid, and even necrotic. Transgression of the cortex with soft tissue extension is not uncommon.

Microscopic Characteristics The hallmark of this neoplasm is the formation of fascicles of elongated spindle cells containing tapered nuclei. The fascicles often intersect at acute angles, forming the so-called herringbone pattern. Intercellular collagen production may be abundant, especially in the low-grade examples. In contrast, high-grade fibrosarcoma is characterized by more of the pleomorphic spindle cells with atypical nuclear features. Mitotic activity is brisk. Collagen production may not be discernible. Differentiation of a grade I fibrosarcoma from a desmoplastic fibroma is frequently difficult.

Staging and Treatment

Staging and treatment are similar to those of other spindle cell sarcomas. Low-grade central and peripheral variants are treated by en bloc resection. Axial and fascial lesions should be treated by resection and local radiotherapy. Adjuvant chemotherapy is warranted for high-grade lesions.

Secondary Sarcomas (Paget's Sarcoma and Radiation-Induced Osteosarcoma)

Secondary tumors are neoplasms arising from an underlying pathological process or from another tumor (Table 16-10).[110] Though rare, this diverse group of lesions requires separate consideration. In general, the management of each tumor is similar to that of its primary counterpart.

Approximately 1 percent of patients with Paget's disease will develop a primary bone sarcoma.[192,193] Most patients with this condition present with pain; thus, a patient with known Paget's disease who complains of increasing pain, especially when it is well localized, should be evaluated radiographically. The diagnosis is usually made by plain radiography and confirmed by biopsy. The level of alkaline phosphatase does not help in diagnosis. Histologically, OS is the most common; fibrosarcoma, chondrosarcoma, and MFH also have been described. The anatomic distribution is similar to that of uncomplicated Paget's disease. Traditionally, less than 8 percent of patients survive, and most deaths occur within 2 years.[194] Treatment is similar to that recommended for adolescent patients with osteosarcoma without metastatic disease.

TABLE 16-10   Types of Secondary Tumors

Primary disease	Secondary tumor
Osteochondroma	Peripheral chondrosarcoma
Enchondroma	Central chondrosarcoma
Fibrous dysplasia	Malignant fibrous histiocytoma (MFH), fibrosarcoma
Paget's disease	Paget's sarcoma (usually osteosarcoma), giant-cell tumor (rare)
Irradiated tissue	Radiation-induced sarcoma of the bone[a] or soft tissue (osteosarcoma, MFH, fibrosarcoma)

[a]Approximately 200 cases. Average latent period is 10 to 12 years; range, 4 to 30 years.

The incidence of sarcoma arising in a previously irradiated field is approximately 0.1 percent, with a median latent period of 13 years.[151,195] The sarcoma originates within previously normal tissue, either bone or the surrounding soft tissue, and can be seen with radiation doses as low as 25 Gy. Criteria for diagnosis are as follows:

1. Histologically proven sarcoma
2. Tumor arising in documented previously radiated field
3. Asymptomatic latent period (minimum of 3 to 4 years)

The treatment of radiation-induced sarcoma is wide resection when possible combined with adjuvant chemotherapy. Overall survival ranges from 25 to 35 percent. The unique difficulty for the surgeon is that of operating within a previously irradiated field. Increased local complications can be anticipated.

Small Round Cell Sarcomas of Bone

Round cell sarcomas of bone behave differently and require different therapeutic management than do spindle cell sarcomas.[196,197] Round cell sarcomas of bone consist of poorly differentiated small cells without matrix production. They present radiographically as osteolytic lesions. These lesions are best treated with radiation and chemotherapy; surgery is reserved for special situations. Non-Hodgkin's lymphoma and Ewing's sarcoma are the two most common small cell sarcomas. The differential diagnosis of all round cell sarcomas includes metastatic neuroblastoma, metastatic undifferentiated carcinoma, histiocytosis, small cell OS, osteomyelitis, and multiple myeloma.

Ewing's Sarcoma

Ewing's sarcoma is the second most common bone sarcoma of childhood; it is approximately one-half as frequent as OS. The lesion is characterized by poorly differentiated small round cells with marked homogeneity. The exact cell of origin is unknown. The clinical and biological behavior is significantly different from that of spindle cell sarcomas. Within the past two decades, the prognosis of patients with Ewing's sarcomas has been dramatically improved by the combination of effective adjuvant chemotherapy, improved radiotherapy techniques, and the select use of limited surgical resection.[35,198–200]

Clinical Characteristics Ewing's sarcomas tend to occur in young children, though rarely in those below the age of 5 years. Characteristically the flat and axial bones (50 to 60 percent) are involved.[21,35] When involvement in a long (tubular) bone is seen, it is most often in the proximal or diaphyseal area. In contrast, OSs occur in adolescence (average age 15), most often around the knees, and involve the metaphysis of long bones. Another unique finding with Ewing's sarcoma is the presence of systemic signs (i.e., fever, anorexia, weight loss, leukocytosis, and anemia).[198] All may be a presenting sign of the disease (20 to 30 percent); this is in contrast to the distinct absence of all systemic signs with OS until late in the disease process. In Ewing's sarcoma, pathologic fracture implies a poor prognosis. The most common complaint is pain and/or a mass. Localized tenderness is often present, with associated erythema and induration. These findings, in combination with systemic signs of fever and leukocytosis, closely mimic those of osteomyelitis.

Radiographic Findings Ewing's sarcoma is a highly destructive radiolucent lesion without evidence of bone formation. The typical pattern consists of a permeative or moth-eaten destruction associated with periosteal elevation. Characteristically there is multilaminated periosteal elevation or a "sunburst" appearance (Fig. 16-21). When Ewing's sarcoma occurs in flat bones, however, these findings are usually absent. Tumors of flat bones appear as destructive lesions with large soft tissue components. The ribs and pelvis are most often involved. Pathologic fractures occur secondary to extensive bony destruction and the absence of tumor matrix. The differential diagnosis is osteomyelitis, osteolytic OS, metastatic neuroblastoma, and histiocytosis.

Natural History Ewing's sarcoma is highly lethal and rapidly disseminates. Historically, fewer than 10 to 15 percent of patients remained disease-free at 2 years.[21,201] Many patients present with metastatic disease. The most common sites are the lungs and other bones. It used to be thought that Ewing's sarcoma was a multicentric disease because of the high incidence of multiple bone involvement. Unlike other bone sarcomas, Ewing's sarcoma is associated with visceral, lymphatic, and meningeal involvement, and these must be searched for.

Evaluation and Staging There is no general staging system for Ewing's sarcoma. The musculoskeletal staging system does not apply to the round cell sarcomas of the bone. Because of the propensity of these lesions to spread to other bones, bone marrow, the lymphatic system, and the

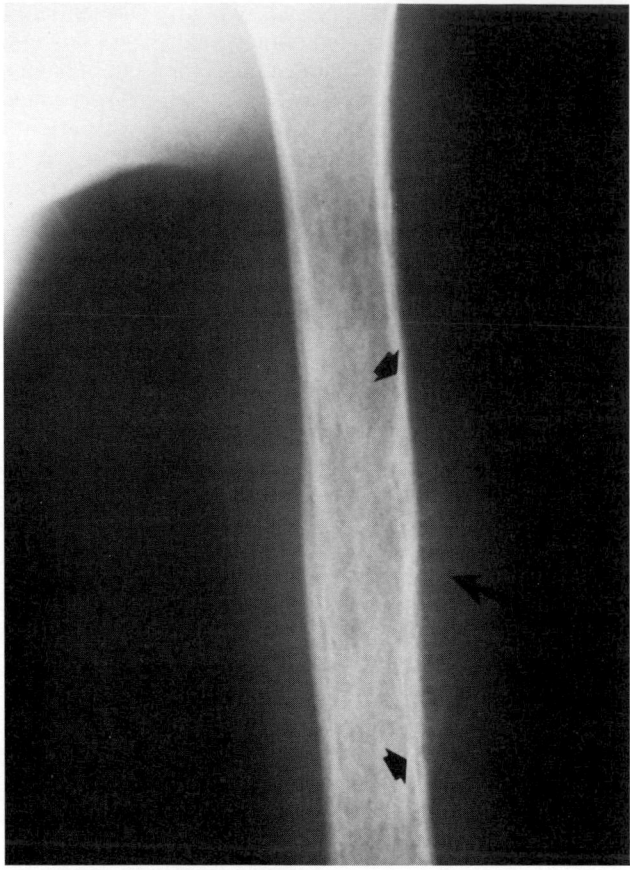

Figure 16-21 Ewing's sarcoma of the humerus. Typical permeative destruction associated with a sunburst appearance (*arrows*). Ewing's sarcoma is often diaphyseal, whereas osteosarcoma tends to be metaphyseal.

viscera, evaluation is more extensive than that for the spindle cell sarcomas. It must include a careful clinical examination of regional and distal lymph nodes and radiographic evaluation for visceral involvement. Liver-spleen scans and bone marrow aspirates are required in addition to CT of the lungs and the primary site. Angiography is required only if a primary resection is planned.

Biopsy Considerations Because of the frequent difficulty of accurate pathologic interpretation and potential problems with bone healing, the following are guidelines for the biopsy of suspected round cell tumors:

1. Adequate material must be obtained for histologic evaluation and electron microscopy. Frozen section analysis should be performed to assure adequate material for interpretation.
2. Routine cultures should be made to aid in the differentiation from an osteomyelitis.
3. Biopsy of the bony component is not necessary and should be avoided; the soft tissue component often provides adequate material. Bone biopsy should be through a *small* hole on the compressive side of the bone. Pathologic fracture through an irradiated bone often does not heal.

Gross Characteristics The tumor appears to arise in the medullary cavity, although permeation into cortical bone and surrounding soft tissues occurs frequently. The mass is soft and gray-white and may contain areas of necrosis and hemorrhage.

Microscopic Characteristics Large nests and sheets of relatively uniform round cells are typical (Fig. 16-22). The sheets of cells are often compartmentalized by intersecting collagenous trabeculae. The cells contain round nuclei with a distinct nuclear envelope. Nucleoli are uncommon, and mitotic activity is minimal. There may be occasional rosette-like structures, although neuroectodermal origin has never been confirmed. In the vicinity of necrotic tumor, small pyknotic cells may be observed. Vessels in these necrotic regions are often encircled by viable tumor cells. The cells often contain cytoplasmic glycogen, although its presence or absence cannot be considered as the only criterion for the confirmation or exclusion, respectively, of Ewing's sarcoma. This neoplasm belongs to the category of small blue round cell tumors, a designation which also includes neuroblastoma, lymphoma, round cell OS, and occasionally osteomyelitis and histiocytosis. When confronted with this differential diagnosis, the pathologist may turn to electron microscopy or immunohistochemistry for additional information.

Treatment Ewing's sarcomas are generally considered radiosensitive. Radiation therapy to the primary site has been the traditional mode of local control. Within the past decade, surgical resection of selected lesions has become increasingly popular. Though detailed management is beyond the scope of this chapter, the following sections summarize some common aspects of the multimodality approach.[35,199,200,202]

Chemotherapy. Doxorubicin, actinomycin D, cyclophosphamide, and vincristine are the most effective agents.[35,201] There are a variety of different combinations and sched-

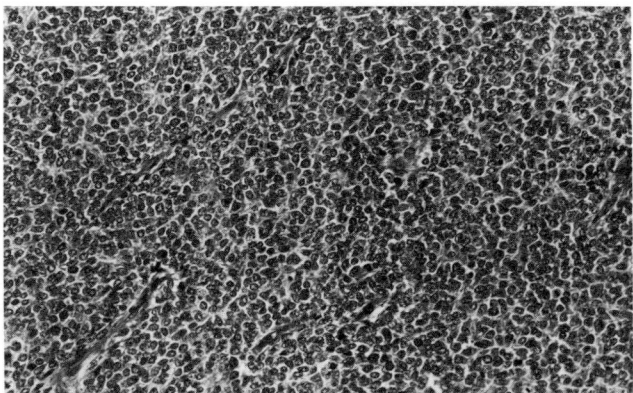

Figure 16-22 Ewing's sarcoma is characterized by sheets of small, round, uniform cells. Application of special stains may disclose cytoplasmic glycogen, although its presence in such cells is not diagnostic. Some cells reveal eccentric nuclei with a paranuclear clear zone—clues to plasma cell differentiation.

ules. All patients require intensive chemotherapy to prevent dissemination. Overall survival in patients with lesions of the extremities now ranges between 40 and 75 percent.

Radiation therapy. Radiation to the entire bone at risk is required. The usual dose ranges between 4500 and 6000 cGy delivered over 6 to 8 weeks. In order to reduce the morbidity of radiation, it is recommended that between 4000 and 5000 cGy be delivered to the whole bone, with an additional 1000 to 1500 cGy to the tumor site.[35,200-202] Sophisticated techniques are required for optimal results: preservation of a strip of unirradiated skin, compensators and/or filters, and simulation and immobilization of the target area. Physical therapy of the affected part is begun during radiation to decrease stiffness and swelling.

There has been increasing concern regarding the development of secondary sarcomas within the irradiated fields in the patients now surviving their primary disease. This is a valid concern, which may favor reduced radiation dosage and increased use of limited surgery.

Surgical treatment. The role of surgery in the treatment of Ewing's sarcoma is currently undergoing change. The Intergroup Ewing's Study recommends surgical removal of expendable bones such as the ribs, clavicle, and scapula.[35,198] In general, surgery is reserved for tumors located in high-risk areas (e.g., ribs, ilium, and proximal femur). *Risk* is defined as an increased incidence of local recurrence and metastases. In general, surgery is considered an adjunct to the other treatment modalities. When surgical resection is performed, a marginal resection only is usually feasible, because of the extensive extraosseous component. Extensive bleeding must be anticipated. Morbidity of surgery is increased secondary to radiation and chemotherapy effects. Primary amputation is often required for lower extremity lesions in a child younger than 10 years of age because of predicted leg-length shortening. Patients presenting with pathologic fractures also often require a primary amputation. Fractures occurring following adequate control of the tumor may heal following immobilization and/or internal fixation. It must be stressed that surgery in conjunction with high-dose radiation and chemotherapy entails significant local morbidity, which in itself may necessitate amputation. There is a significant increase of infection, bleeding, late fracture, and flap necrosis following high-dose radiation and/or chemotherapy.

Recently there has been increased interest in primary resection of Ewing's sarcoma following induction (neoadjuvant) chemotherapy, similar to the treatment of OS. When this is performed, radiation therapy is not given if the surgical margins are negative (wide resection). It is hoped that this approach will increase local control as well as minimize the complications and functional losses that are associated with high-dose radiotherapy.

Lymphomas of Bone

Lymphoma of bone (historically referred to as *reticulum cell sarcoma of bone*) accounts for only 5 percent of all primary bone tumors.[203] In general, lymphoma of the bone is a sign of disseminated (stage IV) disease; only occasion-

ally is it a true solitary lesion (stage IE—involvement of a single extralymphatic organ or site).[203,204] All patients suspected of having a lymphoma of bone should be carefully screened to rule out other sites of disease. Treatment is predominately medical in nature: differentiation between Hodgkin's disease and non-Hodgkin's lymphoma is important for both prognosis and form of treatment. Local radiotherapy can be curative for solitary stage IE lymphoma of bone.[205] Multiagent chemotherapy—combining Adriamycin, alkylating agents, and steroids—has achieved response rates as high as 80 percent, with cure rates of greater than 50 percent.[206,207] Combination of radiotherapy and multiagent chemotherapy has produced 88 to 90 percent survival rates at 8 years.[208,209] Hodgkin's disease, which rarely presents with bone lesions, has a very good prognosis in spite of stage IV disease: an 80 percent 5-year survival can be achieved with combination therapy.[210]

The role of surgery is typically limited to obtaining adequate tissue for diagnosis, treating pathologic fractures, and occasionally resecting expendable bones. The technique of biopsy is important to avoid secondary fracture through potentially irradiated bone. If an extraosseous component exists, there is no need to biopsy the underlying bone. Biopsy of a suspected round cell tumor should always include a frozen section and collect additional material for electron microscopy, tissue cultures, and other special studies. Patients presenting with a pathologic fracture typically will require fixation. To prevent late fracture, all patients treated with radiotherapy should be protected with a brace until reossification occurs. Radiotherapy should be given through a whole bone field as well as to adjacent or involved lymph nodes.[211]

Gross Characteristics The tumor tends to fill the marrow cavity and extend through the cortex and into adjacent soft tissues. The soft gray-white mass often reveals areas of necrosis and hemorrhage.

Microscopic Characteristics The histologic features of large cell "histiocytic" lymphoma of bone are indistinguishable from those of its primary lymph node counterpart. The tumor cells are large with indistinct cytoplasmic borders and eosinophilic cytoplasm. The nuclei reveal characteristic folded or convoluted nuclear membranes and contain prominent nucleoli. Well-differentiated lymphocytic lymphoma and Hodgkin's lymphoma rarely present with primary bone involvement. If possible, fresh tissue obtained at the time of biopsy should be submitted for immunohistochemical and flow cytometry studies to facilitate accurate subclassification of the lymphoma.

Multiple Myeloma/Plasmocytoma

Multiple myeloma is often referred to as the most common primary malignancy of bone, with an incidence between 2 and 3 per 100,000.[212] It is a disease of older adults and frequently presents with signs and symptoms related to bone marrow suppression, hypercalcemia, and renal failure. Bone pain and spontaneous vertebral fractures are often present. The radiographic hallmark of this disease is multiple osteolytic (punched out) lesions involving both the axial and appendicular skeleton. Bone scans are typically less sensitive than plain radiographs because osteoclast activity predominates in the lytic process.[213] Myeloma should be suspected when routine laboratory studies reveal anemia, increased serum creatinine, elevated calcium, and elevated serum protein. Confirmation can readily be made by demonstrating a monoclonal spike on serum protein electrophoresis (SPEP). Infection and renal failure are the most common causes of death, and the presence of either is a poor prognostic indicator.[214]

The role of the orthopaedic surgeon in the management of this disease is twofold. First, accurate diagnosis and differentiation from other lesions of bone is paramount to the institution of appropriate medical therapy. Second, treatment of impending or actual pathologic fractures should be performed to alleviate pain, improve function, and allow patients greater independence. Techniques of fixation as discussed for metastatic tumors, below, are appropriate in these patients. Large amounts of blood loss and medical complications such as infection, hypercalcemia, and progressive renal failure must be anticipated. Patients with advanced disease are at risk for additional pathologic fractures and should be carefully positioned and transferred in the operating room. Multiple rib fractures may result in respiratory failure and ventilator dependence.

Metastatic Bone Disease and Pathologic Fractures

Approximately 100,000 patients a year in the United States develop metastatic disease. The exact incidence of skeletal metastasis and the fracture rate are unknown. The orthopaedic surgeon is commonly asked to manage patients with skeletal metastases. The operative and nonoperative treatment of metastatic disease is continuously evolving.

Clinical Characteristics

Metastatic carcinoma is the most common bone tumor in patients over 40. Despite the wide variety of carcinomas, the hallmark of skeletal involvement is pain. A patient with a known cancer who develops skeletal pain must be assumed to have a bony metastasis until proved otherwise. Approximately 10 percent of cancer patients present with bony metastasis as the first sign of the disease. Plain radiographs may appear normal for weeks or months after the onset of pain. Thus, clinical suspicion is the key to accurate diagnosis. The most common primary sources of skeletal metastases are the lungs, breast, prostate, pancreas, and stomach.

Bone scans are highly accurate and demonstrate increased uptake early on. The most common sites of involvement are spine (thoracic, then lumbar), pelvis, femur, and ribs. This distribution reflects the pattern of hematogenous spread. Vertebral lesions are thought to be secondary to seeding via Batson's plexus, i.e., the valveless venous plexus that permits retrograde flow. The hip and femur are the most common sites of pathologic fracture. Spinal involvement presents with back pain or neurologic deficit secondary to epidural compression. Laboratory data may show hypercalcemia, reflecting accelerated bone resorption. An elevated alkaline phosphatase level is less common and is due to a secondary osteoblastic attempt to repair the destructive lesion. An elevated acid phosphatase level is pathognomonic of metastatic prostate cancer.

Radiographic Findings

Most metastatic carcinomas tend to be irregularly osteolytic with some osteoblastic response. Characteristically, osteoblastic metastases occur in the breast, prostate, lung, or bladder. In general, most endocrine tumors tend to be osteoblastic, whereas nonendocrine tumors tend to be radiolucent or osteolytic. Between 75 and 90 percent of patients with metastatic disease have multiple lesions at initial presentation. Soft tissue extension is rare for metastatic disease; the major exceptions are hypernephroma and thyroid cancer. These two lesions characteristically present as a ballooning expansile lesion with a soft tissue component; both tend to be extremely vascular. Periosteal elevation is rare except with prostate cancer. Radiographic diagnosis of metastatic disease tends to be simple. Factors favoring metastasis are irregular osteolytic and/or mixed osteoblastic lesion, multiple lesions, and age above 40 years. A few metastatic lesions may mimic a primary sarcoma. Specifically, a metastatic prostate (osteoblastic) lesion may appear as a primary osteosarcoma and a solitary hypernephroma as an osteolytic sarcoma, e.g., MFH of bone.

Staging Studies

Staging studies are similar to those used in the evaluation of primary sarcomas. The information obtained is useful in local evaluation and in therapy.

Bone Scans Bone scintigraphy is the most helpful study in evaluating metastatic disease. Presence of multiple lesions favors the diagnosis of metastatic carcinoma and often suggests that there is involvement of other anatomic areas not suspected from clinical examination. Intraosseous extension beyond the area indicated by the plain radiographs is not unusual; this is due to the propensity of carcinoma cells to permeate between the bony trabeculae. Occasionally, decreased uptake of contrast is noted in rapidly growing lesions, presumably because of tumor necrosis.

Computed Tomography/Magnetic Resonance Imaging Axial studies of the body are not only helpful in the definition of localized skeletal disease but also of great importance in diagnosing the site of primary disease in patients initially presenting with a bone lesion. Computed tomography scans of the chest and contrast-enhanced CT scans of the abdomen and pelvis allow for accurate screening for solid tumors of the major organ systems. Despite this, however, approximately 10 percent of all patients will never have an identifiable site of primary disease. Magnetic resonance imaging has become increasingly useful in patients with spinal, pelvic, and hip lesions. This study often demonstrates extraosseous tumor not suspected on the plain radiographs. If a bone scan is "hot" but the x-ray film is normal, CT scans are best at demonstrating the degree of bony destruction. Thus, both CT and MRI are useful in evaluation of patients with metastatic disease.

Angiography Angiography is useful in specific clinical situations when evaluating metastatic disease, most commonly for preoperative embolization for suspected vascular lesions and for planning preoperative resection of certain pelvic and shoulder girdle lesions. In particular, hypernephromas are extremely vascular and should be embolized prior to surgery.

Biopsy

The principles and techniques of biopsy are similar to those described for primary bone tumors. If a metastatic lesion is strongly suspected, a needle biopsy is often sufficient (90 percent) for a correct diagnosis. Needle biopsies are most useful for confirming metastatic carcinoma in a patient with a known cancer.[153] Conversely, if the primary tumor is unknown, a larger range of material is required for special stains, culture, and electron microscopy. A small incisional biopsy is recommended. Material for hormonal receptor tests (approximately 1 g of tissue is required) must be preserved immediately by freezing in liquid nitrogen.

Pathology

Gross Characteristics Since essentially any viscus can be the origin of osseous metastasis, the gross presentation can be quite variable. The nodules are usually well defined and can show a variable amount of hemorrhage and necrosis. A tan-brown or black lesion suggests melanoma.

Microscopic Characteristics The primary site determines, to a large degree, the histologic appearance of the metastatic focus. Unequivocal epithelial features such as acinar formation, papillae with epithelial lining, or keratin pearl formation indicate that the lesion is not primary in bone; furthermore, based on both the pattern and certain histochemical properties, a likely primary site can be suggested. For example, the presence of epithelial mucins within tumor cell vacuoles suggests lung, gastrointestinal tract, or pancreas, among others, as possible primary sites. The Fontana stain confirms the presence of melanin pigment, as would be expected in malignant melanoma. Immunohistochemical studies, as for thyroglobulin or prostate-specific acid phosphatase, offer an additional means of tumor identification. It can be difficult to determine whether a neoplasm is a metastasis or a primary lesion. Metastatic small cell carcinoma can be misinterpreted as primary bone sarcoma or lymphoma. At the other extreme are metastatic pleomorphic caricnomas, particularly from the kidney, which have been misdiagnosed as primary MFH of bone.

Treatment: General Considerations

Treatment considerations for patients with metastatic skeletal disease differ from those for patients with primary bone neoplasms. In general, overall survival is less than 1 year. The main goals of treatment are relief of bone pain, the prevention of fracture, continued ambulation, and the avoidance of cord compression from metastatic vertebral disease. The treatment for each patient must be highly individualized, but there are certain guidelines:

1. Bone pain can be relieved by analgesics and radiation therapy. Lesions of the lower extremity often require prophylactic fixation to avoid fracture. Closed intramedullary rodding reduces the local morbidity of diaphyseal lesions. Prophylactic fixation is recommended if the lesion is greater than one-third to one-half the width of the bone.
2. If multiple sites are involved, the lower extremity (especially the hips) should be treated early to permit ambulation.
3. Early spinal cord compression should be treated aggressively with radiotherapy. If symptoms persist, early decompression is required. Increasing back pain is an early sign of cord compression.
4. Intramedullary fixation is preferred over screw-and-plate fixation. Endoprosthetic replacement is preferred for the hip in lieu of nail or plate fixation. Polymethylmethacrylate is required to permit immediate stable fixation and to prevent loosening. Recurrent tumor, radiation, and poor bony stock are causes for failure if stable fixation is not obtained. Bone graft is never used for pathologic fractures.
5. Perioperative antibiotics are required because of the increased risk of infection.
6. Hematologic parameters should be carefully evaluated before, during, and after surgery because of the increased risk of bleeding in cancer patients. The platelet count, prothrombin time, and partial thromboplastin time (PTT) are routinely obtained.

BENIGN BONE TUMORS

The orthopaedic surgeon is often called to treat benign bone neoplasms. Some benign bone tumors are difficult to differentiate from their malignant counterparts, have a significant rate of local recurrence, and may undergo malignant transformation. Some can be treated successfully by simple curettage (intralesional procedure), while others require extensive resection (marginal or wide). Treatment is based upon the natural history of the specific entity. Treatment must be individualized; preservation of function is important. The important clinical aspects of these tumors are emphasized in this section. In general, the preoperative staging studies are extremely accurate and the plain radiographs often suggest the correct diagnosis. The biological classification, as discussed, helps determine the ideal surgical procedure.

Solitary and Multiple Osteochondromas (Exostosis)

Osteochondromas are the most common benign bone tumor. They are characteristically sessile or pedunculated, arising from the cortex of a long tubular bone adjacent to the epiphyseal plate. Osteochondromas are usually solitary except in patients with multiple hereditary exostosis. Plain radiographs are usually diagnostic, and no further tests are required. Sessile osteochondromas present difficulty in diagnosis, especially when found in unusual sites such as the distal posterior femur, in which case they must be differentiated from a parosteal OS. Bone scintigraphy and CT are helpful in distinguishing between these two entities.

Osteochondromas grow along with the individual until skeletal maturity is reached; growth of an osteochondroma during adolescence therefore does not signify malignancy. Pain is not a sign of malignancy in children or adolescents, although in an adult it is a significant warning sign. Pain in a child may be due to a local bursitis, mechanical irritation of adjacent muscles, or a pathologic fracture.

Between 1 and 2 percent of solitary osteochondromas undergo malignant transformation; patients with multiple hereditary exostosis are at a higher (5 to 25 percent) risk.[21,145,149] Malignant tumors arising from a benign osteochondroma are usually low-grade chondrosarcomas. Proximal osteochondromas are at a higher risk to undergo malignant transformation than are distal lesions. In general, surgical removal is recommended only for symptomatic osteochondromas or for those arising along the axial skeleton and pelvic and shoulder girdle.

Gross Characteristics The lesion presents as a protuberant mass that can range in shape from sessile to a long-stalked polyp with a cauliflower appearance. The polypoid portion is covered by a cartilaginous cap of relatively uniform thickness, which becomes thinner in the adult years. Either persistence of a thick cartilage cap or the presence of irregular nodular chondroid foci in adults should raise the question of chondrosarcomatous transformation occurring within an osteochondroma. On perpendicular section, the hyaline cartilage cap rests on cortical bone, which blends into that of the underlying bone of origin. Furthermore, the marrow cavity of the osteochondroma is continuous with that of the normal bone.

Microscopic Characteristics The cartilage component consists of mature lacunar chondrocytes, often arranged in clusters or rows reminiscent of epiphyseal cartilage. In the growth phase during adolescence, occasional binucleate chondrocytes may be observed. The osseous element is formed by mature lamellar bone; foci of endochondral ossification can be observed. The marrow space may be predominantly composed of adipose tissue or be filled with hematopoietic elements. It is never fibroblastic; if present, this characteristic may be indicative of a low-grade parosteal osteosarcoma.

Enchondromas

Enchondromas may be solitary or multiple (Ollier's disease). They have been reported in most bones.[21,116,145]

These lesions are often difficult to diagnose radiographically and histologically. The biological potential is often over- or underestimated. Malignant transformations do occur, but the rate is difficult to determine.[151] In general, lesions of the pelvis, femur, and ribs are at higher risk than are more distal sites.[147]

Enchondromas are rarely painful unless a pathologic fracture exists. Otherwise, pain is a sign of local aggressiveness and possible malignancy. Enchondromas of the hands and feet, irrespective of pathologic findings, are benign,[21] whereas cartilage tumors of the pelvic or shoulder girdle are often malignant, despite a benign-appearing histologic appearance. Plain radiographs may be helpful in this differentiation. Radiographic scalloping is a sign of local aggressiveness. Bone scintigraphy is not helpful in differentiating a low-grade chondrosarcoma from an active enchondroma. Age is an important indicator of possible malignancy; enchondromas rarely undergo malignant transformation prior to skeletal maturity. Painful, benign-appearing, proximal enchondromas in an adult are often malignant, despite the histologic findings. The correlation of symptoms, plain radiographs, and histologic findings is crucial in assessing an individual cartilage tumor.

Curettage of enchondromas, with or without bone graft, in a child is usually curative. Pathologic fracture may require internal fixation in addition to curettage. In an adult, curettage has a significant rate of local recurrence; resection or curettage combined with cryosurgery has a high success rate.[155,215]

Gross Characteristics When removed intact, the lesion consists of variably sized lobules of white-gray hyaline cartilage. The tumor usually appears to be well circumscribed. Focal myxoid areas can be encountered. In addition, calcification and ossification, which impart a gritty consistency on cutting, frequently occur.

Microscopic Characteristics When chondroid lesions are under evaluation, histologic features must be correlated with both radiographic changes and clinical setting. There may be variable cellularity, but the chondrocytes tend to remain small and uniform. Nuclear atypia is minimal, and occasional binucleate forms are not inconsistent with the diagnosis of a benign lesion. As a rule, the chondrocytes are situated in individual lacunae. Correlating with the gross findings, foci of calcification and endochondral ossification can be observed. Features such as marked nuclear atypia, motitic activity, myxoid degeneration of matrix, and multiple cells in individual lacunae should raise the strong suspicion of chondrosarcoma.

Chondroblastoma, Osteoblastoma, and Osteoid Osteoma

Chondroblastoma and osteoblastoma are characterized by immature but benign chondroid and osteoid production, respectively. Both may undergo malignant transformation in rare cases, while osteoblastoma can metastasize.[151,216] Osteoid osteomas are small (less than 1 cm), painful, bone-forming tumors that are always benign. Chondroblastomas typically occur in the epiphysis of a skeletally immature child (Fig. 16-23). Although osteoblastomas may be found in any bone, the spine and skull account for 50 percent of all reported cases. The differential diagnosis of chondroblastoma includes GCT, aneurysmal bone cyst, and clear cell chondrosarcoma. Osteoblastoma must be differentiated from osteosarcoma and osteoid osteoma. Clinical correlation of age, site, and histologic finding often points to the correct diagnosis.

Chondroblastomas and osteoblastomas are aggressive benign lesions with a high recurrence rate following simple curettage.[21,116,145,151] Local control can be obtained by primary resection; however, routine resection cannot be recommended for tumors adjacent to a joint. Marcove reports a 5 to 10 percent local recurrence when curettage is combined with cryosurgery.[151] This method has avoided the need for resection and extensive reconstruction in select patients. Osteoid osteomas are treated with simple excision: localization of such small lesions may present a difficult problem.

As surgical removal is the treatment of choice for these benign lesions, the role of radiotherapy is limited. Because it is generally difficult to obtain negative margins in osteoblastomas of the vertebrae, radiotherapy may be required for axial lesions if there is recurrence.

Osteoblastoma

Gross Characteristics These neoplasms have been reported as large as 10 cm and are unusually well circumscribed. This is often a highly vascular tumor which has areas of gritty osteoid formation. The overlying cortical bone can be bulging and minimally sclerotic.

Microscopic Characteristics The basic architecture of this lesion consists of a complex network of osteoid trabeculae that are lined by large but uniform osteoblasts (Fig. 16-24). A variable number of multinucleated giant cells are usually present, on occasion causing confusion with GCT. The intervening stroma, particularly in the younger lesions, is highly vascular. The extent of ossification varies from a few small foci to prominent confluent areas.

Chondroblastoma

Gross Characteristics The tumors are relatively small and almost invariably located in the epiphyseal region. They are firm and vary in color from gray-white to red-brown. Irregular chondroid areas are occasionally present. On section, hemorrhagic foci and small cysts are encountered. Extension into adjacent soft tissue is rare.

Microscopic Characteristics These highly cellular neoplasms are composed of round to polygonal cells with eosinophilic cytoplasm. The nucleus is round to oval and may have a longitudinal groove. Scattered mitotic figures are not uncommon. A variable number of giant cells are almost always present. The vast majority of these tumors contain a variable amount of chondroid matrix that stains pink rather than blue. Some zones

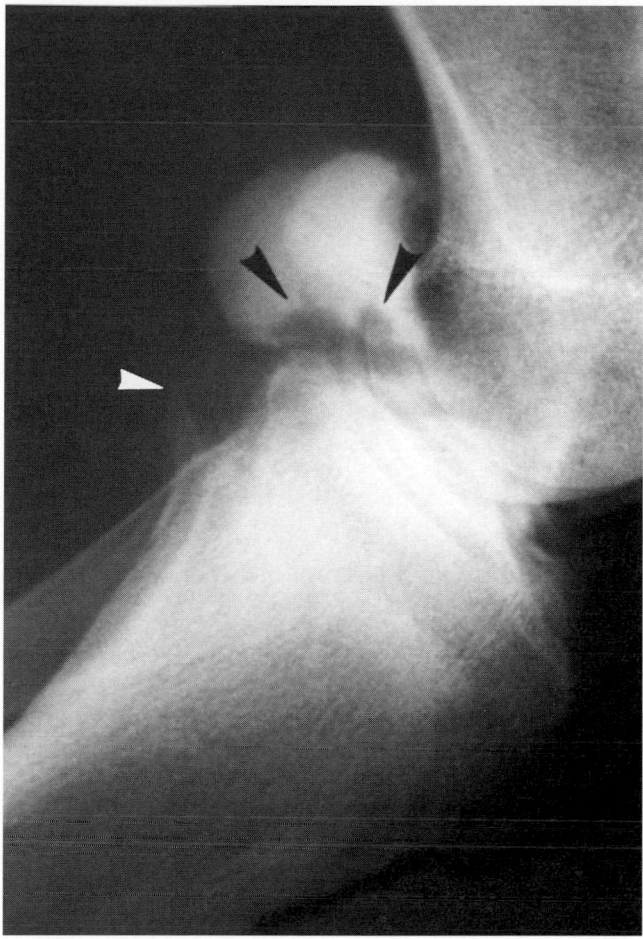

Figure 16-23 Chondroblastoma of the tibia. The contrast material in the radiograph was supplied for arthrography. Arrows outline an expansile lytic lesion of the proximal tibia. Chondroblastomas are always epiphyseal and radiolucent and occur before skeletal maturity. Faint calcifications may be present but often are not seen despite histologic evidence of calcification. The differential diagnosis includes giant-cell tumor, aneurysmal bone cyst, and clear cell chondrosarcoma. (Reproduced with permission from Malawer MM, Abelson HT, Suit HD, in DeVita VT, Hellman S, Rosenberg SA (eds): *Cancer: Principles and Practice of Oncology,* 2d ed. Philadelphia, Lippincott, 1985.)

demonstrate a characteristic lacelike chondroid matrix (Fig. 16-25). These chondroid strands become focally calcified.

Osteoid Osteoma

Clinical Characteristics This lesion has classic symptoms and radiographic appearance in 80 percent of patients affected. Osteoid osteomas are extremely painful (equivalent to a severe toothache) and well localized to the area of bony abnormality. Pain is often worse at night. The pain is relieved by salicylates; narcotics are often not helpful. The response to salicylates is dramatic, occurring in 20 to 30 min with a minimal dose of one or two tablets of regular aspirin. This pain pattern may exist for 6 to 9 months before the appropriate diagnosis is con-

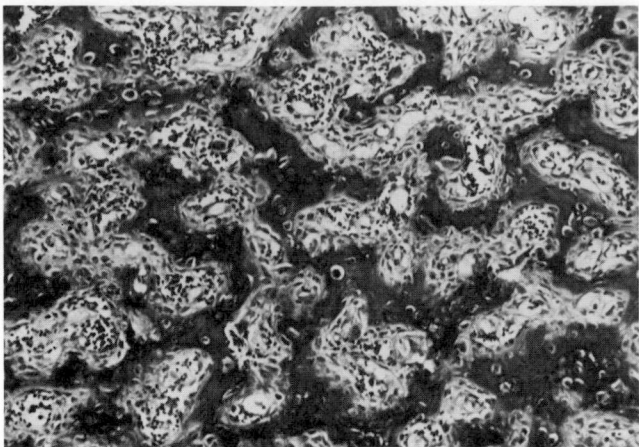

Figure 16-24 Interlacing network of irregular, partially calcified bony trabeculae, as seen in osteoblastoma.

sidered. Occasionally, the pain precedes the appearance of radiographic abnormalities and therefore leads to multiple incorrect diagnoses, including neuroses. The most common anatomic sites are the femur and/or tibia, although any bone—including the skull, spine, and small bones of the hands and feet—can be involved. When the lesion is located near a joint, the symptoms may mimic those of a monoarticular arthritis. Osteoid osteomas of the spine often present as a painful scoliosis mimicking a vertebral osteomyelitis, spinal cord tumor, or abdominal disease. An interlacing network of irregular, partially calcified bony trabeculae, as seen in osteoblastoma, may be present.

Radiographic Appearance and Evaluation The tumor can be found in any portion of a bone. The position relative to the cortex, periosteum, and spongiosa determines

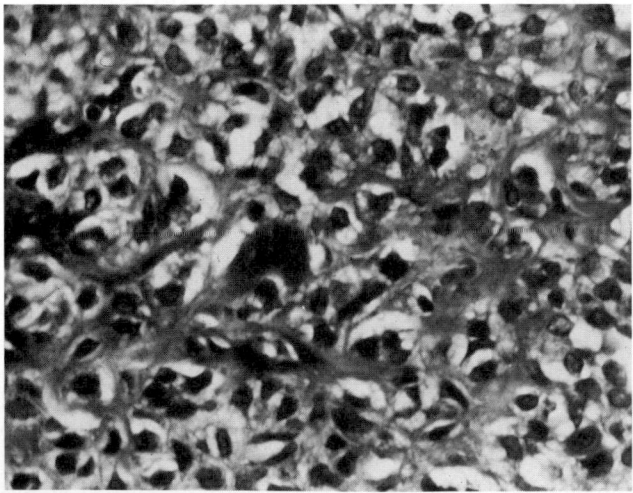

Figure 16-25 Chondroblastoma is characterized by polygonal chondrocytes and scattered multinucleated giant cells enmeshed in a lacelike chondroid matrix.

the radiographic appearance. The most common site is intracortical. Plain radiographs may show the nidus (lesion), which is radiolucent, but it is often obscured by a large amount of dense, white, reactive bone that is stimulated in response to the tumor. When the lesion is intramedullary, there is less sclerotic response. Detection and localization of the lesion are difficult. Bone scintigraphy is the most useful staging study and demonstrates markedly increased uptake of contrast medium. Computed tomography (in a transverse dimension) may demonstrate the nidus and is helpful in determining which portion of the bone is involved. This aids in determining the appropriate surgical approach and the section of bone to be excised. Occasionally CT does not demonstrate the lesion because of the lesion's small size and a partial volume effect. In this case, linear tomography may be more useful. The authors recommend that all the above studies be performed because of the likely difficulty of accurate localization and need for complete surgical removal. In addition, intraoperative scanning of the specimen and the patient is required to assure localization and removal of the lesion.

Treatment Surgical removal of the nidus is required; the sclerotic, reactive bone need not be removed. Pain is dramatically resolved postoperatively if the nidus has been excised. Incomplete removal routinely results in a clinical recurrence. A wide excision of a portion of the reactive bone and area of presumed nidus is often required to accomplish successful removal. Recently, a less aggressive surgical technique, referred to as the *"burr down" method,* has been described.[217] Minimized removal of bone is performed to visualize the nidus, which is then removed under direct vision.

Gross Characteristics Identification of the characteristic nidus is essential to establish a diagnosis of osteoid osteoma. The round, well-delineated nidus rarely measures more than 1.0 to 1.5 cm. It is usually red and can vary from soft and friable to sclerotic.

Microscopic Characteristics The nidus is characterized by an interlacing network of osteoblast-lined trabeculae. Calcification of the osteoid may be prominent, particularly in the center, and cement lines are common. Scattered multinucleated giant cells are commonly noted. The intertrabecular stroma consists of a richly vascular connective tissue, devoid of hematopoietic elements (Fig. 16-26). The bone surrounding the nidus usually reveals nonspecific sclerotic changes. On occasion, it may be exceedingly difficult to differentiate a large osteoid osteoma from an osteoblastoma.

Unicameral (Simple) Bone Cysts

Unicameral bone cysts (UBCs) are benign lesions that occur during growth. They involve the metaphysis and/or diaphysis of a long bone (Fig. 16-27A). They are believed not to be true neoplasms.

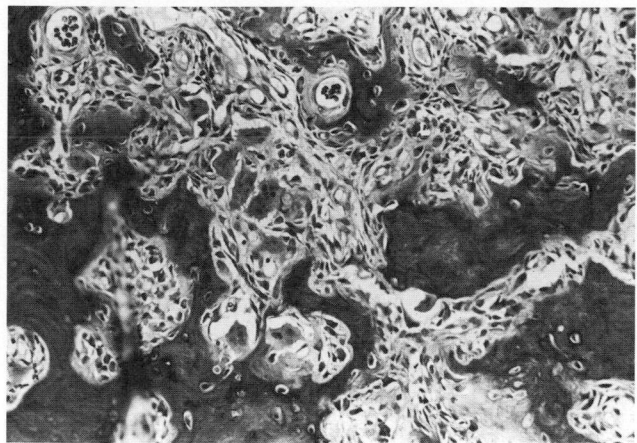

Figure 16-26 High-power micrograph of osteoid osteoma reveals osteoblast-lined trabeculae. Note the richly vascular stroma and scattered multinucleated giant cells.

The most common sites are the proximal humerus (67 percent) and proximal femur (15 percent).[218] These cysts are usually asymptomatic until a fracture occurs. Radiographically, UBCs are radiolucent and slightly expansile with well-defined margins. They are rarely confused with other benign or malignant tumors and are easily diagnosed by plain radiographs when found in the more common locations. Other preoperative staging studies are usually not required. Bone scintigraphy is the most useful study when the diagnosis is in doubt. The bone scan typically shows a photon-deficient area corresponding to the plain radiograph (Fig. 16-27B). A small area of increased uptake of contrast reflects a typical hairline crack that initiates pain and radiographic investigation.

Treatment

The traditional treatment has been curettage. Local recurrence rates have ranged from 35 to 70 percent. Recently, UBCs have been successfully treated by aspiration, flushing, and injection with methylprednisolone acetate. In one series of 40 patients, a second aspiration and injection was required in 27 percent of patients; 95 percent eventually healed.[218] In order to avoid erroneously injecting a bone lesion other than a UBC, four radiographic, nonhistological criteria have been established and are summarized as follows[218]:

1. Typical plain radiograph (and age and location)
2. Positive aspiration (yellow fluid)
3. Typical transduced "arteriolar" pressure curve (range 15 to 28 mmHg)
4. Complete filling of cyst with meglumine diatrizoate (Renografin) following aspiration

In general, UBCs should be treated by aspiration, high-pressure Renografin injection, and intracavitary methylprednisolone. Pathologic fractures should be allowed to heal *before* injection is performed. If the diagnosis is in doubt, a Craig needle procedure or small incisional biopsy should be performed. There may be radiographic recurrence; this can be successfully treated with repeat injections. These lesions should not be left untreated in the hope that they will regress spontaneously. Fewer than 1 percent of UBCs do so; the remainder often become large before the appropriate treatment is undertaken, making definitive treatment more difficult.

Gross Characteristics On section, the UBC usually contains a clear or blood-tinged fluid. Occasionally, the cavity is empty. The wall of the cyst reveals protruding thin-walled septa of variable depth. The cyst lining may be thin and white-gray or may reveal foci of brown-red soft tissue.

Figure 16-27 Unicameral bone cyst. *A.* Typical unicameral bone cyst of the proximal humerus. There is a slight expansion of the cortices without evidence of cortical destruction or periosteal elevation. *B.* Bone scintigraphy. Unicameral bone cysts are classically photon-deficient (cold) lesions (*solid arrows*). In contrast, GCTs and aneurysmal bone cysts routinely show increased uptake. Bone scans are recommended preoperatively only if the diagnosis is in doubt. The epiphyseal plate (*curved arrow*) is noted.

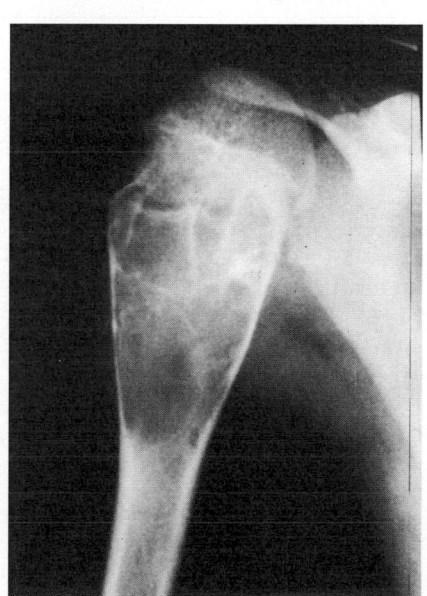

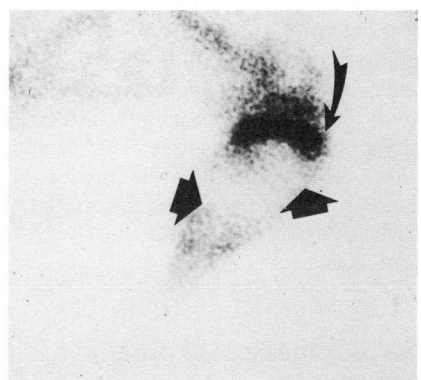

A   *B*

Prior fracture or hemorrhage substantially alters these basic features.

Microscopic Characteristics The cyst lining varies from a thin fibrocollagenous membrane to a thicker, more cellular tissue. The latter foci contain an admixture of giant cells, chronic inflammatory cells, and hemosiderin-laden macrophages. Areas with granulation tissue and reactive bone are occasionally noted.

Eosinophilic Granuloma (Histiocytosis X)

Langerhans' cell histiocytosis is a more descriptive and recently accepted term to describe the disease commonly referred to as histiocytosis X. The solitary or multifocal osseous lesions (Greenberger stage IA and B) were formerly referred to as eosinophilic granuloma (EG).[219] These are solitary destructive lesions arising presumably from the reticuloendothelial system during the first decade of life. There is slight male predominance. Any bone may be involved. The most common sites are the long bones and commonly the periacetabular region. The skull, mandible, ribs, and vertebrae are frequent sites. Multiple bony involvement is common; between 10 and 50 percent of patients develop multiple lesions. Plain radiographs characteristically show a lytic, punched-out lesion with some evidence of cortical destruction; approximately 50 percent of patients have periosteal elevation. The differential diagnosis includes osteomyelitis, Ewing's sarcoma, and lymphoma. The diaphysis and the metaphysis are equally affected. Primary epiphyseal involvement or extension is rare: Leeson reviewed the literature in 1985 and reported 3 new cases; a total of 10 cases have been reported to date.[220]

Good results have been achieved with the use of steroids to treat localized bony EG. The natural history of EG of bone is to spontaneously heal. Curettage or intralesional steroid injection is recommended for documented lesions, especially in a weight-bearing bone. Low-dose radiation therapy (600 to 1000 cGy) is useful for lesions of the jaw, skull, spine, femoral head, recurrent lesions, and lesions associated with diabetes insipidus.[221–224]

Gross Characteristics The curetted tissue is soft and friable and can be pink or yellow.

Microscopic Characteristics Sheets of large histiocytes (Langerhans' cells) characterize this process. These cells have abundant amphophilic cytoplasm and a large vesicular nucleus, which is usually folded or convoluted. There may be inflammatory cells in the background, although abundant eosinophils are almost always present. With this disease it is not possible to predict the extent of the visceral involvement based on the histomorphology of the bone lesions.

Desmoplastic Fibroma

Desmoplastic fibroma is an extremely rare bone tumor. Only 50 cases have been reported.[151] The tumor is characterized by abundant collagen formation and a fibrous stroma without evidence of mitosis or pleomorphism. Radiographically, it presents as an osteolytic lesion with well-defined margins. The basic differential diagnosis is primary fibrosarcoma of bone. Adequate treatment is en bloc resection; curettage has a significant rate of local recurrence.

Gross Characteristics The lesion consists of a homogeneous firm, white-gray, whorled, fibrous tissue.

Microscopic Characteristics The tumor is characterized by intersecting dense collagen bundles containing bland-appearing, uniform spindle cells. Mitotic activity is rare to absent. The histologic picture is essentially indistinguishable from that of soft tissue fibromatosis (desmoid). On occasion, it can be exceedingly difficult to differentiate desmoplastic fibroma from a well-differentiated fibrosarcoma. Furthermore, well-differentiated central osteosarcoma can have features closely resembling desmoplastic fibroma. In these situations, careful clinical and radiologic correlation is necessary to avoid serious misdiagnosis.

REFERENCES

1. Campanacci M, Bacci G, Bertoni F, et al: The treatment of osteosarcoma of the extremity: Twenty years' experience at the Istituto Ortopedico Rizzoli. *Cancer* 48:1569–1581, 1981.
2. Campanacci M, Giunti A, Olmi R: Giant-cell tumors of bone: A study of 209 cases with long-term followup in 130. *Ital J Orthop Traumatol* 1:249–277, 1977.
3. Campanacci M, Picci P, Gherlinzona F, et al: Parosteal osteosarcoma. *J Bone Joint Surg* 66B:313–321, 1984.
4. Chao EYS, Ivins JC: *Design and Application of Tumor Prosthesis for Bone and Joint Reconstruction—The Design and Application.* New York, Thieme-Stratton, 1983.
5. Cortes EP, Holland JP: Adjuvant chemotherapy for primary osteogenic sarcoma. *Surg Clin North Am* 61:1391–1404, 1981.
6. Dahlin DC: The problems in assessment of new treatment regimens of osteosarcoma. *Clin Orthop* 153:81–85, 1980.
7. deSantos LA, Bernardino ME, Murry JA: Computed tomography in the evaluation of osteosarcoma: Experience with 25 cases. *AJR* 132:535–540, 1979.
8. Enneking WF, Spanier SS, Goodman MA: A system for the surgical staging of musculoskeletal sarcoma. *Clin Orthop* 153:106–120, 1980.
9. Malawer MM, Abelson HT, Suit HD: Sarcomas of bone, in DeVita VT, Hellman S, Rosenberg SA (eds): *Cancer: Principles and Practice of Oncology,* 2d ed. Philadelphia, Lippincott, 1985, pp 1293–1343.
10. Malawer MM, Sugarbaker PH, Lambert M, et al: The Tikhoff Linberg procedure: Report of ten patients and presentation of a modified technique for tumors of the proximal humerus. *Surgery* 97:518–528, 1985.
11. Rosenthal DI: Computed tomography in bone and soft tissue neoplasms: Application and pathologic correlation. *CRC Crit Rev Diagn Imaging* 18:243–278, 1982.
12. Enneking WF: *Musculoskeletal Tumor Surgery.* Vol 1. New York, Churchill Livingstone, 1983, pp 1–60.
13. Simon MA, Enneking WF: The management of soft-tissue sarcomas of the extremities. *J Bone Joint Surg* 58A:317, 1976.

14. Enneking WF, Spanier SS, Malawer MM: The effect of the anatomic setting on the results of surgical procedure for soft parts sarcoma of the thigh. *Cancer* 47:1005–1022, 1981.

15. Kruzelock RP, Hansen MF: Molecular genetics and cytogenetics of sarcomas. *Hematol Oncol Clin North Am* 9:513–540, 1995.

16. Eng C, Li FP, Abramson DH, et al: Mortality from second tumors among long-term survivors of retinoblastoma. *J Natl Cancer Inst* 85:1121, 1993.

17. Levine AJ, Momand J, Finlay CA: The p53 tumour suppressor gene. *Nature* 351:453, 1991.

18. Hartley AL, Birch JM, Kelsey AM, et al: Sarcomas in three generations of a family with neurofibromatosis. *Cancer Genet Cytogenet* 45:245, 1990.

19. Henshaw RM, Jones VV, Shmookler B, Malawer MM: Cytogenic abnormalities of malignant and benign tumors. An analysis of 78 consecutive cases. Presented at the Second Annual Meeting of the CTOS, Toronto, Canada, October 1996.

20. Weingrad DN, Rosenberg SA: Early lymphatic spread of osteogenic and soft-tissue sarcomas. *Surgery* 84:231–240, 1978.

21. Dahlin DC: *Bone Tumors: General Aspects and Data on 6,221 Cases,* 3d ed. Springfield, IL, Charles C Thomas, 1978.

22. Marcove RC, Lewis MM, Rosen G, et al: Total femur and total knee replacement: A preliminary report. *Clin Orthop* 126:147–152, 1977.

23. Sim FH, Bowman WE, Chao EYS: Limb salvage surgery and reconstructive techniques, in Sim FH (ed): *Diagnosis and Treatment of Bone Tumors: A Team Approach.* Mayo Clinic Monograph. Thorofare, NJ, Slack Inc., 1983, pp 75–105.

24. Bacci G, Picci P, Calderoni P, et al: Full-lung tomograms and bone scanning in the initial work-up of patients with osteogenic sarcoma: A review of 126 cases. *Eur J Cancer Clin Oncol* 18:967–971, 1982.

25. deSantos LA, Edeiken B: Purely lytic osteosarcoma. *Skel Radiol* 9:1–7, 1982.

26. Goldenberg RR, Campbell CJ, Bonfiglio M: Giant cell tumor of bone: An analysis of two hundred and eighteen cases. *J Bone Joint Surg [Am]* 52:619–664, 1970.

27. Goldstein H, McNeil BJ, Zufall E, et al: Changing indications for bone scintigraphy in patients with osteosarcoma. *Radiology* 135:177–180, 1980.

28. Gray SW, Singhabhandhu B, Smith RA, Skandalakis JE: Sacrococcygeal chordoma: Report of a case and review of the literature. *Surgery* 78:573–582, 1975.

29. Guterberg B, Romanus B, Sterner BL: Pelvic strength after major amputation of the sacrum: An experimental study. *Acta Orthop Scand* 47:635–642, 1976.

30. Hajdu SI, Shin MH, Fortner JC: Tendosynovial sarcoma: A clinicopathological study of 136 cases. *Cancer* 39:1201, 1977.

31. Harwood AR, Krajbich JI, Fornasier VL: Mesenchymal chondrosarcoma: A report of 17 cases. *Clin Orthop* 158:144–148, 1981.

32. Hudson TM, Hass G, Enneking WF, Hawkins EF: Angiography in the management of musculoskeletal tumors. *Surg Gynecol Obstet* 141:11–21, 1975.

33. Malawer MM, Zielinski CJ: Giant cell tumor of bone: Surgical management—cryosurgery and en bloc resection. Analysis of 20 consecutive cases and recommendations for treatment. Presented at the American Academy of Orthopedic Surgeons, Anaheim, California, March 1983.

34. Marcove RC, Rosen G: En bloc resection for osteogenic sarcoma. *Cancer* 45:3040–3044, 1980.

35. Nesbit ME, Perez C-A, Tefft M, et al: Multimodal therapy for the management of primary nonmetastatic Ewing's sarcoma of bone: An intergroup study. *Natl Cancer Inst Monogr* 56:255–262, 1981.

36. Massengill AD, Seeger LL, Eckardt JJ: The role of plane radiography, computed tomography, and magnetic resonance imaging in sarcoma evaluation. *Hematol Oncol Clin North Am* 9:571–604, 1995.

37. Enneking WF, in Enneking WF (ed): *Clinical Musculoskeletal Pathology,* 3d ed rev. Gainesville, FL, University of Florida Press, 1992, p xi.

38. Levine E: Computed tomography of musculoskeletal tumors. *CRC Crit Rev Diagn Imaging* 16:279–309, 1981.

39. McKillop JH, Etcubanas E, Goris ML: The indications for and limitations of bone scintigraphy in osteogenic sarcoma: A review of 55 patients. *Cancer* 48:1133–1138, 1981.

40. Podoloff DA: The role of radionuclide scans in sarcoma. *Hematol Oncol Clin North Am* 9:605–626, 1995.

41. Menendez LR, Fideler BM, Mirra J: Thallium-201 scanning for the evaluation of osteosarcoma and soft tissue sarcoma. *J Bone Joint Surg* 75A:526–531, 1993.

42. Rosen G, Loren GJ, Brien EW, et al: Serial thallium-201 scintigraphy in osteosarcoma: Correlation with tumor necrosis after preoperative chemotherapy. *Clin Orthop* 293:302–306, 1993.

43. Springfield D: Thallium-201 scanning for the evaluation of osteosarcoma and soft-tissue sarcoma. *J Bone Joint Surg [Am]* 75:1880–1881, 1993.

44. Tokuumi Y, Tsuchiya H, Sunayama C, et al: Thallium-201 scintigraphy for diagnosis, evaluation of chemotherapy effects and detection of local recurrence in musculoskeletal neoplasms. *Abstract Book* 1995, p 175.

45. Destouet JM, Gilula LA, Murphy W: Computed tomography of long bone osteosarcoma. *Radiology* 131:439–445, 1979.

46. Sanerkin NG: The diagnosis and grading of chondrosarcoma of bone: A combined cytologic and histologic approach. *Cancer* 45:582–594, 1980.

47. Bohndorf K, Reiaer M, Lochner B, et al: Magnetic resonance imaging of primary tumours and tumour-like lesions of bone. *Skel Radiol* 15:511–517, 1986.

48. Cohen MD, Weetman RM, Provisor AJ, et al: Efficacy of magnetic resonance imaging in 139 children with tumors. *Arch Surg* 121:522–529, 1986.

49. Zimmer WD, Berquist TH, McLeod RA, et al: Bone tumors: Magnetic resonance imaging versus computer tomography. *Radiology* 709–718, 1985.

50. Sundaram M, McGuire MH, Herbold DR: Magnetic resonance imaging of osteosarcoma. *Skel Radiol* 16:23–29, 1987.

51. Malawer MM: Surgical management of aggressive and malignant tumors of the proximal fibula. *Clin Orthop* 186:172–181, 1984.

52. Chuang VP, Benjamin R, Jaffe N, et al: Radiographic and angiographic changes in osteosarcoma after intra-arterial chemotherapy. *AJR* 139:1065–1069, 1982.

53. Carrasco CH, Charnsangavel C, Raymond AK, et al: Osteosarcoma: Angiographic assessment of response to preoperative chemotherapy. *Radiology* 170:839–842, 1989.

54. Mankin HJ, Lange TA, Spanier SS: The hazards of biopsy in patients with malignant primary bone and soft-tissue tumors. *J Bone Joint Surg* 64A:1121–1127, 1982.

55. Mankin HJ, Mankin CJ, Simon MA: The hazards of the biopsy, revisited. *J Bone Joint Surg* 78A:656–663, 1996.

56. Moore TM, Meyers MH, Patzakis MJ, et al: Closed biopsy of musculoskeletal lesions. *J Bone Joint Surg [Am]* 61:375–380, 1979.

57. Schajowicz F, Derqui JC: Puncture biopsy in lesions of the locomotor system: Review and results in 4050 cases, including 941 vertebral punctures. *Cancer* 21:5331–5487, 1968.

58. Barth RJ, Merino MJ, Solomon D, et al: A prospective study of the value of core needle biopsy and fine needle aspiration in the diagnosis of soft tissue masses. *Surgery* 112:536–543, 1992.

59. Ayala AG, Raymond AK, Ro JY, et al: Needle biopsy of primary bone lesions: MD Anderson experience. *Pathol Annu* 24:219–251, 1989.

60. Simon MA, Biermann JS: Biopsy of bone and soft-tissue lesions. *J Bone Joint Surg* 75A:616–621, 1993.

61. Skrzynski MC, Biermann JS, Montag A, Simon MA: Diagnostic accuracy and charge-savings of outpatient core needle biopsy compared with open biopsy of musculoskeletal tumors. *J Bone Joint Surg* 78A:644–649, 1996.

62. Morton DL, Eilber FR, Townsend CM, et al: Limb salvage from a multidisciplinary treatment approach for skeletal and soft tissue sarcomas of the extremity. *Ann Surg* 184:268–278, 1976.

63. Enneking WF, Dunham WK: Resection and reconstruction for primary neoplasms involving the innominate bone. *J Bone Joint Surg [Am]* 60:731–746, 1978.

64. Enneking WF, Shirley PD: Resection-arthrodesis for malignant and potentially malignant lesions about the knee using an intramedullary rod and local bone graft. *J Bone Joint Surg [Am]* 59:223–235, 1977.

65. Francis KC, Worcester JN Jr: Radical resection for tumors of the shoulder with preservation of a functional extremity. *J Bone Joint Surg [Am]* 44:1423–1429, 1962.

66. Janeck CJ, Nelson CL: En bloc resection of shoulder girdle: Technique and indications. Report of a case. *J Bone Joint Surg [Am]* 54:1754–1758, 1972.

67. Mankin HJ, Fogelson FS, Thrasher AZ, et al: Massive resection and allograft transplantation in the treatment of malignant bone tumors. *N Engl J Med* 294:1247–1255, 1976.

68. Marcove RC, Lewis MM, Huvos AG: En bloc upper humeral-intercapsular resection: The Tikhoff-Linberg procedure. *Clin Orthop* 124:219–228, 1977.

69. Watts HG: Introduction to resection of musculoskeletal sarcomas. *Clin Orthop* 153:31–38, 1980.

70. Simon MA, Aschliman MA, Thomas N, Mankin HJ: Limb-salvage treatment versus amputation for osteosarcoma of the distal end of the femur. *J Bone Joint Surg* 68A:1331–1337, 1986.

71. Rosenberg SA, Tepper J, Glatstein E, et al: Adjuvant chemotherapy for patients with soft tissue sarcomas. *Surg Clin North Am* 61:1415–1423, 1981.

72. Lindberg RD, Martin RM, Rohmsdahl MM: Surgery and postoperative radiotherapy in the treatment of soft-tissue sarcomas in adults. *AJR* 123:123, 1976.

73. McNeer GP, Cantin J, Chu F, Nickson JJ: The effectiveness of radiation therapy in the management of sarcoma of the soft somatic tissues. *Cancer* 22:391–397, 1968.

74. Singer S, Antman K, Corson JM, et al: Long term salvageability for patients with locally recurrent soft tissue sarcomas. *Arch Surg* 127:548–554, 1992.

75. Rosen G, Forscher C, Lowenbraun S, et al: Synovial sarcoma: Uniform response of metastases to high dose ifosfamide. *Cancer* 73:2506–2511, 1994.

76. Mertens WC, Bramwell VHC: Adjuvant chemotherapy for soft tissue sarcomas. *Hematol Oncol Clin North Am* 9:801–816, 1995.

77. Eilber FR, Eckardt JF, Rosen G, et al: Neoadjuvant chemotherapy and radiotherapy in the multidisciplinary management of soft tissue sarcomas of the extremity. *Surg Oncol Clin North Am* 2:611–620, 1993.

78. Collins C, Conrad E, Schmidt R, et al: Neoadjuvant chemotherapy of soft tissue sarcomas: Clinical and pathologic correlates of response. *Proc ASCO* 12:470, 1993.

79. Casper ES, Gaynor JJ, Harrison LB, et al: Preoperative and postoperative adjuvant combination chemotherapy and radiation for high grade extremity soft tissue sarcoma. *Cancer* 73:1644–1651, 1994.

80. Eilber F, Eckardt J, Rosen G, et al: Preoperative therapy for soft tissue sarcoma. *Hematol Oncol Clin North Am* 9:817–824, 1995.

81. Demetri GD, Elias AD: Results of single-agent and combination chemotherapy for advanced soft tissue sarcomas. *Hematol Oncol Clin North Am* 9:765–786, 1995.

82. Azzarelli A, Quagliuolo V, Casali P, et al: Preoperative doxorubicin plus ifosfamide in primary soft-tissue sarcomas of the extremities. *Cancer Chemother Pharmacol* 31(suppl 2):S210–S212, 1993.

83. Priebat D, Malawer M, Markan Y, et al: Clinical outcome of neoadjuvant intraarterial cisplatin and continuous intravenous infusion Adriamycin for large high grade unresectable/borderline soft tissue sarcomas of the extremities. *Proc ASCO* 13:473, 1994.

84. Henshaw RM, Valente A, Shmookler BM, et al: Limb salvage, histologic necrosis and disease free survival for unresectable soft tissue sarcomas treated with neoadjuvant intra-arterial chemotherapy and attempted surgical resection. Submitted, AAOS Annual Meeting, San Francisco, 1997.

85. Suit HD, Spiro I: Radiation as a treatment modality in sarcomas of the soft tissue. *Hematol Oncol Clin North Am* 9:733–746, 1995.

86. Bujko K, Suit HD, Springfield DS, et al: Wound healing after preoperative radiation for sarcoma of soft tissues. *Surg Gynecol Obstet* 176:124–134, 1993.

87. Harrison LB, Janjan N: Brachytherapy in sarcomas. *Hematol Oncol Clin North Am* 9:747–764, 1995.

88. Rosenberg SA, Tepper J, Glatstein E, et al: The treatment of soft tissue sarcomas of the extremities. Prospective randomized evaluation of 1) limb sparing surgery plus radiation therapy compared with amputation and 2) the role of adjuvant chemotherapy. *Ann Surg* 196:305–315, 1982.

89. Stinson SF, Delaney TF, Greenberg J, et al: Acute and long term affects on limb function of combined modality limb sparing therapy for extremity soft tissue sarcoma. *Int J Radiat Oncol Biol Phys* 21:1493–1499, 1991.

90. Beech DJ, Pollock RE: Surgical management of primary soft tissue sarcoma. *Hematol Oncol Clin North Am* 9:707–718, 1995.

91. Giuliano AE, Eilber FR: The rationale for planned reoperation after unplanned total excision of soft-tissue sarcomas. *J Clin Oncol* 3:1344–1348, 1985.

92. Noria S, Davis A, Kandel R, et al: Residual disease following unplanned excision of a soft-tissue sarcoma of an extremity. *J Bone Joint Surg* 78A:650–655, 1996.

93. Soule EH, Enriquez P: Atypical *fibrous* histiocytoma, malignant fibrous histiocytoma and epithelioid sarcoma: A comparative study of 65 tumors. *Cancer* 30:128–143, 1972.

94. Weiss SW, Enzinger FM: Malignant fibrous histiocytoma: An analysis of 200 cases. *Cancer* 41:2250, 1978.

95. Weiss SW, Enzinger FM: Myxoid variant of malignant fibrous histiocytoma. *Cancer* 39:1672, 1977.

96. Soslow RA, Moretto JC, Farshid G, Kempson RL: Myxoid fibrohistiocytic tumors (MFTs): A clinicopathologic review of 147 cases. *Lab Invest* 74:13A, 1996.

97. Fletcher CDM: Pleomorphic malignant fibrous histiocytoma: Fact or fiction? A critical reappraisal based on 159 tumours diagnosed as pleomorphic sarcoma. *Am J Surg Pathol* 16:213–228, 1992.

98. Shmookler BM, Enzinger FM: Liposarcoma occurring in children: An analysis of 17 cases and review of the literature. *Cancer* 52:567, 1983.

99. Dei Tos AP, Mentzel T, Newman PL, Fletcher CDM: Spindle cell liposarcoma, a hitherto unrecognized variant of liposarcoma: Analysis of six cases. *Am J Surg Pathol* 18:913–921, 1994.

100. Evans HL: Liposarcoma: A study of 55 cases with a reassessment of its classification. *Am J Surg Pathol* 3:507–523, 1979.

101. Weiss SW, Rao UK: Well differentiated liposarcoma (atypical lipoma) of deep soft tissue of the extremities, retroperi-

toneum and miscellaneous sites: A follow-up study of 92 cases with analysis of the incidence of "dedifferentiation." *Am J Surg Pathol* 16:1051–1058, 1992.

102. Enzinger FM, Weiss SW: *Soft Tissue Tumors,* 3d ed. St. Louis, Mosby, 1995, p 757.

103. Varela-Duran J, Enzinger FM: Calcifying synovial sarcoma. *Cancer* 50:345, 1982.

104. Rosen G, Marcove RC, Caparros B, et al: Primary osteogenic sarcoma: The rationale for preoperative chemotherapy and delayed surgery. *Cancer* 43:2163–2177, 1979.

105. Rosen G, Caparros B, Huvos AC, et al: Preoperative chemotherapy for osteogenic sarcoma: Selection of postoperative adjuvant chemotherapy based upon the response of the primary tumor to preoperative chemotherapy. *Cancer* 49:1221–1230, 1982.

106. Cortes EP, Holland JP: Adjuvant chemotherapy for primary osteogenic sarcoma. *Surg Clin North Am* 61:1391–1404, 1981.

107. Link MP, Goorin AM, Miser AW, et al: The effect of adjuvant chemotherapy on relapse-free survival in patients with osteosarcoma of the extremity. *N Engl J Med* 314:1600–1606, 1986.

108. Eilber F, Giuliano A, Eckardt J, et al: Adjuvant chemotherapy for osteosarcoma: A randomized prospective trial. *J Clin Oncol* 5:21–26, 1987.

109. Malawer MM, McHale KA: Limb-sparing surgery for high grade malignant tumors of the proximal tibia: Surgical technique and a new method of extensor mechanism reconstruction. 4th International Symposium on limb-salvage surgery in musculoskeletal oncology. Kyoto, Japan, 1987.

110. Dahlin DC, Coventry MB: Osteosarcoma, a study of 600 cases. *J Bone Joint Surg* 49A:101–110, 1967.

111. Dahlin DC, Unni KK: Osteosarcoma of bone and its important recognizable varieties. *Am J Surg Pathol* 1:61–72, 1977.

112. Ahuja SC, Villacin AB, Smith J, et al: Juxtacortical (parosteal) osteogenic sarcoma. *J Bone Joint Surg [Am]* 59:632–647, 1977.

113. Wilner D: Osteogenic sarcoma (osteosarcoma), in Wilner D (ed): *Radiology of Bone Tumors and Allied Disorders.* Philadelphia, Saunders, 1982, pp 1897–2095.

114. Francis KC, Kohn H, Malawer MM: Osteogenic sarcoma. *J Bone Joint Surg [Am]* 55:754, 1976.

115. Enneking WF: *Musculoskeletal Tumor Society.* Vol 7. New York, Churchill Livingstone, 1983, pp 1021–1125.

116. Lichtenstein L: *Bone Tumors,* 4th ed. St. Louis, Mosby, 1972.

117. Kurt AM, Unni KK, McLeod RA, Pritchard DJ: Low-grade intraosseous osteosarcoma. *Cancer* 65:1418–1428, 1990.

118. Huvos AG, Rosen G, Marcove RC: Primary osteogenic sarcoma: Pathologic aspects in 20 patients after treatment with chemotherapy, en bloc resection and prosthetic bone replacement. *Arch Pathol Lab Med* 101:14–18, 1977.

119. Jaffe N, Smith E, Abelson HT, et al: Osteogenic sarcoma: Alterations in the pattern of pulmonary metastases with adjuvant chemotherapy. *J Clin Oncol* 1:251–254, 1983.

120. Marcove RC, Mike V, Hajack JV, et al: Osteogenic sarcoma under the age of twenty-one. *J Bone Joint Surg [Am]* 52:411–423, 1970.

121. Rosen G, Holmes CE, Forscher CA, et al: The role of thoracic surgery in the management of metastatic osteogenic sarcoma. *Chest Surg Clin North Am* 4:75–83, 1994.

122. Meyer WH, Schell MJ, Kumar AP, et al: Thoracotomy for pulmonary metastatic osteosarcoma: An analysis of prognostic indicators of survival. *Cancer* 59:374–379, 1987.

123. Skinner KA, Eilber FR, Holmes EC, et al: Surgical treatment and chemotherapy for pulmonary metastases from osteosarcoma. *Arch Surg* 127:1065–1071, 1992.

124. Rougraff BT, Simon MA, Kneisl JS, et al: Limb salvage compared with amputation for osteosarcoma of the distal end of the femur: A long-term oncological, functional, and quality-of-life study. *J Bone Joint Surg* 76A:649–656, 1994.

125. Picca P, Sangiorgi L, Rougraff BT, et al: The relationship of chemotherapy-induced necrosis and surgical margins to local recurrence in osteosarcoma. *J Clin Oncol* 12:2699–2705, 1994.

126. Davis AM, Bell PJ: Prognostic factors in osteosarcoma: A critical review. *J Clin Oncol* 12:423–431, 1994.

127. Harris MB, Cantor AB, Goorin AM, et al: Treatment of osteosarcoma with ifosfamide: Comparison of response in pediatric patients with recurrent disease versus patients previously untreated. A pediatric oncology group study. *Med Pediatr Oncol* 24:87–92, 1995.

128. Patel SR, Hays C, Papadopoulos NE, et al: Pilot study of high dose ifosfamide + G-CSF in patients with bone and soft tissue sarcomas. *Proc ASCO* 14:516, 1995.

129. Cortes EP, Holland JP: Adjuvant chemotherapy for primary osteogenic sarcoma. *Surg Clin North Am* 61:1391–1404, 1981.

130. Muggia F, Catani R, Lee YJ, et al: Factors responsible for therapeutic success in osteosarcoma, in Jones S, Salmon S (eds): *Adjuvant Therapy for Cancer,* 2d ed. New York, Grune & Stratton, 1979.

131. Malawer MM, Buch R, Reaman G, et al: Impact of two cycles of preoperative chemotherapy with intraarterial cisplatin and intravenous doxorubicin on the choice of surgical procedure for high-grade sarcomas of the extremities. *Clin Orthop* 270:214–222, 1991.

132. Pratt CB, Epelman S, Jaffe N: Bleomycin, cyclophosphamide and dactinomycin in metastatic osteosarcoma: Lack of tumor regression in previously treated patients. *Cancer Treat Rep* 7:421–423, 1987.

133. Estrada-Aguilar J, Greenberg H, Walling A, et al: Primary treatment of pelvic osteosarcoma: Report of five cases. *Cancer* 69:1137–1145, 1992.

134. Stephens FO, Stevens MM, McCarthy SW, et al: Treatment of advanced and inaccessible sarcomas with continuous intra-arterial chemotherapy prior to definitive surgery or radiotherapy—A possible alternative to amputation or disabling radical surgery. *Aust NZ J Surg* 57:435–440, 1987.

135. Rosen G, Marcove RC, Huvos AG, et al: Primary osteogenic sarcoma: 8-year experience with adjuvant chemotherapy. *J Cancer Res Clin Oncol* 106(suppl):55–67, 1983.

136. Winkler K, Beron G, Delling G, et al: Neoadjuvant chemotherapy of osteosarcoma: Results of a randomized cooperative trial (COSS-82) with salvage chemotherapy based on histological tumor response. *J Clin Oncol,* in press.

137. Winkler K, Beron G, Kotz R, et al: Neoadjuvant chemotherapy for osteogenic sarcoma: Results of a cooperative German/Austrian study. *J Clin Oncol* 2:617–624, 1984.

138. Giuliano AE, Feig S, Eilber F: Changing metastatic patterns of osteosarcoma. *Cancer* 54:2160–2164, 1984.

139. Edmonson J, Creagan E, Gilchrist G: Phase II study of high dose methotrexate in patients with unresectable metastatic osteosarcoma. *Cancer Treat Rep* 65:5438–539, 1981.

140. Tabone MD, Kalifa C, Rodary C, et al: Osteosarcoma recurrences in pediatric patients previously treated with intensive chemotherapy. *J Clin Oncol* 12:2614–2620, 1994.

141. Unni KK, Dahlin DC, Beaubout SW, Ivins JC: Parosteal osteogenic sarcoma. *Cancer* 37:2466–2475, 1976.

142. Unni KK, Dahlin DC, Beaubout SW: Periosteal osteogenic sarcoma. *Cancer* 37:2476–2485, 1976.

143. Sim FH, Unni K, Beaubout JW, et al: Osteosarcoma with small cells simulating Ewing's tumor. *J Bone Joint Surg* 61A:207–215, 1979.

144. Martin SE, Dwyer A, Kissane JM, et al: Small-cell osteosarcoma. *Cancer* 50:990–996, 1982.

145. Jaffe HL: *Tumors and Tumorous Conditions of the Bone and Joints.* Philadelphia, Lea & Febiger, 1958.

146. Shives TS, Wold LE, Dahlin DC, Beaubout JW: Chondrosarcoma and its variants, in Sim FH (ed): *Diagnosis and Treatment of Bone Tumors: A Team Approach.* Mayo Clinic Monograph. Thorofare, NJ, Slack Inc, 1983, pp 211–217.

147. Marcove RC, Mike V, Hutter RV, et al: Chondrosarcoma of the pelvis and upper end of femur. *J Bone Joint Surg [Am]* 54:561–572, 1972.

148. Pritchard DJ, Lunke RJ, Taylor WF, et al: Chondrosarcoma: A clinicopathologic statistical analysis. *Cancer* 45:149–157, 1980.

149. Garrison RC, Unni KK, McLeod RA, et al: Chondrosarcoma arising in osteochondroma. *Cancer* 49:1890–1897, 1982.

150. Marcove RC: Chondrosarcoma: Diagnosis and treatment. *Orthop Clin North Am* 8:811–819, 1977.

151. Huvos AG: *Bone Tumors: Diagnosis, Treatment and Prognosis.* Philadelphia, Saunders, 1979.

152. Edeiken J: Bone tumors and tumor-like conditions, in Edeiken J (ed): *Roentgen Diagnosis of Diseases of Bone,* 3d ed. Baltimore, Williams & Wilkins, 1981, pp 30–414.

153. Craig FS: Metastatic and primary lesions of bone. *Clin Orthop* 73:33, 1970.

154. Marcove RC: A 17-year review of cryosurgery in the treatment of bone tumors. *Clin Orthop* 163:231–233, 1982.

155. Marcove RC, Stovel IP, Huvos AC, Bullough P: The use of cryosurgery in the treatment of low and medium grade chondrosarcoma: A preliminary report. *Clin Orthop* 122:147–156, 1977.

156. Gitellis S, Bertoni F, Chieti PP, Campanacci M: Chondrosarcoma of bone. *J Bone Joint Surg [Am]* 63A:1248–1257, 1981.

157. Aprin H, Riserborough EJ, Hall JE: Chondrosarcoma in children and adolescents. *Clin Orthop* 166:226–232, 1982.

158. Steel HH: Partial or complete resection of the hemipelvis: An alternative to hindquarter amputation for periacetabular chondrosarcoma of the pelvis. *J Bone Joint Surg* 60A:719–730, 1978.

159. Austin-Seymour M, Munzenrider J, Goitein M, et al: Fractionated proton radiation therapy of chordoma and low-grade chondrosarcoma of the base of the skull. *J Neurosurg* 70:13–17, 1991.

160. Marcove RC, Lyden JP, Huvos AC, Bullough PB: Giant cell tumor treated by cryosurgery: A report of twenty-five cases. *J Bone Joint Surg [Am]* 55:1633–1644, 1973.

161. Unni KK, Dahlin DC, Beaubout JW, Sim FH: Chondrosarcoma: Clear-cell variant. A report of 16 cases. *J Bone Joint Surg [Am]* 57:676–683, 1976.

162. Bjornsson J, Unni KK, Dahlin DC, et al: Clear cell chondrosarcoma of bone: Observations in 47 cases. *Am J Surg Pathol* 8:223–230, 1984.

163. Huvos AG, Rosen G, Dabska M, Marcove RC: Mesenchymal chondrosarcoma: A clinicopathologic analysis of 35 patients with emphasis on treatment. *Cancer* 51:1230–1237, 1983.

164. Dahlin DC, Cupps RE, Johnson EW Jr: Giant cell tumor: A study of 195 cases. *Cancer* 25:1061–1070, 1970.

165. Hutter VP, Worcester JN Jr, Francis KC, et al: Benign and malignant giant cell tumor of bone: A clinicopathological analysis of the natural history of the disease. *Cancer* 15:653–690, 1962.

166. Johnson EW Jr, Dahlin DC: Treatment of giant cell tumor of bone. *J Bone Joint Surg [Am]* 41:895–904, 1959.

167. Johnson EW, Dahlin DC: Treatment of giant cell tumor of bone: An evaluation of 24 cases treated at the Johns Hopkins Hospital between 1925–1955. *Orthopedics* 62:187–191, 1969.

168. Uehlinger E: Primary malignancy, secondary malignancy and semimalignancy of bone tumors, in Grundman E (ed): *Malignant Bone Tumors.* New York, Springer-Verlag, 1976, pp 109–119.

169. Nascimento AG, Huvos AC, Marcove RC: Primary malignant giant cell tumor of bone: A study of eight cases and review of the literature. *Cancer* 44:1393–1402, 1979.

170. Rock MG, Pritchard DJ, Unni KK: Metastases from histologically benign giant-cell tumor of bone. *J Bone Joint Surg* 66A:269–274, 1984.

171. Gitelis S, Mallin BA, Piasecki P, Turner F: Intralesional excision compared with en bloc resection for giant-cell tumors of bone. *J Bone Joint Surg* 75A:1648–1655, 1993.

172. Eckardt JJ, Grogan TJ: Giant cell tumor of bone. *Clin Orthop* 204:45–58, 1986.

173. Bini SA, Gill K, Johnston JO: Giant cell tumor of bone: Curettage and cement reconstruction. *Clin Orthop* 321:245–250, 1995.

174. O'Donnell RJ, Springfield DS, Motwani HK, et al: Recurrence of giant-cell tumors of the long bones after curettage and packing with cement. *J Bone Joint Surg* 76A:1827–1833, 1994.

175. Savino R, Gherlinzoni F, Morandi M, et al: Surgical treatment of giant-cell tumor of the spine. *J Bone Joint Surg* 65A:1283–1289, 1983.

176. Martin NS, Williamson J: The role of surgery in the treatment of malignant tumors of the spine. *J Bone Joint Surg [Br]* 52:227–237, 1970.

177. Sterner BL, Johnson OE: Complete removal of three vertebrae for giant-cell tumor. *J Bone Joint Surg [Br]* 53:278–287, 1971.

178. Marcove RC, Sheth DS, Brien EW, et al: Conservative surgery for giant cell tumors of the sacrum: The role of cryosurgery as a supplement to curettage and partial excision. *Cancer* 74:1253–1260, 1994.

179. Marcove RC, Weiss L, Vaghaiwall M, Pearson R: Cryosurgery in the treatment of giant cell tumor of bone: A report of 52 consecutive cases. *Clin Orthop* 134:275–289, 1978.

180. Malawer MM, Dunham WK, Zaleski T, Zielisnski CJ: The management of aggressive and low grade malignant bone tumors by cryosurgery: Analysis of 40 consecutive cases, in Enneking WF (ed): *Limb-Sparing Surgery for Musculoskeletal Tumors.* New York, Churchill Livingstone, 1987, pp 498–510.

181. Malawer M, Kollander Y, Buch R, Meller I: Cryosurgery in the treatment of giant cell tumor of bone: Analysis of 102 cases. *Acta Orthop Scand* 1996.

182. Bell RS, Harwood AR, Goodman SB, et al: Supervoltage radiotherapy in the treatment of difficult giant cell tumors of bone. *Clin Orthop* 174:208–216, 1983.

183. Bennett CJ, Marcus RB, Million RR, Enneking WF: Radiation therapy for giant cell tumor of bone. *Int J Radiat Oncol Biol Phys* 26:299–304, 1993.

184. Schwartz LH, Okunieff PG, Rosenberg A, Suit HD: Radiation therapy in the treatment of difficult giant cell tumors. *Int J Radiat Oncol Biol Phys* 17:1085–1088, 1989.

185. Huvos AG: Primary malignant fibrous histiocytoma of bone: Clinicopathologic study of 18 patients. *NY State J Med* 76:552–559, 1976.

186. McCarthy EF, Matsuno T, Dorfman HD: Malignant fibrous histiocytoma of bone: A study of 35 cases. *Hum Pathol* 10:57–70, 1979.

187. Spanier SS, Enneking WF, Enriquez P: Primary malignant fibrous histiocytoma of bone. *Cancer* 36:2084–2098, 1975.

188. Bacci G, Springfield D, Picci P, et al: Adjuvant chemotherapy for malignant fibrous histiocytoma in the femur and tibia. *J Bone Joint Surg* 67A:620–625, 1985.

189. Heelen GJ, Koops HS, Kamps WA, et al: Treatment of malignant fibrous histiocytoma of bone: A plea for primary chemotherapy. *Cancer* 56:37–40, 1985.

190. Huvos AG, Higinbotham NL: Primary fibrosarcoma of bone: A clinicopathologic study of 130 patients. *Cancer* 35:837–847, 1975.

191. Wilner D: Fibrosarcoma, in Wilner D (ed): *Radiology of Bone Tumors and Allied Disorders.* Vol 1. Philadelphia, Saunders, 1982, pp 2291–2324.

192. Wick MR, Siegal GP, Unni KK, et al: Sarcomas of bone complicating osteitis deformans (Paget's disease): 50 years' experience. *Am J Surg Pathol* 5:47–59, 1981.

193. Greditzer IIG, McLeod RA, Unni KK, et al: Bone sarcomas in Paget's disease. *Radiology* 146:337–333, 1983.

194. Huvos AG, Woodard HQ, Cahan WG, et al: Postradiation osteogenic sarcoma of bone and soft tissues: A clinicopathologic study of 66 patients. *Cancer* 55:1244–1255, 1982.

195. Amendola BE, Amendola MA, McClatchey KD, and Miller CH Jr: Radiation-associated sarcoma: A review of 23 patients with postradiation sarcoma over a 50-year period. *Am J Clin Oncol* 12:411–415, 1989.

196. Reimer RR, Chabner BAC, Young RC, et al: Lymphoma presenting in bone: Results of histopathology, staging and therapy. *Ann Intern Med* 87:50–55, 1977.

197. Sweet DL, Moss DP, Simon MA, et al: Histiocytic lymphoma (reticulum-cell sarcoma) of bone: Current strategy for orthopedic surgeons. *J Bone Joint Surg [Am]* 63:79–84, 1981.

198. Pritchard DJ, Dahlin D, Dauphine R, et al: Ewing's sarcoma: A clinicopathological and statistical analysis of patients surviving five years or longer. *J Bone Joint Surg [Am]* 57:10–16, 1975.

199. Razek A, Perez CA, Tefft M, et al: Intergroup Ewing's sarcoma study: Local control related to radiation dose, volume, and site of primary lesion in Ewing's sarcoma. *Cancer* 46:516, 1980.

200. Rosen G, Caparros B, Mosende C, et al: Curability of Ewing's sarcoma and consideration for future therapeutic trials. *Cancer* 41:888, 1978.

201. Rosen G, Caparros B, Nirenberg A, et al: Ewing's sarcoma: Ten-year experience with adjuvant chemotherapy. *Cancer* 47:2204–2213, 1981.

202. Perez CA, Razek A, Tefft M, et al: Analysis of local tumor control in Ewing's sarcoma: Preliminary results of a cooperative intergroup study. *Cancer* 40:2864–2873, 1977.

203. Sweet DL, Moss DP, Simon MA, et al: Histiocytic lymphoma (reticulum-cell sarcoma) of bone. Current strategy for orthopedic surgeons. *J Bone Joint Surg [Am]* 63:79–84, 1981.

204. Reimer RR, Chabner BAC, Young RC, et al: Lymphoma presenting in bone: Results of histopathology, staging and therapy. *Ann Intern Med* 87:50–55, 1977.

205. Boston HC, Dahlin DC, Ivins JC, Cupps RE: Malignant lymphoma of bone. *Cancer* 34:1731–1737, 1976.

206. Armitage JO, Fyfe M-A, Leuro J: Long-term remission durability and functional status of patients healed for diffuse histiocytic lymphoma with the CHOP regimen. *J Clin Oncol* 2:898–902, 1984.

207. Laurence J, Coleman M, Allen S, et al: Combination chemotherapy of advanced diffuse histiocytic lymphoma with the six-drug COP-BLAM regimen. *Ann Intern Med* 97:190–195, 1982.

208. Loeffler JS, Tarbell NJ, Kozakewich H, et al: Primary lymphoma of bone in children: Analysis of treatment results with Adriamycin, prednisone, Oncovin (APO), and local radiation therapy. *J Clin Oncol* 4:496–501, 1986.

209. Bacci G, Jaffe N, Emiliani E, et al: Therapy for primary non-Hodgkin's lymphoma of bone and a comparison of results with Ewing's sarcoma: Ten years' experience at the Instituto Orthopedico Rizzoli. *Cancer* 57:1468–1472, 1986.

210. Newcomer L, Silverstein M, Cadman E, et al: Bone involvement in Hodgkin's disease. *Cancer* 49:338–342, 1982.

211. Mendenhall NP, Jones JJ, Kramer BS, et al: The management of primary lymphoma of bone. *Radiother Oncol* 9:137–1137, 1987.

212. National Cancer Survey, 1973.

213. Loeffler RK, DiSimone RN, Howland WJ: Limitations of bone scanning in clinical oncology. *JAMA* 234:1228–1232, 1975.

214. Huvos AG: Multiple myeloma, including solitary osseous myeloma, in Huvos AG (ed): *Bone Tumors: Diagnosis, Treatment, and Prognosis,* 2d ed. Philadelphia, Saunders, 1991, pp 653–676.

215. McKenna RJ, Schwinn CP, Soong KY, Higinbotham NL: Sarcomata of the osteogenic series (osteosarcoma, fibrosarcoma, chondrosarcoma, parosteal osteosarcoma) and sarcomata arising in abnormal bone: An analysis of 552 cases. *J Bone Joint Surg [Am]* 48:1–26, 1966.

216. Merryweather R, Middlemiss JH, Sanerkin NG: Malignant transformation of osteoblastoma. *J Bone Joint Surg* 62B:381–384, 1980.

217. Ward WG, Eckardt JJ, Shayestehfar S, et al: Osteoid osteoma diagnosis and management with low morbidity. *Clin Orthop* 291:229–235, 1993.

218. Malawer MM: The diagnosis, treatment and management of unicameral bone cysts by percutaneous aspiration, hemodynamic evaluation and intracavitary methylprednisolone acetate. *Orthopedic Update Series* IV(26):1–7, 1986.

219. Greenberger JS, Crocker AC, Vawter G, et al: Results of treatment of 127 patients with systemic histiocytosis (Letterer-Siwe syndrome, Schuller-Christian syndrome and multifocal eosinophilic granuloma). *Medicine* 60:311–338, 1981.

220. Lesson MC, Smith A, Carter JR, Makley JT: Eosinophilic granuloma of bone in the growing epiphysis. *J Pediatr Orthop* 5(2):147–150, 1985.

221. Cassady JR: Radiation therapy in less common primary bone tumors, in Jaffe N (ed): *Solid Tumors in Childhood.* Littleton, MA, PSG Publishing, 1979, pp 205–214.

222. Greenberger JS, Cassady JR, Jaffe N, et al: Radiation therapy in patients with histiocytosis: Management of diabetes insipidus and bone lesions. *Int J Radiat Oncol Biol Phys* 5:1749–1755, 1979.

223. Gramatovici R, D'Angio GJ: Radiation therapy in soft-tissue lesions in histiocytosis X (Langerhans' cell histiocytosis). *Med Pediatr Oncol* 16:259–262, 1988.

224. Selch MT, Parker RG: Radiation therapy in the management of Langerhans cell histiocytosis. *Med Pediatr Oncol* 8:151–154, 1990.

II. Neoplasms Affecting the Upper Extremity

Robert M. Henshaw and Martin M. Malawer

TUMORS OF THE SHOULDER GIRDLE, ARM, AND FOREARM

Bone and soft tissue neoplasms occur in the upper extremity only one-third as frequently as in the lower extremity.[1] Despite this, however, the proximal humerus remains the third most common site for osteosarcomas,[2,3] outranked only by the knee region. Cartilage tumors, either benign or malignant, are more common in the shoulder girdle than in the lower extremity. In addition, the proximal humerus is the most common site for unicameral bone cysts (UBCs) and chondroblastomas.[4,5] As in the lower extremity, proximal primary bony neoplasms occur more frequently than distal lesions. Soft tissue tumors, though less common in the upper extremity than in the lower extremity, also tend to favor the shoulder girdle. Although all soft tissue sarcomas may involve the periscapular or proximal humeral musculature, lipomas and liposarcomas are the most common.[1]

Age distribution of tumors in the upper extremity follows the same patterns seen in the lower extremity. Ewing's sarcoma and osteosarcoma, the most common malignant bone tumors of the humerus, occur during adolescence; chondrosarcoma, in contrast, occurs during the third to seventh decades.[6] Characteristically UBCs and chondroblastomas occur prior to skeletal maturity. Metastatic tumors rarely occur below the age of 40 years. Although all carcinomas may involve the shoulder girdle, hypernephroma (renal cell carcinoma) has a unique propensity to involve the proximal humerus. Distal metastatic lesions are rare in general; however, aggressive metastatic lung carcinoma may involve bones distal to the elbow and wrist.

In this chapter, the specific anatomic site and its influence upon the clinical presentation and surgical management of both benign and malignant bone and soft tissue tumors are presented in detail. The surgical staging, indications, and management technique are emphasized.

Scapula and Periscapular Area

Clinical Characteristics

Tumors of the scapula present with pain, a mass, or both. Frequently, these tumors may become quite large before they are brought to the physician's attention. The most commonly encountered malignant bone tumor in childhood is Ewing's sarcoma. Lymphoma and other primary round cell tumors may involve the scapula in adults. Metastatic disease is the most common lesion seen in patients over the age of 40 years. The most common benign lesions are solitary or multiple osteochondromas. When located on the inferior angle or against the chest wall, an osteochondroma may present as a snapping scapula; the location of these lesions often makes diagnosis on standard radiographs difficult. Secondary chondrosarcomas occasionally arise from an underlying osteochondroma. They are a common malignancy in the young adult. Soft tissue sarcomas may involve either the supracapular or the infraspinous musculature; direct involvement of the underlying bone is infrequent. Radiation-induced sarcomas, though rare, may develop in the scapula secondary to radiotherapy for breast carcinoma or mantle radiation for leukemia.

Unique Anatomic Considerations

Tumors arising within the body of the scapula are surrounded by a restrictive cuff of soft tissue in all dimensions during their early stages of development. The natural tendency for sarcoma extension is therefore toward the axilla, where unrestricted growth may occur without detection. Lesions arising from the humeral neck or glenoid often involve the pericapsular tissue and/or the joint itself. This is especially true of malignant cartilage tumors, which may extend along the capsule and rotator cuff to the scapula. Important anatomic areas to evaluate for extension are the axilla and adjacent chest wall as well as the proximal humeral or pericapsular tissue (including the rotator cuff). The base of the axillary nodes should also be carefully examined.

Staging

Staging studies are similar to those used for evaluating tumors elsewhere. Computed tomography (CT) is extremely helpful in evaluating the entire scapula as well as the adjacent chest wall. Magnetic resonance imaging, with images taken in the primary planes of the scapula, can detect involvement of the rotator cuff and periscapular tissue as well as the brachial plexus. Arteriography is important in determining vascular involvement. Displacement is indicative of anterior (i.e., axillary) extension of tumor. Bone scan, although less helpful, may indicate rib involvement.

Biopsy

The biopsy site is a crucial factor in determining the final operative procedure for aggressive and malignant lesions of the scapula. Inadvertent contamination of the neurovascular structures or the chest wall must be avoided. For lesions involving the body of the scapula, a posterior needle biopsy minimizes potential risk of contamination. Similarly, a posterior approach directly through the deltoid and teres minor should be used for lesions of the scapular neck. An anterior approach to the scapula neck should be avoided whenever possible. If an open biopsy is required, it should be in line with the definitive incision. Most operative approaches (see below) involve an incision along the axillary border of the scapula. Therefore, a small medial incision is recommended.

Surgical Management of Tumors of the Scapula

All malignant spindle cell sarcomas of the shoulder girdle have traditionally been treated by forequarter amputation. Radical scapulectomy remains a poor operation for most stage IIB tumors that have extensive soft tissue extension. Today, the Tikhoff-Linberg resection is the preferred operation for high-grade bony sarcomas of the scapula.[7-9] If the staging criteria are met, local control is equal to that of a forequarter amputation. Lower-grade stage IA/B lesions of the scapula can be excised with a curative margin by scapulectomy with removal of an adjacent normal muscle cuff (wide excision–type IIIB; see Fig. 16-31A). Scapulectomy is also useful in the treatment of aggressive lesions such as giant cell tumors and aneurysmal bone cysts. Benign tumors are treated by simple excision or curettage.

Specific Bone Tumors of the Scapula

Osteochondroma

Osteochondromas are benign sessile or pedunculated lesions that may occur as solitary or as multiple lesions. The multiple form of the disease is hereditary, with an autosomal dominant trait of variable expression. Osteochondromas are frequently diagnosed early in life and may grow in size until skeletal maturity is reached. Diagnosis is often made on the basis of their x-ray appearance; however, lesions involving the scapula may be difficult to image even with true scapular lateral (or "Y") views taken along the longitudinal plane of the bone. High-resolution CT scanning excels in detecting osteochondromas of the scapula and may often be the only method of detecting lesions arising of the anterior body. Lesions in this region are often occult and may present solely as a snapping shoulder secondary to impingement with the underlying chest wall.

Secondary chondrocarsarcomas arising from osteochondromas occur more frequently around the shoulder girdle; therefore, frequent evaluation and early intervention is recommended. Computed tomography scanning can measure the overlying cap; caps exceeding 1 cm may indicate the onset of malignant degeneration. In children, osteochondromas of the scapula should be removed by simple excision. Care must be taken to avoid injuring the accessory nerve when removing lesions arising from the upper border near the attachment of the levator scapulae. Osteochondromas of the inferior portion of the scapula may grow quite large and require a partial scapulectomy; this is often seen in multiple hereditary osteochondromatosis (Fig. 16-28). There is no functional loss if the osteotomy is done below the scapular spine. Soft tissue reconstruction is performed by reattaching the rhomboids to the teres major and trapezium. Active motion is begun within a few days. A sling is required for 5 to 7 days.

Giant-Cell Tumor or Aneurysmal Bone Cyst

Giant-cell tumors and aneurysmal bone cysts often cause marked ballooning and destruction of the scapula. Small lesions may be treated by curettage, cryosurgery, or both. If the neck of the scapula is not involved, a partial scapulectomy can be performed with minimal loss of function. Large lesions may require a total scapulectomy. Reconstruction is accomplished by suspending the humerus (see below) from the clavicle by both a static and a dynamic reconstruction.

Chondrosarcoma

Chondrosarcomas of the scapula may arise from an underlying benign osteochondroma[10] (Fig. 16-29); thus, any large cartilaginous lesion of the scapula in a young adult must be approached with a high index of suspicion. These lesions tend to be low grade, stage IB.[11] Extreme caution must be taken in biopsy of a cartilaginous tumor as carti-

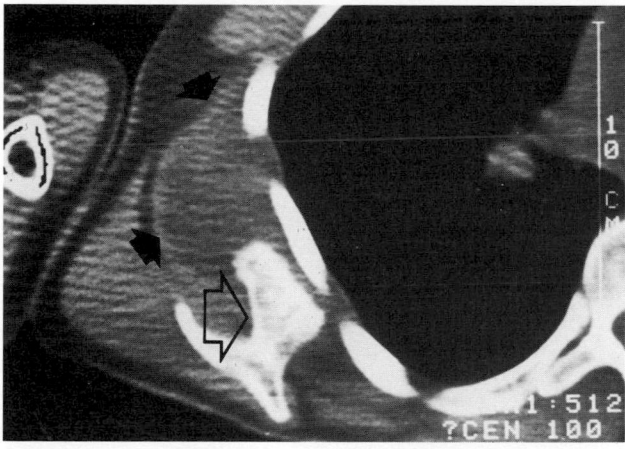

Figure 16-28 Osteochondroma of the scapula. CT of a large osteochondroma (*open arrow*) of the undersurface of the scapula adjacent to the chest wall. There is an associated soft tissue mass (*solid arrows*), suggesting malignant degeneration.

lage can easily be implanted within the soft tissues. Cartilage tumors approaching the glenohumeral joint may directly involve the joint space and readily implant on the articular cartilage. In such cases, an extraarticular resection is generally recommended. A Tikhoff-Linberg resection usually is curative.

Osteosarcoma

Osteosarcoma of the scapula is rare. Curative removal by Tikhoff-Linberg resection or forequarter amputation is required. Adjuvant treatment with chemotherapy is now considered standard for osteosarcomas. The limiting factor in performing a limb-sparing procedure is the size of the extraosseous component. Neurovascular involvement necessitates a forequarter amputation. Chest wall involvement must be evaluated before surgery; if it is present, partial chest wall resection is required en bloc with ablation of the primary tumor. The presence of metastatic disease is not a contraindication to amputation both for palliation as well as achieving local control prior to attempted metastectomy (thoracotomy).

Ewing's Sarcoma

Ewing's sarcoma arising in the scapula is treated by radiation therapy in conjunction with chemotherapy. Functional results are excellent. Recent interest in reducing radiation exposure in young patients has led to the recommendation of partial scapulectomy for lesions limited to the body of the scapula. Total scapulectomy, however, cannot be recommended, since the functional outcome is significantly poorer than in patients treated without surgery. Scapulectomy can be recommended only if it effects a difference in local control of the tumor and thus has an impact on overall survival. This has not yet been demonstrated.

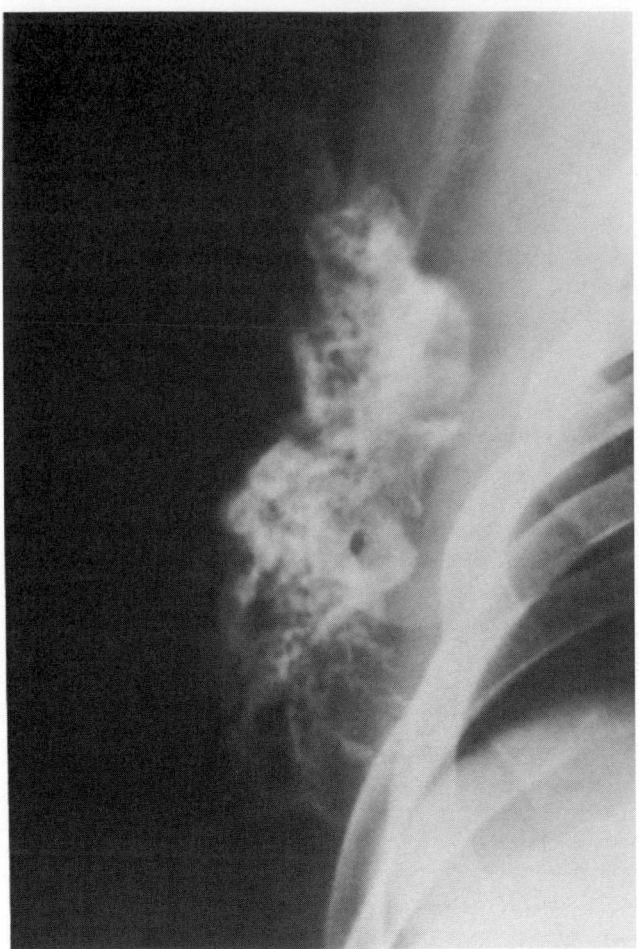

Figure 16-29 Secondary chondrosarcoma. A sessile osteochondroma of the scapula with malignant degeneration in a patient with multiple osteochondromatosis. A partial scapulectomy was performed. Secondary chondrosarcomas tend to be low-grade. (Reproduced with permission from Malawer MM, Abelson HT, Suit HD, in DeVito VT, Hellman S, Rosenberg SA (eds): *Cancer: Principles and Practice of Oncology*, 2d ed. Philadelphia, Lippincott, 1985, pp 1293–1343.)

Periscapular Soft Tissue Sarcomas

Soft tissue sarcomas arising in the periscapular musculature can usually be treated by en bloc removal with wide margins through the adjacent soft tissue and adjuvant radiotherapy. Chemotherapy may be useful for high-grade lesions. Occasionally a soft tissue sarcoma arising from the deeper structures encases the scapula or extends directly into the bone. In these rare situations, scapulectomy is required. Appropriate staging studies indicate the best procedure. If the tumor is distal to the scapular spine, a partial or total scapulectomy may be adequate. Involvement of the suprascapular musculature and/or rotators requires a Tikhoff-Linberg resection.

Surgical Management of Shoulder Girdle Tumors

Tikhoff-Linberg Resection

The Tikhoff-Linberg resection is a limb-sparing procedure for sarcomas arising around the shoulder girdle.[8,9,12] The resection consists of en bloc removal of the scapula, clavicle, and proximal humerus with preservation of a functional arm and hand (Fig. 16-30). Indications for the procedure are low- and high-grade sarcomas of the scapula and peri- and suprascapular soft tissue sarcomas. Conversely, bony sarcomas of the proximal humerus require resection of a large portion of the humerus with preservation of a portion of the scapula. This procedure has been termed a *modified Tikhoff-Linberg resection* and is discussed in detail in the following section.[8,9] A surgical classification of the shoulder girdle resections has recently been established (Fig. 16-31A).

Absolute contraindication to the Tikhoff-Linberg procedure is tumor involvement of the neurovascular bundle and/or chest wall; both types of involvement require a forequarter amputation. Relative contraindications include pathologic fracture, poorly planned biopsy with widespread tumor contamination, and lymph node involvement. Careful preoperative evaluation is required. Computed tomography is useful to determine possible chest wall involvement; MRI may reveal involvement of the brachial plexus. Angiography is crucial to determine axillary vessel involvement. The interval between the tumor and vessels must be carefully evaluated. Venography may be useful in evaluating possible intramural tumor thrombosis occasionally seen with tumors around the shoulder girdle. Bone scan is useful to determine bone and rib involvement.

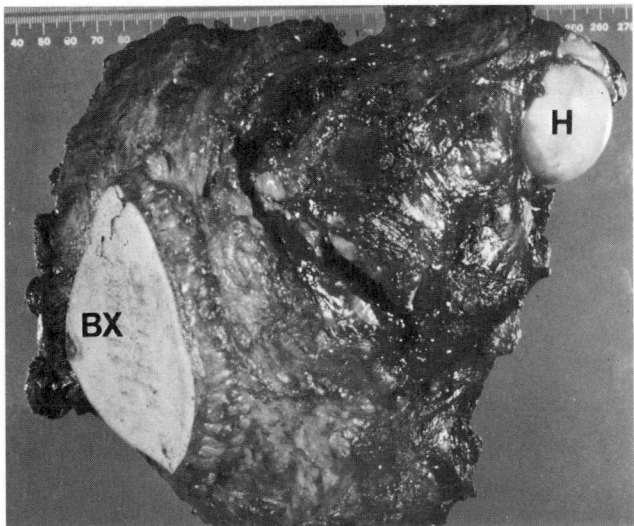

Figure 16-30 Posterior aspect of a gross specimen of a Tikhoff-Linberg resection. All muscles arising and attaching to the scapula are resected en bloc with the entire scapula, glenohumeral joint, and a portion of the distal clavicle. Note the humeral head *H* and the old biopsy site *BX*. The glenohumeral joint has been opened for demonstration purposes.

Prior to surgery, all patients should be informed that a resection may not be possible and that they must be prepared for a forequarter amputation. An anterior incision with large skin flaps is made first to explore the axillary vessels and brachial plexus. If this interval is clear, resection can then proceed. Otherwise, a forequarter amputation should be performed. The most medial margin along the paraspinal muscles and root of the neck should be explored early if there is a question of involvement. These anatomic areas are poorly evaluated by all preoperative studies. It is important to realize that a forequarter amputation cannot improve upon this medial margin. Resection includes all the muscles arising from the scapula and inserting on the proximal humerus, along with an extraarticular resection of the glenohumeral joint. Occasionally the deltoid muscle and the axillary nerve can be preserved; preservation of the deltoid simplifies reconstruction of the resection defect. The goal of reconstruction is to stabilize the remaining arm so that elbow flexion can position the hand in respect to the body. This is accomplished by suspending the proximal humerus from the remaining clavicle using both Dacron tape and muscle transfers. The long and the short heads of the biceps and coracobrachialis are sutured through drill holes to the remaining clavicle. The pectoralis muscle is rotated to cover the defect and to give additional support. A similar maneuver is used following total scapulectomy.

Functional results following a Tikhoff-Linberg resection are the same as those following a total scapulectomy. No active abduction of the shoulder is possible. Patients undergoing a Tikhoff-Linberg resection retain useful hand function and good elbow function. Cosmesis is acceptable and can be improved by the use of a molded shoulder pad. The shoulder should be stable, and no external orthosis is required (Fig. 16-31*B*).

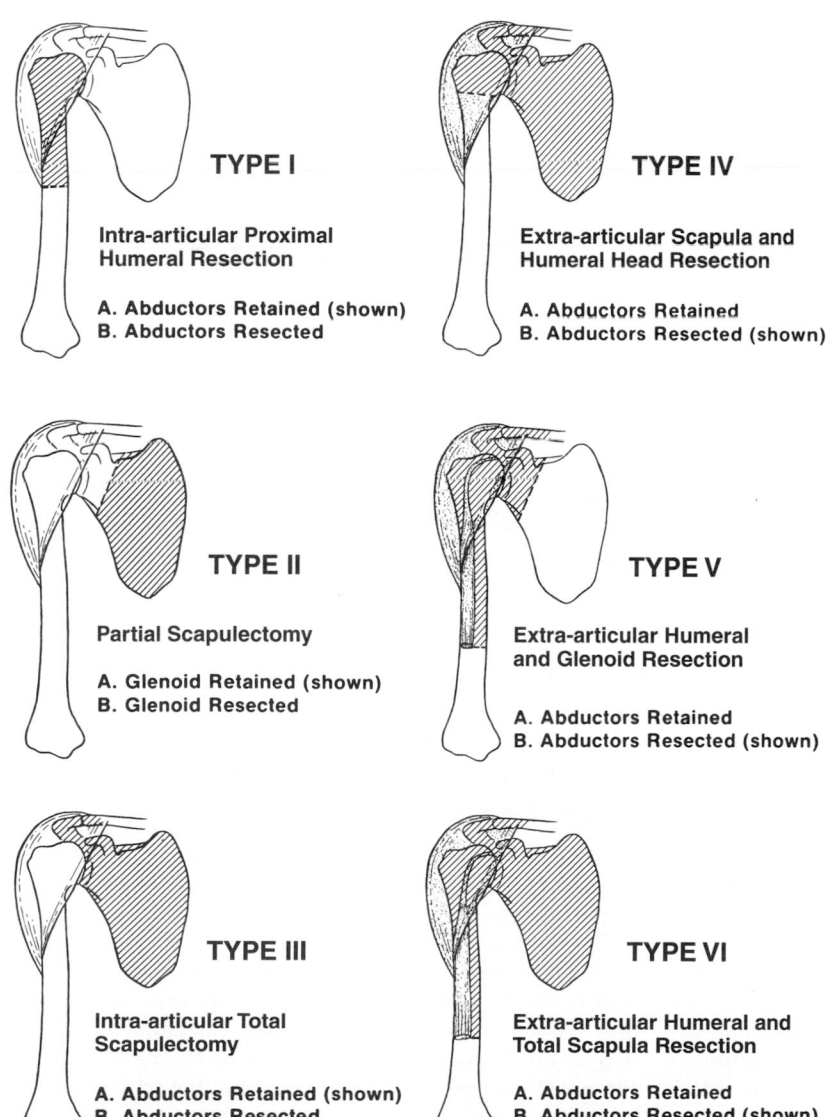

TYPE I

Intra-articular Proximal Humeral Resection

A. Abductors Retained (shown)
B. Abductors Resected

TYPE II

Partial Scapulectomy

A. Glenoid Retained (shown)
B. Glenoid Resected

TYPE III

Intra-articular Total Scapulectomy

A. Abductors Retained (shown)
B. Abductors Resected

TYPE IV

Extra-articular Scapula and Humeral Head Resection

A. Abductors Retained
B. Abductors Resected (shown)

TYPE V

Extra-articular Humeral and Glenoid Resection

A. Abductors Retained
B. Abductors Resected (shown)

TYPE VI

Extra-articular Humeral and Total Scapula Resection

A. Abductors Retained
B. Abductors Resected (shown)

A

Figure 16-31 *A.* Proposed classification of shoulder girdle resections for bone and soft tissue tumors. Types I to III are usually performed for low-grade tumors, whereas types IV to VI are for high-grade tumors. A and B relate to the status of the abductor mechanism: A = intact, B = resected. Types I to III are intraarticular resections and provide a marginal excision. Types IV to VI are extraarticular and accomplish a wide excision. The Tikhoff-Linberg resection is type IVB. (Presented on the 4th International Symposium on Limb Salvage in Musculoskeletal Oncology, Kyoto, 1987.) *B.* Clinical appearance following a classical Tikhoff-Linberg resection. The entire scapula and an extraarticular resection of the proximal glenohumeral joint (type IV resection) was performed for a stage IIB osteosarcoma of the scapula. The shoulder remains stable following reconstruction with normal elbow and hand function.

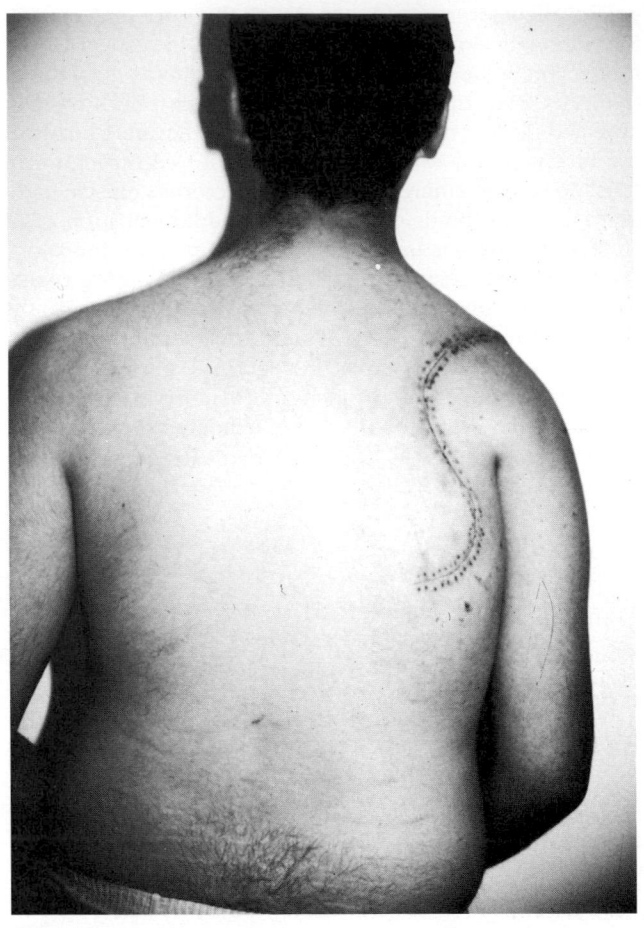

B

Figure 16-31 *(Continued)*

Total Scapulectomy

Total scapulectomy is indicated primarily for stage I or II tumors of the body of the scapula that do not involve the suprascapular region or the glenoid. Preoperative considerations are similar to those for a Tikhoff-Linberg resection: the neurovascular structures and the chest wall must be free of disease. This procedure cannot be recommended for tumors with large soft tissue extensions anteriorly or laterally or for involvement of the glenoid or rotator cuff. The skin flaps are similar to those obtained from the posterior limb during a Tikhoff-Linberg resection. Beginning at the inferior angle, all muscles are transected away from the bone. The neurovascular structures are approached from the back as the scapula is retracted away from the chest cephalad. Care must be taken to avoid injury to the musculocutaneous and axillary nerves near the coracoid and around the subscapularis muscle. One must be prepared to convert this approach to a formal Tikhoff-Linberg resection if the anterior or medial margins are questionable. Soft tissue reconstruction is mandatory to provide stability and to avoid a flail extremity. As with a Tikhoff-Linberg reconstruction, a dual-suspension technique, utilizing Dacron tape to attach the humerus to the clavicle for static support and reattachment of the biceps and triceps

through drill holes in the clavicle, is recommended. The deltoid is then reattached along with the pectoralis major and trapezius to provide additional support and soft tissue coverage. Overall function following total scapulectomy consists of a stable shoulder that allows for useful positioning of the hand via elbow flexion.

Total scapular prosthetic reconstruction may be utilized if significant soft tissue remains following resection.

Partial Scapulectomy

Removal of the scapular body with preservation of the scapular spine leaves a functional shoulder joint. This procedure is indicated for low-grade lesions involving only the body of the scapula. A cuff of infraspinatus, subscapularis, and serratus anterior muscle can usually be preserved. Reconstruction consists of suturing these together to close the dead space and to reconstitute the points of origin and insertion of these muscles. Small tumors involving only the glenoid may be resected with preservation of the medial scapula. Reconstruction following glenoid resection is best accomplished by a primary arthrodesis of the humerus to the remaining scapula. Functional results after partial scapulectomy are superior to those that follow total scapulectomy (Fig. 16-32).

Tumors of the Proximal Humerus

Clinical Characteristics

The proximal humerus is the second most common site for primary bony sarcomas.[2] In the adolescent, such tumors are usually osteochondromas; in the adult, they are primary and secondary chondrosarcomas.[10,11] The proximal humerus is the most frequent site for unicameral bone cysts (UBCs) and chondroblastomas, two common benign bony lesions of childhood.[4,5,13] Bony metastases are common in the adult; they may be confused with a primary sarcoma. Pain is the presenting symptom for most bony lesions. Pathologic fracture is rare except for UBCs, where fracture may be the presenting symptom. Hypernephromas may metastasize to the proximal humerus and simulate a sarcoma. If the plain radiograph suggests a malignant lesion, staging studies should be performed prior to biopsy.

Unique Considerations

Tumors arising within the proximal humerus result in expansion of the head and greater tuberosity. The thin metaphyseal bone and the large metaphyseal vessels permit early extraosseous extension. Malignant tumors often present with large soft tissue components underneath the deltoid medially and under the subscapularis and coracobrachialis muscles. Careful physical examination of the axilla may demonstrate an unsuspected mass. In addition, tumors can develop large posterior extensions that may be hidden by the posterior deltoid and triceps. Pericapsular and rotator cuff involvement occurs early and must be evaluated carefully. Figure 16-33 illustrates the various mechanisms of tumor spread from proximal humeral sarcomas. Large sarcomas arising from the humerus may involve the chest wall directly. Neurologic symptoms from brachial plexus displacement is rare; when it is present, one must suspect possible tumor invasion of the nerve sheaths.

Staging

Staging studies accurately predict resectability of lesions of the proximal humerus. Computed tomography demonstrates extraosseous tumor extension and its relation to the underlying rib cage, while MRI can evaluate the brachial plexus, rotator cuff, and shoulder capsule, as well as the intramedullary extent of the lesion. Angiography can determine the relation of the brachial artery to the tumor and, by inference, of the major nerves to the tumor. Two views are required to determine if there is a clear interval between the lesion and the vessels. Biplane angiography is the single most useful study in this region (Fig. 16-34). Preoperative embolization is usually not feasible for proximal humeral lesions because of the high risk of inadver-

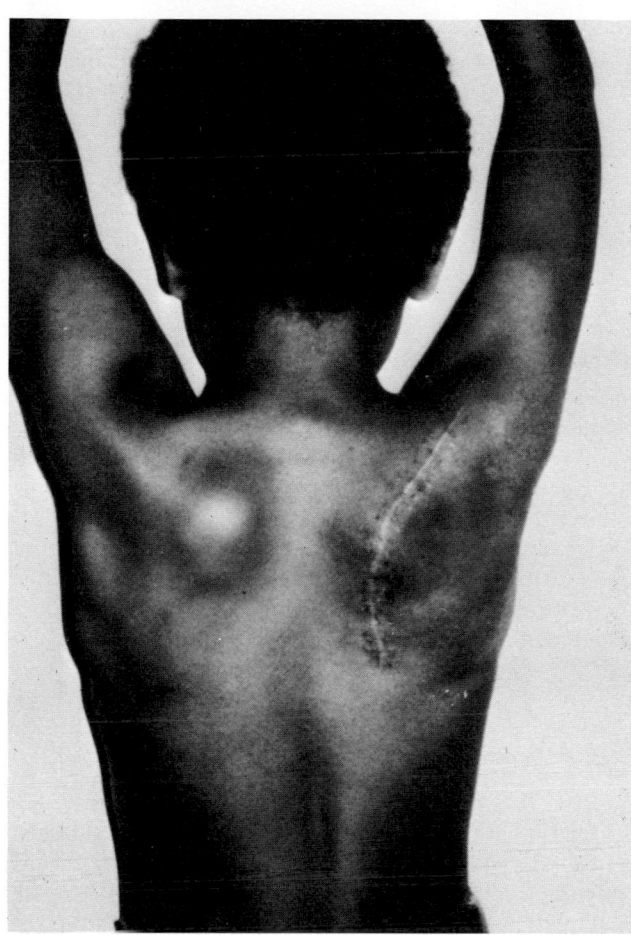

Figure 16-32 Partial scapula (intraspinal) resection. There is a full range of motion following partial scapular resection if the glenohumeral joint is preserved (by contrast, no active abduction follows total scapular Tikhoff-Linberg resection).

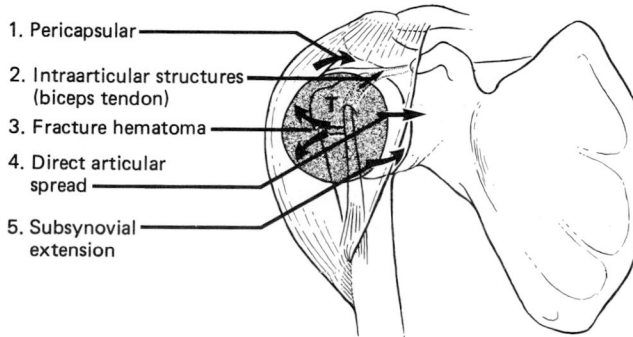

1. Pericapsular
2. Intraarticular structures (biceps tendon)
3. Fracture hematoma
4. Direct articular spread
5. Subsynovial extension

Figure 16-33 Mechanisms of tumor spread of proximal humeral tumors. There are five basic mechanisms. In general, articular involvement by tumor of the shoulder joint is more common than that of the knee joint.

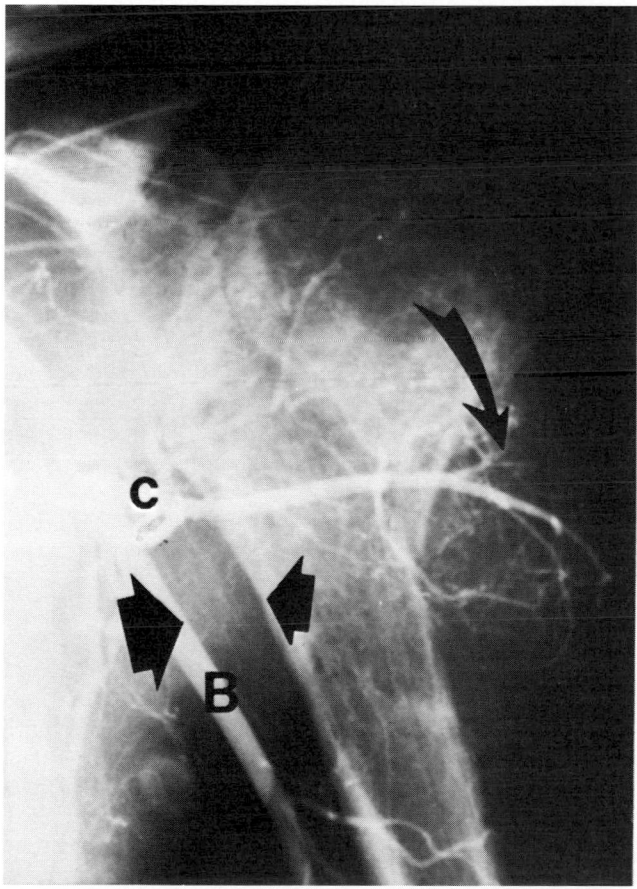

Figure 16-34 Angiography is the most useful staging study for determination of resectability of tumors of the proximal humerus. It demonstrates a lateral soft tissue component (*curved arrow*), with no evidence of tumor medially. If the interval (*solid arrows*) between the brachial artery (*B*) and the humerus is clear, resection is usually feasible. This patient underwent an extended Tikhoff-Linberg resection (see text for classification).

tent embolization of the end arteries of the forearm and hand. Bone scintigraphy determines the intraosseus extent of tumor. Occasionally, a transarticular lesion is noted within the glenoid. Joint involvement is difficult to determine. Arthrography and arthroscopy should be avoided because of the possibility of tumor contamination.

Biopsy

The standard deltopectoral interval should always be avoided when tumors of the proximal humerus are being biopsied. This approach virtually guarantees contamination of the subscapularis and pectoralis muscles and thereby potentially involves the entire brachial plexus and adjacent vessels via extension along the deltopectoral and subscapularis fascia. Malignant tumors biopsied through this approach may then require a forequarter amputation. All lesions of the proximal humerus are readily accessible to a well-placed Craig needle biopsy under fluoroscopic or CT guidance through the anterior or midsection of the deltoid. A small incisional biopsy can be performed through the same approach if necessary. Care should be taken not to involve the joint or the rotator cuff mechanism. It is important to remember the definitive incision for resection.

Treatment

Benign tumors of the proximal humerus are generally treated by curettage or excision. Low-grade (stage IA/B) sarcomas have traditionally been treated by en bloc resection, while high-grade (stage IIB) sarcomas are treated by forequarter amputation. A modified Tikhoff-Linberg procedure (interscapulothoracic resection) can permit salvage of a stable limb with a functional elbow and hand in selected patients. Shoulder joint disarticulation typically cannot achieve wide margins for tumor at this level and is therefore a poor operative choice. Cryosurgery has been successfully utilized for aggressive or recurrent giant-cell tumors, chondroblastomas, and low-grade chondrosarcomas.

Specific Tumors of the Proximal Humerus

Unicameral Bone Cysts

The proximal humerus is the most common site of UBCs (Fig. 16-35). These lesions are usually asymptomatic until a fracture occurs. Diagnosis can usually be made by plain radiographs. UBCs are typically centrally located lytic lesions that expand and thin the surrounding cortex. Two-thirds are active adjacent to the growth plate at the time of diagnosis. Curettage and bone graft were the treatments of choice until the 1970s. Local recurrence following curettage, with or without bone graft, ranged between 35 and 70 percent. The addition of bone graft does not decrease the local recurrence rate. The common belief that UBCs will disappear after fracture is misleading and only leads to unnecessary delays in treatment. Less than 1 percent of UBCs will disappear spontaneously following a pathologic fracture.

Surgery is not indicated in the initial management of a UBC. Percutaneous high-pressure Renografin injection and intralesional methylprednisolone lead to clinical healing in over 90 percent of these patients (Fig. 16-35A and B). Biopsy is recommended only if diagnosis is uncertain. Reossification usually begins within 6 to 8 weeks (Fig. 16-35C). A second aspiration and injection are required in about 30 percent of patients. Rarely are three injections required.

Chondroblastoma (Codman's Tumor)

The proximal humerus is the most common site for chondroblastoma.[14] Epiphyseal location is pathognomonic. Chondroblastomas usually occur before skeletal maturity. Secondary aneurysmal bone cyst formation may confuse the diagnosis. Simple curettage has a recurrence rate of 35 to 50 percent. Cryosurgery is a reliable method of preventing local recurrence. Recurrent chondroblastoma may require a simple excision of the proximal humerus. Arthrodesis is recommended for the young patient.

Chondrosarcoma

The proximal humerus is a common site for central and peripheral chondrosarcomas. Distinction between benign enchondromas and low-grade chondrosarcomas remains a major challenge for both the orthopaedist and the pathologist. The presence of diffuse pain, especially at night, and radiographic evidence of endosteal scalloping are indicators of tumor growth and lead to a clinical diagnosis of chondrosarcoma, even in the absence of malignant features on histologic examination. For this reason, biopsy is not useful and not recommended. Treatment may consist of wide excision or curettage with cryosurgery. These lesions are often referred to as enchondrosarcomas or grade 1/2 chondrosarcomas by various authors. We recommend curettage, cryosurgery, and cementation for low-grade enchondrosarcomas of the proximal humerus.

Stage I tumors of the proximal humerus can be treated by wide excision with minimal functional deficit. High-grade sarcomas require a forequarter amputation or a modified Tikhoff-Linberg resection in carefully selected patients. Intraarticular and synovial involvement seem to be more common with high-grade cartilaginous lesions in the proximal humerus location than with such lesions in other sites. Care must be taken not to contaminate the anterior structures when performing a biopsy. Reconstruction following a marginal resection for a low-grade lesion can be accomplished by prosthesis, allograft, or dual fibula autograft. A primary arthrodesis or an attempt at preserving a functional joint is possible in certain situations. If the rotator cuff and/or deltoid are removed, a primary arthrodesis is favored over attempts at joint reconstruction. Following resection of a high-grade lesion (stage IIB), the functional goal is a painless, stable shoulder with preservation of function in the elbow and hand.

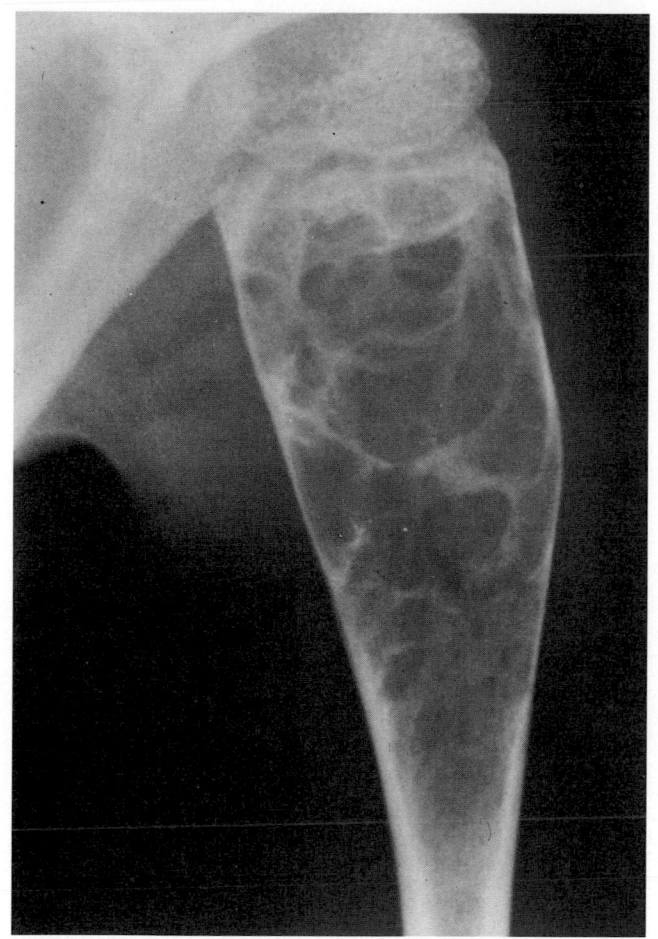

A

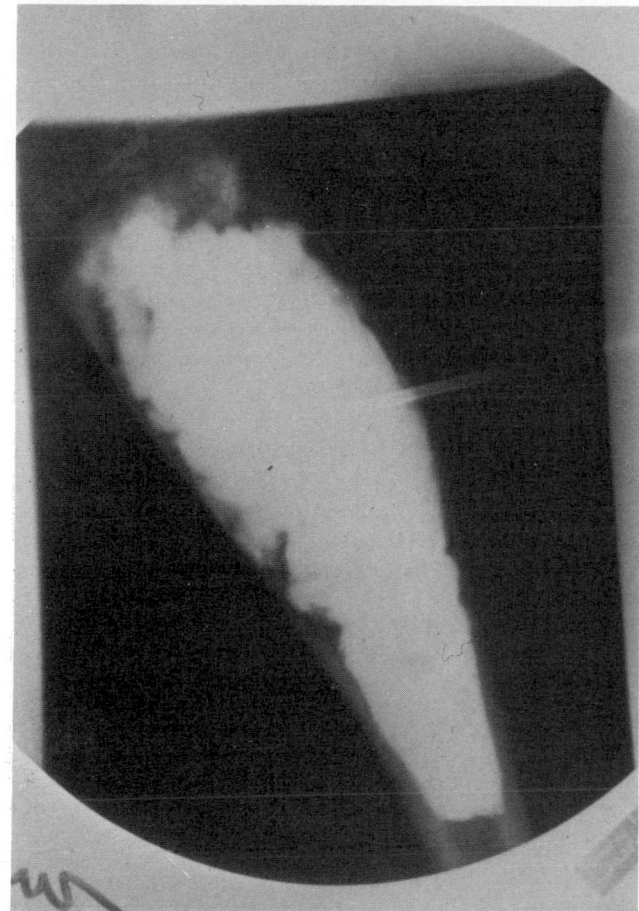

B

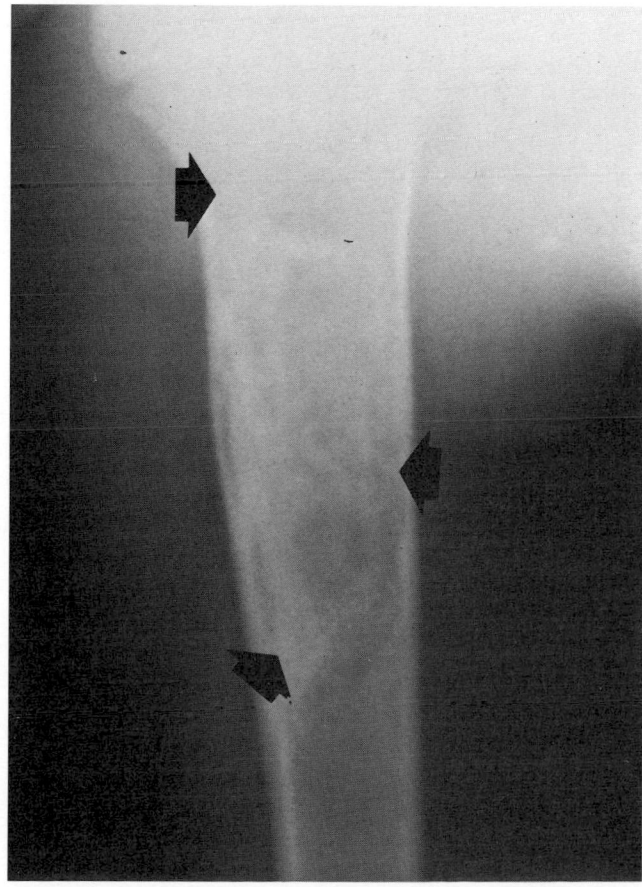

C

Figure 16-35 Unicameral bone cyst (UBC) of the proximal humerus. *A.* Plain radiograph showing a typical UBC with some expansion of the metaphysis and thinning of the cortices. *B.* The patient underwent aspiration, high-pressure Renografin injection, and intralesional methylprednisolone injection under fluoroscopic control. *C.* Ten months following percutaneous treatment, there is complete ossification of the defect (*solid arrows*). Aspiration and injection have replaced curettage as the main treatment of UBCs within the past decade.

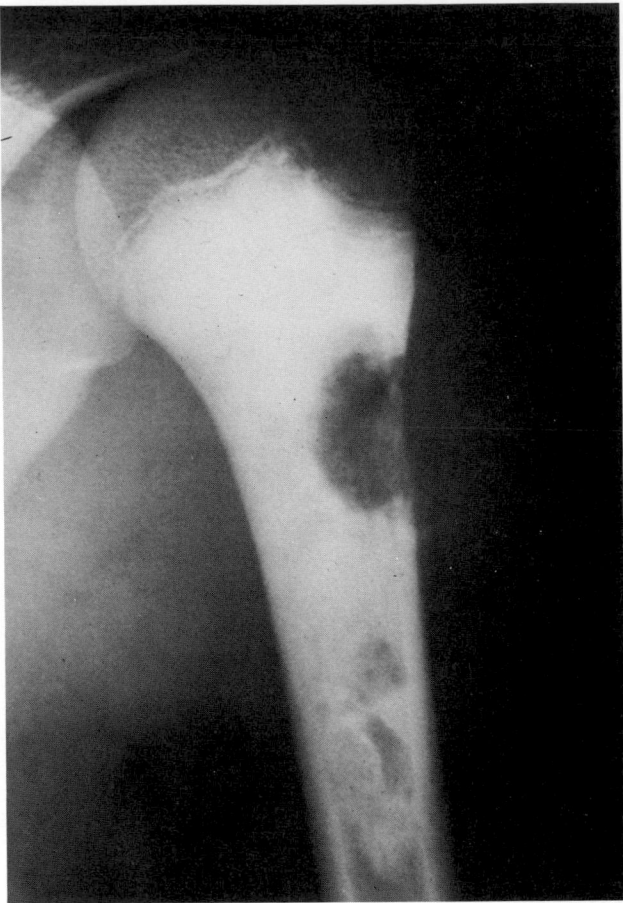

A

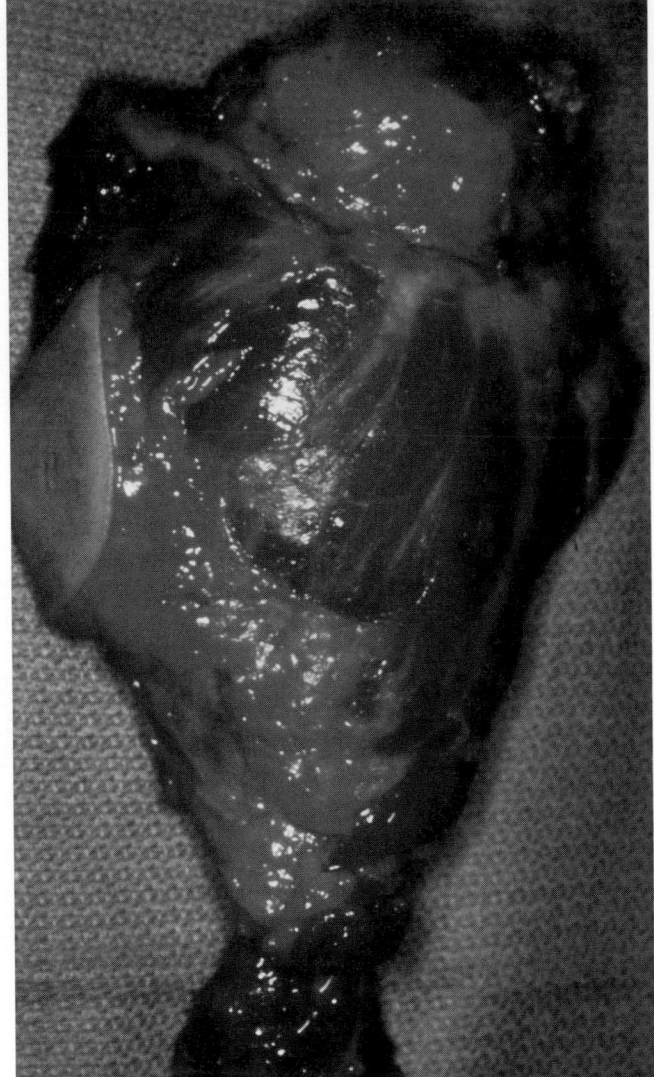

B

Figure 16-36 *A.* Plain radiograph of a sclerosing osteosarcoma of the proximal humerus. (Reproduced with permission from Malawer MM, Abelson HT, Suit HD: Sarcomas of bone, chap. 37 in DeVita VT, Hellman S, Rosenberg SA (eds): *Cancer Principles and Practice of Oncology*, 2d ed, Philadelphia, Lippincott, 1985, pp 1293–1343.) *B.* Intraarticular resection of the proximal humerus, demonstrating excised biopsy site.

Osteosarcoma

The proximal humerus is the third most common site for osteosarcoma (Fig. 16-36*A*), following the distal femur and the proximal tibia.[3,15] Osteosarcomas in the proximal humerus tend to have a poorer prognosis than those around the knee. Plain radiographs often suggest the correct diagnosis. All staging studies should be performed prior to biopsy; biopsy is usually only for confirmation of the diagnosis. Adjuvant or neoadjuvant chemotherapy is now considered standard for treatment of osteosarcomas. On presentation, most osteosarcomas of the proximal humerus will have a significant extraosseous component. Use of neoadjuvent chemotherapy may result in significant reduction of this component, facilitating attempts at limb salvage (Fig. 16-36*B–D*). If the axillary vessels are free of tumor, a limb-sparing procedure is generally indicated, although an extraarticular resection is preferred.[8,9] The majority of osteosarcomas of the proximal humerus can be treated by the modified Tikhoff-Linberg procedure (type V resection per Malawer's classification). Contraindications are neurovascular, chest wall, and/or lymph node involvement. Forequarter amputation is required if resection is not feasible (Fig. 16-37).

Metastatic Carcinoma

All carcinomas can metastasize to the proximal humerus. Hypernephroma has a peculiar predilection for this location and may present a unique problem for surgical management. Hypernephromas are extremely vascular, reflecting their renal origin, and can result in uncontrollable bleeding during surgery. Radiography reveals that hypernephromas cause marked destruction and ballooning, much like an aneurysmal bone cyst or a primary sarcoma. If one encounters a possible hypernephroma, angiography of the humerus and the kidneys is recommended prior to biopsy. Simple biopsy (even with a needle) may lead to severe hemorrhage. Angiography can confirm the diagnosis of a renal lesion and at the same time allow embolization of the skeletal metastasis. Alternatively, temporary occlusion of the axillary artery with a balloon catheter can be performed during surgical procedures. The author prefers to ligate the anterior and posterior circumflex vessels prior to biopsy. These vessels are easily identified at the inferior border of the subcapularis muscle. Care must be taken to identify and protect the axillary nerve within the same interval.

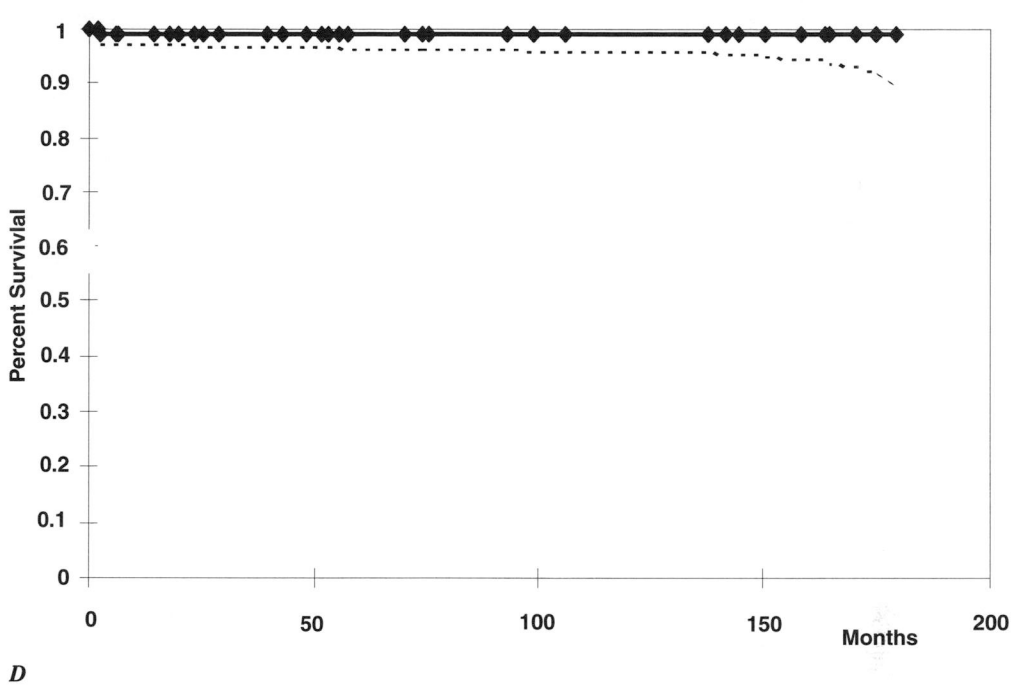

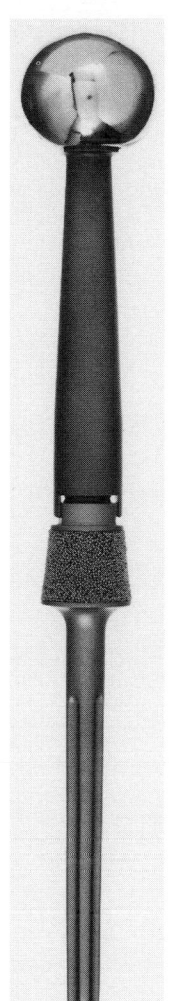

D

C

Figure 16-36 (*Continued*) *C.* Assembled modular endoprosthesis for reconstruction of the proximal humerus. *D.* Kaplan-Meier curve for MSRS survival: analysis of 23 consecutive modular endoprosthetic replacements of the proximal humerus. (Adapted from Henshaw RM, Jones V, Malawer MM: Skeletal reconstruction with non-custom modular endoprostheses. Results of the first 96 consecutive MSRS prosthetic replacements. Presented at the Ninth Annual Symposium of the International Society of Technology in Arthroplasty, Amsterdam, The Netherlands, August 1996.)

Treatment of metastatic carcinoma to the shoulder girdle generally involves radiation to ensure local control of the disease. The goal of treatment should be to reduce pain and maximize the patient's functional independence. A simple and reliable procedure is curettage of the lesion with packing of the humeral head with polymethylmethacrylate and insertion of intramedullary rods through a lateral incision. Prosthetic replacement is safely approached from this direction or alternatively from the anterior approach.

Surgical Procedure for Tumors of the Proximal Humerus

Forequarter Amputation (Interscapulothoracic Amputation)

Forequarter amputation entails removal of the entire upper extremity including the scapula and clavicle.[7] The surgical technique is described in Fig. 16-37. The plane of dissection is between the scapula and clavicle and the chest wall. The main indications for this procedure are high-grade neoplasms involving the shoulder girdle and/or proximal humerus. Two surgical approaches are utilized. The anterior approach (Berger's technique) begins with ligation of

the axillary vessels through an exposure made possible by removal of part of the clavicle. The second approach (Littlewood) is posterior and entails dividing the scapula from the chest wall. The axillary vessels are approached secondarily. The latter is favored because it facilitates vascular ligation and obviates the need to operate through a small anterior incision. These procedures allow for development of a variety of skin flaps; the actual site of the tumor dictates the choice of skin flaps. Wound healing is rarely a problem. The necessity for forequarter amputation has decreased with the increasing popularity of a limb-sparing option, the Tikhoff-Linberg procedure and its modifications, along with the success of neoadjuvant chemotherapy.

Shoulder Girdle Resections (Limb-Sparing Procedures)

There are numerous types of shoulder girdle resections for neoplasms. There is no standard classification. Figure 16-31*A* summarizes the various types of procedures and a proposed classification.

Adequate resection of the proximal humerus for high-grade bony sarcomas can be accomplished by a modified Tikhoff-Linberg procedure (type V).[8,9] This includes en

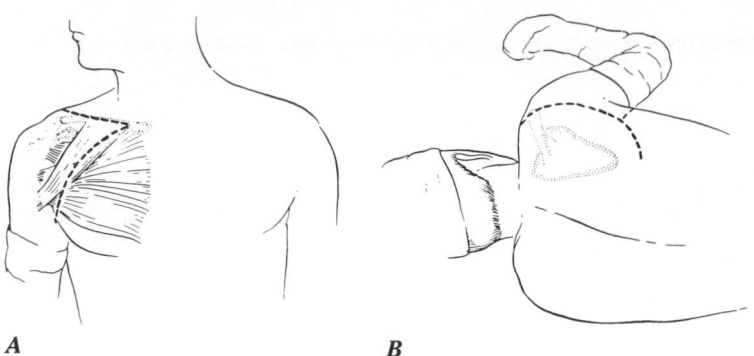

A   *B*

Figure 16-37 Technique of forequarter amputation. *A*. The anterior skin incision. *B*. The posterior skin incision. A lateral position is utilized. *C* and *D*. Posterior dissection. A large posterior, subcutaneous flap is developed. All muscles attaching to the axillary border of the scapula are transected with a cutting cautery including the levator scapulae and latissimus dorsi muscles.

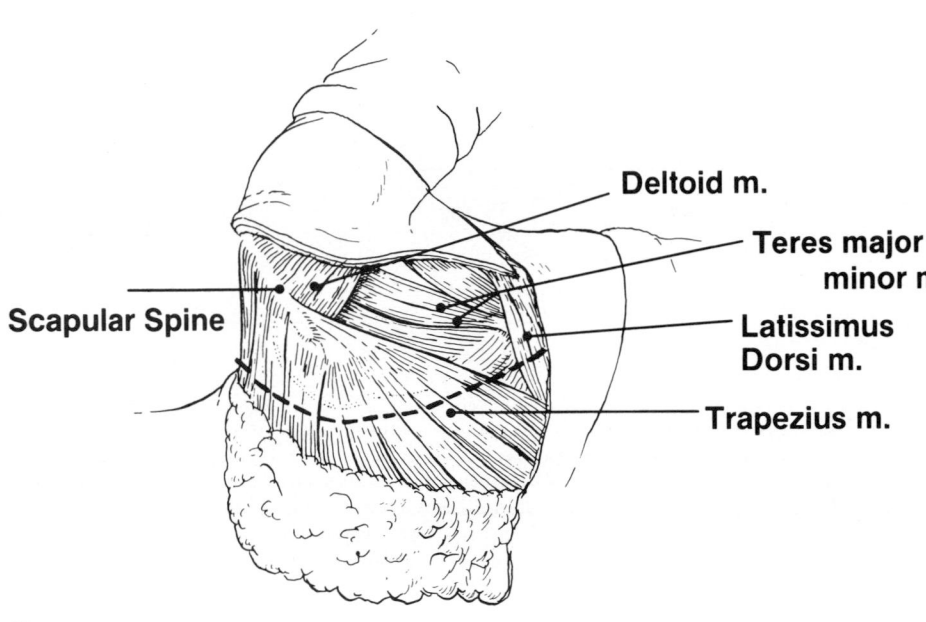

Deltoid m.

Teres major
minor m

Scapular Spine

Latissimus
Dorsi m.

Trapezius m.

C

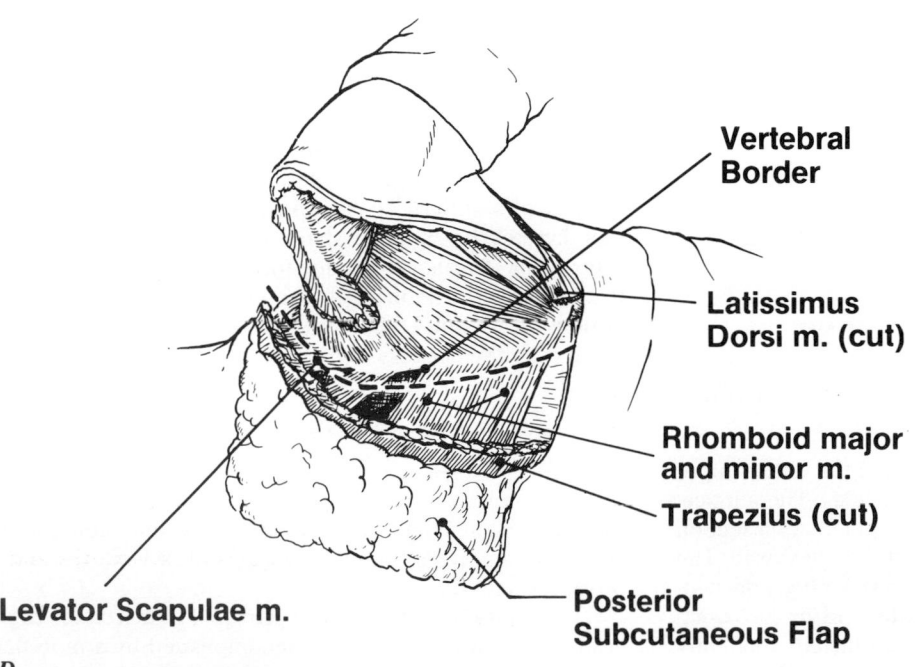

Vertebral
Border

Latissimus
Dorsi m. (cut)

Rhomboid major
and minor m.

Trapezius (cut)

Levator Scapulae m.

Posterior
Subcutaneous Flap

D

Figure 16-37 (*Continued*) *E.* The serratus anterior muscle is transected and the entire scapula is anteriorly rotated. The axillary vessels can now be safely approached from this direction or alternatively from the anterior approach. *F.* Anterior dissection. The pectoralis major and minor muscles are transected. The clavicle is transected at the junction of the proximal one-third. This exposes the axillary vessels and brachial plexus. These structures are now ligated and transected, completing the amputation. *G.* The wound is closed over suction catheters.

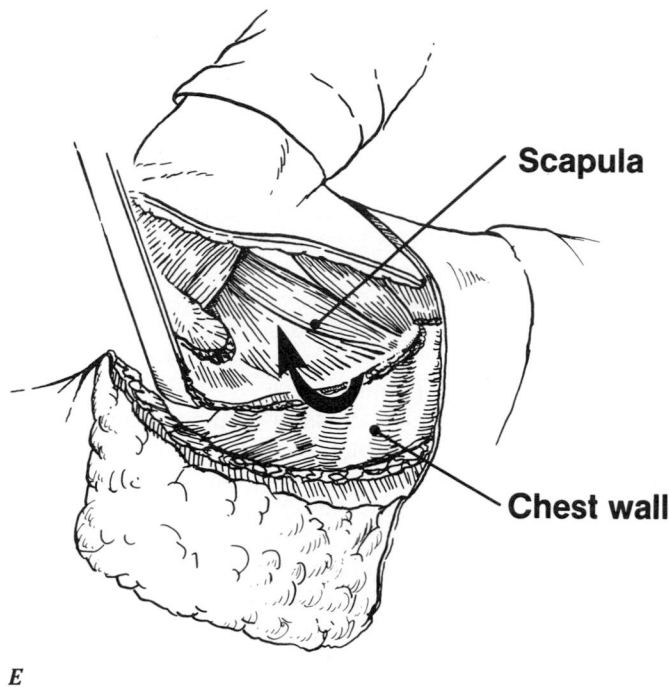

Scapula

Chest wall

E

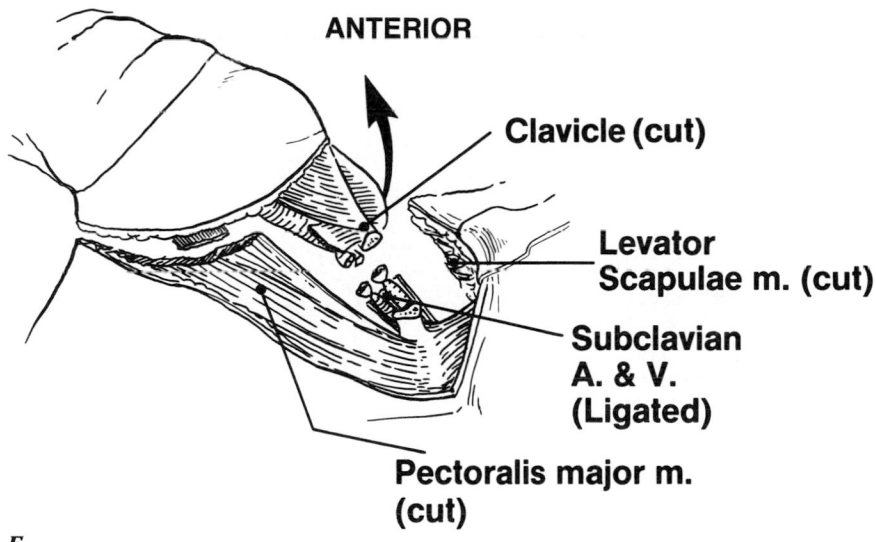

ANTERIOR

Clavicle (cut)

Levator Scapulae m. (cut)

Subclavian A. & V. (Ligated)

Pectoralis major m. (cut)

F

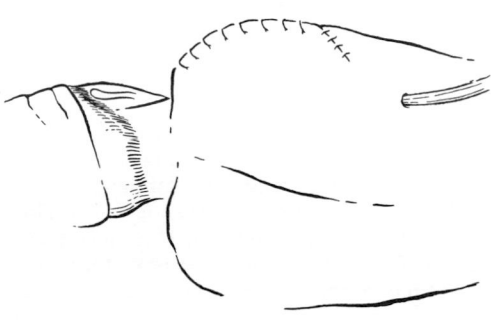

G

bloc removal of 15 to 20 cm of the humerus and shoulder joint with the deltoid, rotator cuff, and portions of the biceps and triceps muscles. The length of bone resection is determined preoperatively from a bone scan. To avoid a positive margin at the site of humeral transection, the distal osteotomy is performed 5 to 6 cm distal to the area of abnormality. Reconstruction involves segmental replacement of the humeral shaft, suspension of the humerus from the clavicle, biceps and triceps motor reconstruction via tenodesis, and transfer of proximal muscles for soft tissue coverage (Fig. 16-38). Approximately 80 to 85 percent of proximal humeral sarcomas can be treated successfully by this limb-sparing option.

The major contraindications to local resection are tumor involvement of lymph nodes, chest wall involvement, pathologic fracture, or massive soft tissue contamination. Resectability is determined by early exploration of the neurovascular structures through an anterior incision with division of the pectoralis major. This approach does not jeopardize formation of an anterior flap in patients who require forequarter amputation. Preservation of the musculocutaneous nerve is extremely important: the short biceps muscle, responsible for elbow flexion, is the most important muscle left after resection. Extraarticular resection of the glenohumeral joint by medial scapulosteotomy is safer than intraarticular resection. In addition, scapular

osteotomy not only removes the potential for tumor contamination of the operative field but also permits medialization of the reconstructured humerus and thus a decrease in bulk of the area to be covered.[9]

A custom or modular proximal humeral prosthesis is used for reconstruction of the humeral shaft. Other options include dual fibula autografts with primary arthrodesis, massive allograft reconstruction, or allograft/prosthetic composite replacement. Irrespective of the selected method of bony reconstruction, soft tissue reconstruction is necessary and is a main determinant of functional outcome. Proximal soft tissue reconstruction and suspension are essential to avoid postoperative pain, instability, and fatigability. This is accomplished by a technique of "dual suspension" through static and dynamic reconstruction. Suspension by Dacron tape and muscle transfers of the pectoralis major, latissimus, and trapezius have proved effective.

Provided that the musculocutaneous nerve is preserved and proximal reattachment of the biceps is performed, function of the elbow will be near normal. This is critical to allow for positioning of the forearm, wrist, and hand following resection. Protection of the brachial plexus is vital to preserving normal hand function. Active shoulder motion is minimal but stable, while scapulothoracic motion provides some useful internal and external rotation. Cosmesis is acceptable and can be enhanced with use of a shoulder pad.

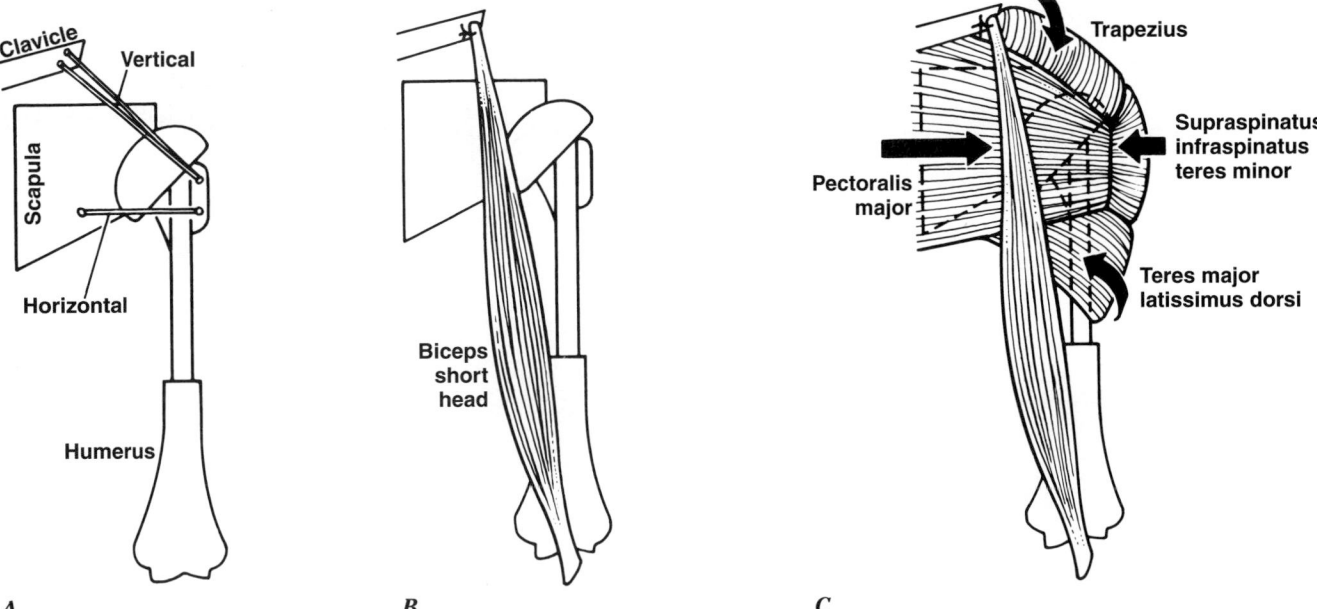

A   *B*   *C*

Figure 16-38 Technique of shoulder girdle suspension and reconstruction following resection (type V) for high-grade osteosarcoma. *A.* Static suspension. Static reconstruction is accomplished by the use of dual Dacron tapes. This protects the muscle transfers until healing occurs. *B.* Dynamic suspension. The short head of the biceps is transferred to the outer edge of the remaining clavicle in order to restore the elbow flexors and permit dynamic suspension. *C.* Motor reconstruction and soft tissue coverage. The entire shoulder girdle and the prosthesis (which acts as a spacer) is covered and suspended by the transferred pectoralis major, trapezius, and latissimus dorsi muscles. Soft tissue reconstruction is mandatory to stabilize and to support the upper extremity following a major resection. External orthoses are rarely required.

BONY TUMORS OF THE ARM AND ELBOW

The humeral shaft is an uncommon site for primary malignant bone tumors. Common benign lesions include unicameral bone cysts (diaphyseal), fibrous dysplasia, and enchondromas. All tend to occur during childhood and adolescence. The elbow is an uncommon site for bony neoplasms; there are no lesions peculiar to this joint. Benign humeral lesions may present with a pathologic fracture or as an incidental radiographic finding. Management of UBCs of the arm and elbow is similar to that of such lesions located elsewhere. Once the correct diagnosis is established, enchondromas and fibrous dysplasia are treated by simple curettage. Fracture through a benign lesion heals readily without the need of internal fixation. Metastatic carcinoma occasionally involves the humeral shaft and elbow and deserves special consideration.

Management of Pathologic Fractures of the Humerus and Elbow

Most metastatic lesions of the humerus do not require surgery. Radiation therapy offers good relief from pain, and reossification of lytic lesions often occurs. Functional bracing during treatment is often well tolerated and does not impede the patient's self-care. If, however, a patient also has metastatic disease of the lower extremities, the upper extremity should receive prompt surgical attention. This allows the patient to use crutches and to remain ambulatory.

Fixation of a pathologic fracture is best performed by open curettage, cementation with PMMA, and intramedullary fixation. For lesions of the proximal two-thirds of the humerus, one small incision is made at the greater tuberosity for rod insertion, and another at the level of the fracture for fracture reduction, curettage of the lesion, and cement insertion. An anterior lateral incision along the humerus is recommended for exposure of the fracture site. The bicep is retracted medially and the brachialis is split anteriorly in order to avoid exposure and possible damage to the radial nerve. Lesions of the distal one-third can be fixed with cross rods inserted through the epicondyles (Fig. 16-39). Plate-and-screw fixation of the humeral shaft following cementation is advocated by some authors to avoid surgical insult to the rotator cuff and to facilitate postoperative rehabilitation.

BONY TUMORS OF THE FOREARM AND WRIST

Lesions of the proximal radius and ulna are unusual. The olecranon may occasionally be the site of a bone tumor but none is specific for this area. The distal radius is a common site for giant-cell tumors; these lesions are often more aggressive than similar lesions in the lower extremity. Osteosarcomas rarely occur in this location. Both tumors in this site present with pain and a mass, whereas pain usually is the sole presenting symptoms when these tumors occur around the knee. Tight anatomic constraints usually do not permit a limb-sparing procedure for stage IIB sarcomas of the distal radius. Thus the rare osteosarcoma necessitates a high amputation across the forearm. In contrast, there are several surgical options for GCT at this site, as listed below. Metastatic carcinoma occasionally occurs in the bones of the forearm; lung carcinoma is the most common source of bony metastasis distal to the elbow.

Giant-Cell Tumors of the Distal Radius
Clinical Aspects

The distal radius is the third most common site for GCTs, following the distal femur and proximal tibia.[16,17] Ten percent of GCTs occur in this location. Giant-cell tumors of the distal radius often present with cortical destruction and soft tissue extension, due to thin cortices and the direct attachment of the pronator quadratus to the bone. Giant-cell tumor of the distal radius is reported to have a higher likelihood of lung metastasis, necessitating staging studies and close radiographic follow-up of these patients. Both CT and MRI can demonstrate the extraosseous extension accurately and the relation of the tumor to the adjacent carpus and the distal ulna. Angiography is extremely useful in planning a surgical approach; the radial artery and in some cases the ulnar artery may be markedly displaced and involved by tumor. In general, the distal radioulnar joint and the carpus must be closely evaluated before and during surgery to determine tumor involvement. Tumor is usually found within the pronator quadratus; this accounts for the significant rate of local recurrence. The articular cartilage of the carpus may also be contaminated by the tumor.

Surgical Management

The recurrence rate following simple curettage of a distal radial GCT is significantly higher than that of a GCT at other sites. Local recurrence is due to the biological aggressiveness of the tumor combined with microscopic extension into the adjacent soft tissues, specifically the pronator quadratus. If the tumor is small and intraosseous, curettage and cryosurgery are recommended. The upper extremity is an ideal location for cryosurgery, since the risk of pathologic fracture is slight.[18–21] Extensive stage 3 or multiply recurrent GCTs are best treated with en bloc resection, including the pronator quadratus, distal radius, distal ulna, and occasionally the proximal row of the carpus (Fig. 16-40). Multiple recurrences can be treated with adjuvant radiation therapy; amputation should be reserved only for cases of malignant degeneration.

Following resection of large lesions, insertion of an autogenous fibula is recommended; allograft replacements have also had good results.[22] In general, a primary arthrodesis is recommended, although attempts at preservation of wrist motion following graft replacement also have yielded good short-term results. Alternatively, following resection, the carpus can be centralized onto the ulna and fused to create a one-bone forearm. This technique avoids the need for either an autogenous fibula or an allograft.

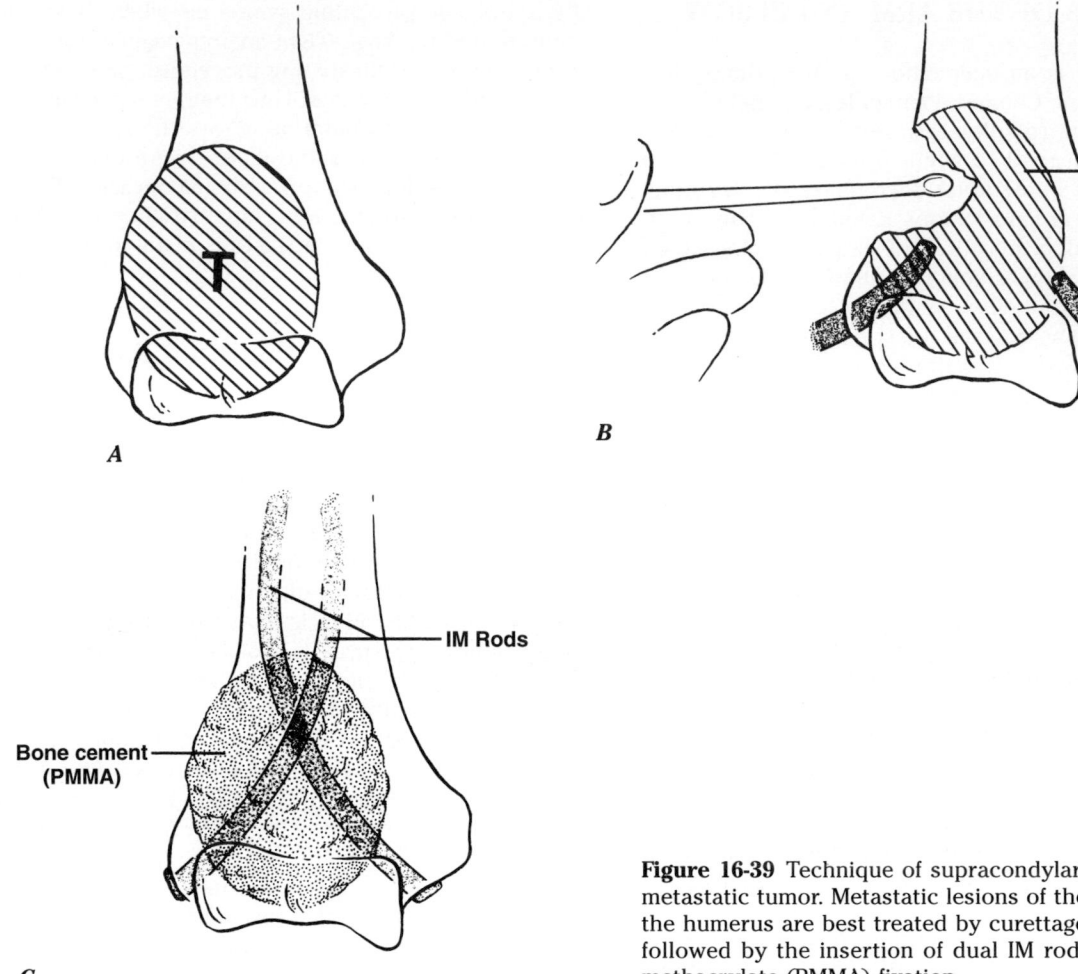

A

B

C

Figure 16-39 Technique of supracondylar reconstruction for metastatic tumor. Metastatic lesions of the distal one-third of the humerus are best treated by curettage of all gross tumor followed by the insertion of dual IM rods with polymethylmethacrylate (PMMA) fixation.

Metastatic Carcinoma

Metastatic cancer sometimes affects the radius and ulna. The occasional patient who presents with a bony lesion of a previously undiagnosed primary carcinoma may be mistakenly diagnosed as having a primary sarcoma. Lesions with predominate osteoblastic features, such as breast or prostate, most commonly mimic a bone-producing sarcoma. Biopsy is necessary to confirm the diagnosis, and staging studies are mandatory to identify the primary site of disease. Radiation therapy offers good results for both palliation and local control of disease. Surgery is rarely indicated; if necessary, intramedullary Steinmann pin fixation combined with cementation for immediate fixation leads to a good result.

SOFT TISSUE SARCOMAS OF THE ARM AND FOREARM

Between 15 and 25 percent of soft tissue sarcomas occur in the upper extremities.[1] Staging studies and principles of treatment are similar to those for such lesions in the lower extremities. The most common error in treatment is to assume that a soft tissue mass is a benign lipoma or ganglion.

Often, the correct diagnosis is made only after an attempted surgical resection that may contaminate vital compartments. All soft tissue masses of the upper extremity should be assumed to be malignant until proven otherwise. All of the previously discussed precautions should be taken regarding the site and timing of the biopsy. Because of anatomic constraints in this area, there is far less room for error in performing a biopsy. Errors such as inappropriate biopsy or prior "shell-out" procedures greatly jeopardize potential limb salvage, more so than in other anatomic sites. The types and grades of soft tissue sarcomas of the upper extremity do not differ from those of the general category of sarcomas. Surgical options are often limited because of previous treatment and anatomic considerations.

Anatomic Considerations

The arm is composed of two well-defined compartments: the anterior compartment (biceps, brachialis) and the posterior compartment (triceps). The brachial artery and the median nerve are contained within the anterior compartment, while the radial nerve and the profunda brachii artery are the main neurovascular structures of the posterior compartment. The ulnar nerve originates in an anterior loca-

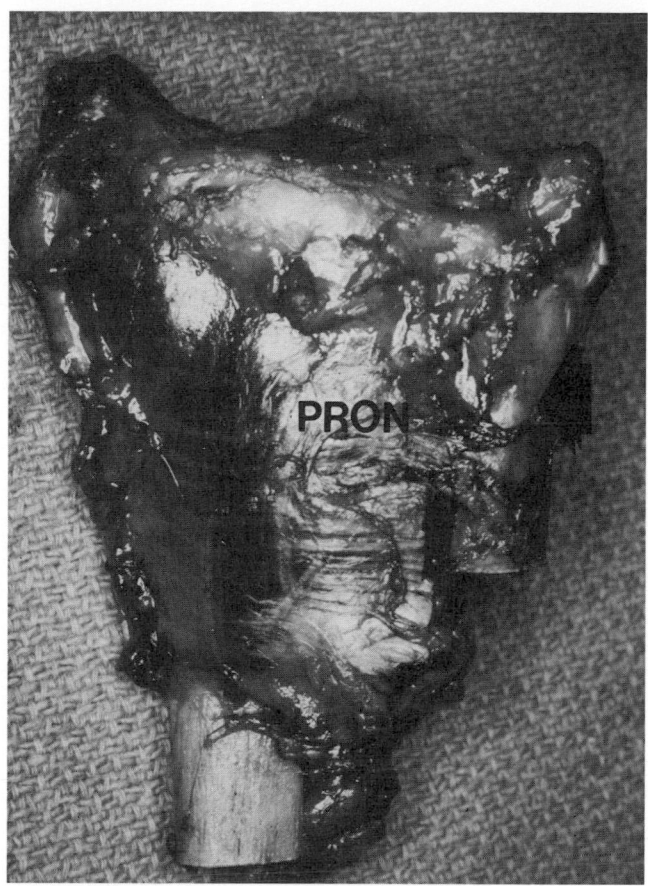

A

B

Figure 16-40 Giant-cell tumor of the distal radius. *A.* Gross specimen following resection of the distal radius. The distal ulna (*solid arrow*) was also removed because of involvement by the tumor. Note that the pronator quadratus (*PRON*) covers the tumor. *B.* Bivalved gross specimen. Note the extraosseous com-

ponent involving the pronator quadratus (*solid arrows*). This is a common finding, which often makes primary resection mandatory. There was direct articular cartilage destruction (in the hand) with synovial involvement. This finding is less common. The proximal row of the carpus was partially resected.

tion and then crosses posteriorly at the origin of the medial intermuscular septum. Similarly, the forearm consists of a volar (anterior or flexor) and dorsal (posterior or extensor) compartment. In general, stage I or IIA tumors remain confined to one compartment until they become quite large. Some lesions, however, are extracompartmental (stage IB or IIB) on presentation. Sarcomas of the arm can often be resected with minimal disability. Portions of muscle, or even entire muscles in each compartment, can be removed without loss of function. The main determinant of function is the degree of involvement of the major nerves. Forearm sarcomas are more difficult to resect as a result.

Staging

Staging studies are similar to those described previously for other sites. Additionally, careful physical examination of the axilla and epitrochlea is required, since sarcomas of the upper extremity may involve the regional lymph nodes. Lymph node involvement is most common with synovial and epithelioid sarcomas, which have a predilection for the forearm and hand.

Biopsy

Because of anatomic constraints in the arm and forearm, all biopsies must be approached with great care. Preoperative planning with the intention of minimizing contamination and for potential removal of the biopsy site en bloc with the lesion is required. Consideration should be given to performing the biopsy with a frozen section and to proceeding with removal in one stage. Such a technique offers the best possibility of avoiding inadvertent contamination and the loss of a limb-sparing option. A small incisional biopsy or needle biopsy is recommended. The biopsy should be done under tourniquet control and be placed longitudinally.

Overall Management

Stage IA/B tumors can be treated safely with surgery alone if negative margins are obtained; otherwise adjuvant radiotherapy is recommended. Stage IIA/B tumors require surgical removal, chemotherapy, and radiotherapy if a marginal or wide excision has been performed. Radiotherapy to the upper extremity requires a high level of expertise to avoid serious sequelae such as fibrosis, contractures, lymphedema, pain, and local recurrence.

Surgical Management

Amputations are often required for sarcomas of the upper extremity: forequarter amputation for tumors of the proximal arm and shoulder disarticulation and above-elbow amputation for lesions of the distal arm and forearm, respectively. Major neurovascular involvement or extensive contamination following a poorly placed biopsy are common reasons for amputation. Limb-sparing surgery is recommended if a functional elbow and hand can be expected. Function varies greatly following this surgery, depending on the location and combination of the nerves involved. In general, sacrifice of the radial nerve is easily compensated for by secondary tendon transfers. Loss of either the median or ulnar nerve leaves some useful function in the hand; however, sacrifice of both nerves results in an unacceptable loss of function.

Specific Anatomic Compartments

Anterior (Biceps)

Angiography will accurately demonstrate the position of the brachial artery and the tumor. If the vessels are clear, removal of the biceps and/or brachialis can be compensated for by a modified Steindler flexorplasty (proximal transfer of the forearm flexors).

Posterior (Triceps)

The triceps can be resected with minimal morbidity. If the radial nerve is involved, it should be removed. Tendon transfers are performed secondarily after recovery of the limb. The triceps itself need not require reconstruction, as extension of the elbow will occur with gravity.

Volar (Forearm Flexors)

This is the most difficult compartment in which to perform a limb-sparing procedure. Deeply situated sarcomas that involve the radius and/or ulna and intermuscular septum may cross over to the extensor group, becoming extracompartmental. Either CT or MRI scanning is helpful in delineating the mass. Bone scintigraphy may determine osseous involvement, which tends to be more common with forearm tumors than with lesions located elsewhere. Biplane angiography is essential to determine the vascular anatomy, which is frequently distorted by the tumor mass. Either the radial or ulnar artery can be sacrificed if there is a patent deep palmar arch. Small tumors can be resected with wide negative margins. The superficial or deep flexors can be entirely removed if necessary. Each lesion must be carefully evaluated in terms of the amount of hand function that will remain. In general, a sensate hand with some function is far superior to a prosthesis.

Dorsum (Forearm Extensors)

The proximal extensors (mobile wad) are a favorite location for soft tissue sarcomas of the forearm. This entire group, along with the posterior interosseous nerve, can be resected without major loss of hand grip; the only deficit is a wrist drop. If the underlying radius is involved, it should be removed en bloc with the lesion. The remaining olecranon is sufficient for elbow stability; there is no need to reconstruct the resected proximal radius. An external orthosis may be required. Tendon transfers are performed secondarily following completion of any planned radiotherapy. In general, tendon transfers following irradiation tend to function mainly as a tenodesis due to radiation fibrosis.

REFERENCES

1. Rosenberg SA, Suit FD, Baker LI: Sarcomas of soft tissue, in DeVita VT, Heilman S, Rosenberg SA (eds): *Cancer: Principles and Practice of Oncology,* 2d ed. Philadelphia, Lippincott, 1985, pp 1243–1293.
2. Dahlin DC: *Bone Tumors: General Aspects and Data on 6,221 Cases,* 3d ed. Springfield, IL, Charles C Thomas, 1978.
3. Dahlin DC, Coventry MB: Osteosarcoma, a study of 600 cases. *J Bone Joint Surg* 49A:101–110, 1967.
4. Malawer MM: The diagnosis, treatment and management of unicameral bone cysts by percutaneous aspiration, hemodynamic evaluation and intracavitary methylprednisolone acetate. *Orthopedic Update Series,* Vol IV, lesson 26. Princeton, NJ, Continuing Professional Education Center, 1986.
5. Neer CS, Francis KC, Kleman HA, et al: Current concepts in the treatment of solitary unicameral bone cysts. *Clin Orthop* 97:40–51, 1973.
6. Marcove RC, Mike V, Hutter RVP, et al: Chondrosarcoma of the pelvis and upper end of femur. *J Bone Joint Surg [Am]* 54:561–572, 1972.
7. Francis KC: Radical amputations, in *Nora's Operative Surgery.* Philadelphia, Lea & Febiger, 1974, pp 1041–1051.
8. Malawer MM: Surgical technique and results of limb-sparing surgery for high grade bone sarcomas of the knee and shoulder: Analysis of 33 consecutive cases. *Orthopedics* 8:597–607, 1985.
9. Malawer MM, Sugarbaker PJ, Lambert PT, et al: The Tikhoff Linberg procedure: Report of ten patients and presentation of a modified technique for tumors of the proximal humerus. *Surgery* 97:518–528, 1985.
10. Garrison RC, Unni KJC, Mcleod RA, et al: Chondrosarcoma arising in osteochondroma. *Cancer* 49:1890–1897, 1982.
11. Gitelis S, Bertoni F, Chieti PP, Campanacci M: Chondrosarcoma of bone. *J Bone Joint Surg [Am]* 63A:1248–1256, 1981.
12. Francis KC, Worcester JN Jr: Radical resection for tumors of the shoulder with preservation of a functional extremity. *J Bone Joint Surg* 44A:1423–1429, 1962.
13. Malawer MM, McKay DW, and Markle B, et al: Analysis of 40 consecutive cases of unicameral bone cysts treated by high pressure Renografin injection and intracavity methylprednisolone acetate: Prognostic factors and hemodynamic evaluation. 52nd Annual Meeting, American Academy of Orthopaedic Surgery, Las Vegas, NV, 1985.
14. Dahlin DC, Ivins JC: Benign chondroblastoma: A study of 125 cases. *Cancer* 30:401–413, 1972.

15. Campanacci M, Bacci G, Bertoni F, et al: The treatment of osteosarcoma of the extremity: Twenty years' experience at the Instituto Orthopedico Rizzoli. *Cancer* 48:1569–1581, 1981.

16. Campanacci M, Giunti A, Olmi R: Giant-cell tumors of bone: A study of 209 cases with long-term follow-up in 130. *Ital J Orthop Traumatol* 1:249–277, 1977.

17. Dahlin DC, Cupps RE, Johnson EW Jr: Giant cell tumor: A study of 195 cases. *Cancer* 25:1061–1070, 1970.

18. Malawer MM, Dunham WK, Zaleski T, Zielinski CJ: Cryosurgery in the management of benign (aggressive) and low grade malignant tumors of bone: Analysis of 40 consecutive cases. Presented at the American Academy of Orthopedic Surgeons (AAOS), New Orleans, February 1986.

19. Marcove RC: A 17-year review of cryosurgery in the treatment of bone tumors. *Clin Orthop* 163:231–233, 1982.

20. Marcove RC, Lyden JP, Huvos AC, Bullough PB: Giant cell tumor treated by cryosurgery: A report of twenty-five cases. *J Bone Joint Surg [Am]* 55:1633–1644, 1973.

21. Marcove PC, Weiss L, Vaghaiwall M, Pearson R: Cryosurgery in the treatment of giant cell tumor of bone: A report of 52 consecutive cases. *Clin Orthop* 134:275–289, 1978.

22. Mankin HJ, Fogelson FS, Thrasher, et al: Massive resection and allograft transplantation in the treatment of malignant bone tumors. *N Engl J Med* 294:1247–1255, 1976.

III. Neoplasms Affecting the Lower Extremity

Robert M. Henshaw and Martin M. Malawer

NEOPLASMS INVOLVING BONE OF THE PELVIS AND LOWER EXTREMITY

The pelvis and lower extremity are the most common sites for benign or malignant bone and soft tissue neoplasms. Overall, the most frequently encountered bone tumors in this region are chondrosarcomas and round cell neoplasms. The distal femur and proximal tibia are the most common sites of osteosarcomas, giant-cell tumors, aneurysmal bone cysts, and malignant fibrous histiocytomas (MFH). Soft tissue sarcomas typically arise around the buttock and thigh or, less frequently, distal to the knee. The quadriceps is the most common anatomic compartment involved by soft tissue sarcomas, although all anatomic compartments and mesenchymal structures can give rise to sarcomas.

The specific anatomic site of the lesion is the predominant feature determining clinical presentation. Techniques for diagnosis and surgical management of bony and soft tissue sarcomas are presented in this chapter according to anatomic site. Emphasis is placed upon surgical staging, surgical indications, and techniques of management. The technique of limb-sparing surgery for each anatomic site is also discussed.

Tumors of the Pelvis

Clinical Characteristics

The pelvis is the most common site for round cell sarcomas and chondrosarcomas. The flat bones that make up the pelvis consist of hematopoietically active marrow within a thin cortical structure; therefore it follows that tumors arising from the marrow (myeloma, lymphoma, and Ewing's sarcoma, as well as metastatic carcinoma) often involve the pelvis. Because of the thin cortical bone, which is easily breached, as well as the large cavity within the true pelvis, these lesions can easily form huge extraosseous intrapelvic components prior to becoming symptomatic. Of the spindle cell sarcomas, chondrosarcoma is the most frequent and is often quite large on presentation.[1–3] Initial complaints are typically nonspecific and can vary greatly, depending upon adjacent structures involved. Dull pain, abdominal fullness, painless abdominal mass, sciatica, hip pain, or occasionally bladder symptoms occurring alone or in combination are typical of the presenting signs. With the exception of large chondrosarcomas, which commonly show new calcification, most tumors of the pelvis are not easily diagnosed by simple radiographs. Therefore, a high degree of clinical suspicion is necessary for early diagnosis. Axial imaging with CT or MRI scans greatly facilitates detection of the extraosseous components and allows for biopsy studies to confirm the diagnosis.

The pelvis consists of three distinct functional regions: the illum, the periacetabulum, and the pubic rami.[4] The region of involvement determines the pattern of tumor growth and therefore the possible surgical options. The extraosseous extent of tumors arising from the ilium is easily underestimated, and they may fill the pelvis without causing many symptoms. This occurs most often with Ewing's sarcomas. Tumors arising from the posterior ilium may involve the sacrum and extend along the sacral nerve roots. Also, the sciatic nerve may become involved, particularly where it crosses the inferior portion of the ilium as it exits via the sciatic notch. Sacral and neurologic involvement must be carefully evaluated prior to surgery. Evaluation of this region has been greatly facilitated by high-resolution MRI. Periacetabular tumors may directly involve the hip joint by extension along the ligamentum teres and/or joint capsule. Tumors of the pubic rami tend to have no clinical signs. Occasionally these tumors enlarge and involve the pubic symphysis and displace the adjacent bladder and urethra. Direct involvement of the urinary system is rare.

Staging Studies

Because of its complicated three-dimensional structure, the pelvis requires thorough radiographic evaluation prior to biopsy or surgical treatment. Although plain radiographs are notorious for appearing "normal" despite obvious neoplasms, a thorough evaluation should still include anteroposterior (AP), obturator and iliac oblique views (as described by Judet), as well as inlet/outlet views. These views are helpful in visualizing the three-dimensional relationships for surgical planning. Computed tomography with intravenous and oral contrast accurately demonstrates possible extraosseous extension, proximity to the sacrum and hip joint, and sciatic nerve involvement.[5–7] In addition, the ureters and bladder can be visualized. Following injection of metrizamide contrast into the epidural space of the spine (CT myelogram), CT scanning is useful if intraspinal tumor extension is suspected. Magnetic resonance imaging excels in visualization of the spinal cord through high-contrast images and the combined use of axial, coronal, and sagittal images.[8] In addition, it has the advantage of being noninvasive. Selection of the imaging modality to be used should be on an individual basis, depending upon the site and radiographic nature of the lesion as well as whether there has been prior surgical intervention. In general, high-resolution CT imaging allows for accurate evaluation of the integrity of cortical bone, while MRI emphasizes the soft tissue extension and involvement of the marrow.

Bone scintigraphy often demonstrates intraosseous spread well beyond that revealed by plain radiographs. It is a very sensitive but nonspecific test for bone involvement and therefore should be done early in patients with pelvic symptomatology to rule out bony disease. Whole-body scanning should always be performed to detect distant bony metastases. Angiography is especially useful to delineate the level of bifurcation of the aorta and the common iliacs if a hemipelvectomy or modified hemipelvectomy is planned. An intravenous pyelogram, cystogram, barium enemas, and sigmoid endoscopy may be required in specific situations. Electromyography is not helpful in determining sacral plexus involvement.

Biopsy

Biopsy of suspected lesions remains necessary to ensure accurate diagnosis and subsequent treatment. Standard orthopaedic approaches to the ilium and acetabulum are unacceptable for biopsy of suspected malignant tumors because they contaminate important tissue planes. The person responsible for the biopsy must have a thorough understanding of the various incisions for hemipelvectomy and the limb-sparing procedures of the pelvis.[9] Trochar biopsy is recommended for the initial biopsy. Iliac lesions should be approached through a small incision that is either parallel to the crest or anterior between the tensor fascia and sartorius muscles. The acetabulum can be approached through the latter incision. The posterior (gluteal) area should always be avoided, since this flap is routinely used for a hemipelvectomy (see below).[9] Care also should be taken to avoid contamination of the hip joint, iliacus, or retroperitoneal areas. The use of fluoroscopic or CT-guided needle biopsy has greatly reduced the need to perform open biopsies in this region. Core needle biopsy minimizes tissue contamination and has been shown to be safe and accurate when performed by a skilled surgeon or radiologist.[10–12] A pathologist should be present at the time of biopsy to ensure that adequate diagnostic material has been collected.

Surgical Management

Malignant spindle cell tumors of the pelvis typically require hemipelvectomy to ensure that adequate surgical margins are obtained. In selected patients, partial pelvic resection may be performed safely with partial preservation of extremity function.[4] Round cell sarcomas and metastatic carcinoma require radiation therapy. Benign tumors are treated by simple curettage. Bone graft or internal fixation usually is not required unless the periacetabulum is involved.

Specific Tumors of the Pelvis

Chondrosarcoma

The pelvis is the most common site for both primary and secondary chondrosarcomas; 33 percent of such tumors arise from this site.[2,13–17] These tumors are typically very large on presentation despite the fact that many are low-grade lesions. Grossly, chondrosarcomas are soft and gelatinous. When cut, they extrude a jelly-like (myxoid material) substance that easily contaminates the entire wound. Extreme care and judgment must be used in undertaking a biopsy. As noted previously, histology alone is not sufficient to establish an accurate diagnosis for cartilage tumors.[18] Use of core needle biopsy is recommended to confirm the presence of cartilage. Adjuvant treatment with either chemotherapy or radiation is of questionable benefit and should be reserved for unresectable disease or local recurrence. Chondrosarcomas of the pelvis can be treated by a limb-sparing resection, although large tumors often require a hemipelvectomy (Fig. 16-41).[17,19,20] Long-term results published by Enneking showed that only 4 percent of lesions will recur if adequate margins are obtained.[4]

Osteosarcoma

Osteosarcoma of the pelvis, approximately 5 percent of all osteosarcomas, continues to have a poorer prognosis than similar lesions located in the extremities. In contrast to chondrosarcomas, most osteosarcomas of the pelvis require a hemipelvectomy in order to obtain safe margins (Fig. 16-42).[4,21,22] Preoperative evaluation is essential to determine whether the sacrum or vertebrae are involved. If the sacrum is involved, an extended hemipelvectomy must be performed, i.e., the amputation passes through the sacral alar rather than the sacroiliac joint. Large osteosarcomas of the pelvis may be unresectable by any means, leading to a dismal prognosis. The University of Florida[23] reported on 25 patients with osteosarcoma of the pelvis treated between 1967 and 1990. Of 18 attempted resections, only 4 achieved negative wide margins, while blood loss exceeding 10 L occurred in 6 cases. A major unexpected finding was that tumor invasion into the large veins of the pelvis was present in about half of these patients. This finding mandates that thorough preoperative evaluation of the iliac vessels be performed prior to attempted resection. Only 1 patient remained disease-free in this study.

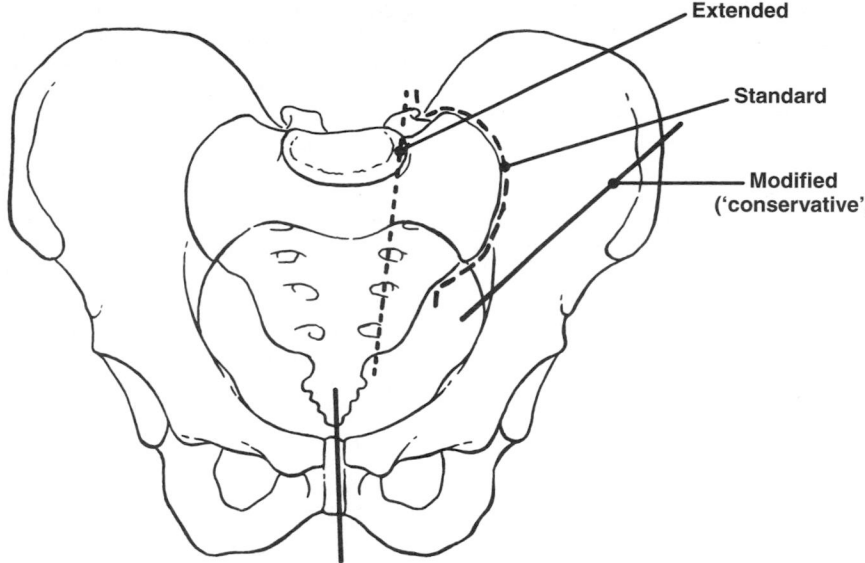

Figure 16-41 Types of hemipelvectomy. The standard (classic) hemipelvectomy is an amputation through the sacroiliac joint and the symphysis pubis with removal of the entire lower extremity and hemipelvis. An extended hemipelvectomy passes through the sacral alar and not the sacroiliac joint. Its main indication is for tumors extending to the posterior ilium and the sacroiliac joint. A modified hemipelvectomy preserves a portion of the ilium as well as the gluteus maximus muscle. A modified hemipelvectomy is utilized only for tumors of the groin and thigh. Its main advantage is to facilitate prosthesis fitting; it aids in sitting and heals more readily than the other modifications.

Tumor response to preoperative chemotherapy may convert an unresectable sarcoma to one that can be treated with a hemipelvectomy. Radiation therapy is effective for short-term palliation. The combination of intraarterial cisplatin and concurrent radiation may provide longer-term control in patients with unresectable disease.[24]

Ewing's Sarcoma

The pelvis is the second most common site for Ewing's sarcoma: 18 to 20 percent of all such lesions occur at this site.[16,25] Classically, Ewing's sarcoma of the pelvis presents as a lytic lesion with a huge extraosseous component. The prognosis for survival varies from 5 to 15 percent. The clinical challenge in treating a pelvic Ewing's sarcoma is to obtain local control and prevent metastatic disease. Experience at the National Cancer Institute shows a 33 percent incidence of local recurrence for "central" Ewing's sarcoma. Of these patients, 57 percent had metastases at the time of presentation.[26,27] Current treatment recommendations combine high-dose radiotherapy (6000 rads) with multidrug combination chemotherapy to improve local control and treat micrometastatic disease. Several centers are now engaged in studies that combine local resection with the above modalities in the hope of improving the prognosis.[28] Dramatic tumor shrinkage of the extraosseous component is often seen with multidrug combination chemotherapy, facilitating limb-sparing resections of the involved portion of the pelvis. In general, amputation should be avoided. Additional experience is needed to determine the optimal combination of treatment modalities.

Metastatic Carcinoma

The pelvis and periacetabular region are common sites for metastatic cancer. It is not unusual for relatively small acetabular defects to be associated with large extraosseous components, which bleed readily when curetted. Preoperative embolization is useful. If the femoral head is not involved, radiotherapy will provide good palliation. In the presence of acetabular disease and femoral head involvement, surgery is often necessary to achieve palliation. Total hip replacement—combined with curettage of the acetabular defect and reconstruction with polymethylmethacrylate (PMMA), protrusio cups, Steinmann's pins, and mesh—yields good short-term results. If the defect is large, a resection arthroplasty (Girdlestone procedure) is a good alternative to a complicated attempt at reconstruction in an individual with a short life expectancy. The saddle prosthesis, which was developed in Europe for treatment of failed total hip arthroplasty, provides a functional palliative procedure in selected patients with periacetabular metastases.[29]

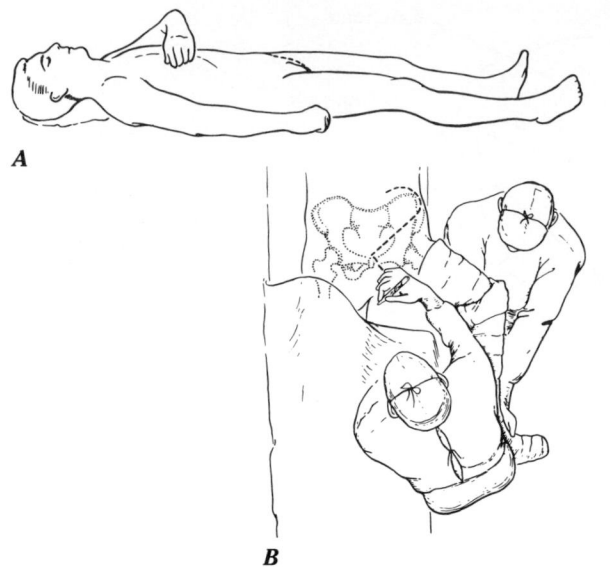

A

B

Figure 16-42 The operation consists of three stages: I, anterior; II, perineal; and III, posterior (see text). *A.* A semisupine position is utilized. The anterior skin incision parallels the inguinal ligament. *B.* The perineal incision follows the adductor crease and extends to the ischium. *C.* The anterior (retroperitoneal) dissection exposes the common iliac vessels and ureter. The common iliac vessels are ligated, and the psoas muscle is transected at the level of the upper sacrum. The bladder is mobilized from the symphysis pubis at this stage. The perineal incision is then made. *D.* The lower extremity is flexed and adducted to expose the buttock. The posterior incision is shown. *E.* A large posterior subcutaneous flap is developed. An osteotome then disarticulates the sacroiliac joint. The remaining pelvic floor structures are transected anteriorly, completing the amputation. *F.* The posterior flap is rotated anteriorly and closed over suction drains.

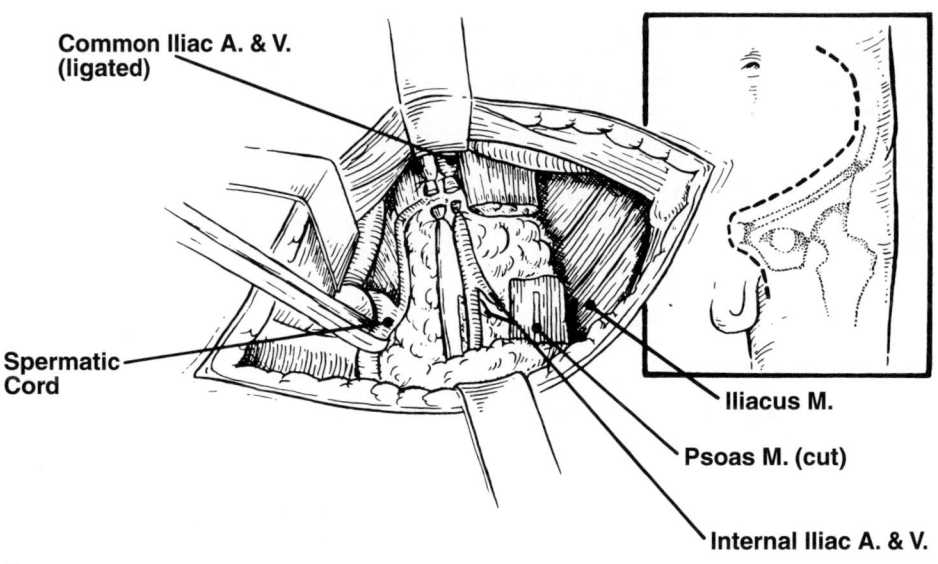

Common Iliac A. & V. (ligated)

Spermatic Cord

Iliacus M.

Psoas M. (cut)

Internal Iliac A. & V.

C

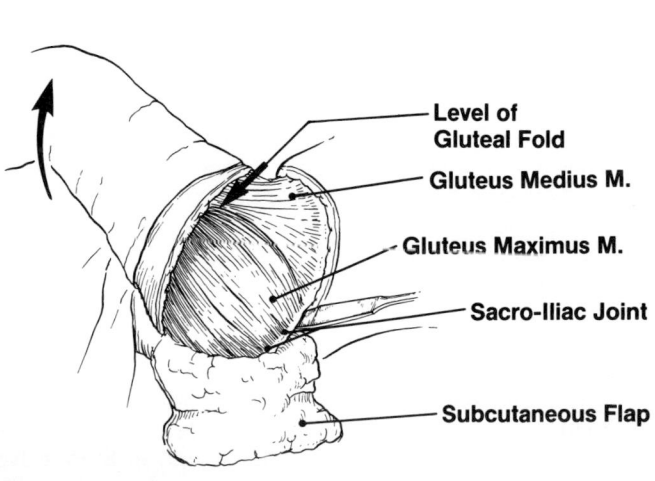

Level of Gluteal Fold

Gluteus Medius M.

Gluteus Maximus M.

Sacro-Iliac Joint

Subcutaneous Flap

D

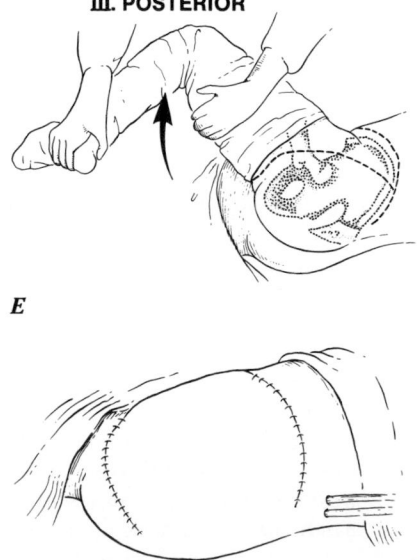

III. POSTERIOR

E

F

Special Surgical Procedures

Hemipelvectomy

Hemipelvectomy is an amputation through the sacroiliac joint and the symphysis pubis in which the entire hemipelvis is removed with the lower extremity.[9,30] The modifications are shown in Fig. 16-41. The dissection is retroperitoneal, with ligation of the common iliac artery and vein and the psoas muscle at the upper level of the sacroiliac joint (see Fig. 16-42). Only the peritoneum, ureter, bladder, and some pelvic floor musculature remain. The classical hemipelvectomy utilizes a large subcutaneous flap of gluteal skin for closure. The major indications for this procedure are neoplasms of the pelvic girdle and buttock sarcomas. Occasionally, hemipelvectomy is necessary for massive pelvic infections and/or irreversible ischemia of the lower extremity following failed attempts at revascularization. Overall mortality for this procedure is less than 5 percent today. The most common surgical problems are hemorrhage, infection, and flap necrosis. A recent modification of this procedure, described by Sugarbaker and Chretien, uses a large anterior myocutaneous flap composed of the quadriceps muscle along with the superficial femoral artery and vein (see Fig. 16-43).[30] This has expanded the indications for this procedure to include certain buttock and iliac lesions that were previously inoperable due to posterior contamination and/or extension.

Figure 16-43 Technique of anterior (myocutaneous) flap hemipelvectomy (see text). *A.* The posterior skin incision. A lateral position is utilized. *B.* Anterior incision. *C.* Elevation of the quadriceps from the femur. Note that the superficial femoral vessels are ligated distally and the profundus femoris vessels are ligated proximally. The entire quadriceps is mobilized on the superficial femoral pedicle. *D.* Rotation and closure of the flap following the amputation.

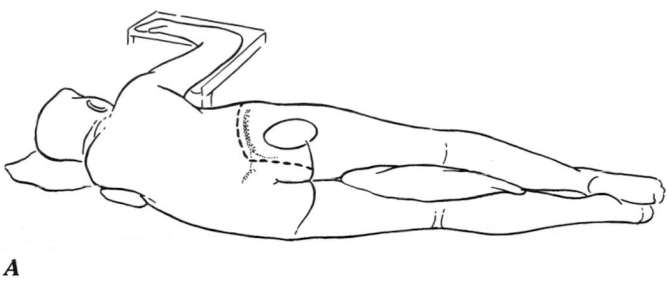
A

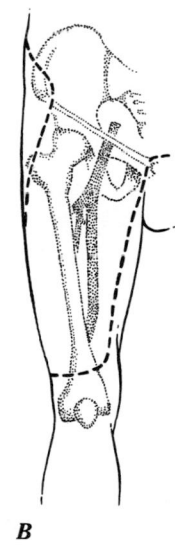
B

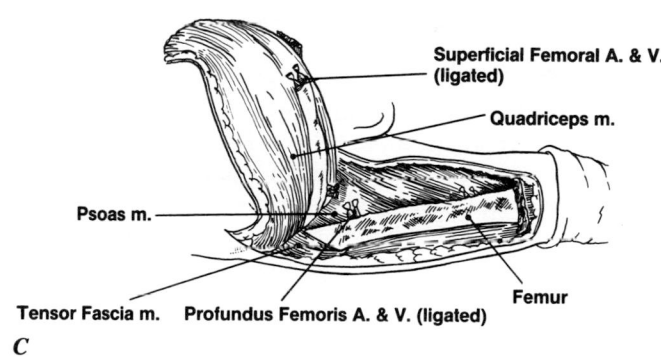
C

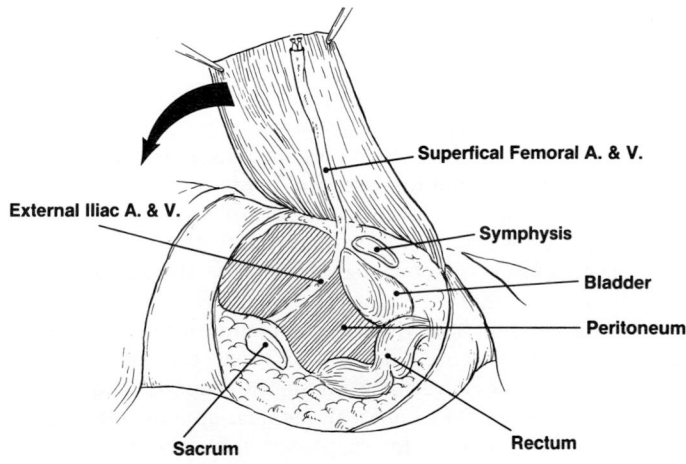
D

Limb-Sparing Surgery: Pelvic Resection

The three regions of the pelvis—the ilium, the periacetabulum, and the pubic rami—may be independently resected.[4,31] Contraindications to resection are vascular, peritoneal, sacroiliac joint, or sacroplexus involvement. A utilitarian incision similar to the anterior, retroperitoneal approach for a hemipelvectomy is used for pelvic resection.[4] The retroperitoneal space is explored first to determine resectability. The potentially limiting structures—iliac vessels, sciatic nerve, femoral nerve, bladder—are explored before proceeding. If the lesion is resectable, a second incision is made that curves distally from the level of the anterior spine to the greater trochanter and then posterior to the sciatic notch. This permits exposure of the sciatic nerve, sacroiliac joint, iliac wing, and hip joint. If resection is deemed unsafe at this point, a hemipelvectomy should be performed.

Following resection of either the ilium or pubic rami, no bony reconstruction is required. However, care must be taken to close muscular defects in order to prevent abdominal hernias and bladder prolapse. Periacetabular resections may be reconstructed as either a deliberate nonunion, primary arthrodesis, or with a saddle prosthesis. Allograft reconstruction is technically demanding and is hampered by difficulties in matching of the graft. Allograft reconstruction as well as reconstruction following autoclaving of the resected bone are associated with a significant incidence of fracture.[32]

Tumors of the Proximal Femur

Clinical Characteristics

The proximal femur is a relatively uncommon site for primary bone sarcomas. Metastatic carcinoma is the most commonly encountered malignant tumor. During childhood, Ewing's sarcomas tend to be more common than osteosarcomas; chondrosarcoma is the most common primary sarcoma at this site among adults. All types of benign lesions may occur in the proximal femur: fibrous dysplasia, enchondromas, and giant-cell tumors are the most common. Because of the mechanical stresses encountered in this region, the most common symptoms are pain or pathologic fracture. A mass is rarely noted. On occasion, "sciatica" due to sciatic nerve compression may be the presenting symptom. In a young patient, plain radiographs of the hip and a routine back series should be performed for sciatic complaints; radiographs are very useful in screening for neoplasms. In the adult, avascular necrosis, early degenerative joint disease, and osteomyelitis may all simulate malignancy. Pathologic fracture, which is more common with metastatic carcinoma than with primary tumors, is usually the factor that prompts orthopaedic intervention.

Tumors arising from the proximal femur often become quite large before being detected. Extraosseous extension of stage II lesions occurs early among the iliopsoas and the abductor muscles. The femoral vessels, specifically the profundus femoris, are often displaced; however, the thick fascia of the femoral triangle and the pectineus muscle prevents direct tumor extension along the common femoral vessels. Direct involvement of the femoral and/or sciatic nerve is rare. The external rotators usually protect the sciatic nerve. Large tumors may involve the retroperitoneal space by extending through the sciatic notch. Acetabular extension may also occur via tumor growth along the ligamentum teres and/or via pericapsular involvement. Because of the distal attachment of the hip capsule, joint contamination occurs early in the presence of pathologic fracture. Extensive osseous involvement is associated with a high risk of pathologic fracture, particularly with metastatic carcinoma and round cell tumors.

Staging Studies

Staging studies are similar to those already discussed. Computed tomography demonstrates extraosseous extent of tumor and is the most useful study in determining intrapelvic extent via the sciatic notch. Bone scans are necessary to demonstrate the extent of intraosseous involvement. They also may reveal acetabular involvement or transarticular skips. Biplane angiography demonstrates the position of the common femoral artery and, more important, the profundus femoris, which may often be markedly displaced. Preoperative embolization or intraoperative ligation may be planned. Preoperative embolization of the profundus femoris is indicated in several tumors, most notably hypernephromas. Intraarticular involvement is difficult to evaluate and a high index of suspicion is therefore necessary. Hip aspiration that reveals bloody fluid is indicative of tumor involvement. Cytologic analysis of the aspirate may demonstrate the presence of tumor cells. Magnetic resonance imaging has been shown to be useful in detecting skip lesions, evaluating the extent of marrow involvement, delineating the soft tissue extension, and evaluating involvement of the hip joint.

Biopsy

A modified Watson-Jones approach is recommended if an open biopsy is required. This avoids contamination of the posterior or anterior structures and conserves the possibility of performing a limb-sparing resection or hemipelvectomy. The standard posterior approaches to the hip should *not* be utilized for biopsy, because this incision contaminates the posterior flap, which is needed if a hemipelvectomy is required. Similarly, a long lateral incision or an anterior Smith-Petersen approach, which involves extensive dissection and contamination, should be avoided. Biopsy of soft tissue tumor extensions allows for accurate diagnosis while minimizing the increased risk of pathologic fracture and wound contamination associated with cortical windows. Craig needle or trephine core biopsy under fluoroscopic or CT control can avoid many of the hazards of open biopsy. Care should be taken to avoid intraarticular contamination. A lateral approach should be used *below* the insertion of the abductors. This avoids contamination of the abductor muscles if a limb-sparing option exists. If the lesion involves the head and neck, a tunnel can be made with a reamer and a small curette can be inserted in the tunnel to withdraw material.

Surgical Management

In order to preserve a functioning joint, benign tumors of the proximal femur should be treated by curettage or minimal excision. Reconstruction of the surgical defect is necessary to prevent secondary fracture. The standard technique of reconstruction combines bone grafting (preferably an autogenous fibular strut or iliac crest graft) with internal fixation. Cortical struts provide increased stability when combined with compression screw fixation. Alternatively, bone cement may be used to fill the defect, eliminating donor site morbidity and providing immediate fixation. Application of liquid nitrogen has been shown to be a useful adjuvant for aggressive or recurrent benign tumors.

Low-grade (stage I) sarcomas may be treated by en bloc resection. High-grade (stage II) sarcomas require wide resection of the hip and result in a loss of a significant portion of the abductors and other muscles attached to the proximal femur. Reconstruction is by endoprosthetic replacement, massive osteoarticular allograft, or allograft-prosthesis composite. The authors favor endoprosthetic replacement because of immediate stability and long-term durability. The recent development of modular endoprosthetic systems allows for intraoperative selection of off-the-shelf components, thus maximizing flexibility in reconstruction of segmental defects. A series of 15 consecutive modular proximal femoral replacements has a 100 percent survival rate at a median follow-up of almost 3 years.[33] Pathologic fractures secondary to metastatic disease usually require tumor resection and reconstruction with a cemented prosthetic replacement. Acetabular involvement often mandates a total hip replacement with additional use of bone cement.

Overall, local recurrence following resection of stage IIB sarcomas of the proximal femur approaches 20 percent.[34] Postoperative radiation may therefore be warranted to improve local control rates. Most high-grade sarcomas of the proximal femur, however, require a proximal amputation, such as a classic or modified hemipelvectomy, particularly if a pathologic fracture has occurred. Hip disarticulation is not recommended for these cases since the soft tissue at risk for local recurrence is not completely removed. An anterior myocutaneous flap hemipelvectomy may be required if the gluteal area has been contaminated by a poorly planned biopsy.[30]

Specific Tumors of the Femur

Unicameral Bone Cysts

The proximal femur is the second most common site for unicameral bone cysts (UBCs); 15 percent of such tumors develop in this location.[35–38] Unlike the case with tumors of the proximal humerus, plain radiographs may not be diagnostic and biopsy may be required. Avascular necrosis and coxa vara are complications of repeated fractures and open management. The author recommends percutaneous, high-pressure Renografin injection and intralesional methylprednisolone followed by cast or brace immobilization.[36,37,39] Treatment options vary for patients who pre-

sent with a pathologic fracture. If the patient is below the age of 10, traction and a spica cast followed by injection and aspiration at 4 to 6 weeks is recommended; adolescents should undergo initial internal fixation combined with curettage.

Chondroblastoma

The proximal femur is the third most common location. Chondroblastomas may arise either in the capital epiphysis or in the epiphysis of the greater trochanter.[40,41] Clear cell chondrosarcoma, a rare entity, may occur in the proximal femur and radiographically and histologically mimic a benign chondroblastoma. Careful evaluation of any atypical features of a presumed chondroblastoma is therefore essential. After diagnosis, treatment should consist of thorough curettage and reconstruction of the resulting defect. Cryosurgery may decrease the local recurrence rate. The capital epiphysis can be approached in three separate ways: an anterior window in the femoral neck, the fovea after careful dislocation of the hip, or through a tunnel from the lateral cortex. Care must be taken to avoid contamination of the synovium; synovial implants occur easily and lead to recurrent disease. Chondroblastoma associated with an aneurysmal bone cyst has a high rate of local recurrence; cryosurgery is recommended for this entity.[42] Recurrent chondroblastoma requires an en bloc resection to achieve local control.

Giant-Cell Tumor and Aneurysmal Bone Cyst

Fewer than 5 percent of giant-cell tumors (GCTs) arise in the proximal femur (Fig. 16-44).[35,43] When they do occur, giant-cell tumors typically involve a large portion of the femoral neck and trochanter and often present with a pathologic fracture. Preoperative angiography allows embolization of the major feeding vessels if curettage is to be performed. Curettage with cryosurgery and internal fixation with PMMA is reasonable for a small lesion.[20,44,45] Large tumors, pathologic fractures, or recurrent tumors should be treated by marginal resection and endoprosthetic replacement. En bloc resection should be reserved for recurrent disease or secondary malignancy.

Fibrous Dysplasia

Fibrous dysplasia commonly occurs in the proximal femur. In the young child, it may cause a varus or shepherd's crook deformity. In the young adult, the plain radiograph is often not diagnostic, for these lesions may simulate other benign or malignant tumors. Bone scans are useful to differentiate other lesions and to detect polyostotic fibrous dysplasia. The goal of surgical management is to prevent progressive deformity and fracture. Local recurrence following curettage ranges from 25 to 35 percent. Thorough curettage and reconstruction of the femoral neck defect by cortical struts (preferably fibular) in addition to plate-and-screw fixation are required. Cementation is useful for large lesions, similar to the treatment of large GCTs. The cortical struts should be placed along the calcar: graft incorporation strengthens the calcar and prevents pro-

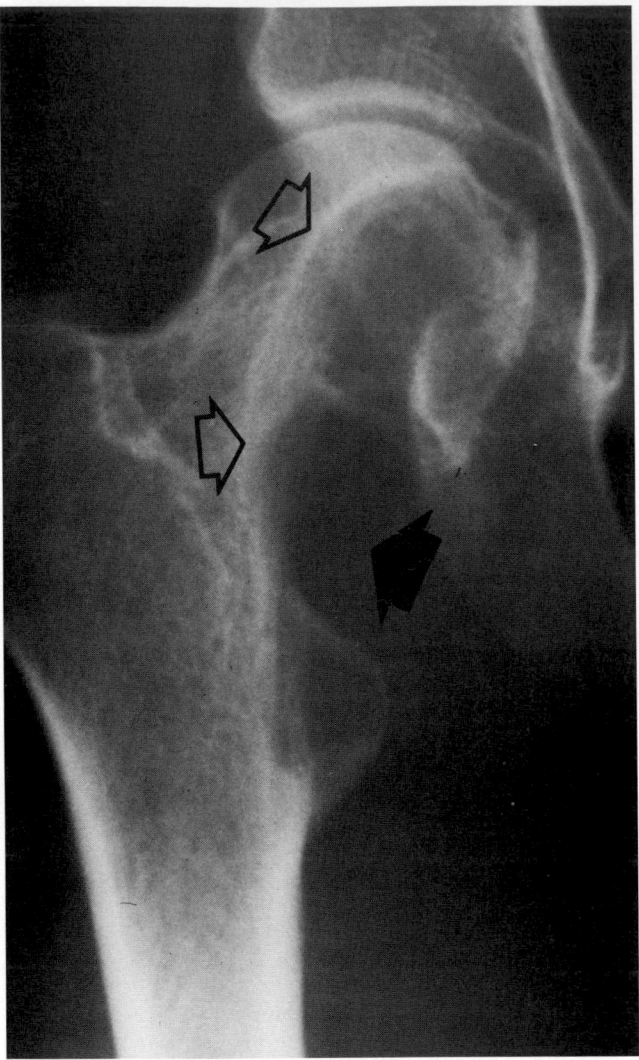

Figure 16-44 Typical giant cell tumor of the proximal femur. Note the sclerotic inner margin (*open arrows*) and the ballooned-out medial cortex (*solid arrow*), which is barely visible. This patient required a primary resection and prosthetic replacement.

gressive deformity and recurrent fracture. Resection is seldom indicated.

Osteoid Osteoma

Twenty-six percent of osteoid osteomas occur in the proximal femur, which is the most common site for these lesions.[35] The surgical problems encountered with osteoid osteomas of the proximal femur are unique. Osteoid osteomas can be intramedullary, intracortical, or subperiosteal. The typical intracortical osteoid osteoma consists of a small radiolucent lesion surrounded by a thickened sclerotic rim, which may obliterate the lytic nidus. Some osteoid osteomas are intramedullary, with minimal adjacent reaction. The least common variant is subperiosteal; these show no response except a small scooped-out defect. The major clinical symptom of os-

teoid osteomas is intermittent, progressive pain that often is worse at night. The pain, which may be alleviated by salicylates, will develop 6 to 12 months before radiographic changes are evident. The differential diagnosis includes monoarticular arthritis, psychoneurosis, and malingering.

Bone scintigraphy in the early stage is abnormal. As the lesion matures, plain radiographs may demonstrate the area of sclerosis; however, the defect itself remains undetected. This makes localization difficult, especially in a constrained anatomic area where minimal bone excision is crucial. Bone scans and tomography combined can localize the nidus. Bone scintigraphy can localize both the nidus and the reactive bone. Tomography may demonstrate the lytic nidus. Computed tomography is essential for evaluating lesions of the femoral neck and can demonstrate in which quadrant the lesion has developed; 1- to 2-mm cuts should be routinely obtained in order to detect the nidus. This information aids in determining the surgical approach. Despite these preoperative studies, it is often difficult to determine if the entire lesion has been resected. Intraoperative bone scintigraphy may be invaluable in this regard (Fig. 16-45).

Treatment consists of removal of the central nidus—there is no need to remove the surrounding sclerotic bone. A "burr down" technique is very useful in minimizing the amount of bone removed. Preoperative localization with a CT-guided needle placement on the day of surgery is recommended to facilitate localization of the nidus intraoperatively. If a large defect is created, a fibular strut is used to reconstruct the area. For anterior lesions, a Watson-Jones approach is recommended; medial calcar lesions require a posterior approach with external rotation of the hip and detachment of the psoas to allow good visualization. Once the lesion has been removed, patients report a complete cessation of pain. Persistent pain following resection indicates that the lesion was not entirely removed. Use of intraoperative bone scanning helps to ensure complete removal. Some authors recommend scanning the excised fragment; we feel that scanning the patient rather than the specimen is more reliable.

Ewing's Sarcoma

The pelvis and femur are the two most common sites for Ewing's sarcoma.[16,26,35,46] As in the pelvis, Ewing's sarcoma of the proximal femur often has a huge soft tissue component. Plain radiographs are highly suggestive of a malignancy, with classic onionskin periosteal reaction present. Management includes combination chemotherapy with radiotherapy. A pathologic fracture in the early course of treatment may necessitate a hemipelvectomy, since localized radiotherapy can no longer be given. Every precaution must therefore be taken to prevent a fracture. The bone need not be biopsied; adequate material can be obtained from the extraosseous component by means of a lateral Craig needle biopsy. In this manner, the flaps for a hemipelvectomy or limb-sparing surgery will not be jeopardized if a spindle cell tumor is encountered. Computed tomography or MRI is used to determine the extraosseous extent of tumor and establish ac-

Figure 16-45 Technique of localization and resection of osteoid osteoma. Localization of a distal femoral osteoid osteoma by a sterile, hand-held scanner. The position of increased counts is marked by a pin. A large-diameter core reamer is then used to remove the suspected area. The patient is then rescanned; if the preoperative area of increased uptake is gone, the osteoid osteoma has been completely removed. It is not necessary to rely on intraoperative plain radiographs or tomography of the specimen.

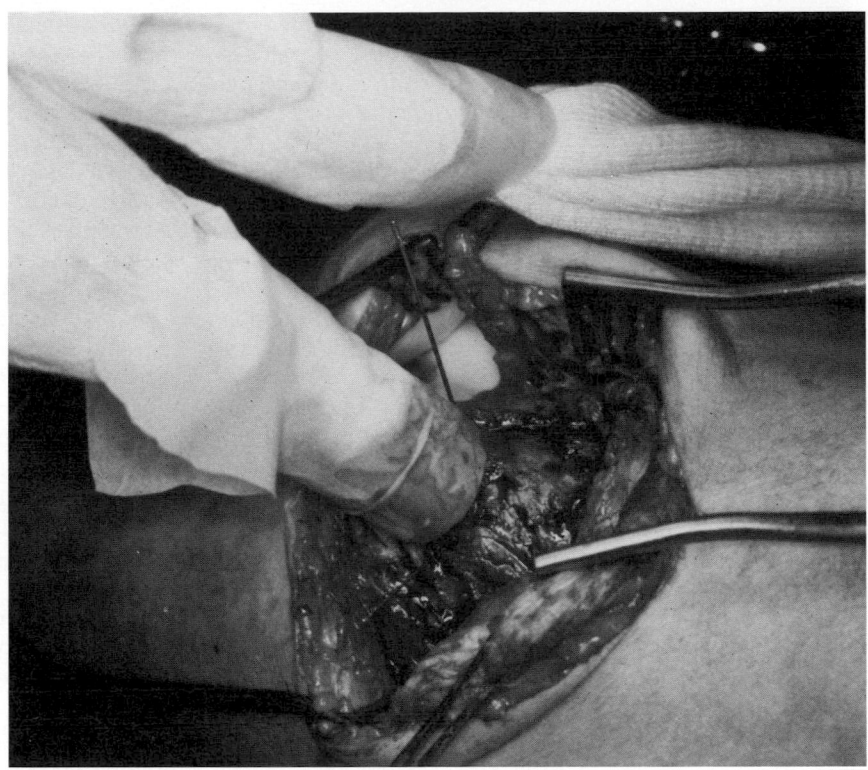

curate radiotherapy ports. Angiography routinely demonstrates a hypervascular lesion. To prevent pathologic fracture, cast or brace immobilization is required until bony reossification is noted. The proximal femur is considered a high-risk location for local recurrence of Ewing's sarcoma. A study at the National Cancer Institute reported a 25 percent rate of local recurrence for proximal lesions.[26,27]

Surgical resection remains controversial for these tumors. At Memorial Sloan-Kettering, resection is recommended whenever feasible, whereas at the National Cancer Institute, it is reserved for large lesions that show poor radiographic response to radiotherapy, or for persistent disease following a combination of radiotherapy and chemotherapy.[47,48] Lesions that respond to chemotherapy and are resectable without undue morbidity should be considered for surgical resection.[49]

Osteosarcoma

Only 4 percent of osteosarcomas involve the proximal femur. Plain radiographs are usually diagnostic; confirmation should be made through a laterally placed needle biopsy. Neoadjuvant chemotherapy followed by surgical resection or amputation is now accepted as standard treatment for all osteosarcomas. Stage IIB osteosarcomas may require either modified or classic hemipelvectomy to achieve adequate margins.[50–52] Low-grade osteosarcoma, tumors with little soft tissue involvement, and the rare parosteal variant can be treated with limb-sparing en bloc resection and prosthetic reconstruction, which is functionally superior to amputation.

Chondrosarcoma

Twelve percent of chondrosarcomas involve the proximal femur; it is the second most common site for such lesions, following the pelvis.[3,19] These lesions tend to be quite large but often are low grade. They contain myxomatous components, which can easily contaminate a wound following biopsy. Care, therefore, should be taken not to contaminate the hip joint when performing the biopsy. In contrast to osteosarcomas in this area, chondrosarcomas may often be treated with limb-sparing resection. All muscle attachments to the proximal femur are removed en bloc with the tumor, necessitating extensive soft tissue reconstruction to maximize function. Functional outcome is superior to amputation.

Metastatic Carcinoma

The hip is a common site of metastasis. Metastatic carcinoma can present with vague pain, pathologic fracture, or minimal symptomatic findings despite a positive routine bone scan during follow-up. A pathologic fracture necessitates surgical intervention; however, many patients with minimal bony destruction and pain can be treated satisfactorily with radiotherapy and protected weight bearing. A lytic lesion involving more than one-third of the cortex should be considered for prophylactic fixation. The "radiosensitive" tumors, especially myeloma and breast carcinoma, tend to reossify. "Radioresistant" tumors (lung, colon, and prostate) tend not to respond to radiotherapy. One must individualize an approach for each patient. Important considerations are contralateral hip involvement (i.e., inability to avoid bearing weight), upper extremity involvement (inability to use crutches), overall extent of disease, progression of pain despite radiotherapy (a sign of tumor progression and/or pending fracture), and quality of nursing care.

Any treatment plan should aim to improve the quality of life of these patients. Palliation of pain and stability of fixation are important to help patients remain ambulatory and independent. In general, metastatic tumors of the proximal femur are best treated by curettage and cemented prosthetic replacement. Evaluation of the remaining femur should be performed to detect distal lesions, which can lead to additional pathologic fractures. The presence of such lesions mandates use of very long femoral stems that bypass the distalmost lesion by at least two femoral diameters. Venting of the femur and avoidance of intramedullary pressurization during reaming and implantation may reduce the risk of fat embolization and sudden intraoperative death. Extensive acetabular involvement usually requires a total hip replacement. Nail-and-plate fixation should be avoided due to a high rate of failure of fixation.

Specific Surgical Procedures

Modified Hemipelvectomy

For selected tumors of the proximal femur, a modified hemipelvectomy can be performed in lieu of a classic hemipelvectomy.[9] A modified hemipelvectomy is an amputation through the sciatic notch and the symphysis pubis. The entire extremity is removed. Unlike the classic hemipelvectomy, it preserves a portion of the wing of the ilium, the gluteus maximus muscle, and the hypogastric (external iliac) vessels as a pedicle. The vascularized posterior flap decreases the problems of flap necrosis, and the residual ilium enhances prosthetic fitting. In general, the patient's ability to function after a modified hemipelvectomy is similar to that following a hip disarticulation and superior to that following a classic hemipelvectomy. Large tumors approaching the sciatic notch are best treated by a classic hemipelvectomy.

Limb-Sparing Resection (Proximal Femoral Resection)

Resection of the proximal femur and adjacent musculature can be performed safely for most stage IA/B and IIA tumors. Despite the size of many stage IB tumors, safe margins can be obtained.[53] Contraindications to resection are involvement of the sciatic nerve or common femoral vessels, intrapelvic extension, and intraarticular and/or acetabular involvement. Careful preoperative evaluation by means of CT, MRI, and bone scan can accurately determine intrapelvic and acetabular involvement.

The surgical procedure consists of resection of the proximal femur (90 to 250 cm); detachment of the abductors, gluteus maximus, and iliopsoas; and removal of the entire capsule from the acetabulum circumferentially. If possible, the greater trochanter is preserved to facilitate reconstruction of the abductors. If the hip joint is involved,

an extraarticular resection is required. The defect can be reconstructed by a modified prosthetic replacement. If the acetabulum remains, a bipolar prosthesis is used. A separate acetabular prosthetic component is required only if the acetabulum has been removed or if insufficient soft tissue remains to create a new joint capsule. A bipolar prosthesis requires a soft tissue "capsule" for stability: if necessary, the iliopsoas and the remaining external rotators are used to reconstruct a hip capsule. If an acetabular cup is required, a horizontal orientation maximizes stability. Alternative methods of reconstruction include massive allografts, allograft-prosthesis composites, or resection with primary fusion to the remaining ischium.

Reconstruction of the abductor mechanism is essential. Reestablishment of the appropriate length and tension of the abductors is facilitated by first suturing them to the prosthesis with 3-mm Dacron tape and then to the remaining fascia lata and vastus lateralis muscles. The tape provides appropriate tension while the adjacent soft tissue heals. If the greater trochanter was preserved, it may be attached to the prosthesis with cerclage wires or cables. The most common complication is dislocation, which may occur in 20 percent of patients. Use of postoperative traction in abduction for 1 to 2 weeks and cast or hip abduction brace immobilization for a minimum of 3 months prevents dislocation during the high-risk period. These patients usually require a cane for stability during the stance phase of ambulation. Occasionally, long-term use of hip abduction bracing is required. Functional results are far superior to those following hemipelvectomy.

Tumors of the Knee

The knee is the most common location for primary tumors of the musculoskeletal system.[35,50] Giant-cell tumors, aneurysmal bone cysts, osteosarcomas, and parosteal osteosarcomas often involve the knee.[14,54–56] Tumors of the distal femur, proximal tibia, and proximal fibula are considered together in this section. The majority of clinical experience with limb-salvage techniques has been obtained in tumors around the knee.[57–63] The techniques and indications for limb salvage are discussed.[53,59,64,65]

Clinical Characteristics

Pain is the most common presenting symptom of benign and malignant tumors of the knee. Malignant tumors often present with a soft tissue mass or fullness. Benign lesions rarely have an extraosseous component. Pathologic fracture, which rarely occurs with osteosarcomas (less than 1 percent), may be seen with GCTs. Effusion is uncommon, despite the size of many lesions. If an effusion is noted, intraarticular involvement should be suspected. In general, all young patients with knee pain of more than 2 to 3 weeks' duration should have a plain radiograph. Occasionally, a patient will present with signs of an internal derangement of the knee. Careful physical examination and plain radiographs will suggest the correct diagnosis. We recommend that all young patients have plain radiographs before undergoing arthroscopy.

With the exception of the gastrocnemius, which originates from the femoral condyles, the distal femur is bare of muscle attachments. The quadriceps forms a portion of the knee capsule but inserts into the tibia. Tumors arising from the distal femur may therefore produce large extraosseous components that displace but do not invade the adjacent muscle. These muscles may, however, harbor microscopic disease, necessitating resection if a limb-sparing procedure is attempted. Tumors can extend posteriorly with minimal resistance and easily involve the popliteal structures. The popliteal artery is the deepest structure within the popliteal fossa. It is leashed to the posterior face of the femur by the geniculate branches. Posterior tumor extension quickly reaches the vascular bundle and may extend to the posterior tibia along the vessels. The knee joint and its extensive capsular reflections may occasionally be transgressed by the tumor. Intraarticular extension occurs by several mechanisms: along the cruciates via the intercondylar notch (most common), by direct extension through articular cartilage (rare), by pericapsular extension, or by pathologic fracture.[66] Synovial implants, which occur occasionally with both malignant and benign tumors, must be evaluated. An effusion should raise clinical suspicion of tumor extension. The proximal fibula is in close proximity to the proximal tibia, and a tumor involving one often involves the other. Lesions of the proximal fibula often present as popliteal masses due to the posterolateral position of this bone.

Staging Studies

Plain radiographs are often diagnostic of tumor.[67] Staging studies for suspected aggressive or malignant tumors of the knee should be performed prior to biopsy.[1,53,68] Bone scans can determine the extent of intraosseous involvement.[69,70] Computed tomography can assist in delineating the extraosseous extent of tumor, detecting small effusions and small pathologic fractures, and evaluating the intercondylar area, which is at high risk for occult tumor extension.[8] Magnetic resonance imaging readily demonstrates the soft tissue extent of the tumor as well as the extent of marrow involvement and the presence of skip metastases.[8] Biplane angiography is crucial for evaluating the popliteal vessels.[71] For tumors of the proximal fibula and proximal tibia, delineation of the vascular anatomy including the takeoff of the anterior tibial artery and identification of possible vascular anomalies is essential.[65] Overall, a combination of studies is required before a decision can be made regarding resectability of an aggressive or malignant lesion. Joint aspiration and cytologic testing should be performed if an effusion is present. A simple transudate denotes a reactive effusion and probably not tumor. Bloody aspirate indicates a fracture and/or synovial implants. Cytologic testing should routinely be performed. Arthrography and arthroscopy are useful for detecting synovial implants in selected patients.

Biopsy

A biopsy should be performed only after appropriate staging studies have been done.[1,53,68] Knowledge of the defini-

tive incision for a limb-sparing procedure is necessary when planning either a trochar or an incisional biopsy. A trochar biopsy will often yield an accurate diagnosis and should be performed prior to an incisional biopsy.[1,72–74]

Most limb-sparing incisions of the distal femur and proximal tibia are longitudinal and near the midline. Care should be taken to avoid contamination of the popliteal fossa, the knee joint, and the sartorial canal. The incision of the proximal fibula is lateral, directly over the fibular head. Extreme caution must be taken to avoid contamination of the peroneal nerve and the tibiofibular joint. Again, soft tissue components should be biopsied in preference to the bony component. If a cortical window is necessary, it should be plugged with PMMA until the definitive procedure is performed in order to decrease the possibility of contamination.

Because the location of biopsy greatly influences the overall outcome and choice of procedure, it should be performed only by the surgeon who is responsible for the definitive care of the patient. Inappropriate biopsy of lesions around the knee contaminates crucial tissue planes and may necessitate an amputation.

Surgical Management

Spindle cell sarcomas of the distal femur and proximal tibia and fibula have traditionally been treated by hip disarticulation or above-knee amputation. In selected patients, limb-sparing preservation can be performed with good functional results and low rates of local recurrence.[22,34,53,58–62,75] To date, this approach is justified only in centers with expertise in this area. All patients with a suspected malignant tumor of the knee should be evaluated for possible limb preservation and should be referred to an appropriate specialist prior to attempted biopsy.

Routine amputation is no longer performed.[22,53,62] The success of adjuvant and neoadjuvant chemotherapy has resulted in the majority of spindle cell sarcomas (stage I and IIA/B) of the knee being treated by limb-sparing surgery. Reported local recurrence ranges from 6 to 20 percent. Reconstruction may be performed by arthrodesis, endoprosthesis, or allograft reconstruction. Amputation may still be recommended for patients with neurovascular involvement, contamination by a poorly planned biopsy, pathologic fracture, or multidirectional soft tissue extension.

Simple benign lesions are treated by simple curettage. Aggressive tumors such as GCTs require extended curettage or resection; amputation is rarely required. Use of local adjuvants such as cryosurgery may help to reduce recurrence rates following curettage. For large lesions around the knee, bone graft and/or bone cement along with internal fixation are often required to prevent fracture.

Specific Tumors of the Knee
Osteoid Osteoma

The distal femur is the third most common location for osteoid osteomas. Plain radiographs are usually diagnostic.

Linear tomography, bone scintigraphy, and CT are essential to localize the lesion and to minimize the amount of bone removal. Surgical excision is curative (Fig. 16-45). Local recurrence, presumably due to incomplete removal, occurs in fewer than 10 percent of all patients.

Nonossifying Fibroma

Nonossifying fibromas around the knee, although common, rarely require treatment. If a pathologic fracture occurs, it should be permitted to heal. Simple curettage is curative; bone graft is not required.

Giant-Cell Tumor

There is a high incidence of local recurrence (40 to 75 percent) following simple curettage.[54,55,76,77] En bloc resection is usually curative, but because of its associated morbidity, it should not be routinely recommended as the initial form of treatment. If the lesion is small, curettage and a local adjuvant such as cryosurgery are preferred.[20,44,78,79] In 102 consecutive cases treated by curettage and cryosurgery, the local recurrence rate has been 7 percent.[45] Complications following cryosurgery include flap necrosis, infection, and pathologic fracture. These have been greatly reduced as experience with cryosurgery has increased. It is now considered essential to reconstruct the defect completely so as to prevent secondary fracture. The authors' preferred technique[45] is autogenous graft along the subchondral bone and intercondylar area supported by bone cement reinforced with intramedullary metal pins (Steinmann, Rush, or supracondylar screw) to provide additional torsional stability and stress transfer.

Every attempt should be made to maintain a functioning joint. If resection is required, reconstruction can be performed by prosthesis, arthrodesis, or allograft replacement. Synovial involvement and soft tissue recurrence can be treated by local excision. Primary en bloc resections are rarely indicated. Multiple local recurrences following intralesional procedures indicate the need for en bloc resection, as the risk of malignant degeneration increases with each recurrence. Radiation therapy is not recommended for lesions that can be treated surgically due to the risk of sarcomatous transformation, which occurs in 10 to 20 percent of all patients.

Giant-cell tumors of the proximal fibula are treated by primary resection with preservation of the peroneal nerve.[65] The lateral collateral ligament and biceps are attached to the lateral joint capsule. Postoperatively, knee function remains normal.

Parosteal Osteosarcoma

The posterior aspect of the distal femur is the characteristic location for parosteal osteosarcomas.[80,81] The plain radiograph is diagnostic.[67] Bone scintigraphy and CT are necessary to determine the portion of the bone to be removed and to evaluate possible intraosseous involvement. Angiography will routinely show displacement of the popliteal vessels; however, upon exploration, the vascular structures are usually found to be free of contamination unless prior surgery or biopsy has been performed. The location of the biopsy is a crucial decision, since a biopsy through the popliteal space contaminates all tissue planes. A needle biopsy along the lateral intermuscular septum can document the lesion prior to resection with minimal contamination.

Treatment consists of surgical resection, which includes the lesion along with a variable portion of the femoral cortex. Large lesions or intramedullary involvement may necessitate excision of the entire distal femur. No experience with preoperative chemotherapy has been reported. The author prefers not to perform a biopsy if a localized resection is to be performed. The resection specimen is the definitive biopsy. Careful evaluation of the cortical margins and the underlying cancellous bone must be performed. If the tumor extends along the posterior capsule, it must be removed with the specimen. Bone graft may be required following local excision. Distal femoral resection can be reconstructed by arthrodesis, prosthesis, or allograft. Local recurrence in the form of vascular encroachment usually necessitates amputation.

Metastatic Tumor

Metastatic carcinoma of the knee can often be satisfactorily treated with radiation therapy. Surgery is required for large lesions or for pathologic fractures. Curettage combined with PMMA and internal fixation will preserve a functional knee. Intramedullary supracondylar rods are preferred to plate fixation to reduce stress-rising effects of screw holes. Prosthetic replacement is rarely required.

Indications and Technique for Limb-Sparing Surgery for Knee Tumors

Tumors of the Distal Femur

Adequate en bloc resection includes 15 to 20 cm of the distal femur, the articular portion of the proximal tibia, and portions of the adjacent quadriceps (Fig. 16-46).[53,59,64] Biopsy must avoid the sartorial canal and the knee joint to prevent contamination. Contraindications to resection are popliteal vessel involvement, extensive soft tissue contamination of the quadriceps resulting from previous biopsy, pathologic fracture, or tumor involvement of the patella or patellar tendon. Large tumors requiring removal of the entire quadriceps and/or hamstring muscles can be adequately reconstructed by an arthrodesis.

The operative procedure begins with exploration and examination of the popliteal vessels. Care should be taken to preserve the sural vessels and the neurovascular pedicle to the gastrocnemius muscles. The corresponding portion of the vastus muscle is removed en bloc, adjacent to the extraosseous tumor component. If an effusion is present, extraarticular resection may be required. If an intraarticular resection is performed, the entire capsule must be removed from its tibial insertion. Care must be taken not to lengthen the extremity, since this may result in arterial thrombosis. Hamstring transfers are required to re-

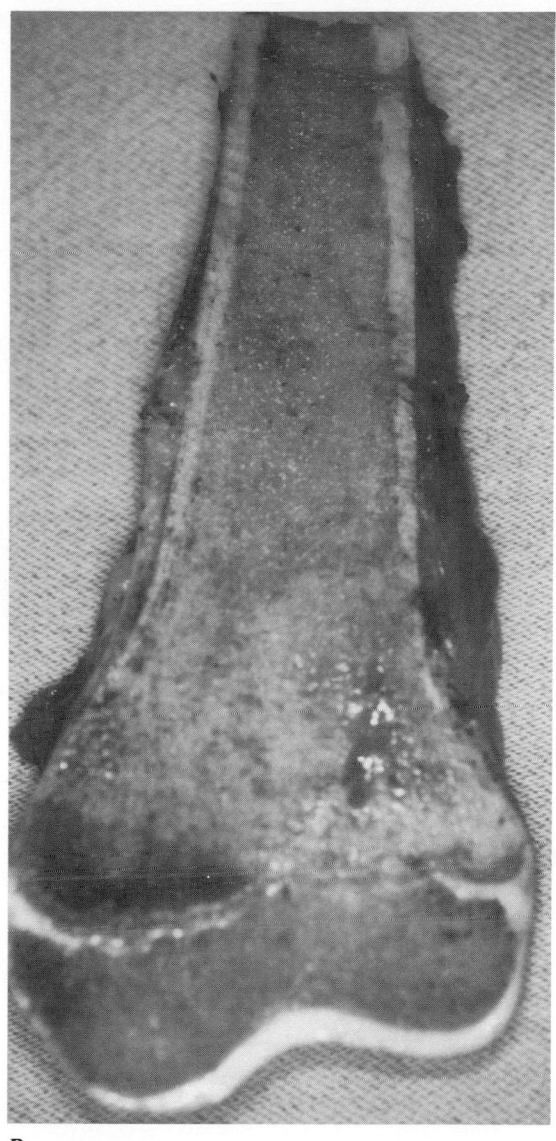

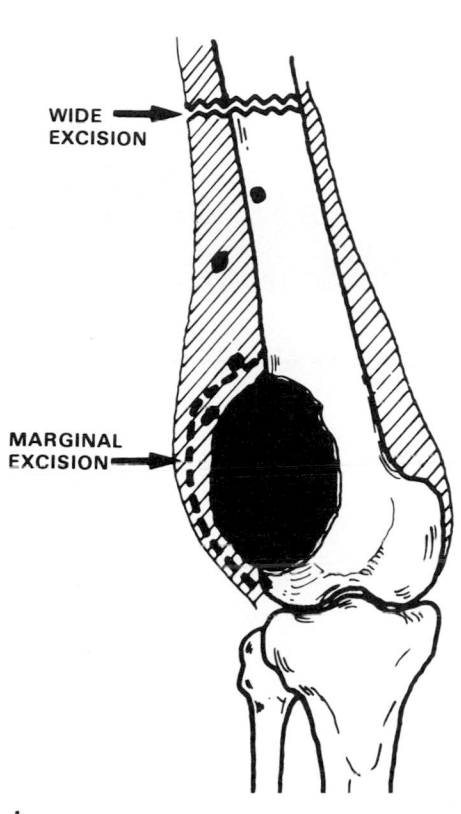

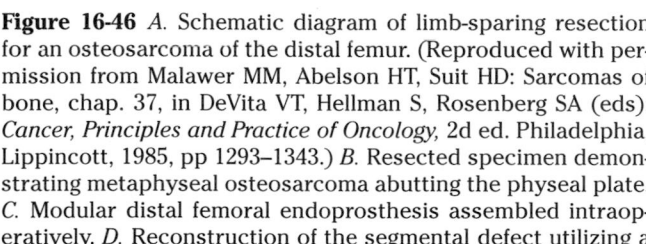

A

B

Figure 16-46 *A.* Schematic diagram of limb-sparing resection for an osteosarcoma of the distal femur. (Reproduced with permission from Malawer MM, Abelson HT, Suit HD: Sarcomas of bone, chap. 37, in DeVita VT, Hellman S, Rosenberg SA (eds): *Cancer, Principles and Practice of Oncology,* 2d ed. Philadelphia, Lippincott, 1985, pp 1293–1343.) *B.* Resected specimen demonstrating metaphyseal osteosarcoma abutting the physeal plate. *C.* Modular distal femoral endoprosthesis assembled intraoperatively. *D.* Reconstruction of the segmental defect utilizing a modular distal femoral replacement and medial gastrocnemius muscle transfer for improved soft tissue coverage. *E.* Kaplan-Meier curve for MSRS survival: analysis of 44 consecutive modular distal femoral replacements. (Adapted from Henshaw RM, Jones V, Malawer MM: Skeletal reconstruction with non-custom modular endoprostheses. Results of the first 96 consecutive MSRS prosthetic replacements. Presented at the Ninth Annual Symposium of the International Society of Technology in Arthroplasty, Amsterdam, The Netherlands, August 1996.)

construct the resected portion of the quadriceps so as to restore extensor strength. A gastrocnemius transposition flap is often used to provide additional muscular coverage and is essential to prevent flap necrosis and secondary wound problems (Figs. 16-46*D* and 16-47).[82] Endoprosthetic reconstruction of segmental defects of the distal femur provides immediate stability and permits full weight bearing without the need for extended periods of immobilization.[64,83] A recently developed modular endoprosthetic system that allows for intraoperative selection and assembly of off-the-shelf components has been shown to have a 97 percent survival at a median follow-up of 32 months (Fig. 16-46*E*).[33] Knee range-of-motion exercise therapy is begun as soon as wound healing has occurred. If an arthrodesis is performed, a long leg cast is required until the grafts are incorporated.[58] In general, hip and ankle motion are normal. A cane and brace are recommended for 12 months following arthrodesis.

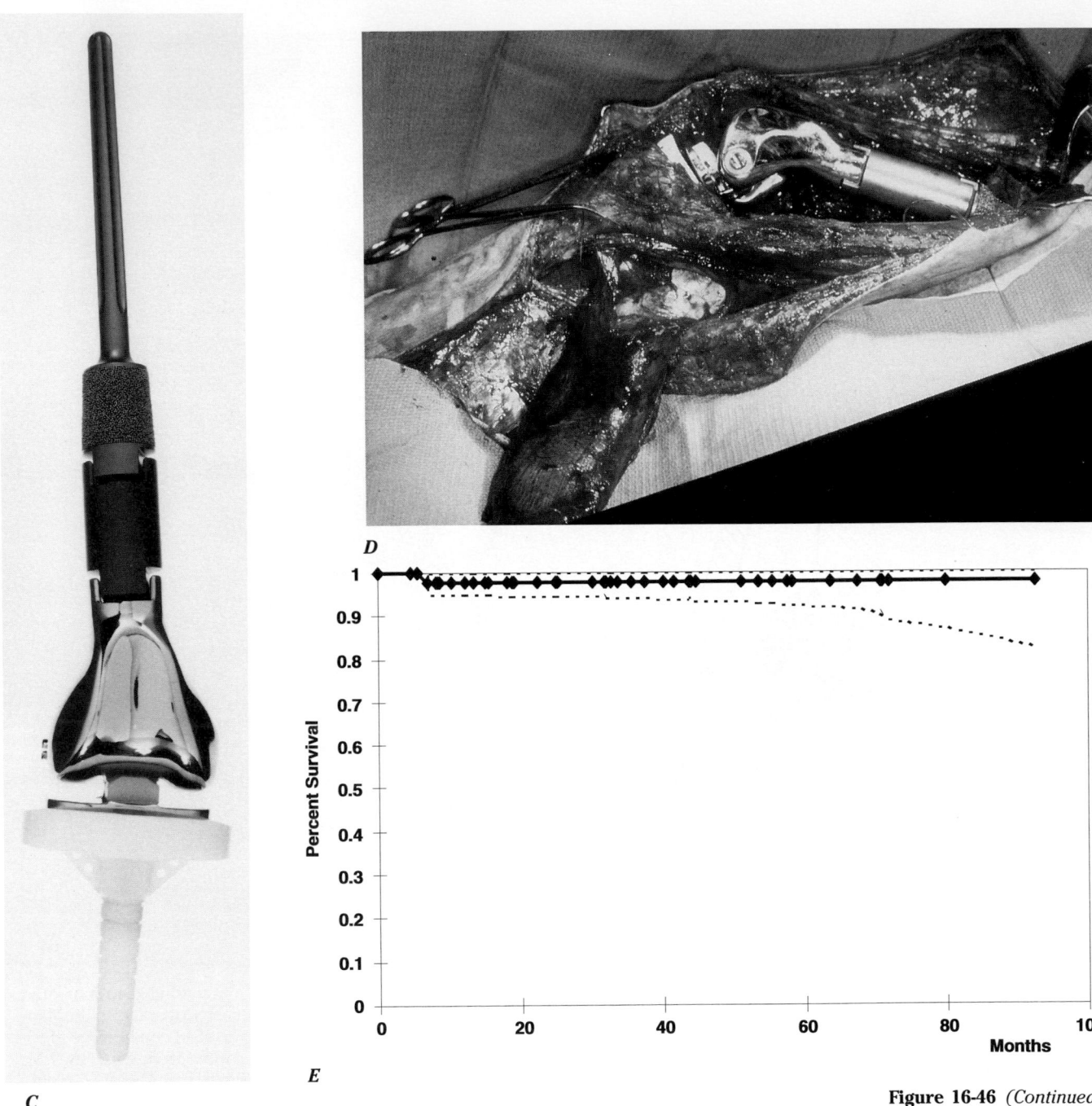

Figure 16-46 *(Continued)*

Tumors of the Proximal Tibia

Limb-sparing procedures are often not feasible for tumors of the proximal tibia because of anatomic constraints of soft tissue coverage and the subcutaneous location of the anteromedial tibia. It is difficult to obtain an adequate margin of resection and a good functional result with these lesions, and they tend to have a higher incidence of local complications than do distal femoral tumors. It is extremely important that the biopsy be small and that it avoid the knee joint. A core biopsy of the medial flare is preferred, so as to avoid contamination of the anterior musculature and peroneal nerve.

The popliteus muscle adjacent to the posterior aspect of the tibia prevents direct tumor involvement of the neurovascular bundle.[40] A large posterior tumor component makes resection ill advised. Lateral angiography can demonstrate this interval, while the AP projection is useful in detecting anomalous vascular patterns. Adequate resection of the proximal tibia requires ligation of the anterior tibial artery and, in most cases, the peroneal artery. The remaining posterior tibial artery leaves a viable extremity in a young individual.[30] An anomalously absent posterior tibial artery, which occurs in 5 percent of all patients, is a contraindication to resection. Tumor extension uniformly involves the tibiofibular capsule. Extraarticular resection of the proximal tibiofibular joint en bloc with the tibia is required to obtain a safe margin; the average resection length is 15 to 18 cm. Reconstruction is by either prosthetic replacement, osteoarticular allograft, or ar-

Figure 16-47 Schematic diagram of gastrocnemius transpositions following limb-sparing resections of sarcomas around the knee. The medial or lateral gastrocnemius muscle is utilized for tumors of the distal femur. In general, the medial gastrocnemius is a larger muscle and is preferred. The medial and lateral gastrocnemius are used following resection of the proximal tibia and proximal fibula, respectively. (Reproduced with permission from Malawer MM, Price WP: Gastrocnemius transposition flap in conjunction with limb-sparing surgery for primary bone sarcomas around the knee. *Plast Reconstr Surg* 73:741–750, 1984.)

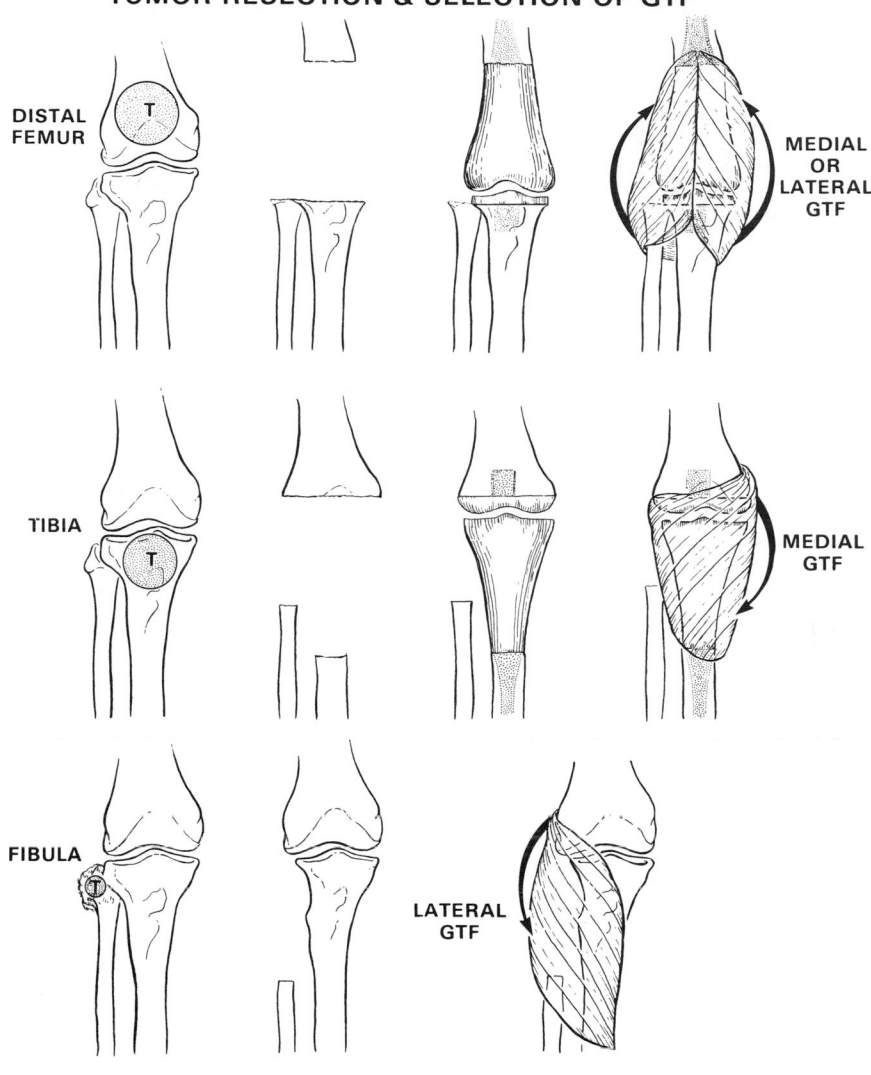

TUMOR RESECTION & SELECTION OF GTF

throdesis. The historical experience of proximal tibial replacement with either allograft or prosthetic replacement has been very discouraging. However, use of a gastrocnemius flap (Fig. 16-47) markedly reduces the risk of flap necrosis and subsequent infection, which usually results in secondary amputation.[82] The medial gastrocnemius is now routinely transferred to provide soft tissue coverage of the reconstructed area. Dacron tape is used to reattach the patellar tendon to the transferred gastrocnemius and prosthesis. This technique, along with development of a modular proximal tibial replacement, has achieved a 78 percent prosthetic survival at median follow-up of almost 2 years.[33] Postoperative management is similar to that for distal femoral resections.

Tumors of the Proximal Fibula

Tumors of the proximal fibula require the same evaluation as do proximal tibial lesions.[65] Unique considerations are early soft tissue extension, proximity to the lateral tibial condyle, necessity of ligation of the anterior and peroneal arteries, potential sacrifice of the peroneal nerve, and tumor infiltration of the tibiofibular joint capsule. Large tumors are often unresectable. The types of resection are shown in Fig. 16-48. Biplane angiography can delineate anomalous vascular patterns and demonstrate vascular displacement. Either CT or MRI is needed to determine involvement of the tibial plateau. Contraindications to resection are direct tibial involvement, an anomalously absent posterior tibial artery, and intraarticular knee joint extension.

Due to the multiple musculotendinous attachments of the proximal fibula, muscle infiltration generally occurs beyond visible borders along muscle planes. Adequate resection includes the fibula, the tibiofibular joint, the anterior and lateral muscle compartments, and portions of the lateral gastrocnemius, the soleus, and the intermuscular septum. Wide excision of all adjacent muscle groups is mandatory. No reconstruction of the bony defect is required. The lateral collateral ligament is reattached to the lateral joint capsule. A lateral upper-gas-

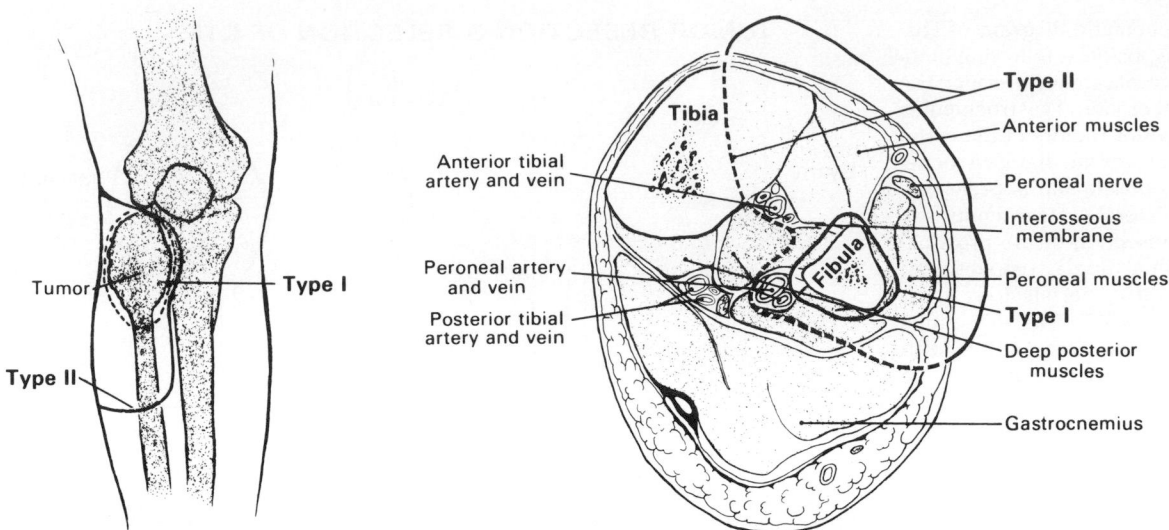

Figure 16-48 Schematic diagram of resection of the proximal fibula. Type I is a marginal excision; type II is a wide excision. (Reproduced with permission from Malawer MM: Surgical management of aggressive and malignant tumors of the proximal fibula. *Clin Orthop* 186:172–181, 1984.)

trocnemius transposition flap is used to close the resultant defect. Knee function is normal following surgery. The only major functional deficit is a drop foot, which is treated by an orthosis initially and subsequently may be electively corrected by tenodesis of the anterior compartment tendons.

Tumors of the Leg

The leg is a less common site for bony or soft tissue tumors than the thigh. Bony tumors arising in the shaft of the tibia and fibula and the muscle compartments are described in this section; tumors of the proximal tibia and fibula were considered in the previous section. Osteoid osteoma and adamantinoma are among the few tumors that have a proclivity for the tibia. Primary sarcomas of the shaft tend to be of round cell origin. Metastatic lesions rarely involve bone distal to the knee.

Clinical Characteristics

Benign and malignant bone tumors of the leg often present with vague aching: a clinical diagnosis of "stress" fracture, muscle tear, or growing pains may be suggested in absence of radiographs. Palpable masses are rare for bone lesions, although soft tissue tumors typically present as painless masses. In general, tumors of the leg tend to be less advanced at the time of detection than their proximal counterparts. Pathologic fracture of the tibia is quite rare.

The medial aspect of the tibia is subcutaneous throughout most of its length. Subcutaneous hemorrhage resulting from biopsy, previous surgery, or pathologic fracture may contaminate large sections of this area. The popliteal artery divides at the lower level of the popliteal muscle, forming the peroneal and posterior tibial arteries. The anterior tibial artery passes through the intermuscular septum and binds this complex to the posterior face of the tibia.[40] This interval must be closely evaluated before attempting any definitive resection. Sacrifice of one or two branches of the popliteal artery leaves a viable extremity in a young patient.[65] Soft tissue tumors may track along the anterior tibial sheath and extend occultly into another compartment through the foramen.

The two major muscle compartments of the leg are the anterolateral and the posterior muscles. Tumors arising within either group tend to remain intracompartmental. Since both groups do attach to the fibula, tumor involvement of the fibula may occur early. Tumors extending posteriorly or medially involve the respective soft tissue compartments. The tibia is the main weight-bearing bone of the leg; the fibula transmits only 15 percent of body weight. Following biopsy or surgery, the tibia must be protected or reconstructed to prevent secondary fractures. The aim of reconstruction is to reestablish an intact tibia; the fibula is expendable and does not require reconstruction proximal to the ankle.

Staging

Plain radiographs are often diagnostic and should always be obtained. If the lesion is benign, further studies may not be required. Bone scan is useful in localizing ill-defined lesions. Rotation views are required to distinguish involvement of the tibia and fibula from soft tissue tumors. Axial CT images clearly demonstrate involvement and loss of cortical bone, while MRI delineates soft tissue extensions and marrow involvement. When soft tissue extension is suspected, biplane angiography is more useful at this site than elsewhere. Evaluation of the arterial trifurcation is mandatory for proximal lesions.

Biopsy

Biopsy of tumors of the tibia and fibula should be performed carefully to avoid contamination of the anterolateral and posterior compartments, prevent pathologic fracture, and avoid excessive subcutaneous contamination. Small tumors of the fibula may be biopsied by primary excision of the lesion. The tibia should be approached through the medial border; the fibula is approached laterally through the peroneal musculature. All incisions should be longitudinal. Core needle or trochar biopsy of the tibia is generally reliable and creates less contamination than do other techniques. If an incisional biopsy is required, PMMA should be inserted into the defect to decrease postoperative hemorrhage and contamination. Muscle contamination must be avoided. If necessary, the skin along the medial border of the tibia can be widely excised and closed by various techniques.[82]

Surgical Management

Benign tumors of the tibia are treated by simple curettage or excisional biopsy. Reconstruction of large defects requires a cortical graft. An autogenous fibular graft provides good material. Aggressive benign or low-grade malignant tumors (stage I) of the shaft of the tibia are treated by limb-sparing resection. Reconstruction is accomplished by dual fibular grafting, allograft, or segmental prosthesis. High-grade spindle cell tumors (stage II), though rare, usually require an above-knee amputation. In selected patients, a limb-sparing resection may be attempted if soft tissue involvement is minimal. Round cell sarcomas are best treated by combination chemotherapy with adjuvant radiotherapy. Metastatic tumors can often be treated nonoperatively with radiotherapy and a brace. Tumors of the fibula can be treated with minimal morbidity by resection of the fibula and the adjacent musculature. Soft tissue sarcomas often can be treated by a limb-sparing procedure; amputations, when necessary, should be performed above the knee.

Specific Tumors of the Leg

Adamantinoma

The tibia is the most common site of this very rare tumor.[16,35] Generally arising from the diaphysis of the tibia, this lesion may also be eccentric and occasionally has a soft tissue component. Plain radiographs often suggest the correct diagnosis. Local recurrence routinely follows curettage; en bloc excision is therefore recommended.[84] Pulmonary metastasis has been reported. Preoperative staging studies are essential to determine the extent of intraosseous involvement and the extraosseous component. The tumor will often extend beyond the plain radiographic margins. Bone scans, CT, and MRI are useful for evaluation of the intramedullary space. Segmental reconstruction is preferred (Fig. 16-49). The defect can be reconstructed by intercalary fibular grafts combined with intramedullary rod fixation, allograft, or intercalary prosthesis. Local recurrence usually requires an above-knee amputation.

Osteoid Osteoma

The tibia is the second most common site for this lesion.[35] Clinically, osteoid osteomas of the tibia present with pain that may be misinterpreted as a symptomatic stress fracture. A helpful clinical distinction is response to immobilization and non-weight-bearing: painful stress fractures improve whereas the pain of an osteoid osteoma persists. Plain radiographs are often diagnostic, and the surgical management is simpler than that of proximal femoral osteoid osteomas. Osteoid osteoma may arise from an intramedullary or cortical location. Resection of the nidus (marginal excision) is recommended. The size of the defect and age of the patient determine whether a graft is necessary. Large defects in young individuals quickly reossify without a graft. Similar defects following skeletal maturity, in contrast, require a fibular graft to ensure healing. Intraoperative bone scintigraphy (see previous discussion) is useful to localize the tumor, decrease the amount of bone resected, and confirm adequate removal.

Metastatic Carcinoma

Bony involvement of the tibia by metastatic carcinoma is unusual and tends to occur late in the course of skeletal dissemination. Pathologic fracture is uncommon. Most metastatic lesions of the tibia can be satisfactorily treated by local radiotherapy and a brace. Curettage, cementation, and internal fixation or intramedullary nailing occasionally is required. Surprisingly, metastatic hypernephroma may cause extensive destruction of the tibia, requiring curettage and reconstruction with PMMA and intramedullary fixation. Preoperative embolization or a tourniquet is required to avoid profuse bleeding.

Specific Surgical Procedures

Resection of Fibula (Diaphysis)

Benign and aggressive tumors of the fibula are treated by resection. Marginal resection along the periosteum is a reliable procedure with minimal morbidity. The fibula is approached through a lateral incision between the peroneus longus and soleus muscles. The peroneal artery and vein, which travel along the medial aspect of the fibula, must be ligated. Fibular excision proximal to within 5 to 6 cm of the lateral malleolus (proximal to the syndesmosis) leaves a stable ankle. To avoid injury to the peroneal nerve, the site of proximal osteotomy should be below the neck of the fibula. Bony reconstruction is not required in this region. For stage I or II sarcomas, a wide excision that includes adjacent muscle, possibly the tibiofibular joint, and occasionally the peroneal nerve is advisable. The technique is similar to that used for sarcomas of the proximal fibula (previously described).

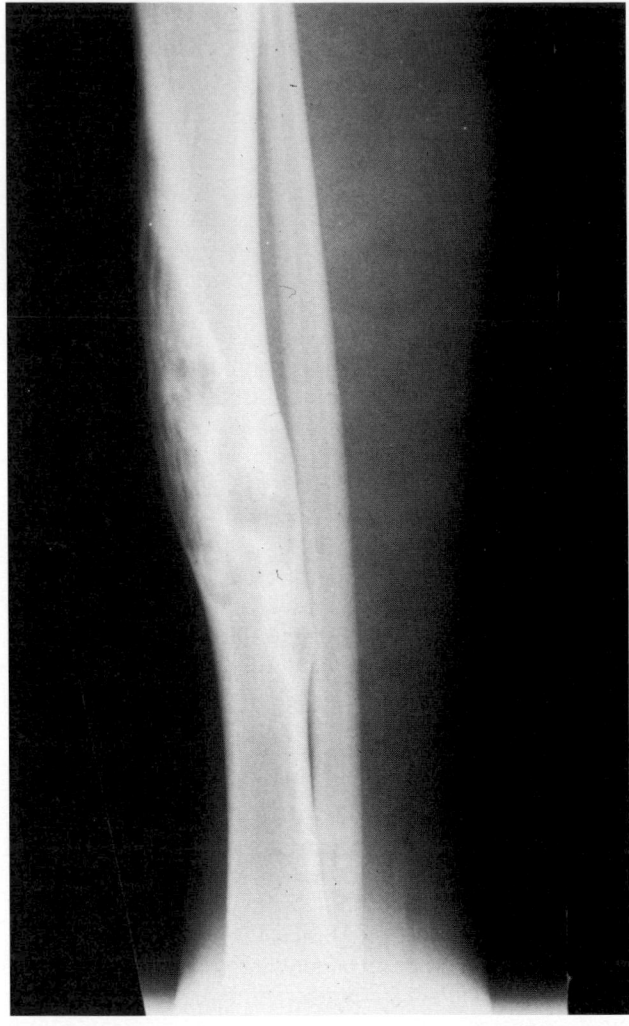

A

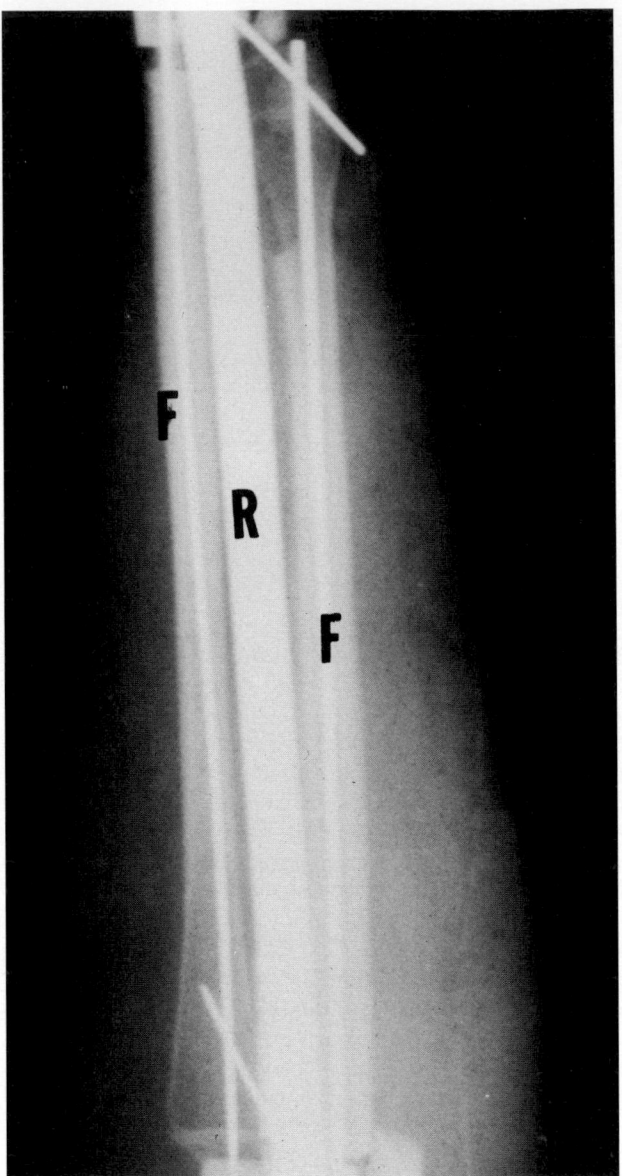

B

Figure 16-49 Adamantinoma. *A.* Typical adamantinoma of the tibia involving a large segment of the diaphysis. *B.* Reconstruction by dual fibular graft (F) and intramedullary rod (R) fixation. Note that the fibular heads are included in the graft, providing cancellous bone for early bony union.

Limb-Sparing Resection of Tibia (Diaphysis)

Resection of the tibia from the insertion of the patellar tendon to the proximal syndesmosis above the ankle, followed by reconstruction, is effective in selected patients. Low-grade (stage I) or aggressive benign diaphyseal tumors with minimal soft tissue extension—e.g., chondrosarcoma and adamantinoma—may be satisfactorily managed in this manner. Bone scintigraphy or MRI is necessary to determine the appropriate level of osteotomy. Reconstruction can be by dual fibular grafting, intercalary allograft, or prosthesis. Recently, procedures involving vascularized fibulas have been performed. A gastrocnemius transposition flap may be necessary to provide soft tissue coverage. A 6- to 12-month period of immobilization is required for graft incorporation.

SOFT TISSUE SARCOMAS OF THE BUTTOCK AND LOWER EXTREMITY

Clinical Characteristics

The lower extremity and the pelvic girdle are the most common sites of soft tissue sarcomas.[85–89] These lesions present clinically as painless masses. Physical examination reveals a firm fixed or mobile mass with discrete borders. The groin should be carefully examined, although lymphatic involvement is rare.[90] All adults presenting with a soft tissue mass must be suspected of having a sarcoma and should undergo the appropriate staging studies. The anatomic compartments of the thigh and pelvis are well delineated. Sarcomas may arise either within compartments (*intracompartmental*) or between them (*extracom-*

partmental). The anterior (quadriceps), posterior (hamstring), and medial (adductor) muscle groups are the most commonly involved. Treatment consists of surgical resection with adjuvant radiotherapy. Based upon success in the treatment of bony sarcomas, adjuvant and neoadjuvant chemotherapy protocols are currently being evaluated by many centers.

Staging Studies

Staging studies are extremely accurate in the lower extremity due to the presence of well-defined anatomic compartments.[85,91] Computed tomography accurately delineates compartmental involvement, proximity to the adjacent bone, suspected extension to a second compartment, and intrapelvic extension; MRI also delineates these features, provides distinct contrast between abnormal and normal tissue, and supplements axial images with sagittal and coronal views. Bone scan is useful in detecting involvement of the underlying bone and periosteum. Uptake into the adjacent bone significantly affects surgical planning. Biplane angiography reveals the position and displacement of the common femoral artery in the groin, the superficial femoral artery in the thigh, and the popliteal vessels in the popliteal space. Displacement of the profundus artery always signifies a deep-seated lesion.

Biopsy

The biopsy of a suspected soft tissue sarcoma should be performed after staging studies have been completed. Large masses may be biopsied easily with a needle or a small incisional procedure. The approach must be in alignment with the potential definitive incision site so that the possibility of resection is not jeopardized. Since all compartments run longitudinally, transverse incisions must always be avoided. Frozen section biopsy at the time of definitive resection is occasionally preferable in difficult locations such as the groin and popliteal space, where the risk of contamination must be minimized. If a soft tissue sarcoma is suspected, the patient should be referred to an institution for biopsy and definitive treatment.

Surgical Management

The primary treatment of a soft tissue sarcoma is surgical removal.[92] The choice of procedure depends upon the stage (grade and anatomic location), previous surgery, contamination, risk of recurrence, and anticipated functional results.[85,91] Low-grade tumors require wide excision; high-grade tumors require either radical resection or wide excision combined with adjuvant therapy. Intracompartmental tumors (stage IA or IIA) are more amenable to a nonablative functional resection than are extracompartmental (either stage IB or IIB) lesions. Extracompartmental tumors frequently involve major neurovascular structures and entail higher surgical morbidity in order to achieve ad-

equate margins. Local contamination by previous excision, poorly placed biopsy, or local recurrence may necessitate an amputation to achieve a satisfactory margin. There is often only one safe opportunity to resect tumors of the groin, popliteal space, and buttock.

If the workup and biopsy are performed correctly, the majority of sarcomas of the lower extremity today can be treated safely with a limb-sparing procedure.[93] Amputation is reserved for those patients in whom a safe margin cannot be obtained by a more limited procedure. The levels of amputation traditionally utilized are hemipelvectomy for buttock and groin tumors, hip disarticulation for midthigh lesions, and high above-knee amputation for distal sarcomas of the thigh and popliteal space. Local recurrence following a low-grade sarcoma usually does not rule out a second attempt at a limb-sparing resection; in contrast, a recurrence following attempted resection of a stage II lesion requires an amputation for local control.

Specific Compartments: Unique Anatomic and Surgical Considerations

Buttock

The buttock is a true compartment (Fig. 16-50). Its anatomic borders are the wing of the ilium (anterior), the gluteal fascia (posterior), and the iliotibial band (lateral). The sciatic nerve passes from the sciatic notch through the buttock and exits between the hamstring muscles. Either CT or MRI is necessary to determine occult retroperitoneal spread via the sciatic notch. Bone scintigraphy is required to determine iliac wing involvement. The approach to biopsy of gluteal tumors should be *lateral* in order to preserve the posterior flap in case a hemipelvectomy is required. Tumor extension through the sciatic notch or involvement of the sciatic nerve often necessitates a hemipelvectomy. Large tumors may involve the sacrum and paraspinal muscles; in this situation, the anterior flap hemipelvectomy is recommended to remove all posterior structures and, if necessary, to permit exploration of the sacral nerve roots.[30] Resection of the gluteus maximus and abductor mechanism results in an abductor lurch and loss of hip extension. A cane is required for ambulation.

Anterior Thigh Compartment (Quadriceps)

The anterior thigh compartment consists of the quadriceps and sartorius muscles and the femoral artery, nerve, and vein (Fig. 16-51).[85] The sartorius, which begins at the apex of the femoral triangle and terminates at the adductor maximus, forms the roof of the femoral canal. This muscle and the femoral canal separate the quadriceps anteriorly from the adductors medially. Dense fascia separates and isolates these two compartments. Tumor involvement of the femoral vessels can be detected with angiography. When such involvement is present, the vessels are resected en bloc with the tumor and replaced with vascular grafts or a contralateral reversed saphenous vein.

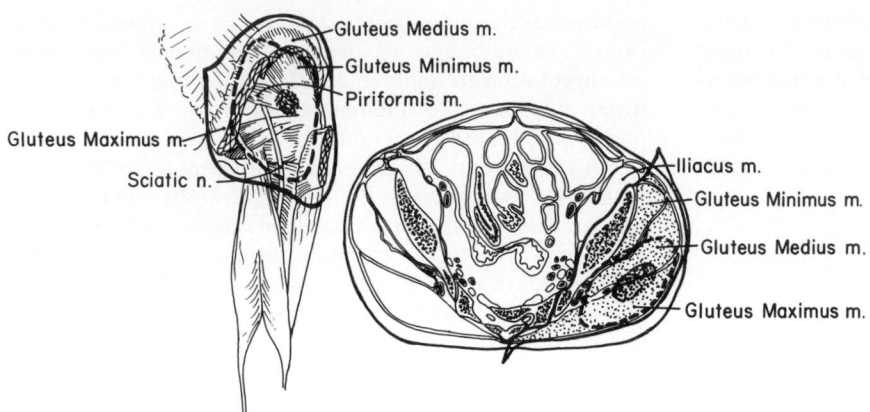

Figure 16-50 Schematic diagram of the buttock compartment. The solid line indicates the entire compartment; its removal would fulfill the criteria of a radical resection or compartmental resection. The dotted line represents a wide or intracompartmental excision, which may preserve the sciatic nerve. (Reproduced with permission from Enneking WF, Spanier SS, Malawer MM: The effect of the anatomic setting on the results of surgical procedures for soft parts sarcoma of the thigh. *Cancer* 47:1005–1022, 1981.)

The vastus intermedius, covering the femur anteriorly and laterally, separates the other vasti from the femur except along the intermuscular septum at the proximal end. Thus, lesions confined to the muscle superficial to the intermedius are one plane removed from the bone and can be resected safely. If the intermedius is involved, resection along the bone will involve the pseudocapsule. Bone scintigraphy is useful to evaluate this plane: increased uptake indicates either direct tumor extension or proximity to the underlying bone, both of which necessitate bone removal. The vastus medialis and the adductor muscles blend at the insertion of the intermuscular septum into the linea aspera. This is the area where a tumor may extend from one compartment to the other.

In general, tumors situated in the distal two-thirds of the thigh remain intracompartmental; their preoperative studies are accurate, and limb-sparing resection is often successful. In contrast, tumors of the proximal third of the thigh tend to spread into the groin, femoral triangle, and adjacent adductor group, or below the inguinal ligament. Preoperative studies may fail to reveal these areas of occult extension. There is a high rate of local recurrence following attempted resection in this region. A modified hemipelvectomy is often required for proximal stage IIB lesions.

The surgical incision extends from the femoral triangle along the sartorius to the level of the knee. Proximal and medial lesions mandate exploration of the femoral vessels. Small lateral and central lesions can be resected by partial muscle resection (myomectomy). Muscle transfers are necessary to cover exposed vessels and bone and to obliterate dead space. Hamstring transfers are required to restore knee extension. Both the semitendinosus and the biceps are mobilized and transferred anteriorly and centrally to recreate a central mechanism.

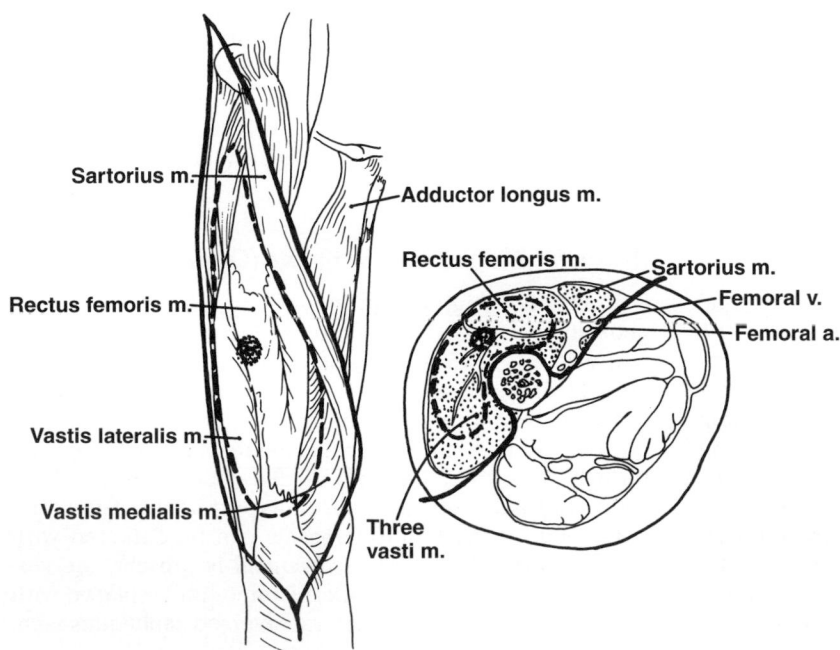

Figure 16-51 Schematic diagram of the anterior thigh compartment. The quadriceps, the sartorius, and the femoral artery, vein, and nerve are contained within the compartment. The solid line indicates a radical (compartmental) resection and the dotted line a wide (intracompartmental) resection. In general, most sarcomas are treated by a wide excision combined with radiotherapy. The femoral vessels are rarely sacrificed. (Reproduced with permission from Enneking WF, Spanier SS, Malawer MM: The effect of the anatomic setting on the results of surgical procedures for soft parts sarcoma of the thigh. *Cancer* 47:1005–1022, 1981.)

Medial Thigh Compartment (Adductor Group)

The medial adductor compartment is a triangular cone located at the top of the thigh (Fig. 16-52). The boundaries are the superior and inferior pubic rami and ischial tuberosity (proximal); the adductor canal and medial intermuscular septum (anterior); the posterior surface of the adductor magnus (posterior); and the deep fascia of the thigh (medial). The medial compartment contains the gracilis; the adductor brevis, longus, and magnus; and the pectineus. The obturator nerve and artery supply this compartment. The profunda femoris artery courses along the pectineus and adductor brevis. Both are intracompartmental and must be sacrificed. All muscles in this compartment take their origin from the pubic rami and ischium by means of short, musculotendinous junctions. Proximal tumors involve these bony structures. The femoral canal lies anterior to the medial compartment, and the location of the lesion may necessitate a vascular graft. The incision should allow for exposure of the femoral canal, ligation of the profundus femoris artery, and access to the interval between the medial hip capsule and the adductors. If possible, the lymphatic vessels along the femoral vessels and in the groin should not be removed. To obtain an acceptable margin, lesions located in the medial aspect of this compartment should be dissected through the medial hamstrings. There is minimal functional deficit following resection of the entire compartment.

Most tumors of the adductor group arise within the proximal muscle mass. Large lesions may extend to the obturator fossa, the linea aspera, or the femoral vessels. Bone scintigraphy and CT demonstrate extension into these areas. Large proximal tumors often extend extracompartmentally into the adjacent hamstrings at their insertion or at the groin, making resection difficult. Involvement of any of these structures may negate a limb-sparing option. Large proximal adductor tumors have a high rate of local recurrence following attempted limb-sparing surgery and may require a modified hemipelvectomy.

Posterior Thigh Compartment (Hamstrings)

The posterior compartment consists of the hamstring muscles, the posterior portion of the adductor magnus, and the sciatic nerve. The anatomic boundaries of this compartment are the lateral intermuscular septum (lateral), the adductor magnus fascia (medial), the ischial tuberosity (proximal), and the musculotendinous junctions of the hamstrings (distal) (Fig. 16-53). The anterior border is formed by the linea aspera and the posterior face of the femur. The sciatic nerve is intracompartmental from the level of the ischial tuberosity to the popliteal space. The usual sites of extracompartmental extension follow the nerve proximally under the gluteus maximus into the buttock or distally into the popliteal space. The incision should allow exposure of the retrogluteal area and popliteal space. Distally, the superficial femoral artery enters the compartment through the adductor canal and crosses over the semitendinosus and semimembranosus muscles to become the popliteal artery. High-grade distal lesions may necessitate arterial resection with vascular grafting or an amputation.

Tumors of the posterior compartment are usually well localized by staging studies. Sciatic nerve involvement is not a definitive indication for amputation. The motor branches to the hamstrings originate in the proximal third of the nerve; thus some knee flexion is preserved following resection of a distal segment of the nerve. A drop-foot orthosis and cane are required. Hemipelvectomy is often required for large lesions of the proximal third with gluteal and/or sciatic nerve involvement. Hip disarticulation is used for midcompartmental lesions involving the femur and/or femoral vessels, while high above-knee amputation is recommended for distal lesions with popliteal extension.

Groin

This extracompartmental space is the proximal extension of the femoral canal. It is bounded by the inguinal ligament

Figure 16-52 Schematic diagram of the medial compartment of the thigh. The medial compartment contains the gracilis; the adductor brevis, longus, and magnus; and the pectineus. The distal two-thirds of the posterior border of this compartment is well defined by the intermuscular septum. The proximal third is poorly defined where the medial hamstrings merge to insert onto the ischium. The solid line indicates a radical (compartmental) resection and the dotted line a wide (intracompartmental) resection. (Reproduced with permission from Enneking WF, Spanier SS, Malawer MM: The effect of the anatomic setting on the results of surgical procedures for soft parts sarcoma of the thigh. *Cancer* 47:1005–1022, 1981.)

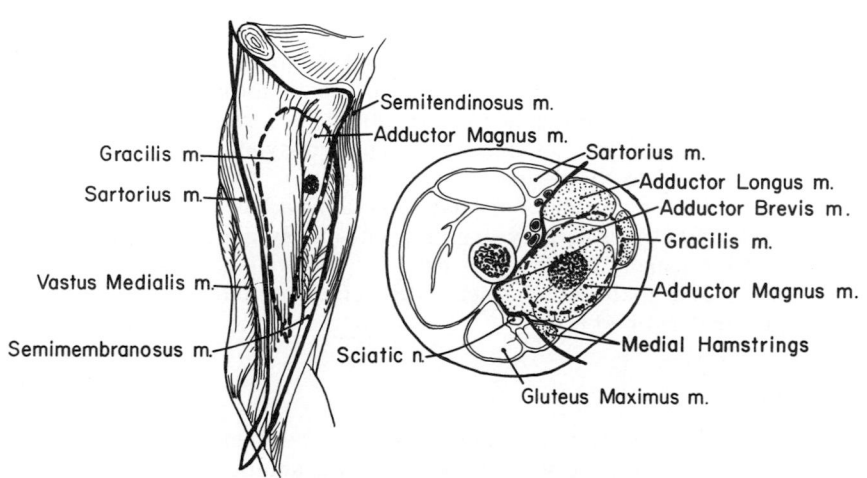

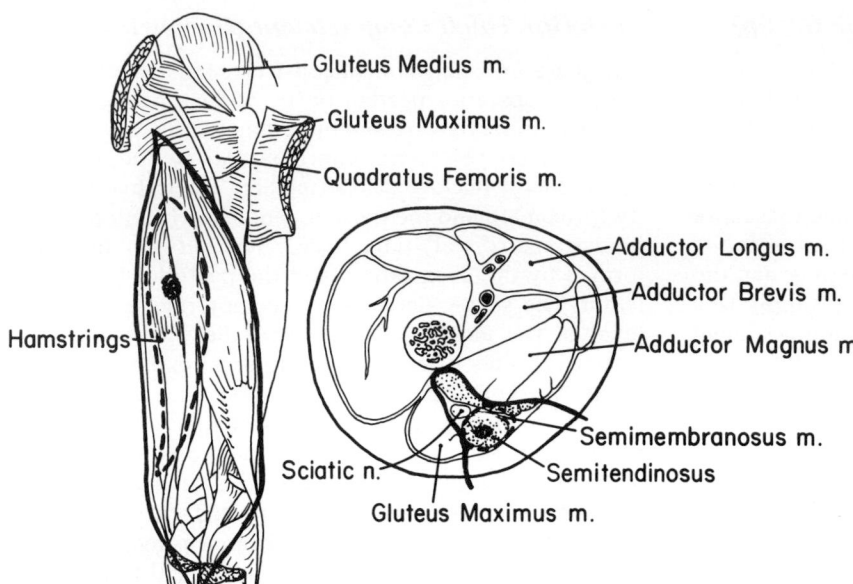

Figure 16-53 Schematic diagram of the posterior compartment. The posterior compartment consists of the hamstring muscles, the posterior portion of the adductor magnus, and the sciatic nerve. The sciatic nerve can often be preserved following a wide excision. The solid line indicates a radical (compartmental) resection and the dotted line a wide (intracompartmental) resection. (Reproduced with permission from Enneking WF, Spanier SS, Malawer MM: The effect of the anatomic setting on the results of surgical procedures for soft parts sarcoma of the thigh. *Cancer* 47:1005–1022, 1981.)

(proximal), the deep fascia (anterior), the iliopsoas and hip capsule (posterior), the tendon of the rectus femoris (lateral), and the pectineus (medial). Tumors may arise from this space or extend directly into it from adjacent compartments. Involvement of the femoral sheath with retroperitoneal spread below the inguinal ligament occurs early. Computed tomography and angiography are often misleading; MRI may be beneficial. Attempted local resection, whether a marginal or wide excision, is difficult in this area. Stage I and/or small lesions may be adequately resected, whereas large lesions or stage II sarcomas require a modified hemipelvectomy. The complication rate following resection, vascular replacement, and postoperative radiation of stage IIA/B lesions is high.

Management of Soft Tissue Sarcomas of the Leg

Some 8 to 12 percent of all soft tissue sarcomas involve the compartments of the leg.[88,89,92] The leg consists of three anatomic compartments: the anterior (extensor), lateral (peroneal), and posterior (extensor) muscle groups. Functionally and anatomically, the first two usually form one compartment. The fibula is a unique structure, forming a border of all three compartments. The biopsy site should be parallel to the definitive line of resection. Like the forearm, the leg permits only one attempt at a limb-sparing resection. Prior surgery, inappropriate biopsy, and contamination usually result in the need for amputation. The clinical and anatomic characteristics of each compartment are described below.

Anterior

The anterior compartment is innervated by the deep branch of the peroneal nerve and consists of the anterior

tibialis, the extensor hallucis longus, and the extensor digitorum communis muscles. The anterior tibial artery, which enters the compartment by passing anteriorly through the foramen in the intermuscular septum and exits distally into the foot, is the major source of blood supply to the compartment. The boundaries of the compartment are the deep fascia of the leg (anterior), the intermuscular septum (posterior), the lateral cortex of the tibia (medial), and the fibula (lateral). The border between the anterior and lateral musculature is the thin fascia, which separates the two compartments. Large and/or high-grade lesions often involve both the anterior and lateral muscle groups; therefore the two compartments functionally are considered as one anterolateral compartment. Bone scan is necessary to determine cortical or fibular involvement. If either shows increased uptake, the adjacent portion of bone should be removed. Angiography is useful in determining involvement of the arterial trifurcation. Exploration of the popliteal vessels and routine ligation of the anterior and/or peroneal branches are necessary for lesions of the proximal muscle groups. A lateral gastrocnemius transposition flap may be required to close the defect. Following resection of the anterior compartment, the only functional deficit is a drop foot, which is treated with an orthosis. Tendon transfers are not done primarily.

Lateral Compartment (Peroneal Group)

The lateral compartment consists of the peroneal muscles and the peroneal nerve. This compartment blends into the anterior musculature medially and into the soleus posteriorly. The medial border is the fibula. Small and stage I lesions can occasionally be treated by resection of the peroneal muscles alone. Larger and high-grade (stage II) lesions often require combined resection of the anterior and lateral compartments, including the fibula and the peroneal nerve, with ligation of the anterior tibial and peroneal arteries. This procedure is termed an *anterolateral resection.* Results are functionally superior to those of an above-knee amputation. The technique is similar to that described for high-grade stage IIB sarcomas of the proximal fibula. However, an extraarticular resection of the tibiofibular joint need not be performed. A lateral gastrocnemius transposition flap is required following this resection.

Posterior Compartment (Flexors)

The posterior compartment consists of the gastrocnemius-soleus complex and the posterior tibialis, flexor hallucis longus, and flexor digitorum communis muscles. The posterior tibial artery and nerve enter the posterior compartment at the popliteal level and exit distally at the ankle, separating the superficial muscles from the deep flexors. The boundaries of the compartment are the intermuscular septum (anterior), the deep fascia of the leg (posterior), the insertion along the tibia (medial), and the insertion around the fibula (lateral). Tumors arising within the superficial muscles, especially the gastrocnemius, can easily be resected. Deep-seated tumors are covered by neurovascular structures, making resection difficult. Most stage I tumors can be treated adequately by a wide excision. Stage II tumors requiring bony and neurovascular resection are best treated by above-knee amputation.

TUMORS OF THE FOOT AND ANKLE

Tumors of the foot and ankle are rare. Overall, fewer than 1 to 5 percent involve this area, though certain bones have a propensity for specific tumors. Giant-cell tumors, aneurysmal bone cysts, simple bone cysts, and characteristically intraosseous ganglion are the most common lesions of the talus, calcaneus, and distal tibia. Most bony tumors are benign: fewer than 1 percent of all osteosarcomas occur in the foot. Similarly, fewer than 2 to 4 percent of soft tissue sarcomas involve the foot and/or ankle. Clear cell sarcoma of the tendon sheath characteristically arises near the ankle and the Achilles tendon. Analogous to the distal distribution in the upper extremity, epithelioid and synovial sarcoma are often found around the foot and ankle. The ankle is the third most common site for pigmented villonodular synovitis. Fibromatosis is the most common benign solid lesion of the foot.[94]

Clinical Characteristics

Bony tumors of the ankle and foot usually present very early in their growth due to early onset of pain, which is often associated with minor trauma. The most common initial diagnosis is ankle sprain. Plain radiographs usually reveal the lesion. Associated soft tissue components are very rare, since most bony lesions in this area are benign. Pathologic fracture is unusual. The rare soft tissue sarcoma usually presents as an asymptomatic mass; clinical

suspicion is necessary for early diagnosis. Most of these sarcomas are small and are considered to be ganglions until removed. Careful physical examination reveals that these are not cystic: aspiration should be performed prior to assuming that a lesion is a ganglion. Therefore, all solid soft tissue masses in unusual locations around the foot or ankle should be carefully staged prior to surgical removal.

Anatomically, there is minimal soft tissue covering the foot and ankle. Thus, all biopsies, surgical procedures, and reconstructions must be carefully planned to avoid inadvertent contamination, wound breakdown, local recurrence, and failure of a reconstructive effort. The ankle and subtalar joints are the most common bones involved by primary bony tumors. Rarely are the posterior tibial vessels and nerve directly involved. Surgical approaches should avoid the neurovascular structures. In general, a lateral approach to the talus, calcaneus, and distal tibia is recommended. The foot, like the hand, has poorly defined anatomic compartments; each ray is best considered as a compartment. The functional aim of all reconstructive efforts is to permit painless weight bearing: motion is of secondary concern. Surgically, this often means resection-arthrodesis or amputation for most aggressive or malignant lesions.

Staging Studies

Plain radiographs are often diagnostic for bony tumors of the foot and ankle. Special views are required to evaluate the calcaneus and subtalar joints. Magnetic resonance imaging delineates soft tissue involvement, while high-resolution CT is invaluable in the evaluation of the calcaneus and talus. Angiography is necessary to determine the location of the posterior tibial vessels for large tumors and helps in the diagnosis of GCTs and aneurysmal bone cysts, both of which show a marked tumor blush. Embolization at this level is not recommended because of the danger to the end arteries of the foot. Additionally, a tourniquet can easily be used proximally for control of hemorrhage. Bone scintigraphy is helpful in determining the extent of the lesion within the larger bones of the foot and distal tibia. However, minor areas of increased uptake may be misleading and may be related to minor trauma and/or disuse, and not to tumor.

Biopsy

Needle biopsy is recommended for suspected aggressive or malignant tumors of the ankle and hindfoot. If an open biopsy is required, the standard anterior and medial incisions should not be utilized due to potential contamination of the anterior and posterior vascular structures and the major tendons. Special care should be taken to avoid contamination of the ankle joint. A small lateral incision through the sinus tarsi is preferred for lesions of the body and neck of the talus. A direct lateral incision avoiding the peroneal muscles is recommended for the calcaneus. Tumors of the forefoot are best approached directly over the lesion, with minimal dissection. For suspected soft tissue tumors of the plantar aspect of the foot, it is the authors' preference to proceed through the most direct route, irrespective of the weight-bearing areas. Incisions through the plantar aspect of the foot heal well and, if necessary, can easily be reexcised if an en bloc resection is required.

Surgical Management

Benign and aggressive bony tumors are treated by curettage and/or resection. Aggressive and recurrent distal tib-

ial lesions can be treated successfully by resection and arthrodesis or cryosurgery (Fig. 16-54).[94,95] Resection of the talus or calcaneus, however, results in a poor functional outcome. The authors prefer curettage and cryosurgery with iliac crest bone grafting and cementation for aggressive lesions of the hindfoot and/or distal tibia.[94,96] Bone graft is usually required following curettage for tumors in this location: fibular struts are preferred for the distal tibia, while iliac corticocancellous struts are used for the calcaneus and talus. Lesions of the metatarsals and phalanges can be successfully treated by curettage,

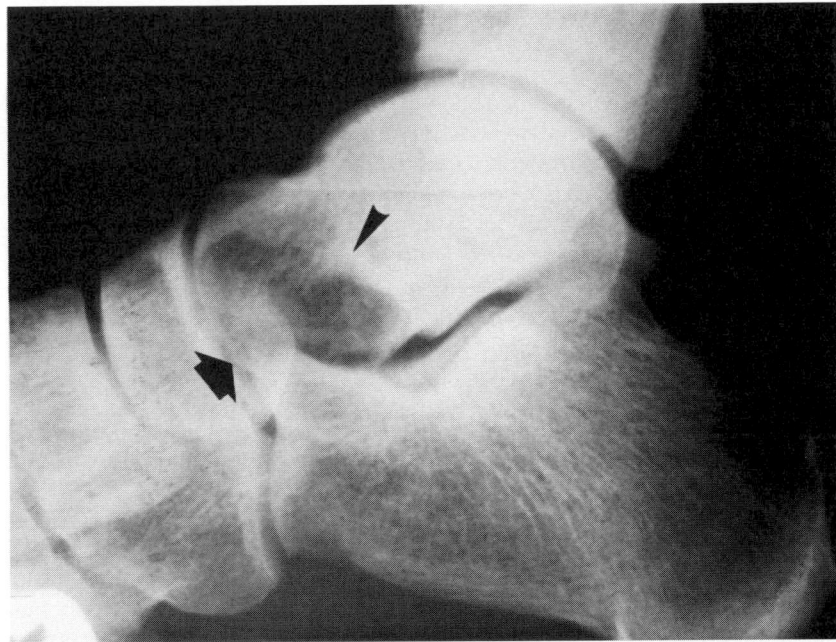

A

Figure 16-54 Giant-cell tumor. *A.* A giant-cell tumor localized to the head of the talus. *B.* Postoperative radiograph 5 years following resection and arthrodesis with bone graft. (Reproduced with permission from Malawer MM, Vance R: Giant cell tumor and aneurysmal bone cyst of the talus: Clinicopathological review and two case reports. *J Foot Ankle Surg* 1:235–244, 1981.)

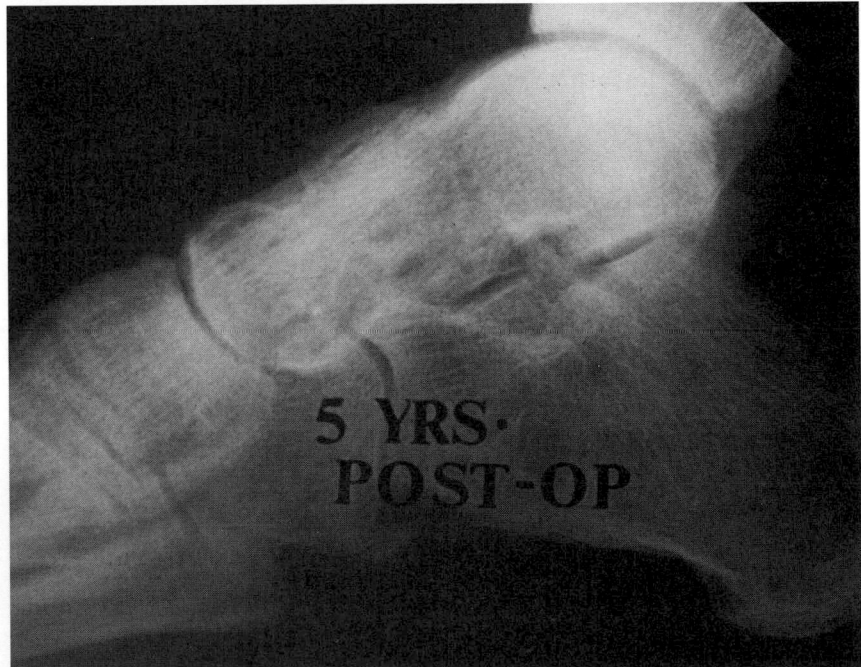

B

resection, and/or cryosurgery. It is difficult to obtain satisfactory margins for high-grade sarcomas (stage IIA/B) while preserving a functional foot: amputation is usually required. Malignant lesions involving the plantar surface also require an amputation. Stage IIA/B tumors of the forefoot are best treated with a Symes amputation, while lesion of the hindfoot or ankle should be treated with a below-knee amputation. Aggressive soft tissue tumors require a wide excision, with adjuvant radiation for high-grade sarcomas. Benign tumors with little tendency to recur (e.g., lipomas or osteochondromas) require only a marginal excision to achieve cure.

Specific Tumors of the Foot and Ankle

Unicameral Bone Cysts

Unicameral bone cysts (UBCs) occasionally occur in the distal tibia (4 percent) and rarely but characteristically in the midportion of the calcaneus. The correct diagnosis is suggested by the plain radiograph correlating with a cold lesion on bone scan. The diagnosis is confirmed by aspiration of yellow fluid and intracavity Renografin (diatrizoate meglumine and diatrizoate sodium) injection.[36] Surgery is not indicated in the initial management. Aspiration and high-pressure Renografin injection, as previously described, is recommended.

Intraosseus Ganglion

The distal tibia, especially the medial malleolus, is the most common (33 percent) location of this rare lesion; second are the tarsal bones. Approximately 100 intraosseous ganglia have been reported. The plain radiograph typically shows a radiolucent defect with a thin rim of sclerosis, suggesting a benign lesion. Bone scintigraphy may show an area of homogeneous uptake or slight decrease in the center. Biopsy routinely demonstrates a thick, fluid-filled cavity with a fibrous lining. Curettage with removal of the lining is often curative. If a direct communication with the joint exists, it should be grafted from within the bony defect. Recurrences are treated by repeated curettage. En bloc excision should be avoided and the joint should be preserved. If the defect is large, an autogenous graft is recommended.

Giant-Cell Tumors and Aneurysmal Bone Cysts

Fewer than 2 percent of all GCTs occur around the ankle or foot. Dahlin reported that 11 percent of 134 ABCs occurred at this region.[35] The most common bone involved by either lesion is the distal tibia and/or talus.[96] The most common primary bone tumor of the talus is the GCT. Plain radiographs show an expansile, lytic lesion without matrix formation. The correct diagnosis is suggested by the marked uptake seen on bone scintigraphy. Angiography is usually not indicated unless soft tissue extension is seen on CT. Computed tomography is necessary to evaluate the amount of bony destruction and the need for bone grafting. Management of distal tibial lesions is similar to that for other anatomic sites—extended curettage, adjuvant cryosurgery, bone grafting of

subchondral margins, and cementation of the main defect. Occasionally, en bloc resection with primary arthrodesis is necessary: amputation is rarely required. Lesions of the talus and calcaneus are similarly treated.[96] Primary resection and/or amputation are rarely required.

Chondrosarcoma

Chondrosarcomas (2 percent), when they occur in the foot, tend to be low grade (stage IA/B) and localized to the hind foot. Local resection and/or cryosurgery can obtain local control. Cartilage tumors of the metatarsals and phalanges, despite an active histologic appearance, are benign enchondromas and should be treated by curettage alone.

Fibromatosis

There is a wide spectrum of fibromatous lesions that tend to involve the foot. They may be classified as one of four types: superficial fibromatosis (e.g., plantar), infantile digital type, infantile (aggressive, desmoid) type, and congenital fibrosarcoma. Diagnosis is based upon clinical and histologic criteria: distinction is necessary for appropriate treatment. Plantar fibromatosis grows slowly and then remains stable. Bilateral foot involvement occurs in about 25 percent of patients. Surgery is required only if they are symptomatic. Removal with normal tissue margins and partial fasciectomy is required. The adjacent digital nerves and flexor tendons should be preserved. Infantile digital fibromatosis presents as small nodules along the toes. Simple excision is usually curative. Conversely, infantile (desmoid-type) fibromatosis and congenital fibrosarcoma are highly aggressive, infiltrative lesions that require wide excision for local control. Congenital fibrosarcoma often arises adjacent to or involves the underlying bony structures. Despite the highly cellular histology of these two lesions, metastases rarely occur, although amputation of the foot is often required after several recurrences in order to obtain local control. Recently, postoperative radiotherapy has been given to aid in local control and so avoid amputation.

Pigmented Villonodular Synovitius

Pigmented villonodular synovitis (PVS) of the ankle presents as a juxtaarticular mass mimicking a sarcoma. Plain radiographs may appear as normal. Marginal excision of the mass and synovectomy should be performed. Local recurrence necessitates reexcision. If local control cannot be obtained, a wide excision, extraarticular resection, and arthrodesis are curative. A trial of radiation therapy to prevent recurrence is recommended prior to consideration of amputation.

REFERENCES

1. Enneking WE: *Musculoskeletal Tumor Surgery.* Vol 1. New York, Churchill Livingstone, 1983.

2. Gitelis S, Bertoni F, Chieti PP, Campanacci M: Chondrosarcoma of bone. *J Bone Joint Surg [Am]* 63A:1248–1256, 1981.

3. Marcove RC, Mike V, Hutter RVP, et al: Chondrosarcoma of the pelvis and upper end of femur. *J Bone Joint Surg [Am]* 54:561–572, 1972.

4. Enneking WF, Dunham WK: Resection and reconstruction for primary neoplasms involving the innominate bone. *J Bone Joint Surg [Am]* 60:731–746, 1978.

5. deSantos LA, Bernardino ME, Murry JA: Computed tomography in the evaluation of osteosarcoma: Experience with 25 cases. *AJR* 132:535–540, 1979.

6. Levine E: Computed tomography of musculoskeletal tumors. *Crit Rev Diagn Imaging* 16:779–309, 1981.

7. Rosenthal DI: Computed tomography in bone and soft tissue neoplasms: Application and pathologic correlation. *CRC Crit Rev Diagn Imaging* 18:243–278, 1982.

8. Massengill AD, Seeger LL, Eckardt JJ: The role of plane radiography, computed tomography, and magnetic resonance imaging in sarcoma evaluation. *Hematol Oncol Clin North Am* 9:571–604, 1995.

9. Francis KC: Radical amputations, in *Nora's Operative Surgery.* Philadelphia, Lea & Febiger, 1974, pp 1041–1051.

10. Barth RJ, Merino MJ, Solomon D, et al: A prospective study of the value of core needle biopsy and fine needle aspiration in the diagnosis of soft tissue masses. *Surgery* 112:536–543, 1992.

11. Skrzynski MC, Biermann JS, Montag A, Simon MA: Diagnostic accuracy and charge-savings of outpatient core needle biopsy compared with open biopsy of musculoskeletal tumors. *J Bone Joint Surg* 78A:644–649, 1996.

12. Simon MA, Biermann JS: Biopsy of bone and soft-tissue lesions. *J Bone Joint Surg* 75A:616–621, 1993.

13. Garrison RC, Unni KK, Mcleod RA, et al: Chondrosarcoma arising in osteochondroma. *Cancer* 49:1890–1897, 1982.

14. Huvos AG: *Bone Tumors: Diagnosis, Treatment, and Prognosis.* Philadelphia, Saunders, 1979.

15. Huvos AG, Rosen G, Dabska M, Marcove RC: Mesenchymal chondrosarcoma: A clinicopathologic analysis of 35 patients with emphasis on treatment. *Cancer* 51:1230–1237, 1983.

16. Jaffe HL: *Tumors and Tumorous Conditions of the Bone and Joints.* Philadelphia, Lea & Febiger, 1958.

17. Pritchard DJ, Lunke RJ, Taylor WF, et al: Chondrosarcoma: A clinicopathologic statistical analysis. *Cancer* 45:149–157, 1980.

18. Sanerkin NG: The diagnosis and grading of chondrosarcoma of bone: A combined cytologic and histologic approach. *Cancer* 45:582–594, 1980.

19. Marcove RC: Chondrosarcoma: Diagnosis and treatment. *Orthop Clin North Am* 8:811–819, 1977.

20. Marcove RC: A 17-year review of cryosurgery in the treatment of bone tumors. *Clin Orthop* 163:231–233, 1982.

21. Dahlin DC, Coventry MB: Osteosarcoma, a study of 600 cases. *J Bone Joint Surg* 49A:101–110, 1967.

22. Marcove RC, Rosen G: En bloc resection for osteogenic sarcoma. *Cancer* 45:3040–3044, 1980.

23. Fahey M, Spanier SS: Osteosarcoma of the pelvis: A clinical and histopathological study of twenty-five patients. *J Bone Joint Surg [Am]* 74:321–330, 1992.

24. Estrada-Aguilar J, Greenburg H, Walling A, et al: Primary treatment of pelvic osteosarcoma: Report of five cases. *Cancer* 69:1137–1145, 1992.

25. Lichtenstein L: *Bone Tumors,* 4th ed. St Louis, Mosby, 1972.

26. Nesbit ME, Perez CA, Tefft M, et al: Multimodal therapy for the management of primary nonmetastatic Ewing's sarcoma of bone: An intergroup study. *Natl Cancer Inst Monogr* 56:255–262, 1981.

27. Perez CA, Razek A, Tefft M, et al: Analysis of local tumor control in Ewing's sarcoma: Preliminary results of a cooperative intergroup study. *Cancer* 40:2864–2873, 1977.

28. Bacci G, Picci P, Gitelis S, Borghi A, Campanacci M: The treatment of localized Ewing's sarcoma. *Cancer* 49:1561–1570, 1982.

29. Aboulafia AJ, Buch R, Mathews J, Li W, Malawer MM: Reconstruction using the saddle prosthesis following excision of primary and metastatic periacetabular tumors. *Clin Orthop* 314:203–212, 1995.

30. Sugarbaker PH, Chretien PA: Hemipelvectomy for buttock tumors utilizing an anterior myocutaneous flap of quadriceps femoris muscle. *Ann Surg* 197:106–115, 1983.

31. Steel HH: Partial or complete resection of the hemipelvis: An alternative to hindquarter amputation for periacetabular chondrosarcoma of the pelvis. *J Bone Joint Surg* 60A:719–730, 1978.

32. Harrington KD: The use of hemipelvic allografts or autoclaved grafts for reconstruction after wide resections of malignant tumors of the pelvis. *J Bone Joint Surg* 74:331–341, 1992.

33. Henshaw RM, Jones V, Malawer MM: Modular endoprosthetic reconstruction of the lower extremity. Results of 73 consecutive cases. To be presented at First International Symposium, Plastic and Reconstructive Surgery in Oncology, Moscow, Russia, March, 1997.

34. Sim FH, Bowman WE, Chao EYS: Limb salvage surgery and reconstructive techniques, in Sim FH (ed): *Diagnosis and Treatment of Bone Tumors: A Team Approach.* Mayo Clinic Monograph. Thorofare, NJ, Slack, 1983, pp 75–105.

35. Dahlin DC: *Bone Tumors: General Aspects and Data on 6,221 Cases,* 3d ed. Springfield, IL, Charles C Thomas, 1978.

36. Malawer MM: The diagnosis, treatment and management of unicameral bone cysts by percutaneous aspiration, hemodynamic evaluation and intracavitary methylprednisolone acetate, in *Orthopedic Update Series.* Princeton, NJ, Continuing Professional Education Center, 1986.

37. Malawer MM, McKay DW, Markle B: Analysis of 40 consecutive cases of unicameral bone cysts treated by high pressure Renografin injection and intracavitary methylprednisolone acetate: Prognostic factors and hemodynamic evaluation. Paper presented at the 52nd Annual Meeting of the American Academy of Orthopaedic Surgeons, Las Vegas, 1985.

38. Neer CS, Francis KC, Kiernan HA, et al: Current concepts in the treatment of solitary unicameral bone cysts. *Clin Orthop* 97:40–51, 1973.

39. Scaglietti Q, Marchetti PG, Bartolozzi NP: The effects of methylprednisolone acetate in the treatment of bone cysts: Results of three years follow-up. *J Bone Joint Surg [Br]* 61:200–204, 1979.

40. Dahlin DC, Ivins JC: Benign chondroblastoma, a study of 125 cases. *Cancer* 30:401–413, 1972.

41. Springfield DS, Capanna R, Gherlinzoni F, et al: Chondroblastoma: Review of seventy cases. *J Bone Joint Surg* 67:748–754, 1985.

42. Biesecker JL, Marcove RC, Huvos AG, Moke V: Aneurysmal bone cysts: A clinicopathologic study of 66 cases. *Cancer* 26(3):615–625, 1970.

43. Goldenberg RR, Campbell CJ, Bonfiglio M: Giant cell tumor of bone: An analysis of two hundred and eighteen cases. *J Bone Joint Surg [Am]* 52:619–664, 1970.

44. Marcove RC, Weiss L, Vaghaiwall M, Pearson R: Cryosurgery in the treatment of giant cell tumor of bone: A report of 52 consecutive cases. *Clin Orthop* 134:275–289, 1978.

45. Malawer M, Kollander Y, Buch R, Meller I: Cryosurgery in the treatment of giant cell tumors of bone: Analysis of 102 cases. *Acta Orthop Scand.* Submitted 1996.

46. Pritchard DJ, Dahlin D, Dauphine R, et al: Ewing's sarcoma. *J Bone Joint Surg [Am]* 57A:10–16, 1975.

47. Rosen G, Caparros B, Mosende C, et al: Curability of Ewing's sarcoma and consideration for future therapeutic trials. *Cancer* 41:888, 1978.

48. Rosen G, Caparros B, Huvos AC, et al: Preoperative chemotherapy for osteogenic sarcoma: Selection of postoperative adjuvant chemotherapy based upon the response of the primary tumor to preoperative chemotherapy. *Cancer* 49:1221–1230, 1982.

49. Neff JR: The current role of surgical therapy in Ewing's sarcoma. *Dev Oncol* 55:210–217, 1988.

50. Campanacci M, Bacci G, Bertoni F, Picci P: The treatment of osteosarcoma of the extremity: Twenty years' experience at the Instituto Orthopedico Rizzoli. *Cancer* 48:1569–1581, 1981.

51. Edeiken J: Bone tumors and tumor-like conditions, in Edeiken J (ed): *Roentgen Diagnosis of Diseases of Bone,* 3d ed. Baltimore, Williams & Wilkins, 1981, pp 5–41.

52. Francis KC, Kohn H, Malawer MM: Osteogenic sarcoma. *J Bone Joint Surg [Am]* 55:754, 1976.

53. Malawer MM, Abelson HT, Suit HD: Sarcomas of bone, in DeVita VT, Hellman S, Rosenberg SA (eds): *Cancer: Principles and Practice of Oncology,* 2d ed. Philadelphia, Lippincott, 1985, pp 1293–1343.

54. Campanacci M, Giunti A, Olmi R: Giant-cell tumors of bone: A study of 209 cases with long-term follow-up in 130. *Ital J Orthop Traumatol* 1:249–277, 1977.

55. Dahlin DC, Cupps RE, Johnson EW Jr: Giant cell tumor: A study of 195 cases. *Cancer* 25:1061–1070, 1970.

56. Dahlin DC, Unni KK: Osteosarcoma of bone and its important recognizable varieties. *Am J Surg Pathol* 1:61–72, 1977.

57. Chao EYS, Ivins JC: *Design and Application of Tumor Prosthesis for Bone and Joint Reconstruction.* New York, Thieme-Stratton, 1983.

58. Enneking WF, Shirley PD: Resection-arthrodesis for malignant and potentially malignant lesions about the knee using an intramedullary rod and local bone graft. *J Bone Joint Surg [Am]* 59:223–235, 1977.

59. Malawer MM: Distal femoral osteogenic sarcoma, principles of soft tissue resection and reconstruction in conjunction with prosthetic replacement (adjuvant surgery), in Chao EYS (ed): *Design and Application of Tumor Prosthesis for Bone and Joint Reconstruction.* New York, Thieme-Stratton, 1983, pp 297–309.

60. Mankin HJ, Fogelson FS, Thrasher AZ, et al: Massive resection and allograft transplantation in the treatment of malignant bone tumors. *N Engl J Med* 294:1247–1255, 1976.

61. Marcove RC, Lewis MM, Rosen G, et al: Total femur and total knee replacement: A preliminary report. *Clin Orthop* 126:147–152, 1977.

62. Morton DL, Eilber FR, Townsend CM Jr, et al: Limb salvage from a multidisciplinary treatment approach for skeletal and soft tissue sarcomas of the extremity. *Ann Surg* 184:268–278, 1976.

63. Watts HG: Introduction to resection of musculoskeletal sarcomas. *Clin Orthop* 153:31–38, 1980.

64. Malawer MM: Surgical technique and results of limb-sparing surgery for high grade bone sarcomas of the knee and shoulder: Analysis of 33 consecutive cases. *Orthopedics* 8:597–607, 1985.

65. Malawer MM: Surgical management of aggressive and malignant tumors of the proximal fibula. *Clin Orthop* 186:172–181, 1984.

66. Simon MA, Hecht JD: Invasion of joints by primary bone sarcomas in adults. *Cancer* 50:1649, 1982.

67. Madewell JE, Ragsdale BD, Sweet DE: Radiographic and pathologic analysis of solitary bone lesions. *Radiol Clin North Am* 19:715–814, 1981.

68. Springfield DS, Goodman MA: Biopsy of musculoskeletal lesions. *Orthopedics* 3:868–870, 1980.

69. Enneking WF, Kagan A: Intramarrow spread of osteosarcoma, in *Management of Primary Bone and Soft Tissue Tumors.* Chicago, Yearbook, 1976, pp 171–177.

70. Goldstein H, McNeil BJ, Zufall E, et al: Changing indications for bone scintigraphy in patients with osteosarcoma. *Radiology* 135:177–180, 1980.

71. Hudson TM, Hass G, Enneking WF, Hawkins EF: Angiography in the management of musculoskeletal tumors. *Surg Gynecol Obstet* 141:11–21, 1975.

72. Craig FS: Metastatic and primary lesions of bone. *Clin Orthop* 73:33, 1970.

73. Moore TM, Meyers MH, Patzakis MJ, et al: Closed biopsy of musculoskeletal lesions. *J Bone Joint Surg [Am]* 61:375–380, 1979.

74. Schajowicz E, Derqui JC: Puncture biopsy in lesions of the locomotor system: Review and results in 4050 cases, including 941 vertebral punctures. *Cancer* 21:5331–5487, 1968.

75. Rosen G, Marcove RC, Caparros B, et al: Primary osteogenic sarcoma: The rationale for preoperative chemotherapy and delayed surgery. *Cancer* 43:2163–2177, 1979.

76. Goldenberg RR, Campbell CJ, Bonfiglio M: Giant cell tumor of bone: An analysis of two hundred and eighteen cases. *J Bone Joint Surg [Am]* 52:619–664, 1970.

77. Hutter VP, Worcester JN Jr, Francis KC, et al: Benign and malignant giant cell tumor of bone: A clinicopathological analysis of the natural history of the disease. *Cancer* 15:653–690, 1962.

78. Malawer MM, Zielinski CJ: Giant cell tumor of bone: Surgical management-cryosurgery and en bloc resection. Analysis of 20 consecutive cases and recommendations for treatment. Paper presented at the 50th Annual Meeting of the American Academy of Orthopedic Surgeons, Anaheim, CA, March 1983.

79. Marcove RC, Lyden JP, Huvos AC, Bullough PB: Giant cell tumor treated by cryosurgery: A report of twenty-five cases. *J Bone Joint Surg [Am]* 55:1633–1644, 1973.

80. Unni KK, Dahlin DC, Beaubout SW, Ivins JC: Parosteal osteogenic sarcoma. *Cancer* 37:2466–2475, 1976.

81. Unni KK, Dahlin DC, Beaubout SW: Periosteal osteogenic sarcoma. *Cancer* 37:2476–2485, 1976.

82. Malawer MM, Price WP: Gastrocnemius transposition flap in conjunction with limb-sparing surgery for primary bone sarcomas around the knee. *Plast Reconstr Surg* 73:741–750, 1984.

83. Malawer MM, Chou L: Prosthetic survival and clinical results with use of large-segment replacements in the treatment of high-grade bone sarcomas. *J Bone Joint Surg* 77A:1154–1165, 1995.

84. Gebhardt MC, Lord FC, Rosenberg AE, Mankin HJ: The treatment of adamantinoma of the tibia by wide resection and allograft bone transplantation. *J Bone Joint Surg [Am]* 69:1177–1188, 1987.

85. Enneking WF, Spanier SS, Malawer MM: The effect of the anatomic setting on the results of surgical procedure for soft parts sarcoma of the thigh. *Cancer* 47:1005–1022, 1981.

86. Hajdu SI, Shiu MH, Fortner JC: Tendosynovial sarcoma: A clinicopathological study of 136 cases. *Cancer* 39:1201, 1977.

87. Lindberg RD, Martin RG, Romsdahl MM: Surgery and postoperative radiotherapy in the treatment of soft-tissue sarcomas in adults. *AJR* 123:123–129, 1976.

88. Weiss SW, Enzinger FM: Malignant fibrous histiocytoma: An analysis of 200 cases. *Cancer* 41:2250, 1978.

89. Weiss SW, Enzinger FM: Myxoid variant of malignant fibrous histiocytoma. *Cancer* 39:1672, 1977.

90. Weingrad DN, Rosenberg SA: Early lymphatic spread of osteogenic and soft-tissue sarcomas. *Surgery* 84:231–240, 1978.

91. Enneking WF, Spanier SS, Goodman MA: A system for the surgical staging of musculoskeletal sarcoma. *Clin Orthop* 153:106–120, 1980.

92. Rosenberg SA, Suit FD, Baker LH: Sarcomas of soft tissue, in DeVita VT, Heilman S, Rosenberg SA (eds): *Cancer: Principles and Practice of Oncology,* 2d ed. Philadelphia, Lippincott, 1985, pp 1243–1293.

93. Morton DL, Eilber FR, Townsend CM Jr, et al: Limb salvage from a multidisciplinary treatment approach for skeletal and soft tissue sarcomas of the extremity. *Ann Surg* 184:268–278, 1976.

94. Chou LB, Malawer MM: Analysis of surgical treatment of 33 foot and ankle tumors. *Foot Ankle Int* 15:175–181, 1994.

95. Malawer MM, Dunham WK, Zaleski T, Zielinski CI: Cryosurgery in management of benign (aggressive) and low grade malig-

nant tumors of bone: Analysis of 40 consecutive cases. Paper presented at the 53rd Annual Meeting of the American Academy of Orthopedic Surgeons, New Orleans, February 1986.

96. Malawer MM, Vance R: Giant cell tumor and aneurysmal bone cyst of the talus. Clinicopathological review and two case reports. *Foot and Ankle* 1:235–244, 1981.

CHAPTER 17

Bone and Joint Infections

Burke A. Cunha, Roger Dee, Natalie C. Klein, and Hormozan Aprin

ACUTE HEMATOGENOUS OSTEOMYELITIS

Osteomyelitis is an infectious process of the bone and its marrow. The term *osteomyelitis* normally refers to infections caused by pyogenic microorganisms but can be used for granulomatous infections, such as tuberculosis and syphilis, or specific viral or fungal infections.

Hematogenous spread from a primary source of infection is the commonest route of infection. Acute osteomyelitis can also be produced by extension of soft tissue infection adjacent to bone, or it can be initiated from an open fracture or a penetrating wound.

Organisms

The most commonly isolated organism in this condition in all age groups remains *Staphylococcus aureus*. This organism is responsible for between 50 and 70 percent of all such infections in children between 1 month and 5 years of age.[1] The second most common organisms are hemolytic streptococci. Both group A and group B streptococci have been implicated in acute hematogenous osteomyelitis, the latter particularly within the first 2 months of life.[1-3] In neonates, *Haemophilus influenzae* is an occasional cause of osteomyelitis but more commonly of septic arthritis. There is often an associated meningitis.[4,5] The wide variety of organisms seen in bone infection following a penetrating wound is not seen in hematogenous infection.

Pathophysiology

Nade quotes the unpublished observations of Emslie and coworkers, who have recently demonstrated that intravenous injection of bacteria may produce abscesses selectively in the bony metaphysis, sparing other organs.[3]

Blood Supply of the Epiphysis and Metaphysis

It is believed that the vascular architecture of the metaphysis, where the nutrient capillaries form sharp loops, predisposes to the establishment of infection following bacteremia.

There are three possible patterns of vascularity.[6] In a child, the nutrient artery terminates in end arteries and capillaries adjacent to the growth plate. An infection of the metaphysis is usually prevented from crossing the growth plate but may progress to septic arthritis depending on the physeal anatomy (Fig. 17-1A). In an adult, the metaphysis and epiphysis are in continuity, and hematogenous osteomyelitis may be primarily metaphyseal or epiphyseal. In an infant, some metaphyseal vessels may penetrate the open growth plate and ramify in the epiphysis. Thus, the infant infection may originate in the metaphysis and have epiphyseal extensions (Fig. 17-1B).[6] It is believed that there is probably a relation between the sites of predilection (proximal tibia, distal femur) and the relative contributions to growth of the physis in those areas.[7] Because of the epiphyseal involvement, secondary intrusion into the joint is more common in the infant and adult than in the child.[6]

The Infectious Process and Its Consequences

The infectious process is characterized by an inflammatory response and the formation of pus within the metaphysis. There is probably impairment of the capillary circulation some 48 h after the beginning of the infection.[8] Pus from the developing metaphyseal abscess gradually finds its way to the subperiosteal region by penetrating through the haversian systems and Volkmann's canals. If the infectious process continues, the subperiosteal abscess strips the periosteum over an extended portion of the diaphysis and circumferentially around the bone (Fig. 17-2). The periosteum may rupture, allowing pus to escape into the adjacent tissues (Fig. 17-1A).

Damage to the metaphyseal blood supply, caused by the release of bacterial toxins and the stripping of the periosteum, results in portions of the bone becoming necrotic. The inner portion of the cortex is supplied by the injured metaphyseal vessels.[6] These portions of dead bone, which are separated from the surrounding viable bone by granulation tissue, are called *sequestra*. The periosteal response is to lay down new bone, called the *involucrum*, which surrounds the infected bone and sequestra (Fig. 17-3). In a fully established infection, defects in the involucrum become *cloacae* through which drainage occurs, establishing sinus tracts. In an advanced case, a major portion of the diaphysis of a long bone may form one large sequestrum, bathed in a lake of subperiosteal pus extending the entire length of the bone. This florid picture is occasionally seen in neonates.

Clinical Features

The first symptom is pain in the region of the infection; the pain is continuous and may be believed to be the result of some recent trauma. There is frequently an association with a recent traumatic injury to the metaphyseal area, which may have predisposed to the infection. Unfortunately, at this stage the child may be given an antibiotic because it is noticed that he or she is febrile. This will in all probability delay timely diagnosis by masking

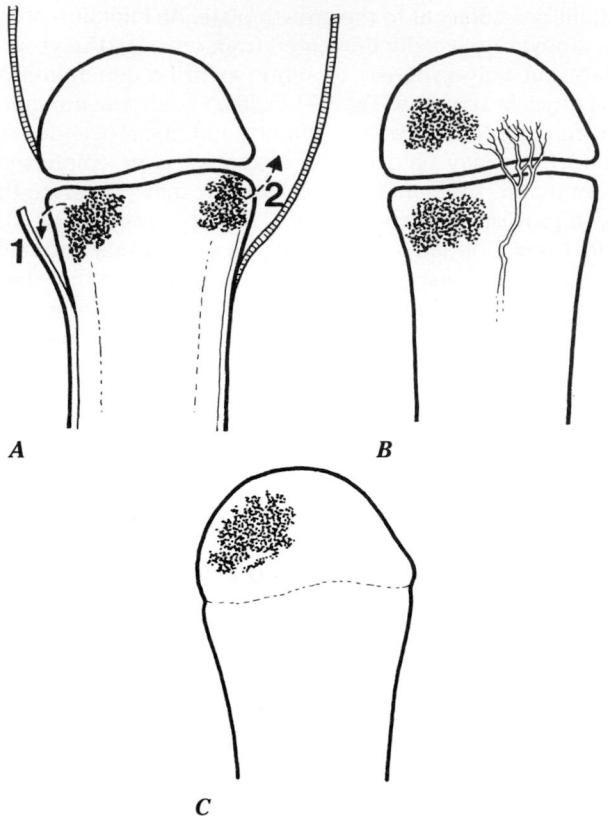

A   *B*

C

Figure 17-1 Sites of hematogenous osteomyelitis of a tubular bone in the child, the infant, and the adult. *A.* In the child, a metaphyseal focus is frequent. From this site cortical penetration can result in a subperiosteal abscess in those locations in which the growth plate is extraarticular (1) or in a septic joint in those locations in which the growth plate is intraarticular (2). *B.* In the infant, a metaphyseal focus may be complicated by epiphyseal extension owing to the vascular anatomy in this age group. *C.* In the adult, a subchondral focus in an epiphysis is not unusual owing to the vascular anatomy in this age group. (Reproduced with permission from Resnick D, Niwayama G: *Diagnosis of Bone and Joint Disorders.* Philadelphia, Saunders, 1981.)

the systemic signs. If antibiotics are not administered, the child will exhibit symptoms and signs consistent with a septic focus. There may be generalized aches and pains, a flushed appearance, and high fever.[3]

The diagnosis is more difficult in neonates and infants who are ill from other causes (e.g., meningitis in the case of *H. influenzae*). These children may be septicemic and have multiple foci of infection, which may be life-threatening. They may need respiratory assistance, be immobile, and be connected to a ventilator. Sometimes the infection is not detected until a large soft tissue abscess is apparent.[2,9,10] They are then at risk for severe long-term complications due to damage to the physis.

Physical Examination

Physical examination shows loss of limb function in all cases. The neonate is observed not to use that limb, and the child holds the limb in a protective attitude. The child

resists motion of the limb, but some movement of the joints can usually be produced with gentle encouragement; this is in contrast with septic arthritis, in which the slightest motion may be excruciating. Local bone tenderness usually points strongly to the diagnosis. It is unusual to be able to elicit fluctuation except in the very late case of untreated disease. There may well be an effusion in the joint, which may indicate a sympathetic reaction in the joint or the complication of coexistent septic arthritis. Soft tissue abscess is accompanied by the usual signs of redness, swelling, and local rise in temperature.

Laboratory Studies

The white blood cell count is usually elevated and the differential shifted to the left, although the count is not as high as that seen in septic arthritis. A range of 7000 to 26,000 was reported by Sullivan et al.[11] A blood smear should be studied to rule out the possibility of leukemia. Mild anemia may be present. The erythrocyte sedimentation rate (ESR) may be normal within the first 48 h but then rises rapidly and may exceed 100 mm/h.[2] The ESR usually remains elevated for weeks. Its gradual decline is an indication of a successful response to treatment.

Blood culture is positive in about 50 to 75 percent of cases.[2,12–15] A positive blood culture can be obtained in 24 h,

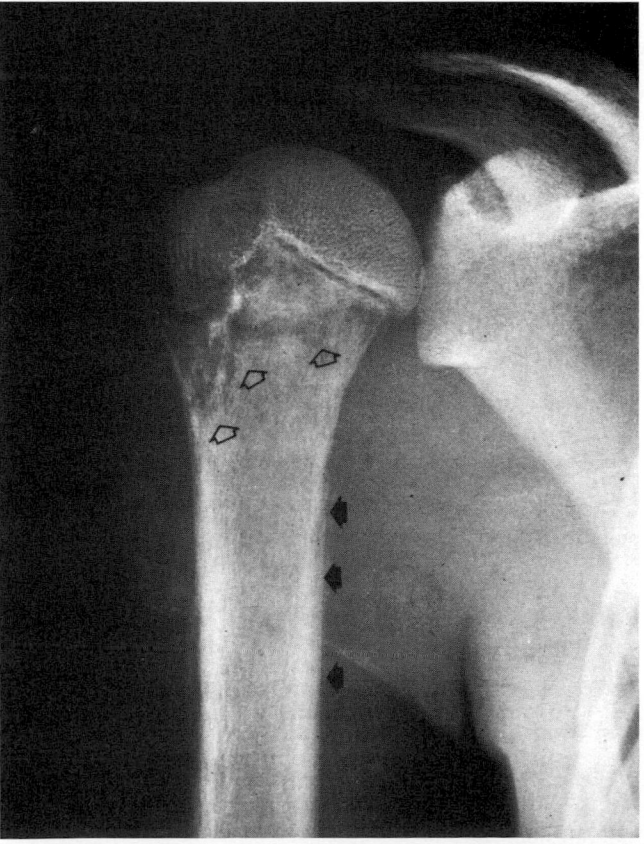

Figure 17-2 Metaphyseal focus in the proximal humerus (*hollow arrows*). Note the periosteal elevation in the diaphysis (*solid arrows*).

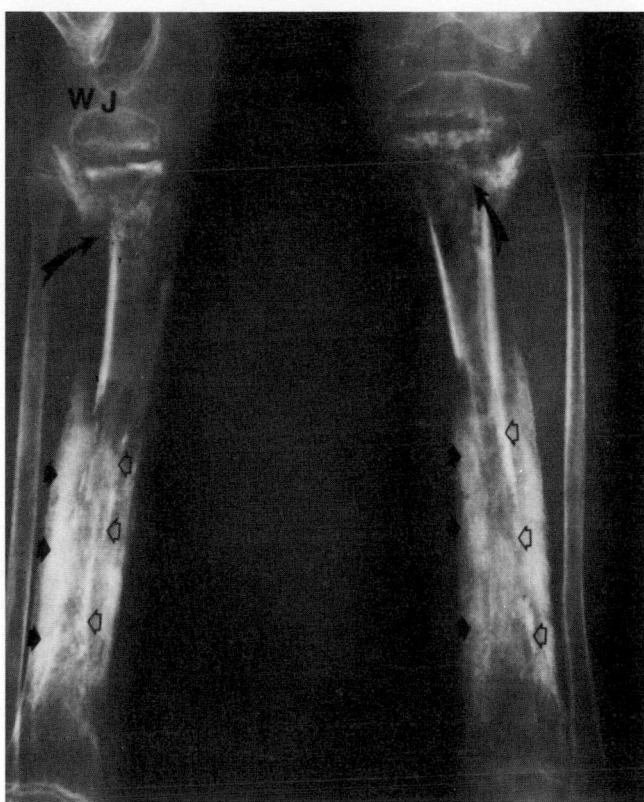

Figure 17-3 Chronic osteomyelitis in a child. The diaphyseal cortex is becoming sequestrated (*hollow arrows*). There is a prominent involucrum (*solid arrows*) and a pathologic fracture proximally (*curved arrows*).

but more time is required for determining specific antibiotic sensitivity. Other tests that may occasionally be helpful include the anti–streptolysin O titer and C-reactive protein. The anti–alpha hemolysin titer is normal in more than 50 percent of patients with staphylococcal osteomyelitis and so is of limited value as a test.[16] Although not a sensitive test for septic arthritis, the detection of antibodies (C-reactive protein) to the teichoic acid cell wall of *S. aureus* has been found valuable for detecting staphylococcal osteomyelitis, especially the acute variety. The test seems to be more sensitive in acute (82 percent) than in chronic (43 percent) osteomyelitis. Gel diffusion technique is used to determine the antibody titer in a specimen of serum that has been found to be positive by counterimmunoelectrophoresis.[17]

Radiographic Studies

Within the first 2 to 3 days, a careful evaluation may show some deep soft tissue swelling in the region of the bone adjacent to the metaphyseal lesion.[18] The soft tissue swelling is identified by displacement of the fat lines that normally parallel the bony surfaces between the muscle planes. Often comparison films are necessary for diagnosis.[3,19] Multiple sites of infection are common in neonates.

Radiographically detectable demineralization does not occur in less than 10 days and is usually first seen as single or multiple areas within the medullary canal, reflecting trabecular destruction. Penetration of the cortex leads to periosteal changes, which may be seen as early as 3 or as late as 6 weeks.[19]

Radionuclide Imaging

Confirmatory bone scan should not be necessary if the diagnosis is clinically obvious, and under no circumstances should appropriate treatment be delayed while awaiting such a test.[3] Technetium 99m–labeled methylene diphosphonate (^{99m}Tc-MDP) can be used to differentiate osteomyelitis from overlying soft tissue lesions. The three-phase bone scan shows a well-defined increase in uptake in the bone on both the blood-pool and the delayed scan. The blood-pool phase (phase 2) shows the relative vascularity of an area, whereas the delayed image phase (phase 3) obtained 3 to 4 h after the injection reflects increased uptake in the skeleton. By contrast with the well-defined bone uptake seen in osteomyelitis, there is rather diffuse uptake in cellulitis and septic arthritis, in the former case into the soft tissue and in the latter case into the region of the joint on blood-pool and delayed scans. Scintigraphy with technetium, although showing positive before the radiographs, nevertheless has only a 77 percent accuracy rate in differentiating between cellulitis, osteomyelitis, and septic arthritis.[11] There may be preferential uptake in periosteal new bone of whatever cause and also in normal physis (which will tend to obscure an adjacent lesion). False positives can occur when changes in bone metabolism or vascularity from other causes lead to increased uptake. Bone scanning often gives false positives in the hands and feet and has been pronounced to be valueless in neonatal osteomyelitis.[10,11]

Because the uptake of gallium citrate labeled with gallium 67 (^{67}Ga) is due to the local accumulation of white cells, particularly polymorphonuclear leukocytes (as well as various labeled serum proteins),[20] this isotope has been used sequentially following the technetium scan to increase the specificity of the test.[21–24] The technetium scan is followed by a 48-h ^{67}Ga gallium citrate scan. An accumulation of both isotopes in the same region of bone is highly suggestive of infection, with an accuracy of 62 percent.[25] However, other conditions, such as a local fracture, can give the same appearance. Patients with septic arthritis show an increased periarticular uptake of ^{99m}Tc-MDP and diffuse gallium concentration around the joint. Patients with cellulitis show an abnormal concentration of gallium in the soft tissue, with minimal uptake of the other isotope.

Gallium citrate has a high sensitivity to infectious inflammatory processes but a variable and unpredictable sensitivity to other inflammatory conditions, which may be noninfective. The ^{67}Ga scan is therefore not helpful if the results are not taken in conjunction with the use of technetium. A problem associated with the use of technetium is the occurrence of "cold spots." These are photopenic areas of diminished activity associated with damaged vascularity of portions of the bone or compression of the vasculature by elevated intraarticular pressures associated with joint effusions.[26] If these are misinterpreted, they will be responsible for false-negative diagnosis.

A third radionuclide scanning method has been employed using leukocytes prepared from a sample of the patient's blood and labeled with indium 111 (^{111}In). This technique avoids the false positives seen with the technetium technique (which may be sensitive to fractures, bone tumors, heterotopic ossification, and arthritis) and the gallium technique (which may give false-positive results in tumors and other forms of inflammatory disease). The initial problem with the indium technique was the length of time that it took to prepare the white cells (not appropriate in a sick child). It is now possible to prepare and reinject ^{111}In-labeled leukocytes in a few hours. This technique appears to be more accurate and easier to interpret than sequential Tc-Ga scanning.[25] Because of the radiation exposure, many pediatricians do not use either the gallium or the indium scan in the diagnosis of acute hematogenous osteomyelitis in children, but the indium scan certainly has great utility in the general area of musculoskeletal sepsis, with a reported sensitivity of 83 percent, specificity of 86 percent, and an accuracy of 83 percent.[25]

Magnetic Resonance Imaging

In the early stage of osteomyelitis, the MRI will show intraosseous and extraosseous changes. These changes are evident before any that may be seen on routine x-ray films. The technique is more useful than other tests such as bone scans and computed tomography (CT) in differentiating the extent of bone marrow abnormalities, but it lacks specificity in determining whether the abnormalities are indeed due to osteomyelitis. The changes are a normal or increased signal intensity on T2-weighted images and a decrease on T1-weighted images as marrow fat is replaced by inflammatory cells.[27–29]

Aspiration and Biopsy

Once the clinical diagnosis of acute osteomyelitis is made, an aspiration of the bone should be performed to identify the pathogen. All material obtained from aspiration should be sent for Gram stain, aerobic and anaerobic culture, as well as fungal and mycobacterial culture in the appropriate clinical setting. Blood cultures should also be obtained. Approximately 80 percent of patients will have a positive aspiration culture and about 50 percent of children will have positive blood cultures.[30,31]

Although aspiration in the early stage of disease may fail to obtain any fluid or pus, it is particularly valuable in obtaining the infecting organism in the presence of a subperiosteal abscess. There is danger that the pus may be so thick that aspiration, even with a fairly large needle, is not productive. A negative aspiration should not rule out the diagnosis. Even a small amount of pus is valuable for culture and Gram stain. A needle bone biopsy is usually not appropriate in acute osteomyelitis unless there is reason to suspect the possibility of malignancy in the differential diagnosis.

Treatment

Resuscitation of a sick, dehydrated child is commenced in the usual way with appropriate intravenous liquids. Blood is sent to the laboratory for the procedure already described.

Oral or parenteral antibiotics in doses adequate to provide satisfactory blood and bone levels are the cornerstones of treatment.[32] The choice of initial antimicrobial agents depends on the most likely organisms encountered, the age of the patient, and whether the patient has any known allergies (Table 17-1). *Staphylococcus aureus* is the most common cause of acute hematogenous osteomyelitis in both children over age 1 and adults; therefore initial therapy should cover this pathogen. Antibiotics with excellent antistaphylococcal coverage include nafcillin, oxacillin, first-generation cephalosporins—i.e., cefazolin—and the third-generation drugs cefotaxime, cefoperazone, ceftizoxime, clindamycin, imipenem, minocycline, or vancomycin. In the penicillin-allergic patient who does not tolerate cephalosporins, clindamycin, imipenem, minocycline, or vancomycin provide safe alternative therapy. Once the culture results become available, the antibiotic is changed according to the sensitivity panel.

In neonates and young infants, the major pathogens are group B streptococci, *S. aureus,* and *Escherichia coli;* therefore empiric therapy with either a combination of oxacillin and gentamicin or any third-generation cephalosporin such as cefotaxime or ceftizoxime should be employed. The most common organisms causing osteomyelitis in children with sickle cell disease are *S. aureus* and *Salmonella,* and empiric use of a third-generation cephalosporin would be appropriate. Quinolones such as ciprofloxacin and ofloxacin have excellent activity against *Salmonella* but should not be used in children. In a recent review of cases of osteomyelitis at a sickle cell anemia clinic, *Salmonella* was the causative agent in 13 of 16 cases of osteomyelitis.[33] The recommended dosage of antibiotics for children and adults for the treatment of acute osteomyelitis is shown in Table 17-2. The minimum duration of therapy for acute osteomyelitis is 4 to 6 weeks, since there is a failure rate of close to 20 percent for children treated for 3 weeks or less.[30] The duration of parenteral therapy is controversial, with a recent trend toward administering a 3-week course of intravenous antibiotics followed by 3 weeks of oral antibiotics.[27] However, if appropriate serum and bone concentrations are obtained using oral antibiotics, there is no need for any particular duration of intravenous therapy.[34] Antibiotics should be continued until there is a successful response to therapy—i.e., the patient becomes afebrile, the white blood cell count returns to normal, the ESR has decreased by 20 percent or more, and there is improvement in local signs and symptoms.

Laboratory facilities must be available for measuring bactericidal levels of antibiotics in the patient's blood after oral administration. Levels are measured after dilution of serum drawn before and after ingestion of oral antibiotic. If bactericidal levels are present in a postdose dilution of 1:8, the dose is thought to be adequate.[5]

Role of Oral Antibiotics

Several papers have documented the treatment of acute osteomyelitis using only oral antibiotics.[34,35] The criteria

TABLE 17-1 Empiric Antimicrobial Therapy for Acute Osteomyelitis

Patient characteristic	Most likely pathogen(s)	Antibiotics
Infant <1 year	Group B streptococcus *Staphylococcus aureus* *Escherichia coli*	Cefazolin *or* cefotaxime *or* ceftizoxime
Children (1–16 years), no underlying disease	*S. aureus* *Streptococcus pyogenes* *Haemophilus influenzae*	Cefazolin *or* ceftizoxime
Sickle cell disease	*S. aureus* *Salmonella*	Cefotaxime *or* ceftizoxime
Penicillin-allergic	*S. aureus*	Clindamycin *or* vancomycin
Adults	*S. aureus*	Nafcillin *or* minocycline *or* clindamycin
	E. coli *Serratia marcescens*	Cefotaxime *or* ceftizoxime
	Pseudomonas aeruginosa	Piperacillin *or* ceftazidime *or* ciprofloxacin *and* gentamicin

TABLE 17-2 Acute Osteomyelitis Antimicrobial Drug Dosage for Parenteral Therapy

Drug	Dose in children	Dose in adults[a]
Nafcillin	100–200 mg/kg per day in 4–6 doses	2 g (IV) q4h
Oxacillin	100–200 mg/kg per day in 4 doses	2 g (IV) q4h
Cefotaxime	100–200 mg/kg per day in 4–6 doses	2 g (IV) q6h
Ceftizoxime	150–200 mg/kg per day in 4 doses	2 g (IV) q8h
Clindamycin	40 mg/kg per day in 3–4 doses	600 mg (IV) q8h
Vancomycin	40 mg/kg per day in 2–4 doses	1 g (IV) q12h
Cefazolin	100 mg/kg per day in 3–4 doses	1 g (IV) q8h
Gentamicin	5.0–7.5 mg/kg per day in 2–3 doses	5–7.5 mg/kg q24h

[a]Assumes normal renal function.

outlined above must be met, particularly the ability to measure minimal inhibitory and bactericidal concentrations of antibiotic in the blood and a certain identification of the appropriate organism. The use of a high-dose cephalexin to treat staphylococcal osteomyelitis following a week of parenteral therapy is a regime that offers many advantages if it can be shown over the long term that the results are as satisfactory as more traditional methods.[35] Oral antibiotics have a role in gram-negative infections, especially those due to *H. influenzae, E. coli,* and *Proteus mirabilis,* where treatment with an oral quinolone provides optimal therapy.[36]

TABLE 17-3   Oral Antibiotic Dosages in Children

Drug	Dosage
Amoxicillin	100 mg/kg per day in 3–4 doses
Cephalexin	150 mg/kg per day in 4 doses
Cefaclor	150 mg/kg per day in 4 doses
Clindamycin	40 mg/kg per day in 3 doses
Penicillin V	125 mg/kg per day in 6 doses

Recommendations of oral antibiotic regimens are shown in Table 17-3. In order to achieve acceptable serum and bone levels with β-lactam antibiotics, the oral dose is often larger than that recommended in the package insert.[30] However, oral and intravenous administration of trimethoprim-sulfamethoxazole, minocycline, quinolones, or clindamycin provide the same blood/tissue levels. This eliminates any advantage to using these drugs intravenously. Moreover, oral regimens are much less costly and are not associated with nosocomial infectious complications, such as infection of the intravenous line.

Immobilization

During treatment, the affected limb is immobilized to diminish pain. A well-padded posterior mold can be used. Occasionally some form of skin traction is required. For ambulant therapy, a cast brace or one-leg hip spica enables the patient to ambulate with the aid of a walker or a pair of crutches. Protective splintage is continued in the upper limb until antibiotic therapy is terminated. In the lower limb, it is continued for an additional 4 to 6 weeks. The average overall length of time for antibiotic therapy is 6 weeks.

Surgical Procedures

Failure to respond to treatment after 36 h probably means that pus is present in the metaphysis and possibly in the subperiosteal region. Occasionally the patient presents late with osteomyelitis that has been ineffectively treated. Radiologic examination may show areas of bony change, and abscess formation or pus may be obtained by aspiration. Surgical drainage of any intramedullary or subperiosteal abscess is required in these patients without further delay.

With the patient under general anesthesia, a pneumatic tourniquet is applied to the affected limb; the tourniquet should be inflated only if absolutely necessary. The extremity should not be exsanguinated with an elastic bandage, as this procedure may release showers of bacteria into the systemic circulation.

If the adjacent joint is swollen, it is aspirated before any surgical incision, since it may be involved and require drainage. Otherwise its contamination must be scrupulously avoided. The bone is exposed at the site of maximum tenderness and swelling, and the periosteum is incised longitudinally. Pus is evacuated, and specimens are obtained for a Gram stain, cultures, and tests for antibiotic sensitivity. Any devitalized soft tissue is excised, and the entire area is then irrigated with several liters of normal saline. Some authors do not recommend drilling the cortex to explore the metaphysis, since it is their view that pus under pressure is rarely found inside the medulla.[2] They believe that the concept of decompressing the medulla and improving the blood flow is unlikely to be of much benefit, since, in the presence of a large subperiosteal abscess, any bone death has already occurred. It is, however, worthwhile drilling any obviously soft areas in the cortex or performing intraosseous aspiration.

The skin may be loosely closed but provision made for free drainage through appropriate surgical drains. The value of closed suction drainage with continuous intramedullary irrigation remains to be proved.[37,38] This technique consists of inserting a perforated plastic catheter through a large hole in the medullary canal; the tip of the catheter is then brought up through a separate hole so that its major portion, which is perforated, lies within the medullary cavity. The periosteum is left open, and an additional outflow catheter is placed in the subperiosteal space. The inflow and outflow tubes are brought out through separate stab incisions in the skin, and the skin is closed around these incisions to prevent leakage of fluid. A supply of irrigating fluid is connected to the inflow tube, which provides continuous flow under gravity at a rate of 500 mL each 8-h period. This irrigation is continued for 4 to 5 days. If the outflow tube becomes plugged by debris, however, it is discontinued. In spite of careful precautions, this technique seems to invite the possibility of secondary infection. For this reason it is probably not applicable in acute osteomyelitis, though it certainly may have a place in the treatment of more chronic infections. It is important that the limb be immobilized during this treatment in such a way that the wound may be frequently observed.

Prognosis and Complications

Acute hematogenous osteomyelitis is curable provided there is early diagnosis and prompt treatment with the correct antibiotic for the correct period of time. Any other course of action affects prognosis negatively. Factors such as host resistance and virulence of the infecting organism also play their part.[3]

The risk of recurrence depends on the site of the infection and the time interval between the onset of symptoms and the beginning of appropriate treatment.[35] Metatarsal lesions have the highest rate of failure, with a 50 percent recurrence rate.[32] Failure rates of 20 to 30 percent have been cited for involvement of the metaphysis in distal femur and proximal and distal tibia, with a more favorable outcome for lesions involving the lower end of the fibula and bones of the upper extremity and spine.[32] Cole and coworkers observed that the prognosis for cure is much worse in patients diagnosed late (25 percent) than in those diagnosed early, in whom the cure rate was 92 percent in the authors' series. The risk of recurrence is below 4 percent 1 year following treatment.[39]

In neonates, involvement of an adjacent joint is common in the proximal humerus and shoulder joint because of the anatomy of the vasculature in this age group and also because of the intracapsular position of the physis. Irreversible damage to the physis and joint may result.[2,9,40] Damage to the physis can result in overgrowth as well as growth retardation.[41,42] Leg-length discrepancy and angular deformity can result. Bowing of the forearm or leg may result because of retardation of growth in an affected bone, with relative overgrowth of its parallel companion.

Pathologic fracture may be caused by resorption of bone either in the acute phase or following surgery and decompression by drill holes through the cortex. A preventive splint or cast for an appropriate period of 2 to 3 months is indicated. This complication is seen more often in chronic osteomyelitis.

SUBACUTE OSTEOMYELITIS

In subacute osteomyelitis the patient may present with a painful limp, and radiologic examination unexpectedly reveals a well-established lesion visible in the bone. The patient is not systemically ill and often has had no previous complaints. There may be no local signs of infection.[43,44] Alternatively there may be clinical signs of subperiosteal pus, synovitis, or pus within a joint.[44] There may be an elevation of the white blood cell count and the ESR, but in half the cases laboratory results are normal.[43] The femur and the tibia are by far the commonest bones affected.

Radiographic Findings: Brodie's Abscess

Certain localized radiolucencies in the tibia, developing silently without any systemic signs and without previous febrile illness, were described by Brodie in 1836.[45] They are common in metaphyses of tubular bones, particularly the tibia, but may also occur occasionally in flat bones, vertebral bodies, and even the diaphysis (Fig. 17-4). They are usually manifestations of subacute osteomyelitis classified by Gledhill into four types depending on location and radiographic manifestation.[46] A type I lesion is a solitary metaphyseal-area lesion that may communicate with the epiphysis.[46] The lesion consists of a solitary cavity that has been walled off, so that a ring of sclerotic reactive new bone is seen. A type II lesion is a radiolucent lesion located in the metaphysis not surrounded by reactive sclerotic bone but with adjacent loss of the cortex. A type III lesion is a diaphyseal lesion associated with cortical hypertrophy and periosteal or endosteal new bone. Radiolucent zones within such an area of hyperostosis can be detected by tomography. These lesions may be confused with osteoid osteoma. A type IV lesion is associated with layers of subperiosteal new bone formation, which, on x-ray views, give an onionskin appearance such as that seen in early Ewing's sarcoma. There is cortical hyperostosis, and careful evaluation of the x-ray film may show intramedullary radiolucency.

SUBACUTE EPIPHYSEAL OSTEOMYELITIS

Green and colleagues believe that there is an entity called primary *subacute epiphyseal osteomyelitis.*[43] They point out that the blood supply of the epiphysis has hemody-

Figure 17-4 *A* and *B.* Anteroposterior and lateral radiographs outline a typical appearance of an abscess of the distal tibia due to staphylococci. Observe the elongated radiolucent lesion with surrounding sclerosis (*arrows*). This extends to the closing growth plate. The channel-like shape of the lesion is important in the diagnosis of this condition. (Reproduced with permission from Resnick D, Niwayama G: *Diagnosis of Bone and Joint Disorders.* Philadelphia, Saunders, 1981.)

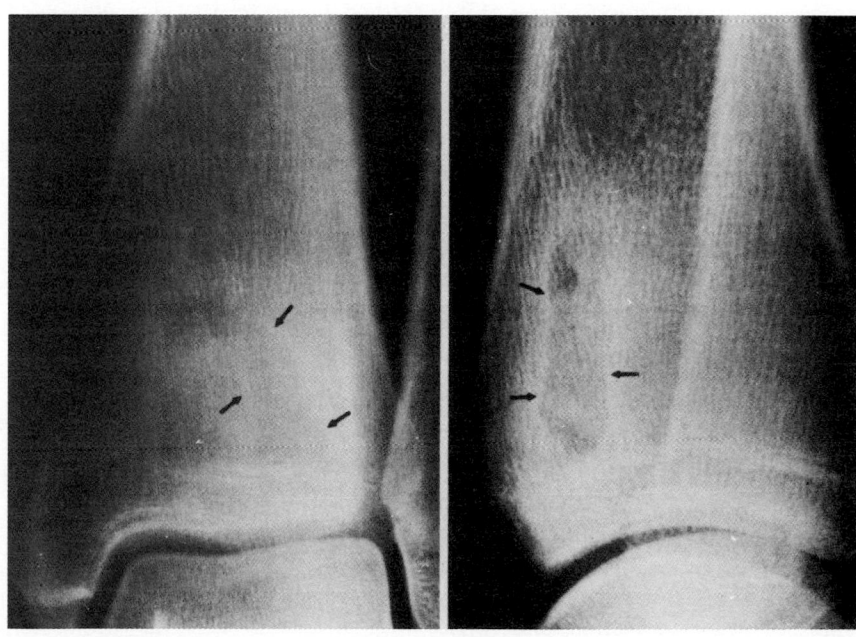

A   *B*

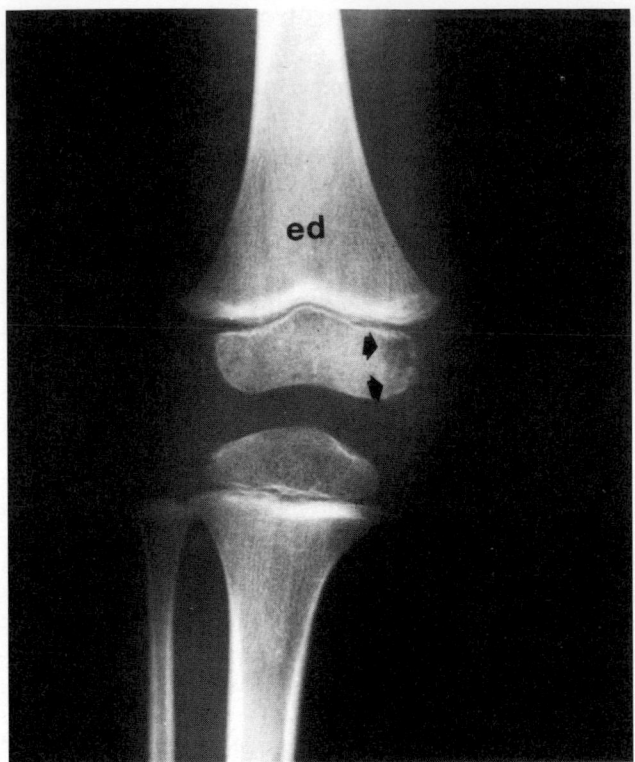

Figure 17-5 Primary epiphyseal subacute osteomyelitis. Note the sclerotic reaction around the lytic focus (*solid arrows*).

namic features, including sluggish blood flow and vascular loops, which make it equivalent to the metaphysis in its susceptibility to infection (Fig. 17-5). They identified lesions of the epiphysis that did not communicate with the metaphysis either radiologically or when examined with a probe during surgery. They pointed out that when a subacute metaphyseal lesion crosses the physis, the communication is always apparent. Ross and Cole also identified some cavities confined to the epiphysis and noted that these were eccentric and were either circular or oval.[44] Half of them had a fine sclerotic margin. Such lesions were occasionally found in the talus, where they sometimes eroded the subchondral bone plate of the ankle joint. Other presentations of this disease identified by these authors were patients with cavities communicating between metaphysis and epiphysis and other patients with aggressive lesions that had clinical, radiologic, and hematologic features indistinguishable from those of primary malignant bone tumors such as Ewing's sarcoma.[44] They stressed the need to exclude such lesions as simple bone cysts, aneurysmal bone cysts, fibrous cortical defect, chondroblastoma, or chondromyxoid fibroma.

Staphylococcus aureus is the only organism causing this pathologic entity. The recommended treatment for these patients without signs of pus in the subperiosteal layer or in the joint is administration of an antistaphylococcal antibiotic and immobilization without operation. Intravenous antibiotics for 48 h followed by oral drugs for 6 weeks is satisfactory.[44] However, in patients who have signs of pus, the lesions should be surgically drained. Green and coworkers described a technique of locating the epiphyseal lesion by using two-plane x-ray views.[43] They first inserted a needle into the lesion and then drilled it from within the joint capsule, avoiding the articular surface and the physis.

Ross and Cole report that opening and gently curetting metaphyseal lesions was successful in healing these cavities. Although the curetted tissue showed the characteristic appearance of osteomyelitis, more than half the patients did not grow an organism. These authors believe that epiphyseal lesions heal without surgery.[44] They gave interesting information on the healing process, noting that there are two observed patterns. In the first, the growth plate grows away from the entire metaphyseal cavity, indicating that it is functioning normally. In the second pattern of healing, the growth plate grows away from the body of the cavity, but a channel-like communication with the physis remains for several months (Fig. 17-6B). Occasionally a small sequestrum persists and prevents complete healing of the cavity (Fig. 17-6C). Growth arrest lines and defects in the epiphysis or metaphysis can result.[44]

CHRONIC OSTEOMYELITIS

Etiology

Inappropriately treated, acute hematogenous osteomyelitis can become chronic in adults and children (Figs. 17-3 and 17-7). Pertinent factors include the degree of bone necrosis, the general nutritional status of the involved tissues, and the nature of the infecting organism. Certain risk categories of patients include the old, the debilitated, and intravenous drug users. Chronic osteomyelitis may also occur following surgery or penetrating trauma. The disease may be a sequel to an open fracture, which may then successfully unite or proceed to nonunion.[47]

The adjacent soft tissues are involved in all forms of osteomyelitis with the exception of the Brodie abscess. The etiologic term *contiguous focus infection* describes the occurrence of bone infection secondary to soft tissue

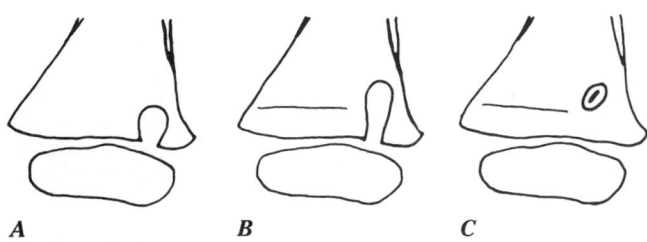

A   *B*   *C*

Figure 17-6 Diagrams to show possible outcomes of treatment of subacute osteomyelitic cavities in the lower end of the femur. *A*. Drawn from a typical preoperative x-ray view following the failure of conservative treatment. Possible sequelae include (*B*), continuing enlargement of the metaphyseal cavity, the mouth of which remains open (there is a growth arrest line), or (*C*), in which case the cavity has failed to heal completely but no longer communicates with the physis. Failure to heal is here associated with presence of a sequestrum. (Reproduced with permission from Ross ER, Coel WG: *J Bone Joint Surg* 67B:443–447, 1985.)

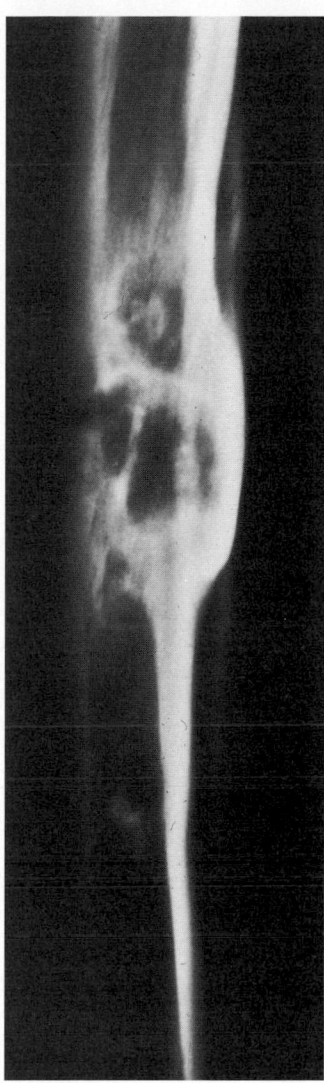

Figure 17-7 Chronic osteomyelitis in an adult tibia, stage IV (see also Fig. 17-8). Note that this multiloculated bony cavity has a sequestrum proximally lying within a separate sclerotic cavity. The separate area of sclerosis distally represents a pin track, which was also infected with gram-negative organisms. Treatment required radical debridement and a free myocutaneous flap.

breakdown.[47] This may occur in patients with vascular disease or other conditions such as diabetes. Steroid therapy, tobacco abuse, immune deficiency, and malnutrition are other factors that predispose to secondary osteitis following soft tissue lesions not initially affecting the bone.[47] However, chronic hematogenous osteomyelitis accounts for at least one-third of the cases of chronic osteomyelitis.[48]

Infecting Organisms

The infecting organism depends on the underlying cause of the chronic osteomyelitis (Table 17-4). Chronic osteomyelitis resulting from nonresolving acute hematogenous osteomyelitis is almost always due to *S. aureus* in both children and adults. Chronic osteomyelitis occurring after trauma, postoperative infection, or soft tissue infections can be polymicrobial, but *S. aureus* still remains an important pathogen. Coagulase-negative staphylococcus (*S. epidermidis*) is a major pathogen causing osteomyelitis in the presence of a prosthetic joint or other foreign material. In the last decade, gram-negative organisms have played an increasing role in the pathogenesis of both acute and chronic bone infection. Gram-negative organisms are now isolated from approximately 50 percent of patients with chronic osteomyelitis.[49] Osteomyelitis secondary to contiguous focus infection in the presence of vascular disease, as in patients with infected diabetic or ischemic foot ulcers, is almost always polymicrobial. Osteomyelitis from an infected sacral decubitus ulcer may also be due to multiple organisms, including streptococcus, *E. coli, Proteus mirabilis,* and *B. fragilis. Pseudomonas aeruginosa* is an important pathogen in osteomyelitis, occurring after a puncture wound of the foot but not in decubitus ulcers in diabetics. A number of unusual gram-negative organisms such as *Pasteurella multocida* or *Capnocytophaga,* along with *S. aureus* and streptococcus, may cause chronic osteomyelitis after a dog or cat bite. An increasing number of joint prosthesis infections are fungal.

Late Complications

Constant drainage in chronic osteomyelitis causes irritation and destruction of the adjacent skin and soft tissues. An eczematous reaction or neoplastic change may follow.[50,51] The skin may become thin, desquamate, and easily traumatized. The epithelium of the skin edge grows inward into the margins of the sinus tract. Epidermoid carcinoma may develop at any point along the fistulous tract and is present in at least 0.5 percent of patients with long-term drainage.[6] Other tumors that may occur include fibrosarcoma, angiosarcoma, rhabdomyosarcoma and adenocarcinoma, basal cell carcinoma, and plasmacytoma. Amyloidosis is a complication that now seems to be infrequent, probably because of improved treatment of this condition.[6]

The prognosis without curative treatment depends upon many factors. A continuously draining sinus and concomitant joint involvement or an infection that has been of long duration is a negative prognostic factor.[52] The sinus tract may close following the spontaneous discharge of a sequestrum, and the disease may be quiescent for a while. However, after a period of stability in the relationship between bacteria and host, following a deterioration in the patient's local resistance or some local trauma, another cycle of activity is initiated, with the formation of another abscess or period of offensive discharge.

Staging

Cierny and Mader and coworkers have classified chronic osteomyelitis into four types.[47,53,54] Type I is medullary osteomyelitis, in which the infected nidus is endosteal. Type II is superficial osteomyelitis, secondary to a breakdown in the soft tissue envelope overlying the bone which is re-

TABLE 17-4 Most Likely Pathogens Causing Chronic Osteomyelitis

Etiology	Infecting organisms	Initial empiric therapy
Acute hematogenous osteomyelitis	*Staphylococcus aureus*	Nafcillin *or* oxacillin
Posttraumatic	*S. aureus* Streptococci Gram-negative bacilli	Cefotaxime *or* ceftizoxime *or* ampicillin-sulbactam
Postoperative infection	*S. aureus* Gram-negative bacilli	Cefotaxime *or* ceftizoxime
Prosthetic device infection	*Staphylococcus epidermidis* *S. aureus* Gram-negative bacilli	Vancomycin *and* gentamicin
Soft tissue infection	*S. aureus* Streptococci Anaerobes Gram-negative bacilli	Cefotaxime *or* ceftizoxime *or* ampicillin-sulbactam
Puncture wound of foot	*Pseudomonas aeruginosa* *S. aureus*	Ciprofloxacin *or* ceftazidime *and* gentamicin
Dog/cat bites	*Pasteurella multocida* *Capnocytophaga* (DF2) *S. aureus* Streptococci	Ampicillin-sulbactam *or* imipenem
Diabetic ulcer	*S. aureus* Streptococci Enterococci Gram-negative bacilli Anaerobes	Ceftizoxime *or* cefotaxime *or* ampicillin-sulbactam *or* clindamycin *plus* gentamicin *or* clindamycin *plus* ofloxacin
Infected decubitus ulcer	*S. aureus* *Proteus mirabilis* *Enterobacter* *E. coli* Streptococci Anaerobes	Cefotaxime *or* ampicillin-sulbactam
Sickle cell disease	*Salmonella* *S. aureus*	Ofloxacin *or* cefotaxime
Intravenous drug users	*S. aureus* *P. aeruginosa* *Serratia marcescens*	Nafcillin *and* gentamicin
Human bites/clenched fist injury	*Eikenella corrodens*	Ampicillin-sulbactam *or* imipenem

fractory to treatment (Fig. 17-8). There is involvement of the periosteum and cortex. In type III disease, there is localized involvement of both the medulla and cortex of a segment of bone with or without soft tissue involvement. There may be a fistulous tract and cloacae in the bone. In type IV osteomyelitis, the bone is diffusely involved, and the bone or limb is unstable or becomes so at the conclusion of the debridement treatment procedure.[54]

It is important to identify those factors in the host, both local and systemic, that will alter the treatment plan and are of significance in the prognosis. Patients may be categorized as "A host," "B host," or "C host." An A host is a normal, otherwise healthy patient who can tolerate the treatment proposed. A C host, by contrast, has numerous factors that may lead to a decision to amputate or suppress the infection and not aggressively seek to eradicate

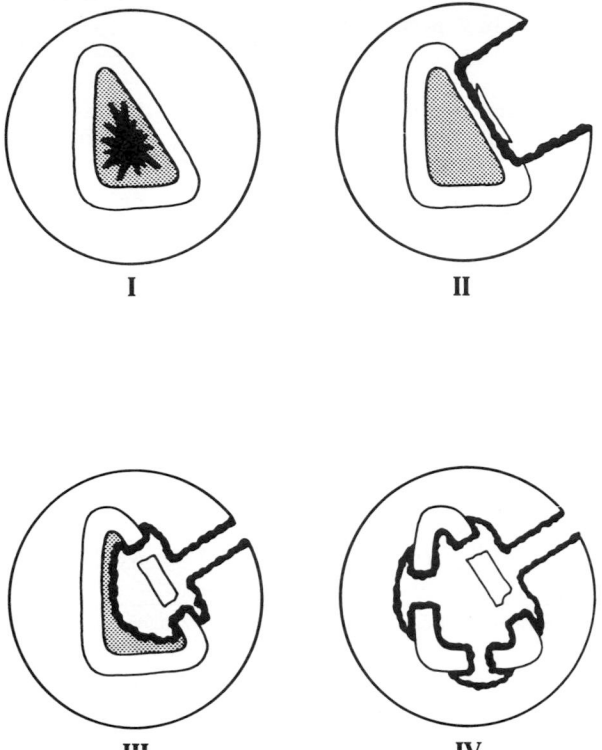

Figure 17-8 The four types of chronic osteomyelitis shown diagrammatically. (Reproduced with permission from Cierny G III, Mader JT: *Orthopaedics* 7:10, 1984.)

it by other means. The B host is also compromised by systemic or local factors that will make treatment more difficult. Compromised hosts may demonstrate adverse local factors such as major vessel disease, extensive scarring, chronic lymphedema, or venous insufficiency. There may be adverse systemic problems such as a past or present history of smoking, malnutrition, or immune deficiency. Other adverse systemic conditions are chronic hypoxia, diabetes, renal failure, malignancy, old age, and so on.[54]

Surgical Debridement

The first stage of surgical treatment following biopsy and culture is a thorough debridement to remove all devitalized and infected material. Good intraoperative tissue biopsies are obtained for reliable culture, so that the appropriate antibiotic may be selected. In type I disease, cortical unroofing is usually required to remove the infected medullary material. The bone deficiency may create a dead space requiring closure, perhaps with a local muscle flap (see later in this chapter). In type II, a shallow decortication of partial thickness of the cortex is sufficient, together with renewal of all damaged overlying soft tissue.[53] It is important that any cortical bone remaining is viable and can be seen to bleed during the surgical procedure. In type II infections, the integrity of the bone is usually preserved. Local transpositions and free tissue transfers may be required to obtain soft tissue coverage.

In the type III situation, the medullary component of the disease must be thoroughly eradicated, as well as the overlying infected soft tissues. Saucerization of the bone by removal of a generous piece of cortex is required to allow access to the medulla, and all sequestra are also removed. Following completion of the debridement, the area is thoroughly irrigated. If there is risk of the residual bone fracturing and of producing future instability, it may be necessary to stabilize the bone by use of an external fixator. In type IV disease, the infected area is usually excised en bloc.[53,54] There is often instability at the conclusion of the aggressive debridement (which unfortunately is essential if one is to have any chance of curing these well-established infections). Stabilization can again be achieved with an external fixator. Antibiotic-impregnated beads may be placed into the defect as a temporary measure before subsequent definitive attempts to close the defect. Once the area is cured of osteomyelitis by such aggressive surgery, the limb bones and joints can be reconstructed safely using intramedullary (IM) rods, custom prostheses, and even structural allografts in the appropriate host (Cierny G III: personal communication).

Management

Bacterial Investigation in Chronic Osteomyelitis

Sinus tract cultures do not usually reflect the bacteria infecting the bone. The depths of the wound or sinus at the very least should be curetted, but bone biopsy is preferable. Aerobic and anaerobic cultures are necessary. Superficial, subcutaneous biopsies may be performed on an ambulant basis. Additionally, material obtained during surgical debridement is invaluable. Histologic preparations are useful. They identify secondary neoplasms and fungal and granulomatous infections. If the histologic findings are consistent with chronic infection but the culture is negative, it may be that the organism was lost during the attempt at culture, it may be an anaerobe, or there may have been some technical error. If the biopsy material and histologic findings do not suggest infection, a positive culture on meat broth medium alone may well be the result of a contaminant. Histologic examination of intraoperative frozen sections from periprosthetic tissue is a reliable method for diagnosing active infection during revision total joint arthroplasty. More than five polymorph nuclear leukocytes per high-power field in such sections is presumptive evidence of infection, but false positives may be obtained in inflammatory joint disease such as rheumatoid arthritis.[55]

Antibiotic Therapy

Antibiotic selection should be based on the antimicrobial susceptibility panel of the infecting organism. Since prolonged therapy is necessary in the treatment of chronic osteomyelitis, the antibiotic chosen should be nontoxic, convenient to administer, and cost-effective.[56]

The antibiotic should penetrate bone in a sufficient concentration to inhibit the infecting pathogen.[49] Since

TABLE 17-5 Infected Bone Concentrations after Antibiotic Administration in Experimental *Staphylococcus aureus* Osteomyelitis

Antibiotic	Serum, μg/mL	Infected bone, μg/g	Percent of serum levels
Clindamycin (70 mg/kg)	12.1 = 0.6	11.9 ± 1.9	98.3
Vancomycin (30 mg/kg)	36.4 = 4.6	05.3 ± 0.8	14.5
Nafcillin (40 mg/kg)	21.8 = 4.6	02.1 ± 0.3	09.6
Tobramycin (5 mg/kg)	14.3 = 1.3	01.3 ± 0.1	09.1
Cefazolin (15 mg/kg)	67.2 = 2.6	04.1 ± 0.7	06.1
Cefazolin (5 mg/kg)	45.6 = 3.2	02.6 ± 0.2	05.7
Cephalothin (40 mg/kg)	34.8 = 2.8	01.3 ± 0.2	03.7

Source: Reproduced with permission from Mader JT, Calhoun J: Osteomyelitis, in Mandell GL, Bennett JE, Dolin R (eds): *Principles and Practice of Infectious Diseases,* 4th ed. New York, Churchill Livingstone, 1995, pp 1039–1051.

drug concentration in cortical bone is less than serum concentration of antibiotic, high serum levels must be maintained for long periods.[57] Ideally, the serum concentration should be at least eight times the minimal bactericidal concentration (MBC).[58] Appropriate oral or intravenous antibiotics should be administered a minimum of 4 to 6 weeks in adults; however, in some cases, the total period of antibiotic administration may be as long as 3 months. In children, a shorter period of antibiotics may be adequate.

Initial antibiotic choice should be based on the most likely pathogen (Table 17-4); however, ongoing therapy may need to be altered once culture results are obtained. There are no standardized methods for measuring bone concentrations of antibiotics; however, in a rabbit model for *S. aureus* osteomyelitis, clindamycin attained the highest bone-to-serum ratio, followed by vancomycin, nafcillin, tobramycin, cefazolin, and cephalothin[56,59] (Table 17-5).

Under certain circumstances, closed irrigation suction methods may have their place in the treatment of this disease. Kawashima and Tamura, who recommend their use when septic emboli, thrombi, or necrosis have contributed to the infection, describe an 88.3 percent success rate.[38] They measured the blood concentration levels of antibiotics during the procedure and observed that absorption of antibiotics from the wound was insignificant. Postoperative bleeding is, however, an important complication.[38] Continuous suction drainage removes exudate from the wound and does not have the complications of the local antibiotic irrigation treatments, which remain controversial. Although acute osteomyelitis is usually easily treated by antibiotic therapy alone, surgical debridement remains the key factor, along with antibiotic therapy, in the treatment of chronic osteomyelitis.

Closure of the Dead Space

Local Flaps A second procedure is required to repair the bone defect and close the dead space following debridement. It should be remembered that fracture through a large bone defect is an important late complication of chronic osteomyelitis. However, if the bony defect is small and does not compromise present or future stability, no additional bone work is required and the dead space may be obliterated with a soft tissue flap. Such techniques as the cross-leg flap are not now recommended because they require prolonged immobilization of both lower extremities and expose the normal limb to the infected area. In recent years the techniques of local muscle flap and free vascularized muscle flap have changed the treatment of chronic osteomyelitis. A muscle flap enhances the healing of the lesion by bringing in a blood supply and can fill an irregularly contoured cavity.

Myocutaneous Flaps If a local muscle flap is inadequate, consideration may be given to bringing a free myocutaneous flap from a distant site and using microsurgical techniques to revascularize it locally. Integrity of the bony structure is a requirement for using either of these techniques. In general, lesions involving the middle and proximal thirds of the tibia are more suitable for coverage than those in the distal third of the tibia and regions of the ankle joint and foot. Coverage is easier in the thigh. The rate of success varies from 79 to 100 percent.[61–64] Complications include sloughing of the muscle flap,[60,65] persistence of infection in the cavity, and fracture of the bone through the saucerized area.[66]

Weiland and coworkers noted major complications in 41 percent of free tissue transfers performed for chronic osteomyelitis.[67] More than half the patients in whom this operation failed subsequently underwent amputation. Thus, although this procedure has advantages when it succeeds (a free latissimus dorsi flap can cover an area as large as 25 to 35 cm), the authors note that it is doomed to failure if the transfer is to tissue that is still infected.

When treating the infected unstable defect or one so large that future pathologic fracture and consequent instability seem likely, the techniques of open cancellous bone grafting, vascularized bone graft, and bypass graft have been utilized.

Open Cancellous Bone Grafting

Open cancellous bone grafting was first used by Rhinelander[68] and later by Papineau.[69,70] A careful description of the necessary protocol has been given by Sachs and Shaffer.[71] It is useful in bone deficiencies of less than 4 cm.

After the debridement, the defect in the bone is filled with autogenous cancellous iliac bone chips. The timing of surgery depends upon the appearance of the wound some 3 weeks following the initial debridement. If nonviable sclerotic bone remains, a second debridement precedes the bone graft procedure. Following the application of the graft, a Zenoform dressing is applied. This is changed every few days, while any necrotic bone is debrided from the surface intermittently. This process is continued until the bone graft is covered with healthy granulation tissue. The defect is then ready for coverage. This can be achieved by allowing the wound to epithelialize, but preferably flap coverage is achieved. Split skin coverage on the graft usually fails.[71] It is important that free drainage be permitted following the initial grafting procedure, since pressure from retained infected tissue exudates may compress fine capillaries and prevent the cancellous bone chips from revascularizing. Contraindications include segmental defects greater than 4 cm, especially in the diaphyseal area. If the quality of the bone and soft tissue or its location is such that bony stabilization cannot be achieved, some other treatment must be used. If an external fixator is applied for stability, it is important that attention be paid to care of the pin site as well as the grafted area.

Vascularized Bone Graft

The vascularized bone graft technique involves the isolation and transfer of a bony segment with its nutrient vascular pedicle. With this technique, the healing process is similar to that of a segmental fracture rather than the process of creeping substitution that occurs when the cancellous bone graft is used.[74] The vascularized bone graft provides immediate and adequate blood flow to the involved area; this is very important and may also increase local antibiotic penetration.

The procedure is usually indicated where there is a bony defect more than 6 cm long and minimal soft tissue loss.[64,73–76] However, the technique can be modified, and an appropriate bony segment can be transplanted with attached muscle or skin if there is also major soft tissue loss.[74] This procedure allows a generous resection of all suspicious or equivocally viable bone in patients having chronic and complex infection with extensive bony involvement. The procedure can be performed within 1 to 2 weeks after complete debridement without intervening wound closure, or it can be performed after completion of soft tissue wound healing.

The fibula and the iliac crest are the most common bones used for vascularized bone transfer. There are other bones that can be transferred with their vascular pedicle, but these are less useful in orthopaedic reconstruction. The technique of harvesting these grafts is well described.[73–75] The fibula is the most useful bone for replacement of a long segment. A length of 6 to 35 cm can be obtained with a fibular graft, while the iliac crest is most useful for defects shorter than 8 cm.[76,77] The vascular supply to the fibula is from branches of the peroneal vessels, which enter the bone in the middle third. The graft can be obtained in three ways: bone with a thin cuff of muscle, bone with a substantial muscular flap, or bone with a combined musculocutaneous flap. The segment of the iliac crest commonly used has multiple nutrient arteries, which are branches of the deep circumflex iliac vessels and enter the bone through the inner cortex.[77] The complications of free vascularized bone grafting include failure of vascularity in the graft, recurrence of infection, and delayed union or nonunion of the segment. In their experience with patients who had vascularized bone transfer for an established chronic osteomyelitis, Wood and Cooney had 1 patient with immediate vascular failure. Infection was controlled in 11 patients (84.6 percent), with no evidence of recurrence of the sepsis, but 5 patients (38.4 percent) developed nonunion, which required further bone grafting.[76]

Bypass Grafts

Bypass grafting involves the establishment of cross union between the tibia and fibula proximal and distal to a defect (Fig. 17-9). This technique offers some protection to the reconstituting bone in a large defect that has been separately grafted and does not impair its blood supply.[78]

Use of the Ilizarov Technique

Using the Ilizarov frame, large bony defects (more than 4 cm) remaining at the conclusion of debridement can be successfully closed. This technique is an alternative to free bone flaps and can be used even in a type B host. In this technique, the limb is acutely shortened to obliterate the defect after debridement, being stabilized with the circular Ilizarov fixator. On day 5, one or two percutaneous cortical osteotomies are made above and/or below the defect and then, after a lag phase, the proximal and distal segments are slowly distracted. Bone forms spontaneously in the osteotomy gaps, and the original length is restored. Ancillary techniques are occasionally used with this method, such as additional bone grafts to the debrided area and free tissue transfers to cover any accompanying

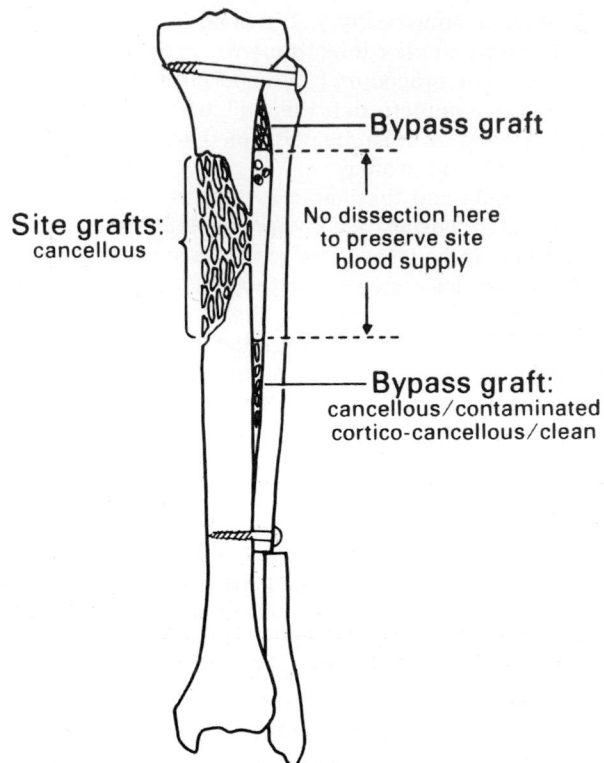

Figure 17-9 A technique of bone bypass grafting following open cancellous bone grafting to a large infected defect. This technique avoids further impairment of the blood supply to the vascularizing graft in the infected bony defect. (Reproduced with permission from Cierny G III, Mader JT: *Orthopaedics* 7:10, 1984.)

soft tissue defects that expose important structures such as vessel, nerve, or tendon.[79]

Amputation

Failure to successfully manage a limb with segmental bony defects, persisting instability, and infection leads to amputation. This is particularly unfortunate if such an outcome follows a long period of painful, expensive treatment, during which the patient's morale may steadily deteriorate. It is important that all the options be placed before the patient and the possibility of failure explained. In some cases, such as that of the type C host, the patient is wise to choose early ablation. A successful outcome will also be jeopardized without informed consent and the patient's determination to stay the course.

CHRONIC SCLEROSING OSTEOMYELITIS

Chronic sclerosing osteomyelitis was described by Garré in 1893. Patients have no necrosis or purulent exudate and little granulation tissue but show intense proliferation of the periosteum, leading to bony deposition.[6,77] It is a condition that mainly affects children and young adults.[80–82]

The average age at onset was 16 years in a series reported by Collert and Isacson.[83] The etiologic basis of sclerosing osteomyelitis is unclear, and routine aerobic cultures may not disclose any organism.[83,84] With more sophisticated techniques, it is possible to incriminate anaerobic organisms such as *Propionibacterium acnes.*[83] Histologic examination shows a nonspecific chronic inflammation with new bone formation and areas of necrosis.

The disease has an insidious onset, with local pain and tenderness of the affected bone and a moderately elevated ESR. The most common site of involvement is the shaft of the long bones, but involvement of other bones such as the mandible has also been reported.[60,85,86] Fifty percent of the cases reported by Collert and Isacson developed similar lesions at a different site after an average of 5.5 years.[83] The roentgenograms show pronounced sclerosis with small cystic areas (Fig. 17-10).

The sclerosis may become progressively more dense even in patients who have not been symptomatic for a long time.[83] Clinically and radiographically, it is difficult to distinguish this lesion from osteogenic sarcoma.[83] There are other conditions that should also be differentiated. These include Ewing's sarcoma, osteoid osteoma, osteoblastoma, and Paget's disease. The symptoms recur at intervals for several years and then gradually subside. There is no satisfactory treatment to eradicate chronic sclerosing osteomyelitis. Fenestration and curettage provide temporary relief. Prolonged antibiotic therapy does not change the clinical course of the disease.[83]

OSTEOMYELITIS IN THE HANDS AND FEET

Osteomyelitis in the distal phalanx follows tardily treated pulp space infection, though such an outcome is uncommon in developed countries. Puncture wounds and human and animal bites, however, remain important sources of infection in the hand. Inappropriate suturing of a small laceration on the hand after it has delivered a blow to the mouth may result in the loss of a digit. The metacarpophalangeal joint is particularly vulnerable in the closed fist. Either septic arthritis or osteomyelitis may occur, with a whole variety of organisms including anaerobes being involved.

Puncture wounds of the foot by foreign bodies may inoculate bone or joint. Bacterial osteomyelitis may result. In many of the reported cases, *P. aeruginosa* has been isolated.[87–90] Local pain and swelling persist, but there may be surprisingly few systemic symptoms. There is often delay in diagnosis.[91] Additional studies such as scintigraphy are helpful. Aspiration may produce diagnostic fluid.

The treatment consists of antibiotic therapy similar to that described for other areas of chronic osteomyelitis combined with appropriate adequate debridement. These wounds are common in children. It is noteworthy that *P. aeruginosa* has an apparent propensity to infect cartilage as well as bone. Parenteral antibiotic therapy for 3 to 6 weeks with aminoglycoside and a broad-spectrum penicillin or an antipseudomonal third-generation cephalosporin (e.g., ceftazidime, cefoperazone, or cefepime is effective against this organism) is recommended.

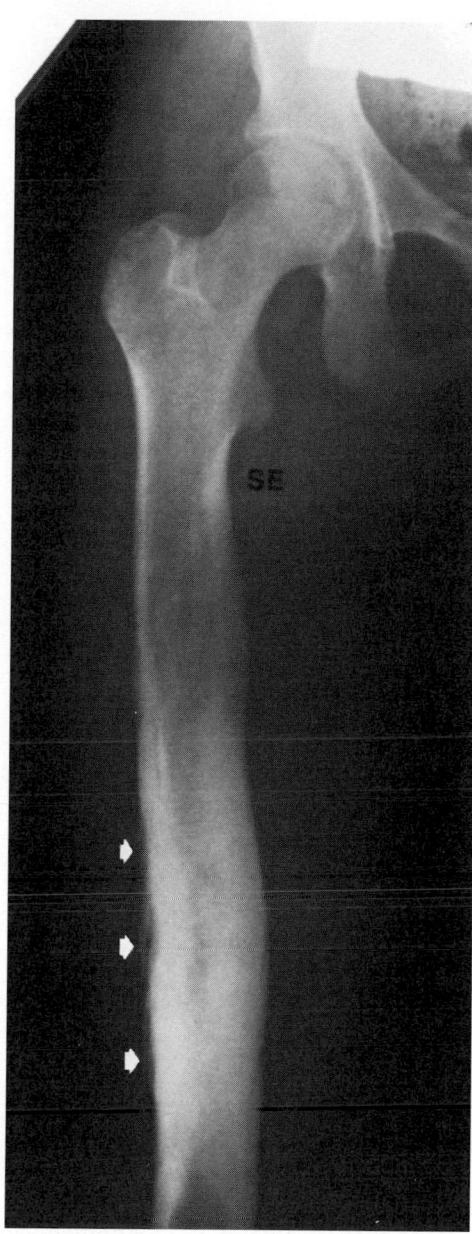

Figure 17-10 Chronic sclerosing osteomyelitis (Garré). Note the area of cortical irregularity and sclerosis (*solid arrows*).

The calcaneus has a firmly attached periosteum, and elevation and subperiosteal abscess formation is less likely. Extraosseous extension occurs usually by perforation of the periosteum. The principles of treatment are similar to those outlined for other bones. The approach through the plantar surface of the heel devised by Gaenslen is useful in extensive chronic osteomyelitis.[92]

PELVIC OSTEOMYELITIS

Osteomyelitis of the pelvis may simulate other disease processes. Acute septic arthritis or sciatica associated with discitis may be suspected in children. There may be an ab-

dominal-type presentation resembling the acute abdomen.[93] Blood culture is positive in about 70 percent of acute cases. *Staphylococcus aureus* is again the most common organism.[94] Computed tomography and appropriate scintigraphy are helpful in this region. Because of the excellent blood flow to the pelvis, antibiotic therapy alone may be adequate to cure the infection if early diagnosis is made. The differential diagnosis of a cystic or sclerotic lesion may include such conditions as eosinophilic granuloma, metastatic neuroblastoma, leukemia, or Ewing's sarcoma.[94]

COMPLICATIONS OF INTRAVENOUS DRUG USERS

Septic arthritis and osteomyelitis are well-recognized complications of intravenous drug abuse. *Pseudomonas aeruginosa* and *S. aureus* are common infecting agents. In addition *Serratia marcescens* may produce multifocal osteomyelitis in these patients. Areas commonly involved are in the axial skeleton, particularly the lumbar vertebrae and sacroiliac joints.[95]

OSTEOMYELITIS CAUSED BY OTHER ORGANISMS (see Table 17-6)

Brucella Osteomyelitis

The various types of *Brucella* can involve the joints and also produce osteomyelitis (frequently chronic) of the flat or tubular bones. Sometimes secondary invasion by staphylococci follows.[6] Of the four *Brucella* species that affect human beings, *B. abortus* is the most common species seen in the United States, and it is the type most likely causing bone infection. Vertebrae, especially the lumbar spine, are the most common sites of involvement.[96,97] The diagnosis requires a high index of suspicion. *Brucella* osteomyelitis is often an occupational disease of young adults in the meat trade.[94,98]

Treatment follows the general principles already outlined for other bone infections, with splintage, antibiotics, and surgery when appropriate. Doxycycline alone is effective, but streptomycin or gentamicin with doxycycline may be more effective. Trimethoprim-sulfamethoxazole (TMP-SMX) combined with gentamicin can be used in children less than 8 years of age.

Salmonella Osteomyelitis

Patients with major sickle cell hemoglobinopathies have a high incidence of *Salmonella* osteomyelitis, and when bone infection occurs in sickle cell disease, *Salmonella* is the causative organism in 74 percent of cases.[5] A photopenic area on bone scan, following the onset of pain, is more consistent with infarction than with infection. On the other hand, an early finding of increased uptake of ^{99m}Tc-MDP is much more likely to represent osteomyelitis.[5]

TABLE 17-6 Unusual Organisms Causing Osteomyelitis

Pathogen	Therapy of choice	Alternative therapy
Brucella	Doxycycline *and* gentamicin	Trimethoprim-sulfamethoxazole
Salmonella	Third-generation cephalosporin *or* quinolone	Trimethoprim-sulfamethoxazole
Bacteroides spp.	Clindamycin *or* metronidazole	Ampicillin-sulbactam *or* imipenem
Blastomyces	Amphotericin B	Itraconazole
Cryptococcus	Amphotericin B	Fluconazole
Coccidioides	Amphotericin B	Ketoconazole *or* itraconazole
Actinomyces	Penicillin G	Minocycline
Actinomadura	Dapsone *and* streptomycin	Trimethoprim-sulfamethoxazole
Nocardia	Trimethoprim-sulfamethoxazole	Minocycline
Mycobacterium tuberculosis	Isoniazid, rifampin, ethambutol, pyrazinamide	Streptomycin

Besides sickle cell disease, patients with other hemoglobinopathies, systemic lupus erythematosus, neoplasms, or immunosuppression are at increased risk of *Salmonella* osteomyelitis.[99] Antibiotics active against *Salmonella* include third-generation cephalosporins and TMP-SMX; however, resistance may occur. Ciprofloxacin and ofloxacin have excellent activity against this pathogen but should not be used in children.

Infections with Anaerobic Organisms

Increasing numbers of cases of chronic osteomyelitis in which anaerobic bacteria are isolated reflect an increased recognition of the appropriate precautions that must be taken in collecting and transporting biopsy material. Cultures of drainage material of open wounds and sinus tracts are often contaminated and may give misleading results.[100,101] A surgical procedure may be performed to obtain bone or tissue biopsy, or a closed aspiration may obtain fluid. Fluid should be drawn into a syringe and handled rather like a blood gas specimen. The usual indications of anaerobic infections, such as putrid exudate and foul odor, are unfortunately not always present. Swabs are not recommended because of problems of inadequate sampling. If a few milliliters of pus or a piece of tissue or bone can be sent to the laboratory, avoidable loss of microorganisms due to exposure to oxygen can be prevented. If transportation is to be delayed more than 20 min, a specific transport system that will keep anaerobes viable for as long as 24 h should be used.[100]

In postsurgical infections, anaerobes are probably introduced into the surgical wound from the skin, where they form part of the normal flora.[102] Although clostridial rods may infect open wounds, anaerobic cocci, particularly the gram-positive peptostreptococci (*Peptococcus magnus*) are frequently isolated from wound cultures. *Bacteroides fragilis* may also be isolated from wounds, particularly in patients with debilitating conditions and vascular disease who develop bone or joint infection. These organisms are usually treated with clindamycin, cefoxitin, ampicillin-sulbactam, or metronidazole.[103] Because of the development of resistant strains, appropriate sensitivity tests should be performed.[61,104,105]

GRANULOMATOUS INFECTIONS OF BONE

Fungal Infections

Blastomycosis

Blastomycosis is endemic to the southeastern and midwestern parts of the United States but not in the southwestern and western regions.

Most systemic infections are caused by hematogenous spread from pulmonary portals of entry. A proportion of these patients have involvement of bone and joint. Osseous lesions are multiple and involve the epiphyseal and metaphyseal ends of long bones. Lesions may also be seen in the small bones of the hands and feet and over bone prominences. Diagnosis is by culture from biopsy material.

Amphotericin remains the treatment of choice for blastomycosis in the immunosuppressed patient with life-threatening disease.[106] Itraconazole has excellent in vitro and in vivo activity and has become an alternative therapy for treatment of mild-to-moderate disease in the immunocompetent patient. Therapy with itraconazole should be continued for at least 6 months.

Coccidioidomycosis

The fungus *Coccidioides immitis* is endemic to the southwestern United States and also to Central America and parts of South America. The infectious spores are inhaled, and the primary lung disease is accompanied by weight loss, eosinophilia, skin lesions, and occasionally an associated arthritis. Osseous lesions resemble blastomycosis in their distribution (Fig. 17-11). Necrosis and caseation produces abscesses, which may involve joints.

Skin tests are specific but may be negative in disseminated disease. Complement fixation tests are available; a titer of 1:64 or higher is positive for systemic disease.[14] Curettage, ablation, or fusion may be required, combined with intravenous amphotericin B in doses of 1 to 1.5 mg/kg up to 2 to 4.6 mg/kg total. Renal and bone marrow function should be closely monitored. Aplastic anemia can occur as a complication of the drug. Synovectomy may be required for joint involvement.

Actinomycosis

In actinomycosis, involvement of mandible and the facial bones commonly occurs because the organism is usually introduced through the oral cavity. Bone involvement is a secondary event following the soft tissue infection. The extremities are infrequently involved. Actinomycotic colonies can be observed in granules (called *sulfur granules*), which may be recovered from the abscesses. The granulomas may be seen in biopsy material. Pencillin G is the drug of choice given intravenously for 6 weeks and then orally for up to 1 year. For the penicillin-allergic patient, tetracycline or minocycline, clindamycin, or erythromycin may be used.

Cryptococcosis

Skeletal cryptococcosis tends to produce radiolucent lesions, and periosteal reaction is unusual.[14] All bones of the skeleton have been reported to be involved, and the disease has been reported from all parts of the world. Cryptococcal meningitis should be particularly suspected in a patient with leukemia, acquired immunodeficiency syndrome (AIDS), Hodgkin's disease, sarcoidosis, or diabetes who has a fever of unknown origin or central nervous system disorder.[106] The drug of choice is amphotericin B or fluconazole.

Mycetoma

Cutaneous fungal infections can occur from direct implantation following a minor breach of the skin and lead to disseminated disease that may also affect bone. Sporotrichosis is a common example.[107] Itraconazole or amphotericin B is the treatment for extracutaneous sporotrichosis.

Fungi may enter the body via an opening in the skin, such as a compound fracture or puncture wound.[108] These fungi may infect bone and soft tissues, producing tumoral enlargements called mycetomas. There are two groups of organisms causing mycetoma: the aerobic *Actinomyces* causing actinomycetoma, and the true fungi *(Eumycetes)* causing eumycetoma.[108] The management depends on the type of the organism.

Actinomycetoma can be effectively treated with a combination of streptomycin and dapsone or TMP-SMX. Mycetoma secondary to *Nocardia* can be treated with TMP-SMX alone.

For most of the eumycetomas, however, surgery is indicated because of resistance to ordinary antibiotic therapy. Iodide and radiation therapy have not been effective.[109–110] Although amphotericin B, griseofulvin,

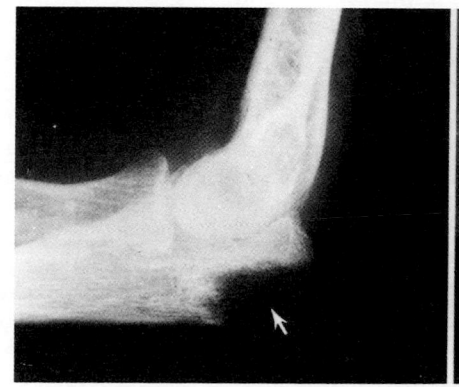
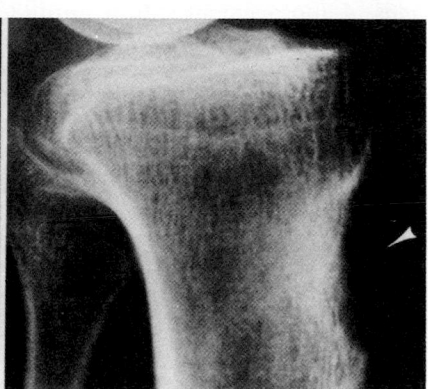

Figure 17-11 Coccidioidomycosis: osteomyelitis. Involvement of bony protuberances such as the olecranon (*A*) and the tibial tubercle (*B*) is frequent. These are discrete lesions with surrounding sclerosis. (Reproduced with permission from Resnick D, Niwayama G: *Diagnosis of Bone and Joint Disorders.* Philadelphia, Saunders, 1981.)

A   *B*

miconazole, and ketoconazole have been effective against the systemic and cutaneous fungal infections,[111] they are less effective or even ineffective for eumycetoma without aggressive surgical drainage.[108–110]

Once the diagnosis of osteomyelitis with eumycetoma has been established, especially when the cause is *Petriellidium boydii* or *Madurella mycetomi,* a radical resection of all the infected bone and soft tissue is necessary. Any spores that remain in the wound will continue to grow and cause recurrence of the infection. Recurrent drainage and spread of the infection with decrease or loss of the function is an indication for amputation.[108]

Syphilis of the Bones

Bone syphilis may be congenital (intrauterine infection) or acquired (postnatal infection). Infection that is blood-borne is caused by the spirochete *Treponema pallidum.* The infection is localized in the metaphyseal and diaphyseal region and does not spread to the joints. With better prenatal supervision and the sensitivity of the spirochete to penicillin, syphilis of the newborn is now less common.

Congenital Syphilis

In early congenital syphilis, the infant is irritable and restless and may have a large, tender swelling around the involved joint. The limb is held immobile. Other signs of syphilis such as skin lesions, mucous patches, and keratitis may be present.

Radiographs demonstrate widening of the metaphysis with marginal density and an indentation on its epiphyseal border. The metaphysis looks osteoporotic or may have patchy areas of radiolucency. There is usually diffuse periostitis, seen as periosteal elevation with layers of new bone formation (Fig. 17-12).

The affected bones may assume a spindle shape, and the medullary outlines become indistinct. With proper preparation, the spirochete can be identified in histologic sections. It is important to remember that in an infant with congenital syphilis, the serologic tests are not positive in the first 3 months because of the infant's inability to produce sufficient antibodies.

The infection responds rapidly to antibiotic therapy. If the child has an adequate defense mechanism and survives the early days after birth, there will be progressive signs of improvement with resorption of the exudate and healing of the bone within a few months. Following successful treatment of the infection, the bone architecture returns to normal.[112]

The late stage of congenital syphilis usually occurs in the second or third year. It is characterized by osteoblastic activity producing a condensing osteitis, which occurs mainly in the tibia, femur, and skull. Subperiosteal bone formation causes a prominent border along the anterior margin of the tibia without any bowing.

In an untreated patient or when the infection is particularly virulent, there may initially be erosion of the cortex, which then progresses to the typical increased densities of osteoblastic activities on x-ray views. The child may

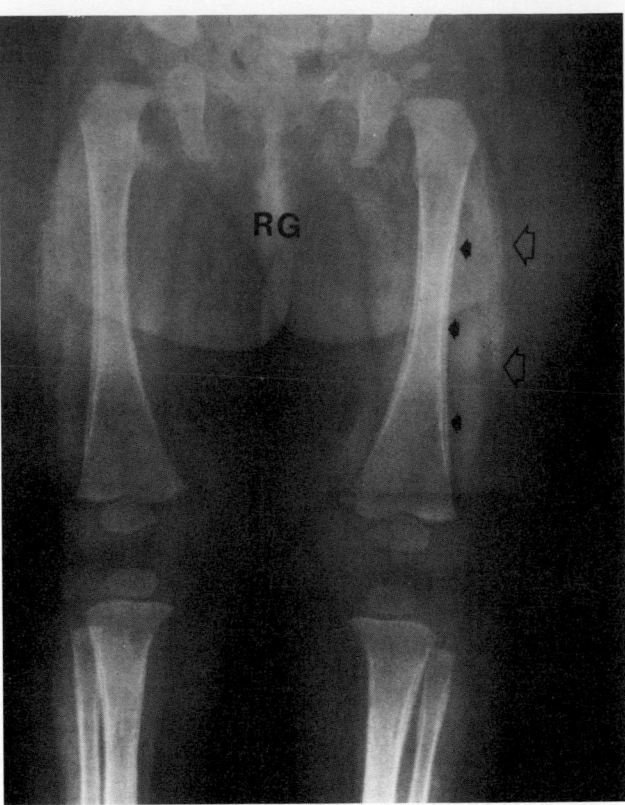

Figure 17-12 Congenital syphilis. There is bilateral diaphyseal periostitis (*solid arrows*). There is also swelling of the soft tissues (*hollow arrows*).

eventually show other signs of syphilis such as interstitial keratitis, deformed incisor teeth, and auditory nerve palsy.[51]

Clutton's Joints

In the late stage of congenital syphilis, between the age of 8 and 18, patients may develop large, bilateral, painless effusion of the knee. This is called *Clutton's joints.* The condition is an intermittent recurrent effusion of the knees. The x-ray examination is negative, and the examination of the joint fluid reveals a high content of mononuclear cells.

Syphilis in Adults

In adults, involvement of bone and joint occurs in the late or tertiary stage of the disease. The patient manifests painless, nontender swelling of a long bone or the skull. Occasionally there are localized gummatous lesions of bones. These may be diffuse sclerosing periostitis, suggesting Paget's disease. Radiographs reveal soft tissue swelling in the region of the gummas, which represents an extraosseous extension of the infection. The relative or absolute absence of pain is one of the characteristic features of syphilitic lesions due to peripheral neuropathic changes (Charcot's joints). Also, normal motion of the joint is often preserved.[51]

Yaws

Another spirochetal infection that is endemic in some tropical countries is yaws. It is common in equatorial Africa, India, and southeast Asia. The primary phase consists of maculopapular lesions. The secondary skin eruption of papillomas begins a few months later. The late tertiary stage, which not all patients develop, consists of nodular lesions that ulcerate, spread, and may penetrate deeply into underlying tissues, involving muscles, joints, and bones. These lesions cause gross deformities by producing contractures and ankylosis.[113] They resemble the gummas seen in syphilis. The introduction of penicillin into affected areas has reduced the incidence of this serious infection.[113]

Tuberculosis of Bones and Joints

Tuberculosis is a chronic granulomatous infection caused by *Mycobacterium tuberculosis.* Involvement of the bones and joints is most often secondary to the hematogenous spread, but occasionally local extension from the lungs, kidneys, or lymph nodes may occur. The spine is the most common site of bony involvement. The other sites of involvement in decreasing order of frequency are knee, hip, ankle, wrist, sacroiliac joint, pubic symphysis, and small bones of hand and foot (tuberculous dactylitis).[114]

The disease is slowly progressive, and the degree of local and general reaction depends on the intensity of the infection and the patient's general condition and resistance. Immunosuppression, which accompanies AIDS and some treatments for rheumatoid arthritis, predisposes to tuberculous infection.

Diagnosis

In the mild granular type of infection, the white blood cell count and ESR may be normal. In the exudative form, caseous material is produced, and there is leukocytosis and an elevated ESR accompanied by general symptoms.

The tuberculin skin test is an allergic inflammatory reaction to the purified protein derivative (PPD) antigen. It is positive in 80 to 90 percent of active cases. A positive reaction indicates that the patient has at some time been infected but does not have diagnostic value for present activity of the disease. A positive reaction in a person who previously had a negative test has diagnostic importance.

Microscopic studies of a smear of material from infected bone or joint fluid usually show the acid-fast bacilli. The culture of any pus obtained will be positive, but it takes 5 to 30 days to grow the organism. Intraperitoneal inoculation of the pus in guinea pigs will show tubercles in 5 to 8 weeks. A microscopic study of biopsy material or sometimes a local enlarged lymph node demonstrates typical tubercles showing epithelioid cells, an encircling ring of round cells and fibrous tissue, and the characteristic Langhans' giant cell. There may be central caseation.

Tuberculous Osteomyelitis

Tuberculous osteomyelitis rarely originates in a long bone, but metaphyseal foci can occur in children; also, the disease may originate in an epiphysis and spread into a neighboring joint.[6] It can be difficult if not impossible to differentiate radiologically between tuberculosis and ordinary pyogenic osteomyelitis of bone.

Tuberculous Dactylitis

Tuberculous dactylitis presents with multiple soft tissue swelling of the digits and diffuse lytic areas of the phalanges and metacarpals associated with periostitis (Fig. 17-13).

Tuberculous Arthritis

In joints, subchondral osteoporosis and cystic changes associated with narrowing of the joint space are common (Fig. 17-14). Differential diagnosis includes rheumatoid arthritis and pigmented villonodular synovitis. Occasionally the con-

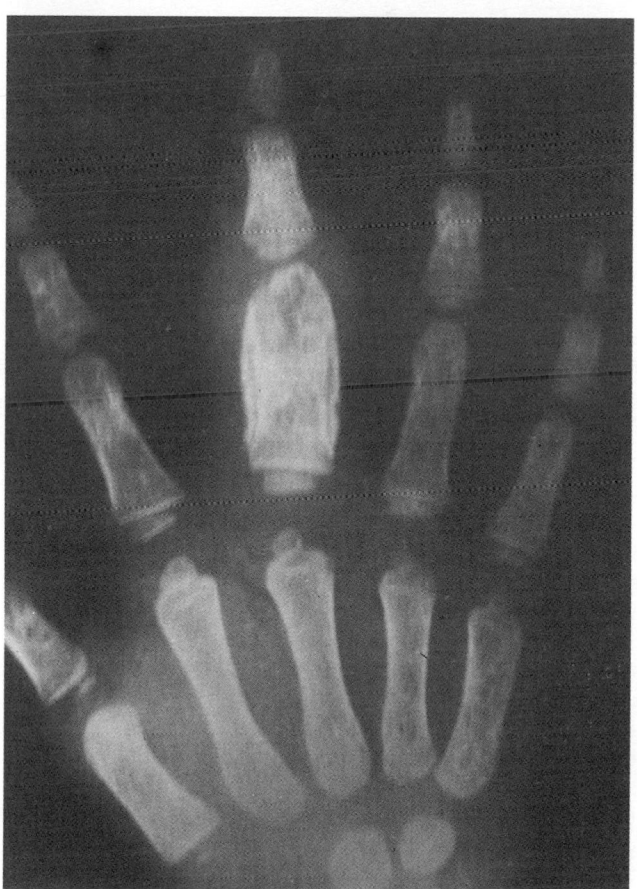

Figure 17-13 Tuberculous dactylitis. Radiographic findings in this child include soft tissue swelling of multiple digits, lytic lesions of several middle and proximal phalanges and metacarpals, and exuberant periostitis and enlargement of the proximal phalanx of the third finger. (Reproduced with permission from Resnick D, Niwayama G: *Diagnosis of Bone and Joint Disorders.* Philadelphia, Saunders, 1981.)

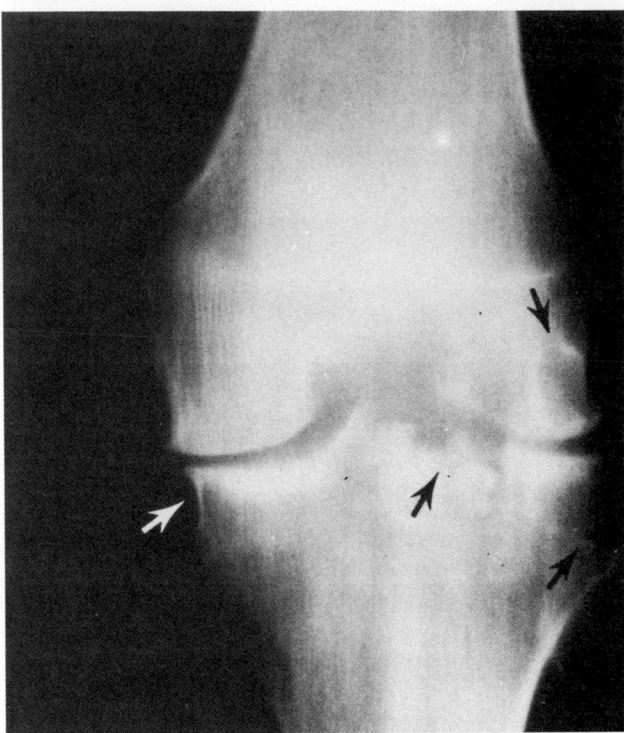

Figure 17-14 Tuberculous arthritis of the knee joint. This tomogram shows typical marginal and central osseous erosions (*arrows*). Osteoporosis is not prominent. (Reproduced with permission from Resnick D, Niwayama G: *Diagnosis of Bone and Joint Disorders.* Philadelphia, Saunders, 1981.)

dition may be confused with reflex sympathetic dystrophy because of the patchy osteoporotic appearance of the bone. Marginal erosions at the corner of the articulating surface are common.[6]

Treatment

In the management of bone and joint tuberculosis, it is important to improve the patient's general condition and nutritional status.

The principles of the treatment of chronic osteomyelitis caused by tuberculosis are identical to those of other granulomas. Drainage is usually not necessary in most cases. The most effective chemotherapeutic drugs include isoniazid, rifampin, ethambutol, pyrazinamide, and streptomycin. Because of the possibility of resistant tuberculosis, therapy is initiated with four antituberculous drugs. Treatment regimens may have to be adjusted once sensitivity patterns are obtained.

Early Disease

Early bone and joint involvement can be controlled with drug therapy. The joints are splinted and gently mobilized as the disease abates and the local signs diminish. The result in early disease should be a mobile joint free from infection.

Surgical Joint Clearance

Joint clearance is recommended for a joint that remains irritated with persisting effusion, thickened synovium, and other local signs of persisting activity. All debris and infected synovium are removed. This operation helps the antibiotics to penetrate and sterilize the joint and permits its eventual mobilization.

Arthrodesis

Arthrodesis is now rarely required in tuberculous arthritis but, performed extraarticularly, it was the standard operation prior to the discovery of antibiotics. It was felt that arthrodesis rendered a joint safe from repeated flare-ups of infection. Before antibiotic therapy became available, it was impossible to be certain that the organisms had been completely overcome and that a flare-up was not a possibility at some point in the future, despite clinical remission. Nowadays, with adequate treatment, joint infection can be cured without obliterating the joint. Indeed, total hip replacement may be performed after an interval of many years in healed tuberculous arthritis. If arthrodesis is chosen, it is for mechanical and pain-relieving reasons rather than to assist in controlling the infection. Nevertheless, the earlier practice is worth remembering in the event of resistant organisms.

Arthroplasty

Arthroplasty has no role in the treatment of active disease and is performed only as salvage surgery after the infection has been eradicated.

Atypical Mycobacterial Infections

A number of species, including *Mycobacterium avium-intracellulare, M. marinum, M. fortuitum,* and *M. gordonae,* can produce ostearticular infection. Infection by atypical mycobacteria usually affects the tendon sheaths and spreads later to the joints of the knee, ankle, and elbows. The role of antituberculous therapy is controversial, since many of these infections respond well to surgery alone.[115]

SEPTIC ARTHRITIS

Septic arthritis can be produced by hematogenous spread to the synovium or by the extension of osteomyelitis involving the epiphysis or an intracapsular metaphysis (Fig. 17-15). Direct contamination of the joint can follow diagnostic or therapeutic aspiration and has been described following venipuncture in the groin.

Clinical Features

Both children and adults with bacterial arthritis typically present with fever, swelling, and limitation of joint motion.

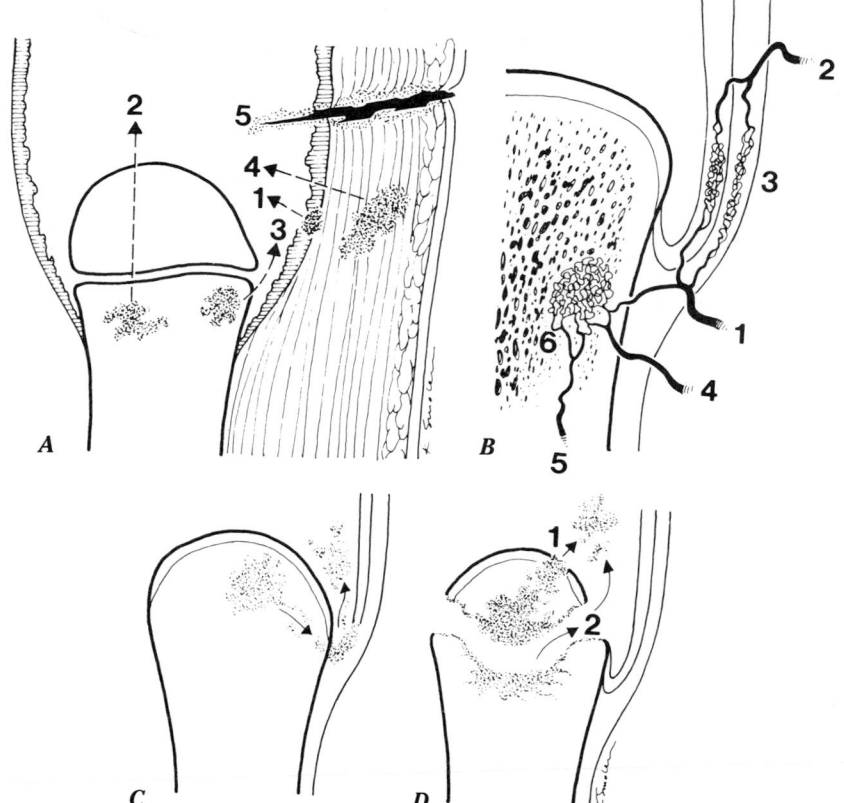

Figure 17-15 Septic arthritis: potential routes of contamination. *A.* Hematogenous spread of infection to a joint can result from direct lodgement of organisms in the synovial membrane (1). Spread into the joint from a contiguous source can occur from a metaphyseal focus that extends into the epiphysis and from there into the joint (2), from a metaphyseal focus with extension into the joint when the growth plate is intraarticular (3), or from a contiguous soft tissue infection (4). Direct implantation following a penetrating wound (5) can also lead to septic arthritis. *B* and *C.* Hematogenous spread of infection to a joint can also occur due to vascular continuity between the epiphysis and synovial membrane. In (*B*), the vessels shown include arterioles (1), venules (2), and capillaries (3) of the capsule; periosteal vessels (4); the nutrient artery (5); and metaphyseal-epiphyseal anastomoses (6). In this fashion, the synovial membrane may become infected from an osseous focus before the joint fluid is contaminated. In (*C*) this sequence of events is diagrammed. *D.* Spread from a contiguous osseous surface can result from penetration of the cartilage (1) or pathologic fracture with articular contamination (2). In this situation, synovial fluid may become infected before the synovial membrane. (Reproduced with permission from Resnick D, Niwayama G: *Diagnosis of Bone and Joint Disorders*. Philadelphia, Saunders, 1981.)

Usually there is monoarticular involvement, and a synovial effusion is visible. The knee is the most common joint affected in all age groups, followed by the hip.

In adults, close to 50 percent of patients have a history of preexisting arthritis and about 30 percent have a history of trauma.[116] Patients with rheumatoid arthritis may have multiple joint involvement.[117] The sternoclavicular and sacroiliac joints are often affected in intravenous drug users.[118]

Septic Arthritis in Children

The infection can occur at any age, but 50 percent of the cases occur in children under 3 years of age and 30 percent occur in children less than 2 years of age.[119–121] In infants, the hip joint is most commonly affected, whereas knee joint involvement is more common in older children.

Some 10 percent of childhood cases may have involvement of more than one joint.[119]

In the neonate, septic arthritis may occur in a child already seriously ill with septicemia and other focal infections. Alternatively, the child may fail to thrive and run a fever. It is only with a high index of suspicion and considerable clinical acumen that the area of infection is localized. Pain on motion of the affected joint or lack of function may be all that is apparent. Later in the disease, the hip may become dislocated or, in the case of other joints, a soft tissue abscess may form. The diagnosis is then facilitated but unfortunately somewhat belated. Unilateral swelling of an extremity may also be a valuable clue. In an older child, the presentation may be with an acutely painful joint held rigidly, not permitting even the slightest motion.[119] In the hip, there may be a fixed flexion deformity associated with intense muscle spasm. In such cases bumping into the bed or cot inadvertently is sufficient to cause the child to cry out in pain, since the joint is exquisitely sensitive to motion. The need to search for a skin lesion or a focus of infection elsewhere in the body should not be overlooked.

Etiology

The bacterial etiology of septic arthritis differs among age groups (Table 17-7). In children, *S. aureus* and streptococci are the predominant pathogens.[121] *Haemophilus influenzae* type B is the most common gram-negative bacillus causing infection in children under the age of 2 in past series; but with the advent of universal immunization of infants against invasive type B infections, the incidence of this pathogen has markedly decreased. Other gram-negative bacilli such as *E. coli, Proteus* species, *Salmonella,* and rarely *Pseudomonas* continue to cause some cases of septic arthritis in infants and children.

In young, sexually active adults, *Neisseria gonorrhoeae* is the most common cause of septic arthritis, while *S. aureus* continues to be a major pathogen in both younger and older adults. Gram-negative bacteria including *E. coli, Proteus, Klebsiella,* and *Pseudomonas* may account for up to 15 percent of the cases of septic arthritis in adults. *Staphylococcus epidermidis* is an important pathogen in patients with prosthetic joints.

Other organisms causing septic arthritis include *M. tuberculosis, M. kansasii, M. marinum, P. multocida, Borrelia burgdorferi, Sporothrix schenckii, Coccidioides immitis, Candida* species, and *Pseudoallescheria boydii;* these are usually associated with specific risk factors (Table 17-8). Mycobacteria typically produce chronic, slowly progressive disease. *Mycobacterium marinum* joint infection should be suspected if there is a history of exposure to a tropical fish aquarium or marine life, while *P. multocida* infections occur after a dog or cat bite. *Candida albicans* septic arthritis usually occurs from hematogenous spread but may occur after trauma or intraarticular steroid injection.[122]

Radiographic Studies

Displacement of the muscles around the joint may be seen as asymmetrical soft tissue shadows compared with the opposite side. In addition, lateral displacement, some upward subluxation of the femoral head, or even frank dislocation may be observed in the hip.

In adults, destruction of subchondral bone and articular cartilage may produce considerable subchondral bone and joint space narrowing at a relatively early stage of the disease.

Late radiologic sequelae in children include infarction and sequestration of the epiphysis. Arthrography may be helpful in the unossified nucleus to ascertain whether or not it has been destroyed by the infective process. Infants with previous knee joint infections may present with an established genu valgum deformity. This fact plus the x-ray appearance may lead one to believe that the physis and part of the distal femoral epiphysis have been permanently damaged. Under these circumstances, careful clinical examination and palpation will reveal the presence of the portion of epiphysis considered to have been destroyed. Similarly, the examination may indicate that the range of motion is well preserved. This is not the case if a large portion of the intraarticular epiphysis has been destroyed and sequestrated.[122]

In the child's hip, areas of translucency appearing approximately 1 month following infection may resemble a pseudoarthrosis of the femoral neck. Provided that the capital epiphysis still remains within the acetabulum, this does not, however, necessarily indicate a fracture, and recalcification of the area often follows with resolution of the illness. Delay in appearance of the ossific nucleus in these cases also does not mean that it has been destroyed. Arthrography is a valuable study in these hips.[122]

Although bone, indium, and gallium scans are usually positive in septic arthritis, routine imaging is rarely necessary unless osteomyelitis is suspected. Computed to-

---

TABLE 17-7 Bacterial Etiology of Septic Arthritis

	<2 years of age	2–16 years of age	16–30 years of age	>30 years of age
Most common	*Haemophilus influenzae* *S. aureus*	*Staphylococcus aureus* *Streptococcus pyogenes*	*Neisseria gonorrhoeae* *S. aureus*	*S. aureus* Streptococci
Less common	Group B streptococci *S. pneumoniae* *Streptococcus pyogenes* *E. coli* *Proteus* *Pseudomonas*	*Streptococcus pneumoniae* *Escherichia coli* *Proteus* *Haemophilus*	*S. pneumoniae* *E. coli* *Proteus* *Klebsiella* *Pseudomonas* *Bacteroides*	*Staphylococcus epidermidis* *E. coli* *Proteus* *Klebsiella* *S. pneumoniae* Polymicrobial
Unusual	*Bacteroides* *N. gonorrhoeae* *N. meningitidis*	*Neisseria meningitidis* *Pseudomonas* Polymicrobial	*Bacteroides* *N. meningitidis* Polymicrobial	*Bacteroides* *H. influenzae* *N. gonorrhoeae* *N. meningitidis*

TABLE 17-8   Risk Factors Associated with Pathogens Causing Septic Arthritis

Pathogen	Risk factor
Neisseria gonorrhoeae	Sexual activity
Streptococcus pneumoniae	Sickle cell disease
Gram-negative bacilli	Urinary tract infections
Eikenella corrodens	Human bite
Pasteurella multocida	Cat/dog bite
Borrelia burgdorferi	Tick exposure
Sporothrix schenckii	Gardeners
Mycobacterium marinum	Tropical fish or marine life exposure
Candida species	Trauma, steroid injections
Pseudoallescheria	Trauma

mography, MRI, and sonography are all more sensitive than plain films in detecting joint effusions.

Diagnostic Aspiration

Synovial fluid analysis is required at the earliest possible moment, and fluid should be obtained by aspiration in all suspected cases. It is important that the needle be placed accurately within the joint, and fluoroscopic control may be called for, with a light general anesthetic if necessary.

The joint fluid should be sent for bacteriologic studies and also for white blood and differential blood cell counts. In well-established septic arthritis, an average of 100,000 cells/mm³ (range, 25,000 to 250,000) is commonly found. Septic arthritis is strongly suspected when there are more than 50,000 cells/mm³ with 90 percent polymorphs, even if no organisms are grown on culture.[119,123] A Gram stain should also be performed and may give some guidance concerning the most effective antibiotic before the results from sensitivity tests are available. Blood cultures and cultures from other septic areas must be obtained prior to the commencement of any antibiotic therapy.

The glucose concentration in the synovial fluid is usually less than blood levels, and the protein concentration may be up to 6 or 8 g/dL, with an electrophoretic pattern resembling that of plasma. Examination of the fluid for urate or calcium pyrophosphate crystals is important in differential diagnosis, particularly in adults.

Differential Diagnosis

It is unlikely that bacterial arthritis will be confused with a periarticular condition such as bursitis. In children, transient synovitis of the hip, which is the commonest cause of irritable hip in children under 10 years of age, may cause confusion. Children with this self-limiting aseptic inflammatory process may also present with a painful joint and

a slight limp. Examination of the hip in these children also reveals a diminished range of motion with some fixed flexion deformity. However, the child is usually apyrexial and laboratory studies are normal. Aspiration of the joint usually settles the diagnosis. An MRI scan may be employed to exclude Perthes' disease.

Acute osteomyelitis must be differentiated from septic arthritis in the manner already described. Cellulitis, similarly, is unlikely to cause confusion, although it is important that any aspiration of the joint not be performed through such an infected area. Other conditions in the differential diagnosis include crystal deposition disease, acute rheumatoid arthritis, and chronic arthritis. In children, acute rheumatic fever, hemophilia, and Henoch-Schönlein purpura may occasionally be encountered. In adults with septic arthritis, consideration should also be given to the presence of associated infective conditions such as bacterial endocarditis.

Treatment

Treatment with parenteral antibiotics should be commenced immediately upon admission provided that all the necessary culture material has been obtained. The type of antibiotic chosen is based on the natural history of the disease, the age of the patient, and the result of the Gram stain.[118,120]

For children under the age of 5 years, empiric therapy should be directed against S. aureus, streptococci, and H. influenzae. Cefotaxime or ceftizoxime are excellent for initial treatment. In a sexually active adult with septic arthritis, ceftriaxone would be a good choice if the Gram stain is suggestive of the gonococcus. In an older patient with a prosthetic joint, empiric therapy should be directed against both S. epidermidis and S. aureus, with a combination of vancomycin and gentamicin.

Once the results of synovial fluid or other cultures are available, it may be necessary to change to a more specific antibiotic. Antibiotics are administered parenterally at first. Oral antibiotics may be used when the infection is under control, using the criteria already described for osteomyelitis. Therapy is monitored by measurement of bactericidal or bacteriostatic levels in the serum and maintaining levels eight times the minimal microbicidal concentration to ensure satisfactory kill rates. The usual length of therapy is from 2 to 3 weeks.

Surgical Drainage

Although serial aspiration appropriately performed can be relatively pain-free and accompanied by minimal risk of introducing additional contaminating organisms into the joint, open drainage and surgical irrigation with large quantities of fluid is often preferred.

Controversy about surgical drainage of septic arthritis still continues, however. There are those who believe that open drainage should now rarely be used[118] and, by contrast, those who concur with Lloyd-Roberts that "the misguided conservation of the needle should yield to the conservation of the knife."[124]

In the hip joint, relief of the capsular distension produced by incision not only prevents lateral migration of the head, leading to dislocation, but has a profound and immediate beneficial effect on the patient's clinical status. By the anterolateral approach, the hip joint can be exposed without cutting any muscle fibers. The proximal portion of this approach is relatively avascular, and the capsular distension makes it possible to find the hip joint rapidly, so that the procedure lacks substantial morbidity. If the posterior approach is used, there is the advantage of gravitational drainage. Once the capsule is freely opened, it is not necessary to leave the wound open; the skin may then be closed after appropriate irrigation. It is advisable to insert a subcutaneous drain through a separate stab incision following the surgical procedure. Similar principles are observed in surgical drainage of other involved joints. The authors have no experience with closed drainage systems using suction irrigation, and no control study has been performed with these methods. The problem with continuous irrigation of fluid into the joint remains the possibility of additional contamination. All authorities agree that instilling antibiotics locally into the joint is not helpful and may be harmful.[8,119,125]

In superficial joints such as the knee, lavage using the arthroscope is an alternative that may effectively drain a joint and irrigate it without a large incision. However, there may be continuing anxiety that free drainage has not been established without incision of the joint capsule and synovium.

Immobilization

Although it is traditional to immobilize the joint to relieve pain during the acute phase of the disease, Salter and coworkers believe that motion of the joint should be established as soon as possible. They advocate use of a continuing passive motion machine. From their experimental study on rabbits, they believe that this improves nutrition of the cartilage, prevents adhesions, and enhances clearance of lysosomal enzymes and purulent exudate from the infected joint while at the same time stimulating the chondrocytes to synthesize matrix components.[126]

Complications

Lloyd-Roberts has commented that despite the alarming x-ray changes, which may give a false impression of the extent of damage to the joint, the prognosis may in fact be relatively good and that a favorable outcome can be predicted with confidence in many of these children.[122] He also points out that the final shape of the articulating surface is not dependent upon the degree of decalcification of the ossific nucleus (epiphysis) or even the metaphysis but upon the damage caused to the physis. Such damage cannot be seen in an early radiograph. The same author suggests that the hip joint be manipulated and explored if the radiographic and physical signs suggest either that dislocation has occurred or that there is so much damage that dislocation may occur in the future. In favorable cases, the hip may be relocated and thereby stabilized.[122]

With modern treatment, substantial mortality and morbidity no longer follow this disease. In general, it can be said that growth disturbances such as coxa magna and those associated with destruction of the femoral capital epiphysis relate to the duration of symptoms before appropriate diagnosis and correct treatment were instituted.[118]

In cases of chronic septic arthritis, there may be an occasional indication for synovectomy as part of a general debridement. At the same time, appropriate cultures may be obtained by biopsy of synovium and bone. Biopsy is rarely required in pyogenic infections. The procedure would seem to be particularly indicated following traumatic injuries to joints and in those cases where the infection is superimposed upon an underlying chronic arthritis.

PROPHYLAXIS AGAINST INFECTION IN BONE AND JOINT SURGERY

Elective total joint surgery and open reduction of fractures are indications for prophylaxis. There is controversy about which antibiotic should be used, most authors recommending a first-generation cephalosporin such as cefazolin.[127]

Vancomycin should be used for patients allergic to penicillins or cephalosporins and for hospitals in which *S. epidermidis* or methicillin-resistant *S. aureus* is a frequent cause of postoperative infection.[128] A single 1- to 2-g dose of cefazolin or 1-g dose of vancomycin given slowly over 60 min just before the surgical procedure should provide adequate tissue concentrations throughout the operation. If surgery is prolonged, a second dose of antibiotic may be required; however, postoperative prophylactic antibiotics are generally not necessary.[128]

REFERENCES

1. Jackson MA, Nelson JD: Etiology and medical management of acute suppurative bone and joint infection in pediatric patients. *J Pediatr Orthop* 2:313, 1982.
2. Cole WG, Dalziel RE, Leitl S: Treatment of acute osteomyelitis in childhood. *J Bone Joint Surg* 64B:218, 1982.
3. Nade S: Acute hematogenous osteomyelitis in infancy and childhood. *J Bone Joint Surg* 65B:109, 1983.
4. DiLiberti JH, Tarlow S: Bone and joint complications of *Haemophilus influenzae*. *Clin Pediatr* 22:7, 1983.
5. Kasser JR: Hematogenous osteomyelitis. *Postgrad Med* 76:79, 1984.
6. Resnick D, Niwayama G: Osteomyelitis, septic arthritis and soft tissue infection, in Resnick D, Niwayama G. (eds): *Diagnosis of Bone and Joint Disorders.* Vol III. Philadelphia, Saunders, 1981, pp 2042–2129.
7. Ogden JA: Pediatric osteomyelitis and septic arthritis: The pathology of neonatal disease. *Yale J Biol Med* 52:423, 1979.
8. Bobechko WP: Infections of bones and joints, in Lovell WW, Winter RB (eds): *Pediatric Orthopaedics.* Philadelphia, Lippincott, 1978.
9. Ekengren K, Bergdahl S, Eriksson M: Neonatal osteomyelitis. *Acta Radiol [Diagn]* 23:305, 1982.

10. Ash JM, Gilday B: The futility of bone scanning in neonatal osteomyelitis: Concise communication. *J Nucl Med* 21:417, 1980.

11. Sullivan JA, Vasileff T, Leonard JC: An evaluation of nuclear scanning in orthopaedic infections. *J Pediatr Orthop* 1:73, 1981.

12. Anderson JR, Orr JD, MacLean DA, Scobie WG: Acute hematogenous osteitis. *Arch Dis Child* 55:953, 1980.

13. Blockey NJ, Watson JT: Acute osteomyelitis in children. *J Bone Joint Surg* 52B:77, 1970.

14. O'Brien T, McManus F, MacAuley PH, Ennis JT: Acute hematogenous osteomyelitis. *J Bone Joint Surg* 64B:450–453, 1982.

15. Winters JL, Cohen I: Acute haematogenous osteomyelitis. *J Bone Joint Surg* 42A:691, 1960.

16. Black CH, Shelswell JH: A serological test in the diagnosis of staphylococcal infection. *J Bone Joint Surg* 37B:135, 1955.

17. Tuazon CU: Teichoic acid antibodies in osteomyelitis and septic arthritis caused by *Staphylococcus aureus*. *J Bone Joint Surg* 64A:762, 1982.

18. Ferguson AB: *Orthopaedic Surgery in Infancy and Childhood,* 4th ed. Baltimore, Williams & Wilkins, 1975.

19. Bonakdar-Pour A, Gaines VD: The radiology of osteomyelitis. *Orthop Clin North Am* 14:21–37, 1983.

20. Berkowitz ID: Normal technetium bone scans in patients with osteomyelitis. *Am J Dis Child* 114:828, 1980.

21. Handmaker H: Acute hematogenous osteomyelitis: Has the bone scan betrayed us? *Radiology* 135:787, 1980.

22. Handmaker H, Giammona A: The "hot-joint"—Increased diagnostic accuracy using combined 99mTc-phosphate and 67Ga citrate imaging in pediatrics. *J Nucl Med* 17:554, 1976.

23. Handmaker H, Leonards R: The bone scan in inflammatory osseous disease. *Semin Nucl Med* 6:95, 1976.

24. Merkel KD, Fitzgerald RH Jr, Brown ML: Scintigraphic evaluation in musculoskeletal sepsis. *Orthop Clin North Am* 15:401, 1984.

25. Merkel KD, Brown ML, Dewanjee MK, Fitzgerald RH Jr: Comparison of indium-labelled leukocyte imaging with sequential technetium gallium scanning in diagnosis of low grade musculoskeletal sepsis. *J Bone Joint Surg* 67A:465, 1985.

26. Murray IPC: Photopenia, skeletal scintography of suspected bone and joint infection. *Clin Nucl Med* 7:13, 1982.

27. Dormans JP, Drummond DS: Pediatric hematogenous osteomyelitis: New trends in presentation, diagnosis and treatment. *J Am Acad Orthop Surg* 2:333–341, 1994.

28. Wegener WA, Alavi A: Diagnostic imaging of musculoskeletal infection. *Orthop Clin North Am* 22:401–418, 1991.

29. Unger E, Moldofsky P, Gatenby R, et al: Diagnosis of osteomyelitis by MR imaging. *Am J Roentgenol* 150:605, 1988.

30. Dick PQ, Nelson JD, Haltalen KC: Osteomyelitis in infants and children: A review of 163 cases. *Am J Dis Child* 129:1273, 1975.

31. Syriopoulou VP, Smith A: Osteomyelitis and septic arthritis, in Feigin RD, Cherry JD (eds): *Textbook of Pediatric Infectious Diseases,* 3d ed. Philadelphia, Saunders, 1992, pp 727–746.

32. Gillespie WJ, Mayo KM: The management of acute haematogenous osteomyelitis in the antibiotics era: A study of the outcome. *J Bone Joint Surg* 63B:126, 1981.

33. Pichl FC, Davis RJ, Prugh SI: Osteomyelitis in sickle cell disease. *J Pediatr Orthop* 13:225, 1993.

34. Nelson JD, Bucholz RW, Kuzmiesz H, Shelton S: Benefits and risks of sequential parenteral-oral cephalosporin therapy for suppurative bone and joint infections. *J Pediatr Orthop* 2:255, 1982.

35. Thompson RL, Wright AJ. Antimicrobial therapy in musculoskeletal surgery. *Orthop Clin North Am* 15:547, 1984.

36. Cunha BA: The use of penicillins in orthopaedic surgery. *Clin Orthop* 190:36, 1984.

37. Anderson LD, Horn LG: Irrigation suction technique in treatment of acute hematogenous osteomyelitis, chronic osteomyelitis and acute and chronic joint infections. *South Med J* 63:745, 1970.

38. Kawashima M, Tamura H: Topical therapy in orthopaedic infection. *Orthopaedics* 7:1592–1598, 1984.

39. Cole WG, Dalziel RE, Leitl S: Treatment of acute osteomyelitis in childhood. *J Bone Joint Surg* 64B:218–223, 1982.

40. Mok PM, Reilley BJ, Ash JM: Osteomyelitis in neonates: Clinical aspects and the role of radiography and scintigraphy in diagnosis and management. *Radiology* 145:677, 1982.

41. Gilmour WN: Acute haematogenous osteomyelitis. *J Bone Joint Surg* 44B:841, 1962.

42. Roberts PH: Disturbed epiphyseal growth at the knee after osteomyelitis in infancy. *J Bone Joint Surg* 52B:692, 1970.

43. Green NE, Beauchamp RD, Griffin PP: Primary subacute epiphyseal osteomyelitis. *J Bone Joint Surg* 63A:107, 1981.

44. Ross ERS, Cole WG: Treatment of subacute osteomyelitis in childhood. *J Bone Joint Surg* 67B:443, 1985.

45. Brodie B: *Pathological and Surgical Observation on the Diseases of the Joints,* 4th ed. London, Longman, 1836.

46. Gledhill RB: Subacute osteomyelitis in children. *Clin Orthop* 96:57, 1973.

47. Cierny G III, Mader JT: Adult chronic osteomyelitis. *Orthopaedics* 7:1557, 1984.

48. West WF, et al: Chronic osteomyelitis: Factors affecting the results of treatment in 186 patients. *JAMA* 213:1837, 1970.

49. Gentry LO: Antibiotic therapy for osteomyelitis. *Infect Dis Clin North Am* 4:485, 1990.

50. Phemister DB: Chronic fibrous osteomyelitis. *Ann Surg* 90:756, 1929.

51. Turek SL: Bone infections, in *Orthopaedics: Principles and Their Application.* Philadelphia, Lippincott, 1977, p 207.

52. Kelly PK: Osteomyelitis in the adult. *Orthop Clin North Am* 6:983, 1975.

53. Cierny G III: Chronic osteomyelitis: Results of treatment. AAOS *Instr Course Lect* 39:495–508, 1990.

54. Patzakis MJ, Calhoun JH, Cierny G III, et al: Symposium: Current concepts in the management of osteomyelitis. *Contemp Orthop* 28:157–185, 1994.

55. Feldman DS, Lonner JH, Desai P, Zuckerman JD. The role of intraoperative frozen sections in revision total joint arthroplasty. *J Bone Joint Surg* 77A:1807–1813, 1995.

56. Mader JT, Calhoun J: Osteomyelitis, in Mandell GL, Bennett JE, Dolin R (eds): *Principles and Practice of Infectious Diseases,* 4th ed. New York, Churchill Livingstone, 1995, pp 1039–1051.

57. Hughes SPF, Anderson FM: Penetration of antibiotics into bone. *J Antimicrob Chemother* 15:517, 1985.

58. Quintiliani R, Nightingale C: Principles of antibiotic usage. *Clin Orthop* 190:31, 1984.

59. Mader JT, Adams KR: Experimental osteomyelitis, in Schlossberg D (ed): *Orthopaedic Infection.* New York, Springer-Verlag, 1988, pp 39–48.

60. Jacobsson S, Hollender L, Lindberg S, Larsson A: Chronic sclerosing osteomyelitis of the mandible. *Scint Radiogr Find Oral Surg* 45:167, 1978.

61. Hall BB, Fitzgerald RH Jr, Rosenblatt JE: Anaerobic osteomyelitis. *J Bone Joint Surg* 65A:30, 1983.

62. Mathes SJ, Alpert BS, Chang N: Use of muscle flap in chronic osteomyelitis: Experimental and clinical correlation. *Plast Reconstr Surg* 69:815, 1982.

63. May JW Jr, Gallico GG III, Lukash FN: Microvascular transfer of free tissue for closure of bone wounds of the distal lower extremity. *N Engl J Med* 306:253, 1982.

64. Weiland AJ, Moore JR, Daniel RK: Vascularized bone autografts: Experience with 41 cases. *Clin Orthop* 174:87, 1983.

65. Gorbach S, Partlett JG: Anaerobic infections: Parts I, II and III. *N Engl J Med* 290:1177, 1237, 1289, 1974.

66. Ruttle PE, Kelly PJ, Arnold PG, et al: Chronic osteomyelitis treated with a muscle flap. *Orthop Clin North Am* 15:451, 1984.

67. Weiland AJ, Moore JR, Daniel RK: The efficacy of free tissue transfer in the treatment of osteomyelitis. *J Bone Joint Surg* 66A:181, 1984.

68. Rhinelander FW: Minimal fixation of tibial fractures. *Clin Orthop* 107:188, 1975.

69. Papineau LJ, Alfageme A, Delacourt JP, Pilon L: Osteomylitie chronique: Excision et greffe de spongieux a l'air libre après mises á plat extensive. *Int Orthop* (SKOT) 3:165, 1979.

70. Papineau LJ: L'excision-greffe avec fermeture retardée deliberée dans l'ostomyelite chronique. *Nouv Presse Med* 2:2753, 1973.

71. Sachs BL, Shaffer BW: A staged Papineau protocol for chronic osteomyelitis. *Clin Orthop* 184:256, 1984.

72. Zammit F: Undulant fever spondylitis. *Br J Radiol* 31:683, 1958.

73. Taylor GI, Miller GDH, Ham FJ: The free vascularized bone graft. *Plast Reconstr Surg* 55:533, 1975.

74. Weiland AJ: Current concepts review: Vascularized free bone transplant. *J Bone Joint Surg* 63A:166, 1981.

75. Weiland AJ, Kleinert HE, Kutz JE, et al: Free vascularized bone graft in the surgery of the upper extremity. *J Hand Surg* 4:129, 1979.

76. Wood MB, Cooney WP: Vascularized bone segment transfers for management of chronic osteomyelitis. *Orthop Clin North Am* 15:461, 1984.

77. Taylor GI, Townsend P, Corlett R: Superiority of the deep circumflex iliac vessels as the supply for free groin flaps: Experiment work. *Plast Reconstr Surg* 64:595, 1979.

78. Colville J, Brady PG, Regan BF: Acute hematogenous osteomyelitis in children with emphasis on treatment. *J Ir Med Assoc* 69:200, 1976.

79. Cierny G III, Zorn K: Segmental tibial defects: Conventional and Ilizarov methodologies. Etiology and medical management of acute suppurative bone and joint infection in pediatric patients. *J Pediatr Clin Orthop* 301:118–123, 1994.

80. Garré C: Über besondere Formen und Folgerzustande der akuten infektiosen Osteomyelitis. *Beitr Klin Chir Tubing* 10:241, 1893.

81. Jones SF: Sclerosing non-suppurative osteomyelitis as described by Garré. *JAMA* 24:985, 1921.

82. Meyerding HW: Chronic sclerosing osteitis (sclerosing non-suppurative osteomyelitis of Garré). *Surg Clin North Am* 24:762, 1944.

83. Collert S, Isacson J: Chronic sclerosing osteomyelitis (Garré). *Clin Orthop* 164:136, 1982.

84. Kopits SE, Debuskey M: Primary sclerosing osteomyelitis. *Johns Hopkins Med J* 140:241, 1977.

85. Ellis DJ, Winslow JR, Indovina AA: Garré's osteomyelitis of the mandible. *Oral Surg* 44:183, 1977.

86. Johannsen A: Chronic sclerosing osteomyelitis of the mandible. *Acta Radiol [Diagn]* 18:360, 1977.

87. Brand RA, Black H: *Pseudomonas* osteomyelitis following puncture wounds in children. *J Bone Joint Surg* 56A:1637, 1974.

88. Hagler, DS: *Pseudomonas* osteomyelitis: Puncture wounds of the feet. *Pediatrics* 48:672, 1971.

89. Johannsen PH: *Pseudomonas* infection in the foot following puncture wounds. *JAMA* 204:262, 1968.

90. Riegler HF, Rouston FW: Complications of deep puncture wounds of the foot. *J Trauma* 19:18, 1979.

91. Green NE: *Pseudomonas* infection of the foot following puncture wounds. *Instr Course Lect* 32:43, 1983.

92. Gaenslen FJ: Split-heel approach in osteomyelitis of the os calcis. *J Bone Joint Surg* 13:759, 1931.

93. Morgan A, Yates AK: The diagnosis of acute osteomyelitis of the pelvis. *Postgrad Med J* 42:74, 1966.

94. Highland TR, LaMont RL: Osteomyelitis of the pelvis in children. *J Bone Joint Surg* 65A:230, 1983.

95. Chan DPK, Kammell WM, Caky D, et al: Multifocal hematogenous *Serratia marcescens* osteomyelitis in a drug user: Case report and review of the literature. *Contemp Orthop* 2:344, 1980.

96. Lowbeer L: Brucellotic osteomyelitis of the spinal column in man. *Am J Pathol* 24:723, 1948.

97. Zvetina JR: *Mycobacterium kansasii* infection of the elbow joint. *J Bone Joint Surg* 61A:1099, 1979.

98. Del Rio MDLA: *Brucella* osteomyelitis. *Pediatr Infect Dis* 2:50, 1983.

99. Cohen JI, Bartlett JA, Corey GR: Extraintestinal manifestations of *Salmonella* infections. *Medicine* 66:349, 1987.

100. Hall BB, Rosenblatt JE, Fitzgerald RH Jr: Anaerobic septic arthritis and osteomyelitis. *Orthop Clin North Am* 15:505, 1984.

101. Mackowsiak PA, Jones SR, Smith JW: Diagnostic value of sinus-tract cultures in chronic osteomyelitis. *JAMA* 239:2772, 1978.

102. Fitzgerald RH, Rosenblatt JE, Tenney JH, Bourgault AM: Anaerobic septic arthritis. *Clin Orthop* 164:141, 1982.

103. Chow AW, Montgomerie JZ, Guze LB: Parenteral clindamycin therapy for severe anaerobic infections. *Arch Intern Med* 134:78, 1974.

104. Murray PR, Rosenblatt JE: Penicillin resistance and penicillinase production in clinical isolates of *Bacteroides melaninogenicus*. *Antimicrob Agents Chemother* 11:605, 1977.

105. Salaki JS, Black R, Tally FP, Kislak JW: *Bacteroides fragilis* resistant to the administration of clindamycin. *Am J Med* 60:426, 1976.

106. Pritchard, DJ: Granulomatous infections of bones and joints. *Orthop Clin North Am* 6:1029, 1975.

107. Duran RJ, Coventry MB, Weed LA, Kierland RR: Sporotrichosis: A report of twenty-three cases in the upper extremity. *J Bone Joint Surg* 39A:1330, 1957.

108. Peterson HA: Fungal osteomyelitis in children. *Instr Course Lect* 32:46, 1983.

109. Lang AG, Peterson HA: Osteomyelitis following puncture wounds of the foot in children. *J Trauma* 16:993, 1976.

110. McCall RE: Maduromycosis *Allescheria boydii* arthritis of the knee: A case report. *Orthopaedics* 4:1144, 1981.

111. Check WA: Oral antifungal agent effective even for widespread infections. *JAMA* 244:2019, 1980.

112. Tachdjian MO: *Pediatric Orthopaedics.* Philadelphia, Saunders, 1972, p 352.

113. Sengupta A: Musculoskeletal lesions in yaws. *Clin Orthop* 192:193, 1985.

114. Davies PDO, Humphries MJ, Byfield SP, et al: Bone and joint tuberculosis: A survey of notifications in England and Wales. *J Bone Joint Surg* 66B:326, 1984.

115. Marchevsky A, Damsker B, Green S, et al: The clinicopathological spectrum of nontuberculous mycobacterial osteoarticular infection. *J Bone Joint Surg* 67A:925, 1985.

116. Cooper C, Cawley MID: Bacterial arthritis in an English health district: A 10-year review. *Ann Rheum Dis* 45:458, 1986.

117. Gardner GC, Weisman MH: Pyarthroses in patients with rheumatoid arthritis: A report of 13 cases and a review of the literature from the past 40 years. *Am J Med* 88:502, 1990.

118. Philips PE: Bacterial arthritis: Uncovering the underlying cause. *J Musculoskel Med* 1:14, 1984.

119. Nade S: Acute septic arthritis in infancy and childhood. *J Bone Joint Surg* 65B:234, 1983.

120. Nade S, Robertson FW, Taylor TKJ: Antibiotics in the treatment of acute osteomyelitis and acute septic arthritis in children. *Med J Aust* 2:703, 1974.

121. Nelson JD, Koontz WC: Septic arthritis in infants and children: A review of 117 cases. *Pediatrics* 38:966, 1966.

122. Lloyd-Roberts GC: Suppurative arthritis in infants. *J Bone Joint Surg* 42B:706, 1960.

123. Ward J, Cohen AS, Bauer W: The diagnosis and therapy of acute suppurative arthritis. *Arthritis Rheum* 3:522, 1960.

124. Lloyd-Roberts GC: Septic arthritis in infancy. *Aust Pediatr J* 15:41, 1979.

125. Compere EL, Metzger WI, Mitra RN: The treatment of pyogenic bone and joint infections by closed irrigation (circulation) with a non-toxic detergent and one or more antibiotics. *J Bone Joint Surg* 49A:614, 1967.

126. Salter RB, Bell RS, Keeley FW: The protective effect of continuous passive motion of living articular cartilage in acute septic arthritis: An experimental investigation in rabbit. *Clin Orthop* 159:223, 1981.

127. Williams J-L, Gustilo RB: The use of preventive antibiotics in orthopedic surgery. *Clin Orthop* 190:83–88, 1984.

128. Antimicrobial prophylaxis in surgery. *Med Lett Drugs Ther* 37:79, 1995.

CHAPTER 18

Amputations and Prosthetics

Ernest M. Burgess, David A. Boone, and Joan T. Gold

I. Amputations and Prosthetics in Adults

Ernest M. Burgess and David A. Boone

AMPUTATION

General Considerations

Historically, trauma and infection have been responsible for most amputations. Pyogenic infections associated with open trauma, in particular gas gangrene, required amputation as a lifesaving measure. War surgeons have measured their skill in terms of speedy and lifesaving limb ablation.

Congenital amputations and severe congenital limb deficits are recorded in the earliest medical history. They occur in all countries. The thalidomide experience provided a remarkable opportunity to observe the influence of exogenous agents as a cause of limb teratogenesis. A majority of these limb deficits can be fitted with appropriate prosthetic devices and do not require surgical revision. Surgical conversion or amputation when indicated often necessitates considerable ingenuity.

Tumors of the extremities continue to require amputations. While connective tissue malignancies of the limbs are few and—with modern oncology management—require amputation less frequently than in the past, they have continued to be responsible for a small percentage of limb loss. As we approach the twenty-first century, the profile of persons requiring amputation is radically changing in the developed countries. Several circumstances are responsible for the change. The first of these is the control of local and systemic infection. Gas gangrene, tuberculosis, leprosy, and other similar scourges are being managed effectively. Following trauma and tumor resection, highly refined limb salvage surgery involving microvascular reconstruction, composite tissue grafting, and prosthetic replacement techniques now saves many limbs that formerly would have come to amputation.

The most important factor changing the profile of limb loss is increasing longevity, with greater numbers of elderly patients developing limb ischemia. Circulatory diseases are responsible for 80 percent or more of major amputations in civilian life today. Approximately half of these individuals suffers from diabetes.[1–3]

Revascularization can prolong viability of the ischemic limb with acceptable comfort and function. This treatment is, however, by its nature, only palliative. The underlying disease processes are not arrested or eliminated by vascular reconstruction, and most end-stage vascular disease requires amputation usually involving the lower limbs. The majority of these patients are 65 years of age and older. The systemic nature of their vascular disease and associated chronic disease states make rehabilitation with restoration of a useful degree of pain-free mobility following amputation a challenge involving many health care disciplines. The changing indications for amputation and remarkable improvements in surgical management have rendered obsolescent many time-honored concepts.[4,5] Long-established sites of election have become obsolete with improved understanding of limb viability,[6] the great progress in prosthetic limb substitutes, and scientific rehabilitation. Staged amputations in the presence of infection have been radically modified as a result of antibiotics. The amputation has become a reconstructive surgical exercise, the reconstruction of a terminal motor and sensory end organ which, through a prosthetic substitute, will interface with the environment.

Surgery

Amputation surgery has been considered dull, professionally unrewarding, and requiring modest technical skills. Surgical training programs often use amputation as a source of basic training in surgical technique to be performed by the most junior member of the house staff, often inadequately supervised. The surgery is further diminished by many surgeons' inadequate knowledge of prosthetic substitution. The surgeon's involvement must continue beyond the period of wound healing to effective rehabilitation. Not only is this a professional requisite, but it gives the surgeon the opportunity to see the patient relieved of pain, with mobility restored and an improved quality of life.

Preoperative Evaluation When the need for amputation has been established and the patient's condition is amenable to surgery, a level of amputation must be established. The tissues must be able to heal at the selected level, and the amputation site must be tolerant of its interface with the prosthesis. An additional requirement is the availability of a suitable prosthesis to fit the residual limb created by the level of amputation.

Detailed physical examination and objective limb viability measurements distate the most distal level of amputation that can be expected to heal. A working knowledge of modern limb substitutes consolidates the decision.

Wound healing is particularly critical in determining the level of amputation for end-stage vascular disease. One of the most significant advances in amputation surgical technique for ischemia relates to an improved understanding of limb viability, allowing more accurate amputation level determination.[6,7] Consequently the number of more distal amputations in the lower limb, i.e., below the knee, has dramatically increased in the last decade and a half. This change is reflected in the improved performance of elderly amputees whose knee joint is preserved and who may thereby maintain functional independence.

A number of laboratory procedures are designed to assist in determining the level of amputation preoperatively. Some of these tests are "borrowed" from the vascular review of limbs by surgeons planning reconstruction. Unfortunately, most of the tests that outline the vascular tree of the limb are not specific indicators of the ability of the tissues, particularly the skin, to heal primarily at the amputation level selected.

While none of the laboratory procedures are completely indicative of appropriate levels of amputation, they do add useful information, especially in questionable cases. The physical examination—including sensibility, ischemic pain levels, etc.—is still the most valuable contribution to level selection preoperatively.

There continues to be a good deal of work to identify limb viability more specifically. These studies should soon delineate appropriate levels of amputation in a high percentage of cases. Objective data are particularly valuable to assist the surgeon who only occasionally performs an amputation and is not as astute in assessing wound healing potential as the operator who is seeing and performing amputations frequently.

The Operation With few exceptions, all prostheses today totally contact the residual limb. The basic principles of plastic and reconstructive surgery apply in the same manner that they are used in surgery of the hand and the foot. Since the amputation site becomes the end organ of the limb contacting the environment, each structure is carefully treated at surgery to permit uneventful healing. Surgical conservation of tissues is the rule. This means in most instances preservation of limb length.

The surgeon seeks a well-healed, nonadherent, painless scar. The surrounding skin should be healthy, with retained sensation. Since the prosthetic socket totally contacts the stump, placement of the scar is relatively unimportant.[1,8]

Muscles make up the bulk of the limb at the site of a major amputation. The contractile function of the muscle is lost when skeletal attachment has been severed. Under these circumstances, muscles atrophy and residual limb function is diminished. Muscles can be stabilized at or near the site of amputation by suturing the muscle itself or its ligamentous and tendinous insertion into bone.[1] This technique (myodesis) is most effective in above-knee and through-knee amputations in the lower limb and in above-elbow and through-elbow amputations in the upper limb. The suturing of muscles to periosteum and distally to each other (myoplasty) is also effective provided that the sutured muscle groups do not form a sling over the end of the severed bone. A fixed attachment is necessary to allow physiologic muscle function and also to prevent the formation of painful bursae. In the presence of ischemia, when primary wound healing is of critical importance, the added surgery for muscle stabilization can compromise wound healing. Fascial closure is used in these conditions.

The treatment of nerves sectioned by amputation has been controversial for centuries. All sectioned nerves form neuromas. Surgical attempts to minimize neuroma formation and to limit or diminish stump pain and/or phantom limb pain include burying the ends of the nerves in bone, cauterizing, crushing, injection with a variety of chemical agents, and ligation. Current practice dictates ligation only with the nerve moderately retracted to allow the sectioned end to retract into the soft tissues away from the site of prosthetic interface pressure. Ligation confines the neuroma and tends to prevent outgrowth. Hemorrhage from the blood vessels contained within the nerve is also controlled by the ligation. Gentle handling of tissues is essential for minimal scar formation. Blood vessels are ligated and cautery is used on the small vessels only.

Proper surgical management of the bone is of great importance. With diaphyseal amputations, the bone is divided with a sharp saw and the cortex well rounded using a saw or file. Good soft tissue coverage is necessary to avoid pressure-sensitive skin problems. With children, the periosteum is removed 0.5 cm from its distal end to diminish or prevent bone regeneration and spur formation. With the adult and particularly the elderly, the periosteum should be left long to be drawn over the end of the sectioned bone and sutured, closing off the medullary canal.

A number of significant improvements and innovations in techniques of amputation surgery have been developed. Muscle stabilization, myodesis, and myoplasty were described above. Angulation osteotomy, tibiofibular synotosis, and cineplasty are among others.[1,4]

Immediate Postoperative Care Important recent improvements in postoperative wound management include the use of rigid dressings, controlled environment chambers, and early mobilization systems.[9a,9b] The amputation presents a unique opportunity for postoperative physical wound management. The wound being terminal, the dressings can apply pressure to control edema. This permits the use or rigid dressings that permit quiet healing, protect the limb, and minimize pain and trauma. As wound healing progresses, the cast or other rigid dressing material can be used as temporary sockets to which a terminal device is applied for limited weight bearing in the lower limb and dexterous hand substitution in the upper limb. The skills required to apply appropriate rigid dressings are precise but easily acquired. Immediate postoperative soft compression dressings are still extensively used but are less effective than rigid dressings in providing an ideal wound healing environment. They displace easily and pressures are difficult to control, especially with elastic wrapping. Frequent reapplication is usually needed.

The Amputation Team The health care skills requisite for amputee rehabilitation are surgical, prosthetic, and rehabilitative. No single discipline encompasses these basic needs, and wartime experience suggests that a dedicated amputation center with an integrated team is the best approach.[2] Although the amputation team functions best in such a setting, it is possible to achieve good communication between the surgeon, the prosthetist, and the therapist operating independently. Absence of a fully integrated team need not preclude many of the benefits of team care.

Rehabilitation

Clinical rehabilitation following amputation is generally carried out by the physical therapist, corrective therapist, and others under the direction of the surgeon or physiatrist. Emphasis is on early, progressive restoration of function. As wound healing progresses, the initial or subsequent rigid dressings can serve as early, temporary prostheses. As soon as wound healing is sound, a provisional or preparatory limb is prescribed.[5,10] As the tissues mature and stabilize in size and pressure tolerance, a definitive limb can be provided. Early progressive rehabilitation has largely eliminated stump and phantom pain as a source of significant long-term disability.

Kinesiologists including those specializing in gait, and a considerable number of people involved in rehabilitation research are contributing to improved, rapid amputee function. Amputee seminars, amputee recreation groups, and physical competition among amputees have combined to enhance social adjustment to achieve performance levels that are often remarkable.

Complications of Amputation Surgery

Complications following amputation are those generally related to wound healing and observed in all types of limb surgery. These include primary wound infections, ischemic necrosis, wound dehiscence, pain, edema, and dysfunction and deformity of proximal structures, especially joints.[1,8]

As the amputation wound is terminal, there are no tissues beyond the site of the surgery to require postoperative management; the wound itself can be subjected to a controlled postoperative physical environment. This environment includes pressure gradients, wound immobilization, thermal and humidity parameters, and sterility.

Postoperative wound infections are handled in the usual manner, with adequate drainage, debridement, and antibiotics. Secondary closure or reamputation may be required. Wound complications secondary to ischemia may involve the skin, the deeper tissues, or both. Ischemic wound dehiscence with or without infection is characteristically seen where determination of the level at which the limb is viable has been inadequate prior to surgery and the amputation is performed through tissues incapable of healing the surgical insult primarily. When local ischemia and necrosis are present, there is usually no chance for secondary healing to occur with local or skin graft coverage. The ischemia related to the wound breakdown militates against there being sufficient healing capacity of those local tissues to close by secondary intent. Reamputation is usually required.

Postsurgical amputee pain in a phenomenon differing from the pain ordinarily experienced following limb surgery. When all structures of the limb, including major and minor nerves, are sectioned transversely, subsequent immediate and long-range pain phenomena are often unique to the amputation alone. This subject is covered in

more depth later in this chapter. Edema and ischemia result in pain. Early postsurgical wound management is directed toward minimizing these normal inflammatory responses following the trauma of surgery. Controlled and carefully monitored postsurgical pressure dressings, whether rigid or soft, are essential. Terminal edema by proximal constriction must be avoided. Skilled application of the rigid dressings, and proper bandaging of the stump postoperatively, are essential ingredients to management preventing these complications. Hematomas can be a very serious complication, especially when the amputation has been performed for ischemia. They can be avoided by adequate hemostasis and careful closure of the dead space. Their prompt recognition postoperatively allows early evacuation of their contents.

Regional Considerations

The amputation is by nature destructive. The whole or a part of a functioning organ is removed and replaced by an inert artificial device, the prosthesis. Since the prosthesis is applied specifically to restore function, it is necessary to understand the functional characteristics of what has been removed and to duplicate them as completely as possible with the artificial limb—that is, functional substitution. This implies that the surgeon has a detailed working knowledge of the function that has been lost. The amputation carries with it the additional loss of body form. The social and psychological outcomes of this loss of body image are in many ways quite unique. The specifics of functional loss and the priorities related to prosthetic substitution are covered in the discussion of the levels of limb loss.

Amputation, Lower Limb

The basic physiologic/mechanical function of the lower limb is to provide stability in stance and gait. This requirement carries over directly into prosthetic substitution. An amputee can stand on a well-secured rigid pylon with no intervening articulations. As the sophistication of prosthetic design progresses, an enlarged range of functional capability and cosmesis is achieved. Today many unilateral lower-limb amputees, even including those with amputations at high, above-knee levels, can walk with little or no perceptible limp. Below-knee amputees, including those with Syme's amputations, not only may have a normal gait but can perform many complex functional activities, including running.

Amputations through the Foot

The foot is an articulated platform providing us with important kinesthetic and proprioceptive information. Removal of any portion of the foot including the toes progressively decreases the size of the platform. The amputation also interferes with the motor leverage system, thus impairing gait. Sensory loss following amputation may affect postural balance.[1,11]

Removal of one or more of the lesser toes disturbs gait minimally if at all. No prostheses are required other than minor shoe adjustments and, on occasion, toe fillers for comfort. Amputation of the great toe is more disabling. Balance and push-off are appreciably affected. Loss of great toe function is especially noticeable when the amputee is attempting to walk rapidly or run in ordinary shoes, particularly soft shoes. This deficit can be masked to some degree by firm shoes that have a rocker-bar mechanism on the sole in the metatarsal region. As with the lesser toes, removal of the great toe does not require prosthetic substitution other than an insole with toe filler for comfort and attention to proper shoe mechanics.

Amputation of one or more toes is usually occasioned by trauma and/or peripheral vascular disease. The surgical techniques are standard. Amputations through the foot including the toes should be viewed as reconstructive plastic surgery. Scars are placed to avoid pressure on the weight-bearing surfaces. Tight skin closures are specifically avoided, and underlying rigid structures—i.e., bone and cartilage—are carefully tailored to avoid sources of pressure that could cause pain or breakdown of overlying skin.

Like all amputations in the foot, transverse amputation through the metatarsals or resection of one or more rays requires careful planning to avoid painful scars. Plantar skin, which is anatomically designed for weight bearing, should be used to cover the plantar and distal surfaces where weight-bearing forces are concentrated. Bone surfaces should be free of irregularities, especially in the weight-bearing areas. Muscle rebalancing is not usually required, since the leg muscles that control ankle and foot function are preserved and postsurgical deformities do not develop.

For amputations through the metatarsals, shoe modification and an insole with forefoot space replacement are satisfactory to improve gait and push-off. Most patients with such amputations can then walk well with little or no appreciable limp other than occasionally having a short stride. If the patient attempts to move from slow and average walking speeds to a fast walk and a run, the deficit becomes apparent.

Amputations through the midfoot have been described in past literature by proper names. Lisfranc's amputation is performed at the tarsometatarsal joints, Chopart's amputation is carried out through the midtarsal joints, and in Pirogoff's amputation, the calcaneus is rotated forward, to be fused to the tibia after vertical section through the midportion of the calcaneus. The Boyd amputation consists of talectomy and forward shift of the calcaneus with calcaneotibial arthrodesis. With present surgical and prosthetic management of amputations through the body of the foot, surgical modifications are often required, so that it is now more appropriate to describe the level of amputation anatomically.

Amputations through the tarsometatarsal joints and through the area of the cuneiforms and distal cuboid bone significantly reduce the size of the foot platform. Major long tendon insertions are disturbed. When the blood supply is adequate for primary healing, muscle rebalancing can be accomplished by surgical section or transfer of tendon insertions. These procedures are designed to maintain a plantigrade, controlled residual foot without contractures or deformity.

The common deformity that develops is a fixed equinus and varus due to the overpull of the gastrocnemius-soleus and posterior tibial muscles. Loss of insertion of the peroneus longus and the long toe extensors additionally produces the deformity. Heel cord lengthening or section, transfer of the anterior tibial tendon insertion to the midline on the dorsum of the foot, and section of the tibialis posterior tendon may prevent fixed equinovarus deformity. Tibiocalcaneal arthrodesis, as with the Boyd and Pirogoff operations, provides a stable, direct weight-bearing surface covered by heel skin. In the presence of ischemia, questionable feeling potential, and a tenuous skin envelope, this rebalancing surgery may not be justified. At this amputation level, dynamic imbalance with potential deformity is best managed in the presence of ischemia by simple tendon sectioning. As the surgeon is able to assess skin-healing potential throughout the foot more accurately, more through-foot amputations are being carried out with successful primary healing.

Proximal foot amputation with retention of the talus and calcaneus or preservation of the calcaneus alone is reserved principally for individuals who will not be fitted with a prosthesis and will be able to walk wearing only a simple shoe or boot. This amputation is frequently used in the less developed countries, where prosthetic services are limited. Proximal foot amputations eliminate those muscle insertions responsible for ankle and toe dorsiflexor power as well as inversion and eversion. Plantar flexion deformity can be prevented or corrected by heel cord section.

Prosthetic substitution for midfoot and hindfoot amputations is difficult. The degree of loss of the foot platform causes an unstable gait. Absence of the forefoot lever arm eliminates physiologic push-off. The advantages of full limb length and a distal end-bearing residual limb can be weighed against the improved function available in more proximal levels of amputations such as the Syme's amputations, where prosthetic components that functionally replace the ankle mechanism are available. Ingenuity is required in designing shoes and prostheses for the more proximal foot amputations (Figs. 18-1 and 18-2). If a combination insole support with anterior filler is fitted into a high boot with a stiff sole and an anterior rocker bar, it al-

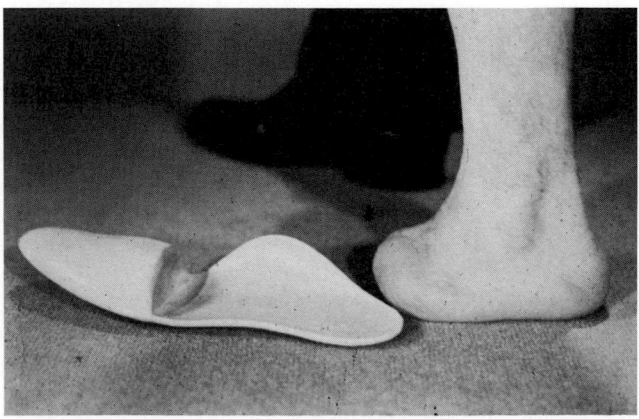

Figure 18-1 Midfoot amputation with the insert prosthesis.

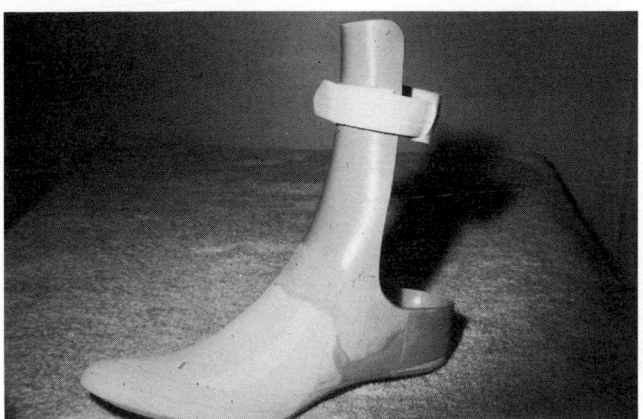

Figure 18-2 Ankle, foot orthosis for amputations through the hindfoot.

lows some gravity push-off as well as increasing stability. Retention of the partial foot in the proper position in the shoe can be a problem. With proper amputee rehabilitation, however, these individuals can enjoy long periods of comfortable function. Modifications of shoes using ski-boot foaming techniques as well as custom-type footwear can enhance function.

The most effective prosthesis for proximal foot amputations extends to just below the knee and blocks the ankle joint, preventing dorsiflexion. In this way gravity push-off gait is regained. Objections to the prosthetic appliance which encompasses the lower leg are outweighed by comfort and enhanced walking capability on the part of the amputee.

Good foot hygiene on the part of the patient is essential. Pressure of shoes and appliances on pressure-sensitive areas, maceration of the skin from retained moisture, and low-grade skin infection can be avoided with proper foot hygiene such as bathing and drying, avoidance of oily and greasy preparations, and the use of lamb's wool and antifungal powder. Individuals with insensitive feet should neither stand nor walk without a protective covering, i.e., a shoe or slipper. The trimming of toenails and calluses in particular, can be a source of acquired infection. Conforming footwear to include relief for pressure-sensitive areas is a necessity.

Amputations through the Ankle: Syme's Amputation

Amputation through the ankle joint as described in 1843[1,12] by the Scottish surgeon James Syme is one of the few operative procedures that has come down through the decades almost unchanged in technique. A landmark treatise by Harris in 1944 emphasized the value of this amputation for many conditions, including trauma and certain types of peripheral vascular disease.[11a] The surgical technique as described both by Syme and Harris involves amputation at ankle joint level with removal of malleoli and a paper-thin removal of the distal articular surface of the tibia. Section of the bones must be at a right angle to the

long weight-bearing axis and parallel to the floor. The calcaneus is carefully removed subperiosteally, avoiding damage to the posterior tibial artery. After the calcaneus and the rest of the tarsal and forefoot bones are removed, the flap is fashioned so as to place skin from the weight-bearing surface of the heel directly over the distal tibia with the skin incision closed anteriorly. This technique is precise. The heel-skin end pad must be centered directly over the distal tibia and stabilized there. The operation can be done in one or two stages, depending upon existing disease. The surgical result is a stable, well-healed, moderately bulbous amputation at ankle level with weight-bearing heel skin over the distal tibial surface.

Earlier Syme's prostheses were unsightly, and breakage of their lateral metal stirrups was common. Women especially objected to the appearance of the prosthesis and requested reamputation to the below-knee level. Modern prostheses are not only much more cosmetic but permit an excellent gait (Fig. 18-3). Several long-term studies of well-performed Syme's amputations indicate the excellent comfort, strength, and quality of function available. Contraindications include poor heel skin and lack of skin-protective sensation.

Patients with bilateral Syme's amputations manage well, often without walking aids.

Amputations through the Leg

Below-knee amputation is statistically the commonest major amputation in the lower limb. Amputations at this level

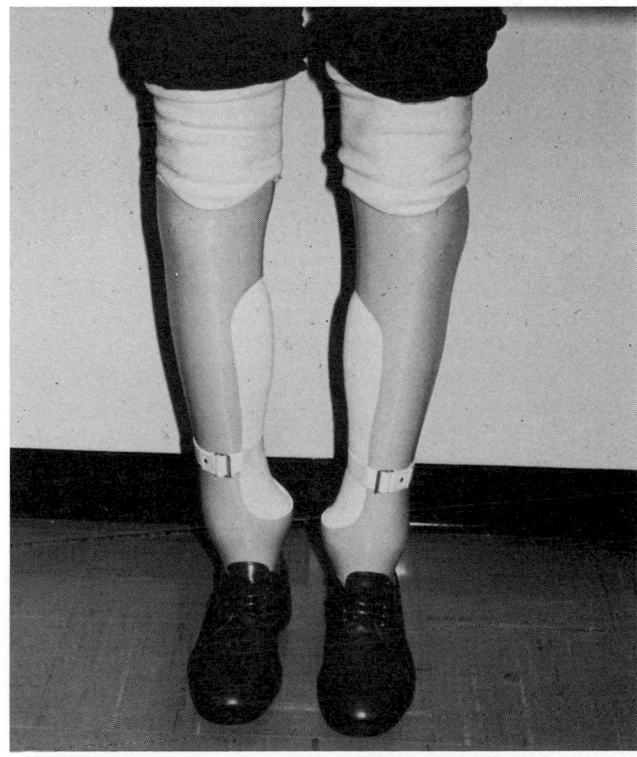

Figure 18-3 Syme's prostheses with medial cutout for donning prosthesis.

heal successfully in the majority of patients with ischemia who require major limb ablation.

Knee function is so critical to prosthetic rehabilitation that every attempt should be made to salvage the knee. Below-knee amputation is a reconstructive procedure requiring careful attention to technical detail. This level is selected on the basis of available healthy tissues, including an understanding of the healing potential present at the below-knee site in the ischemic limb. The site of election is that level where enough soft tissue is available to provide a well-healed, prosthesis-tolerant stump. All length should be saved down to the junction of the middle and lower thirds of the tibia and fibula. Amputations between this site and the ankle joint are avoided because of the difficulty of obtaining appropriate soft tissue coverage. The level limit proximally is just distal to the insertion of the patellar tendon. If significant knee dysfunction is present, the very short below-knee amputation is usually contraindicated and a knee disarticulation or higher amputation is carried out.

Modern technique utilizes a long posterior skin flap with an underlying myofascial flap progressively thinned to its distal end for suture to the anterior periosteum and deep fascia over the anterior tibiofibular area.[1] This myofascial stabilization permits a modest degree of distal muscle fixation to allow contractile activity. Nerves are pulled down gently and ligated high; the anterior tibia is very carefully beveled and rounded, since this is the site of pressure sensitivity within the socket. The fibula is sectioned 1.5 cm higher than the tibia unless one wishes to perform a tibiofibular synostosis, in which event the bones are sectioned at the same level and the osteoperiosteal bridge developed. Routine hemostasis and drainage are used. Postsurgical management likewise must be precise and physiologic. Immediate postsurgical rigid dressings have proved to be the most effective treatment system. These dressings are applied with relief pads placed under the cast for protection of pressure-sensitive areas. The immediate postsurgical rigid dressing is changed, usually 10 to 12 days after the surgery and thereafter as frequently as necessitated by loosening, while the stump matures.

Soft dressings are still frequently used following surgery. They include compression bandaging, which must be carefully monitored to prevent proximal vascular constriction and must be changed frequently to maintain appropriate distal pressure control.

Much of the improvement in below-knee amputation surgery relates to muscle and skin management. The long posterior myocutaneous flap is considered standard. Other techniques are acceptable, including equal sagittal flaps and skewed flaps designed to utilize the healthiest available skin. A wide variety of reconstructive skin coverage procedures may be required to salvage the below-knee level when severe trauma including burns is encountered. These include split-skin grafts, full-thickness grafts, and, on rare occasions, composite grafts.

The surgical goal of the below-knee amputation is the formation of a cylindrical terminal motor and sensory end organ with a degree of muscle stabilization and a nontender, nonadherent scar.

The below-knee amputation is particularly suited for wound management with an immediate postsurgical rigid dressing. The cast can be moderately contoured about the knee for suspension and, with the knee in extension, carried up to the upper one-third of the thigh. Knee flexion contractures are avoided; most patients can be out of bed and in a chair the day following surgery. Progressive early and rapid rehabilitation proceeds to limited weight bearing under supervision. With uneventful wound healing, light, comfortable, temporary prostheses may be used to permit increasing degrees of weight bearing, generally beginning between the fourth and sixth week after surgery. Immediate weight bearing following surgery was recommended by the authors and others in the past but has now been modified. In the elderly, vertical weight loading through the temporary prosthesis and the residual limb is delayed until wound healing is sufficiently advanced that dehiscence will not occur. There is, however, still a place for immediate postsurgical prosthetic fitting and early limited ambulation for children and adults with healthier tissues than the group with peripheral vascular disease. Immediate and early weight bearing should be advised based on the surgeon's observation and experience. There are no exact time guidelines. Uncomplicated primary wound healing is the first priority.

Unhealed and infected wounds have been managed in the past by rigid dressings and limited weight bearing. This treatment was, in essence, an outgrowth of the Orr-Trueta closed-cast management of osteomyelitis. When the infection is well localized and adequately drained and there are no sequestra or bone abscesses, the closed-cast technique, including partial weight bearing, may be used.

Below-knee prostheses are now of a variety of designs, lightweight, comfortable, and easy to clean (Fig. 18-4). Young, active unilateral below-knee amputees can run, jump, engage in most vigorous sports—sometimes at a high level of competition—and enjoy prolonged periods of function as in hiking, mountain climbing, playing soccer, and long-distance running. The functional potential is great and is directly dependent on the quality of surgery and prosthetic rehabilitation.

The fibula is sectioned 1 to 1.5 cm above the level of the tibial amputation. Depending on the length of the below-knee stump, there may be considerable movement between the two bones. The compressive forces of socket fit and weight bearing can irritate interosseus and contiguous structures including branches and neuromas of the peroneal nerve. Arthrodesis of the distal tibia to fibula with bone sectioned at near equal length provides a broad, stable, distal amputation with increased potential for end bearing (tibiofibular synostosis). This surgical technique was developed and popularized by Ertl in Germany and later by Deffer in the United States. A large World War II experience reinforced its value, but it is not indicated when ischemia is present since the additional manipulation of the distal tissues may compromise primary wound healing. The added functional benefit of tibiofibular synostosis is not so important for the elderly, less active person who can be well and comfortably fitted according to the standard below-knee technique. The procedure is justified primarily for the young, active amputee. The synostosis amputation may have to be carried out at a higher level than would otherwise be necessary in order to obtain adequate

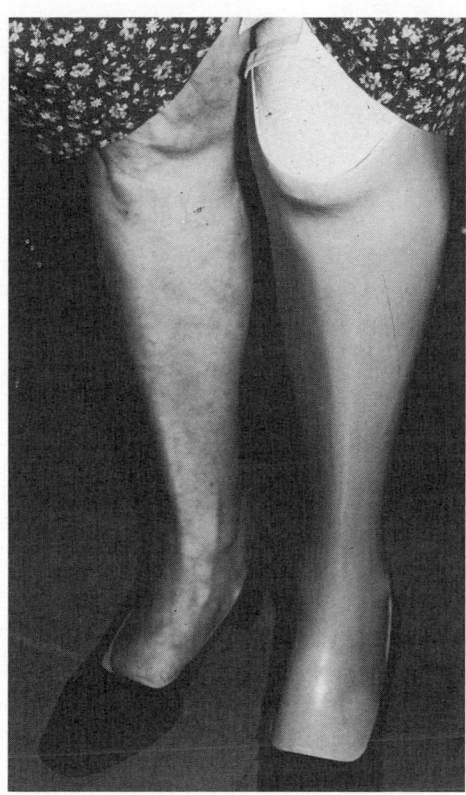

Figure 18-4 Below-knee prosthesis, exoskeletal type, patellar tendon bearing (PTB), total contact socket.

soft tissue closure. If length is critical, the operation is not indicated. The synostosis is accomplished either by interosseus bone graft using a segment of fibula or by an osteoperiosteal tube raised from the distal tibia and sutured transversely across the interosseus space to the distal fibula.

Myodesis (suture of muscle to bone) stabilizing the anterolateral muscles and calf muscles to the distal tibia has been advocated by ourselves and others. Drill holes are placed through the distal tibia to allow firm fixation of the sectioned muscles to bone. Occasional aseptic necrosis of the distal tibia may occur. This complication can be avoided by stabilizing the muscle ends to the distal soft tissues and to each other.

Amputations through the Knee

For many years disarticulation of the knee was popular in the high-risk patient. The surgery could be performed quickly and with minimal blood loss. Surgical mortality and morbidity were considerably lower than for amputation above the knee. As elective surgery in the poor-risk patient has become less threatening, this amputation has been employed less often.

Significant advantages of the knee disarticulation included socket suspension capabilities provided by the bulbous distal femoral stump and good end-bearing capability (Fig. 18-5). In the past, these advantages have been offset by prosthetic difficulties. The bulbous distal stump

necessitated a bulky, unsightly, prosthesis, and intrinsic knee mechanisms could not be incorporated within the limb because of the asymmetrical knee joint level with that of the opposite, intact limb. As with the Syme amputation, women often rejected this amputation for cosmetic reasons.

Modern prostheses have overcome many of these objections. They include hydraulic knee-assist mechanisms and other engineering modifications. Knee disarticulation is now a favored amputation for active persons when the alternative is an above-knee site.

Indications include neoplasms and severe distal trauma or infection where limb salvage or functional prosthetic rehabilitation cannot be obtained with a below-knee amputation. Infections involving the proximal tibia and fibula and also septic arthritis of the knee joint can be treated successfully with this procedure. The soft tissues about the knee and particularly the skin must be adequate for coverage.

Knee disarticulation for limb ischemia is no longer favored. The blood supply to the skin about the knee and in the proximal leg area is such that most patients with ischemia who were treated by knee disarticulation in the past will tolerate a short below-knee amputation using the

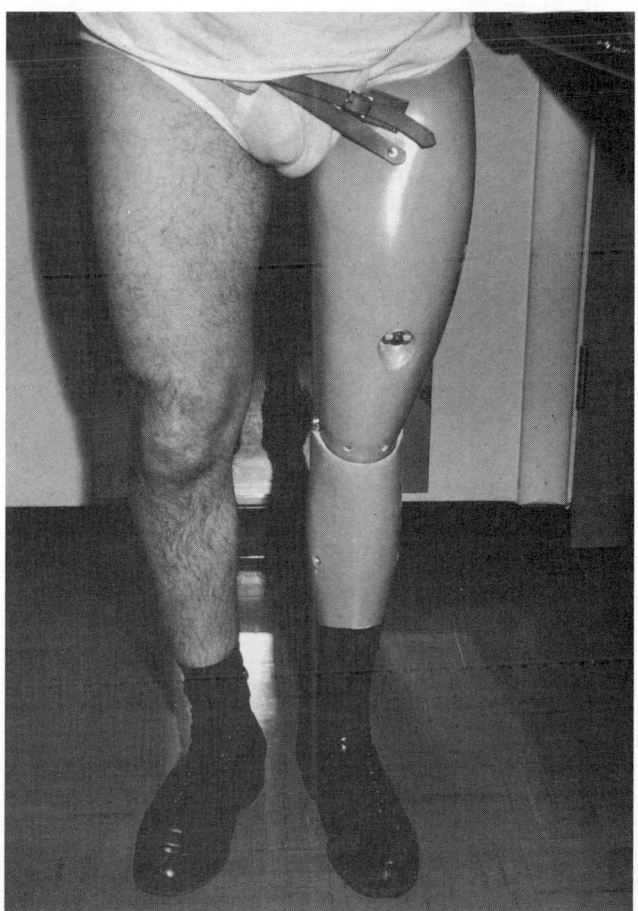

Figure 18-5 Knee disarticulation prosthesis with external knee hinges and rigid thigh socket.

described posterior flap technique. Salvage of a functional knee under these circumstances can generally permit ambulation. If the knee joint cannot be preserved, in most cases the degree of skin ischemia will not allow healing. For this reason knee disarticulation in the presence of severe ischemia is confined to those individuals who are nonambulators but whose tissues will allow skin healing at the knee disarticulation level. Knee flexion contractures are thus avoided, and the long femoral lever arm may be useful in sitting and in patient transfer even though no prosthesis is used.

A sagittal incision with medial and lateral flaps is recommended.[1] The patella is retained and the patellar tendon sutured to the stump of the cruciate ligaments in the femoral intercondylar notch. The biceps femoris tendon and one or more of the medial hamstring tendons are also stabilized by intercondylar suture. A variety of techniques have been described that severely contour the bony femoral condyles. This practice is no longer routinely employed. Radical trimming of the condyles destroys the rotary stability and suspension capability that enhance the value of through-knee amputation. Only modest contouring of ridges and large, bony prominences should be carried out.

The Gritti-Stokes amputation places the patella on the distal end of the femur to accept end-weight bearing. The patella does not normally provide a physiologic weight-bearing surface; rather, weight in the kneeling position is borne on the proximal pretibial area, including the patellar tendon. This circumstance negates much of the possible value of the technique. The Gritti-Stokes amputation gives a longer limb than knee disarticulation, since the patella is placed at the distal end of the femur. Prosthetists find such a stump difficult to fit. The center of axis of the prosthetic knee is well below that of the normal knee. This asymmetry is noted when the patient sits.

A number of low transcondylar techniques have been described that are designed to retain the advantages of knee disarticulation with a slightly shortened femoral lever arm, thus allowing the use of intrinsic prosthetic knee units. Transcondylar amputation more often becomes, in effect, a very long above-knee amputation with partial loss of those very features that make knee disarticulation attractive.

Above-Knee Amputation

Indications for above-knee amputation include trauma, malignancies, congenital limb deficits, and ischemia. Classic sites of election are no longer applicable. The amputation should salvage all femoral length consistent with a painless, well-healed residual limb. Stabilization of the long thigh muscles to prevent their retraction is mandatory when surgical circumstances permit. There is no level of major amputation where muscle stabilization is more important to prosthetic control, even though the surrounding mass of muscles and fascia may prove somewhat difficult to stabilize into the relatively small distal femur. Particularly important is the stabilization under appropriate tension of the adductor muscle group and quadriceps. Weak hamstring function can be partially supplemented by an intact gluteus maximus. During weight bearing, the line of weight transfer from the pelvis through the hip joint

and remaining portion of the femur shifts to the prosthetic socket. Contraction of hip abductors stabilizes the pelvic/femoral segment to prevent trunk sway. When applied to the residual femur of the above-knee amputee, the abductors cause shift of the femur within its soft tissue envelope until it firmly contacts the lateral wall of the above-knee prosthetic socket. If the adductor muscles have not been attached to the distal medial femoral stump so as to oppose this displacement, a lurching Trendelenburg gait results (Table 18-1). Active, stabilized quadriceps muscles assist the hip flexors to propel the prosthesis forward and assist prosthetic toe clearance.

Loss of the knee joint by above-knee amputation significantly compounds the challenge of making the prosthesis functional. Scores of commercially available prosthetic knee mechanisms attest to this engineering challenge. While it is true that a simple peg extension can yield a stable degree of bipedal mobility, refined lower limb function using an above-knee prosthesis requires a complex bioengineering response using gravity-induced energy sources, hydraulics, pneumatics, or mechanical or electrical control systems of great ingenuity to substitute for the lost knee.

The first functional requirement for the above-knee amputee is that the prosthesis be stable in the various phases of weight bearing. Gait training is a key part of rehabilitation, much more so than at lower levels of leg loss. Properly trained, a significant number of geriatric above-knee amputees can learn to walk well with a cane if the opposite limb is intact.

Maximum femoral length is preserved. The length of the residual lever arm is directly related to quality, suspension, alignment, and control of the prosthesis. Energy expenditure also increases as the length of the remaining limb decreases.

The skin incision is dictated by the local circumstances, including previously placed scars from vascular reconstruction or other surgery. Since the stump totally contacts the prosthetic socket, the position of skin scars is far less important than its healing. Free mobility of the skin and subcutaneous tissues, adequate blood supply, sensibility, and lack of tenderness are the important and necessary features.

Skin flaps are fashioned short, using plastic technique to preserve blood supply. The flaps must be planned to avoid a tight skin closure. With the dysvascular amputee, this is the most frequently observed technical error.

The importance of muscle stabilization and means for its accomplishment have been emphasized. The technique of distal attachment of the muscles and fascia depends on the local situation. Ischemic muscles cannot be expected to heal if their blood supply is additionally disturbed by constricting sutures. When the muscle tissue is healthy and well vascularized, as with above-knee amputations for neoplasm, a careful myoplasty and/or myodesis is essential for optimal prosthetic control.

Major nerves are retracted under moderate tension and ligated before being sectioned and allowed to retract.

The bone is divided transversely, the outer cortex moderately rounded to remove sharp edges, and the periosteum purse-string sutured over the cut end of the bone. Routine hemostasis and drainage complete the operation.

TABLE 18-1 Some Commonly Described Abnormalities Requiring Correction by the Prosthetic Team

Abnormality	Definition	Common causes (not exhaustive)
A. Circumduction	Swinging of the entire prosthesis laterally in a wide arc—returning to the line of progression	a. Prosthesis too long b. Inadequate flexion of prosthetic knee c. Hip abductors weak or contracted
B. Valuting or pelvic hike or toe stub	Rising on the toe of the sound foot to permit the prosthesis to swing through without toe stubbing	a. Prosthesis too long b. Inadequate flexion of prosthetic knee c. Excessive plantar flexion d. Toe lever arm too long
C. Medial whip	Inward movement of the prosthetic heel, outward movement of the knee, or initial flexion at the beginning of the swing	a. Knee axis, normally set in 5° of external rotation to compensate for pelvic rotation, excessively rotated b. Varus knee c. Toe break not at right angle to the line of progression d. Weak muscles rotate around the femur
D. Lateral whip	Opposite to movement of medial whip: knee moves inward, heel outward	a. Knee axis *internally* rotated b. Valgus knee c. Toe break not at right angle to the line of progression d. Weak muscles rotate around the femur

Source: Modified and reproduced with permission from Sanders GT: *Lower Limb Amputations: A Guide to Rehabilitation.* Philadelphia, F.A. Davis, 1986.

Rigid immediate postoperative dressings are more difficult to apply and properly suspend at the above-knee level. Accepted practice uses a soft compression dressing carried up as a spica around the pelvis for suspension. If the surgical amputee team is skilled in rigid dressing application at the above-knee level, this technique does offer the advantages previously outlined. Air splints have been used as a postoperative dressing. Lack of equipment and of experience in its use has limited the acceptance of this technique.

Hip Disarticulation

Hip disarticulation is performed infrequently. Indications include severe trauma, malignancies of the more proximal part of the lower limb, and occasionally ischemia. It may be necessary to perform hip disarticulation to control local infection and as a lifesaving procedure. Vascular surgical services are encountering the need for hip disarticulation more and more frequently when repeated vascular reconstructions have failed and little blood supply is present below the renal arteries. Prostheses are not generally indicated with this patient population. Adaptive mobility aids include modified wheelchairs and litters. Some of these patients can be cared for in a home setting; most are institutionalized.

Hip disarticulation for nonischemic disease and specifically trauma and malignancies is occasionally required in young people. The surgical techniques are well standardized.

Excellent prosthetic substitution is available for the young, strong person (Fig. 18-6). Many walk without a cane or other external aid. Remarkable physical achievement with or without a prosthesis is possible. Nonetheless, the inconvenience and learning effort required for use of this heavy prosthesis discourage many individuals. The more rapid and effective the rehabilitation, the more likely that the individual will become an effective regular user of the limb. Without a prosthesis, crutches are required in order to walk or stand for any length of time. Free use of the arms is thus denied.

Hemipelvectomy and Hemicorporectomy

Hemipelvectomy and hemicorporectomy are sometimes required to eliminate malignant tumors about the pelvis,

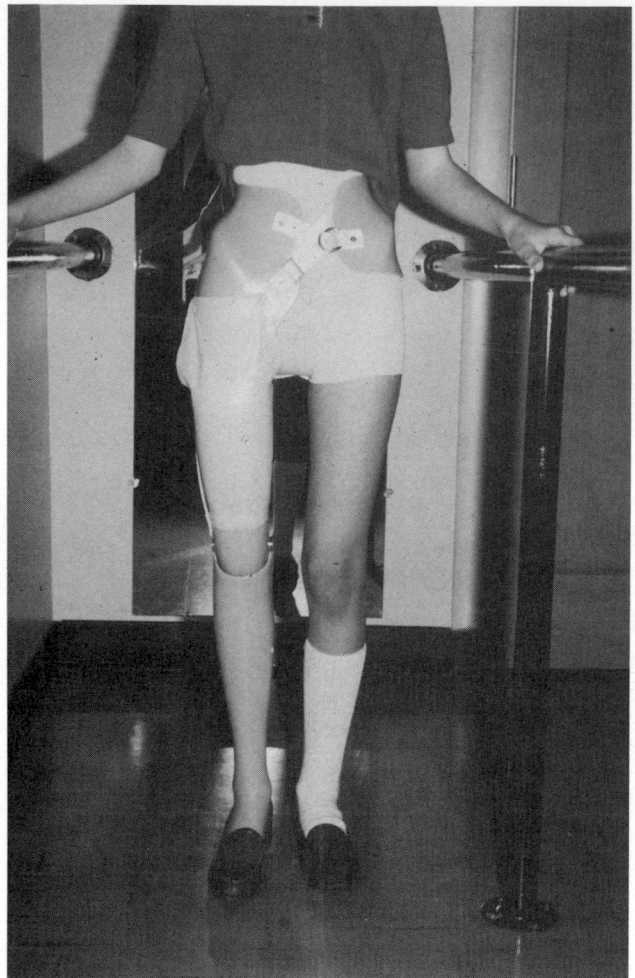

Figure 18-6 Hip disarticulation prosthesis with hydraulic knee mechanism.

but radical local excision and reconstruction with limb salvage, where possible, are much preferred. Weight-bearing prostheses are rarely used after these mutilating procedures. Independent walking without crutches or a walker is not achieved even when a prosthesis can be fitted.

Wrist Disarticulation

Preservation of both forearm bones and the distal radial ulnar articulation provides an excellent amputation result. Pronation and supination are largely preserved. Irregularities in the distal stump contour contribute to the stability and suspension of the prosthesis. Both body and externally powered prostheses allow significant limb rehabilitation. Most wrist disarticulation amputees become skilled prosthetic users and attain a remarkable degree of bimanual function. This level is widely accepted by amputees of both sexes.

Terminal devices (hand substitutes) for the wrist disarticulation amputee include those generally used for loss of the upper limb. In order to maintain comparable length with the intact limb when the amputation is unilateral, it may be necessary to modify the hook or hand substitute.

Prosthetic modification is also required if external power sources such as electricity are used. The residual limb fills the entire socket of the unmodified prosthesis, leaving no room between the end of the amputation and the prosthetic wrist joint in which batteries and electric motor systems may be placed to activate the hook or cosmetic fingers.

Amputations through the Forearm

Amputations at the below-elbow level should conserve all length consistent with proper bone management and soft tissue coverage. Distal muscle stabilization is important, especially when myoelectric signals are to be used for externally powered electric prostheses. Individual muscle fixation is not carried out. The myoelectric signals are obtained from the mass contraction of the flexor and the extensor groups. They should be stabilized by myoplasty to or near the distal ends of both the radius and the ulna.

As the amputation level proceeds proximally from the wrist, voluntary pronation and supination are progressively more limited. The prosthetic socket further restricts rotary movement. Compensation can be partly achieved by body positioning of the limb, primarily through shoulder rotation and elbow flexion/extension. It is also possible, on occasion, to incorporate a small planetary gear within the prosthesis, so as to enhance rotary forearm function.

The short below-elbow amputation is preferred over elbow disarticulation, since the former preserves a useful range of active elbow movement. This implies biceps or brachialis function as well as active extension.

Below-elbow prostheses are conventionally powered by metal or plastic cables activated by body movement, using a fabric axilla loop about the opposite shoulder. The terminal device may also be externally powered by electric batteries encased in the forearm.

Elbow Disarticulation

Amputation through the elbow joint is seldom performed. Prosthetists encounter difficulty fitting the residual limb with an acceptable substitute. This level precludes the use of intrinsic prosthetic elbow mechanisms because of their space requirements. Incorporation of the artificial elbow mechanism disproportionately lengthens the upper arm and shortens the forearm. Limb symmetry can be retained, however, by using external elbow hinges with a number of possible types of elbow control mechanisms.

In spite of these drawbacks, this amputation level does produce the advantage of a long lever arm and an irregular distal contour, making for excellent socket stability. The practice of converting the elbow disarticulation to a low above-elbow amputation is not necessary.

Through-elbow amputation is most often occasioned by trauma, including burns.

Above-Elbow Amputation

There is no site of election for amputations through the upper arm. All length is saved consistent with the creation of a satisfactory residual limb. Even the very short above-elbow level, where only the head of the humerus remains, presents a more normal shoulder contour. The humeral head is not removed unless the shoulder joint is painful or its removal is necessitated by the disease.

Whenever possible, distal muscle stabilization is necessary for the above-elbow amputee to provide strength, prosthetic control, and myoelectric signals for externally powered limbs.

Both functional and purely cosmetic prostheses are available for the above-elbow amputee. Many unilateral above-elbow amputees, particularly those with amputations through the proximal half of the humerus, prefer a nonfunctional, light, cosmetic limb over the heavier, more complicated functional appliance. Three types of functional prostheses are available. The terminal device can be controlled by body movement, by external electric power sources, or by a combination. As technology has improved and electric components have become miniaturized and light, more amputees are being fitted with the combination, or hybrid, prosthesis. As an example, elbow motion is controlled by myoelectric sources with terminal device function accomplished through cables and body movement. Even though suspension of the conventional prosthesis with body-powered harnessing is somewhat uncomfortable and restrictive, both children and adults can be expected to undergo successful prosthetic rehabilitation with daily regular use of the prosthesis. The patience and assisted training necessary to develop skills is outweighed by the great advantage of bimanual function. This is particularly true in the workplace as well as in many recreational activities. Elderly above-elbow amputees are often better served by fitting them with a light, cosmetic device used primarily for dress and social occasions.

Bilateral upper limb loss, whether congenital or acquired, is critically disabling. Infants and children quickly learn to substitute foot function to accomplish daily living needs. Prostheses are often reserved for wear out of the home. When skillfully designed and properly fitted, however, functional prostheses can be successful. Acquired bilateral upper limb loss in adult life makes mandatory the dedicated and intense training for functional prosthetic use.

Immediate postsurgical rigid dressings with prosthetic fitting are particularly successful. The distal compression controls edema, and the immobilization minimizes postsurgical pain. Terminal devices can be fitted to the immediate postsurgical rigid dressing, often within days after surgery. Upper limb amputees rapidly acquire control of the terminal device using this immediate postsurgical system. Myoelectric control electrodes can be placed in the temporary socket for early external powering. Patterns of use carry over to definitive limb use. Under this prompt progressive rehabilitation plan, very few amputees later abandon the use of the prosthesis.

Postamputation physical therapy for all upper limb levels includes particular attention to proximal joint and muscle function. Since the terminal device is generally controlled by active shoulder girdle movement, it is important to prevent contractures and maintain muscle strength.

Assuming normal mobility, the arm amputee moves freely in the environment with or without the prosthesis

and is therefore less challenged than the lower leg amputee to wear the device and improve performance and skills with it. Functional goals should be set high enough to challenge the trainee yet not so great as to be overwhelming and to discourage prosthetic use.

Shoulder Disarticulation and Forequarter Amputation

These radical amputations usually result from malignancy. When they are performed on the immature skeleton, a dorsal scoliosis frequently results. In general, prosthetic substitution is aimed at cosmesis and for the fitting of clothing. Through-shoulder amputation with retention of shoulder girdle muscles results in muscle contractures and "hiking" of the scapula, since the action of the scapular elevator muscles is unopposed by the weight of the part of the arm that has been removed.

Pain following Amputation

Complications aside from a consideration of pain have been discussed earlier. Pain can be associated with the stump itself or experienced in the phantom limb.[1,4] Occasionally both types are present. The diagnosis of these pain patterns must be carried out in a systematic manner. Early postoperative management of the amputation has a considerable influence on their degree and duration. Immediate postoperative rigid dressings, properly applied to control edema and provide wound stability, promote a more comfortable and early healing course. Hematoma or swelling associated with a tight wound closure and wound infection produces severe, persistent pain.

As wound healing progresses, postoperative pain usually subsides and the patient then proceeds to functional rehabilitation. Pain in the phantom limb tends to subside beginning about the fifth or sixth week following amputation. Some phantom sensations including occasional pain usually persist throughout the individual's life. To most persons, this is an annoyance and does not prevent prosthetic wear, call for medication, or significantly influence patterns of daily living.

A greater challenge arises in dealing with chronic pain.[1] These sensations may be regional, phantom, or combined. A thorough history and physical and psychological examination provide a basis for diagnosis. Severe, acute, and chronic preoperative pain predisposes to a carryover of pain patterns following amputation. This is especially true when the pain has been severe and has been present for a significant time prior to surgery. Its preoperative management is also a source of important information. It should include psychosocial assessment of tolerance to previous painful experiences. The physical examination seeks areas of tenderness, particularly in relation to the anatomic position of nerves, neuromas, or underlying bone irregularities. The effects of active muscle contractions on the pain should be assessed as well as the state of the soft tissues, their color, the patient's nutritional and circulatory status, and the presence or absence of edema. Local and regional nerve blockade with local anesthesia using a very small needle may be used to further explain the pain. If additional neurologic information is desired, one then proceeds to a regional nerve block, anesthetizing the remaining limb completely. Persistence of pain indicates its central origin.

Pain due to neurocirculatory dystrophy (Sudeck's atrophy) is occasionally encountered. Not infrequently, pain unrelated to the amputation itself can be overlooked. Sciatica due to a herniated intervertebral disk, arthritic disease in adjacent joints, ischemia, and referred visceral pain need to be ruled out.

Following organized diagnostic screening, one can proceed to treatment. Therapy should be directed toward the diagnosed causative factors. Noninvasive methods are preferred and may include the entire spectrum of pain-abatement measures: electrical, chemical, physical, and psychological. Addictive pain medication and surgical intervention are employed with great caution. Removal of large, tender, adherent neuromas—particularly in the areas of interlace pressure and shear—can have a moderate degree of success. Response to local anesthesia may be the major determinant in deciding upon the local removal of neuromas.

Reamputation to a higher level for pain relief is seldom indicated. Badly scarred, adherent distal tissues with difficult limb fit can benefit from appropriate revision and pain relief, and improved function may follow. Revision with distal muscle stabilization is credited for occasional improvement of severe chronic stump pain. Proximal peripheral and central nervous system surgical intervention such as spinal cord tractotomy has been notoriously unsuccessful. Such intervention involving the nervous system can convert a difficult pain syndrome into a catastrophic one.

The surgical techniques of modern amputation as previously described have reduced to a small number those patients who have chronic, agonizing, intractable pain. These complex problem cases are seen most often at high amputation levels, i.e., hip and shoulder disarticulations. These are best handled by experienced amputation teams cooperating with pain management specialists, including psychiatrists. Fortunately the number of such cases is small.

As many as one-third of congenital amputees who have been surveyed regarding awareness of a phantom limb indicate periods of such awareness. The psychological background for this experience is poorly explained.

Diagnostic Tests for Determination of Amputation Level

Most surgeons rely on a careful history and thorough physical examination to establish the lowest effective amputation level that can be expected to heal without complication. Objective laboratory limb viability studies can assist the surgeon to select amputation levels in the presence of ischemia. Such studies do not replace clinical experience and judgment. These tests do not necessarily correspond to those used by vascular surgeons contemplating surgical reconstruction. In particular, angiography is not generally useful in determining the level of amputation in end-stage disease.

The objective information routinely used at this time by the senior author (E.M.B.) includes skin temperature, Doppler segmental blood pressure with ischemic index and Doppler waveform, transcutaneous P_{O_2}, P_{CO_2}, and laser Doppler flowmetry.[12a] These tests are noninvasive and inexpensive and can be performed by a vascular technician. They permit "limb viability scanning" by multiple-site data accrual.

A number of other examinations used in both the research and clinical settings are fluorescein flowmetry, skin clearance of ^{133}Xe, and nuclear magnetic resonance spectrometry.[6,7,13–17]

An example of the use of these tests can be demonstrated at the below-knee level. Adverse arteriographic findings and the absence of popliteal pulses are not contraindications to below-knee amputation. A segmental Doppler pressure index greater than 0.35 for the nondiabetic patient and 0.45 for the diabetic patient strongly suggests the likelihood of skin healing at that level. Skin oxygen diffusion of 25 to 30 mmHg and higher also delineates an acceptable skin healing potential. Xenon-133 washout of 2.6 mL/100 g, if confirmed with laser Dopper cell velocity, also establishes an adequate level of skin healing.

The most reliable determinant of healing remains the appearance of the tissues at the time of surgery as judged by the experienced surgeon. This applies in particular to the observed vascularity of the skin envelope. With present preoperative diagnostic information and careful observation at surgery, uncomplicated healing rates at the below-knee level are achieved in well over 50 percent of all patients with peripheral vascular disease requiring major limb loss. Of all lower limb amputations for ischemia (which includes amputations involving the foot), 75 to 90 percent should heal primarily at the below-knee level. Reamputation due to failure to heal should not be necessary in more than 6 to 8 percent of this patient population.

PROSTHETICS

General Considerations

Prostheses are as old as recorded amputations. Through the years, artificial limbs have been fabricated by a wide variety of artisans including leather workers, metal workers, woodworkers, medical practitioners, and, in many cases, amputees. Prior to the development of synthetic plastics, most prostheses were constructed from organic material and metals. Leather, linen, cotton, wool, silk, and wood were used in a variety of combinations. These materials combined with steel and aluminum completed the prosthesis.

Prostheses are now primarily modular structures made of plastic and lightweight metals. Composite materials made of carbon and glass fiber in an epoxy or acrylic resin matrix are commonly used. Light, high-strength metals such as titanium or aluminum alloys are used extensively in modular prostheses.[1] Today, prosthetic engineering is pursued by a small group of engineers and design scientists. The demand for modern technology is stimulating increased interest in this area of bioengineering.

The prosthesis is an artificial organ. It should imitate the body segment as nearly as possible in function and appearance. It is composed of three basic components: (1) the socket (the human-machine interface), (2) the terminal device (the physical contact with the environment in the form of the hand or foot portion of either organ), and (3) the body of the prosthesis (the intervening structure).

Comfort is a multifaceted requisite. Fit and material selection of the socket—together with stability, dynamic function, and reliability—are the major components of comfort for the amputee. Cosmesis (natural appearance) is desirable when it can be obtained without compromising overall function. Some amputees will even prefer a strictly cosmetic substitute when they are able to accommodate otherwise for lost physical function.

Suspension refers to the attachment of the prosthesis to the body. The prosthesis is suspended by straps, belts, socket contour, suction, friction, and to some degree by physiologic suspension through muscle control of the stump. Elastic sleeves and socket liners are also commonly used for suspension.

The artificial limb is controlled and manipulated by the body, external power sources, or a combination of both. Residual limb muscles, trunk motion, and gravity ordinarily power lower limb prostheses. The energy requirement for prostheses, particularly in the lower limb, relates to the weight of the artificial limb, its components, its alignment, and the level of amputation. The higher the level of amputation, the greater the energy requirement for limb control. The shoulder girdle, shoulder, and residual limb activate upper limb prostheses. External electric power sources, initiated by simple switches or by myoelectric signals arising in the muscles in the residual limb, are being used increasingly as miniaturization of the electronics has developed. These myoelectric arms are available worldwide for selected users. Indications for the various types of prostheses are described later.

Fabrication

Most prostheses are fabricated over a modified plaster model of the residual limb. After detailed measurements of the limb are made, a plaster wrap cast is taken, removed, and filled with plaster to form a positive model. Precise anatomic measurements are important for checking socket design parameters. Often clear plastic check sockets are used to evaluate fit. Any necessary modifications can be incorporated in the fabrication of a definitive socket. Difficult fitting problems may require several check sockets prior to the final fitting. Foam or alginate gel may be injected to fill areas of noncontact (Fig. 18-7). The definitive socket is then fabricated over the mold, using either thermoplastic or fiber-reinforced resin materials.

Xeroradiography, a process of x-ray imaging, is an effective evaluation tool. This technique demonstrates both soft tissue and bone details not seen in a standard x-ray

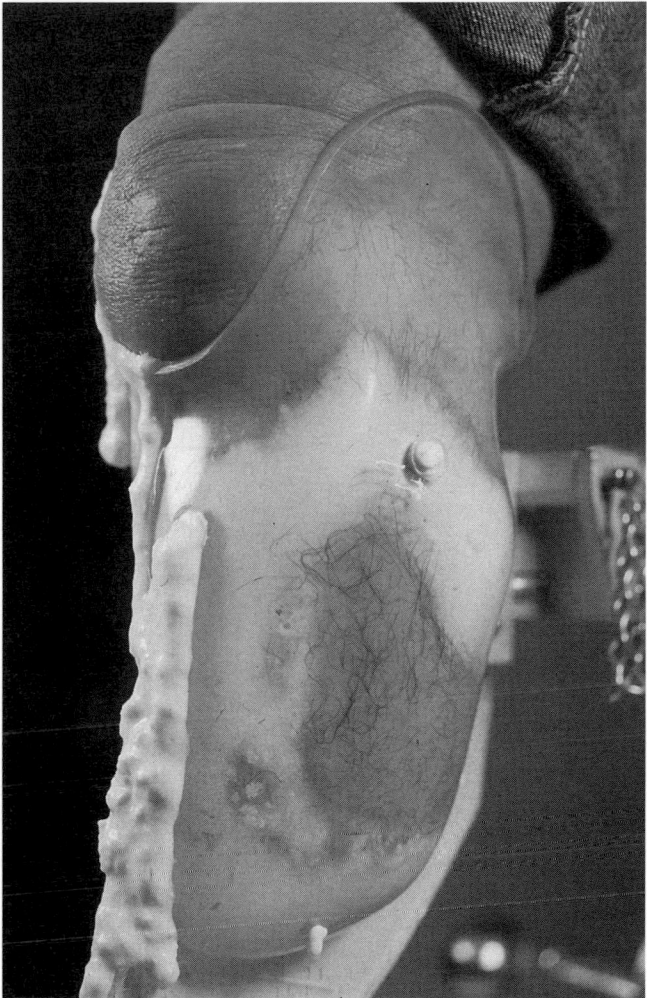

Figure 18-7 Clear plastic check socket with alginate gel providing total contact.

film. Computed tomography, photogrammetry, volume displacement measurements, ultrasound, and laser scanning are research modalities being used to study and improve socket design and fabrication.

Computer-Aided Design and Manufacture

Computed techniques for design and manufacture can rapidly and consistently design, fabricate, align, and digitally store prostheses.[18] The process of computer-aided design and manufacture entails three steps: input of the anatomic form, design of the socket interface, and output of the finished design to an automated fabrication system. Laser or electromechanical digitizers are used to translate the physical features of the residual limb into a three-dimensional numerical model ready for software-based modifications. Design of the socket interface is achieved by the prosthetist through graphical sculpting of the anatomic form on the computer screen. Numerically controlled fabrication machinery duplicates computed design of the

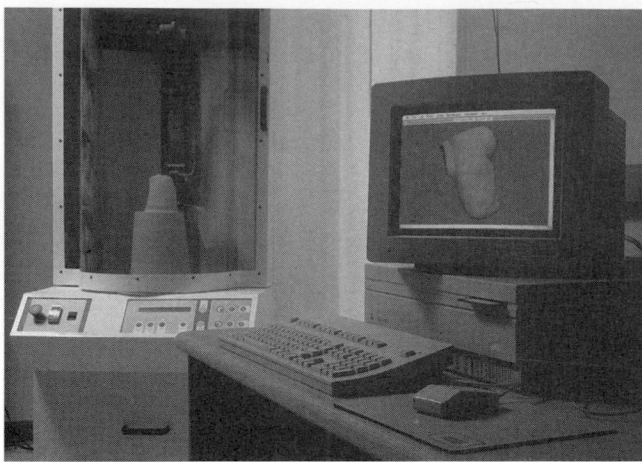

Figure 18-8 System for computer-aided design and manufacture of limb prostheses.

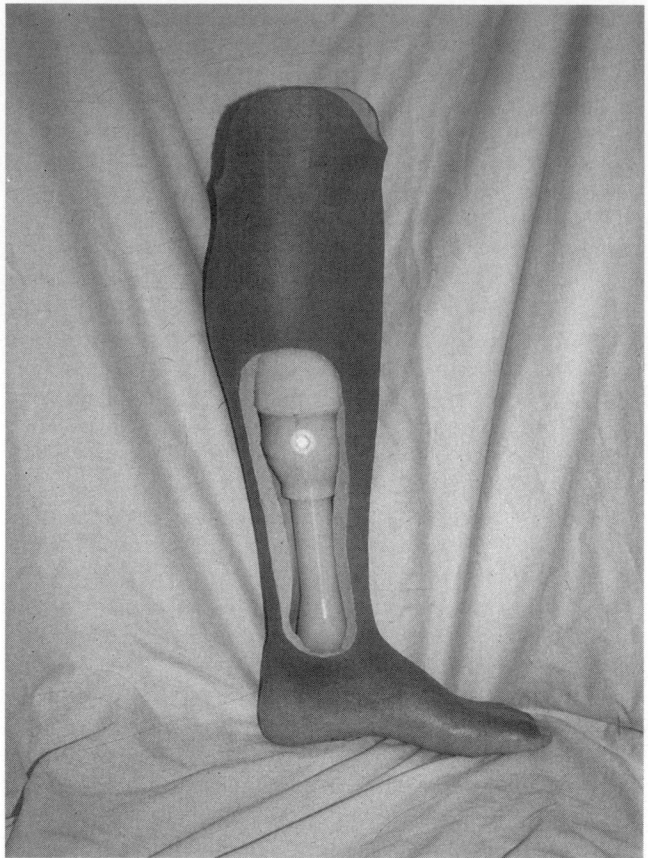

Figure 18-9 Endoskeletal-type below-knee prosthesis with cosmetic cover cut away to reveal structure.

prosthesis (Fig. 18-8). Clinical use of this technology is growing in prosthetics.

Necessary components for completion of the prosthesis are added following socket fabrication. A wide variety of knee, ankle/foot, wrist, and elbow joints are available. These artificial joints range from simple single-axis hinge articulation through polycentric multiple-linkage friction, hydraulic, pneumatic, and electrically controlled devices.

Structural support for the socket and the articulated components is either endoskeletal or exoskeletal. The endoskeletal units are essentially the inner frame of the prosthesis and are constructed of pylons and connectors made of light metals or composite plastics. They are covered by cosmetic synthetic foam simulating the appearance and color of the uninvolved limb (Fig. 18-9). Exoskeletal units are formed in the shape of the normal limb but have no inner structural support. Their strength lies in the rigid shell construction (Fig. 18-4).

Alignment

Prosthetic alignment is critical to proper function. This is especially true on the lower limb, where stability and gait are influenced by the alignment of the socket and articulations relative to the residual limb, the ground, and the line of progression of gait. The prosthetist aligns the limb after careful static and dynamic analysis. A number of alignment tools are used, including jigs, plumb lines, and video recording. Input from the amputee is the final determinant of alignment. Length, stability, control, energy consumption, and comfort relative to discrete variations in alignment can best be appreciated by the amputee.

Prescription Principles

The amputee care team fills its single most important role with limb prescription. The surgeon, prosthetist, and ther-

apist are indispensable when the decision for the type of prosthetic substitute is made. Input from social workers, internists, psychologists, and family may reinforce team judgment, but the three key team members can cooperatively weigh rehabilitation potential, functional capability, and construction options for a new prosthesis. A well-written prescription form avoids overlooking important but less visible needs. The practice of referring the amputee to the prosthetist with a simple request for an artificial limb is insufficient.

Specifics of limb prescription vary depending on the level of limb loss. Recently standardized terminology for describing limb prostheses has been adopted by the International Standards Organization and the American Academy of Orthotists and Prosthetists.[19] In particular, one should note the changes in references to amputations through the long bones: BK (below-knee) has become TT for transtibial, AK is TF for transfemoral, AE is transhumeral, and BE is transradial.

Individual consideration of activities of the amputee will ensure that component construction and selection will match performance requirements of the prosthesis. It is not intended here to outline the numerous variables entering into this process. The following short section condenses these general parameters.

Foot and Ankle Prostheses

Toe, metatarsophalangeal, and transmetatarsal amputations function well with compliant forefoot shoe fillers and shoe modifications. A stiff sole with a forward-placed rocker bar usually further improves gait and push-off.

Amputations through the midfoot, up to and including the Boyd and Pirogoff levels, are best fitted with a high shoe attached to an ankle/foot orthosis (AFO) to block ankle dorsiflexion, allowing push-off against gravity and reducing the flatfoot gait (Fig. 18-2). Syme's amputation requires an entire prosthetic foot rigidly attached to a patellar tendon–bearing type of prosthetic socket. The rigid ankle with heel cushioning and a flexible metatarsophalangeal forefoot section permits many Syme's amputees to walk with a normal gait at ordinary cadence. Walking fast or running elicits a moderately shortened gait pattern and slight limp. The distal Syme's amputation is often bulbous. A flexible insert inside the rigid socket of the prosthesis ordinarily allows entry of the residual limb (Fig. 18-3). Some Syme's amputees need a lateral or posterior replaceable window to allow clearance for stump entry. Enlargement of the prosthesis at ankle level distorts the ankle contour. Women tend to object to this added bulk and thickness. Some are sufficiently sensitive that they request a higher level of amputation through the distal one-third of tibia and fibula to permit fitting with a more cosmetic design.

Suspension of Syme's prosthesis is accomplished by the contour suspension inherent in the bulbous nature of the amputation site (Fig. 18-3). Many users of the prosthesis depend on this feature alone and require no additional suspension system. Additional suspension can be achieved by a strap above the patella attached to the sides of the prosthesis.

Below-Knee Prostheses

The below-knee amputation is the most frequently performed major amputation. Prostheses are designed with a total-contact socket contouring around the entire residual limb up to knee level. Weight is borne generally over the surface of the limb, even including, to a minor degree, the distal end. The patellar tendon area and the proximal and medial faces of the tibia are especially involved in weight bearing. Several variations in socket design are available. The medial and lateral walls can be carried up to the proximal border of femoral condyles and the anterior section brought up over the patella prosthese-tibiale-supra-condylienne (PTS). The classic total-contact patellar tendon bearing (PTB) design does not include the patella, and the trim lines of the socket superiorly lie only slightly above the knee (Fig. 18-4). Suspension of below-knee prostheses can be accomplished by a suspension strap just above the patella and attached to the lateral and medial aspects of the socket. A variety of supracondylar wedges entrap the medial condyle, so that it acts as a suspension point. An additional strap carried up the anterior thigh to a flexible pelvic belt and attached to the medial and lateral socket surfaces can further suspend the limb. When controlled muscle contraction is present in the residual limb

muscles, especially in the gastrocnemius-soleus group, it is possible to obtain some degree of suspension by muscle contraction. This is called physiologic suspension and helps during the swing phase of gait to maintain socket interface stability.

The shank may be either endoskeletal and covered with a cosmetic material or exoskeletal with the leg shell supporting the weight. Ankle/foot mechanisms vary from a single-axis bolt with a fore and aft rubber bumper through a wide variety of mechanical designs some of which incorporate dynamic elastic response. The Seattle foot is a recent development using the latter physical principles (Fig. 18-10).

For many years the below-knee prosthesis was fitted with rigid single-axis knee hinges carried from the medial and lateral proximal socket surfaces up to a thigh lacer, usually encompassing about one-half to two-thirds of the thigh (Fig. 18-11). The total-contact PTB and PTS designs have largely replaced this system (Fig. 18-4). The thigh lacer does provide some additional suspension and stability; however, it largely eliminates rotation of the tibia on the femur when the knee is flexed. Progressive thigh muscle atrophy under the lacer can be expected.

Prescription of this limb is now restricted to long-term users who do not wish to be converted to more physiologic limbs and to people engaged in work and recreation requiring a great deal of stability. Individuals who are up and down ladders and stairs at work, construction workers in high places, and athletes may use a thigh-lacer limb for these specific periods of time when extra stability and control are needed.

Function of the thigh-lacer limb can be marginally improved by polycentric knee joints rather than a single-axis joint. The polycentric hinge simulates the condylar gliding motion of the knee as it flexes and extends.

Knee Disarticulation Prostheses

The knee disarticulation is to a large degree end-bearing. Its bulbous nature provides excellent prosthetic suspen-

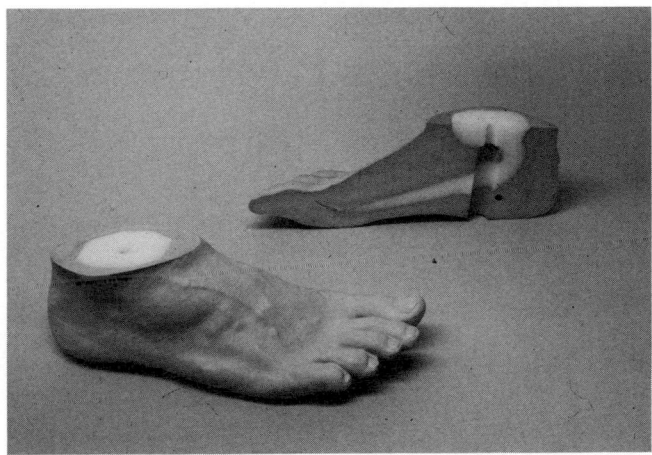

Figure 18-10 Prosthetic foot (Seattle foot) to store gravitational energy and improve physiologic gait.

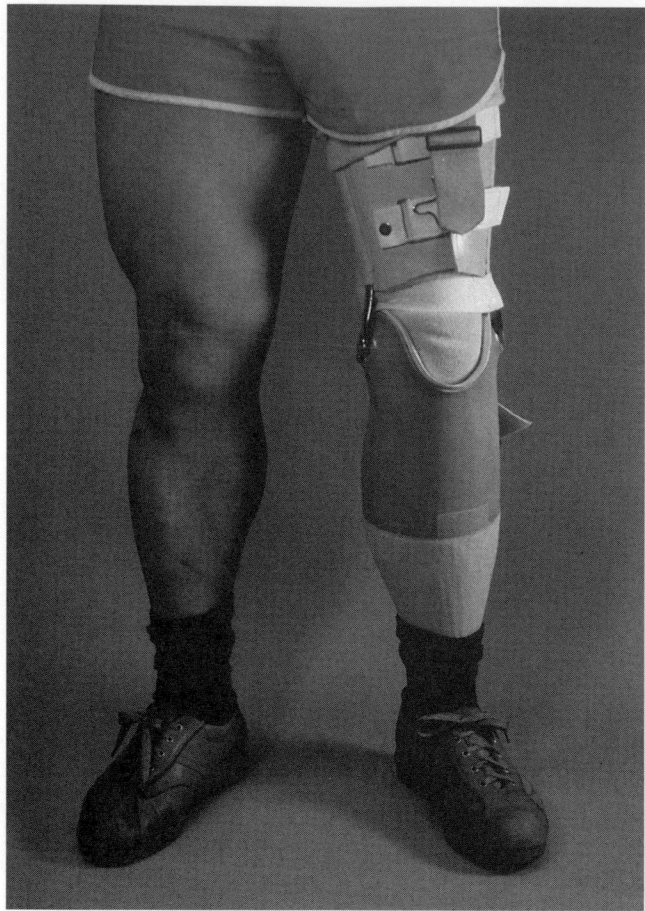

Figure 18-11 Below-knee prosthesis with metal knee joints and leather thigh lacer.

sion. Since the femur is full length, it is necessary to use side joints attached to a thigh component rather than an intrinsic knee mechanism, which would require sufficient space to lengthen the femoral segment excessively and produce significant knee asymmetry when the patient sits (Fig. 18-5). Ingenious intrinsic knee mechanisms have been devised that minimize this length discrepancy. Earlier knee disarticulation prostheses used a thigh lacer of leather. Modern design consists of a semirigid elastic thigh socket in a rigid frame. A rigid, closed thigh section similar to that used for the above-knee prosthesis is also acceptable.

Above-Knee Prostheses

Prosthetic substitution becomes much more complicated without the knee joint. Fitting the socket to the residual limb and the proximally adjacent pelvic structures is technically more difficult than at the through-knee and below-knee levels. Since World War II, the quadrilateral socket has been standard. The brim of the socket posteriorly rests against the ischial tuberosity, and the anteroposterior dimension of the socket is narrowed to maintain the tuberosity on the posterior brim of the prosthesis during weight bearing. Unfortunately, compression in the anteroposterior

plane requires a wider mediolateral dimension to accommodate the tissues, and adductor stability is compromised, accentuating the gluteus medius Trendelenburg lurch.

The present trend departs from the classic quadrilateral design and emphasizes a narrower mediolateral dimension. The ischial tuberosity slides inside the socket and is not the point of major weight bearing. The gluteal structures together with the peritrochanteric area absorb increasing load.

The femoral section of the limb itself may be endoskeletal or exoskeletal and attaches to one of more than 75 available knee mechanisms. These include mechanical, single-axis, and multiple-linkage polycentric knees; a wide variety of hydraulic mechanisms; and pneumatic, gravity friction lock, electronically controlled, and drop-lock designs. The shin and ankle/foot units are those described in the section on the below-knee prosthesis but modified as indicated for particular alignment and individual patient needs. Proper alignment of the above-knee prosthesis following static and dynamic analysis is essential to successful stability and function. Gait abnormalities seen at different phases of the walking cycle give important clues to help the prosthetic team improve prosthetic fitting (Table 18-1).[20]

Suspension is accomplished by suction with a suction valve at the distal end of the socket and also by socket contour. A flexible pelvic belt, a rigid hip joint to a semirigid pelvic belt, and, on rare occasions, shoulder-strap suspension are additional suspension devices that may be used. As with the below-knee residual limb, stump muscle activity enhances suspension in a physiologic manner. Gait training should emphasize the advantages of muscle control of the socket.

Hip Disarticulation and Hemipelvectomy Prostheses

Removal of the hip joint increases the complexity of prosthetic fitting. Most older patients with hip disarticulation prefer not to wear a prosthesis and instead use crutches, walker, and wheelchair. The younger patients can be fitted with a conforming pelvic prosthetic bucket and a mechanical hip joint mechanism carried down to an above-knee type of prosthesis. These prostheses are heavy even when they are made of the lightest available materials. Young, active amputees can use them successfully but generally require an external aid such as a cane for any prolonged walking.

Upper Limb Prosthetics

Prosthetic replacement of upper limb function is far more complicated than that of the lower limb. The hand is such an exquisite motor and sensory organ, so indispensable to the human condition, and so protean as a source of human sensitivity and behavior that even the most sophisticated upper limb prostheses are but crude replicas.

Many engineers have undertaken prosthetic upper limb replacement. As they proceed, their confidence and enthusiasm is replaced by overwhelming awe at the versatility of human upper limbs. Initial disdain of the apparent crude mechanical hooks in common use also is soon overcome by an appreciation of the efficiency of these devices, largely developed by input from the amputee.

The principles of arm prostheses center about the socket, its suspension, the body of the prosthesis, and the terminal device. Like the normal hand, the prosthetic terminal device dominates upper limb function. The shoulder girdle, the shoulder, and the arm down to wrist level assist by positioning the hand or prosthetic substitute in desired positions. The forearm muscles activating hand movement are duplicated in the prosthesis either by substitute muscle groups transferring power/motion mechanically through cables or by external power sources, usually rechargeable batteries and motors housed within the prosthesis.

Wrist Disarticulation Prostheses

Modern sockets are made of composite plastics. The terminal device—hook or hand—is generally fixed firmly to the distal end of the socket without an intervening wrist joint mechanism. The socket extends to the elbow, leaving it free to move in the anteroposterior plane. When the distal radioulnar joint is intact, a considerable degree of pronation and supination is possible. Further rotary assistance in positioning the hand and hook is accomplished by shoulder girdle and shoulder movement. For these reasons, the amputee with wrist disarticulation can operate the prosthesis through a wide spatial area.

Terminal-device control is ordinarily accomplished by a contralateral auxiliary sling controlling a cable across the upper back down to the socket and then attached to the hook or hand. A wide variety of terminal devices are available for general and specific tasks. Excellent function can be accomplished with this prosthetic system. The artificial limb is suspended by shaping its contour to gently grasp the distal radius, ulna, and forearm.

Forearm Prostheses

Since forearm amputations should preserve all available length, the prosthesis is designed to accommodate many amputation levels. Composite plastic material forms the socket, which totally contacts the residual limb. The terminal device is attached to the socket extension, designed with appropriate length for bilateral limb symmetry. The terminal device generally incorporates a mechanical wrist unit to allow prepositioning for rotation, flexion, and extension.

The hand or hook is motivated either by body powering through cables or by myoelectric-activated external energy obtained from a battery and motor housed in the socket space distal to the end of the stump. Electric signals produced by voluntary contraction of the residual forearm stump muscles are amplified to trigger battery/motor energy. The limb is suspended by socket contouring around the remaining forearm and distal humeral condyles. When additional suspension stability is required, elbow hinges are carried from the proximal socket up to an upper arm cuff. Depending upon the length of the residual forearm and stability requirements, a variety of elbow hinges are available including flexible, polycentric, step-up, and single-axis rigid hinges.

Above-Elbow Prostheses

The need for elbow substitution confronts the user with a much greater challenge. The socket must be stabilized about the shoulder to prevent its rotation with prosthetic use. The substitute elbow must first be placed in a position of desired function and then locked or stabilized in this position to permit terminal-device action. The weight of the forearm and terminal device frequently tires the wearer, causing shoulder and upper back fatigue. Many individuals with amputations at this level forego function and resort to a light cosmetic replacement worn for social occasions.

Early, aggressive training following amputation develops bimanual use patterns motivating the arm amputee to become a successful wearer.

The prosthesis is composed of composite plastic material. Its socket contours the residual limb. This contact is not sufficient for suspension, so added straps are usually necessary over the shoulder to assist in prosthetic support.

A wide variety of elbow mechanisms are commercially available. The prosthetic elbow can be positioned and locked in several flexion-extension modes to stabilize the prosthesis for terminal-device use. Elbow rotation is accomplished by prepositioning the forearm through a friction mechanism using the opposite arm.

Dual-control body-powered cable systems are necessary for (1) elbow positioning and locking and (2) terminal-device function. Active shoulder and shoulder girdle motion motivates the cables.

Ingenious myoelectric prostheses are available. National pride is involved in the development of these appliances, as attested by their names: the Boston arm, the Utah arm, the Canadian arm, and others. Electronics miniaturization has permitted the development of highly sophisticated devices using a variety of initiating sources of energy, including electric muscle signaling, displacement electrodes, and muscle "noise." Hybrid systems consisting of body power and external power sources are available. They are particularly useful for the upper arm prosthesis when the elbow can be controlled by electric power sources and the terminal device by body powering through cables. Bioengineering centers throughout the world are continuing research to improve these systems as well as to improve conventional materials and designs.

CONCLUSIONS

The material presented in this chapter is directed toward an understanding and working knowledge of contemporary amputation management. Since several disciplines are involved in amputation rehabilitation, no single monograph, treatise, or text chapter can provide complete coverage of the field. This in no way relieves or excuses the orthopaedic surgeon from acquiring a firm working knowledge of the various services required for superior management.

Throughout the world, millions of amputees function at a high level of human endeavor. No one except an amputee can fully understand and appreciate what it means to be without a limb or limbs. Even the presence of a functionless, insensate limb has a different psychological impact from that of an empty sleeve or pant leg. Currently, we read of amputees scaling mountains, running across continents, engaging in professional baseball and boxing, and competing in a wide array of other physical activities. Each exhibits a unique profile of courage and inner strength. Orthopaedic surgeons involved in amputee management assume the primary responsibility for providing and directing the professional services that will allow full rehabilitation.

II. Amputations and Prosthetics in Children

Joan T. Gold

Knowledge of infant and child development is essential for the clinician treating the limb-deficient child. An understanding of in utero development helps to explain the mechanisms resulting in such a deformity. Familiarity with normal attainment of fine and gross motor skills permits prescription of prosthetic devices in a timely manner, employing newer components that will allow for optimal function and psychological acceptance of the underlying condition. The child's ability to learn permits earlier provision of and training with a prosthesis. Incorporation of a device into the child's body image results in its improved acceptance and use.[21]

In order to foster normal development, the emotional sequelae of these deficiencies also should be considered. A child viewed by himself or herself as defective or dependent has additional handicaps. These children require the services of an entire team, including a pediatric orthopaedist, a pediatric physiatrist, a prosthetist, physical and occupational therapists, a psychologist, and a social worker in order to maximize their functional outcome.

INCIDENCE

Although the size of the amputee population under the age of 21 years is not known, it is thought to represent 10 percent of the total cases. According to Krebs's survey of 45 pediatric amputee clinics in 1980, there were 4105 children under treatment.[22] This may be an underestimation, as children with less complex deficiencies may not have been referred to these centers. Males outnumbered females 3 to 2. Eighty percent of the deficiencies were unilateral. Congenital amputees were twice as frequent as those whose deficiencies were acquired, and in one recent study the ratio approached 3.7:1.[23] These figures, however, may

undergo a gradual change, as the survival statistics for patients with higher-level amputations due to skeletal neoplasms is improving greatly.

Incidence figures for congenital limb reductions and amputations vary. Recent studies in the United States and Sweden reveal an incidence of approximately 6.3 cases per 10,000 births.[24,25] versus 1.48 per 10,000 births in Australia.[23] The terminal transverse below-elbow amputation is the most common congenital deficiency, occurring in over 50 percent of the congenital cases; the left side is more commonly affected.[26,27] There may be a left-to-right gradient in fetal development which would explain this finding. This may subsequently allow for a higher rate of prosthetic acceptance than would otherwise be seen, as the device does not have to replace the function of a dominant upper extremity.[28]

Of the acquired cases, 60 percent involve the loss of a lower extremity, 30 percent involve an upper extremity, and 10 percent involve multiple extremities. Of unilateral cases, lower extremity amputations are the most likely.[22]

ETIOLOGY

Congenital Amputations and Limb Deficiencies

The causative factors of congenital amputations are mostly unknown. Embryologic studies have implicated an insult to the limb buds occurring from 4 to 8 weeks of gestation.[29,30] After that time, further insults do not result in the failure of formation of parts but rather in alterations in size. As development of the upper extremities precedes that of the lower extremities, involvement of all four extremities implies a pathologic process occurring over time and not a trivial, isolated event. This is especially important in easing the guilt of a mother who had had such an infant.

The thalidomide syndrome is one of the rare exceptions in which cause could be proved. Ingestion of this drug at 34 to 50 days of gestation resulted in children with phocomelia of two to four extremities and associated facial, cardiac, and genitourinary malformations.[31] The mechanism of action is reported to be an embryonic neuropathy that has secondary effects on the mesenchymal tissues. Analysis of the total fascicular area of the sciatic nerves from thalidomide exposed and deformed rabbit fetuses revealed a significant reduction in this area, proportionate to the degree of the deformity. Tibial hypoplasia and aplasia were especially common. These findings imply that there may be some sort of neurotrophic growth substance that is responsible for limb differentiation. This may be further related to quantitative changes in the chromosomal maternal in spinal motor neurons.[32,33]

Other recognized causative factors include maternal diabetes (in association with sacral agenesis),[34] hydramnios, maternal exposure to rubella, amniotic bands, uterine cramping, and chromosomal abnormalities (trisomies 13 and 18).[24] Amniotic or Streeter's band formation results from disruption of initially normal limbs due to constriction. They are usually noted with distal constrictions of the limbs or distal amputations of the longer central fingers and medial two toes, but there can be more severe manifestations such as frank transverse amputations, multiple limb involvement, facial clefting, and encephalocele formation.[35,36] These abnormalities generally occur in a sporadic fashion and without a history of maternal trauma, although animal studies imply an association with amniocentesis, subsequent uterine contractions, and hemorrhagic necrosis in the extremities, and low birth weight.[37] A few number of familial cases also have been cited.[38] The mechanism for band formation itself remains unclear.

Disruption of limbs may also occur in utero in response to compression. Foreshortening of the limbs, absence of distal rays, and syndactyly have been seen in association with a bicornuate uterus, large compressive uterine fibroids, and early loss of amniotic fluid.[37]

A third disruptive force that may result in limb deficiencies is vascular compromise. Deformities of the upper extremities seen in association with the Poland, Klippel-Feil, and Möbius syndromes have been reported. Pathology has revealed placental abruption and infarction of the brachial artery.[39] These vascular findings have been reported in association with pathology of the umbilical cord, rubella, and cytomegalovirus infections and gestational diabetes, although a familial predilection may occur.[40]

There may be an etiologic role for multifactorial inheritance, i.e., certain mothers being genetically more susceptible to a given environmental agent. The role of such agents as oral contraceptives,[41] phenothiazine derivatives (such as meclizine),[42] dioxane, folic acid antagonists (such as aminopterin), anticonvulsants, endocrinopathies, and intercurrent infections has not been substantiated.[43] Smoking and alcohol use may be related to limb reduction defects,[44] with vascular spasm being implicated.[45]

The Child Amputee Prosthetic Project (CAPP) study found that among 159 patients with congenital amputations, 65 percent of the mothers had one or more of the following during their pregnancies: urinary tract infections, pneumonia, viral illnesses, or vaginal bleeding.[46] There was a 12 percent incidence of maternal diabetes. These percentages were much higher than predicted.

Acquired Amputations

Of the acquired cases, over 70 percent are trauma-related, and 90 percent of those involve one limb.[26] The majority of posttraumatic cases occur in males after the age of 8 years, when the child is less likely to be observed at play. Most cases occur as the result of motor vehicle accidents.[47] Other cases follow train accidents,[48,49] accidents with power tools and farm equipment,[50] electrical and chemical burns, falls, and gunshot wounds.[49] Children who are loners, have a history of behavioral disorders, and live in a low socioeconomic setting are at risk for such injuries. These factors have to be assessed in planning the rehabilitation programs of such children, and they have implications for prevention as well.[47–49]

Of the acquired cases, 30 percent represent the sequelae of disease; most are related to neoplasia, principally osteogenic sarcoma. Less commonly, infarctions of the limbs may occur in association with a disseminated intravascular coagulopathy seen with staphylococcal and streptococcal sepsis,[51] pneumococcal sepsis often in the presence of sickle cell disease,[52,53] meningococcal sepsis,[54] and varicella.[55] Other cases may represent end-stage treatment for chronic osteomyelitis or a pseudoarthrosis due to neurofibromatosis.[56] Recently, protein S deficiency in association with arterial thrombosis has been reported with lower extremity loss.[57]

CONGENITAL LIMB DEFICIENCIES

Classification

The Burtch revision[58] of the Frantz and O'Rahilly system[59] is the most common classification used to describe limb deficiencies; its terminology is based upon a description of the absent parts. In this system, *amelia* is defined as a complete absence of a limb and *meromelia* as a partial deficit. Meromelias are further subdivided into those that are terminal (at the end of the limb) and those that are intercalary (in the middle of the limb). Further subgrouping denotes deficiencies in the preaxial (radial or tibial) or postaxial (ulnar or fibular) planes. Last, the missing bones or portions thereof are named.

For example, a residual hand attached to the trunk is an intercalary deficiency with absence of the humerus, radius, and ulna. An isolated absence of the fibula would be considered an intercalary deficiency; the same deficiency associated with absence of the lateral rays would be considered a terminal longitudinal postaxial deficiency. Nomenclature is made more cumbersome when several deformities coexist. A child with a proximal femoral focal deficiency has a partial intercalary transverse femoral deficiency associated with variable degrees of acetabular dysplasia and absence of the fibula.

Although applicable to many deformities, the above system does not readily describe failure of separation of parts, duplications, over- or undergrowths, amniotic band syndromes, and generalized skeletal anomalies. These exceptions are taken into account in the more complex classification system proposed by Swanson.[60] Terminal transverse congenital and acquired amputations can be described by the percentage of limb remaining. Further refinements of classification have been proposed by Kay et al.[61] Often, classification cannot be adequately determined at birth, as ossification is incomplete.[60]

General Considerations

The infant with a congenital limb deficiency requires evaluation for associated anomalies. It is necessary to determine if there is a pattern of deformities constituting a recognizable syndrome, with a definable risk of recurrence in future pregnancies. Associated anomalies of other organ systems have been reported in approximately 30 percent of the population.[24,25] Malformations involving the gastrointestinal, respiratory, cardiovascular, genitourinary, and central nervous systems, the eyes and ears, or associated tumors have been documented.[24] An infant with multiple anomalies and high-level deficiencies may have a perinatal mortality risk as high as 20 percent.[25]

Associated congenital musculoskeletal malformations are common; long bone reductions are associated with anomalies of the hand or the foot.[25] Spinal deformities and scoliosis are prevalent, occurring in 18 percent of all upper extremity amputees. Scoliosis occurs in 100 percent of patients with bilateral upper extremity amelias. No relationship has been demonstrated between the side of the deficiency and the apex of the curve.[62]

Most terminal transverse deficiencies occur in isolation and do not pose a risk of recurrence in future pregnancies. There are some exceptions such as acheiropodia (absence of the hands and feet). Also, most ulnar, tibial, and fibular deficiencies are not inherited. Amniotic bands are nongenetic anomalies but are associated with facial clefts and eyelid and skull anomalies. The infant with the noninherited VATER syndrome, who may display vertebral anomalies, imperforate anus, tracheoesophageal fistula, and/or renal malformations (which name the syndrome), presents also with radial deficiencies.[63] However, many radial anomalies are inherited. The thrombocytopenia–absent radius (TAR) syndrome, the Fanconi syndrome, and the Holt-Oram syndrome can be associated with significant hematologic diseases (including blood dyscrasias), congenital heart disease, and renal disease, respectively. Given the degree and distribution of the deformities, a chest roentgenogram, electrocardiogram, blood count, skeletal survey, renal sonograms, and/or chromosomal analysis may be warranted.

An assessment of the infant's future functional capacities and a treatment plan need to be made for the family shortly after birth. According to Marquardt,[64] this requires consideration of training of potential and residual abilities, correction of dislocations and abnormal postures, provision of orthoprostheses and adaptive equipment, and consideration of surgical procedures to maintain or improve function.

Infant amputees must be handled by their parents as soon as possible and in a normal manner.[65] The defective side should not be swaddled, as this could result not only in limitation in range (usually abduction) of the limb but also in hemisensory neglect (failure to respond to stimuli presented on the affected side). Rudimentary digits should be encouraged to be used for function and to provide sensory feedback; later they can be used to activate a cable system, lock, or switch. Infants with bilateral upper extremity amelia should be engaged in activities that maximize cervical, trunk, and lower extremity range.[65] This permits them to manipulate objects with their feet and later to be independent in dressing and in performing perineal care. Infants with lower extremity amelia should be encouraged to roll, strengthen upper extremity and abdominal musculature, and improve sitting balance.

Associated deformities and contractures may need to be surgically corrected. According to Aitken, the surgical conversion rate for congenital anomalies is 8.3 percent for upper extremities and 45.4 percent for lower extremities.[26]

For example, infants with amniotic bands may require serial Z-plasties. The child with a varus hip in association with a proximal femoral focal deficiency may require an osteotomy in order to attain a valgus position.[66]

Previously, provision of an upper extremity prosthesis was advised at age 4 years, just prior to school entry.[67] Current recommendations advise provision of a passive device to unilateral amputees at 3 to 6 months, when the infants are developing the propping reactions that allow them to sit when placed. The lower extremity unilateral amputee should be provided with a monolithic (unjointed) device at 6 to 12 months, when lower extremity weight bearing and pulling to standing commence.[65] Provision of more sophisticated devices, with greater degrees of freedom, occurs with advancement of developmental milestones. With this regimen, the infant learns normal patterns of movement. Up to 94 percent of lower extremity amputees and 61 percent of upper extremity amputees have been shown to use their prostheses all day at age 21 years, with the highest percentage groups having been fitted at the youngest ages.[21] With early provision of devices, atrophy, osteoporosis, and asymmetries may be avoided.

ACQUIRED LIMB DEFICIENCIES

In order to adequately evaluate the child indicated for an amputation, detailed knowledge of the underlying illness or associated injury is necessary. One should be familiar with the details of the child's medical treatment and any complications. When the child is seen preoperatively, information concerning future medical treatment, prosthetic options, and functional outcome should be communicated to the child and the parents in order to allay fear of the unknown.[68]

Preprosthetic training can be initiated in the interval between the child's initial illness or diagnostic biopsy and limb ablation. Bed rest should be discouraged, as it may sabotage later rehabilitation efforts; a child at rest for 2 to 3 weeks may have up to a 50 percent reduction in muscle power.[69] Range-of-motion exercises and strengthening of selected muscle groups required for prosthetic control should be initiated.[70] For example, in a child who is to undergo an above-elbow amputation, shoulder musculature and trunk flexors should be exercised. Deep-breathing exercises should be performed, as reduction in pulmonary function is associated with higher levels of upper extremity loss.[71] While always respecting the need for appropriate resection margins in neoplastic diseases, as much limb length as possible should be preserved at amputation, especially the epiphyses.[72] A long lever arm is able to generate larger forces with less energy expenditure, and nonstandard stump lengths can be accommodated with modern prosthetics. Preservation of the epiphyses permits additional limb growth while avoiding spur formation.

Immediate postoperative prosthetic fitting can be considered in this group because of its advantages of decreased edema and phantom pain,[68,73] but this should be done with extreme caution. A child may not complain of discomfort, causing serious wound problems beneath the dressing to go unnoticed.[70] The child may not be able to feel pain if there is an associated neuropathy following a burn or chemotherapy. If postoperative fitting is not under consideration, the preoperative exercise program should, nevertheless, be continued; ambulation and self-care training, stump wrapping, and hygiene should be taught.[46,74]

The child with an underlying malignancy will have a more difficult course of rehabilitation. Anemia, immunosuppression, and infection may be the sequelae of chemotherapy and poor food intake. The additional energy requirements for crutch walking and prosthetic use may not be met.

Treatment protocols for osteogenic sarcoma have utilized a variety of adjuvant chemotherapeutic agents including doxorubicin, cisplatin, vicristine, methotrexate, actinomycin D, and/or cyclophosphamide.[75,76] Complications of these drugs include cardiomyopathy with failure and arrhythmias,[77,78] peripheral neuropathies, encephalopathies,[79] fractures,[80] and pulmonary fibrosis.[81] Accordingly, results of electrocardiograms and gated pool studies should be reviewed prior to prescribing an exercise program, and a maximal heart rate should be targeted. Exercises that require Valsalva maneuvers are relatively contraindicated if there is pulmonary disease present with an attendant risk of pneumothorax. Overvigorous upper extremity strengthening exercises may result in a central line's being dislodged. Splinting for a drop wrist or foot may be required in the presence of a neuropathy.[82] If deformities are left untreated, Achilles tendon lengthenings may be required. Scoliosis requiring treatment may arise secondary to the irradiation field or to a leg-length discrepancy.

Medical complications result in fluctuations in the child's weight and stump size. The use of an adjustable lower extremity prosthesis permits training during the period when such fluctuations occur. Training with these devices may begin as early as 10 to 14 days postoperatively.

Vigorous rehabilitation treatment and the provision of prostheses to patients with bone tumors have been criticized as futile and not cost-effective. However, the wearing time for 50 percent of this population is over 5 years[68] and exceeds the wearing time of the elderly, dysvascular amputee by 2 to 3 1/2 years.[83] With survival rates higher than 60 percent at 5 years, aggressive rehabilitation should be considered for all these children.

UPPER EXTREMITY AMPUTEES AND THEIR PROSTHESES

The fabrication, components, and function of a child's upper extremity prosthesis is in many ways similar to that of an adult; unfortunately, this includes its lack of cosmesis and insufficient grasp strength. However, pediatric devices must additionally be simple to use, be light in weight, not restrict motion, and be able to accommodate for longitudinal and circumferential growth.[84,85] Both traditional exoskeletal and modular endoskeletal prostheses are available for both the upper and lower extremities.[84,86]

For patients with distal deficiencies such as absent and/or malformed digits, surgical alternatives may be indicated rather than provision of a prosthetic device.[87,88] Radial clubhand deformities are amenable to splinting and subsequent centralization of the hand, with possible ulnar osteotomy.[88] Other deformities, such as ulnar dysmelia, may require surgical correction, possibly elbow disarticulation, prior to attempting prosthetic fitting.[89] A child with a partial hand deficiency may function quite well if a post for opposition attached to the wrist is provided.[85] Some posts are multipositional to accommodate holding objects of different sizes.[90] As the child gets older, a cosmetic hand may also be requested for social engagements.

A first device is supplied to the below- or above-elbow congenital amputee at 3 to 6 months. If the deficiency is unilateral, that side will be nondominant. If the child has bilateral deficiencies, the longer side will be the dominant one and is fitted first. An exoskeletal, double-walled device anchored with a figure-of-eight harness and a terminal device (TD) is the prototype. A passive mitt can be supplied as the first TD, although a "hook," such as the Dorrance wafer, Dorrance 12 plastisol-coated TD or CAPP TD, with the cable system detached, is preferable. This permits toys to be placed in the TD by the adult, stimulating the infant's interest in the limb and encouraging "two-handed" activities. A new option that is light in weight and can easily be adjusted to accommodate for growth is a temporary prosthetic shell made of polypropylene. Another alternative is a spherical mitt covered with Velcro loop material. Devices with the inactivated terminal devices are anchored by a figure-of-eight harness. For the lighter type, an elastic sleeve may be provided, but this does not allow the infant to accommodate to harness use. Normal developmental activities of rolling, sitting, crawling, pulling to standing, weight shifting, and ambulation should follow, with completion of this sequence by about 15 months.[84] Friction wrist units allow for positioning in passive pronation and supination and facilitate use of the terminal device.[92] Provision of the device at a later date may result in a higher rejection rate. The role of the therapist is to facilitate attainment of these milestones. Time without a device should also be permitted to encourage sensory feedback and stump use. The reader is referred to Blakeslee's text for further details of prosthetic training.[46]

Developmental parameters for activation of the TD include the ability to follow two-step commands, an attention span of about 10 min, and an interest in bimanual activities and toys that come apart; this usually occurs at about 18 months.[84]

Opening of the TD is achieved with flexion of the humerus. This voluntary opening device is advantageous to the younger child, as cause and effect are readily demonstrable. Once the object is grasped, continuous tension need not be maintained by the cable to hold the object in place. This permits the child to manipulate the object with the sound, contralateral extremity. Visual cues are not obscured, as would be the case with a functional hand.[93] Traditionally, hands have been reserved for children of school-entry age, although they are now available in smaller sizes for patients as young as 24 months. CAPP TDs are being used more frequently because of their lighter weight, improved appearance, and ability to hold an object with a less precise grasp due to the larger surface area available.[85,90]

Voluntary closing devices are also fabricated and their mechanism is more like that of a normal hand. As they may more closely simulate physiologic function, they have been activated in infants as young as 6 months.[94] Provision of these devices to older children may result in increased prosthetic usage resulting from improved ability to release objects rapidly. This may be especially helpful when participating in sports activities such as riding a bicycle and holding a bat.[95] Despite reported advantages, these terminal devices are not in common use. Also less commonly employed is the voluntary opening larger CAPP #2 terminal device. It is reported as having the advantages of providing improved grip and static pinch despite its light weight and cosmetically acceptable appearance.[96]

To improve prosthetic purchase around the humeral epicondyles, a preflexed or Munster prosthesis may be required for the child with a short below-elbow amputation.[97] However, this option does not permit full elbow flexion. For the child with an elbow disarticulation, an outside elbow joint may be needed.[97]

As an option to the standard sockets utilized with a variety of terminal devices, the ISNY (Icelandic Swedish New York University) flexible socket may be employed. This was initially a socket developed for above-knee amputees. Users report that comfort is increased and that there is increased sensory feedback due to its ability to change in configuration (but not in volume) with muscle contraction.[98]

An elbow-lock cable is generally added to the prosthesis of an above-elbow amputee at the developmental age of 30 to 36 months. This correlates with the child's desire to lift objects with the artificial limb, although the child cannot lift very heavy loads with it. This second system really functions to preposition the TD in the correct place. Cable locking and release are both controlled by shoulder elevation. The TD will not operate unless the elbow is locked. When the elbow lock is released, elbow flexion may be quite rapid. To prevent the child from being hit in the face with the prosthesis, a flexion stop may be required (Fig. 18-12).[99] Some children with this level of amputation may find prosthetic suspension and rotation problematic. Marquardt has suggested an angulation osteotomy of the humerus as one possible solution for this.[87]

The child with an acquired upper extremity amputation, especially when it is tumor-related, usually requires a shoulder disarticulation or a forequarter amputation. The available devices are the same as those available to a congenital amputee. The distal components are similar to those of the above-elbow prosthesis, and the shoulder joint is positioned passively. Occasionally, an additional shoulder or perineal strap may be required for harnessing. An older child with an underlying medical disorder may reject such a device; a shoulder cap or a passive arm prosthesis may be an acceptable cosmetic alternative. One-handed tools such as a rocker knife or a buttonhook and clothing adaptations should be offered to these patients.

The child who has bilateral deficiencies has more complex problems. When there is bilateral absence of the hands, especially when visual problems coexist, a unilateral Krukenberg procedure may be indicated. By having the forearm split into radial and ulnar portions, the child

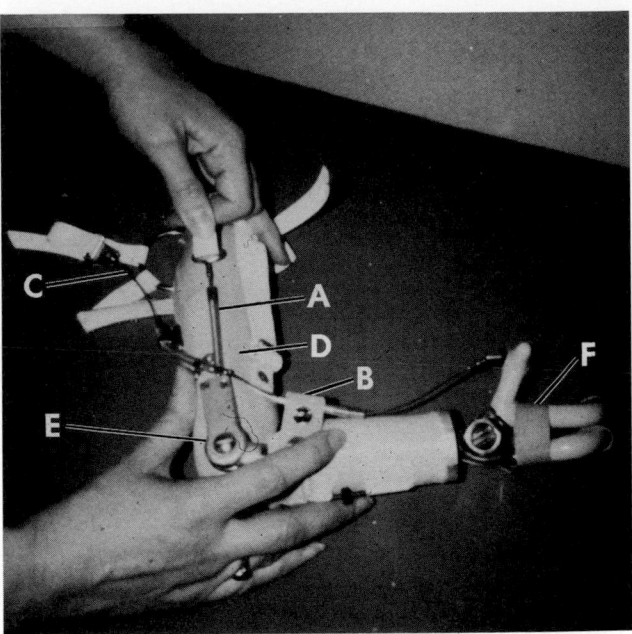

Figure 18-12 A child's standard exoskeletal above-elbow prosthesis. A, elbow lock cable; B, terminal device cable; C, figure-of-eight harness; D, double-walled socket; E, external elbow lock; F, plastisol-coated terminal device.

can grasp objects without a prosthetic device and with direct sensory feedback.[100] Objections to the cosmetic results of the procedure have been raised.

Patients with bilateral amelias are fitted with their first devices at 24 months. Challenor has formulated a developmental timetable for the treatment of such patients.[101] These children may exhibit delays in gross motor skills such as sitting and walking, as the upper extremities cannot be used to improve their balance.[65] Modular components are frequently used because of their lighter weight and ease of replacement.[85,90,102] Regardless of the components, it is essential that at least one wrist unit be positioned in flexion so that midline feeding, dressing, and perineal care activities can be performed. A variety of powered prostheses are also available. Previously, carbon dioxide cartridges were used. Currently, switch-controlled or myoelectric components can be provided,[103] utilizing shoulder girdle movements for activation. Children may prefer to use their feet for activities at home but their prostheses in a social or school setting.[64] Other powered options include a prehension actuator, a motor attached to the TD to enhance grasp strength, and an electric elbow to facilitate the lifting of heavy loads.[85,92]

Myoelectric prostheses are generally reserved for adults with below-elbow deficiencies, with two available muscular control sites to open and close the prosthetic hand. These devices appear more natural, and a suspension harness is not needed. Size constraints in smaller upper extremities have resulted in the development of single-site control systems with opening and closing of the terminal device being in response to the degree of muscular contraction.[104] Recent studies have demonstrated that children as young as 16 months can use these devices effectively.[105] Their cost, their weight, and the need for refitting at 6- to 15-month intervals, in addition to their frequent repairs, have constituted a relative contraindication for prosthetic prescription for some physicians.[85] Although initial preference rates in comparison to body-powered devices may be as high as 78 percent, with time, acceptance may be comparable to that of the more standard devices, and use does not necessarily imply active prehension.[106] While some specific tasks such as donning socks, cutting paper, and bandage application may be faster with a myoelectric hand, grasp and release may be slowed and dropping of objects may be more frequent.[107] It is likely that despite the type of prosthesis and terminal device used, and even in the absence of central nervous system dysfunction, delays in the development of bimanual skills are common in children and not necessarily related to prosthetic wearing or training time.[108]

Upper extremity prostheses need to be replaced about every 2 years; TDs are replaced to keep pace with the size of the contralateral hand. For the Dorrance system of TD components, a size 10P TD is provided at 2 to 3 years, 10X at 3 to 6 years, 99X at 6 to 8 years, 88 at 8 to 13 years, and 5X at 13 years or above.[46] Adjustments for growth can be made by reducing the thickness of the stump socks worn and/or by using a triple-wall socket and removing one layer when growth occurs. Newer developments permit a new customized socket to be fabricated and attached to an existing device by reheating, extending the time that a prosthesis is serviceable.[86]

LOWER EXTREMITY AMPUTEES AND THEIR PROSTHESES

For the child with a below-knee or more distal deficiency, a normal gait and absence of any functional limitations is anticipated if length and fit of the prosthesis is proper.[65] Gait-analysis studies reveal that the center of motion during ambulation remains on the nonprosthetic side of the body throughout the gait cycle[109] and that there is approximately a 15 percent increase in energy expenditure when the patient has such a level of amputation, but neither changes in cadence nor in heart rate are made in response to this.[110] When a child is provided with a prosthesis before 12 months of age, training is a consequence of normal curiosity. Balancing on uneven surfaces, weight shifting, reaching forward to retrieve toys, and even falling down in these attempts are normal precursors to independent ambulation.[46,65] More complex tasks such as kicking a ball, hopping, and jumping should follow.[46]

Shoe fillers have not been particularly successful for children with partial foot amputations. They tend to pull off and/or cause skin irritation and not be cosmetically acceptable. A low-profile prototype device has been designed for use in the presence of Chopart and Lisfranc amputations. It consists of a flexible Silastic liner with an external rigid shell made of polypropylene with a longitudinal arch pad, elastic suspension strap, and a toe extension, the latter acting as a lever arm to assist push-off.[111]

The exoskeletal prosthetic components for children are similar to those supplied to the adult. A single-action,

cushioned-heel (SACH) foot is almost always used; however, regardless of the type of prosthetic foot employed, most of the weight on the prosthetic foot is distributed on the forefoot.[112] More recently, energy storing feet have been made available to children, resulting in a less asymmetric gait for the users. With this modification, moderate changes in push off have been documented with three times the energy return, implying that a reduction in overall energy costs may result.[113,114] This may have an impact on the later development of arthritic changes associated with a prolonged asymmetrical gait pattern.[115] Because of the lack of well-defined contours of the limb, a patellar tendon–bearing device may be unsatisfactory for the younger child and may predispose to complications in adulthood. A thigh cuff may be required to provide additional suspension, to prevent rotation while the child is climbing or engaging in sports, and to prevent genu valgum (Fig. 18-13).[93,116]

The silicone suction socket is a newer device in which an intimately fitting silicone sleeve is rolled onto the limb, providing for improved prosthetic purchase. Close contact is further enhanced by the placement of a retaining pin distally, which locks the socket to the prosthetic shell. It has been utilized in patients as young as 8 months with

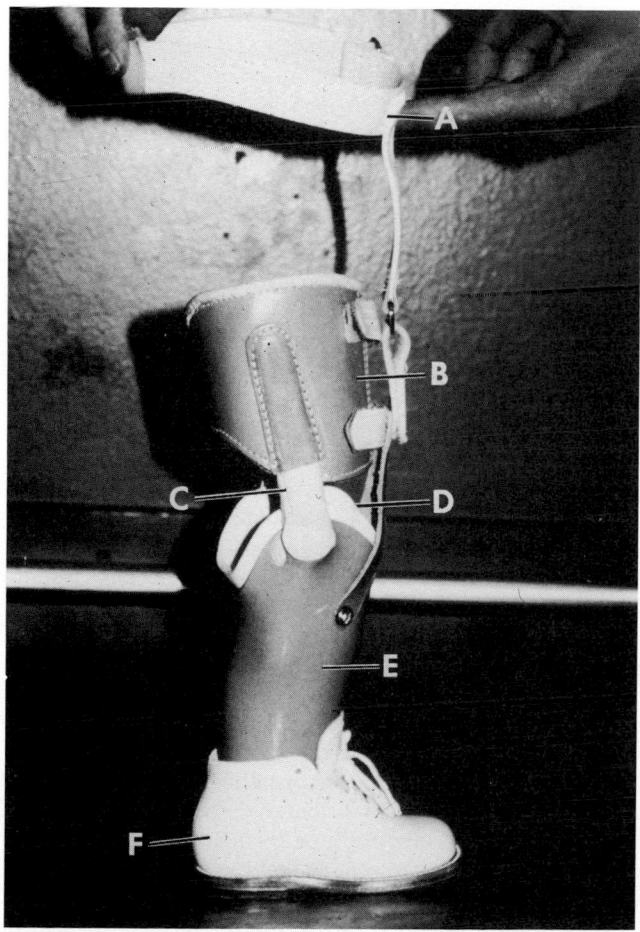

Figure 18-13 Child's standard exoskeletal below-knee prosthesis. A, pelvic belt; B, thigh corset; C, external knee joint; D, removable insert; E, double-walled socket; F, SACH foot (in shoe).

good results, even when the skin on the stump was extremely friable.[117]

Proximally, narrow medial-lateral sockets with high lateral walls and lowered walls in the perineal region have been supplied to children as a biomechanical improvement over the traditional quadrilateral socket.

In order to allow for growth, various strategies are employed, such as supplying a removable plastic liner. The prosthesis may be made intentionally too long and a lift placed on the contralateral shoe; the life is removed when the patient has grown.[97] The shaft of the prosthesis can be lengthened just proximal to the SACH foot and relaminated. With these options, a replacement device needs to be provided every 1 to 2 years up to the age of 12 years and then every 3 to 4 years until the age of 21 years.[21]

Congenital lower limb deficiencies provide more of a challenge than standard surgical amputation levels. A variety of prosthetic and surgical menus have been presented, dependent upon the anticipated amount of limb inequality at the cessation of growth, joint instability above and below the deformity, associated foot deformities and ray abnormalities, and the possible involvement of the contralateral limb.[118] A standard prosthetic device can equalize the leg-length discrepancy associated with congenital absence of the fibula but is suboptimal in dealing with the tibial bowing, valgus foot, talocalcaneal fusion, and ray deficiencies that may be present.[116,118a–120] Considerations as to prosthetic fit and the need for surgical revision are made more complex by the occurrence of bilateral involvement in 25 percent and proximal femoral focal deficiency in 10 percent or more.[30] Some authors have advised soft tissue releases, including Achilles tendon lengthening, posterior capsulotomy, peroneal tendon lengthening, and tibial osteotomies for the correction of such deformities.[118a,119] However, the indications for such procedures have recently been brought into question. An end-weight-bearing ankle disarticulation, or Syme's amputation, is presently considered the treatment of choice for a unilateral deformity of this type.[116,120,121] This is especially true when the foot deformity is severe and a limb-length inequality of over 3 in is predicted. This procedure should be performed before the age of 2 years to lessen the psychological implications of removal of the foot. Unlike the adult who has had a Syme procedure, the child does not have a bulbous stump with prominent malleoli. The Syme procedure is also advantageous because the tibial epiphysis is preserved.[120] Initially, a Syme prosthesis is provided, and with growth, an end-bearing below-knee prosthesis is used. The technically more difficult Boyd procedure, in which the calcaneus is fused to the tibia, also has been used when there is congenital absence of the fibula.[122] Some parents may refuse ablation of a portion of the limb, in which case prostheses that incorporate the residual feet may be fabricated.[123] Surgical procedures in the presence of bilateral involvement should be undertaken with extreme caution, as residual ability to ambulate without prostheses may be impaired.

Congenital absence of the tibia is associated with a shortened limb, a varus foot, and ray deficiencies. Instability of the ankle and knee joints and occasionally congenital hip dislocation or femoral bifurcation may be seen.[124] Classically, either a knee disarticulation and provision of an end-bearing prosthesis or an arthroplasty to retain a below-knee stump (Brown procedure) has been advised to be performed prior to the age of 2 years.[124] If there is good quadriceps function, centralization of the fibular head in the intercondylar notch, with talectomy, and displacement of the lateral malleolus over the calcaneus have been advised to avoid amputation, but this is a much less frequently used alternative[125] due to the progressive knee flexion deformities that develop.[126] For congenital deficiencies where the anticipated length discrepancy is 15 to 20 cm or less, lengthening of the residual bone to facilitate prosthetic fit and function via the Ilizarov technique can be considered; however, it is a lengthy process that must be chosen with caution. Such techniques may also be applied to short posttraumatic residual limbs of the upper and lower extremities.[126,127]

With acquired or congenital above-knee amputations, younger children are first provided with a monolithic device. At the developmental age of 36 to 48 months, when the child would normally negotiate stairs independently, a knee joint is introduced into the system.[93,128] A constant-friction knee that is light in weight but does not adjust to changes in walking speed is most commonly used, often with an elastic anterior knee extension strap. An older child may prefer a heavier hydraulic knee that responds to changes in walking speed.[97] Suction sockets can be used in the older child. With a short above-knee stump, extension of the prosthesis laterally to the pelvic brim may be required to provide additional stability. Pelvic suspension with a Silastic bandage or less commonly with a pelvic band with an external hip joint may also be needed.

Older children with above-knee or higher acquired lesions require more training with balancing, ambulation, and stair climbing and also conditioning and trunk-rotation exercises. Initially, prosthetic fit may be compromised by changes in stump volume and shape associated with cycles of chemotherapy.[129] Accordingly, an adjustable temporary prosthesis must be provided. A temporary device with an adjustable plastic socket, Velcro straps, a manually locking or safety knee, a SACH foot, and an optional cosmetic cover can be provided for use until 5 to 12 months after surgery (Fig. 18-14). As an alternative, the Icelandic-Swedish-New York University (ISNY) above-knee socket, composed of a rigid shell with a flexible interior conforming to changes in shape, may be considered.[130] This has been successfully used in several adolescent patients and permits adjustments for growth. For amputations at the thigh or above, endoskeletal components may be used because of their lighter weight. These devices are more cosmetic but more fragile, as their foam cover may be easily torn. A CAPP endoskeletal above-knee foot with extensions at the heel, toe, and ball of the foot also has been developed.[85,131] With projections that better absorb the torque applied to them rather than transmitting it to the stump, this results in improved stability in the stance phase of gait and better toe clearance. Regardless of the components used, a child with a high-level amputation can be expected to have some gait deviations, such as a Trendelenburg gait or circumduction. Such children not infrequently require a cane or crutch on the contralateral side for ambulation.[93]

foot held in maximal plantar flexion must be provided. For children with relatively stable hip joints (Aitken class A), an Ilizarov lengthening can be considered as an alternative to amputation.[138] Almost one-third of patients with proximal femoral focal deficiency have bilateral involvement.[66] Amputations are usually not performed, as these children can ambulate without prostheses. Such devices may be provided to lessen their significant reduction in height. For others with bilateral, symmetrical deficiencies such as phocomelia, a low-to-ground rocker-bottom prosthesis ("stubby") or swivel walker can be used by the young child to improve balance. These devices can gradually be extended upward. They are provided at about 18 months, but definitive prosthetic fitting may not occur until about 6 years (Fig. 18-15).[65] Similar treatment strategies have been advocated in patients with sacral agenesis or diastrophic dwarfism.[101]

Patients who have hip disarticulations or hemipelvectomies have much more difficulty in ambulating because of their increased energy expenditures and problems with prosthetic fit. Traditionally, a Canadian or bucket type of prosthesis is used, with the younger child requiring a shoulder harness to anchor the prosthesis (Fig. 18-16).[30] This device is also used for patients with phocomelia; the residual foot should not be removed on such patients as it provides a good weight-bearing surface within the prosthesis. Energy for use of the Canadian type of prosthesis comes from the pelvic flexion moment. The use of an anteriorly located broad hip joint, occasionally utilizing a spring-loaded mechanism, helps to minimize energy consumption and maximize stability.[139]

Newer technical developments have included biofeedback devices[140] and computed gait analysis,[141] which facilitate prosthetic adjustments and thereby lessen gait deviations. Many sports prostheses that can hold equipment such as a baseball bat or can be used for swimming have been fabricated. Amputees should be encouraged to participate in sports such as swimming, gymnastics, bicycling, soccer, and skiing with and without their prostheses.[142] For jogging, a lightweight spring-loaded prosthesis with a telescoping shank to prevent vaulting and which will store energy to facilitate push-off has been developed.[143]

The child who is a quadruple amputee requires special considerations that cannot be dealt with in detail in this chapter.[31,102] These children may be quite fragile, being susceptible to fluctuations in body temperature because of their reduced surface area. Some children may do quite well without adaptive devices by utilizing residual limbs with or without digits, by mouthing objects, or by rolling.[31] Other children may benefit from the provision of a motorized cart with a head or a mouth switch control.[90,143a]

COMPLICATIONS

The most common physical complications seen in juvenile amputees are those associated with bone overgrowth and painful spur formation.[144] Spurs arise from appositional bone growth and occur in both the congenital and ac-

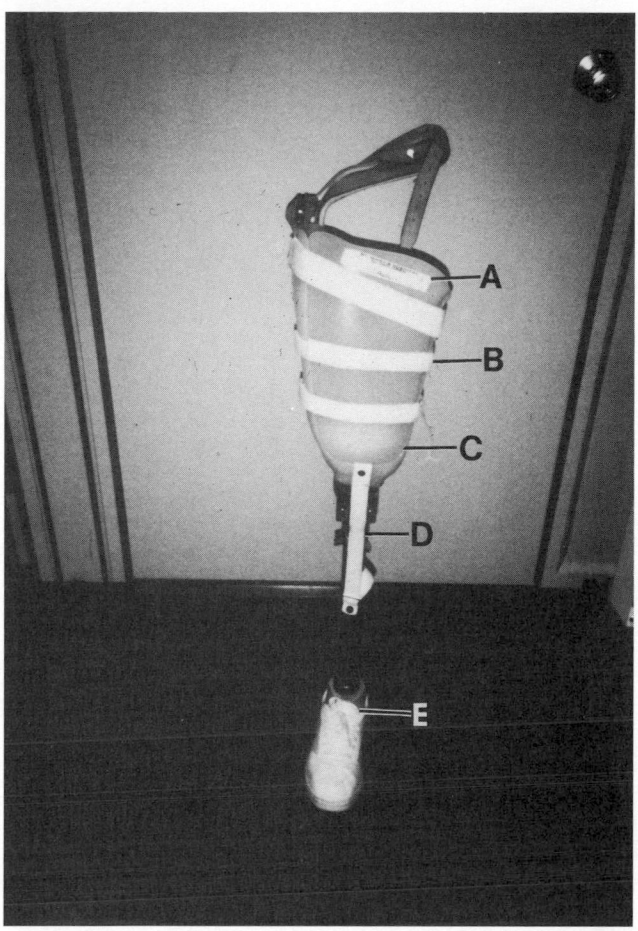

Figure 18-14 Temporary above-knee prosthesis for the adolescent. A, adjustable socket; B, Velcro straps; C, foam end pad; D, manually locking knee joint; E, SACH foot.

Patients with proximal femoral focal deficiency represent a special challenge. There is not only a marked shortening of the limb but also associated anomalies of the femoral head[132] and/or fibular agenesis in 50 percent of the cases.[66,133] Osteotomies to correct the neck-shaft angle or metaphyseal-epiphyseal synostosis to stabilize the joint may be required. Distally, if the fibula is lacking, a Syme amputation with subsequent knee fusion may be indicated. If the potential growth of the patient is calculated correctly, the ankle disarticulation becomes level with the contralateral knee; a knee disarticulation prosthesis is then provided.[66,134] Alternatively, a Van Nes osteotomy with rotation of the tibia 180° can convert the deformity into a type of below-knee deficiency.[135] This rotationplasty is associated with a more energy efficient gait but may not result in any changes in gross motor function.[136] Prosthetic fitting may be difficult secondary to telescoping of the abnormal proximal elements. Even in the presence of a Syme amputation distally, a modified ischial-weight-bearing flexible socket with a high lateral wall may be needed.[137] It may be difficult to convince the family to give consent for ablative surgery even if it will result in improved function; in this case, a relatively uncosmetic prosthesis with the

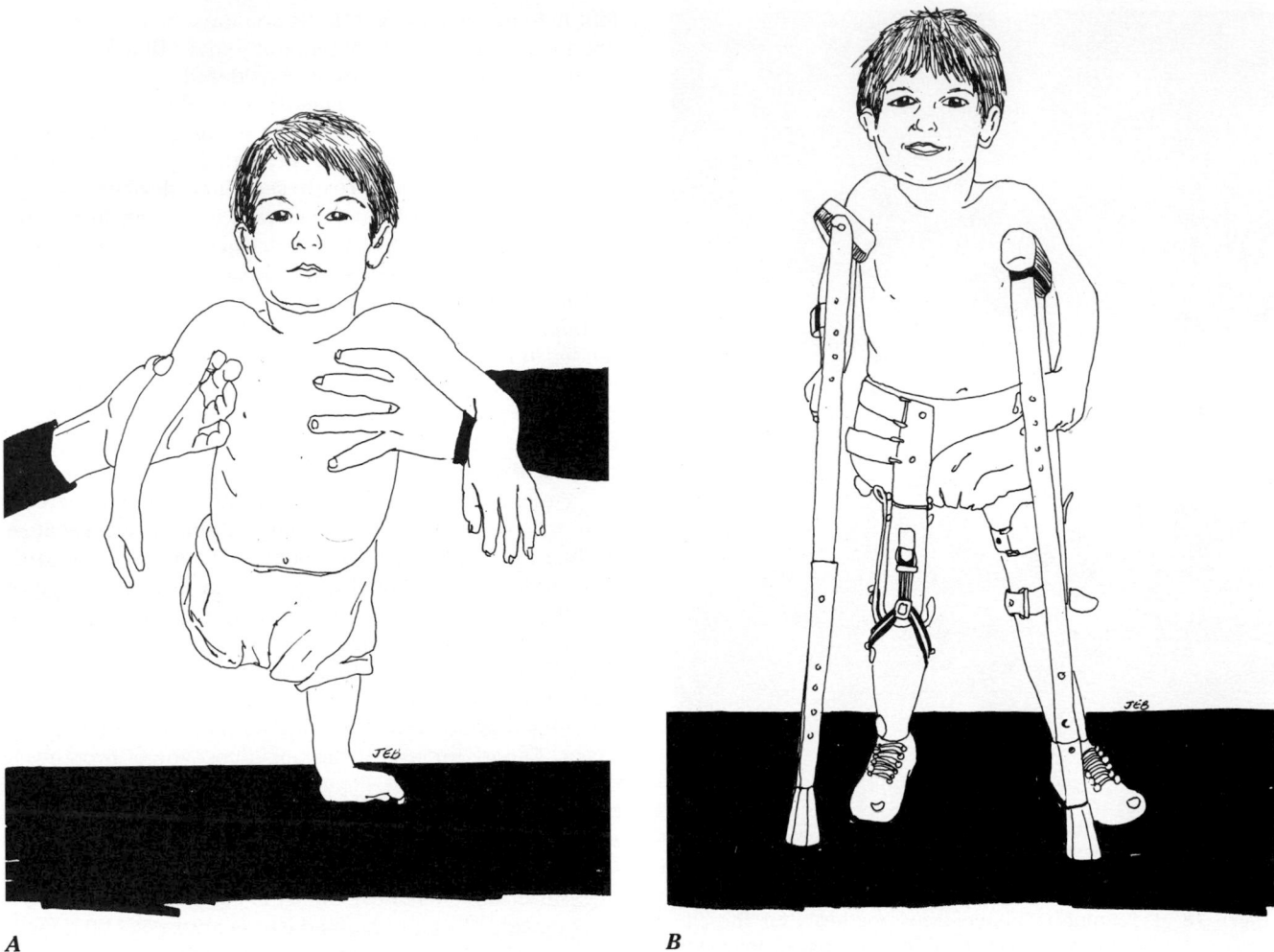

A   *B*

Figure 18-15 *A.* Patient with bilateral phocomelia. Typically one extremity is slightly longer than the other. *B.* Final prosthetic fitting, which may not be accomplished until school age (see text).

quired varieties. The humerus, fibula, and tibia are the bones most commonly requiring surgical revision.[74] Painful bursae may develop in association with bone overgrowth, especially over the fibular head or the tibial tubercle; this is exacerbated by a poorly fitting prosthesis. According to Lambert, the incidence of bursa formation is 8.4 percent.[72] Stump revisions, stump capping utilizing cartilage-cancellous bone grafting,[64] Silastic plugs,[74,145] skin traction, and skin grafting are all methods that can be used to correct this problem. Of these options, stump capping with an autogenous graft appears to be the method associated with the fewest revisions.[146,147] Additional problems which may require surgery include limb length inequalities, especially when the knees are at different levels;[134] contralateral epiphysiodesis may be required. Other surgical procedures may be required for tumor recurrence or release of contractures, as treatment for skin sloughing, for excision[148] or capping of neuromas,[149] or for migration of the posterior heel pad of a Syme amputation.[134,150]

Skin breakdown and infection may occur because of problems with prosthetic fit. The skin around an osteotomy site may be in close proximity to the pelvic band and be susceptible to breakdown. Skin lesions in a child with a neuropathy may go unreported.

Frazier has stated that phantom pain did not occur in congenital amputees or in those whose amputations were acquired under the age of 3 years;[151] others have stated that phantom pain occurred in up to 19 percent of congenital amputees.[152] This may be a gross underestimation, as phantom sensation has been reported in up to 100 percent of patients when they were carefully questioned and phantom pain was noted in the vast majority as well.[153] Preoperative pain, recurrent trauma,[154] and chemotherapy with agents that can cause peripheral neuropathies[155] are predisposing factors. Vincristine induces an axonal neuropathy affecting primarily pain and temperature fibers. Cisplatin neuropathy can cause damage to large proprioceptive fibers; it can affect the nerve roots and spinal cord and is associated with muscle cramping. Such neuropathies may also involve intact limbs and result in relatively unanticipated difficulties with ambulation and the use of walking aids. The mechanism of phantom pain re-

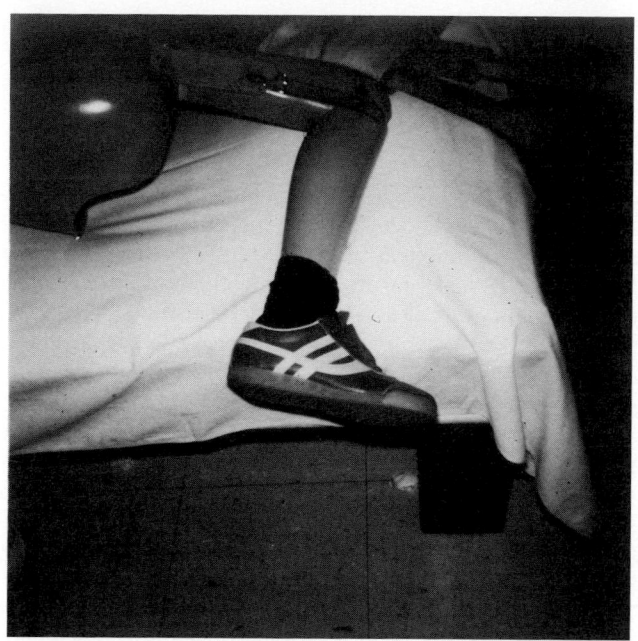
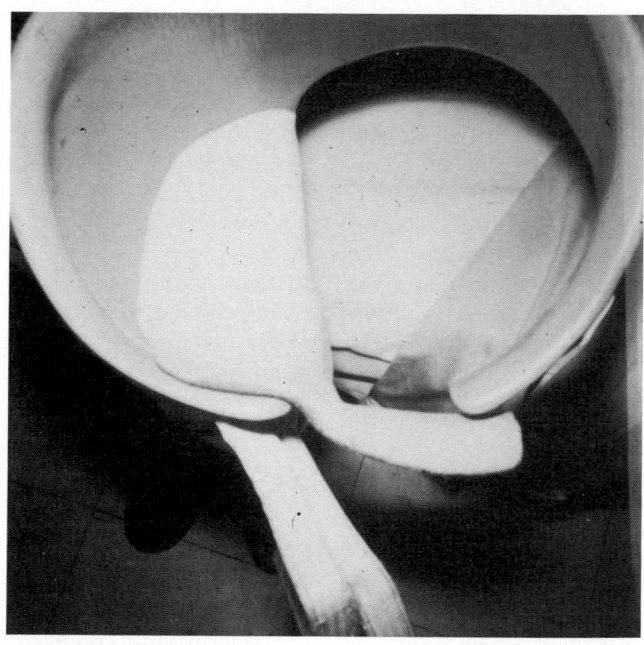

A   *B*

Figure 18-16 *A.* Typical Canadian bucket prosthesis used for patients with a hip disarticulation. *B.* The inside of the bucket must be well padded to protect the often tender surgical site and perineum.

mains unclear but may be associated with increased blood flow in the contralateral primary motor and somatosensory cortices due to altered inhibition of neurochemical transmitters; this suggests that treatment with GABAergic modulating agents may be of help in future treatment.[156] If pain does exist, it is amenable to treatment with transcutaneous nerve stimulation, light massage, and distractions such as play. The option of early prosthetic fitting is generally contraindicated in patients with malignancies who have been given previous chemotherapy with poor tissue healing and a sometimes inconsistent sensory examination. The more invasive treatments of anesthetic nerve blocks, acupuncture, and/or surgical lesioning of the dorsal roots are generally not required in children.

Certain problems are intrinsic to the upper extremity amputee. The intimacy of socket fitting with a myoelectric prosthesis may result in pseudoatrophy of residual muscle groups.[157] Up to a 57 percent reduction in residual limb length may interfere with prosthetic purchase. Perceptual deficits may also be encountered; male children with the less commonly seen right-sided deficiencies have seven times the incidence of learning disabilities when compared to those with left-sided deficits.[158] Children with upper extremity defects may also overestimate the length of their residual limbs, resulting in perceptual errors and attendant functional difficulties.[159] Errors of up to 20 percent may be made in reaching for objects. Therefore, it is essential that a good developmental and school history be obtained in this population, testing performed when indicated, and adaptive strategies initiated when the need is demonstrated.

Up to one-third of adolescent patients with below-knee amputations may develop genu valgum, patella alta,

and patella dislocation.[160] In such patients, the patellar apprehension test is positive and there is pain evoked with knee extension. Patients may need to refrain from strenuous activities. X-ray studies to determine the ratio of patellar height to tendon length, which is normally 1.0, are helpful in identifying this condition. Prosthetic modifications advised include increasing the size of the patellar tendon bar to distribute pressure over a larger area and applying a pad over the anterior tibial crest. For children with associated ligamentous laxity, a more conventional type of device with a thigh cuff may be required. If pain persists despite modifications, lateral release and medial plication of the patella may be indicated.[161]

Prolonged fabrication time and financial problems are significant obstacles that may cause emotional distress for the family.[68]

Emotional problems may arise in the parents of the amputee because of their unwarranted feelings of guilt or their mourning of their anticipated "perfect" child. Children who have acquired deficiencies and/or require surgical revision may experience depression over their loss, changes in body image, perceived social and physical inadequacies, and frequent hospitalizations. When a malignancy occurs, the concern over the side effects of chemotherapy and the fear of death compound the problem.[162]

Psychological support should be anticipatory and occur preoperatively. Intervention should not wait for the symptoms of acting out, depression, or withdrawal to occur. The child's fantasy of being provided with a "bionic" arm or leg must be gently replaced with realistic expectations. Projective play techniques, such as figure drawings or the use of specially made amputee dolls, may be helpful. For older children, prosthetic models and an amputee visitor program may be helpful.[68] Social support is the strongest determinant in avoiding depression, anxiety, and loss of self-esteem, and all efforts to provide same should be made by the treatment team.[163]

Despite the difficulties, the expectations for juvenile amputees are promising if they have had adequate social interaction and education.[21] Cognitive studies have shown them to function at or above the 50th percentile on the average.[164] A Danish study of 74 patients with lower extremity amputations in childhood showed that their marital status and number of children did not deviate from the norm.[148] One-third required assistance, but two-thirds were independent.

ALTERNATIVE TREATMENT TO AMPUTATION

Multiple infectious agents may produce sepsis, shock, and disseminated intravascular coagulopathy with loss of digits or extremities in a child or adult. Treatment of these ischemic changes in a child with meningococcemia with continuous caudal anesthesia has been reported.[165]

The use of a bone graft or an intramedullary rod for the treatment of congenital pseudoarthrosis of the tibia associated with neurofibromatosis and Ehlers-Danlos syndrome may obviate the need for amputation.[166]

With advancements in microsurgical techniques, limb salvage or reimplantation procedures following trauma with restoration of neurovascular, bony, and skin integrity are possible options—for example, in injuries that occur when children use lawn mowers.[167] Once circulation is restored, open reduction, internal fixation, as well as free flap and skin grafting procedures are generally required. With less severe injuries, hospitalization averages 15 weeks, but in more severe cases, up to 30 to 34 weeks of hospitalization may occur. Criteria for poor prognosis include skeletal/soft tissue injury, limb ischemia, shock, and age of under 2 years.[168] Complications include limb-length discrepancies in 50 to 70 percent of cases in patients aged up to 14 years associated with peripheral neuropathies due to crush injuries, nonunions, and the increased risk of thrombosis and septicemia.[169,170] Obviously rehabilitation may be prolonged.

Increased survival of patients with osteogenic sarcoma and soft tissue sarcomas of 66 to 80 percent at 5 years[171,172] has been related to a better definition through imaging studies of surgical margins and control of distant metastases in advance of limb amputation with chemotherapy.[173] Initiation of chemotherapy prior to definitive surgery often allows for tumor shrinkage and technically permits wide resection to be performed in the child who has a low-grade or well-localized malignancy without involvement of the neurovascular bundle and in whom growth is relatively complete.[174] It does not appear that these children have an increased rate of distant metastases or mortality.[174–176]

For a malignancy of the humerus, an en bloc or Tikhoff-Lindberg resection can be performed, leaving a flail upper arm with a functional forearm.[174] For femoral involvement, an en bloc resection can be performed with surgical conversion of the foreleg and the foot, so that a below-knee type of stump can be created, similar to the Van Nes rotationplasty.

Either allografts or custom-made endoprostheses, including ones that are capable of being lengthened and suitable for growing children, can be inserted after an en bloc resection.[177a] Complications include mechanical failure of the endoprosthesis, local recurrence of tumor, and infection, with an overall complication rate of 36 percent.[178] Postoperative precautions are similar to those observed after total joint replacement. Continuous passive range-of-motion exercise is often indicated several days postoperatively to facilitate knee flexion. Muscle groups or the pe-roneal nerve may need to be sacrificed and a knee-ankle-foot orthosis required for a variable period. In a study of 17 children followed for a period of 2 1/2 years following endoprosthetic replacement of the lower extremity, 7 patients did not require orthotics, crutches, or canes. The remainder of patients required a walking aid and/or knee orthosis and a shoe lift to compensate for leg-length discrepancy.[179] The psychological advantages of retaining one's own limb are clear, but advantages in terms of functional status and energy expenditure are less clear. Regardless of the above options, standard amputation surgery for children with osteogenic sarcoma may still be necessary in about 19 percent of cases.[178]

Regardless of the extent of amputation or alternative surgical procedure performed, an understanding of a child's need for exploration of his or her environment with the fewest possible imposed restrictions forms the basic principle of treatment. Prosthetic prescriptions and subsequent training must always be based on this principle so that a physically able and emotionally healthy adult may emerge.

REFERENCES

1. American Academy of Orthopaedic Surgeons: *Atlas of Limb Prosthetics: Surgical, Prosthetic and Rehabilitation Principles*, 2d ed. St Louis, Mosby–Year Book, 1992.
2. Malone JM, Moore WS, Goldstone J, Sandee JM: Therapeutic and economic impact of a modern amputation program. *Ann Surg* 189:798–802, 1979.
3. Porter JM, Baur GM, Taylor LM: Lower-extremity amputations for ischemia. *Arch Surg* 116:89–92, 1981.
4. Kostuik JP (ed) *Amputation Surgery and Rehabilitation. The Toronto Experience.* New York, Churchill Livingston, 1981.
5. Malone JM, Moore WS, Leal JM, Sandee JC: Rehabilitation for lower extremity amputation. *Arch Surg* 116:93–98, 1981.
6. Burgess EM, Matsen FA: Current concepts review: Determining amputation levels in peripheral vascular disease. *J Bone Joint Surg (Am)* 63A:1493–1497, 1981.
7. Moore WS: Determination of amputation level. *Arch Surg* 107:798, 1973.
8. Finch DRA, MacDougal M, Tibbs DJ, et al: Amputation for vascular disease: The experience of a peripheral vascular unit. *Br J Surg* 67:233–237, 1980.
9. Burgess EM, Zettl JH: Immediate postsurgical prosthetics. *Orthop Prosthet* 21:105–112, 1967.

9a. Burgess EM: Wound healing after amputation: effect of Controlled Environment Treatment. *J Bone Joint Surg (Am)* 60A:245–246, 1978.

9b. Kegel B: Controlled Environment Treatment (CET) for patients with below-knee amputations. *Phys Ther* 56:1366–1371, 1976.

10. Friedmann LW: *The Surgical Rehabilitation of the Amputee.* Springfield, IL: Charles C Thomas, 1978.

11. Potts JR, Wendelken JR, Elkins RC, Peytom MD: Lower extremity amputation: Review of 110 cases. *Am J Surg* 138:924–928, 1979.

11a. Harris RI: Amputations. *J Bone Surg (Am)* 26:626–634, 1944.

12. Syme J: Amputation at the ankle joint. *Month J Med Sci* 2:93, 1843.

12a. Matsen FA, Bach AW, Wyss CR, Simmons CW: Transcutaneous P_{O_2}: A potential monitor of the status of replanted limb parts. *Plast Reconstr Surg* 65:732–737, 1980.

13. Burgess EM, Matsen FA, Wyss CR, Simmons CW: Segmental transcutaneous measurements of PO_2 in patients requiring below-knee amputations for peripheral vascular insufficiency. *J Bone Joint Surg (Am)* 64A:378–382, 1982.

14. Holloway GA Jr, Burgess EM: Cutaneous blood flow and its relation to healing of below knee amputation. *Surg Gynecol Obstet* 146:750–756, 1978.

15. Holloway GA Jr, Watkins DW: Laser Doppler measurement of cutaneous blood flow. *J Invest Dermatol* 69:306–309, 1977.

16. Kostuik JP, Wood D, Hornby R, et al: The measurement of skin blood flow in peripheral vascular disease by epicutaneous application of xenon 133. *J Bone Joint Surg (Am)* 58A:833–837, 1976.

17. Lassen NA, Holstein P: Use of radio isotopes in assessment of distal blood flow and distal blood pressure in arterial insufficiency. *Surg Clin North Am* 54:39–55, 1974.

18. Boone DA, Harlan J, Burgess EM: Automated fabrication of mobility aids: Review of the AFMA process and VA/Seattle ShapeMaker design. *J Rehabil Res Dev* 31:42–49, 1994.

19. Schuch CM, Pritham CH: International Standards Organization terminology: Application to prosthetics and orthotics. *JPO* 6:29–33, 1994.

20. Banerjee SN (ed): *Rehabilitation Management of Amputees.* Baltimore, Williams & Wilkins, 1982.

21. Lambert CN, Hamilton RC, Pellicore RJ: The juvenile amputee program: Its social and economic value. *J Bone Joint Surg* 51A:1135–1138, 1969.

22. Krebs DE, Fishman S: Characteristics of the child amputee population. *J Pediatr Orthop* 4:89–95, 1984.

23. Jones LE: The free limb scheme and the limb-deficient child in Australia. *Aust Paediatr J* 24:290–294, 1988.

24. Heinonen OP: Malformations of the musculoskeletal system, in Heinonen, OP et al (eds): *Birth Defects and Drugs in Pregnancy.* Littleton, MA, Publishing Sciences Group, 1977, pp 126–148.

25. Kallen B, Rahmani TM, Winberg J: Infants with congenital limb reduction registered in the Swedish register of congenital malformations. *Teratology* 29:73–85, 1984.

26. Aitken GT: Surgical amputations in children. *J Bone Joint Surg* 45A:1735–1741, 1963.

27. Shurr DG, Cooper RR, Buckwalter JA, Blair WF: Terminal transverse congenital deficiency of the forearm. *Prosthet Orthot Int* 35:22–25, 1981.

28. Corballis MC, Morgan MJ: On the biological basis of human laterality: 1. Evidence for a maturational left-right gradient. *Behav Brain Sci* 2:261–336, 1978.

29. Blechschmidt E: The early stages of human limb development, in Swinyard CA (ed): *Limb Development and Deformity: Problems of Evaluation and Rehabilitation.* Springfield, IL, Thomas, 1969, pp 24–56.

30. Swanson AB: Congenital limb defects: Classification and treatment. *Clin Symp* 33:3–32, 1981.

31. Fletcher I: Review of the treatment of thalidomide children with limb deficiency in Great Britain. *Clin Orthop* 148:18–25, 1980.

32. Mc Credie J, North K, De Longh B: Thalidomide deformities and their nerve supply. *J Anat* 139:397–410, 1984.

33. Pollack ED, Maheras-Rarick NM: Differential limb regeneration in diploid and triploid Rana pipiens larvae with reference to spinal motor neuron development. *J Exp Zool* 254:276–285, 1990.

34. Williamson DAJ: A syndrome of congenital malformations possibly due to maternal diabetes. *Dev Med Child Neurol* 12:145–152, 1970.

35. Askins G, Ger E: Congenital constriction band syndrome. *J Pediatr Orthop* 8:461–466, 1988.

36. Cohen MM: Syndromology: an updated conceptual view: VIII. Deformations and disruptions. *Int J Oral Maxillofac Surg* 19:33–37, 1990.

37. Kennedy LA, Persaud TVN: Pathogenesis of developmental defects induced in the rat by amniotic sac rupture. *Acta Anat* 97:23, 1977.

38. Lubinsky M, Sujansky E, Sanger W: Familial amniotic bands. *Am J Med Genet* 14:81–87, 1983.

39. Hoyme HE, Jones KL, Van Allen MI: Vascular pathogenesis of transverse limb reduction deficits. *J Pediatr* 101:839–843, 1982.

40. Soltan HC, Holmes LB: Familial occurrence of malformations possibly attributable to vascular abnormalities. *J Pediatr* 108:112–114, 1986.

41. Janerich DT, Piper JM, Glebatis DM: Congenital limb-reduction defects. *N Engl J Med* 291:697–700, 1974.

42. Heinonen OP: Antinauseants, antihistamines, and phenothiazines, in Heinonen OP et al (eds). *Birth Defects and Drugs in Pregnancy.* Littleton, MA, Publishing Sciences Group, 1977, pp 322–334.

43. Cohlan SQ: A review of teratogenic agents and human congenital malformations, in Swinyard CA (ed): *Limb Development and Deformity: Problems of Evaluation and Rehabilitation.* Springfield, IL, Thomas, 1969, pp 161–170.

44. Aro T: Maternal diseases, alcohol consumption and smoking during pregnancy associated with reduction limb defects. *Early Hum Dev* 9:49–57, 1983.

45. Altura BM, Altura BT, Carella E: Alcohol produces spasms of human umbilical blood vessels: Relationship to fetal alcohol syndrome. *Eur J Pharmacol* 86:311–312, 1983.

46. Blakeslee B (ed): *The Limb Deficient Child.* Berkeley and Los Angeles, University of California Press, 1963.

47. Galway HR: Traumatic amputations in children, in Kostuik JP, Gillespie R (eds): *Amputation Surgery and Rehabilitation: The Toronto Experience.* New York, Churchill Livingstone, 1981, pp 137–143.

48. Cumming V, Molnar G: Traumatic amputations in children resulting from "train-electric-burn" injuries: A social environmental syndrome? *Arch Phys Med Rehabil* 55:71–73, 1974.

49. Thompson GH, Balourdas GM, Marcus RE: Railyard amputations in children. *J Pediatr Orthop* 3:443–448, 1983.

50. Letts RM, Gammon W: Auger injuries in children. *Can Med Assoc J* 118:520–522, 1978.

51. Rahak JJ, McMahon GE, Weinstein L: Thrombocytopenia and symmetrical peripheral gangrene associated with staphylococcal and streptococcal bacteremia. *Ann Intern Med* 69:35–43, 1968.

52. Bettigole RE: Symmetric peripheral gangrene in pneumococcal sepsis. *Ann Intern Med* 54:335–342, 1961.

53. Stossel TP, Levy R: Intravascular coagulation associated with pneumococcal bacteremia and symmetrical peripheral gangrene. *Arch Intern Med* 125:876–878, 1970.

54. Reinstein L, Govindon S: Extremity amputation: Disseminated intravascular coagulation syndrome. *Arch Phys Med Rehabil* 61:97–102, 1980.

55. Bogumill GB: Bilateral above-the-knee amputations: A complication of chickenpox. *J Bone Joint Surg* 47A:371–374, 1965.

56. Aitken GT: Amputation as a treatment for certain lower-extremity congenital abnormalities. *J Bone Joint Surg* 41A:1267–1285, 1959.

57. Horowitz IN, Galvis AG, Gompertz ED: Arterial thrombosis and protein S deficiency. *J Pediatr* 1212:934–937, 1992.

58. Burtch RL: Nomenclature for congenital skeletal limb deficiencies, a revision of the Frantz and O'Rahilly classification. *Artif Limbs* 10:24–34, 1966.

59. Frantz CH, O'Rahilly R: Congenital skeletal limb deficiencies. *J Bone Joint Surg* 43A:1202–1224, 1961.

60. Swanson AB: A classification for congenital limb malformations. *J Hand Surg* 1:8–22, 1976.

61. Kay HW, Day HJB, Henkel HL, et al: The proposed international terminology for the classification of congenital limb deficiencies. *Dev Med Child Neurol* 34:1–12, 1975.

62. Powers TA, Haher TR, Devlin VJ, et al: Abnormalities of the spine in relation to congenital upper limb deficiencies. *J Pediatr Orthop* 3:471–474, 1983.

63. Lenz W: Genetics and limb deficiencies. *Clin Orthop* 148:9–17, 1980.

64. Marquardt EG: A holistic approach to the limb-deficient child. *Arch Plys Med Rehabil* 64:237–248, 1983.

65. Rosenfelder R: Infant amputees: Early growth and care. *Clin Orthop* 148:41–46, 1980.

66. Rossi TV, Kruger L: Proximal femoral focal deficiency and its treatment. *Orthot Prosthet* 29:37–57, 1975.

67. Aitken GT, Frantz CH: The child amputee. *J Bone Joint Surg* 35A:659–664, 1953.

68. Pritchard DJ: Factors that influence rehabilitation of children who undergo amputation for bone and soft tissue sarcomas: The surgeon's viewpoint. *Natl Cancer Inst Monogr* 56:133–135, 1981.

69. Taylor HL, Henschel A, Brozek J, Key A: Effects of bed-rest on cardiovascular function and work performance. *J Appl Physiol* 2:223–239, 1949.

70. Griffith ER: Rehabilitation of children with bone and soft tissue sarcomas: A physiatrist's viewpoint. *Natl Cancer Inst Monogr* 56:137–143, 1981.

71. Fowler WM, Linde LM, Brooks MB, Jones MH: Pulmonary function and physical work capacity of children who have undergone amputation of an upper extremity. *Arch Phys Med Rehabil* 43:409–413, 1962.

72. Lambert CN: Amputation surgery and the child. *Orthop Clin North Am* 3:473–482, 1972.

73. Romano R, Burgess E: The immediate postsurgical prosthetic fitting technique applied to child amputees. *Interclin Info Bull* 9:1–10, 1970.

74. Shurr DG, Cooper RR, Buckwalter JA, Blair WF: Juvenile amputees: Classification and revision rates. *Orthot Prosthet* 36:22–28, 1982.

75. Rosen G, Caparros B, Huvos AG, et al: Preoperative chemotherapy for osteogenic sarcoma: Selection of postoperative adjuvant chemotherapy based on the response of the primary tumor to preoperative chemotherapy. *Cancer* 49:1221–1230, 1982.

76. Wilbur JR, Sutow WW, Sullivan MP, Gottlieb JA: Chemotherapy of sarcomas. *Cancer* 36:765–769, 1975.

77. Pratt CB, Ranson JL, Evans WE: Age-related cardiotoxicity in children. *Cancer Treat Rep* 62:1381–1385, 1978.

78. Von Hoff DD, Layard MW, Basa P, et al: Risk-factors for doxorubicin-induced congestive heart failure. *Ann Intern Med* 91:710–717, 1979.

79. Fritsch G, Urban C: Transient encephalopathy during the late course of treatment with high-dose methotrexate. *Cancer* 53:1849–1851, 1984.

80. Nesbit M, Krivit W, Heyn R, Sharp H: Acute and chronic effects of methotrexate on hepatic, pulmonary, and skeletal systems. *Cancer* 37:1048–1054, 1976.

81. Tefft M, Lattin PB, Jereb B, et al: Acute and late effects on normal tissue following combined chemo- and radio-therapy for childhood rhabdomyosarcoma and Ewing's sarcoma. *Cancer* 37:1201–1213, 1976.

82. Ryan JR, Emami A: Vincristine neurotoxicity with residual equinocavus deformity in children with acute leukemia. *Cancer* 51:423–425, 1983.

83. Hansson J: Leg amputee: Clinical follow-up study. *Acta Orthop Scand* 69(suppl):1–116, 1964.

84. Clark SD, Patton JG: Occupational therapy for the limb-deficient child. *Clin Orthop* 148:47–54, 1980.

85. Shaperman J, Sumida CT: Recent advances in research in prosthetics for children. *Clin Orthop* 148:26–33, 1980.

86. Hodgins J, Sullivan R, Jain S: A modular below elbow prosthesis for children. *Orthot Prosthet* 36:15–21, 1982.

87. Marquardt E: The operative treatment of congenital limb malformation—part I. *Prosthet Orthot Int* 4:135–144, 1980.

88. Smith RJ, Lipke RW: Treatment of congenital deformities of the hand, part I. *New Engl J Med* 300:344–349, 1979.

89. Ogden JA, Watson HK, Bohne W: Ulnar dysmelia. *J Bone Joint Surg* 58A:467–475, 1976.

90. *Child Amputee Prosthetics Project: Ten Year Report 1967–1977, Research and Development Program.* U.S. Department of Health, Education and Welfare, 1977.

92. Jain S: Rehabilitation in limb deficiency: 2. The pediatric amputee. *Arch Phys Med Rehabil* 77:S9–S13, 1996.

93. Molnar GE, Taft LT: Pediatric rehabilitation part II: Spina bifida and limb deficiencies. *Curr Probl Pediatr* 7:35–54, 1977.

94. Di Cowden MA, Ballard A, Robinette H: Benefit of early fitting and behavior modification training with a voluntary-closing terminal device. *J Assoc Child Prosthet Orthot Clin* 22:47–50, 1987.

95. Crandall R, Hansen D: Clinical evaluation of a voluntary-closing terminal device. *J Assoc Child Prosthet Orthot Clin* 24:70, 1989.

96. Shaperman J, Setoguichi Y: The CAPP terminal device, size 2: A new alternative for adolescents and adults. *Prosthet Orthot Int* 13:25–28, 1989.

97. Downie GR: Limb deficiencies and prosthetic devices. *Orthop Clin North Am* 7:465–473, 1976.

98. Edelstein JE, Berger N, Fishman S: ISNY sockets for upper-limb prostheses. *J Assoc Child Prosthet Orthot Clin* 22:37, 1987.

99. Shaperman J: Learning patterns of young children with above-elbow prostheses. *Am J Occup Ther* 33:299–305, 1979.

100. Swanson AB, Swanson G: The Krukenberg procedure in the juvenile amputee. *Clin Orthop* 148:55–61, 1980.

101. Challenor YB, Rangaswamy L, Katz JF: Limb deficiency in infancy and childhood, in Downey JA, Low NL (eds): *The Child with Disabling Illness.* New York, Raven Press, 1982, pp 409–447.

102. Marquardt EG: The multiple limb-deficient child, in *Atlas of Limb Prosthetics: Surgical and Prosthetic Principles.* St. Louis, Mosby, American Academy of Orthopaedic Surgeons, 1981, pp 595–641.

103. Lamb DW, Scott H: Management of congenital and acquired amputation in children. *Orthop Clin North Am* 12:977–994, 1981.

104. Meredith JM, Uellendahl JE, Keagy RD: Successful voluntary grasp and release using the cookie crusher myoelectric hand in 2 year olds. *Am J Occup Ther* 47:825–829, 1993.

105. Sorbye R: Myoelectric prosthetic fitting in young children. *Clin Orthop* 148:34–40, 1980.

106. Kruger LM, Fishman S: Myoelectric and body-powered prostheses. *J Pediatr Orthop* 13:68–75, 1993.

107. Edelstein JE, Berger N: Performance comparison among children fitted with myoelectric and body-powered hands. *Arch Phys Med Rehabil* 74:376–380, 1993.

108. Thornby MA, Krebs DE: Bimanual skills development in pediatric below-elbow amputation: A multicentric cross-sectional survey. *Arch Phys Med Rehabil* 73:697–702, 1992.

109. Engsberg JR, Tedford KG, Harden JA: Center of mass location and segment angular orientation of below-knee amputee and able-bodied children during walking. *Arch Phys Med Rehabil* 73:1163–1168, 1992.

110. Herbert LM, Engsberg JR, Tedford KG, Grimston SK: A comparison of oxygen consumption during walking between children with and without below-knee amputations. *Phys Ther* 74:943–950, 1994.

111. Pullen JJ: A low-profile paediatric partial foot. *Prosthet Orthot Int* 11:137–138, 1987.

112. Engsberg JR, Tedford KG, Springer MJN, Harder JA: Weight distribution of below-knee child amputee and able-bodied children during standing. *Prosthet Orthot Int* 16:200–202, 1992.

113. Schneider K, Hart T, Zernicke RF, et al: Dynamics of below-knee child amputee gait: SACH foot versus FLEX foot. *J Biomech* 26:1191–1204, 1993.

114. Colborne GR, Naumann S, Eng P, et al: Analysis of mechanical and metabolic factors in the gait of congenital below-knee amputees. *Am J Phys Med Rehab* 71:272–278, 1992.

115. Burke MJ, Roman V, Wright V: Bone and joint changes in lower limb amputees. *Ann Rheum Dis* 37:252–254, 1978.

116. Farmer AW, Lavrin CA: Congenital absence of the fibula. *J Bone Joint Surg* 42A:1–12, 1960.

117. Madigan RR, Fillauer KD: 3-S prosthesis: A preliminary report. *J Pediatr Orthop* 11:112–117, 1991.

118. Damsin JP, Pous JG, Ghanem I: Therapeutic approach to severe lower limb length discrepancies: Surgical treatment versus prosthetic management. *J Pediatr Orthop* 4:164–170, 1995.

118a. Serafin J: A new operation for congenital absence of the fibula. *J Bone Joint Surg* 49B:59–65, 1967.

119. Thompson TC, Straub LR, Arnold WD: Congenital absence of the fibula. *J Bone Joint Surg* 39A:1229–1237, 1957.

120. Wood WL, Zlotsky N, Westin GW: Congenital absence of the fibula. *J Bone Joint Surg* 47A:1159–1169, 1965.

121. Westin GW, Sakai DN, Wood WL: Congenital longitudinal deficiency of the fibula. *J Bone Joint Surg* 58A:492–496, 1976.

122. Eilert RE, Jayakumar SS: Boyd and Syme ankle amputations in children. *J Bone Joint Surg* 58A:1138–1141, 1976.

123. Letts M, Vincent N: Congenital longitudinal deficiency of the fibula (fibular hemimelia). *Clin Orthop* 287:160–166, 1993.

124. Brown FW: Construction of a knee joint in congenital total absence of the tibia (paraxial hemimelia tibia). *J Bone Joint Surg* 47A:695–704, 1965.

125. Wehbe MA, Weinstein SL, Ponseti IV: Tibial agenesis. *J Pediatr Orthop* 1:395–399, 1981.

126. Epps CH, Tooms RE, Edholm CD, et al: Failure of centralization of the fibula for congenital longitudinal deficiency of the tibia. *J Bone Joint Surg* 73A:858–867, 1991.

127. Aronson J, Johnson E, Harp JH: Local bone transportation for treatment of intercalary defects by the Ilizarov technique. *Clin Orthop* 243:71–79, 1989.

128. Baumgartner RF: Above-knee amputation in children. *Prosthet Orthot Int* 3:26–30, 1979.

129. Cole WG: Prosthetic programme after above-knee amputation in children with sarcomata. *J Bone Joint Surg* 64B:586–589, 1982.

130. Kristinsson O: Flexible above knee socket made from low density polyethylene suspended by a weight transmitting frame. *Orthot Prosthet* 37:25–27, 1983.

131. *Child Amputee Prosthetics Project: Progress Report.* U.S. Department of Health, Education, and Welfare, 1980, pp 59–61.

132. Torode IP, Gillespie R: The classification and treatment of proximal femoral deficiencies. *Prosthet Orthot Int* 15:117–126, 1991.

133. Aitken GT: Proximal femoral focal deficiency, in Swinyard CA (ed): *Limb Development and Deformity: Problems of Evaluation and Rehabilitation.* Springfield, IL, Thomas, 1969, pp 456–476.

134. Anderson A, Westin GW, Oppenheim WL: Syme amputation in children: Indication, results, and long-term follow-up. *J Pediatr Orthop* 4:550–554, 1984.

135. Van Nes CP: Rotation-plasty for congenital defects of the femur. *J Bone Joint Surg* 32B:12–16, 1950.

136. Alman BA, Krajbich JI, Hubbard S: Proximal femoral focal deficiency: Results of rotationplasty and Syme amputation. *J Bone Joint Surg* 77A:1876–1882, 1995.

137. Tablada C: A technique for fitting converted proximal femoral focal deficiencies. *Artif Limbs* 15:27–45, 1971.

138. Bryant DD, Epps CH: Proximal femoral focal deficiency: Evaluation and management. *Orthopedics* 14:775–784, 1991.

139. Stoner EK: Management of the lower extremity amputee, in Kottke FJ, Stillwell GK, Lehmann JF (eds): *Krusen's Handbook of Physical Medicine and Rehabilitation.* Philadelphia, Saunders, 1982, p 924.

140. Clippinger FW, Seaber AV, McElhaney JH, et al: Afferent sensory feedback for lower extremity prostheses. *Clin Orthop* 169:202–205, 1982.

141. Sutherland DH: *Gait Disorders in Children and Adolescence.* Baltimore, Williams & Wilkins, 1984, pp 89–106.

142. Galway HR: Recreational activities of juvenile amputees, in Kostuik JP, Gillespie R (eds): *Amputation Surgery and Rehabilitation: The Toronto Experience.* New York, Churchill Livingstone, 1981, pp 211–216.

143. Zazula JL, Foulds RA: Mobility device for a child with phocomelia. *Arch Phys Med Rehabil* 64:137–139, 1983.

143a. Di Angelo DJ, Winter DA, Ghista DN: Performance assessment of the Terry Fox jogging prosthesis for above-knee amputees. *J Biomech* 22:543–558, 1989.

144. Speer DP: Pathogenesis of amputation stump-overgrowth. *Clin Orthop* 159:294–307, 1981.

145. Swanson AB: Silicone-rubber implants to control the overgrowth phenomenon in the juvenile amputee. *Interclin Info Bull* 11:5–8, 1972.

146. Davids JR, Meyer LC, Blackhurst DW: Operative treatment of bone overgrowth in children who have an acquired or congenital amputation. *J Bone Joint Surg* 77A:1490–1497, 1995.

147. Benevenia J, Makley JT, Leeson MC, Benevenia K: Primary epiphyseal transplants and bone overgrowth in childhood amputations. *J Pediatr Orthop* 12:746–750, 1992.

148. Jorring K: Amputation in children: A follow-up of 74 children whose lower extremities were amputated. *Acta Orthop Scand* 42:178–186, 1971.

149. Swanson AB, Boeve NR, Lumsden RM: The prevention and treatment of amputation neuromata by silicone capping. *J Hand Surg* 20:70–78, 1977.

150. Davidson WH, Bohne WHO: The Syme amputation in children. *J Bone Joint Surg* 57A:905–909, 1975.

151. Frazier SH, Kolb LC: Psychiatric aspects of pain and the phantom limb. *Orthop Clin North Am* 1:481–495, 1970.

152. Weinstein S, Sersen EA: Phantoms in case of congenital absence of limbs. *Neurology* 11:909–911, 1961.

153. Krane EJ, Heller LB: The prevalence of phantom sensation and pain in pediatric amputees. *J Pain Sympt Mgt* 10:21–29, 1995.

154. Saadeh ES, Melzack R: Phantom limb experiences in congenital limb deficient adults. *Cortex* 30:479–485, 1994.

155. Smith J, Thompson JM: Phantom limb pain and chemotherapy in pediatric amputees. *Mayo Clin Proc* 70:357–364, 1995.

156. Kew JJM, Ridding MC, Rothwell JC, et al: Reorganization of cortical blood flow and transcranial magnetic stimulation maps in human subjects. *J Neurophysiol* 72:2517–2524, 1994.

157. Weaver SA, Lange LR, Vogts VM: Comparison of myoelectric and conventional prostheses for adolescent amputees. *Am J Occup Ther* 42:87–91, 1989.

158. Dlugosz LJ, Byers T, Msall ME: Relationship between laterality of congenital upper extremity reduction defects and school performance. *Clin Pediatr* 27:319–324, 1988.

159. Mc Donnell PM, Scott RN, Dickison J: Do artificial limbs become part of the user? New evidence. *Rehabil Res Dev* 26:17–24, 1989.

160. Mowery CA, Herring JA, Jackson D: Dislocated patella associated with below-knee amputation in adolescent patients. *J Pediatr Orthop* 6:299–301, 1986.

161. Mc Ivor B, Gillespie R: Patellar instability in juvenile amputees. *J Pediatr Orthop* 7:553–556, 1987.

162. Voute PA, Burgers JMV, Van Patten WJ, Van Dobbenburght OA: Amputations in children: Clinical indications and psychological implications. *Arch Chir Neerland* 25:427–433, 1973.

163. Varni JW, Setoguichi Y, Rappaport LR, Talbot D: Psychological adjustment and perceived social support in children with congenital/acquired limb deficiencies. *J Behav Med* 15:31–44, 1992.

164. Clark S, French R: Can congenital amputees achieve academically? *Am Correct Ther J* 32:7–11, 1978.

165. Tobias JD, Haun SE, Helfaer M: Use of continuous caudal block to relieve lower extremity ischemia caused by vasculitis in a child with meningococcemia. *J Pediatr* 115:1019–1021, 1989.

166. Anderson DJ, Schoenecker PL, Sheridan JJ, Rich MM: Use of intramedullary rod treatment of congenital pseudoarthrosis of the tibia. *J Bone Joint Surg* 74A:161–168, 1992.

167. Love SM, Grogan DP, Ogden JA: Lawn-mower injuries in children. *J Orthop Trauma* 2:94–101, 1988.

168. Helfet DL, Howey T, Sanders R, Johansen K: Limb salvage versus amputation. *Clin Orthop* 256:80–86, 1990.

169. O'Brien B, Franklin JD, Morrison WA, MacLeod AM: Replantation and revascularization surgery in children. *Hand* 12:12–24, 1980.

170. Rich RH, Knight PJ, Erickson DL, et al: Replantation of the upper extremity in children. *J Pediatr Surg* 12:1028–1032, 1977.

171. Meskens M, Burssens A, Hoogmartens M, Fabry G: Osteogenic sarcoma in children: A retrospective study of 58 cases. *Acta Orthop Belg* 59:64–68, 1993.

172. Serpell JW, Ball ABS, Robinson MH, et al: Factors influencing local recurrence and survival in patients with soft tissue sarcoma of the upper limb. *Br J Surg* 78:1368–1372.

173. Picci PM, Sangiorgi L, Rougraff BT, et al: Relationship of chemotherapy-induced necrosis and surgical margins to local recurrence in osteosarcoma. *J Clin Oncol* 12:2699–2705, 1994.

174. Rao BN, Champion JE, Pratt OB, et al: Limb salvage procedures for children with osteosarcoma: An alternative to amputation. *J Pediatr Surg* 18:901–908, 1983.

175. Marcove RC: En bloc resection for osteogenic sarcoma. *Cancer Treat Rep* 62:225–231, 1978.

176. Cara JA, Canadell J: Limb salvage for malignant bone tumors in young children. *J Pediatr Orthop* 14:112–118, 1994.

177. de Bari A, Krajbich JI, Langer F, et al: Modified Van Nes rotationplasty for osteosarcoma of the proximal tibia in children. *J Bone Joint Surg* 72B:1065–1069, 1990.

177a. Imbriglia JE, Neer CS, Dick HM: Resection of the proximal one-half of the humerus in a child for chondrosarcoma. *J Bone Joint Surg* 60A:262–264, 1978.

178. Eckardt JJ, Eilber FR, Rosen G, et al: Endoprosthetic replacement for stage IIB osteosarcoma. *Clin Orthop* 270:202–213, 1991.

179. Frieden RA, Ryniker D, Kenan S: Assessment of patient function after limb-sparing surgery. *Arch Phys Med Rehabil* 71:759, 1990.

Goddard NJ, Hashemi-Nejad A, Fixsen JA: Natural history and treatment of instability of the hip in proximal femoral focal deficiency. *J Pediatr Orthop* 4:145–149, 1995.

PART III

Orthopaedic Trauma

PART III

General Complications and Principles of Treatment

CHAPTER 19

Emergency Treatment of the Trauma Patient

Evan R. Geller

No patient ever died of a broken bone. The fact remains, however, that trauma is the leading cause of death between 1 and 40 years of age.[1] While the expert and expeditious care of orthopaedic trauma directly bears upon the patient's morbidity and eventual functional recovery, the question of patient survival must be addressed prior to any orthopaedic consideration. Often, orthopaedic evaluation and management may occur simultaneously with general surgical evaluation and resuscitation. Indeed, in some instances the emergent intervention of the orthopaedist may be necessary for the successful resuscitation of the severely injured patient. As a rule, however, the initial evaluation and resuscitation of the seriously injured patient must take precedence over all else. It is always in the best interest of both the patient and the consulting orthopaedist that complete general surgical evaluation and resuscitation by accomplished prior to embarking upon complex fracture evaluation and management. While there is no paucity of literature to support the notion that early fracture fixation significantly improves patient outcome, hard experience teaches each of us the price to be paid for the too hasty or overly ambitious orthopaedic intervention in the seriously injured patient.

While by no means a definitive work, this chapter seeks to outline for the consulting orthopaedist those considerations of highest priority for the initial treatment of the trauma victim. It serves well to consider the causes of death following injury. Trunkey described the classic trimodal distribution of patient demise following trauma.[2] A large percentage of patients suffering life-threatening injury will succumb within minutes of their traumatic insult. These patients, having suffered brainstem lacerations, ventricular disruptions, and similar catastrophic injuries, will never become the concern of any physician other than the coroner. The second peak, however, represents the large number of patients who will present to the emergency department alive but have suffered life-threatening injury. During the "golden hour," the patient is steadily deteriorating at a greater or lesser rate. This deterioration is usually due to a developing state of shock from ongoing hemorrhage. Other injuries may also contribute to this deterioration, however, including closed head injury, pulmonary contusion or pneumothorax, or spinal cord injury. During this initial 60 min following injury, it is critical that every effort be expended in the zealous search for life-threatening injuries and in their aggressive treatment. When such a patient is appropriately managed by a skilled trauma team, the potential for survival and functional recovery from serious injury is high. Failure to utilize this initial time wisely inevitably leads to serious morbidity and often to avoidable mortality. This fact is reflected in the third peak of patient mortality seen weeks to months following injury. These patients are dying in the surgical intensive care unit of various multiple organ failure syndromes. Often, these late complications and deaths may be directly attributed to the patient's management during the initial several hours following injury. While these late postinjury deaths are often attributed to sepsis, in reality they reflect the ultimate failure of homeostasis due to overwhelming shock and metabolic insults following injury that were inexpertly diagnosed and inadequately treated. It may be appreciated, therefore, that the initial period of evaluation and treatment of the seriously injured patient is of the highest importance.

INITIAL EVALUATION AND RESUSCITATION

Immediately upon greeting the victim of serious trauma, the physician's primary goal is to ascertain rapidly the presence of life-threatening injury. Priority is given to those injuries that represent an immediate threat to survival. Hemorrhage, while the most common serious threat to the injured patient, rarely represents an immediate threat to life. Compensatory mechanisms allow the patient to sustain vital functions despite ongoing hemorrhage of over 30 percent of total blood volume. For this reason, bleeding infrequently poses an initial threat to the patient. Of immediate concern, however, are any injuries that compromise either the patient's airway or ability to breathe. Such injuries, if not immediately diagnosed and treated, will lead to the patient's demise during the initial minutes of resuscitation.

The first action of the treating physician, therefore, is to ascertain the patency of the patient's airway and the efficacy of air exchange. The most straightforward way of accomplishing this is to question the patient. A patient who is conversant is, by definition, possessed of a patent airway and provided with adequate air exchange. The presence of tachypnea, stridorous respirations, or cyanosis should prompt further investigation. Often, the cause of airway compromise is simply remedied by the clearance of secretions and broken teeth or dentures. Should such simple maneuvers fail, however, it may be necessary to control the airway definitively by endotracheal intubation. The placement of a surgical airway—i.e., cricothyroidotomy—is not indicated unless endotracheal intubation is impossible.

Special note must be made of two classes of trauma patients: those patients who present with a depressed mental status and those who are combative. Poorly responsive or comatose patients require definitive airway management on an urgent basis. Though oxygenation may be adequate early on, the patient's inability to protect his or her airway may lead to aspiration and asphyxiation. Any patient with a depressed mental status should be carefully monitored and consideration given to immediate intubation should this condition deteriorate. Comatose patients (Glasgow Coma Scale < 9) should be intubated for definitive airway management as early during resuscitation as possible.

Conversely, the trauma victim may present as combative and irrational. While at times such behavior may be secondary to intoxication, more frequently the patient will be responding to hypoxia. Attempts at sedation in this setting will only exacerbate the underlying respiratory compromise and may directly contribute to mortality. All combative and uncooperative patients should be carefully assessed for the possibility of hypoxia or shock and aggressive treatment, including the early provision of supplemental oxygen, should be begun. If necessary, early controlled intubation of such combative patients utilizing a rapid-sequence induction may facilitate patient evaluation and decrease mortality. It is necessary to keep in mind that breathing is composed of two functions: ventilation and oxygenation. Resolution of cyanosis and a high saturation on a pulse oximeter with the application of supplemental oxygen by mask is no assurance of adequate respiration. A poorly ventilating patient may develop hypercarbia unless attention is paid to the adequacy of air movement within the chest. Careful auscultation of the chest and observation for symmetry and adequacy of chest wall expansion are required. Diminished breath sounds, palpation of subcutaneous crepitus, or abnormal chest movement requires immediate investigation and treatment. Chest radiography is a necessary adjunct to this evaluation and may reveal the presence of otherwise unsuspected life-threatening chest injury. Often, simple chest tube insertion in a timely manner is sufficient to treat the condition.

The most dangerous period of resuscitation of the injured patient is immediately following intubation.[3] For multiple reasons, cardiac arrest most often occurs during the several minutes following intubation. Care must be taken to optimize the patient's status just prior to intubation. Intubation must be performed expertly by the most qualified individual available. Aggressive evaluation and resuscitation must continue during this period. The trauma patient should never be transported for radiologic studies or left unmonitored during the period immediately following intubation.

Once adequacy of both airway and breathing are determined, the treating physician begins the assessment for the presence of shock. Vital signs cannot be relied upon to make the diagnosis of shock. Shock is defined as inadequacy of perfusion, most often due to hemorrhage following injury. Multiple physiologic compensatory mechanisms serve to preserve blood pressure despite the loss of up to one-third of the patient's blood volume. Beyond this level of blood loss, however, the patient will deteriorate rapidly (Fig. 19-1). It is imperative, therefore, that the clinician recognize shock at its earliest stages. The patient may be quickly categorized as in mild, moderate, or severe shock by palpation of the extremity and pulse (Table 19-1). The presence of unexplained tachycardia and cool extremities is sufficient for the diagnosis of shock. Palpation of the radial artery assures a systolic blood pressure of greater than 80 torr and the classification of mild to moderate shock. Failure to palpate a peripheral pulse should prompt the clinician to immediately determine the presence of either a carotid or femoral pulse. Either of these palpable pulses represents a systolic pressure of at least 60 torr and a severe form of shock. Absent the ability to palpate a central pulse, the clinician must face the decision to begin cardiopulmonary resuscitation (CPR) or consider a diagnosis of death.

Upon diagnosing the presence of shock, the clinician immediately undertakes both presumptive treatment and an aggressive search for the cause of the shock state. Treatment involves the prompt placement of two large-

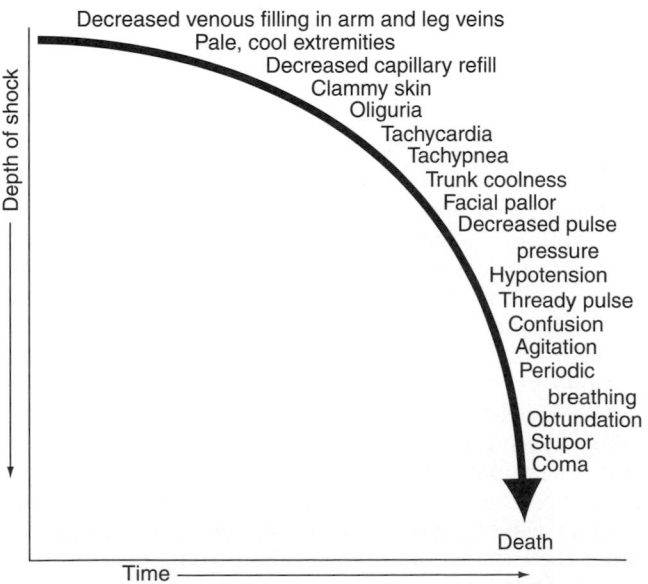

Figure 19-1 Differential diagnosis of shock.

Decreased venous filling in arm and leg veins
Pale, cool extremities
Decreased capillary refill
Clammy skin
Oliguria
Tachycardia
Tachypnea
Trunk coolness
Facial pallor
Decreased pulse pressure
Hypotension
Thready pulse
Confusion
Agitation
Periodic breathing
Obtundation
Stupor
Coma

Death

Depth of shock

Time

TABLE 19-1 Grading of Shock

| Degree of shock | Blood pressure, approx. | Pulse quality | Skin | | | Thirst | Mental state |
			Temperature	Color	Circulation, response to pressure blanching		
None	Normal	Normal	Normal	Normal	Normal	Normal	Clear and distressed
Slight	To 20% decrease	Normal	Cool	Pale	Definite slowing	Normal	Clear and distressed
Moderate	Decreased 20–40%	Definite decrease in volume	Cool	Pale	Definite slowing	Definite	Clear and some apathy unless stimulated
Severe	Decreased 40% to nonrecordable	Weak to imperceptible	Cold	Ashen to cyanotic (mottling)	Very sluggish	Severe	Apathetic to comatose; little distress except thirst

Source: Reproduced with permission from Beecher HK, Simeone FA, Burnett CH, et al: The internal state of the severely wounded man on entry to the most forward hospital. *Surgery* 22:672, 1947.

bore intravenous catheters and the rapid infusion of Ringer's lactate solution. The rationale for this approach lies in the fact that the vast majority of trauma victims will be suffering from hypovolemia as either the sole or a significant contributing cause of shock. In addition, aggressive volume infusion is an effective initial treatment for all other etiologies of shock, including neurogenic, cardiogenic, and cardiac compressive (tension pneumothorax or cardiac tamponade). Ringer's lactate solution has been repeatedly shown to be an effective resuscitative solution.[4] As volume resuscitation is undertaken, the patient's physiologic response is carefully monitored. One of three effects will be rapidly observed. The shock patient may rapidly improve with volume resuscitation, as evidenced by normalization of systolic blood pressure, pulse pressure, and pulse rate. At this point, it is important to slow the rate of infusion and carefully monitor the patient. If the patient remains hemodynamically stable, it may be deduced that he or she had suffered a significant but transient loss of blood volume with no significant active hemorrhage. If, however, the patient again deteriorates, the assumption is that there is an active hemorrhage. Volume infusion should be reinstituted and the source of hemorrhage aggressively sought. This critical diagnostic distinction can be made only by carefully monitoring the patient, with resuscitative infusions slowed. A common error is to assume that normalization of vital signs with resuscitation represents hemodynamic stability. A patient with active hemorrhage, receiving aggressive volume therapy, may well have a normal pulse and blood pressure. The inexperienced clinician may be lulled into a false sense of security, perhaps even allowing the patient to be transported

to radiology or the computed tomography (CT) suite for needed studies. In reality, however, the patient is receiving an exchange transfusion of salt water for blood. While the patient will appear stable for a period of time, the developing anemia will lead to sudden cardiac arrest despite the presence of a normal blood pressure—often on the CT table. Successful resuscitation from such an arrest is exceptionally uncommon.

The third possible response to aggressive volume resuscitation is no response at all. Should the patient fail to improve despite rapid volume infusion, the treating physician must carefully consider the differential diagnosis of persistent shock. This differential consists of either massive ongoing hemorrhage or cardiac compressive shock. Attention is immediately turned to examination of the patient's jugular veins (Fig. 19-2). Flat neck veins suggest massive volume loss, and treatment consists of additional volume therapy and rapid diagnosis of the source of bleeding. Distended neck veins, however, imply the presence of either tension pneumothorax or, less commonly, pericardial tamponade. Absent breath sounds on auscultation and deviation of the trachea confirm the presence of tension pneumothorax and require immediate pleural decompression. The presence of muffled heart tones implies pericardial tamponade (Table 19-2). Pericardiocentesis or immediate surgery is required for successful resuscitation. Either condition, however, may be initially treated with aggressive volume infusion. This treatment will afford additional time for definitive intervention.

From the foregoing, it is obvious that the physician treating the critically injured patient is most often challenged by the need to diagnose hemorrhagic shock rapidly.

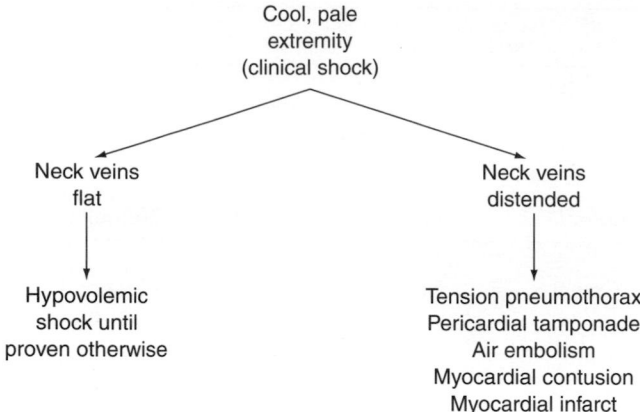

Figure 19-2 Progression of shock: circulation priorities.

The clinican must maintain a high degree of suspicion for the presence of ongoing blood loss. Once significant bleeding is suspected, its source must be aggressively sought. An initial survey for open wounds will reveal obvious sources of hemorrhage. Once identified, bleeding points are controlled with the application of direct pressure. Clamping of vessels or tourniquet application is to be avoided due to the high risk of complication. Scalp lacerations merit special consideration. Due to the rich vasculature deep to the galea, significant hemorrhage may occur. In the pediatric patient, this hemorrhage may become life-threatening. In addition, it is usually not possible to control bleeding from scalp lacerations effectively through any means short of suture closure. Therefore, repair should be undertaken early, preferably before allowing the patient to be transported out of the resuscitation suite. The clinician must also be wary of significant bleeding that may occur beneath the inflated pneumatic antishock garment. A common misconception is that this device is effective in achieving tamponade of bleeding from open extremity injuries. This is frequently not the case. This device is also ineffective as a splint for lower extremity fractures. Indeed, medical antishock trousers (MAST) are most effective in masking underlying significant injury from the attention of the treating physician. As such, the MAST should be removed as soon as aggressive volume resuscitation allows.

In addition to obvious sources of external bleeding, four potential compartments of occult hemorrhage must be considered. Each of these may be the site of fatal hem-

orrhage. The first occult compartment to consider is the thorax. Due to the compressibility of the lung, fatal exsanguination into either hemithorax is possible. Suspicion should prompt rapid portable chest radiography to determine the presence of significant hemothorax. Treatment is initially effected by placement of a chest tube with monitoring of output. Initial drainage of 1500 mL of blood or ongoing drainage of greater than 200 mL of blood per hour in the adult should prompt surgical intervention.

The second occult compartment for consideration is the peritoneal cavity. Physical examination is unreliable in determining the presence of potentially life-threatening hemorrhage in the abdominal cavity. The presence of unexplained shock, therefore, requires adjunctive diagnostic technique to evaluate the peritoneal cavity. In the hemodynamically stable patient, abdominal and pelvic CT scan with both oral and intravenous contrast is highly accurate in diagnosing significant hemorrhage. The ability of CT to detect and characterize injury to solid viscera (liver or spleen), as well as its sensitivity for the presence for significant quantities of intraperitoneal blood, make it an effective adjunct for diagnosis. Hemodynamic instability, or the ongoing need for significant volume infusion to maintain normal blood pressure, precludes transport of the patient to the CT suite. In this event, the patient should rapidly undergo diagnostic peritoneal lavage. This study is highly accurate when utilized to detect the presence of serious intraabdominal hemorrhage following blunt trauma. Standard criteria in this setting for positivity include the detection of greater than 100,000 red blood cells or 500 white blood cells per cubic milliliter of lavage fluid. A negative lavage or CT scan makes the presence of significant intraperitoneal hemorrhage most unlikely.

A negative lavage, however, will not rule out the possibility of retroperitoneal hemorrhage. Life-threatening retroperitoneal bleeding is most often seen in association with posterior pelvic ring disruptions or significant renal injury. It is mandatory, therefore, that patients who have sustained significant blunt force injury undergo pelvic radiography and urine examination for blood. Either of these studies, when positive, may lead the clinician to the diagnosis of potentially fatal retroperitoneal hemorrhage. When possible, CT scan will also make this diagnosis with a high degree of accuracy.

Even the most experienced and astute clinician may neglect to appropriately consider the final compartment of potential occult hemorrhage—the soft tissues. When there is no external hemorrhage, it is easy to overlook the cu-

TABLE 19-2 Differential Diagnosis of Cardiac Compressive Shock

	Trachea	Breath sounds	Heart sounds
Cardiac tamponade	Midline	Normal	Muffled
Tension pneumothorax	Deviated to side opposite pneumothorax	Absent on side of pneumothorax	Normal or quiet

mulative effect of multiple long bone fractures in the seriously traumatized patient. Adults as well as children may bleed to hypotension from a combination of multiple rib fractures and extremity injuries, even in the absence of vascular trauma or obvious hematoma formation. A careful skeletal examination may provide the answer for otherwise inexplicable hemorrhagic shock. Volume resuscitation and fracture immobilization as well as traction and early fixation will effectively reverse this form of shock when employed early.

Before leaving the topic of initial evaluation and resuscitation of the trauma patient, it should be noted that the patient is not in greatest danger upon arrival to the resuscitation room. While the patient may present in a hemodynamically compromised condition, almost every patient will improve with the initiation of therapy as described above. The risk of sudden deterioration and death, however, increases as the patient's compensatory physiology is affected by the clinician's efforts at diagnosis and treatment. The most clear-cut example of this is the fact that the most dangerous period during a trauma resuscitation is immediately following endotracheal intubation. Due to multiple factors (Table 19-3), the 5-min period following this maneuver is the most common time of cardiac arrest. It is critically important that the clinician closely monitor the patient's physiologic responses to the ongoing resuscitative efforts. Deterioration should prompt immediate differential diagnosis of the cause and institution of appropriate resuscitative maneuvers. The patient must not be transported from the resuscitation room or escape the close attention of the treating physician until clear physiologic improvement is evident and hemodynamic stability achieved.

SECONDARY SURVEY

Upon completion of the initial assessment and resuscitation from life-threatening conditions, the physician embarks upon the secondary survey. This phase is primarily concerned with the process of history taking and the completion of a complete physical examination. In addition, however, the astute clinician utilizes this period to reevaluate the patient for response to resuscitation, possible missed injuries, or developing conditions. It is during this phase that the physician will also utilize specific adjunctive diagnostic studies to completely characterize the nature and extent of the patient's injuries.

In order to diagnose the injured patient appropriately, a pertinent history must be obtained. In the relative chaos of the emergency room surrounding the trauma victim, this basic tenet is often abandoned, to the detriment of the patient. It is frequently presumed, often incorrectly, that the patient is incapable of providing any history. The injured patient should be questioned directly regarding the mechanism of injury, preexisting illnesses, and medical allergy. If the patient is indeed incapable of responding, as much information as possible must be obtained from prehospital care providers and relatives. As in all medical care, it is the history that will give the diagnostician the greatest clues regarding diagnosis. In the case of trauma, the critical aspect of the history surrounds the mechanism of injury. Given a specific mechanism of injury, a constellation of associated or probable conditions immediately becomes prominent in the physician's differential diagnosis. As an example, consider the mechanism of an unrestrained driver in a frontal impact collision at high speed. As the patient moves forward, his head strikes the windshield. This is indicated by the prehospital provider's history of a "bull's-eye" pattern on the windshield. Immediately, the physician is suspicious of a possible closed head injury. As the force is conducted down the spine, a possible cervical spine injury is incurred. Therefore, the patient must be fully immobilized and maintained in a cervical collar. The patient's chest strikes the steering wheel, leading to possible myocardial contusion or disruption of the descending thoracic aorta. The clinician will have to order special studies to critically evaluate for each of these subtle injuries. As the patient continues to move forward, his knee strikes the dashboard, leading to posterior hip dislocation or knee injury with possible popliteal artery thrombosis. Finally, the driver's right foot may become entangled in the pedals, leading to right ankle fracture. While a perfectly comprehensive examination of every patient is not possible, the expert physician utilizes his or her knowledge of likely injuries in face of particular injury mechanisms to direct the diagnostic

---

TABLE 19-3   Causes of Cardiac Arrest during or Just after Endotracheal Intubation

---

1. Severe hypoxemia during prolonged attempts at intubation, especially if no preintubation attempted with a bag and mask.
2. Intubation of the esophagus
3. A properly inserted endotracheal tube moving into the right main stem bronchus
4. Excessive ventilatory pressure by hand bagging, raising intrathoracic pressure, and reducing further an already marginal venous return
5. Development of a tension pneumothorax
6. Systemic air embolism, especially if a penetrating lung wound and hemoptysis are present
7. Vasovagal responses—rare unless patient already had inappropriate bradycardia
8. Sudden severe respiratory alkalosis, dropping ionized calcium or potassium levels too rapidly

---

process. In this manner, care is directed in an expeditious fashion and missed injuries are minimized.

In addition to obtaining the history of mechanism of injury, it is necessary to ascertain the presence of preexisting illness. Failure of the patient to respond appropriately to resuscitative efforts may be due to preexisting congestive heart failure rather than ongoing hemorrhage. Similarly, the presence of lateralizing neurologic signs may lead the hapless clinician to extreme measures of diagnosis and treatment should he or she fail to obtain the critical history of a preexisting stroke. Medications affecting the patient's physiologic response to injury, medical allergies, and other historical factors may be critical to the care and treatment of the injured patient.

With the completion of the history and a complete physical examination, the treating physician will now have a list of diagnosed injuries and a longer list of suspected injuries. At this point, specific adjunctive tests are indicated to confirm or rule out particular suspected conditions. Every patient suffering significant blunt-force injury will likely require the standard triad of radiographs of the cervical spine, chest, and pelvis. The anteroposterior (AP) pelvic film is useful in the evaluation of possible significant retroperitoneal bleeding. Also, the presence of significant anterior ring fractures in the male may indicate the presence of urethral injury. Additional radiographs and adjunctive studies such as CT, MRI, or diagnostic peritoneal lavage are ordered selectively as indicated by the clinician's index of suspicion. Evidence of spinal fracture should prompt radiologic survey of the entire spine due to the significant incidence of associated fractures. Bladder and gastric catheters should be placed at this time unless contraindicated.

It is also appropriate at this time to immobilize all fractures. Immobilization not only serves to minimize soft tissue injury and bleeding but also greatly increases patient comfort. This point is worthy of particular emphasis. It is impossible to adequately examine a patient screaming in pain from an overriding femur fracture. Narcotic analgesia will be both ineffective and detrimental to further diagnosis. Care, therefore, should be taken to apply appropriate traction and immobilizing splints to restore alignment and prevent crepitation. This should certainly be accomplished before the patient is moved for additional studies such as CT scanning. Distal pulses should be reevaluated following the application of traction or splints.

During the secondary survey, it is important that the physician continually reassess the patient's physiologic status and response to resuscitation. Vital signs are monitored frequently for possible deterioration. Supplemental oxygen is continued and pulse oximetry instituted. If not contraindicated, placement of a bladder catheter is accomplished and urine is obtained for examination. Appropriate blood work is done, including type and cross-match if indicated. Once satisfied that the patient's condition has been stabilized, the treating physician now takes the opportunity to review the results of the findings to construct a definitive list of the patient's injuries.

DEFINITIVE CARE

Armed with a list of the patient's sustained injuries and a clear idea of the patient's physiologic status following resuscitation, the treating physician must undertake a series of critical decisions. These decisions concern the development of a plan for definitive care of the patient. Primarily, the physician must decide whether the treating institution's resources are capable of providing optimum treatment. A rational and timely assessment of the need for possible transfer is imperative. Any delay in this decision or miscalculation will seriously jeopardize the patient's chances for maximal recovery. Partial treatment is usually inappropriate unless directed toward the most threatening injuries prior to transfer for additional care. At times, operative procedures will be required to effect stabilization of the patient sufficient for transfer to a regional trauma center. These procedures address life-threatening bleeding, airway compromise, or serious head trauma.

Once it is determined that definitive care is to proceed, the treating physician seeks to triage management priorities. As noted in the foregoing, the best of care, if ill timed, can lead to catastrophic consequences. A frequent example is found in the case of the blunt-trauma patient who is brought to the operating room for multiple orthopaedic procedures before full assessment of concomitant injuries is completed. During the course of a lengthy procedure involving fixation of multiple fractures, progressive hypoxia or hypotension is noted by the anesthesiologist. The operating orthopaedist is now in a difficult and dangerous position. Intraoperative diagnosis of the etiology of the patient's deterioration is difficult. The differential diagnosis includes a wide variety of potentially life-threatening conditions, including developing tension pneumothorax and occult bleeding. The most common course is to attempt maximal support and resuscitation while the orthopaedic procedure is hurriedly concluded; often this leads to significant injury to the patient and a compromised orthopaedic repair.

Prioritization of care seeks to address those injuries first which present the most immediate threat to the patient. This does not necessarily correspond with the most serious or difficult injury. A good aphorism to follow overall is: "Blood, brains, bones before the patient goes to bed." Following completion of the primary survey, life-threatening conditions relating to airway and breathing have been addressed. Initial shock resuscitation has been instituted. It is now imperative that bleeding sources be aggressively sought and definitively treated before all else. Any hemodynamically unstable patient must have the cause of shock defined before all else. The patient's response to rapid volume infusion is assessed. When a patient fails to respond to the rapid infusion of 2L of Ringer's lactate solution or demonstrates an ongoing need for rapid volume infusion to maintain pressure, the treating physician initiates transfusion with type-specific packed red blood cells and aggressively seeks the compartment of blood loss. An initial survey for external bleeding is performed. Failing this, an immediate portable chest x-ray is performed to evaluate for possible massive hemothorax. Opacification of the lung field on x-ray is treated with tube thoracostomy. Initial drainage of greater than 1500 mL of blood from the chest tube is an indication for immediate thoracotomy. Lesser amounts of drainage are monitored for continued output.

If chest x-ray does not indicate the source of bleeding and the patient continues to exhibit signs of continuing volume loss, diagnostic peritoneal lavage is undertaken. A CT scan of the abdomen, while diagnostic, is not safely performed in this setting. A positive lavage in the hemodynamically unstable patient requires immediate exploratory laparotomy for control of bleeding. In the blunt trauma patient, an AP portable pelvic radiograph is also obtained to determine the presence of posterior pelvic ring disruption, indicating possible massive retroperitoneal bleeding. Finally, the extremities are examined for multiple fractures possibly contributing to ongoing volume loss.

If the patient remains clinically in shock despite ongoing resuscitation and the above survey fails to identify a compartment of significant blood loss, the examiner must immediately entertain a broader differential diagnosis for persistent shock. As previously mentioned, this differential starts with a search for possible tension pneumothorax or cardiac tamponade. The neck veins are reassessed for possible distension. Initially, neck vein distension may not be apparent in the patient with both volume loss and a cardiac compressive etiology for shock. As the patient's volume is restored, however, jugular vein distension may become apparent. Further evaluation and immediate treatment is performed as previously described.

Also included in the differential diagnosis of persistent shock is the possibility of cervical or high thoracic spinal cord injury. This is quickly ruled out by assessing the patient's ability to move his or her lower extremities. In the comatose patient, this possible diagnosis may be evaluated by the determination of anal sphincter tone and radiologic examination of the spine. Priapism strongly suggests spinal cord injury as a possible etiology of the patient's shock condition.

A last consideration in the patient with persistent shock should be the possibility of cardiogenic failure. The patient may have preexisting cardiac failure contributing to persistent shock or have an acute myocardial infarction that may have led to the accident. Blunt chest trauma may lead to pump failure secondary to myocardial contusion or arrhythmia. This etiology is evaluated by means of emergent 12-lead electrocardiography. Early placement of a pulmonary artery (Swan-Ganz) catheter will aid in the diagnosis of acute cardiogenic shock and should be considered in any persistently hypotensive patient over the age of 40 in whom other causes are not apparent.

The patient in shock is treated for shock before all else. Until the patient is hemodynamically stabilized, all other diagnostic and therapeutic concerns are deferred. Even the possibility of closed head injury must await hemodynamic stabilization prior to CT scanning and treatment. The clinical impression of compartment syndrome must await adequate resuscitation and definitive management of life-threatening hemorrhage prior to evaluation and treatment. The reason for this dogmatic approach lies in the fact that all of these other significant conditions are dramatically worsened by the presence of ongoing shock.[5] Closed head injury, organ injury, and compartment syndrome are best treated initially by assuring adequate perfusion in the form of shock therapy. Definitive control of hemorrhage is the mainstay of shock therapy. If required to effect definitive control of hemorrhage, operative intervention precedes any further care.

Following diagnosis and treatment of shock, the next priority concerns treatment of brain injury. Just as rapid reversal of the shock state is critical to patient survival, it has been repeatedly demonstrated that patient prognosis is directly related to the expeditious definitive care of serious closed head injury.[6] Once hemodynamic stabilization has been achieved, the patient suspected of having sustained a head injury should undergo CT scanning. Initial suspicion of closed head injury is suggested by altered mental status or a deterioration in mental status despite resuscitation. In the current era, neurosurgical intervention requires evaluation with CT scanning. However, the treating practitioner is obliged to begin aggressive therapy at the earliest suspicion of elevated intracranial pressure. If the diagnosis of significant closed head injury is suspected, therapeutic maneuvers aimed at reducing intracranial pressure are instituted pending CT scan. These maneuvers include optimization of perfusion pressure, hyperventilation, and osmotic diuresis with mannitol if the patient's volume status permits. The general approach at the outset should be a "full-court press," utilizing all possible treatment modalities in an aggressive fashion until the diagnosis of elevated intracranial pressure is excluded or definitive care by neurosurgical intervention achieved.

With the completion of evaluation and treatment of both hemorrhage and brain injury, attention is turned to the diagnosis and management of orthopaedic injuries. Many times the patient's condition will allow orthopaedic evaluation and possibly treatment to occur coincidentally with care of hemorrhagic and cerebral insults. At times, orthopaedic intervention will be required in order to effect control of hemorrhagic shock or address neurologic shock due to spinal injury. But even when deferred by the press of life-threatening bleeding or brain injury, proper attention to orthopaedic care must be aggressively pursued as soon as practical. Postponing evaluation and care of significant orthopaedic injuries is associated with significantly higher morbidity and poorer prognosis for functional recovery. In addition, the early aggressive care of lower extremity fractures has been demonstrated to decrease the incidence of pulmonary complications in the seriously traumatized patient.[7]

SPECIAL CONSIDERATIONS

Aortic Injury

Blunt injury to the thoracic aorta accounts for a large percentage of scene deaths following vehicular trauma. While only approximately 10 percent of patients suffering from thoracic aortic injury will survive to present to the emergency department, it is critically important to make an expeditious diagnosis of such injury. The need for timely identification of the injury centers upon the fact that half of the population of patients with this injury will die for each 24 h of delay in diagnosis. Indeed, less than 5 percent of aortic injuries will form a stable pseudoaneurysm.

The diagnosis of blunt thoracic aortic injury is suggested by a history of high decelerative force, either during frontal vehicular impact or as a result of a fall. While interscapular murmur or pulse differential have been described in association with this injury, the majority of patients will lack suggestive symptoms or signs on physical examination. Diagnosis rests with the examining physician's index of suspicion and careful review of the AP chest radiograph in the trauma room. While over a dozen radiologic signs on chest radiograph have been described in association with thoracic aortic injury, few of these have a reliable correlation. Emphasis should be placed on the review of mediastinal width, as the finding of a widened mediastinum (mediastinal width greater than 8 cm) has been repeatedly shown to be almost 100 percent sensitive for thoracic aortic injury. Though this finding is very sensitive, a widened mediastinum is by no means specific, as over 85 percent of aortograms will prove to negative. Nonetheless, the finding of a widened mediastinum on chest film of a patient with a suggestive mechanism of injury should prompt aortography as soon as the patient's condition permits. The treatment of shock, including definitive control of hemorrhage, and the treatment of significant head injury take precedence over the evaluation or treatment of aortic injury.

Pelvic Injury

Significant pelvic injury with hypotension following blunt trauma continues to challenge the most experienced trauma centers. As noted earlier, posterior pelvic ring disruptions may be associated with massive hemorrhage from both arterial and venous sources. In addition, the force required to disrupt the pelvis frequently leads to significant intraperitoneal injury as well. In the hypotensive patient, it can be difficult to determine whether life-threatening hemorrhage is occurring in the peritoneal cavity or in the retroperitoneum secondary to pelvic disruption. Error in prioritizing treatment of these compartments is often associated with the patient's demise. The current recommendation in the setting of a profoundly hypotensive patient with posterior pelvic disruption following blunt trauma is to proceed emergently with diagnostic peritoneal lavage. An initial aspirate of more than 10 mL of gross blood from the peritoneal catheter is indicative of major intraperitoneal blood loss and should prompt immediate laparotomy. If the initial aspirate is negative but the lavage positive by cell count (RBC > 100,000/mL), initial treatment efforts should be aimed at control of hemorrhage from the pelvic fracture and followed by laparotomy for control of intraperitoneal bleeding.[8]

Opinions regarding the best management of pelvic hemorrhage vary. Options include interventional arteriographic embolization, urgent pelvic fixation, and laparotomy for packing with or without open or external fixation of the pelvic ring. While arteriographic embolization effectively controls hemorrhage from arterial injuries, often of the superior gluteal arteries, it is ineffective at controlling the more common problem of massive bleeding from injury to the presacral venous plexus and direct bony hemorrhage. In these cases, fixation is preferred. In addition, arteriographic embolization requires prolonged treatment of a hemodynamically unstable patient in the relatively uncontrolled setting of the radiology suite. For these reasons, it is usually preferred to elect stabilization of the pelvis as an initial approach in the operating room, where aggressive monitoring and resuscitation can continue.

If the treating physician elects to pursue pelvic fixation, one must keep in mind the possibility of associated arterial injury. Injury to the superior gluteal artery, as mentioned, is common. Less common but often life-threatening is the association of blunt-force injury to the iliac or femoral vessels. Continued hemodynamic instability following pelvic fixation should prompt an urgent search for possible arterial injury.

Injury in the Elderly

Special consideration must be given to the elderly patient who has suffered serious blunt trauma. The presence of shock in this setting is difficult to diagnose and often multifactorial. Physiological mechanisms for compensation for acute hemorrhage are inefficient and may be further compromised by the preaccident use of beta-blocking medications. For this same reason, signs and symptoms of significant hemorrhage may be absent. In addition, preexisting cardiac disease may predispose the elderly patient to persistent shock on the basis of pump failure. The relative contribution of volume loss versus cardiogenic shock is difficult to determine.

Due to the difficulty of determining the etiology of shock in the elderly patient, it is often necessary to institute invasive monitoring early in resuscitation in this setting. Early placement of a pulmonary artery catheter is often advantageous in the resuscitation of the severely injured elderly patient. Massive volume resuscitation without invasive monitoring of filling pressures and cardiac function may lead quickly to respiratory embarrassment and further complications.

COMPLICATIONS

Adult Respiratory Distress Syndrome and Systemic Inflammatory Response Syndrome

The most common serious complication of the multiple trauma patient is respiratory failure. This may be due to direct pulmonary trauma, aspiration pneumonitis, or pneumonia. Often, however, such a specific etiology for respiratory compromise is lacking. During the first 3 to 7 days following significant trauma, hypoxia and pulmonary shunting are often detected without obvious cause. These clinical findings are followed by the development of a patchy bilateral infiltrate on chest radiography. Over the course of the next several days, worsening pulmonary function is accompanied by falling pulmonary compliance and extensive whiting out of the lung fields on the radiograph.

While a specific cause may not be obvious, the common denominator for the development of adult respiratory distress syndrome (ARDS) is an overwhelming systemic inflammatory response. Often the cause of this inflammatory response is the severity of the initial trauma itself. If that is the case, the course of the ARDS is often self-limited and recovery expected in the patient with minimal preinjury compromise. Often, however, an ongoing inflammatory focus continues to fuel the pathologic process of ARDS. This inflammatory focus may be obvious, as in the case of a young victim of blunt trauma with overwhelming closed head injury. In this setting, progressive ARDS over the first several days following injury is a common cause of death, even when direct pulmonary injury is lacking. Frequently the cause of the inflammatory stimulus is inapparent. Missed abdominal injuries or aspiration pneumonitis must be considered. In addition, subclinical line sepsis may stimulate this inflammatory cascade. For this reason, all vascular access devices placed in the emergency department or as part of the patient's resuscitation should be replaced during the first 24 h in hospital. Any patient exhibiting worsening ARDS should undergo empiric line replacement as well.

If the cause of inflammation is not discovered and treated, the patient's condition will worsen over the next several days in the intensive care unit (ICU). There, ARDS will progress, requiring increasingly nonphysiologic levels of pulmonary support. Falling compliance and the need to resort to high levels of positive end-expiratory pressure (PEEP) leads to pulmonary barotrauma, itself a cause of ARDS. Barotrauma may also lead to tension pneumothorax, which, if not promptly diagnosed and treated, will rapidly lead to cardiac embarassment and death.

As ARDS progresses, the patient's inflammatory cascade leads to the development of progressive organ failure. Hematopoietic failure and immunologic compromise are often too subtle for detection during these early phases. Soon, however, rising creatinine levels give witness to developing renal failure. This event heralds the development of multiple organ failure. As this systemic inflammatory response syndrome (SIRS) progresses, eventually cardiac failure develops and the patient becomes unsupportable despite massive ventilatory and pharmacologic support.

The SIRS scenario is an all too common one in the ICU following trauma. Often, the patient's worsening course is ascribed to "sepsis," implying a bacteriologic etiology. This misconception arises from the physiologic similarities between SIRS and septic shock, specifically the loss of systemic vascular resistance. Thousands of dollars worth of cultures of every imaginable site are obtained, always positive for multiple organisms having little or nothing to do with the patient's increasingly critical condition. The response to these positive cultures is treatment with broad-spectrum antibiotics, with little therapeutic effect; such treatment also opens the door to fungal infection. The

treating physician's attention would be better spent seeking the inciting inflammatory sources and controlling them. While a bacterial line sepsis or pneumonia may be the cause, one should not overlook the possible etiologies of the untreated abdominal injury or orthopaedic injury. The patient's demise can be averted only by early recognition of this inflammatory cascade, an aggressive search for its source, and prompt treatment.

Fat Embolism Syndrome

Fat embolism syndrome (FES) is a rare complication of trauma, occurring in approximately 1 percent of patients suffering long bone fracture.[9] Risk is greatest in young adults who have suffered multiple blunt trauma with closed long bone fractures. Medullary nailing has been implicated as a possible contributing factor.[10] The specific pathophysiology of the syndrome remains unclear, though support continues for the mechanical embolization theory. Alternatively, a biochemical abnormality in systemic fatty acid metabolism has been implicated.

Clinically, FES usually presents as developing respiratory distress at day 3 to 5 following multiple blunt trauma. The timing of the development of the respiratory compromise is suggestive, occurring later than is usually seen with direct pulmonary trauma and before the usual onset of postinjury pneumonia. Hypoxia and tachypnea may be joined by mental status changes, fever, and tachycardia. Classically, a truncal petechial rash may be observed. Fat droplets on urinalysis may be observed.

Treatment should be both prophylactic and therapeutic. Early immobilization of long bone fractures is felt to reduce the incidence of FES. Controversy exists as to the recommended method of fixation, however, as some feel early internal fixation following multiple trauma may be contributory. Other studies have shown no such increase in the incidence of FES when intramedullary fixation was utilized.[11] Once FES is diagnosed, treatment is generally supportive. Respiratory support is primary. Supplemental oxygen is often all that is required. In addition, intravenous fluid therapy is recommended. While some have advocated heparin and steroid therapies, studies documenting the efficacy of these treatments are lacking. With early diagnosis, fracture stabilization, and aggressive treatment, the condition of FES is often self-limited and recovery is common if other conditions do not supervene.

RECOVERY

Ultimate recovery of the multiply injured patient is dependent upon a number of critical milestones. Initially, aggressive diagnosis and treatment of shock gives the best chance of survival and avoidance of complications in the postinjury course. Appropriate definitive care, including early surgical intervention for both life-threatening hemorrhage and orthopaedic injuries, minimizes the patient's inflammatory response to the trauma. When complications develop, however, careful investigation for a source of on-going inflammation may permit treatment and a return to normal healing. As the patient's condition improves, recovery is completed with a comprehensive program of therapy. In this manner, the patient's fullest ultimate return to function is achieved.

REFERENCES

1. Committee on Trauma Research, Commission on Life Sciences, National Research Council, and the Institute of Medicine: *Injury in America.* Washington, DC, National Academy Press, 1985.
2. Trunkey DD: Trauma. *Sci. Am* 249:28–35, 1983.
3. Wilson, RF: Techniques of resuscitation, in Geller ER (ed): *Shock and Resuscitation.* New York, McGraw-Hill, 1993.
4. Velanovich V: Crystalloid versus colloid fluid resuscitation: A meta-analysis of mortality. *Surgery* 105:65, 1989.
5. Chestnut RM, Marshall LF, Klauber MR, et al: The role of secondary brain injury in determining outcome from severe head injury. *J Trauma* 30:933, 1990.
6. Shackford SR, Baxt WG, Hoyt DB, et al: Impact of a trauma system on outcome of severely injured patients. *Arch Surg* 122:523, 1987.
7. Trafton PG: Lower extremity fractures and dislocations, in Feliciano DV, Moore EE, Mattox KL (eds): *Trauma,* 3d ed. Appleton and Lange, 1996.
8. Gruen GS, Leit ME, Gruen RJ, et al: The acute management of hemodynamically unstable multiple trauma patients with pelvic ring fractures. *J Trauma* 27:998, 1987.
9. Peltier LF, Collins JA, Evarts CM: Fat embolism. *Arch Surg* 109:12–16, 1974.
10. Muller C, Rahn B, Pfister U, et al: The incidence, pathogenesis, diagnosis, and treatment of fat embolism. *Orthop Rev* 107–117, 1994.
11. Pape H-C, Regel G, Dwenger A, et al: Influence of thoracic trauma and primary femoral intramedullary nailing on the incidence of ARDS in multiple trauma patients. *Injury* 23(suppl 3):S82, 1993.

CHAPTER 20

Traumatic Injuries of the Shoulder and Shoulder Girdle

Mark W. Rodosky

FRACTURES OF THE PROXIMAL HUMERUS

Relevant Anatomy

The proximal humerus consists of several anatomic parts including the humeral head (and its articular surface), the lesser tuberosity, the greater tuberosity, the bicipital groove, and the proximal humeral shaft (Fig. 20-1). The anatomical neck of the humerus separates the head from the tuberosities, while the surgical neck lies below the lesser and greater tuberosities. The lesser tuberosity lies at the margin of the humeral head at the anterior aspect of the humerus. It is positioned at the medial aspect of the bicipital groove, serving as the site of attachment for the subscapularis muscle. The greater tuberosity also lies at the humeral head margin, but posteriorly to the bicipital groove; it serves as an attachment site for the supraspinatus, infraspinatus, and teres minor muscles. The long head of the biceps tendon is held in the bicipital groove by the transverse humeral ligament.

Displacement of proximal humeral fractures is influenced by various muscle attachments (Fig. 20-1). The greater tuberosity is generally pulled superiorly and posteriorly by the supraspinatus, infraspinatus, and teres minor muscles. The subscapularis muscle pulls the lesser tuberosity in an anterior and medial direction. The long head of the biceps tendon, which lies between the tuberosity fragments, has the ability to act as a tether, blocking reduction of proximal humeral fractures when it is trapped in the fracture site. However, it serves as a valuable landmark in discerning the lesser from the greater tuberosity in complex proximal humeral fractures. The deltoid is the most powerful muscle of the shoulder and can cause displacement of fractures of the proximal humeral shaft by pulling it proximally. The pectoralis major muscle inserts in the lower portion of the lateral lip of the bicipital groove and tends to displace the proximal shaft in a proximal and medial direction, as is often the case in surgical neck fractures.

The major blood supply to the humeral head comes from the anterior humeral circumflex artery and its branches, which include the arcuate artery.[1] Laing showed that the arcuate artery supplied blood to a very large portion of the humeral head, entering the bone in the area of the intertubercular groove.[2] Blood to the humeral head is also supplied partially from a small contribution by the posterior circumflex artery and from the vascular rotator cuff.[2] Fractures at the level of the anatomic neck disrupt all flow of blood to the humeral head, leading to avascular necrosis (AVN) of the head. Fortunately, most fractures of the proximal humerus occur at the surgical neck, below the level of the tuberosities, and the blood supply to the head remains intact.

Injury to the neurovascular supply of the upper extremity is common with severely displaced proximal humeral fractures. The most commonly injured nerve is the axillary nerve.[3] This nerve crosses the anterior surface of the subscapularis muscle before it dips back posteriorly under the glenoid neck, passing along the inferior border of the capsule of the glenohumeral joint on its way to the quadrangular space. Because it is relatively fixed by the posterior cord of the brachial plexus and deltoid muscle, any abnormal downward motion of the proximal humerus can result in traction and resultant axillary nerve palsy. Its close proximity to the glenohumeral joint also makes it susceptible to injury with anterior fracture dislocations.

Incidence and Etiology

Fractures of the proximal humerus account for 4 to 5 percent of all fractures.[4] Most of these fractures occur in elderly individuals with osteoporosis.[5] The most common mechanism is a fall onto the outstretched hand from a standing height or less.[4] In younger individuals, high-energy trauma such as occurs with motor vehicle accidents is frequently associated. Many of these patients will have fracture dislocations with significant soft tissue disruption and multiple trauma.

Classification

The four-part fracture classification scheme developed by Neer in 1970 is the most logical and commonly used classification system for proximal humeral fractures[6,7] (Fig. 20-2). Before the Neer classification, Codman in 1934 made a very significant contribution to the understanding of proximal humeral fractures. He proposed that fractures be separated into four distinct fragments, including the anatomic head, the greater tuberosity, the lesser tuberosity, and the humeral shaft.[8] Neer based his classification scheme on the ideas of Codman and provided the first truly comprehensive system that considered the anatomy and biomechanical forces, relating these to diagnosis and treatment. The cornerstone of the scheme is the proper identification of the fracture fragments, which can be accomplished only through appropriate radiographs.

Most fractures of the proximal humerus (over 80 percent) are minimally displaced.[5] In the Neer four-part classification scheme, the fracture fragments consist of the articular segment, the greater tuberosity, the lesser tuberosity, and the humeral shaft.[6,7] When any of the four major components is displaced more than 1 cm or angulated more than 45°, the fragment is considered displaced. Nondisplaced components are not considered separate fragments.

Neer also emphasized the term *fracture dislocation*, noting that a fracture dislocation occurs when the humeral

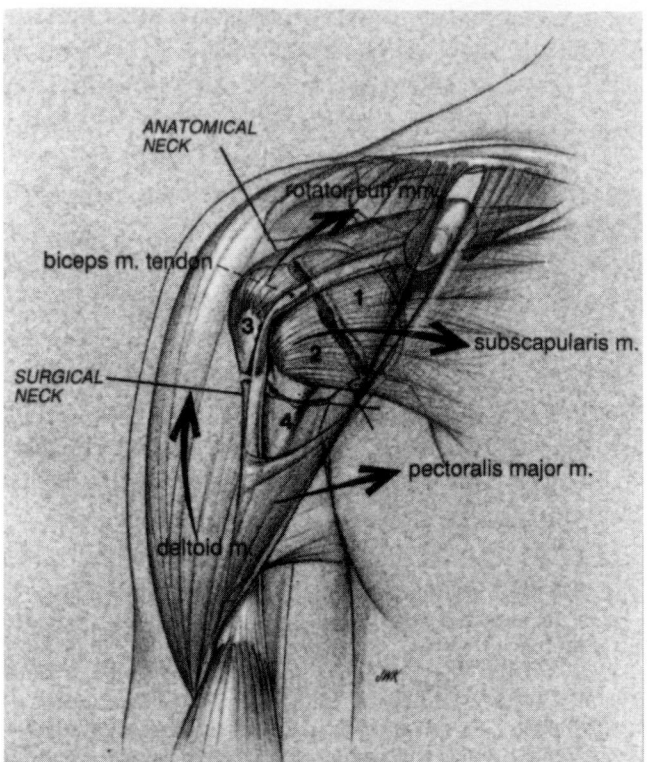

Figure 20-1 The proximal humerus consists of the humeral head (1), the lesser tuberosity (2), the greater tuberosity (3) and the proximal humeral shaft (4). Displacement of the fracture fragments is guided by the direction of muscle pull as shown by the arrows. [Reproduced with permission from Bigliani LU, Flatow EL, Pollock RG: Fractures of the proximal humerus, in Rockwood CA, Green DP, Bucholz RW, et al (eds): *Fractures in Adults, 4th ed.* Philadelphia, Lippincott-Raven, 1996, pp 1055–1107.]

head is dislocated away from the glenoid fossa in association with a fracture. A fracture dislocation can be classified according to direction (anterior or posterior), as well as to the number of fracture fragments (two-part, three-part, or four-part). In addition, the articular surface of the humeral head may be shattered; this is termed a head-splitting fracture. In some instances, an impression fracture may also be present at the humeral head. In this situation, the percentage of the humeral head involved in the impression fracture is calculated for prognostic purposes.

Diagnosis

History and Exam

Most fractures of the proximal humerus present with acute onset of symptoms including pain, swelling, and tenderness about the shoulder, especially at the greater tuberosity. Crepitus may be present, with motion of the fracture fragments. Ecchymosis is generally visible within 24 to 48 h of the injury and may spread to the chest wall and flank as well as down the extremity. A detailed neurovascular evaluation is essential when fracture of the proximal humerus is suspected.

Diagnostic Radiology

A complete and systematic radiographic evaluation is important when a proximal humeral fracture or fracture dislocation is suspected.[6,7] The trauma series is the best initial method for diagnosing a proximal humeral fracture and consists of anteroposterior (AP), Y-scapular, and axillary views. The axillary view is essential, as it allows the examiner to evaluate the degree of tuberosity displacement, the glenoid articular surface, and the relationship of the humeral head to the glenoid cavity. The axillary view can be obtained with the patient either standing, sitting, or in the prone position. The Velpeau axillary view is preferred, as it allows the arm to be left undisturbed in a sling.[9]

In addition to determining angulation of the major fracture line that may be present between the head and shaft, the radiographs are also used to determine displacement of the tuberosity fragments and articular surface. When the amount of displacement or angulation is unclear from the plain radiographs, it is important to obtain a CT scan in order to determine these parameters definitively.

Treatment

Nonoperative Treatment

Sling Immobilization Since most proximal humeral fractures are minimally displaced, they can be satisfactorily treated with sling immobilization and early range-of-motion exercises. Gentle range-of-motion exercises are begun at 7 to 10 days after the fracture, or when the clinician has established that the fracture is clinically stable and moves as a unit. It is important to note that overly aggressive exercises may distract a minimally displaced fracture and result in a malunion or nonunion. Intermittent radiographs are essential in determining whether or not the fracture has displaced.

Closed Reduction *General* Closed reduction of proximal humeral fractures is a suitable and important method of treatment. However, repeated forceful attempts at closed reduction have the potential to complicate a fracture by causing further displacement, fragmentation, or neurovascular injury. For that reason, it is important to understand the type of deformity and forces involved in the fracture prior to attempting a closed reduction. The patient is placed in a supine position and sedated with a muscle relaxant and narcotic. When possible, fluoroscopic control is utilized. The reduction maneuver is performed in a manner that neutralizes the deforming forces. After reduction, the stability of the reduced fracture is evaluated by observing for motion with continuous fluoroscopy.

Two-Part Fractures The types of proximal humeral fractures that are generally amenable to reduction maneuver include displaced two-part surgical neck and two-part greater tuberosity fractures. A truly displaced two-part anatomic neck fracture is infrequent and often unresponsive to treatment with closed reduction maneuvers. On the contrary, in the two-part neck fracture, both tuberosities remain attached to the head, so that it remains in a neu-

Figure 20-2 Neer classification scheme of displaced proximal humeral fractures and fracture dislocations.

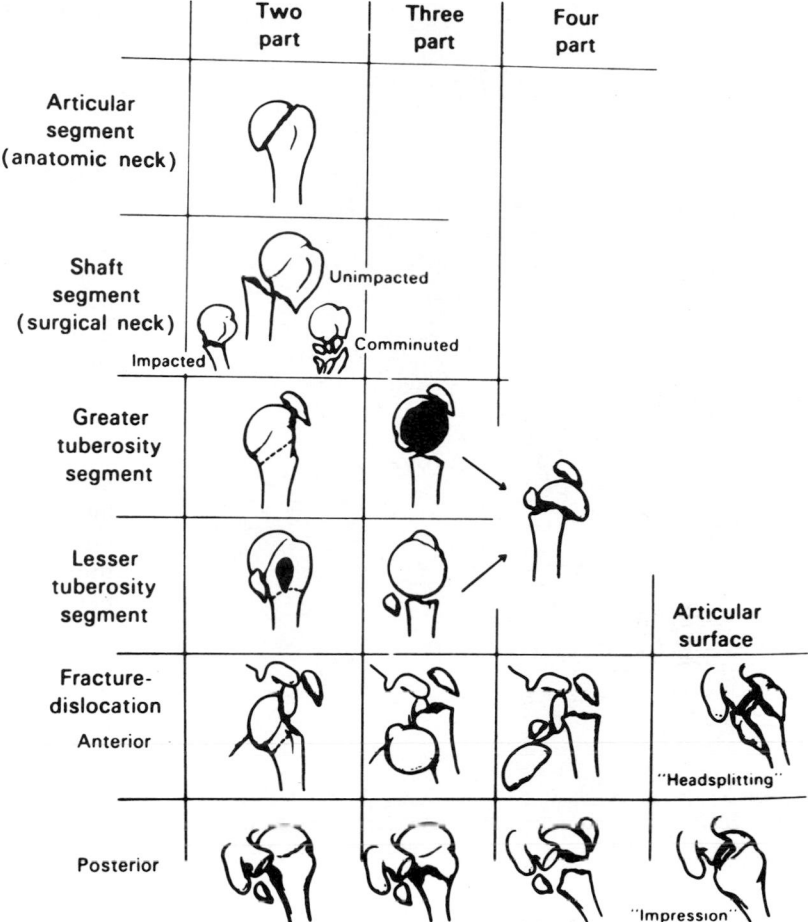

trally rotated position. However, the shaft is usually displaced medially by the pull of the pectoralis major muscle. Therefore, gentle traction with flexion and some adduction is usually all that is necessary to reduce the humeral shaft in order that it can be impacted into the head fragment (Fig. 20-3). One should note that there may be interposition of soft tissue—either muscle, capsular tissue, or the long head of the biceps tendon—that precludes a reduction. In this situation, an open reduction and internal fixation (ORIF) may be needed.

An impacted but angulated two-part surgical neck fracture can also be treated with an attempt at closed reduction. The head should be disimpacted from the shaft and then rereduced with impaction in a less angulated position. A comminuted fracture is generally unstable and will most often require open reduction and internal fixation to properly align and maintain fragment position.

Greater tuberosity fractures are usually retracted in a posterior and superior direction and are difficult to reduce with nonoperative techniques. The exception to this rule is the greater tuberosity fracture that is associated with an anterior dislocation of the humerus. In this situation, a closed reduction of the humerus into the glenoid fossa may often result in reduction of the greater tuberosity fragment. Reduction of the greater tuberosity fragment is generally successful in the absence of a significantly sized ro-

tator cuff tear. When the greater tuberosity fragment is associated with a larger, massive rotator cuff tear, it is difficult to obtain a satisfactory closed reduction. However, even with successful reduction of the greater tuberosity, there is a tendency for the greater tuberosity fragment to displace superiorly and posteriorly after reduction.[10] For this reason, when the reduction is successful, it is important to obtain serial radiographs during the first few weeks after fracture. Isolated greater tuberosity fractures occur with anterior glenohumeral dislocations in 5 to 8 percent of cases.[11]

Two-part lesser tuberosity fractures are far less common and can be successfully treated with closed reduction when the fragment is small and does not block internal rotation. This injury is usually associated with a posterior glenohumeral dislocation and may also be treated by closed means if the articular involvement is minimal. The upper extremity should be immobilized in a neutral position. The fragment should be followed with early serial radiographs, as the pull of the subscapularis may result in further distraction and eventual nonunion.

Three- and Four-Part Fractures Most of the three-part fractures of the proximal humerus are unstable and difficult to treat by closed means. These fractures, by definition, involve a displaced surgical neck fracture as well as

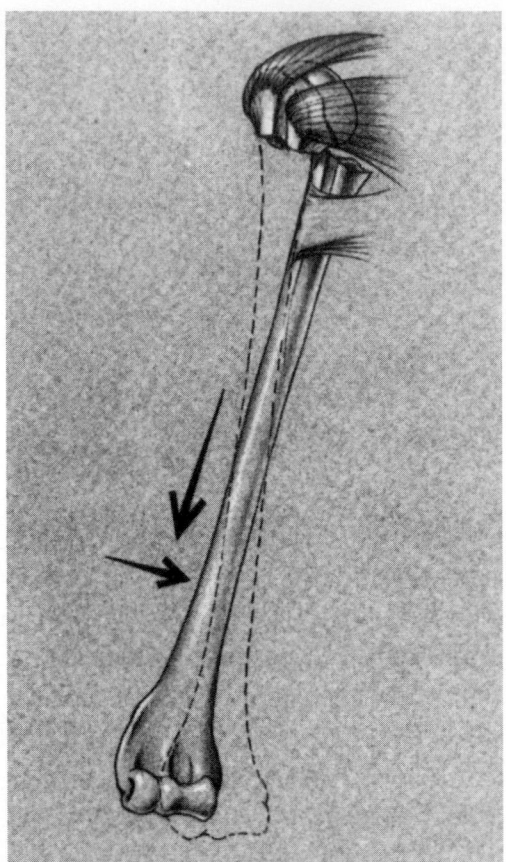

Figure 20-3 Closed reduction of a surgical neck fracture is performed with gentle adduction to lessen the medial pull of the pectoralis major muscle and gentle longitudinal traction to align and impact the fragments. [Reproduced with permission from Bigliani LU, Flatow EL, Pollock RG: Fractures of the proximal humerus, in Rockwood CA, Green DP, Bucholz RW, et al (eds): *Fractures in Adults, 4th ed.* Philadelphia, Lippincott-Raven, 1996, pp 1055–1107.]

a greater or lesser tuberosity fracture. In a three-part fracture, the portion of the rotator cuff that remains attached to the nonfractured tuberosity fragment will serve to rotate the humeral head in the direction of its pull. In addition, the humeral shaft is pulled medially by the pectoralis major muscle. Repeated attempts at closed reduction in three-part greater or lesser tuberosity fractures is not advised, as most of these fractures occur in elderly people with osteopenic bone. The repeated reduction maneuvers may result in further comminution of the fracture.

Four-part fractures of the proximal humerus are associated with an extremely high incidence of avascular necrosis and are not often successfully treated by closed reduction. As described further on, these fractures are generally treated by open means.

Impression Fractures In many instances, impression fractures are associated with unrecognized glenohumeral dislocations. An anterior dislocation results in a posterior impression fracture, and vice versa. Patients with missed dislocations and impression fractures are treated with an attempt at closed reduction when the fracture dislocation is less than 2 or 3 weeks old. If the impression fracture of the humeral head is larger than 20 to 30 percent, operative intervention is generally required.

Operative Treatment

Two-Part Fractures Two-part fractures are treated operatively when the fracture is irreducible by closed means or remains unstable after closed reduction. Anatomic neck fractures are rare and associated with a high degree of AVN of the head fragment. Younger individuals are usually treated with ORIF using cancellous lag screws. Older individuals should be treated with shoulder hemiarthroplasty.

Two-part surgical neck fractures are common and can be successfully treated with closed reduction and sling immobilization in more than 85 percent of cases. When the pull of the pectoralis major continues to displace the fracture in spite of closed reduction, the surgeon can attempt percutaneous pin fixation to hold the reduction. The pins must be placed carefully from lateral, anterior, or superior positions that are precisely located to avoid axillary nerve injury. When tissue interposition precludes reduction, operative intervention is indicated. An anterior approach is utilized, with the surgeon carefully noting the position of the axillary nerve and vessels, as they may be intimately adherent to the displaced shaft fragment. The reduction is held with heavy nonabsorbable sutures placed in a figure-of-eight orientation between the fragments. Wire provides greater stability and may be needed in some cases, but it is generally avoided, as it may later break or migrate and serve as an irritant in the subacromial space. Sutures are placed at the base of the rotator cuff insertions through the greater and lesser tuberosities. For comminuted surgical neck fractures, longitudinal fixation is supplemented with small-diameter intramedullary rods placed in the nonarticular surface just inside the greater or lesser tuberosities (Fig. 20-4). Small incisions in line with the cuff fibers are used to place the nails. Enders rods can be utilized with sutures incorporated through the eyelet in the rod.[12]

Two-part greater tuberosity fractures are often associated with anterior glenohumeral dislocations. After closed reduction, if displacement of the greater tuberosity fragment is greater than 5 to 10 mm, ORIF is indicated (Fig. 20-5). The surgeon should accept very little superior displacement, as patients with 5 mm or more of this may develop impingement. In most instances, displaced fractures are associated with rotator cuff tears.[13] The fracture should be approached through a superoanterior approach in the same way that a rotator cuff tear is approached. In young individuals with strong bone, cancellous lag screws can be utilized. However, in individuals with weaker bone, the fracture reduction can be held more securely with heavy nonabsorbable sutures anchored at the base of the rotator cuff tendons. Rotator cuff repair is an important component of operative treatment (Fig. 20-6).

Displaced lesser tuberosity fractures should be treated with ORIF in the same fashion as greater tuberosity fractures. However, an anterior approach is utilized.

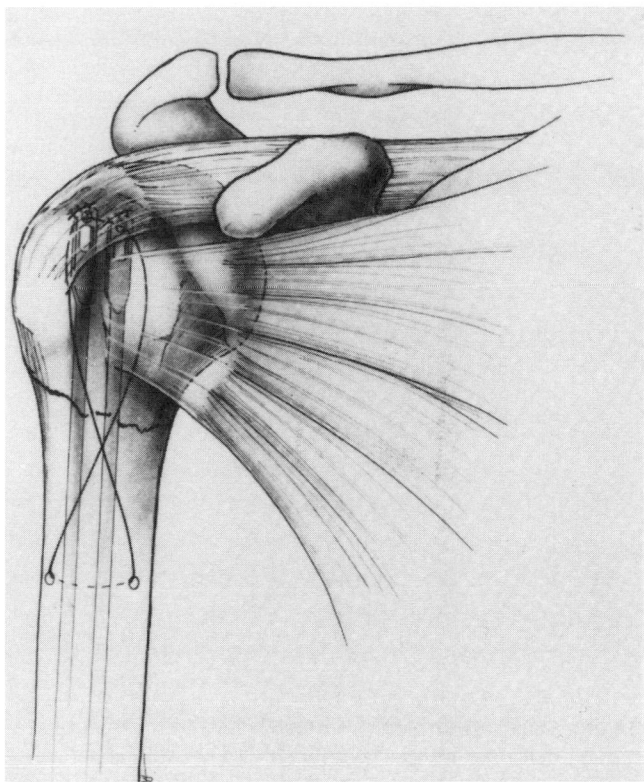

Figure 20-4 Narrow-diameter rods can be used to stabilize unstable surgical neck fractures. The rods are inserted through the cuff tendons. (Reproduced with permission from Bigliani LU, Flatow EL, Pollock RG: Fractures of the proximal humerus, in Rockwood CA, Green DP, Bucholz RW, et al (eds): *Fractures in Adults, 4th ed.* Philadelphia, Lippincott-Raven, 1996, pp 1055–1107.)

Three-Part Fractures   Three-part fractures should generally be treated with ORIF.[12] This includes three-part fracture dislocations, since a closed reduction attempt may convert the three-part to a four-part fracture, disallowing fixation. These fractures are reduced through an anterior approach, with great care taken to preserve soft tissue at-tachments and blood supply. The fragments are held with intramedullary rods and heavy nonabsorbable suture, as described above. The rods may be placed through or nearer the lesser tuberosity when the greater tuberosity fragment precludes placement through it. In patients with osteoporotic bone or significant comminution, prosthetic humeral head hemiarthroplasty is indicated, as described below.

Four-Part and Head-Split Fractures   The treatment of choice for these fractures (Fig. 20-7*A*) is prosthetic humeral head replacement surgery.[7,14] Occasionally in young patients with four-part fractures with lesser displacement, closed reduction and percutaneous fixation with multiple K wires can be attempted. A high incidence of AVN should be expected with this approach.[3]

The hemiarthroplasty is performed through an anterior extended deltopectoral approach. The prosthesis is cemented in the shaft at a height appropriate to maintain proper deltoid tension. The tuberosity fragments are fixed to the proximal humerus and prosthesis with heavy nonabsorbable sutures placed through the shaft prior to cementing (Fig. 20-7*B* and *C*). When intact, the long head of the biceps is preserved in its groove. Cancellous bone graft from the discarded humeral head is placed beneath the tuberosities.

Impacted Valgus Fractures   Jakob et al. have reported that ORIF with multiple pins in a subgroup of patients with valgus impacted fractures can be successful.[15] The fracture pattern is one in which the head is impacted on the shaft and the tuberosities are split but remain in close proximity to the head and shaft. In this group of patients, who do not meet the strict criteria of four-part displacement according to Neer, treatment includes elevating the head and placing the tuberosities beneath it. Jakob et al. reported on 19 patients, with 74 percent satisfactory results and 26 percent failures secondary to AVN.[15]

Impression Fractures   These fractures are usually the result of dislocations. If the head involvement is less than 20 percent of the articular surface and treatment is instituted

Figure 20-5 Anteroposterior (*left*) and Y-scapular views (*right*) showing a displaced greater tuberosity fracture. (Reproduced with permission from Flatow EL, Cuomo F, Maday MG: Open reduction and internal fixation of two-part displaced fractures of the greater tuberosity of the proximal part of the humerus. *J Bone Joint Surg* 73A:1213–1218, 1991.)

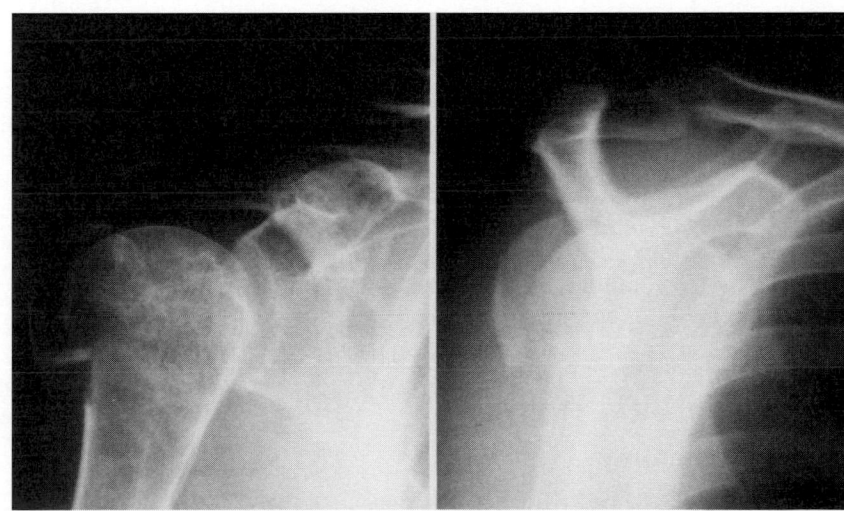

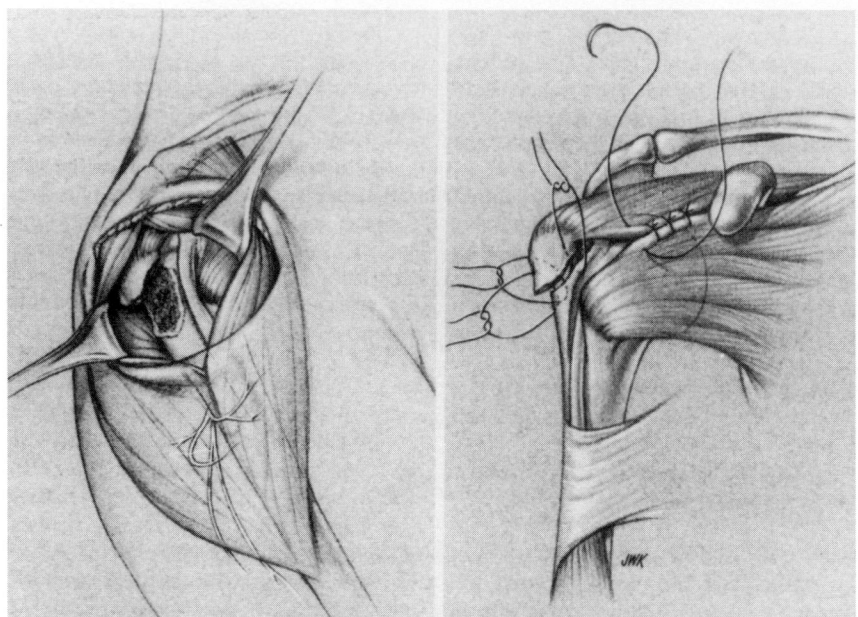

Figure 20-6 Surgical treatment of a greater tuberosity fragment is carried out through a superoanterior approach (*left*) and the fragment and cuff are repaired as shown with nonabsorbable suture (*right*). [Reproduced with permission from Flatow EL, Cuomo F, Maday MG: Open reduction and internal fixation of two-part displaced fractures of the greater tuberosity of the proximal part of the humerus. *J Bone Joint Surg* 73A:1213–1218, 1991.]

within a few weeks of injury, closed reduction is often successful. When 20 to 45 percent of the articular surface is involved, the lesser or greater tuberosity should be transferred into the defect to afford joint stability. For head defects greater than 45 percent or if the dislocation is chronic, leading to softening or degeneration of the head, a prosthetic humeral head hemiarthroplasty is indicated.[3]

Rehabilitation All patients with operative treatment of proximal humeral fractures require early physical therapy to prevent scarring and stiffness. Early passive range-of-motion exercises are begun with forward elevation in the scapular plane and supine external rotation with the arm at the side. Pendulums, pulley exercises, and cane assistance are helpful. At approximately 3 weeks, active assistive exercises are initiated. Active and resistive exercises are begun when the fracture fragments have healed.

Complications

Avascular necrosis is a common complication after anatomic neck displacement. A review of several large series has shown that AVN occurs in 3 to 14 percent of three-part fractures and 13 to 34 percent of four-part fractures.[16] Nonunion is relatively common in displaced surgical neck fractures treated with sling support. It is less frequent in nondisplaced fractures, prompting the surgeon to consider early operative intervention for displaced fractures. Because of the pull of the attached rotator cuff muscles, nonunion is also common in greater and lesser tuberosity fractures treated nonoperatively.[10]

CLAVICULAR FRACTURES
Relevant Anatomy

The clavicle serves as a strut that helps suspend the arm while also serving as a site for muscle attachments, in-

cluding the trapezius and anterior deltoid.[17] Its subcutaneous position renders it vulnerable to open injuries when fractured. It overlies the brachial plexus and subclavian and axillary vessels and therefore provides protection to these structures. However, the close proximity of these neurovascular structures makes them susceptible to blunt or sharp injury with clavicular fractures. Subsequent exuberant callous formation or malunion can compress these structures, leading to thoracic outlet disease.

The clavicle is the first bone in the body to ossify and is the only long bone to form by intramembranous ossification.[18] Although epiphyseal growth plates develop at both ends of the clavicle, the sternal ossification center is responsible for nearly 80 percent of the longitudinal growth. This center usually appears during teenage growth but fails to fuse until ages 22 to 25. Therefore, it is important to keep in mind that in young patients, apparent sternoclavicular (SC) dislocations may actually represent growth plate injury.

The clavicle is shaped like a musical symbol, taking its name from *clavis,* the Latin word for *key.*[17] Its lateral end is flat in cross section and serves as a connection to the upper extremity via the acromioclavicular (AC) joint as well as through the coracoclavicular (CC) ligaments. The CC ligaments connect the coracoid process to the medial aspect of the distal third of the clavicle. These connections serve a suspensory role. Fractures of the distal third of the clavicle, proximal to the CC ligaments, can interfere with this suspensory mechanism. This creates a situation in which the distal fragment can be pulled inferiorly with the upper extremity, which is no longer suspended from the trunk. As a result, the patient may experience brachial plexus symptoms from excess traction or nonunion of the distal clavicular fracture.

The middle third of the clavicle has a more tubular configuration and contains the thinnest cross section. Biomechancial studies have shown that this portion of the clavicle is the weakest.[19] This correlates with clinical ex-

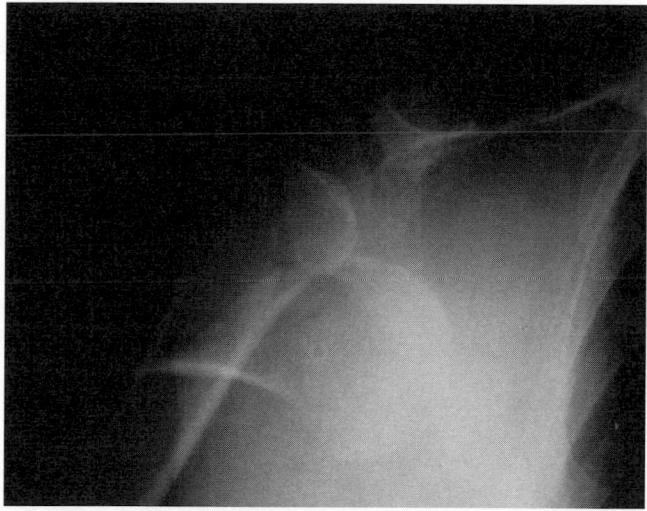

A

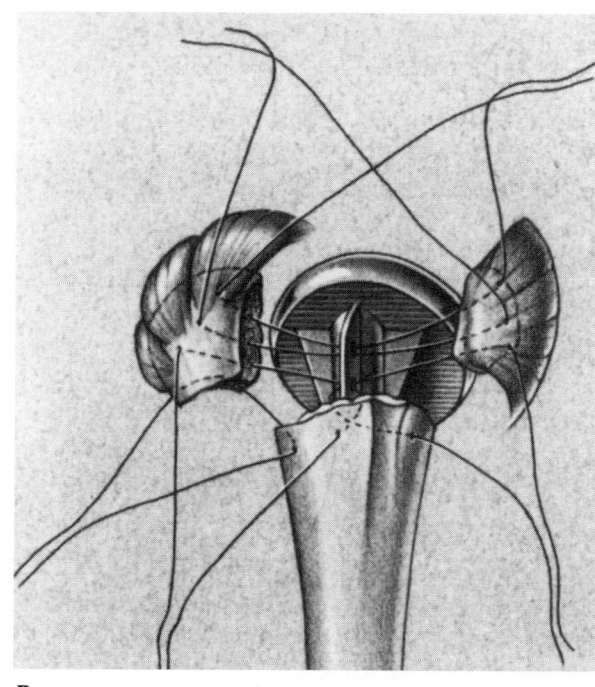

B

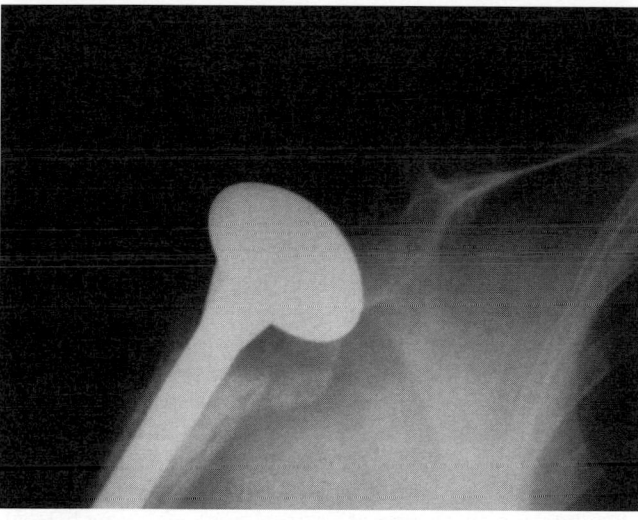

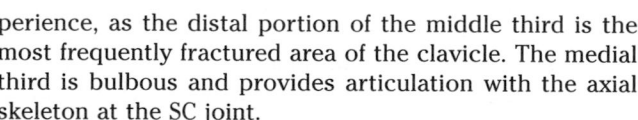

C

Figure 20-7 *A.* Anteroposterior view of a four-part anterior fracture dislocation in an elderly patient. *B.* Schematic of humeral head replacement with tuberosity fixation using heavy nonabsorbable suture. [Reproduced with permission from Bigliani LU, Flatow EL, Pollock RG: Fractures of the proximal humerus, in Rockwood CA, Green DP, Bucholz RW, et al (eds): *Fractures in Adults, 4th ed.* Philadelphia, Lippincott-Raven, 1996, pp 1055–1107.] *C.* Anteroposterior radiograph showing humeral head replacement with healed tuberosity fragments in patient from Fig. 20-7A.

perience, as the distal portion of the middle third is the most frequently fractured area of the clavicle. The medial third is bulbous and provides articulation with the axial skeleton at the SC joint.

Incidence and Etiology

The clavicle is one of the most frequently fractured bones in the human body.[20] The majority of clavicular fractures occur as a result of a fall on the outstretched upper extremity or from a fall or blow on the point of the shoulder. However, high-energy direct trauma, as occurs during motor vehicle accidents, is becoming a relatively frequent cause in adults, with many of the fractures occurring at the lateral end of the clavicle. These high-energy injuries are associated with a higher rate of delayed union or nonunion.[21]

Classification

Fractures of the clavicle have been subdivided into three groups according to location.[21] Group I are the common

middle third fractures; group II are fractures of the lateral third; and group III are medial third fractures, which are often undisplaced (Table 20-1).

The lateral and medial thirds have been further subclassified by Neer and others as is also seen in Table 20-1.[14,22]

Middle-Third Fractures (Group I)

Fractures of the middle third are by far the most common, accounting for 80 percent of all clavicular fractures.[20] Most occur at the lateral aspect of the middle third, where the bone changes shape from tubular to flatter, making this a relatively weaker zone.

Lateral-Third Fractures (Group II)

Fractures of the lateral third account for 12 to 15 percent of all clavicular fractures.[23] Neer recognized that these fractures were unique because of the influence of the CC ligaments and subclassified them with regards to the relative position of the CC ligaments[21,24] (Fig. 20-8). Fractures

TABLE 20-1 Classification of Clavicular Fractures

Group I—middle-third fractures
Group II—distal-third fractures
   Type I—minimal displacement (interligamentous)
   Type II—displacement secondary to fracture medial to the
      coracoclavicular ligaments
   Type III—articular surface fractures
   Type IV—ligaments intact to periosteum (children), with
      displacement of the proximal fragment
   Type V—comminuted, with ligaments not attached
      proximally or distally but to an inferior, comminuted
      fragment
Group III—proximal-third fractures
   Type I—minimal displacement
   Type II—significant displacement (ligaments ruptured)
   Type III—intraarticular
   Type IV—epiphyseal separation (children and young
      adults)
   Type V—comminuted

Source: Reproduced with permission from Craig EV: Fractures of the
clavicle, in Rockwood CA, Matsen FA (eds): *The Shoulder.*
Philadelphia, Saunders, 1990.

that occur lateral to the CC ligaments are type I fractures
and make up the majority of distal clavicular fractures.
The fracture does not displace because the ligaments continue to hold the medial fragment in the proper position
with regard to the lateral fragment. Type II fractures occur
medial to the CC ligaments and are more likely to displace,
since the ligaments are unable to maintain the position of
the medial fragment (Fig. 20-9A). Instead, the weight of the
arm and the force of the muscles pull the distal fragment
away from the medial fragment. Neer pointed out that the
type II fractures are more likely to develop a nonunion because of the deforming forces described above as well as
the high energy generating these injuries. For that reason,
he advocated early ORIF treatment of type II fractures.[24]

Fractures that occur at the very lateral end, involving
the articular surface, are classified as type III fractures.
These fractures almost always heal but can result in degenerative arthritis of the AC joint. Rockwood and others
have added two additional types of distal clavicular frac-

ture.[25] Type IV fractures occur in children. In these fractures, the CC ligaments and periosteal sleeve of the distal
clavicle become avulsed as a result of a growth plate injury. The distal clavicle is not ossified and therefore radiographs appear to show an AC separation. The type V fracture is a rare occurrence in adults and results when the
distal clavicle is severely comminuted. The CC ligaments
lose all sites of attachment to the proximal and distal fragments while remaining attached to an inferior comminuted
fragment.

Medial-Third Fractures (Group III)

Fractures of the medial third of the clavicle account for
only 5 to 6 percent of all clavicular fractures.[23] It is important to remember that these fractures may involve the
growth plate of the medial clavicle, which may not fuse
until early in the third decade of life. The group III fractures can be classified in a fashion similar to the group II
fractures, as shown in Table 20-1.

Clinical Presentation

Clavicular fractures are easily recognized and rarely
missed even in young children. The subcutaneous position
of the bone makes most fractures readily apparent. They
are usually associated with a prominence, with the proximal fragment being displaced superiorly in most instances.
Subcutaneous swelling and ecchymosis occur acutely.
Distal or proximal fractures may present in a fashion similar to AC separations or SC dislocations, respectively.

Physical exam reveals tenderness and crepitus at the
fracture site. The skin is most often intact but must be
carefully assessed to rule out an open fracture. In many instances, the skin may contain abrasions as a result of a fall
on the shoulder. This should be carefully assessed, as it
may interfere with operative treatment when such treatment is indicated. Although most clavicle fractures are not
associated with injuries to surrounding structures, a complete physical examination is necessary to be certain that
a life- or limb-threatening injury is not present.

Associated injuries that must be considered include
lesions to the lung, neurovascular structures, and skin. In
many instances the skin remains intact but becomes se-

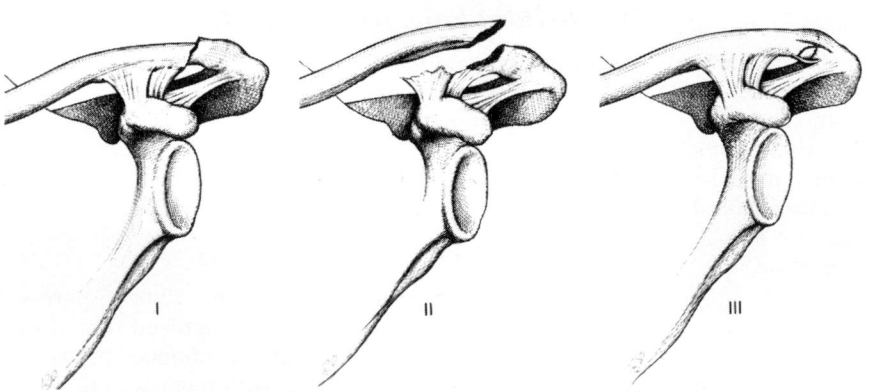

Figure 20-8 Subclassification of lateral (distal) clavicular fractures of types I, II, and III.

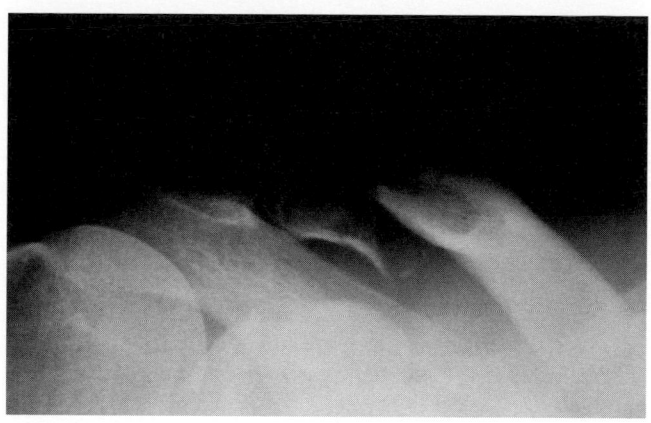

A

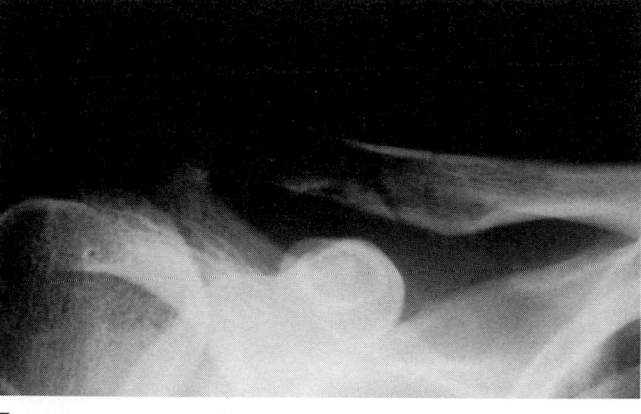

B

Figure 20-9 *A.* Type II distal clavicle fracture in a 22-year-old male after a biking accident. *B.* The fracture was treated with heavy suture fixation to the base of the coracoid and suture cerclage at the fracture site; it healed in good alignment.

verely tented over the fracture site, with the potential for erosion and the development of an open fracture. All of these associated injuries must be addressed and may mandate treatment with ORIF in unstable fractures.

The type of fracture is accurately defined by obtaining proper radiographs. Middle-third fractures are best evaluated with an AP view and a 45° cephalic tilt view. An additional 45° caudal tilt view provides a view that is 90° to the cephalic tilt view and can serve to further quantify displacement. Lateral-third fractures should be evaluated with an AP view with reduced exposure, a lateral Y view, and an axillary view. Medial-third fractures may require computed tomography to determine the extent of injury accurately.

Treatment Methods

Middle-Third Fractures

Nonoperative The great majority of middle-third clavicular fractures heal uneventfully with a variety of closed, nonoperative methods. Most middle-third clavicular fractures are associated with mild shortening and overriding of the fragments. A closed reduction is usually attempted by arching the patient's thoracic spine and pulling the shoulders backward in an attempt bring the distal fragment up and back. The goal of the reduction maneuver is to interdigitate the fragments in hopes of maintaining alignment. Limited immobilization in the form of a figure-of-eight bandage or a sling (with or without swath) is then applied.

The figure-of-eight bandage was introduced to help maintain the position of the reduction.[23] However, in two studies comparing figure-of-eight dressings to sling treatment, it was noted that figure-of-eight dressings were difficult to maintain and that their use was more likely to lead to complications such as neurovascular compression or skin breakdown.[26,27] The authors demonstrated that there was very little difference in outcome, with both groups having similar cosmetic deformities and alignment of the healed fracture virtually unchanged from the initial degree of displacement. With either treatment, it is important to

initiate physical therapy with shoulder motion as soon as symptoms allow.

Operative Operative treatment is indicated when the skin or neurovascular structures are compromised as a result of an unstable midshaft clavicular fracture. Operative treatment consists of ORIF with plate and screws or, less preferably, intramedullary devices. Even though the bone is small, fixation should be carried out with a strong plate, such as a low-contact dynamic compression plate, to withstand the high-level forces experienced at the clavicle. Smaller plates are more likely to break prior to healing of the fracture.[17]

High-energy injuries such as those occurring with motor vehicle accidents are more likely to result in segmental comminution or significant shortening of the fracture. Some series have shown postoperative pain and dysfunction related to shortening greater than 1.5 cm. These high-energy fractures are also associated with a higher rate of nonunion. For these reasons, some surgeons have advocated acute treatment with ORIF in cases with significant shortening.[23]

Lateral-Third Fractures

Group II fractures are treated according to fracture type and displacement. The Neer subcategories of type I and III fractures rarely become displaced and heal well with sling support. Healed type III fractures may produce AC arthritis as a result of incongruity at the joint surface. Type II fractures are generally associated with displacement and a higher prevalence of nonunion. In a recent study, patients with type II fractures treated nonoperatively were found to have a 31 percent rate of pseudoarthrosis.[28] Neer has advocated that these fractures be treated with early ORIF.[24] If the type II fracture is relatively nondisplaced and remains so over a 2- to 3-week period, as documented by serial radiographs, the fracture can be safely treated nonoperatively. Most of these represent type IIB fractures (Table 20-1) in which the fracture is actually located at the site of CC ligament insertion, with some portion of the CC ligaments remaining intact and inserting at the medial fragment.

Operative treatment of displaced type II fractures is carried out in many ways, including pins placed across the AC joint and fracture, screws through the proximal fragment into the coracoid, and suture fixation of the proximal fragment to the coracoid. The suture technique avoids the requirement for later screw removal and the potential for AC arthritis with pin placement. Heavy sutures are placed around the base of the coracoid and through the anterior clavicle, pulling the distal fragment up in alignment with the proximal fragment. An additional cerclage suture around the fracture provides added fixation (Fig. 20-9). The patient is placed in a sling for 4 to 6 weeks with supine shoulder range-of-motion exercises beginning within the first few weeks.

Medial-Third Fractures

Fractures of the proximal clavicle are generally treated with sling support unless there is neurovascular compromise. Whenever possible, ORIF should carried out with a plate and screws, since intramedullary fixation at the medial clavicle has been associated with life-threatening complications.

Complications

Fortunately, the majority of clavicular fractures heal uneventfully. The nonunion rate for group I fractures treated nonoperatively is approximately 1 percent.[29] Type II fractures have a higher rate of nonunion with nonoperative treatment, but this can be reduced to negligible rates with operative intervention. Since middle-third fractures are by far the most frequent type of clavicular fracture, approximately 85 percent of clavicular nonunions occur within this zone. Some 75 percent of patients with clavicular nonunions will develop symptoms of moderate to severe pain. When a painful nonunion develops, operative intervention with autogenous bone grafting and rigid fixation is indicated. In cases with atrophic nonunion and significant shortening, an intercalary bone graft may be necessary to restore length.[23] A success rate greater than 90 percent can be expected using these techniques when rigid fixation is provided by a strong plate or intramedullary device.[23]

Malunion may occur and cause compression of neurovascular structures or significant shortening of the clavicle. The patient may experience pain and dysfunction of the upper extremity. Operative intervention with "bumpectomy" or osteotomy, bone grafting, and internal fixation may be required. Symptomatic posttraumatic arthritis at the SC or AC joints may occur as sequelae from medial or lateral intraarticular fractures involving the respective joints. These are successfully treated with resection of the medial or lateral ends of the clavicle.

SCAPULAR FRACTURES

Relevant Anatomy

The scapula articulates with the humerus at the glenohumeral joint, the clavicle at the acromioclavicular joint, and the thorax at the scapulothoracic joint. Motion at the scapulothoracic and glenohumeral articulations is coordinated in a rhythmic fashion.[17] This coordinated motion is accomplished through the complex interaction of several muscles that envelope the scapula. These include the trapezius, serratus anterior, levator scapulae, and rhomboid muscles, which serve as motors for scapulothoracic motion. It also includes the rotator cuff, deltoid, and teres major muscles, which provide glenohumeral motion.

The suprascapular and axillary nerves are vulnerable to injury with scapular trauma due to their proximity to the scapula. The suprascapular nerve is particularly vulnerable as it traverses the scapular notch to innervate the supraspinatus and further laterally at the spinoglenoid notch prior to innervating the infraspinatus.

The scapula is partially suspended by the clavicle, which connects to the scapula via the AC joint as well as through the CC ligaments between the coracoid and distal clavicle. These connections make up the superior shoulder suspensory complex as described by Goss.[30] Failure of this complex can result in a loss of the suspensory function and a drooping shoulder.

Incidence and Etiology

Scapular fractures are relatively uncommon, representing only 1 percent of all fractures.[30,31] The extensive muscular coverage of the scapula protects it from both direct and indirect trauma. The encapsulating muscles allow the scapula to recoil on impact, dissipating applied force.[14,17] Fractures of the scapula are usually the result of considerable traumatic forces, such as those that would be associated with motor vehicle accidents. For this reason, the treating physician should be alert to the possibility of concomitant injuries such as rib fractures and pneumothorax.[30] In rare cases, the scapula has become avulsed from its muscular attachment to the chest wall. This type of injury is known as a *scapulothoracic dissociation* and is almost universally associated with a neurovascular injury, including disruption of the subclavian artery and/or brachial plexus.[32] Diagnosis is based on the presence of massive soft tissue swelling coupled with neurovascular compromise.

While direct high-energy trauma is the most common way in which a scapular fracture is produced, many indirect forces are also known to contribute to scapular fractures. These include forceful muscular contractions, which may cause fractures of the coracoid. Avulsion fractures may also occur by the same mechanism at the superior scapular angle where the levator scapula inserts, at the inferior angle of the scapula where the serratus anterior inserts, and at portions of the acromial origin of the deltoid muscle.[30] Other indirect causes include stress fractures of the acromion, which may result from overuse in sports or in association with rotator cuff tear arthropathy.[33,34]

Scapular body and spinal fractures account for approximately 50 percent of scapular fractures. Fractures of the neck of the glenoid account for approximately 25 percent of all scapular fractures. The glenoid fossa is involved in only approximately 10 percent of all scapular fractures. Both acromial and coracoid processes are involved in approximately 7 percent of scapular fractures.[30]

Classification

Fractures of the scapula are classified according to anatomic area, including the glenoid fossa, glenoid neck, scapular prominences (i.e., acromion), and scapular body fractures. Glenoid fossa fractures have been further classified by Ideberg into five categories.[35] This scheme has been modified by Goss (Fig. 20-10).[30]

As emphasized by Goss, when classifying the above injuries, it is important to note whether or not there is an associated injury that has compromised the integrity of the superior shoulder suspensory complex (SSSC).[30] The SSSC is a bone–soft tissue ring sitting at the end of the clavicle and the lateral scapular body and spine. The ring consists of the superior glenoid cavity, the coracoid process, the coracoclavicular ligaments, the distal clavicle, the AC joint, and the acromion. If an associated injury is present, it produces the potential for a double disrup-

tion within the complex. Double disruptions, whether they be double fractures or a fracture and a soft tissue disruption, are more likely to result in significant displacements at either or both sites as compared to the situation in which only a single disruption is present.[30] This is particularly true when one of the two injuries is a glenoid neck fracture. In this scenario, the associated injury contributes to instability at the glenoid neck fracture site and results in a floating shoulder.[36,37] This scenario commonly occurs in association with a clavicular fracture. Leung et al. and Herscovici et al. have shown that isolated fixation of the clavicular fracture is an effective treatment for this problem, as it results in an indirect reduction of the glenoid neck fracture in most cases.[36,37]

Clinical Presentation

Scapular fractures are associated with a considerable amount of pain, prompting most patients to hold the arm in an adducted position to protect it from all movements, especially elevation. The fracture results in hemorrhage into the supraspinatus, infraspinatus, and subscapularis muscles, causing spasm and often mimicking a rotator cuff

Figure 20-10 Classification scheme for glenoid cavity fractures: type Ia, anterior rim; type Ib, posterior rim; type III, fracture line through the glenoid fossa exiting at the superior border of the scapula; type IV, fracture line through the glenoid fossa exiting at the medial border of the scapula; type Va, combination of types II and IV; type Vb, combination of types III and IV; type Vc, combination of types II, III, and IV; type VI, comminuted. (Reproduced with permission from Goss TP: Scapular fractures and dislocations: Diagnosis and treatment. *J AAOS* 3:22–33, 1995.)

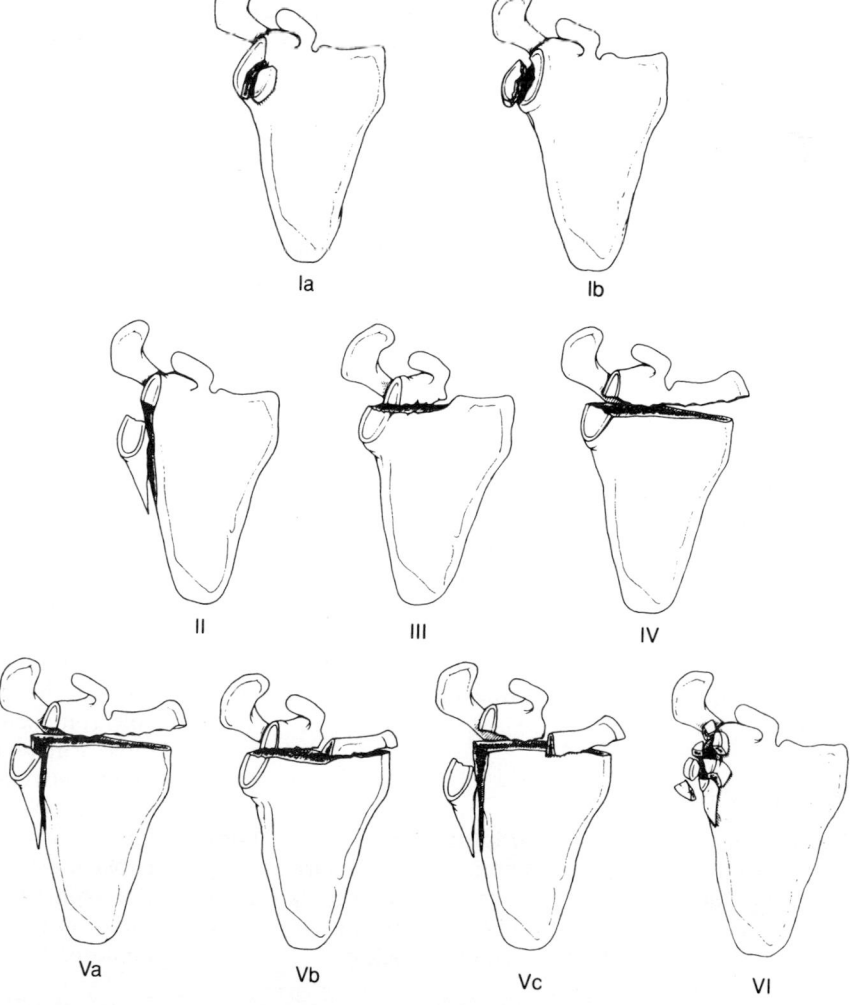

injury. Local pain, crepitus, swelling, and ecchymosis are appreciated. A complete neurovascular exam as well as an exam of the chest and lungs is important to rule out associated injuries.

When a scapular fracture is suspected, it is important to obtain a true scapular AP view as well as Y scapular and axillary views. Once the scapular fracture is verified on plain radiographs, it is important to obtain a computed tomography (CT) scan for comprehensive radiographic evaluation. The complex osseous anatomy of the scapula makes it very difficult to map out the anatomy of the fracture precisely without CT imaging. This is especially important in cases where a glenoid fossa fracture is present or suspected.

Treatment

Glenoid

Fractures of the glenoid rim (type I) are treated nonoperatively when stability of the glenohumeral joint is maintained. When the humeral head subluxates or dislocates because of the fracture, operative intervention is indicated. This can be expected when the fracture is displaced by more than 5 to 10 mm and involves 20 to 30 percent of the articular surface.[30] Small cannulated lag screws are used through either an anterior or posterior approach as dictated by fracture location. Heavy nonabsorbable sutures are employed when comminution precludes the use of a screw.

Fractures of the articular fossa (types II, III, IV, and V) are treated surgically when an articular step-off of 5 to 10 mm or greater exists, particularly when the humeral head is pushed eccentrically as a result of the fracture. In most instances, a posterior approach is utilized. With comminuted type VI fractures, nonoperative management is usually indicated, since fixation is tenuous and may result in extensive soft tissue stripping.[30] The shoulder should be placed in a position that maximizes articular congruity, while allowing early range-of-motion exercises.

Glenoid Neck

Most fractures of the glenoid neck remain relatively nondisplaced and nonangulated; they are treated with sling support and early range-of-motion exercises. When displacement is greater than 10 mm or angulatory deformity greater than 40° in either the transverse or coronal plane, the probability of chronic pain and dysfunction increases.[38] These fractures should be treated surgically through a posterior approach with fixation using a reconstruction plate.

Scapular Body

Fortunately, most scapular fractures occur in the body and are relatively nondisplaced. Owing to surrounding muscle groups, the fractured scapular body heals rapidly with very little residual disability. Early range-of-motion exercises are initiated when symptoms allow.

Scapular Prominences

Most prominence fractures, such as coracoid fractures, remain relatively nondisplaced as a result of the stabilizing effects of surrounding soft tissue structures. These fractures are treated nonoperatively with range-of-motion exercises beginning within the first few weeks, as symptoms allow. Acromion fractures present and behave similarly. However, when angulation or displacement results in considerable narrowing of the subacromial outlet, it is wise to reduce the fracture acutely and stabilize it with a tension-band technique to prevent rotator cuff disease.[14]

Complications

Scapular fractures involving the glenoid articular surface may result in glenohumeral arthritis, especially if articular incongruency exists. Appropriate operative intervention reduces the likelihood of this. Malunited fractures of the scapular body may result in the development of scapular prominences and resultant scapulothoracic bursitis.

DISLOCATIONS OF THE SHOULDER AND SHOULDER GIRDLE

Incidence

In a recent study of 1600 shoulder and shoulder girdle injuries, nearly 25 percent were dislocations, with 84 percent of these being anterior glenohumeral dislocations, 12 percent acromioclavicular, 2.5 percent sternoclavicular, and 1.5 percent posterior glenohumeral dislocations.[39] Although some dislocations of the glenohumeral joint are the result of congenital laxity, Rowe has suggested that greater than 90 percent of all glenohumeral dislocations are related to trauma.[40]

Glenohumeral Dislocations

Etiology

As described elsewhere in this text, the shoulder's basic design sacrifices stability for motion, making it the most commonly dislocated joint in the body. Dislocations of the glenohumeral joint can result from direct trauma, such as a blow to the humeral head, or more commonly from indirect trauma. The more common anterior dislocation is usually the result of excessive combined hyperabduction and external rotation forces. Posterior dislocations can result from axial loading of the abducted and internally rotated arm. Many posterior dislocations are the result of violent muscle contractions secondary to convulsive seizures or electric shock. In this mechanism, the stronger internal rotators (latissimus dorsi, pectoralis major, and subscapularis) overpower the weaker external rotators (infraspinatus and teres minor muscles). Inferior dislocations may result from forced abduction in which the humerus levers against the acromion.

Clinical Presentation

Patients typically present in extreme pain, with the involved arm held immobile. The normal contour of the deltoid is lost, as it is pulled into the void left by the dislocated humeral head. In anterior dislocations, the arm is held in slight abduction and external rotation and internal rotation is blocked. Posterior dislocations are less obvious, with the arm held in adduction and internal rotation. External rotation is blocked with posterior dislocations. In the rare inferior dislocation, or luxatio erecta, the humerus becomes locked in a position of 90° abduction or greater.

The physical examination should include a complete neurovascular exam to rule out the possibility of an associated neurovascular injury. Radiographs including an AP and Y scapular view are extremely important in the definitive diagnosis of glenohumeral dislocations. In most cases, an axillary lateral view should also be obtained, as it will accurately determine whether or not a dislocation is present and in what direction it has occurred.

Treatment

After the dislocation is fully evaluated, initial treatment consists of a closed reduction that is performed as soon as possible. Most dislocations are noted acutely and can be reduced easily in an emergency room setting with muscle relaxation and sedation. If a dislocation is more than 24 h old, it is considered chronic and may require a closed or open reduction in the operating room with general anesthesia. Closed reduction of an acute dislocation can often be facilitated by the administration of local anesthesia using 20 mL of 1% lidocaine injected directly into the glenohumeral joint and subacromial bursa through a lateral approach.[41] Comfort and relaxation are the most important elements to ensure success of closed reduction attempts.

A variety of reduction maneuvers that employ the principles of traction and leverage have been successfully used through the years. Many of the leverage techniques are currently avoided, as they increase the likelihood of neurovascular injury. The most popular method is the traction and countertraction method, in which an assistant stabilizes the torso with a folded sheet wrapped across the chest while the physician applies gentle traction along the involved arm[42] (Fig. 20-11). The traction is applied in line with the deformity and gradually increased, along with gentle internal and external rotation, until the head disengages from the glenoid rim and reduces. If the physician is alone, the Hippocratic method is a successfully utilized maneuver.[42] The same maneuvers are performed, but countertraction is supplied by the examiner's foot, which extends all the way across both anterior and posterior axillary folds with pressure at the chest wall. The neurovascular examination is repeated after the reduction. Once the success of the reduction is verified by an axillary radiograph, the patient is immobilized for a period of time, followed by supervised therapy and a period of restriction from return to full activity. The goal is to provide adequate time for tissue healing in order to minimize the potential for redislocation. Anterior dislocators are placed in a sling and swath.

Posterior dislocators are placed in a brace with the arm at the side in neutral rotation and flexion-extension.

Recurrence of a dislocation is more likely to occur in teenagers than in older individuals. The period of immobilization is controversial. Most authors recommend immobilization for a period of 2 to 4 weeks. Simonet and Cofield found that patients treated in this manner had a redislocation rate that varied with age and activity.[43] Patients younger than 20 years had a recurrence rate of 66 percent, while those between 20 and 40 years had a 40 percent rate. However, the redislocation rate for athletes younger than 30 years was 82 percent. Arciero described similar results and advocates acute surgical intervention with arthroscopic Bankart repair techniques, reducing the redislocation rate to 12 percent. For this reason, he recommends acute arthroscopic repair in athletes younger than 24 years of age.[41]

Complications

Glenohumeral dislocations can result in rotator cuff tears, especially in older individuals. In patients above age 40, the incidence exceeds 40 percent, and it increases to more than 80 percent in patients over the age of 60.[44] The risk of neurologic injury also increases with age. Axillary nerve injury may occur in as many as 35 percent of dislocations. Other common complications include glenoid rim fractures, tuberosity fractures, and humeral head impression fractures. Chronic instability may result after a dislocation. Treatment of this is described elsewhere in this text.

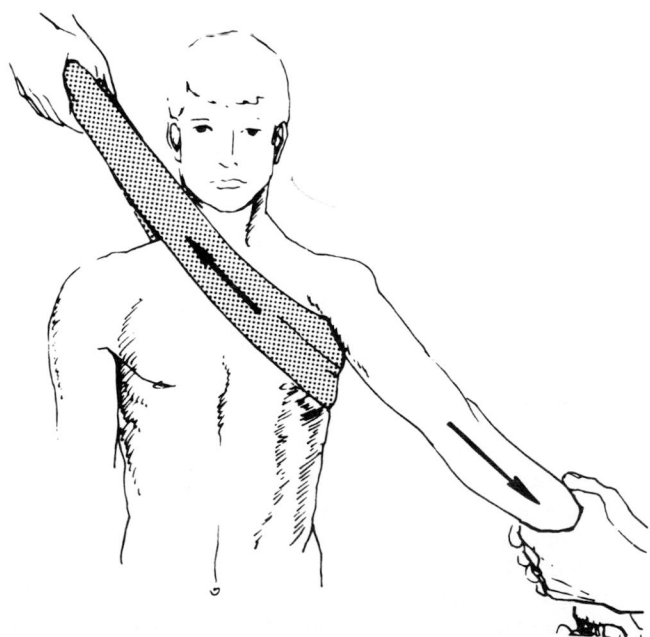

Figure 20-11 Traction-countertraction method for reduction of an anterior dislocation of the shoulder. (Reproduced with permission from Warner JJP, Caborn DN. Overview of shoulder instability. *Crit Rev Phys Rehab Med* 4:145–198, 1992.)

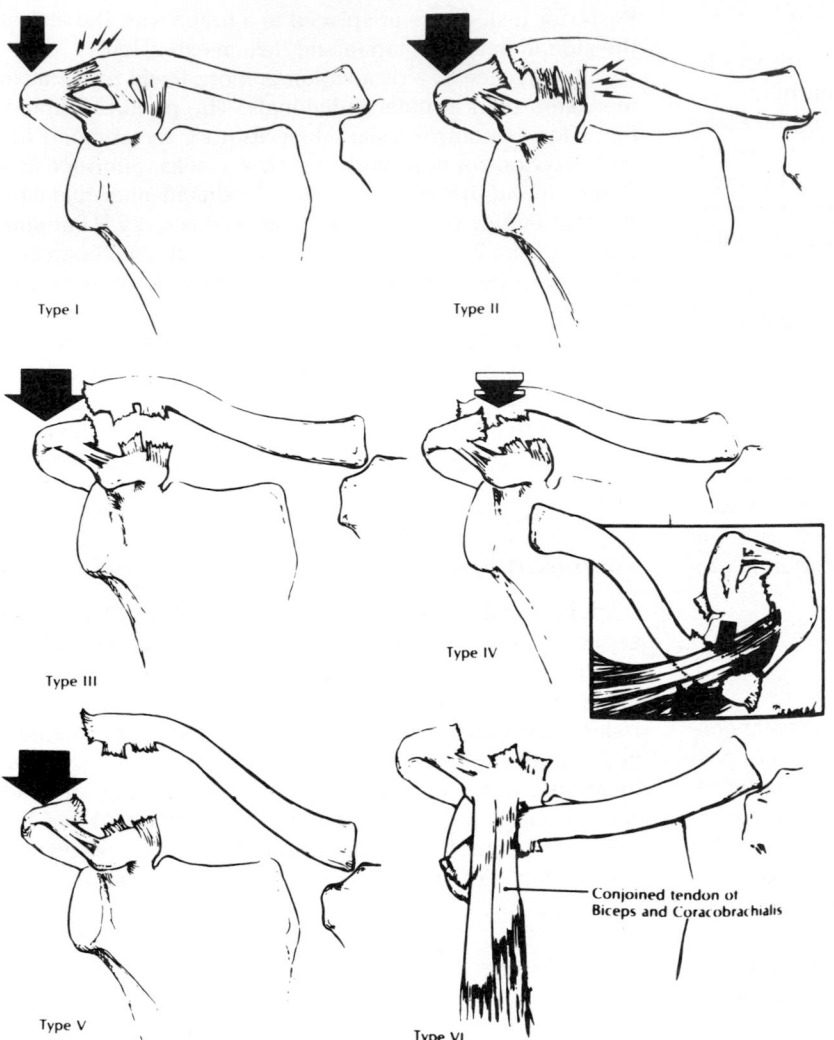

Figure 20-12 Schematic drawings of AC separations. [Reproduced with permission from Rockwood CA, Williams GR, Young DC: Injuries to the acromioclavicular joint, in Rockwood CA, Green DP, Bucholz RW, et al (eds): *Fractures in Adults, 4th ed.* Philadelphia, Lippincott-Raven, 1996, pp 1341–1413.]

Acromioclavicular Separations

Etiology

The stability of the AC joint is maintained by two sets of ligaments: the AC capsuloligamentous complex and the CC ligaments.[17] The most common mechanism of injury is a direct force that occurs from a fall on the point of the shoulder. The weaker AC capsuloligamentous structures fail first, followed by the CC ligaments.[14]

Classification

Acromioclavicular separations are classified according to the severity of the injury, as shown in Fig. 20-12. A mild force results in a sprain or type I injury to the AC capsuloligamentous structures without disrupting the normal alignment. Moderate force results in disruption of the AC joint capsuloligamentous structures and mild sprain of the CC ligaments; it is classified as a type II separation. More severe force results in disruption of both sets of ligaments and a minimum of 100 percent translation of the distal clavicular articular surface and produces types III through VI AC separations.[14] When this occurs, the patient loses the suspensory support of the clavicle and the upper extremity droops downward.

Clinical Presentation

Type I AC separations present with a normal shoulder contour and tenderness at the AC joint. Type II injuries present with an obvious bump at the AC joint and tenderness. Type III through VI separations are identified by drooping of the arm and a prominent, tender deformity at the AC joint. In type IV separations, the distal clavicle lies posteriorly. In type V dislocations, the distal clavicle lies subcutaneously, having pierced the trapezius. In rare type VI separations, the clavicle is palpated beneath the coracoid.[45] With all suspected AC separations, a complete neurovascular exam is important to rule out a traction injury to the brachial plexus.

A complete set of radiographs is important in documenting the severity of the separation. This should include a standing AP view and an axillary lateral view. Comparison views of the contralateral shoulder are taken and the coracoclavicular distance is compared from side to side. Stress radiographs taken with 10- to 15-lb weights hanging from the arms may be helpful in determining severity in borderline cases.

Treatment

Acute Injuries Type I and II injuries are treated with a short period of sling support and early therapy. Full activities are resumed when symptoms allow. Type III injuries are treated in the same fashion. However, some surgeons recommend acute surgical intervention in young overhead athletes or laborers who are likely to develop chronic pain and dysfunction from the loss of their suspensory mechanism. Types IV, V, and VI are treated with acute surgical intervention.

Acute surgical intervention involves open reduction of the AC joint through a superior approach and fixation of the clavicle to the coracoid base, using heavy suture or screws.[46] The patient is kept in a sling for 2 to 6 weeks and range-of-motion exercises are initiated. The patient is instructed to avoid heavy labor or sports for 12 weeks.

Chronic Injuries Type III AC separations that are 3 weeks old are more likely to involve early degenerative AC arthrosis and scarred CC ligaments. Patients appropriate for operative intervention should undergo distal clavicular excision with transfer of the CC ligament into the end of the clavicle in addition to fixation to the coracoid, as above.[14] Patients with nonoperatively treated type III through VI separations who have persistent pain and dysfunction of the shoulder after 3 to 6 months are also candidates for this procedure.

Complications

The most common problem associated with type I and II separations is AC arthrosis requiring AC resection surgery. In some cases, the residual instability present in a type II separation may necessitate stabilization of the distal clavicle by CC ligament transfer into its end. A chronic untreated type III (or higher) AC separation may result in rotator cuff disease from loss of scapulothoracic motion.[14] It may also result in brachial plexus traction symptoms from the loss of the clavicular suspensory function.

Sternoclavicular Dislocations

Etiology and Clinical Presentation

Stability of the sternoclavicular joint is provided by the joint capsule and the costoclavicular and interclavicular ligaments.[17] Most dislocations are the result of indirect trauma from motor vehicle accidents or sports. Anterior dislocations are the most common and are caused by excessive compression along the clavicle when the ipsilateral shoulder is rolled backward. Posterior dislocations occur in the same fashion when the shoulder is rolled forward.[14]

The clinical presentation is that of pain and swelling at the medial clavicle. In many instances it is difficult to determine whether or not the sternoclavicular joint remains dislocated and in which direction. A complete neurovascular exam should be performed to rule out compromise from the displaced medial clavicular pole. The patient may present with hoarseness or dyspnea from pressure against the respiratory tract. Radiologic tests are essential in the diagnosis. Special radiographic views, such as the serendipity view, can be helpful.[47] However, in many cases, plain radiographic views are inconclusive and CT is needed to determine the degree and direction of dislocation accurately.

Treatment

Anterior dislocations are treated with closed reduction under adequate sedation. Closed reduction is performed with the patient lying supine, with a sandbag between the shoulders and posteriorly directed pressure at the SC joint. Many will remain unstable and are usually not improved by open surgical intervention. Posterior dislocations should be reduced in the operating room with general anesthesia. When vascular injury is suspected from the physical exam, vascular studies should be obtained to diminish potential further arterial compromise as a result of reduction maneuvers. A closed reduction is attempted with the patient lying supine with a sandbag between the shoulders while traction is applied along the abducted and extended arm. If this is unsuccessful, a sterile towel clamp is used to pull the clavicle forward. In some cases an open reduction may be required. Once reduced, most posterior dislocations remain stable and are placed in a sling or figure-of-eight dressing for a few weeks, followed by progressive therapy. It is important to remember that many apparent sternoclavicular dislocations in patients less than 17 years of age actually represent growth plate injuries that will remodel without treatment.

Complications

The most severe complications associated with SC dislocations include pneumothorax, neurovascular compromise of the underlying great vessels, and tracheal or esophageal rupture. The long-term sequelae of SC dislocations include the potential for SC arthritis. This can be successfully treated with SC resection.

REFERENCES

1. Kristiansen B, Christensen SW: Proximal humeral fractures. *Acta Orthop Scand* 58:124–127, 1987.
2. Laing PG: The arterial supply of the adult humerus. *J Bone Joint Surg* 38A:1105–1116, 1956.
3. Bigliani LU, Flatow EL, Pollock RG: Fractures of the proximal humerus, in Rockwood CA, Green DP, Bucholz RW, et al (eds): *Fractures in Adults, 4th ed.* Philadelphia, Lippincott-Raven, 1996, pp 1055–1107.
4. Lind T, Kroner TK, Jensen J: The epidemiology of fractures of the proximal humerus. *Arch Orthop Trauma Surg* 108:285–287, 1989.
5. Rose SH, Melton LJ, Morrey BF, et al: Epidemiologic features of humeral fractures. *Clin Orthop* 168:24–30, 1982.
6. Neer CS II: Displaced proximal humeral fractures: I. Classification and evaluation. *J Bone Joint Surg* 52A:1077–1089, 1970.
7. Neer CS II: Displaced proximal humeral fractures: II. Treatment of three-part and four-part displacement. *J Bone Joint Surg* 52A:1090–1103, 1970.
8. Codman EA: *The Shoulder: Rupture of the Supraspinatus Tendon and Other Lesions in or About the Subacromial Bursa.* Boston, Thomas Todd, 1934.
9. Bloom MH, Obata W: Diagnosis of posterior dislocation of the shoulder with the use of the velpeau axillary and angle-up radiographic views. *J Bone Joint Surg* 49A:943–949, 1967.
10. McLaughlin HL: Dislocation of the shoulder with tuberosity fracture. *Surg Clin North Am* 43:1615–1620, 1963.

11. Greeley PW, Magnuson PB: Dislocation of the shoulder accompanied by fracture of the greater tuberosity and complicated by spinatus tendon injury. *JAMA* 102:1835–1838, 1934.

12. Cuomo F, Flatow EL, Maday M, et al: Open reduction and internal fixation of two- and three-part displaced surgical neck fractures of the proximal humerus. *J Shoulder Elbow Surg* 1:287–295, 1992.

13. Flatow EL, Cuomo F, Maday MG: Open reduction and internal fixation of two-part displaced fractures of the greater tuberosity of the proximal part of the humerus. *J Bone Joint Surg* 73A:1213–1218, 1991.

14. Neer CS II: *Shoulder Reconstruction.* Philadelphia, Saunders, 1990.

15. Jakob RP, Miniaci A, Anson PS, et al: Four-part valgus impacted fractures of the proximal humerus. *J Bone Joint Surg* 73B:295–298, 1991.

16. Hagg O, Lundberg B: Aspects of prognostic factors in comminuted and dislocated proximal humeral fractures, in Bateman JE, Welsh RP (eds): *Surgery of the Shoulder.* Philadelphia, Decker, 1984, pp 51–59.

17. Flatow EL: The biomechanics of the acromioclavicular, sternoclavicular, and scapulothoracic joints. *AAOS Instr Course Lect* 42:237–245, 1993.

18. Moseley HF: The clavicle: Its anatomy and function. *Clin Orthop* 58:17–27, 1968.

19. Harrington MA, Keller TS, Seiler JG, et al: Geometric properties and the predicted mechanical behavior of adult human clavicles. *J Biomech* 26:417–426, 1993.

20. Rowe CR: An atlas of anatomy and treatment of midclavicular fractures. *Clin Orthop* 58:29–42, 1968.

21. Neer CS II: Fracture of the distal clavicle with detachment of coracoclavicular ligaments in adults. *J Trauma* 3:99–110, 1963.

22. Allman FL: Fractures and ligamentous injuries of the clavicle and its articulation. *J Bone Joint Surg* 49A:774–784, 1967.

23. Craig EV: Fractures of the clavicle, in Rockwood CA, Matsen FA (eds): *The Shoulder.* Philadelphia, Saunders, 1990.

24. Neer CS II: Fractures of the distal third of the clavicle. *Clin Orthop* 58:43–50, 1968.

25. Rockwood CA: Fractures of the outer clavicle in children and adults. *J Bone Joint Surg* 64B:642, 1982.

26. Anderson K, Jensen PO, Lauritzen J: Treatment of clavicular fractures: Figure of eight bandage vs a simple sling. *Acta Orthop Scand* 57:71–74, 1987.

27. McCandless DN, Mowbray M: Treatment of displaced fractures of the clavicle: Sling vs figure-of-eight bandage. *Practitioner* 223:266–267, 1979.

28. Brunner U, Habermeyer P, Schweiberer L: Die Sonderstellung der lateralen Klavikulafraktur. *Orthopade* 21:163–171, 1992.

29. Neer CS II: Nonunion of the clavicle. *JAMA* 172:1006–1011, 1960.

30. Goss TP: Scapular fractures and dislocations: Diagnosis and treatment. *J AAOS* 3:22–33, 1995.

31. Miller ME, Ada JR: Fractures of the scapula, clavicle and glenoid, in Browner BD, Jupiter JB, Levine AM, et al (eds): *Skeletal Trauma: Fractures, Dislocations, Ligamentous Injuries.* Philadelphia, Saunders, 1992, pp 1291–1310.

32. Ebraheim NA, An HS, Jackson WT, et al: Scapulothoracic dissociation. *J Bone Joint Surg* 70A:423–428, 1988.

33. Dennis DA, Ferlich DC, Claten ML: Acromial stress fractures associated with cuff tear arthropathy. *J Bone Joint Surg* 68A:937–940, 1986.

34. Warner JJP, Port J: Stress fracture of the acromion. *J Shoulder Elbow Surg* 3:262–265, 1994.

35. Ideberg R: Fractures of the scapula involving the glenoid fossa, in Bateman JE, Welsh RP (eds): *Surgery of the Shoulder.* Philadelphia, Decker, 1984, pp 63–66.

36. Herscovici D Jr, Fiennes AGTW, Ruedi TP: The floating shoulder: Ipsilateral clavicle and scapular neck fractures. *J Orthop Trauma* 6:499, 1992.

37. Leung KS, Lam TP: Open reduction and internal fixation of ipsilateral fractures of the scapular neck and clavicle. *J Bone Joint Surg* 75A:1015–1018, 1993.

38. Ada JR, Miller ME: Scapular fractures: An analysis of 113 cases. *Clin Orthop* 269:174–180, 1991.

39. Cave EF, Burke JF, Boyd RJ: *Trauma Management.* Chicago, Year-Book, 1974.

40. Rowe CR: Prognosis in dislocations of the shoulder. *J Bone Joint Surg* 38A:957–977, 1956.

41. Arciero RA: Acute traumatic anterior dislocation of the shoulder, in Bigliani LU (ed): *The Unstable Shoulder.* Rosemont, IL, American Academy of Orthopaedic Surgeons 1996, pp 37–45.

42. Rockwood CA, Wirth MA: Subluxations and dislocations about the glenohumeral joint, in Rockwood CA, Green DP, Bucholz RW, et al (eds): *Fractures in Adults, 4th ed.* Philadelphia, Lippincott-Raven, 1996, pp 1193–1339.

43. Simonet WT, Cofield RH: Prognosis in anterior shoulder dislocation. *Am J Sports Med* 12:19–23, 1984.

44. Pettersson G: Rupture of the tendon aponeurosis of the shoulder joint in antero-inferior dislocation: A study on the origin and occurrence of the ruptures. *Acta Chir Scand Suppl* 77:1–187, 1942.

45. Rockwood CA, Williams GR, Young DC: Injuries to the acromioclavicular joint, in Rockwood CA, Green DP, Bucholz RW, et al (eds): *Fractures in Adults, 4th ed.* Philadelphia, Lippincott-Raven, 1996, pp 1341–1413.

46. Weaver JK, Dunn HK: Treatment of acromioclavicular injuries, especially complete acromioclavicular separation. *J Bone Joint Surg* 54A:1187–1197, 1972.

47. Rockwood CA, Szalay EA, Curtis RJ Jr: X-ray evaluation of shoulder problems, in Rockwood CA Jr, Matsen FA III (eds): *The Shoulder.* Vol 1. Philadelphia, Saunders, 1990, pp 178–207.

CHAPTER 21

Diaphyseal Fractures of the Humerus

Eric T. Johnson
and William G. DeLong, Jr.

Fractures of the humeral shaft account for about 3 percent of all fractures.[1] They may result from any mechanism of injury secondary to either direct or indirect forces.[2] Traditionally, a majority of humeral fractures have been treated by closed or nonoperative methods using splinting or casting techniques. New technology as well as a more critical review of treatment methods and results have increased treatment options to include intramedullary rodding, compression plating, and external fixation. Individual patient variables, mechanism of injury, and a thorough understanding of the regional anatomy each contribute to the formulation of an appropriate treatment plan.

ANATOMY

The humeral diaphysis is defined by the upper border of the pectoralis major proximally and the supracondylar ridge distally.[3] The cross-sectional anatomy varies greatly, from cylindrical proximally to triangular distally, as the shaft widens to form the condyles.[4] Posteriorly, the radial nerve lies within the spiral groove as it courses in a posteromedial to anterolateral direction. Both the endosteum and periosteum are supplied by branches of the brachial artery.[5–7] As discussed later in this section, some of the neurovascular structures about the humerus are at risk as a result of injury and may be placed in danger without thoughtful planning and careful technique in the operative as well as nonoperative management of these fractures.

DIAGNOSIS

Pain, deformity, swelling, and shortening usually make the humeral shaft fractures obvious. However, they may be overlooked or missed during the initial assessment of the multiply injured and/or unconscious patient,[8] thus emphasizing the need for a thorough secondary survey on all trauma patients. When these fractures do occur, the muscles about the shoulder and humerus produce characteristic displacement patterns based on the level of the fracture (Fig. 21-1).[9] Fractures proximal to the pectoralis insertion produce abduction and internal rotation of the proximal fragment by the deltoid and rotator cuff, while the pectoralis major adducts and displaces the distal fragment medially. Fractures occurring distal to the pectoralis insertion but proximal to the deltoid will typically have a medially displaced proximal fragment secondary to the pull of the pectoralis and a laterally displaced distal fragment secondary to the deltoid. When fractures occur distally to both the deltoid and pectoralis insertions, a flexed, abducted proximal fragment is seen, with shortening of the distal fragment.

EXAMINATION

As with any fracture, thorough neurovascular examination and assessment of soft tissue integrity are essential. Doppler examination and measurements of compartment pressure should be included when indicated by clinical exam or an increased index of suspicion. Radiographic evaluation limited to two full-length views of the humerus taken at 90° angles to one another is usually sufficient. The x-ray beam, not the extremity, should be rotated to obtain these studies. Additional studies such as computed tomography (CT), MRI, or bone scans are often indicated in cases involving a pathologic fracture or as a part of tumor staging. Tomograms may be helpful in evaluating humeral shaft nonunions.

CLASSIFICATION

Fractures of the humeral shaft have traditionally been classified by the physical properties of the fracture, such as location, displacement, whether the fracture is open or closed, or if there is associated neurovascular injury. The AO classification (Fig. 21-2)[10,11] represents an organized, logical attempt to classify shaft fractures based on location and the degree of comminution as well as the fracture pattern. As with all long bone fractures, the mechanism of injury of humeral shaft fractures greatly determines the presenting fracture pattern.

Direct blows and bending forces tend to cause more transverse fractures, which may include a butterfly fragment. High-energy or penetrating trauma may result in more comminution and soft tissue injury. Torsional forces or wringing injuries normally result in spiral fracture configurations. This type of fracture, usually seen within the distal third of the humerus, has been noted to occur in throwing athletes as a result of the violent muscle contraction and torsional forces involved in the throwing motion.[12]

TREATMENT

The goal of any treatment for humeral shaft fractures should be bony union without loss of function. With this in mind, the majority of humeral shaft fractures can be treated nonoperatively with favorable results. Union rates of greater than 90 percent have been reported with the use

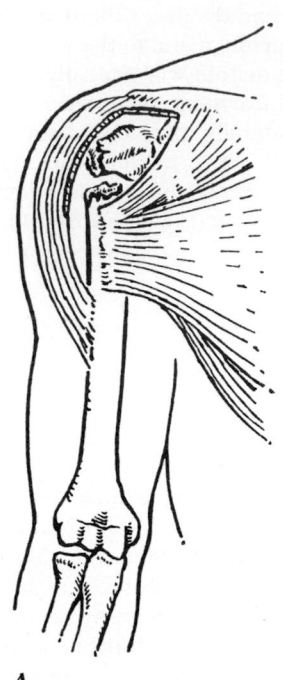
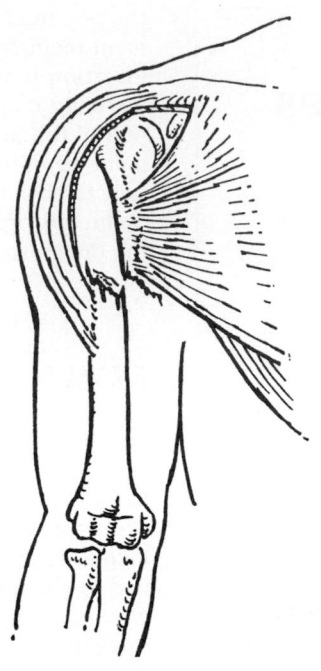
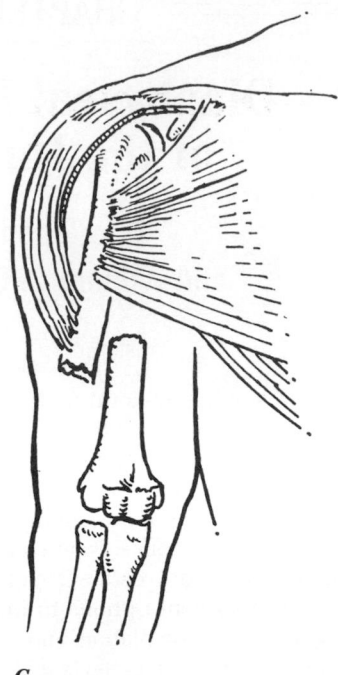

A   *B*   *C*

Figure 21-1 *A*. Fractures proximal to the pectoralis insertion produce abduction and internal rotation of the proximal fragment. *B*. Fractures occurring distal to the pectoralis insertion but proximally to the deltoid will typically have a medially displaced proximal fragment secondary to the deltoid. *C*. When fractures occur distal to both the deltoid and pectoralis insertion, a flexed, abducted proximal fragment is seen, with shortening.

of initial splinting or casting techniques followed by functional bracing within 7 to 10 days.[13]

Closed treatment options include casting, functional bracing, coaptation splinting, abduction splints, or Velpeau sling placement. The degree of mobility within the shoulder joint allows for acceptable deformity of up to 20° of anterior angulation and 30° of varus or valgus and shortening of up to 1 in. Little or no functional disability is to be expected.[14]

The decision to use closed treatment should be accompanied by the understanding that a slight cosmetic deformity may result despite the absence of functional disability and that more frequent follow-up examinations will be required during the initial weeks of treatment. Today, closed treatment remains the treatment of choice for uncomplicated closed humeral shaft fractures. Initial stabilization may be obtained with a U-shaped coaptation splint molded over the deltoid and acromion. The forearm may be supported by either a collar and cuff or a plaster forearm extension with a sling. The splint should hang free of the body and be checked routinely to ensure a well-molded fit, so as to avoid slipping. The patient is instructed on shoulder, elbow, wrist, and hand range-of-motion exercises. The coaptation splint is replaced with a functional brace in 7 to 10 days, allowing time for pain and swelling to subside. Sarmiento et al[15] introduced the principles of functional bracing in 1977, and since then numerous studies[13,16,17] have reported favorable results, with high rates of union, restoration of function, minimal residual angular deformity, and few complications.

In 1933, Caldwell[18,19] introduced hanging casts, which used the weight of the arm and cast to provide traction across the fracture site. Although this technique is not commonly used today, it has proved to be very effective in treating midshaft fractures with shortening, spiral, and/or oblique fracture patterns. Difficulties with this technique include the need to keep the patient in the upright position, fracture distraction (which may lead to delayed union), and the need to monitor the fracture site closely. Hanging casts should not be used in transverse fractures, as they have a high potential for distraction and nonunion. Like coaptation splints, hanging casts may be exchanged for functional braces in 7 to 10 days with good results. When factors unique to the patient or the fracture itself do not allow acceptable alignment to be obtained or maintained, operative options should be considered. If radial nerve function is lost during or after attempts at closed reduction, it could indicate nerve entrapment at the fracture site (Fig. 21-3). If this occurs, expedient exploration of the nerve is warranted.

While the majority of humeral shaft fractures may be treated nonoperatively, this treatment is contraindicated in the following: massive bone or soft tissue loss, flail extremities,[20] unacceptable fracture alignment, definitive surgical indications (Table 21-1), open fractures, and fractures with associated vascular injury.[21] Ipsilateral forearm and humeral shaft fractures have been shown to have a high rate of nonunion or malunion when the humerus is managed by closed means.[22] Ipsilateral intraarticular fractures also do poorly when postoperative joint motion is limited by nonoperative management of humeral shaft fracture. Relative surgical indications may arise based on individual patient variables.

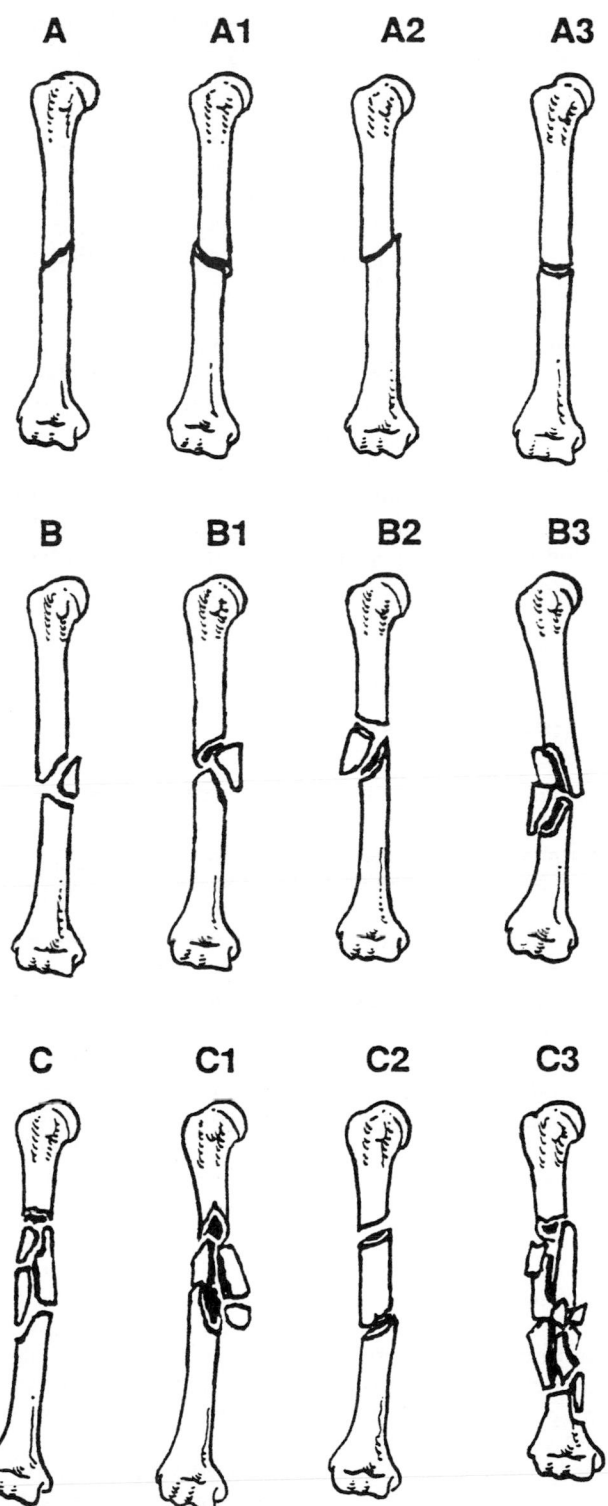

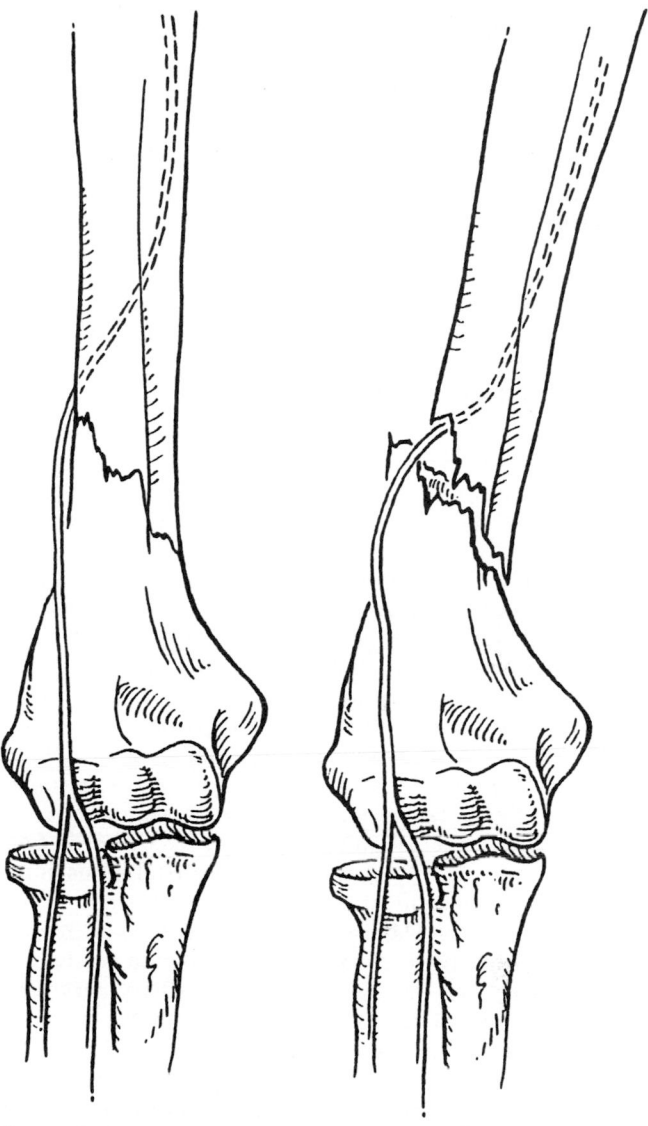

Figure 21-3 Radial nerve entrapment at the fracture site is possible during the course of fracture reduction. Examination may then reveal deterioration of radial nerve function. Acute entrapment at the fracture site should be considered. This warrants rapid surgical intervention.

Figure 21-2 The AO classification: A1, simple fracture, spiral; A2, simple fracture, oblique (>30°); A3, simple fracture, transverse (<30°); B1, wedge fracture, spiral wedge; B2, wedge fracture, bending wedge; B3, wedge fracture, fragmented wedge; C1, complex fracture, spiral; C2, complex fracture, segmental; C3, complex fracture, irregular.

The surgical treatment of humeral shaft fractures has evolved to include compression plating, both flexible and rigid intramedullary rodding, and external fixation. Screw fixation alone does not provide satisfactory torsional stability to prevent failure during healing and rehabilitation.[23–25] The modality selected is determined by the nature of the injury, the condition of the patient, and any associated injuries. The adjunctive use of polymethylmethacrylate with these techniques has been noted to improve fixation and decrease the incidence of pain associated with pathologic fractures.[26]

Plating of the humerus is usually accomplished by one of three approaches. The anterolateral approach appears most beneficial in managing fractures of the proximal and middle thirds of the humerus because the dissec-

TABLE 21-1 Indications for Operative Management of Humeral Shaft Fractures

Open fracture
Associated vascular injury
Floating elbow
Segmental fracture
Pathologic fracture
Bilateral humerus fractures
Humerus fracture in polytrauma patient
Radial nerve dysfunction after fracture manipulation
Penetrating injury with neurologic loss
Fractures with unacceptable alignment
Intraarticular fracture extension

tion exploits the interval between the deltoid and pectoralis major proximally and splits the brachialis muscle distally. The dual innervation of the brachialis muscle (lateral-radial nerve, medial-musculotaneous nerve) allows preservation of function following dissection. Distally, the humerus is exposed between the biceps brachii medially and the brachioradialis laterally. The radial nerve must be respected during this approach, although it is normally protected by the lateral half of the brachialis muscle.

The posterior or triceps splitting approach is best suited for cases involving the middle or distal thirds of the humerus and those in which the radial nerve must be explored. The long and lateral heads of the triceps are bluntly dissected, while the radial nerve and profunda brachii vessels are identified and protected. The axillary nerve and posterior humeral circumflex vessels limit the proximal extension of this approach, and the medial head of the triceps must be divided distally to gain access to the humerus. The anteromedial approach is rarely used in fracture surgery because it puts the median nerve and brachial artery at particular risk.

Humeral plating techniques have resulted in union rates of 96 percent; however, all major studies report radial nerve injury as a small but significant risk.[27–29] Great care must be taken in plating the humerus, as many failures (nonunion or loosening) can be attributed to technical error and lack of attention to detail. The use of a broad 4.5-mm dynamic compression plate with offset screw holes is recommended, although a narrow 4.5- or 3.5-mm plate may be more appropriate for smaller patients. Care must be taken to identify and protect the radial nerve during plate placement and fixation.

Intramedullary fixation can be accomplished with flexible or locked nails.[30–34] Antegrade and retrograde techniques have been described, both resulting in favorable union rates. Intramedullary rodding has been shown to result in higher rates of implant-related complaints and complications, often requiring secondary procedures for hardware removal or failure.

In an effort to avoid postoperative shoulder complaints, great care should be taken with antegrade nailing to avoid compromising the rotator cuff.[35] The proximal starting hole should split the fibers of the deltoid and lie just medial to the greater tuberosity. An effort should also be made to avoid protuberant medial proximal locking screws because of the potential for impingement on the axillary nerve during internal rotation. Anterior to posterior proximal locking screws should not be placed so as to avoid possible harm to the main trunk of the axillary nerve.[36] Retrograde starting holes should be made proximal to the olecranon fossa to avoid causing intercondylar fractures—a potentially devastating complication.

External fixation is usually reserved for injuries with significant soft tissue disruption, bone loss, infection, or burns. It may also serve to provide provisional stabilization until soft tissues or patient concerns allow conversion to other modes of stabilization. Meticulous attention to detail and technique should be taken to avoid pin-tract infection, soft tissue and muscle impingement, neurovascular compromise, and delayed healing.[37] Pins should be placed using the open technique, with blunt dissection down to bone.

COMPLICATIONS

Complications of humeral shaft fractures include radial nerve injury, nonunion, malunion, infection, hardware failure, loss of motion, vascular injury, and painful hardware. Numerous studies have looked at radial nerve injuries in association with humeral shaft fractures,[13,16,38–45] with radial nerve injury occurring in up to 18 percent of the cases presented. Presenting as motor dysfunction, most radial nerve injuries represent a compressive neuropraxia. Recovery can usually be expected to occur spontaneously within 3 to 4 months. When recovery is delayed, neuroelectrophysiologic studies and exploration of the nerve should be performed. Early nerve exploration is indicated in open fractures, because they have been shown to be associated with a greater incidence of nerve laceration or entrapment.[43] Penetrating injuries and palsies secondary to closed reduction remain areas of controversy. While most authors advocate early exploration for these injuries, the exact timing of radial nerve exploration remains unclear, with some studies pointing to similar results between early and delayed nerve exploration. It is also argued that early exploration may place a merely contused nerve at unnecessary surgical risk.[40]

In 1963, Holstein and Lewis described radial nerve injuries associated with distal-third humerus fractures.[43] It should be noted, however, that most fractures with associated radial nerve injury occur in the middle third of the humerus.

Vascular injury represents a surgical emergency as well as an absolute indication for surgical fracture stabilization. Injuries to the brachial artery have been reported to occur in 0.6 to 3 percent of cases.[21] Direct repair in clean lacerations or arterial grafting in cases of severe vessel injury or substance loss should be performed by an experienced surgeon.[46,47]

Nonunion may result secondary to technical error, hardware failure, infection, bone resorption, fracture distraction, soft tissue interposition, inadequate blood supply, or increased motion at the fracture site.[48] Rigid internal fixation with bone grafting is the treatment of choice for nonunion. Both plating and intramedullary techniques have been described,[49-52] some associated with success rates of greater than 95 percent. Complex nonunions require additional planning and attention to detail. Infection in the site of a nonunion should, if possible, be identified and treated prior to stabilization. Avascular nonunions or those associated with a significant bony defect may be treated with plating combined with vascularized fibular grafting.[53,54] Bone cement has also been noted to improve fixation in osteoporotic or diseased bone.[55] Ilizarov techniques may also play a role in managing the complex nonunion.

REFERENCES

1. Christensen S: Humeral shaft fractures: Operative and conservative treatment. *Acta Chir Scand* 133:455, 1967.
2. Fenyo G: On Fractures of the shaft of the humerus. *Acta Chir Scand* 137:221–226, 1971.
3. Williams PL, Warwick R, Dyson M, Bannister LH (eds): *Gray's Anatomy,* 37th ed. New York, Churchill Livingstone, 1989.
4. Hollinshead WH: *Anatomy for Surgeons,* Vol 3. New York, Hoeber-Harper, 1958
5. Laing P: The arterial supply of the adult humerus. *J Bone Joint Surg* 38A:1105, 1956.
6. Carrol SE: A Study of the nutrient foramina of the humeral diaphysis. *J Bone Joint Surg* 45B:176–181, 1963.
7. Hoppenfeld S, De Boer P: *Exposures in Orthopedics.* Philadelphia, Lippincott, 1984, pp 47–75.
8. Ward WG, Nunley JA: Occult orthopaedic trauma in the multiply injured patient. *J Orthop Trauma* 5:308–312, 1991.
9. Zuckerman JD, Koval KJ: Fractures of the shaft of the humerus, in Rockwood CA Jr, Green DP, Bucholz RW, Heckman JD (eds): *Rockwood and Green's Fractures in Adults,* 4th ed, Vol 2. Philadelphia, Lippincott, 1996, pp 1025–1053.
10. Muller ME, Nazarian S, Koch P, et al: *Comprehensive Classification of Fractures of Long Bones.* Berlin, Springer-Verlag, 1990.
11. Muller ME, Allogower M, Schneider R, et al: *Manual of Internal Fixation: Techniques Recommended by the AO-ASIF Group.* Berlin, Springer-Verlag, 1991, pp 118–150.
12. DiCicco JD, Mehlman CT, Urse JS: Fracture of the shaft of the humerus due to muscular violence. *J Orthop Trauma* 7:90–93, 1993.
13. Sarmiento A, Horowitch A, Aboulafia A, et al: Functional bracing for comminuted extra-articular fractures of the distal third of the humerus. *J Bone Joint Surg* 72B:283–287, 1990.
14. Klenerman L: Fractures of the shaft of the humerus. *J Bone Joint Surg* 48B:105–111, 1966.
15. Sarmiento A, Kinman PB, Galvin EG, et al: Functional bracing of fractures of the shaft of the humerus. *J Bone Joint Surg* 59A:596–601, 1977.
16. Mast JW, Spiegel PG, Harvey JP Jr, et al: Fractures of the humeral shaft: A retrospective study of 240 adult fractures. *Clin Orthop* 112:254–262, 1975.
17. Zagorski JB, Latta LL, Emor GA, et al: Dyaphyseal fractures of the humerus: Treatment with prefabricated braces. *J Bone Joint Surg* 70A:607–610, 1988.
18. Caldwell JA: Treatment of fractures in the Cincinnati General Hospital. *Ann Surg* 97:161, 1933.
19. Caldwell JA: Treatment of fractures of the shaft of the humerus by hanging cast. *Surg Gynecol Obstet* 70:421, 1940.
20. Brien WW, Gellman H, Becker V, et al: Management of fractures of the humerus in patients who have an injury of the ipsilateral brachial plexus. *J Bone Joint Surg* 72A:1208–1210, 1990.
21. Gainor BJ, Metzler M: Humeral shaft fracture with brachial artery injury. *Clin Orthop* 204:154–161, 1986.
22. Lange RH, Foster RJ: Skeletal management of humeral shaft fractures associated with forearm fractures. *Clin Orthop* 195:173–177, 1985.
23. Dalton JE, Salkeld SL, Satterwhite YE, et al: A biomechanical comparison of intramedullary nailing systems for the humerus. *J Orthop Trauma* 7:367–374, 1993.
24. Henley MB, Monroe M, Tencer AF: Biomechanical comparisons of methods of fixation of midshaft osteotomy of the humerus. *J Orthop Trauma* 5:14–20, 1991.
25. Zimmerman MC, Waite AM, Deehan M, et al: A biomechanical analysis of four humeral fracture fixation systems. *J Orthop Trauma* 8:233–239, 1994.
26. Vail TP, Harrelson JM: Treatment of pathologic fractures of the humerus. *Clin Orthop* 268:197–202, 1991.
27. Foster RJ, Dixon GL Jr, Bach AW, et al: Internal fixation of fractures and nonunions of the humeral shaft: Indications and results in a multi-center study. *J Bone Joint Surg* 67A:857–864, 1985.
28. Heim D, Heckert F, Hess P, et al: Surgical treatment of humeral shaft fractures: The Beasel experience. *J Trauma* 35:226–232, 1993.
29. Vander Griend R, Tomasin J, Ward EF: Open reduction and internal fixation of humeral shaft fractures: Results using AO plating techniques. *J Bone Joint Surg* 68A:430–433, 1986.
30. Brumback RJ, Bosse MJ, Poka A, et al: Intramedullary stabilization of humeral shaft fractures in patients with multiple trauma. *J Bone Joint Surg* 68A:960–970, 1986.
31. Durbin RA, Gottesman MJ, Saunders KC: Hackenthal stacked nailing of humeral shaft fractures: Experience with 30 patients. *Clin Orthop* 179:168–174, 1983.
32. Hall RF Jr, Pankovich AM: Ender nailing of acute fractures of the humerus: A study of closed fixation by intramedullary nails without reaming. *J Bone Joint Surg* 69A:558–567, 1987.
33. Henley MB, Chapman JR, Claudi BF: Closed retrograde Hackenthal nail stabilization of humeral shaft fractures. *J Orthop Trauma* 6:18–24, 1992.
34. Ingman AM, Waters DA: Locked intramedullary nailing of humeral shaft fractures: Implant design, surgical technique, and clinical results. *J Bone Joint Surg* 76B:23–29, 1994.
35. Robinson CM, Bell KM, Court-Brown CM, et al: Locked nailing of humeral shaft fractures: Experience in Edinburgh over a two year period. *J Bone Joint Surg* 74B:558–562, 1992.
36. Reimer BL, D'Ambrosia R: The risk of injury to the axillary nerve, artery, and vein from proximal locking screws of humeral intramedullary nails. *Orthopedics* 15:697–699, 1992.
37. Neumann HS, Brug E, Winckler S, et al: The surgical treatment of diaphyseal fractures of the humerus: Stabilization with plate osteosynthesis, Hackenthal nailing, locking nail and external fixation. *Int J Orthop Trauma* 3(suppl):25–28, 1993.
38. Bleeker WA, Nijsten MW, ten Duis H-J: Treatment of humeral shaft fractures related to associated injuries: A retrospective study of 237 patients. *Acta Orthop Scand* 62:148–153, 1991.
39. Amillo S, Barrios RH, Martinez-Peric R, et al: Surgical treatment of the radial nerve lesions associated with fractures of the humerus. *J Orthop Trauma* 7:211–215, 1993.
40. Bostman O, Bakalim G, Vainionpaa S, et al: Radial palsy in shaft fractures of the humerus. *Acta Orthop Scand* 57:316–319, 1986.

41. Dabezies EJ, Banta CJ II, Murphy CP, et al: Plate fixation of the humeral shaft for acute fractures, with and without radial nerve injuries. *J Orthop Trauma* 6:10–13, 1992.

42. Foster RJ, Swiontkowski MF, Bach AW, et al: Radial nerve palsy caused by open humeral shaft fractures. *J Hand Surg* 18A:121–124, 1993.

43. Holstein A, Lewis GB: Fractures of the humerus with radial nerve paralysis. *J Bone Joint Surg* 45A:1382–1388, 1963.

44. Samardzic M, Grujicic D, Milinkovic ZB: Radial nerve lesions associated with fractures of the humeral shaft. *Injury* 21:220–222, 1990.

45. Sonneveld GJ, Patlka P, van Mourik JC, et al: Treatment of fractures of the shaft of the humerus accompanied by paralysis of the radial nerve. *Injury* 18:404–406, 1987.

46. Connolly, J: Management of fractures associated with arterial injuries. *Am J Surg* 120:331, 1970.

47. McNamara JJ, Brief DK, Stremple JF, Wright JK: Management of fractures with associated arterial injury in combat casualties. *J Trauma* 13:17–19, 1973.

48. Rosen H: The treatment of nonunions and pseudoarthroses of the humeral shaft. *Orthop Clin North Am* 21:725–742, 1990.

49. Healy WL, White GM, Mick CA, et al: Nonunion of the humeral shaft. *Clin Orthop* 219:206–213, 1987.

50. Rodriguez-Merchan EC: Compression plating versus Hackenthal nailing in closed humeral shaft fractures failing nonoperative reduction. *J Orthop Trauma* 3:194–197, 1995.

51. Barquet A, Fernandez A, Luvizio J, et al: A combined therapeutic protocol for aseptic nonunion of the humeral shaft: A report of 25 cases. *J Trauma* 29:95–98, 1989.

52. Pietu G, Raynaud G, Letenneur J: Treatment of delayed and nonunions of the humeral shaft using the Seidel locking nail: A preliminary report of five cases. *J Orthop Trauma* 8:240–244, 1994.

53. Jupiter JB: Complex non-union of the humeral diaphysis: Treatment with a medial approach, and anterior plate, and a vascularized fibular graft. *J Bone Joint Surg* 72A:701–707, 1990.

54. Wright TW, Miller GJ, Vander Griend RA, et al: Reconstruction of the humerus with an intramedullary fibular graft: A clinical and biomechanical study. *J Bone Joint Surg* 75B:804–807, 1993.

55. Trotter DH, Dobozi W: Nonunion of the humerus: Rigid fixation, bone grafting, and adjunctive bone cement. *Clin Orthop* 204:162–168, 1986.

CHAPTER 22

Fractures and Dislocations Involving the Elbow Joint

Wayne T. Pan, Christopher T. Born, and
William G. DeLong, Jr.,

The elbow is a complex hinged joint consisting of three bony articulations involving the distal humerus and the proximal ulna and radius. Elbow motion is constrained by both its bony architecture as well as by soft tissue restraints. Injury to either component may result in elbow instability. While attention is generally directed at reconstructing the articular surfaces after a traumatic insult, recognition of the important role that the soft tissue structures play in maintaining the congruous articulations within this complex joint is crucial in the successful functional reconstruction of the elbow.

The medial (ulnar) collateral ligament complex consists of three distinct bundles (Fig. 22-1). The anterior bundle (AMCL), the most discrete of the complex, originates posterior to the axis of rotation of the elbow, on the inferior aspect of the medial epicondyle.[1] It inserts near the coronoid process and is a primary stabilizer to valgus stress at the elbow.[2] The AMCL is composed of three fiber components: one which is taut in maximal extension, another which is taut in intermediate positions, and a third fiber component which is always taut and serves as a guiding fiber bundle.[3] The posterior bundle of the medial collateral ligament (PMCL) is less well defined. It appears as a fan-shaped thickening of the posterior capsule extending from the inferior surface of the medial epicondyle and inserting onto the proximal olecranon.[1] Sectioning of the PMCL in experimental studies does not appreciably affect the valgus stability of the elbow.[4] The radial head is a secondary constraint to valgus stability.[2] The third bundle, known as "Cooper's ligament," is a transverse band of tissue spanning the notch between the coronoid process and the olecranon. It does not appear to contribute to elbow stability.[1]

The lateral collateral ligament complex of the elbow is a more varied and less discrete structure[5,6] (Fig. 22-2). It is composed of four parts: the radial collateral ligament (RCL), the lateral ulnar collateral ligament (LUCL), the accessory lateral collateral ligament, and the annular ligament. The RCL originates from the lateral epicondyle and inserts in and around the annular ligament. The LUCL consists of fibers which insert on the ulna at the crista supinatoris. This component is the primary lateral stabilizer of the elbow. Sectioning of this ligament causes posterolateral instability.[7] The accessory lateral collateral ligament arises from the tubercle of the supinator and blends into the annular ligament. The annular ligament is a strong band of tissue that slings around the radial neck, attaching to the anterior and posterior margins of the radial

fossa. It maintains the articulation between the proximal radius and ulna. The anconeus acts as a dynamic stabilizer of the lateral elbow.

Standard radiographic examination of the elbow should include anteroposterior plain films with the elbow in extension and full supination, a lateral view with the elbow at 90°, oblique views with the elbow in extension, and an axial projection of the olecranon process. If a fracture of the radial head and/or capitellum is suspected, then a capitellar view should be performed, angled 45° caudocephalad in the lateral position.[8] Valgus stress views can be helpful with the diagnosis of MCL tears. A gap of more than 0.5 mm as compared to the uninvolved elbow suggests a complete tear of the MCL.[9]

Arthrography is an invasive technique which can be used in identifying complete disruptions of capsular integrity as well as the presence of loose bodies.[8] Arthrograms, however, are useful in diagnosing ligamentous disruptions only if they are obtained early after acute rupture.[10] Partial undersurface tears of the MCL can be identified using a combination of arthrography and computed tomography.[11] Magnetic resonance imaging has been demonstrated to be a highly specific and sensitive tool in the noninvasive evaluation of both partial and complete MCL injuries.[10] Coronal T1-weighted images are best able to demonstrate the AMCL in its entirety. A poorly defined, lax, or irregular AMCL MR signal is highly suggestive of an AMCL injury. Increased signal intensity within and around the MCL on T1- and T2-weighted pulse sequences correspond to the presence of hemorrhage and edema within the MCL.

Soft tissue injury to the elbow can be viewed as a graded spectrum of ligamentous instability beginning with posterolateral rotatory instability (PLRI) and progressing to frank posterior dislocation.[12] The initial stage, stage I, represents disruption of the LUCL and possibly the RCL and posterolateral capsule. Clinically, the patient will complain of recurrent snapping as a result of PLRI. The patient will have a positive lateral pivot-shift sign. The intermediate stage, stage II, is the perched position, with a greater degree of subluxation and disruption of the anterior and posterior capsules and the remainder of the lateral collateral ligaments. The patient will describe symptoms of recurrent subluxation and demonstrate a positive lateral pivot-shift sign as well as varus instability. The reduced elbow will be stable to valgus stress, however, since the AMCL is still intact. Posterior dislocation results in the final two stages, with disruption of the PMCL (stage IIIa) and finally with complete ligamentous disruption including the AMCL (stage IIIb). Clinically, stage IIIa can be distinguished from stage IIIb by demonstration of valgus stability in pronation, whereas stage IIIb dislocations are grossly unstable.

Repair of the LUCL has been successful in restoring stability to recurrent PLRI injuries which have failed conservative treatment.[7]

Medial elbow strains are particularly common in throwing athletes. Evaluation of complaints of pain on the medial side of the elbow following repetitive use should begin with a thorough history followed by an examination focusing on potential medial elbow ligamentous pathology.

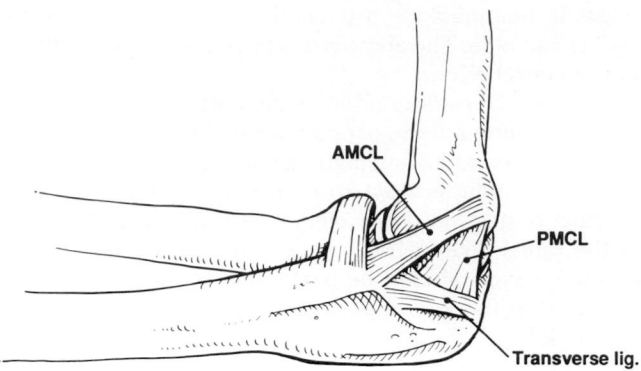

Figure 22-1 The medial (ulnar) collateral ligament complex.

This would include ulnar collateral ligament strains or disruptions, ulnar neuritis or subluxation, medial epicondyle avulsion injuries or epicondylitis, loose bodies, olecranon stress fractures and valgus extension overload syndrome.[13] Appropriate x-rays should be carried out, and MRI scanning should be considered. It is important to note in the history whether the pain has been slow in onset or acute, how the injury occurred, and the character of the pain. Acute ulnar collateral ruptures will frequently be associated with a "pop," whereas ulnar neuritis is much slower in onset and may be described as a "stabbing pain" down the medial aspect of the elbow into the forearm with associated paresthesias. A thorough physical examination with focal inspection and palpation based on a presumed differential diagnosis from the history and the local anatomy of the elbow will usually help to pinpoint the pathology. A full series of plain x-rays should be taken, and consideration should be given to valgus stress views. CT arthrography or MRI with or without arthrography may be helpful to evaluate subtle partial tears of the medial complex. For patients with a complete ulnar collateral liga-

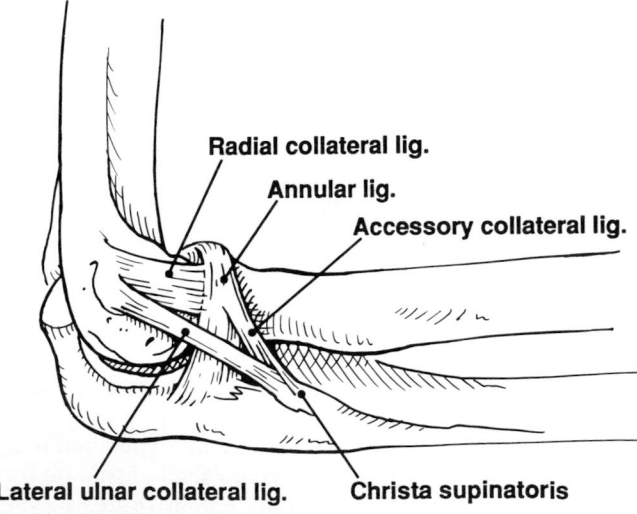

Figure 22-2 The lateral collateral ligament complex.

Radial collateral lig.

Annular lig.

Accessory collateral lig.

Lateral ulnar collateral lig.   Christa supinatoris

ment injury, an ulnar collateral ligament reconstruction can be carried out using the technique described by Job, et al.[14]

SIMPLE DISLOCATIONS

Elbow dislocations are the third most common major joint dislocation after shoulder and patellar dislocations. They occur most often in younger patients, peaking between 5 and 25 years of age, though the median age is 30 in both sexes. Two mechanisms have been proposed: (1) hyperextension of the elbow with levering of the olecranon tip in its fossa and (2) application of valgus and supination forces with axial compression during elbow flexion. Clinical data support the latter mechanism as a unifying concept, which can account for the spectrum of elbow instability from subluxation to frank dislocation.[12]

Elbow dislocations are generally classified with respect to the position of the distal forearm (Fig. 22-3). Posterolateral and direct posterior dislocations are the most common, followed by posteromedial and medial dislocations. Anterior dislocations are extremely rare. Divergent dislocations are elbow dislocations with disruption of the annular ligament and separation of the proximal radius from the ulna. Simple dislocations are those which are not associated with osseous injuries.

Simple elbow dislocations are generally treated in a closed fashion. Posterior dislocations should be reduced with gentle longitudinal traction with the elbow slightly extended and the forearm in a supinated position in order to clear the coronoid process under the trochlea. Pressure on the olecranon can also be applied to assist with the traction. A hanging arm method has also been described in the literature.[15] After reduction, a long-arm splint is applied with the forearm held in neutral rotation and the elbow in 90° of flexion. Early motion is encouraged as soon as pain will allow with initiation of unprotected flexion and extension to begin before 2 weeks.

Ligamentous stability after elbow dislocation should be evaluated following closed reduction. The elbow should be assessed with regard to varus, valgus, and posterolateral rotatory instability. This assessment is usually best performed under general anesthesia. Disruption of the AMCL is present if there is valgus laxity with the forearm in pronation. Varus instability is tested with the shoulder in full internal rotation. Stability is assessed with the elbow fully extended as well as at 30° of flexion. The lateral pivot-shift test is used to evaluate posterolateral rotatory instability. This test involves supination of the forearm with application of a valgus moment and axial compression on elbow flexion. A positive test results in subluxation of the radius and ulna off the humerus, which causes a prominence posterolaterally over the radial head. Further elbow flexion beyond 40° results in a reduction which can be felt as a "clunk."

Surgical treatment of ligamentous injuries following simple dislocations have not been shown to be more effective in restoring elbow function as compared to closed

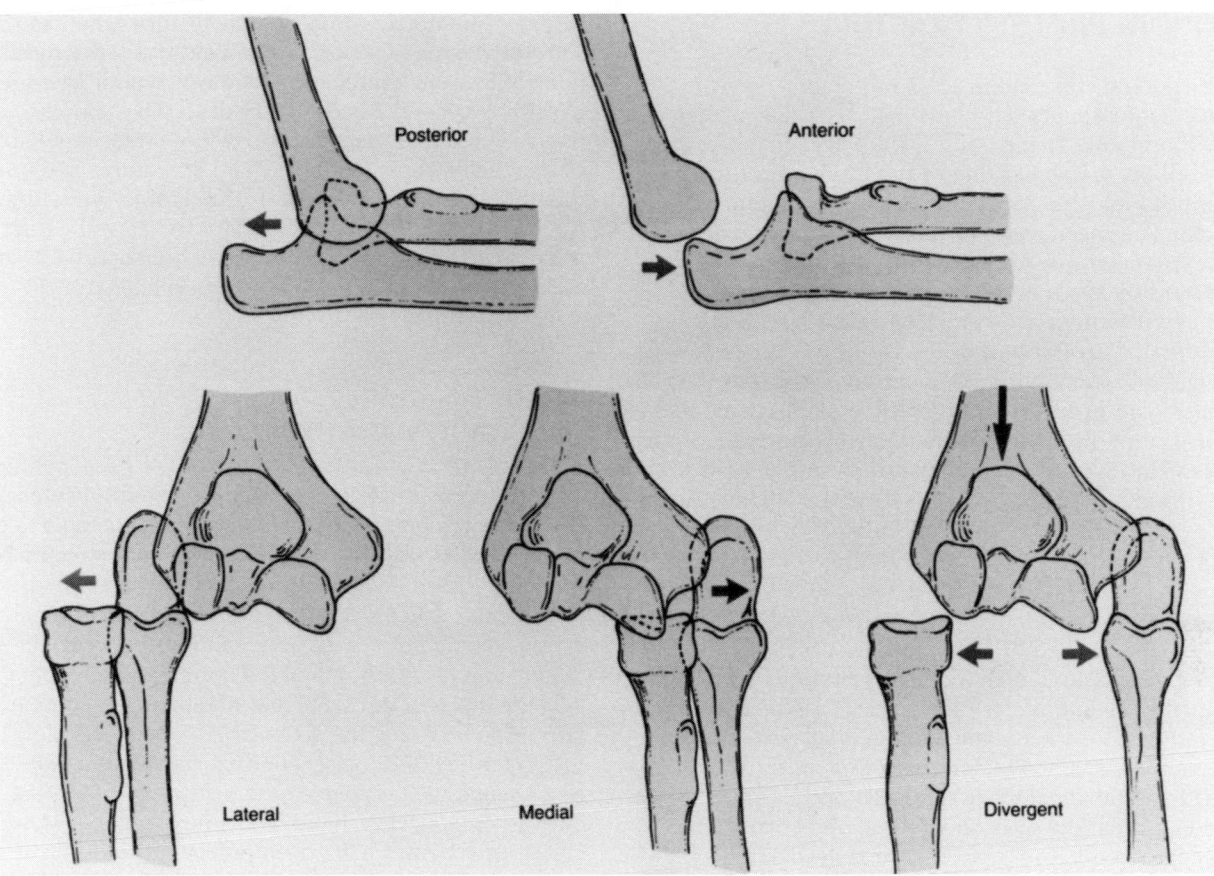

Posterior

Anterior

Lateral

Medial

Divergent

Figure 22-3 An elbow dislocation is defined by the direction of the forearm bone.

treatment.[16,17] Nonoperative management of unstable elbows includes cast brace with an extension block to prevent extension beyond the point of instability. A total of 3 to 6 weeks of bracing with gradual increase in the protected range of motion is usually adequate. However, demonstrated gross ligamentous instability at elbow flexion of 60° or greater should be managed with immediate surgical repair or reconstruction.[18] Late reconstruction of the lateral ulnar collateral ligament is recommended if there is recurrent elbow instability as a result of posterolateral rotatory instability.[19]

Long-term follow-up of patients treated with closed reduction showed 60 percent of patients with some residual symptoms at an average of 34 month follow-up. The most common complaint was residual pain, followed by pain on valgus stress, flexion contracture, and instability. There was a statistically significant correlation between degree of flexion contracture and length of immobilization. The authors of this study recommend that early active motion is the key to successful rehabilitation of the elbow following simple dislocation.[20]

Brachial artery rupture is a rare but potentially limb-threatening complication following simple elbow dislocation. It usually presents with absent radial and ulnar pulses following a dislocation. It can be associated with a compartment syndrome; therefore forearm pressures should be measured if clinically suspicious. The most important procedure is to reduce the elbow first, then reevaluate the radial and ulnar pulses. An arteriogram should be considered with any vascular insufficiency in order to rule out intimal or intramural vascular injuries. Operative management includes fasciotomies as indicated and end-to-end reversed saphenous vein grafting of the injured vascular segment. Ligation of the brachial artery is reserved for patients who are too unstable medically to undergo primary arterial repair.[21–23]

COMPLEX DISLOCATIONS

Fracture dislocations of the elbow are usually associated with greater trauma and an increased incidence of elbow instability, which generally requires treatment with open reduction and internal fixation. Consequently, results after fracture dislocation are not as favorable as after simple elbow dislocations. The general approach to fracture dislocations of the elbow should be to fix bony injuries in order to allow early motion. Repair or reconstruction of the soft tissues should be considered if ligamentous instability disallows elbow motion.[18] Immediate motion is recommended in all injured elbows, treated open or closed.

CORONOID PROCESS FRACTURES

Fractures of the coronoid process of the ulna occur in 2 to 10 percent of patients who have had a posterior dislocation of the elbow. These fractures are associated with recurrent elbow instability due to the insertion of the anterior bundle of the medial collateral ligament at the coronoid. The mechanism of this injury is believed to involve hyperextension of the elbow and a shearing off of the process by the trochlea.

These fractures are classified into three types (Fig. 22-4): type I, chip fracture of the tip of the process; type II, a single or comminuted fragment involving less than 50 percent of the process; and type III, a single or comminuted fragment involving more than 50 percent of the process.[24] Fractures were subclassified into A or B to indicate absence (A) or presence (B) of an elbow dislocation.

A retrospective study from the Mayo Clinic of 35 patients with coronoid fractures demonstrated generally satisfactory outcomes for patients with types I and II fractures treated closed. However, patients with type III fractures, who also had an increased probability of multiple injuries, including additional fractures of the elbow, had a rather poorer outcome, with only 20 percent having a satisfactory result. Patients with simple injuries (subtype A) had statistically better results with respect to arc of flexion, pronation, pain, and overall objective elbow rating as compared to coronoid fractures associated with elbow dislocation. While 64 percent of patients with type I injuries demonstrated asymptomatic calcification of the collateral ligaments, heterotopic ossification which impeded motion was associated with increasing frequency with types II and III injuries. The study also demonstrated a direct correlation between loss of elbow motion and duration of immobilization, which in turn was associated with the degree of severity of injury. Type I fractures were immobilized on average for 13 days; type II fractures, 20 days; and type III fractures, 28 days. The authors recommend closed treatment and early motion for nondisplaced or minimally displaced types I and II fractures and open reduction and internal fixation of unstable types II and III fractures. With severely comminuted type III fractures, fragments should be stabilized with nonabsorbable suture and application of a distraction external fixator.[25]

OLECRANON FRACTURES

The olecranon process of the ulna is located subcutaneously at the elbow joint and is therefore more vulnerable to direct trauma. Along with the coronoid process, it comprises the semilunar (greater sigmoid) notch of the ulna, which serves as the ulnar articulation with the trochlea of the humerus. A transverse line of bare bone midway between the tip of the olecranon and the tip of the coronoid interrupts the articular surface of the semilunar notch. Its recognition is important in restoring the articular surface of the olecranon.

Fractures of the olecranon are usually the result of direct trauma to the posterior aspect of the elbow or a fall onto an outstretched hand with a flexed elbow. Many classification schemes have been published to describe these fractures. This includes those described by Colton,[26] Schatzker,[27] Horne and Tanzer,[28] AO,[29] and the Mayo classification system.[30] While the AO classification is the most comprehensive and thorough, the Mayo classification for olecranon fractures provides the surgeon with a more precise descriptive and functional classification for treatment of these injuries.

The Mayo classification divides olecranon fractures first into nondisplaced (type I) and displaced (>3 mm) fractures. Displaced fractures are then divided into stable (type II) and unstable (type III) fracture patterns. Each fracture type is then further categorized into noncomminuted (A) or comminuted (B) fractures. The treatment algorithm is then based on the classification. Types IA and IB are treated the same: symptomatically for 1 week in a splint, then early range of motion is begun as tolerated.

Type IIA fractures are treated with axial fixation with either tension band wiring or a 6.5 mm AO cancellous screw.[31–33] Type IIB fractures are treated dependent on the age of the patient: below 60 years of age, a 3.5-mm contoured DCP plate; 60 years of age or above and if the fragment makes up less than 50 percent of the articular surface, the fragment is excised and the triceps tendon advanced.[34–37] The triceps tendon should be repaired as closely as possible to the articular surface of the ulna in order to restore the moment arm of the elbow extensor mechanism. Type IIIA fractures are fixed with rigid plates and screws in order to allow for early motion. A distraction external fixator can be added to provide more stability without compromising elbow motion. This device may be beneficial in treating type IIIB fractures, as comminution may compromise rigidity of internal fixation.

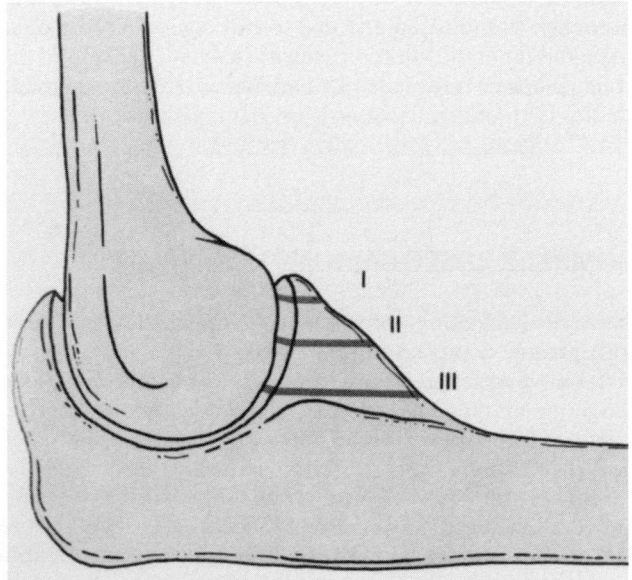

Figure 22-4 The coronoid fracture has been classified into three types by Regan and Morrey.

RADIAL HEAD FRACTURES

Approximately 5 to 10 percent of elbow dislocations are associated with a radial head fracture. The mechanism of injury is usually a fall with the elbow extended and the arm abducted, resulting in a valgus, pronation force applied across the proximal radius. The displaced, and often comminuted radial head fracture can be associated with two distinct soft-tissue injury patterns: (1) a torn medial collateral ligament which creates a grossly unstable elbow to valgus stress and/or (2) an injury to the interosseous membrane and triangular fibrocartilage complex, causing axial instability of the forearm with subluxation of the distal radioulnar joint (Essex-Lopresti dislocation).[38]

Radiographic evaluation of these injuries includes the standard anteroposterior and lateral projections of the elbow. Most radial head fractures can be identified with these two views. A positive "fat pad" sign, in which the normally recessed posterior fat pad becomes visible, may be suggestive of an occult radial head fracture. The radial head-capitellar view can be useful in identifying fractures involving the posterior half of the radial head.[39]

The Mason classification has traditionally been used to characterize radial head fractures (Fig. 22-5). It is a purely radiographic classification, insufficient to guide clinical treatment. The Hotchkiss modification of the Mason classification incorporates the clinical exam and provides guidelines for management of these difficult injuries.[40] Type I fractures have less than 2 mm of intraarticular displacement and there is no mechanical block to forearm rotation. Type II fractures have greater than 2 mm of intraarticular displacement, involve more than the marginal lip of the radial head but are not comminuted. Forearm rotation in type II fractures may be mechanically limited. Type III fractures are severely comminuted, nonreconstructable injuries which cause mechanical limitation to forearm rotation. The AO classification divides radial head fractures into three types: simple (21-B2.1), multifragmentary without depression (21-B2.2), and multifragmentary with depression (21-B2.3).

Minimally displaced fractures seldom require surgical treatment. Closed management includes aspiration of the elbow joint and instillation of anesthetic to provide symptomatic relief, sling for no more than 4 days and immediate elbow motion and forearm rotation as tolerated. Supervised physical therapy is not generally required unless patients fail to progress with elbow range of motion. Most patients can expect good to excellent restoration of elbow function within 2 to 3 months, though they may have some residual pain and loss of extension (<10°).

For Mason-Hotchkiss type II fractures, evaluation of the mechanical block to forearm rotation dictates treatment. Patients who can achieve at least 20 to 140° of elbow flexion and 70° of forearm rotation can be treated nonoperatively with less than 3 weeks of immobilization followed by active range of motion exercises.[25] Patients should be warned that displacement can occur and late radial head excision may be needed for significant pain and loss of motion. In a retrospective study of 21 patients with Mason type II (19 percent) and type III (81 percent) fractures who failed closed treatment, delayed excision of the radial head

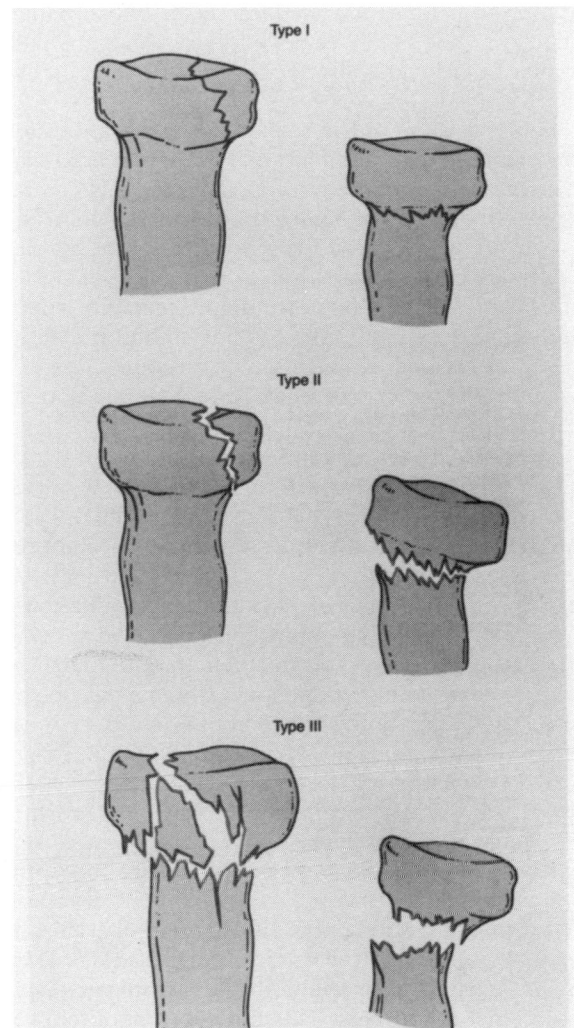

Figure 22-5 The Mason classification system for radial head fractures.

offered improved elbow motion in 81 percent of patients and relief of pain symptoms in 76 percent, with an overall good or excellent result in 77 percent.[41]

In patients with a mechanical block, careful consideration should be given to performing an open reduction and internal fixation of the fracture. Preservation of the radial head should also be attempted when an interosseous membrane injury is suspected or if there is an associated elbow dislocation. Great care must be taken to be sure that implants do not interfere with forearm rotation. A retrospective study of 14 patients with Mason type II (57 percent) and type III (43 percent) fractures treated with open reduction and internal fixation demonstrated 100 percent good or excellent results in patients with Mason type II fractures, whereas only 33 percent good or excellent results were achieved in patients with Mason type III fractures.[42] Injuries with associated elbow dislocation can expect some loss of elbow extension.[42,43] The use of absorbable polyglycolide pins is a feasible alternative to metal implants in patients undergoing open reduction and internal fixation for radial head fractures.[44] Absorbable implants do not need to be removed, thus saving the patient a possible additional operation for symptomatic hardware removal.

Simple excision of the radial head is a viable alternative to open reduction and internal fixation in low-demand patients. Early range of motion postoperatively can be facilitated with the use of a hinged orthosis to minimize valgus stress on the elbow. If the elbow remains unstable following radial head excision, repair of the medial collateral ligament and/or the posterolateral ligament complex should be entertained,[45] though not all authors support ligamentous reconstruction. Morrey recommends use of a distraction-external fixation device to maintain normal elbow motion and stability.[46]

Mason-Hotchkiss type III fractures are usually treated with radial head excision within 48 h of injury unless injury to the interosseous membrane is suspected. Late excision of the radial head in type III injuries does not result in as successful outcome as in type II injuries.[41] In an Essex-Lopresti type injury, consideration should be given to implantation of a large silicone radial head prosthesis in an attempt to preserve radial length and stabilize the distal radioulnar joint.[47] Patients in whom a silicone prosthesis is used should be warned about possible complications resulting from silicone failure and continued proximal axial translation of the radius which may destabilize the wrist.[48] Development of a metal radial head prosthesis, which would presumably avoid the disadvantages of silicone, has shown promising results.[49] Close follow-up of these patients is necessary.

Proximal migration of the radius following radial head excision occurs in 20 to 90 percent of patients.[40] This results in destabilization of the distal radioulnar joint and chronic wrist symptoms. This difficult complication has no satisfactory long-term solutions. Placement of a radial head prosthesis, ulnar shortening, repair of the triangular fibrocartilage complex, and pinning of the distal radio-ulnar joint have all been proposed, though each has its disadvantages.[25,40]

FRACTURES OF THE DISTAL HUMERUS

Fractures of the distal humerus are problematic because of their association with a higher incidence of poor outcomes as compared to other injuries. This is due to our elementary knowledge of the complex interaction of anatomic and soft tissue forces at the elbow joint. The ability to achieve and maintain an anatomic reduction and to resume early active elbow motion are the two key principles which will lead to a good functional result in these injuries.

While many different site-specific classification schemes have been developed for distal humerus fractures, the AO classification, which has been adopted by the Orthopaedic Trauma Association's Committee for Coding and Classification of Fractures, is the most useful in terms of describing what are frequently very complex

injuries (Fig. 22-6). This scheme is based on the columnar concept of the distal humerus, with the integrity of both columns, lateral and medial, determining the osseous stability of the elbow. Type A fractures are entirely extraarticular. These include epicondylar avulsion fractures (A1) as well as supracondylar and transcondylar fractures, subtyped A2 or A3, depending on degree of comminution. Type B fractures involve only a portion of the articular surface, like unicondylar and intercondylar fractures: B1 injuries involve the lateral column, B2 injuries involve the medial column, and B3 injuries affect just the distal articular surface without affecting either osseous columns. Fractures involving the entire distal humeral articular surface are classified as type C: C1 injuries have minimal articular or metaphyseal comminution, C2 injuries have metaphyseal comminution with minimal articular comminution, and C3 injuries are char-

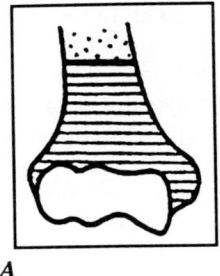

A

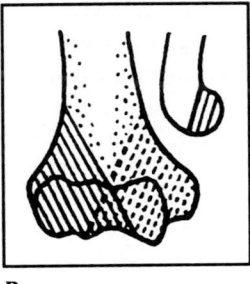

B

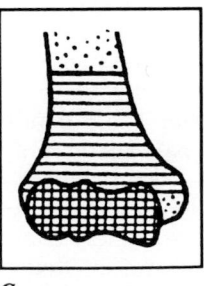

C

Figure 22-6 Basic classification of distal humeral fractures as adopted by the Orthopaedic Trauma Association Committee for Coding and Classification. *A.* Extraarticular fracture. *B.* Partial articular fracture. *C.* Complete articular fracture. Reproduced with permission from *J Orthop Trauma* 10 (suppl 1), 1996.

acterized by bicolumnar osseous injuries with articular comminution.

MEDIAL EPICONDYLE FRACTURES

Extraarticular avulsion fractures of the medial epicondyle (A1) do not disrupt the osseous columns of the distal humerus and therefore are considered stable injuries. Minimally displaced fractures generally do not require surgical intervention and can be treated with short-term immobilization (less than 2 weeks) in a posterior splint with the elbow at 90° and the forearm pronated and wrist flexed, followed by early protected active elbow motion. Surgical intervention is indicated, however, if there is instability resulting from shortening of muscle groups or with associated ligamentous injuries or if the fragment becomes significantly displaced into the joint limiting its motion.

SUPRACONDYLAR/TRANSCONDYLAR HUMERAL FRACTURES

Supracondylar fractures are generally more common among pediatric patients. There are two basic mechanisms of injury: extension-type injury (more than 96 percent of all supracondylar fractures), with the distal fracture fragments displaced posteriorly and flexion-type injury with the distal fracture fragments displaced anteriorly. Since type A2 and A3 fractures affect both the medial and lateral osseous columns, these injuries are considered unstable. Simple metaphyseal fractures (A2) are generally amenable to closed treatment because of the stability of the large fracture fragments. Immobilization should be limited to less than 3 weeks to reduce the incidence of flexion contractures. Functional bracing for an average of 10 weeks has led to union rates of 96 percent with loss of motion no greater than 25°.[50] Alternatively, olecranon pin traction can also be used in the closed management of these injuries.

In unstable or irreducible A2 and the more comminuted A3 fractures, surgical stabilization should be considered. The use of plates and screws is recommended because of the high incidence of fixation failure and nonunion with pins and/or screws alone. The surgical approach to distal humerus fractures can be either direct lateral, medial, or posterior, either with a chevron olecranon osteotomy or a triceps splitting technique.[51,52] Lateral column plates are generally placed posteriorly and medial column plates medially. Early institution of motion is desired following open reduction; stable fixation allowing this must therefore be achieved.

Transcondylar humeral fractures can be viewed as low supracondylar fractures and therefore can be managed in similar fashion. However, because of their more distal location, excessive callus formation, especially in the olecranon and coronoid fossae, can lead to a mechanical block, resulting in decreased elbow motion.

UNICONDYLAR FRACTURES (B1, B2)

While distal humerus fractures affecting only a single osseous column are rare (3 to 5 percent of adult distal humerus fractures), the lateral column (B1) is more often involved than the medial column (B2). The mechanism of injury can be either indirect, via axial transmission of forces from the distal radius/ulna, with the elbow in extension and abduction or adduction, or direct, via forces applied to the posterior aspect of the flexed elbow. The Milch classification is based on the absence (type I) or presence (type II) of the lateral trochlear ridge on the condylar fragment.[53] The AO equivalent fractures are represented with the subtypes B1.1 and B2.1 for Milch type I, lateral and medial condyles, respectively, and B1.2 and B2.2 for Milch type II, lateral and medial condyles, respectively.

Immobilization of minimally displaced or nondisplaced lateral condylar fractures (B1) should be with the elbow flexed at 90°, forearm supinated, and wrist extended. Medial condylar fractures (B2) should be splinted with the elbow flexed at 90°, forearm pronated, and wrist in flexion. With both injuries, immobilization should be limited to less than 3 weeks. A hinged brace can be used to help stabilize the elbow and facilitate early motion. Closed treatment of minimally displaced or nondisplaced fractures can also be supplemented with percutaneous pinning to allow for early elbow motion. Early radiographic follow-up is necessary to monitor for potential fracture displacement.

While some Milch type I fractures can be treated closed, the majority of Milch type II fractures will require an open reduction and internal fixation. The goals of surgical treatment are to restore the trochlear articular congruity and humeral condylar alignment. Repair of collateral ligament tears should be considered if the elbow remains unstable. With medial condylar fractures, the ulnar groove may be involved in the fracture site; therefore an anterior ulnar nerve transposition is recommended.

Another type of unicondylar fracture of the distal humerus has been described which occurs exclusively in adolescents and young adults. The divergent single-column fracture of the distal humerus is characterized by four features: (1) fracture initiation in the trochlear groove from a direct impact on the olecranon, (2) adolescent/young adult population, (3) presence of a large fossa between the coronoid and olecranon fossae, and (4) intact soft tissue constraints. The fracture is considered to be relatively stable and is treated by closed reduction and percutaneous internal fixation.[54]

CAPITELLAR FRACTURES: HAHN-STEINTHAL AND KOCHER-LORENZ FRACTURES (B3)

Capitellar fractures are quite rare, accounting for less than 1 percent of all adult elbow fractures. They are more common in women than in men.[55] They have been classically divided into two types: in type I, the Hahn-Steinthal fracture, the distal fragment, consisting of articular surface and subchondral bone, is displaced anteriorly, whereas in type II, the Kocher-Lorenz fracture, the distal fragment, consisting of just an articular shell, is displaced posteriorly. The proposed mechanism of injury is an axial loading of the radius with impingement of the radial head onto the capitellum. With the elbow in extension, this force creates a lesion on the inferior surface of the capitellum. With subsequent elbow flexion, this piece becomes displaced anteriorly, creating a type I injury. Type II injuries occur with the force applied when the elbow is in flexion, followed by elbow extension and displacement of the fragment posteriorly.

Clinically, type I fractures tend to limit elbow flexion, whereas type II fractures can prevent full elbow extension. Generally, forearm rotation is not limited.[56] Accurate diagnosis of capitellar fractures requires true anteroposterior and lateral views of the elbow. Computed tomography can be helpful, as these fractures may be difficult to identify on plain films. It is important to rule out injuries to the radial head, lateral humeral condyle, and medial collateral ligaments, as they can be associated with this fracture.

Minimally or nondisplaced type I fractures can generally be treated closed. Options for displaced type I fractures include arthroscopic reduction with or without internal fixation, open reduction and internal fixation, or excision of the fracture fragment.[57,58] Internal fixation is difficult because of the size of the fragment, the paucity of bone, and the proximity of the articular surface. The use of small-fragment cannulated screws, Kirschner wires, and/or Herbert screws has been reported, all giving good results.[59] Excision of the fragment has also been shown to result in good elbow motion.[56,60]

Recommended treatment of type II fractures is excision, since the fracture fragment cannot provide any appreciable bony purchase for internal fixation. While short-term return of elbow motion is expected, long-term results are not as favorable with excision as compared with closed reduction or internal fixation.[60]

Regardless of treatment, protected early elbow motion is advised to prevent contractures.

BICONDYLAR FRACTURES (C)

Fractures of the distal humerus which affect both columns are the most common type of distal humerus fracture (62 percent of all distal humerus fractures in one series) and the most difficult to treat.[61] The Riseborough-Radin classification, which is most commonly used in North America, divides these fractures into four types: in type I, fracture fragments are nondisplaced; in type II, fracture fragments are displaced but not rotated; in type III, fracture fragments are both displaced, and rotated; and in type IV, fracture fragments are displaced, rotated and severely comminuted.[62] The AO classification describes these fractures in terms of bicondylar articular involvement (C), with subtypes divided by graded articular and metaphyseal comminution. Neither of these classification systems is adequate in describing the location of the metaphyseal defect, which is important in the planning of internal fixation.

The mechanism of injury is believed to be direct trauma to the olecranon, with impaction of the ulna in the trochlear groove and the elbow either in extension or flexion. Experimentally, bicondylar distal humerus fractures occur with elbow flexion between 115 and 135°.[63] Since these injuries frequently occur with accidents involving high-energy impact, careful evaluation of the soft tissue and neurovascular status will prevent iatrogenic complications.

Evaluation of this injury requires high-quality, true anteroposterior and lateral views. Traction views can be helpful in the visualization of overlapping multiple fragments.

Most bicondylar injuries will require an open reduction and placement of internal fixation (Fig. 22-7). Intraarticular displacement greater than 2 mm, marked metaphyseal comminution and displacement, open injuries, neurovascular compromise, floating elbow, and multiple trauma are all surgical indications. Other factors to be considered include the age of the patient, medical status, degree of osteopenia, condition of the soft tissues, and ability of the surgeon. Careful preoperative planning is imperative for the successful treatment of this fracture. Generally, these fractures are approached posteriorly through an olecranon osteotomy, either extraarticular for C1 fractures or intraarticular for C2 and C3 fractures. Predrilling for the osteotomy and the use of an osteotome to complete the osteotomy will decrease the osteotomy nonunion rate. A protocol designed specifically to address these fractures has been developed by Helfet and Schmeling,[64] which has led to 75 percent good or excellent results. Briefly, the first step is to reduce the articular surface anatomically, being careful not to narrow the trochlea. Next, plate fixation of the condyles to the humeral shaft is achieved. Cancellous bone graft should be used to fill in bony defects and comminution. Once the distal humerus fracture is adequately reduced and secured, repair of the olecranon osteotomy is commenced. Anterior transposition of the ulnar nerve is considered in the event of preoperative ulnar nerve symptoms or if fixation hardware is located near the ulnar groove. Postoperative physical therapy is started within 5 days. The arm remains splinted for 6 to 8 weeks except when supervised range-of-motion exercises are being performed. Indomethacin is prescribed to prevent heterotopic ossification.

With surgical treatment of these fractures, one may be cautiously optimistic as to the clinical results, despite the severity of the injury. It is important to recognize that the surgeon's ability plays a large role in determining the outcome, as this is a technically demanding and unforgiving procedure.

COMPLICATIONS OF ELBOW TRAUMA

Nonunion/Malunion

The incidence of nonunion following internal fixation of distal humerus fractures ranges from 2 to 11 percent. These

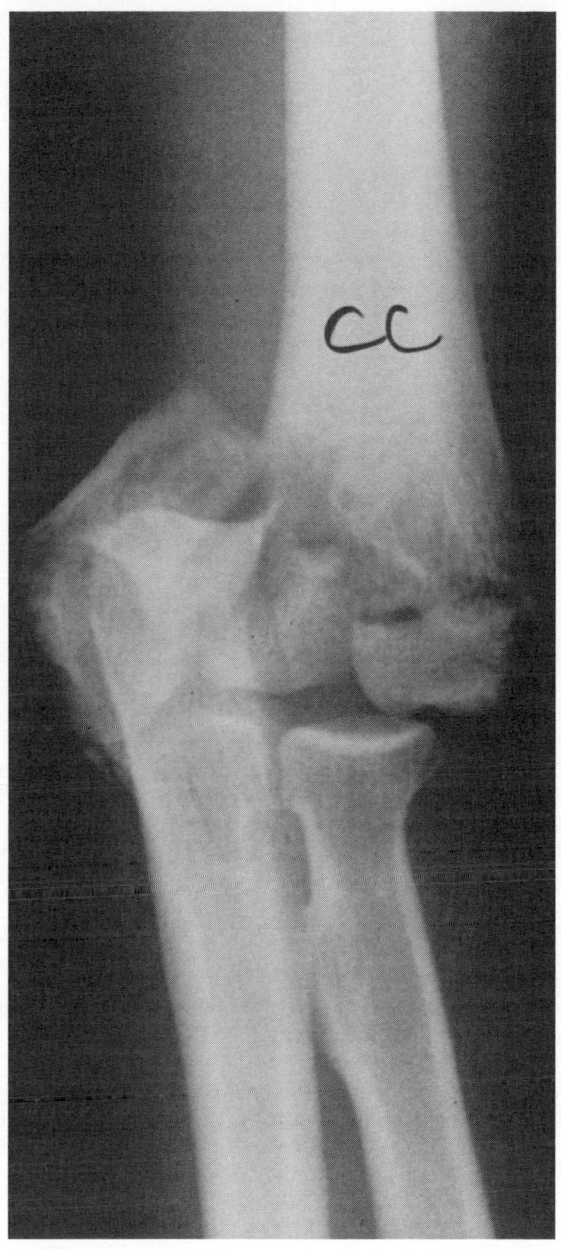

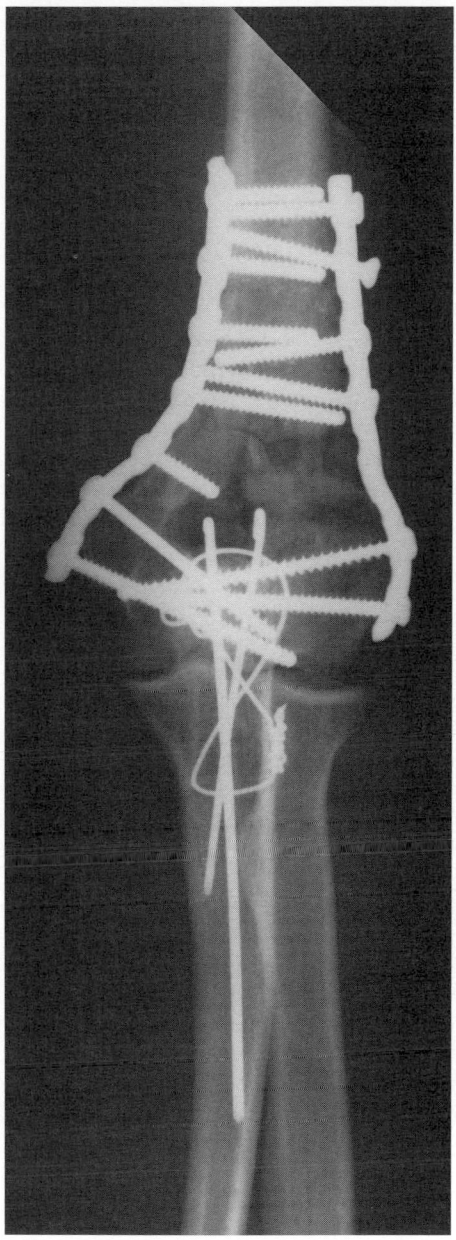

A   *B*

Figure 22-7 Complex bicondylar supracondylar humeral fracture with intraarticular extension (*A*) fixed with bi-column plates and a tension band technique used to repair the osteotomy (*B*).

sequelae generally result from inadequate internal fixation or overly aggressive postoperative rehabilitation. Surgical management of these complications includes corrective osteotomies for malunions, take-down of the nonunion, realignment of the fracture fragments, and placement of stable fixation with bone graft.[65–67] While restoration of complete elbow function is not usually achieved, most patients report diminished pain and improved elbow motion. Alternative treatment includes the use of distal humeral allografts and total elbow arthroplasty, though these methods are less reliable.[68]

Infection/Soft Tissue Coverage

Although, the infection rate in the open treatment of closed elbow fractures is low, infection is nevertheless a devastating complication. Preoperative intravenous antibiotics, meticulous hemostasis, adequate debridement at the time of initial surgery, and gentle handling of the soft tissues all contribute to the prevention of infection. However, once infection is detected, vigorous serial irrigations and debridement procedures are required to control it. Removal of loose hardware is prudent, but well-fixated hardware need not be removed. Should soft-tissue coverage be inadequate, selective use of skin grafts and other soft tissue transfers may be necessary to manage infection successfully.[69,70]

ULNAR NEUROPATHY

Ulnar neuropathy is the most common complication in fractures affecting the medial aspect of the distal humerus, especially in patients with a nonunion or valgus deformity. Treatment of the nonunion, osteotomy of the osseous deformity or removal of hardware with neurolysis, as indicated are all surgical options for this complication. Anterior transposition of the ulnar nerve can reduce nerve irritation and promote resolution of the neuropathy.

ARTHROFIBROSIS/HETEROTOPIC OSSIFICATION

Elbow pain and stiffness are usually the result of prolonged immobilization of the elbow joint. Open or arthroscopic lysis of adhesions can provide some relief of symptoms if performed within one year of the initial surgery.[71,72] Heterotopic ossification (HO) is another cause of elbow pain and decreased motion. The incidence of HO following surgical treatment of distal humerus fractures is 4 percent. The frequency of HO formation appears to be directly correlated with the magnitude of the injury, use of the anterior approach, and delayed surgery. In addition, brain-injured and burn patients have a greater propensity to form HO. Prevention of HO formation includes the use of indomethacin and low-dose radiation. Surgical treatment of symptomatic HO should be delayed until at least 6 months have elapsed from the initial trauma.[73]

REFERENCES

1. Morrey BF, An K-N: Functional anatomy of the ligaments of the elbow. *Clin Orthop Rel Res* 201:84–90, 1985.
2. Morrey BF, Tanaka S, An K-N: Valgus stability of the elbow: A definition of primary and secondary constraints. *Clin Orthop Rel Res* 265:187–195, 1991.
3. Fuss FK: The ulnar collateral ligament of the human elbow joint: Anatomy, function, and biomechanics. *J Anat* 175:203–212, 1991.
4. Søjbjerg JO, Ovesen J, Nielsen S: Experimental elbow instability after transection of the medial collateral ligament. *Clin Orthop Rel Res* 218:186–190, 1987.
5. Morrey BF: Anatomy of the elbow joint, in Morrey BF (ed): *The Elbow and Its Disorders*. Philadelphia, Saunders, 1993, pp 16–52.
6. Guerra JJ, Timmerman LA: Clinical anatomy, histology and pathomechanics of the elbow in sports. *Op Tech Sports Med* 4:69–76, 1996.
7. O'Driscoll SW, Bell DF, Morrey BF: Posterolateral rotatory instability of the elbow. *J Bone Joint Surg* 73A:440–446, 1991.
8. Schwartz ML, Al-Zahrani S: Diagnostic imaging of elbow injuries in the throwing athlete. *Op Tech Sports Med* 4:84–90, 1996.
9. Rijke AM, Goitz HT, McCue FC, et al: Stress radiography of the medial elbow ligaments. *Radiology* 191:213–216, 1994.
10. Mirowitz SA, London SL: Ulnar collateral ligament injury in baseball pitchers: MR imaging evaluation. *Radiology* 185:573–576, 1992.
11. Timmerman LA, Schwartz ML, Andrews JR: Preoperative evaluation of the ulnar collateral ligament by magnetic resonance imaging and computed tomography arthrography: Evaluation in 25 baseball players with surgical confirmation. *Am J Sports Med* 22:26–32, 1994.
12. O'Driscoll SW, Morrey BF, Korinek S, An K-N: Elbow subluxation and dislocation: A spectrum of instability. *Clin Orthop Rel Res* 280:186–197, 1992.
13. Andrews JR, Whiteside JA, Buettner CM: Clinical Evaluation of the Elbow in Throwers. *Operative Techniques in Sports Medicine*, vol. 4, No. 2 (April), 1996, pp 77–83.
14. Job FW, Stark H, Lombardo SJ: Reconstruction of the ulnar collateral ligament in athletes. *JBJS* 68:1158–1163, 1986.
15. Minford EJ, Beattie TF: Hanging arm method for reduction of dislocated elbow. *J Emerg Med* 11:161–162, 1993.
16. Josefsson PO, Gentz C-F, Johnell O, Wendeberg B: Surgical versus nonsurgical treatment of ligamentous injuries following dislocations of the elbow joint. *Clin Orthop Rel Res* 214:165–169, 1987.
17. Habernek H, Ortner F: The influence of anatomic factors in elbow joint dislocation. *Clin Orthop Rel Res* 274:226–230, 1992.
18. O'Driscoll SW: Elbow instability. *Hand Clin* 10:405–415, 1994.
19. Nestor BJ, O'Driscoll SW, Morrey BF: Ligamentous reconstruction for posterolateral rotatory instability of the elbow. *J Bone Joint Surg* 74A:1235–1241, 1992.
20. Mehlhoff TL, Noble PC, Bennett JB, Tullos HS: Simple dislocation of the elbow in the adult: Results after closed treatment. *J Bone Joint Surg* 70A:244–249, 1988.
21. Slowik GM, Fitzimmons M, Rayhack JM: Closed elbow dislocation and brachial artery damage. *J Orthop Trauma* 7:558–561, 1993.
22. Seidman GD, Koerner PA: Brachial artery rupture associated with closed posterior elbow dislocation: A case report and review of the literature. *J Trauma* 38:318–321, 1995.
23. Kharrazi FD, Rodgers WB, Waters PM, Koris MJ: Dislocation of the elbow complicated by arterial injury: Reconstructive strategy and functional outcome. *Am J Orthop* (Suppl) 11–15, 1995.
24. Regan W, Morrey BF: Fractures of the coronoid process of the ulna. *J Bone Joint Surg* 71A:1348–1354, 1989.
25. Morrey BF: Current concepts in the treatment of fractures of the radial head, the olecranon, and the coronoid. *J Bone Joint Surg* 77A:316–327, 1995.
26. Colton CL: Fractures of the olecranon in adults: Classification and management. *Injury* 5:121–129, 1973.
27. Schatzker J: Olecranon fractures, in Schatzker J, Tile M (eds): *The Rational Basis of Operative Fracture Care*. New York, Springer-Verlag, 1987.
28. Horne JG, Tanzer TL: Olecranon fractures: A review of 100 cases. *J Trauma* 21:469–472, 1981.
29. Müller ME, Allgöwer M, Schneider R, Willenegger H: *Manual of Internal Fixation: Techniques Recommended by the AO-ASIF Group*. 3d ed. Berlin, Springer-Verlag, 1991, pp 128–130.
30. Cabanela ME, Morrey BF: Fractures of the proximal ulna and olecranon, in Morrey BF (ed): *The Elbow and Its Disorders*. Philadelphia, Saunders, 1993, pp 405–428.
31. Larsen E, Jensen CM: Tension-band wiring of olecranon fractures with nonsliding pins: Report of 20 cases. *Acta Orthop Scand* 62:360–362, 1991.

32. Rowland SA, Burkhart SS: Tension band wiring of olecranon fractures: A modification of the AO technique. *Clin Orthop Rel Res* 277:238–242, 1992.

33. Wolfgang G, Burke F, Bush D, et al: Surgical treatment of displaced olecranon fractures by tension band wiring technique. *Clin Orthop Rel Res* 224:192–204, 1987.

34. Seiler JG III, Parker LM, Eldridge JC, Starling CC: An isolated depressed intraarticular fracture of the olecranon: Treatment with open reduction and internal fixation. *J Hand Surg* 20A:63–65, 1995.

35. Murphy DF, Greene WB, Dameron TB Jr: Displaced olecranon fractures in adults. *Clin Orthop Rel Res* 224:215–223, 1987.

36. Inhofe PD, Howard TC: The treatment of olecranon fractures by excision of fragments and repair of the extensor mechanism: Historical review and report of 12 fractures. *Orthopedics* 16:1313–1317, 1993.

37. Fern ED, Brown JN: Olecranon advancement osteotomy in the management of severely comminuted olecranon fractures. *Injury* 24:267–269, 1993.

38. Davidson PA, Moseley JB Jr, Tullos HS: Radial head fracture: A potentially complex injury. *Clin Orthop Rel Res* 297:224–230, 1993.

39. Greenspan A, Norman A: Radial head-capitellum view: An expanded imaging approach to elbow injury. *Radiology* 164:272–274, 1987.

40. Hotchkiss RN: Fractures and dislocations of the elbow, in Rockwood CA Jr, Green DP, Bucholz RW, Heckman JD (eds): *Fractures in Adults.* Philadelphia, Lippincott-Raven, 1996, pp 929–1024.

41. Broberg MA, Morrey BG: Results of delayed excision of the radial head after fracture. *J Bone Joint Surg* 68A:669–674, 1986.

42. King GJW, Evans DC, Kellam JF: Open reduction and internal fixation of radial head fractures. *J Orthop Trauma* 5:21–28, 1991.

43. Ebraheim NA, Skie MC, Zeiss J, et al: Internal fixation of radial neck fracture in a fracture dislocation of the elbow: A case report. *Clin Orthop Rel Res* 276:187–191, 1992.

44. Pelto K, Hirvensalo E, Böstman O, Rokkanen P: Treatment of radial head fractures with absorbable polyglycolide pins: A study on the security of the fixation in 38 cases. *J Orthop Trauma* 8:94–98, 1994.

45. Geissler WB, Freeland AE: Radial head fracture associated with elbow dislocation. *Orthopedics* 15:874–877, 1992.

46. Broberg MA, Morrey BG: Results of treatment of fracture-dislocations of the elbow. *Clin Orthop Rel Res* 216:109–119, 1987.

47. Carn RM, Medige J, Curtain D, Koenig A: Silicone rubber replacement of the severely fractured radial head. *Clin Orthop Rel Res* 209:259–269, 1986.

48. Vanderwilde RS, Morrey BF, Melberg MW, Vinh TN: Inflammatory arthritis after failure of silicone rubber replacement of the radial head. *J Bone Joint Surg* 76B:78–81, 1994.

49. Judet T, Garreau deLoubresse C, Piriou P, Charnley G: A floating prosthesis for radial head fractures. *J Bone Joint Surg* 78B:244–249, 1996.

50. Sarmiento A, Horowitch A, Aboulafia A, et al: Functional bracing for comminuted extra-articular fractures of the distal third of the humerus. *J Bone Joint Surg* 72B:283–287, 1990.

51. Bass RL, Stern PJ: Elbow and forearm anatomy and surgical approaches. *Hand Clin* 10:343–356, 1994.

52. Ebraheim NA, Andreshak TG, Yeasting RA, et al: Posterior extensile approach to the elbow joint and distal humerus. *Orthop Rev* 578–582, 1993.

53. Milch H: Fractures and fracture dislocations of the humeral condyles. *J Trauma* 4:592–607, 1964.

54. Kuhn JE, Louis DS, Loder RT: Divergent single-column fractures of the distal part of the humerus. *J Bone Joint Surg* 77A:538–542, 1995.

55. Grantham SA, Norris TR, Bush DC: Isolated fracture of the humeral capitellum. *Clin Orthop Rel Res* 161:262–269, 1981.

56. Alvarez E, Patel MR, Nimberg G, Pearlman JS: Fracture of the capitulum humeri. *J Bone Joint Surg* 57A:1093–1096, 1975.

57. Mosheiff R, Llebergall M, Elyashuv O, et al: Surgical treatment of fractures of the capitellum in adults: A modified technique. *J Orthop Trauma* 5:297–300, 1991.

58. Hamilton WP, Bennett JB: Capitellum osteochondral injury in a football lineman. *Orthopedics* 15:737–739, 1992.

59. Silveri CP, Corso SJ, Roofeh J: Herbert screw fixation of a capitellum fracture: A case report and review. *Clin Orthop Rel Res* 300:123–126, 1994.

60. Dushuttle RP, Coyle MP, Zawadsky JP, Bloom H: Fractures of the capitellum. *J Trauma* 25:317–321, 1985.

61. MacAusland WR, Wyman ET: Fractures of the adult elbow. *Instr Course Lect* 24:165–181, 1975.

62. Riseborough EJ, Radin EL: Intercondylar T fractures of the humerus in the adult. *J Bone Joint Surg* 51A:130–141, 1969.

63. Amis AA, Miller JH: The mechanisms of elbow fractures: An investigation using impact tests in vitro. *Injury* 26:163–168, 1995.

64. Helfet DL, Schmeling GJ: Bicondylar intraarticular fractures of the distal humerus in adults. *Clin Orthop Rel Res* 292:26–36, 1993.

65. Ackerman G, Jupiter J: Non-union of fractures of the distal end of the humerus. *J Bone Joint Surg* 70A:75–83, 1988.

66. McKee MD, Jupiter JB: A contemporary approach to the management of complex fractures of the distal humerus and their sequelae. *Hand Clin* 10:479–494, 1994.

67. Cobb TK, Linscheid RL: Late correction of malunited intercondylar humeral fractures: Intra-articular osteotomy and tricortical bone grafting. *J Bone Joint Surg* 76B:622–626, 1994.

68. Figgie MP, Inglis AE, Mow CS, Figgie HE III: Salvage of nonunion of supracondylar fracture of the humerus by total elbow arthroplasty. *J Bone Joint Surg* 71A:1058–1065, 1989.

69. Bishop AT: Soft tissue loss about the elbow: Selecting optimal coverage. *Hand Clin* 10:531–542, 1994.

70. Chang LD, Goldberg NH, Chang B, Spence R: Elbow defect coverage with a one-staged, tunneled latissimus dorsi transposition flap. *Ann Plast Surg* 32:496–502, 1994.

71. Boerboom AL, deMeyier HE, Verburg AD, Verhaar JAN: Arthrolysis for post-traumatic stiffness of the elbow. *Int Orthop* 17:346–349, 1993.

72. Timmerman LA, Andrews JR: Arthroscopic treatment of post-traumatic elbow pain and stiffness. *Am J Sports Med* 22:230–235, 1994.

73. Hastings H II, Graham TJ: The classification and treatment of heterotopic ossification about the elbow and forearm. *Hand Clin* 10:417–437, 1994.

CHAPTER 23

Forearm Fractures

Thomas M. Reilly
and Christopher T. Born

OVERVIEW

Fractures of the forearm diaphyseal bones, the radius and ulna, can result in significant long-term disability if their primary function, supporting and positioning of the hand, is disrupted. In the adult, the most common mechanism of injury is high-energy trauma, usually in a motor vehicle accident. Therefore, even in apparently isolated injuries, patient evaluation should include a complete systematic musculoskeletal examination.[1,2] Initial radiographic evaluation should include anteroposterior (AP) and lateral views of the forearm, including wrist and elbow joints, as ipsilateral ligamentous and bony injuries are commonly associated with fractures of one or both bones of the forearm and may easily be overlooked.[2]

CLASSIFICATION

Although comprehensive classification systems for diaphyseal fractures have recently been developed by the Orthopaedic Trauma Association and AO/ASIF groups (Fig. 23-1),[4] they have yet to be universally accepted, and their utility remains to be proven.[5] Traditionally, fractures of the forearm have been classified on the basis of the level of the fracture, with the forearm divided into thirds, and the presence of any radioulnar or radiohumeral articular disruption.[3] Specific patterns of forearm injury have been described by several eponyms. Seemingly isolated fractures of the radius may be associated with disruption of the distal radioulnar joint (Galeazzi fracture), while proximal fractures of the ulna may occur in association with radiocapitellar joint dislocation (Monteggia fracture). A direct blow mechanism on the ulna, unlike the radius, may commonly result in an isolated ulnar shaft fracture without associated joint disruption ("nightstick" fracture).

OPEN FRACTURES

Due to the long subcutaneous border of the ulna, the ratio of open to closed fractures is higher in forearm fractures than in any other bone except the tibia.[1,7] The classification system of Gustilo and Anderson may be applied to open forearm fractures for grading of soft tissue injuries,[8] providing a useful prognostic factor for treatment decisions.[9,10]

Initial management consists of prompt operative irrigation and debridement and appropriate broad-spectrum intravenous antibiotics. Recently, immediate open reduction and plating has gained widespread acceptance in the treatment of types I, II, and IIIA open fractures less than 12 to 24 h old.[10,11] Excellent functional outcomes and low infection rates (less than 5 percent) have been documented.[10,11,13]

If interfragmentary compression cannot be obtained due to comminution, autogenous cancellous bone grafting at the time of wound closure has been recommended.[10,12] Type IIIB and IIIC injuries ultimately have poorer outcomes and higher infection rates. Appropriate soft-tissue management requires some form of fixation. Options include external fixation, intramedullary nailing, plating, or delayed conversion to plating from initial external fixation.[13]

In severe injuries, some patients are best served by an early amputation. Scoring systems such as the Mangled Extremity Severity Score (MESS) have been developed as prognostic tools to aid in such decisions.[9]

COMPARTMENT SYNDROME

Forearm compartment syndromes may occur in association with accidental trauma or in the postsurgical setting. Compartment syndromes have even been reported to occur secondary to low-velocity gunshot wounds and other low-energy open fracture injuries.[14] Important early diagnostic indicators include paresthesias and pain on passive extension of the fingers, with absence of the radial pulse occurring later and in only 25 percent.[15] If compartment syndrome is suspected, compartment pressures should be measured, followed by immediate forearm fasciotomy if these are elevated.

TREATMENT OF FOREARM FRACTURES

The primary treatment goal in fractures of the forearm is an anatomic reduction. Healing with angulation of more than 10° has been shown to result in significant limitation of forearm motion, both in cadaver and in clinical studies.[16] Failure to restore the natural bow of the radius can result in loss of motion and grip strength.[17]

Nonoperative

Because of the above factors, closed treatment of adult forearm fractures is usually limited to stable (displaced less than 50 percent of the shaft diameter), isolated fractures of the distal two-thirds of the ulna (nightstick fracture).[18] Long-arm cast immobilization or functional bracing for 8 to 10 weeks yields excellent results, with the latter treatment offering greater patient satisfaction in some

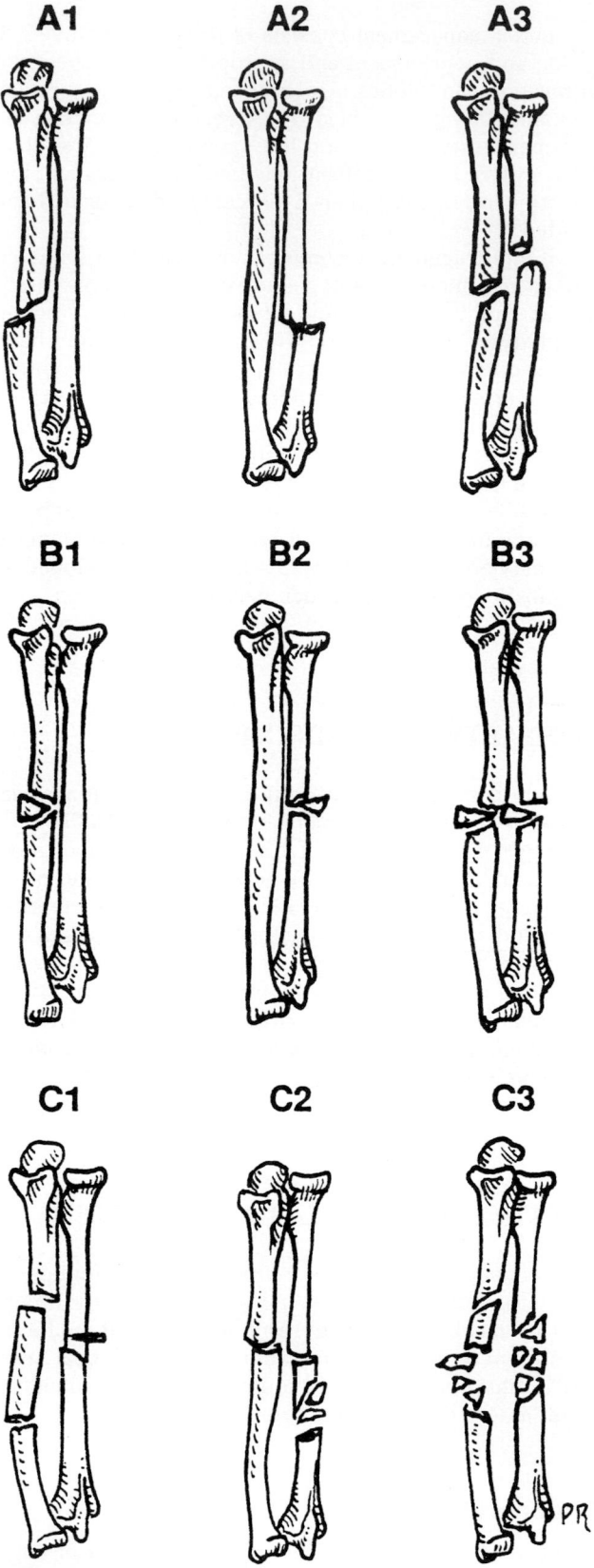

Figure 23-1 AO/ASIF classification of diaphyseal forearm fracture patterns. A1, A2, A3: Simple—of either the radius, ulna, or both. B1, B2, B3: Wedge—of either the radius or ulna or of either bone with the other as a simple or wedge pattern. C1, C2, C3: Complex—of either bone with the other intact/simple/wedge, or comminution of both bones.

studies.[19] Isolated, nondisplaced radial shaft fractures may be amenable to closed treatment if the radial bow is maintained.

Operative

Plate Fixation

Open reduction and internal plate fixation utilizing 3.5-mm dynamic compression plates is the treatment of choice for displaced both-bone diaphyseal fractures of the forearm.[13] Many series have documented union rates greater than 96 percent and good to excellent functional outcomes in 90 percent with this method.[12,13] If more than one-third of the diaphyseal cortex is deficient because of comminution obviating interfragmentary compression, autogenous cancellous bone grafting is recommended.[12,20] The resulting union rates can be similar to those of closed, noncomminuted fractures.[12]

Separate operative approaches should be used for each bone, with surgical exposure of the ulna being best carried out along its subcutaneous border, while the radius may be accessed through either a dorsal Thompson approach or volar Henry approach.

Postoperative management includes protective splinting with early active digital, wrist, and elbow range-of-motion exercises. Most of these fractures will heal within 3 to 4 months, with a loss of less than 25 percent of forearm rotation and 10° of wrist and elbow motion.[1,3,13]

External Fixation

External fixation of forearm diaphyseal fractures is primarily limited to the management of type IIIB and IIIC fractures.[3,21] Indications for its use include fractures associated with severe soft tissue injury, infected nonunions, and maintenance of length in fractures with significant bone loss. However, re-reduction rates may be up to 10 percent,[22] necessitating secondary procedures.[21]

Intramedullary Nailing

Early intramedullary (IM) fixation devices resulted in discouraging results, with high rates of nonunion and healing with angulation due to poor fixation stability.[1] More recent designs include anatomically contoured, fluted IM nails, which offer a more promising biomechanical construct, warranting further investigation into their use in forearm fractures.[23]

COMPLICATIONS
Synostosis

Cross union between the radius and ulna has been reported to occur in 2 to 3 percent of forearm fractures, with a higher incidence in Monteggia fractures.[10,12,24] A classification system based on the anatomic location of the synostosis has been developed: type 1, distal intraarticular portion of the radius and ulna; type 2, diaphyseal; and type 3, proximal one-third.[24] Types 2 and 3 have been found to be the most common. Etiologic factors in cross-union formation include high-energy trauma, infection, open reduction and internal fixation of both bone fractures through a single incision, head-injury, delayed internal fixation (greater than 2 weeks), and fixation screws protruding into the interosseous membrane.[24,25]

Treatment may be conservative if the synostosis develops with the forearm in a functional position. If surgical treatment is required, synostosis resection with interposition of muscle or a silastic sheet may be performed upon maturation of the synostotic bone.[24] Types 1 and 3 lesions have the highest recurrence rate, and type 2, the lowest.[24] Adjunctive postoperative single-fraction, low-dose (800 cGy) irradiation may reduce recurrence rates.[25]

Plate Removal and Refracture

Historically, removal of forearm plates after healing was recommended because of concerns over stress protection under the plate and stress concentration at the end of the plate. However, refracture rates of 4 to 24 percent have been reported after plate removal.[12,17,26,27] Risk factors associated with refracture include use of large (4.5-mm) dynamic compression plates and premature (earlier than 18 months) removal.[12,26,27] Additionally, plate removal has been associated with infection, iatrogenic nerve injury, and failure to relieve symptoms in up to 67 percent of patients with complaints believed referable to the plate.[13,26] Therefore, routine removal of forearm plates is currently discouraged.

GALEAZZI FRACTURE

Classically, this injury is an isolated fracture of the radial diaphysis, usually the distal one-third, along with disruption of the distal radioulnar joint (DRUJ). This uncommon fracture pattern, representing 3 to 6 percent of forearm fractures, is thought to occur through axial loading upon a pronated forearm.[3] Radiographic findings suggesting disruption of the DRUJ include fracture of the ulnar styloid base, widening of the DRUJ space on the AP view, dislocation of the radius with respect to the ulna on a true lateral view, and shortening of the distal radius greater than 5 mm relative to the distal ulna.[28]

Treatment

Open anatomic reduction and plating has yielded the best results for these injuries and may lead to indirect,

stable reduction of the DRUJ.[13,29] If intraoperative examination reveals DRUJ stability after internal fixation of the radius fracture, splinting and early postoperative motion may be started. However, if DRUJ instability is suspected, DRUJ pinning and long arm cast immobilization in supination for 6 weeks is required.[13] Irreducible DRUJ injuries necessitate open reduction to search for soft tissue interposition, such as the extensor carpi ulnaris tendon.

Complications associated with Galeazzi fractures are not uncommon, with some series reporting up to a 39 percent incidence.[6] These include nonunion, malunion, infection, unrecognized DRUJ instability, and iatrogenic nerve injury (usually the dorsal sensory branch of the radial nerve).[6]

MONTEGGIA FRACTURE

The Monteggia lesion describes a fracture of the proximal one-third of the ulna with dislocation of the radial head. This is also an uncommon injury pattern, with an incidence of 1 to 2 percent of all forearm fractures.[1,3] Bado subclassified these injuries based on the pattern of the ulna fracture and radiocapitellar dislocation (Fig. 23-2).[30] Type I injuries are the most common, accounting for 60 to 75 percent of all Monteggia lesions.[31] Normally, a line drawn through the radial shaft and head should intersect the capitellum in any radiographic projection. Radiocapitellar dislocation should be suspected if this is not the case. However, the associated dislocation of the radial head may still be missed in as many as 25 percent of these injuries.[31]

Treatment

In the adult, this injury complex requires open reduction and rigid internal fixation of the ulna, usually by plating.[13,33] Anatomic reduction of the ulna results in reduction of the radial head in over 90 percent of patients. An associated radial head fracture may block reduction, requiring an open reduction and possible internal fixation. Intraoperative stability of the radiocapitellar joint should be assessed throughout flexion, extension, and rotation; if the fracture is stable, splinting and early postoperative range of motion is begun. Long arm cast immobilization for 6 weeks is recommended if instability is suspected.[13]

Complications of Monteggia fracture-dislocations include nonunion, malunion (particularly if the radial head dislocation is missed), infection, and nerve injury. Notably, posterior interosseous nerve injuries may occur in up to 20 percent of patients with Monteggia lesions, particularly the type III pattern. This nerve palsy may be managed conservatively and usually recovers, beginning within 6 to 8 weeks after the injury.[32]

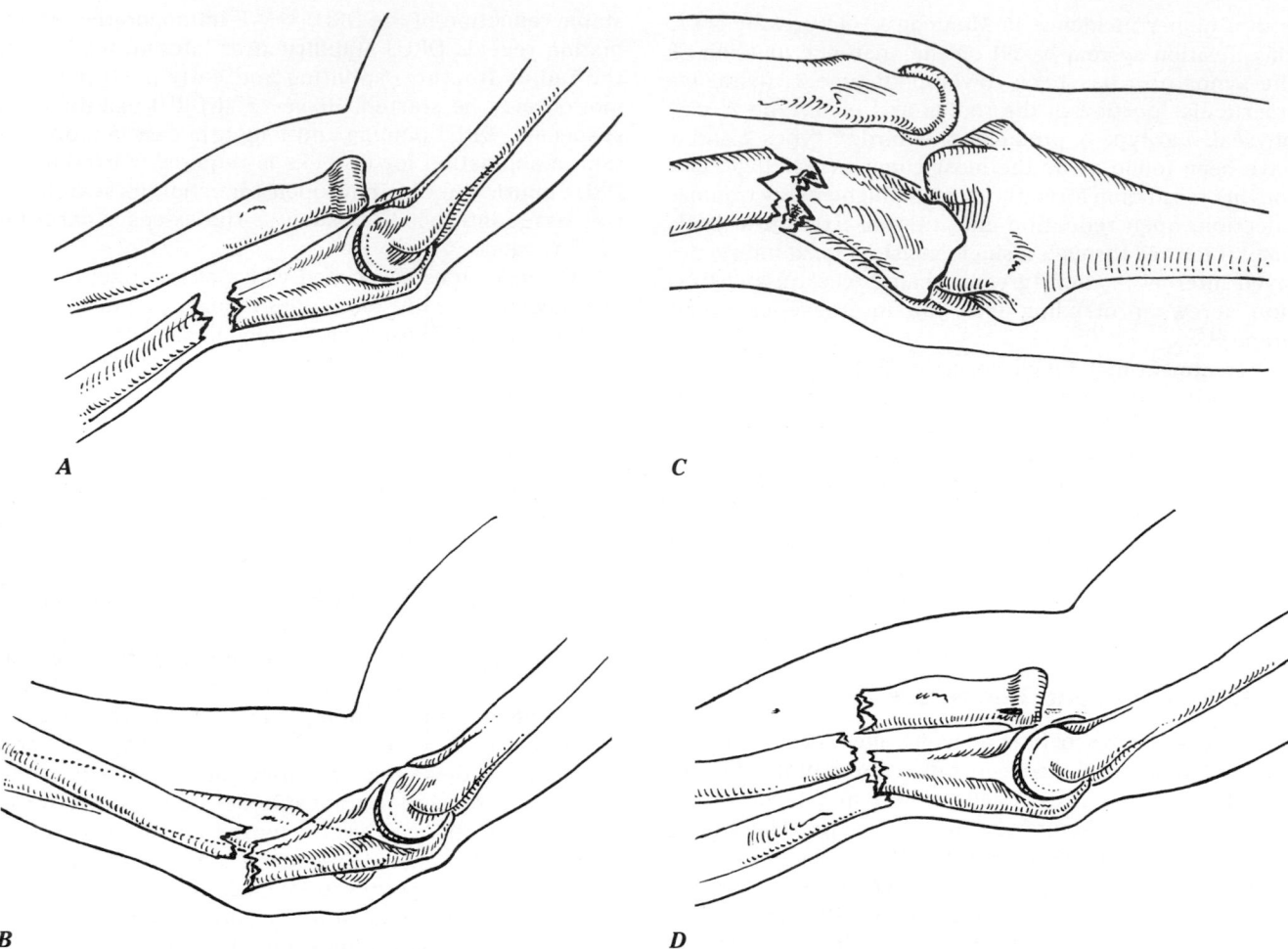

Figure 23-2 Bado classification of Monteggia fractures. *A.* Type 1—ulnar fracture with anterior dislocation of the radial head. *B.* Type II—ulnar fracture with posterior dislocation of the radial head. *C.* Type III—proximal ulnar fracture with lateral dislocation of the radial head. *D.* Type IV—ulnar fracture with anterior dislocation of the radial head and associated fracture of the radial shaft.

REFERENCES

1. Anderson LD, Meyer FN: Fractures of the shaft of the radius and ulna, in Rockwood CA, Green DP, and Bucholz RW (eds): *Fractures in Adults,* 3d ed. Philadelphia, Lippincott, 1991, pp 679.
2. Goldberg HD, Young JW, Reiner BI, et al: Double injuries of the forearm: A common occurrence. *Radiology* 185:223, 1992.
3. Kellam JF, Jupiter JB: Diaphyseal fractures of the forearm, in Browner BD, Jupiter JB (eds): *Skeletal Trauma.* Philadelphia, Saunders, 1992, pp 1095.
4. Muller ME, Nazarian S, Koch P, et al: *Comprehensive Classification of Fractures of Long Bones.* Berlin, Springer-Verlag, 1990, pp 96.
5. Newey ML, Ricketts D, Roberts L: The AO classification of long bone fractures: An early study of its use in clinical practice. *Injury* 24:309, 1993.
6. Moore TM, Klien JP, Patzakis MJ, et al: Results of compression plating of closed Galeazzi fractures. *J Bone Joint Surg* 67A:1015, 1985.
7. Boyd HB, Lipinski SW, Wiley JH: Observations on nonunions of the shafts of the long bones. *J Bone Joint Surg* 43A:159, 1961.
8. Gustilo RB, Merkow RL, Templeman D: Current concepts: Review of the management of open fractures. *J Bone Joint Surg* 72A:299, 1990.
9. Slauterbeck JR, Britton C, Moheb SM, et al: Mangled extremity severity score: An accurate guide to the treatment of the severly injured upper extremity. *J Orthop Trauma* 8:282, 1994.
10. Moed BR, Kellam JF, Foster RJ, et al: Immediate internal fixation of open fractures of the diaphysis of the forearm. *J Bone Joint Surg* 68A:1008, 1986.
11. Jones JA: Immediate internal fixation of high-energy open forearm fractures. *J Orthop Trauma* 5:272, 1991.
12. Chapman MW, Gordon JE, Zissimos AG: Compression plate fixation of acute fractures of the diaphysis of the radius and ulna. *J Bone Joint Surg* 71A:159, 1989.
13. Steyers CM: Elbow and forearm: Trauma, in Kasser JR (ed): *Orthopaedic Knowledge Update 5.* Rosemont IL, American Academy of Orthopaedic Surgeons, 1996, pp 269.
14. Lenihan MR, Brien WW, Gellman H, et al: Fractures of the forearm resulting from low-velocity gun shot wounds. *J Orthop Trauma* 6:32, 1992.
15. Eaton RG, Green WT: Volkmann's ischemia: A volar compartment syndrome of the forearm. *Clin Orthop Rel Res* 113:58, 1975.

16. Sarmiento A, Ebramzaeh E, Brys D, et al: Angular deformities and forearm function. *J Orthop Res* 10:121, 1992.

17. Schemitsch EH, Richards RR: The effect of malunion on functional outcome after plate fixation of fractures of both bones of the forearm in adults. *J Bone Joint Surg* 74A:1068, 1992.

18. Dymond ID: The treatment of isolated fractures of the distal ulna. *J Bone Joint Surg* 66B:408, 1984.

19. Gebuhr P, Hulmich P, Orsnes T, et al: Isolated ulnar shaft fractures: Comparison of treatment by a functional brace and long-arm cast. *J Bone Joint Surg* 74B:757, 1992.

20. Anderson LD, Sisk TD, Tooms RE, et al: Compression plate fixation in acute diaphyseal fractures of the radius and ulna. *J Bone Joint Surg* 57A:287, 1975.

21. Smith DK, Cooney WP: External fixation of high-energy upper extremity injuries. *J Orthop Trauma* 4:7, 1990.

22. Schuind F, Andrianne Y, Burny F: Treatment of forearm fractures by Hoffman external fixation. *Clin Orthop Rel Res* 266:197, 1991.

23. Jones DJ, Henley MB, Schemitsch EH, et al: A biomechanical comparison of two methods of fixation of fractures of the forearm. *J Orthop Trauma* 9:198, 1995.

24. Vince KG, Miller JE: Cross-union complicating fractures of the forearm. *J Bone Joint Surg* 69A:640, 1987.

25. Cullen JP, Pellegrini VD, Miller RJ, et al: Treatment of traumatic radioulnar synostosis by excision and postoperative low-dose irradiation. *J Hand Surg* 19A:394, 1994.

26. Mih AO, Cooney WF, Idler RS, et al: Long-term follow-up of forearm bone diaphyseal plating. *Clin Orthop Rel Res* 299:256, 1994.

27. Beaupree GS, Csongradi JJ: Refracture risk after plate removal in the forearm. *J Orthop Trauma* 10:87, 1996.

28. Moore TM, Lester DK, Sarmiento A: The stabilizing effect of soft tissue constraints in artificial Galeazzi fractures. *Clin Orthop Rel Res* 194:189, 1985.

29. Strehle J, Gerber C: Distal radioulnar joint function after Galeazzi fracture-dislocation treated by open reduction and internal fixation. *Clin Orthop Rel Res* 293:240, 1993.

30. Bado JL: The Monteggia lesion. *Clin Orthop* 50:71, 1967.

31. Boyd HB, Boals JC: The Monteggia lesion. *Clin Orthop* 66:94, 1969.

32. Jessing P: The Monteggia lesions and their complicating nerve damage. *Acta Orthop Scand* 46:601, 1975.

33. Reckling FW: Unstable fracture-dislocations of the forearm. *J Bone Joint Surg* 64A:857, 1982.

CHAPTER 24

Fractures and Dislocations of the Hand and Wrist

Steven P. Sampson, Douglas Wisch, and Edward Akelman

Fractures of the hand are the most common fractures of the skeletal system. Series have shown that hand fractures make up 10 percent of total fractures.[15,44] These injuries often affect people during their wage-earning years and cause significant disability, particularly loss of useful motion.

PHALANGEAL BONES

Fractures of the Distal Phalanx

Fractures of the distal phalanx are the most common fractures of the hand and are frequently complicated by soft tissue loss, severe pulp crush, and nail-bed lacerations. The majority are comminuted but nondisplaced and may be dorsally splinted to immobilize the distal joint. Associated nail-bed lacerations must have thorough irrigation, debridement, and careful repair of the nail bed. Associated subungual hematomas should be drained, permitting the nail to remain intact.[52]

Displaced transverse fractures of the base of the distal phalanx are usually reducible by closed means with the aid of a metacarpal or wrist block. In order to obtain and maintain reduction, flexion of the distal fragment and dorsal splintage of the distal interphalangeal (DIP) joint in slight flexion are often necessary to overcome the flexor profundus pull on the proximal fragment. Displaced fractures may require longitudinal K-wire fixation in order to maintain reduction. Sometimes it may be possible to use an 18-gauge needle to stabilize a fracture in an emergency room setting. Fractures associated with a gap of greater than 2 mm may require open reduction so as to extricate the nail matrix driven into the fracture site.[41]

Dislocations of the Distal Interphalangeal Joint

These dislocations are extremely rare. They are usually dorsal and sometimes open, associated with an innocent-appearing laceration in the region of the DIP joint flexion crease. Following irrigation and debridement of the skin edges, the joint is easily reduced by gentle traction preceded by flexing the wrist and metacarpophalangeal (MCP) joints. A dorsal splint is applied with the DIP joint in slight flexion for approximately 3 weeks, with active proximal interphalangeal (PIP) motion initiated from the onset.[53]

Fractures of the Middle and Proximal Phalanges

Overall skeletal stability of the middle and proximal phalanx is essential for normal PIP function. In this region, fractures will usually displace because of the deforming muscle forces acting on the fracture fragments.[42]

Intracondylar Fractures

Intracondylar fractures of the middle and proximal phalanges are often displaced. These fractures should have an attempted closed reduction utilizing a fracture clamp and percutaneous K-wire fixation (Fig. 24-1). However, more typically, these fractures require an open reduction because of malrotation of the condylar fragment. When these fragments are large enough, 1.5-mm miniscrew fixation may be utilized. Otherwise, transverse K-wire fixation may be adequate with motion of the involved segment delayed for approximately 3 to 4 weeks.[12] Because of the intraarticular nature of these fractures, protected early motion is helpful if fracture stability can be obtained. Dynamic traction techniques are one way to accomplish early motion and maintain reduction of the fragments.[43]

Middle Phalanx Fractures

Extraarticular fractures of the middle phalanx are relatively less common than proximal phalangeal fractures. The displacement of middle phalangeal fractures is usually determined by the relationship of the fracture to the insertion of the flexor digitorum superficialis. Extraarticular fractures of the base of the middle phalanx usually collapse and angulate dorsally. Fractures of the neck, distal to the superficialis insertion, collapse and angulate volarly. Fractures located in the midshaft region between these two extremes may angulate in either direction.[44]

Stable fractures of the middle phalanx may be treated with dorsal splintage, allowing active PIP motion when possible. Because of the increased cortical content of this phalanx, x-ray manifestation of fracture healing will lag about 10 days behind clinical healing. When these fractures are malrotated, displaced, or angulated more than 20°, a closed reduction should be carried out. The hand and wrist should then be placed in a short arm cast incorporating the immediately adjacent digit or digits in such a way as to restore the longitudinal and transverse arches of the hand and wrist. This restoration may be accomplished by placing the hand in an "intrinsic plus" position with the wrist resting in 20° of dorsiflexion, the MCP joints flexed 60 to 70°, and the interphalangeal (IP) joints flexed minimally.[23]

Unstable middle phalangeal fractures may be longitudinally stabilized, avoiding PIP joint fixation (Fig. 24-2). A K wire passed in line with the midaxial skin landmarks will accurately guide pin placement along the midaxis of the bone. Following stabilization, carefully supervised exercises of the PIP joint may be performed during the 4-week splinting period.[12,44]

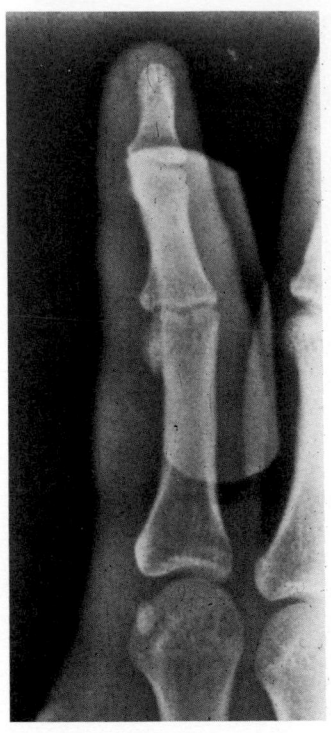
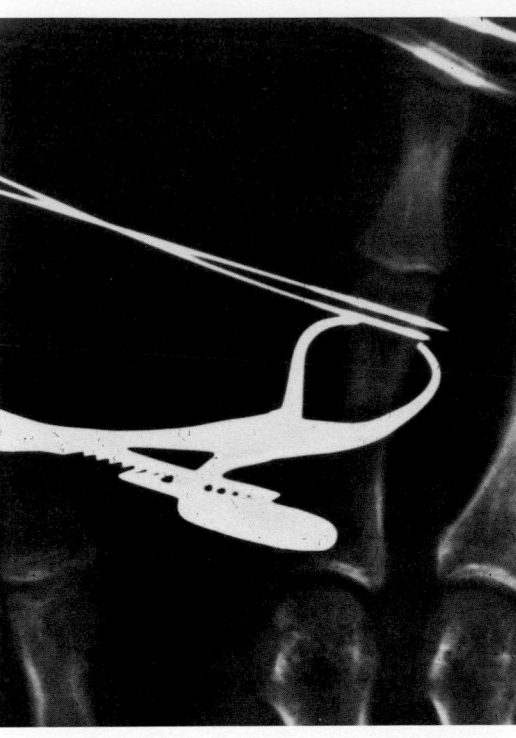

A   *B*

Figure 24-1 *A.* Condylar fracture of the proximal phalanx with an articular stepoff. *B.* Anatomic closed reduction held with percutaneous K-wire pins.

Proximal Phalanx Fractures

Transverse fractures in the proximal third of the midshaft regions of the proximal phalanx collapse with a volar angular deformity. An adequate closed reduction can usually be obtained by traction applied to the middle phalanx while flexing the MCP joint to 90°. This reduction maneuver uses the intact dorsal periosteal sleeve of the proximal phalanx as a hinge. In addition, by flexing the proximal fragment 90°, one overcomes the deforming forces of the intrinsic musculature.[44]

Spiral and oblique proximal phalangeal fractures may be unstable and are usually associated with shortening and malrotation (Fig. 24-3*A* and *B*). These fractures are usually easy to reduce but tend to redisplace in the direction of their prior deformity. Malrotation must be carefully checked by finger flexion and comparison with the opposite hand.

Fractures at the base of the proximal phalanx frequently occur in osteopenic metaphyseal bone and usually deform with the apex volar. These fractures can usually be reduced by similar traction and flexion maneuvers but are usually associated with dorsal comminution and consequently commonly redisplace.[44]

Unstable transverse and short oblique proximal phalangeal fractures can usually be stabilized with a K wire following anatomic closed reduction. The wire is passed into the proximal phalanx in an antegrade fashion with the MCP joint flexed at 60 to 70° and advanced across the fracture to the phalangeal metaphysis but not into the PIP joint. The K wire acts as an "internal suture" allowing provisional stabilization and early PIP joint motion. Incorporation of adjacent digits in plaster helps maintain rotational stability.

The K wire is maintained for approximately 3 weeks, and the pin is then removed. Complications of this technique are avoided by expeditious removal of the K wire.[12,44]

Unstable oblique proximal phalangeal fractures with greater than 45° of angulation may be reduced with a fracture clamp (Fig. 24-3*C*). These fractures can be maintained with the adjacent digit incorporated. Extension block splinting should begin in the early postoperative period in order to allow active PIP flexion. If anatomic closed reduction cannot be obtained, open reduction with K wires or 1.5- to 2.0-mm screw fixation may be considered. Motion of the digit

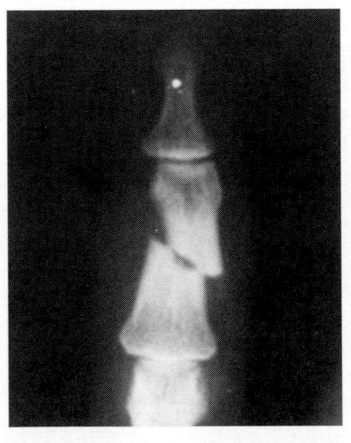
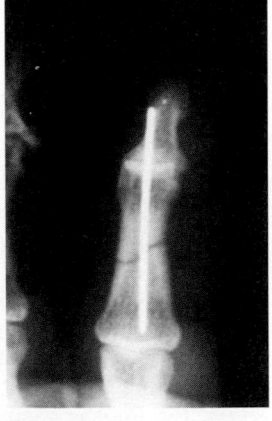

A   *B*

Figure 24-2 *A.* Anteroposterior x-ray view showing angulated fracture of the middle phalanx that failed attempted closed reduction. *B.* Anatomic reduction with K-wire fixation.

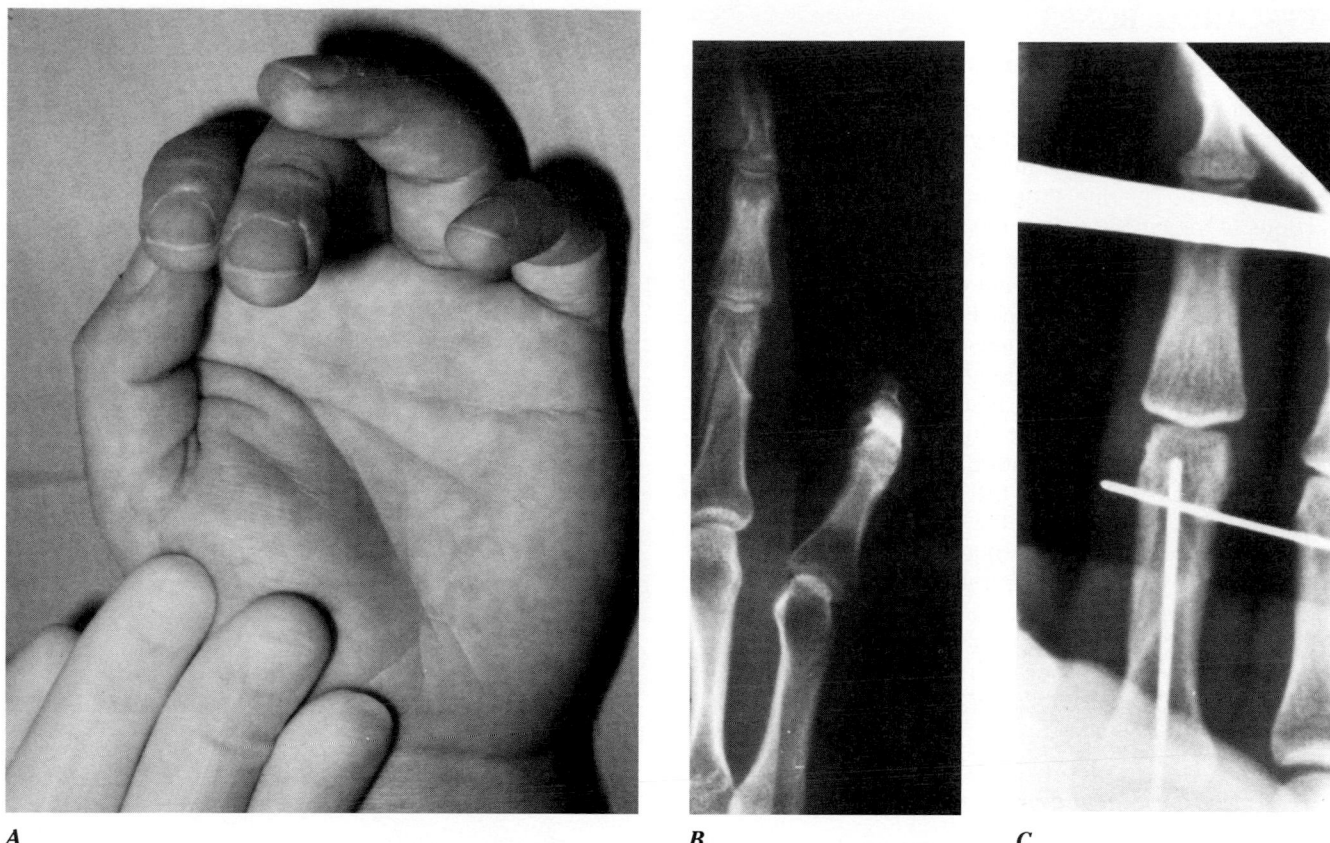

A   *B*   *C*

Figure 24-3 *A.* Malrotation secondary to a spiral oblique fracture of the proximal phalanx. *B.* Shortened spiral oblique fracture of proximal phalanx. *C.* Near anatomic reduction obtained utilizing both longitudinal and transverse K wires.

should be initiated within 48 h of stable operative fixation and a protective splint worn between exercises.[1,7,11,12,44]

Proximal Interphalangeal Dislocations and Fracture Dislocations

Dislocations of the PIP joint are common. Dorsal dislocations with resultant hyperextension injuries to the volar plate are relatively common.[42] Following metacarpal or wrist block anesthesia, these dislocations are usually easy to reduce. Treatment includes dorsal PIP joint splintage in approximately 30° of flexion for approximately 1 week, followed by "buddy" tape splinting to the adjacent digit for the next 6 weeks. Following reduction, all dislocations should be tested for stability with an "active motion test" and a collateral ligament stress test while the patient is under anesthesia. These tests will determine those dislocations that are stable and able to be moved early as opposed to those that will require extension block splinting for more prolonged periods of time.[7,8]

Frequently, intraarticular fractures at the base of the middle phalanx are associated with dorsal dislocation and/or subluxation of the PIP joint. These volar plate fractures are usually stable if less than one-third of the articular surface is involved on examination of a true lateral x-ray view. Fractures with greater than one-third of the articular surface involved are usually unstable because the displaced volar middle phalangeal fragment also contains the distal attachment of the collateral ligament, thereby allowing dorsal displacement. In the acute state, reduction of these subluxations can usually be carried out with flexion of the PIP joint between 60 and 80°. If a closed reduction can be obtained, a 4- to 6-week program of extension block splinting with active PIP joint flexion is carried out. Alternatively, loss of reduction is associated with joint incongruity, necessitating open reduction accompanied by collateral ligament excision, debridement of comminuted volar fragments, and advancement of the volar plate.[7,8,30]

Volar dislocations of the proximal interphalangeal joint are rare injuries. These may be treated conservatively when congruent reduction is obtained with an extension lag of less than 30° actively at the PIP joint. However, these injuries are sometimes irreducible, and they may reveal evidence of joint incongruity due to interposition of the central slip or herniation of the proximal phalangeal condyle through the extensor mechanism with associated rupture of the volar plate and the collateral ligament. These irreducible complex dislocations require open reduction and K-wire pinning of the PIP joint in extension for approximately 2 weeks. Dynamic extension splinting is then used for 2 to 4 weeks. As opposed to dorsal dislocations, volar dislocations of the PIP joint are frequently associated with significant loss of motion.[7,37]

METACARPAL BONES

Fractures of the Metacarpal

Approximately 36 percent of hand fractures involve the metacarpals.[16] Biomechanically, the index and long metacarpals act as the stabilizing central *fixed* unit of the hand and wrist. The ring, little, and thumb metacarpals are portions of the *mobile* unit of the hand. Fracture displacement, angulation, and shortening occurring within the central fixed unit of the hand have dramatically more functional impact than those same injuries sustained in the mobile unit of the hand. Anatomically, the carpometacarpal (CMC) joints of the index and long fingers have stable joint configurations and strong ligamentous attachments, whereas the CMC joints of the ring and little fingers allow flexion, extension, and supination.[17]

The intrinsic muscles are the primary deforming force of fractures occurring within the longitudinal arch of the hand. Instead of flexion occurring at the MCP joint, the intrinsic muscles act to angulate fractures in this region dorsally. Generally, unstable *fixed-unit* metacarpal fractures are evident by compensatory MCP joint hyperextension, whereas metacarpal *mobile-unit* fractures tend to compensate primarily at their mobile CMC joints and then secondarily at the MCP joint.

Intraarticular Metacarpal Fractures

Intraarticular metacarpal head fractures are relatively rare injuries. Sometimes these can be missed if the fracture involves the sides of the metacarpal head. Therefore, a Brewerton view should be added to routine views of the hand.[27] These fractures are most commonly seen in the border digits, the index and little fingers. They may be associated with open osteochondral fractures, and joint sepsis is a key concern. Most fractures in this region are comminuted and are associated with significant soft tissue trauma, including adjacent metacarpal and phalangeal fractures. Large articular fragments should be considered for open reduction and internal fixation, whereas severely comminuted fractures should have controlled early motion initiated, with MCP joint arthroplasty as a salvage alternative. Transverse fractures of the metacarpal head can be associated with avascular necrosis as a late complication.

Intraarticular fractures of the base of the metacarpals are most common in the thumb and little fingers. The most significant clinical problem associated with these injuries is subluxation of the CMC joint. In a *Bennett's fracture,* the strong volar ligament remains attached to the volar-ulnar tubercle of the thumb metacarpal (Fig. 24-4*A*). Due to the continued pull of the abductor pollicis longus, the thumb metacarpal subluxes dorsoradially and the adductor pulls the shaft toward the second metacarpal. Articular congruity must be reestablished with a closed reduction and percutaneous pinning (Fig. 24-4*B*). Closed reduction may be obtained by traction of the thumb metacarpal followed by radial abduction and finally by a pronation rotatory torque, placing the thumb metacarpal in the palmar abduction in opposition to the second metacarpal.[4,44]

Comminuted intraarticular fractures associated with the thumb metacarpal are also known as *Rolando's frac-*

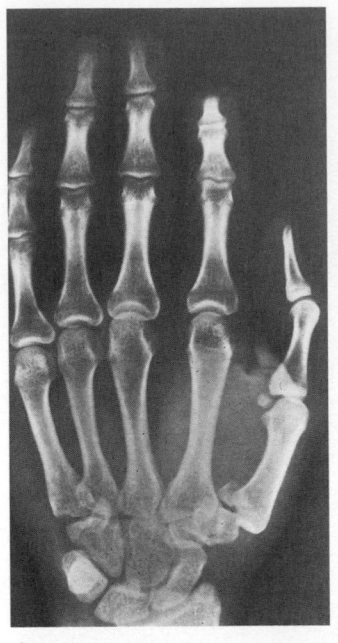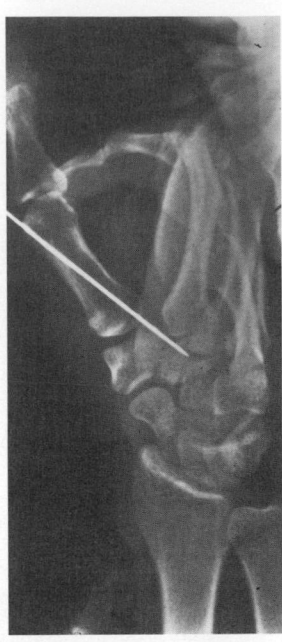

A   *B*

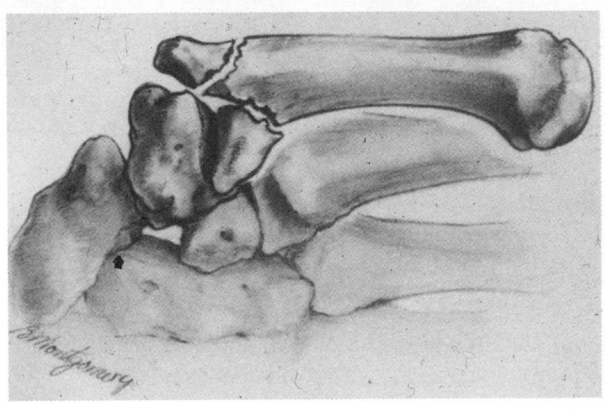

C

Figure 24-4 *A.* Bennett's fracture with subluxation of first metacarpal and loss of joint congruity. *B.* Closed anatomic reduction maintained with an axial K wire. *C.* Rolando's fracture. (Reproduced with permission from Green DP, O'Brien ET: Fractures of the thumb metacarpal. *South Med J* 65:807, 1972.)

tures (Fig. 24-4*C*). These fractures may be initially stabilized in a thumb spica cast with the thumb metacarpal placed in palmar abduction in apposition to the index finger. Early mobilization in 10 to 14 days should be considered, depending upon individual circumstances. Rolando's fractures associated with large intraarticular fragments should be considered for open reduction and internal fixation with either 2.0- or 2.7-mm screws or K-wire stabilization.[4,44]

Fractures of the little metacarpal base simulate Bennett's fracture subluxation of the thumb. Articular congruity must be obtained by a reduction that overcomes the pull of the extensor carpi ulnaris on the metacarpal base and also that of the hypothenar intrinsic musculature. Reduction must be carried out by traction and ulnar abduction of the little finger metacarpal, followed by a slight supination torque. Percutaneous pinning is then car-

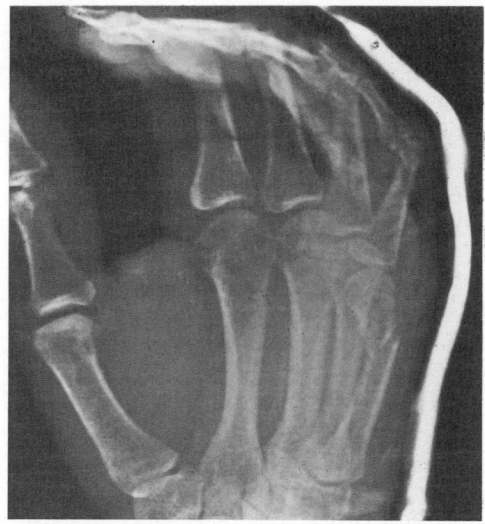
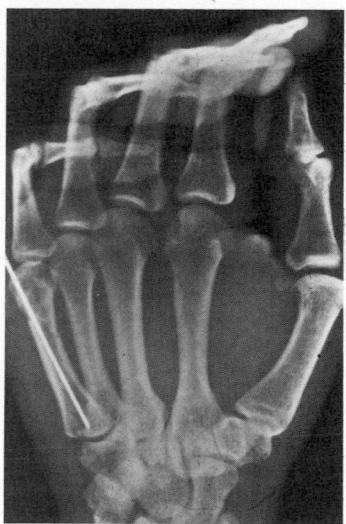

A   *B*

Figure 24-5 *A.* Clawing is evident with MCP hyperextension and PIP flexion in this metacarpal neck-shaft fracture. X-ray films reveal 40° of dorsal angulation. *B.* Anatomic closed reduction held with percutaneous K wire.

ried out, pinning the little to the ring metacarpal and to the hamate. The best x-ray picture taken to visualize reduction of this joint is shot with the forearm pronated 30° from the routine anteroposterior position. Late sequelae of unreduced subluxation dislocations include posttraumatic arthrosis, sometimes requiring ligament interposition arthroplasty, prosthetic arthroplasty, or arthrodesis.[25,38]

Extraarticular Metacarpal Fractures

Fractures of the metacarpal neck are generally unstable injuries because of the concomitant comminution of the volar cortex (Fig. 24-5*A*). Within this region, there is a relatively dramatic transition from thin corticocancellous metaphyseal bone to thickened diaphyseal cortex.[28] Anatomically, the dorsal cortices of the metacarpals are relatively straight in contour, whereas the volar cortices have a concavity corresponding to the contour of the palm. Radiographically, a true lateral of the average metacarpal will reveal a 10 to 15° neck-shaft angulation.

When metacarpal neck fractures are associated with significant dorsal soft tissue swelling following a clenched fist mechanism of injury, the possibility of a human bite infection must be meticulously excluded. Until otherwise proven, any wound over the MCP joint from a human bite is usually associated with an open MCP joint and possibly a defect in the metacarpal head. Aggressive treatment should be initiated—i.e., thorough irrigation and debridement in the operating room and appropriate antibiotics.[45]

Controversy exists as to how much dorsal angulation in the ring and little metacarpal neck fracture is acceptable. Because of compensatory carpometacarpal motion, up to 30 or 40° of dorsal angulation may be acceptable for these mobile-unit neck fractures. This is in contrast to the fixed-unit (index and long) metacarpal neck fractures, in which minimal angulation (10 to 15°) is acceptable.[44]

Closed reduction of metacarpal neck fractures is carried out by traction and disimpaction followed by the Jahss reduction maneuver. This entails 90° of MCP and PIP flexion, thereby controlling the distal metacarpal fragment by the relative tautness of the MCP collateral ligaments. Counterpressure is then applied to the dorsum of the proximal fragment at the fracture site. Typically, reduction is easy to obtain but difficult to maintain.[10] A short arm cast is applied incorporating the adjacent digit to the level just proximal to the PIP joint. The wrist is held in 20° of extension, the MCP joints are held in 60 to 70° of flexion, and the PIP joints are left free. Molding the cast in the 90°–90° reduction position is contraindicated because of the resultant stiffness and potential skin or tendon slough over the dorsum of the PIP joint.[22]

Rowland and Green have described a simple clinical test to identify those patients who may be treated by closed reduction and cast immobilization. Following wrist block anesthesia, those patients who are able to extend the fractured finger fully, without concomitant MCP joint hyperextension and flexion at the PIP joint, may be treated conservatively. If "clawing" or zigzag collapse becomes apparent on this clinical test (Fig. 24-5*A*), then percutaneous pin fixation is recommended to maintain the reduction (Fig. 24-5*B*).[15]

Technically, various methods of percutaneous pin fixation of these metacarpal neck fractures have been described. An anatomic reduction is essential prior to K-wire stabilization paralleling the straight dorsal cortex of the involved metacarpal. In the majority of cases, stabilization of the fracture has occurred by the end of 3 weeks; the K wire is then removed. Removal of the K wire at this time avoids the feared complication of MCP joint arthrofibrosis and sepsis. Following K-wire removal, the involved digits are splinted with buddy tape, usually for 4 to 6 weeks. An additional indication for closed reduction and internal fixation of metacarpal neck fractures is any fracture associated with malrotation or complete displacement.[44]

Fractures occurring in the region of the *metacarpal shaft* may result in similar dorsal angulatory deformities related to the intrinsic muscular forces. Less than 10° of dorsal angulation is acceptable in the index and long metacarpals; 20° is acceptable in the ring and little fingers. The closer a fracture is to the midshaft level, the greater the probability that such a fracture will cause a claw deformity on extension of the digit. Oblique fractures of the metacarpal shaft tend to be unstable and to shorten according to the initial deforming force and to the degree of obliquity at the fracture site. The intervolar plate (deep transverse metacarpal) ligament will usually prevent significant shortening of the central metacarpal (i.e., long and ring fingers). However, greater than 3 or 4 mm of shortening is more likely to occur in the border metacarpals (i.e., index and little fingers and thumb).[16,44]

Unstable metacarpal shaft fractures are treated initially by attempted closed reduction and application of a short arm cast incorporating the adjacent digits to the level just proximal to the PIP joint. Reduction can usually be accomplished by longitudinal traction and extension of the wrist with fixation of the CMC joints, followed by MCP flexion and, finally, "third-point" molding dorsally over the fracture site. If a closed reduction cannot be maintained as swelling subsides, percutaneous K-wire fixation is carried out.

When two adjacent unstable oblique metacarpal fractures occur, a single longitudinal intramedullary K wire is usually inadequate to control angulation, rotation, and shortening. Therefore, besides a longitudinal pin to control dorsal angulation, a distal transmetacarpal pin may be utilized to prevent shortening. This type of treatment may be complicated by delayed union due to overdistraction at the fracture site. Alternatively, unstable oblique fractures of the metacarpal shaft may be treated by open reduction and internal fixation with 2.0- or 2.7-mm screws. Plate fixation may be indicated when the obliquity of the fracture is less than 45 to 60° from the axis of the metacarpal shaft. In general, rigid internal fixation should be reserved for situations in which immediate skeletal stability is required to mobilize joints within the first 48 h.[16,44] However, it should be noted that the majority of hand fractures can be treated with pin fixation. One should always avoid excessive stripping when plating a fracture. One must take into account the effects of soft tissue injury when applying plates and screws versus K-wire fixation.

Metacarpophalangeal Joint Dislocations

Dislocations of the MCP joints of the ulnar four digits are relatively rare injuries. The history is of a significant hypertension injury of either the index or little metacarpal with resultant rupture of the volar plate. Anatomically, the MCP joints are structurally the most unstable phalangeal joints and are dependent on ligamentocapsular restraint to check increased motion. The MCP joints allow abduction, adduction, and some rotation as these joints progress from a flexed to an extended posture. Thus, when forces are applied in the hyperextended position, the collateral ligaments are lax and tension is borne by the volar plate. The central MCP joints of the long and ring fingers are relatively more stabilized by their bordering digits and their respective intervolar plate ligaments.[7,8]

Simple MCP joint dislocations should undergo an attempted closed reduction under wrist block anesthesia. While flexing the wrist, the head of the proximal phalanx is gently grasped. In order to secure reduction, the dorsally displaced proximal phalanx base is gently pushed distally, while the fingers grasping the proximal phalanx are initially hyperextending and then flexing its base. Any overt traction maneuver may convert the simple reducible dislocation into a complex or irreducible one.[7]

The pathognomonic sign of a complex MCP dislocation is the presence of an associated puckering of the skin in the region of the distal palmar crease of the hand.[7] The most common anatomic structure preventing closed reduction is the interposition of the volar plate, which ruptures proximally. This differs from the dorsal dislocations of the PIP joint in which the volar plate usually ruptures distally. Open reduction is carried out after incision of the flexor tendon sheath in the region of the A1 pulley. Care must be taken in using a volar approach because the radial neurovascular bundle may be displaced volarly under tension. Following reduction, the joint is placed in 45° of flexion and a short arm cast is applied incorporating the adjacent digit for approximately 3 weeks, allowing PIP flexion. During the fourth postoperative week, a program of MCP joint extension block splinting is begun.[7,8]

Dislocations of the MCP joint of the thumb are much more common than those seen in the ulnar four digits. They may be simple or complex, and they may be dorsally, volarly, or laterally displaced. The reduction maneuver recommended is as previously described for other MCP joints. Complex dislocations have been attributed to the volar plate, sesamoids, and flexor pollicis longus. Following reduction, a short arm thumb spica cast is applied with the MCP joint in approximately 20° of flexion with the IP joint left free. Few patients develop late collateral ligamentous instability following dorsal and volar dislocations; however, ulnar instability, or a late sequela, must be carefully checked, especially after lateral dislocations.[8,20]

Carpometacarpal Joint Dislocations

Dislocations of the carpometacarpal joints of the ulnar four metacarpals are among the most commonly overlooked dislocations in the hand. These injuries are usually associated with extensive soft tissue swelling, which obscures the true reason for the flattening of the proximal transverse metacarpal arch contour. Dislocations in this region may be dorsal or volar, but most are dorsal with involvement of the fourth and fifth metacarpal bases. As with other ulnar-sided metacarpal injuries, a true lateral radiograph will commonly be difficult to interpret because of the multiple overlapping shadows of the adjacent four metacarpals. Much more information may be derived from lateral x-ray films taken with the forearm pronated 30° from the routine lateral position.[8]

Dislocations of the ulnar four carpometacarpal joints are generally easy to reduce by gentle traction. However, the maintenance of these reductions often requires percutaneous K-wire fixation. When more than one carpometacarpal joint is dislocated, these wires are passed longitudinally following reduction and restoration of the proximal transverse carpal arch. Reductions that are held with transverse K wires at the base tend to flatten this arch, thereby possibly preventing congruous reduction of the CMC joints. A short arm cast is applied with the CMC joints in extension. The involved and the adjacent digits are incorporated with the MCP joints flexed approximately 60°. The pins are removed at 4 weeks, and immobilization is then continued an additional 2 to 3 weeks. Chronic dislocations in this region are associated with pain and loss of grip strength.[21] Either interposition arthroplasty or arthrodesis have been the recommended treatments for this condition.[38]

Carpometacarpal dislocations of the thumb are rare. Again, these dislocations are generally dorsoradial. Generally, reduction is easy to obtain but difficult to maintain. A pin placed longitudinally in a retrograde fashion from the region of the MCP joint across the CMC joint can be used to overcome this difficulty. A short arm thumb spica cast is applied allowing IP motion for approximately 3 to 4 weeks. The pin is then removed and a thumb stabilizer splint is applied for an additional 3 weeks. Chronic CMC dislocations of the thumb usually present with pain, deformity, and weakness of pinch. Treatment is dependent upon the chronicity of the dislocation and the degree of arthrosis found in the basal joint. Treatment options include volar ligament reconstruction, tendon interposition arthroplasty, trapezium arthroplasty, or arthrodesis.[20,33]

CARPAL BONES

A majority of carpal bone fractures occur within the proximal carpal row. Because it is a vulnerable link between the proximal and distal carpal rows, the scaphoid is the most common carpal bone to be fractured, and second only to fractures of the distal radius.[1] Carpal bone fractures usually occur in a relatively young population group and are frequently complicated by severe soft tissue swelling, ligamentous disruption, and/or neurovascular compromise.[19,47]

Scaphoid Fractures

Considerable controversy exists regarding the treatment of scaphoid fractures. A thorough understanding of scaphoid anatomy and its blood supply are important in determining the prognosis for fracture union. Anatomically, this small, boat-shaped carpal bone is almost completely covered with hyaline cartilage. There are two extremely important areas that are devoid of hyaline cartilage. One is the volar insertion of the radioscaphoid-capitate ligament or "sling" ligament, which obliquely crosses the waist of the scaphoid. A second area void of hyaline cartilage lies dorsally along the spiral groove that is coincident with the waist region of the scaphoid. The main intraosseous blood supply to the proximal two-thirds of the scaphoid enters through this dorsal ridge region. Vascular injection studies of the scaphoid have revealed that approximately 13 percent of the specimens would have lost the retrograde blood supplied to the proximal pole following a waist fracture. Vascular variation from individual to individual

contributes to the difficulty in predicting which patients will go on to develop avascular necrosis following similar fractures of the scaphoid.[13,19,36]

Cadaveric studies have demonstrated the mechanism of scaphoid fractures by loading the radial side of the palm, thereby dorsiflexing the wrist beyond its physiologic range (greater than 95°). The wrist then also assumes a posture of radial deviation. This loading position produces a bending moment in the region of the waist of the foreshortened and volar flexed scaphoid, and fracture occurs.[19]

A general guiding principle in the acute management of wrist trauma is that following a fall on the "outstretched" hand and wrist, the presence of any snuffbox tenderness even in the absence of radiographic evidence of a fractured scaphoid should be considered a fracture until proved otherwise. Leslie and Dixon reviewed a series of 222 consecutive patients with acute scaphoid fractures.[29] They included four standard radiographic positions in the wrist trauma series: a posteroanterior (PA) view, a lateral view, a PA view with the wrist pronated 45°, and a similar view supinated 45°. The initial PA and semipronated views enabled these authors to diagnose a clear fracture 98 percent of the time. According to the authors, the remaining 2 percent of fractures became radiographically evident over the ensuing weeks of treatment. These false-negative fractures were incomplete and were located on the compression (concave) side of the scaphoid. The initial lateral radiograph is essential for the diagnosis of concomitant carpal instability.

It is noteworthy that myriad radiographic positions have been devised in an attempt to rule out acute scaphoid fracture. Terry and Ramin have emphasized the adjacent soft tissue planes to the scaphoid, which they call the *navicular* (scaphoid) *fat stripe*. Obliteration or displacement of this soft tissue plane would dictate treatment as an acute fracture. In rare instances, nondiagnostic plain films may be supplemented by bone scan, tomograms, CT scan, or MRI studies. In order to avoid false-negative bone scans, imaging should be delayed at least 48 h following wrist trauma.[19]

Weber and Cooney have developed a radiographic classification based on the degree of initial fracture displacement—i.e., fracture stability. Scaphoid fractures that are nondisplaced and have a fracture gap of less than 1 mm have an intact periosteal hinge and are considered stable fractures. Acute stable fractures, treated in a thumb spica short arm cast with the wrist positioned in slight flexion and radial deviation, had a nearly perfect union rate with an immobilization time of 9 or 10 weeks. Exceptions to the rule of fracture stability were patients whose treatment was delayed, those with concomitant Colles' fracture, and those noted to have a late carpal collapse deformity. The authors have emphasized that the position of the wrist during immobilization may be critical in avoiding late carpal collapse.[19]

A displaced scaphoid fracture with greater than 1 mm of stepoff on any radiographic view, with or without evidence of carpal instability, is considered an unstable fracture. Although Cooney's series was small, approximately 50 percent of such displaced fractures went on to nonunion

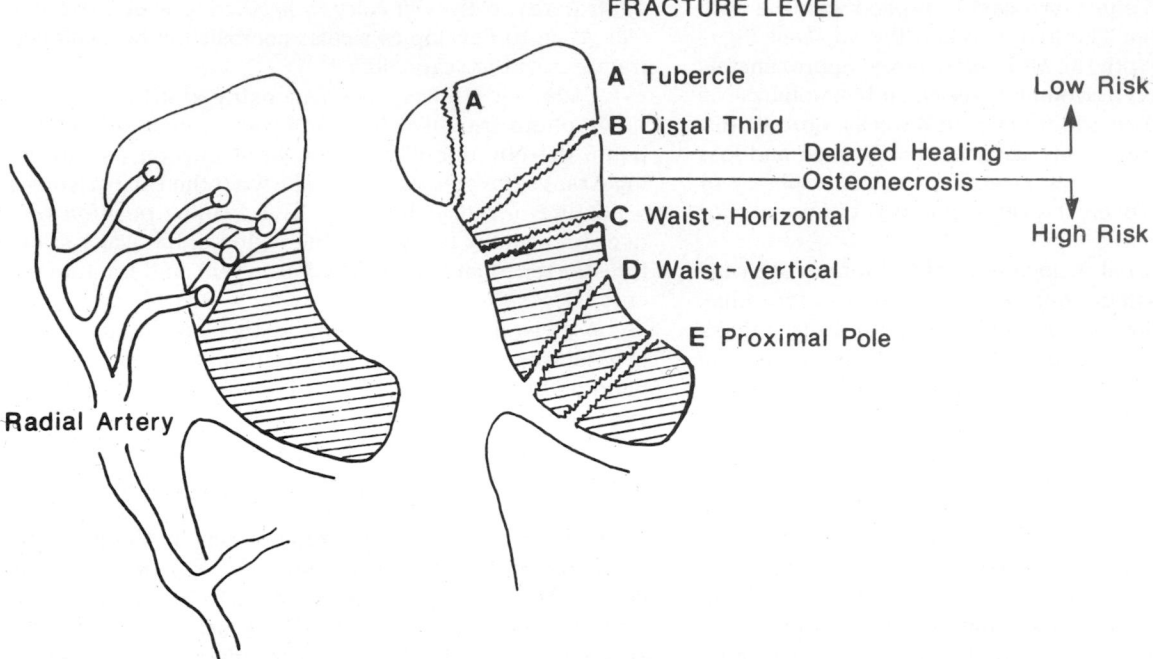

Figure 24-6 Vascular and regional factors affecting prognosis in scaphoid fractures. Fractures within the proximal two-thirds are at high risk for the development of osteonecrosis. (Reproduced with permission from Melone CP: Scaphoid fractures. *Clin Plast Surg* 8:86, 1981.)

despite attempts at closed reduction and casting. The average healing time to union was approximately 4 months in the fractures that healed. Thus, a general recommendation for these displaced fractures is one of attempted closed anatomic reduction with percutaneous K-wire fixation and casting. If an anatomic reduction cannot be obtained, open reduction is recommended, with emphasis on correction of any carpal instability at the time of open reduction.[19]

The prognosis for the management of acute scaphoid fractures is thus based on two important factors: (1) anatomic location of the fracture and (2) fracture stability. Fractures of the proximal and middle thirds of the scaphoid are at high risk for delayed union and avascular necrosis (Fig. 24-6). Since approximately 70 percent of fractures occur in the middle third or waist region and 20 percent within the region of the proximal one-third, it is not surprising that healing time is prolonged. In contrast, fractures of the region of the distal one-third of the scaphoid (approximately 10 percent of scaphoid fractures) go on to uneventful union in approximately 6 weeks. Displaced or unstable fractures are also at high risk for delayed union, malunion, or nonunion. Any fracture offset greater than 1 mm is usually associated with malrotation and thus poor fragment apposition.[1,19,24,32]

High-risk scaphoid fractures may be treated with long arm casting incorporating the thumb to the interphalangeal joint level for 6 weeks, followed by short arm casting with supracondylar extension to limit forearm rotation for 6 more weeks, and finally with a short arm thumb spica cast. The patient is x-rayed in plaster at weekly intervals for 2 weeks from the onset of immobilization and then x-rayed out of plaster at the intervals prescribed above. Fracture healing is determined clinically by the disappearance of snuffbox tenderness and the bridging trabeculae radiographically. Overall, the literature is controversial as to the position of the wrist and thumb during the immobilization period as well as the extension of the cast at or above the elbow level. Those patients who present acutely and adhere to an immobilization protocol will generally go on to uneventful union. Those who are noncompliant, present late, and have sporadic cast immobilization will have a higher rate of nonunion. Distal third fractures and transverse wrist fractures heal in 6 to 8 weeks; oblique wrist fractures in 8 to 12 weeks; proximal pole fractures in 12 to 24 weeks. The more proximal the fracture, the higher incidence of going on to avascular necrosis.[1,19,24]

Open reduction and internal fixation of scaphoid fractures is indicated for unstable fractures or displacement greater than 1 mm, transscaphoid perilunate dislocations, proximal pole fractures less than 25 percent, complete displacement or an avascular fragment, polytrauma, or if a long period of immobilization creates a hardship to the patient. Scaphoid reduction can be maintained using K wires or screw fixation. Volar approaches are more commonly done than dorsal ones, and some advocate arthroscopic techniques, noting that all are technically demanding and should be done by someone with a thorough understanding of the wrist and its anatomy.[19,24,51]

The distinction between delayed union and nonunion is at times extremely arbitrary. A roentgenographic definition of scaphoid nonunion is a fracture that fails to show a progression of fracture healing on three separate monthly examinations after a treatment period of 6 months. Clearly, the pattern of posttraumatic osteoarthritis that extends into the radiocarpal joint over a 20-year period places those individuals with displaced or unstable fractures at high risk. Those displaced scaphoid nonunions should be reduced and bone grafted prior to the onset of pan-scaphoid arthrosis. It remains unclear whether pan-scaphoid arthrosis is inevitable in those patients who have stable nonunions without carpal instability.[1,19,24]

Symptomatic scaphoid nonunions should be treated with some type of either inlay Russe bone graft or an inter-position graft to correct a hump-back deformity. Again, some types of screw fixation may be warranted. Vascularized bone grafts are being used primarily for proximal pole injuries. Salvage procedures include resection arthroplasty with limited fusion, proximal row carpectomy, total wrist fusions, or, in the past, resection and replacement with a silicone implant or now one of titanium.[19,24]

Other Carpal Fractures

Simple fractures are the more common types and are characterized by ligamentous avulsion fracture patterns. The *triquetrum avulsion fracture* is primarily associated with a dorsal fleck of bone with concomitant severe soft tissue swelling over the dorsum of the wrist. Posteroanterior and lateral x-ray films may be nondiagnostic and must be supplemented by 30° semipronated oblique films. The treatment of choice is short arm casting for approximately 4 to 6 weeks. Fractures of the hook of the hamate are associated with a history of athletic injury, especially during baseball, golf, or racket sports. Patients complain of pain radiating to the dorsum of the ulnar side of the wrist associated with hypothenar swelling. On physical exam, there is point tenderness directly over the hook of the hamate palmarly. Once again, standard positioning for x-ray filming is inadequate to reveal the fracture. Acutely, patients may not permit carpal tunnel view positioning due to pain. A CT scan of the hamate will help in the diagnosis of a fracture. The treatment of choice acutely is short arm casting for approximately 4 to 6 weeks. When seen chronically, symptomatic nonunion of hook of the hamate is usually treated by excision of the ununited fragment.[1,24]

Complex carpal bone fractures are rare but extremely disabling injuries. The mechanism of injury usually results from high-energy loading associated with compression and shear. Complex injuries are typified by their concomitant injury to an adjacent joint, which is usually subluxed or dislocated. The extent of osteochondral injury is usually unrecognized and may be associated with late carpal arthrosis. The remainder of the carpal bones have been implicated in this complex pattern of injury. Beginning with the distal carpal row, fractures of the trapezium are often associated with dorsal dislocation of the first metacarpal. Alternatively, compressive loading of the first metacarpal may split the trapezium, requiring open reduction in order to restore the articular congruity of the basal joint. Fractures of the trapezoid are extremely rare and are often associated with fixed-unit disruption of the CMC joints of the index and long fingers. These trapezoid fractures are usually ligamentous avulsion injuries and re-

quire careful reduction of the injured CMC joints. Fractures of the body of the hamate are usually intraarticular in nature and can be associated with CMC dislocations of the ring and little fingers. Closed or possibly open reduction may be the required treatment in order to restore articular congruity. Fractures of the pisiform are extremely rare injuries. A positive grind test may be elicited by gently compressing the pisotriquetral joint surfaces together. Late pisotriquetral arthrosis may be treated by excision of the pisiform. Lunate fractures have been implicated in the pathophysiology of Kienböck's disease. These injuries much more commonly present as a cause of chronic wrist pain. Finally, the most common capitate fracture is associated with fracture of the middle third of the scaphoid. The so-called scaphocapitate fracture syndrome involves a fracture at the level of the neck of the capitate and mal-rotation of the body. These injuries may be associated with avascular necrosis of the head of the capitate nonunion and late carpal collapse. Acutely displaced fractures are treated by open reduction and K-wire fixation.[1,24,49]

Radiocarpal Dislocation

Radiocarpal dislocations are extremely rare and are usually associated with multiple trauma. They are classified according to extent of injury. Type I dislocations are usually associated with dorsal or volar rim distal radial articular fractures. These dislocations are primarily dorsal and are associated with palmar radiocarpal ligament ruptures. Closed reduction followed by immobilization in plaster has been occasionally successful in the management of these injuries. When the closed reduction cannot be maintained or obtained, open reduction is indicated. Type II radiocarpal dislocations are associated with carpal fractures and dislocations. These fractures have uniformly required open reduction and ligament reconstruction. Overall, type I radiocarpal dislocations have a much better prognosis. Posttraumatic arthrosis of the wrist frequently requires arthrodesis.[14,34]

RADIUS
Fractures of the Distal Radius
Classification

Fractures of the distal radius are commonly classified by numerous eponyms such as Colle's, Smith's, Barton's, and reverse Barton's. Confusion in the usage of these eponyms has led to the development of various classification systems. These systems, however, fail to differentiate intraarticular from extraarticular fractures adequately; as a result, they are severely limited in their prognostic value.[35,40]

The authors' modification of Frykman's classification descriptively names each distal radius fracture subtype (Tables 24-1 and 24-2). There are two significant prognostic risk factors: the extent of apparent articular involvement and the presence or absence of fracture stability. Any distal radius fracture may be stable or unstable, dorsally or volarly displaced, and extra- or intraarticular.[35,40]

Table 24-1 Dorsally Displaced Fractures: Distal Radius

Joint involvement	Eponym/description	Position of reduction	
		Wrist	Forearm
Extraarticular[a]			
None	Colles'	V/F[b]	Pronation
Intraarticular[a]			
Radiocarpal (R/C) alone	Dorsal Barton's Dorsal marginal rim Fracture/subluxation	D/F[c]	Pronation
Radioulnar (R/U) alone	Colles' type	V/F[b]	Pronation
Both R/C and R/U	Dorsomedial lunate "Die-punch" fracture	V/F[b]	Pronation

[a]All fractures may be stable or unstable.
[b]V/F = volar flexion.
[c]D/F = dorsiflexion.

Table 24-2   Volar Displaced Fractures: Distal Radius

Joint involvement	Eponym/description	Position of reduction	
		Wrist	Forearm
Extraarticular[a]			
None	Smith's type I Reverse Colles' type	D/F[b]	Supination
Intraarticular[a]			
Radiocarpal (R/C) alone	Volar Barton's Smith's type II Volar marginal rim Fracture subluxation	V/F[c]	Supination
Radioulnar (R/U) alone	Reverse Colles' type Smith's type III	D/F[b]	Supination
Both R/C and R/U	Reverse Colles' type	D/F[b]	Supination

[a]All fractures may be stable or unstable.
[b]D/F = dorsiflexion.
[c]V/F = volar flexion.

Stable fractures are those in which clinically acceptable alignment and joint congruity can be maintained by plaster immobilization with or without a closed reduction. The inherent stability of any closed reduction is primarily dependent upon the presence of fracture comminution and related factors, such as the patient's age and the degree of osteopenia, energy applied, and soft tissue injury. Thus, all unstable distal radius fractures are at high risk for increased morbidity—i.e., loss of motion and strength and the development of posttraumatic arthritis.[24,35,40]

Radiographic Analysis

Van der Linden and Ericson have shown that anatomic displacement of distal radius fractures may reliably be described by two radiographic measurements. A lateral x-ray view of the distal radius shows loss of the normal radial tilt of 11° (dorsal angulation), and the anteroposterior x-ray view shows the presence of a radial shift—an increase in the distance from the long axis of the radius to the most radial part of the styloid process. The presence of any radial shift is usually indicative of a displaced intraarticular fracture. Both the degree of dorsal angulation and radial shift correlate directly with the degree of radial shortening. However, conversely, large radial shifts may be present independent of the degree of dorsal angulation. Thus, both parameters are necessary in order to adequately define and interpret the guidelines and the results of treatment.[26,35,40,50]

Treatment

Dorsally Displaced Extraarticular Fractures Stable extraarticular fractures that require no reduction may initially be placed in a sugar-tong splint and converted, once the initial swelling has subsided, to a short arm cast. If there is any suspicion of latent clinical instability, the patient should be x-rayed again at weekly intervals for the first 2 weeks. From the onset, elevation and full active range of motion of the interphalangeal and metacarpophalangeal joints is emphasized in order to avoid reflex sympathetic dystrophy and arthrofibrosis of the fingers with associated contracture (Table 24-1).[35,40]

Fractures Requiring Reduction Since Colles' first clinical description (1814) of this foreshortened fracture, treatment has focused on the restoration of radial length. Fracture displacement occurs both in the flexion-extension axis of the radiocarpal joint as well as in the rotational axis of the forearm through the head of the ulna. These axial displacements must be taken into consideration when any closed reduction is required.[35,40]

The authors believe that those fractures which present with any degree of dorsal angulation and a resulting loss of radial length require an attempted closed reduction. Under anesthesia, the fracture is disimpacted by applying 10 to 15 lb of longitudinal fingertip traction for approximately 15 min. While traction is maintained, dorsal and rotational displacement may be corrected by pronating the distal radial fragment, thereby "locking" the reduction. In order to correct the dorsal angulation, the final reduction maneuver includes volar flexion and mild ulnar deviation of the wrist as the traction is released. Postreduction x-ray films are obtained following the application and three-point molding of the sugar-tong splint.[35]

Minimal acceptable reduction criteria for extraarticular dorsally displaced fractures are not clearly defined in the literature. Most authors agree that the closer the reduction is to an anatomic one, the better the functional outcome. The possible exception is the elderly, osteopenic, low-demand patient whose functional requirements may be meager in comparison to those of the young adult. Fernandez has analyzed the results of treatment in this latter population following malunited extraarticular fractures of the distal radius.[9] Those patients who presented with a dorsal angulation greater than 25° associated with a loss of radial length greater than 6 mm apparently lost greater than 50 percent of their palmar flexion arc of motion as well as 50 percent of their grip strength. Additionally, a dynamic midcarpal stability has been observed to arise from even smaller magnitudes of dorsal angulation (loss of palmar tilt)—i.e., malunion.[35,40,48]

The authors' prerequisites for an acceptable closed reduction are based upon Cooney's criteria for an unstable extraarticular fracture. These included the inability to maintain fracture reduction without loss of dorsal angulation of more than 5° or with 5 mm of radial shortening.

In order to maintain reduction of these unstable extraarticular fractures, most authors recommend a distraction technique (external fixator or pins in plaster). In addition, sometimes additional internal fixation is needed—i.e., pins, screws, or plates to stabilize the fracture.[2,35,40]

Dorsally Displaced Intraarticular Fractures The closed treatment of dorsally displaced intraarticular fractures of the distal radius (Table 24-1) is not significantly different from that given to extraarticular fractures. However, additionally, the critical prerequisite for an acceptable closed reduction is articular congruity. Knirk and Jupiter found that those fractures that had 2 mm or more of articular depression had a 100 percent incidence of radiographic stigmata of posttraumatic arthritis, whereas those that healed with articular congruity had an incidence of arthritis of only 11 percent.[26,35,40]

Fractures Requiring Reduction Intraarticular fractures of the dorsal rim of the distal radius associated with dorsal subluxation of the carpus are usually inherently unstable fractures. Unlike the case in other dorsally displaced fractures, attempted closed reduction requires dorsiflexion of the wrist in order to reduce the lunate on a stable volar radiocarpal buttress. When reduction cannot be maintained, dorsal rim fractures are usually too comminuted to allow individual fragment fixation. Instead, distraction fixation or dorsal buttress plate fixation may be required.[34,38]

Dorsally displaced intraarticular fractures may involve the radioulnar joint alone. Unstable displaced fractures may be treated by closed reduction and percutaneous pin fixation with or without a fixed distraction apparatus. Rayhack's variation of DiPalma's transulnar pinning is also useful. The ulna is used as an external fixation bar and multiple pins are placed across to the radius. After 3 to 4 weeks of immobilization, monitored flexion and extension exercises can be done in order to prevent or lessen the joint stiffness seen with other external fixation techniques.[39] Late complications of these fractures usually involve pain with a limitation of forearm rotation, which may be treated by a partial distal ulnar excision.[35,40]

Fractures involving both the radiocarpal and radioulnar joints are usually unstable due to the impacted dorsomedial articular fragment—the "die-punch" fracture. If articular congruity cannot be obtained by closed means, open reduction may be required, with elevation of the articular depression and bone grafting or bone grafting substitute for the subchondral defect. Again, reduction may be maintained by pin or screw fixation if the fragment is large enough. Otherwise, distraction fixation or buttress plating may be required. Melone's classification system is very helpful here in understanding the fracture anatomy and therapeutic options.[31]

Volarly Displaced Extraarticular Fractures When someone falls on an outstretched, fixed, and pronated palm (Table 24-2), the extraarticular proximal radial fracture fragment supinates around its rotational axis—i.e., the ulnar head. Ultimately, the distal radius fragment is driven volarward relative to a clinically prominent ulnar head.[35,40]

Fractures Requiring Reduction Under anesthesia, closed reduction may be carried out by disimpaction and supination of the distal radial fragment. When the wrist is dorsiflexed, the volar carpal ligaments become taut, thereby "locking" the reduction. Postreduction x-ray films are obtained following the application and three-point molding of a sugar-tong splint.

Like dorsally displaced extraarticular fractures, reduction criteria for volarly displaced fractures are not clearly defined. As previously mentioned, Fernandez also studied malunions within this fracture displacement subtype. He concluded that those fractures with at least 25° of volar angulation and greater than 6 mm of radial shortening will ultimately have at least a 50 percent loss of dorsiflexion and grip strength.[9,35,40]

The authors consider those volarly displaced fractures that cannot be maintained in a neutral or near-anatomic position as clinically unstable. Following reduction, these unstable fractures may be maintained with the aid of an external fixator or pins-in-plaster treatment. This treatment may be augmented by percutaneously pinning a relatively large distal radial fracture fragment with associated volar cortical comminution. Rayhack's technique of transulnar pinning can also be helpful here.[2]

Volarly Displaced Intraarticular Fractures Intraarticular fractures (Table 24-2) involving the radiocarpal joint are characterized by their instability. Anatomically, the volar carpal ligaments are probably avulsed from the comminuted volar articular rim of the radius. Because this articular rim is insufficient to buttress against the volar shear forces, the wrist subluxes volarly.[35,40]

Fractures Requiring Reduction Attempted closed reduction of the volar rim fracture subluxation should include longitudinal traction followed by supination and slight volar flexion of the wrist. As opposed to the closed reduction maneuver required for other volarly displaced fractures, the volar carpal ligament tether that occurs by dorsiflexing the wrist will have little effect on the avulsed volar rim fracture fragments in this subgroup. Instead, slight volar flexion of the wrist may tend to reduce the volar shear force, thereby preventing redisplacement. Unstable fractures often require open reduction with buttress plating or, at times, an attempt at distraction fixation with an external fixator or pins-in-plaster treatment.

Volarly displaced intraarticular fractures may involve the radioulnar joint alone. These fractures are extremely rare but are more stable than the volar rim fracture subtypes. Closed reduction should be carried out in a similar fashion as described for other volarly displaced extraarticular fractures. Following reduction, unstable fractures may be pinned in order to avoid pain and limitation of forearm rotation.

Fractures involving both the radiocarpal and radioulnar joints clinically have their volar counterpart. In a similar fashion, articular congruity must be restored. Impacted articular fragments depressed more than 2 mm must be elevated and bone-grafted. Volar buttress plating will help maintain this reduction. Techniques using wrist arthroscopy can help in directly visualizing the reduction and fixation in order to make sure that the joint surface is totally congruent. Arthroscopic assisted reduction after bone grafting the under surface of the articular "die-punch" lesion can help prevent fixture incongruity and arthritis development of the joint surface.[51] A small arthrotomy of the wrist can also be used to check the joint surface congruity.

Complications Complications of distal radius fractures are frequent. They include loss of reduction, with malunion; radioulnar joint symptoms; extensor pollicis longus rupture; degenerative arthrosis; reflex sympathetic dystrophy and shoulder-hand syndrome; compressive neuropathy; compartment syndrome; and intrinsic contracture.[6,35,40] It should be noted that clinical research trials are under way using injectable paste of carbonated apatite to treat unstable distal radius fractures. This may help in fracture fixation and in starting to mobilize joints faster (paper presented at the 1996 meeting of the American Academy of Orthopaedic Surgeons in Atlanta, with the permission of J. B. Jupiter, M.D.).

Radial Styloid Fractures

These fractures, originally described as having been caused by sudden reversal of the starter crank, were called *chauffeur's fractures.* Most of these injuries are now caused by forced radial deviation during falls or during motor vehicle accidents. An AP x-ray shows the fracture line best; it usually runs from the scaphoid fossa radially toward the lateral radial cortex. It is, therefore, an intraarticular fracture. Depending on the position of the wrist when the injury occurs, there may be associated radiocarpal ligamentous injuries.[35]

Nondisplaced fractures may be treated by short arm casting for 4 to 6 weeks. If significant displacement is noted, distraction and reduction in an ulnar direction facilitates reduction. Reduction can be maintained by placing the wrist in slight ulnar deviation. Plaster immobilization for 6 weeks is usually sufficient for healing to occur. If the reduction cannot be maintained, open reduction and fixation either with two Kirschner wires or by screw fixation should be done.

ULNAR STYLOID FRACTURES

Ulnar styloid fractures are relatively common injuries. They are often seen in association with distal radius fractures and may also occur as isolated entities. Most are caused by forced radial deviation or dorsiflexion injuries.[3]

The patients present acutely with tenderness at the ulnar styloid. Forearm supination and pronation may cause discomfort. Routine anteroposterior x-ray views allow one to determine whether a fracture is present. Occasionally, one can see an anomalous carpal bone called the *lunula, os styloides,* or *os triangulare.*[3]

Treatment

Treatment of these injuries should be based on the amount of displacement. The triangular fibrocartilage complex (TFCC) attaches to the ulnar styloid. Theoretically, significant displacement may lead to instability of the distal radioulnar joint. It is unclear how much displacement is significant. If the ulnar styloid is minimally displaced, a short arm cast with the wrist in slight ulnar deviation relaxes the TFCC complex and allows the fracture to heal. Healing should take place in 4 to 6 weeks. If the ulnar styloid is significantly displaced and the distal radioulnar joint is subluxed, open reduction and fixation of the ulnar styloid fracture with a Kirschner wire is recommended. The fracture should then be held for 4 to 6 weeks in a long arm cast.[3]

Occasionally one will see a patient with a painful nonunion of the ulnar styloid. Simple excision with repair of the TFCC in selected patients provides excellent results.

RADIOULNAR JOINT DISLOCATIONS

The radioulnar joint is a trochoid, or pivot, joint. The radius rotates around the ulna, with stability achieved by the bony architecture, joint capsule, pronator quadratus, and triangular fibrocartilage complex. This homogeneous complex is made up of the articular disk, the dorsal and volar radioulnar ligaments, the meniscus homologue, the ulnar collateral ligament, and the sheath of the extensor carpi ulnaris. Radioulnar dislocations are not rare injuries. They may be noted as radial fractures and in ulnar styloid fractures. Isolated radioulnar joint dislocations are commonly referred to as ulnar dorsal or ulnar volar, although the ulna is truly the fixed forearm unit. Dorsal dislocations are more frequently seen than volar dislocations. The mechanism of injury of dorsal dislocations is felt to be hyperpronation. Volar dislocations of the radioulnar joint are hypersupination injuries.[3,5]

Most patients with these injuries present acutely with radioulnar joint pain. The pain is reproducible with downward pressure on the joint or by supination and pronation movements of the forearm. A painful "click" or "clunk" may be present. Difficulties in diagnosis may be encountered upon examining x-ray films. Anteroposterior and lateral films of both wrists are helpful for comparison. Anteroposterior views in pronation and supination may help with the determination of injury. Recently, CT has been noted to help make specific diagnoses.[5]

Treatment

Acute injuries, including sprains, are best held in the position that allows ligamentous healing. In dorsal sprains or dislocations, the patient is treated with a long arm cast in supination for 6 weeks. In volar sprains, the patient is treated in hyperpronation in a long arm cast for 6 weeks. Postreduction films are mandatory. If there are any questions as to the position of the reduction, CT scan of the radioulnar joint is recommended. Although rare, a dorsal or volar dislocation may be unstable. An open reduction followed by K-wire stabilization transversely into the radius is carried out. If an open reduction is carried out, an attempt to repair the triangular fibrocartilage complex or to pin the ulnar styloid fragment should be made. The arm is then held in the position of reduction for 6 weeks in a long arm cast.[5]

REFERENCES

1. Amadis PL, Talesnite J: Fracture of the carpal bones, in Green DP (ed): *Operative Hand Surgery,* 3d ed. New York, Churchill Livingstone, 1993, pp 799–860.

2. Cooney WP, Berger RA: Treatment of complex fractures of the distal radius: Combined use of internal and external fixation and arthroscopic reduction. *Hand Clin* 9:603–612, 1993.

3. Bowers WH: The distal radio-ulnar joint, in Green DP (ed): *Operative Hand Surgery,* 3d ed. New York, Churchill Livingstone, 1993, pp 973–1019.

4. Breen TE, Gelberman RH, Jupiter TB: Intraarticular fractures of the basilar joint of the thumb. *Hand Clin* 4:491–501, 1988.

5. Bruchier JD, Alexander AH, Lichtman DM: Acute dislocations of the distal radioulnar joint. *Instr Course Lect* 45:27–30, 1996.

6. Cooney WP, Dobyns JH, Linscheid RL: Complication of Colles' fractures. *J Bone Joint Surg* 62A:613, 1980.

7. Dray GJ, Eaton RG: Dislocations and ligament injuries in the digits, in Green DP (ed): *Operative Hand Surgery,* 3d ed. New York, Churchill Livingstone, 1993, pp 767–798.

8. Eaton RG, Littler JW: Joint injuries and their sequelae. *Clin Plast Surg* 3:85–98, 1976.

9. Fernandez DL: Correction of post-traumatic wrist deformity in adults by osteotomy, bone grafting and internal fixation. *J Bone Joint Surg* 64A:1164–1178, 1982.

10. Ferraro MC, Cappula A, Lippman H, Hurst LL: Closed functional bracing of metacarpal fractures. *Orthop Rev* 12:49–56, 1983.

11. Field LD, Freeland AE, Jabaley ME: Midaxial approach to the proximal phalanx for fracture fixation. *Contemp Orthop* 25:133–137, 1992.

12. Freeland AE, Benviot LA: Open reduction and internal fixation for fractures at the proximal interphalangeal joint. *Hand Clin* 10:239–250, 1994.

13. Gelberman RH, Panagris JS, Taleisnik J, Baumgaertner M: The arterial anatomy of the human carpus: Part I. The extraosseous vascularity. *J Hand Surg* 8:367–375, 1983.

14. Green DP: Carpal dislocations and instabilities, in Green DP (ed): *Operative Hand Surgery,* 3d ed. New York, Churchill Livingstone, 1993, pp 861–929.

15. Green DP, Rowland SA: Fractures and dislocations in the hand, in *Fractures in Adults,* 3d ed. Philadelphia, Lippincott, 1991, pp 441–502.

16. Greene T: Metacarpal fractures, in *The Hand Surgery Update.* Aurora, Colorado, American Society for Surgery of the Hand, 1994, chap 2.

17. Gunther SF: The carpometacarpal joints. *Orthop Clin North Am* 15:259–277, 1984.

18. Hastings H II, Carroll C IV: RE: Treatment of closed articular fractures of the metacarpophalangeal and proximal interphalangeal joints. *Hand Clin* 4:503–527, 1988.

19. Hernedon JH: *Scaphoid Fractures and Complications.* Aurora, Colorado, American Academy of Orthopedic Surgeons Monogram Series, 1994.

20. Hotchkiss RN: Fractures and dislocation of the thumb, in *Hand Surgery Update.* Aurora, Colorado, American Society for Surgery of the Hand, 1994, chap 4.

21. Imbriglia JE: Chronic dorsal carpometacarpal dislocation of the index, middle, ring and little fingers: A case report. *J Hand Surg* 4:343–345, 1979.

22. Jahss SA: Fractures of the proximal phalanges. Alignment and immobilization. *J Bone Joint Surg* 18:726–731, 1936.

23. James JP, Wright TA: Fracture of the metacarpals and proximal and middle phalanges of the finger. *J Bone Joint Surg* 48B:181–182, 1966.

24. Jupiter JB: Scaphoid fractures, in *Hand Surgery Update.* Aurora, Colorado, American Society for Surgery of the Hand, 1994, chap 8.

25. Kiefhaber TR: Intraarticular fractures in joint injuries, in *Hand Surgery Update.* Aurora, Colorado, American Society for Surgery of the Hand, 1994, chap 3.

26. Knirk JL, Jupiter JB: Intra-articular fractures of the distal end of the radius in young adults. *J Bone Joint Surg* 68A:647–659, 1986.

27. Lane CS: Detecting occult fractures of the metacarpal head: The Brewerton view. *J Hand Surg* 2:131–133, 1977.

28. Lazar G, Schulter-Ellis FP: Intra-medullary structure of human metacarpals. *J Hand Surg* 5:477–481, 1980.

29. Leslie IJ, Dickson RA: The fractured carpal scaphoid: Natural history and factors influencing outcome. *J Bone Joint Surg* 63B:225–230, 1981.

30. Malerich MM, Eaton RG: The volar plate reconstruction for fracture-dislocation of the proximal interphalangeal joint. *Hand Clin* 10:251–260, 1994.

31. Melone CP: Articular fractures of the distal radius. *Orthop Clin North Am* 15:217–236, 1984.

32. Melone CP: Scaphoid fractures: Concepts of management. *Clin Plast Surg* 8:83–94, 1981.

33. Miller RJ: Dislocations and fracture dislocations of the metacarpal phalangeal joint of the thumb. *Hand Clin* 4:45–65, 1988.

34. Moneim MS, Bolger JT, Omer GE: Radiocarpal dislocation classification and rationale for management. *Clin Orthop* 192:199–209, 1985.

35. Palmer AK: Fracture of the distal radius, in Green DP (ed): *Operative Hand Surgery,* 3d ed. New York, Churchill Livingstone, 1993, pp 929–971.

36. Panais JS, Gelberman RH, Taleisnik J, Baumgaertner M: The arterial anatomy of the human carpal: Part II. The intraosseous vascularity, *J Hand Surg* 8:375–382, 1983.

37. Peimer CA, Sullivan DJ, Wild DR: Palmar dislocation of the proximal interphalangeal joint. *J Hand Surg* 9A:39–47, 1984.

38. Rowles JGJ: Dislocation and fracture-dislocations at the carpometacarpal joints of the fingers. *Hand Clin* 4:103–112, 1988.

39. Rayhack JM, Lanworthy JN, Belsole RJ: Transulnar percutaneous pinning of displaced distal radial fractures: A preliminary report. *J Orthop Trauma* 3:107–114, 1989.

40. Sanders WE: Distal radius fractures, in *Hand Surgery Update.* Aurora, Colorado, American Society for Surgery of the Hand, 1994, chap 12.

41. Schweider LH: Fractures of the distal interphalangeal joint. *Hand Clin North Am* 10:277–285, 1994.

42. Schenck RR: Classification of fractures and dislocations of the proximal interphalangeal joint. *Hand Clin* 10:179–186, 1994.

43. Schenck RR: The dynamic traction method. *Hand Clin* 10:187–198, 1994.

44. Stern PJ: Fractures of the metacarpals and phalanges, in Green DP (ed): *Operative Hand Surgery,* 3d ed. New York, Churchill Livingstone, 1993, pp 695–758.

45. Stern PJ: Selected acute infection. *Instr Course Lect* 39:539–554, 1990.

46. Strickland JW, Steicher JB, Kleinman WB, et al. Phalangeal fractures. Factors influencing digital performance. *Orthop Rev* 11:39–50, 1982.

47. Taleisnik J: *The Wrist.* New York, Churchill Livingstone, 1985.

48. Taleisnik J, Watson HK: Midcarpal instability caused by fractures of the distal radius. *J Hand Surg* 9A:350, 1984.

49. Vance RM, Gelberman RH, Evans EF: Scaphocapitate fractures: Patterns of dislocation, mechanism of injury, and preliminary results of treatment. *J Bone Joint Surg* 62A:271–276, 1980.

50. Van der Linden W, Ericson R: Colles' fracture: How should its displacement be measured and how should it be immobilized? *J Bone Joint Surg* 63A:1285–1288, 1981.

51. Whipple TL: *Arthroscopic Surgery: The Wrist.* Philadelphia, Lippincott, 1992.

52. Zook EG, Brown RE: The perionychium, in Green DP (ed): *Operative Hand Surgery,* 3d ed. New York, Churchill Livingstone, 1993, pp 1283–1314.

53. Zook EG, Van Beek AL, Wavak P: Transverse volar skin laceration of the finger: A sign of volar plate injury. *Hand Clin* 11:213–216, 1979.

Fractures and Dislocations of the Lower Limb and Pelvis

CHAPTER 25

Pelvic and Acetabular Fractures

M. L. Chip Routt, Jr. and Peter T. Simonian

Pelvic and acetabular fractures remain diagnostic and therapeutic challenges for many reasons. These injuries frequently occur remote from major trauma centers, which makes clinical experience difficult to achieve. Their spherical anatomy as well as the local neurovascular and visceral structures further complicate treatment. Pelvic disruptions and acetabular fractures are quite variable in their severity. Predictable treatment results are dependent on many factors.

PELVIC FRACTURES

General

Disruptions of the pelvic ring are difficult to understand and therefore to treat effectively. Pelvic ring stability relies on bone and soft tissue constraints. Anteriorly, the symphysis pubis articulation is composed of fibrocartilage and ligamentous structures. The symphyseal ligaments surround the cephalad aspect of the symphysis pubis, while the arcuate ligament spans caudally between the inferior pubic rami. The capsular sacroiliac, interosseus, iliolumbar, sacrospinous, and sacrotuberous are regarded as the primary posterior pelvic ligamentous constraints (Fig. 25-1). Clinical and biomechanical investigations to improve our understanding of these and other important pelvic soft tissue constraints are ongoing.

Patient Evaluation

Pelvic fractures and dislocations may be due to a wide variety of traumatic events. Simple low-energy accidents such as a fall from a standing height onto a carpeted floor may produce pelvic injury. These are typically stable and nondisplaced or minimally displaced injuries that require symptomatic treatment alone. High-energy accidents are more likely to cause severely displaced and unstable pelvic ring disruptions with multiple system injuries. Fracture/dislocation displacements result from unopposed muscle pull through the involved fragments.

Spinal precautions are utilized for these patients until the spine is clinically and radiographically cleared. During the initial examination and subsequent evaluations and procedures, the patient is kept warm with blankets and warmed intravenous fluids if necessary. Maintaining the body temperature avoids coagulopathy secondary to hypothermia. Evaluation and treatment occur simultaneously for patients with suspected pelvic disruptions. Hemorrhage may be torrential and can cause death. Exposed cancellous fracture fragments as well as arterial and venous disruptions are the primary early potential sources. The head, thorax, abdomen, and extremities are also carefully evaluated. Lower extremity deformity may result from ipsilateral hemipelvic disruptions. As the history and physical exam are progressing, large-diameter venous catheters are inserted and volume resuscitation begins. Significant intrapelvic bleeding can occur rapidly due to the unstable spherical anatomy of the disrupted pelvis. For this reason, some form of temporary pelvic circumferential support is applied in an attempt to provide fracture stability and prevent further pelvic expansion.

The pelvic clinical evaluation consists of careful skin inspection, including the perineal area, to identify closed degloving or open wounds; a single mechanical assessment of pelvic ring stability; a digital rectal exam; and a bimanual vaginal exam in female patients. The vaginal/rectal exams should include testing for occult blood and in male patients the prostate location. Abnormalities of the bimanual vaginal exam mandate further vaginal inspection with a speculum. Similarly, digital rectal abnormalities are further evaluated with sigmoidoscopy.

Skin violations usually indicate an open injury and may not always be obvious. Extensive perineal wounds with rectal involvement are readily identified, but smaller perineal and posterior pelvic wounds are noted only on careful exam. Large abdominal/flank ecchymoses associated with significant swelling and abraded skin herald a degloving injury. These are frequently seen in patients with massive crush mechanisms of injury.

Assessment of pelvic mechanical integrity is often difficult for medical personnel. A host of excuses to avoid pelvic

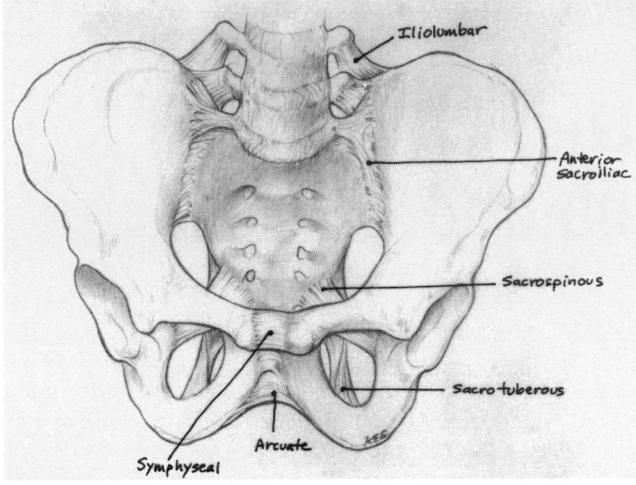

A

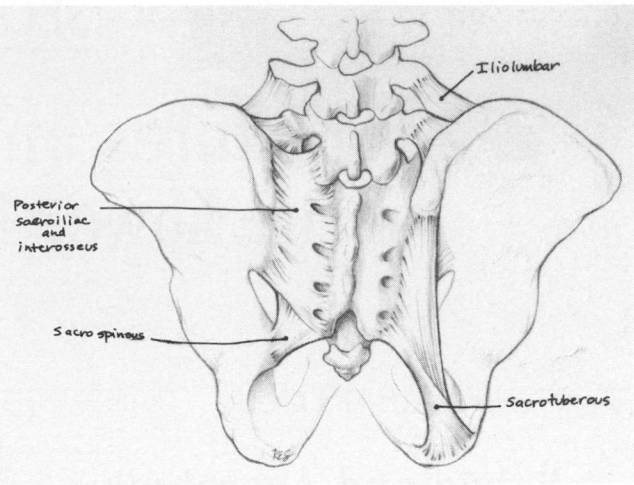

B

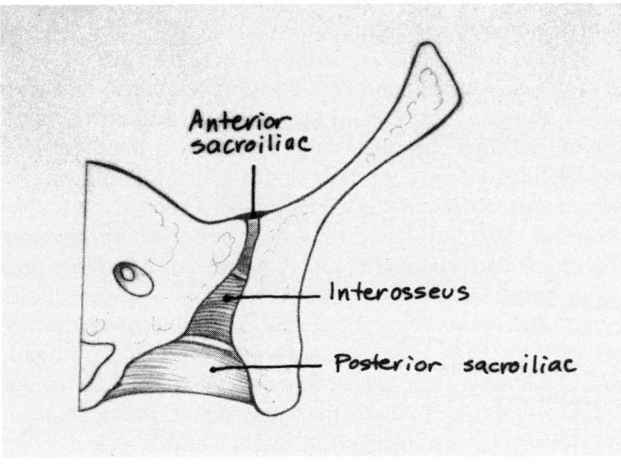

C

Figure 25-1 *A, B,* and *C.* These illustrations identify the primary pelvic ligamentous structures.

Toxic substance screening and nutrition panels may be helpful in certain patients.

Radiology

A screening anteroposterior pelvic plain radiograph is easily and rapidly obtained at patient presentation. This radiograph identifies injuries and gross deformities. Next, orthogonal pelvic inlet and outlet images reveal specific zones of injuries and displacements. Lumbosacral lordosis, pelvic deformities, and other factors make "perfect" inlet and outlet pelvic imaging difficult. Lateral sacral plain radiographs identify certain sacral fractures. Stress radiographs of the pelvis include "push-pull" imaging and may be helpful in unusual situations. Dynamic fluoroscopic pelvic images are possible if the patient will be anesthetized for any surgical procedure. In the operating room, the portable C-arm fluoroscopic unit is used to image the pelvis while a pelvic mechanical exam is performed. Instabilities associated with specific zones of injury are easily noted. This dynamic fluoroscopic assessment of pelvic stability indicates that initially minimally displaced pelvic disruptions can be grossly unstable (Fig. 25-2).

Routine two-dimensional pelvic computed tomography (CT), using contiguous 5-mm axial slices, reveals specific areas of injury and accurately quantifies displacements for most cases (Fig. 25-3A to C).

Three-dimensional pelvic CT scanning is reserved for patients with difficult pelvic malunion/nonunion and those with unusual acute fractures and dislocations that are poorly understood.

Pelvic angiography is indicated in patients with unexplained hemodynamic instability in association with pelvic disruptions. Pelvic arterial bleeding is controlled with strategic embolizations. Certain fractures, such as those involving displacement through the greater sciatic notch,

manipulation include "the patient was too tender to examine" or "she's too obese to get a good exam on." An ideal mechanical evaluation of the potentially unstable pelvic ring should be (1) performed only once, (2) after a review of the screening anteroposterior pelvic radiograph, (3) by the most experienced physician, (4) in a sedated patient, (5) after a detailed neurologic exam is documented, including the lower extremities and perineal/rectal area. Repetitive exams risk early clot disruption and neurologic injury. Careful palpation of the posterior pelvis may reveal focal tenderness.

Urologic consultation is indicated in certain patients with associated bladder and/or urethral disruptions. Gross hematuria strongly correlates with such injuries. Penile urethral meatal bleeding, the inability to urinate, hematuria, and a "high-riding" prostate gland indicate a urethral disruption. Lack of such symptoms does not exclude genitourinary tract injuries, especially in those patients transferred within 1 h after an accident. Urinary catheter insertion may be difficult in these patients and should be done by the consultant whenever possible.

Laboratory evaluations consist of serial hematocrits, a urinalysis, routine serum testing, and arterial blood gas.

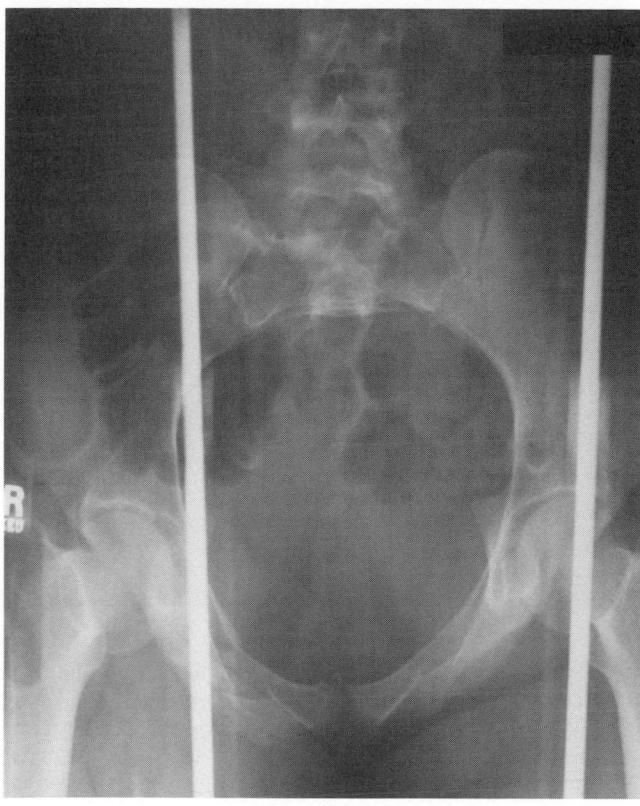

A

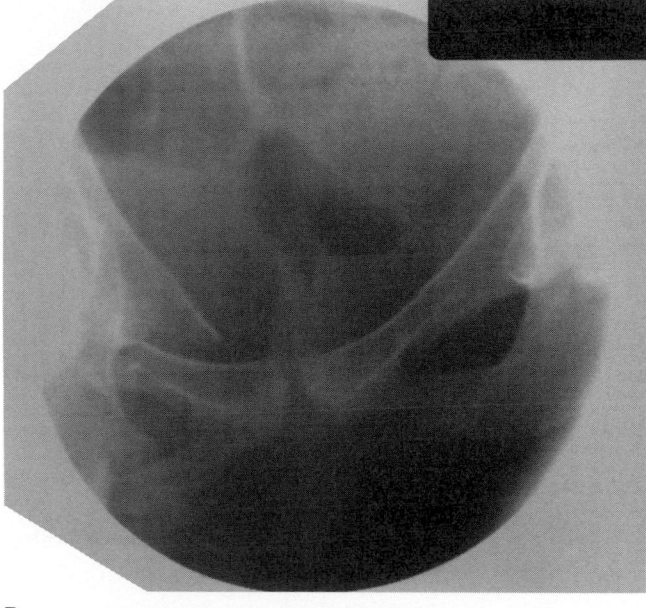

B

Figure 25-2 *A.* This AP plain radiograph of the pelvis demonstrates minimal displacement. The clinical examination for pelvic instability was inadequate in the awake patient due to severe facial trauma and pelvic pain. *B.* The patient was given a general anesthetic for a facial reconstruction. With the patient anesthetized, the pelvic mechanical exam identified significant instability. This intraoperative stress radiograph of the pelvis confirms the instability. *C.* The pelvis was reduced accurately using closed techniques and stabilized percutaneously using an iliosacral screw posteriorly along with an anterior external fixator under the same anesthesia.

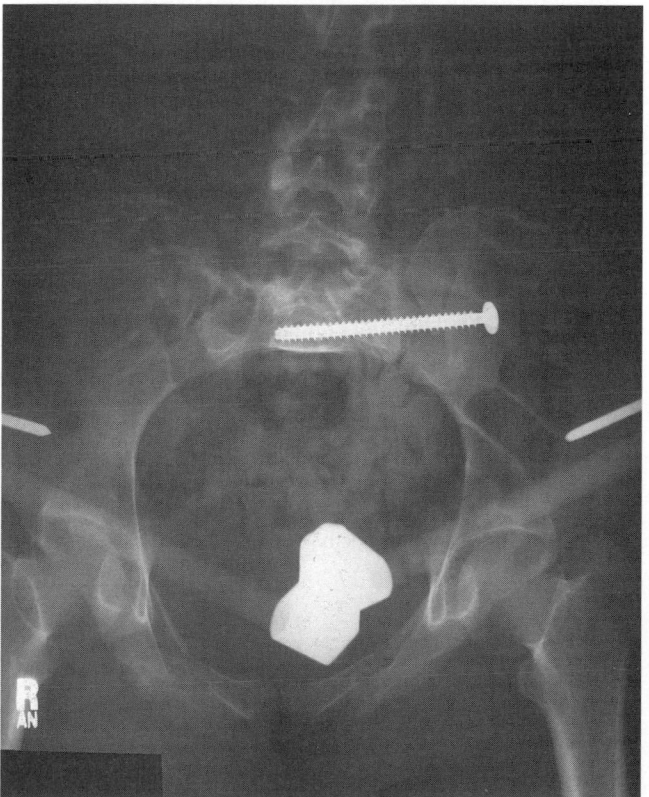

C

are often associated with injuries of the superior gluteal artery and should be evaluated with arteriography, especially if open reduction and internal fixation is planned (Fig. 25-4A to C). New fluoroscopic equipment allows helpful rotational imaging of these complex fractures and dislocations.

The genitourinary system is radiographically evaluated with an intravenous pyelogram, a cystogram, and a retrograde urethrogram as indicated.

Classifications

Several pelvic classification schemes have been described. Each has its advantages. Area of injury, bone deformities, and mechanism of injury have been used in various ways to classify pelvic disruptions. Probably the best way to classify these diverse injuries is to describe the mechanism of injury, identify the skin condition, locate specific fracture/dislocation sites and comminution, include associated visceral injuries, and quantify three-dimensionally the displacement patterns. This is frustrating and, without experience, is very difficult to do accurately and reproducibly. For these reasons a simple and easy-to-remember

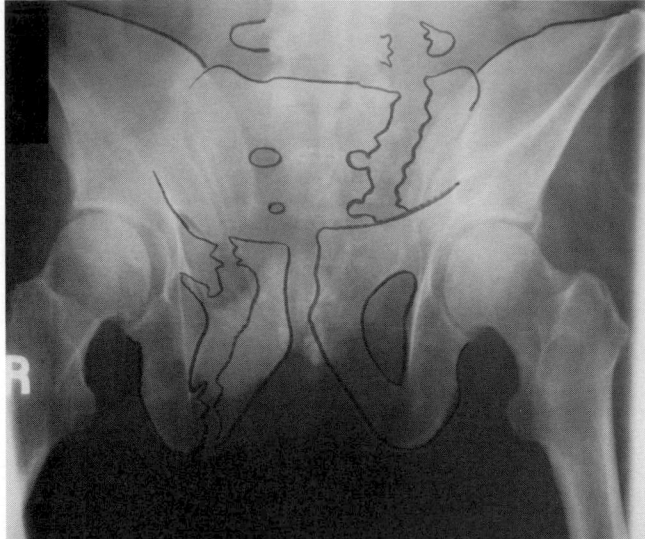

A

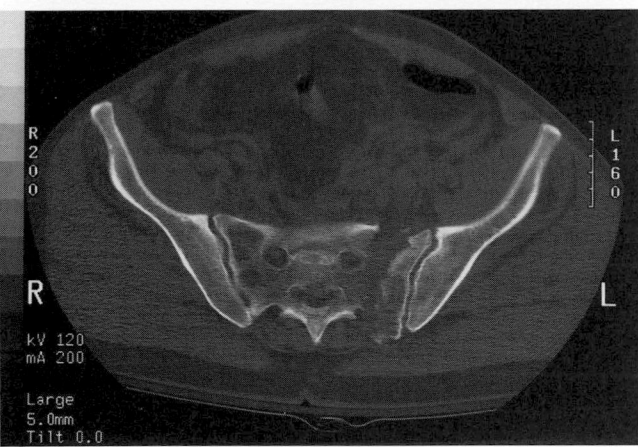

C

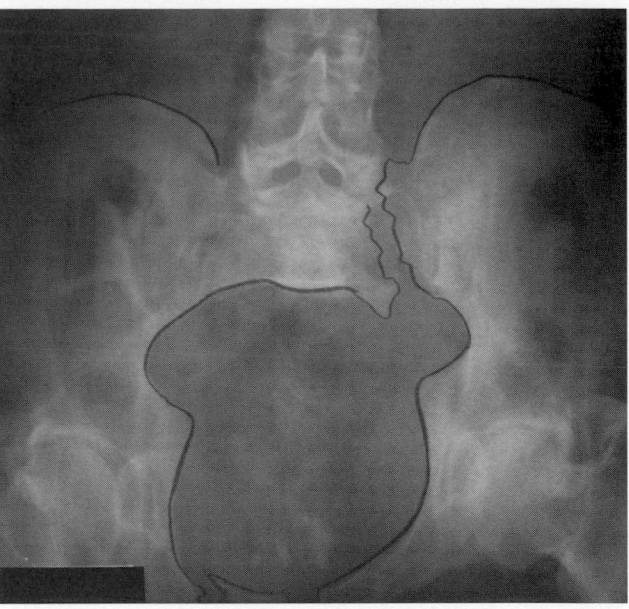

B

Figure 25-3 *A.* This radiograph of the pelvic outlet identifies left-sided fracture of the sacral ala and right-sided fracture of the pubic ramus as well as the pelvic deformity. *B.* The radiograph of the pelvic inlet confirms the displacement. *C.* Routine two-dimensional CT scanning demonstrates the fracture.

pelvic classification system that reproducibly guides treatment and predicts outcome is unlikely.

The pelvis tends to disrupt within certain zones. The symphysis pubis, pubic rami, acetabulum, ilium, sacroiliac joint, and sacrum are injured in many different ways. In most adult pelvic injuries, both anterior and posterior disruptions are linked. Avulsion fractures, direct high-energy loading, and pediatric pelvic injuries may violate this "at least two places on the ring" concept.

Pelvic instability includes a wide range of presentations. Clinical markers include pain and pelvic mobility with manipulative examination, along with focal tenderness. Radiographically, significant pelvic deformity and/or severe displacements are reproducible clues of instability. Some common pelvic instability patterns were identified by Pennal. Distraction ("open-book") and compression ("closed-book") injuries imply isolated rotational pelvic instabilities and are thought to result from anteroposterior compression and lateral compressive loading, respectively. "Vertical shear" pelvic instability indicates a rotational

form of instability coupled with cephalad or caudad hemipelvic displacements. These last injuries reflect more severe and complex pelvic trauma. Pennal's description of pelvic instability neglects, among other things, such important information as hemipelvic flexion and extension deformities. For these reasons, other expanded instability schemes have been described, but they still remain incomplete (Table 25-1).

Treatment—Early

Initial resuscitation secures the airway while maintaining ventilation and circulation. Adequate vascular access allows rapid resuscitation, and the body temperature is maintained. Some form of external support is used to temporarily immobilize the pelvis, such as a vacuum beanbag or circumferential pelvic sheet. Open wound are rapidly debrided and packed aseptically. Firm packing controls bleeding from all but the most extensive wounds.

Treatment—Definitive

Early treatment should be definitive treatment whenever possible. Options include protected activities, traction, spica casting, external fixation, percutaneous internal fixation, and open reduction/internal fixation. Combinations of the above are also possible. The indications for operative and closed managements are widely variable accord-

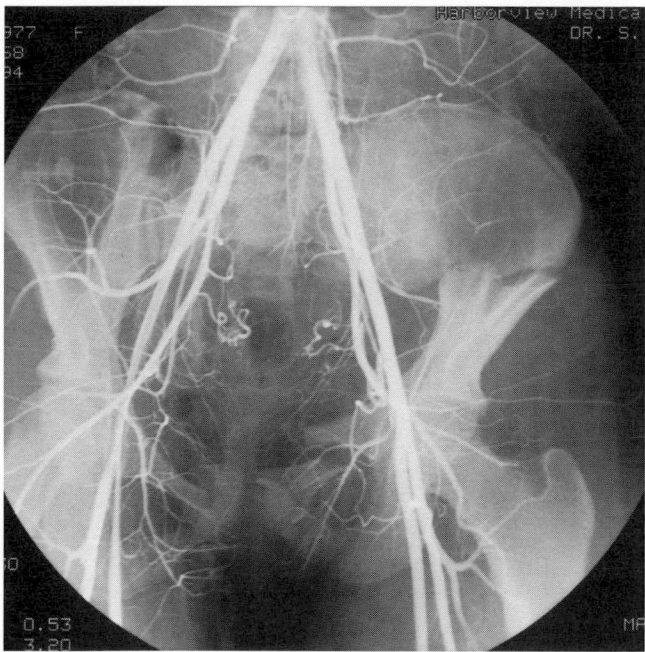

A

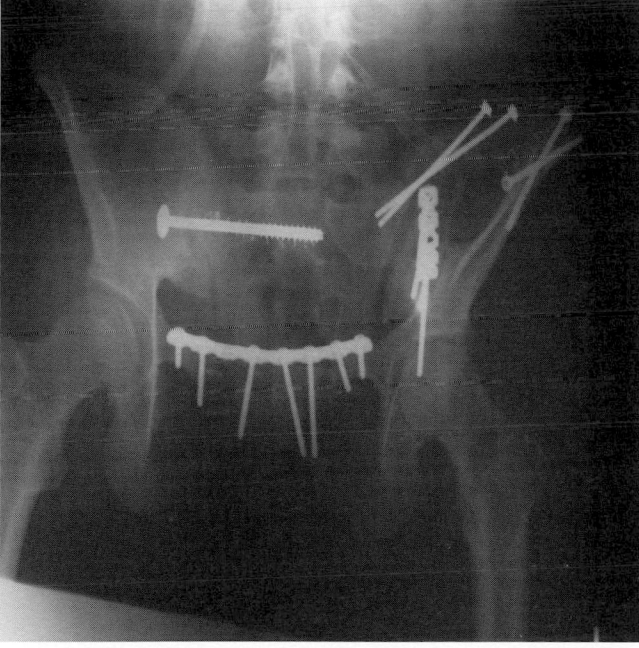

B

Figure 25-4 Fractures involving the greater sciatic notch may injure the gluteal vascular structures. Patients with such injuries are not always hemodynamically unstable. A high index of suspicion is necessary. *A.* This patient jumped from a high window and sustained a severe pelvic injury, including iliac fracture displacement through the greater notch. She was hemodynamically stable, with noted pelvic mechanical instability. Because of the fracture location and its displacement, an urgent pelvic angiogram was obtained, which revealed injury to the gluteal artery. Selective embolization was performed preoperatively. *B.* The patient's pelvic fractures were operatively stabilized on the day of injury.

TABLE 25-1   Classification of Pelvic Injuries

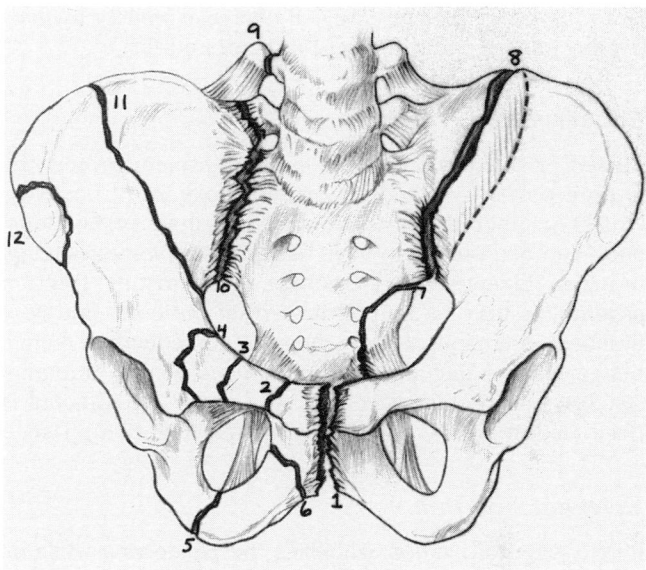

Location

This illustration identifies common areas of pelvic ring disruption.

1. Symphysis pubis dislocation
2. Parasymphyseal ramus fracture
3. Midramus fracture
4. Pubic root fracture
5. Ischial tuberosity fracture
6. Inferior ramus fracture
7. Caudal sacral avulsion fracture
8. Iliac crescent fracture/dislocation
9. Lumbar transverse process avulsion fracture
10. Sacroiliac dislocation
11. Iliac fracture
12. Anterosuperior iliac spine avulsion

Pelvic Instability

Type A—Stable
  A1—Pelvic ring spared, avulsion fracture
  A2—Ring involved, stable fracture (isolated rami)
  A3—Transverse sacral fracture

Type B—Rotationally unstable
  B1—"Open-book" distraction injury (stages 1–3)
  B2—Lateral compression, ipsilateral
  B3—Lateral compression, bilateral

Type C—Rotationally and vertically unstable
  C1—Unilateral
  C2—Bilateral
  C3—Any pelvic ring injury plus acetabular fracture

ing to the severity of the injury, the patient's overall medical status, and the surgeon's experience/preference. Ideal treatment would (1) be inexpensive, (2) be performed acutely, (3) provide anatomic reduction, (4) be minimally invasive, (5) restore pelvic stability to allow early rehabilitation, and (6) prevent chronic and disabling pain to allow full functional recovery. Perhaps one or two "designated pelvic surgeons" are indicated within medical communities to improve patient care and decrease anxiety by maximizing experience with these difficult injuries.

Conservative Treatment

Closed or conservative methods of treatment protect the injured pelvis by avoiding further injury due to activity. Crutch-protected ambulation, bed-to-chair restrictions, and even bed rest have been used for simpler, low-energy injuries. Likewise pelvic slings and various traction assemblies may be helpful in certain patients. Bed confinement is complicated by the systemic effects of recumbency, such as decubitus ulceration and venous thrombosis. Spica casting is successful in pediatric patients but is best used in adults only during the resuscitation phase.

External Fixation

Pelvic external fixation stabilizes the pelvic ring while allowing the patient to be upright. Usually several pins are inserted into the iliac wings and connected by complex frame systems to support the pelvis. Biomechanical comparisons demonstrate deficiencies of pelvic external fixation as compared with internal fixation. Malreduction, fixation failure, and pin-site infection are common associated problems. Pin removal is painful for the awake patient. Recently, simple and low-profile single-pin external fixation frames have been described. A single pin is inserted under fluoroscopic guidance within the tables of the anterior ilium bilaterally. Strategic pin placement allows these simple frames to be durable and mechanically equivalent. Simple frames are routinely used in combination with percutaneous posterior pelvic internal fixation (Fig. 25-5).

Internal Fixation

Open or closed manipulative reductions of the pelvis must be accurate. Various methods of internal fixation have been described in order to stabilize the pelvis after open reduction. Anterior pelvic open reduction is typically achieved using midline laparotomy, Pfannenstiel, ilioinguinal, iliofemoral, or iliac exposures. Posterior pelvic access for open reduction and fixation is accomplished using either vertical paramedian or midline surgical exposures. Plate/screw constructs, tension-band wiring, and medullary lag screws are but a few of the internal fixation devices that have been described to maintain pelvic stability after injury (Table 25-2). Recent reports have demonstrated the safety of early open pelvic stabilization procedures. Blood salvage systems are advocated. Monitoring of somatosensory evoked potentials may decrease the incidence and severity of iatrogenic lumbosacral plexus nerve injuries, especially for displaced transforaminal sacral fractures.

Complications

Numerous complications from pelvic disruptions and their treatments have been described. Malunion and nonunion

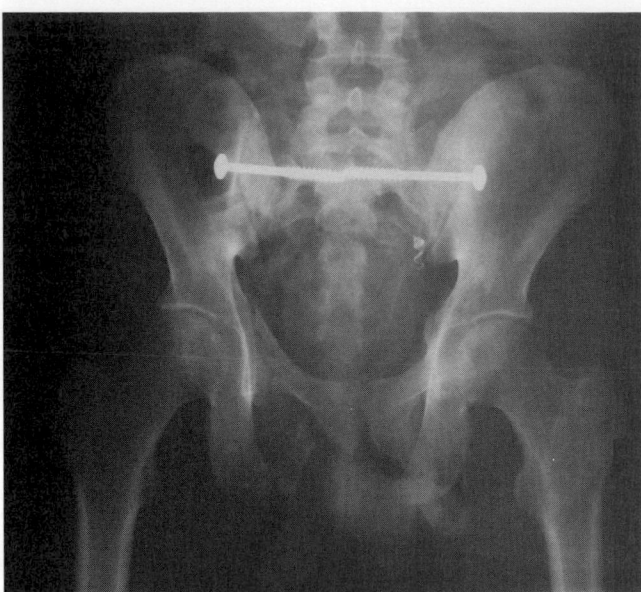

Figure 25-5 A combination of simple two-pin anterior pelvic external fixation and posterior iliosacral lag screws was used emergently to stabilize this open pelvic injury after closed manipulative reduction. Next, an aggressive irrigation and debridement of the perineal wound was followed by urethral realignment and stenting using a large-diameter urethral catheter. Finally, fecal diversion was accomplished with colostomy. Postoperatively, the patient's hematocrit remained labile and a pelvic angiogram identified the gluteal disruption, which was embolized.

of the posterior pelvis are directly related to disabling low back pain in certain patients (Fig. 25-6). Return-to-work rates and functional outcomes are diminished in those patients with more than 2 cm of posterior pelvic malreductions. Anisomelia may also result from malunions. Residual lumbosacral plexus injuries may cause chronic pain and be responsible for genitourinary and sexual dysfunctions. Posterior surgical exposures for fixation have been associated with high complication rates.

ACETABULAR FRACTURES
General

The acetabulum is an unusual anatomic structure situated at the iliac, pubic, and ischial convergence. Except for the fossa acetabulum, it is covered almost entirely with hyaline cartilage. Together with the femoral head, the spherical acetabulum forms the hip joint. The joint is deepened by a peripheral fibrocartilage termed the *acetabular labrum*. The ligamentum teres tethers the fovea capitis of the femoral head to the fossa acetabulum. The surrounding joint capsule contains the majority of femoral head blood supply. Iliofemoral ligaments support the hip joint.

Acetabular fractures occur after a variety of injuries. Typically, an axial load is applied through the femur at the

TABLE 25-2   Internal Fixation Devices and Exposures

Injury zone	Preferred exposure(s)	Implant(s)
Symphysis distraction	Pfannenstiel	3.5-mm 6H malleable plate
Locked symphysis	Pfannenstiel	3.5-mm 6H malleable plate
Pubic ramus	Pfannenstiel Stoppa Ilioinguinal	3.5-mm 6–8H malleable plate
Iliac wing	Iliac Iliofemoral Ilioinguinal	Lag screws 3.5-mm malleable plate(s)

Iliac crescent	Vertical paramedian	Medullary lag screws
		    3.5-mm malleable plate(s),
		    Iliosacral lag screw

SI joint	Iliac	Iliosacral lag screw(s) or
		    Perpendicular 3-4H
		    3.5-mm DC or malleable plates

Sacral-transforaminal	Vertical paramedian	Iliosacral nonlag screw
		    tension band plateor
		    Sacral Bars

knee or pertrochanteric area causing the acetabular fracture to propagate from the joint surfaces into the ilium, ischium, and pubic bones along structurally frail areas. The resulting fracture patterns are determined by the position of the femur at impact, the vector of load application, and bone quality, among other factors. Fracture displacements result from unopposed muscle pull through the fracture fragments.

Until the pioneering work of Letournel and the Judets, acetabular injuries were poorly understood. The investigators divided the acetabulum into two individual columns of bone—the anterior and posterior columns. The anterior column included the superior pubic ramus, anterior acetabular wall, anterior dome, anterior iliac spines, and a portion of the anterior ilium. The posterior column con-

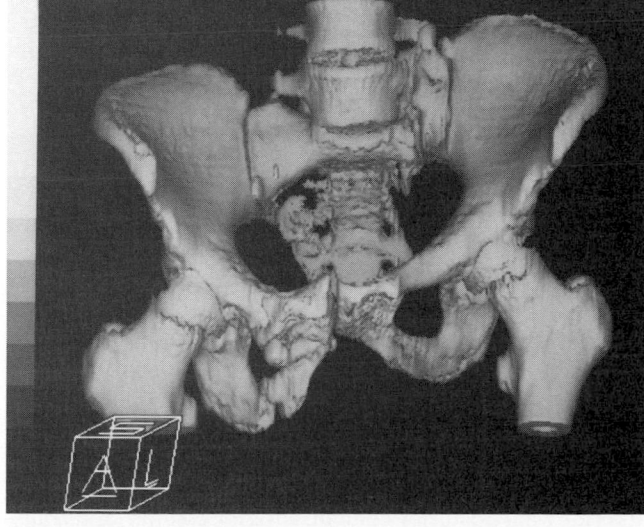

A

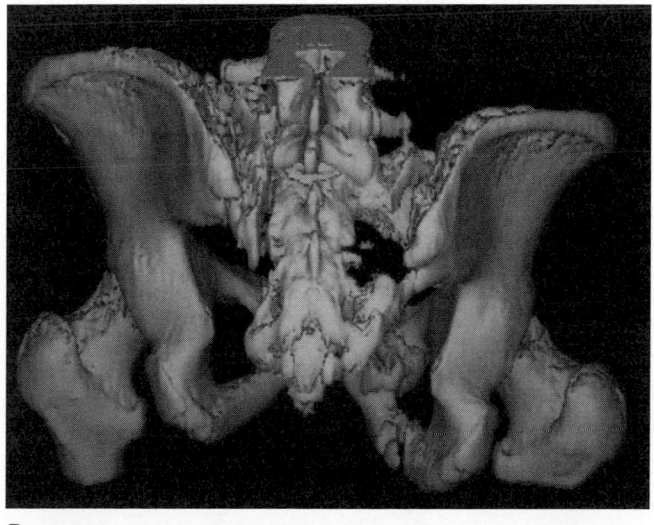

B

Figure 25-6 This patient fell from a standing height and sustained nondisplaced pelvic fractures. She was released from the emergency room on crutches without follow-up. She continued to have pain and presented 8 months later with this pelvic malunion. The 3D CT scan anteriorly (*A*) and posteriorly (*B*).

sisted of the ischium, posterior acetabular wall, posterior dome, and posterior ilium. This bicolumnar division produces the appearance of an inverted Y shape when the acetabulum is viewed directly laterally (Fig. 25-7). The two-column concept is the basis for beginning to understand the acetabulum.

Patient Evaluation

The same principles of simultaneous evaluation and resuscitation apply as described for patients with pelvic disruptions. Open acetabular fractures are rare but do occur, and the skin violations are frequently subtle. Hemodynamic instability is evaluated and treated. Acetabular fractures may be displaced through the greater sciatic notch and injure the gluteal vascular bundle. Range-of-motion examination of the affected hip is painful and therefore avoided.

Deformities are associated with displaced acetabular fracture-dislocations. In addition, ipsilateral lower extremity deformity can be due to a pelvic disruption, femoral neck/intertrochanteric fractures, as well as other lower extremity fracture/dislocation. Rare anterior (or obturator) fracture-dislocation produces a painful abduction/external rotation hip deformity. Much more common are posterior fracture dislocations which result in shortening, adduction, and internal rotation deformities of the ipsilateral lower extremity. A detailed distal neurological exam is documented prior to closed reduction maneuvers. The peroneal division of the sciatic nerve is particularly vulnerable and has a high correlation of injury with posterior fracture-dislocations.

Radiology

The radiographic evaluation of acetabular fracture begins with a good-quality anteroposterior pelvic film. The diagnosis is usually obvious based on this image, especially when significant comminution or displacements occur. The iliopectineal (or iliopubic) line is the cortical density that begins along the pelvic brim and courses to the pubic symphysis, representing the anterior column. The ilioischial line is a similar confluence of cortical densities, also beginning at the pelvic brim but descending to the ischial tuberosity. The ilioischial line represents the posterior column. Special "Judet oblique" images are next obtained to further understand the acetabular fracture. Judet obliques are obtained in the sedated patient by positioning the x-ray beam and cassette exactly as for an anteroposterior (AP) pelvic image. The x-ray source is centered on the injured acetabulum. The patient is then rotated approximately 35 to 45° with the injured hip forward and a soft support or positioning wedge placed beneath the injured side. This "obturator oblique" image places the obturator foramen perpendicular to the x-ray source. The anterior column and posterior wall are identified. The orthogonal "iliac oblique" is obtained by rotating the opposite hemipelvis forward while still centering the radiograph on the injured acetabulum. The positioning wedge is inserted to support the patient once again. The iliac oblique places the x-ray source perpendicular to the iliac fossa and reveals the posterior column and anterior wall. This view is usually obtained in less rotation than the obturator oblique by inexperienced radiology technicians. This position with the injured acetabulum "down" causes pain, and the patient will complain until the image is obtained or the inexperienced technician minimizes the rotation (Fig. 25-8).

Two-dimensional CT is useful to further understand and therefore better classify the acetabular fracture. Contiguous axial slices (5 mm) begin at the iliac crests and continue to the level of the dome. Further 3-mm slices are used through the joint surfaces, followed by 5-mm cuts from the caudal joint surface through the ischial tuberosities. Various technical aspects improve the scan quality. Soft tissue windows are used to better visualize capsular, chondral, and labral structures when indicated. For either associated or variant acetabular fracture patterns, three-dimensional (3D) CT scanning may be beneficial for preoperative planning. High-resolution computer software and narrower axial slices improve 3D images. On-screen viewing and careful correlation with both the plain radiographs and routine CT scan are mandatory to avoid misinterpretation of the 3D CT scan. Three-dimensional acetabular CT scanning is not a substitute for a detailed review of the plain radiographs and routine CT scan preoperatively.

Classification

Acetabular fractures have been included in several hip dislocation, femoral head, and pelvic fracture schemes. Letournel described an acetabular classification based on the two-column acetabular concept. This classification is easy to remember, guides treatment, yet recognizes unusual "variant" fracture patterns. Letournel's classification system is also useful in determining the most beneficial surgical exposure for open reduction and fixation. Acetabular fractures are divided into "elementary" and "associated" patterns. The elementary fractures include posterior wall, anterior wall, posterior column, anterior column, and transverse patterns. It is easy to understand how the single-column and wall fractures are included as elementary, but the transverse pattern's inclusion is confusing, since transverse acetabular fractures involve both the anterior and posterior

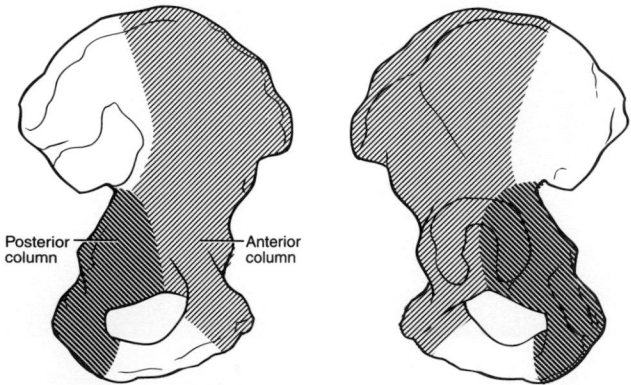

Figure 25-7 The two-column acetabular division according to Letournel separates the anterior and posterior columns, with the dome as the keystone.

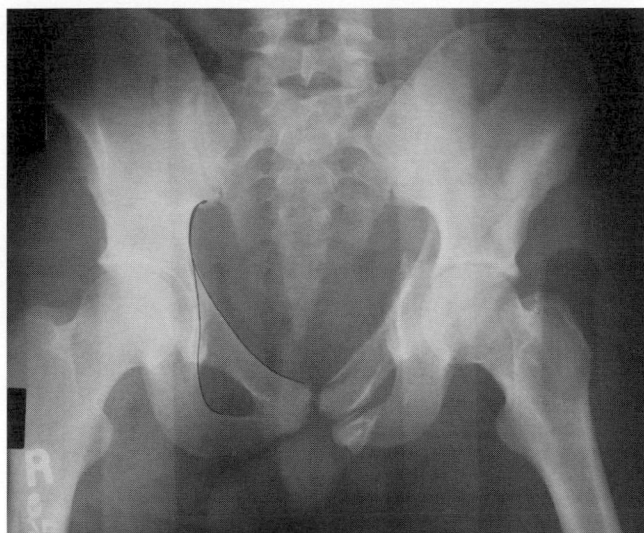

A

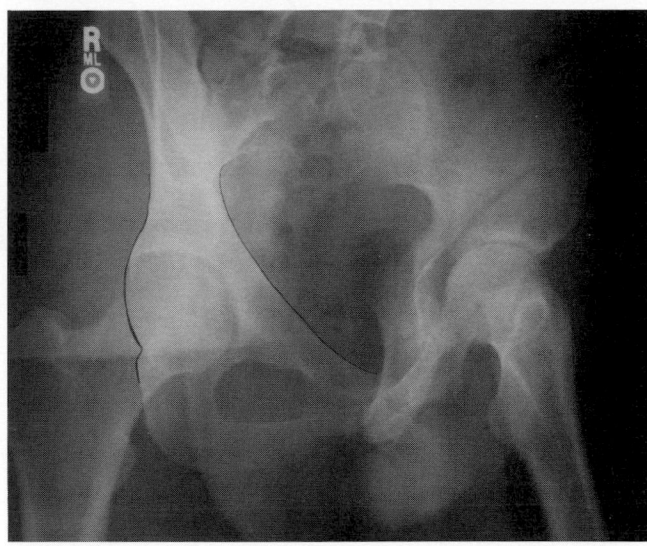

B

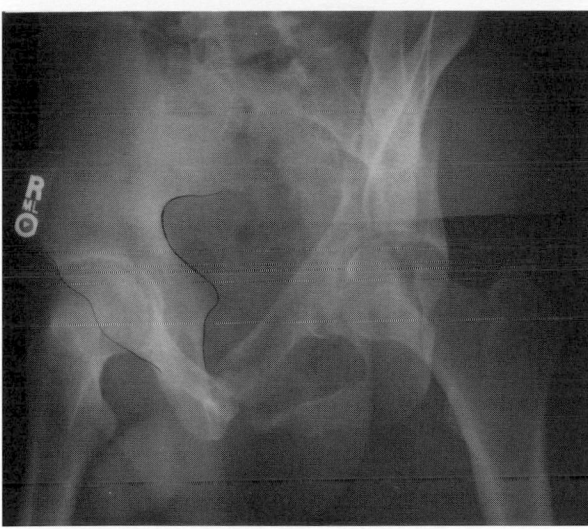

C

Figure 25-8 This anteroposterior pelvic radiograph (*A*) demonstrates the iliopectineal and ilioischial lines. This right-sided obturator oblique radiograph (*B*) is obtained with the patient's right hemipelvis rotated approximately 35 to 45° forward; it identifies the anterior column and posterior wall. The posterior column and anterior wall are best seen on the right-sided iliac oblique image (*C*), obtained with the left hemipelvis rotated similarly. For each oblique view, the patient is turned and the x-ray is centered on the injured acetabulum. In this example, the patient's left acetabulum is fractured. Typically, the Judet oblique is named for the injured side. In this case the obliques are named for the normal side in order to be descriptive.

columns. Letournel included transverse acetabular fractures in the elementary group because of their "purity." Transverse acetabular fractures are simple, despite the fact that they cross the two columns. Transverse acetabular fractures are subdivided according to their dome (or roof/"tectum") involvement. Transtectal fractures split the dome, infratectal fractures disrupt the fossa, and juxtatectal fractures involve the zone between the other two. A transverse acetabular fracture is further defined, therefore, as either transtectal, juxtatectal, or infratectal-transverse.

The associated acetabular fractures include combinations of the elementary patterns. The posterior column with associated posterior wall, transverse with associated posterior wall, T type, anterior column with associated posterior hemitransverse, and both columns are the five associated acetabular fracture patterns. T-type acetabular fractures are transverse fractures with an additional vertical fracture limb that divides the obturator foramen. Anterior column fractures with associated posterior hemitransverse patterns are similar to a T-type fracture, only

with the vertical limb through the lower portion of the anterior column rather than the obturator foramen. The fracture of both columns is a complete dissociation of the articular portions of the acetabulum from the intact hemipelvis. Some describe this pattern as a "floating acetabulum." Confusion frequently arises when Letournel's acetabular classification system is poorly understood, since the transverse, transverse/posterior wall, T-type, anterior column/posterior hemitransverse, and both-columns patterns all involve "both" of the acetabular columns. The true definition of the associated both-columns fracture pattern must not be misinterpreted as a catch-all for any acetabular fracture that disrupts the two acetabular columns (Fig. 25-9).

Treatment Options

Acute Management—Closed Reduction

Dislocations are relocated after patient sedation and prior to further nonemergent evaluations. The femoral head is relocated beneath the residual dome even before the Judet oblique radiographs are obtained. The ipsilateral femoral neck is carefully inspected to rule out an occult fracture prior to closed manipulative reduction of the hip. Prolonged hip dislocation is painful and jeopardizes the

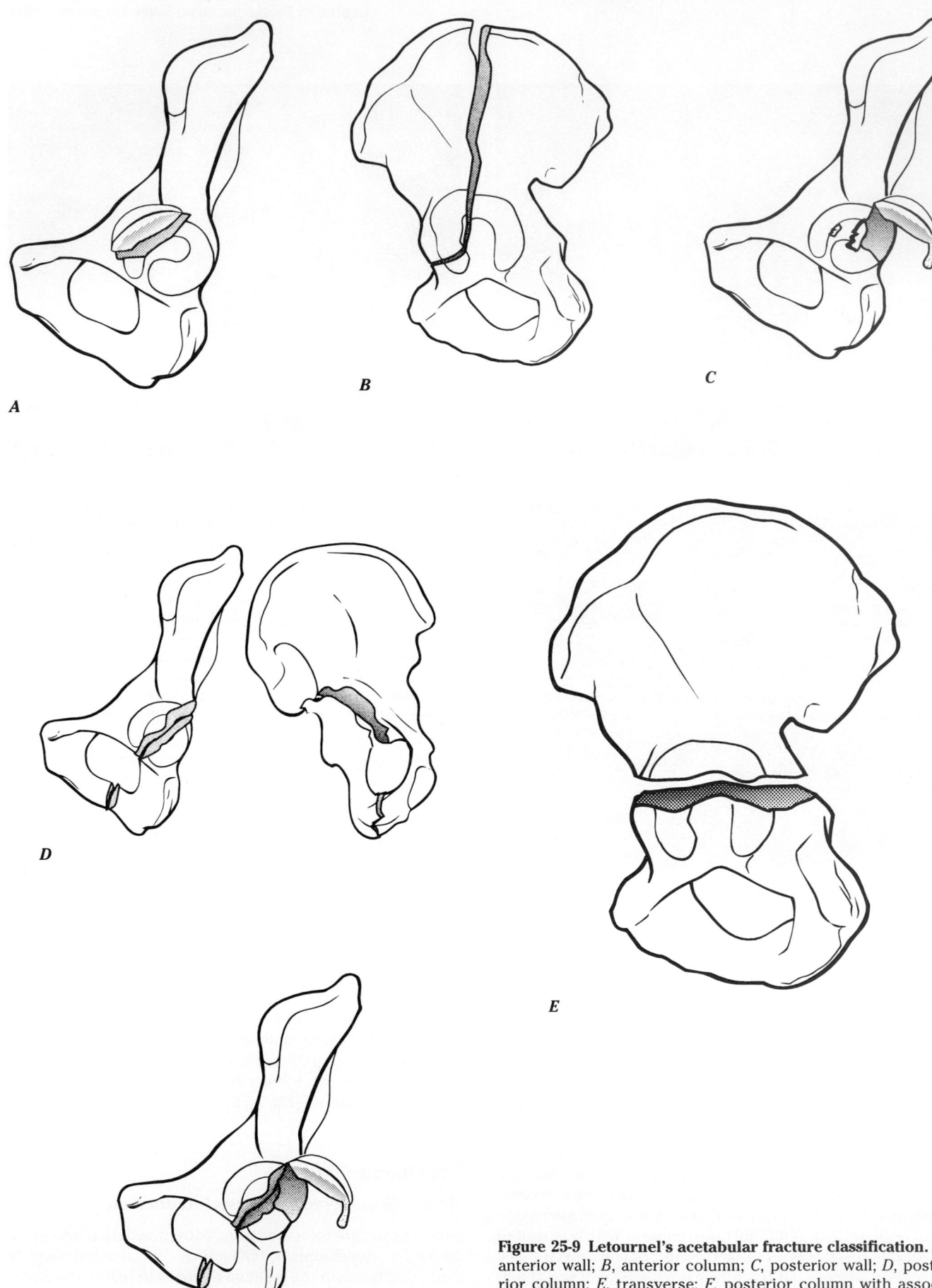

Figure 25-9 Letournel's acetabular fracture classification. *A*, anterior wall; *B*, anterior column; *C*, posterior wall; *D*, posterior column; *E*, transverse; *F*, posterior column with associated posterior wall; *G*, T type; *H*, anterior column associated with hemitransverse; *I*, transverse with associated posterior wall; *J*, both columns.

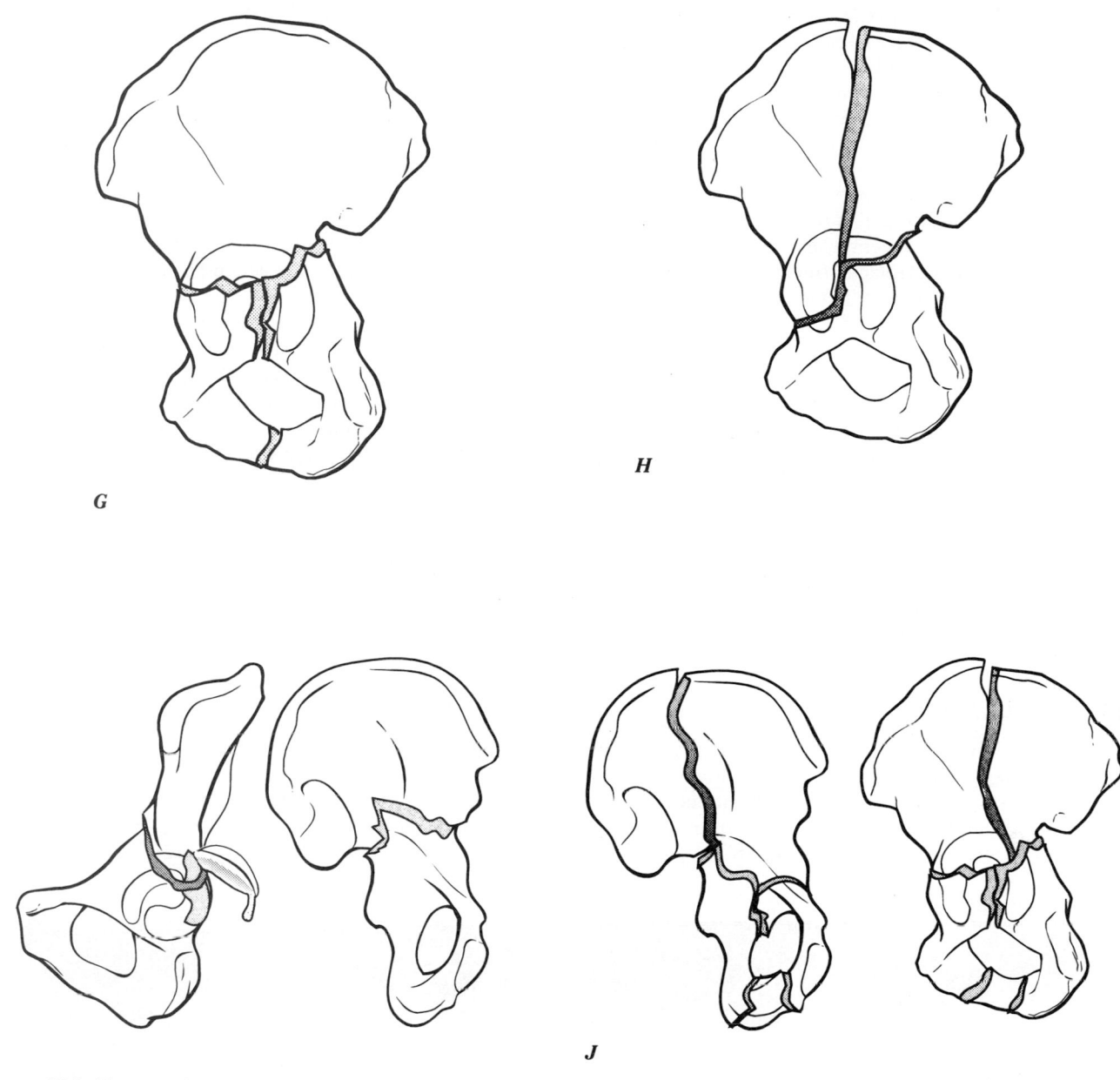

Figure 25-9 (*Continued*)

femoral head's capsular blood supply. Irreducible dislocation may be due to inadequate sedation, soft tissue or loose body interposition, or other causes. Passive hip range-of-motion evaluation after a successful closed reduction is not advocated, since such maneuvers may further injure the femoral head. Certain fracture patterns will produce severe instability even after the reduction is achieved. An irreducible dislocation is not the same entity as this "exploded" acetabular fracture without sufficient residual dome to maintain a reduction. Orthogonal Judet pelvic radiographs demonstrate the hip position after closed reduction. Repeat detailed distal neurologic exam is documented after the reduction. Sciatic or other nerve entrapment within the fracture fragments at the time of re

duction rarely occurs. Redislocation is controversial at this point, but immediate nerve exploration, fracture reduction, and internal fixation may be indicated in such unusual instances.

Conservative Treatment

Some acetabular fractures are treated successfully using closed techniques. Patients with isolated, stable, nondisplaced fractures are mobilized with protected weight bearing. In some acetabular fractures with minimal displacement, distal femoral traction is used together with epidural analgesics and early continuous passive motion devices to improve comfort and healing. Such treatment is most ef fective when the acetabular fracture exhibits "secondary congruence." This indicates that the acetabular fracture fragments have maintained a congruent and spherical relationship with the femoral head. Roof arc angles are also used to quantify femoral head coverage by the dome. These angles are measured using the three plain radiographs. A perpendicular is drawn from a line connecting the ischial tuberosities (assuming no ischial deformity) through the spherical center of the fractured acetabulum. The acetabular spherical center and the femoral head are not the same in some displaced fractures. A second line is then drawn from the spherical center to the fracture edge on each view. The angular measurement is made from the perpendicular to the second line. At least 45° or more of coverage on each view is desired to maximize results after closed management. Excellent sphericity and congruity of the joint should likewise improve outcome. Routine follow-up radiographs are used to assure maintenance of the closed reduction and healing (Fig. 25-10).

Some patients with acetabular fractures have medical and other conditions that preclude operative treatment. Local pelvic skin conditions such as previous surgical exposures, severe degloving injuries, and morbid obesity complicate operative management when they involve the anticipated surgical site.

Internal Fixation

Successful operative management of displaced acetabular fractures is dependent on many factors. Ideal operative management should include (1) proper patient selection; (2) a thorough understanding of the fracture; (3) a complete preoperative plan; (4) an adequate surgical expo-

sure; (5) early, anatomic, and stable fracture reduction; and (6) rapid patient mobilization and joint motion. These goals are likely best accomplished by an experienced surgeon working with a coordinated team approach to these difficult problems (Fig. 25-11A through G).

Emergent open reduction and internal fixation is indicated in those uncommon patients with open acetabular fractures, irreducible fracture/dislocations, and peripheral neurologic changes after closed reductions. Nonconcentric reductions are usually due to intraarticular soft tissues or bone debris and warrant urgent operative management.

The appropriate surgical exposure is dependent on numerous factors but primarily on the fracture pattern. Common surgical exposures for acetabular fractures include the ilioinguinal, Kocher-Langenbeck, and extended iliofemoral. Other surgical approaches for the operative management of acetabular fractures have been described (Table 25-3).

Complications

Complications after acetabular fractures are numerous. Deep venous thromboses should be diminished by sequential compression devices, early patient mobilization, and systemic prophylactic anticoagulation. Routine venous screening evaluations are useful to diagnose asymptomatic thromboses. The development of fatal pulmonary emboli should be avoided by early detection and treatment. Therapeutic anticoagulation and/or vena caval filters are used when indicated.

The incidence of posttraumatic hip arthritis after acetabular fracture is variable. Inaccurate or nonanatomic

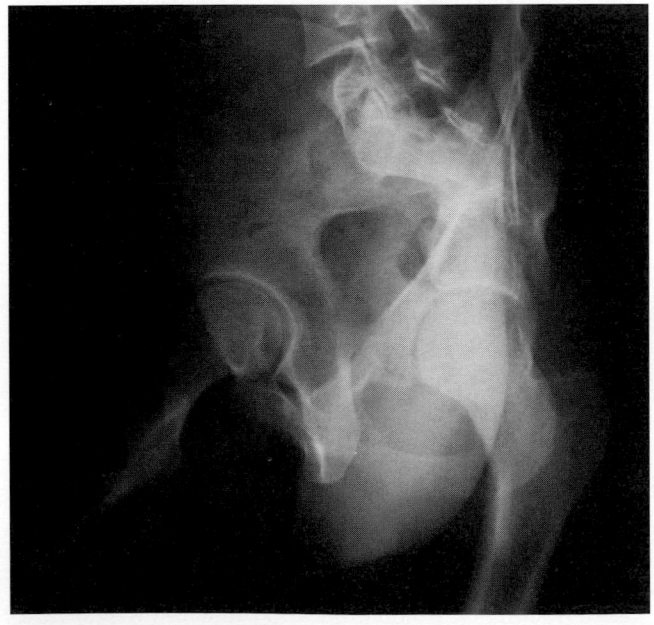

A

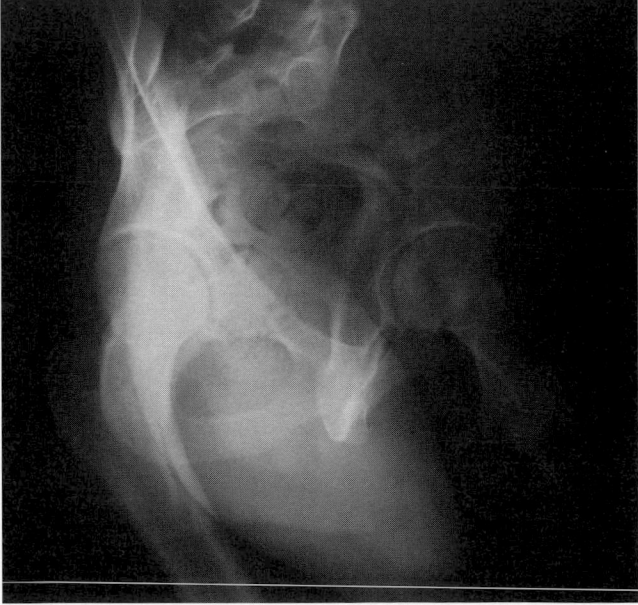

B

Figure 25-10 Closed management was used to treat this patient's left-sided "associated" both column acetabular fracture. *A.* The spur sign is visible on the obturator oblique. *B.* The iliac oblique demonstrates congruity of the joint at the dome and slight malrotation of the posterior column component of the fracture.

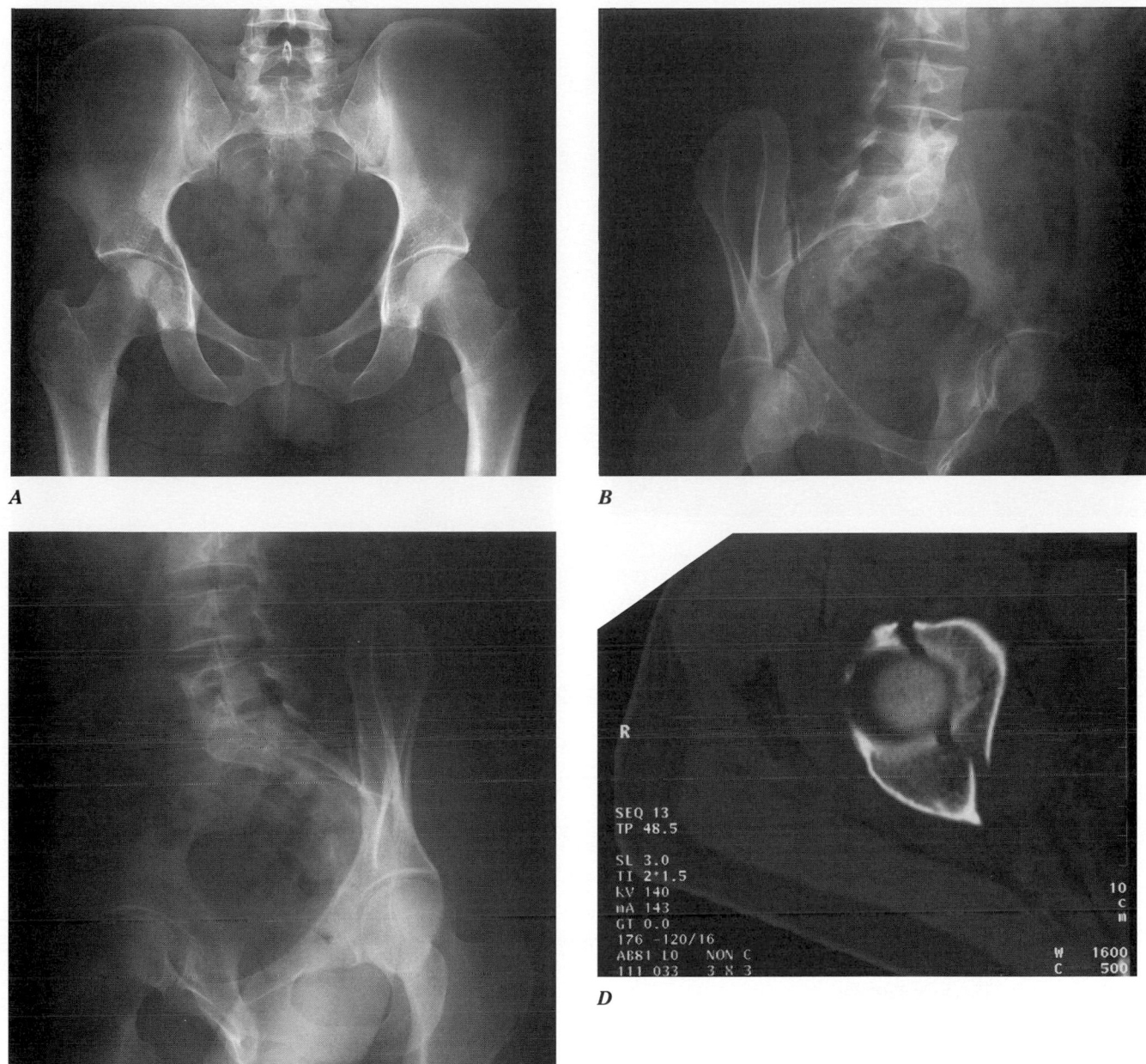

A

B

C

D

Figure 25-11 *A* through *C.* Anteroposterior, obturator oblique, and iliac oblique acetabular plain radiographs were used to evaluate this acetabular fracture. The femoral head is subluxated. *D.* This CT axial image at the dome identifies the lack of articular congruity due to the medially displaced femoral head relative to the stable dome fracture fragment. Despite traction, the femoral head was not maintained beneath the acetabular dome and the roof arc angles also did not support closed management. *E* and *F.* Postoperative radiographs reveal anatomic fracture reduction and joint congruity after a prone Kocher-Langenbeck exposure and open reduction.

fracture reduction is often correlated with such degenerative changes, although numerous factors affect them.

Surgical complications include infection, fixation failure, malreduction, ectopic bone formation, nerve or vascular injury, bladder and spermatic cord injuries, hernia formation, and intraarticular hardware, among many others.

SUMMARY

Pelvic and acetabular fractures are difficult to manage successfully for many reasons. This chapter only begins to introduce and update common concepts and practice methods. The reader is strongly encouraged to investigate these injuries further and in much greater detail.

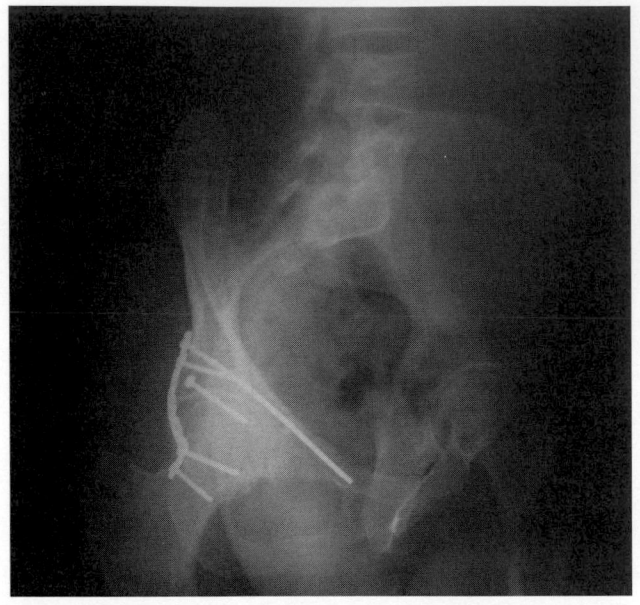

E

Figure 25-11 (*Continued*)

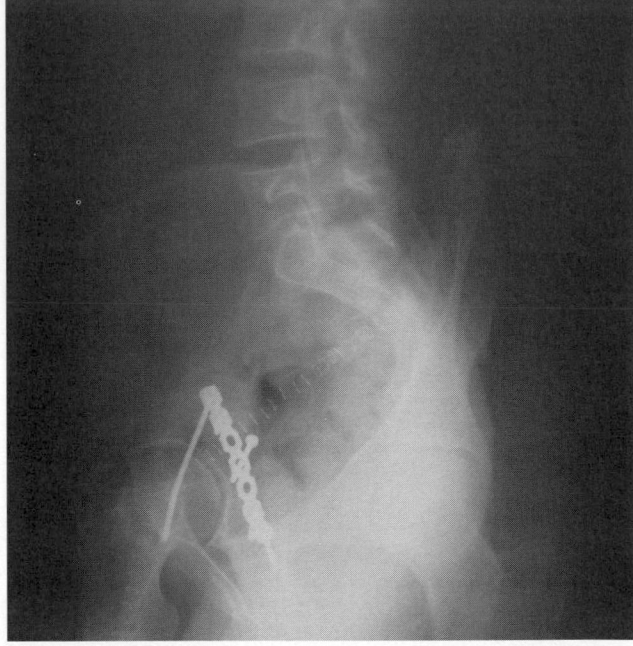

F

TABLE 25-3   Acetabular Fractures and Surgical Exposures

Fracture Pattern	Exposure
Posterior wall	Kocher-Langenbeck
Posterior column	Kocher-Langenbeck (prone)
Anterior wall	Ilioinguinal
Anterior column	Ilioinguinal/iliac
Transverse	Kocher-Langenbeck (prone) Ilioinguinal Extended iliofemoral
Transverse/posterior wall	Kocher-Langenbeck (prone) Extended iliofemoral
Posterior column/posterior wall	Kocher-Langenbeck (prone)
Anterior column/posterior hemitransverse	Ilioinguinal Extended iliofemoral
T type	Extended iliofemoral Ilioinguinal
Both columns	Ilioinguinal Extended iliofemoral

SUGGESTED READINGS

Pelvic Fractures

Classification

Baumgaertel F: Diagnosis, classification, and surgical indications in acetabulum fracture. *Orthopade* 21:427–441, 1992.

Bosch U, Pohlemann T, Haas N, Tscherne H: Classification and management of complex pelvic trauma. *Unfallchirurgie* 95: 189–196, 1992.

Bucholz RW: The pathological anatomy of Malgaigne fracture-dislocations of the pelvis. *J Bone Joint Surg Am* 63:400–404, 1981.

Burgess AR, Eastridge BJ, Young JW, et al: Pelvic ring disruptions: Effective classification system and treatment protocols. *J Trauma* 30:848–856, 1990.

Cryer HM, Miller FB, Evers BM, et al: Pelvic fracture classification: Correlation with hemorrhage. *J Trauma* 28:973–980, 1988.

Dalal SA, Burgess AR, Siegel JH, et al: Pelvic fracture in multiple trauma: Classification by mechanism is key to pattern of organ injury, resuscitative requirements, and outcome. *J Trauma* 29:981–1000; discussion, 1000–1002, 1989.

Eid AM: Fractures of the pelvis. *Postgrad Med J* 59:560–565, 1983.

Euler E, Betz A, Schweiberer L: Diagnosis, classification and indications for surgical treatment of pelvic ring fractures. *Orthopade* 21:354–362, 1992.

Felenda MR, Dittel KK: Classification of unstable pelvic ring injuries—Treatment methods. *Aktuelle Traumatol* 23:263–271, 1993.

Looser KG, Crombie HD Jr: Pelvic fractures: An anatomic guide to severity of injury. Review of 100 cases. *Am J Surg* 132:638–642, 1976.

Mayr E, Braun W, Ruter A: Is there a classification of pelvic ring injuries that takes the trauma mechanism, morphology and stability relations into consideration and thereby gives references for subsequent therapy? *Zentralbl Chir* 119:597–607, 1994.

Messina N: The pelvic bones: II. Classification and mechanics of fractures. *Rass Int Clin Ter* 46:627–643, 1966.

Pennal GF, Tile M, Waddell JP, Garside H: Pelvic disruption: Assessment and classification. *Clin Orthop* 12–21, 1980.

Rommens P, Hartwig T, Wissing H, Schmit-Neuerburg KP: Diagnosis and treatment of unstable fractures of the pelvic ring. *Acta Chir Belg* 86:352–359, 1986.

Rubenstein JD: Radiographic assessment of pelvic trauma. *J Can Assoc Radiol* 34:228–236, 1983.

Sabiston CP, Wing PC: Sacral fractures: Classification and neurologic implications. *J Trauma* 26:1113–1115, 1986.

Serafi A, Vielsacker H, Muller KW: Application of the Isler and Ganz classification of pelvic ring fractures in clinical practice. *Aktuelle Traumatol* 22:197–202, 1992.

Teubner E, Gerstenberger F: Kinematics of the pelvis: Grading and pathomechanical classification of injuries of the pelvic joints and kinematic and clinical consequences of surgical management. *Unfallchirurgie* 95:50–57, 1992.

Tile M, Pennal GF: Pelvic disruption: Principles of management. *Clin Orthop* 56–64, 1980.

Trubnikov VF, Kovalev SI: Classification and treatment of pelvic injuries. *Vestn Khir* 142:75–77, 1989.

Young JW, Burgess AR, Brumback RJ, Poka A: Pelvic fractures: Value of plain radiography in early assessment and management. *Radiology* 160:445–451, 1986.

Young JW, Resnik CS: Fracture of the pelvis: Current concepts of classification. *Am J Roentgenol* 155:1169–1175, 1990.

Radiology

Adam P, Labbe JL, Alberge Y, et al: The role of computed tomography in the assessment and treatment of acetabular fractures. *Clin Radiol* 36:13–18, 1985.

Burk DL Jr, Mears DC, Herbert DL, et al: Pelvic and acetabular fractures: Examination by angled CT scanning. *Radiology* 153:548, 1984.

Dalinka MK, Boorstein JM, Zlatkin MB: Computed tomography of musculoskeletal trauma. *Radiol Clin North Am* 27:933–944, 1989.

Gilula LA, Murphy WA, Tailor CC, Patel RB: Computed tomography of the osseous pelvis. *Radiology* 132:107–114, 1979.

Harris JH Jr, Loh CK, Perlman HC, Rotz CT Jr: The roentgen diagnosis of pelvic extraperitoneal effusion. *Radiology* 125: 343–350, 1977.

Jackson H, Kam J, Harris JH Jr, Harle TS: The sacral arcuate lines in upper sacral fractures. *Radiology* 145:35–39, 1982.

Nelson DW, Duwelius PJ: CT-guided fixation of sacral fractures and sacroiliac joint disruptions. *Radiology* 180:527–532, 1991.

Saks BJ: Normal acetabular anatomy for acetabular fracture assessment: CT and plain film correlation. *Radiology* 159: 139–145, 1986.

Schild H, Muller HA, Klose K, et al: The anatomy, radiology and clinical features of fractures of the sacrum (author's transl). *ROFO Fortschr Geb Rontgenstr Nuklearmed* 134:522–527, 1981.

Vas WG, Wolverson MK, Sundaram M, et al: The role of computed tomography in pelvic fractures. *J Comput Assist Tomogr* 6:796–801, 1982.

White MS: Three-dimensional computed tomography in the assessment of fractures of the acetabulum. *Injury* 22:13–19, 1991.

Young JW, Burgess AR: Use of CT in acute trauma victims (letter). *Radiology* 166:903, 1988.

Young JW, Burgess AR, Brumback RJ, Poka A: Pelvic fractures: Value of plain radiography in early assessment and management. *Radiology* 160:445–451, 1986.

Conservative Treatment

Flory PJ, Trentz O, Buhren V, et al: Management of complex pelvic injuries. *Aktuelle Traumatol* 15:139–144, 1985.

Jurgens C, Wolter D, Kortmann HR: Conservative treatment of spinal and pelvic fractures. *Chirurgie* 61:783–791, 1990.

Tosovsky V, Stryhal F: The conservative treatment of the fractures and dislocations of the extremities in children. *Acta Univ Carol [Med Monogr]* 111:1–145, 1986.

van Gulik TM, Raaymakers EL, Broekhuizen AH, Karthaus AJ: Complications and late therapeutic results of conservatively managed, unstable pelvic ring disruptions. *J Neurosurg (Neth)* 39:175–178, 1987.

External Fixation

Alho A, Horn A: External fixation of pelvic fracture ex vivo. *Ann Chir Gynaecol* 72:308–311, 1983.

Bell AL, Smith RA, Brown TD, Nepola JV: Comparative study of the Orthofix and Pittsburgh frames for external fixation of unstable pelvic ring fractures. *J Orthop Trauma* 2:130–138, 1988.

Bonnel F: External fixation in fractures of the pelvis (author's transl). *Ann Chir* 30:131–134, 1976.

Brown TD, Stone JP, Schuster JH, Mears DC: External fixation of unstable pelvic ring fractures: Comparative rigidity of some current frame configurations. *Med Biol Eng Comput* 20:727–733, 1982.

Buhren V, Marzi I, Trentz O: Indications and technic of external fixation in acute management of polytrauma. *Zentralbl Chir* 115:581–591, 1990.

Castaman E: External fixation of fractures and fracture dislocations of the pelvis. *Ital J Orthop Traumatol* 15:315–329, 1989.

Dahners LE, Jacobs RR, McKenzie EB, Gilbert JA: Biomechanical studies of an anterior pelvic external fixation frame intended for control of vertical shear fractures. *South Med J* 79:815–817, 1986.

Egbers HJ, Draijer F, Havemann D, Zenker W: Stabilizing the pelvic ring with the external fixator. Biomechanical studies and clinical experiences. *Orthopade* 21:363–372, 1992.

Frohlich P, Barnbeck F: External fixation of the pelvis—Indications, assembly and results. *Zentralbl Chir* 112:1501–1507, 1987.

Gylling SF, Ward RE, Holcroft JW, et al: Immediate external fixation of unstable pelvic fractures. *Am J Surg* 150:721–724, 1985.

Havemann D, Egbers HJ: External fixators in treatment of severe fractures of the pelvis. *Langenbecks Arch Chir Suppl II Vehr Dtsch Ges Chir* 445–449, 1989.

Karaharju EO, Slatis P: External fixation of double vertical pelvic fractures with trapezoid compression frame. *Injury* 10:142–145, 1978.

Kellam JF: The role of external fixation in pelvic disruptions. *Clin Orthop* 66–82, 1989.

Lansinger O, Karlsson J, Berg U, Mare K: Unstable fractures of the pelvis treated with a trapezoid compression frame. *Acta Orthop Scand* 55:325–329, 1984.

Liu J, Lai KA, Chou YL: Strength of the pin-bone interface of external fixation pins in the iliac crest: A biomechanical study. *Clin Orthop* 237–244, 1995.

Majeed SA: External fixation of the injured pelvis. The functional outcome. *J Bone Joint Surg Br* 72:612–614, 1990.

Mears DC, Fu F: External fixation in pelvic fractures. *Orthop Clin North Am* 11:465–479, 1980.

Mears DC, Fu FH: Modern concepts of external skeletal fixation of the pelvis. *Clin Orthop* 65–72, 1980.

Molski K: External fixation of multiple injuries of the pelvic bones with metal splint. *Chir Narzadow Ruchu Ortop Pol* 47:139–143, 1982.

Muller J, Bachmann B: Treatment of unstable pelvic girdle fractures with Wagner external fixation. *Helv Chir Acta* 45:59–61, 1978.

Noordeen MH, Taylor BA, Briggs TW, Lavy CB: Pin placement in pelvic external fixation. *Injury* 24:581–584, 1993.

Princic J: Injuries of the pelvic circle treated with external fixation at the Traumatology University Clinic in Ljubljana 1981–1987. *Acta Chir Iugosl* 1:371–373, 1989.

Ravaglia L, Lijoi F: Our experience in the use of external fixation devices. *Chir Organi Mov* 68:425–437, 1982.

Reff RB: The use of external fixation devices in the management of severe lower-extremity trauma and pelvic injuries in children. *Clin Orthop* 21–33, 1984.

Riska EB, von Bonsdorff H, Hakkinen S, et al: External fixation of unstable pelvic fractures. *Int Orthop* 3:183–188, 1979.

Rubash HE, Mears DC: External fixation of the pelvis. *Instr Course Lect* 32:329–348, 1983.

Siemssen SJ, Frandsen PA: Double vertical fractures of the pelvis treated by external fixation. *Ugeskr Laeger* 143:1094–1096, 1981.

Slatis P, Eskola A: External fixation of the pelvic girdle as a test for assessing instability of the sacro-iliac joint. *Ann Med* 21:369–372, 1989.

Slatis P, Karaharju EO: External fixation of the pelvic girdle with a trapezoid compression frame. *Injury* 7:53–56, 1975.

Slatis P, Karaharju EO: External fixation of unstable pelvic fractures: Experiences in 22 patients treated with a trapezoid compression frame. *Clin Orthop* 73–80, 1980.

Vecsei V: Results of biomechanical studies of various external fixation devices of the pelvis. *Aktuelle Traumatol* 18:261–264, 1988.

Wild JJ, Hanson GW, Tullos HS: Unstable fractures of the pelvis treated by external fixation. *J Bone Joint Surg Am* 64:1010–1020, 1982.

Williams RP, Friis EA, Cooke FW, et al: External fixation of unstable Malgaigne fractures: The comparative mechanical performance of a new configuration. *Orthop Rev* 21:1423–1430, 1992.

Internal Fixation

Alho A, Horn A: External fixation of pelvic fracture ex vivo. *Ann Chir Gynaecol* 72:308–311, 1983.

Allgower M, Perren S, Matter P: A new plate for internal fixation—the dynamic compression plate (DCP). *Injury* 2:40–47, 1970.

Bell AL, Smith RA, Brown TD, Nepola JV: Comparative study of the Orthofix and Pittsburgh frames for external fixation of unstable pelvic ring fractures. *J Orthop Trauma* 2:130–138, 1988.

Bonnel F: External fixation in fractures of the pelvis (author's transl). *Ann Chir* 30:131–134, 1976.

Broos P, Vanderschot P, Craninx L, Rommens P: The operative treatment of unstable pelvic ring fractures. *Int Surg* 77:303–308, 1992.

Brown TD, Stone JP, Schuster JH, Mears DC: External fixation of unstable pelvic ring fractures: Comparative rigidity of some current frame configurations. *Med Biol Eng Comput* 20: 727–733, 1982.

Browner BD, Cole JD, Graham JM, et al: Delayed posterior internal fixation of unstable pelvic fractures. *J Trauma* 27: 998–1006, 1987.

Buhren V, Marzi I, Trentz O: Indications and technic of external fixation in acute management of polytrauma. *Zentralbl Chir* 115:581–591, 1990.

Castaman E: External fixation of fractures and fracture dislocations of the pelvis. *Ital J Orthop Traumatol* 15:315–329, 1989.

Cotler HB, La Mont JG, Hansen ST Jr: Immediate spica casting for pelvic fractures. *J Orthop Trauma* 2:222–228, 1988.

Dahners LE, Jacobs RR, McKenzie EB, Gilbert JA: Biomechanical studies of an anterior pelvic external fixation frame intended for control of vertical shear fractures. *South Med J* 79:815–817, 1986.

Duwelius PJ, Van Allen M, Bray TJ, Nelson D: Computed tomography-guided fixation of unstable posterior pelvic ring disruptions. *J Orthop Trauma* 6:420–426, 1992.

Ebraheim NA, Coombs R, Rusin JJ, Jackson WT: Reduction of postoperative CT artifacts of pelvic fractures by use of titanium implants. *Orthopedics* 13:1357–1358, 1990.

Egbers HJ, Draijer F, Havemann D, Zenker W: Stabilizing the pelvic ring with the external fixator. Biomechanical studies and clinical experiences. *Orthopade* 21:363–372, 1992.

Frohlich P, Barnbeck F: External fixation of the pelvis— Indications, assembly and results. *Zentralbl Chir* 112: 1501–1507, 1987.

Goldstein A, Phillips T, Sclafani SJ, et al: Early open reduction and internal fixation of the disrupted pelvic ring. *J Trauma* 26:325–333, 1986.

Goris RJ, Biert J: A single, midline extraperitoneal incision for internal fixation of type C unstable pelvic ring fractures. *J Am Coll Surg* 181:81–82, 1995.

Gylling SF, Ward RE, Holcroft JW, et al: Immediate external fixation of unstable pelvic fractures. *Am J Surg* 150:721–724, 1985.

Havemann D, Egbers HJ: External fixators in treatment of severe fractures of the pelvis. *Langenbecks Arch Chir Suppl II Verh Dtsch Ges Chir* 445–449, 1989.

Hesp WL, van der Werken C, Keunen RW, Goris RJ: Unstable fractures and dislocations of the pelvic ring—Results of treatment in relation to the severity of injury. *Neth J Surg* 37: 148–152, 1985.

Hirvensalo E, Lindahl J, Bostman O: A new approach to the internal fixation of unstable pelvic fractures. *Clin Orthop* 28–32, 1993.

Johnson L: Operative management of unstable pelvic fractures. *Orthop Nurs* 8:21–25, 1989.

Kamhin M, Ganel A, Salai M, Horoszowski H: Rigid fixation in diastasis of symphysis pubis. *J Trauma* 20:523–525, 1980.

Karaharju EO, Slatis P: External fixation of double vertical pelvic fractures with a trapezoid compression frame. *Injury* 10:142–145, 1978.

Kellam JF: The role of external fixation in pelvic disruptions. *Clin Orthop* 66–82, 1989.

Kellam JF, McMurtry RY, Paley D, Tile M: The unstable pelvic fracture. Operative treatment. *Orthop Clin North Am* 18:25–41, 1987.

Lange RH, Hansen ST Jr: Pelvic ring disruptions with symphysis pubis diastasis: Indications, technique, and limitations of anterior internal fixation. *Clin Orthop* 130–137, 1985.

Lansinger O, Karlsson J, Berg U, Mare K: Unstable fractures of the pelvis treated with a trapezoid compression frame. *Acta Orthop Scand* 55:325–329, 1984.

Leenen LP, van der Werken C, Schoots F, Goris RJ: Internal fixation of open unstable pelvic fractures. *J Trauma* 35:220–225, 1993.

Leung KS, Chien P, Shen WY, So WS: Operative treatment of unstable pelvic fractures. *Injury* 23:31–37, 1992.

Liu J, Lai KA, Chou YL: Strength of the pin-bone interface of external fixation pins in the iliac crest: A biomechanical study. *Clin Orthop* 237–244, 1995.

Majeed SA: External fixation of the injured pelvis. The functional outcome. *J Bone Joint Surg Br* 72:612–614, 1990.

Mears DC, Capito CP, Deleeuw H: Posterior pelvic disruptions managed by the use of the Double Cobra Plate. *Instr Course Lect* 37:143–150, 1988.

Mears DC, Fu F: External fixation in pelvic fractures. *Orthop Clin North Am* 11:465–479, 1980.

Mears DC, Fu FH: Modern concepts of external skeletal fixation of the pelvis. *Clin Orthop* 65–72, 1980.

Mears DC, Rubash HE: External and internal fixation of the pelvic ring. *Instr Course Lect* 33:144–158, 1984.

Molski K: External fixation of multiple injuries of the pelvic bones with metal splint. *Chir Narzadow Ruchu Ortop Pol* 47:139–143, 1982.

Muller J, Bachmann B: Treatment of unstable pelvic girdle fractures with Wagner external fixation. *Helv Chir Acta* 45:59–61, 1978.

Nelson DW, Duwelius PJ: CT-guided fixation of sacral fractures and sacroiliac joint disruptions. *Radiology* 180:527–532, 1991.

Noordeen MH, Taylor BA, Briggs TW, Lavy CB: Pin placement in pelvic external fixation. *Injury* 24:581–584, 1993.

Perren SM, Allgower M, Cordey J, Russenberger M: Developments of compression plate techniques for internal fixation of fractures. *Prog Surg* 12:152–179, 1973.

Pohlemann T, Angst M, Schneider E, et al: Fixation of transforaminal sacrum fractures: A biomechanical study. *J Orthop Trauma* 7:107–117, 1993.

Pohlemann T, Bosch U, Gansslen A, Tscherne H: The Hannover experience in management of pelvic fractures. *Clin Orthop* 69–80, 1994.

Pohlemann T, Gansslen A, Kiessling B, et al: Determining indications and osteosynthesis techniques for the pelvic girdle. *Unfallchirurgie* 95:197–209, 1992.

Pohlemann T, Kiessling B, Gansslen A, et al: Standardized osteosynthesis techniques for the pelvic ring: Analysis of a patient sample and surgical technique. *Orthopade* 21:373–384, 1992.

Princic J: Injuries of the pelvic circle treated with external fixation at the Traumatology University Clinic in Ljubljana, 1981–1987. *Acta Chir Iugosl* 1:371–373, 1989.

Ravaglia L, Lijoi F: Our experience in the use of external fixation devices. *Chir Organi Mov* 68:425–437, 1982.

Reff RB: The use of external fixation devices in the management of severe lower-extremity trauma and pelvic injuries in children. *Clin Orthop* 21–33, 1984.

Riska EB, von Bonsdorff H, Hakkinen S, et al: External fixation of unstable pelvic fractures. *Int Orthop* 3:183–188, 1979.

Rommens PM, Vanderschot PM, De Boodt P, Broos PL: Surgical management of pelvic ring disruptions: Indications, techniques and functional results. *Unfallchirurgie* 95:455–462, 1992.

Routt ML Jr, Simonian PT, Ballmer F: A rational approach to pelvic trauma: Resuscitation and early definitive stabilization. *Clin Orthop* 61–74, 1994.

Routt ML Jr, Swiontkowski MF: Operative treatment of complex acetabular fractures: Combined anterior and posterior exposures during the same procedure. *J Bone Joint Surg Am* 72:897–904, 1990.

Rubash HE, Mears DC: External fixation of the pelvis. *Instr Course Lect* 32:329–348, 1983.

Schweitzer G: Open reduction and internal fixation of vertical shear pelvic fractures (letter). *J Trauma* 27:1308, 1987.

Shuler TE, Boone DC, Gruen GS, Peitzman AB: Percutaneous iliosacral screw fixation: Early treatment for unstable posterior pelvic ring disruptions. *J Trauma* 38:453–458, 1995.

Siemssen SJ, Frandsen PA: Double vertical fractures of the pelvis treated by external fixation. *Ugeskr Laeger* 143:1094–1096, 1981.

Simonian PT, Routt ML Jr, Harrington RM, Tencer AF: Internal fixation for the transforaminal sacral fracture. *Clin Orthop* 202–209, 1996.

Simonian PT, Routt ML Jr, Harrington RM, Tencer AF: Internal fixation of the unstable anterior pelvic ring: A biomechanical comparison of standard plating techniques and the retrograde medullary superior pubic ramus screw. *J Orthop Trauma* 8:476–482, 1994.

Slatis P, Eskola A: External fixation of the pelvic girdle as a test for assessing instability of the sacro-iliac joint. *Ann Med* 21:369–372, 1989.

Slatis P, Karaharju EO: External fixation of the pelvic girdle with a trapezoid compression frame. *Injury* 7:53–56, 1975.

Slatis P, Karaharju EO: External fixation of unstable pelvic fractures: Experiences in 22 patients treated with a trapezoid compression frame. *Clin Orthop* 73–80, 1980.

Stocks GW, Gabel GT, Noble PC, et al: Anterior and posterior internal fixation of vertical shear fractures of the pelvis. *J Orthop Res* 9:237–245, 1991.

Stuart PR, Talbot D, Milne DD: Internal fixation of pubic symphysis diastasis with a tension banding technique. *Injury* 21:223–224, 1990.

Trafton PG: Pelvic ring injuries. *Surg Clin North Am* 70:655–669, 1990.

Vander Borght P, Verdonk R, Verstraeten F, Claessens H: Internal fixation of pathologic fractures: A retrospective study. *Acta Orthop Belg* 1:38–41, 1993.

Varga E, Hearn T, Powell J, Tile M: Effects of method of internal fixation of symphyseal disruptions on stability of the pelvic ring. *Injury* 26:75–80, 1975.

Vecsei V: Results of biomechanical studies of various external fixation devices of the pelvis. *Aktuelle Traumatol* 18:261–264, 1988.

Ward EF, Tomasin J, Vander Griend RA: Open reduction and internal fixation of vertical shear pelvic fractures. *J Trauma* 27:291–195, 1987.

Webb LX, Gristina AG, Wilson JR, et al: Two-hole plate fixation for traumatic symphysis pubis diastasis. *J Trauma* 28:813–817, 1988.

Wild JJ, Hanson GW, Tullos HS: Unstable fractures of the pelvis treated by external fixation. *J Bone Joint Surg Am* 64:1010–1020, 1982.

Williams RP, Friis EA, Cooke FW, et al: External fixation of unstable Malgaigne fractures: The comparative mechanical performance of a new configuration. *Orthop Rev* 21:1423–1430, 1992.

Angiography

Barlow B, Rottenberg RW, Santulli TV: Angiographic diagnosis and treatment of bleeding by selective embolization following pelvic fracture in children. *J Pediatr Surg* 10:939–942, 1975.

Baumgartner F, White GH, White RA, et al: Controversies in the management of retroperitoneal hemorrhage associated with pelvic fractures. *J Natl Med Assoc* 87:33–38, 1995.

Ben-Menachem Y: Pelvic fractures: Diagnostic therapeutic angiography. *Instr Course Lect* 37:139–141, 1988.

Brown JJ, Greene FL, McMillin RD: Vascular injuries associated with pelvic fractures. *Am Surg* 50:150–154, 1984.

Flint L, Babikian G, Anders M, et al: Definitive control of mortality from severe pelvic fracture. *Ann Surg* 211:703–706; discussion 706–707, 1990.

Gilliland MG, Ward RE, Flynn TC, et al: Peritoneal lavage and angiography in the management of patients with pelvic fractures. *Am J Surg* 144:744–747, 1982.

Gordon RL, Fast A, Aner H, et al: Control of massive retroperitoneal bleeding associated with pelvic fractures by angiographic embolization. *Isr J Med Sci* 19:185–188, 1983.

Haag C, Wagner G, Blum U: Angiography detection and embolization of a hemodynamically significant hemorrhage from the right dorsal penile artery in symphysis rupture. *Unfallchirurgie* 20:169–173, 1994.

Kadish LJ, Stein JM, Kotler S, et al: Angiographic diagnosis and treatment of bleeding due to pelvic trauma. *J Trauma* 13:1083–1085, 1973.

Kerr WS Jr, Margolies MN, Ring EJ, et al: Arteriography in pelvic fractures with massive hemorrhage. *Trans Am Assoc Genitourin Surg* 64:14–17, 1972.

Klein SR, Saroyan RM, Baumgartner F, Bongard FS: Management strategy of vascular injuries associated with pelvic fractures. *J Cardiovasc Surg (Torino)* 33:349–357, 1992.

Margolies MN, Ring EJ, Waltman AC, et al: Arteriography in the management of hemorrhage from pelvic fractures. *N Engl J Med* 287:317–321, 1972.

Marsman JW, Schilstra SH, van Leeuwen H: Angiography and embolization of the corona mortis (aberrant obturator artery): A source of persistent pelvic bleeding. *ROFO Fortschr Geb Rontgenstr Nuklearmed* 141:708–710, 1984.

Matalon TS, Athanasoulis CA, Margolies MN, et al: Hemorrhage with pelvic fractures: Efficacy of transcatheter embolization. *AJR* 133:859–864, 1979.

Maull KI, Sachatello CR: Current management of pelvic fractures: A combined surgical-angiographic approach to hemorrhage. *South Med J* 69:1285–1289, 1976.

McIntyre RC Jr, Bensard DD, Moore EE, et al: Pelvic fracture geometry predicts risk of life-threatening hemorrhage in children. *J Trauma* 35:423–429, 1993.

Moreno C, Moore EE, Rosenberger A, Cleveland HC: Hemorrhage associated with major pelvic fracture: A multispecialty challenge. *J Trauma* 26:987–994, 1986.

Perlberger RR: Arteriographic localization and treatment of hemorrhage in pelvic fractures. *Ned Tijdschr Geneeskd* 121:9–11, 1977.

Ring EJ, Athanasoulis C, Waltman AC, et al: Arteriographic management of hemorrhage following pelvic fracture. *Radiology* 109:65–70, 1973.

Sundaram M, Patel B, Wolverson MK, Riaz MA: Superior gluteal artery haemorrhage following pelvic features controlled by embolisation. *Clin Radiol* 32:187–190, 1981.

van Urk H, Perlberger RR, Muller H: Selective arterial embolization for control of traumatic pelvic hemorrhage. *Surgery* 83:133–137, 1978.

Wholey MH, Bocher J: Angiography in musculoskeletal trauma. *Surg Gynecol Obstet* 125:730–736, 1967.

Hemorrhage

Agnew SG: Hemodynamically unstable pelvic fractures. *Orthop Clin North Am* 25:715–721, 1994.

Barlow B, Rottenberg RW, Santulli TV: Angiographic diagnosis and treatment of bleeding by selective embolization following pelvic fracture in children. *J Pediatr Surg* 10:939–942, 1975.

Baumgartner F, White GH, White RA, et al: Controversies in the management of retroperitoneal hemorrhage associated with pelvic fractures. *J Natl Med Assoc* 87:33–38, 1995.

Ben-Menachem Y: Pelvic fractures: Diagnostic and therapeutic angiography. *Instr Course Lect* 37:139–141, 1988.

Bosch U, Pohlemann T, Tscherne H: Primary management of pelvic injuries. *Orthopade* 21:385–392, 1992.

Brown JJ, Greene FL, McMillin RD: Vascular injuries associated with pelvic fractures. *Am Surg* 50:150–154, 1984.

Evers BM, Cryer HM, Miller FB: Pelvic fracture hemorrhage: Priorities in management. *Arch Surg* 124:422–424, 1989.

Flint L, Babikian G, Anders M, et al: Definitive control of mortality from severe pelvic fracture. *Ann Surg* 211:703–706; discussion 706–707, 1990.

Flint LM Jr, Brown A, Richardson JD, Polk HC: Definitive control of bleeding from severe pelvic fractures. *Ann Surg* 189:709–716, 1979.

Ganz R, Krushell RJ, Jakob RP, Kuffer J: The antishock pelvic clamp. *Clin Orthop* 71–78, 1991.

Ghanayem AJ, Stover MD, Goldstein JA, et al: Emergent treatment of pelvic fractures: Comparison of methods for stabilization. *Clin Orthop* 75–80, 1995.

Gilliland MG, Ward RE, Flynn TC, et al: Peritoneal lavage and angiography in the management of patients with pelvic fractures. *Am J Surg* 144:744–747, 1982.

Gordon RL, Fast A, Aner H, et al: Control of massive retroperitoneal bleeding associated with pelvic fractures by angiographic embolization. *Isr J Med Sci* 19:185–188, 1983.

Gruen GS, Leit ME, Gruen RJ, Peitzman AB: The acute management of hemodynamically unstable multiple trauma patients with pelvic ring fractures. *J Trauma* 36:706–711; discussion 711–713, 1994.

Haag C, Wagner G, Blum U: Angiography detection and embolization of a hemodynamically significant hemorrhage from the right dorsal penile artery in symphysis rupture. *Unfallchirurgie* 20:169–173, 1994.

Kadish LJ, Stein JM, Kotler S, et al: Angiographic diagnosis and treatment of bleeding due to pelvic trauma. *J Trauma* 13:1083–1085, 1973.

Kerr WS Jr, Margolies MN, Ring EJ, et al: Arteriography in pelvic fractures with massive hemorrhage. *Trans Am Assoc Genitourin Surg* 64:14–17, 1972.

Klein SR, Saroyan RM, Baumgartner F, Bongard FS: Management strategy of vascular injuries associated with pelvic fractures. *J Cardiovasc Surg (Torino)* 33:349–357, 1992.

Margolies MN, Ring EJ, Waltman AC, et al: Arteriography in the management of hemorrhage from pelvic fractures. *N Engl J Med* 287:317–321, 1972.

Marsman JW, Schilstra SH, van Leeuwen H: Angiography and embolization of the corona mortis (aberrant obturator artery): A source of persistent pelvic bleeding. *ROFO Fortschr Geb Rontgenstr Nuklearmed* 141:708–710, 1984.

Matalon TS, Athanasoulis CA, Margolies MN, et al: Hemorrhage with pelvic fractures: efficacy of transcatheter embolization. *AJR* 133:859–864, 1979.

Maull KI, Sachatello CR: Current management of pelvic fractures: A combined surgical-angiographic approach to hemorrhage. *South Med J* 69:1285–1289, 1976.

McIntyre RC Jr, Bensard DD, Moore EE, et al: Pelvic fracture geometry predicts risk of life-threatening hemorrhage in children. *J Trauma* 35:423–429, 1993.

Moreno C, Moore EE, Rosenberger A, Cleveland HC: Hemorrhage associated with major pelvic fracture: A multispecialty challenge. *J Trauma* 26:987–994, 1986.

Mucha P Jr, Farnell MB: Analysis of pelvic fracture management. *J Trauma* 24:379–386, 1984.

Perlberger RR: Arteriographic localization and treatment of hemorrhage in pelvic fractures. *Ned Tijdschr Geneeskd* 121:9–11, 1977.

Riemer BL, Butterfield SL, Diamond DL, et al: Acute mortality associated with injuries to the pelvic ring: The role of early patient mobilization and external fixation. *J Trauma* 35:671–675; discussion 676–677, 1993.

Ring EJ, Athanasoulis C, Waltman AC, et al: Arteriographic management of hemorrhage following pelvic fracture. *Radiology* 109:65–70, 1973.

Sundaram M, Patel B, Wolverson MK, Riaz MA: Superior gluteal artery haemorrhage following pelvic features controlled by embolisation. *Clin Radiol* 32:187–190, 1981.

van Urk H, Perlberger RR, Muller H: Selective arterial embolization for control of traumatic pelvic hemorrhage. *Surgery* 83:133–137, 1978.

Wholey MH, Bocher J: Angiography in musculoskeletal trauma. *Surg Gynecol Obstet* 125:730–736, 1967.

Genitourinary Complications

Agnew SG: Hemodynamically unstable pelvic fractures. *Orthop Clin North Am* 25:715–721, 1994.

Barlow B, Rottenberg RW, Santulli TV: Angiographic diagnosis and treatment of bleeding by selective embolization following pelvic fracture in children. *J Pediatr Surg* 10:939–942, 1975.

Baumgartner F, White GH, White RA, et al: Controversies in the management of retroperitoneal hemorrhage associated with pelvic fractures. *J Natl Med Assoc* 87:33–38, 1995.

Ben-Menachem Y: Pelvic fractures: Diagnostic and therapeutic angiography. *Instr Course Lect* 37:139–141, 1988.

Boone TB, Wilson WT, Husmann DA: Postpubertal genitourinary function following posterior urethral disruptions in children. *J Urol* 148:1232–1234, 1992.

Bosch U, Pohlemann T, Tscherne H: Primary management of pelvic injuries. *Orthopade* 21:385–392, 1992.

Brown JJ, Greene FL, McMillin RD: Vascular injuries associated with pelvic fractures. *Am Surg* 50:150–154, 1984.

Evers BM, Cryer HM, Miller FB: Pelvic fracture hemorrhage: Priorities in management. *Arch Surg* 124:442–424, 1989.

Flint L, Babikian G, Anders M, et al: Definitive control of mortality from severe pelvic fracture. *Ann Surg* 211:703–706; discussion 706–707, 1990.

Flint LM Jr, Brown A, Richardson JD, Polk HC: Definitive control of bleeding from severe pelvic fractures. *Ann Surg* 189:709–716, 1979.

Ganz R, Krushell RJ, Jakob RP, Kuffer J: The antishock pelvic clamp. *Clin Orthop* 71–78, 1991.

Ghanayem AJ, Stover MD, Goldstein JA, et al: Emergent treatment of pelvic fractures: Comparison of methods for stabilization. *Clin Orthop* 75–80, 1995.

Gilliland MG, Ward RE, Flynn TC, et al: Peritoneal lavage and angiography in the management of patients with pelvic fractures. *Am J Surg* 144:744–747, 1982.

Gordon RL, Fast A, Aner H, Floman Y: Control of massive retroperitoneal bleeding associated with pelvic fractures by angiographic embolization. *Isr J Med Sci* 19:185–188, 1983.

Gruen GS, Leit ME, Gruen RJ, Peitzman AB: The acute management of hemodynamically unstable multiple trauma patients with pelvic ring fractures. *J Trauma* 36:706–711; discussion 711–713, 1994.

Haag C, Wagner G, Blum U: Angiography detection and embolization of a hemodynamically significant hemorrhage from the right dorsal penile artery in symphysis rupture. *Unfallchirurgie* 20:169–173, 1994.

Kadish LJ, Stein JM, Kotler S, et al: Angiographic diagnosis and treatment of bleeding due to pelvic trauma. *J Trauma* 13:1083–1085, 1973.

Kerr WS Jr, Margolies MN, Ring EJ, et al: Arteriography in pelvic fractures with massive hemorrhage. *Trans Am Assoc Genitourin Surg* 64:14–17, 1972.

Klein SR, Saroyan RM, Baumgartner F, Bongard FS: Management strategy of vascular injuries associated with pelvic fractures. *J Cardiovasc Surg (Torino)* 33:349–357, 1992.

Livne PM, Gonzales ET Jr: Genitourinary trauma in children. *Urol Clin North Am* 12:53–65, 1985.

Lowenstein SR, Yaron M, Carrero R, et al: Vertical trauma: Injuries to patients who fall and land on their feet. *Ann Emerg Med* 18:161–165, 1989.

Margolies MN, Ring EJ, Waltman AC, et al: Arteriography in the management of hemorrhage from pelvic fractures. *N Engl J Med* 287:317–321, 1972.

Marshman JW, Schilstra SH, van Leeuwen H: Angiography and embolization of the corona mortis (aberrant obturator artery): A source of persistent pelvic bleeding. *ROFO Fortschr Geb Rontgenstr Nuklearmed* 141:708–710, 1984.

Matalon TS, Athanasoulis CA, Margolies MN, et al: Hemorrhage with pelvic fractures: Efficacy of transcatheter embolization. *AJR* 133:859–864, 1979.

Maull KI, Rozycki GS, Vinsant GO, Pedigo RE: Retroperitoneal injuries: Pitfalls in diagnosis and management. *South Med J* 80:1111–1115, 1987.

Maull KI, Sachatello CR: Current management of pelvic fractures: A combined surgical-angiographic approach to hemorrhage. *South Med J* 69:1285–1289, 1976.

McIntyre RC Jr, Bensard DD, Moore EE, et al: Pelvic fracture geometry predicts risk of life-threatening hemorrhage in children. *J Trauma* 35:423–429, 1993.

Meyer PS: Urologic complications associated with pelvic fractures. *Orthop Nurs* 8:41–44, 68, 1989.

Moreno C, Moore EE, Rosenberger A, Cleveland HC: Hemorrhage associated with major pelvic fracture: A multispecialty challenge. *J Trauma* 26:987–994, 1986.

Mucha P Jr, Farnell MB: Analysis of pelvic fracture management. *J Trauma* 24:379–386, 1984.

Patil U, Nesbitt R, Meyer R: Genitourinary tract injuries due to fracture of the pelvis in females: Sequelae and their management. *Br J Urol* 54:32–38, 1982.

Patterson BM: Pelvic ring injury and associated urologic trauma: An orthopaedic perspective. *Semin Urol* 13:25–33, 1995.

Perlberger RR: Arteriographic localization and treatment of hemorrhage in pelvic fractures. *Ned Tijdschr Geneeskd* 121:9–11, 1977.

Richardson JD, Harty J, Amin M, Flint LM: Open pelvic fractures. *J Trauma* 22:533–538, 1982.

Riemer BL, Butterfield SL, Diamond DL, et al: Acute mortality associated with injuries to the pelvic ring: The role of early patient mobilization and external fixation. *J Trauma* 35:671–675; discussion 676–677, 1993.

Rieser C: Diagnostic evaluation of suspected genitourinary tract injury. *JAMA* 199:714–719, 1967.

Ring EJ, Athanasoulis C, Waltman AC, et al: Arteriographic management of hemorrhage following pelvic fracture. *Radiology* 109:65–70, 1973.

Sclafani SJ, Becker JA, Shaftan GW, et al: Strategies for the radiologic management of genitourinary trauma. *Urol Radiol* 7:231–244, 1985.

Sundaram M, Patel B, Wolverson MK, Riaz MA: Superior gluteal artery haemorrhage following pelvic features controlled by embolisation. *Clin Radiol* 32:187–190, 1981.

Uehara DT, Eisner RF: Indications for retrograde cystourethrography in trauma. *Ann Emerg Med* 15:270–272, 1986.

van Urk H, Perlberger RR, Muller H: Selective arterial embolization for control of traumatic pelvic hemorrhage. *Surgery* 83:133–137, 1978.

Weems WL: Management of genitourinary injuries in patients with pelvic fractures. *Ann Surg* 189:717–723, 1979.

Wholey MH, Bocher J: Angiography in musculoskeletal trauma. *Surg Gynecol Obstet* 125:730–736, 1967.

Open Fractures

Costa P, Giancecchi F, Tartaglia I, Fontanesi G: Immediate multiple osteosynthesis in polytrauma. *Ital J Orthop Traumatol* 17:187–198, 1991.

Hanson PB, Milne JC, Chapman MW: Open fractures of the pelvis: Review of 43 cases. *J Bone Joint Surg Br* 73:325–329, 1991.

Niemi TA, Norton LW: Vaginal injuries in patients with pelvic fractures. *J Trauma* 25:547–551, 1985.

Perry JF Jr: Pelvic open fractures. *Clin Orthop* 41–45, 1980.

Reff RB: The use of external fixation devices in the management of severe lower-extremity trauma and pelvic injuries in children. *Clin Orthop* 21–33, 1984.

Rothenberger D, Velasco R, Strate R, et al: Open pelvic fractures: A lethal injury. *J Trauma* 18:184–187, 1978.

Schmit-Neuerburg KP, Joka T: Principles of treatment and indications for surgery in severe multiple trauma. *Acta Chir Belg* 85:239–249, 1985.

van Veen IH, van Leeuwen AA, van Popta T, et al: Unstable pelvic fractures: A retrospective analysis. *Injury* 26:81–85, 1995.

Neurologic Complications

Conway RR, Hubbell SL: Electromyographic abnormalities in neurologic injury associated with pelvic fracture: Case reports and literature review. *Arch Phys Med Rehabil* 69:539–541, 1988.

Costa P, Giancecchi F, Tartaglia I, Fontanesi G: Immediate multiple osteosynthesis in polytrauma. *Ital J Orthop Traumatol* 17:187–198, 1991.

Denis F, Davis S, Comfort T: Sacral fractures: An important problem. Retrospective analysis of 236 cases. *Clin Orthop* 227:67–81, 1988.

Ebraheim NA, Coombs R, Jackson WT, Rusin JJ: Percutaneous computed tomography-guided stabilization of posterior pelvic fractures. *Clin Orthop* 222–228, 1994.

Ellison M, Timberlake GA, Kerstein MD: Impotence following pelvic fracture. *J Trauma* 28:695–696, 1988.

Fisher RG: Sacral fracture with compression of cauda equina: Surgical treatment. *J Trauma* 28:1678–1680, 1988.

Gibbons KJ, Soloniuk DS, Razack N: Neurological injury and patterns of sacral fractures. *J Neurosurg* 72:889–893, 1990.

Goodell CL: Neurological deficits associated with pelvic fractures. *J Neurosurg* 24:837–842, 1966.

Hanson PB, Milne JC, Chapman MW: Open fractures of the pelvis: Review of 43 cases. *J Bone Joint Surg Br* 73:325–329, 1991.

Helfet DL, Koval KJ, Hissa EA, et al: Intraoperative somatosensory evoked potential monitoring during acute pelvic fracture surgery. *J Orthop Trauma* 9:28–34, 1995.

Henderson RC: The long-term results of nonoperatively treated major pelvic disruptions. *J Orthop Trauma* 3:41–47, 1989.

Hersche O, Isler B, Aebi M: Follow-up and prognosis of neurologic sequelae of pelvic ring fractures with involvement of the sacrum and/or the iliosacral joint. *Unfallchirurgie* 96:311–318, 1993.

Majeed SA: Neurologic deficits in major pelvic injuries. *Clin Orthop* 222–228, 1992.

Montesano PX, Jacobs RR: Irreducible sacroiliac dislocation of the pelvic ring with caudal displacement: A case report. *Clin Orthop* 216–218, 1988.

Niemi TA, Norton LW: Vaginal injuries in patients with pelvic fractures. *J Trauma* 25:547–551, 1985.

Patterson FP, Morton KS: Neurological complications of fractures and dislocations of the pelvis. *J Trauma* 12:1013–1023, 1972.

Perry JF Jr: Pelvic open fractures. *Clin Orthop* 41–45, 1980.

Pohlemann T, Gansslen A, Tscherne H: The problem of the sacrum fracture: Clinical analysis of 377 cases. *Orthopade* 21:400–412, 1992.

Rai SK, Far RF, Ghovanlou B: Neurologic deficits associated with sacral wing fractures. *Orthopedics* 13:1363–1366, 1990.

Reff RB: The use of external fixation devices in the management of severe lower-extremity trauma and pelvic injuries in children. *Clin Orthop* 21–33, 1984.

Rothenberger D, Velasco R, Strate R, et al: Open pelvic fracture: a lethal injury. *J Trauma* 18:184–187, 1978.

Schmit-Neuerburg KP, Joka T: Principles of treatment and indications for surgery in severe multiple trauma. *Acta Chir Belg* 85:239–249, 1985.

van Veen IH, van Leeuwen AA, van Popta T, et al: Unstable pelvic fractures: A retrospective analysis. *Injury* 26:81–85, 1995.

Vrahas M, Gordon RG, Mears DC, et al: Intraoperative somatosensory evoked potential monitoring of pelvic and acetabular fractures. *J Orthop Trauma* 6:50–58, 1992.

Mortality

Flint L, Babikian G, Anders M, et al: Definitive control of mortality from severe pelvic fracture. *Ann Surg* 211:703–706; discussion 706–707, 1990.

Gilliland MD, Ward RE, Barton RM, et al: Factors affecting mortality in pelvic fractures. *J Trauma* 22:691–693, 1982.

Gruen GS, Leit ME, Gruen RJ, Peitzman AB: The acute management of hemodynamically unstable multiple trauma patients with pelvic ring fractures. *J Trauma* 36:706–711; discussion 711–713, 1994.

Hesp WL, van der Werken C, Keunen RW, Goris RJ: Unstable fractures and dislocations of the pelvic ring—Results of treatment in relation to the severity of injury. *Neth J Surg* 37:148–152, 1985.

Hossack DW: The pattern of injuries in 470 pedestrians killed in road accidents. *Med J Aust* 1:678–679, 1975.

Lipkowitz G, Phillips T, Coren C, et al: Hemipelvectomy, a lifesaving operation in severe open pelvic injury in childhood. *J Trauma* 25:823–827, 1985.

McAvoy JM, Cook JH: A treatment plan for rapid assessment of the patient with massive blood loss and pelvic fractures. *Arch Surg* 113:986–990, 1978.

McIntyre RC Jr, Bensard DD, Moore EE, et al: Pelvic fracture geometry predicts risk of life-threatening hemorrhage in children. *J Trauma* 35:423–429, 1993.

Patterson FP, Morton KS: The cause of death in fractures of the pelvis: With a note on treatment by ligation of the hypogastric (internal iliac) artery. *J Trauma* 13:849–856, 1973.

Poole GV, Ward EF: Causes of mortality in patients with pelvic fractures. *Orthopedics* 17:691–699, 1994.

Poole GV, Ward EF, Muakkassa FF, Hsu HS, et al: Pelvic fracture from major blunt trauma: Outcome is determined by associated injuries. *Ann Surg* 213:532–538; discussion 538–539, 1991.

Raffa J, Christensen NM: Compound fractures of the pelvis. *Am J Surg* 132:282–286, 1976.

Richardson JD, Harty J, Amin M, Flint LM: Open pelvic fractures. *J Trauma* 22:533–538, 1982.

Riemer BL, Butterfield SL, Diamond DL, et al: Acute mortality associated with injuries to the pelvic ring: The role of early patient mobilization and external fixation. *J Trauma* 35:671–675; discussion 676–677, 1993.

Rossvoll I, Finsen V: Mortality after pelvic fractures in the elderly. *J Orthop Trauma* 3:115–117, 1989.

Rothenberger D, Velasco R, Strate R, et al: Open pelvic fracture: A lethal injury. *J Trauma* 18:184–187, 1978.

Rothenberger DA, Fischer RP, Strate RG, et al: The mortality associated with pelvic fractures. *Surgery* 84:356–361, 1978.

Schmit-Neuerburg KP, Joka T: Principles of treatment and indications for surgery in severe multiple trauma. *Acta Chir Belg* 85:239–249, 1985.

Selivanov V, Chi HS, Alverdy JC, et al: Mortality in retroperitoneal hematoma. *J Trauma* 24:1022–1027, 1984.

Sevitt S: Fatal road accidents. Injuries, complications, and causes of death in 250 subjects. *Br J Surg* 55:481–505, 1968.

Siegel JH, Dalal SA, Burgess AR, Young JW: Pattern of organ injuries in pelvic fracture: Impact force implications for survival and death in motor vehicle injuries. *Accid Anal Prev* 22:457–466, 1990.

Spencer JD, Lalanadham T: The mortality of patients with minor fractures of the pelvis. *Injury* 16:321–322, 1985.

Pulmonary Complications

Atik M, Harkess JW, Wichman H: Prevention of fatal pulmonary embolism. *Surg Gynecol Obstet* 130:403–413, 1970.

Borow M, Goldson H: Postoperative venous thrombosis: Evaluation of five methods of treatment. *Am J Surg* 141:245–251, 1981.

Bosch U, Reisser S, Regel G, et al: Pulmonary fat embolism—An epiphenomenon of shock or a proper mediator mechanism? *Prog Clin Biol Res* 308:37–42, 1989.

Buerger PM, Peoples JB, Lemmon GW, McCarthy MC: Risk of pulmonary emboli in patients with pelvic fractures. *Am Surg* 59:505–508, 1993.

Collins DN, Barnes CL, McCowan TC, et al: Vena caval filter use in orthopaedic trauma patients with recognized preoperative venous thromboembolic disease. *J Orthop Trauma* 6:135–138, 1992.

Fisher CG, Blachut PA, Salvian AJ, et al: Effectiveness of pneumatic leg compression devices for the prevention of thromboembolic disease in orthopaedic trauma patients: A prospective, randomized study of compression alone versus no prophylaxis. *J Orthop Trauma* 9:1–7, 1995.

Knudson MM, Lewis FR, Clinton A, et al: Prevention of venous thromboembolism in trauma patients. *J Trauma* 37:480–487, 1994.

Kozak TK, Diebold R, Beaver RJ: Massive pulmonary thromboembolism after manipulation of an unstable pelvic fracture: A case report and review of the literature. *J Trauma* 38:366–367, 1995.

O'Malley KF, Ross SE: Pulmonary embolism in major trauma patients. *J Trauma* 30:748–750, 1990.

Poole GV, Ward EF, Griswold JA, et al: Complications of pelvic fractures from blunt trauma. *Am Surg* 58:225–231, 1992.

Riseborough EJ, Herndon JH: Alterations in pulmonary function, coagulation and fat metabolism in patients with fractures of the lower limbs. *Clin Orthop* 248–267, 1976.

Rossvoll I, Finsen V: Mortality after pelvic fractures in the elderly. *J Orthop Trauma* 3:115–117, 1989.

Saldeen T: Fat embolism and signs of intravascular coagulation in a posttraumatic autopsy material. *J Trauma* 10:273–286, 1970.

Spencer JD, Lalanadham T: The mortality of patients with minor fractures of the pelvis. *Injury* 16:321–323, 1985.

White RH, Goulet JA, Bray TJ, et al: Deep-vein thrombosis after fracture of the pelvis: Assessment with serial duplex-ultrasound screening. *J Bone Joint Surg Am* 72:495–500, 1990.

Acetabulum
Evaluation

Adam P, Labbe JL, Alberge Y, et al: The role of computed tomography in the assessment and treatment of acetabular fractures. *Clin Radiol* 36:13–18, 1985.

Barnes SN, Stewart MJ: Central fractures of the acetabulum: A critical analysis and review of literature. *Clin Orthop* 276–281, 1976.

Baumgaertel F: Diagnosis, classification and surgical indications in acetabulum fractures. *Orthopade* 21:427–441, 1992.

Fishman EK, Magid D, Drebin RA, et al: Advanced three-dimensional evaluation of acetabular trauma: Volumetric image processing. *J Trauma* 29:214–218, 1989.

Frank CJ, Zacharias J, Garvin KL: Acetabular fractures. *Nebr Med J* 80:118–123, 1995.

Kuhlman JE, Fishman EK, Ney DR, et al: Nonunion of acetabular fractures: Evaluation with interactive multiplanar CT. *J Orthop Trauma* 3:33–40, 1989.

Olson SA, Matta JM: The computerized tomography subchondral arc: A new method of assessing acetabular articular continuity after fracture (a preliminary report). *J Orthop Trauma* 7:402–413, 1993.

Roffi RP, Matta JM: Unrecognized posterior dislocation of the hip associated with transverse and T-type fractures of the acetabulum. *J Orthop Trauma* 7:23–27, 1993.

Rommens P, Wissing H, Serdarevic M: Significance of computerized tomography in the diagnosis and therapy of fractures of the posterior pelvic ring and hip joint. *Unfallchirurgie* 13:32–37, 1987.

Sauser DD, Billimoria PE, Rouse GA, Mudge K: CT evaluation of hip trauma. *AJR* 135:269–274, 1980.

Scott WW Jr, Magid D, Fishman EK, et al: Three-dimensional imaging of acetabular trauma. *J Orthop Trauma* 1:227–232, 1987.

Simonian PT, Routt ML Jr, Harrington RM, Tencer AF: The acetabular T-type fracture: A biomechanical evaluation of internal fixation. *Clin Orthop* 234–240, 1995.

Radiology

Adam P, Labbe JL, Alberge Y, et al: The role of computed tomography in the assessment and treatment of acetabular fractures. *Clin Radiol* 36:13–18, 1985.

Burk DL Jr, Mears DC, Herbert DL, et al: Pelvic and acetabular fractures: Examination by angled CT scanning. *Radiology* 153:548, 1984.

Saks BJ: Normal acetabular anatomy for acetabular fracture assessment: CT and plain film correlation. *Radiology* 159:139–145, 1986.

White MS: Three-dimensional computed tomography in the assessment of fractures of the acetabulum. *Injury* 22:13–19, 1991.

Classification

Adam P, Labbe JL, Alberge Y, et al: The role of computed tomography in the assessment and treatment of acetabular fractures. *Clin Radiol* 36:13–18, 1985.

Baumgaertel F: Diagnosis, classification and surgical indications in acetabulum fractures. *Orthopade* 21:427–441, 1992.

Gill K, Bucholz RW: The role of computerized tomographic scanning in the evaluation of major pelvic fractures. *J Bone Joint Surg Am* 66:34–39, 1984.

Nikodinovski J, Gruev V, Trajkovski L, et al: Therapeutic dilemmas in the care of acetabular fractures. *Acta Chir Iugosl* 2: 203–210, 1982.

Pohlemann T, Gansslen A, Kiessling B, et al: Determining indications and osteosynthesis techniques for the pelvic girdle. *Unfallchirurgie* 95:197–209, 1992.

Saks BJ: Normal acetabular anatomy for acetabular fracture assessment: CT and plain film correlation. *Radiology* 159: 139–145, 1986.

Saterbak AM, Marsh JL, Turbett T, Brandser E: Acetabular fractures classification of Letournel and Judet—A systematic approach. *Iowa Orthop J* 15:184–196, 1995.

Treatment

Baumgaertel F: Diagnosis, classification and surgical indications in acetabulum fractures. *Orthopade* 21:427–441, 1992.

Cole JD, Bolhofner BR: Acetabular fracture fixation via a modified stoppa limited intrapelvic approach: Description of operative technique and preliminary treatment results. *Clin Orthop* 112–123, 1994.

de Ridder VA, de Lange S, Kingma L, Hogervorst M: Results of 75 consecutive patients with an acetabular fracture. *Clin Orthop* 53–57, 1994.

Duquennoy A, Tillie B, Fontaine C, et al: Acetabular fractures and sacroiliac dislocations. *Rev Chir Orthop* 71:311–318, 1985.

Frank CJ, Zacharias J, Garvin KL: Acetabular fractures. *Nebr Med J* 80:118–123, 1995.

Ghalambor N, Matta JM, Bernstein L: Heterotopic ossification following operative treatment of acetabular fracture: An analysis of risk factors. *Clin Orthop* 96–105, 1994.

Leenen LP, van der Werken C, Schoots F, Goris RJ: Internal fixation of open unstable pelvic fractures. *J Trauma* 35:220–225, 1993.

Letournel E: The treatment of acetabular fractures through the ilioinguinal approach. *Clin Orthop* 62–76, 1993.

Matta JM, Anderson LM, Epstein HC, Hendricks P: Fractures of the acetabulum. A retrospective analysis. *Clin Orthop* 230–240, 1986.

Nikodinovski J, Gruev V, Trajkovski L, et al: Therapeutic dilemmas in the care of acetabular fractures. *Acta Chir Iugosl* 2: 203–210, 1982.

Nutz V: Therapeutic problems of acetabulum fracture in polytrauma. *Langenbecks Arch Chir* 370:129–139, 1987.

Pals SD, Brown CW, Friermood TG: Open reduction and internal fixation of an acetabular fracture during pregnancy. *J Orthop Trauma* 6:379–381, 1992.

Pennal GF, Davidson J, Garside H, Plewes J: Results of treatment of acetabular fractures. *Clin Orthop* 115–123, 1980.

Routt ML Jr, Swiontkowski MF: Operative treatment of complex acetabular fractures: Combined anterior and posterior exposures during the same procedure. *J Bone Joint Surg Am* 72: 897–904, 1990.

Ruesch PD, Holdener H, Ciaramitaro M, Mast JW: A prospective study of surgically treated acetabular fractures. *Clin Orthop* 38–46, 1994.

Ruggieri F, Zinghi GF, Specchia L, et al: The treatment of fractures of the acetabulum involving both anterior and posterior columns. *Ital J Orthop Traumatol* 13:27–36, 1987.

Sakaguchi R, Ito T: Surgical treatment of fractures of the acetabulum. *Shujutsu* 23:963–969, 1969.

Tile M, Pennal GF: Pelvic disruption: Principles of management. *Clin Orthop* 56–64, 1980.

Complications

Cooke CPD, Levinsohn EM, Baker BE: Septic hip in pelvic fractures with urologic injury: A case report, review of the literature and discussion of the pathophysiology. *Clin Orthop* 253–257, 1980.

Ebraheim NA, Savolaine ER, Hoeflinger MJ, Jackson WT: Radiological diagnosis of screw penetration of the hip joint in acetabular fracture reconstruction. *J Orthop Trauma* 3: 196–201, 1989.

Frank CJ, Zacharias J, Garvin KL: Acetabular fractures. *Nebr Med J* 80:118–123, 1995.

Frank JL, Reimer BL, Raves JJ: Traumatic iliofemoral arterial injury: An association with high anterior acetabular fractures. *J Vasc Surg* 10:198–201, 1989.

Heppert V, Holz F, Winkler H, Wentzensen A: Necrosis of the rectus abdominis muscle: Complication after ilioinguinal approach. *Unfallchirurgie* 98:98–101, 1995.

Poigenfurst J, Ender HG, Zadra A: Complications in surgical management of pelvic fractures. *Unfallchirurgie* 95:210–213, 1992.

Roffi RP, Matta JM: Unrecognized posterior dislocation of the hip associated with transverse and T-type fractures of the acetabulum. *J Orthop Trauma* 7:23–27, 1993.

Stiehl JB, Harlow M, Hackbarth D: Extensile triradiate approach for complex acetabular reconstruction in total hip arthroplasty. *Clin Orthop* 162–169, 1993.

Vrahas M, Gordon RG, Mears DC, et al: Intraoperative somatosensory evoked potential monitoring of pelvic and acetabular fractures. *J Orthop Trauma* 6:50–58, 1992.

CHAPTER 26

Hip Fractures
and Dislocations

Kenneth J. Koval, Kenneth A. Egol,
and Joseph D. Zuckerman

HIP DISLOCATIONS

Hip dislocations result from high-energy trauma.[1] Severe associated injuries commonly occur and include craniofacial, chest, abdominal, and other musculoskeletal trauma.[1] One must obtain radiographs of the pelvis and entire femur to identify the most commonly associated musculoskeletal injuries. Hip dislocations can be divided into anterior and posterior types; each is discussed separately. Treatment principles for patients with a hip dislocation include (1) careful evaluation to detect associated injuries; (2) immediate gentle closed or, if necessary, open reduction followed by an assessment of hip stability; and (3) careful radiographic evaluation to assess congruency of reduction and associated femoral head or acetabular fracture.

If a concentric, stable reduction can be obtained, the patient is mobilized with protected weight bearing for 4 to 6 weeks. If the reduction is concentric but unstable, without an associated fracture, the extremity is placed in traction for 4 to 6 weeks to allow soft tissue healing. A nonconcentric reduction, as a result of either intraarticular osteochondral fragments, soft tissue interposition, or fracture malreduction, requires open reduction and joint exploration. Associated femoral head or acetabular fracture treatment is dependent upon the size and location of the fracture and joint stability.

Femoral artery and nerve injuries are rare and usually result from an anterior dislocation. Sciatic nerve injury is present in approximately 10 percent of posterior dislocations.[2,3] Osteonecrosis can present up to 5 years after injury; its risk increases with a time delay (more than 6 to 12 h) in reduction.[2,4] It has been reported that simple dislocations have an excellent long-term prognosis if reduced within 6 h of injury.[5] One study, however, documented poor long-term clinical outcome, particularly after posterior dislocation, in a series of hip dislocations without fracture followed for more than 2 years.[6]

Anterior Dislocations

Anterior hip dislocations represent approximately 10 to 18 percent of all hip dislocations and can be classified as either superior or inferior.[5,7–10] Anterior hip dislocations result from abduction and external rotation; superior dislocations occur in extension and the far more common inferior dislocations in flexion.[9] Closed reduction is performed by applying traction in line with the extremity, followed by extension and internal rotation.

An associated femoral head fracture occurs in 22 to 77 of anterior hip dislocations and is classified as either a transchondral or indentation fracture.[7,11] Transchondral fractures that result in nonconcentric reduction require open reduction and either internal fixation or excision, depending on the fragment's size and location.[12] Indentation fractures are usually located on the superior femoral head and require no specific treatment; however, fracture location has significant prognostic implications.[7]

Some 10 percent of anterior dislocations develop osteonecrosis.[2,4,12] Risk factors for osteonecrosis include a time delay in reduction and repeated reduction attempts[13]; risk factors for posttraumatic degenerative arthritis include indentation fracture greater than 4 mm in depth, transchondral fracture, and osteonecrosis.[7,15,16]

Posterior Dislocations

Posterior hip dislocations account for approximately 90 percent of all hip dislocations[2,8] and are classified by Epstein (Table 26-1) based upon the presence or absence of associated acetabular and/or femoral head fracture.[17] Posterior hip dislocations result from an axial force applied to the flexed knee.[2,8,17] If the hip is in a neutral or adducted position, a simple dislocation occurs; if the hip is abducted, there will be a posterior acetabular fracture-dislocation. Closed reduction is performed by applying traction to the adducted and flexed hip. Postreduction radiographs should be evaluated carefully for concentricity of reduction, intraarticular fragments, and associated fractures. Computed tomography (CT) scan is indicated if there is any question concerning the concentricity of reduction on plain radiographs. If closed reduction under general anesthesia is unsuccessful or nonconcentric, an open reduction is required.

Hip stability should be assessed following either closed or open reduction. Computed tomography can be used to help determine stability after reduction of posterior wall fracture-dislocations.[18,19] Stability is inversely related to the size of the posterior acetabular fragment.[18,19]

An acetabular depression fracture is an impacted fragment of the posteromedial acetabulum resulting from a posterior fracture dislocation (Fig. 26-1).[20] This fracture, with a reported 23 percent incidence upon CT evaluation, should be elevated and bone-grafted.[20]

Osteonecrosis of the femoral head is rare (10 percent) after simple posterior dislocation but occurs in over 50 percent of fracture-dislocations.[5,21] The risk of osteonecrosis is related to the severity of the injury, time delay (more than 6 to 12 h) in reduction, and repeated closed reduction attempts.[4,5,22]

Posterior Dislocations
with Femoral Head Fracture

Approximately 10 percent of posterior dislocations have an associated fracture of the femoral head or neck.[23] Pipkin

TABLE 26-1 Thompson-Epstein Classification of Posterior Hip Dislocations

Type I	Pure dislocation with at most an insignificant posterior wall fragment
Type II	Dislocation associated with a large posterior wall fragment
Type III	Dislocation with a comminuted posterior wall
Type IV	Dislocation with an associated acetabular fracture
Type V	Dislocation complicated by a femoral head fracture

Source: Reproduced with permission from Epstein HC: Posterior fracture-dislocations of the hip: Long-term follow-up *J Bone Joint Surg* 56A:1103–1127, 1974.

has further classified these into four types (Table 26-2)[24]: type I, fracture of the femoral head caudad to the fovea; type II, fracture of the femoral head cephalad to the fovea; type III, type I or II plus femoral neck fracture; and type IV, type I, II, or III plus fracture of the acetabular rim. A gentle closed reduction should be attempted for Pipkin types I, II, and IV; type III injuries require open reduction.[25] Postreduction radiographs, including CT scanning should be evaluated for concentricity and reduction of the femoral head fragment.

An unsuccessful or nonconcentric closed reduction necessitates an open reduction. Pipkin types I and II fractures should be reduced from an anterior approach and stabilized using recessed cancellous or Herbert screws.[25] Type III fractures in young, active patients should undergo open reduction and internal fixation of the femoral neck, followed by internal fixation of the femoral head.[25] In the elderly, prosthetic replacement is indicated. Treatment of type IV injuries is dependent upon the stability and concentricity of the reduction.[25] If the reduction is unstable or

nonconcentric, open reduction and internal fixation of both the femoral head and posterior acetabular fracture are indicated.

Pipkin fractures are at increased risk for developing osteonecrosis and posttraumatic degenerative arthritis.[26] Pipkin types I and II are reported to have the same prognosis as a simple dislocation. Pipkin type IV injuries have the same prognosis as posterior fracture-dislocations without a femoral head fracture.[5,27] Pipkin type III injuries have a poor prognosis.[25]

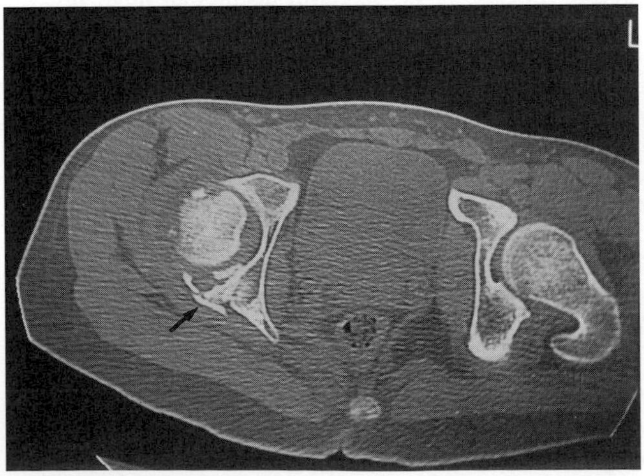

HIP FRACTURES
General Principles

The primary goal of fracture management is to return the patient to his or her prefracture level of function. In most patients with hip fracture, this is best accomplished by operative management, followed by early mobilization.[25] Nonoperative fracture management is appropriate in selected elderly patients who were nonambulators prior to fracture and experience minimal discomfort.[25] These patients require early mobilization to avoid the complications of prolonged bed rest, such as decubiti, urinary tract infections, deep venous thrombosis, and pulmonary complications.[28–31]

Preoperative Assessment—Imaging Studies

The standard radiographic examination of the hip includes an anteroposterior (AP) view of the pelvis and hip and a cross-table lateral. The AP view of the pelvis allows comparison with the contralateral side and may be helpful in identifying nondisplaced and impacted fractures. A cross-table lateral is preferred over the frog lateral because the frog lateral requires abduction, flexion, and external rotation of the affected lower extremity and may result in fracture displacement.[13] An internal rotation view of the hip may be helpful to identify nondisplaced or impacted frac-

Figure 26-1 Fracture-dislocation of the right hip with acetabular depression (*arrow*).

TABLE 26-2   Pipkin Classification of Femoral Head Fracture-Dislocations

Type I	Dislocation with femoral head fracture caudal to the fovea
Type II	Dislocation with femoral head fracture cephalad to the fovea
Type III	Type I or II with associated femoral neck fracture
Type IV	Type I, II, or III with an associated acetabular fracture

Source: Reproduced with permission from Pipkin G: Treatment of grade IV fracture dislocation of the hip. *J Bone Joint Surg* 39A:1027–1042, 1197, 1957.

tures. When a hip fracture is suspected but not apparent on standard radiographs, a technetium bone scan or MRI should be obtained (Fig. 26-2). Although a sensitive indicator of unrecognized hip fractures, a bone scan may require 2 to 3 days to become positive in the elderly patient.[32] Magnetic resonance imaging is as accurate as bone scanning in the assessment of occult fractures of the hip and can be reliably performed within 24 h of injury.[33]

Timing of Surgery

In general, surgery should be performed as soon after injury as possible, after stabilization of all comorbid medical conditions, particularly cardiopulmonary and fluid and electrolyte imbalances.[34,35] In a series of hip fracture patients, Kenzora et al. reported that a surgical delay of less than one week that permitted stabilization of medical problems was not associated with increased mortality.[36]

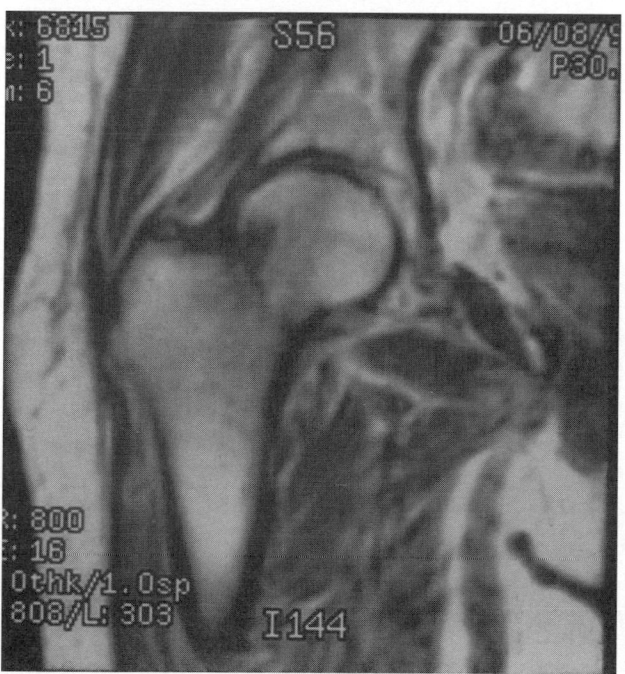

Figure 26-2 Magnetic resonance image of a nondisplaced fracture of the right femoral neck, not visible on plain radiographs.

Interestingly, he found that even healthy patients who underwent surgery within 24 h had a 34 percent mortality at 1 year follow-up, compared to 5.8 percent for those who underwent surgery between the second and fifth days. On the other hand, Sexson and Lehner found that relatively healthy hip fracture patients (up to two comorbid conditions) who had surgery within 24 h after admission had a higher survival rate than those relatively healthy patients who had surgery after 24 h.[31] However, patients with three or more comorbid conditions had a poorer survival rate when operated on within 24 h than those operated upon after 24 h. In a prospective series of 367 elderly hip fracture patients, Zuckerman et al reported that a surgical delay of more than 2 calendar days from hospital admission approximately doubled the risk of the patient dying before the end of the first postoperative year[37]; this relationship was significant when the factors of age, sex, and number of comorbidities were controlled. When these factors were controlled, however, there was also an increase in mortality with surgical delay, although this was not statistically significant.

Considerations of Anesthesia

Although much has been written on the risks and benefits of the different anesthetic techniques, no significant difference in survival rates had been found in elderly hip fracture patients undergoing surgery under regional or general anesthesia.[38] Many anesthesiologists, internists, and surgeons believe that patients "look better" following regional anesthesia. However, studies have documented no difference in postoperative mental status in patients following regional or general anesthesia. Studies have demonstrated the efficacy of regional anesthesia (spinal and epidural) in the prophylaxis of deep vein thrombosis and pulmonary embolus.[39] Since pulmonary embolism is a significant cause of mortality in this population, perhaps regional anesthesia may be preferable, especially if other medical factors compromise utilization of thromboprophylaxis.

Postoperative Mobilization

Postoperative management remains an area of controversy. Some authors have recommended restricted weight bearing until the fracture has healed, while others have shown that unrestricted weight bearing can be started immediately without detrimental effects.[10,40–48] There is little biomechanical justification for restricted weight bearing after hip fracture, since activities such as moving around in bed and use of a bedpan generate forces across the hip approaching those resulting from unsupported ambulation.[49–52] Even foot and ankle range-of-motion exercises performed in bed produce significant loads on the femoral head secondary to muscle contraction. Therefore, attempts at unloading the hip by non-weight-bearing ambulation are not realistic. In addition, geriatric patients have great difficulty ambulating under these conditions. Restricted weight bearing in this patient population will significantly limit their recovery of ambulatory ability. Therefore, it has been our approach to allow weight bearing as tolerated for virtually all geriatric hip fracture patients. Limited weight bearing in younger patients is considered, but at present there are no data to suggest that restricted weight bearing has a beneficial effect on outcome.

FRACTURES OF THE FEMORAL NECK

Anatomy

The femoral neck extends from the distal aspect of the articular surface of the femoral head to the intertrochanteric region. The entire anterior aspect of the femoral neck and the proximal half of its posterior portion are intracapsular. Therefore, femoral neck fractures are considered intracapsular. The blood supply to the femoral head originates from the profunda femoris, which further divides into the medial and lateral femoral circumflex arteries (Fig. 26-3).[53,54] The ascending branch of the lateral femoral circumflex and the medial femoral circumflex make up the extracapsular arterial ring at the base of the femoral neck. This extracapsular ring gives rise to the ascending cervical arteries, which traverse the neck proximally and send small branches into the neck; these anastomose with the

intramedullary nutrient artery of the femur. Once these ascending cervical arteries reach the junction of the head and neck, they form an intracapsular ring. Branches from this ring penetrate the femoral head and provide its primary blood supply. There is also an artery within the ligamentum teres that has only a limited role in adults, providing blood supply to the femoral head.

Mechanism of Injury

Fractures of the femoral neck result from high axial-to-bending load ratios.[49,55] Altered muscle dynamics may increase the risk of hip fracture in the elderly.[55] The energy of a fall, which would be readily dissipated by contracting muscles in younger people, is poorly dissipated by the slower, weaker muscles in the elderly. Muscle contraction in an effort to regain one's balance after slipping may also be sufficiently intense to overload the bone and result in fracture. Falls onto the hip with a direct blow to the greater trochanter may generate an axial force along the neck, creating an impaction fracture.[14] During a severe fall, the lower extremity may rotate externally. At the extremes of external rotation, the femoral neck impinges against the posterior acetabular rim; the associated axial and rotational forces may result in fracture.[56–58]

Classification

The Garden classification of femoral neck fractures is the one most commonly utilized (Fig. 26-4, Table 26-3)[45]; femoral neck fractures are divided into four types, based upon the degree of displacement of the fracture fragments. A type I fracture is an incomplete or valgus impacted fracture. A type II fracture is a complete fracture without displacement of the fracture fragments. A type III fracture is a complete fracture with partial displacement of fracture fragments. A type IV fracture is a complete fracture with total displacement of the fracture fragments, allowing the femoral head to rotate back to an anatomic position. In

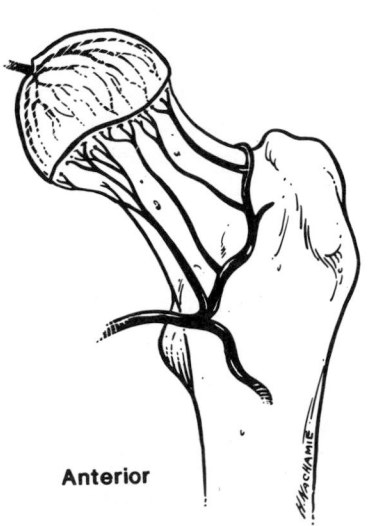

Anterior

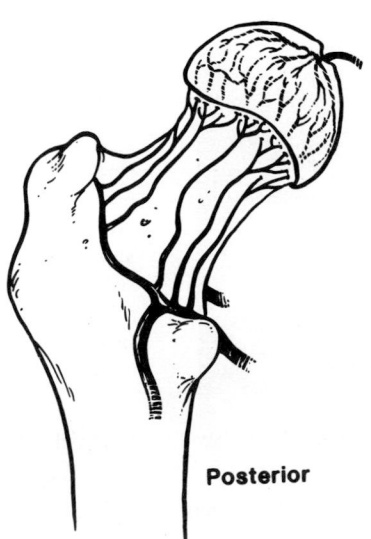

Posterior

Figure 26-3 The blood supply to the femoral head (see text). It is important to note that the blood supply to the femoral head traverses the femoral neck in a distal-to-proximal direction. Therefore, femoral neck fractures that disrupt the ascending cervical arteries deprive the femoral head of its blood supply.

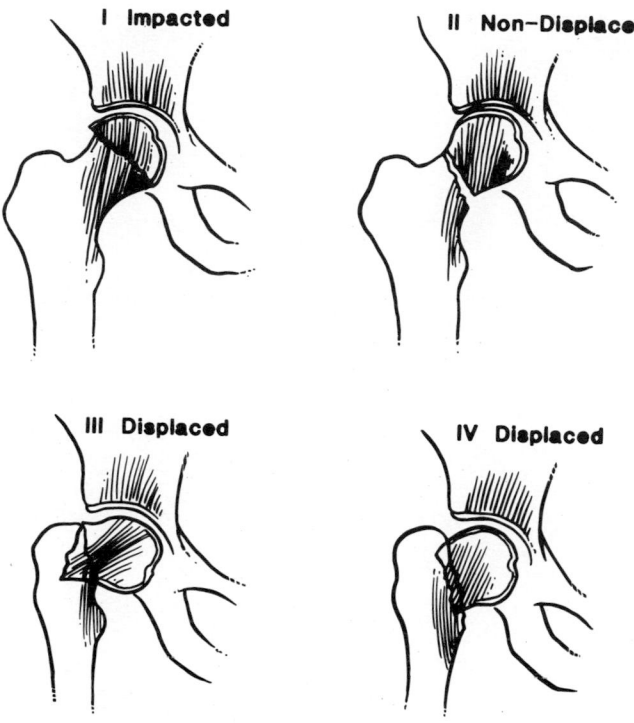

Figure 26-4 The Garden classification (see Table 26-3).

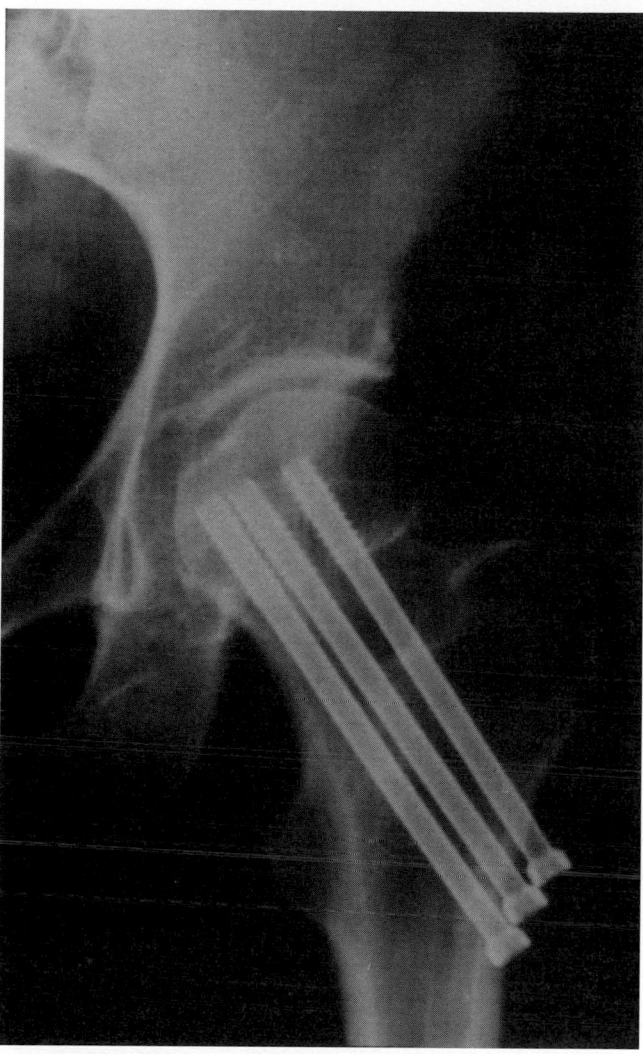

Figure 26-5 Impacted fracture of the left femoral neck stabilized with three cannulated cancellous screws.

practice, however, it is difficult to differentiate the four types of fractures; therefore, it may be more accurate to classify femoral neck fractures as nondisplaced (Garden I and II) or displaced (Garden III and IV).[59–61]

Treatment

Nondisplaced femoral neck fractures (Garden types I and II) should be internally stabilized using multiple lag screws or pins placed in parallel (Fig. 26-5).[62–64] Impacted fractures (Garden type I) have some inherent stability secondary to fracture impaction. Therefore, some authors have recommended nonoperative management.[14] However, Bentley reported a disimpaction rate between 8 and 15 percent in a series of patients.[40,65] Nondisplaced fractures that are not impacted (Garden type II) do not have the inherent stability of impacted fractures and are at higher risk of displacement.[14] There has been no consensus as to the optimal number of pins/screws to use, although most authors report successful treatment using three or four pins/screws for both nondisplaced and displaced fractures.[66] Nonunion and osteonecrosis are un-

TABLE 26-3   Garden Classification of Femoral Neck Fractures

Grade I	An incomplete, impacted fracture in valgus
Grade II	A nondisplaced fracture
Grade III	Incompletely displaced fracture in varus malalignment
Grade IV	Completely displaced fracture with no engagement of the two fragments

Source: Reproduced with permission from Garden RS: Stability and union in subcapital fractures of the femur. *J Bone Joint Surg* 46B:630–647, 1964.

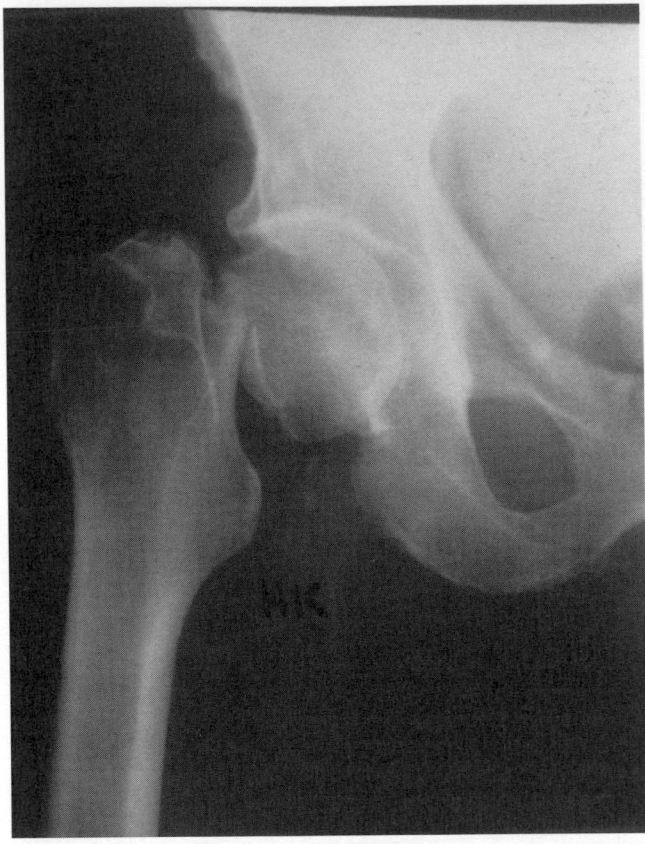

A

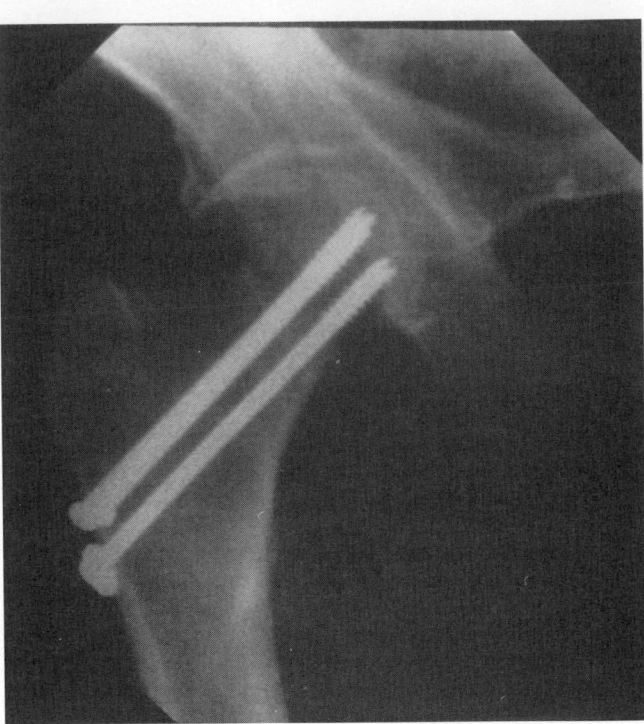

B

Figure 26-6 Displaced right femoral neck fracture (*A*), reduced and stabilized with three cannulated cancellous screws (*B*).

common following nondisplaced fracture, with nonunion occurring in less than 5 percent of cases and osteonecrosis in less than 8 percent.[56,62,63,65,67–70]

Treatment of displaced fractures of the femoral neck is controversial. Most authors advocate closed/open reduction and internal fixation in active, younger patients (Fig. 26-6*A* and *B*), and primary prosthetic replacement in older, less active patients.[25] When internal fixation is utilized, achieving anatomic reduction is probably the most important factor in avoiding healing complications[71,72]; an acceptable reduction may have up to 15° of valgus angulation and less than 10° of anterior or posterior angulation.[60] Prompt reduction of displaced fractures has been advocated but has not consistently been shown to decrease the incidence of nonunion or osteonecrosis.[25] If a closed reduction is unacceptable, open reduction through an anterolateral approach may be required.[25] Internal fixation of displaced fractures most commonly utilizes multiple lag screws or pins placed in parallel.[73,74]

The incidence of nonunion after displaced fracture of the femoral neck ranges from 10 to 30 percent and osteonecrosis from 15 to 33 percent. Capsular distension and increased intracapsular pressure have been implicated as possible causes. Approximately one-third of patients with osteonecrosis and three-quarters of those with nonunion or early fixation failure require additional surgery.[25]

Hemiarthroplasty has been advocated for displaced fractures of the femoral neck in older, less active patients.[25]

Initially only one-piece Austin-Moore or Thompson endoprostheses were available for implantation (Fig. 26-7).[79–84] Although these may be successful in sedentary patients, increased rates of acetabular erosion and loosening of the femoral stem were reported with use of these prostheses.[83,85–88] Use of methylmethacrylate reduced the incidence of femoral stem loosening; however, acetabular wear has remained a problem.[89–94]

The bipolar prosthesis, a self-articulating device, encourages hip motion at a low-friction inner bearing and therefore may decrease the incidence of acetabular erosion (Fig. 26-8).[95–98] Controversy remains however, regarding the indications for use of bipolar prostheses as well as the amount of motion that occurs at the outer and inner surfaces of the prosthesis.[99,100] Lestrange reported that, in a retrospective series of 496 patients with femoral neck fractures, results with cemented bipolar prostheses were better than those with cemented unipolar prostheses.[101] Drinker and Murray, however, in a retrospective series of 261 hip fractures, reported no significant advantages of the bipolar prosthesis over the unipolar prosthesis.[96]

Primary cemented total hip replacement after femoral neck hip fracture has been disappointing.[102–106] At an average follow-up of 56 months, 18 of 37 patients (49 percent) less than 70 years old who had a primary total hip replacement after fracture had undergone or were awaiting revision surgery.[103] A prospective study comparing range of hip motion following total hip replace-

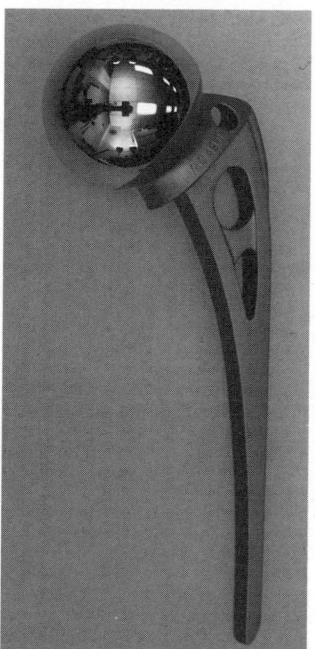

Figure 26-7 Photograph of an Austin-Moore endoprosthesis.

ment for arthritis and fracture reported significantly greater motion in the fracture group,[5] a possible predisposing factor for early loosening and dislocation. Primary total hip arthroplasty is indicated for treatment of acute femoral neck fractures in patients with preexisting acetabular disease (rheumatoid arthritis, osteoarthritis, Paget's disease).[104]

Young Adults

Fractures of the femoral neck in young adults result from high-energy injury (motor vehicle accidents, falls from heights).[64,107,108] Those that occur from a simple fall often have predisposing factors (alcoholism, medication use). Careful evaluation for other injuries should be performed. Specific consideration should be given to the possibility of ipsilateral fractures of the femoral neck and shaft.[109]

Nondisplaced fractures of the femoral neck in young adults should be stabilized by multiple lag screws or pins.[5] Displaced fractures of the femoral neck should undergo open and anatomic reduction.[5] A gentle, closed or open reduction should be performed, followed by fixation with multiple lag screws or pins.[5]

COMPLICATIONS OF FRACTURES OF THE FEMORAL NECK

Complications following internal fixation of fractures of the femoral neck include infection,[7,76,110] loss of fixa-

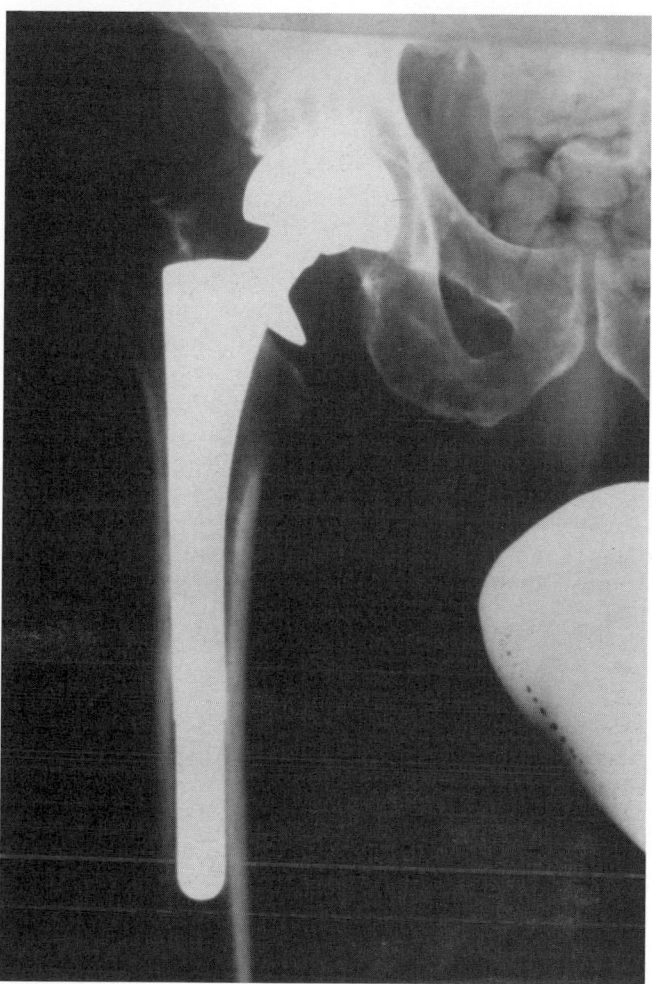

Figure 26-8 Radiograph of a noncemented bipolar endoprosthesis.

tion,[67,111–113] nonunion,[62,63,68] and osteonecrosis.[56,62,63,67–69,8,9,114] Early fixation failure (within 3 months after surgery) occurs in 12 to 24 percent of displaced fractures of the femoral neck.[67,111–113] The most important factors associated with loss of fixation are initial fracture displacement, posterior comminution of the femoral neck, adequacy of reduction, and the patient's age.

The incidence of nonunion is related to fracture type. The nonunion rate after nondisplaced fracture of the femoral neck ranges from 0 to 5 percent[63,67,68,76] and after displaced fractures from 9 to 35 percent.[56,62,67,74–77] Reported risk factors include an inadequate reduction, posterior comminution, and use of a compression hip screw.[52,67,70,76,110,115–117]

The rate of osteonecrosis after nondisplaced fracture of the femoral neck ranges from 5 to 8 percent[56,63,65,67–70] and after displaced fracture, it ranges from 20 to 35 percent.[56,62,63,67–69,89,96,114] Factors associated with an increased incidence of osteonecrosis include a delay in fracture reduction, an inadequate reduction, and use of a sliding hip screw.[67,72,76,114,118]

Complications following primary prosthetic replacement for acute fracture of the femoral neck include infection,[4,79,119,120,131] dislocation,[85,120,122–124] and pain associated with acetabular erosion and prosthetic loosening.[120,125] The incidence of infection has been reported to vary with the surgical approach.[120,126,127] Higher infection rates have been reported when a posterior approach is used.[120,126,127] This probably reflects the risk of fecal contamination because of the proximity of the incision to the perineal area.

The dislocation rate after prosthetic replacement varies from 1 to 10 percent.[85,120,122–124] The posterior approach is associated with a higher dislocation rate than the anterior approach.[120,126–128] Dislocation appears to occur less commonly after bipolar hemiarthroplasty.[122]

The most important prosthesis-related causes of pain are acetabular erosion and prosthetic loosening.[129] Bipolar endoprostheses may result in less acetabular erosion than unipolar hemiarthroplasties.[122,125] Cement fixation of the femoral component reduces the incidence of postoperative pain associated with prosthetic loosening.[122,125]

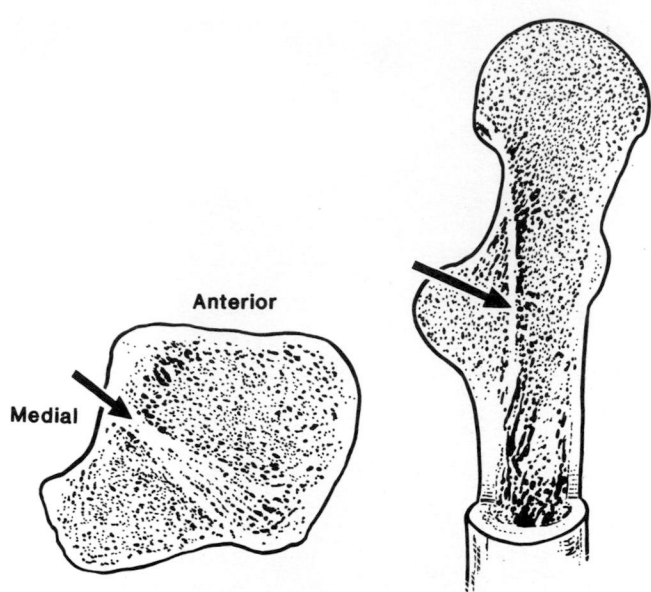

Figure 26-9 The calcar os femorale (*arrows*) is a verticle wall of dense bone that forms an internal trabecular strut within the inferior portion of the femoral neck and intertrochanteric region. It is an important conduit for stress transfer in this area (see text).

INTERTROCHANTERIC FRACTURES

Anatomy

The intertrochanteric region is extracapsular and includes the greater and lesser trochanters and the transitional bone between the femoral neck and shaft. The calcar os femorale is a vertical wall of dense bone extending from the posteromedial aspect of the femoral shaft to the posterior portion of the femoral neck (Fig. 26-9).[14] It forms an internal trabecular strut within the inferior portion of the neck and the intertrochanteric region and acts as a strong conduit for stresses. The cancellous bone in this area is well vascularized.

Epidemiology

Intertrochanteric fractures occur with approximately the same frequency as fractures of the femoral neck in patients with similar demographic characteristics.[30,36,38,131,132] A recent study reported that women who sustain intertrochanteric fractures are more likely to be older, more dependent in activities of daily living, and home ambulators prior to hip fracture compared to those women who sustain femoral neck fractures.[133]

Mechanism of Injury

Intertrochanteric fractures occur as a result of direct or indirect forces transmitted to the intertrochanteric area.[134,135] This may result from a direct blow to the area of the greater trochanter or from indirect forces transmitted along the femoral axis.

Classification

The most commonly used classification system for intertrochanteric fractures was introduced by Evans in 1949 and is based upon the stability of the fracture pattern and the ability to convert an unstable fracture to a stable reduction (Table 26-4).[136] In stable fractures, the posteromedial cortex remains intact and a stable reduction can be obtained. Unstable fracture patterns are characterized by comminution of the posteromedial cortex in the area of the calcar femorale. These fractures are inherently unstable but can be converted to stable reductions if medial cortical opposition can be obtained. Reverse obliquity fractures are inherently unstable because of the tendency for medial displacement of the shaft. Studies, however, have documented poor reproducibility using the Evans classification.[137,138] Therefore, it may be better to classify intertrochanteric fractures as either stable or unstable, depending on the status of the posteromedial cortex (Fig. 26-10). Unstable fracture patterns include those with comminution of the posteromedial cortex, intertrochanteric fractures with subtrochanteric extension, and reverse obliquity fractures.

Treatment

Operative management is the treatment of choice for both nondisplaced and displaced intertrochanteric hip fractures.[14] A sliding hip screw is the implant of choice for most intertrochanteric hip fractures (Fig. 26-11).[139,140] These screws are available in varying plate angles (125 to

TABLE 26-4   Evans Classification of Intertrochanteric Fractures

Type I	Undisplaced two-part fracture
Type II	Displaced two-part fracture
Type III	Displaced three-part fracture with posterolateral comminution
Type IV	Displaced three-part fracture with large posteromedial comminution
Type V	Displaced four-part with comminution involving both trochanters

Source: Reproduced with permission from Evans EM: The treatment of trochanteric fractures of the femur. *J Bone Joint Surg* 31B:190–203, 1949.

155°). Higher-angled devices are more difficult to insert into the center of the femoral head and neck than the 135° device. Therefore, the 135° plate is most commonly utilized. In addition, the insertion point is in metaphyseal bone, which produces less of a stress riser effect than the diaphyseal insertion point required for the 150° device.[139–141]

There seems to be little justification for a formal medial displacement osteotomy with use of the sliding hip screw.[142–146] Because the sliding hip screw allows controlled fracture collapse, anatomically aligned unstable fractures can be expected to collapse spontaneously to a stable and often medially displaced position. This usually results in less shortening of the extremity than a formal medial dis-

placement osteotomy. Clinical studies comparing medial displacement and anatomic reduction for unstable fractures using the sliding hip screw found no advantage of medial displacement over anatomic reduction.[143]

The most important aspect of sliding hip screw insertion is secure placement of the screw within the proximal fragment.[25] The screw should be positioned within 1 cm of the subchondral bone.[25] A central position within the femoral head and neck is most commonly recommended (Fig. 26-12). If a central position is not possible, an inferior position is preferred.[25]

In older patients, posteromedial are usually ignored. In younger patients, an attempt should be made to stabi-

Figure 26-10 Intertrochanteric fractures may be best classified as either stable or unstable, depending on the state of the posteromedial cortex. Stable fractures have an intact posteromedial cortex (*A* and *B*); in unstable fractures, the posteromedial cortex is not intact (*C* and *D*). The reverse obliquity pattern is also considered unstable (*E*).

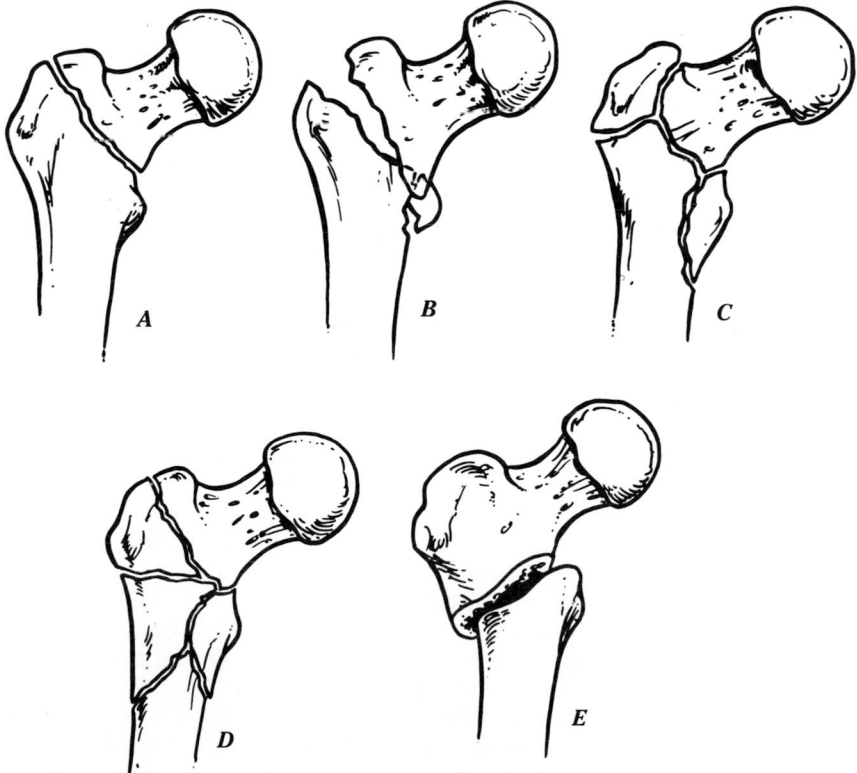

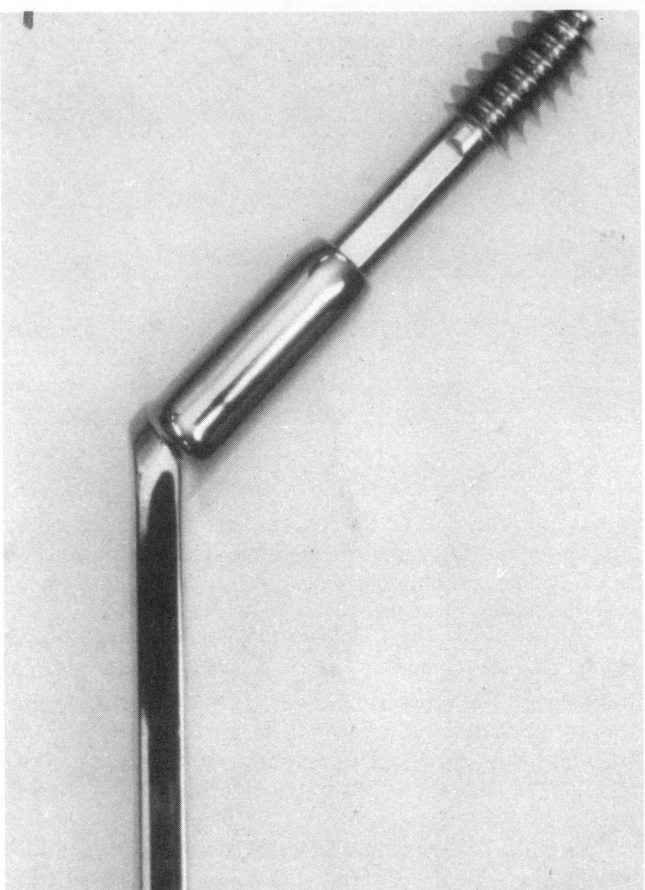

Figure 26-11 Photograph of a sliding hip screw.

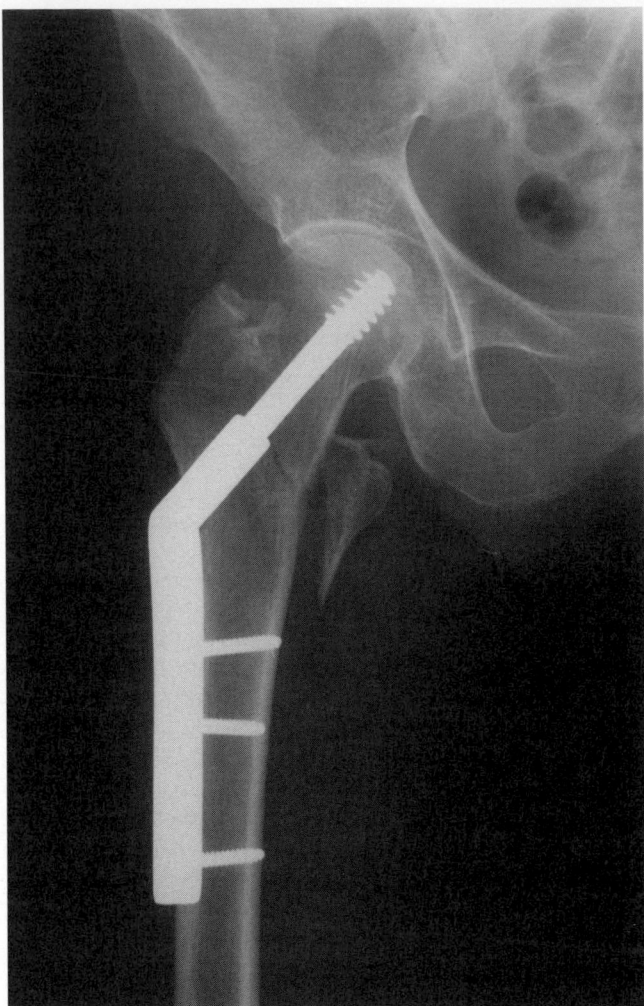

Figure 26-12 An unstable intertrochanteric fracture stabilized with a sliding hip screw; the screw is positioned in the center of the femoral head within 1 cm of subchondral bone.

lize large posteromedial fragments internally in a near anatomic position to prevent excessive screw-barrel slide which would result in fracture and therefore shortening of the extremity. If the patient is positioned on a fracture table, traction is released to mobilize the posteromedial fragment. External rotation of the extremity may be necessary to expose the posteromedial area of the femoral shaft. Fixation of the posteromedial fragment may be difficult, particularly if comminution is present, and involves use of either a lag screw or cerclage wire.

Basicervical hip fractures are located just proximal to or at the intertrochanteric line; nonetheless, they are extracapsular. Insertion of the lag screw into the head and neck may cause the fragment to rotate. Therefore, two guide wires are inserted. One is located in an inferior position and the second is located superior in the femoral head. The sliding hip screw is placed over the inferior guide wire; the proximal guide wire or an inserted cancellous screw prevents rotation of the head and neck fragment during reaming and lag screw insertion.

Reverse obliquity fractures are characterized by an oblique fracture line extending from the proximal medial cortex and exiting the shaft laterally and slightly distally. This results in a tendency toward medial displacement of the distal fragment from the pull of the adductor muscles. Controlled impaction, characteristic of the sliding hip

screw, will not occur secondary to the location and direction of the fracture line (Fig. 26-13). The sliding portion of the device is entirely within the proximal fragment while the plate and screws stabilize the distal fragment. Reverse obliquity fractures are best stabilized with devices used for subtrochanteric fractures, which include intramedullary nails, intramedullary hip screws, and 95° fixed-angle devices.[25]

Intramedullary nail/sliding hip screw devices (Gamma Nail, Intramedullary Hip Screw) have also been used for the treatment of intertrochanteric hip fractures (Fig. 26-14).[147,148] However, studies comparing use of the Gamma nail to a sliding hip screw have found no differences with respect to operating time, blood loss, duration of hospital stay, infection rate or wound complications, implant failure, screw cutout, or screw sliding.[149] Patients treated with the Gamma Nail, however, have had increased rates of femoral shaft fractures at the nail tip or the insertion sites of the distal locking bolts.[149]

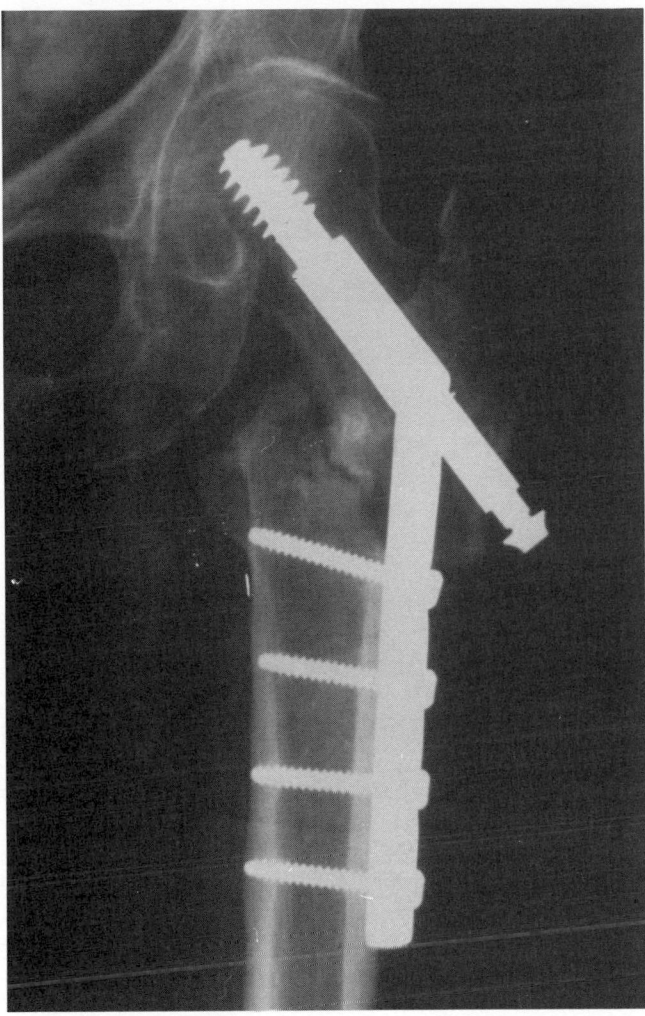

Figure 26-13 Medial shaft displacement resulted with the use of a sliding hip screw for the treatment of a reverse obliquity hip fracture.

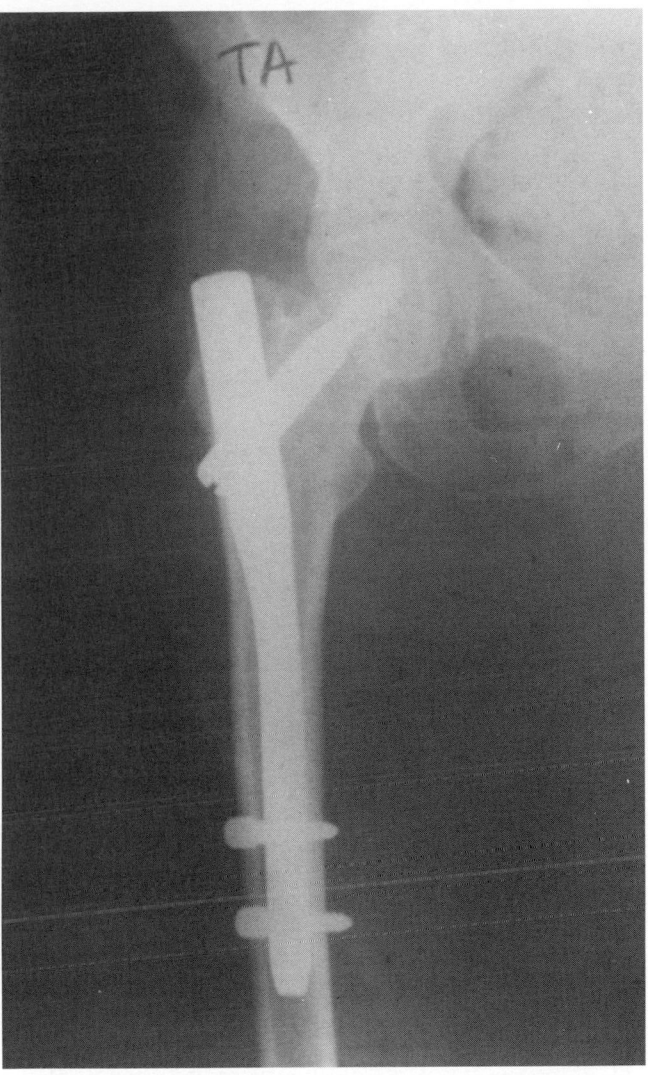

Figure 26-14 Use of an intramedullary hip screw for fixation of a stable intertrochanteric fracture.

Complications

The surgical complications most frequently encountered after intertrochanteric hip fracture are varus displacement of the proximal fragment,[14] malrotation deformity,[14] and nonunion.[150–152] Varus displacement following internal fixation usually occurs in unstable fractures, with the lag screw "cutting out" through the anterosuperior portion of the femoral head.[14] This complication results from (1) placement of the screw into the anterosuperior aspect of the femoral head; (2) inability to obtain a stable reduction; (3) excessive collapse of the fracture such that the sliding capacity of the device is exceeded; (4) inadequate screw-barrel engagement which prevents sliding; or (5) severe osteoporosis, which precludes secure fixation.

Malrotation usually results from internal rotation of the distal fragment at the time of internal fixation. In unstable fractures, the proximal and distal fragments may move independently. In these cases, the distal fragment should be internally fixed in neutral to slight external rotation. Nonunion occurs in less than 2 percent of cases.[139,153–156]

SUBTROCHANTERIC FRACTURES

Anatomy

Subtrochanteric fractures account for approximately 15 percent of all fractures of the proximal femur.[153,155,158,159] These fractures start at or below the lesser trochanter and involve the proximal femoral shaft. The subtrochanteric area experiences some of the highest biomechanical stresses in the body.[160] The medial and posteromedial cortex is a site of high compressive forces, while the lateral cortex experiences high tensile stresses.

Mechanism of Injury

Subtrochanteric fractures occur in three patient groups[25,153,155,158,159]: (1) young patients who are involved in high-energy trauma; (2) older patients with osteopenic bone, whose fracture occurs as a result of a minor fall; and (3) older patients with pathologic fractures from metastatic disease.

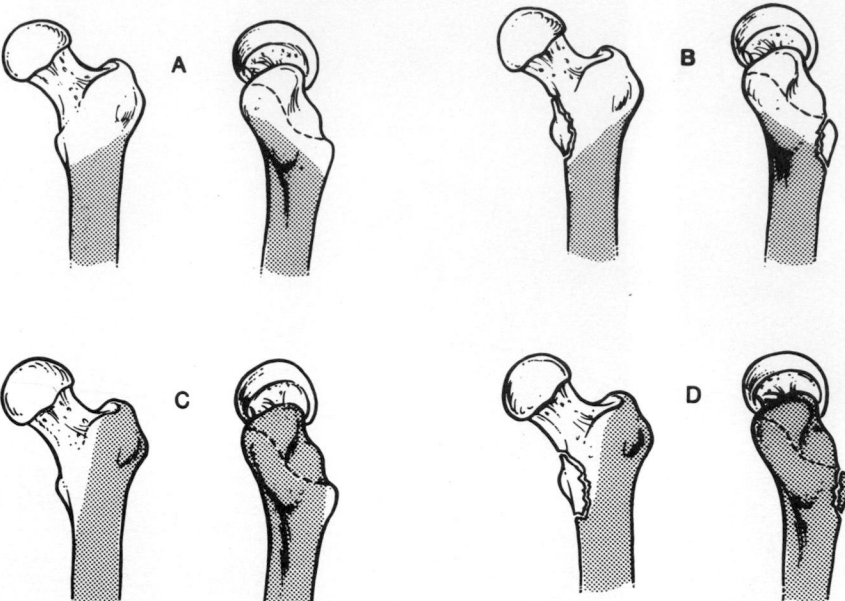

Figure 26-15 The Russell-Taylor classification: (*A*) type Ia, (*B*) type Ib, (*C*) type IIa, (*D*) type IIb (see Table 26-5).

Classification

Various classification systems of subtrochanteric fractures have been proposed.[153,155,161–163] but none has been universally accepted. As with intertrochanteric fractures, fracture stability is based on the presence or absence of a posteromedial buttress.[150,163] In stable fractures, medial and posteromedial cortical support is intact or can be reestablished. In unstable fractures, comminution results in loss of medial cortical continuity. The Russell-Taylor classification is based on the type of internal fixation that allows the best biomechanical construct with the least vascular damage to the fracture site (Fig. 26-15, Table 26-5).[164]

Treatment

The interlocking nail is the implant of choice for subtrochanteric femur fractures (Fig. 26-16).[158–160,165,167–169]

Virtually all nonpathologic subtrochanteric fractures can be stabilized using an interlocked nail, regardless of fracture pattern or amount of comminution.[25] Favorable mechanical characteristics of interlocked nails have eliminated the requirement of surgically reconstituting the medial femoral cortex. High rates of union have been reported in large series of subtrochanteric femur fractures stabilized with both first- and second-generation interlocking nails.[158,170–173]

Screw-plate devices can also be used for the treatment of subtrochanteric fractures. Successful treatment with the sliding hip screw has also been reported, particularly in low-energy subtrochanteric fractures in the elderly[174–177]; one series reported a 95 percent rate of union.[25] Subtrochanteric/intertrochanteric fractures are most suitable for use of a sliding hip screw. Ninety-five degree fixed angle devices, the condylar blade plate or screw, provide improved fixation of the proximal fragment and act as a lateral tension band if the medial cortex is in-

---

TABLE 26-5 Russell-Taylor Classification of Subtrochanteric Fractures

Type Ia	Fracture extension with any degree of comminution from below the lesser trochanter to the isthmus with no extension into the piriformis fossa
Type Ib	Fracture extension involving the lesser trochanter to the isthmus with no extension into the piriformis fossa
Type IIa	Fracture extension into the piriformis fossa; stable medial construct
Type IIb	Fracture extension into the piriformis fossa; no stability of the medial femoral cortex

Source: Reproduced with permission from Garden RS: Reduction and fixation of the subcapital fractures of the femur. *Orthop Clin North Am* 5:683–712, 1974.

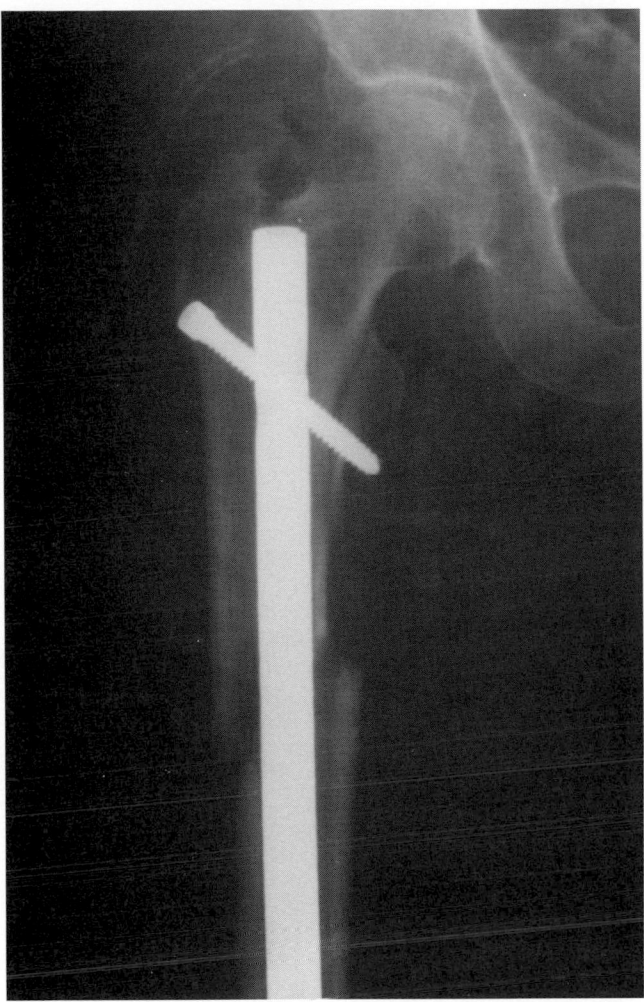

Figure 26-16 Subtrochanteric femoral fracture stabilized with a locked intramedullary nail.

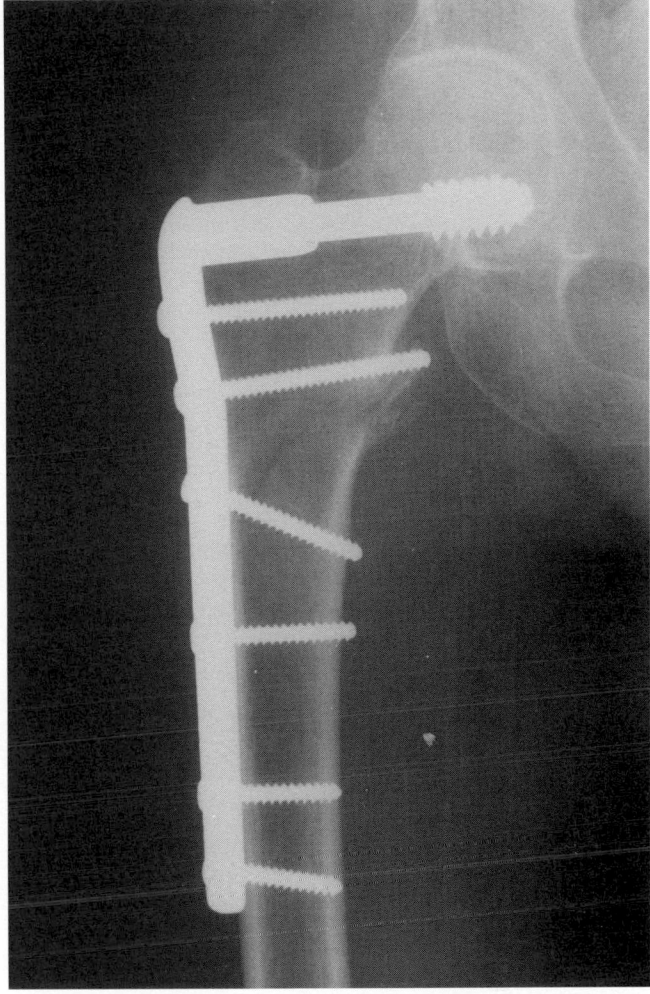

Figure 26-17 Subtrochanteric fracture stabilized with use of a dynamic condylar screw.

tact.[5,160,178–180] The condylar screw is technically easier to insert than the blade plate; one series reported similar results with use of either device for the treatment of subtrochanteric fractures (Fig. 26-17).[181] Complication rates up to 20 percent have been reported with use of these fixed-angle devices, usually related to an inability to restore the medial femoral cortex. One can minimize the risk of healing complications through use of indirect reduction techniques.[5,25,182]

REFERENCES

1. Surachi A: Distribution and severity of injuries associated with hip dislocations secondary to motor vehicle accidents. *J Trauma* 26:458–460, 1986.
2. Epstein HC: Traumatic dislocations of the hip. *Clin Orthop* 92:116–142, 1973.
3. Stewart MJ, McCarroll HR, Mulhollan JS: Fracture-dislocation of the hip. *Acta Orthop Scand* 46:507–525, 1975.
4. Brav EA: Traumatic dislocation of the hip. *J Bone Joint Surg* 44A:1115–1134, 1962.
5. Koval KJ: Trauma, Hip, in Kasser JR (ed): *Orthopaedic Knowledge Update 5.* Rosemont, IL, American Association of Orthopaedic Surgeons, 1996, pp 379–388.
6. Dreinhofer KE, Schwarzkoff SR, Haas NP, Tscherne H: Isolated traumatic dislocation of the hip: Long-term results in fifty patients. *J Bone Joint Surg* 76B:6–12, 1994.
7. DeLee JC, Evans JA, Thomas J: Anterior dislocation of the hip and associated femoral-head fractures. *J Bone Joint Surg* 62A:960–964, 1980.
8. Epstein HC: *Traumatic Dislocation of the Hip.* Baltimore, Williams & Wilkins, 1980.
9. Thompson VP, Epstein HC: Traumatic dislocation of the hip: A survey of two hundred and four cases covering a period of twenty-one years. *J Bone Joint Surg* 33A:746–778, 1951.
10. DeLee JC: Fractures and dislocations of the hip, in Rockwood CA, Green DP (eds): *Fractures in Adults,* 2d ed. Vol 2. Philadelphia, Lippincott, 1984, pp 1211–1357.
11. Brumback RJ, Kenzora JE, Levitt LE, et al: Fractures of the femoral head. Mosby, St. Louis. The HIP Proceedings of the Fourteenth Open Scientific Meeting of the Hip Society, pp 181–206, 1986.

12. Mowery C, Gershuni DH: Fracture dislocation of the femoral head treated by open reduction and internal fixation. *J Trauma* 26:1041–1044, 1986.

13. Scadden WJ, Dennyson WG: Unreduced obturator dislocation of the hip. *S Afr Med J* 53:601–602, 1978.

14. Zuckerman JD, Schon L: Hip fractures, in Zuckerman JD (ed): *Comprehensive Care of Orthopaedic Injuries in the Elderly.* Baltimore, Urban & Schwartzberg, 1990, pp 23–111.

15. Epstein HC, Harvey JP: Traumatic anterior dislocations of the hip: Management and results. An analysis of fifty-five cases. *J Bone Joint Surg* 54A:1561–1562, 1972.

16. Epstein HC, Harvey JP: Traumatic anterior dislocations of the hip. *Orthop Rev* 1:33–38, 1972.

17. Epstein HC: Posterior fracture-dislocations of the hip: Long-term follow-up. *J Bone Joint Surg* 56A:1103–1127, 1974.

18. Calkins MS, Zych L, Borja FJ, Mnaymneh W: Computed tomography evaluation of stability in posterior fracture dislocation of the hip. *Clin Orthop* 227:152–163, 1988.

19. Keith JE, Brashear HR, Guilford WB: Stability of posterior fracture dislocations of the hip: Quantitative assessment using computed tomography. *J Bone Joint Surg* 70A:711–714, 1988.

20. Brumback RJ, Holt ES, McBride MS, et al: Acetabular depression fracture accompanying posterior fracture dislocation of the hip. *J Orthop Trauma* 4:42–48, 1990.

21. Stewart MJ, Milford LW: Fracture dislocation of the hip. *J Bone Joint Surg* 36A:315–342, 1954.

22. Hougaard K, Thansen PB: Coxarthrosis following traumatic posterior dislocation of the hip. *J Bone Joint Surg* 69A:679–683, 1987.

23. Roeder LF, Delee JC: Femoral head fractures associated with posterior hip dislocations. *Clin Orthop* 147:121–130, 1980.

24. Pipkin G: Treatment of grade IV fracture-dislocation of the hip. *J Bone Joint Surg* 39A:1027–1042, 1197, 1957.

25. Zuckerman JD, Koval KJ: Trauma: Hip, in Frymoyer JW (ed): *Orthopaedic Knowledge Update 4.* Rosemont, IL. American Association of Orthopaedic Surgeons, 1983, pp 525–538.

26. Upadhyay SS, Moulton A: The long term results of traumatic posterior dislocation of the hip. *J Bone Joint Surg* 63B:548–551, 1981.

27. Hougaard K, Thansen PB: Traumatic posterior fracture dislocation of the hip with fracture of the femoral head or neck, or both. *J Bone Joint Surg* 70A:233–239, 1988.

28. Agarwal N, Reyes JD, Westerman DA, Cayten CG: Factors influencing DRG 210 (hip fracture) reimbursement. *J Trauma* 26:426–431, 1986.

29. Craxford AO, Stevens J: Proximal femoral fractures in psychiatric patients. *Injury* 11:19, 1979.

30. El-Banna S, Raynal L, Gerbtzop A: Fractures of the hip in the elderly. Therapeutic and medico-social considerations. *Arch Gerontol Geriatr* 3:311–319, 1984.

31. Sexson SB, Lehner JT: Factors affecting hip fracture mortality. *J Orthop Trauma* 1:298–305, 1988.

32. Fairclough J, Colhoun E, Johnson D, Williams L: Bone scanning for suspected hip fractures. *J Bone Joint Surg* 69B:251–253, 1987.

33. Rizzo PF, Gould ES, Lyden JP: Diagnosis of occult fractures about the hip: Magnetic resonance imaging compared with bone scanning. *J Bone Joint Surg* 75A:395–401, 1993.

34. Galasko CS, Rushton S, Sylvester BS, et al: The significance of peak expiratory flow rate in assessing prognosis of elderly patients undergoing operations on the hip. *Injury* 16:398–401, 1985.

35. Schultz RJ, Whitfield GF, Lamura JL, et al: The role of physiologic monitoring in patients with fractures of the hip. *J Trauma* 25:309–316, 1985.

36. Kenzora JE, McCarthy RE, Lowell JD, Sledge CB: Hip fracture mortality. *Clin Orthop* 186:45–56, 1984.

37. Zuckerman JD, Skovron ML, Koval KJ, et al: Postoperative complications and mortality associated with operative delay in older patients who have a fracture of the hip. *J Bone Joint Surg* 77A:1551–1556, 1995.

38. White BL, Fisher WD, Laurin CA: Rate of mortality for elderly patients after fracture of the hip in the 1980s. *J Bone Joint Surg* 69A:1335–1340, 1987.

39. Modig J, Karlstrom G, Maripuu E, Sahlstedt B: Thromboembolism after total hip replacement: The role of epidural and general anesthesia. *Anesth Analg* 62:174–180, 1983.

40. Bentley G: Impacted fractures of the neck of the femur. *J Bone Joint Surg* 50B:551–561, 1968.

41. Jewett EL: One piece angle nail for trochanteric fractures. *J Bone Joint Surg* 23:803–810, 1941.

42. Nieminen S: Early weightbearing after classical internal fixation of medial fractures of the femoral neck. *Acta Orthop Scand* 46:782–794, 1975.

43. Pugh WL: A self-adjusting nail-plate for fractures about the hip joint. *J Bone Joint Surg* 37A:1085–1093, 1955.

44. Ceder L, Stromquist B, Hansen LI: Effects of strategy changes in the treatment of femoral neck fractures during a 17 year period. *Clin Orthop* 218:53–57, 1987.

45. Garden RS: Low-angle fixation in fractures of the femoral neck. *J Bone Joint Surg* 43B:647–663, 1961.

46. Graham J: Early or delayed weight-bearing after internal fixation of transcervical fracture of the femur. *J Bone Joint Surg* 50B:562–569, 1968.

47. Montrey JS, Kistner RL, Kong AY, et al: Thromboembolism following hip fracture. *J Trauma* 25:534–537, 1985.

48. Moore AT: Fracture of the hip joint: Treatment by extra-articular fixation with adjustable nails. *Surg Gynecol Obstet* 64:420–436, 1937.

49. Frankel VH: Biomechanics of the hip joint. *AAOS Instr Course Lect* 35:3–9, 1986.

50. Lygre L: The loads produced on the hip joint by nursing procedures: A telemeterization study. MS thesis. Cleveland, OH, Case Western Reserve University, 1970.

51. Milde FK: Loads on the femoral head during nursing care activities as measured by a telemeterized nail-plate. MS thesis. Cleveland, OH, Case Western Reserve University, 1974.

52. Norden M, Frankel VH: Biomechanics of the hip, in Frankel VH, Norden M (eds): *Basic Biomechanics of the Skeletal System.* Philadelphia, Lea & Febiger, 1980, pp 149–177.

53. Howe WW, Lacey T, Schwartz RP: A study of the gross anatomy of the arteries supplying the proximal portion of the femur and acetabulum. *J Bone Joint Surg* 32A:856–866, 1950.

54. Trueta J, Harrison MHM: The normal vascular anatomy of the femoral head in adult man. *J Bone Joint Surg* 35B:442–461, 1953.

55. Frankel VH: *The Femoral Neck: Function, Fracture Mechanisms, Internal Fixation.* Springfield, IL, Charles C Thomas, 1960.

56. Banks HH: Factors influencing the result in fractures of the femoral neck. *J Bone Joint Surg* 44A:931–964, 1962.

57. Lavell JD: Results and complications of femoral neck fractures. *Clin Orthop* 152:162–172, 1980.

58. Scheck M: The significance of posterior comminution in femoral neck fractures. *Clin Orthop* 152:138–142, 1980.

59. Swiontkowski MF: Intracapsular hip fractures, in Browner BD, Jupiter JB, Levine AM, Trafton PG (eds): *Skeletal Trauma.* Philadelphia, Saunders, 1992, pp 1369–1442.

60. Cardea JA, Kyle RF, Meyers MH, et al: Symposium: Femoral neck fractures. *Contemp Orthop* 17:73–105, 1988.

61. Frandsen PA, Anderson E, Madsen F, Skjodt T: Garden's classification of femoral neck fractures: An assessment of inter-observer variation. *J Bone Joint Surg* 70B:588–590, 1988.

62. Cobb AG, Gibson PH: Screw fixation of sub-capital fractures of the femur: A better method of treatment. *Injury* 17:259–264, 1986.

63. Stappaerts KH, Broos PL: Internal fixation of femoral neck fractures: A follow-up study of 118 cases. *Acta Chir Belg* 87:247–251, 1987.

64. Swiontkowski MF, Winquist RA, Hansen ST: Femoral neck fractures in patients aged 12–49. *J Bone Joint Surg* 66A:837–846, 1984.

65. Bentley G: Treatment of nondisplaced fractures of the femoral neck. *Clin Orthop* 152:93–101, 1980.

66. Swiontkowski MF, Harrington RM, Keller TS, and Van Patten PK: Torsion and bending analysis of internal fixation techniques for femoral neck fractures: The role of implant design and bone density. *J Orthop Res* 5:433–444, 1987.

67. Barnes R, Brown JT, Garden RS, Nicoll EA: Subcapital fractures of the femur. *J Bone Joint Surg* 58B:2–24, 1976.

68. Stromquist B, Hansson L, Nilsson L, Thorngren K: Prognostic precision of postoperative ^{99m}Tc-MDP scintimetry after femoral neck fracture. *Acta Orthop Scand* 58:494–498, 1987.

69. Massie WK: Treatment of femoral neck fractures emphasizing long term follow-up observations on aseptic necrosis. *Clin Orthop* 92:16–62, 1973.

70. Scott WA, Allum RL, Wright K: Implant induced trabecular damage in cadaveric femoral necks. *Acta Orthop Scand* 56:145–146, 1985.

71. Garden RS: Stability and union in subcapital fractures of the femur. *J Bone Joint Surg* 46B:630–647, 1964.

72. Garden RS: Malreduction and avascular necrosis in subcapital fractures of the femur. *J Bone Joint Surg* 53B:183–197, 1971.

73. Madsen F, Linde F, Andersen E, et al: Fixation of displaced femoral neck fractures: A comparison between sliding screw plate and four cancellous bone screws. *Acta Orthop Scand* 58:212–216, 1987.

74. Skinner PW, Powles D: Compression screw fixation for displaced subcapital fracture of the femur: Success or failure? *J Bone Joint Surg* 68B:78–82, 1986.

75. Calandruccio RA, Anderson WE: Post-fracture avascular necrosis of the femoral head: Correlation of experimental and clinical studies. *Clin Orthop* 152:49–84, 1980.

76. Christie J, Howie C, Armoir P: Fixation of displaced femoral neck fractures: Compression screw fixation versus double divergent pins. *J Bone Joint Surg* 70B:199–201, 1988.

77. Soreide O, Molster A, Raugstad TS: Internal fixation versus primary prosthetic replacement in acute femoral neck fractures: A prospective, randomized clinical study. *Br J Surg* 66:56–60, 1979.

78. Harper WM, Barnes MR, Gregg PJ: Femoral head blood flow in femoral neck fractures: An analysis using intraosseous pressure measurement. *J Bone Joint Surg* 73B:73–75, 1991.

79. Carnesale PG, Anderson LD: Primary prosthetic replacement for femoral neck fractures. *Arch Surg* 110:27–29, 1975.

80. Coates R: A retrospective survey of eighty-one patients with hemiarthroplasty for subcapital fracture of the femoral neck. *J Bone Joint Surg* 57B:256, 1975.

81. Kofoed H, Kofoe J: Moore prosthesis in the treatment of fresh femoral neck fractures. *Injury* 14:531–540, 1983.

82. Salvati EA, Artz T, Aglietti P, Asnis SE: Endoprosthesis in the treatment of femoral neck fractures. *Orthop Clin North Am* 5:757–777, 1974.

83. Soreide O, Lillestol J, Algo A, Hvidsten K: Acetabular protrusion following endo-prosthetic hip surgery: A multifactorial study. *Acta Orthop Scand* 51:943–948, 1980.

84. Whittaker RP, Abeshaus MM, Scholl HW, Chung SMK: Fifteen years' experience with metallic endo-prosthetic replacement of the femoral head for femoral neck fractures. *J Trauma* 12:799–806, 1972.

85. D'Arcy J, Devas M: Treatment of fractures of the neck by replacement with the Thompson prosthesis. *J Bone Joint Surg* 58B:279–286, 1987.

86. Gingras MB, Clarke J, Evarts CM: Prosthetic replacement in femoral neck fractures. *Clin Orthop* 152:147–157, 1980.

87. Higgins RW, Hughes JL: Preliminary results of eighty-one replacements with the Bateman endoprosthesis. *Orthop Trans* 7:411–412, 1983.

88. Kwok DC, Cruess RL: A retrospective study of Moore and Thompson hemiarthroplasty. *Clin Orthop* 169:179–185, 1982.

89. Beckenbaugh RD, Tressler HA, Johnson EA: Results after hemiarthroplasty of the hip using a cemented femoral prosthesis: A review of 109 cases with an average follow-up of 36 months. *Mayo Clin Proc* 52:349–353, 1977.

90. Follacci FM, Charnley J: A comparison of the results of femoral head prosthesis with and without cement. *Clin Orthop* 62:156–161, 1969.

91. Obrant KJ, Carlsson AS: Survival of hemi-arthroplasties after cervical hip fractures. *Orthopaedics* 10:1153–1156, 1987.

92. Soreide O, Lerner AP, Thunold J: Primary prosthetic replacement in acute femoral neck fractures. *Injury* 6:286–293, 1974–1975.

93. Welch RB, Taylor LW, Wynne GF, White AH: Results with the cemented hemiarthroplasty for displaced fractures of the femoral neck, in *The Hip, Proceedings of the Fifth Open Scientific Meeting of the Hip Society*. St Louis, Mosby, 1977, p 87.

94. Wrighton JD, Woodyard JE: Prosthetic replacement for subcapital fractures of the femur: A comparative survey. *Injury* 2:287–293, 1971.

95. Bhuller GS: Use of the Giliberty bipolar endoprosthesis in femoral neck fractures. *Clin Orthop* 162:165–169, 1982.

96. Drinker H, Murray WR: The universal proximal femoral endoprosthesis: A short-term comparison with conventional hemiarthroplasty. *J Bone Joint Surg* 61A:1167–1174, 1979.

97. Langan P: The Giliberty bipolar prosthesis: A clinical and radiographical review. *Clin Orthop* 141:169–175, 1979.

98. Long JW, Knight W: Bateman UPF prosthesis in fractures of the femoral neck. *Clin Orthop* 152:198–201, 1980.

99. Chen SC, Badrinath K, Pell LH, et al: The movements of the components of the Hastings bipolar prosthesis: A radiographic study in 65 patients. *J Bone Joint Surg* 71B:186–188, 1989.

100. LaBelle LW, Colwill JC, Swanson AB: Bateman bi-polar hip arthroplasty for femoral neck fractures: A five-to ten-year follow-up study. *Clin Orthop* 251:20–25, 1990.

101. Lestrange NR: The Bateman UPF prosthesis: A 48-month experience. *Orthopedics* 2:373–377, 1979.

102. Coates RL, Armour P: Treatments of subcapital femoral fractures by primary total hip replacement. *Injury* 11:132–135, 1979–1980.

103. Greenough CG, Jones JR: Primary total hip replacements for displaced subcapital fracture of the femur. *J Bone Joint Surg* 70B:639–643, 1988.

104. Sim FH, Stauffer RN: Management of hip fractures by total hip arthroplasty. *Clin Orthop* 152:191–197, 1980.

105. Sim FH, Stauffer RN: Total hip arthroplasty in acute femoral neck fractures. *AAOS Instr Course Lect* 29:9–16, 1980.

106. Taine WH, Armour PC: Primary total hip replacement for displaced subcapital fractures of the femur. *J Bone Joint Surg* 67B:214–217, 1985.

107. Askin SR, Bryan RS: Femoral neck fractures in young adults. *Clin Orthop* 114:259–264, 1976.

108. Tooke SM, Favero KJ: Femoral neck fractures in skeletally mature patients 50 years old or less. *J Bone Joint Surg* 67A:1255–1260, 1985.

109. Swiontkowski MF: Ipsilateral femoral shaft and hip fractures. *Orthop Clin North Am* 18:73–84, 1987.

110. Svenningsen S, Benum P, Nesse O, Furset O: Internal fixation of femoral neck fractures: Compression screw compared with nail-plate fixation. *Acta Orthop Scand* 55:423–429, 1984.

111. Brown T, Court-Brown C: Failure of sliding nail-platefixation in subcapital fractures of the femoral neck. *J Bone Joint Surg* 61B:342–346, 1979.

112. Holmberg S, Kalen R, Thorngren KG: Treatment and outcome of femoral neck fractures. *Clin Orthop* 218:42–52, 1987.

113. Stappaerts KH: Early fixation failure in displaced femoral neck fractures. *Arch Orthop Trauma Surg* 104:314–318, 1985.

114. Linde F, Anderson E, Hvass I, et al: Avascular femoral head necrosis following fracture fixation. *Injury* 17:159–163, 1986.

115. Banks HH: Nonunion in fractures of the femoral neck. *Orthop Clin North Am* 5:865–885, 1974.

116. Arnold WD: The effect of early weight-bearing on the stability of femoral neck fractures treated with Knowles pins. *J Bone Joint Surg* 66A:847–852, 1984.

117. Cassebaum WH, Nugent G: The predictability of bony union in displaced intracapsular fractures of the hip. *J Trauma* 3:421–424, 1963.

118. Manniger J, Kazar G, Gekete G, et al: Avoidance of avascular necrosis of the femoral head following fractures of the femoral neck by early reduction and internal fixation. *Injury* 16:437–448, 1985.

119. Anderson LD, Hamsa WR, Waring TL: Femoral-head prosthesis. *J Bone Joint Surg* 46:1049–1065, 1964.

120. Chan RN, Hoskinson J: Thompson prosthesis for fractured neck of the femur. *J Bone Joint Surg* 57B:437–443, 1975.

121. Hinchey JJ, Day PL: Primary prosthetic replacement in fresh femoral neck fractures. *J Bone Joint Surg* 46A:223–240, 1964.

122. Bochner RM, Pellicci PM, Lyden JP: Bipolar hemiarthroplasty for fracture of the femoral neck: Clinical review with special emphasis on prosthetic motion. *J Bone Joint Surg* 70A:1001–1010, 1988.

123. Johnston CE, Ripley LP, Bray CB: Primary endoprosthetic replacement for acute femoral neck fractures. *Clin Orthop* 167:123–130, 1982.

124. Lunt HRW: The role of prosthetic replacement of the head of the femur as primary treatment for subcapital fractures. *Injury* 3:107–110, 1971.

125. Yamagata M, Chao E, Illstrup D, et al: Fixed-head and bipolar hip endoprosthesis. *J Arthrop* 2:327–341, 1987.

126. Hunter GA: A comparison of the use of internal fixation and prosthetic replacement for fresh fractures of the neck or the femur. *Br J Surg* 56:229–232, 1969.

127. Wood MR: Femoral head replacement following fracture: An analysis of the surgical approach. *Injury* 11:317–320, 1979–1980.

128. Testa NN, Mazur K: Heterotopic ossification after direct lateral approach and transtrochanteric approach to the hip. *Orthop Rev* 18:965–971, 1988.

129. Schon L, Zuckerman JD: Hip pain in the elderly: Evaluation and diagnosis. *Geriatrics* 43:48–62, 1988.

130. Melton LJ, Ilstrup DM, Riggs BL, Beckenbaugh RP: Fifty year trend in hip fracture incidence. *Clin Orthop* 162:144–149, 1982.

131. Miller CW: Survival and ambulation following hip fracture. *J Bone Joint Surg* 60A:930–934, 1978.

132. Dias JJ, Robbings JA, Steingold RF, Donaldson LJ: Subcapital vs intertrochanteric fracture of the neck of the femur: Are there two distinct subpopulations? *J R Coll Surg* 32:303–305, 1987.

133. Koval KJ, Ahronoff G, Rokito A, Zuckerman JD: Femoral neck and intertrochanteric hip fracture patients: Is there a difference? *Clin Orthop.* In press.

134. Lizaur-Utrilla A, Orts AP, Del Campo FS, et al: Epidemiology of trochanteric fractures of the femur in Alicante, Spain 1974–1982. *Clin Orthop* 218:24–31, 1987.

135. Hedlund R, Lindgren U: Trauma type, age and gender as determinants of hip fractures. *J Orthop Res* 5:242–246, 1987.

136. Evans EM: The treatment of trochanteric fractures of the femur. *J Bone Joint Surg* 31B:190–203, 1949.

137. Jensen JS: Trochanteric fractures. *Acta Orthop Scand Suppl* 188:1, 1981.

138. Jensen JS: Classification of trochanteric fractures. *Acta Orthop Scand* 51:949, 1980.

139. Mulholland RC, Gunn DR: Sliding screw plate fixation of intertrochanteric femoral fractures. *J Trauma* 12:581–591, 1972.

140. Wolfgang GL, Bryant MH, O'Neill JP: Treatment of intertrochanteric fracture of the femur using sliding screw plate fixation. *Clin Orthop* 163:148–158, 1982.

141. Meislin RJ, Zuckerman JD, Kummer FJ, Frankel VH: A biochemical analysis of the sliding hip screw: The question of plate angle. Presented at the 1989 Meeting of the American Association of Orthopaedic Surgeons, Las Vegas, February 11, 1989.

142. Dimon JH, Hughston JC: Unstable inter-trochanteric fractures of the hip. *J Bone Joint Surg* 49A:440–450, 1967.

143. Chang W, Zuckerman J, Kummer F, Frankel V: Biomechanical evaluation of anatomic reduction versus medial displacement osteotomy in unstable intertrochanteric fractures. *Clin Orthop* 225:141–146, 1987.

144. Hopkins CT, Nugent JT, Dimon JH: Medial displacement osteotomy for unstable intertrochanteric fractures—Twenty years later. Presented at Annual Meeting of American Academy of Orthopaedic Surgeons, Atlanta, February, 1988.

145. Hofeldt F: Proximal femoral fractures. *Clin Orthop* 218:12–18, 1987.

146. Rao JP, Banzon MT, Weiss AB, Rayhack V: Treatment of unstable untertrochanteric fractures with anatomic reduction and compression hip screw fixation. *Clin Orthop* 175:65, 1983.

147. Gross A, Taglony G: A new device for treatment of trochanteric fractures—The intramediallary gamma locking nail. Presented at the annual meeting of the American Association of Orthopaedic Surgeons, New Orleans, February 10, 1990.

148. Mohamed W, Kellam J, Harrington I, et al: Biomechanical comparison of the gamma nail and sliding hip screw. Presented at the 6th annual meeting of the Orthopaedic Trauma Association, Toronto, November 9, 1990.

149. Bridle SH, Patel AD, Bircher M, et al: Fixation of intertrochanteric fractures of the femur: A randomized prospective comparison of the gamma nail and the dynamic hip screw. *J Bone Joint Surg* 73B:330–334, 1991.

150. Baker HR: Ununited intertrochanteric fractures of the femur. *Clin Orthop* 18:209–220, 1960.

151. Boyd HB, Lipinski SW: Nonunion of trochanteric and subtrochanteric fractures. *Surg Gynecol Obstet* 104:463–470, 1957.

152. Knight WM, DeLee JC: Nonunion of intertrochanteric fractures of the hip: A case study and review. *Orthop Trans* 16:438, 1982.

153. Boyd HB, Griffing LL: Classification and treatment of trochanteric fractures. *Arch Surg* 58:853–866, 1949.

154. Hunter GA: The Results of operative treatment of trochanteric fractures of the femur. *Injury* 6:202–205, 1974–1975.

155. Kyle RF, Gustilo RB, Premer RF: Analysis of 622 intertrochanteric hip fractures: A retrospective study. *J Bone Joint Surg* 61A:216–221, 1979.

156. Mariani EM, Rand JA: Nonunion of intertrochanteric fractures of the femur following open reduction and internal fixation. *Clin Orthop* 218:81–89, 1987.

157. Wilson HJ, Rubin BD, Helbig FEJ, et al: Treatment of intertrochanteric fractures with Jewett nail: Experience with 1,015 cases. *Clin Orthop* 148:186–191, 1980.

158. Bergman G, Winquist R, Mayo K, Hansen S: Subtrochanteric fracture of the femur: Fixation using the Zickel nail. *J Bone Joint Surg* 69A:1032–1040, 1987.

159. Sangeorzan BJ, Ryan JR, Salciccroli GG: Prophylactic femoral stabilization with the Zickel nail by closed technique. *J Bone Joint Surg* 68A:991–999, 1986.

160. Schatzker J and Waddell JP: Subtrochanteric fractures of the femur. *Orthop Clin North Am* 11:539–554, 1980.

161. Fielding JW, Magliato HJ: Subtrochanteric fractures. *Surg Gynecol Obstet* 122:555–560, 1966.

162. Muller ME, Allgower M, Willeneger H: *Manual of Internal Fixation.* New York, Springer-Verlag, 1970.

163. Seinsheimer F: Subtrochanteric fractures of the femur. *J Bone Joint Surg* 60A:300–306, 1978.

164. Garden RS: Reduction and fixation of the subcapital fractures of the femur. *Orthop Clin North Am* 5:683–712, 1974.

165. Beaver RH, Bach PJ: Zickel nail: A retrospective study of subtrochanteric fractures. *South Med J* 71:146–149, 1978.

166. Davis AD, Meyer RD, Miller ME, Killian JT: Closed Zickel nailing. *Clin Orthop* 201:138–146, 1985.

167. Mullen JO, Tranovich M: A simplified technique for Zickel nail insertion. *Clin Orthop* 208:195–198, 1986.

168. Taylor GM, Neufield AJ, Nickel VL: Complications and failures in the operative treatment of intertrochanteric fractures of the femur. *J Bone Joint Surg* 37A:306–316, 1955.

169. Zickel RE: A new fixation device for subtrochanteric fractures of the femur. *Clin Orthop* 54:115–123, 1967.

170. Browner BD, Cole JD: Current status of locked intramedullary nailing: A review. *J Orthop Trauma* 1:183–195, 1987.

171. Kempf I, Gross A, Beck G: Closed locked intra-medullary nailing. *J Bone Joint Surg* 67A:709–720, 1985.

172. Tenser AF, Johnson JD, Johnston WC, Gill A: A biomechanical comparison of various methods of stabilization of subtrochanteric fractures of the femur. *J Orthop Res* 2:297–305, 1984.

173. Wiss DA, Fleming CH, Matta J, Clark D: Commuted and rotationally unstable fractures of the femur treated with an interlocking nail. *Clin Orthop* 212:35–47, 1986.

174. Berman AT, Metzger PC, Bosaco SJ, et al: Treatment of the subtrochanteric fracture with the compression hip nail: A review of thirty-eight consecutive cases. *Orthop Trans* 3:255–256, 1979.

175. DiStefano VJ, Nixon JE, Klein KS: Stable fixation of the difficult subtrochanteric fracture. *J Trauma* 12:1066–1070, 1972.

176. Ruff M, Lubbers L: Treatment of subtrochanteric fractures with a sliding screw-plate device. *J Trauma* 26:75–80 1986.

177. Waddell JP: Femoral head preservation following subcapital fracture of the femur. *AAOS Instr Course Lect* 33:179–190, 1984.

178. Hogh J: Sliding screw in the treatment of trochanteric fractures. *Injury* 14:141, 1982.

179. Kyle RF, Wright TM, Burstein AH: Biomechanical analysis of the sliding characteristics of compression hip screws. *J Bone Joint Surg* 62A:1308–1314, 1980.

180. Waddell JP: Sliding screw fixation for proximal femoral fractures. *Orthop Clin North Am* 11:607–622, 1980.

181. Leung KS, So WS, Shen WY, Hui PW: Gamma nails and dynamic hip screws for peritrochanteric fractures. *J Bone Joint Surg* 74B:345–351, 1992.

182. Kinast C, Bolhofner BR, Mast JW, Ganz R: Subtrochanteric fractures of the femur: Results of treatment with the 95 degree condylar blade plate. *Clin Orthop* 238:122–130, 1989.

CHAPTER 27

Femoral Shaft Fractures

Stephen A. Kottmeier

Fractures of the femoral shaft may occur as a result of high- or low-energy trauma. Additionally, repetitive microtrauma, metabolic disturbance, and neoplastic lesions may compromise osseous integrity, resulting in fracture of the femoral diaphysis.[1–6] Fractures of the femoral shaft in young adults are often the result of high-energy vehicular injury or falls from heights. In such cases, the resultant force is frequently responsible for additional life-threatening injury. Regardless of etiology, the desired outcome is uneventful union of the fracture with preservation of limb alignment, length, rotation, normal hip and knee motion, and, ultimately, satisfactory limb function. These goals must be attained in a fashion that does not compromise the well-being of the patient and ideally in a manner limiting hospitalization and, accordingly, cost of care.

Deformity, shortening, and tenderness to the midthigh region herald the likely presence of a femoral shaft fracture. In the event of labile vital signs, sources of hemorrhage other than the fracture should be investigated. A closed femoral shaft fracture alone or in combination with other minor injuries is an unlikely source of hypotensive shock.[7] Other potentially life-threatening injuries must be identified. Physical examination of the traumatized limb follows a thorough primary survey. The neurovascular and soft tissue envelope status of the extremity are next determined.

Radiographic evaluation of a suspected femoral shaft fracture is initiated with performance of full-length anteroposterior (AP) and lateral views of the entire femur. A pelvis film is reviewed to exclude pelvic ring injury as well as acetabular and proximal femoral lesions. An internal rotation view of the hip is obtained if a femoral neck fracture is suspected but cannot be confirmed with preliminary studies. Quality views of the "joint above and below" must be obtained to identify intraarticular fracture patterns. A full-length radiograph of the contralateral intact femur serves to define femoral length and the dimensions of the medullary canal.

When managing a femoral shaft fracture in a polytraumatized individual, the orthopedic surgeon's role is not simply relegated to that of a peripheral consultant. Early and appropriate management of long-bone fractures has a direct and positive impact on the patient's survival and hospital course. Numerous studies have convincingly demonstrated the physiologic benefits of early operative stabilization of long-bone fractures in multiply injured patients.[8–17] Adherence to this principle dramatically reduces the need for ventilatory support, pulmonary complications (adult respiratory distress syndrome, fat embolism), incidence of multisystem organ failure, hospitalization, and expense of medical care. It greatly facilitates nursing care and mobilization, thereby reducing complications associated with prolonged recumbency. The previously held notion that delay in fracture treatment accelerates union is no longer valid and of obvious detriment in this population.[18–21]

Fractures of the femoral shaft can be described by location and morphologic characteristics. Those patterns involving either end of the shaft have, in the past, been problematic owing to widening within the region of the metaphysis and deforming muscular forces. Newer techniques and implants have made fracture location less of a concern. The classification scheme of Winquist and Hansen emphasizes the importance of comminution and its impact of preferential treatment (Fig. 27-1).[22]

TREATMENT

Nonoperative Treatment

Although nonoperative treatment of femoral shaft fractures utilizing traction and cast-brace techniques may lead to predictable fracture union, this goal alone is inadequate. Limb shortening, angulation, and prolonged hospitalization with such management are not infrequent and are understandably displeasing to the patient. Few indications remain for this method of treatment. In the past, it was employed to treat fractures deemed too comminuted to be satisfactorily managed with conventional intramedullary nailing. Nonoperative methods were instead used as definitive treatment for such injuries or as an adjunct form of therapy to maintain limb length after conventional intramedullary (IM) fixation. In an effort to allow knee motion and patient mobilization, roller traction and early cast-brace application techniques emerged.[23–27] Skeletal traction was exerted through a proximal tibial pin if knee ligaments were intact. Femoral skeletal traction was discouraged if delayed conversion to IM fixation was considered to avoid violation of the canal. At present, its remaining role is one of provisional stabilization for isolated open fractures requiring serial debridement prior to definitive fixation.

Intramedullary Fixation

At present, the standard of treatment for most femoral shaft fractures is IM fixation.[28–33] Location within the IM canal is biomechanically advantageous as compared with the eccentric location of a plate. Bending moment experienced by the implant is diminished and a load-sharing role assumed. In contrast to rigid interfragmentary plate fixation, bony union is accomplished indirectly by initial formation of external callus (Fig. 27-2). This is followed by the ultimate conversion of woven bone into mature lamellar bone.

Antegrade Nailing

Kuntscher introduced the modern-day concept of closed conventional antegrade IM nailing in the early 1940s.[34,35]

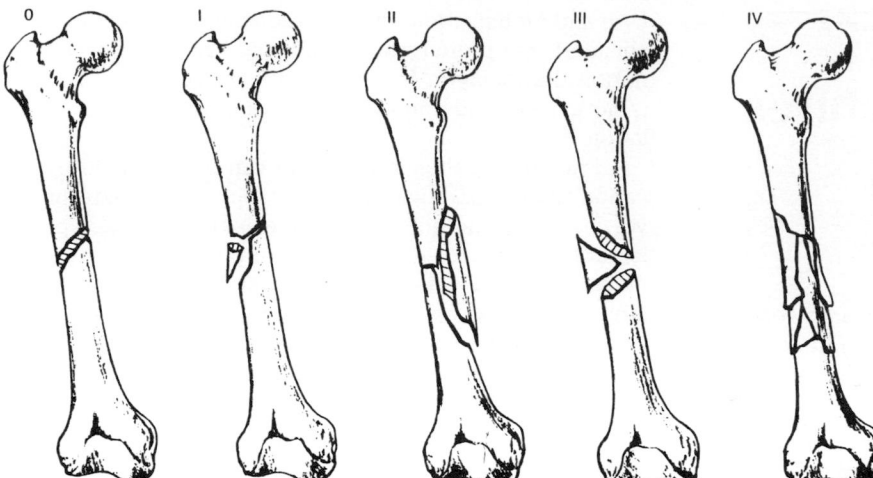

Figure 27-1 Winquist classification of femoral shaft fracture comminution: 0 = no comminution; I = small butterfly; II = 50 percent or more cortical contact remaining; III = less than 50 percent cortical contact remaining; IV = segmental comminution with no cortical contact. (Reproduced with permission from Hansen ST Jr: Femoral shaft fractures, in Hansen ST Jr, Swiontowski MF (eds): *Orthopaedic Trauma Protocols.* New York, Raven Press, 1993, pp 279–290.

Structural limitations of nail design and metallurgy at the time required the insertion of a large-diameter implant to diminish the risk of implant failure. This was accomplished by increasing the internal dimension of the femoral endosteal canal by sequential reaming and inserting the nail through a greater trochanteric starting portal. This portal location, in preference to a more medial one, was selected

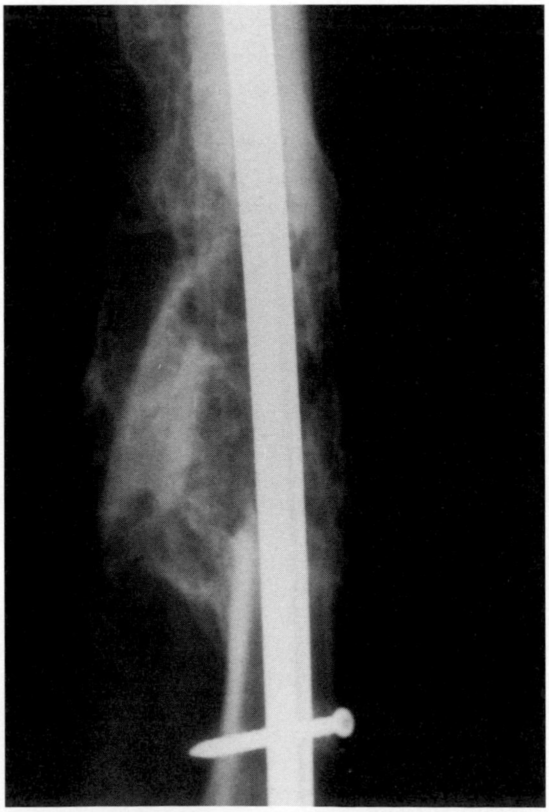

Figure 27-2 Intramedullary stabilization of a femoral shaft fracture with exuberant callus formation (indirect fracture healing).

to avoid intraarticular penetration and potential complications as a result (joint sepsis and avascular necrosis). Direct fracture-site exposure (open nailing) was discouraged so as to preserve fracture hematoma as well as endosteal and periosteal blood supply. These were thought to contribute significantly to fracture union. Earlier indications for this technique were, ideally, limited to simple fracture patterns unlikely to shorten or rotate in the postoperative period. The wide canal of the infraisthmal region did not allow adequate fill with the nail, which contributed to malreduction. This fracture pattern, in addition to comminuted variants, was considered a relative contraindication to this procedure (Fig. 27-3). Alternative forms of treatment, including plate fixation, were accordingly pursued. Expanding the range of fractures managed with conventional IM nailing required the use of adjuvant modalities including traction, external immobilization, and open cerclage of fragments to enhance mechanical stability.[36] Many of the attributes of closed IM stabilization were thus forsaken.

Recent trends in nailing techniques and nail design have evolved in response to a need for improved performance of the device and to manage more complicated fractures and more severely injured patients more effectively. Interlocking nails were developed in response to this demand.[37–45]

Nail Design

The addition of screws in both the proximal and distal limits of the rod expanded indications for IM nailing to include unstable patterns from the lesser trochanter to the supracondylar region. This construct afforded control of both length and rotation. Previous complications encountered with open cerclage techniques, including infection and delayed union, were averted by closed methods of interlocking nailing.[46] Increased forces experienced by these devices in the presence of fracture comminution required changes in design to prevent mechanical failure of the device.[47–50]

Stronger implants, less vulnerable to fatigue failure, were desired. Elimination of a vertical slot (closed-section design) greatly increased torsional rigidity of nails (Fig. 27-4).[51] Wall

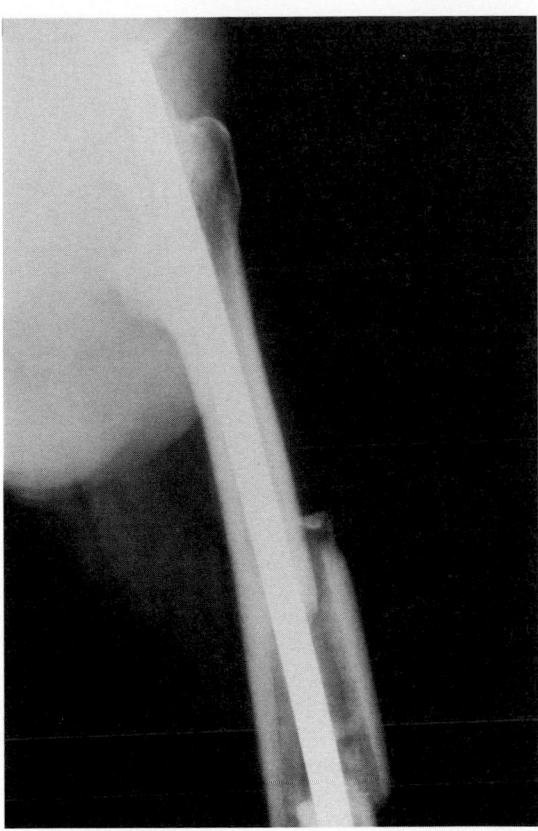

Figure 27-3 Conventional (noninterlocking) intramedullary stabilization of an unstable fracture pattern resulting in limb shortening, with "telescoping" of the implant.

thickness has been increased in some smaller-diameter designs to maintain implant bending properties. Stiffer, smaller-diameter implants with improved resistance to fatigue failure prompted reevaluation of the role of reaming in IM fixation. Increased potential for iatrogenic comminution with insertion of these stiff devices has been recognized as well. Changes in material, including introduction of titanium implants, have introduced another variable in nail design. The intention, with such changes in metallurgy, is to preserve implant flexibility without sacrificing strength. The clinical consequences of some features of nail design modification are as yet uncertain. The contribution of interlocking design is, however, immediately apparent.

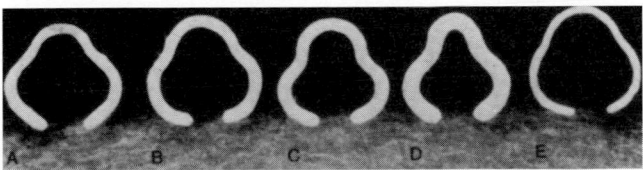

Figure 27-4 Cross section of nails from five different manufacturers. (Reproduced with permission from Johnson KD, Tencer AF, Sherman MC: Biomechanical factors affecting fracture stability and femoral bursting in closed intramedullary nailing of femoral shaft fractures, with illustrative case presentations. *J Orthop Trauma* 1:1–11, 1987.)

Nail Insertion

Operative positioning of the patient for antegrade nailing is dependent upon the presence of associated injury. The supine position is more physiologic and preferred in patients with compromised lung function or axial skeletal injuries. Difficulties encountered with this setup include entry portal access, pudendal nerve palsy,[52,53] and internal rotational deformity. Reduction is facilitated by use of a fracture table, manual traction,[54] and intra-[55,56] or extramedullary devices.[57]

The lateral position allows improved access to the piriformis fossa (nail entry portal). It is reserved for patients with isolated fractures of the femur who are more physiologically tolerant of this position and without contralateral limb injury. A tendency toward external rotational deformity and valgus reduction in infraisthmal fractures must be anticipated and maneuvers executed to prevent malreduction.

According to Winquist, successful closed reduction and entry portal location are the two most important steps in antegrade IM nailing.[58] The piriformis fossa aligns with the longitudinal axis of the medullary canal and is identified with biplanar fluoroscopic control (Fig. 27-5). Excessive anterior positioning of the entry portal results in increased circumferential strain (hoop stress) with nail impaction.[59] This can result in cortical expansion and ultimately bursting of the proximal fragment. A starting portal concentric to the IM canal will allow unresisted insertion of the implant, decreasing the likelihood of iatrogenic comminution. A guide wire is next passed with fluoroscopic assistance and reduction methods and aids as needed.

As mentioned previously, reaming of the IM canal serves several purposes. In the past, the surgical ambition was to insert the largest-diameter implant possible to prevent nail deformation. Additionally, reaming was felt to enhance endosteal contact of the implant, contributing toward stability of fixation. Currently available interlocking nails are inherently stronger and their locking capability eliminates the need for endosteal contact. Studies have demonstrated temporary disturbance to endosteal blood supply with passage of implants and reamers.[60,61] This, however, is readily reconstituted and its temporary absence does not appear to impede formation of external callus. Of current concern are the potentially deleterious effects of reaming in the patient with marginal pulmonary reserve.[62–64] Embolization of fat and marrow contents has been observed.[65,66] The consequences of this, however, have yet to be determined. Presently, reamed interlocking nailing remains the standard of care both for patients with isolated fractures and in the multiply injured. Upon accessing the femoral medullary canal proximally and completion of reaming (if elected), impaction of the nail over a guide wire is performed.

Insertion of screws proximally and distally within an IM nail is termed *static locking*. This mode of fixation imparts rotational and longitudinal stability to the construct (Fig. 27-6). In contrast to dynamic nailing (locking the nail at one end only), load transference through the fracture site though not eliminated, is decreased. It was initially felt that assuming increased load within the device with static

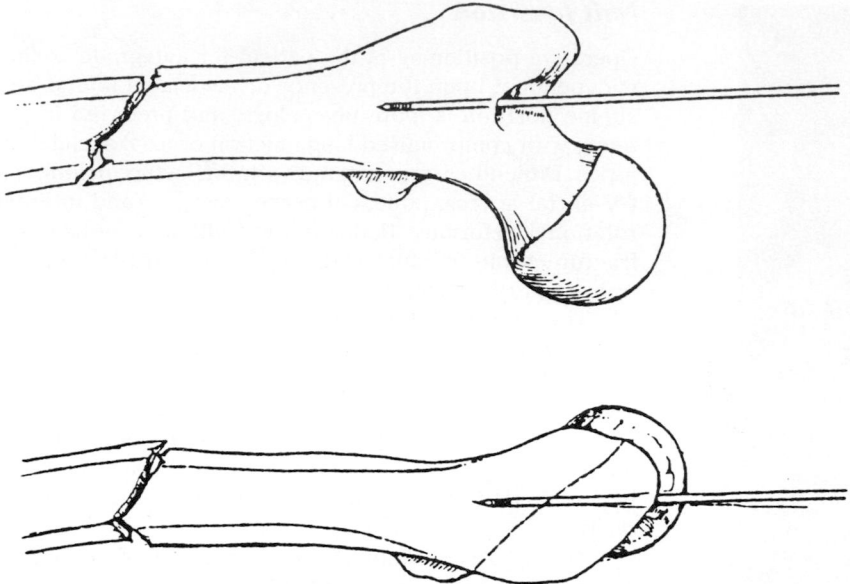

Figure 27-5 The piriformis entry site should align with the medullary canal. (Reproduced with permission from Winquist RA: Locked femoral nailing. *J Am Orthop Surg* 1:95–105, 1993.)

locking would lead to hardware failure and poor consolidation of fracture callus. Dynamization (delayed removal of screws from one end of the nail), after a period of time, was accordingly recommended to remedy these concerns. These complications have, however, been clinically inapparent. Routine static nailing is therefore currently recommended for most acute femoral diaphyseal fracture patterns.[38] Satisfactory union without routine dynamization has been observed in 98 percent of cases.[67] The insertion of a single screw distally appears to be clinically and biomechanically sufficient.[68] However, two screws are recommended in distal fracture patterns requiring sagittal plane stability.

Complications associated with antegrade femoral nailing include iatrogenic comminution and, rarely, femoral neck fracture.[69] IM sepsis, a rare complication, is more common with open techniques involving direct fracture site exposure.[70,71] Malunion is effectively prevented by static interlocking with accurate initial reduction. Implant failure often but not always accompanies nonunion.[72] Both are observed less frequently due to refined methodology and improved implants.[73–75] Heterotopic ossification at

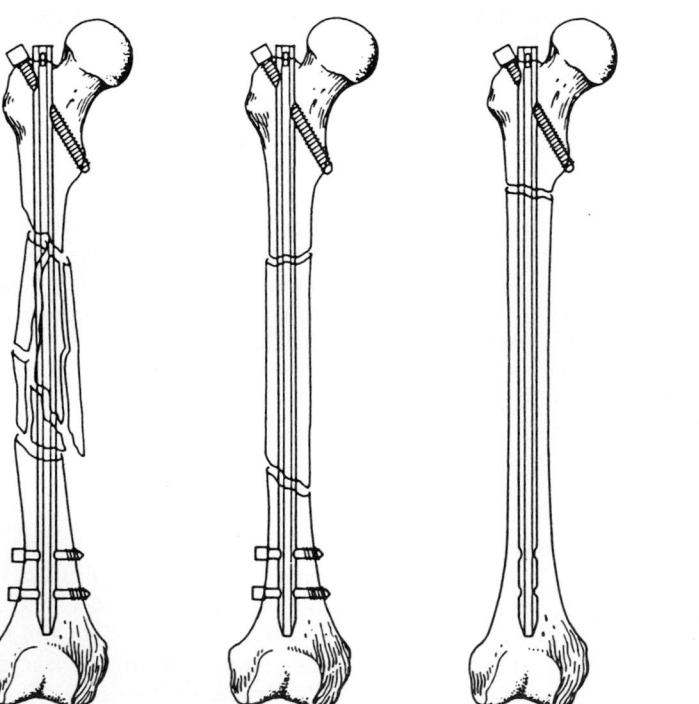
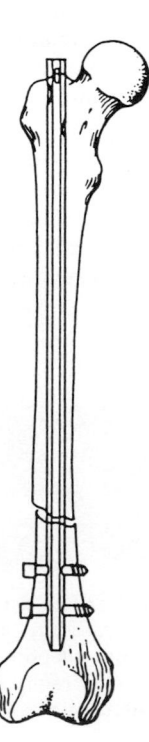

Figure 27-6 Interlocking nailing of femoral shaft fractures—static in comminuted and segmental fractures, dynamic in noncomminuted proximal and distal fractures. (Reproduced with permission from Klemm KW, Borner M: Interlocking nailing of complex fractures of the femur and tibia. *Clin Orthop Rel Res* 212:89–100, 1986.)

the nail insertion site has been described, though functional impairment is uncommon.[76,77]

Retrograde Nailing

Stabilization of IM femoral shaft fractures can be accomplished in retrograde fashion with a variety of implants. Insertion of small-diameter, solid, flexible nails through distal epicondylar portals has been advocated by some investigators.[78–81] They suggest that with skill and small incisions, operative time and blood loss are less than with antegrade nailing. This, however, has not been the experience of others.[82] These devices by themselves will not suffice to manage highly comminuted fractures. Structural inferiority and inability to perform static locking limit current indications for this technique. This method of fracture fixation may prove useful in stabilizing noncomminuted patterns, small canals, fractures below an uncemented prosthesis, and diaphyseal fractures with ipsilateral femoral neck fracture as well as shaft fractures requiring IM stabilization in the skeletally immature with open epiphyseal plates.

Large-diameter devices requiring reaming prior to insertion can also be introduced through the nonarticular portion of the medial femoral condyle[83] or intercondylar notch ("transgenicular" insertion). Interlocking capability extends the indications for this technique beyond those of flexible devices. It is perhaps most appropriately indicated for shaft fractures with coincident fracture of the ipsilateral femoral neck or tibial diaphysis.

Plate Fixation

Several decades ago, IM fixation was reserved by many for those fractures with stable patterns (transverse, short oblique) and was avoided in many instances in infraisthmal fractures. Concern over malreduction and inability to control length and rotation of these patterns prompted use of alternative forms of fixation. Attempts to restore mechanical stability with combined open cerclage generated mixed results. Infection and delayed union were thought to arise as a result of compromised endosteal and periosteal blood supplies. In view of these concerns with IM fixation, plate osteosynthesis remained a popular alternative.[84–87] However, extensive surgical exposure and fracture fragment devitalization associated with plate fixation increased rates of infection and nonunion as well.[88,89] Eccentric location of a plate, unlike an IM device, does not permit load sharing. Weight-bearing restriction and external support were often required in addition to application of medial bone graft to promote union and diminish risk of implant and fixation failure.[90] Bridge-plate osteosynthesis, a form of indirect reduction, has been offered as a means of biological fracture stabilization.[91] This technique emphasizes preservation of osseous fragment viability by limiting stripping and retraction of soft tissues. The soft tissue envelope and physiologic mechanisms of fracture repair are thus preserved.

Present-day indications for plate fixation of the femoral shaft are limited. Interest in this form of fixation has been renewed by concern over the potentially adverse effects of medullary reaming in the traumatized individual with poor pulmonary function.[92] In this setting, plate fixation can fulfill the goals of patient mobilization as well as skeletal and soft tissue stability. Additional (relative) indications include ipsilateral fracture of the femoral neck and vascular injury requiring repair.

External Fixation

There are few remaining indications for external fixation of femoral shaft fractures. Prior to the availability of interlocking nails, it served to secure highly comminuted fractures not amenable to conventional nailing.[93–97] In the event of life- or limb-threatening circumstances, external fixation can be applied expeditiously, providing immediate stability.[98,99] Currently, it is regarded more as a temporizing device to assist in stabilizing dysvascular, extensively contaminated, or infected limbs.[100] Delayed conversion to intramedullary fixation can be considered with caution and only with appropriate measures to prevent intramedullary sepsis. Complications encountered with external fixation of femoral shaft fractures include pin-tract infection, malunion, nonunion, and significant risk of restricted knee motion.

TREATMENT CONCERNS

Open Fractures

The abundant circumferential soft tissue of the thigh accounts for the relative infrequency of open fractures to this region. Consequently, severe high-energy injury is required to cause such a lesion. An open femur fracture in a traumatized patient is therefore frequently associated with additional multiple-system injury. The extensive insult to the soft tissue envelope by itself would tend to contraindicate immediate aggressive operative fixation. Mobilization of the polytraumatized individual is, however, of paramount importance, and immediate skeletal fixation is therefore necessary. Reamed IM fixation, as previously described, is the current standard of care for most closed femoral diaphyseal fractures. If not for increased risk of osseous sepsis, the benefits afforded by it in managing closed injuries could be extended to open fractures. Theoretically, endosteal reaming may further devascularize a segment of bone devoid of periosteal attachment, as is commonly seen with open fractures. Embolization of marrow elements with reaming may be cause for concern as well. The role of unreamed femoral nails in this setting has yet to be conclusively defined. Several studies performed at major trauma centers have demonstrated the safety and efficacy of reamed femoral IM fixation in the treatment of Gustilo grade I and II open fractures of the femur.[101–103] Lhowe suggests immediate stabilization of grade I, II, and IIIA open femur fractures with reamed IM fixation (Fig. 27-7).[104] His recommendation in treating grade IIIB injuries is based upon the patient's status. Reamed nailing is encouraged for those patients requiring immediate mobilization. Traction therapy

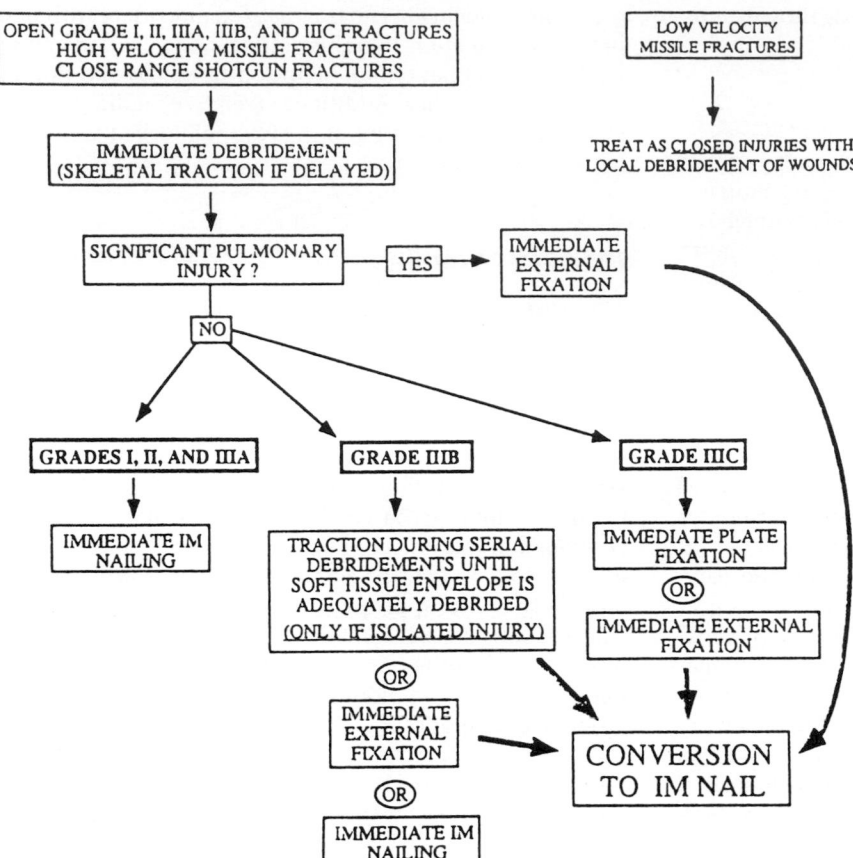

Figure 27-7 Treatment algorithm for open femoral shaft fractures. (Reproduced with permission from Lhowe DW: Open fractures of the femoral shaft. *Orthop Clin North Am* 25:573–580, 1994.)

following operative debridement may initiate fracture treatment in cases presenting with grossly contaminated wounds if the patient is not multiply injured. Delayed definitive treatment is performed when the soft tissue status allows. Similar injuries in severely injured patients should be managed with external fixation. If, later, the pin tracts and soft tissues permit, internal fixation may be executed. Green and Trafton concluded that "immediate internal fixation of type III femoral fractures is only relatively indicated and must be applied with caution."[105] They treated these injuries at different time intervals and with an assortment of devices. The use of internal fixation in cases presenting with severe traumatic wounds was associated with a greater rate of deep infection.

Arterial Injury

Rosenthal observed a 2 percent incidence of arterial injury with femoral fractures secondary to blunt trauma.[106] The association of these two injuries is greater with penetrating trauma. Little argument exists regarding the necessity for operative stabilization of the limb. What remains controversial, however, is the sequence of events and preferred method of fixation.

Injury to the superficial femoral artery occurring as a result of blunt trauma occurs most commonly at the level of the adductor hiatus, where arterial mobility is least (Fig.

27-8). Arterial injury may exist in the absence of clinical signs of ischemia (absent peripheral pulses, cyanosis, pallor, poor capillary refill, decreased peripheral temperature). Penetrating lesions neighboring the vessels should be assessed with proximity angiography if pulses are present and with immediate exploration of the vessels if not. The indications for arteriography in assessing injuries arising as a result of blunt trauma are not as clear. Suspicion of arterial insufficiency associated with distal femoral diaphyseal fractures warrants arteriographic study. Patients with these fracture patterns should be observed frequently to identify intimal lesions that may result in subsequent arterial occlusion. Noninvasive vascular testing (Doppler arterial pressure index) has been reported to reliably exclude such occult arterial trauma in traumatized extremities.[107]

The treatment of arterial injury associated with femoral shaft fracture is determined by ischemic time and the skills of the surgical team. Fracture stabilization may precede arterial repair if performed expeditiously.[108] Delay in presentation or an ischemic time approximating 6 h requires immediate reestablishment of arterial supply. A plate, applied either medially or laterally, or the application of an external fixator is most reliable in executing this, the first phase of limb salvage. Antegrade IM fixation remains an option, though patient position and preparation often disallow this. Retrograde IM fixation has been advocated, since the majority of femoral fractures associated with vascular interruption following blunt trauma are distal in location.[109]

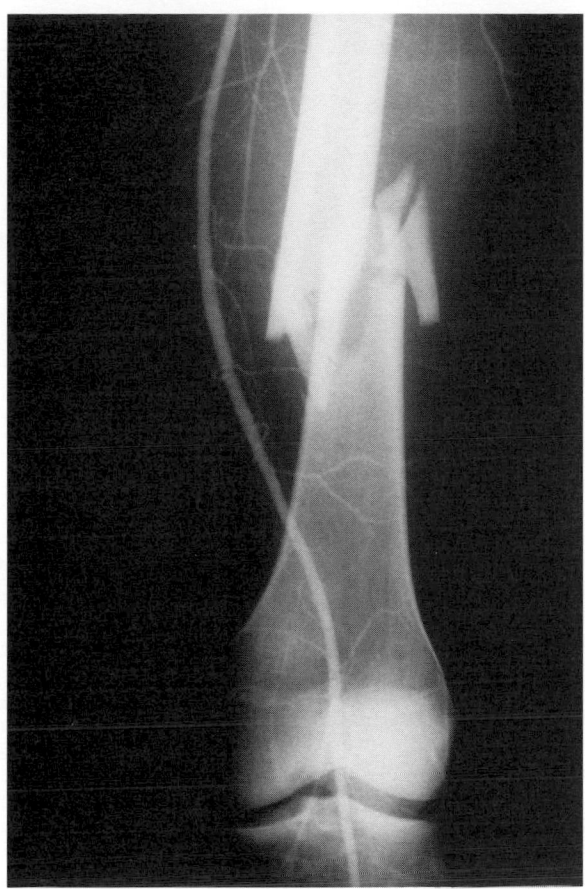

Figure 27-8 Vascular injury associated with femoral shaft fractures occurs most often with distal fracture patterns. The artery in the region of the adductor hiatus is tethered and immobile.

Associated Fractures

The extreme energy required to fracture the femur is often responsible for generating additional osseous injury within the same limb. Of particular concern are ipsilateral fractures of the femoral neck.[110–117] This injury is frequently unappreciated upon initial review of radiographic studies (Fig. 27-9). "Missed" femoral neck fracture can result in delayed treatment and suboptimal treatment. An internal rotation radiograph will most reliably reveal this fracture, which is commonly semivertical and basicervical in character. The femoral shaft fracture is typically located in the middiaphyseal region. In treating this combined injury, priority must be extended to the femoral neck fracture. This is because treatment failure options for the shaft are predictable and straightforward, whereas those for the femoral neck are not. Fixation schemes to address this combined injury pattern involve the use of either a single device or dual devices to manage both fractures. Examples of the former include second-generation "reconstruction" nails or a long side plate and compression screw. Dual-device fixation employs multiple-screw fixation to address the femoral neck fracture and a rod (ante- or retrograde) or compression plate (Fig. 27-10) to manage the shaft fracture. The sur-

geon must prioritize the efforts made to achieve successful fixation of the femoral neck fracture. Acceptable options exist to resolve femoral shaft malunion and nonunion. Avascular necrosis, however, in the young patient, is indeed unfortunate and without predictable remedy.

Ipsilateral fracture of the femoral and tibial shafts ("floating knee") results from high-energy injury. Frequent association with compromised skin integrity renders this a very limb threatening injury. Functional recovery of the limb is best achieved with early stabilization of both fractures, allowing immediate postoperative knee motion.[118–121] Reported studies recommend individualized treatment for each fracture. A more recent protocol describes single-incision retrograde and antegrade nailing for the femur and tibia respectively.

Gunshot Injuries

Diaphyseal fractures resulting from gunshot injuries are managed according to the degree of soft tissue destruc-

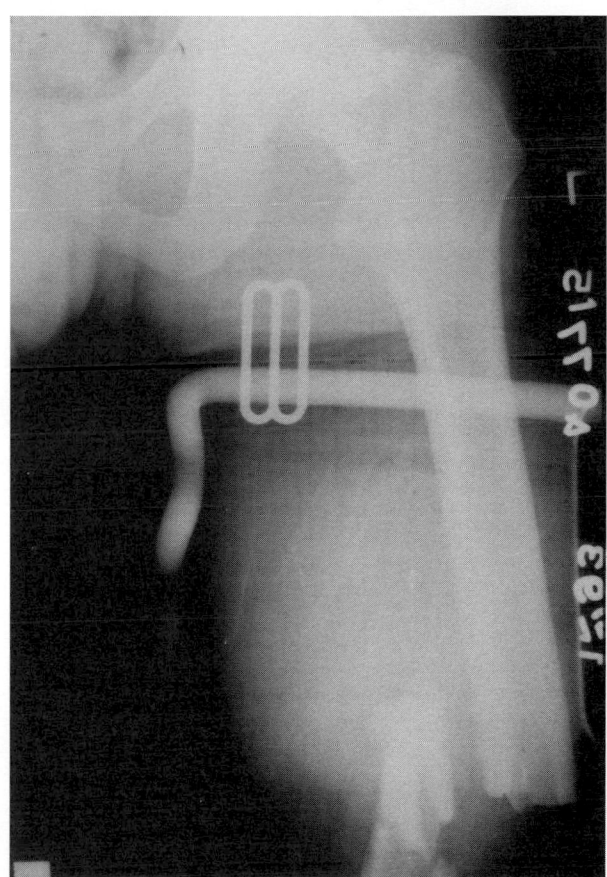

Figure 27-9 Ipsilateral femoral neck and shaft fracture. Identification of the femoral neck fracture requires a better-quality radiograph than that pictured. Repeat performance of the study with internal rotation and proper penetration is recommended if the lesion is suspected. The typical femoral neck fracture in this combined injury is basicervical and semivertical in orientation.

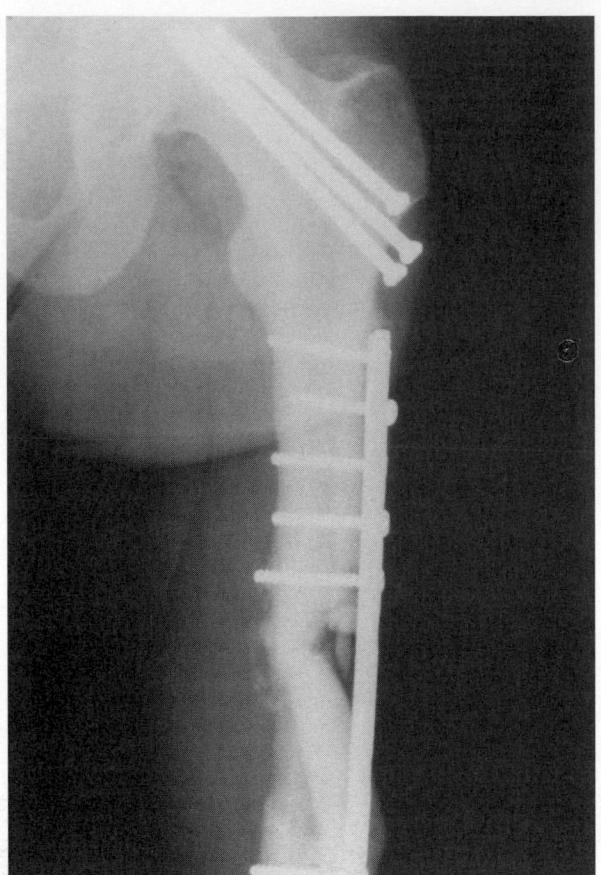

Figure 27-10 Dual device technique to manage an ipsilateral femoral neck-and-shaft fracture combination. Treatment of the femoral neck fracture receives priority.

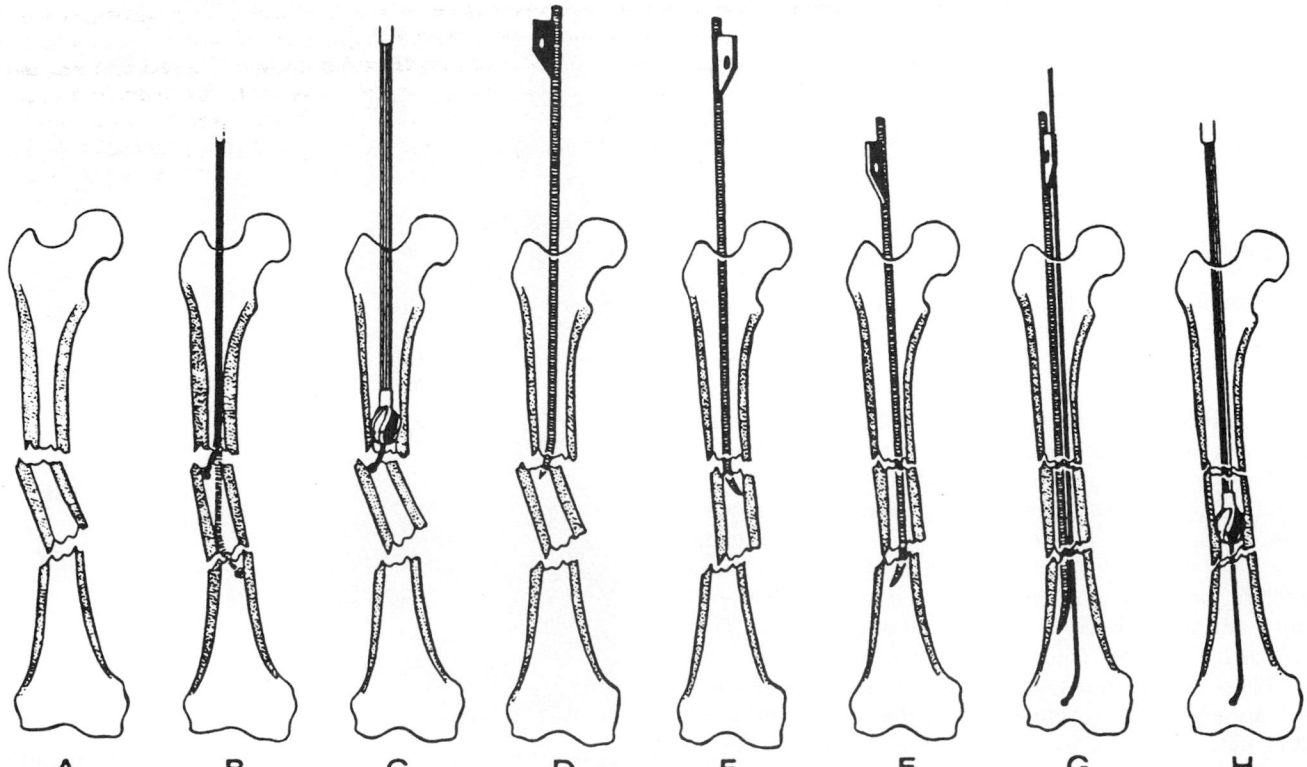

Figure 27-11 *A.* Sequential nailing of a segmental femoral fracture. *B.* Reduction is attempted with bulb-tipped guide. *C.* The diameter of the proximal part of the femoral canal is increased by reaming. *D.* Sharp-tipped guide is passed into middle fragment. *E.* Middle fragment is reduced with the guide. *F.* The guide is passed into the distal fragment. *G.* Bulb-tipped guide is inserted. *H.* Reamer is inserted. (Reproduced with permission from Hansen ST, Winquist RA: Closed intramedullary nailing of fractures of the femoral shaft: Part II. Technical considerations. *AAOS Instr Course Lect* 27:90–108, 1978.)

tion. In the past, low- to mid-velocity gunshot-induced fractures were fixated in delayed fashion in an effort to decrease risk of infection.[122] Several studies have demonstrated uncomplicated fracture union with immediate reamed nailing.[123-125] No detrimental effects were observed and health care costs were considerably reduced. High-velocity gunshot injuries are associated with extensive soft tissue destruction and demand a more conservative approach, initiated by aggressive wound debridement and provisional forms of stabilization or immobilization. Delayed definitive fixation is performed when the soft tissue environment is receptive.

Segmental Fractures

Like open fractures and those femoral fractures associated with ipsilateral fractures, segmental femoral fractures result from high-energy trauma. Intramedullary fixation for segmental fractures is favored over other forms of treatment.[126,127] Closed nailing allows introduction of a load-sharing device without significant surgical dissection or blood loss. It is a technically demanding procedure (Fig. 27-11). Reaming should be performed cautiously at the level of the intercalary fragment to prevent spinning and soft tissue detachment. A large-diameter implant is preferred for those patterns with distal diaphyseal extension to reduce risk of implant failure.[47]

REFERENCES

1. Arneson TJ, Melton LJ III, Lewallen DG, O'Fallon WM: Epidemiology of diaphyseal and distal femoral fractures in Rochester, Minnesota, 1965–1984. *Clin Orthop Rel Res* 234:188–194, 1988.
2. Breen JTF, Jones GS, Seligson D: Fractures of the femoral shaft in a regional hospital setting. *J Trauma* 23:483–487, 1983.
3. Hedlund R, Lindgren U: Epidemiology of diaphyseal femoral fracture. *Acta Orthop Scand* 57:423–427, 1986.
4. Luchini MA, Sarokhan AJ, Micheli LJ: Acute displaced femoral-shaft fractures in long-distance runners: Two case reports. *J Bone Joint Surg* 65A:689–691, 1983.
5. Milgrom C, Giladi M, Stein M, et al: Stress fractures in military recruits: A prospective study showing an unusually high incidence. *J Bone Joint Surg* 67B:732–735, 1985.
6. Spezia P, Brennan R, Brugman JL, Friermood TG: Femur fractures in Alpine skiers. *J Orthop Trauma* 6:443–447, 1992.
7. Ostrum RF, Verghese GB, Santner TJ: The lack of association between femoral shaft fractures and hypotensive shock. *J Orthop Trauma* 7:338–342, 1993.
8. Behrman SW, Fabian TC, Kudsk KA, Taylor JC: Improved outcome with femur fractures: Early vs delayed fixation. *J Trauma* 30:792–798, 1990.
9. Bone LB, Johnson KD, Weigelt J, Scheinberg R: Early versus delayed stabilization of femoral fractures: A prospective randomized study. *J Bone Joint Surg* 71A:336–340, 1989.
10. Browner BD, Burgess AR, Robertson RJ, et al: Immediate closed antegrade ender nailing of femoral fractures in polytrauma patients. *J Trauma* 24:921–925, 1984.
11. Goris RJA, Gimbrere JSF, van Niekerk JLM, et al: Early osteosynthesis and prophylactic mechanical ventilation in the multitrauma patient. *J Trauma* 22:895–903, 1982.
12. Johnson KD, Cadambi A, Seibert GB: Incidence of adult respiratory distress syndrome in patients with multiple musculoskeletal injuries: Effect of early operative stabilization of fractures. *J Trauma* 25:375–384, 1985.
13. Phillips TF, Contreras DM: Timing of operative treatment of fractures in patients who have multiple injuries. *J Bone Joint Surg* 72A:784–788, 1990.
14. Riska EB, von Bonsdorff H, Hakkinen S, et al: Prevention of fat embolism by early internal fixation of fractures in patients with multiple injuries. *Injury* 8:110–116, 1976.
15. Riska EB, von Bonsdorff H, Hakkinen S, et al: Primary operative fixation of long bone fractures in patients with multiple injuries. *J Trauma* 17:111–121, 1977.
16. Riska EB, Myllynen P: Fat embolism in patients with multiple injuries. *J Trauma* 22:891–894, 1982.
17. Seibel R, LaDuca J, Hassett JM, et al: Blunt multiple trauma (ISS 36), femur traction, and the pulmonary failure–septic state. *Ann Surg* 202:283–293, 1985.
18. Eriksson E, Wallin C: Immediate or delayed Kuntscher-rodding of femoral shaft fractures. *Orthopedics* 9:201–204, 1986.
19. Leighton K, Waddell JP, Kellam F, Orrell KG: Open versus closed intramedullary nailing of femoral shaft fractures. *J Trauma* 26:923–926, 1986.
20. Pahud B, Vasey H: Delayed internal fixation of femoral shaft fractures—Is there an advantage? A review of 320 fractures. *J Bone Joint Surg* 69B:391–394, 1987.
21. Wilber MC, Evans EB: Fractures of the femoral shaft treated surgically: Comparative results of early and delayed operative stabilization. *J Bone Joint Surg* 60:489–491, 1978.
22. Winquist RA, Hansen ST, Clawson DK: Closed intramedullary nailing of femoral fractures: A report of five hundred and twenty cases. *J Bone Joint Surg* 66A:529–539, 1984.
23. Hardy AE: The treatment of femoral fractures by cast-brace application and early ambulation: A prospective review of one hundred and six patients. *J Bone Joint Surg* 65A:56–65, 1983.
24. Lesin EB, Mooney V, Ashby ME: Cast-bracing for fractures of the femur: A preliminary report of a modified device. *J Bone Joint Surg* 59:917–923, 1977.
25. McIvor JB, Ross P, Landry G, Davis LA: Treatment of femoral fractures with the cast brace. *Can J Surg* 27:592–594, 1984.
26. Meggitt BF, Juett DA, Smith JD: Cast-bracing for fractures of the femoral shaft: A biomechanical and clinical study. *J Bone Joint Surg* 63:12–23, 1981.
27. Montgomery SP, Mooney V: Femur fractures: Treatment with roller traction and early ambulation. *Clin Orthop Rel Res* 156:196–200, 1981.
28. Hansen ST, Winquist RA: Closed intramedullary nailing of the femur: Kuntscher technique with reaming. *Clin Orthop Rel Res* 138:56–61, 1979.
29. Johnson KD, Johnston DWC, Parker B: Comminuted femoral-shaft fractures: Treatment by roller traction, cerclage wires and an intramedullary nail, or an interlocking intramedullary nail. *J Bone Joint Surg* 66A:1222–1235, 1984.
30. Rothwell AG: Closed Kuntscher nailing for comminuted femoral shaft fractures. *J Bone Joint Surg* 64:12–15, 1982.
31. Webb LX, Gristina AG, Fowler HL: Unstable femoral shaft fractures: A comparison of interlocking nailing versus traction and casting methods. *J Orthop Trauma* 2:10–12, 1988.
32. Weller S, Kuner E, Schweikert CH: Medullary nailing according to Swiss Study Group principles. *Clin Orthop Rel Res* 138:45–55, 1979.
33. Winquist RA, Hansen ST: Comminuted fractures of the femoral shaft treated by intramedullary nailing. *Orthop Clin North Am* 11:633–648, 1980.
34. Kuntscher GBG: The Kuntscher method of intramedullary fixation. *J Bone Joint Surg* 4A:17, 1958.

35. Kuntscher G: Intramedullary surgical technique and its place in orthopaedic surgery: My present concept. *J Bone Joint Surg* 47A:809, 1965.

36. Tscherne H, Haas N, Krettek C: Intramedullary nailing combined with cerclage wiring in the treatment of fractures of the femoral shaft. *Clin Orthop Rel Res* 212:62–67, 1986.

37. Benirschke SK, Melder I, Henley MB, et al: Closed interlocking nailing of femoral shaft fractures: Assessment of technical complications and functional outcomes by comparison of a prospective database with retrospective review. *J Orthop Trauma* 7:118–122, 1993.

38. Cameron CD, Meek RN, Blachut PA, et al: Intramedullary nailing of the femoral shaft: A prospective, randomized study. *J Orthop Trauma* 6:448–451, 1992.

39. Christie J, Court-Brown C, Kinninmonth AWG, et al: Intramedullary locking nails in the management of femoral shaft fractures. *J Bone Joint Surg* 70B:206–210, 1988.

40. Hooper GJ: Closed unlocked nailing for comminuted femoral fractures. *J Bone Joint Surg* 70B:619–621, 1988.

41. Huckstep RL: The Huckstep intramedullary compression nail: Indications, technique, and results. *Clin Orthop Rel Res* 212:48–61, 1986.

42. Kempf I, Grosse A, Beck G: Closed locked intramedullary nailing: Its application to comminuted fractures of the femur. *J Bone Joint Surg* 67A:709–719, 1985.

43. Klemm KW, Borner M: Interlocking nailing of complex fractures of the femur and tibia. *Clin Orthop Rel Res* 212:89–100, 1986.

44. Thoresen BO, Alho A, Ekeland A, et al: Interlocking intramedullary nailing in femoral shaft fractures: A report of forty-eight cases. *J Bone Joint Surg* 67A:1313–1320, 1985.

45. Zuckerman JD, Veith RG, Johnson KD, et al: Treatment of unstable femoral shaft fractures with closed interlocking intramedullary nailing. *J Orthop Trauma* 1:209–218, 1987.

46. Whittaker RP, Heppenstall B, Menkowitz E, Montique F: Comparison of open vs closed rodding of femurs utilizing a Sampson rod. *J Trauma* 22:461–466, 1982.

47. Bucholz RW, Ross SE, Lawrence KL: Fatigue fracture of the interlocking nail in the treatment of fractures of the distal part of the femoral shaft. *J Bone Joint Surg* 69A:1391–1399, 1987.

48. Cook SD, Barrack RL, Renz E, et al: Retrieval and analysis of intramedullary rods: A follow-up study. *Clin Orthop Rel Res* 191:269–273, 1984.

49. Franklin JL, Winquist RA, Benirschke SK, Hansen ST: Broken intramedullary nails. *J Bone Joint Surg* 7A:1463–1471, 1988.

50. Weinstein AM, Clemow AJT, Starkebaum W, et al: Retrieval and analysis of intramedullary rods. *J Bone Joint Surg* 63A:1443–1448, 1981.

51. Russell TA, Taylor JC, LaVelle DG, et al: Mechanical characterization of femoral interlocking intramedullary nailing systems. *J Orthop Trauma* 5:332–340, 1991.

52. Kao JT, Burton D, Comstock C, et al: Pudendal nerve palsy after femoral intramedullary nailing. *J Orthop Trauma* 7:58–63, 1993.

53. Toolan BC, Koval KJ, Kummer FJ, et al: Effects of supine positioning and fracture post placement on the perineal countertraction force in awake volunteers. *J Orthop Trauma* 9:164–170, 1995.

54. Karpos PAG, McFerran MA, Johnson KD: Intramedullary nailing of acute femoral shaft fractures using manual traction without a fracture table. *J Orthop Trauma* 9:57–62, 1995.

55. Baumgaertel F, Dahlen C, Stiletto R, Gotzen L: Technique of using the AO-femoral distractor for femoral intramedullary nailing. *J Orthop Trauma* 8:315–321, 1994.

56. McFerran MA, Johnson KD: Intramedullary nailing of acute femoral shaft fractures without a fracture table: Technique of using a femoral distractor. *J Orthop Trauma* 6:271–278, 1992.

57. Simonian PT, Routt MLC, Harrington RM, Swiontkowski M: Extramedullary skeletal traction for intramedullary femoral nailing. *J Orthop Trauma* 8:409–413, 1994.

58. Winquist RA: Locked femoral nailing. *J Am Acad Orthop Surg* 1:95–105, 1993.

59. Johnson KD, Tencer AF, Sherman MC: Biomechanical factors affecting fracture stability and femoral bursting in closed intramedullary nailing of femoral shaft fractures, with illustrative case presentations. *J Orthop Trauma* 1:1–11, 1987.

60. Kessler SB, Hallfeldt KKJ, Perren SM, Schweiberer L: The effects of reaming and intramedullary nailing on fracture healing. *Clin Orthop Rel Res* 212:18–25, 1986.

61. Whiteside LA, Ogata K, Lesker P, Reynolds FC: The acute effects of periosteal stripping and medullary reaming on regional bone blood flow. *Clin Orthop Rel Res* 131:266, 1978.

62. Pape HC, Regel G, Dwenger A, et al: Influences of different methods of intramedullary femoral nailing on lung function in patients with multiple trauma. *J Trauma* 35:709–716, 1993.

63. Pape HC, Auf'm'Kolk M, Paffrath T, et al: Primary intramedullary femur fixation in multiple trauma patients with associated lung contusion—A cause of posttraumatic ARDS? *J Trauma* 34:540–548, 1993.

64. Pape HC, Dwenger A, Grotz M, et al: Does the reamer type influence the degree of lung dysfunction after femoral nailing following severe trauma? An animal study. *J Orthop Trauma* 8:300–309, 1994.

65. Pell ACH, Christie J, Keating JF, et al: The detection of fat embolism by transoesophageal echocardiography during reamed intramedullary nailing: A study of 24 patients with femoral and tibial fractures. *J Bone Joint Surg* 75B:921–925, 1993.

66. Wenda K, Runkel M, Degreif J, et al: Pathogenesis and clinical relevance of bone marrow embolism in medullary nailing—Demonstrated by intraoperative echocardiography. *Injury* 24(suppl 3):S73–S81, 1993.

67. Brumback RJ, Uwagie-Ero S, Lakatos RP, et al: Intramedullary nailing of femoral shaft fractures: Part 2. Fracture-healing with static interlocking fixation. *J Bone Joint Surg* 70A:1453–1462, 1988.

68. Hajek PD, Bicknell HR Jr, Bronson WE, et al: The use of one compared with two distal screws in the treatment of femoral shaft fractures with interlocking intramedullary nailing: A clinical and biomechanical analysis. *J Bone Joint Surg* 75A:519–525, 1993.

69. Christie J, Court-Brown C: Femoral neck fracture during closed medullary nailing: Brief report. *J Bone Joint Surg* 70B:670, 1988.

70. Green SA, Larson MJ, Moore TJ: Chronic sepsis following intramedullary nailing of femoral fractures. *J Trauma* 27:52–57, 1987.

71. Patzakis MJ, Wilkins J, Wiss DA: Infection following intramedullary nailing of long bones: Diagnosis and management. *Clin Orthop Rel Res* 212:182–191, 1986.

72. Zimmerman KW, Klasen HJ: Mechanical failure of intramedullary nails after fracture union. *J Bone Joint Surg* 65B:274–275, 1983.

73. Chandler RW: Recalcitrant femoral pseudarthrosis healed with a torsionally stiff intramedullary nail: A case report. *J Orthop Trauma* 10:135–137, 1996.

74. Harper MC: Ununited fractures of the femur stabilized with the fluted rod. *Clin Orthop Rel Res* 190:273–278, 1984.

75. Webb LX, Winquist RA, Hansen ST, et al: Intramedullary nailing and reaming for delayed union or nonunion of the femoral shaft: A report of 105 consecutive cases. *Clin Orthop Rel Res* 212:133–141, 1986.

76. Brumback RJ, Wells JD, Lakatos R, et al: Heterotopic ossification about the hip after intramedullary nailing for fractures of the femur. *J Bone Joint Surg* 72A:1067–1073, 1990.

77. Steinberg GG, Hubbard C: Heterotopic ossification after femoral intramedullary rodding. *J Orthop Trauma* 7:536–542, 1993.

78. Mollica Q, Gangitano R, Longo G: Elastic intramedullary nailing in shaft fractures of the femur and tibia. *Orthopedics* 9:1065–1077, 1986.

79. Pankovich AM, Goldflies ML, Pearson RL: Closed ender nailing of femoral-shaft fractures. *J Bone Joint Surg* 61A:222–232, 1979.

80. Pankovich AM: Flexible intramedullary nailing of femoral shaft fractures. *AAOS Instr Course Lect* 36:324–338, 1987.

81. Perry CR, Pankovich AM, Cohn SL: Locked flexible intramedullary nails in treatment of unstable femoral fractures. *J Orthop Trauma* 1:130–140, 1987.

82. Herscovici JD, Scott DM, Behrens F, et al: The use of Ender nails in femoral shaft fractures: What are the remaining indications? *J Orthop Trauma* 6:314–317, 1992.

83. Sanders R, Koval KJ, DiPasquale T, et al: Retrograde reamed femoral nailing. *J Orthop Trauma* 7:293–302, 1993.

84. Cheng JCY, Tse PYT, Chow YYN: The place of the dynamic compression plate in femoral shaft fractures. *Injury* 16:529–534, 1985.

85. Loomer RL, Meek R, De Sommer F: Plating of femoral shaft fractures: The Vancouver experience. *J Trauma* 20:1038–1042, 1980.

86. Magerl F, Wyss A, Brunner C, Binder W: Plate osteosynthesis of femoral shaft fractures in adults: A follow-up study. *Clin Orthop Rel Res* 138:62–73, 1979.

87. Sprenger TR: Fractures of the shaft of the femur treated with a single AO plate. *South Med J* 76:471–474, 1983.

88. Richards RR, Waddell JP, Sullivan TR, et al: Infra-isthmal fractures of the femur: A review of 82 cases. *J Trauma* 24:735–741, 1984.

89. Roberts JB: Management of fractures and fracture complications of the femoral shaft using the ASIF compression plate. *J Trauma* 17:20–28, 1977.

90. Thompson F, O'Beirne J, Gallagher J, et al: Fractures of the femoral shaft treated by plating. *Injury* 16:535–538, 1985.

91. Heitemeyer U, Kemper F, Hierholzer G, and Haines J: Severely comminuted femoral shaft fractures: Treatment by bridging-plate osteosynthesis. *Arch Orthop Trauma Surg* 106:327–330, 1987.

92. Riemer BL, Foglesong ME, Miranda MA: Femoral plating. *Orthop Clin North Am* 25:625–633, 1994.

93. Dabezies EJ, D'Ambrosia R, Shoji H, et al: Fractures of the femoral shaft treated by external fixation with the Wagner device. *J Bone Joint Surg* 66A:360–364, 1984.

94. Gottschalk FAB, Graham AJ, Morein G: The management of severely comminuted fractures of the femoral shaft, using the external fixator. *Injury* 16:377–381, 1985.

95. Marsh CH, Regan MW: Late positional correction of uniting femoral fractures using the Wagner external fixator. *Injury* 17:248–250, 1986.

96. Murphy CP, D'Ambrosia RD, Dabezies EJ, et al: Complex femur fractures: Treatment with the Wagner external fixation device or the Grosse-Kempf interlocking nail. *J Trauma* 28:1553–1561, 1988.

97. Seligson D, Kristiansen TK: Use of the Wagner apparatus in complicated fractures of the distal femur. *J Trauma* 18:795–799, 1978.

98. Coppola JAJ, Anzel SH: Use of the Hoffman external fixator in the treatment of femoral fractures. *Clin Orthop Rel Res* 180:78–82, 1983.

99. Rooser B, Bengtson S, Herrlin K, Onnerfalt R: External fixation of femoral fractures: Experience with 15 Cases. *J Orthop Trauma* 4:70–74, 1990.

100. Alonso J, Geissler W, Hughes JL: External fixation of femoral fractures: Indications and limitations. *Clin Orthop Rel Res* 241:83–88, 1989.

101. Brumback RJ, Ellison PS Jr, Poka A, et al: Intramedullary nailing of open fractures of the femoral shaft. *J Bone Joint Surg* 71A:1324–1330, 1989.

102. Grosse A, Christie J, Taglang G, et al: Open adult femoral shaft fracture treated by early intramedullary nailing. *J Bone Joint Surg* 75B:562–565, 1993.

103. Lhowe DW, Hansen ST: Immediate nailing of open fractures of the femoral shaft. *J Bone Joint Surg* 70A:812–820, 1988.

104. Lhowe DW: Open fractures of the femoral shaft. *Orthop Clin North Am* 25:573–580, 1994.

105. Green A, Trafton PG: Early complications in the management of open femur fractures: A retrospective study. *J Orthop Trauma* 5:51–56, 1991.

106. Rosenthal JJ, Gaspar MR, Gjerdrum TC, Newman J: Vascular injuries associated with fractures of the femur. *Arch Surg* 110:494–499, 1975.

107. Johansen K, Lynch K, Paun M, Copass M: Non-invasive vascular tests reliably exclude occult arterial trauma in injured extremities. *J Trauma* 31:515–522, 1991.

108. DiChristina DG, Riemer BL, Butterfield SL, et al: Femur fractures with femoral or popliteal artery injuries in blunt trauma. *J Orthop Trauma* 8:494–503, 1994.

109. Johnson KD: Femoral shaft fractures, in Browner BD, Jupiter JB, Levine AM, Trafton PG (eds): *Skeletal Trauma.* Philadelphia, Saunders, 1992, p 1576.

110. Friedman RJ, Wyman ET Jr: Ipsilateral hip and femoral shaft fractures. *Clin Orthop Rel Res* 208:188–194, 1986.

111. Geissler WB, Savoie FH, Culpepper RD, Hughes JL: Operative management of ipsilateral fractures of the hip and femur. *J Orthop Trauma* 2:297–302, 1989.

112. Gill SS, Nagi ON, Dhillon MS: Ipsilateral fractures of femoral neck and shaft. *J Orthop Trauma* 4:293–298, 1990.

113. Riemer BL, Butterfield SL, Ray RL, Daffner RH: Clandestine femoral neck fractures with ipsilateral diaphyseal fractures. *J Orthop Trauma* 7:443–449, 1993.

114. Swiontkowski MF, Hansen ST, Kellam J: Ipsilateral fractures of the femoral neck and shaft: A treatment protocol. *J Bone Joint Surg* 66A:260–268, 1984.

115. Swiontkowski MF: Ipsilateral femoral shaft and hip fractures. *Orthop Clin North Am* 18:73–84, 1987.

116. Wiss DA, Sima W, Brien WW: Ipsilateral fractures of the femoral neck and shaft. *J Orthop Trauma* 6:159–166, 1992.

117. Zettas JP, Zettas P: Ipsilateral fractures of the femoral neck and shaft. *Clin Orthop Rel Res* 160:63–73, 1981.

118. Gregory P, DiCicco J, Karpik K, et al: Ipsilateral fracture of the femur and tibia: Treatment with retrograde femoral nailing and unreamed tibial nailing. *J Orthop Trauma* 10:309–316, 1996.

119. Karlstrom G, Olerud S: Ipsilateral fracture of the femur and tibia. *J Bone Joint Surg* 59A:240–243, 1977.

120. Paul GR, Sawka MW, Whitelaw GP: Fractures of the ipsilateral femur and tibia: Emphasis on intra-articular and soft tissue injury. *J Orthop Trauma* 4:309–314, 1990.

121. Veith RG, Winquist RA, Hansen ST: Ipsilateral fractures of the femur and tibia: A report of fifty-seven consecutive cases. *J Bone Joint Surg* 66A:991–1002, 1984.

122. Hollmann MW, Horowitz M: Femoral fractures secondary to low velocity missiles: Treatment with delayed intramedullary fixation. *J Orthop Trauma* 4:64–69, 1990.

123. Bergman M, Tornetta P, Kerina M, et al: Femur fractures caused by gunshots: Treatment by immediate reamed intramedullary nailing. *J Trauma* 34:783–785, 1993.

124. Nowotarski P, Brumback RJ: Immediate interlocking nailing of fractures of the femur caused by low- to mid-velocity gunshot. *J Orthop Trauma* 8:134–141, 1994.

125. Wright DG, Levin JS, Esterhai JL, Heppenstall RB: Immediate internal fixation of low-velocity gunshot-related femoral fractures. *J Trauma* 35:678–682, 1993.

126. Winquist RA, Hansen ST: Segmental fractures of the femur treated by closed intramedullary nailing. *J Bone Joint Surg* 60A:934–939, 1978.

127. Wiss DA, Brein WW, Stetson WB: Interlocking nailing for treatment of segmental fractures of the femur. *J Bone Joint Surg* 72A:724–728, 1990.

CHAPTER 28

Fractures, Dislocations, and Extensor Mechanism Injuries of the Knee

Stephen A. Kottmeier

FRACTURES

Distal Femoral Fractures

Supracondylar fractures of the femur occur at the junction of the distal diaphysis and metaphysis regions. They occur often in combination with articular lesions of the distal femur. The mechanism of injury is often one of axial load imparted on a flexed knee. Analysis of these injuries demonstrates a bimodal distribution. This includes a younger group of patients whose fractures arise as a result of high-energy trauma, often with combined injuries, and an older, osteoporotic group with associated medical concerns. Fracture morphology is determined by injury mechanism, direction of applied force, and bone quality. Treatment of these injuries is frequently complicated by proximity to the knee joint, poor bone quality, and articular comminution. Management remains controversial, although treatment guidelines and options continue to be better defined.

The distal femur encompasses the infraisthmal portion of the distal diaphysis to and including the femoral condyles. An understanding of the osteology of this region is important to enable effective characterization and treatment of distal femoral fractures. The supracondylar region is metaphyseal, presenting a truncated canal with thin cortices and limited bone stock. The condylar region assumes its greatest dimension posteriorly in the coronal and laterally in the sagittal planes. Further distally, the femoral shaft aligns with the anterior half of the condyles. This and the trapezoidal cross-sectional anatomy of the condyles must be appreciated when managing traumatic deformity with insertion of implants.

Muscle insertions of the distal thigh and knee regions produce characteristic fracture deformities. Traumatic shortening of the limb is the result of cocontraction of the quadriceps and hamstrings. The gastrocnemius muscles via their origins produce apex posterior angulation and the perception of anterior displacement of the shaft. They additionally are responsible for rotatory malalignment of the condyles in those fractures possessing a displaced intercondylar component.

Familiarity with the anatomy of the medial distal femur is essential, due to the close proximity of the neurovascular structures. The adductor tubercle offers a point of reference. A cadaveric study defines a zone of up to 8 cm proximal to the tubercle, anterior to the medial intermuscular septum, allowing safe insertion of percutaneous implants.[1]

In treating fractures of the distal femur, one must strive to maintain parallel orientation of the knee joint with the ground. Preservation of the normal anatomic axis (as determined by the contralateral limb) is thus required. This normally has a valgus angulation averaging 9°.

Initial assessment is directed toward the identification and management of potentially life-threatening injury. A secondary survey of the traumatized limb follows. This includes careful scrutiny for deformity, compromise of skin integrity, zones of tenderness, compartment syndrome, and neurovascular impairment. Because the mechanism of injury is often one of axial load, coexistent osseous and soft tissue lesions of the hip, knee, and pelvis must be sought and excluded.

Conventional anteroposterior (AP) and lateral radiographs initiate fracture pattern characterization. Oblique views aid in identification of coronal plane lesions, while traction views serve to assess regions of inter- and supracondylar comminution. Contralateral images for comparison provide a template facilitating restoration of limb alignment and insertion of implants. Computed tomography may better define fracture morphology in complex patterns and help coordinate screw orientation when percutaneous techniques are anticipated. Arteriography is performed when physical examination dictates.

To aid in characterizing and cataloguing these injuries, a practical method of classification is necessary. Several have been proposed, none of which is universally accepted.[2–6] To be effective, a classification scheme should be easy to commit to memory, aid in formulation of a plan of management, and have prognostic application. That proposed by Muller fulfills these objectives effectively (Fig. 28-1).[2]

The goal of treatment of these often complex fractures is return of uncompromised, painless function. This is most predictably achieved by restoration of limb alignment, rotation, length, and articular restoration, followed by early institution of motion. Historically, early operative efforts yielded catastrophic results complicated by fixation failure and infection.[5,6] Traction followed by different forms of external support was accordingly encouraged.[7] This, however, proved ineffective with regard to management of articular incongruity, joint stiffness, and patient mobilization.

Surgical management, during the past three decades, has emerged as the preferred treatment for unstable displaced fractures of the distal femur.[3,8–20] This is due to the evolution of refined operative techniques and devices affording predictable, desired results when executed properly. The patient's age and medical status and the presence of coexistent injuries affect the indication for, timing, and method of osteosynthesis. Absolute indications for surgical management include open lesions, ipsilateral extremity fracture, polytrauma, vascular impairment, and incongruous/irreducible fractures. Contraindications to rigid internal fixation include severe comminution or osteopenia, infection, or severe contamination disallowing adequate debridement.

A surgical tactic is formulated only after the surgeon assesses the "personality" of both the patient and the fracture as well as his or her own skills. This mandates accurate characterization of the fracture as well as selection of

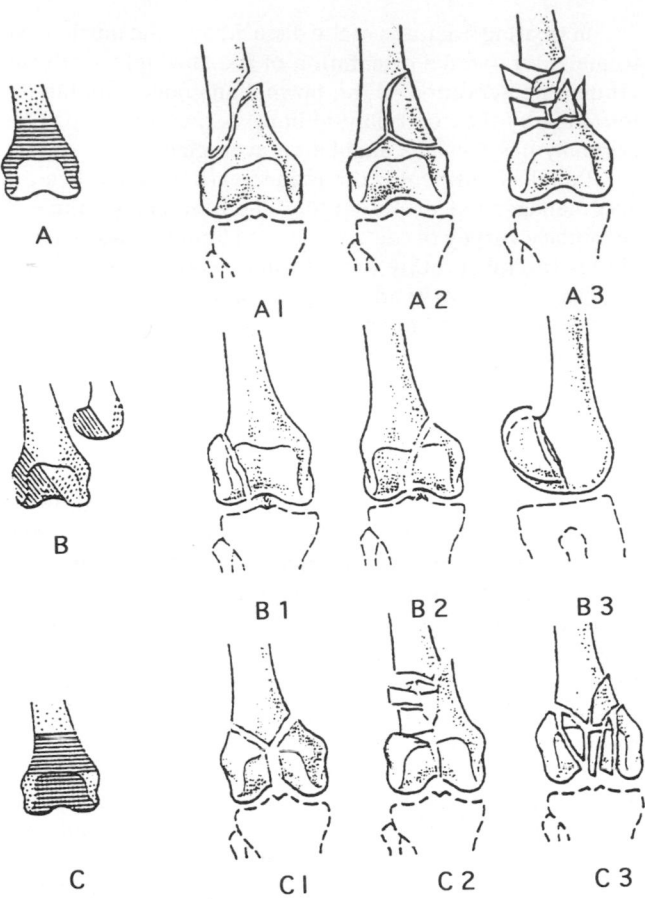

Figure 28-1 The AO/ASIF classification of fractures of the distal femur: type A, extraarticular; type B, unicondylar; type C, bicondylar. (Reproduced with permission from Muller ME, Nazarian S, Koch P, Schatzker J: *The Comprehensive Classification of Fractures of Long Bones.* New York, Springer-Verlag, 1990.)

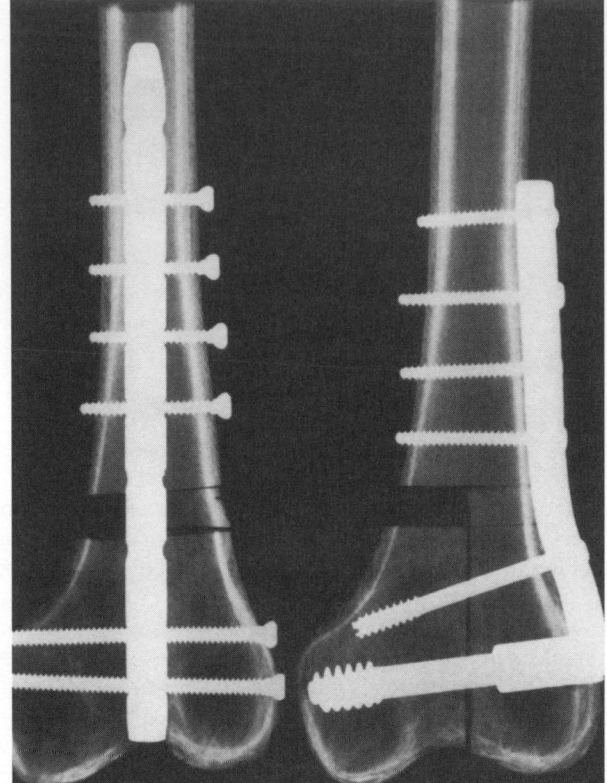

Figure 28-2 Intramedullary and extramedullary (plate) fixation of distal femoral fractures. Bending moment experienced by an intramedullary device is less due to proximity to the femoral bending axis. *Left:* Transgenicular "retrograde" interlocking nail. *Right:* Dynamic condylar screw and side plate. (Reproduced with permission from Firoozbakhsh K, Behzadi K, De Coster TA, et al: Mechanics of retrograde nail versus plate fixation for supracondylar femur fractures. *J Orthop Trauma* 9:152–157, 1995.)

an approach and implant that suits the above. A satisfactory outcome requires adherence to AO/ASIF principles (anatomic articular reduction, rigid fixation, atraumatic handling of soft tissues, preservation of vascular supply, and postoperative rehabilitation of the limb and patient, allowing motion and mobilization).[21]

The sequence of reduction and fixation maneuvers follows a common scheme. Reduction and provisional fixation of the femoral condyles, if an intraarticular component exists, is achieved with a combination of reduction tools and smooth wires. This construct, after definitive fixation with screws, is next secured to the selected implant distally (plate/nail). Correct limb length, alignment, and rotation are then confirmed and proximal fixation performed. Proper implant selection and application are crucial to surgical outcome. No one device is ideally suited for all fractures of the distal femur. Two broad categories (intra- versus extramedullary) exist, distinguished by orientation with respect to the endosteal canal (Fig. 28-2).

Plate fixation remains the operative treatment standard to which other techniques must be compared. Shortcomings of plate fixation include the following: required extensive lateral dissection incurring considerable

potential blood loss, osseous devitalization, and heightened risk of infection. Extensile exposure of the articular surface requires accessory medial exposure or extensor mechanism detachment (tenotomy/osteotomy). The eccentric location of a plate renders it a load-bearing device with increased bending moment. If the opposite cortex is insufficient and cannot withstand compressive forces, fatigue failure of the implant may result. Application of a medial bone graft or adjuvant medial buttress plate may serve to prevent this. Indirect reduction methods, if executed in a skilled "biologically benign" fashion, may obviate this.[22–24] Such technique emphasizes soft tissue preservation and use of the soft tissue envelope for reduction purposes (ligamentotaxis) (Fig. 28-3). High-energy comminuted or open lesions imply traumatic devascularization of osseous segments and may prove inappropriate for this method.

The angled blade plate (Fig. 28-4) is a rigid device possessing a broad surface area of contact and considerable resistance to torsional and bending stresses. Because of its fixed 95° angle when oriented parallel to the distal femoral articular surface, restoration of the femoral axis is assured. Its application is an exacting technique requiring

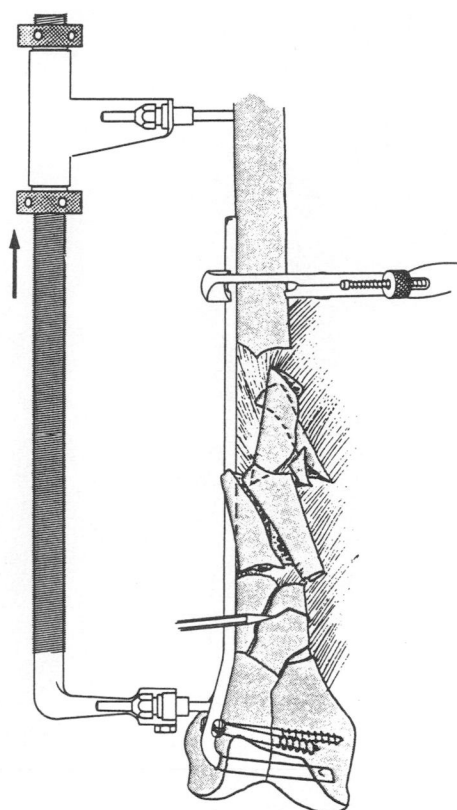

Figure 28-3 Indirect reduction. The soft tissue envelope is preserved and medial dissection and retraction are avoided to preserve the osseous blood supply. Reduction is facilitated by distraction (ligamentotaxis). (Reproduced with permission from Mast J, Jakob R, Ganz R: *Planning and Reduction Technique in Fracture Surgery.* Berlin, Springer-Verlag, 1989.)

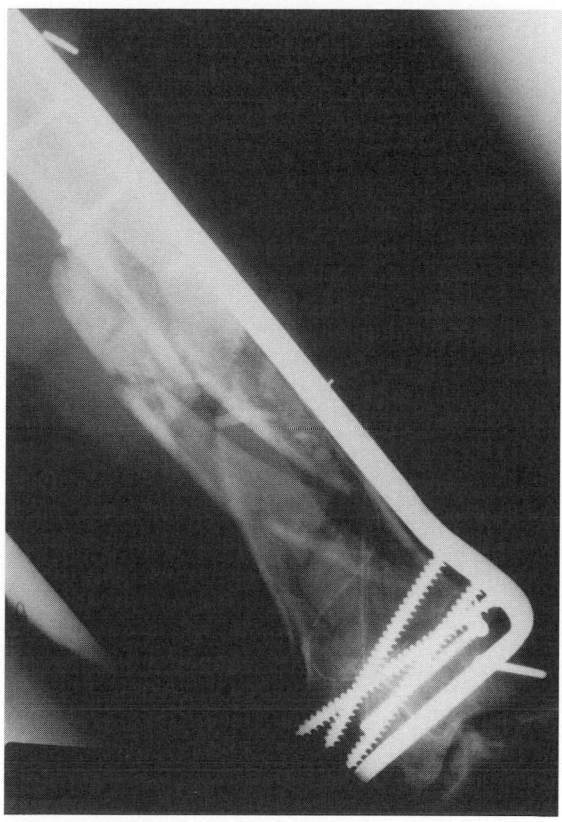

Figure 28-4 This case, demonstrating extensive metaphyseal comminution, was stabilized with a blade plate, employing indirect reduction.

correct insertion in three planes simultaneously.[21,25,26] The dynamic condylar screw (DCS) and side plate (see Fig. 28-2) is less demanding from the standpoint of application.[10,11,13,17] Insertion is facilitated by sagittal plane freedom, modularity, and cannulated screw capability. It is similar to the blade plate and will not adequately address those fracture patterns with multiple, particularly frontal plane, components. Reaming, required for introduction of the screw, results in removal of metaphyseal bone, complicating revision procedures if later required (Fig. 28-5). The condylar buttress plate (Fig. 28-6) allows insertion of multiple distal lag screws with purchase in subchondral bone. This is especially desirable in managing complex fracture patterns in multiple or distal planes, obviating the use of other implants. It suffers from poor mechanical rigidity, demonstrating a tendency toward valgus reduction and varus drift. This is due to inherent structural weakness of the plate itself and the screw/plate interface. It alone is ineffective in neutralizing varus bending forces. If the integrity of the medial cortical buttress is compromised, support in the form of bone grafting or adjuvant plating may be required.[27]

Proximity to the femoral bending axis offers mechanical advantage to intramedullary devices. Bending moment is accordingly diminished, so that there is less risk of implant failure (see Fig. 28-2). This theoretical benefit, however, has not been readily demonstrated with biomechanical testing on cadaveric models.[28] Intramedullary implants, particularly if inserted in a dynamic mode, assume a load-sharing role. In contrast to plate insertion, less fracture site exposure is required, further facilitating union. Flexible intramedullary devices inserted in nonarticular retrograde fashion[9,16,20,29,30] provide little axial and rotational control. These are best reserved for those fractures with no or limited articular involvement and in elderly patients with poor bone quality. More recently, transgenicular intramedullary nailing through the intercondylar notch has been described (see Fig. 28-2).[31–34] This device, versions of which are similar to a conventional antegrade rod, permits static interlocking. Early reports, although encouraging, raise concerns regarding implant failure, nonunion, and synovial metallosis.[35] Conventional antegrade interlocking nailing may suffice for some infraisthmic fractures without significant distal or intraarticular involvement.[36–38] Percutaneous or limited open techniques address simple associated articular patterns. This method is particularly advantageous in managing distal femoral fractures with diaphyseal extension. Centromedullary placement of the nail with insertion of two distal locking screws is required to obtain and maintain acceptable alignment. The use of a large-diameter nail with weight-bearing restriction is encouraged to prevent implant failure.[39]

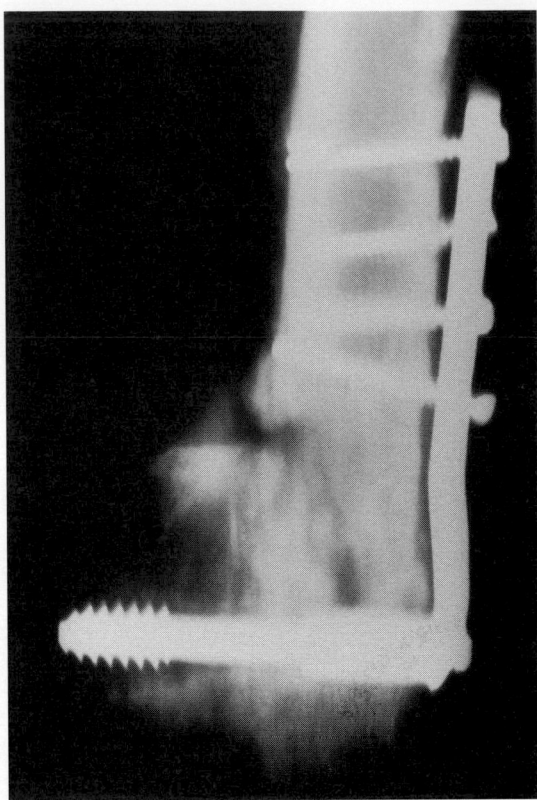

Figure 28-5 A dynamic condylar screw and side plate were used to fixate this distal femoral fracture. Nonunion of the supracondylar component resulted in fixation and implant failure. Bone loss is demonstrated in the region of the compression screw threads. Fixation revision was performed with a condylar buttress plate and bone graft, resulting in satisfactory union (see Fig. 28-6).

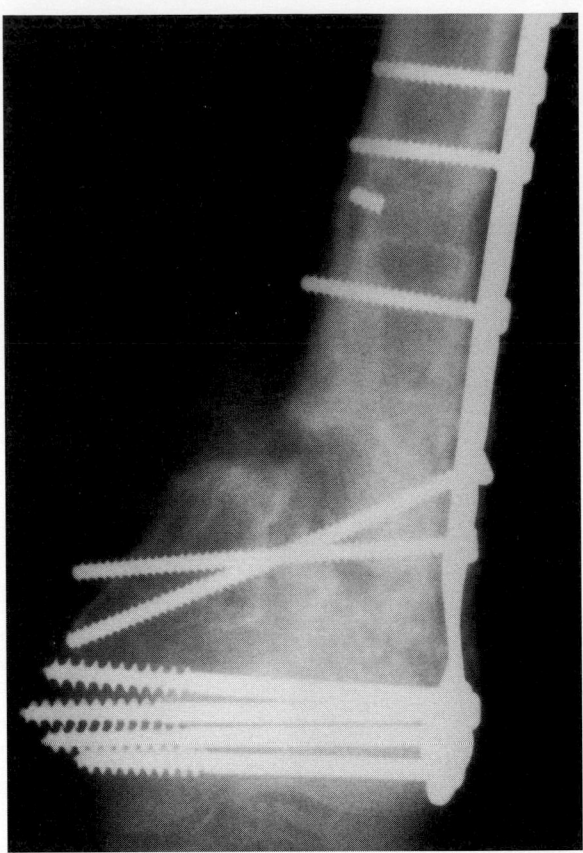

Figure 28-6 Condylar buttress plate. Multiple distal screws can be inserted with this device. This is beneficial in cases demonstrating multiple fracture planes or bone deficit within the region of the condyles.

External fixation of distal femoral fractures is reserved for limbs with severely compromised soft tissues or vascular impairment and for patients with associated life-threatening injury.[40] Its primary purpose is to provide stability to the limb and accordingly to facilitate nursing care. Pins are inserted sagittally into the distal femur if soft tissue and osseous structures allow or into the proximal tibia in "transarticular" configuration if they do not. Immediate stabilization of the articular component with limited fixation may be considered in this setting. Delayed definitive fixation is performed when the patient's condition and the status of the soft tissues improve.

Unicondylar (type B) fractures are subdivided into three types based on anatomic configuration. Displaced fractures demand reduction and fixation using cancellous lag screws to restore joint stability and congruity.[41] Supplemental plating (buttress or antiglide) may be required, depending on bone quality, for type B1 and B2 fractures. Coronal (B3 or "Hoffa") fractures are stabilized with sagittally oriented screws countersunk below the articular surface.

Complications encountered during the course of managing distal femoral fractures may result in significant loss of function.[42] These include infection, nonunion, malunion, fixation and/or implant failure, restriction of knee motion,

and posttraumatic arthritis. Infection and difficulty in achieving union increase in the presence of osseous devitalization. Precipitants of this include high-energy injury and extensive surgical dissection. Recent trends and established protocols support immediate operative treatment of open fractures of the distal femur.[18,43,44] Infection rates are expectedly higher than those associated with closed variants. If the injury is adequately debrided, immediate definitive stabilization appears to afford a better environment for both osseous and soft tissue aseptic recovery and healing. Those presenting with extensive contamination are most predictably managed with limited internal and temporary external fixation restoring joint congruity and limb stability, respectively.

Nonunion, usually involving the supracondylar region, may result from inadequate fixation, infection, or impaired vascular supply to osseous elements. Management is problematic owing to the short length and poor bone quality of the distal segment (see Fig. 28-5). Proximity to the knee joint, often with limited motion, imparts additional stress to the implant and fixation construct. Methods of treatment include fixation revision with either intra- or extramedullary devices,[45–47] a combination of both,[48] and external fixation.[49] Additional surgical alternatives include arthrodesis,[50] arthroplasty, and amputation.[42,51]

Malunion, more common following nonsurgical treatment, presents most often with varus and recurvatum deformities. Postsurgical malunion arising from fixation and/or implant failure is often due to an inadequately addressed deficient medial cortical buttress. Treatment is directed toward restoring the normal mechanical axis, which requires corrective supracondylar osteotomy with stable fixation.

Fixation failure may result from a poorly executed osteosynthesis or a properly indicated and performed procedure complicated by exceedingly poor bone quality and comminution. Postsurgical infection and poor patient compliance with weight-bearing restriction are additional precipitants. These factors are especially evident in the older patient. Treatment of these fractures in the elderly population can be fraught with medical and surgical challenges and complications. Significant functional deterioration in frail individuals, 9 percent of whom required amputation, has been reported.[51] Osteoporotic bone may prove unsuitable for internal fixation, but it does not necessarily contraindicate operative treatment. Fixation-enhancing techniques (deliberate limb shortening,[52] bone cement[53]) and implants (screws with large thread diameters, intramedullary devices[30]) may aid in overcoming stabilization-related obstacles. Primary total knee replacement with a modular distal femoral component has been described for selected osteopenic elderly patients with coexisting gonarthrosis.[54]

Sources of obstructed knee motion include intraarticular adhesions, soft tissue contractures, articular malreduction, and intraarticular protrusion of implants. Treatment of motion restriction is dependent upon the etiology. Salvage procedures (arthrodesis, arthroplasty) may ultimately prove necessary in those cases associated with progressive posttraumatic arthrosis.

Patellar Fractures

The patella is an important component in normal knee function. It serves aesthetic, protective, and functional roles. It increases the mechanical advantage of the quadriceps tendon by displacing it from the axis of knee motion.[55] Dissatisfaction with results in patellectomized knees has encouraged a posture of patellar preservation in managing fractures to this structure.

The patella lies within the quadriceps tendon and receives the trilaminar insertion of the rectus femoris and vastus muscles. The medial and lateral retinacula are derived from aponeurotic fibers of the vastus medialis and lateralus, respectively. The retropatellar articular surface is made up of two facets separated by a vertical ridge. Each is anatomically subdivided into three vertically oriented facets. A single additional longitudinal ridge medially defines the seventh or "odd" facet. Vascular supply to the patella is derived from a dorsal arterial ring arising from geniculate artery contributions. It is received primarily by the central and distal aspects via arterial arcades. This may account for radiographically apparent avascular necrosis of the superior pole in patellar fractures with central involvement.

Patellar fracture types are designated by location, pattern, and degree of displacement. They are thus commonly classified as transverse, polar, comminuted, or vertical. Evaluation should include an adequate history, assessment of soft tissue and extensor mechanism integrity, and radiography. Inability to actively extend the knee suggests retinacular disruption.

Fracture of the patella may occur from direct or indirect mechanisms. High-energy falls or vehicular injuries impart direct impact forces. Resultant fractures are often comminuted and frequently associated with concomitant limb injuries. Tensile forces are accordingly limited, preserving continuity of the extensor mechanism and limiting displacement. Deceleration when falling results in eccentric contraction of the quadriceps. The extensor mechanism fails in tension, often in the form of a transverse patellar fracture. Displacement is considerable and active extension of the knee absent.

Nonoperative treatment, in the form of immobilization, is appropriate for those fractures without articular incongruity or discontinuity of the extensor mechanism. Those injuries failing to meet these criteria are managed operatively. The goal of treatment is to restore satisfactory knee function by reestablishing the integrity of both the extensor apparatus and the retropatellar articular surface. Outcome is most dependent upon initial fracture severity.[56] Surgical treatment options include fixation as well as partial and complete excision of the patella. Earlier enthusiasm toward patellectomy[57–59] has been tempered by more recent reports advocating patellar preservation.[60–63] A well-executed osteosynthesis allowing early range-of-motion offers the best opportunity for restoring knee function.

Stabilization of patellar fractures may be accomplished with open methods of internal[64–66] or external fixation[67] or by closed methods with percutaneous suturing.[68,69] Various fixation constructs have been described, including cerclage, intraosseous wires/sutures, compression screws, and combinations of these. Several of these methods draw upon the principle of tension band fixation. This requires the application of an anteriorly situated wire with proximal and distal pole fixation. Active motion of the knee converts forces of distraction at the fracture site to those of compression. Earlier versions of tension band insertion were of a box configuration with the proximal and distal limits of the band secured through the peripatellar soft tissues. This was later modified by insertion of longitudinal intraosseous wires, which also served as anchors for the band ("modified" tension band) (Fig. 28-7).[66] Anteriorly, the wire may be arranged in a crossed or square ("box") pattern. Proponents of the latter argue that it affords uniform fracture site compression, rotational control, and less implant-related discomfort.

Cerclage fixation alone does not provide sufficient rigidity to allow early motion. Compromise to patellar vascularity is also a concern with this technique. It may, however, serve as adjuvant fixation to other methods in comminuted fracture patterns. Biomechanical analysis of various patellar fixation constructs has been attempted in an effort to define a preferred method. Such studies appear to yield conflicting results due largely to differences

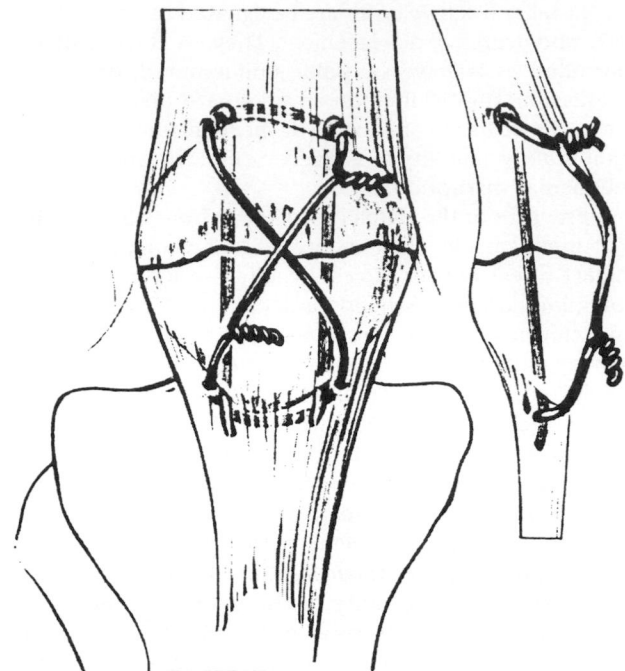

Figure 28-7 Modified tension band. The inclusion of vertical wires enhances stability at the wire loop/bone interface. Anteriorly, the wire may be fashioned in a crossed (as depicted here) or box pattern. (Reproduced with permission from Benirschke SK, Swiontkowski MF: *Knee-Orthopedic Trauma Protocols.* New York, Raven Press, 1993.)

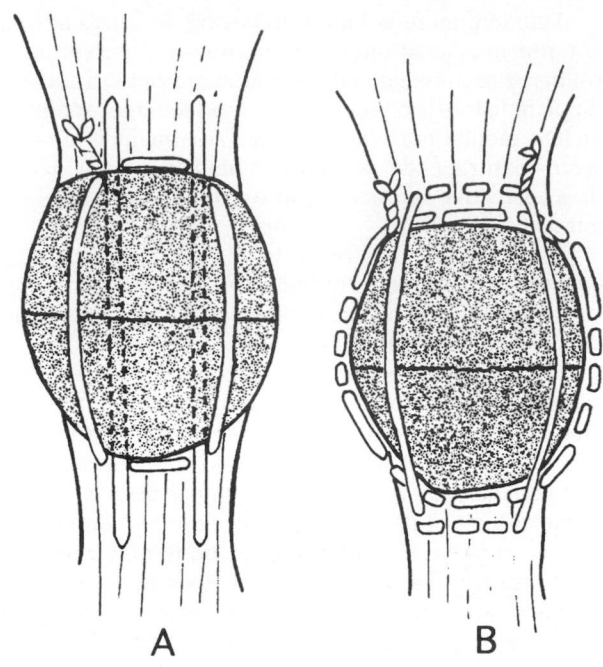

Figure 28-8 *A.* Modified tension band with anterior "box" construct. *B.* Pyrford technique: traditional anterior tension band without vertical intraosseous fixation and peripatellar cerclage. (Reproduced with permission from Curtis MJ: Internal fixation for fractures of the patella. *J Bone Joint Surg* 72B:280–282, 1990.)

in methodology. Weber et al. expressed the importance of inclusion of intraosseous fixation (vertical wires) to improve stability of the interface between the wire loop and bone.[70] They also demonstrated that retinacular repair contributed to fixation stability. Benjamin et al. recommend vertical screws instead of wires in the presence of adequate bone stock.[71] In those cases with comminution and/or osteopenia, the modified tension band with vertical wires was preferred. Curtis suggests that the Pyrford method (anterior tension band and cerclage) offers mechanically superior fixation when compared to the modified tension band (Fig. 28-8).[72]

Most biomechanical studies of patellar fixation have employed models based on a transverse fracture pattern. Treatment directives regarding management of comminuted lesions have evolved "from patellectomy to preservation." Indirect methods of reduction and fixation have been described, emphasizing respect for soft tissue attachments and minimal dissection.[73] Strategically oriented screws as well as circumferential and tension band wires are inserted without violating the blood supply to the individual fragments.

Partial patellectomy should be limited to those patterns with significant comminution in which only one or a few large viable fragments can be retained.[56,61,64,74] These are often inferior-pole fractures, which are largely nonarticular. The tendon margin should approximate the articular edge to prevent patellar tilting. Total patellectomy is re-

served for highly displaced comminuted fractures. Attempts to salvage even small fragments should be considered. Levack and Hobbs, acknowledging superior results with anatomic operative fixation, describe better results with patellectomy in those cases where anatomic reduction could not be achieved.[75]

Postoperative care should permit continuous passive motion as determined by the status of the wound and adequacy of fixation. The insertion of a "neutralization device" (cable/wire) from the superior patellar pole to the tibial tubercle may protect the fixation sufficiently to allow this.[64,76] A rigorous postoperative protocol permitting early motion inhibits formation of intraarticular adhesions and gives better assurance of functional motion.

Complications associated with the management of patellar fractures most frequently include discomfort from the patellofemoral articulation and restriction of motion. Patellofemoral arthrosis may result from articular incongruity. Additionally, change in vertical patellar position, particularly after partial patellectomy, may result in aberrant patellofemoral contact pressure. Tibiofemoral arthrosis, attributed to articular surface trauma sustained at the time of injury, has been observed after fracture of the patella. Postoperative infection, although rare, if refractory to standard modalities, may require soft tissue coverage techniques to resolve.[77] Nonunion may present as a result of an initially neglected fracture[78] or in the postsurgical period.

Proximal Tibial Fractures

Tibial Plateau Fractures

An articular fracture of the proximal tibia presents a potentially complex injury to a large weight-bearing joint. These injuries are often associated with articular surface incongruity, limb instability, and compromise to supportive and periarticular soft tissues. Responsible injury mechanisms include directly (axial) and indirectly (coronal) imparted force combinations of compression and shear. A bimodal distribution exists comprising high-energy injuries in a younger population and low-energy injuries in an older population with osteopenic bone. Common and of considerable concern to the former are associated injuries to the soft tissue envelope, menisci, supporting ligaments, and neurovascular structures. Fracture morphology is dependent upon magnitude and direction of force, bone quality, and knee joint position upon impact. Articular incongruity alone or in combination with ligamentous insufficiency may result in joint instability, limb malalignment, motion restriction, and ultimately traumatic arthrosis. Treatment is focused upon obtaining and maintaining a stable, painless joint with preservation of functional motion. Favorable outcomes are most predictably achieved by adhering to protocols[79,80] emphasizing articular reconstruction, stable fixation, and institution of early motion. This demands and is initiated by an accurate clinical and radiographic assessment. The "personality" of both the fracture and the patient must be considered together. Techniques continue to evolve directed toward achieving goals as described while maintaining respect for periarticular soft tissues and osseous viability.

Anatomic differences between the medial and lateral condyles must be considered when assessing and treating fractures of the proximal tibial articular surface. The medial plateau is larger and concave in the sagittal plane, whereas the lateral is convex and situated more proximally. This observation must be maintained when screws are being inserted from lateral to medial to avoid intraarticular penetration. The greater majority of weight borne by the lateral compartment is received by the lateral meniscus, which covers a relatively larger portion of the articular surface.[81] Medially, however, it is shared equally by the meniscus and articular cartilage. This may account for the seemingly functional and symptomatic tolerance of the lateral compartment to limited radiographic incongruity.[82] The medial condyle offers a stronger osseous foundation. Compromise to this structure is sustained by injury of considerable energy with more potential for soft tissue compromise. The subcutaneous location of the proximal tibia renders it vulnerable to this as well.

Assessment for coexistent closed cavity, axial skeletal, and extremity lesions is performed. The injured extremity must be scrutinized for compromise of the periarticular skin's integrity. Regions of tenderness should be noted and the neurovascular status established. Signs and symptoms of increased intracompartmental pressure should be sought. Assessment of knee stability, under anesthesia if necessary, is performed. A 56 percent frequency of associated soft tissue injuries has been described.[83] The most commonly suspected injury was anterior cruci-

ate ligament insufficiency, which resolved with osseous fixation of the medial plateau fragment. The second most common injury was meniscal (20 percent). Injuries to the ligaments range from osseous avulsion to intrasubstance injuries. Significant injury to collateral and/or cruciate ligaments is implied if operative restoration of articular congruity fails to restore coronal plane stability. Associated ligamentous injury has been suggested to be of significant prognostic importance.[84] Neural injury can range from neuropraxia to neurotmesis and arterial injury from intimal lesions to avulsion. Severe osteoligamentous instability heralds a fracture-dislocation variant for which arterial impairment must be excluded. The injured individual's age, health, expectations, and bone quality serve to define the "personality of the patient." Radiographic delineation of fracture morphology follows to further characterize the "personality of the injury."

Imaging of plateau injuries is initiated with performance of AP, lateral, and 45° oblique conventional radiography. A 10° caudal tilt AP "plateau view" is obtained to better quantify degree of articular depression. Accurate characterization of fracture morphology demands scrutiny of both condyles, cortical rims, posterior condylar components, and fractures involving the central nonarticular region of the tibial eminence. Displacement and/or depression of one or both condyles or components of each is noted and survey for metaphyseal and proximal fibula fracture involvement performed. Rim avulsions and posterior lesions suggest ligamentous compromise and sagittal instability, respectively. An intact proximal fibula may provide support to unicondylar lateral lesions yet contribute to varus deformity in bicondylar or unicondylar medial lesions. Coronal plane radiographic stress testing can better establish osseous versus ligamentous contributions to clinically appreciated instability (Fig. 28-9).[85] Computed tomography with reformatted biplanar images aids in delineating fracture location, depression, and displacement. Information thus obtained may better determine selection of approach, operability, and implant orientation. Magnetic resonance imaging has been suggested to contribute equally reliable information regarding osseous injury in addition to ascertaining the status of meniscal and ligamentous tissues.[86] Angiography or noninvasive methods of arterial study should be employed when potential for vascular insult exists.

Classifications of tibial plateau fractures have historically been founded upon fracture pathomechanics, pathoanatomy, degree of displacement, instability, and integration of location and orientation. The universal classification adopted by the AO group offers a unified method of cataloguing fracture types in order of complexity, allowing effective intra- and interinstitutional communication.[87] The widely utilized classification of Schatzker designates six types, each unique in mechanism, pattern, and approach to management (Fig. 28-10).[80] It offers a logical approach to the characterization of fractures and methods of predictable, effective osteosynthesis. A recent modification of this scheme stresses the importance of associated condylar tilt and its impact on prognosis.[88]

Guidelines regarding treatment of tibial plateau fractures remain inconclusive and without unanimity. This is

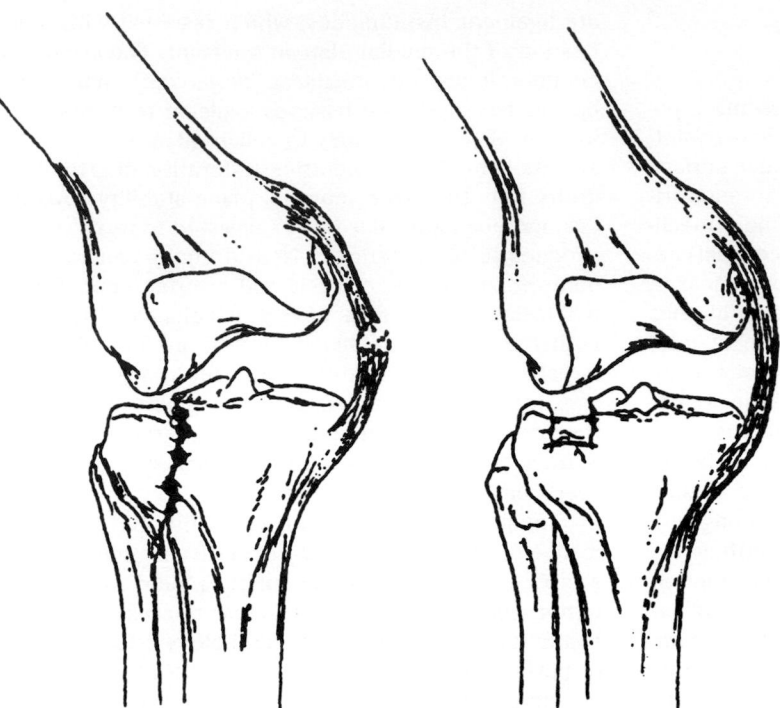

Figure 28-9 Valgus instability may be due to compromise to the osseous foundation *(right),* medial ligaments, or both *(left).* In osteoporotic bone, resistance to axial load is less. The medial collateral ligament is thus spared *(right).* (Reproduced with permission from Koval KJ, Helfet DL: Tibial plateau fractures: Evaluation and treatment. *J Am Acad Orthop Surg* 3:86–94, 1995.)

due primarily to absence of a uniform classification system and inclusion criteria as well as inconsistent radiographic and result-reporting parameters. The goal of therapy in the broadest sense is a painless, stable joint with uncompromised motion and function. Some investigators maintain that ideal joint performance mandates absolute congruency to deter contact stress aberration and subsequent degenerative changes.[80–93] They have determined restoration of anatomic articular congruity to be the single most important factor in predicting the outcome of fractures of the tibial plateau. This, they contend, for all unstable and displaced lesions, is best achieved by open reduction with stable internal fixation and early functional rehabilitation. Others propose that the sole criterion for

operative versus nonoperative treatment depends on knee stability in the coronal plane with full extension.[94–96]

Incongruence to within certain limits has been suggested to be well tolerated without sequelae, owing to meniscal accomodation[97] and fibrocartilage ingrowth.[98] According to some studies, the radiographic appearance does not parallel functional outcome.[99–101] Articular incongruity, if sufficient, may contribute directly to posttraumatic arthrosis or indirectly by disturbing the alignment of the articular axis.[82,89,95,102,103]

Closed treatment is best reserved for those lesions without displacement or signs of osteoligamentous instability.[104] Stability is likely to be dependent upon the fracture location, type, and ligamentous integrity. Preferential

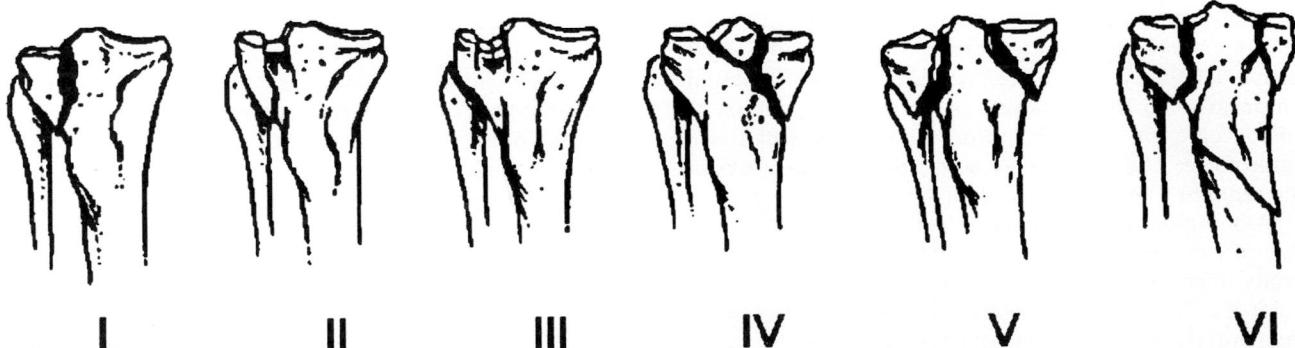

| I | II | III | IV | V | VI |

Figure 28-10 The Schatzker classification of tibial plateau fractures: type 1, wedge fracture of the lateral tibial plateau; type 2, lateral split/depression fracture; type 3, pure central depression fracture; type 4, wedge fracture of the medial condyle; type 5, bicondylar fracture; type 6, metaphyseal/diaphyseal dissociation. (Reproduced with permission from Koval KJ, Sanders R, Borrelli J, et al: Indirect reduction and percutaneous screw fixation of displaced tibial plateau fractures. *J Orthop Trauma* 6:340–346, 1992.)

treatment in such cases consists of early mobilization with restricted weight bearing in a fracture orthosis. Traction therapy is reserved for those cases in which local or systemic host conditions disallow operative treatment when otherwise indicated. Such techniques employing ligamentotaxis are unlikely to reduce impacted fragments devoid of soft tissue attachment. This has been demonstrated with operative distraction techniques as well.[105]

Absolute indications for surgical treatment include those injuries associated with open wounds, compartment syndrome, or vascular compromise. Open fractures require immediate irrigation and debridement of the traumatic wound and administration of parenteral broad-spectrum antibiotics. Initial efforts should be directed toward articular reconstruction. Axial stability is restored by temporary external transfixation of the knee until soft tissues have "stabilized." Alternatively, adhering to a recently established protocol, definitive primary fixation may be considered in managing even complex open fractures.[106] Radiographic criteria for operative treatment continue to evolve based upon fracture location, depression, and impact upon joint alignment.[102] Formulation of an effective treatment strategy is predicated upon the surgeon's clear understanding of the patient, the soft tissue envelope, the fracture pattern, and his or her own abilities. Familiarity with equipment, implants, and reduction techniques are additional prerequisites. Those fractures in which the aforementioned goals are unattainable with closed treatment are managed operatively.

Nondisplaced split fractures may be adequately stabilized with percutaneous screw insertion. Displaced lesions, failing closed reduction, are reduced open or with limited open and/or arthroscopically assisted techniques. Screw fixation alone should suffice in younger patients. Inferior bone quality necessitates the addition of adjuvant limited fixation (antiglide devices) or buttress-plate application.

Fracture patterns demonstrating components of both condylar split and joint depression require articular elevation and reconstitution of the cortical foundation (Fig. 28-11). These efforts are directed toward restoring articular congruity and coronal plane stability. The fracture plane permits access to the region of joint depression. En masse elevation is performed, as disimpaction techniques employing distraction are unlikely to succeed. The resultant void is filled with bone graft or bone graft substitutes. Reduction is preserved utilizing similar fixation methods and implants as for split fractures (Fig. 28-12).

Treatment of pure depression fractures is dependent upon the size and location of the lesion and its impact on knee joint stability. A metaphyseal cortical window is established and joint elevation performed under direct or arthroscopic visualization. The defect is next filled and the graft supported by subchondral screws.

Medial condyle lesions often result from high-energy injury. They are accordingly frequently associated with neurovascular deficit as well as ligamentous and/or os-

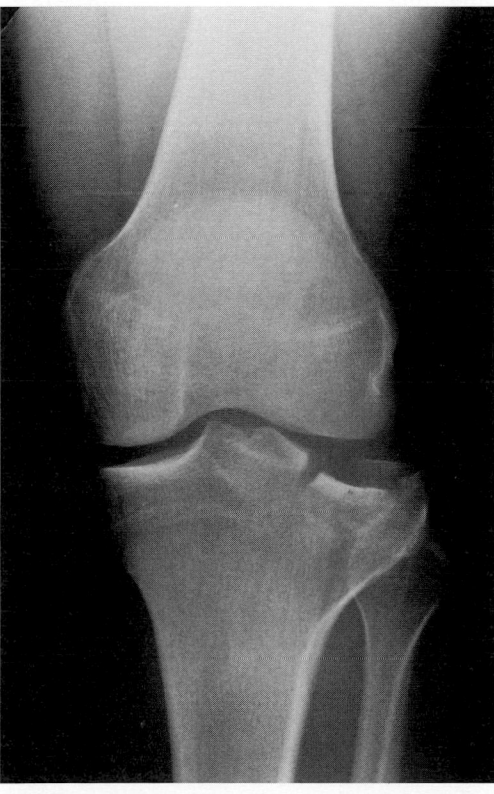

Figure 28-11 A type 2 fracture with lateral condylar split and depression.

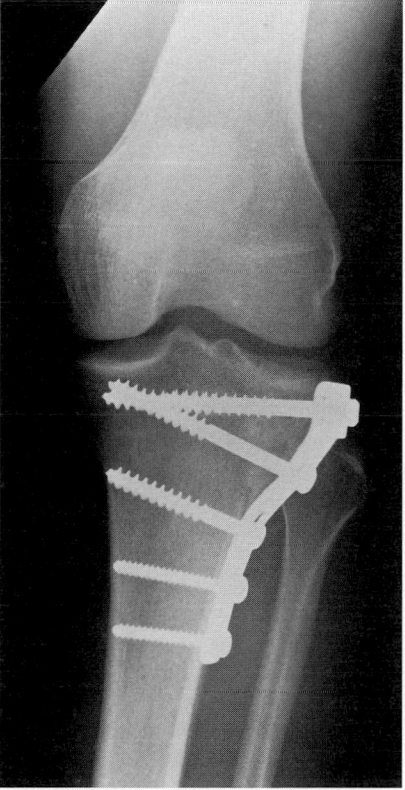

Figure 28-12 Reduction and fixation of a type 2 fracture (see Fig. 28-11) with en masse elevation of the articular surface, application of bone graft, and lateral buttress plate.

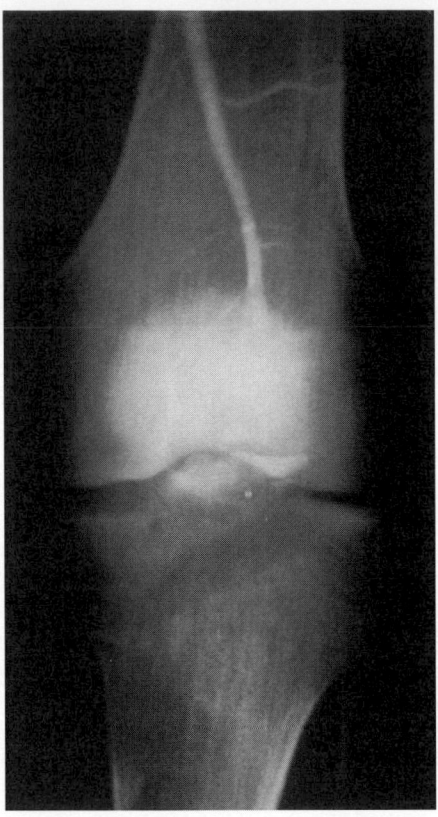

Figure 28-13 A type 4 fracture with associated vascular impairment.

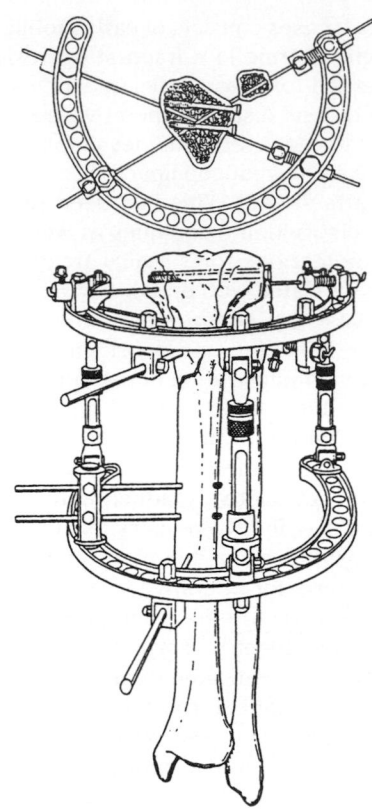

Figure 28-14 Hybrid external fixation. The articular surface is reconstituted and secured to the remainder of the tibia by an external fixator. Small wire transfixion pins are inserted superiorly and unilateral half pins inferiorly. (Reproduced with permission from Stamer DT, Schenk R, Staggers B, et al: Bicondylar tibial plateau fractures treated with a hybrid ring external fixator: A preliminary study. *J Orthop Trauma* 8:455–461, 1994.)

seous instability (Fig. 28-13). Sagittal plane instability may manifest with compromise to intercondylar (cruciate attachment) or posterior condylar regions. Anatomic osteosynthesis with repair of meniscal and ligamentous tissues is the preferred treatment in this often younger patient population. Medial buttress-plate application is required to resist varus forces.

Bicondylar fractures, the product of axial force, pose hazards similar to those of medial lesions. The challenge—particularly in those bicondylar variants with metaphyseal dissociation—is to restore and maintain joint reduction and limb alignment in a fashion that does not compromise soft tissue and osseous viability. Management of these complex lesions continues to evolve from one of absolute rigidity employing dual buttress-plate fixation to a more biological approach emphasizing composite fixation. This trend has demonstrated diminished rates of infection and need for secondary bone grafting. Articular reduction is performed with limited open techniques followed by fixation with screws alone or with unicondylar plate application. The construct is next neutralized by the application of a circular,[107] hybrid circular (Fig. 28-14),[108,109] or contralateral unilateral external fixator[110,111] or a limited antiglide device (Fig. 28-15). This affords anatomic stable fixation without significant surgical trauma or the need for large implants.

The operative approach, based upon the fracture pattern, must afford adequate visualization for reduction and

fixation while maintaining soft tissue and osseous viability. An anterior midline incision with preservation of full-thickness flaps allows for later reconstructive efforts. Unilateral extensile,[112] dual,[113] and posterior[114] approaches have been described as well. Joint inspection is facilitated by a horizontal inframeniscal arthrotomy with cephalad elevation of the meniscus and joint distraction. Alternative techniques to enhance joint visualization include anterior horn meniscal transection,[115,116] sectioning of the iliotibial band, and patellar tenotomy[117] as well as tibial tubercle[118] and proximal fibular osteotomy.[119]

The role of arthroscopic techniques in managing fractures of the tibial plateau continues to be defined.[120–123] In appropriately selected cases, it offers an attractive, less invasive method of assisting reduction and fixation. Its greatest utility is found in assessing the status of additional intraarticular structures. Entrapped meniscal tissues have been observed in fracture patterns with displaced split components.[123] These techniques, however, do not allow effective management of submeniscal, rim avulsion, or metaphyseal lesions.

Complications of tibial plateau fractures, regardless of elected treatment method, can be considerable and with

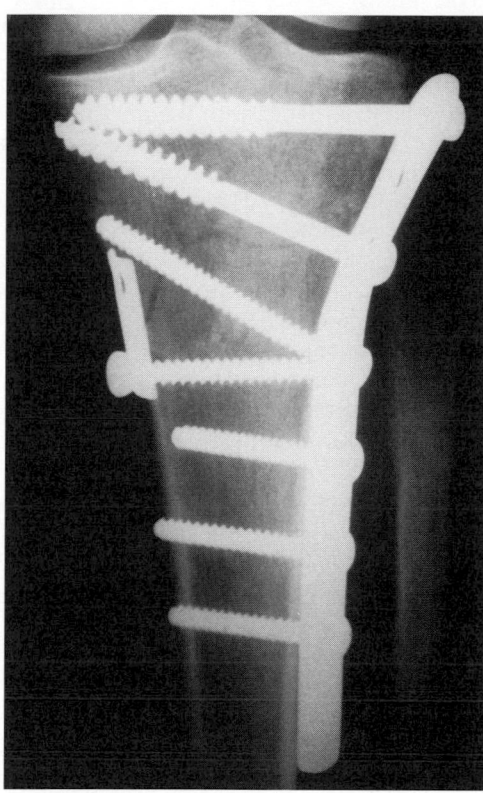

Figure 28-15 This case demonstrates use of a strong plate (lateral tibial condylar buttress plate) in addition to an "antiglide" plate, which was inserted through a small medial wound. This is less threatening to soft tissue and osseous viability than application of large bicondylar implants through a single extensile anterior wound.

serious long-term consequences. Malunion occurs more commonly with nonsurgical treatment. The results of poor open reduction are far worse than the results of poor conservative care.[80] The potential for surgery-related complications increases with fracture severity and extensive operative intervention. Infection rates in complicated bicondylar fractures treated with formal open reduction and internal fixation have been reported to be approximately 25 percent.[80,124] Additional complications include fixation failure, motion restriction, posttraumatic arthrosis, neurovascular injury, compartment syndrome,[125] and nonunion.[126]

Tibial Eminence Fractures

Avulsion fracture of the intercondylar eminence of the tibia may result from knee hyperflexion or due to torsionally and axially imparted loads to a hyperextended joint. Its presence, if displaced, implies incompetence to the anterior cruciate ligament (ACL). Although this is often regarded as an injury of childhood or adolescence, it has been observed with increasing frequency in the adult population.[127–129] Inferior results demonstrated in this latter group may reflect a higher degree of energy yielding additional articular injury (capsuloligamentous, meniscal, articular surface). Uniform agreement regarding treatment of

these fractures has been lacking. Early accurate diagnosis and adequate treatment is essential in achieving a desirable outcome. Reduction, if nonanatomic, may compromise joint motion and stability.[130–133]

The tibial intercondylar eminence consists of the medial and lateral tibial spines. The medial spine is the focus of attachment for the ACL. Avulsion failure in this region occurs through the cancellous bone beneath the subchondral plate.

History obtained upon assessment will often include the perception of a "pop" followed by a rapidly occurring effusion. Initial survey of the limb demonstrates considerable guarding, limited joint motion, and a painful inability to bear weight. Increased excursion and diminished endpoint quality to Lachman testing may be evident. Aspiration of the hemarthrosis may reveal the presence of fat droplets and allow a more detailed physical examination. Coronal plane instability, depending upon skeletal maturity, suggests injury to either collateral ligament or growth plate structures. Conventional radiographic evaluation includes performance of AP, lateral, tunnel, and oblique views to accurately characterize the fracture and identify coexistent lesions. Stress views are of obvious importance if a physeal injury is suspected.

The modified classification scheme of Meyers and McKeever, based upon radiographically appreciated displacement of the fragment, offers a guideline to treatment (Fig. 28-16).[134,135] The role of arthroscopy as a diagnostic aid in the evaluation of tibial eminence fractures continues to be defined. It facilitates accurate fracture type designation and permits assessment for additional intraarticular pathology.[136,137]

Historically, uniform agreement regarding treatment of tibial eminence fractures has been lacking. Neglected, displaced fractures may cause knee motion deficit and laxity.[138,139] Early, accurate diagnosis and adequate treatment are therefore essential. Type 1 lesions with no or minimal displacement are managed conservatively with application of a long leg cast. Closed reduction efforts may be considered in managing displaced lesions. This, however, demands the presence of a sufficiently large fragment that in part opposes the femoral articular surface. Protocols advocating immobilization in hyperextension,[140–142] extension,[137,143] and flexion[130] with closed manipulation have been described. Extreme extension is uncomfortable and may render the ACL taut, contributing to displacement. The latter may occur in the presence of knee flexion as well, due to increased tension within the anteromedial bundle of the ligament. Most current treatment regimens suggest positioning of the joint in 20° flexion with radiographic confirmation of fracture reduction. Irreducible lesions, particularly in the adult population, require operative reduction. Encouraging results with conservatively treated type 3 lesions appear limited to the skeletally immature population and cannot be assured.[144] Obstacles to reduction include interposed hematoma and osteochondral debris as well as incarcerated meniscal tissues.[135,137,145–147] Because of the apparent frequency of this in both type 2 and type 3 lesions, Van Loon and Marti recommend arthroscopic assessment of all such injuries.[136] Operative reduction may be performed by open

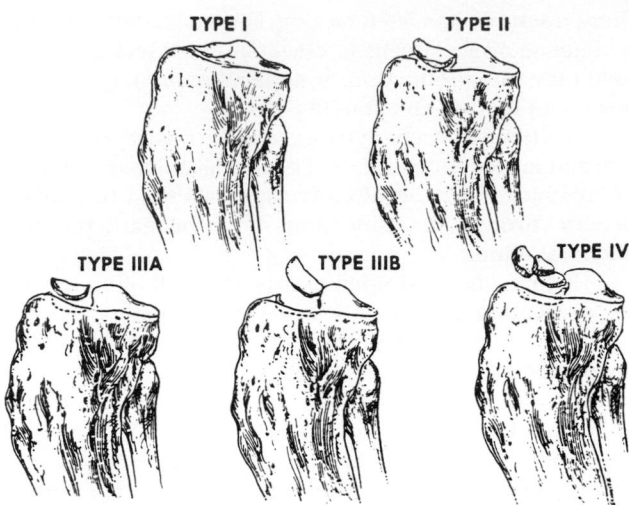

Figure 28-16 Modified Meyers and McKeever classification of fractures of the tibial spine: type I is nondisplaced; type II is hinged with same anterior elevation; type IIIA has complete displacement of the fragment; type IIIB fragment is completely displaced and rotated; and type IV is comminuted and displaced. (Subclassification not depicted: type IIIA, without rotation; type IIIB, with rotation.) (Reproduced with permission from Kendall NS, Hsu SY, Chan KM: Fracture of the tibial spine in adults and children: A review of 31 cases. *J Bone Joint Surg* 59A:1111-1114, 1977.)

arthrotomy[128,130,132,135,145,148] or more recently evolved arthroscopic techniques. Suitable fixation methods are dictated by the skills of the surgeon and the integrity of the fracture fragment. This may be accomplished with wires,[137] staples,[146] or insertion of screws in antegrade[133,149,150] or retrograde fashion.[136] Fragmentation of the eminence is best managed with multiple transosseous sutures.[127,147,151,152]

Despite anatomic reduction, extension deficit and measurable laxity may remain.[143,144,153] This, however, is often of little functional consequence. The combination of associated injuries and a tentative postsurgical rehabilitation program, particularly in the adult patient, may render the joint arthrofibrotic and hence impair motion.[127] Change in the structure of the tibial spine due to incomplete reduction or hypertrophy can block full extension. Enlargement of the intercondylar region (notchplasty) may restore this by accommodating the enlarged eminence.[138,139] Additional complications associated with fractures of the tibial eminence include nonunion[129,154] and chronic meniscal entrapment.[155]

Subcondylar Fractures of the Tibia

Subcondylar fractures of the tibia are commonly the result of high-energy trauma. These have been coined "bumper injuries" by Schatzker.[156] Most are associated with significant bicondylar fracture of the tibial plateau. The subcondylar fracture represents the metaphyseal dissociation component of the injury in such cases. Subcondylar fracture of the tibia without intraarticular extension is rare. Subclassification of these fractures has been proposed to allow distinction between low-energy nondisplaced ex-

traarticular fractures and displaced intraarticular fractures with extensive metaphyseal involvement.[157]

Physical examination and radiographic assessment should follow in accordance with the measures described for fractures of the tibial plateau. Isolated fractures of the subcondylar region are amenable to closed treatment with long leg cast application.[158] Those that are displaced and irreducible or unstable require operative treatment. Classifications for metaphyseal dissociation fractures of the proximal tibia have been proposed based upon the presence or absence of articular involvement and degree of metaphyseal comminution.[157,159] For extraarticular subcondylar fractures, some investigators maintain a preference for external fixation,[157] while others recommend indirect reduction and composite fixation (lateral plate/medial external fixator).[160] Such fractures can be addressed with currently available intramedullary nails as well. The surgeon must, however, recognize technical concerns regarding the nails' entry[161,161a] and orientation as well as design[162] and their impact on reduction.

DISLOCATIONS
Knee Dislocation

Tibiofemoral dislocation is an infrequent but potentially catastrophic injury often resulting in compromise to neurovascular and supportive structures of the knee. Urgent recognition and appropriate treatment are mandatory to avoid limb-threatening complications. The true incidence of this injury is unknown, as spontaneous reduction may occur prior to presentation. The diagnosis, therefore, should not be limited only to those cases in which dislocation is immediately apparent clinically or radiographically. All knees demonstrating significant sagittal plane instability after an acute injury should be evaluated for this occasionally devastating injury.

Knee joint stability is maintained by the conformity of articular surfaces as well as the passive (ligamentous) and dynamic (muscular) supportive structures. The cruciates serve as primary restraints in the sagittal plane and assume secondary roles resisting varus-valgus angulation. The collateral ligaments and posterior corner structures offer primarily coronal plane stability. All act in concert to coordinate the "coupled motions" of the knee, conferring rotational stability. The popliteal artery and vein run within the popliteal fossa in close proximity to the posterior joint capsule. The artery is tethered superiorly by the adductor hiatus and distally by the soleus arch. The geniculate vessels offer only marginal collateral supply and further constrain the artery. The tibial nerve accompanies the popliteal vessels in the popliteal fossa but, unlike the vessels, is not secured proximally, affording more freedom from injury. The peroneal nerve courses behind the biceps femoris muscle and around the fibular neck. Traction injuries to this structure are not infrequent and recovery is unpredictable.

Descriptive terms designating types of knee joint dislocation are based upon direction of displacement, soft tissue wounding (open versus closed), energy of injury (high versus low velocity), and reducibility. Those that present dislocated are described as "complete" and those suggesting spontaneous reduction as "functional." The most common basis for classification is founded upon tibial displacement with respect to the femur.[163] There are thus five major categories: anterior, posterior, medial, lateral, and combined (or "rotatory"). Anterior dislocation, arising from knee hyperextension, is most common (Fig. 28-17). Posterior dislocation, requiring more energy, results from a posteriorly directed force applied to the proximal tibia. Medial and lateral dislocations occur from varus or valgus rotatory moments. These are commonly associated with fractures of the tibial plateau and intercondylar region. Lower rates of associated ligamentous and neurovascular injury as well as more predictable treatment alternatives and outcomes require that they be considered as a separate entity.[164]

Evaluation begins with neurovascular assessment of the limb prior to performance of reduction maneuvers (Fig. 28-18). Anterior dislocation imparts traction injury and posterior dislocation complete avulsion-type tearing of the vessel. Abnormal peripheral pulses in this setting are highly predictive of significant arterial injury. In cases demonstrating absent peripheral pulses, vascular exploration, repair, and fasciotomy must be performed within 6 to 8 h to effect satisfactory limb salvage.[165] The site of injury is generally apparent; arteriography is of little additional benefit and is time consuming. The absence of peripheral signs of

ischemia (cyanosis, delayed capillary refill, absent peripheral pulses, pallor) does not exclude the possibility of arterial occlusion or intimal damage.[166,167] Routine performance of a Doppler arterial systolic pressure index after knee dislocation has been suggested if pulses are identifiable to exclude the presence of nonocclusive lesions.[168]

Reduction should be performed immediately, employing traction in a manner dependent upon direction of dislocation. Anterior dislocations are immobilized in mild flexion with avoidance of extension to prevent redislocation.[169] The opposite holds true for posterior variants. A posterolateral dislocation presenting with a skin dimple medially denotes invagination of the medial joint capsule and, accordingly, irreducibility.[170–172]

Inspection of the soft tissue envelope and neurologic status follows. Open dislocation, denoted by compromised skin integrity, suggests an injury of severe energy and carries a very guarded prognosis for limb viability.[173] Radiographic assessment as necessary is performed to identify coincident fractures or dislocations to the remainder of the limb.[174–176]

Upon assurance of restoration of limb viability, the extent of capsuloligamentous damage is determined. Knee dislocation results in rupture of various combinations of ligaments. The previously held notion that all primary static restraints (both cruciates and both collateral ligaments) must be torn has been disputed.[177,178]

Historically, treatment of ligamentous injury arising from knee dislocation has included cast immobilization,[179] primary repair of all structures,[163,169,180–185] and early versus delayed combinations of repair/reconstruction.[186–189] The literature, when surveyed in an attempt to define preferential treatment, is inconclusive due to absence of uniform reporting criteria and lack of convincing prospective scientifically founded studies. Surgical treatment in the past was often complicated by chronic pain and stiffness. Patients appear more tolerant of moderate instability than restricted motion. It is recommended that surgery be delayed until the second week to allow observation for delayed arterial thrombosis.[189,190] Delay beyond this compromises dissection and identification of structures. Whether the cruciates should be repaired only, repaired and augmented, or reconstructed remains unclear. Avulsion lesions may be amenable to reattachment and, according to one study, are not uncommon with dislocation injuries.[169,191] More recent techniques of ligamentous repair/reconstruction offer a more optimistic attitude and allow for aggressive rehabilitation.

As with treatment of ligamentous injury following knee dislocation, dicta regarding the management of nerve injury are unsubstantiated. Identified transected nerve ends should be tagged for eventual repair, presupposing an understanding of the guarded prognosis. Indication for exploration if surgery is not otherwise undertaken remains vague.

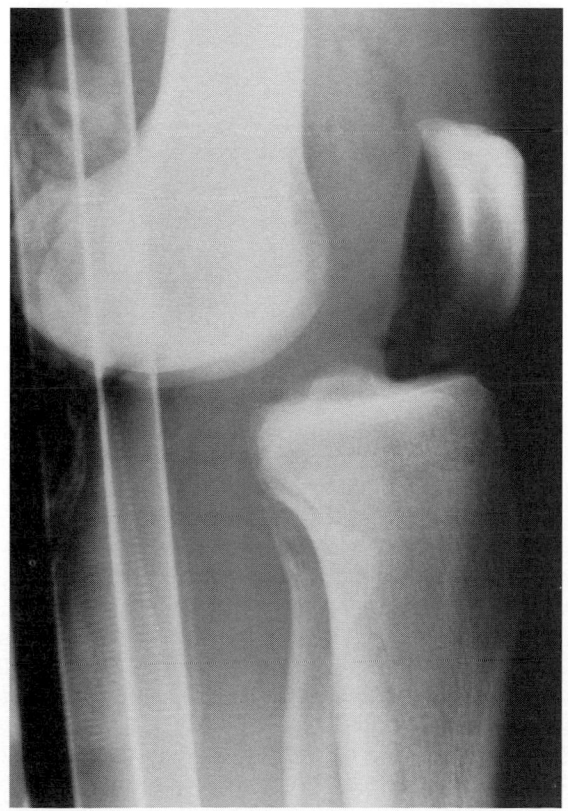

Figure 28-17 Anterior knee dislocation.

Acute Traumatic Patellar Dislocation

Acute traumatic dislocation of the patella occurs primarily in young, active individuals, some of whom may demon-

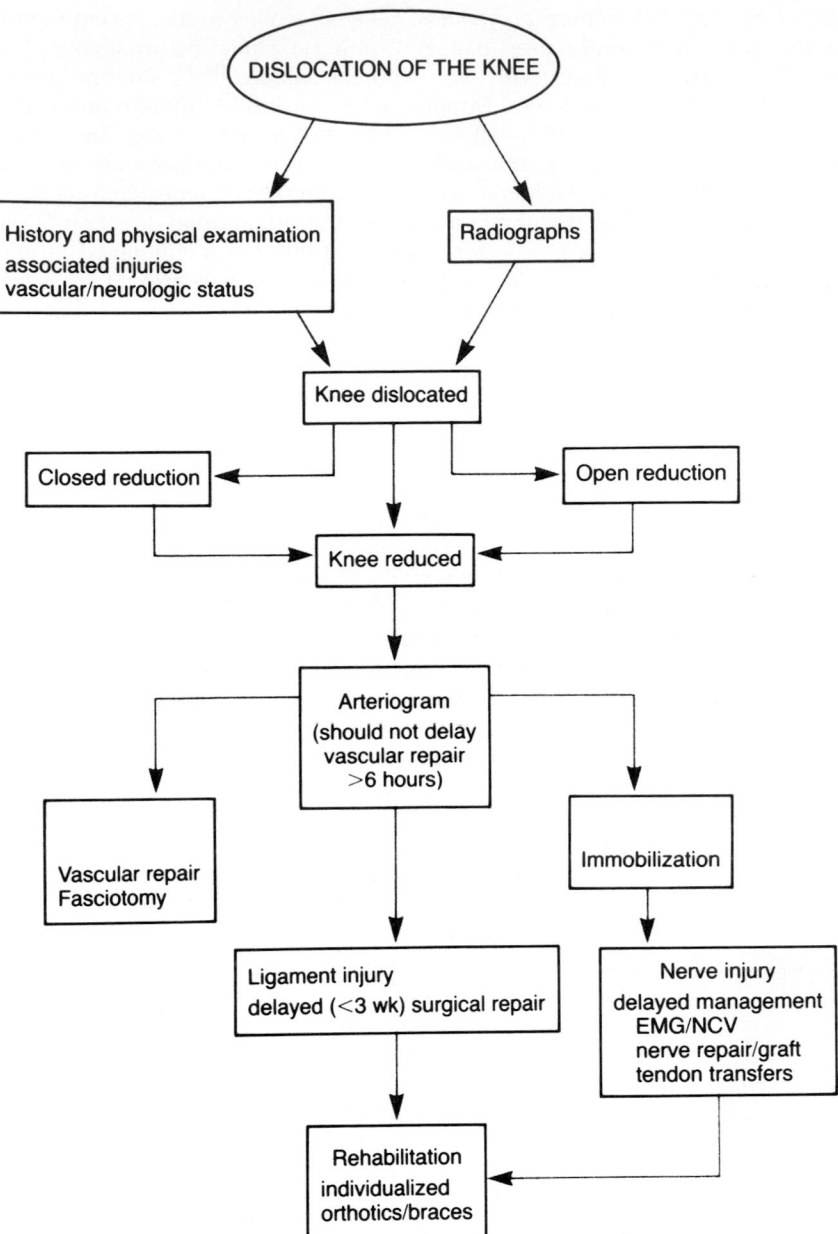

Figure 28-18 Algorithm for dislocation of the knee. [Reproduced with permission from Brown B, Jupiter J, Levine A, et al (eds): *Skeletal Trauma*. Philadelphia, Saunders, 1992, p 1725.]

strate predisposing anatomic factors. Dislocation may occur in the coronal plane or along either the horizontal or vertical axis of the patella. The mechanism of injury is responsible for the variant with which the patient presents. Owing to a tendency to spontaneous reduction, the absence of a clearly apparent dislocation does not exclude the possibility of this diagnosis and complications associated with it. Traumatic patellofemoral dislocation, particularly in the presence of etiologic sources, renders the individual vulnerable to recurrence of injury and chronic symptomatology. Concern for the integrity of the extensor mechanism and the peripatellar retinacular tissues must be maintained and the potential for posttraumatic sequelae (patellar instability, osteochondral injury) kept in mind. Considerable controversy exists regarding the exact location of structural injury and the preferred treatment.

The static stabilizers of the patella consist of the crural fascia and the superficial and deep retinacular layers. Encompassed within the deep layer medially are the medial patellofemoral (MPFL) and patellotibial ligaments. Anatomic variants of the former exist, ranging from robust to absent.[192] The deep fascia of the vastus medialis obliqus (VMO) is adherent to it posteriorly. The MPFL is the principal soft tissue restraint preventing lateral displacement of the patella. Disagreement exists as to its location of traumatic detachment. Some investigators describe ligamentous avulsion from the patella[193,194] while others have observed it to occur from its adductor tubercle origin.[195,196] A negative correlation between patellar tendon length and MPFL integrity has been described.[192] Patella alta accordingly may be associated with a deficient MPFL. Additional anatomic predisposing factors include VMO atrophy, patellar and femoral sulcus morphology, lateral femoral condylar hypoplasia, increased femorotibial angle, femoral anteversion, external tibial torsion, and a history of patellar instability.

Several descriptive terms help distinguish variants of patellar dislocation. These include *location* (intra- versus extraarticular), *direction* (rotational axis), and *degree* (subluxation versus dislocation). Extraarticular dislocation is most common, arising from combined indirect forces of quadriceps contraction, valgus stress, and external rotation of the lower leg. The net result is lateral displacement of the patella with respect to the femur. This is the variant commonly studied in the literature from the standpoints of pathoanatomy, treatment, and outcome. Medial displacement has been described as well but is far less common and often iatrogenic in origin.[197]

Intraarticular dislocation is the result of the patella's rotation about its horizontal or vertical axis while maintaining an anterior position within the knee. Both are subdivided into two categories depending on orientation of the articular surface. Thus, a "horizontal intraarticular" dislocation[198,199] may face superiorly or inferiorly, and a "vertical intraarticular" dislocation[200] medially or laterally. The presence of a horizontal dislocation implies detachment of the knee extensor mechanism at either patellar pole. This, in addition to encountered difficulty with reduction, often necessitates surgical management. Vertical dislocation is the rarest of the two intraarticular subtypes. The likely responsible mechanism is one of a laterally or medially directed force applied to the opposite patellar edge, causing vertical axis rotation. This results in articular surface effacement medially or laterally, respectively. Unlike the case in horizontal types, continuity of the extensor mechanism remains intact, but injury to parapatellar retinacular tissues is likely. Cases of combined lateral dislocation with vertical axis rotational components have been described.[201,202]

Confirmation of patellar dislocation is often reliably made on the basis of inspection and palpation alone. A diagnosis in the reduced state can be made reliably by a history suggesting posttraumatic displacement of the patella, previous patellar instability, presence of medial retinacular tenderness or defect, hemarthrosis, medial epicondylar tenderness (Basset sign),[203] and a positive lateral apprehension sign. The status of the continuity of the extensor mechanism and of the tibiofemoral ligaments is next established. Aforementioned predisposing etiologic factors should be identified clinically and radiographically. Radiographic assessment is initiated with performance of AP, lateral, and tangential views. Quantification of patellar height, sulcus angle, lateral patellofemoral angle, and lateral patellar displacement may offer some insight into patellofemoral dynamics.[204,205] According to some studies of these radiographic observations, statistical significance could be attributed only to sulcus angle[206,207] and asymmetrical lateral displacement.[194] Additional views—including nonoverpenetrated tunnel and oblique images—should be obtained to identify osteoarticular fracture and intraarticular debris. If diagnostic uncertainty exists, MRI may suggest findings consistent with a recent previous patellar dislocation. These include effusion, posterior detachment of the MPFL, retraction of the distal VMO, as well as medial femoral condylar and medial patellar bone bruises.

Presentation in the dislocated state requires reduction. Attempted reduction of intraarticular variants with closed manipulation is appropriate, but it may prove unsuccessful, requiring semiinvasive[200] or open techniques. For the typical lateral dislocation, reduction is achieved closed by applying manual pressure and knee extension, with or without the benefit of systemic or local anesthetic agents. Successful reduction is followed by immobilization or functional rehabilitation.

The potential for the recurrence of injury has prompted some investigators to advocate operative treatment for acute patellar dislocation.[193,203,208–210] It is difficult to define preferential operative treatment because of lack of concurrence regarding the site of the medial lesion (parapatellar versus epicondylar). Sallay et al. describe a surgical repair of the MPFL to its site of femoral detachment.[195] They contend that failures with other techniques result from disregard of this, the "essential lesion." Most authors who favor operative treatment are especially inclined to perform surgery in the presence of preexisting etiologic factors.[211,212] Whether these factors should themselves be addressed directly and remedied remains controversial.

The treatment of associated osteochondral injury begins with its recognition.[207,213] The most common sites of injury are the medial patellar facet and lateral femoral condyle. Plausible mechanisms generating these lesions include injury incurred during the dislocation phase, a fall sustained while in a position of dislocation, and forceful return of the patella to its normal location. Arthroscopy has been offered as a means of identifying suspected lesions not identifiable radiographically. Arthroscopic methods of medial patellar stabilization have been described as well.[214–216]

Proximal Tibiofibular Joint Dislocation

Instability of the proximal tibiofibular joint can be idiopathic or traumatic in origin. Traumatic dislocation results from either direct or indirect mechanisms of injury. It is often unrecognized and erroneously diagnosed as a meniscal lesion or rotatory instability of the knee. Anatomic predisposition may render an individual vulnerable to this injury and complicate treatment. Prompt recognition and an accurate diagnosis are essential to assure a desirable outcome.

The proximal tibiofibular joint is a diarthrodial joint providing articulation between the lateral tibial condyle and the proximal fibula. It has been described as an "accommodatory joint" designed to dissipate torsional stress at the ankle joint.[217] Considerable morphologic variability exists. Ogden describes two types, horizontal and oblique.[218] The latter he suggests to be intrinsically less stable. In addition to vertical inclination, capsuloligamentous structures are responsible for joint support.[219] These are stronger anteriorly than they are posteriorly. Superiorly, support is provided by the lateral collateral ligament;

inferiorly, the interosseous membrane and ankle syndesmotic ligaments provide support. The common peroneal nerve traverses the fibular neck posteriorly and is at risk with posterior dislocation of the joint.

The classification scheme proposed by Ogden describes subluxation—anterolateral, posterolateral, and superior variants.[220] Each is distinguished by unique etiology, complications, and treatment. Subluxation is unassociated with trauma; it is self-limiting and occurs in children and adolescents. Anterolateral dislocation, the most common variant, results from simultaneous hyperflexion of the knee and violent contraction of the anterolateral muscles of the lower leg. A severe direct blow to the anterior aspect of the joint may displace the proximal fibula posteriorly and medially. This type, although infrequent, is most likely to be associated with peroneal nerve deficit. Superior dislocation is usually limited to those injuries with associated fractures or ligamentous lesions to the lower leg.[221–223]

Evaluation begins with obtaining a history of the mechanism of injury. Assessment, particularly with anterolateral dislocation, will demonstrate tenderness and prominence to the proximal fibula as well as incomplete extension of the knee. Radiographs support the diagnosis. If uncertainty exists, however, comparison views may be beneficial.

Adequate treatment of this injury is facilitated by its prompt recognition. Under these circumstances, closed reduction is likely to be successful.[220,224–227] An exception is posteromedial dislocation, for which reduction is often difficult to maintain. Reduction of an anterolateral dislocation requires knee flexion to relax the lateral collateral ligament. Guidelines regarding subsequent weight-bearing restriction and the necessity for immobilization vary. If postreduction instability presents, articular transfixation may be considered. Irreducibility, a problem encountered with delayed treatment, is managed with open reduction and joint transfixation with or without repair of involved ligaments.[228–230] Treatment for chronic dislocation has included fibular head resection[231–234] and arthrodesis of the joint. The former may compromise lateral supportive structures of the knee and the latter impair normal ankle mechanics. Surgical reconstruction of the proximal tibiofibular joint ligaments, in an effort to avoid these problems, has been described.[235,236]

EXTENSOR MECHANISM TENDON RUPTURE

Traumatic disruption of the extensor mechanism of the knee occurs indirectly as a result of rapid contraction of the quadriceps muscle with the knee maintained in flexion. Occasionally, direct (blunt, penetrating) trauma is responsible for interruption of the extensor mechanism. Discontinuity lesions include rupture of the quadriceps or patellar tendons, patellar fracture, and avulsion of the tibial tubercle. Preexistent tendinopathy due to local or systemic conditions may precipitate tendon rupture.[237–240] Additional etiologies include intratendinous injection of corticosteroid agents[241] and chronic repetitive microtrauma sustained by athletes.[242,243] Successful treatment requires early accurate diagnosis followed by surgical reestablishment of extensor mechanism continuity and normal patellar height. Recent trends in management encourage use of autograft or synthetic materials to augment repair, allowing immediate motion of the knee joint.[244–248]

Quadriceps tendon disruption most often occurs in a population greater than 40 years of age. Changes within the quadriceps tendon due to metabolic and collagen disease have been described and implicated in spontaneous rupture (occasionally bilateral).[249] The history obtained is one of acute pain accompanied by giving way of the knee with inability to bear weight to the affected extremity. Physical examination will commonly reveal a palpable defect at the superior patellar pole with inferior displacement of the patella. Attempted active extension of the knee will reveal a lag in contrast to passive extension, which remains uncompromised. Radiographic findings demonstrate superior displacement of the patella, often with concomitant degenerative changes (spurring) at the proximal patellar pole.[250] Magnetic resonance imaging is not normally required to establish the diagnosis unless there is clinical uncertainty (Fig. 28-19).[251]

Quadriceps tendon rupture is most predictably managed by operative repair. Delay in treatment may compromise results owing to quadriceps retraction and fibrosis.[252]

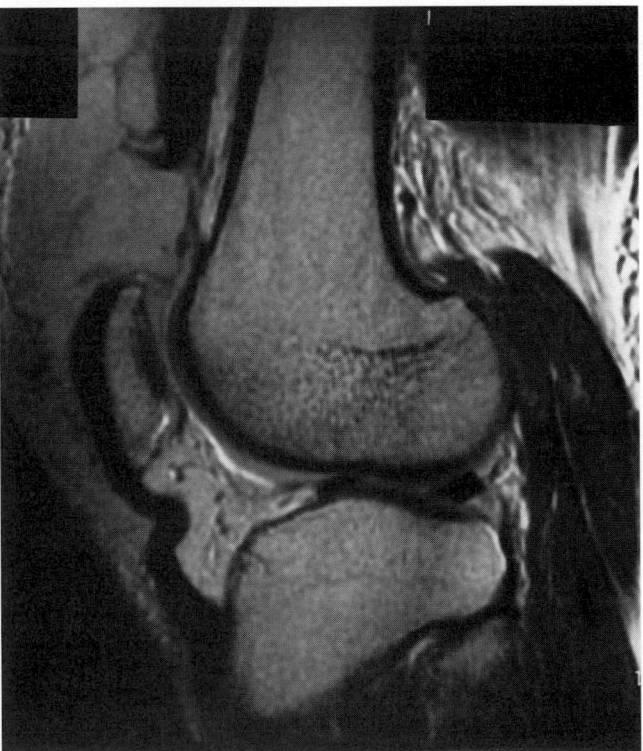

Figure 28-19 Magnetic resonance imaging may be used to support a diagnosis of extensor mechanism injury when clinical uncertainty exists. An example of quadriceps tendon rupture with patella baja (infera) and a patellar tendon "wrinkle" sign.

Figure 28-20 *Left:* Quadriceps rupture repair. Sutures are placed in the tendon; they are passed through three vertical drill holes in the patella and tied at the inferior pole. Retinacular repair is performed. *Right:* Patellar tendon rupture repair. The tendon is repaired directly and augmented with semitendinosus and gracilis tendons. (Adapted with permission from Haas SB, Calloway H: Disruptions of the extensor mechanism. *Orthop Clin North Am* 23:687–695, 1992.)

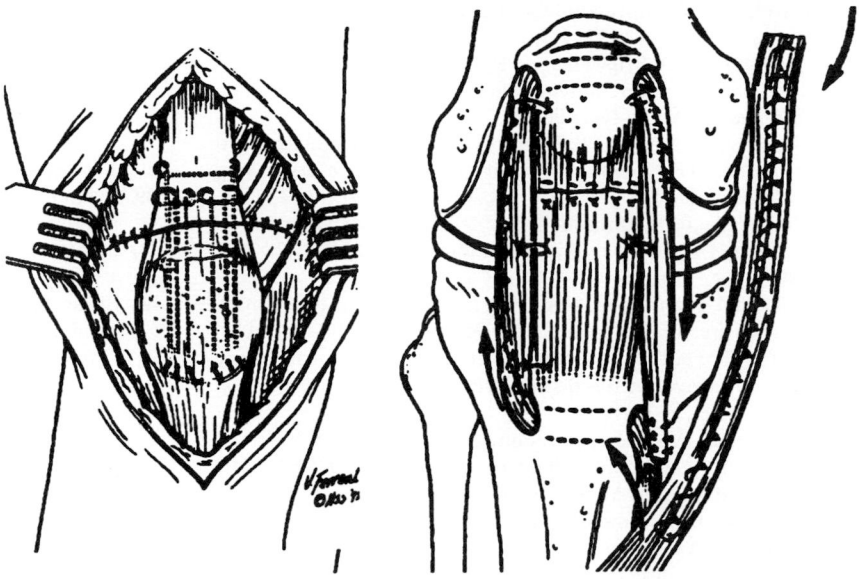

Repair of the acutely disrupted tendon begins with debridement of tendon margins. Direct anastomosis of tendon margins is accomplished and the adequacy of the repair assessed. A distally based triangular flap may be fashioned from the intact portion of the quadriceps tendon to augment the repair.[253] To further neutralize distraction forces, the tendon may be secured with heavy, nonabsorbable suture through vertical osseous tunnels in the patella (Fig. 28-20).[244,254] Postoperative management traditionally has included immobilization in a long leg cast with weight-bearing restriction. Newer protocols advocating surgical reinforcement techniques have evolved, allowing early institution of motion.[247]

Delayed repair of the quadriceps tendon presents difficulties with tendon mobilization. This may necessitate inferior advancement of quadriceps tissues,[253] superior mobilization of the central patellar tendon,[255] or use of synthetic materials.[256] Results are expectedly inferior, emphasizing the need for identification of the lesion upon initial presentation.

Rupture of the patellar tendon tends to occur in a younger, more recreationally active population. The site of the lesion is commonly at the inferior patellar pole. The clinical presentation is similar to that of quadriceps tendon disruption with the exception of direction of patellar displacement (superior). Association with systemic disease, although described, is less common.[257,258] Early repair is performed with insertion of a nonstrangulating suture[259] within the tendon directed through vertically oriented osseous tunnels within the patella. Tension-neutralizing techniques permitting postoperative motion merit consideration (see Fig. 28-20).[244,247] Delayed treatment of neglected patellar tendon ruptures often necessitates reconstruction of the tendon. Techniques include use of autograft tissues[260–263] and synthetic materials.[246,256] Distal mobilization of the patella may prove difficult, requiring preoperative traction or lengthening with tension stress techniques.[264,265]

REFERENCES

DISTAL FEMORAL FRACTURES

1. Olson SA, Holt BT: Anatomy of the medial distal femur: A study of the adductor hiatus. *J Orthop Trauma* 9:63–65, 1995.
2. Muller ME, Nazarian S, Koch P, Schatzker J: *The Comprehensive Classification of Fractures of Long Bones.* New York, Springer-Verlag, 1990.
3. Schatzker J, Lambert DC: Supracondylar fractures of the femur. *Clin Orthop Rel Res* 138:77–83, 1979.
4. Seinsheimer F: Fractures of the distal femur. *Clin Orthop Rel Res* 153:169–179, 1980.
5. Neer CS, Grantham SA, Shelton ML: Supracondylar fracture of the adult femur: A study of one hundred and ten cases. *J Bone Joint Surg* 49A:591–613, 1967.
6. Stewart MJ, Sisk TD, Wallace SL: Fractures of the distal third of the femur. *J Bone Joint Surg* 48A:784–807, 1966.
7. Mooney V, Nickel VL, Harvey JP, Snelson R: Cast-brace treatment for fractures of the distal part of the femur. *J Bone Joint Surg* 52A:1563–1578, 1970.
8. Brown A, D'Arcy JC: Internal fixation for supracondylar fractures of the femur in the elderly patient. *J Bone Joint Surg* 53B:420–424, 1971.
9. Browner BD, Burgess AR, Robertson RJ, et al: Immediate closed antegrade ender nailing of femoral fractures in polytrauma patients. *J Trauma* 24:921–927, 1984.
10. Giles JB, DeLee JC, Heckman JD, Keever JE: Supracondylar-intercondylar fractures of the femur treated with a supracondylar plate and lag screw. *J Bone Joint Surg* 64A:864–870, 1982.
11. Gregory P, Sanders R: The treatment of supracondylar-intracondylar fractures of the femur using the dynamic condylar screw. *Tech Orthop* 9:195–202, 1995.
12. Healy WL, Brooker AF Jr: Distal femoral fractures: Comparison of open and closed methods of treatment. *Clin Orthop Rel Res* 174:166–171, 1983.
13. Mize RD: Surgical management of complex fractures of the distal femur. *Clin Orthop Rel Res* 240:77–86, 1989.
14. Olerud S: Operative treatment of supracondylar-condylar fractures of the femur. *J Bone Joint Surg* 54A:1015–1032, 1972.

15. Pritchett JW: Supracondylar fractures of the femur. *Clin Orthop Rel Res* 184:173–177, 1984.

16. Shelbourne KD, Brusckmann FR: Rush-pin fixation of supracondylar and intercondylar fractures of the femur. *J Bone Joint Surg* 64A:161–169, 1982.

17. Shewring DJ, Meggitt BF: Fractures of the distal femur treated with the AO dynamic condylar screw. *J Bone Joint Surg* 74B:122–125, 1992.

18. Shahcheraghi H, Doroodchi HR: Supracondylar fracture of the femur: Closed or open reduction? *J Trauma* 34:499–502, 1993.

19. Siliski JM, Mahring M, Hofer HP: Supracondylar-intercondylar fractures of the femur. *J Bone Joint Surg* 71A:95–104, 1989.

20. Zickel RE, Fietti VG, Lawsing JF, et al: A new intramedullary fixation device for the distal third of the femur. *Clin Orthop* 125:185–191, 1977.

21. Mueller ME, Allogoewer M, Schneider R, Willeneger H: *Manual of Internal Fixation: Techniques Recommended by the AO Group*, 2d ed. New York, Springer-Verlag, 1991.

22. Bolhofner BR, Carmen B, Clifford P: The results of open reduction and internal fixation of distal femur fractures using a biologic (indirect) reduction technique. *J Orthop Trauma* 10:372–377, 1996.

23. Bone LB: Indirect fracture reduction: A technique for minimizing surgical trauma. *J Am Acad Orthop Surg* 2:247–254, 1994.

24. Mast J, Jakob R, Ganz R: *Planning and Reduction Technique in Fracture Surgery*. Berlin, Springer-Verlag, 1989.

25. Malkani AL, Helfet DL: Blade-plate fixation of supracondylar femur fractures. *Tech Orthop* 9:203–209, 1995.

26. Zehntner MK, Marchesi DG, Burch H, Ganz R: Alignment of supracondylar/intercondylar fractures of the femur after internal fixation by AO/ASIF technique. *J Orthop Trauma* 6:318–326, 1992.

27. Sanders R, Swiontkowsky M, Rosen H, Helfet D: Double-plating of comminuted, unstable fractures of the distal part of the femur. *J Bone Joint Surg* 73A:341–346, 1991.

28. Firoozbakhsh K, Behzadi K, DeCoster TA, et al: Mechanics of retrograde nail versus plate fixation for supracondylar femur fractures. *J Orthop Trauma* 9:152–157, 1995.

29. Zickel RE, Hobeika P, Robbins DS: Zickel supracondylar nails for fractures of the distal end of the femur. *Clin Orthop Rel Res* 212:79–88, 1986.

30. Marks DS, Isbister ES, Porter KM: Zickel supracondylar nailing for supracondylar femoral fractures in elderly or infirm patients. *J Bone Joint Surg* 76B:596–601, 1994.

31. Danziger MB, Caucci D, Zecher SB, et al: Treatment of intercondylar and supracondylar distal femur fractures using the GSH supracondylar nail. *Am J Orthop* 24(9):684–690, 1995.

32. Henry SL, Seligson D: Management of supracondylar fractures of the femur with the GSH supracondylar nail: The percutaneous technique. *Tech Orthop* 93:189–194, 1995.

33. Iannacone WM, Bennett FS, DeLong WG Jr, et al: Initial experience with the treatment of supracondylar femoral fractures using the supracondylar intramedullary nail: A preliminary report. *J Orthop Trauma* 8:322–327, 1994.

34. Lucas SE, Seligson D, Henry SL: Intramedullary supracondylar nailing of femoral fractures: A preliminary report of the GSH supracondylar nail. *Clin Orthop Rel Res* 296:200–206, 1993.

35. Johnson EE, Marroquin CE, Kossovsky N: Synovial metallosis resulting from intraarticular intramedullary nailing of a distal femoral nonunion. *J Orthop Trauma* 7:320–324, 1993.

36. Butler MS, Brumback RJ, Ellison S, et al: Interlocking intramedullary nailing for ipsilateral fractures of the femoral shaft and distal part of the femur. *J Bone Joint Surg* 73A:1492–1502, 1991.

37. Leung KS, Shen WY, So WS, et al: Interlocking intramedullary nailing for supracondylar and intercondylar fractures of the distal part of the femur. *J Bone Joint Surg* 73A:332–340, 1991.

38. Wood EG, Savoie FH, Vander Griend RA: Treatment of ipsilateral fractures of the distal femur and femoral shaft. *J Orthop Trauma* 5:177–183, 1991.

39. Bucholz RW, Ross SE, Lawrence KL: Fatigue fracture of the interlocking nail in the treatment of fractures of the distal part of the femoral shaft. *J Bone Joint Surg* 69A:1391–1399, 1987.

40. Bosse MJ, Sims S, Kellam JF: External fixation of supracondylar femur fractures in the multiple-trauma patient. *Tech Orthop* 9:221–224, 1995.

41. Ostermann PAW, Neumann K, Ekkernkamp A, Muhr G: Long term results of unicondylar fractures of the femur. *J Orthop Trauma* 8:142–146, 1994.

42. Moore TJ, Watson T, Green SA, et al: Complications of surgically treated supracondylar fractures of the femur. *J Trauma* 27:402–406, 1987.

43. Helpenstell T, Hansen JS: The treatment of open distal femur fractures with immediate open reduction and internal fixation. *J Orthop Trauma* 5:235, 1991.

44. Schemitsch E, Waddal J, Kellam J, Powell J: Results of immediate internal fixation of open supracondylar fractures of the femur. *J Orthop Trauma* 5:235, 1991.

45. Koval KJ, Seligson D, Rosen H, Fee K: Distal femoral nonunion: Treatment with a retrograde inserted locked intramedullary nail. *J Orthop Trauma* 9(4):285–291, 1995.

46. McLaren AC, Blokker CP: Locked intramedullary fixation for metaphyseal malunion and nonunion. *Clin Orthop Rel Res* 265:253–260, 1991.

47. Wu CC, Shih CH: Distal femoral nonunion treated with interlocking nailing. *J Trauma* 31:1659–1662, 1991.

48. Matelic TM, Monroe MT, Mast JW: The use of endosteal substitution in the treatment of recalcitrant nonunions of the femur: Report of seven cases. *J Orthop Trauma* 10:1–6, 1996.

49. Koval KJ, Rosen H, Sanders R: Nonunions of the distal femur: Treatment strategies. *J Orthop Trauma* 9(4):285–291, 1994.

50. Beall MS, Nebel E, Bailey RW: Transarticular fixation in the treatment of non-union of supracondylar fractures of the femur: A salvage procedure. *J Bone Joint Surg [Am]* 61:1018–1023, 1979.

51. Karpman RR, Del Mar NB: Supracondylar femoral fractures in the frail elderly. *Clin Orthop Rel Res* 315:21–24, 1995.

52. Meek RN, Boyle MR: Technique for the operative management of supracondylar and intracondylar fractures of the distal femur. *Tech Orthop* 1:39–43, 1986.

53. Struhl S, Szporn MN, Cobelli NJ, Sadler AH: Cemented internal fixation for supracondylar femur fractures in osteoporotic patients. *J Orthop Trauma* 4:151–157, 1990.

54. Freedman EL, Hak DJ, Johnson EE, Echardt JJ: Total knee replacement including a modular distal femoral component in elderly patients with acute fracture or nonunion. *J Orthop Trauma* 9:231–237, 1995.

PATELLAR FRACTURES

55. Kaufer H: Mechanical function of the patella. *J Bone Joint Surg* 53A:1551–1560, 1971.

56. Saltzman CL, Goulet JA, McClellan RT, et al: Results of treatment of displaced patella fractures by partial patellectomy. *J Bone Joint Surg* 72A:1279–1285, 1990.

57. Brooke R: The treatment of fractured patella by excision: A study of morphology and function. *Br J Surg* 24:733–747, 1937.

58. Waston-Jones R: Excision of the patella. *Br Med J* 2:195–196, 1945.
59. West FE: End results of patellectomy. *J Bone Joint Surg* 44A:1089–1108, 1962.
60. Bostman O, Kiviluoto O, Nirhamo J: Comminuted displaced fracture of the patella. *Injury* 13:196–202, 1981.
61. Rink PC, Scott F: The operative repair of displaced patellar fractures. *Orthop Rev* 20:157–165, 1991.
62. Sutton FS Jr, Thompson CH, Lipke J, Kettelkamp DB: The effect of patellectomy on knee function. *J Bone Joint Surg* 58A:537–540, 1976.
63. Wilkinson J: Fracture of the patella treated by total excision. *J Bone Joint Surg* 59B:352–354, 1977.
64. Hung LK, Lee SY, Leung KM, Nicholl LA: Partial patellectomy for patellar fracture: Tension band wiring and early mobilization. *J Orthop Trauma* 7:252–260, 1993.
65. Lotke PA, Ecker ML: Transverse fractures of the patella. *Clin Orthop* 158:180–184, 1981.
66. Muller ME, Allogower M, Schneider R, Willenegger H: *Manual of Internal Fixation: Techniques Recommended by the AO Group.* 3d ed. Berlin, Springer-Verlag, 1991.
67. Quan-Yi L, Jai-Wen W: Fracture of the patella treated by open reduction and external compressive skeletal fixation. *J Bone Joint Surg* 69A:83–89, 1987.
68. Leung PC, Mak KH, Lee SY: Percutaneous tension band wiring: A new method of internal fixation for mildly displaced patella fracture. *J Trauma* 23:62–64, 1983.
69. Ma YZ, Zhang YF, Yeh YC: Treatment of fractures of the patella with percutaneous suture. *Clin Orthop* 191:235–241, 1984.
70. Weber MJ, McLeod P, Nelson CL, et al: Efficacy of various forms of fixation of transverse fractures of the patella. *J Bone Joint Surg* 62A:215–220, 1980.
71. Benjamin J, Bried J, Dohm M, McMurtry M: Biomechanical evaluation of various forms of fixation of transverse patellar fractures. *J Orthop Trauma* 1:219–222, 1987.
72. Curtis MJ: Internal fixation for fractures of the patella. *J Bone Joint Surg* 72B:280–282, 1990.
73. Johnson EE: Part II: Fractures of the patella, in Rockwood DP, Bucholz RW: *Rockwood and Green's Fractures in Adults,* 3d ed. Vol 2. Philadelphia, Lippincott, 1991.
74. Pandey AK, Pandey S, Pandey P: Results of partial patellectomy. *Arch Orthop Trauma Surg* 110:246–249, 1991.
75. Levack BF, Hobbs S: Results of surgical treatment of patellar fractures. *J Bone Joint Surg* 67B:416–419, 1985.
76. Perry CR, McCarthy JA, Kain CC, Pearson RL: Patellar fixation protected with a load-sharing cable: A mechanical and clinical study. *J Orthop Trauma* 2:234–240, 1988.
77. Leung KS, Kevin MH, Shen WY, Leung PC: Reconstruction of extensor mechanism after trauma and infection by transposition of the achilles tendon: Report of techniques and four cases. *J Orthop Trauma* 8:40–44, 1994.
78. Satku K, Kumar VP: Surgical management of non-union of neglected fractures of the patella. *Injury* 21:108–110, 1991.

TIBIAL PLATEAU FRACTURES

79. Anglen JO, Healy WL: Tibial plateau fractures. *Orthopedics* 11:1527–1534, 1988.
80. Schatzker J, McBroom R, Bruce D: The tibial plateau fracture: The Toronto experience 1968–1975. *Clin Orthop Rel Res* 138:94–104, 1979.
81. Walker PS, Erkman MJ: The role of the menisci in force transmission across the knee. *Clin Orthop Rel Res* 109:184–192, 1975.
82. Honkonen SE: Degenerative arthritis after tibial plateau fractures. *J Orthop Trauma* 9:273–277, 1995.
83. Bennett WF, Browner B: Tibial plateau fractures: A study of associated soft tissue injuries. *J Orthop Trauma* 8:183–188, 1994.
84. Delamarter RB, Hohl M, Hopp E Jr: Ligament injuries associated with tibial plateau fractures. *Clin Orthop Rel Res* 250:226–233, 1990.
85. Martin AF: The pathomechanics of the knee joint. *J Bone Joint Surg* 42A:13–22, 1960.
86. Kode L, Lieberman JM, Motta AO, et al: Evaluation of tibial plateau fractures: Efficacy of MR imaging compared with CT. *Am J Roentgenol* 163:141–147, 1994.
87. Muller ME, Allgower M, Schneider R, Willenegger H: *Manual of Internal Fixation,* 3d ed. New York, Springer-Verlag, 1991, pp 142–143.
88. Honkonen SE, Jarvinen MJ: Classification of fractures of the tibial condyles. *J Bone Joint Surg* 74B:840–847, 1992.
89. Blokker CP, Rorabeck CH, Bourne RB: Tibial plateau fractures: An analysis of the results of treatment in 60 patients. *Clin Orthop Rel Res* 182:193–199, 1984.
90. Burri C, Bartzke G, Coldewey J, Muggler E: Fractures of the tibial plateau. *Clin Orthop Rel Res* 138:84–93, 1979.
91. Lachiewicz PF, Funcik T: Factors influencing the results of open reduction and internal fixation of tibial plateau fractures. *Clin Orthop Rel Res* 259:210–215, 1990.
92. Savoie FH, Vander Griend RA, Ward EF, Hughes JL: Tibial plateau fractures: A review of operative treatment using AO technique. *Orthopedics* 10:745–750, 1987.
93. Waddell JP, Johnston DWC, Neidre A: Fractures of the tibial plateau: A review of ninety-five patients and comparison of treatment methods. *J Trauma* 21:376–381, 1981.
94. Duwelius PJ, Connolly JF: Closed reduction of tibial plateau fractures: A comparison of functional and roentgenographic end results. *Clin Orthop Rel Res* 230:116–126, 1988.
95. Lansinger O, Bergman B, Korner L, Andersson GBJ: Tibial condylar fractures: A twenty-year follow-up. *J Bone Joint Surg* 68A:13–19, 1986.
96. Rasmussen PS: Tibial condylar fractures: Impairment of knee joint stability as an indication for surgical treatment. *J Bone Joint Surg* 55A:1331–1350, 1973.
97. Jensen DB, Rude C, Duus B, Bjerg-Nielsen A: Tibial plateau fractures: A comparison of conservative and surgical treatment. *J Bone Joint Surg* 72B:49–52, 1990.
98. Drennan DB, Locher FG, Maylahn DJ: Fractures of the tibial plateau: Treatment by closed reduction and spica cast. *J Bone Joint Surg* 61A:989–995, 1979.
99. Apley AG: Fractures of the lateral tibial condyle treated by skeletal traction and early mobilization: A review of sixty cases with special reference to the long-term results. *J Bone Joint Surg* 38B:699–708, 1956.
100. Volpin G, Dowd GSE, Stein H, Bentley G: Degenerative arthritis after intra-articular fractures of the knee: Long-term results. *J Bone Joint Surg* 72B:634–638, 1990.
101. Weissman SL, Herold ZH: Fractures of the tibial plateau. *Clin Orthop Rel Res* 33:194–200, 1964.
102. Honkonen SE: Indications for surgical treatment of tibial condyle fractures. *Clin Orthop Rel Res* 302:199–205, 1994.
103. Moore TM, Patzakis MJ, Harvey JP: Tibial plateau fractures: Definition, demographics, treatment rationale, and long-term results of closed traction management or operative reduction. *J Orthop Trauma* 1:97–119, 1987.
104. DeCoster TA, Nepola JV, El-Khoury GY: Cast brace treatment of proximal tibia fractures: A ten-year follow-up study. *Clin Orthop Rel Res* 231:196–204, 1988.
105. Koval KJ, Sanders R, Borrelli J, et al: Indirect reduction and percutaneous screw fixation of displaced tibial plateau fractures. *J Orthop Trauma* 6:340–346, 1992.
106. Benirschke SK, Agnew SG, Mayo KA, et al: Immediate internal fixation of open, complex tibial plateau fractures: Treatment by a standard protocol. *J Orthop Trauma* 6:78–86, 1992.

107. Murphy CP, D'Ambrosia R, Dabezies EJ: The small pin circular fixator for proximal tibial fractures with soft tissue compromise. *Orthopedics* 14:273–280, 1991.

108. Weiner LS, Kelley M, Yang E, et al: The use of combination internal fixation and hybrid external fixation in severe proximal tibia fractures. *J Orthop Trauma* 9:244–250, 1995.

109. Stamer DT, Schenk R, Staggers B, et al: Bicondylar tibial plateau fractures treated with a hybrid ring external fixator: A preliminary study. *J Orthop Trauma* 8:455–461, 1994.

110. Ries MD, Meinhard BP: Medial external fixation with lateral plate internal fixation in metaphyseal tibia fractures: A report of eight cases associated with severe soft-tissue injury. *Clin Orthop Rel Res* 256:215–223, 1990.

111. Marsh JL, Smith ST, Do TT: External fixation and limited internal fixation for complex fractures of the tibial plateau. *J Bone Joint Surg* 77A:661–673, 1995.

112. Tscherne H, Lobenhoffer P: Tibial plateau fractures: Management and expected results. *Clin Orthop Rel Res* 292:87–100, 1993.

113. Georgiadis GM: Combined anterior and posterior approaches for complex tibial plateau fractures. *J Bone Joint Surg* 76B:285–289, 1994.

114. De Boeck H, Opdecam P: Posteromedial tibial plateau fractures: Operative treatment by posterior approach. *Clin Orthop Rel Res* 320:125–128, 1995.

115. Perry CR, Evans LG, Rice S, et al: A new surgical approach to fractures of the lateral tibial plateau. *J Bone Joint Surg* 66A:1236–1240, 1984.

116. Karas EH, Weiner LS, Yang EC: The use of an anterior incision of the meniscus for exposure of tibial plateau fractures requiring open reduction and internal fixation. *J Orthop Trauma* 10:243–247, 1996.

117. Schatzker J: *Fractures of the Tibial Plateau: Rationale of Operative Fracture Care.* New York, Springer-Verlag, 1987, pp 279–295.

118. Fernandez DL: Anterior approach to the knee with osteotomy of the tibial tubercle for bicondylar tibial fractures. *J Bone Joint Surg* 72A:208–219, 1988.

119. Gossling HR, Peterson CA: A new surgical approach in the treatment of depressed lateral condylar fractures of the tibia. *Clin Orthop Rel Res* 140:96–102, 1979.

120. Carr DE: Arthroscopically assisted stabilization of tibial plateau fractures. *Tech Orthop* 6:55–57, 1991.

121. Fowble CD, Zimmer JW, Schepsis AA: The role of arthroscopy in the assessment and treatment of tibial plateau fractures. *Arthroscopy* 9:584–590, 1993.

122. Holzach P, Matter P, Minter J: Arthroscopically assisted treatment of lateral tibial plateau fractures in skiers: Use of a cannulated reduction system. *J Orthop Trauma* 8:273–281, 1994.

123. Jennings JE: Arthroscopic management of tibial plateau fractures. *Arthroscopy* 1:160–168, 1985.

124. Young MJ, Barrack RL: Complications of internal fixation of tibial plateau fractures. *Orthop Rev* 23:149–154, 1994.

125. Andrews JR, Tedder JL, Godbout BP: Bicondylar tibial plateau fracture complicated by compartment syndrome. *Orthop Rev* 21:317–319, 1992.

126. King GJW, Schatzker J: Nonunion of a complex tibial plateau fracture. *J Orthop Trauma* 5:209–212, 1991.

TIBIAL EMINENCE FRACTURES

127. Berg EE: Comminuted tibial eminence anterior cruciate ligament avulsion fractures: Failure of arthroscopic treatment. *Arthroscopy* 9:446–450, 1993.

128. Kendall NS, Hsu SY, Chan KM: Fracture of the tibial spine in adults and children: A review of 31 cases. *J Bone Joint Surg* 74B:848–852, 1992.

129. Sullivan DJ, Dines DM, Hershon SJ, Rose HA: Natural history of a type III fracture of the intercondylar eminence of the tibia in an adult: A case report. *Am J Sports Med* 17:132–133, 1989.

130. Meyers MH, McKeever FM: Fracture of the intercondylar eminence of the tibia. *J Bone Joint Surg* 52A:1677–1684, 1970.

131. Clanton TO, DeLee JC, Sanders B, Neidre A: Knee ligament injuries in children. *J Bone Joint Surg* 61A:1195–1201, 1979.

132. Smith JB: Knee instability after fractures of the intercondylar eminence of the tibia. *J Pediatr Orthop* 4:462–464, 1984.

133. Berg EE: Pediatric tibial eminence fractures: Arthroscopic cannulated screw fixation. *Arthroscopy* 11:328–331, 1995.

134. Meyers MH, McKeever FM: Fractures of the intercondylar eminence of the tibia. *J Bone Joint Surg* 41:209–222, 1959.

135. Zarcznyj B: Avulsion fracture of the tibial eminence treated by open reduction and pinning. *J Bone Joint Surg* 59A:1111–1114, 1977.

136. van Loon T, Marti RK: A fracture of the intercondylar eminence of the tibia treated by arthroscopic fixation: A case report. *J Arthrop Rel Surg* 7:385–388, 1991.

137. McLennan JG: The role of arthroscopic surgery in the treatment of fractures of the intercondylar eminence of the tibia. *J Bone Joint Surg* 64B:477–480, 1982.

138. Freedman KB, Glasgow SG: Arthroscopic roofplasty: Correction of an extension deficit following conservative treatment of a type III tibial avulsion fracture. *Arthroscopy* 11:231–234, 1995.

139. Luger EJ, Arbel R, Eichenblat MS, et al: Femoral notchplasty in the treatment of malunited intercondylar eminence fractures of the tibia. *Arthroscopy* 10:550–551, 1994.

140. Clark HO: Fractures of the tibia involving the knee joint: Fracture of the tibial tubercle. *Proc R Soc Med* 28:1043, 1935.

141. Smillie IS: *Injuries of the Knee Joint.* Edinburgh and London, Livingstone, 1962, pp 199–204.

142. Bakalim G, Wilppula E: Closed treatment of fracture of the tibial spines. *Injury* 5:210–212, 1973.

143. Wiley JJ, Baxter MP: Tibial spine fractures in children. *Clin Orthop Rel Res* 255:54–60, 1990.

144. Molander ML, Wallin G, Wikstad I: Fracture of the intercondylar eminence of the tibia. *J Bone Joint Surg* 63B:89–91, 1981.

145. Falstie-Jensen S, Petersen PES: Incarceration of the meniscus in fractures of the intercondylar eminence of the tibia in children. *Injury* 15:236–238, 1984.

146. Kobayashi S, Terayama K: Arthroscopic reduction and fixation of a completely displaced fracture of the intercondylar eminence of the tibia. *Arthroscopy* 10:231–235, 1994.

147. Matthews DE, Geissler WB: Arthroscopic suture fixation of displaced tibial eminence fractures. *Arthroscopy* 10:418–423, 1994.

148. Hayes JM, Masear VR: Avulsion fracture of the tibial eminence associated with severe medial ligamentous injury in an adolescent: A case report and literature review. *Am J Sports Med* 12:330–333, 1984.

149. Lubowitz JH, Grauer JD: Arthroscopic treatment of anterior cruciate ligament avulsion. *Clin Orthop* 294:242–246, 1993.

150. Veselko M, Senekovic V, Tonin M: Simple and safe arthroscopic placement and removal of cannulated screw and washer for fixation of tibial avulsion fracture of the anterior cruciate ligament. *Arthroscopy* 12:259–262, 1996.

151. Carro LP, Suarez GG, Cimiano FG: The arthroscopic knot technique for fracture of the tibia in children. *Arthroscopy* 10:698–699, 1994.

152. Medler RG, Jansson KA: Arthroscopic treatment of fractures of the tibial spine. *Arthroscopy* 10:292–295, 1994.

153. Baxter MP, Wiley JJ: Fractures of the tibial spine in children: An evaluation of knee stability. *J Bone Joint Surg* 70B:228–230, 1988.

154. Keys GW, Walters J: Nonunion of intercondylar eminence fracture of the tibia. *J Trauma* 28:870–871, 1988.

155. Burstein DB, Viola A, Fulkerson JP: Entrapment of the medial meniscus in a fracture of the tibial eminence: A case report. *Arthroscopy* 4:47–50, 1988.

SUBCONDYLAR FRACTURES OF THE TIBIA

156. Schatzker J, McBroom R, Bruce D: The tibial plateau fracture: The Toronto experience 1968–1975. *Clin Orthop Rel Res* 138:94–104, 1979.

157. Yang EC, Weiner L, Strauss E, et al: Metaphyseal dissociation fractures of the proximal tibia: An analysis of treatment and complications. *Am J Orthop* 24(9):695–704, 1995.

158. Hohl M, Johnson EE, Wiss DA: Fractures of the knee: Part I: fractures of the proximal tibia and fibula, in Rockwood DP, Bucholz RW (eds): *Rockwood and Green's Fractures in Adults,* 3d ed. Vol 2. Philadelphia, Lippincott, 1991, p 1756.

159. Muller ME, Nazarian S, Koch P, Schatzker J: *The Comprehensive Classification of Fractures of Long Bones.* New York, Springer-Verlag, 1990.

160. Bolhofner BR: Indirect reduction and composite fixation of extraarticular proximal tibial fractures. *Clin Orthop* 315:75–83, 1995.

161. Freedman EL, Johnson EE: Radiographic analysis of tibial fracture malalignment following intramedullary nailing. *Clin Orthop* 315:25–33, 1995.

161a. Lang GJ, Cohen BE, Bosse MJ, Kellam JF: Proximal third tibial shaft fractures: Should they be nailed?. *Clin Orthop* 315:64–74, 1995.

162. Henley MB, Meier M, Tencer AF: Influences of some design parameters on the biomechanics of the unreamed tibial intramedullary nail. *J Orthop Trauma* 7:311–319, 1993.

KNEE DISLOCATION

163. Kennedy JC: Complete dislocation of the knee joint. *J Bone Joint Surg* 45A:889–904, 1963.

164. Moore TM: Fracture-dislocation of the knee. *Clin Orthop Rel Res* 156:128–140, 1981.

165. Green NE, Allen BL: Vascular injuries associated with dislocation of the knee. *J Bone Joint Surg* 59A:236–239, 1977.

166. McCoy GF, Hannon DG, Barr RJ, Templeton J: Vascular injury associated with low-velocity dislocations of the knee. *J Bone Joint Surg* 69B:285–287, 1987.

167. McCutchan JD, Gillham NR: Injury to the popliteal artery associated with dislocation of the knee: Palpable distal pulses do not negate the requirement for arteriography. *Injury* 30:307–310, 1989.

168. Johansen K, Lynch K, Paun M, Copass M: Non-invasive vascular tests reliably exclude occult arterial trauma in injured extremities. *J Trauma* 31:515–522, 1991.

169. Sisto DJ, Warren RF: Complete knee dislocation: A follow-up study of operative treatment. *Clin Orthop Rel Res* 198:94–101, 1985.

170. Nystrom M, Samimi S, Ha'Eri GB: Two cases of irreducible knee dislocation occurring simultaneously in two patients and a review of the literature. *Clin Orthop Rel Res* 277:197–200, 1992.

171. Quinlan AG, Sharrard WJW: Posterolateral dislocation of the knee with capsular interposition. *J Bone Joint Surg* 40:660–663, 1958.

172. Wand JS: A physical sign denoting irreducibility of a dislocated knee. *J Bone Joint Surg* 71B:862, 1989.

173. Wright DG, Covey DC, Born CT, Sadasivan KK: Open dislocation of the knee. *J Orthop Trauma* 9:135–140, 1995.

174. Freedman DM, Freedman EL, Shapiro MS: Ipsilateral hip and knee dislocation: A case report. *J Orthop Trauma* 8:177–180, 1994.

175. Kreibich DN, Moran CG, Pinder IM: Ipsilateral hip and knee dislocation: A case report. *Acta Orthop Scand* 60:90–91, 1989.

176. Millea TP, Romanelli RR, Segal LS, Lynch CJ: Ipsilateral fracture-dislocation of the hip, knee, and ankle: Case report. *J Trauma* 31:416–419, 1991.

177. Cooper DE, Speer KP, Wickiewicz TL, et al: Complete knee dislocation without posterior cruciate ligament disruption: A report of four cases and review of the literature. *Clin Orthop* 284:228–233, 1992.

178. Meyers MH, Moore TM, Harvey JP: Traumatic dislocation of the knee joint. *J Bone Joint Surg* 57A:430–433, 1975.

179. Taylor AR, Arden GP, Rainey HA: Traumatic dislocation of the knee: A report of forty-three cases with special reference to conservative treatment. *J Bone Joint Surg* 54A:96–102, 1972.

180. Covey DC, Albright JA: Traumatic dislocation of the knee with special reference to complete ligamentous repair. *Orthop Trans* 11:538, 1987.

181. Frassica FJ, Sim FH, Staeheli JW, Pairolero PC: Dislocation of the knee. *Clin Orthop Rel Res* 263:200–205, 1991.

182. Meyers MH, Harvey JP: Traumatic dislocation of the knee. *J Bone Joint Surg* 53A:16–29, 1971.

183. Montgomery JB: Dislocation of the knee. *Orthop Clin North Am* 18:149–156, 1987.

184. O'Donoghue DH: Analysis of end results of surgical treatment of major injuries to ligaments of the knee. *J Bone Joint Surg* 37A:1, 1955.

185. Roman PD, Hopson CN, Zennie EJ: Traumatic dislocation of the knee: A report of 30 cases and literature review. *Orthop Rev* 16:917–924, 1987.

186. Feagin JA Jr: Case study 7: *The Crucial Ligaments*, New York, Edinburgh, London, Melbourne, Churchill Livingstone, 1988.

187. Shelbourne K, Porter D, Clingman J, et al: Low-velocity knee dislocation. *Orthop Rev* 20:995–1004, 1991.

188. Windsor R: Surgery of the knee, in *Dislocation,* 2d ed. New York, Churchill Livingstone, 1993.

189. Merrill KD: Knee dislocations with vascular injuries. *Orthop Clin North Am* 25:707–713, 1994.

190. Kendall RW, Taylor DC, Salvian AJ, et al: The role of arteriography in assessing vascular injuries associated with dislocations of the knee. *J Trauma* 35:875–878, 1993.

191. Burke RL, Schenck RC: Reattachment of ligament avulsions in high energy bicruciate ligament trauma. *Orthop Trans* 16:333, 1992.

ACUTE TRAUMATIC PATELLAR DISLOCATION

192. Reider B, Marshall JL, Koslin B, et al: The anterior aspect of the knee joint. *J Bone Joint Surg* 63A:351, 1981.

193. Sargent JR, Teipner WA: Medial patellar retinacular repair for acute and recurrent dislocation of the patella: A preliminary report. *J Bone Joint Surg* 53A:386, 1971.

194. Vainionpaa S, Laasonen E, Silvennoinen T, et al: Acute dislocation of the patella: A prospective review of operative treatment. *J Bone Joint Surg* 72B:366–369, 1990.

195. Sallay PI, Poggi J, Speer KP, Garrett WE: Acute dislocation of the patella: A correlative pathoanatomic study. *Am J Sports Med* 24:52–60, 1996.

196. Avikainen VJ, Nikk RK, Seppanen-Lehmonen TK: Adductor magnus tenodesis for patellar dislocation: Techniques and preliminary results. *Clin Orthop* 297:12–16, 1993.

197. Hughston JC, Deese M: Medial subluxation of the patella as a complication of lateral retinacular release. *Am J Sports Med,* 16:383–388, 1988.

198. Nsouli AZ, Nahabedian AM: Intra-articular dislocation of the patella. *J Trauma* 28:256–258, 1988.

199. Murakami Y: Intra-articular dislocation of the patella. *Clin Orthop* 171:137–139, 1982.

200. Alioto RJ, Kates S: Intra-articular vertical dislocation of the patella: A case report of an irreducible patellar dislocation and unique surgical technique. *J Trauma* 36:282–284, 1994.

201. Moed BR, Morawa LG: Acute traumatic lateral dislocation of the patella: An unusual case presentation. *J Trauma* 22:516–518, 1982.

202. Carragher AM, Todd A, Blake G: Acute traumatic lateral patellar dislocation. *Ann Emerg Med* 18:1362–1363, 1989.

203. Bassett FH: Acute dislocation of the patella, osteochondral fractures, and injuries to the extensor mechanism of the knee. *Instr Course Lect* 25:40–49, 1976.

204. Laurin CA, Levesque HP: The tangenital x-ray investigation of the patellofemoral joint: X-ray technique, diagnostic criteria and their interpretation. *Clin Orthop* 144:16–26, 1979.

205. Laurin CA, Levesque HP, Dussault R, et al: The abnormal lateral patellofemoral angle: A diagnostic roentgenographic sign of recurrent patellar subluxation. *J Bone Joint Surg* 60A:55–60, 1978.

206. Vainionpaa S, Laasonen E, Patiala H, et al: Acute dislocation of the patella: Clinical, radiographic and operative findings in 64 consecutive cases. *Acta Orthop Scand* 57:331–333, 1986.

207. Nietosvaara Y, Aalto K, Kallio PE: Acute patellar dislocation in children: Incidence and associated osteochondral fractures. *J Pediatr Orthop* 14:513–515, 1994.

208. Ellis JS: Primary dislocation of the patella. *J Bone Joint Surg* 36B:145, 1954.

209. Boring TH, O'Donoghue DH: Acute patellar dislocation: Results of immediate surgical repair. *Clin Orthop* 136:182–185, 1978.

210. Fondren FB, Goldner JL, Bassett FH: Recurrent dislocation of the patella treated by the modified Roux-Goldthwait procedure. *J Bone Joint Surg* 67A:993–1005, 1985.

211. Hawkins RJ, Bell RH, Anisette G: Acute patellar dislocations: The natural history. *Am J Sports Med* 14:117–120, 1986.

212. Cofield RH, Bryan RS: Acute dislocation of the patella: Results of conservative treatment. *J Trauma* 17:526–531, 1977.

213. Rorabeck CH, Bobechko WP: Acute dislocation of the patella with osteochondral fracture. *J Bone Joint Surg* 52B:237–240, 1976.

214. Henry JE, Pflum FA Jr: Arthroscopic proximal patella realignment and stabilization. *Arthroscopy* 11:424–425, 1995.

215. Small NC, Glogau AI, Berezin MA: Arthroscopically assisted proximal extensor mechanism realignment of the knee. *Arthroscopy* 9:63–67, 1993.

216. Yamamoto RK: Arthroscopic repair of the medial retinaculum and capsule in acute patellar dislocations. *Arthroscopy* 2:125–131, 1986.

PROXIMAL TIBIOFIBULAR JOINT DISLOCATION

217. Basmajian JV: *Primary Anatomy,* 6th ed. Baltimore, Williams & Wilkins, 1970, pp 111–112.

218. Ogden JA: The anatomy and function of the proximal tibiofibular joint. *Clin Orthop* 101:186–191, 1974.

219. Eichenblat M, Nathan H: The proximal tibio fibular joint: An anatomical study with clinical and pathological considerations. *Int Orthop* 7:31–39, 1983.

220. Ogden JA: Subluxation and dislocation of the proximal tibiofibular joint. *J Bone Joint Surg* 56A:145–154, 1974.

221. Herscovici D Jr, Fredrick RW, Behrens F: Superior dislocation of the fibular head associated with a tibial shaft fracture. *J Orthop Trauma* 6:116–119, 1992.

222. Andersen K, Lind T: Simultaneous fracture of the ankle and disruption of the superior tibiofibular joint. *Acta Orthop Scand* 62:399–400, 1991.

223. Vigil AB, Barredo PM, Mortera SM: Traumatic luxation of the proximal tibiofibular joint, superior variety: A case report. *Acta Orthop Belg* 49:479–482, 1983.

224. Christensen S: Dislocation of the upper end of the fibula. *Acta Orthop Scand* 37:107–109, 1966.

225. Clews AG: Dislocation of the upper end of the fibula. *Can Med Assoc J* 98:169–170, 1968.

226. Parkes JC, Zelko RR: Isolated acute dislocation of the proximal tibiofibular joint. *J Bone Joint Surg* 55A:177–180, 1973.

227. Thomason PA, Linson MA: Isolated dislocation of the proximal tibiofibular joint. *J Trauma* 26:192–195, 1986.

228. Andersen K: Dislocation of the superior tibiofibular joint. *Injury* 16:494–498, 1985.

229. Crothers OD, Johnson JTH: Isolated acute dislocation of the proximal tibiofibular joint: Case report. *J Bone Joint Surg* 55A:181–183, 1973.

230. Fallon P, Virani NS, Bell D, Hollinshead R: Delayed presentation: Dislocation of the proximal tibiofibular joint after knee dislocation. *J Orthop Trauma* 8:350–353, 1994.

231. Dennis JB, Rutledge BA: Bilateral recurrent dislocations of the superior tibiofibular joint with peroneal-nerve palsy: A case summary. *J Bone Joint Surg* 40A:1146–1148, 1958.

232. Falkenberg P, Nygaard H: Isolated anterior dislocation of the proximal tibiofibular joint. *J Bone Joint Surg* 65B:310–311, 1983.

233. Molitor PJA, Dandy DJ: Permanent anterior dislocation of the proximal tibiofibular joint. *J Bone Joint Surg* 71B:240–241, 1989.

234. Sijbrandi S: Instability of the proximal tibio-fibular joint. *Acta Orthop Scand* 49:621–626, 1978.

235. Giachino AA: Recurrent dislocation of the proximal tibiofibular joint—Report of two cases. *J Bone Joint Surg* 68A:1104–1106, 1986.

236. Weinart CR, Raczka R: Recurrent dislocation of the superior tibiofibular joint: Surgical stabilization by ligament reconstruction. *J Bone Joint Surg* 68A:126–128, 1986.

EXTENSOR MECHANISM TENDON RUPTURE

237. Rascher JJ, Marcolin L, James P: Bilateral sequential rupture of the patellar tendon in systemic lupus erythematosus: A case report. *J Bone Joint Surg* 56A:821–822, 1974.

238. Razzano CD, Wilde AH, Phalen GS: Bilateral rupture of the infrapatellar tendon in rheumatoid arthritis. *Clin Orthop* 91:158–161, 1973.

239. Strejcek J, Popelka S: Bilateral rupture of the patellar ligaments in systemic lupus erythematosus. *Lancet* 2:743, 1969.

240. Peiro A, Ferrandis R, Garcia L, et al: Simultaneous and spontaneous bilateral rupture of the patellar tendon in rheumatoid arthritis: A case report. *Acta Orthop Scand* 47:700–703, 1975.

241. Ismail AM, Balakrishnan R, Rajakumar MK: Rupture of patella ligament after steroid infiltration. *J Bone Joint Surg* 51B:503, 1969.

242. Karlsson J, Lundin O, Lossing IW, Peterson L: Partial rupture of the patellar ligament: Results after operative treatment. *Am J Sports Med* 19:403–408, 1991.

243. Kelly DW, Carter VS, Jobe FW, Kerlan RK: Patellar and quadriceps tendon ruptures—Jumper's knee. *Am J Sports Med* 12:375–380, 1984.

244. Haas SB, Callaway H: Disruptions of the extensor mechanism. *Orthop Clin North Am* 23:687–695, 1992.

245. Larson RV, Simonian PT: Semitendinosus augmentation of acute patellar tendon repair with immediate mobilization. *Am J Sports Med* 23:82–86, 1995.

246. Levin PD: Reconstruction of the patellar tendon using a dacron graft. *Clin Orthop* 118:70–72, 1976.

247. Levy M, Goldstein J, Rosner M: A method of repair for quadriceps tendon or patellar ligament (tendon) ruptures without cast immobilization. *Clin Orthop* 218:297–301, 1987.

248. Lindy PB, Boynton MD, Fadale PD: Repair of patellar tendon disruptions without hardware. *J Orthop Trauma* 9:238–243, 1995.

249. Stern RE, Harwin SF: Spontaneous and simultaneous rupture of both quadriceps tendons. *Clin Orthop* 147:188–189, 1980.

250. Ramsey RH, Muller GE: Quadriceps tendon rupture: A diagnostic trap. *Clin Orthop* 70:161–164, 1970.

251. Kaneko K, DeMouy EH, Brunet ME, et al: Radiographic diagnosis of quadriceps tendon rupture: Analysis of diagnostic failure. *J Emerg Med* 12:225–229, 1994.

252. Siwek KW, Rao JP: Ruptures of the extensor mechanism of the knee joint. *J Bone Joint Surg* 63A:932–937, 1981.

253. Scuderi C: Ruptures of the quadriceps tendon: A study of twenty tendon ruptures. *Am J Surg* 95:626–635, 1958.

254. Miskew NBW, Pearson RL, Pankovich AM: Mersilene strip suture in repair of disruptions of the quadriceps and patellar tendons. *J Trauma* 20:867–872, 1980.

255. Chekofsky KM, Spero CR, Scott WN: A method of repair of late quadriceps rupture. *Clin Orthop* 147:190–191, 1980.

256. Evans D, Pritchard GA, Jenkins DHR: Carbon fibre used in the late reconstruction of rupture of the extensor mechanism of the knee. *Injury: Br J Accid Surg* 18:57–60, 1987.

257. Margles SW, Lewis MM: Bilateral spontaneous concurrent rupture of the patellar tendon without apparent associated systemic disease. *Clin Orthop* 135:186–187, 1978.

258. Webb LX, Toby EB: Bilateral rupture of the patella tendon in an otherwise healthy male patient following minor trauma. *J Trauma* 26:1045–1048, 1986.

259. Krakow KA, Thomas SC, Jones LC: A new stitch for ligament-tendon fixation. *J Bone Joint Surg* 68A:764–766, 1986.

260. Ecker ML, Lotke PA, Glazer RM: Late reconstruction of the patellar tendon. *J Bone Joint Surg* 61A:884–886, 1979.

261. Kelikian H, Riashi E, Gleason J: Restoration of quadriceps function in neglected tear of the patellar tendon. *Surg Gynecol Obstet* 104:200–204, 1957.

262. Mandelbaum BR, Bartolozzi A, Carney B: A systematic approach to reconstruction of neglected tears of the patellar tendon. *Clin Orthop* 235:268–271, 1988.

263. Nsouli AZ, Nsouli TA, Haidar R: Late reconstruction of the patellar tendon: Case report with a new method of repair. *J Trauma* 31:1319–1321, 1991.

264. Ilizarov GA: The tension stress effect on the genesis and growth of tissues. *Clin Orthop* 238:249–281, 1989.

265. Isiklar ZU, Varner KE, Lindsey RW, et al: Late reconstruction of patellar ligament ruptures using Ilizarov external fixation. *Clin Orthop* 322:174–178, 1996.

CHAPTER 29

Tibial Fractures

Paul Tornetta III

ANATOMY

The primary bony landmarks of the tibia and fibula are all easily palpable. These include the fibular head, tibial plateau, and tubercle proximally and the lateral and medial malleolus distally. Most important, the anteromedial surface and crest of the tibia are subcutaneous throughout the entire leg. The muscular envelope surrounding the tibia consists of four compartments, each requiring careful examination in the case of a fracture. The functions of these compartments and their neurovascular contents are listed in Table 29-1.

Adequate vascular supply is necessary for the tibia to unite. Its nutrient artery is a branch of the posterior tibial artery, which enters the proximal tibial shaft posteriorly and courses primarily dorsolaterally within the medullary cavity. Most authors believe that the intramedullary blood supply is the most important, but that the periosteal blood supply has increased significance after fracture.[71,95] This is particularly true in the distal third of the bone.

INCIDENCE AND MECHANISM

Fractures of the tibia are common and occur from a wide variety of mechanisms. In one defined population group, the rate of fracture was 2/1000 per year.[3] Skiing and motor vehicle accidents are common causes of fracture. The disparity in the amount of energy imparted has significant implications for treatment and expected results. Likewise, the mechanism of injury determines the fracture pattern, with rotational mechanisms leading to spiral fractures and direct injuries manifesting transverse or bending fractures with comminution corresponding to the force applied.

DIAGNOSIS

The typical presentation of a patient with an acute tibial fracture is severe pain, deformity, and inability to bear weight after a traumatic episode. The diagnosis can be less clear in cases of stress fracture, incomplete fracture, and when the fibula is intact. In the unconscious patient, the diagnosis can usually be made by feeling displacement or crepitus during routine palpation of the tibial crest from the plateau to the ankle.

EXAMINATION

Physical examination should begin with a complete inspection of the integument circumferentially, looking for wounds that would indicate an open fracture. Any break in the skin at the level of the fracture should be considered indicative of an open fracture. Wounds away from the level of the fracture may also communicate with the fracture, especially in higher-energy injuries. These, too, are considered open. The next step is a careful assessment of the vascular and neurologic status of the leg. Pulses should be compared to those of the contralateral limb. Neurologic examination should consist of muscle and sensory testing of all compartments.

The possibility of compartment syndrome exists in all tibial fractures and must be sought out in every case. This includes open fractures, which may have rates as high as 9 percent.[7] The most sensitive clinical test for increased intracompartmental pressure is pain on passive stretching of the involved compartment.[85] A physical exam consistent with compartment syndrome does not require measurement of intracompartmental pressure before treatment is begun. However, these measurements are recommended in uncooperative or unconscious patients with signs of swelling. Intracompartmental pressure within 30 mm of the patient's diastolic pressure is indicative of compartment syndrome.[80,84]

The knee and ankle should also be palpated for areas of tenderness or joint instability, as concomitant injuries are not uncommon.[68]

Both compartment syndromes and arterial occlusion may present late, and repeat examinations of the patient will help to avoid the catastrophic complications of missed injuries.

IMAGING

In addition to full length anteroposterior (AP) and lateral radiographs of the tibia, formal radiographs of the knee and ankle are required to properly evaluate the fracture pattern and rule out concomitant injury. Oblique views may prove helpful if the fracture extends close to the knee or ankle joint. Repeat radiographs should be obtained after splint or cast placement.

Bone scan or MRI are useful in some cases of stress fracture, particularly if the patient's history is unclear. An arteriogram may be indicated in high-energy injuries with a pulse deficit. The results have implications for healing and possible soft tissue reconstruction, particularly in open fractures.[26] The anterior tibial artery is the most commonly injured.

During follow-up, standard AP and lateral radiographs are usually sufficient to determine union. However, in some cases fibular callus may overlap the tibia on both views. In this situation, a 45° internal rotation view allows for better assessment of the tibia by eliminating the fibular overlap.[29]

The callus that forms in the early stages of healing can be visualized using ultrasonography. This modality has been shown to predict union after nonreamed nailing as

TABLE 29-1 Leg Compartments

Compartment	Function	Nerve	Artery
Anterior	Dorsiflexion of ankle and toes	Deep peroneal	Anterior tibial
Lateral	Eversion of ankle	Superficial peroneal	Peroneal
Superficial posterior	Plantarflexion of ankle	Sural	
Deep posterior	Plantarflexion of ankle and toes	Posterior tibial	Posterior tibial

early as 6 to 9 weeks postoperatively.[83] Secondary procedures have been recommended if a negative ultrasound persisted past 9 weeks.

CLASSIFICATION

Classification of tibial shaft fractures has two purposes. First, the classification gives prognostic information regarding healing time, complication rates, and infection (in open fractures). When this information is applied to specific modes of treatment, these classification systems can help to determine the most appropriate treatment for a given fracture. Tibial fractures are evaluated and stratified by using the degree of soft tissue injury and the bony configuration of the fracture.

Soft Tissue

The degree of soft tissue injury is related to the energy imparted during the injury. Significant muscular injury is possible in both open and closed fractures. It should be understood that classifying the soft tissue injury is an attempt to quantify the physiologic injury to the region of the fracture. Disruption of the periosteum, muscular envelope, and vascular supply of the fracture are the most important factors. Whether the injury is open or closed is of less importance. This understanding has led to more attention being paid to the soft tissues in recent years.[61,96,121]

Tscherne has developed a system for the classification of closed fractures that is prognostically important.[125] This is summarized in Table 29-2. Types 0 and 1 are considered low- or moderate-energy injuries and the soft tissue is not severely damaged. These are usually indirect injuries, such as a twisting injury in a skier. This contrasts with types 3 and 4 injuries, which represent high-energy trauma in which the muscular envelope and periosteum have been badly injured. A common example of a direct mechanism creating a type 3 or 4 injury is a bumper fracture in a pedestrian struck by a car. A great amount of energy is imparted over a relatively small anatomic area.

Open fractures are graded using the system of Gustillo and Anderson.[41] This classification begins with an assess-

TABLE 29-2 Closed Soft Tissue Classification

Grade	Soft tissue damage
0	Absent or negligible
1	Superficial abrasion or contusion from within
2	Deep contaminated abrasion, significant contusion, impending compartment syndrome
3	Crushed skin and severe muscle damage, subcutaneous avulsions, compartment syndrome

Source: Reproduced with permission from Tscherne H, Gotzen L: *Fractures with Soft Tissue Injuries.* Berlin, Springer-Verlag, 1984, pp 5–6.

ment wound size, which should be performed with a ruler for precision and consistency. However, wound size is not the only determinant of grade. Since infection is the primary initial concern in open fractures, the degree of contamination also influences grading. Injuries occurring in severely contaminated environments, such as a farmyard, are considered to be of a higher grade than would be reflected only by the soft tissue disruption. Likewise, an attempt is made to take energy of injury into account. The damage to the muscle and periosteum in segmental fractures and high-velocity gunshot wounds is worse than may be suspected by the size of the wound. These mechanisms, therefore, are considered grade III even if the wound size is small. Thus, the definitive grading should be established only after the operative debridement. Factors such as periosteal stripping, muscle death, and compartment syndrome may not be discernible at the initial inspection in the emergency department. Grade IIIb should be reserved for fractures that require operative reconstruction of the soft tissue envelope. The complete grading scale is reviewed in Table 29-3. It should be noted that several studies have shown poor agreement even among experienced surgeons on the classification of open fractures.[15,50] However, no study that compares grading between surgeons using actual operative inspection has been performed.

Bone

Many methods have been proposed for the classification of the bony injury. Central to these are the pattern and degree of comminution of the fracture. The location within the bone, initial displacement, and status of the fibula are also important.[31,54,120] Shortening of the fracture can be measured on the radiograph. The pattern may be described as transverse, oblique, spiral, segmental, or comminuted. For shaft fractures, the comminution can be described using a system analogous to the Winquist system

for the femur.[46] The location of the fracture is stratified to the proximal, middle, or distal shaft and proximal or distal metaphyseal (extending into the metaphysis). Fractures can be described using the above factors or using complex alphanumeric systems.[86]

Several authors have attempted to consolidate the bony and soft tissue injuries into one system that gives an overall estimate of severity.[31,67,131] In general, the greater the energy of the injury, soft tissue damage, comminution, and initial displacement, the more unstable the fracture, the longer it takes to heal, and the higher the rate of nonunion.

TREATMENT

The primary goals of treatment for a tibial fracture are to obtain union and maintain the relative positions of the knee and ankle joints. Other considerations include an early return to function and the avoidance of stiffness in the knee, ankle, and subtalar joints. Different methods of achieving these goals may be used, depending on the fracture pattern, soft tissue injury, neurologic and vascular status of the leg, concomitant injuries, and individual patient demands. The indications for surgery of fractures with soft tissue injury are well established and are reviewed first.

Open Fractures

The first priority in the treatment of open tibial fractures is to avoid infection. Current protocols include immediate administration of tetanus toxoid and a first-generation cephalosporin. An aminoglycoside and penicillin are added for grade III open fractures or those with significant contamination (e.g., farm injuries). Antibiotics should be continued for 72 h after wound closure. After initial assessment as described above, irrigation in the emergency department is followed by application of a sterile dressing and a splint. This dressing should be removed only in the operating suite. Preoperative cultures do not yield valuable information and are unnecessary. After clearance by the trauma team the patient is brought to the operating room for emergent debridement and irrigation. Debridement within 6 h is recommended to keep the rate of infection as low as possible.[58]

All devitalized tissue and bone must be debrided. The first step in the debridement is to extend the wounds in both directions to obtain full exposure of the fracture and its surrounding soft tissue. Extensions are generally done in a vertical direction, but the need for future flap procedures should be remembered in devising the incisions. The skin is cut back to bleeding edges, necrotic muscle is excised, and all foreign bodies are removed. Bone fragments without significant soft tissue attachments should be discarded.[30] Aggressive bony debridement has been shown to lower the infection rate in high-grade open fractures.[30] The use of laser Doppler has been proposed as

TABLE 29-3 Classification for Open Fractures

Grade	Wound
I	< 1 cm
II	1–10 cm
IIIa	> 10-cm coverage available, segmental, farm,[a] high-velocity gunshot wound
IIIb	Periosteal stripping, requires coverage procedure
IIIc	With vascular injury requiring repair

[a]That is, a highly contaminated environment such as a farmyard.
Source: Reproduced with permission from Gustilo RB, Mendoza RM, Williams DN: Problems in the management of type III (severe) open fractures: A new classification of type III open fractures. *J Trauma* 24:742–746, 1984.

a method of identifying vascularized bone but has not gained wide acceptance. After complete debridement, the wound is irrigated with 10 L of normal saline. Pulsatile lavage is useful in providing mechanical debridement, but the velocity of the spray should not be too great, as this can injure the remaining tissue. Closure of subcutaneous tissue over exposed bone protects it from desiccation and contamination. Formal primary closure, however, should not be performed, as this increases the risk of infection, particularly with clostridia. Alternatively, commercially available occlusive dressings may be used to provide a temporary barrier until the second-look procedure.

The leg is reprepped and draped and new instruments are used for fracture fixation. Stabilization of the fracture is needed to protect the soft tissue from further injury. Ideally, the method of fixation should respect the intramedullary blood supply. Until recently, external fixation with a simple anterior frame was the preferred technique.[5,30,117] This method provides stability and has been shown to have lower infection rates than plates or reamed nails.[6,21] However, pin tract infections remain a common problem requiring treatment, and patient acceptance is low.[127] Additionally, in fractures requiring coverage procedures, the frame is frequently a steric hindrance.

The advent of smaller-diameter interlocking nails has allowed fixation of even unstable fractures without canal preparation, avoiding the thermal necrosis and damage to the intramedullary blood supply caused by reaming. This technique is associated with the same infection rates as external fixation.[104,110,117] Nonreamed nails are more accepted by the patients, allow for easier completion of secondary procedures, and avoid the problem of pin care and pin infection. Treatment of open fractures with nonreamed nails results in a lower rate of malunions, but healing times and infection rates are approximately the same as with external fixation.[104,110,117,123] These findings are consistent with the understanding that the complications encountered in the treatment of open fractures are due to the biological injury.[110,117] Thus, nonreamed nailing is the recommended treatment for grades I to IIIa injuries. Two recent reports have demonstrated comparable results in IIIb injuries and recommended their use for these injuries.[117,123] However, this indication is not universally accepted. The main indications for external fixation are grade IIIb or IIIc injuries in which early amputation is considered a realistic outcome, those in which soft tissue reconstruction may be delayed, and in fractures in which a nail would preclude repeat debridement of an injured posterior compartment. Several authors have also recommended a planned sequence of initial external fixation and then intramedullary nailing within 2 weeks.[6] This is an acceptable choice and is best when the external fixator spans the ankle joint.[137]

Grade I open fractures without soft tissue damage may be allowed to close secondarily. All other fractures require a second-look debridement and irrigation. This procedure is performed 48 to 72 h after the initial debridement. The wound is reopened and systematic evaluation and debridement are again performed. It is normal to find additional muscle necrosis not evident at the first procedure. This process of repeat debridements is continued until there is no nonviable tissue. Only then is it safe to close the wound. The skin should never be closed under tension or stretched, and flap coverage should be utilized liberally.

Many flaps have been described for coverage of exposed bone. In general, gastrocnemius flaps are used in the proximal third, soleus for the middle third, and free flaps for the distal third. Smaller areas may be covered with fasciocutaneous flaps or with the use of relaxing incisions. Delays of more than 2 weeks in the reconstitution of the soft tissue envelope are associated with higher infection rates.[33] Most authors recommend achieving definitive coverage of the wound within the first week.

Low-grade open fractures without bone loss go on to uneventful union in the vast majority of cases. High-grade injuries and those with bone loss, however, should be treated with a prophylactic bone graft or exchange nail to encourage union.[8,23,114,117] Grafting is normally delayed at least 2 weeks after secondary wound closure or 6 weeks after free flap coverage. If it is performed too early, grafting may increase the rate of infection.[5] Posterolateral autogenous bone grafting is the most common method, but direct or central bone grafting can be utilized if the anterior skin is in good condition (Fig. 29-1). Exchange nailing can be used if the initial stabilization was with a nonreamed nail, and it is effective if the bone loss is less than 50 percent of the circumference for a distance of less than 1 cm. If more bone loss is present, an autogenous bone graft is indicated.[23,114] As an unplanned procedure, intramedullary nailing after external fixation is very controversial. At this time, it is recommended as a salvage method only. Solid-core nonreamed nails have been demonstrated to have the lowest infection rates.[96]

Complications of open fractures are many. Compartment syndrome has been demonstrated in 9 percent of open fractures and must be sought out during the initial examination, after stabilization, and during the next 48 h.[7] Infection rates for open tibial fractures range from 0 to 2 percent, 2 to 7 percent, and 10 to 25 percent for grades I, II, and III, respectively. Grade III injuries are divided into types a, b, and c, carrying infection rates of approximately 7 percent, 10 to 50 percent, and 25 to 70 percent. The time to union also varies with the grade of injury. Grade I fractures usually heal in a time frame similar to that of closed fractures. Grade III injuries, on the other hand, heal much more slowly. In one series, only 23 percent of grade III open tibial fractures healed in less than 6 months.[30] The treatment of infections, compartment syndromes, and nonunions is described later.

Amputation is also a well-known complication of open fractures. In particular, grade IIIc injuries have amputation rates as high as 70 percent.[17] The clarification of objective measures that can predict amputation is a current area of research. Several authors have devised scoring systems to aid in the decision to perform a primary amputation.[51,53,102,122] The most widely known is the mangled extremity severity score (MESS).[53] Although all of these scores were found to be accurate by their creators, other authors have found them inaccurate.[9,66] Thus, orthopaedic surgeons should be aware of the scores and are referred to the original references, but they should not apply them rigidly. Warm ischemia time of more than 6 h, infrapopliteal vascular injury, and posterior tibial nerve neurotmesis in the

Figure 29-1 *A.* Lateral radiograph of a grade IIIA open tibial fracture 9 weeks after intramedullary nailing. There is a significant amount of bone loss anteriorly and only a shell of bone posteriorly. At this time the fracture was bone grafted prophylactically. *B.* The same tibia 10 weeks after direct bone grafting shows good incorporation of the graft with union.

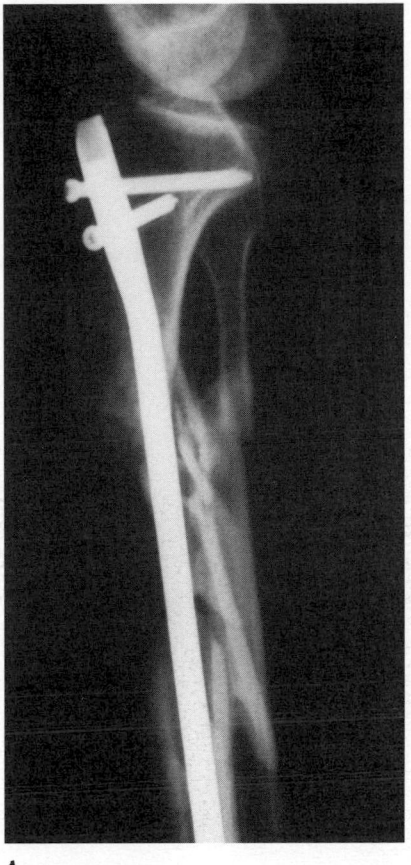

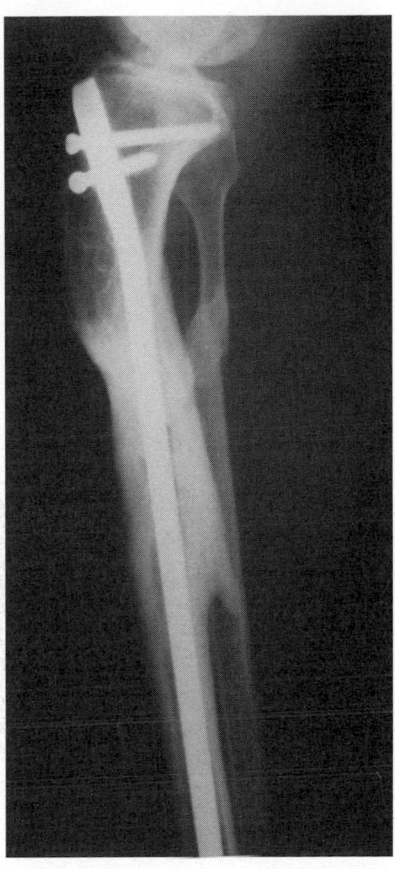

A   *B*

face of a blunt injury are the strongest indications for primary amputation[64,89] (Fig. 29-2). When making this decision, it should be remembered that even technically successful limb salvage in the face of significant soft tissue injury may result in poorer function, longer time out of work, and a more psychologically disturbed patient than an early amputation.[37,93] Patients who have an immediate amputation return to work at a higher rate than those who are reconstructed. Finally, the tremendous cost of prolonged salvage attempts is creating pressure on surgeons to identify those patients who will ultimately benefit from early amputation.[91] This is especially true as nonphysician managed care groups further deplete the resources available to patients.[122]

Compartment Syndromes

All patients with tibial fractures are at risk for compartment syndrome. This includes low-energy injuries as well as high-energy open fractures.[7,79,80] As previously stated, a patient with the physical signs of compartment syndrome does not require direct pressure measurement for confirmation. If measurements are made, a reasonable definition of compartment syndrome is a pressure within 30 mm of diastolic pressure. As the compartment pressure exceeds that level, permanent muscle and nerve damage will occur.[84,85]

Once the diagnosis is made, emergent fasciotomy and stabilization are required. All four compartments should be released. The most common technique is to use two incisions. The anterior and lateral compartments are released through the lateral incision and the superficial and deep posterior compartments through the medial incision. Alternatively, a full release can be performed through a single lateral incision.[42] The fibula should be preserved for stability and possible reconstructive procedures. Regardless of the technique used, the skin incisions should be extensive, as the skin itself may be a barrier to release.[115] Adkison et al.[1a] studied the superficial peroneal nerve in 85 cadaveric limbs. In only 73 percent of the legs did the nerve remain in the lateral compartment from its origin to its exit through the deep fascia between 3 and 18 cm proximal to the lateral malleolus. In 26 percent of the specimens, the nerve passed into the anterior compartment or a portion of it ran in the anterior compartment. These relationships should be respected during the release of the anterior and lateral compartments by entering each from its outer surface and not dividing the intermuscular septum.

After the fascia is released, the injury should be treated as a grade IIIa open fracture. Debridement of nonviable muscle is necessary to avoid infection. Release of the individual muscles' fasciae may also be necessary. Excellent results using a nonreamed interlocked nail for stabilization has been reported, although external fixation is also a good alternative.[38,42] As in the case of open fractures, repeat debridements should be performed until

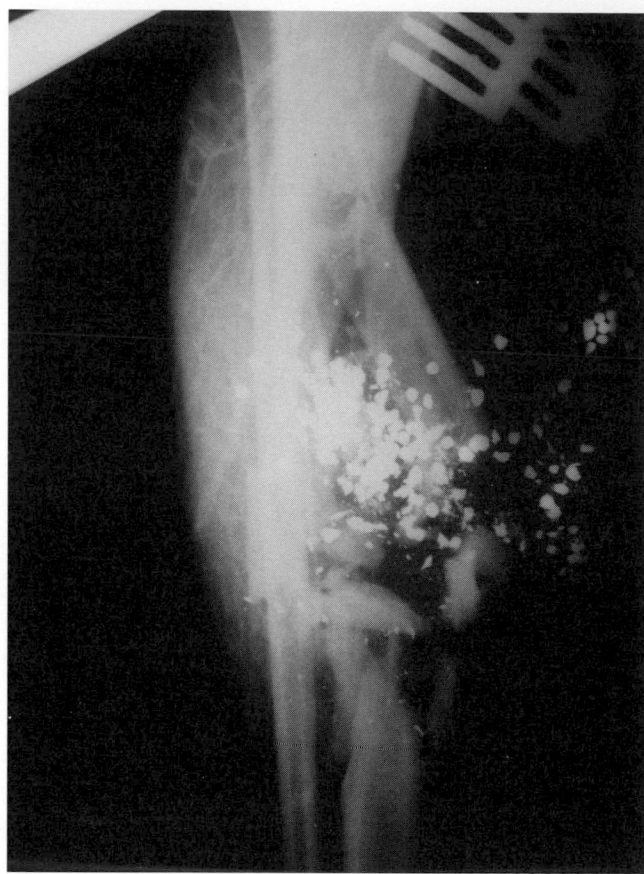

Figure 29-2 Radiograph of a 26-year-old who sustained a shot-gun injury to the tibia with a complete trifurcation injury and loss of the posterior tibial nerve. This limb was amputated acutely.

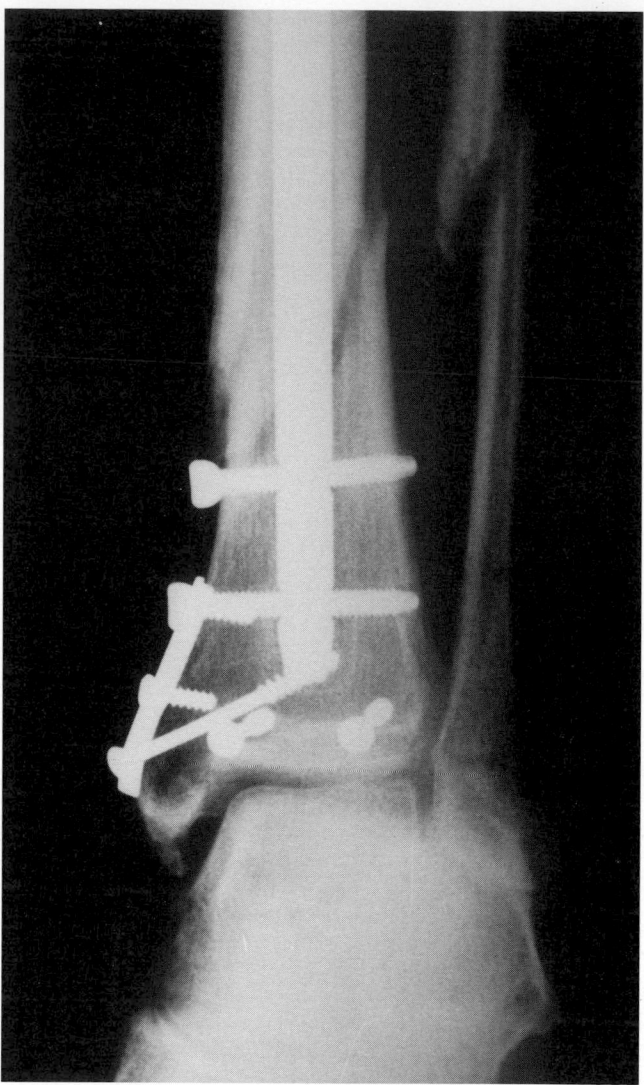

Figure 29-3 Postoperative radiograph of a patient who sustained an inpsilateral ankle and tibial shaft fracture. Fixation of both injuries allows early motion and a better return to function.

there is no nonviable tissue. Delayed primary closure of the medial wound achieves bony coverage. The lateral wound may be dealt with in many ways, including delayed primary closure, skin grafting, relaxing incisions, and gradual closure techniques.[115] More options are available for the lateral wound, as there is good muscle coverage over the bone.

The surgeon should expect that the healing time of a fracture complicated by compartment syndrome will be in the same range as that of a high-grade open fracture.[119] Secondary procedures should be considered as in open fractures. Additional sequelae of compartment syndrome include weakness and contractures secondary to myonecrosis or permanent nerve damage, numbness, foot drop, and deformity. These complications are most common if the release is delayed.[85,98] Missed compartment syndromes represent one of the problems in orthopaedics that can truly be avoided with careful management.

Compartment syndromes may also occur during or after intramedullary nailing; this is discussed later.

Concomitant Injury

Although most closed tibial fractures can be managed nonoperatively, patients with certain concomitant injuries are operative candidates. These include ipsilateral ankle, knee, or femur fractures; segmental tibial fractures; contralateral lower extremity fractures; and multiple injuries (for mobilization).[1,18,57,67,68,76,126] In many of these circumstances, fixation is needed to achieve mobilization of the patient or of an adjacent joint, and the results of fixation are superior to nonoperative management (Fig. 29-3).

Ipsilateral fractures of the femur and tibia create an injury referred to as a "floating knee." Numerous authors have shown superior results with operative treatment of both fractures.[57,126] This allows for early motion of the knee joint and leads to a greater return to the patient's previous occupation.[57]

It takes greater energy to create segmental fractures; therefore these fractures take longer to heal.[106,119] When they are treated nonoperatively, nonunion rates of up to 50 percent have been reported. With intramedullary fixation, segmental fractures have a union rate of better than

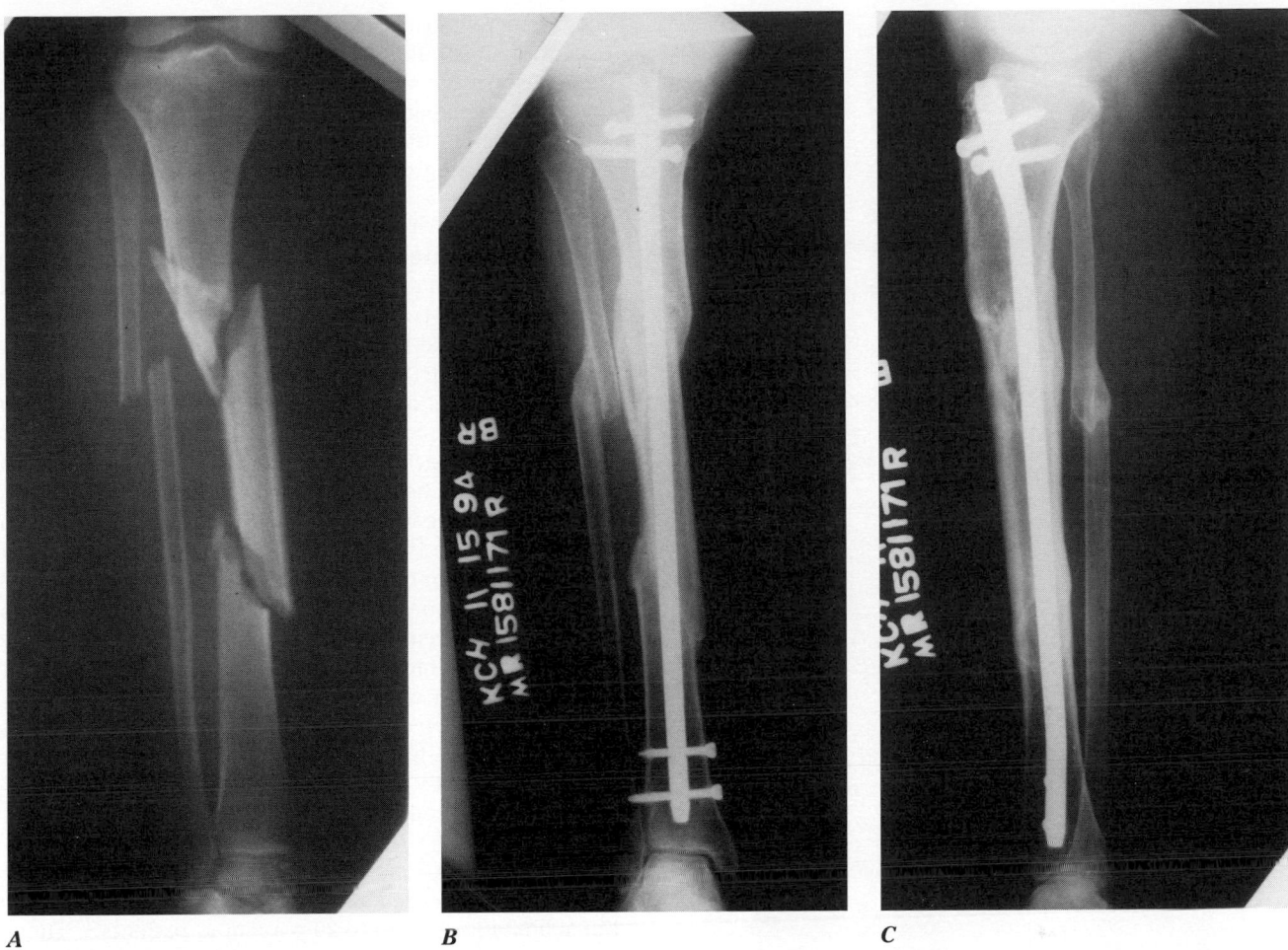

A   *B*   *C*

Figure 29-4   *A.* The preoperative radiograph of a segmental fracture of the tibia in a blunt trauma patient. *B* and *C.* This fracture was treated with a nonreamed IM nail via the semiextended approach; it healed at 16 weeks.

95 percent and heal at a mean of 4.4 months[138] (Fig. 29-4). Segmental fractures also have higher rates of significant soft tissue damage, which are best treated without external pressure from casting.[61]

Closed Fractures

Functional Bracing

With the exceptions noted above, nonoperative management is appropriate for the vast majority of closed isolated tibial fractures without compartment syndrome.[105,106] *Nonoperative,* however, does not imply *nonfunctional.* Several authors have shown that weight bearing within 6 weeks of fracture improves healing.[25,106] Sarmiento et al. described the technique of functional bracing to allow early weight bearing and knee motion during nonoperative management.[105] This treatment method is predicated on the belief that a tibial fracture will not shorten any more than the amount seen on the initial radiograph and that angulation can be controlled without immobilizing the knee or ankle. This technique requires a closed reduction of the fracture and utilizes a long leg cast in extension as the initial immobilization. This is performed under regional anesthesia if significant manipulation will be needed. Weight bearing in the cast is permitted. After 2 to 4 weeks, when the fracture is gaining stiffness and the patient is more comfortable, this is changed to a functional brace (Fig. 29-5). The brace is formed by two overlapping shells and can be made tighter using the straps that hold them together. The patient is instructed to bear weight as tolerated in the brace. When the patient is not walking, the leg is kept elevated and the straps are tightened whenever the brace feels loose. Frequent brace tightening takes full advantage of the hydrostatic forces created by the brace to maintain the fracture in a reduced position. Radiographs are taken in the brace at 2-week intervals for the first month to confirm the reduction. If the reduction is acceptable and stable, monthly visits are sufficient until the fracture is united. Malalignment in the brace may require rereduction. If the alignment or length cannot be maintained, operative intervention is indicated.

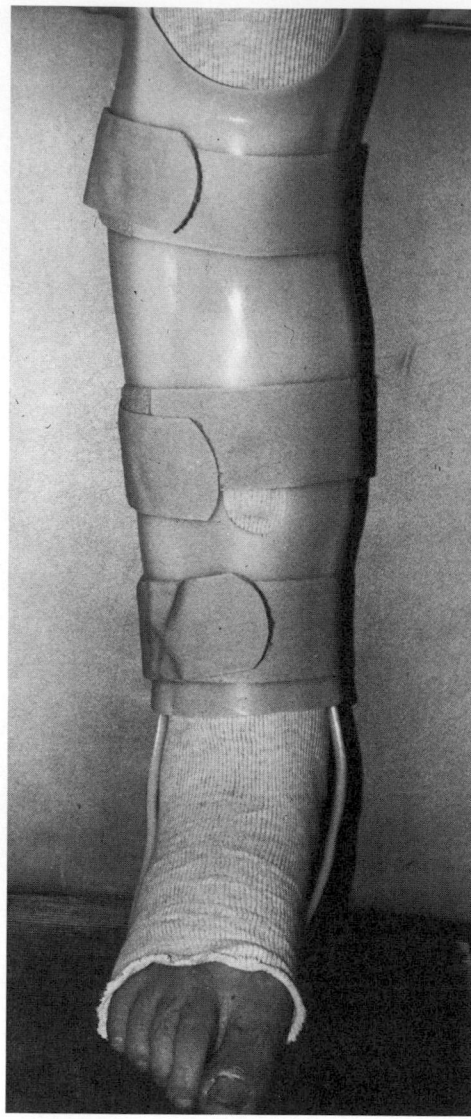

Figure 29-5 Custom-made tibial fracture brace applied after initial treatment in long leg cast.

Sarmiento et al. have recently reported on 943 patients treated with this method.[106] These patients were selected on the basis of acceptable initial shortening, which was considered to be 1.5 cm. If greater than 1.5 cm of shortening is present on the initial radiographs, the fracture is treated operatively. This study demonstrated a nonunion rate of 1.1 percent and a 3 percent dropout rate for loss of reduction. However, final angulation exceeded 6° in over 10 percent of the series. Varus angulation was the most common deformity and was seen in 10 percent. Tibial fractures with an intact fibula healed faster, with less shortening, but were more prone to malalignment. The authors concluded that an intact fibula should be considered a relative contraindication to functional bracing.

Indications for Surgery

The most common indication for surgery in an isolated closed tibial fracture is unacceptable deformity that can-

not be corrected by casting. This includes greater than 1.5 cm of shortening or malalignment in the cast. These fractures are considered unstable and will benefit from operative management. Predictors of instability are degree of comminution, initial translation of more than 50 percent, degree of obliquity, very proximal and distal fractures, and the presence of an intact fibula.[10,13,14,16,27,87]

If the fracture is unstable, proper alignment in the cast cannot be maintained. However, the exact amount of angulation and translation that can be accepted is a source of debate.[14] Small amounts of angulation have progressed to arthrosis of the ankle.[78,92,113] Likewise, arthritic changes have been provoked by tibial malalignment in a rabbit model.[39] Yet at least one major clinical study found no evidence of arthritis in patients with tibial fractures that healed in up to 20° of angulation.[81] Thus, the limits of acceptable angulation are not clear. The closer a fracture is to the knee or ankle, the more effect it has on the contact forces of that joint.[112] The ankle seems more prone to arthritis than the knee. For these reasons, the most commonly quoted limits for an acceptable reduction of the tibia is 5° of varus or valgus, 5 to 10° of anterior or posterior angulation, 1.0 to 1.5 cm of shortening, and less than 50 percent translation. These numbers should be more rigidly applied in more proximal and especially distal fractures. Surgery is indicated if an acceptable reduction cannot be obtained or maintained in a cast.

Additionally, long-term casting has been associated with decreased ankle and subtalar motion, leading to functional limitations in up to 20 percent of patients.[27] Thus, if true functional bracing is not possible, operative management may be indicated. Patient factors must also be evaluated in the decision process. Athletes or patients who require an earlier return to function may choose surgical management despite the risks of surgery. These should be carefully explained when the options for treatment are being discussed with any patient.

If a surgical option is chosen, then several options exist. Intramedullary nailing, plate fixation, and external fixation have all been used successfully in the tibia.[16,20,52,108] Plates allow for anatomic reduction but have an increased incidence of soft tissue complications and do not allow early weight bearing.[52,124] External fixation is safe for the soft tissues but is not preferred by patients and is associated with a high percentage of pin-tract infections.[108,129] Thus, of the available options, intramedullary nailing has become the treatment of choice for acute diaphyseal fractures requiring surgery.[10,20,35,134]

Intramedullary nailing results in union rates near 100 percent for closed injuries.[20,35] However, this procedure is not devoid of complications, both early and late. Early complications include infection (1 to 3 percent), transient neurologic injury (0 to 30 percent), and, most significantly, compartment syndrome (equal to or greater than 1.5 percent).[39,60,79,81,82,92,106] Infection can be kept to a minimum if the fracture site is not opened during the nailing. The risks of neurologic injury and increased compartment pressures are augmented by the use of traction, a posterior post, tourniquets, and reaming.[60,82,109,115] Nonreamed nailing, performed without the continuous traction needed during reaming, has been shown to result in lower compartment pressures that return to normal quickly.[115] By contrast, it takes 72 h for the increased pressures after reaming to dissipate.[80]

Fractures nailed without reaming have demonstrated earlier callus formation than fractures that were reamed.[101] Earlier weight bearing and union have been documented by several authors.[75,76,99] However, these findings are not universal, and others have found secondary procedures to obtain union more common after nonreamed nailing.[24] Static locking (screws placed through the nail proximal and distal to the fracture) with distraction at the fracture site has been shown to delay healing after nonreamed nailing.[11,96] Additionally, hardware failure is higher with narrow, stainless steel, nonreamed implants.[132] Titanium implants, which have a higher ultimate strength, have a significantly lower failure rate.[76,96] Currently, most authors use nonreamed nailing in cases with soft tissue injury and reamed nailing if the fracture is indirect and has only minimal swelling. If reamed nailing is performed in the face of a soft tissue injury or swelling, compartment pressures may be monitored intra- and postoperatively so as to avoid the complication of compartment syndrome.[79]

If nonreamed nailing is chosen and the fracture is statically locked in distraction, then dynamization (removal of the screws on one side of the fracture) is recommended at 6 to 8 weeks.[11] Alternatively, an exchange nailing with a dynamic reamed nail may be performed if union is delayed. These complications are most common in fractures caused by high-energy direct mechanisms.

Proximal Fractures

Several recent reports have questioned the use of intramedullary nailing for fractures of the proximal tibia due to difficulty in obtaining acceptable alignment.[34,63] These injuries occur in an area that is much wider than the nail, and restoration of alignment cannot be expected simply from passing the nail across the fracture. The starting portal is also more difficult to place, and placement that is not central will lead to angulation. Special techniques—including the use of a partial arthrotomy and/or "Pohler" screws—can counteract the problems in nailing proximal fractures[19,61,120] (Fig. 29-4). However, because of the technical difficulty in nailing these fractures, external fixation using a hybrid or standard fixator (depending on the level of the fracture) is a safer option for surgeons less experienced in tibial nailing.

COMPLICATIONS

Complications in the treatment of tibial fractures are most commonly related to the soft tissues. These include compartment syndrome, infection, nonunion, and amputation. The diagnosis and treatment of compartment syndromes were discussed earlier in the chapter. The management of infection is discussed in Chap. 17.

Nonunion

The time to union for a tibial fracture correlates with the energy of the injury and the status of the soft tissues.[31] Functional bracing of closed tibial fractures yields a 90 percent rate of union at 6 months.[105] However, only 23 percent of grade III open fractures are healed at 6 months.[30] The definitions of *delayed* and *nonunion,* therefore, depend on the expected time to union. It is generally held that closed fractures heal by 9 months and open fractures by 1 year. Fractures not healed within these intervals may be considered delayed. The term *nonunion* is best applied to an unhealed fracture with radiographic signs including rounded sclerotic edges (oligotrophic) with resorption (atrophic) or expansile callus with a clear gap at the level of the fracture (hypertrophic or possibly synovial). Infected nonunion is another possibility.

The problem of tibial nonunion is generally managed operatively. The specific methods depend on the fracture pattern, the soft tissues, and the host. These principles are addressed elsewhere in the text.

Malunion

The indications for the treatment of malunion are controversial. Most authors agree that in the absence of large deformities, only symptomatic patients should be treated. Correction of the malunion with an osteotomy and plate fixation is the currently favored method.[45,103,133] Complex multiaxial external fixation is another good option for surgeons with experience in these techniques.[90]

Other Complications

Other problems encountered in the treatment of tibial fractures include knee or ankle stiffness, arthritis, reflex sympathetic dystrophy, refracture, nerve injury, and pain. None of these complications is common, but the clinician should be aware of their possibility.

REFERENCES

1. Adamson GJ, Wiss DA, Lowery GL, Peters CL: Type II floating knee: Ipsilateral femoral and tibial fractures with intra-articular extension into the knee joint. *J Orthop Trauma* 6:333–339, 1992.

1a. Adkinson D, Bosse M, Gaccione D, et al: Anatomical variations in the superficial peroneal nerve. *J Bone Joint Surg* 75A:112–114, 1991.

2. Alho A, Benterud JG, Hogevold HE, et al: Comparison of functional bracing and locked intramedullary nailing in the treatment of displaced tibial shaft fractures. *Clin Orthop* 227:243–250, 1992.

3. Behrens F: *Current Concepts of External Fixation of Fractures.* Berlin, Springer-Verlag, 1982.

4. Behrens F, Searles K: External fixation of the tibia: Basic concepts and prospective evaluation. *J Bone Joint Surg* 68B:246–254, 1986.

5. Bengner V, Ekbom T, Johnell O, et al: Incidence of femoral and tibial shaft fractures. *Acta Orthop Scand* 61:251–254, 1990.

6. Blachut PA, Meek RN, O'Brien PJ: External fixation and delayed intermedullary nailing of open fractures of the tibial shaft: A sequential protocol. *J Bone Joint Surg* 72A:729–735, 1990.

7. Blick, SS, Brumback RJ, Poka A, et al: Compartment syndrome in open tibial fractures. *J Bone Joint Surg* 68A:1348–1353, 1986.

8. Blick SS, Brumback RJ, Lakatos R, et al: Early prophylactic bone grafting of high energy tibial fractures. *Clin Orthop* 240:21–41, 1989.

9. Bonanni F, Rhodes M, Lucke JF: The futility of predictive scoring of mangled lower extremities. *J Trauma* 34:99–104, 1993.

10. Bone LB, Johnson KD: Treatment of tibial fractures by reaming and intramedullary nailing. *J Bone Joint Surg* 68A:877–887, 1986.

11. Bone LB, Kassman S, Stegemann P, et al: Prospective study of union rate of open tibial fractures treated with locked, unreamed intramedullary nails. *J Orthop Trauma* 8:45–49, 1994.

12. Böstman OM: Rotational refracture of the shaft of the adult tibia. *Injury* 15:93–98, 1983.

13. Böstman OM: Spiral fractures of the shaft of the tibia: Initial displacement and stability of reduction. *J Bone Joint Surg* 68B:462–466, 1986.

14. Bridgman SA, Baird K: Audit of closed tibial fractures: What is a satisfactory outcome? *Injury* 24:85–89, 1993.

15. Brumback RJ, Jones AL: Interobserver agreement in the classification of open fractures of the tibia. *J Bone Joint Surg* 76A:1162–1166, 1994.

16. Burwell HN: Plate fixation of tibial shaft fractures: A survey of 181 injuries. *J Bone Joint Surg* 53B:258–271, 1971.

17. Caudle RJ, Stern PJ: Severe open fractures of the tibia. *J Bone Joint Surg* 69A:801–807, 1987.

18. Clough JR: Segmental fractures of the shaft of the tibia. *J Bone Joint Surg* 55B:878–879, 1973.

19. Cole JD: Intramedullary nailing of proximal fourth tibia fractures. Presented at the 11th Annual Orthopaedic Trauma Association Meeting, Tampa, FL, 1995.

20. Collins DN, Pearce CE, McAndrew MP: Successful use of reaming and intramedullary nailing of the tibia. *J Orthop Trauma* 4:315–322, 1990.

21. Court-Brown CM, McQueen MM, Quaba AA, Christie J: Locked intramedullary nailing of open tibial fractures. *J Bone Joint Surg* 73B:959–964, 1991.

22. Court-Brown CM, Keating JF, McQueen MM: Infection after intramedullary nailing of the tibia: Incidence and protocol for management. *J Bone Joint Surg* 74B:770–774, 1992.

23. Court-Brown CM, Keating JF, Christie J, McQueen MM: Exchange intramedullary nailing. *J Bone Joint Surg* 77B:407–411, 1995.

24. Court-Brown CM, Will EM, McQueen MM, et al: Reamed or unreamed nailing in closed tibial fractures: A prospective study. Presented at the 11th Annual Orthopaedic Trauma Association Meeting, Tampa, FL, 1995.

25. DaCosta GIB, Kumar N: Early weight-bearing in treatment of fractures of the tibia. *Injury* 11:123–131, 1979.

26. Dickson K, Katzman S, Delgado E, Contreras D: Delayed unions and nonunions of open tibial fractures: Correlation with arteriography results. *Clin Orthop* 302:189–193, 1994.

27. Digby JM, Holloway GMN, Webb JK: A study of function after tibial cast bracing. *Injury* 14:432–439, 1983.

28. DiStasio AJ, Dogdale TW, Deafenbaugh MK: Multiple relaxing incisions in orthopedic lower extremity trauma. *J Orthop Trauma* 7:27–34, 1994.

29. Ebraheim NA, Savolaine ER, Patel A, et al: Assessment of tibial fracture union by 35–45 degree internal oblique radiographs. *J Orthop Trauma* 5:349–350, 1991.

30. Edwards CC: Staged reconstruction of complex tibial fractures using Hoffman external fixation. *Clin Orthop* 178:130–160, 1983.

31. Ellis H: The speed of healing after fracture of the tibial shaft. *J Bone Joint Surg* 40B:42–46, 1958.

32. Fairhurst MJ: The function of below-knee amputee versus the patient with salvaged grade III tibial fracture. *Clin Orthop* 301:227–232, 1994.

33. Fischer MD, Gustilo RB, Varecka TF: The timing of flap coverage, bone-grafting, and intramedullary nailing in patients who have a fracture of the tibial shaft with extensive soft-tissue injury. *J Bone Joint Surg* 73A:1316–1322, 1991.

34. Freedman EL, Johnson EE: Radiographic analysis of tibial fracture malalignment following intramedullary nailing. *Clin Orthop* 315:25–33, 1995.

35. Gad HF, Abul Kheir IH, Booz MK: Closed nailing of tibial shaft fractures. *Injury* 21:217–219, 1990.

36. Garraway WM, Stauffer RN, Kurland LT, O'Fallon WM: Limb fractures in a defined position: I. Frequency and distribution. *Mayo Clin Proc* 54:701–707, 1979.

37. Georgiadis GM, Behrens FF, Joyce MJ, et al: Open tibial fractures with severe soft tissue loss: Limb salvage compared with below-the-knee amputation. *J Bone Joint Surg* 76:1594–1595, 1994.

38. Georgiadis GM: Tibial shaft fractures complicated by compartment syndrome: Treatment with immediate fasciotomy and locked unreamed nailing. *J Trauma* 38:448–452, 1995.

39. Goodman SB, Lee J, Smith RL, et al: Mechanical overload of a single compartment induces early degenerative changes in the rabbit knee: A preliminary study. *J Invest Surg* 4:161–170, 1991.

40. Gregory P, Sanders R: The treatment of closed, unstable tibial shaft fractures with unreamed interlocking nails. *Clin Orthop* 315:48–55, 1995.

41. Gustilo RB, Mendoza RM, Williams DN: Problems in the management of type III (severe) open fractures: A new classification of type III open fractures. *J Trauma* 24:742–746, 1984.

42. Hak DJ, Johnson EE: The use of the unreamed nail in tibial fractures with concomitant preoperative or intraoperative elevated compartment pressure or compartment syndrome. *J Orthop Trauma* 8:203–211, 1994.

43. Harmon PH: A simplified approach to the posterior tibia for bone grafting and fibular transferral. *J Bone Joint Surg* 27A:496–498, 1945.

44. Heckman MM, Whitesides TE Jr, Grewe SR, Rooks MD: Compartment pressure in association with closed tibial fractures: The relationship between tissue pressure, compartment, and the distance from the site of the fracture. *J Bone Joint Surg* 76A:1285–1292, 1994.

45. Helfet DL, Jupiter JB, Gasser S: Indirect reduction and tension band plating of tibial nonunion with deformity. *J Bone Joint Surg* 74A:1286–1297, 1992.

46. Henley MB: Intramedullary devices for tibial fracture stabilization. *Clin Orthop* 240:87–96, 1989.

47. Henley MB, Meier M, Tencer AF: Influences of some design parameters on the biomechanics of the unreamed tibial intramedullary nail. *J Orthop Trauma* 7:311–319, 1993.

48. Henley MB, Chapman J, et al: Nonreamed nails versus external fixators. Presented at the annual meeting of the Orthopaedic Trauma Society, Los Angeles, CA, 1994.

49. Hooper GJ, Keddell RG, Penny ID: Conservative management or closed nailing for tibial shaft fractures: A randomized prospective trial. *J Bone Joint Surg* 73B:83–85, 1991.

50. Horn BD, Rettig ME: Interobserver reliability in the Gustilo and Anderson classification of open fractures. *J Orthop Trauma* 7:357–360, 1993.

51. Howe HR, Poole GV, Hansen KJ, et al: Salvage of lower extremities following combined orthopaedic and vascular trauma: A predictive salvage index. *Am Surg* 53:205–208, 1987.

52. Jensen JS, Hansen FW, Johansen J: Tibial shaft fractures: A comparison of conservative treatment and internal fixation with conventional plates or AO compression plates. *Acta Orthop Scand* 48:204–212, 1977.

53. Johansen K, Gaines M, Howey T, Helfet DL: Objective criteria accurately predict amputation following lower extremity trauma. *J Trauma* 30:568–573, 1990.

54. Johner R, Wruhs O: Classification of tibial shaft fractures and correlation with results after rigid internal fixation. *Clin Orthop* 178:7–25, 1983.

55. Johnson EE: Acute lengthening of shortened lower extremities after malunion or non-union of a fracture. *J Bone Joint Surg* 76A:379–389, 1994.

56. Johnson KD: Management of malunion and nonunion of the tibia. *Orthop Clin North Am* 18:157–171, 1987.

57. Karlstrom G, Olerud S: Ipsilateral fracture of the femur and tibia. *J Bone Joint Surg* 59A:240–243, 1977.

58. Kindsfater K, Jonassen EA: Osteomyelitis in grade II and III open tibia fractures with late debridement. *J Orthop Trauma* 9:121–127, 1995.

59. Knopp W, Schumm F, Bucholz J, Ekkernkamp A: Functional healing of compartment syndrome of the tibia: An analysis of follow-up results. *Chirurgie* 65:988–991, 1994.

60. Koval KJ, Clapper MF, Brumback RJ, et al: Complications of reamed intramedullary nailing of the tibia. *J Orthop Trauma* 5:184–189, 1991.

61. Krettek C, Schandelmaier P, Tscherne H: Nonreamed interlocking nailing of closed tibial fractures with severe soft tissue injury. *Clin Orthop* 315:34–47, 1995.

62. Kristensen KD, Kiaer T, Blicner J: No arthrosis of the ankle 20 years after malaligned tibial-shaft fracture. *Acta Orthop Scand* 60:208–209, 1989.

63. Lang GJ, Cohen BE, Bosse MJ, Kellam JF: Proximal third tibial shaft fractures: Should they be nailed? *Clin Orthop* 315:64–74, 1995.

64. Lange RH, Bach AW, Hansen ST, Johansen KH: Open tibial fractures and associated vascular injuries: Prognoses for limb salvage. *J Trauma* 25:203–208, 1985.

65. Lawyer RB, Lubbers LM: Use of the Hoffmann apparatus in the treatment of unstable tibial fractures. *J Bone Joint Surg* 62A:1264–1273, 1980.

66. Lazarides MK, Arvanitis DP, Kopadis GC, et al: Popliteal artery and trifurcation injuries: Is it possible to predict the outcome? *Eur J Vasc Surg* 8:226–230, 1994.

67. Leach RE: Fractures of the tibia and fibula, in Rockwood CA Jr, Green DP (eds): *Fractures in Adults*. Vol 2. Philadelphia, Lippincott, 1593–1663, 1984.

68. Lonner JH, Jupiter JB, Healy WL: Ipsilateral tibia and ankle fractures. *J Orthop Trauma* 7:130–137, 1993.

69. Lottes JO, Hill LJ, Key JA: Closed reduction, plate fixation and medullary nailing of fractures of both bones of the leg. *J Bone Joint Surg* 34A:861–877, 1952.

70. MacKenzie DA, Martimbeau C, Mudge K, et al: A prospective study of closed reamed locked intramedullary rods in the early management of open tibial fractures. *J Orthop Trauma* 5:239, 1991.

71. Macnab I, de Haas WG: The role of periosteal blood supply in the healing of fractures of the tibia. *Clin Orthop* 105:27–34, 1974.

72. Markel MD, Chao EY: Noninvasive monitoring techniques for quantitative description of callus mineral content and mechanical properties. *Clin Orthop* 293:37–45, 1993.

73. Matsen F, Mayo K, Krugmire R, et al: A model compartmental syndrome in man with particular reference to the quantification of nerve function. *J Bone Joint Surg* 59A:648–653, 1977.

74. Mawhinney IN, Maginn P, McCoy GF: Tibial compartment syndromes after tibial nailing. *J Orthop Trauma* 8:212–214, 1994.

75. Mayr E, Barnikel C, Braun W, et al: Closed tibial fracture: Reamed or unreamed intramedullary nailing: A clinical study. *Zentrabl Chir* 120:24–30, 1995.

76. McClelland RT, Tornetta III P, Comstock C, et al: Intramedullary nailing of closed tibial shaft fractures. Presented at the AAOS Meeting, Atlanta, GA, 1996.

77. McGraw JM, Lim EVA: Treatment of open tibial-shaft fractures: External fixation and secondary intramedullary nailing. *J Bone Joint Surg* 70A:900–911, 1988.

78. McKellop HA, Llinas A, Sarmiento A: Effects of tibial malalignment on the knee and ankle. *Orthop Clin North Am* 25:415–423, 1994.

79. McQueen MM, Christie J, Court-Brown CM: Compartment pressures after intramedullary nailing of the tibia. *J Bone Joint Surg* 72B:395–397, 1990.

80. McQueen M, Christie J, Court-Brown C: Acute compartment syndrome in tibial diaphyseal fractures. *J Bone Joint Surg* 78B:95–98, 1996.

81. Merchant TC, Dietz FR: Long-term follow-up after fractures of the tibial and fibular shafts. *J Bone Joint Surg* 71A:599–606, 1989.

82. Moed BR, Strom DE: Compartment syndrome after closed intramedullary nailing of the tibia: A canine model and report of two cases. *J Orthop Trauma* 5:71–77, 1991.

83. Moed BR, Watson JT, Goldschmidt P, van Holsbeeck M: Ultrasound for the early diagnosis of fracture healing after interlocking nailing of the tibia without reaming. *Clin Orthop* 310:137–144, 1995.

84. Montava MJ, Whitesides TE, Seiler JG, et al: Determination of the compartment pressure threshold of muscle ischemia in a canine model. *J Trauma* 37:50–58, 1994.

85. Mubarak SJ, Hargens AR, Owen CA, et al: The wick catheter technique for measurement of intramuscular pressure. *J Bone Joint Surg* 58A:1016–1020, 1976.

86. Müller ME: Klassifikation und internationale AO-Dokumentation der Femurfrakturen. *Unfallheilkunde* 83:251–260, 1980.

87. Nicoll EA: Fractures of the tibial shaft: A survey of 705 cases. *J Bone Joint Surg* 46B:373–387, 1964.

88. Olerud S, Karlstrom G: Tibial fractures treated by AO compression osteosynthesis. *Acta Orthop Scand [Suppl]* 1:1–104, 1972.

89. Padberg FT, Rubelowsky JJ, Maldonado JJ, et al: Infrapopliteal arterial injury: Prompt revascularization affords optimal limb salvage. *J Vasc Surg* 16:877–886, 1992.

90. Paley D, Catagni MA, Argnani F, et al: Ilizarov treatment of tibial non-unions with bone loss. *Clin Orthop* 241:146–165, 1989.

91. Pozo JL, Powell S, Andrews BG, et al: The timing of amputation for lower extremity trauma. *J Bone Joint Surg* 72B:288–292, 1990.

92. Puno RM, Vaughan JJ, Stetten ML, et al: Long-term effects of tibial angular malunion on the knee and ankle joints. *J Orthop Trauma* 5:247–254, 1991.

93. Purry NA, Hannon MA: How successful is below knee amputation for injury? *Injury* 20:32–36, 1989.

94. Reckling FW, Waters CH: Treatment of nonunions of fractures of the tibial diaphysis by posterolateral cortical cancellous bone grafting. *J Bone Joint Surg* 62A:936–941, 1980.

95. Rhinelander FW: Tibial blood supply in relation to fracture healing. *Clin Orthop* 105:34–81, 1974.

96. Riemer BL, DiChristina DG, Cooper A, et al: Nonreamed nailing of tibial diaphyseal fractures in blunt polytrauma patients. *J Orthop Trauma* 9:66–75, 1995.

97. Rijberg WJ, van Linge B: Central grafting for persistent nonunion of the tibia: A lateral approach to the tibia, creating a central compartment. *J Bone Joint Surg* 75B:926–931, 1993.

98. Rorabeck CH: The treatment of compartment syndromes of the leg. *J Bone Joint Surg* 66B:93–97, 1984.

99. Rucholtz S, Nast-Kolb D, Betz A, et al: Fracture healing after intramedullary nailing of simple tibial shaft fractures: A clinical comparison of reamed and unreamed procedures. *Unfallchirurgie* 98:369–375, 1995.

100. Ruedi T, Webb JK, Allgöwer M: Experience with the dynamic compression plate (DCP) in 418 recent fractures of the tibial shaft. *Injury* 7:252–257, 1976.

101. Runkel M, Wenda K, Ritter G: Bone healing after unreamed intramedullary nailing. *Unfallchirurgie* 97:1–7, 1994.

102. Russell WL, Sailors DM, Whittle TB, et al: Limb salvage versus traumatic amputation. *Ann Surg* 213:473–481, 1991.

103. Sanders R, Anglen JO, Mark JB: Oblique osteotomy for the correction of tibial malunion. *J Bone Joint Surg* 77A:240–246, 1995.

104. Santoro V, Henley S, Benirschke S, Mayo K: Prospective comparison of unreamed interlocking IM nails versus half-pin external fixation in open tibial fractures. Presented at the Orthopaedic Trauma Association, Toronto, Canada, 1990.

105. Sarmiento A, Sobol PA, Sew Hoy AL, et al: Prefabricated functional braces for the treatment of fractures of the tibial diaphysis. *J Bone Joint Surg* 66A:1328–1339, 1984.

106. Sarmiento A, Sharpe FE, Ebramzadeh E, et al: Factors influencing the outcome of closed tibial fractures treated with functional bracing. *Clin Orthop* 315:8–24, 1995.

107. Schemitsh EH, Kowalski MJ, Swiontkowski MF, et al: Comparison of the effect of reamed and unreamed locked intramedullary nailing on blood flow in the callus and strength of union following fracture of the sheep tibia. *J Orthop Res* 13:382–389, 1995.

108. Schmidt A, Rorabeck CH: Fractures of the tibia treated by flexible external fixation. *Clin Orthop* 178:162–172, 1983.

109. Shakespeare D, Henderson N: Compartmental pressure changes during calcaneal traction in tibial fractures. *J Bone Joint Surg* 64B:498–499, 1982.

110. Singer RW, Kellam JF: Open tibial diaphyseal fractures: Results of unreamed locked intramedullary nailing. *Clin Orthop* 315:114–118, 1995.

111. Stegemann P, Lorio M, Soriano, et al: Management protocol for unreamed interlocked tibial nails for open fractures. *J Orthop Trauma* 9:117–120, 1995.

112. Tarr RR, Resnick CT, Wagner KS, et al: Changes in tibiotalar joint contact areas following experimentally induced tibial angular deformities. *Clin Orthop* 199:72–80, 1985.

113. Teitz CC, Carter DR, Frankel VH: Problems associated with tibial fractures with intact fibulae. *J Bone Joint Surg* 62:770–776, 1980.

114. Templeman D, Thomas M, Varecka T, Kyle R: Exchange reamed intramedullary nailing for delayed union and nonunion of the tibia. *Clin Orthop* 315:169–175, 1995.

115. Templeman D, Tornetta III P: Compartment syndrome and tibial shaft fractures. *J Bone Joint Surg* September 1996.

116. Tornetta III P, Barbera C: Severe heterotopic bone formation in the knee after tibial intramedullary nailing. *J Orthop Trauma* 6:113–115, 1992.

117. Tornetta III P, Bergman M, Watnik N, et al: Treatment of grade IIIb open tibial fractures: A prospective randomized comparison of external fixation and non-reamed locked nailing. *J Bone Joint Surg* 76B:13–19, 1994.

118. Tornetta III P, McClellan RT, Comstock C, et al: Tibial nailing: A multicenter study. *Orthop Trans* 19:483, 1995.

119. Tornetta III P: Segmental tibial fractures treated with a nonreamed nail. Presented at the International Symposium for Minimal Invasive Traumatology. Salzburg, Austria, 1996.

120. Tornetta III P, Collins E: Semiextended position for intramedullary nailing of the proximal tibia. *Clin Orthop* 327:175–179, 1996.

121. Tornetta III P: Technical considerations in tibial shaft fractures. *Inst Course Lect.* In press.

122. Tornetta III P, Olson S: Amputation vs limb salvage. *Inst Course Lect.* In press.

123. Trabulsy PP, Kerley SM, Hoffman WY: A prospective study of early soft tissue coverage of grade IIIb tibial fractures. *J Trauma* 36:661–668, 1994.

124. Trafton PG: Closed unstable fractures of the tibia. *Clin Orthop* 230:58–67, 1988.

125. Tscherne H, Gotzen L: *Fractures with Soft Tissue Injuries.* Berlin, Springer-Verlag, 1984.

126. Veith RG, Winquist RA, Hansen ST: Ipsilateral fractures of the femur and tibia. *J Bone Joint Surg* 66A:991–1002, 1984.

127. Velazco A, Fleming LL: Open fractures of the tibia treated by the Hoffman external fixator. *Clin Orthop* 180:125–132, 1983.

128. Veliskakis KP: Primary internal fixation in open fractures of the tibial shaft: The problem of wound healing. *J Bone Joint Surg* 41B:342–354, 1959.

129. Waddell JP, Reardon GP: Complications of tibial shaft fractures. *Clin Orthop* 178:173–178, 1983.

130. Weckbach A, Blattert TR, Kunz E: Differential indications for intramedullary nailing of the tibia with the reamed and unreamed technique. *Zentrabl Chir* 119:556–563, 1994.

131. Weissman SL, Herold HZ, Engelberg M: Fractures of the middle two-thirds of the tibial shaft. *J Bone Joint Surg* 48A:257–267, 1966.

132. Whittle AP, Wester W, Russell TA: Fatigue failure in small diameter tibial nails. *Clin Orthop* 315:119–128, 1995.

133. Wiss DA, Johnson DL, Miao M: Compression plating for nonunion after failed external fixation of open tibial fractures. *J Bone Joint Surg* 74A:1279–1285, 1992.

134. Wiss DA, Stetson WB: Unstable fractures of the tibia treated with a reamed intramedullary interlocking nail. *Clin Orthop* 315:56–63, 1995.

135. Woll TS, Duwelius PJ: The segmental tibial fracture. *Clin Orthop* 281:204–207, 1992.

136. Wu C, Shih C: Effect of dynamization of a static interlocking nail on fracture healing. *J Can Surg* 36:302–306, 1993.

137. Wu C, Shih C: Complicated open fractures of the distal tibia treated by secondary interlocking nailing. *J Trauma* 34:792–796, 1993.

138. Wu C, Shih C: Segmental tibial shaft fractures treated with interlocking nailing. *J Orthop Trauma* 7:468–471, 1993.

CHAPTER 30

Ankle Injuries

Paul Tornetta III

ANATOMY

The ankle joint is formed by the articulation of the distal tibia and fibula with the talus. The main weight-bearing surface is between the tibial plafond and the dome of the talus. The medial extension of the tibia is called the medial malleolus and articulates with the medial facet of the talus. The distal fibula articulates with the lateral facet of the talus and is referred to as the lateral malleolus. Together, the malleoli and plafond create a "mortise," or constrained joint. The talar dome is wider anteriorly than posteriorly and the mortise is slightly wider anteriorly and superiorly to accommodate the talus.

The mechanical axis of the ankle joint is oriented approximately 20 to 30° externally rotated with respect to the knee axis and 80° to the long axis of the knee. This relationship is more easily understood if the joint is viewed as a cone, with the apex medially and the base laterally.[46] Although the axis of rotation changes slightly during motion, the joint essentially functions as a hinge.

The bony architecture of the ankle is only its framework. The ligamentous supports of the joint provide the strength of its stability. These ligaments are well described and their contributions must be understood by the surgeon treating injuries of the ankle region. There are three regional sets of ankle ligaments: medial, lateral, and syndesmotic. Medially, the deltoid ligament is described as having deep and superficial components. The superficial runs from the anterior colliculus of the medial malleolus to the sustentaculum of the calcaneus, the medial facet of the talus, and to the navicular. The deep portion originates from behind the superficial ligament over the majority of the medial malleolus and inserts on the medial talus. It is the primary restraint to lateral displacement of the talus.[16,24,39,62,67]

There are three ligaments on the lateral side of the ankle. These are the anterior and posterior talofibular and the calcaneofibular. The anterior talofibular ligament runs in an almost transverse direction from the tip of the fibula to the talar neck and is indistinguishable from the capsule in its midportion. Its fibers resist anterior displacement and inversion of the talus from its mortise.[23] The posterior calcaneofibular ligament originates from the posteromedial fibula and inserts on the lateral tubercle of the talus. It is primarily responsible for preventing rotational deformity of the joint. The calcaneofibular ligament is anchored on the tip of the fibula and attaches to a region on the posterolateral calcaneus. It is a stabilizer of the ankle and subtalar joint and resists inversion with the foot in the neutral position.[52]

The final set of ligaments that stabilize the ankle are the syndesmotic ligaments. They act to maintain the relationship between the distal tibia and fibula. The syndesmotic complex is formed by four independent ligaments: the anterior tibiofibular, the posterior tibiofibular, the transverse tibiofibular, and the interosseous. The tibiofibular ligaments run from the tubercles of the tibia adjacent to the fibula to the fibula anteriorly and posteriorly. The transverse ligament lies just inferior to the posterior tibiofibular ligament. The interosseous ligament is the distal extension of the interosseous membrane, which runs between the tibia and fibula throughout their length. Together, these ligaments are quite strong and resist forces that separate the tibia and fibula distally. There is naturally a small amount of motion at the distal tibiofibular joint, which is compensated for by the ligaments.

INCIDENCE AND MECHANISM OF INJURY

Injuries to the ankle are among the most common disorders seen by orthopaedic surgeons. Ankle sprains alone may represent up to 45 percent of athletic injuries in some sports such as basketball.[11,17] Most ligamentous injuries of the ankle occur from an inversion mechanism. The anterior talofibular ligament is the most frequently injured ligament in the body. By contrast, most ankle fractures occur by eversion or external rotation of the foot.

Injuries to the ankle ligament generally occur when the ankle is not fully loaded, as the osseous stability in the loaded joint is difficult to overcome. Indirect ankle fractures may occur with the foot partially loaded as well. The pilon or impaction fractures of the tibial plafond are the most severe form of fracture. They affect the weight-bearing surface and are caused by axial loading until bony failure. These more severe injuries constitute only 1 to 5 percent of all ankle fractures.[13]

DIAGNOSIS

Patients with ankle injuries suffer immediate pain and swelling. They may, however, present in a delayed fashion. Many patients believe that the swelling and pain will resolve in a short time and do not seek help until several days have passed. Acute ligamentous injuries are primarily diagnosed by physical exam. Significant swelling is common, although the patient is usually able to walk on the extremity with a limp. Fractures may present in the same way unless there is associated instability, such as a fracture dislocation. Patients with these more severe injuries come for help on a more urgent basis. Last, patients with neuropathy, such as that caused by diabetes, may present late even after a severe fracture dislocation. The treatment of these patients is different and is discussed later.

EXAMINATION

The physical examination should begin with an inspection of the skin around the ankle joint to rule out open fractures and open joint injuries. A complete neurovascular exam is necessary, as in all extremity injuries. The position of the foot should be noted, as fracture dislocations require urgent reduction. Most commonly, in the case of a dislocation, the foot will be displaced posterolaterally and rotated externally. If this is the case, a closed reduction should be performed (see "Treatment," below).

The difference between ligament injuries and fractures can be made in most cases by a careful exam. The physician should ask the patient which area of the ankle is most painful and examine this area last. The standard exam begins with palpation of the bony anatomy of the ankle, including the malleoli, anterior joint line, syndesmotic region and posterior tibia. Palpation of the entire fibula is necessary, as indirect fractures may involve fractures of the proximal fibula.

Injury to the anterior talofibular ligament is best tested for by palpation over the anterolateral joint line first, followed by stress testing. The anterior displacement of the talus (anterior drawer test) should be performed with the ankle in slight plantarflexion. The syndesmosis may be injured without fracture and may be tested by squeezing the tibia and fibula toward each other in the midcalf region. Pain in the region of the ankle is considered a positive test.

IMAGING

The standard method of imaging for acute ankle injuries is by plain radiographs. Anteroposterior (AP), lateral, and oblique (mortise) views of the ankle are routine. If a fibular fracture is not seen, a full-length radiograph of the tibia should be obtained to rule out a high fibular fracture (Fig. 30-1). Stress radiographs are useful for both ligamentous injuries and fractures (see "Classification," below). Comparison views of the normal ankle are valuable for both diagnosis and preoperative templating. They should be obtained in all cases of pilon fractures. Traction radiographs can remove overlap of fragments and are obtained in high-grade pilon fractures. Computed tomography (CT) has also been used for pilon fractures to help in diagnosing impaction of the articular surface and identifying nondisplaced fracture lines.[92]

Stress views of ligamentous injuries and fractures are described under "Classification."

Magnetic resonance imaging is useful in the diagnosis of occult and chronic injury but has little value in acute cases.

CLASSIFICATION

Ligamentous injuries are graded as mild (I), moderate (II), and severe (III). These ratings are at least partly defined by the results of stress testing, which includes the lateral tilt and anterior drawer tests. Although many definitions of a positive stress test exist, an excursion of 3 mm greater than normal anteriorly and a tilt of 9° greater than on the normal side may be considered positive anterior drawer and talar tilt tests respectively.[14,17,19,23,31,52]

Mild ligamentous injury exists if the ankle is stable and there is only mild swelling. Moderate injury implies diffuse swelling and tenderness, with a positive anterior drawer and negative talar tilt. The patient can generally bear weight, but with pain. The anterior talofibular ligament is torn, but the calcaneofibular ligament is not completely torn. A severe injury is associated with significant pain and swelling. Both the anterior drawer and talar tilt tests are positive and injury to the anterior talofibular and calcaneofibular ligaments is present.

Ankle fractures may be classified in several ways. The most useful of these is the Lauge-Hansen system,[58] it describes one direct injury pattern that is more of a pilon fracture and four indirect injury patterns. The four types of indirect injury are described by letters. The first relates the position of the foot at the time of injury and the second to the external force applied (Fig. 30-2). The foot may be in supination (S) or pronation (P), and the force may be external rotation, adduction, or abduction. The four types of injury are supination-external rotation (SE), supination-adduction rotation (SA), pronation-external rotation (PE), and pronation-abduction (PA). Each pattern has several stages. In each case, the side of the ankle under tension fails first. In supination injuries, the lateral side fails first; in pronation injuries, the medial side fails first. Either the bone or the ligaments of the ankle may fail, depending on the rate and power applied. On the lateral side, either the lateral ligaments tear or the fibula fractures. On the medial side, the deltoid ligament may rupture or the medial malleolus fractures. Fractures that occur in external rotation follow a circular path, and abduction or adduction injuries occur in line with the force. The stages of these injuries are described in Table 30-1. Injuries to the lateral side of the ankle that fracture the fibula above the syndesmosis disrupt the syndesmotic ligaments in addition to the other noted injuries. This implies a loss of stability between the distal tibia and fibula and may require special treatment.

In certain circumstances, it is necessary to perform a stress radiograph to distinguish between stages of injury. The most common example of this is in the case of a fibular fracture from an SE fracture. If the medial malleolus is intact and the medial joint space is not widened on the radiograph, a stress view is indicated to examine the competence of the deltoid ligament. This is performed on the mortise view and an external rotation force is applied. If the medial joint space widens beyond 4 mm, a deltoid ligament injury is present and the fracture is graded as an SE stage 4. If the medial joint space remains normal, the injury is an SE stage 2 injury. Two other circumstances in which a stress view is useful are in distinguishing a direct fibular shaft fracture from an indirect fibular fracture. The ankle is stressed in external rotation and in abduction. Both the medial clear space and the syndesmosis are examined on the radiograph. The normal relationships are shown in Fig. 30-3. Finally, if a medial malleolus fracture is

Figure 30-1 *A.* Anteroposterior view of a dislocated ankle. Note that the syndesmosis is widened (increased space between the distal tibia and fibula) and there is no fibular fracture visible. *B.* The full-length AP of the tibia reveals a high fibular fracture.

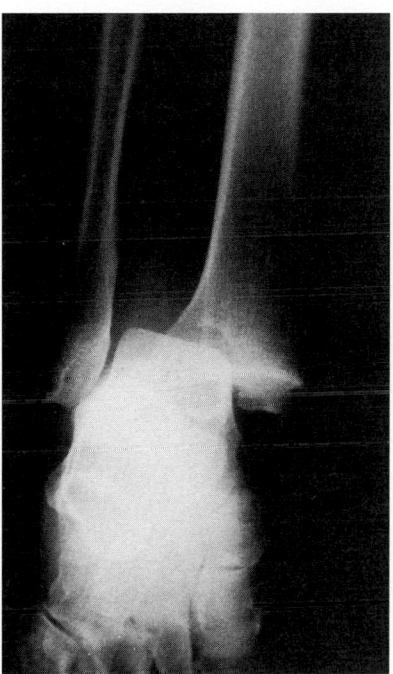

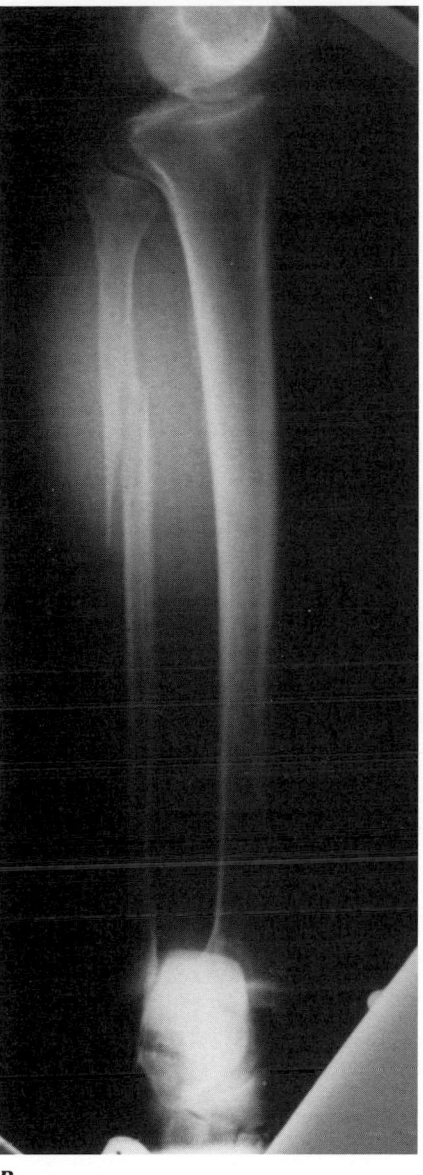

A   *B*

present without fibular fracture, a stress radiograph in external rotation and abduction to examine the syndesmosis will differentiate between a PA stage 1 and 2 or a PE stage 2 and a higher stage (3 or 4). These determinations should be made in the operating room prior to fixation of the medial malleolus.

The final advantage of the Lauge-Hansen system is that the mechanism of the injury is described, allowing for an understanding of the forces needed to reduce the fracture if closed treatment is chosen.

Pilon fractures are graded differently than indirect injuries. They are divided by mechanism and by intraarticular comminution. Ruedi and Allgower separated the fractures into types I, II, and III.[81,82] Type I implies a nondisplaced fracture that extends into the weight-bearing surface of the joint. Type II is a displaced fracture with large fragments and no intraarticular comminution. A type III fracture has comminution at the level of the joint with

significant impaction. These fractures have also been divided on the basis of mechanism by Kellam and Waddell.[51] Rotational injuries are considered type A and axial loading injuries type B. Most of the type B injuries would be classified as a Ruedi type III.

TREATMENT

The management decisions in the treatment of acute ankle injuries is based on the expected outcome of each method and the patient's requirements. The management of a professional athlete may be different from that of a 65-year-old retiree with the same injury. This section first reviews the treatment of ligamentous injuries and then considers fractures.

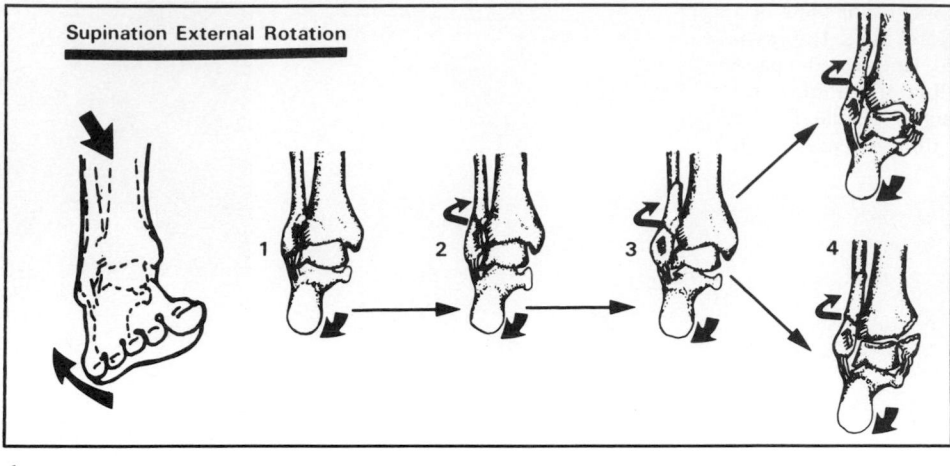

A

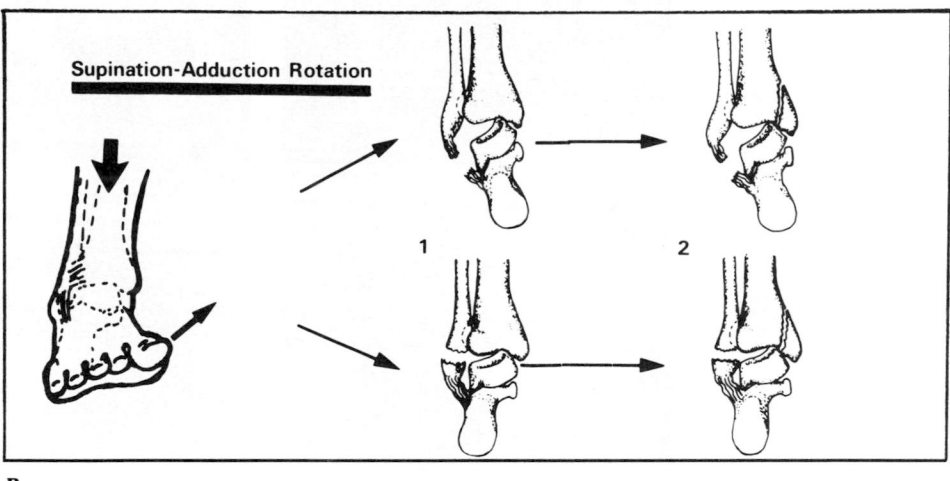

B

Figure 30-2 Five types of injury and the structures that determine their severity, according to a modified Lauge-Hansen classification of ankle injuries. Thick arrows indicate direction of injury forces; thin arrows indicate progression of severity. In every type of injury, the severity is determined by the structures injured. *A.* Supination-external rotation. (1) Rupture of the anterior tibiofibular ligament, (2) spiral or oblique fracture of the lateral malleolus; (3) rupture of the posterior tibial margin, (4) rupture of the deltoid ligament or fracture of the medial malleolus. *B.* Supination-adduction rotation. (1) Traction fracture of the lateral malleolus at or below the level of the ankle joint or rupture of the talofibular ligament, (2) nearly vertical fracture of the medial malleolus. *C.* Pronation-external rotation. (1) rupture of the deltoid ligament or avulsion of the medial malleolus; (2) rupture of the anterior tibiofibular ligament and the interosseous ligament; (3) short spiral fracture of the fibula, typically located 7.6 cm proximal to the ankle joint but not infrequently more proximal; (4) fracture of the posterior tibial margin or rupture of the posterior tibiofibular ligament. *D.* Pronation-abduction. (1) Fracture of the medial malleolus or rupture of the deltoid ligament; (2) rupture of both the anterior and the posterior tibiofibular ligament; (3) bending fracture of the fibula, generally just proximal to the ankle joint, often associated with displacement of the triangular fragment from the lateral surface of the fibula. *E.* Pronation-dorsiflexion. (1) Fracture of the medial malleolus or rupture of the deltoid ligament; (2) fracture of fragment from the anterior articular margin of the tibia caused by the dorsiflexion of the talus; (3) supramalleolar fracture of the fibula; (4) transverse fracture of the posterior lip of the tibial articular surface, this fragment having been avulsed by the dorsiflexion of the talus, which also sheared off the anterior lip of the tibial articular surface. (Reproduced with permission from Petrone FA, Gail M, Pee D, et al. Quantitative criteria for prediction of the results after displaced fracture of the ankle. *J Bone Joint Surg* 65A:667–677, 1983.)

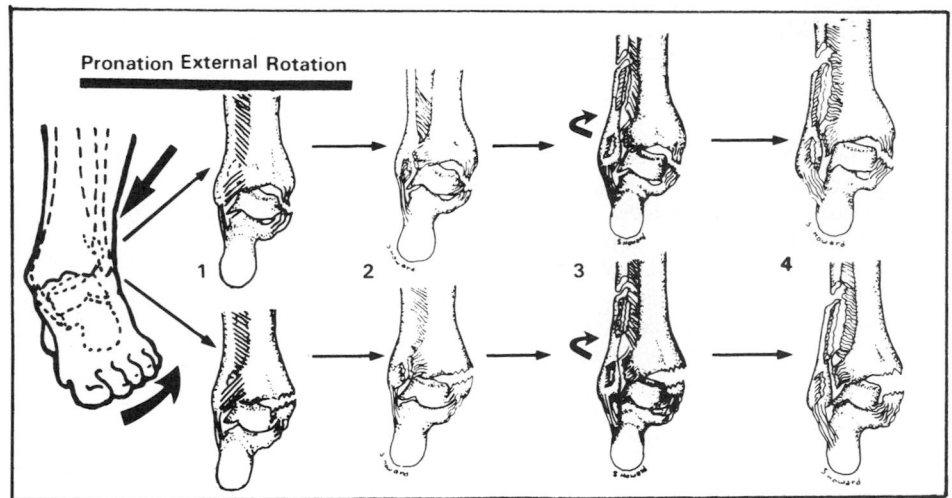

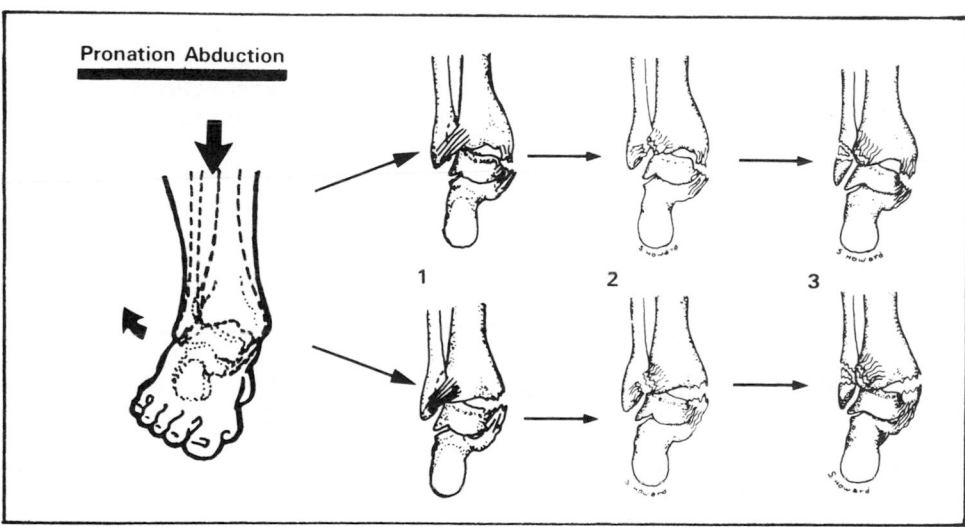

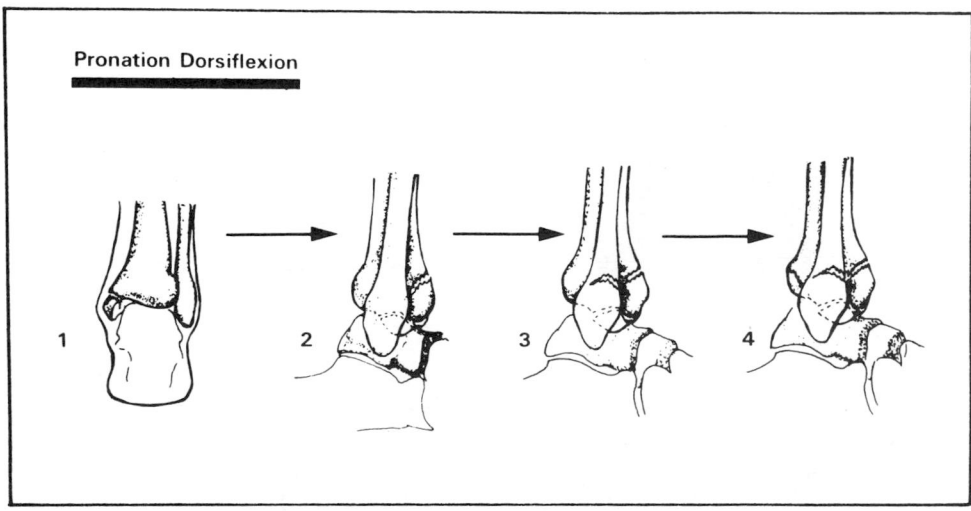

Figure 30-2 *(Continued)*

TABLE 30-1   Lauge-Hansen Classification

Mechanism	Stage	Anatomic injury
SA	1	Low transverse fibular fracture or lateral ligaments
	2	Vertical medial malleolus fracture
SE	1	Anterior talofibular ligament
	2	Anteroinferior to posterosuperior fibula fracture
	3	Posterior talofibular ligament of posterior malleolus fracture
	4	Oblique medial malleolus or deltoid ligament
PA	1	Transverse medial malleolus or deltoid ligament
	2	All syndesmotic ligaments avulsed or ruptured
	3	Transverse fibula 5–7 cm above joint (possibly comminuted)
PE	1	Transverse medial malleolus or deltoid ligament
	2	Anterior talofibular ligament
	3	Posteroinferior to anterosuperior fibula above joint
	4	Posterior talofibular ligament or posterior malleolus

LIGAMENTOUS INJURIES

The mainstay of treatment for acute ligamentous injuries of the ankle is nonoperative. The single exception to this may be in the treatment of a high-level competitive athlete, where an anatomic repair is favored by some authors in an attempt to give greater mechanical stability.[17,18] However, in all other patients, regardless of the degree of sprain, recent literature suggests that early motion and return to weight bearing in a brace yields the best results.[25,48,69] In the immediate postinjury period, elevation and ice are helpful in decreasing the inflammatory re-

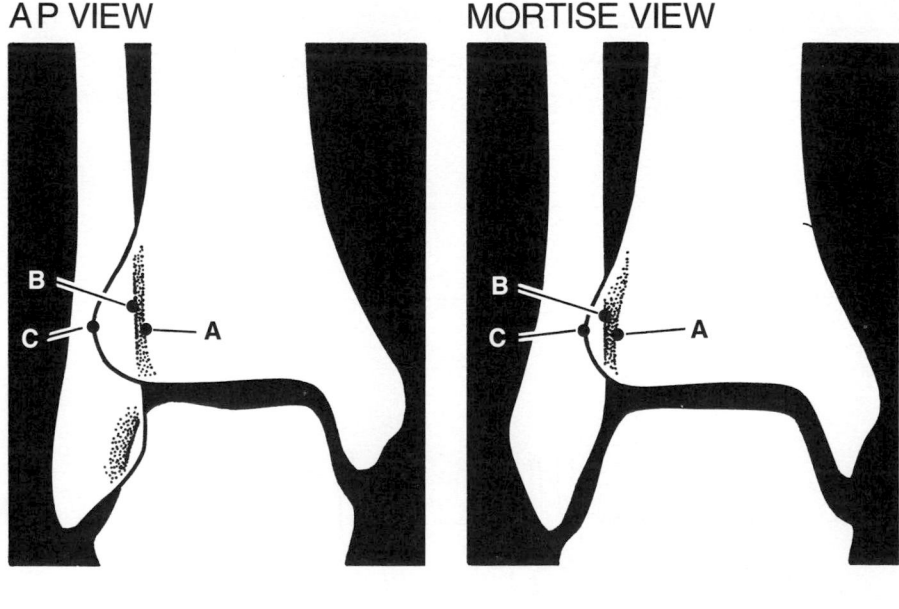
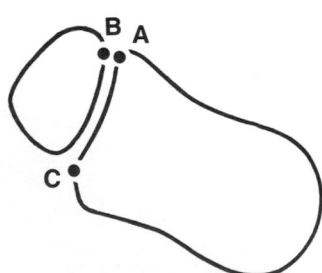
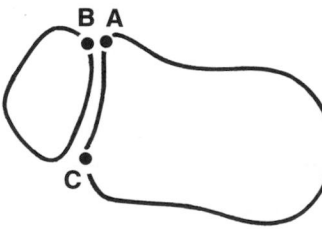

AP VIEW   **MORTISE VIEW**

Figure 30-3 Drawing of an anteroposterior (AP) and mortise views of the right angle and of corresponding cross section at the level of the joint. These show the landmarks used to define the status of the tibiofibular syndesmosis. A, Lateral border of the posterior tibial malleolus. B, Medial border of the fibula. C, Lateral border of the anterior tibial prominence. Disruption of the syndesmosis may be assumed if (1) the distance A–B on the AP view is more than 5 mm; (2) B–C (the overlap of the tibia on the fibula) on the AP view is less than 10 mm; (3) B–C on the mortise view is 1 mm or less. (Reproduced with permission from Pettrone FA, Gail M, Pee D, et al: Quantitative criteria for prediction of the results after displaced fracture of the ankle. *J Bone Joint Surg* 65A:667–677, 1983.)

sponse. After the first 24 to 48 h, mobilization with increasing pressure as tolerated by the patient should be encouraged in a brace. Complete immobilization has been shown to slow return to work and sport.[54] A simple air cast or comparable brace is sufficient. When the patient is able to bear full weight on the ankle (usually at 7 to 10 days), aggressive rehabilitation protocols will help to speed recovery.[17,28] Strengthening of the peroneal musculature and gastrocsoleus complex is paramount in restoring the dynamic constraints of the ankle.[57] Proprioceptive training such as a tilt board helps the patient to regain balance and function.

The patient must understand that, despite aggressive rehabilitation, swelling is part of the natural history after severe ligament injury and may persist for 6 months to a year. The most common problem after low-grade ligamentous injury is not instability but reinjury. For this reason, grade I and II injuries should be aggressively rehabilitated and patients should continue to do strengthening exercises. The results of nonoperative management for grade III injuries is successful in the range of 75 to 100 percent. Some patients may develop late instability requiring surgery, but estimates are no more than 20 percent, even in competitive athletes.

Syndesmotic ligamentous injuries are more severe than other ligamentous injuries about the ankle.[44] Stable injuries (those with no diastasis upon stress testing) are treated like other high-grade ligamentous injuries, with rest and ice followed by functional bracing and rehabilitation.[2] Recovery may take twice as long as with grade III lateral injuries.[11,44,50] If the syndesmosis reveals diastasis on stress radiography in conjunction with a wide medial joint space, the deltoid ligament is presumed injured. In this circumstance, surgical restoration of the distal tibiofibular joint is indicated. If an anatomic reduction is possible, percutaneous placement of a syndesmotic screw is sufficient.[50,88] If the reduction cannot be obtained, then open reduction is required. The syndesmosis is cleaned of any soft tissue blocking the reduction. If anatomic reduction is still not possible, the medial joint space must be cleared of the deltoid ligament. This may be done percutaneously or open. The reduction is then obtained under direct vision and a screw is placed. The screw should be a position screw, not a lag screw, and should be placed with the ankle in neutral position so that the syndesmosis is not overtightened. Overtightening decreases dorsiflexion of the ankle.[70] The syndesmotic screw should be left in place for at least 10 weeks, since removal at 6 to 8 weeks has been associated with loss of reduction. Leaving the screw in for an extended period does not appear to create significant morbidity.[2,50,59,88] Likewise, a synostosis after injury does not cause long-term problems.[1]

INDIRECT FRACTURES

The indications for surgery in the treatment of ankle fractures are dependent on outcome. Long-term results of treatment correspond to the reduction of the talus under the tibia, the mechanical stability of the joint, and the damage to the cartilage that occurs during the initial injury.[4,5,20,22,33,39,47,53,56,61,73,79,94,96,97,99,101–102] An important exception to this rule is in the case of a patient with impaired sensation, such as a severe diabetic. In these cases, the reduction is not important and the patient should be treated in a double upright brace. Other forms of treatment, especially operative, have high rates of complications, and amputation is a significant risk.

A brief review of the biomechanics of ankle fractures justifies obtaining an anatomic reduction of the talus under the plafond of the tibia. Many authors have performed cadaveric studies to examine the changes in contact area and peak pressure. Most of these studies were performed with a static system, which may diminish the clinical applicability of their results.[67] However, it was consistently found that instability can exist in either ligamentous and bony or in purely bony injuries and lead to displacement of the talus from its normal position. Lateral displacement of as little as 1 mm has been associated with an approximate 40 percent reduction in contact area and a corresponding 40 percent increase in peak pressure.[7,26,39,77,88] Although it was originally believed that the talus followed the fibula after injury, it has been demonstrated that this is true only if the medial side of the ankle is injured (medial malleolar fracture or deltoid rupture).[7,68] Thus, injuries that affect both sides of the joint will allow for talar subluxation and increased peak pressures, possibly leading to degeneration of the joint. The treatment of these injuries requires union in an anatomic position in order to avoid these sequelae.

Injuries that do not allow for the subluxation of the talus do not lead to long-term problems with arthritis. The best and most common example of this is an SE stage II fracture of the lateral malleolus. Long-term studies have documented excellent results (95 percent) with nonoperative management consisting of 6 weeks of immobilization.[55,101] With this injury pattern, the relationship of the talus to the malloli and plafond is not affected; therefore, no significant changes in contact area should occur.[68] Operative treatment yields no advantages and bracing is as effective as cast immobilization.[40,89] Fractures rated SA stage 1 do not allow for talar displacement and should also be treated with nonoperative methods.

Injuries that allow for talar subluxation require anatomic restoration of the joint. If an anatomic reduction can be obtained and maintained through union, the expected results are good or excellent in 90 to 95 percent of cases. The guide to the closed reduction of ankle fractures is in understanding the force that caused the injury and reversing it. This is best accomplished with the patient sedated or anesthetized. The classification of Lauge-Hanson describes the mechanism of injury and therefore how to reverse it for the reduction. An SE fracture should therefore be reduced by internal rotation and a PA injury by adduction. The leg must then be casted in this position. However, it is very difficult to maintain an anatomic reduction in an unstable fracture, as the swelling in the leg decreases. Additionally, a long leg cast is required to control rotation, and this may not be well tolerated by older or obese patients. With these factors taken into account, it is easily understood why the results of operative management with an anatomic reduction and internal fixation are superior to closed reduction and casting for unstable fractures.[4,12,33,53,61,73,74,79,96,102] This is especially true in older patients where, because of age and lower activity levels, a suboptimal reduction may be accepted, leading to pain and decreased function.[6] The recommended treatment for unstable ankle fractures is given in Table 30-2.

If operative management of an ankle fracture is undertaken, the goal is an anatomic reduction and stable internal fixation (Fig. 30-4). The fibula is normally fixed using a lag screw and plate for oblique fractures and a plate alone for transverse fractures. Most surgeons place plates laterally and the lag screw from anterior to posterior. However, in patients with poor bone stock and in those who are less reliable, a posterior plate gives stronger fixation in SE-type fractures.[83] This technique is called an *antiglide plate,* because the strong bicortical screws proximal to the fracture allow the plate to resist external rotation of the fibula. The distal screws also get bicortical purchase, as opposed to the unicortical purchase of the distal screws in a laterally placed plate. By contrast, if a younger patient with good bone stock sustains a long oblique fracture, two lag screws are sufficient for a stable construct. Using screws alone is ideal when possible, as problems with painful hardware are diminished. A tension-band technique for the fibula has also been described, but it is useful only in distal transverse patterns, which often do not require fixation at all, as they do not affect the stability of the joint. Finally, if the fibular fracture is sufficiently high, no fixation may be needed if the syndesmosis is reduced and fixed as described above. The distance used for this distinction varies, but if there is room for two syndesmotic screws below the fracture, they are sufficient. In contrast to this approach is the idea that if the medial and lateral malleoli are fixed, the syndesmosis does not require fixation.[7] Likewise, Boden also recommended that the syndesmosis need not be replaced if the fibula is fixed, even if the medial side is not repaired, unless the fibular fracture occurs more than 4.5 cm above the joint. However, this has not been shown to be 100 percent successful in

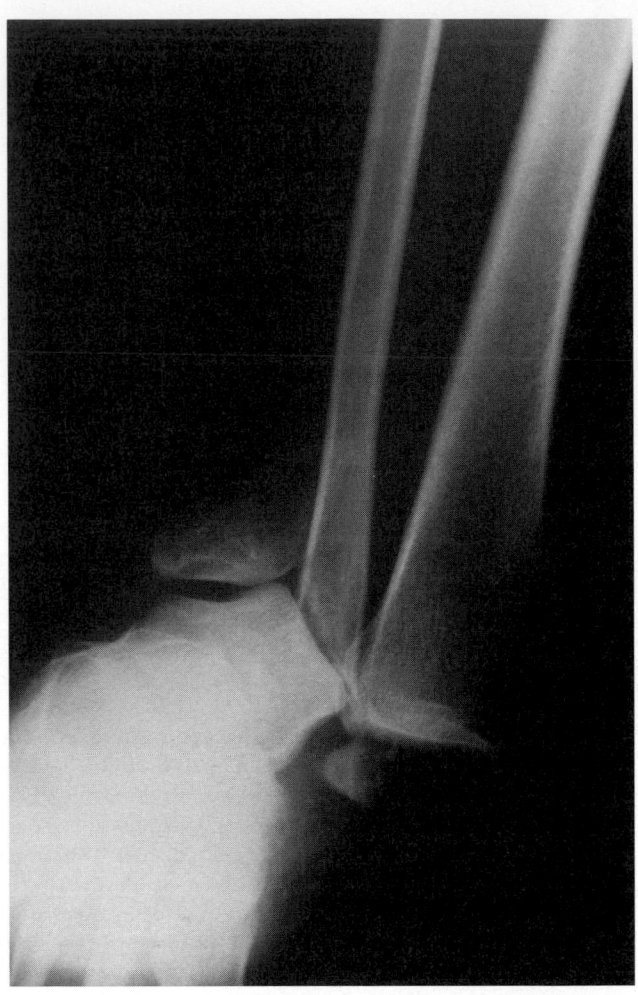

A

Figure 30-4 *A.* The preoperative AP radiograph of a fracture dislocation of the ankle (SE4 type).

TABLE 30-2   Treatment of Ankle Fractures

Mechanism	Stage	Treatment
SA	1	Weight bearing in brace or SLC
	2	ORIF of medial malleolus
SE	1	Treat like ligamentous injury
	2	Weight bearing in brace of SLC
	3	ORIF lateral malleolus, possibly posterior malleolus
	4	ORIF medial and lateral fractures, possibly syndesmotic screw, possibly PM
PA	1	ORIF medial malleolus; if deltoid, treat as ligament injury
	2	ORIF medial malleolus; if deltoid, then syndesmosis fixation
	3	ORIF medial and lateral malleolus
PE	1	ORIF medial malleolus; if deltoid, treat as ligament injury
	2	ORIF medial malleolus; if deltoid, treat as ligament injury
	3	ORIF medial and lateral malleolus
	4	ORIF medial and lateral malleolus

Key: SLC, short leg cast; ORIF, open reduction and internal fixation; PM, posterior malleolus.

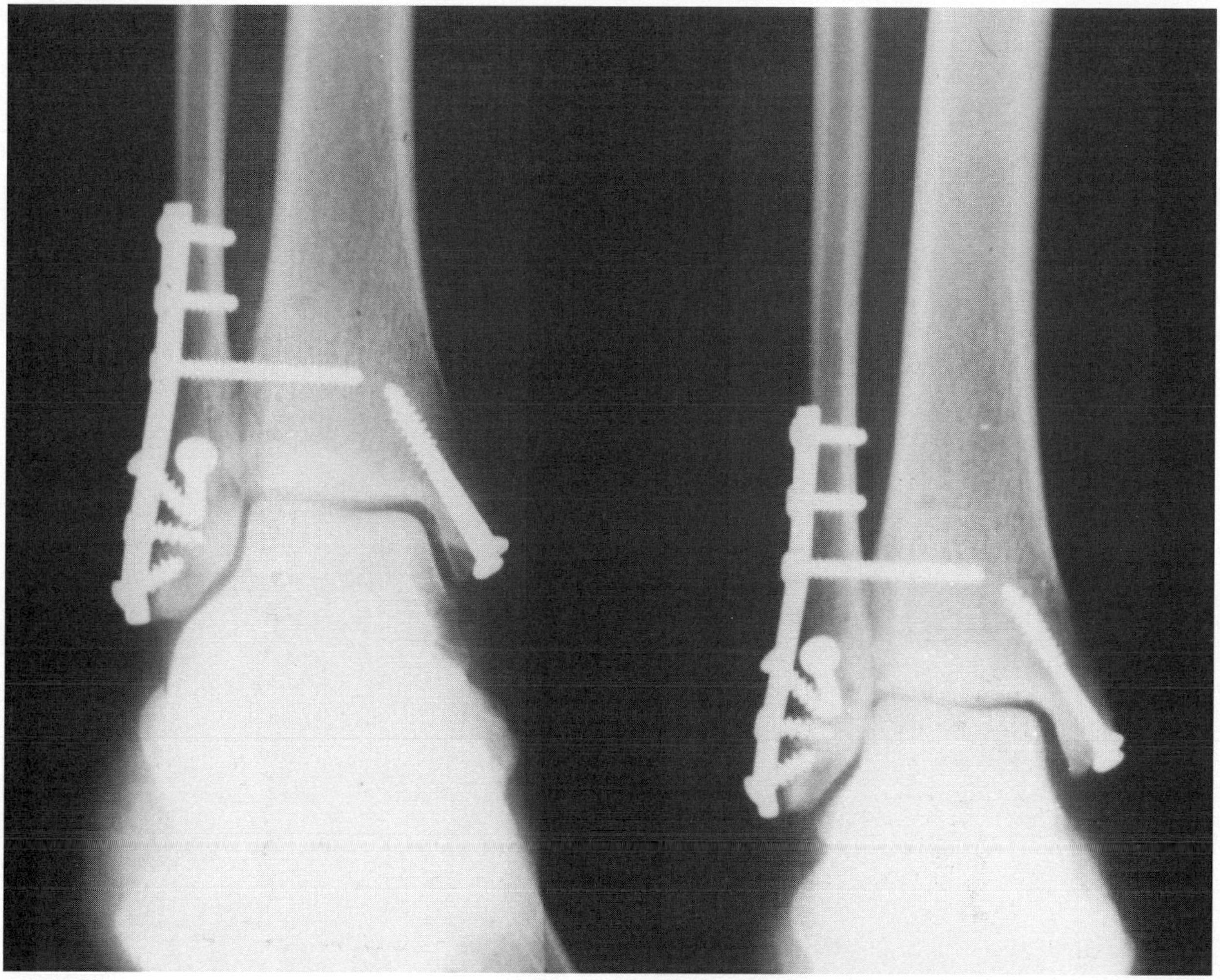

B

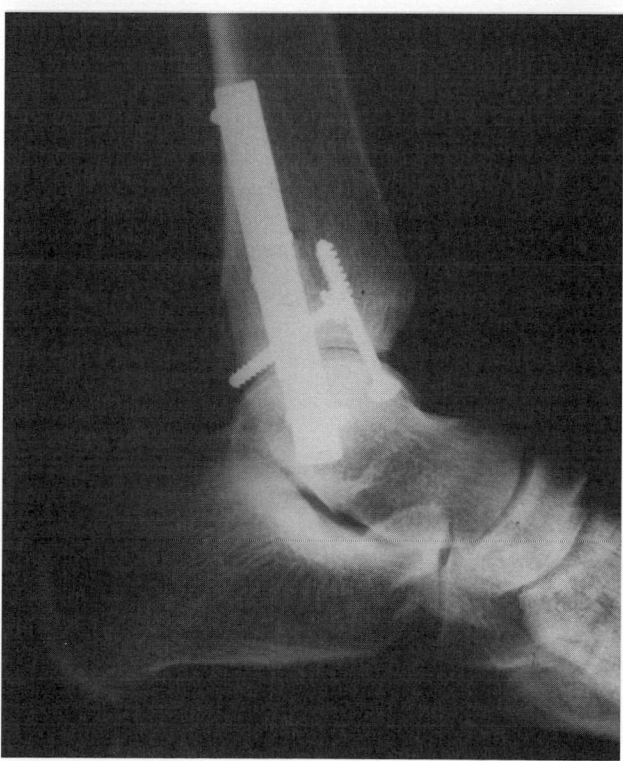

Figure 30-4 *(Continued) B.* The postoperative AP and mortise views showing reduction and fixation of the malleoli and anatomic reconstruction of the mortise. *C.* The lateral view after fixation.

C

maintaining the reduction, and since there is almost no risk to placing a syndesmotic screw, if the syndesmosis can be widened by 2 mm on direct examination in the operating room after all other fixation has been placed, then it should be stabilized with a screw.[1,50,59]

Fixation of the medial malleolus is usually performed using two cancellous lag screws. The addition of an antiglide plate is helpful in a vertical fracture pattern such as an SA injury (Fig. 30-5). Tension-band fixation is useful if the fragment is small. If the medial injury is the deltoid ligament, repair is not necessary if the lateral side of the ankle and syndesmosis are fixed. Prospective evaluation has showed no advantage to medial ligamentous reconstruction.[3,38]

Fixation of the posterior malleolus is rarely necessary. In most cases, the posterior malleolus reduces with fixa-

tion of the other components of the injury. If so, then if the patient is casted, no fixation is required. If the fragment does not reduce and is larger than 25 percent of the articular surface, reduction and fixation are advisable. Likewise, if the fragment does reduce but early motion is to be instituted, a lag screw placed anteriorly will prevent displacement during motion. Regardless of the treatment chosen, it must be clear that the talus is congruent under the tibia on the lateral radiograph. Any posterior displacement of the talus is an indication to reduce and fix the posterior malleolus.

The postoperative management of ankle fractures varies. Recommendations to avoid weight bearing—with early motion, casting, bracing—and immediate motion followed by casting, as well as weight bearing in a cast, can all be justified.[21] The decision must be made on the basis

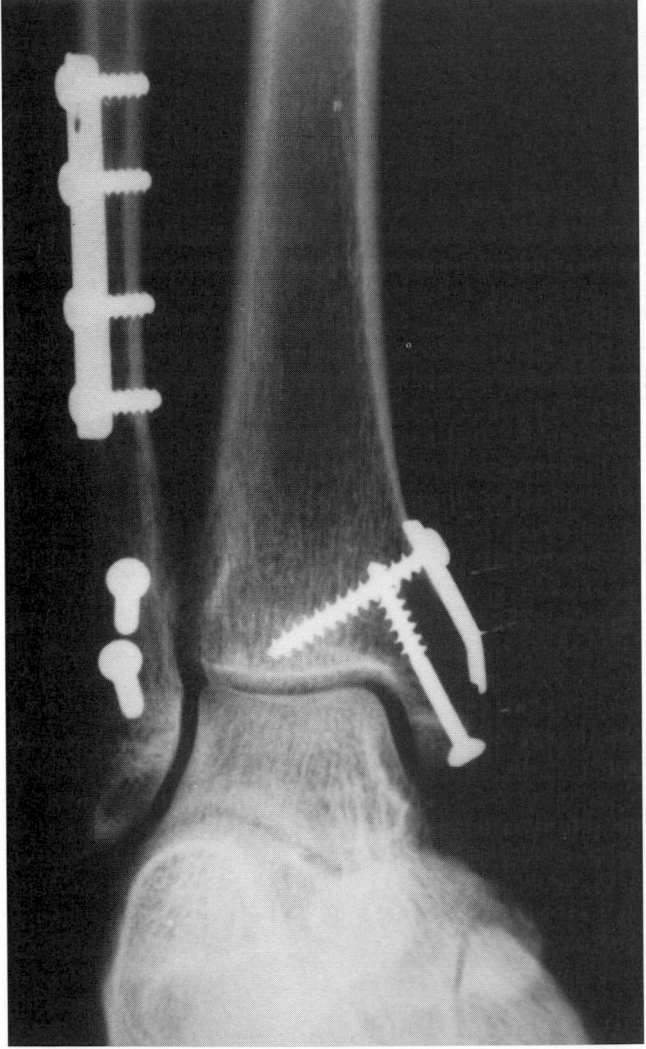

A

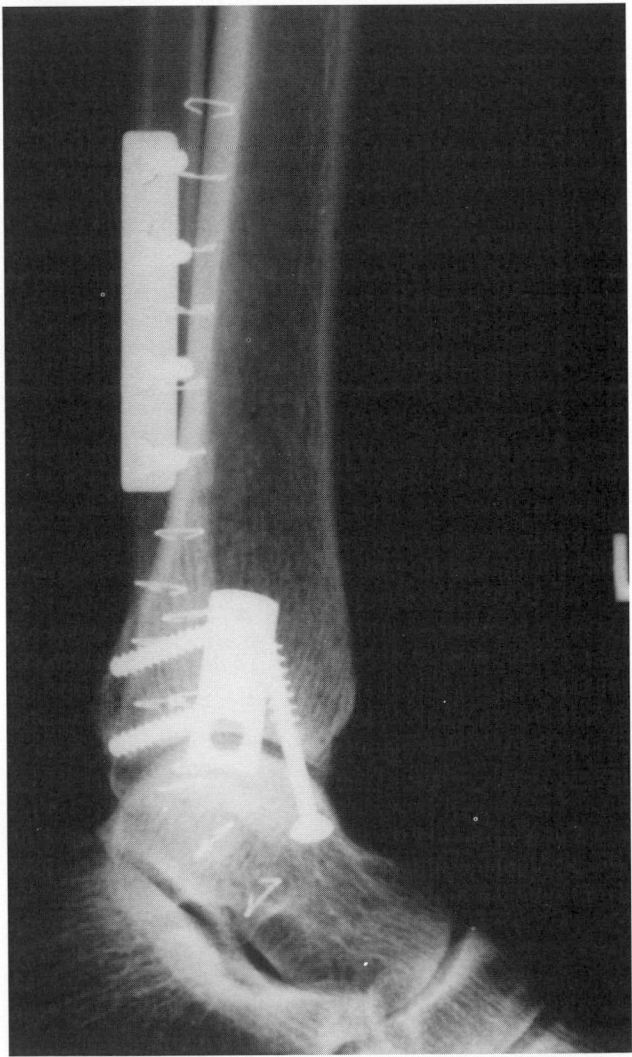

B

Figure 30-5 *A* and *B*. Anteroposterior radiograph after fixation of a complex ankle injury. The medial malleolus was fractured vertically and fixed with an antiglide plate and lag screw. The lateral segmental fracture was fixed with a plate proximally due to comminution and with lag screws alone distally.

of the rigidity of the fixation and the compliance of the patient. In cases of well-motivated patients in whom rigid fixation has been obtained, early motion may be allowed, but without weight bearing. This will allow for an earlier return of motion than other methods. In these same patients, if there is a need for the patient to bear weight early, this may be allowed in a short leg cast with the expectation that the patient will eventually regain 80 to 90 percent of normal motion. If rigid fixation is not obtained, the safest course is to treat the patient in a light short leg cast or prefabricated brace without weight bearing for 6 weeks and then begin weight bearing in a brace. The final consideration is the syndesmosis. If the syndesmosis is fixed, then weight bearing should be delayed for 8 weeks. Some surgeons believe that the syndesmotic screw should be removed before weight bearing ensues, but this is a controversial point. If left in place, it will loosen or break, but it is unlikely to cause pain to the patient. This breakage is caused by the natural motion between the distal tibia and fibula during gait. Further therapy for all ankle fractures regardless of the treatment chosen is the same as that described for ankle sprains.

PILON FRACTURES

The treatment of pilon fractures is more complex than that of indirect ankle fractures. Although the goals of treatment remain an anatomic ankle joint that is held to union, other factors are present that influence treatment. The most important of these is the status of the soft tissue. The strong forces required to cause intraarticular impaction create significant soft tissue damage and concomitant swelling. Surgery performed before the soft tissues have recovered from this injury brings with it an unacceptably high rate of infection and wound breakdown.[90] The traditional teaching with regard to this injury is that open reduction and internal fixation (ORIF) is necessary and should follow the following four steps: fixation of the fibula to regain length, reconstruction of the joint surface, bone grafting for the metaphyseal defect, and finally medial plating to support the metaphyseal-diaphyseal dissociation.[81,82] High rates of soft tissue problems with this technique led some authors to look for alternative methods.[8,9,13,30,72,85,91] The major change invoked by three investigators is the avoidance of periosteal stripping, the use of indirect reduction techniques, and the use of external fixation rather than medial plating for metaphyseal support[8,91,98] (Fig. 30-6). Additionally, the use of computed tomography has been recommended in deciding on the surgical approach.[92] If external fixation is utilized, then fibular fixation is not required. Instead, length is attained in the operating room with the use of the femoral distractor. With these methods, the surgical approach is directly over the major fracture line and periosteal stripping is not needed. Percutaneously placed lag screws maintain the reduction of the joint and graft supports the impacted intraarticular fragments. Once the distal tibia is reconstructed at the level of the joint, the remaining fracture is treated as a distal tibial fracture with external fixation. Both hybrid frames that use tensioned

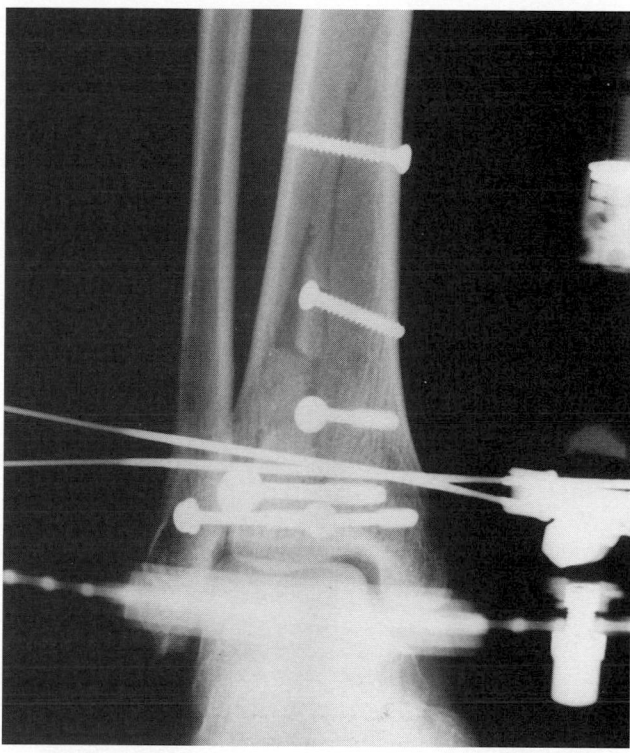

Figure 30-6 Anteroposterior radiograph of a complex pilon fracture after combined limited internal fixation with lag screws and hybrid external fixation.

wires and do not cross the joint and spanning half-pin frames have been recommended. Both techniques have their proponents, and these techniques have been verified by multiple authors.[8,9,13,91,98] The main advantage of this approach is the low rate of soft tissue problems. Some surgeons have also reported lower rates of soft tissue failure using small plates medially and emphasize the need for delaying surgery until the soft tissues have recovered from the initial insult.[10,13,43]

It is clear that these injuries are much more severe than indirect ankle fractures. Likewise, the results of treatment for these injuries are not as good as in simpler fracture patterns. Arthritis, a common finding, occurs in 10 to 40 percent of fractures. The rate of good and excellent results after a type III injury is in the neighborhood of 70 percent even in experienced hands.[8,43,91] One of the causes of early arthritis is the severe direct injury to the cartilage upon impact. There is death at the cellular level that cannot be repaired and may degenerate even in the face of an anatomic reduction.

COMPLICATIONS

The complications after ligamentous injuries of the ankle include reinjury, pain, talar dome injuries, arthritis, and instability. The treatment of chronic problems such as these is discussed elsewhere in the text.

Ankle fractures that unite in an anatomic position generally do well. Late problems with pain, arthritis, hardware, and stiffness occur in 10 to 15 percent of patients. Infection is uncommon and occurs in the range of 1 to 2 percent of operatively treated patients. This is in contrast to pilon fractures, which have high rates of complications. Arthritis occurs in 15 to 60 percent, soft tissue compromise in up to 50 percent, and difficulties obtaining union in up to 40 percent.[72,90,98] Finally, in cases in which external fixators are used, there is a high incidence of pin tract infections.

The treatment of complications must be tailored to the individual. Arthritis is treated symptomatically. When this is severe, arthrodesis is an excellent salvage procedure. It may be performed arthroscopically if there is no deformity in alignment. If malalignment is present, then an open arthrodesis with correction of the axial alignment gives the best results.

Wound slough requires flap coverage in most cases. In this area of the tibia, a free flap is the most common method of obtaining coverage.[72,90,95] If no infection is present and the coverage is obtained early, hardware may be retained. If not, plates should be removed, the bone debrided, and the ankle stabilized with a spanning external fixator. Standard medical treatment of the infection is also necessary. Advanced infections can be treated by the removal of all infected bone and hardware, followed by coverage and fusion. Amputation may be required in the worst of cases, especially if there are severe ipsilateral foot or tibial injuries.

Delays in the union of pilon fractures occur mostly at the metaphyseal fracture site. They are more common if the area is not grafted or if the fracture was open.[13] Delayed direct grafting is the treatment of choice, and union is achieved in more than 80 percent of cases. In patients who refuse grafting, other options such as bone stimulators or percutaneous marrow injection may promote union. It is important to delay weight bearing after the fixation of pilon fractures until after union has been achieved or the fracture is likely to fall into varus. This occurs because the fibula heals before the tibia and provides a lateral strut that resists shortening.

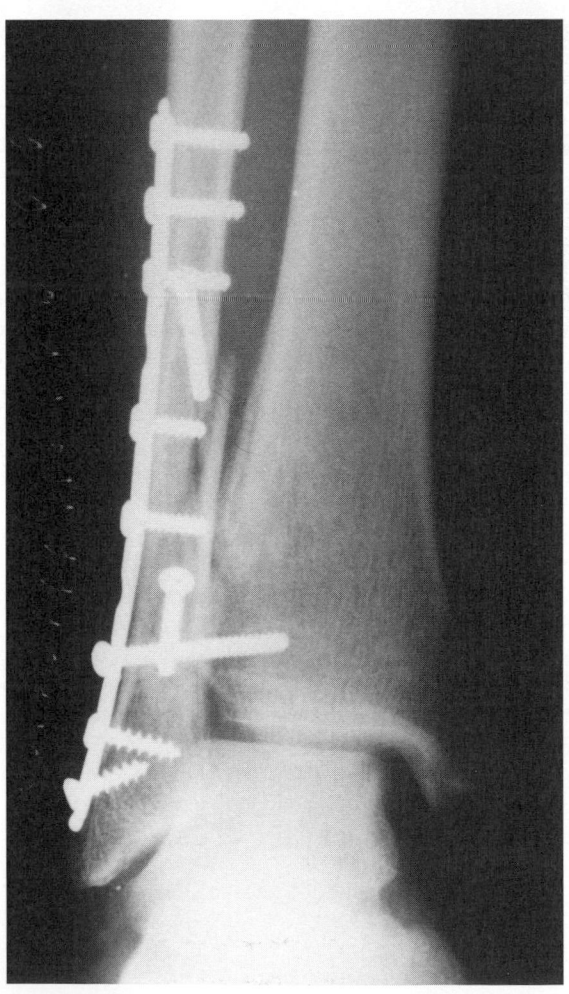

A

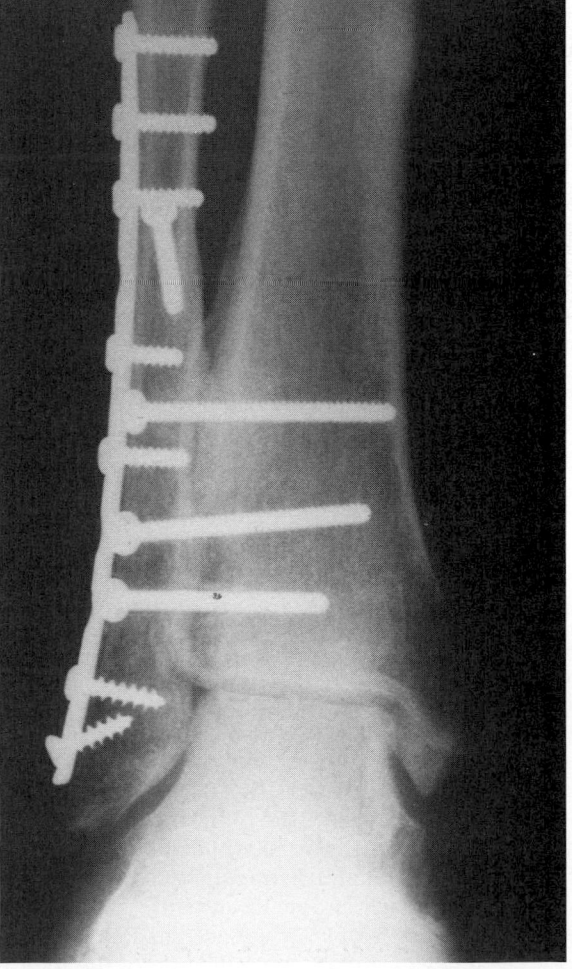

B

Figure 30-7 *A.* Postoperative radiograph of a patient who was bearing weight against advice at 6 weeks. The syndesmotic fixation has failed and the talus has migrated laterally. *B.* The postoperative radiograph after debridement of the medial joint space and syndesmosis followed by rereduction and fixation of the syndesmosis. The joint has been restored.

Pin tract infections should be treated initially by oral antibiotics and local care. If these treatments fail, the pin should be removed. If the fracture is stiff, a cast may be placed; but if there is still instability, the pin should be replaced and the frame kept on. A hybrid frame may be changed to a spanning frame if there is limited access for pin placement.

The final complication in the treatment of ankle fractures is malunion. This is often the result of nonoperative management. The talus is usually laterally displaced, the fibula short and externally rotated, and the medial joint space wide or the medial malleolus displaced. Reconstruction of the mortise is the best option for these patients, even if some joint space narrowing is already present[64,95,100] (Fig. 30-7). The normal ankle is always used as a template for preoperative planning. The preoperative plan should be drawn out to be sure the steps taken and the planned fixation. The first step in the reconstruction is to clean the medial side or free up the medial malunion. The fibula is then osteotomized in as close as possible to the original fracture line. Intraoperative fluoroscopy is done and plain films are obtained after the tentative reduction to confirm the position of the talus with respect to the tibial plafond. Once the position is appropriate, fixation is placed. Bone grafting may be necessary if the fibula does not come together well.

REFERENCES

1. Alberts GHR, DeKort AFCC, Middendorf, PRJM, VanDijik CN: Distal tibiofibular synostosis after ankle fracture. *J Bone Joint Surg [Br]* 78B:250–252, 1996.
2. Amendola A: Controversies in diagnosis and management of syndesmosis injuries of the ankle. *Foot Ankle* 13:44–50, 1992.
3. Baird RA, Jackson ST: Fractures of the distal part of the fibula with associated disruption of the deltoid ligament: Treatment without repair of the deltoid ligament. *J Bone Joint Surg* 69A:1346–1352, 1987.
4. Bauer M, Bergstrom B, Hemborg A, Sandegard J: Malleolar fractures: nonoperative versus operative treatment. *Clin Orthop* 199:17–27, 1985.
5. Bauer M, Jonsson K, Nilsson, B: Thirty-year follow-up of ankle fractures. *Acta Orthop Scand* 56:103–106, 1985.
6. Beauchamp CG, Clay NR, Thexton PW: Displaced ankle fractures in patients over 50 years of age. *J Bone Joint Surg* 65B:329–332, 1983.
7. Boden SD, Labropoulos PA, McCowin P, et al: Mechanical considerations for the syndesmosis screw: A cadaver study. *J Bone Joint Surg* 71A:1548–1555, 1989.
8. Bonar SK, Marsh JL: Unilateral external fixation for severe pilon fractures. *Foot Ankle* 14:57–64, 1993.
9. Bone L, Stegemann P, McNamara K, et al: External fixation of severely comminuted and open tibial pilon fractures. *Clin Orthop* 292:101–107, 1993.
10. Bourne RB, Rorabeck CH, Macnab J: Intra-articular fractures of the distal tibia: The pilon fracture. *J Trauma* 23:591–596, 1983.
11. Boytim MJ, Fischer DA, Neumann L: Syndesmotic ankle sprains. *Am J Sports Med* 19:294–298, 1991.
12. Bray TJ, Endicott M, Capra SE: Treatment of open ankle fractures: Immediate internal fixation versus closed immobilization and delayed fixation. *Clin Orthop* 240:47–52, 1989.
13. Brumback RJ, McGarvey WC: Fractures of the tibial plafond: The pilon fracture. Evolving treatment concepts. *Orthop Clin North Am* 26:273–285, 1995.
14. Bulucu C, Thomas KA, Havorson TL, et al: Biomechanical evaluation of the anterior drawer test: The contribution of the lateral ankle ligaments. *Foot Ankle* 11:389–393, 1991.
15. Burns WD II, Prakash K, Adelaar R, et al: Tibiotalar joint dynamics: Indications for the syndesmotic screw: A cadaver study. *Foot Ankle* 14:153–158, 1993.
16. Calhoun JH, Eng M, Li F, et al: A comprehensive study of pressure distribution in the ankle joint with inversion and eversion. *Foot Ankle* 15:114,125–133.
17. Cass JR, Morrey BF: Ankle instability: Current concepts, diagnosis and treatment. *Mayo Clin Proc* 59:165–170, 1984.
18. Cass JR, Morrey BF, Katoh Y, et al: Ankle instability: Comparison of primary repair and delayed reconstruction after long-term follow-up study. *Clin Orthop* 198:110–117, 1985.
19. Cawley PW, France EP: Biomechanics of the lateral ligaments of the ankle: An evaluation of the effects of axial load and single plane motions on ligament strain patterns. *Foot Ankle* 12:92–99, 1991.
20. Charnley J: *The Closed Treatment of Common Fractures,* 3d ed. Edinburgh, Churchill Livingstone, 1961.
21. Cimino W, Ichtertz D, Slabaugh P: Early mobilization of ankle fractures after open reduction and internal fixation. *Clin Orthop* 267:152–156, 1991.
22. Clarke HJ, Michelson JD, Cox QG, et al: Tibio-talar stability in bimalleolar ankle fractures: A dynamic in vitro contact area study. *Foot Ankle* 11:222–227, 1991.
23. Colville MR, Marder RA, Boyle JJ, et al: Strain measurement in lateral ankle ligaments. *Am J Sports Med* 18:196–200, 1990.
24. Conlin FD, Johnson PG, Sinning JE Jr: The etiology and repair of rotary ankle instability. *Foot Ankle* 10:152–155, 1989.
25. Cox JS: Surgical and nonsurgical treatment of acute ankle sprains. *Clin Orthop* 198:118–126, 1985.
26. Curtis MJ, Michelson JD, Urquhart MW, et al: Tibiotalar contact and fibular malunion in ankle fractures: A cadaver study. *Acta Orthop Scand* 63:326–329, 1992.
27. Danis R: Le vrai but les dangers de l'ostesynthese. *Lyon Chirurg* 51:740, 1956.
28. Diamond JE: Rehabilitation of ankle sprains. *Clin Sports Med* 8:877–891, 1989.
29. DiChristina, Riemer BL, Butterfield SL, et al: Pilon fractures treated with an articulated external fixator: A preliminary report of significant complications. *Orthop Trans* 18:719–720, 1994.
30. Dillin L, Slabaugh P: Delayed wound healing, infection, and nonunion following open reduction and internal fixation tibial plafond fractures. *J Trauma* 26:1116–1119, 1986.
31. Erickson SJ, Smith JW, Ruiz ME, et al: Imaging of the lateral collateral ligament of the ankle. *AJR* 156:131–136, 1991.
32. Etter C, Ganz R: Long-term results of tibial plafond fractures treated with open reduction and internal fixation. *Arch Orthop Trauma Surg* 110:277–283, 1991.
33. Eventov I, Salama R, Goodwin DRA, Weissman SL: An evaluation of surgical and conservative treatment of fractures of the ankle in 200 patients. *J Trauma* 18:271–275, 1978.
34. Franklin JL, Johnson KD, Hansen ST Jr: Immediate internal fixation of open ankle fractures: Report of thirty-eight cases treated with a standard protocol. *J Bone Joint Surg* 66A:1349–1356, 1984.
35. Goergen TG, Danzig LA, Resnick D, Owen CA: Roentgenographic evaluation of the tibiotalar joint. *J Bone Joint Surg* 59:874–877, 1977.
36. Gould N, Slingson D, Glassman J: Early and later repairing of lateral ligaments. *Foot Ankle* 1:84–89, 1980.

37. Greene TA, Hillman SK: Comparison of support provided by semirigid orthosis and adhesive ankle taping before, during and after exercise. *Am J Sports Med* 18:498–506, 1990.

38. Harper MC: The deltoid ligament: An evaluation of need for surgical repair. *Clin Orthop* 226:156–168, 1988.

39. Harper MC: Talar shift: The stabilizing role of the medial, lateral, and posterior ankle structures. *Clin Orthop* 257:177–183, 1990.

40. Harper MC: An anatomic study of the short oblique fracture of the distal fibula and ankle stability. *Foot Ankle* 4:23–29, 1983.

41. Harper MC: Posterior instability of the talus: An anatomic evaluation. *Foot Ankle* 10:36–39, 1989.

42. Harper MC, Keller TS: A radiographic evaluation of the tibiofibular syndesmosis. *Foot Ankle* 10:156–160, 1989.

43. Helfet DL, Koval K, Pappas J, et al: Intraarticular "pilon" fracture of the tibia. *Clin Orthop* 298:221–228, 1994.

44. Hopkinson WJ, St. Pierre P, Ryan JB, et al: An anatomic study of the ankle. *Foot Ankle* 10:224–228, 1990.

45. Hughes JL, Weber H, Willenegger H, Kuner EH: Evaluation of ankle fractures. *Clin Orthop* 138:111–119, 1979.

46. Inman VT: *The Joints of the Ankle.* Baltimore, Williams & Wilkins, 1976.

47. Joy G, Patzakis MJ, Harvey JP Jr: Precise evaluation of the reduction of severe ankle fractures. *J Bone Joint Surg* 56A:979–993, 1974.

48. Kannus P, Renstorm P: Treatment for acute tears of the lateral ligaments of the ankle: Operation, cast, or early controlled mobilization. *J Bone Joint Surg* 73A:305–312, 1991.

49. Karlsson J, Andreasson GO: The effect of external ankle support in chronic lateral ankle joint instability: An electromyographic study. *Am J Sports Med* 20:257–261, 1992.

50. Kaye RA: Stabilization of ankle syndesmosis injuries with a syndesmosis screw. *Foot Ankle* 9:290–293, 1989.

51. Kellam JF, Waddell JP: Fractures of the distal tibial metaphysis with intraarticular extension: The distal tibial explosion fracture. *J Trauma* 19:593–601, 1979.

52. Kjaersgaard-Andersen P, Wethelund J-O, Neilsen S: Lateral talocalcaneal instability following section of the calcaneofibular ligament: A kinesiologic study. *Foot Ankle* 7:355–361, 1987.

53. Klossner O: Late results of operative and non-operative treatment of severe ankle fractures. *Acta Chir Scand Suppl* 293:1–93, 1962.

54. Konradsen L, Holmer P, Sondergaard L: Early mobilizing treatment for grade III ligament injuries. *Foot Ankle* 12:69–73, 1991.

55. Kristensen KD, Hansen T: Closed treatment of ankle fractures: Stage II supination-eversion fractures followed for 20 years. *Acta Orthop Scand* 56:107–109, 1985.

56. Lantz BA, McAndrew M, Scioli M, et al: The effect of concomitant chondral injuries accompanying operatively reduced malleolar fractures. *J Orthop Trauma* 5:125–128, 1991.

57. Larsen E, Lund PM: Peroneal muscle function in chronically unstable ankles: A prospective preoperative and post operative electromyographic study. *Clin Orthop* 272:219–226, 1991.

58. Lauge-Hansen N: Fractures of the ankle: II. Combined experimental surgical and experimental-roentgenologic investigations. *Arch Surg* 60:957–985, 1950.

59. Leeds HC, Ehrlich MG: Instability of the distal tibiofibular syndesmosis after bimalleolar and trimalleolar ankle fractures. *J Bone Joint Surg* 66A:490–503, 1984.

60. Leone VJ, Ruland RT, Meinhard BP: The management of the soft tissues in pilon fractures. *Clin Orthop* 292:315–320, 1993.

61. Lindsjo U: Operative treatment of ankle fracture-dislocations: A follow-up study of 306/321 consecutive cases. *Clin Orthop* 199:28–39, 1985.

62. McCullough CJ, Burge PD: Rotatory stability of the loadbearing ankle: An experimental study. *J Bone Joint Surg* 62B:460–464, 1980.

63. Maale G, Seligson D: Fractures through the distal weight-bearing surface of the tibia. *Orthopedics* 3:517–521, 1980.

64. Marti RK, Raaymakers EL, Nolet PA: Malunited ankle fractures: The late results of reconstruction. *J Bone Joint Surg* 72B:709–713, 1990.

65. Mast JW, Spiegel PG, Pappas JN: Fractures of the tibial pilon. *Clin Orthop* 230:68–82, 1988.

66. McFerran MA, Smith SW, Boulas HJ, et al: Complications encountered in the treatment of pilon fractures. *J Orthop Trauma* 6:195–200, 1992.

67. Michelson JD, Clarke HJ, Jinnah RH: The effect of loading on tibiotalar alignment in cadaver ankles. *Foot Ankle* 10:280–284, 1990.

68. Michelson JD, Magid D, Ney DR, et al: Examination of the pathologic anatomy of ankle fractures. *J Trauma* 32:65–70, 1992.

69. Moller-Larsen F, Wethelund JO, Jurik AG, et al: Comparison of three different treatments for ruptured lateral ankle ligaments. *Acta Orthop Scand* 59:564–566, 1988.

70. Needleman RL, Skrade DA, Stiehl JB: Effect of the syndesmotic screw on ankle motion. *Foot Ankle* 10:17–24, 1989.

71. Neumann H, O'Shea P, Nielson J-P, et al: A physiological comparison of the short-leg walking cast and an ankle-foot orthosis walker following 6 weeks of immobilization. *Orthopedics* 12:1429–1434, 1989.

72. Ovadia DN, Beals RK: Fractures of the tibial plafond. *J Bone Joint Surg* 68A:543–551, 1986.

73. Pettrone FA, Gail M, Pee D, et al: Quantitative criteria for prediction of the results after displaced fracture of the ankle. *J Bone Joint Surg* 65A:667–677, 1983.

74. Phillips WA, Schwartz HS, Keller CS, et al: A prospective, randomized study of the management of severe ankle fractures. *J Bone Joint Surg* 67A:67–78, 1985.

75. Phillips WA, Spiegel PG: Evaluation of ankle fractures: Non-operative vs operative (editorial comment). *Clin Orthop* 138:17–20, 1979.

76. Procter P, Paul JP: Ankle joint biomechanics. *J Biomech* 15:627–634, 1982.

77. Ramsey PL, Hamilton W: Changes in tibiotalar area of contact caused by lateral talar shift. *J Bone Joint Surg* 58A:356–357, 1976.

78. Rovere GD, Clarke TJ, Yates CS, et al: Retrospective comparison of taping and ankle stabilizers in preventing ankle injuries. *Am J Sports Med* 16:228–233, 1988.

79. Rowley DI, Norris SH, Duckworth T: A prospective trial comparing operative and manipulative treatment of ankle fractures. *J Bone Joint Surg* 68B:610–613, 1986.

80. Ruedi T: Fractures of the lower end of the tibia into the ankle joint: Results 9 years after open reduction and internal fixation. *Injury* 5:130–134, 1973.

81. Ruedi TP, Allgower M: Fractures of the lower end of the tibia into the ankle-joint. *Injury* 1:92–99, 1969.

82. Ruedi TP, Allgower M: The operative treatment of intra-articular fractures of the lower end of the tibia. *Clin Orthop* 138:105–110, 1979.

83. Schaffer JJ, Manoli A II: The antiglide plate for distal fibular fixation: A biomechanical comparison with fixation with a lateral plate. *J Bone Joint Surg* 69A:596–604, 1987.

84. Sclafani SJA: Ligamentous injury of the lower tibiofibular syndesmosis: Radiographic evidence. *Radiology* 156:21–27, 1985.

85. Selah M, Shanahan MD, Fern ED: Intra-articular fractures of the distal tibia: Surgical management by limited internal fixation and articulated distraction. *Injury* 24:37–40, 1993.

86. Siegler S, Wand D, Plasha E, Berman AT: Technique for in vivo measurement of the three-dimensional kinematics and laxity characteristics of the ankle joint complex. *J Bone Joint Res* 12:421–431, 1994.

87. Stasikelis PJ, Calhoun JH, Ledbetter BR, et al: Treatment of infected pilon nonunions with small pin fixators. *Foot Ankle* 14:373–379, 1993.

88. Steihl JB: Ankle fractures with distasis. *AAOS Instr Course Lect*

89. Stuart PR, Brumby C, Smith SR: Comparative study of functional bracing and plaster cast treatment of stable lateral malleolar fractures. *Injury* 20:323–326, 1989.

90. Teeny SM, Wiss DA: Open reduction and internal fixation of tibial plafond fractures: Variables contributing to poor results and complications. *Clin Orthop* 292:108–117, 1993.

91. Tornetta P III, Weiner L, Bergman M et al: Pilon fractures: Treatment with combined internal and external fixation. *J Orthop Trauma* 7:489–496, 1993.

92. Tornetta P III, Gorup J: Axial Computed tomography of pilon fractures. *Clin Orthop* 323:273–276, 1996.

93. Trumble TE, Benirschke SK, Vedder NB: Use of radial forearm flaps to treat complications of closed pilon fractures. *J Orthop Trauma* 6:358–365, 1992.

94. Tunturi T, Kemppainen K, Patiala H, et al: Importance of anatomical reduction for subjective recovery after ankle fracture. *Acta Orthop Scand* 54:641–647, 1983.

95. Ward AJ, Ackroyd CE, Baker AS: Late lengthening of the fibula for malaligned ankle fractures. *J Bone Joint Surg* 72:714–717, 1990.

96. Wheelhouse WW, Rosenthal RE: Unstable ankle fractures: Comparison of closed versus open treatment. *South Med J* 73:45–50, 1980.

97. Wilson FC, Skilbred LA: Long term results in the treatment of displaced bimalleolar fractures. *J Bone Joint Surg* 48A:1065–1078, 1966.

98. Wyrsch B, McFerran MA, McAndrew MA, et al: A randomized, prospective study cvaluating the surgical management of pilon fractures. *Orthop Trans* 18:720, 1994.

99. Yablon IG, Heller FG, Shouse L: The key role of the lateral malleolus in displaced fractures of the ankle. *J Bone Joint Surg* 59A:169–173, 1977.

100. Yablon IG, Leach RE: Reconstruction of malunited fractures of the lateral malleolus. *J Bone Joint Surg* 71A:521–527, 1989.

101. Yde J, Kristensen KD: Ankle fractures: Supination-eversion fractures of stage II: Primary and late results of operative and non-operative treatment. *Acta Orthop Scand* 51:695–702, 1980.

102. Yde J, Kristensen KD: Ankle fractures: Supination-eversion fractures of stage IV: Primary and late results of operative and non-operative treatment. *Acta Orthop Scand* 51:981–990, 1980.

CHAPTER 31

Fractures and Dislocations of the Foot

T. Scott Woll

The foot is a lever for transmission of forces from the hindfoot through the forefoot to the ground; however, it also functions as a flexible foundation to accommodate uneven surfaces and absorb impact load at heel strike. This dichotomy of functions is accomplished by a complex system of osseous, ligamentous, and tendinous structures.[1] Disruptions of these structures by injuries result in severe functional limitations.

Due to their rather rare occurrence, many of these injuries are not familiar to every practitioner. This prompted one author to comment that these injuries are "often neglected, usually unsuspected, frequently undiagnosed and occasionally mismanaged."[2] Incomplete understanding of the pathomechanics and inadequate x-ray in the emergency department have frequently contributed to missed injuries and insufficient treatment. As many as 40 percent are misdiagnosed due mainly to inadequate x-ray.[3] It is rare for these injuries to occur in isolation, due to the complex bony shapes and ligamentous attachments; therefore accompanying injuries must be identified.

Because there are few prospective studies examining treatment outcomes, treatment must be directed by the usual principles of trauma care. Fractures involving articular surface step-offs and those that interrupt mechanical axes are best treated by open reduction and internal fixation, followed by early range-of-motion exercises. A reasonable outcome can be expected utilizing the principles, as practiced in other articular and periarticular injuries.[4] Specific to the foot is the concept of essential and nonessential joints. Normal gait depends on the motion of essential joints, including the ankle, subtalar, transverse tarsal, and metatarsophalangeal joints. Nonessential joints include the intercuneiform and first to third tarsometatarsal joints; these are not mobile joints but provide a stable lever to propel the body forward. The nonessential joints may be bridged by screws to provide additional fixation without the concerns that would arise in a mobile joint. Understanding the biomechanical concept of medial and lateral columns of the foot will aid in restoring the mechanical alignment of the fore and hindfoot.[5]

Indirect reduction techniques utilizing small external fixators and minidistractors are helpful in restoring mechanical alignment.[6] Mini- and small-fragment screws and plates have been the workhorses of reconstructing the foot injured by trauma.[7] Newer devices such as cannulated screws that minimize dissection to already compromised bony and soft tissue structures are also helpful.[8] Liberal bone grafting techniques possibly utilizing artificial bone substitutes will aid in providing union for these fractures with small surface areas.

Compartment syndromes of the foot are well-recognized problems; recent articles have clearly defined the various compartments and their decompression.[9] Early diagnosis and release remain the best ways to prevent the residuals of an ischemic contracture that produces a clawfoot.[7]

At times, the severely traumatized foot with open injury is not reconstructible. This needs to be considered before embarking on a complex reconstruction that may be unsuccessful and may affect the individual's life adversely. Severe IIIC open injuries may be best treated by early amputation.[10,11]

FRACTURES OF THE TALUS

The word *talus* is a shortened form of *taxillus,* the Latin term for dice made from the heel bones of horses. The talus is the second most commonly fractured tarsal bone. It is an extremely complex structure with seven articular surfaces; in fact, 60 percent of the talus is covered by articular surfaces.

The main body of the talus is an intraarticular structure with a limited blood supply from branches from the posterior tibial, anterior tibial and perineal arteries. Its main blood supply comes through the tarsal canal, an anastomosis of the artery of the tarsal sinus and the tarsal canal. Additional blood supplies come from the superior neck vessels and from the minor branches coming from the deltoid branches medially and posteriorly from the posterior tubercle branches. Disruption of this blood supply explains the high incidence of osteonecrosis following displaced fractures and dislocations.[12–14] Anatomically, the talus can be divided into three major parts: the body, neck, and head. The body's superior articular surface articulates in the ankle mortise and is wider anteriorly than posteriorly. Posteriorly there are posteromedial and posterolateral tubercles, with the flexor hallucis longus running between them. The os trigonum is an accessory ossicle that is occasionally attached to the posterolateral process of the talus by strong ligamentous structures. When fused, it is called a Stieda's os or an os trigonal process; often this is a source of injury. The lateral process of the talus articulates with the fibula laterally and with the posterior facet of the subtalar joint inferiorly. Medially, the body articulates with the medial malleolus of the tibia. The neck has a medial inclination articulating with the middle facet of the subtalar joint. The head articulates with the tarsal navicular and the anterior facet of the subtalar joint.

A simple anatomic classification system for fractures of the talus includes body fractures, which are subdivided into posterior process fractures, lateral process fractures, trochlear body fractures, neck fractures, and head fractures.

Talar Body Fractures

The posterior process fracture is also known as Shepherd's fracture.[15] These fractures can represent a spectrum of injuries from small avulsions of the posterior capsular ligaments to nutcracker-type compression injuries of the posterior process, with large fragments involving the subtalar and/or ankle joint. These injuries are usually seen after a forced plantar flexion injury or a hyperdorsiflexion avulsion type of injury. Pain is usually located in the area anterior to the Achilles tendon and is frequently augmented by dorsiflexion of the great toe. Small avulsions or nondisplaced fractures respond to approximately 4 to 6 weeks of immobilization in a short leg weight-bearing cast. Displaced fractures involving significant articular surfaces with more than 2 mm displacement require open reduction and internal fixation either through a posteromedial or posterolateral approach, depending on location and the surgeon's preference. Persistent symptoms may require excision of malunited or nonunited fractures.[16,17]

Lateral process fractures represent a spectrum of injuries from avulsions of capsular ligaments to intraarticular injuries involving either the subtalar and/or ankle joints. The usual mechanism is a dorsiflexion inversion type of injury.[18] These are commonly seen in snowboarding injuries, where they are mistaken for ankle sprains by individuals unfamiliar with their pathoanatomy. Early diagnosis and treatment gives the best result. They are diagnosed by pain and tenderness localized to the region of lateral process and confirmed by oblique x-ray views of the subtalar joint. Computed tomography (CT) is helpful in both posterior and lateral process injuries to assess displacement and size of the fragment. Acute treatment is directed to anatomic restoration of displaced fractures; fractures with greater than 2 mm displacement or involving large components of the ankle or subtalar joint require open reduction and internal fixation with mini- or small-fragment lag screws. Frequently there is comminution or debris that requires debridement. Nondisplaced injuries heal with short leg walking casts within 6 weeks. Nonunion or severely comminuted injuries are best treated by excision at a later date.[19–21]

Fractures of the trochlea or body proper include crush, horizontal, coronal, and sagittal shearing injuries (Fig. 31-1). A subclassification of transchondral fractures of the dome has also been described.[22] They usually result from a high-energy injury due either to a fall from a height or to a motor vehicle accident. These fractures involve both ankle and subtalar joints and uniformly have a poor prognosis, with approximately 50 percent developing posttraumatic arthritis.[23,24] Depending on location and displacement, 25 to 100 percent of talar body fractures undergo osteonecrosis. Fortunately, this is rarely global but rather patchy in its distribution.[25,26]

Treatment for these injuries depends on open wounds, fracture displacement, and location. Standard exposures include either anteromedial or anterolateral ankle arthrotomies; frequently medial malleolar osteotomies are needed. Distractors from the tibia into the calcaneus frequently aid in distracting the joint and elevating fragments by ligamentotaxis, particularly in the compression or crush type of injury. Principles in dealing with these complex fractures include immediate closed reduction, emergent open reduction of unreduced fractures, provisional fixation with K wires followed by interfragmentary lag screw fixation, in which the screws are countersunk below the articular cartilaginous surface (Fig. 31-2). Titanium screws should be considered if MRI scans are to be obtained to diagnose osteonecrosis. One should try to preserve the body of the talus whenever possible, even if it is avascular. This will preserve height and bone stock, which can revascularize, providing viable bone for a later reconstruction.[27]

Osteochondral lesions of the talar dome have been described previously by numerous authors. These lesions are included in the category of osteochondrosis and are located on the anterolateral or posteromedial talar dome. Lateral lesions are thought to be secondary to trauma. Medial lesions have been thought to be more typical of osteochondrosis. These lesions have been classified by stage

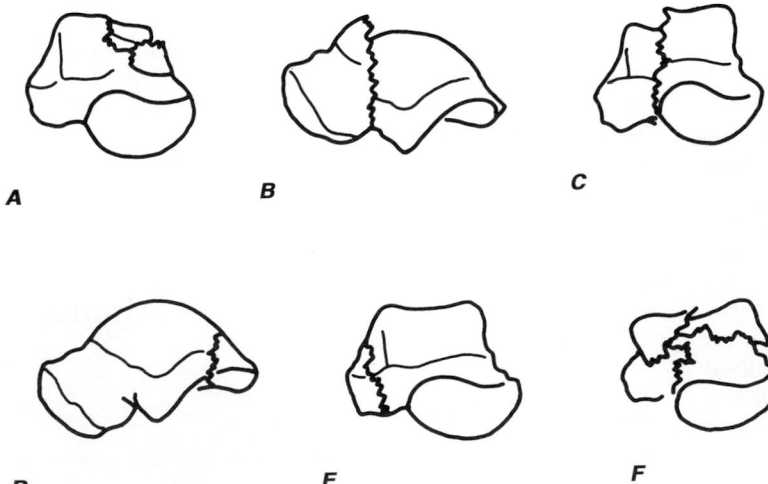

Figure 31-1 Types of talar body fractures. *A.* Compression fracture. *B.* Coronal shearing fracture. *C.* Sagittal shearing fracture. *D.* Fracture in the posterior tubercle. *E.* Fracture in the lateral tubercle. *F.* Crush fracture.

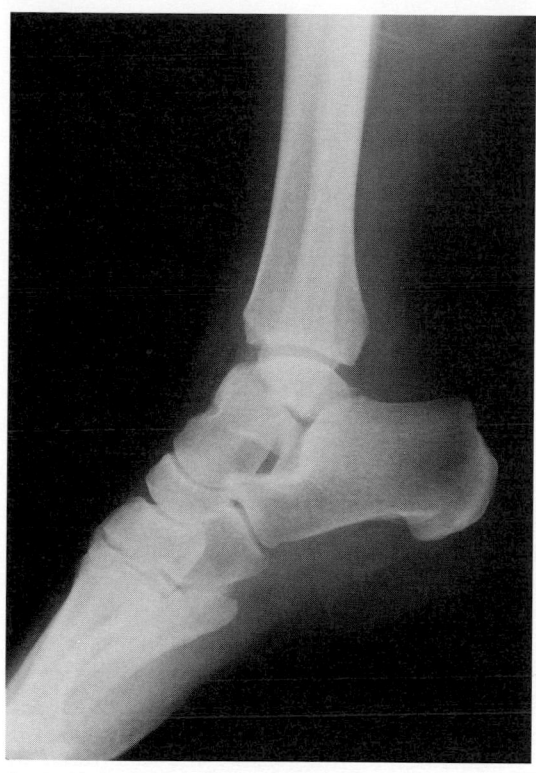

A

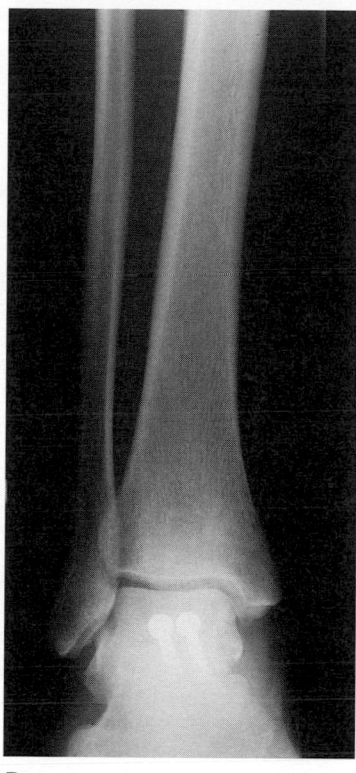

B

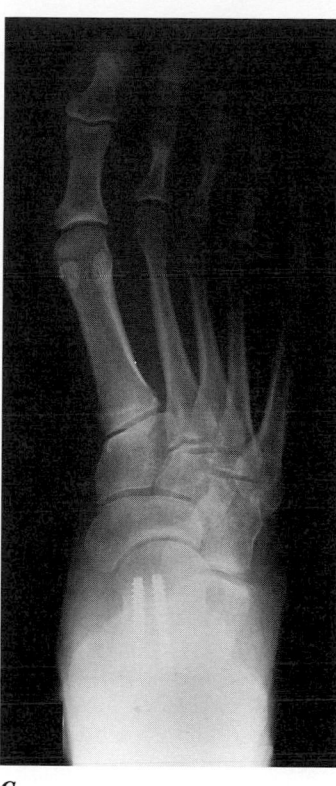

C

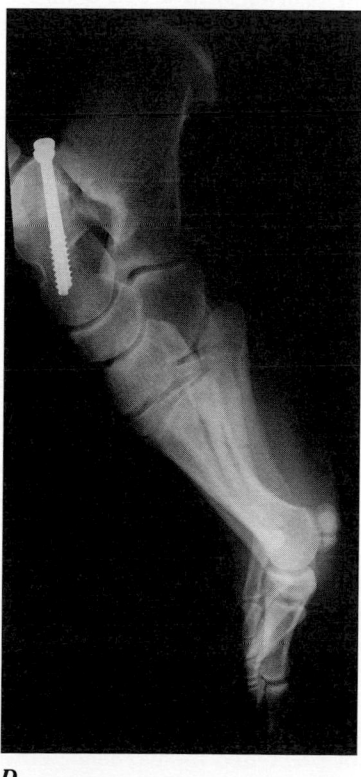

D

Figure 31-2 Talar body coronal shear fracture.

I through IV based on plain radiography.[28,29] Stage I lesions represent subchondral trabecular compression with the lesion. Stage II represents an incomplete separation of the subchondral fracture. Stage III represents undisplaced complete osteochondral lesions, and stage IV lesions involve displaced free-floating fragments. Treatment is directed by stage; stage I and II lesions are best treated by placement in a non-weight-bearing cast for 6 to 12 weeks. Early stage III lesions are treated similarly. Stage III lesions that have not healed by 12 to 16 weeks and stage IV lesions require surgical treatment. If the lesion is small, it may be excised, with the defect being debrided to a stable rim and the subchondral defect drilled with a small K wire or drill. Lesions involving one-third or more of the talar dome require replacement of the fragment into the defect with or without bone grafting and internal fixation. This can be performed with K-wire, lag-screw, or Herbert-screw fixation. Most lesions are amenable to arthroscopic debridement with standard anterolateral and anteromedial portals. Occasionally a posterolateral portal is required.[30] Frequently, posteromedial and posterolateral lesions require a medial malleolar osteotomy.[31] Immobilization usually continues from 2 to 4 weeks, depending on whether an osteotomy is required. Avoidance of weight bearing is advised for 8 to 12 weeks, with range-of-motion exercises being started as soon as the wound allows.[32]

Fractures of the Talar Neck

Fractures of the talar neck are the most common talar fractures and account for approximately 50 percent of all talus injuries. The same trauma maxims described earlier apply to talar neck fractures, including emergent restoration of anatomy by closed or open means, rigid interfragmentary fixation, and early mobilization. These fractures usually occur during a deceleration type of injury such as a fall or motor vehicle accident. A hyperdorsiflexion type mechanism is applied to the forefoot and results in disruption of the posterior capsular ligaments and impingement of the talar neck on the fulcrum of the anterior rim of the tibia. Fracture occurs and, with continued force, the body of the talus may dislocate. This results in an open injury in 15 to 20 percent of cases. Other injuries include medial malleolar fractures, which occur in 20 to 30 percent of injuries and lumbar spine fractures in 10 to 15 percent. The most accepted classification system for talar neck fractures includes types 1 through 4[33,34] (Fig. 31-3). The fracture type has correlated with outcome.[35,36] Type I is a nondisplaced talar neck fracture usually extending through the middle facet of the subtalar joint or between the middle and posterior facets. Type II includes the previously described fracture and a subluxation or dislocation through the subtalar joint. Type III includes the previously described fracture and a talar body dislocation from the ankle mortise. Type IV represents the addition of dislocation of the distal talar head and neck fragment from the talonavicular joint. Radiographic assessment includes standard anteroposterior (AP) and lateral x-rays of the foot and ankle. Special radiographic views of the talar neck include the "Canale view," which is obtained by placing the ankle in maximum plantar flexion with the foot placed on the x-ray cassette and pronated 15°; the x-ray tube is directed 15° cephalad from the perpendicular. This view is helpful in assessing rotation and displacement, most commonly varus. Complete evaluation with plain x-ray, CT scan, or tomo-grams is critical to early, accurate diagnosis and preoperative planning. Treatment is directed to debridement of open wounds, anatomic reduction, and rigid fixation of the displaced fracture as soon as possible. Early motion is advised to prevent stiffness and arthrofibrosis. Type I fractures, by definition, are nondisplaced; however, these have frequently displaced and reduced spontaneously, resulting in fracture fragments being left in the subtalar joint. Computed tomography is needed to assess this. Fractures without intraarticular fragments that are anatomically reduced can be treated in a below-knee cast with slight equinus for the first 4 weeks, followed by a neutral below-knee cast for approximately 4 to 8 weeks. This usually results in predictable healing with a low incidence of avascular necrosis, up to 13 percent in some reports. Because of joint stiffness following this prolonged immobilization, it may be advisable to fix these injuries internally to allow early motion. Type II fractures represent a more emergent injury and are best treated by open reduction and internal fixation. Displaced injuries require direct visualization of the fracture site and also the debridement of intraarticular debris. Anteromedial and anterolateral exposures are helpful to judge rotation and displacement and to allow debridement of the ankle and subtalar joints[26] (Fig. 31-4). Frequently, the use of a minidistractor aids in disengaging the fracture fragments, allowing easier and less traumatic reduction. Fixation with small-fragment interfragmentary lag screws provides rigid fixation. Posterior-to-anterior lag screw fixation through a posterolateral incision may be useful in anatomically reduced injuries.[37] This technique allows for placement of the screw in dense bone.[38] Postoperative treatment is usually approximately 6 weeks without weight bearing with a below-knee cast. Stage III and IV fractures require immediate closed reduction to avoid soft tissue pressure necrosis. All open injuries need debridement with rigid internal fixation and anatomic reduction. Preservation of bone stock is to be advised, but if the fragments are not available due to loss of bone through an open injury or osteonecrosis, the Blair fusion is the salvage procedure of choice.[39–41] Frequently an external fixator can be used to maintain length until soft tissue control is obtained, so that a Blair anterior sliding tibial graft or a tricortical bone block tibiotalocalcaneal fusion can be performed later. This procedure preserves the normal contour of the hind- and midfoot as well as preserving transverse tarsal joint motion. Type IV injuries frequently require a triple if not a pantalar arthrodesis.[42] Late complications of osteonecrosis occur with regularity in type III and IV fractures. This has been reported in between 33 and 100 percent of cases.[34,36,43] Such complications can be avoided by aggressive early treatment and rigid open reduction with internal fixation.[44,45] The osteoporotic lucent line seen under the subcortical talar dome at 8 to 12 weeks postinjury, also known as the "Hawkins sign," is useful prognostically to exclude the diagnosis of osteonecrosis.[33,43] Since MRI may be helpful in predicting osteonecrosis, this may be a relative indication for titanium hardware.[27] Collapse of the talar dome following avascular necrosis is not prevented by avoidance of weight-bearing forces, thus prolonged avoidance of weight bearing is not

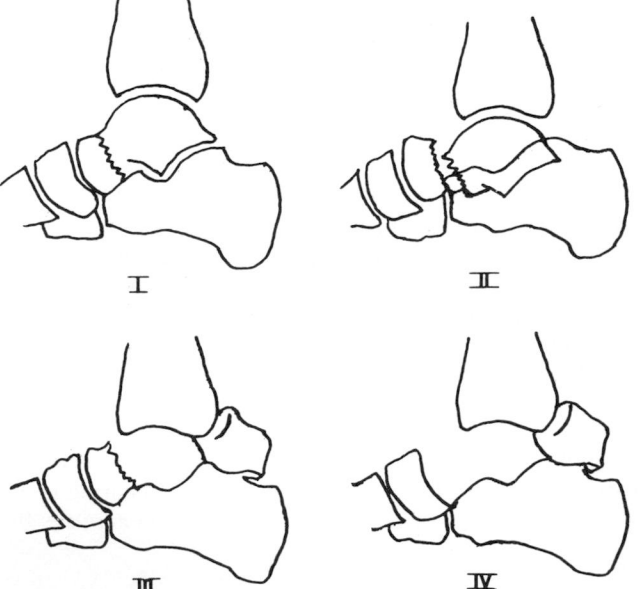

I
II
III
IV

Figure 31-3 Modified Hawkin's classification of talar neck fracture.

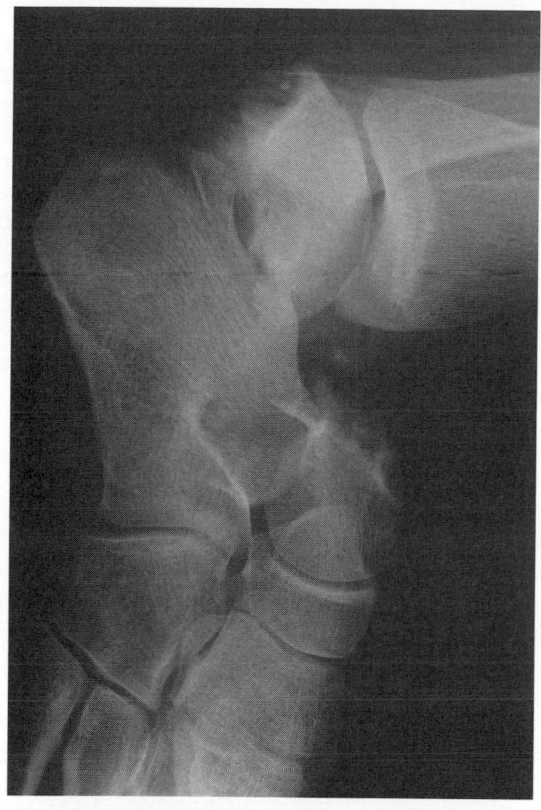

A

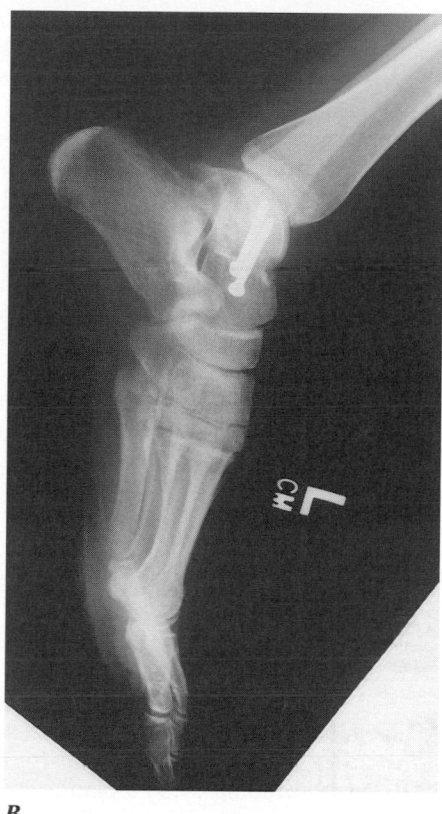

B

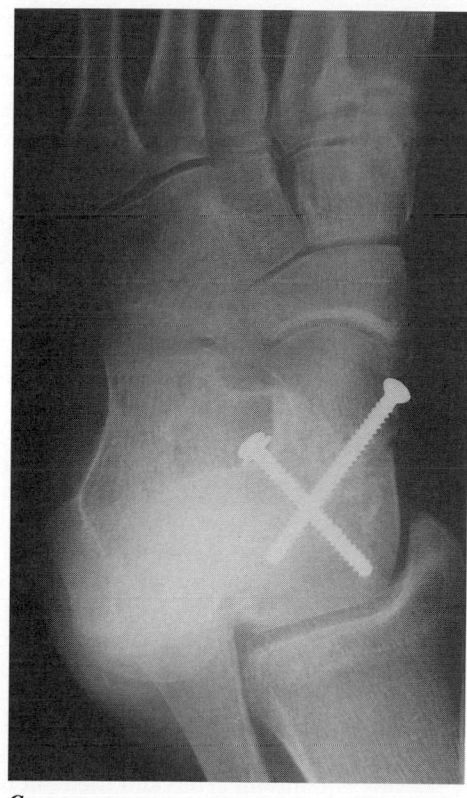

C

Figure 31-4 Talar neck fracture type II; open reduction and internal fixation (ORIF) by anteromedial and anterolateral exposure.

advised.[33] Malunion frequently results from either closed treatment, incomplete reduction, or loss of fixation, leading to loss of the reduction.[23] This results in loss of subtalar joint motion, varus foot position, and posttraumatic arthritis.[46] Other causes of posttraumatic arthritis include collapse of the talar dome secondary to avascular necrosis (AVN) or osteochondral damage at the time of initial injury. This may be treated by arthrodesis of either the ankle and/or subtalar joint.[33,40–42] This can be avoided by thorough preoperative evaluation, early anatomic reduction with rigid fixation through a two-incision technique, and early rehabilitation.[23,27,33,43–45]

Talar Head Fractures

Fractures of the head of the talus are fortunately uncommon. They usually result from longitudinal compression applied to a plantarflexed foot through the metatarsals and the tarsonavicular to compress the talar head.[47] The fracture is frequently missed at the time of initial presentation and will result in instability of the midtarsal joint and arthrosis if it is not anatomically reduced.[48] Canale's pronated oblique x-ray is helpful in defining talar head injuries; however, CT scanning is often necessary to define the fracture.[24] Treatment of a nondisplaced talar head injury involving less than 50 percent of the head and with less than 2 mm displacement usually involves a non-weight-bearing short leg cast for approximately 6 to 12 weeks.

Part of this time may be spent in a removable cast brace to initiate the early range of motion.[48] If it involves more than 50 percent of the head or has significant displacement, open reduction and internal fixation is recommended with K-wire, small-fragment lag-screw, or Herbert-screw fixation.[24,49] These fractures frequently go onto late talonavicular arthritis, which may require isolated arthrodesis. Avascular necrosis of the fragment is rare, and less than 10 percent of patients develop nonunion. This can frequently be treated with simple excision.[50] Other unusual problems observed include interposition of tendons, such as the posterior tibialis or the flexor hallucis longus, and ruptures of the medial structures.

Major talar fractures frequently lead to significant problems in approximately 65 percent of patients.[51] Poor outcomes are seen in the case of open injuries, type 3 and 4 fractures, incomplete reduction, osteonecrosis, and infection as well as in multiple injury patients.[45,52,53]

SUBTALAR JOINT INJURIES

Subtalar joint dislocations are rare injuries that are more properly termed peritalar dislocations of the foot. They are caused by severe trauma when a plantarflexed foot is forced into inversion, resulting in a medial subtalar dislocation. The less common lateral dislocation occurs when the forefoot is forced into everted position.[54] Anterior and posterior dislocations have been described but are exceedingly rare. The mechanism causes a complete disruption of the strong talocalcaneal ligaments as well as the capsuloligamentous attachments of the talocalcaneal facets. Due to the bony architecture of the subtalar joint, lateral process and posterior tubercle process fractures of the talus are frequently associated with these injuries. Additional injury can be seen on the articular surfaces of the subtalar joint, and this contributes to the long-term sequelae of posttraumatic arthrosis. Radiographic analysis, standard AP, lateral, and oblique views of the foot are required for complete evaluation; frequently CT scanning, looking for intraarticular debris and occult talar fractures, is helpful.[55] Treatment is directed to rapid evaluation and reduction of the dislocation to prevent skin breakdown and vascular compromise.[42] Open injuries should be treated prior to reduction with standard irrigation and debridement techniques, as with other open injuries. Closed, isolated subtalar dislocations should be reduced closed as soon as possible, with postreduction CT scanning looking for previously missed intraarticular debris or fracture.[55] General or spinal anesthetic with muscle relaxation is advised to lessen damage to the joint.[56] These fractures are usually intrinsically stable unless there are interposed capsuloligamentous or tendinous structures or there is intraarticular debris. Irreducible dislocation is observed in 10 to 20 percent of cases.[57] This is a result of soft tissues that are buttonholed around the talar head or neck or it can result from an impaction fracture. If this is encountered, open reduction should be undertaken immediately.

These dislocations are usually intrinsically stable. If they are not, transarticular pinning for approximately 4 weeks has been utilized. Cast immobilization is usually limited to 3 to 6 weeks, with early mobilization utilizing physical therapy. Poor prognostic factors include open injuries, delayed reductions, and dislocations involving fractures.[55] There have been sporadic reports of avascular necrosis of the talus following subtalar joint dislocation, but this is rare. Stiffness following these dislocations is common, with a 50 percent loss of subtalar joint motion being expected.[58] Posttraumatic arthritis in the subtalar joint has been reported.[55] This is usually treated by standard techniques with conservative measures, with more advanced arthritis requiring subtalar or triple arthrodesis.

FRACTURES OF THE OS CALCIS

The os calcis is a complex bone, the fracture of which frequently leads to serious, prolonged disability.[59,60] It is reported to be the most commonly fractured tarsal bone.[61] Anatomically it is a very complex structure that supports the subtalar joint, which is made up of a large posterior facet, a middle facet that sits on the sustentaculum of the tali, and an anterior facet that sits on the distal medial aspect of the calcaneus. The anterior process is located at the distal aspect of the lateral calcaneus and is part of the calcaneal cuboid articulation. The thalamic portion of the os calcis is at the area underneath the lateral process of the talus and represents an area of very dense bone. The tuber is the posterior aspect of the calcaneus and is the area of attachment of the Achilles tendon. The medial and lateral tuberosities on the plantar aspect represent apophyseal attachments of the abductor hallucis, flexor digitorum brevis, plantar fascia, and abductor digiti minimi, respectively.[1] Intraarticular involvement is seen in 75 percent of all calcaneal fractures. Basic radiographic evaluation includes an AP ankle, AP and lateral foot, and the axial view of the calcaneus. Radiographic angles include the tuberosity joint angle or Bohler's angle measured from an intersection of lines drawn from the top of the posterior facet to the anterior process and from the top of the posterior facet to the top of the tuberosity. This normally measures approximately 25 to 40°.[62] The critical angle of the Gissane is the angle measuring the angled thalamic portion of the calcaneus immediately below the lateral process of the talus. It normally measures 120 to 145°. Both of these angles are overrated as prognostic indicators.[63] Other views described include Anthonsen's, Broden's, and Isherwood's views and oblique views such as the medial and lateral axial oblique x-rays.[64-67] The medial axial oblique view can easily be obtained intraoperatively, so as to judge posterior facet position. The foot is passively dorsiflexed and inverted and then internally rotated 60° until the foot rests on a 30° wedge. The x-ray beam is then centered approximately 2.5 cm below and anterior to the tip of the lateral malleolus and tilted 10° cephalad. This provides an excellent view of the middle

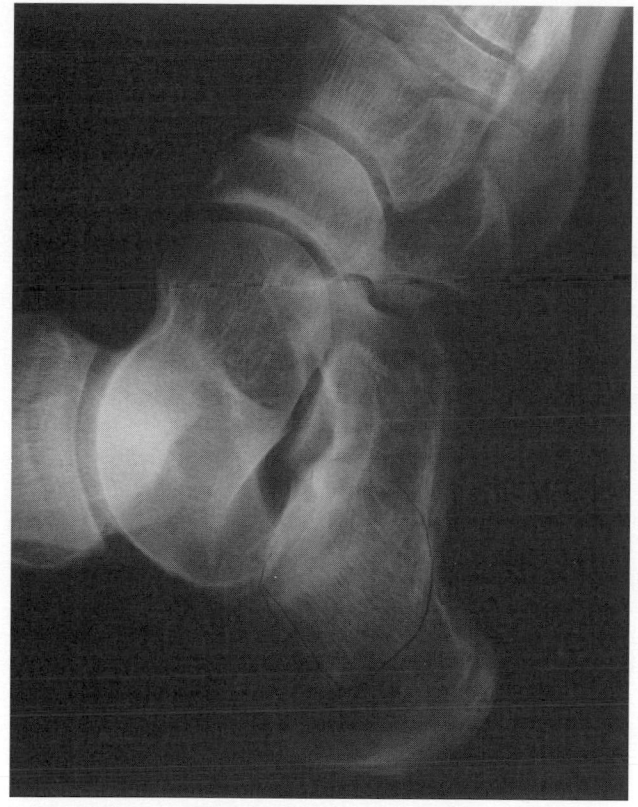

A

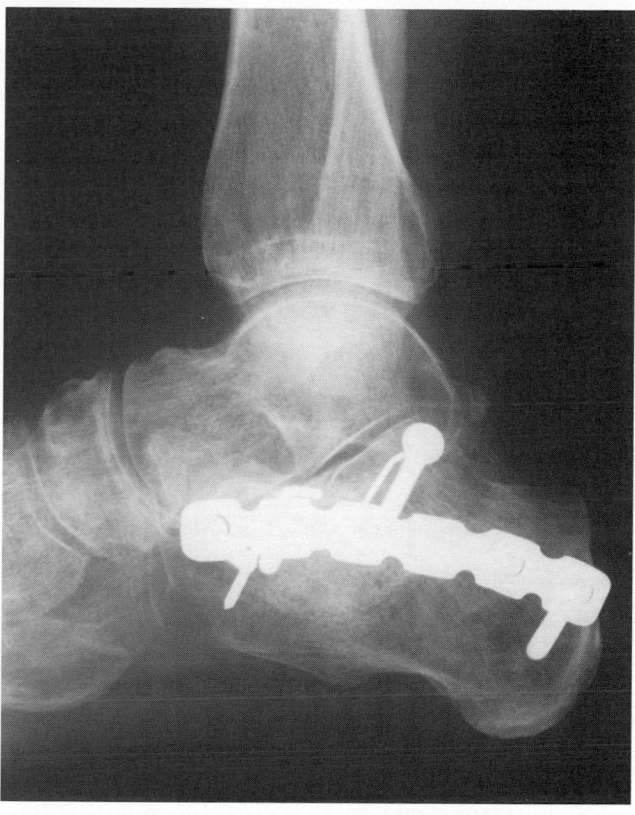

B

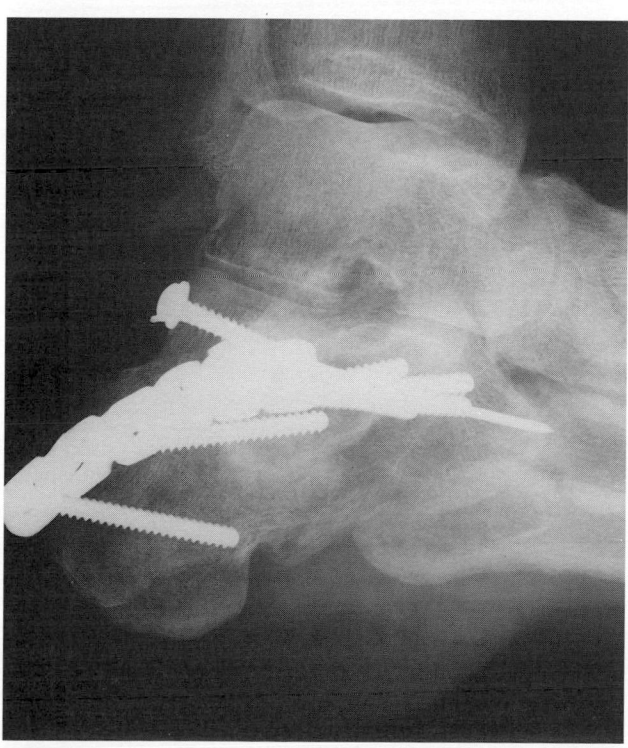

C

Figure 31-5 Joint depression calcaneal fracture, Letournel type II; ORIF by lateral extensile exposure.

and posterior facets and the tarsal canal (Fig. 31-5). The interval between the calcaneus and the fibula, the so-called peroneal tendon gap, is also visualized. The CT scan is the most useful study to evaluate calcaneal morphology.[68,69]

A modified Essex-Lopresti anatomic classification divides calcaneal fractures into extraarticular and intraarticular injuries.[70] Extraarticular injuries include the anterior process, sustentaculum tali, medial and lateral processes, beak and avulsion tuberosities, and body.[64]

Anterior Process Fractures

Anterior process fractures represent an avulsion of either the bifurcate ligament or the calcaneocuboid capsuloligamentous structures or a compression fracture of the distal calcaneal articular surface. These fractures are frequently misdiagnosed as ankle sprains. This injury should not be confused with fracture of the os calcaneus secundarius. Treatment is directed by displacement and size of the fragment. Nondisplaced small injuries are immobilized in a short leg cast for 4 weeks, with good results being obtained. Nonunions with persistent pain are best dealt with by excision.[71] Fractures involving greater than 25 percent of the calcaneal cuboid articulation (if displaced, greater than 2 mm) should be considered for open reduction and internal fixation.[72,73]

Sustentaculum Tali Fractures

Fractures of the sustentacular talus are extremely rare and frequently missed injuries. They are a source of prolonged pain in a misdiagnosed medial ankle sprain. This fracture usually results from landing on an inverted foot. Nondisplaced injuries can be treated with short leg casting for 6 weeks. Displaced injuries may require a closed reduction and casting. Overall, good results can be expected from closed management.[74] Open reduction and internal fixation is rarely needed and reserved for larger fragments. Late excision is used for small nonunions.

Medial and Lateral Calcaneal Process Fractures

Medial and lateral process fractures or vertical tuberosity fractures represent vertical shear fractures, which are produced by a fall on a pronated or supinated heel respectively. Treatment is short leg casting for 4 weeks in nondisplaced injuries. Displaced injuries may require a closed reduction.[75] Shoe modifications or late excision of a prominent displaced process may be necessary for shoe-fitting problems.

Beak and Avulsion Tuberosity Fractures

Beak and the larger avulsion type of fracture represent fractures of the superior aspect of the tuber of the calcaneus. These fractures result from both direct trauma and avulsion of the tendo Achilles. They frequently involve part of the posterior facet. Critical factors to consider are the intraarticular involvement and the degree of displacement, which can lead to dysfunction of the Achilles tendon. Nondisplaced fractures are immobilized in 5 to 10° of plantarflexion for approximately 4 weeks, followed by immobilization in a more neutral cast for an additional 4 weeks. Fractures displaced more than 1 cm are best reduced to restore the length of the Achilles tendon. These may be fixed with interfragmentary wiring or cancellous screws and may be casted for 6 to 8 weeks in a neutrally placed cast.[76–78]

Extraarticular Body Fractures

Extraarticular body fractures result from a fall from a height, causing the posterior aspect of the calcaneus to be driven superiorly. When they are nondisplaced, 4 to 6 weeks of casting followed by early range-of-motion exercises and weight bearing is advised. Displaced injuries result in a wide heel with a limp due to weakness of the gastrocsoleus complex. It is important to reduce Bohler's angle to maintain the length of the Achilles tendon. Closed reduction with medial and lateral compression molding and casting for approximately 6 weeks is successful.[75] Frequently a longitudinal pin or cancellous screw is useful for this.[79,80]

Intraarticular Fractures

Intraarticular fractures represent 75 percent of all calcaneal fractures and 60 percent of all tarsal injuries in general. The usual mechanism of injury is an axial load from a fall from a height or the deceleration of a motor vehicle accident; direct trauma or torsional mechanisms also occur. The fractures are bilateral in approximately 5 to 10 percent of cases, with associated injuries occurring in 25 to 70 percent; 10 percent are associated with fractures of the lumbar spine.[80] The fall causes the superior articular surface of the calcaneus to be driven into the lateral process of the talus, which acts like a splitting wedge and creates the constant separation fracture or primary fracture line of Palmer.[81] This separates the calcaneus into anteromedial and posterolateral fragments. A continued axial load results in collapse into a varus position of the calcaneus and secondary fracture lines, which extend back into the posterior facet and also anteriorly into the calcaneal cuboid joint. The lateral wall expands as the posterior facet joint's depression-type or tongue-type fracture is driven down into the body of the calcaneus (Fig. 31-6). This results in the short, wide heel that is seen with nonoperative treatment.

Several classification schemes based on both x-ray and CT scanning have been described.[68] Letournel has classified these fractures based on plain radiography.[82]

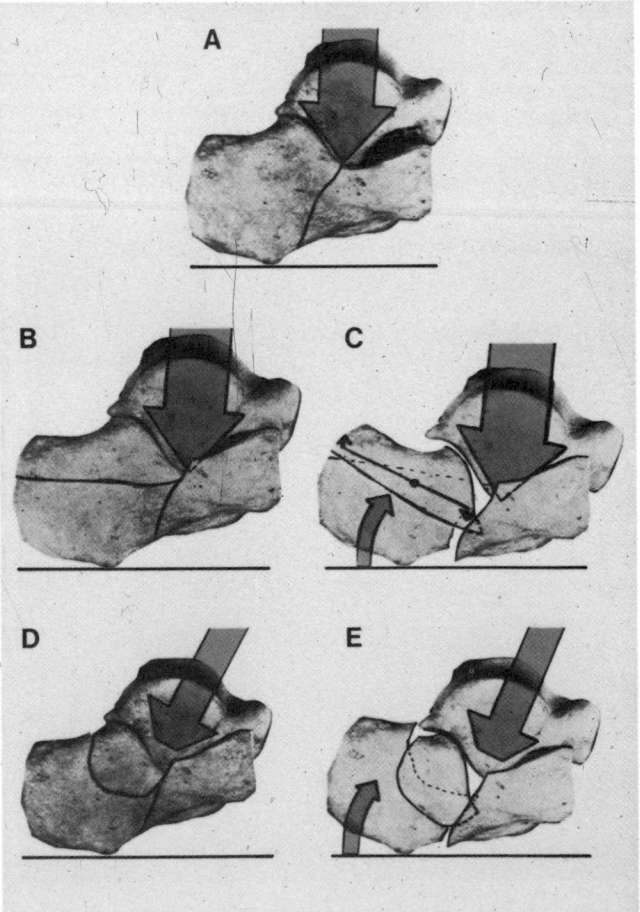

Figure 31-6 Mechanism of intraarticular calcaneus fracture. Primary fracture line (A); tongue type (B, C); joint depression type (D, E).

Type 1 is a two-part fracture of anteromedial and postero-lateral fragments. Type 2 is a three-part fracture that includes the previous fragments but also adds an impaction fracture of the posterior facet either as a joint depression or tongue-type fragment. Type 3 fractures encompass four or more fragments; this includes the previous fragments and additional secondary fracture lines. Sanders has classified these fractures based on coronal CT scanning sections.[69] It is a complex system of four different types based on a lateral, central, and medial column description of the posterior facet. This results in four potential fragments. Type 1 is a nondisplaced fracture regardless of number of fragments or fracture lines. Type 2 is a two-part fracture of the posterior facet; this is subdivided into types A, B, or C depending on location of the primary fracture line. The more medial the fracture line, as in type C, the more difficult the intraoperative visualization. Type 3 encompasses a three-part segmental fracture of the posterior facet with a centrally depressed fragment. Again, these are subdivided into AB, AC, and BC types based on the location of the secondary fracture lines. Type 4 represent highly comminuted four-part fractures with an extremely poor prognosis. Basically the larger the sustentacular fragment and the fewer the number of fragments and articular surfaces involved, the better the prognosis.

There is a great deal of controversy regarding treatment of these complex intraarticular injuries. Treatment is directed at restoration of the three poles of the calcaneus, restoring its height, length, and width. Restoring the morphology of the calcaneus restores the relationships of the tibiotalar, talocalcaneal, calcaneocuboid, and talonavicular joints, all of which are disrupted by displacement. It is important to remember that treatment should be individualized based on the injury and the underlying medical conditions. Nonoperative treatment consists of casting with or without reduction or percutaneous pins, soft compressive dressings, early range of motion to mold the joint, and avoidance of weight bearing for 8 to 12 weeks. The great majority of patients treated nonoperatively have residual hindfoot pain, and these symptoms take up to 3 years to improve.[83] More recent studies have suggested that this results in only a 50 percent satisfactory outcome versus an 80 percent satisfactory outcome with open reduction and internal fixation.[80,84,85]

Operative treatment of these complex fractures is difficult and time-consuming. The prerequisites for open reduction consider the preinjury medical condition, the soft tissue envelope, whether the fracture is reparable, and finally the surgeon's experience with these complex fractures. The relative contraindications include peripheral vascular disease, diabetes mellitus, and inability to cooperate with a postsurgical rehabilitation program. Both medial and lateral approaches have been described.[86–88] The lateral extensile exposure allows a periosteal flap containing the peroneal tendon sheath and sural nerve to be elevated off the lateral aspect of the calcaneus, resulting in direct visualization of the lateral calcaneus and posterior facet.[69,89] The three poles of the calcaneus are reconstructed by reducing fracture fragments to the sustentaculum tali.[82] The posterior facet impaction is gently elevated to its anatomic position relative to the sustentacular

fragment.[90] The use of a Shanz pin as a joystick in the tuberosity aids in recreating the proper height of the tuber, also allowing correction of the varus angulation and the lateral translation. Once anatomic reduction is achieved, provisional K-wire fixation is placed while intraoperative x-ray is obtained to confirm reduction of the posterior facet fragment, medial wall, tuber, and anterior calcaneus. The use of iliac crest bone grafting is controversial but advised for large defects.[82,87] Lag-screw fixation to the sustentaculum tali is performed usually with the aid of a low-profile calcaneal plate (Fig. 31-5). Careful wound closure with suction drain is advised. Avoidance of weight bearing is continued for 8 to 12 weeks postoperatively. A compressive splint is used for the first week. Once the wound is stable, early active range-of-motion exercises of the subtalar and transverse tarsal joints are initiated. The use of primary arthrodesis in calcaneal fractures has been described and is used for severely comminuted fractures with loss of the articular surface.[91,92] Restoration of the morphology is required prior to arthrodesis; frequently these patients need bone grafting.[69] Early complications of open treatment include wound dehiscence and calcaneal osteomyelitis, which should be treated aggressively with debridement, free flap coverage as appropriate, and prolonged intravenous antibiotics. With osteomyelitis, hardware removal and extensive debridements may be required, but ultimately below-knee amputation may provide the most functional alternative. Late complications of posttraumatic arthritis involve both the subtalar and calcaneal cuboid joints. These should be dealt with in the usual fashion with activity modification, anti-inflammatories, bracing, and finally subtalar or triple arthrodesis. Frequently, soft tissue problems such as heel-pad deficiency require the use of a soft cushioning orthotic. Sural nerve neuroma is dealt with by desensitization or proximal resection. Other complications of nonoperative treatment include malunion or lateral wall or peroneal impingement. Lateral wall decompression is useful in relieving lateral hindfoot discomfort.[93] The posterior bone block distraction subtalar arthrodesis corrects the problems of the horizontal talus, fibulocalcaneal abutment, varus heel, and subtalar arthritis with one procedure.[94]

FRACTURES AND DISLOCATIONS OF THE MIDFOOT

The bony midtarsus is the intercalated segment between the transverse tarsal joint and the tarsal metatarsal joint. The ligamentous muscular support for this area is essential in maintaining structural integrity. The tarsal scaphoid and medial cuneiform are keystones in maintaining the medial longitudinal arch and column. The lateral column is bridged by the cuboid. The tarsal scaphoid or navicular receives a blood supply mainly from radially penetrating dorsal and plantar branches of both the dorsalis pedis and posterior tibial vessels.[95] Numerous short plantar and dorsal ligamentous structures play an extremely important and complex role in supporting the midtarsus.[1] Injuries to the midfoot represent a difficult area to image radiographically. Delays in diagnosis of injuries in this area are frequently due to inadequate radiographs.[3] Basic radiographic evaluations should include AP, lateral, and oblique views of the foot with an AP view of the ankle. Additional studies such as cone-down x-ray stress views, comparison views, and CT may be needed to completely define the pathology. Technetium-99m bone scanning is frequently helpful in chronic or poorly defined cases.[96]

TARSAL NAVICULAR FRACTURES

Navicular fractures are the most common midfoot fracture. These injuries have been categorized by a modified Watson-Jones classification.[2,97] The classification defines navicular fractures into a dorsal lip avulsion, tuberosity fractures, and body fractures. Stress fractures represent a subtype of the navicular body fracture that principally occurs in athletic populations.[98]

Tarsonavicular Dorsal Lip Fracture

Fractures of the dorsal lip or avulsion account for approximately 50 percent of all tarsal navicular fractures.[2] They represent an avulsion of the dorsal talonavicular ligaments from a hyperplantar flexion and inversion mechanism. Frequently associated with these are midtarsal subluxations and lateral ankle ligamentous injuries. This injury is best seen on the lateral foot x-ray. Acute treatment is directed to short-term casting of 3 to 4 weeks' duration for nondisplaced minor avulsions. Larger fragments or those with significant portions of the articular surface should be anatomically reduced and internally fixed. Excision is sometimes needed for large hypertrophic fragments resulting in dorsal bossing.[97]

Tarsonavicular Tuberosity Fracture

The navicular tuberosity fracture is generally an avulsion of the posterior tibialis tendon, tibial navicular fibers of the superficial deltoid, and spring ligaments. These injuries account for approximately 25 percent of all navicular fractures.[2] This injury is frequently misdiagnosed as a medial ankle sprain. These fractures need to be distinguished from the accessory ossicle—the os tibialis externum. The accessory ossicle occurs in approximately 15 to 20 percent of the population and is bilateral in approximately 90 percent. The tuberosity fracture is best seen on the AP view of the foot or with tomograms. Treatment is directed by the severity of the pathology. Nondisplaced injuries can be treated conservatively, watching closely for displacement. Immobilization in a well-molded arch-supporting short leg cast is usually required for 4 to 6 weeks. This is often followed by a supportive orthotic. Displaced fractures can result in weak posterior tibial tendon function and prominence in the medial mid-hindfoot. These injuries are dealt with either by excision and advancement of the posterior tibial tendon, with larger frag-

ments being openly reduced and internally fixed. Chronically painful nonunions are often excised with advancement of the posterior tibial tendon into the defect.

Tarsonavicular Body Fracture

Fractures of the body represent approximately 25 percent of all tarsal navicular fractures.[2] They are caused by direct crushing from the dorsal surface or indirectly by compression between the cuneiforms and talus in a nutcracker type of mechanism. These intraarticular fractures represent the most severe injury of the tarsal navicular and are associated with other transverse tarsal joint injuries. These injuries are missed on up to a third of initial films.[3] Nondisplaced fractures are best treated by a short leg cast followed by a supportive orthotic. Many authors have advocated open reduction and internal fixation for displaced fractures.[99] Displaced fractures of the tarsal navicular body have been classified by fracture pattern and comminution.[100] Three fracture patterns are observed. Type 1 is a transverse fracture in the coronal plane best seen on the lateral x-ray. Type 2 is also a transverse fracture, but it runs obliquely from dorsolateral to plantomedial. This type is associated with medially deviated forefoot subluxation. Type 3 represents a fracture with central or lateral comminution with laterally deviated forefoot subluxation. Types 2 and 3 are best seen on the AP x-ray and have a poorer prognosis. Even with open reduction and internal fixation, and 70 percent achieve a satisfactory reduction. About two-thirds have good functional results, and avascular necrosis is noted in approximately 30 percent.[100] Primary arthrodesis of the talonavicular joint has also been advocated, but it should be noted that arthrodesis of this joint will result in severe limitation of supination and pronation of the foot.[101]

Tarsonavicular Stress Fracture

Stress fractures of the tarsal navicular comprise a rare subset of body fractures that occur in the young, athletic male. They are commonly associated with cavus feet, metatarsus adductus, Morton's foot, tarsal coalition, and limited subtalar and ankle motion. Treatment recommendations are controversial, but for uncomplicated nondisplaced fractures, non-weight-bearing casting for 6 to 8 weeks is advised. Open reduction and internal fixation with bone grafting has been recommended for displaced or nonunited fractures that involve more than 50 percent of the width of the tarsonavicular.[98,102]

CUBOID FRACTURES

Fractures of the cuboid represent an uncommon and frequently unrecognized injury. Cuboid fractures are subdivided into capsular avulsions and body fractures.[103] They are caused by direct and indirect mechanisms. A common mechanism is a forced forefoot abduction on a fixed hindfoot. This usually results in a tension failure of the medial column of the midfoot and a compression fracture of the body of the cuboid between the bases of the fourth and fifth metatarsals and the anterior calcaneus.[3] This injury has been described as a "nutcracker fracture."[104] This mechanism is also associated with transverse tarsal and tarsometatarsal joint injuries. Computed tomography is helpful in evaluation and in finding other occult midtarsal joint injuries. Avulsion injuries have a relatively benign course when they occur in isolation. These are best treated as joint sprains with 2 to 4 weeks of casting. Isolated displaced cuboid body fractures with impacted compression of the articular surfaces and subluxation of the midtarsus are best openly reduced and internally fixed with a structural bone graft[105,106] (Fig. 31-7). Postoperative casting for approximately 6 to 8 weeks is followed by supportive orthotics. Salvage procedures include cuboid osteotomy without bone block lengthening or isolated pericuboid or triple arthrodesis.[107]

well.[108] There is usually a dorsal displacement due to the weak dorsal ligament complex. X-ray demonstration of these injuries is difficult; CT is often required to define the pathoanatomy. These injuries are subdivided into avulsions, nondisplaced fractures, and displaced body fractures. The goal of treatment is to reduce midtarsal subluxation and prevent posttraumatic arthrosis. Nondisplaced or avulsion-type injuries are frequently treated successfully with a short leg cast for 4 to 6 weeks with or without weight bearing, depending on the patient's injury. Frequently orthotic management with a steel shank rocker or a full-length rigid insole will return the individual to activities sooner. Displaced fractures are those associated with midtarsal subluxation and usually require anatomic open reduction and internal fixation, with screws frequently being placed into an adjacent tarsal. Salvage of these injuries is that of intertarsal fusion with iliac crest bone graft, frequently tarsometatarsal joint fusion is also required.[109,110]

CUNEIFORM FRACTURES

Fractures of the cuneiform are not similarly quite uncommon. The most frequent mechanism is by direct trauma, which can involve any of the three cuneiforms. These injuries frequently involve the tarsometatarsal joint as

MIDTARSAL JOINT DISLOCATION

Injuries to the midtarsal joints are complex ligamentous disruptions that rarely occur as isolated injuries. These are frequently misdiagnosed and result in a delay in treatment,

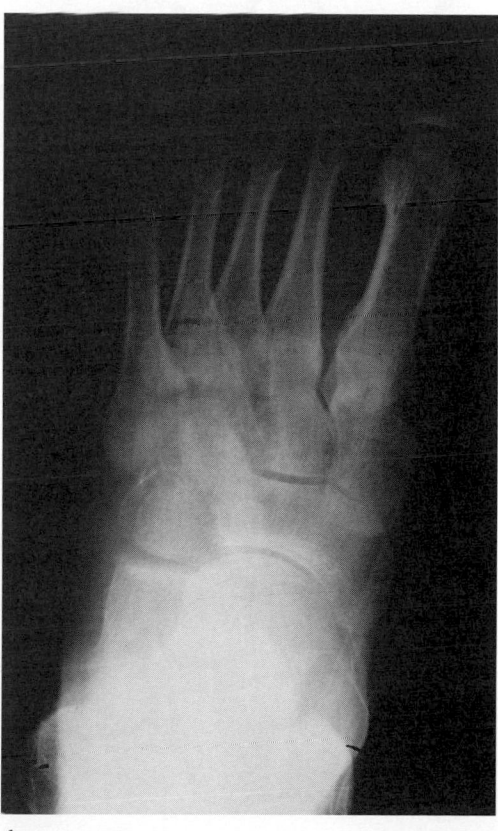
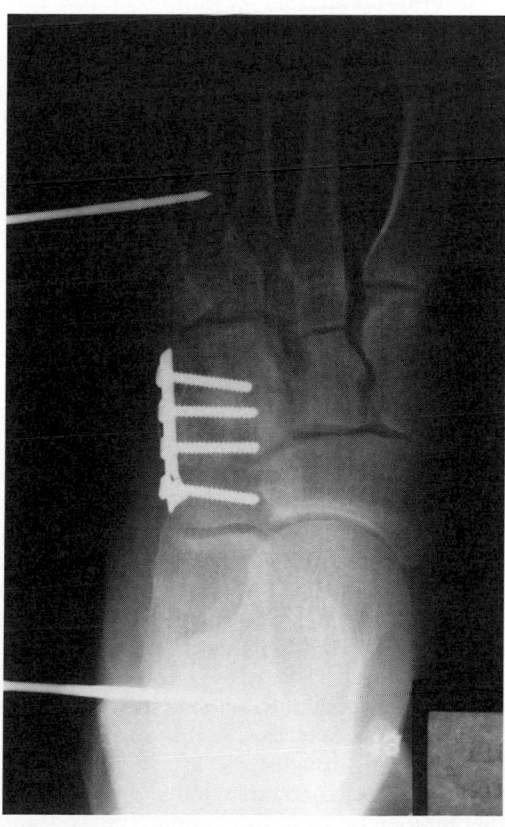

A   *B*

Figure 31-7 Cuboid impaction fracture, ORIF by use of minidistractor and structural bone graft.

with poor results.[3] These injuries have been classified by the direction of the deforming force—medial, longitudinal compression, lateral, plantar, and crush injuries. These are subdivided into fracture/sprains, fracture-subluxation with dislocation, or swivel dislocations. The fracture-sprain is manifest by an avulsion-fracture of the tarsonavicular or cuboid. Fracture/subluxation with dislocation is easily identifiable by a navicular or cuboid body fracture with midtarsal incongruity. Swivel dislocations are recognized by an apparent isolated talonavicular dislocation.

Treatment is directed to reestablishing stability and midtarsal congruity. Satisfactory results can be expected with prompt diagnosis and anatomic reduction with or without internal stabilization.[3] More severe transverse tarsal joint dislocations or body fractures are injuries that carry a poor prognosis if they are not properly treated with aggressive reduction and internal fixation.

FRACTURE/DISLOCATION OF THE TARSOMETATARSAL JOINT

Tarsometatarsal joint fracture/dislocation is an uncommon injury that can result from either high- or low-velocity longitudinal compression or torsion of the forefoot. This injury carries the name of Jacques Lisfranc, one of Napoleon's field surgeons, who reported an amputation through this area for gangrene. The critical anatomy of the area centers on the second metatarsal keystone of the transverse metatarsal arch. The tarsometatarsal joint simulates a Roman arch, with the bones being wider on the dorsal surface than they are on the plantar surface.[111] The stability of the arch comes from the strong plantar tarsometatarsal ligaments. The crucial Lisfranc ligament arises from the medial cuneiform and inserts on the medial base of the second metatarsal (Fig. 31-8). Disruptions of this ligament frequently result in a fleck of bone being avulsed from the base of the second metatarsal. Additional stabilization of the midtarsus and tarsometatarsal joint is provided by the transverse ligaments between the second through fifth metatarsal bases, the anterior tibialis, peroneus longus, plantar fascia, and intrinsic musculature.[1] Due to these strong plantar stabilizers, dorsal dislocation is the most common. The arterial anatomy in this area is a result of the anterior tibialis/dorsalis pedis artery and intermetatarsal branch anastomosis to the plantar circulation with the deep plantar artery. These branches as well as the arcuate artery are disrupted by fracture/dislocations in this area. This can result in a significant hemorrhage, causing the skin slough and/or compartment syndrome. The injury mechanism is usually the result of maximal load applied longitudinally to the forefoot or a direct force applied dorsally over the midtarsal area, resulting in failure through the tarsometatarsal joint. The most commonly used classification is that of Hardcastle, which describes types A through C.[112] Type A describes total incongruity of the tarsometatarsal joint, with an entire lateral or medial tarsometatarsal dislocation. This is described as homolateral. Type B is more common, which is partial incongruity with an isolated medial first metatarsal or the lat-

eral four metatarsals in subluxation or dislocation. Type C is a divergent type with the first metatarsal deviating medially and the lateral four metatarsals laterally. Fractures of the bases of the metatarsals or their necks along with dislocations of the tarsometatarsal joint may also be seen. Radiographic anatomy is visualized by AP, lateral, and 30° oblique radiographs of the foot. On the AP radiograph, the first metatarsal medial cuneiform joint should be congruent and the second metatarsal and middle cuneiform should line up along their medial border. On the oblique x-rays, the lateral border of the third metatarsal base should line up with the lateral border of the lateral cuneiform and the medial border of the fourth metatarsal should line up with the medial border of the cuboid. Telltale signs on x-ray include an avulsion at the base of the medial border of the second metatarsal, greater than 2 mm of widening in this area, and/or an impaction fracture of the distal cuboid at the fourth and fifth metatarsal bases (Fig. 31-9). Sometimes these films are deceptive and stress views are required. Treatment of these injuries is dictated by the soft tissue envelope, the amount of swelling, and whether a compartment syndrome is present. Closed injuries are reportedly treated with closed techniques, with longitudinal traction and percutaneous fixation.[113] If anatomic reduction cannot be achieved, one should proceed directly to open reduction and internal fixation, as there is often interposed soft tissue, tendinous structures, and bony fragments.[114] The longitu-

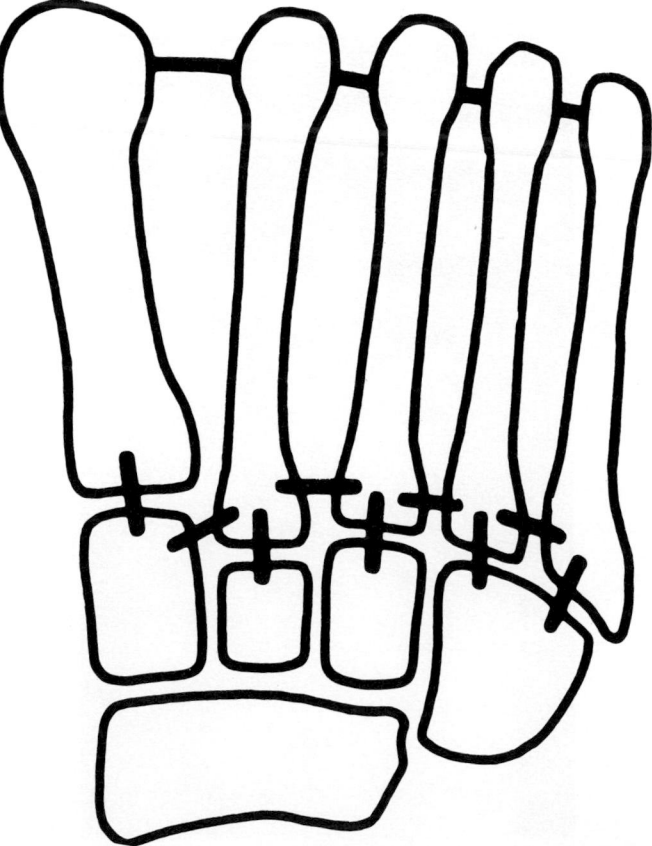

Figure 31-8 Ligamentous attachments of tarsometatarsal joints.

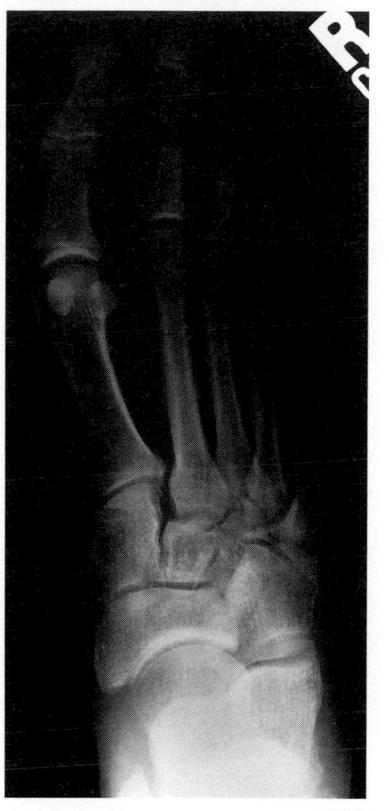

A

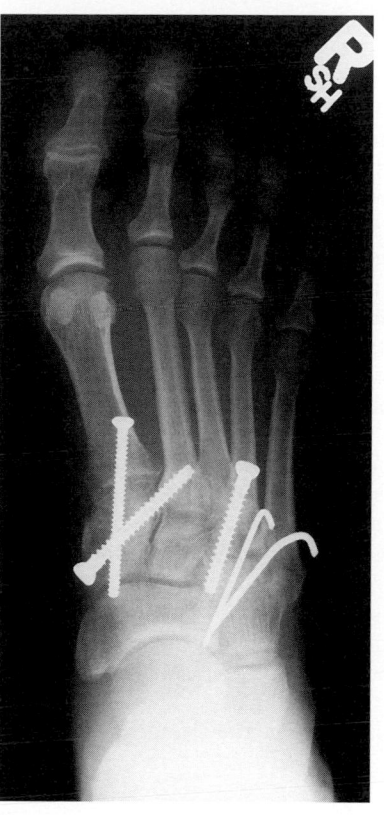

B

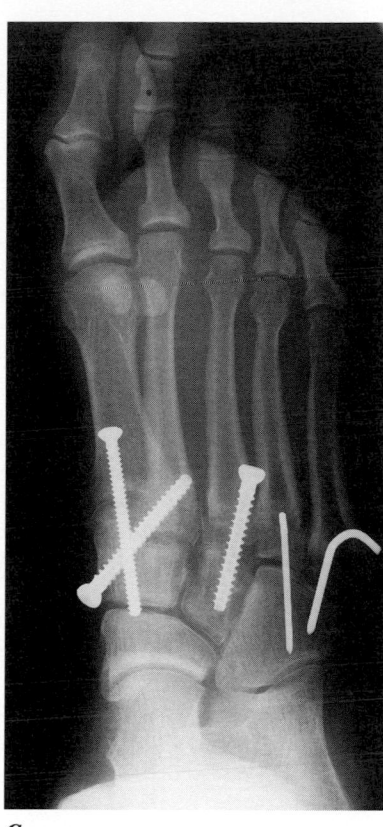

C

Figure 31-9 Lisfranc's fracture-subluxation; ORIF.

dinal incisions are placed dorsally on the lateral border of the first metatarsal so as to expose the first tarsometatarsal joint and the medial aspect of the second tarsometatarsal joint. The second incision is on the medial border of the third metatarsal centered over the tarsometatarsal joint. This allows exposure at the lateral second and the third tarsometatarsal joints. Frequently the fourth and fifth do not require direct exposure but can be percutaneously pinned. Skin incisions should carefully proceed directly to bone without undermining the skin bridge. The joints are debrided and reduction is carried out from a medial to a lateral direction with "positioning" 3.5-mm fully threaded screws holding the first three tarsometatarsal joints and K wires in the fourth and fifth joints (Fig. 31-9).[105] If present, intercuneiform diastasis must be reduced and fixed as well. Care must be taken to inspect the intercuneiform diastasis looking for anterior tibialis interposition. Postoperative care utilizes a non-weight-bearing cast for approximately 8 weeks followed by removable cast bracing and initiation of physical therapy. Physical therapy is helpful in mobilization and desensitization. Hardware removal is routinely performed at 16 to 24 weeks.[115] Frequently longitudinal arch support is used postoperatively. Successful results can be expected in 80 percent of cases. Acute failures include sepsis, which should be prevented by good soft tissue technique and redisplacement, which is usually seen after closed treatment or K-wire fixation.[115] Late complications such as posttraumatic arthrosis may or may not require additional treatment with tarsometatarsal joint arthrodesis.[110] Neuroma formation has been noted and may be dealt with by desensitization or proximal neurectomy.

METATARSAL AND PHALANGEAL FRACTURES

Fractures of the metatarsals can result in abnormalities in the weight-bearing distribution of the forefoot; thus their management must not be ignored. These fractures are often the result of direct trauma from an object dropped onto or run over the dorsum of the foot. Avulsion and stress fractures also cause disability.

Metatarsal Fractures

The majority of isolated metatarsal neck and shaft fractures can be treated nonoperatively provided that the metatarsals adjacent to the fracture are intact to provide stabilization by the intermetatarsal ligaments. Minimally displaced and anatomically reduced fractures can frequently be managed in a short leg non-weight-bearing cast for approximately 4 weeks followed by protected weight bearing, with good results. Reduction is advised for displaced metatarsal fractures with greater than 10° of angulation in the sagittal plane or 3 to 4 mm of displacement, multiple metatarsal fractures, and displaced fractures of the first ray.[116] First metatarsal fractures require an anatomic reduction for a stable medial column to provide plantigrade foot function. If the first metatarsal is elevated, the foot will pronate; if it is plantarflexed, the foot will supinate. Elevation or plantarflexion of a metatarsal head can be evaluated by plantar palpation underneath the metatarsal heads and simulated weight bearing. Displaced fractures of the neck and shaft can be managed with minifragment screws or 1.6-2.0-mm intramedullary K-wire fixation (Fig. 31-10). A dorsal incision is made over the fracture site and the K wire is placed through the distal fragment and driven through the plantar base of the toe, transfixing the metatarsophalangeal joint in the neutral position; the fracture is anatomically reduced and the K wire is driven retrograde back into the proximal fragment.[105,117] This should be protected in the cast for approximately 4 weeks, followed by a stiff-soled shoe after K-wire removal.

Metatarsal head fractures require precise treatment to prevent metatarsophalangeal joint arthrosis. Displaced fractures should be reduced anatomically with the aid of a finger trap providing longitudinal traction; K-wire or interfragmentary minifragment screw fixation provides sta-

ble fixation, allowing early mobilization of the joint with buddy taping to adjacent toes. Delayed unions and nonunions are frequently asymptomatic and rarely require treatment.

Proximal fifth metatarsal fractures are a unique group of fractures, which can be simple tuberosity avulsion fractures by the peroneus brevis/tertius and plantar fascia. These rarely need reduction unless they involve displacement of greater than 50 percent of the fifth metatarsal cuboid articulation or are widely displaced more than 1 cm. Just beyond this is the Jones fracture, located approximately 1 to 2 cm distal to the tip of the fifth metatarsal tuberosity. This fracture carries a rather poor prognosis due to the poor interosseous blood supply to this area of the metaphyseal and diaphyseal anastomosis. These fractures have been extensively written about as being acute, chronic, or stress fractures. Acutely, these fractures can be managed with non-weight-bearing casts for approximately 6 to 8 weeks, but prolonged disability and healing can be expected. Athletic individuals or those with chronic fractures involving medullary sclerosis require intramedullary screw fixation.[118] Late surgery is required in approximately 12 percent of the acute fractures and 50 percent of the chronic fractures treated with conservative measures. Bone grafting may be necessary.[119,120]

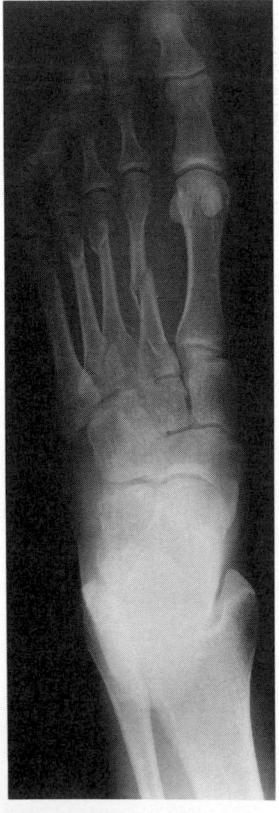
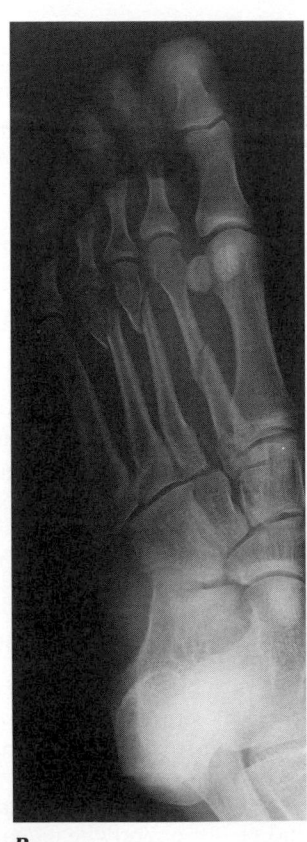
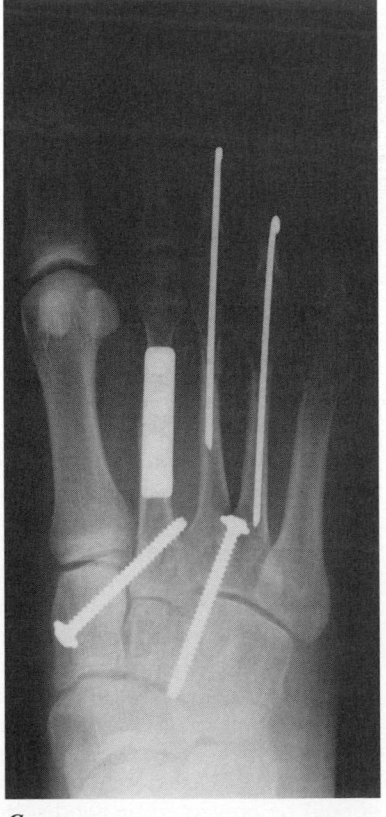

A   *B*   *C*

Figure 31-10 Metatarsal shaft and neck fractures and associated Lisfranc's injury.

Phalangeal Fractures

Phalangeal fractures of the great and lesser toe are usually stubbing type of injuries resulting in condylar fractures.[121] These are usually stable and best treated with buddy taping. If they involve displaced intraarticular surfaces, they should be reduced anatomically and pinned with crossed K wires through dorsal exposures.

The hallux interphalangeal joint is one that frequently has an irreducible dislocation, requiring a plantar incision to remove the plantar plate from the interphalangeal joint along with a frequently observed sesamoid. Repair of the plantar plate through this plantar incision is advised.[122] The use of a short leg cast with a toe plate for approximately 3 weeks followed by buddy taping results in a stable functional joint. Failure to treat these intraarticular injuries aggressively result in posttraumatic arthritis, joint subluxation, and incongruity. Treatment of these delayed complications is usually that of either a resectional arthroplasty or an arthrodesis.

METATARSOPHALANGEAL JOINT DISLOCATIONS

Metatarsophalangeal joint dislocations are most commonly dorsal dislocations, which are usually the result of a longitudinal impact on a dorsiflexed toe. The first metatarsophalangeal joint has an especially unique situation with the sesamoid sling, around which the first metatarsal head can be buttonholed. Type 1 injuries are evident on x-ray, when the sesamoids remain together, an irreducible plantar first metatarsal phalangeal joint dislocation is indicated. These require open reduction with release of the intersesamoidal ligament and reconstruction of the plantar plate. Type 2 injuries reveal separation or fracture of the sesamoids and are reducible by closed means.[123] Both injuries require limited immobilization and early weight bearing.

Lesser metatarsophalangeal joint dislocations are reduced closed fairly simply by hyperextension of the phalanx, distraction, and then plantar flexion. Most are stable and only need buddy taping. If this is unsuccessful, open reduction through a dorsal incision is advised. This may require capsulotomy and deep transverse metatarsal ligament release. Once release is performed, reduction is carried out simply by distraction and flexion.[124] These injuries are usually stable once they are reduced and should be protected for only 3 weeks with a short leg cast with a toe plate. This may be followed by buddy taping for 3 weeks.

SUMMARY

Fracture-dislocations about the foot and ankle can be devastating injuries with prolonged disability. The best results are obtained with early recognition, anatomic reduction, and rigid fixation, allowing early mobilization. The aggressive trauma management of other periarticular injuries can be extended to the foot with goals of restoration of mechanical alignment, articular congruity, and midfoot stability.

REFERENCES

1. Sarrafian SK: *Anatomy of the Foot and Ankle,* 2d ed. Philadelphia, Lippincott, 1993.
2. Eichenholtz SN, Levine DB: Fractures of the tarsal navicular bone. *Clin Orthop Rel Res* 34:142–157, 1964.
3. Main BJ, Jowett RL: Injuries of the midtarsal joint. *J Bone Joint Surg* 57B:89–97, 1975.
4. Allgower M (ed): *Manual of Internal Fixation,* 3d ed. Berlin, Spring-Verlag, 1991.
5. Sangeorzan BJ, Hansen ST: Early and late posttraumatic foot reconstruction. *Clin Orthop* 243:86–91, 1989.
6. Carr JB, Hansen ST, Benirschke SK: Surgical techniques of foot and ankle trauma: Use of indirect reduction techniques. *Foot Ankle* 4:176–178, 1989.
7. Heckman JD, Champine MJ: New techniques in the management of foot trauma. *Clin Orthop* 240:105–114, 1989.
8. Decoster TA, Ferries JF, Shantharam S: Cannulated screw fixation of the foot and ankle. *Tech Orthop* 6:66–68, 1991.
9. Manoli A, Weber TG: Fasciotomy of the foot: An anatomical study with special reference to release of the calcaneal compartment. *Foot Ankle* 10:267–275, 1990.
10. Hansen ST: Overview of the severely traumatized lower limb. *Clin Orthop* 243:17–19, 1989.
11. Lange RH: Limb reconstruction versus amputation: Decision making in massive lower extremity trauma. *Clin Orthop* 243:92–99, 1989.
12. Gelberman RH, Mortensen MD: The arterial anatomy of the talus. *Foot Ankle* 4:64–72, 1983.
13. Peterson L, Goldie IF: The arterial blood supply of the talus: A study on the relationship to experimental talar fractures. *Acta Orthop Scand* 46:1026–1034, 1975.
14. Haliburton RA, Sullivan CR, Kelly PJ, et al: The extraosseous and intraosseous blood supply of the talus. *J Bone Joint Surg* 40A:1115–1120, 1958.
15. Ihle CL, Cochran RM: Fracture of the os trigonum *Am J Sports Med* 10:47–50, 1982.
16. Dimon JH: Isolated displaced fracture of the posterior facet of the talus. *J Bone Joint Surg* 43A:275–281, 1961.
17. Cedell CA: Rupture of the posterior talofibular ligament with avulsion of a bone fragment from the talus. *Acta Orthop Scand* 45:454–461, 1974.
18. Fjeldborg O: Fracture of the lateral process of the talus: Supination-dorsal flexion fracture. *Acta Orthop Scand* 39:407–411, 1968.
19. Hawkins LG: Fractures of the lateral process of the talus. *J Bone Joint Surg* 47A:1170–1175, 1965.
20. Mukherjee SK, Pringle RM, Baxter AD: Fractures of the lateral process of the talus. *J Bone Joint Surg* 56B:263–273, 1974.
21. Heckman JD, McLean MR: Fractures of the lateral process of the talus. *Clin Orthop* 199:108–113, 1985.
22. Berndt AL, Hardy M: Transchondral fractures of the talus. *J Bone Joint Surg* 41A:988–1020, 1959.
23. Sneppen O, Christensen SB, et al: Fractures of the body of the talus. *Acta Orthop Scand* 48:317–324, 1977.
24. Adelaar RS: Fractures of the talus. *Instr Course Lect* 39:147–156, 1990.

25. Kenwright J, Taylor RG: Major injuries to the talus. *J Bone Joint Surg* 52B:36–48, 1970.

26. Mindell ER, Cisek EE, et al: Late results of injuries to the talus. *J Bone Joint Surg* 45A:221–245, 1963.

27. Mayo K: Fractures of the talus: Principles of management and techniques of treatment. *Tech Orthop* 2:42–54, 1987.

28. Berndt AL, Harty M: Transcondral fractures of the talus. *J Bone Joint Surg* 41A:988–1020, 1959.

29. Canale ST, Belding RH: Osteochondral lesions of the talus. *J Bone Joint Surg* 62A:97–102, 1980.

30. Van Buecken K, Barrack RI, et al: Arthroscopic treatment of transchondral talar dome fractures. *Am J Sports Med* 17:350–355, 1989.

31. Ove N, Bosse MJ, et al: Excision of posterolateral talar dome lesions through a medial transmalleolar approach. *Foot Ankle* 9:171–175, 1989.

32. Shea MP, Manoli A: Osteochondral lesions of the talar dome. *Foot Ankle* 14:48–55, 1993.

33. Hawkins LG: Fractures of the neck of the talus. *J Bone Joint Surg* 52A:991–1002, 1970.

34. Canale ST, Kelly FB: Fractures of the neck of the talus: Long term evaluation of seventy one cases. *J Bone Joint Surg* 60A:143–156, 1978.

35. Santavirta S, Seitsalo S, et al: Fractures of the talus. *J Trauma* 24:986–989, 1984.

36. Peterson L, Goldie IF, et al: Fracture of the neck of the talus. *Acta Orthop Scand* 48:696–706, 1977.

37. Lamire RG, Bustin W: Screw fixation of fractures of the neck of the talus. *J Trauma* 20:669–673, 1980.

38. Swanson TV, Bray TJ: Talar neck fractures: A mechanical and histomorphometric study of fixation. *Clin Orthop*

39. Blair HC: Comminuted fractures and fracture dislocations of the body of the astragalus. *Am J Surg* 59:37–43, 1943.

40. Morris HD, Hand WL, Dunn AW: The modified Blair fusion for fractures of the talus. *J Bone Joint Surg* 53A:1289–1297, 1971.

41. Lionberger DR, Bishop JO, Tullos HS: The modified Blair fusion. *Foot Ankle* 3:60–62, 1982.

42. McKeever FM: Treatment of complications of fractures and dislocations of the talus. *Clin Orthop* 30:45–52, 1963.

43. Penny JN, Davis LA: Fractures and fracture-dislocations of the neck of the talus. *J Trauma* 20:1029–1037, 1980.

44. Grob D, Simpson LA, Weber BG: Operative treatment of displaced talus fractures. *Clin Orthop* 199:88–96, 1985.

45. Szyszkowitz R, Reschauer R, Seggl W: Eighty-five talus fractures treated by ORIF with five to eight years follow-up study of 69 patients. *Clin Orthop* 199:97–107, 1985.

46. Daniels T, Smith JW: Varus talar neck malunion: Its influence on foot position and subtalar motion. *Foot Ankle* 14:302, 1993.

47. Coltart WD: Aviator's astragalus. *J Bone Joint Surg* 34B:545–566, 1952.

48. Pennal GF: Fractures of the talus. *Clin Orthop* 30:53–63, 1963.

49. Mallon WJ, Wombwell JH, et al: Intra-articular talar fractures: Repair using the Herbert bone screw. *Foot Ankle* 10:88–92, 1989.

50. Schrock RD: Fractures of the foot. *Instr Course Lect* 9:361–368, 1952.

51. Mindell ER, Cisek EE, et al: Late results of injuries to the talus. *J Bone Joint Surg* 45A:221–245, 1963.

52. Frawley PA, Hart JA, et al: Treatment outcomes of major fractures of the talus. *Foot Ankle* 16:339–345, 1995.

53. Marsh JL, Saltzman CL, et al: Major open injuries of the talus. *J Orthop Trauma* 9:371–376, 1995.

54. Dunn AW: Peritalar dislocation. *Orthop Clin North Am* 5:7–18, 1974.

55. Delee JC, Curtis R: Subtalar dislocation of the foot. *J Bone Joint Surg* 64A:433–437, 1982.

56. O'Brien ET: Injuries of the talus. *Am Fam Physician* 12:95–105, 1975.

57. Leitner B: Obstacles to reduction in subtalar dislocation. *J Bone Joint Surg* 36A:299–306, 1954.

58. Monson ST, Ryan JR: Subtalar dislocation. *J Bone Joint Surg* 63A:1156–1158, 1981.

59. Conn HR: Fractures of the os calcis: Diagnosis and treatment. *Radiology* 62:228–235, 1926.

60. Lindsay WRN, Dewar FP: Fractures of the os calcis. *Am J Surg* 95:555–576, 1958.

61. Cave EF: Fractures of the os calcis: The problem in general. *Clin Orthop* 30:64–66, 1963.

62. Bohler M: Diagnoses, pathology, treatment of fractures of the os calcis. *J Bone Joint Surg* 13:75–89, 1931.

63. Gaul JS, Greenburg BG: Calcaneus fractures involving the subtalar joint: A clinical and statistical survey of 98 cases. *South Med J* 59:605–613, 1966.

64. DeLee JC: Fractures and dislocations of the foot, in Mann RA, Coughlin MJ (eds): *Surgery of the Foot and Ankle,* 6th ed. St. Louis, Mosby, 1992.

65. Anthonsen W: An oblique projection for roentgen examination of the talo-calcaneal joint, particularly regarding intra-articular fracture of the calcaneus. *Acta Radiol* 24:306–310, 1943.

66. Broden B: Roentgen examination of the subtaloid joint in fractures of the calcaneus. *Acta Radiol* 31:85–91, 1949.

67. Isherwood I: A radiological approach to the subtalar joint. *J Bone Joint Surg* 43B:566–574, 1961.

68. Crosby LA, Fizgibbons T: Computerized tomography scanning of acute intra-articular fractures of the calcaneus: A new classification system. *J Bone Joint Surg* 72A:852–859, 1990.

69. Sanders R: Intraarticular fractures of the calcaneus: Present state of the art. *J Orthop Trauma* 6:252–265, 1992.

70. Essex-Lopresti P: The mechanism, reduction technique, and results in fractures of the os calcis. *Br J Surg* 39:395–419, 1952.

71. Degan TJ, Morrey BF: Surgical excision for anterior process fractures of the calcaneus. *J Bone Joint Surg* 64A:519–524, 1982.

72. Hunt DD: Compression fracture of the anterior articular surface of the calcaneus. *J Bone Joint Surg* 52A:1637–1642, 1970.

73. Jahss MH, Kay BS: An anatomic study of the superior process of the os calcis and its clinical applications. *Foot Ankle* 3:268–281, 1983.

74. Carey EJ, Lance EM: Extra-articular fractures of the os calcis. *J Trauma* 5:362–372, 1965.

75. Schottstaedt ER: Symposium: Treatment of fractures of the calcaneus. *J Bone Joint Surg* 45A:863–864, 1963.

76. Protheroe K: Avulsion fractures of the calcaneus. *J Bone Joint Surg* 51B:118–122, 1969.

77. Lowy M: Avulsion fractures of the calcaneus. *J Bone Joint Surg* 51B:494–497, 1969.

78. Lyngstadaas S: The treatment of avulsion fractures of the tuber calcanei. *Acta Chir Scand* 137:579–581, 1971.

79. Geckeler EO: Comminuted fractures of the os calcis. *Arch Surg* 61:469–476, 1950.

80. Rowe CR, Sakellarides HT, et al: Fractures of the os calcis: A long term follow-up study of 146 patients. *JAMA* 184:920–923, 1963.

81. Carr JB, Hamilton JJ, et al: Experimental intra-articular calcaneal fractures: Anatomic basis for a new classification. *Foot Ankle* 10:81–87, 1989.

82. Letournel E: Open reduction and internal fixation of calcaneal fractures, in Spiegel P (ed): *Topics in Orthopedic Surgery.* Baltimore, Aspen, 1984, pp 173–192.

83. Pozo JL, Kirwan EOG, Jackson AM: The long term results of conservative management of severely displaced fractures of the calcaneus. *J Bone Joint Surg* 66B:386–390, 1984.

84. Lance EM, Carey EJ, Wade PA: Fractures of the os calcis: A follow-up study. *J Trauma* 4:15–56, 1964.

85. Simpson LA, Schulak DA, et al: Intra-articular fractures of the calcaneus: A review. *Contemp Orthop* 6:19–28, 1983.

86. Burdeaux DB: Reduction of calcaneal fractures by the McReynolds medial approach technique and its experimental basis. *Clin Orthop* 177:87–103, 1983.

87. Palmer I: The mechanism and treatment of fractures of the calcaneus: Open reduction with the use of cancellous grafts. *J Bone Joint Surg* 30A:2–8, 1948.

88. Stephenson JR: Treatment of displaced intra-articular fractures of the calcaneus using medial and lateral approaches, internal fixation, and early motion. *J Bone Joint Surg* 69A:115–130, 1987.

89. Benirschke SK, Sangeorzan BJ: Extensive intra-articular fractures of the foot: Surgical management of calcaneal fractures. *Clin Orthop* 292:128–134, 1993.

90. Zwipp H, Tscherne H, et al: Osteosynthesis of displaced intra-articular fractures of the calcaneus: Results in 123 cases. *Clin Orthop* 290:76–86, 1993.

91. Dick IL: Primary fusion of the posterior subtalar joint in the treatment of fractures of the calcaneum. *J Bone Joint Surg* 35B:375–380, 1953.

92. Thompson KR: Treatment of comminuted fractures of the calcaneus by triple arthrodesis. *Orthop Clin North Am* 4:189–191, 1973.

93. Braly WG, Bishop JO, et al: Lateral decompression for malunited os calcis fractures. *Foot Ankle* 6:90–96, 1985.

94. Carr JB, Hansen ST, et al: Subtalar distraction bone block fusion for late complications of os calcis fractures. *Foot Ankle* 9:81–86, 1988.

95. Waugh W: The ossification and vascularization of the tarsal navicular and their relationship to Kohler's disease. *J Bone Joint Surg* 40B:765–777, 1958.

96. Morrey BF, et al: The foot and ankle, in Berquist TH (ed): *Imaging of Orthopedic Trauma and Surgery.* Philadelphia, Saunders, 1986, pp 407–498.

97. Watson-Jones R: *Fractures and Joint Injuries,* 4th ed. Vol 2. Baltimore, Williams & Wilkins, 1955.

98. Torg JS, Pavlov H, et al: Stress fractures of the tarsal navicular. *J Bone Joint Surg* 64A:700–712, 1982.

99. Nyska M, et al: Fractures of the body of the tarsal navicular bone. *J Trauma* 29:1448–1451, 1989.

100. Sangeorzan BJ, et al: Displaced intra-articular fractures of the tarsal navicular. *J Bone Joint Surg* 71A:1504–1510, 1989.

101. Fogel GR, et al: Talonavicular arthrodesis for isolated arthrosis: 9.5 year results and gait analysis. *Foot Ankle* 3:105, 1982.

102. Fitch KD, et al: Operation for nonunion of stress fracture of the tarsal navicular. *J Bone Joint Surg* 71B:105–110, 1989.

103. Hillegass RC: Injuries to the midfoot: A major cause of industrial morbidity, in Bateman JE (ed): *Foot Science.* Philadelphia, Saunders, 1976, pp 266–271.

104. Hermel MB, Gersham-Cohen J: The nutcracker fracture of the cuboid caused by indirect violence. *Radiology* 60:850–854, 1953.

105. Hansen ST, et al: Foot, in Muller ME, Allgower M, Schneider R, Willenegger H (eds): *Manual of Internal Fixation,* 3d ed. New York, Springer-Verlag, 1991, pp 613–626.

106. Sangeorzan BJ, Swiontowski MF: Displaced fractures of the cuboid. *J Bone Joint Surg* 72B:376–378, 1990.

107. Dewar FP: Occult fracture-subluxation of the midtarsal joint. *J Bone Joint Surg* 50B:386–388, 1968.

108. Sanders JO, et al: Intermediate cuneiform fracture-dislocation. *J Orthop Trauma* 4:102–104, 1990.

109. Johnson KA: Arthrodeses of the foot and ankle, in Johnson KA (ed): *Surgery of the Foot and Ankle.* New York, Raven Press, 1989, pp 151–208.

110. Sangeorzan BJ, et al: Salvage of Lisfranc's tarsometatarsal joints by arthrodesis. *Foot Ankle* 4:193–200, 1990.

111. Aitken AP, Poulson D: Dislocations of the tarsometatarsal joints. *J Bone Joint Surg* 45A:246–260, 1963.

112. Hardcastle PH, Reschauer R, et al: Injuries to the tarsometatarsal joint: Incidence, classification, and treatment. *J Bone Joint Surg* 64B:349–356, 1982.

113. Cassebaum WH: Lisfranc fracture dislocations. *Clin Orthop* 30:116–128, 1963.

114. Gissane W: A dangerous type of fracture of the foot. *J Bone Joint Surg* 33B:535–538, 1951.

115. Arntz CT, Veith RG, Hansen ST: Fractures and fracture-dislocation of the tarsometatarsal joint. *J Bone Joint Surg* 70A:173–181, 1988.

116. Shereff MJ: Complex fractures of the metatarsals. *Orthopedics* 13:875–882, 1990.

117. Sammarco GJ, Carrasquillo HA: Intramedullary fixation of metatarsal fracture and nonunion: Two methods of treatment. *Orthop Clin North Am* 26:265–272, 1995.

118. Kavanaugh JH, Brower TD, et al: The Jones fracture revisited. *J Bone Joint Surg* 60A:776–782, 1978.

119. Torg JS, Balduini FC, et al: Fractures of the base of the fifth metatarsal distal to the tuberosity: Classification and guidelines for nonsurgical and surgical management. *J Bone Joint Surg* 66A:209–214, 1984.

120. Josefsson PO, Karlson M: Jones fracture: Surgical versus nonsurgical treatment. *Clin Orthop* 299:252–255, 1994.

121. Jahss MH: Stubbing injuries to the hallux. *Foot Ankle* 1:327–332, 1981.

122. Yasuda T, Fujio K, et al: Irreducible dorsal dislocation of the interphalangeal joint of the great toe: Report of two cases. *Foot Ankle* 10:331–336, 1990.

123. Jahss MH: Traumatic disorders of the first metatarsophalangeal joint. *Foot Ankle* 1:15–21, 1980.

124. Rao JP, Banzon MT: Irreducible dislocation of the metatarsophalangeal joints of the foot. *Clin Orthop* 145:224–226, 1979.

CHAPTER 32

Fractures and Dislocations in Children

Roger Dee, Wesley Carrion, Stuart Polisner, and Matthew F. Halsey

GENERAL CONSIDERATIONS

Fractures and fracture/dislocations are more common in children than ligament disruptions and uncomplicated dislocation. The skeletal tissues are more likely to fail. This tendency gradually reverses through the period of adolescence and no longer applies at physeal closure.

Children's bone is more porous and has wider haversian canals than adult bone and consequently has different biomechanical properties. Also, in children the periosteum is thicker and more elastic; therefore it may prevent completion of a tension fracture or limit displacement of bone in a complete fracture.[28,29] It provides a strong soft tissue hinge that helps maintain reduction. Occasionally a fragment of bone can become buttonholed through this strong periosteum, and this then impedes reduction. Juvenile periosteum creates ample callus.[28]

Classification

Certain unique modes of failure result after trauma in children (Fig. 32-1). Increased metaphyseal porosity permits the buckling typical of the *torus* fracture, which occurs as a result of compressive load. The localized outward buckling of the cortex may require several x-ray views for adequate visualization. Another pattern of children's fractures is the *greenstick* type, in which there is an incomplete fracture on the tension side of the bone but the cortex and periosteum remain intact on the compression side. Yet another pattern is *plastic deformation,* which occurs when the elastic limit is exceeded and an irreversible deformation occurs. This takes the form of a gentle bowing of the bone rather than a localized angulation. In the case of the forearm, the diagnosis may be missed, since one bone may be bowed and the other not. This contrasts with the char-

acteristic angular deformation usually seen with fractures of both bones of the forearm. None of these fracture types occurs in adult bone.[22,23,28,29]

Treatment

Angulated greenstick fractures may be reduced by appropriate manipulation. A slight manipulative overcorrection, stretching the intact periosteum, is used by some surgeons, who consider that there is otherwise a tendency to underreduce these fractures. The authors' preference is to reduce to a neutral position and then prevent subsequent recurrence of the deformity with the use of a well-molded cast. In the case of displaced or overriding fractures, it is necessary to have a very cooperative and relaxed patient. Regional blocks or local anesthesia with general analgesia is adequate in a calm patient. Usually, however, general anesthesia is required; this is also true for dislocations in children, when an atraumatic reduction is essential.

The usual techniques of manipulative reduction are used. These include, when necessary, the application of longitudinal traction to disimpact fragments. Sometimes an exaggeration of the deformity to hitch the ends of a fracture is helpful before the angulation is corrected and reduction achieved (Fig. 32-2). Rarely, an open reduction may be required in long bone fractures if good alignment is not achieved. This may be the case when a fragment is buttonholed through the periosteum or when there is plastic deformation. In the latter case, osteotomy and internal fixation in the corrected position may be required. This is occasionally the case in forearm bone fractures in older children. Use of the external fixator has been described, particularly in fractures of the lower limb, and the device is useful when skin loss or burns are associated.

As in adult fractures, cast wedging is an effective way of correcting minor degrees of malalignment.[6] Plastic wedges are commercially available in various sizes.[5] During the initial period of any cast immobilization, the neurovascular status of the extremity should be checked at regular intervals and immediately following any report of increasing discomfort. Unstable fractures should have serial x-ray examinations on a weekly basis for at least 3 weeks in the case of physeal injuries and for at least 6 weeks in diaphyseal fractures. Immobilization is continued until union is secure enough for ordinary gentle daily activities. A rule of thumb is that physeal healing requires approximately half the healing time required for the adjacent diaphysis to heal.[5] In general, for secure healing of physeal fractures, toddlers require 3 weeks, children 4

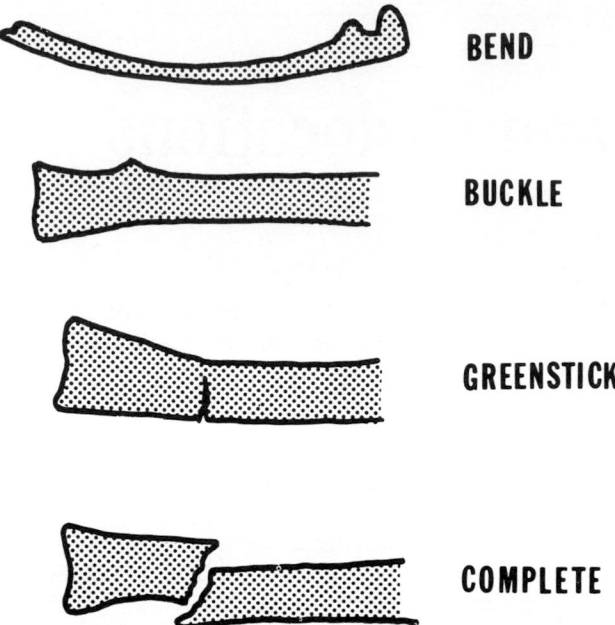

BEND

BUCKLE

GREENSTICK

COMPLETE

Figure 32-1 Patterns of injury in children's bones. From above downward they are plastic deformation, torus-type compression injury (buckling), greenstick fracture, and complete fracture. (Reproduced with permission from Rang M: *Children's Fractures,* 2d ed. Philadelphia, Lippincott, 1983.)

weeks, and adolescents 5 weeks of immobilization. These times may be approximately doubled for diaphyseal fractures, but the final determination is made by visualizing adequate bone callus on the x-ray film.

It may be hazardous to let young children use crutches because of their limited strength and coordination. If crutches are required, a three-point touchdown with partial weight bearing is safer and easier to perform than avoidance of weight bearing. Walkers and walkerettes are preferable, particularly in younger children.

Factors Affecting Fracture Healing in Children

Age The younger the child, the more rapid the healing[3,25,29] and the more complete the bony remodeling.[32] Furthermore, the younger the child, the greater the capacity to correct deformities (e.g., malunions) through growth.[32]

Nutrition Although malnutrition may retard healing, enhanced nutrition has not been proved to be an accelerator of healing.[5] A routine, well-rounded diet is adequate to allow normal healing. In children, calcium stores in the body are generally adequate to heal even multiple fractures. Supplemental calcium may promote hypercalciuria and the formation of kidney stones. Vitamin supplements in recommended daily doses are an innocuous adjunct if dietary deficiencies are suspected.

Mechanism of Injury The rate of healing is generally inversely proportional to the violence of the injury (e.g., the greater the violence, the slower the rate of healing).[6]

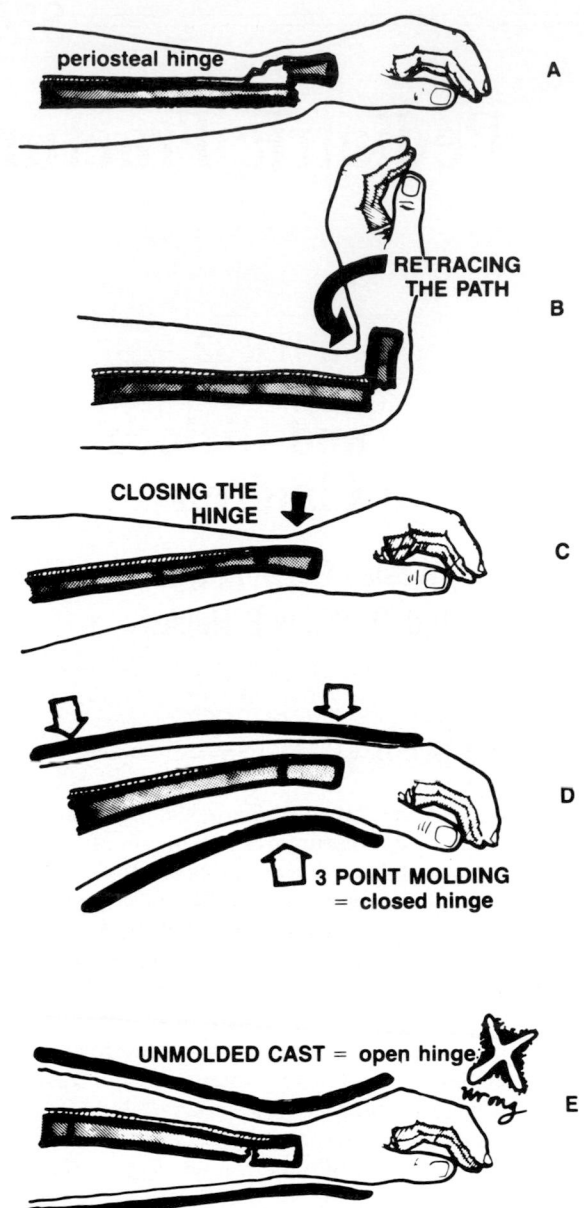

Figure 32-2 Use of intact soft tissue hinge to obtain and maintain reduction. *A.* The periosteum is usually intact on one side of a fracture, and it may prevent reduction when simple traction alone is attempted. *B* and *C.* Achieving reduction by retracing the path of the fracture, followed by closing the periosteal hinge. *D.* The cast should be applied with three-point molding in order to keep the periosteal hinge in tension and the fracture reduced. *E.* Failure to properly mold the cast allows the periosteal hinge to open, and loss of reduction may then occur. (Reproduced with permission from Rang M: *Children's Fractures,* 2d ed. Philadelphia, Lippincott, 1983.)

Type of Fracture Oblique and spiral fractures with relatively large areas of bone contact achieve functional union more quickly than transverse fractures. Separation of fracture fragments slows healing, although children fill in bony gaps faster than adults. With multiple or segmental fractures, healing tends to be slower in at least one fracture site.

Adjacent Injury The less the local soft tissue damage and damage to blood supply of bone and periosteum, the more rapid the healing.

Location of Fracture The closer the fracture is to a growth center, the more rapid the healing, the less abundant the callus, and the greater the remodeling potential. Conversely, the middiaphysis is the slowest-healing portion of the bone.[17]

Head Injury When a severe head injury accompanies the fracture, especially if spasticity or convulsions are associated, healing is rapid and callus abundant. Thus, realignment of the fracture without delay by closed or open means is essential to avoid malunion.

External Fixation External fixation of fractures appears to have a significant effect in delaying the healing of diaphyseal fractures. This may be associated with stress shielding of the fracture site and is more of a problem with a rigid frame than in a fixator that permits dynamization.[21] The negative effect on union is less apparent in children than in adults.[1]

Child Abuse

Green has pointed out the importance of identifying certain fracture patterns commonly associated with child abuse.[10] The child should be generally inspected for signs of bruising, burns, or lacerations, and any suspicion of abuse demands hospitalization. Evidence of multiple fractures throughout the body at different stages of healing is usually confirmatory of the diagnosis. Green points out that epiphyseal-metaphyseal fractures can be almost diagnostic of child abuse, but true physeal injuries are uncommon in child abuse except in the distal humerus, proximal humerus, and proximal femur. Fracture separation of the distal humeral physis, however, may occur in the newborn as a result of obstetric delivery.[2] Child abuse was documented or suspected in 6 of 16 distal humeral fractures seen in the series of Delee and coauthors.[7] Other injuries that should raise suspicion of child abuse include Salter type I injuries of the capital physis of the proximal femur with separation of the capital epiphysis and also a modified Salter type II injury to the proximal tibia. Instead of the usual triangular metaphyseal (Thurston-Holland) fragment there may be a semilunar type of slice taken off the rim of the metaphysis together with the epiphyseal separation. These "corner" or "bucket handle" fractures are associated with torsional as well as traction forces. Green points out that in the tibia, fractures of the diaphysis associated with direct blows are often transverse as opposed to the typical toddler's fracture, which is usually a spiral. In the infant femur, fractures of the shaft associated with child abuse may be transverse or spiral. If the fracture occurs in a child under the age of 1 year, there should be a strong suspicion of child abuse. In contrast, fractures of the tibial diaphysis are commonly associated with accidental falls.

Skeletal survey may reveal rib fractures or skull fractures, which may be multiple, further confirming the diagnosis.

Fracture Remodeling in Children

Children form rapid and abundant callus during closed fracture healing.[33] Callus formation is most impressive in the diaphysis of the bone. In subcutaneous loci (e.g., clavicular, tibial, metacarpal, and phalangeal shafts) where there is little soft tissue covering the exuberant fracture callus, the patient and parents should be forewarned of the visibility, and palpability, of the impending callus formation. This callus is often mistaken for a tumor or a malunion. Preparation of the family reduces unwarranted fears.

The younger the child, the more rapidly and completely the callus dissipates during the remodeling process. The majority of this remodeling occurs within the first 2 years after fracture healing. In prepubertal children, the callus generally disappears completely. In adolescents, the callus matures, smooths, and shrinks, leaving some permanent bony enlargement at the fracture site.[33] Remodeling is controlled by factors that determine the final shape and size of bones during growth. The following are important aspects of the remodeling process.

Bone Length Physeal stimulation causes a long bone to overgrow in length within the first 2 years after fracture.[13,32] This is probably due to the hyperemia of healing, which stimulates the adjacent growth plates.[11] In general, 0.5 to 1 cm of overgrowth can be expected,[8,13,24,31] although 2 cm of gain in length is common and there have been sporadic reported cases of 3 cm or more of overgrowth.[12,29] Overriding of the fracture ends of 1.5 cm can be compensated for in the femur; overgrowth is greatest for fractures in the proximal one-third, indicating that location is important.[14]

Angulation In prepubertal children, deformity of up to 30° may correct spontaneously in the sagittal plane (which is in the same plane as the movement of the adjacent joint), and up to 20° of correction may be achieved in the coronal plane.[14]

Rotation Although rotational correction does occasionally occur, it is generally minimal. Rotational correction is not to be expected with fracture remodeling in children.[18,32]

Translocation Partial side-to-side displacement or complete (bayonet) translocation corrects extremely well in growing children, especially in those who are prepubertal. This deformity generally remodels within 1 to 2 years after fracture, leaving no residual cosmetic or functional disability.

Physeal Injuries

Classification

Several anatomic classifications of physeal injury have been suggested. Such classifications are valuable in relating the anatomy of the fracture to the specific nature of the injury and they also offer some guide to prognosis.

The most commonly quoted classification is that of Salter and Harris.[27] They described five types of injury (Fig. 32-3):

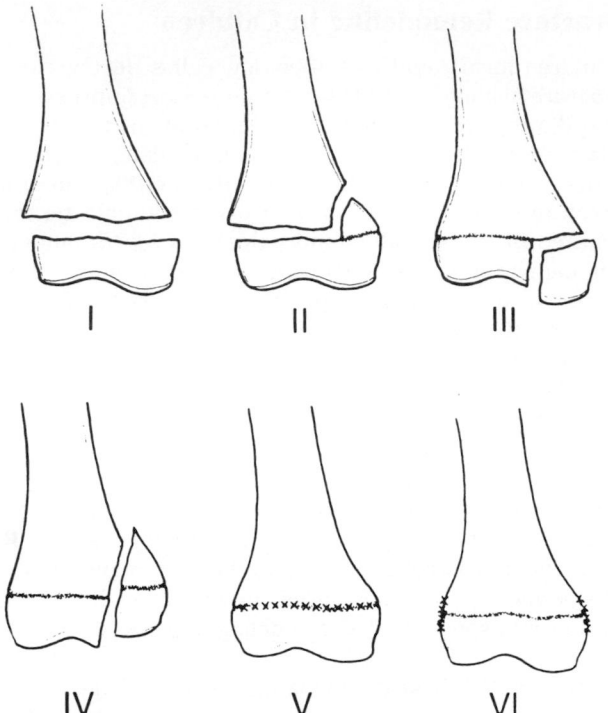

Figure 32-3 Salter's classification of physeal injuries with Rang's type VI added.

   Salter I: The fracture extends through the physis only.

   Salter II: The fracture extends through the physis and part of the metaphysis.

   Salter III: The fracture extends through the physis and the epiphysis.

   Salter IV: The fracture extends through the metaphysis, physis, and epiphysis.

   Salter V: Crush injury to the physis.

   Rang VI: Fracture through the perichondral ring.

(Reproduced with permission from Denton JR: *Orthop Rev* 12:130, 1983.)

1. Type I is a fracture in which a complete separation of the epiphysis from the metaphysis has occurred.
2. Type II is a fracture in which the fracture separation extends into the metaphysis and a triangular metaphyseal bony fragment remains attached to the epiphysis. The x-ray appearance of this fragment, of varying size, is termed the *Thurston-Holland sign*.
3. Type III is a fracture through the epiphysis from the articular surface.
4. Type IV is a vertical fracture through the epiphysis, the physis, and the metaphysis.
5. Type V is radiologically normal, a compression-type injury being inferred by delay or cessation of subsequent growth.

Rang suggests a sixth type (Fig. 32-3) when localized physeal injury to the perichondral rim (zone of Ranvier) occurs.[22]

   While the classification has been of great value, Ogden has suggested that it requires amplification to include additional important patterns of injury. The salient features of Ogden's categorization are summarized in the legend to Fig. 32-4.

Prognostic Considerations in Physeal Injuries

Injuries in this region may be complicated by subsequent growth abnormalities or joint incongruity. Growth may be temporarily or permanently retarded. Alternatively, a bony bar may form across a localized area of physeal damage either centrally or peripherally, causing the development of an angular growth deformity. If the bar is central, cupping of the metaphysis occurs, with relative shortening of the bone.[19]

   The Salter-Harris type IV injury is likely to lead to formation of a bony bar if it is displaced and unreduced. A similar potential, however, exists for type III fractures.[12,19,27] Although Blount believed that open reduction was rarely required in physeal injuries,[3] several modern authors believe that open reduction and anatomic reduction are essential for success in most type III and IV injuries that are displaced.[5,12] Kling and coworkers believe that type III fractures, particularly in the distal tibial physis, should be treated identically to type IV fractures with regard to the need for absolutely accurate reduction.[12] These authors believe that any residual gap, even the 2 mm often cited as acceptable, is too much to accept and may lead to subsequent growth abnormalities. These authors point out that in the region of the ankle, displacement in type II fractures may also be unacceptable and open reduction may be necessary. If reduction of a physeal fracture is delayed beyond 5 to 7 days, some authors recommend that it be permitted to heal, since operative intervention at that stage may interfere with early union between the cartilaginous portions of the physis and consequently encourage nonunion.[5]

   Even if one accepts the position of a type III fracture that is undisplaced, there is always the tendency to subsequent displacement during closed cast treatment, so repeated observation is necessary, particularly over the critical first week after the injury. If 2 mm is too much displacement, there is certainly little margin for error, and any displacement of an undisplaced injury indicates the need for open reduction, particularly in the region of the ankle joint.

   One of the problems is accurate assessment of the nature of the injury, and for this purpose standard radiographs are inadequate. For a fracture to be accepted as undisplaced or in a satisfactory position after closed reduction, not only must the physeal gap be closed but also any malrotation of the fragment must be restored.[12] Computed tomography (CT) and MRI have been recommended as useful in assessing these fractures.[34] Hypocycloidal tomography performed at 0.25- to 0.5-cm intervals with a growth plate perpendicular to the plane of the film is a useful technique for the early detection of a bony bar. Because of the configuration of the physis, both false-positive and false-negative findings may be obtained with standard tomography when looking for a bony bar.[19]

   The development of growth abnormalities can occur following all five types of Salter-Harris injury. Peterson has questioned whether in fact the type V injury ever occurs, pointing out that many factors can be responsible for the growth arrest following injury in the region of the physis. He believes that alterations in local blood flow associated with immobilization are of particular importance. He also

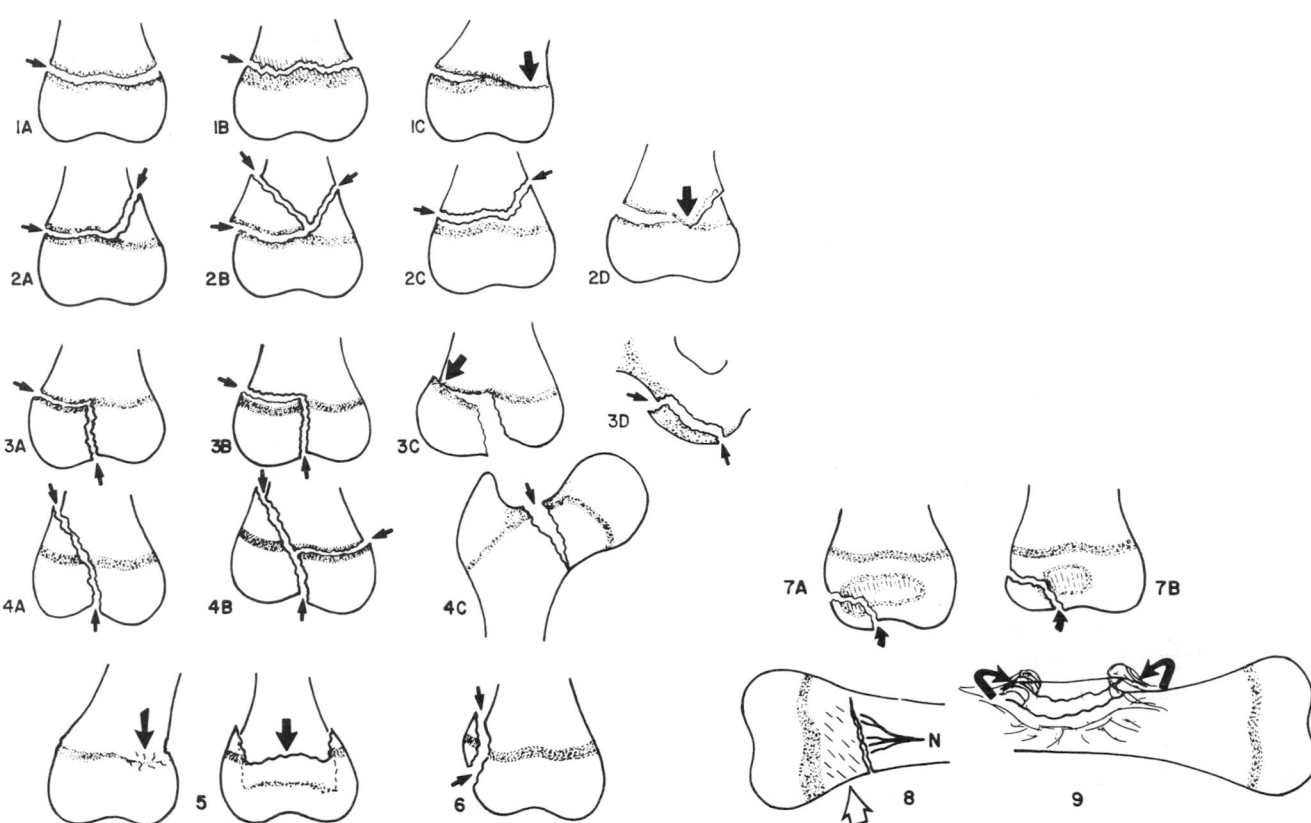

Figure 32-4 The revised classification of injuries in the region of the growth plate proposed by Ogden.

Type 1. This is a fracture through the hypertrophic zone and the zone of provisional calcification. In type 1B the fracture extends more deeply into the degenerating myeloproliferative diseases. In type 1C there is associated local damage to the germinal layer of the physis.

Type 2. This injury shows a large metaphyseal fragment (2A). The presence of this fragment is called the Thurston Holland sign. The periosteum is intact on the compression side. In type 2B there is a free metaphyseal fragment. In type 2C there is a smaller piece of metaphysis than in type 2A. In type 2D associated localized damage to the physis has occurred.

Type 3. This has a transverse fracture line through the physis at the same level as in type 1A. In type 3B this transverse fracture is through the primary spongiosa. In type 3C there is localized damage to the physis, and in type 3D a nonarticular epiphysis is avulsed from the metaphysis.

Type 4. This shows a vertical failure through all layers plus the secondary center of ossification when present. In type 4B there is in addition a transverse fracture causing an accompanying type 3 injury. In type 4C, commonly seen in the neck of the femur, there is a fracture through nonarticular cartilage, an injury which extends from the conjoint physis into the metaphysis.

Type 5. This shows a direct compression injury in which the radiographic appearance is normal but there may be disruption of the germinal layer. Other etiologies have been proposed to explain the consequent growth retardation (see text). It is possible for the metaphysis to be driven through the growth plate into the epiphysis.

Type 6. In this type there is involvement of the peripheral margin of the growth plate in the region of the zone of Ranvier. A localized contusion or slicing laceration may cause this lesion, which can produce a peripheral osseous bridge.

Type 7. This injury is a completely intraepiphyseal injury involving the secondary center of ossification. Type 7B is similar but extends entirely through cartilage and is consequently difficult to diagnose on x-ray films.

Type 8. This is a specialized type of injury in which there is interference with the metaphyseal growth and remodeling region associated with vascular damage. Epiphyseolysis may follow as a result of the temporary metaphyseal ischemia.

Type 9. In type 9 injury there is damage to the diaphyseal growth mechanisms that control appositional membraneous new bone formation. Direct trauma to the periosteum is the cause. (Reproduced with permission from Ogden JA: *J Pediatr Orthop* 2:371, 1982.)

points out that bony bars may develop following many types of physeal injury, e.g., electrical burns, frostbite, metabolic abnormality (vitamin A intoxication), infection, tumors, or irradiation, following the insertion of metal crossing the physis.

The Salter classification of the individual fracture is particularly important when internal fixation is required following open reduction. If there is a metaphyseal frag-

ment, it can be fixed without using pins that cross the physis. Transepiphyseal fixation can also be used. In the case of an unstable type I or type II fracture, as Bright points out, transphyseal pins are unfortunately inevitable, but they should be smooth, not threaded, and should be removed as soon as possible.[5,12] Removal of the metaphyseal fragment to permit visualization of the physis and its accurate reduction has been recommended.[5,12]

Other important facts concerning bony bars have been summarized by Peterson. He points out that although the distal radius is the most frequently injured physis, it is an uncommon site of a bony bar. The proximal tibia and distal femur account for only 3 percent of all physeal injuries but are responsible for the majority of bars. He suggests that the contour of the physis and its rate of growth or its size may be of significance and points out that at the knee, the physes are large in area and irregular in contour, accounting for most of the growth of their respective bones.[19]

The age of the patient and the proximity to skeletal maturity are important. Most type III fractures occur near skeletal maturity and, according to Peterson, they therefore rarely produce bony bars with much clinical deformity.[19] In a younger patient, with more growth remaining, the deformity may be considerable and require such measures as corrective osteotomy, leg lengthening, or contralateral epiphyseodesis for its control.

The treatment of leg-length inequality is dealt with elsewhere in this volume. With regard to the excision of bony bars, the technique varies depending on whether the bar is peripheral or central. A central bar may be approached through an opening in the metaphysis. A transepiphyseal approach is not used because it means transgressing the joint. Accurate localization using the techniques described is first necessary. The bar is best removed with a motorized burr (techniques have been well described by Peterson[19]).

Rehabilitation

A young child is usually his or her own best therapist.[5,22] However, range-of-motion exercises to the surrounding joints, followed by a stretching program and a progressive resistive strengthening program are useful in rapidly restoring normal function in the older child. With fractures that are prone to growth disturbance, degenerative joint changes, or avascular necrosis, reexamination with repeat x-ray films is indicated at 6-month intervals for approximately 2 years after injury.[5] Some surgeons recommend that physeal injuries be followed until skeletal maturity.

UPPER LIMB
Fractures of the Distal Radius and Ulna

The radius is the most commonly fractured bone in the child.[9] Three-quarters or more of these fractures involve the distal third because of the relative weakness of the distal radial metaphyseal bone.[12,71]

These fractures differ from their adult counterparts in that they are rarely intraarticular. Additionally, they usually do not show the radial collapse or radioulnar joint dysfunction that often results from similar adult fractures.[71]

Ossification

The distal radial epiphysis ossifies at 1 to 2 years and fuses at 16 to 18 years of age. The distal ulnar epiphysis ossifies at 5 to 7 years and fuses at 16 to 18 years of age.

Seventy-five percent of the radial and 80 percent of the ulnar longitudinal growth occurs at the distal end.[80]

Mechanism

The mechanism of injury is generally a fall on the outstretched hand with the wrist dorsiflexed.[8] Occasionally, the wrist is palmarflexed upon impact.[12,87]

Clinical Features

Nondisplaced torus or greenstick fractures exhibit tenderness over three-fourths the circumference of the distal radial metaphysis. Swelling is usually present, but it may be minimal. Displaced epiphyseal fractures are obvious and usually appear as a "silver fork" deformity, which may simulate a wrist dislocation. The skin should be carefully inspected for puncture wounds, which may communicate with the fracture. The neurovascular status should be assessed and documented prior to treatment.[71]

Radiologic Characteristics

Subtle fractures may be difficult to diagnose. Soft tissue (pronator quadratus) fat pad swelling may be the only obvious radiologic finding.[19] A torus fracture appears as a cortical bulge, often visible on only one x-ray view. Greenstick fractures may also reveal mild cortical angulation on one view only. The x-ray views in undisplaced physeal fractures may demonstrate only mild, asymmetrical widening of the physis (Fig. 32-5). Where there is doubt, oblique views and/or comparison x-ray views of the opposite wrist should be taken.

Treatment

Nondisplaced or nonangulated fractures are treated in a well-molded short arm cast for 6 weeks in teenagers (less in young children). In the case of infants, obese forearms, or potentially unstable fractures, a cast extending above the elbow is preferable.[45,72]

Fractures with an unacceptable degree of angulation (see "Complications," below) are treated by closed reduction. Hematoma infiltration anesthesia is usually adequate. If one elects to break the intact cortex, controlled force is used to avoid displacement of the fragments.[71] If the displacement of the epiphysis is in a pronated position, it should be splinted in supination after reduction. Usually the converse is the case.

Displaced (overriding) fractures are treated by closed reduction, usually under general anesthesia with muscle relaxation. Gentle traction is applied while the deformity is exaggerated to hook the ends together.[71,72,79] When end-to-end contact is established, angulation can be readily corrected. Displacement of less than 50 percent is acceptable. More should be reduced or the fracture will be prone to redisplacement. Somewhat more latitude is permissible in the child under 5 years of age, in whom general anesthesia is unwise and remodeling will occur.

Epiphyseal displacement should be reduced by applying gentle traction and then realigning the fragment,

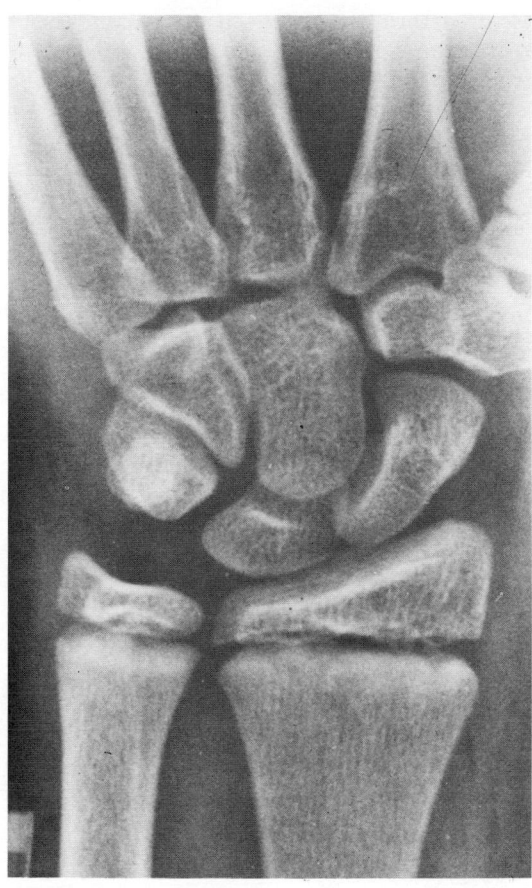

A

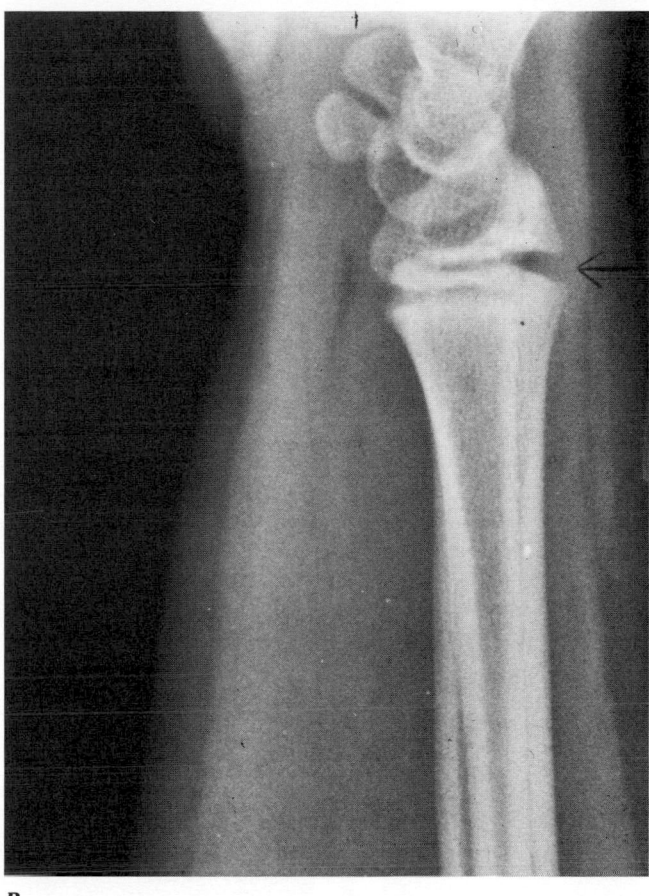

B

Figure 32-5 *A.* Anteroposterior x-ray view of a Salter I injury to the distal radial physis, which appears normal on this projection. The patient had pain, moderate swelling of the wrist, and ring tenderness over the distal radial physis. *B.* Widening of the dorsal aspect of the distal radial physis (*arrow*) on this lateral projection confirms the clinical diagnosis of a Salter I injury.

utilizing thumb pressure to correct the dorsal displacement. Pronation of the fragment is helpful. A long arm cast in some pronation and mild wrist flexion with good three-point molding is indicated for 2 to 3 weeks, followed by a short arm cast until the fracture is healed. Undisplaced physeal fractures are protected in a short arm cast until united.

Open reduction is rarely indicated. Occasional case reports of irreducible fractures have involved interposition of tendons (e.g., extensor pollicis longus)[85] and buttonholing of the distal radial metaphysis through the volar wrist supports.[60] These special fractures required open reduction and internal fixation.

Complications

Strength and motion are usually restored with simple rehabilitation. Growth disturbances are rare.[94] Deformity in the place of motion of the wrist joint usually remodels completely if it is less than 45° in very young children, less than 30° in prepubertal children,[94] and less than 15° in growing teenagers.[72] Fractures of the distal radius correct at approximately 1° per month or about 10° per year

as a result of epiphyseal realignment during growth. Radial or ulnar angulation has less remodeling capacity. Rotational deformities have little or no remodeling potential.[33–35] In summary, the younger the child and the closer the fracture to the physis, the greater the remodeling capacity.

Fractures of the Radial and Ulnar Diaphysis

Mechanism

The mechanism of injury is usually a fall on the outstretched hand,[48] often with a rotatory component. Direct contusion is a less common cause.[90] Propagation of diaphyseal fractures requires greater force than propagation of metaphyseal or physeal fractures.

Clinical Features

There is usually considerable pain and swelling. Clinical deformity is usually obvious. Undisplaced fractures and those caused by plastic deformation (bowing) may go undiagnosed.[54]

Radiologic Characteristics

Care should be taken to assess the fracture site as well as the adjacent joints. Ipsilateral fractures of the distal end of radius and ulna or of the navicular may be overlooked.[54,72]

The bicipital tuberosity reveals the rotational alignment of the proximal radius, while the distal radius can be assessed clinically or radiographically.[72,79] Dissimilar shapes and diameters of opposing bone ends suggest rotational malalignment.[54]

Treatment

Cosmesis and function are both important. Functional recovery includes full restoration of wrist and elbow motion, forearm rotation, and upper extremity strength.

Nondisplaced greenstick fractures require a well-molded long arm cast until healed. When firm but cautious manipu-

lation is used, the angulated greenstick fractures can be corrected without separating the remaining intact cortex and rendering the fracture unstable.[20,44,77,91] The cast must be applied with good three-point molding to prevent reangulation. The elbow is maintained at 90° and the forearm supinated if the angulation is dorsal and pronated if volar.

Complete fractures (overriding) require gentle traction and exaggeration of the deformity to hook the ends; then correction of the angulation and rotation is attempted. The distal fragments are rotated to match the rotation of the proximal fragments.[32,54] Adequate anesthesia with relaxation of the patient is essential. The normal radial curve must be maintained (the ulna is relatively straight) to provide forearm shape and rotation. Casts with a flat ulnar borders avoid gravitational sag of the ulna.

In prepubertal children, bayoneted positioning is compatible with a satisfactory result as long as alignment and rotation are normal[79] and the interosseous space is maintained on at least one view.[32] Such is not the case in ado-

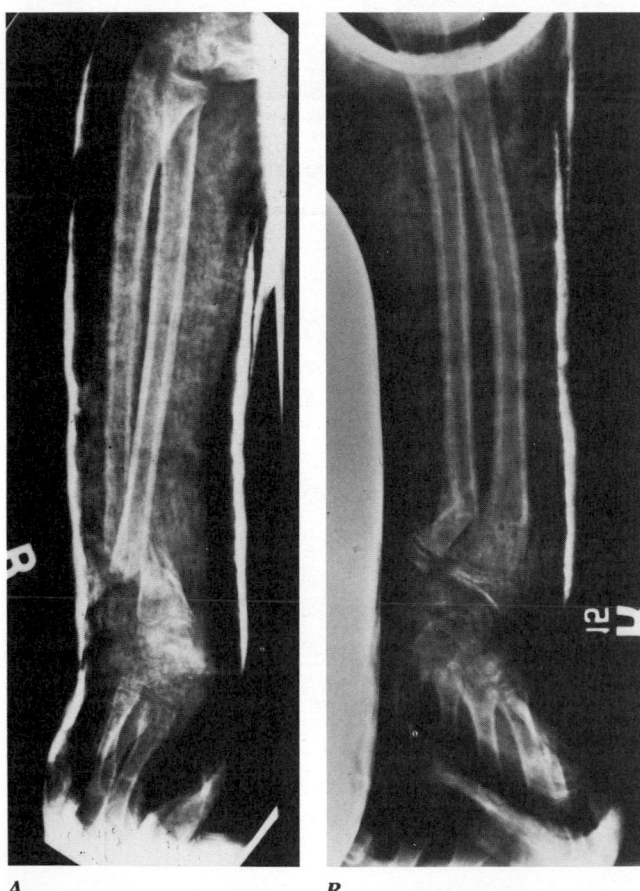

A

B

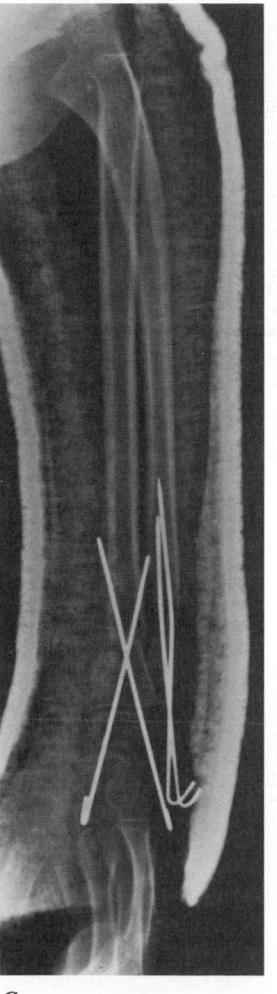

C

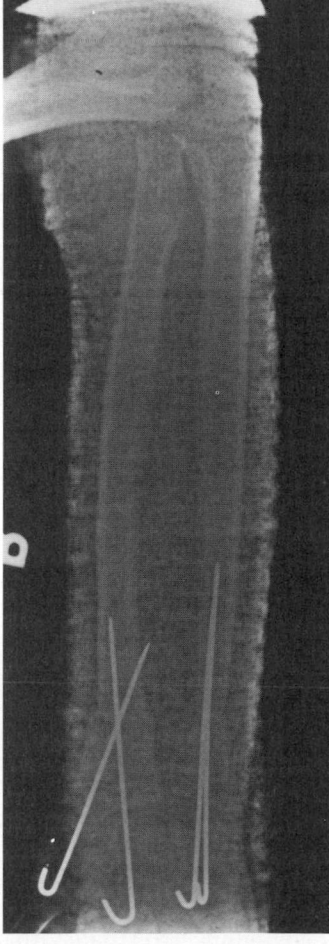

D

Figure 32-6 *A* and *B*. This 10-year-old patient was referred 3 weeks after reduction with fracture of both bones of the forearm. There is considerable volar displacement, and ulnar angulation exceeds 20°. *C* and *D*. Additional closed manipulation

at this stage was not indicated. Open reduction and percutaneous pinning maintained alignment, the pins being removed at 3 weeks. A cast was applied for a total of 6 weeks. Excellent forearm rotation was restored.

lescents who, with little or no growth remaining, will lose some forearm rotation unless reduction is excellent. This is particularly the case in the proximal radius, where any angulation will probably impair motions in the older age group. Weekly follow-up with radiographs and excellent cast maintenance is necessary.

If acceptable reduction is not achieved or maintained, open reduction and internal fixation are recommended in patients over the age of 10 years. There is a high incidence of failure of closed treatment beyond prepuberty[51] (Fig. 32-6). Other indications for open reduction include open fractures with severe soft tissue injury.

In a heavily contaminated open fracture or in the presence of severe soft tissue loss, the external fixator is an alternative. When early stabilizing callus is present, the fixator may be removed and replaced with a well-molded long arm cast until healed. Amit et al. report on the successful use of closed intramedullary nailing of this fracture in adolescents.[4]

Special Types of Forearm Fractures

Plastic Deformation

These "bent bones" without cortical buckling or obvious fracture occur only in prepubertal children and are often overlooked. Occasionally only one bone bows, the other bone of the forearm remaining perfectly straight, or alternatively the accompanying bone is fractured (or the radial head dislocates).

The mechanism of injury is a fall creating a slowly applied, low-energy force causing the bone to bend beyond its elastic limits.[48] The force terminates prior to the propagation of a fracture line, resulting in an abnormally curved bone that deforms the forearm (Fig. 32-7).

Pain, tenderness, and subtle deformity of the forearm are typically present. Pronation and supination may be limited by pain or degree of deformity. Swelling may be minimal.

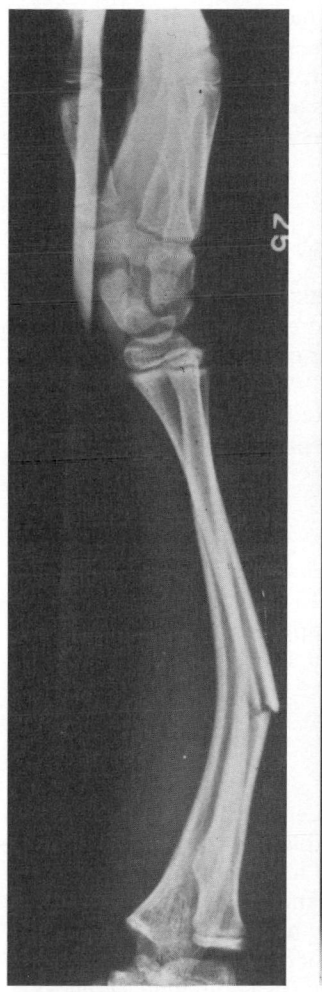
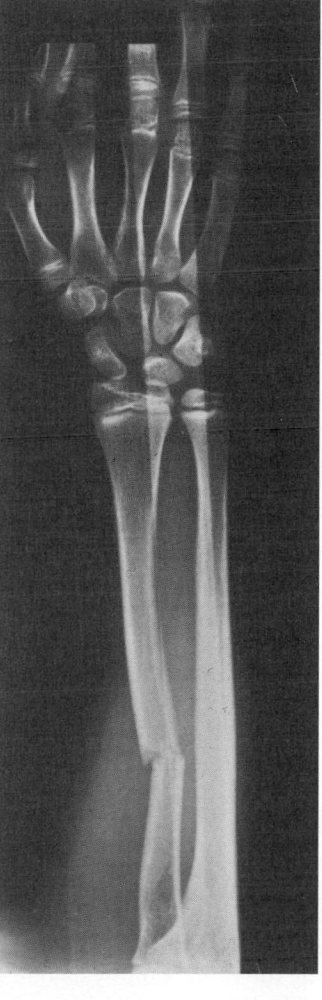
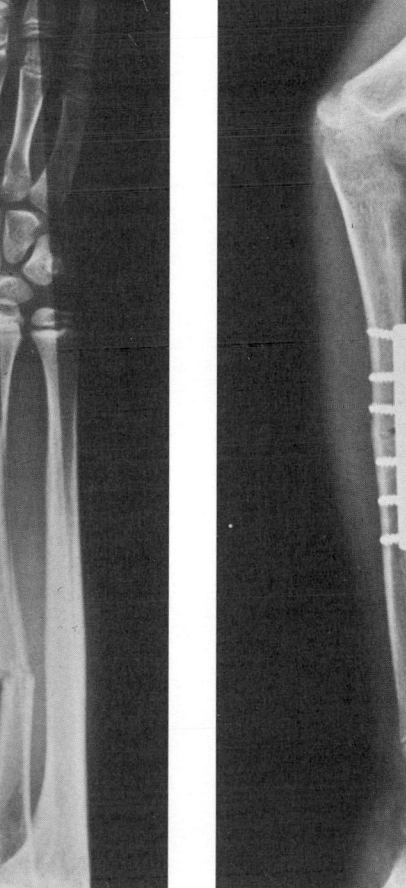
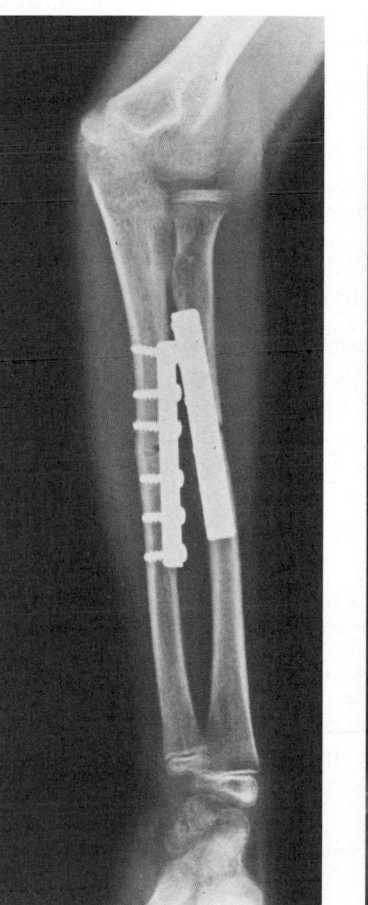
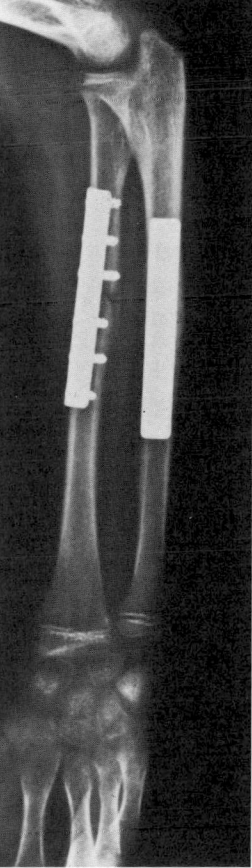

A   B   C   D

Figure 32-7 *A* and *B*. Plastic deformation of the ulna associated with midshaft fracture of the radius in a 10-year-old. Note that ulna looks straight on the oblique AP view (*B*), but the radial fragments are rotated and the interosseous space is lost.

C and *D*. Closed osteoclasis consisting of gentle slow pressure applied for several minutes did not correct bowing. Open osteotomy and internal fixation were required.

If there is doubt, comparison views of the opposite forearm in the same rotation are helpful. X-ray views should include the elbow and wrist to rule out associated injuries. A positive bone scan differentiates an acute bowing from residual deformation following previous injury.[63] During healing, periosteal reaction may be minimal or absent. At 4 to 6 weeks, cortical thickening may be evident on the concavity of the bowed bone.

If the deformity is obvious or if there is restriction of forearm rotation, reduction is indicated. With the patient under anesthesia, a corrective force is applied progressively over several minutes, preferably over a firm fulcrum. Children under 4 years of age usually remodel mild to moderate degrees of bowing spontaneously.[81] Parents should be forewarned that fracturing the bone may be necessary in order to achieve a reduction. In older children, osteotomy may sometimes be required (Fig. 32-7). Usually correction can be achieved by osteotomizing at one level only, at the point of maximal bowing. A small wedge of bone is removed to correct the angulation, and internal fixation may be necessary.

Monteggia's Fracture/Dislocation

This lesion, describe in 1814 by Monteggia, is a proximal ulnar fracture with an associated radial head dislocation.[79] Bado's classification of this fracture is shown in Table 32-1. In children, the Bado type I injury is most common.[31] Also, a "Monteggia equivalent" injury has been reported in children; it consists of a proximal ulnar fracture associated with a lateral humeral condylar fracture.[81] Another equivalent consists of anterior radial head dislocation and plastic bowing of the ulna.

Treatment If the ulnar fracture is transverse, closed reduction and above-elbow casting in the position of radial

---

TABLE 32-1   Bado's Classification of Monteggia Fracture Dislocations

---

Type I
  a. Anterior radial head dislocation
  b. Fracture of the ulnar shaft at any level with anterior angulation

Type II
  a. Posterior or posterolateral radial head dislocation
  b. Fracture of the ulnar shaft with posterior angulation

Type III
  a. Lateral or anterolateral radial head dislocation
  b. Fracture of the ulnar metaphysis

Type IV
  a. Anterior radial head dislocation
  b. Fracture of the proximal radius and ulna at the same level

---

Source: Reproduced with permission from Bado JL: *Clin Orthop* 50:71–86, 1967.

head stability is sufficient. Open reduction is necessary for oblique fractures that are unstable, with plate or K-wire fixation.[31] In late cases corrective osteotomy of the ulna, cleaning out of the radial notch, annular ligament reconstruction, and K-wire stabilization of the radial capitellar joint may be necessary.[31]

Galeazzi Lesion

The true Galeazzi lesion, which is a fracture of the distal shaft of the radius with a dislocation of the distal radioulnar joint, is rare in children. When it occurs in young children, it can be treated by closed reduction and casting, while open reduction is required in adolescents.

Complications of Children's Forearm Fractures

Malunion of fractures is unfortunately a common complication. With adequate immobilization and avoidance of rotational or angular malalignment, union may be expected without functional loss.[51] Refracture of both bones at the same site is common (7 percent) during the first 6 months after fracture.[98] Nerve injuries have been reported and are usually transitory. Compartment syndromes may occur and must be diagnosed and treated immediately. If this is not the case, ischemic necrosis of the forearm muscles will produce Volkmann changes, resulting in a claw hand.

Fractures of the Proximal Radius

Fractures of the proximal radius usually involve the radial neck at the physis but may be greenstick fractures through the metaphysis in very young children. Several patterns are possible (Salter types I to IV), but a type II Salter fracture is most common.[103] Related fractures occur simultaneously about the elbow in 50 percent of cases.[79]

Ossification

The proximal radial epiphysis ossifies at 4 to 5 years and fuses at 14 to 15 (female) and 15 to 17 (male) years of age. The proximal ulnar apophysis appears in the eight to tenth year and fuses at about 12 to 14 (female) and 14 to 15 (male) years of age.[95]

Mechanism

The mechanism of injury is generally a valgus force to the elbow, creating a radiocapitellar impaction. The resulting deformity of the head may be angulation or displacement. With this mechanism, it tilts laterally and displaces outward. In another mechanism, a posterior subluxation of the elbow occurs and then reduces, leaving the radial epiphysis behind the capitellum, often with a 90° backward tilt. Some fractures occur in association with other injuries, such as damage to the medial collateral ligament of the elbow or medial humeral condyle. The whole injury and its mechanism must be carefully evaluated.

Clinical Features

Nondisplaced fractures are often diagnosed and treated late. The parents may be unimpressed with the appearance of the arm or the magnitude of the complaints, and the pain is often referred to the wrist. Proximal radial pain is elicited while gently pronating and supinating the forearm or during active wrist dorsiflexion.

Radiologic Characteristics

X-ray views should include the entire elbow, forearm, and wrist to rule out associated fractures and dislocations. Oblique and/or comparison views are often helpful in diagnosing undisplaced fractures.[38] When the radial head is nonossified, the only radiographic sign may be irregularity of the adjacent metaphyseal border.[70] If a displaced, unossified radial head fracture is suspected, an arthrogram using a few drops of dye may be indicated. Magnetic resonance imaging may prove useful in difficult cases.

Treatment

When the appropriate treatment is selected, the degree and type of displacement, presence of associated injuries, age of the patient, and time elapsed from injury should be taken into consideration.[70,100,103]

A long arm cast is adequate for most nondisplaced or nonangulated fractures. Slings, collar cuffs, and posterior splints are usually inadequate for immobilization in children.

Manipulative closed reduction is indicated for angulated (or translocated) fractures.[89] Although untreated fractures angulated up to 45 to 60° will generally remodel to a remarkable degree in the prepubertal child,[13,101] angulations over 30° should be corrected manipulatively.[72,103] Manipulative technique is based on application of a varus stress to open the lateral side of the joint. The forearm is pronated and supinated to palpate the radial head at its maximum prominence, then digital pressure is applied to the radial head. A well-molded long arm cast is applied with the elbow at 90°. The amount of pronation or supination is determined by the position of stability and the radiographic appearance of the radiocapitellar joint. When in doubt, one uses moderate pronation, as this is the motion that is generally lost after healing.

Open reduction is required for completely displaced fractures or when closed reduction is considered inadequate. Internal fixation can be avoided if a stable reduction is obtained. When required, oblique K wires that do not cross the radiocapitellar joint should be used.

Complications

Radial head excision should be avoided in growing children, since complications include stiffness, proximal radioulnar synostosis, cubitus valgus, and distal radioulnar joint derangement.[72,89,101,103]

Other complications following this injury include growth abnormalities such as overgrowth or premature physeal closure. Posterior interosseous nerve palsy may follow use of K wire. Pin breakage or migration may follow use of radiohumeral transfixion wires to maintain reduction. Heterotopic calcification, myositis ossificans, and proximal radioulnar synostosis have also been reported.

Fractures of the Proximal Ulna

Fractures of the proximal ulna are extremely rare in isolation. They are usually associated with other fractures or dislocation at the elbow.

Ossification

The proximal ulnar apophysis appears in the eighth to tenth year and fuses at 14 to 15 (female) and 15 to 17 (male) years of age.

Mechanism

The mechanisms of injury are direct trauma to the point of the elbow and indirect forces that occur during a fall on the hand with the elbow extended.

Classification

Apophyseal fractures (Fig. 32-8) are rare, since the triceps expansion protects this area, attaching distally beyond the apophysis. A Salter type II physeal separation may occur and not be visible radiographically before 10 years of age. Careful palpation may reveal the metaphyseal irregularity. The fracture line may extend through the cartilage of the proximal ulna, so that the coronoid is also part of the proximal fragment.

The varieties of *metaphyseal* fractures depend on elbow position at injury.

In flexion, the triceps posteriorly and the brachialis anteriorly apply tension, while the distal humerus is the fulcrum over which the ulna breaks.

In extension, if an abduction or adduction force occurs with the olecranon locked in its humeral fossa, the proximal ulna may fail. With associated valgus stress, this olecranon fracture is associated with a radial neck or medial humeral epicondylar fracture. With varus stress in extension, an olecranon fracture occurs with radial head displacement.[103] The olecranon fracture is commonly an angulated greenstick fracture.

Coronoid fractures are rare in children. They are usually associated with elbow dislocations and are thus seen in older children. As an isolated fracture, they occur as a result of an avulsion of the brachialis tendon. Radiographically, the radial head may overlay the coronoid process, necessitating oblique views for diagnosis.

Clinical Features

Physical examination reveals a palpable olecranon gap if displacement has occurred. Extension may be weak or absent if the triceps tendon is injured or interrupted.

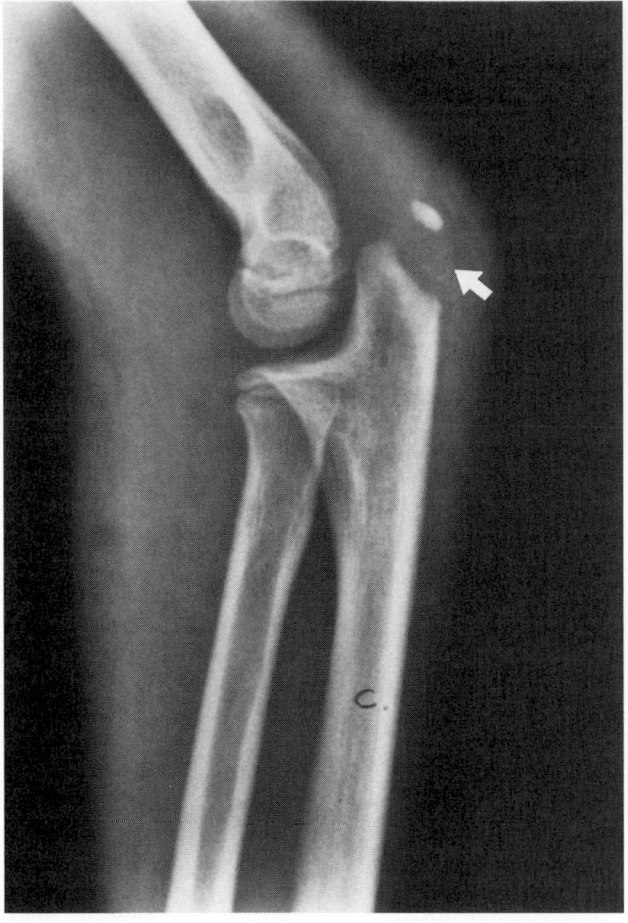

A

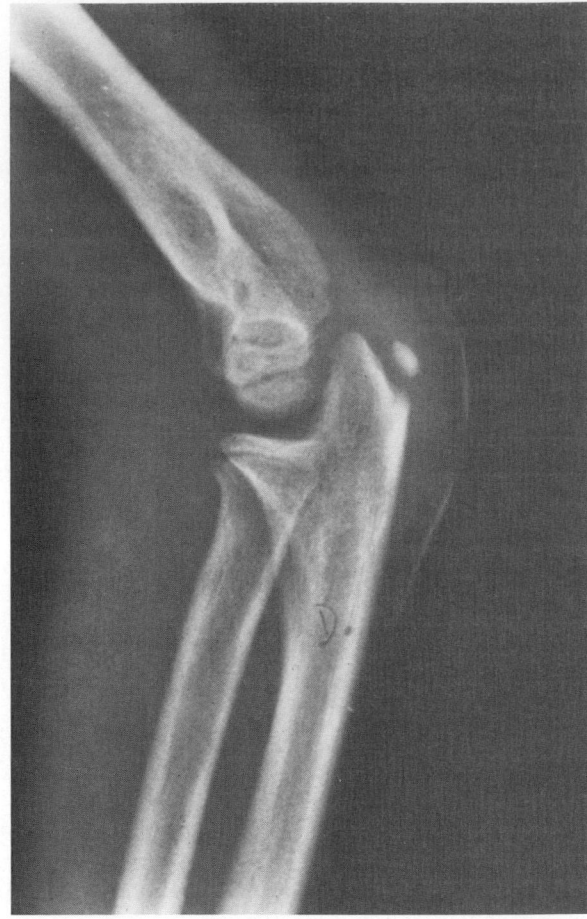

B

Figure 32-8 *A.* A young boy fell with his elbow extended and sustained an avulsion fracture of the olecranon apophysis. Despite some proximal displacement, triceps function remained intact. Note metaphyseal flake (*arrow*). *B.* The fracture was reduced by extension of the elbow with direct thumb pressure. A long arm cast was then applied with the elbow in mild flexion. A pressure pad was used over the tip of the olecranon within the cast.

Radiologic Characteristics

Associated elbow fractures and dislocations must be ruled out. Oblique x-ray and comparison views of the opposite elbow are helpful. When the olecranon apophysis is nonossified (before age 10 years), the diagnosis must be made clinically. A small metaphyseal spike may be palpable.

Treatment

Apophyseal fractures, if undisplaced or mildly displaced, are immobilized in a long arm cast in moderate extension (30 to 45°) to avoid triceps or capsular tension. If the fracture is displaced significantly, open reduction and internal fixation with axial pins and compression wires are indicated.

Metaphyseal fractures are treated with consideration given to the mechanism of injury. Flexion at the fracture reduces any greenstick angulation caused by hyperextension. Varus or valgus angulation is corrected by manipulation with the elbow in full extension, locking the olecranon. Varus deformity and radial head dislocation have a tendency to recur; close observation and follow-up are necessary. With moderate or no displacement, a well-molded long arm cast is applied with elbow flexion of no more than 60°. Displacement of more than 2 mm at the joint surface requires open reduction and internal fixation. Repair of the aponeurosis and tension banding are sufficient to maintain reduction. Crossing the physis with fixation pins should be avoided.

Coronoid fractures are immobilized in a long arm cast with the arm at 90°. This fracture may indicate the presence of a spontaneously reduced elbow dislocation. A careful watch for heterotopic new bone is indicated, and rehabilitation should be gentle and unhurried.

Dislocation of the Elbow

Elbow dislocation is a common injury in children. Children rarely develop a pure dislocation of the elbow or radial head without an associated fracture. Most common is a fracture of the medial epicondyle, which may become entrapped in the joint, blocking reduction.

Classification

The most common mechanism of injury is a valgus force in extension. This disrupts the medial collateral ligament or avulses the medial epicondyle, permitting valgus angulation. Posterior dislocation then occurs, the forearm bones usually being displaced posterolaterally. There is associated stripping of the capsule from the posterior distal humerus.[61] Occasionally the elbow is disrupted by a varus or medial displacement force and the forarm bones lie posteromedially. In both types the lateral ligament complex and medial collateral ligament are disrupted.

Anterior dislocation is unusual but can occur and is associated with the highest incidence of complications. Dislocation of the elbow joint can occur, associated with disruptions of the superior radioulnar joint ("divergent" type).

Clinical Features

The elbow is held semiflexed. With posterior dislocation, there is an undue prominence of the olecranon.[72] The dislocation is then obvious. Prior to radiologic evaluation, this may be confused with a displaced supracondylar fracture, especially when there is considerable swelling.

Radiologic Characteristics

Pre- and postreduction x-ray views should be closely examined for associated avulsion fractures and fragments that have become trapped in the joint.[30,77] Increased joint space indicates probable interposed fragments.

These dislocations should be considered unstable, and weekly x-ray films should be taken for the first month to confirm reduction. The radial head must oppose the capitellum on all views, or subluxation is present.[59,75]

Treatment

Most elbow dislocations can be reduced closed with adequate anesthesia and relation. Reduction should be performed expeditiously to avoid vascular compromise. Open reduction may be required because of fragment entrapment or continuing instability.

Posterior dislocations are reduced by applying gentle traction with the forearm supinated, avoiding full extension, which may cause further soft tissue injury anteriorly. Digital pressure over the posterior olecranon may be added to help direct the ulna anteriorly onto the humerus, while distal humeral pressure is directed posteriorly. Finally, pronation and supination may assist in and confirm location of the radial head. Following reduction, the elbow should be casted in flexion at 100°.[77]

Anterior dislocations have the highest incidence of complications. Reduction is by flexing the elbow, applying gentle traction, and using the forearm as a lever to reduce the proximal radius and ulna posteriorly. Posterior support under the distal humerus is helpful. Postreduction immobilization is at minimal flexion (approximately 45°), since this is a flexion injury.

True medial or lateral dislocations are extremely rare in children. Longitudinal traction is utilized to dislodge the proximal radius and ulna while regaining proper length. Medial or lateral force is then applied to restore proper positions. Correction is maintained by careful molding in the cast with the elbow at 90°.

Divergent dislocations are also extremely rare in children. Reduction is effected by longitudinal traction on the semiextended elbow, correcting the divergence by gentle compression. The position is held with cast molding and the elbow at 90°. Open reduction and internal fixation may be required.[18]

Meticulous casting techniques with close follow-up are important in order to maintain the reduction. The elbow is usually immobilized for 3 to 4 weeks, but a recent study has recommended a shorter period of immobilization.[16]

Complications

Among possible complications,[19,29,49,77–79,103] vascular injuries are uncommon in children. Recurrent dislocation is quite rare. Neurologic injuries are common (particularly of the ulnar nerve). Myositis ossificans is fortunately uncommon but is a disastrous complication. Overenthusiastic physiotherapy and particularly manipulation and passive motion are traditionally thought to contribute in some cases. Such prescriptions are best avoided. Residual stiffness or posterior blocking of full extension by heterotopic new bone often improves dramatically with time and *gentle* but active use.

Isolated Dislocation of the Radial Head

Isolated dislocation of the radial head in children is uncommon, especially in those over 10 years of age. The traumatic dislocation in children is usually anterior (Fig. 32-9).

Mechanism

The usual mode of injury is a fall on the outstretched hand with the forearm locked in pronation. Occasionally, isolated radial head dislocation is produced by a direct blow to the proximal forearm. The common mechanism is believed to be similar to that which occurs during Monteggia's fracture/dislocation.[40] Wiley's anatomic studies led him to believe that the annular ligament is the most important structure torn in isolated dislocations of the radial head.[102] There may be occult plastic deformation of the ulna, and some cases of "congenital" radial head dislocation are possibly sequelae of injuries overlooked in early childhood.

Clinical Features

Localized swelling and tenderness over the anterior or posterolateral aspect of the elbow are present, depending on the direction of dislocation. Elbow motion may be limited, especially rotation of the forearm. The radial head may be palpable in the antecubital space in cases of anterior dislocation.

Radiologic Characteristics

In the absence of an obvious fracture line, a radial head dislocation may easily be missed. A line through the radial

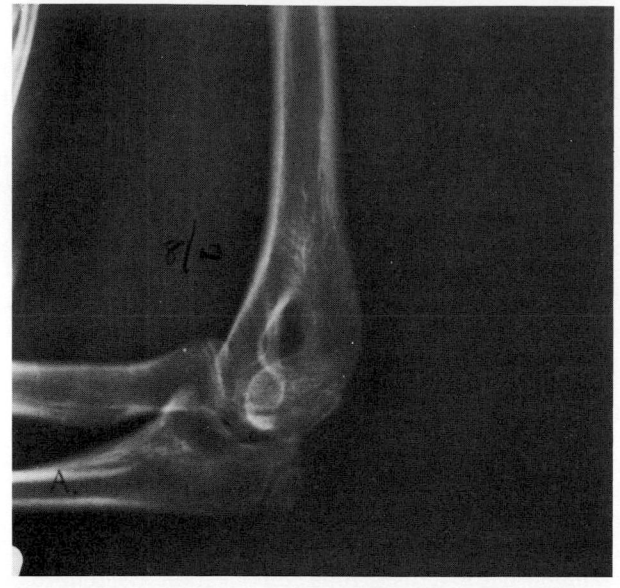

A

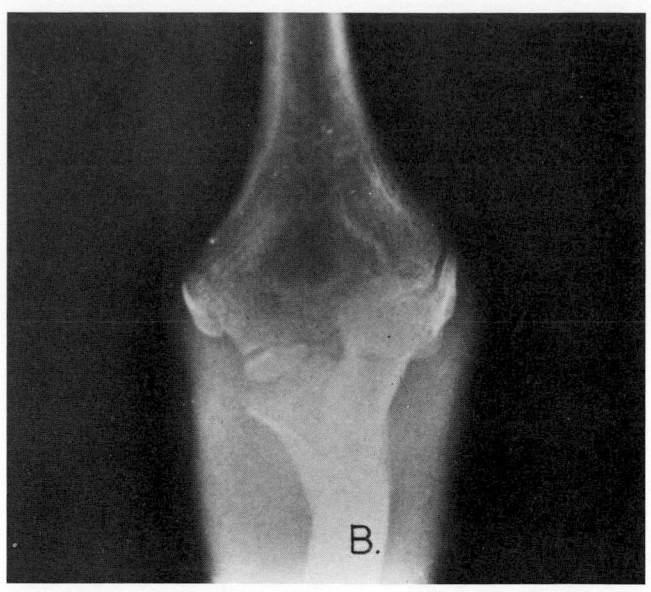

B

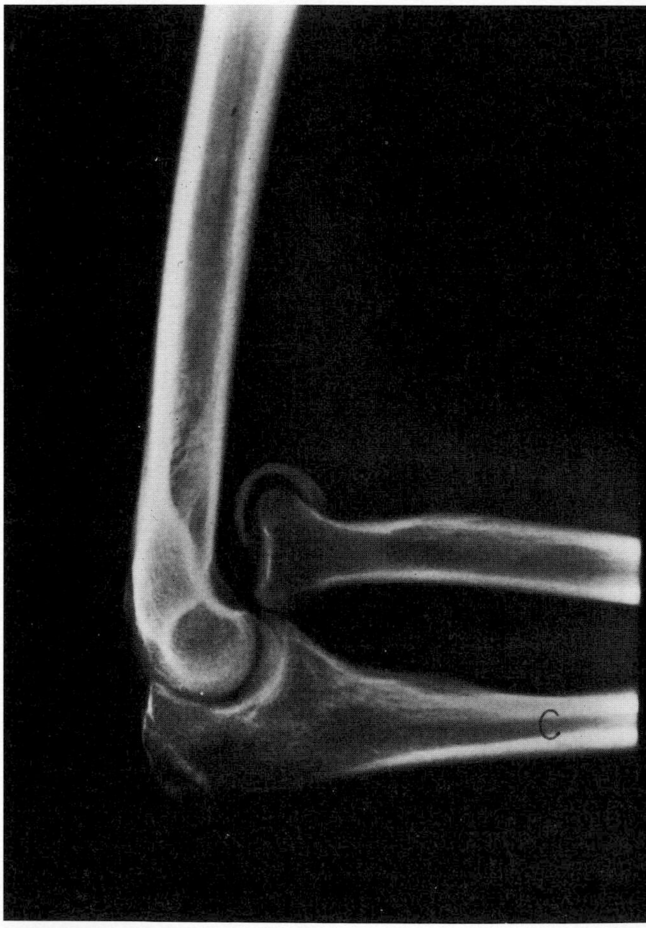

C

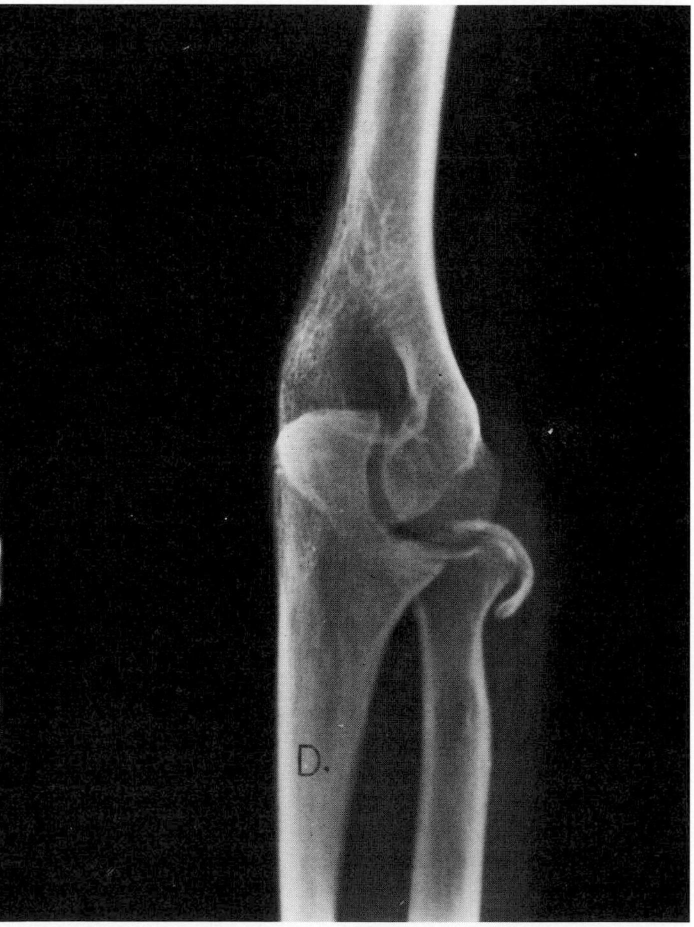

D

Figure 32-9 Anterior radial head dislocation in an 11-year-old girl who sustained a direct blow to the posterior aspect of the upper forearm and elbow. *A* and *B*. Anterior dislocation of the radial head was overlooked on these initial radiographs. If the radiocapitellar line were to be drawn through the radial shaft, it would cross superior to the capitellum. The patient was not seen by an orthopaedist until several months later and was minimally symptomatic. *C* and *D*. At 2 years after injury, the patient remained only mildly symptomatic. Note the ringlike calcification of the soft tissues overlying the dislocated radial head.

shaft should normally pass through the capitellum on every x-ray view.[59,75] If this radiocapitellar line is disrupted, a subluxation or dislocation of the radial head is present (Fig. 32-9A and C). An associated occult fracture of the proximal ulna may not be apparent until healing callus is detected 2 to 3 weeks later.

Treatment

Acute anterior dislocation of the radial head is generally reducible by supination of the forearm with traction on the extended elbow. Downward (anterior to posterior) pressure against the radial head will assist a difficult reduction. The elbow should then be immobilized, flexed slightly less than 90°, and the forearm supinated. In cases where treatment is delayed a week or more, open reduction is indicated if closed reduction fails. Open reduction is worth the attempt even late, at 6 to 8 weeks, but then reconstruction of the annular ligament may be required.

Complications

If the dislocation is untreated, restriction of joint motion may result, but often there is little functional loss. In preadolescents, shortening of the radial side of the forearm may occur, with distal radioulnar joint distortion. The anteriorly displaced radial head may articulate with the distal humerus, creating a localized pseudarthrosis (Fig. 32-9C and D).

Pulled Elbow

Pulled elbow, nursemaid's elbow, radiocapitellar subluxation, subluxation of the radial head, and temper-tantrum elbow are among 18 names for this entity as listed by Salter and Zaltz in 1971.[88] It is probably the commonest musculoskeletal injury in children under 5 years of age. It is found more commonly in boys and more often affects the left elbow.

Mechanism

The mechanism of injury is forcible traction on the pronated hand or wrist with the relaxed elbow extended. Frequently, the traction force occurs when the child suddenly decides to pull away from the parents or drop to the ground. Often a click or snap may be felt or heard.

Pathologic Characteristics

Salter and Zaltz found experimentally that if traction is applied to a pronated forearm with the elbow extended, a transverse tear of the distal attachment of the annular ligament results, allowing partial escape of the radial head.[88] Subluxation of the radial head occurs only in pronation, which is the position where the diameter of the radial head is the narrowest in the anteroposterior plane. Supination of the forearm with some flexion of the elbow allows instantaneous reduction of the radial head.

Clinical Features

The child may be tearful, and the arm hangs limply with the elbow extended and the forearm pronated. Pain, if localized, is sometimes referred to the wrist. There is tenderness over the radial head but no obvious swelling or deformity. Mild flexion and extension are painless, but supination is resisted.

Radiologic Characteristics

X-ray studies are invariably negative but should still be obtained to rule out fracture or other abnormality.

Treatment

Frequently, pulled elbow reduces spontaneously when the elbow is placed in a sling or when the x-ray technician attempts to position the forearm in extension. Reduction is accomplished by firmly supinating the forearm, applying downward (anterior to posterior) radial head pressure, then flexing the elbow to slightly beyond 90°. If reduction is successful, within a few minutes, when the child's confidence returns, full elbow motion and forearm rotation are present. In older children (e.g., 3 to 5 years), or when the elbow had been subluxed for many hours, a sling or cast should be applied in the position noted above for several days, since all the discomfort will not resolve immediately. In a rare resistant case, the child does not respond in the predicted manner. Usually spontaneous reduction occurs within a few days, however, without further intervention.

In cases of recurrent subluxation, a splint or cast may be used for several weeks to encourage stability. The parents should be counseled to avoid longitudinal traction strains on the child's arms by not pulling on the hands or wrists.

Regardless of the number of recurrences, the ability to subluxate usually disappears by 5 or 6 years of age, leaving a normal elbow.[77] One may suspect an occult cartilaginous or bony fracture if the history, physical examination, or response to treatment is not typical.

Supracondylar Fractures of the Humerus

A supracondylar fracture propagates transversely across the thin region of metaphysis proximal to the distal humeral transverse physis. Commonly occurring between 3 and 10 years of age, these troublesome fractures constitute 50 to 60 percent of children's elbow injuries.[65]

Mechanism

The mechanism of injury is a fall on the outstretched hand with transmission of indirect force to the distal humerus. Most commonly, since the elbow is in extension, the distal humeral fragment angulates or displaces posteriorly, with varying degrees of posterior tilt or displacement. Depending on the precise nature of the injury, there may be a pure extension deformity or, alternatively, associated abduction or adduction of the fragment. There is also the possibility of rotational deformity. The adducted fragments (posteromedial fracture pattern) are sometimes internally rotated, and abducted fragments (posterolateral fracture pattern) are often externally rotated. If the elbow is in flexion, the distal humeral fragment angulates or displaces anteriorly. This uncommon type of supracondylar fracture may also have associated rotational or tilt deformity of the fragment, but usually neurovascular injury does not occur.

Classification

One may describe these injuries as being of the flexion or extension category. The extension fractures may be further subdivided into those showing a posterolateral fracture pattern and those with a posteromedial fracture pattern. Alternatively, one may speak of type I (undisplaced), type II (angulated but with one intact cortex), or type III fracture, which is completely displaced, type IIIA being displaced posteromedially and type IIIB being displaced posterolaterally.

Clinical Features

If the bone is posteriorly displaced, there is an S-shaped or zigzag deformity when it is viewed from the side or in the lateral projection. The anterior prominence represents the distal end of the humeral shaft. If this anterior spike approaches the skin, ecchymosis appears in the antecubital space. An antecubital wound implies puncture by the distal humerus and an open fracture. A dimple or puckering in the antecubital space indicates that the humeral shaft has penetrated the anterior compartment musculature and lies beneath the skin. These fractures are difficult to reduce closed.[72]

Swelling depends upon the severity of the displacement and the time elapsed between injury and presentation. The neurovascular status must be well documented prior to treatment. A careful neurologic assessment will include testing for flexion of the terminal joints of the index finger and thumb, which may be impaired if the anterior interosseous branch of the median nerve has been injured by the fracture. This is not uncommon, particularly in the type IIIB injury. Radial nerve injury is more common in the type IIIA injury.

Injury to the brachial artery has been associated with the posterolateral displacement in the extension-type fracture. Vascularity may be estimated by the use of oxygen saturation measurement or Doppler studies, in addition to clinical detection of capillary refill in the nail beds and palpable pulses.

Associated fractures in the ipsilateral extremity must be ruled out before deciding on the plan of treatment, and supracondylar fracture must be clearly differentiated from other injuries in the region of the elbow joint. The diagnostic features are described further on in this chapter.

Radiologic Characteristics

In addition to standard views, oblique and comparison views may be required for full understanding of a fracture.

A positive posterior "fat-pad sign" on a true lateral x-ray view suggests the presence of a fracture in a child (Fig. 32-10). Careful assessment of the mechanism and the nature of any tilt, rotation, or displacement is essential prior to reduction. Adequacy of reduction should be evaluated by measurement. The humerotrochlear angle and Baumann's angle (Figs. 32-10, 32-11, and 32-12) are recorded. The latter, which is around 15°, varies with sex. It is related but not equal to the carrying angle.[105] The angle is a good predictor of final carrying angle.[105] It is also useful to compare the member with the opposite elbow. However, care must be taken to align the x-ray tube not more than 10° off the axis of the forearm, at right angles to the axis of the humerus and not tipped caudally.[106] Biyani and coauthors have observed that the medial epicondylar epiphyseal line can be drawn along the straight, medial, and distal border of the lower humeral metaphysis and will intersect the long axis of the humerus, yielding the medial epicondylar epiphyseal angle (MEE). This angle can also be utilized to assess the accuracy of reduction after supracondylar fracture.

Treatment

Undisplaced fractures require a well-molded long arm cast, with balancing collar and cuff, or a sling. Although some authors still recommend posterior splint,[46] the authors have found them unreliable in children. Any complete cast above the elbow in a fresh injury must, however, be used with utmost care to avoid circulatory embarrassment, and it is prudent to widely monovalve (or bivalve) it down to skin. Antecubital pressure must be avoided.

Manipulative Reduction Mild amounts of sagittal plane angulation (Fig. 32-10) have been reported to correct themselves during growth and remodeling but are nevertheless best corrected initially.[46] Severe posterior displacement requires a logical approach to treatment, with attention to basic principles: (1) reduction must be adequate, (2) position must be maintained, and (3) neurovascular status must be closely observed for possible compromise. Reduction involves gradual, gentle longitudinal traction with the elbow extended, while mildly exaggerating the deformity to hook the bone ends together. Posterior thumb pressure is applied to push the distal fragment anteriorly until hitched, and then the reduction is stabilized by gradually flexing the elbow. It is helpful to have an assistant holding a posteriorly directed force against the distal shaft. Medial or lateral displacement and rotation are then corrected. The elbow is flexed to 90 or 100° degrees (provided that circulation remains adequate) and the cast applied. The forearm is maintained in the pronated position if the distal fragment is displaced medially, or it is supinated if the distal fragment is displaced laterally.[103] Forearm position maintains tension on the elbow ligaments and any intact periosteal hinge to maintain reduction and is therefore very important.

Anterior placement, due to a flexion-type injury, is generally easier to reduce. Traction is applied in a 90° flexed position while using the forearm as a lever to push the distal fragment posteriorly. Thumb pressure may assist in reduction. Any mediolateral displacement or angu-

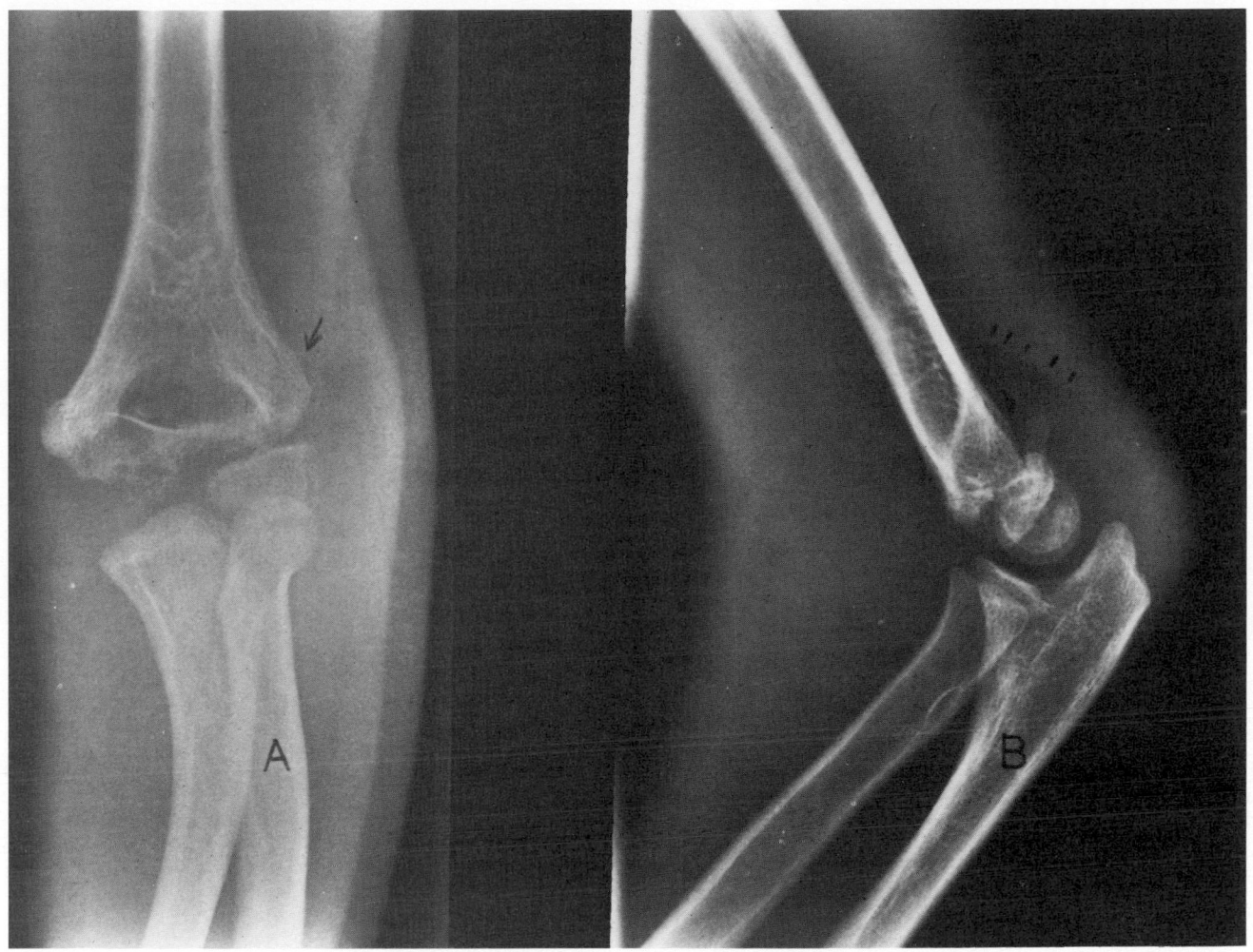

Figure 32-10 *A* and *B*. Mildly displaced extension type of supracondylar fracture of the humerus. The humerotrochlear angle is reversed on the lateral view (*B*) (compare Fig. 32-11*A*). A large intraarticular effusion is present with a markedly en-

larged posterior fat-pad sign (*arrow*). A closed reduction with the elbow immobilized in 110° of flexion restored the normal anterior inclination of the condyles.

lation is then corrected. The long arm cast is applied in relative extension (around 30°)[72,77] and should be well molded, taking care to avoid antecubital compression.

Treatment of Displaced Fractures

Although reduction of a type II displaced fracture can usually be satisfactorily obtained, failure to achieve or maintain anatomic reduction will result in the development of malalignment deformity, usually cubitus varus. If the fracture redisplaces during splintage, malunion will result. In the severely unstable type III fracture, it is exceedingly difficult to obtain and maintain an acceptable reduction. Reduction may be achieved by skeletal traction applied via a horizontal K wire or olecranon traction screw. It is important to avoid injury to the ulnar nerve when these devices are being inserted and they should be placed in the bone fairly distally (at the level of the coronoid portion of the ulna at least 2 cm from the point of the elbow). The screw is probably safer than transverse K wire in avoiding the nerve. The humerus may subsequently be aligned horizon-

tally (Dunlop's method) or vertically (overhead method). The elbow is maintained at the desired degree of flexion by skin traction applied to the forearm (Fig. 32-13). Baumann's angle should be monitored. This is done by aligning the x-ray tube at 90° to the humerus, staying no more than 10° medial or lateral to the axis of the forearm.[105,106] This method gives good results, with, however, some risk of cubitus varus. This may be minimized if x-ray monitoring is performed.[98] It is particularly useful when there is soft tissue swelling or when, after the fracture is reduced by closed methods, it is impossible to flex the elbow to a stable position without compromising the blood flow to the forearm. When the swelling is reduced, traction can often be discontinued, and cast immobilization then maintains the reduction. Alternatively, traction may be maintained for 2 weeks until early callus has stabilized the fracture.[106]

Another method of achieving and maintaining reduction in unstable and displaced fractures has been open reduction and fixation with pins. The surgical approach may be lateral or, alternatively, by some form of triceps-splitting approach. Pin fixation is then performed, using some

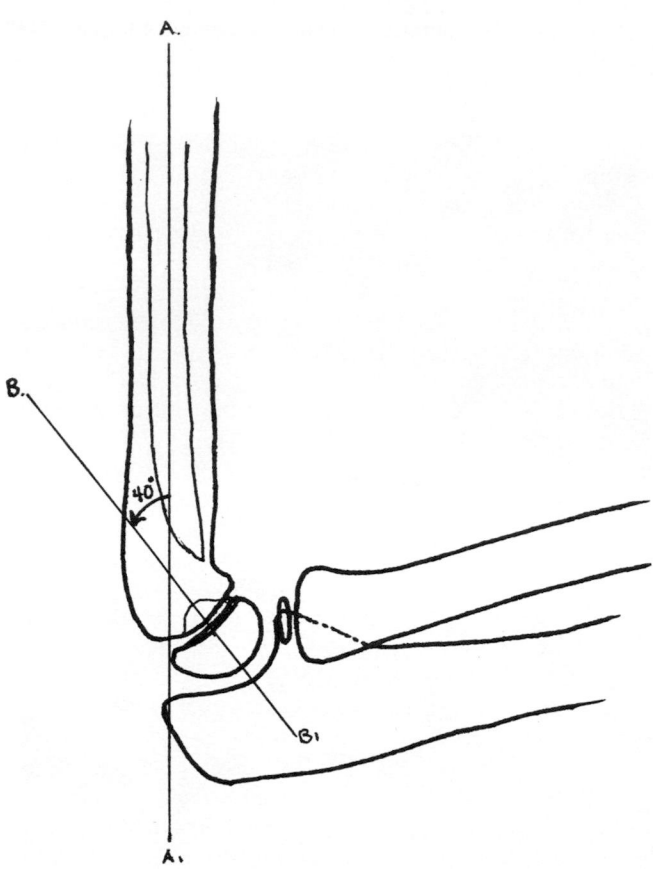

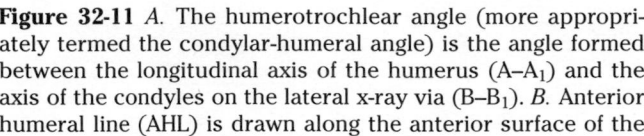

A

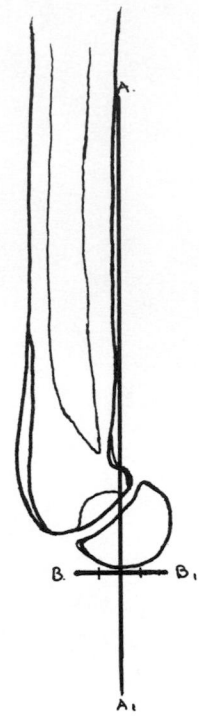

B

Figure 32-11 *A.* The humerotrochlear angle (more appropriately termed the condylar-humeral angle) is the angle formed between the longitudinal axis of the humerus (A–A₁) and the axis of the condyles on the lateral x-ray via (B–B₁). *B.* Anterior humeral line (AHL) is drawn along the anterior surface of the distal humerus (A–A₁) extending through the capitellum. Another line (B–B₁) is drawn perpendicular to AHL from the posterior to the anterior margin of the capitellum. This line is divided into thirds. AHL should normally pass through the middle third of the capitellum.

combination of medial and lateral pins inserted under direct vision. The disadvantage of skeletal traction includes injury to the ulnar nerve during insertion of the traction pin and the possibility of the development of a pin-track infection, in addition to a prolonged hospital stay. Open reduction may also result in subsequent elbow stiffness.

Closed reduction and percutaneous pinning has become the method of choice in the treatment of type III fractures and is also utilized by some authors in type II fractures because they believe an anatomic reduction is more likely to be achieved and maintained by this method and is preferable to closed reduction. The technique is quite demanding, however. It is important to monitor the reduction radiologically by careful positioning of the fluoroscope. Aronson and Prager[4a] would only accept the result of the procedure if the radiograph demonstrated that Baumann's angle was equal to or less than 4° compared with the normal side and in this way avoided a cubitus varus as a complication in these difficult fractures. The technique of pin insertion is also important. Kallio and coauthors recommend two divergent pins inserted from the lateral side but not parallel. They point out that divergent pins do not cross at the fracture site, which would render the fracture unstable, and since they diverge from a narrow entry point, it is not necessary to place one of the pins in a position that compromises the articular surface. They also point out the importance of accurate positioning of the pins on the lateral radiography. The pins should be aimed proximally and posteriorly at an angle of 10° to the axis of the diaphysis.[50] Some authors recommend a pin also inserted from the medial side, but it is difficult to be sure that one will avoid the ulnar nerve when inserting this pin, particularly if there is any swelling around the elbow.

Complications

Vascular Vascular compromise leading to Volkmann's ischemia is the most devastating complication of this injury. The vascular status of the arm assumes priority over all treatment. Palpable pulses do not rule out the presence of a compartment syndrome. Severe pain exacerbated by active finger flexion or passive finger extension or poor nail bed capillary filling are important clinical indications for immediate action. Patients with evidence of vascular compromise should have any cast or circumferential padding or stockinette split to the skin and opened up. If there is no immediate improvement, compartmental pressures should be measured, the operating room prepared, and the vascular surgeon consulted. Some authors recommend closed reduction and percutaneous pinning at this point. If there is then return of adequate vascularity as defined by a palpable pulse, a Doppler-demonstrated pulse, normal capillary refill, and normal oxygen saturation, the patient may be treated by observation. However, if there is evidence of

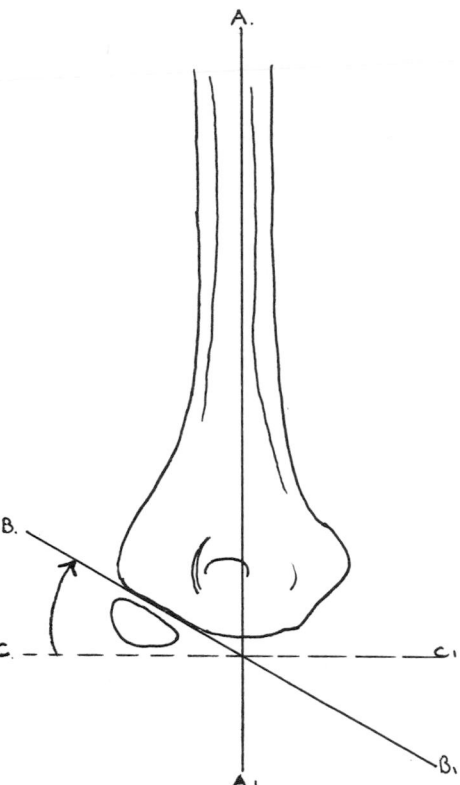

Figure 32-12 Baumann's angle. This measurement, which is obtained from an anteroposterior radiograph of the distal humerus, allows the determination of the alignment of a supracondylar fragment to the humeral shaft. Measurement of Baumann's angle of the injured elbow must be compared with that of the normal elbow in order to determine the exact degree of cubitus varus (or valgus). Baumann's angle is formed by a line (C–C1) perpendicular to the humeral shaft and a line parallel to the physis of the lateral condyle (B–B1).

compartment syndrome or failure to achieve adequate vascular flow into the forearm, forearm fasciotomy is required and the brachial artery must be explored and appropriate procedures performed on the vessel.[17]

Neurologic The incidence of nerve injuries after supracondylar fracture is approximately 5 to 10 percent.[46] The median nerve is more commonly injured in posterolateral displacement and was found to be the nerve most commonly injured in a recent series (52 percent of injuries).[17] The radial nerve was involved in 28 percent of patients in the same series. Ulnar nerve injuries, which are least common, are associated with flexion-type supracondylar fractures, which constitute less than 5 percent of all supracondylar fractures. The nerve may also be injured as part of the treatment if pins are inserted into the proximal ulna.

Nerve recovery is generally spontaneous and complete.[91] Signs of recovery are usually present by 6 to 8 weeks. If recovery is delayed, electrodiagnostic studies are indicated and exploration may subsequently be considered. In the immediate perioperative period, exploration of the nerve is not indicated if anatomic reduction is achieved unless there is anxiety that a medially placed pin may have transfixed the nerve or otherwise compromised it. Late exploration (at 5 months from injury) has successfully improved function following neurolysis, which can be an effective procedure, and lacerations of the nerve will also be identified at this time.[21] If the nerve is found to be in continuity when explored at 5 months, the prognosis after neurolysis is excellent.

Loss of Mobility Given time for proper rehabilitation and growth, most children regain most or all of their motion. Fewer than 5 percent lose flexion or extension over 5°. Few have flexion contractures or hyperextension up to 30°.[43] Loss of flexion is due to posterior angulation or translocation of the distal fragment or the result of rotational defor-

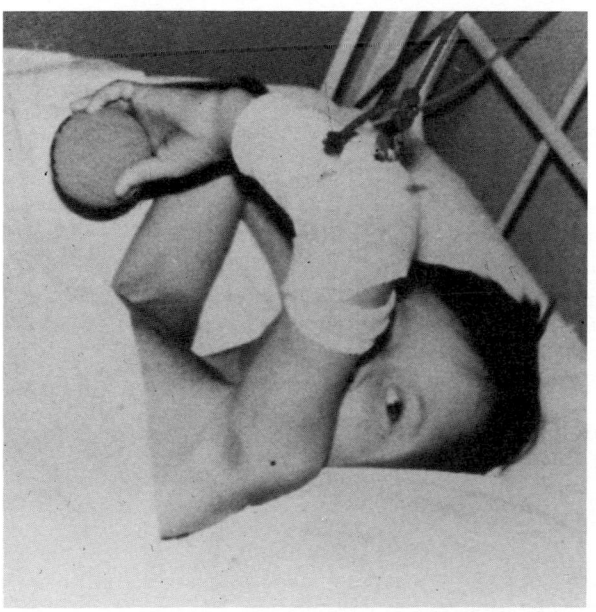

A

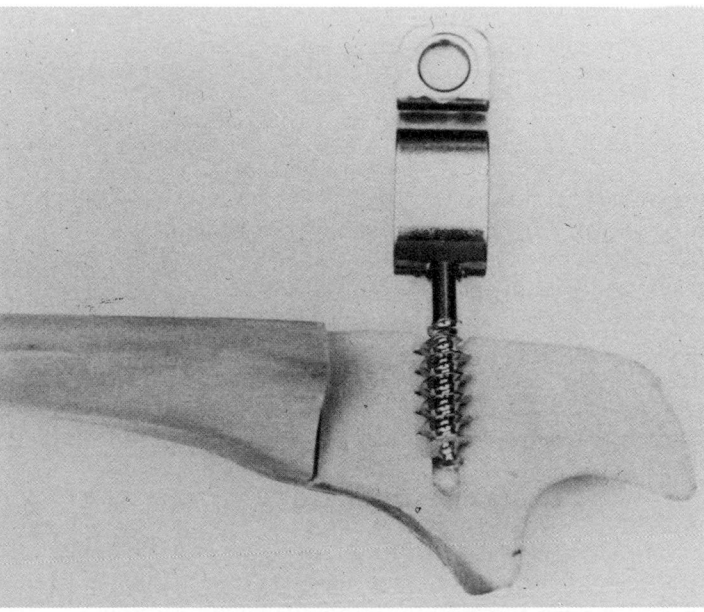

B

Figure 32-13 *A.* A child with a supracondylar fracture treated by overhead traction. Note the neutral position of the forearm. *B.* Ideal position of an olecranon traction screw. Several types of olecranon traction screws are commercially available. (Reproduced with permission from Worlock PH, Colton CL: *Injury* 15:316, 1984.)

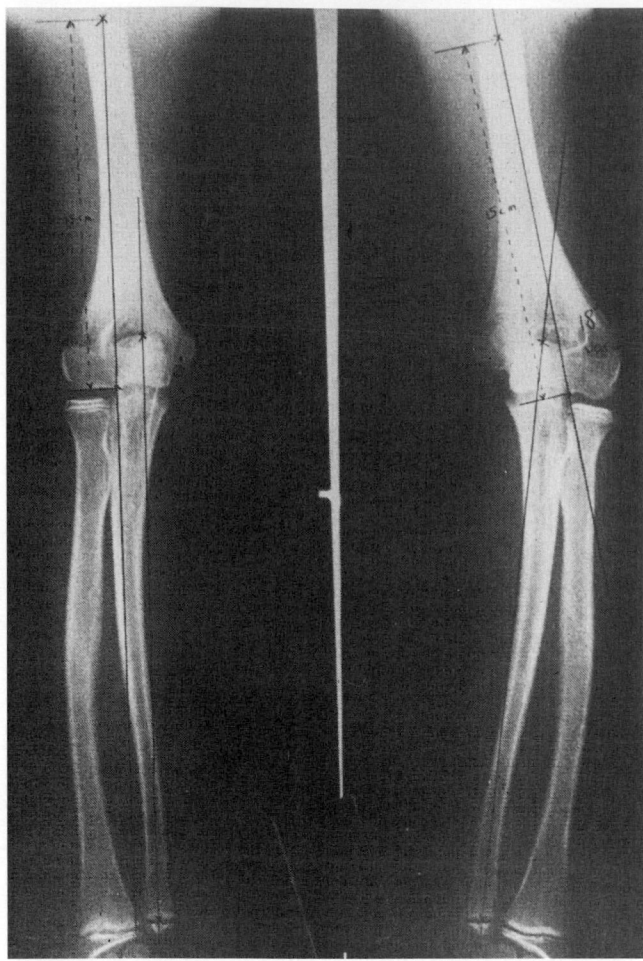

Figure 32-14 Anteroposterior x-ray view of a 12-year-old girl with cubitus varus deformity of her left elbow; both elbows in full extension and supination. The carrying angle is measured by the intersection of lines drawn through the humerus and ulna. The left elbow measures 18° of varus malunion. (Reproduced with permission from Kirz PH, Marsh HO: *Orthop Rev* 10:85, 1981.)

mity leaving an anterior spike. Prepubertal children, through growth, remodel the fracture site, resulting in spontaneous improvement in motion for years after injury.[46]

Myositis ossificans is rare but has been reported to occur after either closed or open reduction. Repeated attempts at manipulative reduction may encourage its formation. Any attempts to force further motion by vigorous physiotherapy should cease if the condition is noticed and an expectant attitude be adopted, since spontaneous improvement may occur.

Angular Deformities Current authors agree that coronal plane—i.e., mediolateral (varus-valgus)—angular deformities do not remodel to a significant degree. Mild amounts of sagittal plane or anteroposterior angulation do remodel, although the amount is perennially debated.[46,57,79] These deformities, although basically cosmetic rather than functional,[43] create much unhappiness among patients and frequently generate litigation.

Cubitus Varus Cubitus varus, or gun-stock deformity (Fig. 32-14), is the commonest deformity to follow supracondylar fracture in children, with a reported incidence ranging from zero to 60 percent.[46] It is associated with a medially displaced fragment and does not occur with the posterolateral fracture pattern. The maximum amount of varus is often not appreciated until the elbow extends fully. Careful radiologic monitoring is therefore crucial from the earliest moment, whatever the treatment method.[106] However, in 40 percent of patients with this fracture, the carrying angle decreases with subsequent growth, even after perfect reduction. Growth disorders are certainly responsible in some cases.[48] The role of uncorrected rotation is disputed but is not as important as that of varus tilting. If the cubitus varus deformity is cosmetically unacceptable, surgical correction is performed by wedge[10,37] supracondylar osteotomy with internal fixation. The procedure should be performed at skeletal maturity in order to eliminate the risk of physeal disturbance.

In some cases of cubitus varus, there is a significant element of internal rotation. In such cases, accurate assessment of the degree of rotation is necessary prior to surgical correction. A simple and useful clinical method has been described comparing the degree of internal humeral rotation bilaterally with the arm in the "arm lock" position behind the back.[107]

Cubitus Valgus Cubitus valgus is rare and is associated with a posterolateral fracture pattern. Cosmetically less objectionable than cubitus varus, it accentuates the normal carrying angle. Functionally, it is frequently associated with loss of full extension. A late concern is the development of tardy ulnar nerve palsy. In contrast to cubitus varus, cubitus valgus has a much greater incidence of associated functional loss in the extremity. The treatment recommended by Langenskiold and Kirilaakaso is a medial closing wedge osteotomy with anterior transposition of the ulnar nerve.[57]

Associated Ipsilateral Fractures

The average incidence of associated ipsilateral fracture is 10 percent (in 150 cases). Most of these lesions involve the forearm or distal radius and occur with severe trauma with ipsilateral fractures. There is then a higher incidence of late cubitus varus, but the incidence of neurovascular complications does not appear to be increased.[82]

Condylar and Epicondylar Fractures of the Humerus

Lateral Epicondylar Fracture

This fracture is relatively uncommon in children as an isolated injury.[67] It may occasionally be associated with an elbow dislocation.[79]

Osteologic Characteristics The lateral epicondyle ossifies at approximately 11 (female) to 12 (male) years of age and fuses with the lateral condyle during puberty.

Clinical Features Since this structure is subcutaneous, local tenderness and swelling over the lateral epicondyle can readily be appreciated.

Radiologic Characteristics Prior to approximately 12 years of age, the lateral epicondyle is nonossified, rendering x-ray films unhelpful except to rule out adjacent injuries. Ossification is often irregular and may be confused with an avulsion fracture between the ages of 12 and 14 years. Comparison views of the opposite elbow in the same projection may be helpful, but often the clinical evaluation makes the diagnosis.

Treatment Generally 3 to 4 weeks of casting is adequate.[67] If displacement exceeds 3 mm, open reduction and internal fixation are indicated.[72]

The risk of growth arrest is minimal, as these fractures occur near skeletal maturity. Fibrous union may occur. The fragment may be excised if the patient is symptomatic.

Lateral Condylar Fractures

These injuries usually occur between the ages of 3 and 14 years, with the peak between 6 and 10 years. These fractures constitute about 18.5 percent of distal humeral fractures in children.[85]

Ossification of the Distal Humerus

The metaphysis of the distal humerus is ossified at birth. Four centers of ossification appear subsequently in the cartilaginous epiphysis. The secondary ossification nuclei, by their growth, permit enlargement of the contours of the articular surface of the humerus. The nucleus for the capitellum and lateral ridge of the trochlea has usually appeared by the age of 6 months, but its appearance may be delayed up to 2 years. The nucleus for the medial epicondyle occurs between the ages of 5 and 8 years and remains separate. However, after the nucleus for the trochlea has appeared, around age 8 to 10 years, and the lateral epicondylar center has appeared, around the age of 8 or 9 years, the centers for the capitellum trochlea and lateral epicondyle fuse and form a single center. Fusion of the capitellum and trochlea is usually complete at the age of 12 years, forming a single center, and this center fuses with the metaphysis in adolescence, usually around 14 (female) and 17 (male) years of age.[95]

Mechanism

The mechanism of injury is thought to be either a varus stress combined with avulsion of the lateral condyle by the lateral ligament or, alternatively, a compression injury causing a vertical shear fracture. Milch characterized fractures of the lateral condyle of the distal humerus in adults, indicating the difference in stability between a Milch type 1 fracture, where the vertical fracture line entered the joint space lateral to the ridge between the capitellum and the trochlea, and a Milch type 2 fracture pattern, where the portion of sheared-off bone was somewhat larger and the

vertical fracture line reached the articular surface within the trochlear groove, permitting instability and, consequently, lateral dislocation of the ulna[62] (Fig. 32-15). In children, the fracture may be classified according to its degree of displacement. In a type I fracture, the obliquely disposed fracture line, passing through the metaphyseal bone, crosses the physis of the distal humerus at some variable point, medially or laterally, to the capitellar-trochlear sulcus, but it may not completely penetrate through the cartilaginous epiphysis and into the articular surface. Such an incomplete fracture is, therefore, undisplaced and has been classified by Jakob and coauthors[47] as a type I fracture. In this type of fracture, it follows that the articular surface is unblemished. In the Jakob classification, a complete fracture is a type II fracture in which there may be some separation of the fragments, but the fragment is not displaced out of the elbow joint. A type III fracture in this classification is completely displaced from the joint. In the case of a Jakob type III fracture, the fragment may be displaced and rotated through 90° in two planes. The fragment maintains its attachment to the radial collateral ligament but has a somewhat tenuous blood supply, which is an important consideration during subsequent surgical treatment. Care should be taken to avoid further devascularization of the fragment during any surgical procedure.

Diagnosis

Clinical examination is important in making the diagnosis. It may be possible to localize the tenderness primarily to the lateral side, but often swelling of the elbow makes clinical diagnosis difficult. If the condyle is ossified, the diagnosis of a displaced fracture is obvious. However, undisplaced fractures or displaced fractures with nonossified epiphyses are difficult to diagnose. Fortunately, however, the capitellum is usually ossified at the age at which this fracture commonly occurs (see Fig. 32-18). It is possible, however, that only a small bony flake may be present with a large portion of separated cartilaginous epiphysis. Oblique views of the elbow are recommended, plus comparison x-ray views of the opposite elbow; occasionally, stress radiography may be helpful. Single contrast arthro-

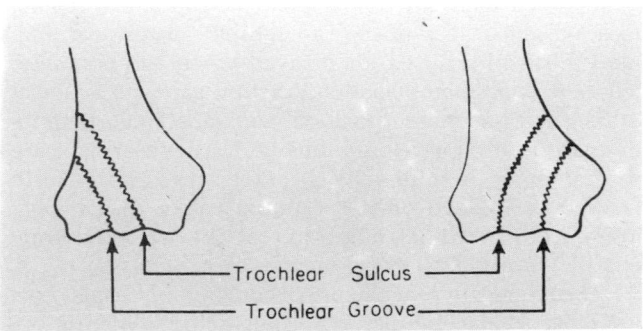

Figure 32-15 Milch classification of condylar fractures. At the left is a lateral condylar fracture. At the right is a medial condylar fracture. (Reproduced with permission from Milch H: *J Trauma* 4:591–607, 1964.)

grams with only 0.5 mL of dye will help visualize the joint surfaces and outline joint cartilaginous fragments.[2] Ultrasound and MRI may also be used in differentiating these injuries from other lesions, such as dislocation of the elbow or fracture separation of the entire physis.

Treatment

Undisplaced fractures may be immobilized in a long arm cast with the elbow flexed to 90°. Immobilization for 6 to 8 weeks is necessary.[28] Displacement during healing is a distinct possibility, so that serial x-ray studies with the arm removed from the cast are necessary, and cast checks should be meticulous in the early stages of healing. Union should be confirmed by anteroposterior (AP), lateral, and oblique x-ray views before the limb is mobilized. Satisfactory results may be expected with closed treatment with fractures displaced less than 2 mm. If there is more displacement, open reduction and internal fixation are indicated, since the fracture is essentially a Salter type IV injury. Displaced Jakob type II and III fractures usually require such intervention. A Monteggia equivalent has been reported involving fracture of the lateral condyle associated with fracture of the proximal ulna.[81] Various types of surgical approaches have been recommended but the modified Kocher approach to the elbow will enable the anterior joint surface to be accurately visualized during reduction. Again, it must be stressed that care should be taken not to further devitalize the fragment by unnecessary stripping of soft tissue attachments. Some Jakob type II fractures will have a large cartilaginous fragment, which must be accurately reduced if subsequent growth arrest is not to follow. Perfect reduction must precede pin fixation with two smooth Kirschner pins, which are usually removed at 3 to 4 weeks from surgery.

Delayed union after 8 weeks is also an indication for open reduction/internal fixation and probable bone grafting in the older child. For malunited fractures, this treatment should be deferred until after skeletal maturity.[28]

Complications

Fishtail deformity of the distal humerus and cubitus valgus occurs when malreduction is present. Functional results are good, regardless of the radiographic or clinical findings.[28] Probable causes for delayed union and nonunion include lack of immobilization, fracture gap with synovial bathing, soft tissue interposition, and, most important, inadequate reduction. Nonunions and growth arrests are more common in minimally displaced fractures than in markedly displaced ones.[77] Cubitus valgus may evolve slowly from proximal migration of the ununited fragment.[53,77] Tardy ulnar palsy may result.[53,67,77]

Premature physeal closure is common but usually occurs close to skeletal maturity. Thus deformity is not obvious.[79] Rutherford reviewed 39 cases with only 1 physeal closure, despite malreduction in 10.[85] Overgrowth or enlargement of the lateral side of the elbow is common. Rang reported 15 of 27 cases and observed that this cosmetic deformity is especially obvious in thin patients.[80]

Medial Condylar Fractures

Medial condylar fractures are rare in children, constituting less than 3 percent of children's elbow fractures. Displaced fractures usually occur in older children.[11]

Osteological Characteristics The medial condyle (and medial trochlea) ossifies at 8 (female) to 9 (male) years of age and fuses with the lateral condyle during puberty. The entire epiphysis then fuses with the humeral shaft in adolescence, at 14 (female) to 17 (male) years.[95]

Mechanism The mechanism of injury is generally considered to be an avulsion injury during a valgus force to the elbow. A second mechanism is a fall onto the point of the flexed elbow.

Clinical Features Tenderness, swelling, and ecchymosis are present over the medial side of the elbow.

Radiologic Characteristics This fracture is generally a Salter type IV injury,[11] although Ogden observes that type III injuries may also occur.[72] During adolescence, it may occur as part of a T-condylar type of fracture. In young children whose medial condyle has yet to ossify, an arthrogram may be necessary to establish the diagnosis.

Treatment Undisplaced fractures may be treated by immobilization in a long arm cast until the fracture is healed. Displaced fractures (more than 2 mm) require anatomic reduction, usually by open reduction and internal fixation.[11,72]

Complications Complications are infrequent. Avascular necrosis may occur with extensive surgical dissection, so such dissection should be avoided during open reduction.[68] The blood supply to the medial condyle is of the terminal type.[11] Nonunion is a mild risk, especially in neglected fractures. Limited motion (especially flexion/extension) often resolves slowly and incompletely. Growth injury may occur, leading to cubitus varus.[11]

Medial Epicondylar Fractures

Medial epicondylar fractures (Fig. 32-16) usually occur in patients who are 7 to 15 years of age. They constitute about 10 percent of children's elbow fractures.[72]

Osteologic Characteristics The medial epicondyle ossifies at about 5 (female) to 7 (male) years of age. It remains separate from the common growth center and fuses to the shaft in adolescence, at 15 (female) to 18 (male) years.[95]

Mechanism The mechanism of injury is a valgus strain combined with forceful contraction of the flexor muscles. Fifty percent of these fractures occur with an elbow dislocation.[67,77,79]

Clinical Features The physical findings of tenderness, swelling, ecchymosis, and crepitation over the medial

Figure 32-16 *A* and *B*. Adolescent female gymnast with displaced avulsion fracture of the medial epicondyle. Note the radial neck fracture. A closed reduction was performed by thumb pressure over the epicondylar fragment, flexion of the elbow and wrist, and long arm cast immobilization (with a medial pressure pad). The fracture went on to fibrous union, but the patient was asymptomatic, and the elbow joint is clinically stable.

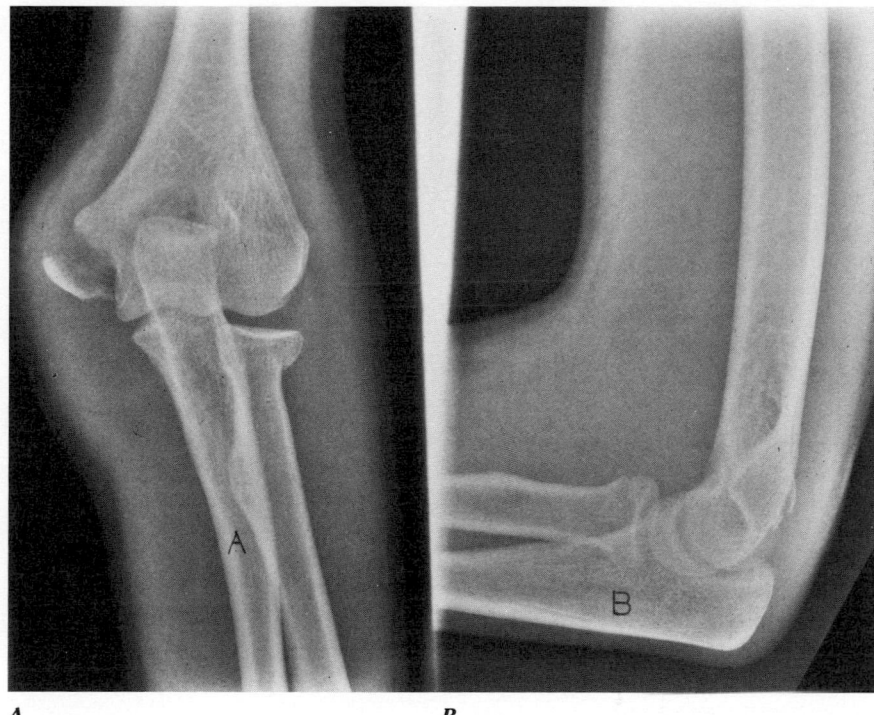

A   *B*

prominence of the lower humerus strongly suggest the diagnosis of a medial epicondylar fracture. If this injury occurs in association with an elbow dislocation, the area may be markedly swollen, thereby obscuring the diagnosis.

Radiologic Characteristics Radiographic diagnosis can be difficult before ossification of the apophysis. Comparison x-ray views may be helpful. Associated fractures and dislocations are common and should be anticipated. Clinical correlation is critical in children under the age of 5 years. The epicondyle should be sought on all appropriate x-ray views, particularly following severe trauma such as dislocation. Its apparent absence may be explained by its entrapment within the joint. In young children, the only radiographic sign may be joint widening compared with the opposite elbow. In older children, oblique views may provide needed information. An arthrogram is useful in difficult cases.[2]

Treatment Undisplaced and minimally displaced fractures require a long arm cast for protection until healed.[77,79] A trapped intraarticular medial epicondylar fragment can occasionally be disimpacted by a valgus stress to the elbow while supinating the forearm. Closed reduction is often unsuccessful, indicating the need for arthrotomy to remove the epicondyle and then open reduction with internal fixation. With fragment entrapments, displacement over 5 mm, or associated medial instability of the elbow joint, open reduction is indicated.[72] Stabilizing the fragment also restores function of the medial collateral ligament, which is a critically important supporting structure for the elbow joint. Accurate repair is important, particularly in the throwing athlete. Pin fixation may not be suitable in the older child, and a long

threaded cancellous screw will avoid redisplacement after surgery.

Complications Motion often recovers slowly, and some degree of permanent stiffness may result. Nonunion occurs, and fragments may be excised if symptomatic. Median nerve entrapment may occur, requiring surgical extrication.[79] Ulnar entrapment may develop months or years later.[72]

T-Condylar Fractures of the Distal Humerus

T-condylar fractures of the distal humerus are rarely seen in the pediatric age group. However, it has been pointed out that the nature of the injury may be overlooked in very young children.[76] In younger children, the fracture line is vertical and extends through the epiphysis, but it may not extend completely through the thick articular cartilage. Near skeletal maturity, the fracture fragments completely separate, as in adults. Open reduction via a posterior triceps-splitting approach and fixation with K wires is recommended and achieves good results if reduction is accurate.[76] Rehabilitation may be difficult and prolonged.

Fracture Separation of the Distal Humeral Physis

Transphyseal separation is relatively uncommon in children, although many feel that this fracture may occasionally be mislabeled as elbow dislocation. It can also be confused with fracture of the lateral condyle. The injury is usually a Salter type I or type II injury (Figs. 32-17 and 32-18C). Diagnosis is particularly difficult in the first year of life if the ossification center for the lateral condyle has not yet appeared.

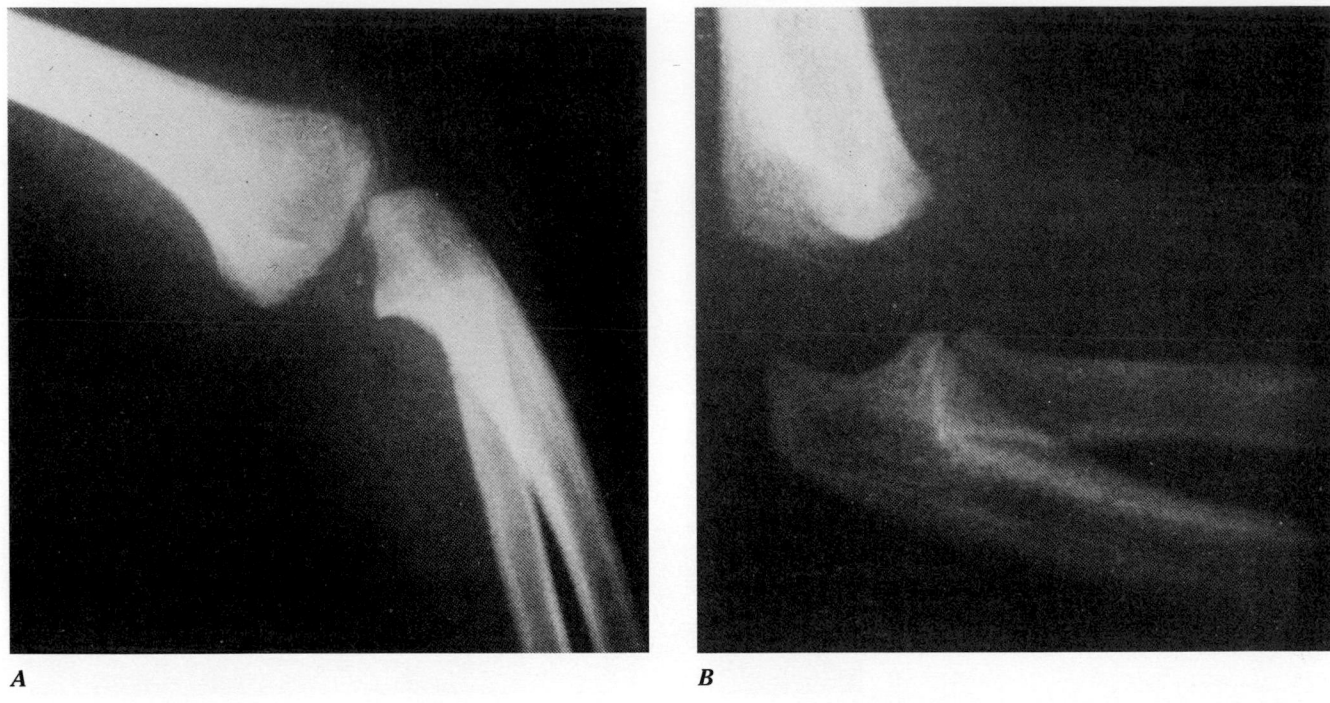

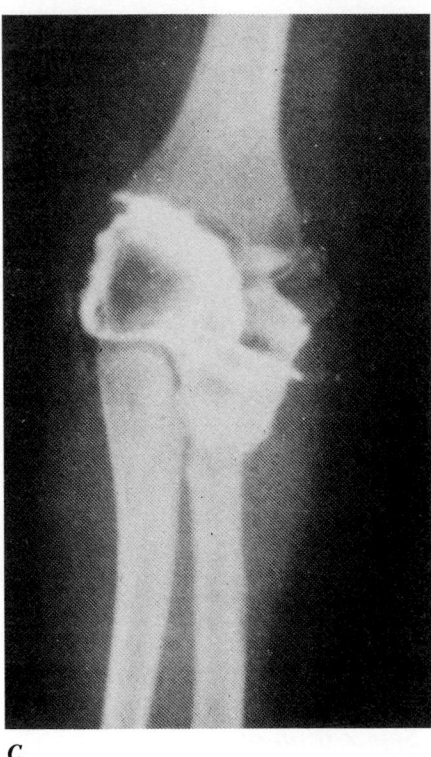

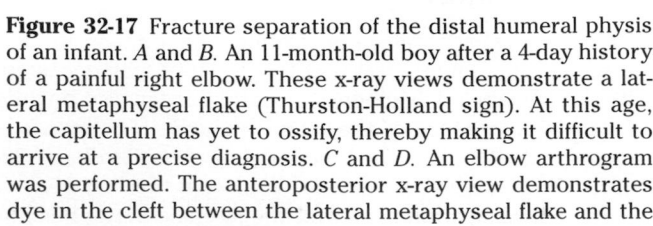

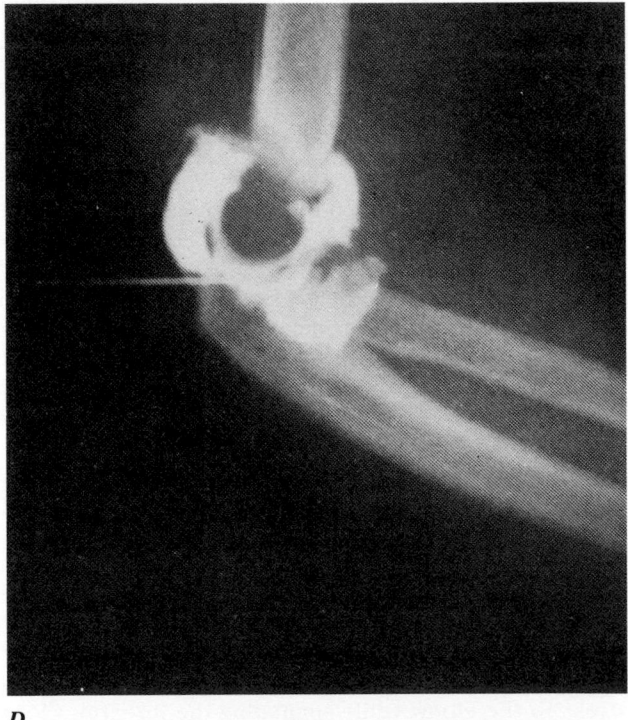

Figure 32-17 Fracture separation of the distal humeral physis of an infant. *A* and *B.* An 11-month-old boy after a 4-day history of a painful right elbow. These x-ray views demonstrate a lateral metaphyseal flake (Thurston-Holland sign). At this age, the capitellum has yet to ossify, thereby making it difficult to arrive at a precise diagnosis. *C* and *D.* An elbow arthrogram was performed. The anteroposterior x-ray view demonstrates dye in the cleft between the lateral metaphyseal flake and the remainder of the metaphysis, with extension medially across the humerus. The lateral view completely outlines the trochlea, which is displaced posteriorly. This arthrogram confirmed the diagnosis of a distal humeral fracture separation (type II physeal injury) and ruled out the existence of the more serious type IV physeal injury. (Reproduced with permission from Hansen PE, Barnes DA, Tullos HS: *J Pediatr Orthop* 2:569, 1982.)

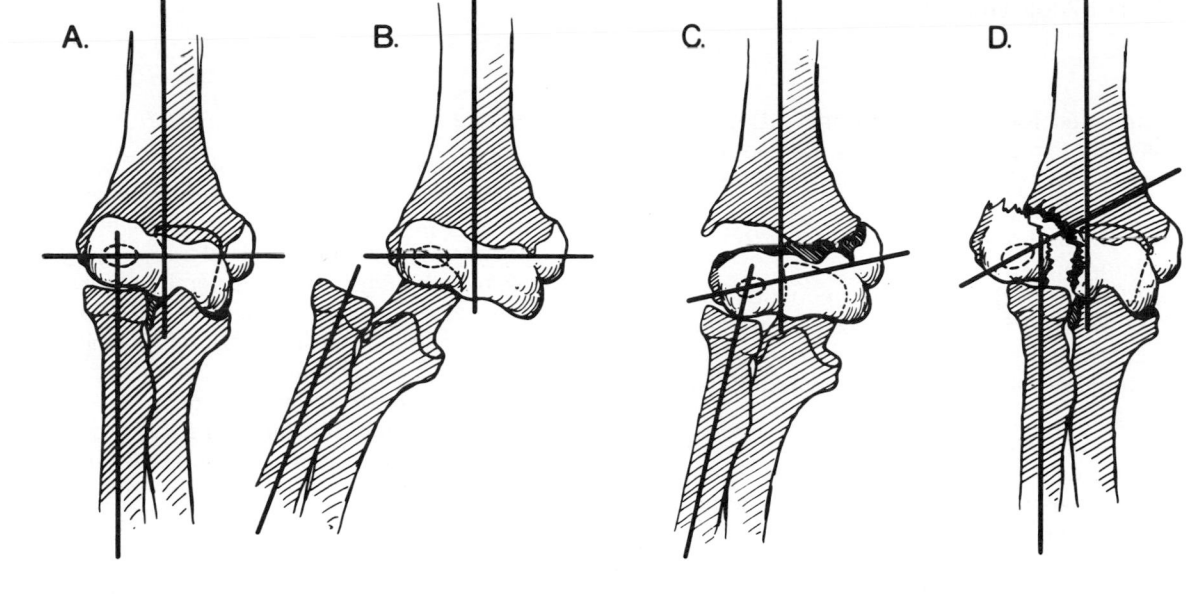

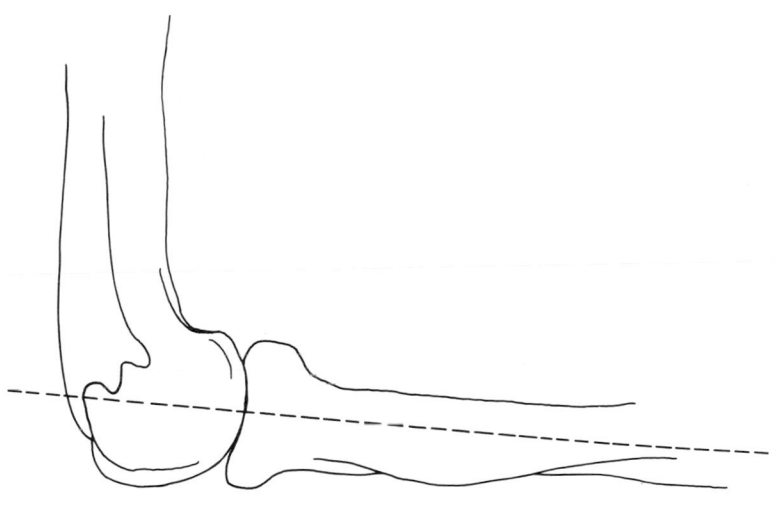

Axis of radius

E

Figure 32-18 Radiographic method of differentiating a fracture separation of the distal humeral epiphysis from other pediatric elbow injuries that may occur in a very young child before the distal humeral epiphysis ossifies. Lines are drawn through the longitudinal axis of the humerus and the radial shaft, and a transverse line is drawn through the distal humeral epiphysis. The capitellum can be used as a reference point if it is ossified. *A.* Unaffected elbow. Normal radiocapitellar and humerocapitellar alignment. *B.* Elbow dislocation. Normal humerocapitellar alignment, altered radiocapitellar alignment. *C.* Salter type II epiphyseal injury. Normal radiocapitellar alignment, altered humerocapitellar alignment. *D.* Salter type IV epiphyseal injury. Altered radiocapitellar and humerocapitellar alignment. *E.* The radiocapitellar line. (*A–D* are reproduced with permission from Hansen PE, Barnes DA, Tullos HS: *J Pediatr Orthop* 2:569, 1982. *E* is modified from Lee J et al: *J Bone Joint Surg* 62A:46, 1980.)

Mechanism The mechanism of injury may be a direct blow or an indirect transmitted force from a fall on the hand. It may be associated with child abuse.[61] Two newborn cases associated with difficult delivery have been reported.[6]

Clinical Features Physical findings vary according to the severity of the trauma and the degree of swelling or displacement. There is usually deformity and instability.[64] Palpable crepitus has been described as "muffled crepitus" and thought to be diagnostic of this injury and caused by the distinct sensation of cartilage rubbing on cartilage. Elbow flexion and extension is limited and painful.

Radiologic Characteristics This injury can be difficult to differentiate from other pediatric elbow injuries, especially since it more commonly occurs at an age prior to appearance of the condylar ossification centers. Multiple x-ray views and comparison x-rays of the opposite elbow may help establish the diagnosis, *but an arthrogram* is commonly needed for definitive diagnosis (Fig. 32-18).[2] The

distal epiphysis may be displaced posteriorly, laterally, or anteriorly. With an elbow dislocation, the relation between the radial head and the lateral condylar ossification center are altered, since the radius and ulna are usually displaced laterally. In an epiphyseal separation, the radius and ulna are usually displaced medially (Fig. 32-18*C*), but the radiocapitellar line on the lateral x-ray view remains intact.[21,64] With displaced fractures of the lateral condyle, the relation of the condylar center to the radial head is altered, but the axial relations of the long bones are normal (Fig. 32-18*D*).[64]

Treatment Closed reduction is performed with initial traction, followed by correction of the medial tilt and varus angulation of the distal fragment. Any residual rotational deformity should then be corrected bimanually. Utilizing the intact medial periosteal hinge for stability, the elbow is flexed to 90° and the forearm pronated.[72] A long arm cast is applied with three-point molding, creating a mild valgus force at the elbow. If the swelling is extensive, the circulation precarious, or the family unreliable, hospitalization is indicated for circulatory observation for the first few days. In extreme cases, with marked swelling, overhead traction may be utilized initially. Because of the degree of swelling, some authors recommend posterior splinting, but the authors have found this extremely unreliable in children.

Most authors consider that open reduction is rarely necessary. However, it has been advocated as the treatment of choice by Mizuna et al.[64] Medial and lateral K wires are appropriate for fixation, augmented by postoperative casting.

If there is a treatment delay of 2 or more weeks, significant healing will already have occurred. Reduction should not then be attempted, since iatrogenic physeal damage may occur.[109] Subsequent supracondylar osteotomy may be necessary to correct deformity.

Complications Cubitus varus occurs less frequently than after supracondylar fractures. Growth disturbances as a consequence of this injury have not been reported. Neurovascular complications are infrequent.[72]

Fractures of the Humeral Shaft

These fractures are uncommon in children and are usually associated with severe trauma or occasionally fracture through cystic lesions.

Osteologic Characteristics

Ossification begins at about 42 days in utero, and the entire diaphysis is ossified at birth.[23]

Mechanism

The most common mechanism of injury is direct, severe trauma, creating a transverse or short oblique fracture. A heavy fall on the outstretched hand occasionally produces torsional forces that create a spiral fracture.[79]

Clinical Features

Infants usually present with irritability and pseudoparalysis of the upper arm. Older children with undisplaced fracture may be remarkably free of symptoms. With displaced or angulated fractures, the diagnosis is obvious. The neurovascular status, especially radial nerve function, should be carefully evaluated prior to manipulative treatment.

Radiologic Characteristics

Birth fractures show callus at 1 to 2 weeks. Metaphyseal fractures should be evaluated for underlying cysts.

Standard radiographic views usually confirm the diagnosis. In cases with equivocal x-ray findings or if a metaphyseal fracture is suspected near the proximal or distal humeral growth plates, comparison x-ray views of the opposite extremity are indicated.

Treatment

Closed treatment is generally indicated. Posterior splints, U or sugar-tong splints, and long arm casts with collar and cuff are all reportedly adequate methods of treatment. In recumbent patients, skin or skeletal traction may be used.[74] The use of a shoulder spica is generally excessive and unnecessary. Hanging casts, if used, should be fabricated of lightweight synthetic casting material to avoid distracting the fracture. As the pain subsides, isometric exercises assist humeral realignment and healing.

Open reduction and internal fixation are indicated rarely to maintain position but are occasionally required for soft tissue interposition with complete displacement in an adolescent.

Complications

Healing and remodeling are excellent in these fractures. Associated radial nerve injuries usually recover spontaneously. Vascular complications are uncommon. Overgrowth of 1 cm can be expected.

Fractures of the Proximal Humeral Metaphysis

The proximal humeral metaphysis is particularly susceptible in the 5- to 11-year-old age group.[72] Compression type (torus) and greenstick fractures occur. Closed treatment is the rule, and displacement requiring reduction is rare. Pathologic fractures through benign cystic lesions (e.g., simple bone cyst) are treated identically to ordinary fractures, definitive treatment of the lesion being delayed until union has occurred.

Fractures of the Head of the Humerus

Fractures and traumatic epiphyseal separations of the proximal humerus represent only 3 percent of all epiphyseal injuries.[69]

Osteologic Characteristics

Ossification of the humeral head appears between birth and 6 months of age; the greater tuberosity ossifies between 7 months and 3 years of age; and the lesser tuberosity ossifies approximately 2 years after the greater tuberosity. The physes close by the age of 17 (females) or 18 (males) years. The proximal physis accounts for 80 percent of the growth of the humerus. The medial portion of the physis and a few millimeters of the medial metaphysis are intraarticular.[23]

Classification

Fractures in this region are usually Salter type I or type II, the latter producing a medial metaphyseal spike of variable size attached to the head fragment. Neer and

Horowitz's classification is based upon the degree of displacement of the epiphysis.[69]

Grade 1: Less than 5 mm of displacement
Grade 2: Displacement up to $\frac{1}{3}$ of the width of the shaft
Grade 3: Displacement up to $\frac{2}{3}$ of the width of the shaft
Grade 4: Displacement over $\frac{2}{3}$ of the width of the shaft (and complete displacement)

Mechanism

The mechanism of injury is generally a fall backward onto the outstretched arm with the elbow extended and the wrist dorsiflexed. Neonates usually sustain a Salter type I fracture, while older children develop Salter type II fractures. The fracture line involves only the metaphysis in 90 percent. In 10 percent, it is metaphyseodiaphyseal.[49] The metaphyseal spike may entrap the long head of the biceps and render the fracture irreducible. Salter types II and IV fractures are very rare[7] and are usually due to direct trauma. Salter type V injuries have not been reported.[7,23]

Clinical Features

In young children, pseudoparalysis of the upper extremity is a common presentation. Painful limitation of shoulder motion, swelling, and deformity (in displaced fractures) are seen in older children.

Radiologic Characteristics

The diagnosis is difficult in neonates, since 80 percent of these children have an unossified epiphysis. They are often diagnosed as having a birth palsy or shoulder dislocation.

Treatment

About 70 percent of children sustain grade 1 or 2 fractures and require only simple support, such as a sling and swathe or Velpeau's bandage for 3 to 4 weeks followed by early motion and rehabilitation.[79] Even with severe displacement, the capacity for remodeling makes excellent functional results possible. The same is true for moderate degrees of varus. Severe varus can be corrected by gentle manipulation under general anesthesia. However, Baxter and Wiley found that manipulation of displaced fresh fracture did not improve the final outcome in their hands.[7] The manipulative maneuver involves longitudinal traction combined with abduction of the arm. For varus angulation, Kohler and Trilland recommend abduction greater than 90° with flexion and external rotation, followed by traction. For valgus angulation, they recommend reduction in adduction.[55]

"Statue of Liberty" spica casting to control the fracture has been used[19] but is awkward and may create complications, including prolonged stiffness and nerve injury.[79] Others recommend the salute position with abduction to 130° for 4 to 5 weeks.[55] If the arm cannot be immobilized at the side of the body after reduction, since the reduction is unstable, inpatient traction in the abducted position is preferred by some authors. This may achieve reduction and maintain it long enough for the arm to be brought down without losing position. Hanging plasters are not recommended.[55]

Surgery consisting of open reduction with internal fixation (with K wires or screws) is rarely indicated.[23] It should be reserved for those nonimpacted irreducible fractures that are completely unstable and with suspected bicipital tendon interposition.[23,55] Surgery should be done only in an adolescent at the end of the growth period.[55]

Complications

This fracture usually heals and remodels well with full return of motion, strength, and appearance. The physis may occasionally close prematurely.[23] Neer and Horowitz found up to 3 cm of shortening in 10 percent of cases with undisplaced fractures and in 40 percent with severely displaced fractures.[69] Smith reported shortening in 20 percent of cases, regardless of the method of treatment, but the discrepancy usually remains unnoticed by the patient.[92a] Others have observed the final shortening at about 2 cm.[7]

Fractures of the Clavicle

Clavicular fractures are among the commonest fractures in children. They almost always heal well, without complications or disability.

Osteologic Characteristics

The clavicle is the first bone to ossify. Primary ossification centers appear at about day 42 in utero (19 mm). One occurs at the junction of the middle and lateral thirds of the bone; the second is at the junction of the middle and medial thirds. The shaft is established by membranous bone formation.[23]

The ends of the clavicle develop by endochondral ossification centers at each end. The acromial end often remains nonossified or appears briefly before fusing at about 19 years of age. The sternal end appears variably at 12 to 19 years of age. Fusion occurs at 22 to 35 years of age. This epiphysis is difficult to see on plain x-ray films.

Mechanism

The mechanism of injury may be direct or indirect. Indirect injury is the more frequent, occurring by a fall on the hand or against the outer shoulder.

Birth fractures occur in about 0.5 percent of vertex and 16 percent of breech deliveries, when the shoulders are compressed during passage through the narrow pelvic inlet. They are generally greenstick fractures and are more common in babies with high birth weights and with the use of forceps.[23]

Clinical Features

In infants and young children, symptoms may be minimal. The diagnosis is often made days later, when the parent notices swelling over the clavicle. Neonates may present with pseudoparalysis due to pain or associated birth palsies. This injury must be differentiated from proximal humeral injury, septic shoulder, and osteomyelitis.

Physical examination reveals localized tenderness, swelling, and often ecchymosis or crepitus. The subcutaneous location of the clavicle greatly facilitates diagnosis.

Fractures of the Medial End of the Clavicle

Until the age of 25 years, the medial physis may separate at the time of injury, with the sternoclavicular ligaments remaining intact. Displacement may be anterior, posterior, or superior. A Rockwood view (45° upshot), AP x-ray views, tomograms, CT, and/or MRI scan assist in diagnosis, which is often obvious on clinical examination. Reduction and its maintenance are difficult. Only rarely is displacement significant and open reduction and suturing or internal fixation required. Posteriorly displaced fragments are adjacent to the great vessels. A vascular surgeon should be in attendance.

Fractures of the Outer End of the Clavicle

This lesion is often mistaken for acromioclavicular dislocation, which, however, is uncommon except in adolescents. In young children, the outer end of the clavicle can sustain Salter type I or II epiphyseal separation, since the acromioclavicular and coracoclavicular ligaments are stronger than the physis. Fracture healing occasionally produces reduplication of the clavicle in the inferiorly displaced periosteal sleeve. Infrequently, it may be necessary to trim away the excess of the "old" clavicle.[73] These displaced distal clavicular physeal injuries can be reduced and percutaneously pinned if detected early.[73] The author has found that excellent healing and remodeling generally make pinning unnecessary.

Differential Diagnosis of Clavicular Injury

Congenital pseudarthrosis occurs in the lateral end of the middle third of the clavicle. A history of trauma is absent. The pseudarthrosis is often asymptomatic. It is usually discovered between 2 and 4 years of age because of the bony prominence at the pseudarthrosis site. Usually occurring on the right side, it is presumed to be due to prenatal compression of the clavicle by the subclavian artery, which is more cephalad on the side opposite the heart. If the lesion is left-sided, one may suspect the presence of dextrocardia. Bilateral cases are associated with cervical ribs. Cleidocranial dysostosis should also be considered in the differential diagnosis.[23,36,90]

Treatment

A figure-of-eight harness is adequate for immobilization of the majority of these fractures. It may be fabricated or purchased. This basically provides protective padding over the fracture site and diminishes shoulder-clavicle motion during healing. Axillary care with powder and absorbent pads avoids chafing. Bilateral hand (gripping) exercises minimize swelling and maintain forearm strength. A sling may also be used for added comfort during the early painful period and for protection around other children.

Complications

The clavicle heals well in spite of respiratory and upper extremity movement. Healing may occur with displacement and angulation, which remodels in children within 1 to 2 years. The family should be forewarned of the possibility of a visible "bump" over the healed fracture site.

Superior angulation is common, and any effort to depress the bone should be avoided, since the major neurovascular structures are directly subjacent. Rarely, subclavian vein compression (with upper extremity edema) occurs because of an inferiorly angulated fracture of the clavicle. It may be treated by closed reduction with or without a spica cast or by bed rest with the arm comfortably elevated. Open reduction is rarely required in children. Infection and nonunion occur only after open reduction.

Occasionally, a comminuted fracture spikes into the subcutaneous tissue, tenting the skin. If an attempt at cautious closed reduction is unsuccessful, the safest treatment is to allow the fracture to heal and to remove the spike electively, under local anesthesia, if the patient remains symptomatic.[23]

Dislocation of the Acromioclavicular Joint

Acromioclavicular joint dislocations, for practical purposes, do not occur in preadolescents. The clavicle usually fails first. If the fracture line is not visible, it has propagated through the cartilaginous lateral epiphysis, which is radiolucent. Adolescents sustaining acromioclavicular separations should be treated as adults.

Dislocations of the Sternoclavicular Joint

Sternoclavicular joint dislocations are rare in children and adolescents, as the medial epiphysis may fuse as late as the age of 25 years. Before fusion, the physis fails before the sternoclavicular ligaments, creating a fracture with or without displacement. Fractures generally heal and remodel satisfactorily, while true medial dislocations require attempted closed reduction, with possible open reduction if not successful.

A recent study of retrosternal clavicular dislocations concluded that all cases under age 25 should be considered displaced Salter type I fractures. If closed reduction was unsuccessful, open reduction and suturing was indicated. Pin fixation is dangerous because of potential migration into the chest.[90]

Dislocations of the Glenohumeral Joint

Dislocations of the glenohumeral joint are extremely rare in prepubertal children, but the condition becomes more prevalent in adolescence. The force that dislocates an adult shoulder fractures the child's proximal humerus. One should be alert for congenital anomalies of the articular surfaces or for the presence of predisposing factors such as joint laxity, Ehlers-Danlos syndrome, or neuromuscular disease. The treatment is similar to that described for adults elsewhere in this book.

Voluntary shoulder dislocation is occasionally encountered, especially in pubertal females and nervous children. Treatment should remain within the realm of counseling, as surgery is often unsuccessful.[84]

LOWER LIMB

Fractures of the Pelvis

Although there is no gross anatomic difference between the pediatric and adult pelvis, the presence of the triradiate cartilage and the apophyses allows for growth and remodeling of the immature pelvis but also renders the pelvis vulnerable to growth disturbances following injury. The child's pelvis is able to accommodate more energy prior to fracture than the adult pelvis; however, the soft tissue pelvic contents are more susceptible in the child because the energy absorbed is transmitted to them. A plastic deformation or greenstick fracture can occur, as in other children's bones, within the pelvis, and ligamentous laxity enables the pelvis to suffer single fractures in the pelvic ring, which is not the case in the adult. The child clearly has more ability to remodel fractures than does the adult.[88] The mechanism of injury is usually a road traffic accident, when the child is exposed to considerable violence. Approximately 60 percent of these injuries occur in children who are struck as pedestrians and 30 percent as crash occupants; the remainder are usually injuries sustained during falls. Pelvic fractures accounted for 2.4 percent of children admitted consecutively for blunt trauma to a regional trauma center, and the mortality rate is around 11 percent in patients with this injury.[88]

Classification

Ossification of the pelvis occurs from three primary centers: the ilium, ischium, and pubis. The *ilium* appears at the second fetal month, the *ischium* at the third fetal month, and the *pubis* at the fourth fetal month. The ischium and pubis fuse inferiorly at 6 to 7 years. The three centers meet at the triradiate cartilage and fuse at about 16 to 18 years.[257]

The secondary ossification centers include the iliac crest, ischial apophysis, anterior inferior iliac spine, pubic tubercle, pubic angle, ischial spine, and lateral wing of the sacrum. The iliac crest appears at 13 to 15 years and fuses at 15 to 17 years. The ischial tuberosity appears at 15 to 17 years and fuses at age 19 or older. The anterior inferior iliac spine appears at 14 years and fuses at 16.

Classification

Numerous classifications exist for these injuries. The one described by Pennal and Tile (Table 32-2) is based on the mechanism of injury and is most useful in describing treatment options.[197,246] In this classification, type A injuries are injuries caused by anteroposterior compression. They include avulsion-type fractures, such as the rectus femoris pulling off the anterior inferior iliac spine or the sartorius avulsing the apophysis of the anterior superior iliac spine (these are A1 injuries, where the fracture does not involve the pelvic ring). Injuries classified as A2 are stable fractures, where anteroposterior violence causes minimally displaced stable fractures of the ring, such as minimally displaced fractures of the ischium and pubis anteriorly without posterior injury.

In this classification, type B injuries are those produced by lateral compression. Unlike type A injuries, which are stable, these injuries are rotationally unstable but vertically stable. A type B1 injury is the classic open-book type of injury, with more than 3 cm of disruption of the pubic symphysis and tearing of the anterior portion of the ligaments of the sacroiliac joints. In type B2 injuries, the lateral compression occurs on only one side. This may produce a combination of injuries, including fractures of the sacral ala and perhaps an associated fracture of the ischial and pubic rami. In a type B3 injury, the lateral compressive force has produced injury on the contralateral side of the pelvis, damaging the pelvic ring in two places, so that there may be an unstable bucket-handle type of pelvic fragment with anterior and posterior disruption. In type C injuries, the fracture is both rotationally and vertically unstable, and this may be the case on one side (C1) or both sides (C2) of the pelvis. There may be total disruption of the sacroiliac joint, with vertical and rotational displacement of one side of the pelvis and anterior disruption either at the symphysis or across the rami of the pubis and ischium. Type C3 injury involves a similar disruption of the pelvic ring anteriorly and posteriorly, which is rotationally and vertically unstable, but on this occasion the anterior injury is associated with an acetabular fracture.

TABLE 32-2   Classification of Pelvic Disruption

Type A	Stable
	A1—Fractures of the pelvis
	    not involving the ring
	A2—Stable, minimally displaced
	    fractures of the ring

Type B	Rotationally unstable, vertically stable B1—Open book B2—Lateral compression: ipsilateral B3—Lateral compression: contralateral (bucket handle)
Type C	Rotationally and vertically unstable C1—Unilateral C2—Bilateral C3—Associated with an acetabular fracture

Source: Reproduced with permission from Tile M: Pelvic ring fractures—should they be fixed? *J Bone Joint Surg* 70B:3, 1988.

Another classification by Torode and Zieg has been used and may give some guidance, in the case of pelvic fractures, as to the likelihood of associated injuries and expected outcomes.[249] In this classification, a type 1 injury is an avulsion fracture, such as may occur associated with avulsions of the iliac apophyses. A type II fracture is a simple fracture through the iliac wing or the iliac apophysis, which is disrupted from the metaphysis. In type III injury, there is a simple ring fracture. This group includes patients with fractures involving the pubic rami or disruptions of the pubic symphysis, but in no case is there clinical instability. The authors note that a large diastasis of the pubic symphysis can occur in children without instability of the sacroiliac joints posteriorly because of the elasticity of the sacroiliac ligaments.

In Torode and Zieg's classification, type IV is reserved for those injuries that involve ring disruption fractures with an unstable segment of pelvic ring. Included in this category are bilateral fractures of the pubic rami, (straddle) fractures involving the symphysis or rami anteriorly with disruption of the sacroiliac joint posteriorly, and also fractures where the anterior break in the ring occurs through the acetabulum. Essentially the type IV fracture of Torode and Zieg corresponds to the Pennal type C classification. The authors were able to correlate, in a retrospective study of 141 patients, the majority of the associated neurologic injuries with a type III and type IV fracture. Both type III and type IV patients experienced equal numbers of genitourinary injuries, but the most severe injuries were seen in the type IV group. The incidence of the necessity for laparotomy increased progressively through types II, III, and IV pelvic fractures. There was a markedly increased incidence of genitourinary injuries in type III compared with type II. There was also a less marked but significant increase in the number of associated musculoskeletal injuries and the transfusion requirements in the type III as compared with type II injury. The authors believe that this classification is useful as a guide to the expectation of associated injuries in children's pelvic fractures.

Bond and coworkers were also able to demonstrate that the fracture pattern/location in pelvic fractures was strongly associated with the probability of abdominal injury. Thus 80 percent of children in their series with multiple pelvic fractures had concomitant abdominal or genitourinary injury, as compared with only 33 percent of those with fractures of the ilium or pelvic rim and 6 percent of children with isolated pubic fractures.[28] McIntyre and coworkers were also able to correlate the geometry of pelvic fracture with the risk of life-threatening hemorrhage in children.[174] They observed no significant difference between the fracture groups with regard to age, injury severity score (ISS), and revised trauma score (RTS). They noted that the transfusion requirements were increased considerably in patients requiring external skeletal fixation and particularly in those with disruption of the anterior and posterior pelvic ring unilaterally or bilaterally. In the former group, 35 percent required the application of an external fixator; in the latter group, 50 percent required an external fixator, mostly in an attempt to stabilize the fracture and control the hemorrhage.

Clinical Features

The clinical picture varies with minor pelvic fractures such as avulsion or an apophysis. The patient usually presents with a localized area of tenderness, swelling, and ecchymosis. For the type B and C fractures described in Pennal's classification to occur, the child must generally sustain multiple injuries and presents severely shocked, suffering from life-threatening trauma.

Diagnostic Evaluation and Treatment

The evaluation and the resuscitation of a patient with multiple injuries is the same for a child as it is for an adult, and it is only when critical lifesaving measures have been taken that radiographic evaluation can be attempted at the discretion of the trauma team. On the other hand, urgent fixation of an unstable pelvic fracture may diminish hemorrhage and be a critical lifesaving maneuver. The orthopaedist should preferably accompany the patient to the x-ray department and assist in the positioning for specific radiographic views. Standard AP x-rays of the pelvis should be supplemented with inlet and outlet views of the pelvis, with caudal and cephalad orientation of the tube at 45°. If the patient's condition permits, oblique Judet views taken with the pelvis rotated in the coronal plane at 45° oblique are useful in evaluating associated acetabular injuries. Elevating the injured hip will give an excellent view of the anterior column and anterior wall, whereas elevating the contralateral side will give an oblique Judet view, which will allow assessment of the posterior column. Before definitive treatment of the disrupted sacroiliac joint or complex acetabular fracture is initiated, CT may be necessary, but this should not be performed in the polytrauma patient during the acute period of treatment but rather only when the patient has been stabilized. Physical examination of the pelvis may identify those injuries where there is anteroposterior or rotational instability; it will also indicate the need for urgent stabilization of the pelvis in the presence of polytrauma and hemorrhage.

McIntyre and his group recommend diagnostic peritoneal lavage as a critical triage tool and advise selective laparotomy immediately when the initial aspirate yields 10 mL of blood if the patient is physiologically unstable. However, if the patient shows positive lavage results only by laboratory criteria, i.e., red blood cells (RBC) more than 100,000/mm³ and white blood cells (WBC) more than 500/mm³—they recommend further evaluation with abdominal CT scanning and external skeletal fixation of the pelvic fracture prior to any laparotomy.[174] In this way, critical lifesaving laparotomy to prevent hemorrhage is facilitated, and yet unnecessary laparotomy—which may lead to mortality when the intraabdominal hemorrhage is uncontrolled—is avoided and the critical application of the external fixator to control the pelvic bleeding is performed instead. Angiography is performed if there is inadequate response to external fixation (vital signs do not normalize and there is a continuing high fluid requirement and failure of hemoglobin level to stabilize).[174] The ipsilateral and contralateral hypogastric arteries are catheterized in this protocol and selective arteriograms enable embolization of any identified arterial hemorrhage with Gelfoam coils.

The type B injury can usually be stabilized with a simple external fixator with a pin inserted into the ilium bilaterally and an anterior frame. Alternatively, where laparotomy is to be performed, open reduction and internal fixation with a 3.5-mm dynamic compression plate can stabilize the symphysis. For type C fractures that are vertically unstable, open reduction and internal fixation is now preferred.[166,167] In addition to all type C fractures, some lateral compression fractures that are widely displaced (type B2 and B3 fractures) may also require open reduction. In addition to anterior fixation, it is necessary to stabilize the disrupted sacroiliac joint. This may be performed by the posterior approach by placing screws posteriorly from the iliac wing into the body of the sacrum traversing the joint, using the same technique as that used in adults.[166,167] Alternatively, in smaller children, it is possible to stabilize the joint using a two-hole 3.5-mm dynamic compression plate with one screw in the sacrum and one in the iliac wing.[238]

Complications

Bucholz et al. reported on nine patients with triradiate physeal cartilage injury. He observed two basic injury patterns, a shearing injury and a crushing injury.[35] The shearing injury, due to a blow to the pubis, ischial ramus, or proximal femur, produces a type I or II physeal injury, causing the acetabulum to split into a superior third and an inferior two-thirds. Since the germinal layer of the physis is unaffected, the prognosis is generally good and premature closure of the triradiate cartilage is not usually seen. A crushing injury to the acetabulum produces a type V physeal injury that results in the formation of a medial osseous bridge with resultant premature closure of the triradiate cartilage. With further growth, progressive acetabular dysplasia results, but symptoms may not appear for years after injury, so follow-up until skeletal maturity is necessary. Bucholz et al. found that children under 10 years of age appear to be at higher risk of developing premature closure of the triradiate cartilage.

Accurate anatomic reduction of children's displaced acetabular fractures is important to minimize incongruity of the acetabulum and prevent subsequent degenerative arthritis of the hip. A knowledge of the location of the apophyses is needed in order to avoid confusing them with avulsion fractures.[176] In questionable cases, comparison with the opposite side of the pelvis may be helpful.

Premature fusion of the sacroiliac joint is a problem that may be expected to occur depending on the fracture pattern. The incidence of leg-length inequality should be minimized by accurate reduction of the displaced posterior ring during definitive treatment. Definitive reconstruction of complex posterior ring disruptions and acetabular fractures will probably be performed a few days following the acute injury, when the patient is more stable and the risk of operative intervention provoking a life-threatening hemodynamic instability is minimal. Unlike adults with pelvic fractures, where 60 percent of the deaths result entirely from the pelvic fracture itself, it has been found that children

with pelvic fractures usually die because of associated head injury.[28] In a recent series 77 percent of the mortalities of children with pelvic fracture were due to this cause. It is observed that, overall, pelvic fractures in children are less likely to bleed than in adults, and some authors have speculated that this may be because the periosteal envelope is more adherent to the underlying bone in the child and that this limits the displacement of the fracture components.[28] They also believe that the children's vessels may be more vasoreactive, helping to limit the hemorrhage in the smaller vessels. However, avoidable mortality associated with the life-threatening hemorrhage that can occur in a proportion of the more serious fractures can be minimized by the type of emergency treatment protocol described.

Dislocation of the Hip

Traumatic hip dislocations are more prevalent in children than fractures in the hip region. As in adults, posterior dislocations are 7 to 10 times more common than anterior dislocations.[209]

Mechanism of Injury

Under the age of 5, the acetabulum consists of pliable cartilage. Dislocation can occur from a seemingly trivial injury, especially if ligamentous laxity is present.[85,187] After 5 years of age, the magnitude of the trauma required to dislocate the hip increases. In older children there is often an associated fracture (femoral or acetabular). Associated sciatic nerve palsy is present in 20 percent.[90]

Clinical Features

The clinical picture is one of acute distress and immobility. With a posterior dislocation of the hip, the leg is flexed, adducted, and internally rotated; with an anterior dislocation, it is extended, abducted, and externally rotated.

Radiologic Examination

Standard radiographic studies will usually differentiate a hip dislocation from a displaced fracture. Combined CT and arthrography may further delineate an obscure lesion.[142]

Treatment

A dislocation of the hip should be treated as an orthopaedic emergency in order to minimize the risk of avascular necrosis.[187] Closed reduction is generally successful and is accomplished by gentle yet firm traction. Hip flexion and internal rotation are then added if the hip is posteriorly dislocated, while hip extension and external rotation are utilized if the hip is anteriorly dislocated. The leg may be gently rocked into mild abduction and adduction to disengage the femoral head and help coax it into the acetabulum. After reduction, the hip should move freely, without crepitus. Stability should be checked in all positions. X-ray examination should reveal restoration of the normal relationship between the femoral head and the acetabulum. If the joint space is widened, capsule,[187] limbus, or fracture fragments may be interposed and an attempt should be made to gently redislocate the hip and once again reduce it. If joint space widening persists, then open reduction and removal of interposed tissue or fragments may be required.

Postreduction treatment generally consists in a few days of skin traction followed by application of a single spica cast for 4 to 6 weeks in the young child in order to allow soft tissue (especially capsular) healing. Follow-up x-ray films should be taken every 3 to 4 months for a year in younger children and for up to 2 years in older children in order to watch for the development of avascular necrosis. If avascularity is suspected and routine x-ray films are inconclusive, bone scanning may be utilized for early diagnosis. Scanning by MRI has been found to be highly diagnostic, as it differentiates avascular bone marrow from normal marrow.

Complications

Avascular necrosis is related to the severity of trauma[186] and delay in reduction.[12,13] The average reported incidence is 10 percent.[90] At follow-up, coxa vara or magna is present in 13 to 47 percent.[187] Any trapped intraarticular fragments must be removed. These may be purely cartilaginous and only identified with a high index of suspicion. Arthrography or MRI may be diagnostic. Recurrent dislocation is rare except in Down's syndrome.[89,142]

Delayed (posterior) fracture dislocation has been reported.[87]

Physeal fracture may result in displacement of the femoral neck into the acetabulum.

Osteoarthritis is usually limited to older children.[12,13,200]

Voluntary Dislocation

Occasionally teenage girls boast that they can make their hip snap or "jump out of the socket." This is generally done by shifting the weight onto one hip and snapping the tensor fascia lata over the greater trochanter. However, the hip joint itself remains stable.[209]

Rarely, a child may be seen, usually a prepubertal female, who can voluntarily subluxate or frankly dislocate the hip by sitting down with the hip flexed, rotating the hip and contracting various muscles. This is followed by spontaneous and immediate reduction upon relaxation. Treatment consists in an appeal to the parents and child to cease this activity, counseling them about the potential complications (e.g., arthritis and instability) and the difficulty of treating these major problems. If this fails, spica casting for an arbitrary 3- to 4-month period may decrease the patient's ability to subluxate. Furthermore, the inconvenience of 3 to 4 months in a spica cast may discourage the child from persisting in this activity.[199]

Fractures of the Proximal Femur

These injuries occur infrequently in the immature skeleton.[114,183,207] The age predilection is 11 to 18 years.[118] Such fractures may occur at birth and must be differentiated from congenital hip dislocation.[189,207,242] Fractures of the proximal femur may also be associated with child abuse. The mechanism of injury in children, unlike adult hip fractures, is usually severe trauma. Since considerable force is required to produce these fractures in children, associated injuries are common. If the fracture has been caused by minor trauma, a pathologic fracture should be suspected.

Ossification

The secondary ossification center in the femoral head ossifies at about 5 to 6 months after birth. The greater trochanteric apophysis appears between 2 and 5 years, while the lesser trochanter ossifies between 9 and 13 years. The shaft has already ossified by the eighth week in utero. The lesser trochanter, greater trochanter, and femoral head epiphysis fuse in that order to the shaft after puberty.

Classification

These fractures may be subdivided into four categories (Fig. 32-19): type I, transepiphyseal fractures (with or without femoral head dislocation); type II, transcervical fractures; type III, basal neck fractures; and type IV, intertrochanteric fractures.

In addition to the usual fracture patterns outlined above, one may identify a proximal femoral separation (epiphysiolysis), sometimes termed transepiphyseal separation of the proximal femoral epiphyses, which is seen in

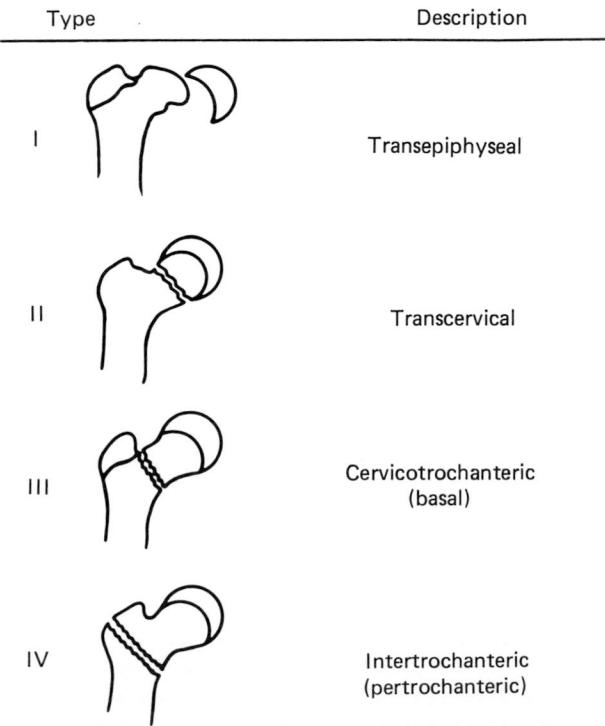

Type	Description
I	Transepiphyseal
II	Transcervical
III	Cervicotrochanteric (basal)
IV	Intertrochanteric (pertrochanteric)

Figure 32-19 Types of femoral head and neck fracture in children. (Reproduced with permission from Morrissy R: *Clin Orthop* 152:202–210, 1980.)

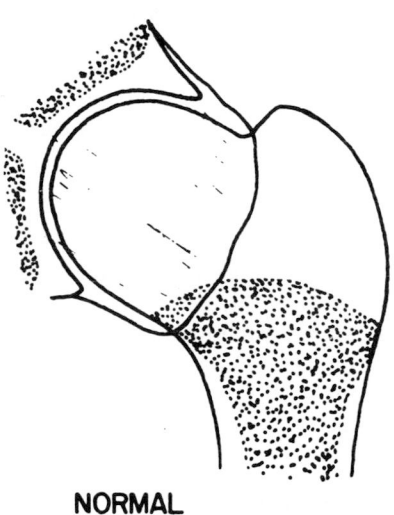

NORMAL

NEONATAL PATTERN

Figure 32-20 Pathologic anatomy of a proximal femoral separation in the neonate. It is usually a type I physeal injury beneath the chondroepiphyses of the capital femur, greater trochanter, and lesser trochanter. The arrows demonstrate the typical displacement pattern, with the shaft displacing laterally and the epiphysis displacing into a varus position. Arthrography confirms the diagnosis and allows differentiation from infection. (Reproduced with permission from Ogden JA, Lee KE, Rudicel SA, Pelher RR: *J Pediatr Orthop* 4:285–292, 1984.)

the newborn infant and is associated with obstetric delivery and injury to the chondroepiphyses (Fig. 32-20).

Clinical Features

Hip pain with or without radiation into the thigh and inability to bear weight are the usual symptoms of proximal femoral fractures in children. If the fracture is displaced, there may be shortening and external rotation of the involved extremity.

Radiologic Examination

Displaced fractures are easily diagnosed with standard radiographic views. Subtle fractures may require additional views, including obliques, comparison views, and tomographic scans. A bone scan may be helpful. If the diagnosis is still unclear in neonates, ultrasonography, MRI, or arthrography of the hip may be needed in order to differentiate a hip dislocation from traumatic transepiphyseal separation of the proximal femoral epiphysis (Fig. 32-20).

Treatment

Because of the rarity of children's hip fractures, most of the reported series contain limited numbers of cases with varying recommendations as to the type of treatment. In general, however, nondisplaced fractures of the hip in children, irrespective of type, may be treated nonoperatively by cast immobilization until healed. Careful follow-up is important, since loss of reduction significantly affects the final outcome. If the patient or family is unreliable and follow-up cannot be arranged as needed, then internal fixation of a nondisplaced transcervical fracture (type II) is recommended.[165]

Displaced type I (transepiphyseal) fractures without associated femoral head dislocation and displaced type II (transcervical), type III (cervicotrochanteric), and type IV (intertrochanteric) fractures should undergo closed reduction with internal fixation.[123,183,202] However, some authors prefer traction, reduction, and spica casting at 3 to 4 weeks for displaced type IV injuries in children and adolescents between the ages of 6 to 12 years.[100,106] Similarly, some authors recommend closed reduction and spica casting alone for type IV fractures in very young children (up to age 6).[114,123,146] They reserve open reduction and internal fixation for older children. The physician should be alert for ischemic syndromes or loss of position when spica cast treatment is chosen.[120] Loss of position is an indication for open reduction and internal fixation.

If closed manipulation of a displaced hip fracture does not produce a satisfactory reduction, then open reduction with internal fixation is necessary. This is almost always required in type I fractures with associated femoral head dislocations. Cancellous bone screws or K wire and cerclage may be used in type III and IV injuries.[120] Threaded pins or a compression hip screw for the older child or adolescent is also acceptable. If the capital physis is to be crossed, as in the treatment of type I fractures, then only smooth, fine pins should be used.[207]

Complications

Avascular necrosis (AVN) is the most feared complication. Unfortunately it is also the most frequent, with an incidence as high as 40 percent in type II injuries.[44] AVN appears earlier in children than in adults, usually within a year of injury.[123] A bone scan or MRI may be helpful in establishing an early diagnosis. Traumatic AVN is often more severe and extensive than that seen in Perthes' disease. The remodeling process may continue for up to 5 years and may be incomplete. The younger the child, the better the result because of the greater remodeling potential. The treatment of AVN is similar to that for Perthes' disease, i.e., limitation of activity and weight bearing, preservation of motion, and containment with an orthosis if needed.

Coxa vara may result from inadequate reduction or immobilization or from asymmetrical and premature physeal closure.[120,188] It causes shortening, abductor lurch, and subsequent degenerative changes in the hip joint. Corrective subtrochanteric valgus osteotomy may be indicated.

Nonunion has been reported in up to 13 percent of cases. Canale and King observe that a lower rate of nonunion follows the use of internal fixation after closed reduction.[44] The treatment for nonunion is subtrochanteric valgus osteotomy and bone grafting.

The incidence of premature physeal closure reportedly ranges from 9 to 61 percent. Since the proximal femoral physis contributes 15 percent of the overall leg length, the shortening is determined by the age of the patient at injury.[207]

Fractures of the Femoral Diaphysis

The femur contributes approximately 26 percent of the adult height. A major part of this growth occurs at the distal physis.[232]

Ossification

Ossification of the femoral shaft begins at the eighth week in utero. The femoral shaft is the second bone to ossify. (The clavicle is the first, ossifying by membranous bone formation.) A secondary ossification center develops in the distal femur during the last 2 months in utero. It fuses to the shaft around age 20.

Mechanism of Injury

Direct trauma often creates a transverse fracture, but there may be a butterfly fragment. Indirect trauma often has a rotational component, creating a spiral fracture. Associated injuries such as Waddell's triad (injury to the femur, chest, and head) may occur in multiple trauma such as that seen in motor vehicle injury. Multiple injuries also occur in child abuse.

Classification

Fractures may be classified according to location as subtrochanteric fractures; fractures of the proximal, middle, or distal third of the diaphysis; or supracondylar fractures. Qualifying terms may describe the fracture as open or closed; may indicate the direction of the fracture and the amount and direction of angulation, displacement, or shortening; or may characterize the fracture according to its complexity—e.g., the amount of comminution and

whether it is segmental or associated with a butterfly fragment.

It is important to recognize fractures that are pathologic or are the result of child abuse (see previous section in this chapter on child abuse, above).

Clinical Features

This is a severely disabling and extremely painful injury. Significant blood loss may occur. The diagnosis is usually so obvious that the ambulance attendants will already have applied a traction splint before arrival at the emergency room. The child should be carefully examined for associated injuries, and the neurovascular status of the limb should be accurately documented.

Radiologic Examination

During overall assessment and stabilization of the patient, the injured extremity should be immobilized. Good-quality portable x-ray films are appropriate if available. X-ray views should include at least the pelvis, hip, and knee joints, to rule out associated ipsilateral fractures and/or dislocations. This fracture is so painful that it will often mask less severe or less painful associated injuries.

Treatment

Treatment of the uncomplicated fracture of the femoral shaft is age-dependent. There is general consensus that in children up to the age of 2, immediate spica casting is the simplest and most comfortable method of managing this fracture. No such consensus, however, is associated with treatment of these fractures in any of the other age groups, and a wide variety of treatment modalities—including external and internal fixation (which includes plating and antegrade and retrograde rodding)—has been advocated. Each has its drawbacks and advantages.

Curtis and coauthors compared two random groups of patients in the 2- to 10-year age group, one treated traditionally by 3 weeks in traction followed by spica casting and a second group treated only for a few days in traction and then with 90°/90° traction pins in plastic spica.[62] The spica was a $1\frac{1}{2}$ spica cast of fiberglass incorporating a large, smooth, distal femoral traction pin applied with the leg in traction from the ceiling at 90° of hip and knee flexion. They attempted to achieve 0.5 to 1.5 cm of shortening during the procedure to compensate for subsequent overgrowth of the physis, which often accompanies the healing of this fracture in this age group. They were subsequently able to remove the anterior half of the distal portion of the cast to allow flexion extension of the knee joint. Pin removal was performed at the fourth week and the spica removed at the eighth week if appropriate. Curtis et al. achieved excellent short- and long-term results with no malalignment of the fracture and an average shortening of only 12 mm. An essential part of the technique was the use of a prefabricated wooden pontoon which was incorporated beneath the tibial region of the leg to prevent cast breakdown.[62]

Buehler and associates have developed criteria for the prospective identification of patients who can be safely and dependably treated with early spica casting without excessive shortening of the fracture fragments.[36] They describe performing a "telescope test," which consists of gentle manual compression applied under general anesthetic across the fractured femur until a distinct endpoint is reached. If the measured shortening during the telescope test is less than 30 mm, patients can be treated with a standard spica cast, whereas if the shortening exceeds 30 mm, treatment in their hands included the incorporation of a distal femoral metaphyseal pin into the spica cast, skeletal traction, or some other method such as external fixation to achieve greater stabilization minimizing the risk of the excessive shortening that might otherwise occur. They concluded that children between 2 and 10 years of age with uncomplicated femoral shaft fractures and a negative telescope test can be safely treated with early spica casting and have a 95 percent chance of having a successful outcome with this treatment.[36] These authors were, however, careful to point out that if children in this age group present with multiple injuries, serious head injury, or open fracture, an alternative method of treatment is recommended rather than spica casting. In these cases external fixation, skeletal traction, or internal fixation is to be preferred.

Early reports of the use of external skeletal fixation in children's fractures indicated that there was a high incidence of drainage from the pins and a high refracture rate after removal of the device.[247] Subsequently, however, there have been several studies showing that this is a satisfactory method of treating femoral fractures that can be employed in all age groups but is probably more suitable for patients between the age of 4 and 12. This is the age group recommended for this method by Aronson and Tursky.[7] They reported success in 44 femoral fractures, none of which developed bone infection. Only 38 percent of these patients had bone overgrowth, and this only averaged 5.8 mm. Similar satisfactory results with external fixation have been reported by other authors.[79,97] It may be necessary to maintain the fixator in position for up to 3 months in adolescents. In children younger than 8 years of age, the fixator should be in place for approximately 6 weeks, but the decision to remove it will depend upon the appearance of healthy bridging callus. If the fixator is removed too early, there is a risk of losing position.

Although external fixators are relatively simple and efficient alternatives for the treatment of femoral fractures, permitting rapid patient mobilization and good control of alignment, it is important that pin care be maintained during the period of application of the frame. If the bone becomes infected, subsequent intramedullary fixation is prejudiced. Another complication of this method has been the development of refracture, probably associated with the stress-shielding effect of rigid frames.[205] External fixation has been recommended in patients with severe head injuries or polytrauma, permitting rapid stabilization of femoral diaphyseal fractures in these situations. It is also particularly useful in the case of open fractures.[20,204] In the younger age group, compression plating of the femur has been recommended in the polytrauma patient or in those patients who may have an associated severe head injury. In these severely injured children, the need to expedite mobilization or rehabilitation requires a more aggressive approach. The major problems associated with plate fixation are the size of the incision and the degree of soft tissue stripping necessary to apply the plate. A higher risk of infection and plate breakage or delayed fracture of the femur after removal of the plate and screws are additional complications of this method. Ward and coauthors believe that intramedullary nailing is a better option for the child above age 12 where the medullary canal and the piriformis fossa are large enough to accept a small nail and are therefore suitable for antegrade nailing.[255] These authors, however, experienced few negative complications in their series of 25 plated femoral fractures, with only one delayed fracture through a screw hole associated with a second injury and with minimal leg-length discrepancy. Similar results with the use of plates in children with polytrauma or head injury have been reported by Kregor and associates, whose 15 patients averaged age 8 years of age.[144a] One problem with the use of the external fixator and also closed intramedullary nailing is the evaluation of rotation, particularly in more proximal fractures, when the proximal fragment is quite often externally rotated.[45] Certainly, this problem is not present with the application of plates. It should be noted, however, that the removal of the plate in itself may cause additional stimulation to the growth plate with further overgrowth of the injured limb, particularly in patients over age 6.

An alternative to external fixation in the younger group where inpatient traction and spica fixation is not an option and where the medullary cavity is too small for antegrade rodding is the use of retrograde flexible nailing. This may be preferred over a period of inpatient traction because of the incidence of malalignment associated with the latter course of treatment and also because of anxiety about health care costs and also the psychosocial effects for the child of several weeks in the hospital, away from parents and school.[36] Good results have been reported in patients of all age groups using elastic (flexible) intramedullary nails inserted through portals in the distal metaphysis of the femur.[81,152] There are no problems in achieving union and leg-length discrepancy is insignificant. In fact, the procedure seems to be remarkably free of complications.

In children above age 10, antegrade intramedullary rodding may be considered as an alternative to distal retrograde flexible nail fixation. In a prospective study, Reeves et al.[213] compared the results of traction and subsequent casting with rigid internal fixation using rigid intramedullary rods introduced in an antegrade fashion. They observed that the group treated with traction and casting had a mean hospital stay of 26 days, whereas the operative group had a mean hospital stay of only 9 days and had fewer complications. They believe that this treatment results in shorter hospitalization, which has psychological, educational, and social advantages (in addition to the monetary savings) over inpatient traction and delayed casting.

Beaty and coauthors similarly report that intramedullary nailing is a reasonable alternative for the treatment of isolated femoral shaft fractures in older adolescents and in young adolescents with multiple trauma.[19] However, they report one case of segmental avascular necrosis of the femoral head, and a similar complication has been reported by O'Malley et al.[191] Another problem with this method has been premature epiphysiodesis of the greater trochanteric physis as a consequence of placement of the rod.[208] To avoid the complication of damage to the blood vessels supplying the femoral epiphysis, some authors[191] believe that rigid intramedullary rods inserted proximally near the piriformis fossa should be avoided entirely in skeletally immature patients. In view of the low incidence of this complication, however, it is now recommended that dissection be limited to the base of the femoral neck and the junction of the piriformis fossa and the greater trochanter and that it not extend into the posterior aspect of the capsule of the midportion of the femoral neck. Thus the blood vessels to the femoral head may be preserved (Fig. 32-21). Another suggestion is that the posterior third of the tip of the greater trochanter be removed and the nail then inserted at the junction of the fossa with the base of the greater trochanter.

In using the technique of femoral nailing with interlocking screws (which enable stabilization without shortening of the more difficult fracture), it is important to avoid transgression of the distal femoral epiphysis with the nail. This often means that the distal interlocking screws have to be inserted somewhat higher than optimal unless special nails are provided for pediatric use in which the interlocking portal in the nail is located somewhat more distally than in the adult design.[45] Complications of intramedullary nailing are similar to those in the adult, including rotational malalignment. Increased femoral neck valgus may occur as a consequence of premature closure of the greater trochanteric physis.

Leg-Length Discrepancy and Angular Deformity

A leg-length discrepancy of 1 cm or less is generally not detectable by the patient or the family; a discrepancy of 1 to 2 cm may be noted by the parents, and a difference greater than 2 cm will usually be noticeable to the patient as well. After fracture healing in children, growth is stimulated. Below age 12, the amount of overgrowth is not related to age.[175] Overgrowth declines in adolescence. It is significantly greater in boys than in girls.[55] Most of the overgrowth occurs during the first 6 months after injury, but it may continue for as long as several years.[223] Meals reported an inverse relationship between the amount of overgrowth and the degree of overriding of the fracture fragments.[175]

With the expectation of overgrowth, prepubertal children should have the femoral fracture reduced with 1.5 to 2 cm of overriding, while femoral fractures in pubertal and early adolescent children should be reduced with about 1 cm of overriding. In adolescence, the femoral fracture should be allowed to heal as close as possible to normal length. Distraction should be avoided.

The amount of angular deformity that is acceptable depends on the patient's age, the location of the fracture, and the plane of the deformity. In general, the younger the patient and the closer the fracture to the physis, the greater the remodeling potential. Varus or valgus angulation has far less remodeling potential than anterior or posterior angulation, and more than 10° of varus or valgus deformity should be avoided.[232] Below age 12, however, up to 20° may occasionally correct satisfactorily.[158] In the sagittal plane, up to 30° of angular deformity will remodel under

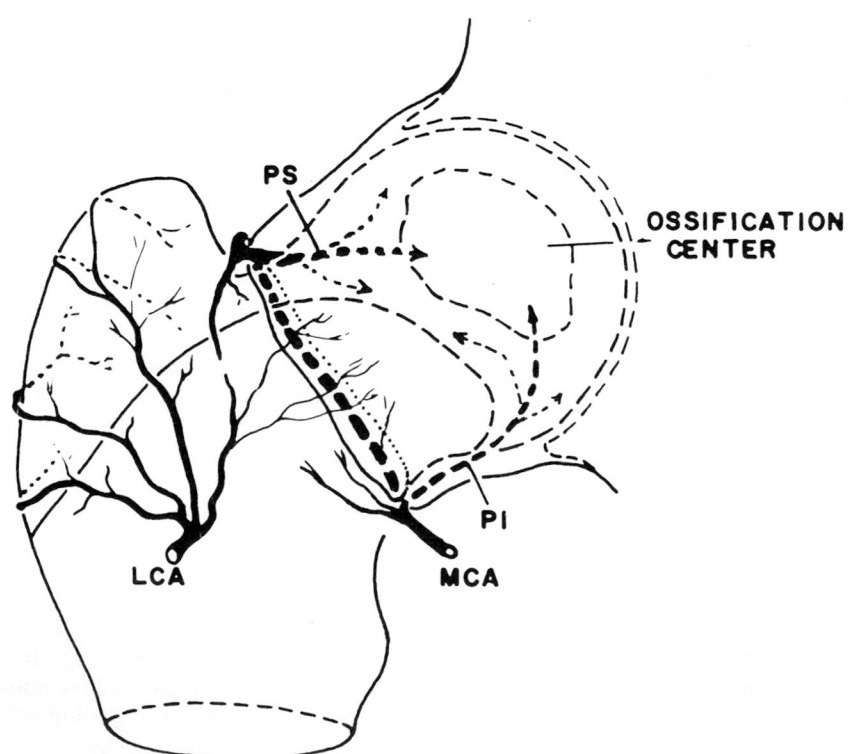

Figure 32-21 Arterial supply to the femoral epiphysis at age 3. The entire capital femoral epiphysis and growth plate are supplied by the medial circumflex artery (MCA) through two retinacular systems—the posterosuperior (PS) and posteroinferior (PI). The contribution of the lateral circumflex artery (LCA) is to the great trochanter and its portion of the proximal femoral growth plate but effectively zero to the capital femoral epiphysis. (Reproduced with permission from Ogden JA: Changing patterns of proximal femoral vascularity. *J Bone Joint Surg* 56A:941–950, 1974.)

age 12; in newborns, as much as 45° of anteroposterior deformity that is in line with knee motion of the distal femur will correct spontaneously. By contrast, 10° of anteroposterior deformity in a slender 13-year-old female may be cosmetically unacceptable and may not remodel adequately.

Clinically obvious rotational deformity is uncommon. By radiologic measurement, rotational deformity is less than 10° in most patients.[158]

Supracondylar Fracture

A supracondylar fracture is located just above the point of gastrocnemius origin; the distal fragment may consequently flex at the knee joint. Complete displacement of this fracture is uncommon in children. Generally, 90°/90° traction with proximal tibial pin fixation is the safest and most effective method of reducing these fractures (care must be taken that the tibial pin is not inserted into the proximal tibial physis or apophysis). A common problem is failure to adequately appreciate the varus alignment of the fracture because of the difficulty in getting long leg films with the knee flexed at 90°. This problem may be avoided by inserting a second traction pin into the metaphyseal fragment and applying a vertical force to this region. This arrangement permits the knee to be slowly extended without loosening of position and facilitates better radiologic monitoring of the fracture alignment. Open reduction and internal fixation runs the risk of physeal injury.[232] Any pin inserted into the distal femoral fragment should be at least 1 cm away from the growth plate. In very small children, crossed Steinmann pins may be used. In older children, an external fixator may be applied without prejudicing the physis.

Special Considerations

Floating knee injuries where there is an associated fracture of the femur and tibia in the same limb may conveniently be managed with an external fixator. These fractures have a tendency to overgrow considerably because of the double injury. The external fixator may actually span the knee joint, since permanent knee stiffness in children is unusual if the joint is uninjured.[45]

Fracture of the Distal Femoral Epiphysis

Originally termed *cartwheel injuries* (resulting from catching a leg in the spokes of a wagon wheel), distal femoral physeal fractures are often caused today by contact sports, falls, or vehicular accidents. In horse-and-buggy days, these injuries often resulted in amputation or death.[3,188,225]

The distal femoral epiphysis is the first to ossify (39th week in utero) and the last to fuse at maturity.[41] This physis contributes 70 percent of the femoral growth and 37 percent of the overall growth of the lower extremity.[48,61] Its rate of growth averages 3/8 in. per year, slowing measurably at age 13 years in girls and 15 years in boys. Local growth rates have been charted by Green-Anderson. The distal femoral physis is considered to be extraarticular

even though anteriorly the suprapatellar pouch extends proximal to the metaphysis.

Mechanism of Injury

The injury is usually a result of direct contusion. Ogden has grouped the etiologic mechanisms into four categories:[188] (1) The abduction type occurs from a blow to the lateral side of the femur. This creates a Salter-Harris type II physeal injury with a lateral metaphyseal spike. The epiphysis may be displaced laterally. (2) Adduction injuries are caused by a medial blow to the femur, creating a type I or II physeal injury with or without medial displacement of the epiphysis. (3) With hyperextension injuries, the distal shaft may be driven into the popliteal structures as the epiphysis displaces anteriorly. (4) Rare hyperflexion injuries result from an anteriorly applied force to the flexed knee, causing posterior displacement of the distal epiphysis.

Classification

Salter types I and II physeal injuries are relatively common. Type I may be undisplaced, or the physeal displacement may be anterior, posterior, medial, or lateral. This type is frequently seen in child abuse. Type II injuries are the most common and may also be displaced in any direction. Types III and IV injuries are uncommon and usually involve the medial or lateral condyle; infrequently, the posterior condylar elements are involved.[248] With type IV injuries, there is often proximal displacement of the fragment. If both condyles are involved, they may also be split apart. Type V injury is rare, its presence usually being revealed only by subsequent observation of partial growth arrest.

Clinical Features

There is a history of severe injury with pain and inability to bear weight. The knee joint and distal femur are markedly swollen and tender. The neurovascular status should be evaluated and documented. These injuries are often misdiagnosed as knee ligament injuries.[182,253] Oblique or tunnel views, a few CT cuts, or MRI may be helpful to establish the diagnosis.[253] A widened physis may be an indication of an undisplaced type I injury. Stress views may then be particularly valuable and will also differentiate these injuries from those of the knee ligaments.

Treatment

The method of closed reduction is based on the mechanism of injury and/or the direction of displacement. Gentle but firm longitudinal traction is followed by reversal of the deforming force or gradual reduction of the displaced distal fragment. Appropriate anesthesia and a good assistant are required in order to achieve as untraumatic a reduction as possible so as to avoid further physeal damage.

If adequate closed reduction is not achieved or if the fracture is unstable or the leg too obese for casting, closed reduction with percutaneous pinning or skeletal traction may be employed. If reduction still cannot be obtained or maintained, then open reduction and internal fixation are required. This is usually the case with type III and IV injuries but may also occur with displaced types I and II with soft tissue interposition. Pins or cancellous screws may be used for fixation but should not cross the physis.

Alternatively, a single spica cast may be needed to maintain reduction with an extremely unstable fracture or an obese or short thigh. Often a well-molded long leg cast is adequate. In nondisplaced fractures, a long, snug cylinder cast will suffice. The knee is usually maintained in 20 to 30° of flexion for stability, although with hyperflexion injuries, full extension is appropriate.

Complications

Distal femoral fractures in children are associated with frequent complications, including vascular injury, peroneal nerve injury, recurrent displacement, progressive angulation, symmetrical or asymmetrical growth arrest resulting in shortening [214,235] or angulation, and knee stiffness. The patient and parents should be forewarned.[215]

Fractures of the Tibia and Fibula

Fractures of the tibia and fibula are the most common lower extremity fractures in children. The fracture patterns are dependent on the age of the patient and the mechanism of injury. The majority of fractures are the result of low-energy trauma. The substantial periosteum tends to limit displacement, improves the ability to achieve an acceptable closed reduction, and leads to rapid healing. High-energy injuries resulting from falls from heights and motor vehicle accidents may result in severely comminuted and open fractures and present the same difficulties and complications as adult tibial fractures.

Ossification The tibial shaft ossifies from a primary center in the eighth fetal week. The proximal epiphysis ossifies shortly after birth, fusing with the shaft at 16 to 19 years, and the distal epiphysis appears by 1 to 2 years, fusing with the shaft at 17 to 18 years. The apophysis (tubercle) appears at puberty and coalesces with the rest of the proximal epiphysis before it fuses in adolescence. The fibular shaft ossifies in the eighth fetal week. The fibular proximal epiphysis appears in the fourth year and fuses at 16 to 20 years, and the distal epiphysis ossifies at 1 to 2 years, fusing at 17 to 18 years.[148,188]

Radiologic Examination The entire tibia and fibula should be included on one x-ray cassette for both the AP and lateral projections. Oblique x-ray views are sometimes necessary if clinical suspicion is high and standard projection views are negative. Children with multiple injuries and/or head trauma should have routine pelvic films to rule out those injuries which are less clinically evident than the obvious fractures of the tibia and fibula.

Fracture of the Intercondylar Eminence of the Tibia

Avulsion injuries are reportedly rare in those under age 10; they are most commonly seen in children 10 to 14 years of age. The Lachman test should be performed on all children with acute knee injuries. This will detect the pure cartilaginous avulsion that is not radiographically evident as well as the much less common midsubstance tear of the anterior cruciate ligament. The anterior cruciate ligament may also be stretched at the time of injury; consequently, even after the anatomic reduction, some laxity may persist in the joint.

Classification Meyers and McKeever are credited with the most commonly utilized classification system (Fig. 32-22).[177,178] Their classification is based on the amount of displacement detected on the lateral roentgenogram. Type I is minimally displaced; in type II, one-third to one-half of the eminence is elevated and hinged on its posterior insertion; type III and type III+ are completely displaced and may be rotated.

Treatment Type I injuries may be treated in a long leg cast or well-molded cylinder cast with the knee in extension for 6 weeks. Most investigators believe that type II injuries can be adequately reduced by bringing the knee into hyperextension. Postreduction films should be obtained to ascertain that the fragment has been adequately reduced.

Type III avulsions, as well as inadequately reduced type II fractures, should be treated by open reduction and internal fixation, particularly in the over-10 age group.[101]

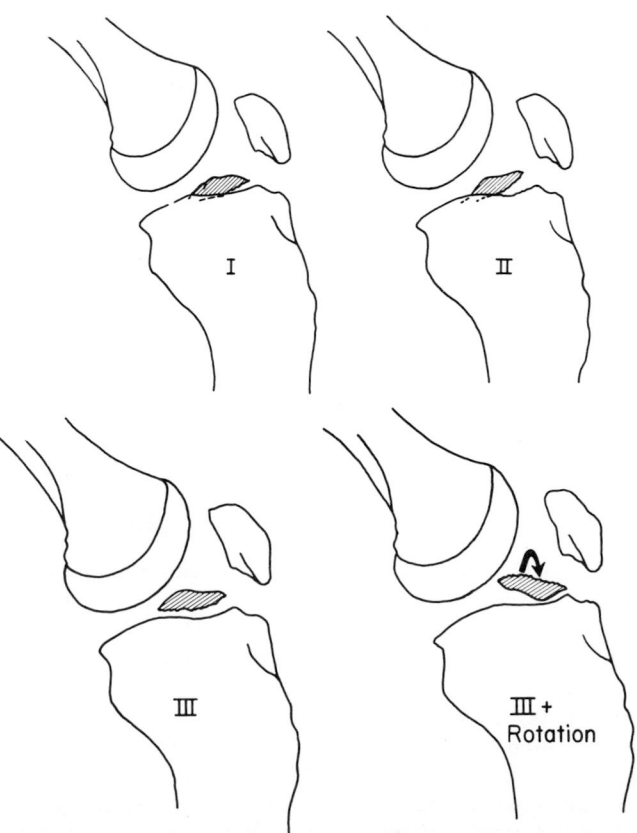

Figure 32-22 Types of intercondylar eminence fracture of the tibia in children according to Meyers and McKeever's classification. (Reproduced with permission from Meyers JH, McKeever FM: *J Bone Joint Surg* 41A:214, 1959.)

Sutures are drawn through drill holes in the fragment as well as through the substance of the anterior cruciate ligament. These sutures are then brought out through drill holes in the anterior tibia. Absorbable suture material is used so as not to have a permanent restraint crossing the proximal tibial epiphysis. Arthroscopic reduction and internal fixation has also been described.[17] Postoperatively, casting is continued for 6 weeks after fixation.

Fractures of the tibial eminence are avulsions of the tibial insertion of the anterior cruciate ligament. These injuries are often thought to be tibial spine fractures; however, intraoperative exploration often reveals complete anterior cruciate avulsion with a large, broad cartilaginous base. The injury has become more common in recent years as organized sports have become more popular among the adolescent age group.

Fracture of the Proximal Tibial Epiphysis

Fracture of the proximal tibial epiphysis occurs infrequently, constituting about 0.5 percent of epiphyseal injuries. This may be because the epiphysis receives no attachment from either the medial or lateral collateral ligaments of the knee.[37] The proximal tibial physis is the second largest growth plate and is well protected by the fibula laterally, the extension of the tibial tubercle anteriorly, the superficial portion of the medial collateral ligament medially, and the semimembranosus posteromedially. The trauma may be direct, indirect, or passive (breech delivery, manipulation, child abuse).[215,244] The injury occurs more frequently in teenagers than in younger children.

Classification These fractures are usually Salter-Harris type II injuries. Type III and type IV injuries are next in order of frequency and then type I. Type V is rare.[37,215] The type I injury occurs in a younger age group. The type IV injury is often seen in lawn mower injury.[37] The metaphysis most commonly displaces posterolaterally or posteromedially.[96]

Clinical Features The child with this injury is most commonly a boy between the ages of 12 and 14[77] who presents with a stiff, swollen, tender knee that may feel unstable because of motion of the fracture site. In adolescents, this injury is often misdiagnosed as a collateral ligament tear. Neurocirculatory assessment is imperative, as popliteal artery and peroneal nerve injury may occur. The use of Doppler and arteriography may be indicated, and there is a potential for the development of a compartment syndrome. The commonest mechanism of injury is a valgus-type force that may be associated with child abuse. Alternatively, the injury may be of the hyperextension type, in which case vascular injury is more likely.

Treatment Salter-Harris type I and II fractures of the proximal tibial epiphysis are treated with closed reduction and application of a well-molded long leg cast for 3 to 5 weeks, depending on the age of the patient. If the fracture is unstable, percutaneous pinning may be required after closed reduction. If the fracture is irreducible, ligament, cartilage, or tendon may be interposed and open reduction may then be necessary.[244] Salter type III and IV fractures require anatomic reduction of the articular surface and the physis. Open re-

duction and internal fixation with pins or lag screws oriented parallel to the physis are indicated in these cases. The prognosis for this injury is usually good; however, growth arrest may subsequently occur[110,188,194] and is inevitable in open type IV injury.[37] All these patients should be followed for at least 1 year, and a scanning micrograph is then advisable.[37]

Fracture of the Proximal Tibial Apophysis

Acute fractures of the proximal tibial apophysis are quite rare, the incidence ranging from 0.4 to 2.7 percent.[96,188] Chronic or subacute lesions such as Osgood-Schlatter's disease are quite common. The broad, fanlike expansion of the insertion of the extensor mechanism, which also inserts into the more distal periosteum and adjacent soft tissues, protects the tibial tubercle apophysis from complete avulsion. These injuries usually occur in athletic males between 14 and 16 years old.[188]

Mechanism of Injury The mechanism of injury is a traction force applied via the quadriceps that is strong enough to overcome the combined strength of the apophyseal plate and the broad distal attachment of the patellar ligament. Preexisting Osgood-Schlatter lesions in the ipsilateral or contralateral knee are common in these cases.

Classification Watson-Jones originally described three types of tibial apophyseal injury.[256] These have been redefined by Ogden and associates (Fig. 32-23):

Type 1: Elevation of the distal part of the tuberosity
    1A: The tuberosity ossification center shows mild anterior separation but is essentially undisplaced
    1B: The fragment is separated from the metaphysis and/or epiphysis
Type 2: Separation of a larger osteocartilaginous fragment representing the entire tuberosity from the metaphysis and remainder of the epiphysis
    2A: The distal tuberosity is separated and angulated anteriorly
    2B: The tuberosity is also fragmented
Type 3: Major separation of fragments with propagation into the knee joint
    3A: Displaced fragment is unitary
    3B: Comminution of the fragments

Clinical Features Since the tibial apophysis is virtually subcutaneous in location, localized tenderness and swelling over the anterior proximal tibia are obvious. With extension of the fracture into the knee joint (type 3), hemarthrosis will also be present. Hamstring spasm will further flex the knee. Active extension of the knee may not be possible in displaced fractures. Clinical examination may also reveal a high-riding patella.[215]

Treatment Minimally displaced fractures may be treated with closed reduction by thumb compression over the apophysis with extension of the knee. All displaced fractures (types 1B, 2A and 2B, 3A and 3B) require open reduction and internal fixation with threaded pins or a screw. The anatomic restoration of the articular surface as well as the tibial apophyseal or epiphyseal centers is impor-

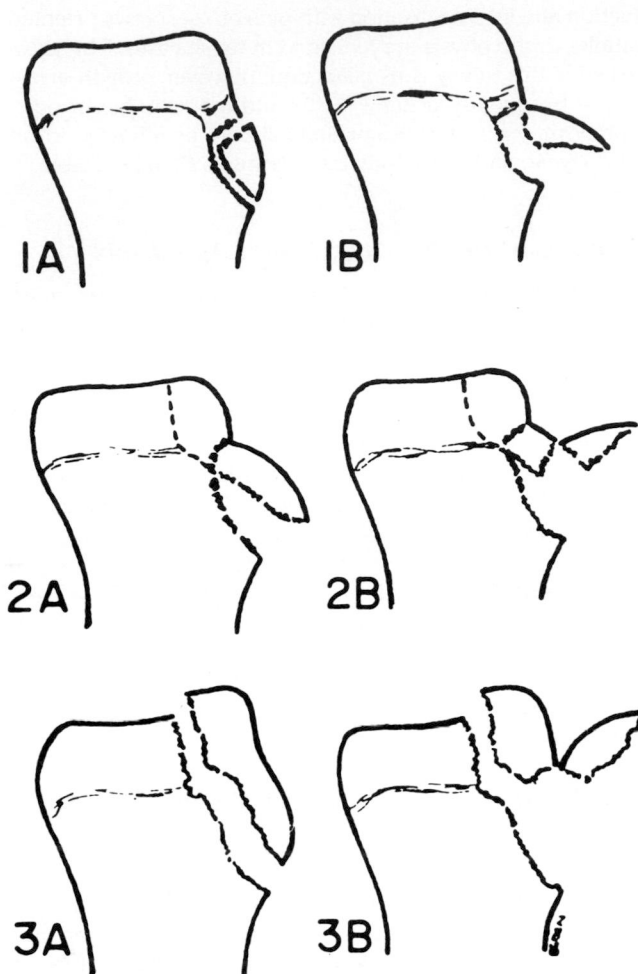

Figure 32-23 Types of fracture of the tibial tuberosity in the Watson-Jones classificaion as modified by Ogden. (Reproduced with permission from Ogden J, Tross RB, Murphy MJ: *J Bone Joint Surg* 62A:205–214, 1980.)

tant. Immobilization should continue for 4 weeks, followed by partial protection with gentle quadriceps isometrics and range-of-motion exercises for 2 weeks. Whenever possible, fixation devices should avoid crossing the physis, and they should be removed early. There may be associated ligamentous damage to knee ligaments, which should not be overlooked.

Fracture of the Proximal Tibial Metaphysis

These simple-looking, complication-ridden fractures usually occur in children from 3 to 6 years.[71,188] Rang aptly divides them by potential complications (arterial hazard and valgus greenstick types).[209] The usual greenstick type of fracture results from indirect trauma through loading of the distal tibia or foot.

Classification Metaphyseal fractures are of torus (compression) or greenstick (tension) types. Displaced (complete) fractures occur more commonly in adolescents.

Clinical Features The subcutaneous location of the proximal tibial metaphysis facilitates diagnosis by observation and palpation. Neurocirculatory watch is important! X-ray diagnosis in subtle fractures may be difficult. Oblique, coned-down, or magnified views may help. The typical fracture is a greenstick type with slight medial opening and mild lateral angulation of the distal fragment. The fibula often remains intact or sustains a subtle tension fracture or mild plastic deformation.[188]

Treatment The angulation is corrected by manual reduction. Completion of the greenstick fracture on the compression (concave) or lateral side may be necessary to attain correction.[188] Mild displacement will remodel as long as axial alignment is good. Reduction should be checked at weekly intervals by full tibial x-ray films to detect recurrent valgus angulation.

Complications Valgus deformity may occur following metaphyseal fracture (Fig. 32-24). This self-limiting phenomenon usually develops within 5 months, then stabilizes. Two major causes are proposed: inadequate reduction and medial tibial overgrowth.[95]

Treatment is prefaced by warning the family that this complication may occur in spite of adequate treatment. Radiographs must be taken with the knee in full extension to adequately assess alignment. Any valgus angulation must be corrected under adequate anesthesia. If the condition is correctable, some authors recommend open reduction and extraction of interposed tissues.[216,253] The long leg cast should be well molded with the knee in extension. Weekly follow-up may show recurrent valgus deformity, indicating the need for cast wedging or cast change after repeat closed reduction. Long leg valgus-correcting orthoses are of disputed value. Late residual valgus over 10 to 15° may be slightly overcorrected by varus osteotomy, although spontaneous correction is likely within 3 years.[116,226]

Tibial and Fibular Diaphyseal Fractures

Diaphyseal fractures of the tibia and fibula in children are easier to treat, heal much faster, and have fewer complications than their adult counterparts. The fibula often remains intact, which helps to minimize tibial displacement. The child's thicker periosteum also helps to reduce the amount of displacement.

Assessment The majority of children's tibial fractures result from low-energy trauma. Depending on the age of the child, the fracture patterns are usually of a torus, greenstick, or spiral type. Bumper injuries as well as other direct trauma create oblique, transverse, and comminuted fracture patterns. The child's age (and remodeling potential), the mechanism of the fracture, and the degree of injury to associated soft tissues should be considered in assessing these injuries.

Clinical Features In very young children with occult spiral fractures and no history of trauma, the diagnosis can be quite difficult. The "toddler's" fracture occurs between

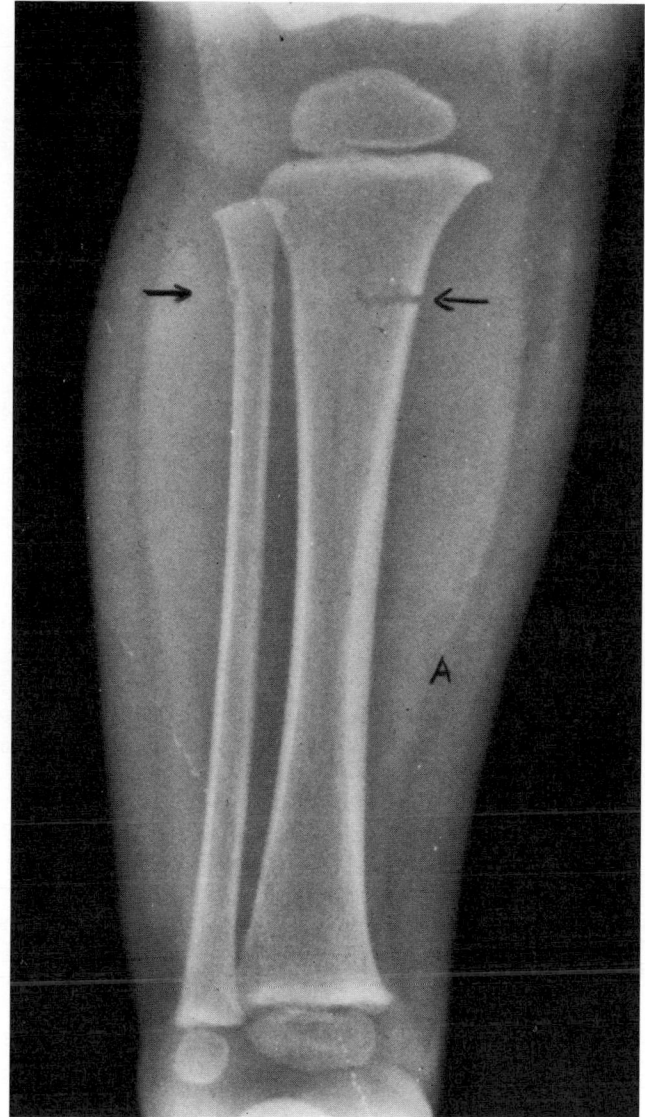

A

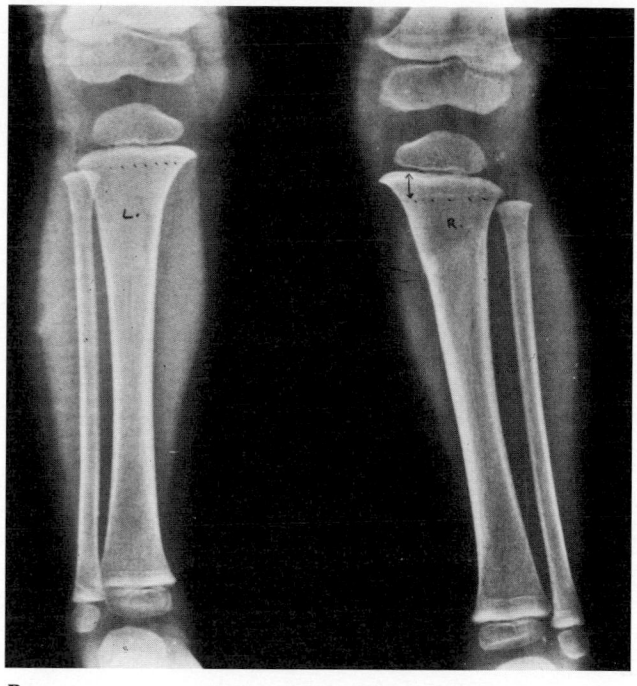

B

Figure 32-24 *A*. A young child sustained this fracture of the proximal tibial metaphysis and proximal fibula. *B*. At 1 year after injury, valgus deformity of the affected extremity is evident.

9 months and 6 years[238] and is an oblique fracture of the distal tibial diaphysis without fibular fracture. A history of sudden crying and inability to bear weight, combined with slight swelling of the lower leg, should arouse suspicion of the toddler's fracture. If standard AP and lateral x-ray films do not reveal a fracture, coned-down and oblique views may help diagnose an occult fracture, or alternatively, a technetium bone scan may reveal increased uptake in the region of the fracture.

Inclusion of the knee and ankle joints will help rule out angular malalignment and ipsilateral concomitant injuries. In major trauma, pelvic x-rays are also important to rule out a pelvic or hip fracture and/or dislocation.

Treatment The majority of children's diaphyseal fractures may be successfully treated by closed manipulation and a long leg cast. Vascular and neurologic injuries are rare, but documentation is important because the complication of compartment syndrome does occur. The oblique, isolated tibial fracture tends to drift into varus position because of the rotational effect of the ankle and toe flexors coupled with an intact fibula. Consequently Dias advises knee flex-

ion and some degree of ankle equinus position during early immobilization to help control the fracture.[71] The author has satisfactory experience casting the limb with the knee extended and the ankle in neutral position. With both bones fractured, shortening with or without angular malalignment becomes the problem. Proper length must be attained at closed reduction; any mild residual angulation may be controlled with cast wedging or cast change and remanipulation.

Open reduction of tibial shaft fractures is rarely indicated. The primary indication is open fracture. Open reduction is also indicated in patients who require open treatment for vascular repair or fasciotomy. Weber also mentions brain injury, cerebral palsy, and facilitation of nursing care as indications,[259] while Dias has found these rarely applicable.[71] Hemophiliac patients may require open reduction and stable internal fixation. Stabilization decreases the incidence of rebleeding, thus reducing the need for prolonged factor replacement.

With extremely unstable fractures or in cases where there is difficulty in obtaining or maintaining reduction, external fixation is an alternative to open reduction and internal fixation and does not disturb the fracture site environment. This method is recommended in the polytrauma patient with head injury and spasticity or when there is cerebral irritation; it is also of use when there are burns or severe soft tissue loss. Prolonged use of fixation or distraction of the fracture fragments may lead to delayed union or nonunion. Needless to say, the fixation pins must be well placed to avoid the physeal region or neurovascular penetration.

Complications There seems to be less remodeling potential in angular malalignment of the tibia than in that of the femur or forearm. Varus or valgus deformity may disrupt normal knee and ankle mechanics and has little or no remodeling potential. Over 5° of varus or valgus angulation should not be accepted. Anterior or posterior angulation has a better capacity to remodel, and up to 10° of angulation may be acceptable. Anterior angulation tends to be more cosmetically undesirable, as the tibial crest is subcutaneous. Rotational malalignment will usually not remodel. External rotation deformity will cause outtoeing, overloading the medial aspect of the ankle and foot, while internal rotation results in intoeing with forced foot pronation or compensatory external rotation at the knee.

Upper tibial physeal closure has been reported but is rare. At this physis, the physeal closures that have been reported have been anterior, resulting in recurvatum deformity of the upper tibia.

Leg-length discrepancy requires correction in tibial fractures, as less overgrowth can be expected at the tibia than in femoral fractures. Younger children may gain some length, but in adolescents overgrowth cannot be relied upon, hence end-to-end apposition at the time of reduction is mandatory. Growth retardation has even been reported.[98]

Delayed union and nonunion are extremely rare in children. Factors leading to deficient union are incorrect application of internal fixation, infection, soft tissue stripping (by trauma or surgery), inadequate immobilization, and distraction secondary to pins and plaster or external fixation.

Vascular injuries are quite rare. They are most often associated with proximal tibial fractures, especially near the metaphysis, resulting in injury to the anterior tibial artery near the trifurcation.

Compartment syndromes are infrequent in children. However, when they are suspected because of unusual pain and verified by intracompartmental pressure testing, four-compartment open fasciotomy is indicated. An interstitial pressure of more than 30 mmHg in any one of the four compartments of the leg is an indication for decompression.[35a]

Fracture of the Fibular Shaft

Isolated fibular shaft fractures in children are uncommon and relatively unimportant, as the fibular shaft is basically a point of muscle attachment. The mechanism of injury is most commonly a direct contusion. Twisting injury may occasionally cause the fibula to fail, creating a spiral fracture.

Classification These fractures are almost always tension (greenstick) types, ranging from the more common trans-

verse fracture to an oblique or spiral fracture line. The presence of an intact tibia rarely allows the development of a compression (torus) fracture of the fibula. Plastic deformation (bowing) is occasionally seen in isolation or, more frequently, in association with a tibial shaft fracture.[163]

Diagnosis is often difficult, as occult fracture may not be evident on initial x-ray films, but its presence may be suspected from a limp and vague fibular shaft pain with twisting of the knee or ankle. Swelling is usually minimal.

Treatment aims to provide support and comfort. Generally, a lightweight short leg walking cast is required for mid- to distal fibular shaft fractures. Proximal fractures may be treated by a cylinder cast and restricted activity.

Complications are rare with this injury.

Fracture of the Distal Tibial Metaphysis

Distal metaphyseal injuries are similar to the proximal fractures except that they are not at risk for the development of valgus angulation. More severe injuries tend to collapse anteriorly, creating a recurvatum deformity at the fracture site. The mechanism of injury may be a tension (tilting) or compression (jamming) force.

Classification These fractures range from minimal compression (torus) to angulated tension (greenstick) fractures. The fracture line is usually transverse or a short oblique. Complete fractures do occur, but displacement is usually minimal because of the intact thick investing periosteum.

Diagnosis of some occult fractures in young children may be difficult. Localized tenderness over the distal tibial metaphysis and difficulty with weight bearing may suggest the diagnosis.

Treatment With undisplaced and stable fractures, a short leg walking cast is appropriate. Angular deformity, especially valgus or varus deformity, requires accurate reduction.[188] Moderate amounts of anterior and posterior angulation, ranging from 10 to 15° in young children and somewhat less in growing adolescents, will probably correct with remodeling. Partial to complete displacement requires closed reduction; if this is unsuccessful, open reduction is indicated. Small amounts of translocation (less than one-quarter to one-third of the metaphyseal width) will also correct during remodeling.

Fracture of the Distal Fibula

Distal fibular fracture occurs in association with abduction or adduction injuries of the distal tibia. However, isolated injury of the distal fibula is a not uncommon type of ankle injury in children.[117] It is often misdiagnosed as ankle sprain.

The mechanism of injury is usually an abduction-eversion injury which drives the talus and os calcis against the fibular epiphysis. Adduction injuries may occur but are less prevalent.

These fractures are generally Salter-Harris type I or type II growth plate injuries, often occurring near skeletal maturity as the physis is closing (cf. the Tillaux fracture of the distal tibia, discussed below).

Diagnosis is often difficult, as displacement is usually minimal. Direct palpation of bony tenderness on the subcutaneous fibula is the best sign of fracture. Oblique and comparison views may be helpful. An irregular surface or sharp edge differentiates a fracture from a normal ossicle, which is smooth.

Treatment The treatment is immobilization for 6 to 8 weeks until there is clinical and radiologic evidence of union.

Posttraumatic perifibular ossicles are common, especially in young athletes, and should be differentiated from fracture fragments by their more regular outline. Although they appear to be floating (*joint mice*), they are usually contained within ligaments or a joint capsule. They are usually asymptomatic and rarely require excision.

Fibrous union occasionally occurs in the tip of the fibula. If the fracture occurs below the level of the ankle plafond, it is usually asymptomatic, as the stresses are reduced and the ankle is stable. Surgery is rarely required.

With displacement, closed reduction should be performed under appropriate anesthesia. The articular surface should be restored as anatomically as possible. Open reduction and pin fixation are rarely required in children.

Complications Complications are unusual, but if the diagnosis is delayed and there is continued use of the leg in spite of pain and swelling, epiphysiolysis may occur.[188]

Ankle Injuries

Classification

Using the Lauge-Hansen guidelines, which form the basis for classification of ankle injuries in adults, Dias and Tachdjian devised a classification for these injuries in children. This classification incorporates the Salter-Harris classification but takes into account the direction of the force and also the position of the foot at injury.[73] In the individual categories of this classification, the position of the foot is indicated first and the nature of the deforming force second.

In the first category, *supination-inversion* injury, two stages are recognized. In stage 1 (Fig. 32-25A) the injury is commonly to the fibula. It is usually a Salter I or Salter II type of physeal injury. Alternatively, there may be a flake avulsion from the tip of the malleolus, associated with ligamentous injury in older children. In stage 2 injuries, in addition to the fibular fracture, a Salter type III or type IV injury to the tibial epiphysis is produced on the medial side. On rare occasions there may be Salter I or II injury.

A *plantarflexion* force with the foot in *supination* (Fig. 32-25B) produces a Salter type II injury of the tibial epiphysis with posterior displacement. Occasionally a Salter I injury occurs. The fibula remains intact. In *supination–external rotation* (Fig. 32-25C), the classification of Dias and Tachdjian again recognizes two stages.[73] In stage 1, a spiral fracture is identifiable, commencing at the lateral margin of the physis and running proximally and medially. When even more violence is applied, stage 2 injury occurs and there is an accompanying spiral fracture of the fibula, which commences immediately and runs superiorly and

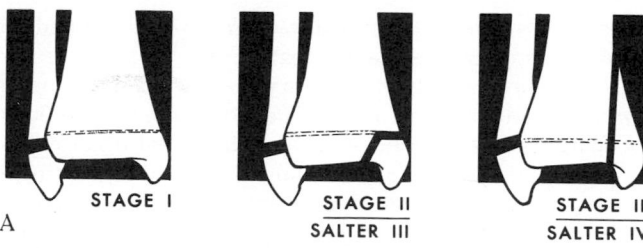

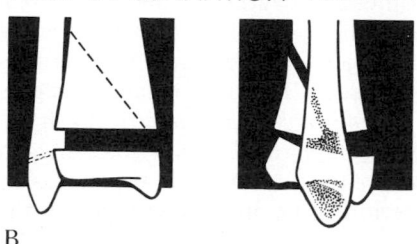

FOOT IN SUPINATION · PLANTAR FLEXION FORCE

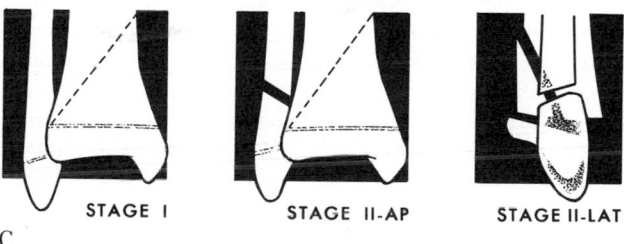

FOOT IN SUPINATION · EXTERNAL ROTATION FORCE

FOOT IN PRONATION

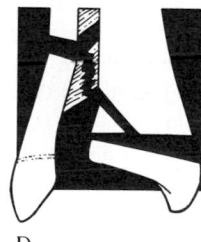

Figure 32-25 *A.* Supination-inversion injury stage I is a Salter I or Salter II physeal injury of the fibula. Stage II consists of the fibular injury seen in stage I plus a Salter III or Salter IV injury of the tibial physis. Only rarely is there a Salter I or Salter II injury of the tibial epiphysis. *B.* Supination-plantarflexion injury. This is a Salter II injury of the tibial physis with posterior displacement and a posterior metaphyseal fragment. The fibula is usually intact. Occasionally a Salter I injury may be produced. *C.* Supination–external rotation injury. Stage II shows anteroposterior and lateral views. Note the direction of the spiral fracture of the lower tibia. The epiphyseal displacement and the position of the metaphyseal fragment are posterior. *D.* Pronation-eversion injury. In this injury the fibular fracture is somewhat higher than in the other types and may be up to 4 in from the tip of the lateral malleolus. (Redrawn, modified, and reproduced with permission from Dias LS, Tachdjian MD: *Clin Orthop* 136:230–233, 1978, and Landin LA, Danielsson LG: *Acta Orthop Scand* 54:634–640, 1983.)

posteriorly. The metaphyseal fracture is posterior, and the tibial epiphysis is displaced posteriorly.[73]

Yet another pattern of injury occurs when the foot is *pronated* and subjected to an *eversion* force (Fig. 32-25*D*). A Salter-Harris type II fracture of the distal tibial epiphysis is the most common result of this injury, with the metaphyseal fragment located laterally or posterolaterally. An associated short oblique fracture of the fibula is located more proximally on the shaft than in other fibular injuries.

Ossification The ossification centers of the distal tibial and fibular epiphyses both appear in the first few years of life. Epiphyseal fusion begins at about age 8 to 12 in girls and age 13 in boys. It is usually complete by age 15 in girls and age 17 in boys. Fusion occurs asymmetrically. It begins in the area of the center of the tibial dome-shaped physis. The medial part of the plate next closes, and fusion then progresses posteriorly. The anterolateral part of the plate fuses last of all.[156]

Transitional Fractures

During the period of incomplete fusion, if the epiphysis is subjected to compressive or shear stresses at injury, a portion of the plate may have already fused while another portion remains open. This fact accounts for the production of certain special, and somewhat complicated, fractures which occur in this age group. It is only over the age of 10 years that an incomplete epiphyseolysis can occur, producing these transitional fractures.[254]

The Juvenile Tillaux Fracture Kleiger and Mankin described the Tillaux fracture in 1974.[141] They indicated their belief that it follows the application of a lateral rotary stress to an epiphysis during an age-related vulnerability period associated with medial plate closure while the lateral portion of the plate remains open. They believed that the inferior tibiofibular ligament also played a part in pulling the epiphyseal fragment from its bed and displacing it. The vertical fracture line in the epiphysis, produced by compressive stresses, changes direction when it

reaches the physis and shears the fragment, which is then more easily displaced from its bed (Fig. 32-26).

Triplane Fracture In another form of transitional fracture, the so-called triplane fracture, a number of variants have been recognized by CT scanning.[128,131,254] Interpretation of ordinary x-ray films may be difficult with this complicated fracture, since there are fracture lines in three planes, as clearly described in the initial report by Marmor.[159] Interpretations of the complex anatomy without CT scanning have given conflicting accounts of the nature of the triplane fracture.[58,72,159] However, CT scanning indicates that there are triplane fractures which consist of two to four fragments.[128,254]

Von Laer has attempted a classification into type I and type II triplane injuries.[254] In his type I lesion, the metaphyseal portion of the fracture ends in the physis (Fig. 32-27*A*), while in type II triplane lesions the metaphyseal portion of the fracture line extends through the physis into the epiphysis and the joint (Fig. 32-27*B*). It should be noted that the triplane fracture is a combination of different Salter-type injuries. Thus, the Von Laer type I triplane

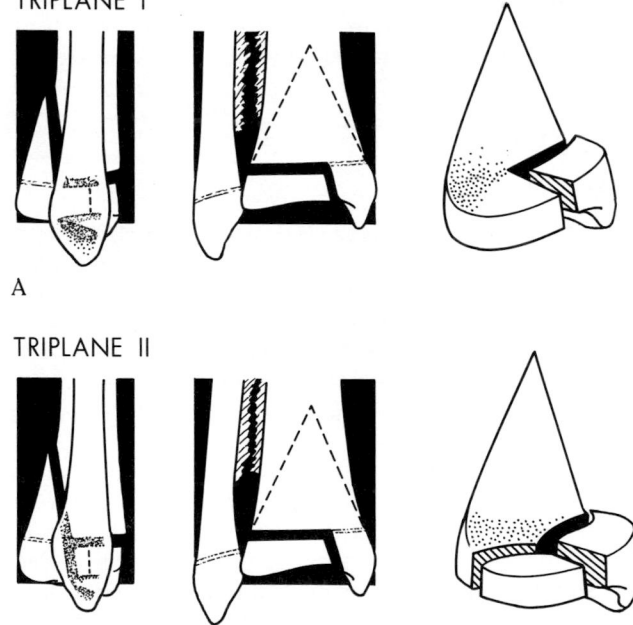

TRIPLANE I

A

TRIPLANE II

B

Figure 32-27 *A.* A triplane fracture type I (Von Laer classification). On the anteroposterior film the fracture (*solid line*) is seen in the medial part of the epiphysis. It may occur also through the malleolus or more centrally. On the lateral radiograph the metaphyseal fragment is clearly seen but the epiphyseal fragment (*dotted line*) may be only just detectable. *B.* Von Laer type II triplane fracture. The anteroposterior radiograph is identical to the middle drawing; however, the Salter IV component of this complex fracture is clearly seen to extend through the physis and epiphysis on the lateral radiograph. The exploded view is constructed from CT scans of the metaphyseal and epiphyseal regions. (Redrawn, modified, and reproduced with permission from Von Laer L: *J Bone Joint Surg* 67A:687–698, 1985.)

TWO PLANE

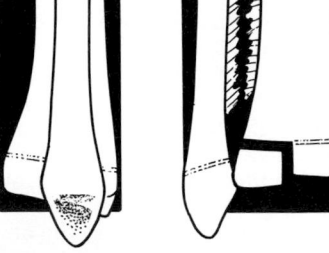

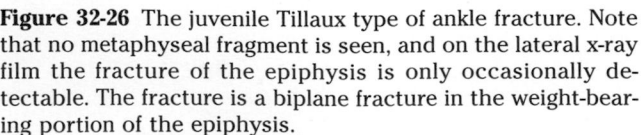

Figure 32-26 The juvenile Tillaux type of ankle fracture. Note that no metaphyseal fragment is seen, and on the lateral x-ray film the fracture of the epiphysis is only occasionally detectable. The fracture is a biplane fracture in the weight-bearing portion of the epiphysis.

injury is a combination of a Salter type II physeal injury (with a metaphyseal fragment) with a Salter type III injury of the epiphysis. A Von Laer type II triplane injury has a Salter type IV fragment combined with a type III injury. As Karrholm and associates pointed out, even with CT scanning, the true state of affairs may not be revealed until operation because certain fracture lines are undisplaced.[131] Recent CT studies have also shown that, on occasion, the fracture line may be intramalleolar through the medial malleolus.[254] Von Laer believes that the precise location of the fracture line reflects the state of fusion of the epiphysis rather than the nature of the injury.[254]

Clinical and Radiologic Examination It goes without saying that careful clinical examination is as important as accurate perusal of the x-ray film. Type II injuries to the fibular physis may be unsuspected without careful clinical examination and may be difficult to identify on radiographs without a high index of suspicion. Letts and Giveault have pointed out that in the Tillaux injury the fracture may be partially hidden by the fibula, so oblique views are essential.[150] The age of the patient, the mechanism of injury, and the direction of the fracture line should facilitate classification. In complex transitional fractures, CT or MRI scans of the metaphysis and the epiphysis may be required.

Treatment Displaced fibular fractures usually respond to closed reduction with few complications. However, occasionally a displaced fibular fracture may prevent reduction of an attached tibial fragment, and in such a case, even at open operations, the fibular fracture may have to be reduced first.[230]

Although it has generally been believed that Salter type III and type IV tibial fractures with less than 2 mm of displacement do not require open reduction,[58,72,230] this view has been challenged in a study by Kling and coworkers, who suggest that *anatomic* reduction of type III and type IV fractures is necessary and may decrease the incidence of gross physeal disturbances, including limb shortening and angulation.[143] They recommend open reduction using smooth K wires drilled from one epiphyseal fragment into the other and not crossing the physis. These pins either diverge or converge, thereby preventing the fragments from slipping or rotating. An alternative method is to secure the metaphyseal fragment, also without crossing the physis, but this may be difficult if the physis is small.

When the fragment is small, care must be taken that the fracture is not confused with a Salter type II injury, which, although generally believed to have a better prognosis, may also cause disturbances in growth.[143,230] The type II fracture is unpredictable.[58,230] It may occur in a younger age group, so that when growth problems arise they are more serious than those occurring, say, in a triplane fracture or a Tillaux fracture within a year or so of complete closure of the epiphysis. Patients with little or no displacement in Salter type II fractures also seem to develop complications as readily as those in whom there is considerable displacement.[58,230] They are usually held in good position, however, after closed reduction. The Salter-Harris classification, in itself, cannot be used to accurately prognosticate in individual fractures.[135]

With regard to treatment of the Tillaux and triplane fractures, the incidence of growth disturbance is not an indication for surgery, since the remaining growth in this age group is small.[131] Displacement of a fragment of epiphysis in these transitional fractures, however, is an indication for reduction. The reason for this is that the residual incongruity of the articular surfaces is unacceptable and will produce symptoms.[131] Consequently, if, following closed reduction, careful assessment indicates more than 2 mm of displacement or continuing incongruity, open reduction is advised. The particular surgical approach depends to a large extent upon accurate preoperative assessment. Two incisions may be required to explore different aspects of this circumferential injury.

Complications Salter type III and type IV fractures carry a high risk of complications, especially if there is more than 2 mm of displacement.[230] These fractures commonly affect the medial side, with premature fusion leading to varus angulation.

Treatment of posttraumatic physeal bars associated with partial closure depend on the amount of residual growth and the size and location of the bar.[47,132,135] Alternatives to excising the bar include fusing the rest of the plate in a child near maturity, perhaps combined with epiphysiodesis on the contralateral side.[47] In a young patient with considerable growth potential remaining, repeated osteotomy may be required plus such additional procedures as leg lengthening and contralateral epiphysiodesis. Ipsilateral fibular epiphysiodesis may also be required.[47] Karrholm and associates have identified a compensatory mechanism associated with proximal or distal sliding of the fibular shaft along the tibia which can compensate in part for growth disturbances in the distal tibia or fibular growth plate.[132] This mechanism should be taken into account when planning any interference with either growth plate. It is advisable to read their paper in full.[132]

Foot Fractures

Fractures of the Talus

The talus is a rare site of fracture in children. Although Trott points out that the prognosis in the displaced talar fracture is considerably better in children than in adults (a fact which he believes may be in part due to the strong periosteum, which helps maintain a blood supply to the disrupted fragments and thus diminishes the incidence of avascular necrosis), the undisplaced talar fracture seems to fare worse.[251]

Undisplaced (type I) fractures are associated with a high proportion of good results in adults.[43,111,241] Letts and Giveault, who observed the higher-than-expected incidence of avascular necrosis in undisplaced fractures of the talar neck in children, also pointed out that in their studies of the children admitted to Winnipeg Children's Hospital with talar fracture over an 18-year period, all the fractures were type I, which indicates that this is probably the most common presentation in children.[150]

The etiologic factors usually are falls from a height or motor vehicle trauma.[150] In these circumstances an undisplaced fracture may be missed, since the cortical defect is often overlooked. This is important, since it seems possible that protected weight bearing may permit the avascular segment to heal and give a good prognosis. However, once flattening of the talus has occurred, a stiff ankle results. Although there have been some attempts to use technetium scans as a prognostic guide or for guidance concerning a return to weight bearing, there may be no significant changes in such a bone scan.[150] Magnetic resonance imaging may turn out to be more useful.

The other types of talus fracture are uncommon. In type II fractures there is subluxation of the subtalar joint associated with separation of the fragments, which may lead to necrosis. In type III fractures, there is also dislocation of the body of the talus, and the prognosis is thought to be exceptionally poor, avascular necrosis being almost certain.

Fractures of the talar dome may elude diagnosis despite routine x-rays.[269] The CT scan is helpful. The lesion is common in adults and may also occur in adolescents. A posteromedial lesion and also a lateral lesion have been identified, associated with plantarflexion and inversion and with dorsiflexion and inversion types of injury, respectively. The latter more often requires surgery and has a worse prognosis.

When the clinical symptoms suggest a loose fragment within the joint with catching or locking, then a conservative regimen should probably be replaced by surgical intervention. When in doubt, arthroscopic evaluation may indicate whether there is a mobile flap of articular cartilage. Large fragments may be drilled and pinned back into the crater after freshening the sclerotic floor (using smooth-bored pins buried beneath the surface of the articular cartilage). The most common procedure is removal of the fragment, which is often small and unsuitable for reattachment. The base of the deficit should, nevertheless, be drilled to promote fibrocartilaginous healing. Early mobilization is advisable after surgery. Transmalleolar osteotomy may be necessary for posteromedial lesions, but lateral lesions can usually be approached through the anterolateral ankle joint capsule. It is not uncommon to find lateral ligamentous insufficiency associated with these lesions. Alexander and Lichtman recommend that the ligament should not be definitively repaired at the time that the intraarticular lesion is treated, since postoperative immobilization is required following the ligamentous repair. They suggest that a second subsequent procedure is preferable.[4] If a combined procedure is elected, the ligament repair should be protected while the ankle is mobilized by using a flexion-extension ankle-foot orthosis (AFO).

Fracture of the Calcaneus

Children represent approximately 5 percent of the population of patients who sustain calcaneal fractures, and although in the prepubertal years the incidence in the two sexes is roughly equal, after the age of 11 males predominate approximately 3 to 1.[220] The most common mechanism of injury is a fall from a height. The two next most common causes are motor vehicle accidents and injuries from lawn mowers (particularly in younger children).[220] One in three children will have sustained additional fractures in the accident, with a significant incidence of associated lower extremity and spine fractures.[220,251] Schmidt and Weiner were able to gather the histories of 59 children with calcaneal fractures and classified them in six types, using a modification of the Essex-Lopresti classification.[220] Types I, II, and III are varieties of extraarticular fracture, whereas types IV and V represent fractures into the subtalar joint. Type VI fractures involve significant bone loss together with loss of the Achilles tendon insertion. In this series 63 percent were extraarticular and 37 percent intraarticular. Between the ages of 1 and 7 years 92 percent of the fractures were extraarticular. However, among teenagers the situation was quite different, with intraarticular fractures predominating (62 percent). These facts probably reflect the increased vulnerability of younger children to injury other than falling from a height and also the fact that they are better able than older children to absorb the stress from compression loading if a fall occurs.[220]

In toddlers, fractures of the calcaneus may be overlooked, and a high index of suspicion is required in a child who presents with a painful heel.[266] Early radiographs may be unhelpful, and bone imaging may be required to detect the fracture.[168,234]

In general, the prognosis even for the displaced fracture seems to be better in children than in adults. For treatment of the displaced intraarticular fracture in adolescence, the guidelines discussed in detail in the adult section on the treatment of calcaneal fractures should be followed. It should be noted that stress fractures of the os calcis have also been reported in a child.[34]

Tarsometatarsal Joint Injuries

Wiley has described this injury in children and identified the common mechanism of injury as acute forced plantarflexion of the forefoot combined with rotation.[265] He also points out that a fracture of the base of the second metatarsal (normally locked in place by the ligaments and surrounding tarsal bone) is a sentinel feature of tarsometatarsal joint injury. Inevitably with this injury there is a fracture of the base of the second metatarsal and usually fracture or fracture dislocation of the third, fourth, and fifth metatarsals. Often the tarsus-to-first-metatarsal joint remains intact. In Wiley's series, all seven fractures were reduced by closed reduction but required K-wire fixation to maintain alignment. The pins were removed 1 month later, and the functional results were excellent, although it was anticipated by the author that future degenerative changes would inevitably occur.[265]

Metatarsal Injuries

At the base of the first metatarsal is an important physis, damage to which causes angulation or growth arrest. It may be injured in crush-type injuries. A Salter type I injury following a fall has also been described.[250] Closed reduction and plaster casting are usually sufficient to obtain and maintain reduction.

An avulsion-type injury of the base of the fifth metatarsal commonly produces a Salter type I injury. It is generally believed that the peroneus brevis tendon is responsible for the avulsion,[251] but other views incriminate the plantar aponeurosis and the abductor digiti minimi tendon.[104] The lesion should be differentiated from the occasional sesamoid bone found in this region.[240] Six weeks in a cast is usually sufficient to heal a lesion. Displacement requiring reduction is unusual.[251] Growth disturbances are also uncommon, but when they occur consist usually in bone overgrowth with production of a localized bony prominence that may give problems in fitting footwear. The fracture should be differentiated from the Robert Jones fracture, which is a transverse fracture of the proximal part of the diaphysis usually occurring in adolescents and with a high incidence of nonunion. Bone grafting[64] and intramedullary lag-screw fixation may be required.[104,136]

Phalangeal Fractures

Phalangeal fractures are treated according to the same general principles as fractures of other long bones. Fractures of the proximal phalanx of the hallux have given rise to a greater incidence of osteomyelitis than might be expected. A high index of suspicion should accompany any small breach of the skin. Trauma to the physeal plate at the base of the proximal phalanx may also lead to asymmetrical or retarded growth, and angular deformities may then occur. Residual stiffness, which is a common sequel after injury to the first metatarsophalangeal joint, should be fully rehabilitated. For infected phalangeal fractures, debridement and delayed closure may save many great toes, according to Trott, for which amputations have been considered.[251] This is particularly the case in very young children. Trott also points out that in open fractures of the foot in children caused by severe injuries, there is so much swelling and tissue damage that adequate debridement is the first requirement. Primary closure should never be attempted. Skin grafting should be performed as required. Patients with these severe injuries are at high risk of growth disturbance.[251]

REFERENCES

General Considerations

1. Aronson J, Tursky EA: External fixation of femor fractures in children. *J Pediatr Orthop* 12:157–163, 1992.
2. Barrett WP, Almquist EA, Staheli LT: Fracture separation of the distal humeral physis in the newborn. *J Pediatr Orthop* 4:617–619, 1994.
3. Blount WP: *Fractures in Children.* Baltimore, Williams & Wilkins, 1955.
4. Bowen A: Plastic bowing of the clavicle in children: A report of two cases. *J Bone Joint Surg* 65A:403–405, 1983.
5. Bright RW: Physeal injuries, in Rockwood CA Jr, Wilkins KE, King RE (eds): *Fractures in Children.* Vol III. Philadelphia, Lippincott, 1984.
6. Charnley J: *The Closed Treatment of Common Fractures,* 3d ed. Edinburgh, Churchill Livingstone, 1974.
7. Delee JC, Wilkins KE, Rogers LF, et al: Fracture separation of the distal humeral epiphysis. *J Bone Joint Surg* 62A:46–51, 1980.
8. Denton J: Trauma to the growing skeleton. *Orthop Rev* 12:129–133, 1983.
9. Godfrey JD: Trauma in children. *J Bone Joint Surg* 46A:422–446, 1964.
10. Green NE, Swionkowski MF (eds): *Skeletal Trauma in Children.* Vol. 3. Philadelphia, Saunders, 1994, pp 517–531.
11. Karrholm J, Hansson LI, Svennson K: Prediction of growth pattern after ankle fractures in children. *J Pediatr Orthop* 3:319–325, 1983.
12. Kling TF, Bright RW, Hensinger RN: Distal tibial physeal fractures in children that may require open reduction. *J Bone Joint Surg* 66A:647–657, 1984.
13. Langenskiold A: Consideration of growth factors in the treatment of fractures of long bones in children, in Chapchal G (ed): *Fractures in Children.* New York, Thieme-Stratton, 1981, p 16.
14. Malkawi H, Shannak A, Hadidi S: Remodeling after femoral shaft fractures in children treated by modified Blount's method. *J Pediatr Orthop* 6:421–429, 1986.
15. Neer CS II, Horwitz BS: Fractures of the proximal humeral epiphyseal plate. *Clin Orthop* 41:24–31, 1965.
16. Ogden J: The uniqueness of growing bone, in Rockwood CA Jr, Wilkins KE, King RE (eds): *Fractures in Children.* Philadelphia, Lippincott, 1984, pp 1–86.
17. Ogden JA: *Skeletal Injury in the Child.* Philadelphia, Lea & Febiger, 1982.
18. Ogden JA: Skeletal growth mechanism injury patterns. *J Pediatr Orthop* 2:371–377, 1982.
19. Peterson HA: Partial growth arrest and its treatment. *J Pediatr Orthop* 4:264–268, 1984.
20. Peterson HA, Burkhart SS: Compression injury of the epiphyseal growth plate: Fact or fiction. *J Pediatr Orthop* 1:377–384, 1981.
21. Probe R, Lindsey RW, Hadley MA, et al: Refracture of adolescent femoral shaft fracture: A complication of external fixation. A report of two cases. *J Pediatr Orthop* 13:102–105, 1993.
22. Rang M: *Children's Fractures,* 2d ed. Philadelphia, Lippincott, 1983.
23. Reed MH: Fractures and dislocations of the extremities in children. *J Trauma* 17:351–354, 1977.
24. Reynolds DA: Growth changes in fractured long-bones: A study of 126 children. *J Bone Joint Surg* 63B:83–88, 1981.
25. Ryoppy S: Characteristics of the growing skeleton from the traumatological point of view, in Chapchal E (ed): *Fractures in Children.* New York, Thieme-Stratton, 1981, pp 6–7.
26. Salter R: *Textbook of Disorders and Injuries of the Musculoskeletal System.* Baltimore, Williams & Wilkins, 1983.
27. Salter RB, Harris RW: Injuries involving the epiphyseal plate. *J Bone Joint Surg* 45A:587–622, 1963.
28. Seharli AF: General observations, in Chapchal G (ed): *Fractures in Children.* New York, Thieme-Stratton, 1981, pp 1–2.
29. Sharrard WJW: *Paediatric Orthopaedics and Fractures.* Vol II. London, Blackwell, 1979.
30. Smith DG, Geist RW, Cooperman DR: Microscopic examination of a naturally occurring epiphyseal plate fracture. *J Pediatr Orthop* 5:306–308, 1985.
31. Staheli LT: Femoral and tibial growth following femoral shaft fracture in childhood. *Clin Orthop* 55:159–163, 1967.
32. Tachdjian MO: *Paediatric Orthopaedics.* Philadelphia, Saunders, 1972.
33. Weber BG: Fracture healing in the growing bone and in the mature skeleton, in Weber BG, Brunner CH, Freuler F (eds): *Treatment of Fractures in Children and Adolescents.* New York, Springer-Verlag, 1980.

34. Yao J, Huurman WW: Tomography in juvenile Tillaux fractures. *J Pediatr Orthop* 6:349–351, 1986.

Upper Limb

1. Agins JJ, Marcus NW: Articular cartilage sleeve fracture of the lateral humeral condyle capitellum: A previously undescribed entity. *J Pediatr Orthop* 4:620–622, 1984.
2. Akbarnia B, Siberstein MJ, Rende RJ, et al: Arthrography in the diagnosis of fractures of the distal end of the humerus in infants. *J Bone Joint Surg [Am]* 68:599–601, 1986.
3. Almquist EE, Gordon LH, Blue AI: Congenital dislocation of the head of the radius. *J Bone Joint Surg [Am]* 51:1118–1127, 1969.
4. Amit Y, Salai M, Chechik A, et al: Closed intramedullary nailing for the treatment of diaphyseal forearm fractures in adolescence: A preliminary report. *J Pediatr Orthop* 5:143–146, 1985.
4a. Aronson DD, Prager BI: Supracondylar fractures of the humerus in children. *Clin Orthop* 219:174–184, 1985.
5. Barnett LS: Little League shoulder syndrome: Proximal humeral epiphysealysis in adolescent baseball pitchers. *J Bone Joint Surg [Am]* 67:495–496, 1985.
6. Barrett W, Almquist EA, Staheli LT: Fracture separation of the distal humeral physis in the newborn: A case report. *J Pediatr Orthop* 4:617–619, 1984.
7. Baxter MP, Wiley JJ: Fractures of the proximal humeral epiphysis. *J Bone Joint Surg* 68B:570–573, 1986.
8. Bayne O, Rang M: Medial dislocation of the radial head following breech delivery: A case report and review of the literature. *J Pediatr Orthop* 4:485–487, 1984.
9. Beekman F, Sullivan JE: Some observations on fractures of the long bones in children. *[Am] J Surg* 51:722–728, 1941.
10. Bellemore GC, Barrett IR, Middleton RWD, et al: Supracondylar osteotomy of the humerus for correction of cubitus varus. *J Bone Joint Surg [Br]* 66:566–572, 1984.
11. Bensahel H, Csukonyi Z, Badelon O, Badaoui S: Fractures of the medial condyle of the humerus in children. *Pediatr Orthop* 6:430–433, 1986.
12. Biyani A, Gupta SP, Sharma JC: Determination of medial epicondylar epiphyseal angle for supracondylar humeral fracture in children. *J Pediatr Orthop* 13:94–97, 1993.
13. Blount WP: *Fractures in Children.* Vol 75. Baltimore, Williams & Wilkins, 1964, pp 58–59.
14. Bohler J: Wire osteosynthesis of supracondylar humerus fractures in children, in Chapchal G (ed): *Fractures in Children.* New York, Thieme-Stratton 1983, p 147.
15. Buckerfield CT, Castle ME: Acute traumatic retrosternal dislocation of the clavicle. *J Bone Joint Surg [Am]* 66:379–384, 1984.
16. Buhl O, Hellberg S: Displaced supracondylar fractures of the humerus in children. *Acta Orthop Scand* 53:67–71, 1982.
17. C[am]pbell CC, Waters PN, Emans JB, et al: Neurovascular injury and displacement in type III supracondylar humerus fractures. *J Pediatr Orthop* 15:47–52, 1995.
18. Carey RPH: Simultaneous dislocation of the elbow and the proximal radio-ulnar joint. *J Bone Joint Surg [Br]* 66:254–256, 1984.
19. Carlioz H, Abobs Y: Posterior dislocation of the elbow in children. *J Pediatr Orthop* 4:8–12, 1984.
20. Catterall A: Fractures in children, in Wilson JN (ed): *Watson-Jones Fractures and Joint Injuries,* 5th ed. Edinburgh, Churchill Livingstone, 1976.
21. Culp RW, Osterman AL, Davidson R: Neural injuries associated with supracondylar fractures of the humerus in children. *J Bone Joint Surg* 72A:1211–1215, 1990.
22. Curtis DJ, et al: Importance of soft tissue evaluation in hand and wrist trauma. *[Am] J Radiol* 142:781–788, 1984.

23. Dameron TB Jr, Rockwood CA Jr: Fractures and dislocations of the shoulder. Vol 3, in Rockwood CA Jr, Wilkins K, King RE (eds): *Fractures in Children.* Philadelphia, Lippincott, 1984, pp 577–607.
24. DeLee JC, et al: Fracture separation of the distal humeral epiphysis. *J Bone Joint Surg* 62A:46–51, 1980.
25. Edman P, Lohr G: Supracondylar fractures of the humerus treated with olecranon traction. *Acta Chir Scand* 126:505–516, 1963.
26. Erne P, Fricker U, Muller HP, et al: Late results of supracondylar fractures of the humerus in children, in Chapchal G (ed): *Fractures in Children.* New York, Thieme-Stratton, 1981.
27. Evans E: Pronation injuries of the forearm with special attention to the anterior Monteggia fractures. *J Bone Joint Surg [Br]* 31:578–588, 1949.
28. Foster DE, Sullivan A, Gross RH: Lateral humeral condylar fractures in children. *J Pediatr Orthop* 5:16–22, 1985.
29. Fowles JV, Kassab MT, Douik M: Untreated posterior dislocation of the elbow in children. *J Bone Joint Surg [Am]* 66:921–926, 1984.
30. Fowles JV, Kassab MT, Moula T: Untreated intra-articular entrapment of the medial humeral epicondyle. *J Bone Joint Surg [Br]* 66:562–565, 1984.
31. Fowles JV, Sliman N, Kassab M: The Monteggia lesion in children. *J Bone Joint Surg [Am]* 65:1276–1283, 1983.
32. Freuler F, Weber BG, Brunner CH: Shaft fractures in the forearm, in Weber BG (ed): *Treatment of Fractures in Children and Adolescents.* New York, Springer-Verlag, 1980, pp 179–202.
33. Friberg KSI: Remodeling after distal forearm fractures in children: I. The effect of residual angulation on the spatial orientation of the epiphyseal plates. *Acta Orthop Scand* 50:537–546, 1979.
34. Friberg KSI: Remodeling after distal forearm fractures in children: II. The final orientation of the distal and proximal epiphyseal plates of the radius. *Acta Orthop Scand* 50:731–739, 1979.
35. Friberg KSI: Remodeling after distal forearm fractures in children: III. Correction of residual angulation in fractures of the radius. *Acta Orthop Scand* 50:741–749, 1979.
36. Gibson DA, Carroll N: Congenital pseudarthrosis of the clavicle. *J Bone Joint Surg [Br]* 52:629–652, 1970.
37. Graham B, Tredwell SJ, Beauchamp RD, Bell HN: Supracondylar osteotomy of the humerus for correction of cubitus varus. *J Pediatr Orthop* 10:228–231, 1990.
38. Greenspan A, Norman A: The radial head, capitellum view: Useful technique in elbow trauma. *[Am] J Radiol* 138:1186–1188, 1982.
39. Gruber M, Hudson O: Supracondylar fractures of the humerus in childhood: End result study of open reduction. *J Bone Joint Surg [Am]* 46:1245–1252, 1964.
40. H[am]ilton W, Parkes JC: Isolated dislocation of the radial head without fracture of the ulna. *Clin Orthop* 97:94–96, 1973.
41. Harvey S, Tchelebi H: Proximal radio-ulnar translocation. *J Bone Joint Surg [Am]* 61:447–449, 1979.
42. Hellinger J: Supracondylar fractures of the humerus, in Chapchal G (ed): *Fractures in Children.* New York, Thieme-Stratton, 1981, pp 141–147.
43. Henrickson B: Supracondylar fractures of the humerus in children. *Acta Chir Scand* (suppl):369, 1966.
44. Howorth MB, Baab O: Orthopaedic disorders: Fractures involving the elbow, in Howorth MD (ed): *Orthopaedic Conditions Due to Trauma.* p 571.
45. Hughston JC: Fractures of the forearm in children. *J Bone Joint Surg [Am]* 44:1678–1693, 1962.
46. Ippolito E, Caterini R, Scola E: Supracondylar fractures of the humerus in children. *J Bone Joint Surg [Am]* 68:333–344, 1986.

47. Jakob R, Fowles JV, Rang M, et al: Observations concerning fractures of the lateral humerus condyles in children. *J Bone Joint Surg* 57B:430–436, 1975.

48. Jarvis JG, D'Astous JL: The pediatric T-supracondylar fracture. *J Pediatr Orthop* 4:697–699, 1984.

49. Jaefsson PO, Hohnell O, Gentry CF: Long-term sequelae of single dislocation of the elbow. *J Bone Joint Surg [Am]* 66:927–930, 1984.

50. Kallio PE, Foster BK, Paterson DC: Difficult supracondylar elbow fractures in children: Analysis of percutaneous pinning technique. *J Pediatr Orthop* 12:11–15, 1993.

51. Kay S, Smith C, Oppenheim WL: Both bone midshaft forearm fractures in children. *J Pediatr Orthop* 6:306–310, 1986.

52. Kekomaki M, Luoma R, Rikalainen H, Vilkki P: Operative reduction and fixation of difficult supracondylar extension fractures of the humerus. *J Pediatr Orthop* 4:13–15, 1984.

53. Keyl W, Wirth CJ, Munchen: Residual deformities after supracondylar humeral fractures, in Chapchal G (ed): *Fractures in Children.* New York, Thieme-Stratton, 1981, pp 179–183.

54. King RE: in Rockwood CA, Wilkins K, King RE (eds): *Fractures in Children.* Vol 3. Philadelphia, Lippincott, 1984, chap 5.

55. Kohler R, Trilland JM: Fracture and fracture separation of the proximal humerus in children: Report of 136 cases. *J Pediatr Orthop* 3:326–332, 1983.

56. Kuhn D, Rosman G: Traumatic, nonparalytic dislocation the shoulder in a newborn infant: Case report. *J Pediatr Orthop* 4:121–122, 1984.

57. Langenskiold A, Kirilaakaso R: Varus and valgus deformity of the elbow following supracondylar fracture of the humerus. *Acta Orthop Scand* 38:313–321, 1967.

58. Last RJ: *Anatomy: Regional and Applied.* London, J. and A. Churchill, Radius and Ulna-Artic, 1963, pp 164–165.

59. Lusted LB, Keats TE: Elbow measurements, in *Atlas of Roentgenographic Measurement,* 2d ed. Chicago, Year Book, 1867, pp 119–121.

60. Manoli A II: Irreducible fracture-separation of the distal radial epiphysis. *J Bone Joint Surg [Am]* 64:1095–1096, 1982.

61. McRae R, Freeman PA: The lesion in pulled elbow. *J Bone Joint Surg [Br]* 47:808.

62. Milch H: Fracture dislocations of the distal humeral condyles. *J Trauma* 4:592–607, 1964.

63. Miller JH, Osterkamp JA: Scintigraphy in acute plastic bowing of the forearm. *Radiology* 142:742, 1982.

64. Mizuno K, et al: Fracture separation of the distal humeral epiphysis in young children. *J Bone Joint Surg* 61A:570–573, 1979.

65. Morrissy R, Wilkins KE: Deformity following distal humeral fracture in childhood. *J Bone Joint Surg [Am]* 66:557–562, 1984.

66. Moseley HF: The clavicle: Its anatomy and function. *Clin Orthop* 58:17–27, 1968.

67. Muller HP, Erne P: Condylar fractures of the elbow region, in Chapchal G (ed): *Fractures in Children.* New York, Thieme-Stratton, 1981, pp 166–168.

68. Neviaser RJ, LeFeure W: Irreducible isolated dislocation of the radial head. *Clin Orthop* 80:72–74, 1971.

69. Neer CS, Horowitz BS: Fractures of the proximal humeral epiphyseal plate. *Clin Orthop* 41:24–31, 1965.

70. Nussbaum A: The off-profile proximal radial epiphysis: Another potential pitfall in the x-ray diagnosis of the elbow trauma. *J Trauma* 23:40–46, 1983.

71. O'Brien ET: in Rockwood CA Jr, Wilkins K, King RE (eds): *Fractures in Children.* Vol 3. Philadelphia, Lippincott, 1984.

72. Ogden JA: *Skeletal Injury in the Child.* Philadelphia, Lea & Febiger, 1982.

73. Ogden JA: Distal clavicular physeal injury. *Clin Orthop* 188:68–73, 1984.

74. Osterwalder C, Thur CH, Wagener G, et al: Open reduction and fixation with two crossed pins in supracondylar fractures of the humerus in children: Indications, technique, results, in Chapchal G (ed): *Fractures in Children.* New York, Thieme-Stratton, 1981, pp 178–179.

75. Ozonoff MD: *Pediatric Orthopaedic Radiology.* Philadelphia, Saunders, 1979.

76. Papavasiliou VA, Beslikas TA: T-condylar fractures of the distal humerus during childhood. *J Pediatr Orthop* 6:302–305, 1986.

77. Pollen AG: *Fractures and Dislocations in Children.* Baltimore, Williams & Wilkins, 1973.

78. Pritchett JW: Entrapment of the medial nerve after dislocation of the elbow. *J Pediatr Orthop* 4:752–753, 1984.

79. Rang M: *Children's Fractures,* 2d ed. Philadelphia, Lippincott, 1982.

80. Rang M: *The Growth Plate and Its Disorders.* London, Livingstone, 1969.

81. Ravessoud FA: Lateral condylar fracture and ipsilateral ulnar shaft fracture: Monteggia equivalent lesions? *J Pediatr Orthop* 5:364–366, 1985.

82. Reed FE, Apple DF: Ipsilateral fractures of the elbow and forearm. *South Med J* 69:149–151, 1976.

83. Riordan DC, Bayne LG: The upper limb, in Lovell WW, Winter RB (eds): *Pediatric Orthopedics,* 2d ed. Philadelphia, Lippincott, 1986, pp 649–702.

84. Rowe CR, Pierce DS, Clark JG: Voluntary dislocation of the shoulder. *J Bone Joint Surg [Am]* 55:445–459, 1973.

85. Rutherford A: Fractures of the lateral humeral condyle in children. *J Bone Joint Surg [Am]* 67:851–856, 1985.

86. Rydholm V, Nilsson JE: Traumatic bowing of the forearm. *Clin Orthop* 139:121–124, 1979.

87. Salter RB: *Textbook of Disorders and Injuries of the Musculoskeletal Structure,* 2d ed. Baltimore, Williams & Wilkins, 1983.

88. Salter RB, Zaltz C: Anatomic investigations of the mechanism of injury and pathologic anatomy of "pulled elbow" in young children. *Clin Orthop* 77:134–143, 1971.

89. Schubert J: Dislocation of the radial head in the newborn infant. *J Bone Joint Surg [Am]* 47:1019–1023, 1965.

90. Selesnick FH, Jablon M, Frank C, Post M: Retrosternal dislocation of the clavicle. *J Bone Joint Surg [Am]* 66:287–291, 1984.

91. Sharrard WJW: *Paediatric Orthopaedics and Fractures.* Vol 2. London, Blackwell, 1979.

92. Shinley JL, Lesnick DS: Distal radius fracture with tendon entrapment. *Orthopaedics* 5:1330–1332, 1982.

92a. Smith FM: Fracture separation of the proximal humeral epiphysis. *Am J Surg* 91:627–635, 1956.

93. Stimson LA: *A Practical Treatise on Fractures and Dislocations.* Philadelphia, Lea Brothers, 1900.

94. Stuhmer KG: in Weber BG (ed): *Treatment of Fractures in Children and Adolescents.* New York, Springer-Verlag, 1980, pp 201–217.

95. Tachdjian MO: *Pediatric Orthopedics.* Vol 2. Philadelphia, Saunders, 1972.

96. Tarr RR, Garfinkel AS, Sarmiento A: The effects of angular and rotational deformities of both bones of the forearm. *J Bone Joint Surg [Am]* 66:65–70, 1984.

97. Thometz JG: Techniques for direct radiographic visualization during closed pinning of supracondylar humerus fractures in children. *J Pediatr Orthop* 10:555–558, 1990.

98. Tredwell K, Van Peteghem K, Clough M: Pattern of forearm fractures in children. *J Pediatr Orthop* 4:604–608, 1984.

99. VonLaer L: Fractures and luxations around the elbow in children and adolescents, in Chapchal G (ed): *Fractures in Children.* New York, Thieme-Stratton, 1981, pp 149–154.

100. VonLaer L: The fracture of the proximal end of the radius in adolescence. *Arch Orthop Traum Surg* 99:167–174, 1982.

101. Wedge JH, Robertson DE: Displaced fractures of the neck of the radius. *J Bone Joint Surg [Br]* 64:256, 1982.

102. Wiley JJ, Pegington J, Horwich JP: Traumatic dislocation of the radius in the elbow. *J Bone Joint Surg [Br]* 56:501–507, 1974.

103. Wilkins K, Rockwood CA, et al (eds): *Fractures in Children.* Vol 3. Philadelphia, Lippincott, 1984, pp 363–575.

104. Worlock PH, Colton C: Displaced supracondylar fractures of the humerus in children treated by overhead olecranon traction. *Injury* 15:316–321, 1984.

105. Worlock P: Supracondylar fractures of the humerus: Assessment of cubitus varus by the Baumann angle. *J Bone Joint Surg* 68B:755–757, 1986.

106. Worlock PH, Colton C: Severely displaced supracondylar fractures of the humerus in children: A simple method of treatment. *J Pediatr Orthop* 7:49–53, 1987.

107. Yamamoto I, Ishii S, Usui M, et al: Cubitus varus deformity following supracondylar fracture of the humerus. *Clin Orthop* 201:179–185, 1985.

108. Yates C, Sullivan JA: Arthrographic diagnosis of elbow injuries in children. *J Pediatr Orthop* 7:54–60, 1987.

109. Yoo CBI, Suh JT, et al: Avascular necrosis after fracture separation of the distal end of the humerus in children. *Orthopaedics* 15:959–963, 1992.

110. Zimmerman H: Fractures of the elbow, in Weber BG (ed): *Treatment of Fractures in Children and Adolescents.* New York, Springer-Verlag, 1980, pp 158–178.

Lower Limb

1. Abbott LC, Gill GG: Valgus deformity of the knee resulting from injury to the lower femoral epiphysis. *J Bone Joint Surg [Am]* 24:97–113, 1942.

2. Abraham E, Ansari A, Huang TL: Fracture of the distal medial femoral epiphysis with subluxation of the knee joint. *J Trauma* 20:339–341, 1980.

3. Aitken AP, Magill HK: Fractures involving the distal femoral epiphyseal cartilage. *J Bone Joint Surg [Am]* 34:96–108, 1952.

4. Alexander AH, Lichtman DM: Surgical treatment of transchondral talar dome fractures: Long-term follow-up. *J Bone Joint Surg [Am]* 62:646–652, 1980.

5. Allen B, Schock EP, Emory FE: Immediate spica cast system for femoral shaft fractures in infants and children. *South Med J* 71:18–22, 1978.

6. Allende G, Lezama LG: Fractures of the neck of the femur in children: A clinical study. *J Bone Joint Surg [Am]* 33:387–394, 1951.

7. Aronson J, Tursky EA: External fixation of femur fractures in children, *J Pediatr Orthop* 12:157–163, 1992.

8. Ashley RK, Larsen LJ, James PM: Reduction of dislocation of the hip in older children: A preliminary report. *J Bone Joint Surg [Am]* 54:545–550, 1972.

9. Balthazar DA, Pappas AM: Acquired valgus deformity of the tibia in children. *J Pediatr Orthop* 4:538–541, 1984.

10. Banagale RC, Kuhns LR: Traumatic separation of the distal femoral epiphysis in the newborn: Case report. *J Pediatr Orthop* 3:396–398, 1983.

11. Barquet A: Traumatic anterior dislocation of the hip in childhood. *Injury* 13:435–440, 1982.

12. Barquet A: Avascular necrosis following traumatic hip dislocation in childhood. *Acta Orthop Scand* 53:809–813, 1982.

13. Barquet A: Natural history of avascular necrosis following traumatic hip dislocation in childhood. *Acta Orthop Scand* 53:815–820, 1982.

14. Barquet A: Recurrent traumatic dislocation of the hip in childhood. *J Trauma* 20:1003–1006, 1980.

15. Barquet A: Traumatic hip dislocation with fracture of the ipsilateral femoral shaft in childhood. *Arch Orthop Trauma Surg* 98:69–72, 1981.

16. Barquet A: Traumatic hip dislocation in childhood: A report of 26 cases and a review of the literature. *Acta Orthop Scand* 50:549–554, 1979.

17. Baxter MP, Wiley JJ: Fractures of the tibial spine in children and evaluation of knee stability. *J Bone Joint Surg* 70B:228–230, 1988.

18. Beals RK, Tufts E: Fractured femur in infancy: The role of child abuse. *J Pediatr Orthop* 3:583–586, 1983.

19. Beaty JH, Austin SM, Warner WC, et al: Interlocking intramedullary nailing of femoral shaft fractures in adolescence: Preliminary results and complications. *J Pediatr Orthop* 14:178–183, 1994.

20. Behrman SW, Fabian TC, Kudsk KA, Taylor JC: Improved outcome with femur fractures early versus delayed fixation. *J Trauma* 30:792–797, 1990.

21. Benum P, Ertresvag K, Hoiseth K: Torsion deformities after traction treatment of femoral fractures in children. *Acta Orthop Scand* 50:87–91, 1979.

22. Bernhang AM: Simultaneous bilateral traumatic dislocation of the hip in a child. *J Bone Joint Surg [Am]* 52:365–366, 1970.

23. Bertin KC, Goble EM: Ligament injuries associated with physeal fractures about the knee. *Clin Orthop* 177:188–195, 1983.

24. Berndt AL: Hardy M: Transchondral fractures (osteochondritis dissecans) of the talus. *J Bone Joint Surg [Am]* 41:988–1020, 1959.

25. Blatter R: Fractures of the pelvis and acetabulum, in Weber BG, Brunner CH, Freuler F (eds): *Treatment of Fractures in Children and Adolescents.* Berlin, Springer-Verlag, 1980, pp 244–253.

26. Blount WP: *Fractures in Children.* Baltimore, Williams & Wilkins, 1964.

27. Boitzy A: Fractures of the proximal femur, in Weber BG, Brunner CH, Freuler F (eds): *Treatment of Fractures in Children and Adolescents.* Berlin, Springer-Verlag, 1980, pp 254–267.

28. Bond SJ, Gotschall CS, Eichelberger MR: Predictors of abdominal injury in children with pelvic fracture trauma. *J Pediatr Orthop* 31:1169–1173, 1991.

29. Bonnemaison MFE, Henderson ED: Traumatic anterior dislocation of the hip with acute common femoral occlusion in a child. *J Bone Joint Surg [Am]* 50:753–756, 1968.

30. Broudy AS, Scott RD: Voluntary posterior hip dislocation in children: Report of two cases. *J Bone Joint Surg [Am]* 57:716–717, 1975.

31. Brouwer KJ, Molenaar JC, VanLinge B: Rotational deformities after femoral shaft fractures in childhood: A retrospective study 27–32 years after the accident. *Acta Orthop Scand* 52:81–89, 1981.

32. Brunner CH: Fractures in and around the knee joint, in Weber BG, Brunner CH, Freuler F (ed): *Treatment of Fractures in Children and Adolescents.* Berlin, Springer-Verlag, 1980.

33. Bryan WJ, Tullos HS: Pediatric pelvic fractures: Review of 52 patients. *J Trauma* 19:799–805, 1979.

34. Buchanan J, Greer RB III: Stress fractures in calcaneus of a child. *Clin Orthop* 135:119–120, 1978.

35. Bucholz RW, Ezaki M, Ogden JA: Injury to the acetabular triradiate physeal cartilage. *J Bone Joint Surg [Am]* 64:600–609, 1982.

35a. Buckley SL, Smith G, Sponseller PD, et al: Open fractures of the tibia in children. *J Bone Joint Surg* 72A:1462–1469, 1990.

36. Buehler KC, Thompson JD, Sponseller PD, et al: A prospective study of early spica casting outcomes in the treatment of femoral shaft fractures in children. *J Pediatr Orthop* 15:30–35, 1995.

37. Burkhart SS, Peterson HA: Fractures of the proximal tibial epiphysis. *J Bone Joint Surg [Am]* 61:996–1002, 1979.

38. Burks RT, Sutherland DH: Stress fracture of the femoral shaft in children: Report of two cases and discussion. *J Pediatr Orthop* 4:614–616, 1984.

39. Burkus JK, Sella EJ, Southwick WO: Occult injuries of the talus diagnosed by bone scan and tomography. *Foot Ankle* 4:316–324, 1984.

40. Buxton RA: Rupture of the urethra in a female child with a fractured pelvis: A case report. *Injury* 9:209–211, 1978.

41. Caffey J, Madell SH, Royer C, Morales P: Ossification of the distal femoral epiphysis. *J Bone Joint Surg [Am]* 40:647–654, 1958.

42. Canale ST, Bourland WL: Fracture of the neck and intertrochanteric region of the femur in children. *J Bone Joint Surg [Am]* 59:431–443, 1977.

43. Canale ST, Kelly FB Jr: Fractures of the neck of the talus. Long term evaluations of 71 cases. *J Bone Joint Surg [Am]* 60:143–156, 1978.

44. Canale ST, King RE: Fractures of the hip, in Rockwood CA Jr, Wilkins K, King R (eds): *Fractures in Children.* Vol. 3. Philadelphia, Lippincott, 1984, pp 733–843.

45. Canale ST, Tolo VT: Fractures of the femur in children. *Instr Course Lect* 44:255–274, 1995.

46. Cannon SR, Pool CF: Traumatic separation of the proximal femoral epiphysis and fracture of the mid-shaft of the ipsilateral femur in a child: A case report and review of the literature. *Injury* 15:156–158, 1983.

47. Cass JR, Peterson HA: Salter Harris type IV injuries of the distal tibial epiphyseal growth plate with emphasis on those involving the medial malleolus. *J Bone Joint Surg [Am]* 65:1059–1070, 1983.

48. Cassebaum WH, Patterson AH: Fractures of the distal femoral epiphysis. *Clin Orthop* 41:79–91, 1965.

49. Cehner J: Fractures of the tarsal bones, metatarsals and toes, in Weber BG, Brunner CH, Freuler F (eds): *Treatment of Fractures in Children and Adolescents.* Berlin, Springer-Verlag, 1980, pp 385–393.

50. Chapman HG, Galway HR: Os calcis fractures in childhood. *J Bone Joint Surg [Br]* 59:510, 1977.

51. Charnley J: *The Closed Treatment of Common Fractures.* London, Churchill Livingstone, 1974.

52. Childress HM: Distal femoral 90–90 traction: For shaft fractures of the femur in children. *Orthop Rev* 8:45–50, 1979.

53. Christie MJ, Dvonch VM: Tibial tuberosity avulsion fracture in adolescents. *J Pediatr Orthop* 1:391–394, 1981.

54. Craig CL: Hip injuries in children and adolescents. *Orthop Clin North [Am]* 11:743–753, 1980.

55. Clement DA, Colton CL: Overgrowth of the femur after fracture in childhood: An increased effect in boys. *J Bone Joint Surg [Br]* 68:534–536, 1986.

56. Colonna PC: Fracture of the neck of the femur in children. *[Am] J Surg* 6:793, 1929.

57. Coltart WB: Aviatiors astragalus. *J Bone Joint Surg [Br]* 34:545–566, 1952.

58. Cooperman DR, Spiegel PG, Laros GS: Tibial fractures involving the ankle in children. *J Bone Joint Surg [Am]* 60:1040–1045, 1978.

59. Crawford AH: Fractures about the knee in children. *Orthop Clin North [Am]* 7:639–655, 1976.

60. Criswell AR, Hand WL, Butler JE: Abduction injuries of the distal femoral epiphysis in rabbits II. *J Bone Joint Surg [Am]* 40:887–896, 1958.

61. Criswell AR, Hand WL, Butler JE: Abduction injuries of the distal femoral epiphysis. *Clin Orthop* 115:189–194, 1976.

62. Curtis JF, Killian JT, Alonso JE: Improved treatment of femoral shaft fractures in children utilizing the pontoon spica cast: A long-term follow-up. *J Pediatr Orthop* 15:36–40, 1995.

63. Czitrom AA, Salter RB, Willis RB: Fractures involving the distal epiphyseal plate of the femur. *Int Orthop* 4:269–278, 1981.

64. Dameron TB: Fractures and anatomical variation of the proximal portion of the fifth metatarsal. *J Bone Joint Surg [Am]* 57:788–792, 1975.

65. Dameron TB Jr, Thompson HA: Femoral-shaft fractures in children: Treatment by closed reduction and double spica cast immobilization. *J Bone Joint Surg [Am]* 41:1201–1212, 1959.

66. Damholt V, Dravkovic D: Quadriceps function following fractures of the femoral shaft in children. *Acta Orthop Scand* 45:756–763, 1974.

67. Danielsson LG: Avulsion fracture of the lateral malleolus in children. *Injury* 12:165–167, 1980.

68. Denton JR, Fischer SJ: The medial triplane fracture: Report of an unusual injury. *J Trauma* 21:991–995, 1981.

69. Devas MB: Stress fractures in children. *J Bone Joint Surg [Br]* 45:528–541, 1963.

70. Devas MB: Stress fractures in children. *J Bone Joint Surg [Br]* 45:528–541, 1963.

71. Dias LS: Fractures of the tibia and fibula, in Rockwood CA Jr, Wilkins K, King R (eds): *Fractures in Children.* Vol 30. Philadelphia, Lippincott, 1984, pp 983–1042.

72. Dias LS, Giegerich CR: Fractures of the distal tibial epiphysis in adolescence. *J Bone Joint Surg [Am]* 65:438–443, 1983.

73. Dias LS, Tachdjian MO: Physeal injuries of the ankle in children. *Clin Orthop* 136:230–233, 1978.

74. Dickason JM, Fox JM: Fracture of the patella due to overuse syndrome in a child. *[Am] J Sports Med* 10:248–249, 1982.

75. Donoghue V, Daneman A, Krajbich I, Smith CR: CT appearance of sacroiliac joint trauma in children. *J Comput Assist Tomogr* 9:352–356, 1985.

76. Edvardsen P, Syversen SM: Overgrowth of the femur after fracture of the shaft in childhood. *J Bone Joint Surg [Br]* 58:339–342, 1976.

77. Edwards PH Jr, Grana WA: Physeal fractures about the knee, *J [Am] Acad Orthop Surg* 3:63–69, 1995.

78. Epstein HC: Fractures and dislocations of the hip and fractures of the acetabulum: Treatment anterior and simple posterior dislocations of the hip in adults and children. *Instr Course Lect* 22:115–144, 1973.

79. Evanoff M, Strong ML, McIntosh R: External fixation maintained until fracture consolidation in the skeletally immature. *J Pediatr Orthop* 13:98–101, 1993.

80. Feigenberg Z, Pauker M, Levy M, et al: Fractures of the femoral neck in childhood: Results of conservative treatment. *J Trauma* 17:937–942, 1977.

81. Fein LH, Pankovich AM, Spero CM, et al: Closed flexible intramedullary nailing of adolescent femoral shaft fractures. *J Orthop Trauma* 3:133–141, 1989.

82. Ford LT, Canales GM: A study of experimental trauma and attempts to stimulate growth of the lower femoral epiphysis in rabbits III. *J Bone Joint Surg [Am]* 42:439–446, 1960.

83. Ford LT, Key JA: A study of experimental trauma to the distal femoral epiphysis in rabbits. *J Bone Joint Surg [Am]* 38:84–92, 1956.

84. Freeman GE Jr: Traumatic dislocation of the hip in children: A report of seven cases and review of the literature. *J Bone Joint Surg [Am]* 43:401–406, 1961.

85. Funk FJ Jr: Traumatic dislocation of the hip in children: Factors influencing prognosis and treatment. *J Bone Joint Surg [Am]* 44:1135–1145, 1962.

86. Fyfe IS, Jackson JP: Tibial intercondylar fractures in children. *Injury* 13:165–169, 1981.

87. Garvan JD: Delayed presentation of posterior fracture dislocation of the hip in a child. *Aust NZ J Surg* 53:493–496, 1983.

88. Garvin KL, McCarthy RE, Barnes CL, Dodge BM: Pediatric pelvic ring fractures. *J Pediatr Orthop* 10:577–582, 1990.

89. Gaul RW: Recurrent traumatic dislocation of the hip in children. *Clin Orthop* 90:107–109, 1973.

90. Glass A, Powell HDW: Traumatic dislocation of the hip in children: An analysis of forty-seven patients. *J Bone Joint Surg [Br]* 43:29–37, 1961.

91. Godshall RW, Hansen CA, Rising DC: Stress fractures through the distal femoral epiphysis in athletes: A previously unreported entity. *[Am] J Sports Med* 9:114–116, 1981.

92. Goergen TG, Venn-Watson EA, Rossman DJ, et al: Tarsal navicular stress fractures in runners. *AJR* 136:201–203, 1981.

93. Goldberg I, Reusso I, Tiqua P: Voluntary habitual dislocation of the hip. *J Bone Joint Surg [Am]* 66:1117–1119, 1984.

94. Goldman AB, Jacobs B: Femoral neck fractures complicating Gaucher disease in children. *Skel Radiol* 12:162–168, 1984.

95. Green NE: Asymmetrical overgrowth of the tibia. *J Pediatr Orthop* 3:235–237, 1983.

96. Greenfield GQ Jr: Proximal tibial epiphyseal fracture. *Orthopaedics* 3:747–750, 1980.

97. Gregory RJH, Cubison TCS, Pinder IN, et al: External fixation of lower limb fractures in children. *J Trauma* 33:691–693, 1992.

98. Greiff J, Bergmann F: Growth disturbance following fracture of the tibia in children. *Acta Orthop Scand* 51:315–320, 1980.

99. Griffin PP: Fractures of the femoral diaphysis in children. *Orthop Clin North [Am]* 7:633–638, 1976.

100. Griffin PP, Anderson M, Green WT: Fractures of the shaft of the femur in children: Treatment and results. *Orthop Clin North [Am]* 3:213–224, 1972.

101. Gronkvist H, Hirsch G, Johansson L: Fracture of the anterior spine in children. *J Pediatr Orthop* 4:465–468, 1984.

102. Gross R: Fractures and dislocations of the foot, in Rockwood CA Jr, Wilkins K, King R (eds): *Fractures in Children.* Vol 3. Philadelphia, Lippincott, 1984, pp 1049–1103.

103. Gross RH, Davidson R, Sullivan JA, et al: Cast brace management of the femoral shaft fracture in children and young adults. *J Pediatr Orthop* 3:572–582, 1983.

104. Gross RH, Stranger M: Causative factors responsible for femoral fractures in infants and young children. *J Pediatr Orthop* 3:341–343, 1983.

105. Hagglund G, Hansson LI, Norman O: Correction by growth of rotational deformity after femoral fracture in children. *Acta Orthop Scand* 54:858–861, 1983.

106. Haliburton RA, Brockenshire FA, Barber JR: Avascular necrosis of the femoral capital epiphysis after traumatic dislocation of the hip in children. *J Bone Joint Surg [Br]* 43:43–46, 1961.

107. Hallel T, Salvati EA: Premature closure of the triradiate cartilage: A case report and animal experiment. *Clin Orthop* 124:278–281, 1977.

108. H[am]melbo T: Traumatic hip dislocation in childhood. *Acta Orthop Scand* 47:546–548, 1976.

109. H[am]dan JA, Taleb YA, Ahmed MS: Traction-induced hypertension in children. *Clin Orthop* 185:87–89, 1984.

110. Harries TJ, Lichtman DM, Lenon WD: Irreducible Salter-Harris II fracture of the proximal tibia. *J Pediatr Orthop* 3:92–95, 1983.

111. Hawkins LG: Fractures of the neck of the talus. *J Bone Joint Surg* 52A:991–1002, 1970.

112. Hedlund R, Lindgren U: The incidence of femoral shaft fractures in children and adolescents. *J Pediatr Orthop* 6:47–50, 1986.

113. Heikkinen ES, Sul[am]aa M: Recurrent dislocation of the hip: Report of two children. *Acta Orthop Scand* 42:58–62, 1971.

114. Heiser JM, Oppenheim WL: Fractures of the hip in children: A review of forty cases. *Clin Orthop* 149:177–184, 1980.

115. Henderson OL, Morrissy RT, Gerdes MH, McCarthy RE: Early casting of femoral shaft fractures in children. *J Pediatr Orthop* 4:16–21, 1984.

116. Herring JA, Moseley C: Instructional case: Post-traumatic valgus deformity of the tibia. *J Pediatr Orthop* 1:435–439, 1981.

117. Hoeksema HD, Olsen C, Rudy R: Fracture of femoral neck and shaft and repeat neck fracture in a child: Case report. *J Bone Joint Surg [Am]* 57:271–272, 1975.

118. Hoekstra HJ, Binnendijk B: Incidence and sex distribution of proximal femoral fractures in children and adolescents. *Netherlands J Surg* 35:69–72, 1983.

119. Hoekstra HJ, Binnendijk B: Restrictions in sports activities after a hip-fracture in a child or adolescent: Criteria for the medical examination. *Int J Sports Med* 5:10–12, 1984.

120. Hoekstra HJ, Lichtendahl D: Pertrochanteric fractures in children and adolescents. *J Pediatr Orthop* 3:587–591, 1983.

121. Hovelius L: Traumatic dislocation of the hip in children. *Acta Orthop Scand* 45:746–751, 1974.

122. Humberger FW, Eyring EJ: Proximal tibial 90–90 traction in treatment of children with femoral-shaft fractures. *J Bone Joint Surg [Am]* 51:499–504, 1969.

123. Ingram AJ, Bachynski B: Fractures of the hip in children: Treatment and results. *J Bone Joint Surg [Am]* 35:867–887, 1953.

124. Irani RN, Nicholson JT, Chung SMK: Long-term results in the treatment of femoral-shaft fractures in young children by immediate spica immobilization. *J Bone Joint Surg [Am]* 58:945–951, 1976.

125. Ireland DCR, Fisher RL: Subtrochanteric fracture of the femur in children. *Clin Orthop* 110:157–166, 1975.

126. Iwaya T, Tahatori Y: Lateral longitudinal stress fracture of the patella: Report of three cases. *J Pediatr Orthop* 5:73–75, 1985.

127. Johnson GF: Pediatric Lisfranc injury: "Bunk bed fracture." *AJR* 137:1041–1044, 1981.

128. Kärrholm J, Hansson LI, Laurin S: Supination, eversion injuries to the ankle in children: A retrospective study of radiographic classification and treatment. *J Pediatr Orthop* 2:147–159, 1982.

129. Kärrholm J, Hansson LI, Laurin S: Incidence of tibio-fibular and ankle fractures in children. *J Pediatr Orthop* 2:386–396, 1982.

130. Kärrholm J, Hansson LI, Laurin S: Post traumatic growth disturbance of the ankle treated by the Langenskiold procedure. *Acta Orthop Scand* 54:721–729, 1983.

131. Kaarholm J, Hansson LI, Laurin S: Computed tomography of intra-articular supination-eversion fractures of the ankle in adolescents. *J Pediatr Orthop* 1:181–187, 1981.

132. Kaarholm J, Hansson LI, Selvik G: Changes in tibiofibular relationships due to growth disturbances after ankle fractures in children. *J Bone Joint Surg [Am]* 66:1198–1210, 1984.

133. Kaarholm J, Hansson LI, Selvik G: Roentgen stereophotogrammetric analysis of growth pattern after pronation ankle injuries in children. *Acta Orthop Scand* 53:1001–1011, 1982.

134. Kaarholm J, Hansson LI, Slevik G: Roentgen stereophotogrammetric analysis of growth patterns. *J Pediatr Orthop* 2:271–279, 1982.

135. Kaarholm J, Hansson LI, Svensson K: Prediction of growth pattern after ankle fractures in children. *J Pediatr Orthop* 3:319–325, 1983.

136. Kavanaugh JH, Brower TD, Mann RV: The Jones fracture revisited. *J Bone Joint Surg [Am]* 60:776–782, 1978.

137. Kay SP, Hall JE: Fracture of the femoral neck in children and its complications. *Clin Orthop* 80:53–70, 1971.

138. Kennedy JC, Weinberg HW, Wilson AS: The anatomy and function of the anterior cruciate ligament as determined by clinical and morphological studies. *J Bone Joint Surg [Am]* 56:223–235, 1974.

139. Keret D, Reis ND: Voluntary habitual dislocation of the hip joint in a child: Case report. *J Pediatr Orthop* 6:22–223, 1986.

140. Key JA, Conwell HE: *Management of Fractures, Dislocations, and Sprains.* St Louis, Mosby, 1951.

141. Kleiger J, Mankin HJ: Fracture of the lateral portion of the distal tibial epiphysis. *J Bone Joint Surg [Am]* 46:25–32, 1974.

142. Klein A, Sumner TE, Volberg FM, Orbon RJ: Combined CT-arthrography in recurrent traumatic hip dislocation. *AJR* 138:963–964, 1982.

143. Kling TF, Bright RW, Hensinger RM: Distal tibial physeal fractures in children that may require open reduction. *J Bone Joint Surg [Am]* 66:647–657, 1984.

144. Kohan L, Cumming WT: Femoral shaft fractures in children: The effect of initial shortening of subsequent limb overgrowth. *Aust NZ J Surg* 52:141–144, 1982.

144a. Kregor PJ, Song KM, Routt MLC, et al: Plate fixation of femoral shaft fractures in multiply injured children. *J Bone Joint Surg* 75A:1774–1779, 1993.

145. Lam SF: Treatment of fractures of the neck of the femur in children. *Orthop Clin North [Am]* 7:625–632, 1976.

146. Lam SF: Fractures of the neck of the femur in children. *J Bone Joint Surg [Am]* 53:1165–1179, 1971.

147. Landin LA, Danielsson LG: Children's ankle fractures (classification and epidemiology). *Acta Orthop Scand* 54:634–640, 1983.

148. Last RJ: *Anatomy, Regional and Applied.* London, Churchill, 1963.

149. Letts RM: The hidden adolescent ankle fracture. *J Pediatr Orthop* 2:161–164, 1982.

150. Letts RM, Giveault D: Fractures of the neck of the talus in children. *Foot Ankle* 1:74–77, 1980.

151. Leung PC, Lam SF: Long-term follow-up of children with femoral neck fractures. *J Bone Joint Surg [Br]* 68:537–540, 1986.

152. Ligier JN, Metasiziau JP, Prevot J, et al: Elastic stable intramedullary nailing of femoral shaft fractures in children. *J Bone Joint Surg* 70B:74–77, 1988.

153. Litton LO, Workman C: Traumatic anterior dislocation of the hip in children. *J Bone Joint Surg [Am]* 40:1419–1422, 1958.

154. Lombardo SJ, Harvey JP Jr: Fractures of the distal femoral epiphyses: Factors influencing prognosis: A review of thirty-four cases. *J Bone Joint Surg [Am]* 59:742–751, 1977.

155. Lynn MD: The tri-plane distal tibial epiphyseal fracture. *Clin Orthop* 86:187–190, 1972.

156. MacNealy GA: Injuries of the distal tibial epiphysis. *AJR,* 138:683–689, 1982.

157. Malkawi H: Traumatic anterior dislocation of the hip with fracture of the shaft of the ipsilateral femur in children: Case report and review of the literature. *J Pediatr Orthop* 2:307–311, 1982.

158. Malkawi H, Shannak A, Hadidi S: Remodeling after femoral shaft fractures in children treated by the modified blount method. *J Pediatr Orthop* 6:421–429, 1986.

159. Marmor L: An unusual fracture of the tibial epiphysis. *Clin Orthop* 73:132–135, 1970.

160. Marti R, in Chapchal G (ed): *Fractures of the Talus and Calcaneus.* New York, Thieme-Stratton, 1981.

161. Marti R: Fractures of the lower leg, in Weber BG, Brunner CH, Freuler F (eds): *Treatment of Fractures in Children and Adolescents.* New York, Springer-Verlag, 1980, pp 330–349.

162. Marti R: Fractures of the talus and calcaneus, in Weber BG, Brunner CH, Freuler F (eds): *Treatment of Fractures in Children and Adolescents.* New York, Springer-Verlag, 1980.

163. Martin W III, Riddervold HO: Acute plastic bowing fractures of the fibula. *Radiology* 131:639–640, 1979.

164. Martin-Ferrero MA, Sanchez-Martin MM: Prediction of overgrowth in femoral shaft fractures in children. *Int Orthop* 10:89–93, 1986.

165. Mason ML: Traumatic dislocation of the hip in childhood: Report of a case. *J Bone Joint Surg [Br]* 36:630–632, 1954.

166. Matta JM, Mehne OK, Roff R: Fractures of the acetabulum: Early results of a prospective study. *Clin Orthop* 205:241–250, 1986.

167. Matta JM, Saucedo T: Internal fixation of pelvic ring fractures. *Clin Orthop* 242:83–97, 1989.

168. Matteri RE, Frymoyer JW: Fractures of the calcaneus in young children. *J Bone Joint Surg [Am]* 55:1091–1094, 1973.

169. McCarthy RE: A method for early spica cast application in treatment of pediatric femoral shaft fractures: Technique. *J Pediatr Orthop* 6:89–91, 1986.

170. McCollough NC III, Vinsant JE Jr, Sarmiento A: Functional fracture-bracing of long-bone fractures of the lower extremity in children. *J Bone Joint Surg [Am]* 60:314–319, 1978.

171. McCullough CJ, Venugopal V: Osteochondritis dissecans of the talus: The natural history. *Clin Orthop* 144:264–268, 1979.

172. McDonald GA: Pelvic disruptions in children. *Clin Orthop* 151:130–134, 1980.

173. McDougall A: Fracture of the neck of femur in childhood. *J Bone Joint Surg [Br]* 43:16–28, 1961.

174. McIntyre RC, Bensard DD, Moore EE, et al: Pelvic fracture geometry predicts risk of life threatening complications in children. *J Trauma* 35:423–429, 1993.

175. Meals RA: Overgrowth of the femur following fractures in children: Influence of handedness. *J Bone Joint Surg [Am]* 61:381–384, 1979.

176. Metzmaker JN, Pappas AM: Avulsion fractures of the pelvis. *[Am] J Sports Med* 13:349–358, 1985.

177. Meyers MH, McKeever FM: Fracture of the intercondylar eminence of the tibia. *J Bone Joint Surg [Am]* 41:209–222, 1959.

178. Meyers MH, McKeever FM: Fracture of the intercondylar eminence of the tibia. *J Bone Joint Surg [Am]* 52:1677–1684, 1970.

179. Miller PR, Welch MC: The hazards of tibial pin replacement in 90–90 skeletal traction. *Clin Orthop* 135:97–100, 1978.

180. Miller WE: Fractures of the hip in children from birth to adolescence. *Clin Orthop* 92:155–188, 1973.

181. Mir D, Lustig KA: Femoral neck fractures in children: Case report and discussion. *Contemp Orthop* 9:47–52, 1984.

182. Moran MC, Dvonch VM: Subtle Salter type II: Distal femoral epiphyseal fracture. *Orthopedics* 8:1414–1416, 1985.

183. Morrissy RT: Hip fractures in children. *Clin Orthop* 152:202–210, 1980.

184. Morrissy RT: Fractures of the hip: Part VIII. Fractured hip in childhood. *Instr Course Lect* 33:229–241, 1984.

185. Nevelos AB, Colton CL: Rotational displacement of the lower tibial epiphysis due to trauma. *J Bone Joint Surg [Br]* 59:331–332, 1977.

186. Nicastro JF, Haupt HA: Probable stress fracture of the cuboid in an infant. *J Bone Joint Surg [Am]* 66:1106–1108, 1984.

187. Offierski CM: Traumatic dislocation of the hip in children. *J Bone Joint Surg [Br]* 63:194–197, 1981.

188. Ogden J: *Skeletal Injury in the Child.* Philadelphia, Lea & Febiger, 1982.

189. Ogden JA, Lee KE, Rudicel A, Pelker RR: Proximal femoral epiphysiolysis in the neonate. *J Pediatr Orthop* 4:285–292, 1984.

190. Ogden JA, Tross RB, Murphy MJ: Fractures of the tibial tuberosity in adolescents. *J Bone Joint Surg [Am]* 62:205–214, 1980.

191. O'Malley DE, Mazur JM, Cummings RJ: Femoral head avascular necrosis associated with intramedullary nailing in an adolescent. *J Pediatr Orthop* 15:21–23, 1995.

192. O'Rahilly R, Gertner E, Gray DJ: The skeletal development of the foot. *Clin Orthop* 16:7–14, 1960.

193. Orenstein E, Dvanch V, Demos T: Acute traumatic bowing of the tibia without fracture. *J Bone Joint Surg [Am]* 67:965–967, 1985.

194. Pappas AM, Anas P, Toczylowski HM Jr: Asymmetrical arrest of the proximal tibial physis and genu recurvation deformity. *J Bone Joint Surg [Am]* 66:575–581, 1984.

195. Pearson DE, Mann RJ: Traumatic hip dislocation in children. *Clin Orthop* 92:189–194, 1973.

196. Peiro A, Aracil J, Martos F, Mut T: Triplane distal tibial epiphyseal fracture. *Clin Orthop* 160:196–200, 1981.

197. Pennal GF, Tile M, et al: Pelvic disruption: Assessment and classification, *Clin Orthop* 151:12–21, 1980.

198. Peterson HA: Operative correction of post fracture arrest of the epiphyseal plate. *J Bone Joint Surg [Am]* 62:1018–1020, 1980.

199. Peterson CH, Peterson HA: Analysis of the incidence of injuries to the epiphyseal plate. *Trauma* 12:275, 1972.

200. Petrini A, Grassi G: Long term results in traumatic dislocation of the hip in children. *Ital J Orthop Traumatol* 9:255–230, 1983.

201. Pforringer W, Rosemeyer B: Fractures of the hip in children and adolescents. *Acta Orthop Scand* 51:91–108, 1980.

202. Piggot J: Traumatic dislocation of the hip in childhood. *J Bone Joint Surg [Br]* 43:38–46, 1961.

203. Pollen AG: *Fractures and Dislocations in Children.* Baltimore, Williams & Wilkins, 1973.

204. Porat S, Milgrom C, Nyska N: Femoral fracture treatment in head injured children: Use of external fixation. *J Trauma* 26:81–84, 1986.

205. Probe R, Lindsey RW, Hadly NA, Barnes DA: Re-fracture of adolescent femoral shaft fractures: A complication of external fixation. A report of two cases. *J Pediatr Orthop* 13:102–105, 1993.

206. Quinlan WR, Brady PG, Regan BF: Fracture of the neck of the femur in childhood. *Injury* 11:242–247, 1980.

207. Raju KK, Tepler M, Dharapak C, Perlman HS: Trans-epiphyseal fracture of the hips in children. *Orthop Rev* 13:33–45, 1984.

208. Raney EM, Ogden JA, Grogan DP: Premature greater trochanteric epiphysiodesis secondary to intramedullary femoral rodding. *J Pediatr Orthop* 13:516–520, 1993.

209. Rang M: *Children's Fractures,* 2d ed. Philadelphia, Lippincott, 1983.

210. Ratliff AHC: Fractures of the neck of the femur in children. *Orthop Clin North [Am]* 5:903–924, 1974.

211. Ratliff AHC: Fractures of the neck of the femur in children. *J Bone Joint Surg [Br]* 44:528–542, 1962.

212. Ratliff AHC: Traumatic separation of the upper femoral epiphyses in young children. *J Bone Joint Surg [Br]* 50:757–770, 1968.

213. Reves RB, Ballard RI, Hughes JL: Internal fixation versus traction and casting of adolescent femoral shaft fractures. *J Pediatr Orthop* 10:592–595, 1990.

214. Riseborough EJ, Barrett IR, Shapiro F: Growth disturbances following distal femoral physeal fracture-separations. *J Bone Joint Surg [Am]* 65:885–893, 1983.

215. Roberts J: Fractures and dislocations of the knee, in Rockwood CA Jr, Wilkins K, King R (eds): *Fractures in Children.* Philadelphia, Lippincott, 1984, pp 891–982.

216. Rooker GD, Salter RB: Prevention of valgus deformity following fracture of the proximal metaphysis of the tibia in children. *J Bone Joint Surg [Br]* 62:527, 1980.

217. Ryan JR: 90–90 skeletal femoral traction for femoral shaft fractures in children. *J Trauma* 21:46–48, 1981.

218. Salter RD: Injuries of the ankle in children. *Orthop Clin North [Am]* 5:147–152, 1974.

219. Saxer U: Fractures of the shaft of the femur, in Weber BG, Brunner CH, Freuler F (eds): *Treatment of Fractures in Children and Adolescents.* Berlin, Springer-Verlag, 1980.

220. Schmidt TL, Weiner DS: Calcaneal fractures in children. *Clin Orthop* 171:150–155, 1982.

221. Schwartz DL, Haller JA Jr: Open anterior hip dislocation with femoral vessel transection in a child: Case report. *J Trauma* 14:1054–1059, 1974.

222. Scott J, Wardlaw D, McLauchlan J: Cast bracing of femoral shaft fractures in children (a preliminary report). *J Pediatr Orthop* 1:199–201, 1981.

223. Shapiro F: Fractures of the femoral shaft in children: The overgrowth phenomenon. *Acta Orthop Scand* 52:649–655, 1981.

224. Shelton WR, Canale ST: Fractures of the tibia through the proximal tibial epiphyseal cartilage. *J Bone Joint Surg [Am]* 61:167–173, 1979.

225. Sideman S: Traumatic separation of the lower femoral epiphysis. *J Bone Joint Surg [Am]* 25:913–915, 1943.

226. Skah SV: Valgus deformity following proximal tibial metaphyseal fracture in children. *Acta Orthop* 53:141–147, 1982.

227. Slavik M, Dungl P, Sprindrich J, Stedry V: Recurrent traumatic dislocation of the hip in a child: Significance of early hip arthrography. *Arch Orthop Trauma Surg* 104:385–388, 1986.

228. Solheim K: Fracture of the femoral neck in children. *Acta Orthop Scand* 43:523–531, 1972.

229. Spak I: Fractures of the talus in children. *Acta Chir Scand* 107:553–566, 1954.

230. Spiegel PG, Cooperman DR, Laros GS: Epiphyseal fractures of the distal ends of the tibia and fibula. *J Bone Joint Surg [Am]* 60:1046–1050, 1978.

231. Splain SH, Denno JJ: Immediate double hip spica immobilization as the treatment for femoral shaft fractures in children. *J Trauma* 25:994–996, 1985.

232. Staheli LT: Fractures of the shaft of the femur, in Rockwood CA Jr, Wilkins K, King R (eds): *Fractures in Children.* Philadelphia, Lippincott, 1984, pp 845–889.

233. Staheli LT, Sheridan GW: Early spica cast management of femoral shaft fractures in young children (utilizing bilateral fixed skin traction). *Clin Orthop* 126:162–166, 1977.

234. Starshak RJ: Occult fracture of the calcaneus—Another toddler's fracture. *Pediatr Radiol* 14:37–40, 1984.

235. Stephens DC, Locus DS: Traumatic separation of the distal femoral epiphyseal cartilage plate. *J Bone Joint Surg* 56:1383–1390, 1974.

236. Stephens NA: Fracture dislocation of the talus in childhood: A report of two cases. *Br J Surg* 43:600–604, 1956.

237. Suman RK: Treatment of fractures of the femoral shaft with early cast bracing. *Injury* 13:239–243, 1981.

238. Swiontkowski MF: Greene, Swiontkowski MF (eds): *Fractures and Dislocations about the Hip and Pelvis in Skeletal Trauma in Children.* Vol 3. Philadelphia, Saunders, 1994, pp 307–326.

239. Swiontkowski MF, Winquist RA: Displaced hip fractures in children and adolescents. *J Trauma* 26:384–388, 1986.

240. Tachdjian MO: *The Child's Foot.* Philadelphia, Saunders, 1985.

241. Tenny JN, Davis LA: Fractures and fracture dislocations of the neck of the talus. *J Trauma* 20:1029–1037, 1980.

242. Theodorou SD, Ierodiaconon MN, Mitsou A: Obstetrical fracture-separation of the upper femoral epiphysis. *Acta Orthop Scand* 53:239–243, 1982.

243. Thomas HM: Calcaneal fractures in childhood. *Br J Surg* 56:664–666, 1969.

244. Thompson GH, Gesler JW: Proximal tibial epiphyseal fracture in an infant. *J Pediatr Orthop* 4:114–117, 1984.

245. Tile M: Pelvic ring fractures: Should they be fixed? *J Bone Joint Surg* 70B:1–12, 1988.

246. Tile M, Pennal GF: Pelvic disruption: Principles of management. *Clin Orthop* 151:56–64, 1980.

247. Tolo VT: External skeletal fixation in children's fractures. *J Pediatr Orthop* 3:435–442, 1983.

248. Torg JS, Pavlov H, Morris VB: Salter-Harris Type-III fracture of the medial femoral condyle occurring in the adolescent athlete. *J Bone Joint Surg [Am]* 63:586–590, 1981.

249. Torode I, Zieg D: Pelvic fractures in children. *J Pediatr Orthop* 5:76–84, 1985.

250. Trafton PG: Epiphyseal fracture of the base of the first metatarsal, a case report. *Orthopedics* 2:256–257, 1979.

251. Trott AW: Fractures of the foot in children. *Orthop Clin North [Am]* 7:677–686, 1976.

252. Verbeek HOF, Bender J, Sawidis K: Rotational deformities after fractures of the femoral shaft in childhood. *Injury* 8:43–48, 1976.

253. Visser JD, Veldhuizen AG: Valgus deformity after fracture of the proximal tibial metaphysis in childhood. *Acta Orthop Scand* 53:663–667, 1982.

254. Von Laer L: Classification, diagnosis and treatment of transitional fracture of the distal part of the tibia. *J Bone Joint Surg [Am]* 67:687–698, 1985.

255. Ward WT, Levy J, Kay A: Compression plating for child and adolescent femur fractures. *J Pediatr Orthop* 12:626–632, 1992.

256. Watson-Jones R: *Fractures and Joint Injuries,* 4th ed. Edinburgh, Livingstone, 1955–1956.

257. Watts HG: Fractures of the pelvis in children. *Orthop Clin North [Am]* 7:615–624, 1976.

258. Weber GH: Fibrous interposition causing valgus deformity after fracture of the upper tibial metaphysis in children. *J Bone Joint Surg [Br]* 59:290–292, 1977.

259. Weber BG: Fractures of the proximal tibial metaphysis, in Weber BG, Brunner CH, Freuler F (eds): *Treatment of Fractures in Children and Adolescents.* Berlin, Springer-Verlag, 1980, pp 324–329.

260. Weber BG, Süsenback F: Malleolar fractures, in Weber BG, Brunner CH, Freuler F (eds): *Treatment of Fractures in Children and Adolescents.* Berlin, Springer-Verlag, 1980, pp 350–372.

261. Weiner DS, O'Dell HW: Fractures of the hip in children. *J Trauma* 9:62–76, 1969.

262. Welch PH, Wynne GF: Proximal tibial epiphyseal separation. *J Bone Joint Surg [Am]* 45:782–784, 1963.

263. Wenger DR, Jeffcoat BT, Herring JA: The guarded prognosis of physeal injury in paraplegic children. *J Bone Joint Surg [Am]* 62:241–246, 1980.

264. Wilchinsky ME, Pappas AM: Unusual complications in traumatic dislocation of the hip in children. *J Pediatr Orthop* 5:534–539, 1985.

265. Wiley JJ: Tarso-metatarsal joint injuries in children. *J Pediatr Orthop* 1:255–260, 1981.

266. Wiley JJ, Profitt A: Fractures of the os calcis in children. *Clin Orthop* 188:131–138, 1984.

267. Wilson DW: Traumatic dislocation of the hip in children: A report of four cases. *J Trauma* 6:739–743, 1966.

268. Wilson JC: Fractures of the neck of the femur in childhood. *J Bone Joint Surg [Am]* 22:531–546, 1940.

269. Yvars MF: Osteochondral fractures of the dome of the talus. *Clin Orthop* 144:185–191, 1976.

270. Zaricznyj B: Avulsion fracture of the tibial eminence: Treatment by open reduction and pinning. *J Bone Joint Surg [Am]* 59:1111–1114, 1977.

271. Ziv I, Rang M: Treatment of femoral fracture in the child with head injury. *J Bone Joint Surg [Br]* 65:276–278, 1983.

PART IV

Pediatric Orthopaedics

CHAPTER 33

Orthopaedic Management of Cerebral Palsy

M. Mark Hoffer

CLASSIFICATION

The cerebral palsies are a group of diseases whose common etiology is brain damage, either intrauterine or soon after birth. Excluded from the strict definition of cerebral palsy are familial and progressive congenital problems and problems acquired in childhood as a result of head injuries. So far as the orthopaedic surgeon is concerned, however, as long as the brain damage is static, the treatment is essentially the same. In the patient with acquired brain damage, it takes at least 2 years to reach such a static state. Brain-damaged children can be roughly classified into groups, depending on the type of involvement the patient has and the geographic distribution of the involvement on the body (Table 33-1). In general, there are three types of cerebral palsy: spastic, motion disorder, and mixed. The child with spasticity has hyperactive reflexes, tends to develop contractures, and may benefit from orthotic and surgical therapeutic approaches. A child with motion disorder (athetosis, chorea, tremor, etc.) has major problems with control of limb position and limb balance. These patients rarely benefit from orthopaedic and orthotic measures; however, therapists have a major impact on their lives in terms of self-care and occupation programs. Many children have a mixed picture of spasticity and motion disorder. It is important to identify these children because the extent to which the patient is disabled by a motion disorder affects the outcome of many surgical procedures.

The geographic distribution of the disability in the cerebral-palsied or head-injured individual has a profound effect on function and the need for orthopaedic care. The *hemiplegic* patient has involvement predominantly on one side. It is not uncommon to see the opposite lower limb slightly involved in the hemiplegic patient. The hemiplegic patient tends to have more involvement distally, that is, in the hands and feet, than proximally. Nearly all hemiplegic cerebral palsy patients eventually walk and talk. This is not necessarily true of those with acquired hemiplegia. The most common deformities in the spastic hemiplegic child are equinovarus and the pronated flexed forearm, wrist, and finger combination.

The *spastic diplegic* patient has involvement predominantly of the lower extremities, although there is practically always some involvement in the upper extremities, and there may in fact be strabismus associated with this spastic diplegia. These patients have more problems with their hips than their feet. They may be ambulatory if they develop balance reactions by 3 years of age. This means that they will have lost the perinatal reflexes prior to that time, usually in a gradual fashion. Thus, the examination for asymmetrical tonic neck reflex (perinatal reflex) versus parachute reaction (early balance reaction) is a key factor in estimating a prognosis for eventual balance and ambulation (Table 33-2). These are the patients who frequently decrease their ambulation as they grow larger in late adolescence. Those patients with radiologically stable hips who demonstrate no progressive loss of femoral head coverage in childhood (and are community ambulators) may undergo rapid hip subluxation in adolescence if they have ventriculoperitoneal shunt dysfunction and unrecognized hydrocephalus.[1] Persistent contractures and dislocated hips also tend to decrease ambulatory ability in this group of patients.

The *totally involved* patient (called *spastic quadriplegic* by some; we would rather reserve the term *quadriplegia* for a spinal palsy) has involvement in all four extremities, but in addition has significant problems in balance, swallowing, and communication. These patients rarely ambulate and most of them have great problems with activities of daily living (ADL). These patients have a higher incidence of scoliosis and dislocating hips.

TABLE 33-1 Classification of Cerebral Palsy

Type
  Spastic
  Motion disorder
  Athetoid ataxia, etc.

Geographic distribution
  Quadriplegia
  Diplegia
  Hemiplegia

Reflex level
  Brainstem: Symmetrical tonic reflexes
  Midbrain: Parachute reaction
           Upright balance

Motor testing
  Contractures, joint or myotendon
  Myotendinous tone, spasticity
  Pattern posture
  Selective control

Sensory testing
  Object identification
  Two-point discrimination

Intelligence

Communication
  Verbal
  Nonverbal

TABLE 33-2 Reflex Testing

Brainstem reflex level: Present normally to 6 months of age; when obligatory thereafter, diagnostic of cerebral palsy. If persistent past 3 years, walking doubtful. If persistent past 6 years, independent sitting doubtful.
  1. Asymmetrical tonic neck reflex—occiput-side extremities flex, face-side extremities extend.
  2. Symmetrical tonic neck reflex—upper extremities flex, lower extremities extend with neck flexed; upper extremities extend, lower extremities flex with neck extended.
Midbrain reflex level: Present normally at 4 to 6 months and throughout life.
Signs of balance reaction:
  1. Parachute—arms and legs abduct and extend when prone child is lowered a few inches.
  2. Upright balance—arms and trunk balance with sideward challenge.

GENERAL ORTHOPAEDIC APPROACH AND MANAGEMENT

Types of Deformities

Deformities that the orthopaedic surgeon is asked to deal with in these spastic patients may be of three varieties. First, there is the dynamic deformity that accompanies abnormal muscle tone. The degree of tone is difficult to estimate unless the patient is totally asleep, and then one may also see how much fixed deformity there is. Second, many deformities that are initially dynamic eventually develop fixed contractures of the musculotendinous structures. Third, fixed joint contractures may develop, and the joints may eventually dislocate.[2,3] Decision making is difficult, but some suggest multiple simultaneous procedures,[4] while others would temporize using botulinum toxin[5] or the still unproven dorsal rhizotomy.

In the totally involved cerebral palsy patient and in the spastic diplegic patient who has not developed balance, hip and knee deformities may become a problem in sitting and ability to transfer.[6] Surgical procedures are usually not performed on deformed feet in nonambulatory patients because of the unpredictability of such procedures.

Deformities and Ambulation Potential

Dynamic deformities in potentially ambulatory children rarely prevent ambulation, although they may make gait less efficient. Thus, these dynamic deformities should be addressed after the patient begins ambulating and when therapist and surgeon perceive that a plateau has been reached that cannot be overcome by therapy and orthotic devices.[7] On the other hand, fixed deformities can interfere with the onset of ambulation in individuals with balance problems and either spastic diplegia or spastic hemiplegia. This is especially true of hip flexion contractures in excess of 45°, adduction contractures prohibiting 30° of abduction, and knee flexion contractures greater than 20°.

Fixed deformities of the foot rarely interfere with the onset of ambulation, although they may affect the efficiency of gait. To estimate where the knee and foot deformities have an effect on ambulatory ability, one should see if the patient can ambulate by knee walking.

Pelvic Obliquity and Scoliosis

The child with scoliosis and pelvic obliquity has instability of the high-side hip.[8–10] It is debatable whether the scoliosis causes this instability or the unstable hip causes the scoliosis.[11–13] Most now believe that the two cannot be separated in a cause-and-effect relation. In terms of treatment, however, the pelvic obliquity must be eliminated before the hip is dealt with. Thus, a spine fusion is necessary when there is fixed pelvic obliquity, and a release of the abducted opposite side is necessary if there is dynamic pelvic obliquity.

Hip Subluxation and Dislocation

Several authors have attempted to correlate the available information and propose guidelines for the treatment of hip instability.[14,15] Fixsen points out that although modern neonatal care has reduced the mortality of low birth weight premature infants, the incidence of brain damage leading to cerebral palsy has not been reduced. In the severely affected nonambulant group, quality of life is the most important issue, and a stable straight spine and stable hips are now considered critical to provide a pain-free patient with good sitting balance.[14] In nonambulators over half will develop progressive hip subluxation, and up to 20 percent will dislocate if untreated.[16] Scrutton[15] points out the importance of the age at which the child pulls to the standing position. Radiologic monitoring of the hips can be carried out by using such measurements as the center edge (CE) angle of Wiberg (Fig. 40-3) or the migration percentage (MP) of Reimers.[12] The migration percentage of Reimers measures the percentage of femoral head uncovered by the acetabulum.[12] Scrutton observed that almost all children who pulled to stand by age 3 had a migration percentage of less than 50. There was a slightly higher incidence of dislocation among children who pulled to stand between 3 and 7 years of age, and after 7 years of age no child learned to pull to stand.[15] Less than 2 percent of hips were a continuing serious problem in those patients who achieved this ability. However, among those children who never pulled to stand, Scrutton observed that 31 percent had a MP of greater than 50; and of these, 20 percent went on to dislocate. Reimers[12] indicates that the hip dislocates rapidly when the MP exceeds 50. He further believes that operation should be carried out without delay as soon as the MP reaches 33.

Advantageous acetabular remodeling is less likely after the age of 4; and for soft tissue surgery alone to be successful, it should be done before the age of 5.[17] Another indication that soft tissue surgery should be performed early was provided by Vidal, who found that acetabular obliquity appears only when migration had reached 20 percent and that it did not appear in children until 30 months of age.[18] In summary, then, early soft tissue surgery performed before displacement of more than 50 percent can be successful, but once there is more than 50 percent displacement or significant acetabular dysplasia, additional bony procedures are required.[14]

Close monitoring of these patients and early preventative surgery to prevent the calamity of dislocation is, therefore, recommended. Soft tissue operations include adductor release or lengthening, obturator neurectomy, and psoas release or lengthening (see below).

When the MP exceeds 50, a combination of femoral osteotomy and soft tissue release may be required. If there is significant acetabular dysplasia, this will be combined with some form of acetabuloplasty. If the hip is already dislocated, open reduction and femoral shortening will be the first step, followed by derotation varus osteotomy of the femur and some form of acetabular osteotomy. Using this kind of approach to the dislocated hip, Root and his coworkers[19] were able to reduce and stabilize the dislocated hip and halt progression in the subluxated variety. Despite femoral shortening to relieve pressure on the femoral head, however, 25 percent of patients displayed some signs of avascular necrosis following these combined procedures, usually leading to premature closure of the growth plate of the femoral head. These authors concluded, however, that the results justified this extensive operation. They point out that once the hip has dislocated, some kind of acetabuloplasty is necessary to stabilize it after reduction. They make the important point that prevention or reduction of dislocation of the hip is desirable to improve the quality of life in patients who are bedridden or confined to a wheelchair, since the dislocated hip interferes with peroneal hygiene and predisposes to a high prevalence of fractures of the lower extremity. They also point out that a large number of these dislocated hips will be painful if left unreduced even in patients who are nonambulators. They performed various types of pelvic osteotomy using the Salter procedure in patients under 12 years of age with a more mobile pelvis (Fig. 40-8) and the Chiari procedure in older children (Fig. 40-13). The Sutherland double osteotomy was carried out in patients who were most severely dysplastic (Fig. 40-11). Their technique was to perform an open reduction procedure through an anterior incision, and a second lateral incision was used for the femoral osteotomy. After the osteotomy was completed and the femoral head reduced into the acetabulum, the femoral fragments were allowed to overlap and the excess femur then removed. They thus shortened these femora by up to 3 cm to reduce the pressure on the relocated femoral head. In some cases, muscle releases of the psoas and adductor tendons were performed at the same time. Blade plate fixation was used to fix the femur following the varus derotation osteotomy, which corrected the excessive anteversion of the femoral head. Other authors report similar success with a combined hip procedure, including varus derotation osteotomy, open reduction, adductor or iliopsoas releases, and pelvic osteotomy.[20]

Release of Hip Deformities

Adduction contractures prohibiting abduction of 30° and hip flexion contractures of 45° or greater should be released, especially when they are increasing in younger children. This is advised even when x-ray views of the hip are normal. It is not necessary, however, in older adolescents with normal-appearing hips.

Adductor Release

Indications

In ambulatory patients, overactivity of the adductors tends to decrease the width of the gait.[21–24] Overactive adductors may cause hip dislocations, especially in the nonambulatory patient. Releases of the adductor longus and the gracilis are the easiest and most proven procedures to decrease this width of gait when tone alone is the problem. When there is a fixed contracture prohibiting 30° of abduction, lengthening of the brevis should be carried out in addition. If there is concern about subluxation, obturator neurectomy should be added.[25,26] Overzealous adductor lengthenings and obturator neurectomies can result in an abducted hip. This penalizes gait and even makes it difficult for patients to sit. Furthermore, it may force the opposite hip to adopt an adducted position in sitting.

Surgical Technique

The adductors are approached through a transverse incision 1 cm beneath the groin crease. The length of the incision should be 3 to 5 cm, and care should be taken to avoid the femoral triangle laterally. The adductor longus can easily be located because it is tendinous and is released in its entirety. The gracilis is a thick band just medial to the adductor longus; it is also released in its entirety. The brevis lies beneath these two muscles, and on the surface of the brevis one can see the anterior branch of the obturator nerve. If an obturator neurectomy is to be carried out, it should be performed upon this branch alone. The brevis is released to the extent of allowing abduction to 50°. The wound is closed with interrupted sutures. Abduction is maintained utilizing two long-leg plasters and a bar with the thighs adducted 45° from each other. In the hip that is stable, this is all that is necessary and it is utilized for only 3 weeks, after which it is utilized as a night splint for another 3 to 4 weeks. In children over age 8, an abduction pillow is better tolerated.

Flexor Release

Indications

Flexed hip postures in the ambulatory patient may cause a lumbar lordosis and a compensatory knee flexion posture. Overactive hip flexors may cause hip dislocations, especially in the nonambulatory patient. There is some discussion in the literature about whether the psoas or all the other flexors cause this problem.[18,27–29] The only definite way to find which is the offending muscle is an ambulatory electromyogram.[30] In general we have found that the psoas tends to be the main problem in this posture. Lengthening of the psoas is advised, especially when an increased sacral femoral angle is seen on a standing lateral view and there is a fixed contracture of the hip exceeding 45°. Overzealous psoas lengthenings may be a problem, especially in patients with "extensor thrust" (tendency to a spastic extensor posture of knees and hips). In these patients an extension contracture of the hips may result, which makes sitting even more difficult.[31] Finally, a rare complication of the extensor posture of the hip may be an anterior dislocation. Therefore, these hip flexor lengthenings should be performed only on patients with fixed contractures who have defined flexed hip postures documented by lateral sacral femoral views.

Surgical Technique

Psoas lengthening is best performed through an anterolateral hip approach and not through the groin. This is because the groin approach releases the psoas from its insertion but the degree of lengthening is difficult to ascertain. Through the anterior approach using either the traditional Smith-Petersen or a more transverse "bikini" skin incision, the sartorius is located and released. Beneath the sartorius, the first muscle encountered is the psoas. Care should be taken to avoid the femoral vessels and also the femoral nerve, which lies within the psoas sheath itself. We generally perform a partial myotomy of the psoas, although a formal psoas recession as described by Bleck may also be performed.[27] The patient is managed postoperatively with a prone program, and no plaster is necessary. The patient is permitted to ambulate whenever he or she is comfortable enough.

Hamstring Release

Indications

The internally rotated thighs pose problems in gait for the ambulatory patient.[32] The stride angle is decreased and the patient may trip. There are many causes for dynamic, internally rotated thigh when there is adequate passive external range. The gait electromyogram can help differentiate the muscle imbalance.[33,34] Generally, hamstring overactivity is the cause for this dynamic posture.[35] When such exists, especially when there is a fixed knee flexion contracture, tenomyotomy of the hamstrings is advised.[36] If there is a dynamic internally rotated gait with adequate external rotation of the hip in the absence of a knee flexion contracture, transfer of the medial hamstring laterally may improve the gait. In that case the semitendinosus alone is transferred. This prevents a recurvatum from occurring[37] as a consequence of decreasing the overall hamstring tone. Another approach to this problem is the anteromedial transfer of the greater trochanter, thus allowing the abductors of the hip to act as external rotators.[38] Tenomyotomy of the hamstrings is the commonest of these procedures and is described in the next section.

The knee-flexed position in the ambulatory patient may be due to a postural problem involving either the hip or the ankle. When there is no fixed contracture, attention should be given to these other joints before dealing with the knee itself. If this precaution is not taken and hamstring lengthenings are carried out, recurvatum may be the result. Proximal hamstring lengthenings have been advocated in the past for this problem, but they may give patients profound weakness in hip extension. Proximal hamstring lengthening should not be performed except in the rare patient with extensor thrust and hip extension posture.[13,39–41] Extensor thrust is that pattern of tone involving hip and knee extensors in uncontrolled overactivity. In ambulatory or nonambulatory patients with knee flexion contractures of greater than 20°, hamstring lengthening is a safe and appropriate procedure. In addition, hamstring procedures may be necessary to balance an internally rotated gait, as noted above. In both cases, the identical approach is taken.

Surgical Technique

The patient is placed prone and a sterile tourniquet is used. A longitudinal incision is made across the middle and distal thirds of the thigh. This incision should avoid the popliteal space. The hamstrings and sciatic nerve are located and the sciatic nerve protected. The semitendinosus may be transferred through the lateral hamstring incision in the case of the internally rotated gait. In the case of a fixed contracture, tenomyotomies may be carried out to allow the knee to extend fully. In general, it is wise to keep at least one hamstring intact during this procedure unless there is fixed contracture of all. Then distal releases of all tendons through transverse popliteal incisions can be performed. Long leg plaster is placed and utilized for at least 3 weeks. Care is taken in the extension of the knee prior to closure of the wound to ensure that the sciatic nerve is not unduly stretched, so that peroneal palsy will be avoided. In children over 8 years of age, a removable knee immobilizer may be better tolerated.

Femoral Osteotomy

Indications

When there is a fixed internal rotation of the thigh, it is usually due either to contracted muscles, as noted above, or to anteversion.[42] This is evaluated clinically by examining the patient in the prone position and rotating the hip internally until the greater trochanter lies parallel to the table. The radiologic examination by anteroposterior and horizontal lateral views or by CT scan may also be utilized. The involved contracted muscles should then be released and derotation osteotomy carried out. If this is an ambulatory child, such a set of procedures is appropriate and may improve the stride angle and gait. In nonambulatory patients, such procedures are necessary only when the hip is subluxed. There are therefore two separate situations when proximal femoral derotation osteotomy is required: (1) anteversion with a dislocated hip in an ambulatory patient and (2) anteversion with a subluxed hip in an ambulatory or nonambulatory patient. When a combination of valgus and anteversion is associated with a subluxed hip, a proximal varus derotation osteotomy should be performed.[34,43,44]

Distal Derotation Femoral Osteotomy

Surgical Technique

Through a lateral incision in the distal thigh using a sterile tourniquet, the bone is approached subperiosteally, and an osteotomy is performed with guide pins in place to note the amount of rotation.[45] Usually, 30 to 45° of derotation is carried out. Then parallel pins are placed and the patient is placed in long leg plaster. Of necessity these pins lie close to the wound. Therefore, a modification of this procedure has been carried out by Rosenfeld. He advises a medial approach, placing the pins through both cortices in the corrected position. Then, after the osteotomy, the pins lie parallel to one another and are driven through the lateral cortex and out the skin. The medial wound is closed and the pins are incorporated in the plaster. Others have utilized the external fixators.[46]

Proximal Varus Derotation Osteotomy

Surgical Technique

A routine lateral hip incision is carried out. The incision is carried down to the subperiosteum. A transverse osteotomy is carried out between the greater and lesser trochanters. The hip is carried into external rotation of 30° and a varus position of approximately 110°. This is done by use of an opening wedge and cross pinning in children from 3 to 8 years of age. In children over age 8, a closing wedge with excision of the medial wedge gives better stability than either smooth pins across the osteotomy site or a nail-plate combination. Nail-plate combinations, especially in younger children, do not allow a great deal of freedom for both the varus and the derotation necessary in this procedure. These are more appropriately used in the older adolescent.

Pelvic Osteotomy

Indications

When there is lateral displacement of the head associated with valgus and/or anteversion, a varus derotation osteotomy as described above is necessary to hold the hip in the acetabulum.[47,48] However, if there is inadequate acetabular coverage, cartilage-sparing pelvic osteotomies (Pemberton, double innominate,[49] triple innominate[50]) or buttress support osteotomies (shelf osteotomy,[51] Chiari osteotomy) may be carried out. The cartilage-sparing osteotomies and the shelf procedure may be effective in the relatively mildly subluxed hip that can be well contained. In the problem hip, however, the author believes the Chiari osteotomy is the most effective procedure. Dietz and Knutsen[52] report that when performed without concomitant femoral osteotomy, Chiari osteotomy will provide for a painless hip at 7 years of age in 80 percent. However, 29 percent of hips will show a migration percentage of greater than or equal to 30 percent. Most of these resubluxations occur in the first year after the operation. The authors comment that longer-term studies are necessary to determine optimal surgical procedures. Multiple simultaneous procedures may be required, as described earlier.[53,54]

Surgical Procedure: Chiari Osteotomy

The Chiari osteotomy is carried out through an anterolateral (Smith-Petersen) approach, the incision being carried farther back posteriorly than usual, exposing the anterior half of the iliac crest. Dissection proceeds subperiosteally to the hip capsule and the sciatic notch. X-ray films are taken with a pin just above the hip joint in the direction of 15° posterosuperiorly. This verification is needed, because too high an osteotomy gives a poor buttress. A curved hemostat is placed in the sciatic notch to protect the structures therein. A motor saw is utilized to get the proper angle all along the interval between the pin below the anteroinferior iliac spine and to approximately 1 in. above the sciatic notch. Then a Gigli saw is placed in the notch and an osteotomy performed from the notch to the original saw cut. The hip is abducted, and this should allow displacement of about half the iliac crest. A pin is then placed to fix the osteotomy and x-ray films are taken to verify its position.

On rare occasions, in the younger child with a high dislocation, an open reduction of the hip and shortening varus osteotomy are helpful. However, it is not wise to perform this procedure in children over 8 years of age or when there is cartilage irregularity. Then one should avoid surgery until the patient has pain.[9,55] If pain becomes a problem, especially if it limits sitting, a head and neck resection of femur can be carried out. This is not always a benign procedure, and many of these children have residual discomfort and heterotopic bone postoperatively.[3,56]

Treatment of the Extended Knee Deformity

The extended knee posture results in recurvatum of the knee during gait in the ambulatory patient and also presents difficulty in sitting in the nonambulatory patient. It is difficult for the hip to flex when the knee is not flexed. The stiff, extended knee in the cerebral palsy patient is due to either overactivity of the quadriceps mechanism, overlengthening of the hamstrings, or overactivity of the triceps surae mechanism. In the ambulatory patient, it is important to control the ankle equinus deformity or tip the tibia forward with an ankle brace or a heel raise to overcome the straight knee position. If the triceps surae mechanism does not prove to be the basic problem, a rectus femoris lengthening may be required.[57] It is advisable to obtain a preoperative gait electromyogram to verify that the other quadriceps muscles are active in stance, so that the rectus femoris may be lengthened without causing a flexed knee posture. The rectus femoris lengthening is also helpful in the stiff knee posture of a sitting patient to help flex the knee and allow the hip thus to flex. If the rectus femoris is active by gait study in swing, then its transfer to act as a knee flexor is advised.[58]

Rectus Femoris Transfer

Surgical Technique

A longitudinal incision is made over the distal third of the thigh. The rectus femoris is located and released just above its insertion in the patella. The tendon is then transferred subcutaneously to the tendon of the semimembranosus through a separate incision.

Treatment of Foot and Ankle Deformities

Talipes Equinus Deformity

Indications for Surgery The foot in cerebral palsy is most commonly involved in the spastic hemiplegic patient. Of the various deformities, equinus is seen most often. In general, equinus deformities, even when fixed, should not be operated upon unless it can be demonstrated that they interfere with the patient's gait. Stretching exercises and even sequential plasters should be tried first. Then triceps surae lengthening procedures should be performed.[39] The two-joint muscle tests to differentiate between gastrocnemius and soleus spasticity are probably not a valid differential. A gait electromyogram is necessary to note precisely which of the two muscles is hyperactive. In most cases it is the soleus; therefore a heel cord lengthening is required.[30,59] Overzealous lengthening of the Achilles tendon can result in calcaneus deformities.[40,60] Thus, care in lengthening and postoperative management are advised.[61]

Surgical Technique: Heel Cord Lengthening A small percutaneous tenotomy with a no. 11 blade is carried out at the Achilles tendon insertion, incising the medial half of the tendon; another incision at the musculotendinous junction severs the middle half of the tendon; a third tenotomy incision between the two incises the lateral half of the Achilles tendon. Then the foot is dorsiflexed, gaps are palpated in the regions of the three tenotomies, and plaster is placed with the ankle in slight equinus. The patient is permitted to walk whenever comfortable. The cast is kept on for 6 weeks followed by a brace for 6 months; then the orthosis may be continued as necessary.

Talipes Varus Deformity

Indications for Surgery Varus foot deformities are also frequent, especially in hemiplegics.[62,63] When these deformities are fixed, they interfere with bracing and ambulation and become rapidly progressive. When this varus deformity is fixed, a posterior tibial tendon lengthening is necessary.[64] The dynamic deformity is more complex to analyze and can be evaluated by gait analysis. Either the posterior or anterior tibial muscles may be the deforming force.[65,66] If it is felt that the posterior tibial muscle is the deforming force, the inferior half of its tendon may be split and one of the split portions transferred laterally into the peroneus brevis tendon.[2,67] On the other hand, if it is felt that the anterior tibial muscle is the deforming force, its tendon may be split and transferred laterally.[68]

Surgical Technique: Split Anterior Tibial Tendon Transfer Three incisions are made: one over the insertion of the anterior tibial tendon, another in the distal third of the tibia over the anterior tibial tendon, and a third over the dorsum of the cuboid. All three incisions are longitudinal. In the first incision, the anterior tibial tendon is located and split. An umbilical tape is placed in the split, and the tape is passed up into the second incision. The lateral half of the tendon is released and carried into the second wound. The tendon is then passed subcutaneously into the third wound, and a drill hole is placed in the cuboid in tunnel fashion. The tendon is driven through the drill hole and sutured to itself. A short leg plaster is placed and the patient is allowed to walk whenever comfortable. The cast is used for 6 weeks. A brace is utilized thereafter for at least 6 months.

Talipes Valgus Deformity of the Foot

Indications for Surgery Valgus deformities are common in ambulatory spastic diplegic patients. Here tendon transfers fail to control the deformity, and eventually the deformity may become fixed and painful. In addition, the forefoot may develop a painful hallux valgus. On the other hand, many of these valgus feet are asymptomatic. When the deformity is progressing, it is wise to utilize a polypropylene ankle-foot orthosis (AFO) to hold the foot and hindfoot in neutral as much as possible. When this becomes difficult, a hindfoot stabilization is advised.[69–71] If a fixed deformity is permitted to occur, the only remedy is to wait until the child is 12 or 13 years of age and perform a triple arthrodesis. Some very mild flexible deformities may respond to opening wedge osteotomies of the calcaneus between its middle and posterior facet, which lengthens the lateral bony aspect of the foot.[72]

Surgical Technique: Alban-Grice Hindfoot Stabilization[73] An oblique incision is made over the dorsolateral aspect of the foot halfway between the lateral malleolus and the fifth metatarsal base and in line with skinfolds. The extensor and the peroneal tendons are located and protected. The incision is carried down to the sinus tarsi, which is debrided. Another portion of the incision distal to the peroneal tendons is developed over the lateral aspect of the heel. A Cloward drill, usually size 12, is placed in the sinus tarsi. This drill cleans out the perichondral tissues while the foot is held in a corrected position. A larger Cloward dowel cutter, usually size 14, is placed in the heel, and a block is removed from the calcaneus. The size 14 dowel of bone is then transferred into the size 12 gap created in the sinus tarsi. A staple is placed across the gap, which also holds the foot in position. The postoperative management is by plaster immobilization for 8 weeks and weight bearing in a polypropylene AFO for at least 6 months thereafter. At the same time, if there is a developing bunion deformity, a release of the adductor hallucis should be carried out and a smooth pin placed across the great toe to be removed at 4 to 6 weeks.

GAIT ANALYSIS IN CEREBRAL PALSY

Motion systems, force-plate studies, and dynamic electromyography are the three modalities of gait analysis that have been utilized to evaluate ambulatory cerebral palsy patients.[74] The motion system analysis documents trunk, thigh, leg, and foot segments throughout the gait cycle, so that one can compute the various joint positions and more accurately assess the inappropriate postures throughout the gait cycle. Force-plate studies generate information about the reaction of the foot on the ground in the cerebral palsy patient and thus can estimate the efficiency of gait. Dynamic electromyography usually utilizes fine wire electrodes in muscles whose activity is in question. The patient is then allowed to ambulate, and one can see which muscles are working in an appropriate phase of the gait cycle. A number of complex postures have been analyzed by gait analysis, and the answers found are unique for the individual tested. In the hip-flexed posture, gait analysis can separate overactivity of the rectus from that of the iliopsoas. In the internally rotated hip posture, the medial hamstrings can be separated from the other internal rotators. In the adducted posture, the gracilis and adductor longus can be separated from the less commonly overactive adductors. In the patient with a flexed knee posture, active hamstrings can be separated from postural reaction to hip or ankle position.[75] Patients with varus ankle and hindfoot in gait can be separated into those who have inappropriate activity of the tibialis posterior and those with hyperactivity of the anterior tibial muscle. Patients with equinus ankle and gait can be separated into groups with overactivity of the gastrocnemius, of the soleus, or both.

Utilizing the information obtained from clinical and gait laboratory assessments, simultaneous multiple operations can now be planned in spastic diplegia. Using an energy expenditure index such as the physiologic cost index (PCI) rehabilitation potential, a probable outcome of such surgery can be predicted and its benefits demonstrated in the gait laboratory[76]:

$$PCI \text{ (beats per meter)} = \frac{WHR - RHR}{\text{speed in meters per minute}}$$

where WHR is the heart rate at the end of the set distance (beats per minute) and RHR is the resting heart rate (beats per minute).

For a further discussion of the gait laboratory and its role in evaluating gait, see Chap. 38.

REFERENCES

1. Little DG, Aiona M, Sussman M: Late hip subluxation in spastic diplegia associated with unrecognized hydrocephalus. *J Pediatr Orthop* 15:368–371, 1995.
2. Kling T, Hensinger R: Results of split posterior tibial tendon transfer in children with cerebral palsy. *Orthop Trans* 7:100–107, 1983.
3. Koffman M: Proximal femoral resection or total hip replacement in severely disabled cerebral-spastic patients. *Orthop Clin North Am* 12:91–100, 1981.
4. Nenc AV, Evans GA, Patrick JH: Simultaneous multiple operations for spastic diplegia: Outcome and functional assessment of walking in 18 patients. *J Bone Joint Surg* 75:488–494, 1993.
5. Koman LA, Mooney JF, Smith B, et al: Management of cerebral palsy with botulinum-A toxin: Preliminary investigation. *J Pediatr Orthop* 13:489–495, 1993.
6. Rang M, Douglas G, Bennet GC, Koreska J: Seating for children with cerebral palsy. *J Pediatr Orthop* 1:279–287, 1981.
7. Hoffer MD, Koffman M: Cerebral palsy: The first three years. *Clin Orthop* 151:222–227, 1980.
8. Letts M, Shapiro, L, Mulder K, Klassen O: The windblown hip syndrome in total body cerebral palsy. *J Pediatr Orthop* 4:55–62, 1984.
9. McHale KA, Bagg M, Nason SS: Treatment of the chronically dislocated hip in adolescents with cerebral palsy with femoral head resection and subtrochanteric valgus osteotomy. *J Pediatr Orthop* 10:504–509, 1990.
10. Mackenzie IG: Abnormalities of the hip in cerebral palsy. *Dev Med Child Neurol* 17:797–799, 1975.
11. Moreau M, Drummond DS, Rogala E, et al: Natural history of the dislocated hip in spastic cerebral palsy. *Dev Med Child Neurol* 21:749–753, 1979.
12. Reimers J: The stability of the hip in children: A radiological study of the results of muscle surgery in cerebral palsy. *Acta Orthop Scand* 184(suppl):1–100, 1980.
13. Sharrard WJ, Allen JM, Heaney SH: Surgical prophylaxis of subluxation and dislocation of the hip in cerebral palsy. *J Bone Joint Surg* 57B:160–166, 1975.
14. Fixsen JA: Orthopedic management of cerebral palsy. *Arch Dis Child* 71:396–397, 1994.
15. Scrutton D: The early management of hips in cerebral palsy. *Dev Med Child Neurol* 31:108–116, 1989.
16. Howard CB, McKibbin B, et al: Factors affecting the incidence of hip dislocation in cerebral palsy. *J Bone Joint Surg* 67B:530–532, 1985.

17. Kalen V, Bleck EE: Prevention of spastic paralytic dislocation of the hip. *Dev Med Child Neurol* 27:17–24, 1985.

18. Vidal J: The anatomy of the dysplastic hip in cerebral palsy related to prognosis and treatment. *Int Orthop* 9:105–110, 1985.

19. Root L, Laplaza FJ, Brourman SN, Angel DH: The severely unstable hip in cerebral palsy. *J Bone Joint Surg* 77A:703–712, 1995.

20. Atar D, Grant AD, Bash L, Lehman WB: Combined hip surgery in cerebral palsy patients. *Am J Orthop* 24:52–55, 1995.

21. Reimers J, Poulsen S: Adductor transfer versus tenotomy for stability of the hip in spastic cerebral palsy. *J Pediatr Orthop* 1:52–54, 1984.

22. Root L, Spero CR: Hip adductor transfer compared with adductor tenotomy in cerebral palsy. *J Bone Joint Surg* 63A:767–772, 1981.

23. Sharps CH, Clancy C, Steel HH: A long-term retrospective study of proximal hamstring release for hamstring contracture in cerebral palsy. *J Pediatr Orthop* 4:443–447, 1987.

24. Sutherland DH, Davids JR: Common gait abnormalities of the knee in cerebral palsy. *Clin Orthop* 288:139–147, 1993.

25. Banks H, Green WT: Adductor myotomy and obturation neurectomy for correction of adduction contracture of the hip in cerebral palsy. *J Bone Joint Surg* 42A:111–126, 1960.

26. Zuckerman JD, Staheli LT, McLaughlin JF: Acetabular augmentation for progressive hip subluxation in cerebral palsy. *J Pediatr Orthop* 4:436–442, 1984.

27. Bleck EE: The hip in cerebral palsy. *Orthop Clin North Am* 11:79–104, 1980.

28. Bleck EE: Postural and gait abnormalities caused by hip-flexion deformity in spastic cerebral palsy: Treatment by iliopsoas recession. *J Bone Joint Surg* 53A:1468–1488, 1971.

29. Roosth HP: Flexion deformity of the hip and knee in spastic cerebral palsy: Treatment by early release of spastic hip-flexor muscles. *J Bone Joint Surg* 53A:1489–1510, 1971.

30. Perry J, Hoffer M, Antonelli D, et al: Electromyography before and after surgery for hip deformity in children with cerebral palsy: A comparison of clinical and electromyographic findings. *J Bone Joint Surg* 58A:201–208, 1976.

31. Bowen JR, MacEwen GD, Mathews PA: Treatment of extension contracture of the hip in cerebral palsy. *Dev Med Child Neurol* 23:23–29, 1981.

32. Basset FH: Deformities of the foot in cerebral palsy. *Instr Course Lect* 20:35–40, 1971.

33. Chong KC, Vojnic CD, Quanbury AO: The assessment of the internal rotation gait in cerebral palsy: An electromyographic gait analysis. *Clin Orthop* 132:145–150, 1978.

34. Wheeler ME, Weinstein SL: Adductor tenotomy-obturator neurectomy. *J Pediatr Orthop* 4:48–51, 1984.

35. Tohen A, Carmona J, Barrera J: The utilization of abnormal reflexes in the treatment of spastic foot deformities. *Clin Orthop* 47:77–82, 1966.

36. Dhawlikar SH, Root L, Mann RL: Distal lengthening of the hamstrings in patients who have cerebral palsy: Long term retrospective analysis. *J Bone Joint Surg* 74:1385–1391, 1992.

37. Damron TA, Breed AL, Cook T: Diminished knee flexion after hamstring surgery in cerebral palsy patients: Prevalence and severity. *J Pediatr Orthop* 13:188–191, 1993.

38. Steel HH: Triple osteotomy of the innominate bone: A procedure to accomplish coverage of the dislocated or subluxated femoral head in the older patient. *Clin Orthop* 122:116–127, 1977.

39. Banks HH, Green WT: Correction of equinus deformity in cerebral palsy. *J Bone Joint Surg* 40A:1359–1370, 1958.

40. Bradley G, Coleman S: Treatment of the calcaneo cavus foot deformity. *J Bone Joint Surg* 63A:1159–1166, 1981.

41. Sharrard WJ, Allen JM, Heaney SH: Surgical prophylaxis of subluxation and dislocation of the hip in cerebral palsy. *J Bone Joint Surg* 57B:160–166, 1975.

42. Laplaza FJ, Root L, Tassanawipas A, Glasser DB: Femoral torsion and neck-shaft angles in cerebral palsy. *J Pediatr Orthop* 13:192–199, 1993.

43. Eilert RE, MacEwen GD: Varus derotational osteotomy of the femur in cerebral palsy. *Clin Orthop* 125:168–172, 1977.

44. Tylkowski CM, Simon SR, Mansour JM: Internal rotation gait in spastic cerebral palsy: The Frank Stichfield Award paper. *Hip* 1:89–125, 1982.

45. Elmer EB, Wenger DR, Mubarak SJ, Sutherland DH: Proximal hamstring lengthening in the sitting cerebral palsy patient. *J Pediatr Orthop* 12:329–336, 1992.

46. Moens P, Lammens J, Molenaers G, Fabry G: Femoral derotation for increased hip anteversion: A new surgical technique with a modified Ilizarov frame. *J Bone Joint Surg* 77:107–109, 1995.

47. Brunner R, Baumann JUL: Clinical benefit of reconstruction of dislocated or subluxed hip joints in patients with spastic cerebral palsy. *J Pediatr Orthop* 14:290–294, 1994.

48. Pope DF, Bueff HU, Deluca PA: Pelvic osteotomies for subluxation of the hip in cerebral palsy. *J Pediatr Orthop* 14:724–730, 1994.

49. Sutherland DH, Larsen LJ, Mann R: Rectus femoris release in selected patients with cerebral palsy: A preliminary report. *Dev Med Child Neurol* 17:26–34, 1975.

50. Stevenson T, Donovan MM: Transfer of the hip adductor origin to the ischium in spastic cerebral palsy. *Dev Med Child Neurol* 13:247–258, 1971.

51. Zuckerman JD, Staheli LT, McLaughlin JF: Acetabular augmentation for progressive hip subluxation in cerebral palsy. *J Pediatr Orthop* 4:436–442, 1984.

52. Dietz FR, Knutsen LM: Chiari pelvic osteotomy in cerebral palsy. *J Pediatr Orthop* 15:372–380, 1995.

53. Herndon WA, Bolano L, Sullivan JA: Hip stabilization in severely involved cerebral palsy patients. *J Pediatr Orthop* 12:68–73, 1992.

54. Samilson RL: Orthopedic surgery of the hips and spine in retarded cerebral palsy patients. *Orthop Clin North Am* 12:83–90, 1981.

55. Pritchett JW: The untreated stable hip in severe cerebral palsy. *Clin Orthop* 184:169–172, 1983.

56. Root L: Treatment of hip problems in cerebral palsy. *Instr Course Lect* 36:237–252, 1987.

57. Sutherland DH, Schottstaedt ER, Larsen LJ, et al: Clinical and electromyographic study of seven spastic children with internal rotation. *J Bone Joint Surg* 51A:1070–1082, 1969.

58. Ounpuu S, Muik E, Davis RB, et al: Rectus femoris surgery in children with cerebral palsy: Part I. The effect of rectus femoris transfer location on knee motion. *J Pediatr Orthop* 13:325–330, 1993.

59. Tylkowski CM, Rosenthal RK, Simon SR: Proximal femoral osteotomy in cerebral palsy. *Clin Orthop* 151:183–192, 1980.

60. Schultz RS, Chamberlain SE, Stevens PM: Radiographic comparison of adductor procedures in cerebral palsied hips. *J Pediatr Orthop* 4:741–744, 1984.

61. Damron TA, Greenwald TA, Breed AL: Chronologic outcome of surgical tendoachilles lengthening and natural history of gastroc-soleus contracture in cerebral palsy: A two part study. *Clin Orthop* 301:249–255, 1994.

62. Bisslar RS, Lewis HL: Transfer of the tibialis posterior tendon in cerebral palsy. *J Bone Joint Surg* 52A:137–141, 1975.

63. Root L: Transfer of posterior tibial tendon in cerebral palsy. Proceedings of the American Academy of Cerebral Palsy, 1971.

64. Frost HM, Ruda R: Cerebral palsy spastic varus treated by intramuscular posterior tibial tendon lengthening. *Clin Orthop* 79:61–70, 1971.

65. Gitzka TL, Staheli LT, Duncan WL: Posterior tibial transfers through the interosseous membrane to correct equinovarus deformity in cerebral palsy. *Clin Orthop* 89:2201–2206, 1972.

66. Hoffer MD, Perry J: Pathodynamics of gait alterations in cerebral palsy. *Foot Ankle* 4:128–134, 1983.
67. Green NE, Griffin PP, Shiavi R: Splint posterior tibial tendon transfers in spastic cerebral palsy. *J Bone Joint Surg* 65A: 748–754, 1983.
68. Hoffer MM, Rieswig J, Garret AA, Perry J: Split anterior tibial tendon transfer in the treatment of spastic varus hindfoot of childhood. *Orthop Clin North Am* 5:31–37, 1974.
69. Drvaric DM, Schmitt EW, Nakano JM: The grice extra-articular subtalar arthrodesis in the treatment of spastic hindfoot valgus deformity. *Dev Med Child Neurol* 31:665–669, 1989.
70. Grice DS: Extra-articular arthrodesis of the subastragalar joint with paralytic flat foot of children. *J Bone Joint Surg* 34:927–940, 1952.
71. Steel HH: Gluteus medius and minimus insertion advancement for correction of internal rotation gait in spastic cerebral palsy. *J Bone Joint Surg* 62A:919–927, 1980.
72. Koman LA, Mooney JF, Goodman A: Management of valgus hindfoot deformity in pediatric cerebral palsy patients by medial displacement osteotomy. *J Pediatr Orthop* 13:137–140, 1993.
73. Alban S, Alban, H: Subtalar extra-articular arthrodesis with calcaneal bone in children with cerebral palsy. Proceedings, American Academy of Cerebral Palsy, 1975.
74. Abel MF, Wenger DR, Mubarak SJ: Quantitative analysis of hip dysplasia in cerebral palsy: A study of radiographs and 3-D reformatted images. *J Pediatr Orthop* 14:283–289, 1994.
75. Sutherland DA, Greenfield K: Double innominate osteotomy. *J Bone Joint Surg* 59A:1082–1091, 1977.
76. Nene AV, Evans GA, Patrick JH: Simultaneous multiple operations for spastic diplegia. *J Bone Joint Surg* 75B:488–494, 1993.

CHAPTER 34

Orthopaedic Management in Myelomeningocele

Samuel R. Rosenfeld

DEFINITIONS

Myelomeningoceles are congenital defects of the vertebrae with neural element abnormalities. *Spinal dysraphism* is the term that categorizes congenital defects of the neural tube. These congenital abnormalities fall within the newer terminology of caudal regression syndrome, which also includes lumbosacral agenesis syndromes. The term *myelodysplasia* is used to broadly categorize associated congenital defects of the neural elements.

Spina bifida occulta is a localized defect in the arch of one or more vertebrae, with the spinal cord and meninges remaining confined within the canal.

Meningocele is a defect of the vertebral arch with protrusion of the meninges from the canal. The skin remains intact over the protrusion. Some neural tissue abnormality may be present.

Myelomeningocele is a defect with associated neural elements within it, which are usually not covered by epithelium.

Lipomeningocele is a meningocele that includes a lipomatous growth. This is now referred to as a *leptomyelolipoma*. Commonly associated deformities include the Arnold-Chiari malformation, hydrocephalus, hydromyelia, diastematomyelia, and spinal cord tethering.

GENERAL CONSIDERATIONS

The incidence of spina bifida around the world averages 1 in 10,000 live births. The incidence varies with location, race, maternal age, and socioeconomic status. The overall incidence in the United States has been reported as high as 1 or 2 cases per 1000 live births; the incidence of spina bifida in Great Britain may be as high as 4 cases per 1000 live births.

Folic Acid Deficiency as the Etiology for Neural Tube Defects

In 1992, the Centers for Disease Control published recommendations for the use of folic acid to reduce the number of cases of spina bifida and other neural tube defects.[62] Prospective randomized studies were undertaken in Great Britain, Europe, Cuba, and the United States. The data indicated that folic acid can help avoid neural tube defects when given at high dose levels (i.e., 4.0 mg/day). Additional vitamins conferred no extra benefit in avoiding neural tube defects. The Centers for Disease Control concluded that there is a possibility of reducing the number of cases of spina bifida and other neural tube defects in the United States by 50 percent through daily consumption of 0.4 mg of folic acid.[62] Because the neural tube is fully formed by 28 days' gestation, folic acid supplementation must be initiated prior to pregnancy. The small genetic component of spina bifida is most likely related to a genetic inability to properly metabolize folic acid.

Developmental Pathology

Although there are multiple theories, the Gardner hydrodynamic theory explains most of the associated abnormalities.[36] It is postulated that the opening of the fourth ventricle does not occur at its normal time within the first 28 days of gestation and that hydrostatic pressure in the neural tube consequently rises. This pressure causes bulging caudally and cranially. The specific deformity depends on the degree of deformation and its timing. Normally, the central canal closes and disappears as soon as the fourth ventricle opens; in myelomeningocele patients, however, the canal remains patent. Neural cord advancement to birth level L2–L3 frequently does not occur and the cord tends to become adherent to the spinal canal (spinal cord tethering). Additionally, scarring from any attempted surgical closure contributes to tethering during subsequent growth.

Hydrocephalus is frequently associated with myelomeningocele (72 percent), most frequently with higher lesions (83 percent thoracic and upper lumbar) and less so with lower-level lesions (60 percent). The *Arnold-Chiari* malformation is usually present with the hydrocephalus.[59] There is downward elongation of the cerebellar tonsils and vermis into the spinal canal, along with similar displacement of the brainstem. This abnormality explains the often observed motor incoordination, causing spasticity when the lesion is at higher neurologic levels. Other complications occur during growth as a result of tethering-associated hydrocephalus or expansion of the central canal (hydromyelia). Diastematomyelia (split spinal cord) may occur and be an additional cause of tethering.

Lumbosacral dysgenesis or agenesis differs from myelomeningocele in that there is rarely involvement of the central nervous system other than the area directly involved with the deformity. Associated deformities such as meningocele or diastematomyelia occur. Partial sacral agenesis is associated with unilateral neurologic involvement. When lumbar vertebral absence extends to L2, ambulatory potential is poor. The resultant severe hip and knee flexion deformities with pterygium rarely respond to orthopedic intervention. Transarticular knee amputation is frequently necessary.

Etiology of Deformities

Deformities result from muscle imbalance, intrauterine positioning, positional contractures, spasticity, and factors related to growth.[60] Consequences of muscle imbalance are seen about the hips (subluxation and dislocation), knees (hyperextension deformities when no flexors are present at birth), and feet (dorsiflexion, causing calcaneal gait and contractures). Uterine positioning problems are seen with "windswept" deformities of the feet at birth, when no muscle function is present (i.e., convex pes valgus on one foot and forefoot adductus or equinovarus on the other). Talipes equinovarus is frequently seen in infants born with lumbar myelocele, so that only hip flexors, adductors, and knee extensors are functioning. Postural contractures—such as knee and hip flexion contractures—can occur with wheelchair usage. Spasticity brings on rapid deformity and limits overall usage of the extremity. Spasticity may result from the primary neurologic problem of hydrocephalus and Arnold-Chiari malformation or from other acquired factors, such as injury from shunt placement, infection, recurrent hydrocephalus, hydromyelia, or tethering of the spinal cord.[43,67]

Progressive deformities occur during growth, associated with asymmetry of soft tissue forces.[83] Spinal deformity increases during periods of rapid growth. Tethering of the spinal cord increases scoliosis and/or lordosis during growth.[44] Although the spine, pelvis, hips, knees, ankles, and feet are primarily involved, the upper extremities must not be forgotten in the evaluation, as loss of function interferes with activities of daily living (ADL).[99] Upper extremity function may progressively deteriorate secondary to neurologic impairment associated with hydromyelia or hydrocephalus. The extent of any motor weakness and neurologic impairment should be recorded routinely and regularly.

Functional Evaluation

The treatment of spina bifida should be directed toward the patient's future level of functioning. Patients are grouped as potential ambulators or wheelchair-dependent. Ambulators will require a straight spine, a level pelvis, extended hips and knees, and plantigrade feet.[3] On the other hand, wheelchair patients require a straight spine, level pelvis, mobile hips, knee flexion, and shoeable feet for protection. There are additional criteria for ambulation. There must be power in the antigravity muscles. These include hip extensor muscles, which should test greater than a good plus (or 4+), knee extension greater than fair plus (3+), and triceps surae greater than fair plus (3+). Orthotics can compensate for missing muscle function. Hip flexion contractures need to be less than 30°. Knee flexion contractures need to be less than 20°, and the hindfoot must be in a braceable and shoeable position. Even if the patient cannot meet all these requirements, orthotics can frequently be used to compensate for some missing functions provided that the upper extremities are sufficiently functional to utilize crutches. To use crutches, shoulder depressors (teres major, pectoralis major, and latissimus dorsi) need to be greater than good

plus grade (4+). Full extension at the elbow should be present along with good grasp.

Ambulation potential is related to the anatomic level of the lesion.[6] The development of spasticity can greatly reduce the ability to walk. Few patients will walk if spasticity is present in both upper and lower extremities.[57] A gradual onset of spasticity indicates progressive neurologic abnormality. Early treatment of the neurologic problem may obviate the need for orthopedic treatment. Intelligence level does not affect ambulation unless IQ is less than 50.[27] Fractures impair ambulation potential because of adjacent joint stiffness and deformity.[3,24,40] The period of immobilization may also be a factor. Obesity seems to be more important in contributing to cessation of ambulation rather than delaying or preventing its initiation.[3,40]

Anatomic Level of the Lesion

Anatomic levels determine not only the potential for ambulatory activities but also the orthotic requirements (see Table 34-1).[31]

A lesion at T12 or above results in no functioning muscles beyond the pelvis. Ambulation in childhood occurs with a maximal orthosis—i.e., a hip-knee-ankle-foot orthosis (HKAFO) or parapodium-type device. Patients who are beyond adolescence are rarely able to walk, and the wheelchair must be used.

An L1 lesions preserves some muscle function by the iliopsoas, enabling hip flexion; however, significant hip flexion does not occur above the L2 level because both the iliopsoas and sartorius flex the hip. If the lesion is within the L1 segment, the patients function as if the lesion were at thoracic level. These patients require at least an HKAFO, but their trunk support is good. They usually cease ambulation during adolescence.

Preservation of function at the L2 level provides strong hip flexion and weak hip adduction. These patients also require an HKAFO by adolescence. Most of them are not ambulatory.

With function at L3, the quadriceps are grade 3 to grade 4 and hip adductors are strong. No hip abduction is present and there is no active knee flexion. These patients require a knee-ankle-foot orthotic system (KAFO), although some may require an HKAFO to initiate ambulation in early childhood. The majority are wheelchair-dependent as adults or, at best, household ambulators (see definitions in the following section). This is related to the high energy requirement for use of a KAFO.[101] With function preserved at the level of the L4 segment, the tibialis anterior is functioning. There is also a minimal amount of hip abduction. Medial hamstring function occurs primarily from the semimembranosus and some from the semitendinosus. Medial hamstrings provide knee flexion as well as some hip extension. An ankle-foot orthosis (AFO) is now sufficient because of increased knee stability.

With function preserved at the L5 level, foot and ankle function results from functioning tibialis anterior and tibialis posterior muscles and some toe extensors. Community ambulation (see below) is anticipated with an AFO.

Paralysis below the S1 segment involves primarily the intrinsic musculature of the foot, eliminating the need for

TABLE 34-1 Functional Classification of Patients and Their Ambulation Potential

Level	Anatomic (neurosegmental) level of lesion	Significant motor function at level	Common major deformity related to muscle imbalance	Childhood (1) requirements (2) mobility	Adult (1) requirements (2) mobility
Thoracic	T12 or above, L1 (some patients)	(No significant function in lower limbs)	Scoliosis and pelvic obliquity	(1) Standing brace and wheelchair; (2) exercise (nonfunctional) ambulators only	(1) and (2) wheelchair only
High lumbar	L1	Hip flexion	Hip flexion contracture or dislocation[a]	(1) Crutches and long braces with hip support; (2) household ambulators or community wheelchair	(1) Long braces (KAFO) with crutches; (2) 75% of patients wheelchair only; remainder will be household ambulators
	L2	Hip adduction			
	L3, L4 (some patients)	Knee extension			
Low lumbar	L4	Knee flexion (medial hamstrings)			(1) Will require short braces (AFO); crutches may also be needed; (2) 75% of patients will be community ambulators
	L5	Ankle extension, hip abduction	Calcaneus deformity of ankle; foot ulceration[b]	(1) Short braces, crutches for long distances; (2) community ambulator	
	S1 (some patients)	Knee flexion (lateral hamstrings)			
Sacral	S1	Ankle flexion, inversion, and eversion	Claw toes, high arch foot	(1) Supports in shoes; (2) community ambulator	(1) May require shoe supports; (2) 100% will be community ambulators for a limited distance (but for up to 90% of their requirements)
	S2	(Foot intrinsics are nonfunctional)			
	S3, S4	(Motor function essentially intact)	Minimal or no deformity		

[a] Some patients with lesions at this level will also have scoliosis and pelvic obliquity.
[b] Some patients with lesions at this level will also have hip flexion contracture or dislocation.

anything other than a shoe orthosis to walk. Because of impaired sensation in the foot, AFO management is usually recommended for positioning protection of the foot. Surgical intervention should be directed at allowing the foot to be braceable.

Functional Levels

Each nerve is named after the nerve root that leaves the neuroforamen. The anterior horn cells contributing to each spinal nerve root occupy a segment of the spinal cord. The cells innervating any individual muscle or muscle group may occupy several segments. Consequently, the precise pattern of muscle weakness is variable depending on the level and extent of neuronal dysgenesis.

For this reason, patients should be classified into functional levels, based upon the voluntary muscles that move the joints. Patients with *thoracic* level function have no function in voluntary muscles crossing the hip joint.

Patients with *high lumbar level* function have hip flexors and/or hip adductors and/or knee extensors. Patients with *low lumbar* level function have functioning voluntary muscles that flex the knee, dorsiflex the ankle, and/or abduct the hip, while those with *sacral level* function have gluteus maximus and/or ankle and foot plantar flexors.

The majority of thoracic level patients function only in wheelchairs. The upper lumbar level patients, for the most part, required a KAFO and HKAFO in early childhood and are usually wheelchair-dependent by adolescence and adulthood. Low lumbar level patients usually ambulate with an AFO and the majority are community ambulators in adulthood. Sacral level patients are usually community ambulators with or without orthotic management. Orthoses are important to position and protect the foot and alleviate long-term complications.[8]

Ambulation categories as defined by Hoffer et al.[40] are as follows:

1. *The community ambulator.* These patients walk indoors and outdoors for most of their activities and

may need crutches, braces, or both. They use wheelchairs only for long trips out of the community or for greater speed of ambulation.

2. *The household ambulator.* These patients walk only indoors and with apparatus. They are able to get in and out of the chair and bed with little or no assistance. They may use wheelchairs for some indoor activities at home and school and for all activities in the community.

3. *Nonfunctional ambulators.* Walking for these patients is a therapy session at home, school, or the hospital. Afterward, they use their wheelchairs to get from place to place and satisfy all their needs for transportation.

4. *Nonambulators.* These patients are wheelchair-bound but can usually transfer from chair to bed.

Treatment

The goal of treatment is maximal habilitation (Table 34-1). Patients are best treated by the team approach. The therapeutic team should be made up of various physician specialists—including neurosurgeon, urologist, pediatrician, and orthopedist—as well as a physical therapist, orthotist, occupational therapist, psychologist, social worker, and nurse practitioner. Accurate documentation is essential to detect changes secondary to progressive neurologic lesions.[44,67]

The orthopedic surgeon must be familiar with the abnormality involved. Starting from the prognosis made on the basis of neurosegmental level and other associated factors, realistic goals should be set, and surgical, orthotic, and physical therapy treatment should be planned accordingly. Any deviation from the planned achievements must be evaluated, bearing in mind the possibility of progressive complications occurring within the central nervous system. If such neurologic changes are not responsible, other causes must be sought and corrected if possible. Orthotic and physical therapy management should be related to helping the child achieve normal milestones of development. Surgical planning, on the other hand, should be related to anticipated adult needs and designed to facilitate orthotic management.

Treatment is tempered by the maturational needs of the infant and child. Close bonding is necessary for infant security. Children must have the ability to explore, handle, and manipulate objects as well as devices. Trial-and-error experience is self-motivating. Progressive upright experience is necessary. In early childhood, standing and attempts to walk may be gratifying to the child as well as the parents. For older children, life becomes a more painful experience. The children find themselves being left behind by more agile playmates, unable to participate in many activities because their hands are occupied with crutches or a walker and unable to expend the energy required in rapid transport from one classroom to another during the junior high and high school years. In addition, short lower extremities result in short stature. During these years, the wheelchair becomes far more socially acceptable and useful for the patients with thoracic and high lumbar levels of function.

Orthotic Treatment

The basic principle of orthotic treatment is the use of lightweight devices to supply stability to those joints that cannot be adequately controlled otherwise. In later childhood, appearance becomes a more important factor. Improvement of mobility is paramount. Devices such as the caster cart should be provided when needed to aid in crawling or other forms of exploration close to the floor.[15]

When a child is ready to stand but requires full support (thoracic- or upper lumber level patients), a standing orthosis should be utilized.[18] Generally, such a child is between 12 and 18 months of age. Standing devices should be simple and lightweight and allow for growth to age 2 years. Polypropylene-formed orthoses may be used to maintain correct foot positioning after surgery or cast correction even before the child's first attempts at standing or walking. A rigid AFO system may interfere with the child's ability to make the transition from lying to sitting and sitting to pulling to stand.

Orthotics for mobility should be provided when the child demonstrates a desire for ambulation or, in high-level lesions, after age 18 months. Trunk stabilization is required for thoracic level patients without pelvic control. Hip stabilization should be provided for those with adequate trunk control but no knee control (high lumbar level). The parapodium,[15,18] Shrewsbury brace,[76] reciprocating orthosis,[105] or standard HKAFO system can be used in these patients.

The parapodium provides a flat base that allows mobility by pivoting the body from side to side, thereby advancing the patient. Swing gait can be used. The Shrewsbury brace uses the same principle but is spring-loaded, so that shifting one's weight from side to side unloads one side and automatically shifts the brace forward. The reciprocating brace allows alternating hip motion. This device functions best with active hip flexors, although low thoracic level patients can utilize it as long as they are free of hip flexion contractures.

Improved balance associated with increasing age, practice, and strength allows for the use of KAFOs in high lumbar level patients. Low lumbar level patients require ankle stabilization but generally have adequate knee stabilizers. Polypropylene orthoses—vacuum-formed for close fit around the calf, ankle, and foot—provide stability, are lightweight, and are cosmetically desirable. Their disadvantage is that there is no accommodation for growth. Prior to age 3 years, a single upright metal brace with growth adjustments and a double-adjustable locked ankle joint may reduce the expense of replacing orthoses with growth.

Patients with borderline knee extension strength benefit from the posterior-entry type of orthosis (Glancy or floor-reaction brace).[49] Polypropylene AFOs are used in nonambulatory patients for foot and ankle positioning. Sacral-level patients may require shoe orthotics because of foot deformities.

The orthotic management of spinal deformities involves thoracolumbosacral orthoses. These should be low-profile systems that will not interfere with sitting activities and hip flexion. The orthoses can be modified for relief of pressure over a kyphotic deformity. This type of orthosis can also be modified to accommodate a vesicostomy, urostomy, and colostomy. The thoracolumbosacral orthosis can also be modified for suspension. A fitting can be placed on either side of this orthosis to actually suspend the orthosis in a wheelchair, feeding seat, and/or car seat, as appropriate. Orthotic management for scoliosis follows the usual principles; however, progressive scoliosis above the dysraphic spine should be fully evaluated for underlying spinal cord pathology, as previously discussed.

Because of impaired proprioception, articulated ankle joints are usually not indicated in patients with myelomeningocele. Rigid ankle orthoses, positioned in slight ankle plantar flexion, are useful. This type of patient usually has a short fibular that allows excessive ankle dorsiflexion with weight bearing, causing pronation at the foot, valgus at the ankle, and excessive hip and knee flexion posture during stance. Positioning the ankle in slight plantar flexion facilitates posterior movement at the tibia, with associated knee and hip extension. In the older patient with an established crouched gait pattern, an adjustable locked ankle hinge can be utilized to increase ankle plantar flexion very slowly, so that the patient can accommodate to this new knee position.

Surgical Treatment

Surgical treatment should be planned to coordinate with the child's other surgical specialty needs. Menelaus has summarized the principles of orthopedic surgery as follows[58,59]:

1. Surgery should be selected with regard to anticipated adult needs.
2. The least orthopedic surgery that will completely and permanently correct the deformities is required. A single surgical procedure is preferred to multiple partial procedures repeated over a long period of time.
3. As much surgery as possible is performed under a single session of anesthesia, with as little immobilization as possible. Early weight bearing should be carried out with the patient in plaster.
4. Muscle imbalance should be corrected in all circumstances.

Latex Allergy

Significant allergic reactions to latex-containing products have been reported in the medical literature over the last decade.[10,23,45,97] Latex is an organic substance obtained from the rubber tree (*Hevea brasiliensis*). Rubber is produced through a process of purification and heating (vulcanization). Latex products are ubiquitous, not only in the hospital setting but also in the household and community. Children are sensitized to latex during surgical procedures, and the incidence of latex reactions is directly related to the number of previous surgical procedures.[97] Although ventriculoperitoneal shunt material does not usually involve latex products directly, those children who have ventriculoperitoneal shunts with multiple shunt revisions are most at risk for developing latex sensitivity.[45]

There are two types of allergic reactions to latex-containing products. Contact dermatitis or T cell–mediated type IV hypersensitivity has been recognized among nurses and surgeons. This immunologic reaction is usually related to sensitizing chemicals that are added during the manufacturing process, such as mercaptodenzothiazole or tetramethylthiuram. Skin testing will rapidly determine hypersensitivity to these chemicals. There is also an IGE-mediated immediate type I hypersensitivity reaction, which is related to a protein or group of proteins existing as impurities after vulcanization. Clinical reactions include local contact urticaria, systemic urticaria, rhinoconjunctivitis, asthma, and anaphylaxis. Fatalities have been reported in the United States due to this type of reaction.[88,89] The prevalence of IGE-mediated latex allergy in the population is extremely low. The prevalence of latex allergies in children with myelomeningocele has been reported to be as high as 34 percent.[97] Evaluation of patients for IGE-mediated latex allergy can be done with epicutaneous or in vitro testing. Radioallergosorbent testing (RAST) is less sensitive than skin testing; unfortunately, children can convert reactivity at any time and remain at risk for latex allergy reactions during surgical procedures. Latex precautions should be utilized during surgical procedures involving patients with myelomeningocele.[97] A latex-free environment should decrease the rate of conversion among these patients. The high-risk group who either have a history of previous latex allergies or positive tests should have prophylactic premedication with H_1 and H_2 antihistamines and parenteral steroids; maintenance of airway and ventilatory support is as important as with any other anaphylactic reaction.[23]

REGIONAL CONSIDERATIONS

Pelvic Obliquity

Obliquity of the pelvis—caused primarily by scoliosis and also by hip contractures—is a seriously disabling problem for the myelodysplastic patient. Pelvic obliquity makes it difficult for the patient to sit by creating poor balance and predisposing to the development of pressure sores on the lower ischial prominence. The walking patient exhibits leg-length inequality, and dislocation of the hips on the elevated side may occur.

When there is a fixed abduction contracture caused by a tight iliotibial band, the pelvis becomes tilted when the legs are brought together parallel with the body axis. Since the patient cannot ambulate with one leg fully abducted and also tends to lie supine with the legs parallel, the tilted pelvis is the position routinely adopted. The pelvic tilt causes the contralateral hip to adopt an increasingly adducted position. If there is a fixed adduction contracture, there is elevation of the affected side of the pelvis and the contralateral hip takes up an abducted position. Only when the pelvis is leveled by placing the two anterior superior iliac spines in the horizontal plane is the appropriate hip deformity revealed.

Correction of the hip contractures brings about correction of the pelvic obliquity. If the contractures are left long enough, fixed secondary contracture develops in the lumbar spine.[42]

If the pelvic obliquity is caused by scoliosis, rotation of the pelvis occurs in conformity with the lumbar curve. Pelvic obliquity in this situation is fixed and unaffected by the position of the legs. The hip joint on the elevated side of the pelvis adopts a secondary position of adduction. If there is associated weakness of the adductor musculature in the same hip and the obliquity occurs early enough in childhood, hip dislocation will occur.

Methods of evaluating pelvic obliquity have not been well defined. Lindseth described a method of relating the transverse axis of the pelvis to the end plate of the uppermost vertebra of the lumbar curve.[48] We have not found this entirely satisfactory and, instead, use a measurement on the complete spine x-ray film that includes the pelvis. The "weight-bearing line of the spine" is estimated to be from the midpoint of the T1 vertebra to the midpoint of S2. Patients in the sitting position tend to bring this line into a vertical position, thereby creating a functional type of pelvic obliquity (Fig. 34-1). Sitting x-ray views show a similar result, but accurate balance is difficult for these patients to maintain. Many times, patients need their arms for balance and are, therefore, constantly changing the overall weight-bearing line. A good transverse pelvic axis is also difficult to obtain on a sitting film, since the pelvis is frequently obscured. The transverse axis of the pelvis is determined by a line connecting two comparable landmarks on each side. The angle this line makes with the vertical weight-bearing line measures the degree of pelvic obliquity.

Treatment of pelvic obliquity associated with spinal deformity is by the use of a body jacket (TLSO) to reduce progression. A polyurethane cushion with appropriate cutouts has been most successful in reducing the incidence of pressure sores.

When it is clear that the spinal deformity is becoming fixed, spinal fusion is indicated in order to obtain a balanced spine and eliminate pelvic obliquity. If the obliquity remains after spinal fusion, additional surgery may be required. Osteotomy of the spine, which some authors recommend, has a high complication rate, and correction is often inadequate.[34,66] Lindseth recommends the bilateral posterior osteotomy, where there is fixed pelvic obliquity due to uncorrectable lumbosacral scoliosis. A wedge of bone is removed from the posterior ilium on the low side of the obliquity and inserted on the opposite side to maintain the correction (Fig. 34-2).[48] A 41 percent correction of pelvic obliquity and 49 percent correction of trunk list from the midline has been reported, with an acceptable complication rate.[48] Indications for surgery are the occurrence of frequent pressure sores and demonstrate imbalance during sitting, requiring at least one hand to stabilize the individual in the upright position and prevent falling over.

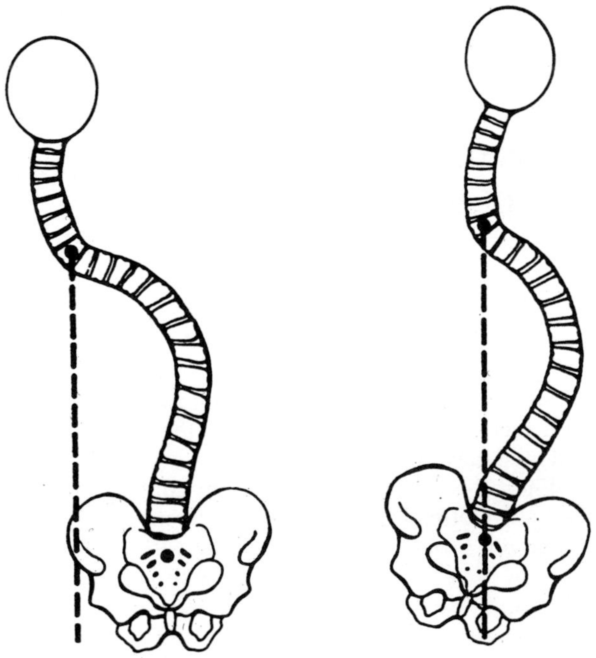

The Hip

Contractures

All patients who have muscle imbalance tend to develop contractures unless these complications have been prevented by appropriate stretching or muscle release.

Release of contractures about the hip is necessary for successful ambulation. In nonambulatory patients, hip flexion contractures are of little concern, but unilateral abduction or adduction contractures that will create pelvic obliquity are important. Both a level pelvis and hip flexion beyond 90° are necessary for appropriate sitting.

Patients with external rotation contractures are treated by extensive posterior release, dividing the short lateral rotators and the posterior hip capsule.[59,60]

Abduction contractures may result iatrogenically from prolonged abduction splinting or postsurgical contractures. If they are the result of a tight iliotibial band, an Ober-Yount procedure provides adequate release. In those older patients who have intraarticular or pericapsular scarring, osteotomy of the proximal femur is appropriate.[99] Similarly, in patients with flexion contracture of greater than 30°, it is necessary either to release all flexion contractures or to perform an extension osteotomy. Patients who are confined to wheelchairs are usually not appropriate candidates for the release of flexion contractures unless the contracture is severe (greater than 50°), as the contractures will readily recur. Pure rotational deformities occurring about the hip in older patients may best be treated by osteotomies, either proximally or distally on the femur.

Figure 34-1 Sitting balance and pelvic obliquity. *Left:* Schematic depiction of person with severe scoliosis placing the pelvis level on a surface. The weight-bearing line would be far to the right, and the person would fall or be required to push with the right arm in order to keep from falling over to the right. *Right:* How the same person would sit by directing the weight-bearing line centrally over the S2 area. Balance would be maintained on one ischium. Unless a sitting x-ray was taken or the entire spine was x-rayed with the pelvis, functional pelvic obliquity would be difficult to determine.

Figure 34-2 Posterior iliac osteotomy for fixed pelvic obliquity. *Left:* After bilateral osteotomy and removal of the wedge of predetermined size from the low side of the obliquity, the pelvis is rotated from the sacrum in the frontal plane by pulling down on the limb on the high side and pushing up on the limb on the low side. This maneuver closes one osteotomy site, where the bone was removed, and opens the one on the opposite side to receive the bone graft. *Right:* The transferred iliac wedge is fixed with two Kirshner wires. While the closed wedge osteotomy is held with nonabsorbable sutures through drill holes, enough of the upward projecting iliac wing is removed to permit two halves of the previously split iliac epiphysis to be approximated back to the top of the iliac wing during closure. (Reproduced with permission from Lindseth RR: Posterior iliac osteotomy. *J Bone Joint Surg* 60A:17, 1978.)

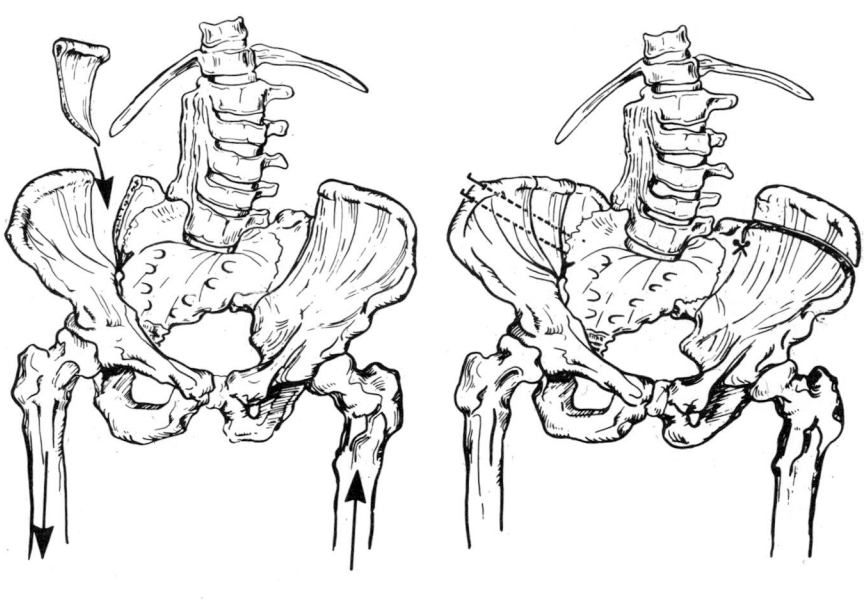

Hip Dysplasia

Hip dysplasia occurs as a result of imbalance of muscle forces in which the flexors and adductors are strong and the abductors and extensors are weak or absent. The result may be a hip at risk for dislocation or one that is already dislocated at birth. The strength of the abductor muscles is the most important factor. Evaluation of patients with poliomyelitis has demonstrated that dislocation does not occur if the abductor muscle power is of better than poor grade.[64] If the opposite hip is in relative abduction, there is an increasing tendency for the adducted hip to dislocate. If other factors are present that tend to place the hip at risk in an adducted position, the individual with no hip muscle imbalance but with a paralyzed (flail) hip joint develops dislocation gradually over a period of time. In a patient with a low lumbar level myelodysplasia, the problem may be a slow subluxation without frank dislocation. The importance of pelvic obliquity due to uncorrected lumbar scoliosis or hip contractures has already been discussed. If such obliquity is present, the adducted upper hip is at particular risk, especially if there is associated acetabular dysplasia and the abductors are weak. To emphasize the role of the adducted position in promoting instability in these circumstances, Somerville stated that "the nearer the angle between the neck of the femur and the horizontal of the pelvis approaches 90°, the more unstable the hip will become" (Fig. 34-3).[91]

In the newborn, the iliopsoas muscle produces a flexed and internal position of the limb.[55] Its contracture is believed to be the predominant cause of the flexion contracture that may be seen in the hip accompanied by a midlumbar myelomeningocele.[7] Under these circumstances, it exerts a bolstering effect the on femoral head, displacing it posteriorly and laterally. The deformity force increases with attempts to relieve the hip flexion contracture by passive hip extension. Breed and Healey point out that, under

these circumstances, it often grooves the femoral head and produces dysplasia of the posterior acetabulum.[7]

The increased valgus of the femoral neck is believed to be due to alteration of bone shape secondary to iliopsoas predominance during the intrauterine and postnatal growth period.[9] In the newborn child, the neck shaft angle at birth approximates 160° ordinarily, diminishing to 120° in adolescence. In the child with myelomeningocele, the valgus may increase. Other factors involved include a lack of stimulation to the activity of the lateral aspect of the growth plate and trochanteric apophysis associated with weak or absent abductor muscles. In addition, lack of weight bearing in the early years may selectively inhibit physeal growth.

The inequality of muscle action may promote torsional deformities. This was shown on the calcified femurs by

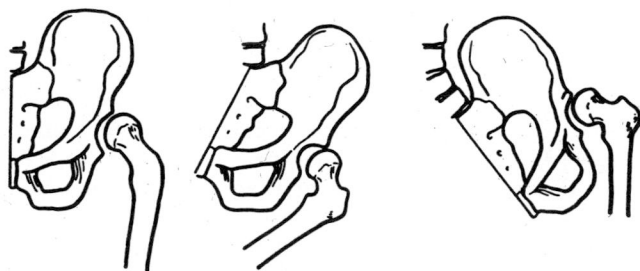

Figure 34-3 Relation between hip stability and femoral neck shaft angle, hip deformity, and pelvic obliquity. *Left:* The neck is in valgus, and the weight-bearing pressures are on the outer aspect of the acetabulum. *Center:* The neck is in normal or even varus position, but the adduction contracture places the weight-bearing pressure on the outer aspect of the acetabulum. *Right:* The femoral angle is normal; however, because of pelvic obliquity, the weight-bearing pressure is again on the outer aspect of the acetabulum.

Brookes and Wardle.[9] They observed that imbalance in flexor over extensor force tends to increase anteversion. The role of the iliopsoas muscle may be more important in the etiology of valgus deformity in the patient with a high lumbar level meningomyelocele (L2 to L3 range) where the adductors are still quite weak but the iliopsoas is at full strength. The presence of a valgus femoral neck with increased anteversion in a joint maintained in an adducted position promotes anterior and lateral acetabular dysplasia, since those portions of the femoral head tend to remain uncovered. The final consequence is hip instability.

Surgical Indications

The ability to walk is more dependent on the neurologic level than upon hip reduction.[31,40] Contractures of the knees, spine, and hips are more important than the reduction status of the hip.

Unilateral dislocations in patients with low lumbar or sacral level deficits should be treated. However, if the muscular deficit is symmetrical, bilateral transfers should be performed, as the opposite hip will undoubtedly sublux and subsequently dislocate. Bilateral subluxations in these patients should also be treated. High bilateral dislocations are best left alone.

Treatment

Treatment of hip dysplasia requires that concentric reduction be obtained and maintained and that the muscle forces be balanced. Various muscle-balancing procedures have been described. Because of the risk that may accompany surgery in a neonate, many authors believe that even if a patient is identified as an appropriate candidate for hip stabilization, no treatment should be carried out until the child is between 12 and 20 months of age. To promote good acetabular development, McKibbin recommends abduction extension splinting of the hip in infants up to 24 months of age who have functional muscles crossing the hip joint.[55] Raycroft also recommends early reduction of the hip by performing adductor and possibly also iliopsoas release and then splinting in a similar position until definitive lateral muscle transfers can be performed at a later date.[76] He describes better long-term hip stability with prompt rather than delayed treatment.

Breed and Healey point out that by 1 year of age, virtually all of the hips of the lumbar level patients are unstable, either with subluxation or dislocation.[7] They recommend the early performance of iliopsoas recession, believing that this procedure is better than splintage alone and must be done early, consistent with their view of the importance of the iliopsoas tendon in maintaining and promoting hip stability and reducing acetabular dysplasia.[7]

Because the Pavlik harness requires active muscle contraction and balance muscle forces, it is not recommended for the child with a myelodysplasia.

As a step toward balancing adductor-abductor forces, it has been recommended that the origins of the adductor longus, brevis, and gracilis be detached from the pelvis and then transferred posteriorly to the ischial tuberosity. In some cases, this procedure is combined with a lateral transfer of the iliopsoas from the lesser to the greater trochanter when the abductors have been severely weakened.[50,64] Any transfer to increased abductor muscle force works only if there is a satisfactory fulcrum—that is, a stable concentric hip joint. Any instability significantly affects the success of such a transfer.

Mustard[63] reported transferring the iliopsoas through a notch in the anterior portion of the ilium to the greater trochanter in paralytic poliomyelitis; Sharrard and Grosfeld[84] then modified the operation by transferring the muscle posteriorly through a foramen made in the ilium. This modification was designed to make up for the lack of extensor muscles as well as the abductor muscles in myelomeningocele and was reported to provide improved extensor strength and a more upright posture in addition to benefiting abduction. Electromyographic studies do not support this contention, and the iliopsoas continues to function with the flexor musculature.[11]

There is a definite place for posterolateral iliopsoas transfer to the greater trochanter in the myelodysplastic patient. In addition to providing lateral muscle power, there is a diminution of the force producing valgus of the femoral neck.[9] There also seems to be improved hip extension from better hamstring function.[7] Patient selection is critical if good results are to be achieved. Jackson et al. noted that factors predisposing to failure are the presence of a dysplastic acetabulum (acetabular index more than 30°), prior hip surgery, limb-length inequality, and a patient over 5 years of age.[43] The presence of strong secondary hip flexors (rectus femoris and sartorius) is critical; otherwise, the patient may lose vital hip flexor function.[92] With good selection and if surgery is performed early, excellent results have been reported.[46,68,69]

The external oblique is a muscle that does not have the bulk of the iliopsoas, but does have a more advantageous position of origin, being further lateral on the trunk and extending straight down to the greater trochanter after transfer.[38] Its transfer may reduce body sway or Trendelenburg lurch during ambulation, but it will not completely eliminate it.[38] This transfer also spares the iliopsoas and allows its use as a flexor. This should not interfere with limb advancement. As discussed, sectioning of the psoas may be an advantage or disadvantage, depending on the individual patient. The external oblique transfer is performed by developing a flap a few centimeters wide, parallel with the fibers of the aponeurosis in the groin. The distal end of the flap is then divided in the region of the pubic tubercle, tubed, and passed subcutaneously to be inserted into the greater trochanter. This operation was first described by Thomas, Thompson, and Straub.[96]

The muscle flap must be dissected proximally to the inferior ribs, so that there is a long enough muscle substance for transfer. Lindseth has recommended also transferring the tensor muscle laterally to help augment abduction strength (Fig. 34-4).[75] The use of both the external oblique and adductor posterior transfer to augment a varus osteotomy is recommended.

Varus Osteotomy

If the child is over 12 months of age and has significant valgus deformity, varus osteotomy should be performed to stabilize the hips. The procedure gives additional cover-

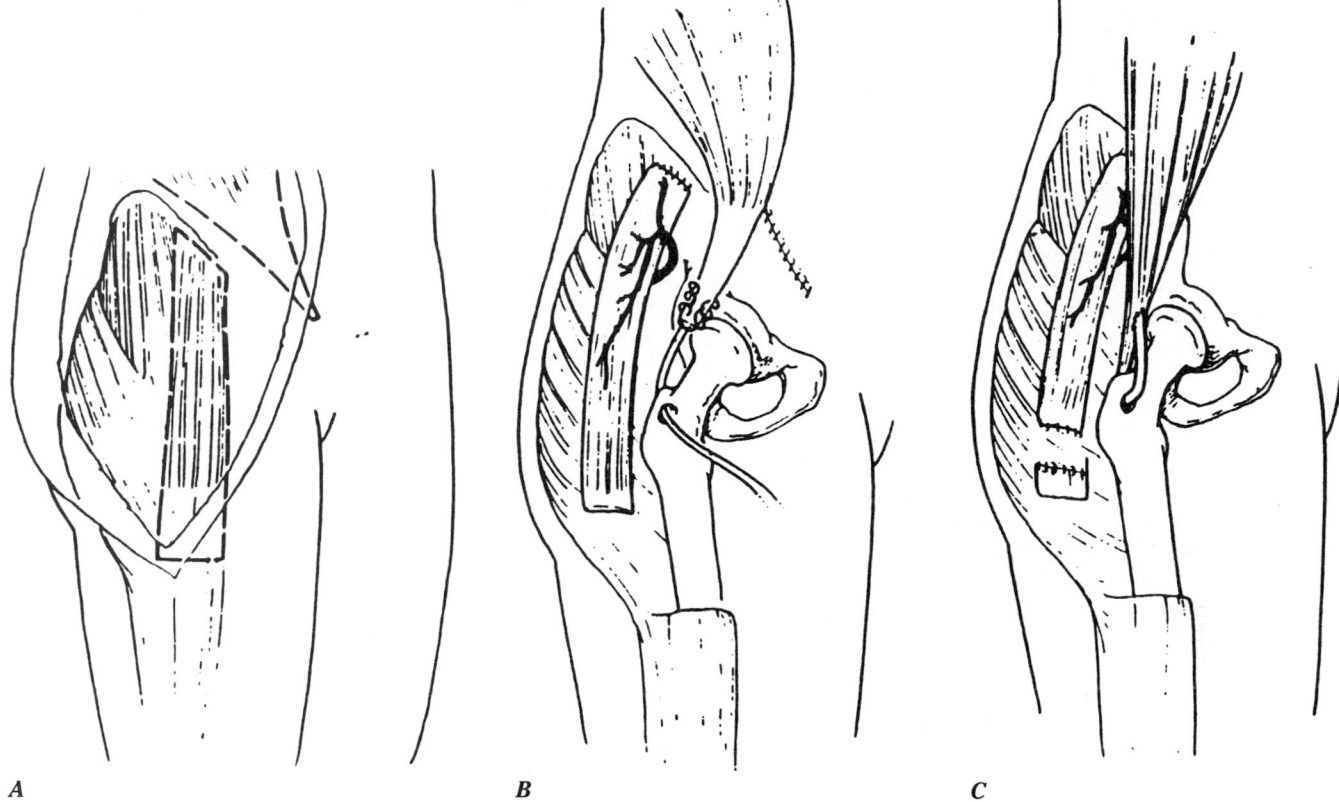

A   *B*   *C*

Figure 34-4 Transfer of external oblique and tensor fascia lata muscles to restore abductor strength. *A*. Skin flaps are elevated to expose the fascia of the leg and the external oblique muscle. *B*. Cut edges of the external oblique muscle and the aponeurosis are folded over and sutured together. The defect in the aponeurosis is sutured closed. The origin of the tensor fascia on the ilium is detached, with care taken to preserve the neurovascular bundle. The remainder of the muscle is prepared for transfer. *C*. The tendon of the external oblique is transferred to the greater trochanter from posterior to anterior, making sure that the muscle reaches the trochanter and that the muscle follows a straight line from the rib cage to the trochanter. The distal end of the tensor fascia lata is woven through the tendon of the gluteus maximus. (Reproduced with permission from Phillips DP, Lindseth RE: Ambulation after transfer of adductors, external oblique and tensor fascia lata in myelomeningocele. *J Pediatr Orthop* 12:712–717, 1992.)

age to the femoral head and may be combined with muscle balancing procedures to augment hip abduction and extension, as discussed above. A closing wedge osteotomy is the most stable.[29] Small anterior plate fixation provides optimal stability of the osteotomy. Spica cast immobilization is used postoperatively. Such immobilization should be limited to 6 weeks postoperatively to help avoid pathologic fractures. Prevention of pathologic fractures is discussed below.

Acetabuloplasty

Acetabular procedures are performed when the acetabulum is deficient in patients over the age of 2 years. The Salter osteotomy is not recommended, as the posterior aspect of the acetabulum may become defective, leading to posterior dislocation.[80] In such cases, more posterior coverage may be obtained by the double osteotomy of Southerland or the triple osteotomy of Steel. Posterior shelf operations, such as the Pemberton, have been performed.[71] This osteotomy has been effective in decreasing the volume of an enlarged acetabulum and brings normal carti-lage over the femoral head. Capsulorrhaphy may be an additional procedure performed with acetabuloplasty.

Good results in stabilizing the hip have been reported with the Chiari osteotomy.[14] Other authors, however, report poor results when Chiari procedures have been combined with iliopsoas transfers.[43] Poor results occur when the iliopsoas transfer acts as a tenodesis, tending to displace the femoral head out of the acetabulum.

Combined Procedures

A combination of procedures to eliminate muscle imbalance and correct skeletal dysplasia is logical. Sharrard used such a combination of procedures and notes that some of his failures were the result of failure to either balance muscles appropriately or obtain good congruent relations between the femoral head and the acetabulum at the time of transfer.[16] Both Carroll and Menelaus strongly recommend capsulorrhaphy for the lax capsule after reduction.[46,60]

Other investigators have also recommended various combinations of bone and muscle procedures for stabilization.[12,50,54,75] Increasing varus of the femur to a neck shaft angle of 100 to 110° is optimal for hip stability in the case of spina bifida.

Complications of Surgical Reduction of the Hips

All the usual surgical complications occur and are to be considered, such as complications of anesthesia, neurologic or vascular complications, and infection. Failure to stabilize the hip can follow even if all of the appropriate measures have been taken.[9,16,43,68] Additionally, postoperative stiffness or contracture with intra- and extraarticular fibrosis can occur.[16,31] Heterotopic bone formation[16,68] or fracture[25,31,68] can compromise the result. Dislocation of the opposite hip may also occur secondary to the treatment of the affected side, and one should be aware of this possibility. Progressive spinal cord pathology—such as hydromyelia, recurrent tethering with Arnold-Chiari malformation, or diastematomyelia—may lead to late dislocation of the previously operative hip.

Fractures following immobilization after hip surgery are a common occurrence in the child with spina bifida. Even if spica cast immobilization can be limited to 6 weeks and weight bearing can be initiated while the patient is in the spica cast, fractures occur frequently. In this author's series, the fracture frequency was 33 percent.[79] Children with spina bifida may have some degree of osteomalacia in addition to disuse osteoporosis. This may account for the increased fracture frequency. The postoperative regimen should include the use of hydroxylated vitamin D (1,25-dihydroxycholecalciferol) in a daily dose of 0.25 μg augmented with calcium supplementation of 400 to 800 mg, depending on the size of the child. This calcium and vitamin D supplementation is continued during spica cast immobilization. With the use of this regimen, subsequent pathologic fractures have been eliminated.[79]

Knee Deformities and Rotational Deformities of the Lower Extremities

Isolating the knee deformities in the patient with myelomeningocele is difficult, as deformities about the hips and ankles influence the knees. Also, any deformity about the knee can accentuate other deformities in the lower extremities.

These deformities may be conveniently discussed as flexion contractures, extension contractures, and varus and valgus deformities. They are directly related to the anatomic level of the patient's lesion and can often be predicted after the neurologic examination. Rotational deformities in the lower extremities are discussed separately. Many knee contractures are secondary to postural contractures and not muscle imbalance. These problems are difficult to deal with and also produce significant functional limitations.

Orthotics

The role of orthotics in the management of knee deformities is straightforward. When there is quadriceps weakness, the orthosis must provide extension support for the knee during weight-bearing activities. Such support can be provided without having the orthosis cross the knee. The ground reaction type of orthosis with the ankle in slight plantar flexion produces a posterior moment on the tibia and is an adjunct for knee extension during stance. In the patient with flexion contractures, orthotics can be used as an adjunct for guided gradual extension of the knee, using an adjustable locked ankle hinge. Care to prevent posterior subluxation of the tibia is essential. Varus and valgus deformities of small degrees can be maintained with double upright metal knee hinges. For rotational problems of the hip joint, twister cables are used to maintain the neutral position in gait. They have limited use with bony deformity to enhance gait while the patient is awaiting surgical correction. In the child under age 3, the use of a twister cable system is appropriate during the time there is spontaneous correction of physiologic tibial torsion. We use lightweight cables attached to a pelvic band and polypropylene AFO or heavier cables attached to KAFO system.

Knee Deformities

Flail knees are present in the patient with myelomeningocele at the thoracic level. These patients are usually not ambulatory; therefore the flail knee is not a clinical problem. These knees can be managed with simple orthoses for positioning. The flail knee frequently develops contractures because of its prolonged or repeated flexion position during full wheelchair usage.[21] When any quadriceps activity is present, extension contractures often result. The management of specific contractures is dealt with in the subsequent section.

Flexion Contractures Flexion contractures about the knee in the patient with spina bifida can be due to intrauterine positioning, positional contractures in the older child, muscle imbalance, and muscle paralysis. Flexion contractures present at birth are secondary intrauterine positioning and often not related to muscle imbalance. With the help of an appropriate exercise program, these contractures demonstrate spontaneous correction within the first 6 months of life. Positional knee flexion contractures are usually secondary to hip flexion contractures, with resultant external rotation of the extremity. These patients are often supine for long periods of time. The hips are flexed and abducted. The lower extremity is subsequently rotated externally and the knees are flexed.

Knee flexion contractures due to muscle imbalance are usually due to increased spasticity from hamstring tone. Hamstring spasticity can be seen in patients with upper or lower lumbar myelomeningocele. Contractures about the knees greater than 15° significantly increase the work load of a possibly weakened quadriceps, and this may lead to progressive contracture.[73]

Treatment of knee flexion contractures is based upon the degree of contracture and the functional level of the patient. In nonambulatory patients who do not bear weight for transfers, knee flexion contractures are rarely a problem. For ambulatory patients with knee flexion contractures of less than 20°, physiotherapy programs for stretching and orthotic management are appropriate.[1,87] In the ambulatory patient with knee flexion contractures above 20°, surgical management is indicated. Depending on the degree of contracture, surgical management commences with specific tendon lengthening. If this does not bring the knee out to less than 20°, posteriorly capsulotomy, carefully protecting the neurovascular structures, is the next step (Fig. 34-5).

With flexion contractures that are not amenable to tendon lengthening of posterior capsulotomy, a distal femoral extension osteotomy should be considered.[81] Osteotomy in the presence of persistent muscle imbalance should not be performed; however, remodeling is rapid and recurrence of the flexion deformity is frequent.[1] Long-term orthotic management postoperatively is indicated. Hamstring transfer to the patellar tendon has been suggested by Abraham et al.,[1] but we have no experience with this procedure in our spina bifida population. These authors also state that surgical management of knee flexion contractures exceeding 30° must precede surgical management of hip flexion contractures.[1] They add that significant mental retardation (IQs of less than 65) combined with arm weakness contraindicate operative management of knee flexion contractures.[1]

Extension Contractures Extension contracture of the knee is frequently associated with ipsolateral hip dislocation. These dislocations are often teratologic, the affected children are born with extension contractures of the knee. Patients with knee extension contractures often have external rotation deformities at the hip, internal tibial torsional deformities of the legs, and talipes equinovarus de-

formities of the hindfoot. The hip dislocation is not reducible until the knee extension contracture is treated. The cause of knee extension contractures is muscle imbalance. This is usually seen in the patient with high lumbar lesions. Unopposed quadriceps activity is present. This leads to quadriceps contracture and resultant fibrosis. Often there is a lateral dislocation of the patella. With progressive extension contracture, knee recurvatum is present. Often this is followed by anterior subluxation of the hamstrings. These abnormal positions of the knee lead to internal derangement of the knee.[81]

Treatment of knee extension contractures has received attention in the literature.[2,21] Attempts at nonoperative management of extension contractures are appropriate prior to any surgical intervention. In the ambulatory patient, knee extension contractures are often helpful in decreasing the amount of orthotic assistance the patient needs for weight-bearing activities. In the nonambulatory patient, extension contractures pose a problem in wheelchair activities. During sitting, the leg is exposed to gravitational forces, and this often helps in the treatment of the contracture. Vigorous physiotherapy should be initiated early on and may obviate the need for surgical management. In the nonambulatory patient with residual extension contracture, simple surgical release of the quadriceps through a transverse incision is appropriate.[2] In the patient with some quadriceps activity, quadriceps function can be maintained with some type of quadricepsplasty (Fig. 34-6).[2,21] Prolonged postoperative splinting is recommended to prevent recurrent extension contracture.[21] We have had little experience with elaborate quadriceps release in our spina bifida population.

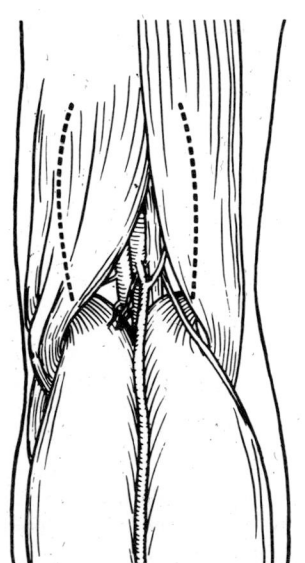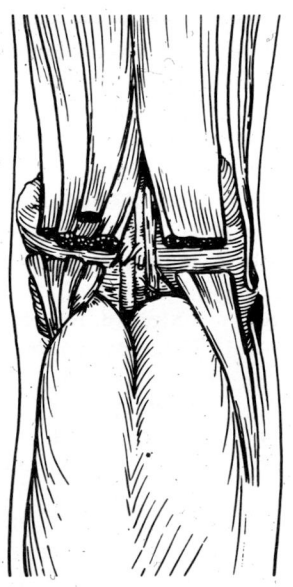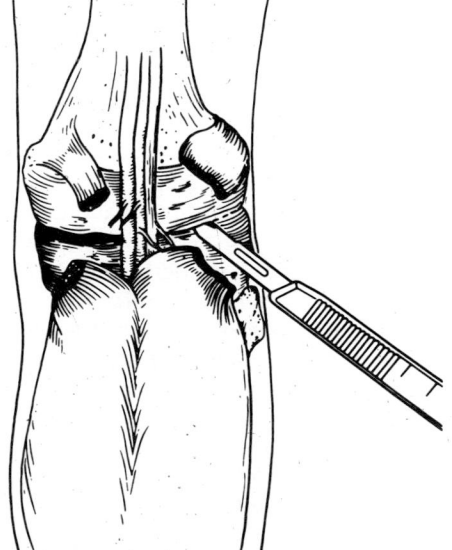

Figure 34-5 Posterior release of knee contracture in myelomeningocele. *Left:* Medial and lateral longitudinal incisions. *Center:* All flexor tendons have been divided and part of the tendons excised. *Right:* The gastrocnemius has been elevated from the femoral condyles. An extensive posterior cap-

sulectomy has been done. The posterior cruciate, medial, and lateral collateral ligaments may be divided when full extension is not obtained after the capsulectomy. (Reproduced with permission from Dias LS: Surgical management of the knee contractures in myelomeningocele. *J Pediatr Orthop* 2:129, 1982.)

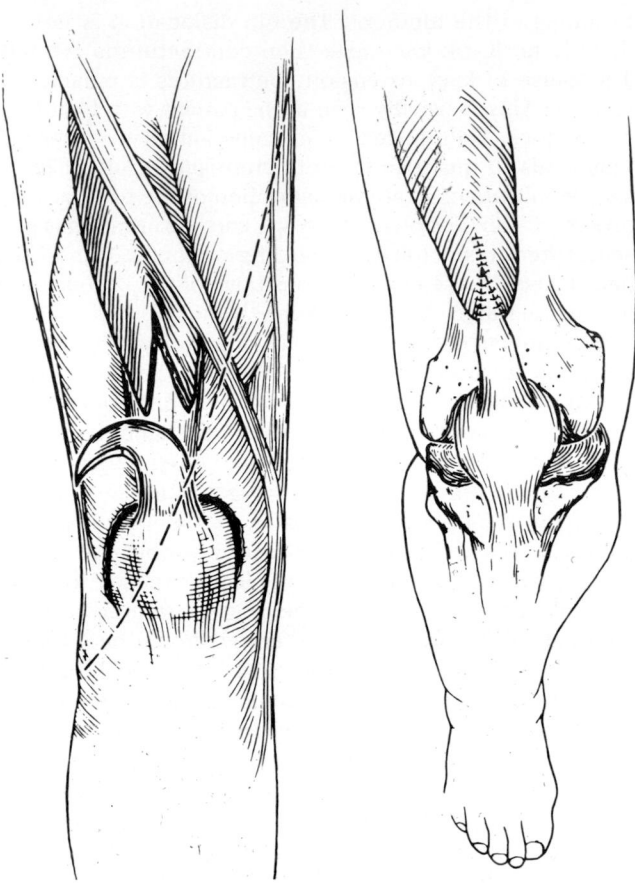

Figure 34-6 V-Y lengthening of the quadriceps mechanism for knee extension contracture in myelomeningocele. *Left:* Medial and lateral release of the knee capsule is performed proximally. *Right:* The quadriceps is sutured with the knee in 45° of flexion. (Reproduced with permission from Dias LS: Surgical management of the knee contractures in myelomeningocele. *J Pediatr Orthop* 2:130, 1982.)

Angular Deformities about the Knee

Varus and valgus deformities about the knee are common in the myelomeningocele patient. The valgus deformity is usually secondary to an iliotibial band contracture.[81] The valgus deformity can also be seen in the rare patient with isolated biceps femoris spasticity. This is commonly seen in association with external tibial torsion and ankle valgus deformities. Valgus deformity about the knee is also common, secondary to malunited fractures of the supracondylar femur. Another group of spina bifida patients who develop progressive valgus deformity of the knee are those ambulatory patients with weak quadriceps who have been bearing weight with no orthotic protection about the knee. These patients often rotate the lower extremity externally and present the medial aspect of the knee forward, allowing the medial collateral ligament to act as the knee stabilizer. With time, this leads to instability of the medial collateral ligament and secondary valgus deformity.

Varus deformities about the knee are less common than other knee deformities. Varus deformity is usually secondary to malunited fractures of the supracondylar femur. The patient with poor quadriceps strength who is ambulating with no orthotic protection may also collapse into a varus knee deformity.

Management of angular deformities about the knee is usually nonsurgical. Appropriate orthotic management, as previously discussed, provides knee stability and prevents future deformity. In the patient with an iliotibial band contracture, a Yount procedure is appropriate and usually successful.[81] Osteotomies about the knee are also successful in correcting the angular deformities. Meticulous preoperative planning is essential for satisfactory results. Care must be taken to protect the distal femoral and proximal tibial epiphyseal plates in the skeletally immature patient.

Angular deformities following fracture about the knee have been addressed above. Residual knee stiffness with limitation of motion is common following fracture about the knee. The limitation of motion is usually established by 6 months after the fracture, and Drabu and Walker found that the majority of contractures secondary to fractures resolve by 3 years after the fracture. These patients usually do not need surgery to regain range of motion.[24] We commonly take advantage of a fracture about the knee to correct any preexisting deformity by manipulation and immobilization.

Torsional Deformities in the Lower Extremities

Torsional deformities in the lower extremities are often difficult to evaluate in view of the multiple deformities present. It is very important to evaluate the patient fully clinically. The foot progression angle should be observed. Orthotic systems may be malaligned because of torsional deformity. The entire mechanical axis of the extremity must be evaluated to check the relation of hip to knee to ankle in a weight-bearing position. The rotational profile of the lower extremity can also be assessed with the patient in a prone position. Internal rotation at the hips with the hips extended gives an indication of femoral torsional deformities. The thigh-foot and intermalleolar axes provide information regarding tibial torsional deformities. Residual talipes equinovarus deformity often masquerades as tibial rotational abnormalities and must be excluded radiographically.

External Torsional Deformities External rotation of the lower extremity may be secondary to femoral or tibial abnormality. Femoral torsional deformities are most commonly postural in the patient with thoracic-level function. Muscle imbalance can be responsible for the production of torsional deformities about the femur. This is most commonly due to contracture of the iliotibial band. Femoral retroversion is also common in these patients. External rotation of the femur is often associated with ankle and foot deformities. These are most commonly calcaneus, calcaneovalgus, calcaneovarus, and abductovarus deformities of the foot.

Treatment of external femoral rotation can be managed temporarily with twister cable. Operative management involves primarily bone, but occasionally soft tissue surgical procedures are required. These have not been successful in our hands. Femoral osteotomy is successful in treatment of femoral torsional deformities. Distal supracondylar femoral osteotomies are preferred.[41] Proximal derotational osteotomies are reserved for those patients who need simultaneous angular osteotomies of the hip.

External rotational deformities about the tibia are also usually secondary to iliotibial band contractures. These patients often have shortening of the fibula.[52] This leads to ankle valgus and external tibial torsion. Commonly, medial malleolar pressure sores are seen in these patients secondary to the use of orthotics. Management for external tibial torsion is with orthotically tempered twister cables. Patients with residual external tibial torsion require tibial osteotomy. My preference has been a proximal oblique tibial osteotomy. Meticulous care to protect neurovascular structures and provide fasciotomies at the time of surgery lessens the potential neurovascular complications. Distal tibial osteotomies often have delayed or nonunion, with recurrent deformity. Distal tibial osteotomy is preferable when angular osteotomy for ankle abnormality is required.

Internal Torsional Deformities Internal torsional deformities about the femur are usually due to excessive femoral anteversion. These are frequently associated with hip dislocation and hip adductor spasticity. These patients often have associated talipes varus, equinovarus, equinus, and cavovarus deformities.[60]

Internal torsional deformities about the tibia are usually secondary to muscle imbalance, with spasticity of the medial hamstrings. They can also occur secondary to muscle imbalance at the ankle, associated with activity of the tibialis posterior muscle. Physiologic internal tibial torsion may also play a role in the younger child.

Internal torsional deformities in the lower extremities can be treated with orthotic management. Twister cables have been successful in the young patient who is beginning to ambulate.

In the older child, surgical management is indicated. We prefer distal femoral and proximal tibial osteotomies unless otherwise indicated.[41] Menelaus has described lateral hamstring transfers.[60] Dias was successful in performing distal tibial osteotomies with transfers of the semitendinosus to the biceps tendon.[22]

In the patients with asymmetrical neurologic levels, "windswept" deformities are common. These deformities must be dealt with individually and obviously pose a considerable management challenge.

Prevention of Neuropathic Knee Deformities in the Adult Patients with Spina Bifida

The degenerative neuropathic knee deformity in adult patients with spina bifida is the single most significant physical impairment that interferes with the ability to maintain ambulatory status. A chronic crouched gait pattern causes weight bearing across a flexed knee and increases the joint reaction forces. Thus, abnormal knee mechanics leads to premature degenerative arthritis and neuropathic knee deformity. The etiologic factors resulting in crouched gait are anatomic (structural), neurologic (paralytic), and due to spinal cord pathology (fluctuating).

The anatomic or structural factors resulting in crouched gait are hip flexion contractures, knee flexion contractures, the short fibula, ankle calcaneal deformity, rotational malalignment, and lumbar kyphosis. The neurologic or paralytic factors resulting in crouched gait are the maintenance of hip flexors and quadriceps strength, with loss of hip extension and power in the triceps surae. The spinal cord pathology leading to fluctuating neurologic status and contributing to a progressive crouched gait include hydromyelia, diastematomyelia, Arnold-Chiari malformation, and spinal cord tethering.

Appropriate orthotic management is the best prevention of the crouched gait and subsequent degenerative arthritis. Appropriate orthotic management for the flexed knee includes a rigid AFO to prevent ankle dorsiflexion and prevention of foot pronation and ankle eversion by keeping the ankle in slight plantar flexion. The ground-reaction AFO helps position the tibia posterior and facilitates knee extension. The orthosis should be extended to the toes for prevention of clawing and protection of insensate skin. A rear walker assistive device will help to prevent crouched gait posture in the child.

Treatment for the knee flexion contracture in the adult includes surgical intervention for contractures exceeding 20°. The surgery includes hamstring lengthening and posterior knee capsulotomy, as discussed above. Gradual orthotic correction should be considered for knee flexion contractures under 20°. The use of an adjustable locked articulated ground reaction AFO system allows gradual increasing of plantar flexion range of the ankle over 3 to 6 months. Hip flexion contracture precludes correction of the knee flexion deformity. In the adult patient with hip flexion contracture, treatment should consider abandonment of the ambulatory program. Surgical intervention should be considered for hip flexion contractures exceeding 30°. The surgical intervention includes tendon lengthening, hip capsulotomy, reduction of unilateral hip dislocation, and augmentation of muscle power with external oblique transfer and adductor posterior transfer, as discussed above. A proning program is beneficial to help correct a hip flexion contracture under 30°, and appropriate orthotic management as discussed above should facilitate knee extension.

There is no satisfactory management of the adult spina bifida patient with established severe degenerative arthritis of the knee. Early aggressive management for the crouched gait is essential to prevent this deformity. Orthotic management should be coincidental with initiation of ambulation in the child. All spina bifida patients regularly need routine, thorough neurologic reevaluation with an interdisciplinary care team. Oral nonsteroidal antiinflammatory medications and arthroscopic debridement do have a role in the adult patient with established degenerative arthritis of the knee.

The Foot

The goal of treatment depends on the patient's functional ability. Patients who are nonambulatory or whose prognosis does not include ambulation require a shoeable foot but not full mobility or a perfectly plantigrade foot. Patients who will be wearing orthotics (KAFO or AFO) do not require full normal mobility of their joints but sufficient mobility that they will be able to accommodate slight changes of position to relieve pressure. Ambulatory patients must have plantigrade feet that do not place excessive pressure on any portion of the plantar surface with weight bearing.

Basic Foot Deformities

The primary types of the deformities seen in the feet of patients with myelomeningocele are talipes equinus, talipes equinovarus or equinovalgus, calcaneus with valgus or varus, valgus foot, convex pes valgus (vertical talus), cavus foot, and toe deformities.

Talipes Equinus Talipes equinus is seen primarily in completely paralyzed legs and is an early deformity. It apparently develops as a contracture of the gastrocsoleus despite the muscle's lack of function. At times, isolated function is present within the gastrocsoleus, and this leads to contracture.

Treatment varies with age group as well as with function. In the nonfunctioning gastrocsoleus, tendon lengthening can be done by subcutaneous tenotomy at a very early age. Frequently, there is no sensation in the area and the procedure may be carried out (as done by Menelaus in 1976) without anesthesia in infants during the first few weeks of life.[58]

Subcutaneous tenotomy is performed by cutting the medial half of the tendon just at the heal level, the lateral half about 2 cm proximal and the medial half for a second time 2 cm proximal to the lateral cut.

In older patients with rigid ankle joints or those who would not benefit from tendon and posterior capsule releases, anterior base wedge osteotomies of the distal tibia have been successful in providing a plantigrade foot. Extreme deformities have been overcome with this method. In children with growing distal tibial epiphyses and fixed equinus, Sharrard and Grosfeld describe posterior soft tissue release followed by anterior tibiofibular ligament release, permitting widening of the mortise and enabling the talus to be brought back up into neutral from its plantar-flexed position.[85]

Talipes Equinovarus Talipes equinovarus appears to occur more frequently in paralysis above the L4 level. Treatment schedules are variable. Other than early release of the Achilles tendon through subcutaneous tenotomy, cast correction is utilized during the early months of life and surgical correction is delayed until the patient is at least 6 months of age. Most patients require complete posteromedial plantar and lateral releases of the foot. Postoperative pinning in the corrected position is necessary. Resection of all tendons at the time of this surgery prevents recurrent foot deformity. The anterior tibial, posterior tibial, flexor digitorum longus, flexor hallucis longus, Achilles, and both peroneal tendons should be resected at the time of this release. Insensate feet must be carefully protected against excessive or localized cast pressure. For

this reason, casting should be used only to protect the foot from outside deformity forces after full correction has been achieved surgically.[28] Cast immobilization for 12 to 16 weeks followed by brace immobilization in the corrected position is required. In the child with talipes equinovarus deformity that does respond to a serial casting program, a forced dorsiflexion lateral x-ray should be obtained to determine whether full bone correction has been achieved; if the lateral talocalcaneal angle is less than 30° after a minimum of 3 months of serial casting, then surgical intervention for complete posteromedial release, as described above, may be considered. Without full hindfoot correction, recurrent deformity is common.

Recurrent deformities undergo repeated releases. In patients who have been neglected or seen late and those patients who have had repeated correction with gross deformity of the talus, talectomy can be considered. This must be done in conjunction with the soft tissue releases and tendon resections discussed above.[60] In recurrent deformities where the lateral column of the foot is longer than the medial column, lateral column shortening is necessary. Evans resection and fusion of the calcaneocuboid joint[26] and Lichtblau distal calcaneal resections[47] are examples.

Adduction and supination deformities in the 5- to 10-year-old age group can be treated by cuneiform-cuboid wedge osteotomy[28] through two vertical incisions over the dorsum of the foot: one over the first cuneiform–second cuneiform area and the other at the third cuneiform–cuboid junction. A lateral base wedge can be removed; this allows derotation of the forefoot as well as correction of the adduction angulation. The advantage of this is that the joints are preserved proximal and distal to the cuneiform, allowing maximum growth of the foot.

Triple arthrodesis is used in more mature feet—in patients over the age of 12 years or the equivalent bone age. Residual deformities in teenagers and young adults that cause ulceration over the proximal portion of the fifth metatarsal are best treated by triple arthrodesis. This surgery is designed only to facilitate bracing and should not be considered as brace replacement surgery.

Calcaneus deformity of the myelodysplastic foot is generally related to excessive dorsiflexion of the ankle. The deformity is benefited by orthotic management, which prevents excessive dorsiflexion; however, the contracture gradually becomes greater and plantigrade stability is lost. Severe deformities defy orthotic management and shoe wear because of lack of posterior heel prominence. Stance is affected and there is no posterior stability. Knee stability is decreased because a knee-flexed position is required to maintain the plantigrade position of the foot. The deformity is secondary to a poor to absent gastrocsoleus and a strong dorsiflexor of the foot. The tibialis anterior is innervated by the highest nerve roots of the muscles crossing the ankle, beginning at about the L4 level; it is the strongest of the L5-level muscles at the ankle. A full-strength tibialis anterior may be present with no gastrocsoleus strength. The peroneus tertius is also frequently functional with lesions at this level. Treatment consists of removing the deforming force—namely, the tibialis anterior—and passing the muscle through the interosseous membrane to the os calcis (Peabody procedure).[39,70,100]

The peroneus tertius, if it is functional, should also be transplanted. Treatment is best carried out between 6 and 24 months of age. Banta et al. demonstrated improved gait with a combined procedure of anterior tibial transplantation and Achilles tenodesis.[5]

Calcaneovarus deformity may be present initially or may occur after transfer if the tibialis posterior was not recognized to be functional.[60] This muscle should be transferred to the os calcis or, if it is relatively weak, may be sectioned. Calcaneovalgus is treated in the same manner with transfers along with the tibialis anterior through the peronei to the heel.

Talipes Valgus Talipes valgus causes instability in weight bearing, since weight is transferred to the medial side of the ankle. Pressure occurs over the medial malleolus and, in an insensate foot, ulcerations occur. Talipes valgus is difficult to control and is usually seen with excessive dorsiflexion of the ankle. Problems appear to become more significant as the child reaches the age of 7 to 10 years and becomes heavier. The earliest and most severe deformities occur from muscle imbalance secondary to strong active lateral muscles, such as the peronei, with absent medial muscles, such as the posterior tibialis. The tibialis posterior muscle is ordinarily innervated by higher levels than the peronei. Spastic peronei may create the problem. Talipes valgus occurs in flaccid feet, secondary to dorsiflexion and eversion. It is necessary in all of these cases to have an absent soleus muscle.[19] The fibula is short compared with a normal fibula and containment of the talus on the lateral aspect is poor.[52] This allows excessive valgus of the joint with wedging of the distal tibial epiphysis.[30] As the weight-bearing center passes more medially, the subtalar joint responds by also going into valgus. The external rotation of the lower extremities further accentuates the problems of pushing foot into valgus.

Treatment of apparent muscle imbalance is necessary with section of the spastic tendons as well as transfers. Weight bearing anterior and posterior radiographs of the ankle joint demonstrate the valgus position of the talus. Computed tomography of the tibial talar joint and subtalar joint, as suggested by Smith and Staples,[90] is helpful in defining whether the subtalar joint is also involved. With the valgus ankle, treatment of the subtalar joint alone is doomed to failure. Treatment of the ankle valgus is carried out in several ways. Patients with no gastrocsoleus function and excessive dorsiflexion can have a tenodesis of the distal portion of the Achilles tendon into the fibula.[104] This provides a blockage of dorsiflexion past neutral. In addition, it applies stress to the fibula with each step, pulling the fibula distalward as the patient rolls forward off the foot. It has been noted that the fibula is stimulated and does pull down to the talus, and the distal tibial epiphysis loses its wedging.[30] Patients with significant eversion of the subtalar joint may require a subtalar fusion. Patients who have ankle problems above the age of 10 years, with remaining growth potential in the distal tibia, undergo medial epiphyseal stapling to allow growth of the lateral side, thereby straightening out the valgus ankle.[13]

Supramalleolar osteotomy has been used in patients who are approaching or have already achieved closure of their distal tibias epiphyseal plates.[87] In these patients, definitive corrective treatment is achieved. The wedge of bone that is removed can be utilized for subtalar fusion if that is desired. Achilles tenodesis can be utilized along with any of the other procedures mentioned to prevent excessive dorsiflexion. Patients with eversion of the subtalar joint and abduction of the midfoot require the stabilization of the triple arthrodesis, as described by Williams and Menelaus.[105] Distal tibial rotational and wedge osteotomies can be performed at the same time.[65]

Paralytic Vertical Talus This deformity consists of a dislocation of the foot around the talus, bringing the foot into valgus. The os calcis is in equinus. The navicular sits on the neck of the talus and thee is convexity at the plantar surface of the calcaneocuboid joint. There is marked rockering at the weight-bearing surface, placing pressure around the head of the talus and at the calcaneocuboid joint. The muscular imbalance is associated with strong dorsiflexors and everters along with weakness of balancing toe flexors, tibialis posterior, and intrinsics. A tight Achilles tendon is present but is not necessarily functioning. Intrauterine position as well as muscle imbalance may be a cause of the development of this type of foot deformity.[60] This diagnosis is confirmed with a forced plantar flexion lateral x-ray, which should demonstrate the inability to reduce the talonavicular joint. Treatment is surgical and requires placing the tibialis anterior into the neck of the talus after reduction.[82] Dias[20] has demonstrated that patients over the age of 4 years require subtalar fusion, and Menelaus recommends subtalar fusion in patients without a functioning anterior tibial muscle.[60]

Talipes Cavus Cavus foot is primarily seen in patients with sacral-level function and is due to the absence of intrinsics with all the other muscles being present. The toes are also clawed. Early treatment consists of sectioning the plantar fascia and lengthening the tibialis posterior tendon to provide relief for the high arch. In older children and adults, a metatarsal osteotomy may be performed. Clawing of the toes has been adequately treated in our patients by the performance of the Taylor-Girdlestone[95] transfer, placing the long toe flexors into the extensor hood. The extensor tendon is lengthened or resected and a dorsal capsulotomy performed. The long toe extensors may be placed into the necks of the metatarsals if forefoot equinus is present. Sharrard recommended a flexor tenodesis of the first toe.[86]

Spastic intrinsic muscles create a cavus foot with extended toes. In patients with no foot sensation, sectioning of the posterior tibial nerve and release of the plantar ligament cures the problems. In patients who have sensation about the bottom of the foot, selected sectioning of the motor branches in the plantar surface of the foot is appropriate.[35]

Talipes cavus may also result from imbalance of the toe flexors, which substitute for the paralytic gastrocsoleus. These patients need AFO management to compensate for the paralytic gastrocsoleus. Usually, the toe clawing and talipes cavus resolve with appropriate orthotic management.

Ulcerations Plantar pressure sores are usually the result of residual deformity, causing prominences on the plantar surface of the foot. Occasionally, ulcerations occur in an insensitive foot because the patients have walked barefoot. The use of protective casts brings about rapid closure of the ulcerations[6]; however, if this problem is due to a bony prominence, the prominence itself must be treated. Determination must be made whether it is a localized prominence of whether the entire foot deformity must be corrected. If there is infection around the metatarsal head, causing persistent drainage and ulceration, it is necessary to resect the head of the metatarsal before healing can occur. A rocker-bottom shoe helps prevent additional ulcerations. Wheelchair patients may suffer ulcerations if they do not wear shoes. (Severe foot deformity may prevent the donning of shoes.) In those cases, surgical correction is required to make the foot shoeable for protection. A long-term review of the sacral-level patients at Rancho Los Amigos Medical Center showed that more than 40 percent of these patients developed osteomyelitis of the foot and over 30 percent required surgical amputation above the midfoot level.[8] These findings reinforce the need for appropriate orthotic management in any patient who has impaired plantar foot sensation.

REFERENCES

1. Abraham E, Verinder DGR, Sharrard WJW: The treatment of flexion contracture of the knee in myelomeningocele. *J Bone Joint Surg* 59B:433–438, 1977.
2. Aprin H, Kilfoyle R: Meningocele: Extension contracture of the knees in patients with myelomeningocele. *Clin Orthop* 144:260–263, 1979.
3. Ascher M, Olson J: Factors affecting the ambulatory status of patients with spina bifida cystica. *J Bone Joint Surg* 350–356, 1983.
4. Baker LD, Dodelin R, Bassett FH: Pathological changes in the hip in cerebral palsy. *J Bone Joint Surg* 44A:1331–1342, 1962.
5. Banta LD, Sutherland DH, Wyatt M: Anterior tibialis transfer to os calcis with Achilles tenodesis for calcaneal deformity in myelomeningocele. *J Pediatr Orthop* 1:125–130, 1981.
6. Brand PW: The insensitive foot, in Jahss MH (ed): *Disorders of the Foot.* Philadelphia, Saunders, 1982.
7. Breed AL, Healey PM: The mid lumbar myelomeningocele hip: Mechanics of dislocation and treatment. *Pediatr Orthop* 2:15–23, 1982.
8. Brinker MR, Rosenfeld SR, Feiwell E, et al: Myelomeningocele at the sacral level: long term outcomes in adults. *J Bone Joint Surg* 76A:1293–1300, 1994.
9. Brookes M, Wardle EN: Muscle action and the shape of the femur. *J Bone Joint Surg* 44B:398–411, 1962.
10. Bubak ME, Reed CE, Fransway AF: Allergic reactions to latex among health care workers. *Mayo Clin Proc* 67:1075–1079, 1992.
11. Buisson JS, Hamblen DL: Electromyographic assessment of the transplanted iliopsoas muscle in spina bifida cystica. *Dev Med Child Neurol* 14:29–33, 1972.
12. Bunch WH, Hakala MW: Iliopsoas transfers in children with myelomeningocele. *J Bone Joint Surg* 65A:224–227, 1984.
13. Burkus JK, Moore DW, Raycroft MD: Valgus deformity of the ankle in myelodysplastic patients. *J Bone Joint Surg* 65A:1157–1162, 1983.
14. Canale ST, Hammond NL, Cotter JM, Snedden HE: Pelvic displacement osteotomy for chronic hip dislocation in myelodysplasia. *J Bone Joint Surg* 57A:177–182, 1975.
15. Carroll N: The orthotic management of the spina bifida child. *Clin Orthop* 102:108–114, 1974.
16. Carroll ND, Sharrard WJW: Long-term follow-up of posterior iliopsoas transplantation for paralytic dislocation of the hip. *J Bone Joint Surg* 54A:551–560, 1972.
17. Compere EL, Garrison M, Fahey JJ: Deformities of the femur resulting from arrestment of growth of the capital and greater trochanteric epiphyses. *J Bone Joint Surg* 22:909–914, 1940.
18. DeSouza LJ, Carroll N: Ambulation of the braced myelomeningocele patient. *J Bone Joint Surg* 58A:1112–1118, 1974.
19. Dias LS: Ankle valgus in children with myelomeningocele. *Dev Med Child Neurol* 20:627–633, 1978.
20. Dias LS: Vertical talus. Presented at the Foot and Ankle Society Annual Meeting, Las Vegas, 1984.
21. Dias LS: Surgical management of the knee contractures in myelomeningocele. *J Pediatr Orthop* 2:127–131, 1982.
22. Dias LS, Jasty MJ, Collins P: Rotational deformities of the lower limb in myelomeningocele, evaluation and treatment. *J Bone Joint Surg* 66A:215–223, 1984.
23. Dormans JP, Templeton JJ, Edmonds C, et al: Intraoperative anaphylaxis due to exposure to latex (natural rubber) in children. *J Bone Joint Surg* 67A:1688–1691, 1994.
24. Drabu KJ, Walker G: Stiffness after fractures around the knee in spina bifida. *J Bone Joint Surg* 67B:266–267, 1985.
25. Drummond DS, Morequ M, Cruess RI: Post-operative neuropathic fractures in patients with myelomeningocele. *Dev Med Child Neurol* 23:147–150, 1981.
26. Evans D: Relapsed club foot. *J Bone Joint Surg* 43B:722–733, 1961.
27. Feiwell E: Selection of appropriate treatment for patients with myelomeningocele. *Orthop Clin North Am* 12:101–106, 1981.
28. Feiwell E: The foot in myelodysplasia, in Mann RA (ed): *Surgery of the Foot,* 4th ed. St. Louis, Mosby, 1985.
29. Feiwell E: The unstable hip: Infra-acetabular osteotomy, in McLaurin R (ed): *Myelomeningocele.* New York, Grune & Stratton, 1977.
30. Feiwell E, Miller G: Valgus of the foot in myelodysplasia. Presented at the *American Orthopaedic Foot Society, 13th Annual Meeting,* Anaheim, CA, 1983.
31. Feiwell E, Sakai D, Blatt T: The effect of hip reduction of function in patients with myelomeningocele. *J Bone Joint Surg* 60A:169–173, 1978.
32. Ferguson AB Jr: Primary open reduction of congenital dislocation of the hip using a median adductor approach. *J Bone Joint Surg* 55A:671–689, 1973.
33. Fleming JL: Biopsoas transplant and femoral osteotomy for paralytic dislocation. *J Bone Joint Surg* 39A:697, 1957.
34. Floman Y, Penny JN, Micheli LJ, et al: Osteotomy of the fusion mass in scoliosis. *J Bone Joint Surg* 64A:1307–1316, 1982.
35. Garceau GJ, Brahms MA: A preliminary study of selective plantar-muscle denervation for pes cavus. *J Bone Joint Surg* 38A:553–562, 1956
36. Gardner WJ: Hydrodynamic mechanism of syringomyelia: Its relationship to myelocele. *J Neurol Neurosurg Psychiatry* 28:247–259, 1965.
37. Hall PV, Lindseth RE, Campbell RL, Kalsbeck JE: Myelodysplasia and developmental scoliosis—A manifestation of syringomyelia. *Spine* 1:48–56, 1976.
38. Hammesfohr R, Topple S, Yoo K, et al: Abductor paralysis and the role of the external oblique transfer. *Orthopedics* 6:315–321, 1983.
39. Hayes JT, Gross HP, Dow S: Survey for paralytic defects in myelomeningocele. *J Bone Joint Surg* 46A:1577–1597, 1964.

40. Hoffer MM, Feiwell E, Perry R, et al: Functional ambulation in patients with myelomeningocele. *J Bone Joint Surg* 55A:137–148, 1973.

41. Hoffer MM, Prietto C, Koffman M: Supracondylar derotational osteotomy of the femur for internal rotation of the thigh in the cerebral palsied child. *J Bone Joint Surg* 63A:389–393, 1981.

42. Irwin CE: The iliotibial band: Its role in producing deformity in poliomyelitis. *J Bone Joint Surg* 31A:141–146, 1949.

43. Jackson RD, Padgett TS, Donovan MM: Posterior iliopsoas muscle transfer in myelodysplasia. *J Bone Joint Surg* 61A:40–45, 1979.

44. Jackson R, Feiwell E: Functional decline due to occult neurological changes in older children with myelomeningocele. *Presented at the Western Orthopedics Meeting,* Houston, TX, October 1985.

45. Kwittken PL, Sweinberg SK, Campbell DE, Pawlowski NA: Latex hypersensitivity in children: Clinical presentation in detection of latex specific immunoglobulin E. *Pediatrics* 95:693–699, 1995.

46. Lee EH, Carroll NC: Hip stability and ambulatory status in myelomeningocele. *J Pediatr Orthop* 5:522–527, 1985.

47. Lichtblau SA: A medial and lateral release operation of club foot. *J Bone Joint Surg* 55A:1377–1384, 1973.

48. Lindseth RR: Posterior iliac osteotomy for fixed pelvic obliquity. *J Bone Joint Surg* 60A:17–22, 1978.

49. Lindseth R, Glancy J: Polypropylene lower extremity braces for paraplegia due to myelomeningocele. *J Bone Joint Surg* 56B:556–563, 1974.

50. London JT, Nichols O: Paralytic dislocation of the hip in myelodysplasia. *J Bone Joint Surg* 57A: 501–506, 1975.

51. Madigan RR, Worrall VT: Paralytic instability of the hip in myelomeningoceles. *Clin Orthop* 125:57–64, 1977.

52. Makin M: Tibio-fibular relationship in paralyzed limbs. *J Bone Joint Surg* 47B:500–506, 1965.

53. McCall R, Douglas R, Richtor N: Surgical treatment in patients with myelodysplasia before using the LSU reciprocation-gait system. *Orthopedics* 6:843–848, 1983.

54. McKay DW: McKay hip stabilization in meningo-myelocele. Presented at the American Academy of Orthopaedic Surgeons, Las Vegas, NV, 1977.

55. McKibbin B: The action of the iliopsoas muscle in the newborn. *J Bone Joint Surg* 50B:161–165, 1968.

56. McKibbin B: The use of splintage in the management of paralytic dislocation of the hip in spina bifida cystica. *J Bone Joint Surg* 56B:163–172, 1973.

57. Mazur JM, Stillwell A, Menelaus M: The significance of spasticity in the upper and lower limbs in myelomeningocele. *J Bone Joint Surg* 68B:213–218, 1986.

58. Menelaus MB: Orthopaedic management of children with myelomeningocele: A plea for realistic goals. *Dev Med Child Neurol* 18(suppl 37):3–11, 1976.

59. Menelaus MB: The hip in myelomeningocele. *J Bone Joint Surg* 58B:448–452, 1976.

60. Menelaus MB: *The Orthopaedic Management of Spina Bifida Cystica.* Edinburgh, Churchill Livingstone, 1980.

61. Mooney V, Einbond MJ, Rogers JE, Stauffer ES: Comparison of pressure distribution qualities in seat cushions. *Bull Prosthet Res* 10:129–143, 1971.

62. *MMWR* 41:34–63, 1992.

63. Mustard WT: Iliopsoas transfer for weakness of the hip abductors. *J Bone Joint Surg* 34A:647, 1952.

64. Nickel V, Perry J, Garrett A, Feiwell E: Paralytic dislocation of the hip. *Proc AAOS* 48A:1021, 1966.

65. Nicol RO, Menelaus MB: Correction of the combined tibial torsion and valgus deformity of the foot. *J Bone Joint Surg* 65B:641–645, 1983.

66. O'Brien JP, Dwyer AP, Hodgson AR: Paralytic pelvic obliquity. *J Bone Joint Surg* 57A:626–631, 1975.

67. Park TS, Cail WS, Maggio WM, Mitchell DC: Progressive spasticity and scoliosis in children with myelomeningocele. *J Neurosurg* 62:367–375, 1985.

68. Parker B, Walkers G: Posterior psoas transfer and hip instability in lumbar myelomeningocele. *J Bone Joint Surg* 57B:53–58, 1975.

69. Parsch K, Goessens H: Surgical treatment of spinal column and hip deformities in spina bifida. *Acta Orthop Belg* 37:230–239, 1971.

70. Peabody C: Tendon transplantation in the lower extremity. *AAOS Instr Course Lect* 6:178–188, 1949.

71. Pemberton PA: Pericapsular osteotomy of the ilium for treatment of congenital subluxation and dislocation of the hip. *J Bone Joint Surg* 47A:65–86, 1965.

72. Perlik PC, Westin G, Marafioti RL: A combination pelvic osteotomy for acetabular dysplasia in children. *J Bone Joint Surg* 67A:842–850, 1985.

73. Perry J, Antonelli D, Ford W: Analysis of knee joint forces during flexed knee stance. *J Bone Joint Surg* 57A:961–967, 1975.

74. Peterson M, Adkins H: Measurements and redistribution of excessive pressures during wheelchair sitting. *J Am Phys Ther Assoc* 62:990–994, 1982.

75. Phillips DP, Lindseth RE: Ambulation after transfer of adductors, external oblique and tensor fascia lata in myelomeningocele. *J Pediatr Orthop* 12:712–717, 1992.

76. Raycroft F: Abduction splinting of the hips of infants with myelodysplasia. *Second Symposium of Spina Bifida—A Multidisciplinary Approach.* Cincinnati, November 1984.

77. Rose GK, Sankarankutty M, Stallard J: A clinical review of the orthotic treatment of myelomeningocele patients. *J Bone Joint Surg* 65B:242–246, 1983.

78. Rose GK, Henshaw JT: A swivel walker for paraplegics: Medical and technical considerations. *Bio Med Eng* 7:420–425, 1972.

79. Rosenfeld SR, Gorab R: Prevention of Postoperative Fractures in Myelomeningocele, Unpublished data.

80. Salter RB: Innominate osteotomy in the treatment of congenital dislocation and subluxation of the hip. *J Bone Joint Surg* 43B:426–444, 1964.

81. Schafer MF, Dias LS: *Myelomeningocele, Orthopaedic Treatment.* Baltimore, Williams & Wilkins, 1983.

82. Sharrard WJW: Paralytic convex pes valgus, in McLauren R (ed): *Myelomeningocele.* New York, Grune & Stratton, 1977.

83. Sharrard WJW: Paralytic deformities in the lower limb. *J Bone Joint Surg* 49B:731–747, 1967.

84. Sharrard WJW: Posterior iliopsoas transplantation in the treatment of paralytic dislocation of the hip. *J Bone Joint Surg* 46B:426–444, 1964.

85. Sharrard WJW, Grosfeld I: Management of foot deformities in myelomeningocele. *J Bone Joint Surg* 50B:456–465, 1968.

86. Sharrard WJW, Smith TWD: Tenodesis of flexor hallucis longus for paralytic clawing of the hallux in childhood. *J Bone Joint Surg* 58B:224–226, 1976.

87. Sharrard WJW, Webb J: Supramalleolar wedge osteotomy of the tibia in children with myelomeningocele. *J Bone Joint Surg* 56:458–461, 1974.

88. Slater JE: Allergic reactions to natural rubber. *Ann Allergy* 68:203–209, 1992.

89. Slater JE: Rubber anaphylaxis. *N Engl J Med* 320:1126–1130, 1989.

90. Smith RW, Staple TW: Computerized tomography (CT) scanning technique for the hindfoot. *Clin Orthop* 177:34–38, 1983.

91. Somerville EW: Paralytic dislocation of the hip. *J Bone Joint Surg* 41B:279–288, 1959.

92. Stevens PM, Coleman SS: Coxa breva: Its pathogenesis and a rationale for its management. *J Pediatr Orthop* 5:515–521, 1985.

93. Stillwell A, Menelaus MB: Walking ability after transplantation of the iliopsoas. *J Bone Joint Surg* 66B:656–659, 1984.

94. Stillwell A, Menelaus MB: Walking ability in mature patients with spina bifida. *J Pediatr* 3:184–190, 1983.

95. Taylor RG: Treatment of claw toes by multiple transfer flexors to extensor tendon. *J Bone Joint Surg* 33B:539–542, 1951.

96. Thomas LI, Thompson TC, Straub L: Transplantation of the external oblique muscle for abductor paralysis. *J Bone Joint Surg* 32A:207–217, 1950.

97. Tosi LL, Slater JE, Shaer C, Mostello LA: Latex allergy in spina bifida patient—Prevalence and surgical implications. *J Pediatr Orthop* 13:709–712, 1993.

98. Trumble T, Banta JV, Raycroft JF, Curtis BH: Talectomy for equinovarus deformity in the myelodysplasia. *J Bone Joint Surg* 67A:21–29, 1985.

99. Turner A: Hand function in children with myelomeningocele. *J Bone Joint Surg* 67B:268–272, 1985.

100. Turner J, Cooper R: Posterior transposition of tibialis anterior through the interosseus member. *Clin Orthop* 79:71–74, 1971.

101. Waters RL, Lunsford RPT: Energy cost in paraplegic locomotion. *J Bone Joint Surg* 67A:1245–1249, 1985.

102. Weissman SL, Torok G, Khermosh OJ: Intertrochanteric osteotomy in fixed paralytic obliquity of the pelvis. *J Bone Joint Surg* 43A:1135–1154, 1961.

103. Werler MM, Shapiro S, Mitchell AA: Periconceptional folic acid exposure and risk of occurrent neural tube defects. *JAMA* 269:1257–1261, 1993.

104. Westin GW, Dingeman RD, Gausewitz SH: The results of tenodesis of the tendo-Achilles to the fibula for paralytic pes calcaneus. *J Bone Joint Surg* 70A:320–328, 1988.

105. Williams PF, Menelaus MB: Triple arthrodesis by inlay graft—A method suitable for underformed or valgus foot. *J Bone Joint Surg* 59B:333–336, 1977.

106. Yngve DA, Douglas D, Roberts JM: The reciprocation gait orthosis in myelomeningocele. *J Pediatr Orthop* 4:304–310, 1984.

CHAPTER 35

Muscular Dystrophies and Other Neuromuscular Diseases

John D. Hsu

The child suffering from neuromuscular disease often does not exhibit motor weakness at birth. The parents may seek medical advice when, subsequently, they observe the child delayed in achieving developmental milestones. Parents also notice that the child's physical activity varies from that of the peer group.[1] For instance, the child may consistently arise from a seated position in an unusual or different way. Alternatively, the affected child may be perceived to stand or walk with feet spread, exhibit some other abnormal gait, be slow in athletic competition, or be the last one in the group to run up a flight of stairs.

When symptoms first manifest in the young adult, they may also be nonspecific. The manifestations of motor weakness occur subtly, and develop over many years. Some patients may complain of increasing fatigue. Tasks that were easily performed in the past require more effort and certain activities must be discontinued. Adults generally adapt to a slowly progressive loss of function and accommodate to increasing disability.

Classification

Our current knowledge of the cause and management of childhood and adult neuromuscular diseases is rapidly changing. Even our classification is being reevaluated. This is because many advances are being made in molecular biology and genetics.[2,3] The clinical laboratory can distinguish and identify very sophisticated changes in gene structure and DNA sequencing and identify the location of abnormalities.[4,5] Incorporating new knowledge, reclassification of the various types of neuromuscular conditions can now be expected more in line with the differences and abnormalities in the genetic makeup. As we develop this new scientific knowledge, there will be an improvement in our understanding of the subtle differences observed in the various clinical syndromes.

The *myopathies* are the group of neuromuscular disorders where the primary abnormality is in the muscle cell. In the *neuropathies*, the muscle changes are secondary to abnormalities or disorders that occur in the anterior horn cell, peripheral nerve, or neuromuscular junction (Table 35-1).

Diagnosis

A complete and accurate clinical history is very important. In a child, information about developmental milestones and the rate of progression of the disorder is critical; a complete family history should also be taken.

The clinical examination will usually give important clues as to the diagnosis. Proximal weakness can be seen in a child with Duchenne muscular dystrophy at a very early age. If the history indicates that this is progressive, it may serve to differentiate this disease from the similar clinical picture presented in spinal muscular atrophy, which is relatively nonprogressive. The distribution of weakness around the face and shoulder girdle may lead to the suspicion that one is dealing with a case of facioscapulohumeral muscular dystrophy (FSHD). Fasciculations or tremors observed in the muscles may suggest neurogenic origin.

Specific diagnosis has usually relied upon measurement of level of muscle enzymes (creatine phosphokinase and aldolase), electrodiagnostic studies (electromyography and nerve conduction tests), and muscle biopsy.[6]

Muscle biopsy of involved muscle groups, usually performed under regional or general anesthesia, depends upon removing a small section of muscle under direct vision through a small incision and keeping the muscle at its normal resting length by clamping the tissue in a special clamp, just over a centimeter in diameter, prior to its removal. The muscle is submitted for light or electron microscopy (see Table 35-2).

MUSCULAR DYSTROPHIES

Duchenne Muscular Dystrophy

Duchenne muscular dystrophy (DMD) is a progressive disease affecting male children and adolescents. The inheritance pattern is X-linked recessive, affecting males severely. Approximately 30 percent of the cases may not have a family history and arise as new mutations. Female carriers of the disease may be normal or only mildly affected and have a normal life span. It is presently the second most common lethal genetic disorder in humans and affects approximately 1 in 3300 live male births.

TABLE 35-1 Motor Unit Disorders

Neuropathies
   Spinal muscular atrophy (SMA)
   Charcot-Marie-Tooth disease (CMT)
   Viral neuropathy: Poliomyelitis, echovirus, coxsackievirus

Myopathies
   Duchenne muscular dystrophy (DMD)
   Becker muscular dystrophy (BMD)
   Facioscapulohumeral dystrophy (FSHD)
   Limb-girdle dystrophy (LGMD)
   Emery-Dreifuss muscular dystrophy (EDMD)
   Myotonic dystrophy
   Congenital myopathy (see Table 35-3)

TABLE 35-2 Enzyme Level and Muscle Biopsy Diagnostic Features in Muscle Disease

CPK level	Diagnosis
↑ X20 to X200 (but falls in late adolescence)	DMD BMD
↑ X10	LGD
↑ X mildly elevated	FSHD EDMD

Muscle biopsy Light microscopy	Frozen in liquid nitrogen within minutes
H & E	General morphology (atrophy? hypertrophy? degeneration? fibrosis? inflammation? infiltration?)
ATPase	Fiber type (grouping? disproportion?)
Nicotinamide adenine dinucleotide–tetrazolium reductase	Fiber type, cellular architecture (e.g., central core)
Gomori trichrome	Connective tissue elements (e.g., nemaline rods)
Periodic acid–Schiff	Glycogen
Oil red O	Lipid

Electron microscopy	Fixed in the operating room in 4% gluteraldehyde

Selected patients to confirm a structural myopathy and assess lipid or glycogen storage and mitochondria

Source: Data from Shapiro F, Specht L: Current concepts review: The diagnosis and orthopedic treatment of inherited muscular diseases of childhood. *J Bone Joint Surg* 75A:439–454, 1993.

Studies have shown a gene defect in the Xp21 locus in the human genome. A protein, *dystrophin,* the product of the DMD gene, is absent from the muscle. Although the specific function of dystrophin is not entirely known at this time, it is a component of the cell membrane cytoskeleton and is believed to protect the muscle cell. Without dystrophin, appropriate substances—including creatine phosphokinase (CPK)—necessary for cell function leak out, and deterioration of the muscle occurs.[7] Dystrophin testing to differentiate DMD from Becker's dystrophy and other diseases is now available on frozen muscle biopsies. Analysis of DNA mutations also provides accurate diagnosis, identifies carriers, and permits prenatal diagnostic testing from blood and amniotic fluid.[8,9]

Clinical Characteristics

Affected males may show mild delay in the early motor milestones or may toe-walk, but they are usually diagnosed between the ages of 3 to 5 years, when they begin to lose skills that have already been acquired. Lumbar lordosis is universally present at this stage and a classic pseudohypertrophy of the calf muscles is common. The muscle weakness is steadily progressive, with the proximal musculature being more affected than the distal. It is because of this proximal weakness that these boys exhibit a positive Gowers' sign (using the hands to climb up the legs) on arising from the floor (Fig. 35-1). Less prominently observed are secondary areas of hypertrophy around the scapulae and in the shoulders. Recurrent respiratory infections, including pneumonia, become more common as the child grows older and respiratory function deteriorates. Cardiomyopathy also becomes prominent. Death usually ensues before the end of the second decade, with three-quarters being pulmonary deaths and approximately one-quarter cardiac deaths.

There is a very high level of serum CPK, particularly in the first year of life, before the disease manifests itself. If this test is normal at this age, it is strong evidence against

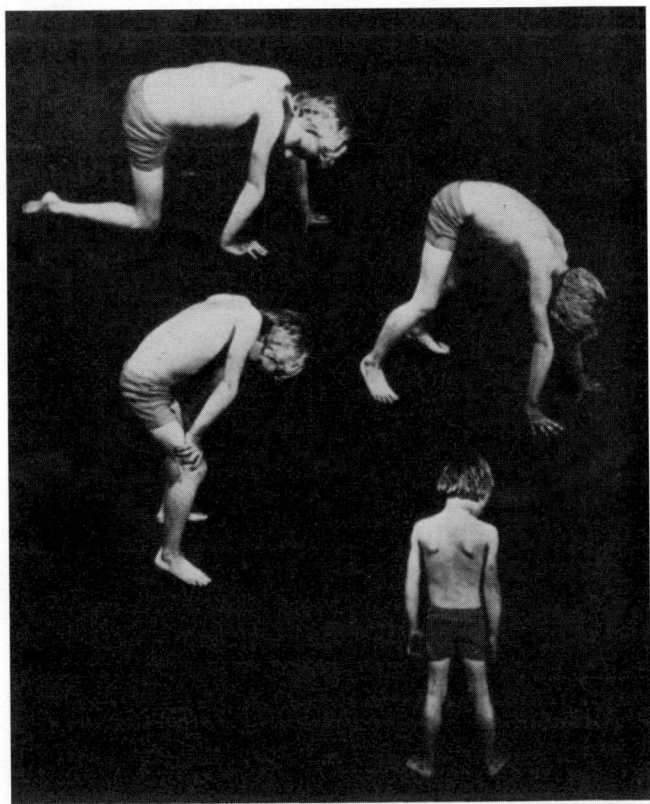

Figure 35-1 Duchenne's muscular dystrophy in a 6-year-old boy. Gowers' sign is present (see text). There is enlargement of the calf muscles and atrophy of the shoulder muscles with scapular winging. (Reproduced with permission from McComas AJ: *Neuromuscular Function and Disorders.* Butterworth, London, 1977.)

the possibility of the disease. The CPK level identifies a female as a carrier and is a useful screening test, but even three negative tests do not entirely rule out the carrier state; the more sophisticated dystrophin and DNA tests, already described, are more definitive. The muscle biopsy shows foci of necrosis with phagocytosis and interstitial infiltration by connective tissue (Fig. 35-2). There is an increase in the amount of connective tissue, which has been identified as type 3 collagen. An increased number of undifferentiated, large, type IIC muscle fibers are present. There are also other abnormalities, such as multisegmented hypotrophied fibers, lateral sarcoplasmic masses, and ringlike structures known as annulets. However, these changes seen on light microscopy are characteristic of various forms of muscular dystrophy and are not specific for DMD. On the electromyogram (EMG), one may occasionally see low-amplitude polyphasic potentials with fibrillation associated with muscle necrosis.

Orthopaedic Treatment

As muscle weakness increases, changes in body alignment during standing and walking are seen.[10,11] The base of support may be widened and there is an increase in lateral swing of the arms and lean of the trunk to compensate for gluteus medius weakness. Hyperlordosis may develop to compensate for a developing flexion or flexion-abduction contracture of the hips, and these patients may also develop flexion contractures of the knees. Postural adjustment to increasing muscle weakness may lead to toe walking, and muscle imbalance may lead to the development of fixed equinus or equinovarus deformities in the ankle and foot. Surgery is indicated if it will prolong the ability to ambulate even for 2 or 3 years, since this is valuable to the patient and family. Surgery is commonly used for this purpose, followed by postoperative bracing to consolidate the functional gain. Generally, hip flexion contractures can be stretched by pronation, But surgical release of the rectus and tensor fascia lata as described by Soutter[12] is sometimes indicated. Various types of hamstring lengthening have been proposed to release knee flexion contractures that cannot be adequately overcome by simple casting.[13] Equinus contractures of the ankle can be released by lengthening of the tendo Achillis or by calf muscle[14] release. In the event of equinovarus deformity, accurate muscle testing will often reveal that the posterior tibial muscle is the strongest remaining muscle in the foot and ankle. Rebalancing of this deforming muscle force may be achieved by lengthening the tendon or rerouting it anteriorly through the interosseous membrane.[15–19]

With the patient sitting all day long, contractures of the upper extremity occur; these consist mainly of abduction contractures of the shoulder and flexion contractures of the elbow, wrist, and finger joints. A ranging program on a daily basis is encouraged to limit the development of these contractures, with the occasional use of an orthotic for the hand and wrist.[20] Prevention of hand and finger deformities is important for wheelchair control.

Spinal collapse occurs in over 60 percent of permanently seated DMD patients.[21] These neuromuscular curves can be rapidly progressive, and several surgeons recommend that a spinal fusion be performed even with a curve of only 10 or 20°.[17] Luque instrumentation has made these operations more feasible.[22–28]

Preoperative surgical assessment is critical for these patients; Shapiro and Specht recommend that operation be performed only in those patients who have a forced vital capacity in excess of 40 percent of normal and have had a careful preoperative cardiac assessment to exclude cardiomyopathy. The same authors point out that although spinal arthrodesis eliminates or greatly minimizes the development of pelvic obliquity and allows the patient to sit more comfortably in the wheelchair, the progressive deterioration and diminishing respiratory function are almost exclusively related to muscle weakness and not to spinal deformity. Therefore, the results of spinal fusion with regard to pulmonary function and longevity have been somewhat disappointing.[7]

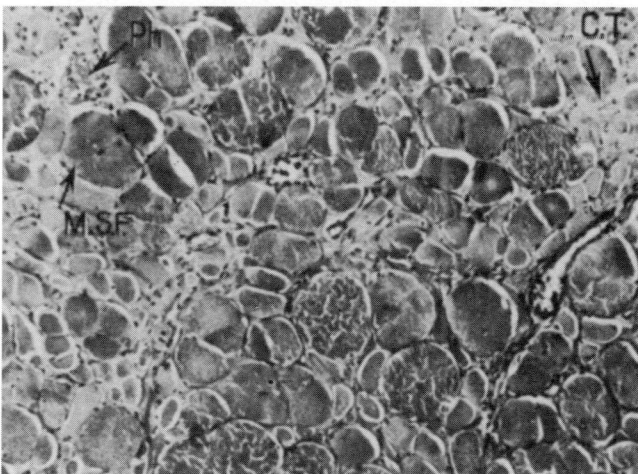

Figure 35-2 Muscular dystrophy. There is irregularity in the size of the muscle fibers; there are also some abnormally large and multisegmented fibers (MSF), loci of necrosis with phagocytosis (Ph), and interstitial infiltration by connective tissue (CT). (H&E.) (Reproduced with permission from Escourelle R, Poirier J: *Manual of Basic Neuropathology.* Philadelphia, Saunders, 1978.)

Becker's Muscular Dystrophy

In Becker's muscular dystrophy (BMD), dystrophin is either produced in insufficient amounts or the molecule itself is abnormal and not fully functional.[29] Again, the disease is a severe X-linked myopathy related to the gene on the Xp21 region of the X chromosome.[7] An affected male will have no sons with the disorder, but all his daughters will be carriers. There is a 50 percent chance that the son of a female carrier will have the disorder and a 50 percent chance that her daughter will be a carrier.

Milestones are often delayed and there is a progressive increase in muscle weakness. Patients can be independent ambulators, but they usually have to give up walking by 30 years of age and often die around the fourth decade. There is, however, significant intrafamilial variability.[30,31]

Because BMD patients ambulate longer, severe spinal curvatures are less commonly seen and spinal fusion is usually unnecessary. Similarly, lower extremity contractures can be minimized in these patients. Clinically, these patients are often confused with patients suffering from limb-girdle dystrophy; however, a very high CPK level and degenerative changes seen on the muscle biopsy (Table 35-2), together with the presence of pseudohypertrophy, point to BMD as the correct diagnosis. The cause of death in these patients is usually respiratory or cardiac failure, since they often have cardiomyopathy.

Facioscapulohumeral Dystrophy

This autosomal dominant myopathy is quite variable in its presentation. The earliest symptom is usually facial weakness, causing difficulty in closing the eyelids tightly, pursing the lips, or puffing out the cheeks. Scapular weakness, however, is frequently the most disabling component of the disorder, causing difficulty in abducting the arms and inability to adequately stabilize the scapula against the thoracic cavity.[32] The patient adapts by using substitute motions and functional aids to compensate for the winging of the scapula and the limited abduction of the arm. Stabilization of the scapula to the ribs as described by Letournel and coworkers has been shown to improve upper limb function.[33] Several other types of surgical corrections are described.[34] The disease is compatible with a normal life span, but there is often later lower limb involvement with proximal weakness and occasional footdrop.

Limb-Girdle Muscular Dystrophy

This condition (LGMD) is an autosomal recessive disorder affecting males and females equally. The onset may be in the first decade or as late as the fourth. It is a slowly progressive disease and proximal musculature is more affected than distal.[32,35,36] The patient will often show a positive Gowers' sign. The CPK is generally only mildly elevated and the muscle biopsy shows a dystrophic picture. Electromyographic changes are also those of a myopathy. A dystrophin study is necessary to differentiate the disease from BMD or a carrier state of DMD. Life span is not shortened by the disease and scoliosis is seldom seen.

Emery-Dreifuss Muscular Dystrophy

This syndrome (EDMD) is now identified as different from LGMD and BMD. Both these conditions have to be ruled out of the differential diagnosis, as also does DMD.

The muscle biopsy is nonspecific, suggesting a myopathy, and the CPK level is only mildly elevated. Dystrophin studies will rule out BMD and DMD. The condition is X-linked recessive and, like other dystrophies, presents in a nonspecific way, with muscle weakness in the first few years of life. With the subsequent development of deformities, heel cord lengthening and posterior tibial tendon transfer may be required. There is significant abnormality of the muscle, leading to extension contraction of the neck. The paraspinal muscles become so rigid that although there is accompanying scoliosis, which may be severe, it is not of the collapsing neuromuscular type and therefore may be nonprogressive and not require surgery. Heart lesions are often fatal.[7]

Congenital Myopathies

This is a group of rarely seen muscle disorders (Table 35-3) exhibiting specific pathologic changes in the ultrastructural appearance of the muscle biopsy, which leads to classification and nomenclature. The terminology is therefore not related to specific clinical or molecular markers of the disease. In some cases, there may be no recognizable abnormality in the muscle structure and the diagnosis is nonspecific. If necrosis and fibrosis are seen, these patients are often categorized as having a congenital muscular dystrophy.[35,37,38] Orthopedic treatment must be individualized and directed to prevention and release of contractures. Dynamic deformities should be balanced and dislocation (especially of the hips) avoided. Spinal deformity is common. Bracing and careful follow-up are needed and occasionally fusion of the spine is required.

Central Core Disease

This is an autosomal dominant congenital myopathy whose hallmark is a muscle fiber with an amorphous central zone devoid of enzymatic activity and therefore not stained using histochemical methods (Fig. 35-3). The fibers affected are predominantly type 1, and a predominance of type I

TABLE 35-3 Congenital Myopathies

Structural
  Central core disease
  Nemaline myopathy
  Congenital fiber-type disproportion
  Myotubular myopathy
  Abnormalities of other subcellular organelles
  Congenital dystrophy

Metabolic
  Glycogenoses
    Acid maltase deficiency (type II glycogenosis)
    Phosphorylase deficiency (McArdle disease, type V glycogenosis)

Lipid disorder
  Carnitine deficiency

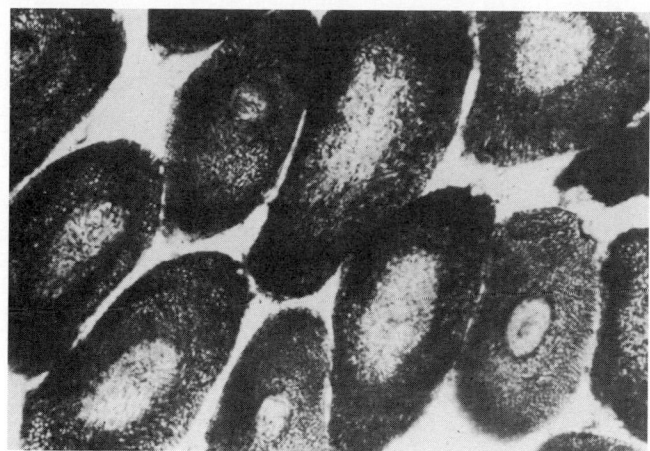

Figure 35-3 Central core disease. The central portion of each muscle fiber contains a zone of absent oxidative activity (succinic dehydrogenase). (×450.) (Reproduced with permission from Banker BQ: Neuropathologic aspects of arthrogryposis multiplex congenita. *Clin Orthop* 194:30–43, 1985.)

fibers is seen in the biopsy. Progressive scoliosis, foot deformity, and congenital dislocation of the hip are all orthopedic problems commonly seen with this disorder. Malignant hypothermia is the most feared complication of central core disease. In this condition, exposure to succinylcholine, halothane, and various other anesthetic agents may induce tachycardia, muscle contracture, and a considerable rise in body temperature. Unless appropriate treatment is undertaken immediately, death is likely. Treatment consists of immediate cessation of anesthesia, changing all anesthetic tubings still contaminated by anesthetic agents, administration of 1 mg/kg sodium bicarbonate and 2.5 mg/kg of dantrolene sodium, icing of the patient, and immediate closure of the incisions. Dantrolene lowers the sarcoplasmic calcium levels and is thought to act on the coupling between the sarcoplasmic reticulum and the T systems in the muscle. Malignant hypothermia may be inherited as an autosomal dominant trait and can be detected by a caffeine-tested muscle biopsy.

Nemaline Myopathy

This autosomal dominant myopathy is characterized by mild, usually nonprogressive weakness. Muscle biopsy will show rodlike structures in a small percentage of fibers, best seen with Gomori trichrome stain. Progressive scoliosis, chest wall deformity, and foot deformities are frequently seen; 90 percent of these patients die in the first few years of life.[7,35]

Congenital Fiber-Type Disproportion

Hypotonia is the hallmark of this disorder and is sometimes noted to be progressive in early life. The most common orthopedic problems include progressive scoliosis, torticollis, congenital dislocation of the hips, and multiple joint contractures of the hands and feet. The biopsy is characterized by a relative disproportion of the size and number of type I and II muscle fibers, with the type I fibers

being smaller than normal and relatively increased in number. The type II fibers seem to be relatively large.[35]

Myotubular Myopathy

This condition, sometimes called *centronuclear myopathy,* is characterized by a muscle fiber appearance superficially resembling that of the myotubes seen in the developing fetus. When the ATPase histochemical stain is used, a central pale area resembling a donut is seen on muscle fiber biopsy. Patients with this disorder show generalized weakness, which is either nonprogressive or slowly progressive. Probably more than one disorder is characterized by this histologic appearance, as differing patterns of inheritance are seen.[35,39]

Mitochondrial Myopathies

This is a group of disorders characterized by ragged red fibers, which are disrupted red-staining fibers seen with Gomori trichome staining. On electron microscopy, the mitochondria are typically abnormal in size and shape. Similar abnormalities are seen in other disorders, including cardiomyopathies and lipid storage disorders such as carnitine deficiency.

Congenital Dystrophy

In this autosomal recessive congenital myopathy, characterized by severe hypotonia in the newborn, type II fibers are completely absent in the muscle biopsy. However, little progression occurs after the first few years of life. Congenital dystrophy is one cause of multiple congenital contractures. Orthopedic abnormalities include scoliosis, talipes equinovarus, and infantile dysplasia with hip dislocation.

Electrodiagnostic Testing in Congenital Myopathies

The normal motor unit potential (MUP) has a duration of 3 to 15 ms, with a peak amplitude up to 3 mV. In myopathy, the number of functioning muscle cells is reduced and the MUP is characteristically small in amplitude and of short duration. By contrast, in denervation disorders, the MUP is usually increased, a development associated with collateral sprouting from residual intact nerve axons[40] (Fig. 35-4).

Using the technique of single fiber electromyography, the average fiber density in a motor unit can also be calculated and is seen to be typically increased in primary myopathies.[41]

Myotonia

In this group of diseases, the muscle fiber membrane is hyperexcitable. Changes in the resting membrane potential have been detected, which render the membrane more easily depolarized.[42] Needle EMG shows waxing and wan-

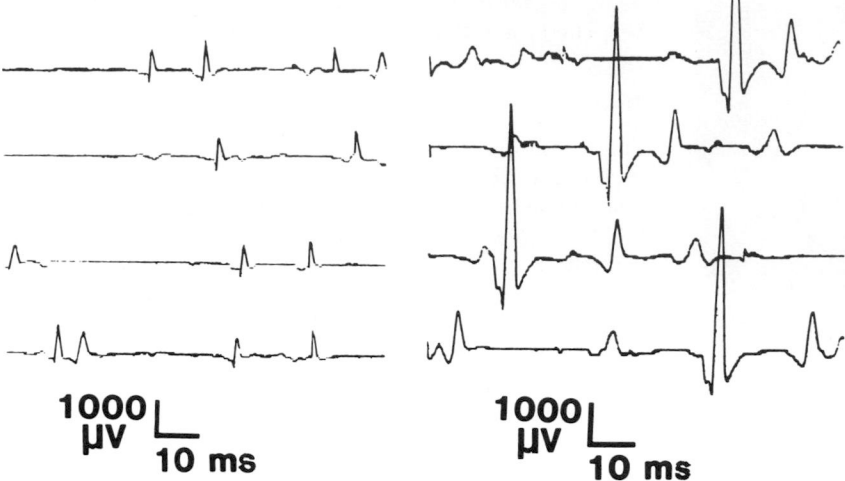

Figure 35-4 The motor unit potential (MUP) in patients with denervation and myopathy. *Left panel:* Small, short MUP in myopathy. *Right panel:* Long, high-amplitude MUP in the denervation process. (Reproduced with permission from Oh SJ: *Clinical Electromyography.* Baltimore, University Park Press, 1984.)

ing in frequency and amplitude. When a loudspeaker is used to monitor the EMG activity, the sound is like that of a dive bomber or a motorcycle revving up.

Steinert's Myotonic Dystrophy

This is a progressive systemic illness characterized by distal weakness, frontal baldness, heart disease, mental deficiency, cataracts, and infertility. It is inherited as an autosomal dominant trait. It is unusual in that patients whose mothers were also affected by the disorder have more severe illness, which manifests itself in early childhood, than do those patients who inherit the disorder from their fathers.[43] Patients with maternally inherited disease may present with congenital symptoms in the newborn nursery, with failure to thrive, respiratory distress, and marked hypotonia.[44] There may be accompanying cataracts, male frontal baldness, gonadal atrophy, heart disease, and endocrine abnormalities. The course is steadily downhill. These patients are often severely retarded, have numerous deformities in the extremities, and walk very late.

Some 50 percent of patients with the congenital form of Steinert's myotonic dystrophy have talipes equinovarus and often present with relapsed clubfoot after serial casting. Soft tissue releases are of little use in treating these feet, and triple arthrodesis may be required in early adolescence. There are often deformities of the hallux, which also require surgical intervention. It is necessary to be aware of the risks of abnormal heart rhythm and pulmonary hypoventilation during anesthesia.

Patients with the congenital form may also be more prone to congenital dislocation of the hips as well as scoliosis, as opposed to patients with the so-called adult form of the disorder (paternally inherited). A defective gene has been localized to chromosome 19 and prenatal diagnostic testing is available.[7]

It should be noted that in infants with the congenital form, hypotonia, not myotonia, is the presenting problem. The characteristic myotonia appears only late in the first or early in the second decade.

The CPK level is only mildly elevated in this disorder, but diagnosis is facilitated by the characteristic electrodiagnostic changes. Muscle biopsy shows an increase in connective tissue and variation of fiber size, the nuclei tending to lie in a more central position. Type I fibers are selectively involved in about half the cases (Fig. 35-5).

Myotonia Congenita (Thomson's Disease)

In spite of the similarity of terms, this disease is distinct from the congenital form of myotonic dystrophy. Thomson's disease is an autosomal dominant condition in which myotonia is most marked on an initial movement and decreases with repetition. The disorder usually ap-

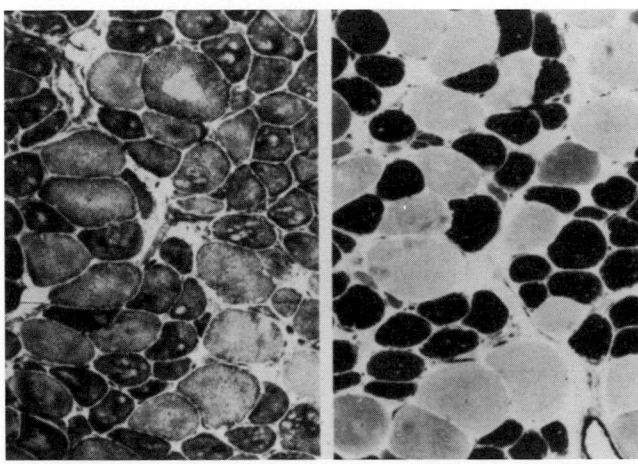

Figure 35-5 Myotonic dystrophy. *A.* NADH tetrazolium reductase preparation. Numerous atrophied fibers with changes in their sarcoplasm. *B.* ATPase preparation at pH 4.35. All atrophied fibers are of type I; most type II fibers are hypertrophied. (×80.) (Reproduced with permission from Escourelle R, Poirier J: *A Manual of Basic Neuropathology.* Philadelphia, Saunders, 1978.)

pears in childhood but is compatible with a normal life span. Frequently there is hypotrophy of the musculature. There are no associated systemic abnormalities.

The EMG is useful in diagnosis, and the defect in the condition seems to be abnormal calcium permeability in the muscle fiber membrane. Muscle biopsy reveals an absence of type IIB fibers.[45] These patients may appear to be normal but show difficulty in relaxing their grip and manifest a painful stiffness, which is accentuated by rest and cold and relieved by activity.

Paramyotonia Congenita (Eulenburg's Disease)

Paramyotonia congenita is an autosomal dominant condition characterized by episodes of myotonic paralysis precipitated by exposure to cold. The disorder particularly affects the hands and face. Frequently there is a hypertrophy of the musculature of these patients.[46]

MYASTHENIA GRAVIS

This is an uncommon disease with no particular pattern of inheritance and several separate presentations. Approximately 1 person in 5000 contracts it at some time in life. Among young adult patients, females predominate by a ratio of 3:1; whereas at an older age, males predominate. Transient neonatal myasthenia occurs in 15 percent of children born to myasthenic mothers; this is thought to be due to passive transfer of antiacetylcholine receptor IgG from mother to fetus. This condition generally improves spontaneously after 2 to 4 weeks and does not recur, but neostigmine treatment may be required.

Clinical Features

The increased fatigability of the muscle characteristic of this disease commonly affects the ocular muscles or the muscles involved in speaking and swallowing. Approximately 1 in 5 patients experiences generalized weakness of the limbs.[45]

Juvenile Myasthenia Gravis

Juvenile myasthenia gravis generally develops after the age of 10 years and initially involves the ocular muscles. Weakness may be restricted to the facial muscles, in which case spontaneous remission may occur. Alternatively, the weakness may extend to the extremities, in which case the myasthenia is usually most marked in the proximal upper extremities.

Congenital or Infantile Myasthenia

Congenital or infantile myasthenia is probably an autosomal recessive condition characterized by ptosis, ophthal-moplegia, and sometimes generalized muscle weakness. There may sometimes be episodes of respiratory distress.

Diagnostic Tests

It is considered that this disease is due to a humorally mediated autoimmune condition that blocks the acetylcholine (Ach) receptors of the neuromuscular junction. Although one finds antibodies in these patients that bind to the Ach receptors (and in animals such antibodies are capable of producing systemic manifestations when passively transferred), their titer correlates poorly with the severity of the disease. There is often a correlation with other autoimmune diseases, and 10 percent of patients have a thymoma.

The response to neostigmine or edrophonium (both of which relieve the symptoms) is a useful diagnostic test.

The muscle biopsy is not as helpful as the EMG but does show some type II fiber atrophy. The easy fatigability of the muscle is demonstrated electromyographically by the repetitive nerve stimulation (Jolly) test.[40] At low rates of repetitive stimulation, a decremental response is seen in involved muscle. Raising the rate of stimulation often abolishes the response. When single-fiber EMGs are used, characteristic changes are also seen in these patients.[40]

Treatment

Thymectomy is valuable in selected candidates and can give long-term relief. Curiously enough, the results are not as good if the patient has a thymic tumor. Emergency treatment may require the administration of neostigmine. Pyridostigmine, which has a longer duration of action, has been used in maintenance therapy. Plasmapheresis as well as steroids and immunosuppressive drugs such as azathioprine have also been utilized.

DISEASE OF THE MOTOR NEURONS
Spinal Muscular Atrophy
Classification

Spinal muscular atrophy is a collection of disorders characterized by degeneration of the anterior horn cells and in some cases of the bulbar motor nuclei.[47,48] The more severe infantile form, characterized by poor head control, inability to obtain sitting balance, and early death, is usually called *Werdnig-Hoffmann disease*. The other well-known form, characterized by later onset—usually in the late first or early second decade and with slower progression—is known by the eponym *Kugelberg-Welander disease* (juvenile spinal muscular atrophy). Both these disorders appear to be autosomal recessive conditions, but there are other spinal muscular atrophies that appear to be dominantly inherited. Subclassification is frequently difficult and based more on clinical criteria than on specific neurochemical classification. Dubowitz and Brooke suggest the following classification of the childhood spinal muscular atrophies: (1) severe—unable to sit unsupported; (2) intermediate—able to sit unsupported but unable to stand or walk unaided; (3) mild—able to stand and walk.[45] In the group with severe spinal muscular atrophy, or Werdnig-Hoffmann disease, children may either be affected from birth or may show weakness within the first few months of life. There are frequently decreased tendon reflexes, and tongue fasciculations are common. Generalized hypotonia, poor head control, swallowing difficulties, and recurrent upper respiratory infections are common. Survival past 1 year of life is rare.

In the intermediate group, children commonly develop normally for the first few months of life and frequently achieve the ability to sit unaided. Nevertheless, these patients are commonly unable to crawl or walk and show progressive motor weakness. The tendon reflexes are decreased, and tongue fasciculations may be seen. Survival may extend into the teenage years or early adulthood and severe, progressive scoliosis is common. Children with mild (Kugelberg-Welander) disease commonly achieve the early milestones but, beginning in the late first decade or early second decade, have difficulty keeping up with their peers. They frequently use a Gowers' maneuver to get up from the floor. Some may have normal reflexes, but commonly most reflexes are depressed. Many of these patients are in wheelchairs by their mid-thirties.[48–50]

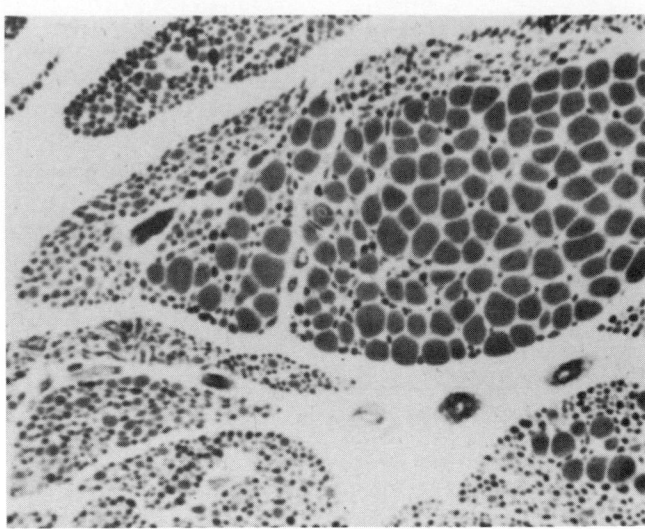

Figure 35-6 The muscle biopsy findings in infantile spinal muscular atrophy show characteristics of "denervation"-type muscle biopsies. There are large numbers of round atrophic fibers. Fiber-type groupings are seen here as clumps of hypertrophic type I fibers. This uniform histochemical type is well shown (ATPase reaction, pH 9.4). (Reproduced with permission from Brooke MA: *A Clinician's View of Neuromuscular Disease.* Baltimore, Williams & Wilkins, 1977.)

Diagnosis

In Werdnig-Hoffmann disease, the muscle biopsy may show clumps of hypertrophic type I fibers with grouping which is fairly characteristic of this disease when it is evaluated with the histochemical ATPase reaction (Fig. 35-6). In this condition, however, CPK levels may be normal, and the EMG is often difficult to interpret, although fibrillation potentials are common.[45]

In Kugelberg-Welander disease, the biopsy shows the fiber-type grouping characteristic of neurogenic atrophy. Instead of the usual mosaic distribution of motor units, there is a tendency for muscle fibers of the same type to group themselves together; type II fibers predominate and CPK levels may be mildly elevated. The EMG changes are consistent with the muscle biopsy and show a mixed pattern of denervation and reinnervation.[45]

Orthopedic Treatment

The orthopedic management of the most severe form (Werdnig-Hoffmann) should these patients survive early childhood, is directed at bracing the spine and neck using a body jacket with a neck extension device. Provision must be made to permit diaphragmatic breathing. Since the patient has no potential for ambulation, lower limb contractures are acceptable provided that they do not interfere with normal seating.

In the less severe type, the children may stand but generally do not walk. Prevention of contractures in the lower extremity by bracing is therefore important, since standing is desirable to maintain muscle tone and prevent

osteoporosis. Scoliosis greater than 20° occurs in over 90 percent of patients. If it is progressive, then surgical intervention and spinal fusion may be necessary.[50,51]

Osteoporosis is common in these patients and fractures can occur easily, especially when there are contracted joints. They are generally undisplaced and can be treated by splinting. Open reduction and internal fixation is occasionally necessary.[52]

Exercise may be beneficial to these patients but should not be overly vigorous or resistive. Assistive devices corresponding with the patients particular needs should be assessed by the occupational therapist. As in the treatment of all these neuromuscular diseases, a comprehensive multidisciplinary team of therapist, social workers, and other health care professionals is necessary, along with the close cooperation of the parents. Mobility in the form of wheelchairs, assistive devices, vehicle modifications and functional adaptations may assist such a patient to maintain maximum independence and to function in the community.[53]

ARTHROGRYPOSIS

It is now recognized that there are many varieties of multiple congenital contractures and that arthrogryposis is not a single disease entity but a large number of specific entities having a similar clinical picture. Over 150 specific known causes of this condition have been identified.[54] It is mentioned here, since the primary disorder may be neurogenic or myopathic. A careful neurologic evaluation together with assessment of muscle enzymes and muscle biopsy may be required to identify a specific neuromuscular disease.[55] However, only a few of these patients have congenital muscular dystrophy or central core disease. The orthopedic treatment of this condition is described elsewhere in this volume.

CHARCOT-MARIE-TOOTH DISEASE

Charcot-Marie-Tooth disease (CMT) represents an inherited neuropathy. It is one of a group of diseases known as hereditary motor and sensory neuropathies (HMSN), a heterogeneous group of inherited diseases of peripheral nerve, and is a fairly common neuropathy affecting both children and adults. There is an estimate that 1 in 2500 persons has a form of CMT, which can frequently lead to significant neuromuscular impairment. A majority of CMT patients have an autosomal dominant form of inheritance.[5]

Clinical Features

Distal muscle weakness and atrophy is seen in both the upper and lower extremities. There is diminished sensation, especially in the hands and feet. Abnormally hypoactive deep tendon reflexes at the ankle occur, and in those cases involving hypertrophic demyelinating neuropathy (onion bulbs), there is reduced nerve conduction velocity. Calf muscle wasting leads to thin "stork legs."

Muscle imbalance causing dynamic deformities in the child, adolescent, or adult can develop because of the underlying neuromuscular condition. When this is persistent and uncorrected, fixed deformities will ensue. The hands and feet are most commonly affected.[56,57] Occasionally, hip dysplasia is reported.[58] Spinal deformity (scoliosis or kyphoscoliosis) is seen in approximately 50 percent of the patients. Although, fortunately, this is not generally severe, severe scoliosis and kyphoscoliosis may require surgery if pulmonary function is compromised.[59] A severe spinal deformity also leads to pain. Deformities in the ankles and feet can give rise to pain and limitation in standing and walking. Weakness and foot deformities interfere with gait.

Young children with CMT disease may present as toe walkers. After the diagnosis is confirmed, toe walking can be corrected by serial casting. When such correction has been effective, it can be maintained by the use of high-top shoes and lightweight ankle-foot orthoses. Surgical correction such as lengthening of the tendo Achillis is not usually indicated. Because of intrinsic muscle weakness of the foot and also peroneal weakness, the characteristic pes cavus can occur, producing a foot that has a high arch with prominent metatarsal heads and abnormal areas of weight bearing. The deformity can progress to an equinovarus foot with claw toes.[60,61] Coleman's test may reveal deformity secondary to tight plantar fascia, requiring surgical correction.[62] Rebalancing the foot by transfer of the posterior tibial tendon may become necessary and claw

toes may also require surgical correction if ranging and stretching have not been effective.[5,56]

With further foot and ankle dorsiflexion weakness, frequent ankle sprains may occur. As the peroneal muscle becomes weaker, calluses develop on the lateral side of the midfoot.

Fixed foot deformities can occur with long-standing muscle imbalance. These are generally seen in the adolescent and older patient. Soft tissue releases and tendon transfers may no longer be sufficient or effective. Dwyer calcaneal osteotomy or wedge resection of the calcaneus may be required to correct the varus deformity of the heel. Midfoot and hindfoot deformities can be corrected by triple arthrodesis followed by muscle rebalancing.[63,64] Careful neurologic assessment and the use of a well-padded cast or a well-molded padded orthosis is important in the perioperative period and during postoperative care.

REFERENCES

1. Brooke MH: *A Clinician's View of Neuromuscular Diseases.* Baltimore, Williams & Wilkins, 1976.
2. Stedman H, Sarkar S: Molecular genetics in muscular dystrophy research: Revolutionary progress. *Muscle Nerve* 11:683, 1988.
3. Koenig M, Monaco AP, Kunkel LM: The complete sequence of dystrophin predicts a rod-shaped cytoskeletal protein. *Cell* 53:219, 1988.
4. Mendell JR, Sahenk Z, Prior TW: The childhood muscular dystrophies: Disease sharing a common pathogenesis of membrane instability. *J Child Neurol* 10:150, 1995.
5. Chance PF, Hsu JD: Inherited neuropathies. *Curr Opin Orthop* 6:100, 1995.
6. Shapiro F, Specht L: Current concepts review: The diagnosis and orthopedic treatment of inherited muscular diseases of childhood. *J Bone Joint Surg* 75A:439–454, 1993.
7. Iannaccone ST: Current status of Duchenne muscular dystrophy. *Pediatr Clin North Am* 39:879, 1992.
8. Blau HM, Springer ML: Molecular medicine—Muscle-mediated gene therapy. *N Engl J Med* 333:1554, 1995.
9. Specht LA, Kunkel LM: Duchenne and Becker muscular dystrophies, in Rosenberg RN, Prusiner SB, Dimauro S, et al (eds): *The Molecular and Genetic Basis of Neurological Disease.* Boston, Butterworth Heinemann, 1993, pp 613–631.
10. Hsu JD, Furumasu J: Gait and posture changes in the Duchenne muscular dystrophy child. *Clin Orthop Rel Res* 288:122, 1993.
11. Sutherland DH, Olshen R, Cooper L, et al: The pathomechanics of gait in Duchenne muscular dystrophy. *Dev Med Child Neurol* 23:3, 1981.
12. Soutter R: A new operation for hip contractures in poliomyelitis. *Boston Med Surg J* 170:380–381, 1914.
13. Bonnet I, Burgot D, Bonnard C, Glorion B: Surgery of the lower limbs in Duchenne muscular dystrophy. *French J Orthop Surg* 5:160–168, 1991.
14. Siegel IM, Miller JE, Ray RD: Subcutaneous lower limb tenotomy in the treatment of pseudohypertrophic muscular dystrophy. *J Bone Joint Surg* 50A:1437, 1968.
15. Spencer GE Jr: Orthopedic considerations in the management of muscular dystrophy. *Curr Pract Orthop Surg* 5:279, 1973.
16. Roy L, Gibson D: Pseudohypertrophic muscular dystrophy and its surgical management: Review of 30 patients. *Can J Surg* 13:13, 1970.

17. Hsu JD: Management of foot deformity in Duchenne's pseudo-hypertrophic muscular dystrophy. *Orthop Clin North Am* 7:979, 1976.

18. Hsu JD, Hoffer MM: Posterior tibial tendon transfer anteriorly through the interosseous membrane. *Clin Orthop* 131:202, 1978.

19. Melkonian G, Cristofaro R, Perry J, Hsu JD: Use of dynamic gait electromyography in neuromuscular disease patients. *Foot Ankle* 1:78, 1980.

20. Hsu JD, Taylor D: Upper extremity deformities in Duchenne muscular dystrophy patients, in Fredricks D, Brody GS (eds): *Symposium on the Neurological Aspects of Plastic Surgery.* St Louis, Mosby, 1978.

21. Hsu JD: The natural history of spinal curve progression in the non-ambulatory Duchenne muscular dystrophy patient. *Spine* 7:771, 1983.

22. Luque ED, Cardoso A: Sequential correction of scoliosis with rigid internal fixation. *Orthop Trans* 1:136, 1977.

23. Hsu JD: The development of current approaches to the management of spinal deformity for patients with neuromuscular disease. *Semin Neurol* 15:24, 1995.

24. Siegel IM: Spinal stabilization in Duchenne muscular dystrophy: Rationale and method. *Muscle Nerve* 5:417, 1982.

25. Sakai D, Hsu JD, Bonnett C, Brown JC: Stabilization of the collapsing spine in Duchenne muscular dystrophy. *Clin Orthop Rel Res* 128:256, 1977.

26. Hsu JD: Spine care of the patient with Duchenne muscular dystrophy. *Spine* 4:161, 1990.

27. Smith AD, Koreska J, Moseley CF: Progression of scoliosis in Duchenne muscular dystrophy. *J Bone Joint Surg* 71A:1066, 1989.

28. Granata C, Merlini L, Cervellati S, et al: Long term results of spine surgery in Duchenne muscular dystrophy. *Neuromusc Disord* 6:61, 1996.

29. Hoffman EP, Fischbeck KH, Brown RH, et al: Characterization of dystrophin in muscle biopsy specimens from patients with Duchenne's or Becker's muscular dystrophy. *N Engl J Med* 318:1363, 1988.

30. Hoffman EP, Kunkel LM, Angelini C, et al: Improved diagnosis of Becker muscular dystrophy by dystrophin testing. *Neurology* 39:1011–1017, 1989.

31. Dennan JC: *Orthopedic Management of Neuromuscular Disorders.* Philadelphia, Lippincott, 1983.

32. Shapiro F, Bresnan MJ: Orthopedic management of childhood neuromuscular disease: Part III. Diseases of muscle. *J Bone Joint Surg* 64A:1102, 1982.

33. Letournel E, Fardeau M, Lytle JO, et al: Scapulothoracic arthrodesis for patients who have facio-scapulo-humeral muscular dystrophy. *J Bone Joint Surg* 72A:78–84, 1990.

34. Ketenjian AY: Scapulocostal stabilization for scapular winging in facio-scapulo-humeral muscular dystrophy. *J Bone Joint Surg* 60A:478–480, 1978.

35. Dubowitz V: *Muscle Disorders in Childhood,* 2d ed. London, Saunders, 1995.

36. Chyatte SB, Vignos PJ Jr, Watkins M: Early muscular dystrophy: Differential patterns of weakness in Duchenne, limb-girdle and facioscapulohumeral types. *Arch Phys Med Rehabil* 47:499, 1966.

37. Dubowitz V: *Color Atlas of Muscle Disorders in Childhood.* Chicago, Year Book, 1989.

38. Shy GM, Magee KR: A new congenital non-progressive myopathy. *Brain* 79:610, 1956.

39. Spiro AJ, Shy GM, Gonatoas NK: Myotubular myopathy: Persistence of fetal muscle in an adolescent boy. *Arch Neurol* 14:1–14, 1966.

40. Oh SJ: *Clinical Electromyography.* Baltimore, University Park Press, 1984.

41. Stalberg E: The motor unit: Electromyography, in Swash M, Kennard C (eds): *The Scientific Bases of Clinical Neurology.* Edinburgh, Churchill Livingstone, 1985.

42. Mastaglia FL: Structure and function of skeletal muscle, in Swash M, Kennard C (eds): *Scientific Basis of Clinical Neurology.* Edinburgh, Churchill Livingstone, 1985.

43. Harper PS, Dyken PR: Early onset dystrophia myotonica: Evidence supporting a maternal environmental factor. *Lancet* 2:53–55, 1972.

44. Vignos PJ, Spencer GE, Archibald KC: Management of progressive muscular dystrophy in childhood. *JAMA* 184:89, 1963.

45. Dubowitz V, Brooke MH: *Muscle Biopsy: A Modern Approach.* London, Saunders, 1973.

46. Von Eulenburg A: Uber eine familiare durch 6 Generationen verfolgbare Form congenitaler paramytonia. *Neuro Zentralbl* 5:265, 1886.

47. Evans GA, Drennan JC, Russman BS: Functional classification and orthopaedic management of spinal muscular atrophy. *J Bone Joint Surg* 63B:516, 1981.

48. Hsu JD: Grollman TB: Orthopedic care of the spinal muscular atrophy child. *J Neurol Orthop Surg* 1:47, 1979.

49. Schwentker EP, Gibson DA: The orthopedic aspects of spinal muscular atrophy. *J Bone Joint Surg* 58A:32, 1976.

50. Granata C, Merlini L, Magni E, et al: Spinal muscular atrophy: Natural history and orthopedic treatment of scoliosis. *Spine* 14:760, 1989.

51. Daher YH, Lonstein JE, Winter RB, Bradford DS: Spinal surgery in spinal muscular atrophy. *J Pediatr Orthop* 5:391, 1985.

52. Hsu JD: Extremity fractures in children with neuromuscular disease. *Johns Hopkins Med J* 145:89, 1979.

53. Furumasu J, Swank SM, Brown JC, et al: Functional activities in spinal muscular atrophy patients after spinal fusion. *Spine* 14:771, 1989.

54. Hall JG: Genetic aspects of arthrogryposis. *Clin Orthop* 194:44–53, 1985.

55. Thomsen GH, Bilenker RM: Comprehensive management of arthrogryposis. *Clin Orthop* 194:6–14, 1985.

56. Hsu JD: *Orthopedic Care for Children and Adolescents with Charcot-Marie-Tooth Disorders: Pathophysiology, Molecular Genetics, and Therapy.* New York, Wiley-Liss, 1990.

57. Brown RE, Zamboni WA, Zook ET, Russell RC: Evaluation and management of upper extremity neuropathies in Charcot-Marie-Tooth disease. *J Hand Surg Am* 17:523, 1992.

58. Kumar SJ, Marks HG, Bowen JR, MacEwen GD: Hip dysplasia associated with Charcot-Marie-Tooth disease in the older child and adolescent. *J Pediatr Orthop* 5:511, 1985.

59. Hensinger RN, MacEwen GD: Spinal deformity associated with heritable neurological conditions: Spinal muscular atrophy, Friedrich's ataxia, familia dysautonomia and Charcot-Marie-Tooth disease. *J Bone Joint Surg* 58A:13, 1976.

60. Sabir M, Lyttle D: Pathogenesis of pes cavus in Charcot-Marie-Tooth disease. *Clin Orthop Rel Res* 175:173, 1983.

61. Holmes JR, Hansen ST: Foot and ankle manifestations of Charcot-Marie-Tooth disease. *Foot Ankle* 14:476, 1993.

62. Coleman SS, Chestnut WJ: A simple test for hindfoot flexibility in the cavovarus foot. *Clin Orthop* 123:60, 1977.

63. Mann DC, Hsu JD: Triple arthrodesis in treatment of fixed cavovarus deformity in adolescent patients with Charcot-Marie-Tooth disease. *Foot Ankle* 13:1, 1992.

64. Chance PE, Hsu JD: Inherited neuropathy: Genetics and orthopaedic aspects. *Curr Opin Orthop* 6:100, 1995.

CHAPTER 36

Arthrogryposis

Dennis P. Grogan

Arthrogryposis is a nonspecific term describing conditions characterized by congenital, nonprogressive limitation of movement due to soft tissue contractures affecting two or more joints.[1] This clinical finding is known to have many causes.[2]

NOMENCLATURE

The term *arthrogryposis* was coined by Stern, who first called this condition *arthrogryposis multiplex congenita*.[1] Today, however, the term *arthrogryposis* has been extended to refer to a spectrum of clinical presentations with congenital soft tissue contractures. Unfortunately, the orthopaedist, the neurologist, and the geneticist see these children and tend to recognize and concentrate on different portions of this spectrum of conditions, so that the term *arthrogryposis* has come to mean different things to different medical specialists.[3] The genetic literature lists as many as 150 conditions under the term *arthrogryposis*.[2] Multiple pterygium syndrome, congenital contractural arachnodactyly, Larsen syndrome, Freeman-Sheldon whistling face syndrome, and diastrophic dysplasia are examples of arthrogrypotic syndromes.

The most common presentation is most accurately referred to as *amyoplasia* and represents approximately 40 percent of patients with arthrogryposis as delineated by studies of large populations in clinical genetics clinics.[1] These children present with extensive contractures of both the upper and lower extremities and represent the classic description of the child with arthrogryposis seen in the pediatric orthopaedic clinic. Amyoplasia was first defined as this specific arthrogrypotic condition by Hall, Reed, and Driscoll in 1983.[1]

The typical child with amyoplasia presents with adduction–internal rotation of the shoulders, fixed flexion or extension contractures of the elbows, rigid palmar flexion–ulnar deviation or dorsiflexion–radial deviation deformities of the wrists, thumb-in-palm deformity, rigid interphalangeal joints, flexion-abduction–external rotation hip contractures with dislocation of one or both hips, fixed extension or flexion contractures of the knees, and severe, rigid bilateral foot deformities, most commonly clubfoot (Fig. 36-1). Normal skin creases are absent and the limbs have a rather tubular appearance. Dimples are commonly present over the joints. Intelligence is within the normal range.

Distal arthrogryposis refers to a specific autosomal dominant disorder characterized by predominant involvement of the distal aspects of both the upper and lower extremities, with preservation of good muscle development in the upper arm and leg (Fig. 36-2). These children often have deformities of the hands and feet similar to those of children with amyoplasia but less of the other typical findings listed above; they also have normal intelligence. Distal arthrogryposis type I has hand involvement in 98 percent of cases, with a typical flexed-fist deformity with overlapping fingers and adduction of the thumb, with simian creases and absent distal interphalangeal creases. Growth, occupational therapy, and use are said to improve function for these upper extremity deformities. The feet are found to be involved in 87.5 percent of cases, with typical calcaneovalgus, equinovarus, vertical talus, or planovalgus deformities that most often require surgical correction.[4] Type II distal arthrogryposis has additional features involving other systems and body parts and has been further classified into five subtypes.[4]

PATHOLOGY

The muscle tissue in the affected areas is replaced partially or completely by fibrofatty tissue. This lack of normally elastic muscle tissue causes the soft tissue contractures and the restricted joint motion, making restoration of joint motion difficult and recurrence of the deformity so common. It is also responsible for the doughy appearance of the soft tissues of these children.

ETIOLOGY

Because of the variety and heterogeneity of the clinical presentations, no one cause is accepted for all children with arthrogryposis. Most authors agree that a diminution of intrauterine movement is the final common pathway leading to arthrogryposis.[3] Shapiro and Specht[3] have divided the causative factors into *intrinsic* and *extrinsic* factors; the time of occurrence during the pregnancy, the regions involved, and the intermittent or continual nature of the causative factors would appear to contribute to the degree of involvement.

Intrinsic causes, or abnormalities of the embryo, are divided into those secondary to neuropathic, myopathic, or fibropathic causes. Neuropathic disorders comprise brain or spinal cord anomalies. Myopathic disorders include the congenital myopathies or congenital muscular dystrophy. The fibropathic abnormalities are those contractural connective tissue syndromes with normal nerve and muscle when examined in areas away from the fibrotic regions. These intrinsic events can also include injury to the spinal cord or muscles due to a virus, a teratogen, a local uterine environmental factor, or a metabolic disorder, among others.[5]

Extrinsic causes are abnormalities of the uterine environment, such as oligohydramnios or structural uterine abnormalities such as a bicornuate uterus, that cause a diminution of movement of an otherwise normally developing embryo. Prenatal diagnosis of arthrogryposis by ultrasonography in the second trimester is now possible, and several cases have been reported.[6,7]

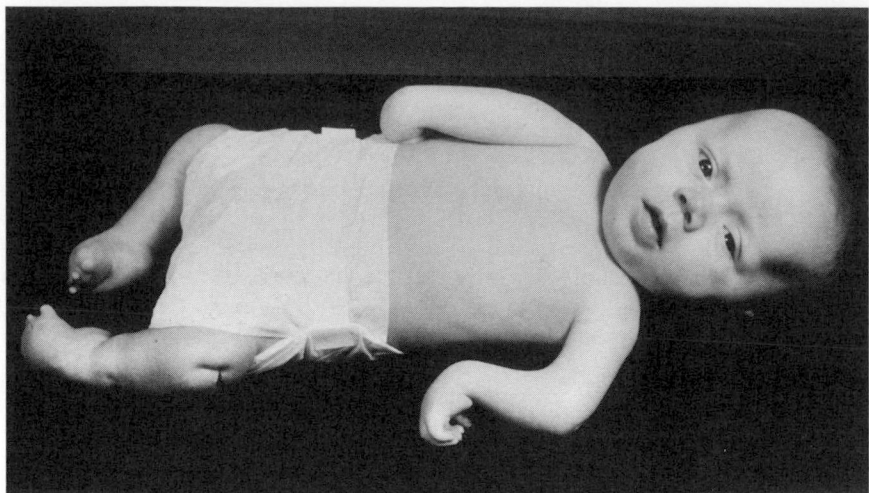

Figure 36-1 Photograph of a 6-month-old infant with amyoplasia. Note the typical elbow, wrist, and hand deformities with bilateral rigid clubfeet and toe deformities. There is a deep dimple over his left knee.

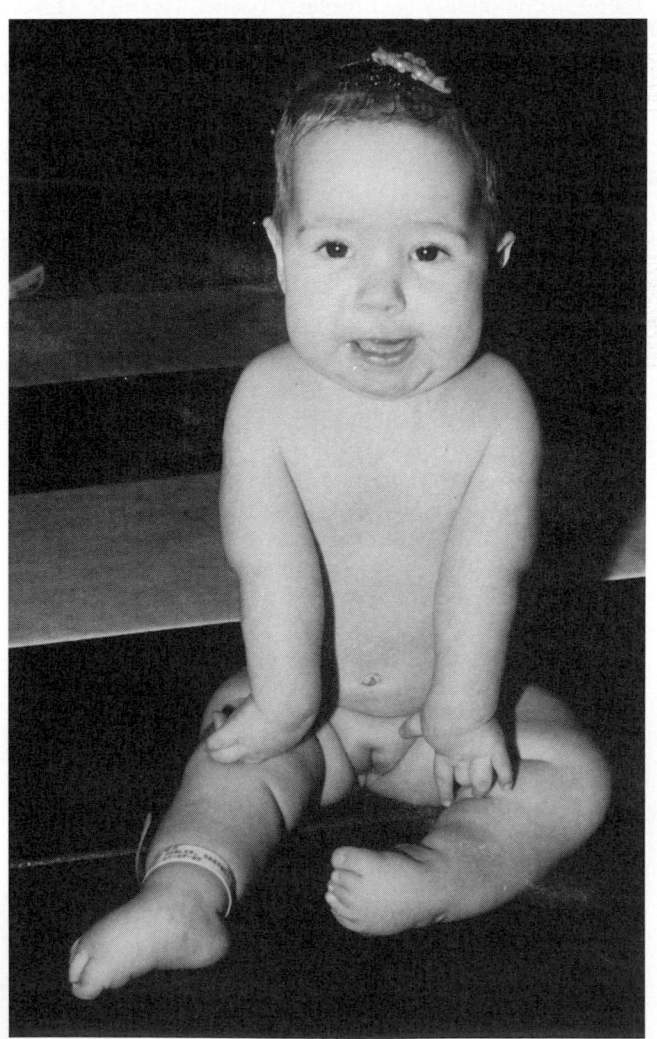

Figure 36-2 Fifteen-month-old child with distal arthrogryposis. Note typical flexed wrists, right planovalgus foot, and a left equinovarus foot deformity.

INHERITANCE PATTERNS

Amyoplasia, the most common form of arthrogryposis, is considered a sporadic condition. There have been no reports of involvement in first-degree relatives of affected children,[1] and affected persons have borne normal children. Distal arthrogryposis (both types I and II) is considered an autosomal dominant condition with variable expressivity.[8]

INITIAL EVALUATION

A complete physical examination and history is important. The history should include gestational, birth, and family history. An evaluation by a clinical geneticist is beneficial to the parents, so that they can better understand the condition and be better informed regarding future pregnancies and family planning, particularly for those types of arthrogryposis with known inheritance patterns (i.e., distal arthrogryposis). A pediatric neurological consultation can be helpful to evaluate the associated hypotonia and weakness and evaluate any underlying neuromuscular causes. The neurologist can then determine the degree of neurologic workup needed in each individual child. This information can be helpful in defining the diagnosis more accurately.

ORTHOPAEDIC TREATMENT
General

The overall goal of treatment should be to maximize the potential for function in each individual child. This goal can best be met through a team approach that includes physical and occupational therapy, splinting, casting, bracing (often long term), and surgical intervention on both the soft tissues and the bony elements. Although many children will be able to walk with the appropriate intervention and assistance, this should not necessarily be the ultimate goal in all affected children. The degree of involvement along with any other associated anomalies, particularly central nervous system abnormalities, will determine each child's potential degree of function. Treatment is aimed at improving the child's ability to perform activities of daily living (ADLs), so as to allow as much independence as possible.

Fractures

At the time of birth, the rigid joint contractures often make for a difficult delivery, which makes the incidence of birth-related fractures higher. The relative disuse and decreased weight bearing in these children during infancy and early childhood make their bones more susceptible to fracture secondary to the disuse osteopenia. Standard techniques of fracture treatment are utilized with some modification, depending on the degree of function in the affected bone or limb. Most fractures can be treated with closed reduction as needed, followed by splinting or casting until healing is achieved.

Spine

Scoliosis is seen in up to one-third of patients with amyoplasia. The curve is often first seen quite early in life, but it can present in childhood or adolescence. The scoliosis is neuromuscular in pattern and behavior and is not usually associated with congenital skeletal abnormalities. As with all of the other deformities noted, the curve is often rigid. Bracing is indicated within the usual parameters but is often unsuccessful in preventing progression of the deformity.[9] If surgical intervention is indicated, posterior fusion with or without anterior release and fusion is appropriate, with instrumentation dependent on the curve pattern and the age of the child.

Upper Extremities

Everything should be done to maximize the child's functional independence. This should be the goal of any therapy—splinting, bracing, or surgery on the child's upper extremities. Passive stretching program is of benefit.[10] It is also important to consider the compensatory mechanisms these children develop in their upper extremities and the fact that function must not be diminished for the sake of appearance.[3]

The shoulder is typically adducted and internally rotated. Deltoid weakness adds to the decreased function. Extension contractures of the elbow with weakness of the biceps and brachialis are common findings and can be a significant limitation to the child's ability to get the hands

to the mouth and face, or for other ADLs. The wrist is most commonly flexed and ulnarly deviated, with stiff finger joints in moderate degrees of flexion.

Although surgical procedures have often been recommended for these deformities, each child must be evaluated individually, with a heavy emphasis on improving function and/or independence before recommending a specific surgical treatment. Rotational osteotomies of the proximal humerus can correct the internally rotated shoulder. Posterior capsulotomy of the elbow can release the extension contracture with either tenotomy, lengthening, or transfer of the triceps tendon, depending on its strength and function. Mennen[11] has recommended a rather aggressive surgical approach to these deformities, his best results having been achieved with surgery at 3 to 6 months of age. He recommends a proximal row carpectomy and transfer of the wrist flexors to the extensor surface of the metacarpals to achieve wrist extension, transfer of the triceps to the neck of the radius, and a posterior capsulotomy of the elbow joint. Again, careful and individual evaluation of each child should occur before this or any other surgical intervention is recommended. Due to the nature of the deformities and the inelasticity of the soft tissues in these children, the response to surgical intervention meant to increase motion or function is often unpredictable. Occupational therapy and prolonged splinting must be a part of the long-term treatment of all these children. Assistive devices provided by the occupational therapist or physiotherapist can often make a large difference in the ability of these children to function independently.

Hips

Soft tissue contractures about the hip are seen in nearly all patients with arthrogryposis, most commonly involving flexion, abduction, and external rotation. The goal of treating such problems should be to obtain a functional position for the hip that will accommodate the child's maximal potential and not be a deterrent to future independence. Passive stretching can often improve the functional range of motion.[10] Soft tissue releases can then supplement this improvement. Alignment can be improved with extension osteotomies of the proximal femur with varus-producing osteotomies to decrease the abduction.

The incidence of hip dislocations in children with amyoplasia has been reported to be between 14 and 42 percent in various series.[12] The child with a unilateral hip dislocation should be treated with open reduction and appropriate releases and/or osteotomies. Either a medial or an anterolateral surgical approach may be used. Given the high rate of failure, increased stiffness, and ischemic necrosis reported with attempts to replace both hips into the acetabulum, bilateral dislocations are often better treated with soft tissue releases done to improve motion and function.

Knees

Knee involvement is common, documented in 89 of 104 patients by Thomas et al.,[13] in 40 of 82 patients by Gibson

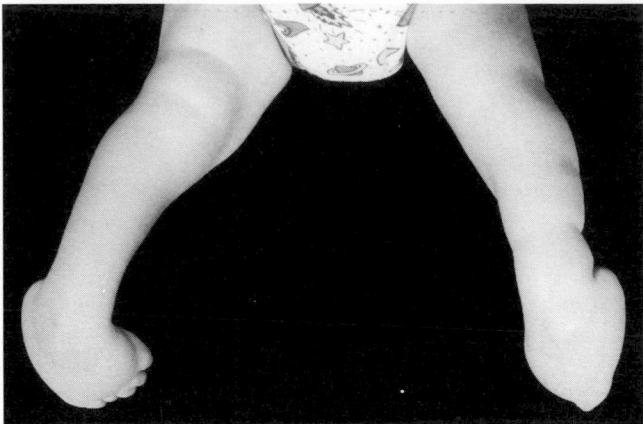

Figure 36-3 Bilateral knee extension deformities with bilateral rigid equinovarus foot deformities in an 8-month-old infant.

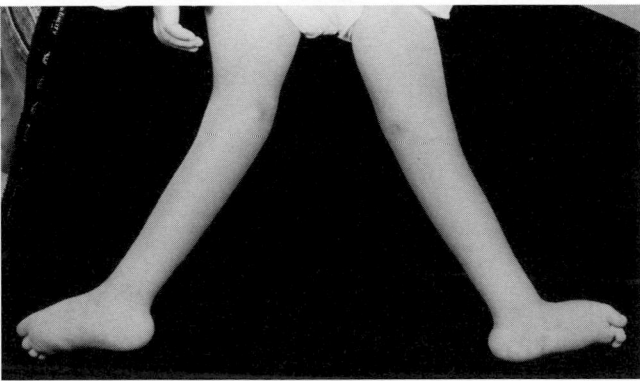

Figure 36-4 Bilateral knee extension deformities with bilateral planovalgus foot deformities in a 2-year-old child. The genu valgum due to the tight iliotibial band and the loss of normal skin creases can also be appreciated.

et al.,[14] and in 30 of 50 patients by Sodergard and Ryoppy.[15] The deformity is either a flexion or extension contracture (Figs. 36-3, 36-4, and 36-5). The extension deformity appears to be slightly more common, but the flexion contracture appears to be the more difficult to correct and maintain correction. Muscle imbalance has been postulated as the cause of this deformity.[15,16]

Initial treatment of the extension contracture should consist of serial manipulation into flexion, physical therapy, and serial casting as necessary. This approach led to a good result in 11 of 17 children in both the early and late evaluation of these patients.[15] A relationship has also been noted between the extension contracture and patella alta, with an increased incidence of chondromalacia patella.[15] A possibly increased incidence in degenerative changes of the articular surfaces of the knee joint was also noted. Whether this was related to the contracture itself or the forceful manipulations that were often performed in these knees was not clear.[15]

Extension contractures that are resistant to nonsurgical treatment can be corrected with a V-Y quadricep-

splasty.[16] This will include sectioning of the iliotibial band, if needed, for correction of the concomitant valgus tethering. Postoperative casting followed by a knee-ankle-foot orthosis (KAFO) will allow for the best maintenance of the correction obtained surgically. Time spent in the KAFO should be split between maximal flexion and extension to maintain the full range and not substitute one deformity for another. Flexion contractures will often require a complete posterior release of the popliteal fossa, including the medial and lateral hamstrings, the adjacent soft tissues, and the knee joint capsule. This procedure will again require long-term bracing postoperatively.

Feet

Foot deformity is seen in a majority of patients with arthrogryposis and the foot is considered the site of the most common deformity in these children. It is also likely to be the dominant orthopaedic deformity during the first year of life.[17] Treatment of these foot deformities is indicated to maximize the child's potential for standing and walking. The most common type of foot deformity is a clubfoot. Planovalgus foot deformity and vertical talus deformities are also frequently seen in these children. All of these conditions are rigid and ultimately resistant to nonoperative treatment. However, the initial treatment remains serial manipulation and casting in order to stretch the soft tissues as much as possible, with the knowledge that operative intervention will likely be necessary, particularly for the clubfoot and the vertical talus. The parents should be advised of this situation early on in the treatment, so that they understand the goal of each aspect of treatment.

Clubfoot

A flexible, nonpainful, plantigrade foot that accommodates an orthosis and/or regular shoes should be the goal of

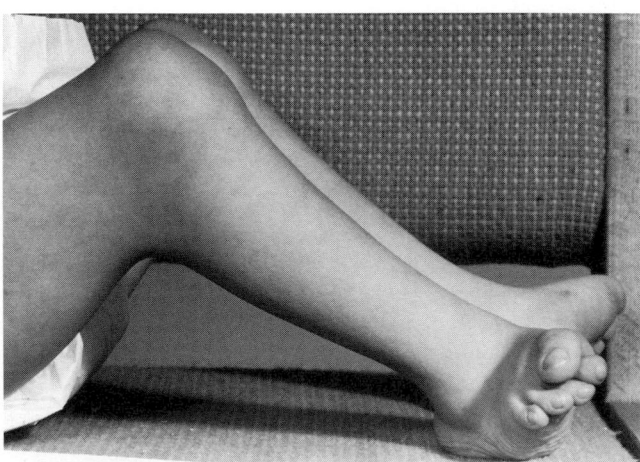

Figure 36-5 Bilateral knee flexion deformities with bilateral planovalgus foot deformities and overlapping toes in a 3-year-old child.

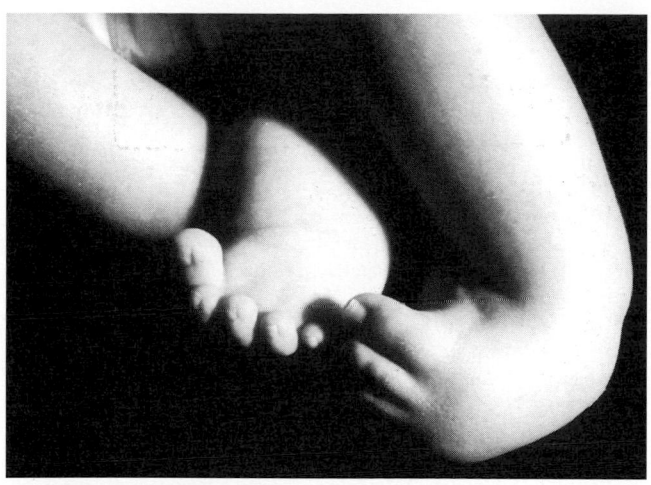

Figure 36-6 Rigid bilateral equinovarus foot deformities with lack of normal skin creases. Note smooth, doughy-appearing soft tissues.

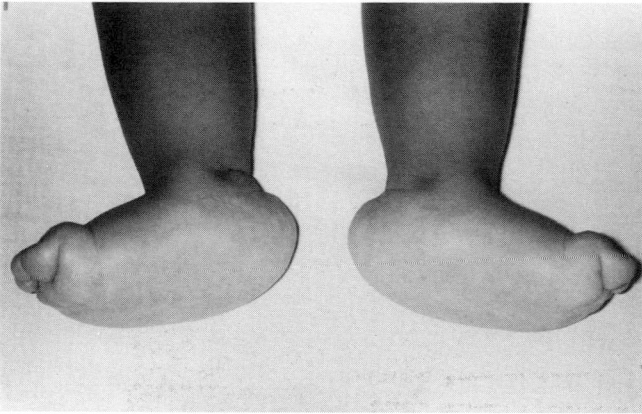

Figure 36-7 One-year-old child with bilateral vertical talus deformities. Note the typical rocker-bottom appearance to the plantar aspect of the feet.

treatment of these rigidly deformed feet. The foot should be manipulated and casted out of its equinovarus position as soon after birth as possible. The rigidity of the soft tissue contractures makes this difficult (Fig. 36-6). Although correction of the hindfoot deformities is usually not obtained, improvement of the forefoot adductus can be seen. Besides the typical contractures seen in an idiopathic clubfoot, these children have an increased amount of midfoot and forefoot equinus or cavus with significant flexion deformity of the toes. After a period of several months of serial manipulation and casting, surgical correction is indicated in nearly all of these children. A soft tissue release with correction of the posterior, medial, plantar, and lateral deformities is recommended. Most often those tendons that are usually lengthened in an idiopathic clubfoot should be released and not repaired. These tendons are often nonfunctional in these feet and can act as a future soft tissue tether to increase the chance of recurrent deformity. Often significant deformity of the talus is also encountered, again more than that seen in the idiopathic clubfoot. If this extensive soft tissue release yields a plantigrade foot, postoperative casting for a period of 3 to 4 months to allow for cartilaginous and bony remodeling is recommended, followed by long-term control with an ankle-foot orthosis (AFO). If the deformities are not corrected satisfactorily after this procedure, a talectomy or talar enucleation is indicated. Previous studies have obtained satisfactory results with these procedures.[17–19] Solund et al.[17] reported 14 of 17 patients with satisfactory feet after a mean follow-up of 13 years posttalectomy. All but one of these patients had soft tissue releases prior to talectomy. Older children or adolescents with persistent deformity may require a triple arthrodesis.

Vertical Talus

The child with a vertical talus deformity should receive the same initial manipulation and casting treatment as the child with a clubfoot. All of these children will, however, require soft tissue release after this initial soft tissue stretching (Fig. 36-7). The age for surgical treatment will be determined by the surgeon's experience and preference. The author prefers surgery at 8 to 9 months of age, so that, after the 3 to 4 months of postoperative casting, the child will be ready to do some weight bearing with either standing or walking. The anterolateral and posterior soft tissue release described and popularized by Coleman et al.[20] has shown proven ability to correct the multiple deformities in these feet. If the correction is not attempted until after the child is past 24 months of age, Coleman et al. recommends a subtalar bone block (extraarticular talocalcaneal arthrodesis) in addition to the soft tissue release and bony realignment.[20] Resistant or recurrent deformities may require a talectomy to obtain a plantigrade foot. All children will require long-term orthotic control of the corrected deformity for the best chance of maintaining correction. Older children or adolescents with persistent deformity may require a triple arthrodesis.

SUMMARY

Although the term *arthrogryposis* has been firmly ensconced in the orthopaedic terminology, most of the classically affected patients seen in the orthopaedic clinic setting would be better described as having amyoplasia, one of the many arthrogrypotic conditions. Children with distal arthrogryposis or one of the many other conditions with arthrogrypotic features will have problems similar to those of children with amyoplasia, but they will have fewer deformities or their deformities will be in association with other medical problems. These children and young adults have a variety of orthopaedic disorders that can be improved with the appropriate intervention, but always with the goal of improving their function and ultimately their independence. Careful evaluation and treatment by a team of medical specialists—including the orthopaedic surgeon and other health-care providers—can provide significant assistance for these children and their families (Fig. 36-8).

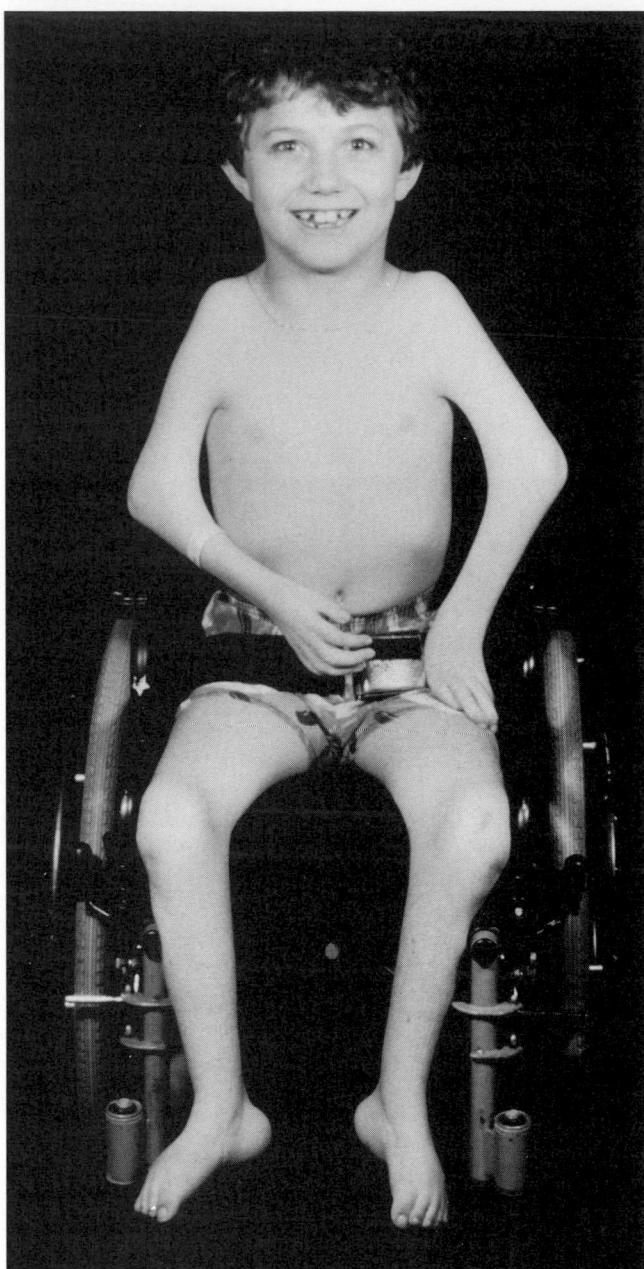

Figure 36-8 Ten-year-old boy with amyoplasia. Internal rotation at the shoulders, webbing at the elbows and knees, and a repaired clubfoot deformity can be seen. This young man is quite functional in his power wheelchair and uses reciprocal gait orthoses to ambulate.

ACKNOWLEDGMENT   The author would like to thank Linda Pugh, RN, Claire Kenneally, MS, Janet Barber, Patti Barber, and the Media Resources Department, all of the Shriners Hospital, Tampa, Florida, for their assistance with the preparation of this manuscript.

REFERENCES

1. Hall JG, Reed SD, Driscoll EP: Part I. Amyoplasia: A common, sporadic condition with congenital contractures. *Am J Med Genet* 15:571–590, 1983.
2. Hall JG: Genetic aspects of arthrogryposis. *Clin Orthop* 194:44–53, 1985.
3. Shapiro F, Specht L: Current concepts review: The diagnosis and orthopaedic treatment of childhood spinal muscular atrophy, peripheral neuropathy, Friedreich ataxia, and arthrogryposis. *J Bone Joint Surg* 75A:1699–1714, 1993.
4. Hall JG, Reed SD, Green G: The distal arthrogryposes: Delineation of new entities—Review and nosologic discussion. *Am J Med Genet* 11:185–239, 1982.
5. Sarwark JF, MacEwen GD, Scott CI: Current concepts review: Amyoplasia (a common form of arthrogryposis). *J Bone Joint Surg* 72A:465–469, 1990.
6. Baty BJ, Cubberley D, Morris C, Carey J: Prenatal diagnosis of distal arthrogryposis. *Am J Med Genet* 29:501–510, 1988.
7. Bui T-H, Lindholm H, Demir N, Thomasen P: Prenatal diagnosis of distal arthrogryposis type I by ultrasonography. *Prenat Diagn* 12:1047–1053, 1992.
8. McCusick MK, Coppola-McCormack PJ, Lee MI: Autosomal dominant inheritance of distal arthrogryposis. *Am J Med Genet* 6:163–169, 1980.
9. Daher YH, Lonstein JE, Winter RB, Moe JH: Spinal deformities in patients with arthrogryposis: A review of 16 patients. *Spine* 10:609–613, 1985.
10. Palmer PM, MacEwen GD, Bowen JR, Mathews PA: Passive motion therapy for infants with arthrogryposis. *Clin Orthop* 194:54–59, 1985.
11. Mennen U: Early corrective surgery of the wrist and elbow in arthrogryposis multiplex congenita. *J Hand Surg* 18B:304–307, 1993.
12. Staheli LT, Chew DE, Elliott JS, Mosca VS: Management of hip dislocations in children with arthrogryposis. *J Pediatr Orthop* 7:681–685, 1987.
13. Thomas B, Schopler S, Wood W, Oppenheim WL: The knee in arthrogryposis. *Clin Orthop* 194:87–92, 1985.
14. Gibson DA, Urs NDK: Arthrogryposis multiplex congenita. *J Bone Joint Surg (Br)* 52:483–493, 1970.
15. Sodergard J, Ryoppy S: The knee in arthrogryposis multiplex congenita. *J Pediatr Orthop* 10:177–182, 1990.
16. Curtis BH, Fisher RI: Congenital hyperextension with anterior subluxation of the knee: Surgical treatment and long-term observations. *J Bone Joint Surg* (Am) 51:255–269, 1969.
17. Solund K, Sonne-Holm S, Kjolbye JE: Talectomy for equinovarus deformity in arthrogryposis. *Acta Orthop Scand* 62:372–374, 1991.
18. Guidera KJ, Drennan JC: Foot and ankle deformities in arthrogryposis multiplex congenita. *Clin Orthop* 194:93–98, 1985.
19. Sodergard J, Ryoppy S: Foot deformities in arthrogryposis multiplex congenita. *J Pediatr Orthop* 14:768–772, 1994.
20. Coleman SS, Stelling FH, Jarrett J: Pathomechanics and treatment of congenital vertical talus. *Clin Orthop* 70:62–72, 1970.

CHAPTER 37

Skeletal Dysplasias and Dwarfism

Dennis P. Grogan and Abraham Ganel

Over 125 different disorders form the group of human skeletal dysplasias. Most of these produce disproportionate short stature and associated skeletal deformities. A list of all known common and uncommon disorders can be found in various sources (see "Recommended Reading" at the end of this chapter). There is also a computer software program that enables the clinician to follow a methodical step-by-step process toward making a diagnosis of a particular syndrome or dysplasia in any child with a known set of abnormalities based on clinical and radiographic findings.[1] The purpose of this chapter is to discuss the more common skeletal dysplasias and to focus on currently known orthopaedic and/or medical treatment recommendations. Included is current knowledge on the treatment of short stature and current data on prenatal diagnosis of bone dysplasias.

BIOCHEMICAL MARKERS OF SKELETAL DYSPLASIAS

Biochemical studies are of diagnostic value in only a few of the skeletal dysplasias. Until recently, the basic biochemical defect had been discovered in only the mucopolysaccharidoses, mucolipidoses, and certain of the mineralization defects, such as hypophosphatasia, hypophosphatemic rickets, and vitamin D–dependent rickets.[2] Abnormalities in proteoglycan chemistry have been demonstrated in pseudoachondroplasia.[3] Structural abnormalities in the various collagens have been demonstrated in several of the dysplasias. Mutations along the COL 1A1 and COL 1A2 procollagen genes have been demonstrated in all four types of osteogenesis imperfecta.[4] Mutations in the COL 2A1 procollagen gene result in achondrogenesis, type II hypochondrogenesis, the spondyloepiphyseal dysplasias, Stickler syndrome, and precocious familial osteoarthropathy.[5-8] The gene for achondroplasia and hypochondroplasia (4p) as well as the gene causing multiple epiphyseal dysplasia (MED) or pseudoachondroplasia (19q) have recently been mapped; the gene and the two specific mutations causing achondroplasia have also been characterized in more detail.[2] These developments and other genetic work currently in progress will allow further exploration of these genes, their role in producing these disorders, improved prenatal diagnosis, and possibly eventual treatment options.

MANAGEMENT OF THE PATIENT WITH A SKELETAL DYSPLASIA

It is important to realize, and to convey to the parents, that at this time there is no known cure for any of these conditions. Orthopaedic, neurologic, and other systemic signs and symptoms must be recognized as early as possible in order to maintain function and minimize morbidity. Shohat and Rimoin have defined effective management of these children to include precise diagnosis, prompt recognition of specific skeletal and nonskeletal complications, appropriate orthopaedic and rehabilitative care, emotional support, and psychosocial and genetic counseling.[2] Prenatal diagnosis is now available for many of the skeletal dysplasias. The length of the femurs at 18 weeks may be used as an indicator of the more severe dysplasias. An atlas of normal fetal skeletal radiology has been published, and the number and types of dysplasias recognizable by ultrasound is increasing rapidly.[9,10]

ACHONDROPLASIA

Achondroplasia is the most common form of disproportionate short stature with rhizomelic (proximal) shortening of long bones. Its prevalence is estimated to be between 0.5 and 1.5 per 10,000 live births.[11]

Achondroplasia is an autosomal dominant condition, although most instances (around 80 percent) represent new mutations. Thus the risk of recurrence in a family with one affected child who represents a sporadic mutation is far below 1 percent.[12] The gene for achondroplasia (4pl6.3) has been mapped[13] and evidence points to mutations in the transmembrane domain of fibroblast growth factor receptor 3 (FGFR 3).[14]

In recent years prenatal diagnosis of achondroplasia has been possible based on ultrasound determination, at 18 weeks gestation, of femoral and humeral length.[9,15] Final patient height averages 131 cm in males and 129 cm in females. In Japan, similar figures were found for males with achondroplasia, whereas the female height averaged 124 cm.[16] Clinical features include typical facial changes such as macrocephaly, frontal bossing, saddle nose, maxillary hypoplasia, and mandibular prognathism. Short, broad hands with a wedge-shaped gap between the third and fourth fingers (trident hands), lumbar lordosis, and progressive genu varum are typical. Most individuals with achondroplasia have normal intelligence and normal life expectancy.[12] The characteristic radiographic features include a large calvarium, short base of skull, square-shaped pelvis, small sacrosciatic notch, short vertebral pedicles, and decreasing interpedicular distances in the lumbosacral spine. A typical V-shaped distal femoral epiphysis develops by midchildhood and the long bones are short and broad (Fig. 37-1A). Children with achondroplasia or other short-limb disorders may have difficulties in performing their activities of daily living and suffer from associated psychological stresses due to their extreme shortness of stature and limb disproportion.[17]

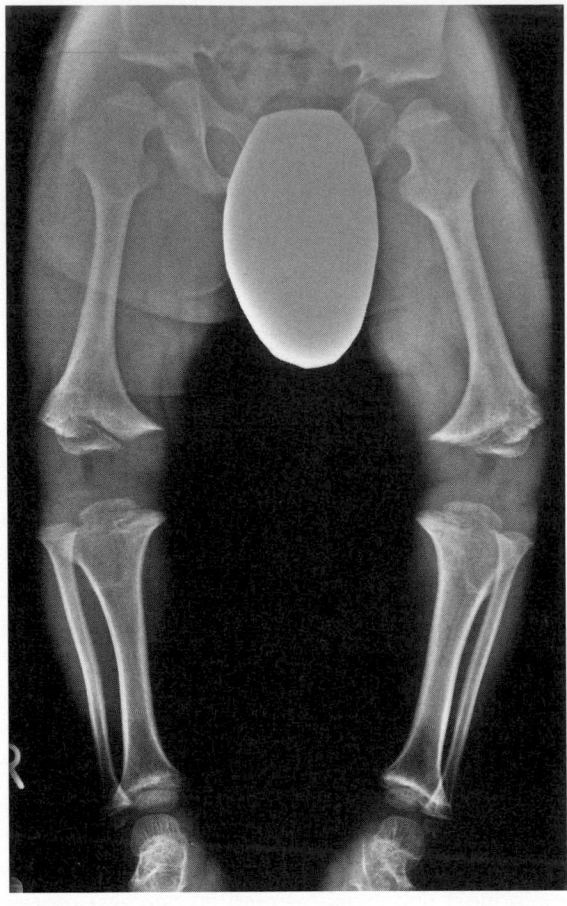

A

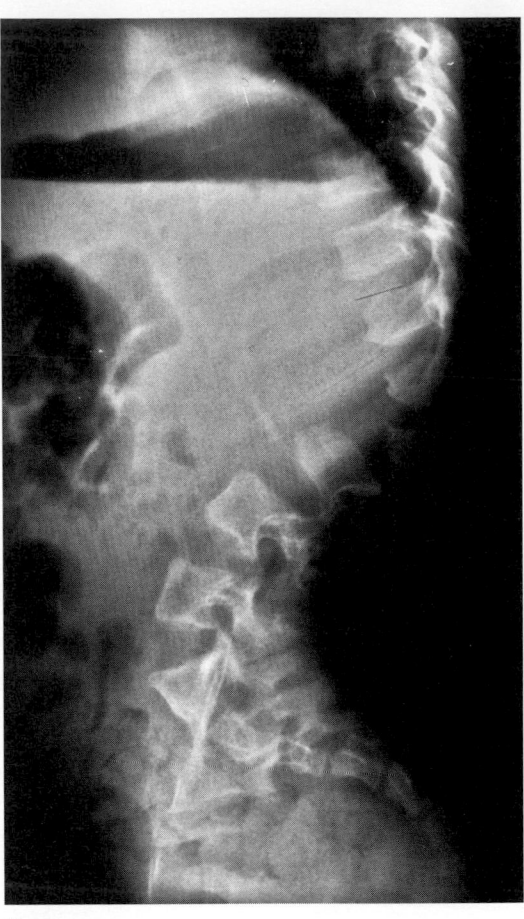

B

Figure 37-1 *A*. Four-year-old child with achondroplasia. The squared-off pelvis, typical V-shaped distal femoral epiphysis, genu varum, and relatively longer fibula can be seen. *B*. Three-year-old child with achondroplasia. Note the anterior wedging of the thoracolumbar vertebral bodies with kyphosis.

Treatment with human growth hormone (HGH) has been tried in achondroplasia, and a short-term beneficial effect has been reported. A multicenter study on HGH treatment for achondroplasia in which various doses of HGH were subcutaneously administered demonstrated that the effect of HGH on height gain is prominent in the first year but declines over time. No beneficial effect can be expected after 5 years of treatment. The expected height gain from HGH treatment over 5 years is approximately 7.5 cm. However there is a large variance in HGH's effect on individual patients.[16]

Surgical limb lengthening has been successfully applied for many years to patients with achondroplasia in Israel and Europe.[18] Various methods of elongation using different distraction devices have demonstrated the ability to correct body disproportion between limbs and trunk, correct axial deviation, and improve appearance. Experience with elongation of femurs, tibiae, and humeri have made it possible to accumulate data on expected complications and surgical strategies.[19,20] Studies have demonstrated that limb lengthening operations can have a positive impact on both body image and self-esteem in adolescents and young adults with achondroplasia.[21] This experience has not yet been embraced in North America.

In addition to decreased height and axial deformities of the lower extremity, many patients with achondroplasia suffer from symptoms related to the spine.[22] Narrowing of the foramen magnum can lead to constriction of the upper cervical cord and edema and or gliosis of the cervical-medullary cord secondary to bony compression,[23] sometimes requiring decompression of the foramen magnum. If thoracolumbar kyphosis remains greater than 40° by 5 or 6 years of age and is associated with a single wedge-shaped apical vertebra, surgery is advised[24] (Fig. 37-1*B*). Cervical and/or lumbar stenosis may also become symptomatic in young adults. The onset of symptoms in cases of spinal stenosis is usually slow, marked by progressive lower extremity weakness and intermittent claudication with or without neurologic deficit. Multiple-level laminectomies over the stenotic area are therapeutic and will usually relieve symptoms and prevent further neurologic compromise. Posterolateral fusion with or without spinal instrumentation may be required if spinal instability results.[24]

HYPOCHONDROPLASIA

Hypochondroplasia is an autosomal dominant condition with clinical findings similar to those of mild achondroplasia. It is a distinct skeletal dysplasia, however. The distinguishing clinical features of hypochondroplasia include later age at diagnosis due to the milder findings, greater adult height than achondroplasia, normal head and facial appearance, normal hand shape, and lack of neurologic problems in adulthood. The lumbar lordosis and bowing of the lower extremities may be present but are much milder than in achondroplasia.[25] There is a reported preponderance of affected females, a high incidence of spontaneous mutation, and higher than expected incidence of mental retardation.[25]

Roentgenographic findings include flaring at the metaphyseal-epiphyseal junction of the long bones, with squaring off of the epiphyses, and normal growth plates. The interpedicular distance is often narrower than normal but not as narrowed as in children with achondroplasia, and it is not associated with any neurologic changes in the cauda equina. The ankle is typically in varus with a long distal fibula.[26] These radiographic changes are mild and not as evident in infancy or early childhood, making the diagnosis not evident until later childhood.

PSEUDOCHONDROPLASIA (PSEUDOACHONDROPLASTIC DYSPLASIA)

This form of rhizomelic dwarfism has clinical characteristics of achondroplasia, with a normal-appearing head and face. It has also been referred to as the pseudoachondroplastic type of spondyloepiphyseal dysplasia (SED) and actually has characteristics of both SED and achondroplasia. Genetic transmission has been documented via both autosomal dominant and autosomal recessive patterns, with considerable variability of expression. Development is usually normal initially, but by 2 to 3 years the growth retardation and short stature become apparent. The child has a relatively long trunk, short extremities, increased lumbar lordosis, and radiographic evidence of platyspondyly. Epiphyseal and metaphyseal changes are widespread, but most notable at the proximal and distal femoral ossification centers. The resulting joint incongruity results in premature degeneration, and reconstructive surgery is often necessary.

THANATOPHORIC DYSPLASIA

This disorder was described by Maroteaux et al. in 1967[27] and named to emphasize the fact that affected patients usually die shortly after birth (*thanatophoric* is from the Greek meaning "death-bringing"). These infants have a severe growth deficiency, with short, bowed long bones and a narrowed thorax with short ribs, leading to pulmonary insufficiency. It is considered a sporadic dominant new mutation. No medical intervention toward survival is usually recommended.[28]

JEUNE'S THORACIC DYSTROPHY SYNDROME

This autosomal recessive condition has also been referred to as *asphyxiating thoracic dysplasia* due to the narrow thorax, short ribs, and frequent respiratory distress during the newborn period that often leads to death.[29] Some children do survive the newborn period and demonstrate progressive improvement in growth of the thoracic cage.[30] Radiographic abnormalities include short ribs with irregular costochondral junctions, a narrow thoracic cage, hypoplastic iliac wings with horizontal acetabular roofs, irregularities of the epiphyses and metaphyses, and shortening of the ulna and fibula (Fig. 37-2). Polydactyly of the feet and hands can be present.

SHORT RIB–POLYDACTYLY SYNDROME

The Majewski type of short rib–polydactyly syndrome is considered an autosomal recessive short-limb dwarfism that is incompatible with life. Death is secondary to pulmonary insufficiency shortly after birth. Pre- and postaxial polysyndactyly of both hands and feet; ovoid, short-

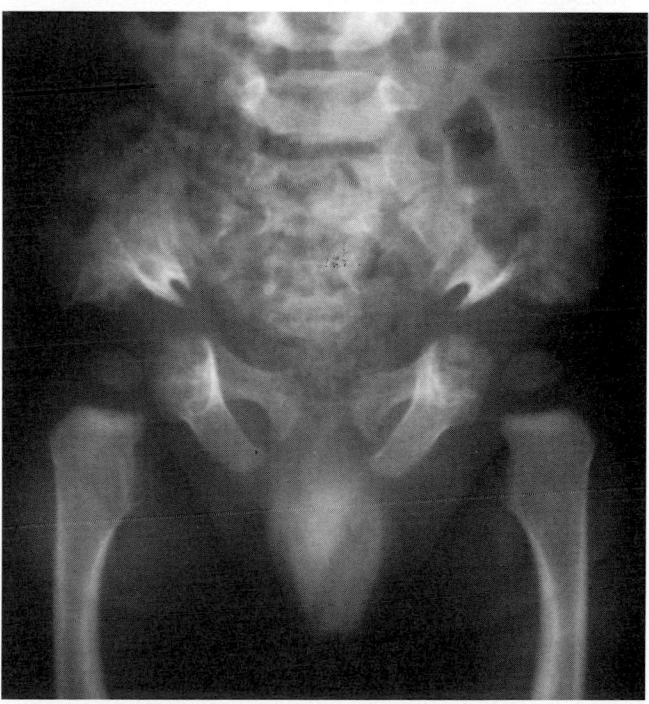

Figure 37-2 One-year-old child with Jeune thoracic dystrophy. Radiographic findings include the hypoplastic iliac wings with horizontal acetabular roofs.

ened tibiae; short, rounded metacarpals and metatarsals; a narrow thorax; and short, horizontal ribs are typical.[31]

SPONDYLOEPIPHYSEAL DYSPLASIA (CONGENITA AND TARDA)

Spondyloepiphyseal dysplasia congenita (SEDC) is an autosomal dominant dysplasia with variable phenotypic expression resulting in short-trunk dwarfism. The clinical variability of SEDC is probably the result of spot mutation affecting different loci of the type II collagen gene. Clinical features include a short trunk, barrel chest, increased thoracic kyphosis, marked lumbar lordosis, and short limbs with relatively normal hands and feet. Axial deviation of either genu varum or genu valgum, muscular hypotonia, a waddling gait, and early degenerative changes in the hips are common. Clubfoot and cleft palate may also present and require treatment. Myopia, retinal degeneration, and retinal detachment constitute the eye problems often encountered in these patients.[32] (Type II collagen is specific for cartilage and vitreous; this probably explains the above clinical features.)

Prenatal diagnosis has been reported—utilizing the ultrasound findings in the second and third trimesters of pregnancy—to include short long bones, flat hypoplastic vertebrae, and a small thorax.[33]

The radiographic appearance of the skeletal system includes delayed ossification of the pubis and the proximal and distal femoral epiphyses, pear-shaped vertebral bodies in infancy, flattening and irregularity of ossification centers in childhood, and severe vertebral flattening by adulthood. Dysplasia of the femoral head with progressive degeneration often requiring replacement arthroplasty is common (Fig. 37-3). Hypoplasia of the odontoid process may lead to cervical instability with spinal cord compression.

The orthopaedic evaluation of SEDC should include a careful neurologic assessment as well as flexion-extension lateral radiographs of the cervical spine to detect atlantoaxial instability, which can be a cause of cervical myelopathy in these children. The usual presentation is generally one of slowly progressive loss of motor strength. In these cases, stabilization of the cervical spine is required to prevent progressive neurologic loss or to facilitate neurologic recovery.[34]

The kyphosis and lumbar hyperlordosis are potential problems and require continued observation. Growth curves for height[35] enable prediction of the final height at the end of growth and raise the issue of limb lengthening. Axial deviations (angular deformities of the lower limbs) require either repeated corrective osteotomies or gradual corrections with the Ilizarov technique that can be combined with lengthening.[36,37] Severe coxa vara with neck shaft angles measuring 100° or less and epiphyseal dysplasia of the femoral head predispose to significant flattening of the femoral head and incongruity of the hip joint. Lateral extrusion and hinge abduction often result. To prevent early degenerative changes of the hip, valgus intertrochanteric femoral osteotomy should be considered.[38] Total hip arthroplasty is often required in the adult.

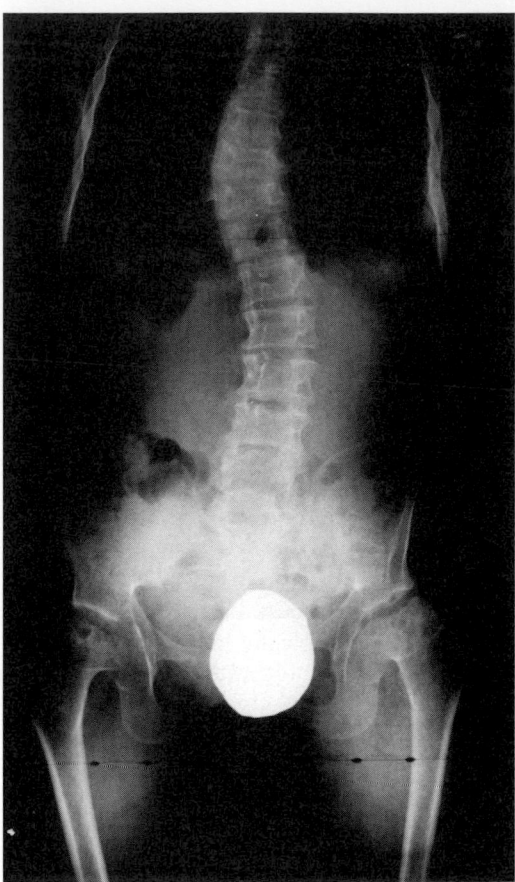

Figure 37-3 This 22-year-old woman with spondyloepiphyseal dysplasia congenita had mild scoliosis and significant degenerative changes in both hips. She underwent bilateral total hip arthroplasty 1 year after this radiograph.

Spondyloepiphyseal dysplasia tarda is usually diagnosed in adolescence and is considered to be an X-linked recessive condition.[39] Clinical manifestations include short stature, mainly short trunk; dorsal kyphosis and lumbar hyperlordosis; and back and hip pain associated with progressive limitation of joint range of motion, mainly hip flexion contractures. Radiographic appearance includes platyspondyly with a hump-shaped deformity in the posterosuperior aspect of the vertebral bodies seen on the lateral view. Mild epiphyseal dysplasia with short femoral neck and coxa vara can be seen with early degenerative changes in the hips. Total hip replacement with a custom-designed prosthesis can be required.[40]

MULTIPLE EPIPHYSEAL DYSPLASIA

Multiple epiphyseal dysplasia is considered to be an autosomal dominant dysplasia. The disorder has been mapped to the pericentromeric region of chromosome 19[41] as well as to chromosome 1.[42] The disorder may not become clinically evident until the patient is 5 to 10 years of age. The radiographic appearance is usually quite normal at birth.[43]

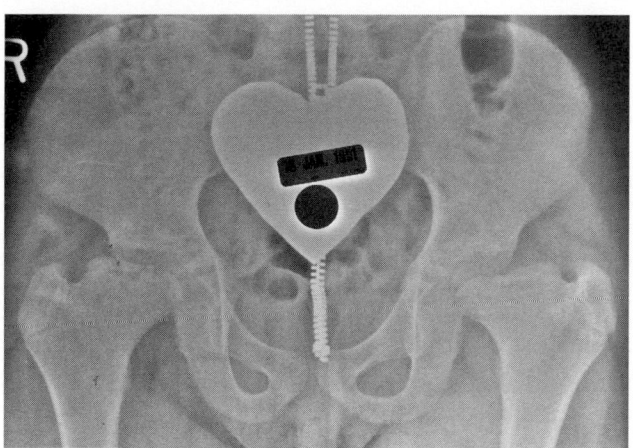

Figure 37-4 Anteroposterior pelvis of a 10-year-old with multiple epiphyseal dysplasia. Note the changes in the proximal femoral epiphyses of both hips.

Presenting symptoms include development of a limp or waddling gait or difficulty in climbing stairs or running.[44] There is mild short stature, short broad hands and thumbs, and normal facies. Valgus deformities of the knees and ankles are common. Joint pain and limitation of motion may occur in the large joints of both upper and lower extremities.

Radiographic appearance includes delayed appearance of the secondary centers of ossification, including the proximal femoral ossification center. There is often a patchy, irregular ossification of the involved epiphyses, which is often symmetrical on both sides. The epiphyses gradually enlarge and the irregular areas coalesce. There is a delay in the appearance of all secondary ossification centers of the tubular bones, including the hands and wrists.

Based on the radiographic appearance of the pelvis and femoral heads, the disorder can be confused with bilateral Legg-Perthes disease or less frequently with Meyers dysplasia (Fig. 37-4). However, MRI studies have shown that most patients do have changes compatible with a superimposed avascular necrosis. The natural history of hip development in these patients demonstrates that all incongruent hips are osteoarthritic by 20 years of age.[45] Those patients with minor epiphyseal abnormalities of the shoulder have been shown to often develop painful osteoarthritis in middle age, but they retain shoulder movement until the degenerative changes are advanced. Those with a significantly deformed "hatchet head" radiographic appearance of the humeral head were shown to have minimal glenohumeral movement from an early stage, and this condition often became painful by the fifth and sixth decades.[46]

The severe form of the disease is known as the Fairbank type, whereas the milder form, in which the hips are primarily involved, is known as the Ribbing type.

METAPHYSEAL CHONDRODYSPLASIA

Metaphyseal chondrodysplasia is a heterogeneous group of disorders, each with its own distinct clinical and genetic

characteristics but with similar radiographic findings. The Schmid type is the most common form and is transmitted as an autosomal dominant condition. The patients have mild to moderate short stature with genu varum and may present with leg pain, which gradually improves with development. The metaphyseal changes are present in all of the tubular bones, with widening and scalloping of the metaphyseal region that may resemble changes seen in children with vitamin D–resistant rickets. The epiphyseal regions and the articular surfaces remain unaffected (Fig. 37-5).

The Jansen type of metaphyseal chondrodysplasia is considered to be autosomal dominant, with most cases being fresh mutations.[28] The radiographic features have been noted to change with development.[47] At birth, the metaphyses of the long bones show areas of diffuse radiolucency and irregularity. Later in childhood, the metaphyses become cupped, with a wide zone of irregular calcification. By adulthood, the large calcified masses in the metaphyses ossify, resulting in bulbous deformities at the ends of short, bowed long bones. They often present with hip and knee flexion deformities and a waddling gait.

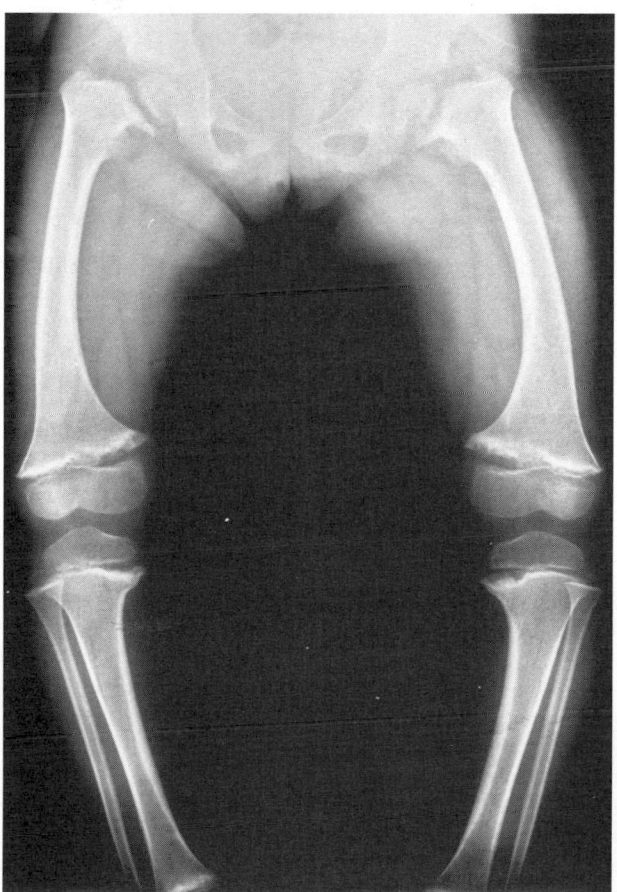

Figure 37-5 Three-year-old girl with metaphyseal chondrodysplasia, Schmid type. Note the changes in the metaphyseal areas, genu varum, and preservation of the epiphyseal areas.

The McKusick type of metaphyseal chondrodysplasia, also known as cartilage-hair hypoplasia, is considered to be an autosomal recessive disorder. This is a progressive disorder characterized by significant shortening of the long bones caused by abnormal development of long bone cartilage. The disorder has been mapped to chromosome 9,[48] and a generalized defect in cellular proliferation has been suggested. Decreased cell-mediated immunity and an increased rate of malignancy have been described. Various pathogens, including the varicella virus, can cause death of these patients.[49] The adult height is about 120 cm (107 to 147 cm). There is fine, sparse hair on the head, eyebrows, and eyelashes. There is often intestinal malabsorption in infancy.

The disorder is most often diagnosed in Finland and in Amish communities in the United States, but it also appears from new mutations at the same genetic locus.[50] A DNA marker–based analysis has been suggested to provide a useful method for early prenatal testing for this disorder.[51]

Radiographically, the metaphyseal regions of the tubular bones are widened, scalloped, and irregularly sclerotic in childhood. Mild scoliosis can occur in about 25 percent of the patients.[52] The long bones are relatively short, with mild bowing, and the tibia is short in relation to the fibula. Congenital hypoplastic anemia and macrocytosis occur during childhood in most affected children[53]; spontaneous recovery occurs before adulthood.

METAPHYSEAL DYSPLASIA

Metaphyseal dysplasia or Pyle disease is an autosomal recessive disorder that was originally described in 1931.[54] The characteristic findings include an Erlenmeyer flask–like flare of the distal femur and the proximal tibia, with similar but lesser involvement of other distal long bones, cortical thinning and osteoporosis, genu valgum, and flexion contractures of the elbows.

SPONDYLOMETAPHYSEAL DYSPLASIA (OF KOZLOWSKI)

Spondylometaphyseal dysplasia represents a group of disorders with spinal and metaphyseal abnormalities. There are several varieties, but the Kozlowski type is the most common and best known.[28] Radiographic findings include odontoid hypoplasia, platyspondyly, thoracic kyphosis, pectus carinatum, and irregular rachitic-like metaphyseal changes, particularly of the proximal femur. A waddling gait with joint limitations as well as early degenerative changes are common.[55] Most cases are felt to represent spontaneous mutations of an autosomal dominant condition.[28]

DIAPHYSEAL DYSPLASIA (CAMURATI-ENGELMANN SYNDROME)

Diaphyseal dysplasia is a rare hereditary skeletal dysplasia that produces typical radiographic changes in the diaphyseal regions of the long bones as well as a typical clinical presentation. It is considered to have an autosomal dominant inheritance pattern, with sporadic mutations responsible for a significant number of new cases. The diaphysis is widened, especially in the midshaft area, with sclerosis and thickening on both the endosteal and periosteal surfaces. The metaphyses are less affected and the epiphyses remain unaffected. The progressive nature of the diaphyseal thickening effectively narrows the medullary cavity. The diaphyses assume a fusiform shape, with a lack of normal bony contours and without evidence of remodeling with growth. The femurs and tibias appear to be most commonly affected, but other tubular bones and the skull are often involved. The age of clinical onset is usually within the first decade of life. Patients present with limb pain, a waddling gait or difficulty in walking or running, decreased muscle mass and subcutaneous fat, and muscular weakness. The muscle weakness may improve with age and may even disappear in adult years, but the bone changes persist. The clinical presentation may resemble a neuromuscular condition, requiring long bone radiographs for differentiation.[56] Laboratory values are usually within normal limits with the exception of an increased sedimentation rate. Corticosteroid treatment has been attempted and may benefit the limb pain, but it does not seem to affect the radiographic changes.[57,58] Orthopaedic surgery is rarely necessary. Life expectancy is normal. The differential radiologic diagnosis includes craniodiaphyseal dysplasia, osteopetrosis, fibrous dysplasia, infantile cortical hyperostosis, melorrheostosis, myelosclerosis, hypervitaminosis A, Paget's disease, and hyperphosphatasia.[56,59]

SCHWARTZ-JAMPEL SYNDROME (CHONDRODYSTROPHICA MYOTONIA)

This autosomal recessive condition combines myotonia with skeletal changes.[60] Fragmentation and flattening of the femoral epiphyses are typical, along with platyspondyly. A progressive myotonia with a sad, fixed facies, slow linear growth, and delayed motor function are usual. Ocular findings include blepharophimosis and myopia.

KNIEST DYSPLASIA (OR SYNDROME)

Disproportionate short-trunk dwarfism with flat atypical facies and enlarged joints with stiffness and contractures are hallmarks of Kniest dysplasia.[61] It is considered an autosomal dominant condition with most cases representing sporadic mutations.[63] Kyphoscoliosis, platyspondyly, and delayed ossification of the femoral heads are common, and atlantoaxial instability may occur. The growth plates of children with Kniest dysplasia have demonstrated evidence of defects in proteoglycan synthesis or processing.[62] Joint contractures develop early in these children, and aggressive physiotherapy is indicated. Early degenerative arthritis has been demonstrated.

CHONDRODYSPLASIA PUNCTATA

Chondrodysplasia punctata has become recognized as a spectrum of disorders rather than as a single condition. Each of these disorders is characterized by small focal calcifications in the articular, epiphyseal, and other types of cartilage in infancy, with the subsequent development of epiphyseal dysplasia and associated anomalies of the facies, eyes, and skin.[64] Conradi-Hunerman syndrome is the most frequent form of chondrodysplasia punctata. It is inherited as an autosomal dominant disorder with considerable variability in expression and a high incidence of spontaneous mutation. Scoliosis is the most common orthopaedic problem in these children and is often seen early in life and related to congenital skeletal abnormalities. Delay in appearance of the secondary centers of ossification as well as limb-length discrepancy are commonly seen.[64,65] A more severe form of chondrodysplasia punctata is transmitted as an autosomal recessive condition in which death is the rule within the first 2 years of life.[66]

DIASTROPHIC DYSPLASIA

Diastrophic dysplasia is an autosomal recessive condition characterized by extreme short-limb disproportionate dwarfism. It has also been called diastrophic dwarfism. The clinical presentation includes marked short stature and several rather typical deformities. Rigid clubfeet are common. The "hitchhiker thumb," or a thumb that is proximally set, abducted, and hypermobile with a shortened first metacarpal, is a classic finding. Symphalangism of the proximal interphalangeal joints of the hands may be seen. Calcification of the cartilage in the ear pinnae is responsible for the "cauliflower ear" seen in most of these children. Severe, progressive kyphoscoliosis and soft tissue flexion contractures of the elbow, knees, and hips are common. As with many of the children with skeletal dysplasias, cervical stability should be assessed. Respiratory problems early in life lead to increased infant mortality, but if the children survive this period, their life expectancy appears normal.[67]

CAMPTOMELIC DYSPLASIA

Maroteaux et al.[68] used the term *camptomelique* or *bent limb* to describe the characteristic anterior bowing of the tibia seen in these children. The dysplasia is considered to be autosomal recessive and most children do not survive the neonatal period. There is often dimpling over the anterior bow of the tibia, shortening of the fibula, bowing of the femur, and clubfoot deformities. Abnormal ribs, scapulae, and cervical vertebrae are seen, often accompanied by severe central nervous system abnormalities. Secondary ossification centers of the distal femur, proximal tibia, and talus are usually absent at birth.[69]

CHONDROECTODERMAL DYSPLASIA (ELLIS–VAN CREVELD SYNDROME)

In 1940, Ellis and van Creveld described an association of four congenital abnormalities: ectodermal dysplasia affecting the hair, teeth, and nails; polydactyly; chondrodysplasia; and congenital morbus cordis.[70]

These children have extremely short limbs in relation to the relatively long trunk. Height remains within the normal range due to maintenance of trunk height. Postaxial polydactyly is most common, with the hand more often involved than the feet. Teeth are rudimentary and peglike. All of the long bones are shortened. Radiographs reveal short, thick bones. The distal phalanges of fingers and toes are poorly developed. The nails of the fingers and toes are small and dystrophic, resembling small scales. The hair is fine and sparse, with scanty eyebrows.

APERT'S SYNDROME (ACROCEPHALOSYNDACTYLY)

Apert's syndrome is recognized as an autosomal dominant condition, with the vast majority of cases representing fresh mutations. The recurrence risk for the unaffected parents of a child with Apert's syndrome is negligible, whereas the recurrence risk for the offspring of the affected individual would be 50 percent.[28] The cranium has a shortened anteroposterior diameter, high full forehead, and flat occiput; craniosynostosis is present, particularly of the coronal suture. The face is flattened with hypertelorism, strabismus, a small nose, and maxillary hypoplasia.[71] Simple or complex syndactyly is present, often with complete fusion of the second, third, and fourth fingers and/or toes (Fig. 37-6). Distal thumbs and distal great toes are broad. Accompanying congenital defects of other organ systems are also common and should be searched for. Correction of the craniosynostosis, reconstruction of the facial cosmetic deformities, and hand surgery to improve both function and cosmesis are usually recommended.

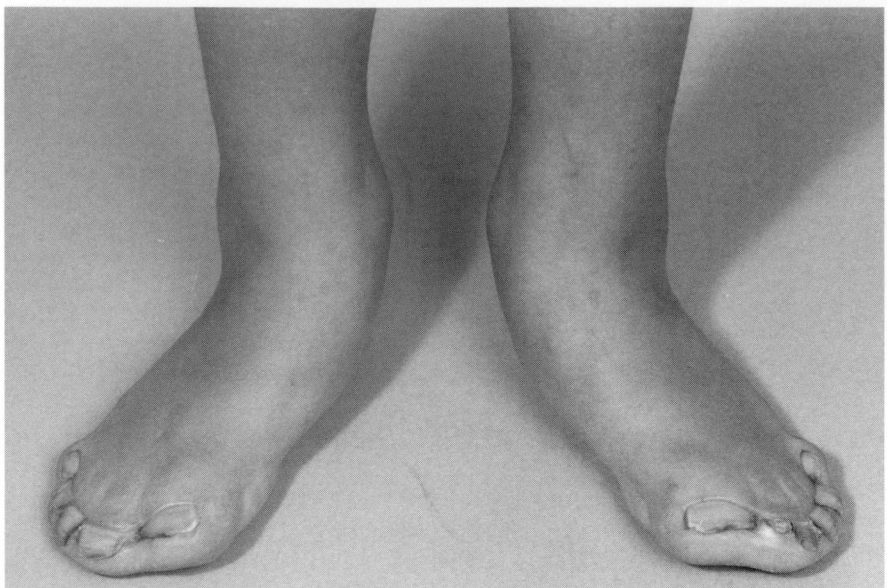

A

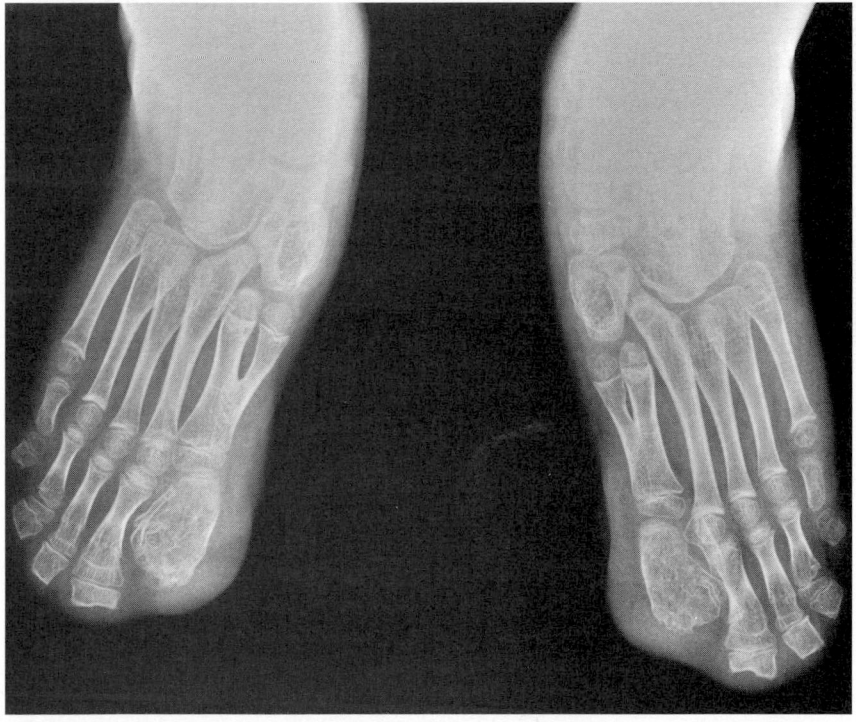

B

Figure 37-6 *A* and *B*. Anteroposterior photograph and radiograph of the feet of a 9-year-old boy with Apert syndrome. Note the complete webbing of both feet as well as the bony duplication. His hands had a similar appearance and have undergone multiple procedures to deepen the web space.

MUCOPOLYSACCHARIDOSES

The mucopolysaccharidoses (MPS) are a group of disorders resulting from lysosomal enzyme deficiencies that alter the ability to metabolize various glycosaminoglycans, resulting in their accumulation. Multiple orthopaedic problems are typical for all of these conditions.

Mucopolysaccharidosis I (MPS I, Hurler's, and Sheie's Syndromes)

Mucopolysaccharidosis I is an autosomal recessive condition that has two clinical presentations. Hurler's syndrome, or MPS I H, was described first.[72] The primary defect is an absence of lysosomal α-L-iduronidase in all tissues. The pathologic result is an accumulation of mucopolysaccharides in parenchymal and mesenchymal tissues and the storage of lipids within neuronal tissues.[28] Diagnosis is by the physical appearance (coarse facies with full lips, hypertelorism, hazy corneas, joint limitation, kyphosis, and thoracolumbar gibbus); diaphyseal broadening of short misshapen bones radiographically; the excretion of dermatan sulfate and heparan sulfate in the urine; and the absence of α-L-iduronidase in cultured fibroblasts.

Sheie's syndrome, or MPS IS, has the same enzymatic deficiency and dermatan sulfate in the urine and can be differentiated from MPS IH only on the basis of the clinical course and phenotype. Joint stiffness is similar. There is little if any impairment of intelligence.[28]

Mucopolysaccharidosis II (MPS II, Hunter's Syndrome)

This condition is the only MPS that is X-linked recessive. The primary defect is a deficiency of iduronate sulfatase with excess dermatan sulfate and heparan sulfate in the urine. Coarse facies plus mental and neurologic deterioration are typical. The clinical phenotype may vary from mild to severe, even in the same sibship. There is limitation of joint motion and coxarthrosis. In contrast to Hurler's syndrome, these children have clear corneas, less severe gibbus, no affected females, and more gradual onset of features.[28]

Mucopolysaccharidosis III (MPS III, Sanfilippo's Syndrome)

This, apparently the most common mucopolysaccharidosis, was described in 1963.[28,73] Slowing mental development by 1 to 3 years of age followed by deterioration in mental and physical functioning are typical. These children will become wheelchair-dependent early and become difficult to manage. Many children die of pulmonary problems by 10 to 20 years of age. There are four subtypes (A, B, C, and D), each having a slightly different enzymatic deficiency but all excreting excess heparan sulfate in the urine and having identical clinical appearances.

Mucopolysaccharidosis IV (MPS IV, Morquio's Syndrome)

This is an autosomal recessive condition with perhaps the most severe orthopaedic problems and a normal mental capacity. Type IV A is caused by a deficiency of N-acctylgalactosamine-6-sulfatase, whereas type IV B is related to a deficiency of β-galactosidase. Identification of an excessive excretion of keratan sulfate in the urine or a deficiency of the enzyme in cultured skin fibroblasts or leukocytes will confirm the diagnosis.[28] Marked platyspondyly, genu valgum, shortening of the long bones, coxa vara, corneal clouding, and generalized growth limitation are typical. Odontoid hypoplasia and generalized ligamentous

laxity may lead to C1-2 instability and should be searched for in these patients and treated.

Mucopolysaccharidosis VI (MPS VI, Maroteaux-Lamy syndrome)

This condition is caused by a deficiency of arylsulfatase B and has been divided into a mild subtype (where patients survive until the second to third decade and succumb to cardiac disease) and a severe subtype (where patients deteriorate rapidly, with serious deformity by 3 to 6 years of age). These children have a milder clinical appearance than those with Hurler's syndrome and mental deterioration is not typical. They do have mild stiffness of the joints, a thoracolumbar kyphosis with platyspondyly, broad ribs, genu valgum, and odontoid hypoplasia.[74]

CLEIDOCRANIAL DYSPLASIA

Cleidocranial dysplasia is considered an autosomal dominant condition, with primary involvement of those bones that form by intramembranous ossification and less of those formed by endochondral ossification. Typical findings include hypoplasia to aplasia of the clavicles, increased transverse enlargement of the cranium, retarded ossification of the fontanelles, dental abnormalities, and delayed or absent ossification of the pubic symphysis.[75] The most common deformity of the clavicle is an absence of the midsection, with a rudimentary sternal and clavicular stub.[76] These deformities are relatively asymptomatic. Associated congenital abnormalities are common.

NAIL-PATELLA SYNDROME

Osteoonychodysostosis, or nail-patella syndrome, is an autosomal dominant condition with a genetic linkage to the ABO blood group locus. The involved family members have the same blood type, but no blood group has been found to have a higher rate of association with the syndrome. The disorder has been mapped to the long arm of chromosome 9.[77] Most involved patients will be identified at birth, but diagnosis is often delayed, particularly in a child born to a family with no previous history of the syndrome. Patients remain ambulatory despite the multiple orthopaedic abnormalities. The nails are hypoplastic or absent, with more involvement on the radial aspect of the hand and the ulnar side of each nail. Most patients have foot abnormalities, ranging from pes planus to clubfoot, but the toenails are less affected than the fingernails. Iliac horns (asymptomatic bony projections from the posterior ilium visible on the radiograph of the pelvis) are known to occur only in this syndrome and were present in 33 of 44 patients in a report.[78,79] Hip subluxation or dislocation may occasionally be seen. Most patients will demonstrate subluxation or dislocation of the radial head, which may be present with flexion contracture of the elbow, loss of supination, or a cubitus valgus deformity. All patients have patellar abnormalities ranging from hypoplasia to complete absence and varying degrees of subluxation. Genu valgum, flexion contracture of the knee, and other radiographic abnormalities of the knees are common. Associated spinal abnormalities may be present. Orthopaedic surgical procedures are often required for the knee and foot.[78]

HYPOPHOSPHATEMIC RICKETS

Hypophosphatemic, or vitamin D–resistant, rickets is a sex (X)-linked dominant inherited condition. All children with this condition require evaluation and treatment by an endocrinologist. Oral phosphate and pharmacologic doses of vitamin D will improve the abnormal physiologic response and improve the child's ability to calcify the nonossified cartilaginous matrix. The most common orthopaedic condition that requires treatment is the genu varus deformity. Osteotomy of the femur and/or the tibia is often required to correct this malalignment. Delayed healing of the osteotomy site may be seen.

HYPOPHOSPHATASIA SYNDROME

This invariably lethal condition was first noted in 1948 as an autosomal recessive disorder.[80] These infants are stillborn or die in early infancy due to respiratory insufficiency. Their condition suggests severe rickets, with short stature, poor mineralization of bone, bowing of extremities, short ribs with a rachitic rosary, anemia, and hypercalcemia. They are also noted to have a decreased serum alkaline phosphatase and an increased urinary phosphoethanolamine. A milder autosomal dominant form has since been described. Prenatal diagnosis has been reported.[81]

FIBROUS DYSPLASIA

Fibrous dysplasia is a benign pathologic condition that affects skeletal development[82] and is considered to be sporadic. In 1937 Albright et al. described an association between fibrous dysplasia, the typical skin changes, and endocrine dysfunction that has since been referred to as McCune-Albright syndrome.[82] Lichtenstein and Jaffe classified fibrous dysplasia as a congenital anomaly that is manifest by a malfunction of bone-forming mesenchyme.[84] Patients are often initially seen during the

first two decades of life, with progressive deformities and pathologic fractures due to the compromised structural integrity of the affected bones that this condition produces. Although the histologic appearance of fibrous dysplasia is relatively stable, the radiographic appearance has been documented to progress both before and after puberty.[85] Radiographically, the bone has a ground-glass appearance, often with expansion of the cortex, with evidence of decreased remodeling. Frequent fractures, microfractures, and bowing deformities are common, with the "shepherd's crook deformity" of the proximal femur often a result. The café au lait pigmentation changes in the skin have an irregular border and resemble "the coast of Maine."

Stephenson et al.[82] reviewed a series of skeletal lesions caused by fibrous dysplasia. Those in the upper extremity were successfully treated in 88 percent of cases, usually by closed means. Minimal functional morbidity was noted due to these lesions. This is in contradistinction to lesions in the lower extremity. Patients over age 18 years did satisfactorily with closed treatment in 8 of 9 cases and in both of the cases treated with curettage and bone grafting. However, patients under age 18 years usually had an unsatisfactory outcome with either closed treatment or curettage and bone grafting. These failures were usually attributed to resorption of the graft and recurrence of the disease. These cases point to the fact that this lesion is extremely difficult to eradicate completely by intralesional curettage. Wide local excision, radical resection, and amputation are the only definitive means of total ablation of these lesions.[82] The results of internal fixation of lesions in the lower extremity were satisfactory in 86 percent of the cases, independent of the patient's skeletal maturity or the number of bones involved. The mechanical support of the structurally compromised bone appears to be the significant difference, rather than any alteration in the basic disease process.

CAFFEY'S DISEASE (INFANTILE CORTICAL HYPEROSTOSIS)

The original clinical presentation and radiographic findings of infantile cortical hyperostosis were described by Caffey and Silverman in 1945.[86] The typical child is 9 weeks of age and most commonly under 6 months of age, presenting with irritability, fever, tenderness of involved bones, leukocytosis, anemia, and radiographic cortical thickening of some combination of the long bones, clavicle, or mandible. Laboratory findings include elevated erythrocyte sedimentation rate and alkaline phosphatase levels. Exacerbations and remissions are common throughout the process. The incidence has been estimated at 3 cases per 1000 patients under the age of 6 months.[87] The etiology remains unclear, but evidence exists for genetic transmission as well as transmission via an infectious agent with a long latency period.[88]

MULTIPLE CARTILAGINOUS EXOSTOSES (HEREDITARY MULTIPLE EXOSTOSES, OSTEOCHONDRODYSPLASIA)

This autosomal dominant condition is one of the most common of the skeletal dysplasias and is characterized by numerous osteocartilaginous exostoses that grow from the juxtaepiphyseal region of the tubular bones and away from the joint.[89] The stalk of the exostosis is bone, with a cap of hyaline cartilage. The growth of these bones is related to the activity of the associated growth plate and therefore should cease with skeletal maturation. Growth after this time or pain from such a lesion should cause concern. Malignant degeneration of the cartilaginous cap may occur. Most commonly these lesions may require excision when they impinge on local structures (tendons, nerves, or vessels), cause a mechanical or cosmetic problem for the child, or when they are associated with longitudinal or angular deformities of the long bones or adjacent joint. The latter is often the case with disturbed or asymmetrical growth of the radius and ulna or of the tibia and fibula, with resultant deformity of the wrist or ankle, respectively (Figure 37-7). Reconstructive surgery is often required to correct these deformities.[90]

MULTIPLE ENCHONDROMATOSIS SYNDROME (OLLIER'S DISEASE)

This sporadic condition involves multiple areas of hyaline cartilage, which replace normal areas of metaphyseal and diaphyseal bone (Fig. 37-8). It may be unilateral but is often bilateral but asymmetrical. Asymmetrical growth is often noted during early childhood.[91] The longitudinal growth of the involved long bones is affected, often with angular deformities. Radiographic abnormalities range from typical areas of cartilaginous enchondromata to areas of longitudinal cartilaginous streaking within the involved long bones and pelvis. A low risk of malignant degeneration of these areas exists. Osteotomy is commonly required to correct the angular deformities. Fractures through these involved areas are treated in usual fashion, but they may increase a preexisting deformity.

MAFUCCI'S SYNDROME

Multiple enchondromata of the hands, feet, and tubular long bones combined with multiple cutaneous hemangiomata comprise Maffucci's syndrome[92] (Fig. 37-9). Hemangiomata may be capillary, cavernous, or phlebectasic and usually appear during the first 4 years of life. Multiple surgical procedures including amputation may be required, and the risk of fracture through the enchondromata is good. Malignant degeneration of the cartilaginous tumors is higher than in Ollier's disease and has been reported at 15 to 18 percent.[93]

DYSPLASIA EPIPHYSEALIS HEMIMELICA

Dysplasia epiphysealis hemimelica is a type of osteochondromatosis involving the epiphysis. It has also been referred to as Trevor's disease and most commonly involves the epiphyses of the distal femur and proximal tibia or the distal tibia and talus (Fig. 37-10). It is essentially an osteocartilaginous overgrowth affecting the medial or lateral half of one or more epiphyses on one side of the body. It does not appear to be inherited and is of unknown etiology.[94] Boys appear to be more often affected. The overgrowth of the osteocartilaginous tissue becomes quiescent after skeletal maturity. Angular (i.e., varus or valgus) deformity may occur at the affected knee or ankle, or limb length discrepancy may develop. Biopsy is not needed for diagnosis, which can be made based on radiologic appearance. Malignant degeneration has not been reported. Skeletal survey for other sites is indicated.

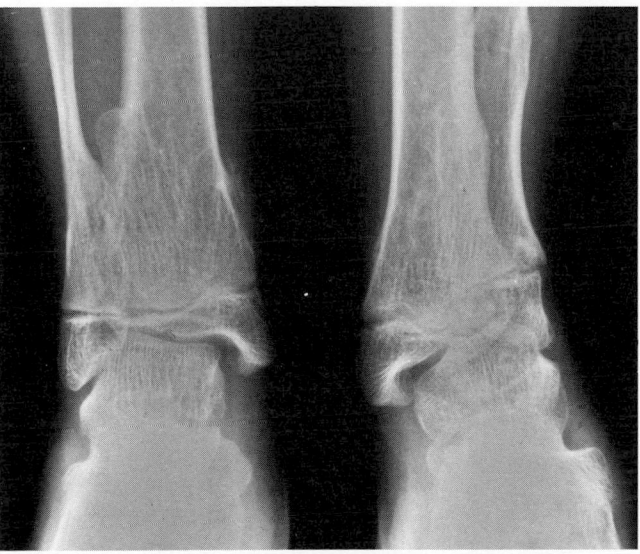

Figure 37-7 Standing anteroposterior radiograph of the ankles of a 13-year-old boy with multiple cartilaginous exostoses. He has bilateral ankle valgus, worse on the left, with fibular shortening and exostoses of both the distal tibia and fibula.

FIBRODYSPLASIA OSSIFICANS PROGRESSIVA (MYOSITIS OSSIFICANS PROGRESSIVA)

Fibrodysplasia ossificans progressiva is considered an autosomal dominant condition with a high mutation rate.[95] Soft tissue swelling, often with pain and fever, develops in aponeuroses, fasciae, and tendons of the neck, dorsal trunk, and proximal limbs, with eventual ossification. The sternocleidomastoid is frequently involved. A shortening

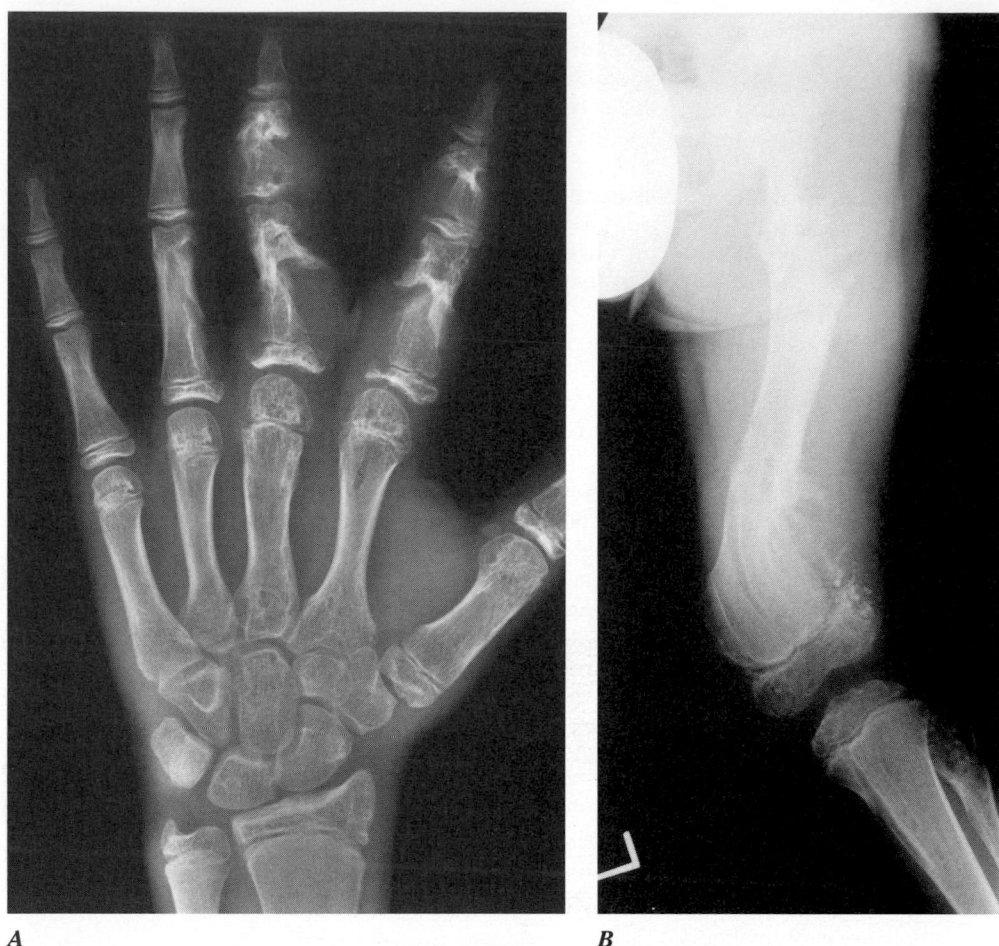

A   *B*

Figure 37-8 Ollier disease (multiple enchondromatosis). *A.* Anteroposterior radiograph of the left hand of a 14-year-old boy. Note the cartilaginous lesions in the metacarpals and the phalanges, with irregular areas of bony growth around them. *B.* Anteroposterior radiograph of the left lower extremity of a 4-year-old boy. Note the large cartilaginous lesion in the distal lateral femur, which is causing a valgus deformity. The proximal femur and proximal tibia and fibula are also affected.

Figure 37-9 Six-year-old girl with Mafucci syndrome. The multiple cartilaginous enchondromata in the bones as well as the multiple hemangiomas in the soft tissues can be appreciated.

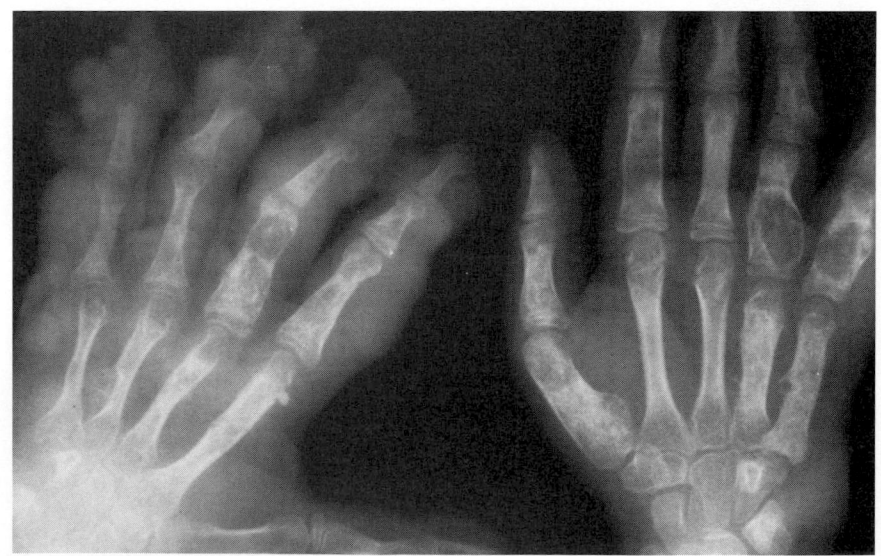

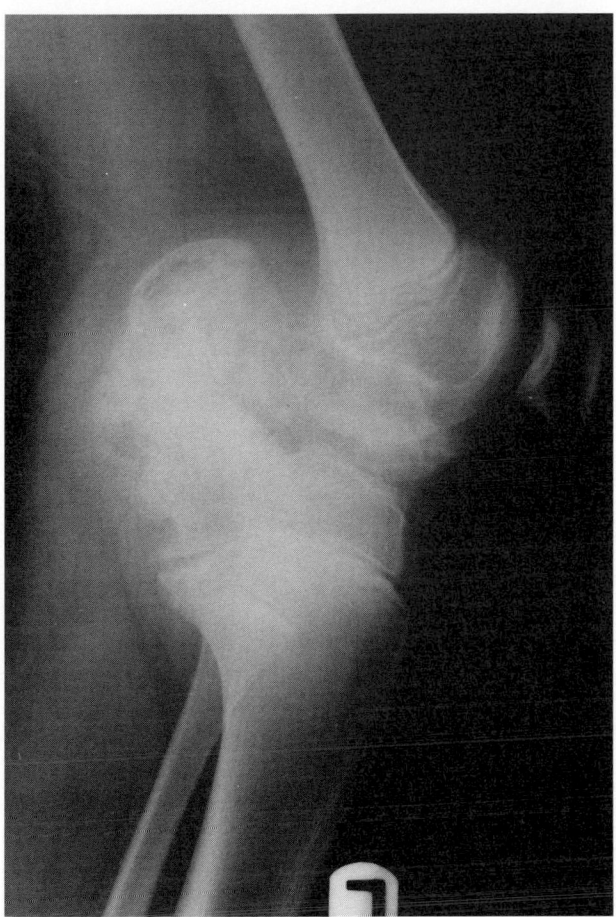

Figure 37-10 Eleven-year-old boy with dysplasia epiphysealis hemimelica involving the distal femur and proximal tibia. He has 90° of knee flexion and is relatively asymptomatic.

of the great toe with hallux valgus is characteristic of this condition. Onset is usually in early childhood. Death usually occurs secondary to pulmonary complications in the second to third decades. No effective treatment has yet been found to halt the ectopic ossification. Biopsy of the areas should be interpreted with caution due to the cellular atypia and potential malignant appearance.

MELORHEOSTOSIS

Melorheostosis is a rare, nonfamilial condition. It was initially reported by Leri, Loiseleur, and Lievre in 1930[96] and was named by combining two Greek words meaning "limb" and "flowing" to describe the radiographic appearance of the hyperostosis resembling molten wax running down the cortex of the bone. This is not usually a painful condition in children but is often painful in adults.

The most common complaint in these children is soft tissue contracture causing often severe and rigid joint deformities (Fig. 37-11). Most children have only one affected limb, but this dysplasia can be present in up to all four extremities. Limb length inequality is common. The overlying soft tissues of the affected area are often described as woody, with thickening and puckering of the skin and deep fascia. Average age at diagnosis is 9 years, although signs and symptoms are present much earlier, indicating the usual delay before diagnosis is made. Histology of the affected bone demonstrates dense cortical bone, with otherwise nonspecific changes, and thickened dense fibrosis of the soft tissues.

Radiographs of the affected limb demonstrate the dripping waxy appearance of the bony sclerosis. Although in adults this hyperostosis appears to be on the outside of the diaphysis of the bone, in children it more commonly appears as endosteal sclerosis. It can have a streaky or mottled appearance, particularly in the small bones. The progression of the pediatric radiographic appearance of endosteal sclerosis to the adult periosteal distribution has been documented in several patients followed into adulthood.[97]

Treatment most often requires radical surgical soft tissue releases, followed by long-term bracing during growth. Conservative or nonoperative means of correcting these deformities have proven ineffective.[98] Osteotomy may be needed to achieve an acceptable degree of correction. Recurrent deformity with growth is common. Amputation

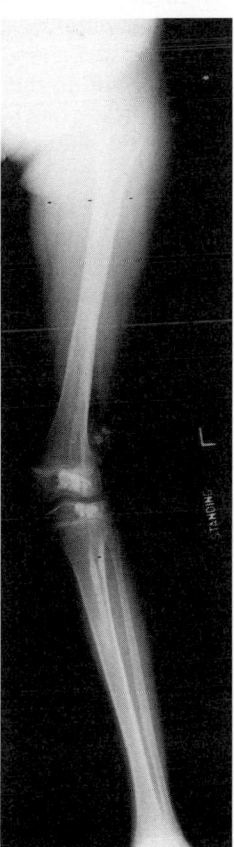

Figure 37-11 Ten-year-old girl with melorheostosis. Note the "dripping wax" appearance along the femur, tibia, and patella, with significant rigid valgus deformity of the knee and lateral dislocation of the patella.

may be required as an ultimate salvage procedure for significant, recurrent deformity and/or inequality.[98]

LARSEN'S SYNDROME

Larsen et al. initially described 6 cases of children with multiple congenital dislocations of various joints, with typical facial changes consisting of flattened facies, prominent forehead, depressed nasal bridge, and wide-spaced eyes.[99] The elbows, hips, and knees are most often dislocated (or subluxated). Foot deformities are common, typically equinovarus or equinovalgus. Abnormal segmentation of the spine, cylindrical fingers that do not taper normally from base to tip, an increased number of ossification centers of the wrist, and palate abnormalities have also been observed in these children.[99,100] The presence of two ossification centers of the calcaneus that coalesce with skeletal maturation has been reported.[100]

Larsen's syndrome is now recognized as being an autosomal dominant condition.[101] The orthopaedic problems center around the treatment of the multiple joint dislocations and foot deformities. As with other children with both dislocations of the knee and the hip, the knee should be reduced first, followed by the hip. The knee dislocation may be reduced with serial manipulation and casting into progressive flexion, but it often requires surgical reduction. Fibrotic replacement of the vastus lateralis muscle and contracture of the iliotibial band add to the deformity. Chronic knee instability is common. The dislocated hips can sometimes be reduced with closed reduction and casting, but they often require open reduction. The dislocations of the radial head usually do not require treatment; if they are symptomatic after skeletal maturation, resection can be considered, with the usual indications and possible sequelae. The foot deformities can be treated with early manipulation and serial casting, with surgical intervention as necessary for the specific deformity. Most of these children will be ambulatory but may require orthoses and assistive devices.

OSTEOGENESIS IMPERFECTA SYNDROME

Osteogenesis imperfecta, or "brittle bone disease," is said to have both clinical and genetic heterogeneity, but all affected children demonstrate multiple fractures due to skeletal fragility. Several previous classification systems have proved inadequate. Although no current system provides a clear delineation of each possible variant with which these children may present, the four categories of Sillence[102] are accepted as the current standard. The patients with Sillence type I and type IV are the autosomal dominant forms and therefore the milder types. Children with type II are often stillborn or die shortly after birth due to the vast number of fractures and resulting pulmonary insufficiency. Children with type III are usually considered to have an autosomal recessive form of the disease and have the most significant orthopaedic problems. Multiple fractures lead to bowing

and angular deformities of the limbs. Multiple osteotomies and intramedullary rodding[103] may control the deformities, minimize the number of future fractures, allow the child to participate in ambulation and/or physiotherapy, and promote neuromotor development. Scoliosis is common. The multiple fractures are treated with standard therapy for pediatric fractures. Healing is within the normal time frame, but with the same abnormal bone.

The biochemical defect has been localized to one or more mutations in the genes COL 1A1 and COL 1A2 encoding the α-1 and α-2 chains of type I collagen. Various point mutations producing substitutions of glycine residues result in procollagen with poor structural properties.[104] Although much genetic and biochemical investigation has been done in this area, much more work will be needed before the specific abnormality in each child can be elucidated. A better-defined classification scheme with possible diagnostic and treatment implications will be possible when the biochemical abnormalities are better understood in this heterogeneous group of patients.

OSTEOPETROSIS

Two forms of osteopetrosis can occur: a more severe, often lethal autosomal recessive form and a milder autosomal dominant form that is often diagnosed incidentally after radiographs are taken for other reasons and which allows a normal life span.[105] The autosomal recessive form is considered a remodeling/reabsorption defect, probably involving the osteoclast function. Dense-appearing but fragile bone results. Lack of development of a medullary canal with decreased ability to form the normal bone marrow components of blood leads to a pancytopenia. Lack of remodeling of the bone canals through which the cranial nerves pass may lead to blindness and cranial nerve palsies. Death is usually in early childhood secondary to complications of anemia and infection. Recent trials of bone marrow transplantation have proven quite effective in providing bone marrow reconstitution and correction of the metabolic and neurosensory abnormalities.[106]

ACKNOWLEDGMENT

The authors would like to thank Linda Pugh, R.N., Claire Kenneally, M.S., Janet Barber, Patti Barber, the Media Resources Department, all of the Shriners Hospital, Tampa, Florida, for their assistance with the preparation of this manuscript.

RECOMMENDED READING

Bailey JA II: *Disproportionate Short Stature: Diagnosis and Management*. Philadelphia, Saunders, 1973.

Beighton P (ed): *McKusick's Heritable Disorders of Connective Tissue*, 5th ed. St. Louis, Mosby, 1993.

Goldberg MJ: *The Dysmorphic Child—An Orthopaedic Perspective.* New York, Raven Press, 1987.

Greenfield GB: *Radiology of Bone Diseases*, 5th ed. Philadelphia, Lippincott, 1990.

Horan F, Beighton P: *Orthopaedic Problems in Inherited Skeletal Disorders.* Berlin, Springer-Verlag, 1982.

Taybi H: *Radiology of Syndromes and Metabolic Disorders*, 2d ed. Chicago, Year Book, 1983.

Thoene JG: *Physicians' Guide to Rare Diseases*, 2d ed. Montvale, NJ, Dowden, 1995.

Wynne-Davies R, Hall CM, Apley AG: *Atlas of Skeletal Dysplasias.* Edinburgh, Churchill Livingstone, 1985.

REFERENCES

1. *POSSUM (Pictures of Standard Syndromes and Undiagnosed Malformations).* Melbourne: Murdoch Institute, 1990.
2. Shohat M. Rimoin DL: Genetics and classification of bone dysplasia, in Laron Z, Mastragostino S, Romano C (eds): *Limb Lengthening—For Whom, When and How?* London, Freund, 1995, pp 41–53.
3. Hirata S, Rimoin DL, Poole AR: Biochemical and immunochemical studies of pseudoachondroplasia: Abnormalities in post-translational processing. *Trans Orthop Res Soc* 15:303, 1990.
4. Byers P: Disorders of collagen biochemistry and structure, in Scriver C, Beaudet A, Sly W, Valle D (eds): *The Metabolic Basis of Inherited Disease,* 6th ed. New York, McGraw-Hill, 1989.
5. Murray LW, Bautista J, James PL, Rimoin D: Type II collagen defects in the chondrodysplasias: I. Spondyloepiphyseal dysplasias. *Am J Hum Genet* 45:5–15, 1989.
6. Lee B, Vissing H, Ramirez F, et al: Identification of the molecular defect in a family with spondyloepiphyseal dysplasia. *Science* 244:978–980, 1989.
7. Ala-Kokka L, Baldwin C, Moskowitz RW, Prockop D: Single base mutation in the type II procollagen gene (COL2A1) as a cause of primary osteoarthritis associated with a mild chondrodysplasia. *Proc Natl Acad Sci USA* 87:6565–6568, 1990.
8. Tiller GE, Rimoin DL, Murray LW, Cohn DH: Tandem duplication within a type II collagen gene (COL2A1) exon in an individual with spondyloepiphyseal dysplasia. *Proc Natl Acad Sci USA* 87:38–43, 1990.
9. Lachman RS, Rappaport V: Fetal imaging in the skeletal dysplasias. *Clin Perinatol* 17:703–722, 1990.
10. Ornoy A, Borochowitz Z, Lachman R, Rimoin DL: *Atlas of Fetal Skeletal Radiology.* Chicago, Year Book, 1988.
11. Orioli IM, Castilla EE, Barbosa-Neto JG: The birth prevalence rates for skeletal dysplasias. *J Med Genet* 23:328–332, 1986.
12. Seashore MR, Cho S, Desposito F, et al: Health supervision for children with achondroplasia: Committee on Genetics. *Pediatrics* 95:443–451, 1995.
13. Velinov M, Salugenhaupt SA, Stoilov, I, et al. The gene for achondroplasia maps to the telomeric region of chromosome 4p. *Nature Genet* 6:314–317, 1994.
14. Shiang R, Thompson LM, Zhu Y-Z, et al: Mutations in the transmembrane domain of FGFR3 cause the most common genetic form of dwarfism, achondroplasia. *Cell* 78:335–342, 1994.
15. Goncalves L, Jeanty P: Fetal biometry of skeletal dysplasias: A multicentric study. *J Ultrasound Med* 13:767–775, 1994.
16. Kida K, Kaino Y, Ito T, et al: Growth hormone treatment in achondroplasia—Expected final height, in Laron Z, Mastragostino S, Romano C (eds): *Limb Lengthening: For Whom, When and How?* London, Freund, 1995, pp 55–60.
17. Galatzer A: Psychological aspects of short stature, in Laron Z, Mastragostino S, Romano C (eds): *Limb Lengthening: For Whom, When and How?* London, Freund, 1995, pp 125–129.
18. Ganel A, Hozoszowski H: Twenty years experience with leg elongation for short stature, in Laron Z, Mastragostino S, Romano C (eds): *Limb Lengthening: For Whom, When and How?* London, Freund, 1995, pp 177–179.
19. Cattaneo R, Catagni MA, Stanitski D, et al: Limb lengthening in dwarfism by the Ilizarov method, in Laron Z, Mastragostino S, Romano C (eds): *Limb Lengthening: For Whom, When and How?* London, Freund, 1995, pp 153–159.
20. Ginebreda I, Villarrubias JM: Monolateral technique for lengthening of the upper and lower limbs, in Laron Z, Mastragostino S, Romano C (eds): *Limb Lengthening: For Whom, When and How?* London, Freund, 1995, pp 169–176.
21. Galatzer A, Ganel A: Psychological aspects of limb lengthening, in Laron Z, Mastragostino S, Romano C (eds): *Limb Lengthening: For Whom, When and How?* London, Freund, 1995, pp 239–243.
22. Kahanovitz N, Rimoin DL, Sillence DO: The clinical spectrum of lumbar spine disease in achondroplasia. *Spine* 7:137–140, 1982.
23. Dominguez R, Talmachoff P: Diagnostic imaging update in skeletal dysplasias. *Clin Imaging* 17:222–234, 1993.
24. Tolo VT: Spinal deformity in short-stature syndromes. *Instr Course Lect* 39:399–405, 1990.
25. Specht EE, Daentl DL: Hypochondroplasia. *Clin Orthop* 110:249–255, 1975.
26. Beals RK: Hypochondroplasia: A report of five kindred. *J Bone Joint Surg* 51A:728, 1969.
27. Marotcaux P, Lamy M, Robert JM: Le nanisme thanatophore. *Presse Med* 75:2519, 1967.
28. Jones KL: *Smith's Recognizable Patterns of Human Malformation,* 4th ed. Philadelphia, Saunders, 1988.
29. Jeune M, Beraud C, Carron R: Dystrophie thoracique asphyxiante de caractere familial. *Arch Fr Pediatr* 12:886–891, 1955.
30. Herdman RC, Langer LOP The thoracic asphyxiant dystrophy and renal disease. *Am J Dis Child* 116:192–201, 1968.
31. Majewski F, Pfeiffer RA, Lenz W, et al: Polysyndaktylie, verkurzte Gliedmassen und Genitalfehlbildungen: Kennzeichen eines selbastandigen Syndroms? *Z Kinderheilkd* 111:118–138, 1971.
32. Ikegawa S, Iwaya T, Taniguchi K, et al: Retinal detachment in spondyloepiphyseal dysplasia congenita. *J Pediatr Orthop* 13:791–792, 1993.
33. Lachman RS: Fetal imaging in skeletal dysplasia: overview and experience. *Pediatr Radiol* 24:413–417, 1994.
34. Svensson O, Aaro S: Cervical instability in skeletal dysplasia: Report of six surgically fused cases. *Acta Orthop Scand* 59:66–70, 1988.
35. Horton WA, Hall JG, Scott CL, et al: Growth curves for height for diastrophic dysplasia, spondyloepiphyseal dysplasia congenita and pseudoachondroplasia. *Am J Dis Child* 136:316–319, 1982.
36. Herzenberg JE, Paley D: Methods and strategies in limb lengthening and realignment for skeletal dysplasia, in Laron Z, Mastragostino S, Romano C (eds): *Limb Lengthening: For Whom, When and How?* London, Freund, 1995, pp 181–199.
37. Prevot J, Guichet JM. Bilateral leg lengthening for short stature: 26 cases treated by the Ilizarov technique, in Laron Z, Mastragostino S, Romano C (eds): *Limb Lengthening: For Whom, When, and How?* London, Freund, 1995, pp 201–211.

38. Bassett GS: Lower extremity abnormalities in dwarfing conditions. *Instr Course Lect* 39:389–397, 1990.

39. Ikegawa S: Spondyloepiphyseal dysplasia tarda: The autosomal recessive form in two sisters. *Arch Orthop Traum Surg* 113:49–52, 1993.

40. Huo MH, Salvati EA, Lieberman JR, et al: Custom designed femoral prosthesis in total hip arthroplasty done with cement for severe dysplasia of the hip. *J Bone Joint Surg* 75A:1497–1504, 1993.

41. Oehlmann R, Summerville GP, Yeh G, et al: Genetic linkage mapping of multiple epiphyseal dysplasia to the pericentromeric region of chromosome 19. *Am J Hum Genet* 54:3–10, 1994.

42. Briggs MD, Choi H, Warman ML, et al: Genetic mapping of a locus for multiple epiphyseal dysplasia to a region of chromosome 1 containing a type IX collagen gene. *Am J Hum Genet* 55:678–684, 1994.

43. Beals R, Horton W: Skeletal dysplasias: An approach to diagnosis. *J Am Acad Orthop Surg* 3:174–181, 1995.

44. Rimoin DL, Lachman RS: Genetic disorders of the osseous skeleton, in Beighton P (ed): *McKusick's Heritable Disorders of Connective Tissue*, 5th ed. St Louis, Mosby, 1993, pp 622–625.

45. Treble NJ, Jensen FO, Bankier A, et al: Development of the hip in multiple epiphyseal dysplasia—Natural history and susceptibility to premature osteoarthritis. *J. Bone Joint Surg* 72B:1061–1064, 1990.

46. Ingram RR: The shoulder in multiple epiphyseal dysplasia. *J Bone Joint Surg* 73B:277–279, 1991.

47. Jansen M: Uber atypische Chondrodystrophie (Achondroplasia) und uber eine noch nicht beschriebene agneborene Wachstumsstorung des Knochensystems: Metaphysare Dysostosis 2. *Orthop Chir* 61:253, 1934.

48. Sulisalo T, Francomano CA, Sistonen P, et al: High resolution genetic mapping of the cartilage hair hypoplasia gene in Amish and Finnish families. *Genomics* 20:347–353, 1994.

49. deSilva LM, Bale P, deCourcy J, et al: Renal failure due to BK virus infection in an immunodeficient child. *J Med Virol* 45:192–196, 1995.

50. Sulisalo T, Van der Burgt I, Rimoin DL, et al: Genetic homogeneity of cartilage-hair hypoplasia. *Hum Genet* 95:157–160, 1995.

51. Sulisalo T, Sillence D, Wilson M, et al: Early prenatal diagnosis of cartilage-hair hypoplasia with polymorphic DNA markers. *Prenat Diagn* 15:135–140, 1995.

52. Makitie O, Sulisalo T, de la Chapelle A, et al: Cartilage-hair hypoplasia (review). *J Med Genet* 32:39–43, 1995.

53. Makitie O, Rajantie J, Kaitila I: Anemia and macrocytosis—Unrecognized features in cartilage-hair hypoplasia. *Acta pediatr* 81:1026–1029, 1992.

54. Pyle E: A case of unusual bone development. *J Bone Joint Surg* 13:874, 1931.

55. Kozlowski K, Maroteaux P, Spranger J: La dysostose spondylometaphysaire. *Presse Med* 75:2769, 1967.

56. Stenzler S, Grogan DP, Frenchman SM, et al: Progressive diaphyseal dysplasia presenting as neuromuscular disease. *J Pediatr Orthop* 9:463–467, 1989.

57. Allen DT, Saunders AM, Northway WH, et al: Corticosteroids in the treatment of Engelmann's disease. *Pediatrics* 46:523–531, 1970.

58. Naveh Y, Alon U, Kaftori JK, Berant M: Progressive diaphyseal dysplasia: Evaluation of corticosteroid therapy. *Pediatrics* 75:321–323, 1985.

59. Naveh Y, Alon U, Kaftori KJ, et al: Progressive diaphyseal dysplasia: Genetics and clinical radiologic manifestations. *Pediatrics* 75:399–405, 1984.

60. Schwartz O, Jampel RS: Congenital blepharophimosis associated with a unique generalized myopathy. *Arch Ophthalmol* 68:52, 1962.

61. Kniest W: Zur abgrenzung der dysostosis enchondralis von der chondrodystrophie. *Z Kinderheilkd* 70:633–640, 1952.

62. Stanescu V, Stanescu R, Maroteaux P: Pathogenic mechanisms in osteochondrodysplasias. *J Bone Joint Surg* 66:817–836, 1984.

63. Rimoin DL, Siggers DC, Lachman RS, Silberberg R: Metatropic dwarfism, the Kniest syndrome and the pseudoachondroplastic dysplasias. *Clin Orthop* 114:70–82, 1976.

64. Spranger JW, Opitz JM, Bidder U: Heterogeneity of chondrodysplasia punctata. *Humangenetik* 11:190–212, 1971.

65. Silengo MC, Luzzatti L, Silverman FN: Clinical and genetic aspects of Conradi-Hunerman disease. A report of three familial cases and review of the literature. *J Pediatr* 97:911–917, 1980.

66. Manzke H, Christophers E, Wiedemann H-R: Dominant sex-linked inherited chondrodysplasia punctata: A distinct type of chondrodysplasia punctata. *Clin Genet* 17:97–107, 1980.

67. Kopits SE: Orthopaedic complications of dwarfism. *Clin Orthop* 114:153–179, 1976.

68. Maroteaux P, Spranger J, Opitz JM, et al: Le syndrome camptomelique. *Presse Med* 79:1157–1162, 1971.

69. Khajavi A, Lachman R, Rimoin D, et al: Heterogeneity in the campomelic syndromes. *Radiology* 120:641–647, 1976.

70. Ellis RWB, van Creveld S: A syndrome characterized by ectodermal dysplasia, polydactyly, chondro-dysplasia and congenital morbus cordis: Report of 3 cases. *Arch Dis Child* 16:65–84, 1940.

71. Apert E: De l'acrocephalosyndactylie. *Bull Soc Med* 23:1310, 1906.

72. Hurler G: Ueber einen typ multipler abartungen, vorwiegend am skelettsystem. *Z Kinderheilkd* 24:220, 1919.

73. Sanfilippo SJ, Podosin R, Langer L, Good RA: Mental retardation associated with acid mucopolysacchariduria (hepartin sulfate type). *J Pediatr* 63:837, 1963.

74. Maroteaux P, Lamy M: Hurler's disease, Morquio's disease, and related mucopolysaccharidoses. *J Pediatr* 67:312, 1965.

75. Marie P, Sainton P: Sur la dysostose cleido-cranienne hereditaire. *Rev Neurol* 6:835, 1898.

76. Dore DD, MacEwen GD, Boulos MI: Cleidocranial dysostosis and syringomyelia: Review of the literature and case report. *Clin Orthop* 214:229–234, 1987.

77. Campeau E, Watkins D, Rouleau GA, et al: Linkage analysis of nail patella syndrome. *Am J Hum Genet* 56:243–247, 1995.

78. Guidera KJ, Satterwhite Y, Ogden JA, et al: Nail patella syndrome: A review of 44 orthopaedic patients. *J Pediatr Orthop* 11:737–742, 1991.

79. Sartoris DJ, Resnick D: The horn, a pathognomonic feature of pediatric bone dysplasias. *Aust Pediatr J* 23:347–349, 1987.

80. Rathbun JC: Hypophosphatasia: A new developmental anomaly. *Am J Dis Child* 75:822, 1948.

81. Warren RC, McKenzie CF, Rodeck CH: First trimester diagnosis of hypophosphatasia with a monoclonal antibody to the liver/bone/kidney isoenzyme of alkaline phosphatase. *Lancet* 2:856–858, 1985.

82. Stephenson RB, London MD, Hankin FM, Kaufer H: Fibrous dysplasia: An analysis of options for treatment. *J Bone Joint Surg* 69:400–409, 1987.

83. Albright F, Butler AM, Hampton AO, Smith P: Syndrome characterized by osteitis fibrosa disseminata, areas of pigmentation and endocrine dysfunction, with precocious puberty in females: Report of five cases. *N Engl J Med* 216:727–746, 1937.

84. Lichtenstein L, Jaffe HL: Fibrous dysplasia of bone. *Arch Pathol* 33:777, 1942.

85. Harris WH, Dudley HR, Barry RJ: The natural history of fibrous dysplasia: An orthopaedic, pathological, and roentgenographic study. *J Bone Joint Surg* 44:207–233, 1962.

86. Caffey J, Sllverman WA: Infantile cortical hyperostosis: Preliminary report on a new syndrome. *Am J Roentgenol* 54:1–16, 1945.

87. Cayler GG, Peterson CA: Infantile cortical hyperostosis. *Am J Dis Child* 91:119–125, 1956.

88. Bernstein RM, Zaleske DJ: Familial aspects of Caffey's disease. *Am J Orthop* 24:777–781, 1995.

89. Shapiro F, Simon S, Glimcher MJ: Hereditary multiple exostoses: Anthropometric, roentgenographic, and clinical aspects. *J Bone Joint Surg* 61A:815–824, 1979.

90. Snearly WN, Peterson HA: Management of ankle deformities in multiple hereditary osteochondromata. *J Pediatr Orthop* 9:427–432, 1989.

91. Ollier L: De la dyschondroplasia. *Bull Soc Chir (Lyon)* 3:22, 1899.

92. Maffucci A: Di un caso di encondroma ed angioma multiplo: Contribuzione alla genesi embrionale dei tumor. *Mov Med Chir* 3:399, 1881.

93. Sun T-C, Swee RG, Shives TC, Unni KK: Chondrosarcoma in Maffucci's syndrome. *J Bone Joint Surg* 67A:1214, 1985.

94. Azouz EM, Slovic AM, Marton, D, et al: The variable manifestations of dysplasia epiphysealis hemimelica. *Pediatr Radiol* 15:44–49, 1985.

95. Rogers IG, Geho WB: Fibrodysplasia ossificans progressiva. *J Bone Joint Surg* 61:909–914, 1979.

96. Leri A, Loiseleur, Lievre J-A: Une nouvelle observation de melorheostose: Etude clinique, anatomique et experimentale. *Bull Mem Soc Med Hôp Paris* 54:1210–1217, 1930.

97. Campbell CJ, Papademetriou T, Bonfiglio M: Melorheostosis: A report of the clinical, roentgenographic, and pathological findings in fourteen cases. *J Bone Joint Surg* 50A:1281–1304, 1968.

98. Younge D, Drummond D, Herring J, Cruess RL: Melorheostosis in children. *J Bone Joint Surg* 61B:415–418, 1979.

99. Larsen LJ, Schottstaedt ER, Bost FC: Multiple congenital dislocations associated with characteristic facial abnormality. *J Pediatr* 37:574–581, 1950.

100. Steel HH, Kohl EJ: Multiple congenital dislocations associated with other skeletal anomalies (Larsen's syndrome) in three siblings. *J Bone Joint Surg* 54A:75–82, 1972.

101. Latta RJ, Graham CB, Aase J, et al: Larsen's syndrome: A skeletal dysplasia with multiple joint dislocations and unusual facies. *J Pediatr* 78:291–298, 1971.

102. Sillence D: Osteogenesis imperfecta: An expanding panorama of variants. *Clin Orthop* 159:11–25, 1981.

103. Sofield HA, Millar EA: Fragmentation realignment and intramedullary rod fixation of deformities of the long bones in children. *J Bone Joint Surg* 41A:1371–1391, 1959.

104. Sztrolovics R, Glorieux FH, Travers R, et al: Osteogenesis imperfecta: Comparison of molecular defects with bone histological changes. *Bone* 15:321–328, 1994.

105. Beighton P, Horan F, Hamersma H: A review of the osteopetroses. *Postgrad Med J* 53:507–516, 1977.

106. Solh H, Da Cunha AM, Giri N, et al: Bone marrow transplantation for infantile malignant osteopetrosis. *J Pediatr Hematol Oncol* 17:350–355, 1995.

CHAPTER 38

Normal and Abnormal Gait in the Pediatric Patient

Roger Dee

NORMAL GAIT

Independent ambulation usually begins between the ages of 12 and 18 months but is usually wide-based and stiff-kneed, reflecting poor balancing skills and relative muscle weakness. At about age 3, the child's gait more closely resembles that of the adult. When walking with an adult, the child has to take more steps per minute to keep up (increased "cadence"). As the child matures, stride length increases and the cadence falls.

The description of gait that follows is based upon the published work of those authors who have been responsible for bringing the study of gait in the gait laboratory into the mainstream of clinical practice. By using this instrument to analyze normal and pathologic gait, they have provided additional insight into the treatment of patients with locomotor disorders.[1-6]

Newton's third law states that for every action there is an equal and opposite reaction. During ambulation, *ground-reactive forces* (*GRF*) produce moments around the joints of the lower limb and pelvis; these moments are resisted by internal joint moments produced by the muscles and ligaments crossing the joints. By measuring the GRF (using a force plate) and also by setting up a system that will measure positions, velocities, and accelerations of all segments of the lower limb (plus anthropometric data), it is possible to calculate the forces and moments acting at the lower limb joints.[5] Three-dimensional kinematic data are obtained in the gait laboratory using a motion measurement system that involves several television cameras and passive retroflected markers placed at strategic points on the lower limb. From the marker locations, the three-dimensional joint kinematics for the lower extremity and pelvis can then be calculated. At the same time, electrical activity is recorded from the muscles of the lower limb, so that muscle activity may be observed during concentric (shortening), eccentric (lengthening), or isometric (neutral) types of contraction.

The principal characteristics of normal gait have been defined as (1) stability in stance, (2) foot clearance in swing, (3) pre-positioning of the foot for initial contact, (4) adequate step length, and (5) energy conservation.[6,7] The normal gait cycle is divided into two major phases—*stance* and *swing* (Fig. 38-1). Stance phase begins with initial contact (heel strike) and ends at toe-off, when swing phase commences. Stance phase makes up the first 60 percent of the cycle and swing phase the remaining 40 percent. The first 10 percent of stance phase is termed

the *loading response.* This is a period of deceleration when the limb absorbs the impact of contact with the floor. This corresponds to a period of preswing on the contralateral leg. This is one of the two periods when both limbs contact the ground (double support). Similarly, at a point between 50 and 60 percent of the cycle, there is a 10 percent period known as preswing that terminates stance phase. This is another period of double support corresponding to loading response on the other leg. The middle 40 percent of stance phase is divided equally into midstance and terminal stance. The swing phase of gait is divided similarly into three periods: initial swing, midswing, and terminal swing.

Using gait laboratory data, it is possible to plot joint *kinematics* for each of the major joints of the lower limb and also to measure the motion of the pelvis in the sagittal, coronal, and transverse planes. In addition to this information about joint motion, the laboratory has the ability to plot the joint *kinetics* (moments) in these various planes for each of the joints and to graph these as flexion or extension moments. If the GRF pass in front of a joint like the knee joint, the external moment generated by the ground reactive force will tend to extend that joint. Internal moments generated either by muscles or ligaments will be required to counteract those dynamic forces on the limb. Finally, the gait laboratory permits us to calculate the *power* generated by muscles across joints. The moment of a force across a joint, it will be recalled, is the product of the magnitude of the force multiplied by the perpendicular distance to the point of action of the force (see Chap. 14). Power generated around a joint in this context is measured as the product of the moment and the angular velocity (muscle force × perpendicular distance × angular velocity = power). The ability to plot the major power phases at each of the joints of the lower limb is valuable. Data from the gait laboratory can measure power generation when muscles are actively accelerating the body during locomotion, but it can also indicate when power is being absorbed by muscles as they contract eccentrically to control excessive joint motion or decelerate segments of the limb (Fig. 38-2).

The Ankle

During the loading response at the ankle, the GRF initially pass posterior to the ankle joint so that an external plantarflexion moment is generated at the ankle (Fig. 38-3).

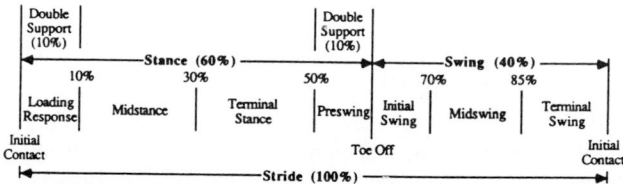

Figure 38-1 Phases of the normal gait cycle. (Reproduced with permission from Ounpuu MS, Gage JR, Davis RB: Three-dimensional lower extremity joint kinetics in normal pediatric gait. *J Pediatr Orthop* 11:334, 1991.)

685

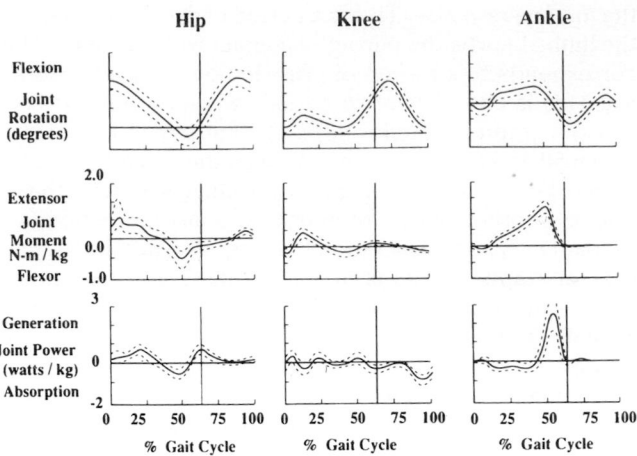

Figure 38-2 The graphic output of sagittal plane moments and powers used at Newington and Gillette Children's Hospitals. From left to right, the top row shows the kinematics of the hip, knee, and ankle, with the gait cycle displayed on the axis and the degrees of motion on the abscissa. The middle row displays the moment of force around each of these joints in newton-meters per kilogram, and the bottom row displays the joint power in watts per kilogram, which is the product of the moment of the joint multiplied by its angular velocity. The solid curves represent the mean and the dotted curves show one standard deviation. (Reproduced with permission from Gage JR: The clinical use of kinetics for evaluation of pathological gait in cerebral palsy. *J Bone Joint Surg* 76A:627, 1994.)

This is counteracted by eccentric contraction of the ankle dorsiflexors (tibialis anterior, extensor digitorum longus, etc.), which gradually permit the foot to come into full contact with the floor. This is called the *period of first rocker*. When the foot is flat on the floor, as locomotion proceeds, the GRF now passes anterior to the ankle joint and an extensor moment is generated. There is eccentric contraction of the plantarflexors as the ankle continues to dorsiflex during what is known as the *period of second rocker*. At the onset of terminal stance, the soleus and gastrocnemius cause concentric plantarflexion, which promotes heel rise, and power generation is now occurring in the calf muscles through the remainder of the stance phase during what is known as the *period of third rocker* (Fig. 38-4). During swing, the anterior tibial muscles concentrically lift the plantarflexed foot in preparation for first contact at the beginning of the next gait cycle.

The Subtalar Joint

Kelikian[8] noted that the medial process of the cuboid lies in a slot beneath the sustentaculum tali, engaging it like a cog in gear and "locking up" the midtarsal joint during inversion of the os calcis. At the onset of stance phase, as body weight is transferred onto the heel at heel strike, internal rotation occurs at the tibia, which simultaneously everts the subtalar joint due to the obliquity of that joint (Figs. 38-5 and 38-6). This has been called the *mitered-hinge*

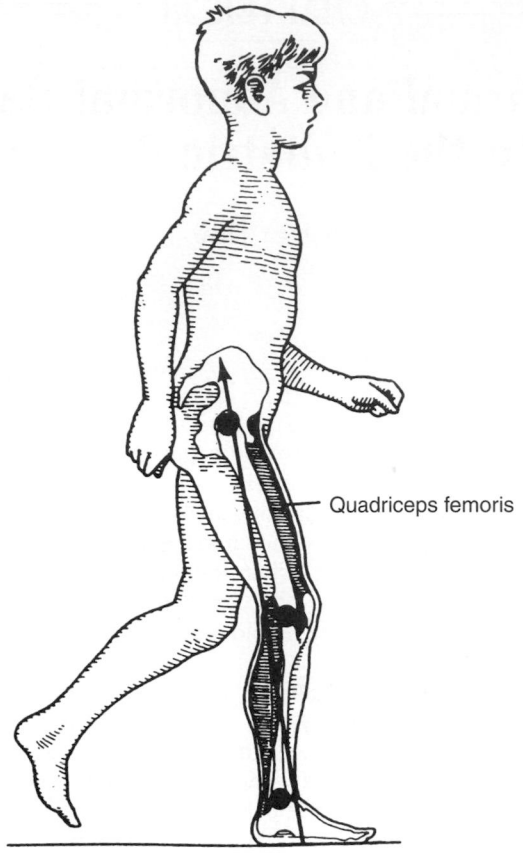

Quadriceps femoris

LOADING RESPONSE

Figure 38-3 The loading response is a period of shock absorption controlled by eccentric contraction of the anterior tibial musculature at the ankle and the quadriceps at the knee. This is the period of the first rocker. (Reproduced with permission from Gage JR: An overview of normal walking. *AAOS Instr Course Lect* 39:297, 1990.)

effect.[9] The eversion of the os calcis unlocks the transverse tarsal joint, so that it becomes more flexible as it approaches the ground during first rocker and is fully planted.[9,10] Once the forefoot contacts the floor, there is a gradual reversal of this motion and inversion is seen to occur as the heel rises during terminal stance, producing an appropriately more rigid foot.

The Knee Joint

Just prior to first contact, the knee flexors are starting to contract eccentrically to slow the extension of the knee in preparation for first contact. At first rocker, the knee is flexed to approximately 15°, which helps absorb some of the impact of first contact and also minimizes the amount of vertical motion of the body's center of mass. During the loading response, the GRF pass posterior to the knee joint and there is therefore an external flexion moment, which is resisted by eccentric action of the quadriceps muscles. Thus the knee is prevented from collapsing into flexion. As the limb moves over the planted foot during midstance,

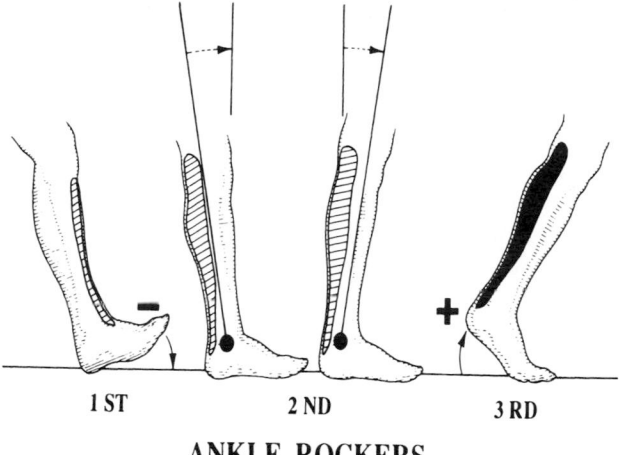

ANKLE ROCKERS

Figure 38-4 Illustration of the three rockers of the ankle in stance. The first two are deceleration rockers, so the respective muscles are acting eccentrically—that is, doing negative work (−) by undergoing a lengthening contraction with energy absorption. The third rocker is an acceleration rocker, so the plantarflexors must act concentrically—that is, produce positive work (+). The point of application of the GRF is forced to move forward with each successive rocker, thus allowing the center of mass to move forward with it. The hatched areas represent eccentric muscle power and the solid areas concentric muscle power. (Reproduced with permission from Gage JR: The clinical use of kinetics for evaluation of pathological gait in cerebral palsy. *J Bone Joint Surg* 76A:625, 1994.)

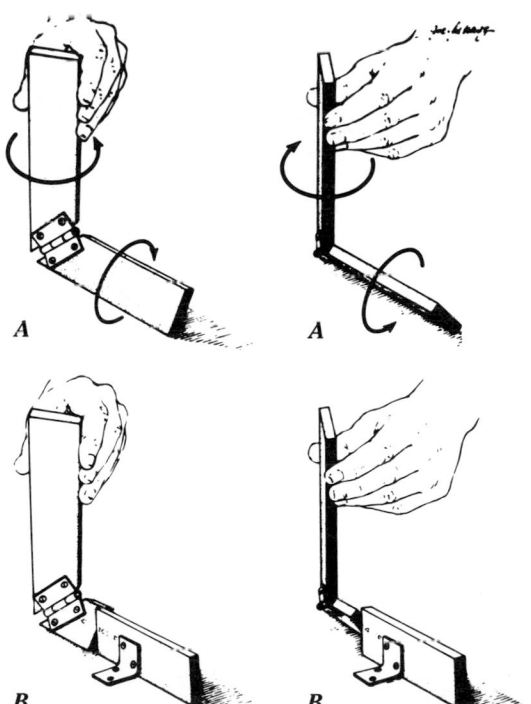

Figure 38-5 *A.* Schematic of the mitered hinge illustrates effect of tibial rotation. *B.* A mobile pivot (representing the calcaneus) when inserted into the model is rotated into eversion during internal tibial rotation. The horizontal member bolted to the floor represents the foot in stance phase. (Reproduced with permission from Inman VT, Mann RA: Biomechanics of the foot and ankle, in *DuVries Surgery of the Foot,* 4th ed. St Louis, Mosby, 1978.)

the GRP moves anterior to the knee joint, so that an external extensor moment is now generated, which is resisted in full extension by a flexor moment generated by ligaments at the back of the knee joint. At heel rise (third rocker), the knee starts to flex and the GRF move posterior to the knee joint, so that an extensor flexor moment is then generated. Power is absorbed as the quadriceps eccentrically contract to counteract this (Fig. 38-7). The knee flexion continues and reaches approximately 45° at toe-off. During swing phase, excessive flexion is controlled by eccentric contraction of the rectus femoris, absorbing power at the knee. This muscle is generating power by proximally accelerating hip flexion concentrically at the same time as it lengthens distally to control excessive knee flexion. Muscles that cross two joints have important but complex functions in controlling locomotion. During terminal swing, as the knee starts to extend again, the rate of extension is now controlled by eccentric contraction of the hamstrings, counterbalancing concentric quadriceps contracture.

The Hip

At first contact, the hip is at approximately 35° of flexion but beginning to extend due to the power generation in the hip extensor muscles, including the gluteus maximus, gluteus medius, and the hamstrings. These power-generating concentric contractions of the hip extensors continue until midway through stance (Fig. 38-2). These muscles also act to prevent the hip joint from collapsing into flexion, since the GRF at this time pass anterior to the joint. During midstance, the GRF move posterior to the hip and the hip extensors still continue to contract concentrically, generating power and pushing the body forward. Electromyography shows that there is little activity in the flexor muscles at this point, energy being absorbed by liga-

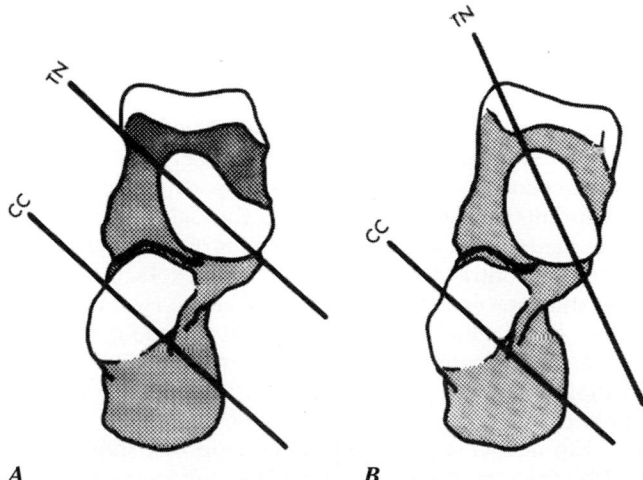

Figure 38-6 Axes of rotation in talonavicular (TN) and calcaneocuboid (CC) joints. These are parallel during eversion (*A*) but not so during inversion (*B*). (Reproduced with permission from Mann RA, in *AAOS Atlas of Orthotics,* 2d ed. St Louis, Mosby, 1985.)

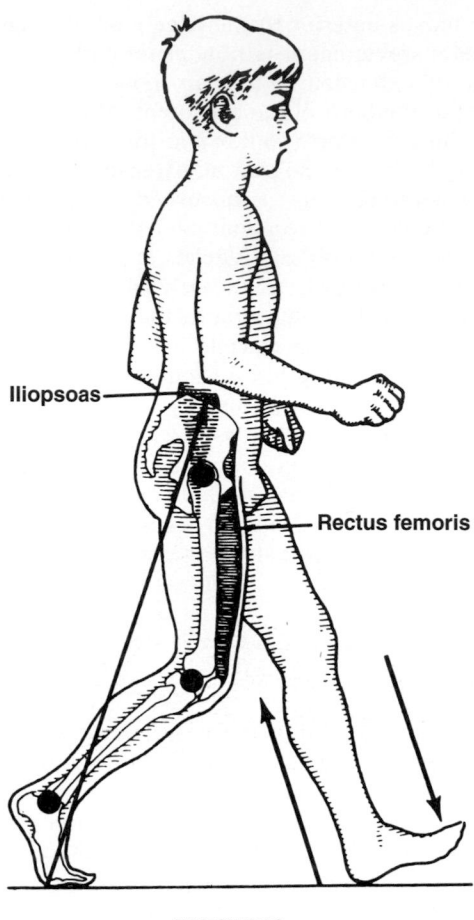

PRESWING

Figure 38-7 Preswing is marked by the onset of double support. As weight is unloaded onto the contralateral foot, concentric action of the iliopsoas accelerates the thigh. Meanwhile, the GRF has fallen behind the knee, creating a strong flexion moment at the joint. Excessive knee flexion is controlled by the rectus femoris, which transfers superfluous kinetic energy from the shank to the pelvis. (Reproduced with permission from Gage JR: An overview of normal walking. *AAOS Instr Course Lect* 39:299, 1990.)

ments and passive muscle stretching in the anterior hip region. However, by terminal stance, the flexor muscles of the hip are eccentrically contracting to absorb power and decelerate hip extension until halfway through the gait cycle at the onset of preswing (double support), at which point concentric contraction begins in the hip flexors, once again generating power and accelerating the limb forward through preswing and initial swing (Fig. 38-7). At the end of terminal stance, the concentric action of the gastrocnemius and the position of the GRF flexes together drive the knee forward and into flexion coincidentally with the hip flexion contracture. Hip flexion is produced by the iliopsoas and accelerated by the rectus femoris, which is simultaneously undergoing eccentric contraction to control excessive knee flexion at the start of preswing and initial swing. Peak hip flexion is reached in midswing. During terminal swing, there is little power generation at the hip, which finally begins to extend in preparation for first contact.

Motion at the Pelvis

During initial contact, the GRF generate adduction moments at the hip and knee, which is resisted by the hip abductors. The adductor magnus muscle supports hip extension and also rotates the pelvis externally toward the forward leg (Fig. 38-8). By midstance, the pelvis has depressed some 5° on the unsupported side and the varus moment is counteracted at the hip by the abductors and at the knee joint by the lateral ligaments and the iliotibial band. By midstance, the hip abductors are contracting concentrically and the unsupported side of the pelvis begins to rise.

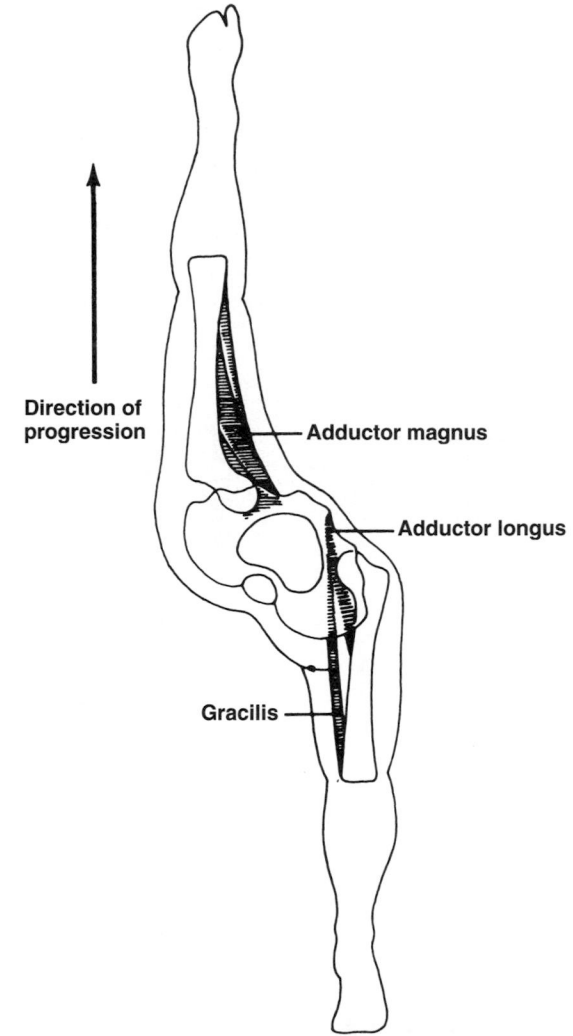

Figure 38-8 A schematic drawing of the transverse plane. Because the front foot is fixed, concentric contraction of the adductor magnus will produce internal rotation of the pelvis and extension of the hip. Concentric contraction of the superficial adductors on the trailing side advances the trailing limb along the line of progression. (Reproduced with permission from Gage JR: An overview of normal walking. *AAOS Instr Course Lect* 39:295, 1990.)

Power Generation

During the cycle, there are phases of power generation and power absorption. These should be noted in Fig. 38-2. The ankle and hip muscles are responsible for the majority of positive work performed during walking (54 percent of the hip and 36 percent at the ankle). The positive power output from the hip is mainly due to the action of the hip extensors during hip extension just after initial contact with another burst of activity associated with the activity of the hip flexors at toe-off. At the ankle, the positive work occurs during the gait cycle in terminal stance and preswing. The knee contributes the majority of negative work (56 percent) associated with the requirement to decelerate segments of the body in a controlled fashion while simultaneously positive work may be done by the same muscles acting across other joints.

PATHOLOGIC GAIT

Each of the attributes of normal walking described under normal gait may be compromised in disease states, particularly neuromuscular conditions. Abnormalities of the foot may influence the pre-positioning of the foot at first contact and stability in stance. Adequate step length may be affected by knee flexion contracture, so that the knee is unable to extend the stride. The ability of the foot to clear the ground in swing may be adversely affected by a stiff knee or a foot that is plantarflexed due to weakness in the dorsiflexors or overactive calf muscles. Any of these abnormal gait patterns will adversely effect energy conservation. Energy consumption may be doubled in a patient with severe gait abnormalities who is using assistive devices.

Widely varying abnormalities of gait are seen in cerebral palsy, where there may be a combination of muscle spasticity together with lack of coordination and balance. There will be abnormalities not only of muscle tone but also of the timing of muscle actions, particularly affecting those muscles that cross two joints. There may be proprioceptive or sensory defects adversely affecting reflex postural balance. The gait laboratory provides, for the first time, consistent explanations for these abnormalities. It has been shown that the results of gait laboratory analysis are reproducible in the same patient when studied in different laboratories.[11] Proponents of gait analysis believe that it provides information that cannot be obtained simply by the clinical examination or visual observation of gait.[7,12] Perry points out that observational analysis requires considerable practice and a systematic approach to train the mind and eye to see deviations from normal. She recommends that if this method is chosen, the clinical analysis should focus on one segment at a time.[13] For example, one would observe the pattern of foot contact with the floor and then, in turn, study the actions throughout the stride of the ankle, knee, hip, pelvis, and trunk. This is good advice for the average clinician, who may not have the resources of a gait laboratory available.

Instrumentation undoubtedly records more action consistently and in greater detail. Clinical examination can certainly evaluate spasticity, and there are many well-known clinical tests for the study of the common muscles found to be overactive in cerebral palsy. However, these examinations give no information about the dynamic activity of these muscles during the gait cycle; only by the use of instrumentation can such critical information be detected and the possibility of an error of surgical judgment thereby minimized or eradicated. An error in surgical judgment involving these patients may mean that a marginal ambulator will become unable to ambulate. Abnormal muscle action may be associated with true shortening of the muscle, there may be spasticity in the muscle, or, alternatively, the problem may simply be due to the weakness of antagonists.

Developmental abnormalities affecting the bone and joints may also adversely affect gait. At the hip, a valgus or short femoral neck (coxa valga or breva) will shorten the moment arm of the abductor muscles. Hip subluxation may also disrupt normal coronal plane gait patterns. Clinically, such problems manifest themselves as a positive Trendelenburg gait with compensatory lurching of the trunk toward the stance leg. Persistent anteversion of the femoral neck associated with a dysplastic hip will manifest itself as an intoeing gait. This abnormality and other lower limb rotational deformity (e.g., tibial torsion) will place the forefoot in a more medial and slightly posterior position at first contact. The GRF adduction moment at the hip and knee will thereby be exaggerated, requiring more counterbalancing activity by the hip abductors. There will be a cost in terms of energy expenditure for all of these problems.

Sagittal Plane Abnormalities

Perry has given a clear exposition of some of the problems in the region of the hip that are commonly seen particularly in cerebral palsy.[13] There may a flexion contracture of the hip or spasticity of the flexor muscles. Alternatively, the hip may be unable to extend normally during gait because of increased knee flexion or plantarflexion of the ankle. There may be primary weakness of the extensor muscles. There will be compensatory lumbar lordosis in midstance and terminal stance in an effort to adapt to the lack of hip extension. If there is limited lumbar spine motion, on the other hand, the trunk cannot compensate but instead will lean forward and require some kind of support, such as a walker or crutches. Sometimes the knee will flex in response to the compensatory hyperlordosis and thus will preserve a neutral alignment of the pelvis in the sagittal plane (Fig. 38-9). However, in the resulting "crouch" position, there is tremendous pressure on the quadriceps muscles, which may exceed their ability to adapt, so that the patient cannot ambulate.

Lack of hip flexion results in a limited ability to advance in swing and also causes toe dragging because the knee cannot flex. Sometimes out-of-phase hamstring contraction is the primary cause of the weak hip flexion.[13] The body will adapt by using the trunk muscles to elevate that side of the pelvis, producing a pelvic hike or circumduction gait.

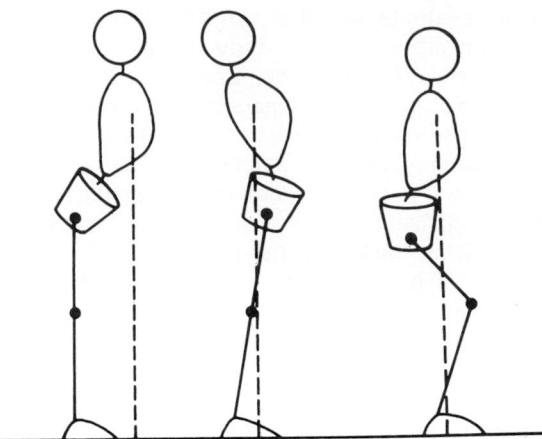

Figure 38-9 Excessive hip flexion: Interference with standing balance and the postures used to realign the body vector over the foot. Lordosis is sufficient to place trunk center posterior to the hip joint. Knee flexion restores a level pelvis. (Reproduced with permission from Perry J: Pathologic gait. *AAOS Instr Course Lect* 29:325–331, 1990.)

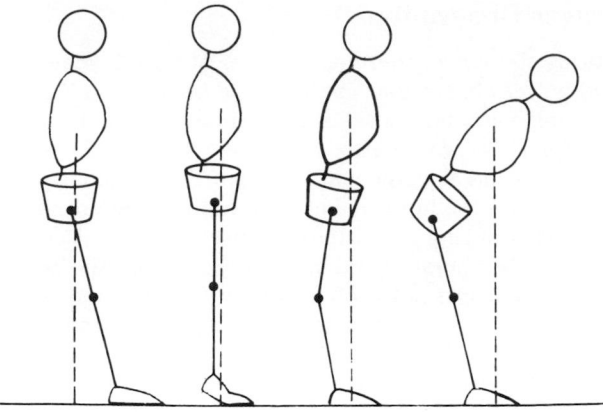

Figure 38-10 Ankle plantarflexion: Interference with standing balance and the postures used to realign the body vector over the foot. Early heel-off. Knee recurvatum. Forward trunk lean. Dotted line indicates body vector. (Reproduced with permission from Perry J: Pathologic gait. *AAOS Instr Course Lect* 29:325–331, 1990.)

Increased knee flexion during gait can be caused by a flexion contracture, spasticity of the knee flexors, or occasionally inadequate power in the quadriceps. The GRF will pass posterior to the knee, and if the quadriceps or the hip extensors are not strong enough to compensate, the knee may collapse further during stance. Other compensatory actions that must take place are increased ankle dorsiflexion and a premature contraction in the rectus femoris, which may impair its normal eccentric action to slow flexion of the knee. It may instead contract concentrically, so that range of motion in the knee joint during swing is impaired.

At the ankle, common gait errors are due to excessive plantarflexion or dorsiflexion. Occasionally there may be a bony deformity affecting ankle joint motion (varus or valgus). If there is an equinus contracture or gastrocsoleus spasticity producing excessive plantarflexion, the heel will not strike the ground at first contact and the GRF will, therefore, be well anterior to their usual position (Fig. 38-10). The normal knee flexion is lost and instead a knee extension moment is produced. The normal first rocker action is not seen and forward progression is therefore limited. The gastrocnemius muscle contracts prematurely, being stretched at both the knee and the ankle, but knee hyperextension nevertheless still develops during terminal stance. During swing, increased flexion of the hip and knee is required to enable the foot to clear the ground. Excessive ankle dorsiflexion may be caused by an ill-advised lengthening of the Achilles tendon or a weak soleus muscle, or it may be secondary to excessive hip flexion, as previously described in the "crouch" gait.

Coronal Plane Abnormalities

Abnormalities of the subtalar joint can be either varus or valgus. The valgus deformity is often associated with weakness of the tibialis posterior muscle, and the gastrosoleus. Varus deformity may not be as important functionally as

any associated equinus provided that the foot drops into a neutral position after it is planted.[13] However, if the foot remains in a position of varus, internal rotation and forefoot adduction during stance phase GRF are abnormally directed and will influence the gait pattern. Overactivity of the tibialis posterior (and occasionally tibialis anterior) plus the long flexors of the toes and hallux contribute to a varus foot deformity. Calcaneovalgus deformity is commonly seen in severe cerebral palsy and may then be associated with weak inverters or spasticity in the peroneal muscles.[7,13]

Varus and valgus deformities of the knee similarly will affect the external moment generated by GRF in the coronal plane. Compensatory valgus deformities commonly develop secondary to long-standing adduction in the hip, and varus deformities of the knee will commonly follow a long-standing hip abduction contracture.

Transverse Plane Abnormalities

The important role of tibial torsion and femoral bony rotational abnormalities in pathologic gait has been emphasized. Identification of the correct cause of transverse plane abnormalities is critical, so that an incorrect surgical procedure is not performed. DeLuca[14] has shown the importance of transverse plane kinematic data in interpreting internal rotation gait abnormalities of the limb in spastic type diplegia (Fig. 38-11). In evaluating transverse plane (rotational) abnormalities of gait, it is important to know whether the pelvis is internally or externally rotated, particularly if one is evaluating femoral anteversion or some other torsional abnormality.

Gait Analysis and Therapeutic Intervention

Gait analysis has been used in other neuromuscular diseases to provide a rational basis for surgical intervention.

Gait analysis has been found useful in studying the gait alterations that occur in muscular dystrophy.[15] In spina bifida, the techniques are being used to predict future ambulatory status.[16] In cerebral palsy, the information obtained has been used to evaluate patients before and after surgical intervention. Furthermore, some authors have suggested that objective criteria can be identified upon which a decision to lengthen the Achilles tendon may be based and the surgical results evaluated in a reproducible manner.[17] Rose and associates have used kinematic and kinetic data to evaluate the response to lengthening of the gastrocnemius fascia. They show by their gait studies that this operation does not result in weakness of the triceps surae at push-off, which may be the case in other procedures used to correct the equinus deformity in spastic cerebral palsy.[18]

Hoffinger and coworkers have used the gait laboratory to study the function of the hamstrings in patients with cerebral palsy crouch gait who in the past have been treated by hamstring lengthening. Their data has enabled them to counsel caution in performing this procedure in some of these patients. They have isolated those patients in whom the hamstrings are doing positive work during gait by aiding hip extension or by exhibiting isometric eccentric lengthening, stabilizing the hip. They point out that clinically detectable tight hamstrings do not necessarily mean short hamstrings and hamstring "weakness" may indeed be an indicator of hip flexion contraction, which should be dealt with instead.[19]

In summary, it should be noted that a great deal of important work is now being performed to delineate accurately and with precision the multiple causes of abnormal gait in children handicapped by muscle or neurologic diseases. The value of this information in improving our surgical practice has now been demonstrated. Gait analysis has also demonstrated its value in adult orthopaedic practice. Andriacchi has measured peak adduction moments at the knee during walking in patients with osteoarthritic varus deformity. He believes, based on the results of his pre- and postoperative studies, that these data can be used to determine more accurately which patients will benefit the most from tibial ostectomy.[20] Gait analysis has also been used to compare the results of knee arthroplasty using different types of prostheses and to study the effect of removing the posterior cruciate ligament at arthroplasty.[21,22]

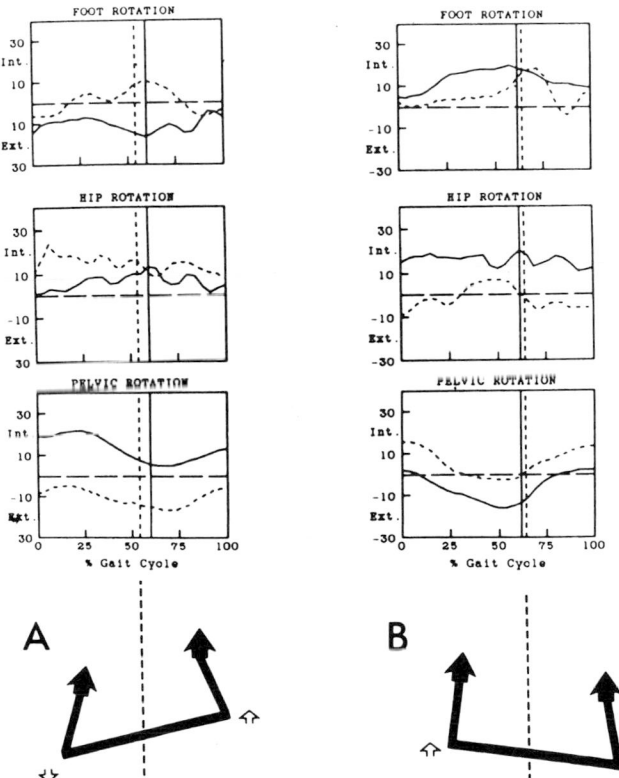

Figure 38-11 Transverse plane kinematic data of (*A*) case 1 (*left column*) and (*B*) case 2 (*right column*). The solid and dotted lines represent rotations of the patients' right and left sides, respectively. Both patients have a diagnosis of asymmetric spastic diplegia and visually have an internal rotation of the left limb. The data for case 1 demonstrate that both hips have excessive internal rotation secondary to femoral anteversion. The left side is more involved and the left pelvis is seen to rotate externally as a compensation. Although the right side of the pelvis is rotated inward, the foot rotation is seen to be external and, in this case, is due to excessive external tibial torsion. Case 2 has excessive right femoral anteversion. The right side of the pelvis is rotated externally as a compensation. In this case, the left foot inward rotation is due to the internal rotation of the pelvis. (Reproduced with permission from DeLuca PA: Gait analysis in the treatment of the ambulatory child with cerebral palsy. *Clin Orthop* 264:68, 1991.)

ACKNOWLEDGMENTS

The author wishes to acknowledge those whose writings form the basis for the information presented in this chapter (see References) and recommends the two excellent CD-ROMs produced by the Gillette Children's Hospital in St. Paul, Minnesota, on normal and pathological gait in cerebral palsy, as invaluable sources of more detailed information.

REFERENCES

1. Gage JR: An overview of normal walking. *AAOS Instr Course Lect* 39:291–305, 1990.
2. Ounpuu S, Gage JR, Davis RB: Three dimensional lower extremity joint kinetics in normal pediatric gait. *J Pediatr Orthop* 11:341–349, 1991.
3. Gage JR: The clinical use of kinetics for evaluation of pathological gait in cerebral palsy. *J Bone Joint Surg* 76A:622–631, 1994.
4. Perry J: "*Phases of Gait*" *Gait Analysis: Normal and Pathological Function.* Thorofare, NJ, Slack, 1992, pp 9–16.
5. Winter DA: *The Biomechanics and Motor Control of Human Gait,* 2d ed. Waterloo, Ontario, Canada, University of Waterloo Press, 1991.

6. Gage JR: Normal Walking: An Overview Based on Gait Analysis. St Paul, MN, Gillette Children's Hospital, 1996 (CD-ROM).

7. Gage JR, DeLuca PA, Renshaw TS: Gait analysis: Principles and applications with emphasis on its use in cerebral palsy. *Instr Course Lect* 45:491–507, 1996.

8. Kelikian A: *Disorders of the Ankle.* Philadelphia, Saunders, 1985.

9. Mann RA: Biomechanics of the foot, in Bunch WH, Keagy R (eds): *AAOS Atlas of Orthotics,* 2d ed. St Louis, Mosby, 1985, pp 112–126.

10. Perry J: Anatomy and biomechanics of the hind foot. *Clin Orthop* 177:9–15, 1983.

11. Kirkpatrick M, Wytch R, Cole G, Helms P: Is the objective assessment of cerebral palsy gait reproducible? *J Pediatr Orthop* 1414:705–708, 1994.

12. Gage JR: The role of gait analysis in the treatment of cerebral palsy. *J Pediatr Orthop* 14:701–702, 1994.

13. Perry J: Pathologic gait. *AAOS Instr Course Lect* 39:325–331, 1990.

14. DeLuca PA: Gait analysis in the treatment of the ambulatory child with cerebral palsy. *Clin Orthop* 264:65–75, 1991.

15. Sutherland DH: Gait analysis in neuromuscular diseases. *AAOS Instr Course Lect* 39:333–341, 1990.

16. Swank M, Dias LS: Walking ability in spina bifida patients: A model for predicting future ambulatory status based on sitting balance and motor level. *J Pediatr Orthop,* 14:715–718, 1994.

17. Etnyre B, Chambers CS, et al: Preoperative and postoperative assessment of surgical intervention for equinus gait in children with cerebral palsy. *J Pediatr Orthop* 13:224–231, 1993.

18. Rose SA, DeLuca PA, et al: Kinematic and kinetic evaluation of the ankle after lengthening of the gastrocnemius fascia in children with cerebral palsy. *J Pediatr Orthop* 13:727–732, 1993.

19. Hoffinger SA, Rab GT, Abou-Ghida H: Hamstrings in cerebral palsy crouch gait. *J Pediatr Orthop* 13:726–732, 1993.

20. Andriacchi TP: Evaluation of surgical procedures and/or joint implants with gait analysis. *AAOS Instr Course Lect* 39:343–349, 1994.

21. Andriacchi TP, Galante JO, Fermier RW: The influence of total knee replacement design on walking and stair-climbing. *J Bone Joint Surg* 64A:1328–1334, 1982.

22. Wilson SA, McCann PD, Gotlin RS, et al: Comprehensive gait analysis in posterior-stabilized knee arthroplasty. *J Arthrop* 11:359–367, 1996.

CHAPTER 39

Femoral Deficiencies

Roger Dee
and Martin A. Gruber

Femoral deficiencies are characterized by a reduction in the osseous material of the bone, producing leg-length discrepancy. They fall into two main groups: those with total or partial deficiencies of the bone and those where there is simply proportional hypoplasia of the femur. Numerous classifications have been attempted, all of which have merit.[1–8]

CLASSIFICATION

The nine classes of congenital abnormality described by Pappas[9] include distal femoral deficiencies (class VI), which are often not included in other classifications. His classification describes a continuum of abnormalities ranging from proximal femoral focal deficiencies to the hypoplastic femora seen in classes V to IX (Fig. 39-1).

EMBRYOLOGIC CONSIDERATIONS

The limb buds first appear in the 5-mm embryo at about 4 weeks.[10–12] The pelvis, acetabulum, and femur are related in their development. The first evidence of acetabular development occurs at 5 weeks. At the same time the mesenchymal condensation representing the proximal femur appears.[6] If a teratologic agent affects development at this point, both the proximal femur and the acetabulum may be completely absent. Between 5 and 6 weeks, the pelvis and femur form two separate cellular mosaics, but the head of the femur develops as part of the pelvic mosaic.[7] Between the sixth and eighth weeks, the chondral model of the femoral shaft is completed and the diaphysis then proceeds to ossify. Also, between the seventh and eighth weeks, joint cavitation occurs. Ossification extends proximally and distally to the level of the metaphysis by the 12th week of intrauterine life. Vascularization and ossification extend into the femoral neck and head region between the 15th and 40th weeks. Interference with the normal process of chondrification or endochondral ossification will produce a varying pattern of congenital lesions, depending on the timing and severity of the noxious agent.[7]

CLINICAL PRESENTATION

When the child is born, the extremity is obviously shortened and there is a typical posture, but the precise nature of the individual deformity remains to be elucidated. Common to all is a position of flexion of hip and knee. There may be associated abnormalities distally in the limb (see Fig. 39-1).

Accurate diagnosis in the neonatal period is extremely important in devising an early management plan.[3,7] Gillespie and Torode believe that, from the point of view of clinical management, there are two principal groups of patients. Group 1 patients have a congenitally short femur but a stable hip joint (i.e., the cartilaginous head, neck, and greater trochanter are present but may not be apparent on early x-rays, since they are radiolucent) (Fig. 39-2). In group 2, according to these authors, the clinical problem is totally different in that there is a true proximal focal femoral deficiency. In group 2 cases, the authors indicate that the thigh segment is considerably shorter and they note that the leg is held in abduction and lateral rotation. They also note that the flexion contractures of the hip and knee are fixed and severe in degree and do not resolve with simple corrective stretching, as they do in children with a group 1–type clinical picture. A group 1 case would correspond to the Pappas classes V to IX, whereas a group 2 deficiency would probably belong to classes I through IV in the Pappas classification.

RADIOLOGIC CHARACTERISTICS

Separating those patients who have the potential for developing a proximal portion of the femur from those where there is a true focal deficiency (classes I through IV) is obviously valuable prognostically, and Fixsen and Lloyd-Roberts[13] have observed several important clues visible on early radiographs (although the proximal femur appears to be absent in all cases). They noted that when the acetabulum appears normal, the femoral head is always present, although its ossification may be delayed. This has been also confirmed by other authors, notably Amstutz,[2] King,[14] and more recently Goddard et al.[15] and Sanpera and Sparks.[8] They also noted that when the proximal end of the distal femoral stump is truly bulbous on the initial x-ray, continuity of the head, neck, and greater trochanter always follows (Fig. 39-3). Fixsen and Lloyd-Roberts indicate that in this kind of abnormality, which they call type I, the hip will become stable proximally, though a pseudarthrosis may develop at the subtrochanteric level.[13] They note that if a tuft or cap of ossification occurs separated from the proximal end of the shaft (which is usually blunt in configuration) by an area of translucency by the age of 1 year, the hip is likely to be unstable. They term this variety type 2. Indeed, whether or not there is a tuft or cap of ossification, if the proximal end of the ossified shaft is blunt, irregular, or pointed, instability is likely (type 3). Additionally they point out that examination of

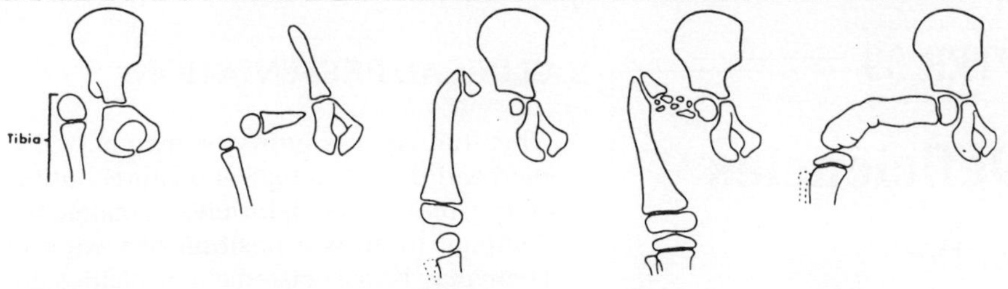

Figure 39-1 The nine classes of congenital abnormalities of the femur are shown here diagrammatically. Information is given regarding the natural history of each and the aim of treatment. (Reproduced with permission from Pappas AM: Congenital abnormalities of the femur and related lower extremity malformations: Classification and treatment. *J Pediatr Orthop* 3:48–49, 1983.)

	Class I	Class II	Class III	Class IV	Class V
Diagram	Tibia				
Femoral shortening (%)	—	70–90	45–80	40–67	48–85
Femoral-pelvic abnormalities	Femur absent Ischiopubic bone structures underdeveloped and deficient Lack of acetabular development	Femoral head absent Ischiopubic bone structures delayed in ossification	No osseous connection between femoral shaft and head Femoral head ossification delayed Acetabulum may be absent Femoral condyles maldeveloped Infrequent irregular tuft on proximal end of femur	Femoral head and shaft joined by irregular calcification in a fibro-cartilaginous matrix	Femur incompletely ossified, hypoplastic, and irregular Mid–shaft of femur abnormal
Associated abnormalities	Fibula absent	Tibia shortened Fibula, foot, knee-joint, and ankle-joint abnormal	Tibia shortened 0–40% Fibula shortened 5–100% Patella absent or small and high riding Knee-joint instability frequent Foot malformed	Tibia shortened 0–20% Fibula shortened 4–60% Knee-joint instability frequent Foot small with infrequent malformations	Tibia shortened 4–27% Fibula shortened 10–100% Knee-joint instability frequent Severe malformations of the foot frequent
Treatment objectives	Prosthetic management	Pelvic-femoral stability through prosthetic management	Union between femoral shaft and hip for hip stability Prosthetic management	Union between femoral head, neck, and shaft Prosthetic management	Prosthetic management

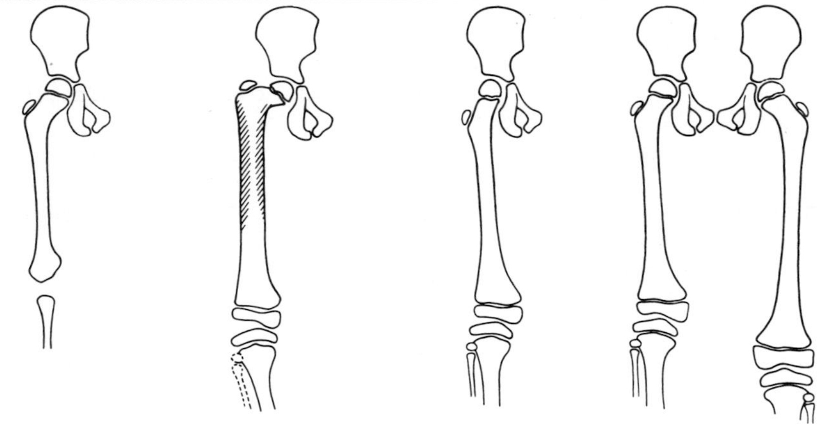

	Class VI	Class VII	Class VIII	Class IX
Diagram				
Femoral shortening (%)	30–60	10–50	10–41	6–20
Femoral-pelvic abnormalities	Distal femur short, irregular, and hypoplastic Irregular distal femoral diaphysis	Coxa vara Hypoplastic femur Proximal femoral diaphysis irregular with thickened cortex Lateral femoral condyle deficiency frequent Valgus distal femur	Coxa valga Hypoplastic femur Femoral head and neck smaller Proximal femoral physis horizontal Abnormality of femoral condyles frequent with associated bowing of shaft and valgus of distal femur	Hypoplastic femur
Associated abnormalities	Single bone lower leg Patella absent Foot malformed	Tibia shortened <10–24% Fibula shortened <10–100% Lateral and high riding patella frequent	Tibia shortened 0–36% Fibula shortened 0–100% Lateral and high riding patella frequent Foot malformed	Tibia shortened 0–15% Fibula shortened 3–30% Additional ipsilateral and contralateral malformations frequent
Treatment objectives	Prosthetic management	Extremity length equality Improved alignment of (a) proximal and (b) distal femur	Extremity length equality Improved alignment of (a) proximal and (b) distal femur	Extremity length equality

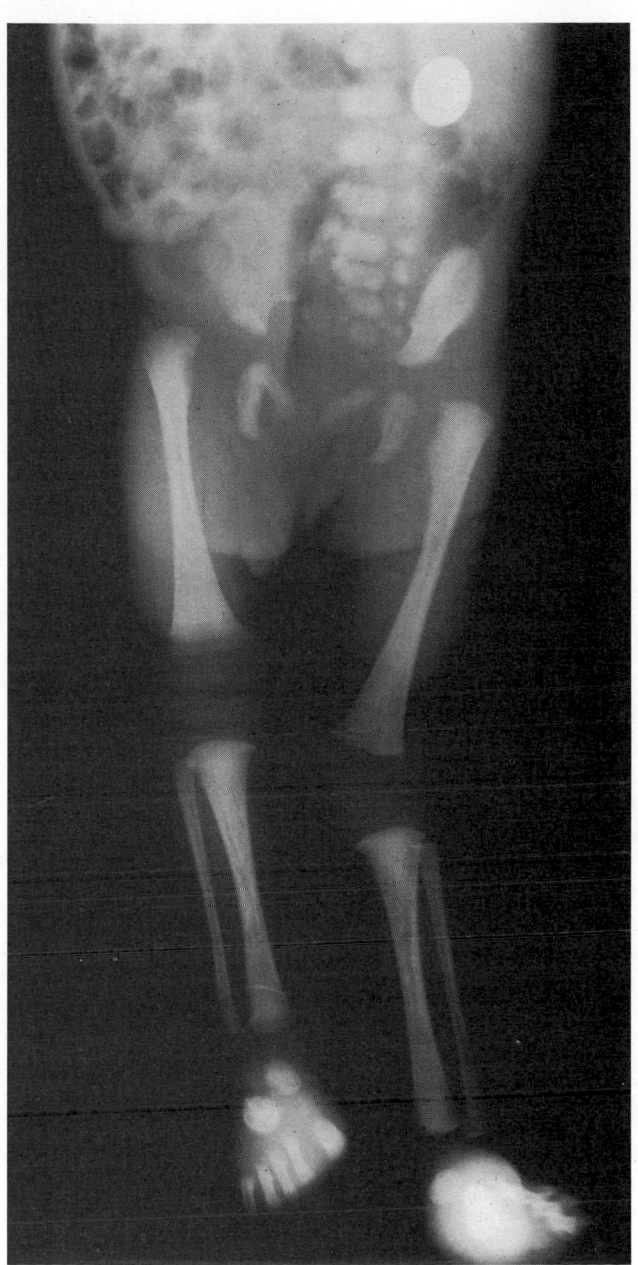

Figure 39-2 Radiograph of hypoplastic femur with coxa vara (class VII).

the nature of the sclerosis in the femoral shaft can give important clues as to the probable underlying defect. In stable defects (that is, those with a proximal cartilaginous model capable of reossification to form a femoral head, neck, and trochanteric region), the sclerosis occurs well down the shaft distal to its most proximal end and nearer its midportion. In the unstable types 2 and 3, however, the sclerosis is always more proximal, indicating that it is immediately distal to the site of any pseudarthrosis or angulation. Additionally, it has the appearance of an inverted V[13] (Fig. 39-3). It would seem that, radiologically, types 2 and 3 (the unstable types) fall within the Pappas classes II through IV. Radiologic interpretation is important because a proximal cartilaginous model that is slow to ossify should,

if possible, be protected and prevented from developing into a pseudarthrosis.[17] Because it is difficult to arrive at an accurate radiologic diagnosis at birth, Fixsen suggests waiting until about 15 months of age before attempting a definitive classification[15] (see treatment of class IV, below).

Magnetic resonance imaging has been studied by Pirani and by Hillman. This technique allows earlier classification by visualizing the cartilaginous anlage of the femoral head before ossification.

GENERAL CONSIDERATIONS OF TREATMENT

If the nature of the individual defect is correctly assessed, a logical plan of treatment can be developed.[3,7,9,18–20]

Decision Making

Epps[19] has observed that the four major biomechanical losses in these children requiring treatment are (1) leg-length inequality, (2) malrotation, (3) instability of the hip joint, and (4) inadequacy of proximal musculature. Also, prophylactic surgery can improve the biomechanical situation and prevent the development of a pseudarthrosis in a patient with coxa vara.

Leg Lengthening

In selected patients, leg-length inequality may be managed in a case classified in classes VII through IX by femoral lengthening, sometimes combined with contralateral epiphysiodesis.[3,5,7] Amstutz pointed out that the percentage of growth inhibition in the congenital segment is fairly constant over time compared with the normal side.[2] This was confirmed by Kalamchi et al.,[5] who observed that variation from the predicted growth was not in excess of 2.4 percent. On the other hand, Pappas believes that congenital abnormalities of the femur in classes II through VI do not follow a proportionate growth rate pattern, although this may be the case for patients in classes VII, VIII, and IX. He believes that abnormal femora grow at a much slower rate in the former group.[9] All authors agree that to project the estimated discrepancy accurately, serial measurements are required, rather than relying on the single radiography.[7,21]

Gillespie and Torode used leg lengthening aggressively, even in patients with a predicted final leg-length discrepancy of 20 cm. They used the Wagner leg-lengthening technique, avoiding delayed union by early rigid internal fixation and bone grafting. These techniques of multiple lengthenings and contralateral epiphysiodesis were associated with a high incidence of complications; therefore other authors[22] feel that lengthening of more than 20 cm is contraindicated. Lengthening the femur beyond 20 percent encourages posterior subluxation of the knee joint, since in these patients the knee joint is commonly abnormal.[3] Sanpera et al.[23] noted that all knees are not unstable

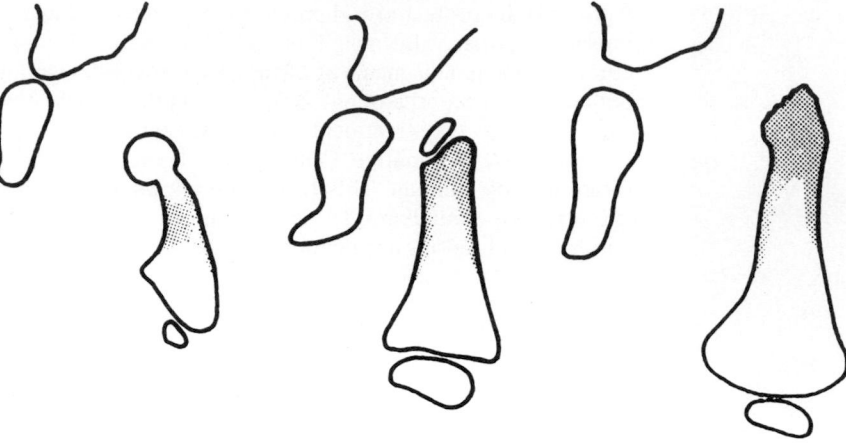

Figure 39-3 Diagram from tracings of radiographs showing the typical early appearance of the bones in the stable and unstable types of proximal femoral dysplasia. Note the bulbous proximal end of the stable type seen on early radiographs. Also observe the shaded area which represents the different patterns of sclerosis seen in the stable and unstable types of dysplasia. (Reproduced with permission from Fixsen JA, Lloyd-Roberts GC: The natural history and early treatment of proximal femoral dysplasia. *J Bone Joint Surg* 56B:91, 1974.)

Type 1 (stable)   Type 2 (unstable)   Type 3 (unstable)

and that the degree of knee instability is variable, so that individual careful evaluation of knee stability is essential. In some children, lengthening beyond 20 percent can be accomplished without knee dislocation. Occasionally, lengthening the femur by 20 percent combined with ankle disarticulation permits a below-knee prosthesis to be fitted. This option is particularly valuable in patients with associated fibular hemimelia (commonly associated with congenital femoral shortening[24] and deformity of the foot) where the Van Nes rotation-plasty (see below) is unsuitable.[3] Because of the severe femoral shortening, however, knee fusion is usually indicated, and the child is then treated like an above-knee amputee. Pappas points out that the repair potential of this bone is not normal and supplemental bone graft and extremely long periods of hospitalization and immobilization may be required after leg lengthenings.

Hip Stability

Hip stability is particularly important for patients in classes III and IV who may have a normal acetabulum. The recognition of an acetabulum on early x-rays helps to identify this group and to differentiate them from class II patients. Initially, prosthetic management should be used to stabilize the hip joint (this is the only available option in class II cases). Later on, in class III and IV patients, metaphyseal-epiphyseal synostosis can be accomplished. Goddard et al. noted that fusion occurs in about 30 percent of cases.[15] In the remainder, operative intervention is needed. This involves obtaining fusion between the femoral stump and the femoral epiphysis. A tibial or fibular graft may be placed across the abnormal area from the ossified femur to the cartilaginous femoral head. Occasionally, it may be necessary to impact the end of the ossified shaft into the epiphysis, particularly if there are two pseudarthroses and the intermediate piece of ossified fragment is not worth preserving.[13]

In a class IV patient, Pappas recommends excising the disorganized fibro-osseous material between the shaft and the epiphysis as an aid to procuring synostosis. He ad-

vises surgery after the femoral head has begun to ossify and when the intermediate region has declared itself, often revealed by the essence of dense, speckled calcification.[9] At this point surgery should probably not be delayed. In obtaining union and stabilizing the hip in these patients, it should be remembered that the degree of shortening produced at surgery is not so important. Subsequent procedures will be performed distally to achieve appropriate prosthetic fitting.

Often, the results of stabilizing surgery to repair a pseudarthrosis around the hip are not entirely satisfactory. Although the x-ray appearance is improved, the gait pattern will often remain disappointing, with a persistent Trendelenburg gait due to inadequacy of the abductor mechanism.[3] Additionally, there may be joint stiffness, rendering prosthetic rehabilitation less satisfactory.[19] Usually, however, the benefits outweigh the disadvantages when successful union is achieved.

Stability may also be achieved by means of an iliofemoral fusion.[25] Steel et al. reported good results after a follow-up of more than 5 years with this procedure. The femur was shortened sufficiently to place the knee at the level of the triradiate cartilage, so that it might act as a hip joint. Secondary procedures including a rotational osteotomy and Symes amputation improved function. Stabilizing procedures should not be performed until the ossification of the femoral shaft and head has developed to a point where there is sufficient satisfactory bone to achieve union. If it is attempted prematurely, a satisfactory result will not be achieved.[7]

Femoral osteotomy to correct the angle of the neck shaft will often be required for the coxa vara of the class VII deformity.[5,9] Rotational deformities may also require attention.

Additional Procedures

Knee arthrodesis is often performed in these patients. Instability of the knee due to soft tissue imbalance is thereby corrected and an appropriate portion of bone can be conveniently resected to achieve the required leg length.[9] This often means excision of both knee epiphyses. Consideration must be given to whether a patient is to be managed as an above-the-knee or below-the-knee amputee.[18]

The alternatives include ablation of the foot by either a Boyd- or Syme-type amputation, both of which give good end-bearing stumps suitable for the prosthesis. The knee joint can be initially stabilized within the socket of the prosthesis until the appropriate time for knee fusion.[19] Many of these patients will be treated by Van Nes tibial rotation-plasty combined with leg shortening, knee fusion, and foot preservation. In this procedure the lower limb is rotated 180°. The ankle joint is adjusted to the same level as the contralateral knee joint and will simulate knee function when fitted with a modified below-the-knee prosthesis.[19,21,26,27] This option is not available if there is a foot deformity associated with fibular hemimelia.

In a patient with proximal local femoral deficiency (e.g., classes II, III, or IV), leg shortening is not usually required to perform the Van Nes rotation-plasty. Early surgery in these cases is usually knee fusion, the foot being preserved until the rotation is performed at a later age.[12] There is a high incidence of patients requiring reoperation, as the tibia spontaneously rerotates with growth. Thus some authors prefer to postpone the procedure until after age 12.[26] For patients in classes VII, VIII, and IX with a lesser degree of shortening and no proximal focal deficiency, the Van Nes option may be chosen if leg-length inequality cannot be appropriately corrected by lengthening procedures and contralateral epiphysiodesis. At the time of the Van Nes procedure, leg shortening will then be required, together with knee fusion. Alman compared the efficiency of Symes amputation and knee fusion with rotation-plasty, using physical appearance, gross motor function, and energy efficiency as criteria. His group found that rotation-plasty was more energy-efficient and that there was no difference in motor function or perceived physical appearance between the two groups.[28]

Van Nes Rotation-Plasty

This procedure is shown in Fig. 39-4. The popliteal artery is permitted to rotate by opening up the distal end of the adductor canal and releasing the insertion of the adductor magnus to the distal femur. The common peroneal nerve is mobilized. The origins of the medial and lateral heads of the gastrocnemius are divided at the knee. Osteotomy is performed through the proximal tibia and the proximal tibial segment is then rotated at the knee joint through approximately 140° or more. If necessary, the additional 40° of rotation may be achieved at the tibial osteotomy site. The position is stabilized with the use of an intramedullary rod.[21]

It is important that the child have normal neurovascular structures, a stable and functional ankle, and a normal foot configuration.[7] The patient and family should be made fully aware of the appearance to be expected following this procedure, preferably by meeting another person who has had the operation. Opinions are divided on the appearance of the limb, and the disturbance level upon

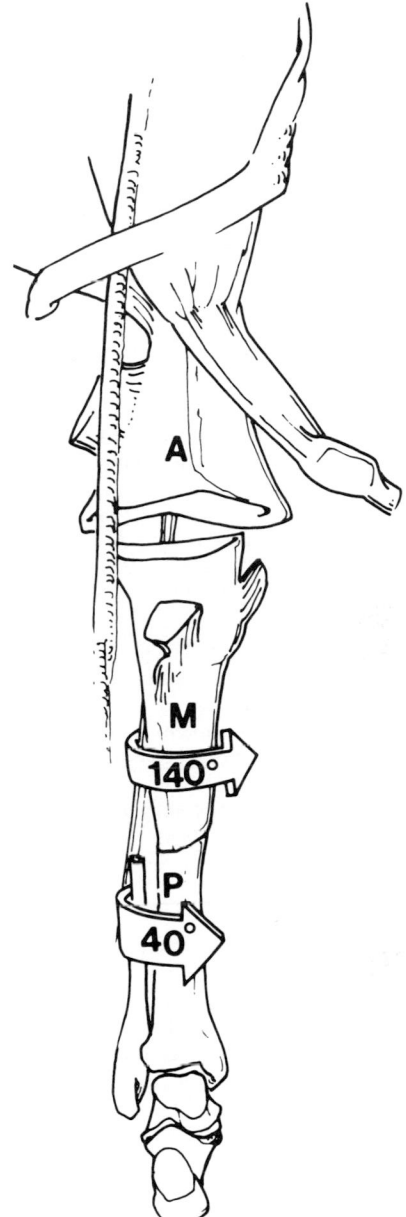

Figure 39-4 The operation of Van Nes rotation-plasty. Portions of the distal femur and proximal tibia have been removed, allowing rotation of the proximal tibia. The proximal tibial segment is rotated as much as possible (140° in this example) and the remaining rotation obtained at the tibial shaft osteotomy. (A, anterior; M, medial; P, posterior anatomical bone surfaces.) (Reproduced with permission from Torode IP, Gillespie R: Rotation-plasty of the lower limb for congenital defects of the femur. *J Bone Joint Surg* 65B:571, 1983.)

viewing the limb certainly varies between individuals. Functional performance following this procedure is good and these children can walk at speeds that are comparable to those of normal children.[28,29] They can also run and climb stairs and participate in many recreational activities. From the functional point of view there are definite advantages over the end bearing of an above-knee amputation in having a joint that functions as a knee joint.[7,9] For detailed management of each of the categories shown in Fig. 39-1, the reader is referred to Pappas.[7]

REFERENCES

1. Aitken GT: Proximal femoral focal deficiency—Definition, classification and management, in Aitken GT (ed): *Proximal Femoral Focal Deficiency: A Congenital Anomaly.* Washington, DC, National Academy of Sciences, 1969.
2. Amstutz HC: The morphology, natural history and treatment of proximal femoral focal deficiencies, in Aitken GT (ed): *Proximal Femoral Focal Deficiency: A Congenital Anomaly.* Washington DC, National Academy of Sciences, 1969.
3. Gillespie R, Torode IP: Classification in the management of congenital abnormalities of the femur. *J Bone Joint Surg* 65B:557–562, 1983.
4. Hamanishi C: Congenital short femur: Clinical, genetic and epidemiological comparison of the naturally occurring condition caused by thalidomide. *J Bone Joint Surg* 62B:307–320, 1980.
5. Kalamchi A et al: Congenital deficiency of the femur. *J Pediatr Orthop* 5:129–134, 1985.
6. Lange DR, Schoenecker PL, Baker C: Proximal femoral focal deficiency: Treatment and classification in forty-two cases. *Clin Orthop* 135:15–25, 1978.
7. Pappas AM: Congenital abnormalities of the femur and related lower extremity malformations: Classification and treatment. *J Pediatr Orthop* 3:45–60, 1983.
8. Sanpera I Jr, Sparks LT: Proximal femoral focal deficiency: Does a radiologic classification exist? *J Pediatr Orthop* 14:34–38, 1994.
9. Murray MP et al: Functional performance after tibial rotationplasty. *J Bone Joint Surg* 67A:392–399, 1985.
10. Felts WJL: The prenatal development of the human femur. *Am J Anat* 94:1–41, 1954.
11. Gardiner E, Gray DJ: The prenatal development of the human hip joint. *Am J Anat* 87:163–211, 1950.
12. Gardiner E, Gray DJ: The prenatal development of the human femur. *Am J Anat* 129:121–140, 1970.
13. Fixsen JA, Lloyd-Roberts GC: The natural history and early treatment of proximal femoral dysplasia. *J Bone Joint Surg* 56B:86–95, 1974.
14. King RE: Some concepts of proximal femoral focal deficiency, in Aitken CT (ed): *Proximal Femoral Focal Deficiency: A Congenital Anomaly.* Washington DC, National Academy of Sciences, 1969.
15. Goddard NJ, Hashemi-Nejad A, Fixsen JA: Natural history and treatment of instability of the hip in proximal femoral focal deficiency. *J Pediatr Orthop* B4:145–194, 1995.
16. Pirani S, Beauchamp RD, Li D, Sawatzky B: Soft tissue anatomy of proximal focal femoral deficiency. *J Pediatr Orthop* 11:563–570, 1991.
17. Hillmann JS, Mesgarzadeh M, Revesz G, et al: Proximal femoral focal deficiency: Radiologic analysis of 49 cases. *Radiology* 165:769–773, 1987.
18. Amstutz HC, Wilson PD: Dysgenesis of the proximal femur (coxa vara) and its surgical management. *J Bone Joint Surg* 44A:1–23, 1962.
19. Epps CH Jr: Current concepts review: Proximal femoral focal deficiency. *J Bone Joint Surg* 65A:867–870, 1983.
20. Van Nes CP: Rotation-plasty for congenital defects of the femur: Making use of the shortened limb to control the knee joint of a prosthesis. *J Bone Joint Surg* 32B:12–16, 1950.
21. Torode IP, Gillespie R: Rotation-plasty of the lower limb for congenital defects of the femur. *J Bone Joint Surg* 65B:569–573, 1983.
22. Damsin JP, Pous JG, Ghanem I: Therapeutic approach to severe congenital lower limb length discrepancies: Surgical treatment versus prosthetic management. *J Pediatr Orthop* B4:164–170, 1995.
23. Sanpera I Jr, Fixsen JA, Sparks LT, Hill RA: Knee in congenital short femur. *J Pediatr Orthop* B4:159–163, 1995.
24. Sorge G, Srdito S, Genuardi M, et al: Proximal femoral focal deficiency (PFFD) and fibular A/hypoplasia (FA/H): A model of a developmental field defect. *Am J Med Genet* 55:427–432, 1995.
25. Steel HH, Lin PS, Betz RR, et al: Iliofemoral fusion for proximal femoral focal deficiency. *J Bone Joint Surg* 69A:837–843, 1987.
26. Kostuik JP, Gillespie R, Hall JE, Hubbard S: Van Nes rotational osteotomy for treatment of proximal femoral focal deficiency and congenital short femur. *J Bone Joint Surg* 57A:1039–1046, 1975.
27. Kritter AE: Tibial rotation-plasty for proximal femoral focal deficiency. *J Bone Joint Surg* 58A:927–934, 1977.
28. Alman BA, Krajbich JI, Hubbard S: Proximal femoral focal deficiency: Results of rotationplasty and Syme amputation. *J Bone Joint Surg* 77A:1876–1882, 1995.
29. Friscia DA, Moseley CF, Oppenheim WL: Rotational osteotomy for proximal femoral focal deficiency. *J Bone Joint Surg* 71A:1386–1392, 1989.

CHAPTER 40

Infantile Hip Dysplasia (Congenital Dislocation of the Hip)

Martin A. Gruber, Donald M. Kastenbaum, Douglas G. Avella, and Wallace B. Lehman

INCIDENCE

The incidence of all forms of hip instability has been reported in the United States to be between 1 and 6 cases per 1000 births.[14,50,92,135] The left hip is affected about twice as frequently as the right.

Risk Factors

Infants at highest risk for developmental hip dysplasia are firstborn girls. Next in importance is family history.[2] Other factors include breech presentation, torticollis, scoliosis, or some other musculoskeletal abnormality.[21,64,65]

Of 11 children with congenital torticollis, 2 had associated hip dysplasia.[65] Calcaneovalgus feet have been reported in association with congenital dislocation of the hip in 25 percent of cases in South Australia.[113] The incidence has been reported to be 10 times greater than normal in children with idiopathic scoliosis.[64]

ETIOLOGY

The hip develops when the block of condensed mesenchymal cells that will form the hip separates by the formation of a cleft at about the 11th postgestational week. True hip dislocation may occur at any time from this point until the postnatal period.[155] Dislocations caused by known neuromuscular disorders present at birth are called *teratologic dislocations* and are discussed elsewhere in this volume. Long-standing deformations within the uterus produce structural changes that are present at birth.

In the more typical form of hip dysplasia, genetic, hormonal, and mechanical factors have each been reported to be significant. A familial tendency to dislocation is demonstrated by studies of families in which more than one child has been shown to have infantile hip dysplasia. The chance of a second child being affected in such a family is about 10 times the expected risk in the general population. Wynne-Davies, Carr, and others[19,158] found that a higher proportion of children with infantile hip dysplasia were lax-jointed as compared with the control population. The degree of joint laxity was in no way different than that exhibited by many normal children, however, and could not in itself be sufficient to explain why the abnormality was present. There was also a higher proportion of lax-jointed individuals among the first-degree relatives of these patients, who were also lax-jointed compared with the control population. The second familial tendency noted was with regard to acetabular dysplasia. The apparently normal parents of children with dislocations had a shallower acetabulum than was found in a control population. Acetabular dysplasia may well be inherited as a multiple gene system, separating this group of cases from those where the joint laxity is primary. This leads to the conclusion that there are two groups, one born with a propensity for acetabular dysplasia at birth and another with joint laxity (who may later develop acetabular dysplasia due to mechanical factors).

Dunn, observing that dislocation of the hip in the neonate was often associated with other musculoskeletal deformities, believed that intrauterine molding was an important factor in their production. Mechanical factors associated with packing disorders in the uterus will greatly increase the incidence of dislocation. There is a greater incidence of congenital dysplasia of the hip (CDH) in primiparous deliveries, in which the uterine and abdominal walls may be tight.[47] The importance of the breech presentation and its effects in the uterus have been confirmed by the finding that infants in breech position born by cesarean section are prone to hip dislocation. Fetal intrauterine limb position is the critical factor. In the breech position, when the knees are hyperextended, there is a delay in developing the flexed knee position that ordinarily helps stabilize the hips of newborns. Associated with the hyperextended knees and the hyperflexed hips are hamstring tightness and iliopsoas contractures.

Three periods in prenatal life during which the hip is at risk have been identified by Stanisavlijevic.[135] At the beginning of the 12th week, the first risk period arises, when medial flotation of the limb occurs. The newly formed labrum is vulnerable at this time and the hip must be very stable during this period. Any deficiency in growth of the labrum (limbus) will result in instability and early dislocation around the 18th week of fetal development. The second risk period arises when active motion of the hip joint begins. Any structural abnormality such as underdevelopment of the anterior capsule, the reinforcing ligament of Bigelow, or the overlying rectus muscle will predispose to dislocation at this time. The initial period of risk is during the last 4 weeks of fetal development. It is at this time that factors such as the breech position, associated with other hormonal or hydrodynamic abnormalities (e.g., oligohydramnios), may suffice to produce congenital hip pathology. Hormonal abnormalities were believed by Andren and Borglin[3] to induce capsular laxity. They reported an increased urinary excretion of estrone and 1 7,8-estradiol during the first week of life, which they believed was due to an inborn error of metabolism. However, this work has not been confirmed by assays performed by other works.[1,144] Wilkinson successfully produced hip dislocation in young rabbits by administering estrogen, but he also splinted the hindlimbs in the breech position.[156] At this time the role of maternal hormones in the last trimester is not thought to be any more than a contributing factor in the multifactorial etiology of this condition. Many children with unilateral hip dysplasia have pelvic obliquity with a fixed abduction deformity on the "normal" side.[47] This abnormality of the contralateral hip places the affected hip in a relatively adducted position. Although the intrauterine position of marked flexion usually found in the fetus will protect these hips, as the hips assume a more extended position at birth, the pelvic obliquity will persist and the adducted hip will be at risk for dislocation. It is interesting that the left hip is more commonly adducted and dysplastic with pelvic obliquity, which is in conformity with the general overall statistics for all hip dysplasia.[47] Dunn showed that the fetus is usually positioned in the uterus with its back toward the mother's left side, this being the position in which the posterior extremity would be more likely to be abducted.[29,30]

PATHOLOGIC ANATOMY

The role of mechanical factors in neonatal hip instability has been studied in the laboratory by loading autopsy specimens. It has been found that deformation of the joint cartilage occurs when neonatal hips are loaded with moderate force for a period of approximately 3 h and that, after loading, marked joint laxity persists.[63] A classification scheme based primarily on the configuration of the acetabulum and whether or not the limbus was inverted or everted was devised by Dunn.[30] He differentiated type I, a hip showing positional instability, from type II, a sublimed hip, and type III, a dislocated hip. The teratologic hip at birth will usually be type II or type III.

Ogden has stressed the dynamic pathobiologic changes responsible for these differences.[110] In a type III hip dysplasia, posterosuperior dislocation occurs with an everted labrum and a false acetabulum. The ligamentum teres is elongated and pulls on the transverse acetabular ligament, further compromising acetabular volume. All these factors, together with the hourglass deformity of the capsule, which is formed by constriction of the psoas tendon, may prevent reduction. This type of deformity will also occur progressively if there is delay in treating the type II hip, which may be only subluxed at birth. Normally at birth, a type I pattern is seen in the overwhelming proportion of cases.[110] The positionally unstable hip (type I) will show only marginal changes in the acetabulum. To casual observation, the acetabulum is not dysplastic. Precise measurements, however, may show values that fall outside the standard deviation for normal subjects.[154] If not detected at birth, a type I patient with associated joint laxity may progress to a type II pattern. Then there will be definite subluxation, loss of femoral head sphericity, and progressive eversion of the labrum together with superior and posterior marginal deformities of the acetabulum.[110]

Additional changes that may be seen progressively in type II and III deformities include flexion and adduction contractures and increasing dysplasia of the anterior acetabular margin (the acetabulum will not develop normally unless there is congruent reduction); also, an increasing degree of femoral anteversion may occur, associated with failure of joint congruency. Limitation of rotation of the femur in the subluxed and dislocated position may also contribute to the femoral anteversion.[94]

Primary *anterior* infantile hip dislocation is exceedingly rare. It can be diagnosed in infancy as a distinct entity. There is a visible and palpable fullness in the femoral triangle associated with marked limitation of abduction and sometimes a severe pelvic obliquity. In these patients, stable reduction is in the position of flexion abduction and internal rotation.[91]

DIAGNOSIS

Physical Assessment

In 1962, Barlow[5] and Von Rosen[152] reported the use of a little-known procedure described by Ortolani, an Italian pediatrician, as a screening test for congenital dislocation of the hip.[111] In Ortolani's test, the baby lies supine with its hips and knees fixed. The pelvis is stabilized with the examiner's hand. The involved hip is examined with a special grip, the thumb being placed in the region of the lesser trochanter on the medial side, the web space of the examiner's hand being placed over the proximal tibia and the long finger over the greater trochanter. The hip is then abducted at 90° of flexion. At the same time gentle, anteriorly directed pressure is applied to the greater trochanter to lift the femoral head, if dislocated, into the acetabulum (Fig. 40-1A). Ortolani's test is positive when the head of the femur is felt to slip back into the acetabulum; therefore it is a test for the dislocated hip.[111]

Barlow described an additional test which he said was more sensitive than the Ortolani test. This is now termed *Barlow's test* and is part of the routine physical examination in the neonate. In this test pressure is applied backward and inward with the thumb on the inner side of the thigh. Once again the infant's hips and knees are flexed (Fig. 40-1B). If the femoral head is unstable, it is gently dislocated by this maneuver and then reduced again with the Ortolani test. Thus, the Barlow test is a test for a *dislocatable* hip.[5] It is important that the test be performed with the baby relaxed and with a sufficient degree of gentleness that pain is not produced, which will make the examination unreliable. Particular care must be taken that the thumb not be pressed hard into the groin. An audible click is *not* the endpoint of these tests. It is instead a *palpable* clunking feeling as the hip dislocates and reduces. Clicks may be produced by ligamentous or fascial structures around the hip and therefore are usually of no significance.

According to Catterall, between the extremes of true dislocation and severe dysplasia on the one hand and a normal hip on the other, there lies a "spectrum of dysplasias" whose clinical feature is a limitation of abduction of the hip flexed to 90°.[20] He points out that radiologic findings in these patients are also variable. The development of real-time ultrasonographic visualization of the hip has facilitated a more precise analysis of this spectrum.[8,33,89,146]

Figure 40-1 *A*. Ortolani reduction test—child is placed on a flat surface. Hips and knees are flexed to 90°. Long finger is placed on the greater trochanter and the thigh is lifted and abducted. *B*. Barlow dislocation test—child's thighs are adducted with gentle downward pressure. Dislocation is felt as the femoral head slips out of the acetabulum (see text).

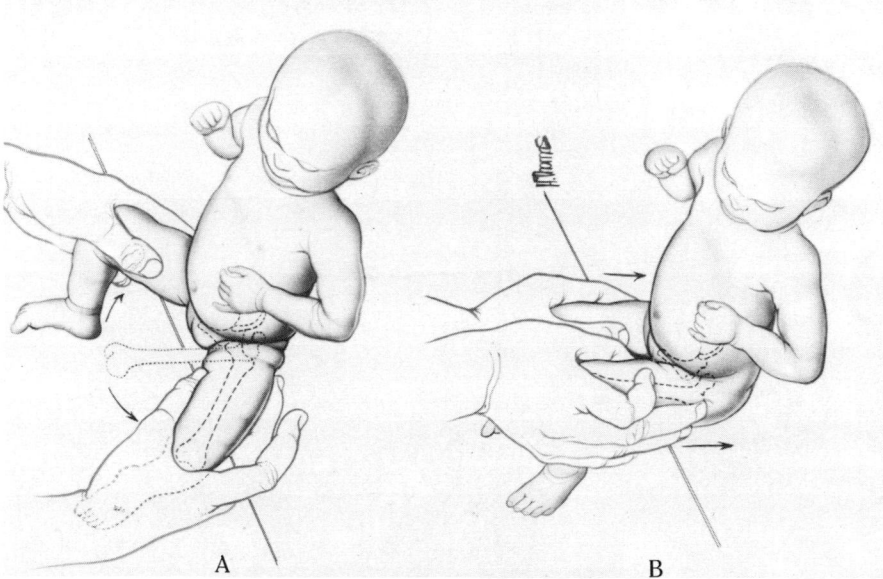

A   B

McKinnon and his coworkers found that 1.61 percent of screened newborns who were examined in the usual way had what the authors identified as *subluxatable* (but not dislocatable) hips. When assessed by the examiner using Barlow's test, they tested negative. The profile of this group was similar to that of patients with dislocated hips. There was consequently an increased frequency of females and breech presentations, left-sided involvement, and associated postural deformities. Significantly, even when treated with an abduction brace, some patients showed acetabular dysplasia or persistent hip laxity at long-term follow-up.[95] It has been shown that many of these patients can be diagnosed by ultrasound.[55,89,146] Some of them may appear as late-diagnosed cases in spite of competent screening programs.[58,69,145]

Radiologic Assessment

An accurate anteroposterior x-ray may show diagnostic features even in the neonate, but a "normal" film does not exclude the diagnosis of instability.[24]

Figure 40-2 and its accompanying legend explains some of the routine measurements that may be valuable. The D and H measurements described and indicated in this figure are of value in a unilateral case but not helpful in bilateral dysplasia.[24] Measurements of the acetabular index, "Hilgenreiner's acetabular angle,"[9,56,57] is particularly unreliable in newborns, since any rotation of the pelvis will render the measurement inaccurate.[9,24] The Von Rosen view taken in 45° bilateral abduction and internal rotation was believed by its author to be a method of showing the dislocated position in the neonate. A line was drawn along the axis of the shaft of the femur. According to Von Rosen, it passes through the lateral margin of the acetabulum in the undislocated hip but through the anterosuperior spine in the dislocated position.[152] Unfortunately, this position will often reduce the positionally unstable hip, so that these radiographs are not reliable for excluding the diagnosis.[24] Catterall has pointed out that apparent pelvic obliquity detected on some early x-rays may also be a result of postural rotational anomalies of the pelvis.[20]

The thickness of the acetabular floor and also the horizontal diameter of the femoral head have been measured and found to be abnormal in older patients with CDH (averaging 27 months). The increased bony thickness of the acetabular floor is probably a reflection of abnormal molding caused by the absence of the femoral head from within it.[112] Thus, the observed lateralization of the femoral head identified in the unreduced hip indicates soft tissue obstruction plus some increased size of the femoral head and increased acetabular thickening. Details of intraarticular pathology and "false lateralization" are well shown with both arthrography and ultrasonography.[131]

In some children, acetabular dysplasia begins to be noted at 6 months or so. Gross points out that such dysplasia is not detectable at birth, and this may be another reason for late diagnosis.[49] Therefore, the use of the terminology *developmental hip dysplasia* is to be preferred to the term *congenital dislocation of the hip,* since the former correctly indicates that some hips dislocate after birth and are therefore not congenital.

Attempts have been made to correlate measurements of acetabular dysplasia with the long-term prognosis of a particular hip joint. This is important in predicting acetabular development following open or closed reduction and in deciding when acetabuloplasty may be advisable. The upper limit of normal values for Hilgenreiner's angle (acetabular index) is 30° (up to 1 year), 25° (1 to 3 years), and 20° (3 years to adult).[57] These numbers are useful in assessing the severity of acetabular dysplasia (Fig. 40-2). Also useful in assessment of the future of the joint is the center-edge (CE) angle of Wiberg. This is measured from the center of the head to the superolateral edge of the acetabulum[9] (Fig. 40-3). Bos et al. utilizing MRI, has described a group of children with apparent acetabular dysplasia on

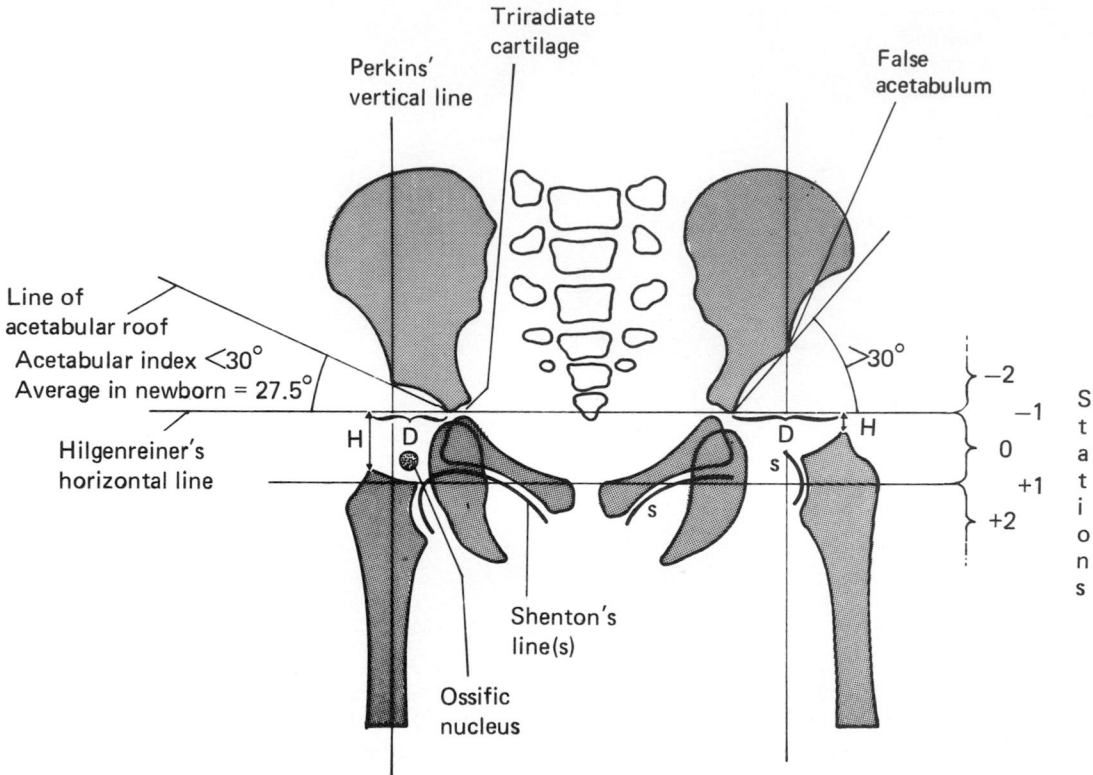

Figure 40-2 Measurements used for radiologic evaluation: Hilgenreiner's line (Y line)—horizontal line drawn through the uppermost portion of both triradiate cartilages. Perkins's line—line drawn from the most lateral ossified margin of the roof of the acetabulum perpendicularly downward through the Y line to form quadrants. In a normal hip, the ossific nucleus of the femoral head is below the Y line and within the lower medial quadrant. Hilgenreiner's angle (acetabular index)—line is drawn from the lateral-most portion of the triradiate cartilage at its intersection with the Y line and extending to the most lateral ossific margins of the roof of the acetabulum. The angle between this line and the Y line is measured. Measurement should be 27 to 30° at birth and decreases to approximately 20° by 2 years of age. Acetabular dysplasia associated with a measurement usually greater than 30°. Shenton's line—line is drawn between the medial border of the femoral neck and the superior border of the obturator foramen. A normal hip reveals a continuous line while a dislocated hip reveals a disrupted line. H = Distance from the highest point of the femoral neck to Hilgenreiner's line. D = Distance from the triradiate cartilage to the intersection of H with Hilgenreiner's line. This distance is increased in hip dislocation and measures lateralization. Hip stations—the medial metaphyseal line is drawn, at the level of the contralateral medial metaphysis and parallel to Hilgenreiner's line. The position of the medial metaphysis on the affected side is determined. If it falls between the two lines, then the station is 0. If the medial metaphysis is at Hilgenreiner's line, then the station is −1. If the medial metaphysis of the abnormal hip is at the medial metaphyseal line, then the station is +1.

conventional radiography who had merely delayed ossification of a normal acetabulum and therefore did not require surgical correction.[12]

The contralateral hip may also show developmental anomalies such as subluxation. Using a combination of measurements such as acetabular depth and acetabular diameter together with the CE angle, it is possible to predict hips that are at risk from the age of 2 years.[9]

Use of Computed Tomography

Information is now being made available concerning acetabular deficiency in both congenital and paralytic hip instability using computed tomography (CT).[16,31,53,115,151] This methodology should not be used for routine evalua-

tion, but it is particularly useful for patients in plaster casts or when plain films are equivocal. Each cut of a CT normally involves 3 or 4 rad.[115] To reduce exposure, a double-cut tomographic technique producing two slices 1 cm apart has been recommended instead of CT.[79]

Information regarding the nature of acetabular dysplasia is still controversial. McKibbin believed from his dissections of the infant pelvis that acetabular anteversion was present in children with hip dysplasia.[94] Browning et al., using CT scan, also concluded that acetabular anteversion played an important role.[16] However, Gugenheim and coworkers found that there is anterior acetabular deficiency in congenital hip instability (and also in the paralytic hip instability of cerebral palsy) and that a torsional disorder such as acetabular anteversion is not the cause of the dysplasia.[50] O'Sullivan has developed a classifica-

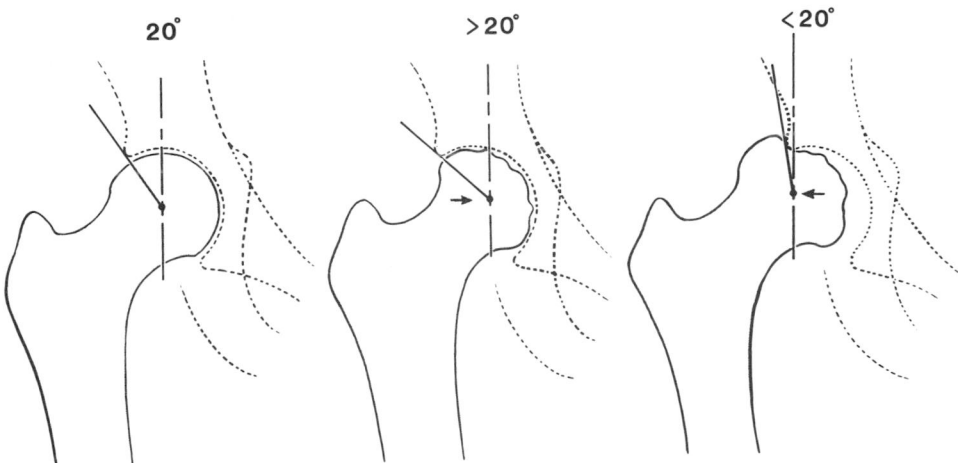

Figure 40-3 Center-edge (CE) angle of Wiberg. Any angle less than 20° indicates lateral subluxation of the hip.

tion system for primary acetabular dysplasia, which he differentiates from developmental dislocation.[106]

More recently, Edelson and others, using CT evaluation, have shown that there is a defect in the posterior ischium associated with the dislocated position of CDH, which they believe to be lateral, superior, and slightly anterior. This defect forms part of the false acetabulum. They noted that true posterior dislocation (Fig. 40-4) is extremely unusual and confirmed that anteversion of the acetabulum was found only occasionally and is only marginal. The children studied were from all age groups between 3 months and 2 1/2 years. Teratologic cases were not included in this study.[31]

One surprising new finding from these CT studies is the fact that the expected increased femoral anteversion on the involved side is not confirmed in this age group.[31,151] Computed tomography can also accurately document the adequacy of reduction (Fig. 40-4).[16,31] Visualization of the soft tissues hindering reduction—such as the hypertrophied pulvinar, a tight iliopsoas tendon, infolding capsule, and labrum—are better visualized by MRI.[10–12,51]

Sonography

Real-time, high-resolution sonography now plays a major role in the diagnosis and treatment of developmental hip dysplasia. Sonography can define an osseous dysplasia of the acetabular rim and also show the presence of a satisfactory acetabular roof when that structure is cartilaginous. This is useful in differentiating true acetabular dysplasia from a condition where there may be delayed ossification of the cartilaginous roof.[46] The technique has been developed and refined by many workers. Suzuki has differentiated three different types of femoral head displacement utilizing ultrasound.[141] In type A, the femoral head is lateralized but aligned with the acetabulum; in type B, the femoral head sits on the posterior acetabular rim; and in type C, the femoral head lies behind the ac-

etabulum. Only cases with type A and some cases with type B displacement are amenable to conservative treatment. The use of sonography for screening all newborns is controversial. Some[8,26,89] are convinced that ultrasound is much more accurate than clinical examination, while others are concerned that its reliability has been exaggerated.[28] Valuable as ultrasound may be, its cost has now become a factor that must be considered.[55]

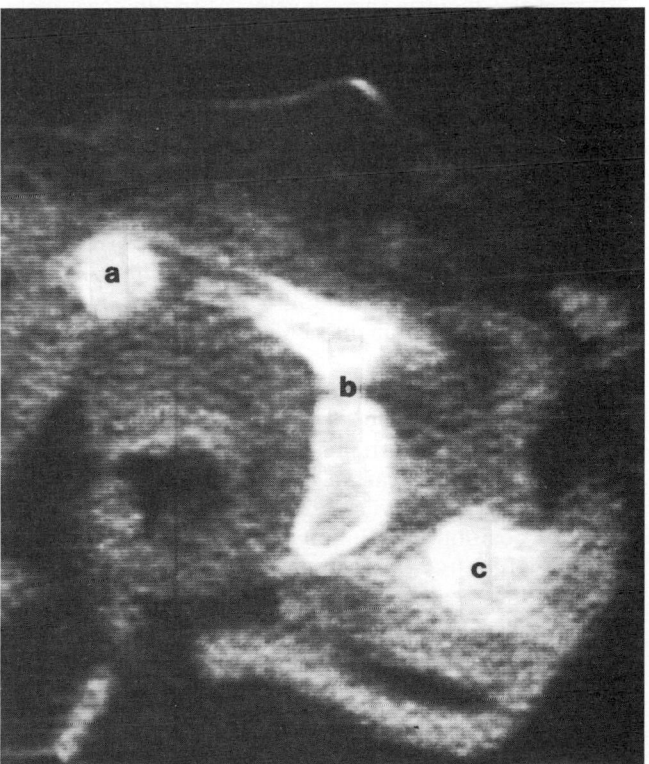

Figure 40-4 This is a posterior hip dislocation of the left hip as visualized with CT scan. *a,* symphysis pubis; *b,* acetabulum; *c,* femoral head.

Magnetic Resonance Imaging

Magnetic resonance imaging does not produce ionizing radiation. It can yield three-dimensional images and is more accurate than CT in the visualization of specific blocks to closed reduction of the hip (adhesion of the capsule of the hip to the ilium, inverted limbus, displaced transverse acetabular ligament). In addition, it can show details of the cartilaginous acetabulum that cannot be seen by any other technique.[10–12]

TREATMENT

Closed Treatment

Treatment of the unstable hip varies with the patient's age group. The most important factor determining the outcome of closed treatment of CDH is the quality of the initial reduction.

Treatment is designed to achieve congruent reduction and maintain the hip in that position until stability is restored. This process is usually accompanied by diminishing capsular laxity and improvement in such objective radiologic criteria as the acetabular index and the CE angle. Race and Herring have identified the criteria for a satisfactory reduction as follows: (1) Shenton's line intact with the legs in neutral position, (2) less than 2 mm of discrepancy (between the affected hip and the contralateral hip) of the distance measured from an acetabular cortex to the medial corner of the femoral metaphysis, (3) the femoral metaphysis directed toward the triradiate cartilage on abduction radiograms, and (4) a clinically stable reduction not requiring an extreme of position to maintain abduction.[119]

In a poor reduction, Shenton's line will be broken and there will often be a discrepancy of more than 5 mm in the lateralization measurement compared with the other side. Additionally, the femoral metaphysis will not be directed toward the triradiate cartilage, and clinically the reduction will be felt to be unstable, requiring an extreme position of flexion or adduction to maintain it. An intermediate position where the reduction may be regarded as adequate but there is mild lateralization was also identified by these authors. There is then a slight break in Shenton's line and a discrepancy of 2 to 5 mm in the measurement of lateralization. In these cases the femoral metaphysis is directed toward the triradiate cartilage on abduction radiographs, and the reduction is clinically stable within reasonable extremes of position. It is important that extremes of position not be required to maintain the position of reduction, since this has been shown repeatedly to be a factor promoting development of avascular necrosis.[72,74,92,120] Race and Herring also noted that, following congruent reduction, the acetabular angle decreased an average of 1.6° per month during treatment. The CE angle also improved as the reduced chondroepiphysis of the femoral head produced its molding effect on the acetabulum. Their criteria for desirable radiographic findings at the conclusion of treatment was an acetabular index less than 25°, a CE angle of more than 20° (Fig. 40-3), an intact Shenton's line, and no avascular necrosis.[119]

From Birth to 6 Months

Except in teratologic dislocation, newborn patients do not demonstrate secondary adaptive change. Consequently, reduction of the dislocated hip (Ortolani) is infrequently resisted by adductor tightness. Maintenance of the reduced position is always required. Similarly, in the positionally unstable or dislocatable hip, what is required is maintenance of the hip in the reduced position until the instability is no longer present. An additional requirement, however, is that some mobility be permitted when the hip is in the reduced position, so as to minimize the risks of avascular necrosis.

It has been argued that treatment of all degrees of hip instability is not worthwhile, since a large number of positionally unstable (subluxatable) hips diagnosed at birth will resolve spontaneously. However, in view of the work of McKinnon and coworkers, to which we have already referred, indicating the profile of the subluxatable hip to be similar to that of true infantile dislocation of the hip, it may be wiser to treat all these patients, acknowledging that many of them will stabilize rapidly within the first few weeks of treatment.[77,95] It is important, however, that any method of treatment adopted not run the risk of causing new problems, especially to infants who may have a condition that would resolve spontaneously without morbidity. It has been pointed out that the most severe forms of avascular necrosis (AVN) occur in patients in whom treatment has begun between birth and the age of 6 months.[72]

Hensinger has reviewed the various devices available, separating them into simple positioning devices and those he classifies as "secure restraints." He points out that the former category includes the Freyka pillow and the use of triple diapers, both of which have the potential for permitting dislocation. It is therefore important that the parent be taught the Ortolani test to be certain that the femoral head is reduced each time the child requires a diaper change.[59] The Craig or Ilfeld splint is a better positional device, since perineal care can be accomplished with it in place.[59,77] Under the heading of secure restraint, the most popular device is the Pavlik harness (Fig. 40-5). The use of this device has been described in detail by many authors.[40,66,67,74,101] The harness has several advantages. It allows active hip motion but at the same time the hip remains reduced within safe limits, which do not impose undue stresses on the chondroepiphysis and thus induce avascular changes. It is important that for each hip the safe zone be determined between that position of adduction (at 90° of flexion) at which the hip will dislocate and the position of maximum abduction. Neither of these two extremes is acceptable. In a patient with limited abduction, there may be a narrower range of safety than in another child who has a good range of abduction[92,120] (Fig. 40-6).

It may be necessary to perform an adductor tenotomy, particularly in a child older than 3 months, before applying the harness in the safe zone. The harness consists of an abdominal strap, two shoulder harnesses, and two leg stirrups. The posterior strap is adjusted so that the thigh will not enter the zone of dislocation but hip motion within the safe zone of reduction is possible. The posterior strap

Figure 40-5 Pavlik harness. *A.* Anterior view of child in a Pavlik harness. Anterior flexion strap can be seen. Hips must be kept at 90° or more of flexion. *B.* Posterior view of the child in a Pavlik harness showing the abduction straps. These straps should not keep the child in more than 60° of abduction; more than this may lead to avascular necrosis.

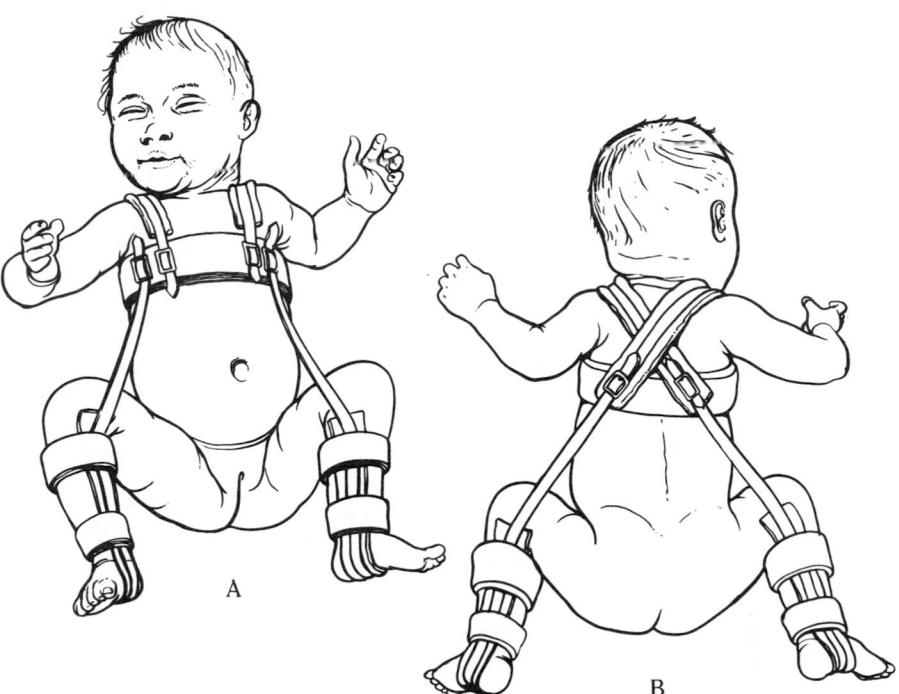

prevents the thigh from adducting further. Its improper use in the past, compressing the vessels of the femoral head, has led to a high incidence of avascular necrosis and produced femoral nerve palsy.[59] Kalamchi and MacFarlane recommend adjusting the posterior strap to prevent adduction and stop the lower limb from crossing the midline, but not using it to achieve abduction.[74] The anterior strap is used to keep the hips in the desired degree of flexion and to limit extension. At least 90° of flexion is the usual position. Radiographs are taken at the beginning of treatment to confirm satisfactory position.

Patients are maintained in the harness for several months until the hips are clinically and radiographically stable. The average treatment period, including weaning from the harness, is 3.6 months in patients aged up to 1 month; 7 months total in babies 1 to 3 months of age; and 9.3 months in those between 3 and 6 months of age.[120] Weaning from the harness is begun when clinically and radiographically there is no evidence of subluxation or lat-

eralization. Recently ultrasound has emerged as a guide to discontinuance to the use of the Pavlik harness.[141] Weaning usually consists of reducing the time in the harness over a period of 4 to 8 weeks.

The majority of children over the age of 3 months will demonstrate some degree of adductor tightness and shortening and there may be other secondary changes preventing concentric reduction. Many surgeons will treat these patients by preliminary traction for a few weeks, followed by a period in a hip spica cast within the safe zone of reduction (for example, 45° of abduction and 90° of flexion). After a satisfactory concentric reduction has been achieved by this method, the child may be placed in the Pavlik harness. However, a number of studies have used the Pavlik harness in this group believing that the harness will itself gently achieve reduction.[40,74] A relatively simple anatomic mechanism makes the harness effective in reducing the hip. When the hip is flexed, the femoral head moves from its superior position to a more posteroinferior

Figure 40-6 Safe zone of Ramsey—any further abduction may cause avascular necrosis. More adduction of the hip may lose stability.

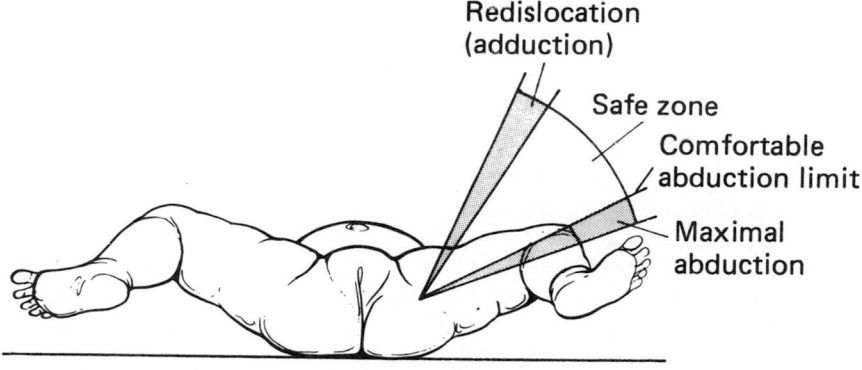

Redislocation
(adduction)

Safe zone

Comfortable
abduction limit

Maximal
abduction

position within the acetabulum, where it is maintained by adductor muscle contraction.[66] All authors agree that for patients with dislocated hips, this treatment should not persist beyond 4 weeks if a stable concentric reduction does not occur. The alternative of closed or even open reduction is then recommended if necessary. It is also generally accepted that the optimal age limit for the use of the harness is about 8 or 9 months.[40,74,88] If the harness is used to *reduce* a dislocation, it is important that adequate hip flexion be obtained in the harness.[40,101,120]

From 6 to 18 Months

Although a preliminary period of traction has traditionally been recommended, several studies have demonstrated no benefit from this.[15,41,71,118] The great majority of hips in this age group can be reduced by a gentle Ortolani maneuver under general anesthesia in the operating room. It is important that absolutely no force be used or manipulation performed. Adductor tenotomy is usually required. The hip is then placed in the safe zone of reduction and a hip spica cast applied. An arthrogram is desirable to confirm reduction and identify any soft tissue obstruction to reduction or to suggest the necessity for open reduction. If concentric reduction is achieved and confirmed radiographically in the cast, satisfactory restoration of stability and improvement in the contours of the acetabulum will usually (but not necessarily) be achieved.[56,119] Immobilization in a hip spica cast for 6 weeks to 6 months is needed. As stability improves in the hip, it may be possible to remove the spica cast and use an abduction splint for part of this time.

From 18 Months to 3 Years

With increasing age and progressive weight bearing, the soft tissue contractures will have become more rigid. In addition, the contour of the acetabular socket may have become more abnormal and there may be increased anteversion of the proximal femur, which must be taken into consideration. Occasionally a gentle closed reduction after an adductor and psoas tenotomy may be possible. Such an outcome is less likely with increasing age, however, an open reduction together with surgery of the acetabulum or proximal femur (see below) is more likely to be required. Indeed, some investigators feel that the risk of avascular necrosis is less with open reduction than closed reduction.[27,37] Good acetabular development is seen in 19 percent of hips reduced between ages 2 and 3 and in only 7 percent of those reduced after age 3.[88] It is generally agreed that closed reduction should probably not be attempted after age 3.[34]

Further surgery to femur or pelvis will be required in 66 percent of hips reduced closed and 30 percent of those reduced by open operations.[88] Williamson et al. found that the incidence of avascular necrosis was reduced from 25 to 10 percent if femoral and pelvic osteotomy were combined at the time of open reduction.[157]

Age Limits for Treatment

Williamson et al. believe that open reduction with both femoral and pelvic osteotomy is indicated in all children with dislocated hips over the age of 3 years.[157]

In patients over 10 years of age with a unilateral dislocation, reduction should probably not be attempted because of the risk of producing a painful hip. Bilateral dislocations should not be treated in these older children, since these untreated hips are usually painless well into adulthood.

Surgical Procedures and Approaches

Open Reduction

Indications for open reduction include those occasions when extreme position of abduction is required to maintain reduction and also when the safe arc of reduction is less than after adductor tenotomy. If the femoral head still remains above the triradiate cartilage, is laterally placed, or remains lateralized (in the "intermediate position"), this usually indicates some degree of soft tissue interposition which will require open reduction and excision of the offending tissue.

Arthrographic Assessment

Various arthrographic findings have been well described in literature.[97,106,121] The pulvinar, ligamentum teres, or transverse ligament may prevent the head from entering the acetabulum. The infolded limbus produced by the pressure of the capsule against the superior acetabular labrum, an hourglass constriction of the joint capsule, or a contracted iliopsoas tendon can also produce an obstruction to reduction visualized on arthrography (Fig. 40-7). False lateralization may be caused by such conditions as eccentric epiphyseal ossification, redundancy of the hip joint capsule, synovitis with excessive fluid in the hip joint, or excessive femoral anteversion. Such errors of interpretation can be clarified by arthrography.

A properly performed open reduction is less likely to damage the chondroepiphysis than are repeated attempts at closed reduction. Some authors believe that open reduction is always preferable to closed reduction.[27,37] Certainly, surgery is preferable to maintaining reduction under tension by placing the hip beyond the safe zone or risking loss of position by splinting near the edge of the safe zone of reduction.

The most conventional approach to a hip for open reduction is the Smith-Petersen approach. At present most pediatric orthopaedic surgeons use a transverse "bikini" incision, which produces a nearly invisible scar with equal surgical visualization. This approach can be extended proximally to perform pelvic osteotomy as described by Salter[124,125] and medially to allow a triple innominate osteotomy. The medial approach first described by Ludloff[85] has been used successfully by several authors.[38,79,90] Kalamchi and McEwen point out that in their hands damage to branches of the medial circumflex artery and accompanying veins was almost inevitable using the medial

Figure 40-7 Soft tissue obstruction to reduction seen on arthrography: *a,* inverted limbus; *b,* "hourglass" deformity of capsule; *c,* iliopsoas tendon; *d,* femoral head.

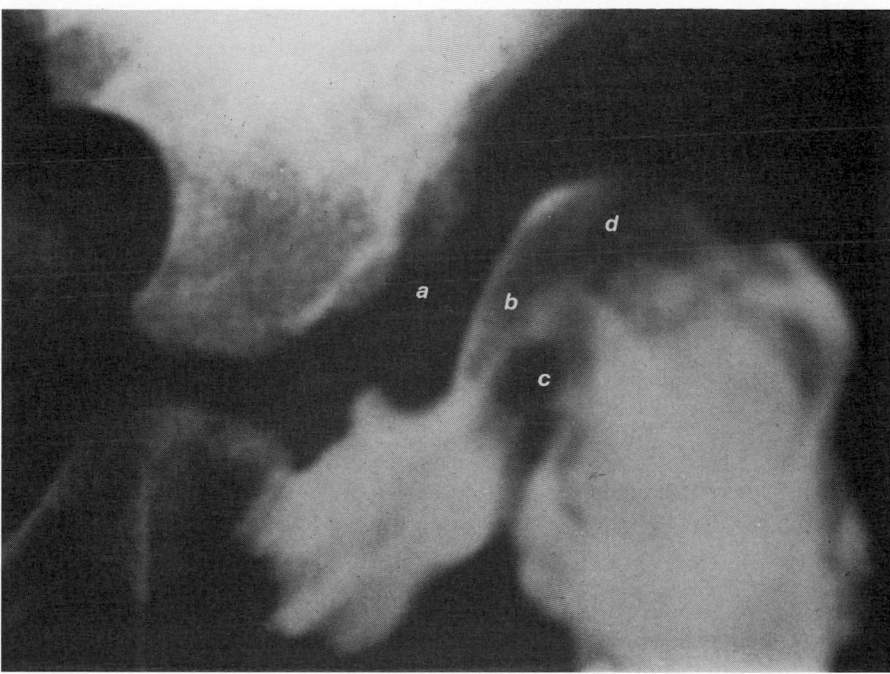

approach of Ludloff. In their series, there was an incidence of AVN of 67 percent with this approach. They note that there is a problem in visualizing these important vascular structures and consequently they reverted to the standard anterior iliofemoral (Smith-Petersen) approach and abandoned the medial approach.[73] The medial circumflex artery is located within close proximity of the tendon of the iliopsoas. Its importance as a source of blood supply to the capital femoral epiphysis is described elsewhere; however, it should be noted here that a collateral circulation does exist at this level. (The medial femoral circumflex is not an end artery. On the other hand, Mankey, Arntz, and Staheli reviewed 66 open reductions performed by the Ludloff approach and considered it to be a safe and effective procedure in children under the age of 24 months.[87]

Posterior approaches to the hip are rarely used for open reduction because they place the blood supply to the capital femoral epiphysis in jeopardy. An alternative method for those familiar with the approach is to expose the hip joint capsule between the abductors and the tensor fascia lata, an approach frequently used for total hip arthroplasty. This approach, however, cannot be extended proximally for pelvic osteotomy. A summary of the surgical approaches for open reduction has been given by Simmons.[132]

The capsule is exposed after reflecting the rectus femoris muscle inferiorly. The iliopsoas tendon is usually lengthened or sectioned. The capsule is incised and the anterior and inferior portions are released, along with the transverse acetabular ligament. The acetabulum is then cleared of any excess fibrous fatty tissue (pulvinar).

Redundant ligamentum teres is excised and any obstructing limbus is incised and reflected or partially removed. The transverse acetabular ligament must be sectioned. It should be possible then to gently reduce the hip.

Some authors claim that when the medial approach is used, preliminary traction is unnecessary prior to open reduction.[123] Others argue that preliminary traction may promote AVN of the femoral head. A comparative study by Schoenecker and Strecker of patients treated by preoperative traction compared with those treated by femoral shortening would seem to favor the latter opinion.[128] These authors believe that the inferior results following traction are attributable to the excessive forces generated on the femoral head when reduction is achieved after discontinuation of traction. They believe that femoral shortening performed at the same time as open reduction avoids any residual compressive force and the development of AVN. They also believe that redislocation is less likely with this method compared with open reduction following traction. It seems from this study that femoral shortening may decompress the hip more successfully than preliminary traction.[128]

Femoral shortening may be combined with femoral derotation if excessive femoral anteversion is apparent. After reduction, intraoperative assessment of femoral head coverage and femoral anteversion will indicate the need for any secondary procedures. These may include acetabuloplasty, acetabular osteotomy, or a femoral procedure. The femoral procedure will occasionally be performed synchronously with the open reduction. Derotation osteotomy of the femur may be indicated when femoral anteversion is in excess of 60°.[6]

Immobilization in a cast is required for a period of 3 months or so following open reduction. The affected hip is usually maintained in some 90° of flexion and 30° of abduction. A degree of internal rotation is usually required for congruous reduction, by contrast with the position following closed reduction. This is probably associated with the increased amount of femoral anteversion or anterior acetabular deficiency. Full internal rotation must be avoided, since it may constrict the posterior blood supply to the femoral head. If derotation is performed as a second stage, it is usually done 6 weeks following the open reduction procedure.

Acetabular Osteotomy

Acetabular dysplasia often not apparent at birth becomes more obvious in older children and can be assessed using the radiologic measurements that have been described. Although radiography will not outline the cartilaginous elements of the acetabular roof, arthrography, sonography, or MRI can provide additional information.[6,7,9] When congruous reduction is achieved, the dysplasia may correct spontaneously.[119] On the other hand, the acetabulum may be so deficient in the older child that the socket is inadequate and the femoral head is not well covered. Radiologic assessment is valuable, but some authors recommend that the decision on whether to perform pelvic osteotomy either immediately or at some later date be made by direct observation of the degree of acetabular coverage seen at open reduction.[6] Salter recommends that, after the age of 18 months, open reduction and innominate osteotomy be combined in the same operation.[127]

The Salter Innominate Osteotomy

The Salter innominate osteotomy was designed to correct anterior and superolateral acetabular deficiency. The head must be concentrically reduced in the acetabulum. If it is not, this procedure will fail.[44,127]

The operation is performed through an extended iliofemoral approach (Fig. 40-8). It is important that the operative technique described by the originator be followed precisely.[124,125] It is probably unwise to do the procedure in a child less than 18 months of age, when the acetabulum has good potential to remodel and fixation of the pelvis is difficult. The accompanying open reduction must be meticulously performed so that the femoral head is well seated. In addition, the psoas tendon must be lengthened or levered and the capsule plicated as described by Salter.[124,125] Subsequent derotation of the femur for excessive anteversion observed during the first procedure may be required. Since the rotation occurs at the symphysis pubis in this operation, the lateral coverage achieved is occasionally inadequate. The osteotomy tends to lengthen the extremity by about 1 cm.[92] Leg-length problems have been noted in 27.7 percent of one series, but AVN, on the other hand, occurred in only 5 percent.[44]

Indications for Innominate Osteotomy

Mardam-Bey and McEwen achieved good to excellent results in 86 percent of osteotomies when the surgery was done for dysplasia but in only 58 percent when this procedure was performed for subluxation. They observed that Salter osteotomy is a better procedure than femoral os-

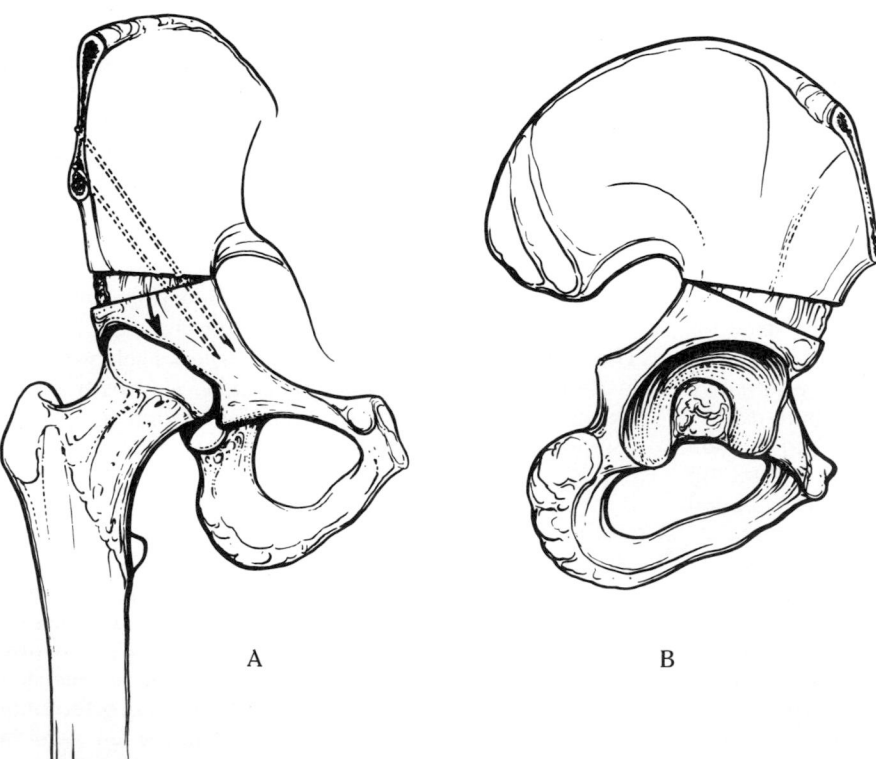

A   B

Figure 40-8 Salter innominate osteotomy. *A.* Procedure includes rotation of the distal fragment over the femoral head anteriorly and superiorly. *B.* Lateral view—the osteotomy enters the greater sciatic notch. Wedge of bone taken from anterior part of ilium.

Figure 40-9 Pemberton periacetabular osteotomy. Procedure is an incomplete osteotomy (does not enter sciatic notch) with bone graft. It allows for anterior and superior coverage. Anteroposterior and lateral views. Hinges on the triradiate cartilage (not shown).

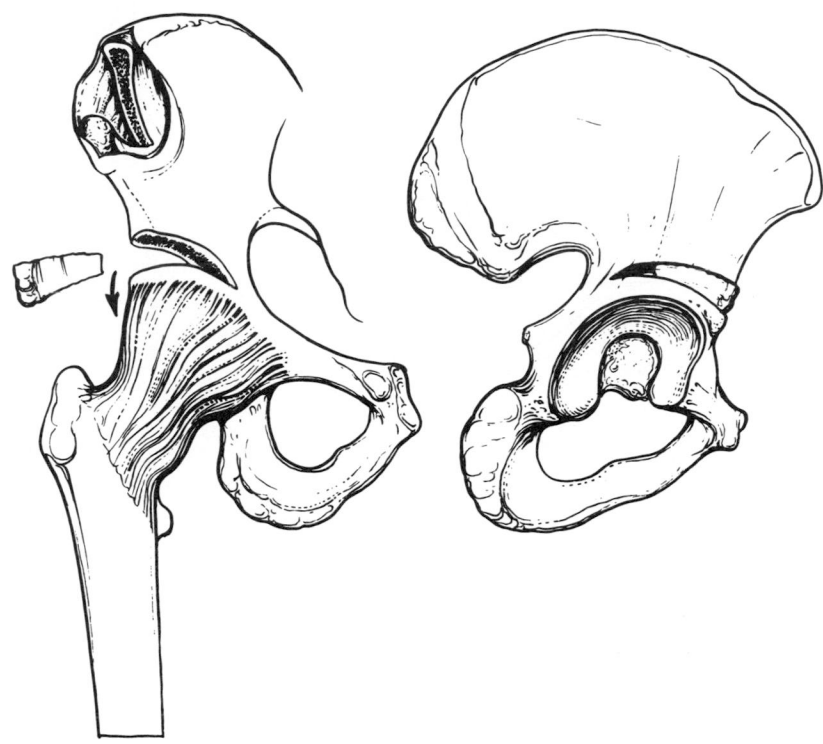

teotomy for the correction of acetabular dysplasia in children below age 6. They recommend that the operation not be delayed beyond the age of 6, because postsurgical remodeling ability markedly decreases after that age. Beyond age 6, they suggest that varus derotation osteotomy may be preferable. If arthrography shows a normal *cartilaginous* acetabular model and the hip is not subluxed, a decision on whether to perform Salter osteotomy can wait until the child is as old as age 7, because the bony acetabulum may reconstitute and the procedure may be avoided.[92] Lindstrom et al. also recommend postponing acetabuloplasty until age 8.[84] If congruent reduction is achieved later than age 4 or 5, the risk of developing a dysplastic acetabulum is increased. The acetabular remodeling and growth response seen in children under 4 years of age with congruent reduction continued in most patients to age 8 and even beyond.[52,54,57]

Pemberton Osteotomy

Requirements for this procedure are an open triradiate cartilage, a skeletal age of less than 7 years, and an acetabulum with considerable remodeling capacity.[35,93,114,148,150] Thus, this procedure does not have the versatility of the Salter osteotomy, which can be done at any age through skeletal maturity. In this procedure (Fig. 40-9), the direction and shape of the roof of the acetabulum is changed by hinging it downward at the triradiate cartilage. The acetabuloplasty is performed by first creating a pericapsular osteotomy into the anterolateral and anteromedial cortex of the ilium in a child with a hip concentrically reduced. This double cut permits the whole roof of the acetabulum to descend and cover the femoral head, both medially and laterally. The position is

maintained by bone graft (either autograft or allograft). The procedure may also be combined with open reduction.[35] The technique of the operation should be read in full before this procedure is attempted.[35,114]

Trevor and associates used bank rib graft or autogenous wedged iliac bone graft and described "timber stacking" the grafts in position.[148] They suggest that improved results require that the acetabuloplasty be accompanied or preceded by open reduction. Even following these principles, however, they observed some deterioration is likely to occur with time, coxa magna being the most common abnormality. They believed that this complication is related to vascular change, but whether this was caused by increased pressure placed on the femoral head at surgery or whether it could be related to attempts at closed reduction was uncertain. It is apparent that by bringing the roof down on the triradiate cartilage, some deformity is created in the shape of the acetabulum. Therefore, it is necessary that the operation be performed while there is still some remodeling potential. Since the procedure is often combined with open reduction, it is important that postoperative immobilization be kept to a minimum to avoid stiffness of the hip. McKay has pointed out that AVN was much more frequent (17.5 percent) in his cases of pericapsular osteotomy but infrequent following the Salter procedure. By contrast, redislocation was infrequent following the pericapsular procedure, but there was a redislocation rate of 11 percent after the Salter osteotomy.[93]

Steel and Sutherland Osteotomy

Other innominate osteotomies have been introduced to overcome the limitations of rotating the fragments solely

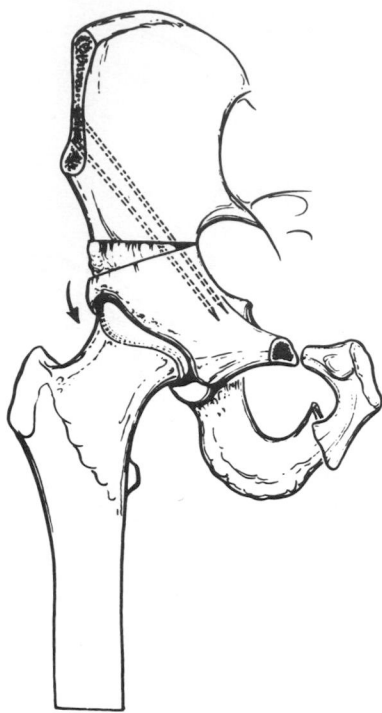

Figure 40-10 Steel's triple innominate osteotomy. Procedure includes iliac, pubic ramus, and ischial osteotomies, rotation of the distal fragment over the femoral head, bone graft, and pin fixation.

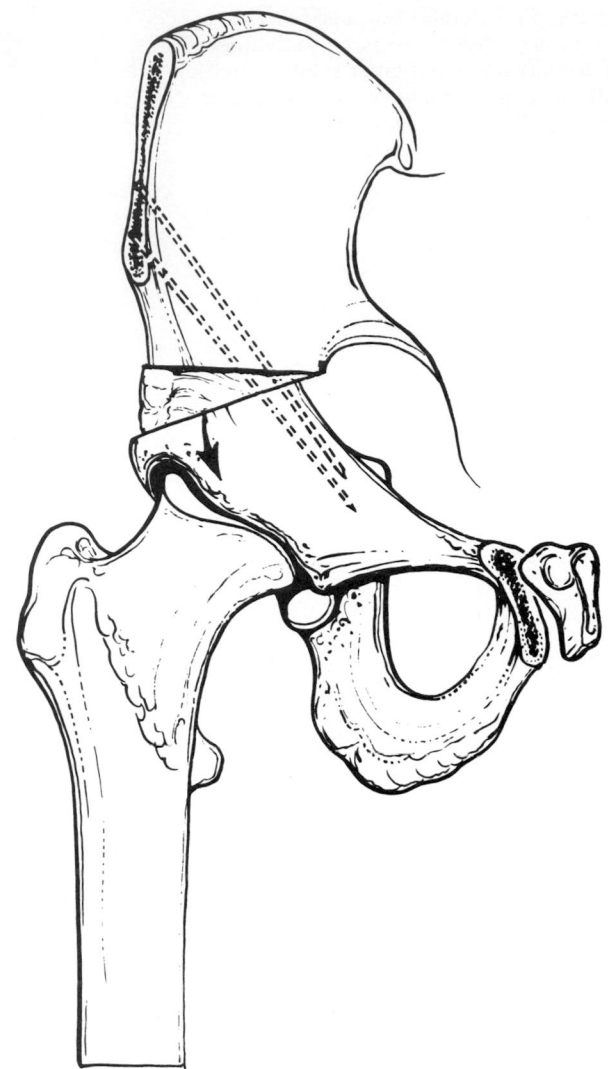

Figure 40-11 Sutherland's double innominate osteotomy. Procedure includes osteotomy of the ilium, osteotomy at the junction of the pubis and ischium lateral to the symphysis pubis, rotation of the distal fragment over the femoral head, graft, and pin fixation.

at the pubis symphysis. In the Steel[136] procedure, the acetabular fragment is rotated after a triple osteotomy is performed (Fig. 40-10). The osteotomy of the ilium is similar to that performed by Salter but somewhat more oblique. Additional osteotomies are performed through the superior pubic ramus and the body of the ischium close to the hip joint immediately behind and *below* the acetabulum. Although Steel performed the ischial osteotomy through a separate posterior incision with the hip flexed, more recent modifications permit the entire procedure to be performed through a single anteriomedial "Bikini" incision.[136] Another modification is the double osteotomy of Sutherland[139] (Fig. 40-11). Osteotomy is performed through the pubis at a site between the obturator foramen and the symphysis. The second osteotomy is made through the ilium. This is an easier procedure than the triple osteotomy.

Rotational Osteotomy

Other, more radical procedures are described for restoring acetabular architecture for the severely dysplastic hip. In these procedures, the acetabulum is rotated into a more horizontal position after being totally freed from the surrounding pelvis by a dome-shaped osteotomy, usually performed with a curved osteotome[45,103,153] (Fig. 40-12). These operations are surgically the most difficult but promise the best coverage of the femoral head. A combined anterior and posterior approach to the acetabulum and con-

siderable experience in hip surgery is required to undertake these formidable operations. They are indicated for patients whose hips show such incongruity that degenerative arthritis is inevitable. They may also be used in adolescent patients whose hips are in an early stage of degenerative arthritis. They must therefore be regarded as salvage procedures.

Chiari Osteotomy

Another alternative in this group is the Chiari pelvic osteotomy[23] (Fig. 40-13). In this procedure, an osteotomy is made just superior to the hip joint capsule and the fragments are displaced to produce a horizontal shelf. Great care is required if the sciatic nerve is not to be compromised or the joint violated. The direction of the osteotomy

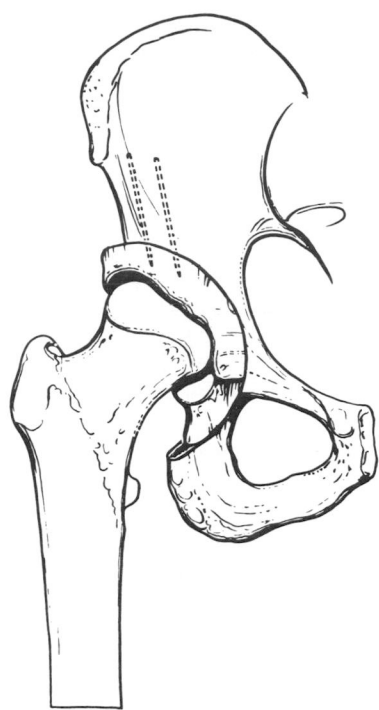

Figure 40-12 Periacetabular osteotomy ("dial" osteotomy). Procedure includes rotation of the acetabulum with pin fixation.

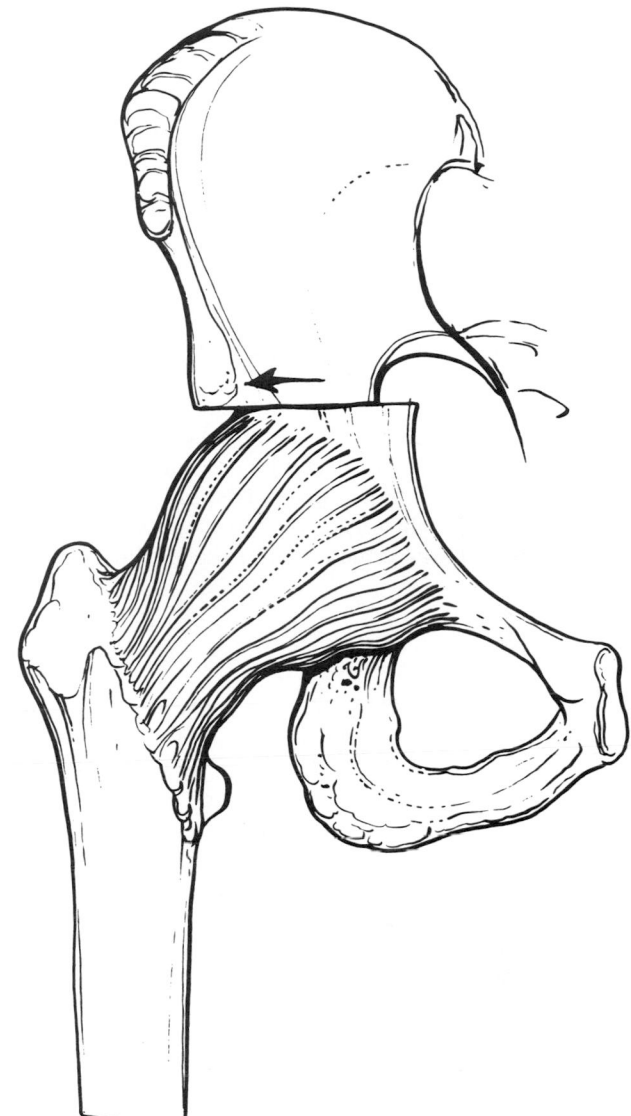

Figure 40-13 Chiari's osteotomy. Procedure includes slightly oblique osteotomy immediately superior to the capsule and medial displacement of the hip.

is slightly upward and medial—not truly horizontal—to enable the displacement of the fragments to occur. There is therefore a little shortening accompanying the procedure. It is important that the capsule not be violated, since the procedure depends upon the superior joint capsule lining the inferior surface of the new horizontal shelf and so preventing postoperative stiffness. The operation may be used for salvage if there is coxa magna, but it is doubtful that this procedure will give an excellent result. The results are better if the CE angle is restored to below 20°.[86] Sciatic nerve damage is also unfortunately all too common.[76,86] Histologic evaluation has shown that if the capsule is interposed between the femoral head and the new acetabulum, well-vascularized connective tissue is produced, suitable for its new function as an interposition membrane.[98] Lack found 75 percent good results in a long-term study of this procedure performed for hip dysplasia.[81]

Femoral Osteotomy

The role of derotation osteotomy and of femoral shortening in maintaining reduction has been described. Varus osteotomy is an additional procedure that may be necessary if, during surgical assessment, it is shown that femoral abduction is required in addition to internal rotation to stabilize the hip joint following open reduction.[92] The age of the patient is an important factor in determining the outcome of varus derotation osteotomy. It is recommended that this procedure be restricted to patients younger than

8 years of age without preexisting AVN. Beyond 8 years, there is little potential for acetabular improvement and little gain from the remodeling effect of improved femoral head position. Varus osteotomy as an isolated procedure has almost no role in the treatment of hip dysplasia.[75] Some caution must also be exercised in performing this operation in the child under 3 years of age, because the neck shaft angle will rapidly return to normal. Thus, there is not enough time for the remodeling effect upon the acetabulum (due to the new femoral alignment) to take place.[92]

Femoral osteotomy, and particularly derotation osteotomy,[7] when combined with innominate osteotomy at the time of open reduction has been shown to produce an improvement in long-term results.[37,157]

COMPLICATIONS

Avascular Necrosis

The etiology of this complication and its relative frequency have already been mentioned. Four types of change have been identified by Kalamchi and McEwen. A classification of AVN is important in predicting the natural history of the condition.[18,72]

Type I

There is delay in appearance of the ossific nucleus or mottling of the cartilaginous model, followed by some flattening and fragmentation with revascularization. The sequel to this type of change affecting the ossific nucleus is that the head will usually regain its spherical shape, usually with a good long-term prognosis and only minimal loss of residual height or coxa magna. Acetabular development is usually not affected and excellent function exists long term.

Type II

This is the group with the most unpredictable outcome; there is localized damage to the lateral part of the physis in addition to type I changes. Localized growth arrest may lead to the development of a valgus neck and subluxation of the head. This may be temporary or permanent. Premature physeal closure may not occur until the pubescent growth spurt, emphasizing the need for long-term follow-up. The resulting valgus configuration of the proximal femur will uncover the femoral head in the acetabulum.[18] Problems that may have to be dealt with in addition to the valgus angulation include relative overgrowth of the greater trochanter and limb-length discrepancy. Treatment must be individualized.

Type III

The damage to the growth plate is more centrally located, so that there is symmetrical slowing or cessation of growth of the femoral neck. This will produce marked growth abnormalities, including relative overgrowth of the greater trochanter compared with the femoral neck and significant leg-length discrepancy.

Type IV

There is total involvement of the head and physis, with coxa magna and irregularity and flattening of the head. Medial breaking occurs together with irregularity, widening, and shortening of the metaphysis. There will be true varus angulation of the femoral neck.[17,72] Ogden has attempted to correlate these changes with interference with the specific components of the vascular supply to the region. Particularly important in his thesis is the fact that the medial circumflex artery may be subjected to compression as the hip is abducted.[107,109,110] Such impingement of the artery between the iliopsoas and the adductor and pectineus muscles may persist for a long period of time in an immobilization device. This fact provides an anatomic basis for not splinting children at the limit of abduction and for the concept of safe zones of reduction.

Treatment of Avascular Necrosis

Chiari osteotomy may be more appropriate than Salter osteotomy as a salvage for patients with AVN, since they often do not have a congruous joint at this stage.[95] In a long-term study of patients who developed AVN following treatment for congenital dislocation of the hip, Cooperman et al. observed that 24 out of 30 hips had moderate or severe osteoarthritis, accompanied in the majority of cases by significant pain or loss of function by the time they were 42 years old.[25] These authors point out that, wherever possible, attempts should be made to prevent lateral and proximal subluxation of the femoral head and to correct these abnormalities, if possible, as soon as they occur. Another study by Robinson and coworkers was more pessimistic. They found that of 51 patients who developed AVN, neither femoral nor pelvic osteotomy produced satisfactory long-term results. Even total hip replacement did not result in long-term success.[122]

Coxa Brevis

Premature proximal femoral physeal arrest may produce different deformities depending upon whether it is symmetrical or asymmetrical. Symmetrical closure will produce a near normal neck shaft angle with shortening of the femoral neck (coxa brevis), relative overgrowth of the greater trochanter, and a short limb. Asymmetrical lateral physeal closure will result in a tilting of the femoral epiphysis externally on the femoral neck. There will also be an associated relative overgrowth of the greater trochanter, producing a short leg and coxa brevis.[13]

In patients less than 7 years of age, trochanteric epiphysiodesis may be recommended for this deformity. In older patients, lateral and distal transfer of the greater trochanter is preferable.[137] Leg-length discrepancy may require epiphysiodesis.[13,145]

Coxa Valga

Valgus angulation occurred in 35 percent of these patients, with lateral physeal arrest in the series reported by Kalamchi and McEwen.[72] Coxa valga may also occur as a complication of varus osteotomy for congenital dislocation of the hip. The coxa valga is subcapital and may be associated with physeal damage. Alternatively, it has been suggested that relative increase of the activity of the medial side of the physis may contribute to the deformity.[70] Uncorrected coxa valga leads to a continuing uncovering of the femoral head, especially if there is any persisting acetabular dysplasia.

REFERENCES

1. Aarskog D, et al: Urinary estrogen excretion in new born infants in congenital dysplasia of the hip joint. *Acta Pediatr Scand* 55:394, 1966.
2. Albinana J, Quesada JA, Certucha JA: Children at high risk for congenital dislocation of the hip: Late presentation. *J Pediatr Orthop* 13:268–269, 1993.
3. Andren L, Borglin WE: Disturbed urinary excretion pattern of oestrogens in newborns with congenital dislocation of the hip. *Acta Endocrinol* 37:423, 1961.
4. Azuma H, Taneda H, Igarashi H: Evaluation of acetabular coverage: Three-dimensional CT imaging and modified pelvic inlet view. *J Pediatr Orthop* 11:765–769, 1991.
5. Barlow TG: Early diagnosis and treatment of congenital dislocation of the hip. *J Bone Joint Surg* 44B:292–301, 1962.
6. Berkeley ME, et al: Surgical therapy for congenital dislocation of the hip in patients who are 12 to 36 months old. *J Bone Joint Surg* 66A:412–420, 1984.
7. Blockey NJ: Derotation osteotomy in the management of congenital dislocation of the hip. *J Bone Joint Surg* 66B:485–490, 1984.
8. Boeree NR, et al: Ultrasound imaging and secondary screening for congenital dislocation of the hip. *J Bone Joint Surg* 76B:525–533, 1994.
9. Bolton-Maggs BC, Crabtree SD: The opposite hip in congenital dislocation of the hip. *J Bone Joint Surg* 65B:279–284, 1983.
10. Bos CF, Bloem JL: Treatment of dislocation of the hip, detected in early childhood, based on magnetic resonance imaging. *J Bone Joint Surg [Am]* 71:1523–1529, 1989.
11. Bos CF, Bloem JL, Obermann WR, Rozing PM: Magnetic resonance imaging in congenital dislocation of the hip. *J Bone Joint Surg [Br]* 70:174–178, 1988.
12. Bos CF, Bloem JL, Verbout AJ: Magnetic resonance imaging in acetabular residual dysplasia. *Clin Orthop* 265:207–217, 1991.
13. Bowen JF: Abnormal growth and development of the pediatric hip, in Stauffer ES (ed): *MOS Instructional Course Lectures.* Vol 34. St Louis, Mosby, 1985, pp 423–433.
14. Bower C, Stanley FJ, Kricker A: Congenital dislocation of the hip in Western Australia: A comparison of neonatally and postneonatally diagnosed cases. *Clin Orthop* 224:37–44, 1987.
15. Brougham DI, Broughton NS, Cole WG, Menelaus MB: Avascular necrosis of the hip following closed reduction of congenital dislocation of the hip: Review of influencing factors and long-term follow-up. *J Bone Joint Surg [Br]* 72B:557–562, 1990.
16. Browning WH, et al: Computed tomography in congenital dislocation: The role of acetabular anteversion. *J Bone Joint Surg* 64A:27–31, 1982.
17. Buchanan JR, et al: Management strategy for prevention of avascular necrosis during treatment of congenital dislocation of the hip. *J Bone Joint Surg* 63A:140–146, 1981.
18. Carey TP, Guidera KG, Ogden JA: Manifestations of ischemic necrosis complicating developmental hip dysplasia. *Clin Orthop* 281:11–17, 1992.
19. Carr AJ, Jefferson RJ, Benson *MKD*: Joint laxity and hip rotation in normal children and in those with congenital dislocation of the hip. *J Bone Joint Surg* 75B:76–78, 1993.
20. Catterall A: What is congenital dislocation of the hip? (editorial). *J Bone Joint Surg* 66B:469–470, 1984.
21. Chapple C, Davidson D: A study of the relationship between fetal positions and certain congenital deformities. *J Pediatr Orthop* 18:483, 1941.
22. Chen IH, Kuo KN, Lubicky JP: Prognosticating factors in acetabular development following reduction of developmental dysplasia of the hip. *J Pediatr Orthop* 14:3–8, 1994.
23. Chiari K: Medial displacement osteotomy of the pelvis. *Clin Orthop* 98:55–71, 1974.
24. Coleman SS, McEwen GD: Congenital dislocation of the hip in infancy, in Stauffer ES (ed): *MOS Instructional Course Lecture.* Vol 21. St Louis, Mosby, 1972, pp 155–166.
25. Cooperman DR, et al: Post reduction avascular necrosis in congenital dislocation of the hip. *J Bone Joint Surg* 62A:247–258, 1980.
26. Dahlström H, et al: Stabilization and development of the hip after closed reduction of late CDH. *J Bone Joint Surg [Br]* 72:186–189, 1990.
27. Dhar S, Taylor JF, Jones WA, Owen R: Early open reduction for congenital dislocation of the hip. *J Bone Joint Surg* 72B:175–180, 1990.
28. Diaz JJ, Thomas IH, Lamont AC, et al: The reliability of ultrasonographic assessment of neonatal hips. *J Bone Joint Surg* 75B:479–482, 1993.
29. Dunn PM: Congenital postural deformities. *Br Med Bull* 32:71–76, 1976.
30. Dunn PM: Perinatal observations on the etiology of congenital dislocation of the hip. *Clin Orthop* 119:11–22, 1976.
31. Edelson JG, et al: Congenital dislocation of the hip and computerized axial tomography. *J Bone Joint Surg* 66B:472–477, 1984.
32. Edelstein J: Congenital dislocation of the hip in Bantu. *J Bone Joint Surg* 48B:397, 1964.
33. Engesaeter LB, Wilson DJ, Nag D, Benson MKD: Ultrasound and congenital dislocation of the hip: The importance of dynamic assessment. *J Bone Joint Surg [Br]* 72:197–201, 1990.
34. Eyre-Brooke AL: Treatment of congenital dislocation or subluxation of the hip in children over the age of three years. *J Bone Joint Surg* 48B:682–692, 1966.
35. Eyre-Brooke AL, et al: Pemberton's acetabuloplasty for congenital dislocation or subluxation of the hip. *J Bone Joint Surg* 60B:18–24, 1978.
36. Faciszewski T, Coleman SS, Biddulph G: Triple innominate osteotomy for acetabular dysplasia. *J Pediatr Orthop* 13:426–430, 1993.
37. Fairbank JC, et al: Relationship of pain to the radiological anatomy of the hip joint in adults treated for congenital dislocation of the hip as infants: A long term follow-up of patients treated by three methods. *J Pediatr Orthop* 6:381–385, 1986.
38. Ferguson AB Jr: Primary open reduction of congenital dislocation of the hip using a medial adductor approach. *J Bone Joint Surg* 55A:671–689, 1973.
39. Ferris B, Leyshon A, Catterall A: Congenital hip dislocation or dysplasia with subluxation: A radiologic study. *J Pediatr Orthop* 11:614–616, 1991.
40. Fipipe G, Carlioz H: Use of the Pavlik harness in treating congenital dislocation of the hip. *J Pediatr Orthop* 2:357–362, 1982.
41. Fish DN, Herzenberg JE, Hensinger RN: Current practice in use of prereduction traction for congenital dislocation of the hip. *J Pediatr Orthop* 11:149–153, 1991.
42. Fisher R, O'Brien TS, Davis KM: Magnetic resonance imaging in congenital dysplasia of the hip. *J Pediatr Orthop* 11:617–622, 1991.
43. Gage J, Winter R: Avascular necrosis of the capital femoral epiphysis as a complication of closed reduction of congenital dislocation of the hip. *J Bone Joint Surg* 54A:373, 1972.
44. Gallien R, et al: Salter procedure in congenital dislocation of the hip. *J Pediatr Orthop* 4:427–430, 1984.
45. Ganz R, Klaue K, Vinh TS, Mast JW: A new periacetabular osteotomy for the treatment of hip dysplasias. *Clin Orthop* 232:26–36, 1988.
46. Graf R: New possibilities for diagnosis of congenital hip joint dislocation by ultrasonography. *J Pediatr Orthop* 3:359, 1983.

47. Green EN, Griffin PP: Hip dysplasia associated with abduction contracture of the contralateral hip. *J Bone Joint Surg* 64A: 1273–1281, 1982.

48. Grill F, Bensahel H, Canadell J, et al: The Pavlik harness in the treatment of congenital dislocating hip: Report on a multicenter study of the European Paediatric Orthopaedic Society. *J Pediatr Orthop* 8:1–8, 1988.

49. Gross RH: Congenital hip dysplasia in infants. *Orthop Surg Update* 3(10):2–7, 1984.

50. Gugenheim JJ, et al: Pathologic morphology of the acetabulum in paralytic and congenital hip instability. *J Pediatr Orthop* 2:397–400, 1982.

51. Guidera KJ, Einbecker ME, Berman CG, et al: Magnetic resonance imaging evaluation of congenital dislocation of the hips. *Clin Orthop* 261:96–101, 1990.

52. Gulman B, Tuncay IC, Dabak N, Karaismailoglu N: Salter's innominate osteotomy in the treatment of congenital hip dislocation: A long term review. *J Pediatr Orthop* 14:662–666, 1994.

53. Guyer B, et al: Dosimetry of computerized tomography in the evaluation of hip dysplasia. *Skel Radiol* 12:123–127, 1984.

54. Hansson G, et al: The Swedish experience with Salter's osteotomy in the treatment of congenital subluxation and dislocation of the hip. *J Pediatr Orthop* 10:159–162, 1990.

55. Harcke HT, Kumar SJ: The role of ultrasound in the diagnosis and management of congenital dislocation and dysplasia of the hip. *Curr Concepts Rev J Bone Joint Surg [Am]* 73:622–628, 1991.

56. Harris NH, et al: Acetabular development in congenital dislocation of the hip. *J Bone Joint Surg* 57B:46–52, 1975.

57. Harris NG, et al: Acetabular growth potential in congenital dislocation of the hip and some factors upon which it may depend. *Clin Orthop* 119:99–121, 1976.

58. Heikkala E, et al: Late diagnosis in congenital dislocation of the hip. *Acta Orthop Scand* 55:256–260, 1984.

59. Hensinger RN: Congenital dislocation of the hip: Treatment in infancy to walking age, in Stauffer ES (ed): *AAOS Instructional Course Lecture.* Vol 34. St Louis, Mosby, 1985, pp 434–456.

60. Hernandez RJ, et al: Ultrasound diagnosis of neonatal congenital dislocation of the hip: A decision analysis assessment. *J Bone Joint Surg* 76B:539–543, 1994.

61. Hernandez RJ, et al: Hip CT and congenital dislocation: Appearance of tight iliopsoas tendon and pulviner hypertrophy. *AJR* 139:335–337, 1982.

62. Hernandez RJ, et al: Hip CT in congenital dislocation: Appearance of tight iliopsoas tendon and pulvinar hypertrophy. *AJR* 139:335–337, 1982.

63. Hjalmstedt A, Aplund S: Congenital dislocation of the hip: A biochemical study in autopsy specimens. *J Pediatr Orthop* 3:491–497, 1983.

64. Hooper G: Congenital dislocation of the hip in infantile idiopathic scoliosis. *J Bone Joint Surg* 62B:447–448, 1980.

65. Hummer CD, McEwen GD: Torticollis and hip dysplasia. *J Bone Joint Surg* 55B:665, 1973.

66. Iwasaki K: Treatment of congenital dislocation of the hip by the Pavlik harness: Mechanism of reduction and usage. *J Bone Joint Surg* 65A: 760–767, 1983.

67. Johnson AH, et al: Treatment of congenital hip dislocation and dysplasia with the Pavlik harness. *Clin Orthop* 155:26–29, 1981.

68. Jones DA, Powell N: Ultrasound and neonatal hip screening: A prospective study of high risk babies. *J Bone Joint Surg [Br]* 72:457–459, 1990.

69. Jones D: An assessment of the value of examination of the hip in the newborn. *J Bone Joint Surg* 59B:318–322, 1977.

70. Jones DA: Subcapital coxa valga after varus osteotomy for congenital dislocation of the hip. *J Bone Joint Surg* 59B:152–158, 1977.

71. Kahle WK, Anderson MB, Alpert J, et al: The value of preliminary traction in the treatment of congenital dislocation of the hip. *J Bone Joint Surg [Am]* 72:1043–1047, 1990.

72. Kalamchi A, McEwen GD: Avascular necrosis following treatment of congenital dislocation of the hip. *J Bone Joint Surg* 62A:876–888, 1980.

73. Kalamchi A, McEwen GD: Congenital dislocation of the hip: Open reduction by the medial approach. *Clin Orthop* 169:127–232, 1982.

74. Kalamchi A, MacFarlane R: The Pavlik harness: Results in patients over three months of age. *J Pediatr Orthop* 2:3–8, 1982.

75. Kasser JR, et al: Varus derotation osteotomy in the treatment of persistent dysplasia in congenital dislocation of the hip. *J Bone Joint Surg* 67A:195–202, 1985.

76. Katz JF: The Chiari osteotomy in the older child with congenital hip subluxation and acetabular dysplasia. *Orthopaedics* 1:109–113, 1978.

77. Kepley RE, Weiner DS: Treatment of congenital dysplasia-subluxation of the hip in children under one year of age. *J Pediatr Orthop* 1:413–418, 1981.

78. Kershow CJ, Ware HE, Pattinson R, Fixsen JA: Revision of failed open reduction of congenital dislocation of the hip. *J Bone Joint Surg* 75B:744–749, 1993.

79. Kling, TF Jr, Hensinger RN: Double cut tomography in the management of congenitally dislocated hips. *J Pediatr Orthop* 2:195–197, 1982.

80. Klisic PJ: Congenital dislocation of the hip—A misleading term: Brief report. *J Bone Joint Surg [Br]* 71:136, 1989.

81. Lack W, Windhager R, Kutschera HP, Engel A: Chiari pelvic osteotomy for osteoarthritis secondary to hip dysplasia: Indications and long-term results. *J Bone Joint Surg [Br]* 73:229–234, 1991.

82. Lehman WB, et al: Hospital for joint diseases traction system for preliminary treatment of congenital dislocation of the hip. *J Paediatr Orthop* 3:104–107, 1983.

83. Lennox IAC, McLauchlan J, Murali R: Failures or screening and management of congenital dislocation of the hip. *J Bone Joint Surg* 75B:72–75, 1993.

84. Lindstrom JR, et al: Acetabular development after reduction in congenital dislocation of the hip. *J Bone Joint Surg* 61A:112–118, 1979.

85. Ludloff K: The open reduction of the congenital hip dislocation by anterior incision. *Am J Orthop Surg* 10:438–454, 1913.

86. Malefijt MC, DeWaal, et al: Chiari osteotomy in the treatment of congenital dislocation and subluxation of the hip. *J Bone Joint Surg* 64A:996–1003, 1982.

87. Mankey MG, Arntz CT, Staheli LT: Open reduction through a medial approach for congenital dislocation of the hip: A critical review of the Ludloff approach in sixty-six hips. *J Bone Joint Surg Am* 75A:1334–1345, 1993.

88. Mardam-Bey TH, MacEwen GD: Congenital hip dislocation after walking age. *J Pediatr Orthop* 2:478–486, 1982.

89. Marks DS, Clegg J, Al-Chalabi AN: Routine ultrasound screening for neonatal hip instability: Can it abolish late-presenting congenital dislocation of the hip? *J Bone Joint Surg* 76B:534–538, 1994.

90. Mau H, et al: Open reduction of congenital dislocation of the hip by Ludloff's method. *J Bone Joint Surg* 53A:1281–1288, 1971.

91. McCarroll HR, McCarroll HR Jr: Primary anterior congenital dislocation of the hip in infancy. *J Bone Joint Surg* 62A:554–556, 1980.

92. McEwen CD, Ramsey PL: The hip, in Lovell WW, Winter RB (eds): *Pediatric Orthopedics.* Vol 1. Philadelphia, Lippincott, 1978, pp 721–799.

93. McKay DW: A comparison of the innominate and the pericapsular osteotomy in the treatment of congenital dislocation of the hip. *Clin Orthop* 98:124–132, 1974.

94. McKibbin B: Anatomical factors in the stability of the hip joint in the new born. *J Bone Joint Surg* 52B:148–159, 1970.

95. McKinnon B, et al: Congenital dysplasia of the hip: The lax (subluxatable) newborn hip. *J Pediatr Orthop* 4:422–426, 1984.

96. Miranda L, et al: Prevention of congenital dislocation of the hip in the newborn. *J Pediatr Orthop* 8:671–675, 1988.

97. Mitchell GP: Arthrography in congenital displacement of the hip. *J Bone Joint Surg* 45B:88–95, 1963.

98. Moll FK Jr: Capsular change following Chiari innominate osteotomy. *J Pediatr Orthop* 2:573–576, 1982.

99. Mooney JF III, Kasser JR: Brachial plexus palsy as a complication of Pavlik harness use. *J Pediatr Orthop* 14:677–679, 1994.

100. Morel C, Briard JL: Progressive gradual reduction of the dislocated hip in a child after walking age, in Tachdjian MO (ed): *Congenital Dislocation of the Hip*. New York, Churchill Livingstone, 1982, pp 373–383.

101. Mubarak S, et al: Pitfalls in the use of Pavlik harness for treatment of congenital dysplasia, subluxation, and dislocation of the hip. *J Bone Joint Surg* 63A:1239–1247, 1981.

102. Naumann T, et al: Comparing the rate of femoral head necrosis of two different treatments of congenital dislocation of the hip. *J Pediatr Orthop* 10:780–785, 1990.

103. Ninomiya S: Rotational acetabular osteotomy for the dysplastic hip. *J Bone Joint Surg* 66A:430–436, 1984.

104. Noritake K, Yoshihashi Y, Hattori T, Takayuki M: Acetabular development after closed reduction of congenital dislocation of the hip. *J Bone Joint Surg* 75B:737–743, 1993.

105. Novack G, et al: Sonography of the neonatal and infant hip. *AJR* 141:639–645, 1983.

106. O'Sullivan ME, O'Brien T: Acetabular dysplasia presenting as developmental dislocation of the hip. *J Pediatr Orthop* 14:13–15, 1994.

107. Ogden JA: Anatomic and histologic study of factors affecting development and evolution of avascular necrosis in congenital dislocation of the hip, in *The Hip: Proceedings of the Second Open Scientific Meeting of the Hip Society*. St Louis, Mosby, 1974, pp 125–153.

108. Ogden JA: Changing patterns of proximal femoral vascularity. *J Bone Joint Surg* 56A:941, 1974.

109. Ogden JA: Normal and abnormal circulation, in Tachdjian MO (ed): *Congenital Dislocation of the Hip*. New York, Churchill Livingstone, 1982, pp 59–92.

110. Ogden JA: Dynamic pathobiology of congenital hip dysplasia, in Tachdjian, MO (ed): *Congenital Dislocation of the Hip*. New York, Churchill Livingstone, 1982, pp 93–144.

111. Ortolani M: Un segno poco noto e sua importanza per la diagnosi precoce di prelussazione congenita dell'anca. *Pediatria* 45:129, 1937.

112. Papavasiliou VA, Piggot H: Acetabular floor thickening and femoral head enlargement in congenital dislocation of the hip: Lateral displacement of femoral head. *J Pediatr Orthop* 3:22–27, 1983.

113. Paterson D: The early diagnosis and screening of congenital dislocation of the hip, in Tachdjian MO (ed): *Congenital Dislocation of the Hip*. New York, Churchill Livingstone, 1982, pp 145–157.

114. Pemberton PA: Pericapsular osteotomy of the ilium for the treatment of congenitally dislocated hips. *Clin Orthop* 98:41–54, 1974.

115. Peterson HA, et al: The use of computed tomography in dislocation of the hip and femoral neck anteversion in children, in Tachdjian MO (ed): *Congenital Dislocation of the Hip*. New York, Churchill, Livingstone, 1982, pp 263–282.

116. Pool RD, Foster BK, Paterson DC: Avascular necrosis in congenital hip dislocation: The significance of splintage. *J Bone Joint Surg [Br]* 68B:427–430, 1986.

117. Powell EN, Gerratana FJ, Gage JR: Open reduction for congenital hip dislocation: The risk of avascular necrosis with three different approaches. *J Pediatr Orthop* 6:127–132, 1986.

118. Quinn RH, Renshaw TS, DeLuca PA: Preliminary traction in the treatment of developmental dislocation of the hip. *J Pediatr Orthop* 14:636–642, 1994.

119. Race C, Herring JA: Congenital dislocation of the hip and evaluation of closed reduction. *J Pediatr Orthop* 3:166–172, 1983.

120. Ramsey PL, et al: Congenital dislocation of the hip. *J Bone Joint Surg* 58A:1000–1004, 1976.

121. Renshaw TS: Inadequate reduction of congenital dislocation of the hip. *J Bone Joint Surg* 63A:1114–1121, 1981.

122. Robinson HJ Jr, et al: Avascular necrosis in congenital hip dysplasia: The effect of treatment. *J Pediatr Orthop* 9:293–303, 1989.

123. Roose PE, et al: Open reduction for congenital dislocation of the hip using the Ferguson procedure. *J Bone Joint Surg* 61A:915–921, 1979.

124. Salter R: Innominate osteotomy in the treatment of congenital dislocation and subluxation of the hip. *J Bone Joint Surg* 43B:518, 1961.

125. Salter RB: An operative treatment for congenital dislocation and subluxation of the hip in the older child, in Apley JC (ed): *Recent Advances in Orthopaedics*. London, Churchill, 1969.

126. Salter RB, Kostuik J, Dallas S: Avascular necrosis of the femoral head as a complication of treatment for congenital dislocation of the hip in young children: A clinical and experimental investigation. *Can J Surg* 12:44, 1969.

127. Salter RB, Dubos JP: The first fifteen years personal experience with innominate osteotomy in the treatment of congenital dislocation and subluxation of the hip. *Clin Orthop* 98:72, 1974.

128. Schoenecker PL, Strecker WB: Congenital dislocation of the hip in children: Comparison of the effects of femoral shortening and skeletal traction in treatment. *J Bone Joint Surg* 66A:21–27, 1984.

129. Schuler P, Feltes E, Kienapfel H, Griss P: Ultrasound examination for the early determination of dysplasia and congenital dislocation of neonatal hips. *Clin Orthop* 258:18–26, 1990.

130. Sharp IK: Acetabular dysplasia: The acetabular angle. *J Bone Joint Surg* 43B:268–272, 1961.

131. Simons GW, Flatley TJ, Sty JR, Starshjak RJ: Intra-articular osteocartilagenous obstruction to reduction of congenital dislocation of the hip: Report of three cases. *J Bone Joint Surg* 70A:760–768, 1988.

132. Simons GW: A comparative evaluation of the current methods for open reduction of the congenitally displaced hip. *Orthop Clin North Am* 11:161–181, 1980.

133. Skirving AP, Scaddan WJ: The African neonatal hip and its immunity from congenital dislocation. *J Bone Joint Surg* 61B:339–341, 1979.

134. Staheli LT, et al: Congenital hip dysplasia. *Instr Course Lect* 33:350–363, 1984.

135. Stanislavlijevic S: Etiology of congenital hip pathology, in Tachdjian MO (ed): *Congenital Dislocations of the Hip*. New York, Churchill Livingstone, 1982, pp 27–33.

136. Steel HH: Triple osteotomy of the innominate bone. *J Bone Joint Surg* 55A:343, 1973.

137. Stevens PM, Coleman SO: Coxa breva: Its pathogenesis and a rationale for its management. *J Pediatr Orthop* 5:515–521, 1985.

138. Sutherland DH, Moore M: Clinical and radiographic outcome of patients treated with double innominate osteotomy for congenital hip dysplasia. *J Pediatr Orthop* 11:143–148, 1991.

139. Sutherland DH, Greenfield R: Double innominate osteotomy. *J Bone Joint Surg* 59A:1082, 1977.

140. Suzuki S, Yamamuro T: Avascular necrosis in patients treated with the Pavlik harness for congenital dislocation of the hip. *J Bone Joint Surg [Am]* 72:1048–1055, 1990.

141. Suzuki S: Ultrasound and the Pavlik harness in CDH. *J Bone Joint Surg* 75B:483–487, 1993.

142. Tanaka T, Yoshihashi Y, Miura T: Changes in soft tissue interposition after reduction of developmental dislocation of the hip. *J Pediatr Orthop* 14:16–23, 1994.

143. Tavares JO, Gottwald DH, Rochelle JR: Guided abduction traction in the treatment of congenital hip dislocation. *J Pediatr Orthop* 14:643–649, 1994.

144. Thieme WT, Wynne-Davies R: Clinical examination and urinary oestrogen assays in newborn children with congenital dislocation of the hip. *J Bone Joint Surg* 50B:546–550, 1968.

145. Thomas CL, et al: Treatment concepts for proximal femoral ischemic necrosis complicating congenital hip disease. *J Bone Joint Surg* 64A:817–828, 1982.

146. Tonnis D, Storch K, Ulbrich H: Newborn screening for CDH with and without sonography and correlation of risk factors. *J Pediatr Orthop* 10:145–152, 1990.

147. Tredwell SJ, Bell MH: Efficacy of neonatal hip examination. *J Pediatr Orthop* 1:61–65, 1981.

148. Trevor D, et al: Acetabuloplasty in the treatment of congenital dislocation of the hip. *J Bone Joint Surg* 57B:167–174, 1975.

149. Tucci JJ, Kumar SJ, Guille JT, Rubbo ER: Late acetabular dysplasia following early successful Pavlik harness treatment of congenital dislocation of the hip. *J Pediatr Orthop* 11:502–505, 1991.

150. Utterbanks T, McEwen D: Comparison of pelvic osteotomies for the surgical correction of the congenital hip. *Clin Orthop* 98:104, 1974.

151. Visser JD, et al: Hip joint measurements with computerized tomography. *J Pediatr Orthop* 2:143–146, 1982.

152. Von Rosen S: Diagnosis and treatment of congenital dislocation of the hip joint in the newborn. *J Bone Joint Surg* 44B:284–291, 1962.

153. Wagner H: Experiences with spherical acetabular osteotomy for the correction of the dysplastic acetabulum, in Weil VH (ed): *Acetabular Dysplasia: Skeletal Dysplasias in Childhood—Progress in Orthopaedic Surgery.* New York, Springer-Verlag, 1978, pp 131–145.

154. Walker JM: Comparison of normal and abnormal human fetal hip joints: A quantitative study with significance to congenital hip disease. *J Pediatr Orthop* 3:173–183, 1983.

155. Weinstein SL: Natural history of congenital hips dislocation (CDH) and hip dysplasia. *Clin Orthop* 225:62–76, 1987.

156. Wilkinson JA: Prime factors in the etiology of congenital dislocation of the hip. *J Bone Joint Surg* 45B:268–283, 1963.

157. Williamson DM, Glover SD, Benson MKD: Congenital dislocation of the hip presenting after age three years: A long term review. *J Bone Surg [Br]* 71:745–751, 1989.

158. Wynne-Davies R: Acetabular dysplasia and familial joint laxity: Two etiological factors in congenital dislocation of the hip. *J Bone Joint Surg* 52B:704–716, 1970.

CHAPTER 41

Coxa Vara

Roger Dee and Martin A. Gruber

At birth the proximal femur has a composite chondroepiphysis for the greater trochanter and the head of the femur.[1] By the fourth to sixth month, secondary ossification occurs in the capital epiphysis as two foci that rapidly coalesce. This development is followed by longitudinal growth in the neck of the femur, separating the regions of the greater trochanter from the femoral head, the latter then establishing a discrete capital femoral physis. Ogden points out that the subsequent development of the femoral neck provides for a continued susceptibility to vascular damage.[1] At 1 year there is still cartilaginous continuity between the femoral neck and the trochanteric region, but only posterosuperiorly. Secondary ossification centers for the greater trochanter coalesce and form one center, which then proceeds to ossify at 3 to 4 years. Over the subsequent growth period the neck shaft angle depends upon the relative contributions of the medial and lateral physeal growth rates of the capital physis but is influenced also by the rate of growth in the trochanteric physeal region. Since the capital femoral physis is responsible for longitudinal growth, it is sometimes called the *longitudinal growth plate*.[1] The ultimate shape of the proximal femur is determined not only by its growth but also by the integrity of the structure of the femoral neck isthmus between the two and its ability to resist physiologic and pathologic stresses.[2,3] At the end of the period between 5 and 8 years, the final anatomic contours of the proximal femur have formed.[4] The normal neck shaft angle of the femur is approximately 150° at birth but diminishes to 142° by the age of 5 years. There is further reduction of only a few degrees up to adult developments.

CLASSIFICATION

These patients have been well classified by Weinstein et al.[5] True congenital coxa vara may occur in association with a hypoplastic femur and together with other associated limb deficiencies. Coxa vara may also be associated with proximal femoral focal deficiencies. Patients in these groups have been discussed in Chap. 39.

Another group of patients may have coxa vara associated with congenital skeletal dysplasias (e.g., multiple epiphyseal dysplasia, spondylometaphyseal dysplasia,[6,7] familial osteopetrosis, achondroplasia, cretinism).

Yet another group may have an *acquired* etiology for coxa vara, due perhaps to injury in early childhood, the development of rickets, or associated with Perthes disease or congenital dislocation of the hip and the treatment of these conditions. Adolescent coxa vara is associated with slipped capital femoral epiphysis and is described in Chap. 43.

This still leaves a category of patient with isolated coxa vara in whom there is no associated congenital abnormality or traumatic or metabolic cause to explain a deficiency in the femoral neck or the growth plate. These patients do not show shortening at birth. The diagnosis is not made until weight bearing begins and progressive deformity is noticed. This group of patients is sometimes referred to as having *infantile coxa vara* or *developmental coxa vara*. The precise etiologic factors responsible in this group of patients remain undetermined. The disease is also sometimes still referred to as *congenital coxa vara*. It is possible that the potential for dysplasia may be present in the femoral neck at birth and that therefore this condition is truly congenital, but the deficiency does not manifest itself in terms of structural failure until the child begins to walk. Unfortunately, this is by no means certain.[8,9] The possibility exists that in some cases the condition may be entirely acquired (e.g., traumatic), so that the use of the term *congenital* is in error. From here on we will refer to this condition as *infantile coxa vara*.

INFANTILE COXA VARA

The incidence of this condition has been assessed at only 1 in 25,000 births.[10] Occasionally there is a familial incidence that can be traced through several generations.[2,11]

Etiology

That there may be a vascular abnormality in the developing neck predisposing this area to dysplasia has been suggested by several workers.[12,13] Certainly, in older children at corrective surgery, a well-established disturbance of endochondral ossification can be shown.[14,15] Other authors have believed that the condition is probably triggered by intrauterine trauma or injury sustained shortly after birth.[1,16] Hoyt and coworkers have summarized the conflicting evidence in a recent review.[8] Ogden has stressed the vulnerability of the blood vessels on the posterosuperior femoral neck, since they pursue a variable intracartilaginous course and are susceptible to damage if fracture occurs through the midcervical regions.

A triangular piece of bone is noted in the inferior portion of the neck associated with the increasing varus deformity. This metaphyseal fragment of bone seems to reflect abnormal metaphyseal bone formation by the medial physis after it has assumed the more vertical orientation associated with the increasing varus. This fragment is seen as the neck calcifies. The medial side of the fragment is separated from the epiphysis by the medial physis. On its lateral side the triangular fragment is separated from the rest of the metaphysis by an oblique fissure, which probably represents a pseudarthrosis (Figs. 41-1 and 41-2). On x-ray, both the fissure and the medial physis are seen as

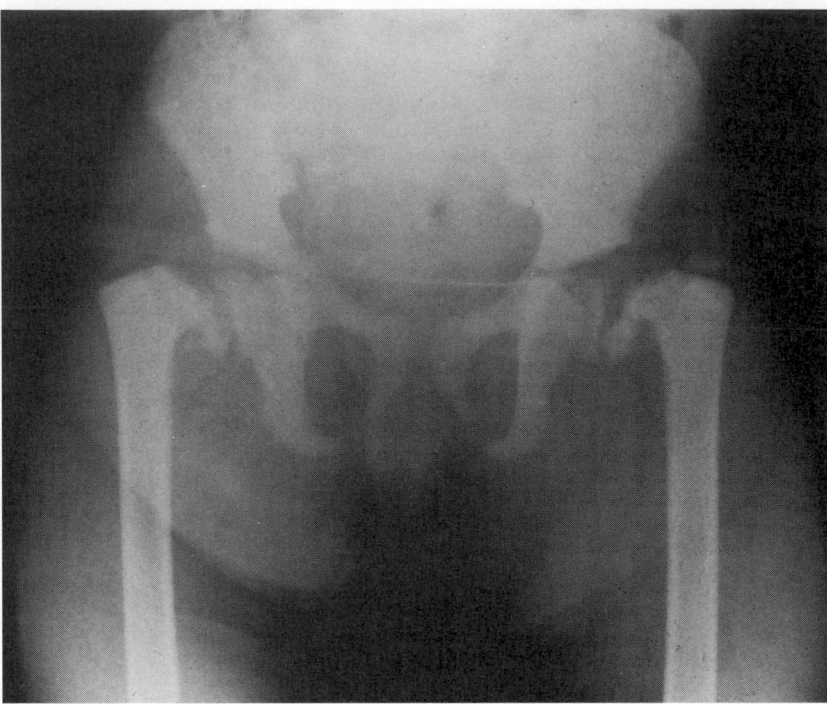

Figure 41-1 Infantile coxa vara (bilateral). This case probably does not require osteotomy. For explanation, see text.

zones of radiolucency that meet at the superior corner of the triangular fragment and then continue superiorly along the line of the lateral portion of the capital physis. If the fragment is large, the major portion of the defect in the neck (i.e., the fissure or pseudarthrosis) lies some way distant from the subcapital physis. By contrast, if the fragment is small, the major portion of the fissure defect runs through the subcapital physeal plate, resulting in a greater deformity.

Other bony abnormalities are seen associated with the deformity. Schmidt and Kalamchi[3] showed that the teardrop configuration of the medial acetabular wall was abnormal in those cases of coxa vara when the neck shaft angle was less than 110° (Fig. 41-2). On the other hand, the acetabulum developed normally if the neck shaft angle was corrected to 140° or more. Correction to less than

135°, however, did not result in normal acetabular development. Hoyt and coworkers have shown that the enlargement of the greater trochanter which often accompanies progressive coxa vara deformity seems to be worse in those patients where there is a small triangular fragment.[8]

Clinical Presentation

The earliest diagnosis of coxa vara may occur during ultrasonographic screening for hip dysplasia. Haake and coworkers have reported a false-positive ultrasound suggesting a dysplastic hip caused by the superiorly displaced greater trochanter in children with a congenital coxa vara.[17] Occasionally a limp or waddling gait is noticed

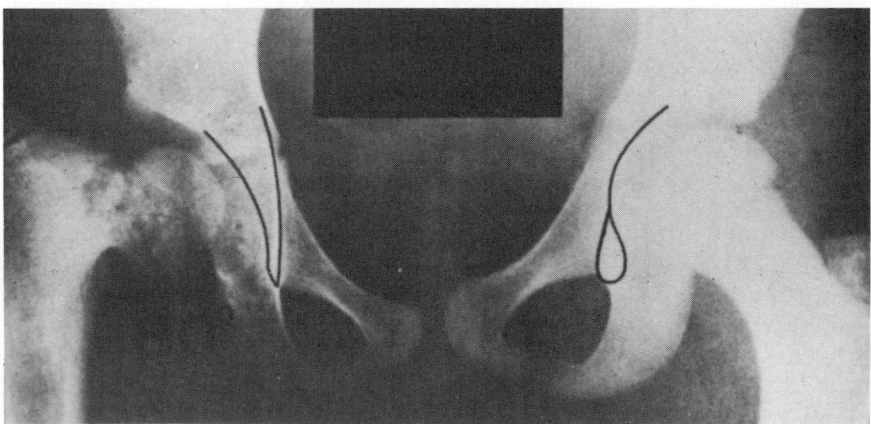

Figure 41-2 The teardrop configuration of the acetabulum is outlined normally on the left hip. The right hip demonstrates lack of development of normal teardrop configuration of the medial acetabular wall. This reflects the acetabular dysplasia seen in association with coxa vara. The acetabulum appears flattened with widening of the opening to the acetabulum. (Reproduced with permission from Schmidt TL, Kalamchi A: The fate of the capital femoral physis and acetabular development in developmental coxa vara. *J Pediatr Orthop* 2:535, 1982.)

when the child first begins to walk, but often it may not be until the age of 3 or 4 years that sufficient abnormality is noted and advice sought.

There is usually no history of significant injury.[18] Weinstein and coworkers[5] observed that 70 percent of their patients presented with a limp; 25 percent of patients with bilateral involvement presented with a waddling gait; and only 5 percent presented with back and leg pain. All patients were observed to have a positive Trendelenburg sign and most had decreased abduction and limitation of internal rotation on physical examination. A leg-length discrepancy of more than 2 cm was unusual.[5] Pain in the hip appears to be an unusual presentation.[18] It usually follows some recent incident of trauma. The limp is characteristically painless.

Radiologic Characteristics

X-ray evaluation requires normal views of the hip and also scanograms to assess any leg-length discrepancy. Skeletal survey may be required to exclude generalized dysplasias. Abnormalities such as proximal focal femoral deficiency and congenital shortening of the femur are associated with a more severe degree of shortening and do not show the characteristic physeal changes of infantile coxa vara. These changes are seen early in the disease before there is calcification in the neck and the typical triangular fragment of bone appears. There is a progressive change of the alignment of the subcapital physis toward vertical, associated with a decreasing neck shaft angle.[19,20] Later on the characteristic fissure appears. The fissure originates superiorly in the region of the physeal plate but then breaks away at a variable point from the line of the physis,

traversing the metaphysis at varying degrees of obliquity to emerge in the region of the calcar. The characteristic triangular fragment is therefore enclosed within the limb of an inverted V- or Y-shaped radiologic lucency (Fig. 43-1, open arrow). The apex of the V or the single limb of the Y shape always originates, however, in the region of the superior portion of the subcapital physis. The work of Schmidt and Kalamchi[3] using radiologic assessment to study the relationship between acetabular dysplasia and the degree of deformity has been described.

Magnetic resonance imaging has revealed a widened growth plate with expansion of the cartilage medio-distally between the capital femoral epiphysis and the metaphysis.[21] Weinstein and coworkers have sought methods of radiologic assessment that can be used in decision making as to the need for corrective osteotomy.[5] They have not found the neck shaft angle to be useful in this situation and regard it as unreliable. They prefer to use the Hilgenreiner epiphyseal (HE) angle. This angle is measured between Hilgenreiner's line and a line drawn through the metaphyseal side of the defect, corresponding with the abnormally orientated growth plate (Fig. 41-3). They indicate that if the HE angle is greater than 60°, corrective surgery should be performed. If the angle is less than 45°, spontaneous correction will occur without surgery. Between 45 to 60°, the outcome is uncertain and careful observation is required before any decision is made[5] (Fig. 41-4).

Treatment

In appropriately selected cases, the objective of surgical treatment is to correct deformity and at the same time to

Figure 41-3 Measurement of the Hilgenreiner epiphyseal angle using Hilgenreiner's line as the horizontal axis and a line through the defect adjacent to the metaphysis axis. (Reproduced with permission from Weinstein JN et al: Congenital coxa vara: A retrospective review. *J Pediatr Orthop* 4:71, 1984.)

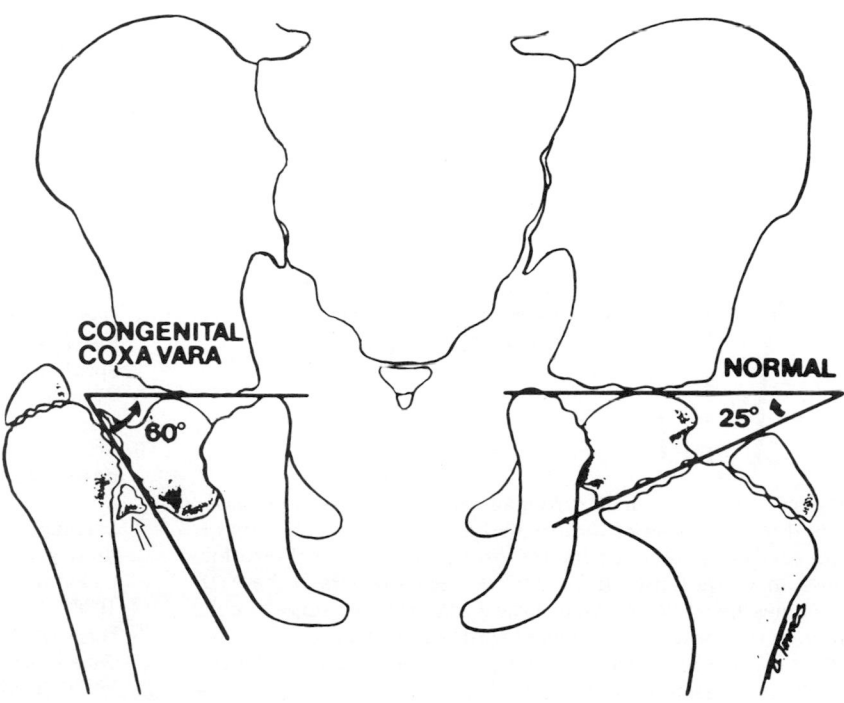

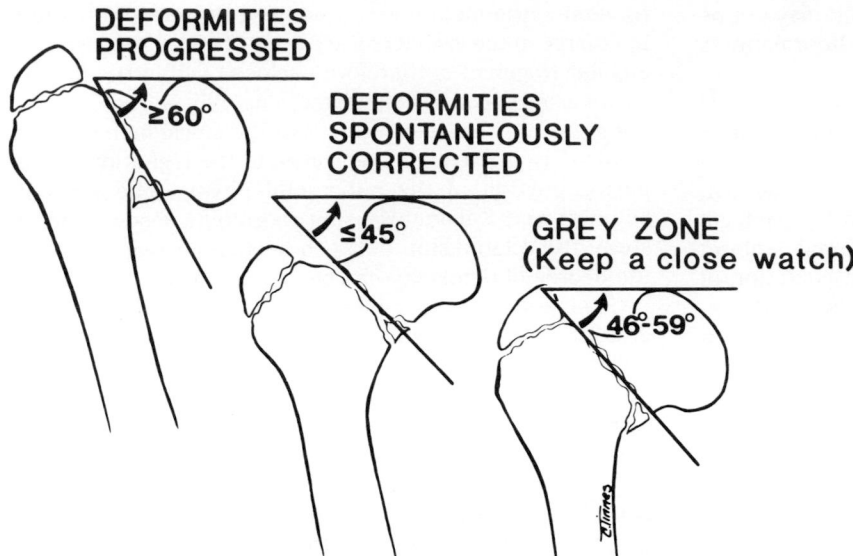

Figure 41-4 When the HE angle is 60° or greater all patients will have progression of their coxa vara deformity. At 45° or less all will correct spontaneously. Between the two is a zone in which patients need careful serial observation. (Reproduced with permission from Weinstein JN et al: Congenital coxa vara: A retrospective review. *J Pediatr Orthop* 4:76, 1984.)

promote ossification. Bowen stressed the importance of correcting femoral retroversion, which commonly accompanies the deformity. For this reason he favors an oblique intertrochanteric osteotomy of the MacEwen-Shands type, which will correct the version and the coxa vara.[12a,22,23] This procedure has also been used for the correction of coxa valga. Cordes and coworkers prefer the Pauwels' Y osteotomy and have reported excellent long-term results.[24] A postoperative HE angle of 35° or less and a head shaft (HS) angle of 130° or more gives consistently satisfactory results with no recurrence, irrespective of the age at surgery. Premature closure of the capital femoral epiph-ysis will occur in approximately 90 percent of hips having valgus osteotomy.[3]

For those patients who do not require surgery or who will remain under observation, conservative therapy should be offered, including gait training and abductor muscle strengthening.[21] Similar guidelines for surgical treatment may be usefully employed in dealing with causes of coxa vara other than the infantile variety. The objective should be to improve the HE angle and restore more normal biomechanics to the affected hip joint. Associated trochanteric overgrowth or coxa brevis may require trochanteric epiphysiodesis or transplantation[9] (Fig. 41-5).

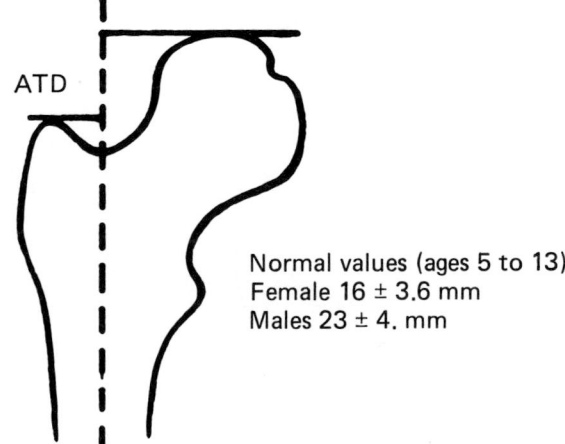

Normal values (ages 5 to 13)
Female 16 ± 3.6 mm
Males 23 ± 4. mm

Figure 41-5 The articular trochanteric distance (ATD) is measured from the top of the ossified femoral head to the tip of the ossified greater trochanter. Normal values are shown for girls and boys between the age of 5 and 13 years. If the ATD becomes negative the coxa brevis may require surgical correction (see text). (Reproduced with permission from Stevens PM, Coleman SS: Coxa breva: Its pathogenesis and a rationale for its management. *J Pediatr Orthop* 5:516, 1985.)

REFERENCES

1. McDougall A: Fracture of the neck of the femur in childhood. *J Bone Joint Surg* 43B:16, 1961.
2. Say B et al: Dominant congenital coxa vara. *J Bone Joint Surg* 56B:78–85, 1974.
3. Schmidt TL, Kalamchi A: The fate of the capital femoral physis and acetabular development in developmental coxa vara. *J Pediatr Orthop* 2:534–538, 1982.
4. Ogden JA: Trauma, hip development and vascularity, in Tronzo RG (ed): *Surgery of the Hip Joint.* 2d ed. Vol 1. New York, Springer-Verlag, 1984, pp 145–180.
5. Weinstein JN et al: Congenital coxa vara: A retrospective review. *J Pediatr Orthop* 4:70–77, 1984.
6. Kozlowski K, Napiontek M, Beim ER: Spondylometaphyseal dysplasia, Sutcliffe type: A rediscovered entity. *Can Assoc Radiol J* 43:364–368, 1992.
7. Lachman RS, Rimoin DL, Spranger J: Metaphyseal chondrodysplasia, Schmid type: Clinical and radiographic delineation with a review of the literature. *Pediatr Radiol* 18:93–102, 1988.
8. Hoyt WA Jr et al: Congenital coxa vara, in Tronzo RG (ed): *Surgery of the Hip Joint,* 2d ed. Vol 1. New York, Springer-Verlag, 1984, pp 203–224.

9. Stevens PM, Coleman SS: Coxa breva: Its pathogenesis and a rationale for its management. *J Pediatr Orthop* 5:515–521, 1985.
10. Johanning K: Coxa vara infantum: II. Treatment and results of treatment. *Acta Orthop Scand* 22:100, 1952.
11. Almond HC: Familial infantile coxa vara. *J Bone Joint Surg* 38B:539–544, 1956.
12. Chung S, Riser W: The histological characteristics of congenital coxa vara. *Clin Orthop* 132:71, 1978.
12a. Desai SS, Johnson LO: Long-term results of valgus osteotomy for congenital coxa vara. *Clin Orthop* 294:204–210, 1993.
13. Nilsonne H: Contributions as to the knowledge of congenital coxa vara. *Acta Radiol* 3:383, 1924.
14. Pylkkanen PV: Coxa vara infantum. *Acta Orthop Scand* 48(suppl):1, 1960.
15. Serafin J, Szulc W: Coxa vara infantum, hip growth disturbances, etiopathogenesis, and long-term results of treatment. *Clin Orthop* 272:103–113, 1991.
16. Blockey NJ: Observations on infantile coxa vara. *J Bone Joint Surg* 51B:106–111, 1969.
17. Haake M, Wirth T, Griss P: False-positive sonographic hip examinations in newborns with congenital varus deformity of the proximal femur. *Arch Orthop Trauma Surg* 114:274–277, 1995.
18. LeMesurier AB: Developmental coxa vara. *J Bone Joint Surg* 30B:585–605, 1948.
19. Fairbank T: *An Atlas of Generalized Affections of the Skeleton.* Edinborough, Churchill Livingstone, 1951.
20. Pavlov H et al: Infantile coxa vara. *Radiology* 135:631–640, 1980.
21. Bos CF, Sakkers RJ, Bloem JL, et al: Histological, biochemical, and MRI studies of the growth plate in congenital coxa vara. *J Pediatr Orthop* 9:660–665, 1989.
22. Bowen R: Abnormal growth and development of the pediatric hip. *AAOS Instr Course Lect* :423–433, 1985.
23. MacEwen GD, Bunnell WP, Ramsey PL: The hip, in Lovell WW, Winter RB (eds): *Pediatric Orthopaedics.* Vol 2. Philadelphia, Lippincott, 1986, pp 736–738.
24. Cordes S, Dickens DR, Cole WG: Correction on coxa vara in childhood: The use of Pauwels' Y-shaped osteotomy. *J Bone Joint Surg* 73B:13–16, 1991.

CHAPTER 42

Legg-Calvé-Perthes Disease

James T. Guille
and J. Richard Bowen

Legg-Calvé-Perthes disease is a condition whereby the immature capital femoral epiphysis undergoes varying degrees of necrosis, for unknown reasons. The disease is actually a cascade of events that begins with necrosis of the capital femoral epiphysis followed by subsequent fragmentation and ends with the eventual reossification and remodeling of the femoral head. This cycle may be repeated several times.

In 1910, the condition was described independently by Legg of the United States, Calvé of France, and Perthes of Germany.[1-3] In the early 1900s, Phemister showed histologically that the condition was osseous necrosis, and Waldenström introduced the term *coxa plana* to describe the appearance of the femoral head after deformation.[4-8]

Legg-Calvé-Perthes disease affects boys four times more commonly than girls. Some believe that girls have a poorer prognosis than boys, most likely because girls reach skeletal maturity earlier than boys and therefore have less remodeling potential. The frequency of left and right hip involvement is almost equal, and both hips are involved in approximately 10 to 15 percent of cases. Typically, symptoms begin between the ages of 4 and 8. Various studies from around the world have reported differing incidences of Legg-Calvé-Perthes disease in their populations: one in 1200 in Massachusetts, one in 1400 in British Columbia, one in 4750 in South Wales, one in 12,500 in England, and 8.5 per 100,000 in Uppsala.[9-12]

ETIOLOGY

The etiology of Legg-Calvé-Perthes disease remains an enigma. Trauma, inflammation, endocrinopathies, inadequate nutrition, and genetic transmission have been proposed as possible causes.[11,13,14] Significantly increased levels of IgG and IgM have been reported, as well as decreased levels of insulinlike growth factor I (IGF-I) and somatomedin C.[15-17] An antecedent toxic synovitis of the hip (irritable hip syndrome) has been associated with subsequent Legg-Calvé-Perthes disease in some series, with an incidence of approximately 1 to 12 percent; however, this has not been shown consistently by other investigators. Vascular compromise, whether venous hypertension or arterial flow deficiencies, has been shown by some authors to cause Perthes-like changes in the hip.[18,19] More recently, hypofibrinolysis, protein C and protein S deficiencies, and

elevated lipoprotein "a" levels have been postulated to result in thrombotic venous occlusion, leading to venous hypertension and osteonecrosis.[20] Legg-Calvé-Perthes disease in patients with hemophilia is said to stem from increased intracapsular pressure secondary to hemarthrosis.[21] Other factors such as short stature and delayed maturation, as demonstrated by bone age, have been associated with Legg-Calvé-Perthes disease.[22-24] A correlation between Legg-Calvé-Perthes disease and attention deficit hyperactivity disorder has recently been proposed.[25] An increased incidence of breech presentation, low birthweight, genitourinary anomalies, pyloric stenosis, and congenital heart disease have also been noted.[26-28] The role, if any, of environmental factors has yet to be determined. Other possible etiologies include socioeconomic factors and increased parental age.

DIFFERENTIAL DIAGNOSIS

Many disease processes can mimic the clinical presentation and roentgenographic appearance of Legg-Calvé-Perthes disease (Table 42-1). Concurrent symmetrical involvement of both hips should alert one to the possibility of multiple epiphyseal dysplasia or hypothyroidism, both of which more commonly present with bilateral hip involvement. When both hips are afflicted with Legg-Calvé-Perthes disease, which can occur in 10 to 15 percent of cases, each hip is usually at a different stage in the course of the disease.

The most difficult of these conditions to differentiate include infection, transient synovitis of the hip, and epiphyseal dysplasia. When the roentgenograms of the hip appear normal, infection and toxic synovitis need to be ruled out. If the leukocyte count, sedimentation rate, or protein C levels are elevated and infection is suspected, the hip must be aspirated under arthrographic control. In cases of toxic synovitis, approximately 50 percent of the

Table 42-1 Differential Diagnosis

Meyer dysplasia
Hypothyroidism
Multiple epiphyseal dysplasia
Minimal slipped capital femoral epiphysis
Eosinophilic granuloma
Osteoid osteoma
Lymphoma
Pigmented villonodular synovitis
Chondroblastoma
Sickle cell disease
Gaucher disease
Tuberculosis
Rheumatologic diseases
Toxic synovitis (irritable hip syndrome)

hips will have radiographic signs of increased inferomedial joint space and lateral bulging of the joint capsule. In patients with epiphyseal dysplasia, the typical sequential changes of Legg-Calvé-Perthes disease are absent, roentgenograms of other epiphyses will frequently show involvement, and other family members may have the condition.

CLINICAL FEATURES

Early in the course of Legg-Calvé-Perthes disease, the most frequently presenting complaints are groin or anterior thigh pain and limp, both of which are usually insidious in onset and exacerbated by increased activity. The limp is typically antalgic, the pelvis dips on the involved side, and the stride is short. The involved lower limb may show some degree of thigh and buttock atrophy. At rest, the limb is held in mild flexion, adduction, and external rotation. The hip will generally have a mild flexion contracture, as shown by the Thomas test, and limited abduction. Loss of internal rotation is an early and sensitive sign.

Most patients present early in the course of the disease. In a series reported earlier from our institution, 75 percent of patients presented during the necrosis or fragmentation phase, 18 percent presented during the reossification phase, and 7 percent presented at or near skeletal maturity.[29] The most frequently reported complaints of those patients presenting late in the course of the disease are limp, which may be of the antalgic, short-leg, stiff-hip, or Trendelenburg type; pain, usually in the hip area; and stiffness of the hip that functionally limits activity.

STAGES OF DISEASE

Phemister showed histologically that the pathologic process in Legg-Calvé-Perthes disease was osseous necrosis of the capital femoral epiphysis, with the overlying articular cartilage remaining essentially unaffected. Around the same time, Waldenström divided the course of Legg-Calvé-Perthes disease into four stages: necrosis, resorption (fragmentation), reossification, and remodeling. The length of time for each stage varies considerably; in general, the necrotic and resorptive stages each last approximately 6 months, reossification may last from 1½ years to 3 years, and remodeling occurs until skeletal maturity.[29] Compensatory changes in the hip joint may continue into adulthood.

Necrotic Stage

The earliest roentgenographic sign of Legg-Calvé-Perthes disease, which is rarely seen, is bulging of the capsule of the hip secondary to synovitis. A small, round osteopenic area in the medial metaphysis of the femoral neck may

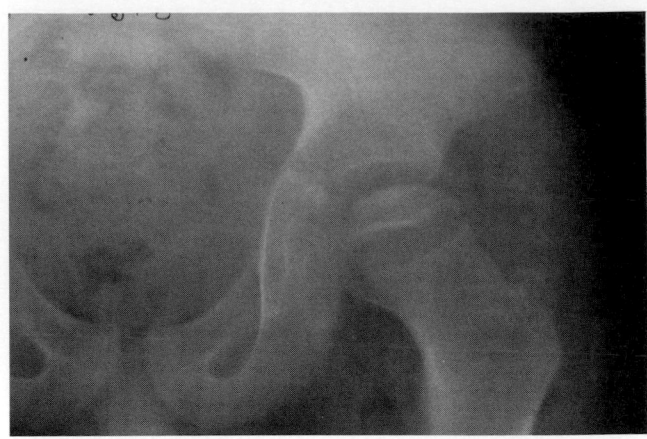

Figure 42-1 Necrosis stage. Note widening of the cartilage space and the small, dense capital femoral epiphysis.

also be observed. In the early stages of the disease, part or all of the epiphysis is infarcted, but the articular cartilage, which receives its nourishment from the synovial fluid, continues to grow. The asymmetrical growth leads to increased thickness over the medial and lateral aspects of the femoral head. Roentgenographically, these changes are demonstrated as a small capital epiphysis and an apparent increased thickening of the articular cartilage that gives the impression of subtle subluxation (Waldenström's sign) (Fig. 42-1). Subsequently the necrotic portion of the femoral head becomes roentgenographically dense. This may be due to relative osteopenia of the viable bone, increased calcification of necrotic epiphyseal bone, or apposition of new bone on necrotic trabeculae (creeping substitution). Theoretically, the initial infarction heals when the woven bone is applied over the necrotic lamellar bone. Repeated infarctions result in necrosis of woven bone, causing thickening of the trabeculae. Metaphyseal osteopenia frequently develops directly under the physeal plate and adjacent to the area of epiphyseal necrosis. Histologically, there are areas of fatty replacement of marrow and occasional areas of cellular infiltrate of lymphocytes and plasma cells.

As mechanical stress is continually applied across the hip joint, the avascular bone becomes unable to support the load and a vertical compression of trabeculae occurs. The height of the bony epiphysis is reduced by this subchondral fracture. Frequently, the fracture of the necrotic bone is seen radiographically as a lucent line, parallel to the joint surface (the crescent sign), best seen on the frog-leg lateral roentgenogram. Continued stress across the hip joint may cause further mechanical disruption and extrusion of the epiphysis, generally in the anterolateral direction.

Resorption (Fragmentation) Stage

As continued stress is applied across the hip, the necrotic bone will be crushed, osteoclasts will remodel the distorted trabeculae, and fibrocartilage will fill in the defect.

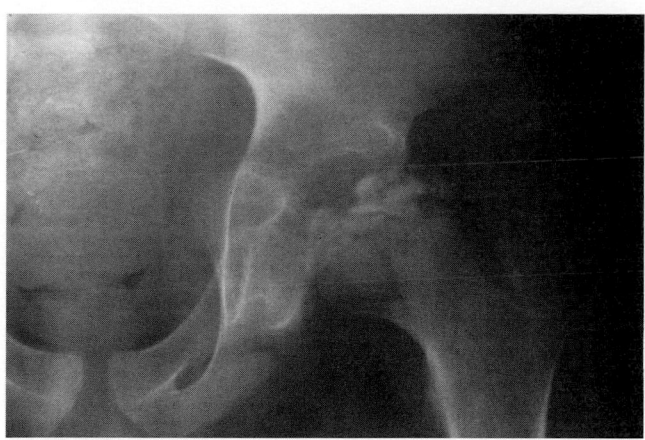

Figure 42-2 Fragmentation stage. The capital femoral epiphysis is irregular, secondary to revascularization by creeping substitution.

The fibrovascular tissue generally begins at the periphery of the epiphysis, replacing the necrotic bone in an irregular manner (Fig. 42-2). Occasionally, lysis of bone occurs at the superolateral portion of the femoral neck (Gage's sign). Extruded cartilage and fibrocartilage may calcify lateral to the acetabulum, giving roentgenographic evidence of femoral head extrusion. In the late necrotic stage and throughout the entire fragmentation stage, the femoral epiphysis may deform, with the femoral neck widening in response to this deformity.

Hinge subluxation is a condition whereby lateral extrusion, flattening, and enlargement of the femoral head prevent normal motion about the hip (Fig. 42-3A through D). When the hip is brought into abduction, this deformity allows the femoral head to abut and pivot on the superolateral margin of the acetabulum, causing limitation of abduction and further incongruity. When attempted internal rotation of the deformed femoral head impinges on the anterior margin of the acetabulum, blocking further internal rotation, the condition is known as anterior impingement. Both conditions perpetuate the joint incongruity and predispose the hip to early degenerative joint disease.

Older patients with Legg-Calvé-Perthes disease do not develop the marked thickening of articular cartilage seen in younger patients. Weight bearing on necrotic avascular bone leads to vertical compression and collapse. Continued stress across the hip may lead to extrusion of the crushed epiphysis, generally in an anterolateral direction, producing an oval-shaped femoral head. Contraction of the hip muscles in flexion, adduction, and external rotation potentiates this deformity. When the lower limb is held in adduction and external rotation, the hip will flex and extend freely; however, abduction and internal rotation are limited. Forced abduction of the lower limb causes the superolateral margin of the acetabulum to impinge on the extruded portion of the femoral epiphysis. This maneuver, which is often painful, leads to widening of the medial joint space and is pathognomonic for hinge subluxation. In some patients, the crushed epiphysis deforms and extrudes anteriorly. This is often seen in patients in whom the lower limb is held in marked exter-

nal rotation during the necrosis and resorptive stages. These patients will ambulate with the lower limb in external rotation. Forced internal rotation causes pain and can lead to subluxation as the femoral head impinges on the anterior margin of the acetabulum. Osteochondritis dissecans of the femoral epiphysis has been reported in this area.

Reossification Stage

Following fragmentation, reossification of the fibrovascular tissue will occur. The reossification generally begins at the margins of the epiphysis and progresses until the entire epiphysis is reossified (Fig. 42-4). This is termed *paraphyseal reossification*. Occasionally, reossification through the growth plate may result in the creation of a bony bridge between the metaphysis and the epiphysis, resulting in growth arrest of the femoral neck (transphyseal reossification).[30]

Remodeling Stage

Once the femoral epiphysis has reossified, the femoral head continues to remodel until the patient reaches skeletal maturity (Fig. 42-5).[31] Further adaptive compensatory changes may take place in the hip joint throughout the patient's life.

MEDICAL IMAGING EVALUATION
Roentgenograms

The initial imaging study to be done on the child suspected of having Legg-Calvé-Perthes disease is a standing, weight-bearing anteroposterior and lateral roentgenogram of the pelvis. These views will not only aid in excluding other diagnoses but also show the stage of disease and extent of involvement. Typically, serial anteroposterior roentgenograms of the hip are made at 1- to 2-month intervals during the active phases of the disease. All of the current classification schemes are based on findings on these views.

Sonograms

Sonography may be used in the initial evaluation of the patient suspected of having Legg-Calvé-Perthes disease to differentiate it from other conditions.[32,33] The nonspecific early findings of synovitis (bulging of the hip capsule) can usually be found. One should remember that in true synovitis, there is a synovial effusion, whereas in Legg-Calvé-Perthes disease, there is thickening of the synovial membrane.

Arthrograms

Arthrograms are useful in assessing the cartilaginous model of the femoral head, and studies have recently shown them

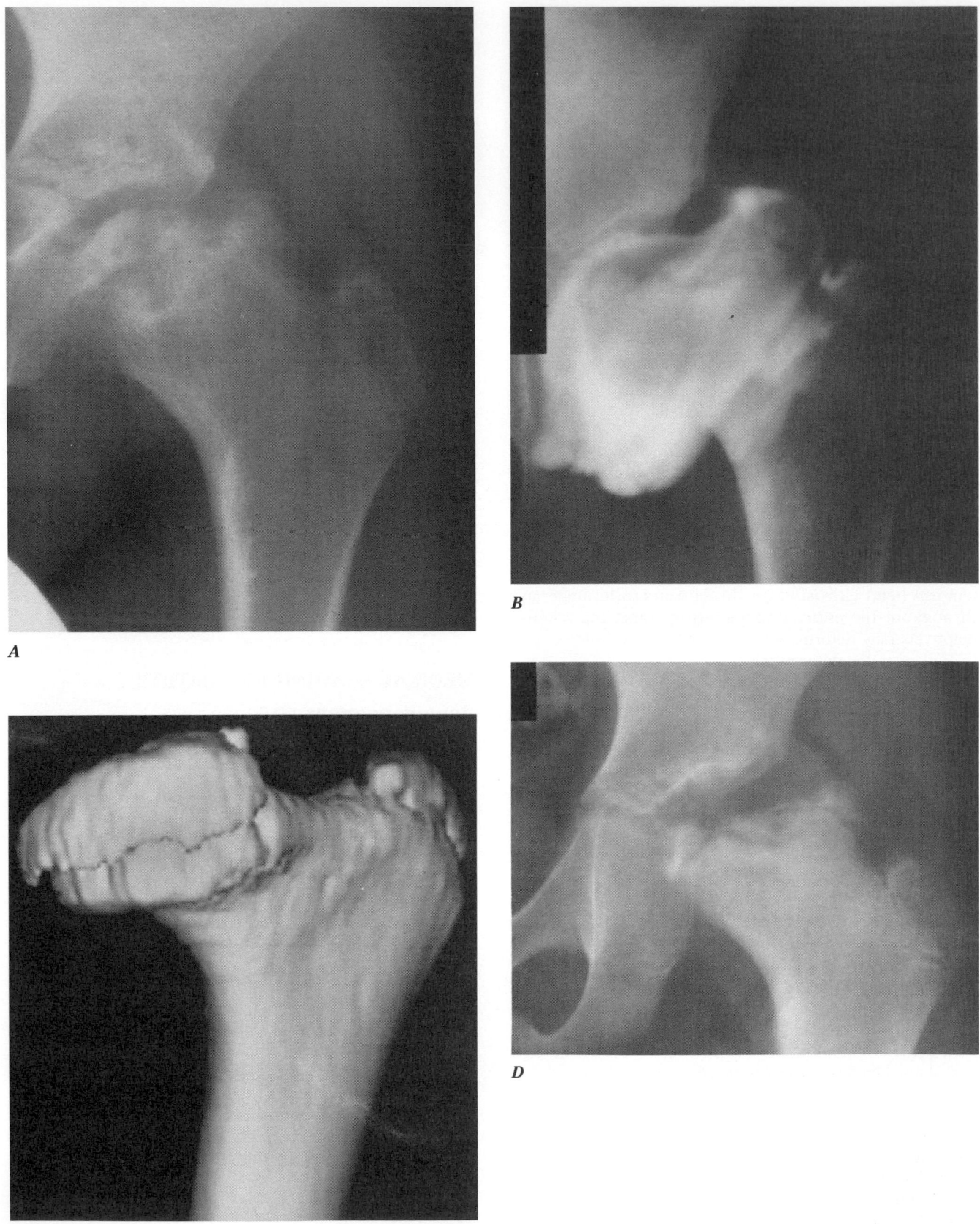

Figure 42-3 Components of hinge subluxation. *A.* Extrusion and flattening of the femoral head. *B.* Three-dimensional computed tomogram showing deformity. *C.* Arthrogram showing area of hinge abduction on lateral corner of acetabulum. *D.* Subluxation with break in Shenton's line.

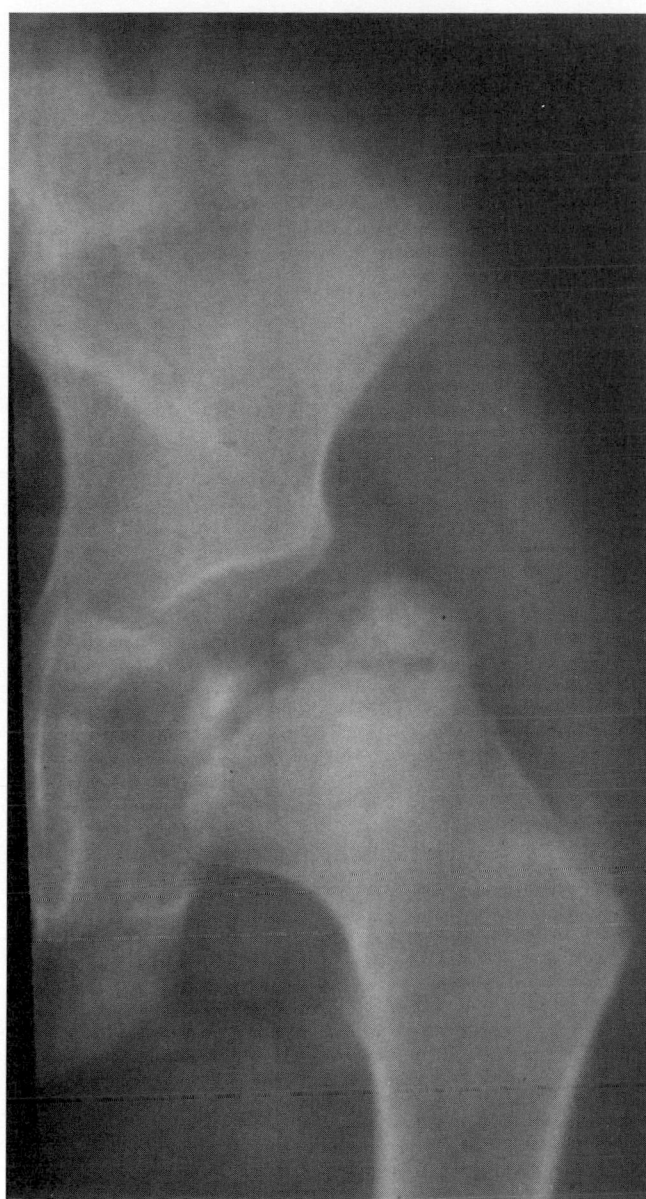

Figure 42-4 Reossification stage. Note area of new bone in the area of the lateral pillar. Treatment may be discontinued at this stage.

to be as good as or superior to magnetic resonance images.[34] Later in the course of the disease, when the necrotic femoral epiphysis collapses and deforms, the hip joint can become noncongruent. Arthrography allows one to appreciate the extent and pattern of deformity as well as to determine the presence of hinge subluxation when the hip is put through its range of motion. Arthrography can also be helpful in planning of operative treatment.

Bone Scans

The precise role and indications for use of bone scintigraphy remain to be determined. Some authors believe that

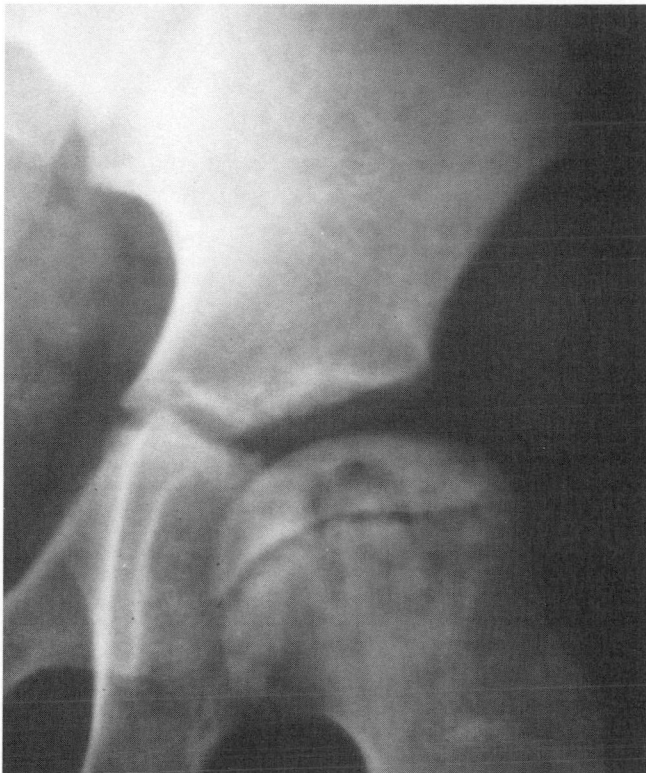

Figure 42-5 Remodeling stage. Note changes in femoral head and greater trochanter from physeal growth.

bone scintigraphy is more sensitive than roentgenograms in detecting subtle vascular changes in the early stages of the disease.[35] Other authors have used this modality to determine the vascularity and viability of the capital femoral epiphysis during the different stages of the disease.[36]

Magnetic Resonance Images

In recent years, MRI of the hip with Legg-Calvé-Perthes disease has gained popularity.[37] Its proponents claim superior advantages in evaluating the extent of necrosis and detecting signs of revascularization.[34,38] While we do not disagree with these conclusions, these findings have not had a great influence on us in determining treatment.

CLASSIFICATION SCHEMES

Catterall Classification

Anteroposterior and frog-leg lateral roentgenograms of the hip are both evaluated (Fig. 42-6*A* through *D*).[39] Group I hips have involvement of the anterior portion of the capital epiphysis with no collapse or sequestrum. Group II hips have up to 50 percent involvement with sequestrum formation. Group III hips have approximately 75 percent involvement with collapse and sequestrum formation.

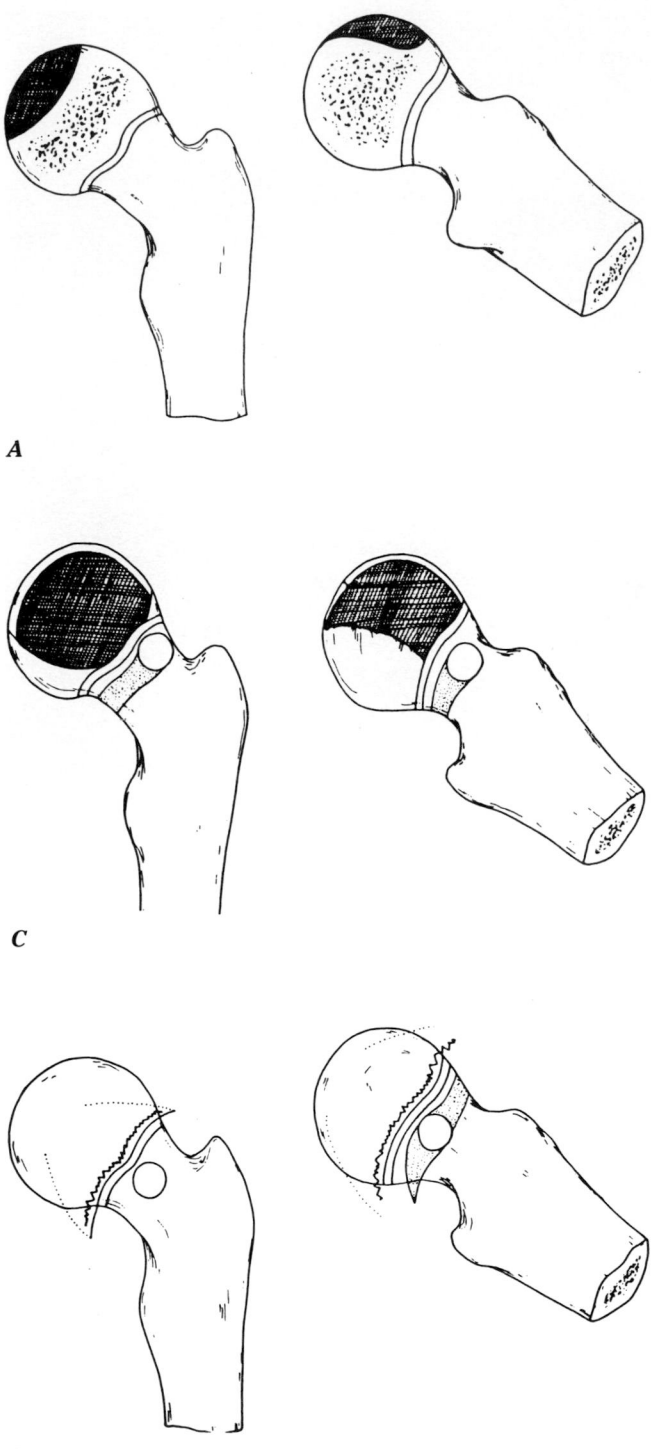

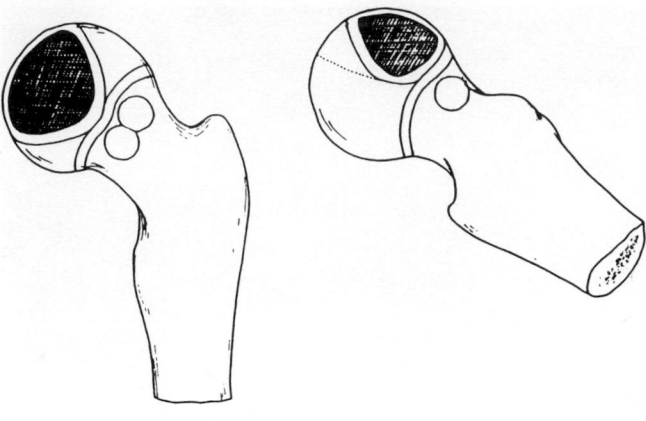

A

B

C

D

Figure 42-6 Catterall classification. *A.* Class I hips show anterior involvement with no sequestrum or metaphyseal involvement. *B.* Class II hips show anterolateral involvement of approximately 50 percent with sequestrum and metaphyseal lesions. The lateral column is intact. *C.* Class III hips show approximately 75 percent head involvement with large sequestrum, metaphyseal involvement, and lateral column involvement. *D.* Class IV hip shows whole head involvement with metaphyseal lesions. (Reproduced with permission from Weinstein SL: Legg-Calvé-Perthes disease, in Morrissy RT (ed): *Lovell and Winter's Pediatric Orthopaedics,* 3d ed. Philadelphia, Lippincott, 1990, pp 851–883.)

Group IV hips have involvement of the entire capital epiphysis. There are two flaws with this classification: (1) a hip can change from one group to another as the disease progresses, especially if the hip was classified prior to the fragmentation stage, and (2) significant inter- and intraobserver error can occur.[40] In his initial report, Catterall also introduced the "head at risk" signs, which include the Gage sign, calcification lateral to the epiphysis, metaphyseal reaction, lateral subluxation, and a horizontal physis.

Salter-Thompson Classification

This two-part classification system is based on the percentage of extent of the subchondral fracture, which the originators claim predicts the ultimate location and involvement of the femoral head.[41,42] Group A is less than 50 percent, whereas group B is greater than 50 percent. Prognosis is generally good in group A (as in Catterall groups I and II), with a poorer prognosis seen in group B (Catterall groups III and IV). The major drawback of this system is that the subchondral fracture is not always seen, as many patients present late in the disease process.

TREATMENT OF HIPS DURING NECROSIS AND FRAGMENTATION STAGES

Various methods of treatment exist for the patient with Legg-Calvé-Perthes disease. Age at onset and extent of the disease process are probably the two most important factors in determining the type and principle of treatment. A general rule of thumb used at our institution is that the majority of children less than 6 years of age or who have less than 50 percent involvement usually do not require treatment other than preservation of motion.[43] The determination of treatment should include factors that are based not only on the patient's medical condition but also on his or her psychosocial situation. A recent report from our institution showed that five different methods of treatment used for five statistically similar groups of patients revealed statistically similar results at follow-up—an outcome suggested by many authors.[44,45] Treatment has traditionally been divided into containment and noncontainment methods, with the former most popular today.[46–51] Rarely is no treatment prescribed.[52] In general, treatment can be discontinued once reossification of the lateral pillar is evident.[53,54]

Motion Therapy

Range-of-motion therapy is usually reserved for children less than 6 years old or those with less than 50 percent involvement of the capital femoral epiphysis. It consists of a physical therapy program in the hospital or at home with proper instruction. If the hip remains stiff following this treatment regimen, further options include trial periods of traction, casting, or adductor tenotomy. We do not believe that motion therapy should be synonymous with noncontainment, as the majority of patients receiving this form of treatment have a well-seated femoral head within the acetabulum.

Containment

We define containment as the location of the capital femoral epiphysis within the acetabulum, with the physeal line medial to the borders of the acetabulum (Fig. 42-7). The theory behind this philosophy is that the acetabulum will act as a mold for the deformed femoral head while it is undergoing reossification and remodeling. Containment treatment is usually reserved for the following patients: those older than 6 years, those with greater than 50 percent involvement or severe collapse of the capital femoral epiphysis, and those with hinge subluxation. Methods of containment treatment include casts, braces, and osteotomies.

Abduction Casts

Bilateral long-leg abduction casts have been used to provide fixed abduction and reduction of subluxation, with

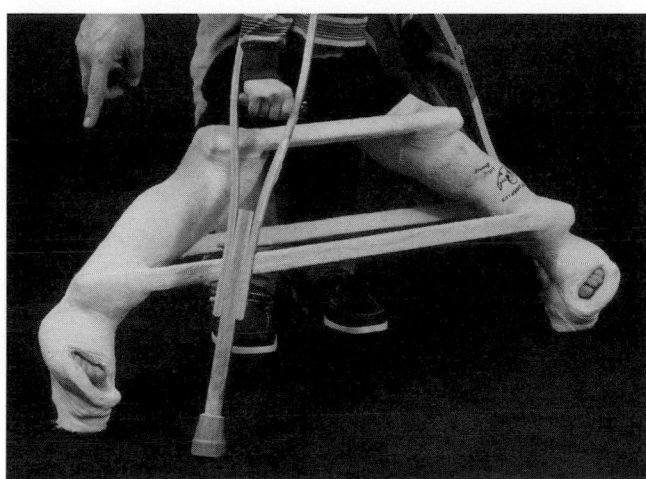

Figure 42-8 Abduction cast. The lower limbs are in abduction and internal rotation. Crutch ambulation is permitted.

the added advantage that they cannot be removed by the patient, thus ensuring compliance.[55,56] The lower limbs are placed in abduction and internal rotation, and containment is verified by an anteroposterior roentgenogram of the hip. The child is then allowed to ambulate with crutches (Fig. 42-8). Kinematic gait analysis has shown that Petrie casts improve lateral and anterior coverage of the femoral head during ambulation.[57] Generally, casts are changed every 6 to 8 weeks and treatment can last over a year. Although generally good results have been reported following this form of treatment, the use of casts has fallen into disfavor because of their awkwardness and the difficulty in regaining knee and ankle motion once the cast has been removed.[58]

Abduction Braces

Due to the aforementioned problems with cumbersome abduction casts, abduction braces have become a popular method of containment.[59–61] Most abduction braces hold the lower limbs in abduction and external rotation (Fig. 42-9). Kinematic gait analysis has shown that the Atlanta brace, for example, increases posterior and slightly increases lateral coverage of the femoral head during ambulation (the area of necrosis in most instances in anterolateral).[57] The long-term results of abduction orthoses have come into question, with unsatisfactory results having been reported.[62,63] A report recently published from our institution showed that sphericity of the femoral head was significantly worse at follow-up after Atlanta brace treatment compared with similar hips treated by other methods.[44]

Proximal Femoral Varus Osteotomy

Proximal femoral varus osteotomy may be undertaken in an effort to reposition the femoral head within the con-

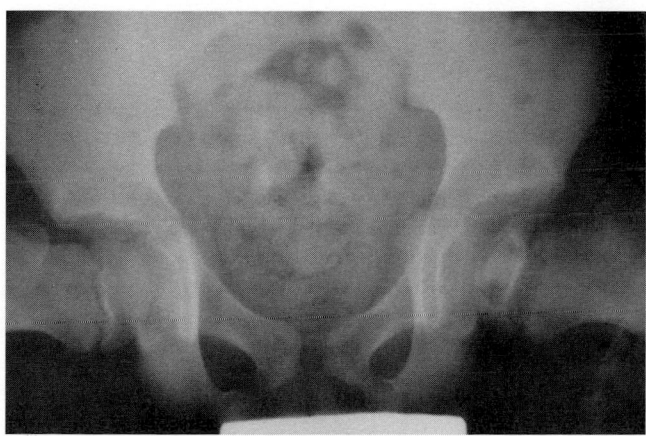

Figure 42-7 Containment. Anteroposterior roentgenogram showing well-seated femoral heads with the hips in abduction.

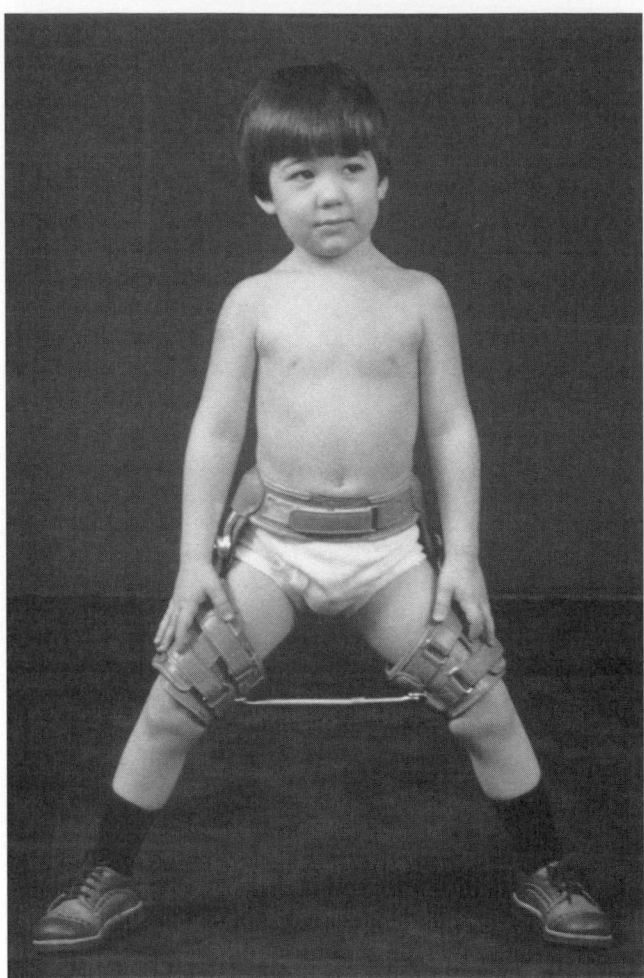

Figure 42-9 Abduction brace. The lower limbs are held in abduction.

fines of the acetabulum, and good results have been reported, especially when this is done early (Fig. 42-10).[64–67] However, the precise role of varus osteotomy remains to be determined. Problems that can occur include elevation of the greater trochanter, shortening, and abductor limp. Varus subtrochanteric osteotomy should not be done with the sole intention of increasing blood flow.[68]

Innominate Osteotomy

Innominate osteotomies can be performed to provide increased coverage of the affected femoral head (Fig. 42-11). The Salter osteotomy increases coverage in an anterolateral direction, which is usually the site of femoral head involvement. Salter reported good results with this procedure when the precise indications for the operation were followed; however, good results have been reported by other authors who did not follow Salter's strict criteria for patient selection.[69] Many patients experience stiffness about the hip postoperatively following immobilization in a spica cast. The precise indication for innominate os-

teotomy has yet to be demonstrated in the literature. The Salter osteotomy may be combined with the varus osteotomy in selected hips.[70]

TREATMENT OF HIPS DURING REOSSIFICATION AND REMODELING STAGES

Shelf Arthroplasty

The shelf operation may be used to increase the volume of the acetabulum in an effort to accommodate the enlarged deformed femoral head.[71,72] The bony buttress that is built also prevents the femoral head from subluxating and avoids the deforming forces transmitted across the edge of the acetabulum, which can cause the pivot seen in hinge subluxation (Fig. 42-12). Ideally, subluxation of the femoral head is corrected prior to performing the operation. A long-term study from our institution showed beneficial results when the procedure was performed late in the disease. We have recently begun performing this procedure during earlier stages and await adequate follow-up for evaluation of our results.

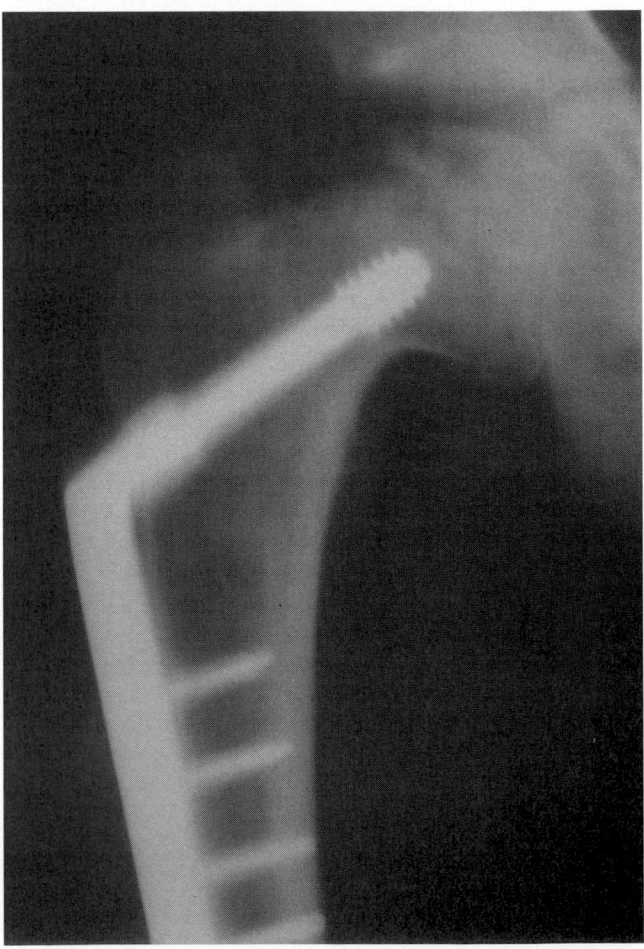

Figure 42-10 Anteroposterior roentgenogram following varus osteotomy.

Garceau Procedure and Chiari Osteotomy

Both of these operations may be done as salvage procedures late in the course of the disease or afterwards.[77–78] In the Garceau procedure, or cheilectomy, the lateral third of the extruding capital femoral epiphysis is removed to alleviate hinge subluxation. Currently, these are not popular treatment options because they do not appear to delay a progressive degenerative arthrosis.

DETERMINING OUTCOME AND NATURAL HISTORY

Mose Classification

The Mose template of concentric circles is superimposed over the anteroposterior and lateral roentgenograms of the femoral head to determine sphericity.[79,80] Mose stated that if the outline of the femoral head in both projections is identical, the result was graded as good. If the deviation is less than 2 mm, then the result is rated fair. If the devi-

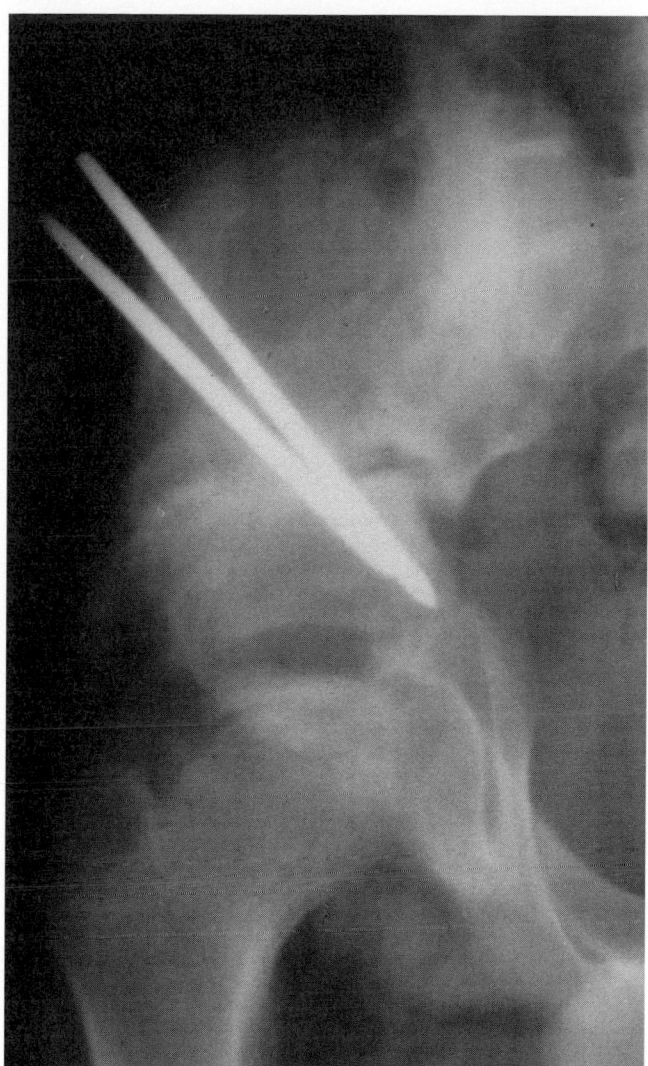

Figure 42-11 Anteroposterior roentgenogram following innominate osteotomy.

Proximal Femoral Valgus Osteotomy

Proximal femoral valgus osteotomy is done to reposition the necrotic weight-bearing area of the femoral head and alleviate hinge subluxation. Roentgenograms of the hip taken in adduction should be performed to determine if the medial area of the femoral head will provide a more suitable weight-bearing surface. The procedure should not be performed in hips with unresolved subluxation. Limb length can be gained and compensate for a mild limb length discrepancy.

Arthroscopy

Arthroscopy may be used to remove loose bodies in hips demonstrating osteochondritis dissecans and impingement.[73–76]

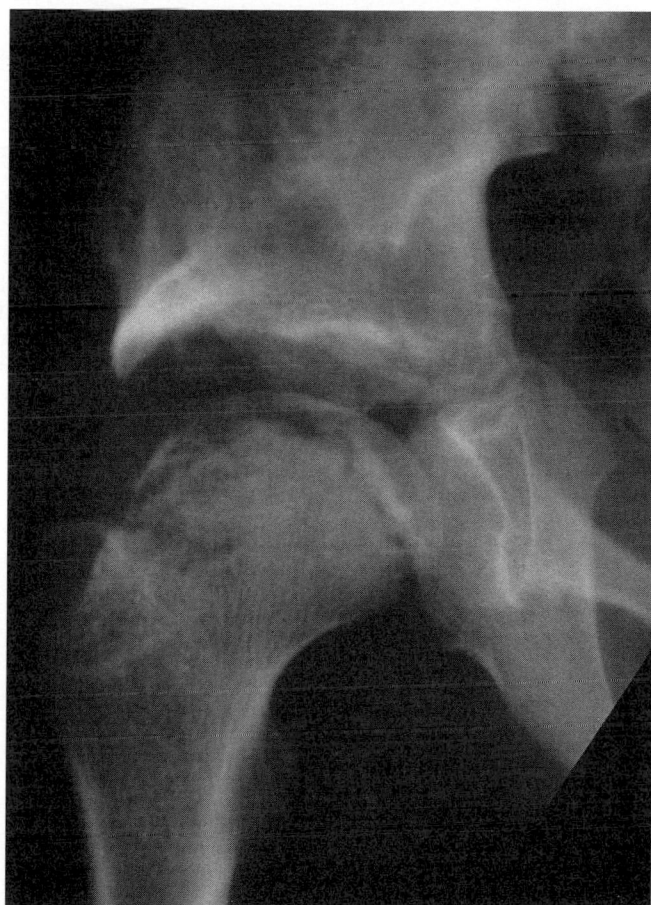

Figure 42-12 Anteroposterior roentgenogram following shelf arthroplasty. Note that the acetabulum has been enlarged to accommodate the coxa magna, providing a larger surface area for remodeling.

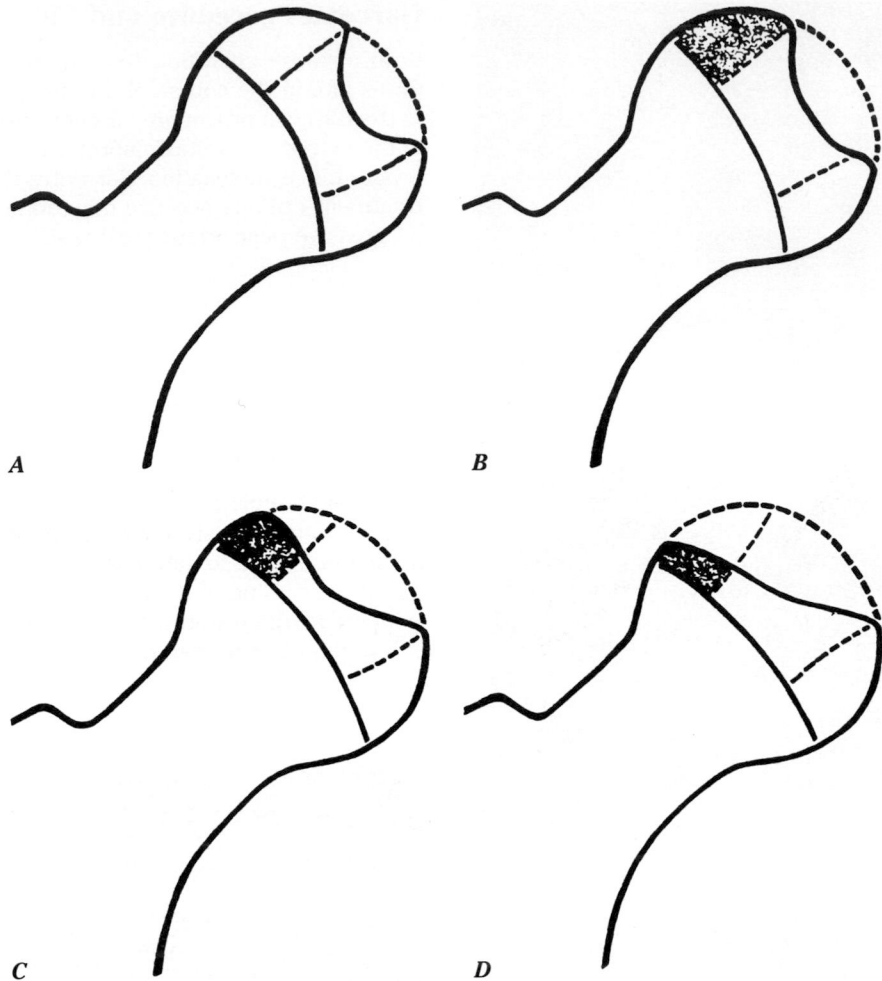

Figure 42-13 Lateral pillar classification. *A.* The femoral head pillars. *B.* Group A shows normal height of lateral pillar. *C.* Group B shows that greater than 50 percent of the lateral pillar height has been maintained. *D.* Group C shows that less than 50 percent of the lateral pillar height has been maintained. (Reproduced with permission from Herring JA, Neustadt JB, Williams JJ, et al: The lateral pillar classification of Legg-Calvé-Perthes disease. *J Pediatr Orthop* 12:143–150, 1992.)

ation is greater than 2 mm on any one projection, the result is rated as poor. Many authors do not agree that Mose sphericity is an accurate predictor of long-term outcome, whereas others have used this system as their sole criterion for success of treatment.[81–83] A general rule of thumb is that a good or fair Mose rating will yield a good result, but a poor Mose rating does not necessarily ensure a poor result.

Lateral Pillar Classification

The lateral pillar classification utilizes a well-taken anteroposterior roentgenogram of the hip.[84] The capital epiphysis is divided into lateral, central, and medial pillars (Fig. 42-13A through D). Group A hips have no involvement of the lateral pillar. Group B hips have more than 50 percent of the lateral pillar height maintained. Group C hips have less than 50 percent of the lateral pillar height maintained. This is a new classification that has yet to stand the test

of time, albeit preliminary reports are favorable.[85] A high correlation in predicting the amount of coxa plana at maturity is reported, and when combined with age at onset, this has been said to predict the natural history of the disease.

Classification of Stulberg and Coworkers

The classification of Stulberg et al. is based on the concepts of sphericity and congruity.[81] The classification is applicable to patients who have reached skeletal maturity and additionally takes into consideration size of the femoral head, trochanteric height, the acetabular angle of Sharp, and the percentage of femoral head coverage. Class I hips have a normal femoral head. Class II hips have a spherical femoral head with a shortened femoral neck and coxa magna, or an increased acetabular index. Class III hips have a nonspherical or ovoid femoral head that is not flat. Class IV hips have a flat femoral head with a flat acetabular roof. Class V hips have a flat femoral head with a normal acetabulum. Class I and II hips are considered to demonstrate spherical congruency and do not develop arthrosis later in life. Class III and IV hips are considered to demonstrate aspherical congruency and develop mild arthrosis later in life. Class V hips are said to have aspherical incongruency and develop severe arthrosis before the age of 50 years.

REFERENCES

1. Legg AT: An obscure affection of the hip joint. *Boston Med Surg J* 162:202, 1910.
2. Calvé J: Sur une forme particuliére de pseudo-coxalgie greffeé sur les deformations caractéristiques de l'extremité superieure du femur. *Rev Chir* 42:54, 1910.
3. Perthes GC: Über arthritis deformans juvenilis. *Dtsch Z Chir* 107:111, 1910.
4. Phemister DB: Operation for epiphysitis of the head of the femur (Perthes' disease): Findings and result. *Arch Surg* 2:221, 1921.
5. Phemister DB: Repair of bone in the presence of aseptic necrosis resulting from fractures, transplantations, and vascular obstruction. *J Bone Joint Surg* 12:769, 1930.
6. Waldenström H: Coxa plana, osteochondritis deformans coxae, Calvé-Perthessche Krankheit, Legg disease. *Zentralbl Chir* 47:539, 1920.
7. Waldenström H: On coxa plana, osteochondritis deformans coxae juvenilis: Legg's disease, maladie de Calvé, Perthes Krankheit. *Acta Chir Scand* 55:577, 1923.
8. Waldenström H: The first stages of coxa plana. *J Bone Joint Surg* 20:559, 1938.
9. Barker DJP, Dixon E, Taylor JF: Perthes' disease of the hip in three regions of England. *J Bone Joint Surg* 60B:478, 1978.
10. Gray IM, Lowry RB, Renwick DH: Incidence and genetics of Legg-Perthes disease (osteochondritis deformans) in British Columbia: Evidence of polygenic determination. *J Med Genet* 9:197, 1972.
11. Wynne-Davies R, Gormley J: The aetiology of Perthes' disease: Genetic, epidemiological and growth factors in 310 Edinburgh and Glasgow patients. *J Bone Joint Surg* 60B:6, 1978.
12. Moberg A, Rehnberg L: Incidence of Perthes' disease in Uppsala, Sweden. *Acta Orthop Scand* 63:157, 1992.
13. Harper PS, Brotherton BJ, Cochlin D: Genetic risks in Perthes' disease. *Clin Genet* 10:178, 1976.
14. Wynne-Davies R: Some etiologic factors in Perthes' disease. *Clin Orthop* 150:12, 1980.
15. Neidel J, Schonau E, Zander D, et al: Normal plasma levels of IGF binding protein in Perthes' disease: Follow-up of previous report. *Acta Orthop Scand* 64:540, 1993.
16. Neidel J, Zander D, Hackenbroch MH: No physiologic age-related increase of circulating somatomedin-C during early stage of Perthes' disease: A longitudinal study in 21 boys. *Arch Orthop Trauma Surg* 111:171, 1992.
17. Joseph B: Serum immunoglobulin in Perthes' disease. *J Bone Joint Surg* 73B:509, 1991.
18. Sanchis M, Zahir A, Freeman MAR: The experimental simulation of Perthes disease by consecutive interruptions of the blood supply to the capital femoral epiphysis in the puppy. *J Bone Joint Surg* 55A:335, 1973.
19. Liu SL, Ho TC: The role of venous hypertension in the pathogenesis of Legg-Perthes disease: A clinical and experimental study. *J Bone Joint Surg* 73A:194, 1991.
20. Glueck CJ, Crawford A, Roy D, et al: Association of antithrombotic factor deficiencies and hypofibrinolysis with Legg-Perthes disease. *J Bone Joint Surg* 78A:3, 1996.
21. Pettersson H, Wingstrand H, Thambert C, et al: Legg-Calvé-Perthes disease in hemophilia: Incidence and etiologic considerations. *J Pediatr Orthop* 10:28, 1990.
22. Burwell RG, Dangerfield PH, Hall DJ, et al: Perthes disease: An anthropometric study revealing impaired and disproportionate growth. *J Bone Joint Surg* 60B:461, 1978.
23. Harrison MHM, Turner MH, Jacobs P: Skeletal immaturity in Perthes' disease. *J Bone Joint Surg* 58B:37, 1976.
24. Fisher RL: An epidemiological study of Legg-Perthes disease. *J Bone Joint Surg* 54A:769, 1972.
25. Loder RT, Schwartz EM, Hensinger RN: Behavioral characteristics of children with Legg-Calvé-Perthes disease. *J Pediatr Orthop* 13:598, 1993.
26. Catterall A, Roberts GC, Wynne-Davies R: Association of Perthes' disease with congenital anomalies of genitourinary tract and inguinal region. *Lancet* 1:996, 1971.
27. Hall DJ, Harrison MHM, Burnwell RG: Congenital abnormalities and Perthes' disease: Clinical evidence that children with Perthes' disease may have a major congenital defect. *J Bone Joint Surg* 61B:18, 1979.
28. Molloy MK, Macmahon B: Birth weight and Legg-Perthes disease. *J Bone Joint Surg* 49A:498, 1967.
29. Bowen JR, Foster BK, Hartzell CR: Legg-Calvé-Perthes disease. *Clin Orthop* 185:97, 1984.
30. Bowen JR, Schreiber FC, Foster BK, Wein BK: Premature femoral neck physeal closure in Perthes' disease. *Clin Orthop* 171:24, 1982.
31. Herring JA, Williams JJ, Neustadt JN, Early JS: Evolution of femoral head deformity during the healing phase of Legg-Calvé-Perthes disease. *J Pediatr Orthop* 13:41, 1993.
32. Futami T, Kasahara Y, Suzuki S, et al: Ultrasonography in transient synovitis and early Perthes' disease. *J Bone Joint Surg* 73B:635, 1991.
33. Eckerwall G, Hochbergs P, Wingstrand H, Egund N: Sonography and intracapsular pressure in Perthes' disease: 39 children examined 2–36 months after onset. *Acta Orthop Scand* 65:575, 1994.
34. Kaniklides C, Lonnerholm T, Moberg A, Sahlstedt B: Legg-Calvé-Perthes disease: Comparison of conventional radiography, MR imaging, bone scintigraphy and arthrography. *Acta Radiol* 36:434, 1995.
35. Sutherland AD, Savage JP, Paterson DC, Foster BK: The nuclide bone-scan in the diagnosis and management of Perthes' disease. *J Bone Joint Surg* 62B:300, 1980.
36. Danigelis JA, Fisher RL, Ozonoff MB, Sziklas JJ: 99m-topolyphosphate bone imaging in Legg-Perthes disease. *Radiology* 115:407, 1975.
37. Hoffinger SA, Henderson RC, Renner JB, et al: Magnetic resonance evaluation of "metaphyseal" changes in Legg-Calvé-Perthes disease. *J Pediatr Orthop* 13:602, 1993.
38. Uno A, Hattori T, Noritake K, Suda H: Legg-Calvé-Perthes disease in the evolutionary period: Comparison of magnetic resonance imaging with bone scintigraphy. *J Pediatr Orthop* 15:362, 1995.
39. Catterall A: The natural history of Perthes' disease. *J Bone Joint Surg* 53B:37, 1971.
40. Hardcastle PH, Ross R, Hamalainen M, Mata A: Catterall grouping of Perthes' disease: An assessment of observer error and prognosis using the Catterall classification. *J Bone Joint Surg* 62B:428, 1980.
41. Salter RB, Thompson GH: Legg-Calvé-Perthes disease: The prognostic significance of the subchondral fracture and a two-group classification of the femoral head involvement. *J Bone Joint Surg* 66A:479, 1984.

42. Simmons ED, Graham HK, Szalai JP: Interobserver variability in grading Perthes' disease. *J Bone Joint Surg* 72B:202, 1990.

43. Schoenecker PL, Stone JW, Capelli AM: Legg-Perthes disease in children under 6 years old. *Orthop Rev* 22:201, 1993.

44. Wang L, Bowen JR, Puniak MA, et al: An evaluation of various methods of treatment for Legg-Calvé-Perthes disease. *Clin Orthop* 314:225, 1995.

45. Wenger DR, Ward WT, Herring JA: Legg-Calvé-Perthes disease. *J Bone Joint Surg* 73A:778, 1991.

46. Brotherton BJ, McKibbin B: Perthes' disease treated by prolonged recumbency and femoral head containment: A long-term appraisal. *J Bone Joint Surg* 59B:8, 1977.

47. Gower WE, Johnston RC: Legg-Perthes disease: Long-term follow-up of thirty-six patients. *J Bone Joint Surg* 53A:759, 1971.

48. Poussa M, Yrjonen T, Hoikka V, Osterman K: Prognosis after conservative and operative treatment in Perthes' disease. *Clin Orthop* 297:82, 1993.

49. Yrjonen T: Prognosis in Perthes' disease after noncontainment treatment: 106 hips followed for 28–47 years. *Acta Orthop Scand* 63:523, 1992.

50. Ratliff AHC: Perthes' disease: A study of thirty-four hips observed for thirty years. *J Bone Joint Surg* 49B:102, 1967.

51. Ratliff AHC: Perthes' disease: A study of sixteen patients followed up for forty years. *J Bone Joint Surg* 59B:248, 1977.

52. Norlin R, Hammerby S, Tkaczuk H: The natural history of Perthes' disease. *Int Orthop* 15:13, 1991.

53. Ferguson AB, Howorth MB: Coxa plana and related conditions at the hip: Part I. Classification and correlation of these conditions. Part II. A study of seventy-five cases of coxa plana. *J Bone Joint Surg* 16:781, 1934.

54. Thompson GH, Westin GW: Legg-Calvé-Perthes disease: Results of discontinuing treatment in the early reossification phase. *Clin Orthop* 139:70, 1979.

55. Petrie GJ, Bitenc I: The abduction weight-bearing treatment in Legg-Perthes' disease. *J Bone Joint Surg* 53B:54, 1971.

56. Richards BS, Coleman SS: Subluxation of the femoral head in coxa plana. *J Bone Joint Surg* 69A:1312, 1987.

57. Rab GT, Wyatt M, Sutherland DH, Simon SR: A technique for determining femoral head containment during gait. *J Pediatr Orthop* 5:8, 1985.

58. Kiepurska A: Late results of treatment in Perthes' disease by a functional method. *Clin Orthop* 272:76, 1991.

59. Bobechko WP, McLaurin CA, Motloch WM: Toronto orthosis for Legg-Perthes disease. *Artif Limbs* 12:36, 1968.

60. Purvis JM, Dimon JH III, Meehan PL, Lovell WW: Preliminary experience with the Scottish Rite Hospital abduction orthosis for Legg-Perthes disease. *Clin Orthop* 150:49, 1980.

61. Tachdjian MO, Jouett LD: Trilateral socket hip abduction orthosis for treatment of Legg-Perthes disease, in proceedings of the American Academy of Orthopaedic Surgeons. *J Bone Joint Surg* 50A:1272, 1968.

62. Meehan PL, Angel D, Nelson JM: The Scottish Rite abduction orthosis for the treatment of Legg-Perthes disease: A radiographic analysis. *J Bone Joint Surg* 74A:2, 1992.

63. Martinez AG, Weinstein SL, Dietz FR: The weight-bearing abduction brace for the treatment of Legg-Perthes disease. *J Bone Joint Surg* 74:12, 1992.

64. Axer A: Subtrochanteric osteotomy in the treatment of Perthes' disease: A preliminary report. *J Bone Joint Surg* 47B:489, 1965.

65. Hoikka V, Poussa M, Yrjonen T, Osterman K: Intertrochanteric varus osteotomy for Perthes' disease: Radiographic changes after 2–16-year follow-up of 126 hips. *Acta Orthop Scand* 62:549, 1991.

66. Weiner SD, Weiner DS, Riley PM: Pitfalls in treatment of Legg-Calvé-Perthes disease using proximal femoral varus osteotomy. *J Pediatr Orthop* 11:20, 1991.

67. Coates CJ, Paterson JMH, Woods KR, et al: Femoral osteotomy in Perthes' disease: Results at maturity. *J Bone Joint Surg* 72B:581, 1990.

68. Lee DY, Seong SC, Choi IH, et al: Changes of blood flow of the femoral head after subtrochanteric osteotomy in Legg-Perthes' disease: A serial scintigraphic study. *J Pediatr Orthop* 12:731, 1992.

69. Paterson DC, Leitch JM, Foster BK: Results of innominate osteotomy in the treatment of Legg-Calvé-Perthes disease. *Clin Orthop* 266:96, 1991.

70. Crutcher JP, Staheli LT: Combined osteotomy as a salvage procedure for severe Legg-Calvé-Perthes disease. *J Pediatr Orthop* 12:151, 1992.

71. Kruse RW, Guille JT, Bowen JR: Shelf arthroplasty in patients who have Legg-Calvé-Perthes disease: A study of long-term results. *J Bone Joint Surg* 73A:1338, 1991.

72. Willett K, Hudson I, Catterall A: Lateral shelf acetabuloplasty: An operation for older children with Perthes' disease. *J Pediatr Orthop* 12:563, 1992.

73. Bowen JR, Kumar VP, Joyce JJ III, Bowen JC: Osteochondritis dissecans following Perthes' disease: Arthroscopic-operative treatment. *Clin Orthop* 209:49, 1986.

74. Kamhi E, MacEwen GD: Osteochondritis dissecans in Legg-Calvé-Perthes' disease. *J Bone Joint Surg* 57A:506, 1975.

75. Schindler A, Lechevallier JJ, Rao NS, Bowen JR: Diagnostic and therapeutic arthroscopy of the hip in children and adolescents: Evaluation of results. *J Pediatr Orthop* 15:317, 1995.

76. Snow SW, Keret D, Scarangella S, Bowen JR: Anterior impingement of the femoral head: A late phenomenon of Legg-Calvé-Perthes disease. *J Pediatr Orthop* 13:286, 1993.

77. Bennett JT, Mazurek RT, Cash JD: Chiari's osteotomy in the treatment of Perthes disease. *J Bone Joint Surg* 73B:225, 1991.

78. Garceau G, Rapp G, Lidge RT: Coxa plana (a surgical approach), in Proceedings of the American Academy of Orthopaedic Surgeons. *J Bone Joint Surg* 55A:1313, 1973.

79. Mose K: *Legg-Calvé-Perthes Disease: A Comparison Between Three Methods of Conservative Treatment.* Aarhus, Universitetsforlaget i Aarhus, 1964.

80. Mose K: Methods of measuring in Legg-Calvé-Perthes disease with special regard to the prognosis. *Clin Orthop* 150:103, 1980.

81. Stulberg SD, Cooperman DR, Wallensten R: The natural history of Legg-Calvé-Perthes disease. *J Bone Joint Surg* 63A:1095, 1981.

82. McAndrew MP, Weinstein SL: A long-term follow-up of Legg-Calvé-Perthes disease. *J Bone Joint Surg* 66A:860, 1984.

83. Herring JA: The treatment of Legg-Calvé-Perthes disease: A critical review of the literature. *J Bone Joint Surg* 76A:448, 1994.

84. Herring JA, Neustadt JB, Williams JJ, et al: The lateral pillar classification of Legg-Calvé-Perthes disease. *J Pediatr Orthop* 12:143, 1992.

85. Ritterbusch JF, Shantharam SS, Gelinas C: Comparison of lateral pillar classification and Catterall classification of Legg-Calvé-Perthes' disease. *J Pediatr Orthop* 13:200, 1993.

CHAPTER 43

Slipped Capital Femoral Epiphysis

Merv Letts

Slipped capital femoral epiphysis (SCFE) is one of the commonest causes of hip pain in boys age 12 to 14 and girls age 10 to 12. In Caucasian children, the incidence of SCFE is 1 to 3 per 100,000.[1-4] Black males have a higher incidence (7 to 8 per 100,000). The incidence in black females is also high (up to 6 to 7 per 100,000 in some geographic localities).[3] Predisposing factors include obesity, rapid growth spurts, and endocrinopathies such as hypothyroidism and renal rickets.

ETIOLOGIC FACTORS

Certain anatomic and structural features contribute to the shear strength of the normal physis and resist separation of the epiphysis. Particularly important is the concave shape of the undersurface of the epiphysis and the presence of the mammillary processes on the metaphyseal side of the zone of provisional ossification, which have an interlocking effect.[5] The perichondral complex is also thought to contribute effectively to resistance to shear stresses.

Mechanical Factors

Changes in the biomechanical orientation of the growth plate have been shown to reduce its resistance to shear stress. Gelberman et al. showed that there is a significant reduction in femoral anteversion and, indeed, there may be actual retroversion in hips with SCFE compared with normals.[6] When normal biomechanical forces are applied to a hip that is retroverted 10° more than normal, the growth plate will experience 20 percent more shear stress.[7]

Some 50 percent of these patients weigh at or above the 95th percentile for their age and at or above the 97th percentile for their height.[8] Three-dimensional force analysis has showed that because of this, the average shear load to produce failure is three to four times body weight in SCFE patients, which is 15 percent less than the shear load to failure in normal patients.[7] Such loads are reached during normal activity (Fig. 43-1). Measurements of the slope of the proximal femoral physis using a method that corrects for different degrees of anteversion showed statistically significant increases in the measured slope of the growth plate (Fig. 43-2) in children with unilateral SCFE.[9] These increases were measured on the affected and unaffected sides and compared with aged matched controls.

The resulting data also confirm earlier observations that there is a normal progression in the slope of the proximal femoral growth plate between the ages of 1 and 18 years as part of normal development, with a maximal increase occurring between the ages of 9 and 11 years.[5,10]

Arthroscopy of hips in SCFE has disclosed erosions of the acetabular cartilage in the anterosuperior region and damage to the posterolateral aspect of the acetabular labrum (Fig. 43-3). Intraarticular hematoma is commonly found, and these changes have led to the hypothesis that traumatic factors predominate in the etiology of this condition.[11]

Maturation Factors

Loder and coworkers have shown that patients with SCFE all have a relatively uniform skeletal age (which may vary from their chronological age). These authors could not confirm the findings of earlier workers that there is skeletal immaturity across the range of patients with this condition, observing instead that the younger children were skeletally advanced in age, whereas the older children were borderline immature. In girls, SCFE occurs almost exclusively before menarche. Loder and coworkers believe there is a narrow window of skeletal age during which SCFE is most likely to occur.[12] They suggest that this period is when the perichondral ring complex of the proximal femur decreases in size but the epiphyseal plate is still thick. Increase in the thickness of the physis reduces its resistance to shear. They further suggest that beyond the age of this narrow window in skeletal development, a few of the mammillary processes fuse and makes slipping thereafter impossible.

Ultrastructural Changes

Core biopsies taken during epiphysiodesis indicate that the hypertrophic zone of the physis is considerably widened and the orderly columnar array of cells disorganized in SCFE. There is less collagen in the extraterritorial matrix of the cells and in the longitudinal septa of the hypertrophic zones and an increase in cellular degeneration and chondrocyte death.[13,14]

Endocrine Influences

The frequency of bilateral hip involvement is different in those patients without associated endocrine abnormalities compared with patients who have an endocrine-associated slip. By contrast with uncomplicated SCFE, where bilateral involvement occurs in up to 25 percent or less of patients at first clinical presentation, initial bilateral hip involvement may approach 70 percent in patients with endocrinopathy.[15] Some authors, therefore, recommend that all patients with SCFE should be screened for hypothyroidism by measuring T4 and TSH levels. Pituitary deficiency should be considered in children who are short for their age and have hypogonadism. Any proven endocrine deficiencies is an indication for prophylactic pinning of the uninvolved hip in such patients, since bilaterality eventually will approach

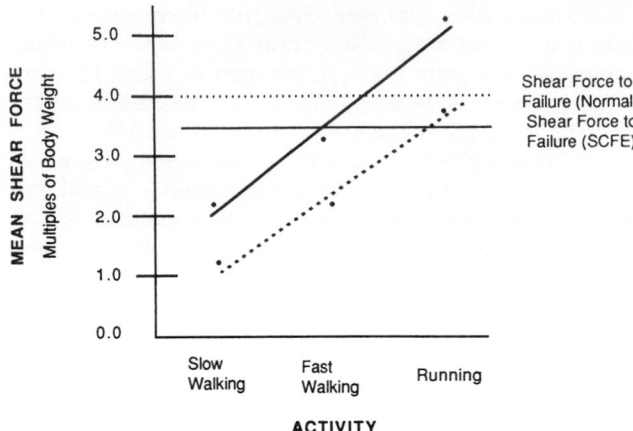

Figure 43-1 Increase in shear force on the proximal femoral growth plate as a function of activity for patients with normal (*dotted line*) and slipped (*solid line*) epiphysis. (Reproduced with permission from Pritchett JW, Perdue KD: Mechanical factors in slipped capital femoral epiphysis. *J Pediatr Orthop* 8:385–388, 1988.)

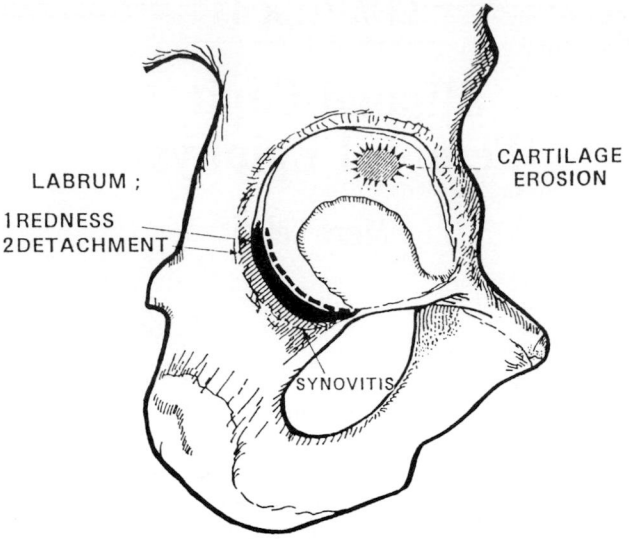

Figure 43-3 Acetabular lesions of slipped capital femoral epiphysis. (Reproduced with permission from Futami T, Kasahara Y, et al: Arthroscopy for slipped capital femoral epiphysis. *J Pediatr Orthop* 12:592–597, 1992.)

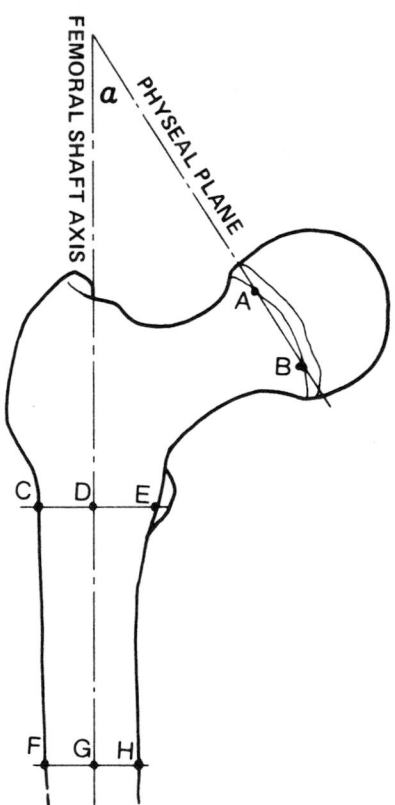

Figure 43-2 Measurement of physeal slope angle (α) defined by the intersection of the physeal plane (A-B) and the axis of the femoral shaft (D-G). (Reproduced with permission from Mirkopulos N, Weiner DS, Askew M: The evolving slope of the proximal femoral growth plate: Relationship to slipped capital femoral epiphysis. *J Pediatr Orthop* 8:268–273, 1988.)

100 percent if SCFE is left untreated. Loder and coauthors[16] have shown that most of the hypothyroid children will have the endocrine diagnosis made at presentation of the first SCFE, whereas, in growth hormone–deficient children, the endocrine diagnosis is usually made before the first slip, which then usually occurs during supplemental hormonal therapy for the growth hormone deficiency.

Wilcox and coauthors[17] found that T3 levels were low in 25 percent and testosterone markedly depressed in 76 percent of their patients with SCFE, while 87 percent had low hormone levels. However, in a subsequent prospective study of plasma levels of such hormones as T3, T4, TSH, testosterone, and growth hormone, Mann and coauthors reported that abnormal values were found in only 4 of 140 patients, and none showed clinical evidence of endocrinopathy.[18] These authors recommend that routine hormonal testing in patients without clinical evidence of endocrinopathy is, therefore, not indicated.

Morrissey and coauthors identified immune complexes in the synovial fluid of patients with SCFE and elevation in the IGM fraction in the serum of those patients that had chondrolysis. The etiologic significance of these findings remains to be elucidated.[19,20]

In summary, then, this condition is a consequence of an imbalance between those forces that tend to stabilize the epiphysis and the normal mechanical forces that may tend to displace it. At the ultrastructural level, changes in the structure of the physis may widen it and impair its ability to resist mechanical shear stresses. Alterations in its slope or in the anteversion of the femur, particularly in an obese individual, may be sufficient to cause failure. The triggering event may be traumatic or related to the activity of the individual patient. In a small subset of patients, a generalized hormonal imbalance may be an important underlying cause. The role of hormonal imbalance as an etiologic factor in patients without clinical endocrinopathy, however, remains unclear.

CLINICAL PRESENTATION

It is usual to describe the displacement of the femoral epiphysis relative to the metaphysis, since the epiphysis actually stays within the acetabulum. Aronsson[21] has suggested that it is actually the femoral neck that displaces anteriorly, creating a retroversion deformity of the proximal femur. The result of the displacement is, however, the same in that there is effectively a posterior displacement of the femoral head relative to the metaphysis. The retroversion deformity is greater than the varus component. It is important to recognize that there is a relative extension deformity between the epiphysis and the rest of the femur, which is why a flexion component is built into any corrective osteotomy. Paradoxically, on physical examination, these patients often demonstrate a fixed flexion deformity due to muscle spasm.

The presentation can vary depending upon the acuity of the slip. In some cases the process is a slow one, developing over several weeks or months and characterized by chronic pain in the groin, in the anterior thigh, or even along the medial aspect of the knee. It must again be emphasized that a child presenting with a painful knee must have an examination of both hips, since this may be the only symptom in some children presenting with this condition.

The clinical presentations have been traditionally described and classified as follows:

1. *Preslip.* This should be suspected when an 11- to 14-year-old child presents with pain in the hip, thigh, or knee associated with a slight limitation of internal rotation of the hip. The radiograph shows widening of the physis by comparison with the contralateral hip. Indeed, there may be an obvious slip on the opposite side. A bone scan may illustrate increased uptake in the involved physis.

2. *Acute slip.* This usually follows a significant trauma, such as being tackled in a football game or falling in some sporting event. The child has an acute pain that prevents ambulation, and acute symptoms have been present for less than 3 weeks. There may have been some prodromal symptoms of pain or a slight limp prior to the acute incident. This type of slip is analogous to a Salter-Harris type 1 fracture through the physis.

3. *Chronic slip.* A child with chronic slip has experienced leg pain in the thigh or knee for a period of more than 3 weeks, and the correct diagnosis may have been overlooked. There may be muscle spasm with limitation of internal rotation and a fixed flexion deformity of the hip. Flexion of the hip is often accompanied by external rotation. The radiograph will show some rounding off of the superior portion of the uncovered metaphysis and new bone formation along the inferior and medial aspects of the femoral neck. Patients with chronic slip represent 60 percent of all cases.

4. *Acute-on-chronic slip.* These patients also have a history of pain for over 3 weeks, like patients with chronic slip. However, they present with an acute onset of severe pain that may or may not be associated with a traumatic

event. Some 20 percent of all SCFE presentations fall into this category. The radiologic changes are similar to those of chronic slip except in degree. Displacement of the epiphysis is usually considerable (Fig. 43-4A and B).

DIAGNOSTIC IMAGING
Plain Radiographs

Most of the pathology of SCFE can be identified with plain films of good quality. In addition to an anteroposterior (AP) view, a frog lateral view is recommended. Care must, however, be taken in patients with acute slips. Further displacement may be provoked by this position and true lateral ra-

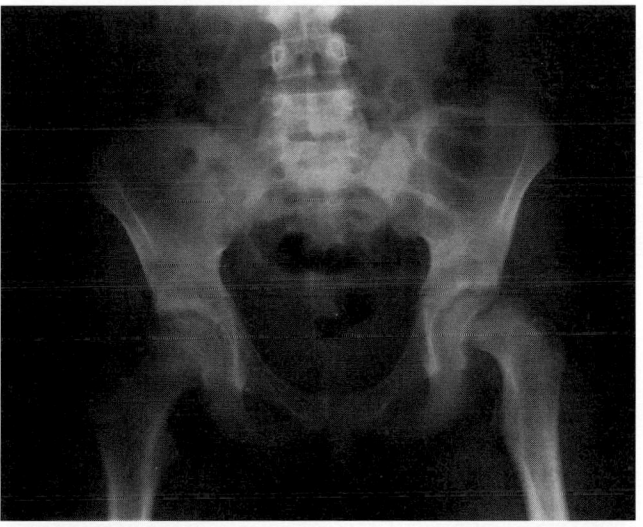

A

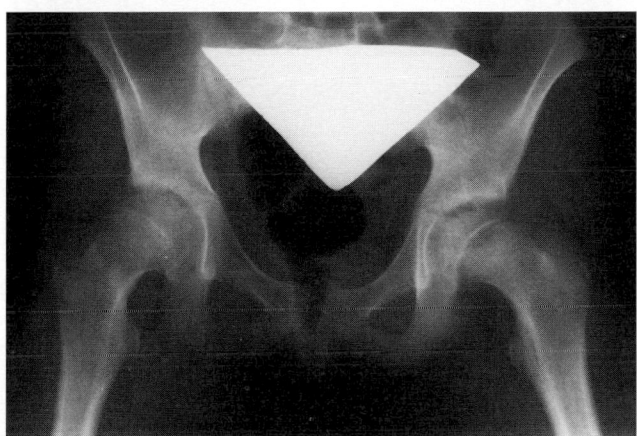

B

Figure 43-4 *A.* Acute-on-chronic grade II slip (*left*) and a grade I slip (*right*) in an 11-year-old girl. *B.* Following 24 h of Buck's traction, the grade II slip has been reduced to grade I. Notice the features of chronicity of rounding off of the superolateral aspect of the metaphysis and a small amount of new bone formation inferomedially.

diographs may then be preferable. Both hips should always be evaluated. Widening of the physis may be subtle but can usually be detected by comparison with the normal hip.

Many of the classic radiographic signs are due to the malposition of the epiphysis. These are (1) a decreased height of the epiphysis when compared to the normal side. (2) The metaphyseal blanch sign, which is a dense area seen in the proximal part of the metaphysis. It is thought by some to represent superimposition of the posteriorly rotated head on the metaphysis. Other authors have considered it part of a healing response.[22] (3) A line described by Klein[23] drawn along the superior border of the femoral neck usually passes through the superior corner of the epiphysis but will no longer do so after a slip (Fig. 43-5). A similar line may be drawn on the AP and lateral view and compared with the contralateral side.

Radiologic Diagnosis of Chondrolysis

A decrease in the width of the joint space of more than 2 mm compared with the contralateral hip has been used by some authors as an indication of the onset of chondroly-

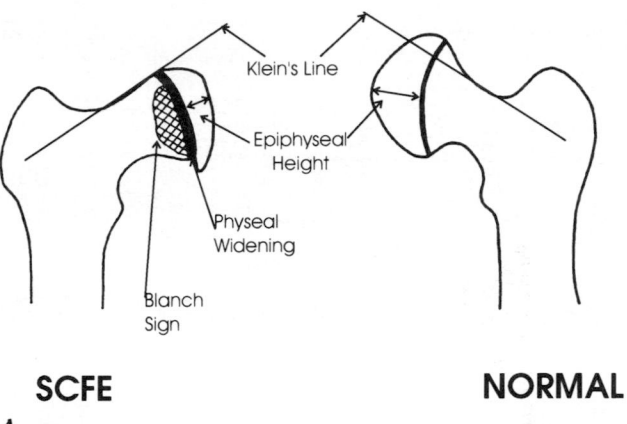

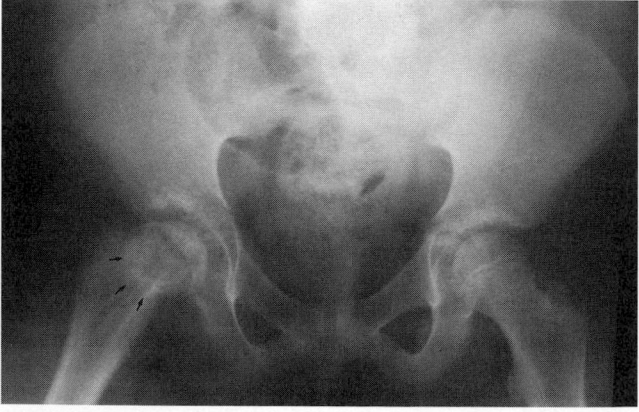

Figure 43-5 *A.* Schematic showing signs of SCFE observed on plain radiographs. Note diminution of epiphyseal height, physeal widening, and blanch sign. Also shown is Klein's line on normal and abnormal sides. *B.* Radiograph showing an 11-year-old girl with a grade II slip. Observe blanch sign (*arrowed*).

sis; in bilateral cases, chondrolysis has been defined as a decrease in the joint space to a width of 3 mm or less.[24]

Other Diagnostic Modalities

Reconstruction by computed tomography (CT) has been used as a guide prior to internal fixation in cases with marked displacement and for patients where corrective osteotomy of the three-dimensional deformity is contemplated.[25] Magnetic resonance imaging adds little diagnostic information, although it can depict marrow changes associated with avascular necrosis at an early stage.

Bone scintigraphy has been found helpful by the author in the diagnosis of preslip. Increased uptake around the physis compared with the contralateral hip is highly suggestive of this diagnosis in doubtful cases. Its usefulness for evaluating the blood supply of the femoral head has been queried because of the incidence of false-positive results for avascularity.[26]

Kallio and coauthors[27] believe that serial sonography is more sensitive than radiography in showing epiphyseal displacement and position. They point out the accuracy of this modality in also evaluating joint effusion and metaphyseal remodeling (Fig. 43-6), which they believe to be useful prognostic indicators (see below).

STABLE AND UNSTABLE SCFE

The traditional classification of SCFE, previously described, is based on duration of symptoms and x-ray appearance. Kallio et al. suggested that SCFE patients may be more accurately classified based upon objective sonographic data.[27] They believe that the presence of a joint effusion indicates physeal instability or recent progression, whereas, by contrast, remodeling is a sign of chronicity. An acute SCFE, characterized by a demonstrable effusion is in their opinion unstable and therefore may be improved with treatment using either gentle manipulation or traction. The position of a chronic slip (without an effusion) on the other hand, cannot be improved, and any form of reduction is contraindicated. Kallio et al. believe that the acute component of an acute or acute-on-chronic slip (characterized by the presence of both joint effusion and remodeling) may also be partially reduced. The presence of joint effusion they also believe to be an indication for operative fixation of an unstable epiphysis.

Loder and coauthors have also suggested a new classification of SCFE into stable and unstable categories based upon the type of clinical presentation.[24] They point out that patients with unstable slips are unable to tolerate any kind of weight bearing on the affected hip, whereas the stable group can ambulate. They further stress the satisfactory prognosis in the stable group in their series (96 percent compared with 47 percent for the unstable group) and the low incidence of avascular necrosis (zero percent compared with 50 percent). Of special significance is their observation that there is a significant difference in the prognosis of patients who would fall within a single category under the traditional classification (e.g., acute on chronic, acute, etc.), when these patients are reclassified as stable or unstable (see Table 43-1). All their patients were treated

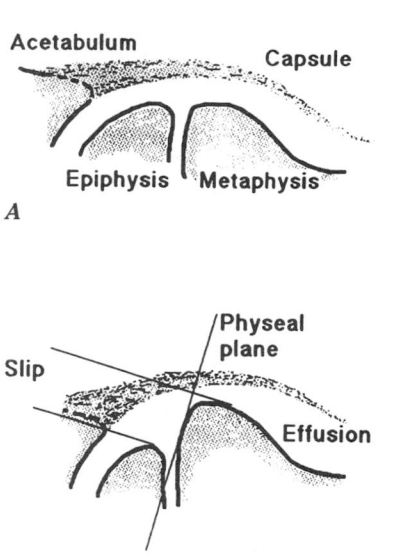

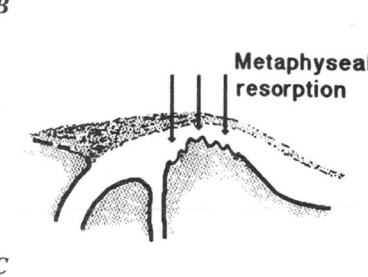

Figure 43-6 *A.* Anatomic structures of the adolescent hip joint as seen in sonographic examination. *B.* The posterior displacement of the proximal femoral epiphysis and effusion in acute SCFE. *C.* Irregular and rounded metaphyseal outline indicating metaphyseal resorption in early remodeling. (Reproduced with permission from Kallio PE, Paterson DC, Foster BK, Lequesne GW: Classification in slipped capital femoral epiphysis. *Clin Orthop* 294:196–203, 1993.)

with internal fixation, and the development of avascular necrosis did not correlate statistically with the severity of the slip, the use of preoperative traction, the degree of reduction, or the number of pins used for fixation.

Severity of the Slip

The severity of the slippage of the femoral head may be quantitated on the basis of the percentage of epiphyseal displacement relative to femoral neck diameter. If one-third or less of the metaphysis is uncovered, it is classified as a grade I slip (mild). If the slippage is up to two-thirds of the diameter of the metaphysis, it is classified as grade II (moderate). When more than two-thirds of the metaphysis uncovered, it is classified as grade III (severe). Another method described by Southwick is to draw a line across the physeal margins of the epiphysis and then draw a perpendicular to this line. Where the perpendicular intersects, a line is drawn along the long axis of the femoral shaft and the angle is measured. The angle for the normal hip is then subtracted from the affected side. A severe slip will have an angular difference in excess of 60°; a moderate slip, between 30° and 60°;

and a mild slip, 30° or less. In bilateral slips where both epiphyses may be displaced, an arbitrary 10° (representing the normal angle) may be subtracted on both sides to give a measurement of the degree of displacement[21] (Fig. 43-7).

TREATMENT

Treatment of a child with SCFE begins as soon as the diagnosis is made. The child is then kept from further weight bearing, since even in patients with stable SCFE, gradual continuing slippage is the rule unless treatment is instituted to prevent it. These children should be put on crutches immediately or kept in a wheelchair and not allowed to bear weight. In most instances, they should be admitted to a hospital as soon as possible. General physical examination is important to exclude any accompanying clinical endocrinopathy, which, if left untreated, will prejudice the treatment of the SCFE.

Although there are differing views regarding the value of traction, it is certainly of value in the child with an acutely painful hip who may have an associated flexion contracture and synovitis. Also, in acute slips, a significant improvement in the displacement of the epiphysis is often observed, and there is some evidence that preliminary traction reduces the incidence of avascular necrosis.[22,28,29]

Traction does not have to be elaborate; Buck's traction is usually sufficient. In an acute slip, 8 to 10 lb of Buck's traction may be sufficient to improve the position of the slip dramatically over the next 24 h (see Fig. 43-4*A* and *B*). In a patient with a stable slip who can ambulate and move the leg freely, preliminary traction is neither efficacious nor necessary, and the same goes for those patients who have only a moderate degree of slip who can be pinned in situ.

Manipulation

Forceful manipulation of a displaced epiphysis is contraindicated and has been shown to be associated with a high risk of avascular necrosis.[30,31] Any form of manipulation is also contraindicated in chronic slips. Kallio and coworkers have suggested that joint effusion shown by sonography in an acute or acute on chronic SCFE indicates instability. In such cases these authors believe that the position of the physis may be improved either by gentle manipulation or traction. They believe that the acute component of an acute on chronic slip identified by their criteria may also be partially reduced, but that attempts to go beyond that and achieve complete reduction of the chronic component of the slip will carry an increased risk of avascular necrosis.[27]

In the operating room, merely positioning the patient on the fracture table will improve the position if the epiphysis is acutely displaced. Any maneuver in the operating room that compromises the posterior retinacular vessels of the femoral epiphysis will lead to disaster. The high incidence of avascular necrosis associated with femoral manipulation of the acute slip (up to 25 percent) should always be borne in mind and the temptation to achieve an anatomic reduction avoided.[32]

TABLE 43-1 Comparison of Patients with Stable SCFE and Those with Unstable SCFE[a,b]

	Stable	Unstable	p value
Age (years)	13 ± 1.4	12 ± 1.5	0.34
Sex	12 F, 13 M	16 F, 14 M	0.90
Race†	10 W, 13 B, 2 H	21 W, 7 B, 4 H	0.07
Obesity (yes/no)	19/6	18/12	0.33
Side of slip	11 R, 14 L	12 R, 18 L	0.98
Trauma (yes/no)	6/19	27/3	<0.0001
Acute/acute-on-chronic	21/4	17/13	0.06
Severity of slip			
Mild/moderate/severe	12/7/6	2/9/19	0.001
Degrees	35 ± 21	51 ± 14	0.002
Duration of symptoms (days)	12 ± 6.1	4 ± 4.6	<0.0001
Time from presentation to operation (days)	2 ± 1.6	4 ± 3.8	0.004
Time from onset of symptoms to operation (days)	14 ± 6.3	8 ± 7.0	0.002
No. of pins or screws (1/≥2)	18/7	7/23	0.0008
Duration of follow-up (years)	3 ± 0.8	3 ± 2.0	0.80
Avascular necrosis (yes/no)	0/25	14/16	0.0003
Result (satisfactory/unsatisfactory)	24/1	14/16	0.0003

[a]Continuous data are expressed as the average and standard deviation.

[b]Note that there were 21 cases of acute slip in the stable category and 4 cases of acute-on-chronic slip, yet no cases of avascular necrosis. Compare the figures for the unstable SCFE patients. It can be seen that classifying patients as acute or acute-on-chronic did not have prognostic significance in this series.

Key: W, non-Hispanic white; B, black; H, Hispanic.
Source: Reproduced with permission from Loder RT, Richards BS, Shapiro PS, et al: Acute slipped capital femoral epiphysis: The importance of physeal stability. *J Bone Joint Surg* 75A:1134–1140, 1993.

Pinning in Situ

Most grade I and II slips (and preslips) are managed by percutaneous pinning in situ (see Fig. 43-10). Treatment is intended to prevent further slippage and to promote closure of the physis. In the past, multiple pins were used, but each pin inserted has the potential to damage the acetabular articular cartilage. The incidence of the subsequent complication of chondrolysis has been substantially reduced by using a single fixation pin or screw and locating it in the central portion of the head at least 5 mm from the articular border.[33,37] It is important that the fixation device avoid the superolateral corner of the epiphysis because of the risk of segmental necrosis occurring due to compromise of the artery of Brodetti.[34]

Since fixation is primarily a radiographic technique, extreme care must be taken to ensure good lateral and AP views to ensure a central position of the screw. The insertion site should start anteriorly on the femoral metaphysis, directing the guidepin posteriorly toward the center of the inferiorly and posteriorly positioned epiphysis (Figs. 43-9 and 43-10). For fixation, a cannulated screw is preferred, since it is important to get a good purchase on the epiphysis to avoid continual physeal growth.[35,36,38] The ideal is shown in Fig. 43-10. Continued physeal growth after pinning of the epiphysis is a complication that can be avoided by using a cannulated screw inserted in this fashion and is more likely when Steinman or Knowles pins are utilized.[39]

In stable slips, the frog-lateral position is satisfactory for identification of pin direction. If the slip is acute, however, the pinning should be done on a fracture table and the hip not moved until the fixation device is in position in the epiphysis. At the end of the procedure, the hip's motion should be visualized using the image intensifier in real time through a full range of motion. This will permit assessment of any protrusion into the hip joint. Care should be taken that the fixation screw device is not inserted too distally in the shaft, as this will predispose to fracturing of the femur during its removal.[40–42] The complications of fixation device removal are not inconsequential and problems occur with both stainless steel and titanium devices that have been implanted for more than 1 year. Indeed, titanium devices are so problematic with regard to their removal that they are no longer recommended.[42]

Postoperatively, the child is ambulated with crutches on the first day. Crutches are used until the synovitis subsides, usually within 4 to 6 weeks. In stable slips, it may be possible to discard the crutches within a few weeks; but in unstable and severely displaced slips, some authors advise protected weight bearing for between 6 and 12 weeks. The reported results for SCFE fixation with a single screw

Figure 43-7 Measurement of the head shaft angle using Southwick's method. *A.* Normal measurement on AP view (*left*). Line A is drawn across the epiphyseal margin. Line B is perpendicular to A and is extended to intersect line C, which is the shaft axis. The angle between B and C is the head shaft angle (normally about 145°). A similar construction (*right*) produces an angle of 110° in a moderate slip. *B.* Similar calculations on the frog lateral (*left*) produce a normal angle of 10 to 12°. This is greatly increased in a moderate slip (*right*).

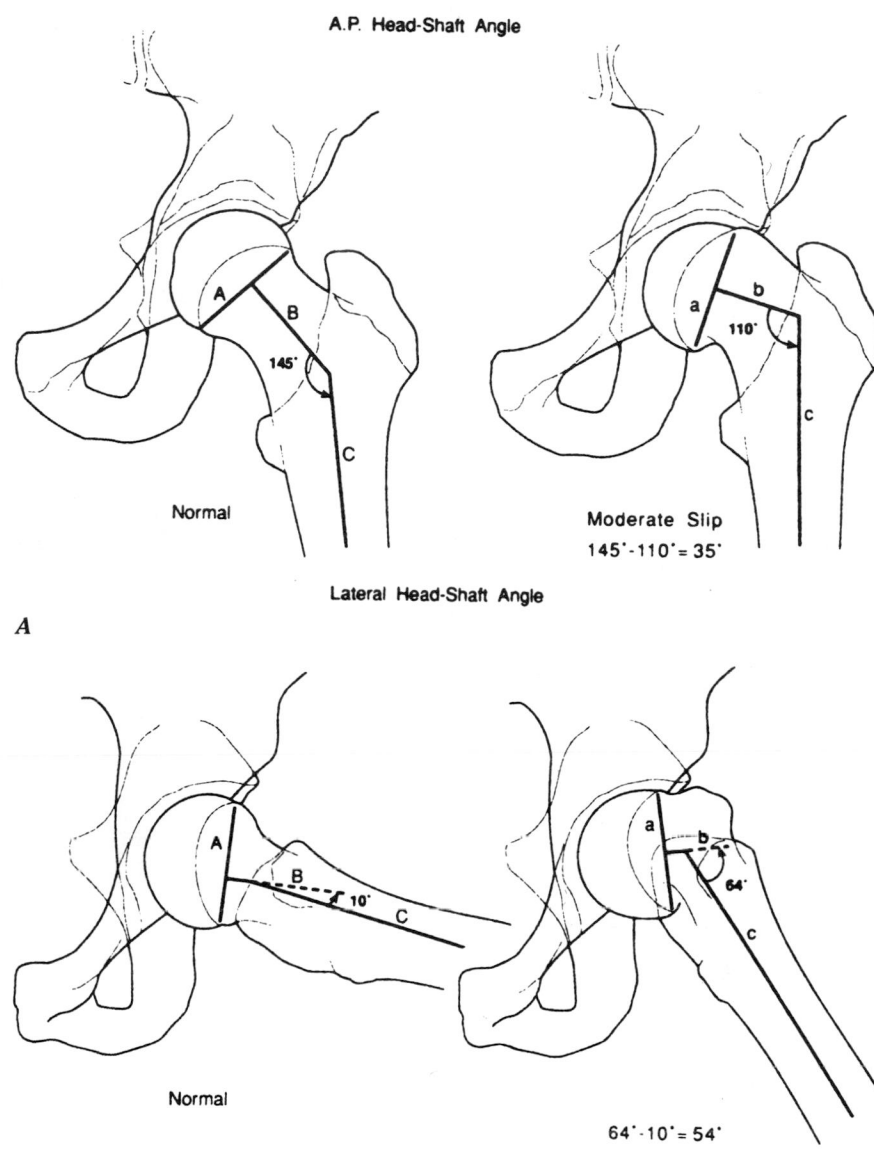

A.P. Head-Shaft Angle

Normal   Moderate Slip 145°-110°= 35°

Lateral Head-Shaft Angle

A

Normal   64°-10°= 54°

B

have been encouraging, with only a low incidence of chondrolysis and avascular necrosis.[43,44]

Bone Graft Epiphysiodesis

This operation has been advocated to avoid the reported complications of pinning and to promote physeal fusion, particularly in severe slips. In this procedure, performed through an anterior or anterolateral approach, a tunnel is created across the physis into the epiphysis using a burr introduced through a cortical window in the metaphysis. Along the tunnel so created is driven a corticocancellous iliac crest bone graft. This can be a technically demanding procedure with a significant morbidity. It was originally introduced by Howorth, who reported no cases of chondrolysis or avascular necrosis among 200 patients.[45] Good results of the procedure were subsequently reported by Herndon and Heyman.[46] Recent reports have been disap-

pointing. Ward and Wood describe graft fixation problems in almost half of their cases and have abandoned this procedure.[47] More recently Rao and Crawford and their coworkers reported on 64 cases, 44 of which had subsequent heterotopic ossification. Because of this and other associated morbidity, these authors also no longer recommend this operation for stable slipped capital femoral epiphysis (see Table 43-2). They reserve it for unstable slips, using it in conjunction with internal fixation.[48] One of the described advantages of this procedure is the associated removal of the protuberant metaphyseal bone anterolaterally, which sometimes impinges on the acetabulum and prevents internal rotation in the chronic slip.[46]

Osteotomy

Several authors have attempted to correct the anatomic abnormality that exists in severe slip by some form of cor-

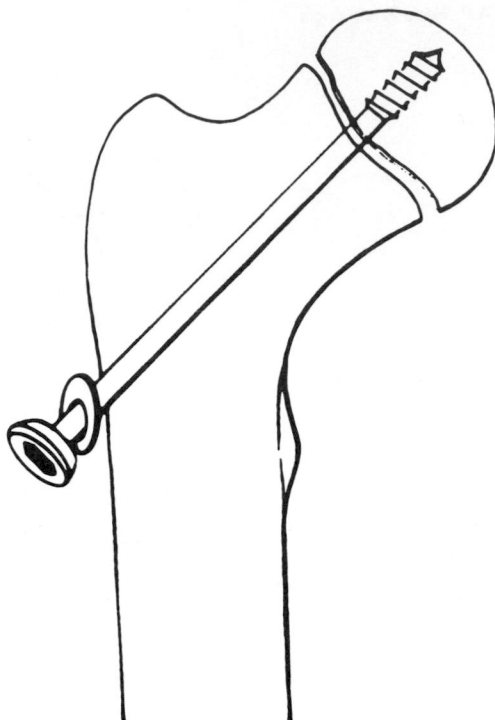

Figure 43-8 The principles of prophylactic dynamic screw fixation of the contralateral hip. All threads engage the head, but they do not penetrate the joint. The screw protrudes laterally 1.5 to 2 cm to allow for physeal growth. (Reproduced with permission from Kumm DA, Schmidt J, et al: Prophylactic dynamic screw fixation of the asymptomatic hip in slipped femoral epiphysis. *J Pediatr Orthop* 16:249–253, 1996.)

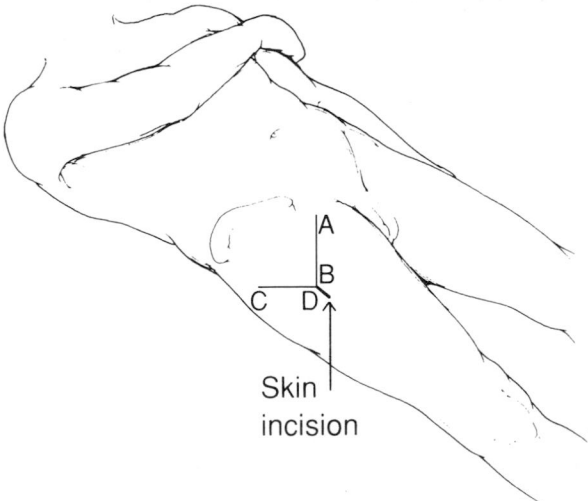

Figure 43-9 Technique and landmarks used to mark the position of the skin incision for pin placement. A-B represents the line overlying the femoral head and neck (bisecting the femoral head and lying perpendicular to the physis) as visualized on an AP fluoroscopic image. C-D represents the line overlying the femoral head and neck (also bisecting the femoral head and lying perpendicular to the physis) as visualized on a lateral image. (From Aronsson DD, Karol LA: Stable slipped capital femoral epiphysis: Evaluation and management. © 1996, American Academy of Orthopaedic Sugeons. Reprinted from the *Journal of the American Academy of Orthopaedic Surgeons.* 4:173–181, 1996, with permission.)

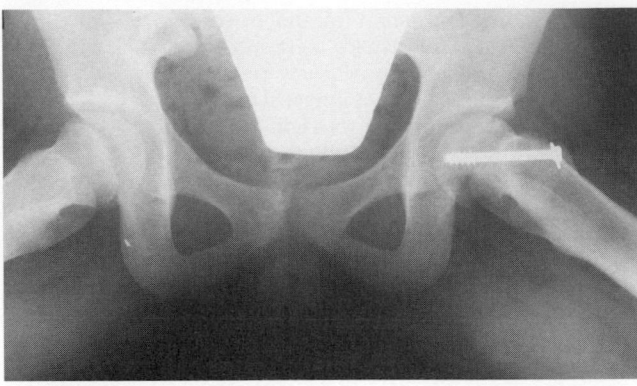

A

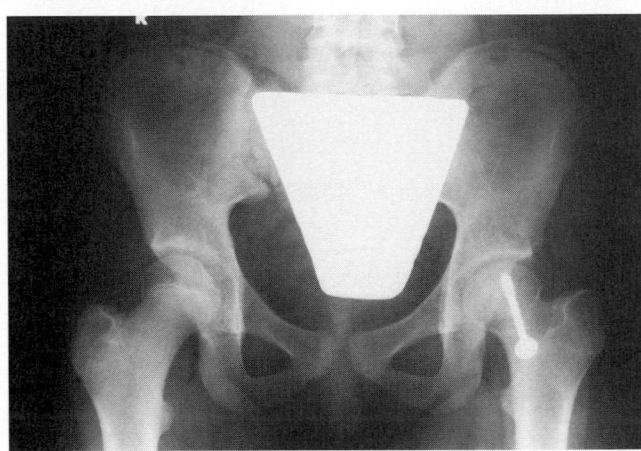

B

Figure 43-10 *A and B.* This grade I SCFE has been pinned with a single screw. Note obliquity of screw.

rective osteotomy. The posterior tilt of the head and the external rotation and varus deformity of the femur produce an exaggerated retroverted position of the upper femur, and the altered anatomy and biomechanics predispose to the subsequent development of osteoarthritis.[49]

Osteotomy through the Femoral Neck

The problem with intracapsular correction of the deformity is that although it is anatomically the most logical and direct correction, it is difficult to see how it can be achieved without compromising the retinacular blood vessels to the epiphysis, thus increasing the incidence of avascular necrosis. This has been the historical experience with this procedure as described in the literature.[50,51,53]

The operation was described by Dunn and Angel via a direct transtrochanteric approach.[50] A T-shaped incision was made in the capsule, with the horizontal limb at the acetabulum. The synovium was incised superiorly along the line of the neck at the vascular watershed and the metaphysis delivered into the wound. The posterior (vascular) synovium was gently dissected from the metaphysis subperiosteally and remained in situ with the epiphysis. A trapezoidal portion of metaphysis was then removed and

TABLE 43-2   Reported Results of Open Bone Peg Epiphysiodesis

Authors	Number of hips	AVN	CL	Other complications	Healing
Howorth (1957)[45a]	200	0	0	One graft absorption, three failure to bridge physis	12 weeks
Herndon and Heyman (1963)[46]	49	0	0	0	6–10 weeks
Miscellaneous (Howorth, 1966)[45]	152	1	0	0	
Zahrawi et al. (1983)[46a]	28	0	0	Four infection, two graft failure, one progression of slip	
Irani et al. (1985)[46b]	48	1	0	Four infection, three graft failure, two failed to heal, one intraarticular penetration	4.6 months
Bloom and Crawford (1985)[46c]	22	0	0	Eleven ectopic bone	12 weeks
Weiner et al. (1984, 1988, 1989)[46d,e,f]	232	3	1	Two graft failure, six progression of slip, two infection	10 weeks
Ward and Wood (1990)[47]	17	0	0	Eight graft failures, 10 anterolateral thigh hypesthesia, five failure to heat, three myositis ossificans	20 weeks (12 cases)
Rao et al (1996)[48]	64	4	3	Three infection, four serous drainage, seven anterolateral thigh hypesthesia, 44 heterotopic ossification, 12 progression of slip	17 weeks

Key: AVN, avascular necrosis; CL, chondrolysis.
Source: Reproduced with permission from Rao SB, Crawford AH, et al: Open bone peg epiphysiodesis for slipped capital femoral epiphysis. *J Pediatr Orthop* 16:37–48, 1996.

the shortened neck reduced back into the hip and pinned to the epiphysis. The shortening of the neck was thought to prevent tension on the posterior retinacular blood vessels.

Recently the procedure has been performed with some modification by Fish, using an anterior closing wedge, but because of the attendant risks, this modification has also failed to find favor.[52] The rate of avascular necrosis with these procedures varied but was approximately 25 percent.

Extracapsular Base-of-Neck Osteotomy

This operation has been described as being safer than intracapsular osteotomy, with no cases of avascular necrosis in a small series[54] (Fig. 43-11). A two-plane wedge osteotomy is performed along a line from the greater to lesser trochanter at the edge of the joint capsule. The procedure is carried out using a standard anterolateral approach. Careful preoperative planning on good AP and frog-lateral radiographs is essential. The base of the wedge posteriorly is extracapsular; therefore, if it is accurately placed, damage to the epiphyseal vessels is avoided. The authors point out that removal of a wedge larger than 2 cm in width not only compromises adequate length of the femoral neck but may increase femoral anteversion to an excessive degree. They note that there are additional technical difficulties in pinning across the osteotomy site if one attempts to correct deformities of more than 55°. However, in general the osteotomy makes

the placing of the screw across the growth plate easier than with in situ pinning for moderate to severe slips. At the conclusion of the osteotomy, after closing of the wedge, three or four cannulated screws are placed across the osteotomy site, but only one longer screw is placed across the physis into the epiphysis if the physis is still open. The authors note that the supralateral quadrant of the head of the epiphysis must be avoided when the screw is placed. They also point out the potential for significant limb-length discrepancy in unilateral slips and recommend contralateral distal femoral epiphysiodesis of the normal femur if the discrepancy exceeds 15 mm. Although these authors do not perform prophylactic in situ pinning of the normal contralateral hip, prophylactic dynamic screw fixation of the asymptomatic hip is enthusiastically recommended by others (Fig. 43-8).[55] This has been shown to be a procedure with few if any perioperative complications, unaccompanied by the complications of avascular necrosis or chondrolysis. It is certainly to be recommended in patients with endocrine disorders, as previously described.

Intertrochanteric Osteotomy

Newman[56] described intertrochanteric osteotomy to correct the biomechanical abnormalities of severe SCFE. Distal correction avoids the complication of avascular necrosis but may result in significant shortening. Southwick developed the procedure and described a method for accurate

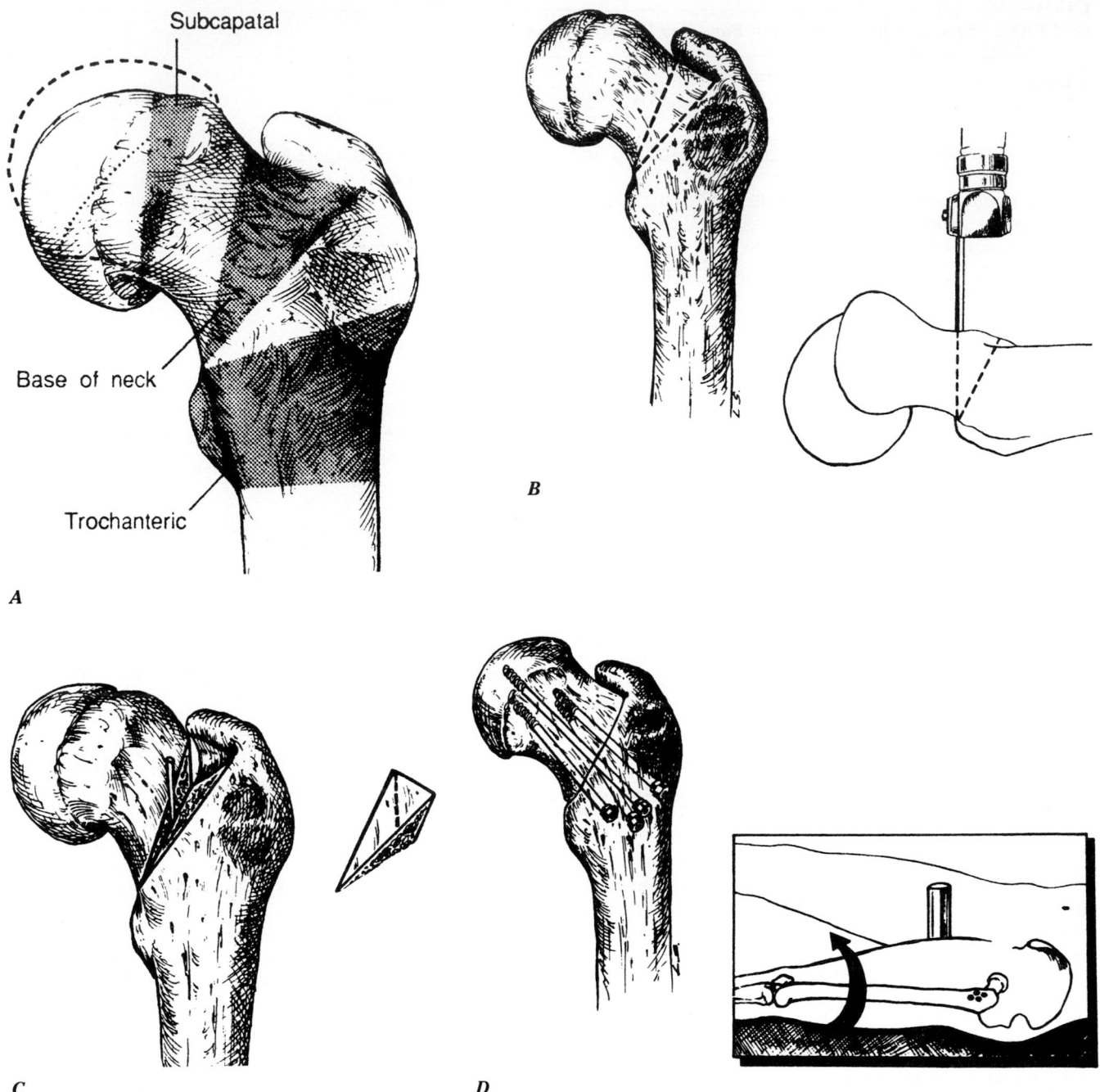

Figure 43-11 Base-of-neck osteotomy. *A.* The site of the osteotomy compared with other procedures for SCFE. *B.* The plane of the osteotomy is obtained by fully rotating the femur internally on the fracture table and using a short length of K wire along the intertrochanteric line with fluoroscopy. *C.* A triangular wedge of bone approximately 15 to 20 mm in width is removed. The bone removed is triangular in two planes. *D.* Internally rotating the leg closes the wedge, and pinning (see text) completes the procedure. (Reproduced with permission from Abraham E, Garst J, Barmada R: Treatment of moderate to severe slipped capital femoral epiphysis with extracapsular base of neck osteotomy. *J Pediatr Orthop* 13:249–302, 1993.)

preoperative planning.[57,58] He identified on both anteroposterior and frog-lateral x-rays the angular correction required to correct the head shaft angle and used intraoperative templates developed from his radiographs. He utilized internal fixation of the osteotomy after the anterolateral wedge was closed. Both Newman and Southwick performed a flexion, valgus, and internal rotation os-

teotomy to correct the posterior tilt and the external rotation and varus deformity of the femur.

Concern has arisen about the difficulty of performing total hip arthroplasty following the Southwick procedure should the need arise in later life. Also, a surprisingly high incidence of chondrolysis has been reported with this procedure.[59]

COMPLICATIONS OF SCFE

Chondrolysis

The rapid, progressive narrowing of the hip joint secondary to the loss of articular cartilage that characterizes this condition can occur even without treatment but is more frequent after multiple pin fixation. The incidence of chondrolysis in black children with SCFE has been reported previously to be many times greater than that in white children. However, these retrospective studies were inconsistent. Recent studies have concluded that pinning in situ for SCFE in black children is safe and effective treatment provided that intraarticular pin penetration is avoided. If this is the case, then the complication rate is comparable to that of the general population.[60] Single central screw fixation has been shown to lead to excellent results in this subset of the population.[61,62]

Treatment of chondrolysis consists of ensuring that the hip is kept in a good functional position. It is especially important to avoid the development of a hip flexion contracture. A period of traction may be required to reduce flexor spasm prior to gentle physical therapy to restore hip motion. The use of a continuous passive motion (CPM) machine to maintain range of motion is recommended.

Avascular Necrosis

This devastating complication has occurred less frequently since formal manipulation of the patient with SCFE has been abandoned. Avascular necrosis is not seen in stable SCFE but occurs in 47 percent of unstable hips.[24] It is probable that unstable slips have more risk of damage to the posterior retinacular vessels, which accounts for the increased frequency of avascular necrosis. In the past, it has been considered that there may be a relationship between delay in initiating treatment (particularly reducing acute displacement) and the development of avascular necrosis. Although, when one considers the anatomy of the blood supply to the epiphysis, this might seem intuitively likely, such a relationship has not in fact been clearly demonstrated. Some authors believe that preoperative traction minimizes the incidence of the avascular necrosis that may follow subsequent hip manipulation procedures in the operating room.[29] A risk factor for the development of avascular necrosis is overreduction of the slip by enthusiastic manipulation, particularly into the dangerous position of valgus reduction.[62] Some authors have concluded that the fate of the epiphysis may already be predetermined in some cases by the time the patient presents, particularly in the case of acute slips.[63,64] The relationship between manipulation and avascular necrosis is complex because manipulative reduction is usually attempted in the most severe slips. The MRI scan is now most commonly used to diagnosis early avascular necrosis. Upon the establishment of this diagnosis, the child should be kept in a non-weight-bearing status in an attempt to minimize the risk of head collapse. Any remaining internal fixation device should be removed prior to head collapse to prevent its subsequent intrusion into the joint. The treatment of this complication is described in Chap. 40.

REFERENCES

1. Henrickson B: The incidence of slipped capital femoral epiphysis. *Acta Orthop Scand* 40:365, 1969.
2. Jacobs B: Diagnosis and natural history of slipped capital femoral epiphysis. *AAOS Instr Course Lect* 21:224, 1972.
3. Kelsey J, Keggi K, Southwick W: The incidence and distribution of slipped capital femoral epiphysis in Connecticut and the Southwestern United States. *J Bone Joint Surg* 8:53, 1926.
4. Loder RT, Aronson DD, Greenfield ML: The epidemiology of bilateral slipped capital femoral epiphysis: A study of children in Michigan. *J Bone Joint Surg* 75A:1141, 1993.
5. Speer DP: The growth plate: Structure and function, in Dee R, Mango DR, Hurst LC (eds): *Principles of Orthopaedic Practice.* New York, McGraw-Hill, 1988.
6. Gelberman RH, Cohen MS, Shaw BA, et al: The association of femoral retroversion with slipped capital femoral epiphysis. *J Bone Joint Surg* 68A:1000–1007, 1986.
7. Pritchett JW, Perdue KD: Mechanical factors in slipped capital femoral epiphysis. *J Pediatr Orthop* 8:385–388, 1988.
8. Kelsea J, Southwick WO: Etiology, mechanism, and incidence of slipped capital femoral epiphysis. *AAOS Instr Course Lect* 21:182–185, 1972.
9. Mirkopulos N, Weiner DS, Askew M: The evolving slope of the proximal femoral growth plate: Relationship to slipped capital femoral epiphysis. *J Pediatr Orthop* 8:268–273, 1988.
10. Beer DP: Experimental epiphyseolysis: An etiologic mode of slipped capital femoral epiphysis. *Trans Orthop Res Soc* 3:47–55, 1978.
11. Futami T, Kasahara Y, et al: Arthroscopy for slipped capital femoral epiphysis. *J Pediatr Orthop* 12:592–597, 1992.
12. Loder RT, Farley FA, et al: Narrow window of bone age in children with slipped capital femoral epiphysis. *J Pediatr Orthop* 13:290–293, 1993.
13. Ippolito E, Mickelson MR, Ponsetti IV: A histochemical study of slipped capital femoral epiphysis. *J Bone Joint Surg* 67A:1109–1113, 1981.
14. Agamanolis DP, et al: Slipped capital femoral epiphysis: A pathological study. *J Pediatr Orthop* 5:40–58, 1985.
15. Wells D, King JD, Rowe TF, Kaufman FR: Review of slipped capital femoral epiphysis associated with endocrine disease. *J Pediatr Orthop* 13:610–614, 1993.
16. Loder RT, Wittenberg B, Desilva G: Slipped capital femoral epiphysis associated with endocrine disorders. *J Pediatr Orthop* 15:348–356, 1995.
17. Wilcox PG, Weiner DS, Leighley B: Maturation factors in slipped capital femoral epiphysis. *J Pediatr Orthop* 8:196–200, 1988.
18. Mann DC, Weddington J, Richton S: Hormonal studies in patients with slipped capital femoral epiphysis without evidence of endocrinopathy. *J Pediatr Orthop* 8:543–545, 1988.
19. Morrissy RT, Aalderon AE, Gerdes MH: Synovial immunofluorescence in patients with slipped capital femoral epiphysis. *J Pediatr Orthop* 1:55, 1981.
20. Morrissy RT, Steele RW, Gerdes MH: Localized immune complexes and slipped capital femoral epiphysis. *J Bone Joint Surg* 65:574, 1983.
21. Aronsson DD, Karol LA: Stable slipped capital femoral epiphysis: Evaluation and management. *J Am Acad Orthop Surg* 4:173–181, 1996.
22. Crawford AH: Current concepts review: Slipped capital femoral epiphysis. *J Bone Joint Surg* 70A:1422–1427, 1988.
23. Klein A, Joplin R, et al: Roentgenographic features of slipped femoral capital epiphysis. *AJR* 66:361, 1951.
24. Loder RT, Richards BS, Shapiro PS, et al: Acute slipped capital femoral epiphysis: The importance of physeal stability. *J Bone Joint Surg* 75A:1134–1140, 1993.

25. Ebraheim NA, Rusin JJ, et al: Percutaneous computed tomography, stabilization of moderate to severe slipped capital femoral epiphysis. *Orthopedics* 14:859–864, 1991.

26. Smergel EM, Harcke HT, Pizzutillo PD, et al: Use of bone scintigraphy in the management of slipped capital femoral epiphysis. *Clin Nucl Med* 12:349–353, 1987.

27. Kallio PE, Paterson DC, Foster BK, Lequesne GW: Classification in slipped capital femoral epiphysis. *Clin Orthop* 294:196–203, 1993.

28. Casey EH, Hamilton HW, Bobechko WP: Reduction of acutely slipped upper femoral epiphysis. *J Bone Joint Surg* 54B:607–614, 1972.

29. Green N, et al: The treatment of acute slipped capital femoral epiphyses: Meeting highlights. *J Pediatr Orthop* 11:126, 1991.

30. Fahey J, O'Brien E: Acute slipped capital femoral epiphysis. *J Bone Joint Surg [Am]* 47:1105, 1965.

31. Fairbank JT: Manipulative reduction in slipped upper femoral epiphysis. *J Bone Joint Surg [Br]* 51:252, 1969.

32. Boyer DW, Mickelson MR, Ponsetti IV: Slipped capital femoral epiphysis: Long-term follow-up study of 121 patients. *J Bone Joint Surg* 63A:85–95, 1981.

33. Stanitsky CL: Acute slipped capital femoral epiphysis: Treatment alternatives. *J Am Acad Orthop Surg* 2:96–106, 1996.

34. Brodetti A: The blood supply of the femoral neck and head in relation to the damaging effects of nails and screws. *J Bone Joint Surg* 42B:794–801, 1960.

35. Morrisy RT: Slipped capital femoral epiphysis: Technique of percutaneous in situ fixation. *J Pediatr Orthop* 10:347–350, 1990.

36. Aronsson DD, Carlson WE: Slipped capital femoral epiphysis: A prospective study of fixation with a single screw. *J Bone Joint Surg* 74A:810–819, 1992.

37. Riley PM, Weiner DS, Gillespie R, Weiner SD: Hazards of internal fixation in the treatment of slipped capital femoral epiphysis. *J Bone Joint Surg* 72A:1500, 1990.

38. Kibiloski LJ, Doane RM, Karol LA, et al: Biomechanical analysis of single- vs double-screw fixation in SCFE at physiological load levels. *J Pediatr Orthop* 14:627, 1994.

39. Laplaza FD, Burke SW: Epiphyseal growth after pinning of slipped capital femoral epiphysis. *J Pediatr Orthop* 15:357, 1995.

40. Baynham GC, Lucie RS, Cummings RJ: Femoral neck fracture secondary to in situ pinning of SCFE: A previously unreported complication. *J Pediatr Orthop* 11:187, 1991.

41. Greenough CG, Bromage JD, Jackson AM: Pinning of the slipped upper femoral epiphysis: A trouble-free procedure? *J Pediatr Orthop* 5:657, 1985.

42. Lee TK, Haynes RJ, Longo JA, Tchu JR: Pin removal in slipped capital femoral epiphysis: The unsuitability of titanium devices. *J Pediatr Orthop* 16:49–52, 1996.

43. Ward WT, Steko J, Wood KB, et al: Fixation with a single screw for slipped capital femoral epiphysis. *J Bone Joint Surg* 74A:799–809, 1992.

44. Aronsson DD, Peterson DA, Miller DV: Slipped capital femoral epiphysis the case for internal fixation in situ. *Clin Orthop* 281:115–122, 1992.

45. Howorth B: The bone pegging operating for slipping of the capital epiphysis. *Clin Orthop* 48:79–87, 1966.

45a. Howorth B: The bone pegging operation for slipping of the capital femoral epiphysis. *Clin Orthop* 10:148–173, 1957.

46. Herndon CH, Heyman CR: Treatment of slipped capital femoral epiphysis by epiphysiodesis and osteoplasty of the femoral neck. *J Bone Joint Surg* 45A:999–1012, 1963.

46a. Zahrawi FB, Stephens TL, Spencer GE Jr, et al: Comparative study of pinning in situ and open epiphysiodesis in 105 patients with slipped capital femoral epiphysiodesis. *Clin Orthop* 177:160–168, 1983.

46b. Irani RN, Rosenzweig AH, Cotler HB, Schwentker EP: Epiphysiodesis in slipped capital femoral epiphysis: A comparison of various surgical modalities. *J Pediatr Orthop* 5:661–664, 1985.

46c. Bloom ML, Crawford AH: Slipped capital femoral epiphysis: An assessment of treatment modalities. *Orthopedics* 8:36–40, 1985.

46d. Weiner DS, Weiner SD, Melby A, Hoyt WA Jr: A 30 yr experience with bone graft epiphysiodesis in the treatment of slipped capital femoral epiphysis. *J Pediatr Orthop* 4:145–152, 1984.

46e. Weiner DS, Weiner SD, Melby A: Anterolateral approach to the hip for bone graft epiphysiodesis in the treatment of slipped capital femoral epiphysis. *J Pediatr Orthop* 8:349–352, 1988.

46f. Weiner DS: Bone graft epiphysiodesis in the treatment of slipped capital femoral epiphysis. *AAOS Instr Course Lect* 38:263–272, 1988.

47. Ward WT, Wood K: Open bone graft epiphysiodesis for slipped capital femoral epiphysis. *J Pediatr Orthop* 10:14–20, 1990.

48. Rao SB, Crawford AH, et al: Open bone peg epiphysiodesis for slipped capital femoral epiphysis. *J Pediatr Orthop* 16:37–48, 1996.

49. Ordeberg G, Hansson LI, Sandstrom S: Slipped capital femoral epiphysis in southern Sweden: Long term result with no treatment or symptomatic primary treatment. *Clin Orthop* 191:95–104, 1984.

50. Dunn DM, Angel JC: Replacement of the femoral head by open operation in severe adolescent slipping of the upper femoral epiphysis. *J Bone Joint Surg* 60B:394–403, 1978.

51. Clark HJ, Wilkinson JA: Surgical treatment for severe slipping of the upper femoral epiphysis. *J Bone Joint Surg* 72B:854–858, 1990.

52. Fish JB: Cuneiform osteotomy of the femoral neck in the treatment of slipped capital femoral epiphysis. *J Bone Joint Surg* 76A:46–59, 1994.

53. Broughton NS, Todd RC, Dunn DM, et al: Open reduction of the severely slipped upper femoral epiphysis. *J Bone Joint Surg* 70B:435–439, 1988.

54. Abraham E, Garst J, Barmada R: Treatment of moderate to severe slipped capital femoral epiphysis with extracapsular base of neck osteotomy. *J Pediatr Orthop* 13:249–302, 1993.

55. Kumm DA, Schmidt J, et al: Prophylactic dynamic screw fixation of the asymptomatic hip in slipped capital femoral epiphysis. *J Pediatr Orthop* 16:249–253, 1996.

56. Newman PN: The surgical treatment of slipping of the upper femoral epiphysis. *J Bone Joint Surg* 42B:280, 1960.

57. Southwick WO: Osteotomy through the lesser trochanter for slipped capital femoral epiphysis. *J Bone Joint Surg* 49A:807–833, 1967.

58. Southwick WO: Compression fixation after biplane intertrochanteric osteotomy for slipped capital femoral epiphysis. *J Bone Joint Surg* 55A:218, 1973.

59. Frymoyer JW: Chondrolysis of the hip following Southwick osteotomy for severe slipped capital femoral epiphysis. *Clin Orthop* 99:120–124, 1974.

60. Spero CR, Masciale JP, Tornetta P III, et al: Slipped capital femoral epiphysis in black children: Incidence of chondrolysis. *J Pediatr Orthop* 12:444–448, 1992.

61. Aronsson DD, Loder RT: Slipped capital femoral epiphysis in black children. *J Pediatr Orthop* 12:74–79, 1992.

62. Bishop JO, et al: Slipped capital femoral epiphysis: A study of 50 cases in black children. *Clin Orthop* 135:93–96, 1978.

63. Hagglund G, et al: Vitality of the slipped capital femoral epiphysis: Pre-operative evaluation by tetracycline labelling. *Acta Orthop Scand* 56:215–217, 1965.

64. Gelfand MJ, et al: Bone scintigraphy in slipped capital femoral epiphysis. *Clin Nucl Med* 8:613–615, 1983.

CHAPTER 44

Rotational Deformity of the Lower Extremity in Children

Kenneth Keller

Rotational abnormalities of the lower limb in children often present as marked toeing in or toeing out. This may result from rotational deformity about the femur, tibia, foot, or a combination of these. The child is commonly presented to the orthopedist by parents and primary care physicians who are concerned that the child's feet are excessively turning in or out. Although surgical treatment for rotational deformity is only occasionally required, toeing in and toeing out are frequently encountered in office practice. It is necessary for the orthopedist to understand the causes and consequences of rotational deformity and to diagnose and treat pathologic deformity. Although most cases of excessive toeing in and toeing out are significant only cosmetically and as a source of familial anxiety, more severe deformity may result in functional impairment, including gait disturbance, knee pain, and arthritis.[11,13,27,44,57,67] Rotational deformities are also commonly associated with neuromuscular disorders and hip disease.[35,62]

Definitions

The terms *version* and *torsion* are commonly used in the orthopedic literature to describe rotational alignment about the long axis of the femur and tibia. They are often used interchangeably, and *version* is more often used with respect to the femur, whereas *torsion* usually pertains to the tibia. Eckhoff and Winter have suggested clarification of this terminology by referring to *version* of the femur and tibia when the rotational alignment is within the normal range and to *torsion* when the deformity is abnormal (beyond two standard deviations).[12] Femoral version is the angle between the transcondylar axis distally and the axis of the femoral neck and head proximally. The plane of the head and neck axis is normally anterior to the transverse plane of the distal condyles, and this is termed *anteversion* (Fig. 44-1). *Retroversion* is torsional deformity of the femur where the plane of the head/neck axis is posterior to that of the femoral condyles.

NORMAL DEVELOPMENT

Retroversion of up to 26° is normally seen in the early fetus, but this develops into anteversion before birth. Femoral version varies with age and decreases from about 40° at birth to 24° at age 10 and to about 16° of anteversion by mid- to late adolescence.[53]

The version of the tibia is commonly determined by comparing the plane of the longitudinal axis of the proximal tibia to the plane of the transmalleolar axis distally. The early fetal tibia has a negative (internal or medial) version, which progressively changes to a more positive (external or lateral) rotation. At birth, the normal tibial version is −15° (range −50 to +4°); this increases to +5° of external rotation by the end of the first year, +10° by mid-childhood, and 20 to 24° of lateral rotation in adulthood.[52,54] It is important to note that there is a wide variation of normal.[52] In addition, significant racial differences may exist. For example, Chinese have 10 to 15° more toeing out than non-Chinese.[6]

TOEING IN

Excessive toeing in is far more common than toeing out. The incidence of internal tibial rotation is about 4 percent among adults.[26] An evaluation of 1320 children demonstrated rotational problems in 13.6 percent, where 174 were related to toeing in and only 6 to toeing out.[41] Excessive toeing in and toeing out is most commonly idiopathic but may also be seen in association with neuromuscular disorders, hip deformity, and fracture malunion. The etiology of idiopathic toeing in is multifactorial and results from a deviation in the natural progression to normal version. This can present as torsion of the femur with excessive anteversion, torsion of the tibia with lack of lateral rotation, or foot deformity with metatarsus adductus or varus. Intrauterine positioning and heredity may be important factors affecting rotational alignment.[22,55]

Internal Tibial Torsion

In the toddler toeing in is common and results from the relative medial version of the tibia and anteversion of the femur compared to that seen in the older child and adult. Internal tibial torsion is believed to be the most significant cause of toeing in in this age range. Because of the significant variation in normal values for hip rotation and femoral and tibial version, even marked toeing in among infants and toddlers should be considered a normal variant until sufficient time is allowed for spontaneous correction. Marked correction of toeing in should be seen by mid-childhood. The average orientation is 4.2° of toeing out for children 4 to 16 years of age. However, up to 8° of toeing in is within two standard deviations from this value and should be considered normal.[38] An increase in toeing in or failure to observe a progression toward correction should prompt investigation to rule out possible underlying pathology such as cerebral palsy or hip dysplasia or instability. One exception to this is that toeing in may appear to worsen somewhat at about the time the child begins to walk. This occurs as the hip loses the flexion and external rotation contractures resulting from "intrauterine packaging" that

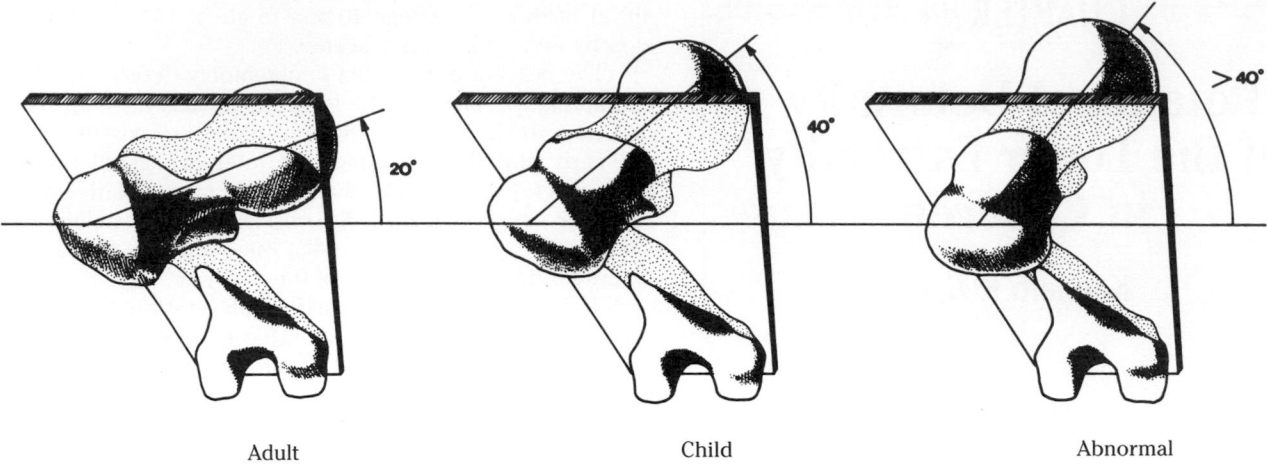

| Adult | Child | Abnormal |

Figure 44-1 Femoral anteversion. The relationship between the transcondylar axis (at distal femur) and the axis of the femoral neck in various groups.

are normally present during the first year of life. The hip moves into a position of more internal rotation as the soft tissues relax, thereby exacerbating the degree of toeing in. It is helpful to explain this phenomenon early on to avoid further anxiety among family members who are awaiting spontaneous improvement in the child's toeing in.

Femoral Antetorsion

The most common cause of idiopathic toeing in seen in midchildhood is increased or persistent femoral anteversion (sometimes known as femoral antetorsion). Fabry et al. studied a series of such children and found that 70 percent of the cases were attributed to femoral torsion (increased anteversion) and 30 percent to internal tibial torsion. The toeing in corrected spontaneously in 65 percent of the cases, and the initial deformity in 83 percent of the spontaneous corrections was femoral antetorsion. However, of those with femoral torsion who spontaneously corrected their toeing in, only 20 percent demonstrated a decrease in femoral anteversion. These data have shown that the correction of the toeing-in gait in the majority of cases with femoral torsion resulted from a compensatory external rotation of the tibia and not from correction of the underlying femoral deformity.[17] There is little correction of femoral anteversion after the age of 8, but compensatory lateral tibial rotation may progress into adolescence. This condition of femoral antetorsion associated with compensatory external torsion of the tibia has been coined "torsional malalignment syndrome" and may require osteotomy for correction.[9] The development of a tibial rotational deformity to compensate for an opposite rotational deformity in the femur is concerning from a biomechanical viewpoint, and a number of studies have associated lateral rotation of the tibia with anterior knee pain, patellofemoral disease, and altered mechanics about the knee.[9,28,64,36]

Miscellaneous Causes

Severe toeing in may be associated with cerebral palsy and other neuromuscular diseases. The rotational deformity worsens the functional impairment caused by the underlying disease. Derotational osteotomy significantly improves gait mechanics and decreases the energy required for ambulation. The reader is referred to Chap. 33 for further discussion.

Toeing in may result from forefoot adduction deformity, including metatarsus adductus and varus. Isolated forefoot adduction deformity corrects spontaneously in 90 percent of cases[55] and also responds well to serial casting. Forefoot adduction deformity is discussed in detail in Chap. 48.

Rotational deformity resulting from fracture malunion is common, occurring in 20 to 30 percent of lower extremity long bone fractures.[8] Deformity up to 25° is tolerated without symptoms. Unlike angular deformity in children with fracture malunion, rotational deformity is poorly corrected with remodeling.[8] Osteotomy should be considered in cases of posttraumatic torsional deformity with marked cosmetic or functional impairment. If intramedullary nail fixation is used either in primary fracture fixation or for corrective osteotomy, care should be taken to assure proper rotational alignment. Femoral torsional deformity of greater than 15° has been reported to occur in about 14 percent of femur fractures treated with intramedullary nailing.[4] However, less than half of these patients had complaints related to their deformity. Intramedullary techniques are not recommended in children under the age of 10 or 12.[3]

TOEING OUT

The foot is normally positioned in external rotation relative to the longitudinal plane of the tibia. Rotational deformity from excessive toeing out is encountered far less frequently than from toeing in. McSweeny's study of rotational deformity in children found only 3 percent attributed to toeing out.[41] The average toeing out for normal children 4 to 5 years old is 2.8°; this increases to 7.3° by age 16 with a range (two standard deviations) of 8.8°.[38] Several studies have found the degree of toeing out to be greater on the right side, for unclear reasons.[20,38] Toeing out has been found to be more pronounced in heavier children.[38] External torsion of the tibia is more often seen in the older child or adolescent and usually occurs in compensation for excessive or persistent femoral anteversion. Toeing out resulting from diminished femoral anteversion is less common and is more pronounced when found in combination with lateral torsion of the tibia. Toeing out may also be seen in neuromuscular diseases such as cerebral palsy, where it is often associated with severe femoral antetorsion and valgus deformity of the foot. Toeing out is also seen as a manifestation of slipped capital femoral epiphysis, where the femur displaces from the epiphysis anteriorly and slips into external rotation.

The point at which excessive toeing out is pathologic is unclear. The lever function of the foot remains intact with up to 60° of external rotation, but gait function may be affected beyond this extent.[56] Excessive toeing out may be cosmetically unappealing and has been associated with patellofemoral problems and anterior knee pain.[9,28,36,64]

CLINICAL EVALUATION

General

Evaluation of the child with lower extremity rotational deformity begins with a careful history. The family's concerns should be discussed and complaints of clumsiness, difficulties with running or walking, and cosmetic appearance noted. Moreover, the child may have significant emotional stress with such difficulties. Prenatal and birth history are important, as complications may be associated with neuromuscular disorders. Oligohydramnios has been associated with a number of limb deformities related to problems with the child's intrauterine position. An increased incidence of toeing out and external tibial torsion has been found among children born preterm and may be related to persistent prone positioning in the neonatal intensive care unit.[28] Family history is also important, as torsional deformity may often run in the family.

The physical exam should include close observation of the child while he or she is standing, sitting, walking, and running. Gait abnormalities are often enhanced by running. While standing, the limb with femoral antetorsion will have an in-turning patella. This may or may not be associated with toeing in or out, depending on the tibial version and the presence of compensatory lateral tibial rotation. The child with significant femoral antetorsion often sits in the "W" position, with the legs out to the side and hips internally rotated. Neuromuscular disease may be present in the child with rotational deformity and must be ruled out at physical exam. Rotational deformity may also

be seen with hip deformity, and evaluation for dysplasia and instability or dislocation should be included.[35]

The child with significant femoral antetorsion has increased internal rotation of the hip and decreased external rotation when examined in extension. However, external rotation is restored when examined in 90° of flexion. This finding clinches the diagnosis of excessive femoral anteversion. The limited lateral rotation is thought to result from a taut anterior joint capsule, which is relaxed in flexion, thereby allowing external rotation of the hip.[59] The knee should be evaluated for patellofemoral pain and instability. The patella points inward when excessive femoral anteversion is present and outward with diminished anteversion. The Q angle should be noted and is increased with increased femoral anteversion or lateral tibial rotation. The foot should be examined, since toeing in may result from adduction deformity of the forefoot and toeing out can be associated with valgus foot deformity. Abnormalities of gait associated with rotational deformities and the role of the gait laboratory in diagnosis are discussed in Chap. 38.

Rotational Profile

The diagnosis of specific rotational deformity of the lower limb is addressed by Staheli's rotational profile[55] (Fig. 44-2). This involves determination of the foot progression angle, medial and lateral hip rotation, the thigh-foot angle, and the presence of foot deformity. This information allows the examiner to attribute the rotational deformity to torsion of the femur, torsion of the tibia, forefoot adduction, or a combination of these. The foot progression angle (FPA) is the angle between the longitudinal axis of the foot and the direction of gait progression (Fig. 44-2D). The FPA is a general measure of the degree of toeing in or out and is influenced by femoral version, tibial version, and foot adduction deformity. The average FPA for children 4 to 16 years of age is +4.2° with a normal range of −8 to +16°.[38] However, rotational deformity may exist despite a normal foot progression angle, as can be seen in cases of excessive femoral anteversion with compensatory lateral tibial rotation. Femoral version and hip internal and external rotation are assessed with the patient prone and the knees flexed 90° (Fig. 44-2C). In this position the hip is rotated by moving the leg medially and laterally while palpating the greater trochanter. The leg is then positioned to the point when the trochanter is most prominent, which brings the head/neck axis to the horizontal. The femoral version is estimated by the degree of hip rotation required to bring the head/neck axis to the horizontal and is represented by the angle between the leg and the true vertical. Medial and lateral hip rotation should be symmetrical. Internal rotation of the hip greater than 70° indicates excessive femoral anteversion.

Tibial rotation is determined by measuring the thigh-foot angle or the transmalleolar angle. The thigh-foot angle is the angle between the longitudinal axes of the thigh and foot when observed from behind with the knee flexed 90° (Fig. 44-2A). The transmalleolar angle is assessed with the patient in the same position and is the angle between

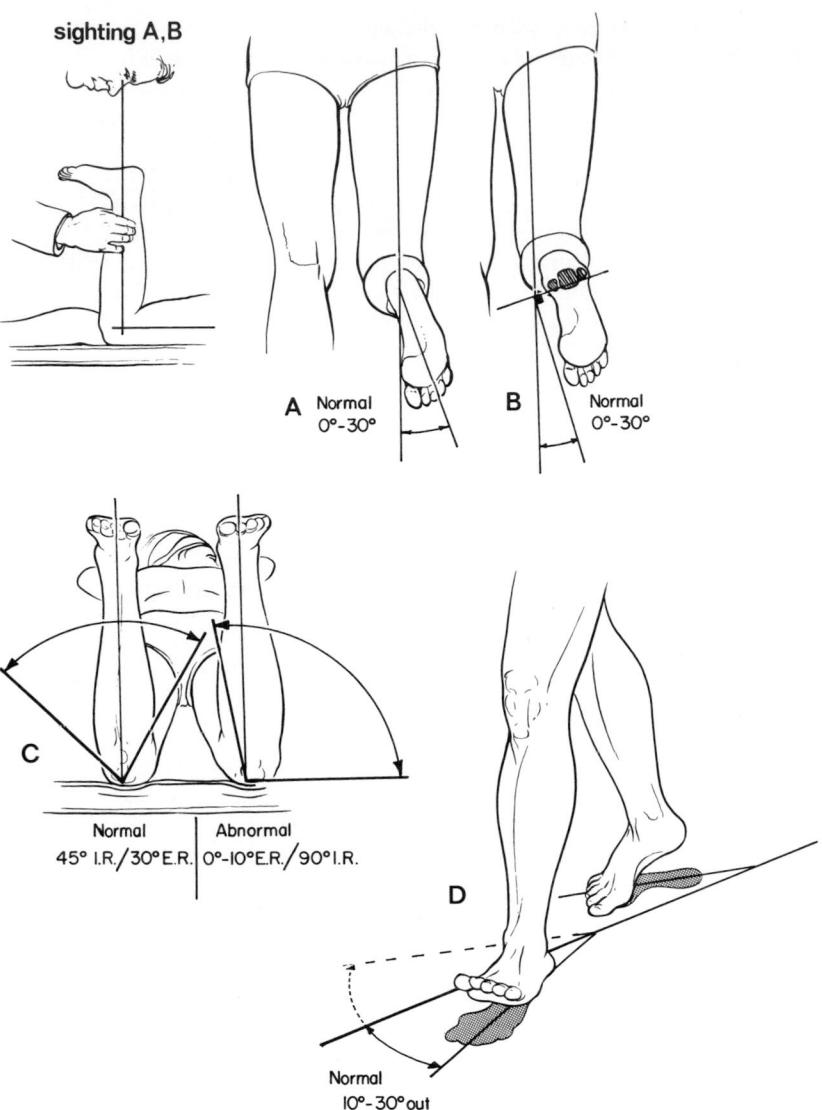

sighting A,B

A Normal
0°-30°

B Normal
0°-30°

C

Normal
45° I.R./30°E.R.

Abnormal
0°-10°E.R./90°I.R.

D

Normal
10°-30°out

Figure 44-2 The rotational profile. The upper left figure demonstrates the clinical method for estimating both *A* and *B*. *A*. Measurement of the thigh-foot angle. *B*. Measurement of the angle of the transmalleolar axis. *C*. Measurement of hip internal and external rotation. *D*. Foot progression angle. Approximate normal ranges are noted for each measurement.

the axis of the thigh and a line perpendicular to the transmalleolar axis (Fig. 44-2*B*). The transmalleolar angle is a more accurate method when foot deformity is present.

The foot is evaluated for forefoot adduction deformity by assessing the position of the forefoot with respect to the midline axis of the hindfoot. The hindfoot axis should normally project to the interspace between the second and third toes and is displaced laterally in metatarsus adductus and varus.[55]

IMAGING

Imaging studies help to confirm the clinical diagnosis and are particularly helpful in preoperative planning and in cases with complex deformity such as the torsional malalignment syndrome. Assessment of lower limb torsional deformities has been described using plain radi

ography,[10,25,39] fluoroscopy,[7] computed tomography (CT),[11,14,44,49,50,61] ultrasonography,[1,5,42,46,61] and MRI.[61] Computed tomography scanning is the most commonly used technique and has been considered the most accurate method for defining the type and degree of rotational deformity. The degree of femoral torsion as measured by CT is the difference between the head/neck axis and the transverse axis of the posterior femoral condyles[11] (Fig. 44-3). Tibial torsion is quantified by measuring the angle between the transverse axis of the proximal tibia and the transmalleolar axis[14] (Fig. 44-4). Recent advances in ultrasound imaging of torsional defects have demonstrated accuracy paralleling that obtained by CT.[1,42,61] The use of MRI in defining torsional deformity is not widespread but results comparable to those of CT imaging have been reported.[51,61] Both MRI and ultrasound are particularly appealing in that they avoid exposure to radiation. Conventional radiography for the evaluation of rotational deformities has been replaced by these other more accurate imaging modalities.

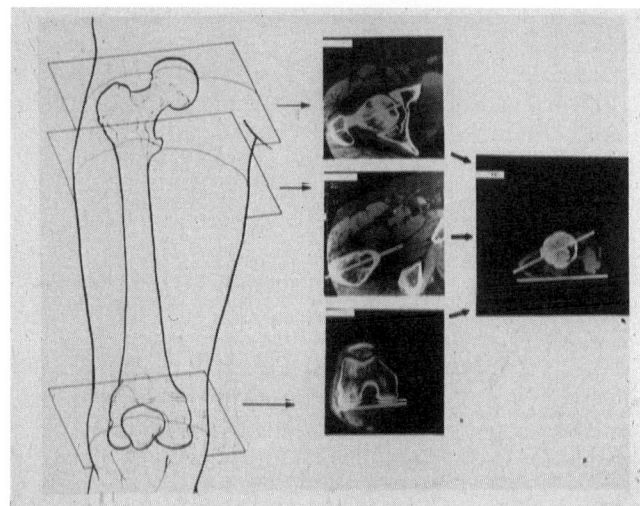

Figure 44-3 A CT torsion scan with axes illustrated. The proximal axis of the femur is determined by the line joining the center of the head and center of the shaft at the level of the lesser trochanter when the top two cuts are superimposed. The distal axis of the femur is determined by the line joining the two most posterior points of the condyles. The anteversion is measured from the angle between the proximal and distal axes when all three cuts are superimposed. (Reproduced with permission from Eckhoff DG, Montgomery WK, Kilcoyne RF, Stamm ER: Femoral morphometry and anterior knee pain. *Clin Orthop Rel Res* 302:64–68, 1994.)

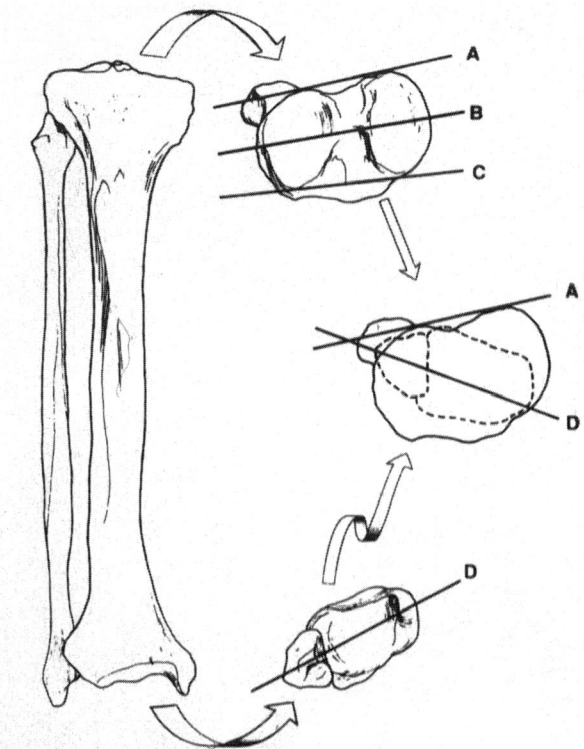

Figure 44-4 Tibia, illustrating the axes selected for comparison. A, posterior tibial axis; B, transtibial axis; C, anterior tibial axis; and D, malleolar axis. Tibial rotation is the angle between the proximal and distal axes when the two are superimposed (*center right*). (Reproduced with permission from Eckhoff DG, Montgomery WK, Kilcoyne RF, Stamm ER: Femoral morphometry and anterior knee pain. *Clin Orthop Rel Res* 302:64–68, 1994.)

TREATMENT

The principal treatment for the vast majority of children with lower limb rotational deformity is observation and reassurance. Staheli estimates that less than 1 percent of cases will require surgical correction.[55] Mild toeing in is rarely problematic. In fact, a recent study has demonstrated that it may provide an athletic advantage. A higher incidence of toeing in was found among a series of successful sprinters.[18] Most cases of toeing in from femoral or tibial torsion will correct spontaneously by the age of 8. Liu et al. have suggested that spontaneous correction occurs by remodeling of the epiphyseal plate in response to altered ground-reactive forces.[37] However, it should be kept in mind that over 50 percent of those with femoral torsion will correct by compensatory lateral rotation of the tibia.[17]

Conservative

Conservative methods such as splinting (e.g., Dennis-Browne splint), twister cables, and shoe orthotics have not been successful in the treatment of femoral or tibial torsion. Although used widely in the past, these methods have been abandoned by most authors, as a number of studies have disproved their effectiveness.[23,31,32,34,55,60,66] A prospective study by Heinrich et al. found that the correction of rotational deformity from splinting was no different from that seen in an untreated control group.[23]

Barlow and Staheli demonstrated that night splinting failed to produce rotational changes in the femur or tibia in an animal model.[2] Moreover, the use of splinting devices may produce abnormalities about the knee, including marked external tibial torsion, valgus deformity, and ligamentous problems.[16,21,23,31]

The role of behavior modification in the treatment of torsional deformity is unclear. It has often been common practice to instruct the toeing-in child to avoid sitting in the "W" position or sleeping prone with the toes turned in. However, in light of the poor results obtained from the splinting studies, the effectiveness of modifying particular behaviors seems questionable.

In contrast to femoral and tibial torsion, toeing in resulting from forefoot adduction deformity responds well to conservative treatment. Both flexible and rigid forefoot adduction deformities are treatable with splinting or casting techniques. Approximately 90 percent of metatarsus adductus cases will correct spontaneously. Splinting or casting can therefore be withheld until failure to progress toward correction is documented. The reader is referred to Chap. 48 for further discussion of metatarsus adductus.

Surgical

The definitive treatment for problematic rotational deformity of the lower extremity is derotational osteotomy. The indications for surgical correction of lower limb rotational deformity are not well defined. Asymptomatic patients with toeing in who tolerate their cosmetic appearance are not considered for surgery. Derotational osteotomy is reserved for those cases with functional gait abnormalities, intolerable cosmetic deformity, or pain resulting from torsional deformity of the femur and/or tibia. Surgery is generally performed after the age of 8 in the child with idiopathic rotational deformity.[55,60] This maximizes the chance for spontaneous correction. However, in the child with coexistent neuromuscular disease, the deformity is often severe and may progress. Such patients should preferably be assessed in the gait laboratory to analyze this complex problem (see Chap. 38). In these patients, derotational osteotomy may be performed at an early age and is often done in conjunction with a hip stabilization procedure, as hip instability is also common in this patient population. Derotational osteotomy in patients with neuromuscular disease significantly improves gait mechanics and decreases the energy requirement for ambulation.[19]

Femoral Osteotomy

Femoral osteotomy is indicated for patients with torsional deformity of the femur. The candidate for surgery should demonstrate at least 80° of internal hip rotation and have at least 50° of femoral antetorsion.[55,60] Intertrochanteric and supracondylar osteotomies have been described. Supracondylar osteotomies have 15 percent complication rate.[47,58] In the series of Payne and Deluca, intertrochanteric osteotomy with blade-plate fixation demonstrated no significant complications and enable more accurate correction of the deformity with decreased requirements for postoperative immobilization.[47] The correction of femoral rotational deformity has been successfully achieved using Ilizarov techniques.[24] Excellent results with closed femoral intramedullary osteotomy followed by intramedullary nail fixation has also been reported.[15] This technique affords the quickest return to full weight-bearing activity and eliminates the need for postoperative immobilization. However, intramedullary techniques should be avoided in children under the age of 12 to avoid the risk of avascular necrosis of the femoral head.[3]

Tibial Osteotomy

Derotational osteotomy of the tibia is performed for the correction of severe torsional deformity of the tibia. The child who is a candidate for tibial osteotomy should demonstrate less than −10° of internal tibial torsion or more than 35 to 40° of external tibial torsion as measured by the thigh-foot angle.[55,60] However, tibial osteotomy may be indicated for less extreme values of tibial torsion when coexistent femoral torsion is present. Proximal and distal osteotomies have been described with or without con-

current fibular osteotomy. Distal osteotomy with pin fixation and long leg cast immobilization is preferred for pure rotational deformity, and proximal osteotomy is preferred if simultaneous correction of an angular deformity is desired.[33] Khermosh et al. recently described a serrated type of osteotomy for the femur or tibia for the simultaneous correction of torsional and angular deformities.[29] Krengal et al. demonstrated a 13 percent complication rate associated with proximal osteotomy and no serious complications with distal supramalleolar osteotomy.[33] Fibular osteotomy is suggested for proximal osteotomies[60] but is not necessarily required for correction by distal osteotomy.[48] A decreased complication rate has been found for distal tibial osteotomy without fibular osteotomy compared to the two procedures when performed together.[40] Fixation of tibial osteotomies usually involves Steinman pins or external fixators, with equally good results.[45] Ilizarov techniques have also been described for tibial derotation.[24]

ARTHRITIS AND PATELLOFEMORAL DISEASE

A growing body of evidence has associated rotational deformity of the femur and tibia to painful disorders of the hip and knee. Torsional deformity of the femur of more than 30° has been shown to produce altered and increased patellofemoral contact pressures.[36] Insall et al. have suggested an association between excessive femoral anteversion and chondromalacia.[27] Femoral antetorsion and internal tibial torsion have been implicated in osteoarthritis of the knee.[13,44,63,64,67] The torsional malalignment syndrome consists of femoral antetorsion with marked compensatory external rotation of the tibia.[9] These patients demonstrate toeing out with an in-turning patella and frequently have anterior knee pain and an awkward gait. Delgado et al. recently reported successful treatment of this syndrome with femoral and/or tibial osteotomies.[9] Studies have failed to relate femoral antetorsion to arthritis of the hip.[30] However, a syndrome of diminished femoral anteversion has been described that appears to be associated with osteoarthritis of the hip.[62] The patients in this study had an average femoral version of 8.5° (normal = 12 to 16°) and developed pain between the ages of 12 and 30. Approximately 18 percent showed early signs of osteoarthritis of the hip. Derotational femoral osteotomy successfully alleviated pain. Further studies are needed to address the question of whether derotational osteotomies should be indicated for the prevention of arthritis and patellofemoral disease in patients with rotational deformity of the lower limb.

REFERENCES

1. Aamodt A, Terjesen T, Eine J, Kvistad KA: Femoral anteversion measured by ultrasound and CT: A comparative study. *Skel Radiol* 24:105–109, 1995.

2. Barlow DW, Staheli LT: Effects of lateral rotation splinting on lower extremity bone growth: An in vivo study in rabbits. *J Pediatr Orthop* 11:583–587, 1991.

3. Beaty JH: Femoral shaft fractures in children and adolescents. *J Am Acad Orthop Surg* 3:207–217, 1995.

4. Braten M, Terjesen T, Rossvoll I. Torsional deformity after intramedullary nailing of femoral shaft fractures: Measurement of anteversion angles in 110 patients. *J Bone Joint Surg [Br]* 75:799–803, 1993.

5. Butler-Manuel PA, Guy RL, Heatley FW: Measurement of tibial torsion—A new technique applicable to ultrasound and computed tomography. *Br J Radiol* 65:119–126, 1992.

6. Cheng JCY, Chan PS, Chiang SC, Hui PW: Angular and rotational profile of the lower limb in 2630 Chinese children. *J Pediatr Orthop* 11:154–161, 1991.

7. Clementz BG: Assessment of tibial torsion and rotational deformity with a new fluoroscopic technique. *Clin Orthop* 245:199–209, 1989.

8. Davids JR: Rotational deformity and remodeling after fracture of the femur in children. *Clin Orthop Rel Res* 302:27–35, 1994.

9. Delgado ED, Schoenecker PL, Rich MM, Capelli AM: Treatment of severe torsional malalignment syndrome. *J Pediatr Orthop* 16:484–488, 1996.

10. Dunlap K, Shands AR, Hollister, et al: A new method for determination of torsion of the femur. *J Bone Joint Surg* 35A:289, 1953.

11. Eckhoff DG, Montgomery WK, Kilcoyne RF, Stamm ER: Femoral morphometry and anterior knee pain. *Clin Orthop Rel Res* 302:64–68, 1994.

12. Eckhoff DG, Winter WG: Femoral and tibial torsion: Editorial comment. *Clin Orthop Rel Res* 302:2–3, 1994.

13. Eckhoff DG, Kramer RC, Alongi CA, VanGerven DP: Femoral anteversion and arthritis of the knee. *J Pediatr Orthop* 14:608–610, 1994.

14. Eckhoff DG, Johnson K: Three-dimensional computed tomography reconstruction of tibial torsion. *Clin Orthop Rel Res* 302:42–46, 1994.

15. Eyres KS, Douglas DL, Bell MJ: Closed intramedullary osteotomy for the correction of deformity of the femur. *J R Coll Surg Edinb* 38:302–306, 1993.

16. Fabry G, MacEwen GD, Shands AR: Torsion of the femur: A follow-up study of normal and abnormal conditions. *J Bone Joint Surg* 55A:1726, 1993.

17. Fabry G, Cheng LX, Molenaers G: Normal and abnormal torsional development in children. *Clin Orthop Rel Res* 302:23–26, 1994.

18. Fuchs R, Staheli LT: Sprinting and intoeing. *J Pediatr Orthop* 16:489–491, 1996.

19. Gage JR: *Gait Analysis in Cerebral Palsy.* London, MacKeith Press, 1991.

20. Germain P, le Damany M: Technique of tibial tropometry. *Clin Orthop Rel Res* 302:4–10, 1994.

21. Griffin PP: The lower limb, in Morrissy RT, Weinstein LT (eds): *Lovell and Winter's Pediatric Orthopedics.* Philadelphia, Lippincott, 1978.

22. Guidera KJ, Ganey TM, Keneally CR, Ogden JA: The embryology of lower extremity torsion. *Clin Orthop Rel Res* 302:17–21, 1994.

23. Heinrich SD, Sharps C: Lower extremity torsional deformities in children: A prospective comparison of two treatment modalities. *Orthop Trans* 13:554–555, 1989.

24. Herzenberg JE, Smith JD, Paley D: Correcting torsional deformities with Ilizarov's apparatus. *Clin Orthop Rel Res* 302:36–41, 1994.

25. Hoeffel JC: A simple roentgenographic measurement of femoral anteversion. A short note (letter; comment). *J Bone Joint Surg [Am]* 76:313, 1994.

26. Hutter CG, Scott W: Tibial torsion. *J Bone Joint Surg* 31A:511, 1949.

27. Insall J, Falvo KA, Wise DW: Chondromalacia pattellae: A prospective study. *J Bone Joint Surg* 58A:1, 1976.

28. Katz K, Krikler R, Wielunsky E, Merlob P: Effect of neonatal posture on later limb rotation and gait in premature infants. *J Pediatr Orthop* 11:520–522, 1991.

29. Kermosh O, Wientroub S: Serrated (W/M) osteotomy: A new technique for simultaneous correction of angular and torsional deformity of the lower limb in children. *J Pediatr Orthop Part B* 4:204–208, 1995.

30. Kitoaka HB, Weiner DS, Cook AJ, et al. Relationship between femoral anteversion and osteoarthritis of the hip. *J Pediatr Orthop* 9:396–404, 1989.

31. Kling TF, Hensinger RN: Angular and torsional deformities of the lower limbs in children. *Clin Orthop* 176:136–147, 1983.

32. Knittel G, Staheli LT: The effectiveness of shoe modifications for intoeing. *Orthop Clin North Am* 7:1019–1025, 1976.

33. Krengel WF III, Staheli LT: Tibial rotation osteotomy for idiopathic torsion: A comparison of the proximal and distal osteotomy levels (review). *Clin Orthop Rel Res* 283:285–289, 1992.

34. Kumar SJ, MacEwen GD: Torsional abnormalities in children's lower extremities. *Orthop Clin North Am* 13:629–639, 1982.

35. Laplaza FJ, Root L: Femoral anteversion and neck-shaft angles in hip instability in cerebral palsy. *J Pediatr Orthop* 14:719–723, 1994.

36. Lee TQ, Sanford HA, Bennett KA, et al. The influence of fixed rotational deformities of the femur on the patellofemoral contact pressures in human cadaver knees. *Clin Orthop Rel Res* 302:69–74, 1994.

37. Liu XC, Fabry G, Van Audekercke R, et al. The ground reaction force in the gait of intoeing children. *J Pediatr Orthop Part B* 4:80–85, 1995.

38. Losel S, Burgess-Milliron MJ, Micheli LJ, Edington CJ: A simplified technique for determining foot progression angle in children 4 to 16 years of age. *J Pediatr Orthop* 16:570–574, 1996.

39. Magilligan DJ: Calculation of the angle of anteversion by means of horizontal lateral roentgenography. *J Bone Joint Surg* 38A:1231, 1956.

40. Manouel M, Johnson LO: The role of fibular osteotomy in rotational osteotomy of the distal tibia. *J Pediatr Orthop* 14:611–614, 1994.

41. McSweeny A: A study of femoral torsion in children. *J Bone Joint Surg* 53B:90–95, 1971.

42. Miller F, Merlo M, Liang Y, et al. Femoral version and neck shaft angle. *J Pediatr Orthop* 13:382–388, 1991.

43. Moens P, Lammens J, Molenaers G, Fabry G: Femoral derotation for increased hip anteversion: A new surgical technique with a modified Ilizarov frame. *J Bone Joint Surg [Br]* 77:107–109, 1995.

44. Moussa M: Rotational malalignment and femoral torsion in osteoarthritic knees with patellofemoral joint involvement: A CT scan study. *Clin Orthop Rel Res* 304:176–183, 1994.

45. Mylle J, Lammens J, Fabry G: Derotation osteotomy to correct rotational deformities of the lower extremities in children: A comparison of three methods. *Act Orthop Belg* 59:287–292, 1993.

46. Pasciak M, Stoll TM, Hefti F: Use of ultrasonography for measurement of femur anteversion and tibial torsion. *Chir Narzad Ruchu Ortop Polska* 59:279–283, 1994.

47. Payne LZ, Deluca PA: Intertrochanteric versus supracondylar osteotomy for severe femoral anteversion. *J Pediatr Orthop* 14:39–44, 1994.

48. Rattey T, Hyndman J: Rotational osteotomies of the leg: Tibia alone versus both tibia and fibula. *J Pediatr Orthop* 14:615–618, 1994.

49. Reikeras O, Hoiseth A: Torsion of the leg determined by computed tomography. *Acta Orthop Scand* 60:330–333, 1989.

50. Sayli U, Bolukbasi S, Atik OS, Gundogdu S: Determination of tibial torsion by computed tomography. *J Foot Ankle Surg* 33:144–147, 1994.

51. Schneider B, Laubenberger J, Wildner M, et al: NMR tomographic measurement of femoral antetorsion and tibial torsion. *Rofo Fortschr Geb Rontgenstr Neuen Bildgeb Verfahr* 162:229–231, 1995.

52. Schwarze DJ, Denton RJ: Normal values of neonatal lower limbs: An evaluation of 1000 neonates. *J Pediatr Orthop* 13:758–760, 1993.

53. Shands AR, Steele MK: Torsion of the femur. *J Bone Joint Surg* 40A:803, 1958.

54. Staheli LT, Engel GM: Tibial torsion: A method of assessment and a survey of normal children. *Clin Orthop* 86:183, 1972.

55. Staheli LT: Rotational problems in children. *AAOS Instr Course Lect* 43:199–209, 1994.

56. Staheli LT: Symposium: Torsional abnormalities. *Contemp Orthop* 10:80–111, 1985.

57. Stroud KL, Smith AD, Kruse RW: The relationship between increased femoral anteversion in childhood and patello-femoral pain in adulthood. *Orthop Trans* 13:555, 1989.

58. Svenningsen S, Apelset K, Terjesen T, Anda S: Osteotomy for femoral anteversion: Complications in 95 children. *Acta Orthop Scand* 60:401–405, 1989.

59. Tachdjian MO: The foot and leg, in *Pediatric Orthopedics,* 2d ed. Philadelphia, Saunders, 1990, p 2803.

60. Tolo VT: The lower extremity, in Morrissy RT, Weinstein LT (eds): *Lovell and Winter's Pediatric Orthopedics,* 4th ed. Philadelphia, Lippincott-Raven, 1996.

61. Tomczak R, Gunther K, Pfeifer T, et al: The measurement of the femoral torsion angle in children by NMR tomography compared to CT and ultrasound. *Rofo Fortschritte Geb Rontgenstr Neuen Bildgeb Verfahr* 162:224–228, 1995.

62. Tonnis D, Heinecke A: Diminished femoral antetorsion syndrome: A cause of pain and arthritis. *J Pediatr Orthop* 11:419–431, 1991.

63. Turner MS: The association between tibial torsion and knee joint pathology. *Clin Orthop Rel Res* 302:47–51, 1994.

64. Turner MS, Smillie IS: The effect of tibial torsion on the pathology of the knee. *J Bone Joint Surg* 63B:396–398, 1981.

65. Verbeek HOF, Bender J, Sawidis K: Rotational deformities after fractures of the femoral shaft in childhood. *Injury* 8:43, 1976.

66. Weseley MS, Barenfield PA, Eisenstein AL: Thoughts on intoeing and outtoeing: Twenty years experience with over 5000 cases and a review of the literature. *Foot Ankle* 2:49–57, 1981.

67. Yagi T: Tibial torsion in patients with medial-type osteoarthrotic knees. *Clin Orthop Rel Res* 302:52–56, 1994.

CHAPTER 45

Limb-Length Discrepancy in Children

Kenneth J. Guidera, John A. Ogden, and Timothy M. Ganey

Limb-length discrepancy is a frequent and complex problem in pediatric orthopaedics. A unilateral deficiency of growth potential in a limb has both present and future clinical implications. Limb-length inequality is more than simple skeletal shortening. The adjacent soft tissues, including neurovascular structures, are all involved and have to be carefully considered in contemplating a corrective procedure.[1] In the growing child the measured inequality may increase as the limb elongates. Fortunately, there are tools to assist in the prediction of future discrepancy in most patients.

The etiology of shortening is also quite variable and may include traumatic, infectious, or congenital origin.[2,3] Infrequently tumors or the treatment of a malignancy may affect growth. Each of these conditions affects physical growth differently. The postinfectious patient may have an incompletely destroyed growth plate on either side of a joint or in multifocal areas. Concomitant joint involvement is common. The possibility of recurrence is present if there is residual infection, such as a chronic metaphyseal or epiphyseal abscess. Hip instability after septic avascular necrosis of the proximal femur is common and may complicate any attempts to lengthen the shortened femur. Residual joint damage will affect lengthening. Posttraumatic discrepancies may have associated soft tissue injuries such as muscle loss, scarring, or joint inquiry with restriction of motion. Congenital deformities frequently have associated muscular anomalies. An example of this is fibular hemimelia, in which there may be dysplasia and soft tissue contractures about the ankle with absent rays on the lateral border of the foot (Fig. 45-1). Alternatively, some congenital deformities have overgrowth as a phenomenon, rather than shortening.[4] These cases tend to have varied responses to lengthening or shortening procedures and should be approached with caution, since the growth potential may be unpredictable.

The anticipated actual and potential effects of the limb-length discrepancy on the child must be evaluated. Future stature and limb growth need to be extrapolated. Genetics and family height are important determinants of treatment, as are social issues. For example, dwarfs are much more accepted in the United States then in Europe and actually have a strong lobbying group against lengthening in this country. Other issues, such as previous surgeries and hospitalizations, should be taken into account. Children with limb-length discrepancies and their families may carry significant psychological scarring and stress related to the deformity and any previous surgery. Some patients simply cannot tolerate the extended time of the lengthening procedure and should be guided toward a less invasive and shorter treatment option. Amputation may often be the treatment of choice and requires psychological preparation for the patient and family, with pre- and postoperative counseling.

It is imperative that the treating orthopaedic surgeon be cognizant of all the ramifications of the morphologic discrepancy in the specific patient, including etiology, associated anomalies, growth potential, and the patient's and family's stability. A team approach is the best way to deal with these complex patients; this includes the surgeon, pediatrician, physical and occupational therapist, orthotist, social worker, and nurse. The team should work together closely to individualize treatment for each patient, realizing that surgery is not required for every case and is only a part of the treatment spectrum.

THE GROWTH OF LONG BONES

The sequence of growth in long bones is well established histologically.[1] Growth may be both an asset and a detriment with regard to limb-length discrepancy. Growth may worsen a deformity or alternatively equalize minor differences. There are two primary methods of bone growth in children.[1,3] Membranous growth involves the maturation and condensation of immature mesenchymal tissues. There is a progressive calcification of a bony matrix on a fibrous network spreading laterally from a central focus. This is the method primarily found in flat bones, but it is an essential component in the growth of all bones.

Elongation of long bones occurs through enchondral bone formation. This occurs through the epiphysis and the physis, which initially are completely cartilaginous. Secondary ossification develops within this cartilaginous region. The histologic pattern of endochondral growth is as follows: Cell columns develop longitudinally and are divided into zones based on physiological activity. There is progressive maturation through the zones of growth and maturation. This is an active area involving both growth and remodeling. The physis has sites of vascular ingrowth and responds to chemical influences (paracrine, endocrine). For example, estrogen may slow down new bone formation through its effect on collagen cross linking, or growth hormone may stimulate elongation.[1] Any injury or infectious process to the physis may result in full or partial growth arrest with shortening or angular deformity (Fig. 45-2). Metabolic diseases such as rickets, developmental processes such as Blount's disease, and congenital anomalies such as hemiepiphyseal dysplasia may all result in partial or complete growth arrest or alteration.

PATIENT EVALUATION

Any child with a limb-length discrepancy requires a thorough evaluation. The initial screening should consist of a careful physical examination and radiographic analysis.

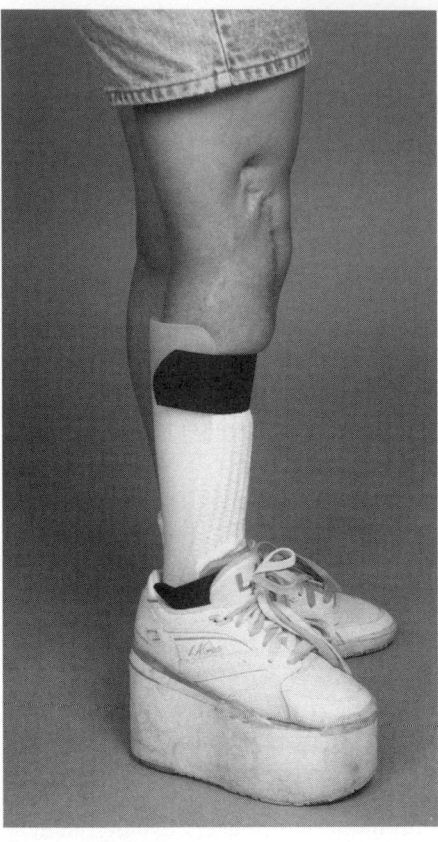

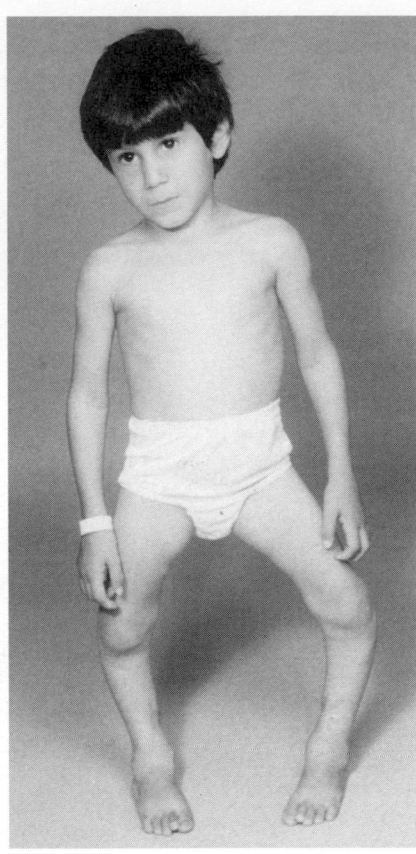

A

B

Figure 45-1 *A.* An example of posttraumatic shortening with soft tissue and osseous injury involving both the growth plate and the joint. Scarring and joint contracture may complicate attempts at lengthening in cases such as this. *B.* Congenital anomalies as in this case of spondyloepiphyseal dysplasia may require both angular correction and lengthening. There are frequently associated anomalies that may have to be addressed prior to any surgical procedure.

The surgeon must remain cognizant of the implications of future growth, since any congenital or acquired deformity or shortening may be affected by future growth. In general, the situation worsens progressively as the limbs continually elongate, albeit in a disparate manner. It is therefore imperative for the treating physician to understand the etiology of the shortening and the child's future growth pattern. Serial examinations are essential, as a one time evaluation is not sufficient to plan a treatment scheme for a limb length discrepancy. At least two subsequent assessments should be made after the initial visit in order to plot the child's growth pattern and determine the nature of the discrepancy or deformity with regard to future growth.

At each subsequent visit, a careful analysis of limb lengths, joint motion, angular deformity, and related posttraumatic or congenital anomalies should be made. The limb lengths may be measured by either the tape or block methods.[2,5] With the former technique, one measures with the patient supine from the anterior iliac spine to the medial malleolus, comparing lengths with the contralateral side. There is a risk of measurement error if the knee or hip is flexed or if there is inexact placement of the tape over the bony cutaneous landmarks. With the block method, the patient stands on measured blocks (under the short-sided foot) until the pelvis appears to be level. The examiner determines this by placing a finger on each iliac crest and observing any differences in height.

Radiographic evaluation should include anteroposterior (AP) and lateral views of the involved long bones, scanograms of the involved upper or lower extremities, wrist films for bone age, and tomograms or computed tomography to evaluate growth plate disturbances. Scanograms should be obtained serially, at least once a year in cases of long-term follow-up (Fig. 45-3). This permits the computed plotting of limb lengths and makes possible a reasonable prediction of future growth patterns. At least three evaluations are required, separated by an average of 6 months. Scanograms are taken with both lower extremities on a long radiographic cassette, with x-ray beams centered over each joint and a radiopaque ruler between the extremities. The upper limbs are measured on separate cassettes. The distance between each joint is measured, giving the relative lengths of each long bone and of the entire limb. An assessment can be made as to how much each long bone contributes to the overall discrepancy, which is an important factor when surgical intervention is being contemplated. The lengths obtained should be recorded and serially plotted on growth charts. A common problem with scanograms is a joint flexion deformity or inappropriate placement of the limb on the x-ray cassettes, which may result in inaccurate measurements.

Wrist films are obtained periodically to determine bone age. The films are compared with standards in the Greulich and Pyle atlas[6] and used to plot coordinates on the growth chart. There is some subjectivity to this inter-

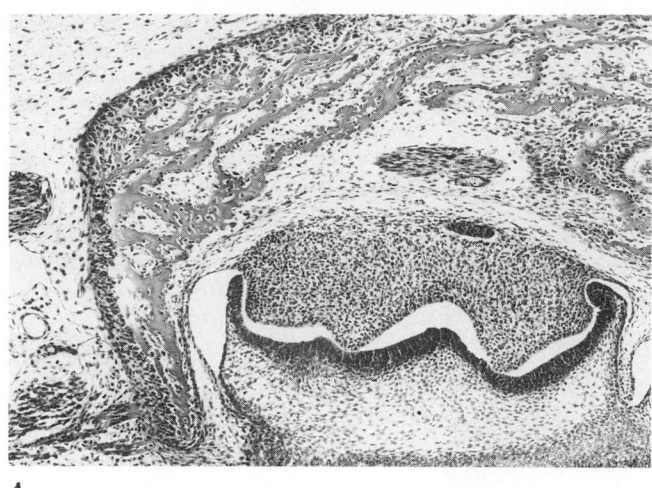

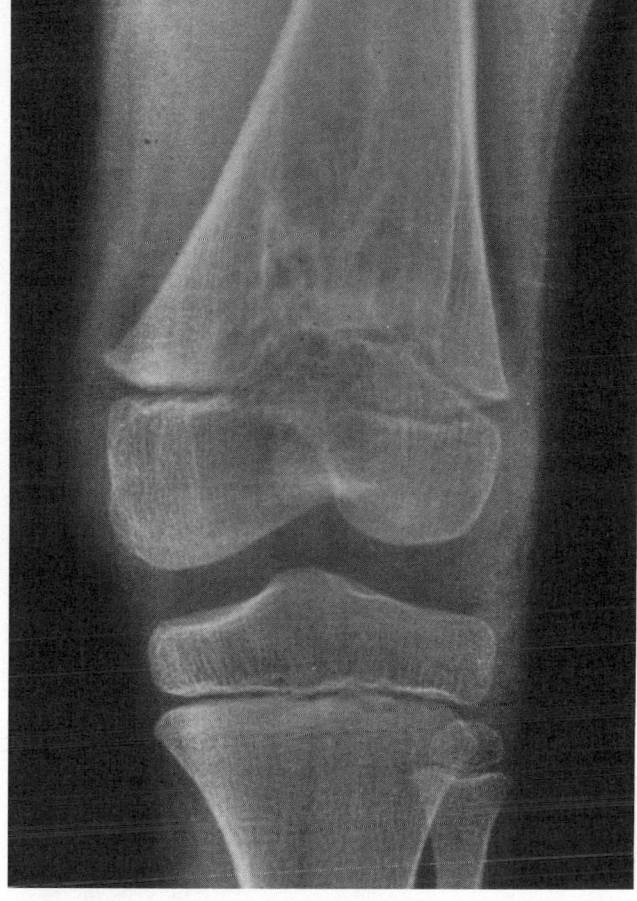

Figure 45-2 *A.* An example of both membranous and enchondral growth seen in a rat embryo. The former is more common in the flat bones and the latter in the physis of long bones. *B.* An area of central growth arrest after a physeal injury. This may result in shortening or angular deformity. Physeal bridges under 50 percent may be resected if there is enough growth remaining.

pretation. The standards were developed using a population of white Anglo-Saxon children; therefore they may not be applicable to other population groups.

Growth Charts

In order to follow and predict growth accurately, objective measurements and guides are necessary. Growth tables that allow the plotting of data and prediction of future growth for both boys and girls are readily available. The Green-Anderson chart[7] presents both a prediction of future growth and timing for epiphysiodesis. As with other methods, several evaluations are required to accurately predict these values.

Moseley[8,9] converted the Green-Anderson tables into a straight-line graph. This method requires three reference points of length. Using the bone age (from hand films), the points are plotted, giving predictions of the final lengths of both the long and short limbs. One may then calculate the timing and appropriateness of an intervention. This chart has been reproduced and is available for placement into the patient's medical records. Moseley has refined this system into a computer model that allows sequential insertion of the data and returns predictions and recommendations for timing of epiphysiodesis (Fig. 45-3). It ana-

lyzes past and future growth, predicts epiphysiodesis, and suggests timing to achieve equality. Although this and other tools simplify the evaluation, the surgeon should not consider these a substitute for careful clinical and radiographic analysis.

TREATMENT

Not all limb length discrepancies require operative treatment. Observation is frequently the best option. This should be carefully explained to the parents, so that they will not feel the problem is being ignored. This is analogous to the situation of families with children who have torsional deformities that will be likely to correct spontaneously with growth. Careful follow-up should be provided to ensure that the discrepancy does not increase and to intervene when appropriate. Many parents worry that the spine or hips will be out of alignment due to minor limb-length discrepancies. One frequently encounters adults who have up to 1 in of shortening and either did not realize it or were never symptomatic. With this in mind, the surgeon should recommend no intervention for children having a 1- to 2-cm limb-length discrepancy. However, one

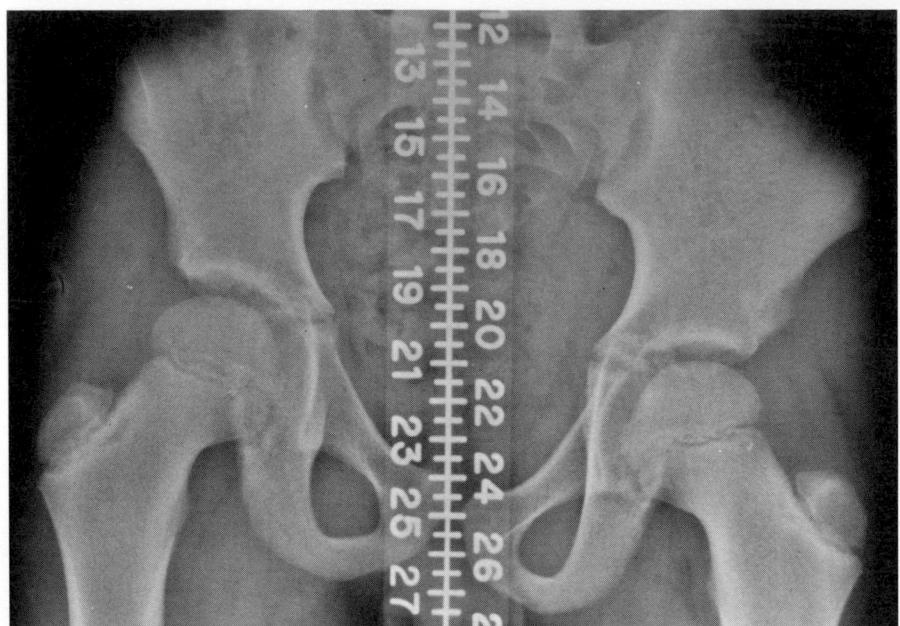

A

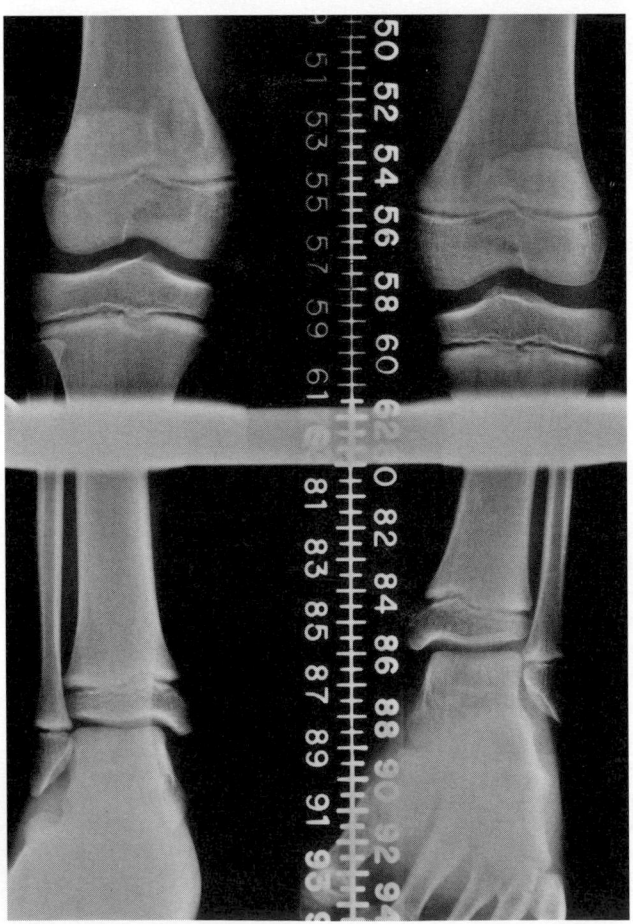

B

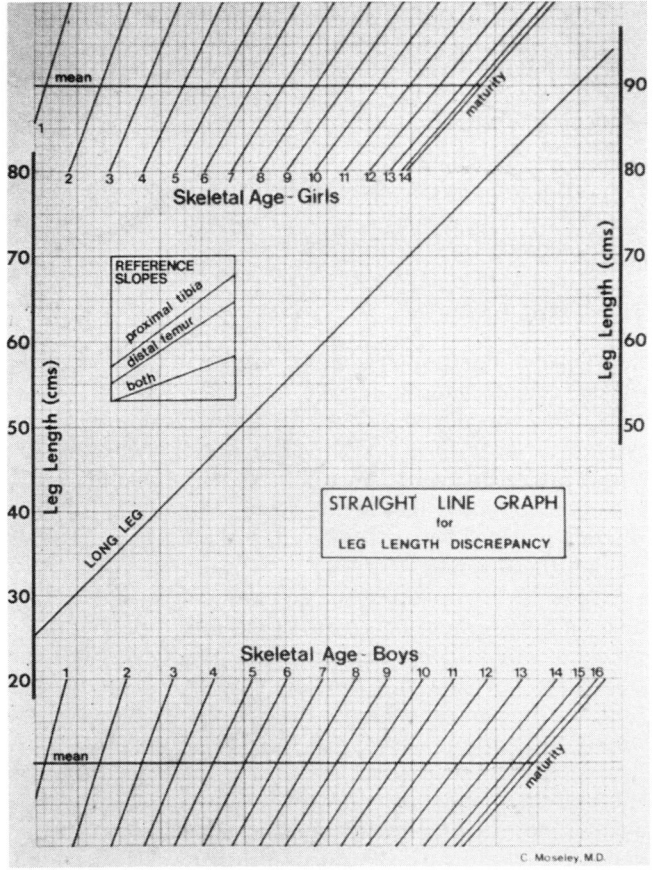

C

Figure 45-3 *A* and *B.* A scanogram provides radiographic evaluation of the length discrepancy by measuring between all three joints of the lower extremity. Malposition or joint contractures may yield unreliable results. *C.* At least three reference points from scanograms are required in order to plot the growth discrepancy and the time for intervention on the Moseley chart, which is reproduced and placed in the medical record.

must be cognizant of future growth potential, as this small amount of shortening may change.

Shoe lifts may be prescribed for children with discrepancies under 3 cm. A lift of up to 1 cm may go inside the shoe and the rest can be placed outside, along the sole. Some children may not tolerate lifts due to their clumsiness (e.g., those with neuromuscular abnormalities such as cerebral palsy) or cosmetic appearance. A large lift may be used as a temporizing measure in patients awaiting a definitive procedure, whether elective amputation or lengthening.

PHYSEAL DAMAGE

Following various types of physeal trauma or infection, a segment of the growth plate may be sufficiently damaged such that it develops a traversing column of sclerotic bone that restricts growth. The overall effect may be decreased longitudinal growth, increasing angulation at the level of the physis, or both. Correction of the length discrepancy by diaphyseal or metaphyseal corticotomy does not address the specific etiology. If feasible, the sclerotic bone bridge should be resected and replaced with an interposition material that may prevent reformation of the bridge.

The objective of surgical excision is the complete removal of the bone bridging between the metaphyseal and epiphyseal ossification centers while preserving as much of the physeal cartilage as possible. Appropriate preoperative planning is essential. This entails various techniques such as hypocycloid tomography or CT scans (especially with three-dimensional reconstruction and subtraction potential) to determine the size of the bridge, its peripheral contour, and its exact location. A bridge greater than 40 percent of the overall physeal area probably should not be resected, as the potential for a desirable result (namely, restoration of longitudinal growth) would be limited.

There are three basic types of bone bridge. Type 1 is a peripheral bridge extending from the edge of the metaphysis inward. There is focal damage to the zone of Ranvier. Type 2 is a linear bridge that extends from one metaphyseal focus to another. The medial malleolus is a common site for such linear bridges. Type 3 is a central lesion, with the bridge being surrounded by physeal tissue. There is no peripheral involvement and the zone of Ranvier is intact. The type 3 lesion tends to become conical (pointed toward the metaphysis) as the surrounding physis attempts to grow longitudinally and latitudinally.

A peripheral bridge (type 1) should be approached directly, using fluoroscopy to select the initial resection site. The sclerotic bone contrasts with normal metaphyseal trabecular bone. Overlying periosteum is completely resected. The estimated bridge is then roughly resected as a block. Under direct vision, the remaining sclerotic bone is carefully removed to expose the physis and contiguous trabecular bone of both the metaphyseal and epiphyseal ossification centers. The physis should be exposed to the point where it merges with the unossified cartilage of the periphery of the epiphysis.

A linear bridge (type 2) is resected as a "tunnel," with the direction being carefully planned through preoperative imaging. Following resection, two "parallel" physes should be evident, with a peripheral hole at each end of the tunnel.

The central bridge (type 3) may be approached through a metaphyseal window or by the removal of a wedge of metaphyseal bone that can be replaced at the end of the procedure. The sclerotic bone is progressively resected, following it into the epiphyseal ossification center. A "circular" physis should be evident all around the resection cavity.

Fat and methylmethacrylate are the most commonly used interposition materials. The surgical defect should be packed with the material. Periosteum should not be placed across any peripheral defect that includes metaphysis, physis, and epiphysis. Angular deformities may be corrected by concomitant osteotomy, especially if they are not in the plane of motion of the joint. Alternatively, the patient may be followed for 3 to 6 months to see if a bridge starts to reform. The osteotomy may be factored into any subsequent surgical needs.

An interesting approach is to use distraction epiphysiolysis (chondrodiastasis). Progressive distraction across the physis may fracture the bridge and the surrounding trabecular bone. This method may be used to lengthen the limb, correct the angular deformity, and "break" the bridge. Because premature epiphysiodesis occurs following chondrodiastasis, the procedure should be done shortly before growth would normally be expected to cease. Also, the bridge is not resected. Accordingly, reformation of bridge bone from the neoosteogenesis is a possibility.

Children treated with bridge resections must be followed closely to monitor responsive growth and to treat the limb-length inequality until equilibration. Further, the damaged physis subjected to bridge resection has a great propensity to premature overall closure.

Epiphysiodesis

With limb-length discrepancies of up to 4 to 5 cm, epiphysiodesis is a prudent surgical intervention. This procedure is basically the surgical interruption of the physiology of the growth plate. In much the same way that a traumatic insult may result in an osseous bridge, which leads to growth arrest, the surgical disruption results in premature closure, or fusion, of the physis. This is done at a predetermined time to stop the growth of the longer limb and to reasonably equalize both sides by the end of limb growth.[2] The techniques of this procedure are relatively simple. The variable aspects are adequate preparation, prediction, and timing. Growth may be temporarily stopped by placing staples across the growth plate; these may be removed later when it is desired for growth to resume.[5] This may be done unilaterally or bilaterally. This technique is unpredictable; growth after staple removal may not proceed at the rate previously anticipated. Other methods of epiphysiodesis include the Phemister and White techniques, in which a bone block is removed from each side of the growth plate, rotated, and reinserted to create an osseous bridge on each side of the physis.[10,11] A cast is applied for 6 weeks, and the consolidation is usually complete within 2 to 3 months. Since the area may be unstable and prone to fracture during the healing period, it must be protected following surgery.

A less invasive method of epiphysiodesis is done percutaneously using an image intensifier.[12] This involves small lateral and medial incisions over the physis with drill placement into the growth plate under C-arm visualization (Fig. 45-4). The physis is then drilled or reamed, destroying the growth potential of the area and stimulating the formation of an osseous bridge. The surgeon must be cognizant of the undulating nature of the physis; therefore simple, straight, transverse drilling should not be performed. The drill position must be checked periodically with the C arm to assure complete physeal obliteration. Breakage of the drill bit may occur. A hazard with this technique is increased radiation exposure when the image intensifier is used excessively. Postoperatively, the patient may bear partial weight on an immobilized knee and be allowed early range-of-motion exercises. The patient must be followed postoperatively both clinically and radiographically to evaluate the progress of the epiphysiodesis. The surgeon should be aware that although this procedure is not technically difficult, the timing is crucial in order to equalize the limb lengths reasonably.

Another method to achieve limb equality is a shortening procedure. This may be done as a femoral or tibial osteotomy with a closed or open technique. It should be performed either at or near the end of growth. The calculated amount of bone to be removed from the long side is excised and the ends are plated with the open technique or removed with special intramedullary osteotomies and

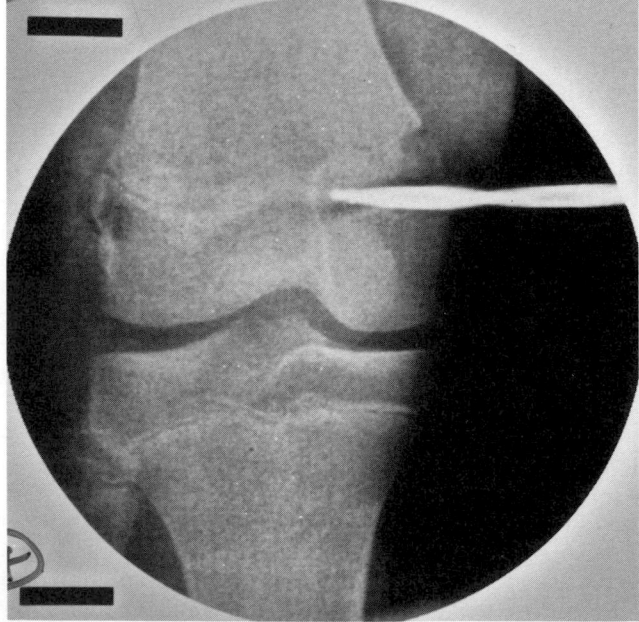

Figure 45-4 A percutaneous epiphysiodesis may be done through two small incisions with no postoperative cast required. The technique is simple but the correct timing is essential.

supported by an intramedullary rod with the closed technique.[13] This latter method is more technically demanding but less invasive and is associated with lower morbidity. Many parents are averse to shortening the normal, longer side, but with proper patient selection, this may be an excellent tool for the correction of a limb-length discrepancy. This method may be used on inequalities ranging from 3 to 5 cm. At the upper end of this scale there may be significant soft tissue bulkiness after the shortening, and motor weakness, especially of the quadriceps mechanism, may be a problem.

Limb Lengthening

This intervention is generally reserved for limb-length discrepancies greater than 4 to 5 cm. The procedure should be approached with caution, patience, and a thorough understanding of the techniques, biology, and psychological aspects of lengthening a child's limb, since there are frequent complications throughout every lengthening procedure. A team approach should be used in the preoperative evaluation of the patient and family. The patient is evaluated by the surgeon as well as by nursing, social services, and physical therapy, with each discipline making its appropriate evaluation. Other procedures may be more appropriate for patients or families that may not be able to tolerate a prolonged lengthening procedure.

Limb lengthening is not a new procedure. Codilla and others attempted this technique in the 1920s using one-stage lengthening.[14] This was basically a cut-and-stretch technique, not allowing the soft tissues or bone to accommodate to the new length temporarily. There were some good results but also many failures and complications. In the 1940s, Anderson popularized a device that allowed for stable osseous fixation with single-stage lengthening. This device resembled some of the current methods of fixation, but the single lengthening mode, again, carried a high complication rate.[15]

The standard for lengthening procedures was introduced by Wagner.[16,17] This technique has been highly successful over many years and is still popular in numerous countries. The Wagner method involves a latterly placed unipolar fixator held with large Schanz screws combined with a diaphyseal osteotomy. There is a latency period after the osteotomy of 5 to 7 days before single daily distractions are begun at a rate of 1 mm per day[14] (Fig. 45-5). Once the length is achieved, the fixator is locked and a plate and screws are applied to the bone, holding it out to length. Bone grafts are frequently added to the defect as an adjunct to regenerate the bone. After radiographic consolidation, the plate may be removed. This is a large, thick plate which frequently leaves a significant stress riser when removed. There has been a high rate of fracture after plate removal, and for this reason many surgeons loosen the plate prior to complete removal.[18] This is done as a separate operative procedure, removing some of the screws and loosening others to dynamize the plate and new bone. In our series, patients had greater than four operations each and a 100 percent completion rate, but with adequate length achieved in each case. Some of the pitfalls

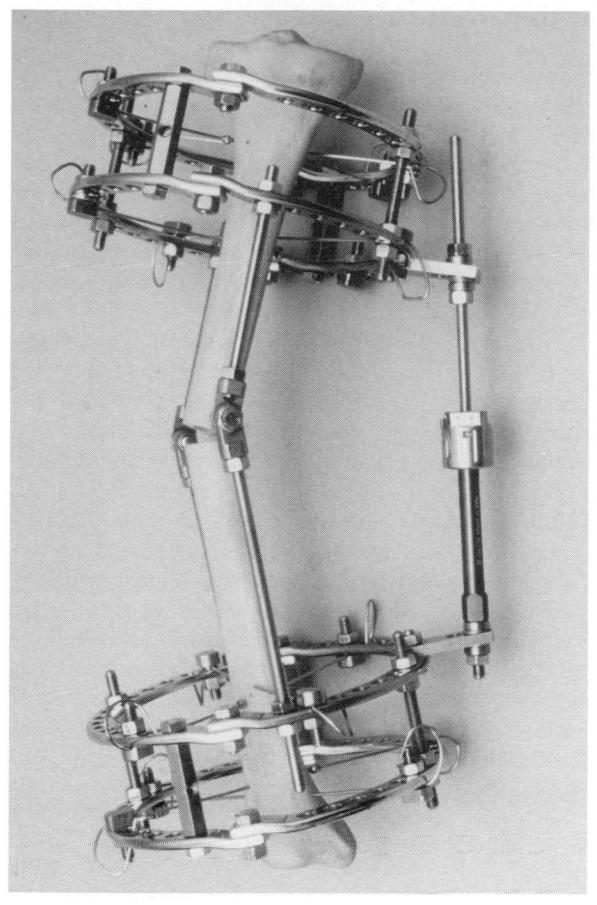

C

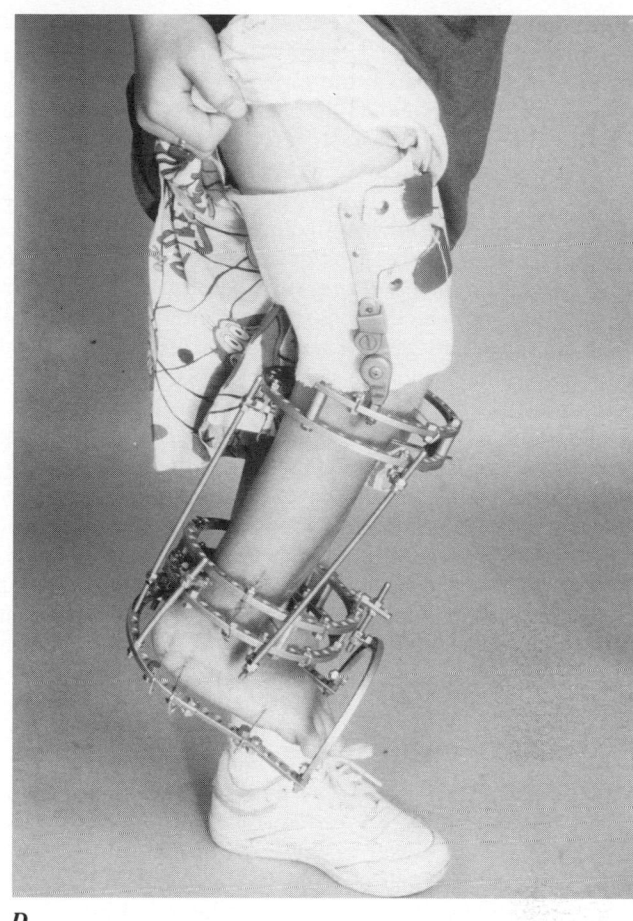

D

Figure 45-6 (*Continued*)

and joint stabilization. This technique allows fixation above and below a joint and simultaneous lengthening of both the femur and tibia. It can be applied to the upper extremity or the foot to correct residual angular deformity or shortening (Fig. 45-6).

Despite its advantages, the Ilizarov method has a significant complication rate, *as do all lengthening techniques.* In our experience, we have seen fractures above and below the fixator, pin-tract infections, joint stiffness, and cyst formation in the lengthened bones.[31] The procedure is technically demanding, requiring close follow-up and supervision. The family and patient must be educated in pin care and a range-of-motion exercise program. Formal physical therapy is beneficial during the lengthening and maturation processes. Frequent adjustments are needed, as there may be some shifting of the frame. When dealing with children, we have found removal of the apparatus best performed in the operating room. This allows the surgeon to stress the regenerate bone under fluoroscopy and to make a decision about removal or further dynamization. Following removal, an orthosis is fabricated to give additional protection while the callus strengthens. We cast the extremity while the brace is being constructed. Following complete consolidation and callus maturation, the orthosis is discontinued. Range-of-motion exercises and a strengthening program are continued during this period. The patient may bear full weight with the device on, but

few children in our experience do. Most use either partial weight bearing or a swing-through gait on crutches.

We have gained over 15 cm of length, or up to 20 to 22 percent of bone length. With the larger discrepancies, it is preferable to stage the procedure or to do a simultaneous lengthening of the femur and tibia. The knee and ankle must be protected and continual range-of-motion exercises maintained during the lengthening process. This is essential. The two constructs may be connected across the knee to provide stability and assist in the range-of-motion exercises. Orthotics may be custom-fabricated and attached to the frame to control the joint above or below the lengthening. The Italians and Russians have reported excellent results with the Ilizarov method and reports from American surgeons are encouraging but lacking in long-term follow-up.[32–34]

Chondrodiastasis

A technique that may gain some length toward the end of growth is chondrodiastasis.[35–37] This involves distraction through the growth plate using an external fixator. The physis, being the relatively susceptible area, is split apart by mechanical force progressively applied by the same rate and rhythm as callostasis lengthening. This results in new metaphyseal bone formation but also with closure of the growth plate. Ganel, however, described a 10-year-old patient who achieved lengthening through this technique and then continued to grow through the physis.[38] This type of lengthening is more popular outside of the United States. Two problems with chondrodiastasis are the placement of the epiphyseal pins, which may be intraarticular, and the amount of pain when the physis separates. It is, however, a valuable adjunct method for lengthening. The procedure must be done just prior to epiphysiodesis, since the "complication" is premature fusion of the widened physis.

With these available techniques, the surgeon has varied options for the correction of limb-length discrepancies. Numerous similar modalities are available, each of which incorporates the basic principles of either the Wagner, DeBastiani, or Ilizarov technique. It is not within the scope of this chapter to recommend one technique over another. The key is for the surgeon to choose patients carefully, educate them and their parents, have a good multidisciplinary team for backup, and anticipate complications. One should have more than one technique available and follow the biological principles presented by Ilizarov and DeBastiani.[20,21,25,27]

Upper-Extremity Lengthening

Limb-length discrepancy in the upper extremity generally requires less surgical intervention than that in the lower limb. Patients adapt quite well to this type of inequality, since there is no effect on gait or trunk balance. However, with a marked discrepancy or significant bilateral shortening, a lengthening procedure may enhance function. There is much less experience with this area as compared to the lower extremity. Cattaneo et al. have reported excellent results with lengthening of the humerus, radius, and ulna (generally for congenital defects), achieving an average of 9 cm in the humerus without major complications.[39,40] Frequently there are associated angular deformities of the hand and wrist, such as those seen with thrombocytopenia–absent radius syndrome, radial club hand, and congenital absence of the radius, which may be corrected simultaneously with the lengthening.[41,42] Occasionally wrist arthrodesis is necessary for stabilization. Either the Orthofix device or Ilizarov device is quite amenable to upper extremity lengthening and hand or wrist alignments (Fig. 45-7). There are hand adaptations to the Orthofix which allow finger and metacarpal lengthening. When these techniques are combined with soft tissue releases, skin grafting, and osteotomies, the results for hand and upper extremity alignment are good. With congenital anomalies of this area, the soft tissues are frequently quite resistant to stretching. Contractures of the digits are common and are best treated with splinting and a vigorous range-of-motion program. If the contractures become resilient, cessation of lengthening or soft tissue release may be necessary. Contractures of the hand and wrist tend to recur and are best treated with a long-term splinting or bracing program. The surgeon should be aware of these potential problems when lengthening the upper extremity, and considerations of cosmesis should not overcome regard for function.[43,44]

Correction of Angular Deformity

Many cases of congenital anomaly are amenable to combined lengthening and deformity correction. These include proximal focal femoral deficiency, Blount's disease, spondyloepiphyseal dysplasia, and tibial or fibular hemimelia. In each of these conditions, there may be a length discrepancy *plus* an angular deformity. Both the Ilizarov and Orthofix devices are designed to facilitate the process of dual deformity correction. Lengthening may be achieved primarily or simultaneously with angular correction. The Ilizarov apparatus has a system of hinges that allow this procedure; these should be placed over the area of deformity correction rather than at the site of the osteotomy.[24] The hinge placement may be adjusted laterally or medially to provide distraction along with angular correction. Improper hinge placement may result in displacement of the osteotomy and loss of correction. In Blount's disease, the surgeon may osteomize medially, leaving the lateral cortex intact. The proximal pins must be placed quite proximally, avoiding the joint space. Generally the physis is nearing closure at the time of this procedure. If it is not, care must be taken to avoid this area unless the medial physis is completely involved, in which case a lateral epiphysiodesis should be added. The frame is removed when there is adequate osseous consolidation, followed by casting or bracing. These patients are frequently quite heavy and prone to recurrence of their deformity and thus should be protected with an orthosis for an extended period.

In spondyloepihyseal dysplasia or multiple epiphyseal dysplasia, the deformity may involve the medial and lateral sides of the growth plate and both sides of the joint. There may be significant varus or valgus deformities with or without shortening that are amenable to surgical correction using an external fixator. The same principles as presented above apply and correction of both femoral and tibial deformity may be achieved simultaneously. Long-term bracing is again recommended to decrease the risk of future recurrence.

With proximal focal femoral deficiency, there is variable absence of the proximal femur along with shortening of the entire femur. Any lengthening procedure must address the femoral shortening, bowing, possible proximal instability, and muscular abnormalities, especially in the tensor fascia lata. In addition, there may be associated anomalies of the tibia, fibula, and foot. These problems may be treated simultaneously or serially but must be considered prior to any lengthening procedure or angular correction. Particularly, knee instability is a significant problem. Most patients have hypoplasia of the lateral femoral condyle and absence of one or both cruciate ligaments. This may lead to posterior displacement of the tibia during lengthening.

Congenital pseudarthrosis of the tibia is a condition involving tibial diaphyseal nonunion, which may be associated with neurofibromatosis. Various modalities have been proposed for the treatment of this resilient condition, including bone grafting, intramedullary rodding, vascularized fibular grafting, and amputation. Congenital pseudoarthrosis may be treated with the Ilizarov device,

Figure 45-7 Both the Orthofix (*A*) and the Ilizarov (*B*) devices are useful in upper extremity lengthening and angular deformity correction. Maintenance of digital range of motion is very important and may be assisted with outriggers, splints, and an aggressive occupational therapy program.

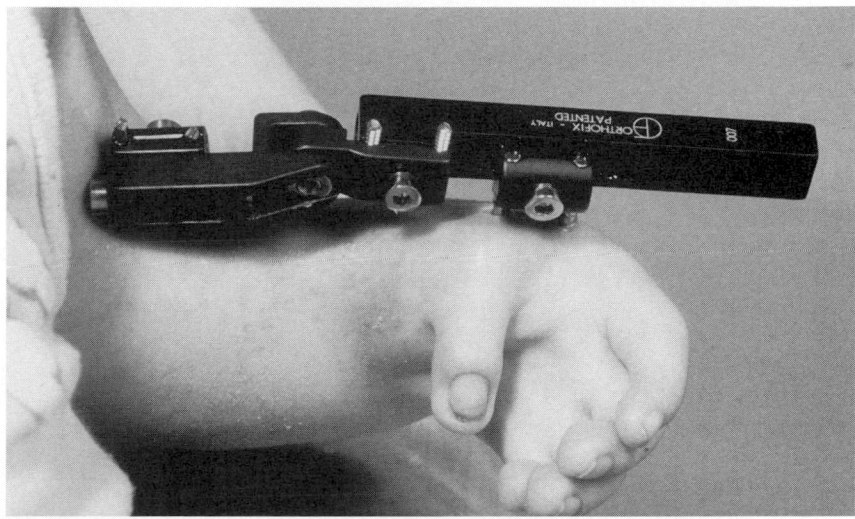

A

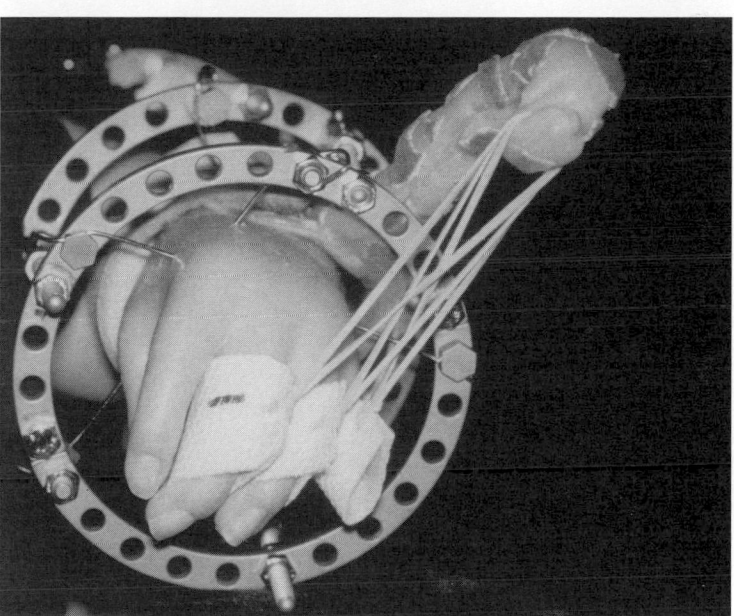

B

using compression across the pseudarthrosis site with distraction above for lengthening if needed.[45] Angular correction may also be applied simultaneously, and the ends of the pseudarthrosis are resected if they are atrophic. The ends are transported gradually to decrease swelling. Once the ends are docked, compression is applied until there is healing. With this technique, we had 9 of 11 patients heal. Two went on to amputation, which is an alternative when the applied techniques fail.[46]

Certain conditions may preclude lengthening procedures. These include active infections, generalized debilitation, psychosis, and spasticity. Conditions that require too much lengthening, such as shortening over 25 to 30 percent of limb length, should be treated instead with amputation and prosthetic fitting. Amputation should always be considered as a treatment option in conditions that in-

volve significant foot or limb deformities precluding adequate function even in the face of a successful lengthening procedure. An example of this may be a short fibular hemimelia with severe foot and ankle deformities or a significant joint contracture associated with shortening in arthrogryposis. Also, many posttraumatic patients have joint injuries with either instability or contracture. Our lengthening attempts have failed in cases of congenital insensitivity to pain, where osteomyelitis developed; postradiation syndrome, which precluded new bone formation; and upper extremity amelia, in which the lengthening procedure severely hindered activities of daily living (Fig. 45-8).

A condition with questionable indications for lengthening is achondroplasia. These individuals have no functional impairment and lengthening is cosmetic. The aesthetic procedure involves six lengthenings; bilateral humeri, femurs,

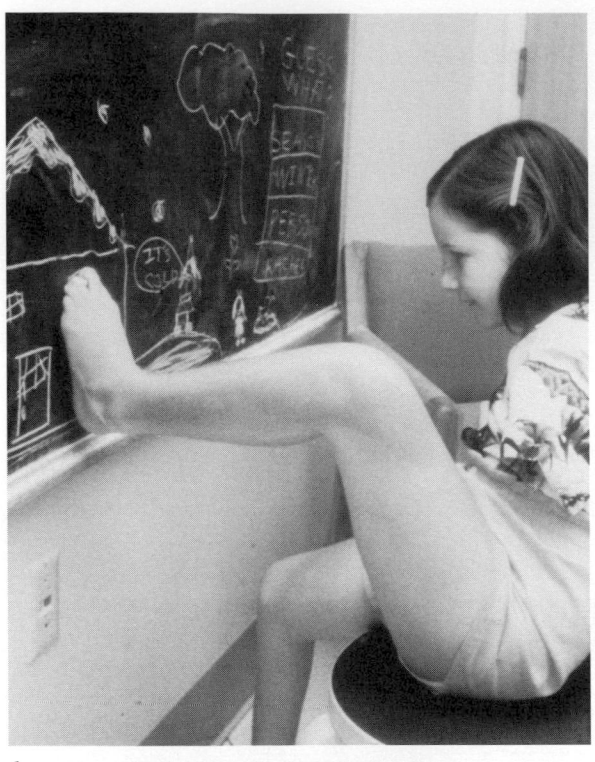

A

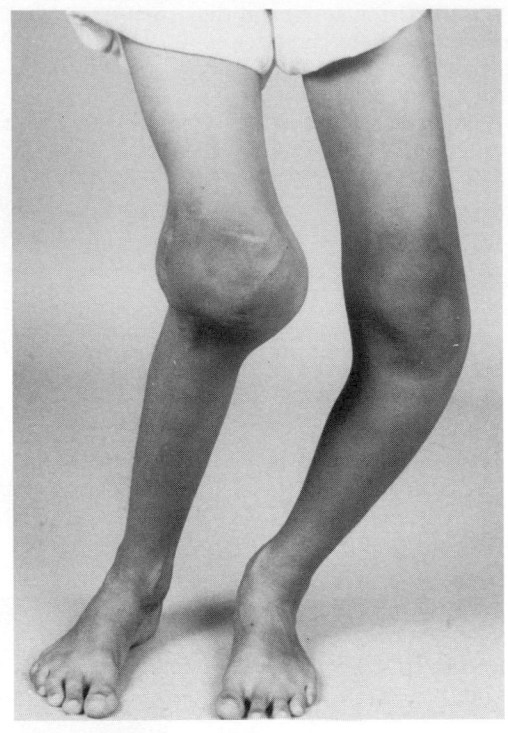

B

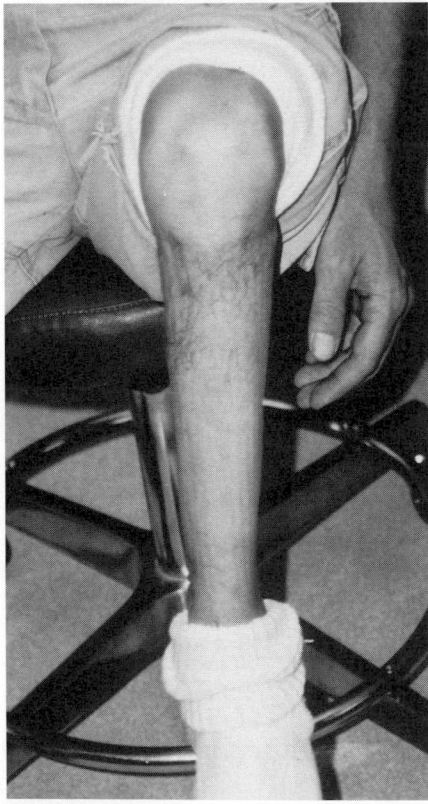

C

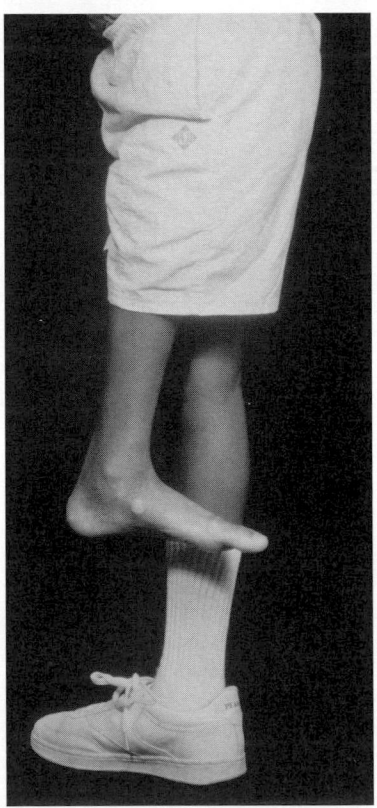

D

Figure 45-8 Examples of cases that may best be treated without lengthening due to the potential for complications. *A.* Upper extremity amelia with proximal femoral deficiency. This lower extremity discrepancy is best left alone, since these limbs perform upper extremity function. *B.* Congenital insensitivity to pain carries a high risk for soft tissue complications and infection. A pin tract infection developed into osteomyelitis in the patient we attempted to lengthen with this condition. *C.* Postradiation syndrome with minimal soft tissue and osseous regeneration potential. *D.* Proximal focal femoral deficiency with severe length discrepancy. A Van Ness derotational osteotomy was used in this case.

and tibias. These must be staged over an extended period of time. Italian surgeons have achieved good results with this approach, but it is not widely accepted in the United States.[47,48] The lack of acceptance is partly related to the strong opposition of the organization representing these patients. Furthermore, there is increased acceptance of this condition in America as opposed to Europe.

Complications

Complications are a frequent occurrence in limb lengthening (Fig. 45-9). Paley has labeled them "problems, obstacles and complications," with a rating scheme.[49] The Russian literature reports a very low rate, but the North American literature documents a significant incidence.[50] Mosca reported a 100 percent incidence using the Wagner device, and we had a significant complication rate using the Orthofix.[19] Other reports with the Ilizarov device describe high complication rates.[22,34] No matter what technique is used, there will be a high complication rate involving *both* the osseous and soft tissues.

All pins eventually cause some drainage. If this is clear and nonpurulent, it should be treated with local cleansing, skin tension release, and oral antibiotics (eg., cephalosporins) for 3 to 5 days. This is different from a true pin-tract infection with overt purulent drainage. These pa-

tients may develop fever, pain, and erythema; eventually, a ring sequestrum may form if the infection extends to the bone. Skin release, antibiotics, and incision and drainage are frequently necessary. We had one major pin-tract infection that developed into fulminant osteomyelitis. Pin problems should be treated vigorously, as they may rapidly progress to deeper, more dangerous infections.

Joint stiffness and loss of motion are common sequelae of lengthening procedures. There may be preexisting joint anomalies or posttraumatic changes. With osseous lengthening, the soft tissues are stretched, frequently resulting in joint contracture. This includes the muscles and ligamentous structures, which may atrophy or undergo fibrosis. The overlying skin becomes thin and shiny. The knee is frequently involved with both femoral and tibial lengthening and the ankle with tibial procedures. In upper extremity lengthening, the below, wrist, and fingers frequently develop contractures.

Prevention is the best treatment for soft tissue contractures. A vigorous stretching program should be initiated early during the treatment process, along with bracing or splinting of the joint above or below the lengthening. If the contractures worsen, the distraction should be slowed or discontinued for a short period. Occasionally, soft tissue surgical releases are necessary during or after the procedure, but with an adequate rehabilitation program, most children regain their motion postoperatively.

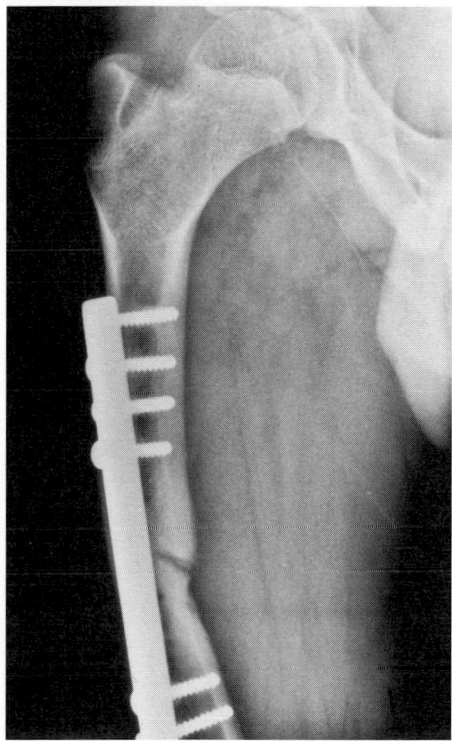

A

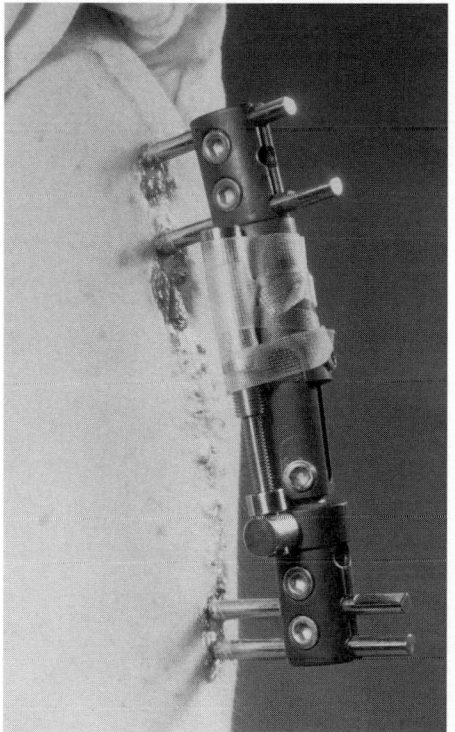

B

Figure 45-9 Complications are common in any lengthening procedure, regardless of the method used. Nonunions may occur after plating a diaphyseal Wagner lengthening, increasing the risk of plate fracture (*A*). The large pins of an Orthofix device may have significant drainage and possibly become infected (*B*). Cysts in the foot (*C*) or fractures (*D*) may develop after Ilizarov device removal. These may be treated with traction (*E*) or orthoses (*F*) applied directly to the frame.

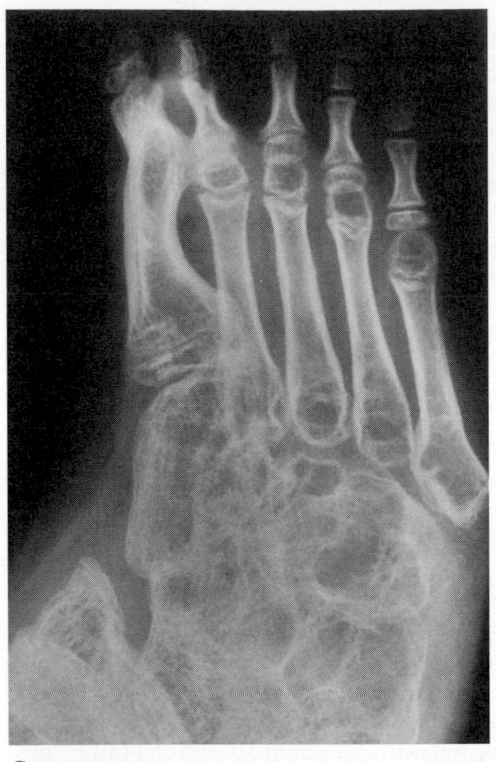

C

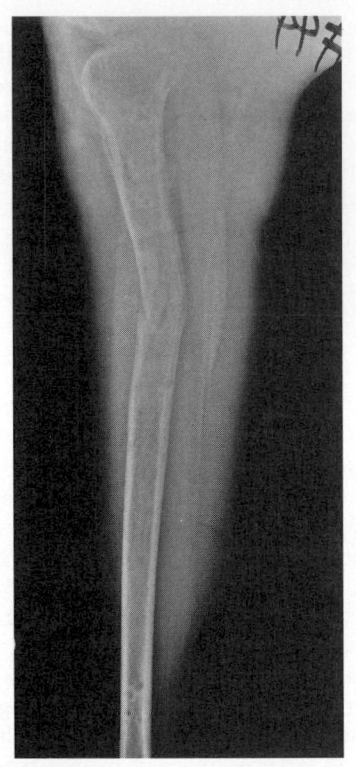

D

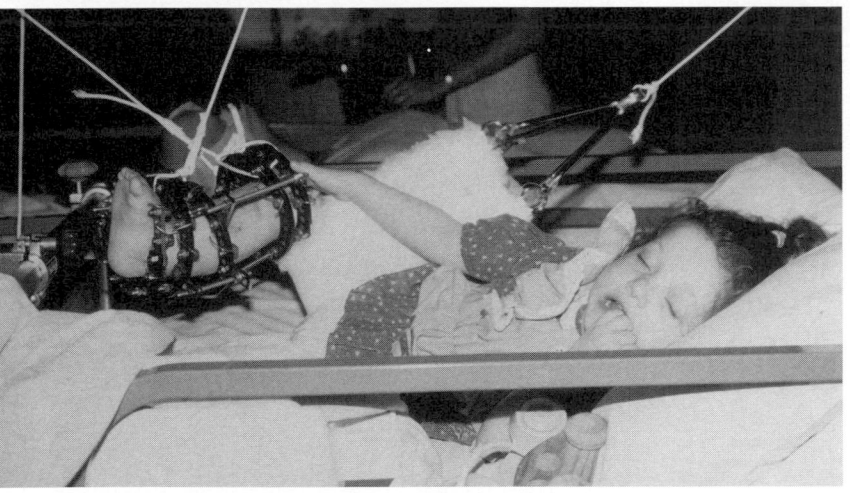

E

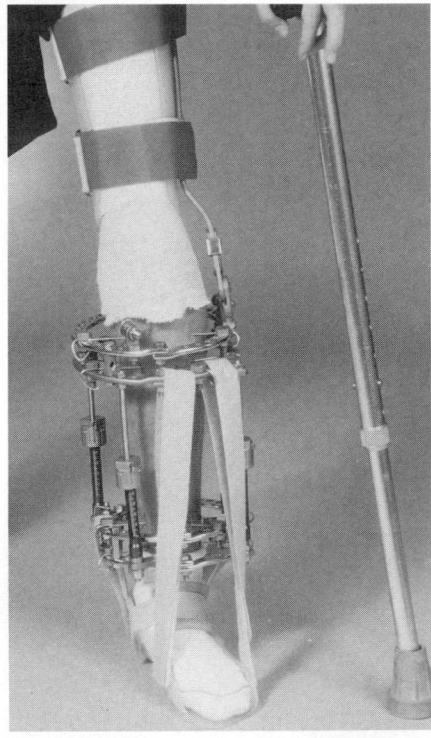

F

Figure 45-9 *(Continued)*

Fractures are a common occurrence during and after the lengthening process. They may occur above or below the lengthened area or through the maturing regenerate bone. Fractures may occur at the pin sites secondary to weakening in that area. They may occur either around the pin or at that site after removal. They are more common with large bone pins such as the Ilizarov half pins, the Wagner screws, or the Orthofix tapered pins.

During distraction, the limb may be weakened by disuse osteopenia or the metabolic demands of the adjacent elongation. Fractures due to minor falls or trauma may occur, similar to those seen in the paralytic population. We have had posttreatment fractures occur up to 2 years after lengthening, and there are reports of fractures occurring as long as 8 years after the procedure.[18,19,51] The treatment of fractures may be either conservative or operative. We have found the Ilizarov device to be quite amenable to the attachment of orthotics for fracture stabilization. Fractures may be avoided with prolonged bracing (average 6 months) after the lengthening device is removed and with an adequate exercise program.

Angulation, malunion, and premature consolidation may also occur with lengthening. Corrective osteotomy or bone grafting may be required. Early consolidation may occur as a result of a slow distraction rate and, if noted early, can be remedied by an increase in the distraction rate or by a closed manipulation.

Neurovascular complications may occur as these structures stretch during the distraction. The neurovascular bundles are frequently contracted or encased in the scar tissue. Both the stretch phenomenon and subclinical neuropraxia have been reported at rates varying from 5 to 30 percent.[52,53] This problem is generally self-limiting and resolves with slowing or discontinuation of the lengthening process. Vascular problems—including deep vein thrombosis, edema, and compartment syndrome—have all been reported.[54,55] The last of these requires emergent compartment release and the former is treated in the usual manner with anticoagulants but does not require routine prophylaxis.

Mechanical failures may also complicate the lengthening procedure. Long osseous pins may fracture or become displaced, the frame may shift, or the bone ends may translate. These complications may be avoidable with close follow-up and should be adjusted immediately upon presentation. Hypertension has been reported and also has been our experience with lengthening, especially in arthrogrypotic patients.[56] It is a rare occurrence and most likely is an autonomic phenomenon secondary to stretching of the sciatic nerve. Other possible etiologies include changes in renal blood flow or increased catecholamine release.[57–59] The treatment is to slow the distraction rate and prescribe beta blockers or other antihypertensive agents.

Psychological and emotional complications are common in children undergoing lengthening. This results from the combined aspects of congenital or traumatic deformity, multiple prior surgical procedures, and a long treatment time that frequently involves pain, keeping them from home and school. The symptoms include depression, regression, acting out, hyperventilation, and even attempted suicide.[60,61] At our institution, the patients and family are screened prior to surgery in order to identify potential problems. During the lengthening procedure, a pain team and support staff are available. Several patients have required psychological counseling and antidepressant medication.

Physical Therapy

Physical therapy is an important adjunct to any lengthening. The joints above and below the distraction site may initially be contracted or tend to tighten further during distraction. An active range-of-motion and strengthening

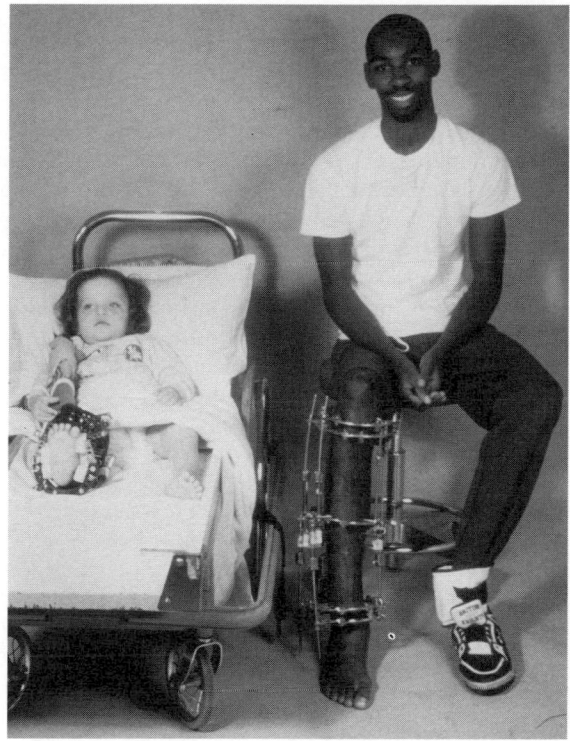

A

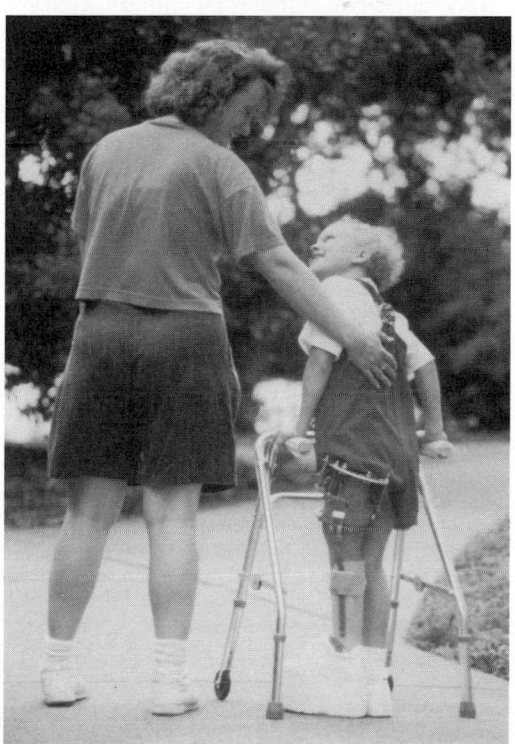

B

Figure 45-10 Patient selection and close follow-up are the keys to a successful lengthening procedure. *A.* There are no size or age limits. *B.* A team approach involving the family is the best way to achieve a good outcome.

program is essential for a successful outcome.[62] The patients need encouragement to bear weight and increase independence. This not only enhances strength but also leads to maturation of the distraction callus. Shoe lifts are used to enable weight bearing and are gradually shortened as the length increases. Orthoses are attached to the frame and frequently adjusted as the range of motion changes. Occupational therapy is an important modality for lengthening of the upper extremity, working on activities of daily living, and range-of-motion exercises. The patients are evaluated and started on a home program postoperatively. During the lengthening, they work directly under a therapist's supervision and gradually progress back to a home program. A team approach involving the therapist facilitates the entire lengthening process.

SUMMARY

Limb-length discrepancy is a common occurrence in pediatric orthopaedics. The treatment may be conservative or surgical and requires careful patient evaluation. Observation, shoe lifts, epiphysiodesis, and osseous shortening are all viable methods of treatment. Lengthening procedures should be considered in the child or adolescent who has significant shortening or angular deformity. This type of surgery may yield good results but involves a long treatment time and a high complication rate. The patients and families must be selected carefully and involved in any decisions. A multidisciplinary team approach offers a better chance of success. With these guidelines and much patience, this complex problem can be treated successfully (Fig. 45-10).

REFERENCES

1. Ogden JA: Anatomy and physiology of skeletal development, in *Skeletal Injury in the Child,* 2d ed. Philadelphia, Saunders, 1990, pp 23–63.
2. Moseley CF: Leg-length discrepancy, in Morrissy RT (ed): *Lovell and Winter's Pediatric Orthopaedics.* Philadelphia, Lippincott, 1990, pp 767–813.
3. Guidera KJ, Grogan DP, Carey TC, et al: The biology of skeletal development and maturation, in Menelaus MB (ed): *The Management of Limb Inequality.* Edinburgh, Churchill Livingstone, 1991, pp 9–35.
4. Guidera KJ, Brinker MR, Kouseff BG, et al: Overgrowth management in Klippel-Trenaunay-Weber and proteus syndromes. *J Pediatr Orthop* 13:459–466, 1993.
5. Tachdijian MO: *Pediatric Orthopaedics,* 2d ed. Vol 4. Philadelphia, Saunders, 1990, pp 889–2892.
6. Greulich W, Pyle S: *Radiographic Atlas of the Skeletal Development of the Hand and Wrist.* Stanford, CA, Stanford University Press, 1959.
7. Anderson M, Green WT, Messner MB: Growth and predictions of growth in the lower extremities. *J Bone Joint Surg Am* 45:1–14, 1963.
8. Moseley CF: A straight line graph for leg length discrepancies. *J Bone Joint Surg* 59A:174–179, 1977.
9. Moseley CF: A straight line graph for leg length discrepancies. *Clin Orthop* 136:33–40, 1978.
10. Phemister D: Operative assessment of longitudinal growth of bodies in the treatment of deformities. *J Bone Joint Surg* 15:1–15, 1933.
11. White J, Stubbins SJ: Growth arrest for equalizing leg lengths. *JAMA* 126:1146, 1944.
12. Timberlake RW, Bowen JR, Guille JT, et al: Prospective evaluation of fifty-three consecutive percutaneous epiphysiodeses of the distal femur and proximal tibia and fibula. *J Pediatr Orthop* 11:350–357, 1991.
13. Winquist R: Closed intermedullary osteotomies of the femur. *Clin Orthop* 212:155–164, 1986.
14. Peterson HA: The evolution of femoral lengthening: Concepts and techniques, in de Pablos J, Canadell J (ed): *Bone Lengthening, Current Trends and Controversies.* Pamplona, Spain, Universidad de Navarra, 1990, pp 15–18.
15. Anderson WET: Leg Lengthening. *J Bone Joint Surg [Br]* 34:150, 1952.
16. Valenti J, de Pablos J: The Wagner's device, in de Pablos J, Canadell J (eds): *Bone Lengthening, Current Trends and Controversies.* Pamplona, Spain, Universidad de Navarra, 1990, pp 45–51.
17. Wagner H: Operative lengthening of the femur. *Clin Orthop* 136:125–142, 1978.
18. Luke DL, Schoenecker PL, Blair VP, et al: Fractures after Wagner limb lengthening. *J Pediatr Orthop* 12:20–24, 1992.
19. Mosca V, Moseley C: Complications of the Wagner leg lengthening and their avoidance. *Orthop Trans* 10:462, 1986.
20. DeBastiani G, Aldegheri R, Renzi-Brev L, et al: Limb lengthenings by callus distraction (callotasis). *J Pediatr Orthop* 7:129–134, 1987.
21. Paley D: Current techniques of limb lengthening. *J Pediatr Orthop* 8:73–92, 1988.
22. Guidera KJ, Hess WF, Highhouse KP, et al: Extremity lengthening: Results and complications with the Orthofix system. *J Pediatr Orthop* 11:90–94, 1991.
23. Sprout JT, Price CT: Recent advances in limb lengthening: Part I. Clinical advances. *Orthop Rev* 21:307–314, 1992.
24. Ilizarov GA, Deviatov M: Operative elongation of the leg with simultaneous correction of the deformities. *Ortop Travmatol Protez* 30:32–37, 1969.
25. Ilizarov GA, Deviatov M: Operative elongation of the leg. *Ortop Travmatol Protez* 32:20–25, 1971.
26. Maiocchi AB: Historical review, in Maiocchi AB, Aronson J (eds): *Operative Principles of Ilizarov.* Baltimore, Williams & Wilkins, 1991, pp 3–8.
27. Fleming B, Paley D, Kristiansen T, et al: A biomechanical analysis of the Ilizarov external fixator. *Clin Orthop* 241:97–105, 1989.
28. Bell DF, Boyer MI, Armstrong PF: The use of the Ilizarov technique in the correction of limb deformities associated with skeletal dysplasia. *J Pediatr Orthop* 12:283–290, 1992.
29. Mezhenina EP, Roulla EA, Pechersky AG, et al: Methods of limb elongation with congenital inequality in children. *J Pediatr Orthop* 4:201–207, 1984.
30. Rajacich N, Bell DF, Armstrong PF: Pediatric applications of the Ilizarov method. *Clin Orthop* 280:72–80, 1992.
31. Ganel A, Grogan DJ, Guidera KJ, et al: Residual bone cysts following correction of severe foot deformities using the Ilizarov technique. *J Pediatr Orthop,* 1996. In press.
32. Atar D, Lehman WB, Grant AD, et al: New method of limb deformities correction in children. *Bull NY Acad Med* 68:447–469, 1992.
33. Bonnard C, Favard L, Sollogoub I, et al: Limb lengthening in children using the Ilizarov method. *Clin Orthop* 293:83–88, 1993.

34. Dahl MT, Gulli B, Berg T: Complications of limb lengthening: A learning curve. *Clin Orthop* 301:10–18, 1994.

35. Monticelli G, Spinelli R: Distraction epiphysiolysis as a method of limb lengthening: III. Clinical applications. *Clin Orthop* 154:274–285, 1991.

36. DeBastiani G, Aldegheri R, Renzi Brivio L, et al: Chondrodiatasis—Controlled symmetrical distraction of the epiphyseal plate. *J Bone Joint Surg* 68B:550–556, 1986.

37. Aldegheri R, Giampaolo T, Lavini F: Epiphyseal distraction. *Clin Orthop* 241:117–127, 1989.

38. Ganel A, Heim M, Farine I: Asymmetric epiphyseal distraction in treatment of Blount's disease. *Orthop Rev* 15;4:81–84, 1986.

39. Cattaneo R, Catagni M: Lengthening of the humerus, in Maiocchi AB, Aronson J (eds): *Operative Principles of Ilivarov.* Baltimore, Williams & Wilkins, 1991, pp 325–334.

40. Cattaneo R, Catagni MA, Guerreschi F: Applications of the Ilizarov method in the humerus: Lengthenings and nonunions. *Hand Clin North Am* 9:729–739, 1993.

41. Cattaneo R, Catagni M: Lengthening of the forearm, in Maiocchi AB, Aronson J (eds): *Operative Principles of Ilizarov.* Baltimore, Williams & Wilkins, 1991, pp 335–343.

42. Catagni MA, Szabo RM, Cattaneo R: Preliminary experience with Ilizarov method in late reconstruction of radial hemimelia. *J Hand Surg (Am)* 18:316–321, 1993.

43. Seik WH, Dobyns JH: Digital lengthening with emphasis on distraction osteogenesis in the upper limbs. *Hand Clin North Am* 9:699–706, 1993.

44. Ogino T, Kato H, Ishii S, et al: Digital lengthening in congenital hand deformities. *J Hand Surg (Br)* 19:125–129, 1994.

45. Paley D, Catagni M, Argnani F, et al: Treatment of congenital pseudarthrosis of the tibia using the Ilizarov technique. *Clin Orthop* 280:81–93, 1992.

46. Guidera KJ: Congenital pseudarthrosis of the tibia treated by the Ilizarov method. Presented at the American Academy of Orthopaedic Surgeons meeting, New Orleans, Feb 7, 1994.

47. Martinez-Lotti G, Gil J, de Pablos J, et al: Limb lengthening in symmetrically short bones (dwarfisms), in de Pablos J, Canadell J (eds): *Bone Lengthening: Current Trends and Controversies.* Pamplona, Spain, Universidad de Navarra, 1990, pp 375–396.

48. Villa A: Lengthening of the limbs in achrondroplastic dwarfism, in Maiocchi AB, Aronson J (eds): *Operative Principles of Ilizarov.* Baltimore, Williams & Wilkins, 1991, pp 344–351.

49. Paley D: Problems, obstacles and complications of limb lengthening by the Ilizarov technique. *Clin Orthop* 250:81–104, 1990.

50. Velasquez RF, Bell DF, Armstrong PF, et al: Complications of use of the Ilizarov technique in the correction of limb deformities in children. *J Bone Joint Surg* 75A:1148–1156, 1993.

51. Faber FWM, Keessen W, van Roermard PM: Complications of leg lengthening: 46 procedures in 28 patients. *Acta Orthop Scand* 62:327–332, 1991.

52. Galardi G, Comi G, Loza L, et al: Peripheral nerve damage during limb lengthenings: Neurophysiology in five cases of bilateral tibial lengthenings. *J Bone Joint Surg* 72B:121–124, 1990.

53. Weber E, Daube J, Coventry M: Peripheral neuropathies associated with total hip arthroplasty. *J Bone Joint Surg* 58A:66–69, 1976.

54. Eldridge JC, Bell DF: Problems with substantial limb lengthening. *Orthop Clin North Am* 22:625–631, 1991.

55. Vizkelety TL, Marschalko P: Limb lengthening operations. Acta Chir Hung 33:55–77, 1993.

56. Helal A, Guidera KJ, Campos A, et al: Hypertension following orthopaedic surgery in children. *J Pediatr Orthop* 13:773–776, 1993.

57. Taleb YA, Hamdan J, Ahmed M: Orthopaedic causes of hypertension in pediatric patients. *J Bone Joint Surg* 64A:291–292, 1982.

58. Whitehall ZH, Hakala MW: The hypertension of femoral lengthening: A canine experimental model. *Surg Forum* 27:525–526, 1976.

59. Yosipovitch ZH, Palti Y: Alterations in blood pressure during leg lengthening: A clinical and experimental investigation. *J Bone Joint Surg* 49A:1352–1358, 1967.

60. Hrutkay JM, Eilert RE: Operative lengthening of the lower extremity and associated psychological aspects: The children's hospital experience. *J Pediatr Orthop* 10:373–377, 1990.

61. Kusalic M, Fortin C, Gauthier Y: Psychodynamic aspects of dwarfism: Response to growth hormone treatment. *Can Psychiatr Assoc J* 17:29–34, 1972.

62. Green SA: Physiotherapy during Ilizarov fixation. *Tech Orthop* 5:61–65, 1990.

CHAPTER 46

Congenital Dislocation of the Knee, Congenital Dislocation of the Patella, and Discoid Lateral Meniscus

Robert E. Eilert

POPLITEAL CYST

Popliteal cysts occur as tumorous swellings on the posterior aspect of the knee; they are cystic structures filled with gelatinous fluid. A popliteal cyst is usually located on the medial side of the popliteal fossa just distal to the flexion crease of the knee, under the medial head of the gastrocnemius. The condition is about twice as common in boys as in girls and usually occurs in only one knee. The popliteal cyst is often called by the eponym *Baker's cyst* because of the description by Baker, in which he proposed that these tumors developed as herniations of the knee joint capsule.[1]

The clinical presentation of a popliteal cyst in children is nearly always the presence of a mass behind the knee. At times there may be some stiffness and local pain, but the mass is usually asymptomatic. The swelling becomes prominent when the knee is straightened and disappears with knee flexion. This cystic mass is firm and characteristically can be transilluminated. Typically, this lesion tends to resolve spontaneously. MacMahon and Dinham[2,3] reviewed the natural history of popliteal cysts and showed that they tend to resolve over a mean period of about 20 months. In contrast, cysts that are treated surgically have an incidence of spontaneous recurrence as high as 50 percent.

The danger of the situation is that a tumor may be mistaken for a popliteal cyst. In adults, these cysts tend to be associated with internal derangement of the knee, particularly tear of the posterior horn of the medial meniscus.[4] Large cysts have been demonstrated in cases of rheumatoid synovitis, which may extend down into the calf.[5] In children, these tend to be spontaneous occurrences of cystic swelling that spontaneously disappear.

One should be concerned if the cyst does not arise in the medial part of the popliteal fossa or, if the cyst has a solid component, ultrasonography may be used to differentiate between a fluid-filled cyst and a solid mass. Computed tomography (CT) or MRI may be used in the unusual case.

If the cyst transilluminates and is otherwise typical but the family remains concerned, an aspiration biopsy may be performed. A needle with a fairly large bore, such as 18 gauge, is used; it removes the gelatinous material. When this material is squirted from the syringe onto a 4- by 4-in gauze pad, both surgeon and parents can be reassured that this asymptomatic mass is indeed benign and that the cyst can be expected to progress to spontaneous resolution.

There is no evidence that the instillation of hydrocortisone will prevent recurrence of the cyst once it is aspirated. Indeed, the swelling usually recurs fairly promptly but should be expected to resolve spontaneously in 10 to 20 months.

Some people recommend surgical excision of cysts that are symptomatic or that do not regress over time.

The cyst tends to lie under the inner border of the medial head of the gastrocnemius; it may extend transversely over the gastrocnemius and semimembranosus muscles and then be reflected onto the articular capsule of the knee joint. When the cyst is removed, it should always be examined histologically, looking for evidence of a more serious tumor, but the usual type of cyst has a fibrous wall with some changes that may be inflammatory, or it may have synovial characteristics.[6]

DISCOID MENISCUS

A discoid meniscus is disk-shaped rather than semilunar in form. The pathology is that of a solid mass of fibrocartilage, roughly circular in shape, which extends from the peripheral margin of the joint to the intercondylar notch. The upper surface of the involved tibial plateau is almost completely covered by the discoid meniscus.[7,8] The lateral meniscus is involved in the overwhelming majority of cases, although the condition occasionally occurs in the medial meniscus. The clinical presentation is usually one of a snapping or click in the knee, with vague symptoms of pain and giving way of the knee.[9] The knee may also present with a fixed flexion contracture.

The physical findings of an unstable meniscus include a palpable loud thunk, which is audible and palpable during the last 15 to 20° of extension.

Other causes of a snapping knee must be ruled out, such as a meniscal cyst, snapping of the popliteus tendons or other tendons about the knee joint, or even a clicking in the proximal tibiofemoral joint.

Commonly the central portion of the meniscus is abnormal and demonstrates a mucinoid degeneration, often with tears or buckling in this area.

The variations in the discoid meniscus have been variously described in the literature. Watanabe[10] has described an incomplete attachment posteriorly, so that there is some degree of hypermobility of the posterior portion of the meniscus, which he called the *Wrisberg ligament type*. Alternatively, there may be a complete or incomplete covering of the compartmental surface, representing variations of the same type.

Arthroscopically, a wave of meniscus is seen, which is produced by a folding of the central portion. This frequently causes the snapping. The posterior detachment may actually be a tear along the margin posteriorly.[11]

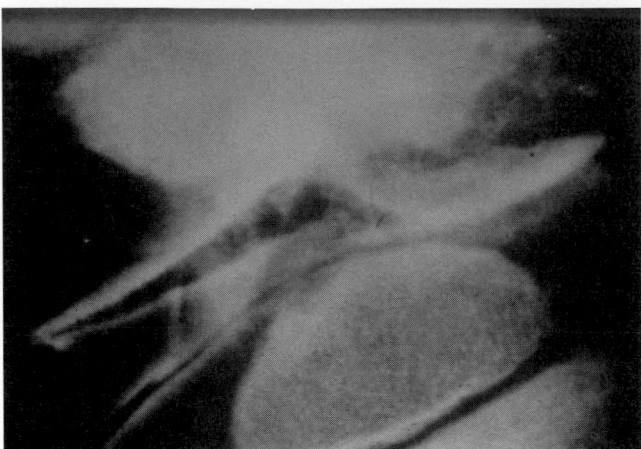

Figure 46-1 Discoid meniscus clearly demonstrated by arthrogram of the knee.

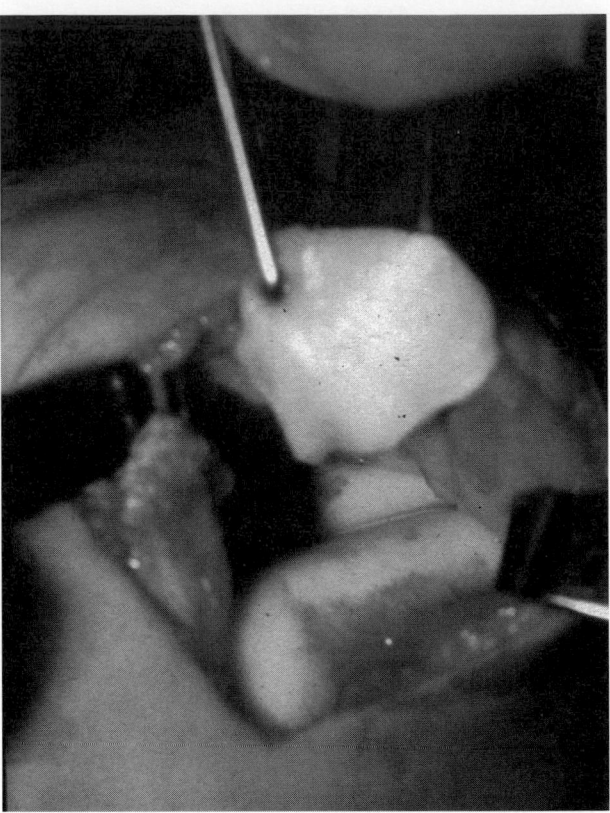

Figure 46-2 Discoid meniscus. The abnormal central portion was removed by arthrotomy, leaving a stable rim. This surgery can be done arthroscopically as well.

The mere presence of discoid meniscus does not cause disability, and it may be asymptomatic throughout life. However, symptoms frequently appear between the ages of 6 and 8 years.

Findings on plain x-ray film may demonstrate some widening of the lateral joint space or even slight flattening of the lateral condyle. Contrast arthrography (Fig. 46-1) can demonstrate the discoid meniscus clearly, but arthrography has recently been replaced by MRI.[12] Magnetic resonance imaging is usually successful but not infallible, as the lateral compartment is somewhat more difficult to visualize accurately by this technique.

Treatment consists of removing the unstable portion of the meniscus, which can usually be done with preservation of the rim of the meniscus. Excision of the central part of the meniscus can usually be done arthroscopically; if this is not possible, however, open arthrotomy should be performed (Fig.46-2).[13]

In rare instances, the entire meniscus must be removed because it totally unstable. The knee may then be prone to early degenerative changes, because the meniscus acts as a template for growth and development of the femoral condyle. Complete removal of the meniscus also removes its functions of providing stability, cushioning, and lubrication to the joint.

RECURRENT SUBLUXATION OR DISLOCATION OF THE PATELLA

Dislocation of the patella is nearly always lateral. It may be congenital, developmental, or posttraumatic. Congenital dislocation of the patella is dealt with in a separate section further on.

Recurrent subluxation of the patella is a more common occurrence than dislocation and is commonly seen in adolescent girls. There is a hereditary tendency for recurrent subluxation of the patella.

Various physical findings may contribute to recurrent subluxation of the patella. The first is general laxity of the ligaments. In these children, hyperextension of the knee and elbow are possible (Fig. 46-3). The lateral soft tissues may be contracted, with shortening of the patellar retinaculum and the patellofemoral ligaments. A weakness of the vastus medialis, particularly its oblique portion, causes a relative muscle imbalance, because the vastus medians is the primary dynamic medial stabilizer of the patella.[14,15] Patella alta also predisposes to subluxation of the patella and is often associated with hypoplasia of the lateral femoral condyle. If the angle between the quadriceps and the patellar ligament is increased such that the patella is exposed to a valgus vector of muscular force, this tends to promote lateral subluxation. Twisting-type injuries may damage the medial capsule of the knee and lead to subluxation.

The usual presentation of recurrent lateral subluxation is a complaint of pain about the anterior knee, which is precipitated by physical activity. The patient is frequently a teenage girl who suffers from some impingement of the patella against the lateral femoral condyle with flexion.

The knee may give way or there may be locking and and a sensation of popping of the knee. It is unusual to see a recurrent effusion unless the patella dislocates completely. The more severe form of this problem is lateral displacement of the patella as an acute episode. The pa-

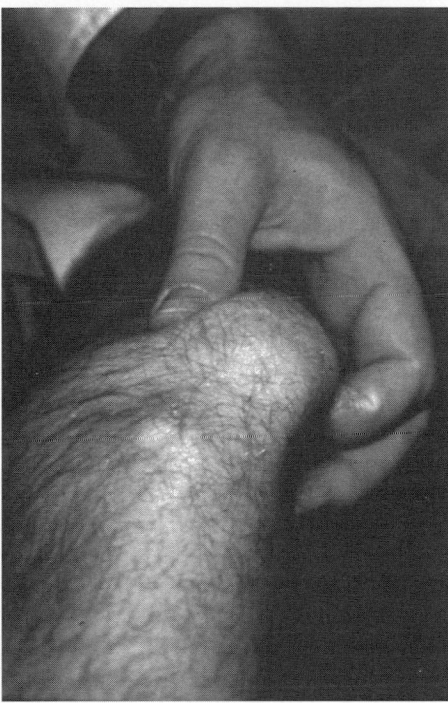

Figure 46-3 Recurrent dislocation of the patella. Lateral hypermobility associated with recurrent dislocation.

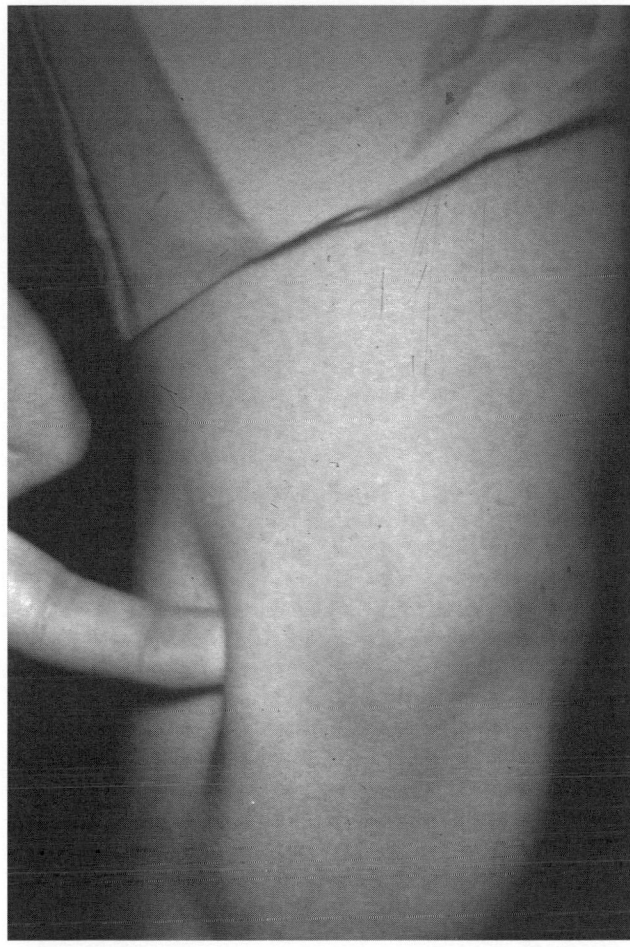

Figure 46-4 Recurrent subluxation of the patella. Lateral overhang demonstrated by placing finger on lateral femoral condyle beneath the patella.

tient's knee may give way completely, resulting in a fall. There is intense pain with an effusion of the knee.

When there is simple subluxation of the patella, there is a sensation that the patella moves laterally and feels uncomfortable, but it does not completely displace.

On examination with the knee flexed 90°, the patella points more toward the ceiling than its normal straight-ahead position (patella alta). With medial pressure applied against the patella, the unstable patella may be moved so far laterally that it may overhang the lateral condyle as much as the width of the thumb (Fig. 46-4). As the tracking of the patella is noted, there is frequently a "J sign": as the patella moves more medially in full extension, it follows a path like the letter "J." Often there is a palpable deficiency of the vastus medians obliquus as the patella shifts toward the lateral side. This can be demonstrated clinically by displacing the patella medially and having the patient contract the quadriceps vigorously, and then repeating this with lateral displacement comparing the muscular pull medially and laterally. The Q angle[15] is defined by a line from the the midpoint of the patella and the insertion in the tibial tubercle and a line from the anterior superior iliac spine and the center of the patella. If this angle is more than about 20°, the resultant valgus force may contribute to recurrent subluxation.

The radiographic findings have been variously described,[17] showing tilt of the patella or incongruency between the patella and the sulcus of the trochlear notch. These radiographic views are all taken under static conditions and provide only relative information, with the large overlap between the normal and symptomatic groups.

Dynamic testing of the patella during motion is the most valuable diagnostic maneuver, along with a careful review of the history. For chronic or habitual subluxation of the patella, the treatment is a vigorous exercise program to try to balance and strengthen the muscles about the knee, the use of bracing to support the patella is also helpful.[18,19]

Lateral retinacular release divides the contracted lateral tissue surgically. It is useful when the subluxation can be demonstrated to be caused by decreased lateral excursion of the patella associated with patellar tilt and symptoms of subluxation. Lateral retinacular release should be approached with caution and works best in patients who cooperate with a good preoperative program of exercise and activity modification. Lateral subluxation of the patella alone is not an indication for lateral release, which should be reserved for the most resistant cases. Lateral release can be performed through a small incision using subcutaneous release of the retinaculum and synovium after arthroscopic confirmation[20–22] of maltracking and patellar tilt. If complete dislocation of the patella is present, both medial stabilization and lateral release will be needed.[23]

Balance may be obtained by medial plication; in the loose jointed individual, however, medial augmentation is often necessary. This can be accomplished by use of the semitendinosus tendon, according to the method of Galeazzi-Dewar.[24,25]

OSTEOCHONDRITIS DISSECANS

Osteochondritis dissecans of the knee is characterized by impending or actual separation of osteochondral fragments from the cartilaginous surface. As these fragments "dissect" free, loose bodies are released into the joint; these produce symptoms of locking, swelling, and pain.

The etiology of the fragment separation is not completely agreed upon, but the fragments are fractured off of their base.[26] Microscopic examination reveals avascular necrosis in the bone of the fragment (Fig. 46-5). Therefore, some combination of trauma and disturbance in blood supply are the most popular and likely explanations. There is seldom a history of major trauma, repeated but minor trauma in physically active children has been postulated to cause the process in a susceptible individual. The femoral condyles are not an area of end arteries, but an underlying larger area of osteonecrosis may be demonstrated in some patients by MRI.

Because the original lesion heals in the majority of skeletally immature patients, the myth exists that this is a completely benign disease in children.[27,28] This is a misconception, as in all reported series there is a 25 to 50 percent[29] incidence of true fragmentation even in the skeletally immature. This misunderstanding has led surgeons to be unusually persistent in waiting for lesions to heal nonoperatively and allowing them to progress to frank separation.

Fragmentation leads to premature degenerative arthritis, although these degenerative changes occur over a very long period of time. The report of Linden,[30] who carefully tracked a group of patients with osteochondritis dissecans, showed that they developed degenerative arthrosis prematurely in the compartment in which the fragment separation had occurred. This natural history was compared to that of the normal aging process, and Linden determined that patients who had fragmentation developed degenerative changes approximately 10 years earlier than the normal degeneration attributed to the aging process. These changes require about 20 years to develop, so that a surgeon who is following such a patient over a shorter time span may fail to notice them.

Spontaneous healing does occur in 50 to 75 percent of skeletally immature individuals. The treatment then is simply observation and some restriction of activity, and this will generally lead to an excellent result. On the other hand, because of the risk of late degenerative changes, it is important not to wait for fragmentation. A lesion that heals without fragmentation may leave a small bone scar on x-ray, as a normal knee would not.

Children who are being followed for osteochondritis dissecans need regular follow-up. When healing occurs with time and restriction of activities, the line defining the osteochondral fragment will gradually blur and fill in, just as a fracture line does in a fracture of a long bone. This healing usually occurs in 3 or 4 months and is accompanied by a decrease in pain in the knee. When such healing does not occur in an orderly fashion, arthroscopy is indicated. Initially, the disease can be diagnosed by radiologic examination. The key view for detection of the lesion is the tunnel view. In about 25 percent of patients, the tunnel view is the only one that demonstrates the lesion clearly. There is some tendency for ossification defects and irregularities to develop posteriorly in the condyles in young children. These are islands of ossification that coalesce without symptoms. These changes on x-ray were described by Caffey[31] and are usually incidental findings. The lesions that tend to cause more trouble by fragmentation are classically posterior to Blumensaat's line, which defines the superior margin of the intercondylar notch on the lateral view (Fig. 46-6). The classic lesion occurs just anterior to this line in the medial femoral condyle, which is immediately adjacent to the insertion of the posterior cruciate ligament.

Arthroscopy can define those lesions that do not appear to be healing on x-ray or are still producing symptoms after 3 to 4 months. In the first stage, as seen at arthroscopy, there is intact cartilage over the lesion, which is usually somewhat softened and may be slightly different in color.[32,33] If the second stage of the disease has been reached, the cartilage itself will be cracked; this defect will communicate with the underlying fracture line in the bone, and there may or may not be some displacement of the fragment. In the third stage, a free fragment is present, as full separation of the osteochondral fragment has occurred.

Treatment depends upon the findings at arthroscopy.[34] Certainly in a child who has the anticipated benign course, no arthroscopy is necessary. Neither a cast nor severe restrictions of activity is needed. Casts in these patients can produce atrophy, stiffness, and severe psychological problems, particularly if the disease is bilateral, which is the case about 50 percent of the time.

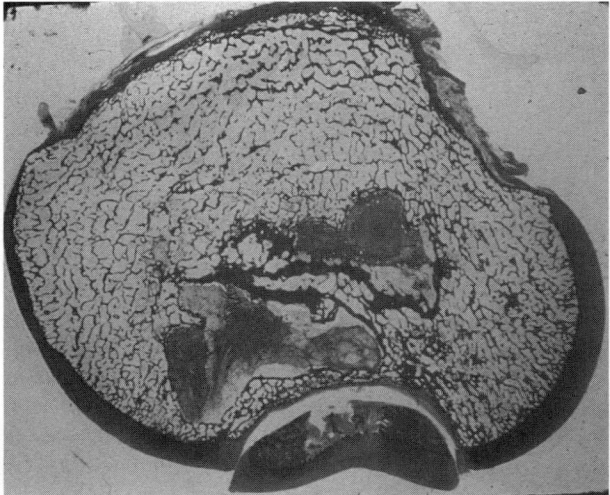

Figure 46-5 Histopathologic section through the condyle of a 13-year-old boy who died in an auto accident. The osteonecrosis in the underlying bed of the lesion is apparent.

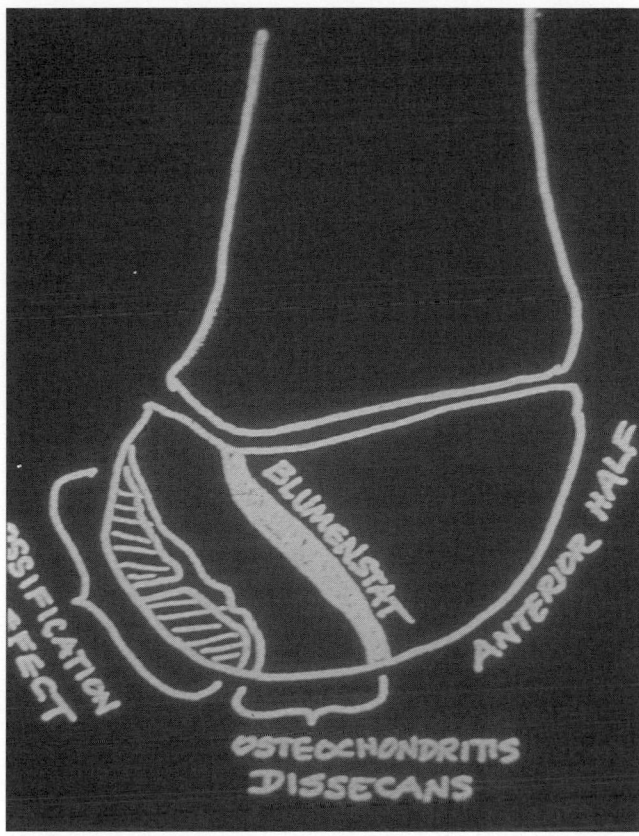

Figure 46-6 Diagram showing typical location of osteochondritis dissecans relative to Blumensaat's line.

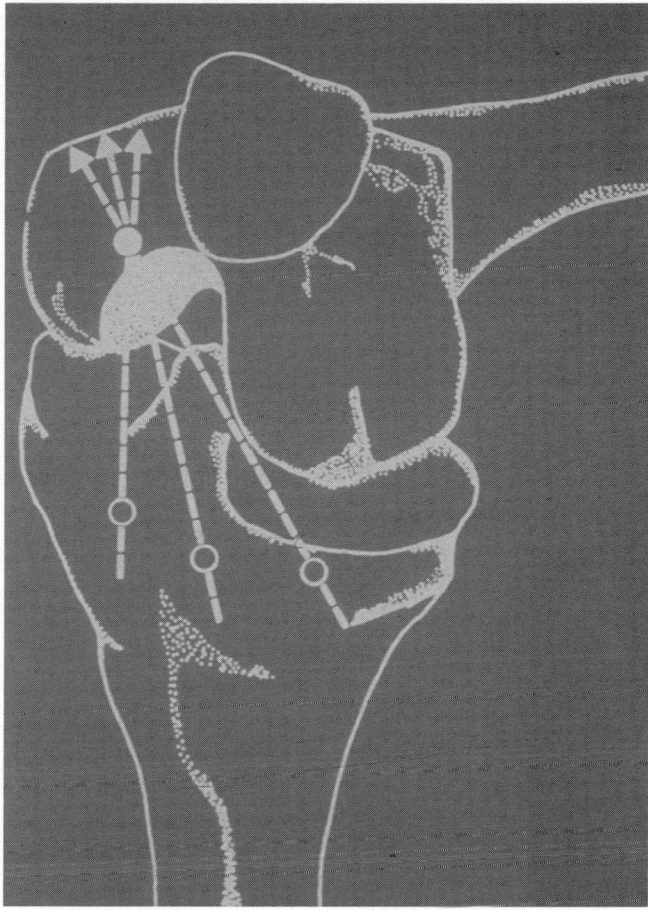

Figure 46-7 Diagram showing drilling technique using a single small portal in the articular cartilage by redirecting the pin through multiple skin punctures.

When symptoms are severe or healing is delayed, arthroscopy is indicated.[35] The basic principle of treatment is that fragmentation should be prevented if possible. In a skeletally immature patient who has stage 1 disease with intact articular cartilage, drilling the lesion through a single portal in the cartilage, using multiple skin portals, can encourage the blood supply to penetrate from the underlying bone and for the fragment to heal (Fig.46-7). Simple drilling, however, is not applicable in patients in a later stage of the disease with impending fragmentation or in a patient who is skeletally mature.

In these patients, internal fixation of some type is indicated.[36] The use of Kirschner wires requires immobilization of the joint, because these wires must be left long to permit removal. We have found cannulated compression screws to be very useful. They can be positioned by fluoroscopy during arthroscopy and are utilized to stabilize the fragment for fracture healing (Fig. 46-8). Early motion is permitted, and the screws can be easily retrieved after healing, at a later date, by using the arthroscope.

Magnetic resonance imaging can define an underlying osteonecrosis if present (Fig. 46-9); some feel that grafting of this area under fluoroscopic guidance is appropriate. Bone scan may be useful to define the original lesion but has not proved accurate in determining whether separation of the fragment will occur.[37,38] If the lesion does not heal promptly (3 or 4 months), an aggressive attitude to-

ward preventing the separation of fragments should be the philosophy in treating children.

When there is a free fragment, it should be replaced if at all possible. If it is so misshapen that it cannot be re-

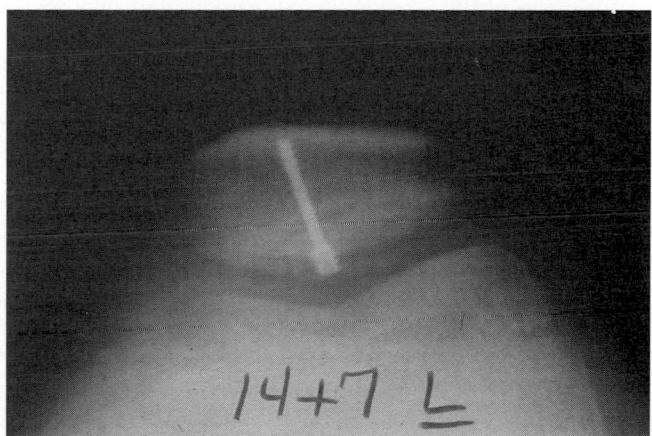

Figure 46-8 Patellar lesion of osteochondritis dissecans stabilized with a Herbert screw.

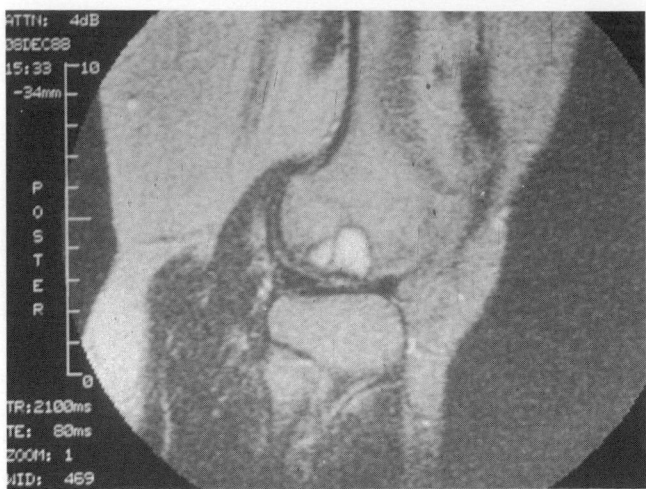

Figure 46-9 Osteochondritis dissecans of the medial femoral condyle demonstrated by MRI.

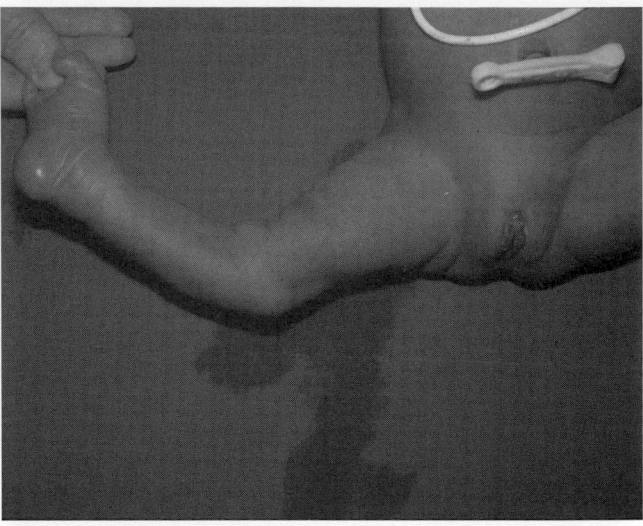

Figure 46-10 Congenital dislocation of the knee: appearance in a newborn.

placed because of growth of the free fragment in the synovial fluid, then the fragment must be removed.

Grafting of either osteochondral plugs or grafts of cultivated cartilage cells or periosteal free grafts has been advocated for filling in these osteochondral defects, which may range from 1 to 3 cm in diameter; these techniques seem to be most applicable here. In long-term follow-up of these patients, widespread skill in applying these techniques should develop over the next few years.

CONGENITAL DISLOCATION OF THE KNEE

In congenital dislocation of the knee, the proximal tibia is displaced anterior to the distal femur. Breech birth and congenital dislocation of the hip are frequently seen in association with dislocation of the knee. Clinically, the knee is hyperextended beyond neutral, producing a striking deformity that is immediately apparent at birth (Fig. 46-10).

Flexion of the knee is limited initially but may be regained by splinting or casting of the knee progressively into more flexion. The knee joint is gently manipulated into flexion and an anterior splint is applied, extending from the groin to the ankle. Treatment should begin in the newborn nursery, as the deformity is the least rigid at birth.[39] The splint is changed daily. As the amount of flexion of the knee increases, the angle of the splint is increased to match. If the deformity corrects easily in a few weeks, the presumption is that the etiology was intrauterine malpositioning and the prognosis is excellent.[40]

When the hip is also dislocated, the knee dislocation should be reduced first and the hip dislocation should be treated secondarily. This process may be facilitated by applying a Pavlik harness once the knee flexion has reached 45° or so. The Pavlik harness can then be used to treat the two dislocations simultaneously.[41]

When a congenital knee dislocation does not reduce with progressive splinting, surgical release and realignment are indicated.[42,43] Early surgical reduction of congenital knee dislocation has produced the best results in reported series.[44]

The pathology that may be encountered at operation includes fibrosis of the quadriceps muscle, anterior displacement of the hamstring tendons, hypoplasia of the cruciate ligaments, and lateral displacement of the patella associated with contracture of the fascia lata or the lateral intermuscular septum. Patients who require surgical correction frequently have a generalized musculoskeletal syndrome such as arthrogryposis.[45]

CONGENITAL DISLOCATION OF THE PATELLA

The patella may be displaced laterally as part of a congenital abnormality of the quadriceps mechanism. The dislocation may be persistant or obligatory. In a persistant dislocation, the patella is tethered in a position lateral to the femoral condyle by a contracture of the lateral retinaculum.[46,47] When the contracture is less severe, the patella is drawn laterally out of the trochlear groove when the knee flexes. This obligatory dislocation reduces during extension. The reverse pattern also occurs, in which the patella is reduced in flexion and dislocated in extension with each cycle of flexion and extension.

Congenital dislocation of the patella is frequently a component of a syndrome such as chondrodysplasia or Down's syndrome. The anomaly may also be present in an otherwise normal child who presents with a knee flexion contracture or difficulty walking.[48] In bilateral cases there may be a delay in walking due to the abnormality.

Figure 46-11 Congenital dislocation of the left patella: MRI showing unossified patella in a persistent lateral dislocated position in 11-month-old child. Right knee is normal.

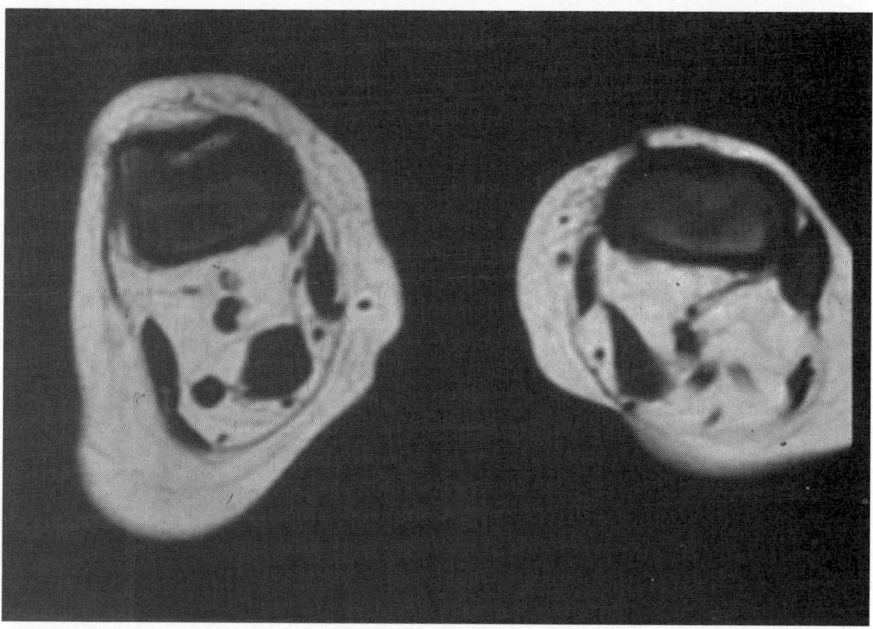

In the young child, a clinical diagnosis by physical examination may be unclear. The child presents with a flexion contracture or inability to walk. Although one can suspect dislocation of the patella by palpation, the patella is smaller than usual and difficult to define in its displaced lateral position. The MRI provides an excellent diagnostic image, as the patella ordinarily is not ossified until 3 to 5 years of age, so that it is not visible on an ordinary roentgenogram (Fig. 46-11). Obligatory dislocation of the patella usually presents at a later age and is a spectacular finding on physical examination. The patella moves in and out of the trochlear notch each time the patient flexes and extends the knee, and the patient complains of instability of the knee.

There is no effective nonoperative treatment. If the deformity is left untreated, ambulation is impaired and arthritis develops prematurely.[49]

The quadriceps mechanism is laterally displaced with a tethering of the fascia lata and shortening of the quadriceps muscle. The medial retinaculum and muscle are drawn over the anterior joint and are usually adherent to the articular cartilage. The trochlear groove is absent and the end of the femur looks like a bald head. The insertion of the patellar ligament may displace laterally as much as 45°. An associated posterior contracture prevents full extension of the tibiofemoral joint. A valgus deformity is common due to contracture of the fascia lata.

Surgical treatment requires lateral release, medial plication, lengthening of the quadriceps, and reinsertion of the patellar ligament.[50] Therefore, the entire alignment of the patella may have to be repositioned. Releasing the flexion contracture is also important, as this element of the deformity will not resolve spontaneously and the persistent contracture will compromise the result. When congenital dislocation of the patella is corrected surgically in an older child, femoral osteotomy may be required for the secondary bony deformity of genu valgum. Obligatory dislocation can be realigned with less extensive operation, but the procedure must be tailored to the pathology that is present. If there is deficiency of the medial quadriceps muscle in the older child, the semitendinosus may be transferred to the patella by the technique of Galeazzi for stabilization.

REFERENCES

1. Baker WM: On the formation of synovial cysts in the leg in connection with disease of the knee joint. *St Bart Hosp Rep* 13:245, 1877.
2. MacMahon EB: Baker's cysts in children—Is surgery necessary: *J Bone Joint Surg* 55A:1311, 1973.
3. Dinham JM: Popliteal cysts in children. *J Bone Joint Surg* 57B:69, 1975.
4. Childress HM: Popliteal cysts associated with undiagnosed posterior lesions of the medial meniscus. *J Bone Joint Surg* 36A:1233, 1954.
5. Burleson RJ, Bickel WH, Dahlin DC: Popliteal cyst: A clinico-pathological survey. *J Bone Joint Surg* 38A:1265, 1956.
6. Gristina AG, Wilson PD: Popliteal cysts in adults and children: A review of 90 operative cases. *J Bone Joint Surg* 45A:1552, 1963.
7. Dickhaut SC, DeLee JC: The discoid lateral meniscus syndrome. *J Bone Joint Surg* 64A:1068, 1982.
8. Cave EF, Staples OS: Congenital discoid meniscus: A cause of internal derangement of the knee. *Am J Surg* 54:371, 1941.
9. Beals RK: The "snapping knee" of infancy. *J Bone Joint Surg* 60A:679, 1978.
10. Watanabe M, Takeda S, Ikeuchi H: *Atlas of Arthroscopy,* 2d ed. Tokyo, Igaku Shoin, 1969.
11. Ikouchi H: Arthroscopic treatment of the discoid lateral meniscus: Technique and long-term results. *Clin Orthop* 167:19, 1982.

12. Hall FM: Arthrography of the discoid lateral meniscus *AJR* 128:993, 1977.
13. McGinty JB, Geuss LF, Marvin RA: Partial or total meniscectomy. *J Bone Joint Surg* 59A:763, 1977.
14. Cofield RH, Bryan RS: Acute dislocations of the patella: Results of conservative treatment. *J Trauma* 17:526, 1977.
15. Fox TA: Dysplasia of the quadriceps mechanism: Hypoplasia of the vastus medians muscle as related to the hypermobile patella syndrome. *Surg Clin North Am* 55:199, 1975.
16. Brattstrom H: Shape of the intercondylar groove normally and in recurrent dislocation of the patella: A clinical and x-ray anatomical investigation. *Acta Orthop Scand* (suppl 68): 1964.
17. Merchant AC, Mercer RL, Jacobsen RH, Cool CR: Roentgenographic analysis of patellofemoral congruence. *J Bone Joint Surg* 56A:1391, 1974.
18. Henry, JH, Crosland JW: Conservative treatment of patellofemoral subluxation. *Am J Sports Med* 7:12, 1979.
19. Fulkerson JP: The etiology of patellofemoral pain in young, active patients: A prospective study. *Clin Orthop* 179:129, 1983.
20. Grana WA, Hinkley B, Hollingsworth S: Arthroscope evaluation and treatment of patellar malalignment. *Clin Orthop* 186:122, 1984.
21. Metcalf RW: An arthroscope method for lateral release of subluxating or dislocating patella. *Clin Orthop* 167:9, 1982.
22. Larson RL, Cabaud HE, Slocum DB, et al: The patellar compression syndrome: Surgical treatment by lateral release. *Clin Orthop* 134:158, 1978.
23. Hughston JC: Reconstruction of the extensor mechanism for subluxating patella. *J Sports Med* 1:6, 1972.
24. Baker RH, Carroll N, Dewar FP, Hall JE: The semitendinosus tenodesis for recurrent dislocation of the patella. *J Bone Joint Surg* 54B:103, 1972.
25. Hall JE, Micheli LJ, McNamara GB Jr: Semitendinosus tenodesis for recurrent subluxation or dislocation of the patella. *Clin Orthop* 144:31, 1979.
26. Aichroth P: Osteochondral fractures and their relationship to osteochondritis dissecans of the knee: An experimental study in animals. *J Bone Joint Surg* 53B:448, 1971.
27. Green WT, Banks HH: Osteochondritis dissecans in children. *J Bone Joint Surg* 35A:26, 1953.
28. Lofgren L: Spontaneous healing of osteochondritis dissecans in children and adolescents. *Acta Chir Scand* 106:460, 1953.
29. Hughston JC, Hergenroeder PT, Courtenay BG: Osteochondritis dissecans of the femoral condyles. *J Bone Joint Surg* 66A:1340, 1984.
30. Linden B: Osteochondritis dissecans of the femoral condyles. *J Bone Joint Surg* 59A:769, 1977.
31. Caffey J, Madell SH, Royer C, Morales P: Ossification of the distal femoral epiphysis. *J Bone Joint Surg* 40A:647, 1958.
32. Bots RA, Stood TJ: Arthroscopy in the evaluation of operative treatment of osteochondrosis dissecans. *Orthop Clin North Am* 10:685, 1979.
33. Casscells SW: The place of arthroscopy in the diagnosis and treatment of internal derangement of the knee: An analysis of 1000 cases. *Clin Orthop* 151:135, 1980.
34. Eilert RE: Arthroscopy in children. *Op Arthrosc* 7:55, 1991.
35. Guhl J: Arthroscopic treatment of osteochondritis dissecans: Preliminary report. *Orthop Clin North Am* 10:671, 1979.
36. Lindholm S, Pylkkanen P, Oesterman K: Fixation of osteochondral fragments in the knee joint. *Clin Orthop* 126:256, 1977.
37. Cahill BR, Berg BC: 99m-Technetium phosphate compound joint scintigraphy in the management of juvenile osteochondritis dissecans of the femoral condyles. *Am J Sports Med* 11:329, 1983.
38. Yeung DW: Radionuclide imaging in osteochondritis dissecans. *Clin Nucl Med* 6:122, 1981.
39. Ahmadi B, Shahriaree H, Silver CM: Severe congenital genu recurvatum. *J Bone Joint Surg* 61A:622, 1979.
40. Curtis BH, Fisher RL: Heritable congenital tibio-femoral subluxation. *J Bone Joint Surg* 52A:104, 1970.
41. Nogi J, MacEwen GD: Congenital dislocation of the knee. *J Pediatr Orthop* 2:509, 1983.
42. Curtis BH, Fisher RL: Congenital hyperextension with anterior subluxation of the knee: Surgical treatment and long-term observations. *J Bone Joint Surg* 51A:255, 1969.
43. Eikelaar HR: Congenital luxation of the knee. *Arch Chir Neerl* 23:201, 1971.
44. Austwick DH, Dandy DJ: Early operation for congenital subluxation of the knee. *J Pediatr Orthop* 3:85, 1983.
45. Jacobsen K, Vopalecky F: Congenital dislocation of the knee. *Acta Orthop Scand* 56:1, 1985.
46. Stanislavjevic S, Zernenick G, Miller D: Congenital, irreducible, permanent lateral dislocation of the patella. *Clin Orthop* 116:190, 1976.
47. Torisu T: Neglected congenital permanent dislocation of the patella. *Clin Orthop* 155:136–140, 1981.
48. Green JP, Waugh W: Congenital lateral dislocation of the patella. *J Bone Joint Surg* 50B:285, 1968.
49. Zeier FG, Dissanayake C: Congenital dislocation of the patella. *Clin Orthop* 148:140–146, 1980.
50. Jones RDS, Fischer RL, Curtis BH: Congenital dislocation of the patella. *Clin Orthop* 119:177, 1976.

CHAPTER 47

The Pediatric Leg

Ronald J. Turker
and James C. Drennan

PEDIATRIC LEG DEFORMITIES

Genu Varum

Parents commonly bring their children to an orthopaedist for a consultation concerning a lower extremity deformity, which can involve rotational, coronal, and sagittal planes. This section discusses coronal plane deformities centered at the level of the knee. The term *genu varum* applies to a bowleg attitude of the knee, while *genu valgum* refers to a knock knee position.

Physiologic Genu Varum

Salenius, Staheli, and Cheng each assessed large numbers of children in three different cultural populations to determine normal coronal plane alignments.[1–3]

These studies show a progressive decrease in the physiologic genu varum of infancy by 18 to 24 months of age, followed by an increasing genu valgum to age 3 or 4 years (Fig. 47-1). This is followed by a slow return toward neutral tibiofemoral alignment with a mild residual valgus commonly persisting after 6 years of age. Cheng used clinical weight-bearing assessment of the tibiofemoral angle, while Staheli employed a technique using measurements of standing clinical photographs. The Chinese population studied by Cheng returned closer to a neutral tibiofemoral angle than the other two populations. He reported that after 7 years of age, a slight genu varum position was considered to be within normal limits when two standard deviations were employed. This differs from the results with the Caucasian children examined by Staheli. Any degree of clinical varus between the ages of 2 and 11 years in his study group was considered abnormal (Fig. 47-1). This discrepancy could represent different clinical methods of measurement or an actual propensity for Chinese people to have a normal slight varus alignment.

PATHOLOGIC GENU VARUM (TIBIA VARA)

Incidence and Etiology

Tibia vara, or Blount disease, is a relatively rare disorder primarily involving the medial proximal tibial metaphysis, physis, and epiphysis. The disorder was originally described by Erlacher in 1922. Blount, in 1937, reported 15 cases from the literature coupled with 13 cases in his personal series. He distinguished two clinical forms differentiated by age at presentation: infantile (less than 3 years of age) and the less common adolescent or late-onset form.[4] Thompson et al. later proposed adding a juvenile category because of the significant rate of recurrent deformity in their patients between 3 and 10 years of age and the absence of recurrence in patients who presented after 10 years of age.[5]

Infantile Tibia Vara

Tibia vara appears to have a multifactorial etiology. Theories have been advanced based on the natural history of the disease, histologic assessment, and mechanical analysis of the lower extremities. Repetitive weight-bearing trauma and preexisting infantile varus alignment in the lower extremity appear to play a role in the development of this disease. Cook et al. used finite element analysis and proposed that 20° of varus in a 2-year-old child of normal weight would produce sufficient force to retard the medial tibial growth plate, in accordance with the Heuter-Volkman principles.[6]

Ligamentous laxity may also contribute to the deformation of the tibia. Children under 3 years of age with a weight-bearing lateral thrust of the knee and genu varum have an increased propensity to develop Blount disease.[7] The disease has a genetic predisposition but no true Mendelian inheritance pattern. Greene reviewed the literature and found that 9 to 43 percent of the patients with the infantile form of tibia vara had an affected sibling or parent.[8] There is a predilection for the disease in the African American population, females, early walkers, and obese toddlers, but it has not been possible to establish a true incidence of Blount disease in the general population.[7–9] In Blount's original series, 60 percent of the patients had bilateral involvement. Other authors report that 48 to 68 percent of these patients presented with bilateral deformities.[4,10–12]

Adolescent Tibia Vara

Blount's original review of 37 patients included 9 with adolescent tibia vara, which is a milder and less common form of the disease.[4] It is often unilateral. Wenger et al. suggested that these children had a history of incompletely resolved infantile genu varum that progressed during the prepubertal adolescent growth spurt to adolescent tibia vara.[13] Henderson and Greene, however, presented two cases of adolescent tibia vara who had previous radiographs documenting normal mechanical axes prior to the onset of the disease.[14] Henderson et al. examined more than 1100 teenage boys undergoing routine physical examinations for football. Of the 140 boys who weighed more than 210 lb (greater than the 95th percentile), 7 had clinical evidence of knee vara, but only two demonstrated radiographic evidence of tibia vara. Both of these boys weighed more than 280 lb.[15]

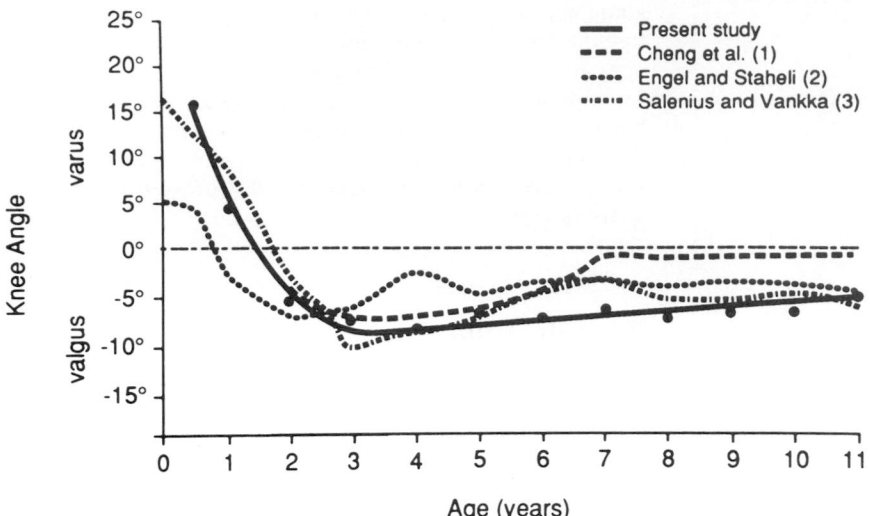

Figure 47-1 Graph showing the mean clinical measurements of normal tibiofemoral angles. The dark line represents the study of Heath and Staheli. Note that the children in Cheng's group returned closer to a neutral position than those in the other reports. (Reproduced with permission from Heath CH, Staheli LT: Normal limits of knee angle in white children. *J Pediatr Orthop* 13:261, 1993.)

Histology

The histology of the proximal tibia physis of both infantile and adolescent tibia vara has been studied. Despite the historical name of *osteochondrosis deformans* used to describe tibia vara, no histologic evidence of avascular necrosis has been reported. Blount and Langenskiöld obtained infantile physeal specimens from the medial physeal metaphyseal beak.[4,10] Wenger et al. analyzed medial physeal tissue from patients with adolescent tibia vara. They found that despite radiographic evidence of bone bridging, the histologic specimens examined showed no true osseous connection.[13] Carter et al. procured specimens of the entire physis from patients with adolescent tibia vara at the time of corrective osteotomy through the proximal tibial physis. They demonstrated abnormal histology resembling the pathologic changes found in the proximal femoral physis of patients with slipped capital femoral epiphysis.[16] Lovejoy and Lovell reported two cases in boys who had

tibia vara associated with slipped capital femoral epiphyses.[17] The pathologic changes of tibia vara included severe disorganization of cartilage cells, which was more pronounced on the medial side of the physis but extended into the lateral side.[16] Additional histologic features included islands of acellular fibrosis, islands of densely packed hypertrophic cartilage, and transphyseal blood vessels.[4,10,13,17]

DIFFERENTIAL DIAGNOSIS

Infantile Tibia Vara

The most common cause of genu varum in the first two years of life is "physiologic bowlegs." This condition shares many clinical characteristics with tibia vara, including internal tibial torsion (Fig. 47-2). An anteroposterior radi-

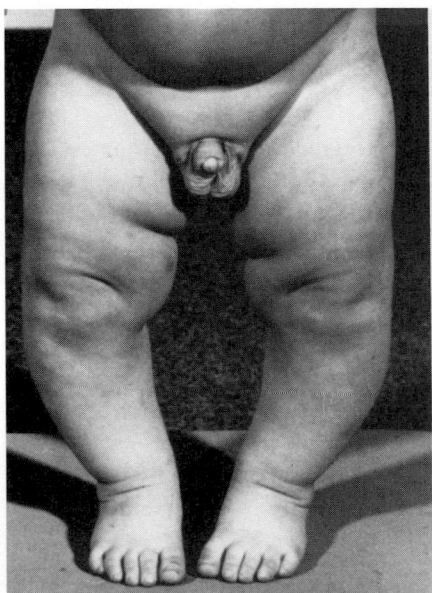
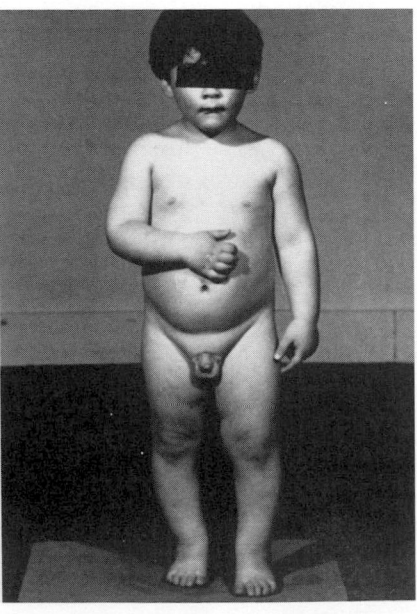

Figure 47-2 An 18-month-old toddler with physiologic bowlegs is seen on the left. Note the degree of internal tibial torsion. Spontaneous resolution by 3 years of age is shown.

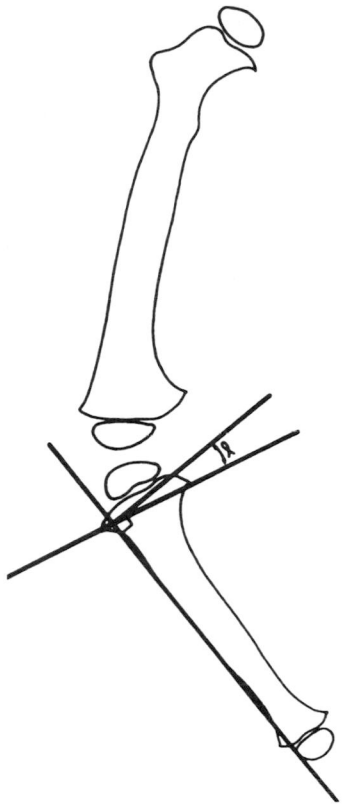

Figure 47-3 The metaphyseal-diaphyseal angle as described by Levine and Drennan. A line perpendicular to the lateral border of the tibia is compared to a line drawn through the metaphyseal flares. An angle greater than 12° is cause for concern. (Reproduced with permission from Feldman MD, Schoenecker PL: Use of the metaphyseal-diaphyseal angle in the evaluation of bowed legs. *J Bone Joint Surg* 75A:1603, 1993. Adapted with permission from Levine AM, Drennan JC: Physiological bowing and tibia vara. *J Bone Joint Surg* 64A: 1159, 1982.)

ograph may be helpful in distinguishing between physiologic and pathologic conditions. Levine and Drennan described the radiographic measurement of the metaphyseal-diaphyseal angle of the proximal tibia as a helpful tool to distinguish between physiologic bowing and true tibia vara at 18 months (Fig. 47-3). They reported that only 3 of 58 extremities with a metaphyseal-diaphyseal angle 11° or less developed tibia vara. All children in this study whose metaphyseal-diaphyseal angle was greater than 12° developed true tibia vara.[18] Henderson et al. showed an interobserver difference of 2° and a possible error of 2.8° secondary to rotation with this radiologic measurement.[19] Feldman and Schoenecker compared 106 children with physiologic bowing to 19 patients with Blount disease. They concluded that there was a "gray" zone between 9 and 16° that produced both false-positive and false-negative results when the diagnosis was based on a single radiograph. The metaphyseal-diaphyseal angle became a more accurate indicator of true tibia vara when serial ra-

diographs were used. Using linear regression analysis, they were able to demonstrate a clear correlation between physiologic bowing with a decreasing metaphyseal-diaphyseal angle over time as opposed to a progressively increasing angle associated with Blount disease.[20]

Other less common causes of bowlegs include generalized or local skeletal dysplasias. Focal fibrocartilaginous dysplasia, metaphyseal and epiphyseal dysplasias, and osteogenesis imperfecta may all be clinically confused with tibia vara. Distinguishing focal fibrocartilaginous dysplasia from Blount disease is important, since the former condition is likely to improve spontaneously.[21–23] Its critical radiographic feature is a focal cortical defect below the physis in the metaphyseal region (Fig. 47-4). Metabolic conditions causing bowlegs include renal osteodystrophy as well as dietary and hypophosphatemic rickets. Infection, trauma, and tumor can also result in the development of bowleg deformity. Clinical history, appropriate radiographs, and blood tests may be needed to rule out these other causes before treatment is initiated.

Classification

The most widely accepted classification of infantile tibia vara was proposed by Langenskiöld and Riska; it considers both radiographic appearance and age. The six stages demonstrate progressive deformity over time (Fig. 47-5). Various papers have attempted to correlate the Langenskiöld stages with prognosis and treatment recommendations.[10,11,24–26] However, many of these studies lack sufficient intra- and interobserver concordance. Stricker et al. noted that interobserver reproducibility of Langenskiöld's classifi-

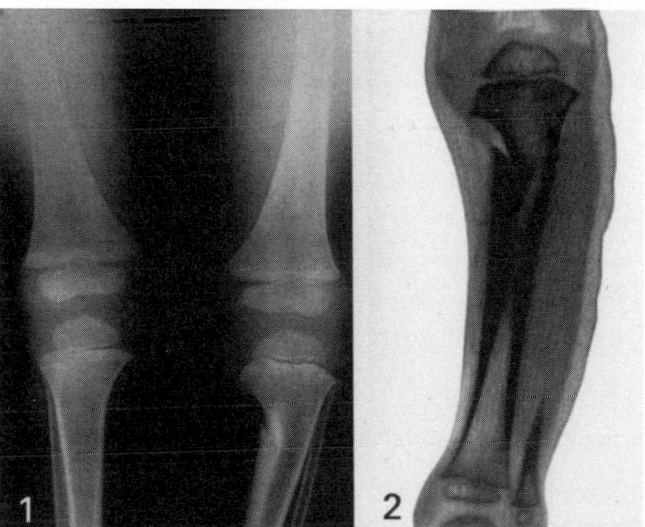

Figure 47-4 The left tibia displays a varus-producing defect just below the metaphysis. Plain radiograph and tomographic reconstruction images reveal no physeal involvement. This osseous defect and varus alignment can be managed by observation. (Reproduced with permission from Cockshott WP et al: Focal fibrocartilaginous dysplasia and tibia vara: A case report. *Skel Radiol* 23:334, 1994.)

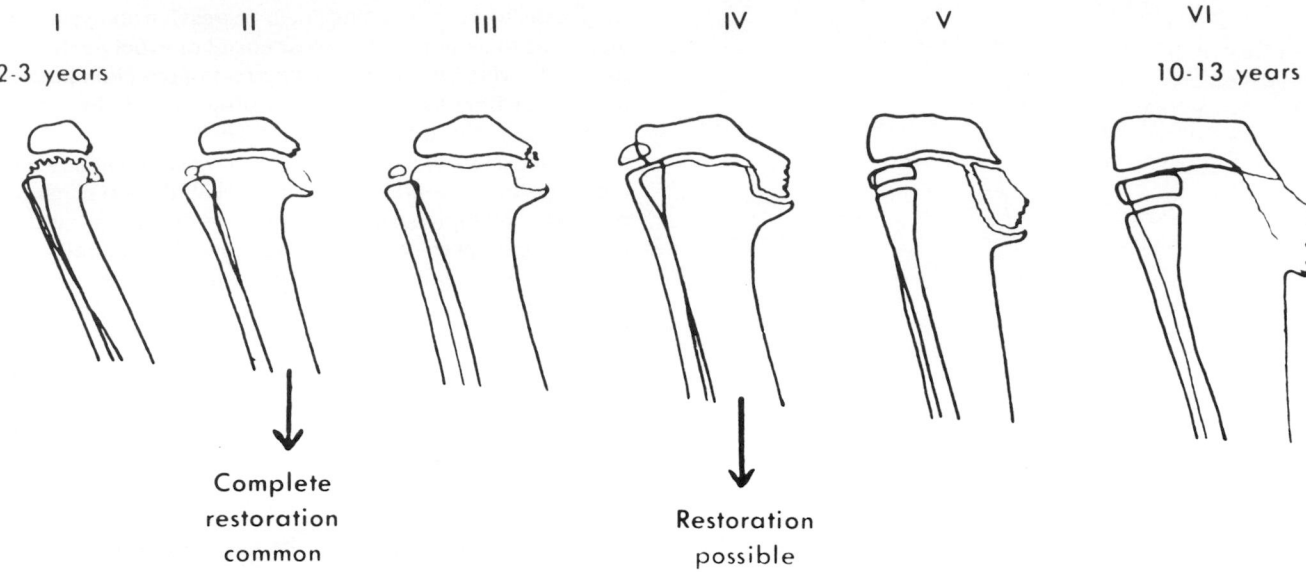

Figure 47-5 The Langenskiöld and Riska classification of infantile tibia vara. Note the association of progression of the patient's age with the severity of the deformity. (Reproduced with permission from Langenskiöld A: Tibia vara (osteochondrosis deformans tibiae): A survey of 23 cases. *Acta Chir Scand* 103:9, 1952.)

cation is difficult even when the reference articles are available to the examiner.[27] There are a number of studies showing that the older the patient with infantile tibia vara is at the time of initial presentation, the more likely he or she is to have a poor prognosis and recurrence.[10,11,24,28] Clinical outcomes from the same radiographic stages may differ with racial populations. Studies reported by Langenskiöld and Loder disagree on the clinical outcome for patients with radiographic stages II and III.[25,26] Langenskiöld reported that one-third of patients in a predominantly white Scandinavian population who had adequate surgical realignment by stage III had favorable outcomes. Loder's predominantly African American population with stages II and III had disease progression despite adequate realignment.[10,26]

TREATMENT
Infantile Tibia Vara

Differentiation between tibia vara and physiologic bowing in infancy is difficult; treatment must be delayed until a diagnosis can be established. After the diagnosis of tibia vara has been established, treatment should begin. The form of management will vary depending upon the age at presentation and severity.

Under 3 Years of Age

Bracing has been reported to be effective in 50 to 80 percent of cases.[12,26] Brace treatment initiated before 3 years of age permits adequate assessment of the effectiveness of

treatment.[11,26] Both single and double upright as well as full hip-knee-ankle-foot orthosis (HKAFO) braces have been advocated. Since biomechanical weight-bearing forces seem to play a role in the pathophysiology of tibia vara, daytime wear should suffice. As the deformity improves, the brace is progressively molded into increasing valgus.[29] Correction to a neutral tibiofemoral angle that can be maintained outside of the brace is the endpoint for brace wear.[26] Proximal tibial osteotomy is recommended if a neutral tibiofemoral axis has not been achieved after 1 year of treatment. It is important that the osteotomy be performed before the age of 4 to 5 years because of a higher recurrence rate when surgery is postponed to a later age.

Over 4 Years of Age

Many different types of osteotomies have been recommended, including opening wedge, chevron, and dome osteotomies.[4,10,29] Significant internal tibial torsion must be corrected at the time of surgical treatment. We prefer the Rab oblique osteotomy, which addresses both the varus as well as the internal tibial rotation (Fig. 47-6). Rab presented an excellent nomogram that depicts an optimal angle of inclination for the osteotomy, depending on the magnitude of the two deformities being corrected. The osteotomy is performed through a transverse incision, which is more cosmetic and can be crossed without avascular compromise at a later date if needed. The osteotomy also has the capability of postoperative manipulation, since single screw fixation is used.

This is beneficial in overcoming the technical problem of inadequate length of intraoperative radiographs, especially in the typical case of an obese child with a relatively

Figure 47-6 The operative technique of the Rab oblique osteotomy. Note the transverse incision and fixation with a single screw lateral to the tibial apophysis. The osteotomy can be manipulated in the cast if necessary. (Reproduced with permission from Rab GT: Oblique tibial osteotomy for Blount's disease. (tibia vara). *J Pediatr Orthop* 8:717, 1988.)

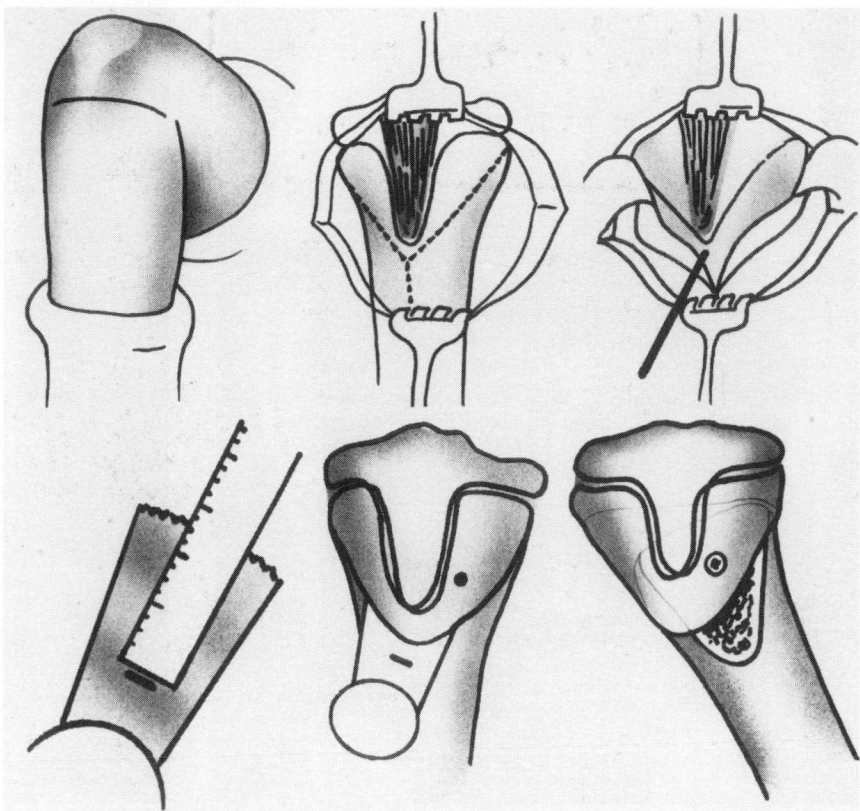

short leg (Fig. 47-7*A, B,* and *C*). At the completion of the procedure, the surgical drapes can be removed, appropriate radiographs obtained, and manipulation performed before applying the long leg cast. Rab strongly recommends that a prophylactic anterior compartment fasciotomy accompany the proximal tibial osteotomy.[30] Steele et al. reported that "neurologic" postoperative complications actually resulted from compartment syndrome.[31]

Patients with Rab type of osteotomy are immobilized in a single hip spica cast for 6 weeks. The amount of radiographic callus determines the possible need for continued immobilization in a single long leg cast. Formal rehabilitation of the knee is generally not needed in this young population. Plating to a predetermined angle has been described for older children, but this requires more extensive exposure and the possible need for plate removal at a later date.[32] External fixation devices have also been utilized and are discussed under the management of late-onset Blount disease.[33,34] The Ilizarov technique offers a slower and safer correction of the soft tissues for extremely severe cases. Occasionally the medial tibial plateau becomes severely depressed in untreated cases and also in patients who have progressed despite early surgical intervention. Combined medial plateau elevation and proximal tibial osteotomy have been described.[12,35] Results are mixed, but these deformities are extreme. These procedures should be considered salvage in nature. Physeal bridge resection can be added to a valgus osteotomy in severe infantile cases. Small series have reported encouraging results.[36,37]

LATE-ONSET TIBIA VARA

Adolescent Tibia Vara

The differential diagnosis of adolescent tibia vara includes trauma, tumor, and infection, but it is less likely to include the metabolic and skeletal dysplasias discussed above. Both juvenile and adolescent groups are considered together. The younger patients have a greater chance of recurrence.[5,38] The variety of osteotomies previously discussed can also be applied to these groups. With a markedly obese child, an external fixation device has the advantage of allowing full weight bearing in the early postoperative period. Weight bearing is encouraged as soon as the patient is comfortable. If a plate is used, the weight bearing is limited to touchdown for at least 6 weeks. No cast is used in this group because these patients are extremely obese (Fig. 47-8). Price et al. described the use of a dynamic axial fixator for all age groups, which permitted correction of both the varus and internal tibial torsion components of the deformity.[33,34] They also recommended an intraoperative radiologic technique using the electrocautery cord to assess the mechanical axis of the limb without having to remove the drape. The cord is aligned with the center of the femoral head as well as the center of the ankle. The knee joint can then be examined by fluoroscopy to see if the cord bisects it in its central portion after correction. The fixator can be manipulated if the hip-knee-ankle alignment is unsatisfactory (Fig. 47-9).

Associated distal femoral deformity adds to the genu varum. In infantile tibia vara, the distal femur is often in

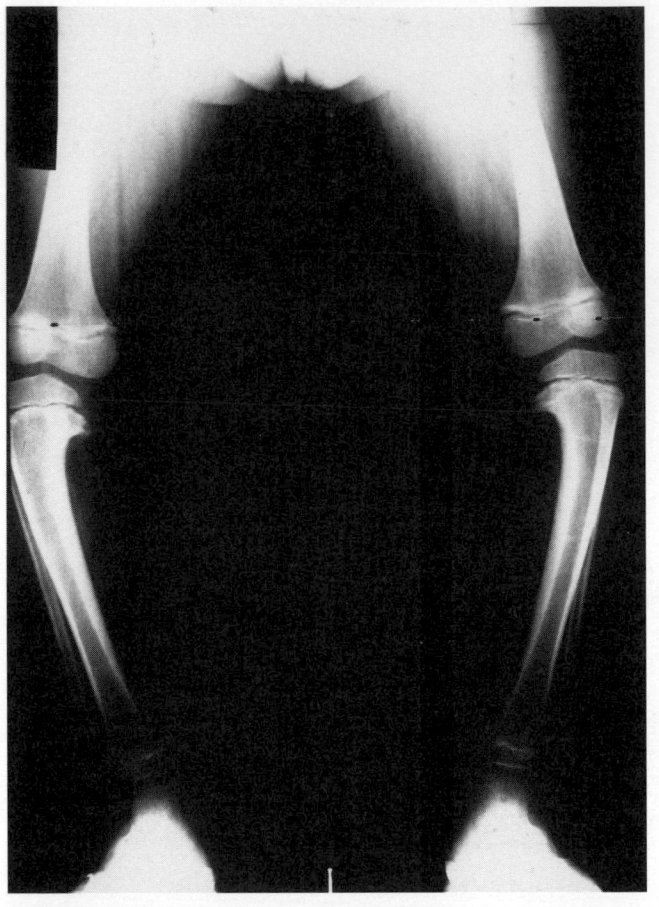

A

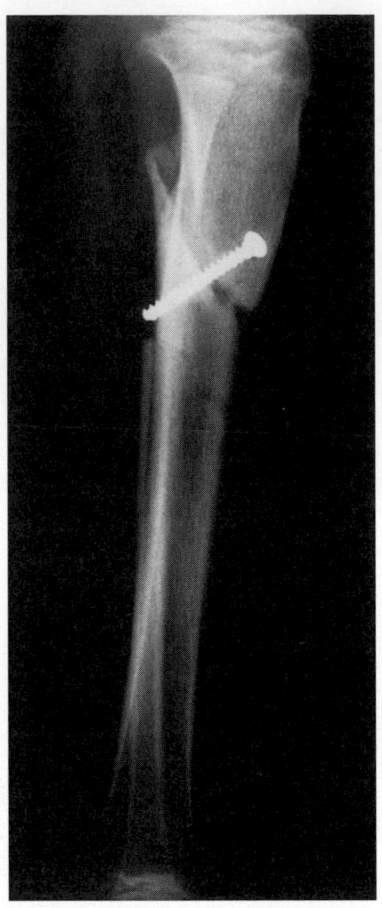

B

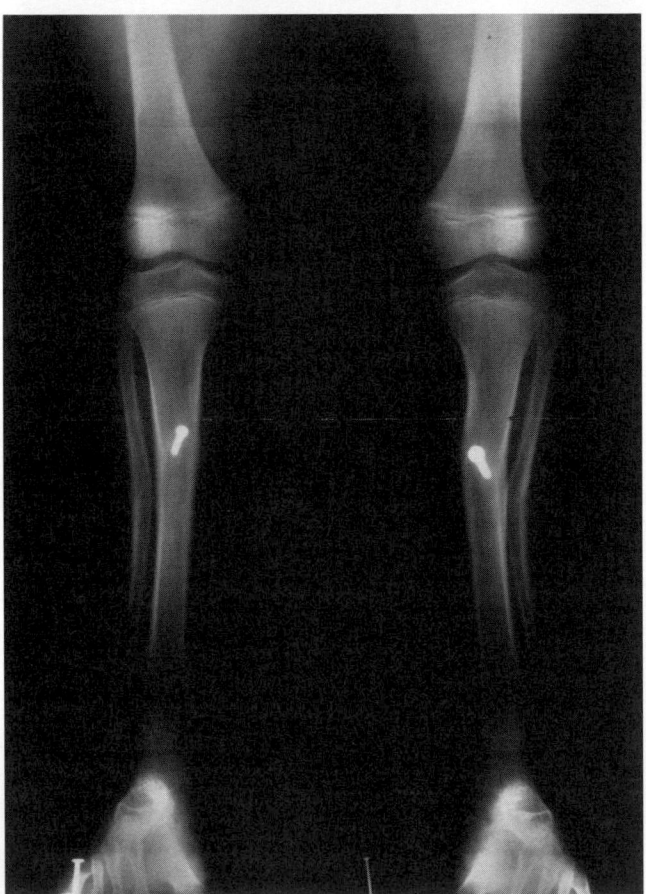

C

Figure 47-7 *A*. A 4-year-old girl with bilateral infantile tibia vara. *B*. The patient was treated with a Rab osteotomy; the lateral film demonstrated a 45° oblique osteotomy. *C*. Follow-up at 2 years shows excellent correction. The screws were subsequently removed.

786

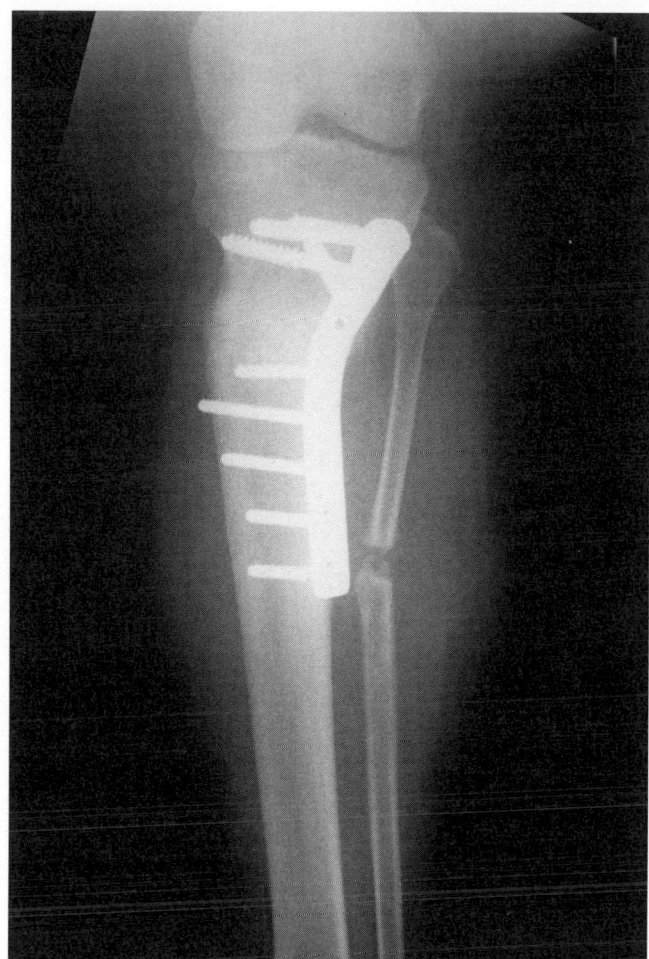

Figure 47-8 To obviate ligamentous laxity of the knee, a plate can be prebent to the appropriate angle with measurements obtained from a standing mechanical axis film.

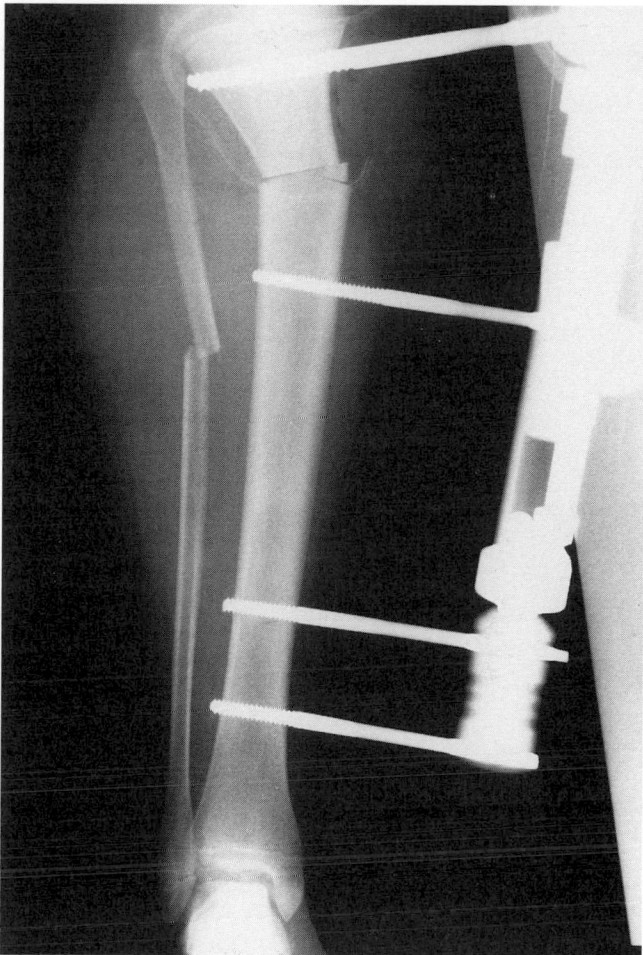

Figure 47-9 An opening/closing wedge osteotomy was performed on a 12-year-old male. The dynamic external fixator allows both postoperative weight bearing and correction if needed. It provides excellent fixation in obese patients.

valgus with an overgrowth of the medial femoral condyle. This may limit the amount of potential elevation of the medial tibial plateau needed in severe cases (Fig. 47-10). The femur often assumes a varus posture in the adolescent form.[12,39,40] Occasionally, the distal femur requires an osteotomy in order to obtain a knee joint surface that is parallel with the ground.[12] Preoperative planning that visualizes deformities of the distal femur, proximal tibia, and the internal tibial rotation components are critical to successful outcome.

GENU VALGUM

Genu valgum, or "knock knees" is another common condition of the lower extremities that often prompts parents to seek evaluation by a physician. Most children undergo normal physiologic changes from birth to 6 years of age that produce a maximum valgus angulation of 10 to 15° by 3 to 4 years of age. The tibiofemoral angulation decreases

over the next 2 years to the typical adult position of 7° of valgus (Fig. 47-1). Cheng has shown that the Chinese population has a propensity toward slightly more varus than the Caucasian population studied by Staheli.[1,2] Most patients who present with genu valgum fall under the category of "normal physiologic variant," but some have an underlying pathologic process that needs to be addressed.

PATHOLOGIC GENU VALGUM

Incidence and Etiology

Pathologic genu valgum may have either a systemic or focal etiology, like genu varum. It is usually unilateral as opposed to physiologic valgus, which is always symmetrical (Fig. 47-11). Pathologic genu valgum can be divided into one of several categories; idiopathic, posttraumatic, congenital, neuromuscular, and metabolic. All forms of severe genu valgum lead to an increased Q angle and lateralizing forces on the patella. This may predispose the patient to

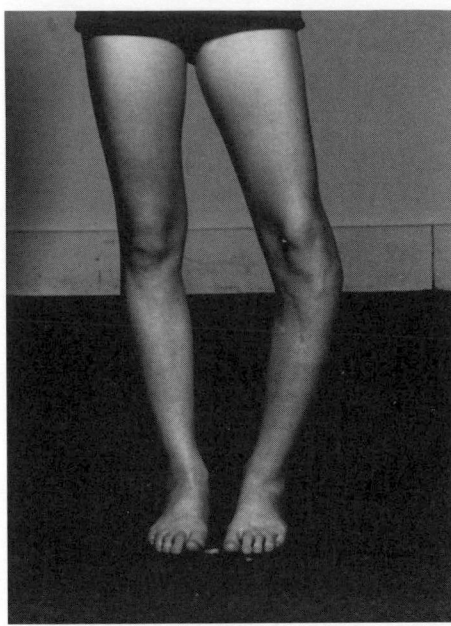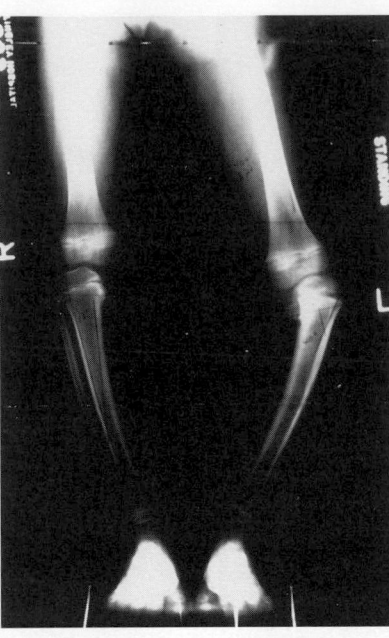

Figure 47-10 Adequate reconstruction of the mechanical axis of the limb must address the lateral subluxation of the tibia and overgrowth of the medial condyle of the distal femur. The patient is an 11-year-old girl.

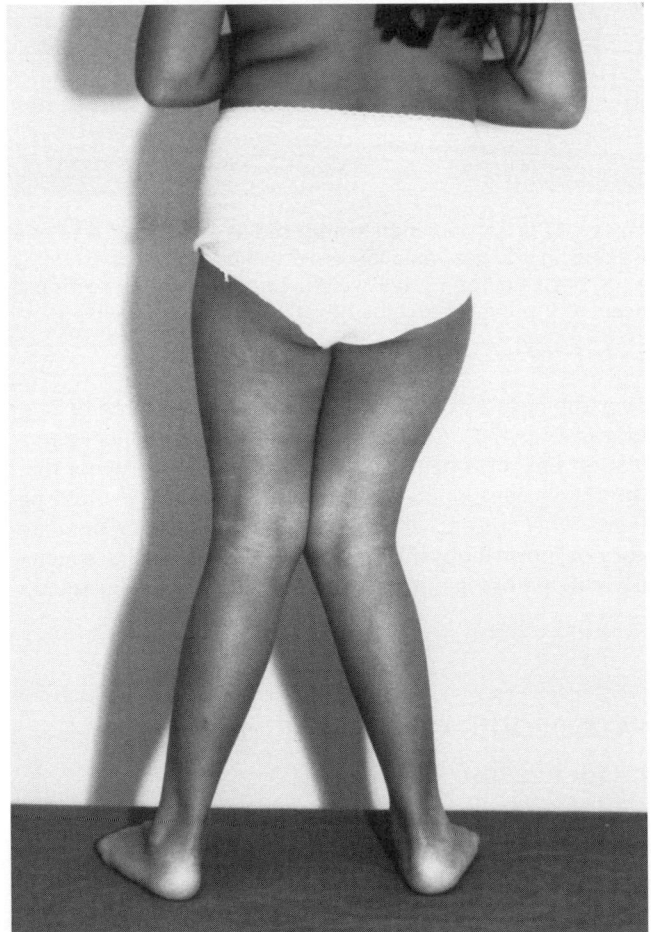

Figure 47-11 This 6-year-old girl has a bilateral valgus deformity, which is considerably greater on the right limb, raising the suspicion that this may represent a pathologic deformity.

chondromalacia, subluxation, or even patellar dislocation. Idiopathic cases are often the residua of an unresolved physiologic genu valgum and are, by definition, more than two standard deviations from the mean. The patients are usually obese, with pes planus and lax ligaments, and may represent a process similar to adolescent tibia vara with retardation of physeal growth secondary to abnormal forces on the limb. The iliotibial band may be contracted in these patients. Femoral hypoplasia has been reported in associated with idiopathic genu valgum.[41] Local trauma is probably the most common pathologic cause of genu valgum. Incomplete ("greenstick") fracture of the proximal tibia in a young child has long been known to carry the risk of a progressive valgus deformity despite adequate osseous union. Skak et al. reported that, in a series of 40 patients, a valgus deformity developed in 15 patients with complete and greenstick fracture, but no deformity developed in patients with buckle fractures.[42] Balthazar and Pappas reported that maximal tibial valgus was reached at 2 years postfracture.[43] Differing opinions as to the etiology of this deformity have been reported in the literature. Some authors felt that a relative medial tibial overgrowth was responsible for the deformity; others felt that it is a combination of the former and an inadequate reduction.[44–46] If a gap is seen in the medial portion of the fracture, there is a possibility that the pes anserinus is trapped in the fracture site.[47]

Fractures of the distal femoral physis are associated with a high incidence of physeal injury and subsequent deformity. The initial fracture pattern and direction of displacement are not predictive of the subsequent direction of deformity and may lead to either a varus or valgus deformity that will not resolve spontaneously.[48]

Hereditary causes of genu valgum include osteochondrodysplasias such as multiple epiphyseal dysplasia and pseudoachondroplasia but rarely achondroplasia, which is almost exclusively associated with genu varum.

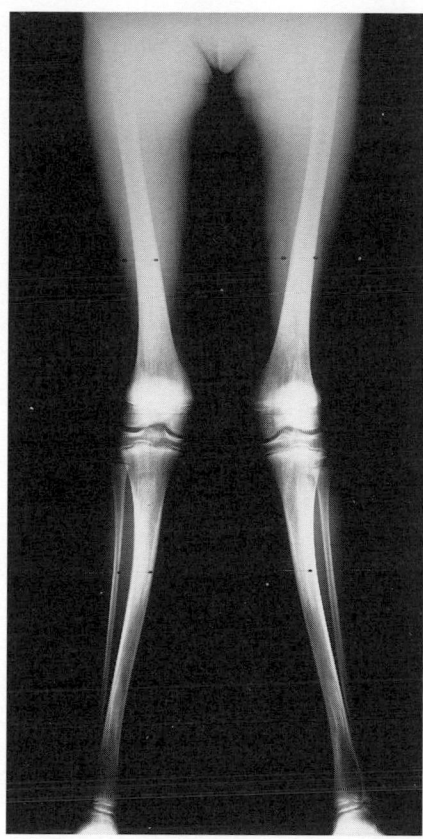

Figure 47-12 A 12-year-old girl with a history of painless knock knees. Radiographs reveal that deformity is in the proximal tibial diaphysis with increased cortical thickness in the area of angulation. Subsequent endocrine workup revealed that the patient had pseudohydroparathyroidism.

Metabolic conditions such as hypophosphatemic rickets, pseudohypoparathyroidism, and renal rickets are often accompanied by an acquired valgus deformity of the knee (Fig. 47-12). Neuromuscular disease such as cerebral palsy, myelomeningocele, and poliomyelitis may also be accompanied by genu valgum. In the paralytic conditions, a tight iliotibial band is thought to be the deforming force.

TREATMENT
Posttraumatic

Acute treatment of the fracture should include objective assessment of the fracture for malalignment. Even a small amount of valgus is unacceptable and should be reduced. Salter and Best recommend that the limb be held in full extension when casting to allow accurate postreduction assessment and avoid malreduction. The typical position of a flexed long leg cast is not sufficient to hold a reduction in the varus/valgus plane.[44] Parents should be informed at the time of fracture that there is a possibility of delayed deformity. Sometimes the valgus deformity following a proximal tibial fracture will resolve spontaneously over a period of 1 to 2 years in the older child and as much as 5 or 6 years in the 3-year-old (the time of maximum physiologic valgus). A period of observation is therefore prudent. Some rebound valgus can be expected after tibial osteotomy and slight overcorrection is advisable.

Idiopathic Genu Valgum

An excellent form of treatment for this condition is slow, gradual correction by physeal stapling of the proximal tibial, distal femur, or both depending on the level of deformity (Fig. 47-13). This gradual correction avoids the potential neurovascular complications that have been reported in acute correction with an osteotomy.[31] Obviously, the patient must be skeletally immature and have enough remaining growth potential to correct the entire deformity. Bowen et al. developed nomograms based on the Green/Anderson growth charts that allows estimation of correction based on physeal width and bone age.[49]

Osteotomies

In skeletally mature patients or those with osteodystrophies, an osteotomy is often necessary. The mechanical axis of the limb must be the prime concern of the surgeon undertaking osteotomies about the knee. A valgus deformity puts the weight-bearing axis in the lateral compartment, but it belongs in the medial portion of the intercondylar notch. If a distal femoral osteotomy is necessary, then care must be taken to avoid medialization of the distal fragment, as this moves the weight-bearing axis back toward the lateral compartment. Both varus or valgus ankle deformities may accompany genu valgum. Preoperative assessment of the ankle position will preclude the possibility of aggravating these deformities. Occasionally, a dual-level osteotomy is necessary.

The peroneal nerve can be stretched during correction of a significant valgus deformity. Stable fixation is necessary so that the postoperative cast can be flexed to alleviate some of the tension on the peroneal nerve.

Ilizarov Device

In the case of a shortened limb with genu valgum secondary to either trauma or fibular hemimelia, a concomitant correction and lengthening may be considered. The considerations of the mechanical axis discussed above also apply here (Fig. 47-14).

CONGENITAL TIBIAL BOWING

Congenital tibial bowing can present with anterior, anterolateral, or posteromedial deformity. All types present potential long-term problems for the growth and development of the involved extremity.

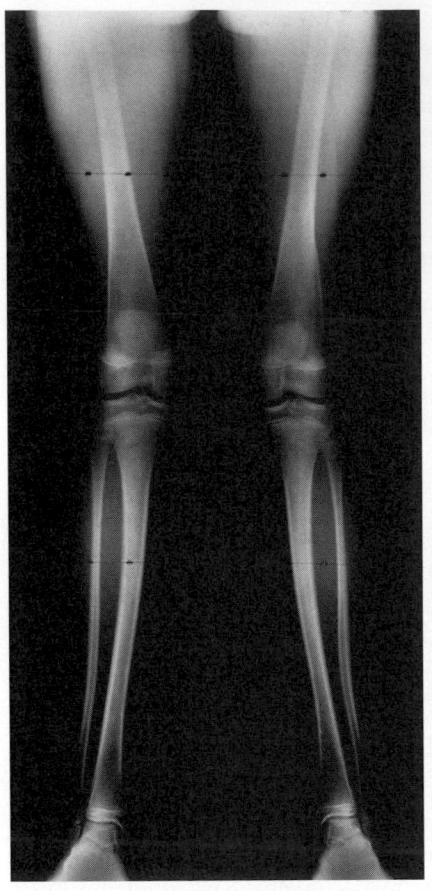

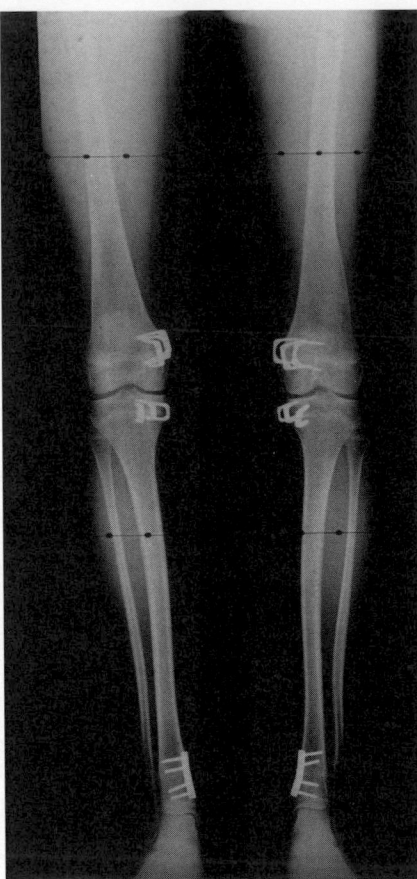

Figure 47-13 *A.* This 12-year-old girl had genu valgum and internal tibial torsion. *B.* One year later, full correction of both deformities has been achieved by epiphyseal stapling and supramalleolar derotational osteotomies.

A

B

Posteromedial Bowing

The etiology of congenital posteromedial bowing has not been established. Earlier authors implicated abnormal positioning in utero. The clinical posterior angulation is localized at the junction of the middle and distal thirds of the leg (Fig. 47-15). Bone, muscle, and subcutaneous tissue are all involved in this rare unilateral condition. The foot is normal but is hyperdorsiflexed and nestled into a concavity on the anterolateral aspect of the tibia. The newborn dorsiflexion contracture can be passively plantar flexed only to neutral. There is persistent decreased plantar flexion of the affected foot throughout life, even after the osseous bowing spontaneously resolves.

Pappas found that the initial radiographic posterior bow decreased, particularly in the first 6 months of life, but that the clinical correction of the deformity lagged behind. The most noticeable clinical improvement took place between 6 and 18 months. Mild residual medial bowing persisted.[50]

A progressive leg-length discrepancy can be expected as the child grows. Pappas reported 33 patients with posteromedial bowing who had an average of 4.1 cm of leg-length discrepancy at maturity (range, 3.3 to 6.9 cm). He showed that the distal tibial physis is the pathologic region of the bone responsible for this discrepancy. The absolute discrepancy increased over time, but the proportionate difference in lengths could be established by 1

year of age. This concept allows for an accurate early estimate of the final discrepancy at maturity.

Treatment

The early treatment of posteromedial bowing includes observation and passive plantar flexion. This may be supplemented with casting or splinting if the soft tissue contracture fails to resolve spontaneously. The absolute and proportionate limb-length discrepancy should be plotted over time, so that the final amount of discrepancy can be predicted. Less than 2 cm of predicted discrepancy should be treated by observation or a shoe lift. Between 2 and 5 cm can be corrected by an appropriately timed contralateral tibial epiphysiodesis. A leg-lengthening procedure may be considered when the discrepancy is predicted to be greater than 5 cm.

INFANTILE TIBIAL NONUNION

Incidence and Etiology

Anterolateral bowing of the tibia and fibula is ominous and should raise strong suspicion that a pathologic process, especially a prepseudarthrosis lesion, may be present.

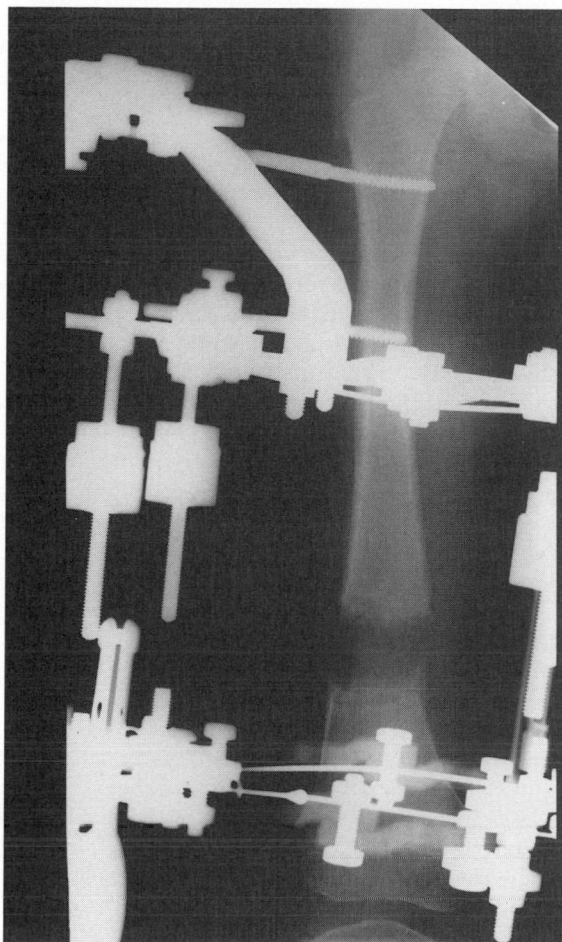

Figure 47-14 This 5-year-old patient underwent a lengthening and varus-producing callotasis for a congenitally short femur with lateral femoral hypoplasia and a partial fibular hemimelia. Note that the distal fragment is slightly lateralized to avoid the medial translation that often accompanies distal femoral varus osteotomies.

Infantile nonunion of the tibia represents a rare pathologic fracture. It more commonly presents in childhood and has a poor prognosis for healing even with prolonged immobilization. A leg-length discrepancy usually accompanies the deformity, which cannot be fully explained by the nonunion and is probably related to abnormal growth of the involved tibia.[51]

The term *congenital pseudarthrosis* is commonly used to describe this condition. This is a misnomer, since the fracture is rarely present at birth. More often the nonunion develops in the first or second year of life and therefore is not truly "congenital."[52,53] The term *pseudarthrosis* describes a true synovial filled space between two segments of the same bone. Most infantile nonunions are filled with a hamartomatous fibrous tissue and are therefore not true pseudarthroses. Based on this reasoning, Bassett et al. used the more accurate term *infantile nonunion* to describe this condition.[54]

The etiology of pseudarthrosis is unknown. It is frequently associated with neurofibromatosis and occasionally with fibrous dysplasia. More than 50 percent of patients with pseudarthrosis have clinical signs of neurofibromatosis.[52,55–58] However, only 13 percent of patients with neurofibromatosis in the large series of Crawford et al. had tibial pseudarthrosis.[58]

Anderson reported an incidence of 1 in 140,000 live births in the Scandinavian population.[52] This rarity leads to small series, which decreases the statistical validity of any single study and increases the likelihood that treatment will be based on the preference of the treating physician.

Clinical Presentation

Most of the patients who develop infantile nonunion of the tibia have had a visible antecedent anterolateral bowing of the distal third of the tibia (Fig. 47-16). This may be less

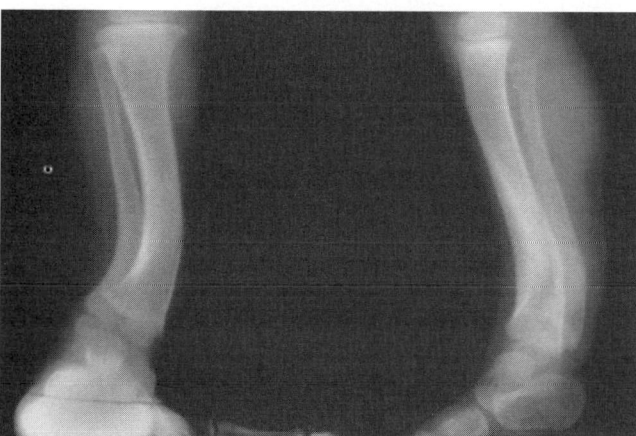

Figure 47-15 Anteroposterior and lateral radiographs demonstrate congenital posteromedial bowing in a 15-month-old toddler. The deformity is localized to the distal third of the leg and can be expected to improve with observation. Anisomelia is a common residual problem.

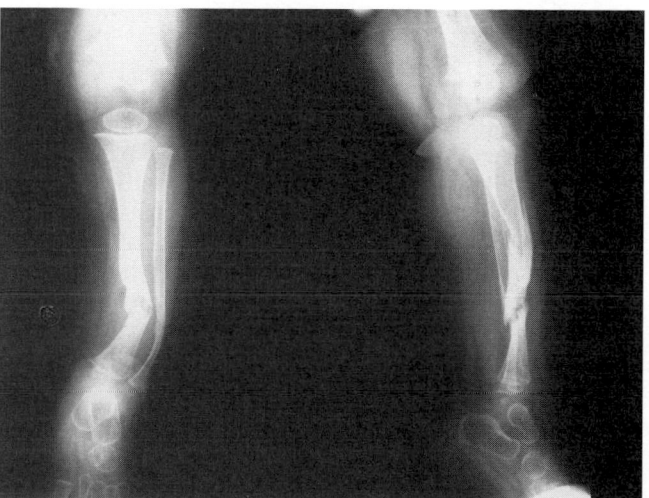

Figure 47-16 Anterolateral bowing, tapering, and sclerosis are all evident in this case of a 4-month-old boy with infantile nonunion of the tibia.

visible in chubby infants. There is a small group of patients who present at an older age, with a fracture after minor trauma, without any obvious premorbid clinical angular deformity. Radiographs at that time, however, may reveal dysplastic changes in the area of fracture, such as sclerosis, cortical tapering, or cyst formation. These patients have been reported to have a more favorable prognosis than those who fracture through a clinically abnormal tibia (anterolateral bowing). Roach et al. reported that 10 of 11 patients who presented in this manner achieved union.[59]

Histology

Histologic studies of the nonunion site only rarely reveal a neurofibroma.[60,61] More often a thickened cuff of periosteum and a proliferation of fibrous tissue is encountered. The fibrous tissue often undergoes metaplasia into disorganized, poorly formed bone.[60]

Classification

Boyd's radiographic classification included six groups:

Type I: Born with anterior bowing and a defect of the tibia (rare).

Type II: Born with anterior bowing and hourglass constriction at the junction of the middle and distal thirds of the diaphysis. This form is often associated with neurofibromatosis. Spontaneous fracture usually occurs before 2 years of age.

Type III: Fracture through a bone cyst in the distal third of the tibial diaphysis. Anterior diaphyseal angulation may precede or follow fracture.

Type IV: Stress fracture arises from a sclerotic segment of the tibia without diaphyseal narrowing.

Type V: Is associated with dysplasic fibula.

Type VI: Is associated with an interosseous neurofibroma or schwannoma (very rare).

Treatment

Earlier literature reported a dismal treatment outcome for this difficult problem, with a high rate of nonunion and eventual amputation.[51,62,63] More recently, the prognosis has become more optimistic, with successful union rates currently approaching 75 percent of cases reported.[55,57,64,65] Results using the Williams intramedullary rodding techniques are good and have the added advantage of a long-term internal splint to help prevent refracture after cortical union has been achieved. The more recently described techniques using either the Ilizarov apparatus or a free vascularized fibular transfer have also reported similar high rates of union.[55,56]

The treatment of infantile nonunions can be laced with difficulty and frustration. Parents should be informed that this is an ongoing problem and that orthopaedic treatment may be required throughout the child's growing years. Some patients need more than one procedure to achieve union.[57,65,66] Recurrent fractures can be particularly disappointing to the patients, family, and physician alike, and these can be as recalcitrant to treatment as the original fracture. The maintenance of union over time is just as important as the initial surgical management. Parents should also be informed that in some cases, an amputation may provide better function than persistent unsuccessful attempts to achieve union.

A number of surgical principles have been developed that increase the chances for primary and long-term union. Realignment of the long axis of the tibia should be a major goal of surgery whenever possible. Residual angulation results in unsatisfactory intrinsic and extrinsic biomechanical forces across the fracture site and increases the risk of refracture. The strength of a tubular object increases by the fourth power of the radius (R^4). Therefore, the diameter of the healed fracture site has great clinical significance. A variety of methods have been recommended to achieve a wider osseous profile at the union site. Bone grafting, side-to-side anastomosis of the spindled ends of bone, and insertion of the spindled proximal segment into the distal segment have all been utilized (Fig. 47-17).

Other factors that must be considered in weighing treatment options include the amount of leg-length discrepancy at the time of treatment as well as the predicted anisomelia at maturity. The affected dysplastic region of bone must be resected at the time of surgery. This can sometimes involve a major segment of the diaphysis and may result in a significant increase in the leg-length discrepancy. However, this should not be the sole criterion determining whether a limb remains salvageable or whether amputation would lead to a better clinical outcome. Patterson and Simonis stated that there is an intrinsic potential for accelerated bone growth after union is achieved in the affected tibia. They felt that up to 10 cm of discrepancy could possibly be made up simply by relying on this accelerated potential growth period,[64] which diminishes after 13 years of age. Another alternative would be the use of the Ilizarov apparatus to compress the nonunion site while performing a concomitant lengthening in the proximal tibial (Fig. 47-17).

Prophylactic Treatment of Bowing

Prophylactic treatment of anterolateral bowing deformities remains controversial. Bypass grafting of severe anterolateral bowing is a technique originally described by McFarland.[67] Tachdijian recommended a delayed bone grafting technique from the contralateral tibial as well as prophylactic curettage and bone grafting of a cystic type of lesion.[68] Staheli wrote that a severe anterolateral deformity should be protected with an orthosis without surgical intervention unless fracture occurred. Mild deformity could be managed by using a flexible intramedullary rod passed retrograde to act as an internal splint.[69] Morrisey et al. reported that prophylactic bone grafting did not alter the outcome in the 7 cases of anterolateral bowing in their series of 40 pseudarthroses. They felt that prophylactic bracing or casting did not prevent fracture or preclude the need for eventual surgery.[51]

Figure 47-17 Resection of the nonunion combined with proximal tibia lengthening can be used to increase tibial diaphyseal radius and length. (Reproduced with permission from Paley D, Catagni M, Argnani F, et al: Treatment of congenital pseudarthrosis of the tibia using the Ilizarov technique. *Clin Orthop* 280:81–93, 1992.)

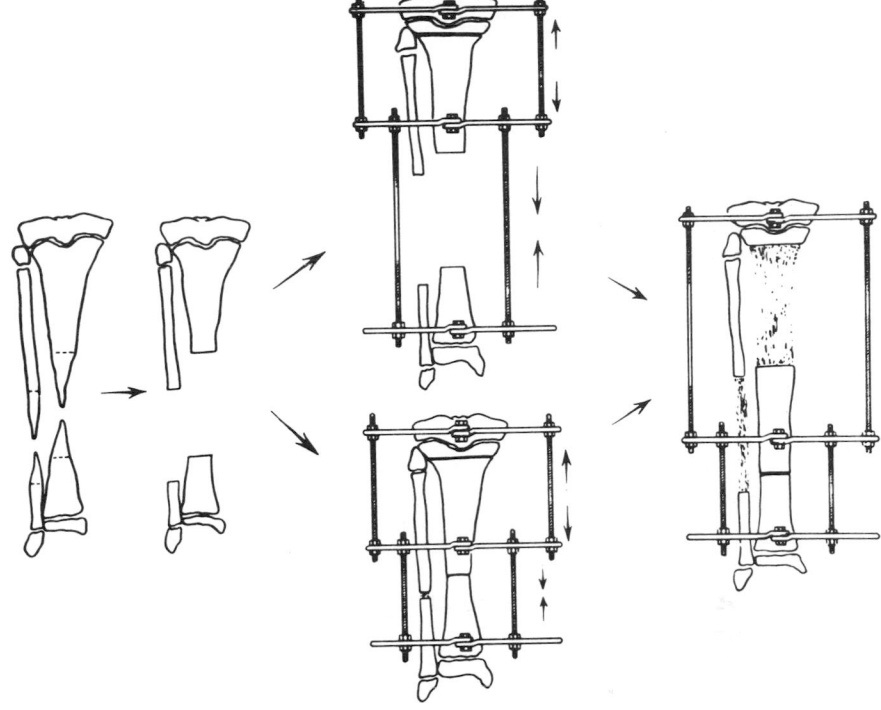

Established Nonunion

Treatment options for nonunion include the following:

1. Resection of the dysplastic bone; intramedullary rodding, and bone grafting
2. Resection of the dysplastic bone and vascularized fibular bone graft (contralateral versus ipsilateral technique)
3. Ilizarov compression of the nonunion with concomitant proximal tibial lengthening (with or without resection of the dysplastic bone)

Intramedullary Rodding

Intramedullary rodding combined with bone grafting, a traditional form of treatment, is still commonly used. The dysplastic portion of the tibial diaphysis is resected to expose a patent proximal and distal medullary canal with bleeding bone surfaces both proximally and distally. A Williams female rod with a threaded male introducer is passed antegrade through the small distal tibial fragment, the talus, and the calcaneus, to exit through the heel pad (Fig. 47-18). The tibial fragments are then realigned and the rod is passed into the proximal fragment of the tibia. The introducer is then disengaged at the level of the plantar surface of the calcaneous after the position is confirmed on anteroposterior (AP) and lateral radiographs. This technique utilizes the cortices of both the talus and calcaneus to help control the small distal tibial fragment. The tibiotalar and subtalar joints are essentially immobilized until continuing growth permits the rod to migrate into the tibia, thus permitting restoration of motion to the ankle and subtalar

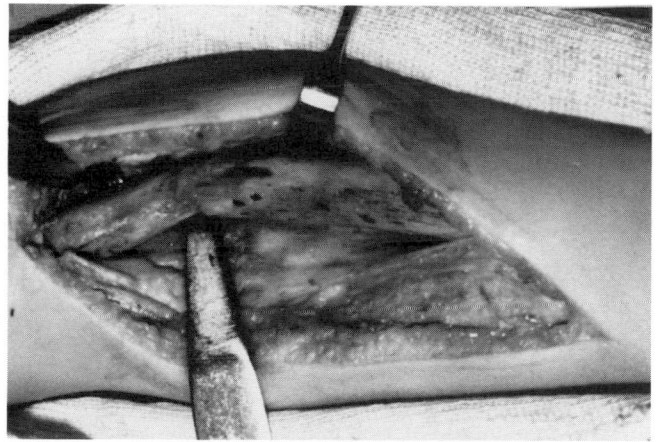

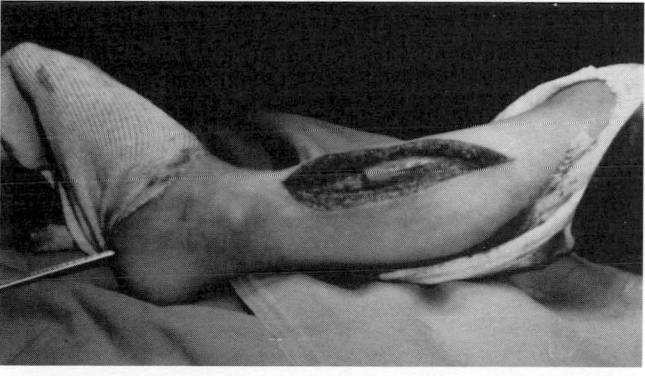

Figure 47-18 *Top:* Fibrous nonunion at the tip of the retractor. *Bottom:* Retrograde Williams rod insertion after resection of the nonunion.

joints. The growth of the distal tibial physis is already affected by the disease and the passage of a smooth rod through its center does not interfere with its growth potential. Care must be taken to correct any accompanying valgus deformity at the ankle when placing the rod. Onlay cancellous or corticocancellous grafts may be used at the fracture site and the patient should be placed into either a bent-knee long leg or spica cast to discourage weight bearing.[58] The patient is placed into a knee-ankle-foot orthosis (KAFO) with a free knee joint for protection after there is radiographic evidence of union. Distal migration of the rod is an occasional complication that can be treated with advancement or reintroduction of a new rod. Reported union rates with this technique exceed 70 percent.

Dual onlay grafts without intramedullary fixation have had limited success because of technical difficulties of obtaining fixation of the graft to the small distal fragment as well as problems with fracture distal to the graft.[57]

Free Vascularized Fibular Transfer

Improvements in microvascular surgical techniques have increased the popularity of this technique. The contralateral limb usually serves as the donor site, since the ipsilateral fibula is often affected by the same dysplastic process as the tibia. Weiland et al. reported an eventual union rate of 95 percent in 19 patients with 10 tibiae left with persistent residual or progressive valgus; 5 of these patients required additional bone grafting to obtain complete union. There was a delayed refracture rate of 10.5 percent and only one amputation was required.[66] Union was achieved in 9 of 11 patients in the series of Simonis et al., with the other two patients requiring amputations. Both the vascular supply of the graft and the initial osseous stabilization of the tibiofibular construct influence the outcome of this procedure. The vascularity of the graft depends on the microvascular surgical anastomosis. There may be considerable technical difficulty in obtaining initial osseous stability because of the size discrepancy between the tibia and fibula. Simonis et al. recommend the use of an external fixator to supplement the internal fixation when the two bones are not well matched in size and firm fixation with screws cannot be accomplished. They suggest a free vascularized fibular transfer as the primary procedure for both tibial lesions with a defect of greater than 3 cm and also for shortening of the leg greater than 5 cm. Approximately 2 cm of shortening can be recovered acutely at the time of this type of surgery. They also recommend free vascularized transfer as a salvage procedure after failure of only one "conventional orthopaedic procedure." For lesions less than 3 cm, they advocate the use of intramedullary rodding, bone grafting, and an implantable electrical stimulator.[56]

The Ilizarov Method

Results utilizing the Ilizarov technique are comparable to the use by Weiland et al. of the free vascularized fibular graft.[66] Technical advantages include the lack of donor site morbidity and the ability to perform a concomitant proximal tibial lengthening as well as increasing the cross-sectional diameter of the tibia at the site of the union, thereby reducing the possibility of refracture. This can be achieved at the nonunion site by overlapping the two tapered segments or inserting one tapered end into the split opposite fragment with supplemental bone graft. The width of the proximal portion of the tibia is maintained by lengthening through the wide metaphyseal region just below the physis. The Ilizarov technique decreases reliance on the concept of "accelerated growth" of the tibia to correct leg-length discrepancies after radical resection of the dysplastic bone. The disadvantages of the technique include pin-tract infection, pain, possible stress concentration at the previous wire sites after fixator removal, and the difficulty of patient tolerance with external fixation for prolonged periods of time.[55]

Amputation

Amputation remains an acceptable functional salvage procedure for this difficult problem. Timing of the procedure still poses a dilemma. An amputation should be considered when it become clear that reconstruction attempts are unsuccessful and before the patient and surgeon develop an emotional commitment to salvage the limb at all costs. Both the Symes and Boyd types of amputation have been recommended. Herring et al. and Epps and Schneider have reported that the orthopaedic function and psychological adjustments of these types of amputations have been excellent.[70,71] Following amputation, patients with a persistent nonunion will require a patellar tendon–bearing, below-knee prosthesis, which differs biomechanically from the prosthesis for an end-bearing amputee.[70,71]

A true below-knee amputation through the pseudo-arthrosis should never be performed because of the vascular insufficiency resulting from scar tissue from previous surgeries and the even more common problem of diaphyseal overgrowth. There is an isolated report of a tibia healing after a Boyd amputation.[57]

Adjuvant Therapy

Pulsed electromagnetic fields (PEMFs) have been added to the armamentarium in the treatment of infantile nonunion; this serves as an adjunctive treatment to operative procedures.[54,57,64,72] Bassett et al. reported that the efficacy of surface-coil PEMFs is dependent on the specific type of lesion being treated. They reported better results in the patient with a gap of less than 5 mm at the nonunion site.[54] Their three part classification in their PEMF outcome report included the following:

Type I: A transverse tibial fracture, a gap less than 5 mm, a significant sclerosis of the medullary canal, and bowing of the tibia

Type II: A fracture gap less than 5 mm with a cystic lesion at the fracture site with or without bowing

Type III: A fracture gap greater than 5 mm with atrophic, spindled bone ends

Of the 28 patients with types I and II lesions seen before operative intervention, 23 (82 percent) healed. Only 6 of 31 patients with type III lesions healed the PEMFs. Patterson and Simonis reported good results using an implantable bone stimulator; this eliminated the need for surface coils to be placed for long periods (12 h per day) on active children.[64] It will be years before the long-term results of some of the newer techniques are known, but the early results are encouraging. As the armamentarium to treat infantile nonunion of the tibia increases, the need for amputation will hopefully diminish.

TIBIAL HEMIMELIA

Etiology and Incidence

Tibial hemimelia is a rare, longitudinal intercalary limb deficiency involving the osseous and soft tissue components of the medial portion of the leg. It has an estimated incidence of 1 in 1 million live births. The term *melia* is derived from the Greek word *melos,* meaning limb. *Amelia* denotes absence of the entire limb and *hemimelia* refers to the loss of half the limb. Frantz and O'Rahilly defined an intercalary defect as missing a forearm or leg segment with a "more or less complete" hand or foot.[73] The foot in tibial hemimelia may appear clinically complete but generally has osseous abnormalities.[74-78]

The specific cause of tibial hemimelia remains unknown. Limb bud development begins approximately 4 weeks postovulation and continues until the end of the embryonal period at approximately 8 weeks. Mechanical or chemical insult during this period can cause a variety of different congenital deformities. Since proximal limb bud development influences the growth of the distal limb, disruption in early embryonal development could lead to increased severity of the distal deformity. Hootnick et al. proposed that a persistence of the fetal pattern of limb circulation, dependent on a single main artery, puts the developing leg at risk because of decreased collateral flow.[75] Whatever the cause, it is clear that the development of the entire sclerotome is affected.

Tibial hemimelia is the only skeletal deficiency with a Mendelian pattern of inheritance. Both autosomal dominant and recessive patterns have been described.[79-83] Most patients with associated hand anomalies follow an autosomal dominant transmission.[83,84] There is a report of two unrelated families involving four children with tibial hemimelia, femoral bifurcation, and ectrodactyly ("lobster claw deformities") of the hands who had an autosomal recessive pattern of inheritance.[79]

Most cases of tibial hemimelia have associated musculoskeletal anomalies, including scoliosis, hip dysplasia, bifurcation of the femur, and ray reduction or polydactyly of the feet (Fig. 47-19). There may be associated defects of cardiac, genitourinary, and gastrointestinal systems.

Several theories attempt to explain the association of the bifurcated femur with tibial hemimelia. Ehrlich, quoted by Wolfgang, stated that the tibial anlage fuses to the distal femur and continues to grow as an exostosis.[85]

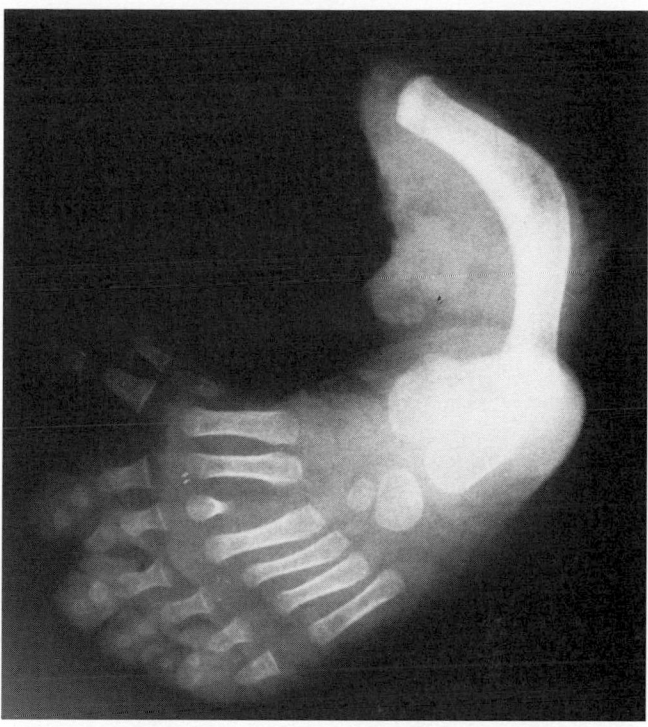

Figure 47-19 Dissection of the amputated specimen revealed multiple tarsal coalitions and polymetatarsia.

Clinical Presentation

Tibial hemimelia presents in the newborn period with severe supination of the foot and concomitant shortening of the involved lower leg. There is often an adherent dimple of skin attached to the distal lateral aspect of the fibula in complete absence of the tibia. A flexion contracture of the knee is usually seen in more severe cases.

Classification

The Jones classification distinguishes between complete and near complete tibial hemimelia. Type I-B is distinguished radiographically from type I-A by the development of the distal femoral physis. However, more recent evidence disputes this radiographic distinction. Williams states that the radiographic presence of a distal femoral physis is not a reliable indicator of the presence of a cartilaginous tibial anlage.[77]

In 1985, Kalamchi and Dawe presented a pragmatic classification based on radiographic and clinical appearance and the functional status of the quadriceps mechanism (Figs. 47-20*A, B,* and *C*). Average age at presentation in their series was 6 months.[87]

Their classification included the following:

Type 1: Patients born with greater than 45° flexion contracture of the knee. Initial radiographs reveal total absence of the tibia associated with significant total proximal migration of the fibula. No active quadriceps function is present.

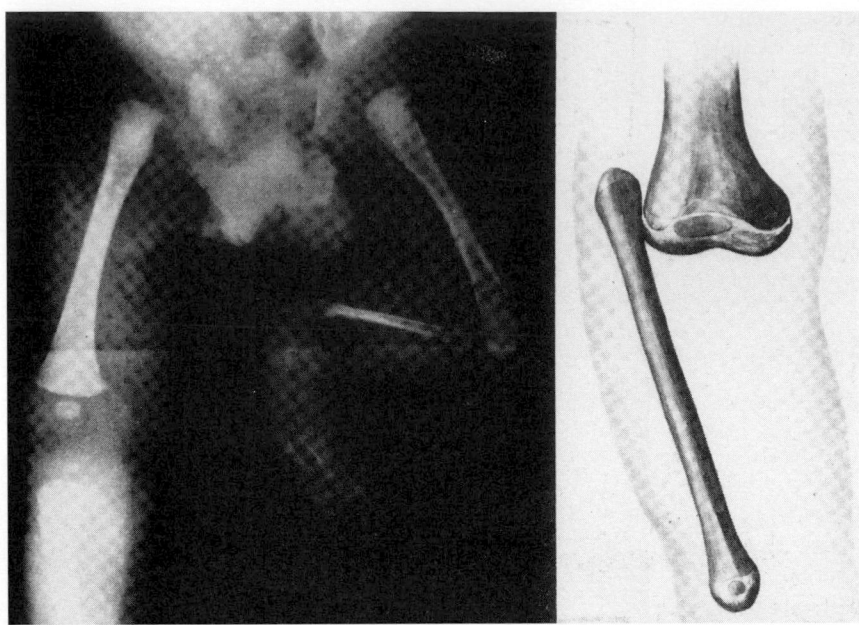

A

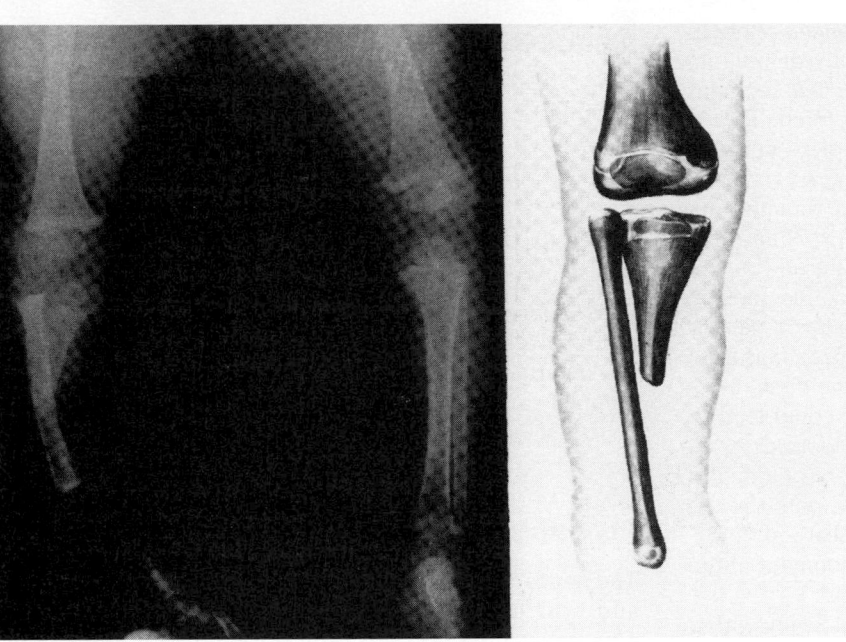

B

Figure 47-20 *A.* Radiograph and diagram of type I deformity demonstrating total absence of the tibia. The radiograph also shows the foot deformity, with missing medial rays, and the absence of the distal femoral epiphysis. *B.* Radiograph and diagram of type II deficiency. The proximal tibia is present and the knee is well preserved. There is less proximal migration of the fibula, but the foot is displaced. *C.* Radiograph of a child with type III deformity showing hypoplasia of the distal tibia and diastasis of the tibiofibular syndesmosis. (Reproduced with permission from Kalamchi A, Dawe RV: Congenital deficiency of the tibia. *J Bone Joint Surg* 67B:581–584, 1985.)

Type 2: Patients born with a knee flexion contracture of 25 to 45°. Initial radiographs reveal a proximal tibial anlage that has a normal relationship with the distal femur. Active quadriceps contraction could be elicited and proximal fibular migration was less pronounced.

Type 3: Radiographs reveal that most of the tibia is present but is dysplastic distally. A distal tibiofibular diastasis is present. Patients are born with a normal knee and a well-developed quadriceps mechanism.

Treatment

The treatment of tibial hemimelia is directed toward giving the child a functional extremity that will provide long-term weight bearing with a minimal amount of surgical intervention. Attempts at salvaging the foot in the presence of complete tibial aplasia are usually unsuccessful. Talocalcaneal coalitions exist universally, even when they are not visible on early radiographs.[74–78] Other tarsal coalitions may be present, which prohibit the foot from transferring energy efficiently to the leg and increase biome-

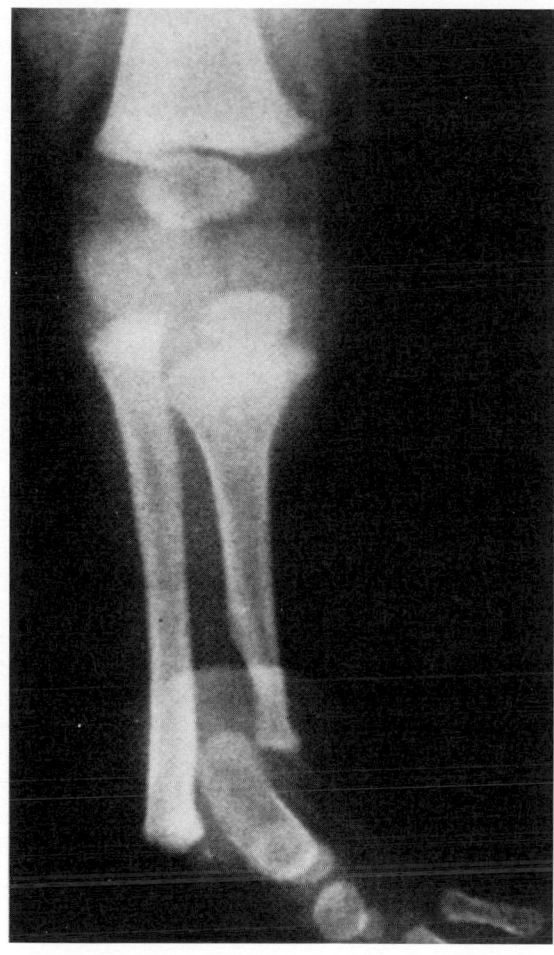

C

Figure 47-20 (*Continued*)

chanical stress on the more proximal limb.[74,78] The involved leg always has shortening, which cannot be corrected by current limb-lengthening techniques. The discrepancy is usually too great to be corrected by contralateral epiphysiodesis. Therefore, most functional reconstructions are based on some form of amputation, with through-knee disarticulation and Syme's amputation forming the basis of current treatment.

Despite the fact that the absolute leg-length discrepancy of an infant may be small and a foot may appear "normal," the discrepancy will increase with age and salvage procedures on the foot are usually futile. Parents do not have the advantage of knowing the natural history of this deformity. They might benefit by meeting other families who have undergone a similar experience. A team approach using a psychologist and a prosthetist to help the family with the decision is highly recommended. A number of authors stress the need for psychological preparation of the patients and their families when ablation of part of a leg or a foot is being considered.[70,88,89] Herring et al. showed that orthopaedic outcome directly correlated with the psychological function of patients with Syme amputations.[70]

Kalamchi and Dawe recommend that type 1 patients be managed by early knee disarticulation and fitting with a pylon-type of prosthesis.[87] The child is ready for this surgical reconstruction when standing is initiated, usually at about 12 to 15 months of age.

Patients with type 2 deformity can be managed by proximal tibiofibular fusion to obtain stability of the knee joint. A modified centralization procedure placing the fibula into the proximal tibial remnant has been successful when done at an early age. At an older age, the authors recommended that a side-to-side tibiofibular synostosis be performed.[87,90] Ablation of the foot is performed at a later date. A calcaneofibular fusion is recommended for those patients with type 3 deformity so as to stabilize the hindfoot and improve function. When this is not technically possible, talectomy and modified Boyd amputation are indicated. Placing the distal fibula into the calcaneus attempts to preserve longitudinal growth and avoid the heel pad migration seen in some Syme amputations.[87,90] Other authors feel that this migration is not a significant functional problem.[70] When there is marked instability between the two leg bones, proximal tibiofibular synostosis is recommended.[87,90]

The length of the femoral segment should be assessed when a through-knee disarticulation is being considered. If the femoral segment is short enough to make prosthetic fitting difficult, the surgeon may consider a femorofibular fusion to increase the length of the residual limb segment.[71,87]

The Brown fibular centralization procedure for complete tibial aplasia is plagued by late recurrent knee contractures that make prosthetic fitting more difficult. Long-term results are generally unsatisfactory, and some patients are functionally improved following a secondary ablation through the knee.[71,87,90–92]

Above-knee and below-knee diaphyseal amputation should always be avoided because of problems with overgrowth of the residual diaphysis.

FIBULAR HEMIMELIA

Incidence and Etiology

Fibular hemimelia is the most common congenital long bone deficiency and represents a spectrum of soft tissue and osseous defects ranging from mild to severe. The exact etiology is unknown. Studies in animal models suggest that fibular development in the embryonal period can be disrupted by radiation and chemical insults. Lewin and Opitz noted the developmental association between the fibula, pubis, proximal femur, anterior cruciate ligaments, and the lateral rays of the foot. This has clinical significance, since fibular hemimelia is frequently associated with defects in these structures (e.g., proximal femoral focal deficiency).[93,94]

Fibula hemimelia is usually a sporadic congenital defect but may be associated with rare hereditary syndromes such as pseudothalidomide syndrome and Volkman's syndrome. These syndromes are associated with other skeletal anomalies, including ulnar deficiencies.[84]

Clinical Presentation

Fibular hemimelia is usually unilateral and presents in the neonatal period, with the affected foot fixed in an equinovalgus position. The lateral rays may be missing. Patients with fibular hypoplasia and lateral deficiencies of one or two pedal rays have less limb-length discrepancy and deformity than those with complete fibular aplasia.[95] Occasionally, the infant presents with antero*medial* bowing of the tibia and a skin dimple over the apex of the associated tibia. This bowing should be distinguished from a prepseudarthrosis, which presents with an antero*lateral* bow. Fibular hemimelia is often associated with genu valgum, which may result from a hypoplastic lateral femoral condyle, a valgus deformity of the proximal tibia, or both. The ankle is often affected in fibular hypoplasia. In the more severe cases, the ankle may assume a valgus position due to the more proximal position of the lateral malleolus. A "ball-and-socket" ankle joint may be seen on radiographs, indicating the presence of a tarsal coalition.[94,96] There may be no radiographic evidence of subtalar coalitions in younger patients, but eventually the hindfoot anomaly becomes evident.[97]

A leg-length discrepancy is always associated with fibular hemimelia. The absolute amount of shortening at maturity is predictable after the first year or two of life. Although the clinical discrepancy will increase with age, the percentage of discrepancy is relatively constant throughout the growth.[76]

Coventry and Johnson proposed a three-part classification based on the degree of fibular dysplasia and whether the deformity is bilateral or unilateral.[98] We prefer the four part classification of Letts, which emphasizes the amount of shortening predicted at maturity and includes the following:

Type A: Unilateral, less than 6 cm of shortening, minimal foot deformity, minimal femoral shortening
Type B: Unilateral, 6 to 10 cm of shortening, minimal foot deformity, minimal femoral shortening
Type C: Unilateral, more than 10 cm of shortening, major foot deformity, and/or major femoral shortening
Type D: Bilateral[89]

Treatment

The treatment of fibular hemimelia is directed toward the achievement of a normal gait pattern and retention of the functional foot when possible. The two main problems that must be addressed are the leg-length discrepancy and the deformity at the ankle and foot. A Syme or Boyd amputation should be considered when a predicted discrepancy at maturity is greater than 20 percent of the limb segment or the congenital deformity of the foot is not compatible with reasonable function (e.g., one- or two-ray foot). An amputation and early prosthetic fitting can often restore function and length more reasonably than multiple operations and needless physical and psychological trauma to the patient and the family. Amputations and prosthetic fitting should be timed to correlate with the de-

velopmental walking age of the child. Herring et al. showed that Syme amputations have excellent long-term physical and psychological outcomes.[64] Letts and Vincent stated that family acceptance of treatment is not problematic on either end of the spectrum of fibular hemimelia. Patients with type C deformities and relatively normal feet create the greatest dilemma for the family unit.[89] Family acceptance is of utmost importance in the outcome of the patient when amputation is deemed necessary.[70,89] Occasionally, the family will not give permission for an amputation in a case that clearly will not respond to lengthening and reconstruction. In these cases, Letts and Vincent use a custom prosthesis that places the foot in a plantarflexed position.[89] This form of treatment may be accepted by younger children, but often, by the time adolescence is reached, the patient's body image needs are not met by a bulky prosthesis. The patient's foot can still be ablated, but the patient and family have a more difficult time adjusting to the amputation psychologically.

In the more severe cases of fibular hypoplasia, the tibia may have an anteromedial bow. This deformity generally corrects spontaneously. Persistence of deformity may have to be addressed surgically, even after ablation, because angular deformity can interfere with prosthetic fitting. Severe bowing can essentially change an end-bearing Syme or Boyd amputation into a patellar tendon–bearing construct.

Medial femoral physeal stapling is an excellent alternative to osteotomy when correction of genu valgum is necessary in patients with amputations.[99]

Ilizarov Method

The Wagner limb-lengthening technique for fibular hemimelia had poor results in a comparative study of lengthening versus amputation.[100] Recent widespread use of Ilizarov's principles has permitted the retention of legs previously deemed unsalvageable.[101–103] Sometimes a decision must be made between having a lengthened leg with a stiff foot that is proprioceptive and a modern prosthesis, which can function remarkably well. The series of Herring et al. included a high percentage of amputees participating actively in high school athletic programs.[70] Nonetheless, it would seem that limb salvage of a sensate foot should still be the surgical goal when feasible.[102]

A number of concepts must be entertained in considering limb-lengthening procedures for these patients. Congenital hypoplastic extremities do not respond as well to lengthening procedures as do limbs that have an acquired shortening or deformity. Osseous regeneration can be slow and refracture is more common. Parents should be made aware of the increased difficulties of performing these procedures for their children. Frequently there is an accompanying hypoplasia of the femur associated with fibular hemimelia. This may often be equal to and sometimes greater than the tibial discrepancy. Consideration should be given to lengthening both bones, either at the same time or in stage procedures. This is critical if the patient's knees are to be kept the same height. The true mechanical axis must be considered in the treatment of this

Figure 47-21 Simultaneous correction of valgus and leg length is possible in a patient with fibular hemimelia and a short femur. (Reproduced with permission from Catagni MA: Management of fibular hemimelia using the Ilizarov method. *AAOS Instr Course Lect* 41:431–434, 1992.)

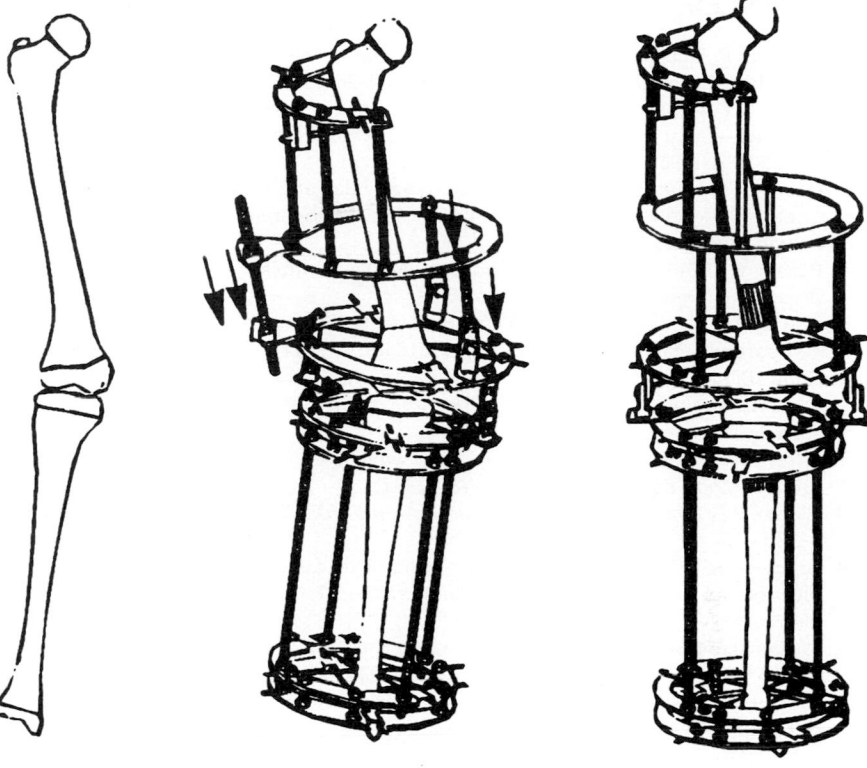

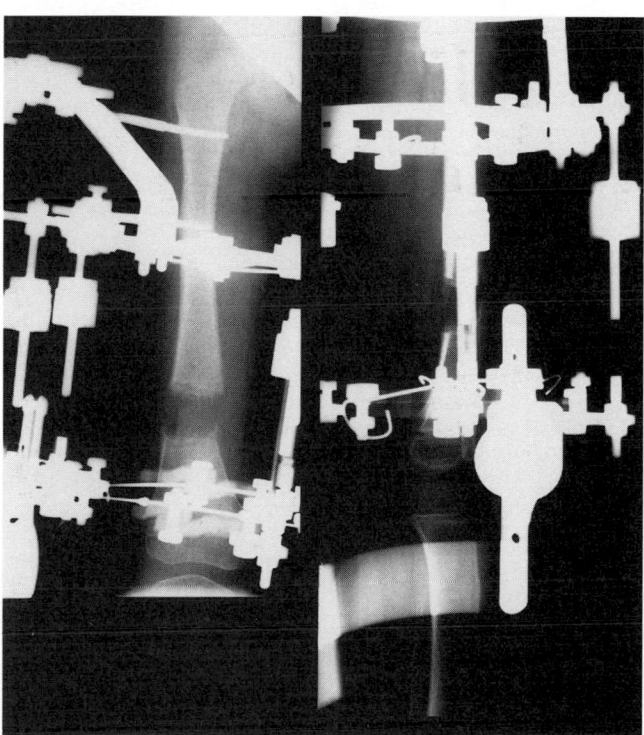

Figure 47-22 A femoral lengthening and correction of genu valgum is being undertaken in this patient with fibular hemimelia and a congenitally short femur. Note the apparatus extending below the distal ring. This spring-loaded device holds the tibia forward during lengthening in this patient who has clinical deficiency of the anterior cruciate ligament.

deformity. Genu valgum should be assessed preoperatively for location (distal femur and/or proximal tibia) and can be corrected simultaneously by a modification of the lengthening construct (Fig. 47-21). Ankle valgus associated with a proximal station of the lateral malleolus can be corrected by placing a single wire through the distal fibula and transporting it more distally than the tibia during the lengthening process.[104]

The integrity of the knee and hip joints must be carefully assessed preoperatively. Acetabular dysplasia may lead to hip subluxation during femoral lengthening. Once subluxation occurs, it is extremely difficult to manage, and treatment may result in loss of part or all of the length gained during lengthening. A prophylactic acetabular augmentation is recommended before lengthening is begun. Hypoplasia of the cruciate ligaments can result in knee flexion contractures and posterior tibial subluxation during femoral and more often tibial lengthening. It is important to maintain the leg in extension during the lengthening procedure. Options to accomplish this include dynamic extension splinting attached directly to the frame or a static Plastizote splint (Fig. 47-22). The latter form is efficient when used with unilateral fixators but can be very difficult to apply when a ring fixator is used. After fixator removal, a knee extension contracture is easier to overcome with physical therapy than a fixed flexion contracture. If posterior subluxation occurs during lengthening, the fixator can be extended above or below the knee joint to permit correction of the problem.

REFERENCES

1. Salenius P, Vankka E: The development of the tibiofemoral angle in children. *J Bone Joint Surg [A]* 57:259–261, 1975.
2. Heath CH, Staheli LT: Normal limits of knee angle in white children—Genu varum and genu valgum. *J Pediatr Orthop* 13:259–262, 1993.
3. Cheng JCY, Chan PS, Chiang SC, Hui PW: Angular and rotational profile in the lower limb in 2,630 Chinese children. *J Pediatr Orthop* 11:154–161, 1991.
4. Blount WP, Tibia vara: Osteochondrosis deformans tibiae. *J Bone Joint Surg* 19:1–29, 1937.
5. Thompson GH, Carter JR, Smith CW: Late-onset tibia vara: A comparative analysis. *J Pediatr Orthop* 4:185–194, 1984.
6. Cook SD, Lavernia CJ, Burke SW, et al: A biomechanical analysis of the etiology of the tibia vara. *J Pediatr Orthop* 3:449–454, 1983.
7. Kling TF Jr: Angular deformities of the lower limbs in children. *Orthop Clin North Am* 18:513–527, 1987.
8. Greene WB: Infantile tibia vara. *J Bone Joint Surg* 75A:130–143, 1993.
9. Bradway JK, Klassen RA, Peterson HA: Blount disease: A review of the English literature. *J Pediatr Orthop* 7:472–480, 1987.
10. Langenskiöld A: Tibia vara (osteochondrosis deformans tibiae): A survey of 23 cases. *Acta Chir Scand* 103:1–22, 1952.
11. Ferriter P, Shapiro F: Infantile tibia vara: Factors affecting outcome following proximal tibial osteotomy. *J Pediatr Orthop* 7:1–7, 1987.
12. Schoenecker PL, Johnston R, Rich MM, Capelli AM: Elevation of the medial plateau of the tibia in the treatment of Blount disease. *J Bone Joint Surg* 74A:351–358, 1992.
13. Wenger DR, Mickelson M, Maynard JA: The evolution and histopathology of adolescent tibia vara. *J Pediatr Orthop* 4:78–88, 1984.
14. Henderson RC, Greene WB: Etiology of late-onset tibia vara: Is varus alignment a prerequisite? *J Pediatr Orthop* 14:143–146, 1994.
15. Henderson RC, Kemp GJ, Hayes PRL: Prevalence of late-onset tibia vara. *J Pediatr Orthop* 13:255–258, 1993.
16. Carter JR, Leeson MC, Thompson GH, et al: Late-onset tibia vara: A histopathologic analysis. A comparative evaluation with infantile tibia vara and slipped capital femoral epiphysis. *J Pediatr Orthop* 8:187–195, 1988.
17. Lovejoy JF, Lovell WW: Adolescent tibia vara associated with slipped capital femoral epiphysis: A report of two cases. *J Bone Joint Surg* 52A:361–364, 1970.
18. Levine AM, Drennan JC: Physiological bowing and tibia vara. *J Bone Joint Surg* 64A:1158–1163, 1982.
19. Henderson RC, Lechner CT, Demasi RA, Green WB: Variability in radiographic measurement of bowleg deformity in children. *J Pediatr Orthop* 10:491–494, 1990.
20. Feldman MD, Schoenecker PL: Use of the metaphyseal-diaphyseal angle in the evaluation of bowed legs. *J Bone Joint Surg* 75A:1602–1609, 1993.
21. Bradish CF, Davies SJM, Malone M: Tibia vara due to focal fibrocartilaginous dysplasia: The natural history. *J Bone Joint Surg* 70B:106–108, 1988.
22. Cockshott WP, Martin R, Friedman L, Yuen M: Focal fibrocartilaginous dysplasia and tibia vara: A case report. *Skel Radiol* 23:333–335, 1994.
23. Husien AMA, Kale VR: Case report: Tibia vara caused by focal fibrocartilaginous dysplasia. *Clin Radiol* 40:104–105, 1989.
24. Langenskiöld A: Tibia vara: Osteochondrosis deformans tibiae. Blount's disease. *Clin Orthop* 158:77–82, 1981.
25. Langenskiöld A: Tibia vara (editorial). *J Pediatr Orthop* 14:141–142, 1994.
26. Loder RT, Johnson CE II: Infantile tibia vara. *J Pediatr Orthop* 7:639–646, 1987.
27. Stricker SJ, Edwards PM, Tidwell MA: Langenskiöld classification of tibia vara: An assessment of interobserver variability. *J Pediatr Orthop* 14:152–155, 1994.
28. Golding JSR, McNeil-Smith JDG: Observations on the etiology of tibia vara. *J Bone Joint Surg* 45B:320–325, 1963.
29. Greene WB: Genu varum and genu valgum in children. *AAOS Instr Course Lect* 43:151–159, 1994.
30. Rab GT: Oblique tibial osteotomy for Blount's disease (tibia vara). *J Pediatr Orthop* 8:715–720, 1988.
31. Steel HH, Sandrow RE, Sullivan PD: Complications of tibial osteotomy in children for genu varum or valgum. *J Bone Joint Surg* 53A:1629–1635, 1971.
32. Price CT: Unilateral fixators and mechanical axis realignment. *Orthop Clin North Am* 25:499–508, 1994.
33. Martin SD, Moran MC, Martin TL, Burke SW: Proximal tibial osteotomy with compression plate fixation for tibia vara. *J Pediatr Orthop* 14:619–622, 1994.
34. Price CT, Scott DS, Greenberg DA: Dynamic axial external fixation in the surgical treatment of tibia vara. *J Pediatr Orthop* 15:236–243, 1995.
35. Gregosiewicz A, Wosko I, Kandzierski G, Drabik Z: Double-elevating osteotomy of tibiae in the treatment of severe cases of Blount's disease. *J Pediatr Orthop* 9:178–181, 1989.
36. Beck CL, Burke SW, Roberts JM, Johnston CE: Physeal bridge resection in infantile Blount disease. *J Pediatr Orthop* 7:161–163, 1987.
37. Birch J: Physeal bar resection. Presentation at the 26th annual Carrie Tingley Winter Seminar, Albuquerque MN, January 1996.
38. Thompson GH, Carter JR: Late-onset tibia vara (Blount's disease): Current concepts. *Clin Orthop* 255:24–35, 1990.
39. Beskin J, Burke SW, Johnston C II, Roberts JM: Clinical basis for a mechanical etiology in adolescent Blount's disease. *Orthopaedics* 9:365–370, 1986.
40. Kline SC, Bostrum M, Griffin PP: Femoral varus: An important component in late-onset Blount's disease. *J Pediatr Orthop* 12:197–206, 1992.
41. White GR, Mencio GA: Genu valgum in children: Diagnostic and therapeutic alternatives. *J Am Acad Orthop Surg* 3:275–283, 1995.
42. Skak SV, Jensen TT, Poulsen TD: Fracture of the proximal metaphysis of the tibia in children. *Injury* 18:149–156, 1987.
43. Balthazar DA, Pappas AM: Acquired valgus deformity of the tibia in children. *J Pediatr Orthop* 4:538–541, 1984.
44. Salter RB, Best TN: Pathogenesis of progressive valgus deformity following fractures of the proximal metaphyseal region of the tibia in young children. *AAOS Instr Course Lect* 41:409, 1992.
45. Jordan SE, Alonso JE, Cook FF: The etiology of valgus angulation after metaphyseal fractures of the tibia in children. *J Pediatr Orthop* 7:450–457, 1987.
46. Taylor SL: Tibial overgrowth: A cause of genu valgum. *J Bone Joint Surg Am* 45:659, 1963.
47. Weber BG: Fibrous interposition causing valgus deformity after fracture of the upper tibial metaphysis in children. *J Bone Joint Surg* 59B:290–292, 1977.
48. Riseborough EJ, Barrett IR, Shapiro F: Growth disturbances following distal femoral physeal fracture separations. *J Bone Joint Surg* 65A:885–893, 1983.
49. Bowen JR, Leahey JL, Zhang ZZ, MacEwen GD: Partial epiphysiodesis at the knee to correct angular deformity. *Clin Orthop* 198:184–190, 1985.
50. Pappas AM: Posteromedial bowing of the tibia and fibula. *J Pediatr Orthop* 4:525–531, 1984.
51. Morrisey RT, Riseborough EJ, Hall JE: Congenital

pseudarthrosis of the tibia. *J Bone Joint Surg* 63B:367–375, 1981.

52. Anderson KS: Congenital angulation of the lower leg and congenital pseudarthrosis of the tibia in Denmark. *Acta Orthop Scand* 43:539–549, 1972.

53. Anderson KS: Radiological classification of congenital pseudarthrosis of the tibia. *Acta Orthop Scand* 44:719–727, 1973.

54. Bassett CAL, Caulo N, Kort J: Congenital "pseudarthroses" of the tibia: Treatment with pulsing electromagnetic fields. *Clin Orthop* 154:136–149, 1981.

55. Paley D, Catagni M, Argnani F, et al: Treatment of congenital pseudoarthrosis of the tibia using the Ilizarov technique. *Clin Orthop* 280:81–93, 1992.

56. Simonis RB, Shirali HR, Mayou B: Free vascularized fibular grafts for congenital pseudarthrosis of the tibia. *J Bone Joint Surg* 73B:211–215, 1991.

57. Baker JK, Cain TE, Tullos HS: Intramedullary fixation for congenital pseudarthrosis of the tibia. *J Bone Joint Surg* 74A:169–178, 1992.

58. Crawford AH, Bagamery N: Osseous manifestation of neurofibromatosis in childhood. *J Pediatr Orthop* 6:72–88, 1986.

59. Roach JW, Shindell R, Green NE: Late-onset pseudarthrosis of the dysplastic tibia. *J Bone Joint Surg* 75A:1593–1601, 1993.

60. Boyd HB, Sage FP: Congenital pseudoarthrosis of the tibia. *J Bone Joint Surg* 40A:1245–1270, 1958.

61. Greene WT, Rudo N: Pseudarthrosis and neurofibromatosis. *Arch Surg* 46:639–651, 1943.

62. Kuo et al: Congenital pseudarthrosis of the tibia. *J Pediatr Orthop* 4:775, 1984.

63. Masserman RL, Peterson HA, Bianco AJ: Congenital pseudarthrosis of the tibia. *Clin Orthop* 9:140–145, 1974.

64. Patterson DC, Simonis RB: Electrical stimulation in the treatment of congenital pseudarthrosis of the tibia. *J Bone Joint Surg* 67B:454–462, 1985.

65. Anderson DJ, Schoenecker PL, Sheridan JJ, Rich MM: Use of intramedullary rod for the treatment of congenital pseudarthrosis of the tibia. *J Bone Joint Surg* 74A:161–168, 1992.

66. Weiland AJ, Weiss AP, Moore JR, Tolo VT: Vascularized fibular grafts in the treatment of congenital pseudarthrosis of the tibia. *J Bone Joint Surg* 72A:654–662, 1990.

67. McFarland B: Pseudarthrosis of the tibia in childhood. *J Bone Joint Surg* 33B:36, 1951.

68. Tachdijian MO: "Congenital" Pseudarthrosis of the tibia, in Tachdijian MO (ed): *Pediatric Orthopaedics* 2d ed. Philadelphia, Saunders, 1990, pp 656–685.

69. Staheli L: The lower limb, in Morrisey RT (ed): in *Pediatric Orthopaedics*, 3d ed. Philadelphia, Lippincott, 1990, pp 741–766.

70. Herring JA, Barnhill B, Gaffney C: Syme amputation: An evaluation of the physical and psychological function in young children. *J Bone Joint Surg* 68A:573–578, 1986.

71. Epps CH, Schneider PL: Treatment of hemimelias of the lower extremity. *J Bone Joint Surg* 71A:273–277, 1989.

72. Bassett AL, Schink-Ascani M: Long-term pulsed electromagnetic field (PEMF): Results in congenital pseudarthrosis. *Calcif Tissue Int* 49:216–220, 1991.

73. Frantz CH, O'Rahilly R: Congenital skeletal limb deficiencies. *J Bone Joint Surg* 43A:1202–1223, 1961.

74. Miller LS, Armstrong PF: The morbid anatomy of congenital deficiency of the tibia and its relevance to treatment. *Foot Ankle* 13:396–399, 1992.

75. Hootnick DR, Packard Ds, Levinsohn EM, Cady RB: Soft tissue anomalies in a patient with congenital tibial aplasia and talo-calcaneal synchondrosis. *Teratology* 36:153–162, 1987.

76. Hootnick D, Boyd NA, Fixsen JA, Lloyd-Roberts GC: The natural history and management of congenital short tibia with dysplasia or absence of the fibula. *J Bone Joint Surg* 59B:267–271, 1977.

77. Williams L, Wientroub S, Getty CJM, et al: Tibial dysplasia: A study of the anatomy. *J Bone Joint Surg* 65B:157–159, 1983.

78. Turker RJ, Mendelson S, Ackman J, Lubicky JP: Anatomical considerations of the foot and leg in tibial hemimelia. *J Pediatr Orthop* 16:445–449, 1996.

79. Kohn G, Shawwa RE, Grunebaum M: Aplasia of the tibia with bifurcation of the femur and ectrodactyly: Evidence for an autosomal recessive type. *Am J Med Genet* 33:172–175, 1989.

80. McKay M, Clarren SK, Zorn R: Isolated tibial hemimelia in sibs: An autosomal-recessive disorder? *Am J Med Genet* 17:603–607, 1984.

81. Pfeiffer RA, Correll J: Hemimelia in Brachmann–de Lange syndrome (BDLS): A patient with severe deficiency of the upper and lower limbs. *Am J Med Genet* 47:1014–1017, 1993.

82. Pavone L, Viljoen D, Ardito S, et al: Two rare developmental defects of the lower limbs with confirmation of the Lewin and Opitz hypothesis of the fibular and tibial development fields. *Am J Med Genet* 33:161–164, 1989.

83. Rambaud-Cousson A, Dudin AA, Zuaiter AS, Thalji A: Syndactyly type IV/hexadactyly of feet associated with unilateral absence of the tibia. *Am J Med Genet* 40:144–145, 1991.

84. Lenz W: Genetics and limb deficiencies. *Clin Orthop* 148:9–17, 1980.

85. Wolfgang GL: Complex congenital anomalies of the lower extremities: Femoral bifurcation, tibial hemimelia, and diastasis of the ankle. Case report and review of the literature. *J Bone Joint Surg* 66A:453–458, 1984.

86. Jones D, Barnes J, Lloyd-Roberts GC: Congenital aplasia and dysplasia of the tibia with intact fibula: Classification and management. *J Bone Joint Surg* 60B:31–39, 1978.

87. Kalamchi A, Dawe RV: Congenital deficiency of the tibia. *J Bone Joint Surg* 67B:581–584, 1985.

88. Davidson WH, Bohne WHO: The Syme amputation in children. *J Bone Joint Surg* 57A:905–909, 1975.

89. Letts M, Vincent N: Congenital longitudinal deficiency of the fibula (fibular hemimelia). *Clin Orthop* 287:160–166, 1993.

90. Schoenecker PL, Capelli AM, Millar EA, et al: Congenital longitudinal deficiency of the tibia. *J Bone Joint Surg* 71A:278–287, 1989.

91. Loder RT, Herring JA: Fibular transfer for congenital absence of the tibia: A reassessment. *J Pediatr Orthop* 7:8–13, 1987.

92. Brown FW: Construction of a knee joint in congenital total absence of the tibia (paraxial hemimelia tibia). *J Bone Joint Surg* 47A:695–704, 1965.

93. Lewin SO, Opitz JM: Fibular a/hypoplasia: Review and documentation of the fibular developmental field. *Am J Med Genet* 2:215–238, 1986.

94. Achterman C, Kalamchi A: Congenital deficiency of the fibula. *J Bone Joint Surg* 61B:133–137, 1979.

95. Maffulli N, Fixsen JA: Fibular hypoplasia with absent lateral rays of the foot. *J Bone Joint Surg* 73B:1002–1004, 1991.

96. Pistola F, Ozonoff MB, Wintz P: Ball-and-socket ankle joint. *Skel Radiol* 16:447–451, 1987.

97. Ogden JA: Ipsilateral femoral bifurcation and tibial hemimelia. *J Bone Joint Surg* 58A:712–713, 1976.

98. Coventry MB, Johnson EW: Congenital absence of the fibula. *J Bone Joint Surg* 34A:941, 1952.

99. Boakes JL, Stevens PM, Moseley RF: Treatment of genu valgus deformity in congenital absence of the fibula. *J Pediatr Orthop* 11:721–724, 1991.

100. Choi IH, Kumar J, Bowen JR: Amputation or limb-lengthening for partial or total absence of the fibula. *J Bone Joint Surg* 72A:1391–1399, 1990.

101. Bell DF: Letter to the editor. *J Bone Joint Surg* 73A:1273, 1991.

102. Herring JA: Symes amputation for fibular hemimelia: A second look in the Ilizarov era. *AAOS Instr Course Lect* 41:435–436, 1992.

103. Saleh M: Letter to the editor. *J Bone Joint Surg* 73:1272–1273, 1991.

104. Catagni MA: Management of fibular hemimelia using the Ilizarov method. *Instr Course Lect* 41:431–434, 1992.

CHAPTER 48

The Pediatric Foot

Norris C. Carroll

THE CLUBFOOT

Historical Review

Clubfoot or talipes equinovarus is the most common congenital orthopaedic anomaly, with an incidence of approximately 1.24 per 1000 live births. Clubfoot is less common in Orientals (0.6 per 1000) and higher in Hawaiians (6.8 per 1000). There is also a high incidence in East Africans.[1] Children with untreated clubfoot are still seen in underdeveloped countries. The deformity can be quite severe, with the sole of the foot pointing backward. The dorsum of the foot becomes the weight-bearing surface, so that the child walks on the head and neck of the talus. The word *talipes* (Latin for *clubfoot*) is derived from *talus* (Latin for *ankle*) and *pes* (Latin for *foot*). With a severe untreated talipes equinovarus, a child walks on the ankle instead of the sole of the foot, the heel is in equinus pointing down like a horse's hoof, and the front of the foot is in varus, twisted toward the midline.

Clubfoot is mentioned in the old Indian prayer book *Yajur-Veda* from the tenth century B.C.[2] Hippocrates (460–377 B.C.) has provided us with the oldest written description of clubfoot and its treatment. He used manual manipulation and bandaging to achieve and maintain correction.[3] Following Hippocrates, there is a gap in clubfoot literature until the sixteenth century.

In 1575, Ambroise Paré described the deformity; he thought that it was caused by pregnant women sitting for too long with their legs crossed.[4] His treatment, too, consisted of manipulations and bandaging. In 1743, Nicholas Andry treated clubfeet with wet dressings to soften the ligaments, daily manipulations, and fixation in splints of cardboard, wood, or iron.[5] Jean André Venel (1740–1791) of Switzerland designed a boot to correct clubfoot.[2] Toward the end of the eighteenth century, Verdier and Tiphaine in France and Jackson in England published descriptions of various therapeutic splints.[2] Brückner, a pupil of Venel, improved his teacher's apparatus in 1796 and was said to have effected many cures.[6] In 1798 Wantzel, another pupil of Venel who himself had been treated by Venel for clubfoot, described the anatomy of clubfoot.[7]

The first detailed description of a clubfoot orthosis was published by Antonio Scarpa in 1803.[8] This was an ankle-foot orthosis. A metal bar went up the lateral aspect of the leg to a cuff that went around the proximal calf and another cuff that went around the leg just above the malleoli. A spring was attached at right angles to the upright portion of the ankle-foot orthosis. A cup gripped the hindfoot, and the spring on the lateral side of the foot was attached to a cuff that produced a pronation and abduction force on the forefoot.

In 1784, Lorenz performed the first Achilles tenotomy.[9] Other reports of Achilles tenotomy were published by Sarotorius in 1806, Michaelis in 1809, and Delpech in 1816.[2] In the early part of the nineteenth century Delpech, in describing the pathoanatomy of clubfoot, likened the hindfoot to the hull of a boat.

Some of the early Achilles tenotomies were followed by infection. In 1831, Stromeyer published a report of several successful cases.[10] He gained fame by doing the procedure on the English physician Little. In 1841, Dieffenbach reported the use of Achilles tenotomy on 350 clubfeet.[11] Allegedly, the French poet Gustave Flaubert was inspired by Stromeyer's operation on Little when he described the treatment of a clubfoot by Achilles tenotomy and subsequent traction therapy in the novel *Madame Bovary*. In 1834, Dieffenbach was the first to use a plaster cast in the treatment of clubfeet.

The treatment of clubfeet was revolutionized by the advent of anesthesia in 1846. In 1854, Solly performed the first osteotomy, resecting almost the entire cuboid bone in a 21-year-old male with severe bilateral clubfeet.[12] In 1872, Lund treated severe bilateral clubfeet in a 7-year-old child by excision of the talus.[13] In 1884, Phelps reported the results of 18 clubfeet that he had treated by extensive soft tissue releases.[14]

Toward the end of the nineteenth century, forceful manipulation became popular. This was supported by König in 1890 and Lorenz in 1895, and in 1889 Gibney reported the results of treatment by a Thomas wrench.[2]

In 1902 Ogston introduced a new form of surgical treatment.[15] He advocated excision of the ossific nucleus of the talus, cuboid, and calcaneus. This procedure made the foot soft and pliable, so that it could be manipulated into a corrected position. In 1913, Vulpius described posterior capsulotomy of the ankle in addition to Achilles tenotomy.[16] The first report of a rotational osteotomy of the tibia was by Pürckhauser in 1911.[17]

Browne described his special splint for the treatment of clubfoot in 1930.[18] At about the same time, Kite was using wedged plaster casts with encouraging results.[19] Wisbrun described his new manipulation technique in 1932, paying particular attention to the supination deformity of the hindfoot.[20] In 1931, Contarygis recommended extensive soft tissue surgery as soon as possible after birth.[21] During the past 40 years, an ever-increasing number of surgeons have advocated early soft tissue releases.[2,22–28]

Inheritance

In the review of the genetic aspects of clubfoot, Cowell and Wein concluded that idiopathic talipes equinovarus is primarily caused by a multifactorial inheritance system that is modified by intrauterine environmental factors and possibly is affected by a gene acting in a dominant fashion.[29] Wynne-Davies's studies indicate that the pattern of inheritance is polygenic.[30,31] Dietz believes that complex segregation analyses support the concept that a single major gene contributes significantly to the likelihood of having clubfoot.[32]

As mentioned above, the overall incidence of talipes equinovarus in the general population is 1.24 per 1000 live births. The incidence in first-degree relatives (siblings and parents) is 2.4 per 1000. The incidence in second-degree relatives (aunts and uncles) is 0.61 per 1000 and the incidence in third-degree relatives (cousins) is 0.2 per 1000. If one monozygotic twin has clubfoot, the second twin has a 1 in 3 chance of having the disorder. When a boy is born with a clubfoot, the chances are 1 in 40 that a subsequent brother will be affected and low that his sister will be affected. When a girl is born with a clubfoot, the probability of a clubfoot in her brother is about 1 in 16 and that in a sister 1 in 40. If both a parent and the child have clubfeet, the chances are 1 in 4 that a subsequent child will be affected.[29] A child can be born with a clubfoot as a part of a syndrome complex on a strictly genetic basis. Freeman-Sheldon syndrome, also known as whistling face syndrome and cranio-carpal-tarsal dysplasia, are examples of autosomal dominance inheritance of clubfoot deformity. Diastrophic dwarfism, Larsen's syndrome, and Smith-Lemli-Opitz syndrome all involve autosomal recessive inheritance of clubfoot. Clubfoot has been reported as part of the Pierre Robin syndrome in cases involving X-linked recessive inheritance. Children with Goldenhar syndrome (oculoauriculovertebral dysplasia) can also have clubfoot deformities.

An increased incidence of clubfoot has been reported in association with oligohydramnios and congenital annual bands.[33]

Theories of Pathogenesis

Germplasm Defect

Irani and Sherman dissected 11 clubfeet and noted that the consistent defect in each foot was a deviation of the anterior part of the talus.[34] They thought that this was the primary cause of the deformity and that all other changes were secondary. They found no abnormalities of vessels, nerves, muscles, or tendon insertions. They concluded that the abnormality in the talus was a result of a defective cartilaginous anlage, which is dependent on a primary germplasm defect.

Developmental Arrest Theory

This theory was postulated in Bohm's article in 1929. He noted that in a 17-mm embryo, the development of the lower limb bud is such that the foot part is a direct extension of the lower leg, and that its long axis, that is, the mediolateral breadth of the lower leg, lies in the same plane as the foot plate.[35] A longitudinal section taken through the lower limb and foot at this stage demonstrates adduction as a result of the medial inclination of the calcaneus and talus. The navicular is near the medial malleolus and the metatarsals are adducted. Toward the end of the second month, the plane of the foot rotates into supination, so that at the beginning of the third month, it is right angles to the plane of the lower leg. With the ankle joint as an axis, the foot then flexes cranially along its medial border. This continues until the middle of the third month, when the long axis of the foot is perpendicular to the plane of the lower leg. By the fourth month, the foot is rotated toward pronation until the planes of the foot and the lower leg are in the relative positions as seen in the human adult.

Bohm postulated that the cause of a clubfoot was an arrest in embryonic development in the first stage. He believed that the talus and calcaneus maintained the position of the fifth week. This interfered with the normal sequence of events. The developing foot was unable to bend up toward the lower leg and correction of the adduction and supination did not occur.

Victoria-Diaz and Victoria-Diaz[35a] have expounded on this theory. They pointed out that at the 15-mm stage the foot of the embryo is in a straight line with the leg (initial position), but by the 30-mm stage has passed into an exaggerated equinovarus and adductus position (the embryonic position). By 50-mm, the foot is changed to a position of slight equinovarus and adductus (fetal position). The change from the initial to the embryonic position is brought about by a fibular phase of rapid growth between 21 and 30 mm, and the change from the embryonic to the fetal position by a subsequent growth spurt of the skeletal elements of the medial side of the foot during what may be described as a "tibial phase" of rapid growth. They suggest that if a teratogenic agent acts during the last half of the tibial phase, a mild clubfoot will result. However, if the interference occurs during the first half of the tibial phase, the foot will remain in a permanent and marked equinovarus-adductus position and a severe clubfoot will result.

Fetal Theory

This theory suggests a mechanical block to development—extrinsic pressure in utero—as popularized by Dunne.[36]

Neurogenic Theory

This theory suggests a primary defect in the nerve supply to the muscles. Martin et al. demonstrated reduced motor unit counts in the distribution of the common peroneal nerve as a consistent finding in neurogenic talipes equinovarus.[37] These findings correspond to clinically demonstrated muscle weakness. The findings of Martin et al. suggested a neuropathic etiology, but the investigators were unable to identify the level and nature of the neuropathy.

Isaacs and associates took biopsies of the posteromedial and peroneal muscle groups in 60 patients with clubfeet.[38] They found histochemical anomalies in 92 of 111 specimens, and all specimens were abnormal at the ultramicroscopic level. The investigators concluded that the shortening of the posterior muscles resulted from a small increase of fibrosis owing to minor changes in innervation occurring in intrauterine life and that there was a dominant neurogenic factor in the cause of clubfoot. Handelsman and Badalamente reported similar findings.[39] They also noted a dominant type I fiber population and a type I fiber grouping. There was a correlated increase in type I neuromuscular junctions, which are neurogenically determined changes. Handelsman and Glasser, reporting on a further study of muscle biopsies, again demonstrated the type I fiber grouping.[40] Gray and Katz found an increase in type I muscle fibers in the soleus of children with clubfoot who were less than 6 months old.[41]

Myogenic Theory

This theory postulates that the primary defect is in the muscle. Atrophy of the leg is a constant sign in congenital clubfoot.[2] There is more atrophy in the peroneal muscles than in the muscles holding the foot in the deformed position.[42] Muscle fiber counts indicate that the number is the same on the clubfoot side and the normal side, so that the atrophy is due to a decrease in the size of the individual muscle fibers. The growth of the muscles during the second half of intrauterine life consists of an increase in size of the individual fibers, not an increase in the number of fibers. The peroneal muscles are more atrophied than the other muscles and therefore are unable to balance the foot. Sodre et al. reported a 15.3 percent incidence of two primary muscle anomalies in patients with congenital talipes equinovarus (CTEV): the accessory soleus muscle and the flexor digitorum accessorius longus muscle.[43] They postulate that these anomalous muscles may play an important role in clubfoot deformity, depending on their insertion and dynamic action.

Vascular Theory

Hootnick et al. have described the arterial development in the limb bud.[44] They have found that the majority of limbs with CTEV are associated with diminution of the anterior tibial artery and its derivatives, a pattern that resembles most closely that seen in the embryo between 14 and 18 mm (5.7 to 6.3 weeks of development). They hypothesize that this abnormal arterial pattern in developing limbs could result in malformation. The diminution of the anterior tibial artery and its derivatives could result in medial tethering secondary to scarring or talar anlage dysplasia, thus leading to CTEV.

Theory of Retracting Fibrosis

Ippolito and Ponseti studied 5 clubfeet and 3 normal feet of fetuses aborted at 16 to 20 weeks of gestation.[45] In clubfoot, the authors found an alteration in the shape, size, and relationship of the tarsal bones. There was a decrease in the size and number of fibers in the distal third of the muscles of the posteromedial aspect of the leg as well as increased fibrous connective tissue in these muscles, their tendon sheaths, and the adjacent fascia and shortening of the triceps surae. There was thickening of the distal parts of the Achilles tendon and the posterior tibial tendon. The ligaments on the posteromedial aspect of the ankle joint were pulled into the joint by the severe plantar flexion and varus displacement of the talus and marked shortening and thickening of the talonavicular and plantar calcaneonavicular ligaments. The investigators concluded that a retracting fibrosis may be the primary etiologic factor of the clubfoot deformity. This theory has to some extent been substantiated by Zimny and colleagues, who did an electron microscopic study of the fascia from the medial and lateral sides of clubfeet.[46] Two cell types were observed in

the fascia from the lateral side of the clubfoot. These were two different types of fibroblasts. Three cell types were observed in the fascia from the medial side of the clubfoot (typical fibroblast, cells resembling myofibroblasts, and mast cells). It was postulated that the contracture of the medial side of a clubfoot may be due to the myofibroblastlike cells, and that this contracture may be enhanced by histamine released from the mast cells.

Pathoanatomy

In a clubfoot, the entire lower limb can be shorter. This shortening can involve the femur, the tibia, and the fibula. Shortening of the fibula is more common than shortening of the femur or tibia. The shortening is more common in females with clubfoot.[47] Unilateral cases of clubfoot invariably show growth inhibition of the affected foot.

The Author's Pathoanatomy Studies

From clinical studies, dissections, surgical observations, serial sections, and three-dimensional computer analysis of clubfeet, the author has drawn the following conclusions about the pathoanatomy of a severe clubfoot:

1. When the patella points forward, the lateral malleolus is posterior.
2. There is a cavus component that can be corrected only by lengthening the plantar fascia and intrinsic muscles.
3. The navicular is subluxated medially against the medial malleolus.
4. There is medial displacement of the distal portion of the medial column and, therefore, medial displacement of the distal portion of the lateral column. This means that the cuboid is displaced medially on the os calcis.
5. With the cavus and medial displacement of the cuboid, there is a contracture of the long and short plantar ligaments.
6. The long axis of the os calcis and the body of the talus are parallel (this can be demonstrated by anteroposterior and lateral radiographs of the hindfoot).
7. The os calcis is in equinus.
8. The talus is in equinus.
9. The triceps surae, tibialis posterior, flexor hallucis longus, and flexor digitorum longus are all short.
10. There is a contracture of the posterior capsule and the collateral ligaments of the ankle.
11. Correction of the equinus requires lengthening of the Achilles tendon plus release of the posterior capsule of the ankle and subtalar joints, including the calcaneofibular ligament and the posterior talofibular ligament.
12. There is medial and plantar deviation of the neck of the talus and external rotation of the body of the talus in the ankle mortise.
13. There is medial rotation and supination of the os calcis.
14. There is adductus and supination of the forefoot (Figs. 48-1 and 48-2).[48]

Reconstructions of clubfeet by computed tomography (CT) in older children demonstrate these same pathoanatomic relationships.

Nonoperative Treatment

Manipulation and Casting

Because there are degrees of severity of clubfoot, the treatment must be individualized in each instance. My preference is to begin treatment with manipulation and casting. The baby must be relaxed and comfortable. (A bottle of formula is a good distraction for a hungry baby.) The foot is manipulated to stretch tight muscles and ligaments and to restore the bony architecture. The plaster cast is used to maintain the position obtained by the manipulation, but it does not produce the correction.

Technique of Manipulation

The thumb is placed on the lateral side of the foot to stabilize the talus in the ankle mortise. Traction is applied to the first ray to stretch the tight tibialis posterior and to correct the forefoot supination and adduction. As the forefoot correction progresses, one attempts to reduce the talonavicular joint. If the talonavicular joint reduces, this means that one is beginning to correct some of the parallelism between the talus and os calcis. At that point, one can begin correction of the equinus by pulling the heel away from the lateral malleolus and by pushing laterally and upward on the front of the os calcis (Fig. 48-3A and B). That is to say as the equinus is corrected, the back of the os calcis is moved medially while the front of the os calcis is moved laterally. One must avoid attempting to correct equinus by pushing up on the metatarsals. This can result in a rocker-bottom deformity. Once manipulation is complete, the skin is covered with tincture of benzoin and a thin layer of cotton flannelette bandage is used for padding. The bandage is trimmed to expose the toes and then plaster is applied. One should use cool water so that there is sufficient time to mold the plaster properly. The molding should be designed to maintain the correction of the forefoot supination and adduction and the medial rotation and equinus of the os calcis. The end of the plaster bandage is

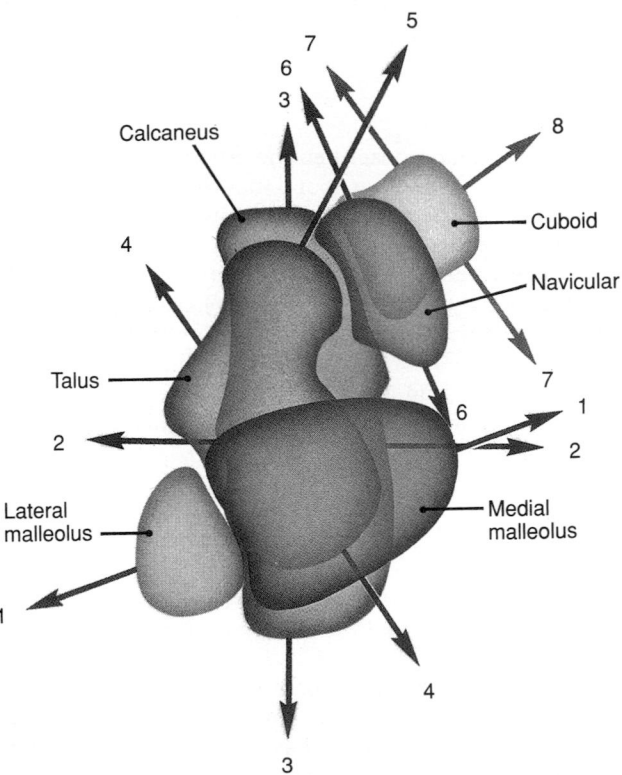

Figure 48-2 Illustration of the computer model of a left clubfoot (*superior view*). The transection has gone across the distal tibia and fibula. There is medial rotation of the os calcis, the body of the talus is externally rotated, the head of the talus demonstrates medial deviation, and the navicular is subluxated toward the medial malleolus. The cuboid is displaced medially as well. Transmalleolar axis (1), transverse axis of os calcis (2), longitudinal axis of os calcis (3), longitudinal axis of body of talus (4), longitudinal axis of head and neck of talus (5), transverse axis of navicular (6), transverse axis of cuboid (7), longitudinal axis of cuboid (8). [Reproduced with permission from Carroll NC: Surgical technique for talipes equinovarus. *Oper Tech Orthop* 3(2):119, 1993.]

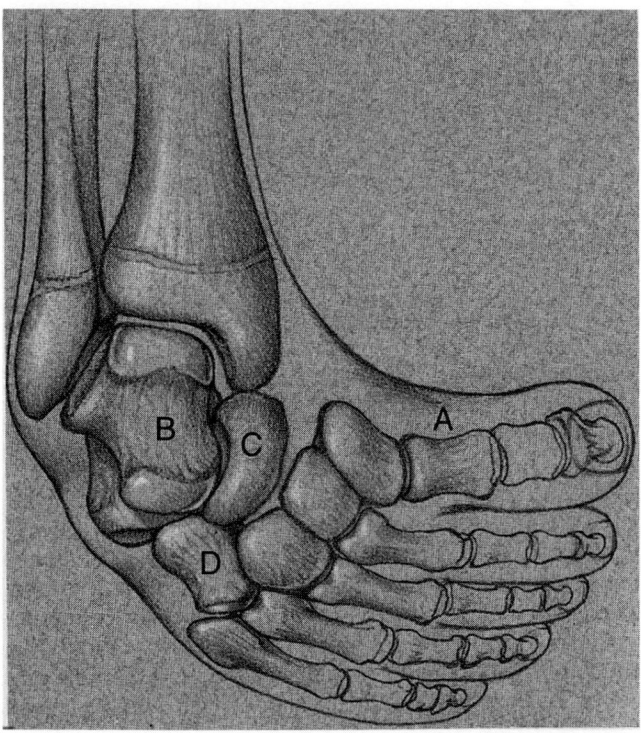

Figure 48-1 Anterior view of right clubfoot of a newborn. A, adduction and supination of forefoot; B, anterior extrusion of talus with increased plantar and medial inclination of talar neck; C, medial subluxation of navicular toward medial molleolus; D, medial subluxation of cuboid in relation to anterior end of os calcis. [Reproduced with permission from Carroll NC: Surgical technique for talipes equinovarus. *Oper Tech Orthop* 3(2):115, 1993.]

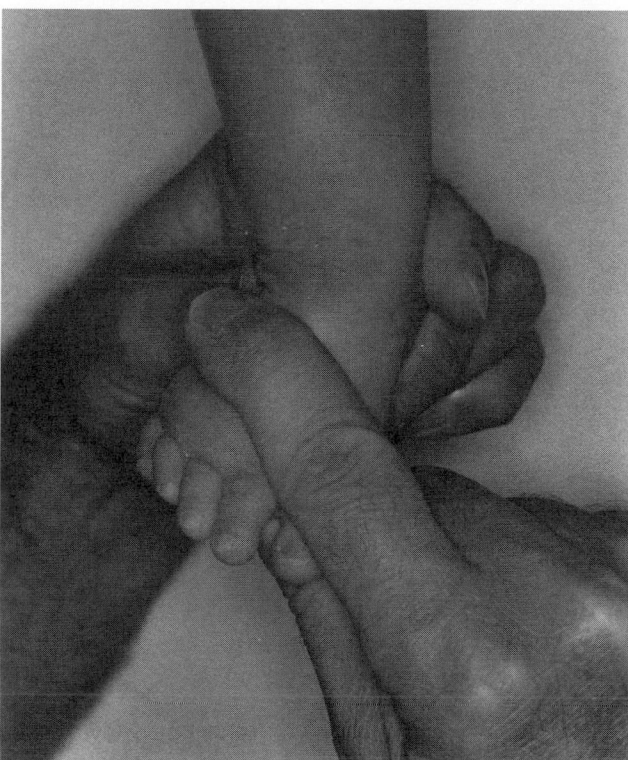

A

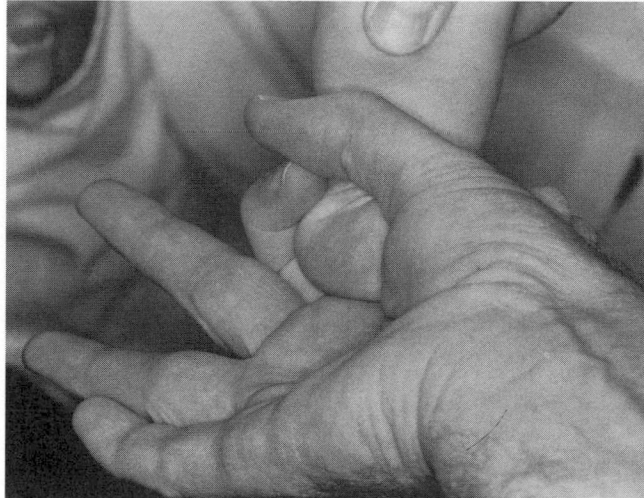

B

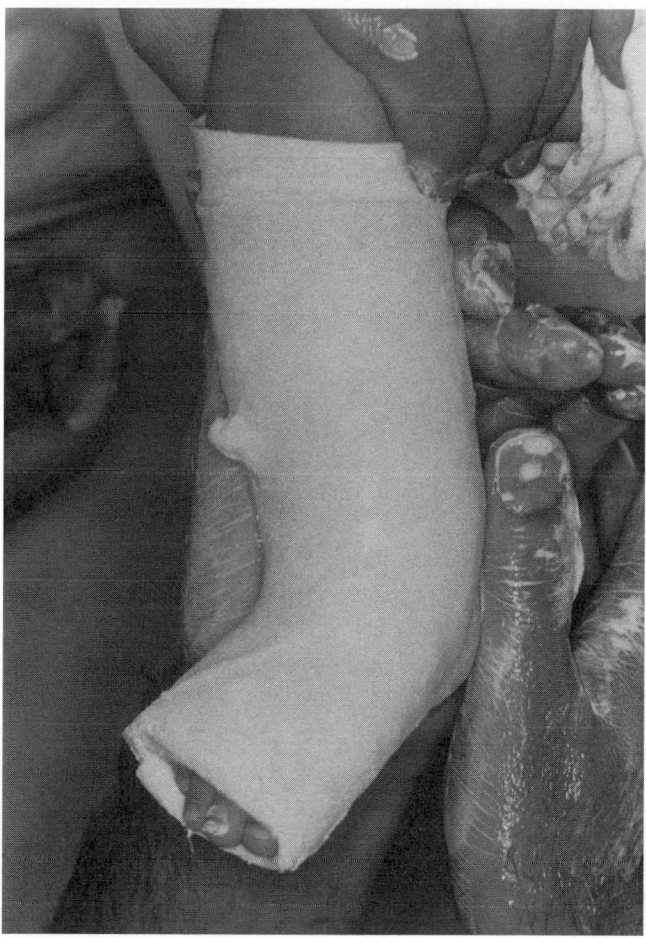

C

Figure 48-3 *A.* Manipulating a right clubfoot. The surgeon's left thumb is pushing the head of the talus medially while the right hand is being used to correct the adductus and supination. *B.* If the navicular will move away from the medial malleolus and if divergence is restored between the talus and calcaneus, the equinus can be corrected by pushing up on the front of the calcaneus with the base of the first metacarpal and by pulling the calcaneus down and away from the fibula. (The medial rotation is corrected along with the equinus.) *C.* A plaster has been applied to maintain the position obtained with the manipulation. The little knob at the front of the cast is the end of the plaster roll.

rolled into a little knob so that the parents can soak and remove the plaster before the next visit (Fig. 48-3*C*).

Other forms of nonoperative treatment are adhesive strapping, tapping on a Denis-Browne splint, orthoses, and special footwear. In assessing the results of nonoperative treatment, I have found that in addition to the clinical assessment of the foot (see later), it is useful to measure the Beatson-Pearson talocalcaneal index[49] and to measure the calcaneotibial angle on a forced dorsiflexion lateral view (Fig. 48-4).[50] Once a correction is achieved with manipulation and casting, the correction is maintained by having the child wear an ankle-foot orthosis (AFO) during his or her unattended hours. The parents should exercise the foot and ankle regularly to prevent stiffness and maintain ankle motion. For nonoperative treatment to be effective, progressive improvement should be possible with each manipulation and cast. If a good correction is not obtained by 3 months, it is increasingly unlikely that nonoperative treatment will be effective.[51]

Operative Treatment

Timing of Surgery

When should the child have surgery? This is controversial. Some surgeons prefer to intervene early, between the ages

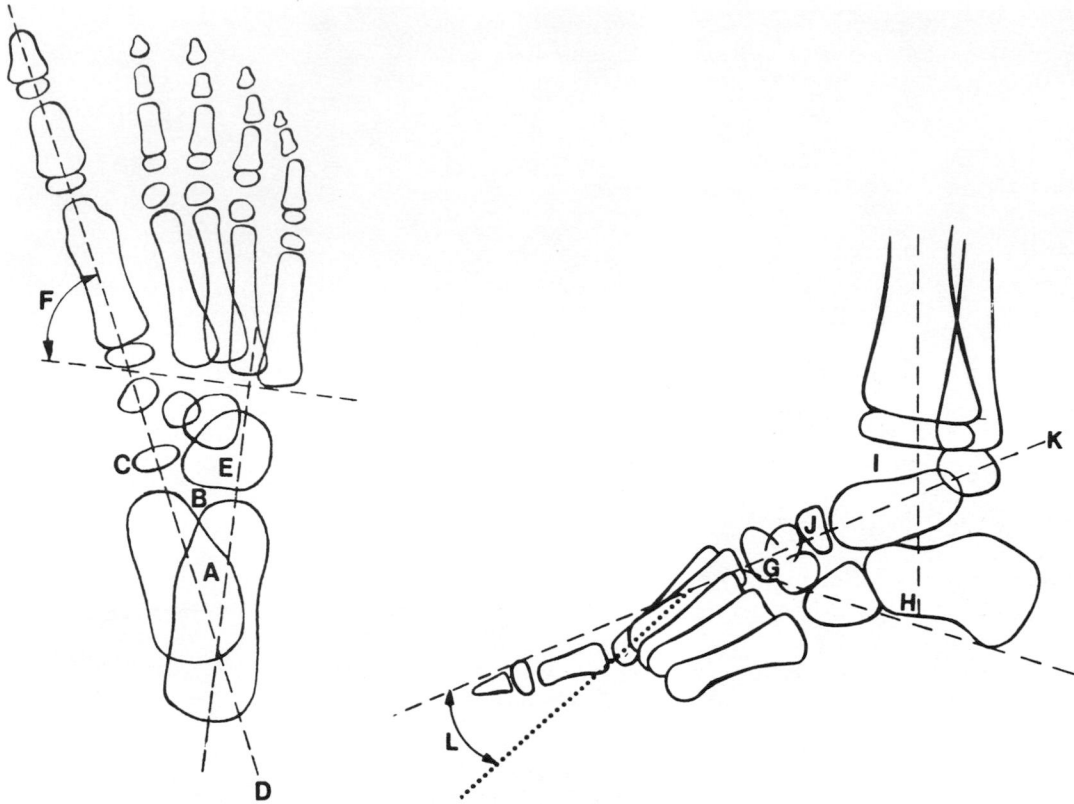

Figure 48-4 Radiographic measurements in the anteroposterior view of a child less than 5 years of age. These include the talocalcaneal angle (A), the talocalcaneal divergence (B), the navicular position (C), the talar axis (D), the cuboid position (E), and the first ray angle (F). Radiographic measurements for the lateral radiograph include the lateral talocalcaneal angle (G), the tibiocalcaneal angle (H), the tibiotalar angle (I), the navicular position (J), the talar axis (K), and the talar–first metatarsal angle (L). [Reproduced with permission from Thompson GH: Congenital talipes equinovarus (clubfeet) and metatarsus adductus, in Simons GW (ed): *The Child's Foot and Ankle.* New York, Raven Press, 1992, pp 927–957.]

of 3 and 6 months,[52–55] while others prefer to delay surgery until the child is 9 to 12 months old.[56–58] There is a lot of growth in the foot during the first year of life and therefore great potential for remodeling. If the bony architecture is properly aligned at an early age, this should promote congruous development of the subtalar calcaneocuboid and talonavicular joints. Early surgery demands a thorough understanding of the pathoanatomy and meticulous surgical technique to prevent excessive scarring and damage of cartilage. Simons states that the size of the foot is more important than the age of the child and recommends surgery when the foot is equal to or greater than 8 cm in length.[59,60] Surgeons who prefer to perform the surgery later feel that anesthesia is safer when the child is older and the pathoanatomy is more apparent—also that early weight bearing on the corrected foot will help to maintain the correction. It is the author's preference to perform the surgery any time after 3 months if the child weighs at least 12 pounds and is thriving.

Percutaneous Tenotomy of the Tendo Achillis

There is controversy as to the role of a simple percutaneous tenotomy of the tendo Achillis. In the Ponsetti treat-

ment of clubfoot, this tenotomy is performed when 15° of dorsiflexion has not been obtained with manipulation and casts, which is true in 95 percent of the feet.[61] The author does not use this technique. At the time of surgery, division of the tendo Achillis does not correct the deformity because of the tight posterior capsule and tight posterior talofibular and calcaneofibular ligaments.

Should Every Clubfoot Have the Same Surgery?

Some surgeons believe that every clubfoot should have a release of the talonavicular joint, the subtalar joint, and the posterior ankle capsule.[59,62–64] Other surgeons believe that the extent of the surgery should be matched to the complexity of the clubfoot deformity. Bensahel calls this the "à la carte" approach.[65] The author agrees with Bensahel's view.

What Should Be Released?

Each clubfoot should have a careful preoperative clinical and radiographic assessment. One of the most difficult problems in the overall management of a clubfoot is the clinical assessment. In order to compare the effectiveness of various forms of treatment objectively, one must have a method of describing the severity of the condition. Dimeglio describes four basic categories of CTEV, as follows[66]:

1. Stiff (irreducible)
2. Severe (slightly reducible)
3. Mild (partially reducible)
4. Postural (totally reducible)

He feels that the amount of reducibility is more significant than the deformity itself. Catterall (Table 48-1) has also tried to define the various types of CTEV.[67] He describes a postural resolving type in which there is no fixed deformity but dorsiflexion above the right angle is not necessarily present. Then there is a tendon contracture type in which the tight structures are mainly posterior, with no fixed deformity in the midtarsus or forefoot. Finally, there is a joint contracture type in which there is fixed deformity in both the hindfoot and the forefoot. Another method of classifying the severity of a clubfoot is to look for the following:

Calf atrophy
The position of the bimalleolar axis
Creases (medial, posterior, and anterior)
Curved lateral border
Cavus
Fixed equinus
Navicular fixed to medial malleolus
Os calcis fixed to fibular
Midtarsal mobility
Forefoot supination

Each of these assessment criteria, if present, can be given one point on a 10-point scale.

At the time of surgery, the author obtains anteroposterior (AP) and lateral radiographs of the foot in the operating room after the child is anesthetized (Fig. 48-5A and B). The foot is held in a position of maximal correction. The AP and lateral films are assessed for the talo-calcaneal angle, the alignment of the first ray in relation to the talus on the lateral view, and the alignment of the cuboid in relation to the os calcis on the AP view. For the past 16 years, we have been paying close attention to the alignment of the cuboid in relation to the long axis of the calcaneus. Simons has provided us with a radiographic grading system for calcaneocuboid malalignment (Fig. 48-6).[68] Since the ossific nucleus of a tarsal bone does not necessarily represent its central portion, we studied 13 clubfeet in 10 patients with preoperative radiographs and MRI. We found that there was a good correlation between the MRI findings and Simons's classification.[69] The degree of equinus is assessed by looking at the long axis of the calcaneus in relation to the long axis of the tibia (Fig. 48-4). The question must then be asked: What must be done to restore the bony architecture to normal and to balance the muscle forces acting on the foot? If, on clinical examination, the first ray is not in equinus and on the lateral x-ray film the talus is aligned with the first ray, the child does not need a plantar release. If, on clinical examination, the lateral border of the foot is straight and if the AP x-ray demonstrates that the cuboid is aligned with the long axis of the os calcis, the child does not need a calcaneocuboid release. If, on clinical examination, the forefoot supination has been corrected, there is midtarsal mobility, and one can feel a space between the navicular and medial malleolus, a medial release is not indicated.

The author believes that in a true clubfoot there is always a posterolateral tether with a contracted calf, a tight posterior capsule, and shortened posterior calcaneofibular and talofibular ligaments. Tables 48-2 and 48-3[70] compare the Turco, Carroll, McKay, Simons, and Bensahel procedures.

Operating Room

The temperature of the operating room should be safe for the baby and comfortable for the surgeon. The child should

---

TABLE 48-1   Clinical Types of Congenital Talipes Equinovarus

Type	Resolving pattern or postural/soft foot	Tendon contracture or fibrous foot	Joint contracture or stiff foot	False correction
Hindfoot				
Lateral malleolus	Mobile	Posterior	Posterior	Posterior
Equinus	No	Yes	Yes	Yes
Creases				
Medial	No	No	Yes	No
Posterior	No	Yes	Yes	Yes
Anterior	Yes	No	No	Yes
Forefoot				
Lateral border	Straight	Straight	Curved	Straight
Mobile	Yes	Yes	No	Yes
Cavus	±	±	±	No
Supination	No	No	Yes	No

Source: Reproduced with permission from Catterall A: Clinical assessment of clubfoot deformity, in Simon GW (ed): *The Clubfoot.* New York, Springer-Verlag, 1994, p 93.

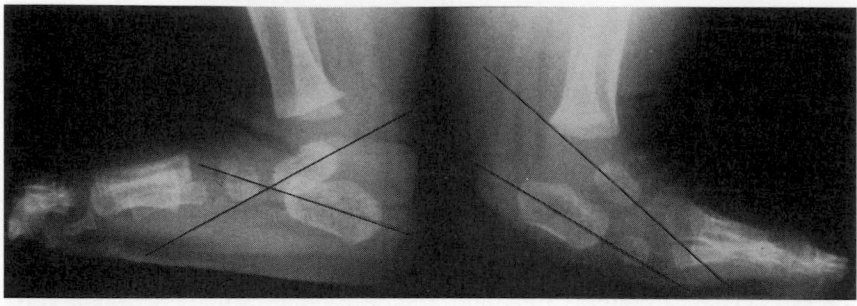

A

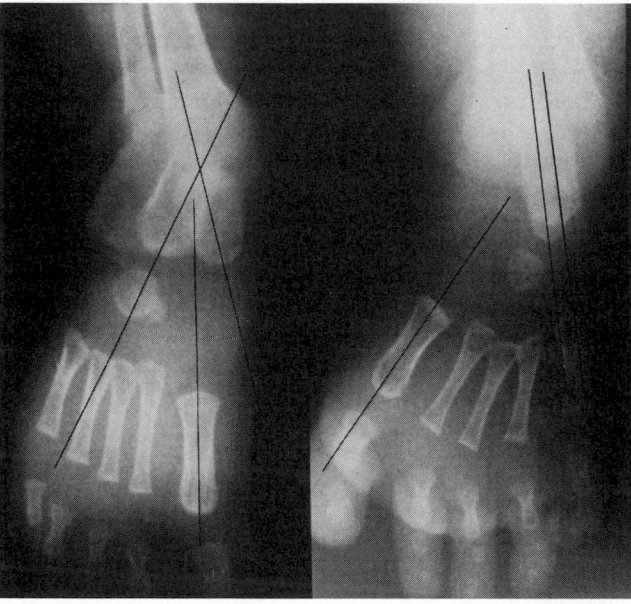

B

Figure 48-5 *A.* Lateral radiographs of a 6-month-old baby with a left clubfoot demonstrating equinus and parallelism between the long axis of the talus and the calcaneus. There is also a rocker-bottom deformity from the conservative treatment. *B.* Anteroposterior view of both feet. Note the parallelism between the long axis of the talus and calcaneus on the left foot (the right side of the x-ray). The navicular will align with the long axis of the first ray and it is displaced toward the medial malleolus. Note also that the cuboid is displaced medial to the long axis of the calcaneus.

Position of the Patient

The position of the patient will be determined by the type of incision or incisions used. With the Cincinnati incision and the present author's two-incision technique, the child is positioned prone. With the Turco incision, the child is positioned supine.

Incisions

Turco[71–73] uses a single medial incision extending from the first metatarsal proximally under the medial malleolus to the tendo Achillis (Fig. 48-7*A* and *B*).[72] The problems with this incision are that it crosses skin creases on the medial side of the ankle, exposure of the plantar fascia is difficult, and the structures in the posterolateral corner—the cal-

be placed on a heating pad and covered with Saran wrap to prevent heat loss. A comfortable surgeon is capable of a more meticulous technique. The surgeon should sit, have a knowledgeable assistant, use delicate instruments, and perform the surgery by sharp dissection.

Anesthesia

General endotrachial anesthesia should be used. The child must be adequately hydrated and monitored. A one-dose caudal anesthetic will keep the baby comfortable in the immediate postoperative period.

Technique for Tourniquet Application

A young baby has a cone-shaped thigh. To prevent skin necrosis due to uneven pressure under the tourniquet, it is recommended that the conical thigh be made cylindrical by pulling the skin and fat distally toward the knee and wrapping the thigh with a flannelette bandage prior to the application of the tourniquet. The tourniquet should be set to inflate to a pressure equal to the child's systolic pressure plus 100 mmHg.

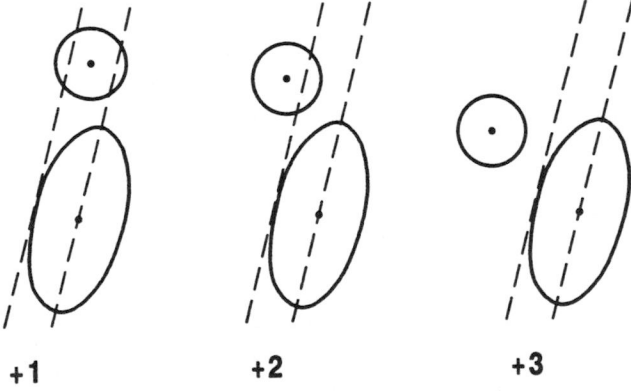

+1   **+2**   **+3**

Figure 48-6 Grading system for calcaneocuboid deformity on the AP or PA radiograph. The midpoint (normal) of the cuboid ossification center lies on the midlongitudinal (long) axis of the calcaneus: +1, midpoint of the cuboid ossification center lies between the long axis of the calcaneus and a line along the medial border of the calcaneus (medial tangent) parallel to the long axis of the calcaneus; +2, the midpoint of the cuboid ossification center lies medial to the medial tangent; +3, the midpoint of the cuboid ossification center lies proximal to the distal end of the ossification center of the calcaneus. The measurements are essentially the same on the AP and PA views. [Reproduced with permission from Simons GW: Calcaneocuboid joint deformity in talipes equinovarus: An overview and update. *J Pediatr Orthop Part B* 4(3):25, 1995.]

TABLE 48-2   Posterior Release

Procedure	Turco[58] Posteromedial release	Carroll[48] Medial and posterolateral release	McKay[63,64] Subtalar rotational and talar release	Simons[59,60] CSTR	Bensahel[65] "À la carte"
Muscles					
Achilles	Z-plasty	Z-plasty	Coronal Z-plasty	Z-plasty	Z-plasty (optional)
FHL	Leave	2 Level intramuscular recession	Transfer to PL (optional)		Z-plasty, suture
FDL					
Capsules					
Ankle	Capsulotomy posteriorly	Capsulotomy posteriorly	Incised posterior, medial, and lateral	Incised posterior and medial	Incised posteriorly
Subtalar	Capsulotomy posteriorly	Capsulotomy posteriorly	Incised posterior, medial, and lateral	Incised posterior and medial	Not opened
Ligaments					
Posterior talofibular	Transected	Incised	Incision (optional)	Incised	
Posterior part of deltoid	Incised	Incised	Partial incision, (optional)	Incised	
Tibiofibular	Incised		Incised (optional)		

Key: FHL, flexor hallucis longus; FDL, flexor digitorum longus; PL, peroneus longus.
Source: Reproduced with permission from Weintroub S, Khermosh MD: Comparative evaluation of initial surgical procedures in clubfoot. *J Pediatr Orthop Part B* 3:171–179, 1994.

caneofibular and talofibular ligaments—are difficult to see. Crawford has popularized the Cincinnati incision (Fig. 48-8).[74] This incision extends from the medial aspect of the foot in the region of the navicular cuneiform joint, curving beneath the distal end of the medial malleolus to the Achilles tendon. It continues in a gentle curve over the lateral malleolus to a point just distal and slightly anterior to the sinus tarsi on the lateral aspect of the foot. It can be extended either medially or laterally. The incision provides excellent exposure. When this incision is used, great care must be exercised to preserve the vessels that supply the heel flap. Loss of the heel flap will mean not only loss of correction but exposure and infection of the calcaneus. Two other problems with the Cincinnati incision are exposure of the plantar fascia to correct a cavus deformity and difficulty exposing enough of the tendo Achillis to do a Z-plasty with good overlap of the two portions of the tendon. The author prefers a two-incision technique, which is described further on.[48]

What Manipulation Should be Performed of the Bones of the Hindfoot Complex?

Goldner believes that the talus and os calcis should be rotated externally to achieve correction.[75] McKay and Turco rotate the calcaneus externally through the subtalar joint.[58,63,64,71–73] The author[48] as well as Howard and Dias[62] believe that the talus should be rotated internally and the calcaneus rotated externally to restore normal divergence.

Pin Fixation

How many pins should be used and across which joints? The number of pins used will be determined by the severity of the deformity and the surgical technique. If there has been a complete release of the subtalar joint, as advocated by Howard and Dias[62] as well as Simons,[59] it will be necessary to stabilize the subtalar joint with one or two pins. When the talonavicular joint has been released and the navicular has been repositioned in relation to the head of the talus, it should be secured with a talonavicular pin. If there is a tendency for a released calcaneal cuboid joint to subluxate out of normal alignment, this joint should be pinned as well.

The following paragraphs describe the author's preferred technique for a severe clubfoot that requires a plantar, medial, lateral, and posterior release.

The Author's Surgical Technique

The author's surgical technique[48,51] is designed to correct the bony architecture of the foot and to balance the muscle forces so that the correction obtained at surgery will be maintained as the child grows.

The skin incisions used by the author have been designed to (1) give excellent exposure of the entire anatomy; (2) allow protection of the neurovascular structures; (3) preserve the tendon sheaths for the tibialis posterior, flexor hallucis, and flexor digitorum; and (4)

TABLE 48-3   Medial Release

Procedure	Turco[58] Posteromedial release	Carroll[48] Medial and posterolateral release	McKay[63,64] Subtalar rotational and talar release	Simons[59,60] CSTR	Bensahel[65] "À la carte"
Muscles					
Posterior tibial	Tenotomy or resection	Z-plasty in calf	Z-plasty	Z-plasty (optional)	Z-plasty
FDL	Z-plasty	2-level intramuscular recession	Z-plasty (optional)	Z-plasty (optional)	
Abductor hallucis	Reflect down	Origin release	Origin release	Origin release	Origin release
Plantar release	Release (>3 yr)	Optional	Optional	Optional	
Tibialis anterior		Retraction			
Capsules					
Talonavicular	Capsulotomy	Capsulotomy: medial, dorsal, volar, and lateral	All around capsulotomy: dorsal, volar, and mesiolateral	Capsulotomy: medial, dorsal, and posterior	Capsulotomy: medial, dorsal, and volar
Subtalar	Capsulotomy	Medial, posterior, and lateral	Release: lateral, posterior, and medial	Release: medial, posterior, and lateral	Not opened
Calcaneocuboid	Medial capsulotomy	Medial, dorsal, and volar	Capsulotomy: plantar and medial	Circumferential release (optional)	
Naviculocuneiform	Capsulotomy				
Cuneiform-metatarsal	Capsulotomy (optional)				
Ligaments					
Talocalcaneal-interosseous	Incised	Intact	Incised lateral, cut partial (optional)	Incised lateral, cut total or partial (optional)	Intact
Anterior part of deltoid	Sectioned	Anterior, deep posterior intact	Incised	Incised	
Calcaneonavicular (spring)	Sectioned	Sectioned	Incised	Incised	
Naviculocuneiform	Incised (optional)				
Henry's knot	Excised	Sectioned	Excised	Freed	
Mass of scar on medial side of talonavicular joint	Excised	Excised	Excised	Excised	
Age	6 months–8 years (most cases >3 years)	>3 months	2 months–15 years	8 cm foot, up to 9 years	3 months–7 years
Position	Supine	Prone	Prone	Prone	Supine
Incision(s)	Medial, transverse	Two incisions: medial and posterior	Cincinnati	Cincinnati	Transverse medial
Fixation	1 to 2 K wires	1 or 2 K wires	2 K wires	2 or 3 K wires	2 K wires

Key: FDL, flexor digitorum longus.
Source: Reproduced with permission from Weintroub S, Khermosh MD: Comparative evaluation of initial surgical procedures in clubfoot. *J Pediatr Orthop Part B* 3:171–179, 1994.

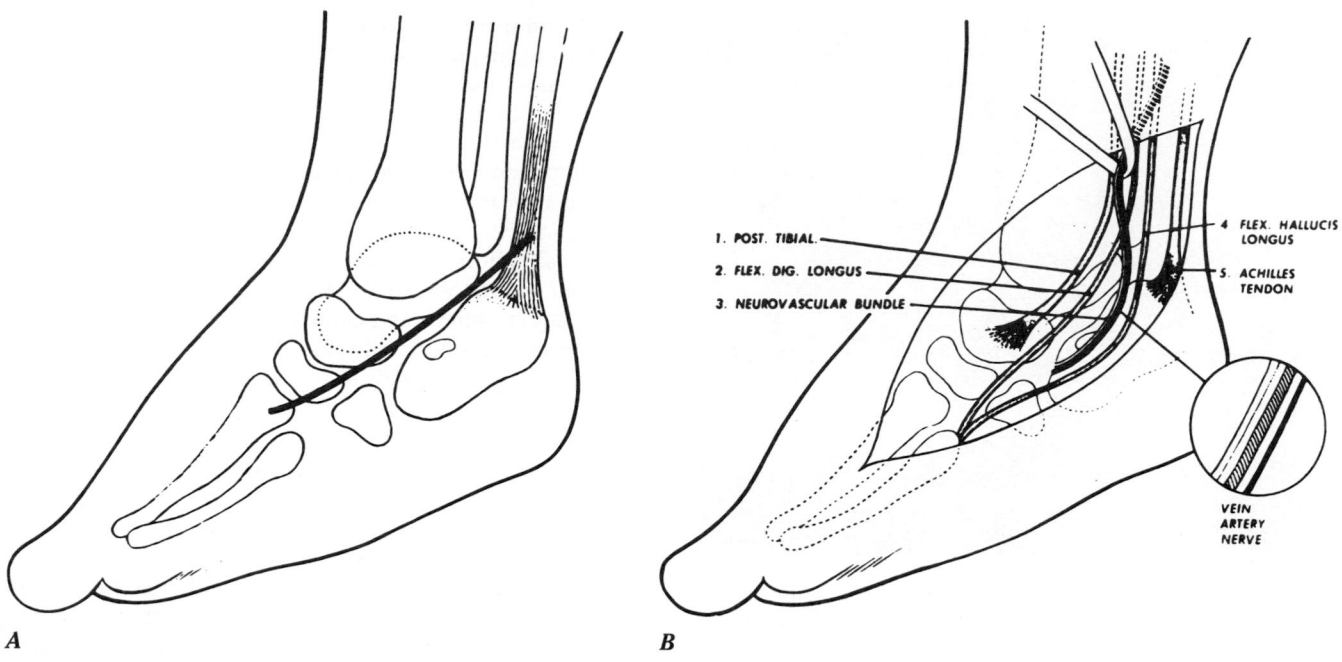

A   **B**

Figure 48-7 *A.* Turco's incision. [Reproduced with permission from Turco VJ: Present management of idiopathic clubfoot. *J Pediatr Orthop Part B* 3(2):149, 1994.] *B.* Important anatomic structures. [Reproduced with permission from Turco VJ: Surgical correction of the resistant clubfoot—One-stage posteromedial release with internal fixation. *J Bone Joint Surg [Am]* 53:477, 1971.]

promote good healing with minimal scarring and good cosmesis.

Two incisions are used; a curvilinear medial incision (Fig. 48-9) and a posterior lateral incision. The landmarks for the medial incision are the center of the os calcis, the front of the medial malleolus, and the base of the first metatarsal. These three points define a triangle. The incision is parallel with the base of the triangle but curved in the plantar direction proximally and over the dorsum of the foot distally. The posterior lateral incision runs obliquely from the midline of the distal calf posteriorly to a point midway between the tendo Achillis and the lateral malleolus.

Through the medial incision, the abductor hallucis is exposed and freed proximally from the os calcis. The deep fascia is opened to expose the medial plantar artery and

nerve and the lateral plantar artery and nerve. A plane is developed between the plantar fascia and the fat beneath the sole of the foot. The lateral plantar nerve and artery form a tunnel that passes toward the lateral side of the foot. The plantar fascia, flexor digitorum brevis, and abductor digiti minimi are freed from the os calcis by placing one blade of the scissor in the tunnel for the lateral plantar nerve and artery and one blade superficial to the plantar fascia (Fig. 48-10).[48]

At the tip of the medial malleolus, the sheath of the flexor digitorum longus is opened and followed distally to Henry's knot, where the flexor hallucis longus is identified. Both of these tendons are protected while the dissection is continued distally. The tibialis anterior is identified on the dorsum of the foot and traced to the base of the first

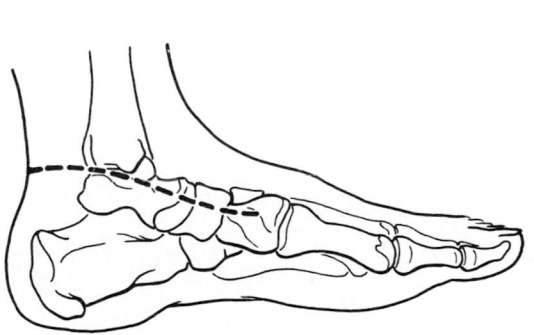

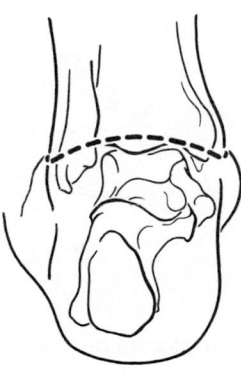

Figure 48-8 A line drawing, superimposed over the tarsal bones and malleoli, showing the possible medial extensions of the Cincinnati incision. The incision may be extended laterally to the same extent as medially, depending on the needs of the surgeon. (Reproduced with permission from Crawford AH, Marxen JL, Osterfeld DL: The Cincinnati incision: A comprehensive approach for surgical procedures of the foot and ankle in childhood. *J Bone Joint Surg [Am]* 64:1335, 1982.)

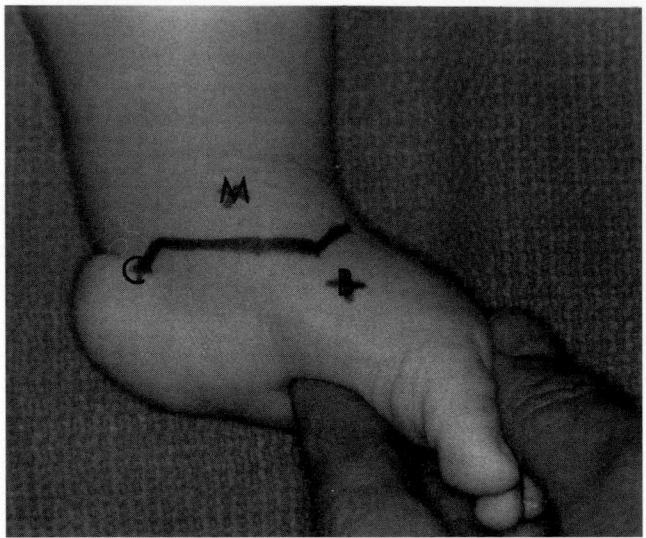

Figure 48-9 Medial incision on left clubfoot: C, center of calcaneous; M, front of medial malleolus; B, base of first ray.

metatarsal. The flexor hallucis and flexor digitorum, together with the neurovascular bundles, are retracted in the plantar direction. The sheath of the peroneus longus tendon is identified and opened; the tendon is traced proximally to the point where it curves around the lateral border of the foot. The peroneus longus tendon is protected while the long and short plantar ligaments are divided. The calcaneocuboid joint is opened by dividing the superior, medial, and plantar capsule (Fig. 48-11).[48] In a child over 8 months old, it may be easier to identify a severely displaced calcaneocuboid joint by making a third incision laterally over the joint.

Through the posterior incision, the sural nerve and short saphenous vein are identified and protected by retraction in a lateral direction. The tendo Achillis is exposed and divided in the sagittal plane, separating the distal, medial half from the os calcis and the proximal, lateral half from the triceps surae. The deep fascia overlying the flexor hallucis longus and neurovascular bundle is opened, the bundle is freed distally, and the flexor hallucis longus tendon is exposed distally to the level of the subtalar joint. In the lateral part of the wound, the peroneus longus and brevis tendons are identified and retracted laterally to expose the posterior calcaneofibular ligament (Fig. 48-12).[48]

Dissection is continued medially and the fascia overlying the flexor digitorum longus and tibialis posterior is opened. The tibialis posterior tendon is identified, divided by means of a Z-plasty, and a suture is attached to the distal portion of the tendon. A narrower retractor is placed underneath the flexor hallucis longus, neurovascular bundle, and flexor digitorum longus. The tip of the long, narrow retractor is brought out through the medial incision. The posterior capsule of the ankle and subtalar joint is opened and the tight posterior calcaneofibular and posterior talofibular ligaments are divided. The posterior portion of the deltoid ligament is divided behind the flexor digitorum longus. At this point, it should be possible to reduce the body of the talus into the ankle mortise (Fig. 48-13).[48]

The distal portion of the tibialis posterior tendon is pulled down through the sheath. The navicular is dissected

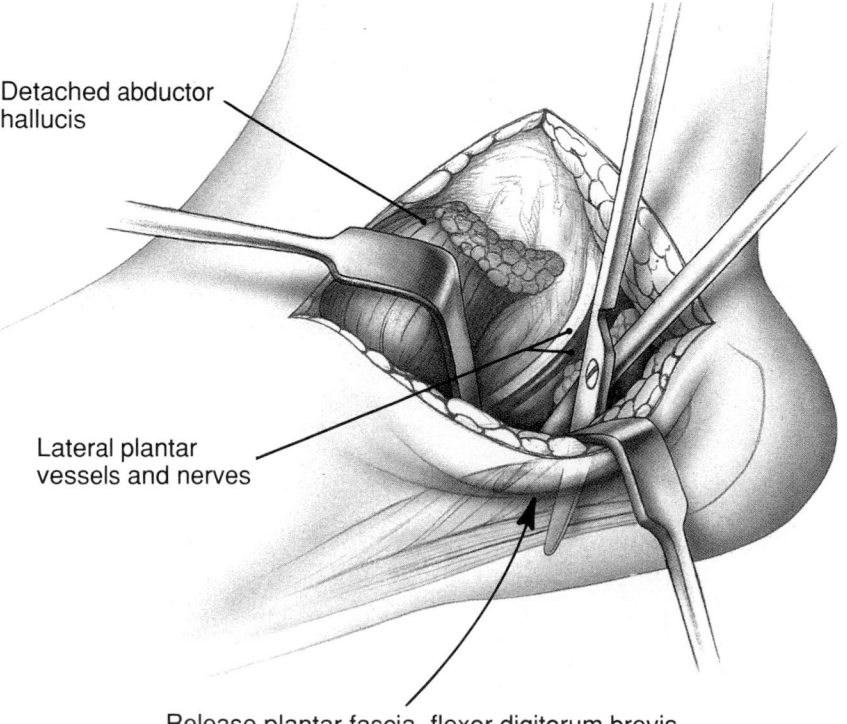

Detached abductor hallucis

Lateral plantar vessels and nerves

Release plantar fascia, flexor digitorum brevis and abductor digiti quinti

Figure 48-10 Medial incision in a right clubfoot demonstrating lateral plantar vessels and nerves and technique of plantar release. [Reproduced with permission from Carroll NC: Surgical technique for talipes equinovarus. *Oper Tech Orthop* 3(2):115, 1993.]

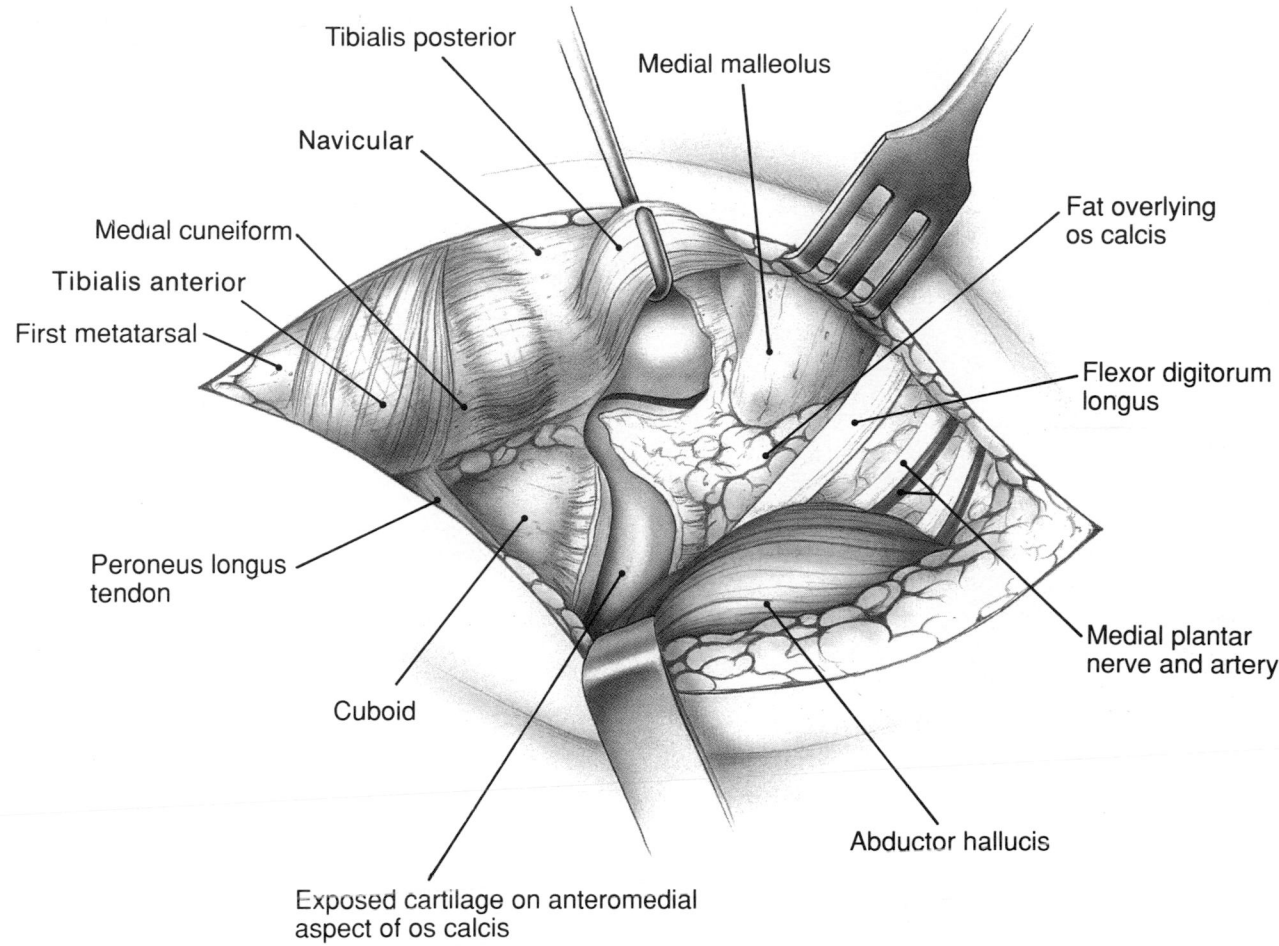

Tibialis posterior

Navicular

Medial cuneiform

Tibialis anterior

First metatarsal

Peroneus longus
tendon

Cuboid

Medial malleolus

Fat overlying
os calcis

Flexor digitorum
longus

Medial plantar
nerve and artery

Abductor hallucis

Exposed cartilage on anteromedial
aspect of os calcis

Figure 48-11 Medial incision in a right clubfoot (heel to right, toes to left). Note the exposed cartilage on the anteromedial aspect of the os calcis as the cuboid swings laterally to correct the medial subluxation. [Reproduced with permission from Carroll NC: Surgical technique for talipes equinovarus. *Oper Tech Orthop* 3(2):115, 1993.]

away from the medial malleolus, and the talonavicular joint is opened circumferentially. The slips of the tibialis posterior that run forward to attach to the undersurfaces of the cuneiforms and bases of the second through fourth metatarsals are divided. A small, curved, blunt elevator is placed in both the talonavicular and calcaneocuboid joints. The joints are opened, so that any residual restricting soft tissue between the anteromedial portion of the os calcis and navicular can be divided.

As can be seen through the posterior wound, the body of the talus is externally rotated in the ankle mortise. After a K wire is inserted posteriorly, the body of the talus is internally rotated in the ankle mortise and the os calcis is rotated externally. When the body of the talus has been reduced into the ankle mortise and divergence has been restored between the long axis of the talus and os calcis, supination and adduction of the forefoot are corrected. The K wire previously inserted in the talus is advanced across the reduced midtarsal joint and through the skin on the dorsum of the forefoot proximal to the bases of the phalanges. The K wire is advanced so that the back of the wire is flush with the cartilage at the back of the talus. The

distal portion of the K wire is cut against the retracted skin on the dorsum of the foot, so that the wire is covered when the skin is pulled back into position. In children older than 8 months of age and in the severely deformed foot, it is advisable to place a second K wire across the reduced calcaneocuboid joint.

The cavus component must be corrected; the heel must align with the long axis of the tibia; the lateral border of the foot must be straight; and the talonavicular and calcaneocuboid joints must be accurately reduced. If the plantar release is inadequate, the navicular will shift anterolateral to the head of the talus, and this will lead to a recurrent deformity. Displacing the navicular too far laterally results in an overcorrected valgus foot.

With the foot in a plantigrade position, the great toe is usually pulled into flexion. This is corrected by performing a two-level recession of the intramuscular portion of the flexor hallucis longus tendon. With the foot held plantigrade the tendo Achillis is repaired and the tibialis posterior is pulled back through its sheath and repaired. A small Hemovac drain is placed in the medial incision, the wounds are closed, and a compressive dressing is ap-

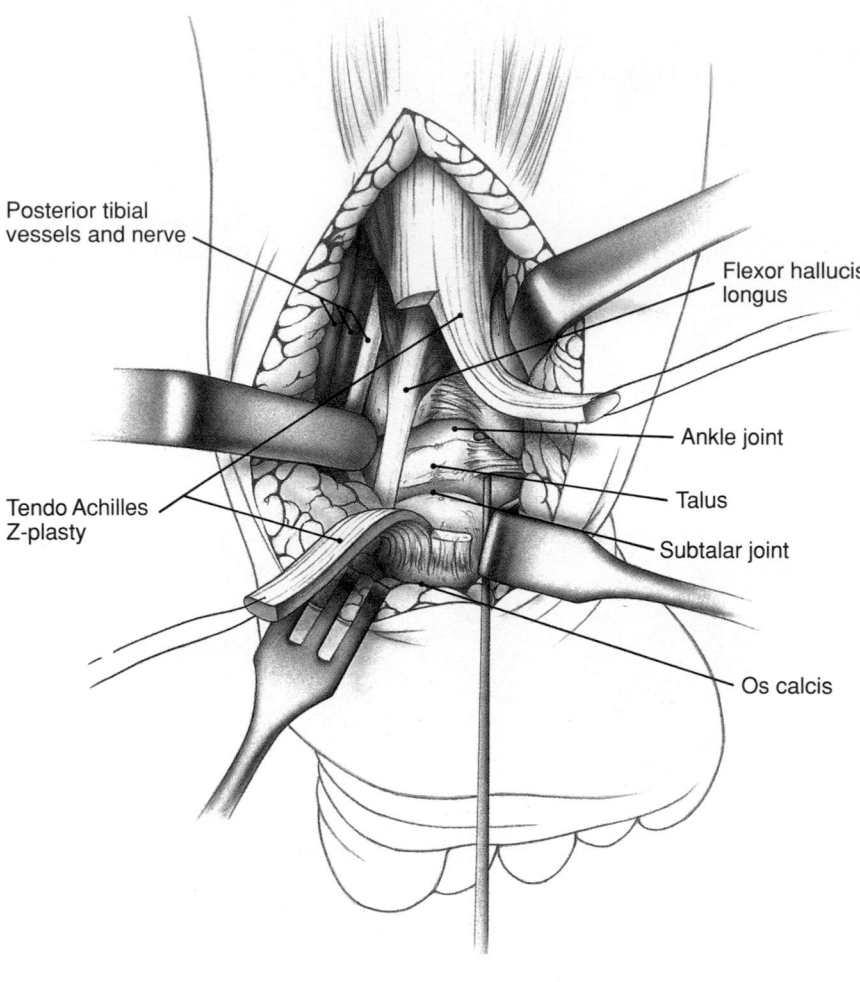

Posterior tibial vessels and nerve

Flexor hallucis longus

Ankle joint

Talus

Tendo Achilles Z-plasty

Subtalar joint

Os calcis

Figure 48-12 Posterior incision in a right clubfoot demonstrating the neurovascular bundle, the Z-plasty of the tendo Achillis, and the subtalar and ankle joints. The cuts of the Z-plasty should be going in the opposite direction. [Reproduced with permission from Carroll NC: Surgical technique for talipes equinovarus. *Oper Tech Orthop* 3(2):115, 1993.]

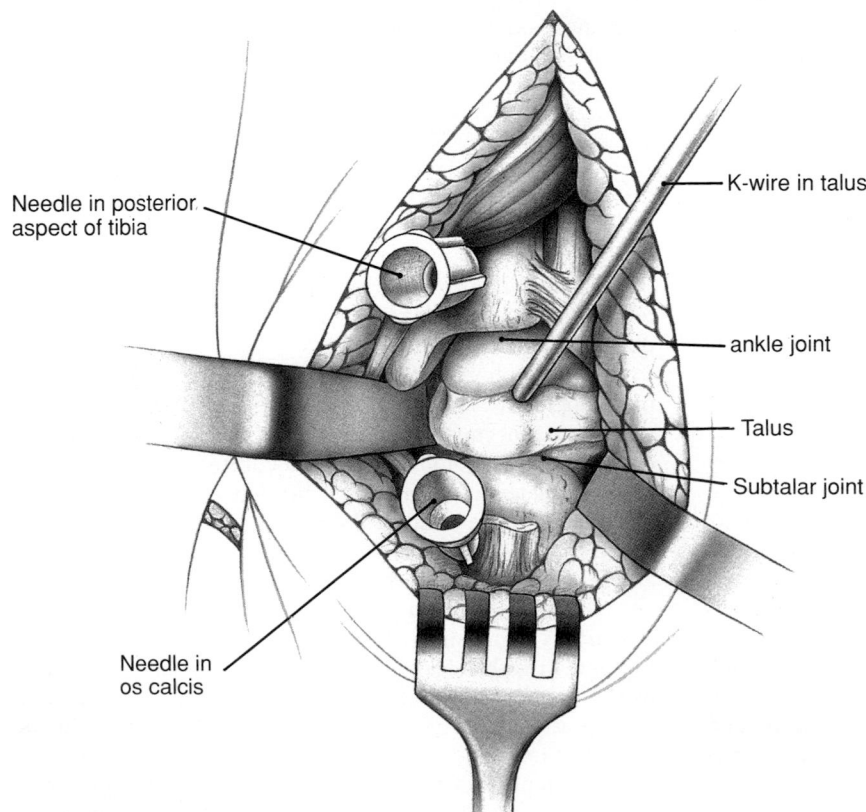

Needle in posterior aspect of tibia

K-wire in talus

ankle joint

Talus

Subtalar joint

Needle in os calcis

Figure 48-13 Posterior view of a right clubfoot demonstrating medial rotation of the talus and external rotation of the os calcis thus restoring divergence between these two bones. [Reproduced with permission from Carroll NC: Surgical technique for talipes equinovarus. *Oper Tech Orthop* 3(2):115, 1993.]

plied that extends from the toes to the hip. The knee is extended in the immediate postoperative period to facilitate venous drainage.

The child is discharged on the second postoperative day and is brought back to surgery 1 week later for cast application. The limb is treated in an above- or below-knee cast for a period of 8 weeks, with cast changes every 3 to 4 weeks. When the cast is removed, the foot is treated in an orthosis until the child is walking and there is clinical and radiographic evidence of a plantigrade foot.

Overcorrection of the clubfoot deformity can be avoided by preserving the anterior deep portion of the deltoid ligament and the interosseous ligament between the talus and os calcis, by being careful not to overdisplace the navicular laterally, and by not overlengthening the tibialis posterior and tendo Achillis. Finally, when the postoperative cast is applied, the foot must not be placed in an overcorrected position.

In summary, the steps in the surgical procedure are as follows: (1) a plantar release; (2) a release of Henry's knot; (3) identification of the tibialis anterior, which will facilitate the identification of the peroneous longus tendon; (4) protection of the peroneus longus tendon while the long and short plantar ligaments are divided to expose the calcaneocuboid joint, (5) a Z-plasty of the tendo Achillis; (6) a Z-plasty of the tibialis posterior tendon; (7) a posterior capsulotomy of the ankle and subtalar joints with release of the calcaneofibular and posterior talofibular ligaments; (8) open reduction of the talonavicular joint; (9) placement of a K wire into the talar body with correction of its anterior extrusion and external rotation; (10) correction of medial rotation of the calcancus; (11) correction of forefoot adduction and supination; (12) K wire fixation of the midtarsal joint; and (13) repair of tendons with the foot held in a plantigrade position[76,77] (Tables 48-2 and 48-3).[70]

Results of Treatment

Morcuende et al. have reported their results with the Ponseti method of manipulation and casting. All components of the clubfoot deformity must be corrected simultaneously, not in sequence, except for equinus, which should be corrected last. A percutaneous Achilles tenotomy may be needed to facilitate correction of the equinus. To prevent recurrences, the corrected feet must be maintained in outward rotation and open shoes attached to a bar for many months. The authors report an 89 percent satisfactory long-term functional result, which has lasted into the fifth decade of the patient's life.[61]

Most institutions have been unable to match these results and have resorted to surgical treatment when the initial nonoperative treatment has failed.

Turco[71] reports that with nonoperative treatment, he has been able to correct permanently only 35 percent of the feet that he has treated from birth. He reports 83 percent satisfactory results, 12 percent fair results, and 5 percent failures with his surgical treatment.

At the end of the 1970s, we reviewed our results of surgical treatment and found that 81 percent of the patients had a satisfactory result. Cavus and adductus was the most common residual deformity; in most of these feet, the plantar fascia was not released and there was residual calcaneocuboid subluxation.

Yngve et al., whose procedure involves clubfoot release without wide subtalar release, report that 82 percent of their surgeries resulted in a satisfactory functional rating.[78]

Thompson et al. divided resistant CTEV patients into three groups: group I, which had incomplete releases; group II, which had failed incomplete releases (leading to subsequent one-stage complete posteromedial release without internal fixation); and group III, which had the Turco-type complete release procedure with internal fixation.[57] The results were different in the various groups. Group I had only 42 percent excellent or good results, group II had 79 percent excellent or good results, and group III had 86 percent excellent or good long-term results assessed both clinically and radiographically. In the case of a resistant clubfoot after failed conservative management, it is important to release all deforming components and to use internal fixation.

Howard and Dias[62] report 87 percent satisfactory results with a posteromedial and lateral release. Their results improved when they used a K wire as a joy stick to derotate the talus and made sure that the calcaneocuboid joint was properly reduced.

Residual Deformity following Initial Surgery

When a child has had an initial surgical procedure to correct a clubfoot deformity and presents with continuing deformity, the question arises whether this continuing deformity represents residual uncorrected deformity or recurrent deformity. In this situation, it is vital to make sure that there is no neurologic cause for the "recurrence." A thorough neurologic examination is mandatory to rule out such causes as a tethered cord. As part of the initial workup of all babies with a clubfoot deformity, we recommend an ultrasound examination of the lower spinal canal. Having ruled out a neurologic cause for the deformity, one must then decide whether the initial surgery was adequate. That is, was a correction obtained, and if the correction was initially obtained, why was it not maintained? Perhaps there was inadequate follow-up or inadequate cast and orthotic care in the postoperative period. To answer these questions, one must make an accurate clinical assessment. One must also make an accurate motor assessment. Is there an imbalance between the functions of the tibialis anterior and peroneus longus? Is there uncorrected pathology in the hindfoot? Is there uncorrected pathology in the forefoot? Are the two columns of the foot balanced (Fig. 48-14)?[79] Is the medial column too short? If so, is there inadequate growth in the dysplastic talus, or is there dorsolateral subluxation of the navicular? Is the lateral column of the foot too long?

One must always consider the age of the patient and the amount of scarring from the initial operative procedure. A decision must then be made as to whether the pathology can be corrected by means of a repeat soft tissue operation or whether a bony procedure is required.

A common cause for persisting cavus, forefoot adduction, and a curved lateral border to the foot is that in the

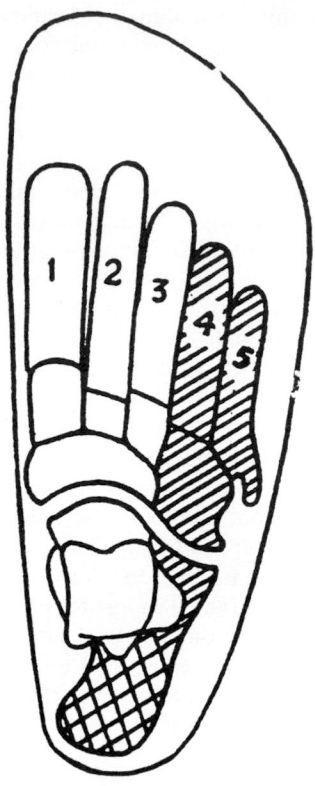

Figure 48-14 Grant described the two columns of the foot. The lateral column consists of the calcaneus cuboid and the fourth and fifth rays. The medial column consists of the talus, navicular, cuneiforms, and first three rays. (Reproduced with permission from Grant JC Boileau: *A Method of Anatomy.* Baltimore, Williams & Wilkins, 1952, p 447.)

initial posteromedial release the plantar fascia was not lengthened, the long and short plantar ligaments were not divided, and the cuboid was not properly positioned on the end of the os calcis. We reviewed the records and radiographs of 125 children with 159 clubfeet that required additional surgery for residual deformity after the initial operative repair. Forefoot adduction and supination were the most common persistent deformities (present in 95 percent of the feet). These deformities resulted from undercorrection at the time of the primary operation. Undercorrection resulted from not releasing the calcaneocuboid joint and plantar fascia and failure to recognize residual forefoot adduction on the interoperative radiographs at the primary operation.[80] An inadequate or omitted plantar release is often associated with dorsolateral subluxation of the navicular. The navicular can be placed in the corrected position, but if there is not enough length in the plantar structures, it will be extruded dorsolaterally with growth.

The cause of persisting intoeing, slight equinus, and apparent varus of the heel can be an inadequate release of the posterolateral tether—that is, the calcaneofibular and talofibular ligaments.

Residual Dynamic Deformity

After the initial clubfoot release, some children present with residual adduction and supination that is completely correctable passively. The adduction and supination become quite apparent during the swing phase of gait. The deformity results from dysfunction of, or incoordination between, the anterior tibial and the posterior tibial muscles as invertors and the peroneal muscles as evertors of the foot.[81] This deformity can be corrected by a tibialis anterior tendon transfer. Garceau and Manning's indication for transposition of the tibialis anterior was supination occurring with dorsiflexion.[81] They transposed the tibialis anterior to the base of the fifth metatarsal. In some instances there was overcorrection, and the tendon had to be moved back. I prefer to do a split transfer of the tibialis anterior so that there is still some dorsiflexion force on the medial side of the foot.[82]

Gartland has recommended a tibialis posterior tendon transfer through the interosseous membrane anteriorly to the third cuneiform to correct residual clubfoot deformity.[83] In my opinion this approach has a very limited role.

Residual Fixed Deformity

A child over 3 or 4 years of age who has persisting or recurrent deformity may have residual parallelism between the long axis of the talus and os calcis (Beatson-Pearson index less than 40°).[49] After the child reaches age 3 or 4, it is almost impossible to achieve an anatomic reduction of the hindfoot complex, especially when considerable scarring exists. Some type of bony procedure may be required to achieve proper alignment. In this type of foot there is often residual medial displacement of the cuboid with a curve to the lateral border of the foot. If there is not too much scarring, it may be possible to repeat the medial release and totally free the midtarsal joint—that is, free all the structures straight across the foot between the talus and navicular and between the os calcis and cuboid, so that the forefoot can be rotated and translated to a position that will help compensate for the residual hindfoot deformity. Sometimes it is possible to translate the cuboid by just releasing the tight structures on the plantar and medial sides of the calcaneocuboid joint. In the older child, however, the capsule may be stuck to the anterolateral portion of the os calcis and a separate lateral incision over the calcaneocuboid joint will be required. If the tight capsule on the medial side of the calcaneocuboid joint is not incised, it will be necessary to remove bone laterally to make the lateral border of the foot straight. This tight, unreleased capsule serves as a tether or a hinge, which makes it impossible to get a straight lateral border of the foot unless bone is excised.

Forefoot Deformity

Berman and Gartland used metatarsal osteotomies to correct forefoot adduction.[84] Residual adduction of the forefoot in most clubfeet is due to residual deformity in the tarsus. It is rare in my experience to have an actual varus deformity of the metatarsals per se. In performing metatarsal osteotomies, one is creating a secondary deformity in the metatarsals to compensate for a primary deformity in the tarsus. Metatarsal osteotomies therefore are rarely indicated as treatment for a clubfoot deformity. Longitudinal incisions are preferable for metatarsal osteotomies, making it easier to protect the dorsal veins. The corrected position should be maintained by pin fixation. This is a dangerous operation accompanied by much forefoot edema.

Heyman and colleagues recommended mobilization of the tarsometatarsal and intermetatarsal joints for correction of residual adduction of the forepart of the foot in congenital clubfoot.[85] This procedure may damage the joint surfaces and I have not used it.

Correction of Adductus

Cuboid Decancellation

If, after a medial release in an older child, there is still residual curvature of the lateral border of the foot, the lateral border can be shortened by a decancellation of the cuboid, as described by Johanning.[86]

Decancellation of a medially displaced cuboid will shorten the lateral column of the foot, but it will not straighten its lateral border. The calcaneocuboid joint should be released so that the cuboid can be placed in its proper position on the end of the os calcis. Decancellation of a reduced cuboid will shorten the lateral column of the foot and also straighten the lateral border.

Calcaneocuboid Fusion

Dillwyn Evans preferred to delay clubfoot surgery until the child was 4 years old. His procedure consisted of a medial and posterior release together with an excision and a fusion of the calcaneocuboid joint.[87] This procedure should not be done in a very young child, because much of the growth cartilage will have to be excised from the anterior end of the os calcis; with further growth, there will be a tendency for the two columns of the foot to become unbalanced and the forefoot may actually become abducted.

The Dillwyn Evans procedure should be reserved for children 4 years of age or older who are presenting for repeat surgery and have severe scarring of the medial side of the foot, a short medial column, a curved lateral border, and residual parallelism between the os calcis and the talus.

Lichtblau has described resection of the anterior end of the os calcis.[88] Again, I caution that this procedure should not be done in a young child, as one may be interfering with the growth of the lateral column of the foot and end up with an abducted forefoot. It may take 5 or 6 years for this deformity to appear.

Another possible way of shortening the lateral column of the foot is to remove some bone from the anterior portion of the calcaneus between the anterior and middle facets but to preserve the growth cartilage on the anterior end of the calcaneus (the reverse of the reverse Dillwyn Evans procedure).

Correction of a Short Medial Column

In some feet the recurrence of the deformity, especially the recurrent adduction, is due to insufficient growth of the medial column of the foot. This is not surprising, because

the most consistent anomaly described in congenital clubfoot is the increase in the medial and plantar inclination of the neck of the talus (see previous discussion). The effect of the increased inclination is to foreshorten the talus. An obvious method of correcting this deficiency in the length of the medial column of the foot is to do an osteotomy of the neck of the talus. This procedure has been described in the Japanese literature,[89] and Roberts has also reported his experience with this procedure.[90] A fear in doing an osteotomy of the neck of the talus is that one may produce an avascular necrosis. One should avoid dissection laterally, preserve the capsule of the talonavicular joint, and perform the osteotomy between the vessels entering the neck from the lateral side and those entering the talus more distally. This procedure will require more study before it is universally accepted.

Another method of lengthening the medial column of the foot is by means of a cuneiform osteotomy, as described by Hoffman and colleagues.[91] This procedure can be better applied to a metatarsus primus varus with a sloped first metatarsal cuneiform joint than to clubfoot.

Correction of Residual Hindfoot Deformity

If there is residual varus of the hindfoot, it probably means that correction of the medial rotation of the os calcis as described by McKay was incomplete.[63,64] The hindfoot can be realigned by a variety of osteotomies. A small varus heel can be corrected and lengthened by a medial open-wedge osteotomy. Kumar et al.[92] reported on a 27-year follow-up of 36 feet on which Dwyer performed this procedure. In 94 percent, the heel was in neutral or valgus, and 86 percent of the feet were plantigrade; 83 percent of the feet had a good range of ankle and subtalar motion. The problem with this procedure is that adequate skin closure may be quite difficult to achieve. A varus heel can also be corrected by resecting a wedge of bone from the os calcis laterally. The disadvantage of doing this procedure in a child with a clubfoot is that the heel is already small. Another alternative is to do an osteotomy of the os calcis and simply shift it laterally without resecting bone. This is my preferred technique, because bone stock is preserved and wound closure is not a problem.

Talectomy

A talectomy is practically never necessary to correct an idiopathic clubfoot. This procedure is more likely to be required in an arthrogrypotic foot or in a severe neurogenic clubfoot; for example, a child with spina bifida. Removing the talus shortens the medial column of a clubfoot, and the medial column is already shortened. Anytime a talectomy is performed, I prefer also to remove the cuboid to help balance the two columns of the foot. If the cuboid is not removed, the lateral border of the foot develops a banana shape.

Wedge Tarsectomy

It is not uncommon to have a preadolescent who has had several previous soft tissue procedures appear with a residual clubfoot deformity. Correction of the hindfoot deformity may be partial, but forefoot adduction and supination are still present. There may be some residual cavus, and the lateral border of the foot is curved. Usually, on the lateral radiograph of such a foot, there is dorsolateral extrusion of the navicular. I find a wedge tarsectomy to be a good way of dealing with this deformity. The piece of bone removed is wider superiorly and laterally. With a wedge tarsectomy, the forepart of the foot can be pronated, abducted, and brought up out of the equinus. Unless there is severe hindfoot deformity, I prefer this procedure over a triple arthrodesis.

Triple Arthrodesis

An adolescent with residual hindfoot, midfoot, and forefoot deformity may be a candidate for a triple arthrodesis. Classic descriptions of triple arthrodesis have been provided by Hoke and Dunn.[93,94] However, these procedures were initially prescribed for stabilizing paralytic feet. Instability is usually not the problem in a clubfoot, in which the foot is rigid in a deformed position. Very few children with clubfeet should require a triple arthrodesis. A child with clubfoot already has a relatively small heel, and when more bone is excised to correct the deformity, the malleoli are brought down even closer to the ground. This makes it difficult to find a shoe that fits properly. In addition, cosmesis is poor, with a bulbous ankle and a small foot.

Except in the most severely deformed feet, I prefer to correct the hindfoot deformity with a sliding osteotomy of the os calcis and to correct the midfoot and forefoot deformity by means of a wedge tarsectomy, as described previously.[51]

There have been recent reports in the literature on the use of the Ilizarov frame to correct residual clubfoot deformity.[95,96] One of the disadvantages of this technique is that the foot may become stiff and painful.

FLATFOOT

Normal Foot Development

Arch development in children was studied by Morley.[97] He showed that the footprint changes with advancing age from a flatfoot pattern to one showing a longitudinal arch. Engel and Staheli supported his findings.[98] In 1987, Staheli et al.[99] reported on a study of both feet of 441 normal subjects who ranged in age from 1 to 80 years. They found that flatfoot is usual in infants, common in children, and within the normal range of observations made in adult feet. Documentation and observation is the recommended management of the flexible flatfoot that falls within the normal range (Fig. 48-15).[99]

Gould et al.[100] observed 125 subjects for 4 years during early childhood. Arch development proceeded independently of the type of footwear worn.

All of these studies demonstrate that the longitudinal arch develops spontaneously during infancy and childhood. This occurs naturally and does not depend on shoes, boots, or orthoses.

Vanderwilde et al.[101] in 1988 described the radiographic changes in a developing child's foot. They found that the radiographic parameters commonly associated with flatfoot—that is, talar inclination and talometatarsal angle—change with age. The range of normal was very broad and included values previously considered diagnostic of pes planus.

The bare foot has been studied by several investigators. Hoffman described the feet of 186 natives of the Philippines and Central Africa who had not worn shoes.[102] He noted that all feet showed excellent mobility, thickening of the plantar skin, and wide variability in the height of the arch. Eversion of the foot was rare and all of these feet were pain-free. Engle and Morton studied the bare feet of Belgian Congo natives.[103] They did not find any "static foot deformities." When James studied the footprints of natives of the Solomon Islands, he found no static foot deformities.[104] Sim-Fook and Hodgson[105] found that the feet of barefoot subjects showed greater mobility and fewer of the deformities seen in those wearing shoes when they compared 118 shoe-wearing with 107 non–shoe-wearing Chinese. These studies all showed that the unshod human foot is characterized by (1) excellent mobility, especially of the forefoot; (2) thickening of the plantar skin; (3) creases in both the plantar and dorsal surfaces of the foot due to the flexibility of the midtarsal joints; (4) alignment of the phalanges with the metatarsals, causing the toes to spread; (5) variability in arch height; and (6) an absence of static deformity.

Flexible Flatfoot

Flexible flatfoot is present in most infants, many children, and about 15 percent of adults. Staheli (Fig. 48-16)[106] describes two basic forms. The developmental flatfoot occurs in infants and children as a normal stage of development. The hypermobile flatfoot persists as a normal variant. This form of flexible flatfoot can be inherited. Harris and Beath,[107] in a classic Canadian army foot study, showed that the flexible flatfoot in the adult is a benign condition. A more recent Israeli[107a] army study showed fewer stress injuries in individuals with low arches. Flexible flatfoot is common, benign, and should be considered a variation of normal. Wenger et al.[108] in a 3-year study of 129 children found no difference between flexible flatfoot treated with a variety of corrective shoes and flatfoot with normal flexible footwear. Gould et al. studied 125 children for 5 years.[109] Four types of footwear were prescribed for flatfoot, and arch development occurred regardless of the type of footwear. In these two prospective controlled studies, corrective shoes did not affect the development of the child's longitudinal arch.

The literature suggests that treatment of flexible flatfoot in a child is probably both unnecessary and ineffective.[110] Staheli has described ideal shoes for infants and children with normal feet. The shoes should be the proper size.[111] Shoes that are too short compress the toes and create deformity. Shoes that are too long make it difficult for the child to walk.[109] Shoes should be quadrangular to conform to the normal foot configuration, with (1) abun-

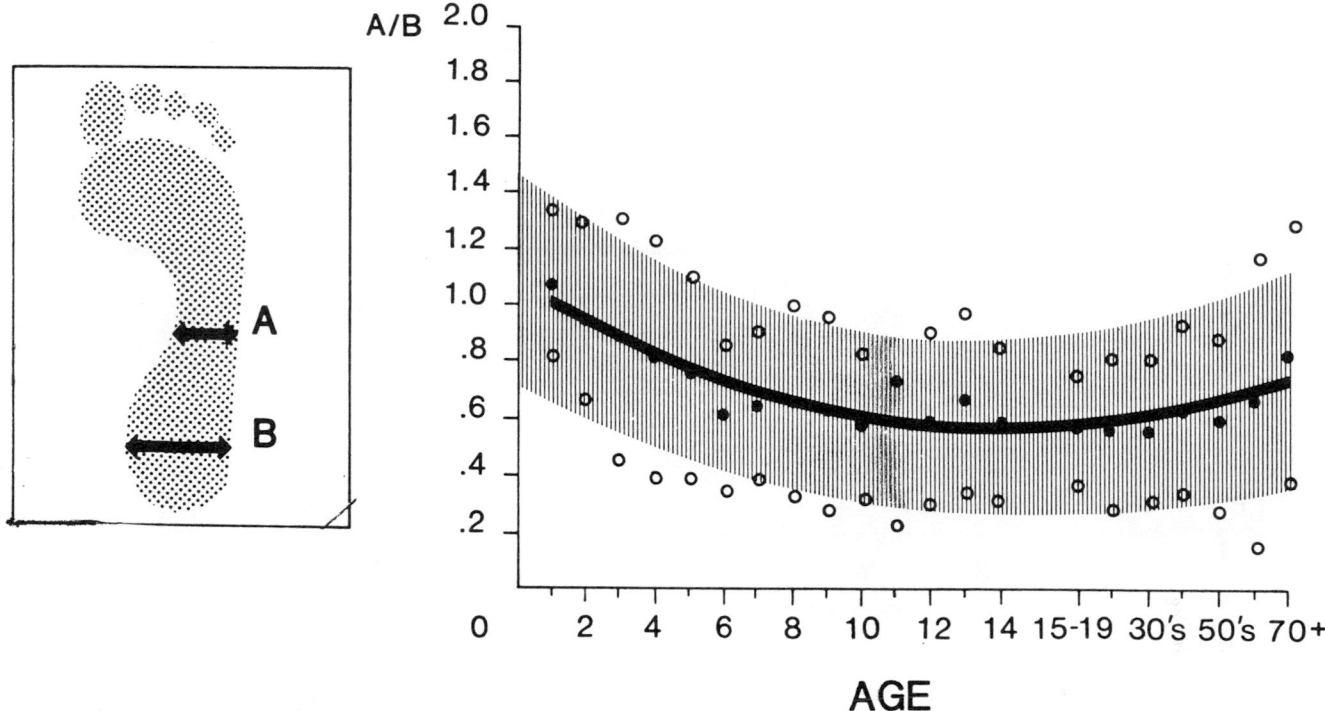

Figure 48-15 A footprint was recorded by chalking the sole of the foot and then making an impression of it on paper. The width of the foot in the area of the arch and the width of the heel were measured, and the former number was divided by the latter to calculate the arch index for each foot. The average of the two feet was used because there was a significant linear relationship between the right and left arch indices ($r = 0.93$). The graph illustrates mean values for the arch index and two standard deviations for each of the 21 age groups. The solid line shows the mean changes with age; the shaded area shows the normal ranges. The actual values for each age group are represented by solid circles for the mean and open circles for two standard deviations. (Reproduced with permission from Staheli LT, Chew DE, Corbett M: The longitudinal arch: A survey of 882 feet in normal children and adults. *J Bone Joint Surg* 69a:426, 1987.)

dant space for the toes[112–114]; (2) flexibility, to allow free foot movement[115,116]; (3) flat soles without elevation of the heel[117]; (4) porous uppers made of leather or unsealed fabric to avoid skin maceration; (5) a sole that provides friction equivalent to that of the bare foot; (6) light weight, to reduce energy expenditure; (7) extent above the ankle in the toddler to prevent the shoe from slipping off during running[118]; (8) acceptable appearance; and (9) a reasonable price. Shock-absorbing footwear with cushioned soles or foam inserts may be helpful in managing overuse syndromes such as heel or shin pain related to sports activities in children and adolescents.

In the clinical examination of a child with a presumed diagnosis of hypermobile flatfoot, one must make sure that the child does not have muscle weakness or a neurologic condition. Over the years, I have seen a number of children sent to the clinic with presumed flatfoot who in fact had muscular dystrophy. When a child is not bearing weight, a flexible flatfoot appears normal; but when the child stands, the midfoot sags toward the ground, the heel goes into valgus, and the foot appears externally rotated in relation to the leg. The weight-bearing axis tends to fall medial to the midaxis of the foot. The parents may complain about the ankles going in or about the heel going out. When the child is asked to walk tiptoe, the longitudinal arch reconstitutes and the heel pulls into varus. The lon-

gitudinal arch can also be formed by forcing the great toe into hyperextension. This maneuver was originally described by Jack.[119] Hicks explained this "windless action."[120] The plantar fascia originates from the calcaneus and inserts into the plantar aspect of the great toe through multiple interconnections. As the great toe is dorsiflexed, the plantar fascia is pulled under the head of the first metatarsal. This brings the calcaneus toward the head of the first metatarsal, thus creating an elevated medial longitudinal arch. It is important to check to make sure that the child with a flexible flatfoot does not have a tight tendo Achillis. With the knee extended and the forefoot supinated to hold the subtalar joint in a neutral position, the child should still have 10 to 15° of dorsiflexion beyond neutral. It is very important to stabilize the subtalar joint, otherwise one will miss the tightness in the heel cord.

Children with flexible flatfoot will have other signs of ligamentous laxity. The knees and elbows may hyperextend, and these children can often oppose their thumbs to the volar surfaces of their forearms.

Hypermobile Flatfoot with Tight Heel Cord

When a child with a contracture of the triceps surae stands, the heel is pulled into valgus. When the heel

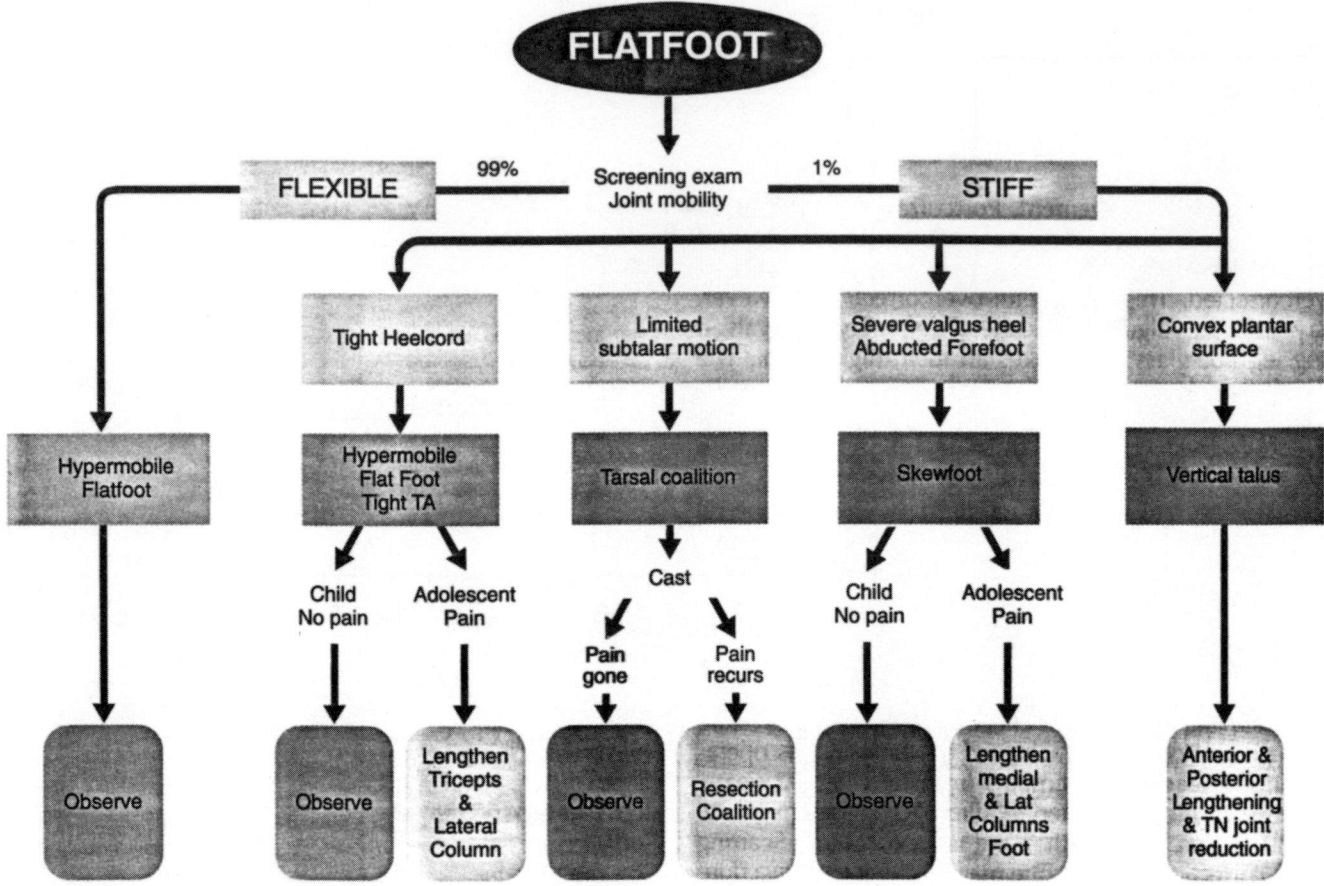

Figure 48-16 This algorithm, devised by Staheli well outlines the evaluation and management of flatfoot. (Reproduced with permission from Staheli LT: *Fundamentals of Pediatric Orthopaedics.* New York, Raven Press, 1992, p 514.)

pulled into valgus, the forefoot follows the hindfoot, and this initially brings the first ray into contact with the ground. Over time, the forefoot will supinate, so that there is even weight bearing over the metatarsal heads with the hindfoot still in valgus. When the heel is brought into neutral alignment with the leg, one can see this forefoot supination. Childhood activities with a normal foot produce dorsiflexion of the ankle; but with a tight heel cord and a flexible foot, there is a break in the midfoot. These feet with altered mechanics can be painful. When they are examined with the heel in neutral and the subtalar joint stabilized in a neutral position, one will see that the whole foot is in equinus and that there is no ankle dorsiflexion.

Initial treatment for this condition consists of stretching exercises. The child should toe in and put a block under the head of the first metatarsal to keep the forefoot supinated and then do a runner's stretch of the heel cord. If the stretching exercises are not successful in relieving the pain, it is worthwhile to give the child a trial of stretching casts. If all else fails, one could consider doing a heelcord and lateral column lengthening, but this is rarely necessary (Fig. 48-16).[106]

RIGID FLATFOOT

Tarsal Coalitions

One of the main causes of a rigid peroneal spastic flatfoot is a tarsal coalition, which is defined as a congenital bony cartilaginous or fibrous connection between two or more tarsal bones. The condition was first described by Buffin in 1750.[121] The first radiographic demonstration of a tarsal coalition was in 1898. Calcaneonavicular and talocalcaneal tarsal coalition are the most common forms. In 1880, Holl proposed a possible connection with flatfoot. In 1897, Sir Robert Jones described peroneal spastic flatfoot.[122] Slomann linked this condition with cases of calcaneonavicular coalition,[123] and then in 1948 Harris and Beath reported a correlation between talocalcaneal coalition and peroneal spastic flatfoot.

Tarsal coalition results from failure of differentiation and segmentation of primary mesenchyme in the developing fetus.[124] It is frequently seen in children with proximal femoral focal deficiency and fibular hemimelia.[125] Leonard concluded that tarsal coalition was a multifactorial disorder of autosomal dominant inheritance with very nearly full penetrance.[126] The incidence of tarsal coalition in the general population is probably less than 1 percent.[127-129] Males tend to be affected more often than females. The most common coalitions are between the calcaneus and talus and between the calcaneus and the navicular. In my own practice I have seen more calcaneonavicular coalitions than any other type. Some 60 percent of calcaneonavicular coalitions are bilateral, compared to 50 percent of talocalcaneal coalitions. The two types can occur in the same foot, so that when one is working up a child with an obvious calcaneonavicular bar, as demonstrated on x-ray, it is wise to look at the width of the posterior facet of the subtalar joint. A narrowed facet may indicate a coexisting talocalcaneal bar. Coalitions tend to be fibrous or cartilaginous during the first years of life and only later start to ossify. A nonossified bar may allow sufficient joint motion to prevent symptoms; however, as the bar ossifies and motion is restricted, the foot may become painful. It has been reported that different coalitions ossify at different times; talonavicular between 3 and 5 years, calcaneonavicular between 8 and 12 years, and talocalcaneal between 12 and 16 years. The most common bridge between the talus and calcaneus involves the middle facet. Harris classified middle-facet coalitions into four types[129a,129b]: (1) a continuous bony bridge; (2) an incomplete form where the medial talus and sustentaculum tali are separated by a thin plate of cartilage or fibrous tissue; (3) rudimentary types, where there is a bony projection extending from the medial talus; and (4) where there is a bony projection from the calcaneus. All four types can be symptomatic.[130]

The normal subtalar joint has a rotatory and gliding motion during walking. At initial stance, the calcaneus is in valgus and external rotation. In terminal stance, the calcaneus is in internal rotation and varus.[122] Tarsal coalitions restrict subtalar motion and produce peroneal spasm. The calcaneus is held in valgus and the navicular overrides the head of the talus, putting traction on the joint capsule and the dorsal talonavicular ligament.

Tarsal coalitions may be asymptomatic, but often children with tarsal coalitions present with pain during the second decade of life as the bar progressively ossifies. The adolescent with a calcaneonavicular bar often complains of pain in the sinus tarsi and on the lateral side of the foot. Talocalcaneal coalitions are associated with a deeper pain below the ankle joint. On clinical examination, the longitudinal arch of the foot is flattened and the heel is in valgus. When the child walks tiptoe, the heel does not pull into varus and the child is unable to walk on the lateral side of the foot. Any forcible attempt to correct the hindfoot valgus or to invert the foot is associated with more peroneal spasm and pain.

If one suspects that a child has a tarsal coalition, a standing AP and lateral x-ray should be ordered plus an axial view of the hindfoot and an oblique view of the foot (Fig. 48-17*A* through *D*). If, from these studies, one suspects a talocalcaneal bar, this is best demonstrated by CT or MRI (Fig. 48-18*A, B,* and *C*).

It is important to remember that in addition to tarsal coalitions, any condition that produces an inflammation of the subtalar joint can result in a peroneal spastic flatfoot (Table 48-4). The initial treatment for a symptomatic tarsal coalition is conservative. The pain may be relieved by an in-shoe orthosis and activity limitation or a period of cast immobilization. I have found, however, that active children with significant pain and peroneal spasm often require a resection of the bar. The technique of resecting a calcaneonavicular bar is illustrated in Fig. 48-19.[122] I prefer to use fat as the spacer, which is held in position by a resorbable suture threaded into Keith needles so that it can be brought out and tied on the medial side of the foot. Following the resection of a calcaneonavicular bar, the foot is held inverted and a cast is applied. This is removed in 2 to 3 weeks, but weight bearing is restricted until the child has regained a full range of subtalar motion.

The surgical treatment of talocalcaneal coalitions is more controversial. It used to be felt that these were best managed with a triple arthrodesis, but Olney[122] and Scranton[122a] reported good results with excision of the coalition (Fig. 48-20).[122] In making the decision whether or not to excise the coalition, one should look at the extent of the bar and the thickness of the cartilage in the posterior facet. If there is a very large bar and very thin cartilage, it is unlikely that the bar excision will produce a good result. I have found that it is sometimes possible to avoid a triple arthrodesis with a sliding osteotomy of the calcaneus to restore the mechanical axis and by lengthening the spastic peroneal muscles.

Calcaneovalgus Deformity

It is not uncommon to have a newborn present in the clinic with the heel in valgus and the foot dorsiflexed to the point where the dorsum of the foot will make contact with the anterolateral part of the distal leg. This calcaneovalgus position results from intrauterine pressure. The plantar flexors and tibialis posterior are overstretched while the dorsiflexors and peronei are shortened. A careful clinical

---

TABLE 48-4 Peroneal Spastic Flatfoot

Coalitions
  Calcaneonavicular (common)
  Talocalcaneal
    Anterior facet (rare)
    Middle facet (common)
    Posterior facet (rare)

Inflammation
  Rheumatoid arthritis
  Hemophilia with bleeding into subtalar joint
  Posttraumatic
  Septic arthritis
  Tuberculosis

Tumor
  Osteoid osteoma (talus)
  Aneurysmal bone cyst (calcaneus)

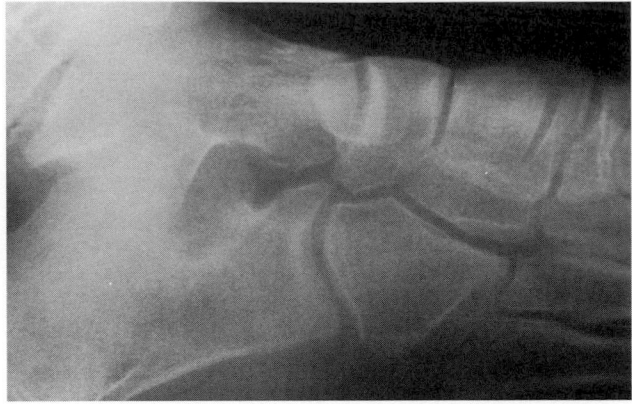

A

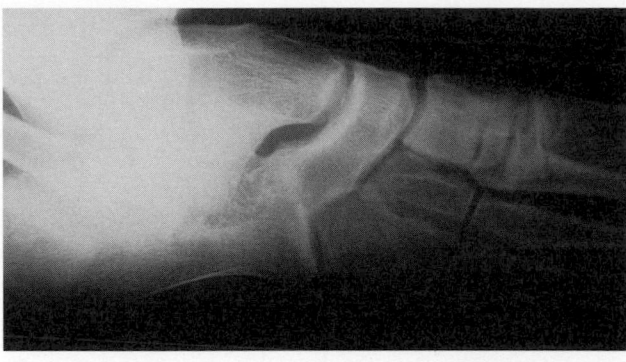

B

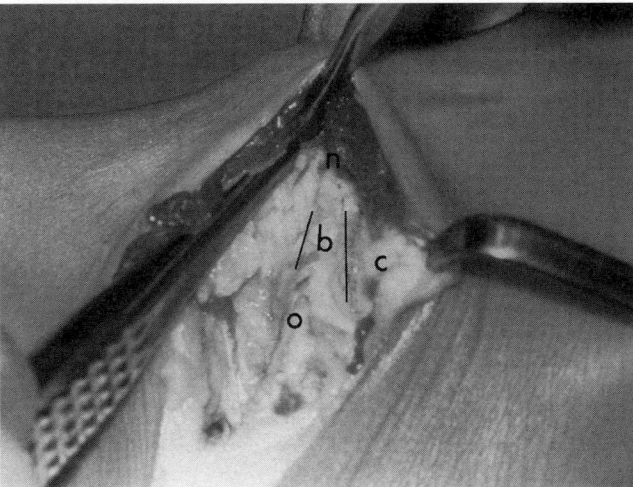

C

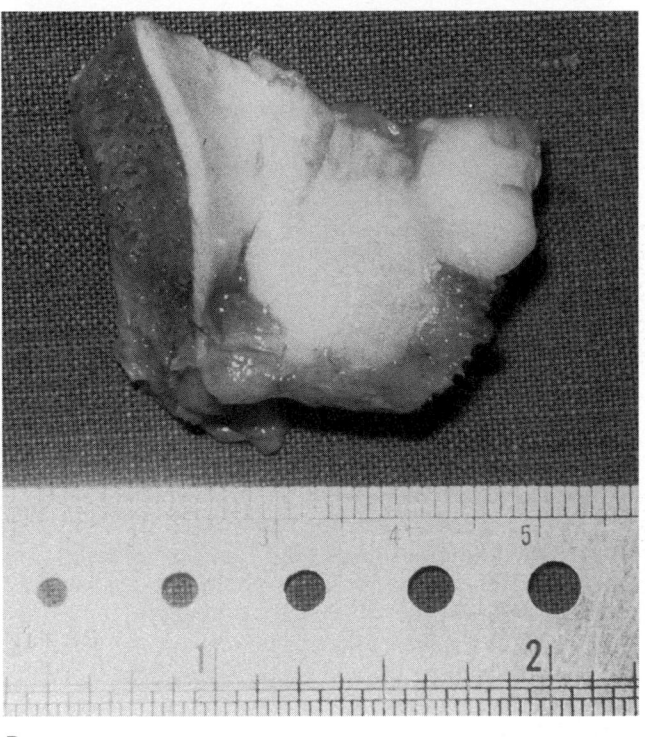

D

Figure 48-17 *A.* Oblique x-ray of a foot demonstrating an incomplete calcaneonavicular bar. This was sufficient to produce a peroneal spastic flatfoot. *B.* A large, completely ossified calcaneonavicular bar. *C.* The black lines outline a large calcaneonavicular bar: o, os calcis; n, navicular; c, cuboid; b, bar. *D.* The excised bar.

examination will demonstrate that all motor groups are functioning. A simple exercise in which the foot is plantarflexed and inverted may speed recovery, but as calcaneovalgus is a positional deformity, it resolves spontaneously and no other treatment is indicated.

CONGENITAL FLATFOOT

Congenital Vertical Talus

In this condition the talus is in a vertical position and there is dorsal dislocation of the navicular, so that it rests on the neck of the talus. This is a rigid dislocation and should be distinguished from an oblique talus, which can be seen with severe ligamentous laxity and in certain neurologic disorders. With a true congenital vertical talus, it

is impossible to reduce the navicula onto the head of the talus. With an oblique talus, a forced plantar flexion lateral x-ray of the foot will demonstrate that the forefoot will align with the long axis of the talus.

Congenital vertical talus can be an isolated finding or may be associated with neurologic conditions such as myelomeningocele, sacral agenesis, or lipoma of the cauda equina.[131–135] Children with muscle abnormalities such as arthrogryposis may have fixed vertical tali. A vertical talus can also be part of a genetic syndrome.[135]

Pathoanatomy

Some authors believe that the dislocation of the transverse tarsal joint can be limited to the talonavicular joint,[135] but in my experience, in a true congenital vertical talus, there is always some dorsolateral displacement of

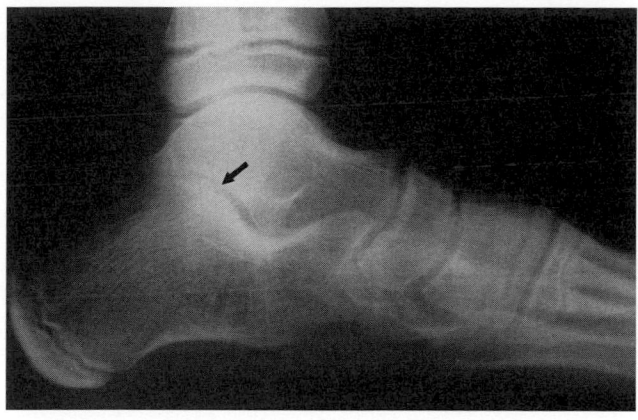

A

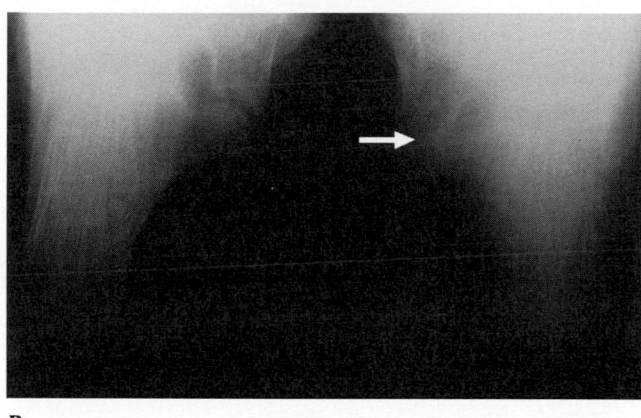

B

Figure 48-18 *A.* Lateral x-ray of the foot of a child with peroneal spasm. Note the narrow posterior facet (*arrow*). *B.* The Harris view demonstrates obliteration of the medial facet of the right foot (*arrow*). *C.* The CT scan demonstrates a bar bridging the medial facet.

C

the calcaneocuboid joint. In this condition, only the posterior third of the talar dome articulates with the tibial plafond. The calcaneus is in severe plantar flexion, the sustentaculum tali is hypoplastic, all of the ligaments on the undersurface of the transverse tarsal joint are attenuated, and those on the dorsal surface are contracted. The triceps surae, tibialis anterior, long toe extensors, and peronei are contracted. The tibialis posterior tendon is subluxated anteriorly. The peronei are also subluxated anteriorly. Since the tibialis posterior and peronei no longer have their fulcrums of the medial and lateral malleoli respectively, they become dorsiflexors of the forefoot.

On clinical examination, the heel is in equinus, the medial column of the foot is convex, and the forefoot is abducted; the head of the talus is palpable in the sole of the foot and it is impossible to correct the deformity by passive manipulation. It is important to remember that a congenital vertical talus in an otherwise normal child will not delay walking. Every severe flatfoot in a toddler should be carefully examined.

Typical radiographic findings are shown in Fig. 48-21. To confirm the diagnosis of a congenital vertical talus, lateral radiographs are made with the foot in maximal plantar flexion and maximal dorsiflexion. In the maximal plantar flexion view, one can see that the midfoot dislocation

is not corrected; the maximal dorsiflexion view will demonstrate the persistent equinus of the calcaneum (Fig. 48-22*A*, *B*, and *C*).

I was taught to do the surgical correction in two stages. The first stage was an open reduction of the talonavicular and calcaneocuboid joints so that the forefoot could be aligned with the hindfoot. To do this, it was often necessary to lengthen the dorsiflexors. Six weeks later, the equinus of the hindfoot was corrected. The problem with the two-stage technique is that, often following the correction of the hindfoot, the lengthened dorsiflexors were too long, and some of these children had difficulty clearing the forefoot during the swing phase of gait. For the last 25 years, I have preferred the one-stage correction, which can be performed at 6 months of age. One can use a medial incision to reduce the talonavicular joint, a lateral incision to reduce the calcaneocuboid joint, and a vertical incision to lengthen the tight heel cord, or one may use the Cincinnati incision.

In the surgical correction, I initially identify the talonavicular joint on the medial side of the foot. To do this, the tibialis posterior is identified at the back of the medial malleolus and followed distally (Fig. 48-23*A*). The talonavicular joint is completely released. Next, a capsulotomy is performed of the calcaneocuboid joint on the lateral side of the foot (Fig. 48-23*B*). The anterior neurovascular

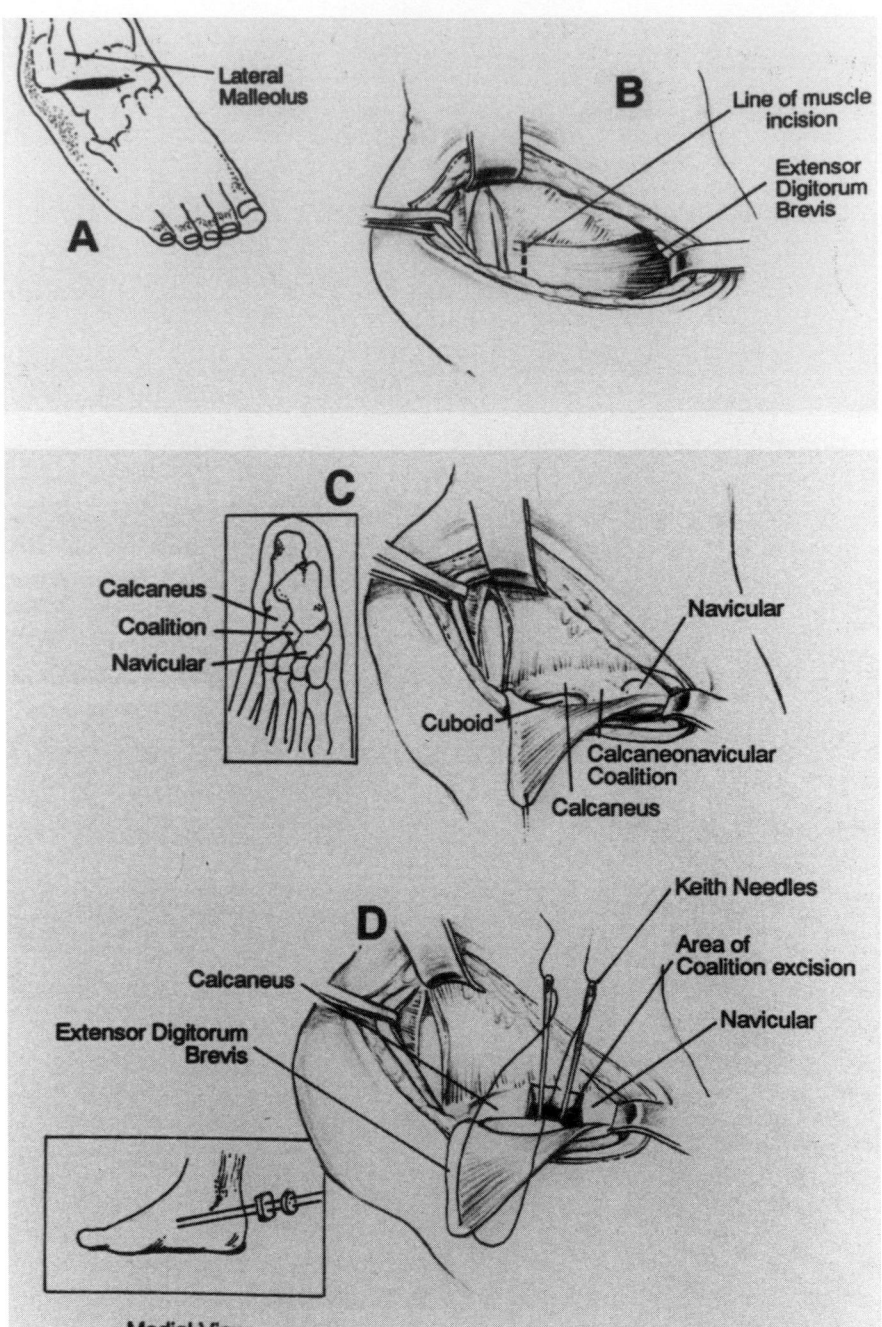

Figure 48-19 Technique of excision of calcaneonavicular coalition (see text). *A.* An oblique incision is made over the lateral aspect of the dorsal hindfoot. *B.* The peroneal tendons and sural nerve are retracted in the lower aspect of the incision. *C.* The extensor digitorum brevis is sharply elevated off the calcaneus to expose the coalition. The coalition is resected with two parallel cuts in the bone. *D.* Absorbable sutures are attached to the extensor digitorum brevis muscle and passed through the coalition resection to the medial aspect of the foot on Keith needles. When the sutures are tied over a button, the muscle is pulled into the void left by the coalition resections. [Reproduced with permission from Olney BW: Tarsal coalition, in Drennan JC (ed): *The Child's Foot and Ankle.* New York, Raven Press, 1992, p 178.]

bundle and the extensor tendons are elevated and any residual tight capsular structures on the dorsal part of the transverse tarsal joint are divided. One then can attempt to assess the severity of the hindfoot contracture by ele-

vating the head of the talus while the forefoot is plantarflexed. Next, the tendo Achillis is lengthened by Z-plasty, but in this instance the distal limb is removed from the lateral side of the calcaneus. The posterior capsule of the an-

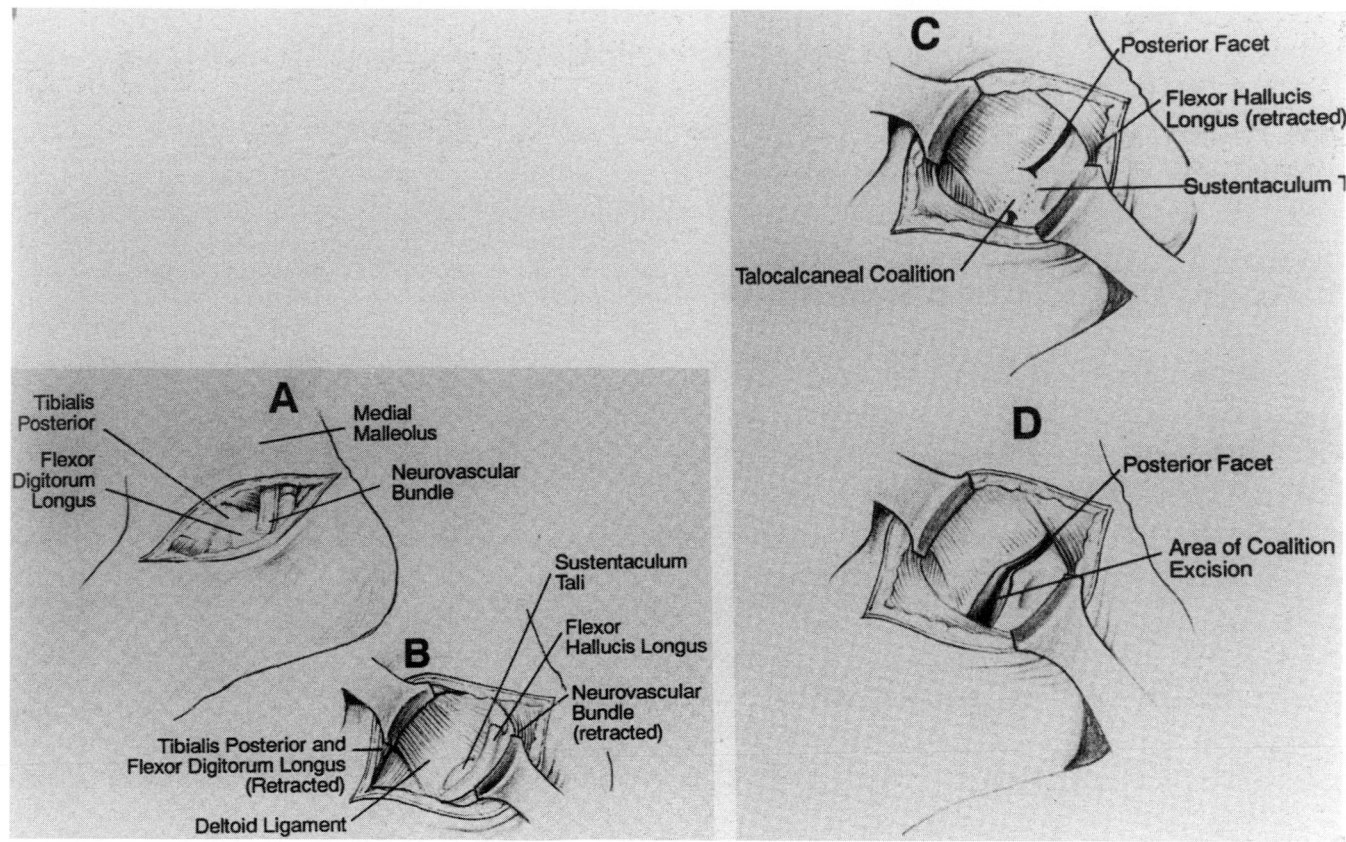

Figure 48-20 Technique of excision of talocalcaneal middle facet coalition (see text). *A.* An incision is made over the middle aspect of the hindfoot, centered over the sustentaculum tali. *B.* The tibialis posterior and flexor digitorum longus tendons are dissected off the coalition and retracted dorsally. The neurovascular bundle is retracted plantarward. *C.* The middle facet coalition is identified just above the sustentaculum tali. *D.* The coalition is resected until there is free motion across the subtalar joint. [Reproduced with permission from Olney BW: Tarsal coalition, in Drennan JC (ed): *The Child's Foot and Ankle.* New York, Raven Press, 1992, p. 178.]

kle and subtalar joint is divided so that the talus can assume its normal position in the ankle mortise and the equinus and valgus of the calcaneus can be corrected. I find it useful to put a K wire in the long axis of the talus from behind to perform this maneuver. The forefoot can then be reduced on the hindfoot and the talonavicular and calcaneocuboid joints pinned. In short, one is following the same plan as in treating a clubfoot. One restores the bony architecture to normal and then attempts to balance the muscle forces. It will always be necessary to lengthen the tendo Achillis and the peronei. I have not routinely lengthened the tibialis anterior and posterior and I have not performed tendon transfers as part of the initial correction. Transferring the tibialis anterior to the neck of the talus can weaken dorsiflexion.

METATARSUS ADDUCTUS

Adduction of the forefoot is the most common foot deformity (Table 48-5).[106] It is characterized by a convexity of the lateral border of the foot and sometimes spreading of the toes. Bleck described the heel bisector method of documenting metatarsus adductus (Fig. 48-24).[136] The weight-bearing surface of the heel forms an ellipse and a line extending the major axis of this ellipse; the heel bisector serves as a reference line. The deformity is considered mild if the line intersects the third toe, moderate if it falls

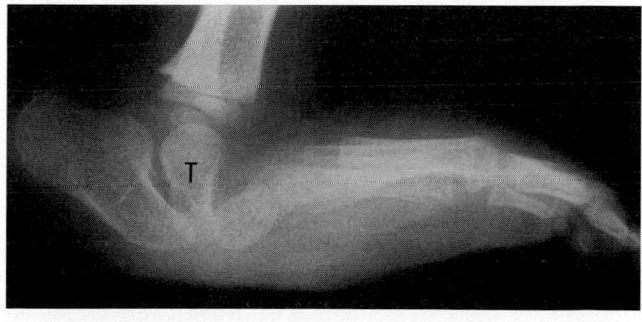

Figure 48-21 Lateral x-ray demonstrating a vertical talus (T) in a child with a rocker-bottom deformity of the foot.

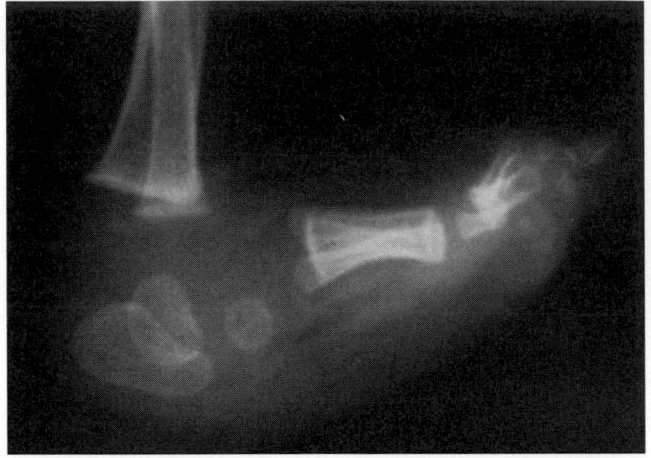

A

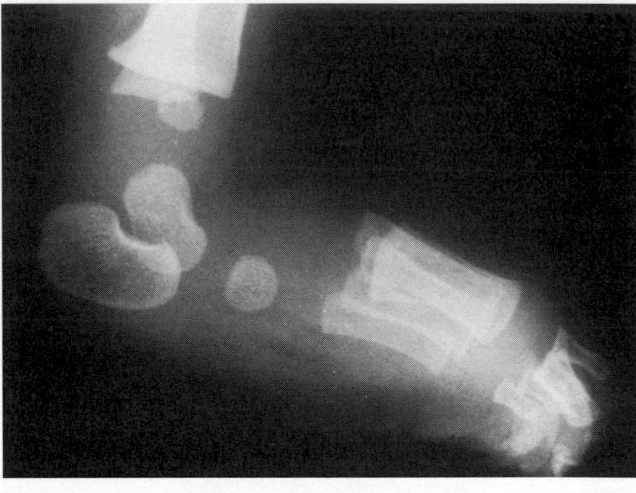

B

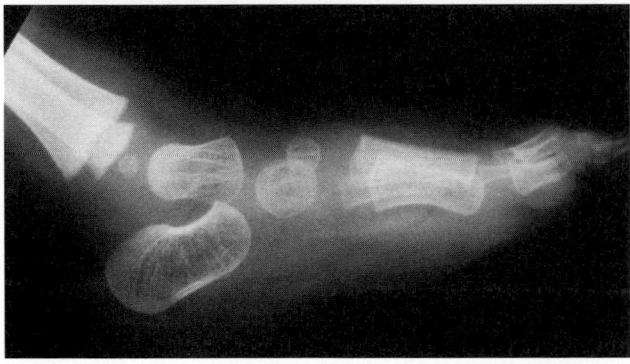

C

Figure 48-22 *A.* Child with a vertical talus in maximal dorsiflexion, demonstrating residual equinus of the os calcis. *B.* After a period of conservative treatment, the midfoot will not reduce with forced plantar flexion. *C.* A dependent film taken 1 year postoperatively demonstrates that the talus and first ray are in alignment.

between the third and fourth toes, and severe if it falls between the fourth and fifth toes. The foot can be further classified as flexible (abduction beyond the midline of the heel bisector), partly flexible (abduction to the midline only), or inflexible (rigid) with no abduction possible. Staheli describes a simple technique of recording the position of the foot by having the baby stand on the copying surface of a standard fixed-base photocopying machine.

Farsetti et al., in yet another classic article from Iowa City, have reported on the long-term functional and radiographic outcomes of untreated and nonoperatively treated metatarsus adductus.[137] They point out that the etiology and pathogenesis of the deformity are unknown and that treatment has been controversial. Some authors have believed that a passively correctable deformity will resolve without treatment, whereas Farsetti et al. recommend manipulation and serial plaster cast when the deformity is rigid.[138–141] Other authors have recommended various operative treatments.[84,85,139,142,143] Thirty-one patients (45 feet) who had metatarsus adductus were evaluated in the Department of Orthopaedic Surgery of the University of Iowa Clinic and were followed for an average of 32 years and 6 months. Of these 31 patients, 21 (31 feet) were examined clinically and radiographically. Information on the remaining 10 patients (14 feet) was obtained by a letter, telephone, or both. Twelve patients (16 feet) who had a passively cor-

rectable deformity, mild or moderate, at the time of the initial presentation had no treatment. Twenty patients (29 feet) who had a partly flexible or rigid deformity, moderate or severe, at the time of initial presentation were managed with serial manipulations and application of plaster casts (one patient who had a bilateral deformity had no treatment on one side and conservative management on the other).

The results were good in all 16 of the untreated feet and in 26 (90 percent) of the 29 feet that had been conservatively treated. There were no poor results. The passively correctable deformities resolved spontaneously. Radiographs showed an obliquity of the medial cuneiform–metatarsal joint in 21 (68 percent) of the 31 feet that were examined clinically and radiographically. Similar findings were observed in 4 of 11 contralateral normal feet. Hallux valgus was not a common outcome and no patient had operative correlation. I concur with Farsetti et al. when they state, "Thus, according to the results we believe that operative treatment is not needed or desirable in patients who have residual mild or moderate deformities."[137]

A child with metatarsus adductus requires careful clinical examination. If the forefoot will correct to or beyond the bisector line of the heel, I encourage the parents to do some simple stretching exercises. The hindfoot is stabilized with the tibia while the forefoot is abducted. The more rigid feet are corrected with serial manipulations and casts (Fig.

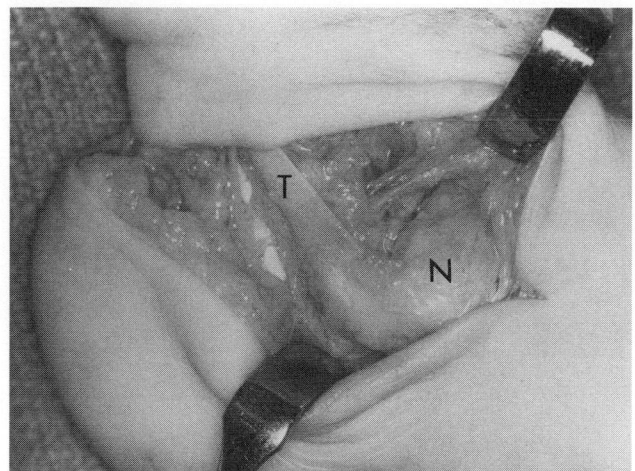

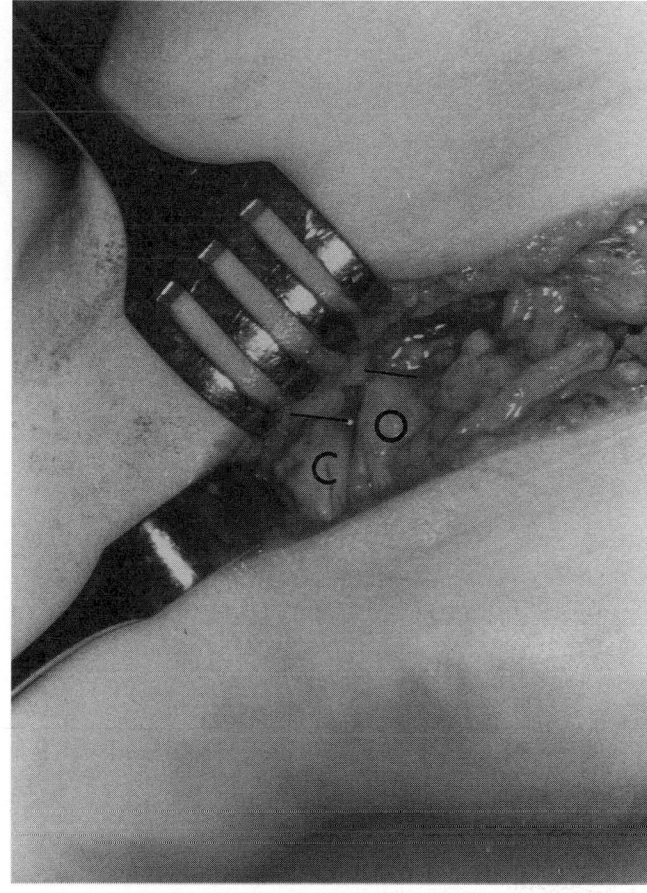

Figure 48-23 *A.* Vertical talus, left foot. Medial incision using the tibialis posterior (T) as the road map to the navicular (N). *B.* Lateral limb of the incision demonstrating that the cuboid (C) moved inferiorly once the calcaneocuboid capsule was released. Before the release, the line on the top of the calcaneus (O) matched the line on top of the cuboid.

B

48-25*A* through *D*). Heyman et al.[85] recommended a tarsal metatarsal capsulotomy for metatarsus adductus for a child between 3 and 7 years of age. Some authors[142] have reported good results with this procedure, while others have been disappointed.[144] In another article,[84] Berman and Gartland reported good results with metatarsal osteotomies.

Patients with severe metatarsus adductus should be carefully evaluated for a skewfoot, which is a condition in which there is valgus of the hindfoot, a short lateral column, lateral subluxation of the navicular in relation to the head of the talus, and metatarsus adductus. This severe foot deformity may require a surgical correction. Mosca[145] has reported good results using a technique consisting of a calcaneal lengthening osteotomy, medial cuneiform opening wedge osteotomy, and lengthening of the tendo Achillis. If one mistakes a skewfoot for a simple metatarsus adduc-

TABLE 48-5 Types of Forefoot Adductus Varus

Type	Etiology	Comment
Metatarsus adductus	Late intrauterine positional deformity	Common form 90% resolves spontaneously
Metatarsus varus	Earlier onset (intrauterine position?)	Often rigid; cast correction necessary
Skewfoot	Familial; generalized joint laxity	Hindfoot valgus Abduction midfoot Adduction forefoot Treatment difficult

Source: Reproduced with permission from Staheli LT: *Fundamentals of Pediatric Orthopaedics.* New York, Raven Press, 1992, p 57.

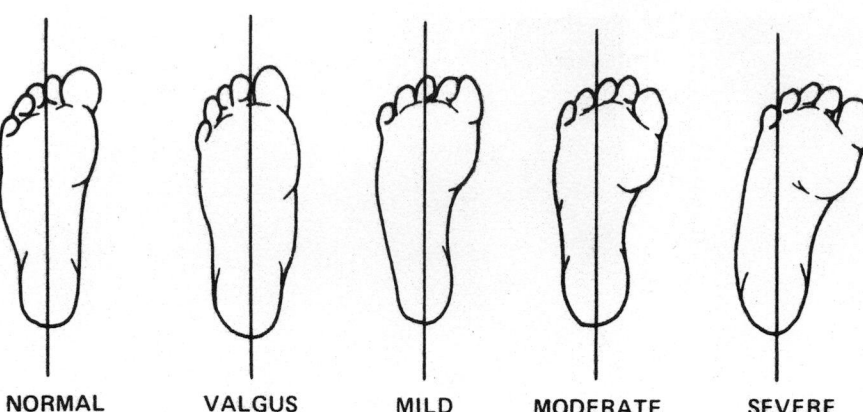

NORMAL VALGUS MILD MODERATE SEVERE

Figure 48-24 The heel bisector, a line extending the major axis of the ellipse of the weight-bearing surface of the heel, defines the severity of the metatarsus adductus. The condition is considered mild if the line intersects the third toe, moderate if it falls between the third and fourth toes, and severe if it falls between the fourth and fifth toes. (Reproduced with permission from Bleck EE: Developmental Orthopaedics III: Toddlers. *Dev Med Child Neurol* 24:533, 1982.)

tus and corrects the metatarsus adductus with metatarsal osteotomies, then the whole foot will be in valgus and the child will walk on the head of the talus.

PES CAVUS

Staheli defines physiologic cavus as a familial condition in which the deformity falls outside of the normal range (beyond two standard deviations of the mean of variability of arch height).[99] This is a relatively stable condition and the children are usually comfortable in shock-absorbing shoewear. True pes cavus is usually due to a muscle imbalance produced by a neuromuscular disorder. It is imperative to do a careful workup on these children to establish a diagnosis and formulate a treatment plan. Sabir and Lyttle define cavus as a fixed equinus deformity of the forefoot on the hindfoot (Fig. 48-26).[146]

Charcot-Marie-Tooth disease is a common cause of the cavus foot. It is a hereditary sensorimotor type I neuropathy.[147,148] This disease presents in the first and second decades of life with early atrophy of the intrinsic muscles of the foot and a cavovarus deformity. Other members of the family may have a similar deformity. One must perform a thorough, complete clinical examination and include a careful neurologic assessment for motor power, sensation, and reflexes. In the detailed examination of the foot, one examines in turn the hindfoot, the midfoot, and then the forefoot and toes and assesses flexibility. A fixed deformity of the hindfoot can be demonstrated by use of the Coleman block test.[149] If the varus of the heel corrects with a block under the lateral side of the foot, there is not a fixed hindfoot varus.[149]

The following imaging studies may be helpful in establishing a diagnosis: standing AP and lateral x-rays of the foot plus an axial view of the os calcis and an oblique view of the foot. It is helpful to x-ray the lumbosacral spine looking for any anomaly that might be missed. Further evaluation will include an electromyogram and nerve conduction studies and possibly a muscle biopsy.[150] Other studies that may be helpful include gait analysis with video motion studies, dynamic electromyography, and force-plate analysis. Sabir and Lyttle[146] have described the pathogenesis of

cavus deformity. Initially there is denervation and weakening of the interossei and lumbricals, which results in a "windlass effect" of the long toe flexors (Fig. 48-27).[146] Next, there is atrophy, fibrosis, and shortening of the short plantar muscles, resulting in a "tie beam" effect. There is then further contracture of the soft tissues and capsules and, finally, complete atrophy and contracture of all of the muscles of the foot, and all deformities become fixed.

In the approach to a cavus deformity, one must first decide if the deformity is correctable or fixed. Then one looks at the hindfoot. Is there heel varus or not? If there is no heel varus but equinus and pronation of the first ray and clawing of the great toe, one should do a plantar release,[151] a first metatarsal osteotomy, and a Jones tendon transfer,[152] with an interphalangeal fusion of the great toe.[153] If there is no heel varus but equinus of several rays and clawing of several toes, it is recommended that the child have a plantar release, metatarsal osteotomies, a Jones transfer, and a transfer of the long toe extensors to the metatarsal necks. If there is fixed heel varus, equinus of the entire forefoot, and clawing of all toes but no structural abnormality on x-ray, the child should have metatarsal osteotomies, a tibialis posterior tendon transfer, correction of the toe deformities, and a calcaneal osteotomy. If there is fixed heel varus, equinus of the entire forefoot, clawing of all of the toes, and structural bony changes on x-ray but still some tarsal movements possible, it is recommended that the foot be treated by a wedge tarsectomy, tibialis posterior tendon transfer, correction of the toe deformities, and a calcaneal osteotomy. If there is fixed heel varus, clawing of all of the toes, equinus of the entire forefoot, structural bony changes on x-ray with all deformities fixed, and the toes dislocated dorsally as well as keratosis, then the child should have a triple arthrodesis, a tibialis posterior tendon transfer, and correction of the toe deformities.

OSTEOCHONDROSES OF THE FOOT
Kohler's Disease

Osteonecrosis of the navicular was first described in 1908 and usually presents with pain along the medial border of

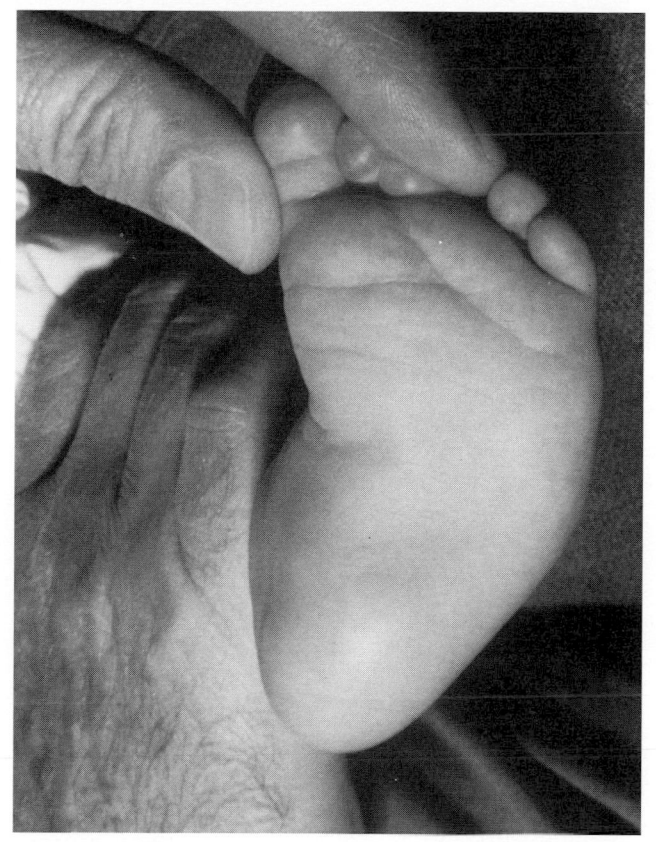

A

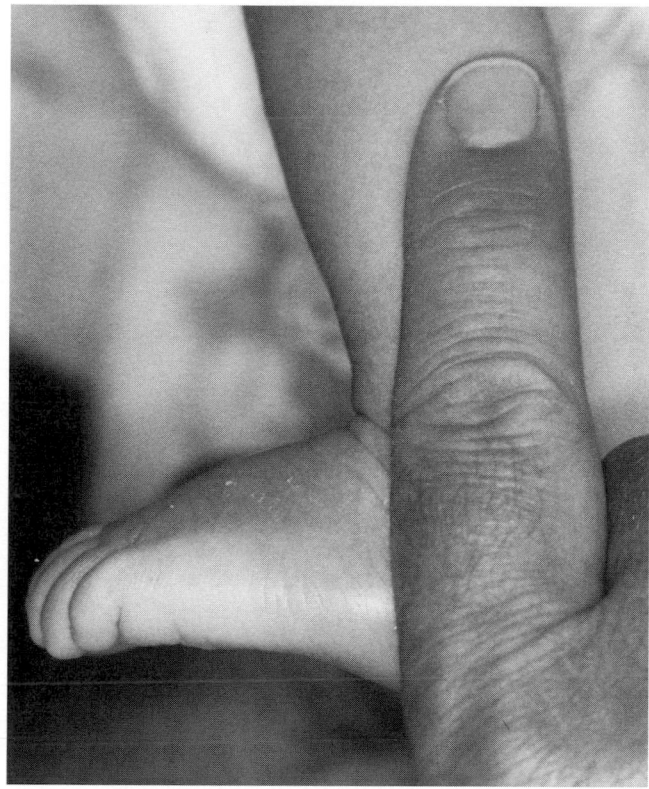

B

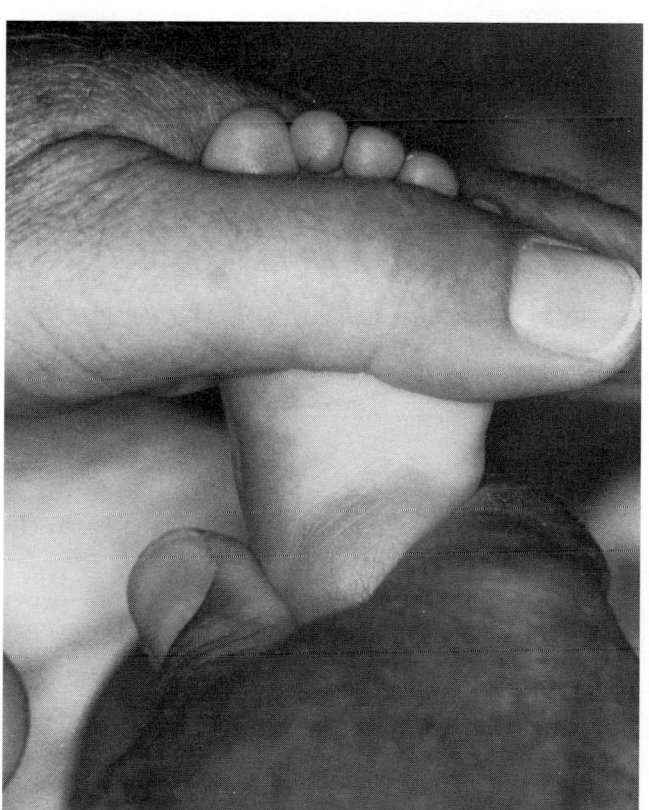

C

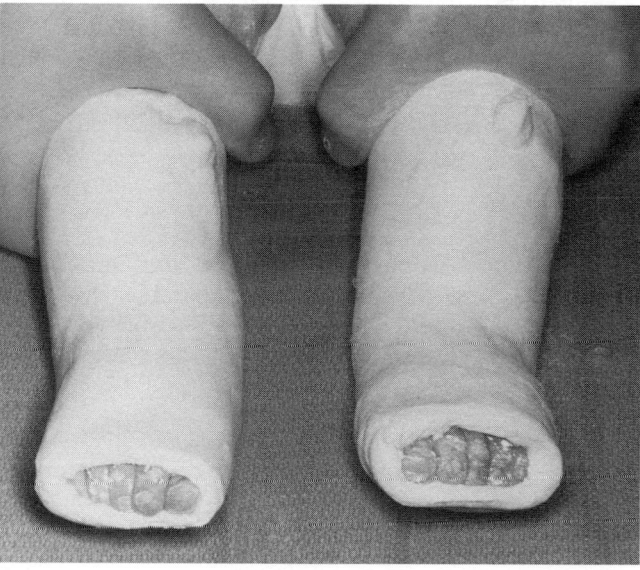

D

Figure 48-25 *A.* A severe metatarsus adductus. *B and C.* The hindfoot is stabilized with the long axis of the tibia while the forefoot is abducted. *D.* Plaster casts have been applied.

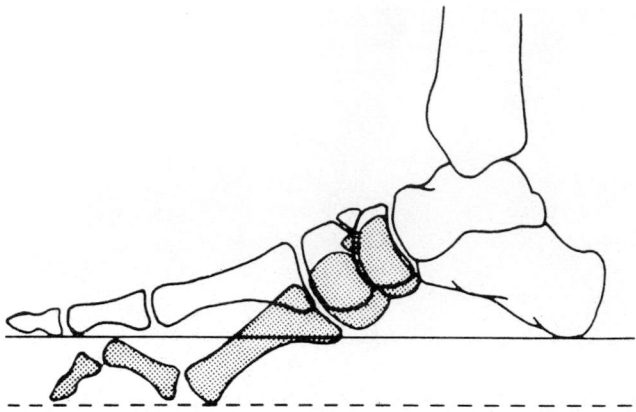

Figure 48-26 Pes cavus—fixed equinus deformity of the forefoot on the hindfoot. (Reproduced with permission from Sabir M, Lyttle D: Pathogenesis of pes cavus in Charcot-Marie-Tooth disease. *Clin Orthop Rel Res* 175:173, 1983.)

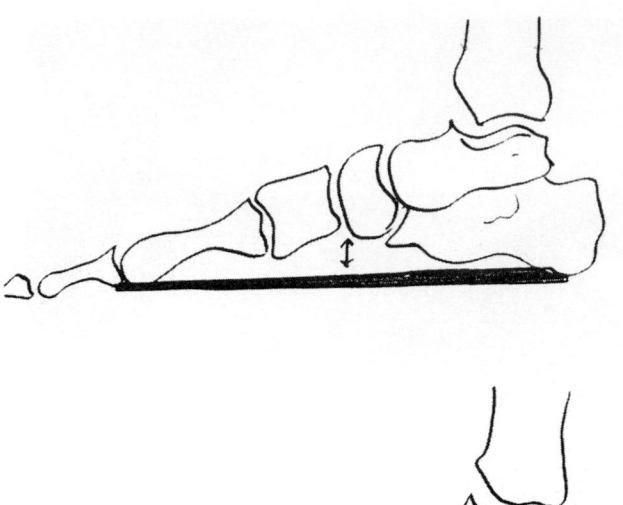

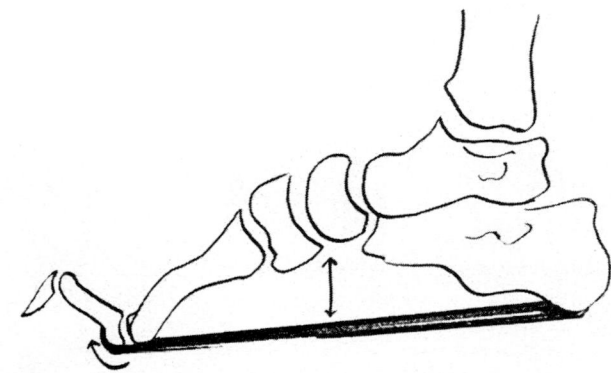

Figure 48-27 "Windlass" effect. (Reproduced with permission from Sabir M, Lyttle D: Pathogenesis of pes cavus in Charcot-Marie-Tooth disease. *Clin Orthop Rel Res* 175:173, 1983.)

the foot. There may be soft tissue swelling, redness, and tenderness over the talonavicular and naviculocuneiform joints. It can occur anytime between the ages of 3 and 10 years and is more frequent in males. The typical radiographic findings are flattening of the navicular with patchy ossification. The navicular begins to ossify between 1 1/2 and 2 years of age in girls and between 2 and 3 years in boys; it is the last of the tarsal bones to ossify completely.[154] The etiology of Kohler's disease is unknown, and various treatments have been prescribed.[155,156] A short leg walking cast until acute symptoms subside may be useful. Afterwards, a high-top running shoe that has good shock absorption will provide comfort. Occasionally it may be necessary to support the talonavicular joint with an orthosis.

Friedberg's Disease

Teenagers with Friedberg's disease complain of metatarsalgia with weight bearing. There is a higher incidence in females. Typically there is point tenderness over the second metatarsal phalangeal joint, but sometimes a third metatarsal phalangeal joint can be involved. The area may be red and swollen. The initial x-rays may demonstrate only joint space widening, but later films will show sclerosis and flattening of the metatarsal head. It is presumed that Friedberg's disease results from repetitive trauma.[157] Smillie has given a four-part classification to the disease process. In stage I, there is a subchondral fissure; in stages II and III, there is progressive resorption of the metatarsal head; and in stage IV there is flattening and severe deformity.[158]

The initial treatment consists of rest; when the acute symptoms subside, the metatarsal head can be protected by the use of a metatarsal pad. If the disease has progressed to the point where there is severe flattening and deformity of the metatarsal head, some form of surgical treatment may be required. The metatarsal head should

not be resected in a child. It may be helpful to remove loose bodies from the joint.[157] Gauthier in 1979 described a dorsally placed closing wedge osteotomy of the metatarsal neck. This shortens the metatarsal a few millimeters and allows the healthier plantar metatarsal articular surface to come in contact with the proximal phalanx.[159]

REFERENCES

1. Porter RW: Clubfoot (congenital talipes equinovarus). *J R Coll Surg Edinburgh* 41(1):66–71, 1995.
2. Reimann I: *Congenital Idiopathic Clubfoot.* Denmark, PJ Schmidt a/s, Vojens, Copenhagen, 1967.
3. Hippocrates: *Oeuvres completes D'Hippocrate* (translated by E Littre). Paris, Baillière, 1844.
4. Paré A: Oeuvres completes (translated by JF Malgaigne). Paris, Baillière, 1840.
5. Andry N: *Orthopaedia* (facsimile reproduction of the first edition in English, London 1743). Philadelphia, Lippincott, 1961.
6. Brückner AD: *Über die Natur Ursachen und Behandlung der einwartsgekrummlen Fusse oder der sogenanten Klumpfusse.* Gotha, 1976, pp 49, 88–135.
7. Wantzel JM: *De Talipedibus varis.* Tubingen, Litteris Fuesianis, 1798, p 17.
8. Dimeglio A: *Le Pied Bot.* Sauramps Medical Avignon, 1985, p 81.

9. Lorenz A: Heilung des Klumpfusses durch des modellierende Redressement. *Wien Klin Wochenschr* 21:289, 1895.

10. Stromeyer L: Division of the tendo Achillis in club foot. *Lancet* 3:648, 1836.

11. Dieffenbach JF: *Über die Durchschneidung der Sehnen und Muskelen.* Berlin, Forstner, 1841.

12. Solly S: Case of double talipes varus, in which the cuboid bone was partially removed from the left foot. *Lancet* 1:478, 1857.

13. Lund E: Removal of both astragali in a case of severe double talipes. *Br Med J [Clin Res]* 2:438, 1872.

14. Phelps AM: *The Treatment of Certain Forms of Clubfoot by Open Incision and Fixed Extension.* Copenhagen, Congress International des Sciences Medicales, 1884, p 132.

15. Ogsten A: A new principle of curing club-foot in severe cases in children a few years old. *Br Med J [Clin Res]* 1:1524, 1902.

16. Vulpius O: Die Behandlung des angeborenen Klumpfusses. *Dtsch Med Wochenschr* 13:585, 1913.

17. Pürkhauser R: Die Torsion der Untershenklknochen bei angeborenen Klumpfussen und ihre Heilung. *Munch Med Wosenschr* 58:571, 1911.

18. Brown D: Modern methods of treatment of club-foot. *Br Med J [Clin Res]* 2:570, 1937.

19. Kite JH: Principles involved in the treatment of congenital clubfoot: The results of treatment. *J Bone Joint Surg* 21:595, 1939.

20. Wisbrun W: Neue Gesichtspunkte zum Redressement des angeborenen Klumpfusses und daraus sich ergebende Schlussfolgerungen bezuglich der Aetiologie. *Arch Orthop Unfall-Chir* 31:451, 1932.

21. Contarygis A: Le traitment operatoire precoce du pied bot congenital chez les nouveau-nes. *Rev Orthop* 18:719, 1931.

22. Bertelsen A: Treatment of congenital club foot. *J Bone Joint Surg [Br]* 39:599, 1957.

23. Bertelsen A: Foddeformiteter og deres behandling. *Manedsskr Prakt Loegegern* 4:153, 1957.

24. Camera U: Mon experience dans le traitment du pied bot congenital. *Rev Chir Orthop* 38:525, 1952.

25. Hirsch C: Observationer vid tidig operation av pes equinovarus congenitus. *Nord Med* 63:425, 1960.

26. Pasilia M, Sulamaa M: Tidlg operation av svar klumpfot. *Nord Med* 66:1274, 1961.

27. Scheel PF: Beobachtungen bei der Behandlung des kongenitalen Klumpfusses. *Zeitschr Orthop* 79:546, 1950.

28. Seyfarth H, Behrens H: Beitrag zur Klumpfossoperation nach Scheel. 96:70–79, 1962.

29. Cowell JR, Wein BK: Genetic aspects of club foot. *J Bone Joint Surg [Am]* 62:1381, 1980.

30. Wynne-Davies R: Family studies in clubfoot. *J Bone Joint Surg* 46B:445, 1964.

31. Wynne-Davies R: Genetic and environmental factors in the etiology of talipes equinovarus. *Clin Orthop* 84:9, 1972.

32. Dietz F: Personal communication.

33. Cowell JR, Hensinger RN: Relationships of clubfoot to congenital annular bands, in Bateman JE (ed): *Foot Science.* Philadelphia, Saunders, 1976, p 41.

34. Irani RN, Sherman SS: The pathological anatomy of clubfoot. *J Bone Joint Surg [Am]* 45:45, 1963.

35. Bohm M: The embryonic origin of clubfoot. *J Bone Joint Surg* 11:229, 1929.

35a. Victoria-Diaz A, Victoria-Diaz J: Pathogenesis of idiopathic clubfoot. *Clin Orthop* 185:14–25, 1984.

36. Dunne PM: Congenital postural deformities. *Br Med Bull* 32:71, 1976.

37. Martin RF, Milo-Manson G, McComas A, Levin S: Neurogenic origin of talipes equinovarus, in Simons GW (ed): *The Clubfoot.* New York, Springer-Verlag, 1994, p 39.

38. Isaacs H, Handelsman JE, Badenhorst M, Pickering A: The muscles in clubfoot—A histological, histochemical and electron microscopic study. *J Bone Joint Surg [Br]* 59:465, 1977.

39. Handelsman JE, Badalamente MA: Neuromuscular studies in club foot. *J Pediatr Orthop* 1:23, 1981.

40. Handelsman JE, Glasser R: Muscle pathology in clubfoot and lower motor neuron lesions, in Simons GW (ed): *The Clubfoot.* New York, Springer-Verlag, 1994. p 21.

41. Gray DH, Katz JM: A histochemical study of muscle in club foot. *J Bone Joint Surg* 63:417, 1981.

42. Adams RD, Denny-Brown D, Pearson CM: *Diseases of Muscle.* New York, Hoeber, 1953, p 224.

43. Sodre H, Bruschini S, Magalhaes AAC, Lourenco A: Anomalous muscles in clubfeet, in Simons GW (ed): *The Clubfoot.* New York, Springer-Verlag, 1994, p 42.

44. Hootnick DR, Packard DR Jr, Levinsohn EM, Wladis A: A vascular hypothesis for the etiology of clubfoot, in Simons GW (ed): *The Clubfoot.* New York, Springer-Verlag, 1994, p 48.

45. Ippolito E, Ponseti IV: Congenital clubfoot in the human fetus: A histological study. *J Bone Joint Surg [Am]* 62:8, 1980.

46. Zimny ML, Willig SJ, Roberts JM, et al: An electron microscopic study of the fascia from the medial and lateral sides of clubfoot. *J Pediatr Orthop* 5:577, 1985.

47. Wynne-Davies R: Talipes equinovarus: A review of eighty-four cases after completion of treatment. *J Bone Joint Surg [Br]* 46:464, 1964.

48. Carroll NC: Surgical technique for talipes equinovarus. *Oper Tech Orthop* 3(2):115, 1993.

49. Beatson TR, Pearson JR: A method of assessing correction in club feet. *J Bone Joint Surg [Br]* 48:40, 1966.

50. Thompson GH: Congenital talipes equinovarus (clubfeet) and metatarsus adductus, in Simons GW (ed): *The Child's Foot and Ankle.* New York, Raven Press, 1992, pp 97–133.

51. Carroll NC: Clubfoot, in Morrissy RT (ed): *Lovell and Winter's Pediatric Orthopaedics,* 3d ed. Philadelphia, Lippincott, 1990, pp 927–957.

52. Carroll NC: Pathoanatomy and treatment of talipes equinovarus. Symposium: current practices in the treatment of idiopathic club foot in the child between birth and five years of age. Parts I and II. *Contemp Orthop* 1 and 2, 1988.

53. DePuy J, Drennan JC: Correction of idiopathic club foot: A comparison of results of early versus delayed posteromedial release. *J Pediatr Orthop* 9:44, 1989.

54. Otremski I, Salama R, Khermosh O, Wientroub S: An analysis of the results of a modified one-stage posteromedial release (Turco operation) for the treatment of club foot. *J Pediatr Orthop* 7:149, 1987.

55. Otremski I, Salama R, Khermosh O, Wientroub S: Residual adduction of the forefoot: A review of the Turco procedure for congenital club foot. *J Bone Joint Surg [Br]* 69:832, 1987.

56. DeRosa GP, Stepro D: Results of posteromedial release for the resistant club foot. *J Pediatr Orthop* 6:590, 1986.

57. Thompson GH, Richardson AB, Westin GW: Surgical management of resistant congenital talipes equinovarus deformities. *J Bone Joint Surg [Am]* 64:652, 1982.

58. Turco VJ: Resistant congenital club foot—One-stage posteromedial release with internal fixation: A follow-up report of 15 years experience. *J Bone Joint Surg [Am]* 61:805, 1979.

59. Simons GW: Complete subtalar release in club feet: Part I. A preliminary report. *J Bone Joint Surg [Am]* 67:1044, 1985.

60. Simons GW: Complete subtalar release in club feet: Part II. Comparison of less extensive procedures. *J Bone Joint Surg [Am]* 67:1056, 1985.

61. Morcuende JA, Weinstein SL, Dietz FR, Ponseti IV: Plaster cast treatment of clubfoot: The Ponseti method of manipulation and casting. *J Pediatr Orthop Part B* 3(2):161, 1994.

62. Howard P, Dias L: Medial rotation of the talus and complete calcaneocuboid release—Its effect on the surgical results in idiopathic clubfoot, in Simons GW (ed): *The Clubfoot*. New York, Springer-Verlag, 1994, pp 209–215.

63. McKay DW: New concept of and approach to clubfoot treatment: Section I. Principles and morbid anatomy. *J Pediatr Orthop* 2:347, 1982.

64. McKay DW: New concept of and approach to clubfoot treatment: Section II. Correction of clubfoot. *J Pediatr Orthop* 3:10, 1983.

65. Bensahel H: Postero-medial approach in clubfoot surgery, in Epeldegui T (ed): *Concepts y Controversias Sobre El Pie Zambo*. Madrid, A. Madrid Vicente, Ediciones, 1993, pp 151–154.

66. Dimeglio A: Classification of talipes equinovarus, in Simons GW (ed): *The Clubfoot*. New York, Springer-Verlag, 1994, p 92.

67. Catterall A: Clinical assessment of clubfoot deformity, in: Simons GW (ed): *The Clubfoot*. New York, Springer-Verlag, 1994, pp 93–96, 1994.

68. Simons GW: Calcaneocuboid joint deformity in talipes equinovarus: An overview and update. *J Pediatr Orthop Part B* 4(1):25, 1995.

69. Grayhack JJ, Zawin JK, Shore RM, et al: Assessment of calcaneocuboid joint deformity by magnetic resonance imaging in talipes equinovarus. *J Pediatr Orthop Part B* 4(1):36, 1995.

70. Wientroub S, Khermosh O: Comparative evaluation of initial surgical procedures in clubfoot. *J Pediatr Orthop Part B* 3(3):171, 1994.

71. Turco VJ: Present management of idiopathic clubfoot. *J Pediatr Orthop Part B* 3(2):149, 1994.

72. Turco VJ: Surgical correction of the resistant clubfoot—One-stage posteromedial release with internal fixation. *J Bone Joint Surg [Am]* 53:477, 1971.

73. Turco VJ: *Clubfoot*. New York, Churchill Livingstone, 1981.

74. Crawford AH, Marxen JL, Osterfeld DL: The Cincinnati incision: A comprehensive approach for surgical procedures of the foot and ankle in childhood. *J Bone Joint Surg [Am]* 64:1335, 1982.

75. Goldner JL: Congenital talipes equinovarus—Fifteen years of surgical treatment. *Curr Pract Orthop Surg* 4:61, 1969.

76. Carroll NC: Congenital clubfoot: Pathoanatomy and treatment. *AAOS Instr Course Lect* 36:117, 1987.

77. Carroll NC: Pathoanatomy and surgical treatment of the resistant clubfoot. *AAOS Instr Course Lec* 37:93, 1988.

78. Yngve DA, Gross RH, Sullivan JA: Clubfoot release without wide subtalar release. *J Pediatr Orthop* 10:473, 1990.

79. Grant JC Boileau: *A Method of Anatomy*. Baltimore, Williams & Wilkins, 1952, p 447.

80. Tarraf YN, Carroll NC: Analysis of the components of residual deformity in clubfeet presenting for reoperation. *J Pediatr Orthop* 12:207, 1992.

81. Garceau GJ, Manning KR: Transposition of the anterior tibial tendon in the treatment of recurrent congenital club foot. *J Bone Joint Surg* 29:1044, 1947.

82. Hoffer MM, Reiswig JA, Garrett AM, Perry J: The split anterior tibial tendon transfer in the treatment of spastic varus hindfoot of childhood. *Orthop Clin North Am* 5:31, 1974.

83. Gartland JJ: Posterior tibial transplant in the surgical treatment of recurrent clubfoot: A preliminary report. *J Bone Joint Surg [Am]* 46:1217, 1964.

84. Berman A, Gartland JJ: Metatarsal osteotomy for the correction of adduction of the forefoot of the foot in children. *J Bone Joint Surg [Am]* 53:498, 1971.

85. Heyman CH, Herndon CH, Strong JM: Mobilization of the tarsometatarsal and intermetatarsal joints for the correction of resistant adduction of the forepart of the foot in congenital club-foot or congenital metatarsus varus. *J Bone Joint Surg [Am]* 40:299, 1958.

86. Johanning K: Exocochleatio ossis cuboidei in the treatment of pes equino varus. *Acta Orthop Scand* 27:310, 1958.

87. Evans D: Relapsed club foot. *J Bone Joint Surg [Br]* 43:722, 1961.

88. Lichtblau S: A medial and lateral release operation for clubfoot: A preliminary report. *J Bone Joint Surg [Am]* 55:1377, 1973.

89. Matsuno S, Kaneda T, Katoh T, Iisaka H: The treatment of congenital clubfoot. *J Jpn Orthop Assoc* 52:101, 1978.

90. Roberts JM: Adjunctive osteotomies to equalize lengths of medial and lateral columns of clubfoot. Presented at the Sixteenth Pediatric Orthopaedic International Seminar, San Francisco, May 1988.

91. Hoffman AA, Constine RM, McBride GG, Coleman SS: Osteotomy of the first cuneiform as treatment of residual adduction of the forepart of the foot in clubfoot. *J Bone Joint Surg [Am]* 66:985, 1984.

92. Kumar PN, Laing PW, Klenerman L: Medial calcaneal osteotomy for relapsed equinovarus deformity: Long-term study of the results of Frederick Dwyer. *J Bone Joint Surg [Br]* 75:967, 1993.

93. Dunn N: Stabilizing operations in the treatment of paralytic deformities of the foot. *Proc R Soc Med* 15:15, 1922.

94. Hoke M: An operation for stabilizing paralytic feet. *Am J Orthop Surg* 3:494, 1921.

95. Grant AD, Lehman WB: Clubfoot correction using the Ilizarov technique. *Bull Hosp Joint Dis Orthop Inst* 51(1):84, 1991.

96. Oganesian OV, Istomina IS: Talipes equinovarus deformities corrected with the aid of a hinged-distraction apparatus. *Clin Orthop Rel Res* 266:42, 1991.

97. Morley AJM: Knock-knee in children. *Br Med J* 2:976, 1957.

98. Engel GJ, Staheli LT: The natural history of torsion and other factors influencing gait in childhood. *Clin Orthop* 99:12, 1974.

99. Staheli LT, Chew DE, Corbett M: The longitudinal arch: A survey of 882 feet in normal children and adults. *J Bone Joint Surg* 69a:426, 1987.

100. Gould N, Moreland M, Alvarez R, et al: Development of the child's arch. *Foot Ankle* 9:241, 1989.

101. Vanderwilde R, Staheli LT, Chew DE, Malagon V: Measurements on radiographs of the foot in normal infants and children. *J Bone Joint Surg* 70A:407, 1988.

102. Hoffman P: Conclusions drawn from a comparative study of the feet of barefooted and shoe-wearing peoples. *Am J Orthop Surg* 3:105, 1905.

103. Engle ET, Morton DJ: Notes on foot disorders among natives of the Belgian Congo. *J Bone Joint Surg* 13:311, 1931.

104. James CS: Footprints and feet of natives of the Solomon Islands. *Lancet* 2:1390, 1939.

105. Sim-Fook L, Hodgson A: A comparison of foot forms among the non-shoe and shoe wearing Chinese population. *J Bone Joint Surg* 40A:1058, 1958.

106. Staheli LT: *Fundamentals of Pediatric orthopedics*. New York, Raven Press, Ltd., 1992, p 5.14.

107. Harris RI, Beath T: *Army Foot Survey: An Investigation of Foot Ailments in Canadian Soldiers*. Ottawa, Ottawa National Research Council of Canada, 1947.

107a. Giladi M, Milgrom C, Stein J, et al: The low arch as protective factor in stress fracture: a prospective study of 295 military recruits. *Orthop Rev* 14:709–712, 1985.

108. Wenger DR, Mauldin D, Speck G, et al: Corrective shoes as treatment for flexible flatfoot in infants and children. *J Bone Joint Surg* 71A:800, 1989.

109. Gould N: Shoes versus sneakers in toddler ambulation. *Foot Ankle* 6:105, 1985.

110. Staheli LT: Philosophy of care. *Pediatr Clin North Am* 33:1269, 1986.

111. Coughlin MF: Fitting children's shoes: What to tell the parents. *J Musculoskel Med* 2(9):39, 1985.

112. Emslie M: Prevention of foot deformities in children. *Lancet* 2:1260, 1939.

113. McKee JJ: Baby needs new shoes! *Hygeia* 20:142, 1942.

114. Bleck EE: The shoeing of children: Sham or science? *Dev Med Child Neurol* 13:188, 1971.

115. Crandon LRG: Flexible balancing shoes. *Boston Med Surg J* CLV: 505–507, 1906.

116. Sofield HA: Care of the feet of normal children. *Illinois Med J* 79:253, 1941.

117. Adams D: Proper shoeing of the child. *JAMA* 92:1753, 1929.

118. Staheli LT, Griffin L: Corrective shoes for children: A survey of current practice. *Pediatrics* 65:13, 1980.

119. Jack EA: Naviculo-cuneiform fusion in the treatment of flat foot. *J Bone Joint Surg [Br]* 35:75, 1953.

120. Hicks JH: The mechanics of the foot: II. The plantar aponeurosis and the arch. *J Anat* 88:25, 1954.

121. Cowell HR: Talocalcaneal coalition and new causes of peroneal spastic flatfoot. *Clin Orthop* 85:16, 1972.

122. Olney BW: Tarsal coalition, in Drennan JC (ed): *The Child's Foot and Ankle.* New York, Raven Press, 1992.

122a. Scranton PE, Jr.: Treatment of symptomatic talocalcaneal condition. *J Bone Joint Surg* 69A:533–538, 1987.

123. Mosier KM, Asher MA: Tarsal coalition and peroneal spastic flatfoot. *J Bone Joint Surg [Am]* 66:976, 1984.

124. O'Rahilly R, Gardner E, Gray DJ: The skeletal development of the foot. *Clin Orthop* 16:7, 1960.

125. Grogan DP, Holt GR, Ogden JA: Talocalcaneal coalition in patients who have fibular hemimelia or proximal femoral focal deficiency. *J Bone Joint Surg* 76A:1363, 1994.

126. Leonard MA: The inheritance of tarsal coalition and its relationship to spastic flatfoot. *J Bone Joint Surg [Br]* 56:520, 1974.

127. Mahaffey HW: Bilateral congenital calcaneocuboid synostosis: Case report. *J Bone Joint Surg* 27:164, 1945.

128. Stormont DM, Peterson HA: The relative incidence of tarsal coalition. *Clin Orthop* 181:28, 1983.

129. Swiontkowski MF, Scranton PE, Hansen S: Tarsal coalition: Long-term results of surgical treatment. *J Pediatr Orthop* 3:287, 1983.

129a. Harris RI: Rigid valgus foot due to talocalcaneal bridge. *J Bone Joint Surg* 37A:169, 1955.

129b. Harris RI: Retrospect—Personeal spastic flatfoot (rigid valgus foot). *J Bone Joint Surg [Am]* 47:1657–1667, 1965.

130. Herzenberg JE, Goldner JL, Martinez S, Silverman PM: Computerized tomography of talocalcaneal tarsal coalition: A clinical and anatomic study. *Foot Ankle* 6:273, 1986.

131. Broughton NS, Graham G, Menelaus MB: The high incidence of foot deformity in patients with high-level spina bifida. *J Bone Joint Surg* 76B:548, 1994.

132. Lamy L, Weissman L: Congenital convex pes valgus. *J Bone Joint Surg* 21:79, 1939.

133. Mau C: Muskelbefunde und ihre Bedeutung beim angeborenen Klumpfussleiden. *Arch Orthop Unfallchir* 28:292, 1930.

134. Sharrard WJW, Grosfield I: The management of deformity and paralysis of the foot in myelomeningocele. *J Bone Joint Surg* 50B:456, 1968.

135. Drennan JC: Congenital vertical talus. *J Bone Joint Surg* 77A:1916, 1995.

136. Bleck EE: Developmental orthopaedics III: Toddlers. *Dev Med Child Neurol* 24:533, 1982.

137. Farsetti P, Weinstein SL, Ponseti IV: The long-term functional and radiographic outcomes of untreated and nonoperatively treated metatarsus adductus. *J Bone Joint Surg* 76A:257, 1994.

138. Hunziker UA, Largo RH, Duc G: Neonatal metatarsus adductus, joint mobility, axis and rotation of the lower extremity in preterm and term children 0–5 years of age. *Eur J Pediatr* 148:19, 1988.

139. Ponseti IV, Becker JR: Congenital metatarsus adductus: The results of treatment. *J Bone Joint Surg* 48A:702, 1966.

140. Reimann I, Werner HH: Congenital metatarsus varus: On the advantages of early treatment. *Acta Orthop Scand* 46:857, 1975.

141. Rushforth GF: The natural history of hooked forefoot. *J Bone Joint Surg* 60B:530, 1978.

142. Kendrick RE, Sharma NK, Hassler WL, Herndon CH: Tarsometatarsal mobilization for resistant adduction of the fore part of the foot. *J Bone Joint Surg* 52A:61, 1970.

143. Lange M: *Orthopädische-Chirurgische Operationslehre.* Munich, Bergmann, 1951.

144. Somppi E, Sulumaa M: Early operative treatment of congenital club foot. *Acta Orthop Scand* 42:513, 1971.

145. Mosca VS: Skewfoot deformity in children: Correction by calcaneal neck lengthening and medial cuneiform opening wedge osteotomies, in Hensinger RN: Meeting highlights. *J Pediatr Orthop* 13:805, 1993.

146. Sabir M, Lyttle D: Pathogenesis of pes cavus in Charcot-Marie-Tooth disease. *Clin Orthop Rel Res* 175:173, 1983.

147. Charcot JM, Marie P: Sur une forme particulière d'atrophie musculaire progressive souvent familial débutant par les pieds et les jambes et atteignant plus tard les mains. *Rev Med [Paris]* 6.97, 1886.

148. Tooth HH: *The Peroneal Type of Progressive Muscular Atrophy.* London, Lewis, 1886.

149. Coleman SS, Chesnut WJ: A simple test for hindfoot flexibility in the cavovarus foot. *Clin Orthop* 123:60, 1977.

150. Basmajian JV: *Muscles Alive.* Baltimore, Williams & Wilkins, 1978.

151. Steindler A: Stripping of the os calcis. *J Orthop Surg* 2:8, 1920.

152. Jones R: The soldier's foot and the treatment of common deformities of the foot: Part II. Clawfoot. *Br Med J* 1:749, 1916.

153. Crenshaw AH (ed): *Campbell's Operative Orthopaedics,* 7th ed. St Louis, Mosby, 1986.

154. Lutter LD: Sports-related injuries, in Drennan JC (ed): *The Child's Foot and Ankle.* New York, Raven Press, 1992.

155. Devane KM: Kohler's osteochondrosis of the tarsal navicular: Case report with 28 year follow-up. *South Dakota G Med* 42:5, 1989.

156. Ippolito PT, Pollini R, Falez R: Kohler's disease of the tarsal navicular: Long term follow-up of 12 cases. *J Pediatr Orthop* 4:416, 1984.

157. Frieberg AH: Infarction of the second metatarsal bone. *Surg Gynecol Obstet* 19:191, 1914.

158. Smillie IPS: Frieberg infarction. *J Bone Joint Surg [Br]* 39:580, 1957.

159. Kinnard P, Lirette R: Dorsiflexion osteotomy in Freiberg's disease. *Foot Ankle* 9:226, 1989.

PART V

Regional Orthopaedics

CHAPTER 49

Inflammatory and Degenerative Disorders of the Hip Joint

Roger Dee, Frank DiMaio, and Robert Pae

CLINICAL FEATURES OF HIP DISEASE

Clinical History

The accurate diagnosis of hip disease depends on a comprehensive and detailed history of the patient's symptoms as well as careful observation and physical examination.

The patient with intraarticular hip disease commonly limps and complains of pain upon weight bearing. The pain is typically experienced about the groin and may radiate to the anteromedial thigh or knee. Complaints of posterolateral hip or buttock pain usually signify some other extraarticular process such as a muscle strain, trochanteric impingement or bursitis, or lumbar radiculopathy. A careful orthopaedic history in these patients should include questions regarding past trauma and fractures as well as any disease of the lumbar spine. Since the lumbar spine is commonly affected secondarily by deformities and disease of the hip joint, distinguishing the origin of symptoms between the two can be difficult. The surgeon should inquire whether the pain occurs at rest or is related to activity; whether this is "start up" pain or the pain begins after a period of activity. Note that patients with hip disease alone do not usually complain of a claudicating type of pain and that such symptoms usually signify the presence of other neurologic or vascular disease. Last, inquiries regarding any recent change in the patient's activities of daily living, as a result of the pain, may assist in determining the source of the pain.

It is particularly important to take a comprehensive history of the genitourinary and digestive systems. A history of abnormal bleeding, change in bowel and urinary habits, or significant weight loss should be sought. Eye symptoms plus sacroiliac joint pain with abnormal urinary or bowel symptoms may suggest one of the spondyloarthropathies. In candidates for surgery, specific inquiry concerning cardiopulmonary status, required medications, and past medical and surgical history is essential.

Physical Examination

The patient with hip pain often demonstrates an *antalgic* gait, characterized by a shortening of the stance phase of the affected limb as the painful joint is protected. In some antalgic gaits, the hip may be held in abduction and progress made by circumducting the affected limb.

Another common pathologic gait disturbance seen in patients with hip disease is the *Trendelenburg gait*. This gait pattern can be characterized by the presence of a sideways lurch of the trunk to bring the patient's body weight over the affected limb. It is classically seen in patients with incompetent hip abductos, including patients with gluteal muscle weakness and trochanteric insufficiency. If this condition is bilateral, then a characteristic "waddling gait" (e.g., of untreated bilateral development hip dysplasia) may be present. Note that many patients with degenerative hip disease may have elements of both antalgic and Trendelenburg gaits, which often confuses the clinical picture.

Other common pathologic gait patterns include the "swing through" gait seen in patients with a fused or ankylosed hip, with motion primarily occurring at the lumbar spine. In addition, patients with a fixed flexion deformity of the hip may demonstrate a hyperlordotic posture of the lumbar spine with a prominence of the buttocks during ambulation. Once the patient has been observed for any abnormal gait patterns, the remainder of the examination should continue.

The patient should be observed for any pelvic obliquity that may be associated with scoliosis. The pelvic obliquity in secondary scoliosis associated with hip joint disease is flexible and will usually resolve when the patent is seated. Persistent scoliosis in the lumbar region while the patient is seated usually indicates a fixed obliquity of the pelvis, which will not correct with a hip procedure.

With the patient lying supine, bony prominences of the pelvis and femur should be palpated. Particular attention is paid to regions of the greater trochanter and the ischium. Soft tissue bursitis in these regions is often confused with serious hip disease. Palpation over the anterior hip joint that elicits tenderness may suggest a local inflammatory process, such as synovitis.

Next, careful assessment of the active and passive range of motion of the patient's hip, knees, and ankles is recommended. Active range of motion should be checked first, followed by a comparative passive range of motion, with manipulation of each joint of each extremity. Degrees of motion should be documented for comparison. Discrepancies between active and passive range of motion should be noted. These discrepancies may be due to pain or weakness, which are important clues to the pathology present.

A complete neurologic examination should be considered in each patient. Strength testing of each significant muscle group of the lower extremity should be performed serially. Neurosensory deficit examination of the L2-S2 dermatomes should be performed bilaterally. In addition, reflex testing and neurotension sign manipulations should be performed to rule out lumbar radiculopathy.

The examination of the patient with hip disease must also include a careful assessment of the vascular status of the limbs. If the history and physical examination give cause for concern, referral to the vascular laboratory is imperative.

Trendelenburg Test

When a patient stands on one leg, the pelvis is normally maintained in the horizontal plane by a mechanism that requires a stable fulcrum at the hip joint as well as functioning abductors in the stance leg. If the pelvis sags, so that the horizontal position of the pelvis is not maintained, the Trendelenburg test is said to be positive. The sagging pelvis during this test is best observed from behind. Careful evaluation of both hips should be performed for comparison. A positive Trendelenburg test typically occurs in patients with hip abductor weakness. Examples include patients who have had multiple hip surgeries and subsequent insufficiency; patients who have neuromuscular diseases, where the abductor musculature is nonfunctional; and patients who have underlying structural abnormalities such as hip dysplasia or trochanteric overgrowth. In addition, the Trendelenburg test may be positive in patients with fixed adduction deformities.

Assessment of Leg-Length Discrepancy

Obliquity of pelvis associated with hip deformity is simple to explain. If there is a fixed adduction deformity, it is impossible, without some adjustment, for the patient to walk without tripping over the adducted leg! Consequently, that side of the pelvis is hitched up by the trunk musculature to compensate and bring the legs into a parallel position. By simulating such a deformity and its correction on oneself, one may easily see that measuring to the medial malleolus on the affected leg from any point in the midline of the trunk will result in a measurement that is shorter than a similar measurement on the contralateral side. This is what is meant by an *apparent* leg-length discrepancy. Similarly, if there is a fixed abduction deformity, then a measurement made from either the xiphisternum, the umbilicus, or the pubic symphysis to the medial malleolus will show apparent lengthening of the abducted leg.

When the patient lies supine on the examination table with the legs in parallel, the apparent leg-length discrepancy is present. In order to unmask this condition, it is necessary to square the pelvis with the long axis of the body, which results in moving the deformed limb into the position that renders the deformity obvious. Thus, to square the pelvis of a patient with a considerable adduction deformity, it may even be necessary to cross the adducted leg over the contralateral extremity. In order to align the pelvis at 90° to the body's long axis (square the pelvis), one must be able to recognize the location of the anterior superior iliac spines, which are then used as reference points. This is often difficult in an obese patient. The best approach is for the examiner to slide his or her thumb upward until it stubs itself on the anterior superior iliac spine. A mark is made on the skin at this point. The sensation is like a boat grounding and, even in an obese patient, it is fairly reproducible and accurate. Once the pelvis is squared, a *true* leg-length determination may be measured from the anterosuperior iliac spine to the medial malleolus. If the one leg has been crossed because it is adducted, then it is important to make the true leg-length measurement of the opposite limb when it lies in a similar position relative to the pelvis, so that the two measurements are comparable.

With the pelvis squared and an appreciation of the fixed abduction or adduction deformity of one or both limbs, it is possible to measure accurately the true abduction and adduction permitted in each limb. It is not at all uncommon to find a fixed adduction deformity in one hip being matched by a fixed adduction deformity in the other. Fixed deformities may be noted in the record by negative values.

Assessment of Flexion Contracture

Patients with progressive degenerative hip and lumbar disease commonly develop flexion contractures about one or both hips. The presence of these contractures usually signifies advanced disease, which may require more aggressive treatment. Documentation of a flexion contracture is important at the time of initial assessment as well as during follow-up examinations. By examining the patient in a prone position, a lack of extension can easily be appreciated. However, the patient with fixed flexion may mask a deformity while lying in the supine position by adopting a hyperlordotic posture while effectively extending the pelvis until the thighs lie flat on the examination table. Unmasking the deformity in a patient with unilateral hip disease is done by asking the patient to clasp the knee of the unaffected limb and bring it up to the chest, thus flexing the pelvis and causing the affected limb to elevate at the hip joint. This test, known as the *Thomas test*, is not satisfactory in the elderly patient who may not be strong enough to perform this maneuver. Patients with bilateral contractures may also have difficulty performing this test. In these patients, the test is simplified by having the examiner gently flexing both hips as far as is comfortable and supporting the weight of the patient's thighs. Next, while maintaining flexion in one hip, the hip joint under scrutiny is gradually extended passively from the fully flexed position. By maintaining flexion in the one hip, the pelvis is fully rotated and any lordosis is obliterated. In the presence of a fixed flexion deformity, as the scrutinized hip descends from the fully flexed position, there will come a point when further descent ceases and the residual deformity can be measured relative to the horizontal plane. One must take care to allow the hip joint being examined to extend from the fully flexed position very slowly while also supporting the weight of the limb. If the point of the flexion contracture is reached abruptly and the limb is not supported, the patient will experience considerable discomfort. The process is repeated for the other limb after fully flexing the hip that has been measured.

Diagnostic Tests

Screening laboratory tests should be considered in patients with hip disease for several reasons. In the first place, patients with hip symptoms often require screening for a host of systemic disorders that may present with hip discomfort. A primary diagnosis of degenerative arthritis cannot be made until other systemic rheumatologic and collagen-vascular disorders are ruled out. Complete blood count (CBC), erythrocyte sedimentation rate, rheumatoid factor, antinuclear antibody (ANA), and systemic lupus erythematosus (SLE) titer determinations should all be considered, especially in young patients. Gout and other metabolic disorders may also need to be excluded. Secondly, baseline determination of liver and kidney function may be required if long-term nonsurgical therapy with anti-inflammatory medications is being considered.

Baseline screening radiographs of the pelvis and hip in question should be evaluated for the presence or absence of normal structural integrity of the pelvis, acetabuli, and proximal femur. Evidence of any previous fractures or surgery should be documented, along with any resultant topographic changes about the hip joints. In addition, many patients may have hip degeneration secondary to underlying structural abnormalities.[1] Measurements of the femoral neck shaft angle, femoral offset, acetabular index, and center edge angle of Wiberg (see Fig. 49-8) are all necessary in making such relationships apparent.

COMMON HIP DISEASES

Osteoarthritis

The osteoarthritic "syndrome" of progressive pain, stiffness, and disability eventually forces the patient to seek medical attention. The insidious history of these symptoms, along with characteristic physical findings, usually precedes any studies that confirm the physician's diagnosis. Note that no specific laboratory test for the diagnosis of osteoarthritis (OA) is known and that this condition is usually confirmed by the patient's clinical course, radiographs, and response to conservative measures.

The most characteristic radiographic finding in patients with osteoarthritis of the hip is the loss of normal joint space. In most patients, bony marginal osteophytes about the joint's periphery will be seen. In addition, bony sclerosis and cyst formation are commonly noted.[2]

Deformation of the femoral head may be a radiographic finding of end-stage disease.

Some authors have subclassified OA into medial, lateral, or global arthritic types.[3,4] Medial OA is identified by loss of medial joint space as the femoral head migrates medially toward the medial wall. The superior joint space is relatively well preserved at first but may become involved at a later stage. In lateral osteoarthritis, progressive loss of the superior joint space in the weight-bearing region of the dome is seen, followed by cyst and osteophyte formation superiorly and laterally. At a later stage, subluxation ensues and medial osteophytes form. In the global type of OA, there is loss of joint space in a diffuse manner medially and laterally; there is little reactive sclerosis in the acetabulum or osteophyte formation. Medial OA has been associated with high rates of acetabular component revision.[4]

Rheumatoid Arthritis

The diagnosis of rheumatoid arthritis (RA) is based upon several criteria described by the American Rheumatism Association regarding the patient's symptom profile as well as physical findings.[5] Morning stiffness, swelling of multiple joints, and pain are common complaints. Nodules upon physical examination of the hands may also be present. Physical evidence of synovitis, bursitis, and soft tissue contracture is more common than in the osteoarthritic patient. Unfortunately, no specific clinical findings about the hip are solely supportive of this diagnosis. In fact, many of the presenting findings in patients with RA of the hip are identical to those of the OA patient. Therefore the surgeon must often rely on positive laboratory studies, such as rheumatoid factor (RF) and ANA to confirm the diagnosis.

Radiographic findings of the rheumatoid hip are often subtle in nature. Osteopenia is seen in a majority of these patients. Loss of the joint space without osteophyte and cyst formation is typical. Evidence of a protrusion deformity is also common and may offer the best radiologic clue to the diagnosis in patients without clinical manifestations of disease, especially in juvenile RA.[6]

Pigmented Villonodular Synovitis

Patients with pigmented villonodular synovitis (PVNS) of the hip are rarely encountered. This disease primarily affects the synovial lining of the joint and usually presents as a recurrent synovitis in a young patient. Discomfort on weight bearing with painful passive range of motion usually warrant an aspiration to rule out septic arthritis in these patients. Radiographic findings similar to those of RA, with cystic changes of the femoral head or acetabulum, may be present. The diagnosis should be suspected if cysts are seen on both sides of the joint but the joint space is well preserved. Tuberculous arthritis sometimes has a similar appearance. The diagnosis of PVNS can be made by MRI, where characteristic hypointense-signal nodular masses are seen on both T1- and T2-weighted images.[7] Characteristic "rust stained" synovium at arthrotomy plus microscopy confirms the diagnosis.

Paget's and Gaucher's Diseases

For diagnostic features of hip disease in Paget's and Gaucher's diseases, see Chaps. 5 and 6.

Osteonecrosis

Osteonecrosis (ON) continues to be one of the most difficult diseases in orthopaedic surgery to treat. In the past, little could be done to limit the natural progression of this condition, but recent management of the disease has focused on early intervention and treatment. The key to improving outcome is now acknowledged to be early detection and timely intervention to arrest the disease at an early stage. Unfortunately, all too often the patient presents to the orthopaedist beyond the point where successful early intervention is possible and nothing less than an arthroplasty can then be considered.

Epidemiology

This disease primarily affects patients between 20 to 50 years of age. Hungerford reported an average age of 38 years in his study of over 200 cases.[8] Males appear to be more commonly affected than females, especially by the idiopathic form of the disease.[9] Generally, the incidence of bilaterality is considered to be approximately 50 percent, but bilateral disease may be encountered in as many as 80 percent of patients in whom corticosteroid use is a predisposing factor.[10]

Etiology

Many factors have been implicated in the etiology of ON (Table 49-1), but an "idiopathic" etiology still remains the most common. Unfortunately no animal model has been found to replicate the pathophysiology of this disease; thus the etiology remains the subject of considerable controversy.

Hip trauma with intracapsular fracture of the femoral neck results in a 15 to 30 percent incidence of ON. Hip dislocation alone is associated with a 10 to 15 percent incidence of this complication. Significant nontraumatic risk factors include alcohol and corticosteroid use. Jones has reported the threshold for ingestion of 100 percent ethyl alcohol to be at least 400 mL per week, with a cumulative dose of 150 L.[11] Dosage levels of prednisolone above 30 mg per day for at least 30 days have been shown to be of etiologic significance.[12]

Pathophysiology

Significant advance in defining the pathophysiology of ON at the cellular and biomechanical levels have recently been reported.[10] Unfortunately, this knowledge has not been matched by significant improvement in patient outcomes.[13] Several theories of ON have been proposed.

1. *Fat embolism theory* One hypothesis considers alterations in lipid metabolism as the cause of ON.[14] The mechanism by which corticosteroids lead to the development of ON may be related to this effect. Systemic corticosteroids produce increased fat stores in the blood, liver, and bone marrow. Variations in steroid dosage or sudden cessation of therapy result in a further increase in hyperlipidemia and subsequent fat mobilization.[15] Fat emboli have been clearly demonstrated both experimentally and pathologically in the subchondral arterioles of the femoral heads in patients with steroid-induced ON and are the suspected cause of the disease in these patients.[14]

2. *Lipocyte hypertrophy theory* Another popular theory suggests that the increased marrow fat concentration and lipocyte hypertrophy that occurs with prolonged steroid intake produce an increased bone marrow pressure within the intraosseous extravascular compartment of the femoral head. A corresponding decrease in the blood flow to the femoral head then occurs, leading to progressive ischemia.[16] The use of lipid-clearing agents has been shown to consistently improve this alteration in blood flow.[17]

It has been suggested that ON represents a compartment syndrome of the femoral head.[10,18] The rigid bony cortex encloses the marrow contents and the collapsible vessels of the intraosseous circulation. This area functions as a closed compartment, and the blood flow through the intraosseous vessels is inversely proportional to the bone marrow pressure within the proximal femur. Any condition that causes an increased bone marrow pressure within the extravascular intraosseous space will produce a decrease in the blood flow to the femoral head. Ischemia will then occur, with subsequent ON.

3. *Accumulative cell stress theory* Proposed by Kenzora and Glimcher, this theory holds that the cause of ON is multifactorial and not the result of a single insult to the femoral head circulation.[19] Various factors including anatomic location, systemic illness and exposure to agents such as alcohol and steroids put more and more stress upon the marrow and the osteocytes until bony necrosis occurs.

TABLE 49-1 Etiologic Factors Associated with Osteonecrosis

Traumatic
 Subcapital fracture of the hip
 Fracture-dislocations of the hip

Nontraumatic
 Idiopathic
 Systemic steroid treatment
 Gaucher's disease
 Hemoglobinopathies
 Irradiation
 Dysbaric osteonecrosis
 Alcoholism
 Hematologic neoplasms (leukemias, lymphomas)
 Hyperlipoproteinemia
 Pregnancy
 Organ transplantation
 Systemic lupus erythematosus
 Chronic kidney failure
 Gout
 Pancreatitis
 Venous occlusion

4. *Intramedullary hemorrhage theory*   In experimental animals, Saito and coworkers[20] were recently able to produce ON in rabbits by giving horse serum (which induced a hypersensitivity reaction with vasculitis) plus steroid. Neither of these agents alone provoked the hemorrhage; ON was produced by the combination. It may be proposed that the serum causes the vasculitis and the steroid then promotes hemorrhage and ON.[20,21]

5. *Acute infarction*   In some situations it seems apparent that acute infarction causes the ON. This is thought to occur in patients who sustain interruption of the femoral head blood supply from fracture, dislocation, or embolism at the time of major trauma to the hip. The infarction is a silent process, and the patient becomes symptomatic when the infarcted segment fails mechanically.[19]

Diagnosis

Patients with ON usually present with a history of insidious groin pain. Typically the pain begins with increased activity and eventually is present at rest. The pain may even wake the patient at night.

In the early stages of the disease, physical examination of these patients may indicate signs of hip synovitis. An antalgic limp is common. Positive physical findings such as apprehension during passive internal rotation of the hip and groin pain with active straight-leg raising may be found. Stiffness and contracture are seen only in the later stages of this disease, when degeneration has occurred.

Once the clinical diagnosis of ON is suspected, radiographs of the pelvis and hip should be obtained. These radiographs are commonly unremarkable in the early stages of this condition but will help to rule out other pathologies in the hip. Hip radiographs should be evaluated for early evidence of ON, including sclerosis, cyst formation, or collapse of the femoral head (Fig. 49-1). Patients with advanced stages of ON are easily identified by plain radiograph. Characteristic early findings include osteopenia, cysts, and subchondral bone collapse or "crescent sign" (Fig. 49-2). More advanced stages include segmental femoral head collapse and acetabular involvement.

Suspected patients with normal radiographs, who may have predisposing factors for ON should be considered for an MRI. The latter technology has been responsible for the earlier and more accurate detection of this disease and is now preferred over radionuclide scanning in the diagnosis of this condition.[22] The hydrogen-rich fat content of the marrow in the femoral head produces a strong MRI signal.[23] Marrow necrosis produces decreased signal intensity in the involved segment of the femoral head early in the course of ON, even before radiographic changes are evident. The accurate detection of this disease early in its course, via MRI, allows the surgeon to choose more conservative surgical measures in an attempt to avoid the need for joint replacement.[24] Examination by MRI should also be considered for the early detection of asymptomatic contralateral hip ON in patients with known disease, since the incidence of bilateral ON is approximately 50 percent (Fig. 49-3).

Indications for alternative reconstructive procedures—including femoral osteotomies—are dependent

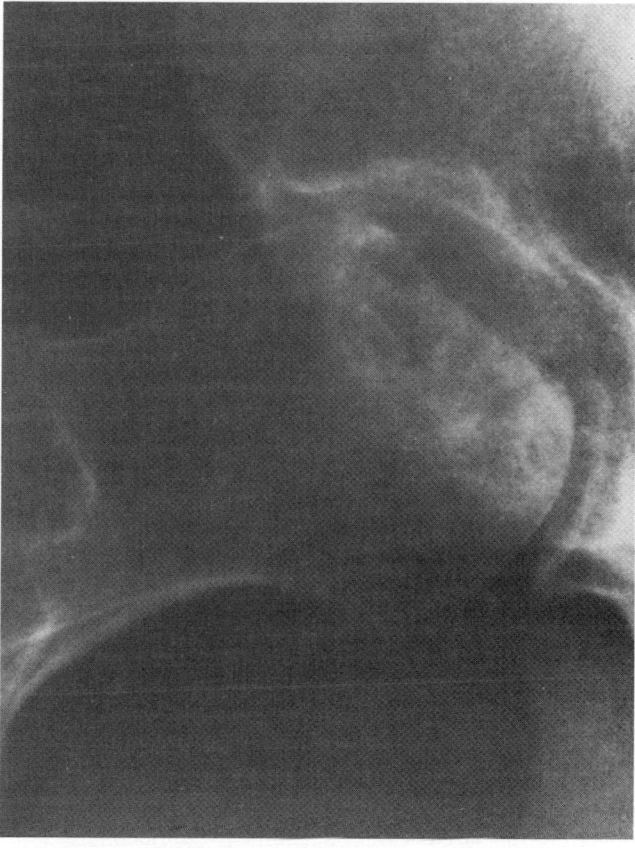

Figure 49-1 Collapse of the avascular segment with disturbance of femoral head congruity in stage IV osteonecrosis. (Reproduced with permission from Hungerford DS: Early diagnosis and treatment of ischemic necrosis of the femoral head, in *Segmental Idiopathic Necrosis of the Femoral Head*. Berlin and Heidelberg, Springer-Verlag, 1981 p. 29.

upon the accurate assessment of the amount of involvement of the femoral head, which can usually be noted on the plain radiograph. More recently, plain and three-dimensional computed tomography scans have also been used for this determination in cases where the extent of involvement is difficult to discern.

Staging

The system originally described by Ficat and Arlet in the early 1980s divided the radiographic progression of ON into four stages that permitted clinical, prognostic, and therapeutic correlation.[25,26] Since that time, several surgeons have successively upgaded this staging system to include more advanced imaging studies (bone scan and MRI) as well as a more thorough description of the necrotic lesion[27,28] (Table 49-2). The international system introduced by the Association Research Circulation Osseous (ARCO) attempts to standardize the approach to the staging of this disease and will also allow for more consistent reporting in the future. Use of this system will hopefully now permit more consistency in reporting the results of therapy at various stages of the disease. In the ARCO stag-

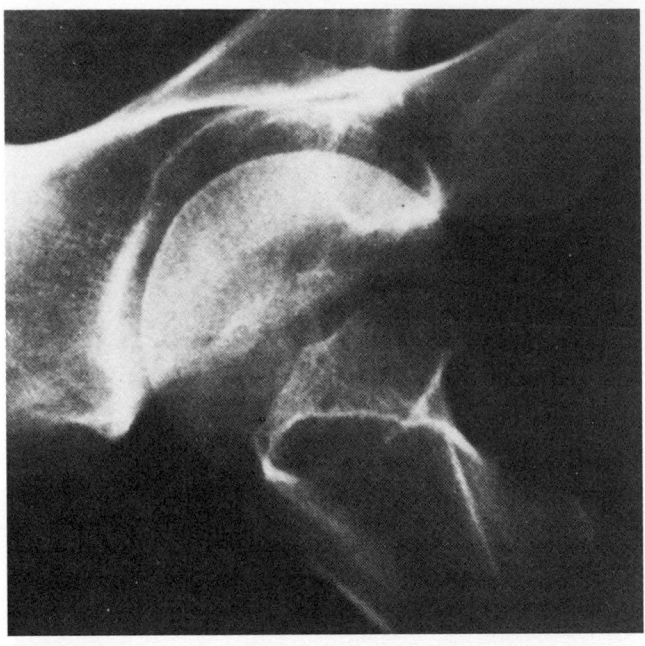

A

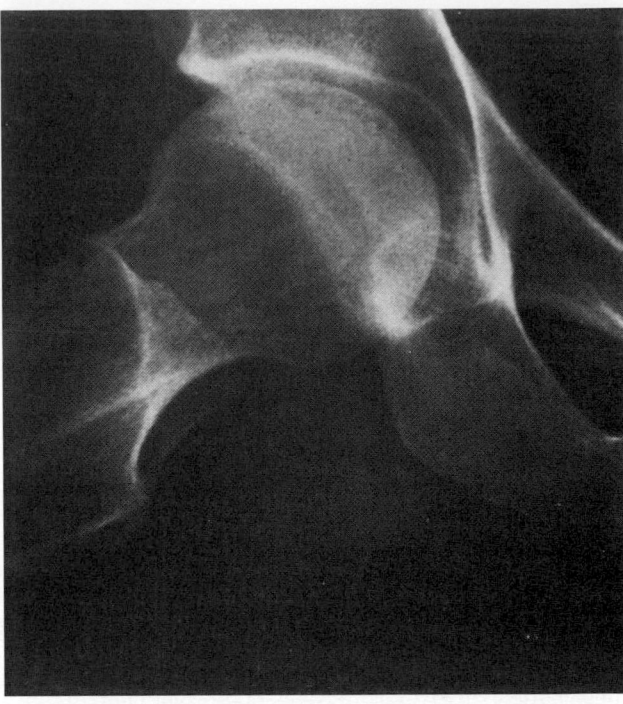

B

Figure 49-2 *A*. Stage II osteonecrosis of the femoral head demonstrating subchondral osteolytic areas. *B*. The "crescent sign" is seen in stage III osteonecrosis. The area of radiolucency is associated with collapse of the subchondral bone.

(Reproduced with permission from Cruess RL: Cortisone induced avascular necrosis of the femoral head. *J Bone Joint Surg [Br]* 59:309, 1977.)

ing system, stage O is when all tests are negative except tissue histology. Stage 1 has a normal radiograph but MRI or some other diagnostic method is positive. Stage 2 shows radiographic evidence of ON but no subchondral collapse. Stage 3 shows collapse but no arthtitis, and stage 4 shows ON with arthritis. The subclassification (Fig. 49-4) quantitates the amount of femoral head involvement, which is important in surgical decision making.[23] More accurate comparisons of various treatment modalities will now be facilitated by this standardization.

Treatment

The likelihood that ON will progress has made early interventions more desirable in the treatment of this disease. Approximately 70 to 80 percent of patients with osteonecrosis will progress within 3 years. There is no place for nonoperative treatment with protected weight bearing, since this will have no effect on the progression of the femoral head destruction.

Core Decompression Ficat and Arlet observed relief of pain and cessation of radiologic progression in a high percentage of patients with early ON who had undergone core biopsy during functional bone investigation.[25] Hungerford, who experienced similar success, subsequently named the procedure *core decompression of the femoral head.*

Wang studied the effects of core decompression on the blood flow in the femoral head in rabbits and found

that the procedure reversed the diminution in blood flow associated with prolonged steroid therapy.[16]

Core decompression has now become a standard option in the treatment of early ON. Currently it is recommended when there is no segmental collapse of the femoral head (stages 1 and 2). The procedure is done under fluoroscopy, and the biopsied bone can then be evaluated histologically to confirm the accuracy of the individual procedure. Smaller lesions have a better prognosis. The efficacy of this procedure has recently been scrutinized. Success rates have varied but appear to be best in the treatment of stage 1 disease. The combined literature suggests that approximately 30 percent of hips with stage 1 or early stage 2 disease treated with core decompression will exhibit radiographic progression despite treatment.[30,31] Worse results can be expected in patients with larger lesions and more advanced stages of the disease (stage 3).

Electrical Stimulation More recently, the application of pulsed electromagnetic fields (PEMFs) with and without core decompression has been shown to curtail the progression of ON. This treatment, used alone and as an adjunct after core decompression, has been attempted.[32–35] Clinical success in approximately 70 to 80 percent of patients with stages 1 and 2 ON was found.[35] No difference in the efficacy of core decompression was noted when PEMFs were used adjunctively.[33,35] Despite these reports, the role of electrical stimulation in the treatment remains to be defined. A variety of different signals, most of which

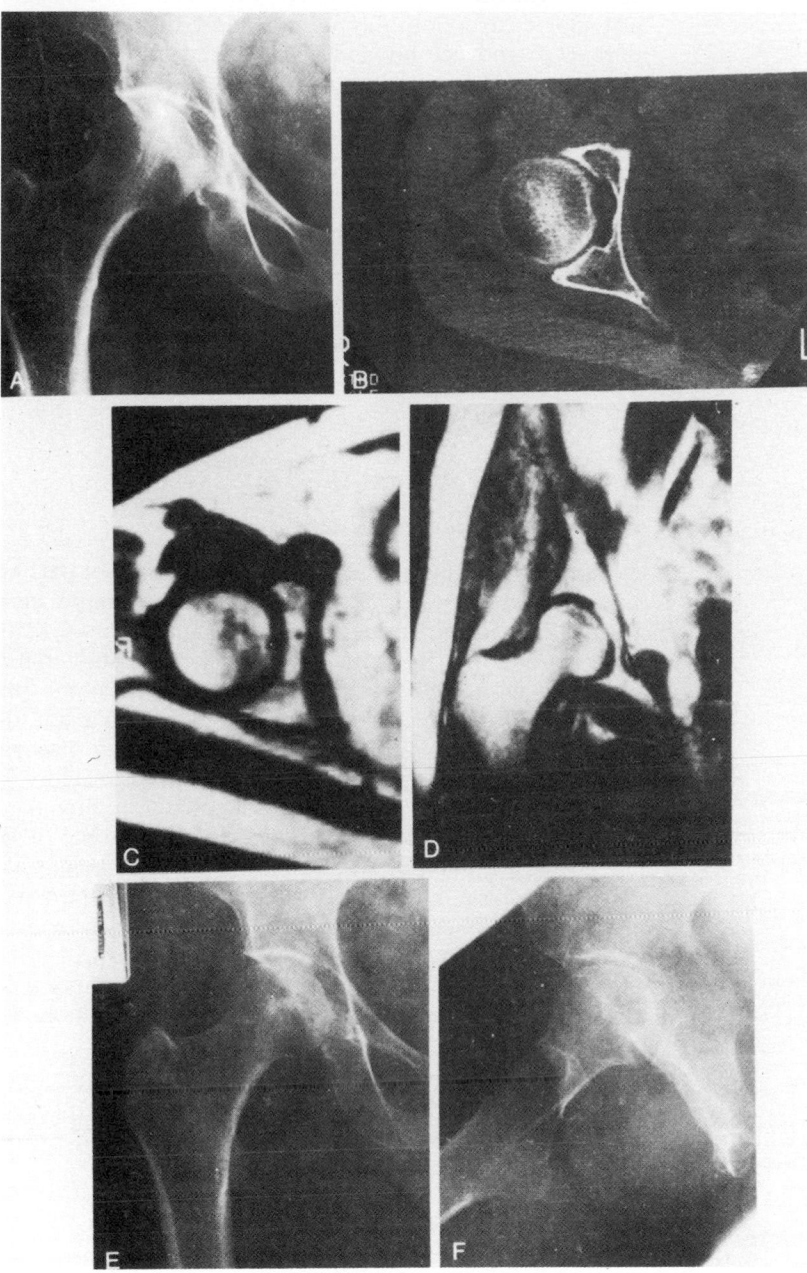

Figure 49-3 The "silent" contralateral hip in a 69-year-old woman with established osteonecrosis in the opposite left hip (stage 0). *A.* The AP radiograph of the asymptomatic right hip appears normal. *B.* Transverse CT section at the level of the fovea reveals normal trabecular bone and a continuous subchondral plate. *C* and *D.* Transverse and coronal MRI images of the left hip demonstrate an area of decreased signal intensity in the antero-superior portion of the femoral head, which is diagnostic of early femoral head necrosis. *E* and *F.* AP and lateral radiographs of the left hip 13 months later, after it became symptomatic. (Reproduced with permission from Jergesen HE, Heller M, Genant HK: Magnetic resonance imaging in osteonecrosis of the femoral head. *Orthop Clin North Am* 16:714, 1985.)

are not yet FDA-approved, as well as a poorly understood mechanism of action, continue to render this modality controversial.

Cortical Bone Grafts Free cortical bone grafts, popularized by Phemister and later by Bonfiglio, involve the use of fibular or tibial cortical struts to provide biomechanical and biological support for the osteonecrotic segment of the femoral head. The rationale is to have the graft support the overlying articular segment before the underlying subchondral bone collapses. Consequently this technique is contraindicated in stage 3 lesions, where collapse has already occurred. Results using this technique have been poor and the number of successes has been limited by technical difficulty.[36] In addition, bone grafting at the time

of osteotomy for stage 3 osteonecrosis has not been shown to improve results.[37]

Osteotomy The use of osteotomy for ON is described later in this chapter.

SURGICAL TREATMENT OF HIP DISEASE

Synovectomy

There are few indications for open synovectomy of the hip joint. A patient rarely presents with rheumatoid arthritis and fulminant synovitis of this joint, which does not re-

TABLE 49-2 Staging Osteonecrosis of the Femoral Head

Stage	Criteria
0	Normal x-ray, bone scan, and MRI
I	Normal x-ray, abnormal bone scan, or MRI A Mild (<15%) B Moderate (15–30%) C Severe (>30%)
II	Sclerosis and/or cyst formation in femoral head A Mild (<15%) B Moderate (15–30%) C Severe (>30%)
III	Subchondral collapse (crescent sign) without flattening A Mild (<15%) B Moderate (15–30%) C Severe (>30%)
IV	Flattening of head without joint narrowing or acetabular involvement A Mild (<15% of surface and <2 mm depression) B Moderate (15–30% of surface or 2–4 mm depression) C Severe (>30% of surface or >4 mm depression)
V	Flattening of head with joint narrowing and/or acetabular involvement A Mild (determined as above plus B Moderate estimate of acetabular C Severe involvement)
VI	Advanced degenerative changes

Reproduced with permission from Steinberg M, Steinberg DR: *Evaluation of avascular necrosis. Semin Arthrop* 2:175–181, 1991.

spond to conservative measures, including limited weight bearing, anti-inflammatory medications, or steroid injection.[6] Patients with rheumatoid arthritis suffering from such a synovitis without radiographic evidence of severe articular destruction may be considered for this procedure. Hip synovectomy and debridement may be considered via anterior or posterior approaches. Theoretical disruption of the blood supply of the femoral head may occur with overzealous dissection or joint dislocation. Results of open synovectomy in rheumatoid arthritis have been discouraging to date.[6,38]

Other indications for synovectomy include pigmented villonodular synovitis, where the procedure may delay the progress of the disease, and eventual arthroplasty. Synovectomy is also part of joint clearance for tuberculous synovitis, but this procedure is exceedingly uncommon nowadays.

Osteotomies around the Hip

General Considerations

Osteotomies around the hip joint are an important part of the contemporary hip surgeon's repertoire. Important lessons have been learned over the past 30 years, which have clarified the role of femoral and pelvic osteotomies in the prevention and treatment of osteoarthritis of the hip in young patients. Most osteoarthritis of the hip is not idiopathic but rather a result of some preexisting disease that predisposes the patient to articular cartilage failure.[39] These preexisting diseases can be identified by the characteristic deformities they produce around the hip. It is the correction of these structural deformities that may alter the progression of the disease and also control the patient's symptoms. In general, an osteotomy performed prior to the progression of osteoarthritis is termed a *reconstructive* osteotomy. Such a procedure hopefully will defer the need for arthroplasty indefinitely. In addition, an

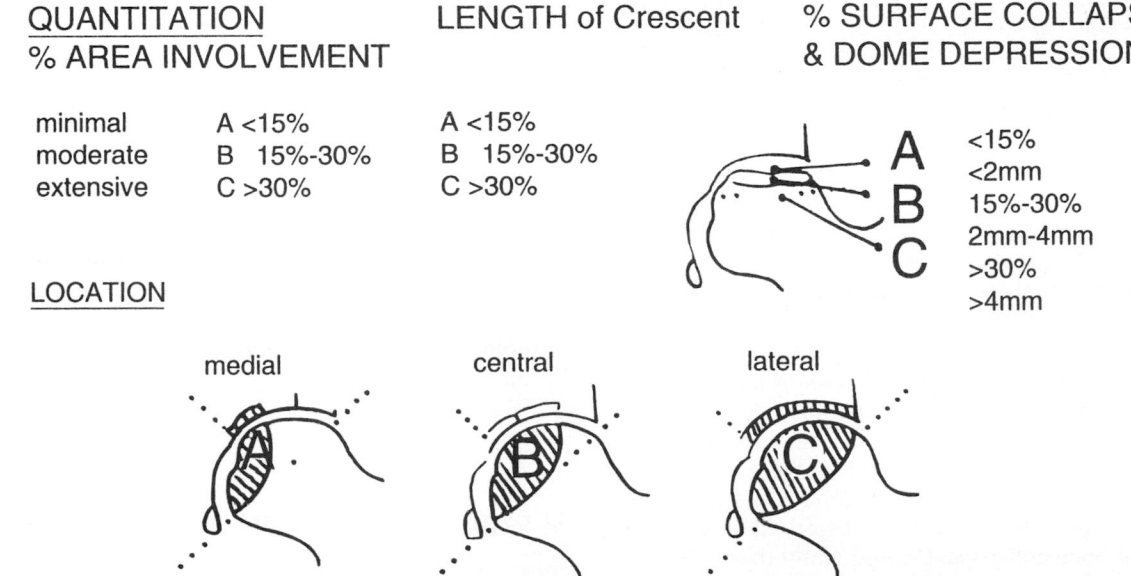

Figure 49-4 The ARCO staging system, which encompasses radiographic subclassification system requiring quantitation of the amount of femoral head involvement. (Reproduced with permission from Stulberg BN: Osteonecrosis. *AAOS Orthopaedic Knowledge Update.* American Association of Orthopaedic Surgeons, Rosemont, IL, 1996, p 92.)

osteotomy can be performed in patients who suffer from advanced stages of osteoarthritis in an attempt to mitigate their symptoms. These *salvage* osteotomies may be used as a method to temporarily halt a young patient's pain until such a time that hip arthroplasty becomes inevitable.

Assessment

A baseline clinical examination should establish the patient's active and passive range of motion. The presence of flexion, abduction, and external rotation contractures should be identified. Moreover, any leg-length discrepancy should be recorded. Also the examination should include multiple passive positionings of the extremity in an attempt to determine whether a definitive *position of comfort* exists.

Radiographic assessment of these patients should begin with independent review of the proximal femur and acetabulum in the anteroposterior (AP) and lateral planes. Femoral problems such as poor bone quality, an abnormal femoral neck shaft angle, incongruity of the femoral head, and unusual trochanteric anatomy should be identified. Evidence of subluxation and joint space narrowing should also be noted. Similarly, the acetabulum should be evaluated objectively for poor bone quality, the presence of cysts and osteophytes, and the degree of any dysplasia, which can be responsible for the lack of femoral head coverage. Once the primary disease is identified, special radiologic studies may be necessary. Functional radiographs (i.e. maximum abduction or adduction AP views) are helpful in establishing which position of the proximal femur will improve the congruency of the hip joint and coverage of the femoral head. These radiographs, depict the proposed change in the relationship of the proximal femur to the acetabulum which will occur after an intertrochanteric osteotomy. For example, an abduction AP view will show the femoral head coverage which may be expected with a varus osteotomy. In addition, a false-profile view of Lequesne[40] (30° oblique) and a von Rosen view, with the leg in maximum abduction and internal rotation, are essential in the planning of a periacetabular osteotomy for hip dysplasia.

Other studies, including a three dimensional CT scan, CT arthrogram, or MRI can also assist in determining the surface anatomy of the joint as well as assessing intraarticular pathology preoperatively.

After this information is gathered, careful analysis by the surgeon is necessary to decide whether a femoral, a pelvic osteotomy, or a combination of the two is indicated in the reconstruction or salvage of the diseased hip. It is important to remember that the indications for these procedures are narrow and that patient understanding and compliance is necessary for their success.

Preoperative Planning

Careful preoperative planning is essential for the successful performance of any osteotomy. Recent advances in computer software technology have relieved some of the burden placed upon the surgeon in this regard. The planning methodology has improved dramatically as a result of these programs and allows the surgeon to decide which type of osteotomy best suits the situation. A digitalizer allows direct transfer of a radiograph to the computer screen and permits the surgeon to accurately rehearse each bone cut and manipulation before the actual procedure. In the case of femoral osteotomy planning, special attention should be given to the relative position of each fragment in anticipation of some future need for total hip arthroplasty and insertion of a femoral stem.

Femoral Osteotomies

The popularity of the femoral osteotomy in the reconstruction and salvage of the hip joint has waxed and waned over the past century. Since McMurray's 1935 description of a medial displacement oblique intertrochanteric osteotomy, many successful variations of the femoral osteotomy have been reported in the treatment of hip osteoarthritis.[41–43] Current indications include the reconstruction and salvage of diseased hips afflicted by primary osteoarthritis as well as secondary arthritis caused by hip dysplasia, Perthes' disease, SCFE, ON, and nonunion of femoral neck fractures. Angular osteotomies are the most common variety, with varus and valgus intertrochanteric osteotomies as the two principal types. True medial displacement osteotomy without some degree of angular correction is not now recommended.[44] Rotational femoral neck (transtrochanteric) osteotomies have also been described in the treatment of ON.

Intertrochanteric Osteotomy of the Femur

As previously discussed, a search for a definitive position of comfort that correlates with one of the previously described functional radiographs will be of positive value in deciding whether or not an osteotomy will be successful. A symptomatic, compliant patient with a minimum of 90° of flexion is a prerequisite. Particular attention to any leg-length discrepancy should be made. This finding certainly may sway the decision away from a varus osteotomy, which may shorten the extremity further.

Careful examination of the radiographs prior to these osteotomies should include evaluation of the pattern of subchondral stress in the acetabulum. The horizontal subchondral density in the superior acetabulum on the AP radiograph, or *sourcil,* is a feature of normal physiologic loading of the hip joint. A vertical sourcil, typically seen in dysplasia, should alert the surgeon to consider a pelvic osteotomy. In addition, there may be increased sclerosis at the edge of the acetabulum in the case of subluxation of the femoral head, indicating lateral overload. One should also inspect the femoral head itself, particularly looking for a large lateral osteophyte that may prevent relocation of a dysplastic hip in abduction. Unless such increased coverage of the head can be shown in functional abduction views preoperatively, a varus osteotomy will not succeed. Inspection may also reveal a large medial osteophyte on the femoral head, which may be subluxing the head superolaterally. This large "capital drop" osteophyte may actually act as a beneficial fulcrum during a valgus osteotomy,

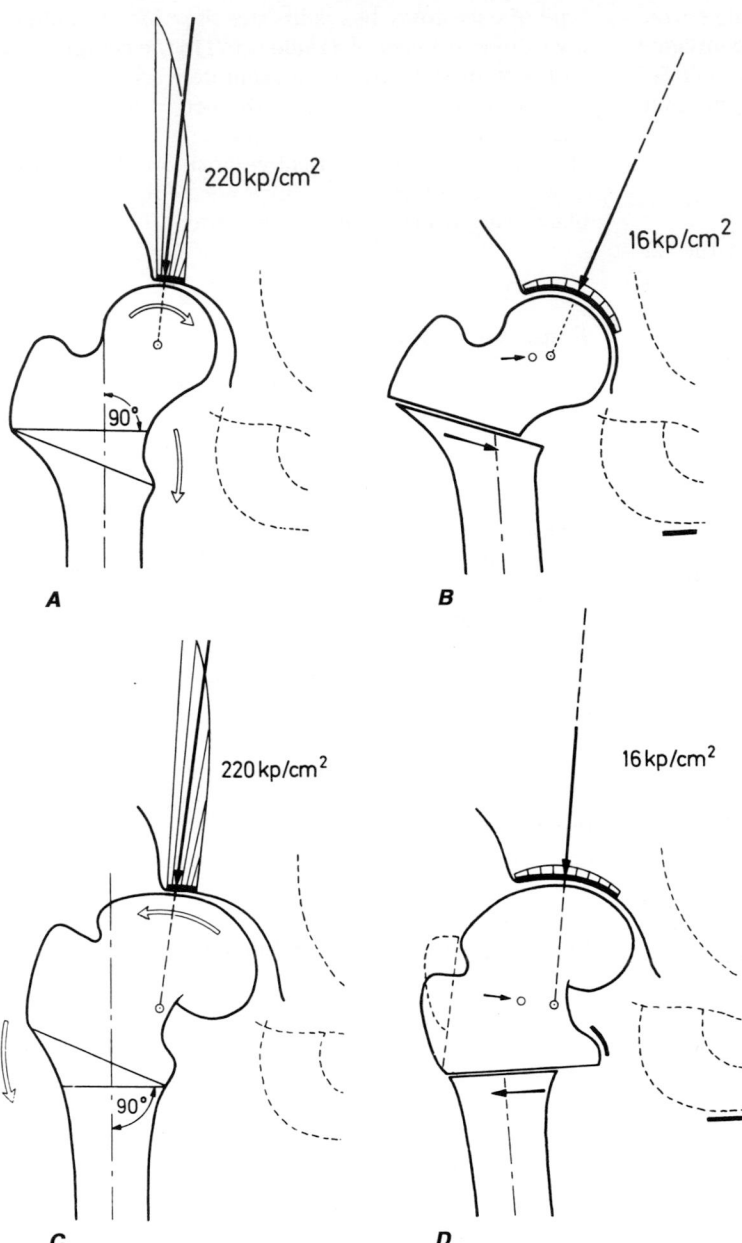

Figure 49-5 Rationale of the various osteotomies aimed at enlarging the weight-bearing surface. *A.* Subluxation of the femoral head: a large compressive force acts near the edge of the acetabulum with localized high stresses. Varus osteotomy is recommended and the varus wedge to be removed is shown. *B.* The compressive force is reduced in magnitude and spread over a wider area after varus osteotomy. *C.* A deformed head with a large capital drop that is also subluxated. Again, there are large localized stresses of high magnitude on a reduced weight-bearing surface. Valgus osteotomy is proposed and the wedge is marked. *D.* After valgus osteotomy, there is an increased weight-bearing surface; the resultant force has moved medially and the stresses, which have been greatly reduced, are more evenly distributed. Pauwels recommends that the shaft fragments be displaced laterally and tenotomy of the adductor and iliopsoas muscles be performed. The greater trochanter is osteotomized and allowed to move proximally, reducing the power of the abductor muscles. [Reproduced with permission from Pauwels F: Biomechanical principles of varus/valgus intertrochanteric osteotomy, in Schatzker J (ed): *The Intertrochanteric Osteotomy.* Berlin and Heidelberg, Springer-Verlag, 1984.]

as the proximal fragment is adducted and the superolateral joint space widens[45] (Fig. 49-5).

Varus Intertrochanteric Osteotomy

In general, a varus osteotomy is indicated in the case of lateral subluxation associated with coxa valga.[45,46] If acetabular dysplasia is also noted, a pelvic osteotomy may be required to complete the reconstruction. It is important that a minimum of 15° of passive abduction be found at the preoperative clinical evaluation. No lateral femoral head osteophyte should be present. Improved femoral head congruency should be observed on the functional abduction view. The varus osteotomy relaxes all the important hip musculature: adductors, abductors, and flexors. According to Muller, a combination of varus angulation of the proximal fragment and medial displacement of

the distal fragment is required to normalize the load at the knee with this procedure (Fig. 49-6).

Complications of a varus intertrochanteric osteotomy can include excessive shortening of the extremity, weak hip abductors, and a Trendelenburg gait. The need for a subsequent distal transfer of the greater trochanter to correct the gait may arise. A postoperative bursitis around the blade plate is the most common complication in the young osteotomy patient. Treatment of this problem may require subsequent hardware removal once remodeling of the osteotomy site has occurred.

Valgus Intertrochanteric Osteotomy

The performance of a valgus intertrochanteric osteotomy for the salvage of an osteoarthritic hip in a young patient was primarily advocated by Pauwels.[45] This procedure is

Figure 49-6 The effects of different types of varus osteotomy and medial displacement on knee joint loading. *A.* The preoperative condition. *B.* Pure varization produces varus overload. *C.* Pure medial displacement produces a valgus overload. *D.* A combination of varization and medial displacement normalizes load conditions of the knee joint. These concepts of M.E. Müller imply that valgization produces valgus overload of the knee joint, which is eliminated by lateralization of the femoral shaft. [Reproduced with permission from Schneider R: Intertrochanteric osteotomy, in Schatzker J (ed): *The Intertrochanteric Osteotomy.* Berlin and Heidelberg, Springer-Verlag, 1984.]

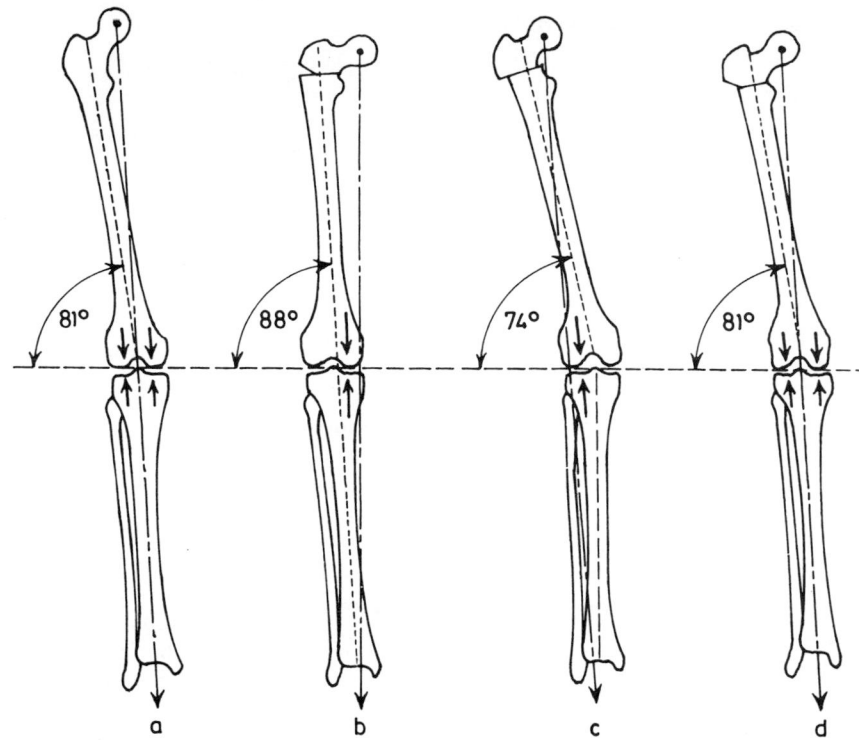

still indicated in young patients with acceptable passive range of motion, including minimum flexion of 90° and adduction of at least 15°. Important preoperative radiologic findings should include an arthritic hip with obvious joint overload superolaterally and an obvious capital drop osteophyte. An elliptical femoral head may also be present. An adduction functional film should show improved congruency of the joint and of widening of the superolateral joint space with the capital drop osteophyte acting as a fulcrum. In addition, the use of this inferomedial osteophyte as a bearing surface enlarges the the load-bearing area of the hip joint and thus diminishes its compressive stresses. Subsequent formation of a "roof osteophyte" may then occur, which further increases the weight-bearing surface and potentially halts the progression of articular degeneration. This salvage osteotomy may even be applied to the situation where a portion of the the femoral head is uncovered. This is possible as long as the functional adduction film shows an improved superolateral joint space when it is compared to a contrasting abduction view. Many surgeons have reported on the incorporation of extension at the intertrochanteric osteotomy site, which can be used to correct flexion contractures up to 20°.[47,48]

The success of this osteotomy "depends not only upon one's skill in patient selection and surgical techniques but also upon the acceptance of its limitations by the patient population."[47] Large series with long-term results by Santore and Bombelli have included overall success rates of 67 and 75 percent in young patients over a minimum follow-up period of 11 years.[47,48]

Valgus Osteotomy and Nonunion of the Femoral Neck

A valgus intertrochanteric osteotomy is an important treatment option for the rare case of fracture of the femoral

neck with nonunion. Again the indication is primarily in the young patient in whom salvage of the hip joint is much more prudent than an arthroplasty.[49] Valgus reorientation of the proximal femur improves the biomechanics of the fracture and promotes subsequent healing. The osteotomy decreases the shear forces as well as maximizing compressive forces at the nonunion site. It is also important to mention that avascular necrosis of the femoral head (ON stages 1 and 2) is not a contraindication to this procedure. Clinical results in young patients with known avascular necrosis prior to valgus osteotomy are similar to those in patients with proven viability of the femoral head.[50]

Proximal Femoral Osteotomies for Osteonecrosis

The long-term failure of total hip arthroplasty in young patients with osteonecrosis (ON) has recently made proximal femoral osteotomies a more popular option.[51–54] The indications for these osteotomies in the reconstruction of an osteonecrotic hip are extremely narrow. Unfortunately, most patients present to the orthopaedist long after their disease has progressed past the point of reconstruction via osteotomy.

In general, these patients must be thoroughly evaluated via an accurate history and physical examination. The etiology of the ON, if any, should be identified, since it may influence the prognosis.[55] In addition, characterizing the patient's pain profile is of utmost importance. An immediate osteotomy is rarely indicated if the patient does not demonstrate significant limiting pain upon the initial evaluation. Particular attention should be paid to determining whether a specific position of comfort soothes the patient during the exam.

Next, routine radiographic studies should be obtained. Anteroposterior and cross-table lateral views are recommended. Tangential views of Schneider (60° obliques) and tomograms can also be obtained.[40] Using these films, the ARCO stage of the disease should be documented. Reconstructive osteotomies are usually recommended for patients with stage 2 or 3 ON. In addition, the position of the lesion within the *quadrants* of the femoral head must be documented. Radiographs should also be used to determine the size of the necrotic lesion in the femoral head, as this has become a key variable in predicting the outcome of any osteotomy. This measurement is performed by drawing two lines from the center of the femoral head to the most peripheral margins of the necrotic sector on both the AP and lateral films. The angles measured are then added together. If this *cumulative necrotic sector angle* is less than 200°, a favorable outcome after proximal femoral reconstructive osteotomy may be expected.[56] An angle greater than 200° may be an indication for a salvage osteotomy in the presence of advanced degenerative disease.

Once the characteristics (stage, position, and size) of the osteonecrotic lesion are documented, the surgeon must decide whether or not an osteotomy is indicated. Classically, small stage 2 or 3 lesions found in the anterolateral quadrant of the femoral head are best suited for reconstruction via osteotomy.

Intertrochanteric osteotomies rely on the reorientation of the intertrochanteric femur to reposition the necrotic lesion of the femoral head away from the weight-bearing forces of the hip joint.[57-59] This repositioning, therefore, allows the normal portions of the femoral head to assume the weight-bearing function. This results in resolution of the patient's pain and also theoretically reduces the chance of further collapse of the necrotic segment. The osteotomy is named by describing the position of the distal fragment with regard to the proximal fragment *after* the intertrochanteric osteotomy has been performed. For example, in the case where there is an anterolateral ON lesion, the surgeon must perform a valgus-flexion intertrochanteric osteotomy. This reorientation allows the normal posteromedial portions of the femoral head to assume the weight-bearing function.

Results

The results of intertrochanteric osteotomies for ON have shown deterioration with time. The surgeon's ability to select indicated patients and to perform these technically difficult procedures certainly plays a role. A recent study reported 76 percent good/excellent results after this type of reconstruction at 11.5 years. Failures were reported in patients with cumulative necrotic sector angles greater than 200° and in patients who continued to receive corticosteroids perioperatively.[60]

The rotational transtrochanteric osteotomy introduced by Sugioka et al. involves rotation of the head and neck of the femur.[61] The osteotomy includes two separate cuts, one vertical and one horizontal, in the intertrochanteric region of the hip. The two cuts meet at an angle slightly more than 90°, allowing for rotation of the proximal fragment and subsequent repositioning of the normal articular surface of the femoral head (Fig. 49-7). The technical difficulty of this operation has made this osteotomy uncommon. Sugioka et al. have published satisfactory long-term results with a 78 percent success rate over a 3- to 16-year follow-up in patients with idiopathic or steroid-induced ON.[62]

Pelvic Osteotomies

Reconstructive Pelvic Osteotomy for Hip Dysplasia

Traditionally, proximal femoral osteotomy has been used in patients with acetabular dysplasia to improve femoral head coverage. But with severe dysplasia, femoral osteotomies may not suffice to achieve this goal. For this reason, attention has recently focused on osteotomy techniques that reconstruct the dysplastic acetabulum via pelvic osteotomy. These osteotomies tend to produce more satisfactory correction of the structural deficiencies associated with hip dysplasia. In addition, they also provide femoral head containment and reestablish a more normal distribution of forces across the hip joint.

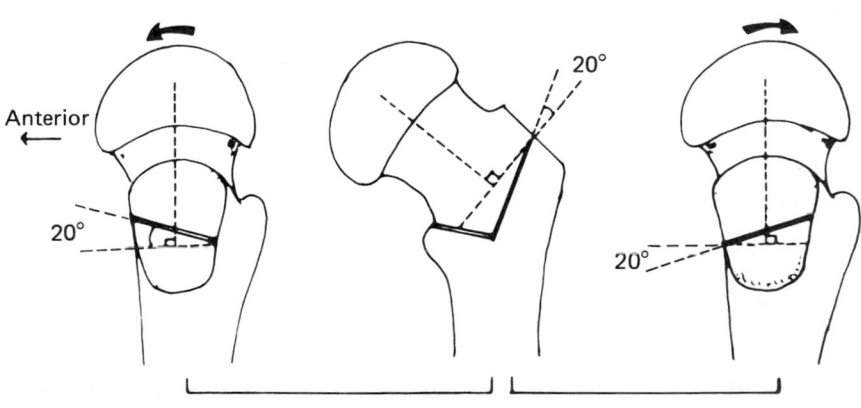

Anterior rotation   Posterior rotation

Figure 49-7 Schematic illustration of the inclination of the osteotomy plane necessary to produce correct rotation and final position of 40° of varus in the Sugioka osteotomy. (Reproduced with permission from Sugioka Y: Transtrochanteric rotational osteotomy in the treatment of idiopathic and steroid induced femoral head necrosis, Perthes' disease, slipped capital epiphysis and osteoarthritis of the hip. *Clin Orthop* 184:12–23, 1984.)

Assessment Patients with mild to moderate hip dysplasia who remain undiagnosed during childhood may function normally into adolescence and adulthood. Many of these patients eventually find themselves in an orthopaedist's office, unaware of their unfortunate predisposition. Young adult patients complaining of hip and groin pain associated with weight bearing and demonstrating hip dysplasia on radiograph should first undergo a trial of conservative treatment. A suitable program will include modification of activities, limited weight bearing, and anti-inflammatory medications. Unfortunately, many of these patients will inevitably fail these conservative modalities and be considered for reconstruction.

The radiographic evaluation of the adult dysplastic hip should begin with standard pelvic, AP, and lateral views. Measurements of an abnormal acetabular index (> 30°), and center-edge angle of Wiberg (< 20°) (Fig. 49-8) are important in determining the grade of dysplasia present. Additional views including the false-profile view of Lequesne are required to determine the amount of anterolateral deficiency present and the acetabular inclination (Fig. 49-9). The false-profile view is an oblique 65° film taken with the patient standing and determines the extent of anterior coverage of the femoral head.[40] The center-edge angle should also be measured on this view. Reconstructive pelvic osteotomies are indicated in adult patients with symptomatic acetabular dysplasia associated with little or no radiographic sign of secondary degeneration. Films illustrating a dysplastic hip joint with a preserved, congruent joint space without femoral head deformity demonstrate the classic indication for pelvic osteotomy. In the event that coxa valga is present, a pelvic osteotomy may be combined with a varus intertrochanteric osteotomy to provide accurate femoral head coverage. This is best determined by evaluating the hip joint radiographically with an AP view in abduction and internal rotation. Once the femoral head has begun to assume an elliptical deformity, the decision making becomes more complex. In many instances, a redirectional pelvic osteotomy is still possible in these cases, though more difficult and less predictable.

A number of different combinations have been described for reconstruction of the dysplastic hip. Single (Salter[63]), double (Sutherland[64]), and triple (Steel[65]) innominate osteotomies, among others, have been used to redirect the dysplastic acetabulum (see Chap. 40). Problems—including hip retroversion, hip center lateralization, insufficient correction, ON, and nonunion—can accompany many of these technically difficult procedures. Despite the potential complications, many of these techniques have been successfully employed in children and adolescents. Unfortunately, the inability to gain complete correction and the need for postoperative cast immobilization has made these methods less popular in adults.[66]

Periacetabular Osteotomy

This "silent" but often significant hip dysplasia is now the subject of much debate. It has been estimated that the rate of end-stage osteoarthritis secondary to dysplasia of the hip may be as high as 43 percent.[40,60]

Often the lateral and anterior acetabular deficiencies present in these patients are too large to be accommodated by a standard redirectional osteotomy. For this rea-

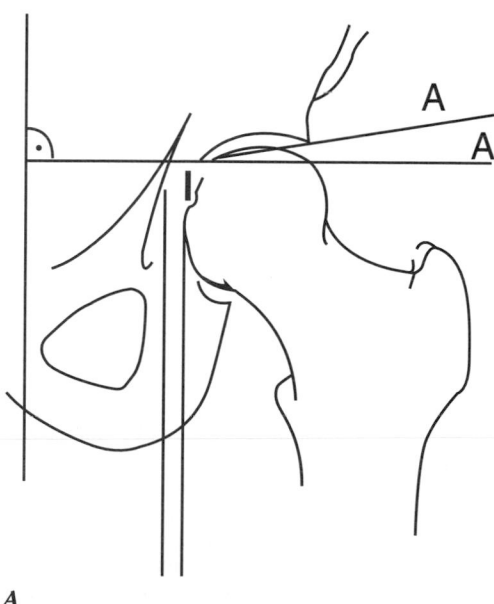

A

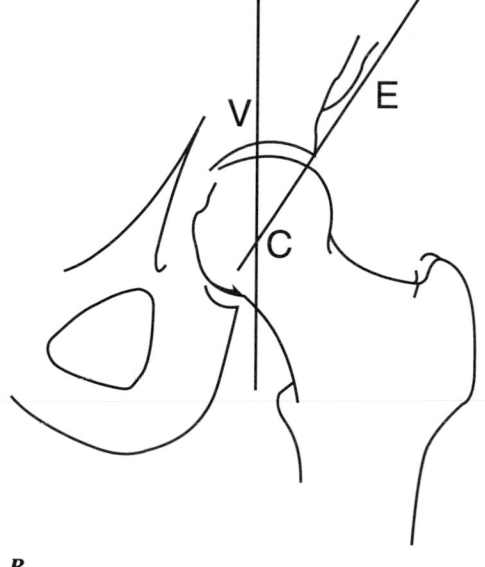

B

Figure 49-8 Schematic diagrams of the measurements obtained preoperatively and postoperatively to evaluate the acetabulum. *A.* The acetabular index angle (AA) is formed between a line parallel to the weight-bearing dome (sourcil) and a line perpendicular to the inter-teardrop line. *B.* The center-edge angle of Wiberg (VCE) is measured as shown. (Reproduced with permission from Trousdale RT, Ekkernkamp A, Ganz R, et al: Periacetabular and intertrochanteric osteotomy for the treatment of osteoarthrosis in dysplastic hips. *J Bone Joint Surg* 77A:73–86, 1995.)

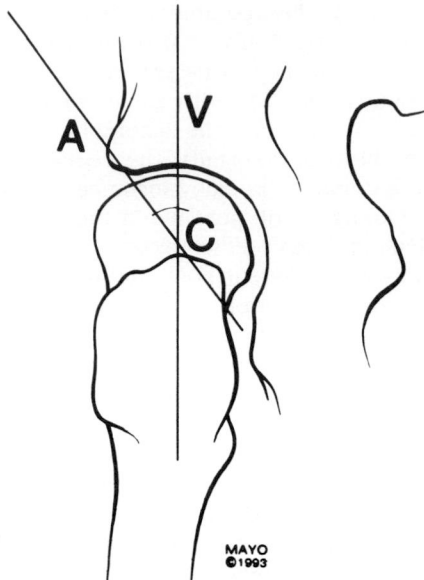

Figure 49-9 The lines used to measure the angle of acetabular ventral inclination (the VCA angle of Lequesne and de Seze). [Reproduced with permission from Trousdale RT, Ekkernkamp A, Ganz R, et al: Periacetabular and intertrochanteric osteotomy for the treatment of osteoarthrosis in dysplastic hips. *J Bone Joint Surg* 77A:73–86, 1995.]

son, early recognition of hip dysplasia in symptomatic adults without evidence of arthritis is important but has been difficult to achieve. Recent development of new periacetabular techniques has improved the prognosis for these patients.[66] By performing extraarticular pelvic osteotomies closer to the acetabulum, greater rotational freedom of the fragments is obtained, allowing for a larger correction. Techniques have been described by a number of surgeons.[40,66,67–69]

Tonnis[67] has described a successful juxtaarticular triple osteotomy for this problem. Unfortunately, the mo-

bility of the osteotomized fragment remains somewhat limited. In addition, ischial nonunions have been reported when major rotational corrections have been attempted.

Spherical or dome osteotomies have also been described.[68,69] The classic dial osteotomy requires the use of a curved osteotome to create a spherical osteotomy in the subchondral dome of the acetabulum. This is an extremely difficult operation and can result in joint penetration and even ON if not performed accurately.

Ganz, et al.[40,66] describe the "Bernese" periacetabular osteotomy, which has recently gained popularity for larger corrections needed in adolescents and adults. This technique includes a series of geometrically arranged osteotomies of the pubis, ischium, and ilium that create a mobile periacetabular fragment as well as large areas of contact between fragments for healing (Fig. 49-10). Moreover, continuity of the posterior column of the pelvis is maintained which provides stability of the osteotomy postoperatively (Fig. 49-11). Early partial weight bearing without immobilization is typical after this surgery.

Despite these advantages, the Bernese osteotomy is a technically demanding procedure that requires expertise in the area of pelvic and acetabular reconstruction. Aberrant intraarticular osteotomies, femoral nerve palsy, pubic nonunion, heterotopic bone formation, and hardware bursitis have all been reported as complications. Preliminary results have been encouraging, with good to excellent results reported in patients with minimal or moderate dysplasia at 5 years. Patients with advanced arthritis or severe dysplasia fared poorly.[40]

Chiari Osteotomy for Salvage

Radiographic findings such as joint incongruity, femoral head subluxation, and advanced osteoarthritis preclude the use of reconstructive osteotomies in many adult patients. A second alternative in these patients is a salvage osteotomy, which may moderate the patient's symptoms and put off the need for a formal hip anthroplasty.

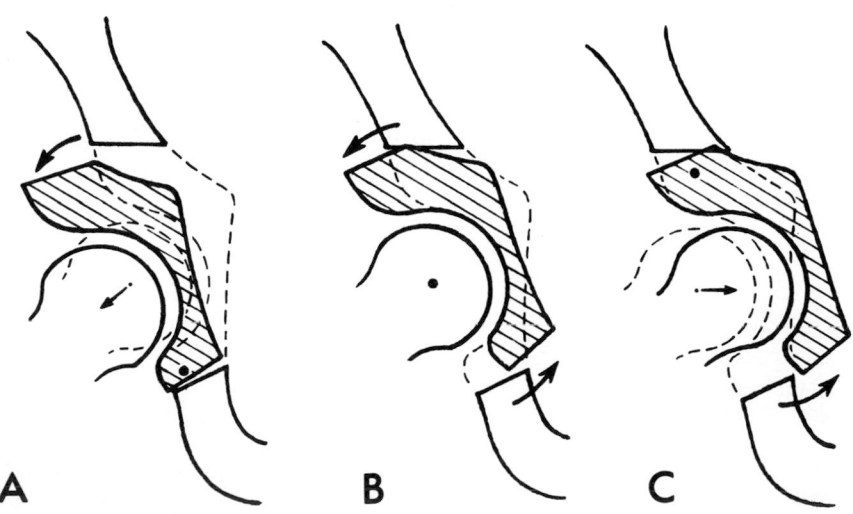

Figure 49-10 Effect of the location of the center of adduction-rotation (indicated by black spot) on mediolateral displacement of the acetabular fragment. *A.* A distal center of rotation with a proximally easily visible correction results in biomechanically undesirable lateral displacement. *B.* If the fragment is rotated around the center of the head, there is neither medial nor lateral displacement. *C.* Proximal location of the center of rotation results in a medial displacement of the femoral head and a barely visible displacement of the supraacetabular osteotomy lines. The medial displacement may be beneficial and intentionally desirable intraoperatively. (Reproduced with permission from Ganz R, Klaue K, Vinh TS, et al: A new periacetabular osteotomy for the treatment of hip dysplasia: Technique and preliminary results. *Clin Orthop Rel Res* 277:111–120, 1992.)

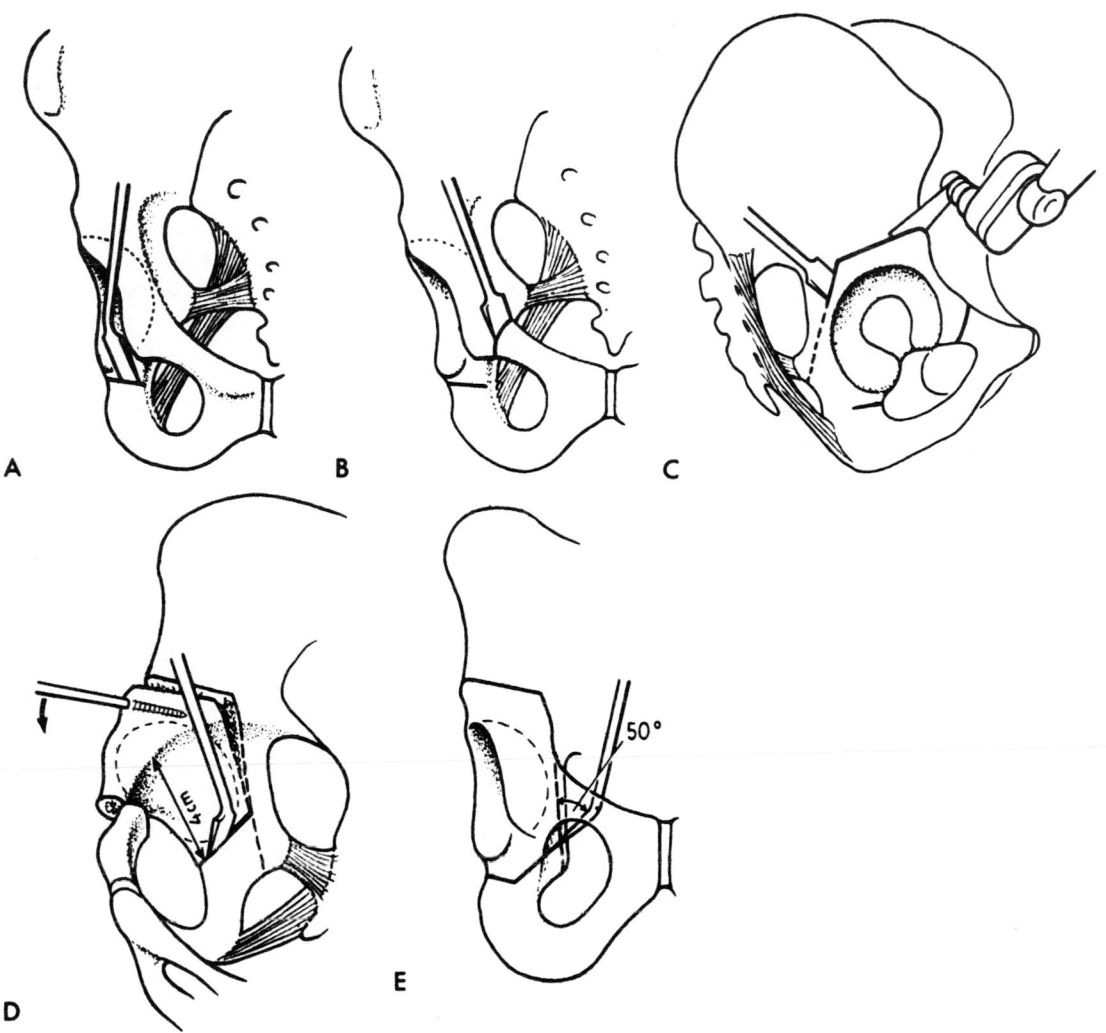

Figure 49-11 *A.* The angled chisel is introduced into the space between the psoas tendon and capsule and the ischium is notched 5 to 10 mm deep at the infracotyloid groove. *B.* Osteotomoy of the pubis immediately adjacent to the acetabulum. *C.* Roof-shaped osteotomy viewed from the outside. The anterior leg of the osteotomy is made with an oscillating saw starting proximal to the anteroinferior iliac spine. The anterior portion of the posterior leg is osteotomized from inside and outside at an angle of 120° using the chisel. The remainder of that osteotomy will break spontaneously toward the ischial spine (*dotted line*). *D.* Introduction of a Schanz screw into the supraacetabular bone tilts the fragment laterally. Osteotomy of the ischium from the quadrilateral surface is done with the angled chisel 4 cm below the well-visualized pelvic brim. The dorsal pillar and sacropelvic connections remain intact. *E.* Using a distance of 4 cm from the pelvic brim, a 50° angle between the blade of the chisel and the quadrilateral surface will result in an osteotomy posterior to the acetabulum. (Reproduced with permission from Ganz R, Klaue K, Vinh TS, et al: A new periacetabular osteotomy for the treatment of hip dysplasia: Technique and preliminary results. *Clin Orthop* 277:111–120, 1992.)

Simmons stated that "The Chiari osteotomy (see also Chap. 40) is a procedure that may be considered a reasonable biologic alternative for the surgical management of dysplasia of the hip joint associated with degenerative arthrosis."[70] This technique, which gained popularity in the treatment of childhood hip dysplasia in the past, still has a place in the treatment of adult hip arthrosis.

The Chiari iliac osteotomy relies on an osseous buttress created after the medial displacement of the distal (acetabular) fragment for superolateral coverage of the femoral head. The osteotomy should be made as close to the capsular attachment of the hip as possible and project proximally toward the posteromedial aspect of the ilium. This technical point allows for a greater buttress effect from the proximal (iliac) fragment and provides a larger osteotomy surface area for healing. Note that an anterior defect may persist after correction with this procedure. The use of an iliac crest bone graft anteriorly may protect against potential persistent instability. Chiari osteotomy can also be performed in conjunction with a proximal femoral osteotomy when warranted.

Results of Chiari osteotomies performed in adults have also been encouraging. Reynolds reported a 90 percent success rate in carefully selected patients at 5 years.[71]

ARTHROPLASTY OF THE HIP

Indications

More than 120,000 total hip arthroplasties are performed annually in the United States.[72] The primary indications for total hip arthroplasty are pain, functional limitation and intraarticular disease confirmed radiographically.[73–76] The National Institutes of Health in a consensus paper in 1994 concluded that indications for total hip arthroplasty are moderate to severe pain and/or disability that is not substantially relieved by an extended course of nonsurgical management in the setting of joint damage on radiographs.[76] A Swedish government consensus panel concluded that instability, loss of mobility, pain with movement, rest pain, and a patient's unwillingness to accept his or her situation are primary indications for total hip arthroplasty.[77] Given the extremely broad nature of these guidelines, the large regional variations in surgical rates in the United States are not surprising.[78] Even within a small geographic area, indications vary widely among various surgeons.[79]

Contraindications both absolute and relative include active infection, younger age, heavy weight, return to high-impact sports or job activities, arterial insufficiency, poor soft tissue coverage, neuromuscular disease, poor hip musculature, severe bone stock loss, substance abuse, mental illness, hostile personality, poor medical condition, limited cooperation, and unrealistic expectations.[79]

It cannot be overemphasized that the presence of severe radiologic degeneration of the hip joint is not an indication in itself to perform total hip arthroplasty. Significant pain and disability must accompany any radiographic changes. A complete evaluation of the patient's overall medical, psychological, and social condition must be performed before total hip arthroplasty is contemplated.

Preoperative Planning

High-quality preoperative radiographs—anteroposterior (AP) of the pelvis and AP and lateral radiographs of the affected hip and proximal femur extending beyond the isthmus—are needed for preoperative templating. The hips should, if possible, be internally rotated approximately 15° to compensate for femoral anteversion, thus placing the femoral head and neck parallel to the radiographic cassette. Since most patients with significant hip disease have limited internal rotation, rolling the patient toward the opposite hip on a radiolucent cushion will have the same desired effect. However, this technique distorts the proximal femur and alters magnification. A second but relatively uncommon technique is to place the patient in the prone position and take a posterolateral x-ray of the hip with the opposite hip elevated. The preferred lateral x-ray is the Lowenstein view. With the patient in almost lateral position, the affected leg is externally rotated toward the x-ray table with the hip and knee flexed close to 90° and the opposite leg extended.[80]

Magnification can be calculated using a magnification marker taped to the thigh at the level of the femur. The marker typically has radiopaque indicators at known distances but can also be an object of known diameter. The marker must be placed at the same distance from the radiographic cassette as the bone to accurately calculate magnification.

The size of both the acetabular and femoral components can be estimated from the manufacturer-supplied templates, which are clear plastic overlays with varying degrees of magnification. The template with magnification closest to that which has been calculated should be used. The acetabulum is best templated from the involved side, while femoral component size is best estimated from the uninvolved hip if only one hip is involved. Once the appropriate femoral component size has been selected, a level for femoral neck resection can be chosen. A transverse line projected medially from the tip of the greater trochanter should pass through the center of rotation of the femoral head. The level of femoral neck resection must be carefully estimated to obtain the proper hip offset and leg length. With a modular femoral head system, a variety of neck resection and femoral head length combinations can be used to create the same leg length but creating different offsets. Restoration of appropriate offset is important in reestablishing the correct muscular and soft tissue tension, which, in turn, affects joint reaction force and strength. Insufficient offset can cause impingement, leading to either limited range of motion or increased likelihood of dislocation.[81,82]

There are benefits to having this knowledge preoperatively. The surgeon avoids intraoperative complications, reduces operative time, identifies the extra equipment or material required (special or custom prostheses, bone graft, etc.), and anticipates correct sizes for both acetabular and femoral implants with the goal of ultimately improving the clinical results.[83–88] The actual benefit of such planning has been poorly quantified in the literature. A limited study of community orthopaedic surgeons shows that intraoperative complications may not be reduced as much as is generally believed by preoperative planning.[89]

If an operation for a cementless prosthesis is being planned, it is important to evaluate the potential for achieving good fit and fill both in the metaphysical and diaphysial regions of the femur. It is necessary to avoid filling the diaphysis with a stem that is too thick (and consequently stiff), leading to stress shielding and cortical osteoporosis. Such will be the case if the canal diameter of the femur is too large at the diaphysis. Dorr advocates measuring the canal diameter at the level of the lesser trochanter and again 10 cm below it. If the distal measurement is greater than 70 percent, of the proximal measurement (canal-to-calcar isthmus or cc ratio), then the medullary canal of the proximal femur lacks the funnel shape necessary to fit a suitable cementless component.[90]

While there is no universal agreement on indications for cemented versus cementless fixation,[91–95] it is generally agreed that the primary indication for cementless total hip replacement is in the young, active individual, usually below the age of 65 physiologically. Hybrid prosthetic replacement (cemented femoral stem and uncemented press-fit metal-backed acetabular cup) is recommended for those over age 65 with more than 10 years of life expectancy remaining. Fully cemented implants are recommended for remaining patients.[96]

Preoperative medical evaluation is of especial importance in patients who are known to have cardiovascular, pulmonary, or diabetic conditions. Although the risk of blood-borne infection (e.g., hepatitis, human immunodeficiency virus) from homologous blood transfusion is fairly small, all patients who are medically capable should donate their own blood prior to surgery. Woolson and Watt have found that the rate of homologous blood transfusion can be brought down to less than 10 percent when an average of 2.6 units of blood are autodonated.[97] General recommendations are autodonation of 2 units of blood for primary hip arthroplasties and 3 to 4 units for revision in adults.

Considerations for Arthroplasty in Other Disease States

Diabetes is a common systemic disease affecting approximately 5 percent of the population. Preoperative cardiac and peripheral vascular evaluations should be carried out routinely. Patients with diabetes have slower healing rates and an increased susceptibility to infection.[98] One study found an increased rate of superficial (9.7 percent) and deep wound (6.5 percent) infections.[99] However, no prophylactic antibiotics were used. In a more recent study where prophylactic antibiotics were used, no increase in infection rate was detected.[100] The overall complication rate was high, at 24.3 percent, with urinary tract infection the most common complication (14.2 percent) and myocardial infarction the most serious one, reinforcing the need for preoperative cardiac evaluation.

Although the rate of successful *renal transplantation* continues to improve, osteonecrosis of the femoral head remains an unfortunate complication, with an incidence between 3 and 41 percent.[101–104] Cemented arthroplasties appear to have a high rate of both early and late complications, with early loosening being the major problem.[105,106] Results appear to be better for cementless hips, at least in short-term follow-up.[107] Care must be exercised in positioning the patient in the lateral decubitus position as inadvertent compression of the renal transplant with patient positioners can cause renal transplant infarction.[108]

In studies of hip arthroplasty in patients with *Gaucher's disease,* increased intraoperative and postoperative bleeding was noted.[109] There was a high rate of loosening in several studies, although overall function and pain relief were excellent.[110,111] (see also Chap. 6).

Osteonecrosis of the femoral head is a well-known complication of *sickle cell disease* and *β-thalassemia.* Preoperative medical and hematologic evaluation is critical. Epidural or spinal anesthesia, good oxygenation, hydration, prophylactic antibiotics, and DVT prophylaxis against deep vein thrombosis are recommended. There is an extremely high complication and failure rate in this group of patients. High intraoperative blood loss, femoral perforation, and fracture secondary to difficulty in reaming a femur with an obliterated femoral canal, infection (16 to 20 percent), and loosening (40 to 60 percent at 5 to 10

year follow-up) are all very common.[112–116] With short term follow-up, uncemented prostheses appear to have lower rates of loosening.

Severe *hemophilic arthropathy* of the hip typically causes valgus deformity and protrusio acetabuli. The most important predictor of long-term outcome is seropositivity for the HIV-I virus, which is in the order of 50 percent in this group of patients. When total hip arthroplasty is considered for a patient with hemophilia, preoperative tests should include determination of the level of factor VIII or IX, presence of inhibitor, a survival study of infused factor concentrate, HIV testing, CD4 lymphocyte count, and intradermal skin testing. According to Greene, a patient with CD4 count of 400×10^9/L and a positive response to an intradermal skin test has little increased risk for infection.[117] In a large multicenter study, there was a 62 percent failure rate of cemented acetabular components and 36 percent failure rate of cemented femoral components at mean follow-up at 8.5 years. The results of arthroplasty with uncemented implants have been excellent, at least in short-term follow-up of 2.7 years.[118]

In *cerebral palsy,* Girdlestone resection has failed to reliably relieve pain from the dislocated or subluxed hip. This option is best reserved for mentally retarded non-ambulators.[119,120] Hip arthrodesis is recommended for nonambulators, those with unilateral involvement, and young, active patients. Because of the high rate of concurrent contralateral hip or spinal deformity, arthrodesis is often contraindicated.[121,122] Cemented arthroplasty is preferred for ambulators with bilateral involvement (see also Chap. 14). In a long-term follow-up study, survivorship was 95 percent at 10 years for loosening and 86 percent with removal for any reason[123]; 94 percent of patients had improved pain and function in this study. Hip spica casts were used routinely to minimize dislocation and trochanteric nonunion for the transtrochanteric approach used in the majority of patients in this series. Others have shown excellent results with low complication rates.[124]

The presence of *psoriasis* is a distinct risk factor for infection, at least in cases where preoperative antibiotic prophylaxis was not used. Menon and Wroblewski[125] have reported a deep infection rate of 5.5 percent and superficial infection rate of 9.1 percent, both significantly higher than for those patients without psoriasis. To date no studies exist examining psoriasis as a risk factor for infection with prophylactic antibiotic use.

As the life span of patients with *osteogenesis imperfecta* has increased, debilitating arthritis is becoming more common in those adults who can walk. Only a small series exists in the literature. Pain relief and functional improvement were excellent at average 7 years follow-up, with one complication of acetabuli protrusio in a patient with a bipolar prosthesis.[126]

It is estimated that six to ten thousand children have marked functional impairment secondary to *juvenile rheumatoid arthritis (JRA).* Short-term results in patients with JRA have shown excellent relief of pain and marked improvement in range of motion and ambulation ability.[127–131] However, long-term studies with cemented components show extremely high rates of loosening (up to 57 percent) of the femoral component.[132–134] In all of these series, early cementing techniques and implants were used. A small number of uncemented implants used in a later study appear to have better survival rates, at least with short-term follow-up.[134] The high rate of failure may be due to the young age of the patients, even though these patients in general have low functional demands.[131] Careful preoperative planning is essential when arthroplasty is being considered in these patients. These patients present complex technical problems that may require reconstruction of femoral and/or acetabular bone deficiencies. Small bone size, osteoporosis, and severe soft tissue disease can make the surgery difficult. Customized miniature or microminiature components may be necessary.[131,135]

Systemic lupus erythematosus is associated with osteonecrosis of the femoral head, usually due to steroid treatment for this immunologic disorder. The risks of performing arthroplasty are poorly defined. The Mayo Clinic experience would suggest that a high complication rate can be expected with such patients. Complications included delayed wound healing in 15 percent, superficial wound infection in 10 percent, and deep infection in about 5 percent of patients.[136] Other studies show negligible increases in perioperative complications, with excellent implant survival.[137,138] Uncemented or hybrid total hip arthroplasties are probably to be recommended for this group of patients.[139,140]

The indications for primary total hip replacement in the setting of *femoral neck fracture* are limited. In the case of pathologic fracture without acetabular involvement, hemiarthroplasty is sufficient. Identification of all lesions in the femoral shaft with MRI is imperative prior to proceeding with surgery, as this will help decrease the risk of femoral fracture. With involvement of the entire proximal femur, a calcar or proximal femoral replacement will be necessary. If the acetabulum is involved, portions of the pelvis may need to be reconstructed with cement, wire mesh, and specialized custom acetabular components. Displaced femoral neck fractures in those patients with rheumatoid arthritis should be treated with prosthetic replacement. This is usually a hemiarthroplasty unless there is some evidence of preexisting acetabular involvement, in which case total replacement is advised. Some studies would suggest that routine hip arthroplasty in this set of patients is warranted.[141] Patients with preexisting osteoarthritis are more likely to sustain intertrochanteric rather than femoral neck fractures, but total hip arthroplasty is indicated in patients with significant preexisting arthritis. The failure rate of primary cemented total hip arthroplasties following displaced femoral neck fracture has been exceedingly high—50 percent at just over 5-year follow-up.[142] The results of secondary replacement were found to be as good as those for primary total hip arthroplasty following displaced femoral neck fracture. However, these were significantly worse results than in patients undergoing primary total arthroplasty for osteoarthritis.

Hip arthroplasty in patients with *osteonecrosis* is associated with higher than normal failure rates. A considerable portion of the difficulties can be attributed to the younger age of these patients. High rates of success can

be found with both cemented and uncemented arthroplasties with 4-year follow-up on average.[144]

Arthroplasty in the setting of neglected *developmental hip dysplasia* poses several problems. Acetabular deficiency with high hip centers has classically been reconstructed with a view to reproducing the anatomic or true hip center, usually with bulk allograft. Initial studies by Harris et al. showed excellent results with bulk allograft in cemented hips, but there was a 47 percent failure rate at 10 years.[145] Engh et al. showed similar failure rates at only 29 months average follow-up in uncemented hips.[146] Reconstruction with a high hip center appears to be a better option as long as the hip center is not displaced laterally.[147] Small acetabular volumes typically require both small acetabular components and smaller than usual 22-mm femoral heads to allow for sufficient polyethylene thickness. Deformity of the proximal femur, typically excessive femoral anteversion with a high neck shaft angle and a small intramedullary canal, may require special or custom femoral components. Extra care must be taken to avoid intraoperative femoral fracture. Limb lengthening is associated with numerous problems (see discussion of neurovascular complications, below). Overall results for neglected developmental hip dysplasia show a 71 percent success rate with long-term follow-up, but many of these patients were quite young. Acetabular deficiency correlated well with acetabular component loosening.[148]

Surgical Procedure

Antibiotic Prophylaxis

Although infection rates have fallen considerably since the first total hip arthroplasties done over thirty years ago, infection remains a persistent problem, occurring in approximately 1 percent of patients over the lifetime of the prosthesis. The use of prophylactic antibiotics is the biggest single factor in the reduction of infection rates. In one series, the rate of infection was 1.3 percent in cases where antibiotics were used compared to 5.8 percent in cases where antibiotics were not used.[149] Because between one-half to two-thirds of implant infections are caused by *Staphylococcus* and other gram-positive organisms,[150,151] prophylaxis usually consists of a first-generation cephalosporin (usually cephalothin or cefazolin) or its equivalent within the hour prior to incision and every 8 h for 24 to 48 h afterwards. Pollard et al.[152] found that 12 h were just as effective as 2 weeks of postoperative antibiotics. Continuing antibiotics beyond a 1- to 2-day period probably helps breed resistant organisms.[151,153]

Although total body exhaust systems, vertical laminar flow systems, ultraclean air systems, and ultraviolet lighting have all had some effect in reducing rates, their exact effect in conjunction with prophylactic antibiotics has yet to be determined. Because infection rates have been brought down to about 0.5 percent with prophylactic antibiotics, the number of patients needed to achieve statistical significance in a prospective, randomized control study is in excess of 10,000 in each group,[154] making it difficult for such a study to be performed.

Surgical Approach

Since Charnley first began performing total hip arthroplasties through the transtrochanteric lateral approach, many different surgical approaches have been described and used for total hip arthroplasty. The choice of surgical approach is dictated by numerous factors, including anticipated exposure requirements, scars from previous surgery or trauma, surgeon comfort and familiarity, and patient size. The anterolateral approach, posterolateral approach, and the direct lateral approach are the most commonly used for primary total hip arthroplasty. Although there are numerous variations for the anterolateral approach, they all approach the hip through the interval between the tensor fascia lata and the gluteus medius muscle. Some portion of the abductor is released from the greater trochanter and the hip is dislocated anteriorly. The anterolateral approach gives excellent acetabular exposure and has a lower dislocation rate than the posterolateral approach.[155,156] Limitations of the anterolateral approach include limited exposure of the femoral canal, especially if significant reaming of the canal is necessary, as in the case of cementless press-fit stems. In working on the proximal femur, either a wafer of bone with the anterior abductors attached can be osteotomized[157] or a trochanteric osteotomy can be done to improve exposure and reduce damage to the abductors. Gore has found decreased abductor strength postoperatively as compared to the posterolateral approach, probably secondary to abductor damage.[158] If the abductors are not securely reattached, significant morbidity from abductor weakness will compromise rehabilitation and the final clinical outcome. Structures posterior to the posterior acetabular rim are also difficult to reach using this approach.

The direct lateral approach, popularized by Harding[159] and subsequently modified, was developed to ensure adequate exposure to the proximal femur as well as to the acetabulum. The major modification from the original anterolateral approach was to leave the posterior portion of the gluteus medius attached to the greater trochanter. Studies using Harding's original approach suggested an increased incidence of abductor weakness, prolonged limp, and increased heterotopic bone formation.[160,161] With modification, these complications can be decreased.[157] This approach allows for ease of orientation of components. Because the posterior soft tissues and capsule are left intact, this approach appears to be particularly useful in noncompliant patients, especially those with neurologic diseases with elements of spasticity, such as Parkinson's disease.

The posterolateral (or posterior) approach gains exposure to the hip by splitting the gluteus maximus muscle, releasing the short external rotators, retracting the abductors anteriorly, and dislocating the femur posteriorly. In one study, desirable neck length, lateral and distal positioning of the greater trochanter relative to the center of the upper head of the femoral component, and equalization of limb length were easier to achieve using the posterior approach.[158] Another study has shown that arthroplasties using the posterior approach are completed in significantly less time and with less blood loss and fewer transfusions than by using the anterolateral approach.[162] The posterior approach is reported to be associated with a higher rate of dislocation, probably due to problems orienting the acetabular component appropriately.[158,163] A technique which repairs a portion of the posterior capsule has been reported to reduce dislocation rates.[164] Decreased surgery time, minimal muscle damage, and the potential for speedy rehabilitation make the posterior approach the method of choice for many surgeons. It is not recommended for patients who are neurologically impaired.

Routine trochanteric osteotomy as originally proposed by Charnley has lost favor for primary arthroplasty. Several studies have shown increases in blood loss and operating time, slower rehabilitation, higher dislocation rates, and increased heterotopic ossification as compared to trochanter-sparing approaches.[165–168] Nonunion and separation of the greater trochanter occur in up to 17 percent of primary surgeries and 13 percent in revision cases.[169] The rate of nonunion is especially high after postoperative hip radiation therapy for heterotopic ossification prophylaxis. Other complications include bursitis associated with wires and wire breakage. Routine osteotomy for revision cases or difficult primary cases (e.g., hip dysplasia) is common, as extended exposure of both the acetabulum and femur is usually required.

Other more specialized extensile approaches have been developed to allow adequate exposure in difficult primary or revision surgeries. These more complicated exposures should be undertaken carefully by the less experienced hip surgeon.

Dislocation

Routine subtotal capsulectomy is done by many surgeons. Capsulectomy is not necessary but can facilitate exposure, especially in patients who have fixed hip contractures. Release of the psoas and gluteus muscles may be necessary to gain adequate exposure in these cases as well. Once the capsulectomy or capsulotomy is accomplished, the hip can be dislocated. Occasionally the removal of large acetabular osteophytes is needed to accomplish this. Under exceptional circumstances, as with ankylosed or fused hips, the femoral neck may need to be osteomized prior to dislocation and the femoral head removed piecemeal.

Leg-Length Measurement

Prior to dislocation, fixed points on the femur and pelvis should be marked with either pins or other devices to allow for accurate assessment of leg-length equality. Various techniques have been described in the literature.[171–174] Care must be taken to reposition the leg in the same amount of flexion, adduction, and rotation when measuring and remeasuring leg length for any of these methods to work accurately. Using a comprehensive approach that gives special attention to leg-length equalization, Woolson reports only 2.5 percent of patients were lengthened more than 6.0 mm.[175] McGee in his study of the problem reported an average of 8.7 mm length discrepancy in hip arthroplasties.[172] These studies show results which are significantly better than previous series.[173,176,177]

The exact effect of leg lengthening is hard to quantify in the literature. Abraham and Dimon[178] emphasize that lengthening of greater than 2.5 cm is associated with increased risk of sciatic nerve palsy. Low back pain, impaired abductor function, and increased dislocation are all suggested to be complications of leg-length inequality. Increased lengthening by as little as 0.5 cm may hasten implant loosening by increasing superolateral acetabular stresses.

Using the appropriate jig supplied with each of the various hip implant systems, the level of femoral neck resection is found as determined by the preoperative plan. Recreation of appropriate offset and leg length is based largely on the level of femoral neck resection.[179]

Acetabular Preparation

Acetabular preparation begins with complete exposure of the acetabulum. Soft tissues must be adequately and safely retracted (see discussion of neurovascular complications, below), and peripheral osteophytes should be removed to allow for adequate visualization of internal landmarks. Although external positioning systems supplied by the various manufacturers are helpful, small changes in patient positioning (especially the lateral decubitus position) can reduce their effectiveness.

Staged hemispherical reamers, typically of the "cheese grater" type, are used to shape the acetabulum. Occluding osteophytes over the haversian gland (pulvinar) and the ligamentum teres are removed to expose the true acetabular floor. Reaming is carried out until a hemispheric contour is achieved, and all cartilage and sufficient subchondral bone is removed to provide for a bleeding cancelleous surface. Loss of subchondral bone weakens the acetabulum and allows for increased micromotion.[180] Cysts are removed and packed with morcellized bone graft. An acetabulum that is not close to being hemispherically shaped before reaming, as in protrusio and hip dysplasia, presents a problem requiring special techniques, some of which are discussed in the final part of this chapter ("Revision Hip Surgery"). An attempt should be made in standard primary hip arthroplasties to ream the acetabulum so that the center of rotation of the hip is nearly anatomic. Superior and lateral positioning of the center of rotation has led to increased rates of loosening.[181] The appropriate-sized component is then impacted into place (cementlessly) or cemented into place taking care to maintain the correct component orientation. McCollum[183] in his study found that optimal position for stability is 30 to 50° abduction and 20 to 40° flexion (anteversion) of the acetabular component. Lewinnek states that for a safe position of the acetabulum, $15 \pm 10°$ anteversion and $40 \pm 10°$ abduction is optimal.[127a] Dislocation rates were four times higher if the cup was oriented outside of the safe zone. Anteversion was found to be more important than abduction for stability. Abduction, on the other hand, appears to be critical to longevity. Lateral containment with complete bony coverage appears to be more important than absolute acetabular abduction positioning in a horizontal position in predicting longevity of an implant.[181,182]

At the current time, most acetabular components are the press-fit, uncemented type. Press-fitting technique involves placing a cup slightly larger (1 or 2 mm) than the size of the last-used acetabular reamer into the prepared acetabulum. This should result in a tight fit around the periphery of the implant. Too large a size mismatch between the implant and reamed acetabulum can cause pelvic fractures when the implant is impacted.

Femoral Preparation

Preparation of the femur typically involves reaming of the femoral canal to remove excess cortical bone in the proximal diaphysis of the femur. This is usually done with non-end-cutting conical or cylindrical power reamers to lessen the likelihood of cortical perforation. Rasps are then used to shape the proximal metaphysis. Care must be taken during the entire process not to fracture the proximal femur. Component orientation should be approximately 15° of anteversion to reproduce normal anatomy. The femoral component is much less critical in preventing dislocation.[183] Shaping the canal to fit an appropriately sized implant is obviously critical for cementless implants, but canal shape and conformity to the implant is also critical in cemented implants. (See below, "Cement Technique.") At this point, trial implants are inserted in their proposed postoperative position and the hip is reduced. The hip is then ranged fully to ensure adequate stability. Adjustments to component orientation and neck length can be accomplished at this time to maximize stability. The majority of current systems in current use are modular to at least some degree which allows for increased options. Modularity is not without complications including dissociation and mismatching of components and increases in fretting, wear debris, and corrosion.[184]

Cement Technique

The original Charnley implants used polymethylmethacrylate (PMMA) as bone cement. Although subtle differences in the chemical and physical properties between the various commercial preparations of PMMA exist, modern PMMA is essentially the same substance as that used over 30 years ago. (See also Chap. 14.) Cementless implants were developed to remove what was theorized to be the instigating factor in premature loosening and osteolysis, or "cement disease." As research has progressed, particulate wear debris has more clearly been defined as the source of implant loosening.

Polymethylmethacrylate is typically supplied in two parts—one powder the other liquid. The powder consists of prepolymerized granules, while the liquid is monomer. Mixing of the two produces the final polymerized product. Improvements in cementing techniques have been made, typically referred to in terms of generations.[185] The "first generation" is the original technique of Charnley, which consisted of hand-mixing of the cement, hand-packing of cement in an unplugged and uncleaned femoral canal and acetabulum. "Second generation" technique consists of plugging the femoral canal with a cement restrictor beyond the implant, pulsatile lavage of bony surfaces, and cement insertion in a retrograde fashion in the femoral canal. "Third generation" techniques currently used include the addition of vacuum and/or centrifuging mixing techniques, pressurization of the femoral canal, and surface modifications of implants.

Properly preparing the femoral canal plays an important part in optimizing the strength of the bone/cement interface. Cleaning the canal with pressurized lavage improves shear strength as compared to standard irrigation or no irrigation.[186] Plugging of the femoral canal allows for increased pressurization. Pressurization improves cement strength, and its use has become routine.[187–189] Complications of pressurization include transient hypotension, cardiac arrest, and sudden death—all caused by the release of cement monomer and fat, air, and marrow emboli into the systemic circulation. These risks are reduced by keeping the patient normotensive and normovolemic during the procedure. A second benefit of plugging the femoral canal is the assurance of a uniform cement mantle distal to the prosthetic tip. Based on Skinner's finite element analysis, the cement restrictor should be placed 2 to 4 cm beyond the end of the stem to decrease the rate of stress change at the tip of the component.[190]

Improved mixing techniques have been shown to decrease air void porosity and thus to increase fatigue strength. Wixson et al.[191] found that vacuum mixing increased fatigue life by a factor of 10. Centrifugation has been found to increase fatigue life by a factor of 5.[192,193] O'Connor found that 70 percent of samples of uncentrifuged cement subjected to the equivalent of 10 years of walking failed, while none of the samples of centrifuged cement failed under the same test conditions.[194]

In a long-term study of cemented femoral components, Sarmiento found that a cement mantle thickness of 2 to 5 mm in the proximal medial region of the femoral component gave the best results. Other studies, such as that of Star et al.,[195] also show increased failure with thin cement mantles. A study of autopsy specimens showed an association of thin, incomplete mantles with cement fragmentation, loosening, and periprosthetic osteolysis.[196] Femoral stems that filled more than half of the femoral canal had lower rates of radiographic loosening than those with less than half the canal filled. Loosening was more common with stems that were oriented in more than 5° of varus as compared to those that were in neutral or valgus.[197] Noble and coauthors have emphasized the value of a distal stabilizer and its role in providing a uniform cement mantle of satisfactory thickness.[198]

Although advanced cement techniques have substantially improved the durability of the cemented femoral component, comparable decreases in acetabular loosening have not been observed.[199]

Prosthesis Design

Crowninshield et al., using finite element analysis, found that implants with broad medial surfaces and rounded corners decrease stresses on the cement mantle.[200] Femoral components made of cobalt-based alloys are superior to those of titanium in reducing proximal cement stress.[201] Titanium femoral components are not usually cemented.

A 28-mm femoral head size is recommended for most prostheses. In a study of polyethylene wear, the greatest volumetric and mean rates of wear were found in patients with 32-mm femoral heads. The greatest linear wear occurred in patients with 22-mm heads. The latter heads are recommended for small acetabuli, so that a minimum of 8 mm of polyethylene thickness can be used for the liner to decrease shear stress on the polyethylene.[202]

Closure

The wound is thoroughly irrigated at this point to remove any loose pieces of bone or cement (if used), which may promote wear or heterotopic ossification, and also to decrease wound bacterial counts to reduce the chance of infection. Layered closure typically with one or two drains is done. No definitive study exists as to the efficacy of drains in preventing postoperative complications such as hematoma. Two studies have failed to show significant differences in arthroplasties with or without drain usage.[203,204]

Postoperative Care

Abduction pillows are typically used postoperatively in cases where either the posterior approach or transtrochanteric lateral approach is used. At the beginning, the abduction pillow is used all the time; later, it is used only at night, when the patient is unable to control his or her leg. For patients whose surgery involved the posterior approach, precautions include no hip flexion past 90° and minimal internal rotation or adduction. Such precautions should be maintained until the pseudocapsule forms, which typically takes about 6 weeks. Where the lateral or anterolateral approach was used, patients must avoid adduction and external rotation for about the same amount of time. When cemented prostheses are used, patients are started on an ambulation program, bearing weight as tolerated on the affected extremity. With ingrowth, practice varies, but some surgeons recommend partial or no weight bearing for the first 6 weeks.

Results

Various outcome measures have been developed to gauge the success of hip arthroplasties. Among the most common in use are the Harris,[205] Mayo,[205a] D'Aubigne,[206] and Iowa[206a] hip scores. These scores weight such measures as pain, function, range of motion, and radiographic evaluation differently. They have not been validated and have been, to date, unable to distinguish differences in outcome based on implant type or fixation.[207] Significant research is being done at the current time to develop outcome measurement tools that will make comparisons of implants and techniques both easier and more reproducible. Kaplan-Meier survivorship analysis allows for direct comparison between the results of various studies.[208] Revision rates are calculated using the remaining survivors in the study as the denominator, with the assumption that the many patients lost to attrition—common in any long-term study—are no more or no less likely to have failed implants.[209] A weakness of such analysis is that not all poorly functioning or painful hips will be revised.

The overall benefit of total hip arthroplasty is less ambiguous. A prospective outcome study has shown that there is dramatic benefit in health-related quality of life, including physical function, social interaction, and overall health.[210]

Cemented Implants. In several studies of cemented implants using first-generation technique with follow-up of approximately twenty years, failure rates tend to be linear and average around 1 percent per year.

The biggest risk of failure is related to the age of patient when total hip arthroplasty is performed. Younger patients in all series have higher rates of loosening and subsequent need for revision. In one long-term series done by the same single surgeon with 20-year follow-up, survivorship was 80 percent for those 65 years old or older and only 68 percent for those 50 years old and younger.[211,212] Kavanagh et al. have shown revision rates of 27 percent for those 59 years old or younger, 13 percent for those aged 59 to 65, and 7.5 percent for those between ages 65 and 70.[213] Other risk factors include increased weight (greater than 75 kg), high activity level, and diagnosis of osteoarthritis or osteonecrosis versus rheumatoid arthritis.[214]

With shorter-term follow-up, fully cemented implants using second-generation techniques have shown lower rates of revision than implants using first-generation technique for a comparable period of time (Tables 49-3 and 49-4). Most of these improvements have come from lower revision rates of the femoral component.

As third-generation cementing techniques are relatively new, follow-up is limited (5 years on average), but the results are encouraging, so far. The results listed in Table 49-5 were achieved with third-generation cement technique for the femur and press-fit uncemented acetabular components (so-called hybrid fixation).

The low failure rates so far are encouraging, especially for the femoral component, as failure and revision rates are linear over time for the femur. Significant failure rates of the acetabulum typically rise exponentially at about 10 years postoperatively.

Uncemented Implants. Because of high failure rates seen in some categories of patients (particularly younger age groups) using early cement techniques, alternatives have been developed. These cementless implants vary greatly in design philosophy. There are proponents of extensively porous coated implants. They believe that the proximal stress shielding seen in the femur associated with distal biological ingrowth and load transmission is a small price to pay for long-term durability of fixation. Others prefer proximally coated femoral components, relying primarily upon metaphyseal fit and fill to stabilize the implant until biological ingrowth occurs. Designs vary, some straight-stemmed, some more anatomic in configuration. There is also considerable variety in surface finish and biological coating among the various available designs.

The problem of thigh pain seen with early cementless designs have now been largely overcome. Recognition of the need for good implant stability to avoid distal micromotion and the avoidance of the use of cementless technology in unsuitable patients has been responsible for this improvement. Patients with stovepipe (cylinder-shaped) femoral canals should be cemented. They would require very large stiff stems to fill the diaphysis, which are more likely to fail if cementless stems are used.

With regard to proximally porous coated stems, there has been concern over the increasing incidence of osteolysis.[215] Extensively porous coated stems probably offer more resistance to the distal migration of particulate wear debris. Most proximally coated porous implants have now been modified so that the coating is circumferential around the area beneath the collar. This was not previously the case, providing smooth pathways for debris to enter the bone/prosthesis interface and migrate distally.

Proximally coated prostheses with uncoated stems load the metaphyseal bone in a more physiologic way than

TABLE 49-3   Results of Implants Using First-Generation Cementing Methods

Location	Number of hips	Age at surgery, range in years	Follow-up, range in years	Revision rate	Radiographic loosening
Iowa[214a]	98	65(29–86)	20(20–22)	10% A; 3% F	22% A; 7% F
Iowa[214b]	58	<50	18(16–22)	13% A; 2% F	50% A; 8% F
Mayo Clinic[214c]	112	65(38–85)	20 minimum	16%	17%
Mayo Clinic[214d]	63	<20	10 minimum	38% A; 25% F	67% A: 19% F
Wrightington[214e]	193	47(23–68 at follow-up)	21(18–26)	7% A; 6% F	
Wrightington[214f]	166	<40	16(10–24)	16% A; 14% F	
Odense, Denmark[214g]	103	62(34–79)	17.6(15–20.6)	10.7%	5% A; 30% F
Odense, Denmark[214h]	37	<55	17.0(15.0–20.6)	11.7%	9% A; 29% F

Key: A, acetabulum; F, femur.

TABLE 49-4   Results of Implants Using Second-Generation Cementing Methods

Location	Number of hips	Age at surgery, range in years	Follow-up, range in years	Revision rate	Radiographic loosening or revised
Massachusetts General Hospital (MGH)[214i]	102	61(21–85)	15	10% A; 2% F	42% A; 3% F
MGH[214j]	50	<50	12(10–14.8)	22% A; 0% F	44% A; 2% F
Iowa[214k]	42	<50	11(10–15)	24% A; 5% F	36% A; 17% F

Key: A, acetabulum; F, femur.

extensively coated components. The stress shielding and femoral bone loss is reduced by comparison. Dorr points out that distal stability is also important.[216] The distal end of the stem should preferably be press-fitted into the diaphysis (the authors underream by 0.5 mm). However, since the distal stem in proximally coated components is uncoated, there is no biological ingrowth distally and no "spot weld" to transfer load distally to the femur and stress shield the proximal bone.

In the largest series to date of extensively porous-coated implants, Engh has followed 166 hips for approximately ten years (6 to 13 years).[217] The overall revision rate was 15 percent: 0.6 percent were revised for femoral loosening while another 1.8 percent appeared radiographically unstable. Thigh pain was 14 percent at the beginning of the series but only 1.2 percent as experience with the implant was gained. Some 4 percent of the patients showed severe bone loss around the implant and 14 percent showed moderate bone loss. Stability of the stem was confirmed by autopsy study. Comparable results with other cementless stems are summarized in Table 49-6.

Metal-Backed Acetabular Prostheses. Metal-backed acetabular components inserted with and without cement were introduced over twenty years ago. Using finite element analysis, several authors predicted decreased stresses and thus lower loosening rates for metal-backed cups.[219–221] Metal-backed components are now in widespread use, far outnumbering the all-polyethylene cups currently implanted. In a comparison of the cups with and without metal backing, Ritter has found statistically significant increases of failure with metal-backed cups (39 versus 25 percent, $p < 0.0001$).[222,223] No other studies are available on the subject at the current time, but if this is reproduced in other studies, return to all-polyethylene acetabular cups will be likely.

Complications
Heterotopic Ossification

Heterotopic ossification (HO) is a relatively common complication of total hip arthroplasty occurring in 20 to 90 percent of all cases.[224] Although usually asymptomatic, heterotopic bone formation can cause major disability in the form of pain and decreased range of motion in up to 7 percent of patients undergoing hip surgery.

TABLE 49-5   Results of Implants Using Third-Generation Cementing (Hybrid) Methods

Location	Number of hips	Age at surgery, range in years	Follow-up, range in years	Revision rate	Radiographic loosening, no revision
Stanford[214l]	121	67(40–88)	6	0% A; 3% F	0% A; 2% F
Mass. General Hospital[214m]	96	61(23–83)	6.5(5–8)	0% A; 1% F	2% A; 1% F
Scripps Clinic[214n]	89	71(41–92)	7(6–8)	1% F	0% A
Rush, Chicago[214o]	109	67(39–85)	5(4–7)	0% A; 0% F	2% A; 2% F

Key: A, acetabulum; F, femur.

TABLE 49-6   Results of Cementless Stems

Location, implant	Number of hips	Age at surgery, range in years	Follow-up, range in years	Revision rate for aseptic loosening, overall revision	Radiograph loosening, no revision	Hip pain
Arlington, VA (AML)[a][214p]	166	?	9.5(6–13)	0.6% (10%)	1.8%	1.2–14%
Washington, DC (PCA)[214q]	91	58(22–81)	5–7	1% (2%)	5%	15–26%
Newcastle upon Tyne (PCA)[214r]	241	47(18–65)	5(2–9)	2%(13%)	27% loose at 8 years (mainly acetabular)	
Rush, Chicago (Harris-Galante)[214s]	121	49(20–70)	5.5(4.5–6.5)	3.3%	9%	
Seoul, Korea (PCA)[214t]	116	48(19–59)	6.3(6.1–7.4)	6%(9%)		

[a]AML (DePUy, Warsaw, IN); PCA (Howmedica, Rutherford, NJ); Harris-Galante (Zimmer, Warsaw, IN).

The exact pathogenesis of HO is poorly understood. Fortunately, risk factors are better understood. The most significant risk factor is previous HO from hip arthroplasty on the same or contralateral leg. Recurrence is very likely and approaches 90 percent in some studies.[226–230] The severity of the recurrence tends to be very similar to that following the original operation. Other risk factors include male sex,[231,232] hypertrophic osteoarthritis,[227,232,233] active ankylosing spondylitis,[234–237] and advanced age.[238,239] There are conflicting data as to the importance of diffuse idiopathic skeletal hyperostosis (DISH) and spinal hyperostosis.[240] Surgical technique also has an influence. Some reports have cited increased incidence of HO in patients with uncemented femoral stems as opposed to cemented stems.[241] The posterior approach also seems to involve lower rates of HO compared to anterolateral and transtrochanteric approaches to the hip.[242,243] However, in a study of 66 arthroplasties there were no significant differences between the cemented and uncemented groups. Surgical approach also did not affect HO rates in this study.[245] Carefully controlling for HO risk factors, Purtill et al.[246] found that there was no significant difference in HO rates between cemented and uncemented arthroplasty groups.

The Brooker system is the most commonly used of the various classification schemes. It is based on the radiographic appearance of the AP pelvis view. Class I represents isolated islands of bone. Class II includes bone spurs with a gap of at least 1 cm between opposing bone surfaces. Class III represents near complete bone bridging with a gap less than 1 cm in size. Class IV is apparent ankylosis.[247]

Two major methods of prophylaxis have evolved. These are medications and radiotherapy. Nonsteroidal anti-inflammatory drugs (NSAIDs) have been shown to de-

crease the incidence of HO. The most studied and used of the NSAIDs is indomethacin. A prospective randomized, double-blinded clinical trial conducted by Schmidt et al.[248] showed no HO in 85 percent of the treated group, while only 25 percent in the patients in the placebo group showed no ossification. More importantly, none of the treated group develop high-grade ossification (i.e., grade III or IV) while 18 percent of the placebo group did. The exact dose and length of treatment with medication is still being investigated. The dosage from the Schmidt study was 25 mg taken three times per day for 6 weeks. A recent study would suggest that 25 mg given three times daily for 2 weeks is just as effective.[236] A number of other medications, such as other NSAIDs[249] and aspirin,[250] have also been investigated. Treatment with aspirin 650 mg twice daily for 6 weeks[236] or with ibuprofen 400 mg three times daily for 6 months[251] appears to produce reductions n HO similar to those of the above-mentioned study. A recent Scandinavian study shows that naproxen taken for as little as 1 week can be effective.[252]

These medications are not without side effects. In one study, as many as 37 percent of patients could not complete the 6-week course of indomethacin because of gastrointestinal side effects, such as gastritis and bleeding.[253] Given that most patients undergoing hip arthroplasty are taking warfarin or low-molecular-weight heparin for deep venous thrombosis, the risk of interaction causing significant bleeding cannot be ignored. There are also studies showing decreased bony ingrowth into porous-coated cementless prostheses in dog femurs.[254] Short-term results in humans do not bear this out, but no long-term studies are available.[255]

Radiotherapy, first proposed in 1981 by Coventry,[256] has become increasingly popular. Current studies show that a single dose of 700 to 800 cGy within 1 to 4 days postoperatively is effective in reducing the incidence of postoperative heterotopic ossification.[257–259] A short-term study suggest that a single preoperative dose of 800 cGy is just as effective as postoperative radiotherapy.[260] Concerns about late malignancy have been expressed, but no malignancy was found in a series of 90 patients followed for 8 years.[257a] The concerns of decreased bony ingrowth raised with NSAID treatment can be avoided by appropriate pretreatment planning, where shields are sized and positioned over these areas as well as trochanteric osteotomy sites.

Because of concern surrounding the side effects of medical treatment and the presumed problem of patient noncompliance with any extended medication treatment, radiotherapy has become the prophylaxis treatment of choice for many surgeons. However, medication, particularly short-course indomethacin, is effective and is the treatment of choice for certain patients, including young women of childbearing age.

Once formed, the character of HO cannot be changed by the above methods of prophylaxis. The timing of surgery remains controversial, but in general excision should be delayed for 6 to 12 months after the original operation.[240,261] Bone scan can be useful to determine the activity of bone formation and thus the appropriate timing so as to reduce the likelihood of bone reformation. Most studies of excision have focused on radiographic criteria for follow-up. Cobb[230a] has examined the functional outcome of excision. Although excision was very effective in increasing range of motion, there was little correlation between radiographs and clinical range of motion. Also, pain relief following excision was extremely variable and again did not correlate with radiographs. Thus, the importance of prevention cannot be understated. Warren[262] followed 12 patients after excision of heterotopic bone; 11 had excellent pain relief and all 12 gained significant motion. As mentioned before, those patients with previous heterotopic ossification are at extreme risk for recurrence, and prophylaxis should be instituted.

Deep Venous Thrombosis

Deep venous thrombosis (DVT) is the most common complication following total hip arthroplasty. DVT rates approach 50 to 70 percent[263] in postarthroplasty patients not treated with thromboembolic prophylaxis. Peak incidence of clinical DVT after arthroplasty occurs at approximately 5 to 10 days after surgery,[264,265] but the period of increased risk is significantly longer—up to three months after surgery.[266,267]

The clinical diagnosis of DVT is unreliable. Its accuracy approaches only 50 percent[268] even with the most experienced clinicians. The "gold standard" for DVT detection remains venography. Contrast dye allergy, superficial vein thrombosis, and patient discomfort limit its usefulness.[269] Duplex Doppler scanning is the most commonly used modality. It has limited effectiveness in detecting thrombi below the popliteal fossa and its accuracy is very dependent on operator technique.[269] The most dangerous sequela of DVT, pulmonary embolism (PE),[270] can be detected by ventilation/perfusion scanning or pulmonary angiography. Postphlebitic syndrome—consisting of pain, swelling, edema, and ulceration—is another serious complication of DVT. In one study following patients 5 years postarthroplasty, postphlebitic DVT was found to affect about one-third of patients and was disabling in about 15 percent of patients despite treatment with full anticoagulation after DVT was detected. Full anticoagulation with intravenous heparin for the treatment of DVT is associated with up to a 45 percent rate of bleeding complication if started within 6 days of surgery.[271]

In general the ideal prophylactic treatment should be effective and well tolerated and have a low complication rate. There are numerous approaches to prophylaxis with varying degrees of efficacy and side effects. There are no reports conclusively showing that one method of prophylaxis is clearly superior to the others, though some are in more widespread use than others.

The different forms of DVT prophylaxis include mechanical devices and various medications. Each agent, of course, has its own advantages, disadvantages, and efficacy. Pneumatic compression devices can bring DVT incidence down to 10 to 20 percent,[272,273] but unfortunately it does a less effective job in preventing proximal vein thrombosis,[274,275] which is more likely to lead to fatal pulmonary embolism.[266] Although originally promising as a prophylactic agent, aspirin does not significantly decrease the rate of DVT following hip surgery.[276,277] A more recent prospective, randomized trial comparing aspirin and warfarin, using both venogram and ventilation perfusion scans, shows no difference between the two groups.[278] Dextran is effective in reducing the incidence of DVT to about 6 percent, but several important side effects such as hypersensitivity and cardiac overload have limited its usage.[279,280] Warfarin (Coumadin) is perhaps the most extensively used form of prophylaxis. Its ability to decrease the incidence of DVT is well documented.[281–284] Postoperative bleeding either at the surgical site or elsewhere continues to be a concern. Careful monitoring is required to maintain therapeutic levels (prothrombin times 1.2 to 1.5 times the control level) without causing excessive bleeding. Fixed minidose warfarin is ineffective.[285] Fixed low-dose heparin (5000 U every 8 to 12 h) has proved to be a failure.[286] On the other hand, subcutaneous heparin administered in adjusted doses (thromboplastin times maintained between 31.5 to 36 s) appears to be quite effective.[287] The newest medication in widespread use is low-molecular-weight heparin (LMWH), which appears to reduce overall DVT incidence to 10.8 percent and proximal DVT to 5.4 percent.[288] In another study, LMWH reduced the risk of DVT by a small amount as compared to warfarin but was accompanied by higher bleeding complications.[289] Although LMWH is more expensive than warfarin, it may be cheaper when all costs are calculated because it requires little monitoring. As compared to fractioned heparin, LMWH appears to be as effective without any increase in bleeding complications.[290] A metaanalysis of randomized trials showed significant differences in the incidence of DVT among studies. The lowest rates of DVT were for LMWH, adjusted-dose heparin, and warfarin, but many regimens had similarly low rates. None, however, reduced the rate to zero.[291] In another metaanalysis, Imperiale and Speroff[292] found that LMWH and compression stockings had the lowest DVT and PE rates (LMWH, 17 percent DVT, 0.7 percent PE; compression stockings, 18 percent DVT, 0.7 percent PE), but compression stockings had a higher proximal DVT rate (13 versus 6 percent). Other methods of prophylaxis such as warfarin (24 percent DVT, 2.7 percent PE, 5 percent proximal DVT) had similar reductions from control (47 percent DVT, 4.0 percent PE, 23 percent proximal DVT).[292] The American College of Chest Physicians has stated that, based on the available literature, LMWH, low-intensity oral anticoagulation with warfarin, and adjusted-dose heparin are the most effective agents for prophylaxis against DVT.[293] Research on DVT prophylaxis has concentrated more on the method of prophylaxis than the duration. The optimal duration of prophylaxis, however, has not been clearly elucidated in the literature. Fitzgerald,[294] in his review of the literature, recommends continuing prophylaxis until "the patient spends the majority of his or her day ambulating with or without assistive devices."

Instability

Postoperative dislocation rates have been reported as varied as anywhere from 1 to 10 percent. Morrey, based on the Mayo Clinic experience, quotes a frequency of 2 to 3 percent. Posterior dislocations typically occur by placing the leg in flexion, adduction, and internal rotation. They make up 60 to 90 percent of postoperative dislocations. Anterior dislocation typically occurs with the leg in the exact opposite position—i.e., extension, abduction, and external rotation—and is more associated with anterior or lateral approaches.[295]

Some 40 to 70 percent of dislocations occur within the first postoperative month. Only 0.4 percent of dislocations first occur more than 5 years after operation, and this is possibly due to capsular stretching.[295] The chance of recurrence is lower if the first dislocation happens within the first month of surgery than if it happens later than 3 months postoperatively.[296]

Many preoperative risk factors have been studied including age, sex, height, underlying diagnosis, and prior surgery. Of these, female predominence in the order $2:1$[156] and prior hip surgery with a more than doubled dislocation rate are statistically significant.[295,297] Intraoperative factors associated with higher rates of dislocation are surgical approach and component orientation. Femoral head size[156,297,298] and myofascial tension have not been associated with higher rates of dislocation. Posterior approach appears to increase posterior dislocation rates by varying degrees (as much as two- to threefold in the Mayo Clinic experience).[156] Of all the risk factors, component, especially acetabular, position is perhaps the most important variable in predicting dislocation. However, component orientation is extremely difficult to evaluate with plain radiographs because of the three-dimensional nature of the orientation.[299,300]

Closed treatment consisting of immobilization in either hip spica cast or brace for 6 to 12 weeks is successful in approximately two-thirds of all cases.[301,302] Approximately 1 percent of all hip arthroplasties will re-

quire surgical revision because of persistent instability.[156] Only about 40 percent of unstable hips will have poor orientation of one or both components.[303–306]

Given that most dislocations happen in a specific direction (i.e., posteriorly), an acetabular liner with an elevated rim would be expected to reduce dislocation rates. In a Mayo Clinic series with 2-year follow-up, dislocation probability was reduced from 3.85 to 2.19 percent using a 10° elevated-rim liner.[307] However, Krushell et al.,[308] in a cadavaric study, found that routine use of elevated-rim liners offered no benefit in cases of correctly positioned components. They recommended the use of elevated-rim liners in cases of instability secondary to poor acetabular cup positioning where the cup position could not be easily changed, as in a cemented acetabular component. Further studies are needed to determine the exact indications and benefits of these components.

Neurovascular Injury

Fortunately, neurovascular injuries are relatively rare. In a series of over 3000 hip arthroplasties, Schmalzried[309] reports injuries in 1.7 percent of all arthroplasties and 1.3 percent of primary arthroplasties. Revision surgery increased nerve palsy rates to 3.2 percent and congenital dysplasia/dislocation increases the rates to 5.2 percent. Limb lengthening only partially accounted for these high rates. The sciatic nerve was overwhelmingly involved. The obturator and femoral nerves are involved less commonly. Partial injuries are more common than complete injuries and are often masked. Combined nerve injury occurs in as many as 20 percent of cases.[310,311] All patients with complete recovery had it by 21 months. Dysesthesias predict poor outcome.[309]

Often the exact cause of nerve palsy is unknown. Known causes of sciatic nerve palsy include direct injury (i.e., via retractor, reamer, cautery, suture, scalpel), postoperative dislocation, bleeding, and lengthening.[278,289,311,312] The femoral nerve can be injured in a similar fashion as well as femoral artery pseudoaneurysm.[313] Obturator nerve injury has occurred secondary to intrapelvic utilization of drills, screws, or cement.

The placement of transacetabular screws for fixation of metal cups has been carefully studied by Wasilewski.[314] Four quadrants are formed by first drawing a line from the anterosuperior iliac spine through the center of the acetabulum to the ischial tuberosity, dividing the acetabulum in half. A second line is drawn perpendicularly to the first line through the midpoint of the acetabulum, thus creating quadrants. The two anterior quadrants are associated with damage to the external iliac artery and vein as well as to the obturator nerve, artery and vein. The anterosuperior quadrant is sometimes termed the "zone of death."

In two retrospective and one prospective studies, the surgical approach used does not appear to affect rates of nerve palsy.[315–317] Use of cortical somatosensory evoked potential (SSEP) which is often done for spinal procedures, was first reported by Stone et al.,[318] who found SSEP monitoring to be extremely useful. However, a more recent study seems to show that SSEP monitoring is not effective in either predicting or preventing sciatic nerve palsy.[319]

Injuries to almost all of the major blood vessels have been described. These include damage to external iliac artery and vein, common femoral vessels, profundus femoral vessels, obturator, superior and inferior gluteal vessels, and internal pudendal vessels. These can occur in any phase of hip arthroplasty including patient positioning, exposure and retraction, leg positioning, and component placement.[320]

Femoral Fractures

Femoral fractures are a rare complication of hip arthroplasty occurring in only about 0.1 to 3.2 percent of cemented arthroplasties.[321–324] Increases in the intraoperative femoral fracture rate have directly paralleled increasing use of uncemented press-fit components, occurring in anywhere between 3 and 28 percent in the literature.[325–329] Cemented hip arthroplasty is associated with significantly lower fracture rates. In revision surgery, fractures tend to occur in weakened areas of bone and can occur in any phase of the surgery.[325]

Intraoperative fractures are best avoided by using careful surgical technique. Not all intraoperative fractures are recognized by the surgeon at time of surgery. In Schwartz's series,[329] only 50 percent of fractures were noted intraoperatively. For fractures above the tip of the planned prosthesis, internal fixation with cerclage wire/cable should be employed. Postoperative rehabilitation is based on the stability of fracture fixation construct. Khan[330] reports excellent results using this method of treatment. Supplemental bone grafting is a useful adjunct which will accelerate healing. Fractures not noted intraoperatively are in general stable and can be treated conservatively with activity modification and hip spica casting/bracing. Schwartz[329] treated fractures not discovered intraoperatively in this fashion and reoperated on displaced fractures. In this series, all fractures healed and the results were equivalent to those without fracture. Others have shown good results from similar treatment methods.[328,331]

Based on an in vivo canine experimental model, cortical perforations near the tip of the proposed prosthesis should be bypassed with a longer stem that extends at least two cortical diameters below the perforation. Femoral strength with the defect bypassed in this manner was about twice that of a femur with a defect not thus bypassed.[332] If the perforation is not noted intraoperatively, conservative treatment may be tried until the defect has filled with bone, but this area is at major risk for periprosthetic fracture. If this does happen, reoperation with removal of cement and bone grafting should be considered.[333,334]

Postoperative periprosthetic fractures are being reported more commonly. The incidence is estimated to be between 1.5 and 4 percent by Duncan and Masri[335] in their review of the literature. Treatment modalities advocated in the literature include conservative treatment with casting/bracing, revision arthroplasty with a longer-stemmed prosthesis, long-stemmed prosthesis with allograft, and open reduction and internal fixation with plates, screws, and wires. Nonoperative treatment risks include malunion and the risks of limited activity in the elderly.[336,337] In cases where the fracture is associated with a loose prosthesis, revision with a long-stemmed prosthesis is advised. Bone grafting or proximal femoral replacement may be necessary. Cement, often used in these cases, should not be allowed to extrude into the fracture site, as this will interfere with fracture healing.[335] For solidly fixed prostheses, especially in younger patients, open reduction and internal fixation (ORIF) is recommended. Various fixation methods have been used. Excellent results for ORIF with standard AO/ASIF hardware and technique were reported by several studies.[338–340] The Ogden plate has been developed to allow for adequate proximal fixation without violating the cement mantle. This plate uses Parham bands proximally for fixation and standard cortical screws for fixation below the femoral stem. Ogden and Rednall,[341] Wang et al.,[342] and Montijo et al.[343] have reported 100 percent union rates with minimal complications. Equally successful results can be achieved with a standard plate and multiple Dahl Miles cables provided that sufficient length of plate is applied proximally and distally (10 to 15 cm). Routine bone grafting has been advocated by many.[339,344–346]

ARTHRODESIS OF THE HIP

Hip arthrodesis remains an acceptable alternative to total hip arthroplasty in certain indicated cases, yet few of these operations are performed. This operation was most applicable in the early part of the century, when antibiotics were nonexistent and tuberculous arthritis was prevalent. At that time, extraarticular hip arthrodesis was considered in such patients to immobilize the infected joint. Now performed by a combination of intraarticular and extraarticular techniques, it remains a viable reconstructive option in young patients in whom hip replacement should be considered as a last resort.

Indications and Contraindications

The indications for hip arthrodesis today are noncontroversial. Arthrodesis should be the first consideration in young, active laborers with unilateral, posttraumatic arthritis of the hip. This is the optimal situation for this procedure, since total hip replacement in these patients has done poorly. Consideration for arthrodesis should also be given to very obese patients as well as patients suffering from painful arthritis as a result of sepsis or tumor. Failed arthroplasty patients may be technically impossible to fuse. Prerequisites include a compliant patient without lumbosacral disease who has a normal ipsilateral knee and contralateral hip.

Contraindications include neuropathic joints and severely compromised bone stock about the hip. Arthrodesis in patients with osteonecrosis of the hip remains controversial and is generally not recommended.

Technique

The ideal position for a fused hip is in 20 to 25° of flexion and neutral rotation. Some 5° of adduction or external rotation is well tolerated. Abduction and internal rotation at the hip should be avoided. Less than 20° of flexion makes sitting difficult and greater than 25° makes ambulation trying and may contribute to back pain.

Recent emphasis on the preservation of the hip abductor mechanism has modified the approach to hip arthrodesis. The possibility of a successful conversion to a total hip arthroplasty after the patient ages makes sparing the abductors an important consideration.

Open preparation of the hip joint through the posterior approach with the patient in the lateral position, followed by rigid internal fixation with an AO Cobra plate, is the most common method used. Intraarticularly, the joint surfaces are congruently reamed to bleeding cancellous bone and any defects are filled with autogenous bone. Rigid fixation from the ilium to the femoral shaft is always preferred and also allows intraoperative compression across the joint through the plate and AO compression device. The classic technique includes a greater trochanteric osteotomy to enhance the exposure as well as to provide bone graft.[347] A concurrent pelvic osteotomy has also been described (see Fig. 49-12). This pelvic osteotomy is no longer recommended, since it may compromise the integrity of the acetabulum if future conversion to arthroplasty is contemplated. Recently the Vancouver technique has been described.[348] It includes the careful preservation of the hip abductors by reattaching the greater trochanter after the fixation has been inserted.

A technique that calls for anterior exposure of the hip joint and anterior internal fixation has recently been described.[349] This method avoids any disturbance of the abductor mechanism by proceeding anteriorly and placing a large dynamic compression plate from the anterior ilium to the anterolateral femur. Difficulty in "bending" the plate to accommodate the flexed hip at the time of fusion may be experienced.

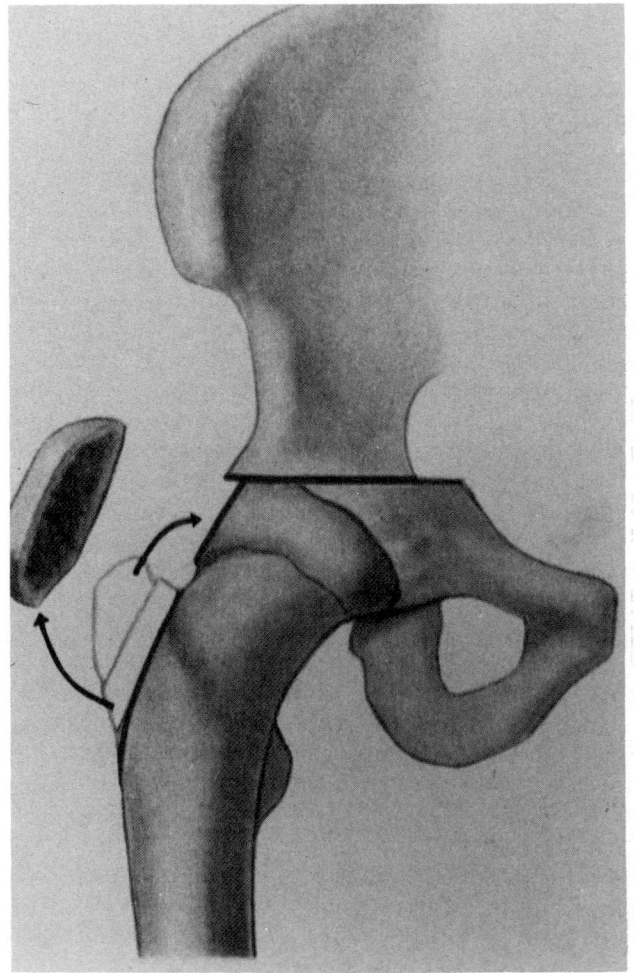

A

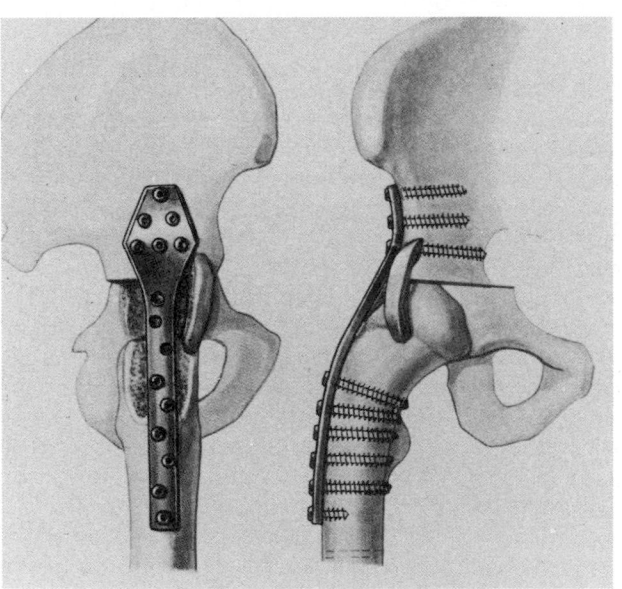

B

Figure 49-12 Arthrodesis of the hip using the Cobra plate. *A.* A pelvic osteotomy has been performed with displacement. Two broad slices of bone are resected from the greater trochanter. One of these will be inserted between the plate and the head. The second will be slotted as a graft anteriorly. *B.* The plate is in situ and compression arthrodesis has been performed (technique of Dr. R. Schneider). (Reproduced with permission from Mueller ME et al: *Manual of Internal Fixation: Techniques Recommended by the AO Group.* Berlin, Heidelberg, and New York, Springer-Verlag, 1979, p 339.)

Results

In the classic report by Sponnseller et al., 78 percent of patients were satisfied with hip arthrodesis after 20 years. Only 13 percent of these patients had undergone a conversion to hip arthroplasty for relief of back or knee discomfort.[350]

In a study by Callaghan et al.,[351] pain in the ipsilateral knee occurred in 60 percent of the patients and back pain in about the same proportion, but not until an average of 23 years later. Laxity of the ipsilateral hip is found in 75 to 80 percent of patients, particularly if fused in abduction.[351]

Duncan reported on 19 patients with an average age of 33 years. Only 1 patient had an unsatisfactory result using a modified hip score.[348]

REVISION HIP SURGERY

The survival rates of both cemented and cementless revision are inferior to those of primary hip surgery. Also the incidence of complications in both the short and long term in association with revision hip surgery exceeds that found in relation to primary arthroplasty.

The reconstruction of these hips, particularly those associated with massive bone loss, is as challenging as any surgical procedure in the orthopaedic repertoire and is not, therefore, for the novice hip surgeon.

Evaluation of the Painful Prosthesis

History and Physical Examination

Before concluding that the patient complaining of symptoms in the region of the hip has a problem with the hip prosthesis, one should carefully consider and eliminate other causes. Spinal canal stenosis can irritate the L5 to S1 nerve roots and give pain that radiates from the outer quadrant of the buttock into the trochanteric region. Occasionally similar pain may be experienced which is of vascular origin or related to a trochanteric bursitis. There may be a trochanteric nonunion associated with broken wires or free-floating hardware.

Pain in the groin or down the front of the thigh on weight bearing associated with a painful limp is strongly suggestive of a hip origin for the pain. If the possibility of sepsis exists, then a past history of a longer than usual period of postoperative drainage from the wound, following the initial arthroplasty, may be significant.[352] Occasionally one may identify an unusual cause of pain around the hip, such as a stress fracture, which does not indicate a serious problem with the prosthesis.[353]

Pain radiating down the front of the thigh has long been known to be a significant indicator of a loose femoral component. However, there are other rarer causes of pain in the thigh, such as obturator nerve entrapment associated with intrapelvic protrusion of cement. Fortunately this kind of complication is now less often seen. Occasionally a patient will give a history of subluxation of the hip with a sponta-

neous reduction. When this occurs in a hip that has been satisfactory for many years, it often indicates failure of the acetabular component or its fixation. Recurrent dislocation is a much more dramatic event, usually associated with repeated visits to the emergency room and a necessity for intervention and reduction under conscious sedation.

When the clinical history and physical examination indicate that the hip prosthesis is most probably the cause of the symptoms, it is important to differentiate sepsis from aseptic loosening of the implant.

Laboratory Investigations

An erythrocyte sedimentation rate (ESR) remaining above 40 mm per hour more than 6 months postoperatively is highly suggestive of the presence of infection.[354] The white cell count (WBC) has no value in diagnosing infection. In acute infection, blood cultures may be positive.

The value of routine aspiration of the hip joint for evaluation of the painful hip prior to revision surgery is controversial. Barrack and Harris[355] recommended that aspiration be performed only for selected patients as determined by clinical history or x-ray changes suggestive of infection. Only 2 percent of hips routinely aspirated prior to revision surgery were determined to be infected in their series. Lachiewicz and his coauthors showed that preoperative aspiration of the hip joint has a sensitivity of 92 percent, a specificity of 97 percent, and an accuracy of 96 percent.[356] These authors also favor a selective approach to aspiration, which they believe to be a valuable and accurate test. They do not recommend aspiration for those hips in which the implant has been in situ for more than 5 years if the patient has a normal ESR. They recommend aspiration for all hips that are painful within 5 years of the arthroplasty and those that have an abnormally elevated sedimentation rate.

In addition to the ESR, the C-reactive protein (CRP) is a laboratory test that is helpful in differentiating the infected joint from the hip with aseptic loosening. This protein is synthesized by hepatocytes and is normally present only in trace amounts. The CRP increases rapidly to 200 to 400 mg/L of plasma within 48 h after prosthetic joint replacement (the normal is 5 to 10 mg/L) but normalizes within 3 weeks. A CRP value in excess of 20 taken in conjunction with an elevated ESR is highly suggestive of periprosthetic infection.[357,358]

Imaging Studies

Radiology Barrack and Harris believe that periostitis, diffuse lysis, and endosteal scalloping are particularly significant radiographic markers for infection, and if these are present they will recommend diagnostic aspiration of the hip. Radiolucent lines in themselves are seen in both septic and aseptic loosening, and endosteal erosions are commonly found in both conditions. The presence of periosteal new bone, however, is specific to the infected hip joint. Unfortunately, however, it is seen in only a small proportion of cases, when it is usually at the junction of the metaphyseal and diaphyseal portions of the femur on the medial side.[352] Rapid progressive bone lysis has always been regarded as significant for osteomyelitis, but particulate wear debris can cause bone destruction, making the differential diagnosis difficult on plain radiographs.

For cemented components, recommended criteria for loosening on plain radiographs have traditionally included (1) a 2-mm or wider bone/cement interface, or progressive widening beyond 2 mm on serial images; (2) a discernible cement prosthesis radiolucency; (3) cement fracture, component migration, or bone destruction.[359]

Using component migration as the only criterion for loosening, O'Neil and Harris correctly predicted the status of 92 percent of their femoral components and 63 percent of acetabular components.[360] Subsequently, Harris has revised his opinion of the significance of radiolucent lines, pointing out that these indicate internal bone remodeling and do not necessarily represent degradation of the bone/cement interface. He points out that laboratory testing of retrieved specimens of implants showing radiolucent lines indicate that these prostheses are often well fixed.[361] It follows, therefore, that it is more important than ever to evaluate migration or subsidence, since these are critical indicators of loose implants. Much attention is, therefore, being paid to radiologic methods of evaluating small changes of position in prosthetic implants. This is necessary for cementless implants, where radiographic evaluation of the painful component is more difficult. Metal markers may be implanted intraoperatively and used for accurate measurement of migration. The use of an acetabular template such as the Muller template is also of value. It has been shown that careful measurements of the migration of cementless components and the detection of early prosthetic micromotion can predict later failure due to loss of fixation.[362,363] The characteristic radiographic signs seen on plain films that distinguish a stable uncemented component from an unstable one have been described. The importance of careful sequential radiologic examination is clear. the presence of progressive implant migration is a major sign of implant instability.[364–366] The absence of reactive lines adjacent to the porous surfaced portion of the implant and the presence of "spot welds" of endosteal new bone contacting the porous surfaces are considered major signs of osteointegration. By contrast, the appearance of a bony pedestal beneath a stem tip, which has some periprosthetic osteolysis around it, is highly suggestive of micromotion and loosening.[364]

Arthrography Arthrography is traditionally performed simultaneously with hip joint aspiration. In and of itself it seems to have limited value, particularly in the evaluation of cementless components. It is doubtful if a needle should be inserted into the joint purely for the purposes of arthrography unless the previously described indications for joint aspiration are also present. Skin flora may be cultured, giving false positives. There is also some risk of introducing infection into the joint by this intervention. Radionuclide arthrography has been claimed to be more accurate than routine arthrography in the detection of loosening (95.5 percent versus 73.3 percent).[367]

Nuclear Medicine Studies The use of scintigraphy in diagnosis of the infected prosthesis has been well reviewed in several publications.[368–370] Indium 111 (^{111}In)–labeled WBC scintigraphy will accurately diagnose sepsis in a much higher proportion of cases than will the earlier technetium gallium techniques, which are not now believed to be effective methods for ruling out sepsis in the painful hip prosthesis.[371,372] After cemented total hip arthroplasty, it takes approximately 1 year for patients to exhibit no significant increase in uptake when they are evaluated with technetium. In the case of cementless components, however, the majority of the patients still have increased uptake around both components as long as 2 years from surgery, although at this time the level of activity is stable or decreasing. Findings have been similar for cementless implants utilizing ^{111}In–labeled WBCs.[373]

Indium 111-labeled human nonspecific polyclonal immunoglobulin (IgG) is a relatively new method of evaluating musculoskeletal infection already being usefully employed in Europe. Fitzgerald suggests it may be particularly important in diagnosing low-grade infections. The same author also points out that a new scintigraphic agent currently undergoing FDA evaluation, technetium 99m (^{99m}Tc monoclonal antibody), may be more accurate than ^{111}In-labeled IgG polyclonal antibody.[352,370]

Both bone scans and sequential radiographs are equally reliable in the diagnosis of simple loosening in the painful hip. However, bone scanning is expensive and is recommended only when the radiographs are inconclusive.[372,374]

The Infected Hip Arthroplasty

Fitzgerald has classified deep periprosthetic infection into three stages.[352,370] Stage 1 sepsis occurs in the immediate postoperative period and is usually the result of infection with *Staphylococcus aureus* or group B streptococcus, perhaps seeding a hematoma. Stage 2 sepsis he defines as the appearance of an infection 6 to 24 months following surgery. In many such cases the organism will often be methicillin-resistant *Staphylococcus epidermidis.* Stage 3 sepsis is characterized by a long latent period before the appearance of the infection (more than 2 years from surgery). Presumably stage 3 infection is the result of hematogenous spread infection from some other source within the body or associated with a serendipitous event, such as a breach of the skin or mucous membrane (e.g., in association with dental work performed without prophylactic antibiotic coverage).

It can be extremely difficult to diagnose early wound infection in the immediate postoperative period, particularly since the patient is on anticoagulants. There is often continuing serous drainage from the wound for several days. If the patient does not exhibit systemic symptoms suggestive of infection or does not have a fever or local pain, local serous drainage is usually innocuous. A subcutaneous hematoma will sometimes produce an area of erythema and perpetuate such drainage, and the diagnosis then is even more difficult. If drainage continues beyond 10 days or so, the temptation to prescribe additional "prophylactic antibiotics" (which is unfortunately a temptation to which many surgeons fall victim) is to be avoided. Instead, it is preferable in these circumstances to take the

TABLE 49-7 Virulence of Causal Microorganisms in Septic Hip Prostheses

Less virulent
 Staphylococcus epidermidis
  (methicillin-susceptible, non-glycocalyx-forming)
 Staphylococcus aureus
  (methicillin-susceptible, non-glycocalyx-forming)
 Anaerobic Gram-positive cocci
 Streptococci (other than enterococci)
More virulent
 Gram-negative bacilli
 Staphylococcus epidermidis
  (methicillin-resistant, glycocalyx-forming)
 Staphylococcus aureus
  (methicillin-resistant, glycocalyx-forming)
 Group D streptococci (enterococci)

Source: From Fitzgerald RH Jr: Infected total hip arthroplasty: Diagnosis and treatment. © 1995, American Academy of Orthopaedic Surgeons. Reprinted from the *Journal of the American Academy of Orthopaedic Surgeons* 3:249–262, 1995, with permission.

patient to the operating room and perform wound irrigation after taking appropriate cultures. If there is a deep hematoma, it can be evacuated and the wound thoroughly irrigated and then closed. If, during exploration, infection is suspected but thought to be entirely superficial, the deep fascia need not then be reopened. If drainage is seen to be coming from the joint deep to the fascia, then the depths of the wound should be reexplored and the prosthesis itself thoroughly irrigated. In a normal host, infections due to a pathogen of low virulence appearing up to 3 weeks following surgery may be treated by such irrigation and appropriate parenteral antibiotics in an attempt to save the implant. Microbiologic factors that should influence the decision include the nature of the infecting organism and its ability to manufacture glycocalyx, a glycoprotein that facilitates the adhesion of the organism to orthopedic implants (Fig. 49-13).[352,370,375]

In stage 2 sepsis, the differential diagnosis from aseptic loosening will be made by the diagnostic methods already outlined. A high ESR and CRP will initiate an aspiration and a positive aerobic or anaerobic culture will establish the diagnosis. There may be additional radiologic features unequivocally suggestive of sepsis. The in-

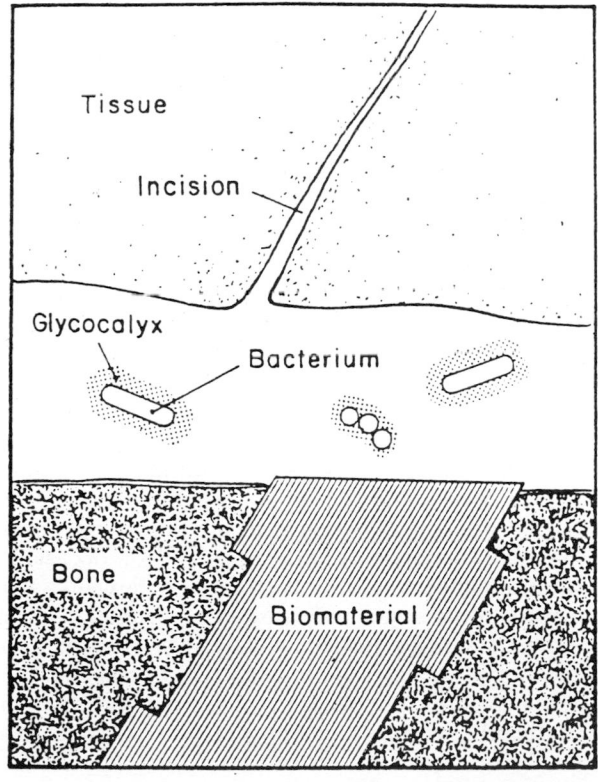

A

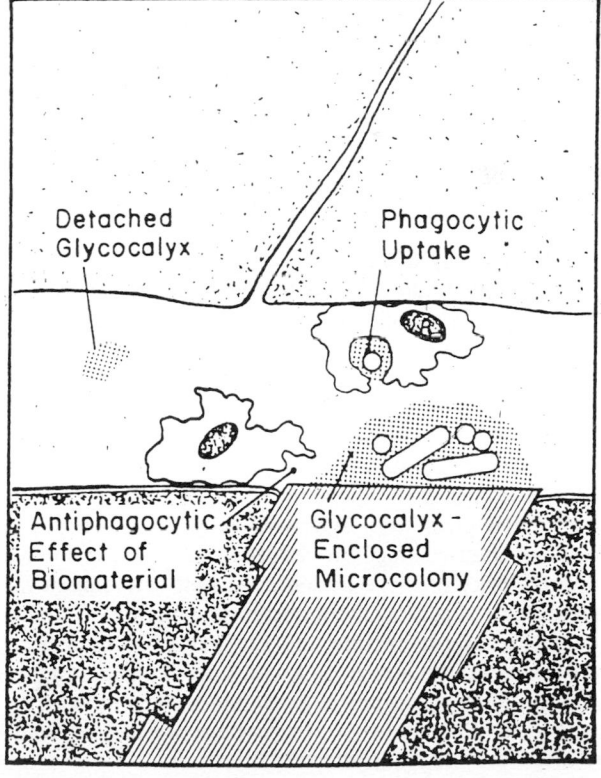

B

Figure 49-13 Diagrammatic evolution of an infection associated with a prosthetic biomaterial. *A.* Initially, bacteria are introduced into the wound. *B.* They express their natural tendency to adhere to an inert surface, on which they are protected by the antiphagocytic effect of the biomaterial and also on which they form as microcolonies within a biofilm that protects them from phagocytic uptake and from nonimmune and immune antibacterial factors. *C.* When the bacterial microcolony has burgeoned to a greater size, the ion-exchange function of its glycocalyx affords a measure of protection from antibiotics and appears to protect the bacteria from bactericidal and opsonizing antibodies. (Reproduced with permission from Gristina AG, Shitata AY, et al: The glycocalyx, biofilm microbes and infection. *Semin Arthrop* 5:160–170, 1994.)

dium bone scan will be confirmatory of infection. In the event that all preoperative studies are inconclusive in differentiating the septic hip, the surgeon is faced with two options, either to perform a small local biopsy (in the case of a well-fixed prosthesis) or, alternatively, to perform a first-stage removal of the implant and use the opportunity to take deep cultures (this will be the case if the implant is radiologically clearly loose). Although intraoperative, Gram stains are of little value,[376] intraoperative cultures by contrast, have been the "gold standard." Recently, however, their value has been reconsidered by Padgett and coauthors, who point out that a positive intraoperative culture may not be predictive of implant sepsis. They recommend permanent histologic analysis as being more reliable.[377]

In a well-fixed prosthesis with little radiologic change, where all preoperative diagnostic tests are negative for infection, the finding of a positive aspirate may raise the question of whether contamination of the specimen has occurred. The culture under these circumstances will merely represent skin flora. In that case, if all other tests are negative for infection, a second aspiration may be performed before deciding whether to revise the loose implant in one stage or alternatively to remove the implant, take deep intraoperative cultures, and perform a second-stage reconstruction. A frozen section taken intraoperatively of the periprosthetic membrane may help in making this decision. Mirra and coauthors have stated that the presence of more than five polymorphonuclear leukocytes per high-power field, pointing to acute inflammation, is the single most reliable indicator of infection at the time of revision surgery.[378] However, this test may not be reliable in inflammatory disease such as rheumatoid arthritis. If it is decided to perform a second preoperative aspiration, then the technique of fine needle aspiration and radiometric culture described by Roberts and coauthors may be useful.[379] This technique takes 2 weeks to give a result, however, and is therefore only applicable in a nonurgent situation.

With perhaps the exception of some early stage 1 infections, where the implant may be preserved, the surgical procedures required are similar for all stages. Although one-stage reimplantation has had some popularity in Europe utilizing gentamicin-impregnated cement, it is not widely used in the United States. One-stage exchange may be considered for low-virulence organisms (e.g., *Streptococcus viridans*), but the two-stage procedure is appropriate and safer in the majority of these patients. At first the implant must be removed, plus all cement and hardware, and there must then be meticulous wound debridement of all infected material. Deep cultures may be taken from tissue, implant, or any fluid present within the joint. It is well to look beneath the psoas and in any other areas where pus may be located and make sure that the wound is thoroughly debrided and irrigated prior to closure.

The techniques for removing all of the cement from the femur usually involves some kind of osteotomy. This may be a standard trochanteric osteotomy or the extended proximal trochanteric osteotomy (described later in the chapter). It is important to remove all of the cement if the infection is to be overcome. It is also important not to devascularize large portions of bone.

Antibiotic beads fabricated from polymethylmethacrylate (PMMA) and impregnated with tobramycin are usually placed in the joint prior to closure over several drains. Several smaller PMMA beads strung on a wire are preferable to one large piece of PMMA because of the relatively larger surface area available for the antibiotic to leach out. Appropriate systemic antibiotics are commenced and modified if necessary when definitive cultures are in hand.

Ideally, one would like to wait up to a year prior to reimplantation, since the recurrence rate is less with a longer interval. In practical terms, however, patients are loathe to tolerate a Girdlestone type of excision arthroplasty for very long. When there is an appropriate organism and the ESR has progressively declined to normal without clinical signs of infection, most surgeons will consider reimplantation as early as 2 months following debridement and implant removal. There may be circumstances relating to host resistance or the nature of the infecting organism which may extend that period considerably. Recently Colyer and Capello have reported an 84 percent success rate using a two-stage reimplantation technique with an interval of only 1 month.[382] They point out that intervals approaching 1 year are a particular hardship on elderly patients. They also stress the importance of a further debridement of the wound at subsequent reimplantation.

Techniques for hip reconstruction following bone loss are described later in this chapter. Fitzgerald points out there may be more than two stages in the treatment of the severe infection with extensive bone loss. It may be necessary to debride the bone extensively to successfully eliminate a virulent infection, so that there is then an even larger bone stock deficiency to be subsequently restored. Such a problem may be appropriately managed utilizing bone grafting as a second stage and then reimplanting the prosthesis as a third procedure after the bone graft has incorporated and matured.[352]

Skin ulceration, chronic disease, or chronic urinary tract infections must be aggressively treated if successful reimplantation is to be achieved. Malnutrition in elderly patients must be reversed. A recent review reported that two-stage reimplantation can be successful in 71 percent of cases when local antibiotics are not used but is successful in 93 percent of patients when local antibiotics supplement the systemic treatment of the infection.[383] On occasion it will be determined with some regret that reimplantation of a new prosthesis is not indicated in a particular patient since the functional gains are unlikely to be rewarding and the risks may be high, due to associated comorbidity. A Girdlestone arthroplasty is occasionally pain-free, particularly if the psoas tendon's femoral attachment is still intact, but for the most part it leads to a poor result.

Aseptic Loosening

The diagnostic features of aseptic loosening have already been described. Particulate wear debris from polyethylene has been shown to be a major factor in the loosening of both cemented and uncemented prostheses.[383] It appears that particulate debris activates macrophages, which then not only stimulate osteoclasts to resorb bone but may themselves play a direct role in osteolysis by the release of proinflammatory cytokines.[384,385] Cytokines present in the periprosthetic membrane in association with a loose implant include interleukin one alpha, one beta, and also interleukin-6 (IL-1 alpha IL-1 beta and IL-6). In addition, the prostaglandins (PGE-2) and tumor necrosis factors (TNF alpha and beta) are also present (Fig. 49-14). These agents can inhibit the synthesis of matrix molecules such as glycosaminoglycans and type 1 collagen. They can also stimulate the release of enzymes that degrade the matrix.[385] Because of the problem of polyethylene wear, it is now recommended that 32-mm heads not be used, since it is important to have an 8- to 10-mm thickness of polyethylene in the acetabular component.[386]

The normal wear of a Charnley polyethylene cup has been estimated to average approximately 0.2 mm per year.[387] Isaac suggests that barium present within small particles of PMMA may scratch the metallic femoral head of a Charnley prosthesis and increase the rate of polyethylene wear.[389] Accelerated wear of the polyethylene has also been associated with the use of titanium femoral heads; the preferred materials now are chrome cobalt or ceramic.

Many other factors that promote accelerated wear in polyethylene are now known. There is an acknowledged relationship with the shelf life of the implant and the use of gamma sterilization techniques.[390,391] Some designs for capturing the polyethylene liner in the metal shell have been flawed, promoting early failure or unacceptable wear rates of the plastic.[392] The use of screws as an adjunct in the fixation of acetabular components should be avoided unless absolutely necessary because of the risk of producing metallic debris when there may be subsequent component migration.

Revision Surgery for Aseptic Loosening

When osteolysis has progressed so far that imminent fracture of the femur is likely, revision surgery is planned with some degree of urgency. Occasionally a patient will appear in the emergency room with a periprosthetic fracture associated with severe osteolysis. The problems of the loose implant and the fracture are then dealt with simultaneously. However, this is a less than optimal setting and these emergency events should be avoided if possible. Timely intervention will permit a more leisurely diagnostic workup and the exclusion of sepsis. Careful serial evaluation of bone loss will produce an appropriate management plan and ensure that revision is performed before osteolysis has progressed too far. Well in advance of revision surgery, the entire operating team should be aware of the nature of the planned reconstruction. This is particularly important when special equipment is required to remove cement or when customized components or allografts must be identified in advance and made available in the operating room.

Techniques of Cement and Implant Removal

Certain situations will mandate that a particular surgical approach be utilized. A posterior column deficiency in the acetabulum will require appropriate exposure of the sciatic nerve prior to reconstruction. This cannot be conveniently performed if the patient is supine or if some of the more anterior approaches are utilized. Occasionally the femoral component is satisfactory and it is only the acetabular component that needs to be revised. Under these circumstances, usually the modular head can be removed from the femoral component to improve exposure and the Morse taper carefully protected with a gauze sponge tied to it. The femur may then be retracted anteriorly or pos-

Figure 49-14 Model depicting the biological events associated with the pathogenesis of aseptic implant loosening after total joint replacement. Mechanical factors contribute to the fragmentation of the implant surface and release of particulate materials. These particles are responsible for the formation of the peri-implant granulomatous reaction. Interaction between the cells present within the granuloma and the particles (contact and phagocytosis) result in the release of a variety of soluble products (cytokines, proteinases, and prostaglandins) that act on bone cells (osteoclast and/or osteoblasts) to directly or indirectly enhance focal bone resorption. These same products may also stimulate fibroblasts to produce increased extracellular matrix proteins and enhanced fibrous tissue deposition. (Reproduced with permission from Wang JT, Harada Y, et al: Biologic mechanisms involved in the pathogenesis of aseptic loosening of total joint replacement. *Semin Arthrop* 7:70–73, 1996.)

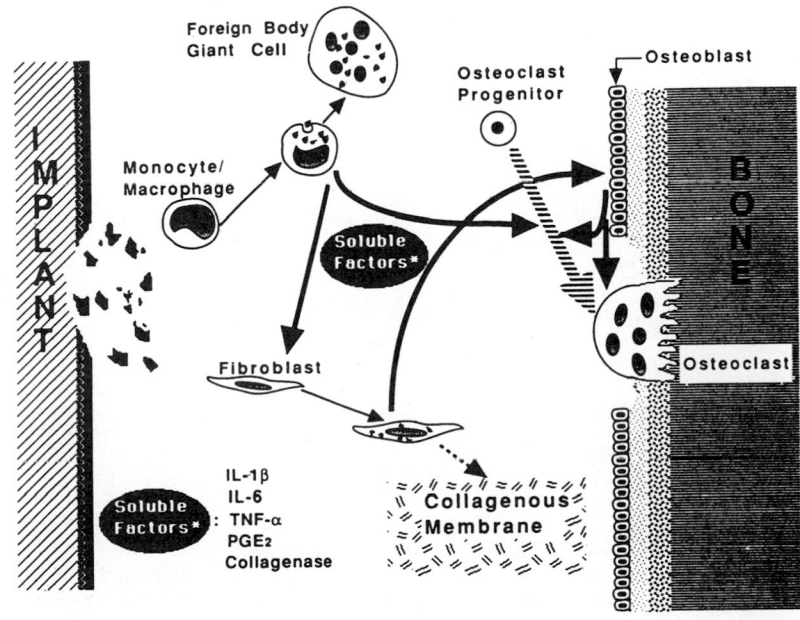

teriorly, depending upon the approach favored by the surgeon. If one chooses a lateral or anterior approach and the femur is retracted posteriorly while the hip is conveniently flexed and adducted to give acetabular access, there is some risk to the common peroneal division of the sciatic nerve. If one elects a posterior approach and retracts the femoral component anteriorly, there is some risk to the femoral nerve. These problems are made worse if the femoral component is nonmodular, so that there is even more restricted access. Trochanteric detachment may improve the access but does not completely solve these problems. In selected cases, the femoral component can be removed from the femur without disrupting the cement mantle; then, after acetabular revision, it can be reinserted into the same cement mantle with a fresh mix of cement interposed.[393] If this is not feasible and good acetabular access is blocked, the femoral component must also be revised.

A well-fixed femoral component can be extremely difficult to remove (Fig. 49-15), particularly if porous-coated or precoated with PMMA. For this reason, some surgeons prefer to use a smooth-textured femoral component for ce-

mented hip arthroplasty and a cementless component that is porous-coated only proximally. If an ultrasonic tool is available for cement removal, trochanteric osteotomy can usually be avoided, since the distal cement can be removed without damaging the femoral cortex.[394] In suitable cases, particularly if the cement mantle is loose, one may employ the technique in which additional cement is placed around a threaded rod and then allowed to cure. After the old cement has adhered to the new cement, the entire mantle and plug can be removed in segments by replacing the threaded rod with the tool provided.[395] Osteotomy of the great trochanter in the classic Charnley fashion will usually give good access and visualization of the cement mantle almost down to the midportion of the stem. In the region of the plug, however, when using a Midas-type tool, most surgeons will want to have either the comfort of fluoroscopic visualization or will alternatively utilize the technique of controlled anterior femoral cortical perforations to complete the removal of cement.[394] Accidental perforation of the femoral cortex, with its associated morbidity, is thus avoided. The elective anterior perforations need be only 5 mm or so in diameter but permit an additional view of the end of the burr as it progresses down the femur (Fig. 49-16). The perforations can also be used to introduce a flexible light into the region of the distal cement. The authors do not favor large cortical windows, which predispose to fracture. It is important for the mechanical integrity of the femur and the success of the subsequent revision that femoral fracture be avoided. Elective cortical perforations must be made anteriorly. The posterior cortex, particularly in the region of the linear aspera, must not be violated.

A variation of the trochanteric osteotomy useful in revision surgery is one in which the trochanter is detached and retracted anteriorly together with the abductor muscles and a variable portion of the vastus lateralis muscle in con-

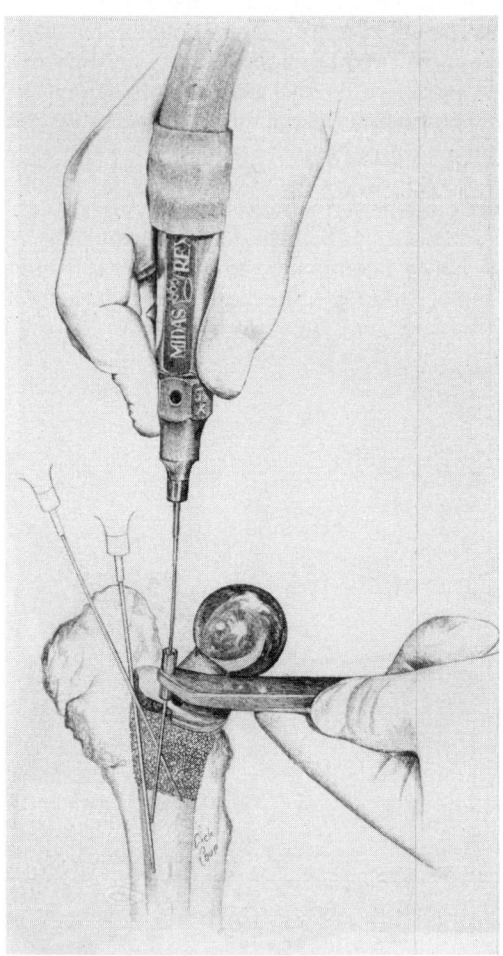

Figure 49-15 Illustration depicting use of flexible Midas Rex AC-1 dissecting tool and guide. The collar of the porous coated femoral component has been partially milled away with a WH-1 or WH-3 dissecting tool. (Courtesy of Richard Coup, EdD, Midas Rex Institute, Fort Worth, TX.)

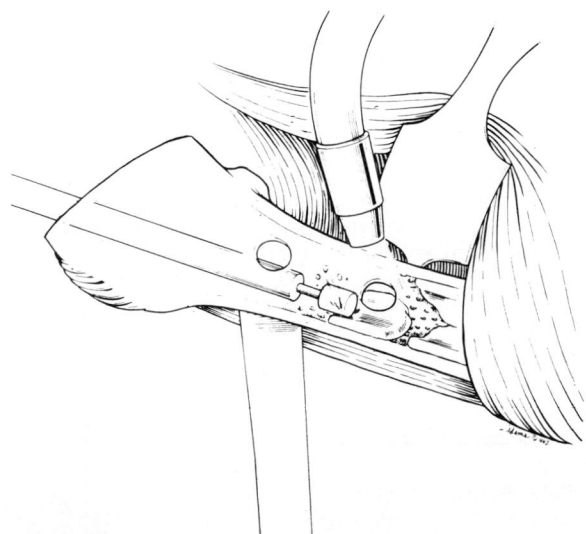

Figure 49-16 Controlled perforation technique for removal of PMMA. (Reproduced with permission from Lombardi AV Jr: Cement removal in revision total hip arthroplasty. *Semin Arthrop* 3:264–272, 1992.

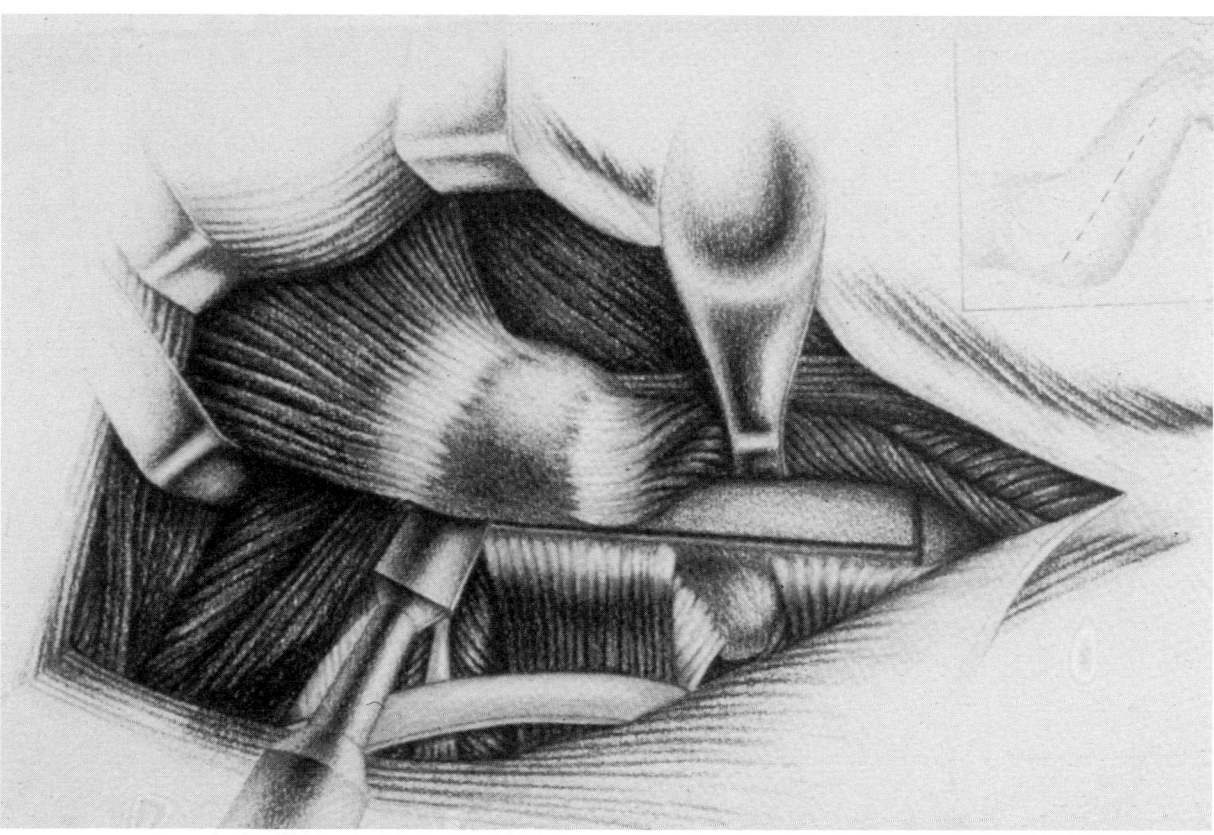

Figure 49-17 Extended proximal femoral head osteotomy. The greater trochanter is removed in continuity with a portion of the anterolateral cortex. (Reproduced with permission from Roberson JR: Proximal femoral bone loss after total hip arthroplasty. *Orthop Clin North Am* 23:291–302, 1992.)

tinuity (thus providing an extensile approach to the anterior and lateral femoral diaphysis, which is useful for performing anterior perforations). Extended proximal femoral osteotomy is another technique that has also been found useful for removal of distally fixed cemented components and cement mantle and also well-fixed distally porous-coated femoral components. In this technique (Fig. 49-17), an anterolateral portion of the proximal femur, approximately one-third of its circumference, is osteotomized along a length of 12 cm or more and hinged open anteriorly with its intact sleeve of periosteum and muscle.[396] None of these osteotomy techniques should be undertaken lightly, and meticulous reconstruction is essential. Conventional trochanteric osteotomy has a nonunion rate that may be over 20 percent in revision surgery.[398] Head and Mallory have described an extensile lateral approach to the hip without trochanteric osteotomy that they believe gives excellent access to the femur and acetabulum for revision total hip arthroplasty.[397] In this procedure, the vastus lateralis is retracted anteriorly in continuity with the anterior fibers of the gluteus minimus and medius. The thick tendinous insertion of the gluteus medius is preserved. A sliver of trochanteric bone is retracted together with the muscle. This procedure is performed with the patient in the lateral position, and the midlateral skin incision inclines slightly posteriorly, so that access to the posterior portion of the joint is also available.

Engh has described the removal of the ingrown fully coated cementless component by cutting through the midportion of the femoral prosthetic stem, having obtained access through a small femoral cortical window. The component is then removed in two portions. The proximal portion can be removed by dividing the prosthesis bone bond using a cutting tool without destroying the metaphysis. The distal portion of the cylindrical stem of this component is then removed using a trephine, which is accurately sized to remove the distal stem with only a minimum amount of bone.[400]

Occasionally, an approach to the anterior column of the pelvis is required to reconstruct the anterior segment of the acetabulum (Fig. 49-18). Under these circumstances, an extensile iliofemoral approach is used.[401] This approach may also be performed as an extension of the anterior limb of a triradiate exposure of the hip, which is favored for difficult revision hip arthroplasty by some authors.[401,402] The triradiate incision is recommended for those cases where obesity, acetabular protrusion, or fragile femoral bone makes safe adequate exposure impossible using a more routine approach. This incision has not been found to cause additional healing problems, but the technique must be followed with precision.[402]

The acetabular component is removed after separation of the polyethylene liner. In the cases of non-metal-

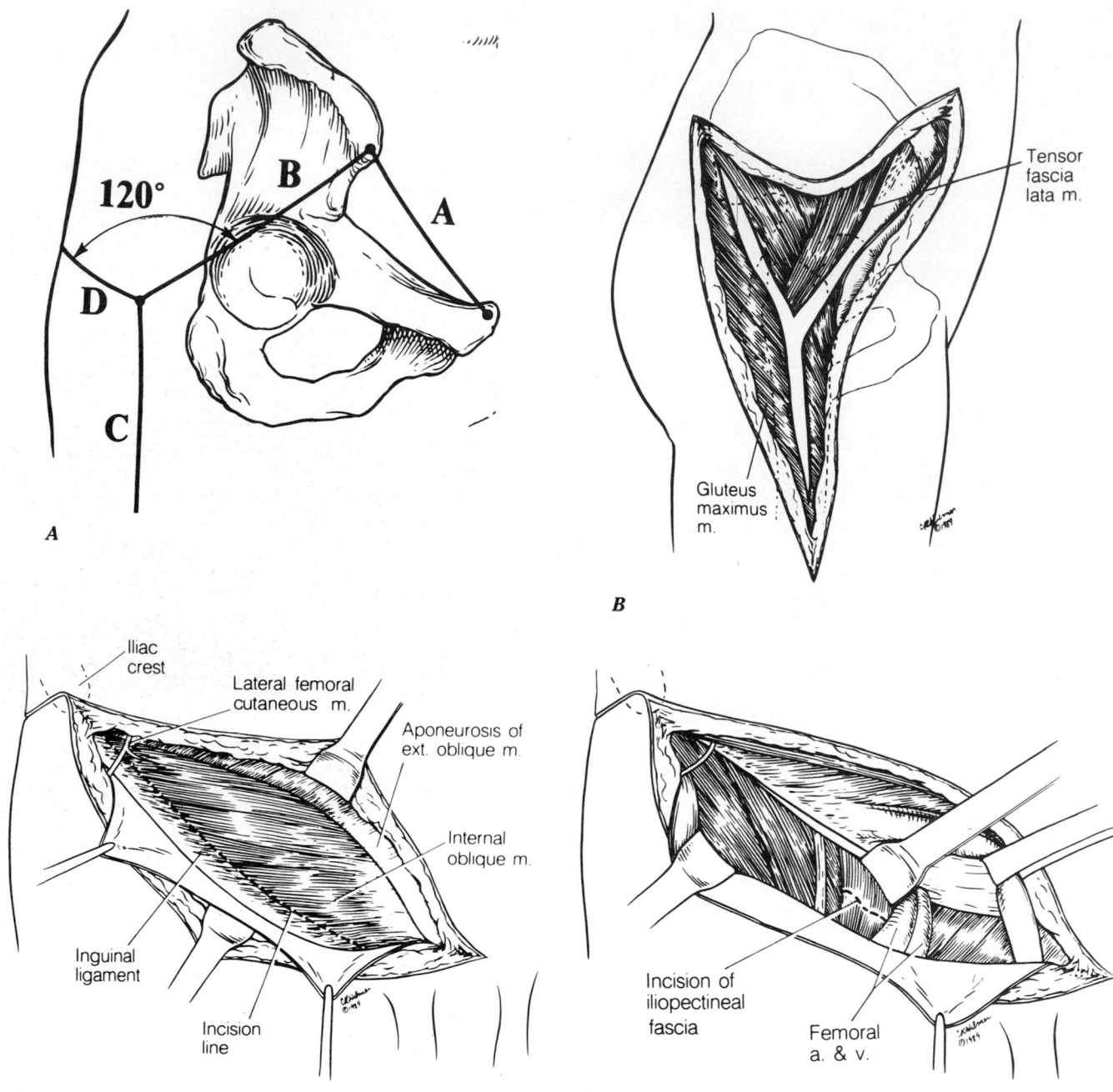

Figure 49-18 *A.* Extensile triradiat incision with 120° superior limbs (B and D) and extension from anterior superior iliac spine to pubis (A). *B.* Muscle dissection. Note that limb B dissection is anterior to tensor fascia lata muscle. *C.* Incision of external oblique muscle aponeurosis 1 cm above liguinal ligament. *D.* Inguinal ligament incised and also iliopectineal ligament lateral to femoral artery. Spermatic cord, femoral artery and vein, and psoas with femoral nerve each encircled with Penrose drains.

E. A difficult reconstruction that will require this surgical approach. There is pelvic disassociation and an anterior column deficiency. *F.* Reconstruction completed. There is an anterior column plate which incorporates bulk allograft to restore the anterior column. This is also a posterior pelvic reconstruction plate from ilium to ischium. (Reproduced with permission from Stiehl JB: Extensile anterior column acetabular reconstruction in revision total hip arthroplasty. *Semin Arthrop* 6:60–67, 1996.

backed polyethylene sockets, these can be cut into quarters using an appropriate cutting tool, such as the Midas, and then removed. After any fixation screws have been carefully removed, a swan-neck type gouge applied closely to the convexity of the metal-backed socket can usually remove even a well-ingrown socket with minimal bone loss.

Classification of Femoral Bone Deficiencies and Their Reconstruction

The various classifications of bone loss in total hip arthroplasty have recently been reviewed.[404] The authors concluded that the classification of the American Academy of Orthopaedic Surgeons (AAOS) hip committee is the most

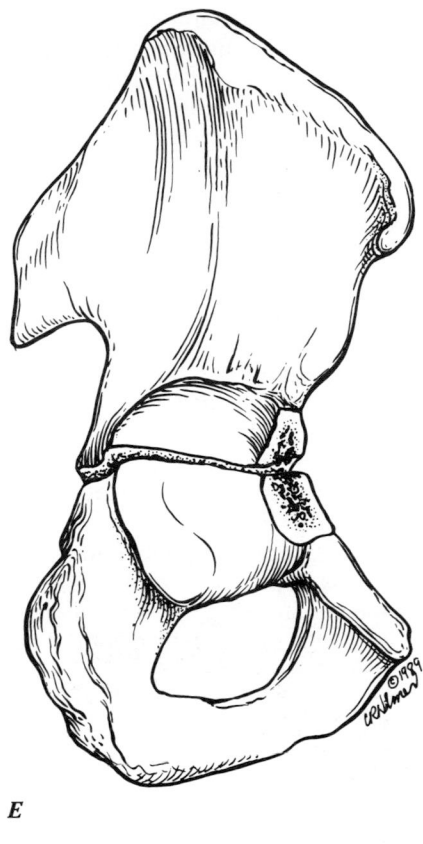

E

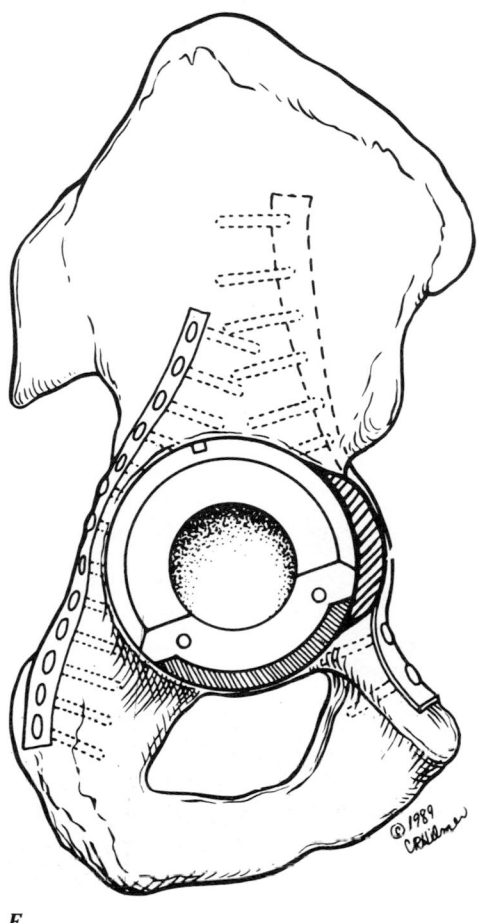

F

Figure 49-18 *(Continued)*

comprehensive and consistent (Table 49-8). This classification identifies *segmental defects,* which are lesions in the supporting cortical shell of the femur, and *cavitary defects,* which are excavations of the cancellous or endosteal cortical bone without violation of the outer shell of the femur. These may be partial or complete and are identified by their anatomic location. A segmental defect surrounded by bone (e.g., a window) is termed an *intercalary defect. Ectasia* is a subclassification referring to an enlargement of the medullary canal without cortical perforation but usually associated with marked thinning of the cortex (a ballooning effect). The classification also includes fractures of the femur (*femoral discontinuity*), which occur occasionally during revision.[403] In addition to the classifications shown in the table, a subclassification also defines the level of bone loss. Level 1 is proximal to the inferior portion of the lesser trochanter, level 2 between the inferior border of the lesser trochanter to 10 cm below it, and level 3 is anything distal to level 2. The classification also grades the amount of bone loss. Grade 1 is minimal bone loss with good host prosthetic contact maintained; no bone grafting is therefore required. In grade 2 bone loss, good support of the prosthesis is still maintained by the host bone but some bone graft may be required. In grade 3 bone loss, there is such loss of host prosthetic contact that structural bone graft is required for the reconstruction.

From the practical point of view, one may be faced with a femur where there is no calcar remaining and the metaphysis cannot support the stresses of load bearing of an implant. There may be a thin, sclerotic cortex unsuitable for cement and similarly unable to provide sufficient mechanical support to the revision prosthesis without augmentation. Implant stability by press-fit is likewise unattainable in such a femur without some additional support measures. Intercalary defects may be present, which predispose to the extrusion of bone cement with the potential for additional complications. The bone is often so thin that it must be carefully handled intraoperatively or the outcome will be further prejudiced by the development of a femoral fracture.

Cemented Revision Femoral Stems   In all femoral reconstructions, it is important that as much host bone as possible be preserved. The revision procedure should certainly not subtract from the complement of host bone and, in cases of severe bone loss, should add to it. In the case of cementless revision, it is critically important that implant stability be obtained at surgery to permit biological ingrowth between the host bone and the porous-coated implant.

Because of anxieties concerning the development of osteolysis, some authors have been loathe to advise cementless revision, particularly using long-stemmed femoral components. They believe that such implants may act as an attractive conduit, allowing particulate wear debris to reach more distal portions of the femur. These authors

TABLE 49-8 The American Academy of Orthopaedic Surgeons Classification of Femoral Deficiencies in Total Hip Arthroplasty

Segmental deficiencies
   Proximal
      Partial
         Anterior
         Medial
         Posterior
      Complete
   Intercalary
   Greater trochanteric
Cavitary deficiencies
   Cancellous
   Cortical
   Ectasia
Combined segmental and cavitary deficiencies
Malalignment
   Rotational
   Angular
Femoral stenosis
Femoral discontinuity

cite substantial improvement in the results of femoral revision with the use of contemporary cementing techniques.[405–409] The failure of cemented revision femoral components has been reported as low as 6 to 11 percent at 10 years and approaching 20 percent at 5 years which is a considerable improvement over the results obtained with early techniques of cement handling.[406,407,409]

One of the problems with cemented revision is that it usually adds no new bone to the patient's femur and acetabulum, so that if a subsequent revision is necessary, there may then be little host bone left to revise. In those cases where there is extensive femoral osteolysis but the cortical tube is still able to provide firm support for a cemented prosthesis without allograft, impaction grafting of morcellized bone into the femur prior to the insertion of cement has facilitated the restoration of bone stock and avoided the necessity of using a long-stemmed component with cement. This technique has been popularized by Ling and associates and its early success in the near term has led to its adoption by other authors.[407–409] The technique involves clearing the marrow cavity of all residual cement debris and fibrous membrane and then occluding the femur distally using a plug placed 2 cm distal to the most distal area of bone lysis. Any cortical defects are covered by fine wire mesh held in position by cerclage wires. Additional support for large proximal defects is provided by reconstruction plates, which, in turn, support mesh, which will help constrain the bone grafts. The canal is then packed with cancellous allograft bone chips prepared from femoral head allografts and morcellized. When the femur is filled with graft, approximately 8 to 10 cm below the tip of the greater trochanter, a tapered femoral trial component is impacted into the chips. This oversized component creates a wedge-shaped envelope within the medullary cavity as it pushes the bone chips up against the wall of the femoral canal (Fig. 49-19). The procedure is repeated until the whole femur has been reinforced internally on its endosteal surface by bone chips vigorously impacted against the cortical shell. The tapered femoral component is then cemented into the envelope created in the proximal femur. It is anticipated that there will be some subsidence of the construct and the cement mantle, but a recent retrieval study demonstrates that this technique restores bone stock in the proximal part of the femur and apparently acts as a barrier to the distal migration of polyethylene particles. Subsidence has been measured, averaging 2.8 mm in 48 percent of these stems within the cement mantle. But only 7 percent of the cement graft composites subsided within the cortical tube at short-term follow-up (31 months).[410] There were no cases of femoral stem revision, which contrasts favorably with the 5-year follow-up results of the tapered stem used as a primary implant.[411,412]

In cementing a revision component, most surgeons favor "going short" as opposed to going long with a long-stemmed component. Short-stemmed components can be removed together with the cement mantle if subsequent further revision becomes necessary. On the other hand, the problem of revising a long-stemmed cemented component is formidable. However, if femoral bone is deficient due to intercalary defects, there is no alternative to inserting a component at revision that has a longer stem than the original implant. If the perforation is less than one-third of the femoral diameter, it is preferable that the revision stem should extend beyond the area by $2\frac{1}{2}$ canal diameters. If the stem is cemented, that is sufficient, and no bone grafting of the defect is required. If the femoral deficiency is greater than one-third of the diameter of the femur, however, additional onlay bone grafting is required.

Authors have reported their results using long-stemmed cemented revision femoral components. In Turner's series of 110 hips evaluated at least 5 years from surgery, 30 percent were rated fair or poor. However, only one-third were rated excellent.[414]

Cementless Revision Femoral Stems Good success has been reported at a minimum of 5 years follow-up using uncemented, extensively coated porous stems and relying on good distal fixation for femoral revision.[415] Significant osteolysis was not observed in this series, and it may be that the large area of bone ingrowth acts as a barrier to polyethylene migration along the long-stemmed uncemented implant. Those who use this technique emphasize that the proximal femur is often a biologically and mechanically poor environment for either proximal porous ingrowth or the use of proximal cement. They believe that extensive porous coating and diaphyseal fixation is a reliable and durable method of femoral reconstruction in these difficult cases.

A different approach has been taken by others who utilize proximal load-bearing cementless prostheses together with cortical onlay strut allografts to restore the structural integrity of a damaged proximal femur.[416] For this technique to succeed, it is essential that the revision porous-coated prosthesis be stabilized at surgery. The deficient femoral bone stock must be augmented by allograft and load must be transferred directly to the proximal fe-

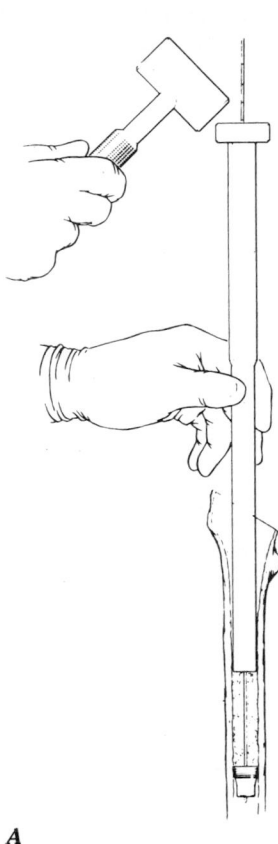

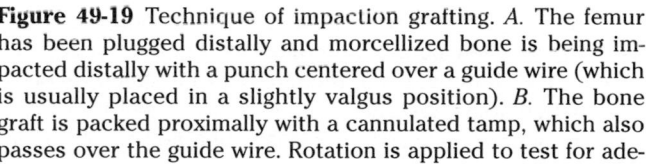

A

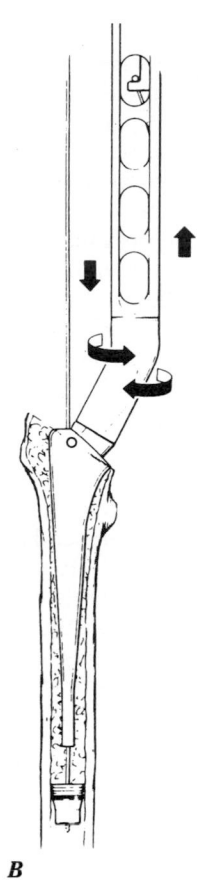

B

Figure 49-19 Technique of impaction grafting. *A.* The femur has been plugged distally and morcellized bone is being impacted distally with a punch centered over a guide wire (which is usually placed in a slightly valgus position). *B.* The bone graft is packed proximally with a cannulated tamp, which also passes over the guide wire. Rotation is applied to test for ade-

quate seating of the tamp as the femur is prepared for cement and prosthesis. (Reproduced with permission from Nelissen RGH, Bauer TW, Weidenhielm LR, et al: Revision total hip arthroplasty with the use of cement and impaction grafting. *J Bone Joint Surg* 77A: 412–422, 1995.)

mur, so that future proximal femoral resorption is minimized. A calcar replacement prosthesis may be used proximally so that load is transferred directly to the region of the lesser trochanter. The area immediately beneath the load-bearing bone in the lesser trochanteric region and distally to it is augmented with cortical strut allografts. The authors of this technique report 3 percent failure at 3-year follow-up, with grafts incorporated in 98 percent of cases adding bone stock to the damaged femora.[416]

Certainly if one attempts to reconstruct a severely deficient femur using a long-stemmed and proximally porous-coated implant, failure is certain unless the implant is stabilized in the metaphysis. Also the metaphysis must be mechanically reinforced, if necessary, to prevent subsidence. Femoral cortical onlay strut allografts have been reported to be satisfactory both from a mechanical and a biological point of view for reinforcement of the deficient metaphyseal region, augmenting the patient's bone stock. Their incorporation into the femur occurs in the majority of cases.[417,418]

A popular porous-coated modular component frequently used for cementless revision because of its functional adaptability is the modular S-Rom.[419,420] This pros-

thesis has a modular conical collar, available in a number of different configurations, that can be positioned so as to obtain support either on the calcar or (if rotated 180°) on the flare of the greater trochanter within the medullary cavity. This modular collar is porous-coated and, when appropriately fitted, can provide a biological seal in the metaphyseal region, which appears to be resistant to the distal migration of polyethylene particles. If the metaphyseal bone is deficient, however, it will again require augmentation and mechanical support. Distal fit is achieved by reaming the diaphysis to receive the long diaphyseal stem of the component, which may then be press-fitted distally. Proximally, the stem is impacted within the collar, where there is a Morse taper fit. This implant, despite anxiety about its modularity and the possible generation of particulate metal debris associated with that fact, has given 69 percent excellent results in a recent reported series, with 11 percent poor results.[420] The follow-up period, however, was only 2 to 6 years. Nevertheless, the results are encouraging.

It is extremely difficult to insert a nonmodular (one-piece) long-stemmed proximally coated cementless femoral revision prosthesis, either straight or curved, into the compromised femoral bone one finds at revision.[419,420] This is particularly the case as one attempts to achieve good fit and fill in both the diaphysis and metaphysis. It is not surprising that a 46 percent incidence of intraoperative femoral fracture is reported and a 20 to 40 percent incidence of subsidence within 5 years has been documented for some of these implants.[421,425]

In cases where the proximal femur is simply too deficient to be reconstructed and, therefore, unable to support any kind of prosthesis, the alternatives are either a custom-made segmental implant that replaces the upper portion of the femur with metal or, alternatively, the use of a major structural allograft.[422,423,426]

The proximal femoral allograft has considerable flexibility, since it can be cut to many configurations. In one technique, a long-stemmed revision component is cemented into the allograft, which is used to replace the upper 6 in or so of the femur, depending on the level of proximal bone damage in the host femur. If the isthmus of the host femus is not completely destroyed, it may be possible to obtain a press-fit distally of the prosthetic stem within the host diaphysis. If this is impossible and the distal stem is cemented into the host femur, it is important to accurately oppose the allograft to the host femur, preventing cement interposition. This is particularly important because union of the structural allograft to the host femur is essential for long-term success. If cement is not used, we prefer to protect the junction between allograft and host femur with a cortical onlay graft banded to the allograft proximally and the host distally. Plates are also available with grooves suitable for cables, which can also be used for this purpose. It is unnecessary to spend a great deal of time fitting the prosthesis into a small allograft; therefore, a good-size allograft should be ordered from the bone bank. It is not necessary to match the size of the allograft to the patient precisely. Chandler recommends using a prosthesis with a fluted stem to resist rotation but does not routinely reinforce the junction with a bone graft or a plate.[423]

Chandler has described other ways of ingeniously using allograft fashioned in customized ways to fit particular applications.[424] He will use a portion of full-thickness iliac crest to form a new calcar, placing it beneath the collar of the prosthesis inside the residual medial metaphyseal bone, so that it is under compression. Alternatively, he may cut a piece of metaphyseal bone shaped like a truncated cone from the cancellous bone of a femoral head or upper tibial metaphysis, using it to fill a large ectasia of the femoral metaphysis. Again, one should stress that the goal is to achieve implant stability, so that allograft bone may subsequently be successfully incorporated or at least unite to the host bone (large structural allografts are not fully replaced by host bone).

Classification of Acetabular Bone Deficiencies and Their Reconstruction

The classification of acetabular deficiencies adopted by the AAOS is shown in Table 49-9. The definition of segmental and cavitary deficiencies is the same as that for the femur.

TABLE 49-9   The American Academy of Orthopaedic Surgeons Classification System for Acetabular Deficiencies in Total Hip Arthroplasty

Type	Description
Type I	Segmental deficiencies
	Peripheral
	Superior
	Anterior
	Posterior
	Central (medial wall absent)
Type II	Cavitary deficiencies
	Peripheral
	Superior
	Anterior
	Posterior
	Central (medial wall intact)
Type III	Combined deficiencies
Type IV	Pelvic discontinuity
Type V	Arthrodesis

Kavanagh et al. reported on 81 acetabular components that had been revised with a cemented component at a mean follow-up period of 4 to 5 years after revision. Of those sockets which had been previously revised for aseptic loosening, 50 percent were again loose.[427] Second and third revisions with cemented acetabular components have even poorer outcomes.[428] The use of cement together with allografting techniques to augment acetabular deficiencies has been found to have a failure rate at 8 years of over 50 percent.[429] It is probable that as the allografts are gradually incorporated by host bone, there is some bone resorption and the cement/bone interface simply cannot take the new additional stresses. Silverton and coauthors observed that the reported rate of failure of cemented acetabular components was between 17 and 60 percent at 2 to 8 years of follow-up. They contrasted this with the results of their cementless acetabular revisions, which showed 87 percent survival at 11 years. However, they also observed a 3 percent rate of progressive radiolucent lines in these latter patients, which may be related to their use of screw fixation to guarantee implant stability.[430] Revision total hip arthroplasty in the acetabulum is now usually performed using a cementless component.[430,431]

However, progressive osteolysis remains a troubling problem. Factors that increase the rate of polyethylene wear or encourage the production of metallic debris have already been described. Also important is the prevention of peripheral areas of poor contact between the prosthesis and the bone. Such gaps may predispose to the migration of debris particles and facilitate osteolysis.[432]

Larger-diameter acetabular components are required in order to obtain stability by rim fit at revision. There is always some bone loss associated with the revision procedure, and the larger component also lowers the center of rotation to partially compensate for a slightly higher position.

Dorr has observed that it is occasionally necessary to medialize the component so that the dome of the cup protrudes into the pelvis. It is often necessary to place the cup in a sufficiently medial position to achieve satisfactory superolateral coverage with host bone in the revision situation. He notes that this breach of the medial wall did not have any negative effects on his results.[434]

Most acetabular revisions can be satisfactorily achieved provided that the anterior and posterior rims are sufficiently preserved to support the implant. If there is sufficient bone medially, a small-diameter reamer may be used at first to medialize in the region of the fovea until the base of the fovea is exposed. At that point the acetabular reamer is quite abruptly redirected from its medially directed path into the appropriate alignment for acetabular placement. At this juncture, the dimensions of the sequential reamers should be increased relatively rapidly to the appropriate size necessary to achieve a rim fit. While this is done, the reamer is gently held in the medialized position but does not penetrate further medially. Care must be taken not to ream out the anterior column. When the reamer fits snugly within the newly fashioned envelope without being able to be displaced in any direction, reaming is concluded and an acetabular component that is undersized by 2 mm will then obtain stable rim fixation. Any remaining superolateral deficiency up to 25 percent of the acetabular area can be confidently filled with morcellized bone graft. If there is anxiety about the stability of the fit, it is usually because the anterior rim has been inadvertently damaged during the procedure. Screws are then advisable, but they must be inserted carefully, avoiding the "zone of death" (see previous discussion of neurovascular injuries under "Complications") or other positions where they may impinge upon important neurovascular structures. Morcellized allograft has been shown to incorporate almost completely some 83 months after insertion.[433] This material is also useful for filling a contained cavitary defect beneath a revision acetabular component that has achieved good rim fixation. Under these circumstances, incorporation of the bone graft may be expected to occur rapidly. Morcellized bone graft may be used to reconstruct contained anterior wall and medial wall defects. Its use with the insertion of a bipolar prosthesis has, however, been shown to lead to a high rate of failure and is not recommended.[434,435]

Reconstruction of Segmental Deficiencies Posterior segmental deficiencies must always be reconstructed, otherwise the acetabular revision will fail. One recommended technique has been to incorporate a femoral head allograft into the posterior rim deficiency. A pelvic reconstruction plate is attached to the ilium, then to the graft, and finally to the body of the ischium. By reaming a convexity within the fixed femoral graft, one then restores the posterior wall of the acetabulum. If there is associated pelvic dehiscence (disassociation), an additional plate is placed posteriorly to the first plate, passing directly from the ilium to the body of the ischium (see Fig. 49-18*F*).

The anterior column may also require plating in complete pelvic disassociation. In such cases and also where there is a segmental bone deficiency of the anterior column, a bulk allograft may be required to fill the segmental deficiency beneath the plate in the region of the iliopectineal eminence. The plate is fixed to the pelvic surface of the ilium and then supports the bulk allograft beneath the psoas. Its medial end is fixed to the pubis adjacent to the symphysis with screws. This technique is similar to that used for pelvic fracture reconstruction (See Fig. 49-18*F*).

Paprosky[438] believes that structural allografts should be used to stabilize a porous-coated acetabular component in a revision situation for that critical period of time during which the implant will achieve biological fixation. Clearly there must be sufficient host bone in contact with the implant for this to occur. Paprosky has classified acetabular deficiencies into three categories to provide a rational basis for surgical intervention. In his classification, a type 1 deficiency is very similar to a primary acetabulum, with perhaps some cement holes present but no major structural defects. Type 2 represents the most common acetabular deficiency, with some distortion of the superior rim associated with lysis and migration but with the anterior and posterior columns still intact, so that a rim fit may still be achieved. Component migration is less than 2 cm superiorly and there is minimal lysis of the ischial region or around the teardrop, indicating an intact posterior rim. Type 2 deficiencies are subdivided by Paprosky into type 2A deficiencies, with superomedial migration; type 2B deficiencies, with superolateral migration; and type 2C deficiencies, with medial migration. Since a rim fit may be achieved in type 1 and type 2 revisions, the potential for successful ingrowth is good. If the superior deficiency is contained, then morcellized bone graft or an oblong acetabular components may be used to fill it. The latter commercially available component has a hemispheric extension on the superior aspect of the component, which can be fitted congruently into an appropriately reamed superior contained cavitary defect.

A Paprosky type 3 acetabular deficiency has a superior migration greater than 2 cm, as measured from the superior obturator line, with severe ischial and medial osteolysis. The recognition of these x-ray signs indicates that the acetabular rim will not support a component without repair. An essential part of the Paprosky subclassification identifying the type 3 deficiency is the status of the implant relative to the ilioischial line of Kohler (Fig. 49-20). If this line is intact, some 30 to 60 percent of the surface porous coating of the component will be in contact with support allograft, and this classifies the deficiency as a type 3A defect (the remainder will be supported by host bone). However, in those patients where component migration has transgressed Kohler's line (which is no longer intact), the classification changes to type 3B. This indicates that over 60 percent of the component will not be supported by host bone but will only be in contact with the support allograft. The type 3B defect is a massive defect in which the failed component has usually migrated 3 cm or more above the upper margin of the obturator foramen and there is severe damage to the anterior and posterior columns and the dome as well.

For the type 3A defect, Paprosky recommends that a distal femoral allograft be cut in the shape of "figure 7" and placed so as to reconstruct the superior rim and cav-

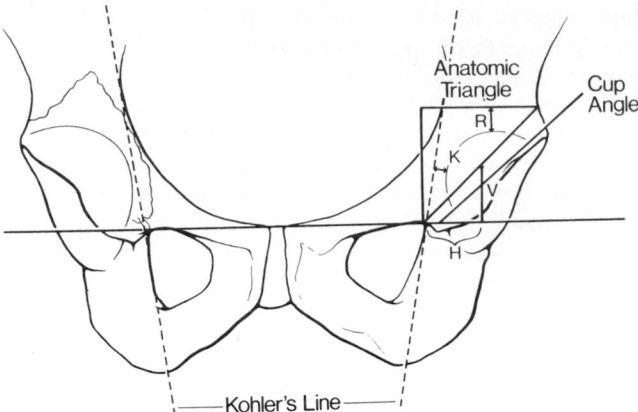

Figure 49-20 Drawing illustrating Kohler's line. This important line is drawn along the medial border of the ilium and ischium. In evaluating the correct placement of the acetabular component, the anatomic triangle of Ranawat is drawn as follows: From a point 0.5 lateral to the intersection of Kohler's and Shenton's lines a vertical line is drawn upward for one fifth the height of the pelvis (about 5 cm). A horizontal line is then drawn for the same distance and the equilateral triangle marking best placement of the acetabular component is completed. Other lines (R, K, V, H) are references off this triangle. (Reproduced with permission from Padgett PE, Kull L: Revision of the acetabular component without cement after total hip arthroplastis. *J Bone Joint Surg* 75A:663–673, 1993.)

itary defect (Fig. 49-21). In these patients, a porous-coated prosthesis can be used with the expectation that about 50 percent or more of the host bone will be in contact with the implant and so permit good long-term biological fixation. In the case of the 3B deficiency (superior migration

more than 2 cm but with Kohler's line no longer intact and severe teardrop and ischial lysis), Paprosky has now abandoned the use of the "figure 7" graft and recommends instead that a total acetabular transplant graft be used and the revision prosthesis cemented into this graft.[438a] The graft is fashioned to fit the defect. This means cutting the ischium and pubic rami away from the graft so that it may abut with the host bone and then be fixed in place with cancellous screws. The iliac portion of the graft is cut to provide a rim of allograft that fits on the external aspect of the host ilium and is likewise attached with screws (Fig. 49-22).

For those severe deficiencies that Paprosky classifies as type 3B, alternative techniques are now available. For many years the Oh-Harris metal reinforcing protrusion shell has been available.[439] It fits on the rim of the acetabulum and substitutes for a severe medial wall deficiency. The revision acetabular component is cemented within it. Similar devices are now achieving a resurgence of interest, mainly because of anxiety about the long-term fate of large structural allografts. They also may offer a solution to the problem of massive combined bone loss in the anterior column and medial and central regions of the acetabulum. However, technically, it appears that their use presents special problems, and careful attention to technique is necessary for success.[440] The Burch-Schneider anti-protrusio cage (APC) has been used in patients with massive acetabular bone deficiency to bridge areas of bone loss and provide support for cement fixation of the acetabular socket (Fig. 49-23). Deep to the cage, the deficiency has been successfully filled with morcellized bone graft. In one series, 76 percent of such cases showed no evidence of failure or loosening at follow-up averaging 5 years.[441] An 80 percent success rate has also been re-

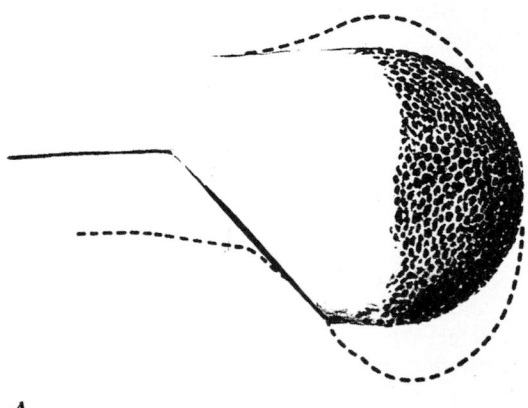

A

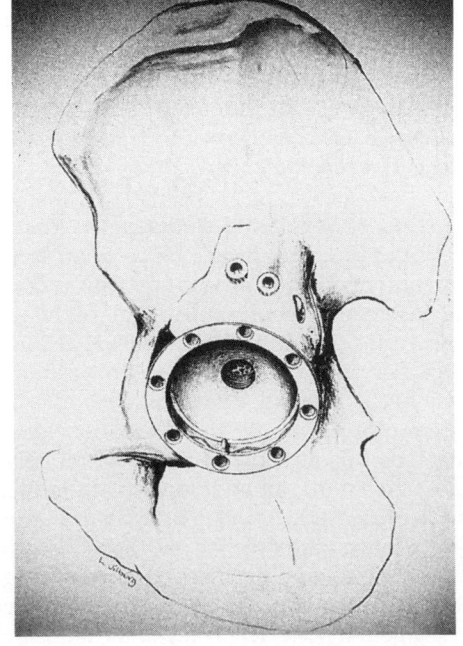

B

Figure 49-21 "Figure 7" reconstruction of a type 3A acetabular deficiency utilizing distal femoral allograft. *A.* The graft is reamed with a large concave reamer to remove extraneous bone from the condyles and match the size of the acetabular ream. The metaphyseal cortex is then cut as shown to remove some cortex posteriorly (a somewhat fanciful resemblance to the figure 7). *B.* The graft is fixed in place with 6.5 mm cancellous screws placed in the normal lines of force of the hip joint and obliquely through the graft. (Reproduced with permission from Paprosky WG, Bradford MS, Jablonski NS: Acetabular reconstruction with massive acetabular allograft. *AAOS Instr Course Lect* 45:149–160, 1996.)

orly that hooks beneath the cortical bone of the cotyloid notch (Fig. 49-25). At the present time the Burch-Schneider APC would seem to be the implant most suitable for medial segmental defects, extensive cavitary defects, and combined deficiencies. These bone defects are best reconstructed with bone graft rather than cement.[441] However, the Burch-Schneider device does cause some problems because of the need to clear a portion of the il-

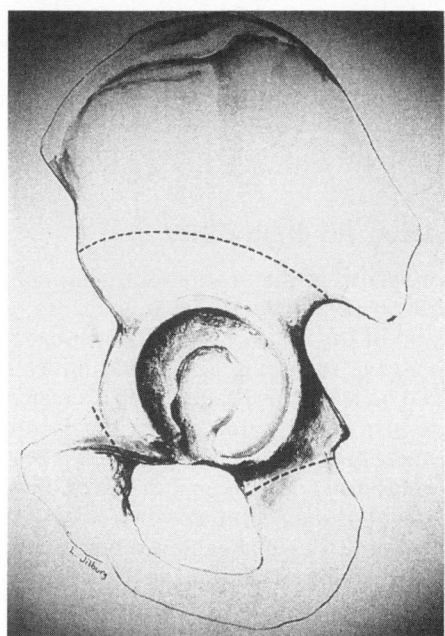

Figure 49-22 Preparation of hemipelvis allograft to reconstruct type 3B defect. Dotted lines indicate where graft is sectioned, but these cuts will vary in individual patients. (Reproduced with permission from Paprosky WG, Bradford MS, Jablonski NS: Acetabular reconstruction with massive acetabular allograft. *AAOS Instr Course Lect* 45:149–160, 1996.)

ported using the Muller support ring. However, a high incidence of nonprogressive radiolucencies of the cement bone interface was observed with the latter device.[442] Both of these APCs are screwed to the ilium. In the case of the Burch-Schneider APC, the ischial flange of the device is driven into the ischium to achieve additional purchase. The Muller device on the other hand does not have this feature (Fig. 49-24). The Ganz APC has a hook inferi-

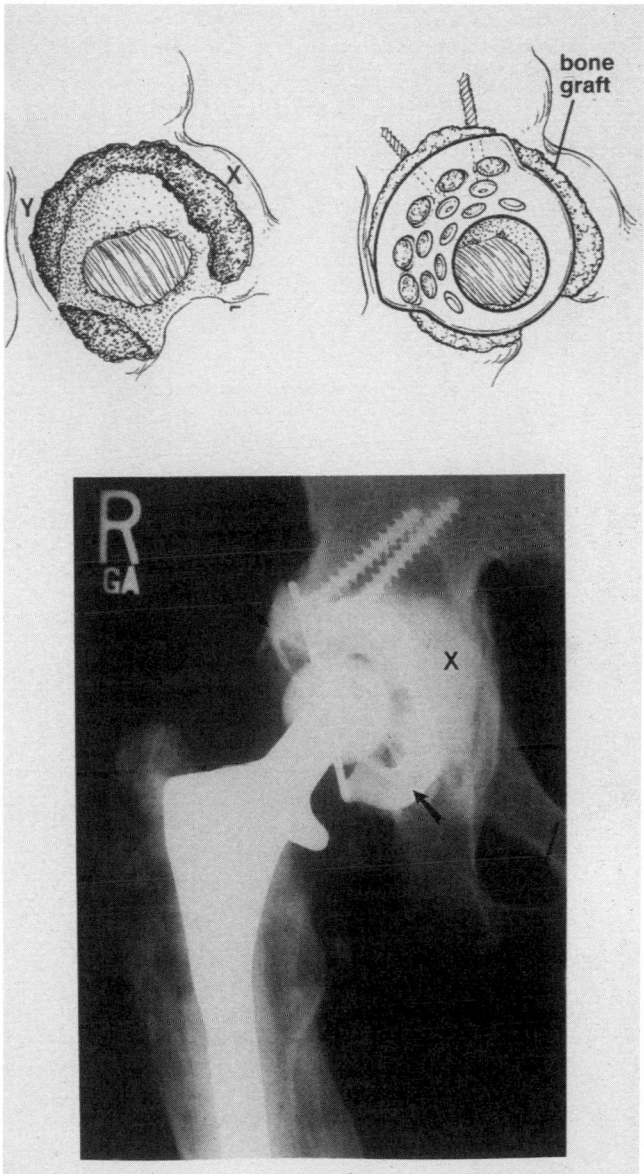

Figure 49-24 *Top left*: This acetabulum has segmental defects including the anterior (*x*) and medial wall (*y*). A rim-fit cup cannot be placed because of lack of supporting bone. *Top right*: A Mueller ring is in place with bone graft behind the ring and screws for additional fixation. *Bottom*: This anteroposterior radiography on a Mueller ring shows cement penetration into cancellous bone graft (*x*). Note the more horizontal position of the cup (*arrows*) relative to the ring placement. (Reproduced with permission from Possai KW, Dorr LD, McPherson EJ: Metal ring supports for deficient acetabular bone in total hip replacement. *AAOS Instr Course Lect* 45:161–170, 1996.)

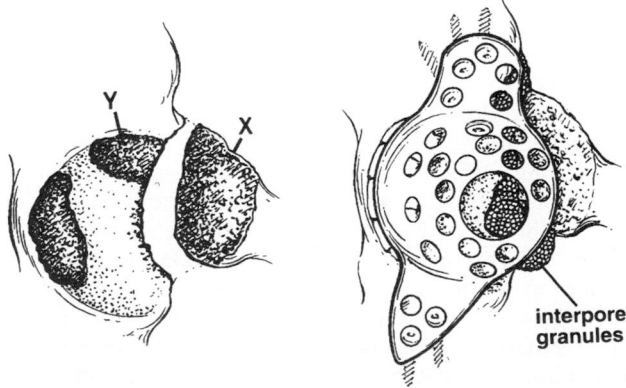

Figure 49-23 *Left:* A AAOS type IV acetabular defect with pelvic discontinuity. These are segmental (X) and cavitary (Y) defects. *Right:* The Burch-Schneider APC has been used with bone graft substitute. (Reproduced with permission from Possai KW, Dorr LD, McPherson EJ: Metal ring supports for deficient acetabular bone in total hip replacement. *AAOS Instr Course Lect* 45:161–170, 1996.)

iac wing for attachment of the flange with screws. There is consequently some interference with abductor function. A high dislocation rate may also be expected unless the device is correctly placed.[438] One of the advantages of the Burch-Schneider cage is that it can be used when there is associated pelvic discontinuity to give further support

to the usual plate applied from the ilium to the ischium. Paprosky now observes that APC devices may be used to augment fixation of whole acetabular replacement allografts in type 3B defects as an alternative to an ilioischial reconstruction plate.

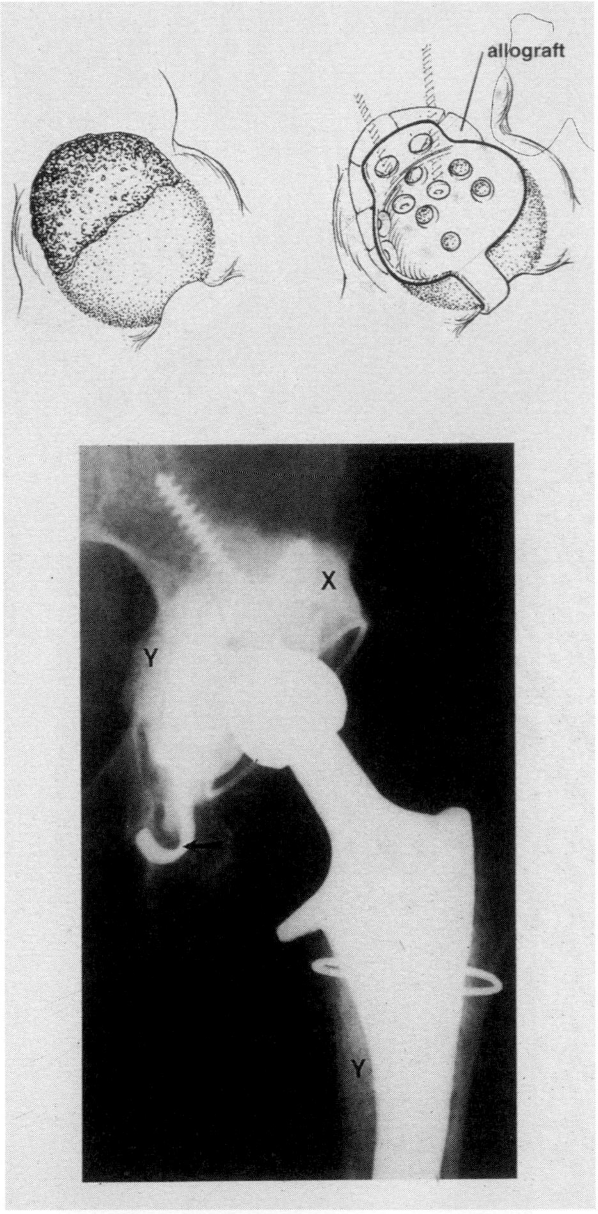

Hip Revision for Instability

Surgery for recurrent dislocation of the hip following total hip arthroplasty depends for its success on correct identification of the cause of the dislocation. As part of the preoperative planning, acetabular anteversion can be evaluated on the lateral radiograph. The angle formed by the intersection of a line across the face of the acetabulum and a line perpendicular to the horizontal plane should be measured.[306] A common cause of dislocation is malalignment of the acetabular or femoral component; an indication of this can be achieved by appropriate preoperative radiologic measurements. Revision of the acetabular component in the presence of a satisfactory femoral component is quite common. It is occasionally possible to rotate a new polyethylene liner into a more suitable position and to stabilize the implant without revising the metal shell. Occasionally impingement may be found as a cause of the recurrent dislocation. This may be a consequence of a too short neck length of the femoral component. Occasionally the acetabular component will have been medialized with inadequate femoral offset. The cause of the impingement may relate to some preexisting deformity of the femur associated with hip dysplasia, perhaps with previous osteotomy. Impinging bone capsule or cement may need to be removed. Frequently there may be an associated disruption of the trochanteric abduction mechanism that requires repair to stabilize the hip.[306]

Figure 49-25 *Top left*: This acetabulum has superior segmental and cavitary defects larger than 2.5 cm. *Top right*: A Ganz ring is positioned with bone graft support and screw fixation. *Bottom*: In this anteroposterior radiograph of a Ganz ring and cemented polyethylene cup, the hook (*arrow*) is hooked into cortical bone of the cotyloid notch. For successful liner position, the superior rim of the liner usually requires cement support (*x*). Interpore granules are visible behind the cup and around the proximal stem (*y*). (Reproduced with permission from Possai KW, Dorr LD, McPherson EJ: Metal ring supports for deficient acetabular bone in total hip replacement. *AAOS Instr Course Lect* 45:161–170, 1996.)

HIP ARTHROSCOPY

Arthroscopic examination of the hip has not achieved the central place in the therapeutic armamentarium that arthroscopy now occupies in the treatment of other joints in the body. However, for the appropriate case, it is a useful intervention, providing opportunities for accurate diagnosis and definitive treatment.

In patients with a suspected loose body in the hip joint, arthroscopy has been shown to be successful in locating and removing the fragment of bone or cartilage. Such bony or osteochondral fragments can be the result of trauma or end-stage disease (e.g., in Perthes' disease).[443] Other causes of loose fragments in the joint are osteochondritis dissecans and synovial chondromatosis; these fragments may also be successfully removed with the arthroscope.[444] Hip arthroscopy has also been found useful in identifying lesions of the acetabular labrum.[445,446] The technique has been used successfully in children to assess the articular cartilage in chondrolysis, avascular necrosis, and juvenile rheumatoid arthritis.[447] Some authors have also used arthroscopic lavage for treating septic arthritis of the hip in children as an alternative to open surgery, following this by suction drainage for 24 h to maintain decompression of the joint capsule.[448] The arthroscope is also a useful instrument for visualizing the synovium and performing biopsy when required.

Technique

The anterolateral portal is usually made at the junction of two lines, one drawn vertically downward from the anterior superior iliac spine and one passing horizontally at the level of the superior border of the symphysis pubis.[445] A spinal needle is then advanced toward the femoral head and into the joint. This needle is angled cephalad 45° from the horizontal (transverse) medial plane and inward at 45° to the vertical (sagittal) plane. The joint is filled with saline in the usual way and the arthroscope enters the joint along the same pathway. Although at first it might seem that a somewhat higher entry point in the region of the greater trochanter would be equally applicable, anterior portals in that portion of the femur (paratrochanteric) tend to be somewhat more dangerous because the arthroscope will be located more anteriorly than is ideal and may consequently damage the femoral neurovascular bundle.[445] On the other hand, if one makes an entry point proximal to the tip of the greater trochanter (the proximal trochanteric portal), this is relatively safe, although again care must be taken that the arthroscope does not drift anteriorly and damage the femoral neurovascular bundle. Posterior portals are described, but the sciatic nerve is always of concern and some authors recommend a miniarthrotomy approach to identify the sciatic nerve and superior gluteal vessels. The arthroscope may then be introduced into the capsule with safety.[445] The patient is usually placed supine for utilization of the anterolateral and anterior paratrochanteric portals but should be in the lateral position for the trochanteric portal or any of the posterior approaches. It would clearly be unwise to perform a posterior approach in a child, where there is risk of damage to the retinacular blood vessels.

Complications

The lateral cutaneous femoral nerve is at risk with the anterolateral portal and there are reports of its division during arthroscopy.[446] Transient pudendal nerve dysesthesia has also been described in hip arthroscopy, as have pressure wounds of the scrotum. These are complications of intraoperative traction table pressure.[449] In examining the anterior portion of the joint, minimal traction is required but McCarthy and coauthors recommend that the hip should be in a position of 45° of flexion and 30° of internal rotation.[445] They also suggest that if traction is limited to approximately 50 lb, there is less risk of complications caused by excessive pressure on soft tissues. The peroneal support should also be well padded. Small arthroscopes such as those used in the ankle should be available.[450]

REFERENCES

CLINICAL FEATURES OF HIP DISEASE AND COMMON HIP DISORDERS

1. Harris WH: Etiology of osteoarthritis of the hip. *Clin Orthop Rel Res* 213:20–33, 1988.
2. Bullough PG, Vigorita VJ: *Atlas of Orthopaedic Pathology with Clinical and Radiographic Correlation.* Philadelphia, Lippincott, 1984, chap 7.
3. Wroblewski BM, Charnley J: Radiographic morphology of the osteoarthritic hip. *J Bone Joint Surg* 64B:568–572, 1982.
4. Bissacotti JF, Cates HE, Keating ME, et al: Survivorship analysis of acetabular revision in medial, lateral and global primary osteoarthritis. *Orthopaedics* 18:1145–1149, 1995.
5. Schumacher (ed): *Primer on the Rheumatic Diseases,* 10th ed. Atlanta, Arthritis Foundation, 1993.
6. Maynard MJ, Ranawat CS, Flynn WF, et al: Total hip replacement arthroplasty in patients with inflammatory arthritis. *Semin Arthrop* 6:145–166, 1995.
7. Weisz GM, Gal A, Kitchener PN: Magnetic resonance imaging in the diagnosis of aggressive villonodular synovitis. *Clin Orthop* 236:303–306, 1988.
8. Hungerford DS: Treatment of ischemic necrosis of the femoral head, in Evarts CM (ed): *Surgery of the Musculoskeletal System.* Vol 6. London, Churchill Livingstone, 1983, pp 16–17.
9. Taylor LJ: Multifocal avascular necrosis after short term high dose steroid therapy: A report of three cases. *J Bone Joint Surg (Br)* 66:431–433, 1984.
10. Ficat RP: Treatment of avascular necrosis of the femoral head, in Hungerford DS (ed): *The Hip* Proceedings, 11th Open Scientific Meeting of the Hip Society. St Louis, Mosby, 1983, pp 279–295.
11. Jones JP Jr: Etiology and pathogenesis of osteonecrosis. *Semin Arthrop* 2:160–168, 1991.
12. Ono K, Sugioka Y: Epidemiology and risk factors in avascular osteonecrosis of the femoral head, in Schoutens A, Arlet J, Gardeniers JW, et al (eds): *Bone Circulation and Vascularization in Normal and Pathological Conditions.* New York, Plenum Press, 1993, pp 243–248.
13. Callaghan JJ, Dennis DA, et al: *Orthopaedic Knowledge Update: Hip and Knee Reconstruction. Osteonecrosis.* Rosemont, IL, American Academy of Orthopaedic Surgery, 1995, pp 87–95.
14. Jones JP Jr: Fat embolism and osteonecrosis. *Orthop Clin North Am* 16:595–633, 1985.
15. Cruess RL, Blennerhassett J, MacDonald FR, et al: The etiology of steroid-induced avascular necrosis of bone. *Clin Orthop* 113:178–182, 1975.
16. Wang GJ, Dughman SS, Reger SI, Stamp WG: The effect of core decompression on femoral head blood flow in steroid-induced avascular necrosis of the femoral head. *J Bone Joint Surg* 67A:121–124, 1985.
17. Wang GJ: Improvement of femoral head blood flow in steroid treated rabbits using lipid-clearing agent, in Brand RA (ed): *The Hip.* Proceedings of the 14th open scientific meeting of the Hip Society. St Louis, Mosby, 1987, pp 87–93.
18. Hungerford DS: Bone marrow pressure, venography, and core decompression in ischemic necrosis of the femoral head, in *The Hip.* Proceedings of the 7th open scientific meeting of the Hip Society. St Louis, Mosby, 1979.
19. Glimcher MJ, Kenzora JE: The biology of osteonecrosis of the human femoral head and its clinical implications: II. The pathologic changes in the femoral head as an organ and in the hip joint. *Clin Orthop* 139:283–312, 1979.
20. Matsui M, Saito S, Ohzono K, et al: Experimental steroid induced osteonecrosis in adult rabbits with hypersensitivity vasculitis. *Clin Orthop* 277:61–72, 1992.

21. Schroer WC: Current concepts on the pathogenesis of osteonecrosis of the femoral head. *Orthop Rev* 23:487–497, 1994.

22. Robinson HJ, Hartleben PD, et al: Evaluation of magnetic resonance imaging in the diagnosis of osteonecrosis of the femoral head. *J Bone Joint Surg* 71A:650–663, 1989.

23. Jefesen HE, Heller M, et al: Magnetic resonance imaging in the diagnosis of osteonecrosis of the femoral head. *Orthop Clin North Am* 16:705–716, 1985.

24. Mitchell DG, Rao VM, et al: Femoral head avascular necrosis: Correlation of MRI, radiographic staging, radionuclide imaging and clinical findings. *J Radiol* 162:709–715, 1987.

25. Ficat RP, Arlet J: *Ischaemia and the Necrosis of Bone.* Baltimore, Williams & Wilkins, 1980.

26. Ficat RP: Idiopathic bone necrosis of the femoral head: Early diagnosis and treatment. *J Bone Joint Surg (Br)* 67:3–9, 1985.

27. Steinberg ME, Steinberg DR: Evaluation and staging of avascular necrosis. *Semin Arthrop* 2:175–181, 1991.

28. Gardeniers JMW: The ARCO perspective for reaching one uniform staging system of osteonecrosis, in Schoutens A, Arlet J, Gardeniers JW, et al (eds): *Bone Circulation and Vascularization in Normal and Pathological Conditions.* New York, Plenum Press, 1993, pp 375–380.

29. Musso ES, Mitchell SN, et al: Results of conservative management of osteonecrosis of the femoral head: A restrospective review. *Clin Orthop* 207:209–215, 1986.

30. Stulberg BN, Bauer TW, Belhobek GH: Making core decompression work. *Clin Orthop* 261:186–195, 1990.

31. Stulberg BN, Davis AW, Bauer TW, et al: Osteonecrosis of the femoral head: A prospective randomized treatment protocol. *Clin Orthop* 268:140–151, 1991.

32. Steinberg ME, Brighton CT, et al: Treatment of avascular necrosis of the femoral head by a combination of bone grafting, decompression, and electrical stimulation. *Clin Orthop* 186:137–153, 1984.

33. Steinberg ME, Brighton CT, et al: Early results in the treatment of avascular necrosis of the femoral head with electrical stimulation. *Orthop Clin North Am* 15:163–175, 1984.

34. Steinberg ME: Osteonecrosis of the femoral head. *Semin Arthrop* 2:159–249, 1991.

35. Rosenberg A, et al: A comparison of electrical stimulation, core decompression, or combined modalities in femoral head osteonecrosis. American Academy of Orthopaedic Surgeons, New Orleans, 1994.

36. Nelson LM, Clark CR: Efficacy of Phemister bone grafting in nontraumatic aseptic necrosis of the femoral head. *J Arthrop* 8:253–258, 1993.

37. Scher MA, Jakim I: Intertrochanteric osteotomy and autogenous bone grafting for avascular necrosis of the femoral head. *J Bone Joint Surg* 75A:1119–1133, 1993.

SURGICAL TREATMENT OF HIP DISEASE

38. Ranawat CS: Surgery for rheumatoid arthritis, lower limb, surgery of the hip. *Clin Orthop* 259:83–91, 1990.

39. Harris WH: Etiology of osteoarthritis of the hip. *Clin Orthop* 213:20–33, 1986.

40. Trousdale RT, Ekkernkamp A, Ganz R, et al: Periacetabular and intertrochanteric osteotomy for the treatment of osteoarthrosis in dysplastic hips. *J Bone Joint Surg* 77A:73–85, 1995.

41. McMurray PT: Osteoarthritis of the hip joint. *Br J Surg* 22:916, 1935.

42. Harris NH, Kirwan E: The results of osteotomy for early primary osteoarthritis of the hip. *J Bone Joint Surg* 46B:477–487, 1964.

43. Pauwels F: Des affections de la lanche d'origine mechanique et de leur traitment par l'osteotomie d'adduction. *Rev Chir Orthop* 37:22–30, 1951.

44. Miegel RE, Harris WH: Medial-displacement intertrochanteric osteotomy in the treatment of osteoarthritis of the hip. *J Bone Joint Surg* 66A:878–887, 1984.

45. Pauwels F: Biomechanical principles of varus/valgus intertrochanteric osteotomy (Pauwels I and II) in the treatment of osteoarthritis of the hip, in Schatzker J (ed): *The Intertrochanteric Osteotomy.* New York, Springer-Verlag, 1984, pp 4–23.

46. Maquet PGJ: *Biomechanics of the Hip.* New York, Springer-Verlag, 1985.

47. Bombelli R: Osteoarthritis of the hip—Classification and pathogenesis, in *The Role of Osteotomy as a Consequent Therapy,* 2d ed. Berlin, Springer-Verlag, 1983.

48. Santore RF, Bombelli R: Long term follow up of the Bombelli experience with osteotomy for osteoarthritis: Results at 11 years. *The Hip. Proceedings of the 11th meeting of the Hip Society.* St Louis, Mosby, 1983, pp 106–128.

49. Maistrelli GL, Gerundini M, et al: Valgus-extension osteotomy for osteoarthritis of the hip: Indications and long term results. *J Bone Joint Surg* 72B:653–657, 1990.

50. Marti R, Schuller H, Raaymakers L: Intertrochanteric osteotomy for non-union of the femoral neck. *J Bone Joint Surg* 71B:782–787, 1989.

51. Dorr LD, Luckett M, Conaty JP: Total hip arthroplasties in patients younger than 45 years: A nine to ten year follow-up study. *Clin Orthop* 260:215–219, 1990.

52. Saitio S, Saito M, et al: Long term results of total hip arthroplasty for osteonecrosis of the femoral head: A comparision with osteoarthritis. *Clin Orthop* 244:198–207, 1989.

53. Solacoff D, Mont MA, Krackow KA: Uncemented total hip arthroplasty in patients less than 45 years with avascular necrosis. *Orthop Trans* 17:1085, 1993–1994.

54. Katz R, Bourne R, Rorabeck C, et al: Total hip arthroplasty in patients with avascular necrosis of the hip: Follow-up observation on cementless and cemented operations. *Clin Orthop* 281:145–151, 1992.

55. Mont MA, Hungerford DS: Current concepts review: Non-traumatic avascular necrosis of the femoral head. *J Bone Joint Surg* 77A:459–474, 1995.

56. Steinberg ME, Bands RE, et al: Does lesion size affect outcome in avascular necrosis? *Orthop Trans* 16:706–707, 1992–1993.

57. Maistrelli G, Fusco U, Avai A, Bombelli R: Osteonecrosis of the hip treated by intertrochanteric osteotomy: A four to fifteen year follow-up. *J Bone Joint Surg* 70B:761–766, 1988.

58. Jacobs MA, Hungerford DS, Krachow KA: Intertrochanteric osteotomy for avascular necrosis of the femoral head. *J Bone Joint Surg* 71B:200–204, 1989.

59. Scher MA, Jakim I: Intertrochanteric osteotomy and autogenous bone grafting for avascular necrosis of the femoral head. *J Bone Joint Surg* 75A:1119–1133, 1993.

60. Mont M, Fairbank AC, Krachow KA, Hungerford DS: Corrective osteotomy for osteonecrosis of the femoral head. *J Bone Joint Surg* 78A:1032–1038, 1996.

61. Sugioka Y, Katsuki L, Hotokebuchi T: Transtrochanteric rotational osteotomy of the femoral head for femoral head osteonecrosis. *Clin Orthop* 169:115–126, 1982.

62. Sugioka Y, Hotokebuchi T, Tsutsui H: Transtrochanteric anterior rotational osteotomy for idiopathic and steroid induced necrosis of the femoral head: Indications and long term results. *Clin Orthop* 277:111–120, 1992.

63. Salter RB: Innominate osteotomy in the treatment of congenital dislocation and subluxation of the hip. *J Bone Joint Surg* 43B:518–539, 1961.

64. Sutherland DH, Greenfield R: Double innominate osteotomy. *J Bone Joint Surg* 59A:1082–1091, 1977.

65. Steel HH: Triple osteotomy of the innominate bone. *J Bone Joint Surg* 55A:343–350, 1973.

66. Ganz R, Klaue K, Vinh TS, et al: A new periacetabular osteotomy for the treatment of hip dysplasia: Technique and preliminary results. *Clin Orthop* 277:111–120, 1992.

67. Tonnis D: *Congenital Dysplasia and Dislocation of the Hip in Children and Adults.* Berlin, Springer-Verlag, 1987.

68. Eppright RH: Dial osteotomy of the acetabulum in the treatment of dysplasia of the hip. *J Bone Joint Surg* 58A:726, 1976.

69. Wagner H: Osteotomies for congential hip dislocation, in *The Hip.* Proceedings of the fourth Open Scientific Meeting of the Hip Society. St Louis, Mosby, 1976, pp 45–66.

70. Simmons EH: Chiari osteotomy—A biologic alternative for the surgical management of dysplasia of the hip joint associated with arthrosis. *Hip* 14–17, 1984.

71. Reynolds DA: Chiari innominate osteotomy in adults: Technique, indications and contraindications. *J Bone Joint Surg* 68B:45–54, 1986.

ARTHROPLASTY OF THE HIP

72. Harris WH, Sledge CB: Total hip and total knee replacement. *N Engl J Med* 323:725, 801, 1990.

73. Quinet RJ, Winters EG: Total joint replacement of the hip and knee. *Med Clin North Am* 76:1235, 1992.

74. Liang MH, Cullen KE, Poss R: Primary total hip or knee replacement: Evaluation of patients. *Ann Intern Med* 97:735, 1982.

75. Liang MH, Katz JN, Phillips C: The total hip arthroplasty outcome evaluation form of the American Academy of Orthopaedic Surgeons. *J Bone Joint Surg* 73A:639, 1991.

76. National Institutes of Health Consensus Development Conference statement: Total hip replacement. September 1994 (draft).

77. Swedish Consensus Conference: Total hip-joint replacement in Sweden. *JAMA* 248:1822, 1982.

78. Peterson MGE, Hollenberg JP, Szatrowski TP: Geographic variations in the rates of elective total hip and knee arthroplasties among Medicare beneficiaries in the United States, *J Bone Joint Surg* 74A:1530, 1992.

79. Mancuso CA, Ranawat CS, Esdaile JM: Indications for total hip and total knee arthroplasties: Results of orthopaedic surveys. *J Arthrop* 11:34–46, 1996.

80. D'Antonio JA: Preoperative templating and choosing the implant for primary THA in the young patient. *AAOS Instr Course Lect* 43:339–347, 1994.

81. Davey JR: Femoral component offset: Its effect on micromotion, strain in the cement, bone, and prosthesis. In proceedings: Controversy in Total Hip Replacement. Boston, 1989.

82. Johnston RC, Brand RA, Crowninshield RD: Reconstruction of the hip, a mathematical approach to determine optimum geometric relationships. *J Bone Joint Surg* 61A:639–652, 1979.

83. Capello WN: Preoperative planning of total hip arthroplasty. *Instr Course Lect* 35:249–257, 1986.

84. DeOrio JK, Bladder KE: Indications and patient selection, in Morrey BF (ed): *Joint Replacement Arthroplasty.* New York, Churchill-Livingstone, 1991, pp 547–559.

85. Engh CA: Recent advances in cementless total hip arthroplasty using the AML prosthesis. *Tech Orthop* 6:3, 1991.

86. Mallory TH, Kraus TJ, Vaughn BK: Intraoperative femoral fractures associated with cementless total hip arthroplasty. *Orthopedics* 12:231, 1989.

87. Schwartz JT, Mayer JG, Engh CA: Femoral fracture during noncemented total hip arthroplasty. *J Bone Joint Surg* 71A:1135, 1989.

88. Woolson ST: Leg length equalization during total hip replacement. *Orthopedics* 13:17, 1990.

89. Knight JL, Atwater RD: Preoperative planning for total hip arthroplasty: Quantitating its utility and precision. *J Arthrop* 7(suppl):403–409, 1992.

90. Dorr LD, Mackel A, Faugere MC: Histologic validation of a new x-ray classification of hip changes in patients with osteoarthritis requiring total hip replacement. *Orthop Trans* 12:464, 1988.

91. Engh CA, Glassman AH, Suthers KE: The case for porous-coated hip implants: The femoral side. *Clin Orthop Rel Res* 261:63–81, 1990.

92. Hungerford DS, Jones LC: The rationale for cementless total hip replacement. *Orthop Clin North Am* 24:617–626, 1993.

93. Welch RB, McGann WA, Rasmussen L: Femoral stem fixation: The case for cement. *Clin Orthop Rel Res* 261:134–139, 1990.

94. Hozack WJ, Rothman RH, Booth RE Jr: Cemented versus cementless total hip arthroplasty: A comparative study of equivalent patient populations. *Clin Orthop Rel Res* 289:161–165, 1993.

95. Wrobleski BM: Cementless versus cemented total hip arthroplasty: A scientific controversy? *Orthop Clin North Am* 24:591–597, 1993.

96. Callaghan JJ: Total hip arthroplasty: Clinical perspectives. *Clin Orthop Rel Res* 276:33–40, 1992.

97. Woolson ST, Watt JM: Use of autologous blood in total hip replacement. *J Bone Joint Surg* 73A:76–80, 1991.

98. Einhorn TA, Boskey AL, Gundberg CM: The mineral and mechanical properties of bone in chronic experimental diabetes. *J Orthop Res* 6:317, 1988.

99. Menon TJ, Thjellesen D, Wroblewski BM: Charnley low-friction arthroplasty in diabetic patients. *J Bone Joint Surg* 65B:580, 1983.

100. Moeckel B, Huo MH, Salvati EA: Total hip arthroplasty in patients with diabetes mellitus. *J Arthrop*; 8:280–284 1993.

101. Bradford DS, Janes PC, Simmons RS: Total hip arthroplasty in renal transplant recipients. *Clin Orthop Rel Res* 181:107, 1983.

102. Cruess RL, Blennerhassett MB, MacDonald FR: Aseptic necrosis following renal transplantation. *J Bone Joint Surg* 50A:1577, 1968.

103. Bewick M, Steward PH, Rudge C: Avascular necrosis of bone in patients undergoing renal allotransplantation. *Clin Nephrol* 5:66, 1976.

104. Hawking KM, Van Den Bosch BF, Wilmink JM: Avascular necrosis of bone after renal transplantation. *N Engl J Med* 294:397, 1976.

105. Devlin VJ, Einhorn TA, Gordon SL: Total hip arthroplasty after renal transplantation: Long-term follow-up study and assessment of metabolic bone status. *J Arthrop* 3:205–213, 1988.

106. Deo S, Gibbons CLMH, Emerton M: Total hip replacement in renal transplant patients. *J Bone Joint Surg* 77B:299–302, 1995.

107. Alpert B, Waddell JP, Morton J: Cementless total hip arthroplasty in renal transplant patients. *Clin Orthop Rel Res* 284:164–169, 1992.

108. Zimmerman CE, Yett HS: Renal transplant infarction during total hip arthroplasty. *Clin Orthop Rel Res* 165:195–196, 1982.

109. Lachiewicz PF: Total hip replacement in Gaucher's disease. *J Bone Joint Surg* 63A:602–607, 1981.

110. Lau MM: Hip arthroplasties in Gaucher's Disease. *J Bone Joint Surg* 63A:591–601, 1981.

111. Goldblatt J, Sacks S, Dall D: Total hip arthroplasty in Gaucher's disease. *Clin Orthop Rel Res* 228:94–98, 1988.

112. Moran MC, Huo MH, Garvin KL: Total hip arthroplasty in sickle cell hemoglobinopathy. *Clin Orthop Rel Res* 294:140–148, 1993.

113. Bishop AR, Roberson JR, Eckman JR: Total hip arthroplasty in patients who have sickle-cell hemoglobinopathy. *J Bone Joint Surg* 70A:853–855, 1988.

114. Clarke HJ, Jinnah RH, Brokker AF: Total replacement of the hip for avascular necrosis in sickle cell disease. *J Bone Joint Surg* 71B:465–470, 1989.

115. Arcurio MT, Friedman RJ: Hip arthroplasty in patients with sickle-cell haemoglobinopathy. *J Bone Joint Surg* 74B:367–371, 1992.

116. Wayne AS, Zelicoff SB, Sledge CB: Total hip arthroplasty in β-thalassemia: Case report and review of the literature. *Clin Orthop Rel Res* 294:149–154, 1993.

117. Greene WB, DeGnore LT, White GC: Orthopaedic procedures and prognosis in hemophilic patients who are seropositive for human immunodeficiency virus. *J Bone Joint Surg* 72A:2–11, 1990.

118. Kelley SS, Lachiewicz PF, Gilbert MS: Hip arthroplasty in hemophilic arthropathy. *J Bone Joint Surg* 77A:828–834, 1995.

119. Baxter MP, D'Astous JL: Proximal femoral resection interpositional arthroplasty: Salvage hip surgery for the severely disabled child with cerebral palsy. *J Pediatr Orthop* 6:681, 1986.

120. McCarthy RE, Simon S, Douglas B: Proximal femoral resection to allow adults who have severe cerebral palsy to sit. *J Bone Joint Surg* 70A:1011, 1988.

121. Cooperman DR, Bartucci E, Dietrick E: Hip dislocation in spastic cerebral palsy: Long term consequences. *J Pediatr Orthop* 7:268, 1987.

122. Bleck EE: The hip in cerebral palsy. *Orthop Clin North Am* 79: 79–104, 1980.

123. Buly RL, Huo M, Root L: Total hip arthroplasty in cerebral palsy: Long-term follow-up results. *Clin Orthop Rel Res* 296:148–153, 1993.

124. Skoff HD, Keggi K: Total hip replacement in the neuromuscularly impaired. *Orthop Rev* 15:154–159, 1986.

125. Menon TJ, Wroblewski BM: Charnley low-friction arthroplasty in patients with psoriasis. *Clin Orthop Rel Res* 176:127–128, 1983.

126. Papagelopoulos PJ, Morrey BF: Hip and knee replacement in osteogenesis imperfecta. *J Bone Joint Surg* 75A:572–580, 1993.

127. Bisla RS, Inglis AE, Ranawat CS: Joint replacement surgery in patients under thirty. *J Bone Joint Surg* 58A:1098, 1986.

127a. Lewinnek GE, Lewis JL, Tarr R: Dislocations after total hip replacement arthroplasties. *J Bone Joint Surg* 60A:217–220, 1978.

128. Colville J, Rannio P: Total hip replacement in juvenile rheumatoid arthritis. *Acta Orthop Scand* 50:197, 1979.

129. Lachiewicz PF, McCaskill B, Inglis A: Total hip arthroplasty in juvenile rheumatoid arthritis. *J Bone Joint Surg* 68A:502, 1986.

130. Ruddlesdin C, Ansell BM, Arden GP: Total hip replacement in children with juvenile chronic arthritis. *J Bone Joint Surg* 68B:218, 1986.

131. Scott RD, Sarokhan AJ, Dalziel R: Total hip and total knee arthroplasty in juvenile rheumatoid arthritis. *Clin Orthop Rel Res* 182:90–98, 1984.

132. Mogensen B, Brattstrom H, Ekelund L: Total hip replacement in juvenile chronic arthritis. *Acta Orthop Scand* 54:422, 1983.

133. Learmonth ID, Heywood AWB, Kaye J: Radiological loosening after cemented hip replacement for juvenile chronic arthritis. *J Bone Joint Surg* 71B:209, 1989.

134. Maric Z, Haynes RJ: Total hip arthroplasty in juvenile rheumatoid arthritis. *Clin Orthop Rel Res* 290:197–199, 1993.

135. Woolson ST, Harris WH: Complex total hip replacement for dysplastic or hypoplastic hips using miniature or microminiature components. *J Bone Joint Surg* 65A:1099–1108, 1983.

136. Hanssen AD, Cabanela ME, Michet CJ: Hip arthroplasty in patients with systemic lupus erythematosus. *J Bone Joint Surg* 69A:807–814, 1987.

137. Huo MH, Salvati EA, Browne MG: Primary total hip arthroplasty in systemic lupus erythematosus. *J Arthrop* 7:51–56, 1992.

138. Low CK, Lai CH, Low YP: Results of total hip replacement in systemic lupus erythematosus. *Singapore Med J* 32:391–392, 1991.

139. Brinker MR, Rosenberg AG, Kull L: Primary total hip arthroplasty using noncemented porous-coated femoral components in patients with osteonecrosis of the femoral head. *J Arthrop* 9:457–468, 1994.

140. Cracchiolo A III, Severt R, Moreland J: Uncemented total hip arthroplasty in rheumatoid arthritis diseases: A two- to six-year follow-up study. *Clin Orthop Rel Res* 277:166–174, 1992.

141. Bogoch E, Oullette G, Hastings D: Failure of internal fixation of displaced femoral neck fractures in rheumatoid patients. *J Bone Joint Surg* 73B:7–10, 1991.

142. Greenough CG, Jones JR: Primary total hip replacement for displaced subcapital fracture of the femur. *J Bone Joint Surg* 70B:639–643, 1988.

143. Franzen H, Nilsson LT, Stromqvist B: Secondary total hip replacement after fractures of the femoral neck. *J Bone Joint Surg* 72B:784–787, 1990.

144. Katz RL, Bourne RB, Rorabeck CH: Total hip arthroplasty in patients with avascular necrosis of the hip: Follow-up observations on cementless and cemented operations. *Clin Orthop Rel Res* 281:145–151, 1992.

145. Kwong LM, Jasty M, Harris WH: High failure rate of bulk femoral head allografts in total hip acetabular reconstructions at 10 years. *J Arthrop* 8:341–346, 1993.

146. Hooten JP Jr, Engh CA Jr, Engh CA: Failure of structural acetabular allografts in cementless revision hip arthroplasty. *J Bone Joint Surg* 76B:419–422, 1994.

147. Russotti GM, Harris WH: Proximal placement of the acetabular component in total hip arthroplasty: A long-term follow-up study. *J Bone Joint Surg* 73A:587–592, 1991.

148. Anwar MM, Sugano N, Masuhara K: Total hip arthroplasty in the neglected congenital dislocation of the hip: A five to 14-year follow-up study. *Clin Orthop Rel Res* 295:127–134, 1993.

149. Nelson JP: The effect of previous surgery, operating room environment, and preventive antibiotics on postoperative infection following total hip arthroplasty. *Clin Orthop Rel Res* 147:167, 1980.

150. Williams DN, Gustilo RB: The use of preventive antibiotics in orthopaedic surgery. *Clin Orthop Rel Res* 190:83–88, 1984.

151. Sanderson PJ: Infection in orthopaedic implants. *J Hosp Infect* 18(suppl A):367–375, 1991.

152. Pollard JP, Hughes SPF, Scott JE: Antibiotic prophylaxis in total joint replacement. *Br Med J* 1:707–709, 1979.

153. Neu HC: Cephalosporin antibiotics as applied in surgery of bone and joints. *Clin Orthop Rel Res* 90:50–63, 1984.

154. Learmonth ID: Prevention of infection in the 1990s. *Orthop Clin North Am* 24:735–741, 1993.

155. Morrey BF: Instability after total hip arthroplasty. *Orthop Clin North Am* 23:237–248, 1992.

156. Woo RYG, Morrey BF: Dislocations after total hip arthroplasty. *J Bone Joint Surg* 64A:1295, 1982.

157. Dall D: Exposure of the hip by anterior osteotomy of the greater trochanter. *J Bone Joint Surg* 68B:382–386, 1986.

158. Gore DR: Anterolateral compared to posterior approach in total hip arthroplasty: Differences in component positioning, hip strength and hip motion. *Clin Orthop Rel Res* 165:180–187, 1982.

159. Harding K: The direct lateral approach to the hip. *J Bone Joint Surg* 64B:17–19, 1982.

160. Callaghan JJ, Dysnet SH, Savory CG: The uncemented porous-coated anatomic total hip prosthesis: Two-year results of a prospective consecutive series. *J Bone Joint Surg* 70A:337–346, 1988.

161. Baker AS, Bitounis VS: Abductor function after total hip replacement: An electromyographic and clinical review. *J Bone Joint Surg* 71B:47–50, 1989.

162. Roberts JM: The comparison of the posterolateral and anterolateral approaches for total hip replacement. *Clin Orthop Rel Res* 187:205–210, 1984.

163. Vicar AJ, Coleman CR: A comparison of the anterolateral, transtrochanteric and posterior surgical approaches in primary total hip arthroplasty. *Clin Orthop Rel Res* 188:152, 1984.

164. Hedley AK, Hendren DH, Mead LP: A posterior approach to the hip joint with complete posterior capsular and muscular repair. *J Arthrop* 5(suppl: S57–S66, 1990.

165. Parker HG, Weisman HJ, Ewald FC: Comparison of preoperative, intraoperative and early postoperative total hip replacements with and without trochanteric osteotomy. *Clin Orthop Rel Res* 121:44, 1976.

166. Parker HG, Weisman HJ, Ewald FC: Comparison of immediate and late results of total hip replacement with and without trochanteric osteotomy. *J Bone Joint Surg* 56A:1537, 1974.

167. Weisman JH Jr, Simon SR, Ewald FC: Total hip replacement with and without osteotomy of the greater trochanter. *J Bone Joint Surg* 60A:203, 1978.

168. Robinson RP: Transtrochanteric and posterior approaches for total hip replacement. *Clin Orthop Rel Res* 147:143–147, 1980.

169. Frankel A, Booth RE Jr, Balderston RA: Complications of trochanteric osteotomy. *Clin Orthop Rel Res* 288:209–213, 1993.

170. Harris WH: Revision surgery for failed, nonseptic total hip arthroplasty: The femoral side. *Clin Orthop Rel Res* 170:8–20, 1982.

171. Knight WE: Accurate determination of leg lengths during total hip replacement. *Clin Orthop Rel Res* 123:22–28, 1977.

172. McGee HMJ, Scott JHS: A simple method of obtaining equal leg length in total hip arthroplasty. *Clin Orthop Rel Res* 194:269–270, 1984.

173. Williamson JA, Reckling FW: Limb length discrepancy and related problems following total hip joint replacement. *Clin Orthop Rel Res* 134:135–138, 1978.

174. Woolson ST, Harris WH: A method of intraoperative limb length measurement in total hip arthroplasty. *Clin Orthop Rel Res* 194:207–210, 1985.

175. Woolson ST: Leg length equalization during total hip replacement. *Orthopedics* 13:17–21, 1990.

176. Rand JA, Ilstrup DM: Comparison of Charnley and T-28 total hip arthroplasty. *Clin Orthop Rel Res* 180:201–205, 1983.

177. Love BRT, Wright K: Leg length discrepancy after total hip replacement. *J Bone Joint Surg* 65B:103, 1983.

178. Abraham WD, Dimon JH III: Leg length discrepancy in total hip arthroplasty. *Orthop Clin North Am* 23:201–209, 1992.

179. Levy RN: The location of the level of femoral neck transection for prosthetic hip arthroplasty. *Clin Orthop Rel Res* 171:51–52, 1982.

180. Morscher EW: Current status of acetabular fixation in primary total hip arthroplasty. *Clin Orthop Rel Res* 274:172–193, 1992.

181. Yoder SA, Brand RA, Pedersen DR: Total hip acetabular position affects component loosening rates. *Clin Orthop Rel Res* 228:79, 1988.

182. Sarmiento A, Ebramzdeh E, Gogan WJ: Cup containment and orientation in cemented total hip arthroplasties. *J Bone Joint Surg* 72B:996–1002, 1990.

183. McCollum DE, Gray WJ: Dislocation after total hip arthroplasty: Causes and prevention. *Clin Orthop Rel Res* 261:159–170, 1990.

184. Barrack RL: Modularity of prosthetic implants. *J Am Assoc Orthop Surg* 2:16–25, 1994.

185. Schmalzried TP, Harris WH: Hybrid total hip replacement: A 6.5-year follow-up study. *J Bone Joint Surg* 75B:608–615, 1993.

186. Majkowki AJ, Miles AW, Bannister GC: Bone surface preparation in cemented joint replacement. *J Bone Joint Surg* 75B:459–463, 1993.

187. Bourne RB: Femoral cement pressurization during total hip arthroplasty: The role of different femoral stems with reference to stem size and shape. *Clin Orthop Rel Res* 183:12–16, 1984.

188. Oh I, Carlson CE, Tomford WW: Improved fixation of the femoral component after total hip replacement using methacrylate intramedullary plug. *J Bone Joint Surg* 60A:608–612, 1978.

189. Oh I, Bourne RB, Harris WH: The femoral cement compactor: An improvement in cementing technique in total hip replacement. *J Bone Joint Surg* 65A:1335–1338, 1983.

190. Skinner HB: Stress changes in bone secondary to the use of a femoral canal plug with cemented hip replacement. *Clin Orthop Rel Res* 166:277–283, 1982.

191. Wixson RL, Lautenshiager EP, Novak MA: Vacuum mixing of acrylic bone cement. *J Arthrop* 2:141–149, 1987.

192. Davies JP, Jasty M, O'Connor DO: The effect of centrifuging bone cement. *J Bone Joint Surg* 71B:39–42, 1989.

193. Davies JP, O'Connor DO, Burke DW: The effect of centrifucation on the fatigue life of bone cement in the presence of surface irregularities. *Clin Orthop Rel Res* 229:156–161, 1988.

194. O'Connor DO, Burke DW, Davies JP: SN curve for centrifuged and uncentrifuged PMMA. *Trans Orthop Res Soc* 10:325, 1985.

195. Star MJ, Colwell CW Jr, Kelman GJ: Suboptimal (thin) distal cement mantle thickness as a contributory factor in total hip arthroplasty femoral component failure. *J Arthrop* 9:143–149, 1994.

196. Jasty M, Maloney WJ, Bragdon CR: The initiation of failure in cemented femoral components of hip arthroplasties. *J Bone Joint Surg* 73B:551–558, 1991.

197. Ebramzadeh E, Sarmiento A, McKellop HA: The cement mantle in total hip arthroplasty: Analysis of long-term radiographic results. *J Bone Joint Surg* 76A:77–87, 1994.

198. Noble PC, Tullos HS, Landon G: The optimum cement mantle for total hip replacement. *Intr Course Lect* 40:145–150, 1991.

199. Mulroy WF, Estok DM, Harris WH: Total hip arthroplasty with use of so-called second-generation cementing techniques. *J Bone Joint Surg* 77A:1845–1852, 1995.

200. Crowninshield RD, Brand RA, Johnston RC: An analysis of femoral component stem design in total hip arthroplasty. *J Bone Joint Surg* 62A:68–78, 1980.

201. Huiskes R, Chao EY: A survey of finite element analysis in orthopedic biomechanics: The first decade. *J Biomech* 16:385–409, 1983.

202. Livermore J, Ilstrup D, Morrey BF: Effect of femoral head size on wear of the polyethylene acetabular component. *J Bone Joint Surg* 72A:518–528, 1990.

203. Beer KJ, Lomardi AV Jr, Mallory TH: The efficacy of suction drains after routine total joint arthroplasty. *J Bone Joint Surg* 73A:584–587, 1991.

204. Ritter MA, Keating EM, Faris PM: Closed wound drainage in total hip or total knee replacement: A prospective randomized study. *J Bone Joint Surg* 76A:35–38, 1994.

205. Harris WH: Traumatic arthritis of the hip after dislocation and acetabular fractures: Treatment by mold arthroplasty. An end-result study using a new method of result evaluation. *J Bone Joint Surg* 51A:737–755, 1969.

205a. Kavanagh BF, Fitzgerald RH Jr: Clinical and radiographic assessment of total hip arthroplasty: A new hip score. *Clin Orthop Rel Res* 193:133–140, 1985.

206. Merle d'Aubigne R, Postel M: Functional results of hip arthroplasty with acrylic prosthesis. *J Bone Joint Surg* 36A:451–475, 1954.

206a. Larso CB: Rating scale of hip disabilities. *Clin Orthop Rel Res* 31:85–93, 1963.

207. Gartland JJ: Orthopaedic clinical research: Deficiencies in experimental design and determinations of outcome. *J Bone Joint Surg* 70A:1357–1364, 1988.

208. Kaplan EL, Meier P: Nonparametric estimation from incomplete observations. *J Am Stat Assoc* 53:457–481, 1958.

209. Dorey F, Amstutz HC: The validity of survivorship analysis in total joint arthroplasty. *J Bone Joint Surg* 71A:544–548, 1989.

210. Laupacis A, Bourne R, Rorabeck C: The effect of elective total hip replacement on health-related quality of life. *J Bone Joint Surg* 75A:1619–1626, 1993.

211. Schulte KR, Callaghan JJ, Kelley SS: The outcome of Charnley total hip arthroplasty with cement after a minimum twenty-year follow-up: The results of one surgeon. *J Bone Joint Surg* 75A:961–975, 1993.

212. Sullivan PM, MacKenzie JR, Callaghan JJ: Total hip arthroplasty with cement in patients who are less than fifty years old: A sixteen to twenty-two year follow-up study. *J Bone Joint Surg* 76A:863–869, 1994.

213. Kavanagh BF, Wallrichs S, Dewitz M: Charnley low-friction arthroplasty of the hip: Twenty-year results with cement. *J Arthrop* 9:229–234, 1994.

214. Schurman DJ, Block DA, Segal MR: Conventional cemented total hip arthroplasty: Assessment of clinical factors associated with revision for mechanical failure. *Clin Orthop Rel Res* 240:173–180, 1989.

214a. Schulte KR, Callaghan JJ, Keley SS: The outcome of Charnley total hip arthroplasty with cement after a minimum twenty-year follow-up: The results of one surgeon. *J Bone Joint Surg* 75A:961–967, 1993.

214b. Sullivan PM, MacKenzie JR, Callaghan JJ: Total hip arthroplasty with cement in patients who are less than fifty years old: A sixteen to twenty-two year follow-up study. *J Bone Joint Surg* 76A:863–869, 1994.

214c. Kavanagh BF, Wallrichs S, Dewitz M: Charnley low-friction arthroplasty of the hip: Twenty-year results with cement. *J Arthrop* 9:229–234, 1994.

214d. Torchia ME, Klassen RA, Bianco AJ: Total hip arthroplasty with cement in patients less than twenty years old: Long-term results. *J Bone Joint Surg* 78A:995–1003, 1996.

214e. Joshi AB, Porter ML, Trail IA: Long-term results of Charnley low-friction arthroplasty in young patients. *J Bone Joint Surg* 75B:616–623, 1993.

214f. Wroblewski BM, Siney PD: Charnley low-friction arthroplasty of the hip: Long-term results. *Clin Orthop Rel Res* 292:191–201, 1993.

214g. Neumann L, Freund KG, Sorensen KH: Long-term results of Charnley total hip replacement. *J Bone Joint Surg* 76B:245–251, 1994.

214h. Neumann L, Freund KG, Sorensen KH: Total hip arthroplasty with the Charnley prosthesis in patients fifty-five yars old and less. *J Bone Joint Surg* 78A:73–79, 1996.

214i. Mulroy WF, Estok DM, Harris WH: Total hip arthroplasty with use of so-called second-generation cementing techniques: A fifteen-year average follow-up study. *J Bone Joint Surg* 77A:1845–1852, 1995.

214j. Barrack RL, Mulroy RD Jr, Harris WH: Improved cementing techniques and femoral coponent loosening in young patients with hip arthroplasty: A 12-year radiographic review. *J Bone Joint Surg* 74B:385–389, 1992.

214k. Ballard WT, Callaghan JJ, Sullivan PM: The results of improved cementing techniques for total hip arthroplasty in patients less than fifty years old: A ten-yer follow-up study. *J Bone Joint Surg* 76A:959–964, 1994.

214l. Woolson ST, Haber DF: Primary total hip replacement with insertion of an acetabular component without cement and a femoral component with cement: Follow-up study at an average of six years. *J Bone Joint Surg* 78A:698–705, 1996.

214m. Schmalzried TP, Harris WH: Hybrid total hip replaement: A 6.5-year follow-up study. *J Bone Joint Surg* 75B:608–615, 1993.

214n. Oishi CS, Walker RH, Colwell CW Jr: The femoral component in total hip arthroplasty: Six to eight-year follow-up of one hundred consecutive patients after use of a third-generation cementing technique. *J Bone Joint Surg* 76A:1130–1136, 1994.

214o. Mohler DG, Kull LR, Martell JM: Total hip replacement with insertion of an acetabular component without cement and a femoral component with cement: Four to seven-year results. *J Bone Joint Surg* 77A:86–96, 1995.

214p. Engh CCA, Hooten JP Jr, Zettl-Schaffer KF: Porous-coated total hip replacement. *Clin Orthop Rel Res* 298:89–96, 1994.

214q. Heekin RD, Callaghan JJ, Hopkinson WJ: The porous-coated anatomic total hip prosthesis, inserted without cement. *J Bone Joint Surg* 75A:77–91, 1993.

214r. Own TD, Moran CG, Smith AR: Results of uncemented porous-coated anatomic total hip relacement

214s. Martell JM, Pierson RH III, Jacobs JJ: Primary total hip reconstruction with a titanium fiber-coated prosthesis inserted without cement. *J Bone Joint Surg* 75A:554–571, 1993.

214t. Kim Y-H, Kim VEM: Uncemented porous-coated anatomic total hip replacement: Results at six years in a consecutive series. *J Bone Joint Surg* 75B:6–14, 1993.

215. Smith E, Harris WH: Increasing prevalence of femoral lysis in cementless total hip arthroplasty. *J Arthrop* 10:407–412, 1995.

216. Dorr LD, cited in Fixation of uncemented stems, discussion. *Orthopaedics Special Edition* 3(5):16, 1994.

217. Engh CCA, Hooten JP Jr, Zettl-Schaffer KF: Porous-coated total hip replacement. *Clin Orthop Rel Res* 298:89–96, 1994.

218. Harris WH: A new total hip implant. *Clin Orthop Rel Res* 81:105–113, 1971.

219. Bartel DL, Wright TM, Edwards D: The effect of metal backing on stresses in polyethylene acetabular components, in *The Hip: Proceedings of the Eleventh Open Scientific Meeting of the Hip Society.* St Louis, Mosby, 1983, pp 229–239.

220. Carter DR: Finite-element analysis of a metal-backed acetabular component, in *The Hip: Proceedings of the Eleventh Open Scientific Meeting of the Hip Society.* St Louis, Mosby, 1983, pp 216–228.

221. Crowninshield DR, Pedersen DR, Brand RA: Analytical support for acetabular component metal backing, in *The Hip: Proceedings of the Eleventh Open Scientific Meeting of the Hip Society.* St Louis, Mosby, 1983, pp 207–215.

222. Ritter AM, Keating EM, Faris PM: Metal-backed acetabular cups in total hip arthroplasty. *J Bone Joint Surg* 72A:672–677, 1990.

223. Ritter MA: The cemented acetabular component of a total hip replacement: All polyethylene versus metal backing. *Clin Orthop Rel Res* 314:69–75, 1995.

224. Charnley J: The long-term results of low-friction arthroplasty of the hip performed as a primary intervention. *J Bone Joint Surg* 54B:61–76, 1972.

225. Thomas BJ, Amstutz HC: Prevention of heterotopic bone formation. Proceedings of the Fourteenth Meeting of the Hip Society. 1986, pp 59–68.

226. DeLee J, Ferrari A, Charnley J: Ectopic bone formation following low friction arthroplasty of the hip. *Clin Orthop Rel Res* 121:53–59, 1976.

227. Ritter MA, Vaughan RB: Ectopic ossification after total hip arthroplasty: Predisposing factors, frequency and effect on results. *J Bone Joint Surg* 59A:345–351, 1977.

228. Kjaersgaard-Andersen P, Stinke MS, Hougaard K: Heterotopic bone formation following hip arthroplasty: A retrospective study of 65 bilateral cases. *Acta Orthop Scand* 62:223, 1991.

229. Nollen AJG, Sloof TJJH: Para-articular ossifications after total hip replacement. *Acta Orthop Scand* 44:230, 1973.

230. Sodemann B, Persson PE, Nilsson O: Periarticular heterotopic ossification after total hip arthropalsty for primary coxarthrosis. *Clin Orthop Rel Res* 237:150, 1988.

230a. Cobb TK, Berry DJ, Morrey BF: Functional outcome of excision of heterotopic ossification after total hip arthroplasty. Presentation at the 61st Annual Meeting of the AAOS, New Orleans, LA, February 1994.

231. Kjaergaard-Andersen P, Hougaard K, Linde F: Heterotopic bone formation after total hip arthroplasty in patients with primary or secondary coxarthrosis. *Orthopedics* 13:1211, 1990.

232. DeLee J, Ferrari A, Charnley J: Ectopic bone formation following low friction arthroplasty of the hip. *Clin Orthop Rel Res* 121:53–59, 1976.

233. Goel A, Sharp DJ: Heterotopic bone formation after hip replacement: The influence of the type of osteoarthritis. *J Bone Joint Surg* 73B:255–257, 1991.

234. Bisla R, Ranawat CS, Inglis AE: Total hip replacement in patients with ankylosing spondylitis with involvement of the hip. *J Bone Joint Surg* 58A:233–238, 1976.

235. Errico TJ, Fetto JF, Waugh TR: Heterotopic ossification: Incidence and relation to trochanteric osteotomy in 100 total hip arthroplasties. *Clin Orthop Rel Res* 190:138, 1984.

236. Kjaersgaard-Andersen P, Ritter MA: Short-term treatment with nonsteroidal anti-inflammatory medications to prevent heterotopic bone formation after total hip arthroplasty: A preliminary report. *Clin Orthop Rel Res* 279:157–162, 1992.

237. Sundaram NA, Murphy JCM: Heterotopic bone formation following total hip arthroplasty in ankylosing spondylitis. *Clin Orthop Rel Res* 207:223, 1986.

238. Hierton C, Blomgren G, Lindgren U: Factors associated with heterotopic bone formation in cemented total hip prostheses. *Acta Orthop Scand* 54:698, 1983.

239. Lazansky MG: Complications revisited: The debit side of total hip replacement. *Clin Orthop Rel Res* 95:96, 1973.

240. Lewallen DG: Heterotopic ossification following total hip arthroplasty. *Instr Course Lect* 43:287–292, 1994.

241. Maloney WJ, Krushell RJ, Jasty M: Incidence of heterotopic ossification after total hip replacement: Effect of the type of fixation of the femoral component. *J Bone Joint Surg* 73A:191–193, 1991.

242. Finerman GA, Brooker AF, Coventry MB, et al: Symposium on heterotopic ossification following total hip arthroplasty. *Contemp Orthop* 5:95, 1982.

243. Morrey BF, Adams RA, Cabanela ME: Comparison of heterotopic bone after anterolateral, transtrochanteric and posterior approaches for total hip arthroplasty.

244. Bischoff R, Dunlap J, Carpenter L: Heterotopic ossification following uncemented total hip arthroplasty. Effect of operative approach. *J Arthrop* 9:641–644, 1994.

245. Duck HJ, Mylod AG: Heterotopic bone in hip arthroplasties: Cemented versus noncemented. *Clin Orthop Rel Res* 282:145–153, 1992.

246. Purtill JJ, Eng K, Rothman RH: Heterotopic ossification: Incidence in cemented versus cementless total hip arthroplasty. *J Arthrop* 11:58–63, 1996.

247. Brooker AF, Bowerman JW, Robinson RA: Ectopic ossification following total hip replacement: Incidence and a method of classification. *J Bone Joint Surg* 55A:1629, 1973.

248. Schmidt SA, Kjaersgaard-Andersen P, Pedersen NW, et al: The use of indomethacin to prevent the formation of heterotopic bone after total hip replacement: A randomized, double-blinded clinical trial. *J Bone Joint Surg* 70A:834, 1988.

249. Gebuhr P, Soelberg M, Orsnes T: Naproxen prevention of heterotopic ossification after hip arthroplasty: A prospective control study of 55 patients. *Acta Orthop Scand* 62:226–229, 1991.

250. Pignaci MJ, Pellicci PM, Salvati EA: Effect of aspirin on heterotopic ossification after total hip arthroplasty in men who have osteoarthrosis. *J Bone Joint Surg* 73A:924, 1991.

251. Elmstedt E, Lindholm T, Nilsson O: Effect of ibuprofen on heterotopic ossification after hip replacement. *Acta Orthop Scand* 56:25, 1985.

252. Gebuhr P, Wilbek H, Soelberg M: Naproxen for 8 days can prevent heterotopic ossification after hip arthroplasty. *Clin Orthop Rel Res* 314:166–169, 1995.

253. Cella JP, Salvati EA, Sculco TP: Indomethacin for the prevention of heterotopic ossification following total hip arthroplasty: Effectiveness, contraindication, and adverse effects. *J Arthrop* 3:229–234, 1988.

254. Longo JA, Magee FP, Hedley AK: The effect of chronic indomethacin on fixation of porous implants to bone, in Transactions of the 35th Annual Meeting of the Orthopedic Research Society. 14:337, 1989.

255. McMahon JS, Waddell JP, Morton J: Effect of short-course indomethacin on heterotopic bone formation after uncemented total hip arthroplasty. *J Arthrop* 6:259–264, 1991.

256. Coventry MB, Scanlon DW: The use of radiation to discourage ectopic bone. 201, 1981.

257. Thomas BJ, Amstutz HC: Prevention of heterotopic bone formation, in Proceedings of the Fourteenth Meeting of the Hip Society. 1986, pp 59–68.

257a. Thomas BJ: Hexerotopic bone formation after total hip arthroplasty. *Orthop Clin North Am* 23:347–358, 1992.

258. Pellegrini VD Jr, Konski AA, Gastel JA: Prevention of heterotopic ossification with irradiation after total hip arthroplasty: Radiation therapy with a single dose of eight hundred centigray administered to a limited field. *J Bone Joint Surg* 74A:186–200, 1992.

259. Healy WL, Lo TC, Covall DJ: Single-dose radiation therapy for prevention of heterotopic ossification after total hip arthroplasty. *J Arthrop* 5:369–375, 1990.

260. Pellegrini VD Jr, Gregoritch SJ: Preoperative irradiation for prevention of heterotopic ossification following total hip arthroplasty. *J Bone Joint Surg* 78A:870–881, 1996.

261. Thomas BJ: Heterotopic bone formation after total hip arthroplasty. *Orthop Clin North Am* 23:347–358, 1992.

262. Warren SB, Brooker AF Jr: Excision of heterotopic bone followed by irradiation after total hip arthroplasty. *J Bone Joint Surg* 74A:201–210, 1992.

263. Silver D: An overview of venous thromboembolism prophylaxis. *Am J Surg* 61:537–540, 1991.

264. Sikorski JM, Hampson WG, Staddon GE: The natural history and aetiology of deep vein thrombosis after total hip replacement. *J Bone Joint Surg* 63B:171–177, 1981.

265. Anderson FA Jr, Wheeler HB: Natural history and epidemiology of venous thromboembolism. *Orthop Rev* 23(suppl 1):5–9, 1994.

266. Lotke PA, Steinberg ME, Ecker ML: Significance of deep venous thrombosis in the lower extremity after total joint arthroplasty. *Clin Orthop Rel Res* 299:25–30, 1994.

267. Trowbridge A, Boese CK, Woodruff B: Incidence of posthospitalization proximal deep venous thrombosis after total hip arthroplasty: A pilot study. *Clin Orthop Rel Res* 299:203–208, 1994.

268. Swayze OS, Nasser S, Roberson JR: Deep venous thrombosis in total hip arthroplasty. *Orthop Clin North Am* 23:359–364, 1992.

269. Salzman EW, Harris W: Prevention of venous thromboembolism in orthopaedic patients. *J Bone Joint Surg* 58A:903–913, 1976.

270. Nielson HK: Pathophysiology of venous thromboembolism. *Semin Thromb Hemost* 17(suppl 3):S250–S253, 1991.

271. Patterson BM, Marchand R, Ranawat C: Complications of heparin therapy after total joint arthroplasty. *J Bone Joint Surg* 71A:1130–1134, 1989.

272. Ishak MA, Morley KD: Deep venous thrombosis after total hip arthroplasty: A prospective controlled study to determine the prophylactic effect of graded pressure stockings. *Br J Surg* 68:429, 1981.

273. Wolson ST, Watt J: Intermittent pneumatic compression to prevent proximal deep vein thrombosis during and after total hip replacement. *J Bone Joint Surg* 73A:507–512, 1991.

274. Gallus A: Venous thrombosis after elective hip replacement: The influence of preventive intermittent calf compression and of surgical technique. *Br J Surg* 79:17–19, 1983.

275. Bailey JP, Kruger MP, Solano FX: Prospective randomized trial of sequential compression devices vs low-dose warfarin for deep venous thrombosis prophylaxis in total hip arthroplasty.

276. Harris WH, Athanasoulis C, Waltman A: High- and low-dose aspirin prophylaxis against venous thromboembolic disease in total hip replacement. *J Bone Joint Surg* 64A:63–66, 1982.

277. Harris WH, Athanasoulis C, Waltman A: Prophylaxis of deep-vein thrombosis after total hip replacement. *J Bone Joint Surg* 67A:57–62, 1985.

278. Lotke PA, Palevsky H, Keenan AM: Aspirin and warfarin for thromboembolic disease after total joint arthroplasty. *Clin Orthop Rel Res* 324:251–258, 1996.

279. Francis CW, Pellegrini V, Marder V: Prevention of venous thrombosis after total hip arthroplasty. *J Bone Joint Surg* 71A:327–335, 1989.

280. Salvati EA, Lachiewicz P: Thromboembolism following total hip arthroplasty. *J Bone Joint Surg* 58A:721–925, 1976.

281. Amstutz HC, Friscia D, Dorey F: Warfarin prophylaxis to prevent mortality from pulmonary embolism after total hip replacement. *J Bone Joint Surg* 71A:321–326, 1989.

282. Coventry MB, Nolan DR, Beckenbaugh RD: "Delayed" prophylactic anti-coagulation: A study of results and complications in 2,012 total hip arthroplasties. *J Bone Joint Surg* 55A:1487–1492, 1973.

283. Francis CW, Marder V, Evarts C: Two-step warfarin therapy: Prevention of postoperative venous thrombosis without excessive bleeding. *JAMA* 249:374–378, 1983.

284. Harris WH, Salzman E, Athanasoulis C: Comparison of warfarin, low-molecular-weight heparin in prevention of venous thromboembolism following total hip replacement. *J Bone Joint Surg* 56A:1552–1562, 1974.

285. Fordyce MJ, Baker AS, Staddon GE: Efficacy of fixed minidose warfarin prophylaxis in total hip replacement. *Br Med J* 303:219–220, 1991.

286. Harris WH, Salzman E, Athanasoulis C: Comparison of warfarin, low-molecular-weight heparin in prevention of venous thromboembolism following total hip replacement. *J Bone Joint Surg* 56A:1552–1562, 1974.

287. Leyvraz PF, Richard J, Bachmann F: Adjusted versus fixed dose subcutaneous heparin in the prevention of deep vein thrombosis after total hip replacement. *N Engl J Med* 309:954–958, 1983.

288. Turpie AGC, Levine M, Hirsch J: A randomized controlled trial of a low-molecular weight heparin (Enoxaparin) to prevent deep-vein thrombosis in patients undergoing elective hip surgery. *N Engl J Med* 315:925–929, 1986.

289. Hull R, Raskob G, Pineo G: A comparison of subcutaneous low-molecular-weight heparin with warfarin sodium for prophylaxis against deep-vein thrombosis after hip or knee implantation. *N Engl J Med* 329:1370–1376, 1993.

290. Colwell CW, Spiro TE, Trowbridge AA: Use of enoxaparin, a low-molecular-weight heparin and unfractionated heparin for the prevention of deep venous thrombosis after elective hip replacement. *J Bone Joint Surg* 76A:3–14, 1994.

291. Mohr DN, Silverstien MD, Murtaugh PA: Prophylactic agents for venous thrombosis in elective hip surgery: Meta-analysis of studies using venographic assessment. *Arch Intern Med* 153:2221–2228, 1993.

292. Imperiale TF, Speroff T: A meta-analysis of methods to prevent venous thromboembolism following total hip replacement. *JAMA* 271:1780–1785, 1994.

293. Clagett GP, Anderson FA Jr, Heit J: Prevention of venous thromboembolism. *Chest* 108:312S–334S, 1995.

294. Fitzgerald RH Jr: Post-discharge prevention of deep vein thrombosis following total joint replacement. *Orthopedics* 19(suppl):15–18, 1996.

295. Morrey BF: Instability after total hip arthroplasty. *Orthop Clin North Am* 23:237–248, 1992.

296. Williams JF, Gottesman MJ, Mallory TH: Dislocation after total hip arthroplasty: Treatment with an above-knee hip spica cast. *Clin Orthop Rel Res* 171:53–58, 1982.

297. Eftekhar NS: Dislocation and instability complicating low friction arthroplasty of the hip joint. *Clin Orthop Rel Res* 121:120, 1976.

298. Fackler CD, Poss R: Dislocation in total hip arthroplasty. *Clin Orthop Rel Res* 151:169–178, 1980.

299. Herrlin K, Selvik G, Pettersson H: Space orientation of total hip prosthesis. *Acta Radiol Scand* 27:619, 1986.

300. Ackland M, Bourne W, Uhthoff H: Anteversion of the acetabular cup: Measurement of angle after total hip replacement. *J Bone Joint Surg* 68B:409, 1986.

301. Dorr LD, Wolf AW, Chandler RW: Classification and treatment of dislocation of total hip arthroplasty. *Clin Orthop Rel Res* 173:151, 1983.

302. Ritter MA: Dislocation and subluxation of the total hip replacement. *Clin Orthop Rel Res* 187:53–58, 1976.

303. Daly P, Morrey BF: Surgical correction of the unstable total hip. Presented at the American Academy of Orthopedic Surgeons. New Orleans, Feb 8–13, 1990.

304. Fraser GA, Wroblewski BM: Revision of the Charnley low-friction arthroplasty for recurrent or irreducible dislocation. *J Bone Joint Surg* 63B:552–555, 1981.

305. Kaplan SJ, Thomas WH, Poss R: Trochanteric advancement for recurrent dislocation after total hip arthroplasty. *J Arthrop* 2:119–124, 1987.

306. Daly P, Morrey BF: Operative correction of the unstable total hip. *J Bone Joint Surg* 74A:1334–1343, 1992.

307. Cobb TK, Morrey BF, Ilstrup DM: The elevated-rim acetabular liner in total hip arthroplasty: Realtionship to postoperative dislocation. *J Bone Joint Surg* 78A:80–86, 1996.

308. Krushell RJ, Burke DW, Harris WH: Elevated-rim acetabular components: Effects on range of motion and stability in total hip arthroplasty. *J Arthrop* 6(Suppl):S53–S58, 1991.

309. Schmalzried TP, Amstutz HA, Dorey FJ: Nerve palsy associated with total hip replacement. *J Bone Joint Surg* 73A:1074–1080, 1991.

310. Solheim LF, Hagen R: Femoral and sciatic neuropathies after total hip arthroplasty. *Acta Orthop Scand* 51:531, 1990.

311. Weber ER, Daube JR, Coventry MB: Peripheral neuropathies associated with total hip arthroplasty. *J Bone Joint Surg* 58A:66, 1976.

312. Harris WH, Salzman E, Athanasoulis C: Comparison of warfarin, low-molecular-weight heparin in prevention of venous

thromboembolism following total hip replacement. *J Bone Joint Surg* 56A:1552–1562, 1974.

313. Wasielewski RC, Crossett LS, Rubash HE: Neural and vascular injury in total hip arthroplasty. *Orthop Clin North Am* 23:219–235, 1992.

314. Wasielewski RC, Cooperstein LA, Kruger MP: Acetabular anatomy and the transacetabular fixation of screws in total hip arthroplasty. *J Bone Joint Surg* 72A:501–508, 1990.

315. Johanson NA, Pellicci PM, Tsairis P: Nerve injury in total hip arthroplasty. *Clin Orthop Rel Res* 179:214, 1983.

316. Robinson RP, Robinson HJ Jr, Salvati EA: Comparison of the transtrochanteric and posterior approaches for total hip replacement. *Clin Orthop Rel Res* 147:143, 1980.

317. Navarro RA, Schmalzried TP, Amstutz HC: Surgical approach and nerve palsy in total hip arthroplasty. *J Arthrop* 10:1–5, 1995.

318. Stone RG, Weeks LE, Hajdu M: Evaluation of sciatic nerve compromise during total hip arthroplasty. *Clin Orthop Rel Res* 201:26, 1985.

319. Rasmussen RJ, Black DL, Bruce RP: Efficacy of corticosomatosensory evoked potential monitoring in predicting and/or preventing sciatic nerve palsy during total hip arthroplasty. *J Arthrop* 9:53–61, 1994.

320. Wasielewski RC, Crossett LS, Rubash HE: Neural and vascular injury in total hip arthroplasty. *Orthop Clin North Am* 23:219–235, 1992.

321. Poss R, Walker P, Spector M: Strategies for improving fixation of femoral components in total hip arthroplasty. *Clin Orthop Rel Res* 235:181–194, 1988.

322. Taylor MM, Meyers MH, Harvey JP: Intraoperative femur fractures during total hip replacement. *Clin Orthop Rel Res* 137:96–103, 1978.

323. Khan MAA, O'Driscoll M: Fractures of the femur during total hip replacement and their management. *J Bone Joint Surg* 59B:36–41, 1977.

324. Scott RD, Turner RH, Leitzes SM: Femoral fractures in conjunction with total hip replacement. *J Bone Joint Surg* 57A:494–501, 1975.

325. Christensen CM, Seger BM, Schultz RB: Management of intraoperative femur fractures associated with revision total hip arthroplasty. *Clin Orthop Rel Res* 248:177–180, 1989.

326. Kavanagh BF, Illstrup DM, Fitzgerald RH: Revision total hip arthroplasty. *J Bone Joint Surg* 67A:517–526, 1985.

327. Stuchin SA: Femoral shaft fracture in porous and press-fit total hip arthroplasty. *Orthop Rev* 19:153–159, 1990.

328. Fitzgerald RH Jr, Brindley GW, Kavanagh BF: The uncemented total hip arthroplasty: Intraoperative femoral fractures. *Clin Orthop Rel Res* 235:61–66, 1988.

329. Schwartz JT, Meyer JG, Engh CA: Femoral fracture during noncemented total hip arthroplasty. *J Bone Joint Surg* 71A:1135–1142, 1989.

330. Khan MAA, O'Driscoll M: Fractures of the femur during total hip replacement and their management. *J Bone Joint Surg* 59B:36–41, 1977.

331. Mont MA, Maar DC, Krackow KA: Hoop-stress fractures of the proximal femur during hip arthroplasty: Management and results in 19 cases. *J Bone Joint Surg* 74B:257–260, 1992.

332. Larson JE, Chao EYS, Fitzgerald RH Jr: Bypassing femoral cortical defects with cemented intramedullary stems. *J Orthop Res* 9:414–421, 1991.

333. Fredin H: Late fracture of the femur following perforation during total hip arthroplasty: A report of two cases. *Acta Orthop Scand* 59:331–332, 1988.

334. Eschenroeder HC Jr, Krackow KA: Late onset femoral stress fracture associated with extruded cement following hip arthroplasty: A case report. *Clin Orthop Rel Res* 236:210–213, 1988.

335. Duncan CP, Masri BA: Fractures of the femur after hip replacement. *Instr Course Lect* 44:293–304, 1995.

336. Johansson JE, McBroom R, Barrington TW: Fracture of the ipsilateral femur in patients with total hip replacement. *J Bone Joint Surg* 63A:1435–1442, 1981.

337. Scott RD, Turner RH, Leitzes SM: Femoral fractures in conjunction with total hip replacement. *J Bone Joint Surg* 57A:494–501, 1975.

338. Stern RE, Harwin SF, Kulick RG: Management of ipsilateral femoral shaft fractures following hip arthroplasty. *Orthop Rev* 20:779–784, 1991.

339. Levenberg R, Iorio R, Gingrich K: Femur fractures associated with total hip arthroplasty. *Orthopedics* 13:1188–1189, 1990.

340. Serocki JH, Chandler RW, Dorr LD: Treatment of fractures about hip prostheses with compression plating. *J Arthrop* 7:129–135, 1992.

341. Ogden WS, Rednall J: Fractures beneath hip prostheses: A special indication for Parham bands and plating. *Orthop Trans* 2:70, 1978.

342. Wang G-J, Miller TO, Stamp WG: Femoral fracture following hip arthroplasty: Brief note on treatment. *J Bone Joint Surg* 67A:956–958, 1985.

343. Montijo H, Ebert FR, Lennox DA: Treatment of proximal femur fractures associated with total hip arthroplasty. *J Arthrop* 4:115–123, 1989.

344. Ruedi TP, Luscher JN: Results after internal fixation of comminuted fractures of the femoral shaft with DC plates. *Clin Orthop Rel Res* 138:74–76, 1979.

345. Kavanagh BF: Femoral fractures associated with total hip arthroplasty. *Orthop Clin North Am* 23:249–257, 1992.

346. Berman AT, Levenberg RJ: Femur fractures associated with total hip arthroplasty. *Orthopedics* 15:751–753, 1992.

ARTHRODESIS OF THE HIP

347. Liechti R: *Hip Arthrodesis and Associated Problems.* Berlin, Springer-Verlag, 1978.

348. Duncan C: Hip disease in young adults. *Can J Surg* 38:S55–S68, 1995.

349. Tornetta P: personal communication, 1996.

350. Sponseller PD, McBeath AA, Perpich M: Hip arthrodesis in young patients. *J Bone Joint Surg* 66A:853–859, 1984.

351. Callaghan JJ: Hip arthrodesis: A long-term follow up. *J Bone Joint Surg* 66A:1328–1335, 1985.

REVISION HIP SURGERY

352. Fitzgerald RH Jr: Infected total hip arthroplasty: Diagnosis and treatment. *J Acad Orthop Surg* 3:249–262, 1995.

353. Oh I, Hardacre JA: Fatigue fracture of the inferior pubic ramus following total hip replacement for congenital hip dislocation. *Clin Orthop* 147:154–156, 1980.

354. Foster IW, Crawford R: Sedimentation rate in infected and uninfected total hip arthroplasty. *Clin Orthop* 168:48–52, 1982.

355. Barrack RL, Harris WH: The value of aspiration of the hip joint before revision total hip arthroplasty. *J Bone Joint Surg* 78A:749–754, 1996.

356. Lachiewicz PF, Rogers GD, Thomason WC: Aspiration of the hip joint in revision total hip arthroplasty. *J Bone Joint Surg* 78A:749–754, 1996.

357. Shih LY, Wu J, Yang DG: Erythrocyte sedimentation rate and C-reactive protein values in patients with total hip arthroplasty. *Clin Orthop* 225:238–246, 1987.

358. Sanzen L, Carlson AS: The diagnostic value of C-reactive protein in infected hip arthroplasties. *J Bone Joint Surg* 71B:68–641, 1989.

359. Phillips WC, Kattapuram SV: Prosthetic hip replacement: Plain films and arthrography for component loosening. *AJR* 138:677–682, 1982.

360. O'Neil DA, Harris WH: Failed total hip replacement: Assessment by plain radiographs, arthrograms and aspiration of the hip joint. *J Bone Joint Surg* 66A:540–546, 1984.

361. Harris WH, Barrack RL: Developments in diagnosis of the painful total hip replacement. *Orthop Rev* April:439–447, 1993.

362. Nivbrant B, Karrholm J, et al: Migration of porous press fit cups in hip revision arthroplasty. *J Arthrop* 11:390–396, 1996.

363. Karrholm J, Borssen B, et al: Early micromotions in cemented femoral stems subsequently revised due to pain or osteolysis. *Trans Orthop Res Soc* 19:246, 1994.

364. Engh CA, Massin P, Suthers KE: Roentgenographic assessment of the biologic fixation of porous surfaced femoral components. *Clin Orthop* 257:107–127, 1990.

365. Barrack RL, Lebar RD: Clinical and radiographic analysis of the uncemented LSF total hip arthroplasty. *J Arthrop* 735:754–762, 1992.

366. Johnston RC, Fitzgerald RH, Harris WH: Clinical and radiographic evaluation of total hip replacement. *J Bone Joint Surg* 72A:161, 1990.

367. Capello WN, Uri BG, Wellmann HN, et al: Comparison of radiographic and radionuclide hip arthrography in determination of femoral component loosening of hip arthroplasties, in *The Hip*. St Louis, Mosby, 1985.

368. Evans BG, Cuckler JM: Evaluation of the total hip arthroplasty. *Orthop Clin North Am* 23:203–310, 1992.

369. Schneider R, Gruen D, Brause B: Diagnosis of infected joint prostheses. *Semin Arthrop* 6:167–175, 1995.

370. Fitzgerald RH Jr, Nasser S: Infection following total hip arthroplasty in hip and knee reconstruction, in Callaghan JJ, Dennis DA, Poprosky WG, Rosenberg AG (eds): *Orthopedic Knowledge Update*. Rosemont, IL, American Association of Orthopaedic Surgeons, 1995, pp 157–161.

371. Merkel KD, Brown ML, Dewanjee MK, et al: Comparison of indium labeled leukocyte imaging with sequential technetium gallium scanning in the diagnosis of low grade musculoskeletal sepsis. *J Bone Joint Surg* 67A:465–475, 1985.

372. Lieberman JR, Huo MH, et al: Evaluation of painful hip arthroplasties: Are technetium bone scans necessary? *J Bone Joint Surg* 75B:475–478, 1992.

373. Osweld SG, Van Nostrand D, Savory CG, et al: The acetabulum, a prospective study of three phase bone and indium white blood cell scintigraphy following coated hip arthroplasty. *J Nucl Med* 31:274, 1990.

374. Levitsky KA, Hozack WJ, et al: Evaluation of the painful prosthetic joint. *J Arthrop* 6:237–244, 1991.

375. Gristina AG, Shitata AY, et al: The glycocalyx, biofilm microbes and infection. *Semin Arthrop* 5:160–170, 1994.

376. Calandruccio R: Arthroplasty of the hip, in *Campbell's Operative Orthopedics,* 7th ed. St Louis, Mosby, 1987.

377. Padgett DE, Silverman A, et al: Efficacy of intraoperative cultures obtained during revision total hip arthroplasty. *J Arthrop* 10:420–426, 1996.

378. Mirra JN, Marder RA, Amstutz HC: The pathology of failed total joint arthroplasty. *Clin Orthop* 170:175–183, 1982.

379. Roberts P, Walters AJ, McMinn DJ: Diagnosing infection in hip replacements. *J Bone Joint Surg* 74B:265–269, 1992.

380. Glassman AH, Engh CA: The removal of porous coated femoral hip stems. *Clin Orthop* 285:164–180, 1992.

381. McDonald DJ, Fitzgerald RH Jr, Ilstrup DM: Two stage reconstruction of total hip arthroplasty because of infection. *J Bone Joint Surg* 71A:828–834, 1989.

382. Colyer RA, Capello WN: Surgical treatment of the infected hip implants. *Clin Orthop* 298:75–79, 1994.

383. Garvin KL: Two stage re-implantation of the infected hip. *Semin Arthrop* 5:142–146, 1994.

384. Cautilli GP, Beight J, et al: A prospective review of 303 cementless universal cups with emphasis on wear as the cause of failure. *Semin Arthrop* 5:25–29, 1994.

385. Maloney WJ, Smith RL: Periprosthetic osteolysis in total hip arthroplasty: The role of particulate wear debris. *Instr Course Lect* 45:171–182, 1996.

386. Lavernia CJ, Hungerford D: Wear in the porous coated anatomic total hip replacement. *Semin Arthrop* 5:20–24, 1994.

387. Wroblewski BM: Direction and rate of socket wear in Charnley low friction arthroplasty. *J Bone Joint Surg* 67B:757–761, 1985.

388. Wang JT, Harada Y, et al: Biologic mechanisms involved in the pathogenesis of aseptic loosening of total joint replacement. *Semin Arthrop* 7:70–73, 1996.

389. Isaac GH, Wroblewski BM, Ackenson JR, et al: Tribological study of retrieved hip prostheses. *Clin Orthop* 276:115–125, 1992.

390. Trieu HH, Avent RT, Paxson RD: Effect of sterilization on shelf aged UHMWPE tibial inserts. *Trans Soc Biomat* 18:109, 1995.

391. Sutula LC, Sum KA, Collier JP, et al: Time dependent oxidation and damage in retrieved and never implanted UHMWPE components. *Trans Orthop Res Soc* 20:118–120, 1995.

392. Collier JP, Mayor MM, et al: Mechanisms of failure of modular prostheses. *Clin Orthop* 285:129–139, 1992.

393. Liebermann JR, Moeckel BH, et al: Cement within cement revision hip arthroplasty. *J Bone Joint Surg* 75B:869–871, 1991.

394. Lombardi A: Cement removal in revision total hip arthroplasty. *Semin Arthrop* 3:264–272, 1989.

395. Schurman DJ, Mallon WJ: Segmental cement extraction and revision: Total hip arthroplasty. *Clin Orthop* 285:158–163, 1992.

396. Younger TI, Bradford MS, Magnes RE, Proposki WG: Extended proximal femoral osteotomy. *J Arthrop* 10:329–338, 1995.

397. Head WC, Mallory TH, Berklacich FM, et al: Extensile exposure of the hip for revision arthroplasty. *J Arthrop* 2:265–273, 1987.

398. Berman AT, Salter FL, Koenig T: Revision total hip replacement without trochanteric osteotomy. *Orthopedics* 10:755, 1987.

399. Glassman AH: Complication of trochanteric osteotomy. *Orthop Clin North Am* 23:321–333, 1992.

400. Glassman AH, Engh CA: The removal of porous coated femoral hip stems. *Clin Orthop* 285:164–180, 1992.

401. Stiehl JB: Extensile anterior column acetabular reconstruction in revision total hip arthroplasty. *Semin Arthrop* 6:60–67, 1995.

402. Krackow KA, Steinman H, Cohn BT, Jones LC: Clinical experience with a triradiate exposure of the hip for difficult total hip arthroplasty. *J Arthrop* 3:267–278, 1988.

403. Christensen CM, Seger BM, Schultz RB: Management of intraoperative femur fractures associated with revision hip arthroplasty. *Clin Orthop* 248:177–180, 1989.

404. Masri BA, Dunkin CP: Classification of bone loss in total hip arthroplasty. *Instr Course Lect* 45:199–208, 1996.

405. Rubash HE, Harris WH: Revision of non-septic loose cemented femoral components using modern cementing techniques. *J Arthrop* 3:241–248, 1988.

406. Estok DM, Harris WH: Long term results of cemented femoral revision surgery using second generation techniques: An average 11.7 year follow-up evaluation. *Clin Orthop* 299:190–202, 1994.

407. Gie GA, Linder L, Ling RSM, et al: Impacted cancellous allografts and cement for revision total hip arthroplasty. *J Bone Joint Surg* 75B:14–21, 1993.

408. Katz RP, Callaghan J, et al: Results of cemented femoral revision total hip arthroplasty using improved cementing technique. *Clin Orthop* 319:178–183, 1995.

409. Callaghan JJ, Goetz DD, Johnston RC: Revision of a failed cemented total hip prosthesis with insertion of an acetabular component without cement and a femoral component with cement. *J Bone Joint Surg* 78A:982–994, 1996.

410. Elting JJ, Mikhail WE, et al: Preliminary report of impaction grafting for exchange femoral arthroplasty. *Clin Orthop* 319:159–167, 1995.

411. Weber KL, Nelissen RGH, Bouer TW, et al: Revision hip arthroplasty with the use of cement and impaction grafting. *J Bone Joint Surg* 77A:412–422, 1995.

412. Rockborn P, Olsson SS: Loosening and bone resorption in Exeter hip arthroplasty. *J Bone Joint Surg* 75B:865–868, 1993.

413. Fowler JL, Gie GA, et al: Experience with the Exeter total hip replacement since 1970. *Orthop Clin North Am* 19:477–489, 1988.

414. Turner RH, Mattingly DA, Scheller A: Femoral revision total hip arthroplasty using a long stem femoral component. *J Arthrop* 2:247, 1987.

415. Moreland JR, Bernstein ML: Femoral revision hip arthroplasty with uncemented porous coated stems. *Clin Orthop* 319:141–150, 1995.

416. Head WC, Vagna RA, Emerson RH: Revision total hip arthroplasty in the deficient femur with proximal load bearing prosthesis. *Clin Orthop* 298:119–126, 1994.

417. Pak JH, Paprosky WH, et al: Femoral strut allografts in cementless revision, total hip arthroplasty. *Clin Orthop* 295:172–178, 1993.

418. Emerson RH, Malinin TI, et al: Cortical strut allografts in the reconstruction of the femur in revision total hip arthroplasty. *Clin Orthop* 285:35–44, 1992.

419. Chandler HP, Ayres DK, et al: Revision total hip replacement using the S-Rom femoral component. *Clin Orthop* 319:130–140, 1995.

420. Cameron HU: The two to six year results with proximally modular noncemented total hip replacement used in hip revision. *Clin Orthop* 298:47–53, 1994.

421. Malkani AL, Lewaller DG, et al: Femoral component revision using an uncemented proximally coated long stemmed prosthesis. *J Arthrop* 11:411–418, 1996.

422. Allan DG, Lavoie GJ, McDonald S, et al: Proximal femoral allografts in revision hip arthroplasty. *J Bone Joint Surg* 73B:235–240, 1991.

423. Chandler HC, Clark J, Murphy S, et al: Reconstruction of major segmental loss of the proximal femur in revision total hip arthroplasty. *Clin Orthop* 298:67–74, 1994.

424. Chandler HC: Intramedullary grafting of the expanded femoral canal in total hip replacement. *Tech Orthop* 7:33–43, 1993.

425. Peters CL, Rivero DP, et al: Revision total hip arthroplasty without cement: Subsidence of proximally porous coated femoral components. *J Bone Joint Surg* 77A:1217–1226, 1995.

426. Malkani AL, Sim FH, Chao EYS: Custom made segmental femoral replacement prostheses in revision total hip arthroplasty. *Orthop Clin North Am* 24:727–733, 1993.

427. Kavanagh BF, Ilstrup DM, Fitzgerald RH Jr: Revision total hip arthroplasty. *J Bone Joint Surg* 67A:517–526, 1986.

428. Kavanagh BF, Fitzgerald RH Jr: Multiple revisions for failed total hip arthroplasty not associated with infection. *J Bone Joint Surg* 69A:1144–1149, 1987.

429. Jasty M, Harris WH: Salvage total hip reconstruction in patients with major acetabular bone deficiency using structural femoral head allografts. *J Bone Joint Surg* 72B:63–68, 1990.

430. Silverton CD, Rosenberg AG, Scheinkopf M, et al: Revision total hip arthroplasty using a cementless acetabular component. *Clin Orthop* 319:201–208, 1995.

431. Hungerford DS, Jones LC: The rationale of cementless revision of cemented arthroplasty failures. *Clin Orthop* 235:12–24, 1988.

432. Maloney WJ, Peters P, Engh CA, et al: Severe osteolysis of the pelvis in association with acetabular replacement without cement. *J Bone Joint Surg* 75A:1627–1635, 1993.

433. Schmalzried TP, Kwong LM, Tasty M, et al: The mechanism of loosening of cemented acetabular components in total hip arthroplasty. *Clin Orthop* 274:76–78, 1992.

434. Dorr LD, Wan Z: 10 years experience with porous acetabular components for revision surgery. *Clin Orthop* 319:191–200, 1995.

435. Heekin RD, Engh CA, Vinh T: Morcellized allografts in acetabular reconstruction. *Clin Orthop* 319:184–190, 1995.

436. Brien WW, Bruce WJ, Salvati EA, et al: Acetabular reconstruction with a bipolar prosthesis and morcellized bone grafts. *J Bone Joint Surg* 72A:1230–1234, 1990.

437. Murrey WR: Acetabular salvage in revision total hip arthroplasty using the bipolar prosthesis. *Clin Orthop* 251:92–99, 1990.

438. Paprosky WG, Magness RE: Principles of bone grafting in revision total hip arthroplasty. *Clin Orthop* 298:147–155, 1994.

438a. Paprosky WG, Bradford MS, Jablonski NS: Acetabular reconstruction with massive acetabular allografts. *AAOS Instr Course Lect* 45:149–160, 1996.

439. Oh I, Harris WH: Design concepts, indications and surgical technique for use of the protrusio shell. *Clin Orthop* 162:175–184, 1982.

440. Possai K, Dorr LD, McPherson EJ: Metal ring supports for deficient acetabular bone in total hip replacement. *Instr Course Lect* 45:161–170, 1996.

441. Berry DJ, Muller ME: Revision arthroplasty using an antiprotrusio cage for massive acetabular bone deficiency. *J Bone Joint Surg* 74B:711–715, 1992.

442. Haentjens P, DeBoeck H, et al: Cemented acetabular reconstruction with the Muller support ring. *Clin Orthop* 290:225–235, 1993.

HIP ARTHROSCOPY

443. Schindler A, Lechevallier JJ, Rao NS, Bowen JR: Diagnostic and therapeutic arthroscopy of the hip in children and adolescents: Evaluation of results. *J Pediatr Orthop* 15:317–321, 1995.

444. Bowen JR, Kumar VP, et al: Osteochondritis dissecans following Perthes disease. *Clin Orthop* 209:49–56, 1986.

445. McCarthy JC, Day B, Busconi B: Hip arthroscopy applications and technique. *J Am Acad Orthop Surg* 3:115–122, 1995.

446. Futami T, Kasahara Y, et al: Arthroscopy for slipped capital femoral epiphysis. *J Pediatr Orthop* 12:592–597, 1992.

447. Holgerrson S, Brattstrom H, et al: Arthroscopy of the hip in juvenile chronic arthritis. *J Pediatr Orthop* 1:273–278, 1981.

448. Chung WK, Slater GL, Bates EH: Treatment of septic arthritis of the hip by arthroscopic lavage. *J Pediatr Orthop* 13:444–446, 1993.

449. Frich LH, Lauritzen J, Juhl M: Arthroscopy in diagnosis and treatment of hip disorders. *Orthopaedics* 12:389–392, 1989.

450. Eriksson E, Arvidsson I, Arvidsson H: Diagnostic and operative arthroscopy of the hip. *Orthopaedics* 9:169–176, 1986.

The Knee

CHAPTER 50

Meniscal and Ligamentous Injuries of the Knee

Jeffrey D. Stone and Freddie H. Fu

MENISCAL INJURIES

Meniscal Function

The menisci serve several functions, all of which play an important role in maintaining a healthy knee joint. These functions include weight bearing or load distribution, shock absorption, maintaining joint stability, lubrication, articular cartilage nutrition, and proprioception. The menisci play an important role in weight bearing. Any load applied to the knee joint is shared by both the articular and meniscal cartilage. The menisci protect the articular cartilage by increasing both the joint congruity and contact area as well as preventing focal concentrations of stress. The structure of the menisci allows them to perform this very important function. When a load is transmitted across the knee joint, the circumferentially oriented collagen fibers within the menisci generate a hoop stress, which resists extrusion of the menisci from between the femoral condyle and tibial plateau.[1] Ahmed and Burke have shown that the menisci transmit approximately 50 percent of the weight-bearing forces across the knee joint in extension and 85 percent at 90° of knee flexion.[2] Furthermore, it has been shown that the medial and lateral menisci bear differential proportions of the loads transmitted across their respective compartments. In the medial compartment, the medial meniscus bears 50 percent of the load across the compartment, while the articular compartment also bears 50 percent of the load; whereas in the lateral compartment, the lateral meniscus carries approximately 70 percent of the load transmitted across its respective compartment.[3,4] Given the significant roles of the menisci in load transmission across the joints, it is evident that there are significant increases in the local contact stress borne by the articular cartilage after meniscectomy.[5] Other studies have shown that the contact area is decreased and load transmission is reduced 50 to 70 percent following meniscectomy.[2,5,6] Consequently it appears that meniscectomy results in a significant increase in the load per unit area within the knee joint, thus contributing to possible damage to and degeneration of the articular cartilage. It also has been demonstrated that partial meniscectomy decreases contact area and increases local contact stresses.[5] In fact, Seedholm and Hargraves demonstrated that even resection of 15 to 34 percent of the meniscus resulted in increased contact pressure by over 350 percent.[7] The menisci can be described as possessing the qualities or characteristics of viscoelasticity. This means that menisci exhibit time- and history-dependent stress-strain behaviors. They display the properties of both stress relaxation and creep. *Stress relaxation* is described as a time-dependent decrease in load when the material is subject to a constant strain. *Creep* is described as a time-dependent increase in elongation that occurs when a viscoelastic material is subject to a constant load. It is these viscoelastic properties that allow the menisci to function as shock absorbers in the knee joint. During gait, viscoelastic deformation of the menisci allows for attenuation of the load transmitted through the knee joint.[7,8] Voloshin and Wosk[8] have demonstrated that meniscectomized knees have approximately 20 percent less shock-absorbing capacity than normal knees. The menisci have also been shown to contribute to joint stability. Levy et al.[9] demonstrated that the medial meniscus is an important secondary restraint to anterior displacement of the knee in anterior cruciate ligament (ACL)–deficient knees. Using a cadaveric model, they showed that without compressive loads, the medial meniscus functions as a secondary restraint to anterior tibial translation. Their evidence demonstrated that the posterior horn of the medial meniscus provides the most significant contribution to resisting anterior tibial displacement.[9] In ACL-deficient knees that had undergone medial meniscectomy, there was significantly greater anterior tibial translation between flexion angles of 30 and 90° than was seen in knees with sectioned ACLs alone. In knees with an intact ACL, however, medial meniscectomy did not influence anterior tibial translation. In another study, Levy et al.[10] demonstrated that lateral meniscectomy in ACL-deficient knees did not increase the amount of anterior tibial translation when compared with ACL-deficient knees alone.[10] Shoemaker and Markolf[11] also used the cadaveric model to study the role of the menisci as secondary restraints to anteroposterior displacement of loaded, ACL-deficient knees. The results of their study demonstrated that when compressive loads were applied to the knee after sectioning of the anterior cruciate ligament, the medial meniscus did restrain anterior tibial translation. They also noted that the greatest contribution to anterior displacement was provided by the posterior horn of the medial meniscus. Furthermore, the magnitude of translation was dependent upon the magnitude of both the compressive load and the applied anterior drawer force. They hypothesized that physiologic anterior tibial forces would most likely overcome the resistive forces of the menisci as a secondary restraint to anterior tibial translation.[11] The role of the menisci as secondary restraints providing stability to the knee joint have been described by other authors as well.[12,13] Furthermore, the menisci increase congruity between the femoral and tibial condyles, thus contributing to overall joint congruity and stability. As the knee moves, there is excursion of the menisci in the anterior and posterior directions along the tibial plateaus. As a result, the menisci act to distribute synovial fluid along the articular surfaces, providing both joint lubrication and distribution of nutrients to the avascular articular cartilage. Finally, it has been suggested by some, based on the presence of types I and II nerve endings in the menisci, that they function in providing proprioceptive feedback for joint position sense.[14,15] The clinical function of the menisci has been inferred from the degenerative changes that have been seen in patients who have undergone partial or total meniscectomy. In 1936, King was the first to identify degenerative arthritis following meniscectomy.[16] Several years later, Fairbank characterized the classic degenerative changes that commonly result from meniscectomy. Characteristic radiographic changes include joint space narrowing, flattening and squaring of the femoral condyle, as well as peripheral ridge or osteophyte formation.[17,18] Despite earlier recognition that meniscectomy can lead to severe degenerative changes, it has been only over the last 10 years that meniscal repair has taken the place of traditional meniscectomy in the treatment of many meniscal injuries. Partial and subtotal meniscectomies are still indicated under certain conditions; however, meniscal repair has become the preferred procedure in order to preserve both the meniscus and the long-term well-being of the knee joint.[19]

Meniscal Anatomy

The menisci are biconcave disks that are thick at their attachments to the joint capsule peripherally and taper to a thin, central free edge. The proximal surfaces of the menisci are concave, thus allowing for increased contact area with the femoral condyles. The flat distal surfaces rest on the tibial plateau.[20]

The medial meniscus is semicircular, measuring approximately 3.5 cm in anteroposterior length, with one thin and one wider posterior horn. The anterior horn of the medial meniscus attaches to the anterior intercondylar fascia of the tibia anterior to the ACL footprint. The posterior horn of the medial meniscus attaches posteriorly to the intercondylar fascia between the posterior cruciate ligament (PCL) tibial footprint and the posterior insertion of the lateral meniscus. The medial meniscus is bound to the joint capsule peripherally; it is bound to the femur and tibia at its midportion by the deep medial collateral ligament.[20] The lateral meniscus is nearly circular in shape and covers a greater area of the tibial-articular surface than does the

medial meniscus. The width of the lateral meniscus is essentially equal as it is followed in the anterior-to-posterior direction. The lateral meniscus attaches anteriorly to the tibial eminence behind the ACL footprint, with which it partially blends. The posterior horn attaches behind the tibial eminence anterior to the posterior edge of the medial meniscus. The lateral meniscus also has variable femoral attachments: the anterior and posterior meniscofemoral ligaments (Humphrey's and Wrisberg's ligaments; Fig. 50-1). Like the medial meniscus, the lateral meniscus is loosely attached to its respective tibial plateau by a capsular apron, also known as the *coronary ligament.* The medial and lateral menisci are connected to each other anteriorly via the transverse ligament.[20] The collagen fibers of the menisci are primarily circumferential, while a few radially and obliquely oriented fibers act to increase the structural rigidity of the meniscus.[1]

A detailed knowledge of the vascular anatomy of the meniscus is necessary to understand the approach to meniscal repair. The first successful meniscal repair was reported by Annandale in 1885.[21] Annandale recognized the potential for significant benefit of preserving the menisci; however, the significance of meniscal blood supply was not elucidated until 1936, when King published his work on meniscal healing in dogs.[22] He determined that communication with the peripheral blood supply from the synovial membrane was absolutely necessary for meniscal healing. Despite King's work, the microvascular anatomy of the meniscus was not completely understood until Arnoczky and Warren published their work based on intravascular India ink injections of the human meniscus in 1982.[23] They demonstrated that the meniscal blood supply originates from the superior and inferior branches of the lateral and medial geniculate arteries. These vessels give rise to a perimeniscal capillary plexus, oriented circumferentially around the periphery of the menisci and supplying the peripheral border of each meniscus. The smaller radial branches supply the peripheral 20 to 30 percent of the medial meniscus and 10 to 25 percent of the lateral meniscus. The remaining central portions of the menisci rely upon the diffusion of nutrients from the synovial fluid, as these portions are avascular.[23] In addition, a 3-mm fringe of synovial tissue extending around the edge of the femoral and tibial articular surfaces functions as a significant source of vascularization and growth during meniscal healing following injury, despite the fact that the synovial fringe does not normally contribute vessels to the meniscus.[23–25]

As discussed, King was the first to suggest the importance of the peripheral meniscus and its vascular supply to the healing of meniscal tears. Using a canine model, he observed that meniscal tears in the avascular portion of the meniscus healed only if they extended to the vascularized meniscosynovial junction. Subsequent studies have confirmed that the peripheral meniscal blood supply is critical for the successful healing of meniscal tears.[22–26] It is the presence of a vascular supply that allows for the characteristic inflammatory response of injury repair.[23,25]

The first response to injury or tearing of the meniscus within the peripheral vascular zone is formation of a fibrin clot, which provides a scaffold for proliferation of vessels from the perimeniscal capillary plexus. This is followed by

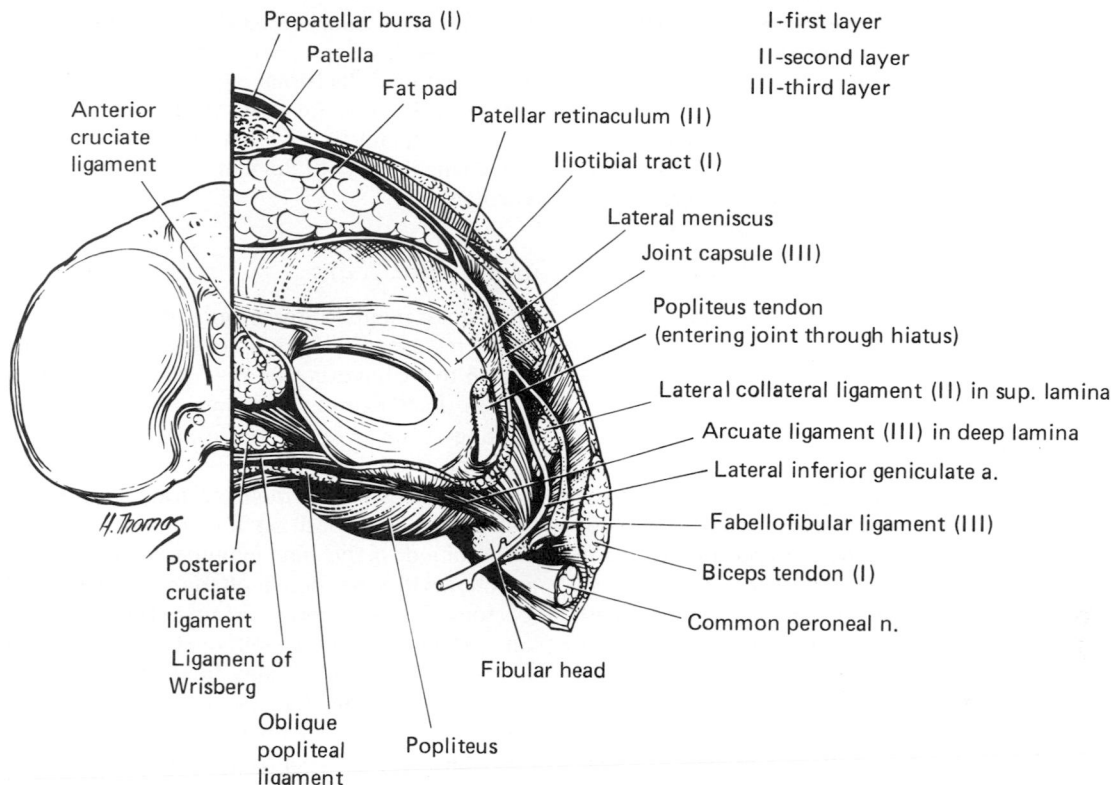

Figure 50-1 A view of the right knee joint from above after removal of the right femur. The three layers of the lateral side of the knee are depicted. The posterolateral portion of the capsule (layer 3) is divided into superficial and deep laminae separated by the lateral inferior geniculate vessels. (Reproduced with permission from Seebacher JR, Inglis AE, Marshall J, Warren RF: The structure of the posterolateral aspect of the knee. *J Bone Joint Surg* 64A:536–541, 1982.)

the influx of undifferentiated mesenchymal cells. Fibrovascular scar tissue then forms, essentially gluing the torn edges together. Vessels from a proliferative vascular pannus extending from the synovial fringe also begin to penetrate the fibrovascular scar tissue, further enhancing the cellular inflammatory response.[23] Radial lesions of the meniscus extending to the synovium can heal with fibrovascular scar tissue in approximately 10 weeks.[23] The strength of this scar tissue is substantially less than that of normal meniscal tissue, and this tissue does undergo further remodeling over the ensuing several months.

Diagnosis of meniscal injury is based primarily on a thorough history and physical examination. In the athletic population, the patient typically describes a twisting injury as the inciting event. Often, with degenerative tears, there is no one known inciting event. If there is an inciting event, swelling frequently develops. The patient may describe clicking or locking as well as loss of motion, which can be secondary to an effusion, pain, or true mechanical block (which is uncommon).

Upon physical examination, effusion is often present with joint-line tenderness, pain with squatting, a positive flexion McMurray test, and positive Apley compression and distraction tests. Plain radiograph should always be a part of the routine evaluation. This includes a 45° pos-

teroanterior weight-bearing view, also known as a Rosenberg view, as well as lateral and axial (for example, Merchant or Sunrise) views.

Preoperative imaging modalities, although not often obtained prior to proceeding with arthroscopy, may include contrast arthrography, computed tomography (CT) arthrogram, or MRI. Arthrography has the advantage of low cost, low morbidity, accessibility, and 83 to 93 percent accuracy. However, it is limited for diagnosis of central or inner-margin tears and lateral compartment pathology.[27–29] Magnetic resonance imaging has also become much more accessible, and it is frequently useful for cases where the diagnosis is not clear; at times, given our health care environment, it may be necessary for definitive diagnosis. The cost of obtaining MRI studies is decreasing significantly and there is no morbidity associated with the MRI. It has been shown to be approximately 89 to 95 percent accurate for meniscal lesions; however, this accuracy is still interpreter-dependent.[30–32] Stoller has developed a grading system that correlates signal intensity on MRI with actual pathologic findings at the time of surgery.[33] His is a four-grade system for defining signal types that correlate with pathologic changes in the menisci. Grade 0 refers to a uniform, low signal intensity corresponding to a normal meniscus. Grade 1 refers to the finding of a globular area of increased intensity within the meniscus that is not contiguous with either articular surface of the meniscus. Grade 2 refers to a linear area of increased signal intensity without communication with either articular surface of the meniscus. The grade 1 and 2 signals represent patterns of mucinous or mucoid degeneration and do not correspond to arthroscopically visualized meniscal tears. A grade 3 lesion refers to a linear, globular, or complex area of increased signal intensity that extends to one or both articular surfaces of the meniscus. This correlates highly with the presence of a meniscal tear that can be visualized during arthroscopy.

Treatment of Meniscal Tears

Treatment options for meniscal tears include no intervention, partial meniscectomy, or meniscal repair. Before a decision can be made with regard to the type of treatment for a particular individual's injury, several variables must be considered. These factors include the patient's age and the chronicity of the injury, activity requirements, and location and length of the tear. In addition, any associated ligamentous injuries must also be defined. Preoperative physical examinations are critical for planning a definitive treatment. The final treatment decision, however, is often not made until the time of arthroscopic evaluation. Consequently, each of the possible options must be outlined with the patient prior to arthroscopic examination, the patient must consent to any possible procedure, and all necessary equipment must be available at the time of initial arthroscopy. Thorough inspection of the knee joint at the time of arthroscopy allows the surgeon to delineate the type of tear present. Often a 70° arthroscope must be inserted in order to visualize the posterior compartment optimally. This arthroscope can be inserted through the intercondylar notch, as described by Gillquist et al.[34] Use of the 70° arthroscope also allows for defining the location of the tear with respect to the meniscosynovial junction and enables the surgeon to prepare the meniscus for any repair.

Given the importance to meniscal healing of the peripheral blood supply, meniscal tears are classified depending on the zone or location of injury. The factors upon which this classification is based include the location of the tear and its morphology, size, and stability. The major morphologic types of meniscal tears include (1) the degenerative, (2) horizontal, (3) radial, (4) oblique (also known as flap or parrot-beaked), (5) vertical longitudinal, and (6) complex, which involve multiple cleavage planes (Fig. 50-2). Vertical-longitudinal and oblique tears are the most common types.

Degenerative Tears

Degenerative meniscal tears are most commonly seen in patients over the age of 40. Individuals with degenerative meniscal tears may frequently have the associated radiographic findings characterized by Fairbank. These include joint space narrowing, squaring of the condyles, and formation of an osteophyte ridge.[17] These associated findings are best visualized on the 45° posteroanterior flexion weight-bearing radiographs described by Rosenberg et al.[35] Treatment decisions regarding degenerative meniscal tears should be made with extreme caution because it can be very difficult to tell whether a patient's symptoms are due to meniscal pathology or the degeneration of articular cartilage.

Horizontal Tears

Horizontal meniscal tears originate near the central edge of the meniscus and extend outward toward the periphery. These tears have both superior and inferior portions or leaves. Joint pain or mechanical symptoms of clicking or locking occur as one of these pieces or portions slides in and out of the joint space. Traditional treatment of these tears involves partial meniscectomy with resection of the flap peripherally until a stable rim of remaining meniscus is obtained. If the tear extends to the meniscocapsular junction with resection, it often requires a near total meniscectomy. If a peripheral portion of the meniscus is left with an unstable horizontal cleft, the tear may continue to propagate and the patient may have recurrence or enhancement of symptoms. Because of the concern for tear propagation or symptom recurrence, one should also avoid resecting only one leaf of the tear.

Radial and Oblique Tears

Radial and oblique tears result in the disruption of the circumferential collagen fibers of the meniscus. If the tear extends to the peripheral portion of the meniscus, thus disrupting the majority of the circumferential collagen fibers, the ability of the meniscus to generate a hoop stress in order to dissipate the force of an applied axial load will be negligible. Traditionally, most surgeons treat radial and oblique tears with partial meniscectomy. The torn portion of the meniscus is trimmed so that a well-contoured, stable, and balanced rim is obtained.[36] Unfortunately, large radial tears of meniscus can result in profound acceleration of degenerative changes, as significant as that seen as the result of total meniscectomy.[37] Because radial tears as well as the traditional treatment—which includes subtotal or total meniscectomy—can result in accelerated degenerative changes in the knees, some surgeons have advocated repair of these large radial tears and have often used a fibrin clot at the time of meniscal repair, citing good rates of healing.[38–40] Healing with scar tissue following meniscal repair does not necessarily result in normal meniscal function. Consequently, there are those who continue to recommend partial or subtotal meniscectomy for large radial tears.[41–43] In our opinion, there are certain cases in which repair of a large radial or oblique tear would be reasonable. In young patients with large radial or oblique tears, particularly those of the lateral meniscus, treatment of the tear by excision, resulting in near-total removal of the meniscus, can lead to very poor long-term outcomes. Consequently, groups have become more aggressive in repairing these large radial or oblique tears in young, active patients. It should be noted, however, that these repairs can often be tenuous and the patient must

Figure 50-2 Diagrammatic representation of the major types of meniscal tears. [Reproduced with permission from Ciccotti MG, Shields CL Jr, El Attrache NL: Meniscectomy, in Fu FH, Harner CD, Vince KG, Miller MD (eds): *Knee Surgery.* Vol 1. Baltimore, Williams & Wilkins, 1994, p 602.]

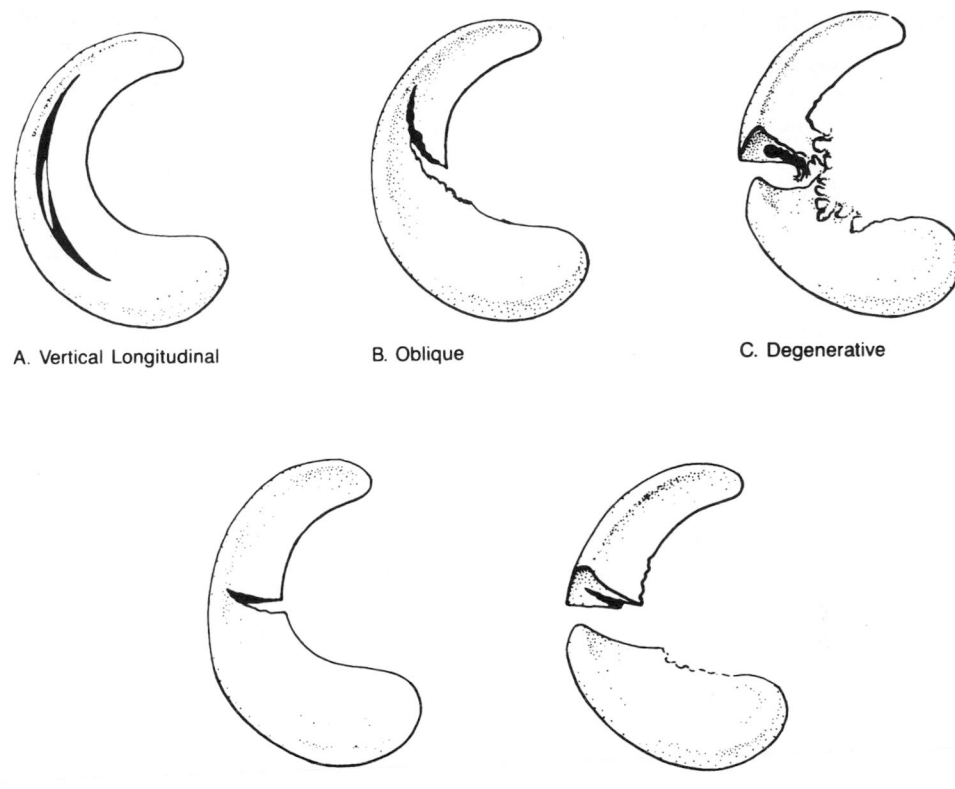

A. Vertical Longitudinal   B. Oblique   C. Degenerative

D. Transverse (Radial)   E. Horizontal

be prepared to accept the increased risk of surgical morbidity and the possible need for further surgery if the repair is unsuccessful and further secondary damage to the knee joint occurs.

Vertical-Longitudinal Tears

Vertical tears are described as being either complete or incomplete. Incomplete tears occur in either the superior or inferior surface of the meniscus, and they have a predilection for occurring in the posterior horns. Complete tears, on the other hand, communicate with both the superior and inferior surfaces of the meniscus. Incomplete tears are frequently seen in conjunction with ACL injuries. During arthroscopy, careful inspection with a probe allows the surgeon to assess the stability of the tear. Stable tears are those noted to be less than 1 to 1.5 cm in length. The stable tear can be abraded with arthroscopic rasps, which are felt to stimulate vascular ingrowth.[36,44] Larger, incomplete tears greater than 1.5 cm in length or tears that show instability with probing should be treated with partial meniscectomy or meniscal repair, as the likelihood of tear propagation and/or secondary cartilage damage is increased.

Small, complete vertical-longitudinal tears can often be difficult to visualize during arthroscopy. Often these are discovered during careful probing of the meniscus. Typically, their small size causes them to appear reduced during arthroscopic visualization in a stationary knee. They may displace only during range-of-motion exercises of the knee and thus cause symptoms only then or during

weight-bearing. It is necessary to probe these lesions thoroughly and carefully to demonstrate any instability. Vertical orientation of these tears as well as the fact that they are common in young individuals make them ideal candidates for meniscal repair procedures. Some feel that the ideal candidate for meniscal repair is a young individual who has sustained an acute longitudinal tear in the periphery of the lateral meniscus measuring 1 to 2 cm in length with associated ACL tear.[40,45] Smaller, stable tears measuring less than 1 cm and occurring in the periphery of the meniscus will most likely heal following abrasion of the edges for vascular ingrowth alone. "Bucket handle" tears are large, vertical-longitudinal tears. Bucket-handle tears are frequently displaced but can also be nondisplaced, which typically occurs in young, active patients, often in conjunction with tears of the ACL. Treatment of bucket-handle or large vertical-longitudinal meniscal tears via partial meniscectomy, which will most likely result in the excision of a very large percentage of the involved meniscus. Consequently, in young, active individuals, this is not an ideal situation, because of the risk of accelerated degenerative joint disease. Therefore, most surgeons advocate repair of bucket-handle tears. The displaced portion of the bucket-handle tear must first be reduced so that the exact nature of the tear can be assessed; only then can it be determined whether the tear would be amenable to surgical repair. Chronically displaced tears can frequently be permanently deformed. Repair of the meniscus in this setting is not indicated when congruent reduction cannot be obtained.

Indications for Meniscal Repair

As previously discussed, many factors need to be considered before the decision to perform meniscal repair is made. These factors include the patient's age; preinjury activity level and expectations for postinjury activity level; chronicity of the injury; type, location, and size of the tear; and the associated ligamentous injuries. Also, the peripheral meniscal blood supply plays a critical role in the healing potential of meniscal tears. Consequently, further classification of meniscal tears has been based on the location of the tear with respect to three anatomic zones based on the vasculature of the meniscus. Each zone carries a different prognosis for the healing of meniscal tears located within that zone (Fig. 50-3). The red zone is at the periphery of the meniscus; it indicates the presence of vascularity. The white zone represents approximately the central two-thirds of the meniscus, indicating its avascular portion. The red-white zone occurs at the transition from the avascular to the vascularized portion of the meniscus. Red-red tears occur within the peripheral vascularized zone of the meniscus. This tear pattern has intact blood supply to both the central and capsular sides of the meniscal tear, and they have an excellent potential for healing. The red-white tears occur at the junction of the avascular and vascular portions of the meniscus, and only the peripheral portion of the tear has a vascular supply. These tears have a relatively good potential for healing following adequate repair, but they are less likely to heal than tears in the red-red zone. Finally, white-white tears have the worst potential for healing, as they occur entirely within the central avascular portion of the meniscus. More recently, however, repair of white-white meniscal tears with the utilization of exogenous fibrin clots has been shown to have somewhat better results.[24,39] There continues to be little agreement with respect to the relative indications for meniscal repair. Most authors agree, however, that

the ideal candidate for successful meniscal repair is the young, active individual who has sustained an acute longitudinal complete tear in the peripheral vascularized meniscus measuring 1 to 2 cm in length, when repair is performed at the same time as ACL reconstruction.[40,45] Beyond this ideal situation, the decision to perform meniscal repair depends greatly on the individual surgeon's personal preference and experience. It should be noted, however, that there is a relative increasing trend among surgeons to preserve the meniscus as much as possible, especially when there is an associated ACL injury and need for reconstruction.

Techniques of Meniscal Repair

Several techniques for meniscal repair have been described. All share basic technical principles: adequate rim preparation, which includes abrasion of both sides of the tear as well as the meniscosynovial junction, and stable suture fixation of the torn fragments or components. The four basic approaches to meniscal repair that have been described include open repair, arthroscopic all-inside repair, arthroscopically assisted outside-in repair, and arthroscopically assisted inside-out repair. As with any procedure, each technique has advantages and disadvantages. The experience of each individual surgeon and his or her expertise will dictate which procedure is best in that individual's hands. Several different suture placements are possible with each technique. The specific meniscal repair technique employed, surgeon preference, as well as the type of needle system available (whether it be double- versus single-lumen cannula) will all dictate the particular suture orientation that it is best for each individual case. Vertically stacked or vertical sutures with divergent superior and inferior limbs have been demonstrated to provide the best opposition of the tear components (Fig. 50-4).[46]

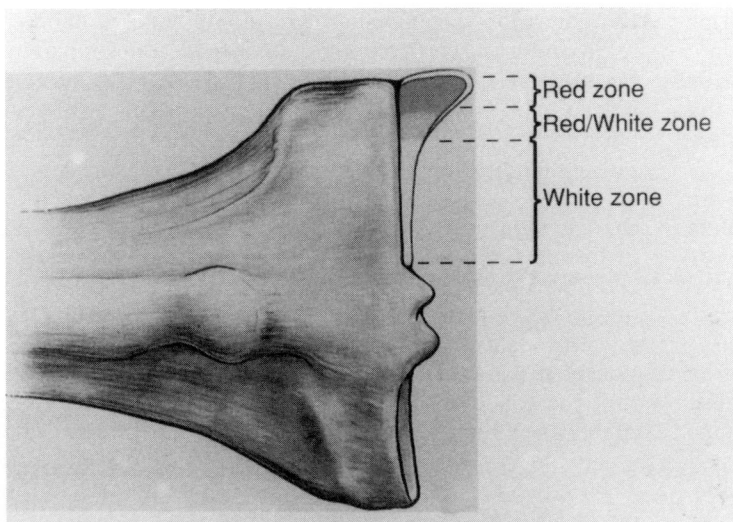

Figure 50-3 Schematic drawing indicating the various zones of the meniscus. Note that red-red and red-white zones are capable of healing and repair is recommended. [Reproduced with permission from Miller MD, Warner JJP, Harner CD: Meniscal repair, in Fu FH, Harner CD, Vince KG, Miller MD (eds): *Knee Surgery.* Vol 1. Baltimore, Williams & Wilkins, 1994, p 616.]

Open Meniscal Repair

Open repair of peripheral meniscal tears was first described by DeHaven and has since been popularized by several other authors.[47–49] Long-term follow-up of 10 years has shown that open meniscal repair is successful.[50] In order to confirm the presence of the tear and assess whether it is amenable to open repair technique, DeHaven and Stone recommended first performing an arthroscopic examination, including visualization of the posterior aspect

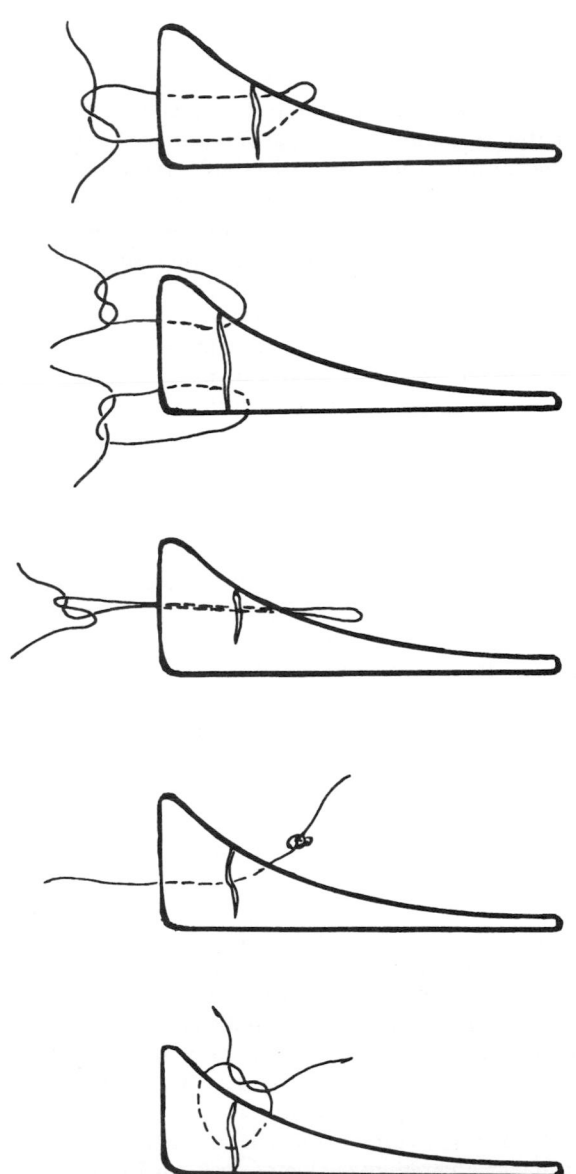

Figure 50-4 Composite diagram demonstrating orientation of sutures used in meniscal repair. From top to bottom: vertical mattress, stacked sutures, horizontal mattress, mulberry knot, suture using all-inside technique. [Reproduced with permission from Miller MD, Warner JJP, Harner CD: Meniscal repair, in Fu FH, Harner CD, Vince KG, Miller MD (eds): *Knee Surgery.* Vol 1. Baltimore, Williams & Wilkins, 1994, p 618.]

of the knee joint before proceeding with the open repair surgery. For repair of the medial meniscus, a 5-cm incision is made over the posterior medial aspect of the knee joint. This is carried down to the posterior medial capsule. The capsule is incised obliquely posterior to the medial collateral ligament in order to expose the torn meniscus. The capsular bed and meniscal rim can be prepared under direct visualization using a curette, followed by use of double-armed sutures to place vertically oriented sutures, which are approximately 3 to 4 mm apart, in order to perform an anatomic repair. Lateral meniscus repair is performed utilizing a 5-cm incision along the posterolateral aspect of the joint posterior to the lateral collateral ligament. The inner tibial band must be split longitudinally to expose the posterolateral capsule. This is then incised obliquely posterior to the border of the popliteus tendon, thus exposing the lateral meniscus. Again, the capsular bed and meniscal rim are prepared with a curette under direct visualization, and this is followed by placement of vertically oriented sutures. The sutures must first be placed from superior to inferior through the meniscus and then through the capsule. The knot is then secured extracapsularly. Open meniscal repair has the advantage of proven results with long-term follow-up. Disadvantages, however, include the tediousness of placing horizontal mattress sutures, the requirement for greater dissection about the popliteal tendon necessary for the repair of posterolateral meniscus tears, and the applicability of the open repair technique to peripheral meniscal tears only.

All-Inside Arthroscopic Repair

The all-inside technique for meniscal repair is performed entirely under arthroscopic control with an intraarticular method of suturing the meniscus. Sutures are placed across the tear with intraarticular knots, utilizing an inoperative cannula. The vertically oriented sutures oppose the components of the meniscal tear only without incorporation of the joint capsule. Indications for the all-inside technique include single vertical-longitudinal tears of the posterior horn and tears of the lateral and medial meniscus located within 3 mm of the meniscocapsular junction. Using the method as described by Morgan and Mulhollan,[51–53] the tear in the posterior horn of the meniscus is observed with a 70° arthroscope, which is advanced anteriorly to posteriorly through the intercondylar notch. The cannula is placed from the posterior corner into the posterior compartment so that instrumentation can be passed. Once the arthroscope and operative cannula are in place, each side of the tear is debrided and abraded using a rasp. A cannulated 16-gauge needle-hook is then used to place the sutures via the posterior cannula. Several cannulated suture hooks are available, with variable terminal hook designs, in order to accommodate various tear geometries and angles of approach. After the suture hook is passed through the posteroinferior stable rim of the meniscus, it is advanced across the tear in an inferior-to-superior direction through the free or mobile fragment or component of the meniscal tear (Fig. 50-5*A*). Following passage of the suture hook, the suture is fastened with the

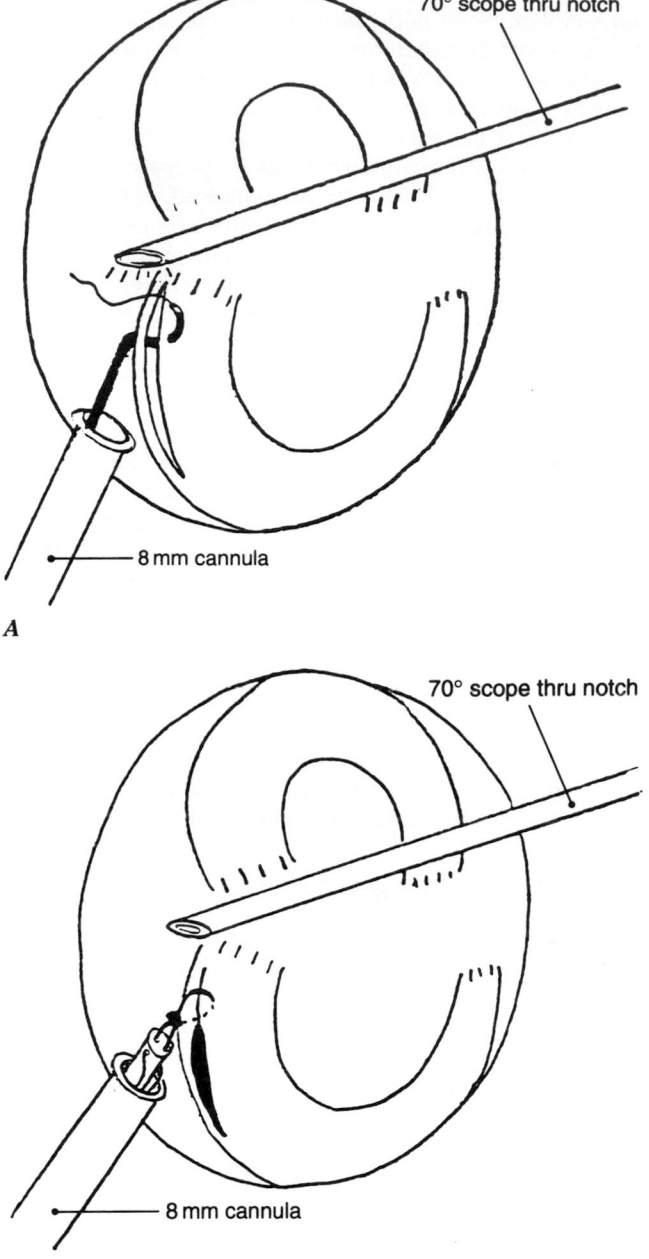

Figure 50-5 *A.* Suture placement through a posterior operative cannula with a suture hook while viewing with a 70° arthroscope advanced through the intercondylar notch. *B.* Knot tying is done with an arthroscopic knot pusher, which advances sequential throws through the posterior cannula while viewing with a 70° arthroscope advanced through the intercondylar notch. (Reproduced with permission from Morgan CD: "All-inside" arthroscope meniscus repair. *Tech Orthop* 8:109, 1993.)

aid of a knot pusher and tied intraarticularly (Fig. 50-5*B*). Advantages of this technique include the ability to place vertically oriented sutures, thus facilitating anatomic opposition of the tear components, and the ability to achieve coaptation of the tear components without entrapping the

posterior capsule. This enables the surgeon to avoid entrapping the posterior capsule and any vital neurovascular structures that might be contained within it. Disadvantages of the all-inside technique include technical difficulty in passing the 70° arthroscope anterior to posterior through the intercondylar notch as well as in placing the posterior operative cannula.

Outside-in Repair The outside-in technique of meniscal repair utilizes various numbers of small (less than 1 cm) vertical incisions made in strategic positions along the joint line. The subcutaneous soft tissues are then bluntly dissected down to the level of the joint capsule. A spinal needle is then passed from outside the knee across the meniscal tear site, using arthroscopic visualization. Suture is passed from outside the knee through the spinal needle and into the knee joint, where it is grasped and brought out of the knee joint through an anterior arthroscopic portal. The suture is then tied into a "mulberry knot," and this is withdrawn back into the joint. The knot is abutted against the meniscus. A series of sutures are placed in this fashion with approximately 3- to 4-mm space between them; they are then tied to one another over the capsule after the soft tissue is bluntly dissected to avoid possible entrapment of vital neurovascular structures.

A variation of this technique involves bringing out two adjacent sutures through the anterior portal, tying them together, and then pulling them back into the knee, thus creating a horizontal mattress suture. The free ends of these sutures are then tied over the joint capsule. A disadvantage of this technique is the difficulty of suturing extremely posterior tears. This can sometimes be circumvented by prebending the needle for greater ease of suture passage. In addition, the needles must be passed under direct visualization to minimize the risk of neurovascular injury when the sutures are tied down to the joint capsule.

Inside-out Repair Currently, the inside-out technique of meniscal repair is the most popular. The very first arthroscopic meniscal repair was performed by Ikeuchi in Tokyo in 1969.[54] Henning was the first to popularize the inside-out technique for meniscal repair.[40,55] Although the Henning technique of meniscal repair is considered by many to be the most difficult, it has become the most common type of repair performed. This technique provides great flexibility, and a variety of commercially available suture delivery systems can be used to perform the Henning procedure. Either a single- or double-barrelled cannula can be used. The single-cannula technique has the advantage of allowing for placement of vertically oriented sutures, which provide better coaptation at the tear site.[56]

In repairing the medial meniscus, the posterior medial joint must be carefully evaluated, using a 70° arthroscope passed anterior to posterior via the intercondylar notch.[34] To facilitate observation of the posteromedial joint, the patient's knee is placed at 90° of flexion and a blunt obturator is introduced via an infralateral portal. It is subsequently passed between the medial femoral condyle and the PCL until it enters the posterior aspect of the knee joint. The standard posterior medial arthroscopic portal is then used for preparation of the perimeniscal synovium and the meniscal tear site. We prefer to use a single-lumen zone-specific cannula system for passage of the needles. The ipsilateral portal is used to view the tear site while the cannula is inserted via the contralateral portal. The advantage of the single-lumen cannulas is that they allow for placement of vertically oriented sutures as well as a variety of other suture types. Utilizing the curve of each cannula, a particular zone of the meniscus can be accessed. We prefer to use braided nonabsorbable 2-0 suture on a double-armed long Beath needle.

All tears must be observed thoroughly with arthroscopic visualization to determine the appropriateness of the surgical repair procedure chosen. Preparation of the tear site is critical for successful repair. A specially designed meniscal rasp or a mechanized shaver is used to abrade the peripheral and central sides of the tear. As previously mentioned, the adjacent meniscosynovial junction is also rasped in order to remove any avascular fibrous tissue in the tear site. In addition, rasping is thought to stimulate the ingrowth of vascular tissue, which is critical for the healing of a meniscal tear. If additional visualization is required during the rasping procedure, an accessory posteromedial or posterolateral portal can be used. In addition, a 70° arthroscope may be utilized to visualize peripheral tears of the posterior horn in either the posteromedial or posterolateral compartments.

Posteromedial skin incisions are used for repair of the medial meniscus tears. These incisions generally measure approximately 3 to 4 cm and are oriented longitudinally at the junction of the knee joint line in the posterior aspect of the femoral condyle with the knee at 90° of flexion. The ideal placement of the incision is with approximately one-third of the incision above the joint line and the remaining two-thirds below the joint line. A 70° arthroscope placed through the intercondylar notch can be used to provide transillumination to facilitate identification and localization of the saphenous vein. The superficial fascia is also incised longitudinally and the pes anserinus is retracted posteriorly in order to protect the saphenous vein and nerve. At this point the posteromedial joint line and underlying meniscus can be palpated. If the meniscus is not palpable, it may be necessary to bluntly dissect the medial head of the gastrocnemius and a portion of the semimembranosus off the joint capsule to facilitate complete exposure.

In order to repair tears of the lateral meniscus, the incision is placed over the posterolateral aspect of the knee. The interval between the iliotibial band and the anterior margin of the biceps tendon is bluntly dissected and the biceps tendon retracted posteriorly with a right-angled retractor of sufficient depth to expose the lateral head of the gastrocnemius and protect the peroneal nerve. The nerve is at risk unless carefully protected. The posterolateral joint line and underlying lateral meniscus are exposed by bluntly dissecting the lateral head of the gastrocnemius from the joint capsule. After the lateral or medial meniscus is adequately exposed, the sutures on the double-armed long Beath needles are passed from inside to outside across the tear site while the needles are retrieved via a posteromedial or posterolateral incision. At the same time, vital neurovascular structures must be protected

from injury during the passage of the needle. All of the necessary sutures are passed across the tear site before they are tied. Following passage of all necessary sutures required to achieve stable fixation, they are tied over the joint capsule. The tear site is packed with clot prior to suture tying so that the clot can be secured within the tear cleft by the sutures. An advantage of the inside-out technique popularized by Henning is that sutures can be placed in a divergent fashion, allowing for containment of a larger amount of meniscal tissue within each suture and thus providing for better apposition of the tear components.[57]

Fibrin Clot Technique for Meniscal Repair

It is generally accepted that meniscal healing depends on an available blood supply, which presumably provides various growth factors that essentially direct the healing process. Because meniscal lesions occurring in the avascular or central portion of the meniscus do not have an intrinsic blood supply, it is believed that an exogenous fibrin clot placed in tears within this region can provide the various as to yet unknown growth factors that support a healing response. The efficacy of using an exogenous fibrin clot to assist in the repair of tears within the avascular zone of the menisci was first demonstrated by Arnoczky et al. in 1986.[58] This idea was initially based on the findings of Arnoczky and Warren, who evaluated the healing of meniscal injuries in a canine model.[23] They observed that following an injury in the vascular zone of the meniscus, a fibrin clot formed at the site of injury, and this clot was felt to act as a scaffold for the ingrowth of new vessels originating from the perimeniscal capsular plexus and the synovial fringe. Furthermore, they noted that lesions or tears within the avascular zone of the menisci did not heal unless they were connected to the peripheral aspect of the meniscus via a vascular channel. Following recognition that lesions or tears within the avascular portion of the meniscus do not heal, various methods of providing a blood supply to the torn regions of the menisci have been investigated. Various methods to introduce a vascular supply to the avascular portion of the meniscus have included the creation of vascular access channels,[23] placement of synovial pedicle grafts over the site of injury,[59] as well as abrasion of the synovial fringe with rasps to create a vascular pannus.[60] In 1986, Arnoczky et al.[58] used a dog model to investigate the application of exogenous fibrin clot to assist in the healing of avascular meniscal tears. They demonstrated that placement of a fibrin clot within a stable lesion occurring in an avascular portion of the meniscus can result in a healing response similar to that seen in the vascularized periphery of the meniscus. The results showed that at 6 months, the healing tissue resembled mature fiber cartilage histologically. Biochemical analysis of the clot revealed that platelet-derived growth factor and fibronectin were present, and these are believed to function in the process of chemotaxis and mitogenesis for other cells, thus activating a repair response. In addition, as observed in normal healing, it was their opinion that the exogenous fibrin clot did serve as a scaffold for the ingrowth of vascular channels. They also utilized radiolabeled sulfate to demonstrate that active matrix synthesis was stimulated by the exogenous fibrin clot. Consequently, their results indicated that an exogenous fibrin clot could either initiate or enhance the healing of meniscal tears in regions of avascularity. The existence of various serum factors that can induce meniscal fibrochondrocytes to proliferate and synthesize matrix was demonstrated by Webber et al.[61] To date, however, the exact identity and nature of the various growth or stimulatory factors within serum that participate in initiating and directing the healing response are not known and certainly require the attention of future studies.

The fibrin clot is prepared from a sample of approximately 60 mL of the patient's blood. This is obtained via venipuncture and then placed in a glass beaker under sterile technique. The blood is then stirred with a glass rod for approximately 5 to 10 min in order to promote coagulation. The sintered inner barrel of a glass syringe is used as the stirring rod. A firm clot forms on the glass rod during this period. The rod is then taken out of the beaker and loose cellular elements are removed by sequential washings with sterile saline followed by gentle blotting with gauze sponges. The fibrin clot remaining on the glass stirring rod is felt to contain the concentrated factors that serve to enhance vascular ingrowth and stimulate or promote the healing process as well as to provide the structural scaffold that supports vascular ingrowth. A plastic tube with a pusher or a syringe with a blunt needle is then used to insert the clot into the meniscal tear.[62,63] The previously placed sutures that are spanning the meniscal tear are then tightened and tied over the joint capsule, securing the clot within the tear. Henning et al.[62] reported an increased incidence in healing for isolated meniscal tears repaired by the inside-out technique with incorporation of the fibrin clot. Prior to use of the fibrin clot, Henning reported healing rates of 59 percent, which improved to 92 percent after he began to use the fibrin clot technique.[62]

Meniscal Transplant

The concept of meniscal transplant can be traced back to Gebhardt and Lexer who, in 1916, performed fat tissue interposition arthroplasty in an attempt to replace a meniscus.[66] The first free meniscus transplants, however, were not performed until 1984, when Milachowski et al. used deep frozen and lyophilized allografts to replace the medial meniscus in 23 patients.[65–67] At the same time and subsequently, others have investigated the use of partial meniscus grafts,[68] infrapatellar fat pad,[69,70] and the patellar tendon,[71] while others have used a reabsorbable collagen scaffold molded into the shape of a meniscus.[72,73] Unfortunately, none of these experimental procedures have had consistently successful results.

Subsequently, groups have attempted to use the quadriceps tendon and the patellar tendon in addition to the infrapatellar fat pad. Results from these experiments have demonstrated that the materials do transform over time into meniscuslike tissues, although they are not structurally or functionally homologous to the native meniscus.[69,70,74,75] Johnson also reported a technique that could be used only if meniscal damage was limited to the posterior horn. In this situation the anterior horn of the same meniscus is substituted for the damaged posterior horn by removing the anterior horn and reinserting it dorsally.[68] Despite the experimentation with numerous meniscal substitutes, the optimal replacement material or tissue has not been found. However, as organ transplantation has left the experimental realm and has now become a common if not routine procedure in many medical centers, cadaveric meniscal transplantation is now becoming more popular. The first essential component of successful meniscal transplantation is the availability of menisci of high tissue quality in various sizes to match various recipients and satisfy the mechanical requirements of a transplanted meniscus.

Generally speaking, menisci do not elicit a host immune response.[76] However, the primary concern, as with all allograft organ and tissue transplantation, is the potential transmission of diseases, especially hepatitis and the human immunodeficiency virus. Consequently, several different techniques of tissue preparation or sterilization have been used, including fresh (not sterilized)-frozen cryopreserved, freeze-dried, and gluteraldehyde-preserved meniscal grafts. Sterilization techniques have included the use of ethylene oxide and gamma irradiation. All forms of storage and sterilization cause some degree of degradation or eradication of ground substance and reduction of fibrochondrocyte viability. The loss of various amounts of ground substance, fibrochondrocytes, and enzymes has some effect on the ability of the graft to incorporate as well as to perform its intended function within the knee joint.

There are no firmly established guidelines for meniscal transplantation; however, there is a general set of indications for meniscal transplants. Meniscal transplantation is considered to be indicated under the circumstances of total meniscectomy in young patients, as these are the most vulnerable to premature and accelerated degenerative joint disease, especially when the lateral patellofemoral joint is involved. In addition, in patients who have sustained complete rupture of the anterior cruciate ligament and have at the same time completely destroyed their medial meniscus or have undergone previous medial meniscectomy, it is felt that medial meniscus transplantation will provide additional joint stabilization and thus help protect the reconstructed ACL. Third, in certain circumstances, meniscal transplant may delay the need for high tibial osteotomy or total knee arthroplasty in middle-aged or elderly patients who have low-grade medial compartment degenerative joint disease. Finally, meniscal transplant may be used in older patients with advanced medial compartment degenerative arthritis in order to enhance the effect of high tibial osteotomy despite the fact that the life expectancy of the meniscal transplant would be shortened secondary to the already present degenerative changes in the joint surfaces.

Technique of Meniscal Transplant Meniscal transplantation can be performed either as an open procedure or arthroscopically. Open meniscal transplantation is generally performed only when other procedures such as ACL reconstruction are being performed at the same time, whereas arthroscopic meniscal transplantation is generally used for transplants of menisci without bone blocks. There are, generally speaking, three different techniques of fixation of the meniscal allograft. First, the allograft meniscus can be sutured to the anterior and posterior remnants of the native meniscus. Second, the anterior and posterior ends of the allograft can be sutured or tagged with sutures that are brought out through the anterior aspect of the tibia through drill holes made through the respective anterior and posterior insertion sites of the native meniscus, exiting via the anterior tibia. These sutures are then tied over the bone bridge between the two tunnels. Third, meniscal allograft can be harvested with bone plugs from both the anterior and posterior insertions. Drill holes can be then made in the anterior and posterior insertion sites of the anterior and posterior horn of the meniscus in the host knee, after which the bone plugs are pulled into the tunnels with sutures. In each situation the meniscal allograft is secured with interrupted absorbable sutures to the trimmed base of the native meniscus. Postoperatively, early mobilization as well as weight bearing are allowed, depending upon surgeon's preference.

Several studies have evaluated meniscal allografts and their incorporation into the knees of dogs, goats, and sheep as well as rabbits. Generally speaking, meniscal allografts transplanted into these animal recipients were noted to develop material properties similar to those of the native menisci over a 3- to 6-month period following transplantation.[77-82]

Given these early results, meniscal transplantation will certainly become more popular and become the subject of future studies. Several questions will need to be addressed. First of all, although fresh meniscal allografts would be the best suited for transplantation, the risks of transmission of diseases such as hepatitis and acquired immunodeficiency syndrome (AIDS) makes the use of fresh tissue an unpleasant or undesirable choice. Therefore, future studies will need to continue to focus upon the most effective and least destructive methods of tissue allocation, preparation, and sterilization. In addition, more exact methods of estimating the size of the meniscus required for transplantation from preoperative x-ray or MRI studies will allow for more economical allotment of donor tissues. Finally, there is the question of the best method of anchoring the meniscal allografts and whether the use of bone blocks versus suturing the free ends provides more anatomic positioning and optimization of the biomechanical functioning of the meniscal allografts. Ultimately, in today's era of cost-conscious medical care, the patients who will most benefit from meniscal transplant must be identified, so that maximal benefit can be obtained from the increasingly scarce health care dollar.

Postoperative Course

There is no consistent agreement as to the best postoperative protocol following meniscal repair. Depending on the particular technique of repair used, each surgeon has his or her own particular views on appropriate protocols with respect to length and position of immobilization, weight-bearing status, restrictions on range of motion, as well as timing for allowing the patient to return to normal activity and athletic activities.[47,51,56,83] One area of consistency, however, is that most surgeons who perform meniscus re-

pair in conjunction with ACL reconstruction will follow the normal post-ACL reconstruction protocol, which allows the patient to begin range-of-motion exercises earlier than with traditional postmeniscal repair protocols.

The general principles behind rehabilitative protocols following meniscal repair are to enhance meniscal healing and facilitate early return to normal levels of activity with normal knee function. Generally speaking, traditional approaches prevent early motion. However, some are beginning motion earlier, especially, as previously mentioned, in the cases of meniscal repair in conjunction with ACL reconstruction. Future studies will need to be performed with regard to the effects of weight bearing, immobilization, and range of motion of the knee on meniscal healing before any definitive statements can be made.[84,85]

INJURIES OF THE ANTERIOR CRUCIATE LIGAMENT

Function and Biomechanics

The ACL is a major stabilizer of the knee. It is an intercapsular ligament that originates in the medial aspect of the lateral femoral condyle and inserts in the anterolateral aspect of the medial tibial plateau. The ACL resists excessive anterior tibial displacement, tibial rotation, and varus-valgus angulation. Many animal studies have established that unlike the medial collateral ligament, the ACL has limited ability to form scar tissue and/or heal. Consequently, a midsubstance tear of the ACL has been observed to be incapable of healing.[86-89] The inability of the midsubstance tear of the ACL to heal is thought to be due to differences in the metabolic activities and/or environment of the ACL cells. However, this is still subject to debate and will require further investigation. The primary function of the ACL is to restrain abnormal anterior displacement of the tibia with respect to the femur by resisting tensile loads. Butler demonstrated that the anterior cruciate ligament encounters approximately 400 to 500 N of force during normal walking and that these forces can be increased up to 1700 N during sudden acceleration or deceleration or sharp cutting activities.[90] As previously mentioned, the ACL is the primary restraint to anterior tibial translation. Several studies have determined that the ACL accounts for approximately 86 percent of this restraining force to anterior tibial displacement.[91-93] Other structures—such as the collateral ligaments, the joint capsule, and the menisci, especially the medial meniscus—account for the remaining secondary restraint to anterior tibial translation. It is also felt that large joint effusions may decrease the objective observation of anterior translation when the Lachman test is performed in acutely injured knees. This can result in a false-negative finding.

Many variables affect the long-term outcome of ACL reconstruction, and much of the orthopaedic literature is focused on some of these variables, which include the structural and mechanical properties of the graft materials, graft selection, graft positioning, graft tensioning and fixation, as well as patient selection and postoperative muscle strength in rehabilitation.[94–98] Numerous investigators have characterized the biomechanical properties of the human femur–patellar tendon–tibia graft.[99–102] A major reason for its widespread use is that the patellar tendon has been found to have the highest tensile strength of the common graft tissues, which also include the semitendinosus, gracilis, iliotibial band, and Achilles tendon. The ultimate load of the patellar tendon is approximately 1.6 times greater than that of the normal ACL. However, the tensile properties of the patellar tendon graft have been found to reach only approximately 33 percent of the tensile properties of the normal ACL at 2-year postoperative follow-up.[103] In the past, the evaluation of ACL reconstruction has focused on the reestablishment of knee stability and the restraint of anterior translation of the tibia with respect to the femur.[104] More recently, a much greater emphasis has been placed on obtaining a greater understanding of knee kinematics under normal mechanical loads and the contribution of the ACL to knee function in situ. It is generally believed that this knowledge is necessary if we are to improve the techniques and outcomes of ACL reconstructive surgery. Recently our laboratory has utilized robotics technology to gain information on the magnitude, direction, and point of application of the in situ forces in the ACL.[105–107] Using 10 porcine knees, the magnitude and direction of the in situ forces in the ACL were noted to change between 1 and 5° of freedom under testing conditions. Under 110 N of anterior tibial drawer, in situ force magnitudes were found to be 116 ± 12 and 110 ± 14 N for the 1° of freedom and 5° of freedom, respectively. The mean direction of the in situ forces in the ACL were found to be 25 and 11° (elevation and deviation) in 1° of freedom and 15 and 60° in 5° of freedom. From these observations we can conclude that the role of the ACL is apparently affected by the way in which motion is controlled during testing. It is believed that the use of testing systems with multiple degrees of freedom will enable us to further understand the mechanics in ACL–deficient knees as well as to validate the efficacy of ACL reconstruction with respect to the biomechanics of the knee joint.

In addition to the soft tissues that guide and help to restrain knee motion, the muscles that cross the knee play a significant role in the physiologic function of the knee. The activity of muscles can introduce large changes in the forces experienced by the ACL or its replacement. Smidt[108] reported that the quadriceps exerts an anterior shear force on the tibia when the knee is flexed between 5 and 60° and a posterior shear force when the knee is flexed between 75 and 90°. Other investigators have also documented the interaction between the quadriceps and the ACL in the initial arc of joint flexion.[93,110–112] In general, quadriceps muscle forces induce increased anterior translation of the tibia, while hamstring muscle forces have the opposite effect. Markolf et al.[112] reported that passive extension of the knee generated forces in the ACL only during the last 10° of extension (at 5° of hyperextension, the mean force was found to be 118 N). When a 200-N force generated through the quadriceps tendon was applied to the knee, the force in the ligament increased at all angles of knee flexion, with the largest changes in the passive case occurring between 5 and 40° of flexion.

In our laboratory we have studied the role of quadriceps in hamstring contractions and the unloading of ACL during knee flexion–extension.[113] Through the use of an "Oxford rig" assembly,[114] unconstrained 5° of freedom and motion was allowed while simulating knee flexion and extension during vertical stance loading. In this study, the muscle forces were applied to a cadaveric knee to simulate a squat exercise with isolated quadriceps activation and then also with quadriceps and hamstrings cocontraction. By testing the knee in intact, ACL-deficient, and ACL-reconstructed states, it was demonstrated that muscle cocontraction has a significant effect on knee kinematics. The introduction of hamstring force with quadriceps force significantly reduces anterior tibial translation in the ACL-deficient knee and also reduces forces in the reconstructed ACL during extension of the knee. The hamstrings have the potential of negating the increased strains in the ACL caused by quadriceps contraction and may indicate the usefulness of closed-chain (cocontraction) kinetic exercises during rehabilitation following ACL reconstruction. From the above discussion, it is clear that muscle contraction significantly alters the kinematics of the knee. These changes may compensate for or accentuate other conditions present in the knee, such as ACL deficiency, and therefore should be considered in a comprehensive treatment regimen. Noyes et al.[115] demonstrated that the site of failure of the ACL was dependent upon strain rate. Utilizing ACLs from nine caged primates and an Instron testing machine, they demonstrated that at high strain rates, the majority of specimens fail in the mid-substance of the ligament; whereas at slow strain rates, failure occurred at the ligament-bone interface. Furthermore, it was demonstrated that following cast mobilization of primate knees, osseous reabsorption occurred beneath the ligamentous insertions, as observed on histologic analysis. Human cadaveric studies of the femur-ACL-tibia complex has demonstrated that there is an age dependence with regard to maximum load to failure of the ACL. In younger patients (age 16 to 26 years of age), specimens yielded loads to failure of 1730 N at fast strain rates versus less than 900 N for older cadaveric specimens 48 to 86 years of age.[116] More recently, Woo et al.[46] have demonstrated that in young patients, loads to failure are as high as 2500 N. Consequently, it is evident that the results of biomechanical evaluation of the ACL as well as other ligaments are dependent upon specimen age, preparation, orientation, and numerous variables inherent to the experimental testing apparatuses.[100,117] A major reason for its widespread use is that the patellar tendon has been found to have the highest tensile strength of the common graft tissues, which also include the semitendinosus, gracilis, iliotibial band, and Achilles tendon. The ultimate load of the patellar tendon is approximately 1.6 times greater than that of the normal ACL.[103] However, the tensile properties of the patellar tendon graft have been found to reach only approximately 33 percent of the tensile properties of the normal ACL at 2 years postoperative follow-up.[103]

Anatomy of the Anterior Cruciate Ligament

The ACL is an intracapsular ligament that originates in the medial aspect of the lateral femoral condyle and inserts in the anterolateral aspect of the medial tibial plateau, the anterior tibial eminence.[118] Like all ligaments, the ACL ligament is composed of primarily type I collagen, with varying amounts of elastin and reticulin. The exact structural organization of these molecules, however, is still the subject of some debate. There are several models primarily based on the findings of light microscopy and scanning electron microscopy of mostly tendons. In general, all of the models agree that the collagen molecules are aggregated into fiber bundles, which are aligned to some degree in a parallel fashion along the long axis of the ligament. They disagree with respect to the basic unit and level of segmentation of the collagen aggregates and fiber bundles.[119–122]

Under polarized light microscopy, the collagen bundles have a sinusoidal wave pattern referred to as "crimp." This crimping allows the ligament to elongate slightly as the bundles straighten when an external load is applied along the axis of the ligament. Despite the lack of complete agreement over the complex structure of ligaments, it is evident that it is uniquely suited to the primary functions of providing joint stability, guiding fluid motion within normal load ranges, limiting excessive motion when excessive loads are applied, and thus protecting the soft tissues and neurovascular structures of the knee. The ACL is generally described as having two bundles, the anteromedial and posterolateral bands. These are named for their anatomic tibial insertion sites.[123] The posterolateral band is taut at knee extension while the anteromedial band tightens with flexion (Fig. 50-6). An anterior load on the tibia will be distributed differently at different flexion angles to these two bundles, thus providing stability throughout the full range of knee motion. The posterolateral band has been observed to be the larger of the two.[118] The major blood sup-

ply for the ACL is derived from the middle geniculate artery, which sends small vessels to the synovial sheath, giving off paraligamentous vessels and providing nutrition and metabolic maintenance to the ACL. The tibial nerve is felt to supply mechanoreceptors to the ACL, which, in turn, are believed to provide proprioceptive information with respect to knee joint position, allowing for compensatory muscle tone around the knee.[124]

Incidence of Injury/Epidemiology

It is estimated that there are 98 knee ligament injuries per 100,000 per year in the general population of the United States.[125] Lesions of the ACL and the medial collateral ligament account for the majority of these injuries. The ACL is the most frequently injured knee ligament. Based on the San Diego Kaiser Knee Clinic Study, injury of the ACL accounts for 48 percent of all knee ligament injuries and approximately, 500,000 clinically significant ACL injuries are sustained in the United States each year.[125,126] The majority of significant knee ligament injuries occur during participation in athletic activities, and injury of the knee is the most common injury of many sports. For example, it is estimated that 100,000 people sustain a lesion of the ACL while skiing each year in the United States, and the relative incidence of these injuries, which is 72 per 100,000 skier days, appears to be on the rise.[127] Football is another sport with a high and apparently increasingly relative rate of ACL injury: 56 per 100,000 player days in college football.[128]

Natural History of Injury to the Anterior Cruciate Ligament

Many animal studies have established that, unlike the medial collateral ligament, the ACL has limited ability to form

Figure 50-6 Schematic drawing representing changes in the shape and tension of the anterior cruciate components in extension and flexion. In flexion, lengthening of small medial band (A-A') and shortening of the bulk of the ligament (B-B'). (Reproduced with permission from Girgis F, Marshal JL, Monajem ARS: The cruciate ligaments of the knee joint: Anatomical, functional, and experimental analysis. *Clin Orthop Rel Res* 106:229, 1975.)

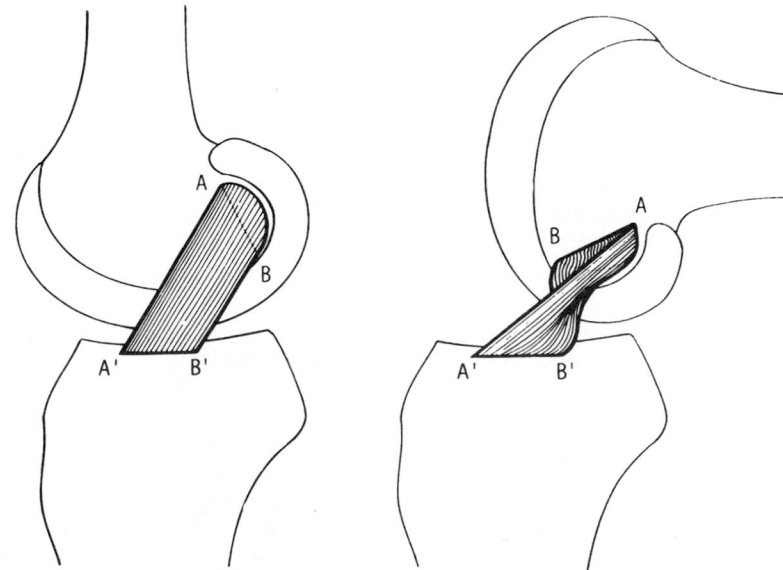

scar tissue and/or heal. Consequently, a midsubstance tear of the ACL is observed to be incapable of healing.[86–89] This is thought to be due to differences in metabolic activity in the environment of the ACL's cells, but it is still subject to debate and will require further biochemical and histologic investigation.

Unrepaired, isolated rupture of the ACL and the resultant abnormal force distribution can lead to progressive deterioration of the knee. The abnormal knee kinematics can further lead to secondary damage of the knee, including meniscal tears as well as injury to the medial collateral ligament and ultimately progressive premature osteoarthritis.[129–134] In addition, many other studies have demonstrated that conservative treatment of an isolated ACL rupture has a poor outcome.[135] Reconstructive surgery for ACL rupture has two primary goals: first, to increase stability and level of function and, second, to halt the progression of osteoarthritis and other secondary damage to the knee joint. There is, however, no conclusive evidence that ACL reconstruction actually slows the progression of degenerative joint disease. In fact, Daniels et al., in a study of 236 patients with documented knee instability who were grouped based on their own decision to undergo reconstructive surgery or be treated nonoperatively, found that those patients who underwent reconstruction had a higher incidence of degenerative joint disease at 5-year follow-up as observed on radiographs and by bone scans.[136] An interesting finding was that the patients in the operative group did have a smaller degree of measured joint instability, but their perceived instability was no different from that of the nonoperative group. It was the general opinion of the investigators that the increased incidence of degenerative joint disease in the reconstructive group was most likely due to a greater incidence of meniscal and/or other soft tissue injury, which had occurred preoperatively. The reconstruction was based on symptoms and instability as well as patient desire for surgery; therefore, there may well have been bias for the worst cases to be placed in the surgical group.

Diagnosis of Injury to the Anterior Cruciate Ligament

A thorough history of the inciting incident must be obtained. Injury of the ACL is most commonly associated with valgus and external rotation, hyperextension, deceleration, and rotational movements of the knee.[137,138] Most commonly, the patient will give a history of low-velocity deceleration or rotational injury to the knee, and often, no physical contact with another player is involved. Athletic shoes and artificial turf often play a role in injury to the ACL. The patient may describe giving way or buckling of the knee and they may also report hearing an audible "pop" at the time of injury. Frequently there is associated swelling within several hours of the injury, indicating hemarthrosis of the knee. Injury to the ACL can occur or has been shown to occur in 70 to 75 percent of all cases of acute hemarthrosis of the knee.[136,138,139]

Physical examination should include evaluation of both the involved and uninvolved knees. Both active and passive range of motion as well as competence of the extensor mechanism should be assessed. The presence or absence of knee effusion should also be determined. The Lachman, anterior drawer, and pivot shift tests are all key components of the physical examination for ACL deficiency. The Lachman test is the most sensitive and reliable test for determining injury to the ACL.[140,141] It is performed with the knee at 25 to 30° of flexion, which allows for maximum anterior translation of the tibia with respect to the femur. Increased anterior translation as compared with the uninvolved knee as well as the absence of a firm endpoint constitute a positive Lachman test, indicating ACL deficiency. The anterior drawer test is performed with the knee at 90° of flexion and again, increased anterior tibial translation with respect to the femur as well as absence of a firm endpoint are indicative of ACL insufficiency. The pivot maneuver is classically described as being performed with the hip in neutral abduction/adduction and the foot in internal rotation while a valgus stress is placed on the knee and the knee and hip are flexed and extended, eliciting an uncontrolled anterior shift as the tibia translates with respect to the femur. It is best performed with the patient under anesthesia, when the results are much more reliable.[140] Bach et al. demonstrated that performance of the pivot shift test while the patient is under general anesthesia and holding the hip in abduction with external rotation of the tibia leads to fewer false-negative results from the pivot shift test.[142] The knee must also be thoroughly examined for evidence of instability of the meniscal and medial collateral ligaments as well as other ligamentous instability such as injury to the posterior cruciate ligament. Arthrometric or instrumented laxity examination of the knee may also be extremely helpful in evaluating an acutely injured knee. A side-to-side difference greater than or equal to 3 mm or a maximum translation of more than 10 mm is highly suggestive of ACL insufficiency.[143]

The physical examination should also include standard radiographs of the knee. An avulsion of the lateral meniscal capsular ligament from the lateral tibial plateau, also known as a Segond fracture, strongly indicates associated injury to the ACL.[144]

Magnetic resonance imaging is also a valuable tool, which has good sensitivity and specificity for ACL injuries as well as associated chondral, meniscal, and additional ligamentous injuries.[145] Often on MRI, there is evidence of bone bruising or edema in the lateral femoral condyle associated with the ACL tear. Although MRI can be very useful in delineating or defining the extent of secondary damage in the knee joint, it is certainly not required for adequate diagnosis of ACL insufficiency in the majority of patients.

Treatment of Injury to the Anterior Cruciate Ligament

In the case of avulsion of the ACL from its tibial insertion site, surgical fixation of the avulsion fracture is recommended. On the other hand, midsubstance tears of the ACL present a much more difficult problem, as they have been shown to be incapable of healing. Consequently, repair of the ACL is no longer advocated. Some physicians believe that many isolated tears of the ACL can be treated nonoperatively with behavioral modification.[146,147] DeHaven and coworkers, however, have provided evidence that reconstruction of the isolated ACL rupture may prevent secondary injury to the meniscus.[148] Despite the fact that universally successful results are not obtained with ACL reconstructive surgery, it remains the mainstay of treatment for isolated rupture of the ACL. However, following diagnosis of injury to the ACL, it is extremely important that the physician and patient discuss and evaluate both the operative and nonoperative treatment options. Factors that must be honestly assessed include the patient's age; preinjury level of activity, both recreational and occupational; expectations for future level of activity; motivation and ability to participate in rehabilitation or physical therapy; and the degree of knee instability and associated ligamentous or meniscal pathology.[149] The patient's activity level, motivation, and ability to comply with pre- and postoperative rehabilitation are the most important factors in the decision concerning surgery. The timing of surgery is of utmost importance once operative treatment has been chosen. Several authors have documented an increased incidence of postoperative stiffness or loss of motion associated with acute surgery performed within 3 to 4 weeks from the time of initial injury versus delayed ACL reconstruction.[150–152] It is generally believed that significant problems can arise when surgery is performed while the knee is still undergoing an acute inflammatory reaction following injury in hemarthrosis. It is felt that surgery can accelerate or exacerbate the inflammatory process, causing further damage or scarring to the knee joint. Therefore, it is strongly recommended that surgery be delayed until the swelling, pain, inflammation, and stiffness subside and full range of motion and muscle function, especially quadriceps function, have returned. Consequently, the patient will be enrolled in a preoperative rehabilitation program consisting of initial symptomatic therapy for pain reduction and reduction of inflammation and swelling utilizing such modalities as rest, ice, and immobilization followed by strengthening and proprioceptive training and range-of-motion exercises.

Surgical Technique for Arthroscopic Reconstruction of the Anterior Cruciate Ligament

Once the patient has been placed under anesthesia, repeat examination is performed on both knees. The Lachman test is performed with the knee between 25 and 30° of flexion and, again, the degree of anterior tibial translation as well as the presence of an endpoint are determined and graded. The pivot shift test is performed with the hip at 20° of abduction and the tibia internally rotated to maximize the pivot shift phenomenon. Bach et al. demonstrated that when the pivot shift test is performed while the patient is under anesthesia, placement of the hip in abduction with external rotation of the tibia leads to fewer false-negative results from the pivot shift test.[142] The integrity of the posterior cruciate ligament is evaluated by performance of the posterior sag, posterior drawer, and recurvatum tests. Evaluation of the integrity of

both the medial collateral and lateral collateral ligaments is performed by testing for varus-valgus laxity at 0 and 30° of knee flexion, while the presence of posterolateral rotatory instability is assessed with the knee at 30 and 90° of flexion. Several authors also recommend performance of the KT-1000 measurement with the patient under anesthesia.[153]

Arthroscopic examination of the knee is then performed. The patient is placed supine on the operating table and positioned in the standard fashion for routine arthroscopic surgery. Standard inferomedial, inferolateral, and superomedial cannula portal sites are used. A tourniquet is placed but not inflated unless needed, and superomedial inflow with gravity flow are the preferred method to avoid rapid extravasation of fluid into the thigh or lower leg. The integrity of the ACL and PCL is evaluated, and all chondral surfaces are carefully assessed. The presence of both medial and lateral compartment chondrosis as well as patellofemoral chondrosis should be determined and documented. In addition, both the medial and lateral menisci should be thoroughly evaluated and the extent of the tear documented. Particular attention should be paid to both the size and location of the tear with respect to the vascular zone of the meniscus to determine the amenability of the tear to repair versus resection. It is generally believed that meniscal repair should be performed at the same time as ACL repair, as the hemarthrosis resulting from surgery increases the presence of fibrin and platelet-derived growth factors, which may enhance meniscal healing. Furthermore, the shape and size of the intercondylar notch should be thoroughly examined.

Choice of Repair Method

Traditionally, operative approaches have included primary repair of the torn ACL; repair plus augmentation by semitendinosus autograph or prosthetic material; reconstruction with autografts with or without prosthetic augmentation; reconstruction utilizing allografts (primarily Achilles tendon allograft) or prosthetic material; and extraarticular reconstruction. The exact details of all of these procedures are beyond the scope of this chapter; however, we will focus on the two most popular techniques of ACL reconstruction at this time—autograft reconstruction of the ACL with bone–patellar tendon–bone autograft and semitendinosus or hamstring autograft. It should be mentioned that no single graft material currently available is absolutely ideal for ACL reconstruction. The ideal graft material for ACL reconstruction would have sufficient tensile strength and biomechanical properties replicating the complex physiologic behavior of the native ACL, minimal associated morbidity due to harvesting of the graft, and avoidance of disease transmission such as HIV and hepatitis; furthermore, the ideal graft would elicit no immunologic response and would show no change in its material and mechanical properties over time.

Technique of Reconstruction of the Anterior Cruciate Ligament with Patellar Tendon Autograft

Bone–patellar tendon–bone autograft reconstruction is the most commonly used graft in ACL reconstruction. The primary advantage of this autograft is its time zero maximum load to failure strength.[103] Noyes[103] demonstrated that a 14- to 15-mm-wide central one-third bone–patellar tendon–bone autograft had a maximum load to failure of approximately 2900 N. This was very similar to values obtained by Cooper for the 10-mm-wide central one-third bone–patellar tendon–bone autograft.[154] A second very significant advantage of this type of graft is the ability to attain rigid fixation due to the bone plugs on each end of the graft within the tibial and femoral tunnels.

Disadvantages of the bone–patellar tendon–bone autograft include residual patellofemoral pain, fracture of the patella, patellar tendon rupture, as well as contracture of the patellar tendon, in addition to advanced arthrofibrosis, osteoarthrosis, and alterations in the biomechanics of the extensor mechanism of the knee.[155–162]

Harvesting and Preparation of the Autograft

Following placement of the tourniquet and of the thigh in a thigh holder so that the foot and lower leg hang freely, the patient is prepped and draped with Betadine in the usual sterile fashion. The tourniquet is then inflated following exsanguination of the extremity with an Esmark. We make a vertical midline incision extending approximately 4 to 6 cm from the inferior pole of the patella down to the medial edge of the superior aspect of the tibial tubercle. The subcutaneous flaps are then sharply developed off of the underlying peritenon of the patellar tendon. Electrocautery is used where necessary to obtain hemostasis, and the peritenon is incised and then sharply dissected free from the underlying patellar tendon. A ruler is then used to measure the width of the patella tendon so that 10 mm or approximately one-third of the patellar tendon width is measured for harvesting. A scalpel is used to harvest the central third of the patellar tendon. The scalpel is inserted in line with the longitudinal collagen fibers of the patellar tendon and the tendon is incised from superior to inferior, marking the bony blocks of the patella as well as the tibial tubercle. Bone blocks, 10 by 10 by 20 mm, are then harvested from the patella then the tibial tubercle utilizing an oscillating saw. Finally, an osteotome is used to free the bone blocks from their cancellous beds (Fig. 50-7). The surgeon must be very careful not to disrupt the articular surface of the patella. Bone graft can be taken from the proximal tibial tubercle to fill in the bony defect in the central donor site of the patella. The graft is then taken to a back table where an assistant utilizes a cylindrical bone-plug sizer as well as a rongeur and Mayo scissors to cylindricize the bone plug to fit a 10-mm tunnel. A drill is then used to place one hole in the patellar bone plug for a #5 Ethibond suture to enable passage of the graft into the femoral tunnel. One drill hole is made in the tibial bone plug, the plug is rotated 90°, and two additional holes are placed for the passage of three #5 Ethibond sutures for tensioning of the graft upon fixation. The graft is then tensioned and curved Mayo scissors are used to remove excess tissue from the tendon and bone surface. The bone-tendon junctions are marked with a marking pen, as are uniformly distanced sites along the tendon surface.

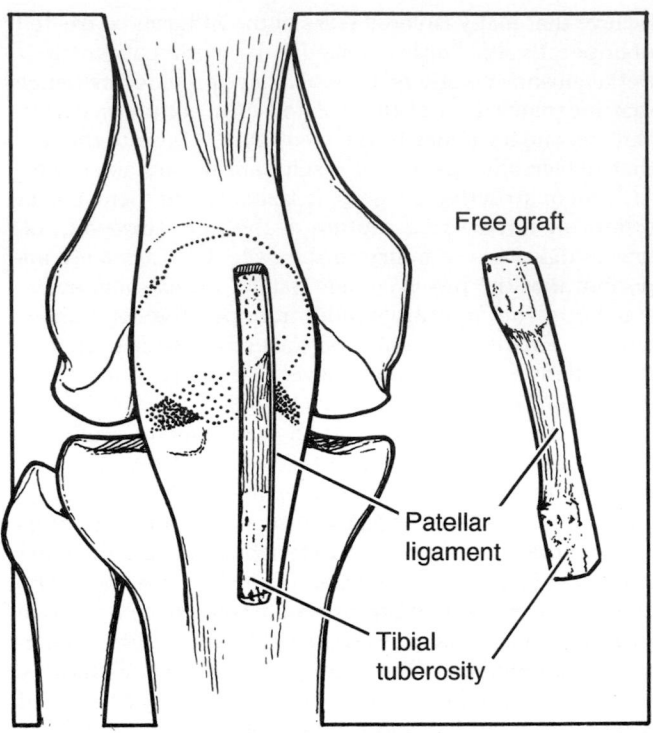

Figure 50-7 Technique for the harvesting of a free, central one-third patellar tendon graft. (Reproduced with permission from Clancy WG Jr, Keene JS, Goletz TH, et al: Treatment of knee joint instability secondary to rupture of the posterior cruciate ligament. *J Bone Joint Surg* 65A:310, 1983.)

This helps to position and rotationally align the bone plug and graft within the tunnels. The graft is then placed in an antibiotic-soaked sponge and put on the back table until the knee is ready for placement of the graft (prepared).

Preparation of the Tibial Tunnel

In order to ensure that both the bone blocks are contained within the femoral and tibial osseous tunnels, the tibial bone–patellar tendon–bone graft with a 25-mm tibial bone plug and a 20-mm patellar bone plug measures anywhere from 90 to 105 mm, whereas the intraarticular portion of the graft measures an average of 30 mm. Consequently, in order to determine the length of the tibial tunnel needed, the length of the femoral tunnel plus 30 mm for the intraarticular portion of the graft is subtracted from the overall length of the graft. Typically, a tibial tunnel of 35 to 50 mm is required to accommodate the majority of grafts. Tibial drill guides are available that enable the surgeon to determine or measure the length of the tibial tunnel prior to drilling. Generally, 5 mm is added to the length of the projected tibial tunnel in order to accommodate the oblique opening of the tunnel at the surface of the tibial plateau so as to minimize the "windshield washer" effect.

The joint is prepared arthroscopically by first using the medial and lateral peripatellar portals. A shaver is introduced via the medial portal to resect synovium, allowing for full visualization of the menisci and the intercondylar notch. Currently we prefer to retain the ACL stump, which serves as a source of graft vascularization and allows for limited notchplasty. Again, the posterior compartment is visualized through the intercondylar notch, and the posterior attachments of the medial meniscus are probed. The integrity of the posterior cruciate ligament is also determined by probing. Valgus stress is then placed on the knee so that the scope can be placed in the medial compartment, and the medial tibial plateau and medial femoral condyles are evaluated for evidence of chondrosis while at the same time the medial meniscus is probed for evidence of tears. Next, the superior patellar pouch is examined in order to evaluate the patellar cartilage. In addition, the knee is flexed and extended in order to observe patellar tracking. The scope is then brought into the lateral compartment, and the posterolateral recess is examined. The lateral condyle as well as the lateral meniscus, popliteal tendon, and lateral tibial plateau are inspected for any signs of damage. Limited notchplasty is performed in the medial aspect of the lateral femoral condyle in order to prevent impingement of the graft (Fig. 50-8). The notch is initially widened anteriorly and then, under observation with the scope, the notch is deepened and extended posteriorly to the articular edge. The desired site in the femoral tunnel is then marked with a burr. While the notchplasty is being performed, it is very important not to mistakenly identify the "resident's ridge," which occurs approximately two-thirds of the way from anterior to posterior along the intercondylar notch, as the

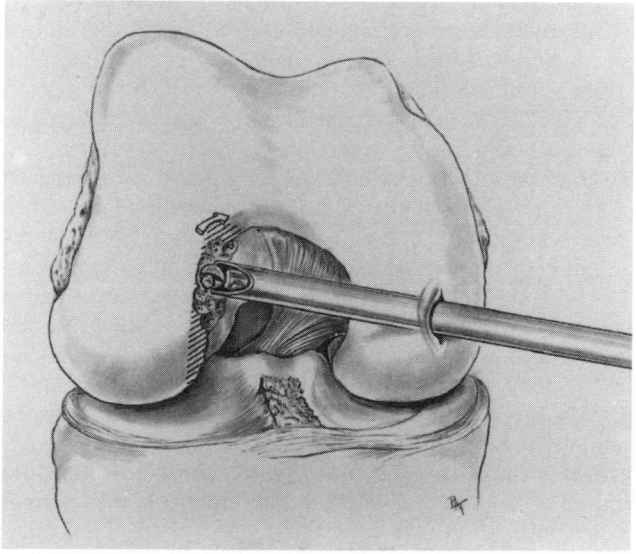

Figure 50-8 A notchplasty is performed with a 5- to 6-mm round motorized abrader to expand the wall so as to minimize graft abrasion postoperatively and to allow arthroscopic visualization of the over-the-top region. The notchplasty is usually performed progressively from anterior to posterior from intercondylar apex to floor. "Notch phimosis" should be avoided. [Reproduced with permission from Nogalski MP, Bach BR Jr: Acute anterior cruciate ligament injuries, in Fu FH, Harner CD, Vince KG, Miller MD (eds): *Knee Surgery.* Vol 1. Baltimore, Williams & Wilkins, 1994, p 707.]

over-the-top position. An adequate notchplasty leads to approximately 2 to 3 mm of clearance for the graft while the knee is in full extension. Following completion of the notchplasty, it is important to probe the over-the-top position to confirm adequate notchplasty and the correct position for placement of the femoral tunnel.

Placement of the Tibial Tunnel

The knee is placed at 90° and the target tip of the tibial drill guide is placed on the lateral slope of the medial tibial spine within the ACL tibial footprint. The ideal site for placement of the tibial drill guide is approximately 1 to 2 mm plus the radius of the desired tibial tunnel, anterior to the posterior wall and PCL fibers at the midpoint of a line drawn between the medial intercondylar eminence and the inner rim of the anterior horn of the lateral meniscus. The surgeon must be very careful not to place the tibial tunnel too anterior, as this results in impingement of the graft by the roof of the intercondylar eminence.[163,164] The anterior skin incision is retracted medially and distally to enable the surgeon to place the 45° angled drill guide medial to the tibial tubercle. Depending on the type of drill guide used, the drill guide can be adjusted to provide for the desired tibial tunnel length (Fig. 50-9). Using the tibial guide, a 3/32 Steinman pin is then passed through the tibia into the intercondylar notch region. Passage of the Steinman pin is performed under arthroscopic visualization. Following placement of the tibial guide pin, the knee is brought into full extension to assure that there is no impingement with the anterior intercondylar notch. A 10-mm cannulated drill bit is then used to drill the tibial tunnel, and, again, drilling of the tibial tunnel is visualized arthroscopically while a curette is placed over the tip of the tibial guide pin to prevent plunging of the drill bit into the joint space as well as advancement of the tibial guide pin into the joint or articular cartilage. The edges of the tibial tunnel are then debrided of bony debris and soft tissue, and the shaver is used to smooth the edges of the tunnel. While this is being performed, the distal aspect of the tibial tunnel can be plugged to prevent outflow of fluid in order to maintain optimal visualization of the joint space.

Placement of the Femoral Tunnel

The proper site of placement of the femoral tunnel is identified by placing the knee at 70 to 90° of flexion. Endoscopically, a point at approximately 10 o'clock in the right knee or 2 o'clock in the left knee is identified along the posterior intercondylar notch. Ideally, the femoral tunnel should have a 1- to 2-mm thick posterior cortical wall so that interference screw fixation can be used on the femoral side. A femoral tunnel placement guide—which essentially consists of a sleeve and a locator that fits over the posterior edge of the intercondylar notch or the "over-the-top" position—allows for accurate placement of the femoral tunnel while also providing for a 2-mm-thick posterior cortical shell. The femoral pin placement guide is passed through the tibial tunnel with the knee at 70 to 90° of flexion. The locator is placed in the "over-the-top" position at approximately 10 o'clock on the right knee or

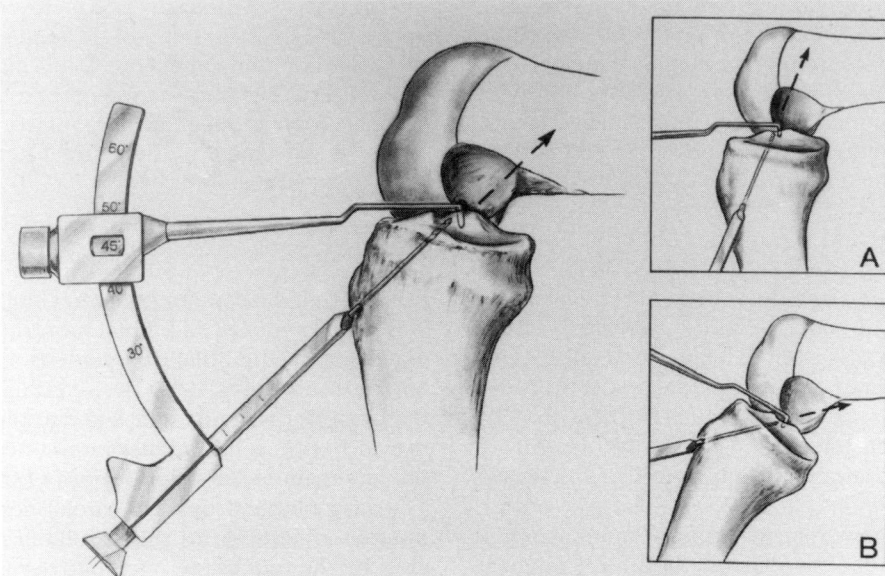

Figure 50-9 Placement of the tibial tunnel guide. This schematic diagram demonstrates the importance of knee flexion position and orientation of the tibial pin. If the tibial tunnel is too steep, the femoral tunnel placement may be made too anteriorly with the knee flexed at 90°. A steep tibial tunnel may necessitate less knee flexion at the risk of violating the posterior cortex. Similarly, if an appropriate tibial tunnel angle is selected (50°) but the knee is inadequately flexed, posterior cortical blowout may occur. [Reproduced with permission from Nogalski MP, Bach BR, Jr: Acute anterior cruciate ligament injuries, in Fu FH, Harner CD, Vince KG, Miller MD (eds): *Knee Surgery.* Vol 1. Baltimore, Williams & Wilkins, 1994, p 721.]

2 o'clock on the left knee. The guide is then used to drill a 3/32 guide wire through the femoral condyle. A ball-tipped, calibrated, cannulated drill is then used to drill the femoral tunnel to a depth of 25 mm (Fig. 50-10). The calibrated, cannulated drill can be used to accurately measure the depth of the femoral tunnel at 25 mm as well as the total end-to-end length between the osseous tunnels, which can be determined from the reading at the distal exit site of the tibial tunnel. Generally a total length 5 mm greater than the length of the graft is desirable. A probe is then used to assure the integrity of the posterior cortical wall; once this has been confirmed, either a 3.2-mm drill bit or the guide pin can be advanced to penetrate the lateral cortex. The graft is then brought from the back table and the suture from the patellar bone plug is attached through the eye of the Beath needle. The Beath needle is utilized to pass the graft from distal to proximal through the tunnels and is passed out through the lateral skin above the knee. Then, under arthroscopic visualization, the patellar bone plug is advanced into the femoral tunnel, utilizing a probe to guide the plug. The cancellous surface of the patellar bone plug is oriented superolaterally and the cancellous surface of the tibial bone plug rotated and oriented posteriorly. The graft is then maneuvered into place utilizing the pen markings at the tendon-bone junction to mark the appropriate depth at which the plug should be pulled into the femoral tunnel. Under arthroscopic visualization, the knee is then brought into extension and any evidence of impingement upon the graft by the intercondylar notch is evaluated. If

there is impingement, the tibial bone plug can be rotated further or a larger notchplasty can be performed. Interference screw fixation is then used to affix the bone plug rigidly within the femoral tunnel. A guide wire is passed through the inferomedial portal and placed between the superolaterally facing cancellous bone of the bone plug and the femoral tunnel. Generally a 7- by 20-mm cannulated interference screw is then passed over the guide wire utilizing a cannulated screwdriver; with the knee flexed to approximately 100 to 110°, the interference screw is passed over the guide wire up to the femoral tunnel. The screw is then advanced until it is just within the femoral tunnel. Following removal of the screwdriver and guide wire, the rigidity and strength of fixation are tested by pulling on the distal sutures of the tibial bone plug. In addition, while maintaining tension on the graft, the knee is taken through several cycles of full flexion-extension to confirm that the femoral bone plug is rigidly fixed and that there is minimal excursion of the tibial bone plug within the tibial tunnel. Less than 3 mm of excursion with full flexion and extension is most desirable. With the knee in full extension, approximately 10 lb of tension is placed on the suture, and a 9- by 25-mm noncannulated interference screw is placed on the posterior aspect of the tibial bone plug between the cancellous bone of the bone plug and the tibial tunnel. The interference screw is passed so that the tip is adjacent to the tip of the bone plug. Adequate placement of the interference screw is then confirmed by placing the arthroscope retrograde through the tibial tunnel. The knee is then

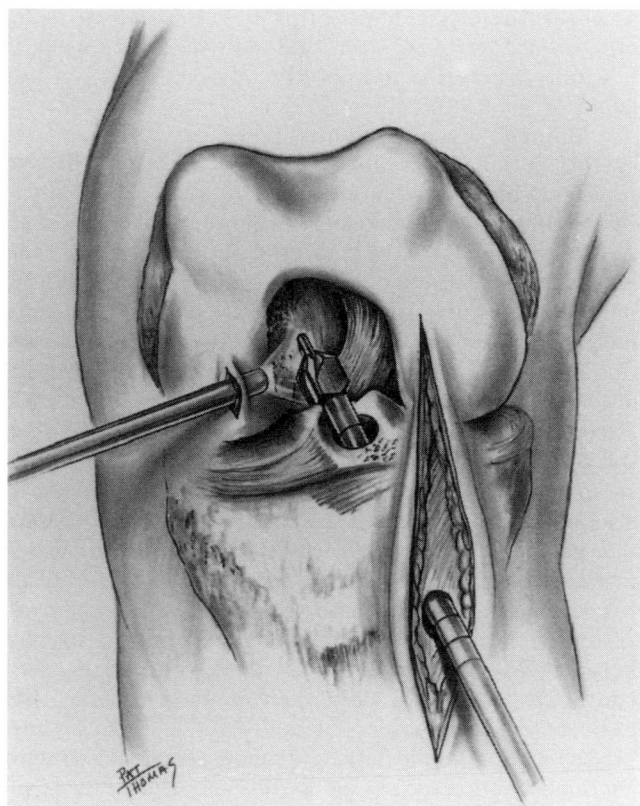

Figure 50-10 A 10-mm endoscopic reamer is manually inserted retrograde through the tibial tunnel up to the femoral region. A "footprint" is created with the reamer tip. This is reamed 5 mm deeper than the longest bone plug length on the patellar tendon construct. [Reproduced with permission from McKernan DJ, Paulos LE: Graft selection, in Fu FH, Harner CD, Vince KG, Miller MD (eds): *Knee Surgery*. Vol 1. Baltimore, Williams & Wilkins, 1994, p 722.]

moved through a full range of motion while the graft is observed arthroscopically for any evidence of excursion or loss of fixation. The Lachman and anterior drawer tests are then performed to assure restoration of knee stability. The tourniquet is then deflated. The bone graft from the tibial tubercle and remnants of bone plugs are then placed within the donor site of the patella; the remaining patellar tendon and peritenon are sutured with running sutures; and the anterior incision is closed in layers, followed by closure of the arthroscopic portals.

Technique of Reconstruction of the Anterior Cruciate Ligament with Semitendinosus and Gracilis Autografts

Following administration of anesthesia, the patient is positioned on the table and prepped and draped in the same fashion as previously described for patellar tendon autograft reconstruction. Again, a thorough examination under anesthesia is performed. The arthroscope is utilized to do a thorough examination of all chondral surfaces as well as the medial and lateral menisci and the PCL and ACL. All lesions of the chondral surfaces as well as menis-

cal lesions are identified and documented, and any reparable lesions of the menisci are repaired prior to performance of ligament reconstruction. A notchplasty is performed with a 12-mm radius resector as described previously.

Attention is then turned to harvesting of the semitendinosus and/or gracilis tendons. First, the insertion of the pes anserinus tendons is identified by palpation in a region medial to the tibial tubercle. A 4- to 5-cm vertical incision is made over the pes anserinus tendons. A scalpel is used to dissect the deep fascia overlying the tendons in a longitudinal direction. The semitendinosus and gracilis tendons are then identified and mobilized with the short blade of army-navy retractors or right-angle clamps. Each tendon is then dissected free from all deep fascial attachments with the use of Metzenbaum scissors. Great care must be taken to remove all of the fascial attachments so that the tendon stripper does not track in the wrong direction, which can result in transection of the tendon before the muscle body is reached. Preparatory experience in the anatomy laboratory is recommended. Once the semitendinosus and gracilis tendons have been mobilized by dissection of all fascial attachments, they are freed from their tibial insertion sites by sharp transection. Ethibond suture (#5) is then used to tag each distal end of the semitendinosus and gracilis tendons. While tension is maintained through these stay sutures, a tendon stripper is used in a distal-to-proximal direction to the level of the distal thigh, thus completely mobilizing each tendon. Typically, a length of 25 to 30 cm of tendon is mobilized. The proximal ends of each tendon are marked and then tagged with a #5 Ethibond suture and the gracilis and semitendinosus tendons are taken to the back table, where they are aligned side by side. They are then looped over a Dacron tape loop, creating a four-strand tendon graft. The Ethibond suture is woven in an ascending then descending baseball stitch fashion to secure the ends of the tendon strands firmly. A graft sizer is then used to determine the required reamer diameter for drilling of the tibial and femoral tunnels. The graft is then placed in gauze moistened with antibiotic solution until the tibial and femoral tunnels have been prepared for passage of the graft.

Using the anterolateral portal, the tip of the tibial drill guide is placed into the anatomic footprint of the native ACL utilizing the landmarks previously described. The medial tibial incision utilized for harvesting of the hamstring grafts are then used as the starting point for the tibial tunnel. A 3/32 Kirschner (K) wire is then drilled into the ACL's tibial insertion site and, following satisfactory replacement of the tibial drill's guide pin, a 9-, 10-, or 11-mm cannulated drill bit is used to ream the tibial tunnel while a curette is placed over the guide pin intraarticularly to prevent the pin or reamer from plunging across the joint. The intraarticular edges of the tibial tunnel are then chamfered and smoothed while residual soft tissue is debrided from the tibial tunnel margin.

Having already performed the notchplasty, the surgeon turns attention to identifying the site of the femoral tunnel. Again, a cannulated femoral drill-pin guide can be placed at the 10 o'clock position in the right knee or the

2 o'clock position in the left knee to place the femoral tunnel guide pin while the knee is flexed to approximately 90 to 100°. The guide wire is drilled from inside the joint through the lateral cortex of the lateral femoral condyle until it can be palpated subcutaneously at the lateral femoral condyle. A scalpel is then used to make a small incision, measuring approximately 3 to 5 cm, over the lateral femoral condyle over top of the femoral guide pin. The fascia lata is sharply cut longitudinally in line with its fibers and the vastus lateralis is elevated. The cannulated reamer is then placed over the guide wire through the tibial tunnel, the distal end of the femoral tunnel is chamfered, and all soft tissue debris is removed. A tendon passer is then passed from the lateral aspect of the femoral condyle through the femoral tunnel by way of the tibial tunnel. The Dacron tape that was looped around the graft is tied around the tendon passer and the graft is then pulled in a retrograde fashion from the tibial tunnel intraarticularly; the Dacron tapes are then pulled out of the femoral tunnel under arthroscopic visualization. The Dacron tape is then threaded through a polyethylene button and, while the distal graft is held under tension via the Ethibond sutures, the Dacron tape is tied over the end button at the lateral femoral condyle. The graft is observed while the knee is moved through complete range of motion to ensure that there is no evidence of impingement of the graft. The knee is then placed at 20° of flexion while a posteriorly directed drawer force is applied to the tibia, and the distal aspect of the graft is fixed with a screw and soft tissue washer. Again, the knee is placed through a full range of motion under arthroscopic examination to assure minimal excursion of the tendon autograft as well as the absence of any signs of impingement. The stability of the knee is tested by performance of anterior and posterior Lachman tests. The lateral femoral and medial tibial incisions are then closed in layers, and the arthroscopic portals are closed. Sterile dressing is then applied to the wound, followed by application of Ted-hose or a full-length Ace wrap. A Cryo-cuff is placed while the patient is still in the operating room, and the patient is encouraged to use the Cryo-cuff for at least 24 to 48 h postoperatively. The extremity is also placed in a rehabilitation knee brace.

Postoperative Rehabilitation

Several authors have demonstrated that immobilization for decreasing the stress on ligaments and tendons results in detrimental effects on the biomechanical properties of ligaments and tendons,[114,164] while other studies have shown that exposure to exercise and stress results in some improvement of the mechanical properties of normal ligaments.[165,167,168] Noyes et al.[169] found that, following 8 weeks of immobilization with a plaster cast, ACL strength in primates was decreased by 39 percent and ACL stiffness decreased by 36 percent. They also noted that it required up to 1 year of activity before the material properties returned to their normal levels.[169]

Despite these findings in native ligament substances, the general consensus today is that graft materials are their strongest on day zero at the time of implantation;

however, there is evidence that they do undergo some process of "ligamentization," during which they begin to take on some of the morphologic characteristics of ligaments.[170–173]

Although one often thinks of postoperative treatment as the initial rehabilitative period, the rehabilitation process truly begins immediately following ACL injury. Due to the early incidence of arthrofibrosis following acute ACL reconstruction, there is now a focus on the attainment of the full range of motion as quickly as possible.[151] Preoperatively, initial work should be done on regaining full range of motion and minimizing the swelling. Acutely, this can be initially achieved by icing of the knee, followed by range-of-motion exercises as well as initiation of strengthening and proprioceptive training exercises once the knee swelling has subsided and the acute pain has resolved. Also during this period, the patient can be instructed and prepared for the intensive physical therapy that will be required postoperatively. Postoperative goals include regaining full range of motion, including full extension; allowing the wound to heal and the swelling to subside; and regaining quadriceps strength and straight-leg raising. With these goals in mind, the patient is encouraged to continue use of the Cryo-cuff and is allowed to bear weight as tolerated with crutches, utilizing a knee brace. In addition, the patient is encouraged to do straight-leg raising and exercises along with heel slides; he or she is also encouraged to work on regaining full extension of the knee, both with active quadriceps contraction and advancement to straight-leg raising as the quadriceps strength returns. Utilization of a pillow under the heel will help to establish full extension of the leg. The patient is also instructed by physical therapy and encouraged to work on flexion to 90° as soon as possible in the first several postoperative days with or without the assistance of continuous passive motion. The patient is discharged home on the night of surgery or in the first several postoperative days, ambulating with crutches and utilizing the brace for ambulation and when outside of the house. Physical therapy is continued, with quadriceps strengthening and range-of-motion exercises, working on full extension and advancing flexion aggressively as tolerated. Upon discharge, the patient is encouraged to continue using the Cryo-cuff and elevation to minimize swelling. As the swelling decreases, the patient is obviously capable of advancing with flexion exercises; however, full flexion to 140 to 145° may not be achieved for 5 to 6 weeks postoperatively. At approximately 2 to 3 weeks postoperatively, the patient can begin with isokinetic or cocontraction exercise, which involves exercises such as leg press and bicycle riding. These exercises allow for cocontraction of the quadriceps and hamstring muscles to minimize the anterior shear force of the tibia with respect to the femur. Following approximately 6 weeks of strengthening exercises, once the patient has regained a strength greater than 75 percent of the unaffected leg, strength training is intensified and the patient may begin activities such as straight-line jogging and more sports-specific types of training at a lower intensity. It is not until the patient has completely regained quadriceps and hamstring strength equal to or greater than those of the unaffected leg that the patient is allowed to begin higher-intensity sports-specific training, which requires up to an additional 4 months before the patient can resume his or her preinjury level of participation with confidence.

It is also very important that the patient undergo neuromuscular or proprioceptive training.[161] Specific modalities that can be used include muscle stimulation and biofeedback, followed by balance exercises that essentially allow patients to reeducate their muscular coordination to maintain joint stability in the absence of the normal mechanoreceptors of the native ACL that would otherwise provide feedback for joint position.

COMBINED INJURIES

Combined Injuries of the Anterior Cruciate Ligament and Medial Meniscus

Spindler et al.[174] evaluated the incidence of meniscal lesions in association with recent tears of the ACL by arthroscopy and MRI. They observed that 56 percent of knees with recent ACL tears had also had associated lateral meniscus lesions. They noted that 53 percent of these meniscal tears were complete, while 47 percent were incomplete. Of the meniscal lesions, 37 percent involved medial meniscal tears, with 95 percent being complete and the remaining 5 percent incomplete. In chronic ACL-deficient knees, the incidence of medial meniscal tears is greater.[175]

Review of the literature reveals that there is an increased failure rate for meniscal repairs performed in ACL-deficient knees.[40,46,65,177] Warren observed that as many as 40 percent of meniscal repairs performed in ACL-deficient knees failed, while nearly 90 percent of meniscal repairs healed when they were performed at the same time as ACL reconstruction.[63] It is generally believed that the instability due to ACL insufficiency results in increased shear forces placed on the meniscus, which can lead to further secondary damage as well as disruption of meniscal repair. On the other hand, if ACL reconstruction is performed at the same time as meniscal repair, the improved stability of the knee as well as the large hemarthrosis that occurs after reconstructive surgery, providing certain unidentified growth factors, may ultimately provide an improved environment for healing and thus account for the improved rate of healing for meniscal repairs. Consequently, we recommend that any reparable meniscal tears be repaired at the time of ACL reconstruction surgery.[177]

The classic (O'Donoghue) triad involves a tear of the ACL, the medial collateral ligament, and the medial meniscus.[178,179] Injuries of this severity result in a significantly unstable knee and thus predispose the patient to premature onset of osteoarthritis of the involved knee.[180–182] The treatment of such combined injuries involving the ACL and the medial collateral ligament (MCL) along with the medial meniscus has evolved over the past several decades. In the 1950s O'Donoghue endorsed surgical repair of all complete ligamentous ruptures in the knee.[178] However, anecdotal evidence has suggested that acute operative treatment of both the ACL and MCL in these combined injuries often results in an unacceptably high incidence of postoperative knee stiffness. Consequently, a great deal of attention has been paid to combined injuries in both the basic science and clinical research areas.

Isolated rupture of the MCL is the second most prevalent significant knee injury.[125] In the past, surgical repair of isolated ruptures of the MCL was the standard of care. More recently, animal studies have demonstrated the healing capability of the MCL.[87,183] Subsequently, many clinical investigators have supported conservative treatment of isolated MCL tears.[184–187] In order to achieve a successful outcome with the nonoperative method, it is critical to first demonstrate unequivocally that one is dealing with an isolated MCL injury without associated injury to the ACL or menisci. Several animal studies have also demonstrated the healing capability of the nonsurgically treated MCL rupture.[188–190]

The value of early mobilization of the injured joint has become increasingly recognized. Early mobilization promotes MCL healing and recovery of function.[191] Studies in rabbits have demonstrated that immobilization slows recovery of normal collagen fiber orientation, adversely affects the mechanical properties of the ligament midsubstance, and weakens the femur-MCL-tibia complex, particularly at the tibial insertion site. The weakening of the insertion site was noted on histologic examination to be secondary to osteoclastic activity, which apparently accounted for the increased failure by avulsion.[190] Several animal and human studies have found that early passive motion and early functional rehabilitation as well as increasing stress and tension are beneficial to the healing of isolated MCL ruptures, having positive effects on the biomechanical, biochemical, and morphologic properties of the ligament.[183,192,193] These studies suggest that an isolated, complete tear of the medial collateral ligament can be treated nonoperatively, with early mobilization and functional rehabilitation while progressively increasing stress; the result is more rapid recovery and relative success as compared with surgical repair. Patients with combined injuries of the ACL and MCL have been found to have a much poorer prognosis regardless of the treatment received.[184,195]

The optimal treatment for the MCL component of these more severe injuries involving combined lesions of the ACL and MCL with and without meniscal injury has yet to be established. Several combination-injury animal models have been used to compare the effects of nonoperative treatment of the combination MCL tear versus the same tear as an isolated injury. These studies have confirmed that the nonoperatively treated MCL of the combination injury had an inferior quality of healed tissue when evaluated biomechanically and histologically.[180,196–198] In 1987, Inoue et al.[199] provided evidence that greater instability results from the increased varus-valgus rotation secondary to ACL deficiency in an MCL-deficient knee, which thus adversely affects MCL healing. Given that combined tears of the ACL and MCL create an adverse environment for MCL healing, the next question to address is whether MCL repair alone should be performed in such a situation. In animals, such surgical repair had no significant benefits over nonrepair in comparing subsequent ligamentous tensile strength and varus-valgus stability.[200,201]

Several authors endorse repair of the MCL plus ACL reconstruction.[182,195] Others simply recommend ACL reconstruction alone, claiming that this converts the combined injury to an isolated MCL injury[203–205] Engle et al.,[206] using a rabbit triad-injury model, tested the hypothesis that surgical reconstruction of the ACL would reduce instability of the knee, improve MCL healing, and slow the progression of osteoarthritis in the knee. The results from this study confirm this hypothesis. Knee joint instability was reduced as initial anterior-posterior translation was restored to the level of the contralateral knees. The reconstructed ACL knees were found to have varus-valgus stability comparable with that of knees with isolated MCL ruptures, but unlike the latter group, varus-valgus stability did not subsequently improve with time. In addition, reconstruction of the ACL was associated with improved healing of the femur-MCL-tibia complex. The improved structural properties of the healing femur-MCL-tibia complex were felt to be primarily due to healing of the tibial insertion site rather than improvement of the mechanical properties of the ligament substance itself, as the modulus of reconstructed ligaments was only 10 percent of the control values. The surgery seemed to delay the early onset of osteoarthritis, as demonstrated by the absence of the severe osteophyte formation, degenerative joint disease, and pronounced synovial proliferation that was found on the ACL-deficient (the nonreconstructed) group.

Based on the finding that ACL reconstruction is beneficial for MCL healing in combined injuries, Ohno et al.[207] attempted to determine the effects of ACL reconstruction with and without MCL repair. They created combined ACL and MCL injuries in adult rabbits by transecting the ACL and creating a mop and tear of the MCL. All rabbits then underwent ACL reconstruction with flexor tendon allografts. They were subsequently divided into surgical and nonsurgical groups to determine whether MCL repair restored the stability, mechanical properties of the healing MCL tissue (i.e., tissue quality), and structural properties of the healing femur-MCL-tibia complex. The findings of this study support surgical repair of MCL tears with ACL reconstruction. This treatment has led to less varus-valgus knee instability and improved healing of the femur-MCL-tibia complexes that were found to have significant greater ultimate load and stiffness. There was, however, no significant difference in either anteroposterior translation or modulus between the repair and nonrepair groups. Follow-up in this study was only 12 weeks; therefore long-term studies are required to further validate these results.

Despite these early findings suggesting that MCL repair along with ACL reconstruction is most beneficial, many physicians today advocate treating the torn MCL conservatively with a period of immobilization initially for pain control followed by early mobilization. They favor delayed operative reconstruction of the ACL and the medial meniscus until the acute inflammatory phase has subsided and full range of motion of the knee has been reestablished. This, they believe, will prevent the development of arthrofibrosis associated with acute reconstruction.[208]

INJURIES OF THE POSTERIOR CRUCIATE LIGAMENT
Anatomy

The PCL is an intraarticular but extrasynovial knee ligament. It has a broad origin that forms a semicircle on the lateral aspect of the medial femoral condyle, and it inserts in a depression or fovea 1 cm inferior to the articular surface on the posterolateral aspect between the medial and lateral tibial plateaus. The PCL is composed of two functional components: the anterolateral and posteromedial bands. These bands are named for the relative positions of their respective insertion sites. The anterolateral fiber group is larger, representing approximately 95 percent of the total PCL substance. It is taut with knee flexion and lax with knee extension. The posteromedial fiber group is smaller, consisting of approximately 5 percent of the total PCL substance; it is lax with knee flexion and taut with knee extension.[209–210] In addition to the anterolateral and posterior medial fiber groups, there are two variable meniscofemoral ligaments. These ligaments arise from the posterior horn of the lateral meniscus and insert on the lateral aspect of the medial femoral condyle. The anterior meniscofemoral ligament, also known as the ligament of Humphrey, runs anterior to the PCL, while the meniscofemoral ligament of Wrisberg runs posterior to the PCL.

Either the anterior or posterior meniscal femoral ligament is present in approximately 70 percent of all knees. The posterior meniscofemoral or Wrisberg's ligament is more common, and its femoral origin has been shown to merge with that of the PCL.[118]

Function and Biomechanics of the Posterior Cruciate Ligament

The posterior cruciate ligament provides 95 percent of the total restraining force to posterior tibial displacement and is the primary restraint to posterior tibial translation. All other ligamentous and soft tissue structures provide the remaining 5 percent of secondary restraint.[91] In addition, along with the ACL, the PCL is believed to facilitate the "screw-home" mechanism as the knee is brought to full extension.[211] Kennedy et al.[212] determined that the ultimate strength of the PCL is twice that of the ACL. Unfortunately, these values may be inaccurate, as Woo et al.[98] have demonstrated that conditions of age, orientation, and loading can influence studies of ligamentous strength and tensile properties. Subsequently, Prietto et al.[213] used young cadaveric knees to determine ultimate loads of the PCL; their values of 1627 ± 491 N were relatively similar to values obtained for the tensile strength of the ACL. Studies have shown that the anterolateral component is approximately twice as strong and stiff as the posteromedial component and the meniscofemoral ligaments.[214,215] It also has been determined that the PCL contributes to posterior rollback of the femur with increasing knee flexion.[216]

Incidence of Injury to the Posterior Cruciate Ligament

According to the literature, injury to the PCL accounts for approximately 3 to 20 percent of all knee ligament injuries.[125,217] The true incidence of PCL injury, however, is not known, because many isolated injuries to the PCL go undetected. Parolie et al.[218] noted that there was a 2 percent rate of PCL injury among asymptomatic college football players in the NFL predraft examinations. However, with improved techniques of physical examination and the increased use of MRI, there has been a heightened awareness as well as an increase in the number of PCL injuries diagnosed. People who sustain injuries of the PCL are most often involved in either athletic activities or trauma, such as motor vehicle accidents. Three common events are associated with injury to the PCL. The first is hyperflexion of the knee with or without an anterior tibial force, such as a fall into a flexed knee with a plantar-flexed foot, or the classic "dashboard" injury in which the impact of the dashboard forces the tibia posteriorly. The second is hyperflexion with downward force on the thigh, and the third is hyperextension of the knee with or without associated varus or valgus force, which can often result in combined ligamentous injury.[219] In the past, the general consensus was that patients with an isolated PCL injury usually do well when treated nonoperatively with quadriceps-strengthening programs.[220–222] Several other authors have challenged this assumption, citing an increased incidence of premature degenerative changes of the medial femoral condyle and patellofemoral joint as well as increased incidence of pain and symptoms or complaints of instability.[223,224] Premature degenerative joint disease of the patellofemoral and medial compartments is felt to be secondary to increased joint contact forces in the PCL-deficient knee.[225,226] Furthermore, like tears of the ACL, midsubstance tears of the PCL heal poorly. Consequently, primary repair of midsubstance tears of the PCL does not consistently produce good stability.[227,228]

Diagnosis of Injury of the Posterior Cruciate Ligament

As for any injury, an initial comprehensive history must be taken. The patient may give a history of involvement in a motor vehicle accident or may describe mechanisms such as hyperflexion or hyperextension of the knee with an associated "pop." On physical examination, it is very important to perform a complete neurovascular examination and assure palpable pulses and intact sensation and motor function of the lower extremity. The posterior drawer test, which is performed with the knee at 90° of flexion with a posterior force directed on the tibia, has been shown to be most sensitive for detecting disruption of the posterior

cruciate ligament.[229] When the posterior drawer test is performed, it is critical to reestablish the normal tibial step-off (8 to 10 mm anteriorly) between the medial tibial plateau on the femoral condyle before applying a posteriorly directed force. If baseline posterior tibial subluxation is not initially recognized, the examiner may have a false impression of ACL disruption. The knee must be further examined for evidence of anterior laxity following restoration of the normal tibial step-off as well as varus-valgus laxity and any evidence of meniscal lesion must be determined by performance of the McMurray or Appley tests. The posterior tibial sag sign is performed by placing the hip and knee at 90° and observing for the normal anterior step-off. If there is absence of the normal anterior tibial step-off with the knee and hip flexed at 90°, the posterior sag sign is positive, indicating posterior subluxation of the tibia with respect to the femur. The knee is also examined for both posterolateral and posteromedial instability. Posterolateral instability is evaluated by performing the posterolateral drawer test, which is the posterior drawer test with the foot externally rotated to 15° (Fig. 50-11). The posteromedial drawer test is performed with the foot internally rotated to 15°. The external rotation recurvatum test is performed with the knee in slight flexion. As the knee is slowly extended by lifting the feet off the table, the examiner feels for recurvatum and external rotation of the tibia (Fig. 50-12). Additional tests include the reverse pivot shift (Fig. 50-13) and quadriceps active test which has been well described by Daniel et al.[230] As for all knee injuries, standard anteroposterior (AP), lateral, and oblique radiographs of the knee should be obtained to detect any possible bony injury or bony avulsion of the PCL. If there is uncertainty with regard to the diagnosis of PCL injury or concern for associated injuries, MRI may provide further information, but it is not absolutely necessary for all cases. Furthermore, technetium bone scans may be obtained in chronic PCL-deficient knees to assess the degree of early degenerative changes not detectable on standard radiographs.

Treatment of Injuries of the Posterior Cruciate Ligament

Most surgeons agree that avulsion fractures of the PCL's tibial insertion should be treated surgically with open reduction/internal fixation of the avulsed fragment with standard screws. In the case of midsubstance tears of the PCL, there is still considerable debate. Generally, however, the current recommendations for treatment of midsubstance PCL tears are as follows. For grade I and II ligament tears (Table 50-1), there is general agreement on conservative treatment consisting of brief immobilization for resolution of pain and swelling followed by a quadriceps strengthening rehabilitation program. For complete or grade III tears of the posterior cruciate ligament, treatment is still debated; however, most currently recommend reconstruction of the PCL in young, active patients with greater than 10 mm of posterior tibial drawer.[231] For grade IV or combined ligamentous injuries, the general consensus is that they should all be surgically repaired.

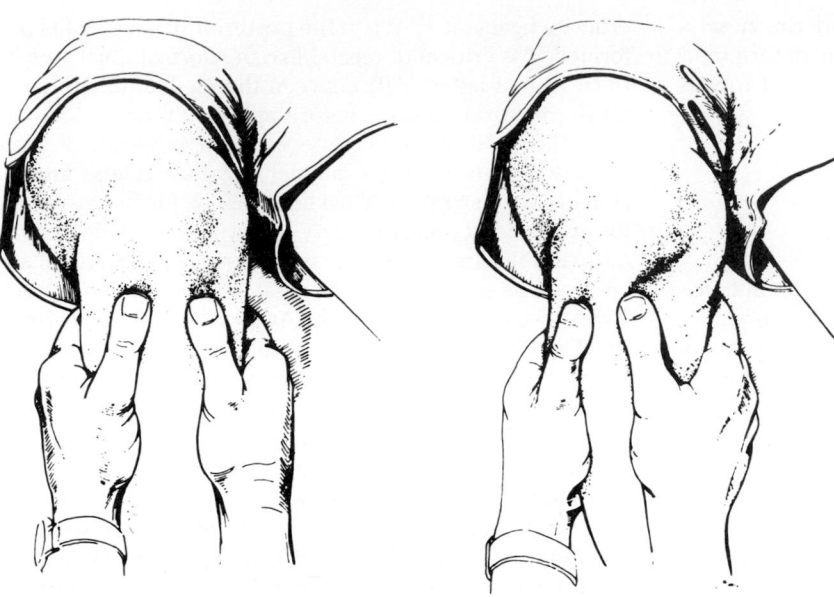

Figure 50-11 Posterolateral drawer test—anterior view. With the knee flexed over the side of the table, the proximal tibia is firmly grasped with the thumbs on either side of the tibial tubercle. A positive posterolateral drawer test is demonstrated by posterior and external rotation of the lateral tibial condyle. (Reproduced with permission from Hughston JD, Norwood LA: The posterolateral drawer test and external rotational recurvatum test for posterolateral rotatory instability of the knee. *Clin Orthop* 133:82–87, 1980.)

The goals of PCL reconstructive surgery are to restore tibial/femoral stability and kinematics, prevent progression of degenerative joint disease, and allow the patient to return to his or her previous level of activity without pain or instability. Either autograft or allograft tissues and open or arthroscopic assisted procedures have been used to reconstruct the PCL. Popular technique stresses anatomic placement of the grafts and most attempt to reproduce the anterolateral band of the PCL, as it is the most substantial of the two bands, both anatomically and functionally.

Arthroscopic Reconstruction of the Posterior Cruciate Ligament with Achilles Tendon Allograft

As with the procedure for ACL reconstruction, prior to the arthroscopic reconstruction, a complete examination is performed under anesthesia. This includes performance of the posterior drawer test with the knee at 90° of flexion, as this has been shown to be the most sensitive for the detection of PCL injury.[229] In addition, the normal 8- to 10-mm tibial step-off between the femoral condyles and

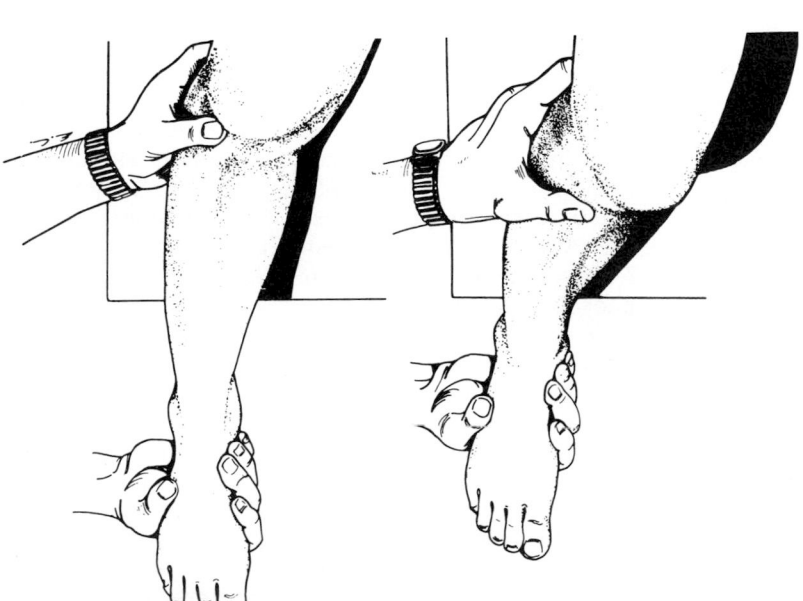

Figure 50-12 External rotational recurvatum test. The knee is held in slight flexion to start (*left*). As the knee is slowly extended, the examiner's hand feels for the external rotation and recurvatum at the posterolateral aspect of the knee. (Reproduced with permission from Hughston JD, Norwood LA: The posterolateral drawer test and external rotational recurvatum test for posterolateral rotatory instability of the knee. *Clin Orthop* 133:82–87, 1980.)

Figure 50-13 Reversed pivot shift sign. The starting position is with the knee flexed and the leg externally rotated. As the knee is extended with a slight axial load in valgus stress, the posterolateral subluxation will reduce. [Reproduced with permission from Jakob RP, Hassler HU, Staeubli H: Observations on rotatory instability of the lateral compartment of the knee. *Acta Orthop Scand* 52(suppl 191), p. 19.]

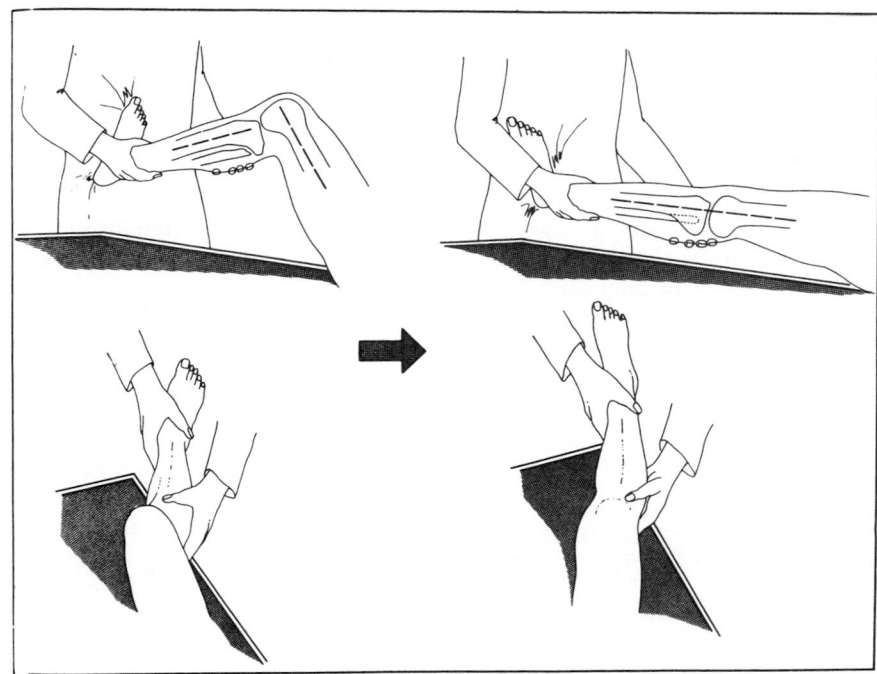

the anterior tibial plateau should be evaluated. If this is absent, then the posterior subluxation of the tibia on the femur is indicative of PCL injury. A thorough examination for evidence of other ligamentous injuries of the knee should also be performed at this time. The integrity of the posterior lateral structures must also be evaluated, as an increased incidence of posterolateral corner injuries is associated with injury of the PCL. These structures are assessed by performing a posterolateral and posteromedial rotation drawer test; varus stress testing is also done, as well as passively rotating the tibia externally with the knee at both 30 and 90° of flexion. These maneuvers are followed by performance of external rotation recurvatum and reverse pivot shift tests. After comprehensive physical examination under anesthesia, the patient is prepared for surgery. The patient is placed in the supine position with the foot of the table dropped and folded under. The nonoperative leg is placed in a well-leg holder while the hip is abducted and externally rotated with the knee and hip flexed at approximately 90°. Careful attention is paid to padding and protecting all bony prominences. Following application of a thigh tourniquet, the operative extremity is then positioned in an arthroscopic leg holder. Following adequate positioning of the patient and protection of all bony prominences, the extremity is prepped and draped in the usual sterile fashion.

Comprehensive diagnostic arthroscopy is then performed, following placement of standard anterolateral and anteromedial portals. A 30° arthroscope is used to perform a thorough examination of the medial and lateral compartments as well as the patellofemoral compartment, observing for any evidence of chondrosis or meniscal pathology. In addition, the knee is taken through a full range of motion to observe patellar tracking. Any associated pathology—including meniscal lesions, damaged ar-

TABLE 50-1 Grading and Treatment of Tears of the Posterior Cruciate Ligament

Grade	Definition	Laxity, mm[a]
Isolated		
I	PCL stretched	<5
II	PCL torn, MF ligamentous intact	5–9
III	PCL and MF ligaments torn	>10
Combined		
IV A	PCL and LCL/posterolateral injury	>12
IV B	PCL and LCL/posteromedial injury	>12
IV C	PCL and ACL torn	>15

[a] Laxity determined by posterior drawer test.
Key: PCL, posterior cruciate ligament; MF, meniscofemoral; LCL, lateral collateral ligament; MCL, medial collateral ligament; ACL, anterior cruciate ligament.
Source: Reproduced with permission from Miller MD, Johnson DL, Harner CD, Fu FH: Posterior cruciate ligament injuries. *Orthop Rev* 12:1201, 1993.

ticular cartilage or meniscal tears—is addressed prior to reconstruction of the PCL. The ACL may not appear damaged, but it may seem to be lax on initial observation due to the posterior subluxation of the tibia on the femur, giving the false impression of a damaged ACL. This can be evaluated by placing an anterior force on the tibia to reestablish the normal anterior tibial step-off. The PCL is inspected thoroughly, as midsubstance injury may be hidden by the anteriorly crossing ACL. Following confirmation of a tear of the PCL, a full-radius resector is used to remove the femoral remnant of the ligament under arthroscopic visualization. A notchplasty and debridement of overhanging osteophytes can be performed with the full-radius resector. Most of the PCL is resected; however, the PCL's femoral footprint on the medial femoral condyle is preserved for assistance with placement of the femoral tunnel.

Placement of the Tibial Tunnel

A 70° arthroscope is placed through the anterolateral portal and passed into the posterior aspect of the intercondylar notch while the knee is at 90° of flexion. Placement of the scope between the medial femoral condyle and the ACL allows for visualization of the tibial insertion site of the PCL. A second posterior medial portal is then created under direct visualization, the posteromedial corner of the knee is transilluminated with the arthroscope, and an 18-gauge spinal needle is placed just anterior to the saphenous vein. A scalpel with a #11 blade is used to make a longitudinal stab incision at the entry point. A periosteal elevator or a curved curette placed through the posterior medial portal is used to elevate the posterior capsule off of the PCL. This allows for full exposure of the entire tibial insertion site as well as protection of the posterior neurovascular structures when the tibial tunnel is drilled. A full-radius resector is then placed through the posterior medial portal to excise the tibial remnant under visualization. The footprint itself is left intact in order to assist with tunnel placement. A 3- to 4-cm longitudinal skin incision is made over the intended tibial tunnel site, which is approximately 1 cm below the tibial tubercle and 3 cm medial to it. Hemostasis is obtained with electrocautery, the tibial periosteum is sharply divided, and medial and lateral flaps are elevated with blunt dissection. Development and preservation of the periosteal flaps is critical for proper closure following completion of the reconstructive procedure. A 55° arthroscopic drill guide is inserted through the anterior medial portal and intercondylar notch and placed in the posterolateral aspect of the PCL footprint. The distal aspect of the drill guide is placed in a position of approximately 1 cm below and 2 to 3 cm medial to the tibial tubercle, and a 3/32 K wire is drilled through the tibia through the guide at an angle that approximates the slope of the tibiofibular joint. The orientation of the drill guide is thus approximately 50° with respect to the tibial shaft. This slope closely approximates the slope of the proximal tibiofibular joint. Under arthroscopic visualization, the K wire is drilled through the tibia until it exits the posterior cortex of the tibia within the posterior PCL's insertion

site. This step is carefully visualized with the arthroscope to avoid plunging of the K wire into the posterior neurovascular structures of the knee. The drill guide is then taken away from the knee, and intraoperative lateral radiographs are obtained to assess the position of the guide wire. The ideal positioning of the guide wire is such that it is parallel with the easily visualized posterior cortical flare of the tibia, exiting at the junction of the distal and middle thirds of the fovea, where the native PCL inserts. Once the guide wire has been placed in the desired position and this has been confirmed with intraoperative radiographs, a cannulated 10- to 12-mm reamer is used to drill the tibial tunnel under direct visualization. The size of the tibial tunnel and thus the reamer is determined by the predetermined size of the graft bone plug. A large curette is placed through the posterior medial portal in order to protect the posterior capsule and vital neurovascular structures while the tibial tunnel is reamed under arthroscopic visualization. The edges of the tunnel are then chamfered and smoothed with a rasp and excess tissue is removed with a shaver. If excess soft tissue is not removed and the tunnel is not chamfered, passage of the graft through the tunnel may be very difficult and the graft may suffer significant abrasion against the sharp bone edges. This is very important, because the graft takes an almost 90° turn as it exits and courses toward the femoral tunnel.

Femoral Tunnel

The medial femoral epicondyle and medial edge of the patella are identified and marked. A 3- to 4-cm longitudinal medial peripatellar incision is then made halfway between the medial femoral condyle and medial edge of the patella and centered over the articular edge of the medial femoral condyle. The vastus medialis obliquus muscle is retracted superiorly while the medial retinaculum and synovium are sharply incised to expose the articular edge of the medial femoral condyle. The tip of a 30° arthroscopic drill guide is then inserted or placed through the anterior medial portal while the knee is at 90° of flexion. As previously mentioned, we attempt to reproduce the anterolateral band of the PCL; therefore the tip of the drill guide is positioned at the anterosuperior portion of the PCL's femoral footprint (Fig. 50-14). This corresponds with a point approximately 8 to 10 mm posterior to the articular cartilage of the medial femoral condyle at the 2 o'clock position in the right knee and at the 10 o'clock position of the left knee within the intercondylar notch. Following satisfactory positioning of the tip of the drill guide, its cannulated portion is then placed against the medial femoral condyle through the medial peripatellar incision. A 3/32 K wire is then drilled through the medial femoral condyle, entering through the anterior aspect of the PCL's anatomic footprint at a site approximately 5 to 10 mm from the articular cartilage. Once the guide wire has been placed in a proper position, a 10- to 12-mm cannulated drill is used to create the femoral tunnel under arthroscopic visualization. Again, the edges of the tunnel are chamfered and beveled with a rasp, while excess tissue is excised with a shaver.

Figure 50-14 Femoral tunnel creation for posterior cruciate ligament repair. *A.* Frontal view demonstrating passage of a Kirschner wire after appropriate positioning of the arthroscopic drill guide on the medial femoral condyle. *B.* Lateral view. Note the close approximation of the guide pin entry site to the articular margin of the medial femoral condyle. (Reproduced with permission from Swenson TM, Harner CD, Fu FH: Arthroscopic posterior cruciate ligament reconstruction with allograft. *Sports Med Arthrosc Rev* 2:125, 1994.)

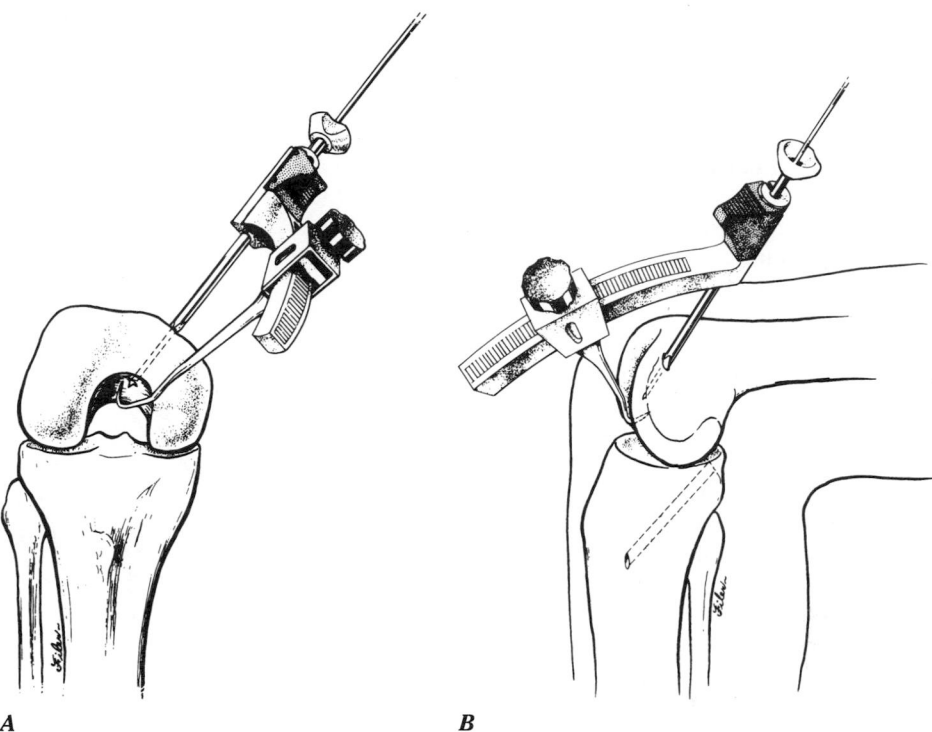

A   *B*

Graft Preparation

We prefer to use fresh-frozen Achilles tendon allograft for PCL reconstruction. Advantages of using this allograft include (1) decreased operative time as compared to use of autograft tissue; (2) decreased surgical trauma; (3) if concomitant ACL reconstruction must be performed, the patellar tendon can be used for ACL reconstruction, while the Achilles tendon can be used for reconstruction of the PCL; (4) Achilles allograft tendon has a bone plug attached to one end, thus facilitating passage of the soft tissue end through the tunnels without significant difficulty; and (5) Achilles tendon allografts have sufficient length for adequate passage of the graft through the tunnel and fixation. There is concern, however, with use of any allograft tissue about the risk of disease transmission, including hepatitis and HIV viruses, as well as about the effects of different sterilization treatments on the integrity of the graft substance.

The fresh-frozen Achilles tendon allograft is prepared at a back table. To facilitate the entire procedure as well as decrease total operative time, the allograft is typically prepared by an assistant while the tibial and femoral tunnels are prepared. Prior to the surgery, the fresh-frozen Achilles tendon allograft is thawed at room temperature (temperatures below 40°C) in order to avoid denaturization of the collagen. We prefer to prepare the Achilles tendon with a 12-mm-diameter bone plug. A 12-mm bone-plug sizer is used as a guide, while a rongeur is used to create a bullet-shaped bone plug. Mayo scissors are used to clean all excess soft tissue from the tendon surface, and #5 Tycron or Ethibond sutures are placed in antegrade and retrograde baseball-stitch fashion in order to tubularize the free end of the tendon. The sutures on the free end are left hanging to facilitate passage, while two holes are drilled at right angles to each other in the bone plug for the passage of two more #5 Ethibond or Tycron sutures for graft passage. The entire allograft is then passed through a graft sizer of the same size as the tibial and femoral tunnels in order to ensure easy passage of the graft during placement in the knee.

Graft Insertion

A looped 18-gauge malleable wire is inserted in a retrograde fashion through the femoral tunnel and grasped with a pituitary rongeur via the tibial tunnel. The wire is then brought out of the distal aspect of the tibial tunnel. The #5 Tycron or Ethibond sutures are then tied around the looped end of the malleable wire; the wire is subsequently withdrawn from the femoral tunnel, pulling the Tycron sutures with it. The graft is then pulled through the tunnels via the sutures. The graft is advanced so that the bone plug remains within the tibial tunnel, and the soft tissue end exits the femoral tunnel. If the edges of the tibial and femoral tunnels have not been properly prepared and beveled, the graft can become frayed during passage. The allograft bone plug is recessed within the tibial tunnel so that its leading edge becomes flush with the posterior cortex of the knee. This is done in order to minimize any undue bending and shearing forces, which can result in abrasion of the graft against the bony edges of the tunnel. Sidles et al.[233] observed large internal graft pressures occurring at the sites of excess graft bending. They thus concluded that incorporation of the graft into the bony tunnels can be hindered at the sites of fixation due to large pressures and bending, which have associated shearing forces on the graft. It is our opinion that graft bending angles and graft abrasion are minimized by placing the bone plug flush against the opening of the tibial tunnel. A 9- by 20-mm interference screw is placed between the cancellous portion of the allograft bone plug and the cancellous bone of the tibial tunnel in order to secure the plug within the tunnel. The arthroscope can be placed directly into the tibial tunnel in order to confirm adequate placement and seating of the interference screw.

The allograft is preconditioned with cyclical tensioning of the free end prior to fixation of the graft within the femoral tunnel. This is accomplished by repeating cycles of full flexion and extension of the knee while tension is maintained on the graft. The knee is then placed at 80 to 90° of flexion while an anterior tibial drawer force of approximately 156 N is placed. The soft tissue portion of the graft is maintained under 80 N of tension while the graft is fixed by utilization of a screw and spiked soft tissue washer. We choose to tension and fix the graft while the knee is at 90° of flexion, because we attempt to recreate the anterolateral band that, in the native PCL, is noted to be taut with knee flexion and lax with knee extension. Other forms of fixation of the femoral portion of the graft include use of staple fixation, sutures tied around a post, and use of a calcaneal strut graft removed from the bony insertion of the Achilles tendon allograft, fashioned into a corticocancellous bone plug of appropriate diameter, and placed in the femoral tunnel. The bone plug is then tamped into the femoral tunnel and advanced so that it is flush with the edge of the tunnel and an interference screw is inserted in the usual fashion between the bone plug and the cancellous bone of the femoral tunnel (Fig. 50-15). Often, additional fixation, consisting of a staple or screw and spiked washer, are added. All excess tissue is then debrided from the allograft and tunnel. The knee is then thoroughly examined for stability and rigid fixation of the graft. The knee is taken through a full range of flexion and extension while the graft is visualized arthroscopically in order to confirm absence of impingement, appropriate tensioning of the graft during knee flexion and during performance of posterior drawer testing. Each incision is then closed in layers. The tibial periosteal flaps are carefully closed over the tibial tunnel and, following wound closure, sterile dressing is applied. Tedhose or Ace wrap is then placed on the entire lower extremity, followed by application of a Cryo-cuff, and the knee is placed in a hinged long-leg brace locked in full extension.

Postoperative Course/Rehabilitation

Immediately postoperatively, the knee is immobilized in a long-leg hinged knee brace locked in extension in order to minimize any gravitational forces acting to sublux the tibia posteriorly on the femur, thus placing the graft under the least amount of tension. The patient is allowed to bear weight as tolerated with the knee brace locked in full extension. Isometric quadriceps-strengthening exercises as well as straight-leg raising are begun on the night of surgery or on postoperative day 1. While the patient is in bed, he or she is encouraged to place a pillow under the tibia to

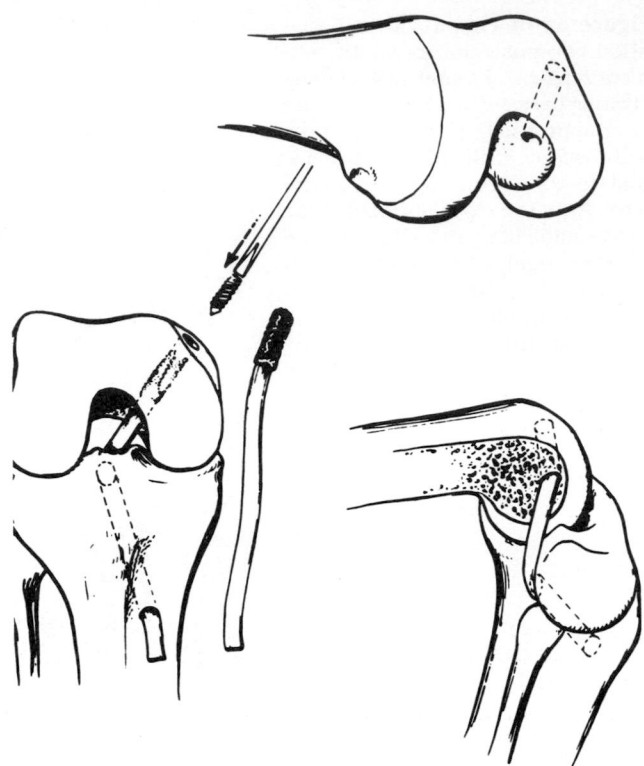

Figure 50-15 Composite of the current technique of PCL reconstruction with Achilles tendon. Note preferred sites of tunnel placement—posterolateral aspect of tibial footprint and anterosuperior aspect of femoral footprint.

prevent posterior subluxation of the tibia due to gravitational forces. The patient is allowed unrestricted weight bearing as tolerated, utilizing crutches with the knee brace locked in full extension. At approximately 2 weeks postoperatively, the patient is begun on range-of-motion exercise, first consisting of passive, then progressing to active assisted, and then to active range-of-motion exercises at approximately 4 weeks postoperatively. If the patient had associated injuries to the ACL, posterior lateral corner, or medial meniscus that also required reconstruction or repair, the patient may be immobilized for a longer period of time with placement of additional restrictions as per the surgeon's preference.

Posterolateral Rotatory Instability

The posterolateral corner is an anatomically complex region of the knee joint. The primary structures of the posterolateral corner include the lateral collateral ligament, popliteofibular ligament, popliteus tendon, patellofibular ligament, arcuate ligament, short lateral ligament, and posterolateral joint capsule. Several studies involving cadaveric dissection have revealed that the posterolateral corner has variable anatomy in both size and presence of these various components in different individuals[234–236] (Fig. 50-1). The posterolateral region of the knee is frequently divided in two primary components consisting of the lateral collateral ligament and the remaining structures, referred to as the posterolateral complex. Selective cutting studies have been utilized to define the contributions of the lateral collateral ligament and the posterolateral corner or complex to overall knee stability.[229,238,239] From these studies, it is evident that transection of the lateral collateral ligament results in smaller increases in varus laxity of the knee at all angles of knee flexion. However, when both the lateral collateral ligament and posterior lateral complex are transected, larger increases in varus angulation and laxity are noted, with maximal increase occurring at 30° of knee flexion. When the PCL is also transected in addition to the lateral collateral ligament (LCL) and posterolateral corner, even larger increases in varus angulation are noted throughout the full range of knee flexion. Gollehan et al.[238] demonstrated that in a normal knee with intact ligaments, application of a posterior drawer force to the tibia results in external rotation of the tibia. They described this as coupled rotation of the tibia. However, when the PCL was transected and the same posterior force is applied, they observed only direct posterior tibial displacement without the coupled external tibial rotation. When the lateral collateral ligament and posterolateral complex are transected and the posterior cruciate ligament is left intact, the amount of coupled external rotation due to a posterior tibial drawer force increases significantly at all angles but the greatest increase occurs at 30° of knee flexion. Transection of the PCL, lateral collateral ligament, and posterolateral corner or complex does not result in any increased coupled external rotation of the tibia as compared with transection of the LCL and posterolateral complex alone. Posterior tibial translation is altered minimally following isolated or combined transection of the LCL and posterolateral complex. It is well documented that transection of the PCL results in a significant amount of posterior translation of the tibia with respect to the femur at knee flexion angles between 0 and 90°, with the greatest degree of displacement occurring at 90° of knee flexion. Transection of the PCL, LCL, and posterolateral complex, however, results in the greatest amount of posterior tibial translation at all angles of knee flexion. Interestingly, Gollehan et al. determined that isolated transection of the PCL does not affect external tibial rotation, whereas transection of the posterolateral complex alone results in a significant amount of increased external rotation at 90° of knee flexion. Furthermore, combined sectioning of the LCL and posterolateral complex resulted in significant increases in external tibial rotation at all angles of knee flexion but maximally at 30° of knee flexion. When the PCL, LCL, and posterolateral complex are all transected, external tibial rotation increases between 60 and 90° of knee flexion.[238] The information gathered by such selective cutting studies has provided the basis for the present-day physical examination used to diagnose disruption of the posterolateral corner. Instability of the posterolateral corner is most frequently found with combined ligament injuries, whereas it is rarely found as an isolated injury alone. Because the peroneal nerve is anatomically very close to the posterolateral corner, any injury to the posterolateral corner must alert the physician to carefully evaluate the patient for any possible injury or deficits of the peroneal nerve.

Following careful and comprehensive history, physical examination includes evaluation of all ligaments of the knee, including the MCL, ACL, and PCL as well as the integrity of the menisci and also complete neurovascular examination. Specific tests designed to assess for injuries to the posterolateral corner include the following: (1) varus stress at 0 and 30° of knee flexion, (2) the external rotation recurvatum test (Fig. 50-12),[240] (3) external tibial rotation at 30 and 90° of knee flexion, (4) the reverse pivot shift test (Fig. 50-13), and (5) the posterolateral drawer test (Fig. 50-11).[240] As with any physical examination of an extremity, comparison of the injured knee with the uninvolved one allows the examiner to correlate any individual variability. Any differences in side-to-side comparisons on physical examination should be noted and documented.

As previously mentioned, isolated injury to the PCL is indicated by increased posterior tibial translation when the posterior drawer test is performed with the knee at 90° of flexion. When the PCL alone is deficient, there should be no observed increase in varus or valgus laxity or any increased external tibial rotation. When the posterolateral corner is disrupted, there is increased varus angulation and increased external tibial rotation at 30° of knee flexion. Furthermore, the examiner may note slightly increased posterior tibial drawer force with the knee at 30° of knee flexion; however, no laxity should be observed at 90° of knee flexion with posterior tibial drawer force.

The presence of a combined posterior lateral corner and PCL injury results in increased varus angulation, external tibial rotation, and posterior translation at all flexion angles tested. The posterolateral drawer test, reverse pivot shift test, and external rotation recurvatum test can also be used to provide additional information if the previous maneuvers are equivocal.

A combined PCL and posterolateral corner injury should be suspected if there is a side-to-side difference of more than 10 mm on performance of posterior drawer testing. Concomitant deficiency of the PCL makes assessment of posterolateral instability difficult due to possible posterior tibial subluxation. Hence, when faced with this situation, the examiner must remember to place an anterior drawer force on the tibia to eliminate the posterior tibial subluxation during evaluation of the posterolateral corner. If placement of anterior tibial drawer force is difficult, the patient can be placed prone on the examining table, thus allowing gravity to reduce the posterior tibial subluxation and facilitate examination for injury to the posterolateral corner.[241] The extent of injury and location of injury to structures can be adequately assessed by carefully noting any side-to-side differences in the amount of posterior drawer and external tibial rotation at 30 and 90° of knee flexion as well as determining the amount of varus angulation present in both full extension and 30° of knee flexion. It is generally held that acute injuries of the posterolateral corner should be surgically repaired within 3 weeks of the initial injury.[242] Ideally, all injured structures should be repaired. In patients with chronic deficiency of the posterolateral corner, it is not always possible to perform direct surgical repair. Consequently, a variety of techniques have been used, including autograft or allograft tissue for augmentation as well as tissue advancement procedures. Currently, there is no optimal procedure for reconstructing the posterolateral corner in situations where direct primary repair is not feasible. This is reflected by the large number of procedures described, and there is no consensus on the most appropriate methods of reconstruction. Certainly in the future this will be the subject of many basic science and clinical research projects that are needed to further improve our understanding of posterolateral corner injuries and, it is hoped, improve surgical techniques and outcomes for posterolateral complex instability of the knee.

PATELLOFEMORAL DISORDERS

Normal function of the patellofemoral joint depends upon the complex and smooth interplay of the dynamic and stable structures of the knee. When faced with the challenge of patellofemoral dysfunction, the physician must differentiate between pain and instability. A thorough understanding of the anatomy and biomechanics of the patellofemoral joint enables the physician to approach patellofemoral disorders in a logical manner.

Patellofemoral Anatomy

The patella is the central component of the patellofemoral joint. Its articular surface is the thickest in the body and can measure up to 4 to 5 mm in its central portion. The median ridge or crest divides the patella into lateral and medial facets. The medial facet can vary anatomically from person to person; it is divided into the medial facet proper and a smaller "odd" facet. A secondary ridge separates the smaller odd facet from the medial facet proper. The odd facet is purely cartilaginous and is felt to develop secondary to forces generated between the lateral aspect of the medial femoral condyle and the medial facet.[243] The odd facet comes into contact with the trochlear portion of the medial femoral condyle at 135° of knee flexion. The medial facet is flat to slightly convex, while the lateral facet is concave as well as larger than the medial facet.[244] Facet hypoplasia and anatomic variations in the patella have been implicated in the etiology of patellar instability. Wriberg[244] and Ficat et al.[245] have classified different patellar morphologies based on radiographic shape and angle created by the medial and lateral facets, respectively, and their relationship to patellar stability. Ficat et al. described that the normal angle created by the medial and lateral facets as between 120 and 140°, with angles greater than 140° being potentially unstable.

The distal femur has both medial and lateral facets, which articulate with their respective facets on the patella. The medial and lateral femoral condyles or facets have a convex shape and form the intercondylar notch distally. The articular cartilage of the femoral facets measures approximately 2 to 3 mm. The articular cartilage of the lateral facet is thicker, and the lateral facet is larger and projects more cephalad and anteriorly than the medial facet.[246] The normal sulcus angle formed by the medial lateral femoral facets is 142°, as determined by Brattstrom.[247]

Underdeveloped condyles and/or sulcus angles of more than 150° can also lead to patellofemoral instability.[248]

The patella derives its primary blood supply from the medial and lateral superior and inferior geniculate arteries in addition to contributions from the supreme geniculate artery and the medial and anterior tibial recurrent arteries. For technical purposes, it is important to remember that the superior lateral geniculate artery is located between the lateral retinaculum and the synovium at the superolateral pole of the patella (Fig. 50-16). Patellofemoral joint stability is provided by the bony architecture of the medial and lateral facets of the patella as well as those of the femur, in addition to the static and dynamic stabilizers about the knee. Static restraints include the lateral peripatellar retinaculum, which is composed of two major components. Connecting the lateral patella to the iliotibial band, the superficial oblique retinaculum is the less significant component, whereas the deep transverse retinaculum is more extensive and substantial. Within its substance is the lateral patellofemoral ligament, the patellotibial band, and the iliopatellar bands. The static restraints on the medial side of the patella include the patellofemoral and patellotibial ligaments as well as a capsular condensation. In addition, the patellar tendon, acting as a restraint in the frontal plane, limits excess patellar displacement proximally to less than 10 mm.[246] The four major components of the quadriceps muscle act as the dynamic stabilizers of the patellofemoral joint. These components include the rectus femoris and vastus intermedialis tendons as well as the vastus medialis and the anatomically distinct vastus medialis obliquus, which originates from the adductor tubercle and inserts on the medial patella at a 55° angle, serving as a primary dynamic stabilizer against lateral translation of the patella.[249] Finally, a portion of the distal aspect of the vastus lateralis muscle inserts onto the lateral patella obliquely, thus providing dynamic stabilization against medial displacement of the patella.[250,251]

Biomechanics of Patellar Tracking and Patellofemoral Contact

The quadriceps muscles act primarily to extend the knee. The patella plays a major role in facilitating the function of the quadriceps muscles by increasing the distance of the quadriceps tendon from the center of rotation of the knee—i.e., increasing the moment arm. This gives the quadriceps tendon a biomechanical advantage, increasing quadriceps force by 33 to 50 percent.[252] Furthermore, the patella provides protection for the knee joint and femoral condyles as well as functioning to guide the quadriceps tendon within the trochlear groove. Thick hyaline cartilage of the patella allows the extensor mechanism to glide smoothly, thus protecting the quadriceps tendon from shear forces that could potentially cause excessive wear on the quadriceps tendon. Under normal circumstances, the articular surface of the patella is subjected to significant forces. Using a mathematical model, Reilly and Martens[253] determined that the patellofemoral joint's reactive force was approximately half body weight during normal walking, and

Figure 50-16 Anastomosis at the front of the knee formed by genicular branches from the popliteal artery and descending branches, which connect the femoral artery proximally with the popliteal and anterior tibial arteries distally. [Reproduced with permission from Insall JN, Kelly MA: Anatomy, in Insall JN, Windsor RE, Kelly MD, et al (eds): *Surgery of the Knee,* 2d ed. New York, Churchill Livingstone, 1993.]

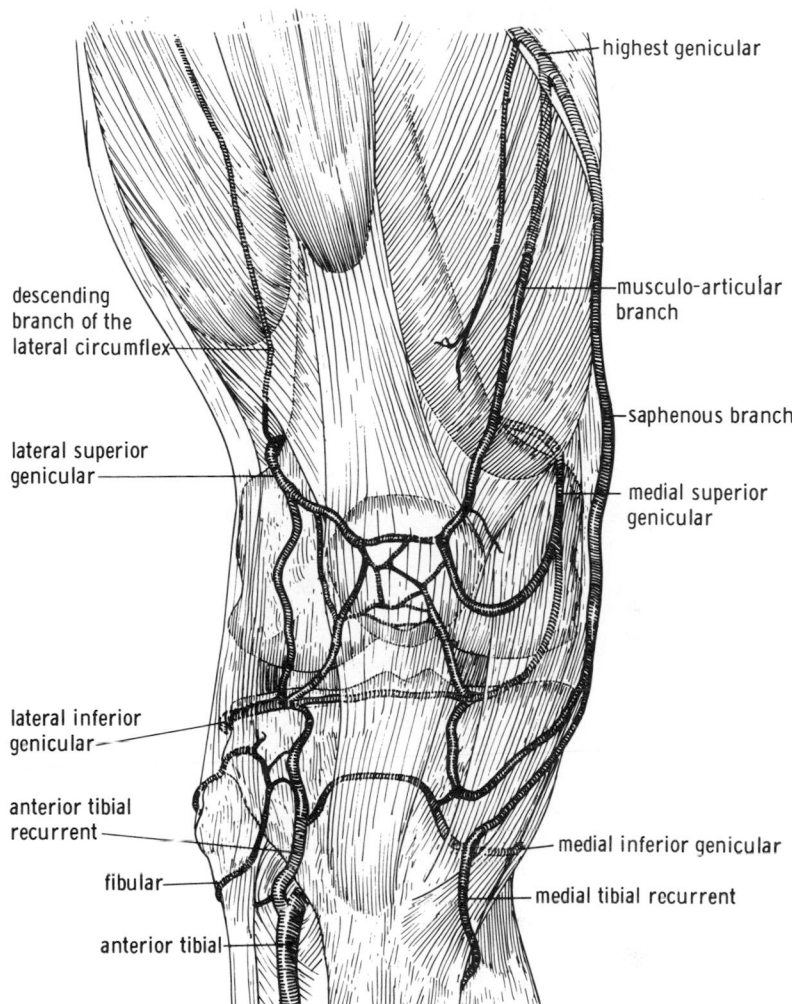

these forces increase to greater than three times body weight with stair climbing. Others have demonstrated that placing a weight around the ankle during knee extension results in significantly greater patellofemoral joint reactive forces, especially in the middle arcs of knee motion.[254–256]

With the knee in full extension, the patella does not come into contact with the trochlea. In a knee with normal patellar tendon length, the patella does not come into contact with the trochlea until the knee has been flexed to 10°. The distal patella is the first portion to come into contact with the trochlea; as knee flexion is increased, the area of contact moves proximally along the patella. Initially the lateral facet is the first to make contact, gliding along the lateral trochlea; at approximately 20° of flexion, the medial facet and medial trochlea begin to articulate, but this does not necessarily occur in some knees until the knee has been flexed to 30 or 40°. The odd facet does not come into contact until the knee has been flexed to 135° (Fig. 50-17). Once the knee has been flexed to 90°, the quadriceps tendon begins to contact the trochlea, thus sharing the compressive load. Furthermore, the patellofemoral contact area increases with increasing knee flexion as this contact area moves proximally along the patella.[255]

Diagnosis of Patellofemoral Disorders

When the examiner is presented with a patient with a patellofemoral disorder, it is imperative first to differentiate between pain and instability and then further to determine whether the knee pain is caused by trauma to the retinaculum or articular surface or whether it is due to patellar malalignment. The first and foremost step in the diagnosis of patellofemoral disorders is a careful history. This includes determination of the onset, duration, and nature of the pain as well as any inciting events such as trauma, athletic activities, or other factors that aggravate the pain or problem. It is key to ask the patient to localize the pain by pointing to the most painful region.

The second and equally important step is a meticulous physical examination. Physical examination should be performed with the patient disrobed and wearing shorts and should include complete examination of the hip as well as the ankle and foot, as referred pain is often a factor. The patient's gait should be evaluated, and the patient should be examined in both the supine and standing positions. The nature of stance and gait as well as overall limb alignment should be noted, and complete sensory, motor,

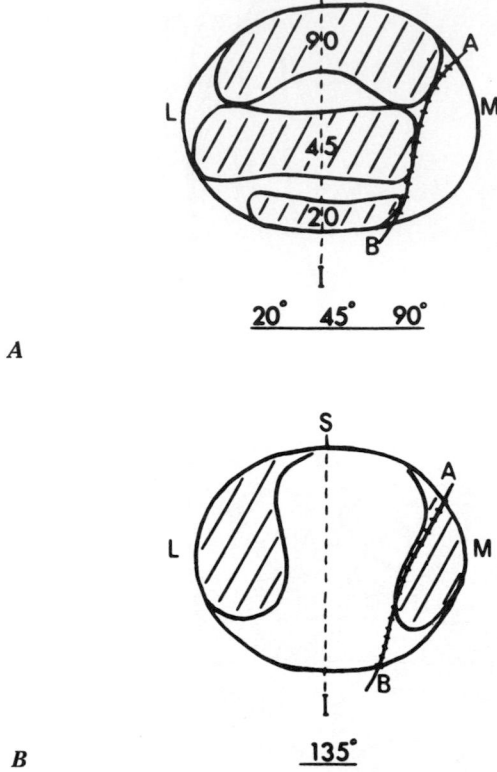

A

B

Figure 50-17 Experimentally determined areas (*cross-hatched*) of patellar contact with femur through varying degrees of knee flexion. *A.* Areas in contact at 20, 45, and 90°; *B.* Two areas in contact at 135°. (Reproduced with permission from Goodfellow J, Hungerford DS, Woods C, et al: Patello-femoral joint mechanics and pathology. *J Bone Joint Surg* 58B:287, 1976.)

maximal quadriceps isometric contraction. If, upon maximal contraction of the quadriceps muscles, the patella is pulled laterally more than proximally, a patellar tracking abnormality is suggested. Next, the passive patellar tilt test is performed by grasping the patella between the thumb and forefinger and elevating the lateral side of the patella. Normally the patella can be passively tilted from 0 to 20° from the horizontal plane. A lateral patellar tilt of less than 0° indicates excessive lateral tightness.[246,259]

The restraint of the lateral and medial soft tissues is assessed by performing the medial and lateral glide tests (Fig. 50-18). The patient is instructed to relax the quadriceps muscle, and the knee is flexed to 30°. A medial and then a lateral force is then applied to the knee, and total excursion of the patella, both laterally and medially, from its passive resting position within the trochlea is measured by the number of quadrants that the patella can be displaced. The normal range of medial glide at 30° of knee flexion if 1 to 2½ quadrants, whereas the normal range for lateral glide at 30° of flexion is ½ to 2½ quadrants. If the lateral glide is greater than 3 quadrants, the integrity of the medial restraints is questionable, suggesting possible subluxability of the patella. A medial glide of 3 to 4 quadrants indicates incompetent lateral restraints.

The joint line, patella, femoral condyles, and tibia as well as all peripatellar retinacular structures are palpated and inspected for evidence of abnormal tightness or laxity as well as tenderness, and the presence of crepitus with range of motion is also determined. Incisions and scars from previous surgery or trauma are also noted at this time. Furthermore, the patella can be compressed while the knee is taken through a full range of motion to determine the presence of articular pain.

and vascular exam should be performed on the lower extremities. Next, attention should be turned to examination of the knee, including evaluations of all ligamentous structures for stability as well as determination of the presence of an effusion and tenderness.

Specific examining tools used to evaluate patellofemoral disorders include the following. The quadriceps muscle angle or Q angle is felt to play a major role in the kinematics of the patellofemoral joint. The Q angle, described by Brattstrom in 1964,[247] describes the extent of lateral pull on the patella by the quadriceps muscle and tendon. This angle was initially measured with the knee in full extension; however, it is now recommended to perform measurements at both full extension and with the knee flexed to 30 and 90°. The Q angle is determined by measuring the angle between a line drawn from the anterosuperior spine to the central portion of the patella and the line between the central portion of the patella and the tibial tubercle. Insall determined that the normal Q angle varies between 8 and 17°.[257] An angle greater than 15° in men and 15 to 20° in women is generally thought to be abnormal.[247,257,258] At this point the quadriceps muscle mass is also assessed, and the position of the patella is observed while the quadriceps muscle is relaxed as well as with

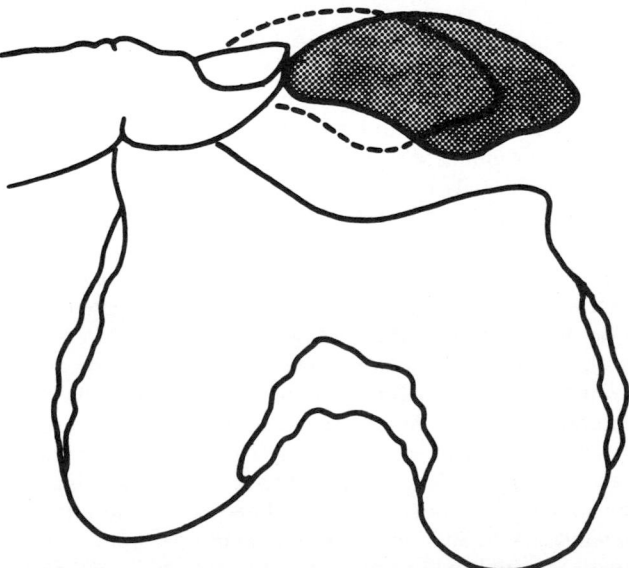

Figure 50-18 Medial glide should be checked as well as lateral glide, particularly in the patient who notes patellar instability after surgery. (Reproduced with permission from Fulkerson JP, Kalenak A, Rosenberg TD, Cox JS: Patellofemoral pain. *AAOS Instr Course Lect* 41:85, 1992.)

Patellofemoral stability can be assessed by performance of the Fairbank or apprehension test. The examiner places the knee at 30° of flexion resting it over a leg or bolster, and with the quadriceps relaxed, a lateral force is applied to the patella. If the patient responds by contracting the quadriceps muscle due to fear of dislocation of the patella, then the test is considered positive. Initial radiographic examination includes the Merchant view, which is taken with the knee flexed to 45° and the beam angled 30° from the horizontal or femoral plane. The Laurin or 20° knee flexion view can also be used to evaluate the patellofemoral joint.[260,261] Further views include a 45° PA flexion weight-bearing radiograph, extension weight-bearing AP, and lateral views of the knee. Ficat and Hungerford have described indirect radiologic signs of excessive lateral pressure (Fig. 50-19A) and excessive lateral ligamentous tension (Fig. 50-19B) on the patella.

The Merchant views can be used to measure several angles that assist in the evaluation of patellofemoral stability. First of all, the sulcus angle, which is a measurement of the angle of the trochlear groove, has a normal range of approximately 140 ± 5°. As previously mentioned, sulcus angles of more than 140° can lead to patellofemoral instability. The congruence angle is measured by bisecting the sulcus angle of the trochlea, then drawing a line to the medial crest of the patella and measuring the angle between the bisected angle of the sulcus and the median patellar crest line. This is the congruence angle. An angle in the medial direction is designated negative, whereas angles in the lateral direction are designated as positive (Fig. 50-20). The normal range is −6 ± 11°. The congruence angle provides a quantitative evaluation of medial or lateral sub-

luxation.[246,260] The lateral patellofemoral angle can also be measured from the Merchant view. This is the angle formed between a line placed along the peaks of the lateral and medial femoral condyles and a second line placed along the lateral facet of the patella. Normally, the lateral patellofemoral angle opens laterally and provides a radiographic measure of resting patellar tilt.[261] On the CT scan, the posterior condylar line can also be used most reliably and its alignment measured relative to the lateral patellar facet.

The lateral knee x-ray can be used to evaluate for patella alta (elevated patella) or patella baja (distal patella or shortened patellar tendon). There are several techniques for assessing the vertical distance of the patella from the tibia. First of all, a radiodense line marking the roof of the intercondylar fossa, also known as Blumenstaat's line, can be used on lateral x-rays of the knee flexed at 30°. If the distal pole of the patella lies above Blumenstaat's line, it is generally held that patella alta is present. Orientation of the proximal pole of the patella below Blumenstaat's line indicates patella baja.[262] Patellar tendon length can also be assessed by using Insall's ratio, which is represented by dividing the length of the patellar tendon by the height of the patella. The normal value for the Insall's ratio index is 1.2.[263]

If there is need for further evaluation, a midpatellar transverse CT scan taken through knee flexion from 15 to 30° provides an assessment of patellar tracking and patellar tilt. Other studies that have been used include MRI as well as kinematic MRI and radionuclide imaging. Generally, however, a standing AP weight-bearing view with the knee in extension, a PA weight-bearing view with the knee at 45°

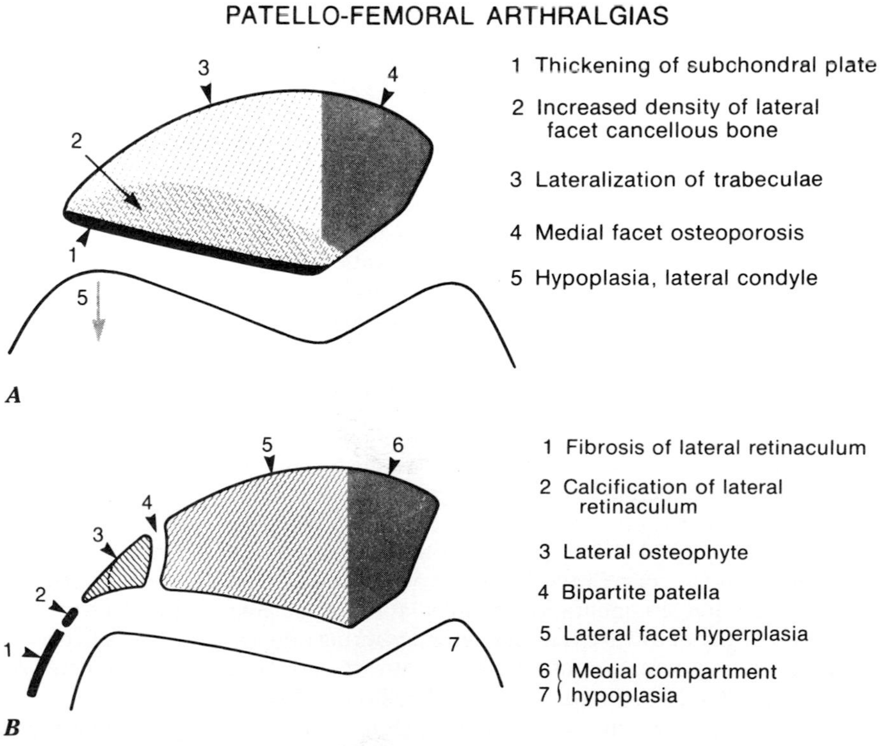

Figure 50-19 *A.* Indirect radiologic signs of excessive lateral pressure. *B.* Indirect radiologic signs of excessive lateral ligamentous tension. (Reproduced with permission from Ficat RP, Hungerford DS: *Disorders of the Patello-Femoral Joint.* Baltimore, Williams & Wilkins, 1977.)

PATELLO-FEMORAL ARTHRALGIAS

1 Thickening of subchondral plate

2 Increased density of lateral facet cancellous bone

3 Lateralization of trabeculae

4 Medial facet osteoporosis

5 Hypoplasia, lateral condyle

A

1 Fibrosis of lateral retinaculum

2 Calcification of lateral retinaculum

3 Lateral osteophyte

4 Bipartite patella

5 Lateral facet hyperplasia

6 ⎫ Medial compartment
7 ⎬ hypoplasia

B

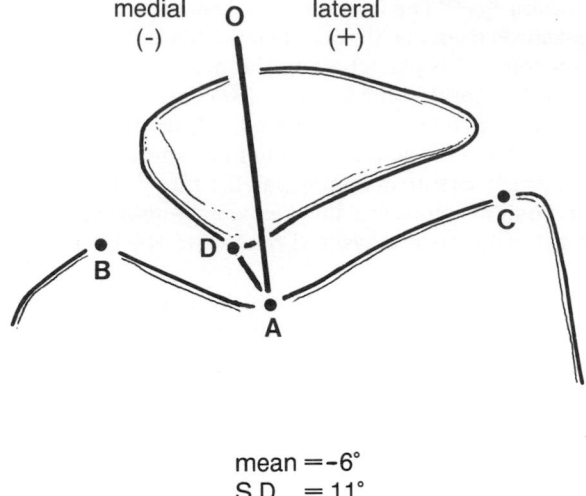

medial O lateral
(-) (+)

mean = -6°
S.D. = 11°

Figure 50-20 The sulcus angle (BAC) is drawn from the highest points on the femoral condyles to the lowest point at A. This angle is then bisected by the line AO. A second line (AD) is drawn from the base of the sulcus angle (point A) to the median ridge of the patella. The angle DAO is the congruence angle. All values medial to the O reference line AO are designated as minus and those lateral as plus. The mean congruence angle equals − 6° with a standard deviation of 11°. (Reproduced with permission from Merchant AD, Mercer RL, Jacobsen RH, et al: Roentgenographic analysis of patellofemoral congruence. *J Bone Joint Surg* 56A:1391–1396, 1974.)

of flexion, a lateral view with the knee in 30° of flexion, and a Merchant view with the knee at 45° of flexion are sufficient for the evaluation of patellofemoral disorders. With these views, the degree of patellofemoral chondrosis, orientation of the patella, gross chondral thickness, and shape of the patella and trochlea can be assessed.

Chondrosis

Chondrosis is defined as anterior knee pain associated with degenerative changes in the articular surface of the patella and/or trochlea. Articular injury can result from patellar instability, trauma, recurrent subluxation, and increased Q angle with lateral pull on the patella, quadriceps muscle imbalance, excessive lateral pressure syndrome, meniscal injury, or inflammatory conditions such as rheumatoid arthritis, recurrent hemarthrosis, synovitis, and alkaptonuria, repeated intraarticular steroid injections, prolonged immobilization, or osteoarthritis.[264] A system has been developed by Outerbridge to classify the degrees of articular cartilage degeneration into four grades. In grade I, there is localized softening and swelling of the cartilage and the changes are in an area of less than or equal to ½ cm. Grade II lesions are characterized by fissuring and fragmentation or fibrillation of an area less than or equal to 1.3 cm in diameter. Fissuring and fibrillation or fragmentation of an area greater than 1.2 cm in diameter is characteristic of grade III lesions, whereas grade IV lesions are characterized by extensive erosion

to bone with the presence of eburnated or sclerotic subchondral bone.[265] Chondrosis of the patellofemoral joint is most often characterized by complaints of anterior knee pain with the presence of crepitus and knee effusion.

Treatment of patellofemoral chondrosis, like that of all patellofemoral disorders, involves an initial 3 to 6 months of conservative therapy, which includes activity modification through which the patient avoids aggravating activities as well as prolonged sitting or kneeling with the knees flexed, as these can result in high patellofemoral joint forces. In addition, physical therapy focuses on quadriceps strengthening and reestablishment of normal balanced strength and flexibility of the knee and peripatellar structures. Conservative management is not intended to reverse the degenerative changes in the articular cartilage but rather to alleviate the resulting soft tissue abnormalities that are a consequence of prolonged abnormal biomechanics and long-standing pain. Nonsteroidal anti-inflammatory medications can be used to treat the inflammatory component of the pain, while specific physical therapy is directed at stretching tight structures such as the lateral retinaculum and iliotibial band and increasing quadriceps muscle flexibility and strength. The exercises should not be painful; if necessary the patient should begin with very gentle stretching and isometric muscle exercises with gradual increase in range of motion and progression to resistive exercises, along with various patellar taping and bracing programs. Gradually the patient is progressed to closed kinetic chain exercises as well as specific exercises directed toward training isolated aspects of the quadriceps such as the vastus medialis obliquus. Disorders of the hip, ankle, and foot can be addressed as well. Surgical treatment for patellofemoral chondrosis is a last-resort measure reserved for patients who have failed a comprehensive 3- to 6-month period of conservative treatment and physical therapy and have persistent, recalcitrant pain. Specific procedures are directed at the damage to the articular cartilage or to effect a change in forces such that the injured surfaces will not have to bear excessive force. These include debridement of fragmented cartilage as well as removal of loose bodies and abrasion of subchondral bone in order to stimulate a fibrocartilaginous healing response. If the goal is to alter the patellofemoral forces, lateral release can be performed as well as possible elevation of the anterior tibial tuberosity to decrease patellofemoral pressures. If there is an alignment, then a proximal or distal realignment procedure alone or in combination can be performed.

Rehabilitation for Patellofemoral Disorders

Once the diagnosis—the primary pain versus primary instability problem—has been determined, it is still necessary to treat both types of patellofemoral disorders with a comprehensive rehabilitation program as the initial course of treatment. A course of at least 3 to 6 months of rehabilitation is absolutely necessary prior to considering surgical intervention.[266–272] The rehabilitation program should be comprehensive, focusing not only on therapeutic exercises and adjunctive modalities but also upon modification of the patient's activity, so that the patient can progress through therapy without any exacerbation of symptoms. The goal of therapy is to obtain strength and flexibility and ultimately to improve endurance through activity-specific training programs. Strengthening is initiated with isometric exercises focusing on quadriceps sets and advancing to straight-leg raising. Quadriceps isometrics and straight-leg raising are begun initially because they produce a lower amount of patellofemoral joint forces than knee extension exercises.[273] Once the patient is able to perform straight-leg raising without pain, he or she is advanced to ankle weights with continued straight-leg raising. Following advancement to straight-leg raising with ankle weights, the patient begins short-arc quadriceps strengthening through knee motions from 20° of flexion to full extension. Specific attention is then focused on the vastus medialis obliquus (VMO), beginning with isometric adduction exercises followed by progressive VMO activation during sitting, standing, and ultimately stair climbing.[274]

Flexibility and muscle stretching are also integral parts of a comprehensive physical therapy program. Specific attention is paid to hamstring muscle flexibility as well as stretching of the gastrocsoleus complex, as these may also lead to increased patellofemoral joint compressive forces. Of further note, the iliotibial band is often implicated in lateral tracking of the patella as well as the syndrome of excessive lateral pressure. The iliotibial band can be stretched by passive medial displacement of the patella as well as pressure-point massage of the lateral retinaculum and iliotibial band. In addition, the patient is instructed on specific active stretching exercises for the iliotibial band as well as the hamstrings, quadriceps, and gastrocsoleus muscles.[266,268]

Once the patient has progressed well with strengthening as well as flexibility, he or she is gradually advanced to endurance training and functional activities directed toward the specific demands and activities of his or her lifestyle. Endurance training is often begun with swimming and utilization of a stationary bike with a high seat position. Once the patient can perform these activities without significant pain or discomfort, he or she is advanced to running and stair climbing and ultimately to more sports-specific activities.

Adjunctive therapy is aimed at decreasing inflammation and joint effusion; nonsteroidal anti-inflammatories, judicious use of ice, and phonophoresis can be used. Sometimes it is helpful to use external support such as bracing or taping to provide support and warmth as well as protection from patellar dislocation or subluxation and to assist in normal patellar tracking.[274–276] McConnell[274] has developed specific taping techniques intended to restore normal patellar alignment and position. She contends that restoration of patellar alignment and position not only significantly decreases pain during training and rehabilitation but in doing so allows for more successful strengthening of the vastus medialis obliquus, in which normal contraction forces can be inhibited by pain stimuli.

Operative Treatment of Patellofemoral Disorders

As previously mentioned, operative treatment of patellofemoral disorders is a last-resort option that should be considered only after the patient has undergone a 3- to 6-month period of a comprehensive rehabilitation protocol. Patellofemoral disorders can be caused by a multitude of individual factors as well as a combination of these factors; similarly, there are multiple surgical approaches to patellofemoral disorders. Cox and Kalenak[259] have developed a useful algorithm for the treatment of various patellofemoral disorders (Table 50-2). The basic procedures, used either alone or in combination, include lateral release, proximal realignment of soft tissue, distal realignment, and bony realignment in conjunction with soft tissue realignment procedures.

The first step for all of the operative procedures includes a thorough examination under anesthesia followed by a thorough patellofemoral arthroscopic examination with arthroscopic evaluation of the entire knee joint. With the patient under anesthesia or appropriate regional block, the knee is examined, testing for all ligamentous laxity and noting patellar tracking and crepitance in the knee. Then diagnostic arthroscopy is performed to evaluate the chondral surfaces as well as the integrity of the menisci and ligamentous structures. Any articular pathology is addressed at this time as well. An arthroscope can be inserted through a portal 4 to 5 cm proximal to either the superolateral or superomedial pole of the patella.[277] The quadriceps muscle is penetrated by use of a sharp trochar; however, a blunt trochar is used to enter the superpatellar pouch in order to avoid accidental injury of the articular cartilage. If feasible, the surgeon can evaluate the dynamic tracking of the patella by stimulating the femoral nerve while the patient is under general anesthesia or by utilizing selective epidural anesthesia, allowing for active quadriceps muscle contraction by the patient, which can also occur with use of local anesthesia. The knee is then systematically inspected beginning with the patellofemoral articular surfaces and the medial and lateral gutters. It is also observed for plicae. All articular surfaces are not only observed but also palpated to determine the extent of articular pathology. Next, the knee is passively flexed and extended, evaluating passive tracking of the patella. If possible, the patient is asked to actively flex and extend the knee to evaluate active patella tracking. The angle of flexion at which the various regions of the patella engage the femoral condyles is noted, as is the pattern of articular chondrosis corresponding with the patellofemoral engagement. Following this, the lateral and medial femoral compartments and their respective menisci as well as the integrity of the cruciate and collateral ligaments are evaluated. Instrumentation is introduced via an inferolateral portal.

Lateral Retinacular Release

There is general consensus that the indication for lateral release include (1) patellofemoral pain with lateral patella tilt, (2) lateral retinacular pain with lateral tilt or lateral patellar position, and (3) tight lateral retinaculum, also

TABLE 50-2 Recommendations for the Management of Patellofemoral Disorders

I. Patellofemoral (PF) arthralgia
  A. No instability, malposition, chondrosis/arthrosis
     No surgery
  B. Malposition (static)
     1. Lateral—lateral release if symptomatic with tilt
     2. Medial (rare)—surgery usually not indicated
     3. Alta—no surgery
     4. Baja—proximal shift only if symptomatic
     5. Lateral compression with tilt—minimal arthrosis—lateral release
  C. Chondrosis/arthrosis
     1. Surgery directed at diseased cartilage
        a. Debridement of fibrillated cartilage
        b. Removal of loose cartilage
        c. Subchondral bone abrasion or drilling to form some protective cartilage
     2. Surgery directed at change in forces
        a. Normal patellar position—anterior tibial tuberosity elevation to decrease PF pressures
        b. Abnormal patellar position
           (1) Anteromedial realignment for decompression and redistribution of forces
           (2) Three-dimensional surgery to also correct patella alta or patella infera
II. PF instability
  A. General principles
     1. Arthralgia may or may not be present
     2. Chondrosis/arthrosis may or may not be present
  B. Subluxation/dislocation
     1. Normal PF position
        a. Medial subluxation/dislocation
           (1) Very rare
           (2) Occasionally traumatic and usually associated with ligamentous injuries of the knee
           (3) Usually iatrogenic
              (a) Follows a lateral retinacular release, particularly when vastus lateralis tendon insertion is detached
              (b) May follow extensor mechanism realignment if anterior tibial tuberosity is shifted too far medially
           (4) Associated occasionally with muscle paralysis (poliomyelitis)
           (5) Surgical treatment for medial subluxation/dislocation of patella
              (a) Difficult problem to correct surgically; get CT or MRI scan to determine tracking
              (b) Determine degree of knee flexion at which medial subluxation occurs
              (c) Surgical realignment with use of femoral nerve stimulation to determine dynamic tracking
        b. Lateral subluxation/dislocation—normal PF position
           (1) Almost always an underlying malalignment problem and/or tight lateral retinaculum
           (2) Watch for ligamentous laxity of the knee, particularly if there is anterior cruciate ligament laxity
           (3) When patella is in normal position in regard to alta or baja, a realignment procedure in itself will usually correct problem
           (4) If chondrosis/arthrosis is present, may also require anterior transfer of anterior tibial tuberosity to decompress forces
     2. Abnormal PF position—try to correct existing problems, such as patella alta, which may be associated with lateral or medial dislocation
        a. When two malalignment factors are present, such as patella alta and in increased quadriceps angle, it may be more difficult to recognize these factors than when the variation appears alone, because in combination each finding is less pronounced
        b. Medial dislocation (rare)—try to correct all existing abnormal problems
        c. Lateral subluxation/dislocation—correct all malalignment problems
        d. Abnormal PF position may require correction of patella infera and patella alta along with medial realignment (three-dimensional tuberosity shift)

Source: Reproduced with permission from Fulkerson JP, Kalenak A, Jacobsen RH, Cool CR: Patellofemoral pain. *AAOS Instr Course Lect* 41:57–72, 1992.

known as excessive lateral pressure syndrome or lateral patellar compression syndrome.[246,278] A combination of lateral release with medial capsular reefing or use of re-alignment of the tibial tuberosity should be employed in cases where there is patellar instability with significant subluxation or dislocation of the patella. Excessive lateral pressure syndrome or lateral patellar compression syndrome is characterized by patellar tilt without associated patellar instability. In this condition, there is lateral tilting of the patella secondary to a tight lateral retinaculum. The Q angle is normal and there is no evidence of patellar subluxation or hypermobility. The objective finding in this condition is a passive patellar tilt of less than 0°.

Patellofemoral pain syndrome of adolescence, advanced patellofemoral arthrosis, and a normally tracking patella are all contraindications for lateral retinacular release. Arthroscopic lateral release is performed through a lateral parapatellar arthroscopic portal, and either a scissors, meniscotome, or electrocautery is used to release the lateral retinaculum.[279] The primary objective of lateral retinacular release is incising the lateral retinaculum approximately 1 cm from the border of the patella. This region is the least vascular region of the lateral retinaculum. Extreme care must be taken to avoid severing the vastus lateralis tendon as well as to identify the superior lateral geniculate vessels and cauterize them. Although the arthroscopic technique of lateral retinacular release probably provides a more cosmetic result, it is our opinion that the open Z-plasty procedure is safer and can be performed through a very small incision.

Following diagnostic arthroscopy, the inferolateral portal is extended with a 2-cm longitudinal incision lateral to the patella. The subcutaneous tissues are then bluntly dissected down to the superficial layer of the lateral retinaculum. All layers of the lateral retinaculum as well as the synovium are incised approximately 1 cm lateral to the lateral border of the patella. This region corresponds to a midway point between the lateral border of the patella and the lateral femoral condyle. The release is extended proximally with sharp dissection, utilizing heavy Mayo scissors, until it has been released 2 to 3 cm above the superior border of the patella along a fatty plane between the vastus lateralis and vastus lateralis obliquus muscles. The superior lateral geniculate vessels are carefully identified and electrocauterized, while extreme care is taken to avoid incision of the vastus lateralis tendon.[280] The release is also extended distally to the tibial tubercle, resulting in release of the patellotibial ligament as well. All synovial adhesions within the infrapatellar fat pad are released, and the anterior portion of the lateral meniscus is carefully protected. Following a successful release, one should be able to evert the patella passively to 90°. Following adequate release, the tourniquet is let down and hemostasis is obtained, with special attention directed toward the lateral superior geniculate vessels to confirm that they have been adequately electrocauterized or ligated, assuring hemostasis. Postoperatively, the patient is placed in a Cryocuff for 48 h, followed by institution of active range-of-motion exercises with gentle progression. Hemarthrosis, often due to inadequate electrocauterization or ligation of the superior lateral geniculate vessels, is the most com-mon complication following a lateral release procedure.[281] Sometimes a medial imbrication of the medial capsule is used in conjunction with lateral retinacular release or other bony transfer procedures.

Medial Realignment

The current version of the Roux-Elmslie-Trillat procedure has evolved over many years.[282–285] This procedure involves release of the lateral retinaculum with medial capsular reefing and transfer of the anterior tibial tuberosity medially. The indications for the Roux-Elmslie-Trillat procedure include recurrent lateral patellar subluxation or dislocation and the presence of an increased quadriceps angle as well as patellofemoral arthrosis with lateral patellar position, lateral patellar tilt, and increased Q angle. The goal of this procedure is to redistribute the forces in the patellofemoral joint and thus relieve the pain of arthrosis. The presence of a normal Q angle or open epiphyseal plates contraindicates the Roux-Elmslie-Trillat procedure.

A 3- to 5-cm lateral longitudinal incision is made on the lateral border of the patella. The prepatellar bursa is then carefully dissected, creating a skin flap. A thin tenosynovial tissue flap is raised laterally, and the lateral retinaculum is released by Z-plasty. The lateral transverse retinaculum is transected and the patellofemoral and patellotibial ligaments are released. Again, the superior lateral geniculate vessels are identified and electrocauterized while the release is extended proximally. Then the release is extended distally to the level of the tibial tubercle. Subsequently, a medial parapatellar incision beginning at the 1 o'clock position extending to the 4 o'clock is used. This is sharply carried down to the synovium on the medial aspect of the knee. Medial capsular reefing is then performed.

Several transverse holes are made through the tibial tubercle in the medial to lateral direction using a 3.5-mm K wire to drill these holes approximately ½ cm posterior to the anterior cortex. In situations where anteriorization of the tibial tubercle is also required, the amount of anteriorization can be determined by the obliquity of the drill holes. From the lateral aspect of the tibial tubercle, an osteotome is placed behind the patellar tendon at the proximal end of the tubercle. The osteotome is then inserted with a mallet distally so that it emerges underneath the periosteum, elevating a thin piece of tibial tubercle with a distal periosteal pedicle. The anterior medial tibial periosteum is elevated using a periosteal elevator and a burr or rasp is used to blunt the sharp edge of the medial tubercle's cortex. Using the periosteal hinge, the tibial tuberosity is rotated medially so that the quadriceps muscle mechanism is realigned through a position allowing for optimal patellar tracking within the femoral trochlea. This is confirmed by flexing the knee from 0 to 90° of flexion and observing patellar tracking. The tibial tubercle can generally be medialized up to 1 cm, while at least 50 percent of the bone overlap is required for adequate fixation. Once the optimal position of the tibial tubercle is determined, guide pins are used to fix the tibial tubercle in its new position, and the knee is then again placed through a full range of motion during which patellar tracking is again observed. Two 4.5-mm cannulated screws are used to secure the tibial tuberosity with bicortical fixation. The periosteal flap is then closed. Finally, medial capsular reefing is performed while the transverse fibers of the lateral retinaculum are sutured, allowing 1 cm of lengthening of the lateral retinaculum.

Postoperatively, the knee is placed in a Cryo-cuff and knee immobilizer or hinged brace with 10° of flexion. The patient begins partial weight bearing as tolerated, utilizing crutches. On postoperative day 1, the patient begins isometric quadriceps contractions with straight-leg-raising exercises. After several days, the patient is allowed to perform active range-of-motion exercises, and at 4 weeks postoperatively he or she begins active assisted range-of-motion and progressive resistive exercises. Specific attention is paid to increasing the strength and bulk of the vastus medialis obliquus muscle. The Roux-Elmslie-Turrat procedure is generally reproducible; use of the lateral longitudinal incision enables the surgeon to avoid injuring the infrapatellar branch of the saphenous nerve, and the extensor mechanism can be realigned without moving the tibial tuberosity further distally or posteriorly. This procedure does not, however, result in reduction of patellofemoral forces for the relief of pain associated with arthrosis.

Anterior Realignment

Anterior realignment is indicated primarily for the relief of patellofemoral pain secondary to chondrosis. This procedure is most successful when the chondrosis is located on the distal articular surface of the patella. Anterior realignment is contraindicated in the presence of a diffuse, advanced patellofemoral arthrosis, especially if there is proximal patellar arthrosis. In 1976 Maquet[286] introduced a procedure in which the anterior tibial tuberosity is elevated in order to reduce patellofemoral joint force. Maquet endorsed elevation of the tibial tubercle by 2 cm or more; however, this has been associated with many complications, leading Ferguson et al., in 1979,[287] to recommend that an elevation of 1.25 cm was sufficient to reduce both patellofemoral joint forces and the complication rate associated with anterior realignment. In addition, Nakamura et al.[288] evaluated contact areas following various magnitudes of elevation of the anterior tibial tuberosity and determined that with elevations of 1 cm or less, the contact area remained essentially unchanged. However, elevation of the tibial tuberosity by 2 cm resulted in significant change in the contact area, while forces were concentrated on the proximal patellar surface. Additional elevation beyond 2 cm resulted in an even greater increase in the patellofemoral forces experienced by the proximal patella. Finally, a 1 cm of elevation, it was found that patellofemoral force was decreased at all angles of flexion while there was negligible change in contract patterns as well as very little decrease in contact area.

A 5-cm incision is made lateral to the tibial tubercle, as this incision enables the surgeon to avoid the infrapatellar branch of the saphenous nerve. An oblique osteotomy of the tibial tubercle of approximately 10 cm is made, and the tibial tuberosity is elevated utilizing an iliac crest or Gerdy's tubercle bone graft from 1 to 1.5 cm. One or two bicortical screws are used for fixation, and the wound is closed in layers. The most common complica-

tions associated with this procedure include possible anterior compartment syndrome and skin necrosis.

Anteromedial Realignment of the Tibial Tubercle

The goal of anteromedial realignment is to realign the extensor mechanism by elevating the tibial tuberosity as well as medializing it. This results in a redistribution of forces toward the proximal patellar surface as well as a decrease in the magnitude of force. Anteromedialization of the tibial tubercle is indicated primarily for patellar chondrosis located on the lateral and/or distal patellar surface and associated with malalignment of the extensor mechanism. Fulkerson et al.[289] recommend that the tibial tubercle be transferred anteriorly to a maximum of 17 mm. The magnitude of anteriorization is controlled by the angle of the tibial tubercle osteotomy. The goal of medialization of the tibial tubercle is to reestablish normal patellar tracking.

Following diagnostic arthroscopy, a longitudinal incision of approximately 15 cm is made from the midlateral patella extending approximately 5 cm distal to the lateral aspect of the tibial tubercle. A lateral release is performed to the level of the patella without violating the vastus lateralis. The anterior compartment is incised along the tibial crest, and the musculature is elevated along with a subperiosteal flap. Exposure is extended to the posterolateral corner of the tibial plateau. The anterior tibial artery, vein, and peroneal nerve are identified and avoided. The borders of the patellar tendon and its insertion into the tibial tubercle are identified. An oblique osteotomy is then planned. The degree of obliquity is determined by the desired degree of tuberosity transfer. The osteotomy is planned and the cut is outlined by scoring the periosteum with a Bovie so that the distal aspect of the fragment tapers to a 3- to 4-mm tip approximately 6 to 7 cm beyond the tibial tuberosity. The periosteum is then elevated from the site of planned osteotomy and a series of at least four to six parallel 4-mm drill holes are placed in the plane of the osteotomy obliquely aligned, entering from the anteromedial tibia and exiting toward the posterolateral tibia. These drill holes are placed under direct vision to avoid damage to the neurovascular bundles. Special care should be taken to confirm that the anterior tibial vessels and peroneal nerves are not damaged from placement of the drill holes. The use of a Hoffman drill guide with drill bits in the superior and inferior positions is very helpful for accurate placement of parallel drill holes. The osteotomy is begun by directing the osteotomy proximally from the posterolateral tibia at the most superoposterior drill hole and extending the osteotomy anteriorly to a level proximal to the insertion site of the patellar tendon. This prevents possible propagation of the osteotomy into the more proximal tibia as well as allowing for anterior medial rotation of the tibial tubercle. The anterior cortex is then cut with a ½-in. osteotome proximal to the tibial tuberosity while the patellar tendon is protected at all times to avoid possible injury. A saw or broad osteotome is used to complete the remainder of the tibial tubercle osteotomy, and the superior and inferior drill bits are used as guides for the plane of osteotomy. It is very important to make sure that a flat osteotomy plane is obtained, as this allows for optimal transfer and fixation following transfer. Following completion of the osteotomy, the tibial tubercle is rotated anteromedially. The knee is then taken through ranges of flexion and extension while patellar tracking is observed. Once the tibial tubercle has been moved to the optimal medialized position, two large-fragment AO cortical lag screws are countersunk and placed through the tibial tubercle and into the posterior cortex. Anteriorization of 12 to 15 mm can be obtained through this procedure without the need for bone graft. If anteriorization of greater than 15 mm is desired, bone graft can be obtained from the lateral tibial metaphysis and used to add further anteriorization of the tibial tubercle (Fig. 50–21). When medialization only of the tibial tubercle is desired or needed, a less oblique osteotomy can be made more in line with the coronal plane. If patellar tracking is not completely or satisfactorily corrected by anterior medialization of the tibial tubercle, the next step is to perform reefing or imbrication of the vastus medialis obliquus muscle. However, this is not usually necessary. Hemostasis is assured where necessary and the wound is irrigated and closed in layers following placement of a drain.

Postoperatively, a Cryo-cuff is used for the first 24 to 48 h with a compression dressing. Drains are removed on postoperative day 1 and the patient is begun on therapy consisting of straight-leg raises and quadriceps strengthening as well as passive range-of-motion exercises with advancement to active and active assisted range of motion. The patient is placed in a knee immobilizer and allowed to bear weight as tolerated; the knee immobilizer is discontinued once the patient is able to perform straight-leg raises without significant discomfort. On follow-up at 6 weeks postoperatively, repeat radiographs are obtained to confirm healing of the osteotomy; if there is adequate evidence of healing, the patient is allowed to discontinue use of the crutches. The patient is also gradually advanced through progressive resistance exercises and continued flexibility training. Once normal strength, range of motion, and flexibility are obtained, the patient is usually advanced to more sport-specific activities at 2 to 3 months postoperatively.

Other Bony Realignment Procedures

For patients with patellar subluxation, dislocation, and patella alta, the anterior tibial tuberosity can be osteotomized and shifted distally to correct patella alta. Normally the tibial tuberosity can be transferred from 1 to 1.5 cm distally without causing excess patellofemoral joint forces. Some 2 in. of anterior tibial crest is osteotomized in continuity with the tubercle and reattached distally with screws. If the patella alta is severe and distal transfer of the tibial tuberosity of greater than 1.5 cm is necessary, then Z-Y plasty of the quadriceps tendon can be performed.[290] For patients with patella baja secondary to contracture of the patellar tendon, the anterior tibial tuberosity is transferred proximally.

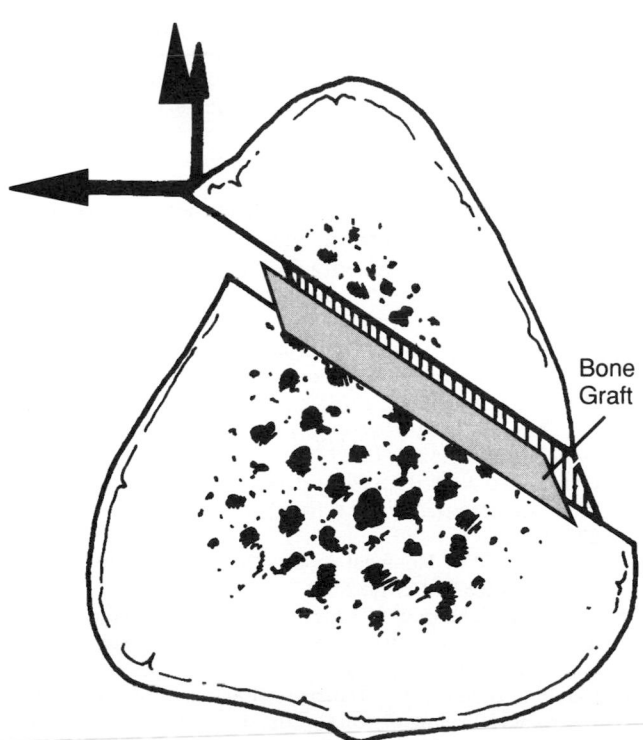

Bone Graft

Figure 50-21 Cross section of the anteromedial tubercle transfer. The obliquity of the osteotomy determines the amount of anterior displacement associated with the medial transfer. [Reproduced with permission from Cox JS, Cooper PS: Patellofemoral instability, in Fu FH, Harner CD, Vince KG, Miller MD (eds): *Knee Surgery.* Vol 1. Baltimore, Williams & Wilkins, 1994, p 980.]

REFERENCES

1. Bullough P, Munuera L, Murphy J, et al: The strength of the menisci of the knee as it relates to their fine structure. *J Bone Joint Surg [Am]* 52B:564, 1970.
2. Ahmed AM, Burke DL: In vitro measurement of static pressure distribution in synovial joints in the tibial surface of the knee. *J Biomech* 105:216–225, 1983.
3. Seedholm B, Wright V: Functions of the menisci. *J Bone Joint Surg* 56B:381, 1974.
4. Walker P, Erkman M: The role of the menisci in transmission across the knee. *Clin Orthop* 109:184, 1975.
5. Baratz M, Fu FH, Mengato R: Meniscal tears: The effect of meniscectomy and repair on intra-articular contact areas and stress in the human knee. *Am J Sports Med* 14:270, 1986.
6. Fukubayashi T, Durosawaw H: The contact area and pressure distribution pattern of the knee: A study of normal and osteoarthritic knee joints. *Acta Orthop Scand* 50:871–880, 1980.
7. Seedholm BB, Hargraves DJ: Transmission of the load in the knee joint with special reference to the role of the menisci: Part 2. *N Engl J Med* 8:220–228, 1979.
8. Voloshin AS, Wosk J: Shock absorption of meniscectomized and painful knees: A comparative in vivo study. *J Biomech* 5:157–161, 1983.
9. Levy I, Torzilli P, Warren R: The effect of medial meniscectomy on anterior-posterior motion of the knee. *J Bone Joint Surg* 64:883, 1982.
10. Levy I, Torzilli, Gould J, et al: The effect of lateral meniscectomy on motion of the knee. *J Bone Joint Surg* 71:401, 1989.

11. Shoemaker S, Markolf K: The role of the meniscus in the anterior-posterior stability of the loaded anterior cruciate deficient knee. *J Bone Joint Surg* 68A:71, 1986.

12. Wang CK, Walker PS: Rotatory laxity of the human knee joint. *J Bone Joint Surg* 56:161–170, 1974.

13. Walker PS, Erkman MJ: The role of the menisci in forced transmission across the knee. *Clin Orthop* 109:184–192, 1975.

14. Wilson AS, Legg PG, McNeur JC: Studies on the innervation of the medial meniscus in the human knee joint. *J Anat Rec* 165:485–492, 1969.

15. O'Conner BL, McConnaughey JS: The structure and innervation of cat knee menisci, and their relation to a "sensory hypothesis" of meniscal function. *Am J Anat* 153:432–442, 1978.

16. King D: The function of the semi-lunar cartilages. *J Bone Joint Surg* 18:1069–1076, 1936.

17. Fairbank TJ: Knee joint changes after meniscectomy. *J Bone Joint Surg* 30:664–670, 1948.

18. Cox JS, Nye CE, Schaeffer WW, et al: The degenerative effect of partial and total resection of the medial meniscus in dogs' knees. *Clin Orthop* 109:178–183, 1975.

19. Cannon W: Arthroscopic meniscal repair, in McGinty J (ed): *Operative Arthroscopy*. New York, Raven Press, 1991, pp 237–251.

20. Arnoczky SP: Gross and vascular anatomy of the meniscus and its role in meniscal healing, regeneration, and remodeling, in *Knee Meniscus: Basic and Clinical Foundations*. New York, Raven Press, 1992, pp 1–14.

21. Annandale T: An operation for displaced semi-lunar cartilage. *Br Med J* 1:779, 1885.

22. King D: The healing of the semi-lunar cartilages. *J Bone Joint Surg* 18:333–342, 1936.

23. Arnoczky SP, Warren RF: Microvasculature of the human meniscus. *Am J Sports Med* 10:90–95, 1982.

24. Arnoczky SP, Warren RF, Spivak J: Meniscal repair using an exogenous fibrin clot: An experimental study in dogs. *J Bone Joint Surg* 70:1209, 1988.

25. Cabaud H, Rodkey W, Fitzwater J: Medial meniscus repairs: An experimental and morphologic study. *Am J Sports Med* 19:129, 1981.

26. Heathley FW: The meniscus: Can it be repaired? An experimental investigation in rabbits. *J Bone Joint Surg* 62:397–402, 1980.

27. Rosenberg TD: Forty-five degree posterior-anterior flexion weight-bearing radiography of the knee. *J Bone Joint Surg* 70:1479–1483, 1988.

28. Dumas JM, Edde DJ: Meniscal abnormalities: Perspective correlation of double contrast arthrography and arthroscopy. *J Radiol* 160:453–456, 1986.

29. Gillies H, Seligson D: Precision of the diagnosis of meniscal lesions: A comparison of clinical evaluation, arthrography, and arthroscopy. *J Bone Joint Surg* 61:343–346, 1979.

30. Fischer SP, Fox JM, Del Pizzo W, et al: Accuracy of diagnoses from MR imaging of the knee. *J Bone Joint Surg* 73:2–10, 1991.

31. Mink JH, Levy T, Crues JV, et al: Tears of the ACL of the knee: MR imaging evaluation. *J Radiol* 167:769–777, 1988.

32. Spindler KP, Schils T, Bergfeld J, et al: Prospective study of osteo, articular and meniscal lesions in recent ACL tears by MR imaging and arthroscopy. *Am J Sports Med* 21:551–557, 1993.

33. Stoller DW, Martin C, Crues JV, et al: Meniscal tears: Pathologic correlation with MR imaging. *J Radiol* 163:731–735, 1987.

34. Gillquist J, Hagberg G, Oretorp M: Arthroscopic examination of the posteromedial compartment of the knee joint. *Int Orthop* 3:313, 1979.

35. Rosenberg T, Paulos L, Parker R, et al: The 45 degree posterior-anterior flexion weight-bearing radiograph of the knee. *J Bone Joint Surg* 70:1479, 1988.

36. Metcalf R: Arthroscopic meniscal surgery, in McGinty J (ed): *Operative Arthroscopy*. New York, Raven Press, 1991, pp 203–236.

37. Shrive N, O'Conner J, Goodfellow J: Load-bearing mode of the knee joint. *Clin Orthop* 131:279, 1978.

38. Henning C, Clark J, Lynch N, et al: Arthroscopic meniscal repair with a posterior incision. *AAOS Instr Course Lect* 37:209, 1988.

39. Henning C, Lynch N, Yearot K, et al: Arthroscopic meniscal repair using an exogenous fibrin clot. *Clin Orthop* 252:64, 1990.

40. Scott G, Jolly B, Henning C: Combined posterior incision in arthroscopic intra-articular repair of the meniscus: An examination of factors affecting healing. *J Bone Joint Surg* 68:847–861, 1986.

41. DeHaven K: Decision-making factors in the treatment of meniscus lesions. *Clin Orthop* 252:49, 1990.

42. DeHaven K: Meniscus repair: Open versus arthroscopic. *Arthroscopy* 1:173, 1985.

43. Newman A, Daniels A, Burks R: Principles in decision making in meniscal surgery. *Arthroscopy* 9:35, 1993.

44. Weiss C, Lundberg M, DeHaven K, et al: Non-operative treatment of meniscal tears. *J Bone Joint Surg* 71A:811–821, 1989.

45. Cannon WD, Vittori JN: The incidence of healing in arthroscopic meniscal repairs in anterior cruciate ligament reconstructed knees versus stable knees. *Am J Sports Med* 20:176–181, 1992.

46. Woo SL-Y, Hollis JM, Adams DJ, et al: Tensile properties of the human femur—Anterior cruciate tibia complex: The effect of specimen age. *Am J Sports Med* 19:217–225, 1991.

47. DeHaven KE: Peripheral meniscal repair: An alternative to meniscectomy. *J Bone Joint Surg* 63:463, 1981.

48. Cassidy R, Shaffer A: Repair of peripheral meniscus tears: A preliminary report. *Am J Sports Med* 9:209, 1981.

49. Hamberg P, Gillquist J, Lysholm J: Suture of new and old peripheral meniscus tears. *J Bone Joint Surg* 65:193, 1983.

50. DeHaven KE, Stone RC: Meniscal repair, in Sahriaree H (ed): *O'Conner's Textbook of Arthroscopic Surgery*. Philadelphia, Lippincott, 1992, pp 327–338.

51. Morgan CD: The "all-inside" meniscus repair: Technical note. *Arthroscopy* 7:120, 1991.

52. Mullhollan J: Inside/inside meniscus repair: Sewing and tying through punctures. 11th Annual Meeting of Arthroscopy Association of North America: Boston, April 1992.

53. Morgan CD: "All-inside" arthroscopic meniscus repair. *Tech Orthop* 8:105–112, 1993.

54. Ikeuchi H: Surgery under arthroscopic control: Proceedings of the Societe Internationale d'Arthroscopie, 1975. *Rheumatology* 3:57–62, 1976.

55. Henning CE: Arthroscopic repair of meniscus tears. *Orthopaedics* 6:1130–1132, 1983.

56. Cannon WD Jr: Arthroscopic meniscal repair, in McGinty JB (ed): *Operative Arthroscopy*. New York, Raven Press, 1991, pp 237–251.

57. Cannon WD Jr: Meniscal repair—The Henning technique. *Tech Orthop* 8:92–98, 1982.

58. Arnoczky SP, McDevitt C, Warren R, et al: Meniscal repair using an exogenous fibrin clot: An experimental study in the dog. *Trans Orthop Res Soc* 11:152, 1986.

59. Gershuni D, Skyhart M, Danzig L, et al: Experimental models to promote healing of tears in the avascular segment of canine knee menisci. *J Bone Joint Surg* 71:1363–1370, 1989.

60. Henning C, Lynch M, Clark JR: Vascularity for healing of meniscus repairs. *Arthroscopy* 3:13–18, 1987.

61. Webber R, Harris M, Haough A: Cell culture of rabbit meniscal fibrochondrocytes: Proliferative and synthetic response to growth factors and ascorbate. *J Orthop Res* 3:36–42, 1985.

62. Henning C, Lynch M, Yearout K, et al: Arthroscopic meniscal repair using an exogenous fibrin clot. *Clin Orthop* 252:64–72, 1990.

63. Warren R: Meniscectomy in the anterior cruciate deficient patient. *Clin Orthop* 252:55–63, 1990.

64. Gebhardt K: *Der bandschaden des Kniegelenkes.* Liepzig: Barth, 1933.

65. Milachowski KA, Weismeier K, Wirth CJ, Kohn D: Meniscus transplantation: Experimental study and first clinical report. *Am J Sports Med* 15:626, 1987.

66. Milachowski KA, Weismeier K, Wirth CJ: Homologous meniscus transplantation. *Int Orthop* 13:1–11, 1989.

67. Wirth CJ, Milachowski KA, Weismeier K: *Rekonstruktive Meniskuschirurgie: Arthroskopische Meniskuschirugie.* Stuttgart, Enke, 1986, pp 11–114.

68. Johnson LL: *Arthroscopic Surgery: Principles in Practice,* 3d ed. St Louis, Mosby, 1986.

69. Milachowski KA, Kohn D, Wirth CJ: Meniskusersatz durch Hoffa'schen Fettkoerper: Erste klinische Ergebnisse. *Unfallchirurgie* 16:190–195, 1990.

70. Milachowski KA, Kohn D, Wirth CJ: Arthroskopische Befunde nach Meniskustransplantatin und Meniskusersatz. *Arthroskopie* 3:57–66, 1990.

71. Kohn D: Der plastische Ersatz des Innen meniscus mit koerpereigenem Gewebe: Eine experimentelle Untersuchung. Thesis at Hannover Medical School, Germany, 1989, p 191.

72. Stone KR, Rodkey WG, Webber RJ, et al: Collagen-based prosthesis for meniscal regeneration. *Clin Orthop* 252:129–135, 1990.

73. Stone KR, Rodkey WG, Webber RJ, et al. Meniscal regeneration with copolymeric collagen scaffolds: In vitro and in vivo studies evaluated clinically, histologically and biochemically. *Am J Sports Med* 20:11, 1992.

74. Wirth CJ: Meniscus replacement. 5th Annual Panther Symposium in Pittsburgh, Pennsylvania, April 2–4, 1992.

75. Kohn D: Autogenous meniscal replacement. Presented at the 14th Symposium of the Italian Club of Knee Surgery, Bologna, Italy, November 1992.

76. Milachowski KA, Weismeier K, Wirth CJ, Kohn D: Meniscus transplantation in surgery, in Mueller W, Hackenbruch W (eds): *Arthroscopy of the Knee.* Berlin, Springer-Verlag, 1988, pp 380–388.

77. Arnoczky SP, Cuzzell JZ, McDevitt CA, et al: Meniscal replacement using a cryo-preserved allograft: An experimental study in the dog. *Trans Orthop Res Soc* 9:220–293, 1984.

78. Milachowski KA: Meniskurefixation-Meniskusteransplantion. Thesis at University of Munich, 1985, p 105.

79. Wesmeier K, Milachowski KA, Wirth CJ: Meniscal transplantation: An experimental study in animals. *Am J Sports Med* 13:422, 1985.

80. Keating EM, Malinin TI, Belchic G: Meniscal transplantation in goats: An experimental study. *Orthop Trans* 13:147, 1988.

81. Zukor DJ, Brooks PJ, Gross AE: Meniscal allografts: An experimental and clinical study. *Orthop Rev* 17:522, 1988.

82. Zukor DJ, Farine I, Brooks PJ, et al: Allo-transplantation of the rabbit medial meniscus. Presented at the 22nd Annual meeting of the Canadian Orthopaedic Research Society, Ottawa, Canada, June 1988.

83. Cooper D, Arnoczky S, Warren R: Arthroscopic meniscal repair. *Clin Orthop* 9:589, 1990.

84. Fowler PJ, Pompan D: Rehabilitation after meniscal repair. *Tech Orthop* 8:137–139, 1982.

85. Buseck MJ, Noyes FR: Arthroscopic evaluation of meniscal repairs after anterior cruciate ligament reconstruction and immediate motion. *Am J Sports Med* 19:489, 1991.

86. Hefti FL, Kress I, Fasel J, Morscher EW: Healing of the transected anterior cruciate ligament in the rabbit. *J Bone Joint Surg* 73A:373–383, 1991.

87. Frank C, Woo SL-Y, Amiel D, et al: Medial collateral ligament healing: A multi-disciplinary assessment in rabbits. *Am J Sports Med* 11:379–389, 1983.

88. Frank CB, Amiel D, Woo SL-Y, Akeson WH: Normal ligament properties and ligament healing. *Clin Orthop Rel Res* 196:15–25, 1985.

89. Murphy PG, Frank CB, Hart DA: The cell biology of ligaments and ligament healing, in Jackson DW, Arnoczky SP, Woo SL-Y (eds): *The Anterior Cruciate Ligament: Current and Future Concepts.* New York, Raven Press, 1993, pp 165–177.

90. Butler DL, Grood ES, Noyes FR, Sodd AN: The interpretation of our ACL data. *Clin Orthop Rel Res* 196:26–34, 1985.

91. Butler DL, Noyes FR, Grood ES: Ligamentous restraints to anterior-posterior drawer in the human knee. *J Bone Joint Surg* 62A:259–270, 1980.

92. Grood ES, Suntay WJ, Noyes FR, Butler DL: Biomechanics of the knee—Extension exercise: Effect of cutting the ACL. *J Bone Joint Surg* 66A:725–734, 1984.

93. Fukubayashi T, Torzilli PA, Sherman MF, Warren RF: An in vitro biomechanical evaluation of anterior-posterior motion of the knee. *J Bone Joint Surg* 64A:258–264, 1982.

94. Beynnon BD, Johnson RJ, Flemming BC: The mechanics of anterior cruciate ligament reconstruction, in Jackson DW, Arnoczky SP, Woo SL-Y (eds): *The Anterior Cruciate Ligament: Current and Future Concepts.* New York, Raven Press, 1993, p 259.

95. Kurosaka M, Yoshia S, Andrish JT: The biomechanical comparison of different surgical techniques of graft fixation in anterior cruciate ligament reconstruction. *Am J Sports Med* 15:225–229, 1987.

96. Woo SL-Y, Adams DJ: The tensile properties of human anterior cruciate ligament ACL and ACL graft tissues, in Daniel DM, Akeson WH, O'Conner TT (eds): *Knee Ligaments: Structure, Function, Injury and Repair.* New York, Raven Press, 1990, pp 279–289.

97. Newton PO, Horibe S, Woo SL-Y: Experimental studies in the anterior cruciate ligament autografts and allografts: Mechanical studies, in Daniel DM, Akeson WH, O'Conner TT (eds): *Knee Ligaments: Structure, Function, Injury and Repair.* New York, Raven Press, 1990, pp 389–399.

98. Woo SL-Y, Hollis JM, Adams DJ, et al: Tensile properties of the human femur—Anterior cruciate ligament–tibia complex: The effect of specimen age and orientation. *Am J Sports Med* 19:217–225, 1991.

99. Butler DL, Kay MD, Stauffer DC: Comparison of material properties in bone-fasicle-bone units from human patellar tendon and knee ligaments. *J Biomech* 19:425–432, 1986.

100. Arnoczky SP, Warren RF, Ashlock MA: Replacement of the anterior cruciate ligament using a patellar tendon allograft. *J Bone Joint Surg* 68A:376–385, 1986.

101. Johnson G, Choi N, Tramaglini D, et al: Visco-elastic properties of the human patellar tendon: Age related changes. 2nd North American Congress on Biomechanics. Chicago, 1992, pp 9–10.

102. Hart RC, Powlson AC: The effect of test environment on cyclic stretching on the failure properties of the human patellar tendon allografts. *J Orthop Res* 8:532–540, 1990.

103. Noyes FR, Butler DL, Grood ES, et al: Biomechanical analysis of human knee ligament grafts used in knee ligament repairs and reconstructions. *J Bone Joint Surg* 66A:334–352, 1984.

104. Markolf KL, Mensch JS, Amstutz HC: Stiffness and laxity of the knee—The contributions of the supporting structures. *J Bone Joint Surg* 58A:583–593, 1976.

105. Fujie H, Livesay GA, Kashiwaguchi S, et al: A new methodology for direct, non-contact determination of in situ forces in soft tissues. 2nd North American Congress on Biomechanics. Chicago, 1992, pp 7–8.

106. Fujie H, Mabuchi K, Woo SL-Y, et al: The use of robotics technology to study human joint kinematics: A new methodology. *J Biomech Eng* 115:211–217, 1993.

107. Woo SL-Y, Livesay GA, Xerogeanes JW, Rudy TA: Biomechanics of the ACL and ACL reconstruction: New concepts and application. Proceedings of the 20th annual meeting of the Japanese Society for Clinical Biomechanics and Related Research, Tokyo, Japan, 1993.

108. Smidt GJ: Biomechanical analysis of knee flexion and extension. *J Biomech* 6:79–92, 1973.

109. O'Conner TT, Biden EN, Bradley J, Fitzpatrick D: The muscle stabilized knee, in Daniel DM, Akeson WH, O'Conner TT (eds): *Knee Ligaments: Structure, Function, Injury, and Repair.* New York, Raven Press, 1990, pp 239–277.

110. Renstrom P, Arms SW, Stanwyck TS, Johnson RJ: Strain within the anterior cruciate ligament during hamstrings and quadriceps activity. *Am J Sports Med* 14:83–87, 1986.

111. Arms SW, Pope MJ, Johnson RJ, Fischer RA: The biomechanics of anterior cruciate ligament rehabilitation and reconstruction. *Am J Sports Med* 12:8–18, 1984.

112. Markolf KL, Gorek JF, Cabo JM, Shapiro MS: Direct measurement of the resultant forces in the anterior cruciate ligament. *J Bone Joint Surg* 72A:557–567, 1990.

113. More RC, Karras BT, Neiman R, Fritschy D: Hamstrings: An anterior cruciate ligament protagonist—an in vitro study. *Am J Sports Med* 21:231–237, 1993.

114. Bidden EN, O'Conner JJ: Experimental methods used to evaluated knee ligament function, in Daniel DM, Akeson WH, O'Conner TT (eds): *Knee Ligaments: Structure, Function, Injury, and Repair.* New York, Raven Press, 1990.

115. Noyes FR, DeLucas JL, Torvik PJ: Biomechanics of ACL failure: An analysis of strain-rate sensitivity, and mechanisms of failure in primates. *J Bone Joint Surg* 56A:236–253, 1974.

116. Noyes FR: Functional properties of knee ligaments and alterations induced by immobilization. *Clin Orthop Rel Res* 123:210–243, 1977.

117. Woo SL-Y, Young CP, Kwan MK: Fundamental studies in knee ligament mechanisms, in Daniel DM, Akeson WH, O'Conner TT (eds): *Knee Ligaments: Structure, Function, Injury and Repair.* New York, Raven Press, 1990, pp 115–133.

118. Girgis F, Marshal JL, Al Monajem ARS: The cruciate ligaments of the knee joint: Anatomical, functional, and experimental analysis. *Clin Orthop Rel Res* 106:216–231, 1975.

119. Danychuk KD, Finlay JB, Kreck JP: Microstructural organization of the human and bovine cruciate ligament. *Clin Orthop Rel Res* 131:294–298, 1978.

120. Kastellic J, Gazleski A, Bauer E: A multi-composite structure of tendon. *Connect Tissue Res* 6:11–23, 1978.

121. Smith BA, Livesay GA, Woo SL-Y: Biology and biomechanics of the anterior cruciate ligament. *Clin Sports Med* 12:637–669, 1993.

122. Clark JM, Sidles JA: The inter-relation of fiber bundles in the anterior cruciate ligament. *J Orthop Res* 8:180–188, 1988.

123. Arnoczky SP: Anatomy of the anterior cruciate ligament. *Clin Orthop* 172:19, 1983.

124. Johansson H, Sjolander P, Sojka P: A sensory role for the cruciate ligaments. *Clin Orthop Rel Res* 268:161–178, 1991.

125. Miyasaka KC, Daniel DM, Stone ML, Hirshman P: The incidence of knee ligament injuries in the general population. *Am J Knee Surg* 4:3–8, 1991.

126. Hirshman HP, Daniel DM, Miyasaka K: The fate of unoperated knee ligament injuries, in Daniel DM, Akeson WH, O'Conner TT (eds): *Knee Ligaments: Structure, Function, Injury and Repair.* New York, Raven Press, 1990, p. 462.

127. Feagin JA, Lambert KL, Cunningham RR: Consideration of the anterior cruciate ligament injury in skiing. *Clin Orthop* 216:13–18, 1987.

128. Hewson GF, Ricky MA, Wang JB: Prophylactic knee bracing in college football. *Am J Sports Med* 14:262–266, 1986.

129. Fetto JF, Marshall JL: The natural history and diagnosis of anterior cruciate ligament insufficiency. *Clin Orthop Rel Res* 147:29–38, 1980.

130. Finsterbush A, Frankle U, Matan Y, Mann G: Secondary damage to the knee after isolated injury of the anterior cruciate ligament. *Am J Sports Med* 18:475–479, 1990.

131. Kannus P, Jarvinen M: Conservatively treated tears of the anterior cruciate ligament. *J Bone Joint Surg* 69A:1007–1112, 1987.

132. Kannus P, Jarvinen M: Post-traumatic anterior cruciate ligament insufficiency as a cause of osteoarthritis in the knee joint. *J Rheumatol* 18:251–260, 1989.

133. Hirshman PH, Daniels DM, Miyasaka K: The fate of unoperated knee ligament injuries, in Daniel DM, Akeson WH, O'Conner TT (eds): *Knee Ligaments: Structure, Function, Injury, and Repair.* New York, Raven Press, 1990.

134. McDaniel WJ Jr, Dameron TB Jr: The untreated anterior cruciate ligament rupture. *Clin Orthop Rel Res* 172:90–92, 1983.

135. Noyes F, Matthews D, Mooar P, Grood ES: The symptomatic anterior cruciate deficient knee: Part I. The long-term functional disability in athletically active individuals. *J Bone Joint Surg* 65A:154–162, 1983.

136. Daniel DM, Stone ML, Dobson BE, et al: Fate of the ACL injured patient: A prospective outcome study. *Am J Sports Med* 22:632, 1994.

137. Hardaker WT, Garrett W, Bassett FH: Evaluation of traumatic hemarthrosis of the knee joint. *South Med J* 83:640–644, 1990.

138. Noyes FR, Bassett RW, Grood ES, Butler DL: Arthroscopy in acute traumatic hemarthrosis of the knee. *J Bone Joint Surg* 62A:687–695, 1980.

139. DeHaven KE: Diagnosis of acute knee injuries with hemarthrosis. *Am J Sports Med* 8:9, 1980.

140. Donaldson WF, Warren RF, Wickiewicz T: A comparison of acute anterior cruciate ligament examinations. *Am J Sports Med* 10:100, 1992.

141. Torg JS, Conrad W, Kalen V: Clinical diagnosis of anterior cruciate ligament instability in the athlete. *Am J Sports Med* 4:84, 1976.

142. Bach BR, Warren RF, Wickiewicz TL: The pivot shift phenomenon: Results and description of a modified clinical test for anterior cruciate ligament insufficiency. *Am J Sports Med* 16:571–576, 1988.

143. Bach BR, Warren RF, Flynn WM, et al: Arthrometric evaluation of knees that have a torn ACL. *J Bone Joint Surg* 72A:1299–1306, 1990.

144. Woods GW, Stanley RF, Tullos HS: Lateral capsular sign: X-ray clue to a significant knee instability. *Am J Sports Med* 7:27–33, 1979.

145. Speer KP, Spritzer CE, Goldner JL, Garrett WE: Magnetic resonance imaging of traumatic knee articular cartilage injuries. *Am J Sports Med* 19:396–402, 1991.

146. Jackson RW, Peters RI, Marczyk RI: Late results of untreated anterior cruciate ligament rupture. *J Bone Joint Surg* 62B:127, 1980.

147. Jackson RW: The torn ACL: Natural history of untreated lesions and rationale for selective treatment, in Feagin JA (ed): *The Cruciate Ligaments,* 2d ed. New York, Churchill Livingstone, 1994.

148. DeHaven K: Meniscus repair in the athlete. *Clin Orthop Rel Res* 198:31–35, 1985.

149. Harner CD, Irrgang JJ, Paul J, et al: Loss of motion following ACL reconstruction. *Am J Sports Med* 20:507, 1992.

150. Mohtadi NGH, Webster-Bogaert S, Fowler PJ: Limitation of motion following ACL reconstruction. *Am J Sports Med* 19:620, 1991.

151. Shelbourne KD, Wilckens JH, Mollabashy A, et al: Arthrofibrosis in acute ACL reconstruction: The effect of timing of reconstruction and rehabilitation. *Am J Sports Med* 19:332, 1991.

152. Noyes F, Matthews D, Mooar P, et al: The symptomatic anterior cruciate deficient knee: II. The results of rehabilitation, activity modification, and counseling on functional disability. *J Bone Joint Surg* 65A:163, 1983.

153. Nogalski MP, Bach BR Jr: Acute anterior cruciate ligament injuries, in Fu FH, Harner CD, Vince KG, Miller MD (eds): *Knee Surgery.* Vol 1. Baltimore, Williams & Wilkins, 1994, pp 700–701.

154. Cooper DE, Arnoczky SP, Warren RF, et al: Tensile strength of the bone-patellar tendon-bone complex. Paper presented at the 59th Annual Meeting of the American Academy of Orthopaedic Surgeons, Washington, DC, February 1992.

155. Bonamo JL, Krinick RM, Sporn AA: Rupture of the patella ligament after use of its central third for anterior cruciate reconstruction: A report of two cases. *J Bone Joint Surg* 66A:1294–1297, 1984.

156. Burks RT, Haut RC, Lancaster RL: Biomechanical and histological observations on the dog patellar tendon after removal of its central one third. *Am J Sports Med* 18:146–153, 1990.

157. Jackson DW, Schefer RK: Cyclops syndrome: Loss of extension following intraarticular anterior cruciate ligament reconstruction. *Arthroscopy* 6:171, 1990.

158. Langan P, Fontanetta AP: Rupture of the patellar tendon after use of its central third. *Orthop Rev* 15:61, 1987.

159. McCarroll JR: Fracture of the patella during a golf swing following reconstruction of the anterior cruciate ligament. *Am J Sports Med* 11:26–27, 1983.

160. Paulos LE, Rosenberg TD, Drawbert J, et al: Infrapatellar contracture syndrome. *Am J Sports Med* 15:331–341, 1987.

161. Roberts TS, Drez D, Banta CJ: Complications of anterior cruciate ligament reconstruction, in Briggs NF (ed): *Complications in Arthroscopy.* New York, Raven Press, 1989, pp 169–177.

162. Sachs RA, Daniel DM, Stone ML, Garfen RF: Patellofemoral problems after anterior cruciate ligament reconstruction. *Am J Sports Med* 17:760–765, 1989.

163. Howell SM, Clark JA, Farley TE: Rationale for predicting anterior cruciate graft impingement by the intercondylar roof: A magnetic resonance imaging study. *Am J Sports Med* 19:276–282, 1991.

164. Yaru NC, Daniel DM, Penner D: The effect of tibial attachment site on graft impingement in an anterior cruciate ligament reconstruction. *Am J Sports Med* 20:217–220, 1992.

165. Woo SL-Y, Gomez MA, Woo Y-K, et al: Mechanical properties of tendons and ligaments: II. The relationships of immobilization and exercise on tissue remodeling. *Biorheology* 19:397–408, 1982.

166. Amiel D, Akeson WH, Harwood FL, et al: Stress deprivation effect on metabolic turnover the medial collateral ligament collagen: A comparison between 9 and 12 week immobilization. *Clin Orthop Rel Res* 172:265–270, 1983.

167. Baud HE, Chatty A, Gildengorin V, et al: Exercise effects on the strength of the rat anterior cruciate ligament. *Am J Sports Med* 8:79–86, 1980.

168. Zuckerman J, Stull GA: Effects of exercise on knee ligament separation force in rats. *J Appl Physiol* 26:716–719, 1969.

169. Noyes FR, Torvik PJ, Hyde WB, et al: Biomechanics of ligament failure: II. An analysis of immobilization, exercise and reconditioning effects in primates. *J Bone Joint Surg* 56A:1406–1418, 1974.

170. Clancy WG, Narechania RG, Rosenberg TD, et al: Anterior and posterior cruciate ligament reconstruction in rhesus monkeys. *J Bone Joint Surg* 64A:1270–1284, 1981.

171. Kennedy JC, Roth JH, Mendenhall I IV, Sanford JB: Intra-articular replacement of the anterior cruciate ligament deficient knee. *Am J Sports Med* 8:1–8, 1980.

172. Puddu J, Ippolioto E: Reconstruction of the anterior cruciate ligament using the semitendinosus tendon: Histological study of a case. *Am J Sports Med* 11:1416, 1983.

173. Viidik A: Elasticity and tensile strength of the anterior cruciate ligament in rabbits influenced by training. *Acta Physiol Scand* 74:372–380, 1968.

174. Spindler K, Schils J, Bergfeld J, et al: Perspective study of osseous, articular, and meniscal lesions in recent anterior cruciate ligament tears by magnetic resonance imaging and arthroscopy. *Am J Sports Med* 21:555, 1993.

175. Wickiewicz TL: Meniscal injuries in the cruciate deficient knee. *Clin Sports Med* 9:681, 1990.

176. Rosenberg T, Scott S, Coward D, et al: Arthroscopic meniscal repair evaluated by repeat arthroscopy. *Arthroscopy* 2:20, 1986.

177. DeHaven KE, Black KP, Griffiths HJ: Open meniscus repair: Technique and two to nine year results. *Am J Sports Med* 17:788–795, 1989.

178. O'Donoghue DH: Surgical treatment of fresh injuries to the major ligaments of the knee. *J Bone Joint Surg* 32A:721–738, 1950.

179. O'Donoghue DH: An analysis of end results of surgical treatment of major injuries to the ligaments of the knee. *J Bone Joint Surg* 37A:1–13, 1955.

180. Anderson DR, Weiss J, Takai S, Ohland KJ, Woo SL-Y: Healing of the medical lateral collateral ligament following a triad injury: A biomechanical and histological study of the knee in rabbits. *J Orthop Res* 10:485–495, 1992.

181. Kannus P: Long-term results of conservatively treated medial collateral ligament injuries of the knee joint. *Clin Orthop Rel Res* 226:103–112, 1988.

182. Larson RL: Combined instabilities of the knee. *Clin Orthop Rel Res* 147:68–81, 1980.

183. Fronek J, Frank C, Amiel D, et al: The effect of intermittent passive motion (IPM) on the healing of the medial collateral ligament. *Transactions of the Orthopaedic Research Society.* Anaheim, CA, 8:31, 1983.

184. Fetto JF, Marshall JL: Medial collateral ligament injuries of the knee: A rationale for treatment. *Clin Orthop Rel Res* 132:206–218, 1978.

185. Reider B, Sathy MR, Talkington J, et al: Treatment of isolated medial collateral ligament injuries in athletes with early functional rehabilitation: A 5-year follow-up study. *Am J Sports Med* 22:22–28, 1993.

186. Hastings DE: Non-operative management of collateral ligament injuries of the knee joint. *Clin Orthop Rel Res* 147:22–28, 1980.

187. Indelicato PA: Non-operative treatment of complete tears of the medial collateral ligament of the knee. *J Bone Joint Surg* 65A:323–329, 1993.

188. Woo SL-Y, Inoue N, McGurk-Burleson E, Gomez M: Treatment of medial collateral ligament injury: II. Structure and function of canine knees in response to different treatment regimens. *Am J Sports Med* 15:22–29, 1987.

189. Weiss JA, Woo SL-Y, Ohland KJ, et al: Evaluation of a new injury model to study medial collateral ligament healing: Primary repair versus non-operative treatment. *J Orthop Res* 9:516–528, 1991.

190. Woo SL-Y, Gomez M, Sites TJ, Newton PO: The biomechanical and morphological changes in the medial collateral ligament of the rabbit after immobilization and remobilization. *J Bone Joint Surg* 69A:1200–1211, 1987.

191. Woo SL-Y, Matthews J, Akeson WH: Connective tissue response to immobility: A correlative study of biomechanical and biochemical measurements of normal and immobilized rabbit knees. *Arthritis Rheum* 18:257–264, 1975.

192. Long ML, Frank C, Schachar NS, Dittrich D: The effects of motion on normal and healing ligaments. *Trans Orthop Res Soc* 7:43, 1982.

193. Gomez MA, Woo SL-Y, Amiel D, Harwood F: The effects of increased tension on the healing medial collateral ligaments. *Am J Sports Med* 19:347–354, 1991.

194. Kannus P: Long-term results of conservatively treated medial collateral ligament injuries of the knee joint. *Clin Orthop Rel Res* 226:103–112, 1988.

195. Warren RF, Marshall JL: Injuries of the anterior cruciate and medial collateral ligaments of the knee: A long-term follow-up of 86 cases (Part II). *Clin Orthop Rel Res* 136:198–211, 1978.

196. Bray RC, Frank CB, Shrive DD, Chimich DD: Joint instability alters scar quantity and quality in healing rabbit ligament. *Trans Orthop Res Soc* 15:58, 1990.

197. Forbes I, Frank CE, Lam T, Shrive N: The biomechanical effects of combined ligament injuries on the medial collateral ligament. *Trans Orthop Res Soc* 13:186, 1988.

198. Woo SL-Y, Young EP, Ohland KJ, Marcin JP: The effects of ACL transection on MCL healing: An experimental study of the canine knee. *J Bone Joint Surg* 72A:382–392, 1990.

199. Inoue M, McGurk-Burleson E, Hollis JM, Woo SL-Y: Treatment of the medial collateral ligament injury (Part I): The importance of anterior cruciate ligament on varus-valgus knee laxity. *Am J Sports Med* 15:15–21, 1987.

200. Hart DP, Dahners LE: Total healing of the medial collateral ligament in rats. *J Bone Joint Surg* 69A:1194–1199, 1987.

201. Bray RC, Frank CB, Shrive NG, Chimich DD: Effects of joint instability and joint mobilization on ACL-deficient MCL healing in the adult rabbit model. *Trans Orthop Res Soc* 16:1935, 1991.

202. Lechner CT, Dahners LE: Healing of the medial collateral ligament in unstable rat knees. *Am J Sports Med* 19:508–512, 1991.

203. Ballmer PM, Ballmer FT, Jakob RP: Reconstruction of the ACL alone in the treatment of combined instability with complete rupture of the MCL. *Arch Orthop Trauma Surg* 110:139–141, 1991.

204. Shelbourne KD, Baile JR: Treatment of combined ACL-MCL injuries. *Am J Knee Surg* 1:56–62, 1988.

205. Shelbourne KD, Porter DA: Anterior cruciate ligament–medial collateral ligament injury: Non-operative management of MCL tears with anterior cruciate reconstruction. *Am J Sports Med* 20:283–286, 1992.

206. Engle CP, Noguchi M, Ohland KJ, Shelley FJ: Rabbit medial collateral ligament healing following an O'Donoghue triad injury: The effects of anterior cruciate ligament reconstruction. *J Orthop Res* 12:357–364, 1994.

207. Ohno K, Pomaybo AS, Schmidt CC: MCL healing following a combined MCL and ACL injury and ACL reconstruction: Repair vs non-repair of MCL tears in rabbits. Accepted for publication. *J Orthop Res.*

208. Shelbourne KD, Patel DV: Management of combined injuries of the anterior cruciate and medial collateral ligaments. *AAOS Instr Course Lect* 45:275, 1996.

209. Girgis F, Marshall JL, Almonajem ARS: The cruciate ligaments of the knee joints: Anatomical, functional, and experimental analysis. *Clin Orthop Rel Res* 106:216–231, 1975.

210. Brantigan OC, Vosnell AF: The mechanics of the ligaments and menisci of the knee joint. *J Bone Joint Surg* 23A:44–46, 1941.

211. Detenbeck LC: Function of the cruciate ligaments in knee stability. *Am J Sports Med* 2:217–221, 1974.

212. Kennedy JC, Hawkins RJ, Willis RB, Danylchuk KD: Tension studies of the human knee ligaments. *J Bone Joint Surg* 58A:350–355, 1976.

213. Prietto MP, Bain JR, Stonebrook SN, Settlage RA, et al: Tensile strength of the human posterior cruciate ligament. *Trans Orthop Res Soc* 34:195, 1988.

214. Harner CD, Livesay G, Choi N, et al: Evaluation of the sizes and shapes of the human anterior and posterior cruciate ligaments: A comparative study. *Trans Orthop Res Soc* 17:123, 1992.

215. Race A, Amis A: Mechanical properties of the two bundles of the human posterior cruciate ligament. *Trans Orthop Res Soc* 17:124, 1992.

216. Fukubayashi T, Torzilli PA, Sherman MF, et al: An in vitro biomechanical evaluation of anterior-posterior motion of the knee: Tibial displacement, rotation, and torque. *J Bone Joint Surg* 64A:258, 1982.

217. Clenendin MB, DeLee J, Heckman J: Interstitial tears of the posterior cruciate ligament. *Orthopedics* 3:764, 1980.

218. Parolie JM, Bergfeld JA, et al: Long-term results of non-operative treatment of isolated posterior cruciate ligament injuries in the athlete. *Am J Sports Med* 14:35–38, 1986.

219. Wascher D, Markolf K, Shapiro M, et al: Direct in vivo measurements of forces in the cruciate ligaments: Part I. The effect of multi-plane loading on the intact knee. *J Bone Joint Surg* 75A:377, 1993.

220. Fowler PJ, Messieh SS: Isolated posterior cruciate ligament injuries in athletes. *Am J Sports Med* 15:553–557, 1987.

221. Satku K, Chew CM, Seow H: Posterior cruciate ligament injuries. *Acta Orthop Scand* 55:26–29, 1984.

222. Parolie JM, Bergfeld JA: Long-term results of non-operative treatment of isolated posterior cruciate ligament injuries in the athlete. *Am J Sports Med* 14:35–38, 1986.

223. Harner CD: Posterior cruciate ligament: Current concepts. Presented at the Panther Symposium, Pittsburgh, May 1992.

224. Clancy WG, Shelbourne KD, Zoellner GB, et al: Treatment of knee joint instability secondary to rupture of the PCL: A report of a new procedure. *J Bone Joint Surg* 65A:310–322, 1983.

225. MacDonald PR, Miniaci A, Fowler PJ, et al: Biomechanical analysis of joint contact forces in the posterior cruciate deficient knee. Presented at the 60th Annual Meeting of the American Academy of Orthopaedic Surgeons, San Francisco, February 1993.

226. Skyhar MJ, Schwartz E, Warren RF, et al: The effects of PCL and posterolateral complex laxity on the articular contact pressures within the knee. *J Bone Joint Surg* 75A:694–699, 1993.

227. Pournaras J, Symeonides PP: The results of surgical repair of acute tears of the posterior cruciate ligament. *Clin Orthop Rel Res* 267:103–107, 1991.

228. Bianchi M: Acute tears of the posterior cruciate ligament: Clinical study and results of operative treatment in 27 cases. *Am J Sports Med* 11:308–314, 1983.

229. Grood ES, Stowers S, Noyes F: Limits of movement in the human knee: Effect of sectioning the posterior cruciate ligament in the posterolateral structures. *J Bone Joint Surg* 70A:88, 1988.

230. Daniel DM, Stone ML, Barnett P, et al: Use of the quadriceps active test to diagnose PCL disruption and measure posterior laxity of the knee. *J Bone Joint Surg* 70A:386, 1988.

231. Swenson TM, Harner CD, Fu FH: Arthroscopic posterior cruciate ligament reconstruction with allograft. *Sports Med Arthrosc Rev* 2:120–128, 1994.

232. Insall JN, Hood RW: Bone block transfer of the medial head of the gastrocnemius for posterior cruciate insufficiency. *J Bone Joint Surg* 64A:691–699, 1982.

233. Sidles JA, Clark JM, Garbini JL: A geometric theory of the equilibrium mechanics of fibers and ligaments in tendons. *J Biomech* 24:943–949, 1991.

234. Maynard MG, Deng X, Wickiewicz TL, et al: The poplite-ofemoral ligament: The "missing link" in posterolateral rotatory instability of the human knee. Program and abstracts: 20th Annual Meeting of the American Orthopaedic Society for Sports Medicine, Palm Desert, CA, 1994.

235. Seebacher JR, Inglis AE, Marshall J, et al: The structure of the posterolateral aspect of the knee. *J Bone Joint Surg* 64A:536, 1982.

236. Sudasna S, Harnsiriwattanagit K: The ligamentous structures of the posterolateral aspect of the knee. *Bull Hosp Joint Dis* 50:35, 1990.

237. Watanabe Y, Moriwa H, Takeshi K: Functional anatomy of the posterolateral structures of the knee. *Arthroscopy* 9:57, 1993.

238. Gollehan D, Torzilli P, Warren R: The role of posterolateral and cruciate ligaments in the stability of the knee: A biomechanical study. *J Bone Joint Surg* 69A:233, 1987.

239. Markolf KL, Wascher DC, Finerman GA: Direct in vitro measurements of forces in the cruciate ligaments: Part II. The effect of sectioning of the posterolateral structures. *J Bone Joint Surg* 75A:387, 1993.

240. Hughston JC, Norwood LA: The posterolateral drawer test and external rotation recurvatum test for posterolateral instability of the knee. *Clin Orthop Rel Res* 147:82, 1980.

241. Harner CD: PCL surgery: Future directions. *Sports Med Arthrosc Rev* 2:174, 1994.

242. Palmer I: The injuries to the ligaments of the knee joint: A clinical study. *Acta Chir Scand* 31 (suppl 53):81, 1938.

243. Ficat P, Hungerford D: *Disorders of the Patellofemoral Joint.* Baltimore, Williams & Wilkins, 1977.

244. Wriberg G: Roentgenographic and anatomic studies on the femoral patellar joint. *Acta Orthop Scand* 12:319–410, 1941.

245. Ficat P, Bizou H: Luxations recidivintes de la rotule. *Orthop Rev* 53:721, 1967.

246. Fulkerson JP, Hungerford DS: *Disorder of the Patellofemoral Joint,* 2d ed. Baltimore, Williams & Wilkins, 1990.

247. Brattstrom H: The shape of the intercondylar groove normally and in recurrent dislocations of the patella. *Acta Orthop Scand* 68(suppl):134–148, 1964.

248. DeJour H, Walch G, Neyret PH, Adeleine P: La dysplasie de la trochlee femorale. *Rev Chir Orthop* 16:45–54, 1990.

249. Lieb FJ, Perry J: Quadriceps function: An anatomical and mechanical study using amputated limbs. *J Bone Joint Surg* 50A:8, 1535–1548, 1968.

250. Hallisey MJ, Doherty N, Bennett WF, et al: Anatomy of the junction of the vastus lateralis tendon in the patella. *J Bone Joint Surg* 69A:545–549, 1987.

251. Suzuki S: The role of the quadriceps muscle for the patellofemoral malalignment syndrome. *J Jpn Orthop Assoc* 61:905–916, 1987.

252. Kaufer H: Patellar biomechanics. *Clin Orthop Rel Res* 144:51–54, 1979.

253. Reilly D, Martens N: Experimental analysis of quadriceps muscle force and patellofemoral joint resultant force of various activity. *Acta Orthop Scand* 43:126, 1972.

254. Huberti HH, Hayes WC: Patellofemoral contact pressures: The influence of Q angle and tendofemoral contact. *J Bone Joint Surg* 66A:715–724, 1984.

255. Hungerford DS, Barry M: Biomechanics of the patellofemoral joint. *Clin Orthop Rel Res* 144:9–15, 1979.

256. Huberti HH, Hayes WC, Stone JL, Shybut GT: Force ratios in the quadriceps tendon and ligamentum patellae. *J Orthop Res* 2:1, 49–54, 1984.

257. Insall J: *Surgery of the Knee.* New York, Churchill Livingstone, 1984.

258. Hughston JC: Subluxation of the patella. *J Bone Joint Surg* 50A:1003–1026, 1968.

259. Fulkerson JP, Kalenak A, Rosenberg TD, Cox JS: Patellofemoral pain. *AAOS Instr Course Lect* 41:57–72, 1992.

260. Merchant AC, Mercer RL, Jacobsen RH, Cool CR: Roentgenographic analysis of the patellofemoral congruence. *J Bone Joint Surg* 56A:1391–1396, 1974.

261. Laurin CA, Dussault R, Levesque HP: The tangential x-ray investigation of the patellofemoral joint: X-ray technique, diagnostic criteria and their interpretation. *Clin Orthop Rel Res* 44:16–26, 1979.

262. Blumenstaat C: Die Haufabweichungen und Verrunkungen der Kniescheibe. *Ergebn Chir Orthop* 31:149–223, 1938.

263. Insall J, Salvati E: Patella position in the normal knee. *Radiology* 101:101–104, 1971.

264. Insall J, Falvo KA, Wise DW: Chondromalacia patellae: A prospective study. *J Bone Joint Surg* 58A:1–8, 1976.

265. Outerbridge RE: Etiology of chondromalacia patella. *J Bone Joint Surg* 43B:752–757, 1961.

266. Brunet ME, Stewart GW: Patellofemoral rehabilitation. *Clin Sports Med* 8:319–330, 1989.

267. Cherf J, Paulos LE: Bracing for patellar instability. *Clin Sports Med* 9:813–821, 1989.

268. DeHaven KE, Dolan WA, Mayer PJ: Chondromalacia patellae in athletes: Clinical presentation and conservative management. *Am J Sports Med* 7:5–11, 1979.

269. Paulos LE, Rusche K, Johnson C, Noyes FR: Patellar malalignment: A treatment rationale. *Phys Ther* 60:1624–1632, 1980.

270. Shelton GL, Thigpen LK: Rehabilitation of patellofemoral dysfunction: A review of the literature. *J Orthop Sports Phys Ther* 14:6, 1991.

271. Steadman JR: Nonoperative measures for patellofemoral problems. *Am J Sports Med* 7:374–375, 1979.

272. Wild JJ, Franklin TD, Woods GW: Patellar pain in quadriceps rehabilitation: An EMG study. *Am J Sports Med* 10:12–15, 1982.

273. Hungerford DS, Lennox DW: Rehabilitation of the knee in disorders of the patellofemoral joint: Relevant biomechanics. *Orthop Clin North Am* 14:397–402, 1983.

274. McConnell J: The management of chondromalacia patellae: A long-term solution. *Austr J Physiother* 32:215–223, 1986.

275. Fischer RL: Conservative treatment of patellofemoral pain. *Orthop Clin North Am* 17:2, 269–272, 1986.

276. Palumbo PM: Dynamic patella and brace: A new orthosis in the management of patellofemoral disorders. *Am J Sports Med* 9:45–49, 1981.

277. Schreiber SN: Proximal superior medial portal and arthroscopy of the knee. *Arthroscopy* 7:246–251, 1991.

278. Kolowich P, Paulos LE, Rosenberg T, Farnsworth S: Lateral release of the patella: Indications and contraindications. *Am J Sports Med* 18:361, 1990.

279. McGinty JB, McCarthy JC: Endoscopic lateral retinacular release. *Clin Orthop Rel Res* 56:120–125, 1981.

280. Hallisey MJ, Doherty N, Bennett JP, Fulkerson JP: Anatomy of the junction of the vastus lateralis tendon in the patella. *J Bone Joint Surg* 69A:545–549, 1987.

281. Small NC: An analysis of complications in lateral retinacular release procedures. *Arthroscopy* 5:282–286, 1989.

282. Roux C: Luxation habituelle de la rotule: Traitement operatoire. *Rev Chir* 8:682–689, 1988.

283. Hauser EDW: Total tendon transplant for slipping patella: A new operation for recurrent dislocation of the patella. *Surg Gynecol Obstet* 66:199–214, 1938.

284. Trillat A, DeJour H, Courette A: Diagnostic traitement des subluxation recidevantes de la rotule. *Rev Chir* 60:813–823, 1964.

285. Hughston JC: Reconstruction of the extensor mechanism for subluxing patella. *Am J Sports Med* 1:6–13, 1972.

286. Maquet P: Advancement of the tibial tuberosity. *Clin Orthop Rel Res* 115:225–230, 1976.

287. Ferguson AB Jr, Brown TD, Fu FH, et al: Relief of patellofemoral contact stress by anterior displacement of the tibial tubercle. *J Bone Joint Surg* 61A:159–166, 1979.

288. Nakamura N, Ellis M, Seedhom BB: Advancement of the tibial tuberosity: A biomechanical study. *J Bone Joint Surg* 67B:255–260, 1985.

289. Fulkerson JP, Meaney JA, Becker GJ, et al: Anteromedial tibial tubercle transfer without bone graft. *Am J Sports Med* 18:490–497, 1990.

290. Scott RD, Siliski JM: The use of modified ZY quadriceps palsy during total knee replacement to gain exposure and improve flexion in the ankylosed knee. *Orthopaedics* 8:45–48, 1985.

291. Swenson TM, Harner CD: Knee ligaments and meniscal injuries: Current concepts. *Orthop Clin North Am* 26:3, 1995.

CHAPTER 51

Intraarticular Knee Lesions in Children

Stuart Cherney

MENISCAL INJURIES IN CHILDREN

In a series of 475 consecutive meniscectomies, Henry and Craven report 2 percent occurring in patients 14 years old or younger.[1] In a retrospective study from the Hospital for Crippled Children in Baltimore, Abrams reported that only 7 cases out of 2500 were performed for true mechanical or developmental lesions of the menisci in the knees of children 12 years of age or younger.[2] Both medial and lateral lesions have been reported, and a locked knee has been reported in a child of 4.[3]

Long-term results following meniscectomies in children are now available.[4–6] One study followed 26 patients with open epiphyseal plates who underwent uncomplicated meniscectomy. Length of follow-up was 8.3 years and only 42 percent demonstrated excellent or good results. Postoperative disorders included ligamentous laxity, early degenerative arthritis, and symptomatic knee pain. Extensive preoperative evaluation and conservative management of selected meniscal lesions in children is recommended by the author.[5] A separate study reviewed 49 children who had undergone meniscectomy with a follow-up period of 7.5 years. A good result was noted in 68 percent of males and 29 percent of females. Only 27 percent of the patients had normal radiographs, with 19 percent demonstrating early osteoarthrosis. Meniscectomy in children, according to the authors, is not a benign procedure and preoperative assessment should include arthroscopy or possibly arthrography.[6]

When other possible causes of knee pain have been excluded, a conservative therapeutic regimen should be prescribed. In children with definite episodes of mechanical locking, arthroscopy is recommended. Peripheral tears that meet the described criteria should undergo surgical repair. Partial meniscectomy should only be carried out in meniscal lesions not amenable to repair.[7,8] However, the long-term results of partial meniscectomy compared to total meniscectomy are not significantly different.

Discoid Meniscus

A discoid meniscus is one characterized by a round rather than crescent shape.[9] Approximately 90 percent of the discoid menisci occur on the lateral side. The overall incidence of the discoid lateral meniscus ranges from 1.4 to 15.5 percent.[9–12] Kaplan reported that the lateral meniscus does not appear in the form of a disk in any stage of development. He concluded that patients with discoid menisci

represent individuals who have a normally shaped lateral meniscus at birth which lacks anatomic attachment of the posterior horn of the lateral meniscus to the tibial plateau. As a result, an abnormal motion of the lateral meniscus develops, leading to a hypertrophy into the discoid form.[19]

In the series reported by Nathan and Cole, pain is the most common complaint. Clicking, swelling, and locking followed in order of frequency. Over one-half of the patients presented with symptoms of less than 6 months duration. Objective findings on physical examination included joint line tenderness and clicking, present in two-thirds of knees examined. Other physical findings included effusion, limited extension, a mass over the lateral joint line, positive grinding test (Apley), limited flexion, and thigh atrophy.[11] The fairly high association with meniscal clicking has led to the description of this entity as the "snapping knee syndrome," and the majority of patients are under the age of 15.[11,14]

Certain radiographic features have been associated with the discoid lateral meniscus. Plain roentgenographic features include (1) widening of the lateral joint space, (2) flattening of the lateral femoral condyle, (3) tilt of the articular surface of the lateral tibial condyle, (4) hypoplasia of the lateral tibial spine, and (5) a more proximal position of the fibular head.[15] Cupping of the lateral aspect of the tibial plateau has also been described.[16] Characteristic features of the lateral discoid meniscus seen on knee arthrography are a wide, wedge-shaped structure with extension into the intercondylar notch.

Arthroscopic management is recommended to allow complete evaluation of the nature of the discoid meniscus and determine the significance of any tears or associated articular surface degeneration. In patients with an intact, complete-type discoid lateral meniscus discovered incidentally, no operative treatment is required. Likewise, a partial tear in the complete-type discoid meniscus which is asymptomatic and stable does not require surgical intervention. When a complete-type discoid lateral meniscal lesion is associated with instability of the inner segment, a partial meniscectomy is advocated provided that the remaining peripheral meniscal rim is stable. This technique has also been referred to as "saucerization." Finally, in the "Wrisberg ligament" type of discoid lateral meniscus attached by that ligament to the femur but lacking any attachment to the tibia, total meniscectomy has been advocated due to the underlying instability of the peripheral attachment of the posterior segment of the meniscus (Fig. 51-1).

In summary, partial meniscectomy with contouring of the remaining meniscal rim to recreate the normal shape of the lateral meniscus is indicated only when the discoid meniscus (1) exhibits slight degeneration or minimal tear, (2) shows no abnormal thickening, (3) is not of the Wrisberg type, (4) is not hypermobile, and (5) has an intact capsular attachment.[17]

Osteochondritis Dissecans

Osteochondritis dissecans, or, more properly, osteochondrosis dissecans, is an intraarticular lesion of the knee which is characterized by disorderly endochondral ossifi-

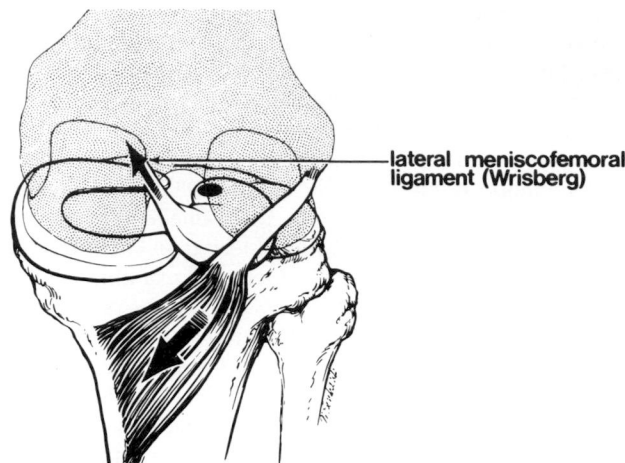

Figure 51-1 Wrisberg-ligament-type discoid lateral meniscus with the knee in extension. The meniscus is displaced into the intercondylar notch by its attachment to the Wrisberg ligament. (Reproduced with permission from Dickhaut S C, and DeLee J C, The discoid lateral-meniscus syndrome, *J Bone Joint Surg*, 64A:1068–1073, 1982.)

cation of epiphyseal growth during childhood. The knee is the most frequently involved of all joints affected by the osteochondroses.[18] The term *osteochondritis dissecans* was first used by Konig in 1888 in describing a lesion that he felt was caused by spontaneous necrosis resulting from trauma.[19] Multiple etiologies have been proposed regarding the osteochondroses. Current theories are that the lesion is secondary to one or more of the following: trauma, ischemia, or abnormal ossification within the epiphysis.[18,20,21] Two separate groups of patients have been identified with this disorder: (1) young patients with a lesion secondary to trauma or irregular ossification centers and (2) adults, resulting from a vascular insult.

Trauma has long been felt to be a major etiologic factor in osteochondritis dissecans. In most series approximately 40 percent of patients presenting with osteochondritis dissecans have a history of prior knee trauma. As a possible factor, Fairbank felt that indirect trauma caused by impingement of the tibial spine on the lateral aspect of the medial femoral condyle during internal rotation was significant.[22] The possibility has been raised that osteochondral fractures which do not unite become indistinguishable from osteochondritis dissecans. Ischemic necrosis secondary to obstruction of end arteries to the femoral condyle has also been suggested as a possible mechanism in the production of osteochondritis dissecans. The etiology of this mechanism is purely speculative, and one study has revealed that the blood supply to the subchondral bone is vast and that ischemic insult is therefore unlikely.[23]

The areas of the knee joint which are most frequently affected include (1) the intercondylar aspect of the medial femoral condyle (75 percent), (2) the weight-bearing surface of medial femoral condyle (10 percent), (3) the weight-bearing surface of the lateral femoral condyle (10 percent), and (4) the anterior intercondylar groove of the patella (5 percent).[24]

Pappas has devised a classification system based on factors that pertain to the natural history and outcome. Category 1 involves children through age of early adolescence (skeletal age 11 for girls, 13 for boys) and is associated with excellent prognosis. Category II includes the age group of skeletal age 12 for girls and 14 for boys to the age of 20 for both. During this period the physes may continue to appear open radiographically, although their contribution to longitudinal growth is minimal. Category III includes patients 20 years of age or older with closed physes. These patients are at risk to develop more significant joint deformation with possible loose fragment formation and extensive articular defects.[18]

The chief symptoms associated with osteochondritis dissecans include pain, stiffness, and swelling. Mechanical symptoms of locking or giving way are also noted. Symptoms are exacerbated in proportion to the level of activity. The physical examination is noteworthy for tenderness over the involved femoral condyle with the knee in full flexion. Wilson's sign may also suggest the presence of an osteochondritis dissecans. This test is performed by internally rotating the tibia with the knee flexed 90° and extending the knee while maintaining internal rotation of the tibia. If positive, pain produced by impingement of the tibial eminence on the lateral aspect of the medial femoral condyle will occur at approximately 30° of knee flexion.[25]

Radiographic evaluation of the knee joint includes anteroposterior (AP), lateral, and patellofemoral views. The tunnel view is mandatory and provides superior visualization of the intercondylar notch. The findings on x-ray may range from a narrow radiolucent separation of the osteochondral fragment to the presence of a loose intraarticular fragment and osteosclerotic crater. A crescent-shaped radiolucent line may be present separating the fragment from the underlying femoral condyle. Arthrography has also been employed to evaluate the integrity of the overlying articular surface.

The objectives of treatment in osteochondritis dissecans are to prevent the formation of a partially attached or free osteochondral fragment and prevent articular surface degeneration.

Management of children who fall into Pappas' category I lesion is nonoperative. Observation, activity restriction, rest, and up to 16 weeks of immobilization are recommended. The severity of the symptoms will dictate whether immobilization is required. Within this category, children may be seen with radiographic changes suggesting a variant of normal ossification; they may not require rest or immobilization. Following category I patients with technetium bone scans has been advocated by Cahill to determine the progress of healing. Repeated scans every 6 to 8 weeks will reveal persistent activity—an indication for surgical intervention.

Category II includes patients between the ages of 12 and 20. An initial treatment program of rest and observation is recommended for lesions which are not progressive. Arthroscopy is indicated in symptomatic lesions over 1 cm in size located in the weight-bearing area. Evidence of progressive osteochondral fragment formation, increasing subchondral osteodensity, or articular changes is significant.

Guhl has proposed an arthroscopic classification of osteochondritis lesions as follows: (1) intact lesions, 1 to 3 cm in diameter with no break in the articular cartilage (surface may be slightly raised or depressed); (2) lesions with early signs of separation, including a break in the articular cartilage with fibrous tissue protruding; (3) partially detached lesions usually held superiorly by a hinge of articular cartilage (these may be completely displaced out of the crater with interposition of fibrous tissue); and (4) craters usually filled with fibrous tissue.[26,27] In cases where the osteochondritic fragment is completely loose, it should be removed. For fragments which have maintained a normal contour, repositioning of the fragment and internal fixation may be attempted. According to the classification system of Guhl, intact lesions are treated with multiple drill holes using a 0.06 Kirschner (K) wire. Lesions showing signs of early separation are drilled, edges are debrided, and fixation is achieved with smooth K-wire pinning. Partially detached fragments are managed with thorough debridement of the undersurface of the fragment and crater prior to reduction, drilling, and pinning.

In category III patients (full skeletal maturity), drilling is used for lesions which are not separated and drilling with pin stabilization for early fragment separation. Large, detached lesions are treated with curettage of the base of the crater and undersurface of the free fragment, followed by stabilization with pins or bone grafting. Bone grafting is advocated in patients with large lesions and x-ray findings of a sclerotic border and radiolucent margin. This includes lesions which exhibit large amounts of protruding fibrous tissue from the fissures in the articular surface. Local cancellous bone graft, corticocancellous cores, iliac matchstick grafts, and freeze-dried allografts have all been used.[26]

Postoperative management in all cases includes casting the knee in a flexed position and keeping the patient non-weight-bearing until radiographic evidence of healing is present. Non-weight-bearing may be required for an additional 2 to 3 months until x-rays reveal evidence of complete healing. Open arthrotomy has been found necessary in the management of large lesions measuring 4 to 5 cm. Fixation and bone grafting can then be carried out.

Results of the various surgical treatment approaches have been reported. Lipscomb et al. reported the use of K wires to reattach loose, osteochondral fragments in eight knees, with successful union in seven.[28] Gillespie and Day used bone pegs to fix 18 defects in 17 patients with union achieved in all cases.[29] Lindholm et al. reported a series of bone pegging in 20 patients with 73 percent good to excellent results in their 5-year followup.[30] In his initial report on 49 knees undergoing arthroscopic procedures, Guhl found 90 percent had healed at an average period of 5 months. Of 15 patients who underwent drilling alone, 14 healed. Eight lesions were drilled, and pinned with all 8 healing. Of the 12 bone grafts, 9 healed. Complications reported in this series included (1) superficial pin erosion through skin, (2) pin breakage, (3) loosening during surgery, and (4) graft displacement.[26,27]

The utilization of autologous chondrocytes cultured in the laboratory to fill articular cartilage defects in animals has been reported by Minas and Spector.[31] Some early results of this technique in humans have been reported in Sweden in patients under age 50 for articular cartilage defects of the femur. However, the long-term success of this procedure is unknown, and it is too early to assess the place such innovative therapies may occupy in our future therapeutic armamentarium.

REFERENCES

1. Henry JH, Craven PR: Traumatic meniscal lesions in children. *South Med J* 74:1336–1337, 1981.
2. Abrams RC: Meniscus lesions of the knee in young children. *J Bone Joint Surg* 39A:194–195, 1957.
3. Schlonsky J, Eyring EJ: Lateral meniscus tears in young children. *Clin Orthop* 97:117–118, 1973.
4. Rozbruch JD, Campbell RC, Insall J: Tibial tubercle elevation (the Maquet operation): A clinical study of 31 cases. *Orthrop Trans* 3:291, 1979.
5. McBride GG, Constine RM, Hofmann AA, Carson RW: Arthroscopic partial medial meniscectomy in the older patient. *J Bone Joint Surg* 66A:547–551, 1984.
6. Zaman M, Leonard MA: Meniscectomy in children: Results in 59 knees. *Injury* 12:425–428, 1981.
7. Grana WA, Connor S, Hollingsworth S: Partial arthroscopic meniscectomy: A preliminary report. *Clin Orthop* 164:78–83, 1982.
8. Gross RH, Grana WA: Meniscus injuries in children. *Adv Orthop Surg* 8:95–99, 1984.
9. Jeannopoulos CL: Observations on discoid menisci. *J Bone Joint Surg* 32A:649–652, 1950.
10. Dickhaut SC, DeLee JC: The discoid lateral-meniscus syndrome. *J Bone Joint Surg* 64A:1068–1073, 1982.
11. Nathan PA, Cole SC: Discoid meniscus: A clinical and pathologic study. *Clin Orthop* 64:107–112, 1969.
12. Smillie IS. *Injuries of the Knee Joint,* 4th ed. Edinburgh, Churchill Livingstone, 1970.
13. Kaplan EB: Discoid lateral meniscus of the knee joint: Nature, mechanism, and operative treatment. *J Bone Joint Surg* 39A:77–87, 1957.
14. Berson BL, Hermann G: Torn discoid menisci of the knee in adults: Four case reports. *J Bone Joint Surg* 61A:303–304, 1979.
15. Haveson SB, Rein BJ: Lateral discoid meniscus of the knee: Arthrographic diagnosis. *Am J Roentgenol* 109:581–585, 1970.
16. Engber WD, Mickelson MR: Cupping of the lateral tibial plateau associated with a discoid meniscus. *Orthopaedics* 4:904–906. 1981.
17. Ferrer-Roca O, Vilalta C: Lesions of the meniscus. Part 2: Horizontal cleavages and lateral cysts. *Clin Orthop* 146:301–307, 1980.
18. Pappas AM: The osteochondroses. Osteochondrosis dissecans. *Clin Orthop* 158:59–69, 1981.
19. Konig F: Euber freie Korper in den Gelenken. *Dtsch Z Chir* 27:90, 1888.
20. Mubarak SJ, Carroll NC: Juvenile osteochondritis dissecans of the knee: Etiology. *Clin Orthop* 157:200, 1981.
21. Petrie PWR: Aetiology of osteochondritis dissecans. Failure to establish a familial background. *J Bone Joint Surg* 59B:366, 1977.
22. Fairbank HAT: Osteochondritis dissecans. *Br J Surg* 21:67, 1933.
23. Rogers WM, Gladstone H: Vascular foramina and arterial supply of the distal end of the femur. *J Bone Joint Surg* 32A:867–874, 1950.

24. Aichroth P: Osteochondritis dissecans of the knee: A clinical survey. *J Bone Joint Surg* 53B:440, 1971.

25. Wilson JN: A diagnostic sign in osteochondritis dissecans of the knee. *J Bone Joint Surg* 49A:477, 1967.

26. Guhl JF: Update in the treatment of osteochondritis dissecans. *Orthopaedics* 7:1744–1751, 1984.

27. Guhl J: Arthroscopic treatment of osteochondritis dissecans. Preliminary report. *Orthop Clin North Am* 10:671, 1979.

28. Lipscomb P, Jr, Lipscom P, Byron R: Readily removable pin fixation in the treatment of osteochondritis dissecans of the knee. *Am Acad Orthop Surg* 1977.

29. Gillespie NF, Day B: Bone peg fixation in the treatment of osteochondritis dissecans. *Clin Orthop* 143:125–130, 1979.

30. Lindholm S, Pylkkanen P: Internal fixation of the fragments of osteochondritis dissecans of the knee by means of a bone pin. *Acta Chir Scand* 140:626, 1974.

31. Minas T, Spector M: New animal, human data reported for autologous chondrocyte transplants. *Orthop Today* 16:18–19, 1996.

CHAPTER 52

Treatment of Inflammatory and Degenerative Conditions of the Knee

Peter Larcom
and Paul A. Lotke

A variety of inflammatory and degenerative disorders may involve the knee. The following sections are devoted to their surgical treatment.

SYNOVECTOMY

Open synovectomy was first performed in the late nineteenth and early twentieth centuries for tuberculous arthritis and a variety of other disorders.[1-4] However, it only became widespread in the 1960s and 1970s, primarily in the treatment of rheumatoid arthritis.[5-11] Recently the indications for synovectomy have become more refined and results of the procedure more clearly established. Nevertheless, the role of synovectomy in the treatment of knee disorders continues to evolve.[12]

Table 52-1 lists the most commonly encountered disorders in which synovectomy is utilized. Traditionally, synovectomy has been performed most frequently for rheumatoid arthritis involving the knee.[13-17] It allows removal of the inflammatory synovium, resulting in rapid relief of pain and the associated swelling.[11,18,19] It is unlikely that synovectomy arrests the progressive joint deterioration associated with rheumatoid arthritis.[18,19,20] The rheumatoid synovium often regenerates following the procedure.[8]

The indications for synovectomy in rheumatoid arthritis are (1) failure of comprehensive medical management following at least a 6-month trial, (2) persistent synovitis, and (3) stage I or II arthropathy as defined by the American Rheumatism Association (i.e., little or no bony involvement). It is contraindicated when significant narrowing of the joint space is present.

The three methods currently available to perform the synovial ablation are open synovectomy, arthroscopic synovectomy, and chemical or radiation synovectomy.

Open Synovectomy

Open synovectomy has been utilized for over 100 years. It allows a subtotal removal of the synovial lining of the knee and is easily performed. Despite its proven efficacy, open synovectomy has several drawbacks that have led to a decline in its usage. Most significantly, it is associated with a

risk of infection, hemarthrosis, and the potential for a permanent loss of joint motion. It requires a formal arthrotomy, necessitating hospitalization.

Technique

Traditionally, open synovectomy was performed via medial and lateral incisions to allow wide exposure of the joint. More recently, an anterior longitudinal skin incision with medial parapatellar arthrotomy has been the approach of choice, because future arthroplasty through this incision may easily be performed and wound healing complications are minimized. A subtotal synovectomy may easily be accomplished with standard orthopaedic instruments. The anterior synovium may often be removed en masse like the rind of an orange (Fig. 52-1). Debridement of the posterior recesses of the knee is difficult by open synovectomy.

Arthroscopic Synovectomy

Arthroscopic synovectomy has gained popularity since its initial results were reported in the 1980s.[9-12] The procedure has evolved quickly with the advent of specialized cameras and motorized instruments. The advantages of arthroscopic synovectomy include its very low risk of infection, hemarthrosis, and loss of motion.[9-12,21] In addition, a more complete debridement is possible than with open synovectomy. The procedure can be performed on an outpatient basis with high patient tolerance. Recent studies indicate that the results of arthroscopic synovectomy rival or exceed those of open synovectomy.[9-12]

Technique

Arthroscopic synovectomy is a technically demanding procedure. Standard portals are utilized initially; however, multiple other portals are usually necessary to allow a near complete removal of joint synovium. Motorized resecting instruments are generally employed.

Radiation and Chemical Synovectomy

Radiation synovectomy represents a potential alternative, nonsurgical means of ablating abnormal synovium. It is currently considered experimental. Attempts at chemical

---

TABLE 52-1 Disorders in Which Synovectomy Is Most Commonly Utilized

Rheumatoid arthritis
Rheumatoid variants associated with proliferative synovitis
Pigmented villonodular synovitis
Synovial chondromatosis and osteochondromatosis
Hemophilic synovitis
Infectious synovitis

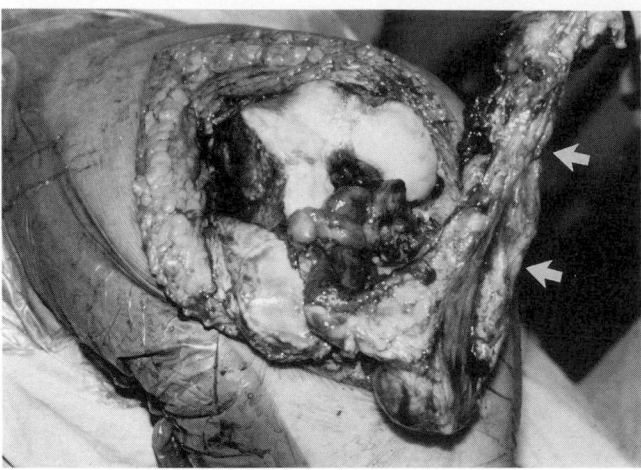

Figure 52-1 Open synovectomy. Rheumatoid synovium is picture being removed en masse from the knee *(arrows)*. Cartilaginous surfaces of the joint demonstrate near normal appearance.

synovectomy, by instillation of caustic alkylating agents such as osmic acid, have largely been abandoned because of the associated damage to articular cartilage. Radiocolloids have been used experimentally in recent years to achieve a complete synovial ablation. Potential advantages of the technique include its lack of surgical morbidity and high patient tolerance. Disadvantages include the potential carcinogenic risk both locally and systemically[22] and its as yet unproved nature. At present the

results of radiation synovectomy appear to be comparable to those of both open[23] and arthroscopic synovectomy.[24]

ARTHRODESIS

Arthrodesis is the creation of an immobile knee through surgical femorotibial bony fusion. The highly successful outcomes of alternative reconstructive procedures have presently relegated arthrodesis to a salvage procedure reserved for a small number of select patients (Fig. 52-2A and B). Orthopaedic surgeons must carefully consider a number of factors, including patient age, reasonable expectation of function, level of demand on the knee, and the various options available and their longevity prior to recommending arthrodesis. More often than not, other treatment modalities that preserve motion and provide satisfactory long-term results are available.

Rationale

It is well recognized that patients often reject arthrodesis despite appropriate indications. Nevertheless, successful arthrodesis creates a stable, pain-free knee that provides the patient with a durable and functional joint over many years. The primary disadvantage of arthrodesis is the abnormal gait following surgery. When surgery is performed correctly, patients are generally satisfied and often avoid subsequent surgeries altogether. In addition, the proce-

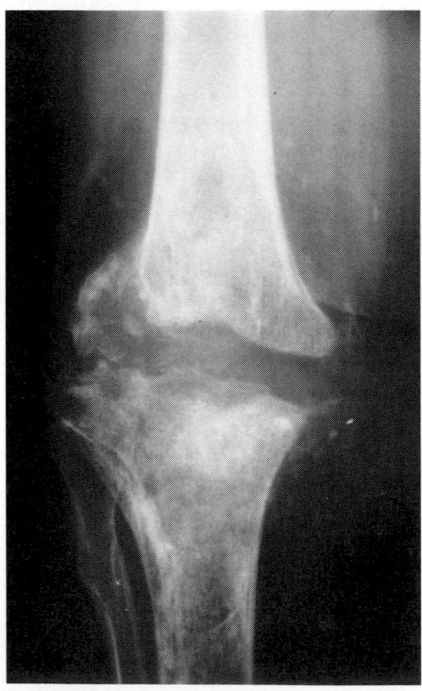

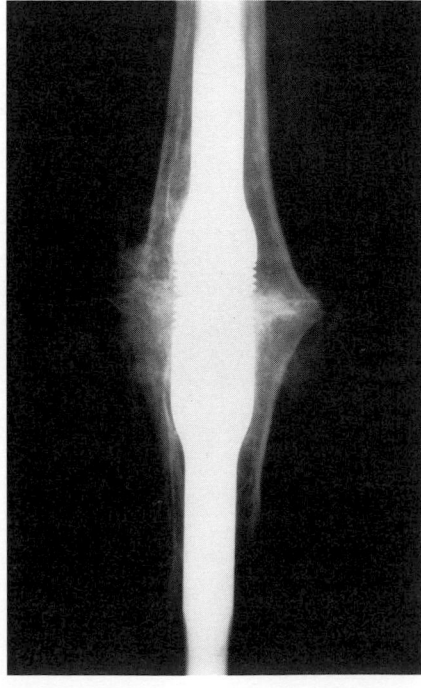

A *B*

Figure 52-2 *A.* Resection arthroplasty of an infected total knee arthroplasty following removal of components and bone loss. Loss of ligamentous structures yields an unstable knee that often requires bracing. *B.* Successful arthrodesis of the knee has been achieved using intramedullary fixation. Bone union is evident.

dure can be beneficial in eradicating sepsis of the knee that has proven recalcitrant to other means of treatment. The energy expenditure for ambulation is increased following athrodesis.[25]

Indications

The most common indication encountered today is a failed arthroplasty in a young, active individual, particularly when accompanied by severe ligamentous instability or infection. In such patients arthrodesis remains the treatment of choice. Attempts at prosthetic revision are ill advised and usually sentence the patient to multiple surgeries, predictable deterioration in results, and more difficult subsequent arthrodesis.

Septic arthritis is an indication for arthrodesis, particularly when multiple attempts at debridement have failed or when the infecting organism is particularly virulent. Long-term antibiotic toxicity or severely immunocompromised states strengthen the indication.

Painful ankylosis of the knee (defined as less than 20° of total motion) is often best treated by arthrodesis. Spontaneous ankylosis of the knee, as occurs in juvenile rheumatoid arthritis, may be considered for arthroplasty because such joints are often relatively pain-free, and motion-sacrificing procedures are contraindicated with involvement of multiple joints.[26,27]

Paralytic conditions such as poliomyelitis often lead to instability of the knee. While varus or valgus instability is often amenable to bracing, severe recurvatum deformities are difficult to brace adequately. This uncommon problem may be an indication for arthrodesis.

Painful Charcot or neuropathic arthropathy, while uncommon, remains an indication for arthrodesis, although achieving bony union may be difficult.[28] Painless joints may or may not be treatable by bracing. There are reports suggesting that arthroplasty may be a viable option; however, the long-term results are unknown.[29]

A deficient extensor mechanism or severe ligamentous incompetence is an indication for arthrodesis. Reconstruction of the extensor mechanism or collateral ligaments has been reported; however, the functional results and long-term outlook of such reconstructions remains unknown.[30]

Malignant or highly aggressive tumors about the knee may necessitate surgical arthrodesis if bone loss or soft tissue insufficiency obviates alternative reconstructive procedures. Rarely, malignant lesions may necessitate total removal of the extensor mechanism. Resultant knee function is often marginal and fusion of the knee provides a more functional extremity.

Contraindications

Contraindications to arthrodesis include ipsilateral hip or ankle disease, severe bone deficiency, and contralateral above-knee amputation or knee fusion.

Arthrodesis of the knee is contraindicated in the individual who may at some later date be considered for arthroplasty. Unlike hip arthrodesis, knee arthrodesis cannot be converted with any reliability to a functional arthroplasty, and complications are common.[31] Recent case reports suggest that at some future date, arthroplasty may be possible following arthrodesis.[32,33]

Technique

Numerous techniques have been utilized to perform arthrodesis. These may be categorized as (1) intramedullary rods,[34-38] (2) plate-and-screw constructs,[39,40] and (3) external fixators.[41-44]

Intramedullary Rod Fixation

Successful arthrodesis utilizing intramedullary rods has been achieved in between 66 and 100 percent of patients.[34-38] The advantages of these devices include rigidity of fixation, ability to bear weight immediately, and overall high patient tolerance. Disadvantages include extensive surgical time and blood loss, difficulty in achieving proper limb alignment, potential foreign material within infected tissue when used in septic knees, and the potential of rod migration, necessitating removal. Intramedullary rod fixation is currently the most effective means of achieving arthrodesis of the knee (Fig. 52-2B).

Plate-and-Screw Fixation

Plate-and-screw fixation has been utilized in the past; however, is not widely recommended at present. Distinct disadvantages include the extensive surgical exposure necessary and consequent tissue devitalization; the large amount of internal hardware required, serving as a potential infectious nidus; difficulty in soft tissue closure over internal hardware; and the inferior rigidity of plate-and-screw fixation as compared with intramedullary and external fixation.

External Fixation

External fixation is the technique of choice in the knee with active infection. Arthrodesis utilizing external frames has been reported to be successful in between 25 and 100 percent of patients.[41-45] Advantages include structural rigidity, ease of application and modification, and avoidance of foreign material within an infected bed. Disadvantages include pin-tract problems necessitating early frame removal, inability to bear weight fully, poor patient tolerance, and long treatment time.

Whatever the technique used, the surgeon should aim to achieve a final alignment of full extension in the sagittal plane and 7° of valgus in the coronal plane. Some have recommended slight flexion of the knee; however, this position tends to functionally shorten the extremity, which has often lost significant length already.

Complications

The most commonly cited complications of arthrodesis of the knee include painful fibrous ankylosis, material failure of implanted hardware, femoral or tibial fractures following arthrodesis, and patient dissatisfaction with gait anomalies and the lack of motion.

RESECTION ARTHROPLASTY

Resection arthroplasty involves debridement of the articular surfaces of the knee or removal of prosthetic implants with maintenance of some motion. Resection arthroplasty may achieve spontaneous arthrodesis in certain cases. Resection arthroplasty has a limited role in the treatment of knee disorders. At the present time it is utilized primarily as a temporary treatment of infected arthroplasty prior to attempted reimplantation of prosthetic components. As a definitive procedure, resection arthroplasty is limited to those individuals who are minimal ambulators or nonambulators prior to implant removal, patients with life-threatening sepsis of the knee, or those with severe rheumatoid arthritis and polyarticular involvement.[46,47]

Resection arthroplasty consists of thorough joint debridement and removal of articular cartilage or implanted devices followed by maintenance of the extremity in a weight-bearing cast for prolonged periods to allow fibrous stabilization of the articulation.[48]

Function following resection arthroplasty is often marked by chronic pain and instability.[48–50] In general, all patients should expect to require walking aids postoperatively, and over two-thirds will need braces.[48]

ARTHROSCOPIC DEBRIDEMENT

Arthroscopic debridement is a procedure advocated for mild arthrosis with or without concurrent mechanical derangement or crystalline-induced inflammation. The precise role of arthroscopic debridement in the treatment of the arthritic knee has been debated since Jackson reported symptomatic improvement following arthroscopic lavage of arthritic knees in 1974.[51] Later reports have confirmed the beneficial effects of arthroscopic debridement; however, the results have often been neither predictable nor long-lasting.[52–55] In general, arthroscopic debridement will provide relief of symptoms in approximately 50 to 70 percent of patients in short-term follow-up.[51–55] The placebo effect of the procedure is unknown.

Rationale

At present, arthroscopic lavage may be recommended as a palliative procedure to relieve the pain associated with early arthritis.[56,57] Proponents of the procedure feel that lavage of the arthritic joint removes inflammatory mediators and arthritic debris, which contribute to pain. No long-term beneficial effect on joint degeneration has been demonstrated. The advantages of the procedure include its low morbidity, high patient tolerance, and its provision of direct access to intraarticular pathology such as loose bodies and meniscal tears, which can cause mechanical symptoms. The disadvantages of the procedure include its unpredictable duration of symptomatic relief following debridement, particularly in poorly selected patients.

Indications

The ideal candidate for arthroscopic debridement is a young individual with mild degenerative joint disease in whom one wishes to delay more extensive surgery.[56,57] Patients with a short duration of discomfort, early degenerative changes on radiographs and on arthroscopic inspection, symptoms secondary to mechanical derangement, and acute onset of crystalline-induced inflammation appear to respond most reliably to arthroscopic debridement.[57,58] Patients with advanced arthritis, a long duration of symptoms, or malalignment of the knee often fail to obtain relief.[55,57,59,60]

Technique

The technique of arthroscopic debridement is relatively straightforward. Visualization and instrumentation are carried out via routine anterior arthroscopic portals. Alternate portals may be utilized if needed to access regions of the knee not accessible by anterior ones. Attempts should be made to debride any obvious mechanical impediments or loose bodies within the joint and to irrigate the knee copiously. Wide synovectomy and abrasion chondroplasty are of no benefit and should be avoided.[60,61]

Complications

Arthroscopic debridement is associated with a very low rate of wound infection, thromboembolic disease, and arthrofibrosis. Occasionally, there is early recurrence of pain, but this is difficult to predict.

DISTAL FEMORAL OSTEOTOMY

Distal femoral osteotomy is a procedure designed to address valgus deformity with lateral gonarthrosis. Because degenerative genu valgum with isolated lateral gonarthrosis is far less common than degenerative genu varum, there are few studies in the literature from which to draw clearcut conclusions regarding the outcomes of varus femoral osteotomy.

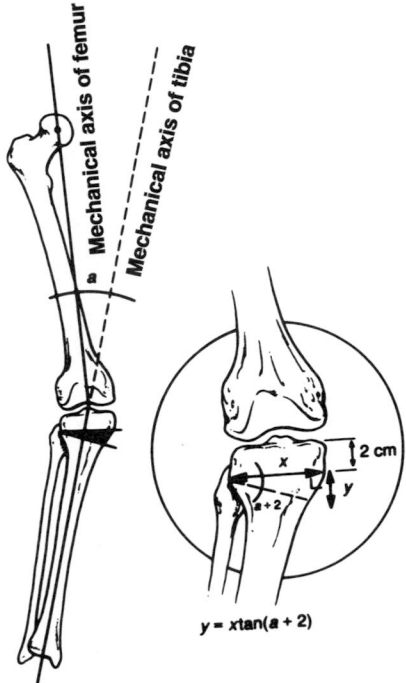

Figure 52-3 Tibial varus osteotomy. Planning-procedure operative tracings based on full-length standing radiographs can be used to calculate a wedge that shifts the mechanical axis to a point just medial to the medial spine (in this case angle "a" plus 2°). (From Murray PB, Rand JA: Symptomatic valgus knee: The surgical options. © 1993, American Academy of Orthopaedic Surgeons. Reprinted from the *Journal of the American Academy of Orthopaedic Surgeons* 1:3 1993, with permission.)

Rationale

Femoral osteotomy is favored over tibial osteotomy because lateral compartmental arthritis is often accompanied by erosion of the lateral femoral condyle, which accentuates the anatomic valgus of the distal femur while maintaining the normal tibial orientation. A medially based osteotomy of the tibia will result in a joint line that is oriented obliquely with respect to the ground. This obliquity, in turn, leads to femorotibial shear during weight bearing, which causes eventual lateral tibial subluxation and progressive arthrosis.

Proximal tibial varus osteotomy, however, may be utilized for a valgus knee deformity (tibiofemoral angle of 12° or less) if preoperative planning (Fig. 52-3) confirms that the final obliquity of the joint line will be less than 10°. Distal femoral osteotomy performed proximal to the joint will avoid any possibility of resultant joint-line obliquity and therefore decrease the likelihood of premature failure of the surgery (Fig. 52-4*A* and *B*).

Indications

The ideal candidate for distal femoral varus osteotomy is a relatively young individual with isolated lateral unicompartmental arthritis and modest activity demands. Patients should have exhausted all means of conservative management, including nonsteroidal anti-inflammatory drugs, use of canes or crutches, and activity modification. Most authorities reserve osteotomy for the individual below 60

Figure 52-4 *A.* Lateral femorotibial arthrosis with valgus alignment of the knee. The joint space has been maintained medially, allowing for realignment osteotomy. *B.* Postoperative view of the knee following distal femoral valgus osteotomy. A blade plate is used to achieve rigid fixation of the osteotomy.

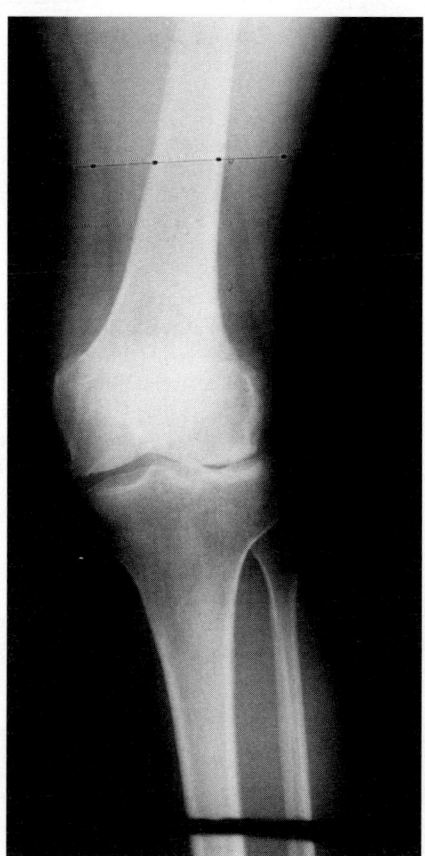

A

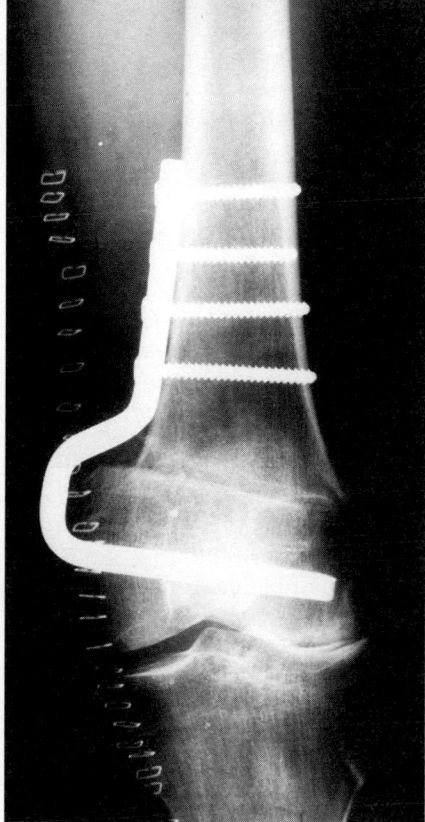

B

years of age, while older individuals are offered arthroplasty. Treatment must be individualized, however, and is based upon factors including the patient's activity level, weight, bone stock, and physician preference.

No specific criteria exist regarding the ideal weight or activity levels suited for osteotomy. Excess weight or activity will potentially cause premature failure of any reconstructive surgery. Many knee surgeons feel that because osteotomy is extraarticular in nature, conversion to an arthroplasty may be performed later, if necessary. For this reason, osteotomy may be preferable in the heavy or highly active patient. To date, there are no long-term studies that document the relative ease of conversion or the durability of total joint arthroplasty following failed distal femoral osteotomy.

Adequate bone stock is a prerequisite for performing osteotomy. Loss of correction has been reported as high as 35 percent[62–64] following distal femoral osteotomy. It is imperative, then, that bone quality be sufficient to maintain internal fixation. Severe osteoporosis is a contraindication to femoral osteotomy.

Slight arthritic involvement of the medial tibiofemoral compartment or of the patellofemoral articulation may be permitted; however, any significant chondral degeneration or exposure of bone within these compartments necessitates total joint replacement. Arthritis secondary to inflammatory, systemic, or crystalline deposition disorders is a contraindication to performing osteotomy regardless of apparent unicompartmental involvement.[65–68]

Stiffness of the knee is a relative contraindication to performing a femoral osteotomy. Most authorities recommend that patients have less than 10° of fixed flexion contracture (which is uncommon in the valgus knee) and that there be more than 90° of flexion. Valgus deformities often exhibit a some degree of recurvatum; in such cases, the varus osteotomy may be combined with slight flexion to optimize the final range of motion.[69]

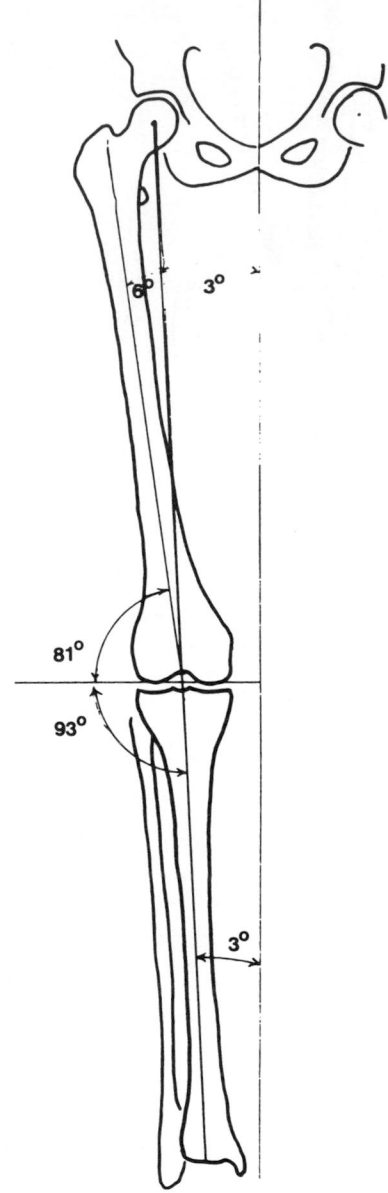

Figure 52-5 A normal limb showing a mechanical axis extending from the center of the femoral head through the medial tibial spine and ending at the center of the ankle; also a tibiofemoral angle of 6° and an inclination of the tibia 3° off from vertical. (Reproduced with permission from Teitge R: Preoperative planning for osteotomy of the proximal tibia. *Semin Arthrop* 7:132, 1996.)

Anatomic and Mechanical Axes

The mechanical axis of the lower limb is described by a line drawn from the center of the femoral head to the center of the ankle joint (talus). This axis usually falls directly through the center of the medial intercondylar tibial spine. The angle between the mechanical axis of the femur and that of the tibia is usually 0°. This mechanical axis is usually at an angle of around 3° to the vertical, since the lower limb inclines slightly medially (Fig. 52-5). Although the axis of the tibial shaft inclines slightly medially, the articular surfaces of both the tibia and femur are horizontal at the knee. The tibiofemoral valgus angle is the angle between the anatomic axis of the femoral and tibial shafts and is around 6° of valgus.

The knee indicated for femoral varus osteotomy should exhibit at least 15° of tibiofemoral valgus and more than 6° of valgus tilt of the joint line (from the horizontal).[70,71] Less than 10° tibiofemoral valgus or transverse orientation of the joint line may still be effectively treated

by femoral osteotomy; however, many experts would suggest that a proximal tibial varus osteotomy is more appropriate in these selected cases.

Subluxation and instability of the femorotibial articulation are considered contraindications to osteotomy. A subluxation of greater than 1 cm is considered by many to represent the limit of acceptability, while others feel that any subluxation whatsoever is unacceptable.

Preoperative Planning

The optimum amount of correction is not known. A final alignment of 0 to 2° of tibiofemoral valgus is believed preferable. Full-length lower extremity films are necessary to template planned bone removal. The anatomic axis is determined using the film. The final anatomic weight-bearing axis should move slightly onto the uninvolved medial side once the osteotomy has been performed. Templates should calculate the final anatomic axis of the limb to lie slightly medial to the tibial spines (Fig. 52-6).

Technique

Several techniques have been described for carrying out varus femoral osteotomy. A medial-based closing wedge osteotomy is commonly utilized with blade-plate fixation (Fig. 52-4B). The use of stepped staples is inadequate to provide secure fixation.[71] A medial longitudinal incision is used. Fluoroscopy is used to confirm that the precise amount of templated bone is removed and that the hardware is appropriately placed. Steinmann pins are used as guides. The lateral cortex and periosteum are left inviolate during bone removal to enhance fixation once the osteotomy has been closed down. A blade plate is used to maintain the correction.

Results

The results of distal femoral osteotomy are documented by a few limited series. Healy et al. and McDermott et al. describe 83 and 88 percent satisfactory results, respectively, at an average of 4 years follow-up.[62,72] Edgerton and associates have found a 71 percent satisfactory result at an average of 8 years.[63] It appears that correction of between 0 and 2° of final valgus offers the best chance of a successful outcome.

Complications

Distal femoral osteotomy is a technically demanding procedure. Nonunion and delayed union occur in between 5 and 10 percent of osteotomies regardless of the type of fix-

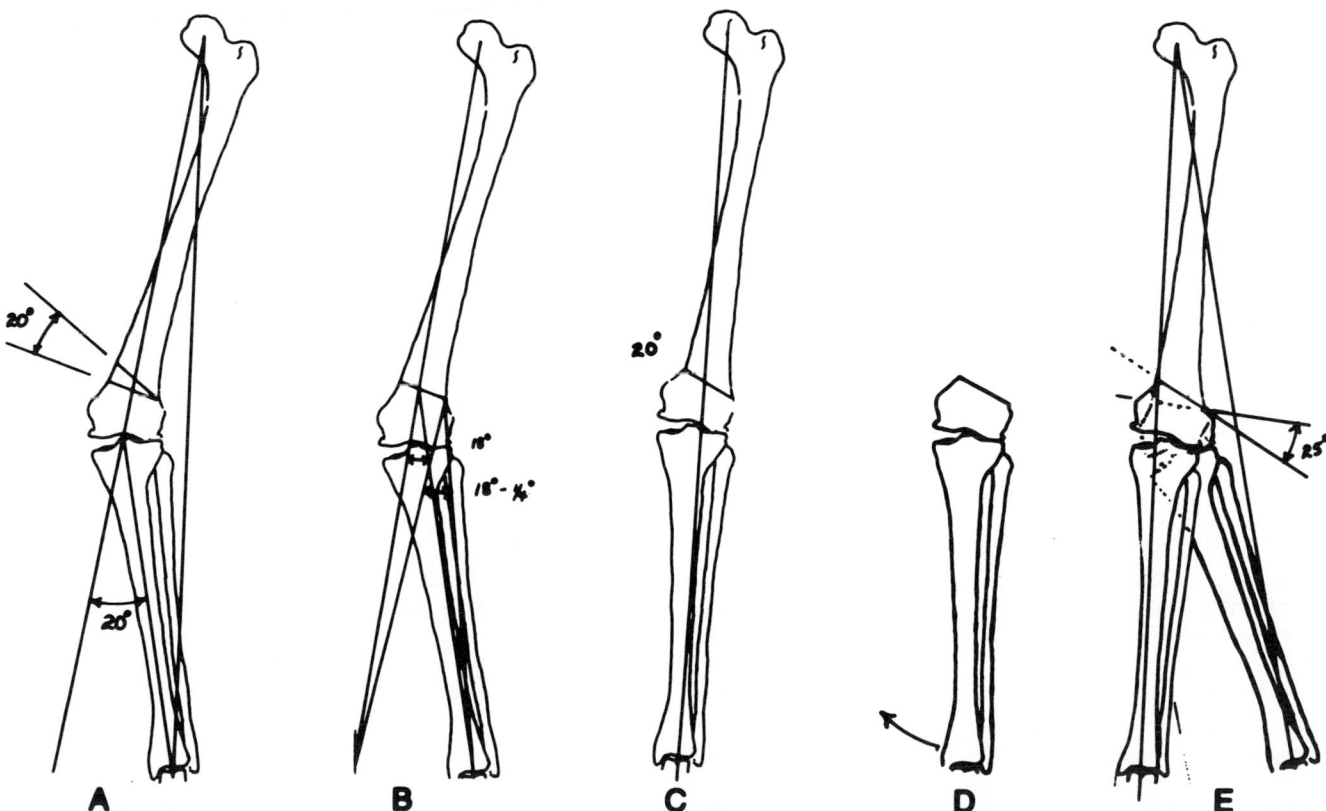

Figure 52-6 Preoperative planning for distal femoral varus osteotomy. Because the center of the knee joint rotates more medially as the wedge is closed, it is necessary to keep a straight edge along the continually changing mechanical axis until the desired correction is obtained. *A.* Twenty degrees of tibiofemoral valgus is measured. *B* and *C.* After 20° of correction, the mechanical axis still falls in the lateral compartment. *D.* Rotation of this segment about the apex of the wedge continues. *E.* Finally, at 25°, a satisfactory new mechanical axis for the limb is established. (Reproduced with permission from Teitge R: Supracondylar osteotomy for lateral compartment osteoarthritis. *Semin Arthop* 7:197, 1996.)

ation used.[62,63,72] Limitation of motion may occur, and early mobilization and motion is encouraged. A low incidence of thromboembolic, neurovascular, and infectious complications associated with distal femoral osteotomy has been documented.

PROXIMAL TIBIAL OSTEOTOMY

Proximal tibial osteotomy was initially developed by Jackson in the 1950s to address medial compartmental osteoarthritis[73,74] and later popularized by Coventry.[75–79] While the development of total knee arthroplasty has eliminated the need for osteotomy in older and more sedentary individuals, it remains a useful operation in young, active individuals with isolated medial compartmental arthritis.

A majority of patients with degenerative arthritis of the knee demonstrate early involvement of the medial compartment with relative sparing of the lateral compartment and patellofemoral articulation. Loss of cartilage leads to a resultant varus alignment of the knee during stance. This varus alignment shifts the limb's weight-bearing axis, with progressively more load being borne in the medial compartment. These loads accelerate the medial wear and lead to worsening varus. Thus a cycle ensues resulting in severe arthritis of the medial compartment with relative sparing of the remainder of the knee.

Rationale

The rationale behind proximal tibial osteotomy is to realign the weight-bearing axis from varus to slightly valgus. The osteotomy produces a shift of the axis laterally into the uninvolved lateral compartment and a reduction in the medial-sided pain. Progressive arthritis of the lateral and patellofemoral compartments may occur with time. Most surgeons are willing to accept this decline in result with the expectation that total knee arthroplasty may be performed at a later time, when the patient's age and activity level are more compatible with arthroplasty.

Indications

The primary indication (Table 52-2) for proximal tibial osteotomy is a relatively young or highly active individual with isolated varus gonarthrosis who wishes to continue an active lifestyle. Most authorities recommend the procedure to individuals below 60 years of age, while older individuals are generally offered total or unicompartmental knee replacement. Cases must be individualized based upon the patient's lifestyle as well as surgeon preference.

Patients should demonstrate less than 10° of fixed flexion of the knee and greater than 90° of active flexion.

Mild lateral compartment osteoarthritis and moderate patellofemoral involvement can be tolerated. Severe change involving either of these compartments is a strict contraindication to tibial osteotomy.

Relative contraindications include subluxation of the tibiofemoral articulation, more than 1 cm of medial bone loss, insufficiency of the anterior cruciate ligament, or incompetence of the medial collateral ligament. The procedure may still be indicated in select individuals.[80]

Preoperative Planning

Planning of the procedure requires a careful physical examination of the knee and proper preoperative radiographs. The patient must demonstrate a mild varus deformity that is passively correctable and should not demonstrate a significant lateral thrust during gait. The medial collateral ligament must be competent.

Preoperative radiographs should include a weight-bearing AP and lateral, and a skyline view to confirm isolated medial compartmental gonarthrosis. A 3-ft standing AP view of the entire extremity should be obtained. The mechanical axis (represented by a line passing from the center of the femoral head to the center of the ankle mortise) will pass through or medial to the medial compartment of the knee.

TABLE 52-2   Indications for Proximal Tibial Osteotomy versus Total Knee Arthroplasty

	Proximal tibial osteotomy	Total knee arthroplasty
Age	<60 years	Any age
Patient characteristics	Heavy or physically active	Ideal weight, relatively sedentary
Arthritic involvement	Unicompartmental medial femorotibial arthritis	Uni-, bi-, or tricompartmental arthritis
Arthritic nature	Degenerative arthritis (idiopathic or posttraumatic arthritis, avascular necrosis, etc.)	Degenerative or inflammatory arthritides
Range of motion	<10° flexion contracture >90° total flexion	Any range of motion

Although many techniques have been described for performing the realignment of the extremity,[81–85,85a] the laterally based closing wedge osteotomy above the level of the tibial tubercle remains the most often employed. Templating x-rays will allow one to determine the appropriate size of the wedge to be removed. The final alignment should create an 8 to 12° degree valgus alignment. The templated mechanical axis should pass through the lateral compartment approximately one-third of the distance between the tibial spines and the peripheral edge of the lateral tibial plateau.[86,87]

To template preoperatively, the planned postoperative mechanical axis is drawn from the center of the femoral head through a point at the knee joint one-third of the distance between tibial spine and the lateral tibial plateau. A second line is drawn from the ankle center along the tibial diaphysis to the medial tibial metaphysis approximately 2 cm below the joint. Finally, a third line connects the mechanical axis at the level of the ankle joint to the point where the second line touches the medial tibial metaphysis. The angle between the second and third lines represents the angle of the osteotomy wedge.

Technique

Surgery is performed with the patient supine. A horizontal lateral transverse incision is commonly used because it will allow future conversion to a total knee arthroplasty with minimal risk of postoperative wound slough. After adequate exposure, a wedge of bone is removed from the lateral side of the proximal tibia several centimeters below the joint line. The proper bony resection will have been templated. The wedge osteotomy may be carried out in freehand fashion or using instrumentation. The medial tibial cortex represents the apex of the bony wedge and should be left intact.

Bone resection may be carried out utilizing either an oscillating saw or sharp osteotomes. Osteotomes may be preferable because they avoid the thermal necrosis of bone associated with the oscillating saw.

Fixation of the osteotomy may be carried out utilizing cast immobilization, stepped staples, or plate-and-screw constructs. The author's preference is for stepped staples. A cylinder cast may be utilized even with internal fixation to protect the fixation. Loss of knee motion is uncommon secondary to cast immobilization if the joint is left inviolate. Some surgeons prefer rigid internal fixation and early mobilization.

A variety of other, less commonly employed techniques such as dome osteotomies, oblique osteotomies, and opening wedge osteotomies have been described[86]; however, none have proven superior to closing wedge osteotomies in final results.

Results

The results of proximal tibial osteotomy support its role as a procedure that provides good function and pain relief. Because it is appropriate for patients who are considered too young for arthroplasty, most surgeons perform proximal tibial osteotomy as a temporizing measure. It should be recognized that there is a decline in satisfactory results with time and that therefore many patients will eventually require conversion to a total knee arthroplasty.

The results clearly depend upon a number of factors, including patient age, weight, activity demands, and proper correction of limb alignment at the time of surgery.

The procedure has less satisfying results in the severely overweight patient.[79] It is felt that obesity leads to excessive force transmission across the knee with a more rapid deterioration in result. Young, active patients may experience premature failure for similar reasons.

The angular correction necessary to achieve optimal results has not been clearly established. Slight overcorrection of the limb appears to correlate with the best long-term results.[88–95] As previously stated, 8 to 12° of final valgus may be optimal.

The published data indicate that a majority of patients may expect 5 to 10 years of satisfactory function[96–99] if the patient characteristics are ideal and postoperative alignment objectives are achieved. A review by Coventry et al. indicates that the procedure may reliably yield very good results for more than a decade.[79]

Complications

Most of the complications of proximal tibial osteotomy result from errors in surgical technique. Careful attention to detail will help to minimize these problems.

The most common complication of proximal tibial osteotomy is inadequate valgus correction at the time of surgery. Various studies document a high incidence of undercorrection.[78–80,86] Most authorities advocate a correction of the tibiofemoral angle to between 8 and 14° of valgus. In other words, a slight increase in the normal alignment of 6° of tibiofemoral valgus appears optimal. Healy and Riley have reported good results in patients corrected to the anatomic axis.[100]

Overcorrection of the osteotomy is uncommon but may lead to poor results. Overcorrection generally results from an overestimation of the true bony deformity due to attenuation of the lateral collateral ligament. Overcorrection leads to poor results because of mechanical patellofemoral derangement (lateral patellar subluxation and patella baja) and overload of the lateral femorotibial compartment (with premature progression of arthrosis). The unappealing cosmetic result associated with overcorrection may lead to patient dissatisfaction despite a satisfactory functional result.

If the osteotomy is performed too close to the joint line or if the apex of the bony wedge does not approximate the medial cortex, an intraarticular fracture may occur when the osteotomy site is closed. To minimize the risk of this complication, the proximal osteotomy should be kept at least 2 cm distal to the joint line.

Avascular necrosis of the tibial plateau is an uncommon complication of proximal tibial osteotomy. Assuring that the osteotomy is appropriately made 2 cm distal to the joint line will help to avoid this complication. It may be helpful to minimize soft tissue dissection about the proximal tibia.

Vascular injuries are fortunately rare complications. Injury most commonly involves the anterior tibial artery. Excessive surgical dissection or internal fixation devices are often to blame. Injury to the popliteal artery has been reported.[101]

Anterior compartment syndrome may occur following proximal tibial osteotomy.[102,103] It may result from postoperative bleeding, particularly when tight circumferential dressings or casts are used. Careful attention to achieving hemostasis, avoiding injury to the anterior tibial artery, use of postoperative suction drainage, and application of loose dressings will prevent this serious complication.

Nerve injury, in particular peroneal nerve palsy, is always a risk when a proximal tibial osteotomy is performed. With fibular osteotomy, the incidence of complications including nerve injuries has been reported to be as high as 14 percent.[86,104,105] For this reason, fibular osteotomy has generally been abandoned. Disarticulation of the proximal tibiofibular joint or fibular head resection under direct observation is currently recommended as a means of protecting the peroneal nerve. Casts and tight circumferential dressings should be used judiciously to minimize the possibility of compression neuropraxia.

Delayed union and nonunion of the osteotomy occur in a small number of cases. Most delayed unions will unite if immobilization is maintained long enough and internal fixation is secure. Prevention of nonunion is minimized by preservation of the medial periosteum (to enhance security of the osteotomy), utilization of secure lateral-sided fixation, creation of broad, flat osteotomy cuts that oppose one another maximally, and avoidance of thermal bone necrosis secondary to the use of high-speed power saws.

Conclusion

Proximal tibial osteotomy is an appropriate procedure for the young, active patient presenting with unicompartmental medial arthrosis and varus deformity. It is easily performed and may provide years of satisfactory function when performed well. There are a number of complications associated with the procedure which generally result from errors in surgical technique.

UNICOMPARTMENTAL KNEE REPLACEMENT

Unicompartmental knee arthroplasty is used to treat unicompartmental femorotibial arthrosis by replacing only the arthritic compartment and preserving the contralateral and patellofemoral articulations. The indications for unicompartmental prosthetic replacement have been evolving for some time. The initial unicondylar prostheses were introduced by McKeever and MacIntosh in the early 1950s.[106,107] These prostheses were metallic interpositional devices inserted into the arthritic compartment without cement.[107–109] The first cemented metal-on-polyethylene unicompartmental knee prosthesis was introduced by Marmor in 1972. Despite nearly 25 years of experience, the role of unicompartmental knee replacement continues to be debated.

Rationale

Unicompartmental knee replacement remains somewhat controversial owing to the disparity of reported results. Many reports suggest good initial and long-term results,[110–115] while others have been less encouraging.[116–119] Most authorities agree that periarticular osteotomies are appropriate for the "younger" patient with unicompartmental disease, while total knee arthroplasty is indicated in the older patient with bi- or tricompartmental arthritis. Unicompartmental knee arthroplasty appears to be indicated in the older patient who has limitation of arthritis to a single compartment (Table 52-3).

Proponents of the unicompartmental knee replacement point out that the procedure has several advantages over osteotomies and total knee replacement. Compared with osteotomies, unicompartmental arthroplasty has higher initial success and fewer early complications.[114,120–122] Weale's results imply that the long-term re-

---

TABLE 52-3 Indications for Unicompartmental Knee Arthroplasty versus Total Knee Arthroplasty

	Unicompartmental knee arthroplasty	Total knee arthroplasty
Age	>60 years	Any age
Patient characteristics	Ideal or light body habitus, sedentary	Any weight, any activity level
Arthritic involvement	Unicompartmental medial or lateral femorotibial arthritis	Uni-, bi-, or tricompartmental arthritis
Arthritic nature	Degenerative arthritis (idiopathic or posttraumatic arthritis, avascular necrosis, etc.)	Degenerative or inflammatory arthritides
Range of motion	<15° flexion contracture >90° total flexion	Any range of motion

sults may be better as well.[123] In addition, because only one compartment is resurfaced, bone stock is preserved, potentially making future revision to total knee arthroplasty easier. Since the anterior and posterior cruciate ligaments are preserved, knee mechanics and proprioceptive appreciation are more natural than following total knee arthroplasty.[124,125]

Indications

Unicompartmental knee replacement is most appropriate in the older, lighter, sedentary patient. Most surgeons reserve the procedure for individuals with a physiologic age greater than 60 years who weigh less than 200 lb (Fig. 52-7*A, B,* and C). Younger, heavy or active patients appear to

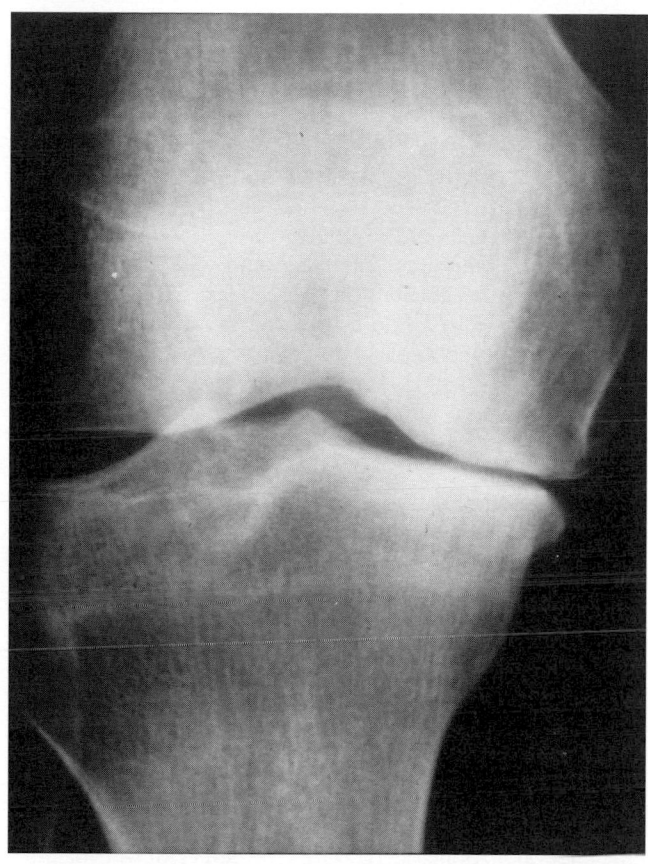

A

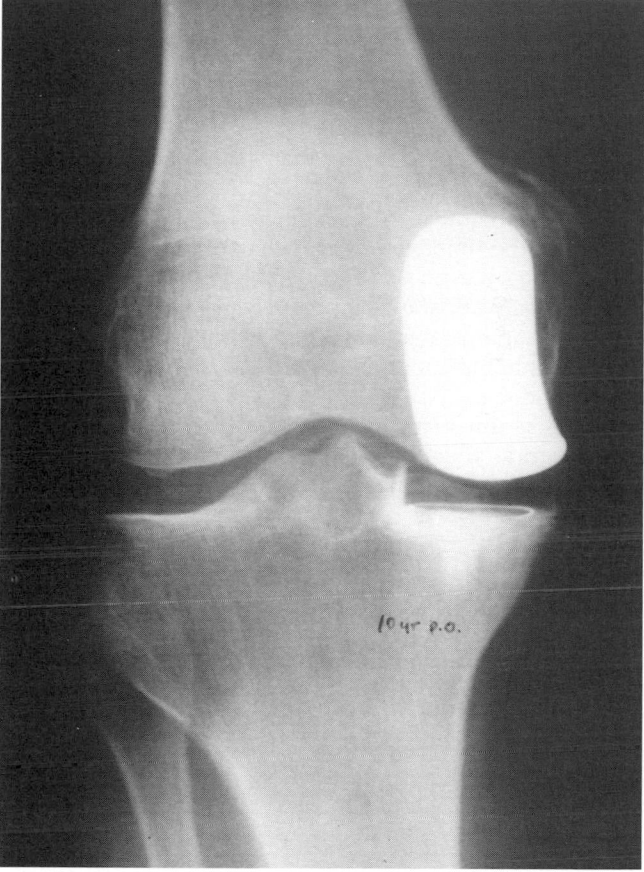

C

Figure 52-7 *A.* Unicompartmental medial femorotibial arthritis in an elderly patient. *B.* Intraoperative view of the knee demonstrates the arthritic medial femoral condyle. *C.* Postoperative view of medial unicompartmental knee replacement 10 years following arthroplasty. There has been no significant progression of lateral arthritis and the arthroplasty is functioning well.

B

be better served by either osteotomies or total knee arthroplasty.[126]

The procedure is appropriate for unicompartmental disease resulting from osteoarthritis, osteonecrosis, or traumatic causes. The procedure may be indicated in knees with mild changes of chondromalacia of the contralateral tibiofemoral or patellofemoral articulations; however, severe cartilage degeneration or exposed subchondral bone warrants total knee replacement.

Patients should demonstrate an adequate range of motion preoperatively. Most surgeons limit the procedure to individuals with less than a 15° flexion contracture and greater than 90° of active flexion.

Deformity in the coronal plane can be accepted if it is moderate. Unicompartmental knee replacement can be performed in knees with less than 10° of varus or 15° of valgus preoperatively provided that these deformities are passively correctable to physiologic alignment. Any subluxation of the tibiofemoral articulation is a contraindication to surgery even with acceptable coronal alignment. This is usually apparent on preoperative radiographs but may not be appreciated until the time of surgery, when tibial spine impingement is noted on the intracondylar femoral surface.

Because unicompartmental knee replacement reproduces normal knee kinematics, ligamentous stability is necessary for long-term success. Insufficiency of the anterior cruciate ligament or significant imbalance of the collateral ligament contraindicates unicompartmental replacement.

Inflammatory or crystalline deposition arthropathies are contraindications to unicompartmental knee replacement. Studies have shown inferior results than when such disorders are treated with tricompartmental prosthetic replacement.[126]

Technique

The superficial dissection is similar to that of total knee arthroplasty. Exposure can be achieved either through a midline anterior, subvastus, or lateral approach. Care is taken during initial exposure to protect the anterior cruciate ligament and anterior meniscal attachment of the contralateral compartment. The intact cartilagenous surfaces should be kept moist to prevent their desiccation during the procedure.

The joint should demonstrate near-normal articular cartilage in the contralateral and patellofemoral articulations. In addition, the anterior cruciate ligament should be intact. Note is made of any cartilaginous erosion on the medial aspect of the lateral femoral condyle secondary to tibial spine impingement. When present, this is an early sign of lateral tibiofemoral subluxation. If the erosion is small, unicompartmental arthroplasty can be performed. If the erosion is large, significant lateral subluxation exists and total knee arthroplasty should be performed instead.

Distal femoral bone resection should be minimal. Excessive removal of the normally dense subchondral bone may predispose to subsidence of the femoral component. In addition, conversion to total knee arthroplasty later is made more difficult by excessive resection of bone. The femoral component must resurface most of the eburnated bone present. It is imperative to position the component so that the anterior flange is slightly recessed below the surface of the remaining cartilage, so as to prevent patellar impingement during knee flexion.

The coronal alignment should strive for reconstitution of the patient's anatomic alignment. This will allow more balanced loading of the femorotibial articulations and prevent overloading of the uninvolved compartment, which can result in progressive arthrosis. Various guides are available to aid in determining the angle of resection of the distal femoral condyle.

The tibial resection should be parallel to the distal femoral cut. In general, 8 to 10 mm of proximal tibial bone is resected during its preparation, and the anatomic joint line is reconstructed. The angle of resection is perpendicular to the long axis of the tibia.

With the components in place and with proper coronal alignment, the normal joint line is recreated in flexion and extension. Care should be taken to avoid excessive posterior bone resection, as this can lead to anterior placement of the femoral component or to instability of the knee in flexion.

If adjustments cannot be made to achieve proper alignment, soft tissue balance, and component positioning, the unicompartmental arthroplasty should be abandoned and total knee arthroplasty performed instead.

Postoperative rehabilitation for unicompartmental knee arthroplasty is similar to that for total knee arthroplasty.

Results

Controversy continues with regard to the long-term durability of unicompartmental replacement as compared to total knee arthroplasty. To date, the survivorship of unicompartmental arthroplasty is lower than that of total knee arthroplasty.[124,125,127–129] Marmor in 1988 reported satisfactory results in only 63 percent of patients followed for 10 to 13 years.[112] He noted that most failures were attributable to excessively thin tibial components, which are generally not used at present. Only 2 of 56 patients required conversion to total knee replacement for progression of arthrosis.

Scott reports somewhat more encouraging results, with a 91 percent survival at 9 years.[115] He predicts an accelerated drop in survivorship following the 10th year, with only 82 percent survivorship expected at 11 years. Other studies agree that the failure rate of unicompartmental replacements is slightly greater than 1 percent per year over the 10 years following surgery.[110,118,130,131]

Proponents of unicompartmental arthroplasty point out that long-term studies are compromised by patients who are no longer considered candidates for the procedure by current standards.[112,126] Modern surgical technique, improved instrumentation, more durable implants, and exacting patient selection may lead to long-term results that are comparable to those of total knee arthroplasty.

Complications

Patellar impingement on the anterior edge of the femoral component is a common complication of unicompartmental replacement. It occurs secondary to inadequate recession of the femoral prosthesis below the surface of the surrounding cartilage. Care should be taken during insertion of the final component to see that patellar tracking is smooth and free of impingement.

Pes anserine bursitis has been estimated to occur in 13 percent of patients following surgery. The presentation of bursitis is often similar to that of failed arthroplasty and care must be taken in identifying that precise etiology of the pain.

Arthritic degeneration of the unresurfaced compartments is low if appropriate coronal alignment is created. Most series report less than 10 percent failure due to progression of arthrosis.

Component loosening, neurovascular injuries, thrombophlebitis, and postoperative infections are reported complications of unicompartmental arthroplasty; however, their incidence appears to be low. The high failure rates in early series were often the result of poor patient selection, improper surgical technique, and deficiencies in prosthetic designs.

Summary

In conclusion, despite over 20 years of experience with unicompartmental knee arthroplasty, the precise role of the procedure continues to evolve. The long-term durability remains less predictable than that of total knee arthroplasty. However, survivorship analysis demonstrate results that appear to be improving.

TOTAL KNEE ARTHROPLASTY

Approximately 130,000 total knee replacements are performed every year in the United States. The indications for this procedure, surgical technique, and issues regarding alignment, soft tissue balance, component orientation, and outcome analysis have been standardized to a large degree. Overall, the results of total knee arthroplasty have proved highly satisfying on long-term review.

Indications

The indications for total knee replacement have changed very little in recent years. In general, patients presenting with pain not relieved by conservative means and with radiographic evidence of severe arthritis are candidates for the procedure. The ideal patient is elderly, modestly active, and of ideal body weight. He or she should have disabling pain, especially with activity, but often including night or rest pain as well. The associated disability should limit the patient in carrying out the activities needed to maintain a satisfying lifestyle. Any candidate should have

exhausted all nonsurgical means of managing the pain, including the use of nonsteroidal anti-inflammatory medications, employment of a cane or crutches, physical therapy, occasional intraarticular steroid injections, and activity modification.

The indications for total knee arthroplasty include severe bi- or tricompartmental gonarthrosis. Patients with rheumatoid arthritis or other inflammatory arthritides are considered candidates for arthroplasty even at a young age. Patients with failed periarticular osteotomies and posttraumatic arthritis are also candidates.

Relative contraindications to total knee replacement include a physiologically young age, severe obesity, or a highly active lifestyle. The excellent long-term results of total knee arthroplasty published in recent years have demonstrated satisfactory results even with these conditions, and arthroplasty is increasingly performed despite these relative contraindications. Such patients must be forewarned that they are at increased risk for premature failure of the procedure and may well require subsequent revision surgery.

A history of prior osteomyelitis about the knee is a relative contraindication, although good results have been reported.[132] Preoperative workup must fail to show any evidence of ongoing subclinical infection.

Other relative contraindications include severe peripheral vascular disease or any medical condition that may seriously risk the patient's ability to withstand the surgery.

Strict Contraindications

Active sepsis of the knee, with the possible exception of tuberculous infection,[133] is an absolute contraindication to total knee arthroplasty. As previously noted, remote sepsis about the knee may not preclude performance of arthroplasty provided that clinical, laboratory, and radiographic workup does not demonstrate ongoing infection.

Solid, painless surgical arthrodesis remains a contraindication for conversion to total knee replacement. Despite reports of successful conversion to arthroplasty[134,135] of surgically or spontaneously fused knees, the surgery is not recommended, as the soft tissue scarring will necessitate insertion of highly constrained devices that are at high risk of loosening. In addition, many patients fail to regain functional motion. Rearthrodesis of a failed constrained device often fails.

Significant genu recurvatum, as seen in long-standing paralytic knee dysfunction (e.g., polio myelitis) or rheumatoid arthritis contraindicates arthroplasty. Unconstrained devices are ineffective in eliminating the deformity; therefore constrained devices are needed. The likelihood of premature loosening with such devices warrants extreme caution. Recently a technique has been described[136] in which the origins of the collateral ligament are transferred to address the recurvatum deformity. The long-term results of this procedure are unknown, and at the present time recurvatum deformities remain better treated by simple bracing or by arthrodesis.

Inability to carry out and maintain active extension generally precludes a functional arthroplasty. Reconstruction of the extensor mechanism has been described[137]; however, the utility of such reconstructions is unknown.

Traditionally, arthroplasty of a neuropathic joint has been considered an absolute contraindication to total knee replacement. This view may be changing. Soundry and colleagues have reported encouraging results of arthroplasty in such patients. However, constrained devices are needed.[138] The durability of these arthroplasties is suspect.

Surgical Exposure

The Anterior Approach

This approach to total knee arthroplasty is generally through an anterior midline longitudinal skin incision and median parapatellar arthrotomy. A description of the specific steps is available in many texts on surgical exposure.

The advantages of the anterior approach include its extensile potential, its wide exposure medially and laterally, and its utilitarian nature. The approach may generally be reutilized without undue difficulty should subsequent surgery be necessary. Disadvantages of the approach include its violation of the quadriceps mechanism, which may contribute to patellofemoral derangement, as well as potential devascularization of the patella, with consequent avascular necrosis (particularly if lateral release is needed).[132–136] Despite these potential problems, the approach is the overwhelming choice of most surgeons for performing total knee arthroplasty.

The Subvastus Approach

The subvastus or Southern approach (Fig. 52-8) is an alternative exposure utilized in total knee replacement surgery. The approach was described in 1945[137]; however, it was largely ignored until recently.[138]

The subvastus approach utilizes the same midline anterior skin incision as the anterior approach. The deep dissection differs proximally in that the quadriceps tendon is not violated. Rather, the vastus medialis is elevated anteriorly and laterally from the femur and medial intermuscular septum. The entire extensor mechanism is lifted anteriorly, allowing the arthrotomy to be created from the suprapatellar pouch to the tibial tubercle. Blunt elevation proximally of the vastus medialis will allow eventual patellar eversion and wide enough exposure to allow arthroplasty to be performed.

The advantages of the subvastus approach include maintenance of the quadriceps mechanism with decreased postoperative pain and earlier functional recovery.[133,139] The possibility of wound dehiscence and patellar subluxation or dislocation are avoided by preserving the quad mechanism. Devascularization of the patella is decreased because the descending, medial superior, and medial inferior geniculate arteries are preserved.[140]

Disadvantages of the approach include its somewhat more limited exposure, particularly laterally. Patellar eversion can be much more difficult to carry out in obese or

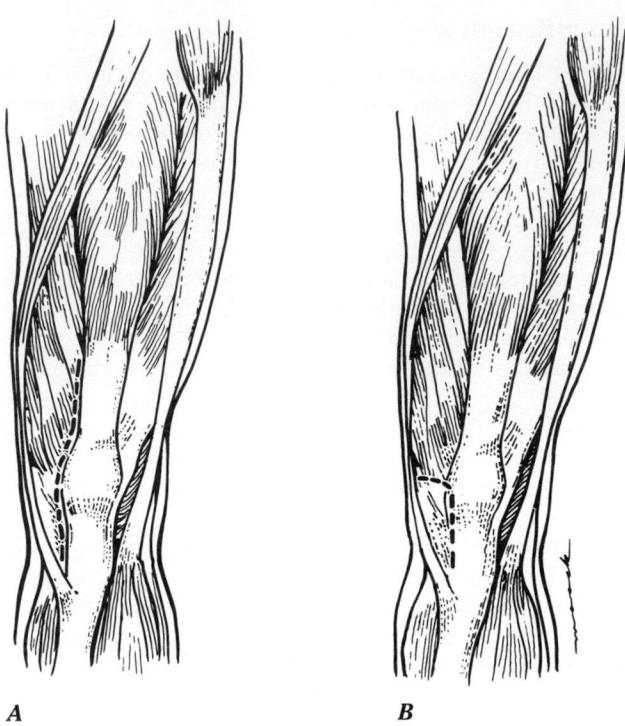

A   *B*

Figure 52-8 *A.* Medial parapatellar arthrotomy. *B.* Subvastus approach. For explanation, see text. (Reproduced with permission from *Surgical Techniques* brochure. Austin, TX, Intermedics Orthopaedics, Inc, 1990, p. 10.)

heavily muscled individuals or in severely arthritic joints. Because any degree of infrapatellar scaring can likewise prevent patellar eversion, this approach is contraindicated in revision arthroplasties, following proximal tibial osteotomy, or following previous major arthrotomy.[138]

The Lateral Approach

A recently described approach to the knee is the lateral approach.[141] Unlike the case with the anterior and subvastus approaches, dissection and arthrotomy are carried out lateral to the patella and through the medial edge of Gerdy's tubercle. The approach allows direct access to the lateral knee structures, including the iliotibial band, the arcuate complex and marginal osteophytes, which may lead to fixed valgus of the knee. For this reason the approach has been advocated specifically for valgus deformities.

Proponents admit that the exposure is more difficult, the anatomy less familiar and patellar displacement more difficult, however they feel that the "clinical results over a nine year period support the lateral approach as a superior method in correction of valgus deformity."[141] More widespread reports of the approach and its outcomes must be awaited before the approach can be recommended.

The Multiply Operated Knee

Occasionally the surgeon is faced with a knee that has seen previous operations. The surgeon must select an approach allowing access to the knee with a minimum of subsequent soft tissue complications. When prior knee incisions are available, they should be utilized or incorporated into new incisions to minimize the possibility of flap necrosis from parallel incisions and interrupted blood supply. If previous incisions cannot be incorporated, then new incisions should be created with a wide skin bridge between the two. One should leave a skin bridge half of the length of the incisions.

One should avoid crossing previous incisions whenever possible. In situations where this is impossible, one should cross incisions at as wide an angle as possible. The blood supply about the knee generally proceeds from lateral toward medial. Therefore when two old incisions of equal length are available, it is often wisest to utilize the lateral one.

Limb Alignment

The technique of total knee arthroplasty varies somewhat depending on the particular prosthesis being implanted. Prior to undertaking surgery, one must familiarize oneself with the recommended technique suggested by the component manufacturers. Despite this, certain principles apply to all knee arthroplasties, such as alignment, implant sizing, ligament balance, etc., which are reviewed briefly below.

The anatomic axis of the femur is defined by the femoral diaphysis. Because of the varus orientation of the femoral neck, the anatomic axis of the bone lies in 5 to 7° of valgus relative to its mechanical axis (Fig. 52-5). The anatomic axis of the tibia is the same as its mechanical axis provided that there is no significant bow to the bone or other malalignment. Most modern arthroplasty designs create femoral and tibial bone cuts that are perpendicular to their mechanical axes, thereby assuring that appropriate alignment is retained or restored. Failure to achieve coronal alignment is associated with an increased incidence of component loosening and wear.[142]

The guide systems responsible for creating the distal femoral and proximal tibial bone cuts are designed in one of two ways. Either they utilize palpable anatomic landmarks for orientation (extramedullary systems), or they are placed within the medullary canals of the respective bones (intramedullary systems). Most manufacturers of prostheses provide both systems to accommodate surgeon preference.

Intramedullary guide systems are somewhat more popular for establishing alignment of the femur because they tend to be more accurate than extramedullary systems. Varus or valgus malalignment of less than 2° of the femoral components can be expected. The proper distal femoral cutting guide is determined preoperatively by measuring the mechanical and anatomic axes of the bone on long-standing radiographs. Jiang and Insall have demonstrated that internal or external rotation of the limb may affect the estimated alignment of the femur.[143] For this reason, many surgeons routinely cut the femur at 5° of valgus relative to the intramedullary rod.

Any significant deformity of the femur secondary to traumatic, congenital, or metabolic causes or ipsilateral total hip arthroplasty with a long-stemmed femoral component may preclude the use of the intramedullary system. An extramedullary system is available for these uncommon cases. Some extramedullary systems utilize a radiopaque reference marker, which is positioned over the femoral head under fluoroscopic guidance prior to draping the extremity. This marker must be palpable beneath the surgical drapes to serve as a landmark for the guide system. This method of determining alignment is more time-consuming and less accurate than intramedullary system and is therefore rarely employed. Newer, more accurate alignment systems are being developed.

Intra- and extramedullary systems are available for determining alignment of the proximal tibia. Because landmarks such as the tibial tubercle, tibial crest, and malleoli are easily palpable, extramedullary guide systems are more easily used. Many surgeons feel that the internal anatomy of the tibia is inconsistent, making intramedullary systems less accurate. Extramedullary guides are therefore somewhat more popular than intramedullary ones. One advantage of most internal guide systems is that they may be checked for accuracy with accompanying external rods.

Implant Sizing

The prosthetic implants should approximate the anatomic dimensions of the femoral and tibial surfaces they are replacing. This may be problematic in cases where significant bone loss has occurred and distorted normal anatomy. Some surgeons favor preoperative templating of radiographs to determine implant sizes. The lateral view of the femur is the most accurate view on which to base the femoral component, while the AP view of the tibia is the most accurate way to estimate tibial component size.

Many surgeons feel that templating films is an inaccurate means of determining prosthetic size and therefore rely upon intraoperative estimates to determine the size of the implants. While some manufacturers of prostheses allow tibial and femoral components of different sizes to be implanted and "matched," this is usually not necessary. Most individuals are consistent in requiring the same-size implants for both the femur and tibia.

In uncomplicated arthroplasties the tibial bone surface is the best means of determining the size of a prosthetic implant. The most appropriate size will be that which most nearly covers the bony surface without overhanging the edge of the tibial plateau. Undersizing of the tibial component predisposes to implant subsidence, while oversizing of the component can lead to irritation of the collateral ligament and chronic pain.

The femoral component will usually be the same size as the tibial. When properly sized, the anterior flange of the femoral component will lie flush with the anterior surface of the femoral shaft, while the posterior condyles of the component recreate the normal condylar dimensions. A femoral component that is too large will "overstuff" the patellofemoral joint and have a similar effect as a patellar component that is too thick.

Implant Constraint

The first generation of knee implants in the 1970s were rigidly constrained hinge joints. Since they accommodated no side-to-side or rotational motion, higher stresses were transmitted to the cement/bone interface, leading to early failure. Because constraint is felt to result in elevated stress at the prosthesis/bone interface, most modern condylar designs incorporate minimal constraint between all implants as a way of potentially increasing longevity of the arthroplasty. Most primary arthroplasties performed will utilize components that rely upon the patient's anatomy to confer stability to the articulation; design modifications of the prosthesis are rarely necessary to substitute for ligamentous stability. Despite 20 years of experience with both posterior cruciate ligament (PCL)-sacrificing and PCL-sparing arthroplasty designs, there is no evidence as yet to suggest that the slight amount of increased constraint seen by the PCL-sacrificing designs result in premature failure. Occasionally in a salvage situation with loss or insufficiency of medial or lateral ligament tissue, a more constrained type of device (such as the constrained condylar) may be required. These devices require longer intramedullary stems to improve fixation because of the increased constraint built into the articulation. The patellofemoral articulation often utilizes minimal constraint to improve the wear characteristic of the implants.

Soft Tissue Balancing

Accurate bone cuts are not sufficient to produce a successful arthroplasty. Equally important is balancing of the soft tissues about the knee.

For valgus or varus deformities, appropriate release of contracted medial or lateral structures will permit the opposite side to be approximately tensioned with the correct size of implant in the majority of cases. Occasionally the soft tissues on the overstretched side are so lax that they must be tightened up or too thick an insert is required.

In the valgus knee sequential release of the popliteus tendon, the iliotibial band, and less commonly the lateral ligament or biceps is performed while the resulting balance is assessed at each step. Various Z-plasty techniques are used. The popliteus and lateral ligament can also be detached from their femoral origins in continuity with a sliver of bone, which can either be left with its soft tissue attachments or reattached with a screw at the new length. If the medial collateral ligament is attenuated, then reefing or preferably ligament advancement on the tibia is required to achieve valgus stability.

In the case of the severely varus knee, the capsular insertion of the ligament into the medial tibial plateau is released around the posteromedial corner above the insertion of the semimembranosus. If the medial side is still too tight, the insertion of the medial collateral ligament into the tibial metaphysis may be stripped inferiorly in continuity with the periosteum without creating instability. In rare cases, the lateral ligament may be tightened by removing and reattaching the lateral ligament (with attached piece of fibula head) using a screw and washer.

Flexion and Extension Gap

One should also achieve flexion-extension balancing. This means that the extension gap between the distal femoral and tibial cuts and the flexion gap between the posterior femoral and tibial cuts, with the knee flexed to 90°, is equal when distraction of the knee is carried out. If the flexion gap is looser than the extension gap, recutting the distal femoral cut should yield appropriate balance. If the flexion gap is tighter than the extension gap, the problem may be addressed either by downsizing of the femoral component or the addition of posterior slope to the tibial cut (usually about 5° is required). If both the flexion and extension gaps are too tight, the proximal tibial cut will have to be lowered to allow components to be implanted. A flexion gap that is too tight becomes apparent during flexion with trial components in place. The front of the tibial trial component will lift up in flexion. Occasionally, simply partial release of the PCL or recession from its femoral origin will solve the problem in the case of PCL-sparing arthroplasty.

It is important that a symmetrical flexion gap be created medially and laterally. Cutting the tibia at 90° to the tibial axis removes more articular surface on the lateral side (Fig. 52-9). This cut parallels the femoral cut in extension, but at 90° of flexion it is necessary to compensate by cutting more bone from the posterior aspect of the medial femoral condyle to create a symmetrical flexion gap. To achieve this, the femoral cutting block is externally rotated (2 to 5°), and this is the position of placement of the femoral component. This position fortunately also improves patellar tracking.

Consideration must also be given to restoring the anatomic joint line. Raising or lowering the joint line leads to alteration of PCL tension and adversely affects patellofemoral joint function.

COMPLICATIONS OF TOTAL KNEE ARTHROPLASTY

Neurologic Complications

Peroneal nerve palsy is the most common neurologic complication of total knee replacement, occurring in approximately 1 percent of surgeries.[144-147] While nerve injury can occur in any knee, the complication is most commonly seen in the valgus knee or when a fixed flexion deformity exists preoperatively.[144-147] Over two-thirds of these are noted within 24 h of surgery; however, they may not be appreciated for several days postoperatively.[144] Prophylactic decompression of the nerve in high-risk knees is unwise and has not been shown to prevent the development of a peroneal palsy postoperatively.[144]

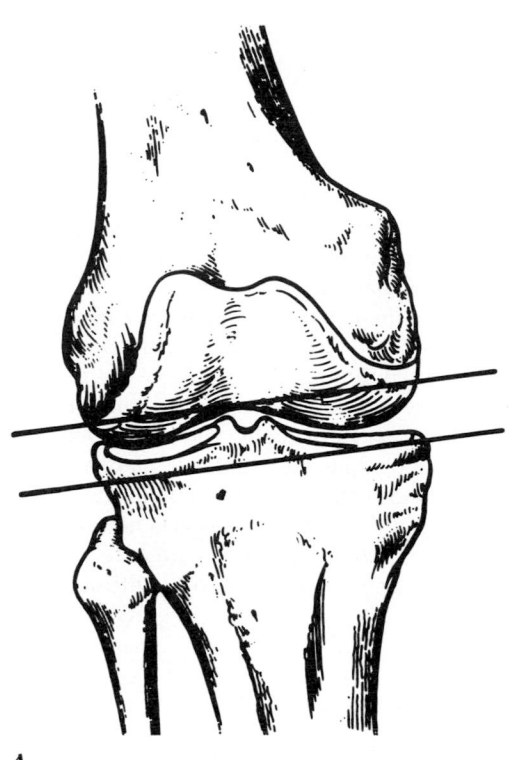

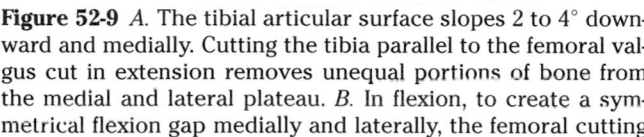

A

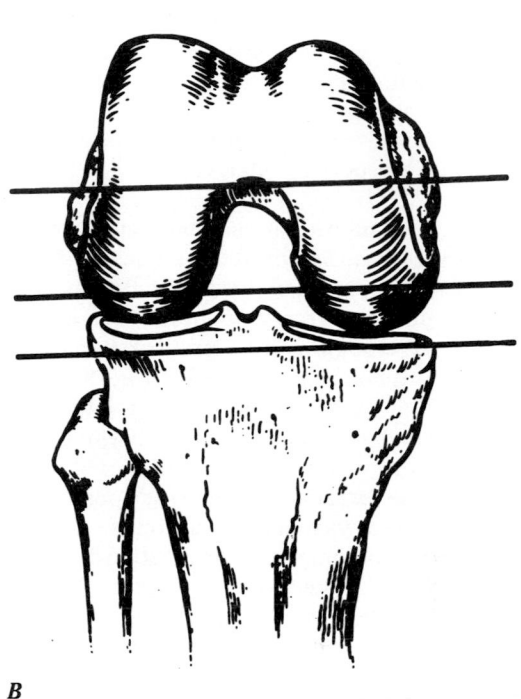

B

Figure 52-9 *A.* The tibial articular surface slopes 2 to 4° downward and medially. Cutting the tibia parallel to the femoral valgus cut in extension removes unequal portions of bone from the medial and lateral plateau. *B.* In flexion, to create a symmetrical flexion gap medially and laterally, the femoral cutting block must be rotated externally up to 5° so that more bone is resected from the back of the medial femoral condyle. (Reproduced with permission from Whiteside LA: Bone preparation techniques for cementless fixation of total knee replacement. *Tech Orthop* 6:10, 1991.)

The injury is felt to arise from indirect causes and likely represents a traction injury sustained during surgery or a compression injury occurring postoperatively. The tourniquet in the operating room should be tested and calibrated regularly to ensure proper function. The varus realignment of the valgus knee and extension of the knee with fixed flexion may lead to injury to the nerve lying in the posterolateral aspect of the joint. Conversely, peroneal nerve palsy may occur postoperatively secondary to tight surgical dressings, perioperative bleeding, and the use of immobilizers.

The outlook for postarthroplasty peroneal palsy has been examined by Asp and Rand.[145] Their experience revealed that two-thirds of injuries were complete while the remainder were incomplete. Among patients treated conservatively, approximately half experienced full neurologic recovery while half experienced partial recovery. Those with complete palsies, however, were less than half as likely to experience full recoveries than those with incomplete palsies. Incomplete neuroplexias overall have a better prognosis.

Treatment

Once a peroneal nerve palsy is identified, prompt removal of all circumferential dressings and flexion of the knee should be carried out. This maneuver alone may provide immediate relief in a number of patients. Treatment otherwise is conservative, with routine rehabilitation of the operated knee and use of an ankle-foot-orthosis to maintain neutral position of the foot in the face of a drop foot. Should the palsy continue beyond several months without improvement, Krackow et al. suggest operative decompression of the nerve. Their results point to marked improvement in peroneal function, even after many months.[148]

Anesthesia

The increasing popularity of continuous epidural and spinal anesthesia for the arthroplasty patient warrants special attention, as patients and their physician are less likely to appreciate and appropriately treat peroneal nerve injuries in the immediate postoperative period secondary to anesthetic sensory and motor blockade.[149]

Vascular Complications

Severe, limb-threatening vascular injury can occur during total knee arthroplasty with an incidence of 0.03 to 0.17 percent.[144,145] Injuries have been noted to the superficial femoral,[148] popliteal,[152,153] and genicular[152,154,155] vessels.

Injuries include direct lacerations, late arteriovenous fistulae, pseudoaneurysms, and acute thromboses.

Direct arterial laceration may be noted at the time of surgery. Often injury is first suspected in the postoperative period, when diminished or absent pedal pulses are noted. Patients at risk include individuals with known peripheral vascular disease or who demonstrate calcific atherosclerosis of the periarticular vessels on routine radiographs.

Although such injuries are uncommon, surgeons must be aware of the potential for serious injuries. Prevention of vascular complications involves consultation with a vascular surgeon prior to surgery whenever severe peripheral vascular disease is identified on preoperative evaluation. Orthopaedic surgeons may choose to perform surgery without the thigh tourniquet in patients with significant disease or in individuals with a past history of vascular reconstructive surgery.[156,157] Careful monitoring of the vascular status of the extremity is necessary postoperatively.

Any suspected vascular compromise noted postoperatively demands immediate evaluation by a vascular surgeon with appropriate vascular studies. The potential of limb loss must be borne in mind. Insall and Haas have noted that 3 of 7 perioperative vascular injuries at their institution necessitated above-knee amputations.[158]

Fat Embolism Syndrome

Fat embolism syndrome (FES) has been a clinically recognized entity since its description by Gurd and Wilson 1974.[159] While most often seen following long bone trauma, its association with total joint arthroplasty of the hip and knee is well established.[160–165] The pathogenetics underlying FES are incompletely understood. It appears that introduction of marrow elements into the systemic circulation and their eventual deposition within the pulmonary vasculature liberates inflammatory mediators that cause the syndrome. Compromised gas exchange and respiratory insufficiency are the end result. If it is severe enough, FES may prove fatal.

That FES complicates total knee arthroplasty has been clearly established,[160–162, 164–166] and the syndrome is felt to complicate 3 percent of total knee arthroplasties. It has been seen in conjunction with intraoperative use of intramedullary drills,[165] rodded guide systems,[162,163] or stemmed prosthetic devices. In addition, simple deflation of the thigh tourniquet may liberate significant amounts of marrow elements and debris and thus cause the syndrome.[166]

Clinically overt FES can be recognized by the triad of respiratory insufficiency, mental status changes (confusion, agitation), and a petechial rash (most notable on the upper trunk, axillae, and subconjunctival regions). In addition, patients may demonstrate fever, tachycardia, retinal changes, and fat globules in the urine and saliva. Because these signs may be absent or unrecognized, the rate of FES associated with lower extremity arthroplasty is likely higher than generally appreciated. Confusion and hypoxia in the posteropertive period are often incorrectly attributed to narcotic administration, atelectasis, or senile "sundowning."

Treatment

The treatment of FES is largely supportive. Mechanical ventilation may be required in severe cases. Intravenous fluid administration, glucose, heparin, dextran, aspirin, and ethanol have been administered with no effect upon the clinical course. Corticosteroids may be beneficial if given early and in large doses[167,168]; however, the potential associated morbidity limits their prophylactic use in the arthroplasty population.

Prevention, then, is the most effective means of avoiding FES. Use of fluted intramedullary guides with lavage of intramedullary contents, overdrilling of guide holes, and slow advancement of intramedullary instruments and prosthetic components are probably the most effective means of avoiding this complication. Some surgeons suggest that bilateral total knee arthroplasty increases the likelihood of this complication[169,170]; however, this is not universally accepted. Recent studies appear to indicate that bilateral arthroplasties may be carried out without increased risk.[171,172]

Thromboembolic Disease

Thromboembolic disease is a well recognized sequella of knee arthroplasties.[173–178] Despite a relatively high incidence of lower extremity thrombi, less than 2 percent of patients develop clinically significant pulmonary emboli and less than 0.5 percent have fatal ones. Controversy continues to surround the diagnosis of lower extremity deep vein thrombosis (DVT) in the postoperative state.

Incidence

A large number of postarthroplasty venous thrombi develop in the popliteal and infrapopliteal vessels. Varying reports suggest that between 40 and 65 percent of patients will develop thrombi within these vessels. Because of their small size, they appear to represent little risk of producing life-threatening embolism. Approximately 5 percent of arthroplasty patients develop DVT proximal to the popliteal veins.[179] If large, these may represent a significant risk. To date, there is no agreement on how large a thrombus must be to pose a significant risk. The only consensus is that the greater the total clot burden, the greater the risk to the patient.

Deep vein thrombosis in situ does not necessarily pose a life-threatening risk to the patient (although little is known regarding the long-term local morbidity of DVT, such as chronic venous insufficiency). When thrombus dislodges, it is carried through the venous system to the lungs, where it is deposited (i.e., pulmonary embolism). The frequency of postoperative pulmonary embolism is probably underestimated. Recent studies using ventilation perfusion scanning in asymptomatic postarthroplasty patients estimate that up to 20 percent of patients experience asymptomatic pulmonary emboli (PE).[179] The clinical significance of these asymptomatic emboli, if any, is unclear.

When the embolus is large, the patient presents with cardiopulmonary embarrassment or arrest. The thrombi leading to such episodes are believed to arise in the major veins of the thigh or pelvis. There is no clear agreement as to whether clinically significant PE result from propagation of small, "insignificant" DVT, or whether small DVT represent a predisposition to larger DVT. Previous studies suggest a 5 to 20 percent rate of proximal propagation.[180,181]

Diagnostic Tests

Much of the confusion regarding thromboembolic disease following arthroplasty arises from the variable results of the various testing modalities. Currently, the two most widely utilized tests for detecting DVT are the contrast venogram and B-mode duplex ultrasonography. Older tests—including clinical examination, iodine-131 labeled fibrinogen scanning, and impedance plethysmography—have largely been abandoned because of their proven inaccuracy.[182,183]

Contrast venography is currently recognized as the gold standard modality for diagnosing DVT. It is felt to be highly sensitive and specific. The test is invasive in nature and is associated with thrombophlebitic, nephrotoxic, and contrast-allergenic reactions.[182,184] It is inconsistent in its ability to visualize the vessels of the pelvis.

Duplex ultrasonography has recently been shown to rival contrast venography in its ability to identify clinically significant DVT, and its use is becoming more widespread.[185–187] Unfortunately, B-mode duplex ultrasonography cannot visualize the vessels above the inguinal ligament and therefore potentially ignores extensive DVT. Its performance is highly technician-dependent.[188–189]

The drawbacks to contrast venography and duplex ultrasonography have led to a search for alternative means of diagnosing clinically significant DVT. At present, no modality has been shown to equal these tests. Magnetic resonance venography is currently being examined for use because it avoids the drawbacks of other screening tests as well as allowing the visualization of pelvic vessels.[190]

Routine postoperative evaluation of patients who have undergone total knee arthroplasty is not widely practiced for several reasons. Because of the infrequency of serious pulmonary embolism following surgery, testing of all patients is not felt to be cost-effective. In addition, the morbidity associated with the diagnostic tests and with various treatment modalities may outweigh the benefits. Finally, because the risk of serious pulmonary embolism remains elevated for up to 2 months postoperatively, the optimal timing of evaluative tests is unknown.

Prophylaxis

The risk of postarthroplasty thromboembolic disease and the best means of identifying the "at risk" patient is not currently known. For these reasons, most surgeons favor the routine use of some form of DVT prophylaxis. Prophylactic regimens may be either mechanical, chemical, or a combination of both.

Mechanical means of DVT prophylaxis include elastic calf or thigh hose, intermittent pneumatic compression stockings, plantar foot compression pumps, early patient mobilization, postoperative continuous passive motion,

and inferior vena cava filters. None of these are proved to decrease the risk of serious or fatal PE. Intermittent pneumatic compression stockings have been shown to decrease the incidence of calf thrombi; however, their effectiveness in preventing more proximal DVT has not been established. Elastic compression stockings, early patient mobilization, and continuous passive motion appear to be ineffective in preventing postoperative DVT. Inferior vena cava filters are invasive to place, require potentially hazardous contrast agents, and are expensive. Their use as a prophylatic measure is discouraged. In summary, mechanical prophylactic measures in and of themselves appear to be insufficient in preventing serious thromboembolic complications.

Chemoprophylaxis includes the administration of continuous intravenous heparin, subcutaneous fractionated low-molecular-weight heparin, oral warfarin, intravenous dextran, and aspirin. Debate continues over the relative effectiveness of one agent over another, and no single agent is clearly superior. It is clear, however, that each of these agents poses a significant risk in and of itself. Postoperative complications—including increased bleeding necessitating transfusion, wound hematomas, hemarthroses, gastrointestinal bleeding, and cerebrovascular hemorrhage—are recognized. It would appear that increasing effectiveness in preventing DVT is associated with increasing risk of bleeding complications. The appropriate risk-benefit from these agents is still being debated.

Treatment of Documented Deep Vein Thrombosis

The patient with known, clinically significant DVT demands treatment. Most surgeons agree that thrombosis above the popliteal level represents a risk. Most popular regimens favor institution of intravenous heparin to maintain the partial thromboplastin time between 1.5 and 2 times control. Oral warfarin is administered concomitantly. Once the PT has been brought to between 1.5 and 2 times control, the heparin is discontinued. Warfarin is then utilized to maintain the level for 6 weeks to 6 months before discontinuance. This regimen should not be initiated without careful consideration, since therapeutic levels of heparin anicoagulation are associated with a 30 to 40 percent risk of bleeding in the perioperative period. The use of therapeutic levels of heparin is also associated with a 0.7 to 1.0 percent risk of death from a bleeding complication.[191]

Infection of Total Knee Arthroplasty

Sepsis of the knee is an uncommon but potentially disastrous complication following arthroplasty. The potential adverse effects upon patient health and function and the high cost of treatment are obvious reasons to avoid this problem. Preventing infection, then, is an integral part of performing the procedure, while early and appropriate treatment of the established infection is of utmost importance.

Early in the evolution of total knee arthroplasty, the incidence of infection was recognized as being unacceptably high, with reports of up to 16 percent septic complications. This generally occurred with early hinged devices. Infection complicating modern total condylar designs is much lower, with most recent reports documenting between a 1 and 2 percent incidence.[191–195] A number of changes in technique and prosthetic design have contributed to this decrease.

Etiology

Infection occurring in the perioperative period is generally the result of contamination at the time of surgery. Late infection may occur in a previously sterile joint that becomes septic secondary to hematogenous seeding of the arthroplasty.

Multiple factors have been identified that increase the risk of infection. These may be exogenous (e.g., resulting from break in technique, etc.) or endogenous (e.g., predisposition resulting from the patient's disease process).

Exogenous factors are generally controlled by the surgeon and therefore must be addressed at the time of surgery. Numerous developments in surgical technique during the past 30 years have resulted in a dramatic decline in the subsequent infection rate. The routine use of broad-spectrum antibiotics perioperatively, laminar-flow operating rooms, use of sterile isolation gowns ("space suits"),[196] limitation of operating room personnel,[197] and modern total condylar designs have all contributed to a decreased incidence of postarthroplasty infection.

A number of endogenous or host factors have been identified that appear to predispose certain patients to septic complications. Diabetes mellitus, rheumatoid arthritis and its variants, corticosteroid use, poor nutritional status, extreme old age, concurrent infections, prior history of septic arthritis, obesity, and prior knee surgeries have all been shown to increase the risk of early and/or late sepsis of the knee.[191,192,194,198–200]

Microbiology

The most common organisms isolated from septic arthroplasties have been *Staphylococcus aureus* and *Staphylococcus epidermidis*. Together these microbes are identified in over half of all infected arthroplasties in a wide range of studies.[191,194,201–210] Nevertheless, a sizable number of infections are known to be caused by gram-negative species, streptococcal species, anaerobes, mixed flora, and other microorganisms.

In selecting perioperative antibiotic coverage, it is important to choose a broad-spectrum agent with antimicrobial action against many of these organisms. A first- or second-generation cephalosporin is often a wise choice, as its antistaphylococcal coverage is excellent, while coverage of other potential pathogens remains good. Intravenous cefazolin is currently the most widely used antibiotic for perioperative prophylaxis.

Diagnosis

Arthroplasties may become infected at any time following implantation of a prosthesis. Patients may present with a variety of complaints, and a high index of suspicion is warranted. The patient with severe pain, erythema, swelling,

fever, or drainage may easily be diagnosed. Often, however, patients complain of mild pain or swelling with no other obvious findings. These patients can pose a diagnostic dilemma and, in the absence of other demonstrable causes, must be considered infected until proved otherwise.

Hematologic tests are often not helpful but may arouse suspicion if abnormal. Routine blood culture in the absence of fever or other septic stigmata is rarely useful. Peripheral leukocyte count may be elevated; however, one study found only one-quarter of infected arthroplasties to have counts greater than $11,000/mm^3$.[207] Another found the average leukocyte count to be normal despite infection of the knee.[210] An elevated erythrocyte sedimentation rate (ESR) is often found; however, inflammatory conditions or recent joint surgery will often yield elevations in this value irrespective of whether the joint is infected or not. One study documents that the ESR value may be normal in patients with infected arthroplasties.[211]

Routine radiographs are often unimpressive early in the infectious process and therefore are unhelpful in establishing a diagnosis (Fig. 52-10A). With time, a osteolytic reaction may develop around the prosthetic components and may heighten suspicion of infection. Technetium bone scanning will generally demonstrate increased periarticular uptake; however, this is nonspecific for infectious processes. Indium-111 scanning of the knee can be a helpful adjunct, with a quoted accuracy of 85 percent in predicting infection.[211] Gallium scanning and contrast arthrography are not beneficial in the diagnosis of sepsis.

Aspiration of the joint may confirm the diagnosis of infection in between 45 and 85 percent of cases in various series.[207,209,210,212,213] Gram's stain will demonstrate the etiologic organism only 25 percent of the time.[214] Aerobic and anaerobic culture, acid-fast staining, and fungal culture should be obtained. In addition glucose level (usually low in infected knees), protein level (usually high in infected knees), and leukocyte count with differential should be obtained. Any leukocyte count above $25,000/mm^3$ or a differential of more than 75 percent polymorphonuclear luekocytes should be considered confirmatory for infection.[215]

New techniques, such as the use of the polymerase chain reaction for DNA amplification are currently being investigated for use in diagnosing infection. This technique has the potential to be highly sensitive and may be used in the future.

Management of Established Infection

Several options are available in the management of the septic arthroplasty. These include antibiotic suppression alone, wide surgical debridement with retention of the prosthesis, resection arthroplasty, implant removal and arthrodesis, and one- or two-stage reimplantation.

Antibiotic Suppression

It is difficult to sterilize an established infection with antibiotics alone. Therefore, long-term suppression with antibiotics is rarely indicated in the treatment of septic total knee arthroplasties. In the rare patient with limited life ex-

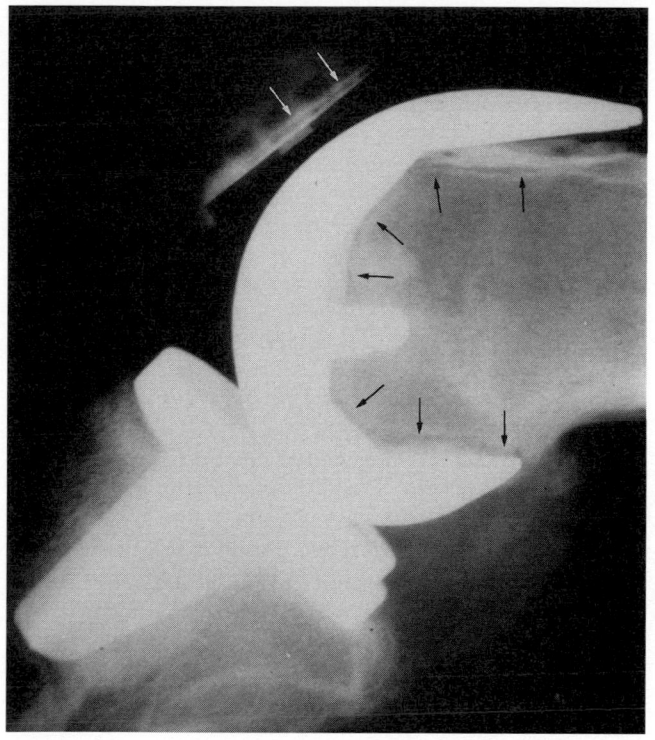

A

B

Figure 52-10 *A.* Infected total condylar design total knee arthroplasty. Arrows demonstrate lucency at the bone/cement interface consistent with long-term infection. *B.* Radiograph following removal of prosthetic components and placement of antibiotic-impregnated polymethyl methacrylate spacer.

pectancy or whose concurrent medical condition obviates surgery, antibiotic suppression may be justified provided that the infecting organism is of low virulence and has known sensitivity to oral antibiotics.

Debridement with Prosthetic Retention

Debridement involves the removal of all infected intraarticular contents with retention of the prosthesis. This is an option provided that the infection is caught early. Arthroplasties that become infected at the time of prosthetic implantation or previously sterile arthroplasties that develop acute hematogenous infections may be considered for debridement.

The reported results of debridement of infected arthroplasties vary widely.[192,194,201,203,207,216,217] It would appear, however, that infections caused by gram-negative organisms or *Staphylococcus aureus,* those occurring in older patients, and those with a longer duration of symptoms are associated with an increased failure rate when such cases are treated by debridement alone. Overall, the results of debridement do not support its routine use as definitive treatment of infected total knee arthroplasties.

Arthrodesis

Removal of components and surgical arthrodesis of the knee is rarely done, but this is a potentially beneficial means of managing infected arthroplasties. The results of arthrodesis tend to be less satisfying than those of revi-

sion arthroplasty; however, it remains the option of choice when satisfactory revision is not expected secondary to severe bony or ligamentous deficiency. It is also the most durable option for the very young or active patient, where premature failure of revision arthroplasty can be expected.

Resection Arthroplasty

Resection arthroplasty plays a very limited role in the treatment of infected prosthetic arthroplasty. It may be used as the first stage of a two-stage exchange arthroplasty (see below). When it is used as a definitive procedure, the results appear to be less satisfying than those of other surgical options. It is, however, considered the most appropriate option available in severe rheumatoid arthritis with multiple joint involvement.

Exchange Arthroplasty

Exchange arthroplasty involves removal of an infected prosthesis with subsequent revision arthroplasty either at the same time or at a later point. When it is feasible, exchange arthroplasty holds the greatest potential for satisfactory knee function of all the available reconstructive alternatives. The candidate for exchange arthroplasty must meet several criteria before this route is selected: (1) he or she must be medically fit to tolerate a long course of treatment with possible multiple surgeries; (2) the infecting organism must be sensitive to antibiotic therapy and the patient must be able to tolerate the potential antibiotic toxicity; (3) the bone and soft tissues must be adequate to provide for a functional revision.

The precise timetable for exchange is determined per surgeon discretion. It appears that immediate or early exchange (Less than 3 weeks following removal of the infected arthroplasty) may be successful in a high percentage of patients. Most series, however, involve a small numbers of patients.[203,204,216,218,219]

Delayed exchange usually implies revision arthroplasty more than 4 to 6 weeks following prosthetic removal. Overall, the results of delayed exchange are encouraging; however, complications are common.[194,215,217,220] The ideal timing for performing the revision arthroplasty has not been determined.

The potential difficulty with delayed exchange is the scar formation and soft tissue contracture that occurs following removal of the prosthesis. In order to prevent this, many surgeons utilize spacers, most often antibiotic-impregnated polymethylmethacrylate, to maintain the joint spaces. Antibiotics are incorporated into the cement during is preparation. Gradual leaching of the antibiotics from the cement will result in high local antibiotic concentrations that theoretically help to eradicate infection and im-

prove the likelihood of successful reimplantation. The disadvantages of using antibiotics include the potential for selection of antibiotic-resistant microorganisms and the possible adverse systemic effects of the antibiotics. The clinical success of such a protocol has not been shown definitely to improve the overall result of subsequent reimplantation over nonantibiotic-impregnated spacers.[221]

Periprosthetic Fractures

A perioprosthetic fracture (Fig. 52-11A) is one that occurs less than 15 cm from the joint line or one that occurs around or in close proximity to the intramedullary stem of a prosthetic component. Periprosthetic fractures complicate approximately 1 percent of knee of arthroplasties. They may occur during surgery or at any time postoperatively. Postoperative fractures may be either traumatic or fatigue fractures. Intraoperative fractures are uncommon. They result from excessive force used in the preparation, trailing, or impaction of final components. They occur most commonly in individuals with poor bone quality and therefore are seen with osteopenic states and in revision situations. On the femoral side, they often occur as a re-

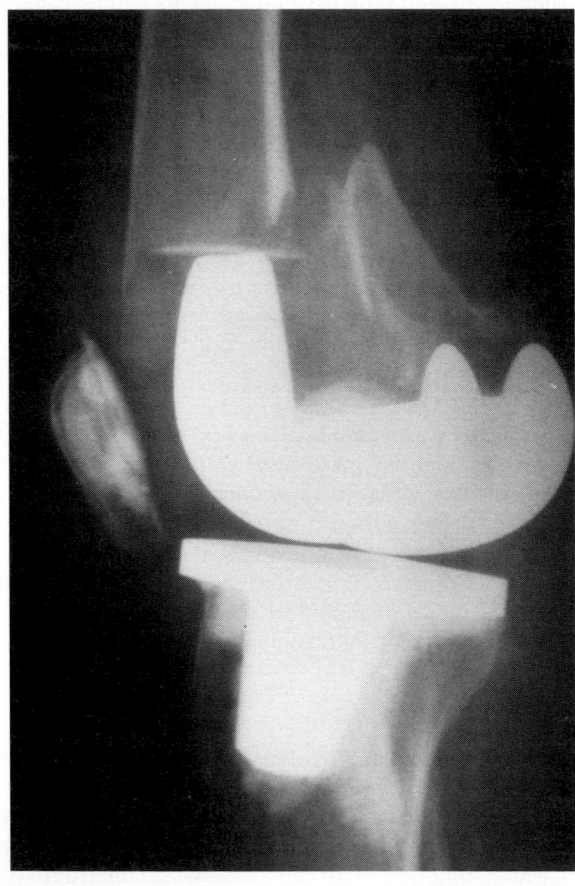

A

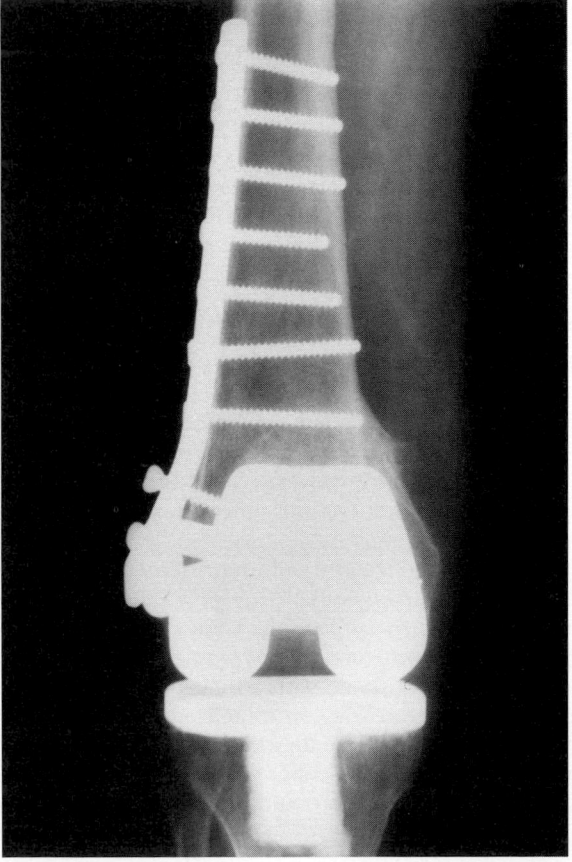

B

Figure 52-11 *A.* Periprosthetic femoral fracture. Such fractures are often caused by low-energy trauma and often occur through bone of inferior quality. *B.* Radiograph of the knee following open reduction and internal fixation with a construct comprising a lag screw and side plate. The alignment of the limb has been restored and the prosthetic component left in place.

sult of insufficient bony resection of the central box in posteriorly stabilized designs, where a longitudinal condylar split develops during trialing or prosthetic component placement. On the tibial side, a fracture of the tibial plateau may occur. Most intraoperative fractures are minimally displaced. Treatment must be individualized and may be conservative, with protective weight bearing until fracture union, use of internal fixation such as screws or wires, or the use of stemmed components to span the fracture site.

Stress fractures are uncommon after total knee arthroplasty. They may occur anywhere in the extremity from the hip to the foot.[192,200,201] Again, treatment must be individualized.

Posttraumatic fractures generally result from a fall or other low-energy injury and are often comminuted and displaced.[193–199] These fractures occur far more commonly in the femur than in the tibia. Osteoporotic states and revision arthroplasty predispose to this complication. Controversy surrounds the potential relative risk of subsequent femoral fracture when the anterior femur is notched at the time of prosthetic replacement. Traditionally, many have felt that such notching predisposes to supracondylar fractures of the femur[193,197]; however, others feel that it is not significantly associated with fracture.[200]

Treatment guidelines have recently been developed.[203] Conservative therapy is recommended as long as limb alignment can be restored and maintained. Increasingly, reports recommending operative treatment of many fractures have been published in recent years. These studies indicate an overall better long-term result with decreased morbidity.[204–206]

It can be difficult to obtain sufficient purchase in the distal femoral fragment, but if a condylar screw can be insinuated anterior to the fixation lugs of the femoral component, then open reduction and internal fixation (ORIF) with a plate can be completed and early motion of the knee joint commenced (Fig. 52-11B). Recently fixation with the intramedullary supracondylar nail has gained favor. This device is inserted intraarticularly through the notch (easier with some femoral component designs and impossible with others) and fixed to the femoral diaphysis and fracture fragment with interlocking screws (Fig. 52-12).

Wound Healing Complications

Wound healing problems, if inappropriately managed, may result in disastrous outcomes in an otherwise appropriately performed arthroplasty. Certain conditions are known to be associated with wound complications. Obesity,[191] poor nutritional status,[192] and diabetes mellitus[193] are all felt to predispose to postoperative wound complications. There are conflicting data regarding the propensity of patients with rheumatoid arthritis to develop problems, with some studies indicating an increased risk[194] while others do not.[191,195,197]

Errors in surgical technique may likewise contribute to wound complications postoperatively. Most are easily avoided if careful attention to detail is maintained.

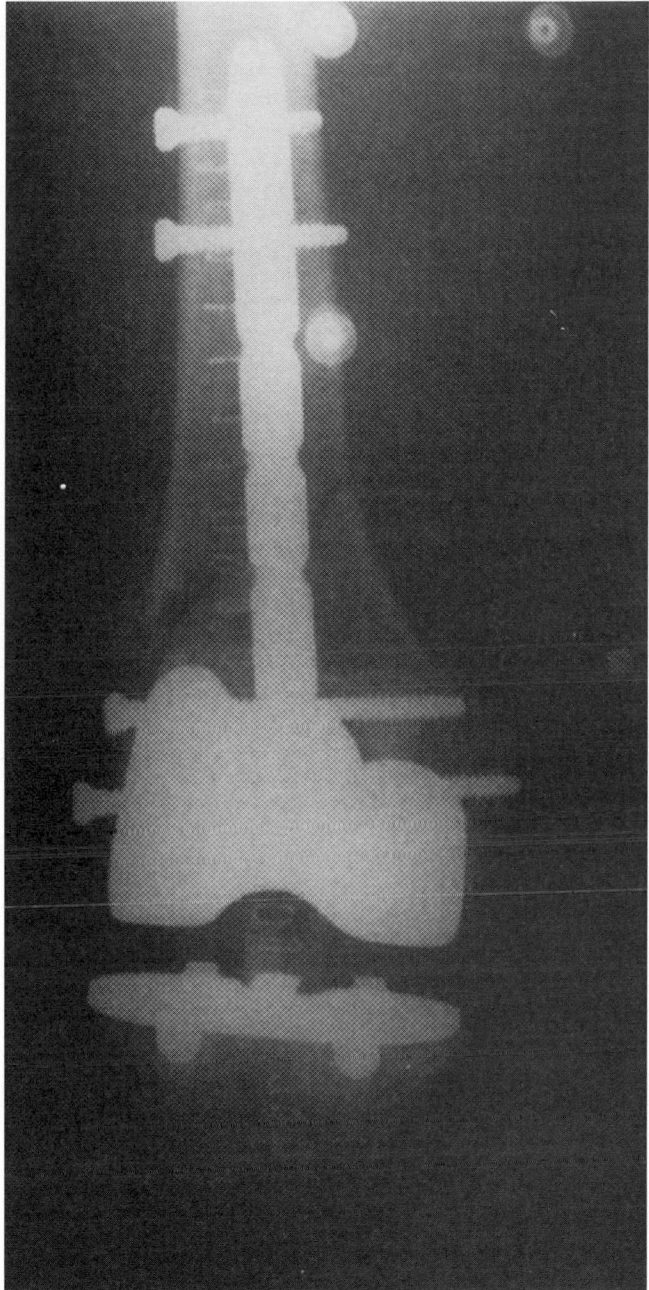

Figure 52-12 Anteroposterior radiograph after fixation of a supracondylar femoral fracture with an intramedullary supracondylar nail. (From Chnell MJ, Moran MC, Scott RD: Periarticular fractures after total knee arthroplasty: Principles of management. © 1993, American Academy of Orthopaedic Surgeons. Reprinted from the *Journal of the American Academy of Orthopaedic Surgeons* 4:112, 1996, with permission.)

Utilization of previous incisions or incorporation of old incisions into new ones will greatly diminish the possibility of wound complications. Often this is not feasible. When old incisions are transverse in nature, they should be crossed at right angles. If a new longitudinal incision is made parallel to a previous one, an adequate skin bridge should be maintained between the two. The bridge should be as wide as possible but should not be less then one-fourth of the length of the longitudinal incisions.

Postoperative hematoma formation may increase the likelihood of wound complications. Hematoma is best prevented by meticulous attention to hemostasis at the time of surgery, gentle handling of the soft tissues during the operation, and tight closure in layers of all potential dead spaces. The benefits of postoperative suction drainage are undocumented, with several recent reports failing to demonstrate their effectiveness.[196,198] The routine use of postoperative thromboprophylactic medications make hematoma formation more likely; therefore all possible attempts should be made to avoid excessive anticoagulation.

The routine use of continuous passive motion in the postoperative period has not been shown to affect the likelihood of wound complications significantly.[199–201] The timing of tourniquet deflation likewise has not been shown to affect subsequent wound healing.

Three types of wound complications are seen following arthroplasty: prolonged wound drainage, superficial wound necrosis, and wound dehiscence.

Prolonged Wound Drainage

The most commonly recognized wound problem following arthroplasty is that of prolonged surgical drainage. Drainage from the incision is expected for several days postoperatively. Continued drainage beyond this time is considered prolonged. The drainage may result from either incomplete deep fascial closure, with synovial fluid tracking to the skin surface, or from poor superficial healing. Whatever the cause, continued drainage may permit bacterial contamination of the subcutaneous tissues and subsequent wound sepsis.

Treatment consists of immobilization of the knee for several days until the drainage ceases. If this proves ineffective in stopping the drainage after several days, the patient should be returned to the operating room for exploration, irrigation, and sound closure of the wound in layers.[206] The role of prophylactic antibiotics during the period of active drainage is not known.

Superficial Necrosis

Fortunately, necrosis of the wound is uncommon. Nevertheless, the complication is potentially serious, as it may easily be overlooked. Because of the relatively thin soft tissue sleeve between the skin and the knee joint itself, even a small area of necrosis may pose the threat of possible exposure and bacterial contamination. Attempts at debridement and primary closure are rarely successful.

Treatment of wound slough is generally by myocutaneous or fasciocutaneous graft coverage.[201–205] The medial or lateral gastrocnemius flap is a common choice, as it provides excellent coverage with a minimum of functional loss.

Wound Dehiscence

Frank dehiscence of the wound is a very rare complication. It usually arises secondary to trauma, obesity, patel-

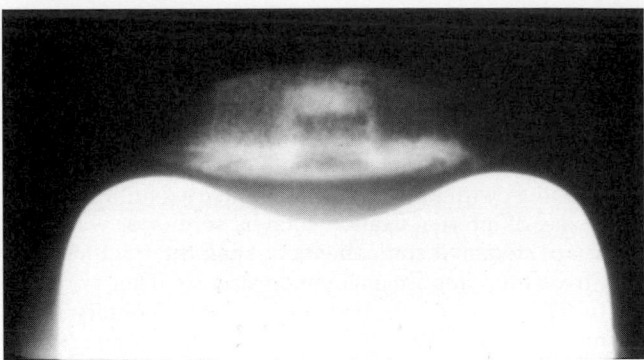

Figure 52-13 Axillary view of the patellofemoral articular following placement of an all-polyethylene cemented patellar component. The patella is centralized within the femoral trochlea.

lar instability, or premature staple or suture removal. Dehiscence should be treated as a surgical emergency, with immediate return to the operating room, copious lavage of the wound, institution of broad-spectrum antibiotics, and closure of the wound with retention sutures.

PATELLAR COMPLICATIONS OF TOTAL KNEE ARTHROPLASTY

Patellar Instability

With modern total condylar designs, patellar instability, either subluxation or dislocation, occurs in less than 1 percent of total knee arthroplasties. Patellar instability is usually secondary to technical errors at the time of surgery, but it may also be due to abnormal patient anatomy or trauma.

The most common cause of patellar instability is failure to assure proper tracking at the time of arthroplasty (Fig. 52-13). Excessive internal rotation of the femoral or tibial components results in relative lateral displacements of the patella, thereby predisposing to subluxation or dislocation. Providing appropriate rotation is relatively straightforward if one takes care to assure appropriate component alignment during surgery.

Femoral Component

Prosthetic manufacturers often provide guide systems for the femoral cutting block that are designed to achieve several degrees of external rotation of the placement of the femoral component. Whether such a system is used or not, one should confirm that, in the absence of preexisting posterior condylar bone loss, slightly more bone has been resected from the posterior medial condyle than from the posterolateral condyle. This will yield a small amount of external rotation of the component to improve patellar tracking as well as fill the flexion gap appropriately (Fig. 52-9).

Tibial Component

The tibial resection is generally made perpendicular to the long axis of the bone. Nevertheless, internal rotation of the component often occurs because the laterally displaced extensor mechanism and the poorly exposed lateral tibial plateau make internal rotation of the component common. To assure that the tibial component's rotation is correct, one should confirm that the intercondylar eminence is aligned with the medial third of the tibial tubercle or with the anterior crest of the tibia. Additionally, it is important that neither the tibial nor the femoral components be medialized, since this affects patellar tracking adversely.

Patellar Component

The patellar component should be positioned centrally upon the patella. In cases of oblong or asymmetrical patellae, one should strive to place the component somewhat medially. This allows a small amount of lateral patellar displacement to occur while permitting the component to track normally. It should never be oversized and overhang the cut surface of the patella. Some surgeons undersize routinely. However, the previous patellar thickness should be restored by the implant. Again, the component should not be too thick, otherwise the final composite will impose painful stresses on the retinaculum and limit motion because it is too tight.

Patellar instability arising from component malrotation is most appropriately treated with revision arthroplasty. Should patellar subluxation or dislocation occur despite correct component orientation, realignment of the extensor mechanism may be performed.[222–224] Realignment procedures may be carried out proximally or distally. Proximal procedures are generally easier and have a lower complication rate; therefore they are most commonly performed.

Lateral retinacular release alone may suffice in correcting the persistent instability despite proper component positioning. This most often occurs in cases of long-standing valgus deformity. These patients often present with a lateral retinacular contracture and concurrent medial retinacular attenuation. Retinacular release may be combined with an advancement of the vastus medialis obliquus and a medial retinacular reefing.

Distal realignment procedures are rarely warranted and are associated with a high incidence of patellar tendon rupture.[222] These procedures generally osteotomize the tibial tubercle and move it medially. They are most appropriate when abnormal tibial anatomy presents a lateralized tibial tubercle position, which cannot be corrected with proximal procedures.

Patellar instability following trauma generally responds to conservative management. Persistent subluxation or dislocation may require operative repair of the torn medial retinaculum.

Results

The treatment of recurrent or chronic patellar instability generally results in satisfactory outcomes in 60 to 100 percent of patients. Two reports note a high complication rate.[222,225] There is an approximately 20 percent rate of re-

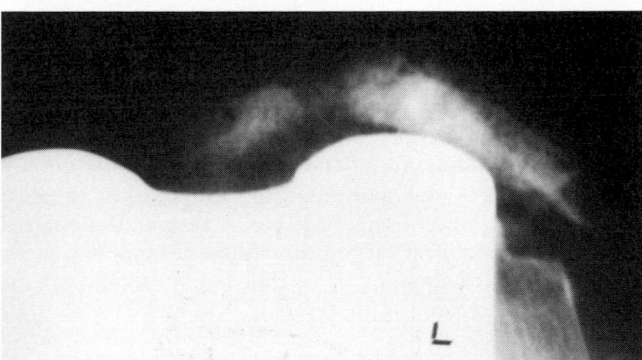

Figure 52-14 Patellar fracture following total knee arthroplasty. Such fractures may be associated with avascular necrosis. The patella is noted to be subluxed laterally; this may result as well from maltracking of the patella following arthroplasty. Such maltracking is often the result of improper tibial or femoral rotation.

current instability. In addition, there is a greater than 10 percent incidence of either patellar tendon or tibial tubercle avulsion and a 5 to 8 percent incidence of deep infection.

Patellar Fractures

Fracture of the patella is a well-known complication of total knee arthroplasty and may occur with or without patellar resurfacing[222–230] (Fig. 52-14). Fractures may occur following direct trauma or, more commonly, secondary to gradual fatigue of the bone. That patellar resurfacing predisposes the bone to fracture may be the result of one or more factors.

Etiology

Bony Resection and Patellar Fixation Excessive resection of bone yields a weakened bone lacking the cortical subchondral bone plate. The result is a weakened, predominantly cancellous bone. Conversely, underresection of bone leaves an abnormally thick patella. The forces transmitted to the thickened patella, particularly in knees with normal range of motion, are excessive. Therefore either under- or overresection of the patella yields bone with inadequate strength. The end result is bony fatigue or fracture. Patellar fixation holes create a stress riser effect on already weakened bone.[222,227]

Careful attention to proper resection of bone will minimize the potential for patellar fracture. A general rule of thumb is to resect precisely the amount of bone that is to be replaced with polyethylene. Some surgeons prefer to utilize patellar components with multiple small fixation lugs rather than a single large central lug to further decrease the chance of fracture.

Component Tracking

Component alignment during total knee arthroplasty is related to patellar fracture later.[223,231,232] Improper patellofemoral mechanics will lead to high patellofemoral contact stresses, most often with the patella tracking laterally in the trochlear groove.[232] This results from malalignment of the femoral or tibial components, long-standing soft tissue contracture, or lateralization of the prosthetic button on the patellar bone surface.

Proper alignment of the femoral and tibial components—in particular avoiding internal rotation of either component, judicious use of lateral retinacular release, and slight medialization of the patellar component on the patellar bone will help to optimize patellofemoral mechanics and prevent bone fatigue.

Avascular Necrosis

Avascularity of the patella has been documented following total knee arthroplasty and is felt by many to predispose to patellar fractures.[222,228–230,233] Routine medial parapatellar arthrotomy sacrifices the supreme geniculate, the superior medial geniculate, and the inferior medial geniculate vessels. The inferior lateral geniculate vessel is often taken during lateral meniscal removal. The superior lateral geniculate artery remains the sole blood supply to the patella. Overexuberant lateral release can easily damage the vessel, leaving a completely devascularized bone. Many surgeons feel that minimizing the extent of the lateral retinacular release and careful protection of the lateral superior geniculate artery will preserve this important arterial source.[222] Others disagree and feel that even these maneuvers are inadequate to assure that the patellar blood supply remains intact.[234,235]

Disruption of the Extensor Mechanism

Fortunately, rupture or avulsion of the patellar tendon is a rare event that complicates less the 0.2 percent of total knee arthroplasties.[223] If this condition is unrecognized or inadequately treated, the outcome can be disastrous, because patients will lose active extension of the knee. Even with appropriate treatment, patients may continue to exhibit incomplete knee extension and ultimately may have unsatisfactory results.[223,228]

Etiology

Avulsion of the patellar tendon most commonly occurs in cases where exposure is difficult, as with previous major arthrotomy (e.g., revision total knee arthroplasties or prior tibial osteotomy), in primary cases where patients exhibit severe range-of-motion deficits, or in cases associated with poor quality of bone or soft tissue (e.g., rheumatoid arthritis). This complication most commonly occurs at the time of surgery but may arise even years later. Avulsion of the patellar tendon at its tibial insertion is the most common location and can occur in as many as 30 percent of difficult revision surgeries.

Prevention

Prevention of this complication is important and a number of intraoperative maneuvers may be performed to mini-

mize its occurrence. A thorough debridement of the lateral gutter of the knee, division of the patellofemoral ligament, and lateral retinacular release may suffice to allow patellar eversion and to relieve tension on the patellar ligament. In cases where further release is needed, a proximal quadriceps "snip," a V-Y turndown,[224] or a distally located tibial tubercle osteotomy[225,226] will generally afford adequate release to protect the extensor mechanism during the arthroplasty. Proximal releases are preferred, because tibial tubercle osteotomy is associated with a high rate of nonunion and proximal migration.

Treatment

The treatment of patellar tendon rupture depends upon when the rupture occurs. Those occurring during or immediately following surgery are best treated by immediate reattachment of the tendon using sturdy, nonabsorbable suture, while bony avulsions may be reattached with screw fixation. Ruptures occurring late after surgery, if recognized early, are treated in similar fashion.

Late recognition of ruptures represents a more challenging reconstructive problem. Quadriceps contracture and patellar tendon scarring make simple reattachment impossible. In these cases, autograft or allograft reconstruction of the patellar tendon has been advocated.[222,223] An article by Emerson et al. reports satisfactory short-term results utilizing an allograft quadriceps tendon, patella, and patellar ligament.[236]

Results

Even the best reported results of repair of a patellar ligament rupture note satisfactory outcomes between zero and 67 percent of patients, depending on the reconstructive technique used.[223,228]

Complications

The most common complication following repair of a disrupted extensor mechanism is a persistent extensor lag. Inability to achieve near total extension results in abnormal gait and difficulty in negotiating stairs or arising from chairs. Rerupture and infection may complicate operative repair.

Patellar Loosening

Isolated loosening of the patellar component is uncommon, occurring in approximately 1 percent of total knee arthroplasties.[222,223] It is most commonly seen in cases of maltracking, patellar bone deficiency, avascular necrosis, asymmetrical bony resection, high patient activity levels, and high degrees of knee flexion.[223]

Loosening of the patellar component may be asymptomatic but generally requires revision of the patellar implant. If bone stock is adequate, the solution is straightforward, with standard patellar bone preparation and recementing of the new patellar component. Often there is a central deficiency following removal of the loose patella.

This deficiency may preclude the use of a standard patellar component. Such cases may be treated with revision to an inset component. If bone stock is inadequate to permit patellar revision, one must either retain the unresurfaced patellar fragment or perform a formal patellectomy.

Metal-Backed Patellae

Numerous reports have recently been published implicating metal-backed patellar designs with a high rate of failure.[222–229] Because of these poor results, many surgeons no longer implant such components and utilize all-polyethylene components instead.

Rationale

The rationale behind the development of metal-backed patellae was a theoretical improvement in stress transfer from the implant to the bone and consequent decrease in deformation and wear rates in the polyethylene. The addition of metal backing results in an increased failure rate from causes not envisioned by the component designers. Metal-backed patellae demonstrate premature polyethylene wear from thinning of the polyethylene over the metallic lugs, polyethylene-metal dissociation, and peg failure.[222–226] A report by Laskin and Bucknell suggests that the poor results of metal backing may not be universal. They report good long-term results using metal-backed patellar components provided that the implant is inset into the patellar bone.[237]

Diagnosis

Diagnosis of patellar component failure may not be obvious. Patients often present with complaints of anterior knee pain, swelling, joint effusion, or patellofemoral crepitus. Symptoms may be sudden in onset or may develop gradually.[222] The diagnosis may be suspected on axial radiographs, which will demonstrate articulation between the patellar backing and the femoral component. On AP and lateral views, metallic debris may be noted within the soft tissue about the joint. Aspiration of the joint, yielding dark synovial fluid, will generally confirm the diagnosis. Microscopic analysis will demonstrate the presence of metallic debris.

Failure of metal-backed patellar components is more likely in knees where there is maltracking of the patella.[225] Other factors that have been implicated include obesity, high activity levels, high degrees of postoperative knee flexion, and excessively thick patellar implants.[222,225,227]

Treatment

Treatment of failed metal-backed patellae usually involves revision of the patellar component to an all-polyethylene one. Tricompartmental revision should be performed at the the time of patellar exchange. A thorough synovectomy, is required if metallic debris is present throughout the joint. Obvious maltracking of the patella may necessitate a tricompartmental revision to correct the problem, even in the absence of metallic burnishing.

Summary

Metal-backed patellae represent a step back in the development of total knee arthroplasty. Despite the abandonment of these implants, a great number of patients are functioning with these implants even today.

CURRENT CONTROVERSIES IN TOTAL KNEE ARTHROPLASTY

Cement versus Cementless

Traditionally, arthroplasties have been implanted with polymethylmethacrylate (PMMA) cement to achieve immediate and secure fixation of the prosthetic components to bone. The long-term survivorship of such implants is excellent at 10 to 15 years.[238–239] Over the past 15 years, theoretical concerns over the long-term durability of PMMA have arisen. Its brittle nature, association with osteolysis, and finite longevity have led to a search for alternative means of achieving prosthesis-bone stability.

Porous coating of metallic implants has been shown to allow the ingrowth of bone and achievement of biological interlock, which is capable of bonding the implant to the surrounding bone. The potential for achieving prosthetic fixation by such ingrowth would obviate the use of PMMA and therefore potentially remove a source of arthroplasty failure. Arthroplasties fixed by bony ingrowth would presumably function identically to cemented arthroplasties.

The clinical results of noncemented arthroplasties to date have been similar to, or slightly inferior to those of cemented arthroplasties.[238,243–246] One study by Collins et al. found similar clinical results between the two designs; however, the incidence of radiolucent lines, loose beads, and tibial component subsidence was more common in the cementless group.[240] Another study documents a higher rate of radiolucent lines with cementless designs than with cemented ones.[240a] The significance of these lines is unclear.

Long-term follow-up indicates increased frequency of persistent pain, patellar failure, and inadequate bony ingrowth into the tibial ingrowth surface. Because of these findings, some surgeons currently favor hybrid arthroplasties with cementless fixation of the femoral component and cemented fixation of the patellar and tibial components. One study demonstrates 93 percent good and excellent results with such a hybrid technique.[240b]

In summary, cemented fixation remains the standard against which cementless fixation must be judged. At this time, cementless fixation has not been shown to equal the long-term results of cemented arthroplasty. Continued design changes of cementless arthroplasties are expected, which may result in superior results.

Total Knee Arthroplasty Either Sparing or Sacrificing the Posterior Cruciate Ligament

The posterior cruciate ligament (PCL) is nearly always intact in knees undergoing primary arthroplasty. In the early 1970s, two schools of thought developed concerning the relative merits of arthroplasty that preserved or sacrificed the PCL. Debate has continued to the present time, and both design types continue to be implanted with overall good and excellent results.[250,250a,252a,253a]

The potential benefits of PCL-sparing arthroplasty include more normal knee kinematics, enhanced proprioceptive control of the joint, and minimal constraint between femur and tibia. Femoral bone stock is preserved to a slightly greater degree than with PCL-sacrificing designs. Proponents feel that these factors result in a more natural "feel" of the knee and diminished prosthesis-bone stress transfer. Improved short- and long-term results are theorized.

Designs sparing the PCL have been shown to recreate a more normal gait pattern, particularly with stair climbing, in a number of studies.[247–249] It is unclear however, whether the noted differences in gait are of any clinical significance.

Advocates of PCL-sacrificing arthroplasty point out that the PCL, while present, is rarely normal in arthritic knees. Therefore its preservation may alter kinematics negatively. In addition, arthroplasty is technically more difficult with PCL-sparing designs. Finally, the PCL may easily be substituted for by design features of the prosthesis. For these reasons proponents of PCL-sacrificing arthroplasty feel that such designs will result in enhanced outcomes.

The controversy regarding PCL-sparing versus PCL-sacrificing designs is unlikely to be resolved in the near future. Long-term follow-up studies demonstrate similar survivorship rates of both design types[250–253] at 10 years and longer. Functional outcome and knee scores appear to be similar as well. One study documents equal preference between the two designs in a group of patients in whom bilateral arthroplasties were performed, with one PCL-sparing implant and one PCL-sacrificing implant.[250a]

In summary, debate continues regarding the superiority of either design type. At 10- to 15-year follow-up, the survivorship and functional results are comparable. At the present time, polyethylene wear appears to be the predominant cause of long-term failure of arthroplasties. It may therefore overshadow much of the controversy regarding the long-term durability of one design over the other.

SPECIAL CONSIDERATIONS

Obesity

Excessive weight has traditionally been considered a relative contraindication to performing arthroplasty procedures on the knee. There is a widely held perception that the perioperative complication rate is elevated and the long-term results are inferior in this population.

Unfortunately, the data regarding the short- and long-term results of total knee arthroplasty in obese patients have been somewhat conflicting and further studies are needed.

Obesity is felt to contribute to the perioperative complication rate. When length of hospital stay was reviewed by Epstein and colleagues, they found an overall increase in days spent in the hospital for obese patients as compared to nonobese patients.[255] In contrast, Stern and Insall have found no significant increase in the incidence of deep venous thrombosis or wound healing complications in their obese patients as compared to a control population.[256] At present it is difficult to determine whether excessive weight contributes to the perioperative risk in total knee arthroplasty; however, it does not appear to elevate the risk enough to deny patients total knee arthroplasty unless other serious medical conditions coexist.

The long-term outlook for total knee arthroplasty in the obese population is controversial as well. Because polyethylene wear and component loosening or fatigue are affected by the forces transmitted across the knee, conventional logic assumes that increased patient weight would accelerate these processes and potentially lead to premature failure. One report has found a significantly higher failure rate in patients weighing over 80 kg as compared to weighing less,[257] while another demonstrated a decreased rate of satisfactory results in morbidly obese women as compared to controls.[258] In contrast, Stern and Insall have found no statistically significant increase in the failure rate of their arthroplasties; however, they did note a statistically significant increased incidence of patellofemoral symptoms in their moderately to severely obese patients.[256] Scott and colleagues have reviewed the results of arthroplasty in their obese population and have failed to demonstrate a difference in postoperative knee scores relative to patient weight.[259]

While the contribution of excessive weight to perioperative morbidity and long-term functional outcome remains unclear, it seems prudent to be cautious in recommending arthroplasty to an obese individual. Retrieval studies continue to implicate excess weight with accelerated wear. Thus obesity remains a relative contraindication to total knee arthroplasty. These patients should be aware of the potential of suboptimal outcome. Weight reduction should be encouraged; however, the success of significant weight loss and the ability of patients to maintain that loss are poor.[257]

Young Patients

Total knee arthroplasty has traditionally been contraindicated in the young patient. A conservative approach—comprising nonsteroidal antiinflammatory medications, use of a cane, weight reduction, and activity modification—is often the first line of treatment. Failing this, the patient may be a candidate for surgery. Usually, procedures other than total knee arthroplasty are indicated. Arthroscopic debridement, periarticular osteotomies, or arthrodesis may be more appropriate than arthroplasty given the particular situation. When an adolescent or young adult has incapacitating pain and severe functional limitation, he or she may be considered for total knee arthroplasty.

Unfortunately, much of the conventional thought about total knee arthroplasty in the young patient has been inferred from the literature on the results of total hip arthroplasty in young patients.[260,261] Relatively little has been written on the long-term results of total knee arthroplasty in the young patient. One recent report notes a cumulative survivorship of 94 percent at 18 years in a series of patients less than 55 years of age.[262] It is hoped that future studies will validate these excellent findings.

In the series reported to date, the results of follow-up studies appear to contradict the presumption that arthroplasty will fail prematurely in young individuals. Most studies demonstrate between 86 and 100 percent satisfactory results at an average of 5 years follow-up.[263–267] Despite these excellent results, caution is needed. Because most follow-up studies of total knee arthroplasty in young patients include a preponderance of rheumatoid or juvenile rheumatoid patients who have lower activity demands than patients with osteoarthritis or posttraumatic arthritis, the results may be less satisfying in these patients. Ranawat has shown that the results of total knee arthroplasty in the young patient with osteoarthritis are inferior to those in patients with rheumatoid arthritis, although a 94 percent satisfactory result was reported at 6 years average follow-up.[267,268]

Most of the results published to date are median length follow-up. It is possible that longer-term studies will demonstrate a more precipitous drop in arthroplasty survivorship in younger patients. Rand and Ilstrup correlate an increase in 10-year survivorship for their patients over 60 years of age as compared to more youthful patients (83 and 77 percent respectively).[253] In addition, increased life expectancy makes failure of the arthroplasty more likely in young patients than in the elderly.

In summary, it would appear that the results of total hip arthroplasty in the young patient may not be extrapolated to total knee arthroplasty in such a patient. Relative youth does not necessarily contraindicate performance of total knee arthroplasty. Predictably good results may be expected in the first 5 to 10 years. Polyethylene wear and not bone/cement stability appears to be the factor responsible for the long-term failure of total knee arthroplasty.

Total Knee Arthroplasty in Hemophilia

Hemophilia is an intrinsic, genetically transmitted deficiency of the normal clotting cascade. Patients with this disorder are predisposed to the development of spontaneous recurrent hemarthroses involving the large joints of the appendicular skeleton. The end result of hemarthroses is articular degradation with resultant severe arthritis and ankylosis. The knee is the most commonly involved joint. The pathomechanics underlying the arthropathy are unclear. Current theory implicates free radical formation secondary to hemoglobin breakdown, which leads to cartilage breakdown.

Treatment is aimed at minimizing the incidence of hemarthroses. Patients with severe hemophilia are maintained on factor VIII therapy to prevent spontaneous bleeding episodes. Hemophiliacs often produce inhibitors to factor VIII, which complicates the prophylaxis of severe bleeding and makes elective surgery unwise.

Joints with recurrent hemarthroses but without joint space destruction or synovitis are treated conservatively. Spontaneous hemarthroses are splinted for comfort for brief periods followed by gradual mobilization with physical therapy. The goals of physical therapy are to maintain a functional range of motion.

The surgical treatment of hemophilia is similar to that for rheumatoid arthritis. Patients presenting with a history of recurrent bleeding episodes and resultant synovitis are candidates for synovectomy. Synovectomy is effective at decreasing the incidence of hemarthroses as well as pain due to the synovitis. Its effect upon joint space degradation has not been established.

Patients with hemophilic arthritis are candidates for tricompartmental arthroplasty. Osteotomy and unicompartmental arthroplasty are contraindicated in hemophilic arthropathy. Arthrodesis is a reasonable treatment option; however, patients usually reject it when reconstruction is also an option. Multiple joint involvement may contraindicate arthrodesis as well.

Hemophiliacs undergoing arthroplasty require careful perioperative monitoring of factor VIII levels. Patients with known factor VIII inhibitors are not candidates for elective surgery. It is recommended that factor VIII levels be maintained above 100 percent for the first 2 to 3 days following surgery. During the following 2 weeks, the patient should be maintained at greater than 50 percent of normal levels. Maintenance of 30 to 50 percent normal levels is continued for up to 6 weeks postoperatively.

The results of total knee arthroplasty in this population appear to be good, at least in the short term.[269,270] The postoperative complication rate has been noted to be greater than 50 percent.[271,272] The long-term outcome of knee replacement surgery appears to be satisfactory; however, more intensive review is necessary.

Universal blood precautions are strictly observed, as up to 70 percent of hemophiliacs who have received untreated pooled factor VIII preparations are currently HIV-positive.

Total Knee Replacement in Paget's Disease

Paget's disease is a relatively common disorder of unknown etiology. It is marked by excessive bone resorption and formation, leading to an enlarged and deformed bone that is densely sclerotic. Because most patients with the disorder are clinically asymptomatic, the diagnosis is often established only when radiographs are taken. Paget's disease in the vicinity of the knee is felt to predispose the joint to degenerative changes similar to those of primary osteoarthritis. The treatment of these knees has been tricompartmental arthroplasty once the patient has failed conservative treatment.

Until recently the long-term outlook for arthroplasty performed for Paget's-associated arthritis has been unclear. Recent follow-up studies of both hip and knee replacement surgery have been encouraging.[273,274] Blood loss and the rate of aseptic loosening does not appear to be significantly different from that of primary osteoarthritis. The presence of sclerotic and cystic bone and femoral or tibial bowing will lead to technical difficulties at the time of operation. A higher than expected rate of varus or valgus prosthetic positioning has been demonstrated.[274]

REVISION OF TOTAL KNEE ARTHROPLASTY

Despite the excellent long-term results of total knee arthroplasty, a predictable decline in outcomes can be anticipated over time. Most reports document a 0.5 to 1 percent failure rate of modern condylar designs with each year following implantation.[275,276] Most failed arthroplasties may be successfully addressed by revision of the arthroplasty. Revision arthroplasties present more complex reconstructive challenges than primary arthroplasty, and the results tend to be less gratifying.

Rationale

Revision total knee arthroplasty is performed with the expectation that patients will achieve acceptable function and good pain relief. Soft tissue integrity and bone stock must be sufficient to permit revision. Minor deficiencies may be addressed by design features of the revision system used (e.g., semiconstrained femorotibial articulation, stems, wedges, etc.); however, if major deficiencies prevent successful revision, alternative procedures are called for.

Indications

The most common indication for revision total knee arthroplasty is aseptic loosening of a prior arthroplasty. Other indications include material failure of the implanted components or severe pain unresponsive to conservative management despite adequate clinical appearance of the knee.

Contraindications to revision surgery include active infection of the knee, severe bony deficiencies, severe ligamentous instability, extensor mechanism incompetence, and extremely poor medical condition.

Preoperative Planning

Prior to undertaking revision arthroplasty, the probable causes of failure must be assessed. Failure usually results from poor patient selection, implant component failure, or suboptimal technique leading to malalignment, instability, or other problems. Failure of the revision surgery is predictable if the cause of prior failed arthroplasty is not identified and appropriately dealt with.

Poor patient selection may lead to premature failure of arthroplasty and may therefore obviate successful revision surgery. Extreme youth and excessive functional demand are the most commonly encountered problems with regard to poor patient selection. Any patient considered to represent a contraindication to primary arthroplasty is also considered unsuitable for revision surgery for obvious reasons.

Material failures were common problems in older, constrained, or hinged devices but are uncommon with modern total condylar designs. Nevertheless, component failures can occur and may led to bony or soft tissue defects, which, if not addressed properly at the time of revision, can predispose the new implant to similar failure.

Failure of technique is the most common cause of failed arthroplasty. Issues such as alignment, component orientation, soft tissue balance, and appropriate kinematics require careful scrutiny preoperatively to identify obvious problems. Any of these problems must be corrected at the time of revision to assure the best results.

Exposure

Exposure of the knee is usually carried out through previous dissection planes. Creation of new incisions is unwise, as it may compromise the superficial blood supply, resulting in soft tissue slough or problems with wound healing. Full-thickness flaps will minimize avascularity. Old transverse scars should be crossed at right angles whenever possible. Any question concerning soft tissue viability mandates consultation with a plastic surgeon.

A standard median parapatellar arthrotomy is usually employed. Eversion of the patella and flexion of the knee is often difficult and the risk of avulsing the patellar tendon must be recognized. A thorough debridement of synovium and scar and lateral retinacular release may be required to allow complete exposure. Uncommonly, a release of the extensor mechanism with either a snip or a quadriceps turndown may be needed.[224]

Implant Removal

Following soft tissue exposure, removal of the implant is carried out. A loose component is usually extracted easily with little concurrent bone loss. A securely fixed component requires meticulous interruption of all possible component/cement or component/bone interfaces prior to attempted removal. The risk of significant bone loss with the component must be borne in mind. Thin, flexible osteotomes usually suffice; however, specialized motorized instruments may be necessary. The femoral component is generally removed first, because extraction of the tibial component is difficult with the femoral implant in place.

Limb Orientation

Limb orientation in revision arthroplasty should recreate the anatomic 5 to 7° of valgus alignment of the knee. Stemmed femoral components often have a 7° orientation of the stem, necessitating equal valgus of the femoral component to ensure that the stem fits easily within the intramedullary canal.

The distal femoral cut is created using an intramedullary guide. Bony resection should be kept at a minimum because of antecedent bone removal and the risk of moving the joint line proximally. Augmentation with metal spacers may be needed.

Rotational orientation of the femoral component is difficult because of a lack of reliable bony landmarks. If proper rotational alignment existed prior to prosthetic failure, it is best to reorient the revision component in the same fashion. In situations where rotational malalignment was likely, the femoral epicondyles may provide reasonable landmarks by which to estimate rotation. The medial femoral epicondyle lies slightly anterior to the lateral femoral epicondyle (Fig. 52-9).

Tibial alignment is more straightforward. The component should be oriented transverse to the long axis of the bone. Intra- or extramedullary alignment systems are used. As with the femur, a minimal bony resection should be taken to preserve remaining bone stock. A slight posterior slope to the tibial cut will often benefit the resultant knee flexion.

Implant Sizing

Estimating the proper size of the femoral component can be difficult due to bone loss from the posterior femoral condyles. This may lead to inadvertent undersizing of the femoral implant. To avoid this error, one should estimate the appropriate size preoperatively from templated radiographs of the opposite knee whenever possible. Size estimations are carried out during surgery by adding augmentation to the posterior flanges to recreate the normal posterior condylar dimensions and to equalize the flexion and extension balancing.

In sizing the tibial implant, the component that most completely covers the tibial bone surface should be selected. Oversizing, particularly medial overhang, should be avoided because it leads to irritation of the collateral ligament and pain. Undersizing may result in component subsidence. Occasionally bony deformity of the proximal tibia precludes "off-the-shelf" tibial components because the tibial keel abuts cortical bone within the metaphysis, which pushes the component into an asymmetrical position. In such cases a custom tibial component with an asymmetrical stem orientation may be needed.

Implant Constraint and Stems

Decreasing the amount of constraint is felt to relieve prosthesis/bone stress transfer, which may in turn result in premature implant loosening. Therefore an unconstrained device should be selected whenever possible. Because of PCL scarring or attenuation, it is rarely possible to reimplant a PCL-sparing device, and a PCL-substituting implant should be chosen. If significant varus or valgus imbalance exists following soft tissue balancing, a more highly constrained device such as the Total Condylar III prosthesis should be selected. It is extremely uncommon that sufficient imbalance exists to necessitate the use of a hinged prosthesis.

Femoral and tibial stems should be considered in any revision with poor bone stock. Stems are useful because they relieve prosthesis-bone stress transmission. Stemmed components transfer stresses to more sound bone proximally in the femur and distally in the tibia.

Controversy exists regarding whether cemented or uncemented stems are optimal. No long-term studies have demonstrated the superiority of one over the other.

Cemented stems are advantageous in that their fixation is immediate and strong. Their disadvantages include the difficulty encountered in removing cement, if necessary, at a later point. Cementless stems are potentially easier to remove; however, their immediate fixation is less secure than that of cemented stems.

There are no data concerning the optimum stem length for femoral and tibial components. It seems prudent to minimize their length whenever possible to less than 150 mm so as to preserve bone stock and limit the extent of stress shielding.

Joint Line Placement

Attempts should be made to recreate the normal joint line at the time of revision. This will help to achieve flexion and extension balancing as well as optimize patellofemoral mechanics. While the normal joint level is difficult to determine at the time of revision surgery, a preoperative review of the AP radiography will allow a reasonable estimate of whether the joint line should fall postoperatively. The anatomic joint line normally lies several millimeters distal to the midpoint between the medial femoral epicondyle and the fibular head, approximately 1.5 cms above the fibular head.

Bone Loss

Bone defects can be classified as either central or peripheral. Central defects constitute bony loss with maintenance of the cortical rim, whereas peripheral defects involve concurrent loss of the cortical rim.

Central defects are usually easier to address and may either be grafted with bone prior to cementing or filled with cement. The choice of one technique over another is discretionary and may depend upon patient age, likelihood of future revisions, the extent of bone loss, or physician preference.

Peripheral defects are somewhat more controversial. They may be addressed by cement, corticocancellous bone graft, metallic wedge augmentation, or customized implants. No clear consensus exists regarding which of these techniques yields the best long-term results. Whatever method is chosen, one should be sure that the prosthesis seats securely and there is no coronal or sagittal malalignment at the time of implantation.

Patellar and Extensor Mechanism

A loose or fractured patellar component requires revision whenever possible. Securely fixed patellar components may or may not require revision at the time of femoral and tibial revision. The decision to revise a well-fixed patellar component must be individualized and depends upon the patellofemoral congruity achieved at revision, the amount of patellar bone remaining to accept a new patellar component, and the symmetry of the original bony resection.

A rule of thumb is that at least 10 mm of patellar thickness must remain if reimplantation is to be contemplated. Less than this amount will obligate either conversion to an unresurfaced bony remnant or a formal patellectomy.

Patellas with a thickness of greater than 10 mm will generally accept a standard patellar button and may be prepared in standard fashion. A frequent scenario encountered at the time of patellar revision is the creation of a concave central defect with adequate peripheral bone remaining. Such cases may be managed with a biconvex patellar component, which effectively fills the central defect while reconstituting adequate thickness.

Prosthetic Fixation

Polymethylmethacrylate (PMMA) cement is utilized for fixation of almost all revision total knee arthroplasties. As noted, intramedullary stems may be cemented or press-fitted. When stems are going to be cemented, the technique used is similar to that for the cementation of femoral stems in total hip arthroplasties. The intramedullary canals are plugged distal to the estimated stem tips and the canals are then lavaged and dried. Vacuum-mixing of PMMA is carried out and the prepared canals are filled in retrograde fashion with a cement gun. It is often time-consuming to place the PMMA and seat the final components; therefore cementing is usually carried out in two stages. Many surgeons prefer to deflate the tourniquet prior to final component implantation in order to achieve hemostasis, which is more difficult with the components in place.

Closure

Closure is carried out in standard fashion, with suction drainage during the first 24 h.

Results

While modern condylar prostheses are felt to yield superior results to older, more constrained devices, the results of all revision total knee arthroplasties are inferior to those of primary arthroplasties, while the complication rate is far higher. Various studies document between 44 and 75 percent satisfactory results (generally at medium-term follow-up)[276–280] using semiconstrained prostheses such as the Total Condylar III and the Kinematic Rotating hinge. Complications occur in approximately 30 percent.

The results of revision arthroplasty using unconstrained condylar prostheses are better yet. At early follow-up, some have reported approximately 90 percent good and excellent results.[281] Jacobs and colleagues note a 68 percent good and excellent result with their series.[282] They note that their results are somewhat less good than they should have been largely because several of their patients were revised for pain of unknown etiology, and this population overall demonstrated poor results.

Complications

The complication rate associated with revision total knee arthroplasty is between 15 and 30 percent. The most frequent complications include patellofemoral malalignment, soft tissue slough, wound healing problems, and sepsis of the arthroplasty.

TOTAL KNEE ARTHROPLASTY FOLLOWING HIGH TIBIAL OSTEOTOMY

The results of proximal tibial osteotomy reflect a decline in results with the passage of time, with approximately 50 percent of patients reporting satisfactory results at 7 to 10 years. Approximately one-quarter of patients having proximal tibial osteotomy require conversion to total knee arthroplasty.[283,284] Proponents of osteotomies feel that conversion to arthroplasty can be performed with relative ease and that the results should approximate those of primary arthroplasty in previously unoperated knees.

Despite osteotomy's extraarticular nature, the procedure does make performance of arthroplasty somewhat more difficult. Several factors are responsible for the difficulties.

Patella infera occurs in approximately 80 percent of proximal tibial osteotomies.[285] This makes surgical exposure more difficult, in particular patellar eversion. Not infrequently, lateral retinacular release or proximal extensor mechanism releases are required.

Lateral compartmental bone loss secondary to the wedge removal or erosion of bone resulting from chronic valgus alignment of the knee can be sufficient to necessitate tibial wedge augmentation or bone grafting. In such knees, the lateral collateral ligament may become contracted and require release to restore the normal alignment.

Alteration of the metaphyseal contour leads to a relatively medialized medullary canal, which may cause asymmetrical prosthetic coverage of the prepared tibia. Occasionally a custom tibial tray may be required to avoid medialization.

Finally, retained hardware may prevent proper placement of the tibial component and removal (often through additional incisions) is necessary.

Results

Despite the increased difficulty in converting proximal tibial osteotomy to arthroplasty, the results appear to be good. Staeheli et al. report similar results of total knee arthroplasty following osteotomy in patients without prior osteotomy.[286] Katz et al. report less satisfactory results in patients having arthroplasty following osteotomy as compared to a control group having primary arthroplasty.[283] Insall reports a 20 percent fair and poor results in patients undergoing conversion.[287]

Complications

The complications of arthroplasty following osteotomy are the same as those following primary arthroplasty. Several complications are more commonly encountered, including extensor mechanism rupture, patellotibial impingement, tibial component malrotation or medialization, and ligamentous imbalance.

TOTAL KNEE ARTHROPLASTY FOLLOWING UNICOMPARTMENTAL KNEE ARTHROPLASTY

Advocates of unicompartmental knee replacement point out that preservation of bone stock and the cruciate ligaments should make revision to total knee arthroplasty relatively easy. The consequent surgical result and complication rate should therefore more closely approximate those of primary arthroplasty than those of revision arthroplasty. To date, the relatively small body of literature fails to clearly support this belief.

Despite sparing of the patella and contralateral femorotibial compartment, revision of failed unicompartmental arthroplasty often presents the surgeon with significant bony deficiencies in the resurfaced compartment. Various studies have documented incidence of significant bone loss between a 50 and 76 percent.[288–289]

The overall complication rate of unicompartmental revision averages 20 percent in these studies. The most common complications encountered include prosthetic loosening, infection, hematoma formation, and patellar complications.

Satisfactory results may be anticipated in between 66 and 84 percent of revised unicompartmental arthroplasties.[288–291]

Despite results that are inferior to those of primary total knee arthroplasty and similar to revision total knee arthroplasty, it should be pointed out that revision of unicompartmental arthroplasties may be advantageous because the surgery may often be revised to an unconstrained total condylar design without the need for extensive augmentation of the arthroplasty. This, in turn, may provide for increased ease of subsequent revision should it become necessary.

REFERENCES

1. Volkman R von. 1877. Quoted on *Clin Orthop Rel Res*, 36:7, 1964.
2. Muller W: Zur Frage der operativen Behandlung der Arthritis deformans und des chronischen Gelenkrheumatismus. *Langenbecks Arch Klin Chir* 47: 1894.
3. Goldthwait JE: Infectious arthritis. *Boston Med Surg J* 150:363, 1904.
4. Sweet PP: Synovectomy in chronic infectious arthritis *J Bone Joint Surg* 5:110, 1923.
5. Aiden HP, Baker LD: Synovectomy of the knee joint in rheumatoid arthritis. *JAMA* 187:4, 1964.
6. Marmor L: Surgery of the rheumatoid knee. *Am J Surg* 111:211, 1966.
7. Conaty JP: Surgery of the hip and knee in patients with rheumatoid arthritis. *J Bone Joint Surg* 55A:301. 1973.
8. Patzakis MJ, Mills DM, Clayton ML, et al: A visual, histological, and enzymatic study of regenerating rheumatoid synovium in the synovectomized knee. *J Bone Joint Surg* 55A:287, 1973.
9. Matsui N, Taneda Y, Ohta H, et al: Arthroscopic versus open synovectomy in the rheumatoid knee. *Int Orthop* 13:17, 1989.
10. Shibata T, Shiraoka K, Takubo N: Comparison between arthroscopic and open synovectomy for the knee in rheumatoid arthritis. *Arch Orthop Trauma Surg* 105:257, 1986.
11. Ogilvie-Harris DJ, Basinski A: Arthroscopic synovectomy of the knee for rheumatoid arthritis. *Arthroscopy* 7:91, 1991.
12. Klein W, Jensen KU. Arthroscopic synovectomy of the knee joint: Indication, technique and follow-up results. *Arthroscopy* 4:63, 1988.
13. Marmor L: Surgery of the rheumatoid knee: Synovectomy and debridement; *J Bone Joint Surg* 55A:535, 1973.
14. Marmor L: Synovectomy of the knee joint. *Orthop Clin North Am* 10:211, 1979.
15. Ranawat CS, Ecker ML, Straub LR: Synovectomy and debridement of the knees in rheumatoid arthritis; *Arthritis Rheum* 15:571, 1972.
16. Ranawat CS, Desai K: Role of early synovectomy of the knee joint in rheumatoid arthritis. *Arthritis Rheum* 18:117, 1975.
17. Verdeck WN, McBeath AA: Knee synovectomy for rheumatoid arthritis. *Clin Orthop Rel Res* 134:168, 1978.
18. Ishikawa H, Ohno O, Hirohata K; Long-term results of synovectomy in rheumatoid patients. *J Bone Joint Surg* 68A:198, 1986.
19. Rydholm U, Elborgh R, Ranstam J, et al: Synovectomy of the knee in juvenile chronic arthritis: A retrospective consecutive follow-up study. *J Bone Joint Surg* 68B:223, 1986.
20. Doets HC, Bierman BT, Soesbergen RM: Synovectomy of the rheumatoid knee does not prevent deterioration: 7-year follow-up of 83 cases. *Acta Orthop Scand* 60:523, 1989.
21. Smiley P, Wasilewski SA: Arthroscopic synovectomy. *Arthroscopy* 6:18, 1990.
22. Doyle DV, Glass JS, Gow PJ, et al: A clinical and prospective chromosomal study of yttrium-90 synovectomy. *Rheum Rehab* 16:217, 1977.
23. Gumpel JM, Roles NC: A controlled trial of intraarticular radiocolloids versus surgical synovectomy in persistent synovitis. *Lancet* 1:488, 1975.
24. Sledge CB, Zukerman JD, Shortkroff S, et al: Synovectomy of the rheumatiod knee using intra-articular injection of dysprosium-165-ferric hydroxide macroaggregates. *J Bone Joint Surg* 69:970, 1987.
25. Mazzetti RF: Effect of immobilization of the knee on energy expenditure during walking. *J Bone Joint Surg* 42A:533, 1960.
26. Montgomery WH, Becker MW, Windsor RE, Insall JN: Primary total knee arthroplasty in stiff and ankylosed knees. *Orthop Trans* 15:54, 1991.
27. Schurman JR II, Wilde AH: Total knee replacement after spontaneous osseous ankylosis: A report of three cases. *J Bone Joint Surg* 72A:455, 1990.
28. Drennan DB, Fahey JJ, Maylahn DJ: Important factors in achieving arthrodesis of the Charcot knee. *J Bone Joint Surg* 53A:1180, 1971.
29. Soudry M, Binazzi, Johanson NA, et al: Total knee arthroplasty in Charcot and Charcot-like joints. *Clin Orthop Rel Res* 208:199, 1986.
30. Emerson RH Jr, Head WC, Malinin TI: Reconstruction of patellar tendon rupture after total knee arthroplasty with an extensor mechanism allograft. *Clin Orthop Rel Res* 260:154, 1990.
31. Naranja RJ, Pagnano MW, Hanssen AD, Lotke PA: Reconstruction of an ankylosed knee to a total knee replacement. Presented American Academy of Orthopaedic Surgeons, Atlanta, GA, February 1996.
32. Holden DL, Jackson DW: Considerations in total knee arthroplasty following previous knee fusion. *Clin Orthop Rel Res* 227:223, 1988.
33. Mahomad N, McKee N, Solomon P, et al: Soft-tissue expansion before total knee arthroplasty in arthrodesed joints: A report of two cases. *J Bone Joint Surg* 76B:88, 1994.
34. Donley BG, Matthews LS, Kaufer H: Arthrodesis of the knee with an intramedullary nail. *J Bone Joint Surg* 73A:907, 1991.
35. Fern ED, Stewart HD, Newton G: Curved Küntscher nail arthrodesis after failed knee replacement. *J Bone Joint Surg* 71B:588, 1989.
36. Puranen J, Kortelainen P, Jalovaara P: Arthrodesis of the knee with intramedullary nail fixation. *J Bone Joint Surg* 72A:433, 1990.

37. Wilde AH, Stearns KL: Intramedullary fixation for arthrodesis of the knee after total knee arthroplasty. *Clin Orthop Rel Res* 248:87, 1989.

38. Griend RV: Arthrodesis of the knee with intramedullary fixation. *Clin Orthop Rel Res* 181:146, 1983.

39. Nichols SJ, Landon GC, Tullos HS: Arthrodesis with dual plates after failed total knee arthroplasty. *J Bone Joint Surg* 73A:1020, 1991.

40. Pritchett JW, Millin BA, Matthews AC: Knee arthrodesis with a tension band plate. *J Bone Joint Surg* 70A:285, 1988.

41. Charnley J, Baler SL: Compression arthrodesis of the knee: A clinical and histological study. *J Bone Joint Surg* 34B:187, 1952.

42. Knutson K, Bodelind B, Lidgren L: Stability of external fixators used for knee arthrodesis after failed knee arthroplasty. *Clin Orthop Rel Res* 186:90, 1984.

43. Charnley J: Arthrodesis of the knee. *Clin Orthop Rel Res* 18:37, 1960.

44. Charnley J, Lowe HG: A study of the end-results of compression arthrodesis of the knee. *J Bone Joint Surg* 40B:633, 1958.

45. Stulberg SD: Arthrodesis in failed total knee replacements. *Orthop Clin North Am* 13:213, 1982.

46. Thornhill TS, Dalziel RW, Sledge CB: Alternatives to arthrodesis for the failed total knee arthroplasty. *Clin Orthop Rel Res* 170:131, 1982.

47. Stulberg SD: Arthrodesis in failed total knee replacement, *Orthop Clin North Am* 13:213, 1982.

48. Falahee MH, Matthews LS, Kaufer H: Resection arthroplasty as a salvage procedure for a knew with infection after a total arthroplasty. *J Bone Joint Surg* 69A:1013, 1987.

49. Rand JA, Bryan RS: The outcome of failed knee arthrodesis following total knee arthroplasty. *Clin Orthop Rel Res* 205:1986.

50. Figgie HE III, et al: Knee arthrodesis following total knee arthroplasty in rheumatoid arthritis. *Clin Orthop Rel Res* 224:237, 1987.

51. Jackson RW: The role of arthroscopy in the management of the arthritic knee. *Clin Orthop Rel Res* 101:28, 1974.

52. Jackson RW, Silver R, Marans H: The arthroscopic treatment of degenerative joint disease. *Arthroscopy* 2:114, 1986.

53. Spague NF III: Arthroscopic debridement for degenerative knee joint disease. *Clin Orthop Rel Res* 160:118, 1981.

54. Timoney JM, Kneisl JS, Barrack RL, et al: Arthroscopy in the osteoarthritic knee: Long-term follow-up. *Orthop Rev* 19:371, 1990.

55. Baumgaertner MR, Cannon WD Jr, Vittori JM, et al: Arthroscopic debridement of the arthritic knee. *Clin Orthop Rel Res* 253:197, 1990.

56. Livesley PJ, Doherty M, Needoff M, et al: Arthroscopic lavage of osteoarthritic knees *J Bone Joint Surg* 73B:922, 1991.

57. Aichroth PM, Patel DV, Moyes ST: A prospective review of arthroscopic debridement for degenerative joint disease of the knee. *Int Orthop* 15:351, 1991.

58. Ogilvie-Harris DJ, Fitsialos DP: Arthroscopic management of the degenerative knee. *Arthroscopy* 7:151, 1991.

59. McLaren AC, Blokker CP, Fowler PJ, et al: Arthroscopic debridement of the knee for osteoarthritis. *Can J Surg* 34:595, 1991.

60. Rand JA: Role of arthroscopy in osteoarthritis of the knee. *Arthroscopy* 7:358, 1991.

61. Bert JM, Maschka K: The arthroscopic treatment of unicompartmental gonarthrosis: A five year follow-up of abrasion arthroplasty plus arthroscopic debridement and arthroscopic debridement alone.

62. McDermott AG, Finkelstein JA, Farine I, et al: Distal femoral varus osteotomy for valgus deformity of the knee. *J Bone Joint Surg* 70A:110, 1988.

63. Edgerton BC, Mariane EM, Morrey BF: Distal femoral varus osteotomy for painful genu valgum: A five- to 11-year follow-up study. *Clin Orthop Rel Res* 288:263, 1993.

64. Miniaci A, Gorssman SP, Jakob RP: Supracondylar femoral varus osteotomy in the treatment of valgus knee deformity. *Am J Knee Surg* 3:65, 1990.

65. Chan RN, Pollard JP: High tibial osteotomy for rheumatoid arthritis of the knee: A one to six year follow-up study. *Acta Orthop Scand* 49:78, 1978.

66. Ahlberg A, Scham S, Unander-Scharin L. Osteotomy in degenerative and rheumatoid arthritis of the knee joint. *Acta Orthop Scand* 39:379, 1968.

67. Morrey BF: Upper tibial osteotomy: Analysis of prognostic features: A review. *Adv Orthop Surg* 9:213, 1986.

68. Coventry MB: Upper tibial osteotomy. *Clin Orthop Rel Res* 182:46, 1984.

69. Healy WL, Barber TC: The role of osteotomy in the treatment of osteoarthritis of the knee. *Am J Knee Surg* 3:97, 1990.

70. Coventry MB: Proximal tibial varus osteotomy for osteoarthritis of the lateral compartment of the knee. *J Bone Joint Surg* 69A:32, 1987.

71. Morrey BF, Edgarton BC: Distal femoral osteotomy for lateral gonarthrosis. *Instr Course Lect* 41:77, 1992.

72. Healy WL, Angler JO, Wasilewski SA, Krackow KA: Distal femoral osteotomy. *J Bone Joint Surg* 70A:102, 1988.

73. Jackson JP: Osteotomy for osteoarthritis of the knee: Proceedings of the Sheffield Regional Orthopaedic Club. *J Bone Joint Surg* 40B:826, 1958.

74. Jackson JP, Waugh W: Tibial osteotomy for osteoarthritis of the knee. *J Bone Joint Surg* 43B:746, 1961.

75. Coventry MB: Osteotomy of the upper portion of the tibia for degenerative arthritis of the knee: A preliminary report. *J Bone Joint Surg* 47A:984, 1961.

76. Coventry MB: Osteotomy about the knee for degenerative and rheumatoid arthritis. *J Bone Joint Surg* 55A:23, 1973.

77. Coventry MB: Upper tibial osteotomy for gonarthrosis: The evolution of the operation in the last 18 years and long-term results. *Orthop Clin North Am* 10:191, 1979.

78. Coventry MB: Upper tibial osteotomy. *Clin Orthop Rel Res* 182:46, 1984.

79. Coventry MB, Illstrup DM, Wallrichs SL: Proximal tibial osteotomy: A critical long-term study of eighty-seven cases. *J Bone Joint Surg* 75A:196, 1993.

80. Jakob RP, Murphy SB. Tibial osteotomy for varus gonarthrosis: Indications, preoperative planning and technique. *Orthop Clin North Am* 25(3):477–483, 1994.

81. Coventry MB: Stepped staple for upper tibial osteotomy. *J Bone Joint Surg* 51A:1011, 1969.

82. Maquet P: Valgus osteotomy for osteoarthritis of the knee: *Clin Orthop Rel Res* 120:143, 1976.

83. Jackson JP, Waugh W: Tibial osteotomy for osteoarthritis of the knee. *J Bone Joint Surg* 43B:746, 1961.

84. Gariepy R: Genu varum treated by high tibial osteotomy. Proceedings of the Joint Meeting of the Orthopaedic Associations of the English-Speaking World. *J Bone Joint Surg* 46B:783, 1964.

85. Hernigou PH, Medevielle D, Debeyre J, Goutallier D: Proximal tibial osteotomy for osteoarthritis with varus deformity. *J Bone Joint Surg* 69A:332, 1987.

85a. Sundaram NA, Hallet JP, Sullivan MF. Dome osteotomy of the tibia for osteoarthritis of the knee. *J Bone Joint Surg* 68B:782, 1986.

86. Fujisawa Y, Masuhara K, Shiomi S: The effect of high tibial osteotomy on osteoarthritis of the knee: An arthroscopic study of 54 knee joints. *Orthop Clin North Am* 10:585, 1979.

87. Jakob RP: Instabilitatsbedingte Gonarthrose—Spezielle

Indikationen fur Osteotomien bei der Behandlung des insta- bilen Kniegelenkes, in Jakob RP, Staubi HU, (eds): *Kniegelenk und Kreuzbander.* New York, Spring Verlag, 1991, p 555.

88. Cass JR, Bryan RS: High tibial osteotomy. *Clin Orthop Rel Res* 230:196, 1988.

89. Jokio PJ, Lindholm TS, Vankka E: Medial and lateral go- narthrosis treated with high tibial osteotomy. A preoperative study. *Arch Otrhop Trauma Surg* 104:135, 1985.

90. Keene JS, Monson DK, Roberts JM, Dyreby JR Jr: The evalu- ation of patients for high tibial osteotomy. *Clin Orthop Rel Res* 243:157, 1981.

91. Kettlekamp DB, Wenger DR, Chao EYS, Thompson C: Results of proximal tibial osteotomy: The effects of tibiofemoral an- gle, stance-phase flexion-extension, and medial plateau force; *J Bone Joint Surg* 58A:952, 1976.

92. Myerts R: High tibial osteotomy with overcorrection of varus malalignment in medial gonarthrosis. *Acta Orthop Scand* 51:557, 1980.

93. Rudan JF, Simurda MA: High tibial osteotomy: A prospective clinical and roentgenographic review. *Clin Orthop Rel Res* 255:251, 1990.

94. Stuart MJ, Grace JN, Ilstrup DM, et al: Late recurrence of varus deformity after proximal tibial osteotomy. *Clin Orthop Rel Res* 260:61, 1990.

95. Odenbring S, Egund N, Knutson K, et al: Revision after os- teotomy for gonarthrosis: A 10–19-year follow-up of 314 cases. *Acta Orthop Scand* 61:128, 1990.

96. Brennan AT, Bosacco SJ, Kirshner S, et al: Factors influencing long-term result in high tibial osteotomy. *Clin Orthop Rel Res* 272:192, 1991.

97. Coventry MB: Proximal tibial osteotomy for gonarthrosis: The evaluation of the operation in the last 18 years and long- term results. *Orthop Clin North Am* 10:191, 1979.

98. Coventry MB, Bowman PW: Long-term results of upper tibial osteotomy for degenerative arthritis of the knee. *Acta Orthop Belg* 48:134, 1982.

99. Ivarrson I, Mynerts R, Gillquist J: High tibial osteotomy for medial osteoarthritis of the knee: A 5 to 7 and an 11 to 13 year follow-up *J Bone Joint Surg* 72B:238, 1990.

100. Healy WL, Riley LH Jr: High tibial valgus osteotomy. A clini- cal review. *Clin Orthop Rel Res* 209:227–233, 1986.

101. Rubens F, Wellington JL, Bouchard AG: Popliteal artery in- jury after tibial osteotomy: A report of two cases; *Can J Surg* 33:294–297, 1990.

102. LeMarc R: Etude comparative de deux series d'osteotomies tibialis avec fixation par lame-plaque ou par cadre de com- pression. *Acta Orthop Belg* 48:157, 1982.

103. Weill D, Schneider M, Simon G: Les osteotomies du genou dans le traitement de 10 ans et de plus 400 interventions. *Rev Chir Orthop* 67(suppl):119–122, 1981.

104. Allen T, Jackson JP, Waugh W: Neuromuscular complications of high tibial osteotomy, cited in Jackson JP, Waugh W (eds): *Surgery of the Knee Joint.* London Chapman and Hall, 1984.

105. Curley P, Eyres K, Bregimora V et al: Common peroneal nerve dysfunction after high tibial osteotomy; *J Bone Joint Surg* 72B:405, 1990.

106. McKeever DC, Elliot RB: Tibial plateau prosthesis. *Clin Orthop Rel Res* 18:86, 1960.

107. MacIntosh DL: The use of hemiarthroplasty prosthesis for advanced osteoarthritis and rheumatoid arthritis of the knee. *J Bone Joint Surg* 40A:1431, 1972.

108. Potter TA: Arthroplasty of the knee with tibial metallic im- plants of the McKeever and MacIntosh design. *Surg Clin North Am* 49:903, 1969.

109. Scott RD, Joyce MJ, Ewald FC, Thomas WH: McKeever metal- lic hemiarthroplasty of the knee in unicompartmental de- generative arthritis: Long-term clinical follow-up and current indications. *J Bone Joint Surg* 65A:203, 1985.

110. Christensen NO: Unicompartmental prosthesis for gonathro- sis: A nine-year series of 575 knees from a Swedish hospital. *Clin Orthop Rel Res* 273:165, 1991.

111. Marmor L: Lateral compartment arthroplasty of the knee. *Clin Orthop Rel Res* 186:115, 1984.

112. Marmor L: Unicompartmental knee arthroplasty: Ten to thirteen year follow-up study. *Clin Orthop Rel Res* 226:14, 1988.

113. Bae KK, Guhl JF, Keane SP: Unicompartmental knee arthro- plasty for single compartment disease: Clinical experience with an average four-year follow-up. *Clin Orthop Rel Res* 176:223–238, 1983.

114. Scott RD, Santore RF: Unicondylar replacement of os- teoarthritis of the knee. *J Bone Joint Surg* 63A:536, 1986.

115. Scott RD, Cobb AG, McQueary FG, Thornhill TS: Unicompartmental knee arthroplasty, eight to twelve year follow-up with survivorship analysis. *Clin Orthop Rel Res* 271:96, 1991.

116. Insall JN, Walker P: Unicondylar knee replacement. *Clin Orthop Rel Res* 120:38, 1976.

117. Insall JN, Aglietti P: A five- to seven-year follow-up of uni- condylar arthroplasty. *J Bone Joint Surg* 62A:1329, 1980.

118. Laskin RS: Modular total knee replacement arthroplasty. *J Bone Joint Surg* 58A:766, 1976.

119. Padgett DE, Stern SH, Insall JN: Revision total knee arthro- plasty for failed unicompartmental replacement. *J Bone Joint Surg* 73A:186, 1991.

120. Broughton NS, Newman JH, Bailey RA: Unicompartmental re- placement and high tibial osteotomy for osteoarthritis of the knee. *J Bone Joint Surg* 63B:447, 1986.

121. Inglis G: Unicompartmental arthroplasty of the knee. *J Bone Joint Surg* 66B:682, 1984.

122. Ivarsson I, Gillquist J: Rehabilitation after high tibial os- teotomy and unicompartmental arthroplasty. *Clin Orthop Rel Res* 266:139, 1991.

123. Weale AE, Newman JH: Unicompartmental arthroplasty and high tibial osteotomy for osteoarthritis of the knee: A com- parative study with twelve to seventeen year follow-up pe- riod. *Clin Orthop Rel Res* 302:134, 1994.

124. Rougraff BT, Heck DA, Gibson AE: A comparison of tricom partmental and unicompartmental arthroplasty for the treat- ment of gonarthrosis. *Clin Orthop Rel Res* 273:157, 1991.

125. Laurencin CT, Zelicof SB, Scott RD, Ewald FC: Unicompart- mental versus total knee arthroplasty in the same patient: A comparative study. *Clin Orthop Rel Res* 273:151, 1991.

126. Thornhill TS, Scott RD: Unicompartmental knee arthroplasty. *Orthop Clin North Am* 20:245, 1989.

127. Ranawat CS, Boachie-Adjei O: Survivorship analysis and re- sults of total condylar knee arthroplasty: Eight to 11-year fol- low-up period. *Clin Orthop Rel Res* 226:6, 1988.

128. Scuderi GR, Insall JN, Windsor RE, et al: Survivorship of cemented knee replacements. *J Bone Joint Surg* 71B:798, 1989.

129. Rand JA, Ilstrup DM: Survivorship analysis of total knee arthroplasty. *J Bone Joint Surg* 73A:397, 1991.

130. Heck DA, Marmor L, Gibson A, Rougraff BT: Unicompartmen- tal knee arthroplasty. A multicenter investigation with long- term follow-up evaluation. *Clin Orthop Rel Res* 286:154, 1993.

131. Stockelman RE, Pohl KP: The long-term efficacy of unicom- partmental arthroplasty of the knee. *Clin Orthop Rel Res* 271:88, 1991.

132. Jerry GJ Jr, Rand JA, Ilstrup D: Old sepsis prior to total knee arthroplasty. *Clin Orthop Rel Res* 236:135, 1988.

133. Kim YH: Total knee arthroplasty for tuberculous arthritis. *J*

Bone Joint Surg 70A:1322, 1988.

134. Schurman JR II, Wilde AH: Total knee replacement after spontaneous osseous ankylosis: A report of three cases. *J Bone Joint Surg* 72A:4550, 1990.

135. Holden DL, Jackson DW: Considerations in total knee arthroplasty following previous knee fusion. *Clin Orthop Rel Res* 227:223, 1988.

136. Krackow KA, Weiss APC: Recurvatum deformity complicating performance of total knee arthroplasty: A brief note. *J Bone Joint Surg* 72A:268, 1990.

137. Emerson RH Jr, Head WC, Malinin TI: Reconstruction of patellar tendon rupture after total knee arthroplasty with an extensor mechanism allograft. *Clin Orthop* 260:154, 1990.

138. Soundry M, Binazzi R, Johanson NA, et al: Total knee arthroplasty in Charcot and Charcot-like joints. *Clin Orthop* 208:199, 1986.

139. Scuderi GR, Insall JN, Windsor RE, et al: SUrvivorship of cemented knee replacements. *J Bone Joint Surg* 71B:798, 1989.

140. Wright J, Ewald FC, Walker PS, et al: Total knee arthroplasty with the kinematic prosthesis: Results after five to nine years: A follow-up note. *J Bone Joint Surg* 72A:1003, 1990.

141. Stern SH, Insall JN: Posterior stabilized prosthesis: Results after follow-up on nine to twelve years. *J Bone Joint Surg* 74A:989, 1992.

142. Jeffery RS, Morris RW, Denham RA: Coronal alignment after total knee replacement. *J Bone Joint Surg* 73B:709, 1991.

143. Jiang C-C, Insall JN: Effect of rotation on the axial alignment of the femur: Pitfalls in the use of femoral intramedullary guides in total knee arthroplasty. *Clin Orthop Rel Res* 248:50, 1989.

144. Rose HA, Hood RW, Otis JC, et al: Peroneal nerve palsy following total knee arthroplasty. *J Bone Joint Surg* 64A:347, 1982.

145. Asp JP, Rand JA: Peroneal nerve palsy after total knee arthroplasty. *Clin Orthop Rel Res* 261:233, 1990.

146. Stern SH, Moeckel BH, Insall JN: Total knee arthroplasty in valgus knees. *Clin Orthop Rel Res* 273:5, 1991.

147. Knutson K, Loden I, Sturfelt G, et al: Nerve palsy after knee arthroplasty in patients with rheumatoid arthritis. *Scand J Rheumatol* 12:201, 1983.

148. Krackow KA, Maar DC, Mont MA, Carroll C IV: Surgical decompression for peroneal nerve palsy after total knee arthroplasty. *Clin Orthop Rel Res* 292:223, 1993.

149. Horlocher TT, Cabenela ME, Wedel DT: Does postoperative epidural analgesia increase the risk of peroneal nerve palsy after total knee arthroplasty. *Anesth Analg* 79:495, 1994.

150. Rand JA: Vascular complications of total knee arthroplasty. *J Arthop* 2:89, 1987.

151. Calligaro KD, Delaurentis DA, Booth RE, et al: Acute arterial thrombosis associated with total knee arthroplasty. *J Vasc Surg* 20:927, 1994.

152. Rush JH, Vidovich JD, Johnson MA: Arterial complications of total knee replacements. *J Bone Joint Surg* 69B:400, 1987.

153. Wilson FC, Fajgenbaum DM, Venters GC: Results of knee replacement with the Walldius and geometric prosthesis. *J Bone Joint Surg* 62A:497, 1980.

154. Dennis DA, Neuman RD, Toma P, et al: Arteriovenous fistula with false aneurysm of the inferior medial geniculate artery: A complication of total knee arthroplasty. *Clin Orthop Rel Res* 222:255, 1987.

155. Stanley D, Cumberland DC, Elson RA: Embolization for aneurysm after total knee replacement: A brief report. *J Bone Joint Surg* 71B:138, 1989.

156. Dalaurentis DA, Levitsky KA, Booth RE, et al: Arterial and ischemic aspects of total knee arthroplasty. *Am J Surg* 164:237, 1992.

157. McPherson EJ, Friedman RJ: Arterial thromboembolism associated with total knee arthroplasty: A report of two cases. *Am J Knee Surg* 5(suppl):94, 1992.

158. Insall J, Haas SB: Complications of total knee arthroplasty, in *Surgery of the Knee,* 2d ed. New York, Churchill Livingstone, 1993.

159. Gurd AR, Wilson RI: The fat embolism syndrome. *J Bone Joint Surg* 56B:408, 1974.

160. Manto RR, Garcia J, Callaghan JJ: Fatal fat embolism following total condylar knee arthroplasty. *J Arthop* 5:291, 1990.

161. Bisla RS, Inglis AE, Lewis RJ: Fat embolism following bilateral total knee replacement with the GUEPAR prosthesis: A case report. *Clin Orthop* 115:195, 1976.

162. Caillouette JT, Anzel SH: Fat embolism syndrome following the intramedullary alignment guide in total knee arthroplasty. *Clin Orthop* 251:198, 1990.

163. Dorr LD, Merkel C, Mellman MNF, Klein I: Fat emboli in bilateral total knee arthroplasty: Predictive factors for neurologic manifestations. *Clin Orthop* 248:112, 1989.

164. Fahmy NR, Chandler HP, Danylchuk K, et al: Blood gas and circulatory changes during total knee replacement: Role of the intramedullary alignment rod. *J Bone Joint Surg* 72A:19, 1990.

165. Hall TM, Callaghan JJ: Fat embolism precipitated by reaming of the femoral canal during revision of a total knee replacement: A case report. *J Bone Joint Surg* 76A:899, 1994.

166. Parmet JL, Horrow JC, Singer R, et al: Echogenic emboli upon tourniquet release during total knee arthroplasty: Pulmonary hemodynamic changes and embolic composition. *Anesth Analg* 79:940, 1994.

167. Lindeque BGP, Schoeman HS, Dommisse GF, et al: Fat embolism and the fat embolism syndrome: A double blind therapeutic study. *J Bone Joint Surg* 69B:128, 1987.

168. Stollenberg JJ, Gustilo RB: The use of methylprednisolone and hypotonic glucose in the prophylaxis of fat embolism syndrome. *Clin Orthop* 143:211, 1979.

169. Lachiewicz PF, Ranawat CS: Fat embolism syndrome following bilateral total knee replacement with total condylar prosthesis: Report of two cases. *Clin Orthop Rel Res* 160:106, 1981.

170. Dorr LD, Merkel C, Mellman MF, Klein I: Fat emboli in bilateral total knee arthroplasty. *Clin Orthop Rel Res* 248:112, 1989.

171. Jankiewicz JJ, Sculco TP, Ranawat CS, et al: One-stage versus 2-stage bilateral total knee arthropalsty. *Clin Orthop* 309:94, 1994.

172. Kolettis GT, Wixson RL, Peruzi WT, et al: Safety of 1-stage ilateral total knee arthroplasty. *Clin Orthop* 309:102, 1994.

173. Cohen SH, Ehrlich GE, Kauffman MS, et al: Thrombophlebitis following knee surgery. *J Bone Joint Surg* 55A:106, 1973.

174. Frances CW, Ricotta JJ, Evarts CM, Marder VJ: Long-term clinical observations and venous functional abnormalities after asymptomatic venous thrombosis following total hip or knee arthroplasty.

175. Hull RD, Rasob GE: Prophylaxis of venous thromboembolic disease following hip and knee surgery. *J Bone Joint Surg* 68A:146, 1986.

176. Stringer MD, Steadman CA, Hedges AR, et al: Deep vein thrombosis after elective knee surgery: An incidence study in 312 patients. *J Bone Joint Surg* 71B:492, 1989.

177. Stulberg B, Insall JN, Hood RW, Williams G: Postoperative thrombosis following total knee arthroplasty. *Trans Orthop Res Soc* 7:291, 1982.

178. Stulberg BJ, Insall JN, Williams GW, Ghelman B: Deep-vein thrombosis following total knee replacement: An analysis of six hundred and thirty-eight arthroplasties. *J Bone Joint Surg* 66A:194, 1984.

179. Haas SB, Insall JN, Scuderi GR, et al: Pneumatic sequential

compression boots compared with aspirin prophylaxis of deep-vein thrombosis after total knee arthroplasty. *J Bone Joint Surg* 72A:27, 1990.

180. Doouss TW: The clinical significance of venous thrombosis of the calf. *Br J Surg* 63:377, 1976.

181. Kakkar VV, Howe CT, Flanc C, Clarke MB: Natural history of postoperative deep-vein thrombosis. *Lancet* 2:230, 1969.

182. Bettmann MA, Robbins A, Braun SD, et al: Contrast venography of the leg: Diagnostic, efficacy, tolerance, and complication rates with ionic and nonionic contrast media. *Radiology* 165:113, 1987.

183. Spritzer CE, Sostamn HD, Wilkes DC, Coleman RE: Deep venous thrombosis: Experience with gradient-echo MR imaging in 66 patients. *Radiology* 177:235, 1990.

184. Albrechtsson U, Olsson CG: Thrombotic side-effects of lower-limb phlebography. *Lancet* 1:723, 1976.

185. Woolson ST, Pottorff G: Venous ultrasonography in the detection of proximal vein thrombosis after total knee arthroplasty. *Clin Orthop Rel Res* 273:131, 1991.

186. Woolson ST, McCrory DW, Walter JF, et al: B-mode ultrasound scanning in the detection of proximal venous thrombosis after total hip arthroplasty. *J Bone Joint Surg* 72A:983, 1990.

187. Froehlich JA, Dorfman GS, Cronan JJ, et al: Compression ultrasonography for the detection of deep venous thrombosis in patients who have a fracture of the hip: A prospective study. *J Bone Joint Surg* 71A:249, 1989.

188. Davidson BL Elliot CG, Lensing AW: Low accuracy of color Doppler ultrasound in the detection of proximal leg vein thrombosis in asymptomatic high-risk patients. *Ann Intern Med* 117:735, 1992.

189. Larcom PG, Lotke PA, Holland GA, et al: Comparison of magnetic resonance venography to standard contrast venography in the diagnosis of deep venous thrombosis following lower extremity joint surgery. Presented at the American Academy of Orthopaedic Surgeons Annual Meeting, Atlanta, 1996.

190. Hull RD, Raskob GE, Rosenbloom D, et al: Heparin for 5 days with 10 days in the initial treatment of proximal venous thrombosis. *N Engl J Med* 322:1260, 1991.

191. Poss R, Thornhill TS, Ewald FC et al: Factors influencing the incidence and outcome of infection following total joint arthroplasty. *Clin Orthop Rel Res* 182:117, 1984.

192. Rand JA, Fitzgerald RH Jr: Management of the infected total knee arthroplasty. *Orthop Clin North Am* 20:201, 1989.

193. Salvati EA, Robinson RP, Zeno SM, et al: Infection rates after 3175 total hip and total knee replacements performed with and without a horizontal unidirectional filtered air-flow system. *J Bone Joint Surg* 64A:525, 1982.

194. Wilson MG, Kelley K, Thornhill TS. Infection as a complication of total knee replacement arthroplasty. *J Bone Joint Surg* 72A:878, 1990.

195. Grogan TJ, Dorey F, Rollins J, Amstutz HC: Deep sepsis following total knee arthroplasty. *J Bone Joint Surg* 86A:226–234, 1986.

196. Ritter MA: Intraoperative controls of bacterial contamination during total knee replacement. *Orthop Clin North Am* 20:49, 1989.

197. Fitzgerland RH, Keely PJ: Total joint arthroplasty: Biologic causes of failure. *Mayo Clin Proc* 4:590, 1979.

198. Gristina AG, Kolkin J: Total joint replacement and sepsis. *J Bone Joint Surg* 65A:128, 1983.

199. Petty W, Bryan RS, Coventry MB, Petersen LFA: Infection after total knee arthroplasty. *Orthop Clin North Am* 6:1005, 1975.

200. Jerry GT, Rand JA, Ilstrup DM: Ancient sepsis prior to total knee arthroplasty. *Clin Orthop Rel Res* 236:135, 1988.

201. Bengston S, Knutson K, Lidgren L: Treatment of infected knee arthroplasty. *Clin Orthop Rel Res* 245:173, 1989.

202. Booth RE Jr, Lotke PA: The results of spacer block technique in revision of infected total knee arthroplasty. *Clin Orthop Rel Res* 248:57, 1989.

203. Borden LS, Gearen RF: Infected total knee arthroplasty: A protocol for management. *J Arthrop* 2:27, 1987.

204. Grogan TJ, Dorey F, Rollins J, Amstutz HC: Deep sepsis following total knee arthroplasty. *J Bone Joint Surg* 86A:226, 1986.

205. Jacobs MA, Hungerford DS, Krackow KA, Lennox DW: Revision of septic total knee arthroplasty. *Clin Orthop Rel Res* 238:159, 1989.

206. Lettin AWF, Neil MJ, Citron ND, August A: Excision arthroplasty for infected constrained total knee replacements. *J Bone Joint Surg* 72B:220, 1990.

207. Morrey BF, Westholm F, Schoifet S, et al: Long-term results of various treatment options for infected total knee arthroplasty. *Clin Orthop Rel Res* 248:120, 1989.

208. Rand JA, Bryan RS, Chao EYS: Failed total knee arthroplasty treated by arthrodesis of the knee using the Ace-Fischer apparatus. *J Bone Joint Surg* 69A:39, 1987.

209. Wilde AH, Ruth JJ: Two-stage reimplantation in infected total knee arthroplasty. *Clin Orthop Rel Res* 236:23, 1988.

210. Windsor RE, Insall JN, Urs WK, et al: Two-stage reimplantation for the salvage of total knee arthroplasty complicated by infection. *J Bone Joint Surg* 72A, 272, 1990.

211. Rand JA, Brown MK: The value of indium-111 leukocyte scanning in the evaluation of the painful or infected total knee arthroplasty. *Clin Orthop Rel Res* 259:178, 1990.

212. Rand JA, Bryan RS: Reimplantation for the salvage of an infected total knee arthroplasty. *J Bone Joint Surg* 65A:1081, 1983.

213. Levitsky KA, Hozack WJ, Balderston RA, et al: Evaluation of the painful prosthetic joint: Relative value of bone scan, sedimentation rate, and joint aspiration. *J Arthrop* 6:237, 1991.

214. Brause BD. Infected total knee arthropalsty. *Orthop Clin North Am* 13:245, 1982.

215. Insall JN: Infection of total knee arthroplasty. *Inst Course Lect* 35:319, 1986.

216. Teeny SM, Dorr L, Murata G, Conaty P: Treatment of infected total knee arthroplasty—Irrigation and debridement versus two-stage reimplantation. *J Arthrop* 5:35, 1990.

217. Walker RH, Schurman DJ: Management of infected total knee arthroplasties. *Clin Orthop Rel Res* 186:81, 1984.

218. Freeman MAR, Sudlow RA, Casewell MW, Radcliff SS: The management of infected total knee replacement. *J Bone Joint Surg* 67B:764, 1985.

219. Goksak SB, Freeman MA: One stage reimplantation for infected total knee arthroplasty. *J Bone Joint Surg* 74B:78, 1992.

220. Insall JN, Thompson FM, Brause BD: Two-stage reimplantation for the salvage of infected total knee arthroplasty. *J Bone Joint Surg* 65A:1087, 1983.

221. Nelson CL, Evans RP, Blaha JD, et al: A comparison of gentamicin-impregnated polymethylmethacrylate beard implantation to conventional parenteral antibiotic therapy in infected total hip and knee arthroplasty. *Clin Orthop Rel Res* 295:93, 1993.

222. Rand JA, Coventry MB: Stress fractures after total knee arthroplasty. *J Bone Joint Surg* 62A:226, 1980.

223. Fipp G: Stress fractures of the femoral neck following total knee arthroplasty. *J Arthrop* 3:347, 1988.

224. Aaron RK, Scott RD: Supracondylar fracture of the femur after total knee arthroplasty. *Clin Orthop Rel Res* 219:136, 1987.

225. Cain PR, Rubash HE, Wissinger HA, McClain EJ: Periprosthetic femoral fractures following total knee arthroplasty. *Clin Orthop Rel Res* 208:205, 1986.

226. Cordiero EN, Costa RC, Carazzato JG Silva JD: Periprosthetic fractures in patients with total knee arthroplasty. *Clin Orthop*

Rel Res 252:182, 1990.

227. Culp RW, Schmidt RG, Hanks G, et al: Supracondylar fracture of the femur following prosthetic knee arthroplasty. *Clin Orthop Rel Res* 224:212, 1987.

228. Figgie MP, Goldberg VM, Figgie HE III, Sobel M: The results of treatment of supracondylar fracture above total knee arthroplasty. *J Arthop* 5:267, 1990.

229. Merkel KD, Johnson EW Jr: Supracondylar fracture of the femur after total knee arthroplasty. *J Bone Joint Surg* 68A:29, 1986.

230. Sisto DJ, Lachiewicz PF, Insall JN: Treatment of supracondylar fractures following prosthetic arthroplasty of the knee. *Clin Orthop Rel Res* 196:265, 1985.

231. Ritter MA, Faris PM, Keating EM: Anterior femoral notching and ipsilateral supracondylar femur fracture in total knee arthroplasty. *J Arthrop* 3:185, 1988.

232. Hardy DC, Delince PE, Yasik E, et al: Stress fractures of the hip: An unusual complication of total knee arthroplasty. *Clin Orthop Rel Res* 281:140, 1992.

233. McElwaine JP, Sheehan JM: Spontaneous fractures of the femoral neck after total replacement of the knee. *J Bone Joint Surg* 64B:323, 1982.

234. DiGioia AM III, Rubash HE: Periprosthetic fractures of the femur after total knee arthroplasty: A literature review and treatment algorithm. *Clin Orthop Rel Res* 271:135, 1991.

235. Hanks GA, Mathews HH, Routson GW, et al: Supracondylar fracture of the femur following total knee arthroplasty. *J Arthrop* 4:289, 1989.

236. Emerson RH Jr, Head WC, Malinin TI: Reconstruction of patellar tendon rupture after total knee arthroplasty with an extensor mechanism allograft. *Clin Orthop Rel Res* 260:154, 1990.

237. Laskin RS, Bucknell A: The use of metal-backed patellar prosthesies in total knee arthroplasty. *Clin Orthop Rel Res* 260:52, 1990.

238. Vince KG, Insall JN, Kelly MA: The total condylar prosthesis, ten-to-twelve year results with a cemented knee replacement. *J Bone Joint Surg* 71B:783, 1989.

239. Volatile TB, Ewald FC, Friedman RS, et al: Ten-year results of 139 duocondylar total knee replacements. *Orthop Trans* 10:491, 1986.

240. Collins DN, Heim SA, Nelson CL, et al: Porous-coated anatomic total knee arthroplasty: A prospective analysis comparing cemented and cementless fixation. *Clin Orthop Rel Res* 267:128, 1991.

240a. Rosenberg AG, Borden RM, Galante JO: Cemented and ingrowth fixation of the Miller-Galante prosthesis: Clinical and roentgenographic comparison after 3- to 6-year follow-up studies. *Clin Orthop Rel Res* 260:71–79, 1990.

240b. Wright RJ, Lima J, Scott RD, et al: Two- to four-year results of a posterior cruciate-sparing condylar total knee arthroplasty with an uncemented femoral component. *Clin Orthop Rel Res* 260:80–86, 1990.

241. Ranawat CS, Flynn WF Jr, Saddler S, et al: Long-term results of the total knee arthroplasty: A 15-year survivorship study. *Clin Orthop Rel Res* 286:94, 1993.

242. Ritter MA, Herbst SA, Keating EM, et al: Long-term survival analysis of a posterior cruciate-retaining total condylar total knee arthroplasty. *Clin Orthop Rel Res* 309:136, 1994.

243. Dodd CA, Hungerford DS, Krackow KA: Total knee arthroplasty fixation: Comparison of the early results of paired cemented versus uncemented porous coated anatomic knee prostheses. *Clin Orthop Rel Res* 280:66, 1990.

244. Moran CG, Pinder IM, Lee TA, et al: Survivorship analysis of the uncemented porous-coated anatomic knee replacement. *J Bone Joint Surg* 73A:848, 1991.

245. Rorabeck CH, Bourne RB, Lewis PL, et al: The Miller-Galante knee prosthesis for the treatment of osteoarthritis: A comparison of the results of partial fixation with cement and fixation without any cement. *J Bone Joint Surg* 75A:402, 1993.

246. Rorabeck CH, Bourne RB, Nott L: The cemented kinematic-II and the non-cemented porous coated anatomic prosthesis for total knee replacement: A prospective evaluation. *J Bone Joint Surg* 70A:483, 1988.

247. Figgie HE, Goldberg VM, Shea K, et al. A clinical kinematic comparison and a mechanical correlation of posterior cruciate retaining versus posterior cruciate-substituting total knee prosthesis. Annual Meeting of the American Academy of Orthopaedic Surgeons, Anaheim, CA, March 1991.

248. Andriacchi TP, Galante JO: Retention of the posterior cruciate in total knee arthroplasty. *J Arthop* 3:S13, 1988.

249. Andriacchi TP, Galante JO, Fermier RW: The influence of the total knee replacement design on walking and stair-climbing. *J Bone Joint Surg* 64A:1328, 1982.

250. Cobb AL, Ewald FC, Wright RJ, Sledge CB: The kinemaic knee survivorship analysis of 1943 knees. Proceedings of the Annual Meeting of the British Orthopaedic Association. *J Bone Joint Surg* 72B:542, 1990.

250a. Becker-Fleugal MW, Insall JN: Bilateral total knee arthroplasty: One cruciate-retaining and one cruciate-substituting. Presented at the Annual Meeting of the Knee Society, New Orleans, Louisiana, February 1990.

251. Epstein AM, Read JL, Heoffer M: The relation of body weight to length of stay and charges of hospital services for patients undergoing elective surgery: A study of two procedures. *Am J Public Health* 77:993, 1987.

251a. Ranawat CS, Boachie-Adjei O: Survivorship analysis and results of total condylar knee arthroplasty: Eight- to eleven-year follow-up period. *Clin Orthop Rel Res* 226:6, 1988.

252. Stern SH, Insall JN: Total knee arthroplasty in obese patients. *J Bone Joint Surg* 72A:1400, 1990.

252a. Scuderi GR, Windsor RE, Insall JN, Moran MC: Survivorship of cemented knee replacements. *J Bone Joint Surg* 71B:798, 1989.

253. Tauber C, Baron AB, Ganel A, Malkin C: The total condylar knee prosthesis: A review of 71 operations. *Arch Orthop Trauma Surg* 104:352, 1986.

253a. Rand JA, Ilstrup DA: Survivorship analysis of total knee arthroplasty: Cumulative rates of survival of 9200 total knee arthroplasties. *J Bone Joint Surg* 73A:397, 1991.

254. Pritchett JW, Bortell DT: Knee replacement in morbidly obese women. *Surg Gynecol Obstet* 173:119, 1991.

255. Scott WN, Rubenstein M, Scuderi G: Results after knee replacement with a cruciate-substituting prosthesis. *J Bone Joint Surg* 70A:1164, 1988.

256. Bisla RS, Inglis AE, Ranawat CS: Joint replacement in patients under thirty. *J Bone Joint Surg* 58A:1098, 1976.

257. Chandler HP, Reineck FT, Wixon RL, McCarthy JC: Total hip arthroplasty in patients younger than thirty years old: A five year follow-up study. *J Bone Joint Surg* 63A:1426, 1981.

258. Diduch P, Insall JN, Scott W, Scuderi G, Rodriguez D: Presented at the AAOS Meeting, Atlanta, 1996.

259. Sarokhan AJ, Scott RD, Thomas WH, et al: Total knee arthroplasty in juvenile rheumatoid arthritis. *J Bone Joint Surg* 65A:1071, 1983.

260. Carmichael E, Chaplin M: Total knee arthroplasty in juvenile rheumatoid arthritis. *Clin Orthop Rel Res* 210:192, 1986.

261. Ewald FC, Christie MJ: Results of total knee replacement in young patients. *Orthop Trans* 11:442, 1987.

262. Stuart MJ, Rand JA: Total knee arthroplasty in young adults who have rheumatoid arthritis. *J Bone Joint Surg* 70A:84, 1988.

263. Ranawat CS, Padgett DE, Ohashi Y: Total knee arthroplasty for patients younger than fifty-five years, *Clin Orthop Rel Res* 248:27, 1989.

264. Stern SH, Bowen MK, Insall JN, Scuderi GR: Cemented total knee arthroplasty for gonarthrosis in patients 55 years old or younger. *Clin Orthop Rel Res* 260:124, 1990.

266. Kjaersgaar-Anderson P, Christiansen SE, Ingersleu J, Sneppen O: Total knee arthroplasty in classic hemophilia. *Clin Orthop Rel Res* 256:137, 1990.

267. Karthaus RP, Novakova IR: Total knee replacement arthropathy. *J Bone Joint Surg* 70A:382, 1988.

268. Figgie MP, Goldberg VM, Figgie HE III, et al: Total knee arthroplasty for the treatment of chronic hemophilic arthropathy. *Clin Orthop Rel Res* 248:98, 1989.

269. Lachiewicz PF, Inglis AE, Insall JN, et al: Total knee arthroplasty in hemophilia. *J Bone Joint Surg* 67A:1361, 1985.

270. Gabel GT, Rand JA, Sim FH: Total knee arthroplasty for osteoarthritis in patients who have Paget's disease of bone at the knee. *J Bone Joint Surg* 73A:739, 1991.

271. McDonald DJ, Sim FH: Total hip arthroplasty in Paget's disease: A follow-up note. *J Bone Joint Surg* 69A:766, 1987.

272. Scuderi GR, Insall JN, Windsor RE, Moran MC: Survivorship of cemented knee replacements. *J Bone Joint Surg* 71B:798, 1989.

273. Vince KG, Insall JN, Kelly MA: The total condylar prosthesis: 10- to 12-year results of a cemented knee replacement. *J Bone Joint Surg* 71B:793, 1989.

274. Rand JA, Chao EYS, Stauffer RN: Kinematic rotating-hinge total knee arthroplasty. *J Bone Joint Surg* 69A:489, 1987.

275. Donaldson WF, Sculco TP, Insall JN, Ranawat CS: Total Condylar III prosthesis: A long-term follow-up study. *Clin Orthop Rel Res* 226:21, 1988.

276. Bush-Joseph CA, Rosenburg AG, Barden R, et al: Total Condylar III knee arthroplasty. Orthop Trans 13:630, 1989.

277. Rand JA: Revision total knee arthroplasty using Total Condylar III prosthesis. *J Arthrop* 6:1, 1991.

278. Insall JN, Dethmers DA: Revision of total knee arthroplasty. *Clin Orthop Rel Res* 170:123, 1982.

279. Jacobs MA, Hungerford DS, Krackow KA, Lennox DW. Revision total knee arthroplasty for aseptic failure. *Clin Orthop Rel Res* 226:78, 1988.

280. Insall JN, Joseph PH, Msika C: High tibial osteotomy for varus gonarthrosis: A long-term follow-up study. *J Bone Joint Surg* 66A:1040, 1984.

281. Scuderi GR, Windsor RE, Insall JN: Observations on patellar height after proximal tibial osteotomy. *J Bone Joint Surg* 71A:245, 1989.

282. Staeheli JW, Cass JR, Morrey BF: Condylar total knee arthroplasty after failed proximal tibial osteotomy. *J Bone Joint Surg* 69A:28, 1987.

283. Katz MM, Hungerford DS, Krackow KA, Lennox DW: Results of total knee arthroplasty after failed proximal tibial osteotomy for osteoarthritis. *J Bone Joint Surg* 69A:225, 1987.

284. Barrett WP, Scott RD: Revision of failed unicondylar unicompartmental knee arthroplasty. *J Bone Joint Surg* 69A:1328, 1987.

285. Padgett DE, Stern SH, Insall JN: Revision total knee arthroplasty for failed unicompartmental replacement. *J Bone Joint Surg* 73A:186, 1991.

286. Lai CH, Rand JA: Revision of failed unicompartmental total knee arthroplasty. Presented at the Annual Meeting of the American Academy of Orthopaedic Surgeons. Anaheim, CA, March 1991.

287. Marmor L: Unicompartmental and total knee arthroplasty. *Clin Orthop Rel Res* 192:75, 1985.

CHAPTER 53

The Ankle, Subtalar Joint, and Surrounding Tissues

Steven P. Sampson, Gregory L. Hung, and Stephen F. Conti

TENDON DISORDERS OF THE FOOT AND ANKLE

Overview

Overuse as well as attritional and traumatic tendon injuries are common in the foot and ankle region. Historically, descriptions of tendon disorders have been imprecise and often confusing, leading to the recommendation of a more standardized scheme based on observed histopathology (Table 53-1).[12,41,57] In one such scheme, *paratenonitis* refers to inflammation of the paratenon (outer sheath that encloses a tendon) (Fig. 53-1). Histologically, paratenonitis is characterized by an inflammatory cell infiltrate in the paratenon and peritendinous tissues. Clinically, there is pain, warmth, swelling, crepitus, and local tenderness of the tendon sheath. On the other hand, *tendinosis* refers to an intratendinous degenerative process that may be associated with aging, microtrauma, or vascular compromise. Histologically, tendinosis is characterized by collagen fiber disorientation, hypocellularity, local necrosis, and calcification.[18] Clinically, an asymptomatic tendon nodule may be present without any associated swelling of the tendon sheath. The presence of *paratenonitis with tendinosis* is a possible intermediate in the spectrum of disorders of tendon inflammation and degeneration.

The alteration of tendon nutrition is thought to play a major role in the pathophysiology of these derangements.[16] Tendon nutrition occurs in a dual manner. Both segmental blood flow and intrasynovial diffusion play key roles in this nutritional process.[35] A zone of hypovascularity exists 2 to 6 cm proximal to most large tendon insertional sites. In addition, intratendinous pathology may be provoked by any marked anatomic directional change of the tendons at the level of the malleoli—e.g., peroneals, posterior tibialis, and flexor hallucis longus (FHL). Osteophytic prominences may also cause mechanical attritional injury to tendons that are held securely by their retinacula—e.g., Achilles, FHL. Overall, intratendinous swelling may significantly alter tendon gliding and lead to a complete loss of tendon excursion. Ultimately, this loss of tendon excursion may result in a crucial imbalance of mechanical forces across an adjacent joint and a relative overpull of the unopposed normal tendon. For example, with posterior tibial tendon dysfunction, there is a loss of midfoot supination and hindfoot inversion, leading to an unopposed pull of peroneal tendons, midfoot pronation, and hindfoot eversion. Although any tendon can become symptomatic, the following discussion outlines the most commonly observed tendon disorders in the region of the ankle.

POSTERIOR TIBIAL TENDON DYSFUNCTION

Overview

Posterior tibial tendon dysfunction (PTTD) refers to a spectrum of disorders that involve varying loss of posterior tibial tendon function as well as secondary capsuloligamentous and joint restraints (Table 53-2). This may progress in "stages" from being dynamically flexible to a condition in which deformities of the medial longitudinal arch, transverse tarsal joints, and subtalar joints are rigid.[16]

Anatomically, the posterior tibial tendon lies posterior to the axis of the ankle—e.g., ankle plantar flexor and medial to the axis of the subtalar joint, e.g., midfoot inverter.[2] The posterior tibial tendon inserts on the navicular and the plantar aspect of the middle three metatarsal bases, the cuneiforms and the cuboid. Typically, posterior tibial tendon swelling occurs 1 to 2 cm distal to the medial malleolus, corresponding to a zone of hypovascularity and high functional load.[5] Holmes and Mann reported that the majority of patients with posterior tibial tendon dysfunction at highest risk are middle-aged women who have a medical history of hypertension, obesity, diabetes, previous trauma to the medial aspect of the foot and/or ankle, or treatment with steroids.[6] Similarly, steroid injections in the region of the posterior tibial tendon are associated with increased risk of rupture and/or insufficiency. Finally, seronegative inflammatory disorders such as ankylosing spondylitis, Reiter's syndrome, and psoriasis have been associated with PTTD.[7] Whereas some authors have also associated rheumatoid arthritis (RA) with PTTD, Meyerson postulated that the flatfoot deformity in RA is more common secondary to synovitis of the talonavicular and subtalar joints.[16]

TABLE 53-1 Classification of Tendon Inflammation and Degeneration

New Term	Definition	Histologic Findings	Clinical Signs and Symptoms
I. Paratenonitis	An inflammation of only the paratenon, either lined by synovium or not	Inflammatory cells in paratenon or peritendinous areolar tissue	Cardinal inflammatory signs: Swelling, pain, crepitation, local tenderness, warmth, dysfunction
II. Paratenonitis with tendinosis	Paratenon inflammation associated with intratendinous degeneration	Same as I, with loss of tendon collagen fiber disorientation, scattered vascular ingrowth, but no prominent intratendinous inflammation	Same as I, with palpable tendon nodule, swelling, and inflammatory signs
III. Tendinosis	Intratendinous degeneration due to atrophy (aging, microtrauma, vascular compromise, etc)	Noninflammatory intratendinous collagen degeneration with fiber disorientation, hypocellularity, scattered vascular ingrowth, occasional local necrosis, or calcification	Often palpable tendon nodule that is *asymptomatic;* swelling of tendon sheath is absent

Source: Reproduced with permission from Saltzman C, Bonar S: Tendon problems of the foot and ankle, in Lutter LD, Mizel MS, Pfeffer GB (eds): *Orthopaedic Knowledge Update: Foot and Ankle.* Rosemont, IL, American Academy of Orthopaedic Surgeons, 1994, pp 269–281.

Staging

Four clinical stages of PTTD have been described based on the severity of the associated adult acquired flatfoot deformity (see Table 53-2).[16] While MRI is very sensitive for detecting intratendinous changes, the clinical diagnosis of PTTD is primarily dependent on a thorough clinical exam as well as standard weight-bearing x-rays of the foot and ankle.[4,23] *Stage I* involves medial ankle and foot pain and swelling without deformity. Tendon excursion is normal. The patient experiences pain but still has the ability to perform a single-limb heel-rise test. During this test, the posterior tibialis tendon inverts and stabilizes the hindfoot as the patient attempts to rise on the forefoot, while the uninvolved foot remains suspended off the ground. Stages II, III, and IV are characterized by posterior tibialis tendon insufficiency with loss of normal tendon excursion. In *stage II,* the flatfoot de-

formity remains flexible. Midfoot pronation and forefoot abduction at the transverse tarsal joint are reducible by the examiner. Functionally, the patient is unable to maintain a standing posture without exhibiting the "too many toes" sign secondary to the above conformational change. In addition, the patient is unable to perform a single-limb heel-rise test. Hinterman has clinically emphasized the importance of the first metatarsal head-rise sign as an adjunctive clinical test for accurately assessing early PTTD.[25] While the patient is bearing full weight on the involved extremity, the examiner rotates the involved leg externally. If, as a result, the first metatarsal head rises from the floor, this test is positive and indicative of PTTD (Fig. 53-2). A dynamic assessment of the patient's gait is also helpful in diagnosing PTTD.

The posterior tibialis tendon's principal role is as an inverter of the subtalar joint. This hindfoot inversion dy-

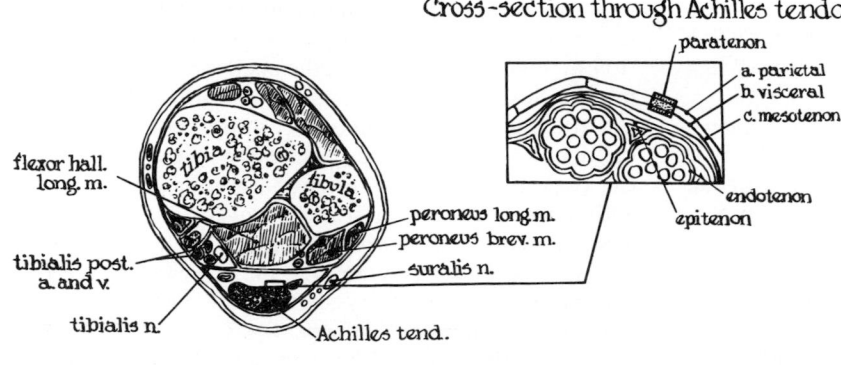

Cross-section through Achilles tendon

Cross-section through distal portion of leg

Figure 53-1 Cross-sectional anatomy of the leg at the level of the Achilles tendon (*left*) with a magnified view of the peritendinous structures (*right*). The paratenon is a double-layer structure that surrounds the tendon. The mesotenon connects the outer, parietal layer to the inner, visceral layer and serves as a passageway for vessels nourishing the tendon. The density of these vessels is highest along the anterior Achilles tendon. [Reproduced with permission from Saltzman C, Bonar S: Tendon problems of the foot and ankle, in Lutter LD, Mizel MS, Pfeffer GB (eds): *Orthopaedic Knowledge Update: Foot and Ankle.* Rosemont, IL, American Academy of Orthopaedic Surgeons, 1994, p 269.]

TABLE 53-2   Treatment of Dysfunction of the Posterior Tibial Tendon

Stage	Characteristics	Treatment	
		Non-Operative	Operative
Tenosynovitis	Acute medial pain and swelling, can perform heel-rise, seronegative inflammation, extensive tearing	Anti-inflammatory medication, immobilization for 6–8 weeks; if symptoms improve, ankle stirrup-brace; if symptoms do not improve, operative treatment	Tenosynovectomy, tenosynovectomy + calcaneal osteotomy, or tenosynovectomy + tenodesis of flexor digitorum longus to posterior tibial tendon
Rupture Stage I	Medial pain and swelling, hindfoot flexible, can perform heel-rise	Medial heel-and-sole shoe wedge, hinged ankle-foot orthosis, orthotic arch-supports	Debridement of posterior tibial tendon, flexor digitorum longus transfer, or flexor digitorum longus transfer + calcaneal osteotomy
Stage II	Valgus angulation of heel, lateral pain, hindfoot flexible, cannot perform heel-rise	Medial heel-and-sole shoe wedge, stiff orthotic support, hinged ankle-foot orthosis, injections of steroids into the sinus tarsi	Flexor digitorum longus transfer + calcaneal osteotomy or flexor digitorum longus transfer + bone-block arthrodesis at calcaneocuboid joint
Stage III	Valgus angulation of heel, lateral pain, hindfoot rigid, cannot perform heel-rise	Rigid ankle-foot orthosis	Triple arthrodesis
Stage IV	Hindfoot rigid, valgus angulation of talus	Rigid ankle-foot orthosis	Tibiotalocalcaneal arthrodesis

Source: Reproduced with permission from Meyerson MS: Adult acquired flatfoot deformity. *J Bone Joint Surg* 78A:783, 1996.

namically locks the transverse tarsal joints, providing more efficient transfer of push-off power during the gait cycle. With PTTD, prolonged heel eversion and forefoot abduction associated with a midfoot collapse (thrust) on push-off is visualized in the medial longitudinal arch region. With repeated abnormal posturing or dynamic collapse of the midfoot, the posterior tibialis tendon loses its normal excursion and tends to elongate structurally, becoming functionally "insufficient." Secondary attenuation occurs in concert with "sagging" of capsuloligamentous structures surrounding the talonavicular complex. Unbalanced "overpull" of the normal peroneal tendon abduction forces exaggerates the loss of posterior tibial tendon function. *Stage III* PTTD involves a rigid flatfoot deformity associated with a hindfoot valgus and loss of subtalar joint motion. A distinguishing feature of this stage is that the patient experiences predominantly anterolateral ankle pain secondary to impingement of the calcaneus on the fibula, not anteromedial ankle or foot pain, as in the earlier stages of PTTD.

Meyerson has emphasized the importance of identifying patients with fixed forefoot supination.[16] These fixed forefoot deformities must be corrected rotationally in order to reduce the transverse tarsal joint properly. A fixed forefoot supination deformity may remain either when the hindfoot valgus position is correctable to neutral (stage II) or when the valgus hindfoot remains fixed (stage III). Finally, *stage IV* PTTD is associated with more significant proximal soft tissue attenuation and loss of the deltoid lig-

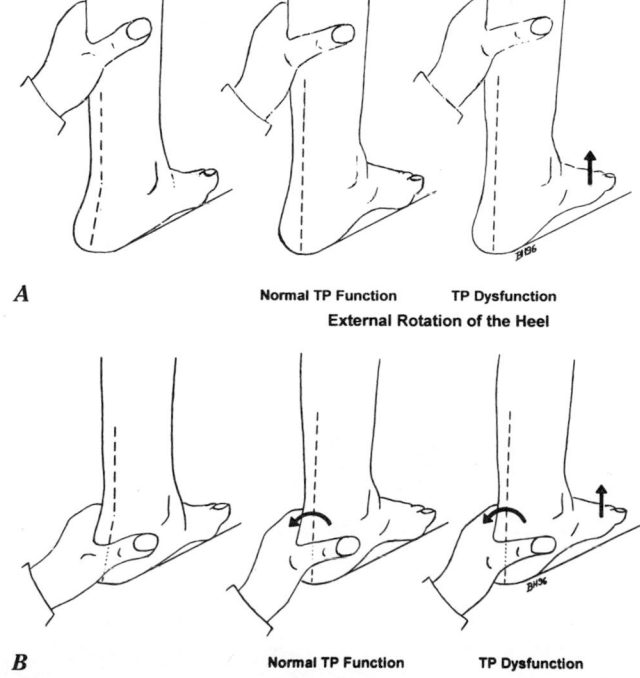

Figure 53-2 First metatarsal rise sign as a test for posterior tibial tendon dysfunction. (Reproduced with permission from Hinterman B, Gachter A: The first metatarsal rise sign: A simple, sensitive sign of tibialis posterior tendon dysfunction. *Foot Ankle Int* 17:236–241, 1996.)

ament support. Resultant valgus angulation of the talus produces abnormal tibiotalar contact forces and leads to early ankle arthrosis.

Treatment of PTTD depends on the stage at presentation.[26,31] Initially, nonsurgical management of stage I should include immobilization in a short leg walking cast.[8,21] Stage II may be managed with a UCBL (University of California Biomechanics Laboratory) type of foot orthosis with a medial longitudinal arch support along with medial hindfoot posting.[14,24] Alternatively, an AFO (ankle-foot orthosis) may be required for patients who are obese or those who have lax ligaments.[16]

The surgical treatment of stage II PTTD remains controversial. The most common soft tissue reconstruction involves transfer of the flexor digitorum longus (FDL) to reconstruct the posterior tibial tendon (Fig. 53-3).[1,2,22] Instead of the FDL transfer, alternative reconstructive procedures have been advocated because of an inability of soft tissues alone to correct the flatfoot deformity predictably. Recent in vitro biomechanical studies have documented better correction of an adult flatfoot model using a rerouted peroneus longus (PL) tenodesis rather than the standard FDL transfer.[15] This intriguing soft tissue approach attempts to rebalance the muscle forces acting on the hindfoot by transferring a major forefoot abductor deforming force.

Two alternative methods of augmentation of medial soft tissue reconstruction have been recommended. First, a medial displacement calcaneal osteotomy is postulated to countershift the pathologic hindfoot valgus posturing by redirecting the strong pull of the gastrocnemius muscle force medial to the axis of the subtalar joint, thereby restoring its normal varus force on the hindfoot (Fig. 53-4).[10]

Second, Sangeorzan et al. have recommended the use of lateral column lengthening at the level of the calcaneocuboid joint.[11,19] The concept of lateral column lengthening attempts both to realign the transverse tarsal joint neutrally and to maintain talonavicular and subtalar joint motion. However, Meyerson feels that lateral column lengthening may be preferred over medial calcaneal displacement osteotomy only when the forefoot does not have a fixed supination deformity.[16] Other authors have also advocated various hindfoot arthrodesis patterns for stage II PTTD, including subtalar, talonavicular, transverse tarsal, or even triple arthrodesis.[3,9,13,20] Stage III PTTD typically requires a subtalar or triple arthrodesis depending on the degree of joint arthrosis, location, and age of the patient—e.g., older patients tend to require arthrodesis.[3,9,13,20,28–30] Finally, in stage IV PTTD, a tibiotalocalcaneal arthrodesis may be required if the tibiotalar joint is incongruent and arthritic.[16,226]

ACHILLES TENDON INJURIES

Overview

Anatomically, the Achilles tendon is the largest and strongest tendon in the body, formed as a conjoint tendon of the gastrocnemius and soleus muscles. The tendon rotates 30 to 150° before inserting on the inferior aspect of the posterior calcaneal surface. The Achilles tendon has no true synovial sheath and its major nutritional supply is by way of blood vessels from the paratenon. Injection studies have shown that the Achilles tendon has a hypovascu-

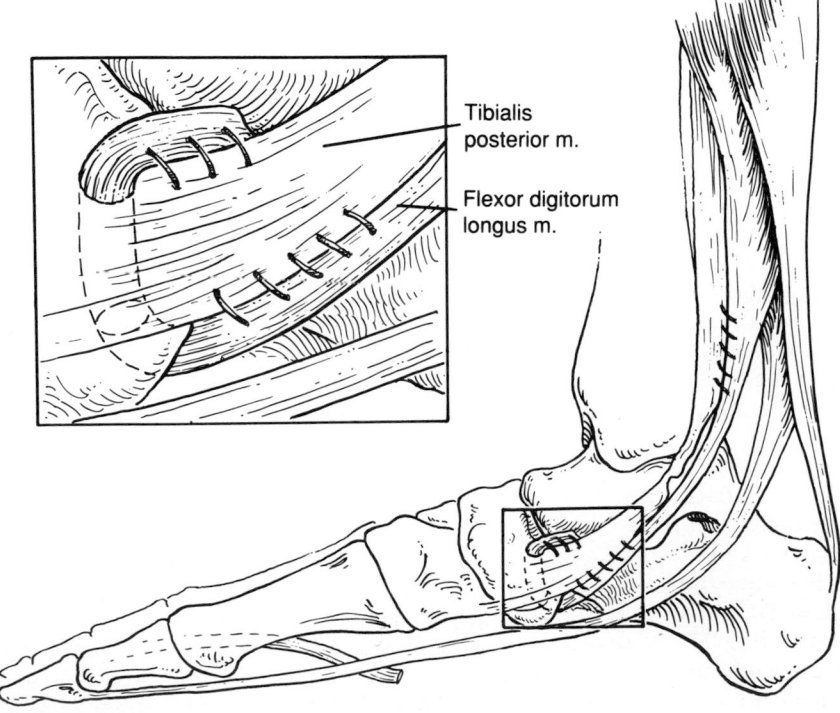

Figure 53-3 Flexor digitorum longus transfer with proximal tenodesis to ruptured posterior tibial tendon. [Reproduced with permission from Johnson KA: Tibialis posterior tendon release-substitution, in Johnson KA (ed): *The Foot and Ankle: Master Techniques in Orthopaedic Surgery.* New York, Raven Press, 1994, p 279.]

Tibialis posterior m.

Flexor digitorum longus m.

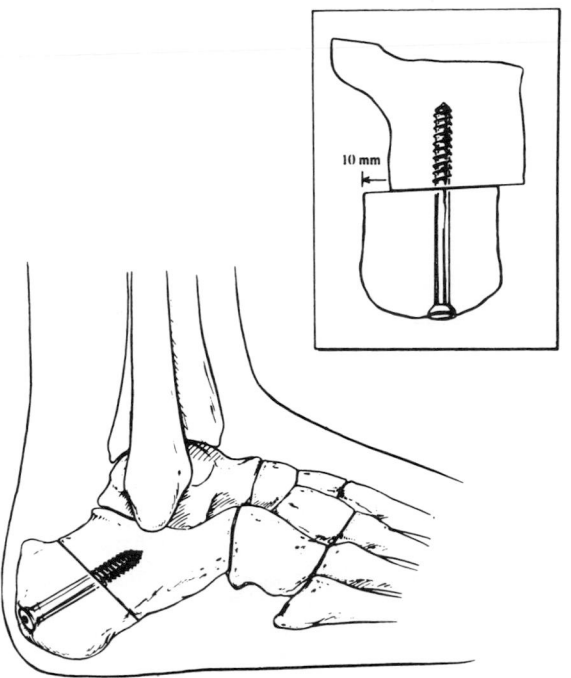

Figure 53-4 Medial displacement calcaneal osteotomy associated with soft tissue augmentation. (Reproduced with permission from Meyerson MS: Adult acquired flatfoot deformity. *J Bone Joint Surg* 78A:784, 1996).

lar zone that corresponds to the region of maximal internal rotation of its tendon fibers, in a region located 2 to 5 cm proximal to its calcaneal insertion.[35,46]

Insertional/Noninsertional Tendinitis

Clinically, Baxter has divided Achilles tendon problems into two groups: insertional and noninsertional.[56,59] Insertional "tendinitis" involves the tendon/bone junctional region, including the area of the posterior superior tubercle of the calcaneus as well as the retrocalcaneal bursa. Insertional Achilles tendonitis has been associated with Haglund's deformity ("pump bump") and retrocalcaneal bursitis.[60,63,64] Clinically, these entities may overlap. The Achilles tendon becomes involved only toward the later stages of attritional injury. Those patients who present with either a cavus type foot or a rigid, plantarflexed first ray will have a predisposition for developing hindfoot varus associated with a prominent posterolateral bursal prominence. Anatomically, Frey has described a horseshoe-shaped retrocalcaneal bursa lying atop the posterosuperior aspect of the calcaneal tuberosity, immediately anterior to the Achilles tendon.[65] Radiographically, Pavlov has described the use of parallel pitch lines to assess the potential for retrocalcaneal bursal impingement on a weight-bearing lateral x-ray of the foot (Fig. 53-5).[60,63,64] Conservative management begins with modification of the patient's heel counter in the region of the prominent bursa by using a heel lift. Additionally, by elevating the heel height

of the shoe, the angle of calcaneal inclination is decreased, which has the overall effect of bringing the posterosuperior calcaneal tuberosity (bursal projection) away from the heel counter. Local steroid injections are discouraged because of the risk of Achilles tendon rupture. If conservative measures fail, surgical management usually includes removal of the posterosuperior calcaneal prominence along with the inflamed retrocalcaneal bursa.[61,62,66] Inspection of the anterior surface of the Achilles tendon should be performed during the limited calcanectomy. Baxter has recommended that the inflamed or degenerated tendon tissue be resected along with any calcified spurs in the immediate vicinity.[59] In recalcitrant cases, a tendon transfer procedure to reinforce the Achilles tendon insertion may be indicated (discussed below).

Additional nonmechanical causes of insertional Achilles tendinopathy may include gout, rheumatoid arthritis, and enthesiopathies provoked by seronegative spondyloarthropathies such as Reiter's syndrome.[172]

Noninsertional Achilles tendinopathy is the prototypical tendon disorder in which any histopathologic stage, as previously discussed, may occur.[41,56] Biomechanically, the Achilles tendon may transmit forces up to 10 times body weight. Intrinsic and extrinsic factors both contribute to the pathophysiology of Achilles tendinopathy. Intrinsically, the pronated foot is at high risk, because midfoot pronation is coupled with an internal rotatory force on the tibia, which is opposite to the normal external rotatory force applied to the tibia during knee extension. These counterrotating forces have been postulated to result in unusually high tensile stresses to this vascularly "at risk" region of the heel cord. Additionally, when exposed to mechanical overloading, any "heel-cord tightness" may predispose the Achilles tendon to interstitial tears and

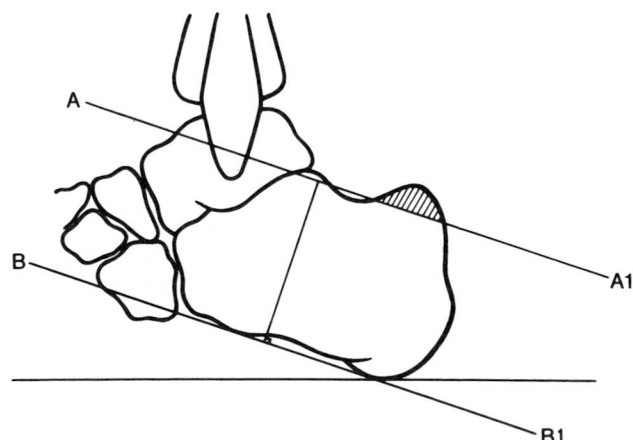

Figure 53-5 Parallel pitch lines for assessment of abnormal bursal projection of the posterior superior calcaneal tuberosity. A perpendicular line is drawn from the lip of the posterior facet of the subtalar (A-A1) to a line that joins the anterior and medial calcaneal tuberosities (B-B1). The shaded bone above A-A1 corresponds to bone impinging on the retrocalcaneal bursa. (Reproduced with permission from Stephens MA: Haglund's deformity and retrocalcaneal bursitis. *Orthop Clin North Am* 25:43, 1994.)

overt rupture in the hypovascular zone. Extrinsically, any sudden alteration in the routine pattern or the intensity level of exercise may also adversely provoke similar Achilles tendon injuries.[62] Steroid injections in this region have been associated with tendon rupture and are contraindicated.[54,58]

Paratenonitis is the most common clinical presentation of noninsertional Achilles tendinitis.[27] Acutely, an inflammatory response is prevalent, with local tenderness and palpable crepitus noted. Acute or chronic paratenonitis presentations are commonly associated with tendinosis or nodular thickening of the heel cord. These findings may be consistent with partially healed Achilles tendon ruptures superimposed on an acute injury. Conservative management consists of rest and ice—as well as a 1- to 2-cm heel lift with a medial longitudinal support to correct any midfoot pronation. James has recommended a "brisement" steroid injection into the Achilles "pseudosheath" to treat the acute inflammation. With this technique, he attempts to break up adhesions mechanically and promote tendon gliding. Extreme caution must be rendered to avoid injecting into the Achilles tendon proper.[27] Instead of brisement, many authors feel that other, less invasive modalities should be utilized, such as phonophoresis, ultrasound, or electrical stimulation. Surgical treatment has been considered as early as 3 months after failure of nonoperative treatment. Magnetic resonance imaging of the Achilles tendon may help to distinguish all the above phases of paratenonitis (peritendinous fluid) with or without tendinosis (nodular thickness).[56] Surgical management includes extensive debridement of the paratenon. Longitudinal resection of intratendinous nodules is indicated if the nodules occupy two-thirds or more of the cross-sectional area of the tendon.[8,27,55] Following nodule excision, augmentation of a peri-insertional defect with a tendon transfer may be required—e.g., FDL transfer (Fig. 53-6).[43] Noninsertional defects may be reconstructed using a local Achilles turndown flap.[27,52]

Acute and Chronic Achilles Tendon Ruptures

Acute Achilles tendon rupture is recognized by most patients as a dramatic event associated with acute pain, swelling, and a palpable defect noted in the region of the rupture. Clinical examination in the prone position reveals a positive Thompson test.[34] When the examiner squeezes the superficial calf muscles, little or no plantarflexion of the ankle is produced. Some patients do not present acutely. Remarkably, up to 25 percent of Achilles tendon ruptures have been missed completely on clinical examination.[44] Active albeit weak plantarflexion of the ankle is still possible through intact toe flexors and peroneals. However, marked plantarflexion weakness associated with tendon rupture does not allow single-limb heel rising. Adjunctive tests such as MRI and ultrasound are not necessary to make a diagnosis. However, these adjunctive tests may be very useful in determining the extent of tendon gap formation.[27,32] There is continuing controversy in the literature about the best way to treat the rupture (Table 53-3).[33,44,57,59] Traditional nonoperative treatment involves initial im-

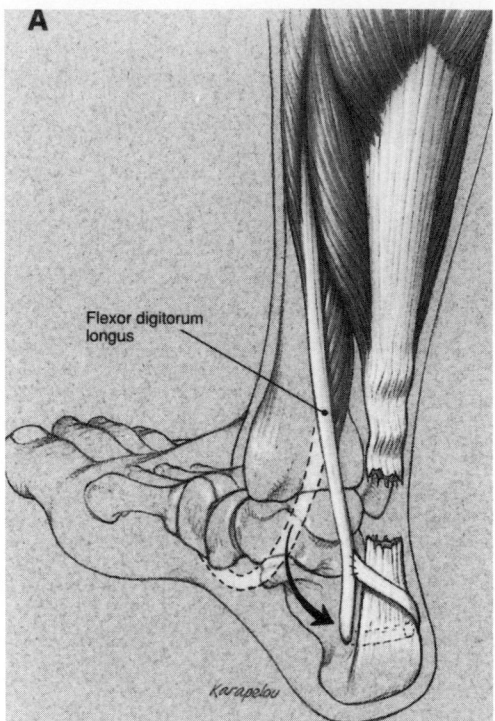

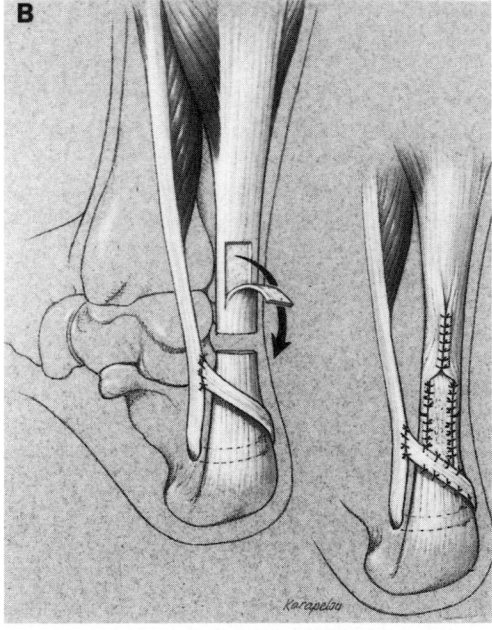

Figure 53-6 Flexor digitorum longus local tendon transfer for Achilles tendon rupture with augmentation. (Reproduced with permission from Mann RA: Achilles tendon reconstruction using the flexor digitorum longus. *Op Techn Orthop* 4:139, 1994.)

mobilization in a long leg non-weight-bearing cast with the foot in a gravity equinus position.[27,40] Once the acute inflammatory period is over, a modified short leg cast or walking orthosis with a 3-cm heel lift may be permitted for a 6- to 8-week period. Saltzman has emphasized that Achilles tendon apposition (i.e., minimal or no palpable defect) is the key to nonoperative treatment.[27,44] He recommends using MRI or ultrasound to document the presence or absence of tendon diastasis in 20° of ankle plantarflexion. The timing of the patient's presentation may also play a key role in the ability to reduce the tendon gap, since the presence of a significant hematoma and/or scar may mechanically block tendon-tendon apposition. If the Achilles tendon scar is subsequently allowed to heal with nontendinous tissue interposition, an elongated and attenuated tendon callous will occur. The net effect is that nonoperative treatment is usually associated with a return of approximately 75 percent of normal function only if the gap is minimized and results in a higher rerupture rate of 10 to 29 percent. Operative management has been proposed for the athletic patient, who requires the strongest functional result—i.e., restoration of physiologic length—and wishes to minimize the incidence (down to 1 or 2 percent) of rerupture with no gaps.[27,37,55] The standard surgical repair uses a straight medial longitudinal incision with a minimal skin flap mobilization in the adjacent incisional region anterior to the Achilles tendon. Acutely, tendon apposition is usually obtained with simple end-to-end approximation and plantaris tendon augmentation. Careful handling of the skin and a tension-free closure are important factors in attempting to avoid complications such as skin necrosis, infection, and fistulas.[44] Percutaneous techniques have been devised to limit soft tissue complications.[50] However, these techniques are associated with a much higher incidence of sural nerve injury and are reported to provide repairs 50 percent weaker than standard open Achilles tendon reconstruction.[36,49]

Chronic rupture has been defined as any rupture of the Achilles tendon with a delay in treatment or diagnosis greater than 4 weeks.[44] Typically, the patient's chief complaint is marked gait weakness associated with walking and stair climbing. An ankle-foot orthosis is recommended for those patients who are medically compromised or unwilling to accept the risks of surgical reconstruction.

The type of surgical reconstruction for chronic ruptures of the Achilles tendon is dependent on the size of the defect.[27,44,51] Most small gaps (1 to 3 cm) are treated by the turndown flap technique of Lindholm.[27,44] A distally based

plantaris graft may augment this reconstruction. Moderate-sized gaps (3 to 8 cm) can usually be treated with V-Y lengthening of the triceps surae aponeurosis (Fig. 53-7).[38] Gabel and Manoli have emphasized the need to make the arms of the V at least $1\frac{1}{2}$ times the length of the gap to be approximated.[44] Also, they have emphasized the fact that this technique requires extensive dissection of the V portion completely through the aponeurosis, essentially making it a free graft. Longitudinal excision of the deep posterior fascia immediately anterior to the Achilles tendon has been proposed to permit vascular ingrowth from the adjacent FHL muscle belly. Local tendon transfers have been described, including the peroneus brevis, FHL, and flexor digitorum longus.[39,42,43,50-52] These tendon transfers attempt to augment severe tendon gaps. Synthetic augmentation materials have been used in attempts to avoid donor site morbidity such as those created by the use of local tendon transfers or free vascularized or nonvascularized tendon transfers (e.g., fascia lata).[45,52]

PERONEAL TENDON INJURIES AND SUBLUXATION/DISLOCATION

Overview

Sobel and Mizel have described two anatomic zones of injury.[88] Zone 1 injuries occur in the vicinity of the lateral malleolus. In this zone, the peroneus brevis and longus tendons travel together in a common sheath with the brevis immediately adjacent to a lateral retromalleolar groove.[97] Because of this anatomic arrangement, peroneus brevis tendon injuries are most common in this zone. Zone 2 injuries involve primarily the peroneus longus tendon; these injuries begin distal to the tip of the fibula along the lateral wall of the calcaneus or within the cuboid tunnel. In this zone, the peroneus longus tendon lies within its own sheath beneath the inferior peroneal retinaculum. Just as the peroneal groove of the distal fibula acts as a ful-

---

TABLE 53-3 Considerations in the Choice of Treatment of Acute Rupture of the Achilles Tendon

Consideration	Type of treatment	
	Nonoperative (casting alone)	Operative (operation and casting)
Morbidity	Decreased	Increased
Surgical risk	None	Increased
Hospital stay (cost)	Decreased	Increased
Dynametric data	Inferior	Superior
Rerupture	10%	2%
Compliance with rehabilitation	Less	More

Source: Reproduced with permission from Plattner PF, Johnson KA: Tendons and bursae, in Helal B, Wilson D (eds): *The Foot.* New York, Churchill Livingstone, 1988, pp 581–613.

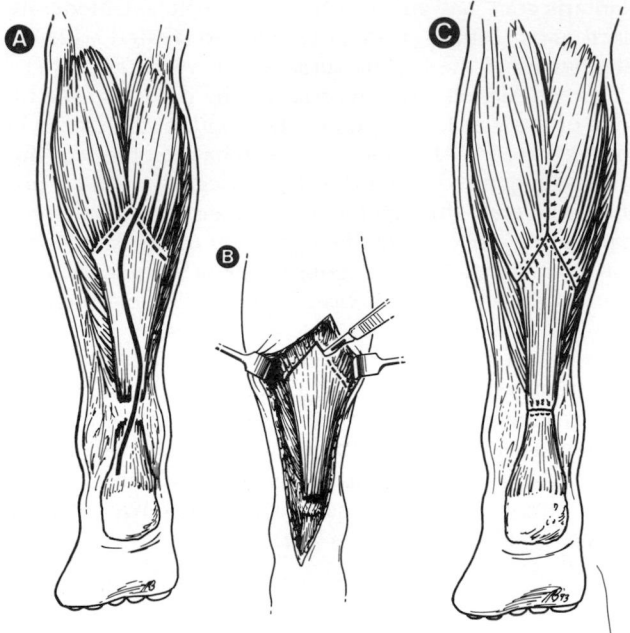

Figure 53-7 Technique of V-Y lengthening of the triceps surae aponeurosis. (Reproduced with permission from Greenfield G, Stanish WD: Tendinitis and tendon ruptures. *Op Tech Sports Med* 2:14, 1994.)

crum for the peroneus brevis, the cuboid (plantar) tunnel acts as a critical fulcrum for the peroneus longus on its way toward its plantar insertion into the base of the first metatarsal and the medial cuneiform.[72] Any swelling of either tendon immediately proximal to its bone fulcrum may prevent normal tendon excursion and therefore produce a stenotic site of tendon entrapment (i.e., stenosing tenosynovitis). While triggering of the peroneus longus tendon may occur in the region of a prominent peroneal tubercle of the calcaneus, tendinosis is a more common cause of triggering.[87,96] The net effect is that when a tendon does not have normal excursion or stops gliding, it is more susceptible to a pathologic injury cycle of interstitial tearing, swelling, healing (tendinosis), and—rarely—rupture. Unique to zone 2, the os peroneum is an (osseous or fibrocartilaginous) sesamoid anatomically located within the peroneus longus tendon within a tunnel formed by the long plantar ligament and a sulcus of the cuboid tuberosity. Sobel et al. have described a spectrum of conditions located in zone 2 that may be responsible for plantar lateral foot pain and have coined the term *painful os peroneum syndrome* (POPS).[72,99]

Zone 1 Injuries

Zone 1 injuries have been associated with attritional splitting of the peroneus brevis tendon (Fig. 53-8).[68,69,74,78,81,84,86,88,97] These splits have been reported in up to 37 percent of cadaveric specimens and—in contradistinction to the microvascular studies of both the

posterior tibial and the Achilles tendons—a critical hypovascular zone was not identified in the region of these splits.[94]

The primary mechanical restraint to peroneal tendon subluxation/dislocation in zone 1 is the superior peroneal retinaculum (SPR), which is formed by two bands originating from the fibula; it inserts superiorly into the lateral border of the Achilles tendon sheath and inferiorly into the posterolateral aspect of the calcaneus (Fig. 53-8).[73] Any laxity in the SPR may dramatically alter gliding of the peroneus brevis tendon and significantly contribute to tendon subluxation/dislocation.[71,75] The bone geometry of the lateral retromalleolar or peroneal groove of the fibula usually provides a stable concave sulcus (82 percent) for tendon gliding. However, a narrow sulcus (18 percent) predisposes a patient to recurrent peroneal tendon subluxation/dislocation, which may provoke subsequent laxity of the SPR restraint.[84,88]

Inversion injuries of the ankle may traumatically avulse the SPR from its fibular origin with or without production of a posterior marginal "rim" fracture of the distal fibula. The location of this fracture is pathognomonic of an SPR avulsion injury.[90,91] Furthermore, the distinction between a lateral ankle sprain and an acute peroneal tendon subluxation may be subtle. Clinically, examination reveals point tenderness and swelling in the region of the anterior talofibular ligament or the retromalleolar regions, respectively. Without a high index of suspicion, peroneal tendon injuries are often mistreated as "the sprain that won't go away."[192] Finally, the presence of anomalous peroneal muscles (i.e., peroneus quartus) has been associated with an increased incidence of peroneus brevis splits.[83,95] These anomalous peroneal muscles may hypertrophy, provoking tendon entrapment in zone 1. The clinical diagnosis and provocation of peroneal tendon dislocation is made by asking the patient to dorsiflex the ankle while the examiner restricts the foot in a plantarflexed and everted position. Pain or frank dislocation may occur with this maneuver.[75]

Peroneal tendinopathy or paratenonitis is a common clinical presentation.[88] The patient complains of posterolateral ankle pain radiating along the lateral border of the foot. As stated previously, peroneal tendinopathy may be clinically confused and/or clinically associated with lateral ankle instability. Alteration in peroneal tendon gliding may provoke retromalleolar crepitus and, rarely, peroneal tendon rupture.[70,85] If acute nonoperative treatment fails, including rest, ice, compression, and elevation (RICE), further diagnostic evaluation may include an MRI and a lidocaine injection test into the retromalleolar region of the peroneal sheath. The lidocaine injection should be performed as a preoperative assessment to help differentiate peroneal tendinopathy from other local pathology (e.g., posterior ankle impingement, sinus tarsi syndrome, subtalar arthrosis).

Upon failure of conservative treatment, surgical exploration in zone 1 may encounter peroneus brevis tears, SPR incompetence, and peroneal tenosynovitis along with aberrant hypertrophic peroneal muscles.[88] Peroneal tendinosis may be treated with nodule excision and repair. Splitting of the peroneus brevis is usually treated with debridement. Advanced irreparable splitting of the brevis is

Figure 53-8 Zone 1 peroneus brevis split is identified after retracting the superior retinaculum posteriorly and the peroneus longus anteriorly. The peroneus brevis split is noted to lie intimately associated with the posterior fibular ridge. [Reproduced with permission from Sobel M, Bohne WHO: Peroneal tendon repair-reconstruction, in Johnson KA (ed): *The Foot and Ankle: Master Techniques in Orthopaedic Surgery.* New York, Raven Press, 1994, p 290.]

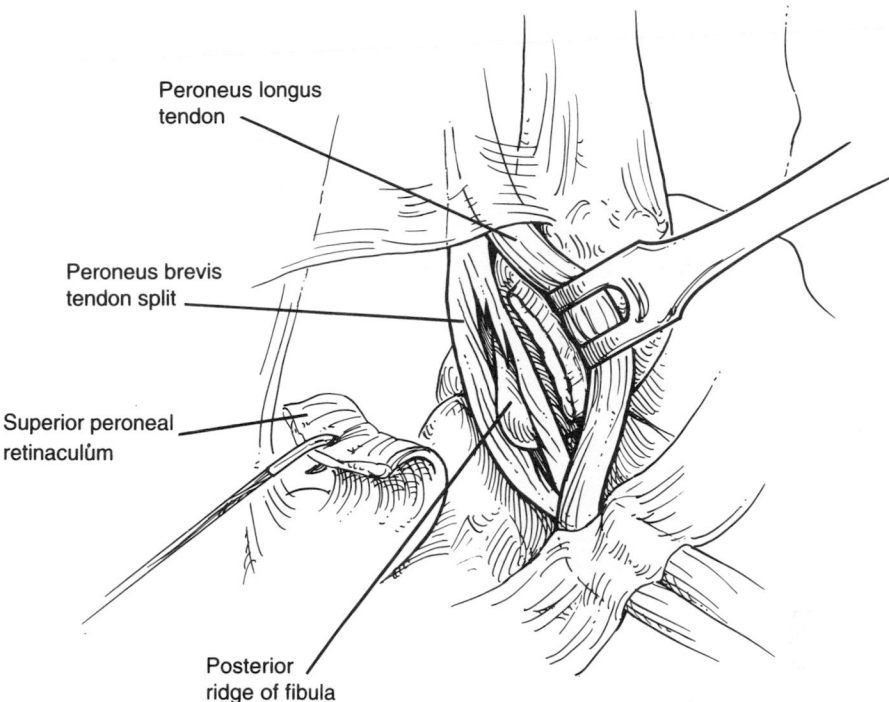

Peroneus longus tendon

Peroneus brevis tendon split

Superior peroneal retinaculum

Posterior ridge of fibula

treated by tenodesing the remaining brevis tendon to the intact peroneus longus, both proximally and distally to the preserved SPR.

Numerous surgical techniques have been devised for reconstruction of SPR incompetence, including (1) direct repair and reattachment to the fibula, (2) local soft tissue augmentation (e.g., slip of the Achilles tendon or osteoperiosteal flap from the fibula), (3) bone block procedures using the fibula, (4) groove-deepening procedures, and (5) rerouting procedures under the adjacent calcaneofibular ligament.[67,76,77,89] A combination of these procedures may be required in an attempt to reestablish "normal" tenodesis (see Fig. 53-9).[88] Postoperatively, any adhesions or stenosis through the reconstructed SPR may lead to poor tendon gliding. Finally, simultaneous lateral ligament reconstruction (e.g., Bröstrom) should be performed at the time of SPR reconstruction when these conditions coexist.[80,83,93]

Zone 2 Injuries

Zone 2 injuries involve primarily the peroneus longus. Painful os peroneal syndrome (POPS) usually results from inversion-type injuries to the ankle that may result in acute or chronic symptoms of os peroneum fracture.[72,88] Acute ruptures of the peroneus longus tendon associated with an os peroneum diastasis may be diagnosed by pain located over the lateral foot associated with weakness noted on an attempted single-limb heel rise. Marked weakness is also noted on attempted plantarflexion of the first metatarsal. Chronic POPS may be associated with repeated episodes of giving way very similar to the clinical presentation of chronic lateral ankle instability. Chronic os peroneum fracture diastasis may present as stenosing per-

oneus longus tenosynovitis.[97,99] Oblique x-rays of the foot may reveal proximal migration of an os peroneum avulsion fracture. A bone scan may help to differentiate a multipartite os peroneum from an acute fracture. Acute repair of the peroneus longus with excision of the os peroneum may be indicated. Chronic attritional tears are initially treated with cast immobilization. Operative exploration in zone 2 should be done through the interval between the peroneus brevis and peroneus longus, with care to avoid injury to the sural nerve. When the distal peroneus longus tendon is irreparable, excision of the os peroneum and tenodesis of the proximal segment of the peroneum longus with the peroneus brevis has been recommended.[79] Absence of peroneus longus function has been reported to be associated with a pes cavovarus deformity in a child.[98] Rupture of both peroneals may cause transverse tarsal joint subluxation secondary to a major tendon imbalance provoked by the unopposed pull of the intact anterior and posterior tibial tendons acting across this region.

ANTERIOR TIBIAL TENDON INJURIES

Anatomically, ruptures of the anterior tibial tendon usually occur between the inferior extensor retinaculum and its tendon insertion on the base of the first metatarsal and medial cuneiform.[100,101,104,106] Like the Achilles tendon, the anterior tibial tendon rotates 90° just prior to insertion. In performing a split anterior tibial tendon transfer (SPLATT), Fennel has technically recommended utilizing the proximal and/or medial portion of the anterior tibial tendon inserted on to the cuneiform to avoid knotting of tendon

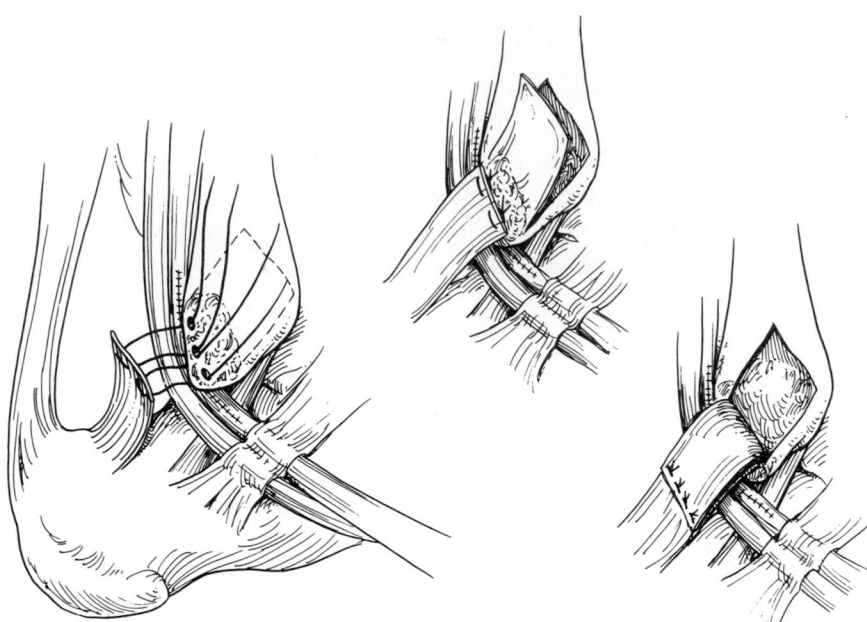

Figure 53-9 Zone 1: Following debridement of peroneus brevis split, superior peroneal retinaculum is reconstructed and reinforced with a local periosteal flap from the distal fibula. Simultaneous deepening of the fibular groove may be performed when a shallow peroneal sulcus is present. [Reproduced with permission from Sobel M, Bohne WHO: Peroneal tendon repair-reconstruction, in Johnson KA (ed): *The Foot and Ankle: Master Techniques in Orthopaedic Surgery.* New York, Raven Press, 1994, p 296.]

proximally.[105] As in the peroneal tendons, no hypovascular zone was noted in the region 1 to 3 cm proximal to the anterior tibial insertion.[103] Anterior tibial tendon attritional ruptures usually occur secondary to a dorsal exostosis at the first metatarsal–medial cuneiform joint. Clinically, a steppage type of gait is noted, with the patient unable to perform tandem heel walking. Conservative management would require a dorsiflexion assist ankle-foot orthosis. Acute tears are amenable to primary repair. Secondary repairs within the first few months have been performed with an extensor tendon transfer or interpositional grafting if the proximal muscle belly has normal excursion.[100–102,104]

OSTEOCHONDRAL LESIONS OF THE TALAR DOME

Various descriptive terms in the literature have been applied to a lesion of the talar dome, including *osteochondritis dissecans, subchondral cyst with osteochondral fracture, transchondral dome fracture, osteochondral fracture,* and *partial talar necrosis.*[110,111,116,125,133] Since Berndt and Hardy's study, most authors have favored a traumatic etiology.[112] However, other presumed etiological factors, possibly associated with remote trauma, may clearly play a role—e.g., aberrant vasculature with spontaneous osteonecrosis as well as endocrine, hormonal, or genetic factors.[107,108,116]

Medial osteochondral lesions (55 percent) are thought to occur with greater frequency than lateral lesions (45 percent). The proposed mechanism of injury of medial (posteromedial location) lesions is an inversion force applied with the ankle in plantarflexion, whereas lateral (anterolateral location) lesions are thought to occur with the

ankle in dorsiflexion.[112] Clinically, a history of acute trauma is recalled in nearly all lateral lesions. However, up to one-third of patients with medial lesions deny any history of trauma. Thus, these lesions are frequently missed on initial presentation. Despite a history of activity-related ankle pain, clinical examination findings are usually nonspecific or may even be within normal limits. As the size and depth of these lesions increase, the patient will usually complain of worsening pain associated with weight bearing and a catching or giving-way sensation. At this stage, an ankle effusion with diminished motion is usually evident, associated with anterolateral or anteromedial joint-line tenderness. All in all, the diagnosis and staging of these lesions are dependent on x-rays, bone scan, computed tomography (CT) and/or MRI, and arthroscopy.[109,112,116–118,122,125] When the lesion is not evident on plain x-ray films, most authors advocate the use of MRI[117] and some prefer ankle arthroscopic staging.[109,117,118,133,136]

Staging

The original Berndt and Harty classification was based on standard anteroposterior (AP) x-ray evaluation of the ankle, as follows:

Stage I—subchondral compression fracture with no visible fragment
Stage II—fragment attached (flap)
Stage III—fragment detached in situ
Stage IV—displaced fragment, loose body (Table 53-4)[112]

At initial clinical presentation, x-ray evaluation will miss up to one-third of stage 1 patients. When they are radiographically visible, AP x-ray evaluation of the ankle in plantarflexion will help to identify posteromedial lesions, while AP mortise views in dorsiflexion will maximize x-ray evalua-

TABLE 53-4   Staging for Characterizing Osteochondral Lesions

	Arthroscopic	MRI	Radiographs (Berndt and Harty[112])
Stage I	Irregularity and softening of articular cartilage; no definable fragment	Thickening of articular cartilage and low signal changes	Compression lesion; no visible fragment
Stage II	Articular cartilage breached, definable fragment, not displaceable	Articular cartilage breached, low signal rim behind fragment indicating fibrous attachment	Fragment attached
Stage III	Articular cartilage breached, definable fragment, displaceable, but attached by some overlying articular cartilage	Articular cartilage breached, high signal changes behind fragment indicating synovial fluid between fragment and underlying subchondral bone	Nondisplaced fragment without attachment
Stage IV	Loose body	Loose body	Displaced fragment

Source: Reproduced with permission from Dipaolo JD, Nelson DW, Colville MR: Characterizing osteochondral lesions by magnetic resonance imaging. *Arthroscopy* 7:101–104, 1991.

tion of anterolateral lesions.[116] When initial and repeat x-ray evaluations are negative, bone scan screening is indicated. In the blood pool phase, bone scanning is 100 percent sensitive. A negative bone scan would avoid the necessity of an MRI. Upon identifying a stage I lesion on bone scan, an MRI evaluation will help determine a *stable* stage II attached fragment lesion (intact cartilage with attachment to subchondral bone) versus an *unstable* stage III detached fragment lesion (fluid interface between fragment/crater junction).[109,116] In the case of lesions initially identifiable on plain films, high-resolution CT scanning has been proposed as the best method to document the coordinates of size and extent of talar dome involvement and is helpful in differentiating stage II from stage III lesions (Fig. 53-10).[133]

Asymptomatic stage I, II, and III lesions do not require treatment.[116] Treatment of symptomatic stage I lesions should include restriction of motion and activities. Symptomatic stage II lesions are usually treated for 6 to 12 weeks with short leg cast immobilization, with weight bearing allowed. Symptomatic stage III lesions are the most controversial. Some authors believe that lateral lesions should have immediate surgical treatment whereas medial stage III lesions should be treated conservatively. Almost all authors agree that chronic stage IV lesions should be excised. Acute stage IV lesions (larger than 1.0 to 1.5 cm) may require open reduction or arthroscopically assisted pinning with no weight bearing allowed postoperatively for at least 3 months.[111,116,125]

Surgical treatment of symptomatic stage II and III lesions that have failed conservative management requires excision of the necrotic sequestrum (osteochondritic dissecans fragment), curettement of the crater, and drilling of the subchondral bone. Drilling of intact stage II lesions has been proposed to promote neovascularization and healing of the avascular fragment.[120,122,133]

Prior to surgical treatment, arthroscopic examination should be performed to assess the quality of the surface of the articular lesion and probe the lesion's stability as compared with preoperative CT or MRI evaluations.[133] Surgical management may be performed by either arthrotomy or arthroscopy. It is important to note that the best surgical outcomes are achieved if conservative management does not continue for longer than 12 months from the time of injury.[114] Postoperatively, early range-of-motion exercises are recommended for debrided fragments whereas immobilization for up to approximately 6 weeks has been recommended for intact stage II fragments that have been pinned.

Arthroscopic Approaches to Osteochondral Lesions

Arthroscopic treatment usually utilizes a 2.7- or 4.0-mm scope with both 30 and 70° angulation.[122,132] A noninvasive soft tissue joint-distracting method, using a strap placed around the heel and midfoot, allows better visualization.[122] Three primary portals have been recommended (Fig. 53-11).[127,128,130–133] The anteromedial portal is made medial to the anterior tibial tendon. Careful blunt dissection helps avoid injury to the greater saphenous vein and saphenous nerve.[123] The anterolateral portal is made lateral to the peroneus tertius and extensor digitorum longus tendons. Careful blunt dissection attempts to avoid injury to the superficial peroneal nerve—the most commonly injured nerve during ankle arthroscopy.[121–124,129] Finally, the posterior portal—the safest being posterolateral—is placed immediately adjacent to the lateral border of the Achilles tendon, approximately 1.2 to 2.5 cm above the tip of the fibula (depending upon the degree of joint distraction). Branches of the lesser saphenous vein and sural nerve are at risk with the posterolateral approach.[126] According to Ferkel, anterolateral lesions are best approached with the scope anteromedial, the inflow posterolateral, and the instrumentation anterolateral. Anterolateral lesions are usually more accessible than their posteromedial counterparts.[122] Stage II lesions can be stabilized with a small joint (needle-scope) cannula and pinned

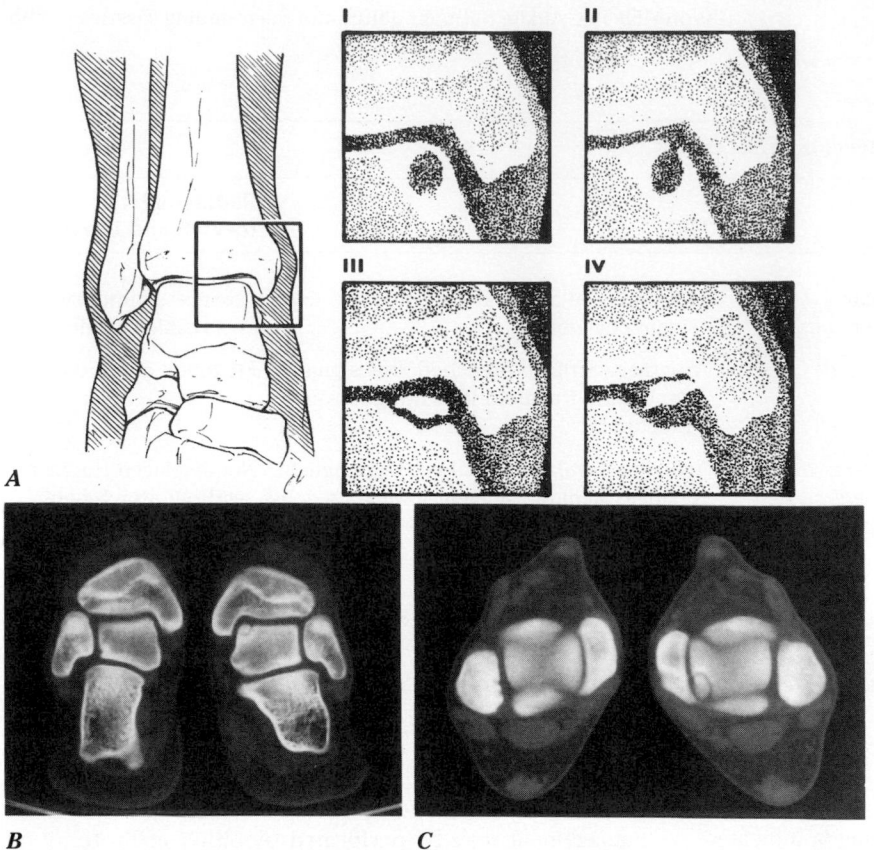

Figure 53-10 *A*. Staging of osteochondral lesions of the talus by CT. Stage I, subchondral cystic lesion with intact roof; stage II, subchondral plate disrupted with lesion extending into joint; stage III, in situ osteochondral lesion with radiolucent "halo" surrounding nidus as seen in coronal (*B*) and axial (*C*) scans; stage IV, displaced osteochondral fragment (osteochondritis dissecans) with distinct radiolucent defect. [Reproduced with permission from Ferkel RD: Arthroscopy of the ankle and foot, in Mann RA, Coughlin MJ (eds): *Surgery of the Foot and Ankle*. St Louis, Mosby, 1993, p 1292.]

A

B   *C*

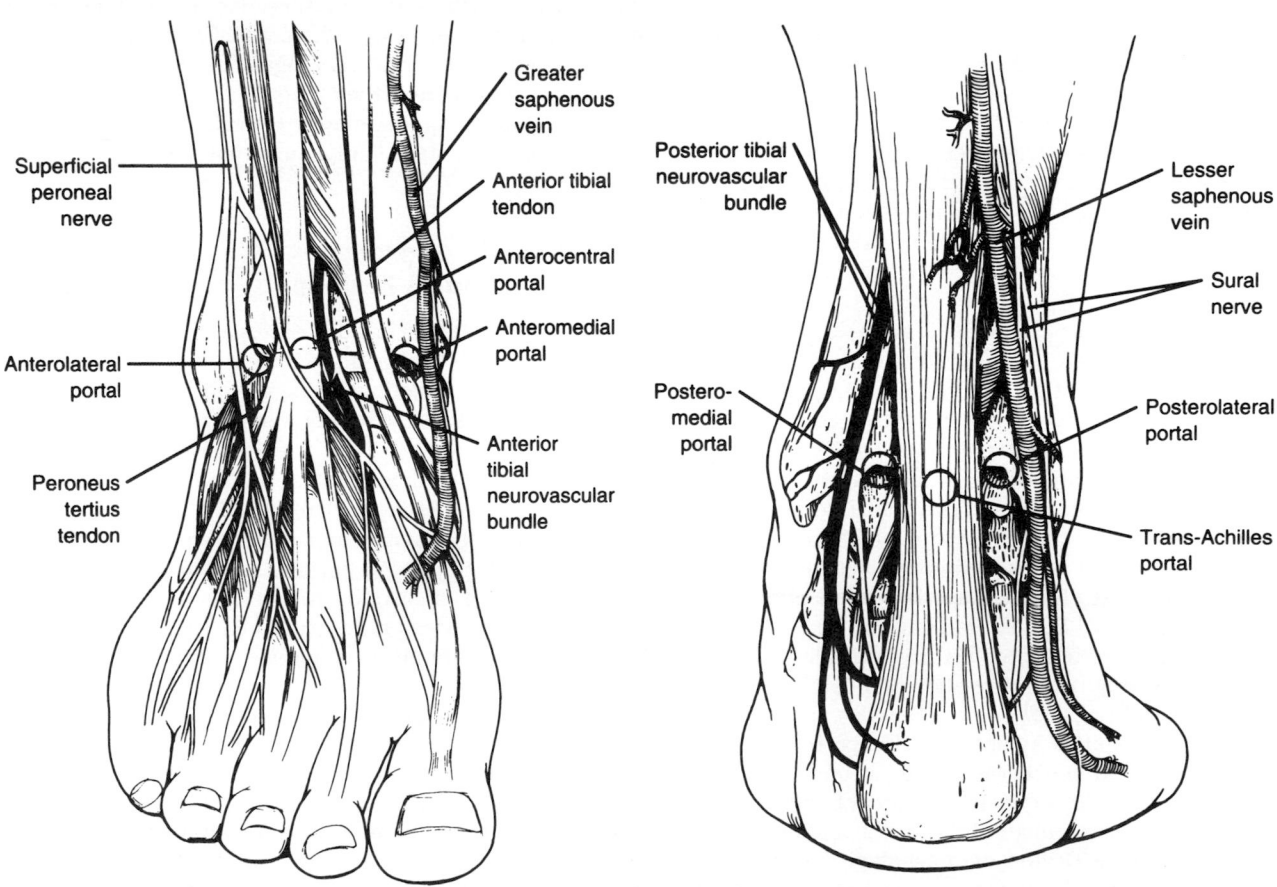

A   *B*

Figure 53-11 Anterior and posterior arthroscopic portal anatomy. (Reproduced with permission from Stetson WB, Ferkel RD: Ankle arthroscopy: I. Technique and complications. *J Am Acad Orthop Surg* 4:19, 1996.)

using two or three absorbable pins. Bone resorption around these pins has been reported as a potential postoperative concern. Posteromedial lesions are usually best visualized with the portal posterolateral, the inflow anterolateral, and the instruments anteromedial. In order to gain access for difficult-to-reach posteromedial lesions, Gould has recommended gouging the anteromedial tibial plafond region.[115] Other authors have advocated transmalleolar drilling if ankle plantarflexion alone does not achieve adequate visualization.[120] Rather than damaging an adjacent articular surface, transtalar drilling has been advocated with a 0.062-in, smooth K wire passing percutaneously into the sinus tarsi from distal to proximal under arthroscopic control[122] (Fig. 53-12). Ferkel has described using a cannulated trephine with this transtalar approach in order to initially debride and then to bone graft the posteromedial osteonecrotic lesion. Finally, most authors have recommended a medial malleolar osteotomy to gain access to large posteromedial lesions.[119] With this open approach, thorough debridement and bone grafting of the debrided necrotic base and crater may be performed. Access to the lesion is obtained along the medial peripheral talar articular margin in order to maintain the greatest possible surface integrity of intact stage II fragments.

Retrospective outcome data for surgical treatment of stage III and IV lesions reveal "good" results in 63 to 88 percent of cases.[111,113,116] A clinical plateau in postoperative improvement may require 18 to 24 months.[114] Long-term follow-up of these lesions is guarded. The development of osteoarthrosis and degenerative joint disease has been documented more commonly in "conservatively" treated stage III and stage IV lesions. Remarkably, no clinical outcome studies have yet correlated the size of the lesion (percent weight-bearing talar dome involvement) and the long-term development of osteoarthrosis.

SOFT TISSUE IMPINGEMENT LESIONS

Differential Diagnosis of Chronic Inversion Sprain Injuries

The most common cause of chronic postinversion sprain symptomatology is anterolateral soft tissue impingement.[136–138] The differential diagnosis of chronic inversion sprain symptoms includes avulsion fractures of the distal fibula (os fibulare) with or without lateral instability, peroneal tendinopathy, posteromedial fibrous talocalcaneal coalition,[150] occult fracture of the posterolateral tubercle of the talus (trigonal or Shepherd's fracture), lateral talar process fracture,[181,182,184] anterior calcaneal process fracture,[151] subtalar instability with or without sinus tarsi syndrome,[134,135] reflex sympathetic dystrophy, and other soft tissue impingement syndromes (syndesmotic and posterior).[147]

Anterolateral Impingement Lesions

The anterolateral impingement syndrome is typically related to scarification located in the lateral talomalleolar recess

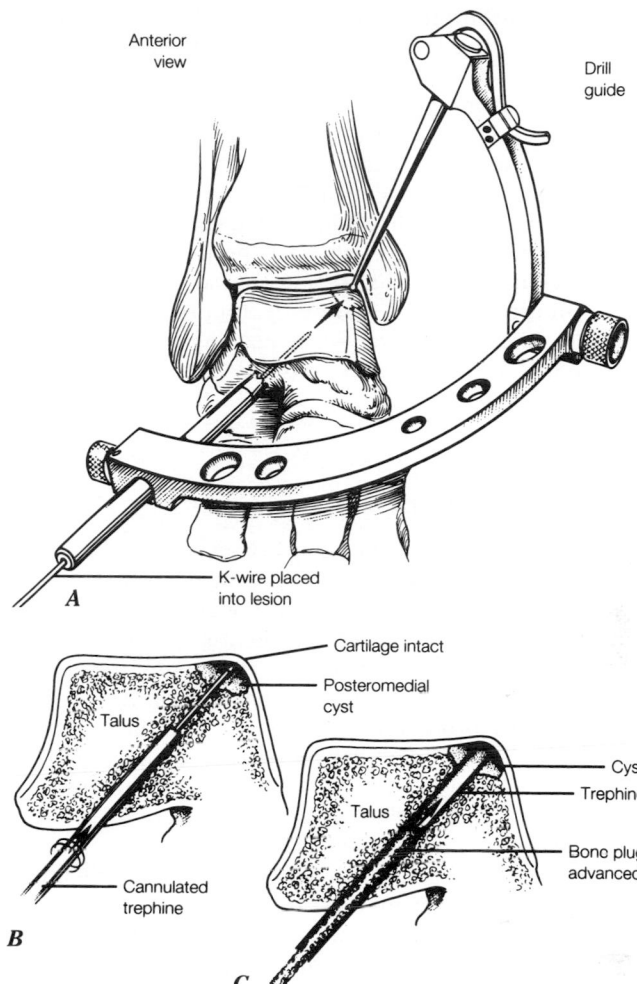

Figure 53-12 Transtalar drilling of an osteochondral defect. [Reproduced with permission from Ferkel RD: Articular surface defects, loose bodies and osteophytes, in Ferkel RD (ed): *Arthroscopic Surgery—The Foot and Ankle.* Philadelphia, Lippincott-Raven, 1996, p 166.]

(lateral gutter). Wolin and others originally described this scar as a "meniscoid" lesion.[144–146] Scarring of the superior portion of the anterior talofibular ligament (ATFL) and distal slip of the anterior inferior tibiofibular ligament (AITFL) may mature into a hyalinized "lesion" associated with localized synovitis. The patients usually complain of anterolateral ankle pain associated with a catching sensation and giving-way episodes. However, stress radiographs of the ankle and/or subtalar joints are usually negative. Following a 4- to 6-month period of refractory nonoperative treatment, a diagnostic attempt to differentiate lateral gutter pathology from sinus tarsi syndrome is made using directed local anesthesia. The sinus tarsi syndrome has a similar clinical presentation as an anterolateral impingement syndrome.[134,135] However, scarring of the fat pad and synovitis occur in sinus tarsi and are thought to occur in conjunction with partial tearing of the calcaneofibular, cervical, or interosseous talocalcaneal ligaments. Debridement of the scarred fat pad in the sinus tarsi has been advocated, with preservation of the cervical and interosseous ligaments advised.

If a differential local anesthetic injection relieves symptoms in the lateral gutter and not the sinus tarsi, arthroscopic debridement of the lateral gutter is indicated.[136,137] It is important to remember that dorsiflexion of the ankle tends to anatomically open the lateral gutter by relaxing the anterior capsule.[138] Ankle distraction in this circumstance will tend to restrict entry and therefore restrict arthroscopic visualization in this region. Complete arthroscopic resection of the intraarticular portion of the AITFL is indicated and will not cause syndesmotic diastasis. However, complete resection of the ATFL should be avoided. According to Ferkel, good to excellent results are achieved in 75 to 90 percent of cases.

Syndesmosis Injuries

Syndesmosis injuries have been called *high ankle sprains* by Hamilton[147,152,192] and are commonly missed.[147,152] The syndesmosis of the ankle is composed of AITFL, the posterior inferior tibiofibular ligament (PITFL), the transverse ligament, and the interosseous membrane (IOM).[138,140,149,152] The mechanism of the syndesmosis injury is usually pronation and external rotation, although some authors have discussed hyperdorsiflexion injuries. Four clinical examination findings have been helpful in the diagnosis of these sprains: (1) direct tenderness in the region of the syndesmosis and IOM proximally; (2) the "squeeze test," performed by compressing the fibula toward the tibia in the midcalf region (a positive test elicits referred pain distally in the region of syndesmosis and IOM tears); (3) the external rotation stress test (Fig. 53-13), which simulates the mechanism of injury (with the knee held in 90° of flexion, an external rotation torque is applied to the foot with the ankle held in neutral position—a positive test reproduces the patient's symptoms and causes pain in the region of the AITFL, PITFL, and IOM); and (4) the Cotton test, performed by stabilizing the calcaneus and talus in a neutral ankle mortise position and attempting to displace the fibula in a medial to posterolateral position.[139] Anteroposterior and mortise stress radiographs of the ankle are performed with an applied external rotated stress.[153,154] If these diagnostic studies are negative, a bone scan will usually identify a "hot spot." High-resolution axial CT scanning through this area may also identify subtle occult avulsion fractures of the syndesmosis ligaments (fracture of Tillaux). Axial CT scanning may additionally identify subtle static rotatory malalignment or subluxation of the inferior tibiofibular joint, especially occurring after a short oblique fibular fracture.[141,142,148]

Soft tissue impingement of the AITFL alone (Bassett's ligament) may occur in the absence of instability of the syndesmosis.[146] Arthroscopic debridement of this ligament and a limited synovectomy have been recommended to help alleviate talar impingement. Complete syndesmosis rupture allows the fibula to shorten and rotate externally, causing ankle incongruency and late arthrosis.[139,140] Reduction of the syndesmosis is mandatory. Extraction

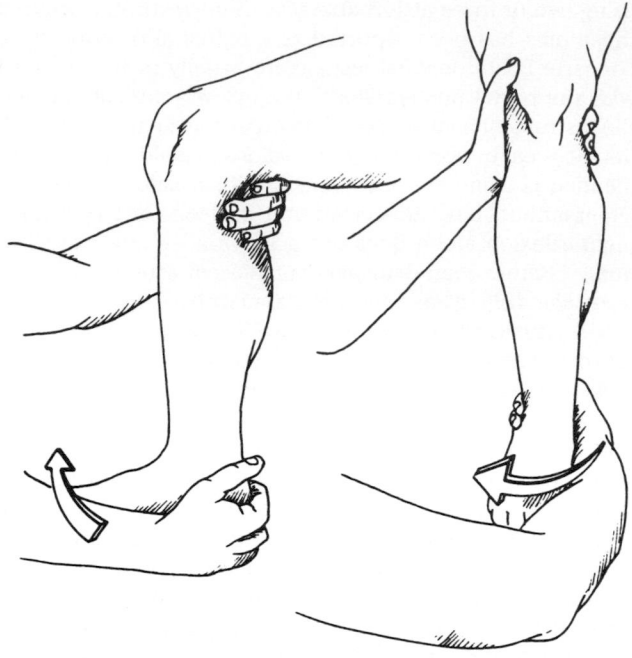

Figure 53-13 The external rotation stress test for syndesmosis sprains. The abduction/external rotation stress test produces extreme pain in syndesmosis sprains and is the method for eliciting latent diastasis by stress radiography. (Reproduced with permission from Clanton TO, Schon LC: Athletic injuries to the soft tissues of the foot and ankle, in Mann RA, Coughlin MJ (eds): *Surgery of the Foot and Ankle*. St. Louis, Mosby, 1993.)

of soft tissue interposition may be required, followed by the placement of a transsyndesmosis screw for a minimum period of 8 weeks. Suture of the AITFL or open reduction and internal fixation of the Tillaux fragment is performed when the fragment is large enough. Late calcification or heterotopic ossification of the IOM may help identify the extent of the injury.[143] Patients with tibiotalar synostosis or more limited IOM heterotopic ossification will complain of pain while bearing weight, especially on the initiation of push-off. Examination will reveal limited ankle dorsiflexion. In selected high-performance athletes, late excision of focal heterotopic ossification sites has been helpful in improving motion and relieving pain.

Posterior Soft Tissue Impingement Lesions

Posterior soft tissue impingement usually provokes posterolateral, not anterolateral, symptoms. However, posterior impingement may present in an isolated form or simultaneously with anterolateral impingement and injuries to the syndesmosis. Scarring usually involves the PITFL, the transverse tibiofibular ligament, and a tibial slip. Hamilton has described a "pseudomeniscus" or labial type of tear in this region, which likewise may be treated with arthroscopic debridement.[192]

SUBTALAR JOINT SPRAIN AND INSTABILITY

Overview

The subtalar joint is subdivided into the anterior talocalcaneonavicular joint and the posterior talocalcaneal joint by the tarsal canal and a lateral opening called the sinus tarsi.[133,161] Harper has also subdivided the ligamentous anatomy of the subtalar complex into three layers: the superficial, containing the calcaneofibular ligament (CFL); the intermediate, containing the cervical ligament (CL); and the deep, containing the talocalcaneal interosseous ligament (TCIL) or ligament of the tarsal canal (Fig. 53-14).[159,161] The symptoms of subtalar instability are difficult to differentiate from chronic lateral ligamentous instability of the tibiotalar joint following an inversion injury or stress.[157,161] Subtalar injuries are usually associated with tenderness in the region of the sinus tarsi. However, ankle and subtalar instability frequently coexist. Various standard ankle stress tests have all failed to identify clear-cut indications for documenting subtalar joint instability, including an AP inversion stress view (talar tilt), a lateral anterior drawer stress view, and a 40° stress Broden's view.[164,165] Sectioning studies have documented the importance of the CFL in stabilizing the posterior talocalcaneal joint.[157] However, Pisani has proposed that the interosseous ligament has not only a strong functional role but also a proprioceptive role, like the anterior cruciate ligament of the knee.[166] The interosseous ligament is strategically positioned in a centralized area between the anterior and posterior portions of the subtalar joint and may function as a significant rotational "pivot" point. Abnormal rotatory instability of the subtalar joint is not examined by our current conventional uniplanar stress tests of the ankle. Pisani has postulated that laxity of the subtalar joint is associated with elongation or rupture of the interosseous ligament and has recommended interosseous ligament reconstruction using a distally based portion of the peroneus brevis. Other authors have more commonly recommended use of the Chrisman-Snook or modified Bröstrom-Gould reconstructions.[155,156,158,160] Both of these latter ankle ligament reconstructions bridge the tibiotalar and subtalar joints in a more posterior and lateral location, attempting to functionally reconstruct the ATFL and CFL, not the interosseous ligament.

Subtalar Arthroscopy

Subtalar arthroscopy has been advocated for assessing the posterior talocalcaneal facet.[161,162] Lateral access to the anterior talocalcaneonavicular joint is prevented by the interosseous ligament, which "guards" this region. Ferkel has described two lateral portals: anterolateral and posterolateral. Posteriorly, the sural nerve and the lesser saphenous vein are at significant risk of injury.[161–163] Surgical indications may include a preoperative assessment of the subtalar joint (posterior facet) prior to ankle arthrodesis. With only anecdotal data available, arthroscopic lysis of adhesions secondary to arthrofibrosis in the posterior facet of the subtalar joint has been attempted.

Figure 53-14 Ligamentous anatomy of the subtalar joint—superficial, intermediate, and deep layers inserting into the dorsal aspect of calcaneous. (Reproduced with permission from Sarrafian SK: *Anatomy of the Foot and Ankle,* 2d ed. Philadelphia, Lippincott, 1993, p 197.)

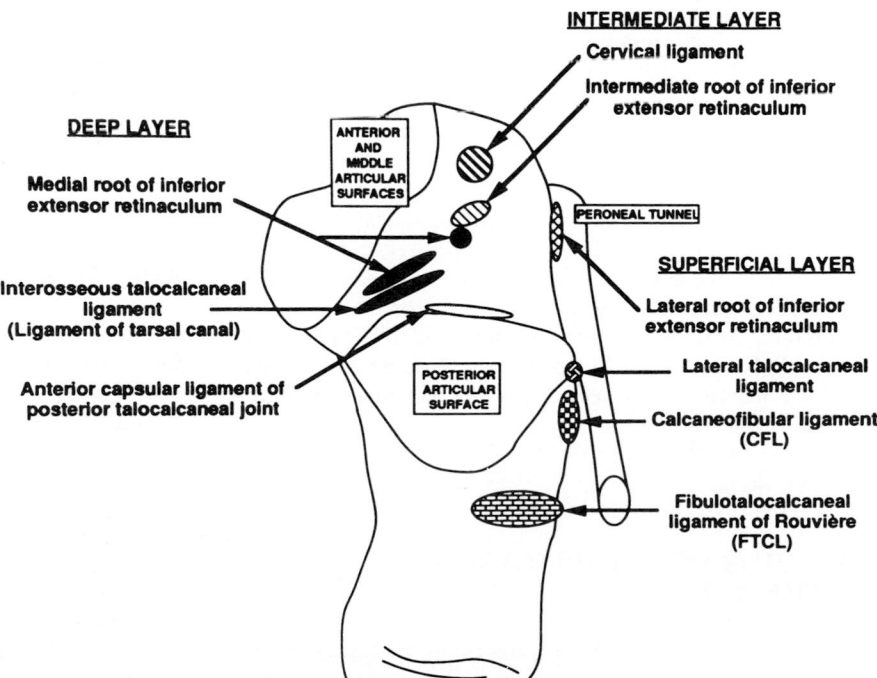

POSTERIOR BONE IMPINGEMENT SYNDROMES

Os Trigonum Syndrome

This syndrome occurs in ballet dancers secondary to full weight in maximum plantarflexion of the ankle (demi-pointe and/or full pointe position).[173,174,188] Another synonym for the os trigonum syndrome is the talar compression syndrome.[167,168,192] The os trigonum is an ununited posterolateral tubercle of talus, which occurs in 7 to 10 percent of the population and has an incidence of 50 percent bilaterally. A fused os trigonum process is called a trigonal (Stieda's) process.[192] Hamilton has stated that posterior impingement is often but not always associated with an os trigonum or trigonal process. Clinically, patients complain of posterolateral ankle pain with tenderness noted behind the peroneals. Pain is exacerbated by forced plantarflexion of ankle (plantarflexion sign).

Flexor Hallucis Longus Tendinopathy

The differential diagnosis of posterior impingement syndrome includes a fracture of the trigonal process (Shepherd's fracture),[180–184,186] FHL tendinopathy (dancer's tendinitis),[187] peroneal tendinopathy, talocalcaneal coalition,[171] and osteoid osteoma.[192] The FHL tendon passes through a fibrocartilageneous retinaculum between the lateral and medial tubercles of the posterior process of the talus, extending to the level of the sustentaculum tali. Swelling or tendinosis of the FHL may initiate triggering of the great toe (hallux saltans) or provoke locking of the FHL nodule behind the medial malleolus (pseudo–hallux rigidus).[192]

Nonoperative treatment of posterior impingement includes modification of activities and possibly a steroid injection following a positive lidocaine injection test placed posterior to the peroneal sheath at the site of posterior talar compression. If conservative treatment has failed, Hamilton has recommended a posterolateral approach between the peroneals and the FHL in order to remove the os trigonum in the absence of FHL tendinopathy.[187–189] However, if the patient has coexisting pain associated with FHL tendinopathy, a medial approach is recommended to identify and protect the neurovascular bundle, as well as decompression of the FHL tendon during os trigonum/posterior talar process fracture excision.[188,190,192] Fracture of the medial tubercle of the posterior process of the talus (Cedell's fracture) has been reported to cause tarsal tunnel syndrome.[169,170,175–180]

ANTERIOR BONE IMPINGEMENT OF THE ANKLE

Anterior ankle osteophytes (spurs) may be intraarticular, intracapsular, or extraarticular and are usually located on either the anterior tibia articular margin and/or the talar neck; they are probably associated with early osteoarthrosis of the ankle.[194] These lesions are thought to be secondary to trauma, induced by extreme dorsiflexion or plantarflexion injuries that cause anterior capsular avulsion and periosteal new bone formation. Symptoms include pain, giving way, marked swelling, and limitation of dorsiflexion. A lateral stress x-ray taken in maximum dorsiflexion may clearly document the region of impingement. Conservative management should include avoidance of impact loading and the use of a heel lift.[192]

Preoperative assessment for anterior cheilectomy of the tibia or talar neck should include a weight-bearing lateral ankle x-ray to determine the amount of osteophytic bone to be resected (Fig. 53-15).[194] Ferkel has emphasized that the normal tibiotalar angle should be 60° or greater. Preoperative planning with an air or contrast CT arthrogram is helpful if symptoms of catching are present and loose bodies are suspected. Additionally, a bone scan that shows uptake *only* in the anterior impingement region is confirmatory, whereas global uptake throughout the tibiotalar and/or subtalar joints is indicative of a more extensive osteoarthritic process. When a more advanced osteoarthritic condition exists, focal, anterior impingement surgical treatment may provide transient postoperative pain relief.[191]

Surgical management for anterior impingement syndrome is dependent on the location and extent of osteophyte formation.[191,193] Isolated beaking lesions of either the anterior tibia or talar neck may be approached arthroscopically. Ferkel has recommended careful identification of the anterior osteophyte and avoidance of injury to the anterior neurovascular bundle while elevating the soft tissue enveloping the osteophyte. Unexpected concomitant intraarticular pathology should be treated simultaneously—i.e., limited synovectomy and removal of loose bodies. When osteophytes are present on both the anterior tibial and talar neck simultaneously, Hamilton has recommended open arthrotomy utilizing an anteromedial approach.[192] An intraoperative lateral x-ray is recommended to ensure adequate osteophyte resection (cheilectomy) and reestablishment of the normal tibiotalar angle.[194]

RHEUMATOID HINDFOOT

The talonavicular, subtalar, and calcaneocuboid joints are the most commonly involved hindfoot joints in rheumatoid arthritis.[195,198,199] Hindfoot involvement appears at a later stage compared to forefoot involvement.[200] The ankle joint is the least involved of all hindfoot joints.[201,203]

The most common clinical presentation of rheumatoid hindfoot disease is a planovalgus deformity.[200,201] This deformity may be secondary to advanced posterior tibial tendinopathy (stage III or stage IV) or talonavicular and/or subtalar synovitis.[195,196,204] Medical management should be supplemented with a UCBL (University of California Biomechanics Laboratory) foot orthosis or an AFO. Treatment of posterior tibial tendon dysfunction (PTTD) should be similar to treatments described previously.

Figure 53-15 Anterior ankle impingement secondary to spur formation: weight-bearing lateral x-ray used to determine tibiotalar angle. *A.* Normal: the normal angle between the distal tibia and talus is 60° or greater. *B.* Bony impingement: osteophytic formation on the distal tibia and/or talar neck with the angle diminished to under 60°. (Reproduced with permission from Ferkel RD: Arthroscopy of the ankle and foot, in Mann RA, Coughlin MJ (eds): *Surgery of the Foot and Ankle.* St. Louis, Mosby, 1993.)

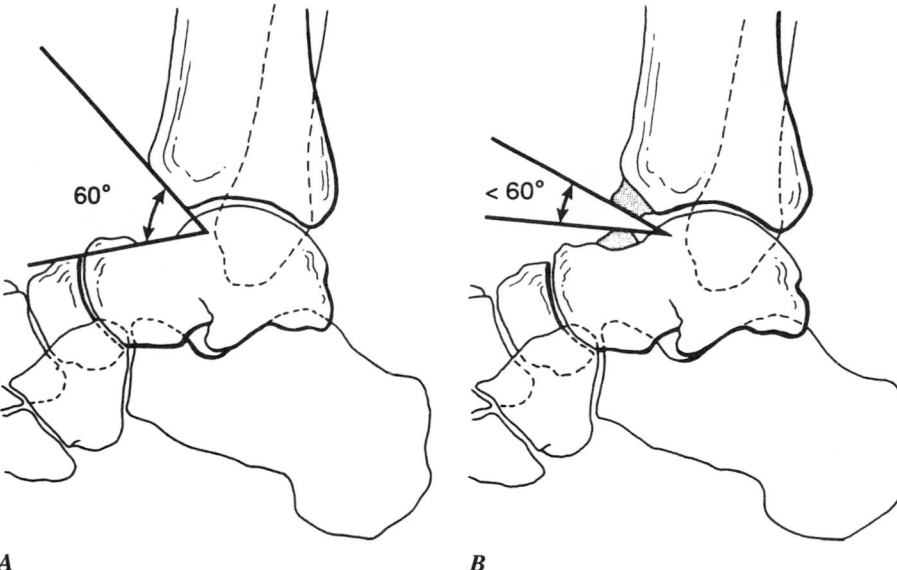

A   *B*

Unfortunately, patients frequently present with fixed hindfoot valgus (stage III) associated with forefoot abduction.[201,203]

Isolated talonavicular synovitis may predominate.[202] Conservative management should include a foot orthosis with medial longitudinal arch support. Isolated talonavicular arthrodesis has been advocated and is thought to possibly prevent or delay the progression of forefoot abduction associated with hindfoot valgus.[202] When involvement of two of the three hindfoot joints occurs and medical management is unsuccessful, triple arthrodesis is indicated.[197,200,227,228]

Insufficiency fracture of the distal third of the fibula may present as hindfoot valgus, whereas similar fractures along the medial aspect of the tibia may cause hindfoot varus. Significant deformities can be avoided only by early recognition and treatment of the insufficiency fracture with an AFO or a short leg cast.[200] A corrective osteotomy may be indicated in rare instances.

ANKLE ARTHRITIS

There are many known causes of tibiotalar arthritis, including (1) trauma initiated by displaced ankle fractures, osteochondral lesions, talar neck fractures with avascular necrosis,[209] and chronic ankle ligamentous instability; (2) degenerative joint disease;[230] (3) inflammation (e.g., rheumatoid); (4) joint sepsis; (5) Charcot neuroarthropathy; and (6) tumor (e.g., osteoid osteoma, synovial chondromatosis).[212]

Conservative management is dependent on etiology. A history of posttraumatic arthritis may not require an extensive workup. However, patients with a sensory neuropathy, infection, or tumor are managed differently. Patients with neuropathy usually have x-ray destruction out of proportion to the complaints of pain. A thorough vascular assessment is required, especially with respect to any plantar ulceration. A patient with any history of previous operative treatment or intraarticular steroid injection must be evaluated for occult joint sepsis with aspiration and appropriate cultures. Tumor involvement may be suggested by a history of night pain. Routine x-ray evaluation may identify "aggressive" or destructive lesions. Appropriate referral of these lesions to a musculoskeletal oncologist for workup and biopsy has been recommended.

Nonoperative management of posttraumatic or degenerative joint disease includes a trial of nonsteroidal anti-inflammatory drugs (NSAIDs) or possible intraarticular steroid injection once sepsis is ruled out.[223] Modification of everyday footwear to shoes with greater shock-absorbing qualities, such as rocker-bottom soles with a solid ankle cushioned heel (SACH), may extend the "life" of an arthritic joint.[225] An AFO is recommended to help control hindfoot position and motion. However, this orthosis or even a patellar tendon–bearing orthosis usually provides insufficient relief of impact loading forces across the tibiotalar or subtalar joints.

Advanced ankle arthrosis that is refractory to medical management and does not allow resumption of activities of daily living because of pain is the most common indication for ankle arthrodesis.[212] Total ankle replacement (TAR) arthroplasty has been attempted. However, the long-term results of TAR remain unacceptable due to recurrent pain, component migration, loosening, and malalignment.[212] Finally, secondary reconstruction following failed TAR arthroplasty is complicated because of a marked deficiency in bone stock following implant removal.[222,223]

Numerous techniques have been described to obtain successful ankle arthrodesis (see References 206–209, 212–214, 217–220, 224, 226, 229, 235). Currently, the technique of choice for ankle arthrodesis most commonly employs rigid internal fixation (Fig. 53-16). With advances in ankle arthroscopy, arthroscopically assisted

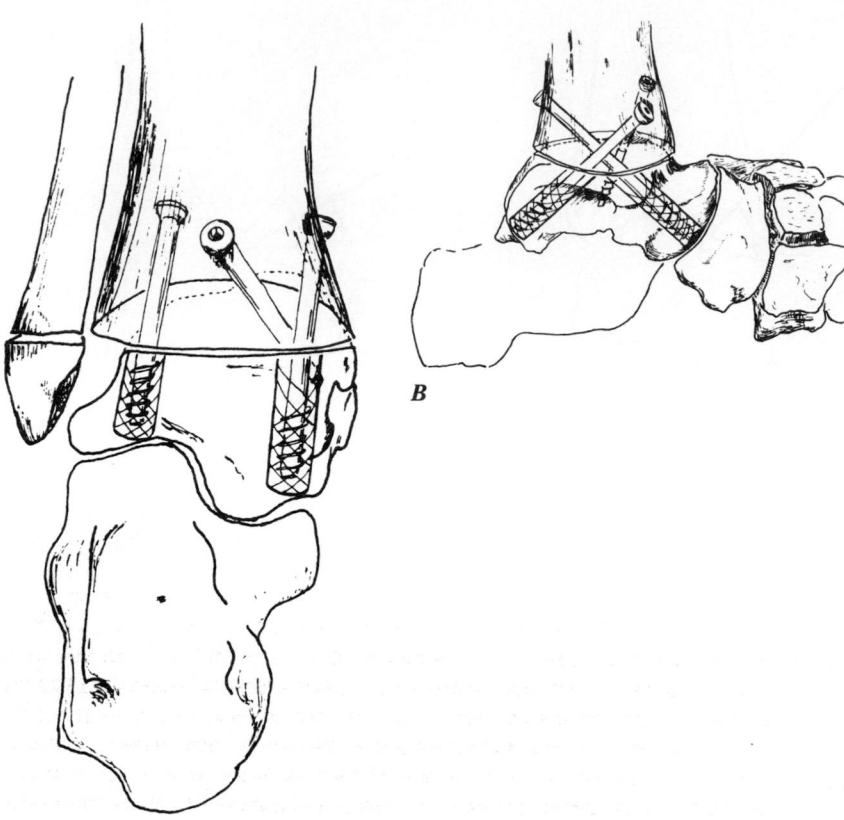

A

B

Figure 53-16 "Square cut" ankle arthrodesis with distal fibular ostectomy performed with cannulated screw internal fixation. *A*. Posterior view of the left ankle. *B*. Medial view of the left ankle. (Reproduced with permission from Kish G, Eberhart R, King T, et al: Ankle arthrodesis placement of cannulated screws. *Foot Ankle Int* 14:223, 1993.)

ankle arthrodesis techniques have achieved as good or better fusion rates in shorter postoperative periods of time: 8 to 9 weeks with arthroscopy versus 3 to 4 months with conventional "square-cut" open arthrodesis.[206,207,210,212] In situ arthroscopic ankle arthrodesis is contraindicated when the patient presents with any hindfoot varus or valgus greater than 15° or any significant rotatory malalignment.[210] The key to obtaining a successful in situ arthroscopic arthrodesis appears to relate to the debridement of only the minimum amount of hyaline cartilage and necrotic bone during the procedure. In so doing, minimal alteration in the general joint conformation is achieved, leaving more bone stock and a broad vascular bed. On the other hand, open ankle arthrodesis is traditionally performed by "squaring off" both the tibial plafond and the talar dome, as in open transfibular realigning arthrodesis techniques (Fig. 53-16). These open techniques are associated with much greater soft tissue stripping and more bone loss. However, Meyerson et al. have reported excellent results with a miniarthrotomy ankle arthrodesis technique, which compares favorably with the in situ arthroscopic arthrodesis and has similar incisions and contraindications.[234] Clearly, this study supports the miniarthrotomy over the arthroscopic technique with respect to a greater degree of operative skill necessary to perform the latter and the significantly greater operative time required for arthroscopically assisted procedures.

Whatever method is employed to obtain ankle arthrodesis, the optimum arthrodesis position appears to be neutral (0°) flexion/extension tibiotalar position; hindfoot valgus of 5 to 10°, external rotation of 5 to 10°, and neutral mediolateral displacement.[211,232] Slight posterior translation (≤ 1 cm) of the talus with respect to the tibia has been recommended to diminish midfoot loading stresses.[212]

Complications reported with ankle arthrodesis include nonunion, malunion, infection, and leg-length discrepancy.[212] Approximately 50 percent loss of inversion and eversion has been reported, with an additional partial loss of subtalar motion.[223] Following ankle arthrodesis, most patients achieve an improved gait pattern secondary to relief of pain; decreased walking speed and shortened stride length are generally noted.[232,233]

REFERENCES

1. Funk DA, Cass JR, Johnson KA: Acquired adult flatfoot secondary to posterior tibial tendon pathology. *J Bone Joint Surg* 68A:95–102, 1986.
2. Mann RA, Thompson FM: Rupture of the posterior tibial tendon causing flatfoot: Surgical treatment. *J Bone Joint Surg* 67A:556–561, 1985.

3. Jahss MH: Spontaneous rupture of the tibialis posterior tendon: Clinical findings, tenographic studies, and a new technique for repair. *Foot Ankle* 3:158–166, 1982.

4. Conti S, Michelson J, Jahss M: Clinical significance of magnetic resonance imaging in preoperative planning for reconstruction of posterior tibial tendon ruptures. *Foot Ankle* 13:208–214, 1992.

5. Frey C, Shereff M, Greenridge N: Vascularity of the posterior tibial tendon. *J Bone Joint Surg* 72A:884–888, 1990.

6. Holmes GB Jr, Mann RA: Possible epidemiological factors associated with rupture of the posterior tibial tendon. *Foot Ankle* 13:70–79, 1992.

7. Meyerson M, Solomon G, Shereff M: Posterior tibial tendon dysfunction: Its association with seronegative inflammatory disease. *Foot Ankle* 9:219–225, 1989.

8. Trevino S, Gould N, Korson R: Surgical treatment of stenosing tenosynovitis at the ankle. *Foot Ankle* 2:37–45, 1981.

9. Southwell RB, Sherman FC: Triple arthrodesis: A long-term study with force plate analysis. *Foot Ankle* 2:15–24, 1981.

10. Meyerson MS, Corrigan J, Thompson FM, Schon LC: Tendon transfer combined with calcaneal osteotomy for treatment of posterior tibial tendon insufficiency: A radiologic investigation. *Foot Ankle Int* 16:712–718, 1995.

11. Deland JT, Otis JC, Lee KT, Kenneally SM: Lateral column lengthening with calcaneocuboid fusion: Range of motion in the triple joint complex. *Foot Ankle Int* 16:729–733, 1995.

12. Jones DC: Tendon disorders of the foot and ankle. *J Am Acad Orthop Surg* 1:87–94, 1993.

13. Miller RA, Hayes W: Subtalar arthrodesis with screw fixation in the adult. *Op Tech Orthop* 4:169–172, 1994.

14. Graves SC, Badwey TH, Graves KO: Biomechanics and orthotics of the foot in athletes. *Op Tech Sports Med* 2:2–8, 1994.

15. Thordarson DB, Schmotzer H, Chon J: Reconstruction with tenodesis in an adult flatfoot model. *J Bone Joint Surg* 77A:1557–1564, 1995.

16. Meyerson MS: Adult acquired flatfoot deformity: Treatment of dysfunction of the posterior tibial tendon. *J Bone Joint Surg* 78A:780–792, 1996.

17. Wapner KL, Hecht PJ, Shea JTR, Allardyce TJ: Anatomy of second muscular layer of the foot: Considerations for tendon selection in transfer for Achilles and posterior tibial tendon reconstruction. *Foot Ankle Int* 15:420–423, 1994.

18. Delmi M, Kurt AM, Meyer JM, et al: Calcification of the tibialis posterior tendon: A case report and literature review. *Foot Ankle Int* 16:792–795, 1995.

19. Sangeorzan BJ, Mosca V, Hansen ST Jr: Effect of calcaneal lengthening on relationships among the hindfoot, midfoot and forefoot. *Foot Ankle* 14:136–141, 1993.

20. Sangeorzan BJ, Smith D, Verth R, Hansen ST Jr: Triple arthrodesis using internal fixation in treatment of adult foot disorders. *Clin Orthop* 294:299–307, 1993.

21. Teasdall RD, Johnson KA: Surgical treatment of stage I posterior tibial tendon dysfunction. *Foot Ankle Int* 15:646–648, 1994.

22. Meyerson MS: Posterior tibial tendon insufficiency, in Meyerson M (ed): *Current Therapy in Foot and Ankle Surgery.* St Louis, Mosby–Year Book, 1993, pp 123–135.

23. Aronson J, Nunley J, Frankovitch K: Lateral talocalcaneal angle in assessment of subtalar valgus: Follow-up of seventy Grice-Green arthrodeses. *Foot Ankle* 4:56–63, 1983.

24. Bordelon RL: Correction of hypermobile flatfoot in children by molded insert. *Foot Ankle* 1:143–150, 1980.

25. Hinterman B, Gachter A: The first metatarsal rise sign: A simple sensitive sign of tibialis posterior tendon dysfunction. *Foot Ankle Int* 17:236–241, 1996.

26. Pedowitz WJ, Kovatis P: Flatfoot in the adult. *J Am Acad Orthop Surg* 3:293–302, 1995.

27. Saltzman CL, Therman H: Achilles tendon problems, in Pfeffer GB, Frey CL (eds): *Current Practice in Foot and Ankle Surgery.* Vol 1. New York, McGraw-Hill, 1993, pp 194–218.

28. O'Malley M, Deland JT, Lee KT: Selective hindfoot arthrodesis for the treatment of adult acquired flatfoot deformity: An in vitro study. *Foot Ankle Int* 16:409–417, 1995.

29. Resnick RB, Jahss MH, Choneka J, et al: Deltoid ligament forces after tibialis posterior tendon rupture and calcaneal displacement osteotomies. *Foot Ankle Int* 16:14–20, 1995.

30. Horton GA, Olney BW: Triple arthrodesis with lateral column lengthening for treatment of severe planovalgus deformity. *Foot Ankle Int* 16:395–400, 1995.

31. Conti SF: Posterior tibial tendon problems in athletes. *Orthop Clin North Am* 25:109–121, 1994.

32. Thermann H, Hoffman R, Zwipp H, Tscherne H: The use of ultrasonography in the foot and ankle. *Foot Ankle* 13:386–390, 1992.

33. Troop RL, Losse GM, Lane JG, et al: Early motion after repair of Achilles tendon ruptures. *Foot Ankle Int* 16:705–709, 1995.

34. Thompson TC, Doherty JH: Spontaneous rupture of tendon of Achilles: A new clinical diagnostic test. *J Trauma* 2:126–129, 1962.

35. Carr AJ, Norris SH: The blood supply of the calcaneal tendon. *J Bone Joint Surg* 71B:100–101, 1989.

36. Hockenbury RT, Johns JC: A biomechanical in vitro comparison of open versus percutaneous repair of tendon Achilles. *Foot Ankle* 11:67–72, 1990.

37. Inglis AE, Scott WN, Sculco TP, et al: Ruptures of the tendon Achilles: An objective assessment of surgical and non-surgical treatment. *J Bone Joint Surg* 58A:990–993, 1976.

38. Leitner A, Voigt C, Rahmanzadeh R: Treatment of extensive aseptic defect in old Achilles ruptures: Methods and case reports. *Foot Ankle* 13:176–180, 1992.

39. Mann RA, Holmes GB Jr, Seals KS: Chronic rupture of the Achilles tendon: A new technique of repair. *J Bone Joint Surg* 73A:214–219, 1991.

40. Nistor C: Surgical and non-surgical treatment of Achilles tendon rupture: A prospective randomized study. *J Bone Joint Surg* 63A:394–399, 1981.

41. Puddu G, Ippolito G, Postacchini F: A classification of Achilles tendon disease. *Am J Sports Med* 4:145–150, 1976.

42. Wapner KL, Hecht PJ: Repair of chronic Achilles tendon rupture with flexor hallucis longus. *Op Tech Orthop* 4:132–137, 1994.

43. Mann RA: Achilles tendon reconstruction using the flexor digitorum longus. *Op Tech Orthop* 4:138–140, 1994.

44. Gabel S, Manoli A II: Neglected rupture of the Achilles tendon. *Foot Ankle Int* 15:512–517, 1994.

45. Lidman D, Nettleblad H, Berggren A, et al: Reconstruction of soft tissue defects including the Achilles tendon with free neurovascular tensor fascia lata flap and fascia lata. *Scand J Plast Reconst Surg* 21:213, 1987.

46. Hattrup SJ, Johnson KA: A review of ruptures of the Achilles tendon. *Foot Ankle* 6:34–38, 1985.

47. Watson TN, Jurist KA, Yang KH, et al: The strength of Achilles tendon repair: An in vitro study of the biomechanical behavior in human cadaver tendons. *Foot Ankle Int* 16:191–195, 1995.

48. Aracil J, Pina A, Lozano J, et al: Percutaneous suture of Achilles tendon rupture. *Foot Ankle* 13:350–351, 1992.

49. Ma GWC, Griffith TG: Percutaneous repair of acute closed ruptured Achilles tendon—A new technique. *Clin Orthop* 128:247–255, 1977.

50. Wapner KL, Pavlock GS, Hecht PJ, et al: Repair of chronic Achilles tendon rupture with flexor hallucis longus tendon transfer. *Foot Ankle* 14:443–449, 1993.

51. Wapner KL, Hecht PJ, Mills RH: Reconstruction of neglected Achilles tendon injury. *Orthop Clin North Am* 26:249–263, 1995.

52. Greenfield G, Stanish WD: Tendinitis and tendon ruptures. *Op Tech Sports Med* 2:9–17, 1994.

53. Gould N, Korson R: Stenosing tenosynovitis of the pseudosheath of the tendo Achilles. *Foot Ankle* 1:179–187, 1980.

54. Wiggins ME, Fadale PD, Ehrlich MG, Walsh WR: Effects of local injection of corticosteroids on the healing of ligaments. *J Bone Joint Surg* 77A:1682–1690, 1995.

55. Roberts DK, Pomeranz SJ: Current status of magnetic resonance imaging in radiologic diagnosis of foot and ankle injuries. *Orthop Clin North Am* 25:61–68, 1994.

56. Saltzman C, Bonar S: Tendon problems of the foot and ankle, in Lutter LD, Mizel MS, Pfeffer GB (eds): *Orthopaedic Knowledge Update—Foot and Ankle*. Rosemont, IL, American Academy of Orthopaedic Surgeons, 1994, pp 269–282.

57. Soma CA, Mandelbaum BR: Repair of acute Achilles tendon ruptures. *Orthop Clin North Am* 26:239–247, 1995.

58. Kleinman M, Gross AE: Achilles tendon rupture following steroid injection: A report of three cases. *J Bone Joint Surg* 65A:1345–1347, 1983.

59. Clain MR, Baxter DE: Achilles tendinitis. *Foot Ankle* 13:482–487, 1992.

60. Pavlov H, Heneghan MA, Harsh A, et al: The Haglund syndromes: Initial and differential diagnosis. *Radiology* 144:83–88, 1982.

61. Schepsis AA, Leach RE: Surgical management of Achilles tendinitis. *Am J Sports Med* 14:308–315, 1987.

62. Scioli MW: Achilles tendinitis. *Orthop Clin North Am* 25:177–182, 1994.

63. Stephens MM: Haglund's deformity and retrocalcaneal bursitis. *Orthop Clin North Am* 25:41–46, 1994.

64. Heneghan MA, Pavlov H: The Haglund painful heel syndrome. *Clin Orthop Rel Res* 187:228, 1984.

65. Frey C, Rosenburg Z, Shereff M, et al: The retrocalcaneal bursa: Anatomy and bursography. *Foot Ankle* 13:203–207, 1992.

66. Angerman S: Chronic retrocalcaneal bursitis treated by resection of the calcaneus. *Foot Ankle* 10:285–287, 1990.

67. Das De S, Balasubramaniam P: A repair operation for recurrent dislocation of peroneal tendons. *J Bone Joint Surg* 67B:585–587, 1985.

68. Sammarco GJ, DiRaimondo CV: Chronic peroneus brevis tendon lesions. *Foot Ankle* 9:163–170, 1989.

69. Sobel M, Bohne WH, Levy ME: Longitudinal attrition of the peroneus brevis tendon in the fibular groove: An anatomic study. *Foot Ankle* 11:124–128, 1990.

70. Thompson FM, Patterson AH: Rupture of the peroneus longus tendon: A report of three cases. *J Bone Joint Surg* 71A:293–295, 1989.

71. Zoellner G, Clancy W Jr: Recurrent dislocation of the peroneal tendon. *J Bone Joint Surg* 61A:292–294, 1979.

72. Sobel M, Pavlov H, Geppert MJ, et al: Painful os peroneum syndrome: A spectrum of conditions responsible for plantar lateral foot pain. *Foot Ankle Int* 15:112–124, 1994.

73. Davis WH, Sobel M, Deland J, et al: The superior peroneal retinaculum: An anatomic study. *Foot Ankle Int* 15:271–275, 1994.

74. Sobel M, Geppert MJ, Olson EJ, et al: The dynamics of peroneus brevis tendon splits: A proposed mechanism, technique of diagnosis and classification of injury. *Foot Ankle* 13:413–422, 1992.

75. Brage ME, Hansen ST Jr: Traumatic subluxation/dislocation of the peroneal tendons. *Foot Ankle* 13:423–431, 1992.

76. Pozo JR, Jackson AM: A rerouting operation for dislocation of peroneal tendons: Operative technique and case report. *Foot Ankle* 5:42–44, 1984.

77. Sarmiento A, Wolf M: Subluxation of the peroneal tendons: Case treated by rerouting tendons under calcaneofibular ligament. *J Bone Joint Surg* 57A:115–116, 1975.

78. Sobel M, Bohne WHO, Markisz JA: Cadaver correlation of peroneal changes with magnetic resonance imaging. *Foot Ankle* 11:384–388, 1991.

79. Peterson DA, Stinson W: Excision of the fractured os peroneum: A report on five patients and review of the literature. *Foot Ankle* 13:277–281, 1992.

80. Sobel M, Warren R, Brourman S: Lateral ankle instability with dislocation of the peroneal tendons treated by the Chrisman-Snook procedure: A case report and literature review. *Am J Sports Med* 18:539–543, 1990.

81. Sobel M, Bohne WHO, DiCarlo E, Collins L: Longitudinal splitting of the peroneus brevis tendon: An anatomic and histologic study of cadaveric material. *Foot Ankle* 12:165–170, 1991.

82. Sobel M, Geppert MJ: Repair of concomitant lateral ankle ligament instability and peroneus brevis splits through a posteriorly modified Brostrom Gould. *Foot Ankle* 13:224–225, 1992.

83. Sobel M, Levy M, Bohne WHO: Congenital variations of the peroneus quartus muscle: An anatomic study. *Foot Ankle* 11:81–89, 1990.

84. Sobel M, Levy M, Bohne WHO: Longitudinal attrition of the peroneus brevis tendon in the fibular groove: An anatomic study. *Foot Ankle* 11:124–128, 1990.

85. Kilkelly FX, McHale KA: Acute rupture of the peroneus longus tendon in a runner—A case report and review of the literature. *Foot Ankle Int* 15:567–569, 1994.

86. Yodlowski ML, Mizel MS: Reconstruction of peroneus brevis pathology. *Op Tech Orthop* 4:146–151, 1994.

87. Zeiss J, Ebraheim N, Rusin J, Loombs RJ: Magnetic resonance imaging of the calcaneus: Normal anatomy and application in calcaneus fractures. *Foot Ankle* 11:264–273, 1991.

88. Sobel M, Mizel MS: Peroneal tendon injury, in Pfeffer GB, Frey CC (eds): *Current Practice in Foot and Ankle Surgery*. Vol 1. New York, McGraw-Hill, 1993, pp 30–56.

89. Steinbock G, Pinsger M: Treatment of peroneal tendon dislocation under the calcaneofibular ligament. *Foot Ankle* 15:107–111, 1994.

90. Ebraheim NA, Zeiss J, Skie MC, et al: Marginal fractures of the lateral malleolus in association with other fractures in the ankle region. *Foot Ankle* 13:171–175, 1992.

91. Eckert WR, Lakes M, Davis EA: Acute rupture of the peroneal retinaculum. *J Bone Joint Surg* 58A:670–673, 1976.

92. Sammarco GJ, DiRaimondo CV: Chronic peroneus brevis tendon lesions. *Foot Ankle* 9:163–170, 1989.

93. Sobel M, Geppert MJ: Repair of concomitant lateral ligament instability and peroneus brevis splits through a posteriorly modified Bröstrom-Gould: Technique tips. *Foot Ankle* 13:224–225, 1992.

94. Sobel M, Geppert MJ, Hannafin JA, et al: Microvascular anatomy of the peroneal tendons. *Foot Ankle* 13:469–472, 1992.

95. Hammerschlag WA, Goldner JL: Chronic peroneal tendon subluxation produced by an anomalous peroneus brevis: A case report and review of the literature. *Foot Ankle* 10:45–47, 1989.

96. Burman M: Subcutaneous tear of the tendon of the peroneus longus: Its relationship to the giant peroneal tubercle. *Arch Surg* 73:216–219, 1956.

97. Sammarco GJ: Peroneal tendon injuries. *Orthop Clin North Am* 25:135–145, 1994.

98. DeLuca PA, Banta JV: Pes cavovarus as a late consequence of peroneus longus laceration. *J Pediatr Orthop* 5:582, 1985.

99. Sammarco GJ: Peroneus longus tendon tears: Acute and chronic. *Foot Ankle Int* 16:245–253, 1995.

100. Ouzounian TJ, Anderson R: Anterior tibial tendon rupture. *Foot Ankle Int* 16:406–410, 1995.

101. Rimoldi RL, Oberlander MA, Waldrop JI, et al: Acute rupture of the anterior tibial tendon: A case report. *Foot Ankle* 12:176–177, 1991.

102. Forst R, Forst J, Heller KD: Ipsilateral peroneus brevis tendon grafting in a complicated case of traumatic rupture of the tibialis anterior tendon. *Foot Ankle Int* 16:440–444, 1995.

103. Geppert MJ, Sobel M, Hannafin JA: Microvasculature of the tibialis anterior tendon. *Foot Ankle* 14:261–264, 1993.

104. Mankey MG: Treatment of tibialis anterior tendon rupture. *Op Tech Orthop* 4:141–145, 1994.

105. Fennel CW, Phillips P III: Redefining the anatomy of the anterior tibialis tendon. *Foot Ankle Int* 15:396–399, 1994.

106. Floyd DW, Heckman JD, Rockwood CA: Tendon lacerations in the foot. *Foot Ankle* 4:8–14, 1983.

107. Wright DG, Adelaar RS: Avascular necrosis of the talus. *Foot Ankle Int* 16:743–744, 1995.

108. Gelberman RH, Mortensen WW: The arterial anatomy of the talus. *Foot Ankle* 4:64–72, 1983.

109. Ferkel RD, Flannigan BD, Elkins BS: Magnetic resonance imaging of the foot and ankle: Correlations of normal anatomy with pathologic conditions. *Foot Ankle* 11:289–305, 1991.

110. Schenk RC, Goodnight JM: Current concepts review— Osteochondritis dissecans. *J Bone Joint Surg* 78A:439–456, 1996.

111. Stone JW: Osteochondral lesions of the talar dome. *J Am Acad Orthop Surg* 4:63–73, 1996.

112. Berdnt AL, Harty M: Transchondral fractures (osteochondritis dissecans) of the talus. *J Bone Joint Surg* 41A:988–1020, 1959.

113. Canale ST, Belding RH: Osteochondral lesions of the talus. *J Bone Joint Surg* 62A:97–102, 1980.

114. Pettine KA, Morrey BF: Osteochondral fractures of the talus: A long term follow-up. *J Bone Joint Surg* 69B:89–92, 1987.

115. Flick AB, Gould N: Osteochondritis dissecans of the talus (transchondral fracture of the talus): Review of the literature and new surgical approach for medial dome lesions. *Foot Ankle* 5:165–185, 1985.

116. Shea MP, Manoli A: Osteochondral lesions. *Foot Ankle* 14:48–55, 1993.

117. Dipaolo JD, Nelson DW, Colville MR: Characterizing osteochondral lesions by magnetic resonance imaging. *Arthroscopy* 7:101–104, 1991.

118. Pritsch M, Horshouski H, Farine I: Arthroscopic treatment of osteochondral lesions of the talus. *J Bone Joint Surg* 68A:862–865, 1986.

119. Ove PN, Bosse MJ, Reinert CM: Excision of posterolateral talar dome lesions through a medial transmalleolar approach. *Foot Ankle* 9:171–175, 1989.

120. Gepstein R, Conforty B, Weiss RE, et al: Closed percutaneous drilling for osteochondritis dissecans of the talus: A report of two cases. *Clin Orthop* 213:197–200, 1986.

121. Adkinson DP, Bosse MJ, Giaccionc DR, et al: Anatomical variations in the course of the superficial peroneal nerve. *J Bone Joint Surg* 73A:112–114, 1991.

122. Ferkel RD: *Arthroscopic Surgery: The Foot and Ankle.* Philadelphia, Lippincott-Raven, 1996.

123. Ferkel RD, Scranton PE Jr: Arthroscopy of the ankle and foot. *J Bone Joint Surg* 75A:1233–1242, 1993.

124. Ferkel RD, Health DD, Guhl JF: Neurological complications of ankle arthroscopy: A review of 612 cases. *Arthroscopy* 9:352, 1993.

125. Stone JW: Ankle arthroscopy, in Lutter LD, Mizel MS, Pfeffer GB (eds): *Orthopaedic Knowledge Update—Foot and Ankle.* Rosemont, IL, American Academy of Orthopaedic Surgeons, 1994, pp 61–72.

126. Lawrence SJ, Botte MJ: The sural nerve in the foot and ankle: An anatomic study with clinical and surgical implications. *Foot Ankle Int* 15:490–494, 1994.

127. Feder KS, Schonholtz GJ: Ankle arthroscopy: Review and long term results. *Foot Ankle* 13:382–385, 1992.

128. Feinell LA: Standard set up and portals for ankle arthroscopy. *Op Tech Orthop* 4:181–183, 1994.

129. Barber FA, Glick J, Britt BJ: Complications of ankle arthroscopy. *Foot Ankle* 10:263–266, 1990.

130. Feinell LA, Frey C: Anatomic study of arthroscopic portal sites of the ankle. *Foot Ankle* 14:142–147, 1993.

131. Guhl JF (ed): *Ankle Arthroscopy: Pathology and Surgical Techniques.* Thorofare, NJ, Slack, 1988.

132. Stetson WB, Ferkel RD: Ankle arthroscopy: I. Technique and complications. *J Am Acad Orthop Surg* 4:17–23, 1996.

133. Ferkel RD: Arthroscopy of the ankle and foot, in Mann RA, Coughlin MA (eds): *Surgery of the Foot and Ankle,* 6th ed. Vol 2. St Louis: Mosby, 1993, pp 1277–1310.

134. Taillaird W, Meyer JM, Garcia J, et al: The sinus tarsi syndrome. *Int Orthop* 5:117–130, 1981.

135. O'Connor D: Sinus tarsi syndrome—A clinical entity. *J Bone Joint Surg* 40A:720, 1958.

136. Stetson WB, Ferkel RD: Ankle arthroscopy: II. Indications and results. *J Am Acad Orthop Surg* 4:24–34, 1996.

137. Ferkel RD, Karzel RP, Del Pizzo W, et al: Arthroscopic treatment of anteriolateral impingement of the ankle. *Am J Sports Med* 19:440–446, 1991.

138. Ferkel RD: Soft tissue lesions of the ankle, in Ferkel RD (ed): *Arthroscopic Surgery—The Foot and Ankle.* Philadelphia, Lippincott-Raven, 1996, pp 121–144.

139. Lofvenberg R, Karrholm J, Selvik G: Fibular mobility in chronic lateral instability of the ankle. *Foot Ankle* 11:22–29, 1990.

140. Amendola A: Controversies in diagnosis and management of syndesmosis injuries of the ankle. *Foot Ankle* 13:44–50, 1992.

141. Harper MC: An anatomic and radiographic investigation of the tibiofibular clear space. *Foot Ankle* 14:455–458, 1993.

142. Harper MC: The short oblique fracture of the distal fibula without medial injury: An assessment of displacement. *Foot Ankle Int* 16:181–186, 1995.

143. Veltri DM, Pagnani MJ, O'Brien SJ, et al: Symptomatic ossification of tibio-fibular syndesmosis in professional football players: A sequela of the syndesmotic ankle sprain. *Foot Ankle Int* 16:285–290, 1995.

144. Stone JW, Guhl JF: Meniscoid lesions of the ankle. *Clinics Sports Med* 10:661–676, 1991.

145. Wolin I, Glassman F, Sideman S: Internal derangement of the talofibular component of the ankle. *Surg Gynecol Obstet* 901:193–200, 1950.

146. Bassett FH III, Gates HS III, Billys JB, et al: Talar impingement by the anterioinferior tibiofibular ligament: A cause of chronic pain in the ankle after inversion sprain. *J Bone Joint Surg* 72A:55–59, 1990.

147. Renström AFH: Persistently painful sprained ankle. *J Am Acad Orthop Surg* 2:270–280, 1994.

148. Harper MC: An anatomic study of the short oblique fracture of the distal fibula and ankle stability. *Foot Ankle* 4:23–29, 1983.

149. Morris JR, Lee J, Thordarson D, et al: Magnetic resonance imaging of acute Maisonneuve fractures. *Foot Ankle Int* 17:259–263, 1996.

150. Kulik SA, Clanton TO: Tarsal coalition. *Foot Ankle Int* 17:286–296, 1996.

151. Jahss MH, Kay BS: An anatomic study of the anterior superior process of the os calcis and its clinical application. *Foot Ankle* 3:268–281, 1983.

152. Hopkins WJ, St Pierre P, Ryan JB, et al: Syndesmosis sprains of the ankle. *Foot Ankle* 10:325–330, 1990.

153. Marder RA: Current methods for the evaluation of ankle ligaments injuries. *J Bone Joint Surg* 76A:1103–1111, 1994.

154. Stephens MM, Sammarco GJ: The stabilizing role of the lateral ligament complex around the ankle and subtalar joints. *Foot Ankle* 13:130–133, 1992.

155. Schon LC, Clanton TO, Baxter DE: Reconstruction for subtalar instability: A review. *Foot Ankle* 11:319–326, 1991.

156. Chrisman OD, Snook GA: Reconstruction of lateral ligament tears of the ankle: An experimental study and evaluation of seven patients by a new modification of the Elmslie procedure. *J Bone Joint Surg* 51A:904–912, 1969.

157. Cranton TO: Instability of the subtalar joint. *Orthop Clin North Am* 20:583–592, 1989.

158. Chrisman GA, Chrisman OD, Wilson TC: Long term results of the Chrisman-Snook operation for reconstruction of the lateral ligaments of the ankle. *J Bone Joint Surg* 67A:1–7, 1985.

159. Harper MC: The lateral ligamentous support of the subtalar joint. *Foot Ankle* 11:354–358, 1991.

160. Hamilton WG, Thompson FA, Snow SW: The modified Broström procedure for lateral ankle instability. *Foot Ankle* 14:1–7, 1993.

161. Ferkel RD: Subtalar arthroscopy, in Ferkel RD (ed): *Arthroscopic Surgery—The Foot and Ankle.* Philadelphia, Lippincott-Raven, 1996, pp 215–230.

162. Frey C, Gasser S, Feder K: Arthroscopy of the subtalar joint. *Foot Ankle Int* 15:424–428, 1994.

163. Mekhail AO, Heck BE, Ebraheim NA, et al: Arthroscopy of the subtalar joint: Establishing a medial portal. *Foot Ankle Int* 16:427–432, 1995.

164. Harper MC: Stress radiographs in the diagnosis of lateral instability of the ankle and hindfoot. *Foot Ankle* 13:435–438, 1992.

165. Louwerens JW, Ginai AZ, VanLinge B, et al: Stress radiography of the talocrural and subtalar joints. *Foot Ankle Int* 16:148–155, 1995.

166. Pisani G: Chronic laxity of the subtalar joint. *Orthopaedics* 19:431–437, 1996.

167. Wredmark T, Carlstedt CA, Bauer H, et al: Os trigonum syndrome: A clinical entity in ballet dancers. *Foot Ankle* 11:404–406, 1991.

168. Hedrick MR, McBryde AM: Posterior ankle impingement. *Foot Ankle Int* 15:2–8, 1994.

169. Ebraheim NA, Padanilam TG, Wong FY: Posteromedial process fractures of the talus. *Foot Ankle Int* 16:734–739, 1995.

170. Meyerson MS, Berger BI: Nonunion of a fracture of the sustentaculum tail causing a tarsal tunnel syndrome. *Foot Ankle Int* 16:740–742, 1995.

171. McHale KA: Resection of tarsal coalition. *Op Tech Orthop* 4:173–180, 1994.

172. Chand Y, Johnson KA: Foot and ankle manifestations of Reiter's syndrome. *Foot Ankle* 1:167–172, 1980.

173. Quirk R: Common foot and ankle injuries in dance. *Orthop Clin North Am* 25:123–133, 1994.

174. Hardaker WT: Foot and ankle injuries in classical ballet dancers. *Orthop Clin North Am* 20:621–627, 1989.

175. Bohay DR, Manoli A II: Occult fractures following subtalar joint injuries. *Foot Ankle Int* 17:164–169, 1996.

176. Stefko RM, Lauerman WC, Heckman JD: Tarsal tunnel syndrome caused by an unrecognized fracture of the posterior process of the talus (Cedell fracture). *J Bone Joint Surg* 76A:116–118, 1994.

177. Kim DH, Hrutkay JM, Samson MS: Fracture of the medial tubercle of the posterior process of the talus: A case report and literature review. *Foot Ankle Int* 17:186–188, 1996.

178. Cedell CA: Rupture of the posterior talotibial ligament with the avulsion of a bone fragment from the talus. *Acta Orthop Scand* 45:454–461, 1974.

179. Ebraheim NA, Padanilam TG, Wong FY: Posteromedial process fracture of the talus. *Foot Ankle Int* 16:734–739, 1995.

180. Veazey BL, Heckman JD, Galindo MJ, et al: Excision of ununited fractures of the posterior process of the talus: A treatment for chronic ankle pain. *Foot Ankle* 13:453–457, 1992.

181. Dimon JH III: Isolated displaced fracture of the posterior facet of the talus. *J Bone Joint Surg* 43A:275–281, 1961.

182. Hawkins LG: Fracture of the lateral process of the talus. *J Bone Joint Surg* 47A:1170–1175, 1965.

183. Ihle CL, Cochran RM: Fracture of the fused os trigonum. *Am J Sports Med* 10:47–50, 1982.

184. Mukherjee SK, Pringle RM, Baxter AD: Fracture of the lateral process of the talus: A report of thirteen cases. *J Bone Joint Surg* 56B:263–273, 1974.

185. Burkus JK, Sella EJ, Southwick WO: Occult injuries of the talus diagnosed by bone scan and tomography. *Foot Ankle* 4:316–324, 1984.

186. Mankey M: Fractures of the talus, in Lutter LD, Mizel MS, Pfeffer GB (eds): *Orthopaedic Knowledge Update: Foot and Ankle.* Rosemont, IL, American Association of Orthopaedic Surgeons, 1994, pp 205–226.

187. Hamilton WG: Tendinitis about the ankle joint in classical ballet dancers: "Dancer's tendinitis." *J Sports Med* 5:84, 1977.

188. Hamilton WG: Stenosing tenosynovitis of the flexor hallucis longus tendon and posterior impingement upon the os trigonum in ballet dancers. *Foot Ankle* 3:74–80, 1982.

189. Trepman E, Mizel MS, Newberg AH: Partial rupture of the flexor hallucis longus tendon in a tennis player: A case report. *Foot Ankle Int* 16:227–231, 1995.

190. Thompson FM, Snow SW, Herson SJ: Spontaneous atraumatic rupture of the flexor hallucis longus tendon under the sustentaculum tali: Case report, review of the literature and treatment options. *Foot Ankle* 14:414–417, 1993.

191. Scranton PE Jr, McDermott JE: Anterior tibiotalar spurs: A comparison of open versus arthroscopic debridement. *Foot Ankle* 13:125–129, 1992.

192. Hamilton WG: Foot and ankle injuries in dancers, in Mann RA, Coughlin MJ (eds): *Surgery of the Foot and Ankle,* 6th ed. Vol 2. St Louis, Mosby, 1993, pp 1241–1276.

193. Oglivie-Harris DJ, Mahomed N, Demazire A: Anterior impingement of ankle treated by arthroscopic removal of bony spurs. *J Bone Joint Surg* 75B:437–440, 1993.

194. Stone JW, Guhl JW, Ferkel RD: Osteophytes, loose bodies and chondral lesions, in Ferkel RD (ed): *Arthroscopic Surgery—The Foot and Ankle.* Philadelphia, Lippincott-Raven, 1996, pp 145–184.

195. Spiegel TM, Spiegel JS: Rheumatoid arthritis in the foot and ankle: Diagnosis, pathology and treatment—The relationship between foot and ankle deformity and disease duration in 50 patients. *Foot Ankle* 2:318–324, 1982.

196. Keenan MA, Peabody TD, Gronley JT, et al: Valgus deformities of the feet and characteristics of gait in patients who have rheumatoid arthritis. *J Bone Joint Surg* 73A:237–247, 1991.

197. Clain MR, Baxter DE: Simultaneous calcaneocuboid and talonavicular fusion: Long term follow-up study. *J Bone Joint Surg* 76B:133–136, 1994.

198. Gold RH, Bassett LW: Radiologic evaluation of the arthritic foot. *Foot Ankle* 2:332–341, 1982.

199. Guerra J, Resnick D: Arthritides affecting the foot—Pathological correlation. *Foot Ankle* 2:325–331, 1982.

200. Thompson FA, Mann RA: Arthritides, in Mann RA, Coughlin MJ (eds): *Surgery of the Foot and Ankle,* 6th ed. Vol 1. St Louis, Mosby, 1993, pp 615–671.

201. Kitaoka HB: Rheumatoid hindfoot. *Orthop Clin North Am* 20:593–604, 1989.

202. Ljung P, Kaji J, Knutson K, et al: Talonavicular arthrodesis in the rheumatoid foot. *Foot Ankle* 13:313–316, 1992.

203. Fitzgibbons TC: Valgus tilting of ankle joint after subtalar (hindfoot) fusion: Complication or natural progression of valgus hindfoot deformity. *Orthopaedics* 19:415–423, 1996.

204. Michelson J, Easley M, Wigley FM, et al: Posterior tibial tendon dysfunction in rheumatoid arthritis. *Foot Ankle Int* 16:156–161, 1995.

205. Michelson J, Easley M, Wigley FM, et al: Foot and ankle problems in rheumatoid arthritis. *Foot Ankle* 15:608–613, 1994.

206. Meyerson MS, Quill G: Ankle arthrodesis: A comparison of an arthroscopic and an open method of treatment. *Clin Orthop Rel Res* 268:84–95, 1991.

207. Oglivie-Harris DJ, Lieberman I, Fitsialos D: Arthroscopically assisted arthrodesis for osteoarthritic ankles. *J Bone Joint Surg* 75A:1167–1174, 1993.

208. Scranton PE Jr: Use of internal compression in arthrodesis of the ankle. *J Bone Joint Surg* 67A:550–555, 1985.

209. Urquhart MW, Mont MA, Michelson JD, et al: Osteonecrosis of the talus: Treatment by hindfoot fusion. *Foot Ankle Int* 17:275–282, 1996.

210. Glick JM, Ferkel RD: Arthroscopic ankle arthrodesis, in Ferkel RD (ed): *Arthroscopic Surgery—The Foot and Ankle.* Philadelphia, Lippincott-Raven, 1996, pp 215–230.

211. Buck P, Morrey BF, Chao EYS: The optimum position of arthrodesis of the ankle: A gait study of the knee and ankle. *J Bone Joint Surg* 69A:1052–1062, 1987.

212. Kitaoka HB, Newman SR: Arthritis and deformities of the hindfoot and ankle, in Lutter D, Mizel MS, Pfeffer GB (eds): *Orthopaedic Knowledge Update—Foot and Ankle.* Rosemont, IL, American Academy of Orthopaedic Surgeons, 1994, pp 382–294.

213. Braly WG, Baker JK, Tullos HS: Arthrodesis of the ankle with lateral plating. *Foot Ankle Int* 15:649–653, 1994.

214. Moore TJ, Prince R, Pachotko D, et al: Retrograde intramedullary nailing for ankle arthrodesis. *Foot Ankle Int* 16:433–436, 1995.

215. Mann RA, Chou LB: Tibiocalcaneal arthrodesis. *Foot Ankle Int* 16:401–405, 1995.

216. Shih LY, Wu JJ, Lo WH: Changes in gait and maximum ankle torque in patients with ankle arthritis. *Foot Ankle* 14:97–103, 1993.

217. Schneider JM, Bono JV, Jacobs RL: Ankle arthrodesis—Techniques and tips. *J Orthop Tech* 2:5–7, 1994.

218. Dohm M, Purdy BA, Benjamin J: Primary union of ankle arthrodesis: Review of a single institution/multiple surgeon experience. *Foot Ankle Int* 15:293–296, 1994.

219. Dohm M, Benjamin JB, Harrison J, et al: A biomechanical evaluation of three forms of internal fixation used in ankle arthrodesis. *Foot Ankle Int* 15:297–300, 1994.

220. Friedman RL, Glisson RR, Nunley JA: A biochemical comparative analysis of two techniques of tibiotalar arthrodesis. *Foot Ankle Int* 15:301–305, 1994.

221. Frey C, Halikus NM, VuRose T, et al: A review of ankle arthrodesis: Predisposing factors to non-union. *Foot Ankle Int* 15:581–584, 1994.

222. Wynn AH, Wilde AH: Long term follow-up of the conaxial (Beck-Steffee) total ankle arthroplasty. *Foot Ankle* 13:303–306, 1992.

223. Kitaoka HB, Patzer GC, Ilstrup DM, et al: Survivorship analysis of the Mayo total ankle arthroplasty. *J Bone Joint Surg* 76A:974–979, 1994.

224. Abdo RV, Wasilewski SA: Ankle arthrodesis: A long-term study. *Foot Ankle* 13:307–312, 1992.

225. Baker PL: SACH heel improves results of ankle fusion. *J Bone Joint Surg* 52A:1485–1486, 1970.

226. Kish G, Eberhart R, King T, et al: Ankle arthrodesis placement of cannulated screws. *Foot Ankle* 14:223–224, 1993.

227. Bennett GL, Graham CE, Mauldin DM: Triple arthrodesis in adults. *Foot Ankle* 12:138–143, 1991.

228. Scranton PE Jr: Results of arthrodesis of the talus: Talocalcaneal, midtarsal and subtalar joints. *Foot Ankle* 12:156–164, 1991.

229. Casaei R, Ruggieri P, Giuseppe T, et al: Ankle resection arthrodesis in patients with bone tumors. *Foot Ankle Int* 15:242–249, 1994.

230. Lee TH, Wapner KL, Mayer DP, Hecht PJ: Computerized tomographic demonstration of the vacuum phenomenon in the subtalar and tibiotalar joints. *Foot Ankle Int* 15:382–385, 1994.

231. Smith EJ, Wood PLR: Ankle arthrodesis in the rheumatoid patient. *Foot Ankle* 10:252–256, 1990.

232. King HA, Watkins TB, Samuelson KM: Analysis of foot position in ankle arthrodesis and its influence on gait. *Foot Ankle* 1:44–49, 1980.

233. Mazur JM, Schwartz E, Simon SR: Ankle arthrodesis long term follow-up with gait analysis. *J Bone Joint Surg* 61A:964–975, 1979.

234. Paremain GD, Miller SD, Meyerson MS: Ankle arthrodesis: Results after miniarthrotomy technique. *Foot Ankle Int* 17:247–252, 1996.

235. Mann RA, VanManen JW, Wapner K, et al: Ankle fusion. *Clin Orthop Rel Res* 268:49–55, 1991.

CHAPTER 54

Miscellaneous Disorders of the Foot and Ankle

Gregory L. Hung, Stephen F. Conti,
and Steven P. Sampson

THE DIABETIC FOOT
Overview

Foot problems, particularly infections, are the major reason for hospitalization of diabetics in the United States.[1] In fact, the leading cause of nontraumatic foot amputations in the western world today is diabetes mellitus and its complications.[35] Disorders of the foot in diabetes have been attributed to the presence of two main factors: (1) peripheral neuropathy[17] and (2) ischemia resulting from large- and small-vessel atherosclerosis. There is also evidence to suggest that an impaired immune system may be present. These factors combine to cause the major foot problems that plague diabetics, namely infection, gangrene, skin ulceration, and neuropathic joint destruction (Charcot fractures).[17–20]

The diabetic foot does not function normally. Collagen is excessively cross-linked in the process of glycosylation, producing tissues that are stiffer than normal. This results in less resilient skin and ligaments, which may restrict joint motion. Bone may be osteopenic, increasing the susceptibility to acute and stress fractures. Neuropathy results in loss of sensibility and proprioception, causing problems with balance and placing the foot at increased risk for injury.[17]

Progress in the management of the diabetic foot has come about largely as a result of a multidisciplinary approach that emphasizes preventive care, patient education, and regular follow-up. Patients should be instructed in proper daily foot care, regular foot inspection, nail care, and well-fitting socks and shoes. Furthermore, diabetic management that includes strict glucose control has been shown to slow the progression of certain complications of diabetes, such as neuropathy.[2,3,18] Proper daily foot care is summarized below.

1. Wash feet daily with a mild soap and warm water. Autonomic neuropathy results in reduced sweat production in diabetics, leading to dry skin. Harsh, perfumed commercial soaps tend to dry out skin, resulting in fissuring and the possibility of infection.[23] Patients with severe neuropathy should test the bathwater with their hands or elbows or a thermometer to prevent placing their foot in extremely hot water, which can scald the skin.

2. Powder should be placed between the toes and a moisturizer over the rest of the foot to the level of the ankle joint. Alpha hydroxyl colloids may be best but are expensive. Vaseline products are very effective and inexpensive.

3. Plain cotton socks should be worn turned inside out, so the toe seams face away from the skin. For young recreational athletes, two pairs of thin cotton socks may be worn simultaneously. This allows shear forces to be dissipated between the layers of the socks rather than against the skin and may help to reduce blister formation (and consequently ulcer formation).

4. Diabetics without significant neuropathy require well-fitting shoes that accommodate all deformities. Athletic sneakers are appropriate and acceptable to most of these patients. Patients with clinically significant neuropathy must be protected in total contact inlays (TCI) and often require extra-depth footwear with rocker soles as well. The TCIs are custom-molded orthoses made of several layers of material and are designed to distribute plantar pressures evenly over the sole of the foot (Fig. 54-1).[37,41]

5. Daily inspection is mandatory.[21,22] The patient or patient's caretaker should visually inspect both feet at least three times a day. Any new blisters or ulcerations should be reported to the physician immediately. Unilateral warmth and swelling should be reported as well. This may represent cellulitis or Charcot fractures and must be dealt with urgently.

Diabetic Foot Infections

Based on clinical experience, there is little disagreement that, compared to nondiabetics, diabetics have a markedly increased risk for developing foot infections. These infections can range from cellulitis and infected superficial ulcers to deep abscesses and osteomyelitis. Decreased pain sensibility from peripheral neuropathy places the diabetic patient at greater risk for infection due to potential skin injury.[17] Skin penetration from sharp objects or ulcer formation from localized pressure is more likely with diminished protective sensation. Dry skin resulting from impaired sweating (another consequence of diabetic neuropathy) may lead to skin fissuring, creating additional portals for bacterial entry. Studies have reported the existence of impaired leukocyte function and mobility in diabetic patients,[4,5] although whether diabetic patients are truly immunologically compromised is disputed in the medical literature. The presence of poor circulation resulting from atherosclerosis further impairs tissue resistance to infection and impedes local antibiotic delivery.

For several reasons, foot infections present diagnostic challenges to the physician caring for diabetic patients. Making an accurate and timely diagnosis may be difficult. Because the signs of infection—such as pain, swelling, and erythema—may be subtle or even unrecognized by patients, there can be a delay in seeking treatment. Patients, particularly those with advanced neuropathy, may present only with complaints of acute swelling of the foot. Deep infections resulting from local extension through injured skin are far more common than deep infections arising from hematogenous seeding. Consequently, a thorough search for penetrating injuries or ulcers should be made whenever deep infections are suspected.

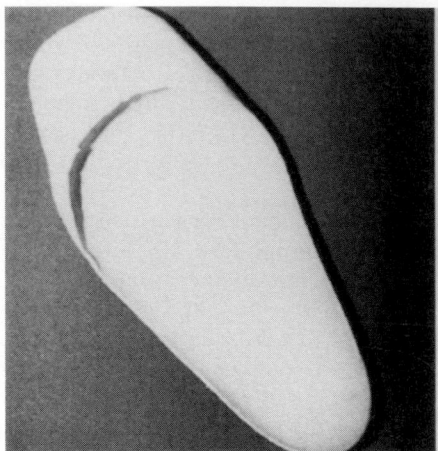 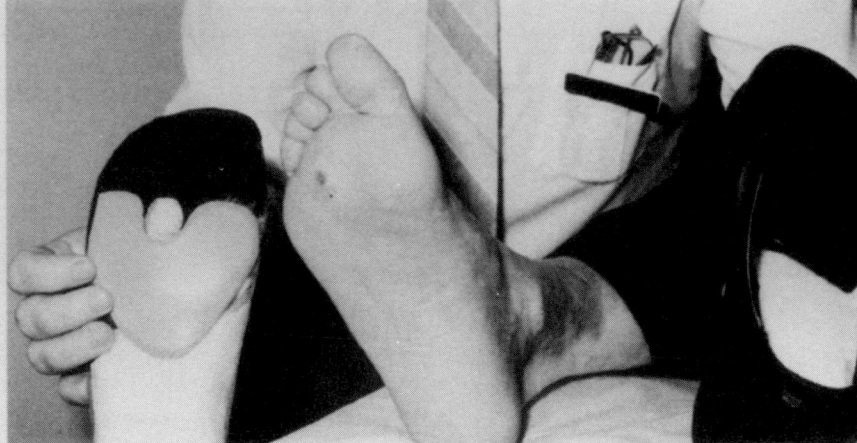

Figure 54-1 Total contact orthoses. *Left:* Toe filler. *Right:* Total contact insole constructed of multiple layers of selected density materials for third metatarsal head ulcer. [Reproduced with permission from McDermott JE (ed): *The Diabetic Foot.* Rosemont, IL, American Association of Orthopaedic Surgeons, 1995, p 21.]

A thorough physical examination includes close inspection of the area between the toes for skin breakdown and the plantar surfaces for evidence of penetrating wounds. Laboratory analysis should always be completed, keeping in mind that in diabetics, leukocytosis may be absent in the face of infection.[6] Superficial wound cultures are often misleading and should be avoided. Plain films should include three views of the foot and be examined for evidence of a foreign body or osteomyelitis. Radiographic abnormalities are often nonspecific and may mimic changes present in neuroarthropathy. CT scans with soft tissue windows and MRI are particularly helpful in localizing abscess cavities and delineating the patterns of loculations. It is not unusual to note extension of the infection to sites distant from a main cavity.

Mild cellulitis may be treated with outpatient oral antibiotics. Diabetic foot infections are frequently polymicrobial; therefore most antibiotic regimens are selected to cover a wide spectrum of aerobic and anaerobic organisms. Combination antibiotic therapy is often indicated to provide this broad coverage. An example of this is the use of clindamycin and ciprofloxacin. Clindamycin offers excellent coverage of gram-positive and anaerobic bacteria, while ciprofloxacin provides complementary coverage of many gram-negative organisms and most *Pseudomonas* species.

Determination of whether an infection is present in a superficial ulcer is often confusing. Obtaining cultures of the uncomplicated superficial ulcer is usually not necessary and only adds to the confusion. The diagnosis of infection in this setting is based on clinical evaluation of the quality and quantity of drainage, the status of the surrounding soft tissues, and laboratory tests. More severe cellulitis or infected superficial ulcers should be treated with hospitalization and a course of intravenous antibiotics followed by oral antibiotics administered on an outpatient basis provided that there is demonstration of response to treatment and no coexistent vascular compromise. The patient's ability to comply with limb elevation and local wound care should be considered.

Chronic nonhealing plantar foot ulcers are a common problem in diabetics and are frequently associated with osteomyelitis. The size and depth of a wound is correlated with the likelihood of underlying osteomyelitis. It has been suggested that an ulcer with a diameter of more than 2 cm has a 94 percent chance of associated osteomyelitis, and an ulcer in which bone is exposed is associated with a 100 percent risk of osteomyelitis.[7] Differentiating osteomyelitis from neuroarthropathic joint destruction may be difficult on plain films and CT, because both conditions may exhibit features of osteopenia, bone destruction, and fragmentation. Bone scintigraphy with technetium-99m (^{99m}Tc) isotopes is very sensitive in identifying areas of increased bone turnover suspicious for osteomyelitis, but it is not specific. It is not possible to differentiate osteomyelitis from fracture or Charcot neuroarthropathy on bone scan. Indium-111 (^{111}In)-labeled leukocyte scanning may be performed in conjunction with bone scanning to increase the specificity for infection.[24,27] MRI has been studied in assessing osteomyelitis, but it too has poor specificity (81 percent) in spite of excellent sensitivity (99 percent).[8,25,26]

When the clinical, laboratory, and radiographic picture suggests the presence of a deep abscess or osteomyelitis, initial treatment should include thorough irrigation and debridement of all necrotic tissue in conjunction with administration of intravenous antibiotics selected on the basis of deep wound cultures. Deep wound cultures are most reliable when obtained through an area of uninvolved skin. Guidelines for the duration of intravenous antibiotic therapy are empirical. Intravenous antibiotics are usually administered for 6 weeks for the treatment of osteomyelitis, although this should be tailored to each individual case.

The role of hyperbaric oxygen therapy in the treatment of diabetic foot infections is unclear. Infection and ischemia are frequently observed in the same foot, making it difficult to assign importance to the roles each plays in the development of gangrene. The increased metabolic requirements necessary to combat infections can lead to gangrene when there is a tenuous baseline circulation. Diabetics frequently have associated atherosclerotic coronary and peripheral vascular disease and consequently have limited capacity to increase blood flow to areas of increased metabolic demand. Neuropathy may result in arteriovenous shunting, further impairing tissue oxygenation.

Amputations

Diabetic peripheral vascular disease accounts for approximately 60 percent of amputations performed in the western world.[9] Amputations of the lower extremity in diabetics are usually performed to remove gangrene and for control of infection. Because of their frequent coexistence, the extent of infection and circulatory compromise must both be assessed preoperatively. The metabolic cost of walking is generally decreased with more distal-level amputations, but the level of amputation should not be selected solely to preserve length without consideration for prompt healing and recovery. The patient's overall health and nutritional status should be evaluated and optimized.[38] Clinical laboratory parameters thought to be necessary for wound healing include a serum albumin level greater than 3.5 g/dL and a total lymphocyte count greater than 1500/mm^3. Total lymphocyte count is calculated by multiplying the white blood cell count (WBC) by the percentage of lymphocytes in the differential.[39] The functional requirements of the patient and activity level should be ascertained. Ultimately, the potential for healing of any amputation depends on the vascular status of the limb, and it may be necessary to obtain a vascular consultation to diminish the amount of tissue removed.

A variety of tests are available to assess the circulation of a limb. These include the ankle-brachial index (ABI), Doppler toe pressures, and transcutaneous oxygen partial pressure (TCPO$_2$).[28–31] The ABI is useful for determining whether a below-knee amputation (BKA) is appropriate but frequently is artificially elevated in the presence of vessel cacification in the lower limbs. An ABI of 0.45 is often quoted as the minimum ratio necessary for healing wounds in diabetics, in contrast to 0.35 in nondiabetics. Low ABIs are indicative of circulatory insufficiency, while normal or elevated indices do not ensure adequate circulation for the reason mentioned above. Since diabetics may have vessel disease distal to the ankle, it is useful to obtain toe pressures. Toe systolic blood pressures of 55 mmHg with pulsatile flow indicated by phasic waveforms are compatible with healing and are useful in predicting healing of transmetatarsal amputations. However, TCPO$_2$ has been found to be the most accurate measurement for predicting wound healing and determining appropriate amputation levels.[10] Normal TCPO$_2$ values fall between 60 and 90 mmHg. Wound healing is less likely with TCPO$_2$ values less than 30, and it is often delayed when less than 40.

A successful amputation depends on the ability to control local infection and ischemia. All necrotic tissues in the gangrenous foot should be aggressively debrided to prevent extension into adjacent normal tissues. It may not be desirable to close an infected wound primarily. Additional smaller, secondary debridements with delayed primary closure may be necessary. All tissues should be handled gently, with care taken to avoid traumatizing skin edges with forceps or overzealous retraction. Wound edges should be closed without tension, using nonabsorbable monofilament suture through skin only, without a separate subcutaneous closure. If a tension-free closure is not possible, split-thickness skin grafts may be fashioned from the amputated part to cover the wound provided that these grafts are not placed on plantar or distal surfaces. Broad-spectrum perioperative antibiotics should be utilized and appropriately adjusted as deep wound cultures and sensitivities become available. There are no absolute guidelines for the duration of postoperative antibiotics, but generally intravenous antibiotics are continued for 10 days, followed by oral antibiotics until the wounds have healed. Drains should routinely be used to evacuate any hematoma. A closed continuous irrigation drain may be fashioned from a Foley catheter and a normal saline infusion used to irrigate the wound out between the sutures.[11]

Amputation of part of a toe is planned around the available soft tissue coverage. Nonviable skin is excised along with infected bone. It is desirable, whenever possible, to leave the base of the proximal phalanx to act as a spacer between the adjacent toes, preventing the toes from migrating into the defect created by excision of an entire toe. When complete amputation of one or more toes is being performed, the ideal level of amputation should be just proximal to the metatarsal neck. A racquet-shaped skin incision is often used, with sufficient skin maintained to perform a tension-free closure. The fifth toe is ideally resected at a slightly more proximal level to avoid a lateral prominence. A single toe should not be left between two amputated toes.

The transmetatarsal amputation is a well-accepted procedure with a high success rate. Patients can learn to ambulate well without the need for bracing. No special shoe modifications are necessary; however, many patients benefit from an extended steel shank added to the sole of the shoe to resist bending of the shoe at the end of the foot during push-off.[32] Toe fillers allow use of a regular shoe.

Lisfranc (tarsometatarsal) and Chopart (midtarsal) amputations have been described in the midfoot but have been unpopular because of the high failure rate from the late development of equinus deformities due to the detachment of the tibialis anterior tendon during the excision of the base of the first metatarsal. However, when the procedure is properly performed, this complication can reliably be avoided. Combining these surgeries with transection of the Achilles tendon and transfer of the tibialis anterior tendon into a drill hole in the talar neck with postoperative bracing minimizes the problem of equinus deformities. Varus deformities can be avoided in Lisfranc amputations by balancing the pull of the posterior tibial tendon with the peroneus brevis. It is useful to leave the fifth metatarsal base to preserve the peroneus brevis insertion. The advantage of these amputations over a Symes (ankle-level) disarticulation is that the retained length permits use of a shoe with a filler instead of a prosthesis.

The Boyd-Pirogoff amputation is a hindfoot amputation in which the heel pad is preserved together with a portion of the osteotomized calcaneus, which is rotated up and apposed to the osteotomized tibial plafond. Internal fixation is required to maintain this bony apposition until union has occurred. This amputation has been particularly useful in the pediatric population, where posterior heel pad migration has been observed with Symes amputations, but is rarely used in the elderly diabetic population because of the greater time required for healing and resumption of weight bearing. In this population, its utility lies mainly in the salvage of a Chopart amputation when there is insufficient skin for closure.

The Symes ankle disarticulation has several advantages over a long BKA.[33,34] Rehabilitation and prosthetic wear is easier with a longer stump. It is possible to ambulate short distances without a prosthesis in emergency situations. This amputation may be performed in two stages, if necessary, when there is extensive infection of the midfoot. In this operation, the calcaneus is shelled out in a subperiosteal fashion to preserve the attachments of the fibrous septa of the heel pad, the Achilles tendon is divided, and the malleoli are osteotomized flush with the plafond and narrowed. The anterior flap of the heel pad is sutured to the anterior tibia through drill holes.

Postoperative care following any amputation should initially include bed rest with limb elevation. Local dressing changes are necessary for open wounds. Otherwise, the limb should be protected and elevated in a non-weight-bearing cast to control edema and hemorrhage and provide soft tissue immobilization. The cast is changed after 4 to 7 days to permit inspection of the wound, and weight bearing is initiated at 3 to 4 weeks. Sutures are left in place until weight bearing because of the delayed healing of diabetic wounds. Casting is relatively contraindicated in the severely ischemic limb, because use of a circumferential dressing may lead to gangrene.

Neuropathic Ulcer

Ulcer formation is an common problem in the diabetic foot and is thought to be primarily related to the presence of a sensory neuropathy associated with focal cutaneous pressure. In the diabetic foot, the plantar aspect of any bone prominence is at high risk for ulceration—e.g., the metatarsal heads secondary to claw-toe formation and the naviculocuneiform region secondary to Lisfranc-Charcot neuroarthropathy. The mapping and documentation of sensory threshold testing along the plantar surface of the foot using Semmes-Weinstein (S/W) monofilaments clearly aids in distinguishing the neuropathic foot at risk for ulceration. Diabetic patients who are unable to quantitatively detect a 5.07 S/W monofilament on the plantar foot surface are at high risk and therefore fail to demonstrate adequate levels of protective sensation. Skin erythema and blister formation are clearly early clinical signs for imminent ulceration. Subcutaneous cavitation may occur beneath hard callosities under shear conditions. By the time skin ulceration is initially noted, these "malperforans ulcers" may rapidly enlarge. It is important to realize that foot ischemia is not as much an issue in causation of the ulcer as in the potential for its healing.[12]

Wagner devised a classification scheme that divides ulcers into five stages based on their depth and the presence of infection or gangrene[39] (Table 54-1). This has been useful as a treatment guideline. Footwear modifications alone are usually successful in treating stage 0 (pressure area at risk for ulceration). The objectives of pedorthotic management include the even distribution of plantar pressures, particularly beneath the metatarsal heads; reduction of shear; accommodation of deformities; and provision of cushioning. Ideal shoewear should accommodate

TABLE 54-1 Wagner Classification and Recommended Management

Stage	Classification	Recommendations
0	Pressure area on foot aggravated by footwear	Footwear modification
I	Open but superficial ulceration	Local treatment Footwear modification
II	Full-thickness ulceration	Occlusive cast Footwear modification
III	Full-thickness ulceration with secondary infection	Debridement Antibiotics
IV	Infected area with local gangrene	Antibiotics Local amputation Hyperbaric O$_2$
V	Ulceration with extensive gangrene, foot and leg	Regional amputation Antibiotics Rehabilitation

Source: Reproduced with permission from McDermott JE (ed): *The Diabetic Foot.* Rosemont, IL, American Association of Orthopaedic Surgeons, 1995, p 18.

deformities such as hammertoes or claw toes with features such as an extra-depth toe box.[41] A blucher opening will permit easier entry into the shoe. A total contact insert is a custom orthosis made to fit the exact contours of an individual's foot and is useful for distributing plantar pressures evenly and reducing weight bearing in problematic areas. External shoe modifications commonly used for the diabetic foot include the rocker sole in conjunction with an extended steel shank, cushioned heel, and medial or lateral wedges, stabilizers, or flares.

Stage I or II ulcers in which there is superficial or full-thickness ulceration usually require initial treatment with total-contact casts to achieve healing followed by appropriate footwear to prevent recurrence. Ulcer debridement at the time of cast changes should be performed to facilitate healing. Careful debridement of the necrotic skin edges, calluses, eschars, or hypertrophic granulation tissue will facilitate ingrowth of the skin edges. Certain stage II ulcers may require wound care consisting of operative debridement, whirlpool treatments, and dressing changes to convert them to ulcers with clean granulation beds prior to total-contact casting.[15,36] Full-thickness ulcers with secondary infection and exposed bone (stage III) require treatment with more formal debridements and antibiotics.

Exposed bone is considered infected and resection may be required.[40,42] Local gangrene (stage IV) or extensive gangrene (stage V) may lead to amputations. Hyperbaric oxygen has been used in the treatment of stage IV ulcers.

Another classification scheme to describe neuropathic ulcers has been described by Brodsky.[12] The depth/ischemia index grades ulcers separately by their depth and the vascular status of the foot (Table 54-2). The advantage of the Wagner classification lies in its simplicity and wide use in clinical practice; however, its limitation lies in its suggestion of a continuum between the depth of an ulcer and the presence of gangrene. The depth/ischemia system more clearly distinguishes these two components in separately assessing the size of the ulcer and the circulation to the foot. This leads to a more accurate assessment and appropriate treatment of the diabetic ulcer.

Neuroarthropathy

Neuroarthropathy (neuropathic joint disease or Charcot fracture) is a chronic but accelerated form of degenerative arthropathy that is thought to be related to decreased sensory innervation of the involved joints.[44] Loss of proprio-

---

TABLE 54-2 The "Depth Ischemia" Classification of Diabetic Foot Lesions

Grade	Definition	Treatment
Depth classification		
0	The "at risk" foot; previous ulcer or neuropathy with deformity that may cause new ulceration	Patient education Regular examination Appropriate shoe wear and insoles
1	Superficial ulceration, not infected	External pressure relief: total contact cast, walking brace, special shoe wear, etc.
2	Deep ulceration exposing tendon or joint (with/without superficial infection)	Surgical debridement → wound care → pressure relief if closes and converts to grade 1 (PRN antibiotics)
3	Extensive ulceration with exposed bone and/or deep infection: i.e., osteomyelitis or abscess	Surgical debridements → ray or partial foot amputation → IV antibiotics → pressure relief if wound converts to grade 1
Ischemia classification		
A	Not ischemic	Adequate vascularity for healing
B	Ischemia without gangrene	Vascular evaluation (Doppler, TCPO$_2$, arteriogram, etc) → vascular reconstruction PRN
C	Partial (forefoot) gangrene of foot	Vascular evaluation → vascular reconstruction (proximal and/or distal bypass or angioplasty) → partial foot amputation
D	Complete foot gangrene	Vascular evaluation → major extremity amputation (BKA, AKA) with possible proximal vascular reconstruction

Source: Reproduced with permission from Brodsky JW: The diabetic foot, in Mann RA, Coughlin MJ (eds): *Surgery of the Foot and Ankle,* 6th ed. St Louis, Mosby, 1993, pp 1361–1367.

ceptive and nociceptive reflexes leads to repeated trauma to the involved joints. With the increased survival of diabetics and the development of effective treatments for syphilis, diabetic neuropathy has surpassed tabes dorsalis as the major etiologic factor for neuroarthropathy.[13] Other etiologies include peripheral neuropathies from other causes (i.e., alcoholism), syringomyelia, and congenital indifference to pain.

Three stages in the natural history of Charcot joints have been described by Eichenholtz.[14,52] Stage I, or the fragmentation stage, is characterized by acute inflammation with the presence of painless swelling, erythema, and warmth. Bony fragmentation and articular destruction may occur in this initial phase. These findings are commonly indistinguishable from infection. In stage II, there is less swelling and warmth, with x-rays demonstrating evidence of periosteal new bone formation and rounding of fractured bone ends. Stage III, or the consolidation phase, reveals a foot with no warmth or swelling and radiographs showing complete bone healing and resolution of osteopenia. A misdiagnosis of infection can lead to inappropriate treatment with antibiotics. The patient with infection will often present with fever, elevated WBC with a left shift, and erythema that does not reduce in intensity with elevation of the foot. The erythema from a Charcot process will significantly reduce if the foot is elevated above heart level for 10 min. Bone scans and ^{111}In-labeled WBC scans may be helpful adjuncts to clinical diagnosis. The clinical acumen of the treating physician, however, is as important as laboratory and radiologic tests in differentiating infection from the Charcot process.

The treatment of neuroarthropathy is primarily nonsurgical, with the goals being attainment of a stable, plantigrade foot that is shoeable and suitable for weight bearing.[47,49,52,53,56,57] Treatment begins with non-weight-bearing immobilization in a total-contact cast until active neuroarthropathy is under control, followed by protected weight bearing. The total-contact cast is useful for protected weight bearing during the subacute stage of bony consolidation and healing.[15] Casting may be discontinued when there is no perceptible temperature difference between the affected and unaffected feet and swelling is significantly reduced. This can take several months to a year. Forefoot and midfoot Charcot with deformity leads to ulceration,[49,53] while hindfoot and ankle Charcot is associated with severe instability.[47] Footwear modifications can accommodate most forefoot and midfoot deformities. Severe midfoot deformities and all hindfoot and ankle deformities require long-term bracing.[51]

Reconstructive procedures including open reduction and arthrodesis have been utilized in treatment of ankle or hindfoot instability not amenable to bracing, but they can be associated with complications.[16,43,45–50,55] Recurrent midfoot ulcers can be managed with surgical reconstruction with good results. Late rigid deformities may be reconstructed with various operations, including ostectomy to prevent the recurrent plantar ulceration associated with midfoot collapse. Amputation is reserved as an option for gangrene or uncontrolled infections.

The indications for closed versus operative treatment of acute fractures in patients with diabetic neuropathy are similar to those present in the normal population. The rec-ommended period of non–weight bearing and cast immobilization, however, is prolonged in diabetics. As a general rule, casting should be continued twice as long as for a nondiabetic with a similar fracture.[43,45,54,56]

HALLUX VALGUS

Normal and Pathologic Anatomy

Hallux valgus is a disorder in which a prominent eminence (bunion) is present on the medial aspect of the first metatarsal head with lateral deviation of the proximal phalanx. Accompanying the disorder, there is frequently medial deviation of the first metatarsal (metatarsus primus varus), subluxation of the sesamoids, and pronation of the great toe. The exact cause of hallux valgus is still unclear, but certain associations have been made. Particularly among women, fashionable footwear has been implicated as a cause of bunions in Western societies. Confining toe boxes and increased heel height seem to predispose to the development of hallux valgus, as evidenced by the nine-to-one greater prevalence in females versus males.[58] Hallux valgus is rare among unshod populations. Heredity, however, seems to play a role, in that features intrinsic to the first ray may predispose susceptible patients to the deforming forces of footwear. These include hypermobility of the first metatarsocuneiform (MC) joint, metatarsus primus varus, a medially slanted first MC joint, atypical first metatarsal length,[74] a rounded first MTP joint, and hyperpronation of the first ray.[59]

Stability of the first metatarsophalangeal (MTP) joint is maintained by a combination of static and dynamic stabilizers[60–62] (Figs. 54-2, 54-3, and 54-4). The strong capsuloligamentous sling of the first MTP joint and the bony shape of the first MTP and MC joints form the key static stabilizers, providing a good compromise between stability and suitability for weight transfer on one hand and motion on the other. Medial and lateral stability of the first MTP joint is provided by the collateral ligaments, located from the metatarsal head to the proximal phalangeal base. Also contributing to stability are the sesamoid ligaments, which connect the metatarsal head to the sesamoids, and the hood ligament, which stabilizes the extensor tendons dorsally. Plantarly, the sesamoids, which are located in the split tendon of the flexor hallucis brevis, are stabilized by the bony configuration of their articulation with the undersurface of the metatarsal head and by the intersesamoidal ligament, the plantar plate, and the transverse metatarsal ligament. Further medial and lateral stability is thought to be provided by the shape of the opposing MTP joint surfaces, with flat surfaces being more inherently stable than round surfaces. Dynamic stabilizers include the abductor hallucis, whose tendinous insertion blends with the medial slip of the flexor hallucis brevis to insert medially on the proximal phalangeal base, and the two heads of the adductor hallucis (transverse and oblique) whose tendinous insertions blend with the lateral slip of the flexor hallucis brevis to insert on the lateral proximal phalangeal base as the conjoined tendon.

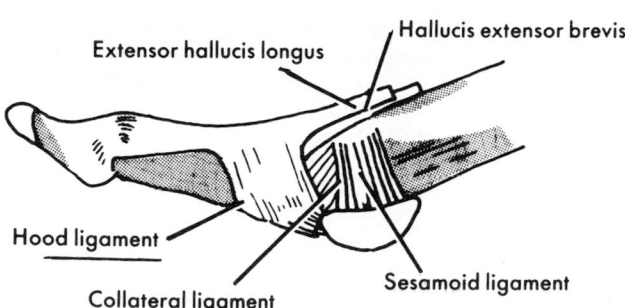

Figure 54-2 Collateral ligament structure and extensor mechanism about the first MTP joint. [Reproduced with permission from Mann RA, Coughlin MJ: Adult hallux valgus, in Mann RA, Coughlin MJ (eds): *Surgery of the Foot and Ankle,* 6th ed. St Louis, Mosby, 1993, pp 167–296.]

In hallux valgus deformity, there is a disruption of the intricate balance previously described. The metatarsal head migrates medially, resulting in metatarsus primus varus, while the proximal phalanx becomes laterally deviated and eventually displaced. The medial capsule and supporting structures become attenuated, and the lateral structures contract. With progressive deformity, the sesamoids may become laterally positioned relative to the first metatarsal head, since they remain attached to the second metatarsal through the intermetatarsal ligament. The sesamoids typically remain with the proximal phalanx and may flatten the crista as they subluxate lateral to the medially displaced metatarsal head. The hallux may become pronated, with the abductor hallucis coming to lie in a more plantar position, where it is less effective in preventing further lateral deviation of the proximal phalanx. The laterally deviated proximal phalanx may push the metatarsal head medially, further accentuating the deformity. The key to understanding hallux valgus is to appreciate that there are both static and dynamic deformities occurring simultaneously in a given patient.

Juvenile hallux valgus occurs in children and adolescents, mostly female, and is notable for larger hallux valgus angles and smaller intermetatarsal angles than the adult counterpart. This is a condition in which heredity predominates over shoewear in etiological significance. Often the first MTP joint is more congruent and the medial eminence less prominent than in adults. Careful assessment of the congruence of the first MTP joint must be made in cases of suspected juvenile hallux valgus, since the distal metatarsal articular angle may be large, giving the false initial impression that the joint is incongruent. Hypermobility of the first metatarsocuneiform joint may be present. Inconsistent results have been reported after surgical correction of juvenile hallux valgus deformities. The recurrence rate is high and

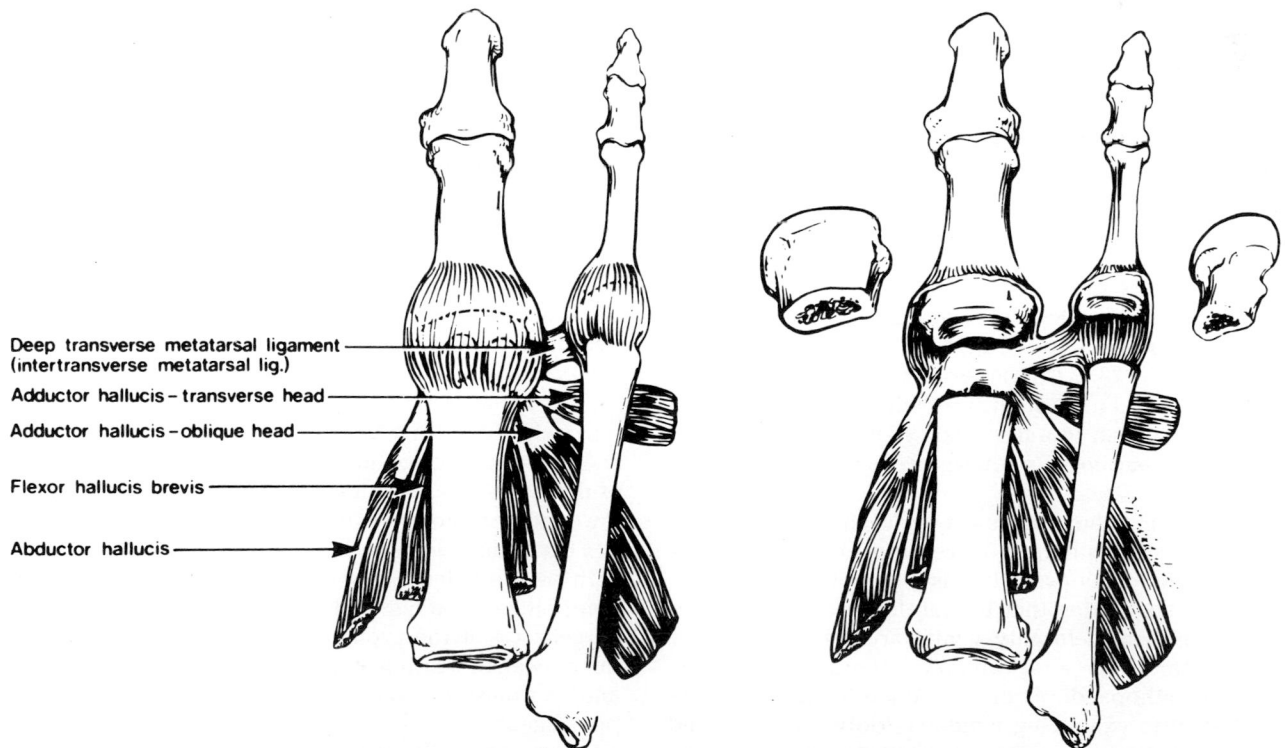

Deep transverse metatarsal ligament
(intertransverse metatarsal lig.)

Adductor hallucis – transverse head

Adductor hallucis – oblique head

Flexor hallucis brevis

Abductor hallucis

Figure 54-3 *Left:* Anatomy of the normal first MTP joint. Note the relationship of the deep transverse metatarsal ligament and the conjoined tendon of the adductor hallucis and lateral head of the flexor hallucis brevis. *Right:* Metatarsal heads removed to improve view. [Adapted from Pedowitz WJ: Deformities of the first ray, in Lutter LD, Mizel MS, Pfeffer GB (eds): *Orthopaedic Knowledge Update: Foot and Ankle.* Rosemont, IL, American Association of Orthopaedic Surgeons, 1994, pp 141–162.]

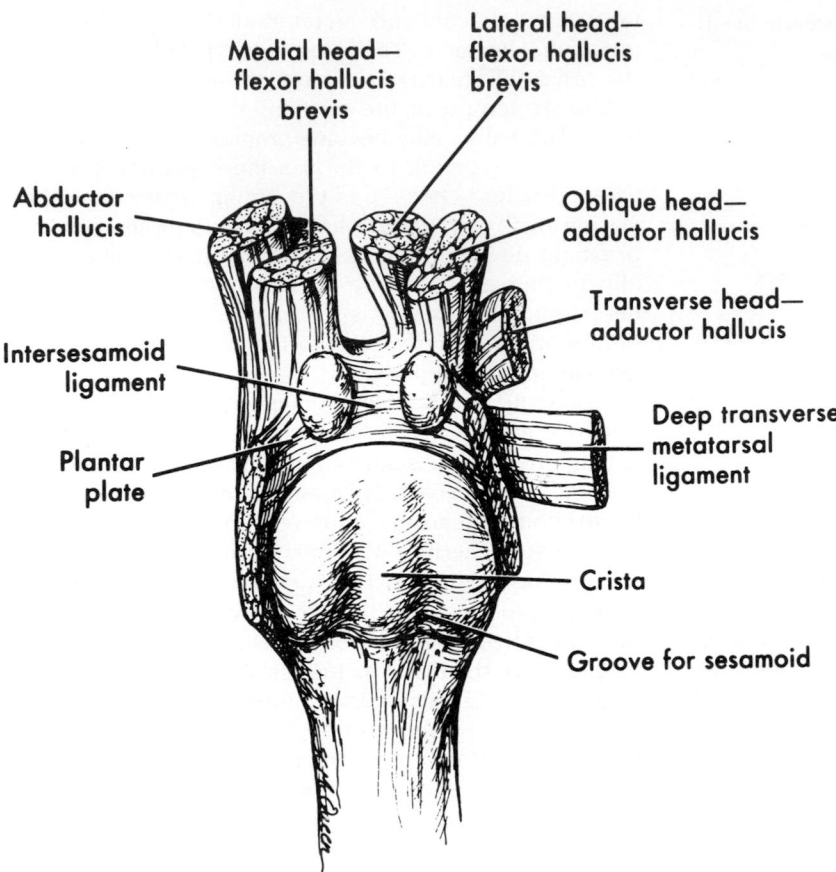

Medial head—
flexor hallucis
brevis

Lateral head—
flexor hallucis
brevis

Abductor
hallucis

Oblique head—
adductor hallucis

Transverse head—
adductor hallucis

Intersesamoid
ligament

Deep transverse
metatarsal
ligament

Plantar
plate

Crista

Groove for sesamoid

Figure 54-4 Plantar surface of the first metatarsal head. [Reproduced with permission from Richardson ER: Disorders of the hallux, in Crenshaw AH (ed): *Campbell's Operative Orthopaedics,* 8th ed. Vol 4. St Louis, Mosby, 1992, pp 2615–2692.]

surgery should be delayed until skeletal maturity in all but the most unusual cases.[72,73] Perhaps the most significant challenge facing the orthopaedist evaluating a patient with bunions is recognizing the juvenile bunion. Although the onset of deformities begins in childhood or adolescence, it is not unusual for patients to first seek treatment in their late twenties or thirties. In one group of adult patients evaluated for hallux valgus deformity, over 50 percent recalled onset in their adolescent years while only 5 percent stated that their bunions appeared after the age of 20.[63] Characteristic findings on history, physical exam, and radiographs will occasionally lead the astute clinician to a diagnosis of juvenile hallux valgus even in patients in their late second and third decades.

Adult-onset hallux valgus may be seen in patients with a genetic predisposition; however, the predominant risk factor is confining footwear. In this group of patients, there is evidence suggesting that lateral deviation of the great toe is the primary deformity, while varus deformity of the first metatarsal is a secondary phenomenon.[64] The American Orthopaedic Foot and Ankle Society has conducted studies examining women's footwear and found that the majority of American women wear shoes that are too narrow, supporting the role of footwear in the development of the much higher prevalence of hallux valgus among women.

Evaluation and Initial Treatment

The patient with symptomatic hallux valgus complains of pain over the medial eminence while wearing shoes, which usually is relieved when the patient is barefoot. This is in contrast to the patient with degenerative arthritis of the first MTP joint, who has pain while bearing weight with or without shoewear. In more advanced cases of hallux valgus, however, the patient may complain of discomfort under the first metatarsal head while walking barefoot as well.

Examination of the patient should occur with and without weight bearing. Overall lower extremity alignment should be noted, particularly coronal plane malalignment of the knees. It is also important to note any deformity of the hindfoot and great toe while the patient is standing. Pes cavus and pes planus are significant findings. Patients with severe valgus knee deformities or planovalgus foot deformities are at high risk for recurrence following bunion surgery. Great toe pronation is usually appreciated only during weight bearing; it is also a risk factor for recurrence and can mask the radiologic appearance of hallux interphalangeus.

Hypermobility of the first metatarsal in the sagittal plane is a significant finding, particularly in association with pes planus. The stability of the first MC joint can be assessed by holding the first MTP joint in one hand and the second MTP joint in the other, comparing the amount of dorsomedial and plantar lateral displacement of the first MTP joint relative to the contralateral foot. Whether hypermobility of the first MC joint can be reproducibly measured by this or any other technique, however, is debatable. The term *hypermobility* should be reserved for cases in which the intermetatarsal angle is greater than 15°, a callus is present beneath the second metatarsal head, and increased sagittal plane motion of the first metatarsal is appreciated on physical exam.

The first MTP joint should be carefully assessed. Proximal phalangeal dorsiflexion of 70 to 90° relative to the metatarsal shaft is usually possible. Loss of motion or pain with range of motion is characteristic of degenerative arthritis.[115,116] Testing of the MTP joint is often performed following reduction of the hallux valgus and metatarsus primus varus deformities. The examiner should compress the first and second metatarsals together and reduce the great toe prior to testing MTP motion. A significant loss of motion occurs in large deformities and serves as a predictor of postoperative motion. Any crepitus in the MTP joint or the metatarsosesamoid joints might indicate arthrosis not yet appreciable on radiographs. Finally, the clinician should assess for the presence of hallux valgus interphalangeus, which is seen as a lateral deviation of the distal aspect of the great toe.

Radiographs of the feet should always be taken in the weight-bearing position. The key measurements of angular deformity[65] are obtained from the anteroposterior (AP) film and include the hallux valgus (HV), intermetatarsal (IM), and hallux interphalangeus angles. These angles are formed by lines that bisect the shafts of the appropriate metatarsals or phalanges (Fig. 54-5). The normal hallux valgus angle is up to 15° and the normal intermetatarsal angle is up to 9°. Small variations in the angle of the x-ray tube, however, can produce great variations in the intermetatarsal angle. The distal metatarsal articular (DMA) angle is frequently increased when a hallux valgus deformity exists with a congruent first MTP joint.[75,76] This angle is defined by a line transversely connecting the proximal edges of the distal metatarsal articular surface and a second line bisecting the metatarsal shaft. There is normally less than 10° of lateral deviation of the distal articular surface of the first metatarsal. The first MTP joint should be assessed radiographically for incongruence, sesamoid subluxation, and the presence of degenerative arthritis. A simulated weight-bearing view of the metatarsal head should be obtained in most cases. An axial view will demonstrate the alignment of the sesamoids under the metatarsal head and aid in the assessment of metatarsosesamoid arthritis.

The initial treatment of hallux valgus is nonoperative and primarily involves modification of footwear to accommodate the deformity. Use of shoes with flexible soles and wide toe boxes made of soft, seamless leather may be helpful. High heels should be avoided. Surgery is indicated with the failure of conservative measures to relieve pain, although radiographic evidence of progression of deformity is arguably a relative indication for surgery.

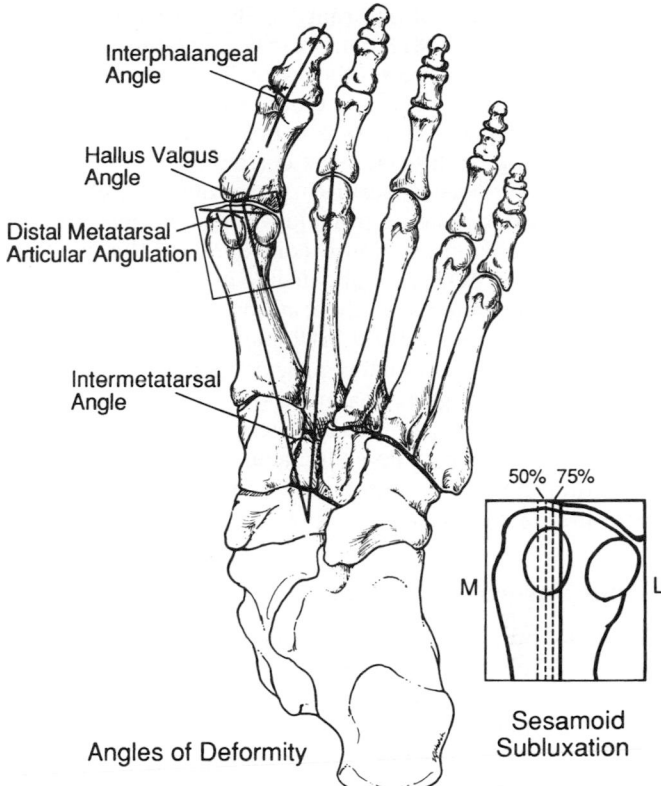

Figure 54-5 Angles of deformity in hallux valgus and assessment of sesamoid subluxation. The tibial sesamoid is considered medial if 75 percent of its width is medial to the central line; lateral, if 75 percent is lateral to the central line. Otherwise, the sesamoid is considered to be centrally located. [Reproduced with permission from Pedowitz W: Bunion deformity, in Pfeffer G, Frey C (eds): *Current Practice in Foot and Ankle Surgery*. New York, McGraw-Hill, 1993, pp 219–242.]

Review of Surgical Procedures

Over 100 procedures have been described for the surgical treatment of hallux valgus, serving as testimony to the variety of presentations of hallux valgus deformity and the care that must be taken in characterizing it and selecting procedures when surgery is contemplated. The goal of any operation should be, foremost, to relieve pain and to produce a shoeable, plantigrade foot. Correction of all elements of the deformity while maintaining motion of the MTP joint is desirable. There are certain situations that are relative contraindications to surgery.[59,65] Spasticity, equinus contracture, gross ligamentous laxity as with Marfan syndrome or Ehler-Danlos syndrome, vascular insufficiency, metatarsus adductus, short first metatarsal, or neurosis are such situations.

Potential complications of surgery are numerous and should always be discussed with the patient. Soft tissue complications such as infection, delayed wound healing, skin slough, adherent scar, or paresthesias of the toe may occur. Shortening, dorsiflexion, plantarflexion, or nonunion of the first metatarsal can occur as well. Inadequate correction, recurrence of deformity, hallux varus deformity, incongruence of the MTP joint, transfer metatarsalgia, and failure to relieve pain are other complications associated with surgery. Many of these complications are minimized if proper preoperative assessment is performed with a thoughtful approach to surgical correction. An algorithm has previously been described that outlines an effective decision-making scheme in hallux valgus surgery[62] (Fig. 54-6). This scheme takes into consideration the congruence of the first MTP joint, the degree of hallux valgus and metatarsus primus varus deformities, whether a hypermobile first MC joint or first MTP joint arthritis is present, and the age and functional requirements of the patient. In spite of proper surgical treatment, there is a tendency for deformities to recur in certain circumstances. These include the presence of juvenile hallux valgus, severe foot pronation deformity, metatarsus adductus, and long or short first metatarsals.

Distal Chevron Osteotomy

The distal Chevron osteotomy is most useful for patients with congruent MTP joints or those with incongruent joints in which the hallux valgus deformity is mild (IM angle <15°; HV angle <30°) and there is no sesamoid subluxation or toe pronation[77,78] (Figs. 54-7 and 54-8). This allows correction of the intermetatarsal angle to less than 10°, which correlates with a good functional result. It is performed by resecting the medial eminence, creating a transverse "V" osteotomy through the metatarsal neck in the coronal plane, and laterally displacing the first metatarsal head. The V osteotomy is typically made with the apex 1 cm proximal to the articular surface of the metatarsal head. The angle of the V should measure 50 to 60° and is fashioned with a longer plantar limb to avoid entering the metatarsosesamoid articulation.[82] Approximately 1° of IM angle correction can be expected with each millimeter of lateral displacement of the capital fragment. The transverse width of the first metatarsal at the level of the osteotomy is approximately 15 mm and the head is displaced about one-third of this distance. Thus, 4 to 5° of IM angle correction can usually be expected.[117] Following manual impaction of the displaced head, fixation can be enhanced with K wires or screws. The medial capsule is then imbricated in a slightly overcorrected fashion to ensure centralization of the sesamoids. If the distal Chevron osteotomy is performed in a patient with a distal metatarsal articular angle greater than 15°, the procedure can be modified by resecting a medial closing wedge

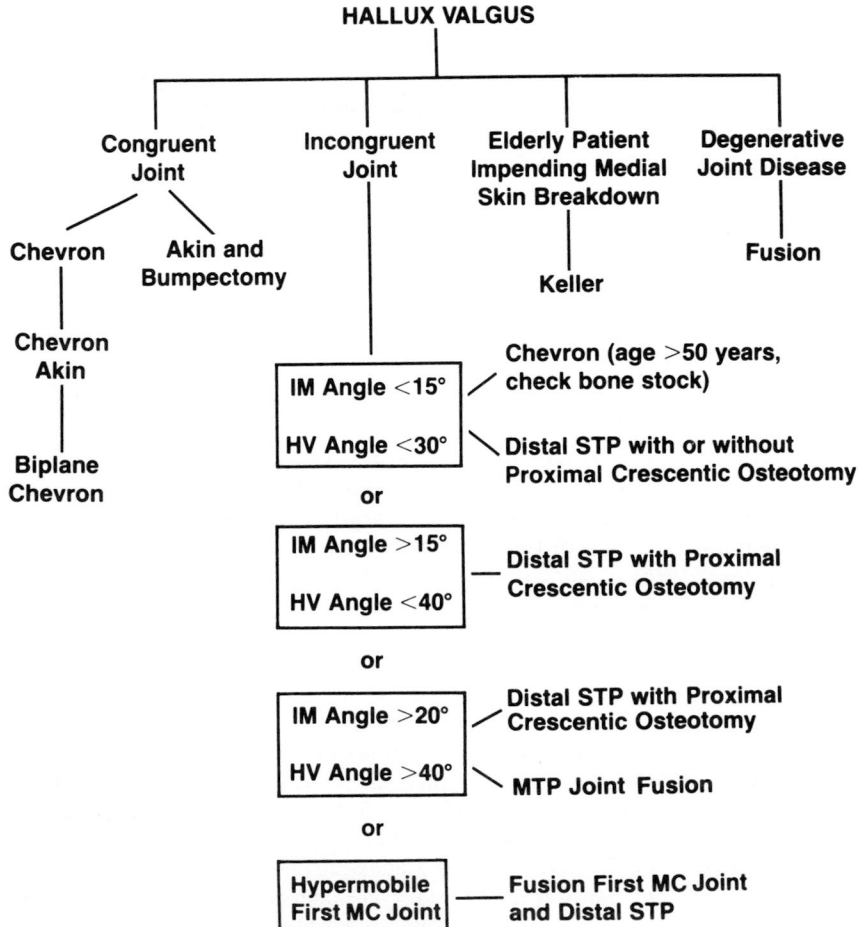

Figure 54-6 Algorithm that presents a scheme for decision making in hallux valgus. *Key:* IM, intermetatarsal; HV, hallux valgus; STP, soft tissue procedure; MTP, metatarsophalangeal; MC, metatarsocuneiform. [Adapted with permission from Mann RA: Decision making in bunion surgery. *Instr Course Lect* 39:3–13, 1990.]

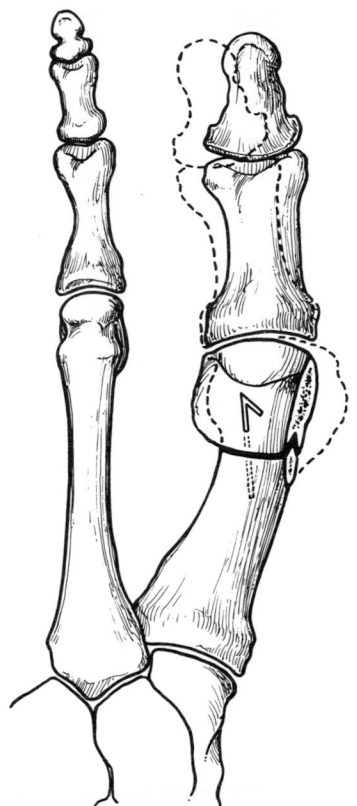

Figure 54-7 Chevron osteotomy. Lateral displacement of the metatarsal head allows the proximal phalanx to correct. [Reproduced with permission from Pedowitz W: Bunion deformity, in Pfeffer G, Frey C (eds): *Current Practice in Foot and Ankle Surgery.* New York, McGraw-Hill, 1993, pp 219–242.]

to reduce the DMA angle (see Fig. 54-8). Some surgeons perform the standard distal Chevron osteotomy and add a separate medial closing wedge osteotomy of the proximal phalanx (Akin procedure) to achieve a similar result (Fig. 54-8).[85] Contraindications to the procedure are an age above 50 years, an IM angle greater than 15°, an HV angle greater than 30°, and pronation of the great toe greater than 15°. The most common complications of the Chevron osteotomy include incomplete reduction and avascular necrosis of the first metatarsal head. Incomplete reduction can be prevented by not stretching the indications for surgery. The incidence of avascular necrosis can be lessened by avoiding excessive lateral stripping of the soft tissues about the first metatarsal head. Since the blood supply to the capital fragment is intraosseous (through the shaft) and extraosseous (entering the head through the dorsolateral soft tissues), it is advisable not to perform a distal soft tissue realignment at the same time.[79–81,83,84] Similarly, excessive lateral penetration of the saw blade should be avoided, since it may damage the lateral capsular circulation to the metatarsal head. Other reported complications include hallux varus secondary to excessive medial eminence resection and arthrosis of the sesamoid articula-

tion if the plantar osteotomy limb is not made sufficiently proximal to this articulation.

Distal Soft Tissue Procedure plus/minus Proximal Metatarsal Osteotomy

McBride described a soft tissue procedure for the correction of hallux valgus in which the adductor hallucis tendon was released, the lateral sesamoid excised, and the medial eminence resected, followed by repair of the medial capsule.[67] This procedure was later modified by Mann to reduce the risk of overcorrection and hallux varus deformity.[68,86] Also known as the modified McBride procedure (Fig. 54-9), the distal soft tissue procedure (DSTP) involves release of the lateral capsule, the adductor hallucis, and the intermetatarsal ligament through a dorsal first-web-space incision. The adductor hallucis tendon is then reattached to the soft tissues between the first and second metatarsal heads. The medial eminence is resected and the medial capsule plicated. This procedure is indicated for incongruent MTP joints only and should never be used for congruent joints, because rotation of the proximal phalangeal base around the metatarsal head can change a congruent joint into an incongruent joint. It may be used alone in mild hallux valgus or in combination with a proximal metatarsal osteotomy in moderate (IM angle >15°; HV angle <40°) or severe (IM angle >15°; HV angle >40°) hallux valgus deformities.[87–89] The distal soft tissue procedure alone usually corrects the intermetatarsal angle 5°. A proximal first metatarsal osteotomy may have to be added when the IM angle is greater than 15°. If a crescentic osteotomy is performed, it should be made through a dorsal incision located over the proximal third of the metatarsal and oriented so that the concavity of the osteotomy is directed proximally, so as to avoid excessive medial displacement and a resulting negative IM angle.[69] Some surgeons prefer to perform a proximal Chevron osteotomy because it is technically easier, with less likelihood of dorsiflexion malunion of the first metatarsal; it increases cancellous bony contact; and it is biomechanically more stable. The decision to perform a distal soft tissue procedure alone is made after intraoperative assessment. The first metatarsal must be passively correctable so that, after the deforming forces on the great toe are surgically rebalanced, correction of the first intermetatarsal angle will be maintained. A facet on the lateral aspect of the first metatarsal base is a radiographic finding that should lead the clinician to suspect that the first metatarsal varus is fixed and not amendable to simple soft tissue release.

The major complication of a poorly performed DSTP with or without a proximal metatarsal osteotomy is hallux varus. This occurs when the lateral tendon of the flexor hallucis brevis is released from the lateral sesamoid at the time the adductor tendon is released. Hallux varus can be avoided by taking care to avoid releasing the lateral slip of the flexor hallucis brevis tendon in performing the soft tissue release and orienting the concavity of the proximal metatarsal osteotomy toward the heel to avoid excessive medial displacement of the base of the first metatarsal. Overzealous medial eminence resection of the first metatarsal is another cause of hallux varus.[90–93]

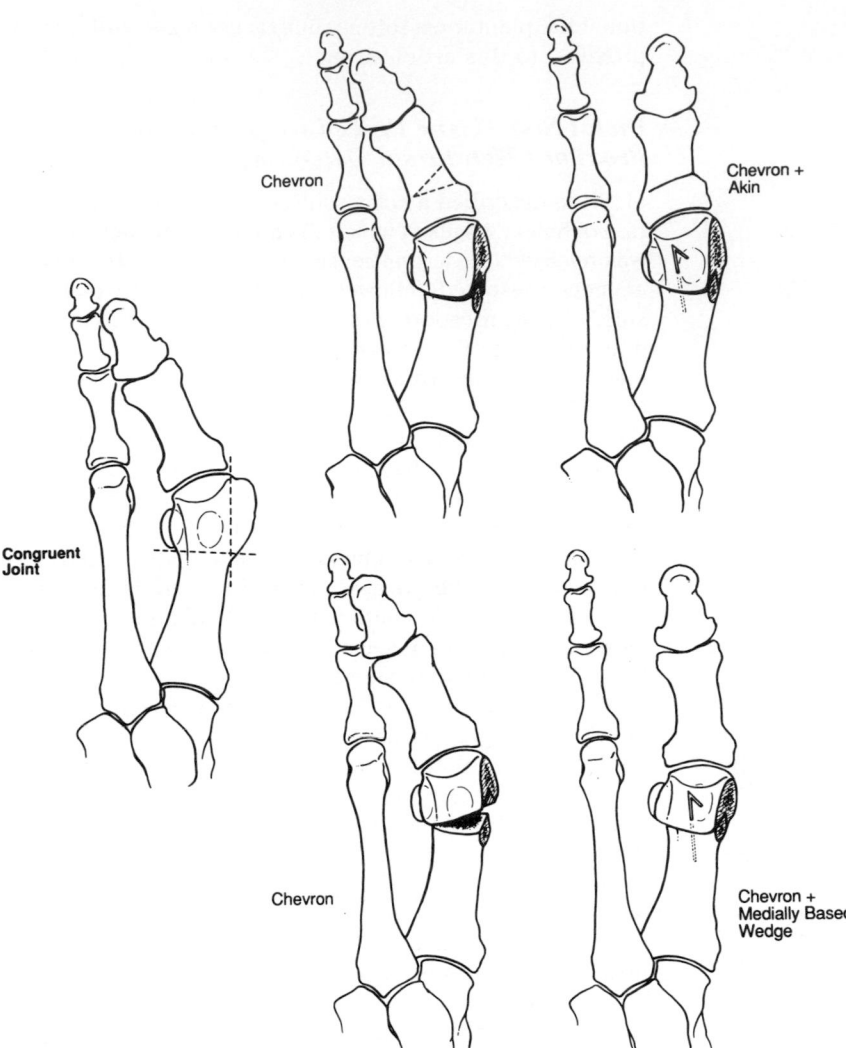

Figure 54-8 Management of the congruent joint with Chevron-Akin and biplane Chevron osteotomies. [Reproduced with permission from Pedowitz W: Bunion deformity, in Pfeffer G, Frey C (eds): *Current Practice in Foot and Ankle Surgery.* New York, McGraw-Hill, 1993, pp 219–242.]

Akin Procedure

The Akin procedure is a medially based closing wedge osteotomy performed at the proximal phalangeal base.[94,95] It is most useful for correcting a lateral deviated great toe in the presence of a congruent joint and is occasionally combined with a distal Chevron osteotomy (see Fig. 54-8). Other uses include correction of hallux valgus interphalangeus and mild recurrent bunion deformity. Technically, the osteotomy is usually performed 8 mm from the proximal articular surface. The lateral cortex of the proximal phalanx is not removed so as to enhance stability of the osteotomy. After gently cracking through the lateral cortex manually, fixation is secured with a K wire, staple, or wire suture. It should never be used as the definitive corrective procedure for a bunion deformity but is commonly used in conjunction with other procedures to optimize the position of the great toe.[85]

Mitchell Procedure

The Mitchell procedure is a double step-cut osteotomy through the neck of the first metatarsal which shortens the metatarsal and displaces and plantarflexes the metatarsal head fragment laterally[96] (Fig. 54-10). The osteotomy may be held in place with the use of K wires. It is technically demanding, and its main indication is moderate hallux valgus deformity with an incongruent MTP joint. Excessive shortening or dorsal displacement of the distal first metatarsal may produce transfer metatarsalgia, which is difficult to salvage surgically.

Arthrodesis

Fusion of the first MTP joint is the procedure of choice for pain relief in the presence of degenerative joint disease in the patient with several hallux valgus or hallux rigidus (Fig. 54-11). It is the preferred treatment for hallux valgus when there is neuromuscular instability or instability of the MTP joint associated with rheumatoid arthritis.[101,150,156] It is also useful as a salvage procedure for recurrent deformity or intractable metatarsalgia.[97] Arthrodesis is usually performed with the proximal phalanx in 15 to 20° of valgus and 10 to 15° of dorsiflexion from the plantar aspect of the foot. Fixation can be main-

Figure 54-9 *Left:* Distal soft tissue procedure with proximal crescentic osteotomy. *Right:* Proximal Chevron osteotomy. [Reproduced with permission from Pedowitz W: Bunion deformity, in Pfeffer G, Frey C (eds): *Current Practice in Foot and Ankle Surgery.* New York, McGraw-Hill, 1993, pp 219–242.]

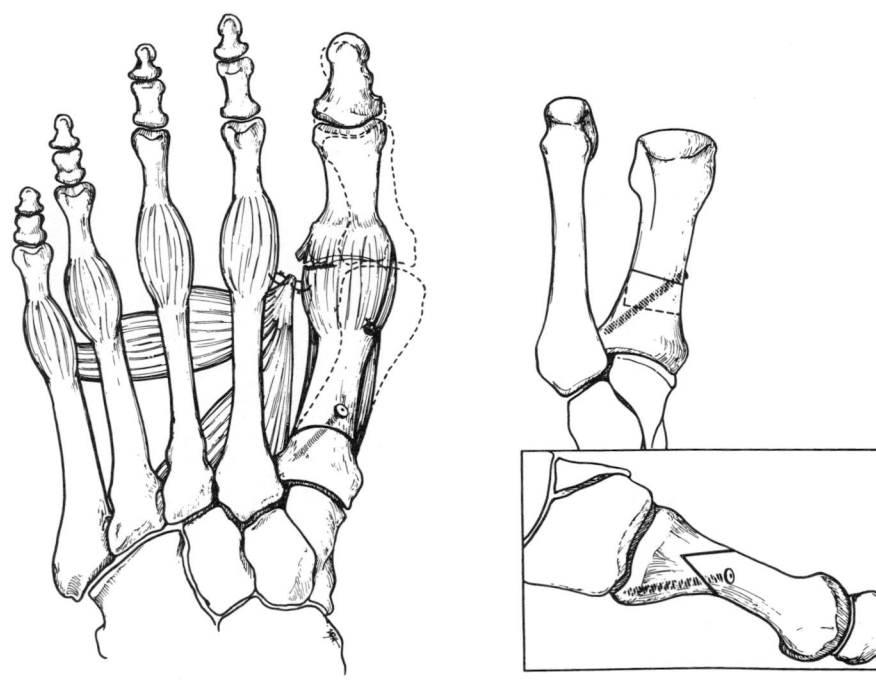

tained with plates and screws or multiple pins if the bone is osteoporotic. Fusion rates of 90 to 95 percent can be expected, although a pain-free fibrous nonunion may be asymptomatic. With long-term follow-up, patients may develop radiographic evidence of interphalangeal (IP)-joint arthritis following MTP joint fusion, but this is seldom associated with significant symptoms.

Lapidus Procedure

The first MC joint may be fused when a hypermobile MC joint exists in conjunction with an increased IM angle[98–100] (Fig. 54-12). Other indications include arthritis of the MC joint and revisions. This is a technically demanding operation for several reasons. The joint is multiplanar and irregular. Rotational malalignment is not well tolerated. Since

the medial column is shortened, the surgeon must estimate the proper amount to plantarflex the first metatarsal during the procedure. Inadvertent dorsiflexion or shortening of the first metatarsal may produce transfer metatarsalgia. Fusion may take several months.

Keller Procedure

Resection of the base of the proximal phalanx with medial eminence excision is indicated for the low-demand, elderly patient or as a salvage procedure for failed surgery in the elderly[102,103] (Fig. 54-13). It is useful in patients with degenerative arthritis of the MTP joint or those with a fixed deformity in which soft tissue releases would be inadequate. Difficulty in reestablishing flexor function of the great toe often results in decreased push-off strength and

Figure 54-10 Mitchell procedure. *Left:* The medial eminence is removed in line with the medial aspect of the metatarsal. A distal cut is then made in the metatarsal. *Center:* Lateral displacement of osteotomy. The degree of lateral displacement depends on the magnitude of the deformity. *Right:* Lateral view demonstrates position of osteotomy site, preferably with slight plantarflexion of distal fragment. (Reproduced with permission from Mann RA, Coughlin MJ: *The Video Textbook of Foot and Ankle Surgery.* St Louis, Medical Video Productions, 1991.)

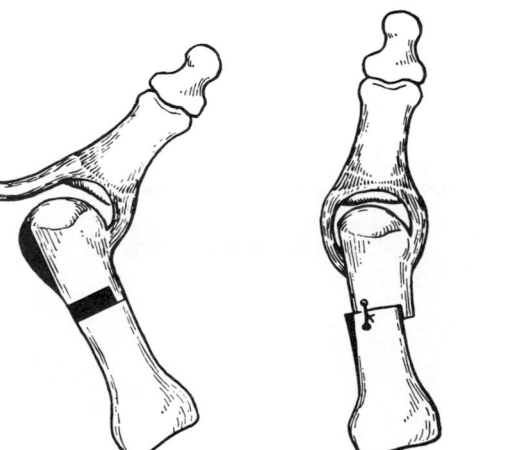
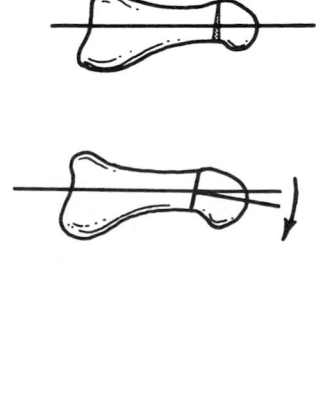

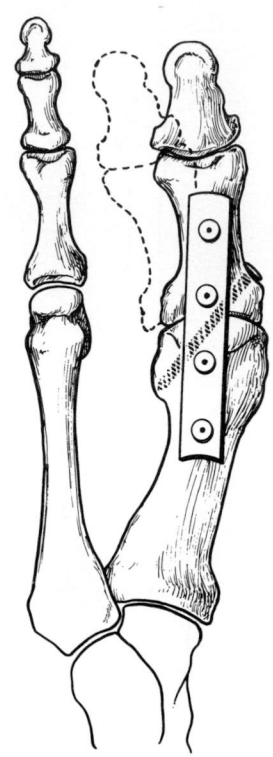

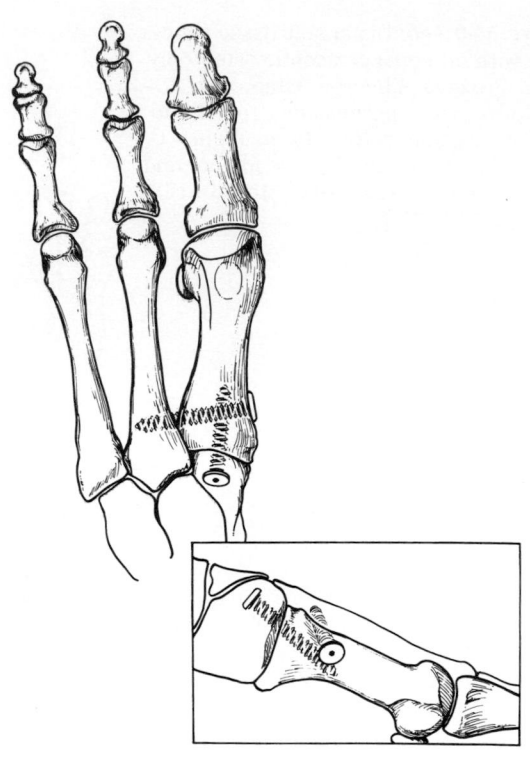

Figure 54-11 MTP arthrodesis. Alignment should be 15° valgus and 10 to 15° dorsiflexion from the plantar aspect to the foot. [Reproduced with permission from Pedowitz W: Bunion deformity, in Pfeffer G, Frey C (eds): *Current Practice in Foot and Ankle Surgery.* New York, McGraw-Hill, 1993, pp 219–242.]

Figure 54-12 Metatarsocuneiform arthrodesis. [Reproduced with permission from Pedowitz W: Bunion deformity, in Pfeffer G, Frey C (eds): *Current Practice in Foot and Ankle Surgery.* New York, McGraw-Hill, 1993, pp 219–242.]

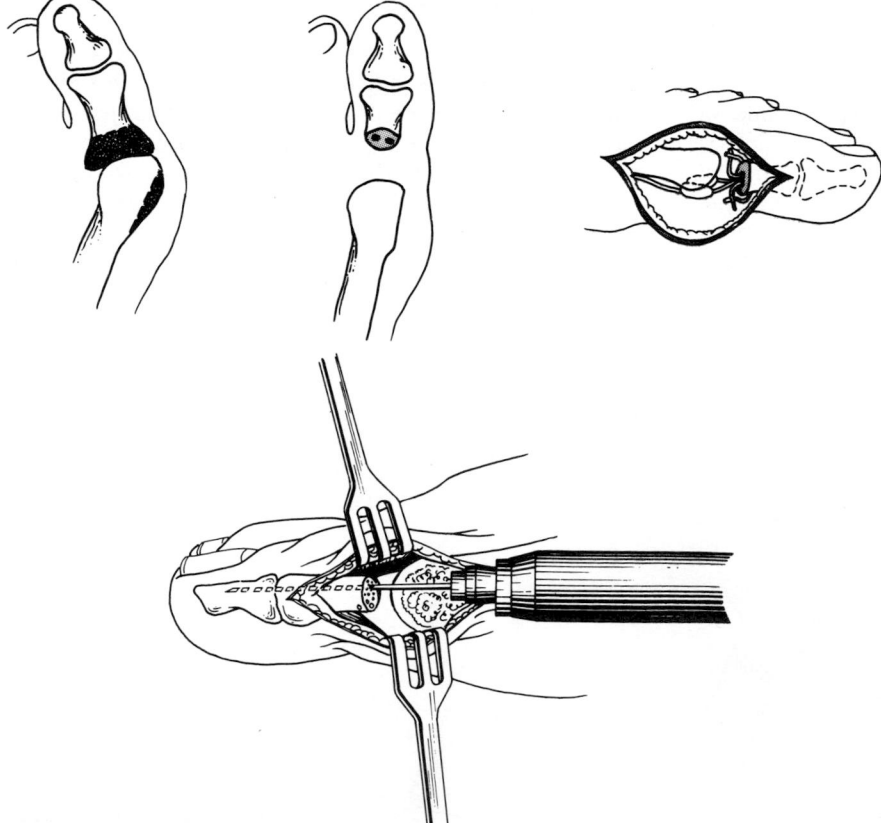

Figure 54-13 Keller procedure. *Top left* and *center:* The medial eminence is removed in line with the medial aspect of the metatarsal shaft. The proximal third of the proximal phalanx is excised. *Top right:* An attempt is made to reapproximate plantar and medial capsular structures to the remaining base of the proximal phalanx. (Reproduced with permission from Mann RA, Coughlin MJ: *The Video Textbook of Foot and Ankle Surgery.* St Louis, Medical Video Productions, 1991.) *Bottom:* Fixation of the MTP joint using 5/64-in Steinmann pin. [Reproduced with permission from Pedowitz WJ: Deformities of the first ray, in Lutter LD, Mizel MS, Pfeffer GB (eds): *Orthopaedic Knowledge Update: Foot and Ankle.* Rosemont, IL, American Association of Orthopaedic Surgeons, 1994, pp 141–162.]

later development of a cockup toe deformity. If the extensor hallucis longus is tight, it may need to be lengthened to prevent this deformity. The plantar plate should be reattached to the base of the proximal phalanx through drill holes and the flexor hallucis longus reattached to the plantar aponeurosis to augment flexor function and avoid cockup toe deformity. There is an increased incidence of transfer metatarsalgia associated with this procedure, and the great toe is shortened.[101]

Other Procedures

Medial eminence resection (Silver bunionectomy) is a minimally invasive procedure that is indicated only for treatment of hallux valgus deformities in very limited situations because of the high rate of recurrence.[104] Inactive elderly patients with impending skin ulceration where the eminence is the primary problem will benefit most from the procedure.

The use of Silastic implants in the MTP joint has been controversial because their durability in the active patient is limited and eventual failure can be expected.[114] The use of single-stem implants to replace the base of a resected proximal phalanx or of flexible double-stemmed implants following resection arthroplasty has been described. Complications related to silicone synovitis, bone resorption, and implant fracture are common.

OTHER DISORDERS OF THE HALLUX

Hallux Rigidus

Hallux rigidus involves a painful loss of motion, particularly dorsiflexion of the first metatarsophalangeal (MTP) joint due to degenerative joint disease.[115,116] It has been associated with long first metatarsals, flat first MTP joints, and prior history of hyperextension injuries of the great toe. In juveniles, it may be associated with avascular necrosis of the first metatarsal head. Patients complain of pain with weight bearing, with or without footwear, particularly during the push-off phase of gait. Physical examination is remarkable for limited first MTP dorsiflexion and dorsal joint tenderness. No tenderness is noted on palpation of the sesamoids. There is minimal crepitus with range of motion of the first MTP joint. This is in contrast to diffuse joint arthrosis, in which there is sesamoid tenderness and crepitus of the first MTP joint. Although radiographs may be normal initially, later changes include osteophytic spurs around the joint, particularly dorsally and laterally, with varying degrees of joint space narrowing.

Initial treatment is nonoperative and involves the use of a stiff-soled shoe to limit dorsiflexion at the first MTP joint. Other shoe modifications include orthoses with a Morton's extension or a rocker-bottom sole. Nonsteroidal anti-inflammatory drugs (NSAIDs) or intraarticular steroid injections may provide temporary relief during acute exacerbations. Operative management depends on the degree of arthrosis present in the first MTP joint. In the early stages of the disease, when the joint space and motion are

well preserved, cheilectomy is a good option. This is performed through a dorsal incision placed just medial to the extensor hallucis longus tendon. The dorsal third of the first metatarsal articular surface is excised with an oscillating saw and all periarticular osteophytes are removed with a rongeur. The goal of surgery is to provide substantial pain relief with ambulation. Patients are rarely completely pain-free. Although many patients will obtain an increase in first MTP motion, this is not a consistently reported result. The addition of a proximal phalangeal dorsal closing wedge osteotomy (Moberg procedure) is helpful in situations where less than 60° of great toe dorsiflexion is obtained intraoperatively. Following the osteotomy, the apparent range of motion of the great toe is increased. Any motion plantar to the plane of the floor can be exchanged for an equal amount of increased dorsiflexion by performing this dorsal closing wedge osteotomy. It is important to carefully assess the first MTP joint range of motion preoperatively to avoid an excessive wedge resection, leading to a great toe that does not contact the floor during stance.

In the presence of advanced degenerative joint disease, cheilectomy is not indicated. Surgical options include arthrodesis, resection of the proximal phalanx (Keller procedure), and Silastic implant arthroplasty. Use of a Silastic implant is limited only to the elderly, low-demand patient and is highly controversial because of potential complications related to the durability of the implant and silicone synovitis. The Keller procedure retains motion but results in weakness during push-off and is contraindicated in the young or middle-aged active person. Long-term complications include a cockup toe deformity, which can interfere with footwear. Arthrodesis is clearly the procedure of choice for the younger, active patient, although loss of motion at this joint may necessitate minor footwear modifications. Theoretically, an arthrodesed hallux should provide a strong, long weight-bearing lever arm and thereby alleviate any excessive preoperative loading of the lesser metatarsals. This has been demonstrated in biomechanical weight-bearing studies but has not been shown consistently during clinical evaluations. Weight bearing on the first metatarsal depends on many factors, such as its length compared with the other metatarsals, the degree of varus angulation, the angle of declination, and sagittal plane flexibility. However, improved first metatarsal weight bearing is generally obtained following an arthrodesis as compared to a Keller procedure.

The optimal position for fusion of the first MTP joint has generally been agreed to be 10 to 15° of dorsiflexion with respect to the floor, 15° of valgus, and neutral rotation, although consideration should be given to the overall foot shape (pes cavus or pes planus), motion at the IP joint, and desired heel height. Fusions should not be performed in more dorsiflexion simply to accommodate higher heels in women because of the greater likelihood of developing pain beneath the sesamoids with greater MTP extension and potential difficulties with fitting the foot inside the toebox of shoes with standard heel heights. Preoperative templating of weight-bearing lateral radiographs taken in the patient's footwear is helpful in planning the amount of dorsiflexion desired. There is less confusion regarding the intraoperative positioning of the hallux in the sagittal plane when the "floor" (horizontal plane) is used as the frame of reference, rather than the first metatarsal shaft. A sterile, hard, flat surface may be used intraoperatively to apply pressure to the sole of the foot and serve as such a frame of reference. With the IP joint extended fully, the head of the proximal phalanx should clear the horizontal surface by 5 to 10 mm.

Hallux Extensus

Cockup deformity of the hallux can be developmental or due to loss of flexor function. This may be iatrogenic, resulting from resection of both sesamoids with failure to reattach the flexor hallucis brevis (FHB). The Jones procedure—transposition of the extensor hallucis longus (EHL) to the first MT neck—or Meyerson's modification using the EHB has been described in treating this deformity.[90–93] Another option involves restoration of MTP joint flexion by releasing the contracted EHL tendon and fusing the IP joint, allowing the flexor hallucis longus (FHL) tendon to act as an MTP joint flexor.

Dorsal Bunion

This deformity is characterized by plantarflexion of the great toe at the MTP joint together with elevation of the first metatarsal. It is observed mostly in children when there is an imbalance between the various tendons acting on the first ray. It is seen with a strong tibialis anterior dorsiflexing the first metatarsal associated with a weakness of the peroneus longus, resulting in loss of first metatarsal plantarflexion. Consequently, the peroneus longus should never be released without tenodesing its distal tendon stump to the peroneus brevis. It may also be seen with a combination of weak toe extensors with strong plantarflexors of the great toe. Its appearance may follow surgery for clubfoot when supination of the forefoot has not been adequately corrected.[70] The development of a dorsal bunion following posteromedial release for clubfoot has also been postulated to result because the patient compensates for weakness of the triceps surae by pushing off with the toe flexors.[71] Surgical treatment involving transfer of the FHL to the neck of the first metatarsal has been recommended, along with a plantar closing wedge osteotomy of the first metatarsal base. McKay has described transfer of the tendons of the short flexor and abductor and adductor hallucis to the first metatarsal neck with first MTP capsulotomy and sesamoidectomy.

Disorders of the Sesamoids

Disorders of the sesamoids include sesamoiditis, fractures,[105] subluxation or dislocation,[110] avascular necrosis,[106,108,109] and arthritis.[113] Generally, the diagnosis is made with a history of painful weight bearing and an exam that is well localized to the area. Sesamoid (axial) ra-

diographic views may be useful. There is a 25 to 30 percent incidence of bipartite sesamoids (85 percent bilateral). Disorders of the sesamoids more frequently involve the medial (tibial) sesamoid and can be documented by bone scanning.[112] Initial treatment includes immobilization, accommodative footwear, orthoses with sesamoid pads, and activity modification. Refractory cases of sesamoiditis, fractures, or arthritis may be treated by excision of the affected sesamoid.[107] Only one sesamoid should be excised because of the late risk of cockup toe deformity due to release of the FHB.[11]

A subhallux sesamoid is a pathologic condition in which a painful sesamoid exists between the plantar aspect of the MTP joint and the FHL tendon. Its presence may be heralded by the presence of a large callus beneath the great toe. Careful clinical examination in conjunction with sesamoid views will allow the diagnosis to be made. The differential diagnosis includes neuritis of the medial plantar digital nerve to the hallux, bursitis beneath the first metatarsal head, or a simple callus. Conservative treatment, similar to that for hallux rigidus, is attempted first. If this is unsuccessful, sesamoidectomy may be required, with precautions taken to preserve the integrity of the FHB tendon and thus avoid a cockup deformity of the great toe.

DEFORMITIES OF THE LESSER TOES
Hammer, Claw, and Mallet Toes

The lesser toes function in balance and weight bearing in the distal lateral aspect of the foot. Normal toe functioning depends on the interplay of the extrinsic and intrinsic flexors and extensors of the toes (Figs. 54-14 and 54-15). There is also a role for static stabilizers (Fig. 54-16), including the plantar aponeurosis (which inserts on the bases of the proximal phalanges), plantar plates, capsules, and collateral ligaments.[127–129] Lesser toe deformities have been associated with multiple risk factors in which this fine balance is disrupted. As with hallux valgus, there is an increased incidence among shod populations, particularly among women. This has been attributed to footwear with confining toe boxes and high heels. These deformities are also more common among the elderly and those with rheumatoid arthritis.

The characteristic deformity in a mallet toe is a flexion deformity of the distal interphalangeal (DIP) joint, with uninvolved MTP and proximal interphalangeal (PIP) joints.[125,130] Hammertoes and claw toes share flexion deformities at the PIP joints.[131] Hammertoes are neutral or extended at the MTP joint and may be in any position at the DIP joint, although extension is more common. Whereas mallet and hammertoe deformities are primarily limited to the IP joints, the essential feature of claw-toe deformities (Fig. 54-17) is MTP hyperextension. Lesser toe deformities are precipitated by an imbalance between the intrinsic and extrinsic muscle tone in the foot with concomitant failure of the static stabilizing structures. The intrinsic muscles of the foot, the lumbricals and interossei,

Figure 54-14 *Top:* Lateral view of the lesser toe, demonstrating insertion of extrinsic and intrinsic tendons. *Below:* A portion of the extensor hood is removed to demonstrate insertion of the interossei into the base of the proximal phalanx. (Reproduced with permission from Coughlin MJ: Subluxation and dislocation of the second metatarsophalangeal joint. *Orthop Clin North Am* 20:535–551, 1989.)

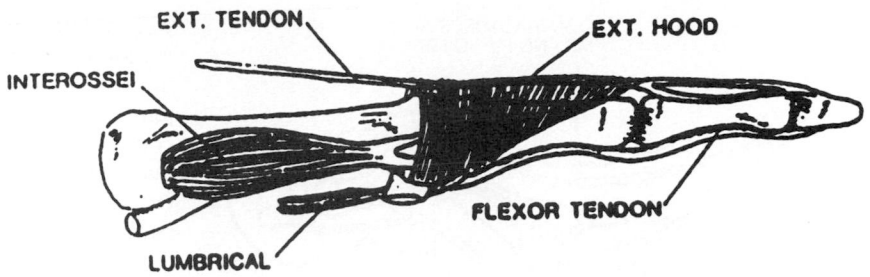

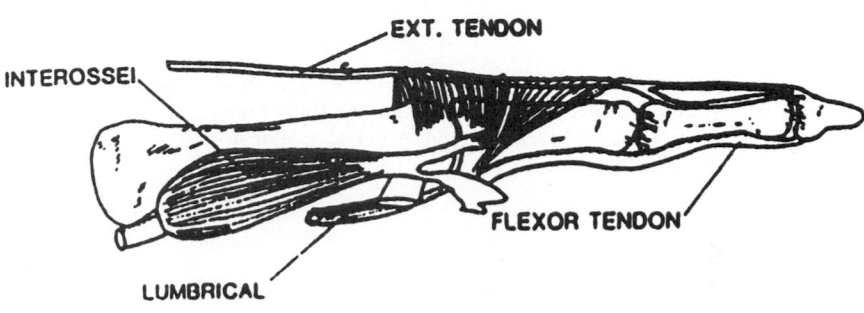

are normally flexors of the MTP joints and extensors of the PIP and DIP joints. In a claw-toe deformity, the function of the intrinsics may be overcome by the extrinsic long flexor or extensor muscles, leading to hyperextension at the MTP joints and flexion deformities at the PIP and DIP joints. With loss of integrity of the MTP joint and dorsal subluxation of the proximal phalanx, the plantar fat pad beneath the metatarsal head may become displaced distally with the proximal phalanx. Development of callosities plantar to the metatarsal heads and dorsal to the PIP joints then ensues. Frequently, all four lesser toes are involved and clawing is present bilaterally. Factors contributing to claw-toe deformities include peripheral neuropathy (diabetes, Charcot-Marie-Tooth disease), lower motor neuron dis-

ease (myelodysplasia), upper motor neuron disease (cerebral palsy, cord tethering, multiple sclerosis, stroke), and sequelae of trauma (compartment syndrome).[140,144]

Paramount to the evaluation and treatment of these deformities is determining whether they are flexible or fixed.[125] Accommodative footwear that may initially be prescribed for the treatment of claw- or hammertoe deformities includes high, wide toeboxes and full-length,

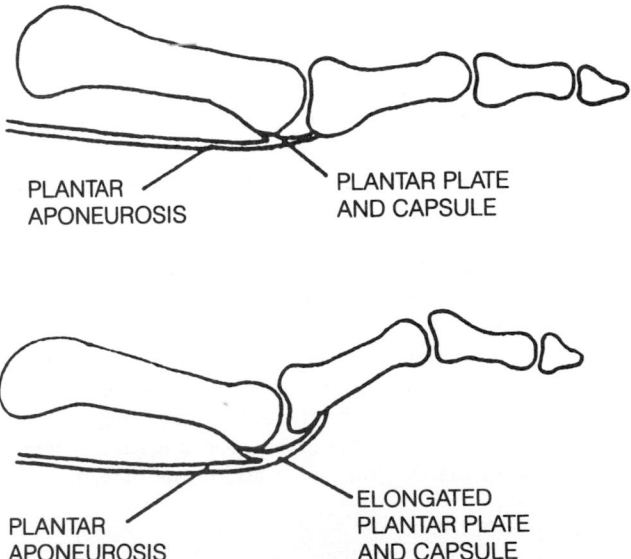

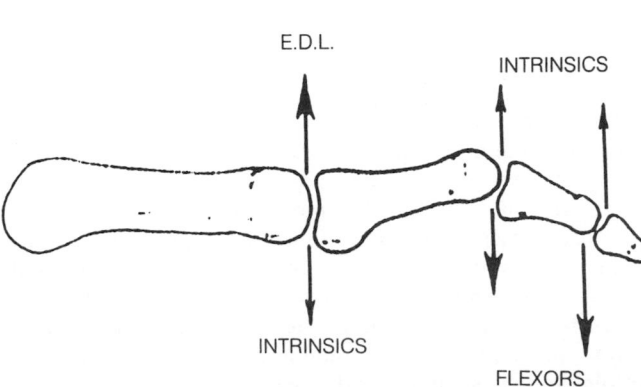

Figure 54-15 Lateral view of the imbalance of extrinsics and intrinsics of the lesser toe. (Reproduced with permission from Coughlin MJ: Subluxation and dislocation of the second metatarsophalangeal joint. *Orthop Clin North Am* 20:535–551, 1989.)

Figure 54-16 Lateral view of the static plantar stabilizers of the lesser toe. (Reproduced with permission from Coughlin MJ: Subluxation and dislocation of the second metatarsophalangeal joint. *Orthop Clin North Am* 20:535–551, 1989.)

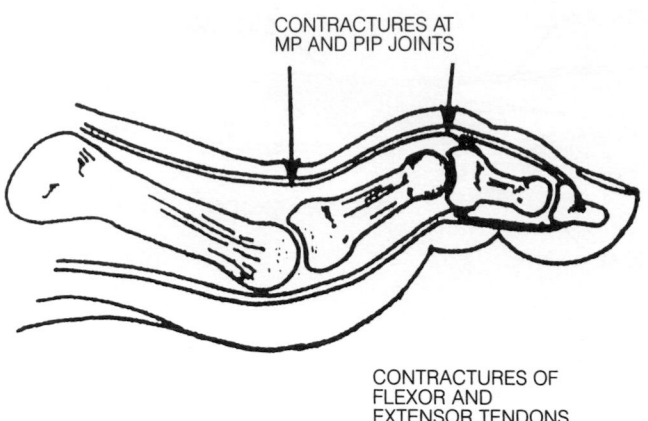

CONTRACTURES AT
MP AND PIP JOINTS

CONTRACTURES OF
FLEXOR AND
EXTENSOR TENDONS

Figure 54-17 Lateral view of claw toe. (Reproduced with permission from Coughlin MJ: Mallet toes, hammer toes, claw toes, and corns: Causes and treatment of lesser toe deformities. *Postgrad Med* 75:191–198, 1984.)

semirigid longitudinal arch supports with metatarsal pads to more evenly distribute plantar pressure. Flexible claw- or hammertoe deformities may be treated surgically with the Girdlestone-Taylor procedure (split FDL transfer to the extensor hood)[118,125,136] (Fig. 54-18). Fixed deformities may be treated with resection of the head and neck of the proximal phalanx[125,135] (Fig. 54-19). It may be necessary to release both flexors and extensors. Alternatively, proximal phalangectomy[132] or PIP joint arthrodesis[133,137] may also be used for treating fixed hammertoes. Contractures of the MTP joint in claw-toe deformity may be corrected by extensor tenotomy. After adequate soft tissue releases about the MTP joint alone, the proximal phalanx may still remain dorsiflexed.[138] In this situation, an MTP arthroplasty may be performed that involves resection of the distal portion of the head of the metatarsal (DuVries arthroplasty)[124] (Fig. 54-20) or the base of the proximal phalanx.[121,132,134] Temporary K-wire fixation is recommended. Resection of the lesser metatarsal heads can decompress the forefoot and allow the plantar fat pads to return to their original positions. Resection of a single metatarsal head should rarely be performed because it will predictably lead to transfer metatarsalgia.

Mallet-toe deformity commonly affects the second toe, although any of the lesser toes may be involved.[136] Accommodative footwear may be prescribed, but is usually not helpful. Surgical options include FDL tenotomy if the deformity is flexible and the extensor digitorum longus tendon is intact. Occasionally fixed and traumatic deformities can occur and may be treated by resecting the middle phalangeal head and neck and performing a flexor tenotomy. Fusion of the DIP joint is an additional option.

Subluxation of the Second-Toe MTP Joint

Crossover deformity most commonly involves the second toe and is frequently accompanied by an adjacent hallux

valgus deformity.[119,120] Hallux valgus may cause a deforming force against the medial aspect of the second toe, leading to dorsal or lateral subluxation of the second MTP joint. Increased pressure from footwear exacerbates the condition. Overlapping of the second toe over the hallux may occur. The static stabilizers of the MTP joint (collateral ligaments and plantar plate) become attenuated, resulting in instability of the joint. Synovitis of the MTP joint may be present.[122] A Lachman-like test (Thompson-Hamilton sign) has been described that demonstrates dorsal instability of the joint.[124] This may be performed by stabilizing the metatarsal with one hand and using the other to dorsally subluxate the proximal phalanx.[123,124,126] Conservative treatment of second-MTP instability includes taping, MT toe pads, or a stiff-soled shoe. Surgical treatment consists of flexor-to-extensor transfers, plantar condylectomies, or MTP joint arthroplasty. When this instability is associated with hallux valgus, correction of the hallux deformity is necessary to prevent recurrence of crossover deformity.

Fifth-Toe Deformities
Cockup and Overlapping Deformities

Cockup and overlapping deformities are two common disorders of the fifth toe. Cockup deformity may be congenital or related to footwear. The resulting deformity can be quite severe and may result in a proximal phalanx that is perpendicular to the metatarsal shaft. As a result, surgery is often necessary to treat the problem. DuVries arthroplasty (partial resection of the distal metatarsal articular surface)[124] or the Ruiz-Mora procedure (excision of the proximal phalanx)[142] with syndactylization of the fourth and fifth toes are two common procedures used to treat this deformity. Overlapping fifth toes are thought to be congenital in origin. Symptoms are exacerbated by shoewear. Several procedures have been devised to correct this problem through release of the MTP and EDL contractures.

Bunionette of the Fifth Metatarsal (Tailor's Bunion)

A bunionette is characterized by a painful prominence of the lateral eminence of the fifth metatarsal head.[143,145] The fifth metatarsal deviates laterally with respect to the fourth metatarsal and the fifth toe moves in a medial direction. Friction between the underlying bony prominence and constricting footwear can lead to the development of a callus over the lateral aspect of the fifth metatarsal head or a plantar lateral callus under the head. Although this condition may superficially resemble a bunion deformity, the etiology, assessment, and treatment are different.[143] Clinical evaluation should take into consideration the overall structure of the foot (i.e., cavovarus deformity) as well as the specific orientation of the fifth toe. Distinction must be made between the directly lateral versus the plantar

Figure 54-18 The Girdlestone-Taylor flexor to extensor transfer. *A.* Lateral view of lesser toe. *B.* Cross-section anatomy through the metatarsal head region. *C.* The FDL tendon has been detached from its insertion and split longitudinally along its raphe. *D* and *E.* The FDL is brought up on each side of the extensor hood through subcutaneous tunnels and sutured to the extensor expansion with the toe in corrected position. [Reproduced with permission from Coughlin MJ, Mann RA: Lesser toe deformities, in Mann RA, Coughlin MJ (eds): *Surgery of the Foot and Ankle,* 6th ed. Vol 1. St Louis, Mosby, 1993, pp 341–411.]

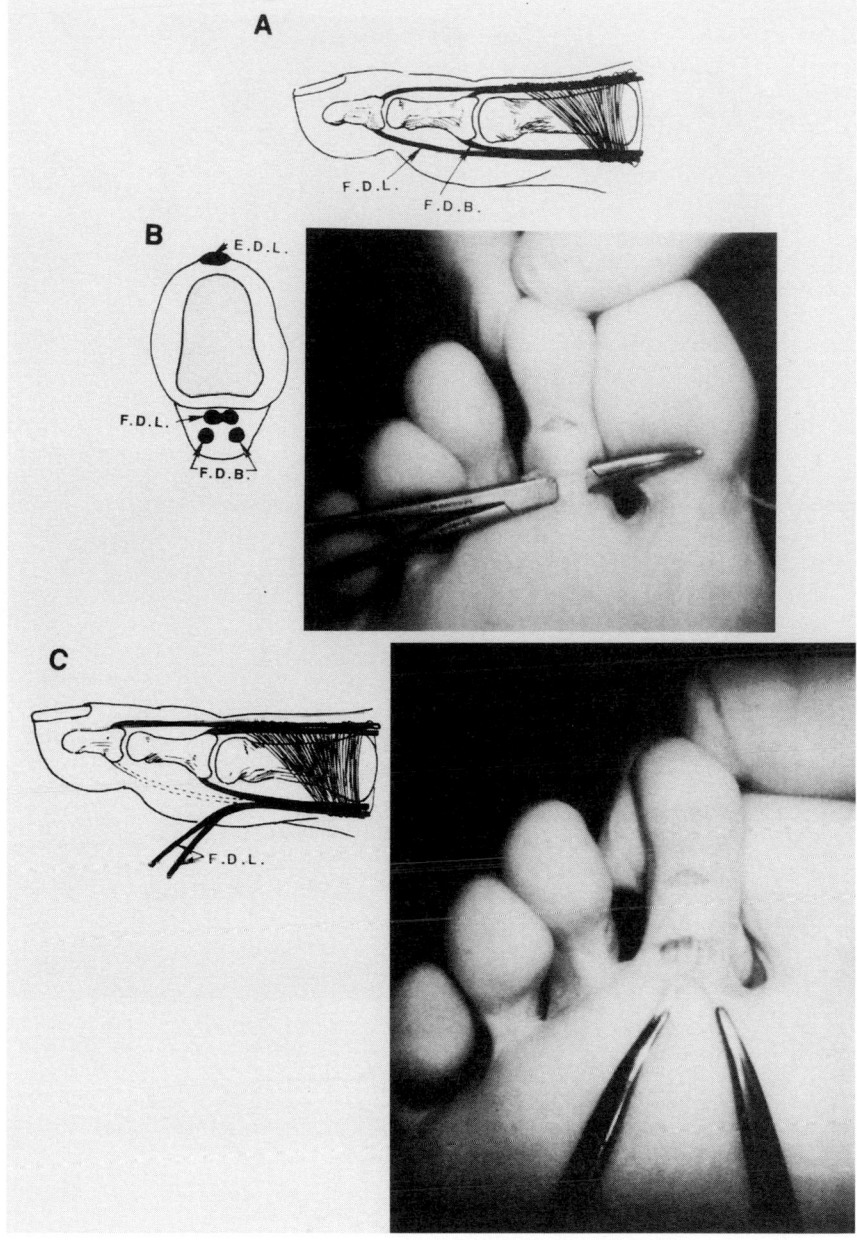

(Fig. 54-18 continues on page 1028)

lateral callous at the fifth metatarsal head. Radiographic assessment should include measurement of the fifth metatarsophalangeal angle and the fourth-to-fifth intermetatarsal angle.[145] Three types of bunionette deformity have been described. A type 1 deformity is characterized by an enlarged fifth metatarsal head. Type 2 deformity involves lateral bowing of the distal fifth metatarsal shaft. An abnormally widened fourth-to-fifth intermetatarsal angle is the feature of a type 3 deformity.

Nonoperative treatment consists of appropriately wide footwear, shaving of the callus, and padding around the bony prominence. Surgical management is guided by the type of deformity present.[143] Type 1 deformity is treated with a lateral/plantar condylectomy of the fifth metatarsal head. Failed cases can be managed with a distal fifth

metatarsal osteotomy or metatarsal head resection.[144,147] Type 2 deformity with lateral callosity should be treated with a distal fifth metatarsal osteotomy. If there is a plantar lateral callus, then an oblique diaphyseal osteotomy is often required.[143,148] Type 3 deformity should be treated with a diaphyseal osteotomy.[146]

The most common complications following surgical treatment of bunionette deformity include malunion, avascular necrosis, recurrence, and incomplete relief of the plantar keratosis. Proximal metatarsal osteotomy, while popular for bunion deformities, is rarely necessary in the treatment of bunionettes.[146] There is a high incidence of delayed healing and nonunion of proximal osteotomies. Floating osteotomies should not be used because of inconsistent results.

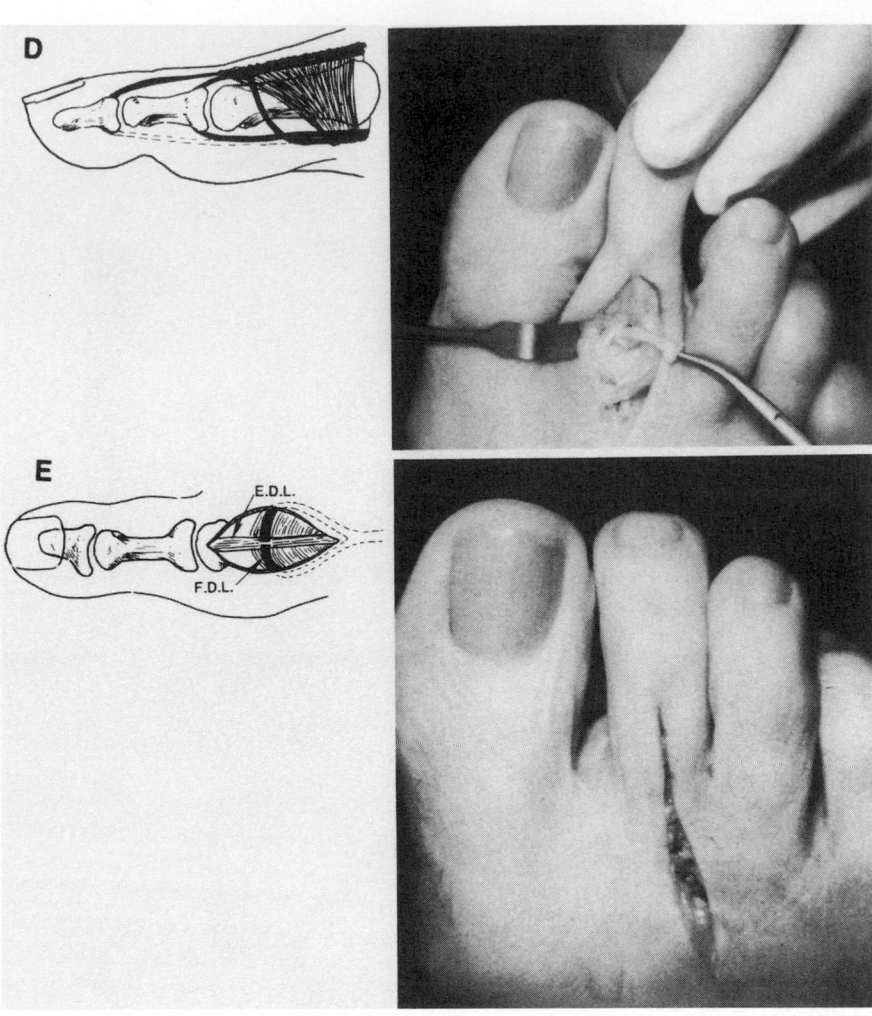

Figure 54-18 (*Continued*)

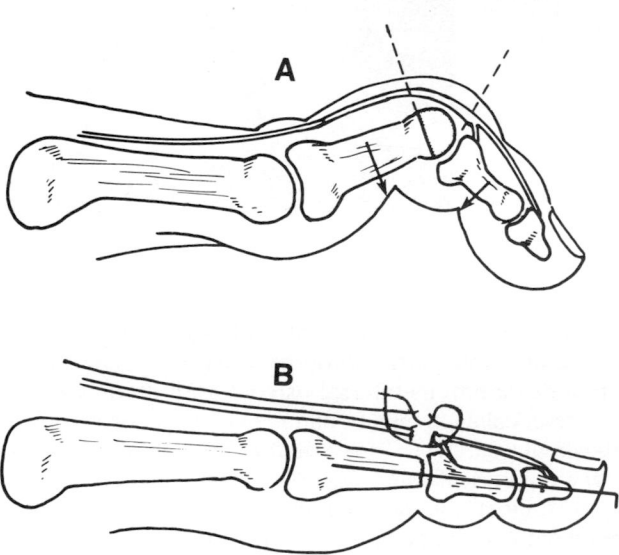

Figure 54-19 Surgical correction of hammertoe deformity through dorsal capsulotomy and proximal interphalangeal joint excisional arthroplasty. *A.* Proposed area of bony resection. *B.* Following bony resection, stabilization with intramedullary K wire. [Reproduced with permission from Coughlin MJ, Mann RA: Lesser toe deformities, in Mann RA, Coughlin MJ (eds): *Surgery of the Foot and Ankle,* 6th ed. Vol 1. St Louis, Mosby, 1993, pp 341–411.]

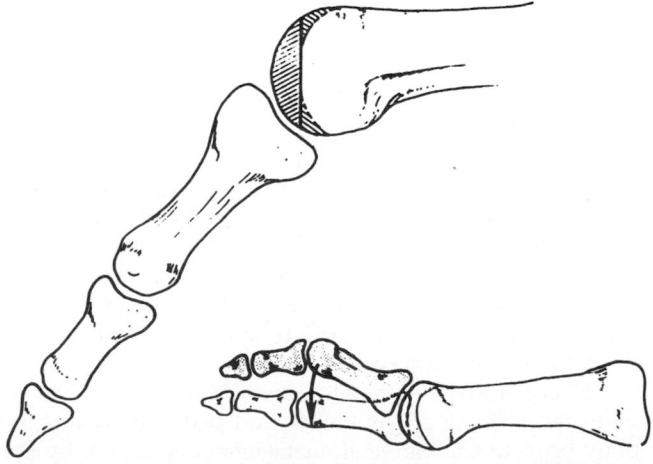

Figure 54-20 The modified DuVries arthroplasty. (Reproduced with permission from Coughlin MJ: Subluxation and dislocation of the second metatarsophalangeal joint. *Orthop Clin North Am* 20:535–551, 1989.)

Rheumatoid Forefoot Deformities

The forefoot is more frequently involved than either the hindfoot or the ankle in rheumatoid arthritis (RA). Recurrent inflammatory MTP synovitis is prototypical of RA and results in instability and deformity in this region.[155,158,159] Static stabilizers such as the collateral ligaments, plantar plate, capsule, and plantar aponeurosis are attenuated by the combination of chronic effusions and direct invasion by pannus. Destruction of articular cartilage by rheumatoid pannus leads to further joint incongruity and instability. Dorsal subluxation of the proximal phalanges leads to distal migration of the plantar fat pads with ensuing metatarsalgia and the development of painful plantar callosities. Claw toes, hammertoes, and hallux valgus deformity may develop. The effects of restrictive footwear further accentuate these deformities.

Following medical evaluation and treatment of the systemic disorder, symptomatic treatment of forefoot problems begins with footwear modifications. These include the use of metatarsal pads or arch supports to reduce weight bearing on the metatarsal heads and depth shoes to accommodate claw- or hammertoe deformities. First MTP fusion is the procedure of choice for treatment of rheumatoid hallux valgus and is frequently performed in conjunction with resection of the lesser metatarsal heads.[150–157] The latter decompresses the MTP joints and may allow relocation of the plantar fat pads to their normal plantar positions. Older and sedentary patients may benefit from Keller resection arthroplasty as an alternative procedure at the first MTP joint. In this instance, the resection arthroplasty has the advantage of a shorter operative time and a faster postoperative recovery period, since the patient may need to refrain from bearing weight for only 4 weeks instead of 6 to 8 weeks with a fusion.[149,155]

DISORDERS OF THE SKIN AND NAILS

Intractable Plantar Keratosis

Plantar keratosis may present as a discrete, well-localized hyperkeratotic proliferation under a single metatarsal head or a diffuse thickening of the skin beneath all the lesser metatarsal heads.[160] The development of either is the result of abnormal pressure, which can arise from a multitude of causes. Discrete plantar keratosis is usually found under a metatarsal head with a prominent fibular condyle. Other causes include metatarsal fractures that heal with a relative plantar prominence of one metatarsal head. Alternatively, a metatarsal fracture that heals with dorsal displacement can lead to a transfer lesion beneath an adjacent metatarsal head. This is particularly true of displaced fractures of the second and third metatarsals. Diffuse plantar keratosis can be found whenever abnormal pressure is present beneath the metatarsal heads. This may be due to altered weight bearing, as in the cavus foot with claw toes, or following subluxation of the MTP joints and the plantar fat pads. Iatrogenic causes include transfer metatarsalgia complicating surgical procedures that shorten or dorsiflex the first metatarsal. This has been observed following the Mitchell

procedure or following first metatarsocuneiform fusions positioned in relative dorsiflexion.

Treatment initially involves relieving pressure and redistributing the plantar forces with metatarsal pads and semirigid full-length longitudinal arch supports. Shaving the prominent callus in the office at regular intervals may be a useful adjunct. Surgical options include basal metatarsal dorsal wedge osteotomy or metatarsal head arthroplasty (DuVries) for discrete plantar keratosis.[161–164] Resection of a single metatarsal head is likely to lead to transfer lesions in the remaining toes and should be avoided. Diffuse metatarsalgia with plantar fat-pad atrophy is a contraindication to surgery. However, Mann has recommended first MTP arthrodesis with resection of the lesser metatarsal heads in an attempt to salvage intractable metatarsalgia.[97]

Plantar Wart

Plantar warts are caused by a papillomavirus infection that produces a painful, discrete, raised lesion, which may be similar in appearance to plantar keratosis. Unlike discrete plantar keratosis, plantar warts may appear anywhere on the plantar skin, including non-weight-bearing surfaces. Further differentiation is possible on clinical examination, since plantar warts are highly vascular and exhibit central punctate bleeding when shaved. The typical presentation is in children and young adults. Some 20 to 60 percent of cases will undergo spontaneous regression over several years without treatment.

Various strategies have been devised to remove plantar warts, none of which are uniformly successful. Most nonsurgical methods employ the use of keratolytic agents, such as salicylic, acetic, or lactic acids. Liquid nitrogen or electrosurgery have also been used. Surgical excision is usually attempted only as a last resort.

Onychomycosis

Fungal infections of the nail are usually caused by one of three dermatophytes. The organism *Trychophyton rubrum* is responsible for the commonly observed distal subungual onychomycosis. The organism first infects the skin, then the subungual nail matrix. The accumulation of subungual keratin leads to separation of the nail plate from the nail matrix. The nail plate is infected only secondarily. The *T. rubrum* fungus is also responsible for the proximal subungual onychomycosis. Superficial onychomycosis, a white discoloration of the surface of the nail plate, is caused by *Trichophyton mentagrophytes*. The presence of pus in association with onychomycosis is almost diagnostic of a candidal yeast infection. Candidal infections are frequently found in association with psoriasis or diabetes mellitus. Treatment of onychomycosis with the oral antifungals, such as griseofulvin, takes as long as $1\frac{1}{2}$ years.

Onychocryptosis (Ingrowing Toenail)

Constricting shoes and socks made of synthetic materials together with poor foot hygiene contribute to the production of ingrown toenails.[165] Microtrauma to the tips of the toes, development of excessive curvature of the nail plate in the older person, and improper trimming of toenails are additional contributory factors. The toenails should be cut straight across rather than cutting off the corners, which encourages symptomatic regrowth into the lateral nail grooves.

Three stages of progression have been described. In stage 1 there is painful irritation about the embedded nail plate, which has penetrated into the lateral nail groove. Stage 2 is characterized by an overt infection with granulation tissue and moist discharge. Stage 3 is identified by the growth of epithelium over the chronic granulation tissue of the deeply embedded nail plate.

Conservative care consists of warm saline soaks twice daily. A cotton pledget is placed under the corner of the nail, elevating it from the lateral groove. The cotton wool is changed frequently and the nail encouraged to grow clear of the embedded area. When it has grown beyond the danger area, it is important that the toenail be cut transversely to prevent recurrence. The nail will grow at a rate of 2 mm per month.

Surgical options include partial ablation of the nail plate, complete ablation of the nail plate with excision of the lateral granulation tissue, partial onychectomy (excision of the lateral germinal matrix responsible for production of the edge of nail that irritates the lateral groove), or complete onychectomy.

Other Nail Disorders

Onychogryphosis is a condition in which the nail becomes thickened and will grow to resemble a ram's horn if left uncut. Trauma is probably the precipitating agent. Radical excision of the nail bed is the treatment of choice.

Subungual exostosis is a benign tumor of bone occurring in the distal phalanx beneath the nail. X-rays confirm the presence of the bony exostosis. There are various theories concerning the etiology of this condition.[166,167] On histologic examination, the lesion resembles an osteochondroma. It occurs a little distal from the nail bed, so that after removal of the nail plate and complete removal of the excess bone, a new nail grows in a satisfactory fashion. If the germinal matrix is involved, however, it has to be reflected away from the tumor during its removal. If this is done with care and the matrix is then replaced, a relatively normal nail is possible.

PES CAVUS AND PES PLANUS

Pes Cavus

Cavus deformities of the foot are characterized by a high longitudinal arch. The two principal cavus deformities are the cavovarus and calcaneocavus deformities. Although there are a number of diseases that produce the cavus foot, the deformities arise as a result of muscular imbalances.

Cavovarus Deformity

The prominent features of a cavovarus foot are plantarflexion of the first ray, pronation and adduction of the forefoot, and hindfoot varus. Weakness of the tibialis anterior relative to the peroneus longus results in plantarflexion of the first ray. Forefoot adduction and hindfoot varus facilitate weight bearing on the lateral foot and hindfoot in the presence of a plantarflexed first ray. Weakness of the peroneus brevis further accentuates the hindfoot varus deformity. Compensation for the weak tibialis anterior by the long toe extensors (acting as an ankle dorsiflexor), in conjunction with weakness of the intrinsics, leads to clawing of the toes. Cavovarus deformities are commonly found in hereditary motor and sensory neuropathy type I (type I Charcot-Marie-Tooth disease), spinocerebellar degeneration (Friedreich's ataxia), cerebral palsy, and as a residual deformity following clubfoot correction or compartment syndrome of the leg. The exact pattern of muscular imbalance that produces the cavovarus deformity differs for each of these conditions.[169,173]

Evaluation of the cavovarus deformity should include assessment of the flexibility of the deformity with manual testing. Hindfoot flexibility may be assessed with the Coleman block test, in which the patient stands with the heel and lateral half of the affected foot supported by a 1-in block, allowing the first metatarsal to hang free. With a flexible hindfoot deformity, the heel varus should correct when the patient is standing on the block.[170]

Nonsurgical treatment of cavovarus deformities with footwear modification is effective only for mild deformities. Selection of surgical treatment depends on the flexibility of the deformity, the age of the patient, and the underlying condition. Soft tissue procedures may be successful in treating flexible deformities. A medial plantar release (abductor hallucis, short toe flexors, and plantar fascia) may be useful in the young patient with a flexible hindfoot varus deformity.[168] Metatarsal osteotomies or the Dwyer (lateral calcaneal closing wedge) osteotomy may be indicated for more rigid deformities. A triple arthrodesis is often necessary in the rigid, mature foot.[168,169,171,172]

Calcaneocavus Deformity

Polio is the most common cause of the calcaneocavus deformity, although other causes include type II Charcot-Marie-Tooth disease and spina bifida. Cerebral palsy and Friedreich's ataxia are associated with both cavovarus and calcaneocavus deformities. Weakness of the triceps surae leads to the calcaneocavus deformity, in which a high longitudinal arch is the result of a dorsiflexed calcaneus and a plantarflexed forefoot. This has been described as a "pistol-grip" deformity. There is frequently associated clawing of toes. Calluses may develop beneath the heel pad. On standing lateral radiographs, the inclination of the calcaneus measured with respect to the floor (calcaneal pitch) measures greater than 30°.

The young, asymptomatic patient without bony deformities will usually progress and ultimately require treatment. Tendon transfers, including the posterior tibialis and peroneals to the os calcis, have been described, although subtalar or triple arthrodeses may be necessary to stabilize the foot.

Pes Planus

Pes planus or flatfoot involves loss of the longitudinal arch and encompasses a variety of disorders in children and adults. Associated deformities include subtalar subluxation, valgus heel, abduction of the midfoot, and forefoot supination. In the pediatric population, congenital vertical talus, tarsal coalition (associated with peroneal spastic flatfoot), and accessory navicular are common causes. Idiopathic flexible pes planus is not uncommmon and may correct spontaneously. Semirigid full-length longitudinal arch supports or orthotics should be utilized only if they provide symptomatic relief. Wenger has prospectively found no significant benefit of either "corrective shoes" or orthotics in treating flexible flatfoot in normal children.[174] Adult-acquired flatfoot is associated with a variety of degenerative conditions including posterior tibial tendon dysfunction, talonavicular arthritis, and diabetic neuroarthropathy. Specific treatment of these entities is discussed in Chap. 53.

METATARSALGIA

Introduction

Metatarsalgia is a descriptive term that refers to the presence of pain beneath the MTP joints of the lesser toes. The etiologies are numerous and encompass a spectrum of disease processes.[160] One common source of metatarsalgia is the development of claw- or hammertoe, which leads to the dorsal subluxation of the proximal phalanges and associated distal migration of the plantar fat pads from beneath the metatarsal heads. Painful plantar callosities may then develop beneath the metatarsal heads. This topic was discussed previously. This section focuses on other common etiologies of metatarsalgia.

Freiberg's Infraction

The second metatarsal head is most commonly the site of avascular necrosis affecting a metatarsal head, attributable to its longer length.[175] There is speculation that repetitive stresses and microfractures lead to compromise of its blood supply.[125] Symptoms include activity-related pain that is localized to the metatarsal head. Painful limitation of motion is usually noted on physical exam. Plain films may be normal early in the disease process, although the more sensitive bone scan or MRI study will reveal changes consistent with avascular necrosis. The natural history of the disease is variable and can range from resolution with little deformity to progressive destruction of the metatarsal head. The resulting head may be irregular or flattened.

Treatment of the acute phase involves immobilization of the joint with a stiff-soled shoe postoperatively or a short leg cast. Intraarticular steroid injections may provide some pain relief. Surgical options include synovectomy, debridement of the MTP joint, DuVries arthroplasty, or a dorsal closing wedge osteotomy through the metatarsal neck if the volar portion of the head is relatively spared.[175,177]

Interdigital Neuroma

The presence of an interdigital (Morton's) neuroma between two of the lesser toes must be considered in the evaluation of metatarsalgia.[160] The most common presenting symptom is burning plantar foot pain in the involved intermetatarsal forefoot region exacerbated by weight bearing.[178] The incidence of Morton's neuroma is highest among middle-aged females, usually presenting unilaterally (85 percent) and occurring in the 3 to 4 interspace (45 percent) more frequently than the 2 to 3 interspace (37 percent).[178,192] The incidence of simultaneous neuromas in the same foot is rare (less than 4 percent).[184,188] Ill-fitting high-heeled shoes provoking increased intermetatarsophalangeal pressures[182] place women at higher risk for the development of a "neuroma" or entrapment of the third branch of the medial plantar nerve (third web space) as it courses beneath the transverse intermetatarsal ligament.[191] Examination should attempt to differentiate MTP and metatarsal head symptomatology from those symptoms originating from the intermetatarsal spaces just proximal to the metatarsal heads.[160] Gentle compression of the foot across the forefoot, simulating a "tight shoe," is used to elicit a Mulder's click or sign, which tends to reproduce the patient's pain dramatically in the involved web space.[190,192] Weight-bearing x-rays are obtained to help exclude other causes of metatarsalgia. While MRI and ultrasonography have been shown to document the location of a neuroma, these studies are rarely indicated.[186] Likewise, electrodiagnostic testing has not proved to be clinically diagnostic. Conservative treatment should include appropriate accommodative footwear that provides an adequate intermetatarsal girth and a relatively rigid sole in an attempt to limit MTP hyperextension on weight bearing. Additionally, a metatarsal bar provided by a soft insert or orthotic is typically used to relieve pressure in the symptomatic intermetatarsal region.[187,192] Intermetatarsal bursal injection of steroids has not proved to be clinically efficacious, noting only a 30 percent "cure" rate at 2 years after a series of injections.[189] Inadvertent steroid injections into the adjacent MTP capsular region may provoke attenuation and rupture of collateral supporting structures of the MTP joint, resulting in toe divergence and metatarsalgia as well as plantar fatpad atrophy.

Should conservative methods fail, a diagnostic lidocaine injection directed into the symptomatic web space is indicated.[192] Both dorsal or plantar longitudinal approaches for primary surgical excision of neuroma and division of the transverse intermetatarsal ligament have been advocated.[178,179] However, most authors favor an initial dorsal approach and a secondary plantar approach only if the patient presents with a recalcitrant stump neuroma.[178,180,181] Plantar digital nerve tethering has been advanced as a potential cause for failure of the stump neuroma to adequately retract proximally after excision of the neuroma.[183,185]

HEEL PAIN

Proximal (Insertional) Plantar Fasciitis

Plantar heel pain may be caused by a variety of conditions, the most common of which is proximal plantar fasciitis (PPF) or heel pain syndrome (Fig. 54-21). The plantar fascia is a dense sheet of connective tissue that originates from the medial calcaneal tuberosity and inserts in multiple slips on the bases of the proximal phalanges and flexor tendon sheaths. This fascia lies immediately plantar to the superficial layers of muscles: the abductor hallucis, the flexor digitorum brevis, and the abductor digiti quinti. The medial and lateral plantar nerves pass between these superficial muscles and the quadratus plantae. The first branch of the lateral plantar nerve innervates the region of the medial calcaneal tuberosity, the site of maximal tenderness.[194,200]

The etiology of plantar fasciitis is not well understood but is generally thought to be related to degeneration and microtearing of the origin of the plantar fascia at the medial calcaneal tuberosity.[193,194] An acute injury may be the precipitating event that initiates the process of inflammation and injury at this location, but frequently no specific traumatic event can be recalled. Patients typically report pain that is worse for the first few steps upon arising in the morning. This is thought to be a result of the equinus posturing of the foot during sleep and the resulting microtearing and inflammation that is reinitiated with the first few steps in the morning. Pain is also worse upon rising after long periods of rest. Obesity, occupations involving prolonged standing, long-distance running, or hyperpronated feet have all been associated with plantar fasciitis.[194] There is no causal relationship between the presence of calcaneal spurs that lie anatomically within the origin of the flexor digitorum brevis muscle and heel pain. Calcaneal spurs, however may form as a result of chronic periostitis of the calcaneus at the origin of the plantar fascia.[194,201]

On physical examination, there is maximal tenderness at the medial plantar aspect of the calcaneal tuberosity. This is the most important finding in making a diagnosis of proximal plantar fasciitis.[193,194] Radiographs may reveal the presence of a calcaneal spur originating from the origin of the flexor digitorum brevis muscle in 50 percent of patients with PPF. A bone scan will frequently be useful in supporting the diagnosis of PPF, although the diagnosis is made primarily on clinical grounds. A two-phase bone scan may show uptake in the area of the medial calcaneal tuberosity in the early phase as a result of the increased blood flow associated with inflammation and in the later phases associated with periosteal reaction.

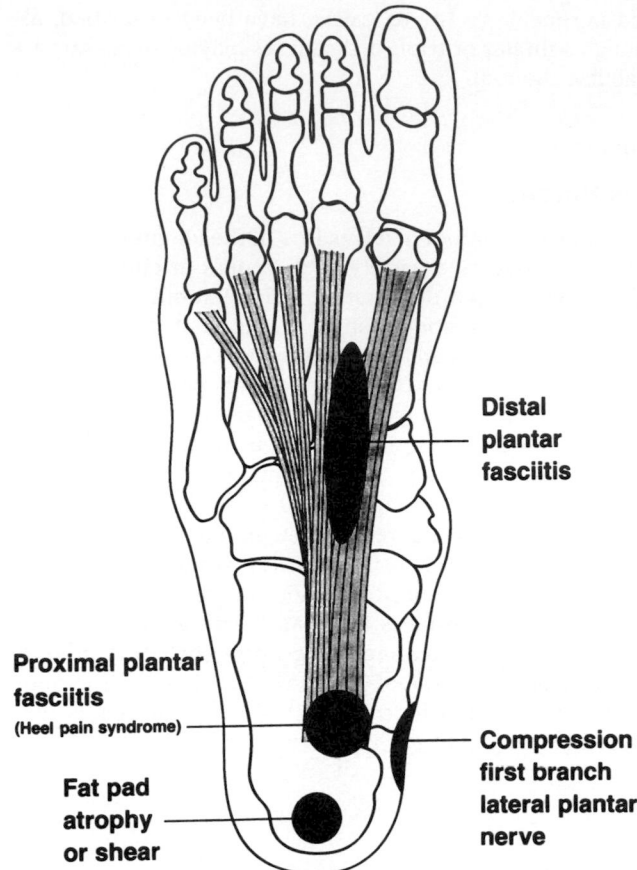

Figure 54-21 Areas of maximal plantar tenderness in plantar heel pain. (Adapted with permission from Dreeben SM, Mann RA: Heel pain: Sorting through the differential diagnosis. *J Musculoskel Med* 9:21–37, 1992.)

Conservative treatment involves the use of multiple modalities including heel cushions, NSAIDs, physical therapy emphasizing stretching the heel cord and plantar fascia, and night splinting. This regimen is effective in treating PPF in 95 percent of cases, although up to a year of conservative therapy may be required to allow the disease to run its course.[202,204] The ineffectiveness of nonsurgical treatment, however, has been noted in a recent outcome study.[210] Steroid injections may be a helpful adjunct to the above regimen, but potential complications include fatpad atrophy from misplaced injections and acute plantar fascial rupture.[199,203,206] The latter may have an effect similar to that of surgical release of the plantar fascia and should be treated with rest and immobilization in a cast. Recalcitrant PPF may be treated with a nighttime AFO positioned in neutral or slight dorsiflexion and/or a short leg walking cast.[197,208,210]

Surgical treatment of PPF is controversial and should be undertaken only after failure of conservative therapy for 6 months to 1 year.[194–196,198,199] The most common surgical procedure is a release of the partial plantar fascia with or without spur excision performed through a medial or oblique incision.[196,198,205,207] A variety of surgical procedures have been described, however, ranging from partial to complete plantar fascia release to resection.[194,200] Removal of 1 cm of the medial slip of the plantar fascia adjacent to the medial calcaneal tuberosity effectively decompresses the nerve to the abductor digiti quinti.[198,209] Complications include flattening of the longitudinal arch, leading to metatarsalgia and injury to the medial calcaneal nerve.[194,199]

Heel-Pad Atrophy

The subcalcaneal heel pad is a fat pad penetrated by an intricate network of fibrous septa running between the periosteum of the calcaneus and the thick plantar skin. These septa contain and support the adipose tissue that protects the inferior calcaneal surface. Atrophy of the heel pad is thought to be a degenerative process that accompanies aging, although it is also a reported complication of local steroid injections.

The pain of heel-pad atrophy is typically worse with walking and standing and is exacerbated with the use of hard-soled shoes. Treatment involves the use of supportive heel cups in an attempt to redistribute and contain the heel pad beneath the calcaneus. Full length semirigid longitudinal arch supports may help redistribute plantar heel pressures.

Tarsal Tunnel Syndrome

Tarsal tunnel syndrome is an entrapment neuropathy of the posterior tibial nerve and its terminal branches beneath the flexor retinaculum or laciniate ligament, which spans from the medial malleolus anteriorly and attaches to the medial wall of the calcaneus posteroinferiorly and the superior fascial border of the abductor hallucis[192,221] (Fig. 54-22). In order to comprehend the anatomic causes of tarsal tunnel syndrome adequately, it is imperative to understand the anterior or dorsal boundary of the tunnel. Proximally, the posterior aspect of the tibia lies along the anterior boundary, including the posterior recesses of the ankle joint and the os trigonum (the unfused lateral tubercle of the posterior talar process). At this level, the medial calcaneal branch is usually given off, which provides sensation to the heel pad. In the hindfoot, the posterior tibial nerve usually divides into medial and lateral plantar nerves at a point within 0 to 2 cm of an imaginary line that connects the tip of the medial malleolus and the calcaneus. Superiorly in this region, the sustentaculum tali lies adjacent to the medial plantar nerve, and the lateral plantar nerve lies inferiorly along the medial border of the calcaneus. Finally, in the midfoot, the anterior/dorsal boundary of the tunnel is formed by the master knot of Henry, which secures the flexor digitorum longus crossing superficially over the flexor hallucis longus to the medial longitudinal arch of the foot.[212,217,218,220]

Typical symptoms of tarsal tunnel syndrome include a diffuse burning pain associated with dysesthesias that radiate along the distribution of the medial and lateral plantar nerves. The symptoms are usually aggravated by weight bearing, especially on a hyperpronated foot.[211,213–215] Any marked varus or valgus posturing of the hindfoot may be associated with conformational changes in the cross-sectional area of the tarsal tunnel. As with carpal tunnel syndrome, patients frequently complain of worsening pain at night. Examination may include a positive Tinel's percussion test over the tarsal tunnel or a positive tunnel compression test. Masses that are palpable should be transilluminated, and an MRI is useful to define the origin and extent of solid masses anatomically.[216] Sensory nerve conduction velocity (NCV) testing of the medial and lateral plantar nerves is probably the most accurate method.[192] Fibrillation potentials in either the abductor hallucis (medial plantar nerve) or the abductor digiti quinti (lateral plantar nerve) muscles would denote a more advanced compression neuropathy. The peroneal nerve should be evaluated by NCV to rule out a more diffuse peripheral neuropathy.

Conservative management is based on treating the provoking cause. An AFO may control any hindfoot varus or valgus posturing. Compression stockings or a mechanical edema pump may control peripheral edema. Space-occupying masses that may require excision include "soft" masses such as ganglia and lipoma or "hard" masses such as nonunited fractures of the sustentaculum tali and posterior process of talus. Surgical decompression is indicated if the clinical complaints, examination, and nerve conduction study all support the diagnosis of tarsal tunnel syndrome.

Alternatively, if two of the above criteria are met, cautious decompression in selected patients may also be beneficial.[192] Clearly, those patients with well-defined anatomic lesions have a more predictably positive outcome than those in whom no specific pathology is identified.[192,221] Reexploration of the tarsal tunnel is seldom beneficial unless it is clear than an inadequate decompression was initially performed.[219]

Other Etiologies of Heel Pain

Calcaneal pain may arise from stress fractures, particularly on the medial side of the plantar aspect of the calcaneus. Such patients will have a positive bone scan. A radiologic technique has also been described to demonstrate the stress fracture. This involves having the patient stand on the cassette and angling the x-ray tube 45° to the cassette on the medial side of the foot.[195] Several grades of stress fracture may be seen, from a slight protrusion or indentation to a complete break. Treatment should involve continuation of conservative measures if a stress fracture has been diagnosed as the etiology of the heel pain.

Haglund syndrome involves painful swelling of the soft tissues of the posterior heel just anterior and superior to the Achilles tendon insertion, associated with lateral calcaneal bursitis and Achilles tendinitis. Radiology confirms a prominent posterosuperior border of the calcaneus. Other factors implicated in this diagnosis have included the presence of a step on the posterior surface of the bone, Achilles tendon calcification, and an increased calcaneal pitch (which brings the prominent posterosu-

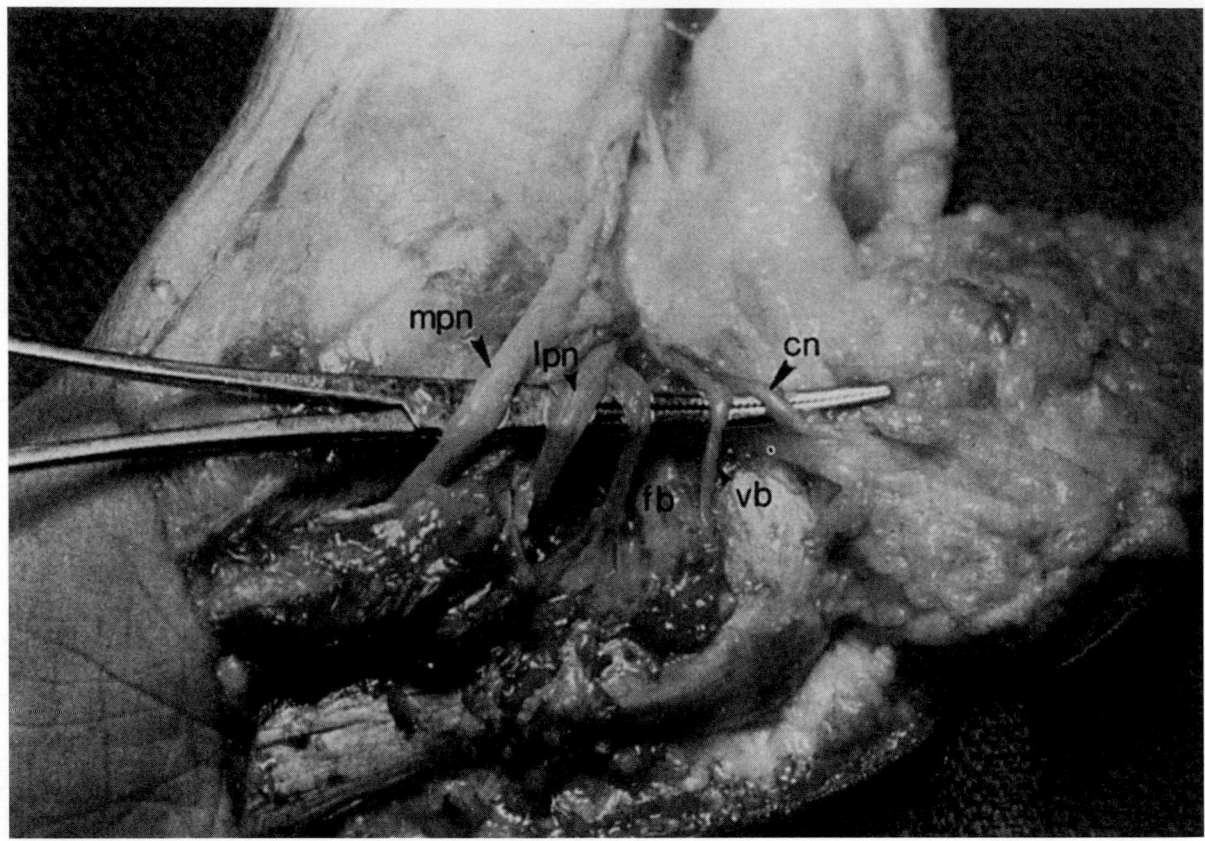

Figure 54-22 The branches of the tibial nerve are demonstrated. Infrequently, a variant branch (vb) is identified. [Reproduced with permission from Schon LC: Plantar fasciitis: Heel pain, in Pfeffer GB, Frey CC (eds): *Current Practice in Foot and Ankle Surgery.* New York, McGraw-Hill, 1993, pp 243–261.]

perior portion of the calcaneus into a position to provoke a retrocalcaneal bursitis). Heel elevation has been advised to relieve this abnormal pitch angle.[222] Excision of the bony prominence is occasionally required (see "Ankle" in Chap. 53).

Sever's disease involves pain in the region of the heel associated with localized tenderness in the region of the calcaneal apophysis, together with x-ray findings of fragmentation and sclerosis. The calcaneal apophysis, which normally develops between the fifth and twelfth years, characteristically does so in an irregular fashion. This region serves as attachment for the Achilles tendon superiorly and for the plantar fascia and short muscles of the sole of the foot inferiorly; it may often be the site of pain and tenderness.[223] An irregular, dense apophysis is a normal finding in healthy children, whether they have painful heels or not. Neither density of the apophysis nor its apparent fragmentation can consequently be related to the cause of heel pain.[224] It has been suggested that a strain in Sharpey's fibers, which attach the tendons and fascia to the calcaneal apophysis, may be responsible for the symptoms.[225] Rest usually relieves symptoms.

Finally, the development of heel pain is common in patients with inflammatory arthritis, particularly seronegative spondyloarthropathy. Some 90 percent of such patients will have evidence of HLA-B27 antigens.[226]

REFERENCES

1. Rieber GE: Diabetic foot care: Financial implications and practice guidelines. *Diabetes Care* 15:29–31, 1992.
2. DCCT Research Group: Diabetes control and complications trial (DCCT) update. *Diabetes Care* 13:427, 1990.
3. Pirart J: Diabetes mellitus and its degenerative complications: A prospective study of 4400 patients observed between 1947 and 1973. *Diabetes Care* 1:168, 1978.
4. Brayton RG, Stokes PE, Schwartz MS, et al: Effect of alcohol and various diseases on leukocyte mobilization, phagocytosis, and intracellular bacterial killing. *N Engl J Med* 282:123–128, 1970.
5. Fortes ZB, Farsky SP, Oliviera MA, et al: Direct vital microscopic study of defective leukocyte-endothelial interaction in diabetes mellitus. *Diabetes* 40:1267–1273, 1991.
6. Leichter SB, Allweiss P, Harley J, et al: Clinical characteristics of diabetic patients with serious pedal infections. *Metab Clin Exp* 37(2 suppl 1):22–24, 1988.
7. Levin S: Digest of current literature. *Infect Dis Clin Pract* 1:49–50, 1992.
8. Wang A, Weinstein D, Greenfield L, et al: MRI and diabetic foot infections. *Magn Reson Imaging* 8:805–809, 1990.
9. American Diabetes Association: *1985 Fact Sheet on Diabetes.* Alexandria, VA, American Diabetes Association, 1985.
10. Karanfilian RG, Lynch TG, Zirul VT, et al: The value of laser Doppler velocimetry and transcutaneous oxygen tension determination in predicting healing of ischemic forefoot ulcer-

ations and amputations in diabetic and nondiabetic patients. *J Vasc Surg* 4:511–520, 1986.

11. Myerson M: Amputations of the midfoot and hindfoot, in Myerson M (ed): *Current Therapy in Foot and Ankle Surgery.* St Louis, Mosby–Year Book, 1993.

12. Brodsky JW: The diabetic foot, in Mann RA, Coughlin MJ (eds): *Surgery of the Foot and Ankle,* 6th ed. St Louis, Mosby, 1993, pp 1361–1467.

13. Gupta R: A short history of neuropathic arthropathy. *Clin Orthop Rel Res* 296:43–49, 1993.

14. Eichenholtz SN: *Charcot Joints.* Springfield, IL, Charles C Thomas, 1966.

15. Myerson M, Papa J, Eaton K, et al: The total-contact cast for management of neuropathic plantar ulceration of the foot. *J Bone Joint Surg* 74A:261–269, 1992.

16. Papa J, Myerson M, Girard P: Salvage with arthrodesis in intractable diabetic neuropathic arthropathy of the foot and ankle. *J Bone Joint Surg* 75A:1056–1066, 1993.

17. Brand PW: The insensitive foot (including leprosy), in Jahss MH (ed): *Disorders of the Foot and Ankle.* Philadelphia, Saunders, 1991, pp 2171–2178.

18. McDermott JE: *The Diabetic Foot.* Rosemont, IL, American Association of Orthopaedic Surgeons, 1995.

19. Laughlin RT, Calhoun JH, Mader JT: The diabetic foot. *J Am Acad Orthop Surg* 3:218–225, 1995.

20. Harrelson JM: Management of the diabetic foot. *Orthop Clin North Am* 20:605–619, 1989.

21. Weaver FM, Bundi MD, Pinzur MS: Outpatient foot care: Correlation to amputation level. *Foot Ankle Int* 15:498–501, 1994.

22. Brodsky JW: Outpatient diagnosis and care of the diabetic foot. *Inst Course Lect* 42:121–139, 1993.

23. Pedowitz WJ: The malodorous foot. *Foot Ankle Int* 17:54–55, 1996.

24. Oyen WJ, Netten PM, Lemmens JA, et al: Evaluation of infectious diabetic foot complications with Indium-111-labeled human nonspecific immunoglobulin G. *J Nucl Med* 33:1330–1336, 1992.

25. Weinstein D, Wang A, Chambers R, et al: Evaluation of magnetic resonance imaging in the diagnosis of osteomyelitis in diabetic foot infections. *Foot Ankle* 14:18–22, 1993.

26. Levine SE, Neagle CE, Esterhai JL, et al: Magnetic resonance imaging for the diagnosis of osteomyelitis in the diabetic patient with a foot ulcer. *Food Ankle Int* 15:151–156, 1994.

27. Johnson JE, Kennedy EJ, Shereff MJ, et al: Prospective study of bone, Indium-111-labeled white blood cells, and gallium-67 scanning for the evaluation of osteomyelitis in the diabetic foot. *Foot Ankle Int* 17:10–16, 1996.

28. Pinzur MS, Sage R, Stuck R, et al: Transcutaneous oxygen as a predictor of wound healing in amputations of the foot and ankle. *Foot Ankle* 13:271–272, 1992.

29. Pinzur MS, Stuck R, Sage R, et al: Transcutaneous oxygen tension in the dysvascular foot with infection. *Foot Ankle* 14:254–256, 1993.

30. Larson J, Apelqvist J, Castenfors J, et al: Distal blood pressure as a predictor for the level of amputation in diabetic patients with foot ulcer. *Foot Ankle* 14:247–253, 1993.

31. Smith DG, Boyd EJ, Ahroni JH, et al: Paradoxical transcutaneous oxygen response to cutaneous warming on the plantar foot surface: A caution for interpretation of plantar $TCPO_2$ measurements. *Foot Ankle Int* 16:787–792, 1995.

32. Garbalosa JC, Cavanagh PR, Wu G, et al: Foot function in diabetic patients after partial amputation. *Foot Ankle Int* 17:43–48, 1996.

33. Laughlin RT, Chambers RB: Syme amputation in patients with severe diabetes mellitus. *Foot Ankle* 14:65–70, 1993.

34. Smith DG, Sangeorzan BJ, Hansen ST, et al: Achilles tendon tenodesis to prevent heel pad migration in the Syme's amputation. *Foot Ankle Int* 15:14–17, 1994.

35. Apelqvist J, Ragnarson-Tennvall G, Larsson J, et al: Long term costs for foot ulcers in diabetic patients in a multidisciplinary setting. *Foot Ankle Int* 16:388–394, 1995.

36. Michelson JD: Treatment of diabetic ulcers by total contact casting. *Op Tech Orthop* 4:190–195, 1994.

37. Slavens ER, Slavens ML: Therapeutic footwear for neurotrophic ulcers. *Foot Ankle Int* 16:663–666, 1995.

38. Larson J, Agardh LD, Apelqvist J, et al: Clinical characteristics in relation to final amputation level in diabetics with foot ulcers: A prospective study of healing below or above the ankle in 187 patients. *Foot Ankle Int* 16:69–74, 1995.

39. Wagner FW Jr: A classification and treatment program for diabetic, neuropathic and dysvascular foot problems. *Instr Course Lect* 28:143–165, 1979.

40. Woll TS, Beals RK: Partial calcanectomy for the treatment of osteomyelitis of the calcaneus. *Foot Ankle* 12:31–34, 1991.

41. Kaye RA: The extra depth toe box: A rational approach. *Foot Ankle Int* 15:146–150, 1994.

42. Jacobs RL, Karmody AM: Treatment of the diabetic foot with exposed os calcis. *Foot Ankle* 1:173–178, 1980.

43. Johnson JTH: Neuropathic fractures and joint injuries: Pathogenesis and rationale of prevention and treatment. *J Bone Joint Surg* 49A:1–30, 1967.

44. Cofield RH, Morrison MJ, Beabout JW: Diabetic neuroarthropathy in the foot: Patient characteristics and patterns of radiographic change. *Foot Ankle* 4:15–22, 1983.

45. Clohisy DR, Thompson RC Jr: Fractures associated with neuropathic arthropathy in adults who have juvenile-onset diabetes. *J Bone Joint Surg* 70A:1192–1200, 1988.

46. Stuart MJ, Morrey BF: Arthrodesis of the diabetic neuropathic ankle joint. *Clin Orthop Rel Res* 253:209–211, 1990.

47. Brodsky JW: Management of Charcot joints of the foot and ankle in diabetes. *Semin Arthrop* 3:58–62, 1992.

48. Myerson M: Arthrodesis for diabetic neuroarthropathy, In Myerson M (ed): *Current Therapy in Foot and Ankle Surgery.* St Louis, Mosby, 1993, pp 116–122.

49. Pinzur MS, Sage R, Stuck R, et al: A treatment algorithm for neuropathic (Charcot) midfoot deformity. *Foot Ankle* 14:189–197, 1993.

50. Bono JV, Roger DL, Jacobs RL: Surgical arthrodesis of the neuropathic foot. *Clin Orthop Rel Res* 296:14–20, 1993.

51. Saltzman CA, Johnson KA, Goldstein RH, et al: The patellar tendon–bearing brace as a treatment for neuroarthropathy: A dynamic force-monitoring study. *Foot Ankle* 13:14–21, 1993.

52. Harrelson JM: The diabetic foot: Charcot arthropathy. *Instr Course Lect* 42:141–146, 1993.

53. Myerson MS, Henderson MR, Saxby T, Short KW: Management of midfoot diabetic neuroarthropathy. *Foot Ankle Int* 15:233–241, 1994.

54. Holmes GB, Hill N: Fractures and dislocations of the foot and ankle in diabetics associated with Charcot joint changes. *Foot Ankle Int* 15:182–185, 1994.

55. Tisdel CL, Marcus RE, Heiple KG: Triple arthrodesis for diabetic peritalar neuroarthropathy. *Foot Ankle Int* 16:332–338, 1995.

56. Schon LC, Marks RM: The management of neuroarthropathic fracture-dislocations in the diabetic patient. *Orthop Clin North Am* 26:375–392, 1995.

57. Alpert SW, Koval KJ, Zuckerman JD: Neuropathic arthropathy: Review of current knowledge. *J Am Acad Orthop Surg* 4:100–108, 1996.

58. Scranton PE Jr: Current concepts review, principles in bunion surgery. *J Bone Joint Surg* 65A:1026–1028, 1983.

59. Pedowitz WJ: Deformities of the first ray, in Lutter LD, Mizel MS, Pfeffer GB (eds): *Orthopaedic Knowledge Update: Foot and Ankle.* Rosemont, IL, American Academy of Orthopaedic Surgeons, 1994, pp 141–162.

60. Miller JW: Acquired hallux varus: A preventable and correctable disorder. *J Bone Joint Surg* 57A:183–187, 1975.

61. Alvarez R, Haddad RJ, Gould N, Trevino S: The simple bunion: Anatomy at the metatarsophalangeal joint of the great toe. *Foot Ankle* 4:229–240, 1984.

62. Mann RA, Coughlin MJ: Adult hallux valgus, in Mann RA, Coughlin MJ (eds): *Surgery of the Foot and Ankle.* Vol 1. St Louis, Mosby, 1993, pp 167–296.

63. Piggott H: The natural history of hallux valgus in adolescence and early adult life. *J Bone Joint Surg [Br]* 42:749–760, 1960.

64. Hardy RH, Clapham JCR: Observations on hallux valgus. *J Bone Joint Surg* 33B:376–391, 1951.

65. Pedowitz W: Bunion deformity, in Pfeffer G, Frey C (eds): *Current Practice in Foot and Ankle Surgery.* New York, McGraw-Hill, 1993, pp 219–242.

66. Mann RA: Decision-making in bunion surgery. *Instr Course Lect* 39:3–13, 1990.

67. McBride ED: The surgical treatment of hallux valgus in bunions. *Am J Orthop* 5:44–46, 1963.

68. Mann RA: Hallux valgus. *Instr Course Lect* 31:180–200, 1982.

69. Jahss MH, Troy AI, Kummer F: Roentgenographic and mathematical analysis of first metatarsal osteotomies for metatarsus primus varus: A comparative study. *Foot Ankle* 5:280–321, 1985.

70. Lapidus PW: Dorsal bunion, its mechanics and operative correction. *J Bone Joint Surg* 22:627–636, 1940.

71. McKay DW: Dorsal bunions in children. *J Bone Joint Surg* 65A:975–980, 1983.

72. Scranton PE, Zuckerman JD: Bunion surgery in adolescents: Results of surgical treatment. *J Pediatr Orthop* 4:39–43, 1984.

73. Coughlin MJ: Juvenile hallux valgus: Etiology and treatment. *Foot Ankle Int* 16:698–704, 1995.

74. Harris RI, Beath T: The short first metatarsal, its clinical incidence and clinical significance. *J Bone Joint Surg* 31A:553–565, 1949.

75. Richardson EG, Graves SC, McLure JH, et al: First metatarsal head shaft angle: A method of determination. *Foot Ankle* 14:181–185, 1993.

76. Vittetoe DA, Saltzman CL, Krieg JC, et al: Validity and reliability of the distal metatarsal articular angle. *Foot Ankle Int* 15:541–547, 1994.

77. Austin DW, Leventen EO: A new osteotomy for hallux valgus: A horizontally directed "V" displacement osteotomy of the first metatarsal head for hallux valgus and primus varus. *Clin Orthop Rel Res* 157:25–30, 1981.

78. Johnson KA: Chevron osteotomy of the first metatarsal: Patient selection and technique. *Contemp Orthop* 3:707–711, 1981.

79. Shereff M, Yang Q, Kummer F: Extraosseous and intraosseous arterial supply to the first metatarsal and metatarsophalangeal joint. *Foot Ankle* 8:81–93, 1987.

80. Johnson J, Clanton T, Baxter D: Comparison of Chevron osteotomy and modified McBride bunionectomy for correction of mild to moderate hallux valgus deformities. *Foot Ankle* 12:61–68, 1991.

81. Peterson DA, Zilberfarb JL, Greene MA, et al: Avascular necrosis of the first metatarsal head: Incidence in distal osteotomy combined with lateral soft tissue release. *Foot Ankle Int* 15:59–63, 1994.

82. Donnelly RE, Saltzman CL, Kile TA, Johnson KA: Modified Chevron osteotomy for hallux valgus. *Foot Ankle Int* 15:642–645, 1994.

83. Pochatko DJ, Schlehr RJ, Murphey MD, et al: Distal Chevron osteotomy with lateral release for treatment of hallux valgus deformity. *Foot Ankle Int* 15:457–461, 1994.

84. Thomas RL, Espinosa FJ, Richardson EG: Radiographic changes in the first metatarsal head after distal Chevron osteotomy combined with lateral release through a plantar approach. *Foot Ankle Int* 15:285–292, 1994.

85. Mitchell LA, Baxter DE: A Chevron-Akin double osteotomy for correction of hallux valgus. *Foot Ankle* 12:7–14, 1991.

86. Mann RA, Rudicel S, Graves SC: Repair of hallux valgus with a distal soft tissue procedure and proximal metatarsal osteotomy: A long term follow-up. *J Bone Joint Surg* 74A:124–129, 1992.

87. Granberry WM, Hickey CH: Hallux valgus correction with metatarsal osteotomy: Effect of lateral distal soft tissue procedure. *Foot Ankle Int* 16:132–138, 1995.

88. Easley ME, Kiebzak GM, Davis WH, et al: Prospective, randomized comparison of proximal crescentic and proximal Chevron osteotomies for correction of hallux valgus deformity. *Foot Ankle Int* 17:307–316, 1996.

89. Dreenan S, Mann RA: Advanced hallux valgus deformity: Long term results utilizing the distal soft tissue procedure and proximal metatarsal osteotomy. *Foot Ankle Int* 17:142–144, 1996.

90. Juliano PJ, Myerson MS, Cunningham BW: Biomechanical assessment of a new tenodesis for correction of hallux varus. *Foot Ankle Int* 17:17–20, 1996.

91. Myerson MS, Komenda GA: Results of hallux varus correction using an extensor hallucis brevis tenodesis. *Foot Ankle Int* 17:21–27, 1996.

92. Tourne Y, Saragaglia D, Picard F, et al: Iatrogenic hallux varus surgical procedure: A study of 14 cases. *Foot Ankle Int* 16:457–463, 1995.

93. Johnson KA, Spiegl PV: Extensor hallucis longus transfer for hallux varus deformity. *J Bone Joint Surg* 66A:681–686, 1984.

94. Frey C, Jahss MH, Kummer FJ: The Akin procedure: An analysis of results. *Foot Ankle* 12:1–6, 1991.

95. McGarvey SR: Internal fixation of the Akin osteotomy. *Foot Ankle Int* 16:172–173, 1995.

96. Blum JL: The modified Mitchell osteotomy-bunionectomy: Indications and technical considerations. *Foot Ankle Int* 15:103–106, 1994.

97. Mann RA, Chou LB: Surgical management for intractable metatarsalgia. *Foot Ankle Int* 16:322–327, 1995.

98. Sangeorzan BJ, Hansen ST: Modified lapidus procedure for hallux valgus. *Foot Ankle* 9:262–266, 1989.

99. Myerson M, Allon S, McGarvey W: Metatarso-cuneiform arthrodesis for management of hallux valgus and metatarsus primus varus. *Foot Ankle* 13:107–115, 1992.

100. Fritz GR, Prieskorn D: First metatarsal cuneiform motion: A radiographic and statistical analysis. *Foot Ankle Int* 16:117–123, 1995.

101. Coughlin MJ, Mann RA: Arthrodesis of the first metatarsophalangeal joint as salvage for the failed Keller procedure. *J Bone Joint Surg* 69A:68–75, 1987.

102. Harper MC: A modified Keller resection arthroplasty. *Foot Ankle Int* 16:236–237, 1995.

103. Vallier GT, Peterson DA, LaGrone MO: The Keller resection arthroplasty: A 13 year experience. *Foot Ankle* 11:187–197, 1991.

104. Kitaoka HB, Franco MG, Weaver AL, et al: Simple bunionectomy with medial capsulorrhaphy. *Foot Ankle* 12:86–91, 1991.

105. VanHal ME, Keenes JS, Lange TA, Clancy WG Jr: Stress fractures of the great toe sesamoids. *Am J Sports Med* 10:122–128, 1982.

106. Pretter Klieer ML, Wanivenhaus A: The arterial supply of the sesamoid bones of the hallux: The course and source of the nutrient arteries as an anatomical basis for surgical approaches to the great toe. *Foot Ankle* 13:7–13, 1992.

107. Mann RA, Hapner KL: Tibial sesamoid shaving for treatment of intractable plantar keratosis. *Foot Ankle* 13:196–198, 1992.

108. Sobel M, Hashimoto J, Arnoczky SP, et al: The microvasculature of the sesamoid complex: Its clinical significance. *Foot Ankle* 13:359–363, 1992.

109. Chamberland PDC, Smith JW, Fleming LL: The blood supply to the great toe sesamoids. *Foot Ankle* 14:435–442, 1993.

110. Rodeo SA, Warren RF, O'Brien SJ, et al: Diastasis of bipartite sesamoids of the first metatarsophalangeal joint. *Foot Ankle* 14:425–434, 1993.

111. Aper RL, Saltzman CL, Brown TD: The effect of hallux sesamoid resection on the effective movement of the flexor hallucis brevis. *Foot Ankle Int* 15:462–470, 1994.

112. Chisin R, Pyer A, Migrom C: Bone scintigraphy in the assessment of the hallucal sesamoids. *Foot Ankle Int* 16:291–294, 1995.

113. Mair SD, Coogan AC, Speer KP, et al: Gout as a source of sesamoid pain. *Foot Ankle Int* 16:616, 1995.

114. Shereff MJ, Jahss MH: Complications of silastic implant arthroplasty in the hallux. *Foot Ankle* 1:95–101, 1980.

115. Hattrup SJ, Johnson KA: Subjective results of hallux rigidus following treatment with cheilectomy. *Clin Orthop Rel Res* 226:182–191, 1988.

116. Mann RA, Chanton TO: Hallux rigidus: Treatment by cheilectomy. *J Bone Joint Surg* 70A:400–406, 1988.

117. Graves SC, Dutkowsky JP, Richardson EG: The Chevron bunionectomy: A trigonometric analysis to predict correction. *Foot Ankle* 14:90–96, 1993.

118. Thompson FM, Deland JT: Flexor tendon transfer for metatarsophalangeal instability of the second toe. *Foot Ankle* 14:385–388, 1993.

119. Coughlin MJ: Second metatarsophalangeal joint instability in the athlete. *Foot Ankle* 14:309–319, 1993.

120. Coughlin MJ: Crossover second toe deformity. *Foot Ankle* 8:29–39, 1987.

121. Daly P, Johnson K: Treatment of painful subluxation or dislocation at the second and third metatarsophalangeal joints by partial proximal phalangectomies and subtotal webbing. *Clin Orthop Rel Res* 278:164–170, 1992.

122. Mann RA, Mizel MS: Monarticular nontraumatic synovitis of the metatarsophalangeal joint: A new diagnosis? *Foot Ankle* 6:18–21, 1985.

123. Deland JT, Sobel M, Arnoczy SP, Thompson FM: Collateral ligament reconstruction of the unstable metatarsophalangeal joint: An in vitro study. *Foot Ankle* 13:391–395, 1992.

124. Coughlin MJ: Subluxation and dislocation of the second metatarsophalangeal joint. *Orthop Clin North Am* 20:535–551, 1989.

125. Mizel MS, Yodlowski ML: Disorders of the lesser metatarsophalangeal joints. *J Am Assoc Orthop Surg* 3(3):166–173, 1995.

126. Fortin PT, Myerson MS: Second metatarsophalangeal joint instability. *Foot Ankle* 16:306–313, 1995.

127. Deland JT, Leckt, Sobel M, et al: Anatomy of the plantar plate and its attachments in the lesser metatarsal phalangeal joint. *Foot Ankle Int* 16:480–486, 1995.

128. Johnston RB, Smith J, Daniels T: The plantar plate of the lesser toes: An anatomical study in human cadavers. *Foot Ankle* 15:276–282, 1994.

129. Yao L, Cracchiolo A, Farahanik, et al: Magnetic resonance imaging of plantar plate rupture. *Foot Ankle Int* 17:33–36, 1996.

130. Coughlin MJ: Operative repair of the mallet toe deformity. *Foot Ankle Int* 16:109–116, 1995.

131. Myerson MS, Shereff MJ: The pathologic anatomy of claw and hammer toes. *J Bone Joint Surg* 71A:45–49, 1989.

132. Conklin MJ, Smith RW: Treatment of atypical lesser toe deformity with basal hemiphalangectomy. *Foot Ankle Int* 15:585–594, 1994.

133. Mulier T, Dereymacker G, Fabry G: Jones transfer to the lesser toes in metatarsalgia: Technique and long term follow-up. *Foot Ankle Int* 15:523–530, 1994.

134. Cahill B, Connor D: A long term follow-up on proximal phalangectomy for hammer toes. *Clin Orthop Rel Res* 86:191–192, 1972.

135. Sarrafian SK: Correction of fixed hammertoe deformities with resection of the head of the proximal phalanx and extensor tendon tenodesis. *Foot Ankle Int* 16:449–451, 1995.

136. Barbari SG, Brevig K: Correction of clawtoes by the Girdlestone-Taylor flexor-extensor transfer procedure. *Foot Ankle* 5:67–73, 1984.

137. Lehman DE, Smith RW: Treatment of symptomatic hammertoe with proximal interphalangeal joint arthrodesis. *Foot Ankle Int* 16:535–541, 1995.

138. Myerson MS, Fortin P, Girard P: Use of skin Z-plasty for management of extension contracture in recurrent claw- and hammertoe deformity. *Foot Ankle Int* 15:209–212, 1994.

139. Thompson FM, Chang VK: The two-boned fifth toe: Clinical implications. *Foot Ankle Int* 16:34–36, 1995.

140. Santi MD, Botte MJ: Volkman's ischemic contracture of the foot and ankle: Evaluation and treatment of establish deformity. *Foot Ankle Int* 16:368, 1995.

141. Bohay DR, Manol A: Clawtoe deformity following vascularized fibula graft. *Foot Ankle* 16:607–609, 1995.

142. Janecki CJ, Wilde AH: Results of phalangectomy of the fifth toe for hammertoe. The Ruiz-Mora procedure. *J Bone Joint Surg* 58A:1005–1007, 1976.

143. Coughlin MJ: Etiology and treatment of the bunionette deformity. *Instr Course Lect* 39:37–48, 1990.

144. Kitaoka HB, Holiday AD: Metatarsal head resection for bunionette: Long term follow-up. *Foot Ankle* 11:345–349, 1991.

145. Nestor BJ, Kitaoka HB, Ilstrup DM, et al: Radiologic anatomy of the painful bunionette. *Foot Ankle* 11:6–11, 1991.

146. Diebold PF: Basal osteotomy of the fifth metatarsal for the bunionette. *Foot Ankle* 12:74–79, 1991.

147. Moran MM, Claridge RJ: Chevron osteotomy for bunionette. *Foot Ankle Int* 15:684–688, 1994.

148. Coughlin MJ: Treatment of bunionette deformity with longitudinal diaphyseal osteotomy with distal soft tissue repair. *Foot Ankle* 11:195–203, 1991.

149. Vahvanen V, Pirainen H, Kettunen P: Resection arthroplasty of the metatarsophalangeal joints in rheumatoid arthritis. *Scand J Rheumatol* 9:257–265, 1980.

150. Mann RA, Thompson FM: Arthrodesis of the first metatarsophalangeal joint for hallux valgus in rheumatoid arthritis. *J Bone Joint Surg* 66A:687–692, 1984.

151. Mann RA, Katcherian DA: Relationship of metatarsophalangeal joint fusion on the inter metatarsal angle. *Foot Ankle* 10:8–11, 1989.

152. Brodsky JW, Sanders M: Footings: Metatarsal head extractor. *Foot Ankle* 10:8–11, 1989.

153. Saltzman CL, Johnson KA, Donnelly RE: Surgical treatment of mild deformities of the rheumatoid forefoot leg partial phalangectomy and syndactylization. *Foot Ankle* 14:325–329, 1993.

154. Graham CE: Rheumatoid forefoot metatarsal head resection without first metatarsalphalangeal joint arthrosis. *Foot Ankle* 15:689–690, 1994.

155. Gedppart MJ, Sobel M, Bohne WHO: The rheumatoid foot. *Foot Ankle* 13:550–558, 1992.

156. Mann RA, Schakel ME: Surgical correction of rheumatoid forefoot deformities. *Foot Ankle Int* 16:1–6, 1995.

157. Levine MJ, Wapner KL, Leeth, et al: Surgical management of the rheumatoid forefoot. *Foot Ankle* 14:303, 1993.

158. Thompson FM, Mann RA: Arthritides, in Mann RA, Coughlin ML (eds): *Surgery of the Foot and Ankle,* 6th ed. St Louis, Mosby, 1993, pp 615–671.

159. Michelson J, Easly M, Wigley FM, et al: Foot and ankle problems in rheumatoid arthritis. *Foot Ankle Int* 15:608–613, 1994.

160. Scranton PE: Metatarsalgia: Diagnosis and treatment. *J Bone Joint Surg* 62A:723–732, 1980.

161. Sclamberg EL, Lorenz MA: A dorsal wedge V osteotomy for painful plantar callosities. *Foot Ankle* 4:30–32, 1983.

162. Leventen EO, Pearson SW: Distal metatarsal osteotomy for intractable plantar keratosis. *Foot Ankle* 10:247–251, 1990.

163. Kitaoka HB, Holiday AD, Campbell DC III: Distal Chevron metatarsal osteotomy for bunionette. *Foot Ankle* 12:80–85, 1991.

164. Harper MC: Dorsal losing wedge metatarsal osteotomy: A trigonometric analysis. *Foot Ankle* 10:299–302, 1990.

165. Dixon GL Jr: Treatment of ingrown toenail. *Foot Ankle* 3:254–260, 1983.

166. Muse G, Raya G: Subungual exostosis. *Orthopaedics* 9:997–998, 1986.

167. Multhopp-Stephens H, Walling AK: Subungual exostosis: A simple technique of excision. *Foot Ankle Int* 16:88–91, 1995.

168. McCluskey WP, Lovell WW, Cummings RJ: The cavovarus foot deformity: Etiology and management. *Clin Orthop* 247:27–37, 1989.

169. Alexander IJ, Johnson KA: Assessment and management of pes cavus in Charcot-Marie-Tooth disease. *Clin Orthop Rel Res* 246:273–281, 1989.

170. Paulos L, Coleman SS, Samuelson KM: Pes cavovarus: Review of a surgical approach using selective soft tissue procedures. *J Bone Joint Surg* 62A:942–953, 1980.

171. Jahss MH: Tarsometatarsal truncated wedge arthrodesis for pes cavus and equinovarus deformity of the forepart of the foot. *J Bone Joint Surg* 62A:713–722, 1980.

172. Mann DC, Hsu JD: Triple arthrodesis in the treatment of fixed cavovarus deformity in adolescent patients with Charcot-Marie-Tooth disease. *Foot Ankle* 13:1–6, 1992.

173. Tynan MC, Klenerman L, Helliwell TR, et al: Investigation of muscle imbalance in the leg in symptomatic forefoot pes cavus: A multidisciplinary study. *Foot Ankle* 13:4898–501, 1992.

174. Wenger DR, Mauldin D, Speck G, et al: Corrective shoes and inserts as treatment for flexible flatfoot in infants and children. *J Bone Joint Surg* 71A:800–810, 1989.

175. Helal B, Gibb P: Freiberg's disease: A suggested pattern of management. *Foot Ankle* 8:94–102, 1987.

176. Stanley D, Betts RP, Rowley DI, et al: Assessment of etiological factors in the development of Freiberg's disease. *J Foot Surg* 29:444–447, 1990.

177. Kinnard P, Lirett R: Dorsiflexion osteotomy in Freiberg's disease. *Foot Ankle* 9:226–231, 1989.

178. Mann RA, Reynolds JC: Interdigital neuroma: A critical clinical analysis. *Foot Ankle* 3:238–243, 1983.

179. Graham CC, Graham DM: Morton's neuroma: A microscopic evaluation. *Foot Ankle* 5:150, 1984.

180. Beskin JL, Baxter DE: Recurrent pain following interdigital neurectomy: A plantar approach. *Foot Ankle* 9:34–39, 1988.

181. Johnson JE, Johnson KA, Unni KK: Persistent pain after excision of interdigital neuroma. *J Bone Joint Surg* 70A:651–657, 1988.

182. Holmes GB: Quantitative determination of intermetatarsal pressure. *Foot Ankle* 13:532–535, 1992.

183. Amis JA, Siverhus SW, Liwnicz BH: An anatomical basis for recurrence after Morton's neuroma excision. *Foot Ankle* 13:153–156, 1992.

184. Thompson FM, Deland JT: Occurrence of two interdigital neuromas in one foot. *Foot Ankle* 14:15–17, 1993.

185. Levitsky KA, Alman BA, Jevgevan DS, et al: Digital nerves of the foot: Anatomic variations and implications regarding the pathogenesis of interdigital neuroma. *Foot Ankle* 14:208–214, 1993.

186. Shapiro PP, Shapiro SL: Sonographic evaluation of interdigital neuromas. *Foot Ankle Int* 16:604–606, 1995.

187. Bennett GL, Graham CE, Mauldin DM: Morton's interdigital neuroma: A comprehensive treatment protocol. *Foot Ankle Int* 16:760–763, 1995.

188. Benedetts; RS, Baxter DE, Davis FL: Clinical results of simultaneous adjacent interdigital neurectomy of the foot. *Foot Ankle Int* 17:264–268, 1996.

189. Greenfield J, Rea J Jr, Ilfeld FW: Morton's interdigital neuroma: Indications for treatment by local injections versus surgery. *Clin Orthop Rel Res* 185:142–144, 1984.

190. Mulder JD: The causative mechanism in Morton's metatarsalgia. *J Bone Joint Surg* 33B:94–95, 1951.

191. Bossley CJ, Cairney PC: The intermetatarsophalangeal bursa: Its significance in Morton's metatarsalgia. *J Bone Joint Surg* 62B:184–187, 1980.

192. Mann RA, Baxter DE: Diseases of the nerves, in Mann RA, Coughlin MJ (eds), *Surgery of the Foot and Ankle,* 6th ed. St Louis, Mosby, 1993, pp 543–573.

193. Dreeben SM, Mann RA: Heel pain: Sorting through the differential diagnosis. *J Musculoskel Med* 9:21–37, 1992.

194. Dreeben SM: Heel pain, in Lutter LD, Mizel MS, Pfeffer GB (eds): *Orthopaedic Knowledge Update: Foot and Ankle.* Rosemont, IL, American Association of Orthopaedic Surgeons, 1994, pp 179–191.

195. Graham CE: Painful heel syndrome: Rationale of diagnosis and treatment. *Foot Ankle* 3:261–267, 1983.

196. Schepsis AA, Leach RE, Gorzyca J: Plantar fasciitis, etiology, treatment, surgical results, and review of the literature. *Clin Orthop Rel Res* 266:185–196, 1991.

197. Wapner KL, Sharkey PF: The use of night splints for treatment of recalcitrant plantar fasciitis. *Foot Ankle* 12:135–137, 1991.

198. Baxter DE, Pfeffer GB: Treatment of chronic heel pain by surgical release of the first brand of the lateral plantar nerve. *Clin Orthop Rel Res* 279:29–236, 1992.

199. Daly PJ, Kitaoka HB, Chao EYS: Plantar fasciotomy for intractable plantar fasciitis: Clinical results and biomechanical evaluation. *Foot Ankle* 13:188–195, 1992.

200. Schon LC, Glennon TP, Baxter DE: Heel pain syndrome: Electrodiagnostic support or nerve entrapment. *Foot Ankle* 14:129–135, 1993.

201. Tanz SS: Heel pain. *Clin Orthop Rel Res* 28:169–177, 1963.

202. Wolgin M, Cook C, Graham C, Mauldin D: Conservative treatment of plantar heel pain: Long-term follow-up. *Foot Ankle Int* 15:97–102, 1994.

203. Sellman JR: Plantar fascia rupture associated with corticosteroid injection. *Foot Ankle* 15:376–381, 1994.

204. Davis PF, Severud E, Baxter DE: Painful heel syndrome: Results of nonoperative treatment. *Foot Ankle Int* 15:531–535, 1994.

205. Hawkins BJ, Langerman RJ, Gibbons T, et al: An anatomic analysis of endoscopic plantar fascia release. *Foot Ankle Int* 16:552–558, 1995.

206. Miller RA, Torres J, McGuine M: Efficacy of first-time steroid injection for painful heel syndrome. *Foot Ankle Int* 16:610–612, 1995.

207. Hofmeister EP, Elliot MJ, Juliano PJ: Endoscopic plantar fascia release: An anatomical study. *Foot Ankle Int* 16:719–723, 1995.

208. Tisdale CL, Harper MC: Chronic plantar heel pain: Treatment with shortleg casting. *Foot Ankle Int* 17:41–42, 1996.

209. Sammarco GJ, Helfrey RB: Surgical treatment of recalcitrant plantar fasciitis. *Foot Ankle Int* 17:520–526, 1996.

210. Gill LH, Kiebzak GM: Outcome of non-surgical treatment for plantar fasciitis. *Foot Ankle Int* 17:527–532, 1996.

211. Kaplan PE, Kernahan WT: Tarsal tunnel syndrome. *J Bone Joint Surg* 63A:96–99, 1981.

212. Dellon AL, MacKinnon SE: Tibial nerve branching in the tarsal tunnel. *Arch Neurol* 41:645–646, 1984.

213. Cimino WR: Tarsal tunnel syndrome: Review of the literature. *Foot Ankle* 11:47–52, 1990.

214. Baxter DE: Functional nerve disorders in the athlete's foot, ankle and leg. *Instr Course Lect* 42:185–194, 1993.

215. Sammarco GJ, Chalk DE, Feibel JH: Tarsal tunnel syndrome and additional nerve lesions in the same limb. *Foot Ankle* 14:71–77, 1993.

216. Frey C, Kerr R: Magnetic resonance imaging and the evaluation of tarsal tunnel syndrome. *Foot Ankle* 14:159–164, 1993.

217. Richli WR, Roger DJ, Carrasco CH, et al: An anatomical study of the tarsal tunnel using low pressure compartmental infusion. *Foot Ankle* 14:257–260, 1993.

218. Baxter DE: Compressive neuropathies of the foot and ankle. *Op Tech Sports Med* 2:18–23, 1994.

219. Skalley TC, Schon LC, Hinton RY, Myerson MS: Clinical results following revision tibial nerve release. *Foot Ankle Int* 15:360–367, 1994.

220. Davis TJ, Schon LC: Branches of the tibial nerve: Anatomical variations. *Foot Ankle Int* 16:21–29, 1995.

221. Lian G: Nerve problems in the foot, in Lutter LD, Mizel MS, Pfeffer GB (eds), *Orthopaedic Knowledge Update: Foot and Ankle*. Rosemont, IL, American Association of Orthopaedic Surgeons, 1994, pp 123–132.

222. Heneghan MA, Pavlov H: The Haglund painful heel syndrome. *Clin Orthop* 187:228–234, 1984.

223. Katz JF: Nonarticular osteochondroses. *Clin Orthop* 158:70–76, 1981.

224. Brower AC: The osteochondroses. *Orthop Clin North Am* 14:99–117, 1983.

225. Gregg JR, Das M: Foot and ankle problems in the preadolescent and adolescent athlete. *Clin Sports Med* 1:131–147, 1982.

226. Spiegl PV, Johnson KA: Heel pain syndrome: Which treatments to choose. *J Musculoskel Med* 1:66–71, 1984.

The Shoulder Joint and Girdle

CHAPTER 55

The Shoulder and the Shoulder Girdle

Mark W. Rodosky and Louis U. Bigliani

FUNCTIONAL ANATOMY OF THE SHOULDER AND SHOULDER GIRDLE

The shoulder and shoulder girdle consists of the bones, capsuloligamentous structures, and muscles of the glenohumeral (GH), acromioclavicular (AC), sternoclavicular (SC), and scapulothoracic (ST) joints (Fig. 55-1). These anatomic structures facilitate the prehensile activity and wide functional motion afforded the human arm.

Development

The structures of the shoulder girdle are the end result of maturation of the upper limb bud, which is first seen opposite the lower six cervical and first and second thoracic segments at the end of the fourth week of gestation.[99] During the fifth week of gestation, the mesodermal cells of the limb bud begin to form the basic structure of the shoulder and shoulder girdle. These developing cells are soon invaded by ectodermal cells that form the brachial plexus.[125] During this week, the humerus begins to form a cartilaginous core and the clavicle becomes the first bone to begin the process of ossification. The clavicle will also be the last bone to complete the ossification process somewhere in the third decade of life. The clavicle forms by intramembranous ossification as opposed to the endochondral process of the humerus and other long bones. By the eighth week, the upper limb has rotated laterally (opposite the rotation of the lower limb) and has taken on the form of the adult upper limb, including formation of the GH, AC, SC, and ST joints.[99,125] The remainder of fetal and childhood development of the upper extremity is mainly concerned with growth of these structures.

At completion of developmental growth, the shoulder drifts inferiorly, with the superior border of the scapula at the level of second rib and the inferior border at the level of the seventh rib. Failure of descent of the scapula secondary to aberrant bony or soft tissue attachments results in Sprengel's deformity.[160] The scapula, which forms via intramembranous ossification, has several ossification centers, including one located at the anterior aspect of the acromion. An unfused apophysis, termed a *mesoacromion,* at this location is not uncommon and can be a cause of impingement.

Bones of the Shoulder and Shoulder Girdle

The clavicle, scapula, and humerus form an intercalated complex, working in concert during motion of the shoulder (Fig. 55-1). The clavicle is S-shaped and serves as a strut that helps to suspend the arm while also serving as a site for muscle attachments, including the trapezius and anterior deltoid. It articulates with the manubrium of the sternum medially at the SC joint. The lateral aspect of the clavicle articulates with the acromion at the AC joint (Fig. 55-1).

The scapula is encased in muscle and therefore has a pseudoarticulation with the chest wall (Fig. 55-2). It overlaps the second through seventh ribs on the posterior thorax. The scapula is tilted obliquely forward at an angle of approximately 30° from the coronal plane and is tilted 3° medially from the sagittal plane[169] (Fig. 55-3). A total of 17 muscles arise or insert on the scapula (Fig. 55-2 and Table 55-1). These muscles are involved in dynamic control of the scapula as well as motion of the GH and elbow joints. The rotator cuff muscles cover the major surfaces of the scapula, with the subscapularis arising from the anterior surface. The supraspinatus and infraspinatus lie in fossae on either side of the scapular spine, as denoted by their names (Fig. 55-2).

The thickened lateral aspect of the scapula forms the glenoid, which serves as an articular platform for the proximal aspect of the humerus. The glenoid is separated from the body of the scapula by the scapular neck. It has an average superior tilt of 5°, which helps control inferior stability. It is generally retroverted with respect to the body of the scapula at an average of 7°[169,172] (Fig. 55-4).

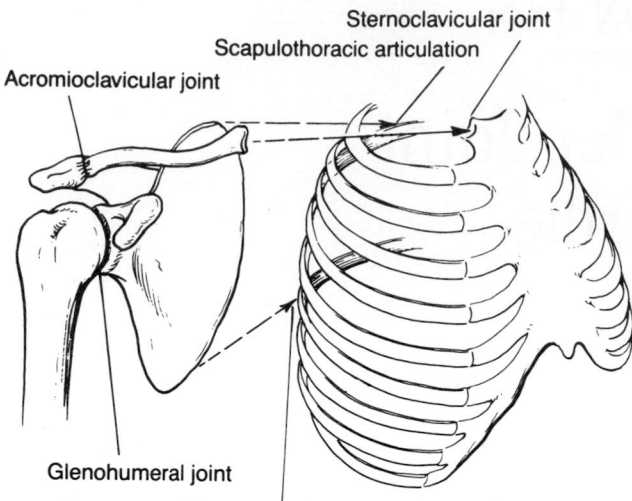

Figure 55-1 The shoulder and shoulder girdle consists of the bones, capsuloligamentous structures, and muscles of the glenohumeral (GH), acromioclavicular (AC), sternoclavicular (SC) and scapulothoracic (ST) joints. (Reproduced with permission from Warner JJP, Caborn DN: Overview of shoulder instability. *Crit Rev Phys Rehabil Med* 4:145–198, 1992.)

The scapula projects two notable prominences. The coracoid process arises from the anterosuperior portion of the scapular neck and protrudes at the anterosuperior aspect of the GH joint (Fig. 55-5A). It serves as the attachment site for the coracoacromial, coracohumeral, and transverse scapular ligaments as well as the pectoralis minor muscle (Fig. 55-5B). The conjoined tendon (short head of biceps and coracobrachialis muscles) originates from the coracoid process. The acromion projects over the humeral head as a broad but flat expansion of the scapular spine. It serves as the major site of origin for the deltoid muscle and articulates with the clavicle at the AC joint (Fig. 55-1).

The proximal aspect of the humerus consists of the humeral head, anatomic neck, and metaphysis. The humeral head has an average retroversion of 30 to 40° relative to the transcondylar axis of the distal humerus. The anatomic neck shaft angle of the proximal humerus averages 130 to 140°[169,172] (Fig. 55-6). The metaphyseal region is often termed the *surgical neck,* as most proximal humeral fractures occur in this region. The greater and lesser tuberosities arise from the metaphyseal region and are located on opposite sides of the bicipital groove. The tuberosities play an important role in shoulder function, as they serve as the attachment site for the rotator cuff tendons, with the subscapularis inserting on the lesser and the supraspinatus, infraspinatus, and teres minor tendons inserting on the greater tuberosity. One of the primary goals in the treatment of comminuted proximal humerus fractures is proper orientation and healing of the tuberosity fragments. The bicipital groove serves as a trochlea for the long head of the biceps tendon, which goes into the glenohumeral joint to insert at the supraglenoid tubercle. The tendon is constrained in the groove by the transverse humeral ligament as well as the rotator cuff insertions into the tuberosities.

Glenohumeral Joint

The GH joint is the major articulation of the shoulder complex. It is formed by the articulation between the surfaces of the hemispherical humeral head and a relatively smaller, shallow glenoid fossae (Fig. 55-1). The radii of curvature of the two surfaces are well matched to within 2 mm of each other.[158] However, a significant mismatch in size between the two leaves the articulation with very little inherent stability. The glenoid fossa is pear-shaped, with average vertical and horizontal dimensions of 35 and 25 mm, respectively.[125] The articular surface of the larger humeral head has an average vertical dimension of 48 mm and an average transverse dimension of 45 mm. The relative area of contact between the two surfaces is analogous to that of a basketball sitting on top of a teacup saucer with only 25 to 30 percent of the humeral head articulating with the glenoid socket at any time. This geometry allows more motion than that of any other joint in the body at the expense of intrinsic stability. Stability of the joint is provided by surrounding soft tissue structures, which can be separated into static and dynamic restraints.

Static Stabilizers

The static restraints consist of the glenoid labrum, joint capsule, GH ligaments, and coracohumeral ligament (Fig. 55-7). The labrum is a fibrous structure that forms a rim around the periphery of the glenoid socket. Its main function is to serve as an anchoring source for the long head of the biceps and the glenohumeral capsule and its thickenings, the GH ligaments. The labrum has a considerable amount of anatomic variability from person to person. This variability is more pronounced in the anterosuperior portion of the glenoid, where it is frequently loosely attached. The posterior and anteroinferior portions of the glenoid labrum are usually tightly attached. Labral detachments in these areas are more likely to represent pathology consistent with instability, while a detachment in the anterosuperior quadrant may simply represent a normal anatomic variant. Other minor roles of the labrum include increasing the depth of the glenoid socket as well as acting as a load-bearing structure for the humeral head. This is analogous to that of a "chock block," which is used to prevent a wheel from rolling on an inclined surface.[82]

The capsuloligamentous structures play a greater role in stability of the GH joint. These structures help to prevent excessive translation and rotation of the humeral head on the glenoid during prehensile activity of the upper extremity. They interact in a complex fashion that varies with differing positions and loading conditions of the GH joint (Fig. 55-8). The structures vary slightly from person to person but can generally be separated into four areas. These include the rotator interval, the middle GH ligament, the inferior GH ligament complex, and the posterior capsule.

Rotator Interval The rotator interval area consists of the wedge-shaped region bordered by the subscapularis inferiorly, the supraspinatus superiorly, and the hood over the bicipital groove laterally (Fig. 55-9). The ligamentous components of this area are the coracohumeral ligament (CHL)

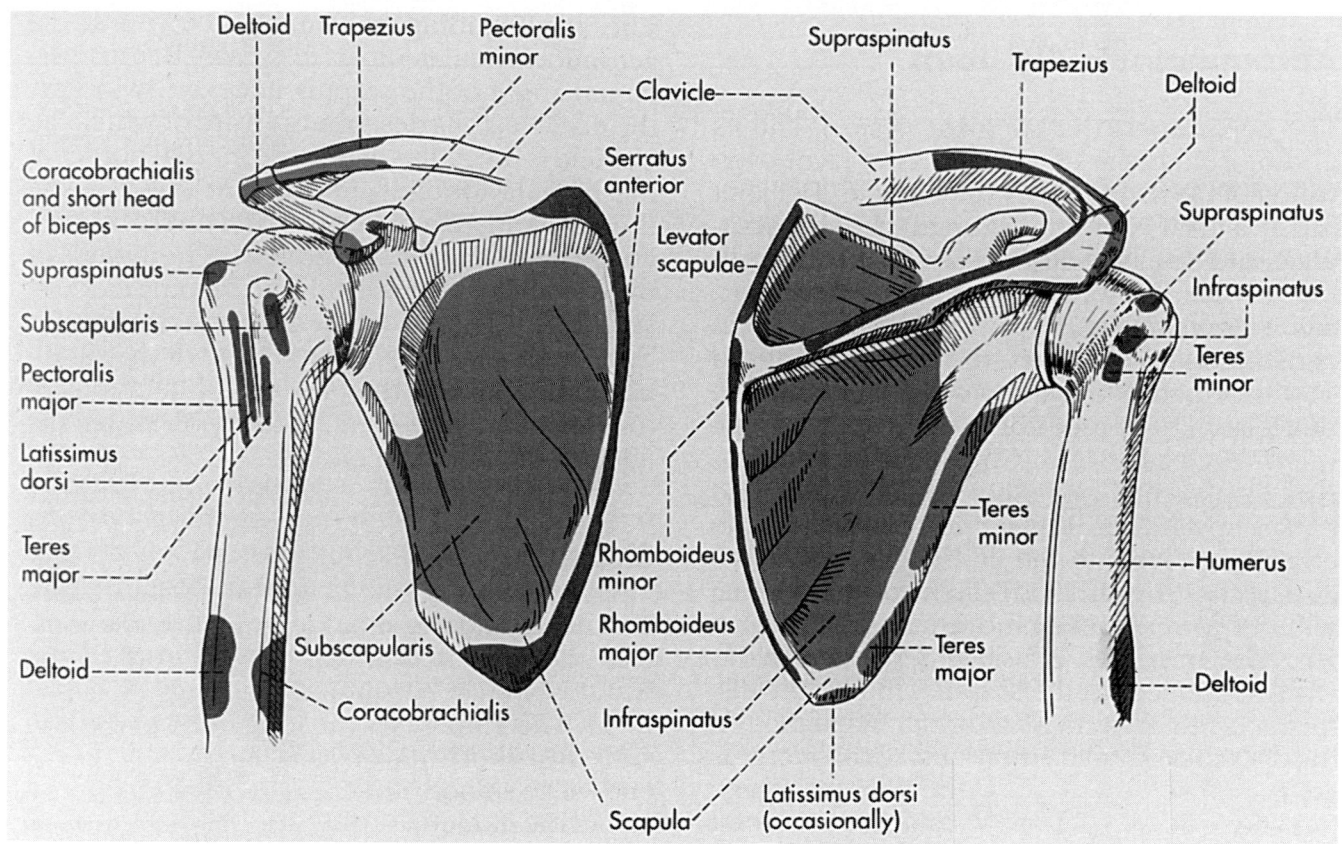

Figure 55-2 Muscles of the shoulder and shoulder girdle. (Reproduced with permission from Jenkins DB: *Hollinshead's Functional Anatomy of the Limbs and Back,* 6th ed. Philadelphia, Saunders, 1991, fig. 5-3.)

and the superior GH ligament (SGHL). The CHL originates from the coracoid process, while the SGHL originates from the superior labrum at the supraglenoid tubercle (Fig. 55-9). Both insert into the most superior aspect of the lessor tuberosity and are consistently found in more than 90 percent of human shoulders.[172] Their primary role is to prevent excessive inferior translation and external rotation with the arm at the side. They may also aid in preventing excessive posterior translation when the shoulder is in a flexed, adducted, and internally rotated position.

Figure 55-3 Orientation of the scapula with reference to the chest wall. (Reproduced with permission from Warner JJP: The gross anatomy of the joint surfaces, ligaments, labrum and capsule, in Matsen FA III, Fu FH, Hawkins RJ (eds): *The Shoulder: A Balance of Mobility and Stability.* Rosemont, IL, American Academy of Orthopaedic Surgeons, 1993, pp 7–27.)

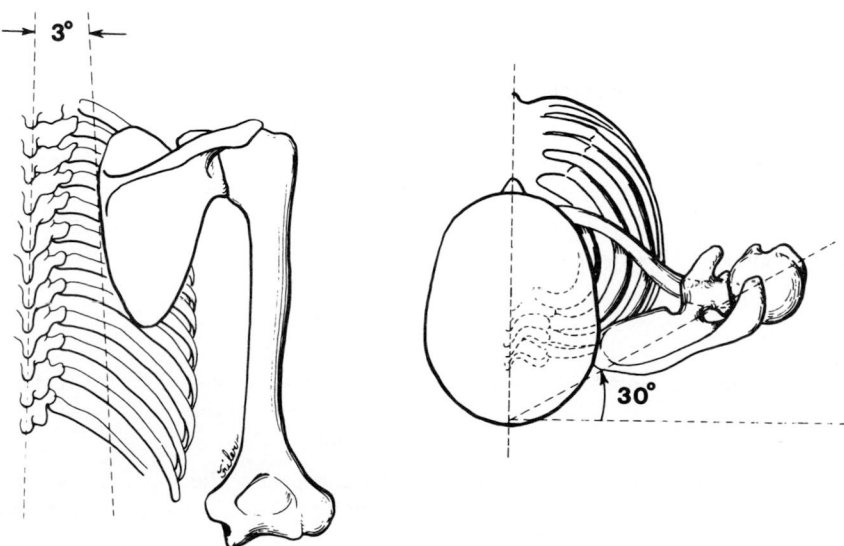

TABLE 55-1   Muscles of the Shoulder and Shoulder Girdle

Muscle	Innervation	Origin	Insertion	Muscle testing
Biceps brachii (long head)	Musculocutaneous	Superior aspect of the glenoid	Radial tuberosity	Resisted flexion with supination of the forearm
Biceps brachii (short head)	Musculocutaneous	Coracoid process	Radial tuberosity	Resisted flexion with supination of the forearm
Coracobrachialis	Musculocutaneous	Coracoid process	Medial half of the humerus	None
Deltoid	Axillary	Lateral third of the clavicle, scapular spine, and acromion	Deltoid tuberosity of the humerus	Resisted motion at 90° of abduction
Infraspinatus	Suprascapular	Infraspinatus fossa of the scapula	Greater tuberosity of humerus	Resisted external rotation
Latissimus dorsi	Thoacodorsal	Spines of vertebrae T6–T12, ilial crest, and ribs 8–12	Medial aspect of the bicipital groove	Resisted posterior inferior motion of the arm palpable at inferior angle of scapula
Pectoralis major	Lateral and medial pectoral	Medial third of the clavicle, sternum, and aponeurosis of the external oblique abdominal muscles	Lateral aspect of the bicipital groove	Resisted adduction with arm at 30° of flexion
Pectoralis minor	Medial pectoral	Ribs 3–5	Coracoid process	None
Levator scapulae	Dorsal scapular	Transverse processes of C1–C4	Medial border of the scapula (superior angle)	Resisted posterior motion of the elbows with hands on hips
Rhomboid major	Dorsal scapular	Spines of vertebrae T2–T5	Inferior medial border of the scapula	Resisted adduction and rotation of the scapula
Rhomboid minor	Dorsal scapular	Spines of vertebrae C7–T1	Base of scapular spine on the medial side	Resisted adduction and rotation of the scapula
Serratus anterior	Long thoracic	Surface of ribs 1–9	Medial border of the scapula	Wall push-up with scapular winging
Sternocleido-mastoid	Spinal accessory	Superior aspect of the sternum to the anterior surface of manubrium and medial third of the clavicle	Mastoid process and lateral half of occipital bone	Head turn to one side against resistance
Subscapularis	Subscapular	Subscapular fossa of the scapula	Lesser tuberosity of the humerus	Gerber lift-off test
Supraspinatus	Suprascapular	Supraspinatus fossa of the scapula	Greater tuberosity of the humerus	Resisted abduction in scaption
Trapezius	Spinal accessory	Occiput and spines of vertebrae C1–T12	Lateral third of clavicle to the spine of scapula and the acromion	Shoulder shrug against resistance
Teres major	Lower subscapular	Lateral border of scapula	Greater tuberosity of the humerus	Resisted posteroinferior motion of the arm palpable at inferior border of scapula
Teres minor	Axillary	Dorsal surface of the lateral border of the scapula	Greater tuberosity of the humerus	Resisted external rotation
Triceps brachii (long head)	Radial	Inferior aspect of the glenoid	Posterior aspect of the olecranon	Resisted extension of the elbow in various positions

Figure 55-4 The glenoid version averages 7° of retroversion and 5° of superior tilt. (Reproduced with permission from Warner JJP: The gross anatomy of the joint surfaces, ligaments, labrum and capsule, in Matsen FA III, Fu FH, Hawkins RJ (eds): *The Shoulder: A Balance of Mobility and Stability.* Rosemont, IL, American Academy of Orthopaedic Surgeons, 1993, pp 7–27.)

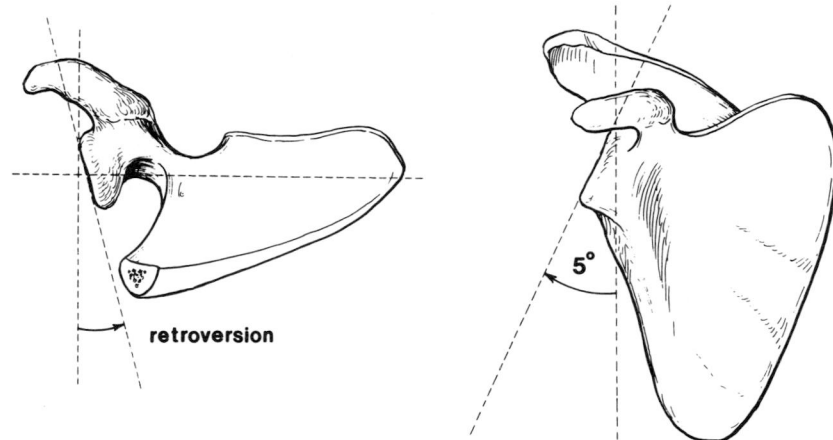

Middle Glenohumeral Ligament The middle GH ligament (MGHL) is a more variable structure, which may be absent in up to 30 percent of people and poorly defined in another 10 percent.[172] When present, it can be found in one of two morphologies: (1) cordlike, with a foraminal separation between it and the anterior band of the inferior GH ligament (IGHL), or (2) sheetlike and confluent with the anterior band of the IGHL. Its principal role is to prevent anterior translation of the humeral head when the shoulder is abducted 45° and externally rotated.[169,172] It also serves to limit external rotation of the adducted shoulder and inferior displacement of the adducted and externally rotated shoulder.[169]

Inferior Glenohumeral Ligament Complex The inferior GHL complex (IGHLC) is the most important static stabilizer of the GH joint.[166] The complex is composed of the in-

ferior capsule or axillary pouch, which is suspended between two ligamentous bands in the same fashion that a hammock is slung between two ropes. These are the anterior and posterior bands of the IGHLC.[126] The posterior band is an inconsistent structure.[162] The IGHLC tightens in a reciprocal fashion depending on the rotation of the humeral head and can act to prevent inferior translation of the abducted shoulder at differing rotational positions (Fig. 55-8). Its primary role is to prevent anteroinferior translation in the abducted and externally rotated shoulder.[166]

Posterior Capsule The posterior capsule is the thinnest portion of the GH capsuloligamentous structures and is located superior to the posterior band of the IGHLC. Its primary function is believed to be in limiting posterior translation of the humeral head. Its overall importance has not been clearly studied[169,172] (Fig. 55-7).

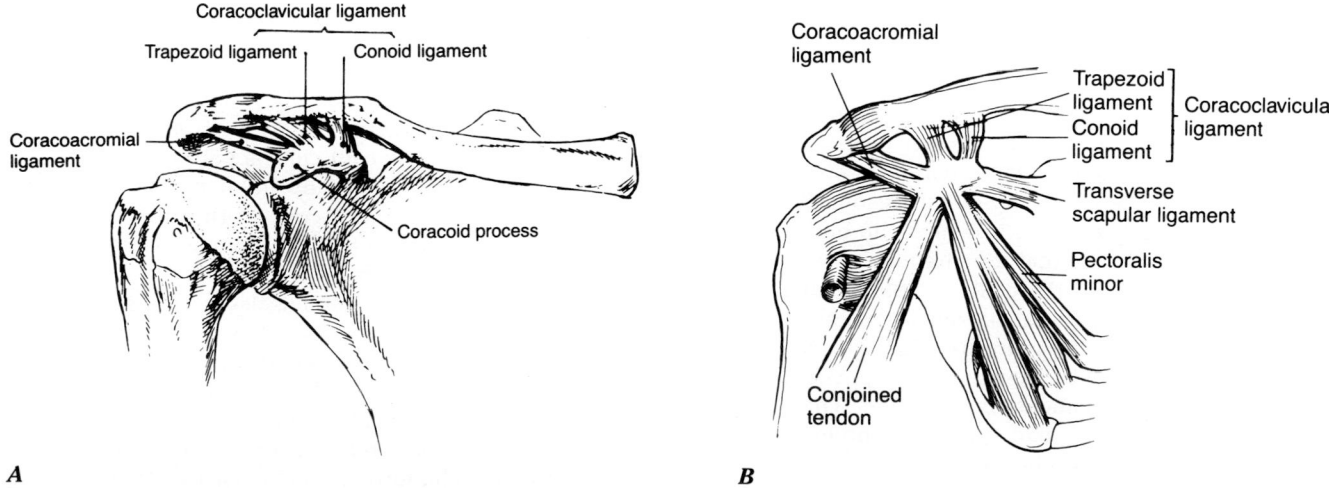

A

B

Figure 55-5 *A.* The coracoid process arises from the superior anteromedial aspect of the glenoid neck, serving as an attachment site for several ligaments. *B.* Muscle and ligament attachments to the coracoid process. (Reproduced with permission from Warner JJP: Shoulder, in Miller MD, Cooper DE, Warner JJP (eds): *Review of Sports Medicine and Arthroscopy.* Philadelphia, Saunders, 1995, pp 113–164.)

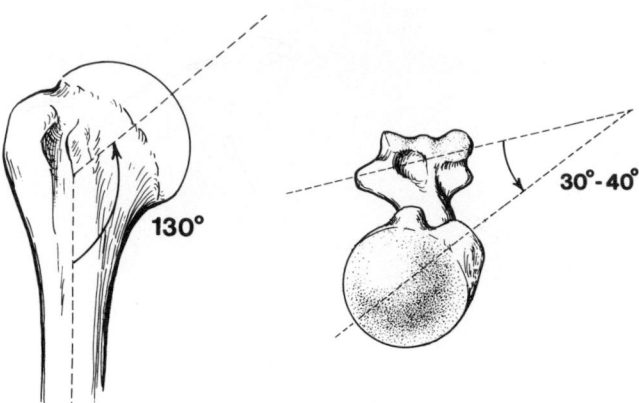

Figure 55-6 Humeral articular orientation averages 130° at the neck shaft and 30 to 40° of retroversion with respect to the transepicondylar axis. (Reproduced with permission from Warner JJP: The gross anatomy of the joint surfaces, ligaments, labrum and capsule, in Matsen FA III, Fu FH, Hawkins RJ (eds): *The Shoulder: A Balance of Mobility and Stability*. Rosemont, IL, American Academy of Orthopaedic Surgeons, 1993, pp 7–27.)

Dynamic Stabilizers

While the static capsuloligamentous structures serve as passive "check reins" at the extremes of motion, the dynamic structures are important stabilizers in the midranges of motion. The dynamic stabilizers of the GH joint consist of the rotator cuff and long head of biceps muscles. These structures cross the GH joint and work in a coordinated fashion to provide functional motion while at the same time preventing excessive translation and rotation of the humeral head. The muscles were traditionally believed to prevent excessive translation in the direction of their position around the GH joint. However, clinical experience has demonstrated that they can also provide stability in the direction opposite their humeral insertion, as evidenced by anterior shoulder dislocations that may occur as a result of superior and posterior rotator cuff tendon rupture.[55] Recent biomechanical studies have verified this clinical experience.[40,147]

The dynamic restraints are hypothesized to work via several means that are currently under investigation. The muscles compress the GH joint creating a concavity-compression effect. The concavity-compression effect is enhanced by a steering effect, in which the muscles work synergistically to ensure that the direction of compressive force is pointed toward the center of the glenoid.[40] They may also serve as an actual barrier to translation when they tighten and become more like rigid structures. In a similar fashion, they may also serve to tighten surrounding labral or capsuloligamentous structures. This theory is supported by biomechanical studies of the long head of the biceps and superior labrum.[147]

Scapulothoracic Articulation

Although the glenohumeral articulation is the principal joint of the shoulder complex, its motion is highly coordi-

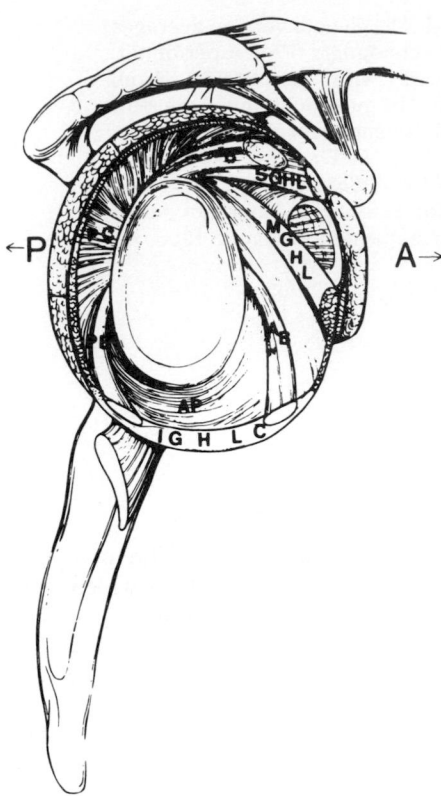

Figure 55-7 Anatomy of the joint capsule and ligaments, viewed from the side with anterior (A) to the right and posterior (P) to the left. The humeral head has been removed to show the superior glenohumeral ligament (SGHL), the middle glenohumeral ligament (MGHL) and the inferior glenohumeral ligament complex (IGHLC). The IGHLC consists of the anterior band (AB), the posterior band (PB), and the interposed axillary pouch (AP). The posterior capsule (PC) is shown posteriorly. (Reproduced with permission from O'Brien SJ, Neves MC, Arnoczky SP, et al: The anatomy and histology of the inferior glenohumeral ligament complex of the shoulder. *Am J Sports Med* 18:449–456, 1990.)

nated with that of the scapulothoracic (ST) articulation. The intricate manner in which the two work together are poorly understood except to state that failure of one or the other leads to significant clinical pathology. Motion at the ST articulation essentially involves sliding of the scapula over the truncated cone of the rib cage.[59] The scapula essentially floats in a bed of muscle, and its stability and motion are controlled by the periscapular muscles. The two most important muscles are the serratus anterior, which holds the medial angle against the chest wall and the trapezius, which serves to rotate and elevate the scapula in synchrony with the glenohumeral joint. The scapula conforms to the shape of the thorax. Any surface irregularities that may result from a fracture or growth such as an osteochondroma can impair its smooth gliding motion.

The GH and ST joints work in synchrony to provide arm motion. Although the ratio of GH to ST motion varies from lower to higher degrees of elevation, there are generally 2° of GH elevation for each 1° of ST elevation.[59]

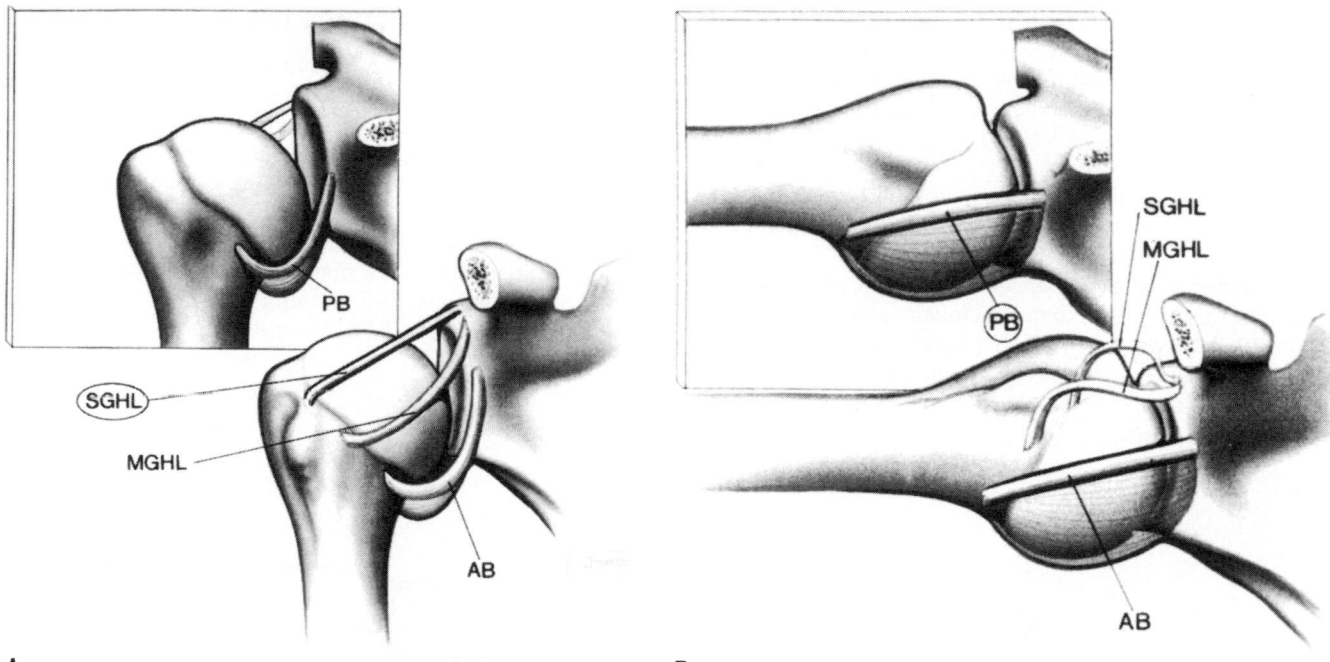

A   *B*

Figure 55-8 *A.* The anterior (AB) and posterior (PB) bands of the inferior gleno-humeral ligament complex are lax with adduction of the shoulder, while the superior glenohumeral ligament (SGHL) and the middle glenohumeral ligament (MGHL) are taut. *B.* In reciprocal fashion, the IGHL tightens with abduction, while the SGHL and MGHL become lax. (Reproduced with permission from Warner JP, Deng XH, Warren RF, et al: Static capsuloligamentous restraints to superior-inferior translation of the glenohumeral joint. *Am J Sports Med* 20:675–685, 1992.)

Throughout the entire range of elevation, the ST muscles are working to lessen the shear at the GH joint by helping to keep the glenoid centered beneath the humeral head. They also work as shock absorbers to absorb impact that might otherwise lead to a material failure (i.e., fracture) of the thin scapular bone.[111]

Sternoclavicular Articulation

The sternoclavicular (SC) joint is formed where the inferior portion of the medial end of the clavicle articulates with the manubrial portion of the sternum (Fig. 55-10). It sits directly in front of the great vessels, resulting in a potentially hazardous situation (see Fig. 55-22) when a pos-

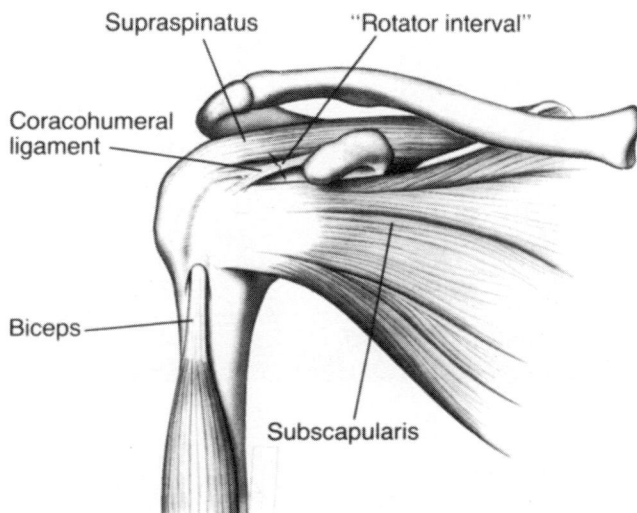

Figure 55-9 The rotator interval area of the shoulder.

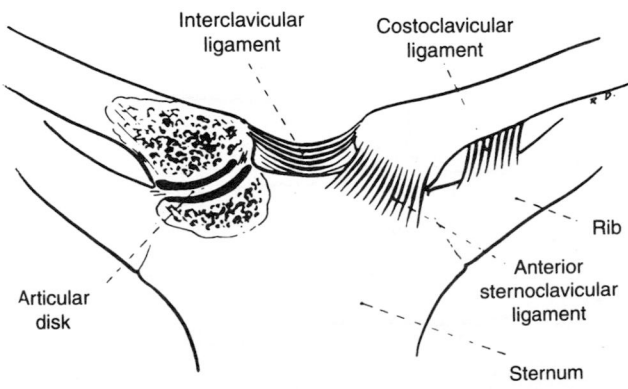

Figure 55-10 The medial clavicle articulates with the sternum and the first ribs; their upper portions make up the sternal notch. The ligaments are shown. (Reproduced with permission from Hollinshead WH: *Functional Anatomy of the Limbs and Back.* Philadelphia, Saunders, 1951, p 89.)

terior dislocation occurs. It is considered a gliding joint with an intervening articular disk and an extensive fibrous envelope. The joint is stabilized by the costoclavicular ligament, the interclavicular ligament, and the anterior and posterior SC ligaments.[111] The proportional role of each is poorly understood except to state that when the medial clavicle is excised for arthritic conditions, it is important to maintain the costoclavicular ligaments to prevent instability of the medial end of the clavicle.[111]

In order to provide essential motion at the scapulothoracic articulation, the clavicle may rotate as much as 60° at the SC ligament.[59] For this reason, it is a well-known fact that metal across the SC joint should be avoided, as it can be extruded and then migrate into the great vessels or deep into the chest.[89,183]

Acromioclavicular Articulation

The acromioclavicular (AC) joint is a diarthrodial joint of varying inclination between the concave surface of the anteromedial aspect of the acromion and the convex surface of the distal clavicle (Fig. 55-11). This inclination is easily seen on radiographs and, when noted, can greatly improve the accuracy of needle placement during injection studies. A fibrocartilaginous disk exists within the joint as an interposed structure. This disk is most often incomplete, projecting downward into the joint as a rim of tissue from the superior capsule.[56,152] There is evidence to suggest

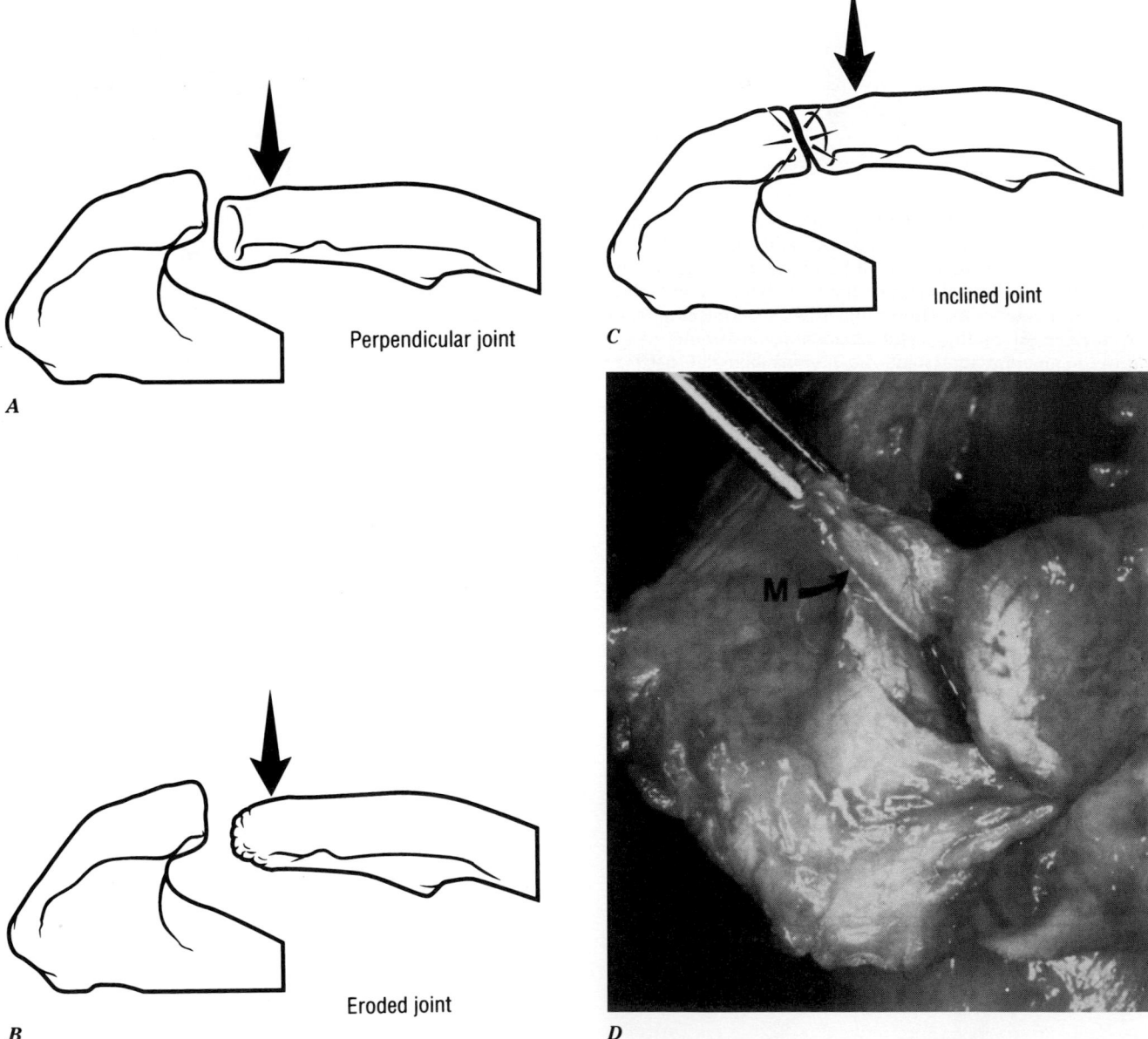

A Perpendicular joint

B Eroded joint

C Inclined joint

D

Figure 55-11 *A* to *C.* The AC joint has varying inclination. *D.* Anatomic dissection demonstrates a reflected superior AC capsule and ligaments with the underlying meniscus (M). (Reproduced with permission from Rodosky MW, Flatow EL: Arthroscopic debridement of the acromioclavicular joint and distal clavicle resection, in McGinty JB: *Operative Arthroscopy.* Philadelphia, Lippincott Raven, 1996, pp 773–783.)

that a complete meniscal disk may protect the cartilaginous surfaces of the AC joint from arthritic degeneration.[131]

The scapula moves in synchrony with the clavicle as it rotates axially, translates horizontally, and elevates superiorly; therefore, very little motion actually occurs at the AC joint. The main function of the AC joint is to serve as a connection between the scapula and clavicle, allowing for support of the shoulder girdle on the chest wall. The forces experienced by the AC joint are predominantly compressive in nature.[59] Because the area of the AC joint is relatively small and the forces transmitted from the chest wall muscles (i.e., pectoralis major) to the humerus are large, the stresses at this articulation can be extremely high. For this reason, it is not surprising to see compressive failure of this joint, especially in weight lifters, who are prone to osteolysis of the AC joint.[38,64]

The stability of the AC joint is maintained by two sets of ligaments: the AC capsuloligamentous complex and the coracoclavicular ligaments (conoid and trapezoid)[59] (Fig. 55-5). The AC ligaments (the inferior and the thicker superior) act as primary restraints to posterior clavicular displacement, controlling 90 percent of posterior motion. The coracoclavicular ligaments (the trapezoid and conoid) provide restraint to superior and anterior displacement of the clavicle. The conoid ligament seems to provide the majority of this support.[68]

SURGICAL ANATOMY OF THE SHOULDER AND SHOULDER GIRDLE

Surgical approaches of the shoulder are designed to allow access to the pertinent pathology while reducing the chance for morbidity from the approach. The shoulder can be approached as a structure that consists of four layers of tissue[53] (Fig. 55-12). The deltoid, trapezius, and pectoralis major muscles serve as the outer layer. The deltoid muscle is the most important muscle of the shoulder and is encountered in almost every type of surgical interven-

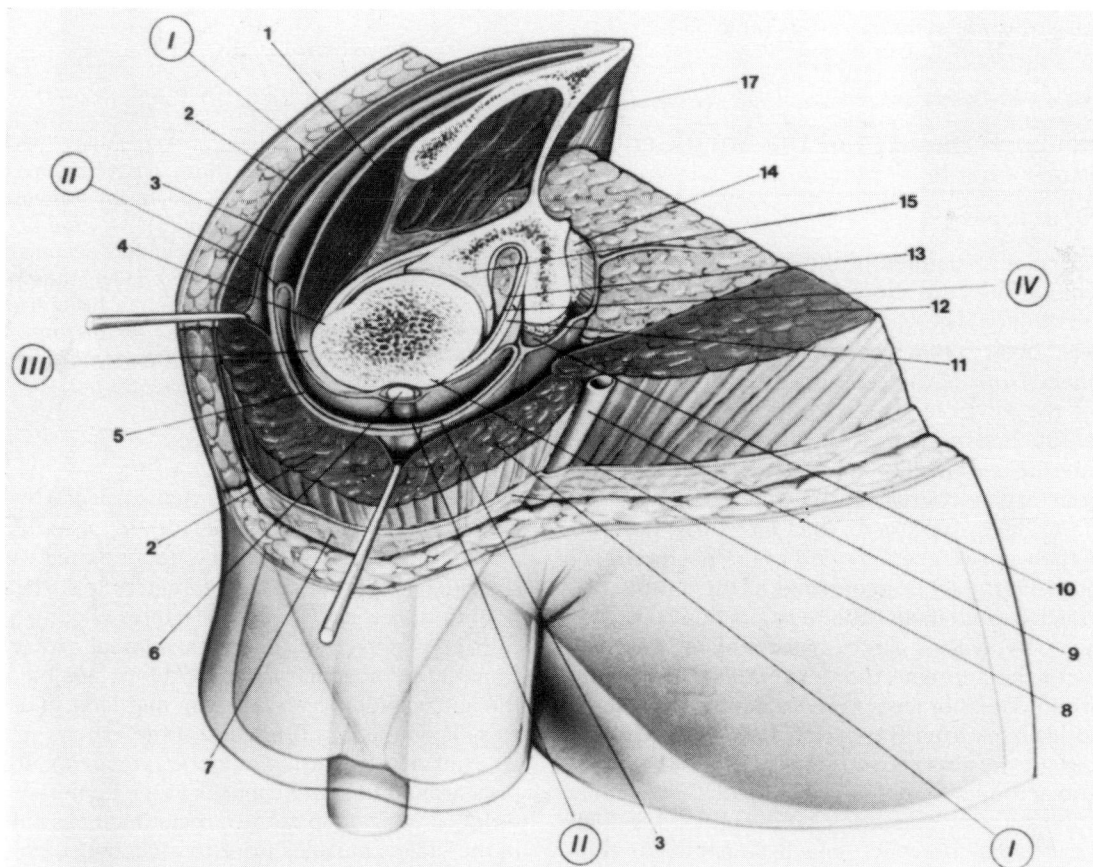

Figure 55-12 Cross-sectional view of the right shoulder at the level of the lesser tuberosity. The shoulder can be divided into four layers: layer I, deltoid (2), pectoralis major (12), fascia (7), cephalic vein (9); layer II, conjoined tendon (10), pectoralis minor (14); layer III, fascia (3), subdeltoid bursa (5), rotator cuff (1, 17), suprascapular neurovascular bundle (not shown); and layer IV, glenohumeral capsule (11), greater tuberosity (4), long head of the biceps (6), lesser tuberosity (8), synovium (13), and glenoid (15). (Reproduced with permission from Cooper DE, O'Brien SJ, Warren RF: Supporting layers of the glenohumeral joint: An anatomic study. *Clin Orthop* 289:144–155, 1993.)

tion involving the shoulder and shoulder girdle. The pennate deltoid muscle can be divided into posterior, middle, and anterior portions, with the anterior being the most important to the overall function of the arm and the segment that is most commonly encountered.

Injury to the deltoid muscle is poorly tolerated and can result in permanent dysfunction of the shoulder. Very little can be done to reconstruct a damaged deltoid muscle. It is important to prevent deltoid damage by making sure that its neurologic supply, the axillary nerve, is protected from injury. In addition, it is important to ensure that the deltoid is properly repaired at completion of the surgical procedure. Being certain that both the deep and superficial fascial layers of the deltoid are grasped with the repair and using direct suturing to the acromion when the overlying fascia is weak are techniques that can be utilized to help prevent catastrophic deltoid damage.

The inner three layers of the shoulder are encountered next and consist of the following, as seen in Fig. 55-12: II, clavipectoral fascia, conjoined tendon, and pectoralis minor; III, rotator cuff and bursae; and IV, GH capsule and ligaments. The various muscles associated with the four layers of the shoulder, as well as other muscles involved with the shoulder girdle, are summarized in Table 55-1.[53]

Neurovascular Structures of the Shoulder and Shoulder Girdle

Arterial Structures

The neurovascular structures of the shoulder girdle pass from the neck through the shoulder girdle on their way to the upper extremity. The vascular structures begin with the subclavian artery, which originates directly from the brachiocephalic trunk in the right upper extremity and directly off of the aorta in the left upper extremity (Fig. 55-13). The subclavian artery then passes between the scalenus anterior and medius muscles, where it becomes the axillary artery as it crosses the outer border of the first rib. The axillary artery is divided into three portions based upon their position with regard to the pectoralis minor muscle: the first part lies cephalad to the muscle, the second part lies behind it, and the third portion continues on caudally.[83] The axillary artery has six main branches, beginning with the supreme thoracic, which arises from the first portion. The thoracoacromial artery is the second branch, and it arises from the midportion of the axillary artery. Although the thoracoacromial artery has several branches, the acromial branch is the one most commonly encountered in surgery. This branch runs upward and laterally adjacent to the coracoacromial ligament and is commonly ligated during dissection of the coracoacromial ligament. The lateral thoracic artery is the next branch off of the midportion of the axillary artery. It passes downward behind the pectoralis minor muscle, running along its inferior lateral border and supplying branches to the pectoralis and serratus anterior muscles.[83]

The subscapular artery is the first branch to arise from the inferior portion of the axillary artery. It is com-

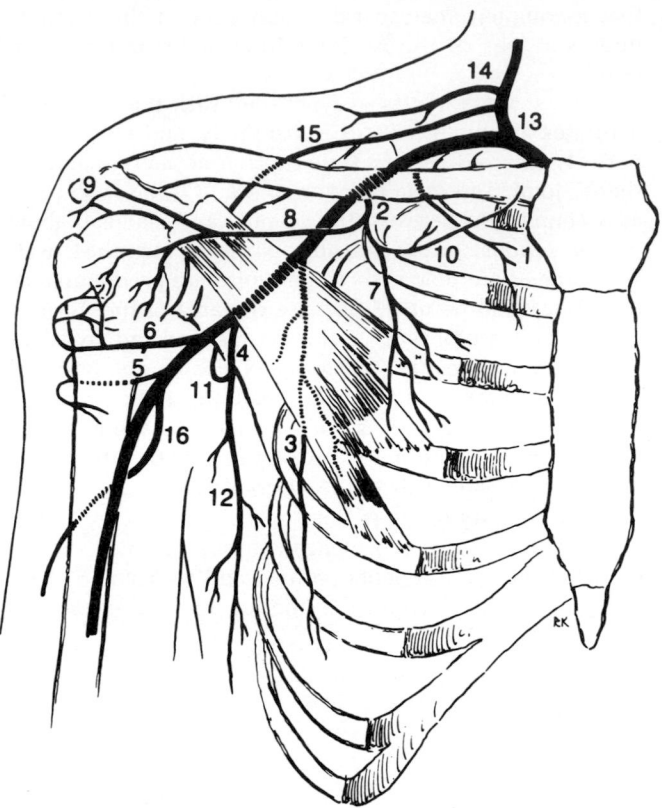

Figure 55-13 Arterial supply of the shoulder. Vessels include the supreme thoracic (1), thoracoacromial axis (2), lateral thoracic (3), subscapular (4), posterior humeral circumflex (5), anterior humeral circumflex (6), pectoral (7), deltoid (8), acromial (9), clavicular (10), circumflex scapular (11), thoracodorsal (12), thyrocervical trunk (13), transverse cervical (14), subscapular (15), and profunda brachii (16). (Reproduced with permission from Jobe CM: Anatomy of the shoulder, in Bigliani LU (ed): *Complications of Shoulder Surgery.* Baltimore, Williams & Wilkins, 1993, pp 1–23.)

monly the largest branch of the axillary artery, giving off two main vessels. These include the scapular circumflex artery, which passes backward around the lower border of the subscapularis muscle and enters the triangular space bordered by the subscapularis, teres major, and long head of triceps muscles. The thoracodorsal artery also arises from the subscapular artery and provides blood supply to the subscapularis, teres major, and latissimus dorsi muscles. The final two branches of the axillary artery are the anterior and posterior humeral circumflex arteries. They pass around the surgical neck of the humerus, with the anterior running deep to the coracobrachialis and short head of the biceps muscles prior to ascending along the tendon of the long head of the biceps to reach the shoulder joint. The posterior humeral circumflex artery runs with the axillary nerve as it passes through the quadrangular space bounded by the subscapularis, teres major and long head of the triceps muscles, and the humerus.[83] It is an important source of blood supply to the proximal humerus. When inadvertently severed in surgery, it can result in a quick and life-threatening source of blood loss which is difficult to coagulate, especially from an anterior approach.

Venous Structures

The major venous structure of the shoulder is the axillary vein, which is a direct continuation of the basilic vein and can be found lying medial to the axillary artery.[83] The vein is supplied by the venae comitantes of the above-mentioned arteries. In addition, the cephalic vein is also an important source of venous drainage into the axillary vein, and it serves as an important landmark due to its constant superficial position between the pectoralis major and deltoid muscles. It is preserved whenever possible to help provide venous drainage of the upper extremity.

Brachial Plexus and Nervous Structures

The nervous structures that supply the upper extremity pass through the shoulder girdle, forming a plexus that intimately surrounds the axillary artery and vein and their branches. This plexus of nerves is known as the *brachial plexus*. The brachial plexus normally arises from the union of the ventral rami of five spinal roots: C5, C6, C7, C8, and T1. Plexi with contributions cephalad to C5 are given the term *prefixed*, while those with caudal contributions below T1 are known as *postfixed*.[92] The brachial plexus is organized in a hierarchical fashion as follows: roots, trunks, divisions, cords, and terminal nerves. The clavicle crosses the brachial plexus at the level of the cords dividing the plexus into supra- and infraclavicular portions. Brachial plexus injuries in the supraclavicular area, proximal to the cords, have a poor prognosis in comparison to infraclavicular injuries, which occur at or beyond the cord level. The entire plexus hierarchy can be simplified beginning with formation of the upper, middle, and lower trunks. The trunks are formed from coalition of the C5 to T1 ventral rami as follows: C5 and C6 form the upper, C7 the middle, and C8 and T1 the lower trunk. This is easily remembered by noting that C7 is the only contribution to the middle trunk. Each trunk then separates into anterior and posterior divisions. The divisions continue on to form the cords, with the posterior divisions of all three trunks forming the posterior cord, the anterior divisions of the upper and middle forming the lateral cord, and the anterior division of the lower trunk forming the medial cord. It is important to note that injuries rarely occur at the division level and that no peripheral nerves originate at this level.[92]

Three peripheral nerves arise in the supraclavicular portion of the plexus, above the level of the anterior and posterior divisions: the long thoracic, the dorsal scapular, and the suprascapular. The dorsal scapular and long thoracic arise from the root level. The suprascapular nerve arises from Erb's point, which is the site of coalition of the C5 and C6 roots forming the upper trunk. When a brachial plexus injury is suspected, noting any dysfunction of the muscles innervated by these three nerves can help localize the site of injury to the supraclavicular portion of the plexus. Injury to the long thoracic and dorsal scapular generally signify a root injury; in many cases, this does not recover.[92]

Supraclavicular plexus injuries are commonly divided into pre- and postganglionic injuries.[92] A general knowledge of the microanatomy of the spinal root is important in understanding the distinction. Preganglionic injuries occur proximal to the dorsal root ganglion. Postganglionic injuries occur along the ventral ramus distal to the origin of the peripheral nerve and the dorsal ramus to the paracervical muscles and distal to the sympathetic ganglion in the case of T1. Preganglionic injuries indicate avulsion of the root from the spinal cord, with virtually no chance for recovery. Postganglionic injury has a better prognosis for recovery. Preganglionic injuries are often indicated by the following exam findings and tests: winging of the scapula, abnormal electromyographic (EMG) studies of the rhomboid and paracervical muscles, Horner's syndrome, normal histamine response test, and the presence of a meningocele on cervical myelography.

The infraclavicular portion of the brachial plexus supplies the remaining peripheral nerves innervating the upper extremity. Nerves arise from the three cords that are named for their position with regard to the axillary artery. Precise localization of infraclavicular brachial plexus injuries is determined by noting deficiencies in upper extremity sensorimotor function and applying that information to the architecture of the brachial plexus. For instance, patients with a proximal posterior cord injury will have deficient function of the upper subscapularis, thoracodorsal, lower subscapularis, axillary, and radial nerves.[92]

Surgical Approaches

Arthroscopic Surgery

General Shoulder arthroscopy has become an important procedure that aids in both the diagnosis and treatment of shoulder pathology. It has several advantages as compared with open techniques, including less invasiveness, improved visualization of intraarticular structures, less morbidity to the deltoid muscle, and quicker rehabilitation. Its disadvantages include the inability to mobilize scarred structures such as retracted rotator cuff tears. The arthroscopic approach is also limited in its ability to shift capsular tissue during instability surgery. As with other areas of the body, arthroscopic surgeons continue to develop improved arthroscopic techniques, which may ultimately replace many open procedures.

Shoulder arthroscopy is a very technically demanding procedure. Setup and positioning of the patient is extremely important to the overall success of any arthroscopic approach. The beach-chair position has become the most preferred method of positioning. The patient is operated upon while sitting upright. This position is advantageous, as it provides a normal vertical orientation of the GH anatomy, free movement of the arm, and the ability to convert to an open procedure easily. In addition, it avoids the use of traction, which can unduly harm the brachial plexus. The lateral decubitus position is an alternative method. The patient is stabilized in a lateral decubitus position and the GH joint is distracted with traction. The arm is positioned in slight abduction and slight forward flexion.

As with other areas of the body, the necessary arthroscopic equipment includes a fiberoptic cable and light source for transmission through a lens connected to a video camera. This provides a magnified view of the areas of interest, primarily the GH joint and subacromial space. These areas are insufflated with arthroscopic fluid, which is either run through the same cannula as the arthroscopic lens or through an additional working cannula. The arthroscopic fluid usually consists of a physiologic solution, such as normal saline, and a dilute quantity of epinephrine to diminish bleeding. A 1-to-300,000 dilution of epinephrine is a safe and effective concentration that can be used. It is helpful to have one of several commercially available working cannulae with a rubber diaphragm that easily maintains the anatomic portal while allowing insertion and removal of arthroscopic equipment.

General anesthesia or a regional anesthesia consisting of an interscalene block can be utilized.[33] Once the patient is anesthetized, it is important always to perform an evaluation under anesthesia, which will help to determine the true passive range of motion and define the stability or instability of the GH joint as compared with the contralateral limb. The patient is then placed in the desired beach-chair or lateral decubitus position. At this point, it is helpful to mark the bony landmarks with a marking pen to assist in identifying safe areas for portal placement.

Portals Several portals are routinely used and are based upon the preoperative diagnosis and planned surgical procedure (Fig. 55-14). The GH joint is routinely examined at the outset, and this can be accomplished through the two most commonly used portals, the posterior and anterior portals. The posterior portal is located at the posterior "soft spot" approximately 2 cm distally and 1 cm medially to the posterolateral corner of the acromion. It is generally found to be at the same level as the tip of the coracoid process, which lies anteriorly. To help determine the proper location of the GH space, it is helpful to translate the humeral head anteriorly and posteriorly between the surgeon's thumb and index finger. A spinal needle is then placed into the GH joint by passing it through the skin portal and aiming straight toward the tip of the coracoid process. Arthroscopic solution can then be placed through the spinal needle into the GH joint, insufflating it with 40 to 60 mL of saline. The surgeon can be sure that the saline is in the GH joint when it flows freely back through the needle under pressure. After the spinal needle properly identifies the line of the GH joint, a scalpel is used to incise skin only; then the arthroscope cannula, fitted with a blunt trochar, is passed through the deltoid, rotator cuff, and joint capsule prior to entering the GH joint. When the above method is used, the cannula generally passes just lateral to the glenoid rim at the junction of the infra- and supraspinatus muscle tendons.

Once the posterior portal is established, an arthroscope is placed through the cannula and arthroscopic fluid flow is initiated through the same cannula. The arthroscope provides direct visualization of the structures in the interior of the GH joint. The anterior portal is then established to provide a means of probing anatomic structures. This portal is located approximately 1 cm lateral to the tip of the coracoid process. A small skin stab wound is made

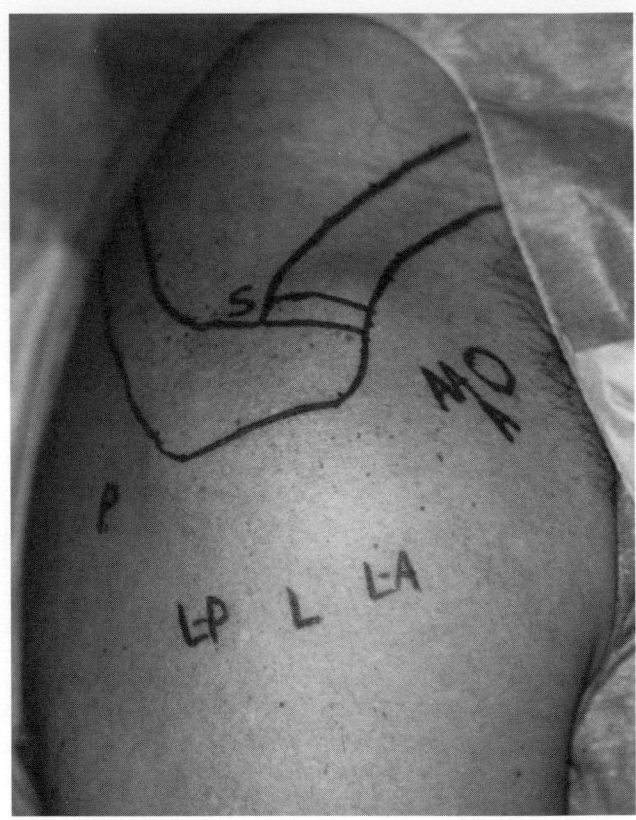

Figure 55-14 The commonly used shoulder arthroscopy portals are shown: anterior (A), accessory anterior (AA), posterior (P), lateral (L), supraspinatus (S), lateral-anterior (L-A), and lateral-posterior (L-P).

vertically and a cannula with a blunt or sharp trochar is passed through the deltoid and then through the rotator cuff interval at the junction of the subscapularis and supraspinatus muscles, directly inferior to the biceps tendon. A disposable cannula is generally placed in this position. The placement of this cannula can be precisely localized by using either a spinal needle under direct visualization or a Wissinger rod. The Wissinger rod technique is carried out by passing the arthroscope tip directly to the portal site from inside the GH joint, then removing the lens while maintaining the position of the cannula and passing a Wissinger rod through the cannula anteriorly, piercing the joint capsule, deltoid muscle, and skin. A cannula is then placed over the Wissinger rod into the GH joint. It is important to ensure that the cannula is placed laterally to the coracoid to prevent any chance of injury to the musculocutaneous nerve.

Glenohumeral When glenohumeral arthroscopy is performed, it is important to establish an ordered sequence of examination so as to ensure a complete diagnostic evaluation. Once the arthroscope is placed into the GH joint through the posterior portal, the humeral head and glenoid surfaces are identified and the long head of the biceps tendon at its insertion into the superior labrum is noted (Fig. 55-15). This will ensure proper orientation of the arthro-

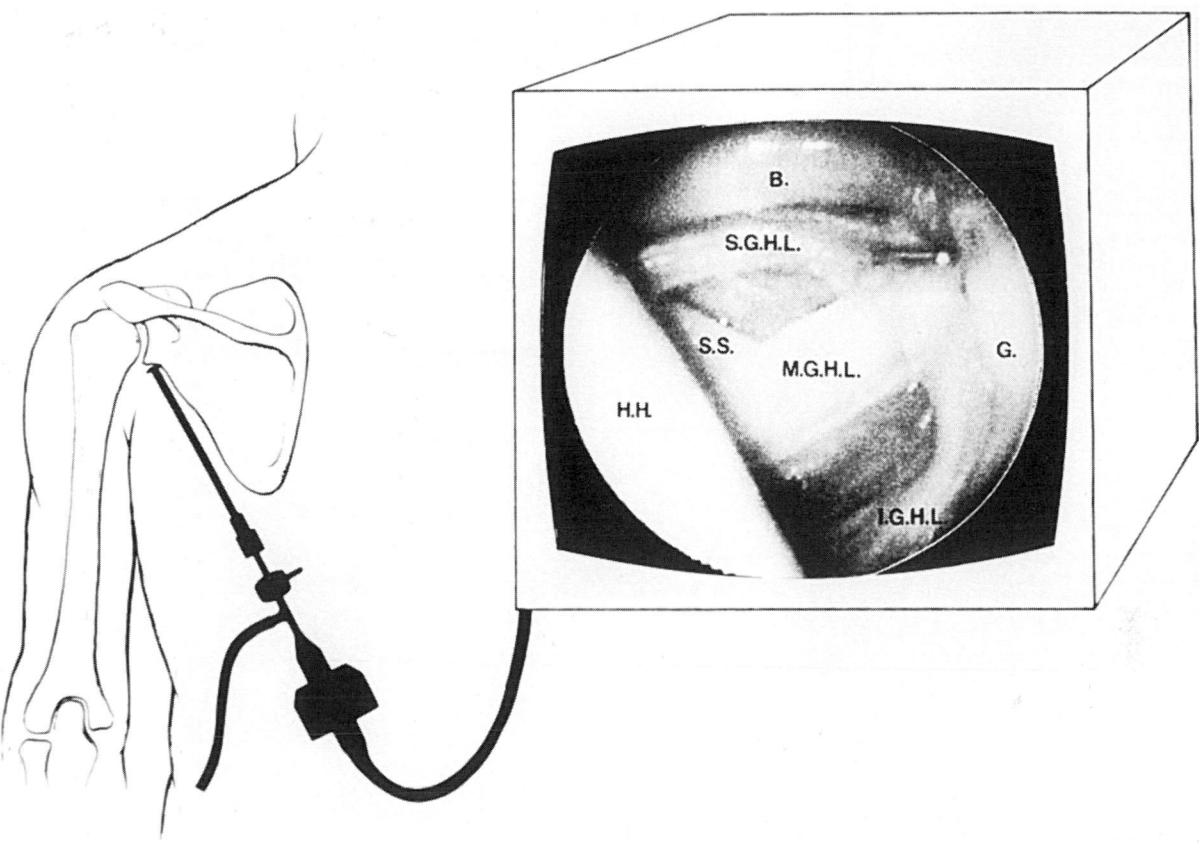

Figure 55-15 Arthroscopic view of the anterosuperior glenohumeral joint showing the humeral head (HH), subscapularis muscle (SS), glenoid cavity (G), long head of the biceps tendon (B), and the glenohumeral ligaments (SGHL, MGHL, and IGHL). (Reproduced with permission from Caborn DNM, Warner JP, Berger R, et al: Dynamic capsuloligamentous anatomy of the glenohumeral joint. *Trans Orthop Res Soc* 17:498, 1992.)

scope. The anterior labral tissue and superior labrum from anterior to posterior are then examined. The GH ligaments are then noted. An attempt is made to sweep the arthroscope between the humeral head and glenoid into the axillary pouch. When this maneuver is easily accomplished, excessive capsular laxity is suspected. The long head of the biceps tendon is then examined from its insertion site at the superior glenoid labrum to its passage into the intertubercular groove. The rotator cuff is fully evaluated while looking superiorly and laterally as it inserts into the greater tuberosity. The arthroscope is then swept posteriorly, looking at the bare area of the humeral head. Significant pitting or compression fractures in the bare area are often representative of anterior instability. Structures are probed to determine their integrity. It is important to move the humeral head in synchrony with the arthroscope, both in rotation and in forward elevation, in order to allow complete visualization of all desired structures.

When arthroscopy is utilized for treatment of anterior instability, it is common to use two anterior portals (Fig. 55-16). In this situation, an additional anterior portal can be used to place tension on capsular labral tissue while an arthroscopic tack or other anchoring device is being utilized. The extraanterior portal also provides an additional

site for visualization with the camera, while the other anterior portal is used for direct instrumentation during preparation and fixation of labral or capsuloligamentous tissue. When an additional anterior portal is placed, the regular anterior portal is placed slightly superiorly; the additional anterior portal is termed an *anteroinferior* portal and is placed 2 cm distal to the regular anterior portal.

Subacromial When subacromial arthroscopy is being performed, the arthroscope is placed into the subacromial space with one cannula while other instruments are placed through an additional lateral portal (Fig. 55-17). This can be accomplished by using the previous posterior portal site for penetration of skin and deltoid and redirecting the arthroscope cannula into the subacromial space. A straight lateral portal is then placed in a similar fashion. This method eliminates the need for additional deltoid penetration. An alternative method is to utilize two lateral portals, with the posterior portal generally being used for the arthroscope and the anteriormost portal being used for instrumentation. In this method, the portals are placed laterally to the anterior and posterior corners of the acromion (Fig. 55-14). This method allows the arthroscope to be positioned in front of the posterior bend of the acromion for

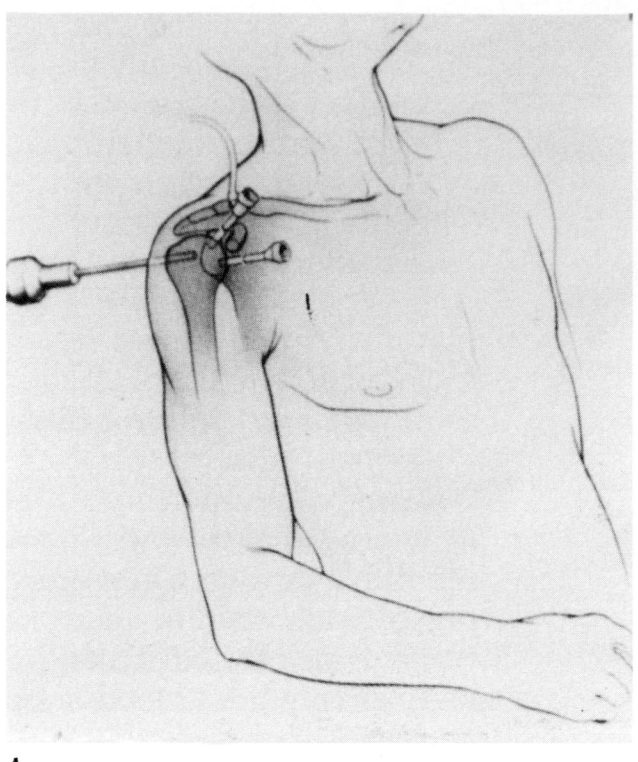

A

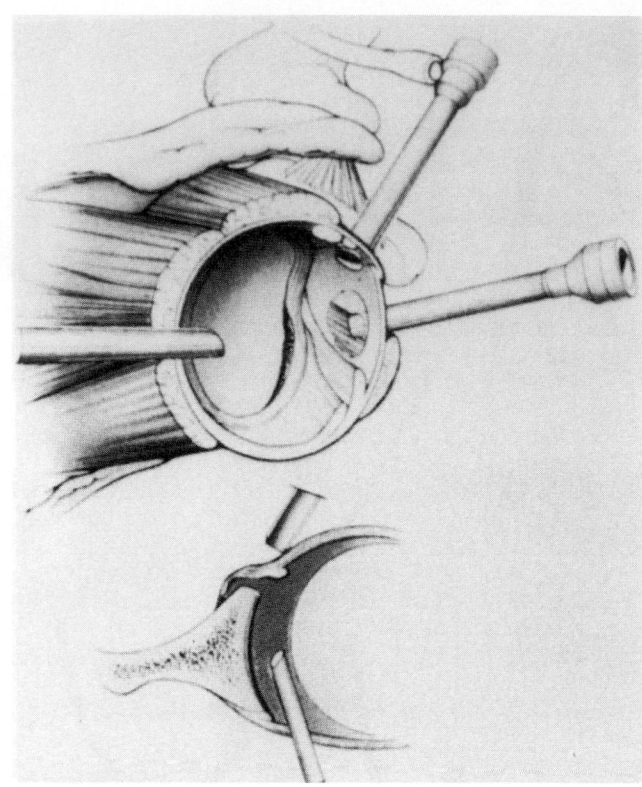

B

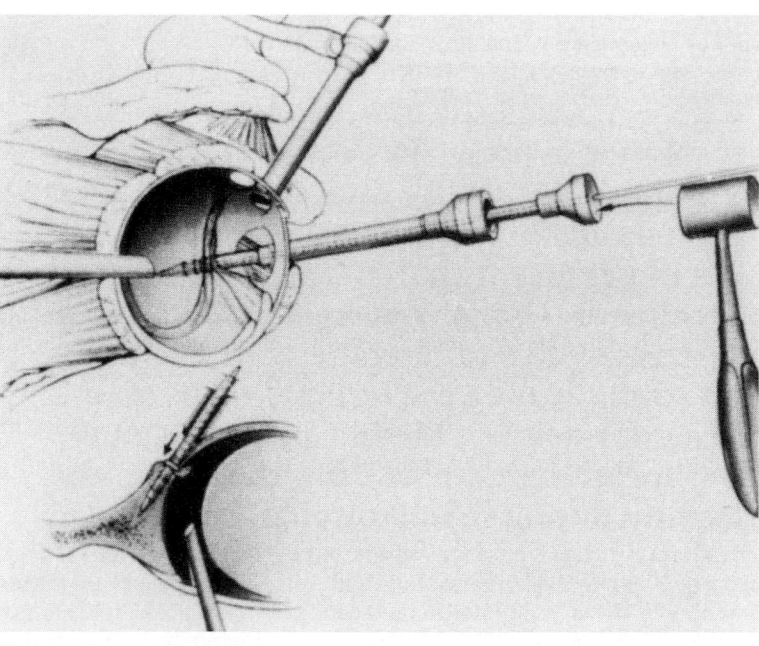

C

Figure 55-16 Arthroscopic Bankart repair with a biodegradable fixation tack: portals (*A*), visualization of the Bankart lesion (*B*), and insertion of the device (*C*). (Reproduced with permission from Warner JJP, Warren RF: Arthroscopic Bankart repair using cannulated, absorbable fixation device. *Op Tech Orthop* 1:192–198, 1991.)

improved visualization of the subacromial space. In order to avoid axillary nerve damage but allow easy passage of arthroscopic equipment beneath the acromial edge, any of the above lateral portals should be placed approximately 3 cm lateral to the acromial edge. To lessen the risk of damage to deltoid muscle fiber, it is helpful to pass the cannulas using first a sharp trochar and then converting

to a blunt trochar once the cannula has been passed through the deltoid muscle. A supraspinatus portal is occasionally used as an adjunct portal for subacromial or GH arthroscopy. This portal is located at the lateral corner of the supraspinatus fossa (Fig. 55-14).

In subacromial arthroscopy, once the posterior or lateral-posterior portal for the arthroscope is established, the

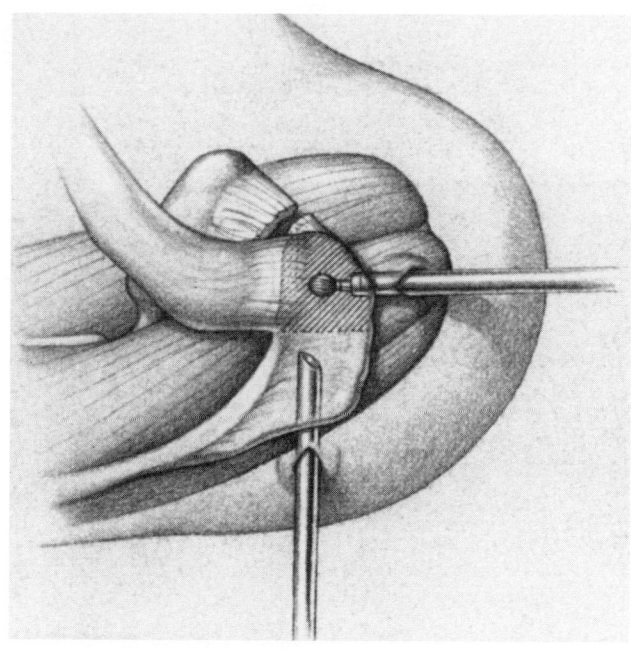

A

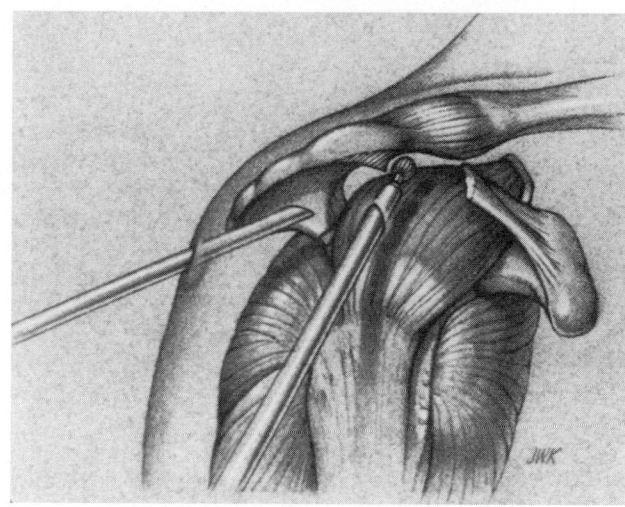

B

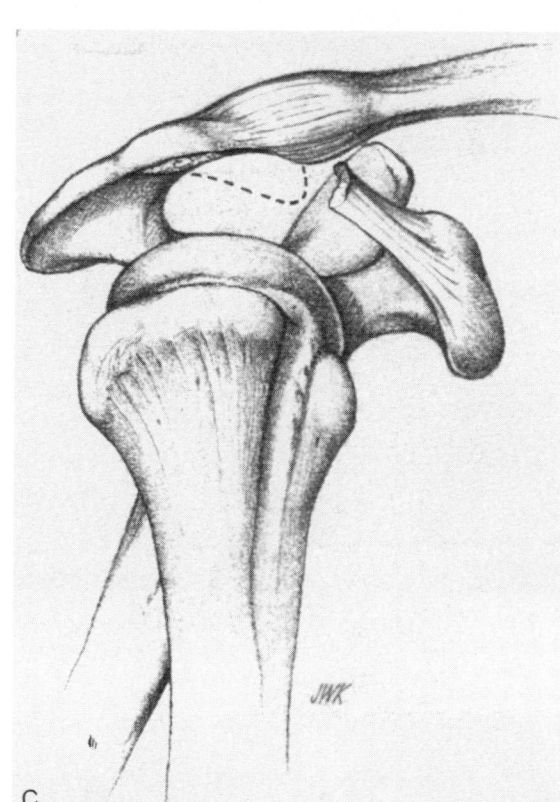

C

Figure 55-17 Subacromial arthroscopy for anterior acromioplasty. *A.* Superior view. *B.* Lateral view. *C.* Acromioplasty and CA ligament resection completed. (Reproduced with permission from Harner CD: Arthroscopic subacromial decompression. *Op Tech Orthop* 1:229–234, 1991.)

second portal is established for use as a working portal. Next, the bursal space is opened by using the shaver to debride bursal tissue. This creates a visualized space. It is important to have electrocautery immediately available to prevent excessive bleeding, which can obliterate the field of view. It is helpful to insufflate the subacromial space with approximately 30 mL of an arthroscopic epinephrine solution at the beginning of such surgery to help constrict any blood vessels that might bleed during subacromial arthroscopy.

Acromioclavicular Acromioclavicular arthroscopy is often performed in conjunction with subacromial ar-

throscopy.[146] In this case, the acromioclavicular joint is entered through the bursal space, and visualization of the distal clavicle is aided by digital pressure on the end of the clavicle (Fig. 55-18). When AC arthroscopy is being performed as an isolated procedure, direct portals can be established for placement of the scope and instrumentation directly into the AC joint (Fig. 55-19). These portals are placed in parallel with the AC joint, approximately 1 cm anteriorly to the anterior edge of the AC joint and 1 cm posteriorly to the posterior edge of the AC joint. In patients with extremely narrow AC joints, it may be necessary to use a wrist arthroscope until the joint space is

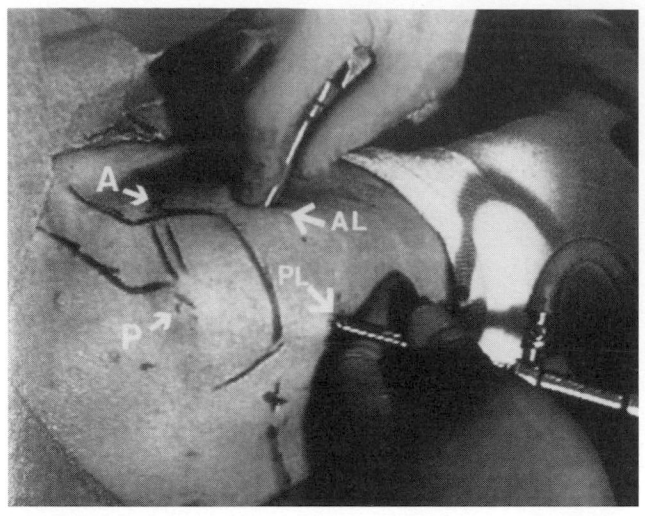

A

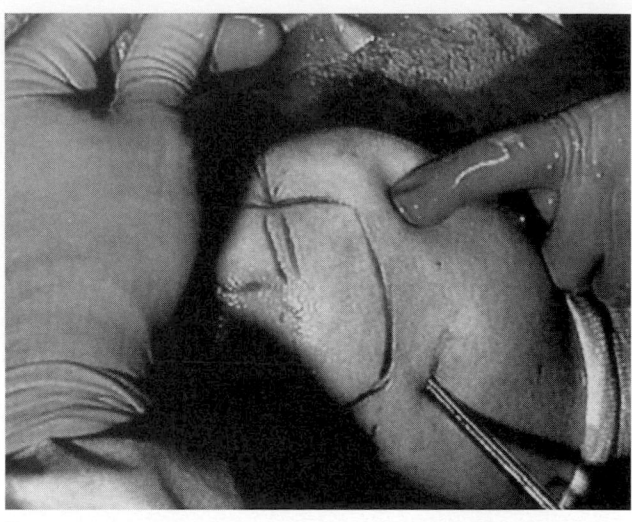

B

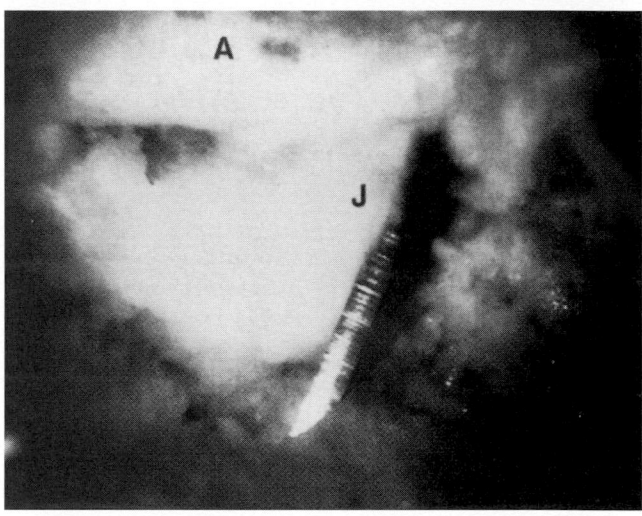

D

C

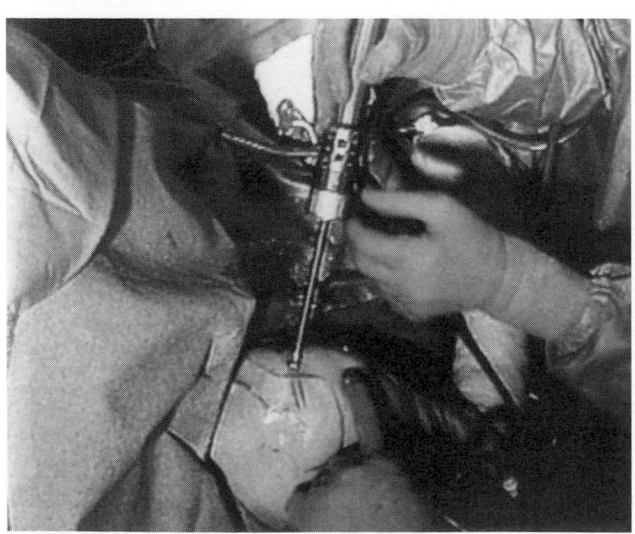

E

Figure 55-18 *A.* Subacromial arthroscopy has been performed through postero- and anterolateral portals in this right shoulder. The anterosuperior (A) and posterosuperior (P) portals for direct access with instrumentation will be used to resect the distal clavicle, while the arthroscope will remain in the subacromial space. *B.* A needle is used to locate the AC joint through the anterosuperior portal. *C.* The needle pierces the AC joint inferior capsule (J) from the anterosuperior aspect of the AC joint (A = acromion). *D.* The knife is used to create the anterosuperior portal (A = acromion, J = AC joint capsule). *E.* The burr is placed through the portal. *F.* Schematic superior view. *G.* Schematic anterior view. (Reproduced with permission from Rodosky MW, Flatow EL: Arthroscopic debridement of the acromioclavicular joint and distal clavicle resection, in McGinty JB: *Operative Arthroscopy.* Philadelphia, Lippincott Raven, 1996, pp 773–783.)

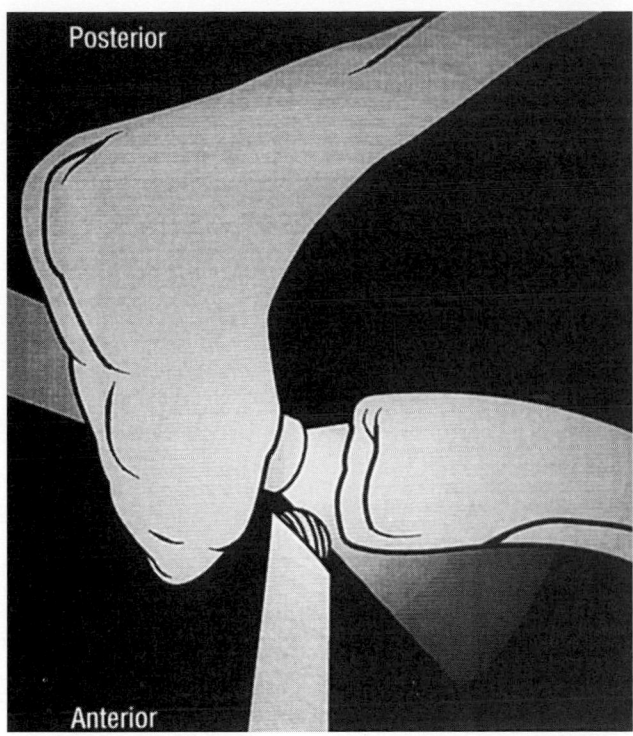

F

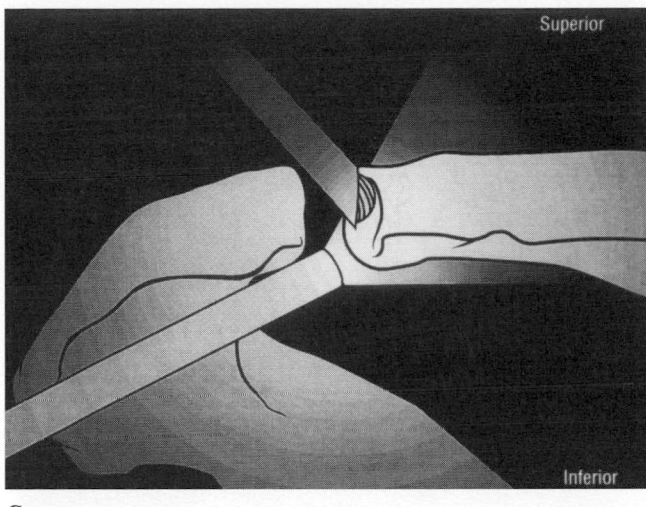

G

Figure 55-18 *(Continued)*

widened with a burr.[60] A single direct portal can also be utilized to aid in resection of the distal clavicle, even when a bursal approach for visualization is being utilized. In addition, the anterior portal can often be used to place instruments into the AC joint. The cannula is simply directed into the subacromial space, and the AC joint is entered inferiorly and anteriorly.[146]

Anterior Approach

The anterior approach to the shoulder takes advantage of the interval between the deltoid and pectoralis major muscles. It is a useful approach for arthroplasties, proximal humeral fractures, and instability repair. The patient is placed in a beach-chair position, with the torso angled from 25 to 70° and the shoulder sitting off the edge of the table. A special head holder is helpful in providing superior access.

For instability repairs, a smaller incision is utilized and is made in line with the axillary crease (Fig. 55-20). This incision can be hidden in the axillary crease in cases where cosmesis is important. For shoulder arthroplasty, a larger incision is utilized. The incision runs from the clavicle to the lateral edge of the coracoid and down to the anterior edge of the deltoid insertion into the humerus (Fig. 55-21). The cephalic vein is identified and used as landmark to locate the deltopectoral interval. It is taken either medially or laterally as the interval between the deltoid and pectoralis major muscles is opened. Next, the conjoined tendon (strap muscles) is identified and retracted medially. The clavipectoral fascia immediately lateral to the short head of the biceps muscle is then incised, gain-

ing exposure to the subscapularis muscle below. Access to the GH joint is then carried out by either splitting the subscapularis muscle along the line of its fibers or incising the subscapularis laterally at the lesser tuberosity.

The vascular structures at greatest risk with this procedure are the anterior humeral circumflex vessels, which lie at the inferior border of the subscapularis tendon. These can be safely ligated to prevent uncontrolled bleeding. Nervous structures at risk include the axillary nerve, which crosses over the body of the subscapularis and runs beneath the anterior humeral circumflex vessels and medial aspect of the axillary pouch on its way through the quadrilateral space. Its position should be noted by palpation, using a tug test in which the index finger is swept beneath the coracoid process over the subscapularis and gently hooks the axillary nerve, or through direct visualization.[61] The musculocutaneous nerve is also at risk as it enters the conjoined tendon as high as 1.5 mm distal to the coracoid process.[63] Excessive force during retraction on the conjoined tendon should be avoided.

Superoanterior Approach

The superoanterior approach is commonly used for rotator cuff surgery.[12,13,23] The deltoid muscle fibers are split to allow access to the front of the acromion and rotator cuff insertion at the greater tuberosity. To lessen postoperative scar, it is helpful to make the skin incision in Langer's lines.[23] The skin incision is typically made from the mid portion of the acromion to slightly posterior and lateral to the coracoid process. It is placed over the lateral edge of the acromion. To help with tissue mobilization, it

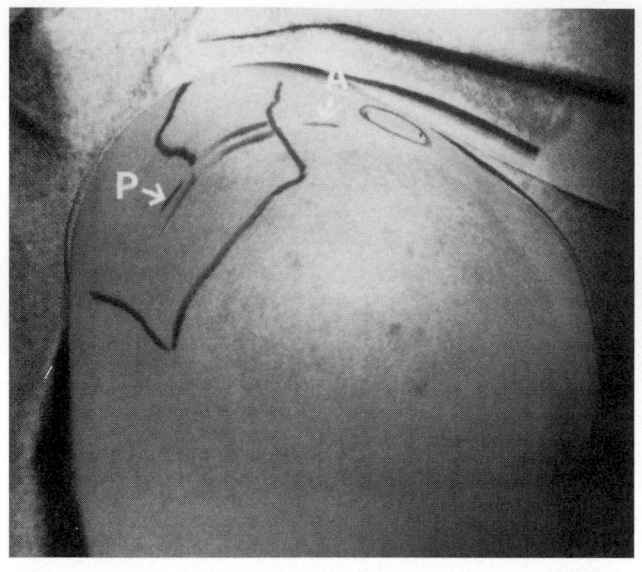

A

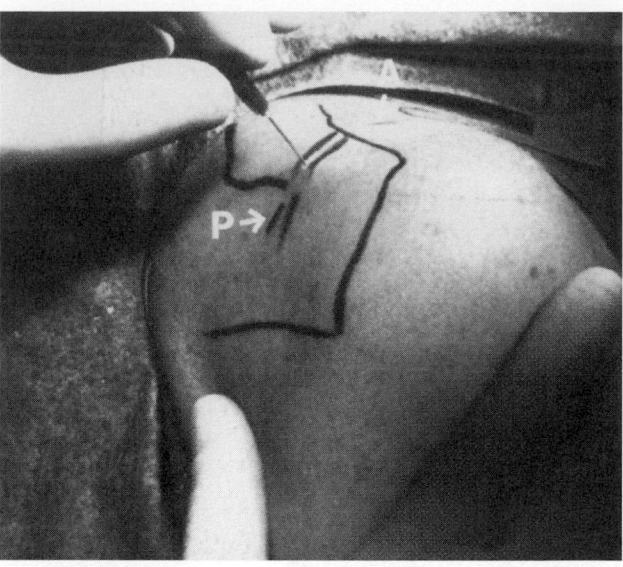

B

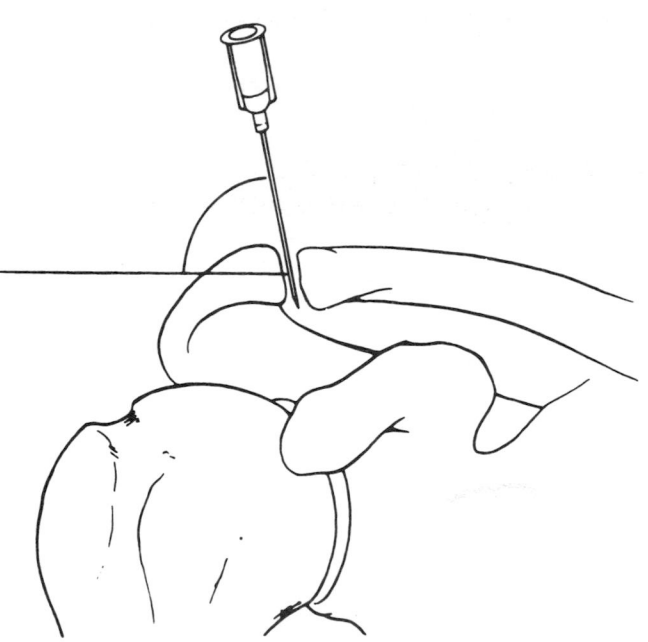

C

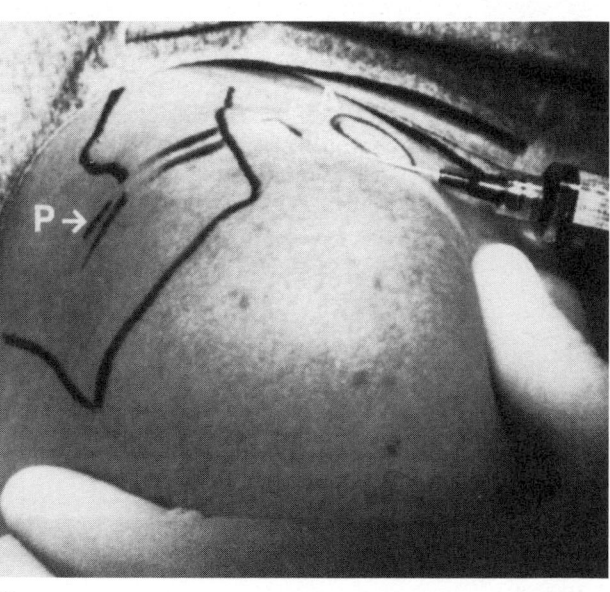

D

Figure 55-19 *A.* Right shoulder prior to arthroscopy of the AC joint with the anterosuperior (A) and posterosuperior (P) portals indicated. *B.* Confirming the position of the AC joint with a needle (A = anterosuperior portal, P = posterosuperior portal). *C.* The needle helps define the precise inclination of the joint. *D.* The portal sites are injected with lidocaine and epinephrine to diminish bleeding (A = anterosuperior portal, P = posterosuperior portal). *E.* The arthroscope and instruments are passed into the joint via the portals as shown. The position of the scope and instruments may be alternated to allow an even resection of bone. *F.* Schematic superior view of direct approach. *G.* Schematic anterior view of direct approach. (Reproduced with permission from Rodosky MW, Flatow EL: Arthroscopic debridement of the acromioclavicular joint and distal clavicle resection, in McGinty JB: *Operative Arthroscopy.* Philadelphia, Lippincott Raven, 1996, pp 773–783.)

Figure 55-19 *(Continued)*

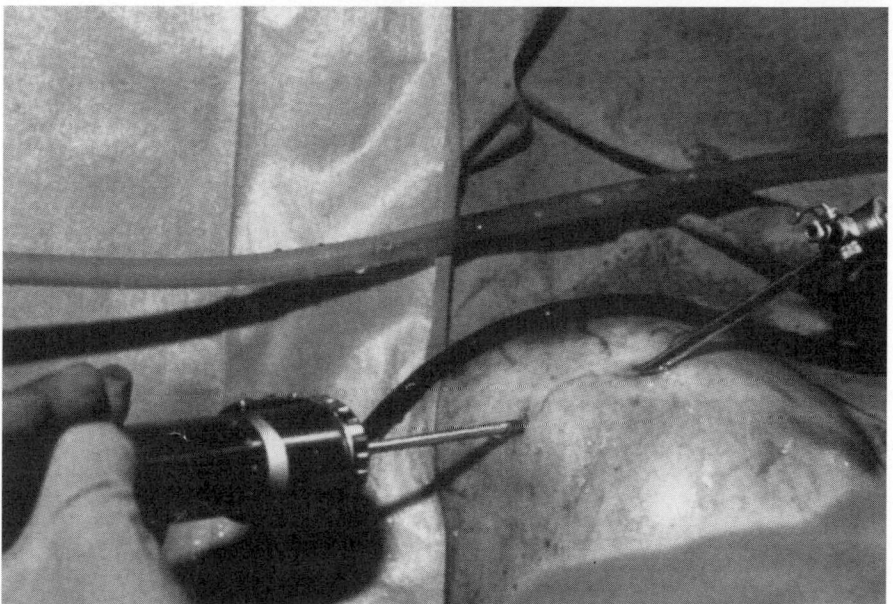

E

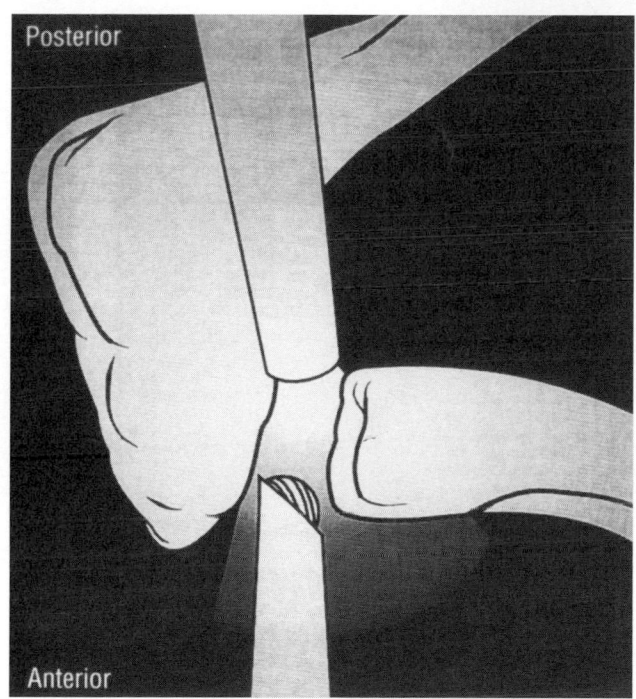

F

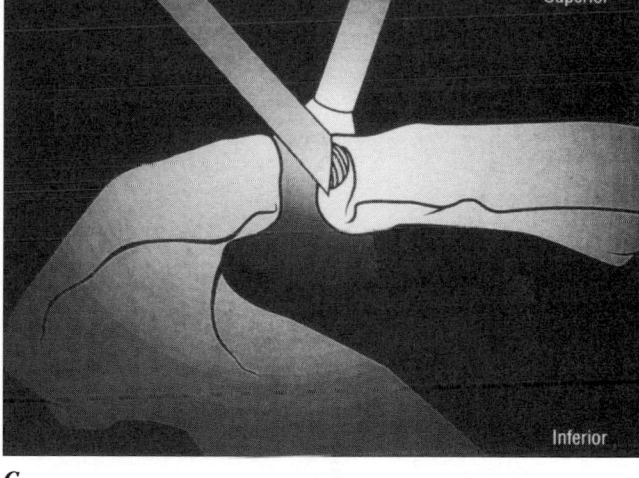

G

is important to undermine the skin at the junction of the subcutaneous tissue and superficial deltoid fascia. This plane is developed to allow access 5 cm lateral to the acromion and medial to the acromioclavicular joint. The deltoid muscle is split in line with its fibers beginning at the medial aspect of the AC joint and extending past the front edge of the acromion. Approximately 5 mm of strong deltotrapezial insertion fascia is left at the front edge of the bone to assist in later closure.[23] The deltoid muscle split can continue on safely to approximately 4 cm lateral to the anterolateral corner of the acromion without injur-

ing the axillary nerve. It is helpful to place a stay suture at the lateral aspect of the split to prevent propagation of the split and potential injury to the axillary nerve. In cases where a large amount of scar and retraction of the posterior aspect of the cuff is expected, it is helpful to make the split as far posteriorly as possible, so that it will be centered over the greater tuberosity. This will make access to the posterior cuff easier. While access to the front edge of the acromion is being gained, the coracoacromial ligament is subperiosteally dissected off the front of the acromion. The subacromial bursal tissue below can then be resected

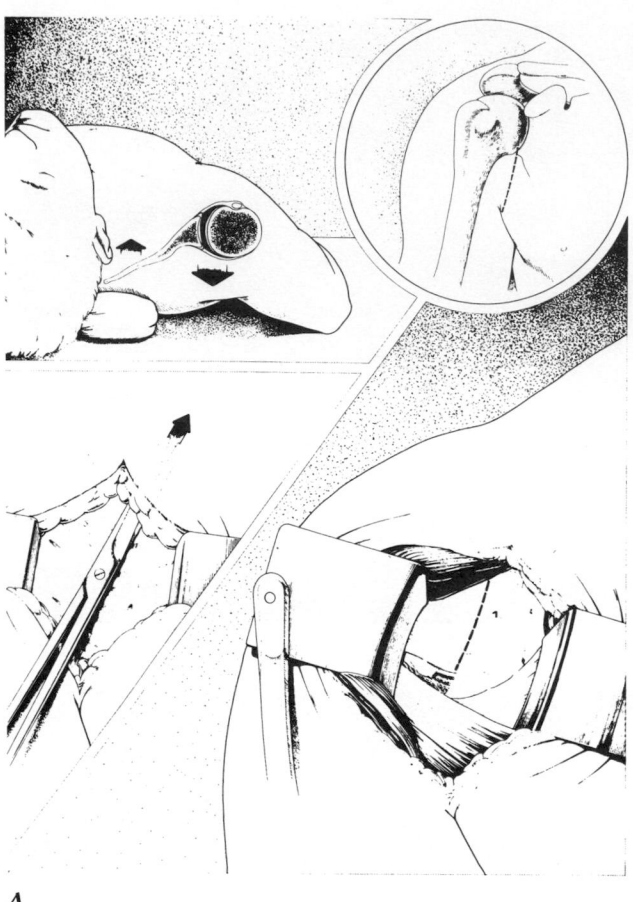

Figure 55-20 *A.* Instability repairs are carried out through a small anterior axillary incision with the deltoid retracted laterally and the pectoralis retracted medially. This exposes the conjoined tendon (1). *B.* With gentle medial retraction of the conjoined tendon (1), the subscapularis muscle (2) comes into view. *C.* The subscapularis (2) is then either incised transversely, as shown or in line with its fibers. *D.* This exposes the undersurface of the subscapularis muscle (3) and the capsule (4). Reproduced with permission from Randelli M, Gambrioli PL, Minola R, et al: *Surgical Techniques for the Shoulder.* Padua, Piccin, 1995.)

A

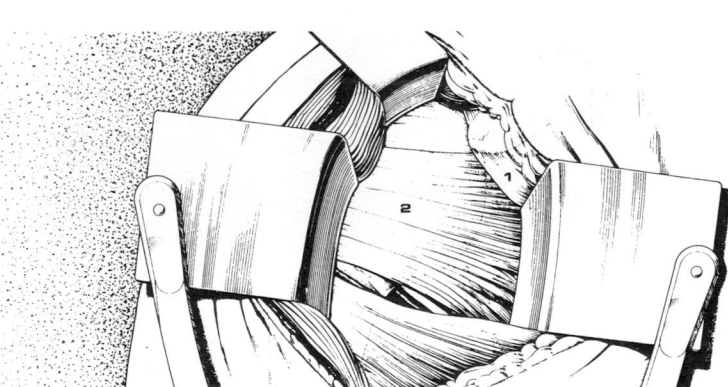

B

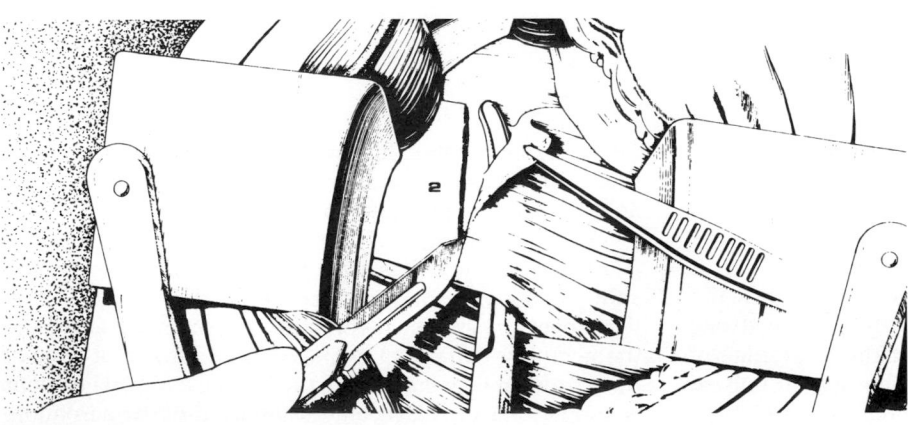

C

Figure 55-20 *(Continued)*

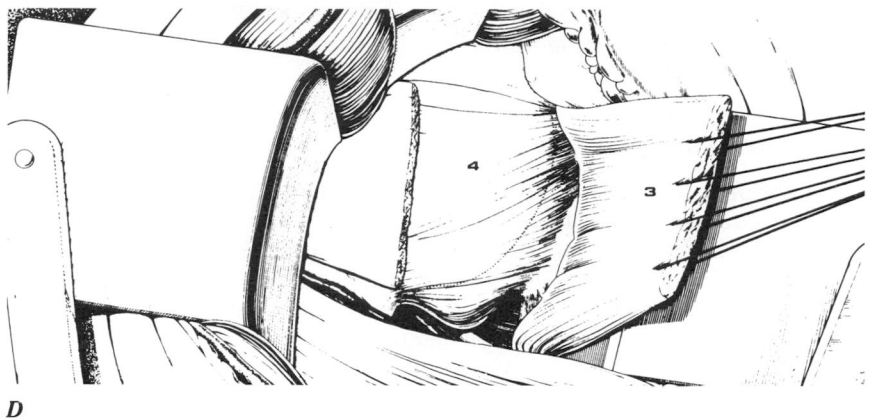

D

to gain visualization of the rotator cuff. Visualization of the posterior cuff tissue is made possible by internally rotating and extending the arm. The lesser tuberosity and subscapularis are made accessible by forward flexion of the

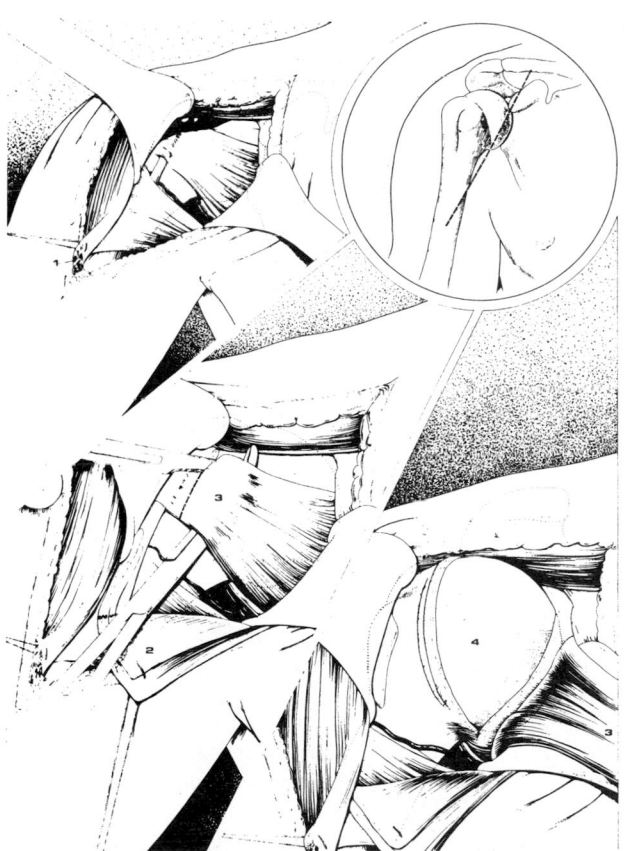

Figure 55-21 The extended deltopectoral approach for total shoulder replacement is carried out by separating the deltoid (1) and pectoralis muscles (2). The pectoralis muscle can be partially resected to aid in inferior visualization. Next, the subscapularis muscle and capsule (3) are incised to expose the humeral head (4). (Reproduced with permission from Randelli M, Gambrioli PL, Minola R, et al: *Surgical Techniques for the Shoulder.* Padua, Piccin, 1995.)

arm. The neurovascular structures at risk for this procedure include the acromial branch of the thoracoacromial artery. This is often encountered when incising the CA ligament. It can be safely coagulated with cautery. The axillary nerve is also vulnerable as it passes posteriorly through the quadrangular space and then wraps around the neck of the humerus on its way to insertion into the deltoid muscle. It penetrates the deltoid muscle generally 5 cm laterally to the lateral edge of the acromion.

Posterior Approach

The posterior approach to the shoulder is useful for instability procedures directed at posterior instability as well as for scapular or posterior glenoid fractures.[10] The skin incision is made in an oblique fashion, running in line with the deltoid fibers from the lateral aspect of the scapular spine to the posterolateral aspect of the shoulder. A small portion of deltoid is then subperiosteally stripped from the lateral aspect of the scapular spine and split from the posterolateral corner of the acromion in line with the deltoid fibers. The deltoid should be split no further than the inferior border of the teres minor muscle in order to prevent injury to the axillary nerve. With medial and lateral retraction of the split deltoid muscle, the posterior rotator cuff structures are easily visualized.

The GH joint can be entered by either splitting the infraspinatus muscle laterally, prior to its insertion into the greater tuberosity, or by transversely opening the interval between the infraspinatus and teres minor muscles. Alternatively, the entire deltoid can be retracted superolaterally. This allows access to the infraspinatus and teres minor muscles more medially over the glenoid rim. It is extremely difficult to gain lateral access to the GH joint using this variation.

Neurovascular structures at highest risk with the posterior approach include the axillary and suprascapular nerves. The axillary nerve passes through the quadrilateral space just beneath the teres minor muscle, which can be used as a landmark to help prevent injury to the axillary nerve. The suprascapular nerve passes beneath the ligament of the suprascapular notch, passing across the supraspinatus fossa and laterally to the scapular spine on its way into the lateral aspect of the infraspinatus fossa. It lies approximately 3 cm medially to the posterior glenoid rim. Retraction or dissection beyond this point can result in significant suprascapular nerve palsy.

Acromioclavicular Approach

The anterior approach to the AC joint can be used for AC reconstruction and excision of the distal clavicle. The skin incision is generally made in Langer's lines and is centered over the AC joint.[83] The AC joint is easily exposed beneath the trapezial-deltoid fascia. In AC reconstruction, the deltotrapezial fascia is incised over the lateral aspect of the acromion, running laterally at the front edge of the acromion to its anterolateral corner. This will provide access to both the CA ligament and the coracoid process. In AC resection surgery, the deltotrapezial fascia is incised directly over the lateral portion of the clavicle and is continued laterally across the AC joint to the medial aspect of the acromion. The fascial insertion into the periosteum and periosteum itself are elevated with an elevator to allow for approximately 1 cm resection of the distal clavicle. T incisions directly over the AC joint can be utilized to help with exposure. The suprascapular muscle and its nerve should be protected when a distal clavicular excision is performed by placing retractors under the distal aspect of the clavicle.

Sternoclavicular Approach

The approach to the SC joint is used primarily for resection of this joint in patients with arthritis or infection or for stabilization of the unstable SC joint. The skin incision is generally made in an oblique fashion, running anterior to the SC joint and perpendicular to the joint surfaces (Fig. 55-22). Soft tissues are incised directly over the SC joint and a capsulotomy is performed. It is important to use blunt elevators and retractors to prevent damage to the great vessels, which lie directly beneath the SC joint.

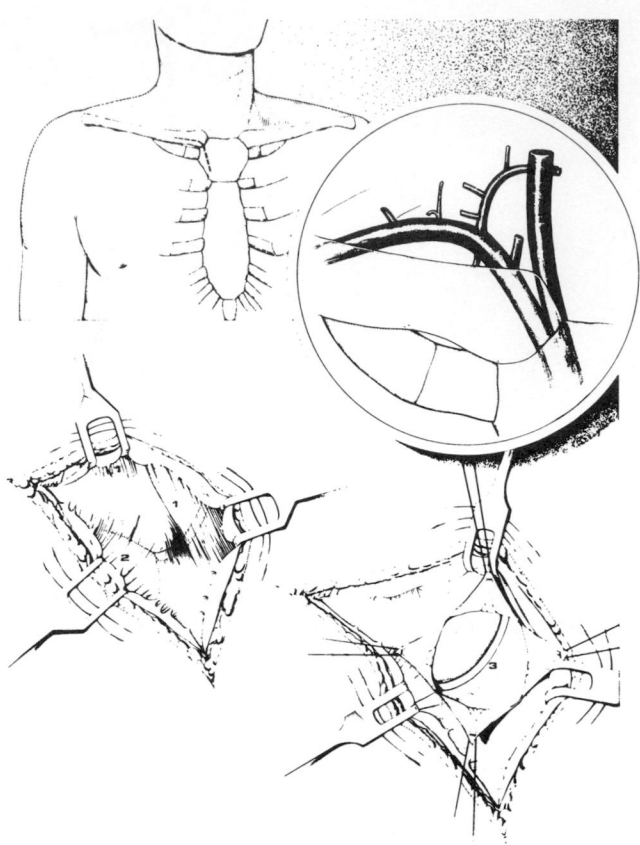

Figure 55-22 To expose the sternoclavicular joint, the tissue overlying the joint and between the sternocleidomastoid (1) and the pectoralis major (2) is incised. This directly exposes the underlying joint (3). (Reproduced with permission from Randelli M, Gambrioli PL, Minola R, et al: *Surgical Techniques for the Shoulder.* Padua, Piccin, 1995.)

HISTORY, PHYSICAL EXAMINATION, AND DIAGNOSTIC MODALITIES

A comprehensive history and physical examination serve as the basis for diagnosis and treatment of shoulder pathology.[15] Diagnostic modalities—including roentgenograms and radiographic studies, laboratory tests, and arthroscopy—serve an important adjunct function and may be necessary to certify the diagnosis. The history and physical examination are performed in a systematic fashion so that each and every important piece of information is included (Table 55-2).

The history begins with age, sex, and chief complaint. Hand dominance, occupation, and functional or athletic activities are noted so as to enable the examiner to understand the past and future functional demands of the shoulder in question. For instance, the differential diagnosis and future goals of an octogenarian are quite different from those of a young throwing athlete. Additionally, there may be a relationship between the patient's activity and the pathology, such as rotator cuff disease in an overhead laborer or osteolysis of the distal clavicle in a weight lifter.[15]

History

The patient's chief complaint can be broken down into categories including pain, weakness, stiffness, and instability. If one or more of these categories applies, it is important to fully understand the proportional relationship. For example, pain and weakness may be related to a rotator cuff tear, whereas pain and stiffness may be caused by a frozen shoulder. Next, it is important to document when the symptoms began, what provoked them, how severe they are, when they occur, and the nature of any exacerbating activities. It is also important to note any known mechanism of injury. It is not uncommon for a patient to have an insidious onset of shoulder symptoms from chronic disease that is exacerbated by an acute injury. For instance, a patient with impingement and partial tearing of the rotator cuff may suffer a hard fall and go from cuff disease to a full-thickness tear.[15]

TABLE 55-2 History

I. Patient
  A. Hand dominance
  B. Occupation
  C. Athletics
    1. Sports
    2. Level of competition
    3. Relation to shoulder problem (e.g., weight-lifting and osteolysis of the distal clavicle)
  D. Other medical disorders (e.g., diabetes, cancer)
  E. Family history (e.g., arthritis, ligamentous laxity)
II. Shoulder disorder
  A. Chief complaint
    1. Pain
    2. Weakness
    3. Stiffness
    4. Instability
  B. Symptom pattern
    1. Duration
    2. Provocation
    3. Severity
    4. Location
  C. Injury
    1. Traumatic
    2. Atraumatic
    3. Repetitive microtrauma
    4. Preexisting condition?
  D. Level of disability
    1. Athletes
    2. Occupation
    3. Daily tasks
III. Related symptoms
  A. Cervical pain
  B. Neurologic
    1. Cervical radiculopathy
    2. Brachial plexus
    3. Peripheral nerve
  C. Chest (e.g., cardiac, lung, herpes zoster)

The pattern of shoulder pain should be fully documented. Recurrent pain that occurs when the arm is in an abducted and externally rotated position may be an indication of anterior instability, whereas a more episodic history of severe pain and inflammation may be related to calcific tendinitis. Rest pain and night pain are often present and can be related to any type of shoulder pathology.[15]

To complete the history, it is necessary to obtain a general medical history. A patient with diabetes mellitus may present with a frozen shoulder, or one with a rheumatologic disease may be suffering from an arthritic shoulder. Past surgical history is also important, especially when it involves the symptomatic shoulder or upper extremity. A family history should be obtained, as it may provide information regarding congenital conditions, such as generalized ligamentous laxity in a patient with multidirectional GH instability.

A review of systems is obtained, with specific attention to adjacent regions, such as the neck, chest, and cardiac system. Pathology in these areas may result in referred pain to the shoulder. It is very common for cervical disease to present with pain referred to the shoulder. However, this pain is most often referred to the posterior shoulder and trapezius and may also be felt more distally into the forearm or hand. Pain from intrinsic shoulder pathology is usually more localized. In addition, pain originating from the neck is often related to the position of the cervical spine and can also result in numbness or tingling throughout the upper extremity. The exception to this rule is a patient with instability of the GH or AC joint, which causes mechanical strain at the brachial plexus.

Physical Examination
Routine Exam

Physical examination of the shoulder is carried out in an orderly sequence of observation, palpation, motion, motor ability, sensation, vascularity, and provocative testing. The patient should be examined with each shoulder fully exposed. This is accomplished by having men disrobe above the waist and having women wear strapless gowns tied beneath their shoulders. Inspection is then performed from the front as well as the back of the patient. The examiner looks for asymmetry of muscle mass and contour as well as prominences or deformity of bone and joint structures. Atrophy of the supraspinatus or infraspinatus muscles, commonly associated with a rotator cuff tear, can easily be seen from the patient's back.[12]

Palpation is initiated while the examiner is standing behind the patient and checking for areas of tenderness. A systematic approach is utilized, beginning with palpation of the AC joint, the clavicle, and the SC joint. Next, the acromion and rotator cuff insertion into the greater tuberosity are palpated for tenderness. The examiner palpates the long head of the biceps tendon as it passes through the bicipital groove by rolling the lesser and greater tuberosities between his or her fingers. Next, the posterior joint line, coracoid process, and anterior joint line are palpated. Other structures are palpated as directed by the history.

Tenderness localized to the rotator cuff insertion into the greater tuberosity or the anterior edge of the acromion is often associated with impingement or rotator cuff disease. Joint line tenderness at the anterior or posterior aspects of the GH joint may be associated with GH instability. Posterior joint line tenderness is also commonly associated with GH osteoarthritis.[111]

Range of motion must be evaluated. This evaluation typically includes forward elevation in the scapular plane (normal, 160 to 180°), abduction (normal, 160 to 180°), external rotation with the arm at the side (normal, 30 to 80°), external rotation with the arm at 90° of abduction (normal, 70 to 90°), and maximal internal rotation. Maximal internal rotation is best evaluated by having the patient reach behind his or her back and placing his or her thumb at the highest possible vertebral level in the midline of the back (normal, T5 to T11). Active motion is tested first, followed by passive motion. True passive range of motion in forward elevation and external rotation is best evaluated by having the patient lie supine, trapping the scapula between the body and the examining table. This helps to eliminate false measurements due to motion at the thoracolumbar spine. The motion that is measured is a combination of both GH and ST motion. When the examiner is suspicious that an abnormal ratio of GH to ST motion (normally 2:1) is present, motion at each of the articulations is carefully evaluated.[111]

Motor strength is assessed using manual muscle strength tests. Specific muscles are isolated in a systematic fashion. When a patient has significant pain, it may be difficult to truly assess motor function due to the patient's inability to sustain maximal muscle force. Since most shoulder pathology involves the rotator cuff muscles, it is common to begin motor testing with the supra- and infraspinatus muscles. These muscles are tested by having the patient resist abduction and external rotation. The supraspinatus is best isolated by having both upper extremities in a position of 90° of forward elevation in the scapular plane.[15] Resistance is applied at the level of the arm as the patient makes a fist, with the thumbs pointing in a cranial direction. The infraspinatus is best isolated by having the patient resist external rotation with the arm at the side. The "French horn" test is an additional and very sensitive test that picks up weakness in either the supraspinatus or infraspinatus musculature. It is performed by having the standing patient place his or her shoulder in 45° of forward elevation in the scapular plane and 45° of external rotation. With the elbows flexed to 90°, a caudally directed force is applied at the forearms. A positive test occurs when the patient is unable to sustain the position against force. When the test is positive, the patient will typically rotate the scapula to compensate for weakness at the GH joint. The scapular rotation results in the forearm assuming a position more or less parallel to the floor, similar to the way a horn is held. Although weakness in external rotation and forward elevation is most often related to rotator cuff pathology, it may also be the result of cervical disease or compromise of the suprascapular nerve.

Weakness of the subscapularis muscle results in a loss of internal rotation strength. However, since there are many other strong internal rotators of the shoulder, including the pectoralis major muscle, it can often be difficult to detect subscapularis muscle deficiency. The "lift off" test of Gerber is a very sensitive test for subscapularis weakness.[73] It is performed by having the patient fully rotate the shoulder internally, placing the dorsal aspect of the forearm directly against his or her backside (Fig. 55-23). The patient with an incompetent or neurologically compromised subscapularis muscle will be unable to lift the hand off of his or her backside.

It is important to remember that weakness as documented by any of the above tests may be related to tearing or incompetence of a muscle tendon unit, or it may be the result of neurologic deficiency. Therefore, it is of paramount importance that a careful neurologic assessment of the entire upper extremity be performed. When it is unclear whether the weakness is related to a structural defi-

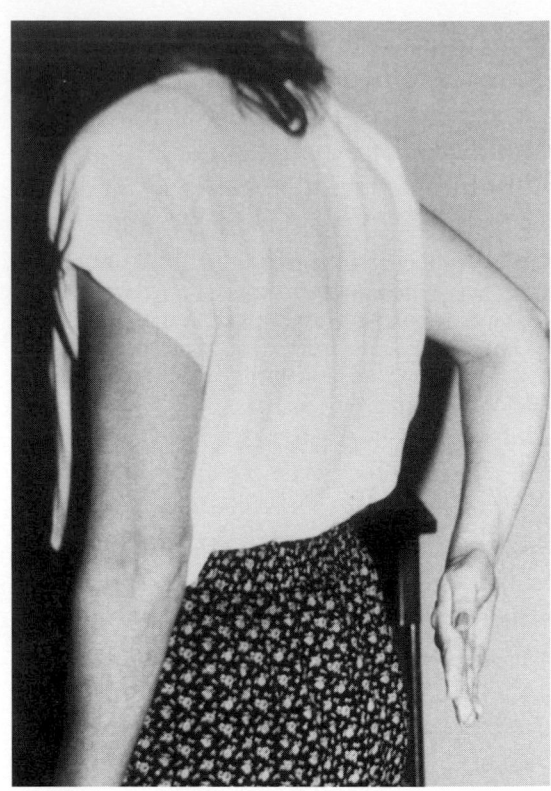

Figure 55-23 The lift-off test. (Reproduced with permission from Bigliani LU, Flatow EL, Codd TP: History, physical examination, and diagnostic modalities, in McGinty JB: *Operative Arthroscopy,* Philadelphia, Lippincott Raven, 1996, pp 635–646.)

ciency of the muscle or tendon versus neurologic insufficiency, an electromyographic analysis is indicated. In some patients, both may be responsible. For example, an elderly patient with an anterior dislocation of the shoulder may have both a rotator cuff tear and an axillary nerve palsy. The motor examination is completed by examining for muscle strength throughout the remainder of the upper extremity.

Sensory and reflex testing complete the neurologic exam and provide additional information to help differentiate structural from neurologic deficiency. It is important to have a general knowledge of sensory dermatomes of the upper extremity, as follows: C5, lateral arm; C6, thumb; C7, middle finger; C8, small finger; and T1, medial aspect of the arm. It is also important to have a general knowledge of specific sensory zones of the arm related to specific nerves, such as the lateral aspect of the shoulder controlled by the axillary nerve and the lateral aspect of the forearm controlled by the continuation of sensory nerves that travel with the musculocutaneous nerve. The reflexes of the biceps (C5), brachial radialis (C6), and triceps (C7) should also be tested and can be helpful in differentiating shoulder pain from a cervical radiculopathy.

The complete shoulder exam includes a vascular examination of the upper extremity. The brachial pulse is palpated at the medial aspect of the arm. Radial and ulnar pulses are palpated distally in the wrist. Complaints of vascular symptoms—such as easy fatigability, cramping, color changes, or paresthesias in the arm—can be related to vascular compression or disease, such as thoracic outlet syndrome. A useful test for suspected thoracic outlet syndrome is the Adson test, in which the arm is placed in an extended, abducted, and externally rotated position, with the neck extended and the head rotated toward the opposite shoulder. The radial pulse is palpated during this maneuver and the intensity of the pulse is compared to that which is present when the arm is placed in a comfortable position at the patient's side. Reduction in the radial pulse or production of the patient's symptoms is considered a positive test result.

Provocative Testing

Provocative tests are useful tools in the diagnosis of shoulder pathology. They should be performed as directed by the routine history and physical exam. The following paragraphs describe the most commonly used provocative tests.

Impingement Rotator cuff disease is most commonly related to impingement of the subacromial bursa or rotator cuff tendons against the acromion or coracoacromial arch. Pain induced by this abutment results in the subacromial impingement syndrome. The presence of this syndrome is verified by subacromial impingement signs and by the subacromial impingement test (Fig. 55-24). Subacromial impingement signs are tested by having the patient elevate the upper extremity in such a fashion as to cause the rotator cuff insertion into the greater tuberosity to abut against the acromion and coracoacro-

mial arch. Impingement signs are considered positive when they result in painful abutment of the rotator cuff against the coracoacromial arch when the shoulder goes beyond 90° of forward elevation in the scapular plane.[111] In patients with subtle findings or most posteriorly located areas of rotator cuff inflammation, it may be necessary to rotate the humerus internally during this provocative test or even to place the arm in true forward elevation and internal rotation at 90° in order to elicit painful abutment of the cuff against the coracoacromial arch.[15] When impingement signs are positive, it is important next to perform the impingement test, which is a repetition of the impingement maneuvers after performing a subacromial injection of lidocaine. Pain elicited by the impingement signs should be relieved during the impingement test, verifying the presence of true impingement syndrome.[111]

Biceps Pathology involving the long head of the biceps tendon is often elicited by palpation directly over the long head of this tendon between the greater and lesser tuberosities, as described above. Other tests include the Yergason test, which involves pain at the long head of the biceps in association with resisted supination of the hand while the elbow is flexed[180] (Fig. 55-25). Alternatively, the

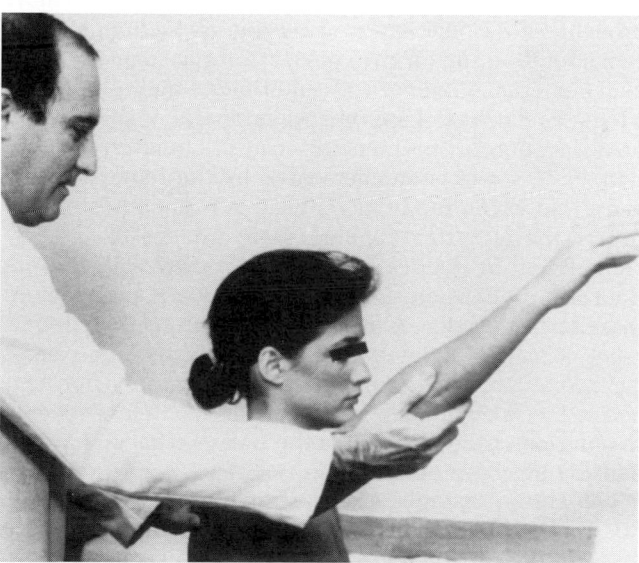

Figure 55-24 The impingement sign in forward elevation. (Reproduced with permission from Bigliani LU, Flatow EL, Codd TP: History, physical examination, and diagnostic modalities, in McGinty JB: *Operative Arthroscopy.* Philadelphia, Lippincott Raven, 1996, pp 635–646.)

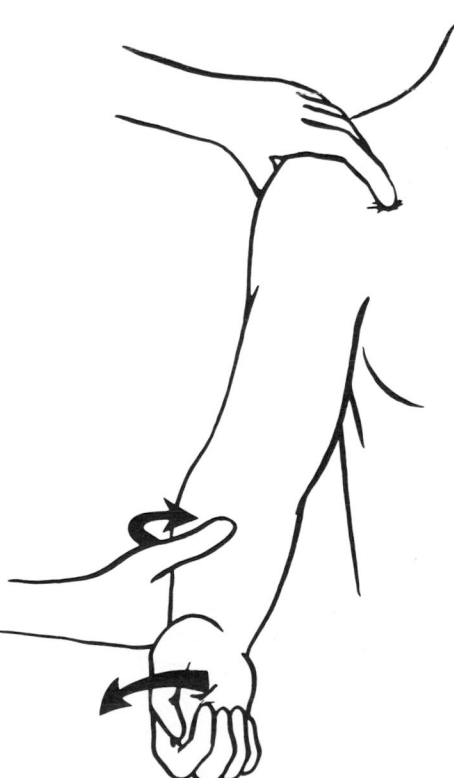

Figure 55-25 Yergason's sign. There is pain felt in the region of the long head of biceps in association with resisted supination (the elbow being in flexion.) (Reproduced with permission from Burkhead WZ Jr: The biceps tendon, in Rockwood CA Jr, Matsen FA III (eds): *The Shoulder.* Philadelphia, Saunders, 1990, pp 791–836.)

Speeds test can be utilized; it involves pain at the long head of the biceps tendon during resisted forward elevation of the upper extremity with the elbow in extension and the forearm in supination[36] (Fig. 55-26). When either of these maneuvers elicits pain localized to the long head of the biceps tendon, the presence of inflammatory changes in the long head of the biceps tendon should be suspected. The biceps instability test may also be helpful in determining whether or not the long head of the biceps tendon is subluxating. In this test, the examiner palpates the biceps tendon in the groove while the arm is placed in an abducted and externally rotated position and subsequently internally rotated. A palpable or audible and painful click may be noted as the biceps tendon reduces and then subluxates, passing over the lesser tuberosity.[36]

Acromioclavicular Joint Pathology at the AC joint is best determined by direct palpation. Patients with arthritis, chondrolysis, or osteolysis will have tenderness to direct palpation. Another test indicative of AC pathology is pain with cross-chest adduction of the upper extremity. This results in compression at the AC joint. However, this test may also be positive as a result of impingement. A more sensitive test for AC pathology is the presence or absence of pain with maximal internal rotation of the GH joint.[146] This maneuver also results in compression at the AC joint and is less likely to overlap with impingement pain.

A differential injection test is often very helpful in differentiating AC pain from impingement pain.[146] A subacromial impingement test is first performed; if complete elimination of symptomatology results, the diagnosis of impingement syndrome is made. If symptoms remain, the AC joint is injected with lidocaine. Relief of AC symptoms verifies the diagnosis of AC pathology. The subacromial injection test is performed first to eliminate the possibility of accidentally injecting the subacromial space during the AC injection, thereby clouding the results of the differential injection.[15]

Instability Instability of the GH joints is one of the most difficult diagnoses to verify.[111] Several provocative tests

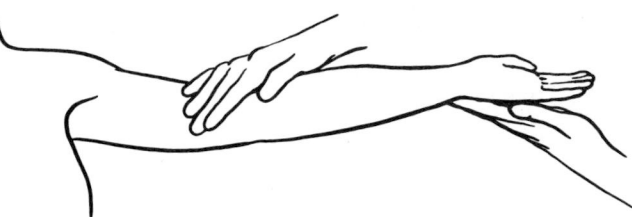

Figure 55-26 Speed's test. There is pain experienced in the region of the long head of biceps during resisted forward elevation of the upper extremity (the elbow being extended and the forearm supinated.) (Reproduced with permission from Burkhead WZ Jr: The biceps tendon, in Rockwood CA Jr, Matsen FA III (eds): *The Shoulder*. Philadelphia, Saunders, 1990, pp 791–836.)

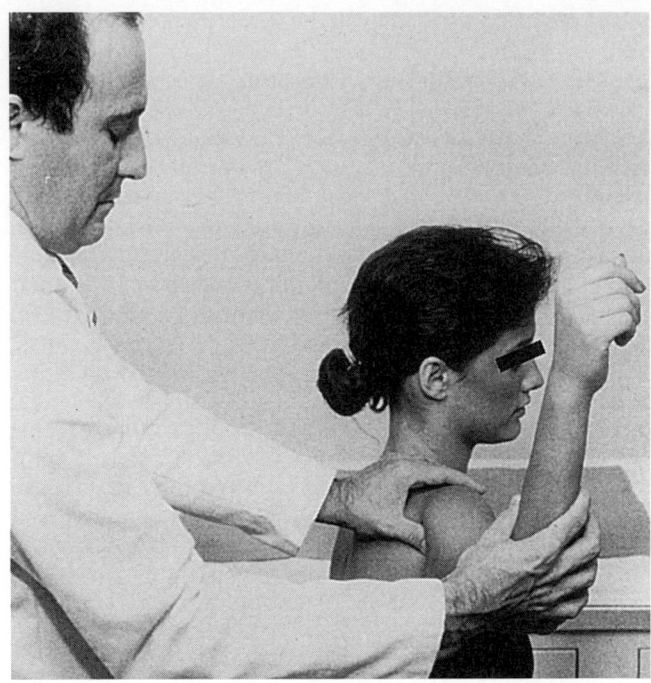

Figure 55-27 The anterior apprehension sign is performed by bringing the arm into a position of abduction and external rotation. The test is positive when the patient demonstrates a feeling of impending doom. (Reproduced with permission from Bigliani LU, Flatow EL, Codd TP: History, physical examination, and diagnostic modalities, in McGinty JB: *Operative Arthroscopy*. Philadelphia, Lippincott Raven, 1996, pp 635–646.)

are available to improve the veracity of the diagnosis. The anterior apprehension sign is the classic provocative test used for anterior instability (Fig. 55-27). The arm is brought into a position of extension, abduction, and external rotation and forward pressure is placed on the proximal humerus. A patient with anterior instability will have a bona fide feeling of apprehension for fear of subluxation or dislocation of the humeral head in an anterior direction.[150] This test is supplemented by the relocation maneuver, in which the humeral head is pushed posteriorly during the test; this eliminates any chance of anterior subluxation or dislocation and does away with the patient's apprehension. In addition to true apprehension, these tests may also be associated with the production or relief of pain associated with anterior instability. Painful symptoms produced by the anterior apprehension test and reduced by the relocation test are much less specific to anterior instability than is the true presence of apprehension.[159]

Posterior instability is much more difficult to verify. Posterior instability is tested with the posterior stress test, in which the patient's upper extremity is placed in 90° of true forward flexion and 90° of internal rotation while a posteriorly directed axial force is applied through the elbow (Fig. 55-28). A positive test occurs when the patient's symptoms are recreated. The scapula must be stabilized during this provocative test.[132]

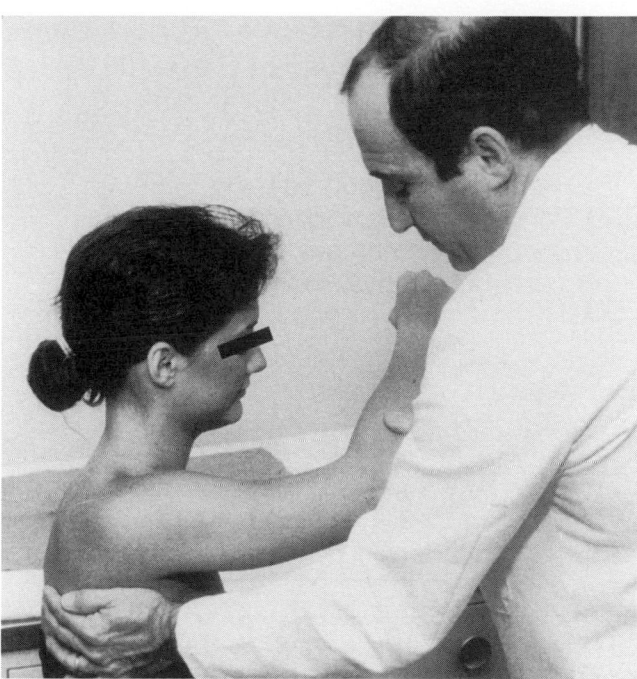

Figure 55-28 The posterior stress test. (Reproduced with permission from Bigliani LU, Flatow EL, Codd TP: History, physical examination, and diagnostic modalities, in McGinty JB: *Operative Arthroscopy*. Philadelphia, Lippincott Raven, 1996, pp 635–646.)

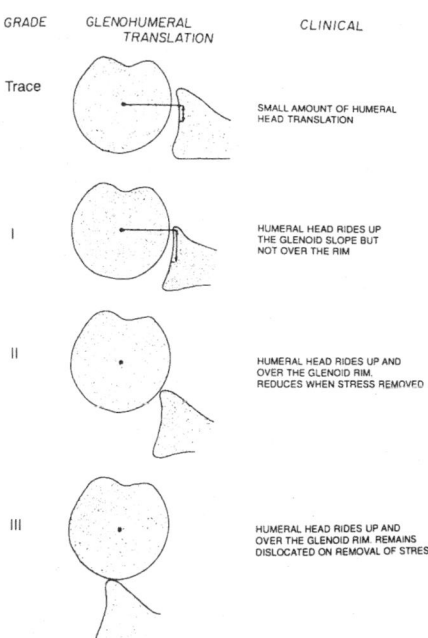

Figure 55-29 Method for documenting translation of the humeral head. (Reproduced with permission from Hawkins RJ, Bokor DJ: Clinical evaluation of shoulder problems, in Rockwood CA Jr, Matsen FA III (eds): *The Shoulder*. Philadelphia, Saunders, 1990.)

When the diagnosis of instability is being considered, it is important to determine whether the patient has generalized ligamentous laxity.[116] This can be evaluated by assessing the patient's ability to place the thumb to the forearm and looking for hyperextension at the metacarpal-phalangeal, elbow, or knee joints. The presence of increased systemic laxity may be indicative of multidirectional instability.[15]

When any of the above tests raises the level of suspicion for the diagnosis of instability, it is important to look for evidence of abnormal translation of the humeral head with respect to the glenoid. This is done by assessing the amount of translation in the anterior, inferior, and posterior directions. Two common schemes are utilized to grade the amount of translation. In one scheme, the percentage of humeral head surface that abnormally translates over the glenoid rim is estimated. In the other scheme, translation is graded as 1, or mild, when the humeral head rides up but not over the rim of the glenoid; moderate, or grade 2, when the humeral head rides up over the glenoid rim but reduces spontaneously when stress is removed; and severe, or grade 3, when the humeral head rides up and over the glenoid rim and remains dislocated on removal of stress[77] (Fig. 55-29). Excessive translation in the inferior direction is also called a *positive sulcus sign*. This relates to widening of the subacromial space, which creates a visible sulcus between the humeral head and the acromion. It is important to note that increased laxity is not necessarily pathologic and that comparisons must be made to the asymptomatic contralateral extremity.[111]

Diagnostic Modalities

Lab Tests

Routine blood tests can be important in the diagnosis of systemic rheumatologic disorders, infections, and tumors that may be causing shoulder pathology. A complete blood count, sedimentation rate, chemistry profile, and rheumatoid factor or latex fixation test are obtained in most cases. Other laboratory tests such as serum protein electrophoresis are indicated when directed by the history and physical examination.[15]

Radiographic Tests

All patients should have a routine radiographic assessment, which will assist in the diagnosis of tumors, fractures, or dislocations.[111] Standard views include a true anteroposterior (AP) radiograph and an axillary lateral. The true AP radiograph is obtained by angulating the body at 30 to 45° from the plane of the thorax (Fig. 55-30). The axillary lateral is performed by abducting the upper extremity to 90°, with the radiograph beam aimed in a cranial direction through the axilla. In cases where trauma is suspected, this view can be obtained with the arm abducted 20° and still provide valuable information about the orientation of the humeral head with respect to the glenoid socket. Although this view can be obtained in almost any patient, the occasional patient who resists efforts to abduct the arm may have alternative views taken to provide similar information. The simplest alter-

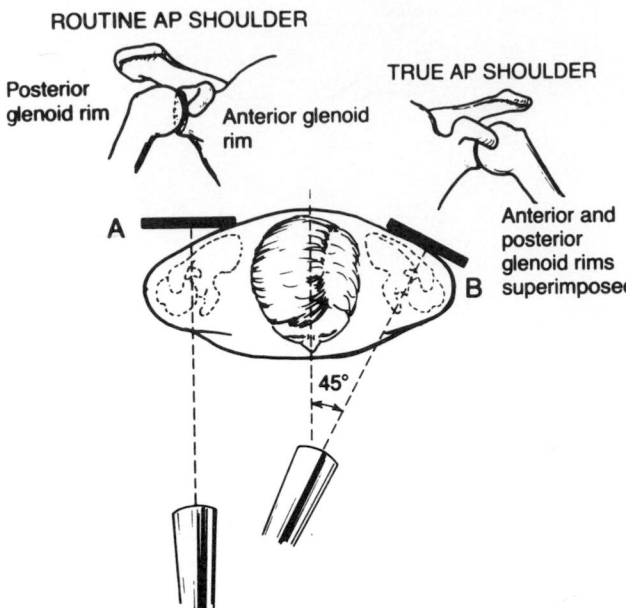

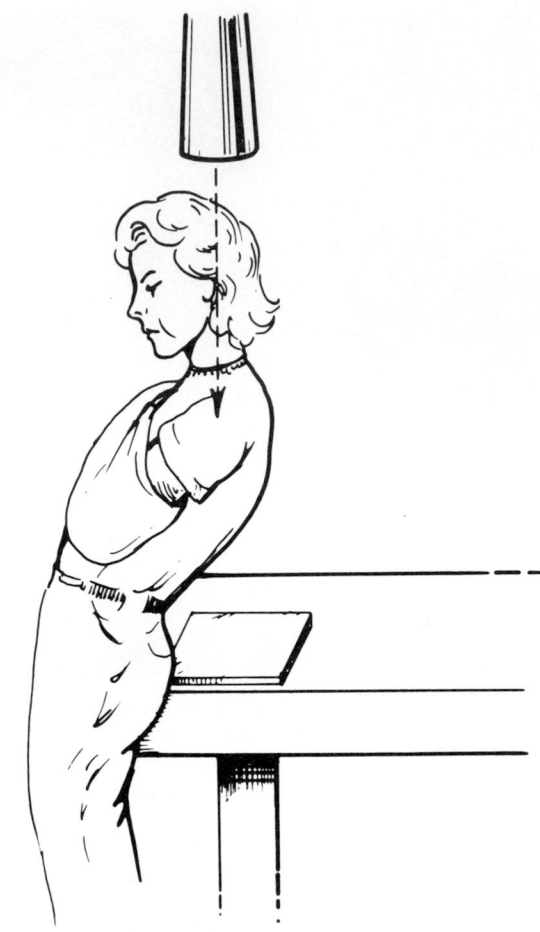

Figure 55-30 True AP radiograph technique. (Reproduced with permission from Warner JJP, Caborn DN: Overview of shoulder instability. *Crit Rev Phys Rehab Med* 4:145–198, 1992.)

Figure 55-31 Velpeau axillary radiograph technique. (Reproduced with permission from Warner JJP, Caborn DN: Overview of shoulder instability. *Crit Rev Phys Rehab Med* 4:145–198, 1992.)

native is to perform a Velpeau or sling axillary lateral, in which the arm remains at the side and the patient is asked to simply lean backward over the edge of the radiography table while the beam is directed from superior to inferior[27] (Fig. 55-31). If the patient is unable to perform this maneuver, a Y-scapular view can be obtained with the beam of the x-ray directed parallel to the spine of the scapula (Fig. 55-32). In this view, the glenoid fossa is located at the intersection of the body of the scapula with the spine of the scapula and coracoid process.

Several specific radiographic views have been developed to assist in diagnosing certain conditions. When calcific tendinitis is suspected, it is helpful to obtain AP radiographic views in internal, neutral, and external rotation. Calcific deposits hidden in one degree of rotation may become apparent in various other degrees of rotation. In addition, the internal rotation AP view may also demonstrate the presence of a Hill-Sachs lesion.[80] The Hill-Sachs lesion is a posterior impression fracture at the anatomic neck of the proximal humerus in association with an anterior dislocation of the GH joint. The Stryker notch view is also helpful in evaluation for a Hill-Sachs lesion[75] (Fig. 55-33). It is obtained with the radiographic beam aimed in an AP direction with 10° of cephalic tilt while the patient lies supine with the affected hand resting on his or her head.

The West Point and Garth views are also helpful when the diagnosis of instability has been considered.[71,149] These views are designed to highlight the anterior and anteroinferior rim of the glenoid socket. The West Point view is similar to an axillary lateral, but the patient lies prone and the beam is placed at a 25° angle to the horizontal in the PA direction and at a 25° angle away from the sagittal plane in a caudal cranial direction.

The supraspinatus outlet view is useful when the impingement syndrome is suspected. This view delineates the morphology of the acromion and is obtained in a similar fashion to the Y- scapular view. The radiographic beam is directed parallel to the spine of the scapula in a posterior-to-anterior direction with 5 to 10° of caudal tilting.

The acromioclavicular joint can be highlighted using an AP view taken with 10° of cephalic tilt. This view should be taken with approximately 50 percent of the voltage of a standard AP shoulder radiograph, as there is very little soft tissue overlying this joint.[142] When an AC separation is suspected, it is useful to obtain an AP radiograph with both shoulders on a wide cassette, so that the coracoclavicular distance can be measured and compared. Differences from side to side can be accentuated with stress views in which 10 to 20 lb weights are suspended from each of the patient's wrists and the comparison is repeated.

Sternoclavicular injuries are often difficult to diagnose and can be viewed with the help of radiographic views designed to eliminate overlap of the joint with the rest of the thorax. The *serendipity view* is a radiographic view taken by directing the radiographic beam at a 40° cephalic tilt while

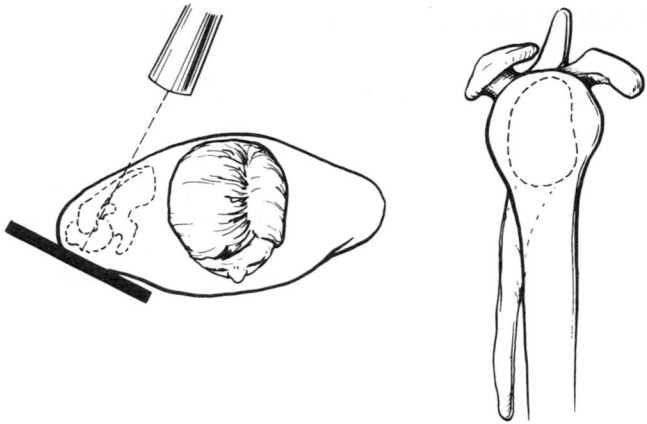

Figure 55-32 Y-scapular radiograph technique. (Reproduced with permission from Warner JJP, Caborn DN: Overview of shoulder instability. *Crit Rev Phys Rehab Med* 4:145–198, 1992.)

the patient is supine.[142] Findings are based on evaluation of the longitudinal axis of the clavicle compared to the contralateral side. Anterior dislocation is suspected in the presence of superior displacement of the clavicle in relationship to the longitudinal access of the clavicle. Posterior dislocation is suspected by inferior displacement in the same fashion. A Hobb's view may also be helpful and is taken with the radiographic beam directed from posterior to anterior while the patient slumps over the radiographic cassette, resting on his or her elbows. In many cases, these views are difficult to interpret, and a computed tomography (CT) scan is required for definitive diagnosis.[142]

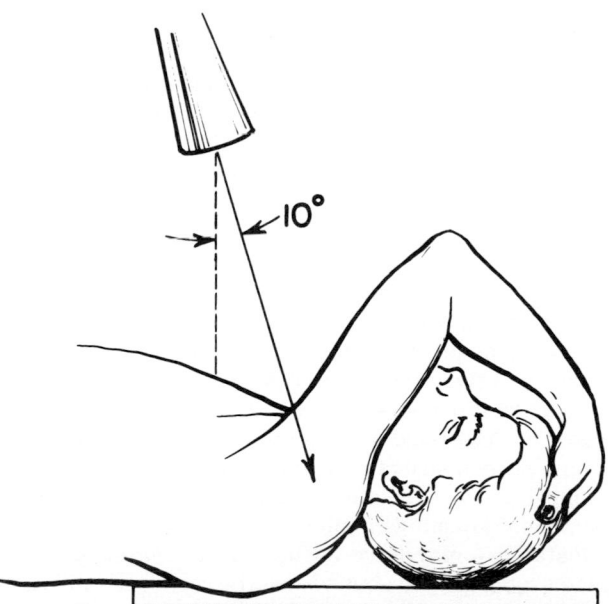

Figure 55-33 Technique for Stryker notch radiograph. (Reproduced with permission from Warner JJP, Caborn DN: Overview of shoulder instability. *Crit Rev Phys Rehab Med* 4:145–198, 1992.)

Special Radiographic Tests

In addition to plain radiographs, many other radiologic tests are extremely valuable in the diagnosis of shoulder pathology. As previously mentioned, CT scans are often essential. They are extremely helpful in the diagnosis of sternoclavicular pathology, especially suspected dislocations. In addition, they can often be helpful in determining the degree of displacement present at the lesser and greater tuberosities in three- or four-part proximal humeral fractures. In many instances, a CT scan is necessary to properly evaluate fractures of the scapula, including the glenoid cavity. Such scans are often needed during preparation for total shoulder arthroplasty to determine the degree and type of bone loss that is present at the glenoid fossa. A CT scan obtained after a radiographic dye has been injected into the GH joint can also provide valuable information about the GH capsuloligamentous structures and their insertion, or lack thereof, into the glenoid rim.[15]

The presence or absence of a rotator cuff tear is easily and inexpensively determined utilizing a conventional arthrogram. The conventional arthrogram is highly accurate in detecting a full-thickness rotator cuff tear and may even detect some deep-surface, partial-thickness tears. However, the arthrogram cannot provide much information concerning the size of the rotator cuff tear or the quality of the rotator cuff tendons and muscle. In addition, it may occasionally give a false-negative result in very rare cases where the rotator cuff tendon has avulsed from the greater tuberosity and the underlying capsule has remained intact. Ultrasonography is also a very cost-effective, noninvasive imaging modality that can be utilized for the diagnosis of rotator cuff tears; however, its reliability is extremely variable and is dependent upon the experience of the operator.

The MRI scan has quickly become the "gold standard" in detecting the presence or absence of soft tissue pathology about the shoulder[15] (Fig. 55-34). It has the advantage of being able to document the presence of both partial- and full-thickness rotator cuff tears as well as showing the size of a tear and the quality of the tendon and muscle structures. Recently, MRI arthrograms have been performed with the use of gadolinium contrast placed into the GH joint. The MRI arthrogram is very useful in delineating labral pathology (Fig. 55-35).

Electromyography and nerve conduction studies are very useful in sorting out peripheral nerve injuries, brachial plexus pathology, nerve entrapment syndromes, and cervical radiculopathies. This type of testing should be performed in any patient in whom a neurologic process is being considered based on the history and physical examination.[15]

ROTATOR CUFF DISEASE

Rotator cuff disease has been recognized for over 100 years, the first description of a rotator cuff tear having been made by J. G. Smith, an English anatomist, in 1834. The first report of a rotator cuff repair was not made until

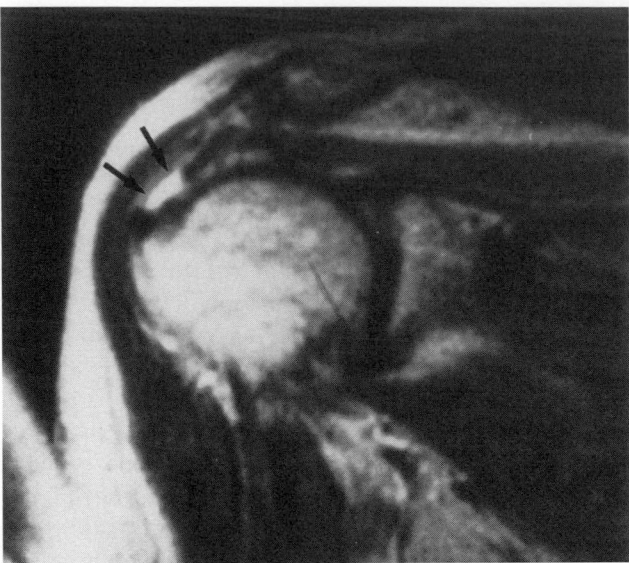

Figure 55-34 This patient has a full-thickness rotator cuff tear as documented by this T2-weighted MRI view showing fluid within a supraspinatus tear *(arrows).*

three-quarters of a century later. Ernest A. Codman presented an initial report on rotator cuff repair in 1911 and followed this with his classic book *The Shoulder* in 1934.[44,45] Since that time, much has been learned about the incidence, etiology, and treatment of rotator cuff disease.[111] Many factors, including the addition of the anterior acromioplasty described by Neer in 1972, have greatly improved the success rate of rotator cuff repair, with most series describing greater than 85 percent good results.[26,107,111,115] Over the past several years, shoulder arthroscopy has had a profound impact on both the evaluation and treatment of rotator cuff disease.[57]

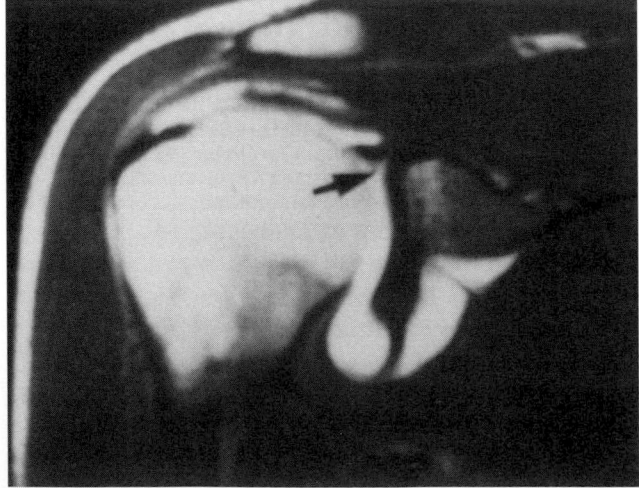

Figure 55-35 This patient has a superior labral tear *(arrow)* as shown by this MRI image with gadolinium enhancement.

Etiology and Pathology

Rotator cuff disease is a continuum of pathology starting with inflammatory changes in the subacromial bursa and rotator cuff tendons, which may continue on to become a rotator cuff tendon rupture or tear.[14] Rotator cuff disease primarily involves the distal aspect of the supraspinatus tendon as it inserts into the greater tuberosity.[111] In more severe cases, the disease may also encompass the infraspinatus and teres minor muscles. The long head of the biceps tendon may also be involved.[111] The subscapularis tendon is less frequently involved.

The supraspinatus insertion into the greater tuberosity passes directly beneath the coracoacromial arch when the upper extremity is elevated to the overhead position.[109] The area beneath the coracoacromial arch is known as the supraspinatus outlet.[111] In some individuals, for a variety of reasons, the rotator cuff insertion may impinge or abut against the coracoacromial arch. When this process is repeated chronically, as may occur in an overhead laborer or athlete, the structures in the supraspinatus outlet (i.e., bursa, rotator cuff, and biceps) may become inflamed.[17] This microtraumatic process can eventually result in pain and/or dysfunction and is called *subacromial impingement.*[107]

Neer pointed out that impingement is most often the result of narrowing of the supraspinatus outlet, commonly caused by a downsloping acromion.[107] Bigliani et al. demonstrated a direct relationship between acromial morphology and the incidence of rotator tears in cadavers.[19,24,122] On the basis of this work, Bigliani developed a classification scheme for acromial morphology in which a type I morphology represents relatively flat acromion, a type II morphology represents a curved acromion, while a type III morphology indicates a prominent hook at the anterior edge of the acromion. Individuals with a type III acromion are more likely to develop impingement than are those with a type I acromion. An anterior acromial traction spur in the course of the coracoacromial ligament is also known to predispose to rotator cuff impingement.[111] Inferior osteophytes at the acromioclavicular joint may also increase the likelihood of impingement in rotator cuff disease[109] (Fig. 55-36). Other less common causes of narrowing of the supraspinatus outlet include an unfused acromial epiphysis that tips inferiorly into the outlet area; a nonunion of a fracture of the base of the acromion, which may result in downward toggling of the acromion; cephalic protrusion of the superior glenoid rim; and anterolateral overhang of the coracoid process.[6,111]

Several other, less frequent causes of impingement exist and are classified as nonoutlet sources.[111] This would include prominence of the greater tuberosity as a result of a congenital or developmental malformation or fracture malunion. Patients with altered GH kinematics as a result of instability may have an increased tendency for the greater tuberosity to abut against the coracoacromial arch. A loss of the suspensory mechanism of the shoulder as a result of a severe AC separation can also be associated with impingement by creating an abnormal downward tilt of the scapula. As a result, during elevation of the arm, the patient must compensate with increased GH motion. The

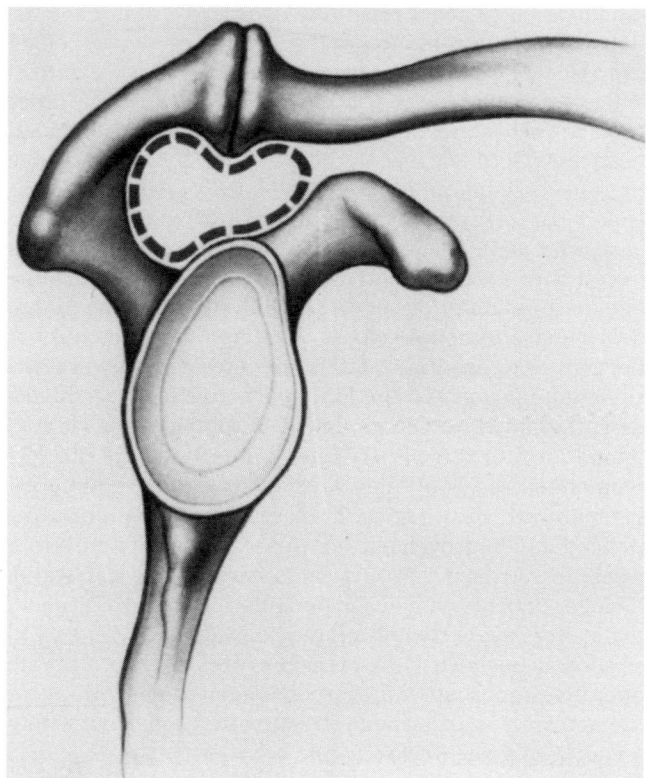

Figure 55-36 Impingement can also result from hypertrophy of the AC joint as well as the commonly found acromial legion.

increased GH elevation can result in an increased potential for abutment of the greater tuberosity against the coracoacromial arch. The same type of mechanism also occurs in patients with trapezius paralysis whom are unable to rotate their scapulas.[21] In a similar fashion, patients with surgical neck malunions in a position of varus must also compensate with an increase in the amount of GH elevation to reach the same degree of forward elevation. Excessive tightness of the posterior capsule is also thought to result in impingement by forcing the humeral head against the coracoacromial arch as the shoulder is elevated.[14]

As described by Neer in the early 1970s, subacromial impingement can be broken down into three stages. In stage I impingement, the microtraumatic process is sufficient to produce edema and hemorrhage in the subacromial bursa and supraspinatus tendon. As the process progresses, it reaches a more severe stage, stage II, in which the edema and hemorrhage go unchecked and eventually result in fibrosis and tendinitis at the distal supraspinatus tendon. In the final stage, stage III, the rotator cuff tendon reaches a point of failure, resulting in a rotator cuff tear.[107,109,111]

The pathologic severity of stage III disease is dependent on tear size, tissue scarring and retraction, and chronicity of the disease. Tear size is generally considered small when it is less than 1 cm, medium when from 1 to 3 cm, large when from 3 to 5 cm, and massive when greater than 5 cm.[138] More severe disease is associated with larger

tears and a higher degree of scarring and retraction. With larger retracted tears of long duration, the greater tuberosity may begin to undergo mechanically induced changes as a result of continuing and worsening impingement. The changes begin with sclerosis and may progress to erosive change, with cartilage and bone loss. The end result is the joint destruction seen in rotator cuff tear arthropathy.

Rotator cuff tear arthropathy is directly related to a deficiency in rotator cuff function.[111,113] This leads to an inability to keep the humeral head in direct contact with the glenoid fossa. Instead, the humeral head migrates proximally to abut the coracoacromial arch, including the undersurface of the acromion and AC joint. In addition, the humeral head may dislocate in an anteroinferior direction from the loss of the stabilizing effects of the posterior aspect of the rotator cuff (i.e., posterior mechanism for anterior instability; see "Instability," above). With time, the continued abutment against the coracoacromial arch and the continued instability subject the humeral head to unusual wear and tear. The end result is cuff tear arthropathy, characterized by an incongruous and distorted humeral head with superior erosion and subchondral collapse as well as erosion of the undersurface of the acromion and AC joint.[111]

Several factors are thought to contribute toward progression to stage III disease. The distal portion of the supraspinatus tendon is known to contain a zone in which vascularity is somewhat limited.[140] Increased contact pressure at the coracoacromial arch may further impede blood flow via increased pressure from direct contact or shear between different fiber bundles.[65,69,107,167] The decrease in blood supply results in attrition and eventual tearing of the rotator cuff tendons. The attritional process has a predilection for the articular side of the cuff tendon over the bursal side. Studies have shown that the shear pressure effects are higher at the articular side than at the bursal side, and this may explain why attrition occurs primarily in this area.[102]

Macrotrauma from a sudden violent incident may occasionally be a cause of rotator cuff disease. The traumatic episode may create an acute area of inflammation in the subacromial bursa or supraspinatus tendon similar in severity to that which may be caused by many years of repetitive microtrauma. The trauma may be so severe as to cause frank rupture of the rotator cuff tendon. In many individuals, acute trauma may be superimposed upon chronic attritional changes at the rotator cuff, resulting in exacerbation of preexisting disease or extension of a partial tear to a complete tear or a small tear to a large tear.

Clinical Presentation

The most consistent symptom present with rotator cuff disease is pain.[15] It is usually centered at the greater tuberosity and anterior acromion but can extend down in the area of the deltoid muscle. There may also be referred pain down the arm to the elbow, medially to the chest wall, or superiorly in the area of the trapezius muscle. If the AC joint is arthritic or involved in the impingement process, it may also be a site of pain. Night pain is very common and either interrupts sleep or does not allow the patient to lie on the affected shoulder. Patients may complain of weakness and loss of function. This may be secondary to pain or to stage III disease, in which a rotator cuff tear is present. The disease primarily interferes with overhead activities.

The physical examination will generally demonstrate tenderness at the greater tuberosity and anterior acromion. The AC joint and biceps tendon may also be tender if they are involved in the impingement process. The most reliable physical signs are impingement signs which are verified by the impingement test. In stage III disease, true weakness in abduction and external rotation will be present due to incompetence of the rotator cuff tendons. When the subscapularis is involved in stage III disease, the Gerber lift-off test will be positive.[73]

Radiographic changes are dependent upon the stage of the disease, with most occurring in advanced stages. Standard radiographs are routinely obtained. Early on, radiographs are used to rule out other disease processes, such as calcific tendinitis. Anteroposterior views in internal, external, and neutral rotation are helpful. The axillary view is important to evaluate for a persistent unfused acromial epiphysis, which can contribute to the impingement process. The outlet view is obtained to look at the morphology of the acromion and acromial spurs. With advanced disease, the greater tuberosity may become sclerotic or develop excrescences. In the presence of a rotator cuff tear, the acromiohumeral distance may narrow as the humeral head migrates proximally. As a result, the undersurface of the AC joint may develop osteophytes or excrescences. As stage III disease progresses to cuff tear arthropathy, the radiographic findings consist of a distorted humeral head with superior erosion and subchondral collapse as well as erosion of the undersurface of the acromion and AC joint.[111]

Ancillary studies are important in the evaluation of rotator cuff disease, with the gold standard currently consisting of MRI evaluation, as discussed earlier in the text (see "Special Radiographic Tests," above). Arthrography still has a role. It can be important in patients with claustrophobia who cannot tolerate an MRI or in a revision situation in which scarring has made interpretation of the MRI difficult. Open-sided MRI tests are often inconclusive. Electromyography should be used when significant weakness exists in the presence of a negative MRI or arthrogram.

Nonoperative Treatment

The treatment of rotator cuff disease is dependent upon the stage of the disease and the severity of symptoms. Some individuals may have significant pain and disability from impingement, while others may have rotator cuff tears of large size with very little symptomatology. In general, the first line of treatment consists of physical therapy alone or in conjunction with a subacromial steroid injection. This approach will be sufficient in the majority of patients with stages I and II disease and in some with stage III disease. The therapeutic approach consists of activity

modification to avoid repetitive overhead use in conjunction with range-of-motion and rotator cuff–strengthening exercises. The goal of the exercises is to promote a normal state of capsular laxity and normal cuff strength in order to minimize or prevent upward migration of the humeral head and abutment against the coracoacromial arch. Once therapeutic intervention is initiated, the patient's progress is carefully assessed. Those patients with stage I or II disease who show no progress or worsening of symptoms over a 6- to 8-week period are studied with an MRI to rule out the possibility of occult stage III disease. The MRI is delayed an additional 6 weeks if a steroid injection has not been given to see if this additional intervention will bring some improvement. If the MRI is negative for stage III disease, therapy in conjunction with steroid injections is continued for 3 to 6 months. Multiple injections are not recommended, as they may weaken the cuff tendons.[111] Patients with known stage III disease who have not experienced any improvement or worsen over the first 6 to 8 weeks are advised that surgical intervention is warranted. Younger patients with suspected full-thickness rotator cuff tears after severe trauma should be evaluated with an MRI as soon as possible. If the presence of a large tear is noted, operative repair should be recommended early to avoid the excessive scarring and retraction that can occur within a matter of a few weeks.

Operative Treatment

Operative treatment is indicated after failure of nonoperative treatment, as mentioned above. In patients with advanced stage III disease, it is often the first line of treatment. Operative treatment can be divided into arthroscopic and open treatment, as described below.

Arthroscopic Treatment

Arthroscopy has become a very important tool in the treatment of the early stages of rotator cuff disease.[57] Although its primary importance is relegated to treatment, it is often very helpful in adding diagnostic information. The arthroscope provides the ability to confirm the preoperative assessment of the extent of rotator cuff tendon damage and to uncover unsuspected pathology that may warrant treatment. For instance, an impending biceps rupture may suggest the need for tenodesis, an unknown full or extensive partial-thickness cuff tear may require an open repair, and early GH arthritis may allow the surgeon to counsel the patient about a less favorable prognosis.

Arthroscopic Treatment of Stage I, Stage II, and Partial-Thickness Stage III Disease Arthroscopic subacromial decompression has become the mainstay of treatment for patients with impingement who have failed nonoperative treatment, as described above. The procedure has a success rate greater than 85 to 90 percent.[57,72,129] It includes a therapeutic anterior acromioplasty combined with an arthroscopic GH evaluation. The GH evaluation allows the surgeon to examine the articular surface of the rotator cuff. After cuff evaluation, an arthroscopic anterior acromioplasty is performed (Fig. 55-17). Neer recognized that the critical area of impingement occurs at the anterior edge of the acromion.[107] Prior to this recognition, many surgeons performed radical or lateral acromionectomies, which weakened the deltoid.[117]

The anterior acromioplasty is performed by first placing the arthroscope into the subacromial space, as previously described (see "Surgical Approaches," "Arthroscopic Approach") (Fig. 55-17). A working portal is established and the bursal surface of the cuff is evaluated. The CA ligament is stripped from the undersurface and anterior edge of the anterior acromion. A burr is introduced through the lateral or lateral-anterior portal and resection of the anteroinferior acromion is accomplished. The goal is to convert the prominent anterior acromion into a thinner, flatter anterior acromion. Since the deltoid origin at the acromion is preserved, postoperative rehab is quickly pushed toward active assistive and strengthening exercises as tolerated. A sling is advised for comfort only during the immediate postoperative period.

When a partial-thickness tear is identified, the area and thickness of the tear are determined. Most are smaller and less than 50 percent of the tendon thickness; they are treated with debridement in conjunction with the arthroscopic decompression. Tears that are more than 50 percent of the thickness of the tendon over a large tendon area are associated with a less favorable prognosis.[175] For this reason, many surgeons advocate excision of the partial tear and repair. In the era before arthroscopy, excision and repair of significant partial tears seemed logical and added little morbidity to the already open procedure.[111] Currently, however, since few studies are available to determine the efficacy of this approach in conjunction with arthroscopy, we generally advocate arthroscopic debridement and decompression.

Arthroscopic Treatment of Full-Thickness Stage III Disease Although open rotator cuff repair is the gold standard, arthroscopy has come into increasing use in the treatment of a broad spectrum of full-thickness rotator cuff disease. This includes unsuspected tears noted during the diagnostic portion of an arthroscopic subacromial decompression as well as known tears, from small to massive. Available options include an arthroscopic subacromial decompression combined with a "mini" open tendon repair, arthroscopic tendon repair, and debridement without repair.

The combination of an arthroscopic subacromial decompression with an open tendon repair through a small deltoid split has become a standard procedure with a high rate of successful results.[7,130,170,175] Arthroscopic localization of the tear allows precise incision placement, and newer suture passing devices have allowed the procedure to be performed with very small incisions. Advantages over open repair include deltoid preservation, quicker rehabilitation, and shorter hospitalization. Small, easily mobilized tears are ideal for this approach. The cuff tear is evaluated for elasticity and mobility. If the torn edge is easily mobilized to the greater tuberosity, the arthroscopic subacromial decompression is completed as planned and the cuff tear is repaired, as described below, through a small or mini open incision, usually by extending one of the portals. The deltoid muscle fibers are split only to the edge of the acromion. The patient is placed in an accelerated rotator cuff repair rehabilitation program, as described later. Tears that cannot be easily mobilized are better treated through conventional open repair techniques.[12]

Despite the low morbidity of mini open repair, efforts have continued to find methods for entirely arthroscopic tendon repair.[128] Arthroscopic techniques using suture anchors have been developed. These are still in experimental stages.[156] Further advancements in this evolving area and analysis of long-term results will facilitate definition of appropriate indications for entirely arthroscopic rotator cuff repair.

Rockwood and others have treated massive rotator cuff tears, with extensive scarring and retraction, with subacromial decompression, debridement, and rehabilitation; they have had good short-term results.[35,143] However, in a recently reported prospective randomized study by Montgomery et al., open surgical repair fared significantly better than arthroscopic debridement.[98] Results from a previous study by Bigliani et al. of rotator cuff repair for large and massive tears would suggest that open treatment offers reliable pain relief, with a high percentage of satisfactory results that do not deteriorate over time.[12] Until further evidence is presented, open decompression and repair rather than debridement should be considered for most patients with massive tears. Arthroscopic debridement is reserved for elderly patients who are infirm and would not be able to comply with postoperative rehabilitation. In this situation, the coracoacromial arch should not be aggressively resected but rather gently contoured, recognizing that it will continue to function as an articulating surface with the superiorly translating humeral head.

Open Surgical Treatment

Open treatment of rotator cuff disease has long been a standard approach, with good long-term results in more than 85 percent of patients.[23,26,47] Although it is no longer the primary treatment advocated for stage I and II disease, it is still an accepted form of treatment. The technique for open subacromial decompression is the same as that utilized during open repair of full-thickness rotator disease, described below. The only difference is that a smaller incision and smaller deltoid split are utilized.

The repair of a rotator cuff tear can be divided into four distinct phases: the approach, the decompression, the actual repair of cuff tissue to bone, and postoperative rehabilitation. The approach consists of the superoanterior approach previously described (see "Superoanterior Approach," above).[23] For this approach, the patient is placed in a beach-chair position, with the torso angled approximately 60° from the horizontal plane. A head rest is used, which allows access to the superior and posterior aspects of the shoulder. The arm is draped free, allowing shoulder rotation, extension, and elevation. With this approach, the split in the deltoid is centered on the greater tuberosity, so that the posterior aspect of the rotator cuff is accessible. Furthermore, the anterolateral aspect of the deltoid is anterior to the incision and does not block access to the posterior cuff. The anterior and posterior aspects of the cuff can be well visualized by rotating the arm in internal or external rotation, since it has been draped free.

The decompression is performed next. To perform an adequate decompression, the CA ligament is released subperiosteally from the front edge and undersurface of the acromion and any anterior acromial spurs are excised. Recent studies have emphasized the importance of the CA ligament as a superior restraint to proximal migration of the humeral head.[66] For that reason, in patients with large or massive rotator cuff tears who may have an element of superior migration postoperatively, it may be prudent to repair the CA ligament at the completion of the repair rather than resecting it. If it is not going to be preserved and reattached, it can be excised close to the coracoid. Following this, the remaining cuff of strong deltoid insertion tissue at the front edge of the acromion is meticulously elevated in a superior direction.

The undersurface of the acromion is cleared of bursal and/or rotator cuff tissue that often adheres to it. The anterior acromioplasty is then performed, using an osteotome or other device such as a burr or microsaw. A wedge of bone is removed with the front edge approximately 7 to 8 mm in thickness and tapering posteriorly, approximately one-third to one-half the length of the acromion.[23] The thickness of the acromion can be measured by palpating it between an index finger and thumb. The piece should consist of the full width of the acromion from the medial to the lateral border. In most cases, a properly performed acromioplasty removes part of the lateral aspect of the AC joint, often leaving the distal clavicle quite prominent, and the rough edges of the undersurface of the distal clavicle should be removed with a rasp. If the entire distal clavicle must be removed, this can be done from underneath with a burr or ronguer. Approaching the AC joint from below prevents violation of the superior AC ligaments, helping to preserve stability of the joint.[59]

Attention is now turned toward mobilizing the torn rotator cuff tissue. The biceps tendon is inspected to see whether it is intact or torn. If intact, the biceps is left in its groove and not transposed posteriorly. If the biceps tendon is torn, the proximal stump is generally resected and, if it has not fully retracted into the arm, the distal stump is tenodesed in the groove. The cuff is then mobilized from medial to lateral in a sequential fashion. Multiple stay sutures are placed at the visible edge of the torn tendons. Internal rotation and extension of the free arm help to provide access to the posterior tissues. It is important to emphasize that the undersurface of the acromion is a common location for cuff and bursal adhesions. This area should be evaluated prior to the acromioplasty, as tissue may be stuck underneath the anterior aspect of the bone. After complete bursal surface release and exposure, the posterior tissues are assessed to determine the full extent of the tear. Often, a portion of the infraspinatus and the teres minor remain attached to the humeral head. The surgeon should be careful not to remove these during attempts at mobilization and release of surrounding tissues.

Attention is then turned toward mobilization and release of the undersurface of the rotator cuff. The undersurface is commonly scarred to the glenoid rim and base of the coracoid. Undersurface release is generally carried out bluntly, but can be done sharply with caution. After a complete and systematic release of the undersurface of the cuff from posterior to anterior, the excursion of the torn tendons are assessed by pulling on the stay sutures. For a successful repair, the edges of the torn tendon should reach the anatomic neck of the humerus with the arm in a functional position of slight forward elevation (10°) and slight abduction (10°).

If sufficient tendon cannot be mobilized to bring the leading edge of the cuff over to the anatomic neck, several maneuvers can be used. The rotator interval may be released to the base of the coracoid. Often the coracohumeral ligament is retracted and stuck down, inhibiting the cuff from being pulled laterally.[119] The complete release of the rotator interval and coracohumeral ligament down to the base of the coracoid is termed *the interval slide* and will allow the supraspinatus to be mobilized, laterally and distally, 1 to 1.5 cm.[12,23] Using this maneuver, we have avoided transfer of the upper portion of the subscapularis. Several authors have reported success with transfer of the upper portion of the subscapularis, but we have found it to be of little help.[46,111] However, if a subscapularis transfer is performed, it is important not to transfer the underlying capsule, as this may lead to instability. If further mobilization is required, further releases can be done along the posterior and medial aspect of the cuff on the glenoid rim. However, this should be done bluntly or cautiously with a scissors, spreading more that cutting. Sharp dissection in this area can injure the suprascapular nerve and should be avoided. In the majority of cases, these maneuvers will provide sufficient mobilization to allow the torn rotator cuff tendons to reach the anatomic neck, with the shoulder in the desired position of 10° of forward elevation and abduction. With mobilization complete, the actual repair of the tissues becomes the next step.

The greater tuberosity is prepared for tendon repair by removing all soft tissue to expose bare bone. A trough is not used, as it increases the amount of tendon mobilization required and has not been found to aid in tendon to bone healing.[23] Multiple drill holes are then placed into the greater tuberosity, starting medially in the anatomic neck. A corresponding lateral tuberosity hole is made, leaving a 1- to 1.5-cm bridge of tuberosity bone between the holes and thereby creating a bony tunnel for suture repair to bone. Number 1 or 0 braided nylon sutures are then passed through the tunnels with a curved needle. During the repair, the arm is held in approximately 10 to 15° of flexion as well as about 10° of abduction and the sutures are tied over the bony bridges formed by the bone tunnels. This allows excellent apposition of the bone and healing cuff edge. If an anterior interval slide has been performed, this should be sutured in such a way as to realign the interval tissue, with the mobilized supraspinatus edge of the interval being brought further lateral with respect to the subscapularis edge of the interval. In addition, if there is a split between the infraspinatus and teres minor, this should also be closed. Generally, this is the apex of the cuff tear. This soft tissue closure at the apex of the cuff should be sutured first. Synthetic material or allografts have been used when sufficient mobilization was unsuccessful, but the results have been poor and their use is not generally advocated.

The deltoid is then meticulously repaired to the cuff of strong deltoid insertion tissue that was previously left, and the stay suture in the distal deltoid split is removed. If the deltoid tissue is of poor quality, drill holes are placed in the acromion and it is repaired to bone. The arm is kept in a sling for the first 4 weeks.

Rehabilitation begins on the first postoperative day. In the first 4 to 6 weeks, only three exercises are done. These include pendulum exercises, supine external rotation with a stick to 30°, and assisted forward elevation to 140 to 160°. These are augmented with pulleys and supine cane exercises to assist with elevation. In large and massive cuff tears, we like to avoid extension and pulley exercises in the first 4 to 6 weeks, as this puts stress across the rotator cuff repair. Isometric and active assistive exercises are usually started during the 6- to 8-week period. These exercises generally begin with supine external rotation, theraband exercises, and active supine forward elevation. Once these exercises are performed, erect forward elevation with the help of a stick can be performed. This is usually done initially with a stick alone, followed with weights from 1 to 5 lb. A weight can then be used in the hand on the supine portion to raise the arm. Weights can be increased to 3 lb. Once these exercises can be performed without difficulty, more active strengthening exercises can be added.

Open Treatment of Isolated Rupture of the Subscapularis Tendon

Tears of the subscapularis tendon are less common and rarely occur in isolation. The patients exhibit a positive Gerber lift-off test and may have an associated subluxated or dislocated long head of the biceps tendon[73] (Fig. 55-23). The pathology is picked up easily with an MRI scan. In patients with symptoms of pain and functional disability, an open repair using an anterior approach is advocated. The tendon is repaired to the lesser tuberosity with sutures directly through bone or with suture anchors. Chronic cases may require extensive mobilization. The axillary nerve becomes particularly vulnerable and should be exposed and protected with retractors. The long head of the biceps tendon should be tenodesed in cases where it has been shortened, damaged, or ruptured. If it is normal, the tendon is replaced in the groove and the transverse humeral ligament is reconstructed. Although large series of results of isolated subscapularis repairs are not yet available, preliminary results are promising.[73]

Open Surgical Treatment of Cuff Tear Arthropathy

Patients with glenohumeral arthritis as a result of long-term cuff deficiency have been difficult to treat.[113] The cuff deficiency is irreparable in most cases. Constrained total shoulder arthroplasty has been attempted but has been associated with a universally high early failure rate.[111] Nonconstrained total shoulder arthroplasty has been utilized with more success but remains with a significant number of glenoid component failures secondary to superior

eccentric loading of the glenoid component.[144,148] The preferred alternative is humeral hemiarthroplasty performed through an anterior approach.[134] The technique is the same as that for GH osteoarthritis with a few exceptions (see "Arthritic and Degenerative Disorders of the Glenohumeral Joint," below.) After the humeral head is resected, the available rotator cuff tissue is mobilized and repaired to the greater tuberosity (Fig. 55-37). The rotator cuff is reconstructed with an emphasis toward anteroposterior stability rather than complete closure of the cuff. The prosthetic head is allowed to articulate with the coracoacromial arch, which permits a new stable fulcrum in the face of altered GH mechanics. Although functional improvements arc modest, pain relief if achieved in a majority of patients.[134]

Complications

Arthroscopic techniques are extremely safe, with relatively few complications.[16] Arthroscopic subacromial decompression is successful, with failure rates generally less than 15 percent. Most failures are related to persistent uncorrected AC joint pain, inadequate decompression, or an untreated full-thickness tear. Complication rates have been low, ranging from 1 to 8 percent. Reported complications include instrument breakage, neuropraxias (especially with lateral positioning), and excessive bleeding requiring conversion to an open technique.

Open rotator cuff repair is successful more than 85 percent of the time. Several factors have been associated with failure of treatment.[13] These include inadequate decompression, unrecognized AC disease, poor tissue quality, and damage to the deltoid origin. Loss of the deltoid origin is a major complication, with devastating consequences.[62] This has become less of a problem since radical or lateral acromionectomies are no longer advocated. Loss of deltoid function can also occur when the axillary nerve is injured. The deltoid split should not be carried more than 4 to 5 cm lateral to the anterolateral edge of the acromion to prevent this complication. The suprascapular nerve can be injured during mobilization of the cuff. Injury results in loss of function of the supraspinatus and infraspinatus muscles, rendering the repair useless. Sharp dissection should be limited to no further than 2 cm medial to the glenoid rim to prevent this unwanted complication. An unrecognized, unfused acromial epiphysis may occasionally cause persistent impingement and pain after cuff repair. An axilllary view is often necessary to make the diagnosis preoperatively.

CALCIFIC TENDINITIS

Etiology and Pathology

Calcific deposits can occur in the rotator cuff tendons and bursa and are usually seen during the fifth and six decades of life.[29,168] They occur equally in men and women. The specific etiology is unclear, but it is generally believed to be the result of local avascular changes in the rotator cuff tendon without systemic involvement. Excessive trauma

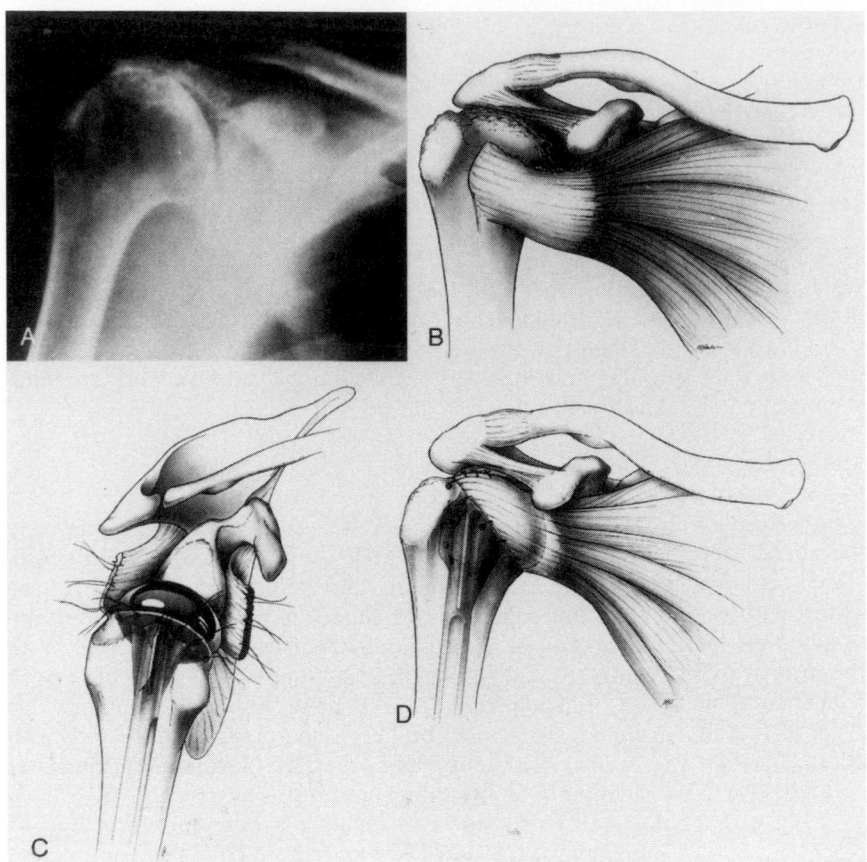

Figure 55-37 *A.* Anteroposterior radiograph of the GH joint in a patient with cuff tear arthropathy. *B.* The rotator cuff deficiency allows proximal migration of the humeral head. *C.* The rotator cuff is mobilized and the humeral head replaced. *D.* The rotator cuff is repaired to bone around the prosthesis with an emphasis toward anteroposterior stability over complete superior coverage. (Reproduced with permission from Rodosky MW, Bigliani LU: Indications for glenoid resurfacing. *J Shoulder Elbow* 5:231–248, 1996.)

or repetitive microtrauma may even play a role. There is degeneration of the collagen in association with calcium salt deposition and a focus of necrotic tissue and inflammation. The calcium is known to take two forms: a semi-liquid, gellike substance usually seen in the acute phase and a granular or chalklike deposit seen chronically. In some individuals, a dormant calcium deposit may be seen on routine radiographic studies and remain asymptomatic. The most common location for a calcium is in the supraspinatus followed by the infraspinatus tendons. Less frequently, deposits may also be noted in the subscapularis and teres minor tendons. The calcium is generally situated in a superficial position adjacent to the subacromial bursa. Perforation of the calcific deposit into the bursa can be beneficial as it may often decompress the blister-like swelling in the rotator cuff–like tissue. The calcium deposit is believed not to rupture into the articular space.

Clinical Features

Calcific deposit can be a very painful condition that ordinarily presents in a fashion similar to impingement. In fact, an unrecognized calcific deposit may be the true cause of shoulder pain in many individuals who fail to respond to a subacromial injection and physical therapy for suspected impingement. However, there is no relationship between a full-thickness rotator cuff tear and a calcium deposit except that occasionally the two may be seen in coexistence.[111]

Clinically, there are generally two stages: acute and chronic. The acute stage is often characterized by excruciating pain, which may radiate down the arm. The examiner may comment that the pain seems to be out of proportion to the stimulus. The patient often holds the arm close to his or her side and is fearful of making even the slightest movement. There may be a great deal of local tenderness to palpation along with a significant degree of inflammation. In the chronic phase, the pain is generally less intense. There is a longer history of pain and of discomfort which is more gradual in onset. With chronicity of the disease, many patients may eventually end up with a frozen shoulder, which severely limits mobility. If the calcium deposit is large enough, subacromial crepitus may be noted as it impinges against the coracoacromial arch.

To verify the suspected diagnosis of calcific tendinitis, it is necessary to obtain a complete series of shoulder radiographs. This should include internal, external, and neutral rotation AP views as well as an axillary and/or a Y-scapular view. The calcific deposit can easily hide behind the humeral head and go unrecognized if appropriate views are not obtained.[15]

Treatment

Treatment of the acute stages of calcific tendinitis includes subacromial steroid injections and anti-inflammatory medications.[111] In this stage, the calcium may be liquid and an attempt should be made to aspirate or lyse the calcific deposit during the subacromial injection. In some instances, the pain may be so severe as to warrant the use of narcotic medications. Range-of-motion exercises should be initiated to treat existing stiffness and avoid further stiffness. A second cortisone injection may be indicated approximately 3 months after the first, but multiple injections should be avoided. This type of nonoperative intervention is generally successful in 80 percent or more of patients.[76] If the patient continues to complain of significant pain after several months using the above intervention, arthroscopic intervention is indicated.

Arthroscopic treatment involves removal of the calcium deposit and decompression of the subacromial space. Subacromial arthroscopy is performed in a routine fashion. A bursectomy is performed to give good visualization of the rotator cuff tendons. Based on careful preoperative planning and adequate radiographs, the suspected position of the calcific focus is needled with an 18-gauge spinal needle. When a calcific deposit is entered with a needle, release of calcium is usually visualized. This occurs as a milky white fluid or powder is emitted into the arthroscopic fluid. In some instances, calcium release is not visualized. This may occur when the calcific deposit is firmer and less granular. In this instance, the surgeon needles those areas in which the calcific deposit is suspected to be positioned in the hope that a slow release of the calcium will occur later. Ark et al. have reported 91 percent good or satisfactory results in 23 patients who underwent arthroscopic decompression and removal of a calcium deposit.[5] Good results have also been reported using open techniques.[95] However, the open techniques necessitate a deltoid split, thereby adding potential morbidity and lengthening the time of postoperative recovery.

BICEPS TENDON DISORDERS

The long head of the biceps tendon serves as a humeral head depressor.[111] Rodosky et al. have shown that the long head of the biceps tendon and its attachment into the superior glenoid labrum may play a role in anterior stability of the glenohumeral joint.[147] A variety of disorders including biceps tendinitis, biceps subluxation or dislocation, and biceps rupture have long been recognized as pathologic entities. With the advent of arthroscopy, pathology at the attachment site of the long head of the biceps tendon into the superior glenoid labrum has been identified.[4] This disorder has been coined the "SLAP lesion," for superior labrum anterior to posterior, by Snyder.[157]

Biceps Tendinitis and Rupture

Biceps tendinitis and rupture is rarely if ever a primary event. It almost universally occurs as a result of concomitant impingement and rotator cuff disease.[111] In rare instances, it may also be the result of arthritic change, with osteophytic growth or stenosis of the bicipital groove. The

physical examination is usually notable for tenderness of the long head of the biceps tendon within the bicipital groove. This is best identified by internally and externally rotating the GH joint while palpating between the lesser and greater tuberosities. The Speed test and Yergason sign, as previously described, can help confirm the diagnosis (Figs. 55-25 and 55-26).

The underlying cause of bicipital tendinitis and rupture is almost universally impingement; therefore, treatment is directed at eliminating the impingement syndrome. This is described elsewhere in the text. In the rare case of primary bicipital tendinitis, treatment is initiated with a steroid injection in the bicipital groove. The tendon itself should not be injected, as this can result in attrition and possible rupture. If this course of intervention fails, then tenodesis of the biceps tendon into the proximal humerus may be indicated. After tenodesis, the long head of the biceps tendon is no longer able to serve as a humeral head depressor. In cases where tendinitis has led to attrition of the tendon and rupture, the proximal stump of the tendon is resected and the remaining distal stump is tenodesed.

Tenodesis can be accomplished through a variety of surgical approaches, including direct suturing to surrounding soft tissues, transosseus sutures, or suture anchors. Prior to tenodesis, the long head of the biceps tendon is resected at its attachment into the superior labrum. Its proximal end is shortened and the surrounding bone is debrided of the soft tissue in order to prepare the site for attachment. A keyhole technique may also be utilized, in which the stump of the biceps tendon is knotted and inserted into a keyhole in the proximal humerus.[67] When using this technique, some protection against loading of the proximal humeral bone should be put into place, as the keyhole serves as a stress riser that can lead to proximal humeral fracture.

Biceps Tendon Subluxation

Subluxation of the biceps tendon often occurs in association with disruption of the subscapularis attachment into the lesser tuberosity. The adjacent transverse humeral ligament is often disrupted in concert with the subscapularis insertion. As a result, the biceps tendon is free to move out of the groove. The most frequent position of translocation is into the intraarticular space. In most cases, a thin layer of connective tissue remains between the lateral aspect of the intertubercular groove and the subscapularis tissue.

Other causes of biceps tendon subluxation include a primary rupture of the transverse humeral ligament associated with impingement. In this case, an extraarticular subluxation occurs. The direction of sublxation can either be toward the subscapularis or toward the infraspinatus tendons. Subluxation of the long head of the biceps tendon may also occur in concert with a fracture of the lesser or greater tuberosity that disturbs the architecture of the intertubercular groove.

When subluxation of the long head of the biceps tendon is suspected, the patient should be carefully examined for evidence of a subscapularis tear. The Gerber lift-off test can be instrumental in making the diagnosis.[73] The biceps instability test may also be helpful in determining whether or not the long head of the biceps tendon is subluxating. In this text, the examiner palpates the biceps tendon in the groove while the patient's arm is placed in an abducted and externally rotated position and subsequently internally rotated. A palpable or audible and painful click may be noted as the biceps tendon reduces and then subluxates passing over the lesser tuberosity.[36]

Operative treatment is generally indicated in association with a rotator cuff tear. The tendon is reduced into the groove and the transverse humeral ligament is reconstructed with local tissue including the subscapularis tendon. If the sublaxation is chronic and the tendon scarred and shortened, it may be prudent to perform a biceps tenodesis in order to prevent a significant postoperative biceps tendinitis.[173]

Superior Labral Lesions

A superior labral lesion is a pathologic abnormality at the site of the long head of the biceps tendons insertion into the superior labrum from both anterior and posterior directions. The superior labral lesion was first noted by Andrews et al. in a series of overhead throwing athletes who complained of pain and symptoms of clicking and popping in the GH joint.[4] An arthroscopic evaluation of these athletes demonstrated abnormalities at the insertion of the long head of the biceps tendon into the superior labrum. Snyder et al. classified the lesion into four types, as shown in the diagram in Fig. 55-38.[157] This is the SLAP lesion, previously described.

Biomechanical studies by Rodosky et al. have shown that the presence of a type II superior labral lesion may adversely influence anterior stability at the glenohumeral joint.[147] The etiology of the superior labral lesion is felt to be related to either repetitive microtrauma secondary to eccentric loading of the tissue or to a compression injury with the humeral head being driven up into the superior labrum.

The diagnosis of a superior labral lesion is difficult to make. The patient often complains of a clicking or popping feeling associated with pain and overhead use of the arm. The physical examination may demonstrate a positive Speed test or Yergason sign. Magnetic resonance imaging may be helpful in making the diagnosis. Unfortunately, a large degree of anatomic variability exists at the superior labrum, which reduces the specificity of an MRI. Radiologists are currently working with gadolinium enhancement in the hopes that the MRI's diagnostic accuracy will be improved (Fig. 55-35). The gold standard for diagnosis is an arthroscopic examination with inspection and probing.

The indications for treatment of a superolabral lesion remain controversial. Debridement of such a lesion has not been very successful.[54] Recent reports have indicated relatively high success rate with arthroscopic reattachment of the superior labral tissue using a variety of techniques including transosseus sutures, biodegradable tacks, and suture anchors.[141] The long-term benefit of these procedures is as yet undocumented. These procedures should be reserved for those individuals who have failed to respond to several months of physical therapy that includes rotator cuff, biceps, deltoid, and pericapular muscle

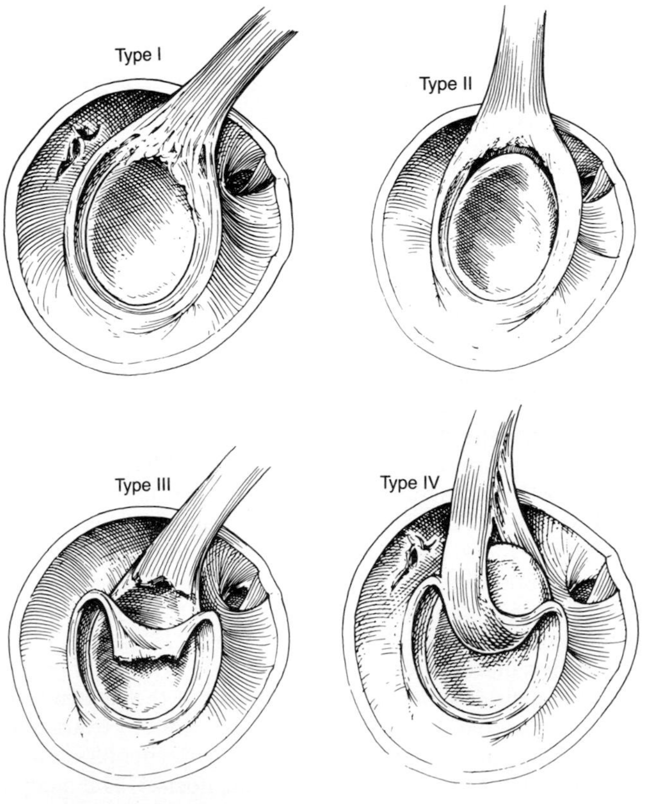

Figure 55-38 Slap lesion classification: type I, fraying with intact anchor; type II, detachment of biceps anchor; type III, bucket-handle tear with biceps intact; and type IV, bucket-handle tear into biceps. (Reproduced with permission from Snyder SJ, Wuh HCK: Arthroscopic evaluation and treatment of the rotator cuff and superior labrum anterior to posterior lesion. *Op Tech Orthop* 1:212–213, 1991.)

strengthening. In many cases, the superior labral pathology may be caused by occult (or micro-) instability. Further work to help define the true etiology and best treatment methods for superior labral lesions is currently ongoing.

ARTHRITIC AND DEGENERATIVE DISORDERS OF THE GLENOHUMERAL JOINT

Arthritic and degenerative disorders of the GH joint result in pain and dysfunction that can greatly interfere with the patient's ability to use the upper extremity for activities of daily living and greatly diminish quality of life. The most prevalent of these conditions include primary osteoarthritis, secondary osteoarthritis, rheumatoid arthritis, cuff tear arthropathy, and avascular necrosis.

Because the upper extremity is subjected to fewer weight-bearing demands and is not required for ambulation (except in individuals with lower extremity pathology), many individuals are able to tolerate advanced stages of disease by compensating with the contralateral upper extremity or by increased compensatory motion at the scapulothoracic and elbow joints. Those individuals are successfully treated with anti-inflammatory medications and activity modification. When these methods of treatment fail, surgical intervention is indicated. The pathologic features common to all arthritic and degenerative disorders of the GH joint include incongruity of the articular surfaces and loss of the GH fulcrum.[111] As in other joints, this pathology has been treated in the past with resection of the painful arthritic surfaces to avoid articular contact; however, this leaves the patient with a resultant flail arm. Arthrodesis has been successful in eliminating pain but leaves the individual with very little rotation and limited motion in forward elevation.[48]

The most dramatic advance in treatment of arthritic and degenerative disorders of the GH joint has been the introduction of replacement arthroplasty.[111] This approach has become the treatment of choice, almost entirely supplanting GH arthrodesis and/or resection. However, both the technique of surgery and the postoperative rehabilitation are made difficult by the unique anatomy of the GH joint. The GH soft tissues must be appropriately reconstructed in order to obtain postoperative stability and motion. When this is accomplished, the postoperative results of shoulder arthroplasties are equal or superior to results of other major joints both in durability and function.[111]

Pathology

Osteoarthritis

Primary GH osteoarthritis is a common condition that should not be confused with the end stages of severe rotator cuff deficiency. Patients with primary GH osteoarthritis almost always have an intact rotator cuff and long head of the biceps tendon. The disease is characterized by limitation of GH motion secondary to incongruity of the articular surfaces. The humeral head becomes en-

larged by marginal osteophytes, the largest of which are located at the inferior margin of the joint, where they cover the calcar area of the proximal humerus. Initially, thinning of the articular cartilage of the humeral head occurs in that area of the head which is in contact with the glenoid cavity when the humerus is in abduction. This results in greater wear on the superior part of the articular surface.[111]

At the glenoid fossa, the wear is more intense posteriorly than anteriorly, resulting in posterior bone loss. In long-standing cases, the excessive posterior glenoid wear results in significant retroversion of the osteoarthritic glenoid. At the same time, the anterior capsular structures and subscapularis become contracted, which ultimately serves to increase the potential for posterior erosion of the glenoid. Osteophytes may form around the glenoid but are generally smaller in size than those of the humeral head. Osteochondral loose bodies may become so numerous as to suggest the presence of osteochondromatosis, and they often become trapped in the subcoracoid recess.

Rheumatoid Arthritis

Rheumatoid arthritis is a systemic disease that involves all the tissues of the GH joint, including the muscles, bursa, and joint surfaces. Rheumatoid pannus formation can result in very significant erosion of GH joint surfaces, with the resultant pathology based on age and severity of the disease. The humeral bone is osteoporotic and easily fractured. The head erodes from invasion of pannus; therefore fewer and smaller humeral head osteophytes are present. In a like fashion, the glenoid cavity becomes eroded, which generally results in a protrusion pattern of destruction (Fig. 55-39). This often leaves the inferior aspect of the glenoid fossa intact, giving the glenoid surface a cephalic tilt. However, in some instances, the erosive pattern may be primarily anterior or primarily posterior, with resultant excessive anteversion or retroversion of the glenoid cavity.[85]

As the disease progresses, the rotator cuff tissue is eroded by pannus, becoming thin and dysfunctional. Erosive tearing of the rotator cuff may be present in 20 to 30 percent of patients with rheumatoid arthritis. With continued loss of the glenoid and humeral head surfaces and thinning of the rotator cuff, the humeral head progressively migrates in a proximal direction, causing impingement erosion of the cuff and furthering the likelihood of a rotator cuff tear.[111]

Avascular Necrosis

Avascular necrosis (AVN) of the humeral head is caused by a lack of blood supply to the bone. In a fashion similar to other major joints, the etiology is multifactorial and includes corticosteroid use, alcoholism, sickle cell disease, and various other causes. The clinical manifestations are similar to those of primary osteoarthritis; however, range of motion is usually maintained well into the late phases of the disease process. The superior portion of the humeral head, which comes in contact with the glenoid at approximately 60 to 90° of abduction, is the area that usually suffers articular surface collapse. The glenoid cavity is rarely

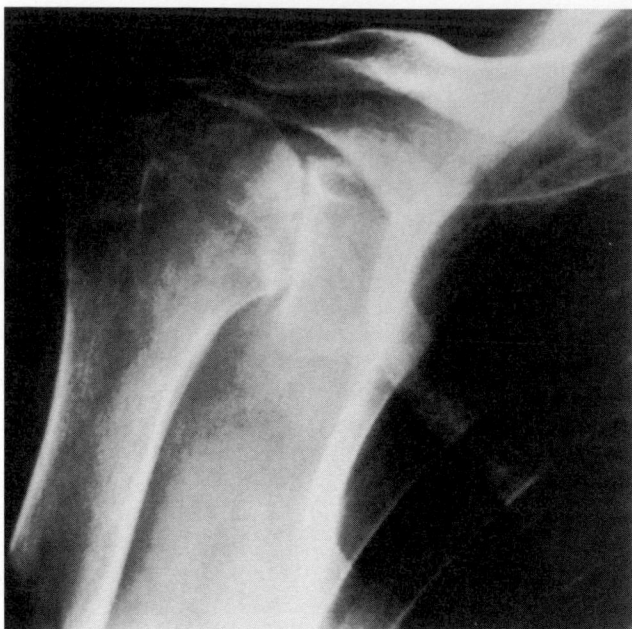

Figure 55-39 Anteroposterior radiograph demonstrating osteoporosis and proximal migration of the humeral head as well as central erosion of the glenoid cavity down to the coracoid base in a patient with long-standing rheumatoid arthritis.

affected to a degree that would require glenoid resurfacing. In most cases, the lesser and greater tuberosities are spared and the soft tissues and rotator cuff do not become significantly contracted. Shoulder arthroplasty in these individuals usually meets with a high degree of success. However, small number of patients with avascular necrosis of the humeral head present with rapid collapse of the head, which may progress to the point of fracturing of the greater and/or lesser tuberosities.[111]

The pathologic changes that are seen are explained by the type of joint contact that occurs at the glenoid fossa. The glenoid contacts the humeral head with maximal pressure at approximately 90° of elevation. This correlates to contact at 60° of GH elevation. This area of contact at the humeral head is the site of collapse. A classification scheme for AVN of the humeral head has been described by Neer with four stages.[111] Stage I shows subtle changes, whereas stage II progresses to a "meniscal sign," representing a small area of subchondral bone changes. In stage III, the disease is characterized by a "step-off" sign with evident collapse of subchondral bone and the overlying cartilage. In stage IV, the collapse continues, resulting in further incongruencies and eventual involvement of the glenoid cavity.

Posttraumatic Arthritis

Posttraumatic arthritis is a broad category encompassing many different pathologic situations caused by a variety of etiologies. The various etiologies include proximal humeral fractures with resultant nonunions or malunions and articular incongruencies, arthritis after recurrent disloca-

tions or subluxations, and arthritis after surgical intervention for instability problems. Soft tissue contractures are universally present in patients with posttraumatic arthritis. The major form of soft tissue contracture includes the coracohumeral ligament and rotator interval tissue, resulting in a significant internal rotation contracture.[111] Malunion of the tuberosity fragments results in an offset of the normal line of action for the rotator cuff muscles. This can result in eccentric loading of the glenoid cavity, compounded by soft tissue contracture. Tuberosity malunion can also result in subacromial impingement or coracoid impingement. Nonunion of the tuberosity fragments can result in extensive contracture of that portion of the rotator cuff which attaches to the nonunited tuberosity. These nonunited tuberosity fragments often scar near or to the axillary nerve.

Cuff Tear Arthropathy

Rotator cuff tear arthropathy is directly related to a deficiency in rotator cuff function. This leads to an inability to keep the humeral head in direct contact with the glenoid fossa. Instead, the humeral head migrates proximally to abut the coracoacromial arch, including the undersurface of the acromion and AC joint. In addition, the humeral head may dislocate in an anteroinferior direction from the loss of the stabilizing effects of the posterior aspect of the rotator cuff (i.e., posterior mechanism for anterior instability; see "Instability," above). With time, the continued abutment against the coracoacromial arch and the continued instability subject the humeral head to unusual wear and tear.[113] The end result is cuff tear arthropathy characterized by an incongruous and distorted humeral head with superior erosion and subchondral collapse as well as erosion of the undersurface of the acromion and AC joint. With advanced disease, the glenoid cavity can become eroded and incongruous.

Infection

Septic arthritis is an infrequent cause of GH arthritis.[43] The infectious process results in rapid destruction of the cartilaginous surfaces, both at the glenoid cavity and the humeral head. If the infection goes unrecognized for a length of time, the subchondral bone may eventually become involved in the disease process, with resultant osteomyelitis. In successfully treated infections of the GH joint, the erythrocyte sedimentation rate is usually found to be normal. In cases where treatment with surgical intervention has been chosen, a frozen section analysis of abnormal tissue encountered during surgery can be helpful in verifying the presence or absence of an active infectious process.

Clinical Evaluation

The patient with GH arthritis presents with shoulder pain and concomitant loss of motion and strength. The pain of GH arthritis is often more intolerable than that of arthritis in the hip or knee, since shoulder pain is not alleviated by recumbency but is in most cases made worse. Recumbency eliminates the distractive force created by the weight of the arm in a non-recumbent position. As GH arthritis progresses, GH motion diminishes and the patient must compensate with increased scapulothoracic motion. Because scapulothoracic movement contributes little to rotation, limitation of external rotation is a more sensitive physical sign than that of loss of forward elevation. Other signs specific to GH arthritis include posterior joint line tenderness and crepitus at the GH joint.[111]

When the clinician suspects that GH arthritis is present, a standard radiographic series should be obtained. This would include an AP view of the GH joint made perpendicular to the plane of the scapula as well as an axillary view. In patients with radiographic findings consistent with significant erosion of the humeral head and/or glenoid cavity, a CT scan can be obtained to allow the clinician to quantify the extent of bone loss precisely. This becomes particularly important when shoulder arthroplasty is being considered. In patients with posttraumatic arthritis, the CT scan can be very helpful in the evaluation of deformity at the greater and lesser tuberosities.

Laboratory studies are an important component of the clinical evaluation of a patient with suspected GH arthritis. These studies include a complete blood count (CBC) with differential and an erythrocyte sedimentation rate to screen for the presence of infection.[43] When these screening studies are positive, an aspiration arthrogram can be used to obtain a fluid specimen for culture and sensitivity. When rheumatoid arthritis is suspected, the specific laboratory studies, as described elsewhere in this text, can be helpful in screening for serologic evidence of the disease.[111]

When a concomitant rotator cuff tear is suspected, it is helpful to obtain an MRI study to verify the diagnosis of cuff disease. Such a study may also have the added benefit of providing information about loss of bone or bone deformity, negating the need for a CT scan. However, because of the significant cost of an MRI scan, the test should be limited to those cases where a potential change in the treatment plan may be indicated by the study.[412]

Glenohumeral Arthroplasty

Indications

The primary indication for shoulder arthroplasty is unremitting pain that has persisted after a course of nonoperative treatment. Loss of function is a secondary indication of surgery. Shoulder arthroplasty is rarely performed to improve range of motion without concomitant pain. The patient should have a stable medical status and should be capable of playing an essential role in the postoperative rehabilitation. Absolute contraindications to arthroplasty of the GH joint include the presence of an active infection and/or paralysis or complete functional loss of both the rotator cuff and deltoid muscles.

Alternatives to Arthroplasty

Arthroplasty is by far the most successful type of treatment for most arthritic involvements of the GH joint.

However, it is important to understand that other forms of surgical intervention are available and may be indicated in select cases. For instance, debridement and soft tissue balancing can be useful in treating young patients with mild or moderate arthritis after instability repair with a concomitant internal rotation contracture. The goal of the treatment is to normalize the biomechanics of the GH joint, therefore ensuring that the GH joint forces will be more evenly distributed throughout the glenoid surface rather than being focused at the posterior aspect of the glenoid cavity.[90]

The use of GH arthroscopy for irrigation and debridement, combined with soft tissue release, has some degree of limited success in patients who are poor candidates for joint replacement. Weinstein et al. found that arthroscopy for GH arthritis provided significant pain relief and increased motion in 78 percent of patients at an average of 2 1/2 years' follow-up.[176] This procedure was not helpful in patients with complete loss of joint space, large osteophytes, or significant posterior humeral subluxation. The long-term value of this type of intervention is as yet undocumented. Open debridement for synovectomy and bursectomy is rarely indicated but can be helpful in the rare patient with rheumatoid arthritis who presents with signs of significant intraarticular inflammation and synovitis and who has maintained congruency of the GH joint without evidence for significant pannus invasion of the humeral head or glenoid.[154]

Humeral head resection can be used as a salvage procedure for a variety of shoulder pathologies.[112] These include resistant infections as well as failed arthroplasties with resultant extensive bone loss. In a recent review, it was noted that one-half to two-thirds of patients achieve satisfactory pain relief after humeral head excision and that motion is limited on average to 40 to 90° of forward elevation with minimal to no active external or internal rotation.[48] After humeral head resection, the patient should be placed in a sling for 6 to 8 weeks and allowed pendulum range-of-motion exercises only, with the aim being to develop scarring that will improve the stability of the proximal humerus and diminish the chances for abutment against surrounding structures.[111]

Prior to the introduction of a shoulder arthroplasty, shoulder arthrodesis was a commonly indicated procedure for GH arthritis.[103,104] The fused shoulder eliminated pain at the GH joint and provided stability and durability, enabling the patient to perform heavy labor. However, many patients with shoulder fusion developed periscapular pain and all have a limited functional range of motion.[78] Currently, shoulder arthrodesis is used primarily for patients with paralysis or compromise of both the rotator cuff and deltoid muscles. The young, active laborer may be better served with a humeral head replacement.[111]

History

Several different prosthetic designs for shoulder arthroplasty have been utilized throughout the years. These have included constrained and nonconstrained designs. The constrained designs were found to have a very high failure rate and have been largely abandoned.[145] Several different nonconstrained designs are currently being used, many with modularity. Modularity primarily involves the ability to use different-sized humeral head components with varying stem sizes. The most commonly used prosthetic components include cemented metal humeral components and cemented polyethylene glenoid components. Glenohumeral arthroplasty is performed with either humeral head replacement alone or humeral head replacement and glenoid resurfacing.[105,106,108]

Humeral Head versus Total Shoulder Replacement

The current indications for glenoid replacement remain similar to those that were put forth by Dr. Neer in the early 1970s: pain due to glenoid incongruity that has failed to respond to conservative treatment in patients with adequate glenoid bone stock, good surgical risk and motivation, the absence of active infection, and the absence of paralysis and/or destruction of both the rotator cuff and deltoid muscles.[110,111,120] However, based on the collective experience of many, these indications have been modified as concerns for glenoid failure have been raised.

Currently, glenoid resurfacing is avoided in patients with rotator cuff deficiency.[42,134] These patients are predominantly those affected by cuff tear arthropathy and chronically torn and scarred rotator cuff muscles. Patients with significant rheumatic or inflammatory disease may have similarly contracted deficient rotator cuff mechanisms, which would place them in the same category. Some of these individuals may also have significantly eroded glenoid bone stock, which, in some instances, may prohibit the use of a glenoid component. However, most individuals with rheumatoid or inflammatory arthritis retain adequate glenoid bone stock and intact functional rotator cuff muscles; they therefore fare better with glenoid resurfacing.[145] A recent report of 10-year follow-up in these types of patients shows that the glenoid revision rate was only 5.6 percent.[86]

The results of glenoid resurfacing in patients with arthritis have been very satisfactory, with a glenoid revision rate of only 5.6 percent at more than 12 years.[64] However, many of the patients developed radiolucencies around their glenoid components; therefore, most shoulder surgeons advocate caution in considering use of a glenoid resurfacing component in a younger osteoarthritic patient. Additionally, patients with posttraumatic arthritis have a higher potential for abnormal GH mechanics secondary to tuberosity deformity and extensive soft tissue contracture. Patients in this category have a higher potential for abnormal subluxation and increased focal eccentric loading of the glenoid postoperatively. This translates into an increased risk for glenoid loosening or failure.[145] Although the earlier literature supports use of glenoid resurfacing in these patients, more recent work suggests that surgeons proceed with caution with regard to glenoid resurfacing in a patients whose soft tissue envelope and tuberosity deformity increase the risk for postoperative instability. For similar reasons, most shoulder surgeons also continue to advocate the avoidance of arthroplasty in patients with neurotrophic arthropathy

who remain unaware of the loading conditions and position of their GH joint.[145]

Patients with painful glenoid incongruity, adequate bone stock, and normally functioning rotator cuff muscles without significant tuberosity deformity are treated with total shoulder replacement, including glenoid resurfacing. Fortunately, the great majority of patients with primary osteoarthritis, posttraumatic osteoarthritis, and rheumatoid arthritis have these characteristics.[111] Patients with avascular necrosis have sparing of the glenoid cavity until the very late phases of the disease; therefore they do not require glenoid resurfacing.

Patients with smaller rotator cuff tears and good-quality tissue are treated with total shoulder arthroplasty and cuff repair. When the cuff tissue is atrophic or the rotator cuff tear is larger, humeral hemiarthroplasty is performed and the rotator cuff is repaired with an emphasis toward anterior/posterior stability of the implant over complete superior coverage.[42,134] Patients with posttraumatic arthritis are evaluated based on the amount of tuberosity deformity and soft tissue distortion. Those with a significant potential for abnormal GH mechanics, including subluxation with eccentric loading of the glenoid, are treated with humeral hemiarthroplasty rather than total shoulder replacement.[145]

Humeral Head Replacement

The technique for humeral head replacement is based on that described by Neer.[111] The patient is anesthetized with general anesthesia or given a region interscalene block, which has the added benefit of pain control in the perioperative period. Appropriate perioperative antibiotics should be administered. The surgery is performed with the patient in a semisitting or beach-chair position with avoidance of neck hyperextension. The shoulder must be brought off the side of the operating table in order to allow full extension of the glenohumeral joint. An extended anterior deltopectoral approach is utilized (Fig. 55-21). This preserves both the origin and insertion of the deltoid. The incision is made from the inferior border of the clavicle, proceeding laterally to the coracoid and obliquely toward the anterior portion of the deltoid insertion. It is recommended that the coracoid not be osteotomized so as to lessen the risk of musculocutaneous nerve damage. The subacromial space must be freed of bursal adhesions. The coracoacromial arch is preserved except in the rare case where there is evidence of significant impingement. The long head of the biceps tendon is preserved. Inferiorly, the leading edge of the pectoralis major insertion may be partially released to enhance exposure.

The axillary nerve is identified by a tug test at the inferior medial border of the subscapularis and protected throughout the operation[61] (Fig. 55-40). The subscapularis and capsule are released together at the most lateral aspect of the lesser tuberosity in order to maintain maximal length. The subscapularis can then later be repaired to the edge of the humeral head resection, effectively lengthening the tendon. This is a necessary step, since most patients with arthritis have some degree of anterior soft tissue contracture and loss of external rotation. To maximize

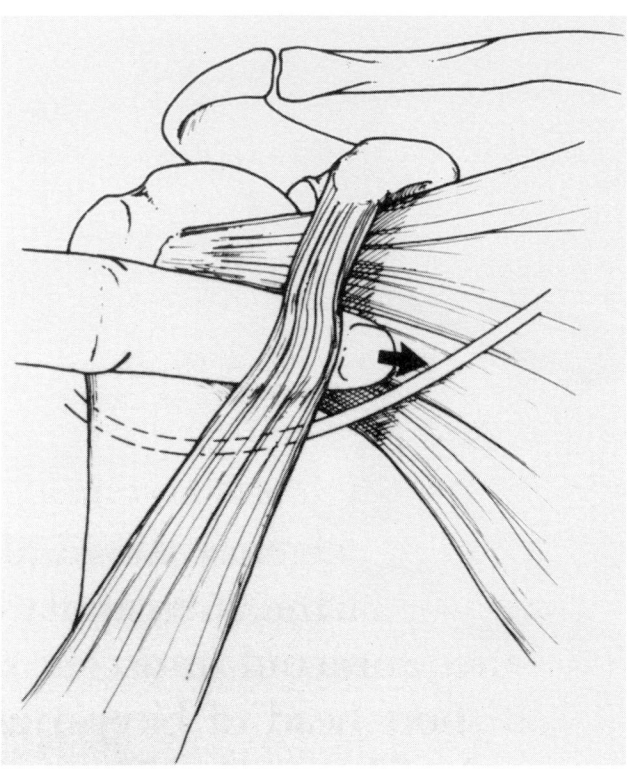 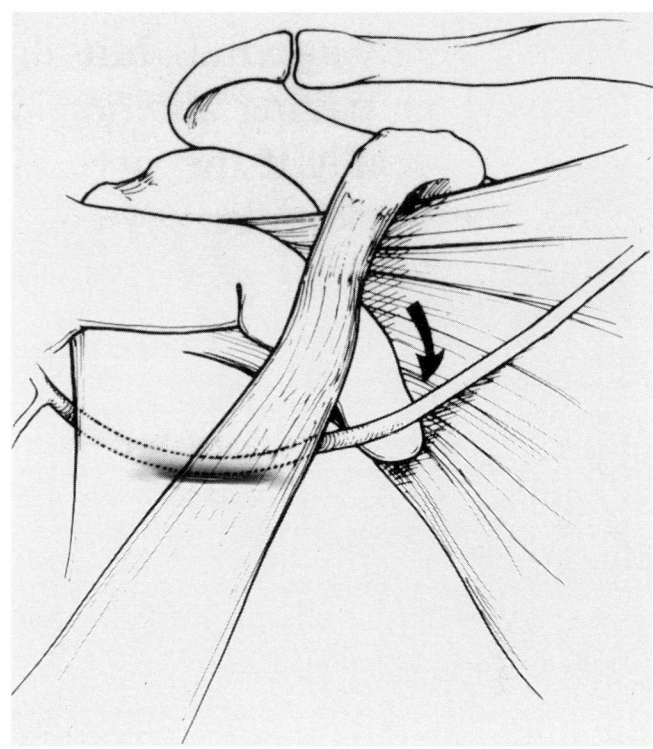

A   *B*

Figure 55-40 *A.* The tug test is used to locate the axillary nerve during anterior shoulder approaches. The index finger is passed directly medially over the subscapularis and under the coracoid. *B.* The finger is then rotated and swept down until the axillary nerve is palpated. (Reproduced with permission from Flatow EL, Bigliani LU: Locating and protecting the axillary nerve in shoulder surgery: The tug test. *Orthop Rev* 21:503–505, 1992.)

excursion of the subscapularis tendon, humeral and glenoid osteophytes must be excised and osteochondral loose bodies removed. These loose bodies may often migrate to the subcoracoid recess beneath the subscapularis. In addition, the anterior glenohumeral capsule must be released from the glenoid margin in order to allow maximal excursion of the subscapularis tendon. If these steps are not taken to eliminate the anterior soft tissue contracture, the patient will remain with tight anterior structures postoperatively, which diminish external rotation and can lead to posterior subluxation of the humeral component. This can result in posterior instability and/or early failure of the glenoid component when it is employed. In some individuals, it may be necessary to lengthen the subscapularis in order to gain adequate anterior soft tissue tensioning (Fig. 55-41). This may be necessary when a patient has had a previous subscapularis shortening procedure for instability.

The humeral head is then dislocated by gently rotating the shoulder externally and extending the humerus. This step is greatly facilitated by adequate release of the inferior and posteroinferior capsule around the humeral neck. At this point, it is necessary to determine the precise location of the posterior cuff insertion into the greater tuberosity in order to avoid damage to the cuff tissue during humeral head resection. Osteophytes along the infe-

rior margin of the head at the calcar area must be removed to better delineate the true articular surface of the humerus. A guide is then used to assist in planning and performing the osteotomy for removal of the arthritic head (Fig. 55-42*A*). It is important to note that in most cases of arthritis, the inferior portion of the head becomes enlarged with osteophytes while its superior portion erodes, giving the illusion that the center of the humeral head is lower than it actually is. The surgeon should recognize this fact in order to prevent excessive removal of the head, which may jeopardize the rotator cuff insertion (Fig. 55-42*B*).

The humeral cut is made orthogonal to the humeral shaft by externally rotating the humerus 30 to 40° and cutting directly parallel or, by using the humeral epicondyles as a landmark, and making a cut approximately 30 to 40° retroverted to them (Fig. 55-42*C*). When the cut is made appropriately, the lateral fin of the humeral prosthesis should lie approximately 5 to 10 mm posterior to the posterior margin of the bicipital groove. The superior aspect of the osteotomy should exit just above the insertion of the posterior cuff. In patients with arthritis after a locked humeral dislocation, the version of the humeral cut is adjusted to compensate for the instability that results from chronic expansion of the soft tissues. In this situation, the retroversion is decreased for posterior instability and increased for anterior instability.

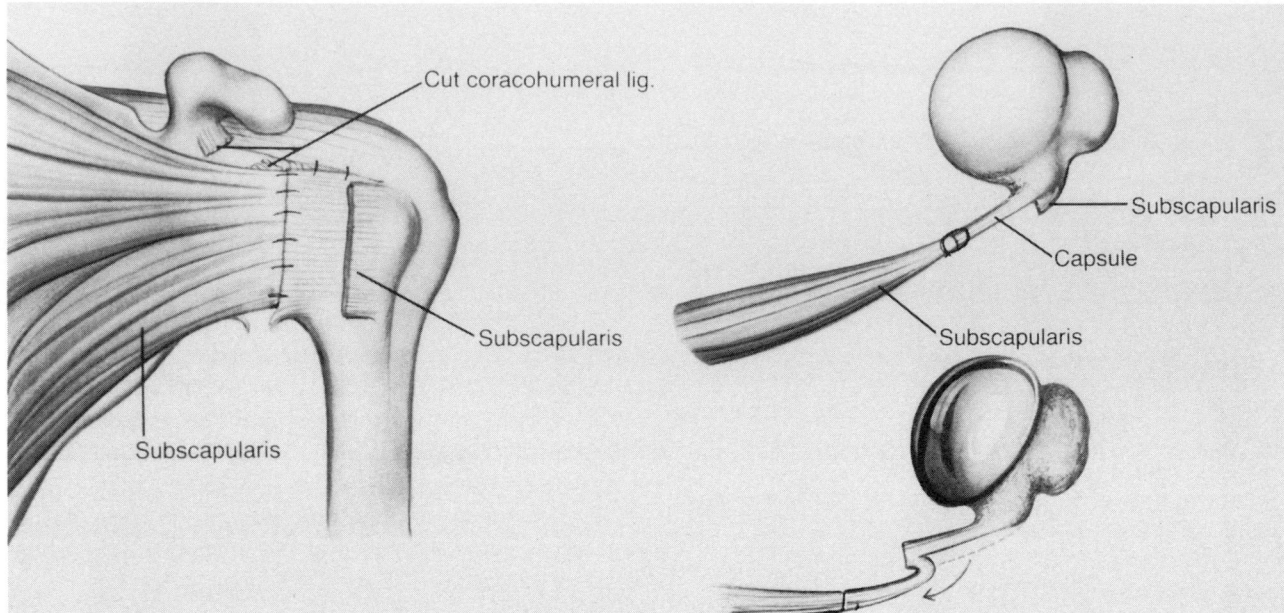

Figure 55-41 Subscapularis lengthening.

Next the medullary canal of the humerus is prepared with progressive manual reaming. A slot is made for the lateral fin of the prosthesis posterior to the bicipital groove. This is carried out with a small rongeur and can be helpful in diminishing the chance of a tuberosity fracture during reaming or placing of trial humeral components. The trial implant is then placed in the humeral canal in the appropriate amount of retroversion and the glenohumeral joint is reduced. Humeral head height must be checked to avoid prominence of the tuberosity, which can lead to impingement. During the trial process, appropriate version and soft tissue balance are assessed. The goal is to have the humeral component translate to approximately 50 percent of the humeral head diameter and allow 45° of external rotation with the arm at the side.

Once appropriate humeral sizing is obtained, the humeral trial prosthesis is removed and the glenoid cavity assessed. At this time, the surgeon verifies that a glenoid resurfacing prosthesis is not indicated and a humeral component of appropriate size is cemented or press-fitted into position. Immediately prior to this, bony drill holes placed at the anterior humeral neck are filled with #2 nonabsorbable braided nylon sutures. These sutures are used to repair the subscapularis tendon. When the humeral component is cemented, a cement plug is recommended in patients for whom elbow arthroplasty may be necessary at a later time. The cement is not pressurized so as to avoid cement extrusion through the humeral bone, which is much thinner and weaker than the femur.

The wound is thoroughly irrigated, followed by closure of the deltopectoral interval and skin. Suction drains may be used between the deltoid and rotator cuff and should be brought out through separate stab incisions. The patient is placed in a sling and swathe and physical therapy is begun on the first postoperative day.

Glenoid Resurfacing

When it has been determined that glenoid resurfacing is indicated, the surgeon proceeds with total shoulder replacement.[111,120] After the humerus has been prepared for prosthetic implantation, attention is focused on the glenoid cavity. The humeral head retractor is placed along the posterior glenoid neck and retracts the humerus in a posterior direction. The arm should be stabilized with an arm holder, arm board, or Mayo stand. Great care must be taken to avoid crushing the exposed proximal humeral bone, especially in patients with rheumatoid arthritis, who often have very soft and osteopenic bone.

Once adequate visualization of the glenoid cavity has been provided with appropriate retraction, soft tissues at the glenoid margin, including labral tissue, are freed and a blunt retractor is placed along the anterior neck of the glenoid. Any remaining labral tissue is sharply resected to allow a complete view of the entire glenoid cavity. Throughout this procedure, the axillary nerve must be carefully protected. At this time, the glenoid is evaluated to make certain that the bone stock is adequate. Also at this time, it is important to verify the type and quantity of bone loss by comparison with that suspected based on preoperative studies. The glenoid cavity is prepared to accept the glenoid component so that the latter will have complete and precise peripheral support of the glenoid prosthesis platform. Past studies of glenoid component loosening have shown that buildup of noncontained cement or incomplete support of the platform by bone can lead to toggling and early loosening of glenoid prostheses.[25,144,145,148]

Erosion of glenoid bone stock resulting from an arthritic process must be recognized and dealt with at the time of glenoid resurfacing. The most common pattern of

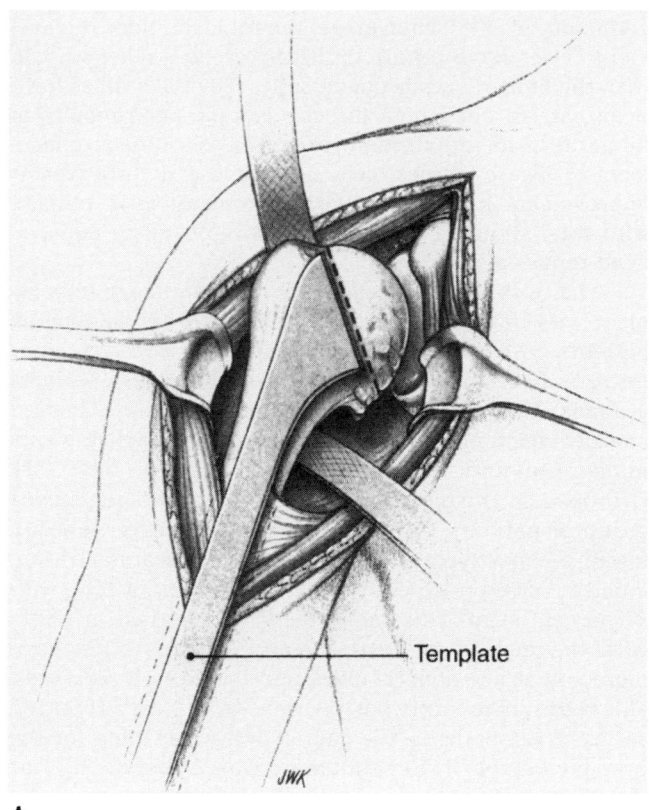

A

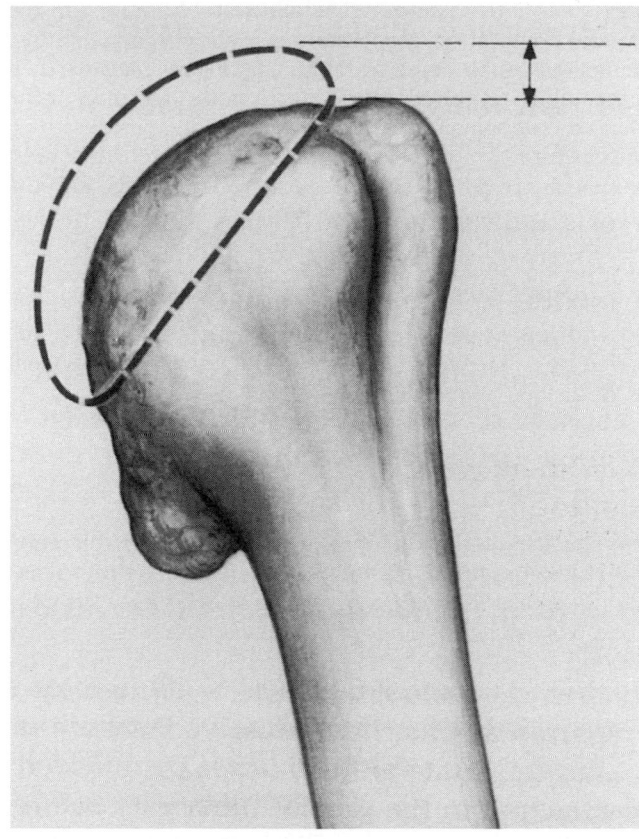

B

C

Figure 55-42 *A.* After exposure and dislocation of the humeral head, osteophytes are removed and a template is used to determine the line of humeral resection. *B.* The surgeon must be sure that the humeral osteotomy is above the level of the tuberosities. *C.* The humeral cut is made orthogonal to the humeral shaft by rotating the humerus externally 30 to 40° and cutting directly parallel or by using the humeral epicondyles as a landmark and making a cut approximately 30 to 40° retroverted to them. (Reproduced with permission from Knetsche RP, Friedman RJ: Cement versus noncement: Humerus. *Op Tech Orthop* 4:210–217, 1994.)

glenoid wear is posterior erosion. In this instance, the surgeon must either lower the anterior surface of the glenoid, recreating a normal glenoid tilt, or lessen the amount of humeral retroversion so that the combined retroversion of the two components is no greater than 30 to 40° of retroversion. For instance, if the glenoid component is left in 10° of retroversion, the humeral component should be left in 20 to 30° of retroversion, so that the combined retroversion is between 30 and 40°. In certain cases, it may be necessary to bone graft the glenoid cavity in order to eliminate abnormal tilt and provide adequate bone stock for a glenoid replacement.[118]

Currently, in most cases, the glenoid component is fixed with methylmethacrylate. Once the glenoid face has been adequately contoured to allow stable seating of the glenoid component, preparation is made for implantation. Hemostasis is obtained by first using pulsatile lavage; then a thrombin- or epinephrine-soaked gauze is placed in the glenoid component stem or peg slots. The cement is then pressurized by a cement gun or syringe and further pressurized by packing the corner of a gauze sponge into the stem or peg slots. A second infusion of cement is then placed and the component is pressed into position with firm digital pressure until the cement cures. Humeral trialing is once again carried out in order to ensure that the appropriate-sized humeral component is implanted, followed by subsequent insertion of the humeral component as described above.

Rehabilitation

Postoperative rehabilitation is an important component in the success of glenohumeral arthroplasty. Rehabilitation after shoulder arthroplasty is based on Neer's three-phase shoulder rehabilitation program, in which phase I emphasizes passive motion in forward elevation and external rotation.[111] Phase II progresses to active assisted and active exercises of the shoulder, generally beginning at 6 to 8 weeks after surgery. In phase III, advanced muscle stretching and progressive resistive strengthening exercises are initiated, usually at 3 months postoperatively; these continue indefinitely. The patient's specific pathology and bone and soft tissue quality direct the timing of the rehabilitation program. Premedication with oral narcotics during the early postoperative phase is necessary.

Nonconstrained Arthroplasty Component Designs

The most successful and most utilized glenohumeral arthroplasty design incudes the use of a cemented metal humeral component and a polyethylene cemented glenoid component. These components have a failure rate of less than 6 percent at 12-year follow-up.[164] Non-porous, press-fit humeral components are known to have a high degree of subsidence over time.[134] Porous, coated humeral components have recently been employed. They avoid the need for cement but have the disadvantage of creating extensive bone loss when revision surgery is necessary. Metal-backed glenoid components have been cemented in the past but have fallen out of favor because of concerns over abnormal stress concentration and the potential for early glenoid loosening. In recent times, several clinical trials with porous ingrowth glenoid components have been initiated. Early designs were fraught with complications, including polyethylene dissociation and screw breakage.[49,50] Longer follow-up is needed to determine whether or not newer designs can improve upon the known success with cemented polyethylene components.

Glenohumeral Arthroplasty Results

The overall results for both humeral head replacement and total shoulder replacement have been very satisfactory. Most series have reported greater than 80 to 90 per-

cent pain relief.[145] On average, the total shoulder replacement series have reported slightly greater relief of pain than the humeral replacement series. Several studies have been carried out which directly compare the results of humeral head replacement with total shoulder replacement.[145] These studies have also found a slightly greater improvement in postoperative symptomatology in patients with total shoulder replacement as opposed to humeral head replacement.

The postoperative results for total shoulder replacement vary depending on the type of arthritis. In general, patients with primary GH osteoarthritis and avascular necrosis have the best functional results. These patients are most likely to have a normal rotator cuff and deltoid muscle, which are the main determinants of active glenohumeral motion. In a recent report from the New York Orthopaedic Hospital Shoulder Service, a homogeneous group of patients with primary osteoarthritis were followed prospectively for an average of 3.3 years and were found to have postoperative active elevation of 160°, with 97 percent significant pain relief.[137] In contrast, patients with rheumatoid or posttraumatic arthritis often have more soft tissue abnormalities and therefore have a variable return of function postoperatively. In Neer's reported series of 194 patients, the gain in active elevation for the primary osteoarthritic shoulders was 77 versus 57° for rheumatoid shoulders and only 33° for the posttraumatic shoulders with old trauma.[111,120]

Complications of Glenohumeral Arthroplasty

Fortunately, the incidence of complications after shoulder arthroplasty has been less than that noted for other major joint reconstructions.[96] As in other areas of the body, many complications can be avoided by utilizing proper indications, technique, and rehabilitation. The incidence of infection after shoulder arthroplasty is extremely low at less than 0.5 percent. This compares very favorably with reported infection rates following other major joint replacements. An early hematogenous infection can often be treated with irrigation debridement and wound closure over a closed drainage system and appropriate intravenous antibiotics. Delayed infections require removal of the prosthesis and all cement, foreign bodies, and sequestra as well as long-term antibiotic therapy. With less virulent organisms such as *Staphylococcus aureus*, the prosthesis can be replaced after adequate treatment of the infection. Where more virulent organisms are involved, it may be advisable to maintain the state of resection arthroplasty and/or perform GH fusion.

Nerve injuries during shoulder arthroplasty are extremely uncommon. These injuries most often result in a neuropraxia, which can be treated expectantly. The axillary nerve is the one most likely to be injured, as it runs on the inferior aspect of the capsule and then curves posteriorly at the undersurface of the deltoid muscle. If there is suspicion that the axillary nerve was lacerated during surgery and electromyography at 6 weeks reveals a complete lesion with no improvement at 12 weeks, early exploration and repair of the axillary nerve may be beneficial. If the lesion is partial and/or improving, observation is indicated.

Intraoperative fractures of the humerus or scapula are uncommon but can occur in osteoporotic bone.[28,31] Fractures are more likely to occur when a press-fit porous component is being inserted rather than a cemented component. When a humeral shaft fracture occurs, a long-stem prosthesis may be utilized to help stabilize the fracture. Tuberosity fragments can also fracture, especially in osteoporotic patients with rheumatoid arthritis. These fragments must be secured by heavy suture after the humeral component is cemented in position. Bone graft from the humeral head can be utilized in the fracture situation.[51]

Fortunately, postoperative instability has been reported to occur in only 1 to 2 percent of patients after shoulder arthroplasty. The stability of an unconstrained implant depends on preservation of humeral length, proper vision of the components, and appropriate soft tissue balance. In Neer's report of 194 total shoulder replacements with an average of 37 months follow-up, there were only 4 dislocations.[111,120] All were treated with closed reduction and immobilization for 3 to 6 weeks and then rehabilitation. Only 1 of the 4 had recurrent subluxations. When the instability is caused by significant abnormalities in the orientation of the humeral or glenoid component, either one or both of the components must be revised to prevent continued instability.

Postoperative tearing of the rotator cuff is one of the most frequent complications following total shoulder arthroplasty, with an incidence of 3 to 4 percent.[51] When the rotator cuff tear results in pain or instability, an open rotator cuff repair should be performed. This can be difficult, especially when very little bone stock is present for transosseous sutures. Subscapularis tendon pull-off occurs when the anterior soft tissues have not been adequately released or when the size of the humeral head component is large and abuts the postoperative subscapularis repair. Failure of the subscapularis repair must be treated early so as to avoid extensive retraction and scarring of the subscapularis. If extensive scarring occurs and significant anterior instability results, insertion of a fascial auto- or allograft may be necessary to prevent anterior instability.[97]

Prosthetic loosening is a rare complication of GH arthroplasty. In the current peer-reviewed literature, the overall glenoid revision rate was 3.2 versus 1.8 percent for humeral components.[145] Loosening of the glenoid component is less likely to occur when the appropriate indications for glenoid resurfacing are followed. When the glenoid component loosens and becomes symptomatic, it is necessary to revise or remove the glenoid component to prevent pain and dysfunction. When the glenoid bone stock is adequate and the glenohumeral mechanics are stable, the component is replaced. When bone stock is inadequate, which may occur after cement removal and/or when there are concerns over the potential for abnormal GH mechanics with eccentric loading of the glenoid, it may be prudent simply to remove the glenoid component and increase the size of the humeral head component.[144] In some cases with extensive glenoid or humeral bone loss following loosening of GH arthroplasty components, it may be necessary to use osteochondral allografts in conjunction with humeral and glenoid prostheses.[51] In a recent report

on surgical treatment of glenoid component failures, relief of pain was successful in 79 percent of patients.[148]

ACROMIOCLAVICULAR ARTHRITIS

Acromioclavicular degenerative arthritis is often the result of trauma, as occurs with damage to the articular cartilage and/or incongruity of the joint surface associated with type III intraarticular fractures of the distal clavicle. More often, the etiology is idiopathic, with an insidious onset. Degenerative arthritis of the AC joint often leads to isolated pain. However, the degenerative process often produces large proliferative osteophytes at the AC joint, which may protrude inferiorly into the rotator cuff and contribute to symptoms of impingement.[111] Osteolysis of the distal clavicle may also follow trauma to the AC joint.[101] There may be loss of subchondral bone detail and cystic resorption with generalized osteoporosis of the distal clavicle. This is often the result of repetitive microtrauma, as occurs with weight-lifting or gymnastics. Other less common etiologies include rheumatoid arthritis and hyperparathyroidism.[111]

Evaluation

Anterosuperior shoulder pain and difficulty sleeping on the affected side are common symptoms of AC joint arthritis. The pain often radiates to the trapezius muscle, which has fascia that is confluent with the superior capsule of the AC joint. This can lead to painful spasm of the trapezius. Tenderness to direct palpation of the joint is the most reliable physical finding on clinical examination. Osteophytic enlargement of the joint may also be appreciated.

Provocative maneuvers that compress the AC joint, such as horizontal adduction of the arm or internal rotation of the shoulder, may also elicit pain. These provocative tests, however, are not entirely specific and may show overlap with other painful conditions, such as those associated with excessive posterior capsular tightness.

The radiographic evaluation should be performed with a standard shoulder series including an AP in the scapular plane with the humerus in neutral, internal rotation, and external rotation, a transscapular lateral, and an axillary view. These views will allow adequate assessment of the shoulder complex but may overpenetrate the distal clavicle. They should be supplemented with an AP radiograph with a 10° cephalic tilt using "soft tissue" technique (reduced penetration) to reveal subtle changes in the distal clavicle. These views will help in assessing the true inclination of the joint space. Magnetic resonance images of the AC joint obtained incidentally during an investigation of rotator cuff pathology can be helpful, as they will reveal soft tissue hypertrophy and synovitis at the AC joint.

Radiographic findings associated with degenerative arthritis of the AC joint include narrowing of the cartilage space, subchondral sclerosis, and marginal osteophytes. It should be recognized, however, that the radiographic appearance of the AC joint undergoes an age-related narrowing that is not necessarily pathologic and that AC symptoms may not correlate with radiographic findings. Radiographic findings indicative of osteolysis include loss of subchondral bone detail, cystic resorption of the distal clavicle, and a generalized osteopenia of the distal clavicle.

The most valuable diagnostic tool that can be utilized to determine whether or not the AC joint is contributing to a patient's shoulder pain is a lidocaine injection into the AC joint. It can help predict the value of possible surgical resection of the distal clavicle and has the added benefit of providing a therapeutic intervention if a steroid preparation is added. Multiple steroid injections should be avoided.

Treatment

The majority of patients will respond to conservative management, which includes nonsteroidal anti-inflammatory medications, activity modifications, and a steroid injection. If the patient does not respond or has a limited response to treatment, operative intervention with resection of the distal clavicle should be considered.

Operative intervention involves resecting the distal end of the clavicle to eliminate the painful articulation. Open resection of the distal clavicle has been a relatively successful operation for AC joint pathology since it was first reported by Gurd and Mumford.[74,100] Open resection, however, requires violation of the deltoid and trapezial fascial insertions at the distal clavicle. This affects the time needed for postoperative rehabilitation. In addition, the superior aspect of the AC capsuloligamentous complex is also incised and stripped for visualization and access to the distal clavicle, and this has the potential to interfere with its important role in preventing posterior translation of the distal clavicle. In contrast, the arthroscopic approaches to distal clavicular excision avoid interference with the distal clavicular insertions of the deltoid and trapezius, and active motion can begin shortly after surgery. Arthroscopic procedures also have the added advantage of preserving the superior aspect of the AC capsuloligamentous complex, making it less likely that abnormal posterior translation will occur after resection.[64,146] The arthroscopic procedure can be carried out via a bursal (Fig. 55-18) or direct approach (Fig. 55-19), as previously described in this text. It is important to remove no more than approximately 1 cm of bone to avoid loss of the coracoclavicular ligaments. The success rate of distal clavicular excision is greater than 90 percent in most series.[20,146]

FROZEN SHOULDER

The basic pathology in all cases of frozen shoulder includes scarring and contracture of the capsuloligamen-

tous structures of the glenohumeral joint. Hence, a loss of passive range of motion is the end result. Frozen shoulder results from a variety of etiologies that can be broken down into primary and secondary causes. Primary frozen shoulder is also known as idiopathic frozen shoulder or adhesive capsulitis. It occurs spontaneously in the absence of a known secondary cause. Systemic disorders such as diabetes mellitus are often present, and immunologic influence is suspected. The secondary type of frozen shoulder is the result of a known cause. This includes intrinsic conditions such as rotator cuff disease or extrinsic conditions such as cervical radiculopathy or posttraumatic capsular adhesions.

Etiology

Primary Frozen Shoulder/Adhesive Capsulitis

An immunologic cause for adhesive capsulitis has been theorized by many researchers. This has been influenced by the fact that many patients with diabetes mellitus are afflicted with adhesive capsulitis, which is often recalcitrant to treatment with physical therapy and/or manipulation under anesthesia. In a recent study by Bridgman, the incidence of frozen shoulder in non-diabetic controls was 2.3 versus 10.8 percent in diabetic patients.[32] Another study identified abnormal glucose tolerance tests in only 12 percent of control patients without shoulder symptoms versus 28 percent of those with clinical evidence for frozen shoulder.[87] As in many other disorders with suspected immunologic etiologies, a direct link for frozen shoulder has yet to be determined.

Secondary Frozen Shoulder

The etiology for secondary frozen shoulder can be directly linked to an intrinsic or extrinsic cause. It is very common for individuals with chronically untreated rotator cuff disease to avoid overhead motion and therefore develop scar and contracture of the capsuloligamentous structures of their GH joints. This includes contracture of the coracohumeral ligament in the rotator cuff interval area, a condition that may be compounded by the presence of a rotator cuff tear. Scarring of the coracohumeral ligament and rotator interval tissue results in loss of external rotation. In addition, when the patients avoid elevation, the inferior capsular pouch may scar and contract, resulting in loss of passive elevation.

Other intrinsic causes include posttraumatic scarring of the capsuloligamentous structures subsequent to fracture at the surgical neck and/or tuberosity segments. The scarring is compounded by lack of adequate physical therapy and/or malunited fractures or joint incongruities. One of the major barriers to successful treatment of patients with malunited proximal humeral fractures can be the associated scarring that occurs in the capsuloligamentous structures and rotator cuff.

Extrinsic causes are produced by disorders resulting in pain and an individual's unwillingness to move his or her shoulder. This can include referred pain from cervical radiculopathy. It can also occur after hand, wrist, or elbow surgery in which a patient is placed in a sling for a long period of time. It has also been known to occur following breast surgery, especially when an axillary node dissection has been performed. Scarring and contracture of the capsuloligamentous structures is a direct result of keeping the arm at the side for an extended period of time, anywhere from a few weeks to several months. It is important to note that there may be overlap between primary and secondary causes and the pathology of frozen shoulder. For instance, an individual with diabetes mellitus and rotator cuff disease may develop extensive scarring and contracture of the GH soft tissues, while another individual without systemic disease may maintain a full passive range of motion in spite of untreated rotator cuff disease.

Pathology

Primary Frozen Shoulder/Adhesive Capsulitis

In a classic description by Neviaser in 1945, the adhesive capsulitis was broken down into four pathologic and clinical stages.[121] The earliest stage is the preadhesive one, in which punctate capillary proliferation of normal synovium is noted. The disease subsequently progresses to stage 2 or the adhesive stage, which is the most painful and initiates loss of motion. Pathologic findings include full-blown capillary proliferation with synovial hypertrophy and capsular adhesions. In the third stage or maturation phase, the synovial capillary changes diminish, leaving capsular contractures. The patient begins to experience less pain during this phase. In the fourth and final stage of the disease, the synovial changes are absent but the capsular contractures remain severe and tight.

Secondary Frozen Shoulder

The pathology and clinical presentation of secondary frozen shoulder is quite different from that of primary frozen shoulder or adhesive capsulitis. There is much less synovial inflammation. The clinical presentation is entirely dependent on the intrinsic or extrinsic cause. These causes almost universally result in the avoidance of range-of-motion activities of the involved glenohumeral joint. The capsuloligamentous structures scar and contract as a direct result of the immobility. Patients with secondary extrinsic causes develop scar and contracture very similar to that found in the final stages of adhesive capsulitis. Patients with intrinsic causes often have additional scar and contracture as a direct result of their disease process. This includes more extensive coracohumeral ligament and interval scarring in patients with chronic rotator cuff deficiency.[119]

Clinical Evaluation

The clinical evaluation begins with a thorough history and physical examination, which should include the cervical spine. It is essential to document both active and passive range of motion accurately in all planes. Routine radiographs and laboratory studies are also carried out.

Ancillary studies such as the subacromial impingement test can be helpful in differentiating intrinsic from extrinsic causes. Arthrography may be helpful in confirming the diagnosis. Positive findings include a reduced joint volume, obliteration of the axillary fold, and a thickened capsule. Magnetic resonance arthrography has the added benefit of giving the clinician the ability to evaluate the soft tissue structures in looking for evidence of intrinsic pathology.

Treatment

Nonoperative

The goals of treatment are to relieve pain and restore motion and function. Pain relief is important, as it will help the patient to participate in a rehabilitation program. The first step in relieving pain is to eliminate any known intrinsic or extrinsic causes. Patients with secondary frozen shoulder may temporarily regain motion but will likely suffer regression if the underlying cause is not eliminated. Patients with primary frozen shoulder or adhesive capsulitis can benefit from nonsteroidal anti-inflammatory medications, which may help to reduce inflammatory changes while also providing direct pain relief. Glenohumeral steroid injections may be helpful during the early inflammatory stages of adhesive capsulitis. However, the clinician is cautioned against the repeated use of steroids, which can contribute to connective tissue breakdown and/or infections of the glenohumeral joint.

Patients are begun on an active and active-assistive range-of-motion rehabilitation program combined with stretching. These exercises are carried out in all planes, including forward elevation, external rotation, and internal rotation. It is important to notify the patient that the first several weeks of therapy may lead to a transient increase in pain, which most often subsides shortly after the therapy session ends. Without this knowledge, many individuals will fail to comply with the therapy regimen for fear that they are causing more harm than good. Compliance on a daily basis is important to the success of the rehabilitation program. The exercises should be done a minimum of twice a day and as much as four to five times each day for more rapid progress. Modalities such as ultrasound and deep heat prior to therapy and ice at its completion may be helpful. However, it is of little benefit to the patient to carry these modalities to excess, resulting in very little time for actual range-of-motion exercises. As a patient progresses, with diminishing pain and improving range of motion, more aggressive stretching is helpful. This includes utilization of body weight by hanging from a door or bar. It also includes pushing one's body weight against a doorway to improve external rotation.

Patients must assume direct responsibility for their own daily therapy. In the first 6 weeks, it is helpful for the patient to see a therapist once a week to verify that the exercises are being performed appropriately and to provide instruction and supervision as well as encouragement.

The patient is encouraged to use the affected arm for activities of daily living as much as possible throughout the day. Most patients will begin to see progress, with diminishing pain and improving range of motion, over the first 6 to 8 weeks of therapy. The patient should be made well aware that it may take 12 to 18 months to regain motion fully. More than 90 percent of patients will respond to physical therapy alone.[111]

Operative Treatment

Manipulation under Anesthesia Patients who worsen or show no response after 3 months of continuous physical therapy usually require an intervention other than physical therapy. Through the years, manipulation under anesthesia has been the mainstay of treatment for patients who fail to respond to physical therapy. Manipulation under anesthesia can also be performed in conjunction with surgical treatment for intrinsic disease in order to provide normal postoperative motion.[111]

Manipulation under anesthesia can be performed under general anesthesia or under an interscalene block. The interscalene block is more advantageous, as a long-acting block can provide pain relief for several hours after the manipulation. This gives the patient a head start in the postmanipulation physical therapy regimen. Manipulation under anesthesia must be performed in a gentle fashion so as not to risk fracture of the humerus. For that reason, it is contraindicated in an individual with significantly osteoporotic bone.[111]

After the patient is anesthetized, he or she is examined to verify the diagnosis of frozen shoulder. With two-finger pressure, the arm is raised to as near full elevation in the scapular plane as possible and then placed in a position of external rotation at the patient's side. This is followed by positioning in abduction with two-finger pressure. In a position of abduction, the shoulder is forced into internal and external rotation. The maneuvers are then repeated in the same order until range of motion is maximized. Palpable and audible breakage of adhesions are often heard at the initial stages of the procedure. The final passive range of motion is recorded. Following the manipulation, passive range of motion is recorded and the exercises described above are initiated. Narcotics are given in the early postmanipulation period to help with pain relief.[111]

Arthroscopic Release Arthroscopy can be extremely helpful in both the diagnosis and treatment of frozen shoulder, particularly when an intrinsic cause is suspected. Arthroscopy allows a direct view of the synovium and capsuloligamentous structures involved in the disease. In addition, it also provides the ability to directly examine the articular and subacromial surfaces of the rotator cuff. Arthroscopy permits an accurate release of contracted capsuloligamentous structures and bursal adhesions as well as distention of the contracted capsule, known as *brisement*. Arthroscopy is currently indicated in patients who have failed manipulation under anesthesia, putting them in the category of resistant frozen shoulder syndrome.[135]

Glenohumeral and subacromial arthroscopy is performed in a routine fashion. The patient is anesthetized with either a general anesthetic or an interscalene block. Once again, the interscalene block has the added advantage of continued postoperative pain relief. An interscalene block has a second advantage: an indwelling catheter can be left in position for 2 to 3 days of repeat injections to aid in postoperative rehabilitation.[41] During arthroscopy, the synovial tissue and glenohumeral capsuloligamentous structures as well as the subacromial bursa are evaluated. The surgeon is then able to directly lyse capsuloligamentous scar and adhesions in a controlled fashion. Once the direct release of scar has been accomplished, the arm is gently manipulated, as described above.

The routine physical therapy regimen as described above is initiated in the early postoperative period. When an indwelling interscalene catheter is left in position, the patient can be either kept in the hospital for repeat blocks over the next 72 h or brought back on an outpatient basis for repeat blocks and supervised physical therapy. Recent reports from the New York Orthopaedic Hospital Shoulder Service and other centers have shown excellent results in patients with resistant frozen shoulder utilizing this approach.[41] At some centers, it is believed that arthroscopic intervention in conjunction with manipulation under anesthesia is safer than manipulation under anesthesia alone, as the capsular adhesions are directly lysed and separated with gentle force rather than being ruptured by force alone. Further work and documentation are necessary to verify or disprove this belief.

Open Release Open release is utilized as a treatment primarily when the disorder results from posttraumatic causes. These include fractures with deformity and malunion or nonunion of the tuberosity fragments as well as scarring after instability repairs. The major advantage of an open surgical release is the ability to intervene in an extraarticular fashion. For example, it may be necessary to release and lengthen the subscapularis tendon after failed instability repairs in which the subscapularis is excessively tightened, resulting in loss of external rotation and elevation and producing posterior subluxation of the humeral head.[111] Other examples include the ability to perform tuberosity osteotomies for malunion, such as may occur after a fracture of the greater tuberosity.

Complications Complications rarely if ever occur after nonoperative intervention. With manipulation under anesthesia, a humeral fracture may result if excessive force is utilized. This is especially true in patients with osteopenia. In these patients, it may be safer to perform an operative release. It is important to obtain full-length humeral films following manipulation under anesthesia so as to verify the presence or absence of a humeral fracture postmanipulation.

Arthroscopic intervention is safe and effective, with very little chance of complications. Open surgical release, especially in the posttraumatic situation, poses the greatest risk in treatment for frozen shoulder. The axillary nerve may be entrapped in scar and must be identified via palpation or direct visualization in order to avoid injury.

GLENOHUMERAL INSTABILITY

Descriptions of shoulder instabilities and their treatment are prevalent in the ancient and medieval literature. In 450 BC Hippocrates provided one of the earliest complete analyses of the subject.[1] Subsequent to these descriptions, little was written until the late eighteenth century, when methods of reduction were well described; later in the nineteenth century, surgical repair became popular. In more recent times, we have learned much about the biomechanics of the GH joint, which has helped a great deal in understanding the etiology of the disease.[172] This has greatly improved our ability to treat the disorder.

Glenohumeral instability occurs in varying degrees from subluxation to unreducible dislocation. A subluxation occurs when the humeral head is partially displaced from the glenoid fossa, whereas dislocation occurs when the humeral head is no longer in contact with the articular surface of the glenoid fossa. Subluxation or dislocation of the humeral head may become recurrent or chronic.

Incidence

The GH joint's proclivity toward motion over stability makes it the most commonly dislocated major joint in the human body. Instability of the GH joint is common, affecting all age groups and both sexes. In a study by Hovelius in Sweden, 1.7 percent of individuals in an age group from 18 to 70 years were noted to have glenohumeral dislocation at some time in their lives.[81] The sex ratio varies with age, with males predominating 9 to 1 in the age group from 21 to 30 years and a female predominance of 3 to 1 in the sixth and seventh decades of life. Anterior dislocation of the glenohumeral joint is much more common, with posterior dislocations accounting for only about 3.8 percent.[94] Multidirectional instability is less common and harder to recognize. Recent data have shown that unrecognized multidirectional instability can be responsible for a large percentage of failed surgeries for anterior instability.[116]

Etiology

In recent years, we have learned much about the biomechanics of the GH joint. This has given us great insight into the varying etiologies of instability. A complete description of the various factors that help stabilize the glenohumeral joint is provided earlier in this text. In brief, stability is provided by the osseous and cartilaginous joint surfaces, the static labral-capsuloligamentous structures, and the dynamic muscular structures. These structures must be competent and must work cooperatively in order to prevent subluxation and/or dislocation of the GH joint.

The osseous and cartilaginous structures serve as a fulcrum for motion of the upper extremity. Past studies have suggested a correlation between congenital flaws in glenoid version and instability of the shoulder. Because of these studies, osteotomy at the glenoid neck became a popular treatment for instability. However, in recent studies, researchers have not been able to identify differences in glenoid or humeral orientation when comparing patients with normal shoulders versus those with recurrent instability problems.[139] It is currently believed that osteochondral abnormalities are important only in cases of significant hypoplasia or with acute loss of substance or orientation secondary to trauma (i.e., glenoid rim fractures, humeral impaction fractures, or malunited glenoid neck fractures).

Defects of the humeral head as a result of abutment against the glenoid rim after a dislocation can occur and contribute to recurrent instability problems. These impression fractures are more frequently seen at the posterior head as a result of an anterior dislocation. They have been well described by Hill and Sachs and are commonly known as Hill-Sachs lesions.[80] A posterior dislocation can result in an anterior head defect and an inferior dislocation can result in a superior head defect. These impression fractures contribute to instability by reducing the effective contact area of the humeral head for articulation with the glenoid.

The static labral-capsuloligamentous structures are more commonly involved in the etiology of instability (Fig. 55-7). These structures become incompetent when they have a high degree of congenital laxity, when they are excessively stretched from acute or micro/repetitive trauma, and when they lose their attachment to bone. Bankart popularized the claim that the essential lesion in anterior posttraumatic instability was the detached anterior glenoid labrum, referred to by subsequent authors as a Bankart lesion.[8] Biomechanical studies have shown that the labral-capsuloligamentous structures must undergo an obligate plastic deformation of at least 10 percent prior to avulsion from bone.[22,163] It is well known that plastic deformation or complete capsular disruption without avulsion from bone can be a primary etiology for instability in any direction. It is further known that excessive laxity is the essential lesion for multidirectional instability.

While the capsuloligamentous structures serve as check reins at the end range of motion, the muscles work to maintain stability through joint compression in midranges of motion. An imbalance in these muscles forces can result in instability. Rotator cuff deficiency is generally seen in older age groups and can result in superior subluxation of the humeral head or superior dislocation if the coracoacromial arch is incompetent. The long head of the biceps helps to counter this effect, but in long-standing cuff disease, it may be incompetent as well. A rotator cuff tear can also contribute to anterior instability and is recognized as a posterior mechanism for the disorder. An anterior mechanism for anterior instability is recognized when the anterior capsuloligamentous structures are defective or detached from bone.

Classification

Glenohumeral instability can be classified as to mechanism, direction, circumstance, and degree[136] (Table 55-3). Acute trauma is recognized as the most common mechanism and generally occurs after a violent injury, such as a fall in sports or a direct blow to the upper extremity while

TABLE 55-3   Classification of Glenohumeral Instability

Mechanism
    Traumatic
    Microtraumatic
    Atraumatic

Direction
    Anterior
    Posterior
    Inferior
    Superior
    Multidirectional

Circumstance
    Acute
    Recurrent
    Chronic
    Involuntary
    Voluntary

Degree
    Subluxation
    Dislocation

in a vulnerable orientation, such as external rotation and abduction. The occurrence is immediately recognized by the patient with noticeable pain and deformity. However, a spontaneous reduction may occur at the time of injury making clinical and radiographic documentation difficult. Furthermore, transient episodes of subluxation may not be associated with any clinical or radiographic findings. The patient suffers a brief episode of excruciating pain, which subsides after the GH joint is reduced. However, the painful symptoms recur with motion.

In both subluxation and dislocation, there must be a concomitant injury to either the osteochondral structures, the capsuloligamentous structures and their attachment into the labrum, or the muscles or their tendons. The extent of the injury varies depending on the type of applied force, the position of the arm, and the age and quality of the tissue structures. In younger individuals, there is a propensity toward avulsion of the capsuloligamentous and labral structures from bone with a small concomitant plastic deformity; in older individuals, there is a penchant for capsuloligamentous stretching or tearing and/or rotator cuff tears. For this reason, it is extremely important to screen individuals over the age of 40 for the possibility of a rotator cuff tear following a GH dislocation.

The microtraumatic transmission of instability is most frequently seen in athletes and laborers involving repetitive-type overhead motions. The common example is the competitive swimmer who has placed repetitive stretch at the anterior GH capsuloligamentous structures over the course of many years. The continued repetitive microtrauma results in gradual stretching and incompetence of the capsuloligamentous structures, resulting in focal or multidirectional instability. The instability may present as recurrent subluxation or dislocation.[116]

The atraumatic mechanism of instability is primarily related to congenital tissue laxity. This can occur in patients with a collagen disease such as Ehlers-Danlos syndrome. Less frequent causes include hypoplasia of the glenoid fossa or humeral head. It can also be seen in neuromuscular disorders, with resultant muscular imbalance.

A dislocation is generally considered acute when it has occurred within 24 h of presentation. After this time, it is generally considered chronic or unreduced. A locked dislocation is one in which the humerus becomes impaled against the glenoid rim. The resultant humeral impression fracture is difficult to reduce except by open means. Acute posterior dislocations have less obvious clinical and radiographic findings and are harder for the uninformed clinician to recognize. Many are missed by the initial examiner and go on to become chronic or locked.

Recurrent instability usually means multiple episodes of documented subluxations or dislocations. However, it can be difficult to determine accurately how many times or in what direction a dislocation or subluxation has occurred, since the only evidence may be the patient's history. For that matter, it can be difficult to differentiate an episode of subluxation from a frank dislocation.[136]

Recurrent dislocation of the GH joint can be either involuntary or voluntary. When it is involuntary, it presents in individuals who have no desire, either consciously or subconsciously, to have the dislocation recur. These individuals may indeed be able to dislocate their shoulders at will, but they do not wish to do so. The voluntary dislocator has both the ability and the desire to dislocate the shoulder. This desire may be either a subconscious or conscious motivation or secondary gain or other psychiatric reasons. A full psychiatric evaluation is indicated for these patients.[136]

Clinical Features

General

Instability of the GH joint can be one of the most difficult diagnoses to make. At the time of examination, the patient may be completely asymptomatic and have very little clinical or radiographic evidence to support the diagnosis. This can be particularly true with subluxation. The patient with subluxation may be difficult to differentiate from the patient with subacromial impingement. Clinical features of instability are best appreciated when the examiner utilizes a systematic directional approach.

Anterior Instability

As previously mentioned, anterior dislocations and their associated tissue disruptions are more frequent than any other forms of dislocation. For this reason, anterior instability is the most frequent form of instability and is most commonly related to incompetence of the anterior labral-capsuloligamentous structures or their attachment to bone.[111] The patient generally presents with complaints of recurrent dislocations when the arm is placed in an externally rotated and abducted position.

The examiner will find that the patient is reluctant to have the arm positioned in abduction and external rotation for fear or apprehension that the GH joint will dislocate. This fear or apprehension can be eliminated by maintaining a posteriorly directed force at the humeral head. These two tests are respectively known as the apprehension and relocation tests (Fig. 55-27). The examiner should be sure to differentiate the feeling of apprehension from symptoms of pain.[159] Although the patient with anterior instability may have pain in the abducted and externally rotated position, this impingement type of symptomatology is generally not specific to anterior instability. In addition, the humeral head will generally be found to translate anteriorly with an anteriorly directed force at the humeral head. The amount of translation should be compared to that of the normal, contralateral shoulder and can be graded by percentage or degree, as previously described in this text. A complete neurovascular exam should be performed to rule out the presence of a neurovascular injury or rotator cuff tear.

A standard radiographic evaluation should be performed with a minimum of an anteroposterior view, a lateral view in the scapular plane, and a true axillary view (Figs. 55-30 and 55-32). These studies should verify reduction of the humeral head in the glenoid fossa and determine whether or not a posterior humeral head impression injury (Hill-Sachs defect) or anterior glenoid rim defect is present. In addition to these views, the Stryker notch view or an AP view with internal rotation can be helpful in looking for a posterior humeral head defect (Fig. 55-33). The West Point axillary view can be useful in evaluation of the anterior glenoid rim.

A CT arthrogram or MRI scan can also be very useful in the diagnosis of anterior instability. These studies can be helpful in documenting the presence of a Bankart lesion and in evaluating bony defects of the glenoid rim or humeral head. Recently, gadolinium-enhanced MRI studies have been introduced; these may greatly increase the sensitivity and specificity of the MRI exam.

Posterior Instability

Posterior instability is less common than anterior instability, as posterior dislocations occur less frequently. Posterior dislocations may result from an electric shock or a seizure. This is secondary to the spasmic contraction of the larger and more numerous internal rotators which overpower the weaker external rotators, thereby pushing the humeral head posteriorly. Repetitive microtrauma can also play a role in posterior instability and should be suspected when indicated by the history. An example of this may be seen in a football linesman whose arms are repeatedly pushed posteriorly in the position of true forward flexion. This results in repetitive microtrauma and stretching of the posterior capsule (Fig. 55-7).

Just as posterior dislocations are harder to recognize, posterior instability is harder to diagnose. Patients often complain of pain and a sense of instability with the arms in a forward flexed and internally rotated position, especially when posteriorly directed axial force is applied. The examiner tests for this by stabilizing the scapula and placing the shoulder in a position of 90° forward flexion and 90° internal rotation while a posteriorly directed force is placed along the axis of the humerus. This test is similar to the anterior apprehension test for anterior instability and is termed the *posterior stress test* (Fig. 55-28). The test is considered positive when symptoms are reproduced. Unlike the anterior apprehension sign, the reproduced symptoms often consist of pain with or without a sense of posterior subluxation or dislocation.[132,133]

Inferior and Superior Instability

Isolated inferior instability is extremely rare. When it is present, it is usually the result of a traumatic dislocation in which the humeral head is pushed in a true inferior direction with resultant plastic deformation of the inferior capsule.[111] Inferior instability is usually an associated finding of other forms of instability and is noted by the sulcus sign. The sulcus sign is positive when the humeral head translates inferiorly with an inferiorly directed force, creating a sulcus at the site of deltoid attachment into the acromion into the humeral head.

Superior instability is easily recognized by direct view or palpation as the humeral head rises through an incompetent coracoacromial arch. It is generally present only in individuals with a deficient rotator cuff and lack of a coracoacromial arch. With attempted elevation of the arm, the deltoid muscle forces the unstabilized humeral head through the arch.

Multidirectional Instability

Multidirectional instability as described by Neer in 1980 is a relatively new concept in instability.[116] Through the years, it has often gone unrecognized and has been a frequent cause of past failures of instability treatment.[123] Multidirectional instability can be one of the most difficult clinical diagnoses to make, since there may be signs of both anterior and posterior instability. The patient may have anterior, posterior, and inferior apprehension or any combination of the above. Patients with multidirectional instability will universally have an inferior component resulting in a positive sulcus sign

Since multidirectional instability has several etiologies, there are many clinical presentations that need to be recognized. The degree of difficulty arises from overlap with pure posteroinferior or pure anteroinferior instability. For instance, a shoulder may dislocate in one direction and subluxate in another direction. The subluxation is less obvious and easier to miss during the clinical exam. The examiner must attempt to quantify the degree of translation in the anterior, inferior, and posterior directions.

The patient with multidirectional instability as a result of collagen laxity may have equal displacement in all three directions. When the degree of displacement becomes symptomatic, the disease processes crosses the line between asymptomatic hyperlaxity and multidirectional instability. Some individuals may encounter a traumatic event that results in increased laxity in one direction on top of asymptomatic hyperlaxity. The traumatic event pushes them over the edge, resulting in multidirectional instability with a more severe component in one direction than in the other two. Other individuals may place repetitive stress on their capsuloligamentous structures to a higher degree in one direction than in the other two directions. This can also result in multidirectional instability, with one directional component being more severe than the other two. In both instances, the patient should be treated as a patient with multidirectional instability. Where the differentiation between uni- or bidirectional instability and multidirectional instability is difficult to make, fluoroscopic examination can be helpful. As will be described later, it may be necessary to perform an examination under anesthesia as well as diagnostic arthroscopy to truly verify the diagnosis.

Occult or Microinstability

In some individuals, instability is present but to a much lesser degree. This occult type of instability generally produces episodes of very mild subluxation. This condition is extremely difficult to differentiate from impingement as the symptoms are very similar. In fact, in many individuals, occult anterior subluxation may be the cause of known impingement. In this scenario, the increased excursion of the humeral head results in abutment against the coracoacromial arch. For this reason, it is prudent to consider the diagnosis of occult instability or microinstability in young patients who present with symptoms of impingement. Many of these individuals may have mild capsuloligamentous defects, such as a superior labral detachment, resulting in mild episodes of subluxation. When the diagnosis of occult or microinstability is considered, a CT arthrogram, MRI, or MRI arthrogram can be helpful. Ultimately, an examination under anesthesia and diagnostic arthroscopy may be necessary to make the diagnosis.

Treatment

Nonoperative Treatment

Patients who have experienced several nonvoluntary dislocations and who present with pain or dysfunction that severely limits their lifestyle are considered for early operative intervention. This is especially true when the dislocations begin to occur with trivial events such as turning in bed. Voluntary dislocators, subluxators, and patients with symptoms of mild instability in spite of a nonvoluntary dislocation should be placed on a strengthening exercise regimen. The program varies with the direction of instability, but several basic principles are followed. These include avoiding provocative activities while at the same time performing a closely supervised rehabilitation program to strengthen the shoulder muscles. The aim of the physical therapy is to regain strength and balance about the shoulder. The therapy is directed primarily at the rotator cuff and biceps muscles. Secondarily, the periscapular muscles and deltoids are strengthened.

Operative Treatment

General When nonoperative treatment has failed or when patients present with a severe disability that is not amenable to conservative therapy, operative intervention is considered. Over the years, numerous surgical procedures have been utilized for instability of the GH joint. In the past, muscular advancement procedures such as the Putti-Plat, Magnuson-Stack, and the Boyd-Sisk have been used.[30,91,127] These function by removing muscles from their normal attachment sites and placing them in a position that will limit GH motion. For example, the Magnuson-Stack procedure moves the insertion of the subscapularis from the lesser tuberosity to the greater tuberosity, thus greatly diminishing external rotation. The trouble with these procedures is that they result in loss of motion and are not truly directed at the underlying cause of the instability. In like fashion, osteotomies of the glenoid, neck, and/or humerus are rarely if ever indicated, as the etiology of GH instability is almost never related to congenital problems with glenoid or humeral version.

Anterior Instability Many different procedures have been described for reconstruction of anterior GH instability. These have included isolated repair of detached labral tissue using sutures or staples; muscle transposition of the subscapularis muscles, as in the Magnuson-Stack procedure; shortening of the subscapularis and anterior capsule, as in the Putti-Plat procedure; transfer of the coracoid, as in the Bristow procedure; osteotomy of the proximal humerus, as in the Weber procedure; osteotomy of the glenoid, as in the Meyer-Burgdorff procedure; and reconstruction with fascia lata grafts, as in the Gallie procedure.[70,79,91,127,151,174] These procedures have had a great deal of success in preventing recurrence of dislocation but have had relatively poor outcomes in terms of function and motion. Procedures that limit external rotation, such as the Putti-Plat and Magnuson-Stack repairs, have caused limitations in activities and therefore have fallen out of favor. Moreover, the resultant restricted motion has been implicated in the production of arthritis.

With increasing knowledge concerning the contribution of anatomic structures toward GH stability, the emphasis has been on restoring normal anatomy. In the case of anterior instability, this is generally either detachment of the capsuloligamentous structures from their insertion on the anterior glenoid rim or excessive laxity of these structures. A number of capsulorrhaphy procedures are currently utilized and address the problem of laxity as well as detachment from bone.[11,18,114] The results from these procedures have been satisfactory in more than 93 percent of cases, with an average loss of external rotation between 5 and 7 percent and a high percentage return to functional activity, including overhead sports.[11]

These type of capsulorrhaphy procedures can be performed in a variety of fashions, with the most common approaches utilizing a vertical incision in the capsule at either the humeral or glenoid sides (Fig. 55-43). The capsule is incised perpendicular to this vertical incision and overlapped in a fashion that allows reduction in laxity and associated joint volume. These procedures also allow simultaneous repair of detached anterior labral tissue from the glenoid rim utilizing transosseus sutures or suture anchors. The subscapularis tendon can either be incised and separated from the underlying capsule or split in line with

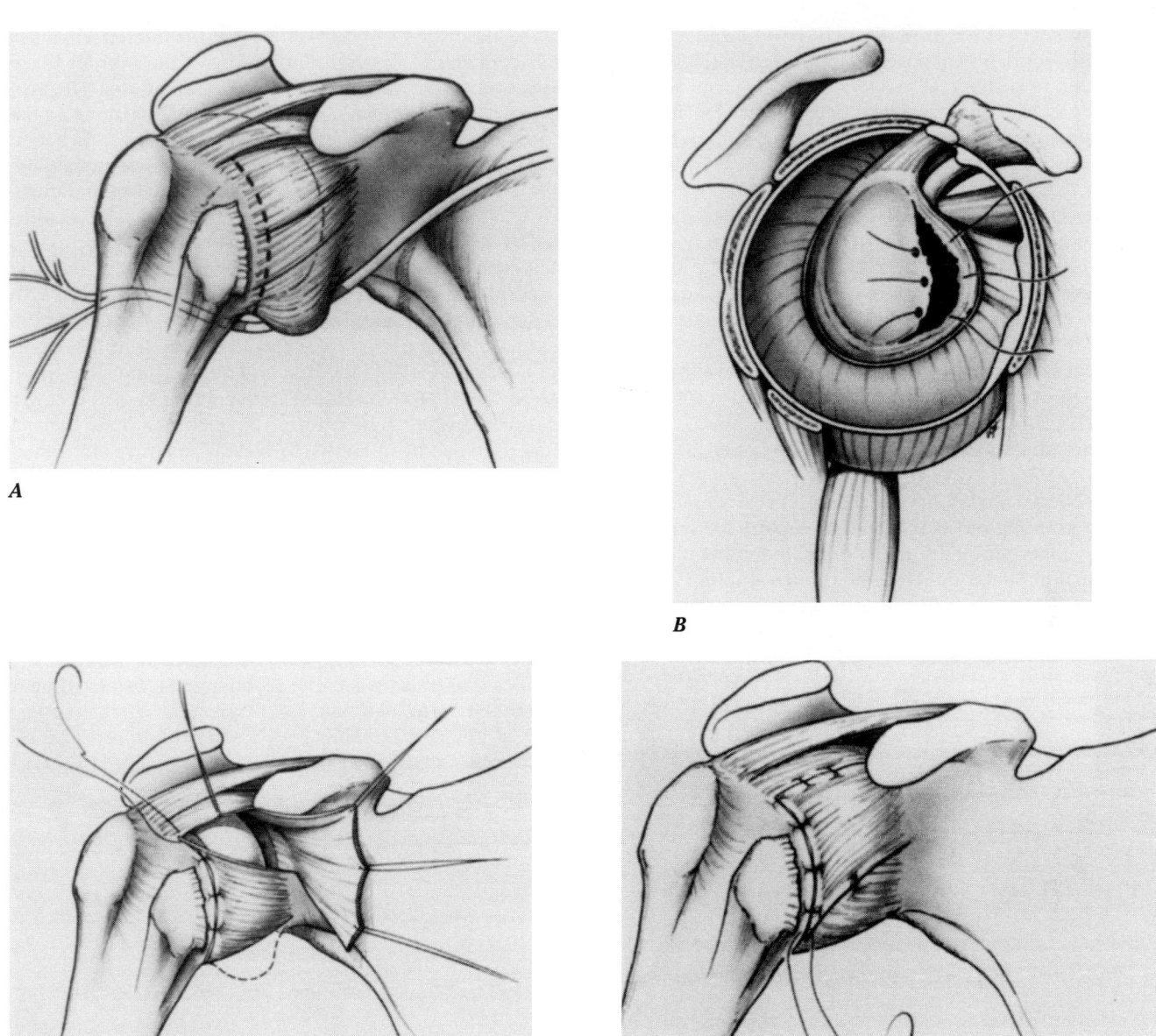

A

B

C

D

Figure 55-43 *A.* The anterior capsular repair is carried out through an anterior approach as previously described in this text. The capsule is exposed and incised. *B.* When a labral detachment is present, it is repaired to bone. *C.* The capsule is divided into flaps. *D.* The flaps are then crossed over and repaired to obliterate laxity.

its fibers. In the latter case, the capsulorrhaphy must be based near the glenoid rim. In all cases, the subscapularis muscle is anatomically repaired without shortening it. Occasionally, the surgeon may encounter unsuspected anterior glenoid bone loss. This can be successfully treated by transferring the coracoid process into the defect.[111]

Posterior Instability A number of different operative treatments have been recommended for the treatment of pure posterior instability; these have varied based on the per-

ceived etiology of the instability.[11,133] In some cases, this has included humeral osteotomies for suspected humeral head retrotorsion, glenoid osteotomies for suspected glenoid retroversion, and posterior labral repair for suspected labral detachment.[153,161] Recent studies have shown that the bony indices at the proximal humerus and glenoid can rarely if ever be implicated in posterior instability of the glenohumeral joint.[139] Posterior labral lesions are rare and are found in less than 10 percent of patients with true posterior instability.[133]

Recent success has been brought by utilizing a capsular shift procedure from a posterior approach[132] (Fig. 55-44). This procedure is aimed at reducing excessive capsular laxity, but it can also address labral detachment. Satisfactory long-term results have been reported in more than 80 percent of cases.[10] In the rare instance when a posterior glenoid bone deficiency is noted, a portion of the scapular spine can be used to graft the defect. In a fashion similar to the anterior approach, posterior capsulorrhaphy can be based off the humeral or glenoid sides. When it is based off the humeral side, the infraspinatus tendon is incised medial to the greater tuberosity and separated from the posterior capsule. When the glenoid approach is utilized, the infraspinatus muscle can be split in line with its fibers, or, alternatively, the interval between the infraspinatus and teres minor can be utilized. Once again, transosseus glenoid rim sutures or suture anchors are utilized to reattach capsule to bone.

Multidirectional Instability Neer and Foster were instrumental in pointing out that standard repairs for unidirectional instability problems are inadequate for treating multidirectional instability of the glenohumeral joint.[116] They fail to reduce the excessive inferior capsular redundancy and tend to overtighten one side, leading to fixed subluxation in the opposite, unaddressed side.

As described by Neer and Foster, the inferior capsular shift procedure allows reduction in volume on all three sides of the joint: anterior, posterior, and inferior. The procedure can be performed either from an anterior or a posterior approach (Figs. 55-43 and 55-44). The choice is based on the major or predominant direction of the instability. This is determined preoperatively with a history and physical examination and is confirmed by diagnostic studies and by examination under anesthesia. In this approach, the vertical capsular incision is placed laterally, near the humeral neck, rather than near the glenoid rim. With humeral rotation and flexion or extension, the surgeon is able to gain access to the capsular tissue that inserts at the inferior aspect of the humeral neck on the side opposite to the approach. This allows tightening of the entire inferior capsule, from anterior to posterior. This type of procedure has been shown to be successful in more than 90 percent of cases.

Arthroscopy Arthroscopy can be used very effectively as a diagnostic tool in conjunction with the examination under anesthesia. The arthroscope can verify the presence of a labral detachment as well as capsuloligamentous stretching or tearing. It can also verify the presence of bony abnormalities at the glenoid fossa and the humeral head.

The use of arthroscopic techniques in the treatment of glenohumeral instability is evolving. In clinical series, isolated anterior instability as a result of anterior labral

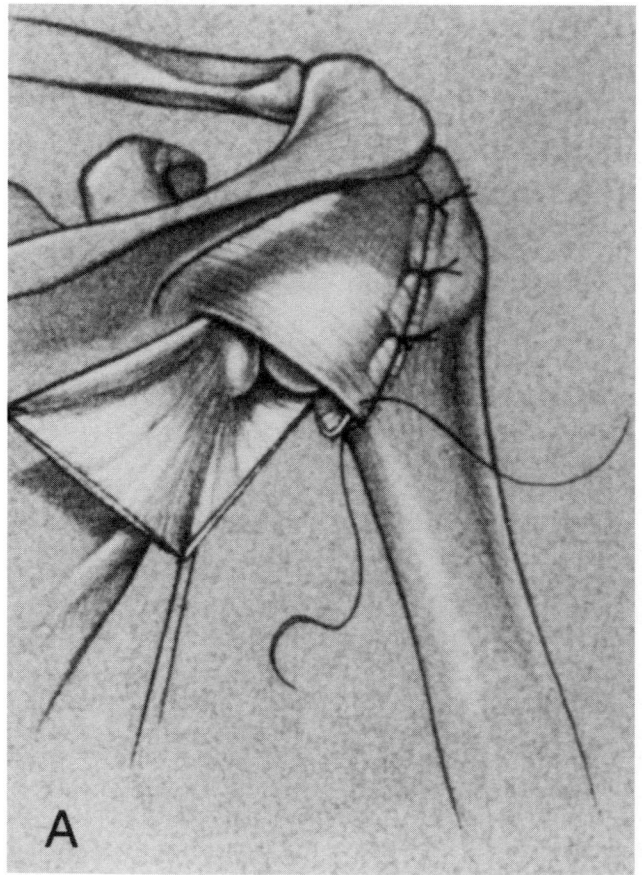

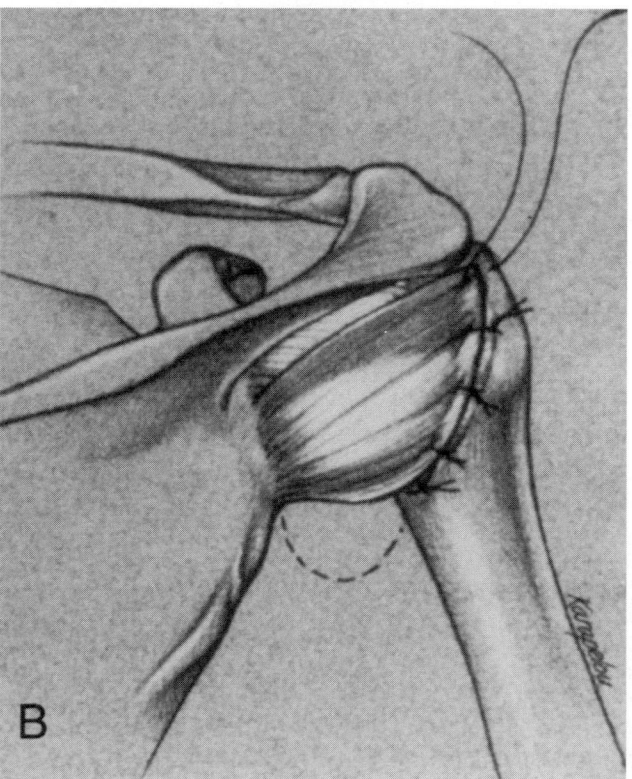

Figure 55-44 *A.* In posterior capsular repair procedures, the posterior capsule is exposed and capsular flaps are created. *B.* The flaps are overlapped to obliterate laxity.

avulsion was successfully treated with arthroscopic surgical techniques.[3] These techniques were successful only when the patients had very little plastic deformation of the anterior capsuloligamentous structures. These techniques have included transglenoid suturing as well as biodegradable tacks (Fig. 55-16). Failures occur when the patients have concomitant, excessive laxity of the anterior capsuloligamentous structures that cannot be easily shifted by the arthroscopic techniques.

Rehabilitation The purpose of the postoperative physical therapy program is to attain strength, motion, and synchronous function of the glenohumeral and scapulothoracic articulations. The ultimate goals are prevention of recurrence of the instability and return to function. The specific therapy protocol is based on the type of instability, quality of the tissue, the type of repair, and the future demands that will be placed on the patient.

After an anterior capsular shift procedure for anterior instability, the shoulder should be protected in a sling for 4 to 6 weeks. The sling must be removed daily for elbow range-of-motion exercises. After approximately 2 weeks, active-assistive range of motion is allowed to 90°, with forward elevation and 10° of external rotation. This is progressed so that at 6 weeks, active-assistive limitations are increased to 160° of forward elevation and 30° of external rotation. Active motion is then begun gently, with the goal being full motion at 3 to 4 months postoperatively. During this period, isometric strengthening is initiated and advanced to isotonic and isokinetic programs. Sports activities are restricted until the patient has regained full motion and strength, typically at 5 to 6 months postoperatively.

In patients with multidirectional instability or unidirectional posterior instability, the shoulder is protected in a brace with the arm positioned at the side in 5 to 15° abduction and neutral rotation, flexion, and extension. This helps to reduce inferiorly directed distractive forces and also serves to protect the infraspinatus repair when a posterior approach is utilized. Range-of-motion exercises are initiated when the patient's brace is removed at 4 to 6 weeks postoperatively. Strengthening exercises are generally begun at 6 to 8 weeks after surgery and are gradually progressed. Return to labor and sports activities is generally allowed at 6 to 9 months postoperatively.

Complications Fortunately, complications as a result of operative intervention in instability problems are rare. The shoulder's high degree of vascularity helps it maintain a degree of resistance against infection. The axillary nerve is the most common neurologic structure to be damaged. Injury to the nerve can be prevented by utilizing the tug test to make sure of its position at all times. It is vulnerable in surgery for both anterior and posterior instability surgery.

The most frequent complications following instability repair are related to a nonanatomic approach or by failing to recognize all components of the patient's instability. In these cases, a glenohumeral joint may be tightened excessively on one side, pushing the humeral head out the other side. This results in chronic subluxation and associated degenerative changes. The end result is arthritis after instability repair. In addition, metal staples and screws often loosen, resulting in articular destruction of the glenohumeral joint. In most cases, the anatomic approaches described above avoid the need for metal fixation and lessen the chance of metal loosening and migration.[123]

NEUROVASCULAR INJURIES AND SYNDROMES

Several well known types of neurovascular injuries or syndromes have been encountered and described. Many are the result of sharp or blunt trauma, and many occur as a result of repetitive trauma in athletes. The following is a brief description of these entities, including etiology, pathology, and treatment.

Axillary Nerve Injury

The axillary nerve is made up of fibers from the fifth and sixth cervical nerve roots. It originates from the posterior cord of the brachial plexus near the level of the coracoid process and passes anterior to the subscapularis muscle and posterior to the axillary artery. The nerve then goes on to course posteriorly and inferiorly at the lower border of the subscapularis, entering the quadrilateral space.

The most common cause of axillary nerve palsy is trauma. It occurs relatively frequently with anterior GH dislocations. The incidence of injury to the axillary nerve following acute anterior dislocations is significant with a range reported in the literature from 9 to 18 percent.[93] The axillary nerve may also be injured by a sharp fracture fragment in a complex proximal humeral fracture, especially when it is associated with a dislocation. Operative intervention is also a significant cause of axillary nerve injury as a result of sharp or blunt trauma.

The axillary nerve must be protected from harm during anterior approaches to the shoulder, such as that utilized for anterior instability and arthroplasty. It becomes particularly vulnerable when the arm is placed in relative abduction and internal rotation, which tightens the nerve and adds to the blunt force of retraction. It is also vulnerable during superoanterior approaches to the shoulder for rotator cuff repair. The axillary nerve lies approximately 5 cm lateral to the anterior lateral corner of the acromion, having come around through the quadrilateral space to innervate the deltoid.[37] The deltoid split must not exceed this level or the axillary nerve will be placed in peril. It can be helpful to place a heavy stay suture at the end of the split to prevent propagation and lessen the likelihood of nerve damage.

Axillary nerve damage can be devastating. The axillary nerve innervates the deltoid, which is the most important muscle of the shoulder. Loss of deltoid function results in significant weakness and loss of motion. When an axillary nerve injury is suspected, it is important to obtain an electromyographic (EMG) evaluation in order to confirm the diagnosis. Where a disruption of the nerve is suspected, surgical exploration is usually considered after 3 to 4 months of no return of function.

Quadrilateral Space Syndrome

The quadrilateral space syndrome is a less frequent cause of axillary nerve compression. In this syndrome, the posterior humeral circumflex artery is also compressed as it passes through the quadrilateral space. Compression is usually the result compression of both the nerve and vessels by fibrous bands when the arm is abducted and externally rotated.[39] The patient generally complains of poorly localized pain and paresthesias in the upper arm without any significant trauma. The pain is often exacerbated by abduction and external rotation of the arm, which may interfere with overhead activities such as throwing.[124] Point tenderness may be localized over the area of the quadrilateral space. Neurologic examination is usually normal. A diagnosis can be made with a subclavian arteriogram, which is performed with the patient's arm at the side and while in an abducted and externally rotated position. The study is considered positive when occlusion of the posterior humeral circumflex artery occurs.

Suprascapular Nerve Injury

The suprascapular nerve originates from the spinal roots of C5 and C6. It branches from the upper trunk of the brachial plexus at Erb's point, running laterally to cross the posterior triangle of the neck. The nerve then passes deep to the omohyoid muscle and trapezial muscle on its way to the suprascapular notch. It passes beneath a thick transverse scapular ligament and enters the supraspinatus fossa, giving off motor branches to the supraspinatus muscle before passing lateral to the scapular spine to enter the infraspinatus fossa, where it provides motor branches to the infraspinatus muscle.

Suprascapular nerve injury is a well-described clinical entity and may result from blunt trauma, anterior dislocation of the shoulder, and fractures at the suprascapular notch.[9,181,182] Excessive traction and injury to the nerve can occur with a fall onto the point of the shoulder or during overhead sports.[58] Iatrogenic causes of suprascapular nerve injury include direct damage with mobilization of rotator cuff muscles or direct injury during decompression procedures. Ganglion cysts are a well-described cause of compression injury to the suprascapular nerve.

The patient with a suprascapular nerve compression may present with poorly localized pain at the superior posterior aspect of the shoulder and/or weakness of external rotation and abduction as a result of supraspinatus and/or infraspinatus compromise. The supraspinatus and/or infraspinatus may be visibly atrophied. Electromyography is an important diagnostic test to rule out the presence of suprascapular nerve pathology. Magnetic resonance imaging can be helpful in looking for evidence of ganglion cyst compression and can also show denervation signal changes in the muscle belly of the supraspinatus and/or infraspinatus muscles. The combined information from the EMG and MRI tests is used to determine the location of the suprascapular nerve compression. This may occur at the suprascapular notch beneath the transverse scapular ligament or more distally as the nerve passes the spinoglenoid notch on its way into the infraspinatus fossa. In considering the diagnosis of the suprascapular nerve injury or entrapment, it is important to rule out the presence of rotator cuff pathology. In that regard, MRI studies are very helpful.

Once the diagnosis of suprascapular nerve injury or entrapment has been confirmed, conservative measures of treatment are initiated. These include rest from stressful physical or athletic activities, analgesics, electrical stimulation, and occasional steroid injections. Traction injuries to the suprascapular nerve due to blunt trauma usually have a favorable prognosis. When the site of injury is located to the suprascapular or spinoglenoid notch by EMG testing or when compression from a ganglion cyst is noted on MRI, conservative measures are often less successful. If no clinical improvement or recovery is noted based on follow-up EMG studies within the first several months, surgical exploration and decompression of the suprascapular nerve are indicated. This involves excision of the transverse scapular ligament with decompression at the suprascapular notch, ganglion cyst removal, or decompression at the spinoglenoid notch.

Injury to the Long Thoracic Nerve

The long thoracic nerve is formed from the spinal roots of C5, C6, and C7. The nerve passes through the scalene muscles, beneath the brachial plexus and clavicle, and dorsal to the axillary vessels. It continues down along the anterolateral aspect of the chest wall, supplying the serratus anterior muscle. The long thoracic nerve is a pure motor nerve, its only function being innervation of the serratus anterior muscle. An injury to this can occur with blunt or sharp trauma as well as with traction on the neck or shoulder.[93] It may also occur as a result of repetitive stretching as is relatively common in competitive swimmers.

The clinical presentation of an injury to the long thoracic nerve consists of a painful aching or burning sensation around the shoulder and winging of the scapula. The patient may have scapular pain and weakness in forward flexion and be unable to raise the arm above the horizontal level. Scapular winging is tested by having the patient flex the shoulders to 90° and extending the elbows while rotating the shoulders internally and pushing against a wall with both hands. Other causes of winging of the scapula, such as trapezius paralysis from a spinal accessory nerve injury or diffuse shoulder girdle weakness, must be ruled out.[21] Once again, an EMG study is paramount in making the diagnosis.

Initial treatment should be conservative, as, more often than not, function of the serratus anterior muscle will return. It may be helpful to fit the patient with a modified thoracolumbar brace with a scapular pad that prevents scapular winging and the recurrent traction of the long thoracic nerve, which may continue and worsen as a result of continued winging. Johnson and Kendall, in a review of 111 cases, reported an overall good response to conservative treatment.[84] However, if the patient's symptoms and paralysis persist and become chronic and disabling, surgery may be indicated. Muscle transfer procedures to substitute for the serratus anterior have been used with success. The most common and successful procedure is transfer of the sternal head of the pectoralis major, using a fascial interposition graft placed through a hole at the inferior angle of the scapula.

Trapezial Paralysis

The trapezial muscle is innervated by the spinal accessory nerve (cranial nerve XI). During its course to innervate the trapezial muscle, the spinal accessory nerve passes superficial to the floor of the posterior cervical triangle. It lies in subcutaneous tissue and is very susceptible to sharp or blunt trauma. Injury to the nerve may occur from a penetrating wound such as a stab or gunshot wound or from blunt motor vehicular trauma.[179] The nerve may also be injured inadvertently during a surgical procedure such as a cervical lymph node biopsy.

Injury to the spinal accessory nerve results in trapezial paralysis. The patient presents with drooping of the shoulder, asymmetry of the neck line, winging of the scapula, and weakness in forward elevation and abduction.[21] Loss of trapezial function interferes with the intricate balance of muscle forces about the scapula, resulting in loss of scapulohumeral rhythm. Pain develops because of muscle spasm and radiculitis caused by traction on the brachial plexus. Electromyographic studies are essential to confirm the diagnosis and will demonstrate denervation of the sternocleidomastoid and the trapezial muscles.

Initial treatment for the disorder includes physical therapy in an attempt to strengthen the levator scapula and rhomboid muscles, so as to help compensate for loss of the trapezius. However, active patients often do poorly with conservative treatment, as the adjacent scapular muscles are unable to substitute fully for the function of the trapezius muscle. Bigliani et al have reported very favorable results using a dynamic transfer of the levator scapulae and rhomboid muscles to substitute for the paralyzed trapezial muscle.[21] Long term follow-up of their patients has demonstrated maintenance of good results with this procedure.[52]

Brachial Plexus Injury

Brachial plexus injuries are common and related to excessive traction on the upper extremity, GH dislocations, and blunt trauma such as may occur with a violent sports injury or as a result of motor vehicle accident. Burners or stingers are a common symptom of brachial plexus injury in football players. The mechanism of injury involves compression of the fixed brachial plexus between the shoulder pad and the superior medial scapula when the pad is compressed into the area of Erb's point, located just superior to the clavicle. Fortunately, these burners or stingers are usually transient, lasting for a matter of seconds.

More serious injuries occur with motor vehicle trauma, especially that resulting from a motorcycle accident. Traction injuries may recover over time. However, more severe injuries such as root avulsions are associated with a poor prognosis. Initial treatment consists of observation for a period of months to determine whether any neurologic return will occur. In the absence of neurologic return, treatment is directed toward substitution of working muscles for nonworking muscles.

Thoracic Outlet Syndrome

Thoracic outlet syndrome is caused by compression of the neurovascular structures that course from the neck to the axilla through the thoracic outlet. Numerous etiologies have been recognized. Cervical ribs may be the most commonly noted bony abnormality. However, less than 10 percent of individuals with a cervical rib will have symptoms consistent with thoracic outlet compression.[34] Following a clavicular fracture, excessive callus formation, malunion, or hypertrophic nonunion may result in thoracic outlet compression due to a decrease in size of the costoclavicular space.

The clinical presentation of thoracic outlet syndrome is dependent upon which neurovascular structures are predominantly involved. There may be venous engorgement, paresthesias down the involved arm, cold intolerance, or a feeling of fatigue secondary to weight of the arm. In athletes, the symptoms are generally associated with a specific motion such as overhead throwing. The Adson-Wright test may be helpful in making the diagnosis.[87]

Initial treatment of thoracic outlet syndrome is conservative, with activity modification, nonsteroidal anti-inflammatory medications, muscle strengthening, and postural training. Surgery is indicated only if rehabilitation fails. Surgical intervention depends on the specific etiology and can include excision of the cervical rib, removal of fibrous bands between the scalene muscles, and surgical treatment of a nonunited or malunited clavicular fracture.[87]

Axillary Artery Occlusion

The axillary artery is a continuation of the subclavian artery where it crosses the outer border of the first rib and is divided into three segments, as previously described.[178] The axillary artery may become transiently occluded due to pressure from the pectoralis minor muscle. This is more apt to occur when the arm is abducted, externally rotated, and extended. Overhead throwing athletes are susceptible to this disorder.[165]

Patients with occlusion of the axillary artery beneath the pectoralis minor present with pain, tenderness to palpation over the pectoralis minor, claudication, fatigue, diminished pulses, and pallor. These symptoms are often aggravated by hyperabduction and external rotation. The diagnosis is dependent upon angiography which will demonstrate the area of thrombosis. Vascular surgery is usually indicated.

Axillary Vein Effort Thrombosis

The axillary vein is a continuation of the basilic vein, beginning at the lower boundary of the teres major muscle. It becomes the subclavian vein at the lateral edge of the first rib. The vein can be compressed at various sites along its track, with the most common area being the costoclavicular space. Compression in the costoclavicular space is aggravated when the patient hyperextends the cervical spine and concurrently hyperabducts the arm. The term *effort thrombosis* refers to the frequent association of axillary vein compression and repetitive vigorous activities. Although, it is a rare disease, the clinician should recognize that overhead throwing athletes are at risk.[2] The symptoms usually occur within 24 to 48 h of the precipitating activity. The patient often complains of a dull, aching pain and a feeling of numbness and heaviness in the upper arm and shoulder. The entire upper extremity may become swollen, cool, and cyanotic. The pulses are initially normal but may diminish with excessive engorgement of the upper extremity.

Treatment initially consists of rest and observation. Heparin followed by warfarin is often indicated during the acute phase of the disorder to inhibit progression of the thrombus. Streptokinase may be used to lyse the clot. Decompression of the costoclavicular space may be necessary. This may include a resection of the first rib.

MUSCLE RUPTURES

Rupture of the Pectoralis Major Muscle

Pectoralis major muscle rupture is infrequent but not rare. It is often unrecognized and most commonly diagnosed after it has become a chronic condition. Acute rupture occurs as a result of mechanical failure of the pectoralis major muscle, either at the musculotendinous junction or at the tendinous insertion into the humerus. The most typical mechanism of injury is weight lifting.

The acute injury presents with swelling, tenderness, and ecchymosis. The diagnosis is difficult to make since, in many cases, there is no apparent asymmetry or palpable defect. Resisted adduction and internal rotation of the arm are generally weak and accompanied by pain. An MRI scan can be helpful in determining where the rupture has occurred. This is important in planning treatment, since ruptures of the muscle belly or musculotendinous junction cannot be repaired surgically.

Partial ruptures, muscle belly ruptures, and musculotendinous junction ruptures are treated conservatively with icing, rest, and therapy. Resistant exercises should be delayed for 6 weeks. Near complete or complete ruptures of the pectoralis major tendon are best treated with surgical repair.[177] The tendon is repaired directly to bone via transosseous sutures or suture anchors. Since there is very little retraction of the muscle, chronic ruptures have been repaired with success as much as 5 years after the injury.

Ruptures of the Deltoid Muscle

Complete traumatic disruption of the deltoid is an extremely rare event. Most injuries to the deltoid muscle are strains and partial injuries that occur as a result of trauma. These injuries usually respond to ice, rest, and therapy. Complete ruptures of the deltoid are more frequently associated with inadequate repair after rotator cuff surgery. When the lesion is caught early, repair can be very successful. However, when the disruption is more than 3 weeks old, reconstruction can be difficult. In these instances, a deltoplasty consisting of mobilization of the middle third of the deltoid anteriorly may provide improved function. However, the best treatment for this disorder is prevention.

REFERENCES

1. Adams F: *The Genuine Works of Hippocrates.* New York, William Wood, vols 1 and 2, 1886.
2. Adams JT, DeWeese JA: Effort thrombosis of the axillary and sublcavian veins. *J Trauma* 11:923–930, 1971.
3. Altchek DW, Skyhar MJ, Warren RF: Shoulder arthroscopy for shoulder instability. *Instr Course Lect* 38:187–198, 1989.
4. Andrews JR, Carson WG Jr, McLeod WD: Glenoid labrum tears related to the long head of the biceps. *Am J Sports Med* 13:337–341, 1985.
5. Ark JW, Flock TJ, Flatow EL, Bigliani LU: Arthroscopic treatment of calcific tendinitis of the shoulder. *Arthroscopy* 8:183–188, 1992.
6. Armengol J, Brittis D, Pollock RG, et al: The association of an unfused acromial epiphysis with tears of the rototar cuff: A review of 41 cases. *J Shoulder Elbow Surg* 3:S14, 1994.
7. Baker CL, Liu SH: Comparison of open and arthroscopically assisted rotator cuff repairs. *Am J Sports Med* 23:99–104, 1995.
8. Bankart AS: The pathology and treatment of recurrent or habitual dislocation of the shoulder joint. *Br J Surg* 26:23–29, 1938.
9. Bateman JE: Nerve injuries about the shoulder in sports. *J Bone Joint Surg* 49A:785–792, 1967.
10. Bigliani LU: Anterior and posterior capsular shift for multidirectional instability. *Tech Orthop* 3(4):36–45, 1989.
11. Bigliani LU: Recurrent anterior instability: Open surgical repair, in Bigliani LU (ed): *The Unstable Shoulder.* Rosemont, IL, American Academy of Orthopaedic Surgeons, 1995, pp 59–67.
12. Bigliani LU, Cordasco FA, McIlveen SJ, Musso ES: Operative treatment of massive rotator cuff tears: Long-term results. *J Shoulder Elbow Surg* 1:120–130, 1992.
13. Bigliani LU, Cordasco FA, McIlveen SJ, Musso ES: Operative treatment of failed repairs of the rotator cuff. *J Bone Joint Surg* 74A:1505–1515, 1992
14. Bigliani LU, Fischer RA, Flatow EL, et al: Pathogenesis, in Iannotti JP: *Rotator Cuff Disorders.* Park Ridge, IL, American Academy of Orthopaedic Surgeons, 1991, pp 1–11.
15. Bigliani LU, Flatow EL, Codd TP: History, physical examination, and diagnostic modalities, in McGinty JB: *Operative Arthroscopy.* Philadelphia, Lippincott Raven, 1996, pp 635–646.
16. Bigliani LU, Flatow EL, Deliz ED: Complications of shoulder arthroscopy. *Orthop Rev* 20:743–751, 1991.

17. Bigliani LU, Kimmel J, McCann PD, Wolfe I: Repair of rotator cuff tears in tennis players. *Am J Sports Med* 20:112–117, 1992.

18. Bigliani LU, Kurzweil PR, Schwartzbach CC, et al: Inferior capsular shift procedure for anterior inferior shoulder instability in athletes. *Am J Sports Med* 22:578–584, 1994.

19. Bigliani LU, Morrison DS, April EW: The morphology of the acromion and its relationship to rotator cuff tears. *Orthop Trans* 10:228, 1986.

20. Bigliani LU, Nicholson GP, Flatow EL: Arthroscopic resection of the distal clavicle. *Orthop Clin North Am* 24:133–141, 1993.

21. Bigliani LU, Perez-Sanz JR, Wolfe IN: Treatment of trapezius paralysis. *J Bone Joint Surg* 67A:871–877, 1985.

22. Bigliani LU, Pollock RG, Soslowsky LJ, et al: Tensile properties of the inferior glenohumeral ligament. *J Orthop Res* 10:187–197, 1992.

23. Bigliani LU, Rodosky MW: Techniques of repair of large rotator cuff tears. *Tech Orthop* 9(2):133–140, 1994.

24. Bigliani LU, Ticker JB, Flatow EL, et al: The relationship of acromial architecture to rotator cuff disease. *Clin Sports Med* 10:823–838, 1991.

25. Bigliani LU, Weinstein DM, Rodosky MW, et al: Surgical treatment of loose glenoid components after total shoulder replacement. *J Shoulder Elbow Surg* 3(1, part 2):S75, 1994.

26. Black AC, Codd TD, Rodosky MW, et al: Surgical management of rotator cuff disease. Presented at the American Academy of Orthopaedic Surgeons 62nd Annual Meeting, February 16–21, 1995, Orlando, FL.

27. Bloom MH, Obata WG: Diagnosis of posterior dislocation of the shoulder with use of Velpeau axillary and angle-up roentgenographic views. *J Bone Joint Surg* 49A:943–949, 1967.

28. Bonutti PM, Hawkins RJ: Fracture of the humeral shaft associated with total replacement arthroplasty of the shoulder: A case report. *J Bone Joint Surg* 74A:617–618, 1992.

29. Bosworth BM: Calcium deposits in the shoulder and subacromial bursitis: A survey of 12,122 shoulders. *JAMA* 116:2477–2482, 1941.

30. Boyd HB, Sisk TD: Recurrent posterior dislocation of the shoulder. *J Bone Joint Surg* 54A:779–786, 1972.

31. Boyd AD, Thornhill TS, Barnes CL: Fractures adjacent to humeral prosthesis. *J Bone Joint Surg* 74A:1498–1504, 1992.

32. Bridgman JF: Peri-arthritis of the shoulder and diabetes mellitus. *Ann Rheum Dis* 31:69–71, 1972.

33. Brown AR, Weiss R, Greenberg C, et al: Interscalene block for shoulder arthroscopy: Comparison with general anesthesia. *Arthroscopy* 9:295–300, 1993.

34. Brown C: Compressed invasive referred pain to the shoulder. *Clin Orthop* 173:55–62, 1983.

35. Burkhart SS: Arthroscopic debridement and decompression for selected rotator cuff tears: Clinical results, pathomechanics, and patient selection based on biomechanical parameters. *Orthop Clin North Am* 24:111–123, 1993.

36. Burkhead WZ Jr: The biceps tendon, in Rockwood CA Jr, Matsen FA III (eds): *The Shoulder*. Philadelphia, Saunders, 1990, pp 791–836.

37. Burkhead WZ Jr, Scheinberg RR, Box G: Surgical anatomy of the axillary nerve. *J Shoulder Elbow Surg* 1:31–36, 1992.

38. Cahill BR: Osteolysis of the distal part of the clavicle in male athletes. *J Bone Joint Surg* 64A:1053–1058, 1982.

39. Cahill BR, Palmer RE: Quadrilateral space syndrome. *J Hand Surg* 8:65–69, 1983.

40. Cain PR, Mutschler TA, Fu FH, et al: Anterior stability of the glenohumeral joint: A dynamic model. *Am J Sports Med* 15:144–148, 1987.

41. Codd TD, Duralde XA, Brown AR, et al: Treatment of resistant and frozen shoulder with indwelling interscalene catheter. 107th Annual Meeting of the American Orthopaedic Association, Sun Valley, ID, June 5–8, 1994.

42. Codd TP, Pollock RG, Flatow EL: Prosthetic replacement in the rotator cuff-deficient shoulder. *Tech Orthop* 1994; 8:174–183, 1994.

43. Codd TP, Yamaguchi K, Flatow EL: Infected shoulder arthroplasties: Treatment with staged reimplantation versus resection arthroplasty. Presented at the American Shoulder & Elbow Surgeons 11th Annual Open Meeting, Orlando, FL, February 1995.

44. Codman EA: Complete rupture of the supraspinatus tendon: Operative treatment with report of two successful cases. *Boston Med Surg J* 164:708–710, 1911.

45. Codman EA: *The Shoulder, Rupture of the Supraspinatus Tendon and Other Lesions in or about the Subacromial Bursa*. Boston, Thomas Todd, 1934.

46. Cofield RH: Subscapular muscle transposition for repair of chronic rotator cuff tears. *Surg Gynecol Obstet* 154:667–672, 1982.

47. Cofield FH: Current concepts review: Rotator cuff disease of the shoulder. *J Bone Joint Surg* 67A:974–979, 1985.

48. Cofield RH: Shoulder arthrodesis and resection arthroplasty. *Instr Course Lect* 34:268–277, 1985.

49. Cofield RH: Uncemented total shoulder arthroplasty: A review. *Clin Orthop* 307:86–93, 1994.

50. Cofield RH, Daly PJ: Total shoulder arthroplasty with a tissue-ingrowth glenoid component. *J Shoulder Elbow Surg* 1:77–85, 1992.

51. Cofield RH, Edgerton BC: Total shoulder arthroplasty: Complications and revision surgery. *Instr Course Lect* 39:449–462, 1990.

52. Compito CA, Duralde XA, Wolfe IN, Bigliani LU: Levator scapulae and rhomboid transfer for trapezius paralysis. *J Shoulder Elbow Surg* 4:S8, 1995.

53. Cooper DE, O'Brien SJ, Warren RF: Supporting layers of the glenohumeral joint: An anatomic study. *Clin Orthop* 289:144–155, 1993.

54. Cordasco FA, Steinman SP, Flatow EL, et al: Arthroscopic treatment of glenoid labral tears. *Am J Sports Med* 21:425–431, 1993.

55. Craig EV: The posterior mechanism of acute anterior shoulder dislocations. *Clin Orthop* 190:212–216, 1984.

56. DePalma AF: *Degenerative Changes of the Sternoclavicular and Acromioclavicular Joints in Various Decades*. Springfield, IL, Charles C Thomas, 1957.

57. Ellman H, Kay SP: Arthoscopic subacromial decompression for chronic impingement: Two- to five-year results. *J Bone Joint Surg* 73B:395–398, 1991.

58. Ferretti A, Cerullo G, Russo G: Suprascapular neuropathy in volleyball players. *J Bone Joint Surg* 69A:260–263, 1987.

59. Flatow EL: The biomechanics of the acromioclavicular, sternoclavicular, and scapulothoracic joints. *Instr Course Lect* 42:237–245, 1993.

60. Flatow EL, Bigliani LU: Arthroscopic acromioclavicular joint debridement and distal clavicle resection. *Op Tech Orthop* 1:240–247, 1991.

61. Flatow EL, Bigliani LU: Locating and protecting the axillary nerve in shoulder surgery: The tug test. *Orthop Rev* 21:503–505, 1992.

62. Flatow EL, Bigliani LU: Complications of rotator cuff repair. *Comp Orthop* 8:298–303, 1992.

63. Flatow EL, Bigliani LU, April EW: An anatomic study of the musculocutaneous nerve and its relationship to the coracoid process. *Clin Orthop* 244:166–171, 1989.

64. Flatow EL, Cordasco FA, McClusky GM, Bigliani LU: Arthroscopic resection of the outer end of the clavicle from a superior approach: A critical, quantitative, radiographic assessment of bone removal. *Arthroscopy* 8:55–64, 1992.

65. Flatow EL, Soslowsky LJ, Ticker JB, et al: Excursion of the rotator cuff under the acromion: Patterns of subacromial contact. *Am J Sports Med* 22:779–788, 1994.

66. Flatow EL, Weinstein DM, Duralde XA, et al: Coracoacromial ligament preservation in rotator cuff surgery. *J Shoulder Elbow Surg* 3:S73, 1994.

67. Fromison AI, Oh I: Keyhole tenodesis of biceps origin at the shoulder. *Clin Orthop* 112:245–249, 1974.

68. Fukuda K, Craig EV, An K, et al: Biomechanical study of the ligamentous system of the acromioclavicular joint. *J Bone Joint Surg* 68A:434–439, 1986.

69. Fukuda H, Hamada K, Nakajima T, Tomonaga A: Pathology and pathogenesis of the intratendinous tearing of the rotator cuff viewed from en bloc histologic sections. *Clin Orthop* 307:60–67, 1994.

70. Gallie WE, LeMesurier AB: Recurring dislocation of the shoulder. *J Bone Joint Surg* 30B:9–18, 1948.

71. Garth WP Jr, Slappey CE, Ochs CW: Roentgenographic demonstration of instability of the shoulder: The apical oblique projection—A technical note. *J Bone Joint Surg* 66A:1450–1453, 1984.

72. Gartsman GM: Arthroscopic acromioplasty for lesions of the rotator cuff. *J Bone Joint Surg* 72A:169–180, 1990.

73. Gerber C, Krushell RJ: Isolated rupture of the tendon of the subscapularis muscle: Clinical features in 16 cases. *J Bone Joint Surg* 73B:389–394, 1991.

74. Gurd FB: The treatment of complete dislocation of the outer end of the clavicle: A hitherto undescribed operation. *Ann Surg* 63:1094, 1941.

75. Hall RH, Isaac F, Booth CR: Dislocations of the shoulder with special reference to accompanying small fractures. *J Bone Joint Surg* 41A:489–494, 1959.

76. Harmon HP: Methods and results in the treatment of 2580 painful shoulders with special reference to calcific tendonitis in the frozen shoulder. *Am J Surg* 95:527–544, 1958.

77. Hawkins RJ, Bokor DJ: Clinical evaluation of shoulder problems, in Rockwood CA Jr, Matsen FA III (eds): *The Shoulder.* Philadelphia, Saunders, 1990.

78. Hawkins RJ, Neer CS: Functional analysis of shoulder fusions. *Clin Orthop* 223:65, 1987.

79. Helfet AJ: Coracoid transplantation for recurring dislocation of the shoulder. *J Bone Joint Surg* 40B:198–202, 1958.

80. Hill HA, Sachs MD: The grooved defect of the humeral head: A frequently unrecognized complication of dislocations of the shoulder joint. *Radiology* 35:690–700, 1940.

81. Hovelius L: Incidence of shoulder dislocation in Sweden. *Clin Orthop* 166:127–131, 1982.

82. Howell SM, Galinat BJ: The glenoid-labral socket: A constrained articular surface. *Clin Orthop* 243:122–125, 1989.

83. Jobe CM, Anatomy of the shoulder, in Bigliani LU (ed): *Complications of Shoulder Surgery.* Baltimore, Williams & Wilkins, 1993, pp 1–23.

84. Johnson JTH, Kendall HO: Isolated paralysis of the serratus anterior muscle. *J Bone Joint Surg* 37A:567–574, 1955.

85. Kelly IG: Surgery of the rheumatoid shoulder. *Ann Rheum Dis* 49:824–829, 1990.

86. Kelly IG: Unconstrained shoulder arthroplasty in rheumatoid arthritis. *Clin Orthop* 307:94–102, 1994.

87. Leffert RD: Thoracic outlet syndrome. *J AAOS* 2:317–325, 1994.

88. Lequesne M, Dang N, Bensasson M, et al: Increased association of diabetes mellitus with capsulitis of the shoulder and shoulder-hand syndrome. *Scand J Rheumatol* 6:53–56, 1977.

89. Lyons FA, Rockwood CA Jr: Current concepts review: Migration of pins used in operations on the shoulder. *J Bone Joint Surg* 72A:1262–1267, 1990.

90. MacDonald PB, Hawkins RJ, Fowler PJ, Miniaci A: Release of the subscapularis for internal rotation contracture and pain after anterior repair for recurrent anterior dislocation of the shoulder. *J Bone Joint Surg* 74A:734–737, 1992.

91. Magnuson PB, Stack JK: Recurrent dislocation of the shoulder. *JAMA* 123:889–892, 1943.

92. McCann PD, Bindelglass DF: The brachial plexus: Clinical anatomy. *Orthop Rev* 20:413–419, 1991.

93. McIlveen SJ, Duralde XA: Isolated nerve injuries about the shoulder, in Bigliani LU (ed): *Complications of Shoulder Surgery.* Baltimore, Williams & Wilkins, 1993, pp 214–239.

94. McLaughlin HL: Posterior dislocation of the shoulder. *J Bone Joint Surg* 34A:584–590, 1952.

95. McLaughlin HL: The selection of calcium deposits for operation: The technique and result of operation. *Surg Clin North Am* 43:1501–1504, 1963.

96. Miller SR, Bigliani LU: Complications of total shoulder replacement, in Bigliani LU (ed): *Complications of Shoulder Surgery.* Baltimore, Williams & Wilkins, 1993, pp 59–72.

97. Moeckel BH, Atlchek DW, Warren RF, et al: Instability of the shoulder after arthroplasty. *J Bone Joint Surg* 75A:492–497, 1993.

98. Montgomery TJ, Yerger B, Savoie FH: Management of rotator cuff tears: A comparison of arthroscopic debridement and surgical repair. *J Shoulder Elbow Surg* 3:70–78, 1994.

99. Moore KL: *The Developing Human.* Philadelphia, Saunders, 1982.

100. Mumford EB: Acromioclavicular dislocation: A new operative treatment. *J Bone Joint Surg* 23:799–801, 1941.

101. Murphy OB, Bellamy R, Wheeler W, Brower TD: Post-traumatic osteolysis of the distal clavicle. *Clin Orthop* 109:108–114, 1975.

102. Nakajima T, Rokuuma N, Hamada K, et al: Histological and biomechanical characteristics of the supraspinatus tendon: Reference to rotator cuff tearing. *J Shoulder Elbow Surg* 3:79–87, 1994.

103. Neer CS II: Articular replacement of the humeral head. *J Bone Joint Surg* 37A:215, 1955.

104. Neer CS II: Indications for replacement of the proximal humeral articulation. *Am J Surg* 89:901, 1955.

105. Neer CS II: Prosthetic replacement of the humeral head. *Surg Clin North Am* 43:1581, 1963.

106. Neer CS II: Articular replacement for the humeral head. *J Bone Joint Surg* 46A:1607, 1964.

107. Neer CS II: Anterior acromioplasty for the chronic impingement syndrome in the shoulder: A preliminary report. *J Bone Joint Surg* 54:41–50, 1972.

108. Neer CS II: Replacement arthroplasty for glenohumeral osteoarthritis. *J Bone Joint Surg* 56A:1–13, 1974.

109. Neer CS II: Impingement lesions. *Clin Orthop* 173:70–77, 1983

110. Neer CS II: Unconstrained shoulder arthroplasty. *Instr Course Lect* 34:278–286, 1985.

111. Neer CS II: *Shoulder Reconstruction.* Philadelphia, Saunders, 1990.

112. Neer CS II, Brown TH, McLaughlin HL: Fracture of the neck of the humerus with dislocation of the head fragment. *Am J Surg* 85:252, 1953.

113. Neer CS II, Craig EV, Fukuda H: Cuff tear arthropathy. *J Bone Joint Surg* 65A:1232–1244, 1983.

114. Neer CS II, Fithian TF, Hansen PE, et al: Reinforced cruciate repair for anterior dislocations of the shoulder. *Orthop Trans* 9:44, 1985.

115. Neer CS II, Flatow EL, Lech O: Tears of the rotator cuff: Long term results of anterior acromioplasty and repair. *Orthop Trans* 12:735, 1988.

116. Neer CS II, Foster CR: Inferior capsular shift procedure for involuntary inferior and multidirectional instability of the shoulder: A preliminary report. *J Bone Joint Surg* 62A:897–908, 1980.

117. Neer CS II, Marberry TA: On the disadvantages of radical acromionectomy. *J Bone Joint Surg* 63A:416–419, 1981.

118. Neer CS II, Morrison DS: Glenoid bone-grafting in total shoulder arthroplasty. *J Bone Joint Surg* 70A:1154–1162, 1988.

119. Neer CS II, Satterlee CC, Dalsey RM, Flatow EL: The anatomy and potential effects of contracture of the coracohumeral ligament. *Clin Orthop* 280:182–185, 1992.

120. Neer CS, Watson KC, Stanton FJ: Recent experience in total shoulder replacement. *J Bone Joint Surg* 64A:319–337, 1982.

121. Neviaser JS: Adhesive capsulitis of the shoulder. *J Bone Joint Surg* 27:211–222, 1945.

122. Nicholson GP, Goodman DA, Pollock RG, et al: The acromion: Morphology and age related changes: A study of 420 scapulae. *Orthop Trans* 17:976, 1993–1994.

123. Norris RS, Bigliani LU: Analysis of Failed Repair for Shoulder Instability—A Preliminary Report, In Bateman JE, Welsh RP (eds): *Surgery of the Shoulder*. Philadelphia, Decker, 1984.

124. Nuber GW, McCarthy WJ, Yao J, et al: Arterial abnormalities of the shoulder in athletes. *J Sports Med* 18:514–519, 1990.

125. O'Brien SJ, Arnoczky SP, Warren RF, et al: Developmental anatomy of the shoulder and anatomy of the glenohumeral joint, in Rockwood CA Jr, Matsen FA III (eds): *The Shoulder*. Vol 1. Philadelphia, Saunders, 1990, pp 1–33.

126. O'Brien SJ, Neves MC, Arnoczky SP, et al: The anatomy and histology of the inferior glenohumeral ligament complex of the shoulder. *Am J Sports Med* 18:449–456, 1990.

127. Osmond-Clarke H: Habitual dislocation of the shoulder: The Putti-Platt operation. *J Bone Joint Surg* 30B:19–25, 1948.

128. Paletta GA Jr, Warner JJP, Altchek DW, et al: Arthroscopic-assisted rotator cuff repair: Evaluation of results and a comparison of techniques. *Orthop Trans* 17:139, 1993.

129. Paulos LE, Franklin JL: Arthroscopic shoulder decompression development and application: A five year experience. *Am J Sports Med* 18:235–244, 1990.

130. Paulos LE, Kody MH: Arthroscopically enhanced miniapproach to rotator cuff repair. *Am J Sports Med* 22:19–25, 1994.

131. Petersson CJ: Degeneration of the acromioclavicular joint: A morphological study. *Acta Orthop Scand* 54:434–438, 1983.

132. Pollock RG, Bigliani LU: Recurrent posterior shoulder instability: Diagnosis and treatment. *Clin Orthop* 291:85–96, 1993.

133. Pollock RG, Bigliani LU: Glenohumeral instability: Evaluation and treatment. *J AAOS* 1:24–32, 1993.

134. Pollock RG, Deliz ED, McIlveen SJ, et al: Prosthetic replacement in rotator cuff deficient shoulders. *J Shoulder Elbow Surg* 1:173–186, 1992.

135. Pollock RG, Duralde XA, Flatow EL, Bigliani LU: The use of arthroscopy in the treatment of resistant frozen shoulder. *Clin Orthop* 304:30–36, 1994.

136. Pollock RG, Flatow EL: Classification and evaluation, in Bigliani LU (ed): *The Unstable Shoulder*. Rosemont, IL, American Academy of Orthopaedic Surgeons, 1995, pp 25–36.

137. Pollock RG, Higgs GB, Codd TP, et al: Total shoulder replacement for the treatment of primary glenohumeral osteoarthritis. *J Shoulder Elbow Surg* 4:S12, 1995.

138. Post M, Silver R, Singh M: Rotator cuff tear: Diagnosis and treatment. *Clin Orthop* 173:78–92, 1983.

139. Randelli M, Gambrioli PL: Glenohumeral osteometry by computed tomography in normal and unstable shoulders. *Clin Orthop* 208:151–156, 1986.

140. Rathbun JB, Macnab I: The microvascular pattern of the rotator cuff. *J Bone Joint Surg* 52B:540–553, 1970.

141. Resch H, Golser K, Thoeni H, Sperner G: Arthroscopic repair of superior glenoid labral detachment (the SLAP lesion). *J Shoulder Elbow Surg* 2:147–155, 1993.

142. Rockwood CA, Szalay EA, Curtis RJ Jr: X-ray evaluation of shoulder problems, in Rockwood CA Jr, Matsen FA III (eds): *The Shoulder*, Vol 1. Philadelphia, Saunders, 1990, pp 178–207.

143. Rockwood CA, Williams GR, Burkhead WZ: Debridement of degenerative, irreparable lesions of the rotator cuff. *J Bone Joint Surg* 77A:857–866, 1995.

144. Rodosky MW, Bigliani LU: Surgical treatment of nonconstrained glenoid component failure. *Op Tech Orthop* 4:226–236, 1994.

145. Rodosky MW, Bigliani LU: Indications for glenoid resurfacing. *J Shoulder Elbow* 5:231–248, 1996.

146. Rodosky MW, Flatow EL: Arthroscopic debridement of the acromioclavicular joint and distal clavicle resection, in McGinty JB: *Operative Arthroscopy*. Philadelphia, Lippincott Raven, 1996, pp 773–783.

147. Rodosky MW, Harner CD, Fu FH: The role of the long head of the biceps muscle and superior glenoid labrum in anterior stability of the shoulder. *Am J Sports Med* 22:121–130, 1994.

148. Rodosky MW, Weinstein DM, Pollock RG, et al: On the rarity of glenoid failure. *J Shoulder Elbow Surg* 4:S13, 1995.

149. Rokous JR, Feagin JA, Abbott HG: Modified axillary roentgenogram. *Clin Orthop* 82:84–86, 1972.

150. Rubenstein DL, Jobe FW, Glousman RE: Anterior capsulolabral reconstruction of the shoulder in athletes. *J Shoulder Elbow Surg* 1:229–237, 1992.

151. Saha AK: *Theory of Shoulder Mechanism: Descriptive and Applied*. Springfield, IL, Charles C Thomas, 1961.

152. Salter EG, Nasca RJ, Shelley BS: Anatomical observations on the acromioclavicular joint and supporting ligaments. *Am J Sports Med* 15:199–206, 1987.

153. Scott DJ Jr: Treatment of recurrent posterior dislocations of the shoulder by glenoplasty: Report of three cases. *J Bone Joint Surg* 49A:471–476, 1967.

154. Simpson NS, Kelly IG: Extra-glenohumeral joint shoulder surgery in rheumatoid arthritis: The role of bursectomy, acromioplasty, and distal clavicle excision. *J Shoulder Elbow Surg* 3:66–69, 1994.

155. Smith JG: Pathological appearances of seven cases of injury of the shoulder joint with remarks. *London Med Gaz* 14:280, 1834.

156. Snyder SJ, Bachner EJ: Arthroscopic fixation of rotator cuff tears: A preliminary report. *Arthroscopy* 9:342, 1993.

157. Snyder SJ, Kanzel RP, Del Pizzo W, et al: SLAP lesions of the shoulder. *Arthroscopy* 6:274–279, 1990.

158. Soslowsky LJ, Flatow EL, Bigliani LU, Mow VC: Articular geometry of the glenohumeral joint. *Clin Orthop* 285:181–190, 1992.

159. Speer KP, Hannafin JA, Altcheck DW, et al: An evaluation of the shoulder relocation test. *Am J Sports Med* 22:177–183, 1994.

160. Sprengel RD: Die Angeborene Verschiebung des Schulterblattes Nach Oben. *Arch Klin Chir* 42:545, 1891.

161. Surin V, Blader S, Markhede G, et al: Rotational osteotomy of the humerus for posterior instability of the shoulder. *J Bone Joint Surg* 72A:181–186, 1990.

162. Ticker JB, Bigliani LU, Soslowsky LJ, et al: Viscoelastic and geometric properties of the inferior glenohumeral ligament. *Orthop Trans* 16:304–305, 1992.

163. Ticker JB, Flatow EL, Pawluk RJ, et al: The inferior glenohumeral ligament: A correlative biomechanical, and histological investigation. *Orthop Trans* 17:721–722, 1993.

164. Torchia ME, Cofield RH, Settergren CR: Total shoulder arthroplasty with the Neer prosthesis: Long-term results. *J Shoulder Elbow Surg* 4:S12, 1995.

165. Tullos HS, Erwin WD, Woods et al: Unusual lesions of the pitching arm. *Clin Orthop* 88:169–182, 1972.

166. Turkel SJ, Panio MW, Marshall JL, et al: Stabilizing mechanisms preventing anterior dislocation of the glenohumeral joint. *J Bone Joint Surg* 63A:1208–1217, 1981.

167. Uhthoff HK, Hammond DI, Sarkar K, et al: The role of the coracoacromial ligament in the impingement syndrome: A clinical, radiological and histological study. *Int Orthop* 12:97–104, 1988.

168. Uhthoff HK, Sarkar K: Calcifying tendonitis, in Rockwood CA Jr, Matsen FA III (eds): *The Shoulder.* Vol 2. Philadelphia, Saunders, 1990, pp 774–790.

169. Warner JJP: The gross anatomy of the joint surfaces, ligaments, labrum and capsule, in Matsen FA III, Fu FH, Hawkins RJ (eds): *The Shoulder: A Balance of Mobility and Stability.* Rosemont, IL, American Academy of Orthopaedic Surgeons, 1993, pp 7–27.

170. Warner JJP, Altchek DW, Warren RF: Arthoscopic management of rotator cuff tears with emphasis on the throwing athlete. *Op Tech Orthop* 1:235–239, 1991.

171. Warner JJP, Caborn DNM, Berger R, et al: Dynamic capsuloligamentous anatomy of the glenohumeral joint. *J Shoulder Elbow Surg* 2:115–133, 1993.

172. Warner JJP, Flatow EL: Anatomy and biomechanics, in Bigliani LU (ed): *The Unstable Shoulder.* Rosemont, IL, American Academy of Orthopaedic Surgeons, 1995, pp 1–24.

173. Warren RF: Lesions of the long head of the biceps tendon. *Instr Course Lect* 34:204–209, 1985.

174. Weber BG, Simpson LA, Hardegger F, et al: Rotational humeral osteotomy for recurrent anterior dislocation of the shoulder. *J Bone Joint Surg* 66A:1443–1450, 1984.

175. Weber SC, Schaefer R: "Mini-open" versus traditional open repair in the management of small and moderate size tears of the rotator cuff. *Arthroscopy* 9:365–366, 1993.

176. Weinstein DM, Bucchieri JS, Pollock RG, et al: Arthroscopic debridement of the shoulder for osteoarthritis. *Arthroscopy* 9:366, 1993.

177. Wolfe SW, Wickiewics TL, Cavanaugh JT: Ruptures of the pectoralis major muscle: An anatomic and clinical analysis. *Am J Sports Med* 20:587–593, 1992.

178. Wright IS: The neurovascular syndrome produced by hyperabduction of the arms. *Am Heart J* 29:1, 1945.

179. Wright TA: Accessory spinal nerve injury. *Clin Orthop* 108:15–18, 1975.

180. Yergason RM: Supination sign. *J Bone Joint Surg* 13:160, 1931.

181. Yoon TN, Grabois M: Suprascapular nerve injury following trauma to the shoulder. *J Trauma* 21:652–655, 1981.

182. Zoltan JD: Injury to the suprascapular nerve in association with anterior dislocation of the shoulder: Case report and review of the literature. *J Trauma* 19:203–206, 1979.

183. Zuckerman J, Matsen F: Complications about the glenohumeral joint related to the use of screws and staples. *J Bone Joint Surg* 66A:175, 1984.

The Elbow Joint

CHAPTER 56

The Elbow Joint

Roger Dee, Christian H. Dee, and Michael D. Ries

BIOMECHANICS OF THE ELBOW

The elbow functions to position the hand in the sagittal plane by flexion-extension and in the transverse plane by pronation-supination. Three articulations consisting of the humeroulnar, radioulnar, and radiocapitellar joints permit this motion. The elbow acts as a fulcrum, thus functioning as a load-bearing joint in actions such as lifting, overhead throwing, and pushing.

Kinematics

The elbow is a trochoginglymus joint, which permits flexion-extension and axial rotation or pronation-supination. The normal range of flexion-extension is from 0 to 146°.[1] Most activities of daily living may be accomplished with a functional arc of 100° from 30 to 130°.[2] Mall[3] found the axis of rotation for elbow flexion at the center of trochlea. This conclusion was supported in three-dimensional analyses done by Morrey and Chao[4] and by Youm et al.[5] using independent coordinate systems for the humerus and ulna on cadaver specimens. This evidence supports the concept that elbow flexion is represented as a uniaxial hinge. In contrast, Ewald[6] and Ishizuki[7] found a changing center of rotation with flexion. London[8] found that the axis of rotation passed through concentric arcs formed by the trochlear sulcus and capitellum. However, at the extremes of flexion and extension, the axis of rotation changed, so that joint motion became a rolling instead of a sliding movement. In addition, Morrey and Chao[4] found that slight internal axial rotation of the ulna occurred during early flexion and slight external axial rotation during terminal flexion. Dempster[9] noted humeral rotation relative to the ulna with joint flexion. Thus it appears that the elbow may not be represented by a uniaxial hinge throughout the flexion-extension range. The changing center of rotation and the sliding movement at the extremes of joint movement

may be related to the high incidence of loosening seen with constrained hinge-type elbow replacements.

The average normal range of pronation-supination is from 71° of pronation to 81° of supination. Most activities of daily living may be accomplished in 100° of forearm rotation from 50° of pronation to 50° of supination.[2]

The axis of forearm rotation is usually considered to pass through the capitellum and head of the radius extending to the distal ulna.[10,11] The rotation axis is oblique to the anatomic axis of the radius and ulna, so that pronation-supination outlines a cone. The head of the radius rotates within the annular ligament, and the distal radius rotates around the ulna in an arc (Fig. 56-1). Ray et al.[12] found slight motion of the distal ulna during pronation and supination about an axis passing through the index finger. The motion of the ulna was opposite to that of the radius in the lateral plane, so that the ulna was abducted during pronation and adducted during supination. Youm et al.[5] found slight distal ulnar motion to be a combination of flexion-extension and abduction-adduction. This motion was noted to be greatest when the axis of pronation-supination was more radial. However, proximal ulnar motion was found to be negligible. Kapandji[13] suggests that the distal ulna is displaced on a small arc consisting of a lateral component and an extension component, whereas the distal radius rotates on a larger arc (Fig. 56-2). The center of both arcs is the point through which the axis of pronation-supination passes.

The axis of the radial head is displaced laterally approximately 2 mm in pronation; this is due to the ovoid shape of the radial head. This lateral displacement permits room for the radial tuberosity to move medially in pronation[13] (Fig. 56-3).

The Carrying Angle

The carrying angle is the angle formed by the long axes of the humerus and the ulna. Potter[13a] first quantitated the carrying angle, reporting an angle of 6.83° in males and 12.65° in females. Others have noted similar differences in the carrying angle between males and females.[3,11,14–16]

The carrying angle changes as the elbow joint is flexed. Thompson[17] described the disappearance of the carrying angle during flexion, although the forearm did not cross the axis of the humerus. Dempster[9] found an oscillatory pattern of change. Amis et al.[18] described a decrease in carrying angle similar to a sinusoidal curve with flexion. Youm et al.[5] found a variation in pattern for different spec-

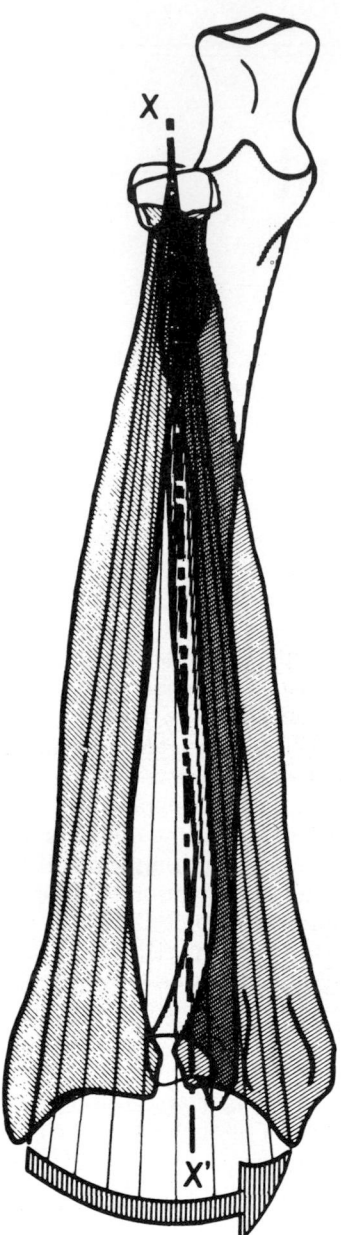

Figure 56-1 Arrow shows the arc formed by the distal radius about a line *X X'* through the heads of the radius and ulna during pronation-supination. (Reproduced with permission from Kapandji IA: *The Physiology of the Joints.* Vol 1. New York, Churchill Livingstone, 1982.)

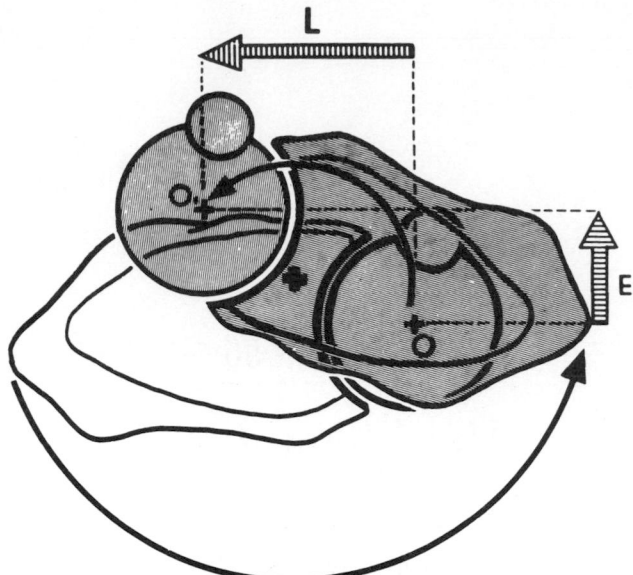

Figure 56-2 The right radius and ulna viewed from distal aspect. Ulna moves in the arc shown during supination but does not rotate on its own axis. Motion consists of a lateral component, L, and an extension component, E. The complementary motion of the radius is also shown, but this bone also rotates as shown in Fig. 56-1. Radius moves in a larger arc. Center of rotation for pronation-supination passes through the point (*cross*) around which both bones move. (Reproduced with permission from Kapandji IA: *The Physiology of the Joints.* Vol 1. New York, Churchill Livingstone, 1982.)

imens, with either a sinusoidal or linear change in carrying angle beyond 90°. Morrey and Chao[4] described a change in the carrying angle from valgus in extension to slight varus in extreme flexion. In contrast, London[8] found the carrying angle to be constant through the flexion range.

An et al.[19] defined the carrying angle in terms of three variables: the angle of joint flexion and the oblique angles of the humerus and ulna. If the carrying angle is defined as the angle between the long axis of the humerus and the projection of the long axis of the ulna on a plane containing the humerus, or if it is defined as the angle between the long axis of the ulna and the projection of the long axis of the humerus on a plane containing the ulna, the carrying angle changes minimally with joint flexion. If, however, the carrying angle is defined as the abduction-adduction angle of the ulna relative to the humerus using Eulerian angles to define the position of the humerus and ulna, the carrying angle decreases with joint flexion. Depending on the values of the oblique angles of the humerus and ulna, the carrying angle may change from valgus in extension to slight varus in flexion.[14]

Elbow Joint Forces

The magnitude and direction of forces acting at the elbow joint may be determined from free body force analysis (Fig. 56-4).

Since the flexor muscles act through a relatively short moment arm, a large muscle force is needed to hold a weight in the hand at a greater distance from the center of the elbow flexion. A large joint reaction force is created to a consequence of the large muscle force, which may predispose the joint to degenerative arthritis. The short moment arm of the muscle force is mechanically inefficient. However, only a short concentric muscle contraction is necessary to achieve a relatively large arc of motion at the hand.

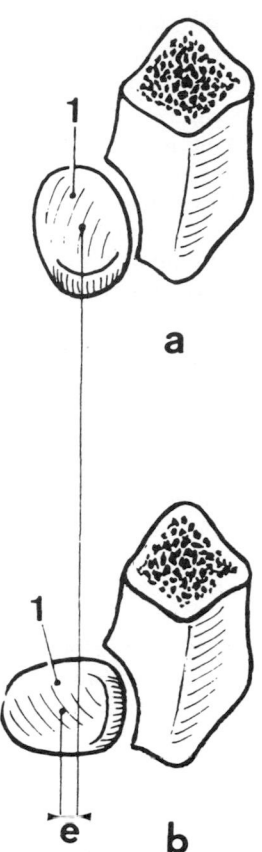

Figure 56-3 Radial head in contact with radial notch of ulna. Due to the ovoid shape of the radial head (1), the axis of the radial head is shifted laterally from **a,** the pronated position, to **b,** the supinated position, by the distance *e.* (Reproduced with permission from Kapandji IA: *The Physiology of the Joints.* Vol 1. New York, Churchill Livingstone, 1982.)

Rapid distal motion of the limb, made possible by short excursions of proximal muscles lying close to the axis of joint rotation, facilitates actions such as throwing.[20] However, because of the large joint reaction forces that occur during these activities, the elbow joint should not be considered as a "non-weight-bearing" joint.

Flexor muscles exert joint compression as well as flexion forces which may be separated by vector addition.[21] The magnitude of these forces will depend upon the angle of joint flexion as the length of the flexor moment arm changes with elbow flexion. Since the flexor moment arm is shortest at full extension, a large muscle force is necessary to cause a flexion component, and the joint compression load at this position is relatively large.[22]

Strenuous forearm adduction against resistance with the elbow flexed at 90° can generate substantial torque across the elbow. This torque is resisted by tension in the medial collateral ligament of up to 1.28 kilonewtons (kN) and a radiocapitellar compressive force of up to 1.84 kN.[22] After total elbow replacement, these torques are transmitted to the stem and cement mantle. Such forces have been considered an additional cause of loosening after total el-

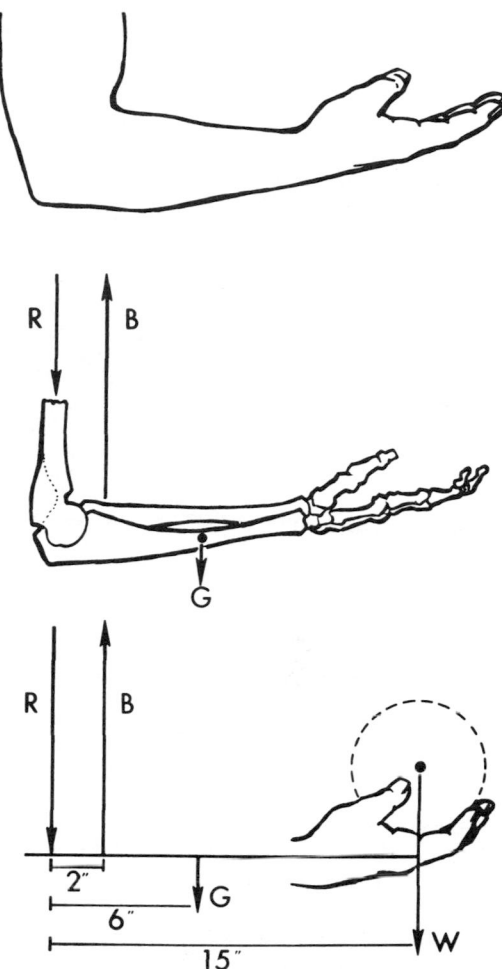

Figure 56-4 Two-dimensional free body force analysis: B = flexor muscle force, G = weight of forearm, W = weight at hand, and R = joint reaction force. Conditions of equilibrium are satisfied by the following equation for the sum of the moments about the center of the elbow joint: $(G \times 6 \text{ in}) + (W \times 15 \text{ in}) - (B \times 2 \text{ in}) = 0$. For a weight W of 20 lb and a forearm weight of 5 lb, $(5 \text{ lb} \times 6 \text{ in}) + (20 \text{ lb} \times 15 \text{ in}) - (B \times 2 \text{ in}) = 0$, or $B = 165$ lb; the sum of forces in the vertical direction must also equal zero. Thus: $R + 5 + 20 - 165 = 0$, or $R = 140$ lb. [Reproduced with permission from Williams A, Lissner B, in LeVeau B (ed): *Biomechanics of Human Movement.* Philadelphia, Saunders, 1977.]

bow replacement.[23,24] Current nonconstrained designs rely more on the ligaments to transmit this torque.

ELBOW JOINT STABILITY

Articular congruity as well as soft tissue constraints contribute to elbow joint stability. The medial aspect of the elbow is supported by the medial collateral ligament complex (MCL). This structure consists of three parts; a strong anterior oblique portion (AMCL), which has an average

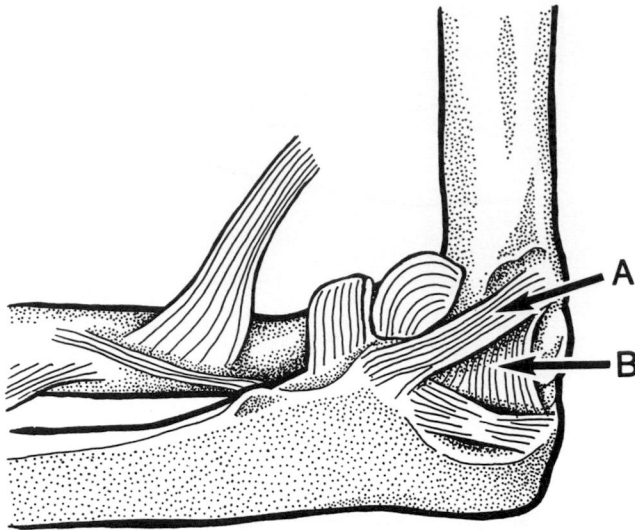

Figure 56-5 The medial collateral ligament showing (*A*) the anterior medial collateral ligament (AMCL) and (*B*) the posterior medial collateral ligament (PMCL). (Reproduced with permission from Sojbjerg JO, Wvesen J, Nielsen S: Experimental instability after transection of the medial collateral ligament. *Clin Orthop* 218:186–190, 1987.)

failure load of 260 N[25]; a weaker posterior oblique portion (PMCL); and a transverse intervening segment (Fig. 56-5).

The lateral ligament complex consists of three components in addition to the annular ligament. There is a fan-shaped radial collateral ligament (RCL), which originates from the lateral epicondyle and inserts into and blends with the annular ligament. Also separately identified is a continuation of the posterior fibers of the RCL, which insert onto the ulna at the crista supinatoris (Fig. 56-6). This structure is now termed the *lateral ulnar collateral ligament* (LUCL). Some additional fibers termed the *accessory collateral ligament* run from the crista to be inserted diffusely over the annular ligament.

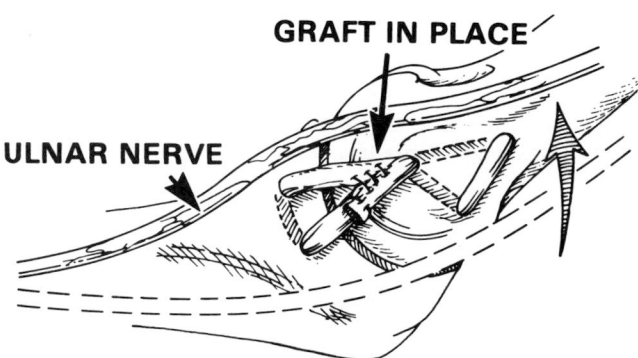

Figure 56-6 Medial ligament reconstruction using a figure-8 palmaris longus graft. Ulnar nerve is anteriorly transposed. (Reproduced with permission from Jobe FW, Stark H, Lombardo SJ: Reconstruction of the ulnar collateral ligament in athletes. *J Bone Joint Surg* 68A:1158–1164, 1986.)

The AMCL and RCL are taut through most of the entire arc of flexion.[25] The PMCL is taut only when the elbow is in a flexed position. The AMCL is the primary stabilizer to valgus stress in cadaver specimens. Stability is maintained when the PMCL is sectioned and the AMCL is left intact. The elbow becomes unstable when the AMCL is sectioned and the PMCL is left intact.[26–28]

Using segmental ligament cutting techniques on cadaver elbows, it was demonstrated that the AMCL is the primary valgus stabilizer, contributing 55 percent of the resistance to valgus stress at 90° of elbow flexion.[29] The remainder is provided by the shape of the articular surfaces and anterior capsule. In full extension, valgus stability is equally divided between the MCL, anterior capsule, and bony articulation. Using a more sophisticated experimental model with simulated active motion and muscle activity, Morrey and coworkers subsequently have shown that absence of the radial head does not significantly affect valgus stability in the presence of an intact MCL.[30] However, if the MCL is absent, the radial head is an important secondary stabilizer.

On the lateral side of the elbow, the RCL fibers maintain consistent patterns of tension in the anterior, middle, and posterior fibers no matter whether varus, valgus, or no force is applied to the elbow joint through the arc of flexion.[25] The lateral ligament contributes only 9 percent of the restraint to varus stress at 90° of flexion, while the capsule contributes 13 percent. The remainder of the joint stability is provided by bony articulation. In extension, the lateral ligament contributes 14 percent of this restraint, with 54 percent provided by joint articulation and 32 percent from the capsule.[29]

Clinical Application

Medial Ligament Deficiency and Valgus Overload

Disruption and chronic attenuation of the MCL are important clinical entities. Valgus stress encountered during overhead throwing activities is associated with rupture of the MCL.[31–35] Secondary valgus deformity occurs in 30 percent of professional baseball pitchers.[26] Throwers with injury to the MCL commonly present with medial pain and difficulty in throwing. The differential diagnosis includes posteromedial olecranon osteophytes, flexor pronator muscle mass injuries, ulnar nerve symptoms, and even stress fractures of the ulna. Valgus instability can be recognized clinically by flexing the elbow to 25° to unlock the olecranon and gently stressing the medial side of the joint.[35] The forearm should be pronated during the test to avoid false positives due to lateral side laxity. Pain during resisted volar wrist flexion and pronation, on the other hand, identifies the flexor muscle injury. However, computed tomography (CT) arthrography is 91 percent specific and MRI 100 percent specific for identification of these lesions.[36] The MCL is difficult to repair primarily and must often be reconstructed. A technique using palmaris longus graft is now most often utilized[35] (Fig. 56-6). Similar surgical technique is used for the chronically attenuated ligament.

In children, overuse conditions of the thrower's elbow can produce separation or fragmentation of the medial epicondyle ("Little League elbow"). Valgus stress views are useful in both children and adults. They are taken with the patient supine and the shoulder at 90° and fully externally rotated, so that the weight of the forearm opens up the medial joint line at the extended elbow. A large epicondylar fragment shown to move with the MCL should be reattached to the humerus.

The adolescent athlete is also at risk for the development of lesions on the lateral side of the elbow thought to be associated with repetitive valgus overload. A localized area of osteochondritis dissecans can occur in the capitellum in teenage athletes, with the development of a subchondral sclerotic infarct surrounded by an area of bone rarefaction. In Panner's disease, fragmentation of the entire ossific nucleus of the capitellum is seen. Initially, the articular cartilage mantle over the infarcts may be normal, but separation of the osteochondral fragments can occur in both conditions, with the development of loose bodies. Arthroscopy is a valuable tool in evaluating the lesion and defining the indications for removal of loose fragments. Restriction from continued throwing activities is essential.

Lateral Ligament Deficiency

Many of the operative procedures to correct chronic instability following dislocation of the elbow have succeeded by repair of lax lateral capsuloligamentous structures.[37,38] Instability after first-time elbow dislocation is unusual in adults,[39–42] even though a complete rupture of both the medial and lateral ligament complexes usually accompanies most if not all acute dislocations of the elbow.[43,44] Risk factors for recurrent dislocation include age of less than 15 years at the time of injury,[45] associated muscle damage,[46,47] or the presence of osseous or osteocartilaginous loose bodies within the joint. A high incidence (39 percent) of associated fractures has been observed in acute elbow dislocation in adults[48]; these include fractures of the capitellum, the coronoid process, and the radial head. Flattening of the capitellum has been observed in chronic elbow dislocation,[37,38] but this is probably adaptational. Protzman believes that a coronoid fracture is the only acute injury that has an effect on the potential stability of the reduction.[48] In some patients, additional factors may be worth consideration; Dryer and coworkers describe four patients with chronic elbow instability after closed traumatic posterior dislocation of the elbow, all of whom had avulsed the insertion of the brachialis and detached the elbow capsule from the coronoid process.[46] A similar lesion has been described by King.[47]

O'Driscoll and coworkers have drawn attention to a spectrum of elbow instabilities with injury of the lateral ligament occurring in the presence of an intact MCL.[49] After sequential section of the lateral ligament and anterior capsule, they have shown that a valgus external rotation force can dislocate the elbow posteriorly, the forearm rotation on the intact MCL. They believe that if valgus stability with forearm pronation is demonstrated after reduction, the AMCL is intact and immediate rehabilitation in a hinged cast brace with the elbow in full pronation can be commenced. The same group

has further defined chronic insufficiency of the lateral ligamentous complex, demonstrating that its ulnar portion in particular, if lax, can create a condition of recurrent posterolateral rotary instability without frank redislocation.[50] Associated with the incident of instability is the appearance of a prominence in the region of the radial head. Spontaneous redislocation is common with a snapping sensation. Some patients may have a complete recurrent dislocation that requires reduction. On other occasions the symptoms may only be those of a recurrent giving way of the arm. The diagnostic test (which is best performed under general anesthesia) is the elbow pivot shift test. With the patient lying supine and the examiner standing above the patient's head, the shoulder is fully externally rotated and the forearm fully supinated as valgus stress is applied. The test commences in a position of full extension while a valgus supination moment and an axial compression force are applied. This produces a rotary subluxation of the ulnohumeral joint, and the radial humeral joint dislocates posterolaterally. As the elbow flexion continues and reaches approximately 40°, the displacement increases to a maximum, but additional flexion will produce a sudden reduction of the joint with palpable and visible "snap." Patients with this condition respond well to operative repair (Fig. 56-7). If the ligament is of good quality, a little stretched, or merely avulsed from the lateral epicondyle, it can be imbricated or advanced back to its origin with a Bunnell suture. Otherwise, a tissue graft using tendon or fascia as a replacement must be used.[51] The same authors recommend that since this lesion occurs in young patients, most commonly secondary to elbow dislocation, patients less than 20 years old should not have their elbows stressed or mobilized too soon after reduction. They recommend that the elbow be immobilized for at least 3 or 4 weeks after a dislocation in patients who are less than 16 years old.[51]

LATERAL EPICONDYLITIS AND ASSOCIATED CONDITIONS

Tennis elbow is the most common elbow affliction of the adult population.[52] Of the many causes postulated to explain the pain and tenderness experienced in the region of lateral epicondyle by these patients, the most common are that it is a tendinitis arising in the region of the insertion of the extensor carpi radialis brevis muscle or, alternatively, that it is associated with entrapment of some branches of the radial nerve.[53,54] A less popular theory of some intraarticular derangement involving the annular ligament or a redundant synovial fold has been the basis for intraarticular operations, which are currently less favored. Some calcification is not uncommon in the region of the extensor carpi radialis brevis, and biopsy of the region will often show fibroangiomatous hyperplasia.[55] Analysis of errors in stroke production or racket grip may relieve the symptoms in tennis players. Although rest and nonsteroidal anti-inflammatory drugs (NSAIDs) may be useful, a local injection of steroid and anesthetic into the point of maximal tenderness is often required. The results are very gratifying, with a high cure rate. Of those few patients who fail conservative treatment, 90 percent will usually respond

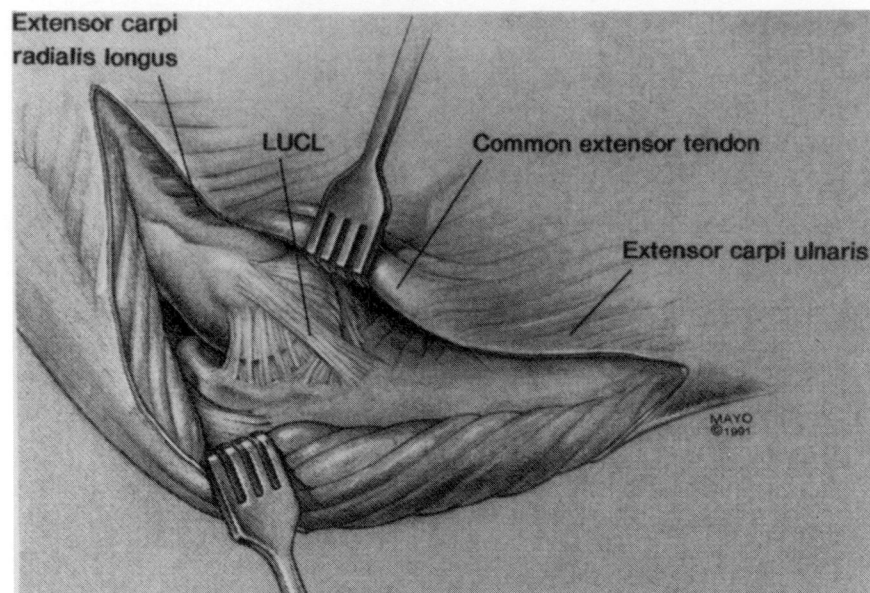

Extensor carpi
radialis longus

LUCL

Common extensor tendon

Extensor carpi ulnaris

MAYO
©1991

A

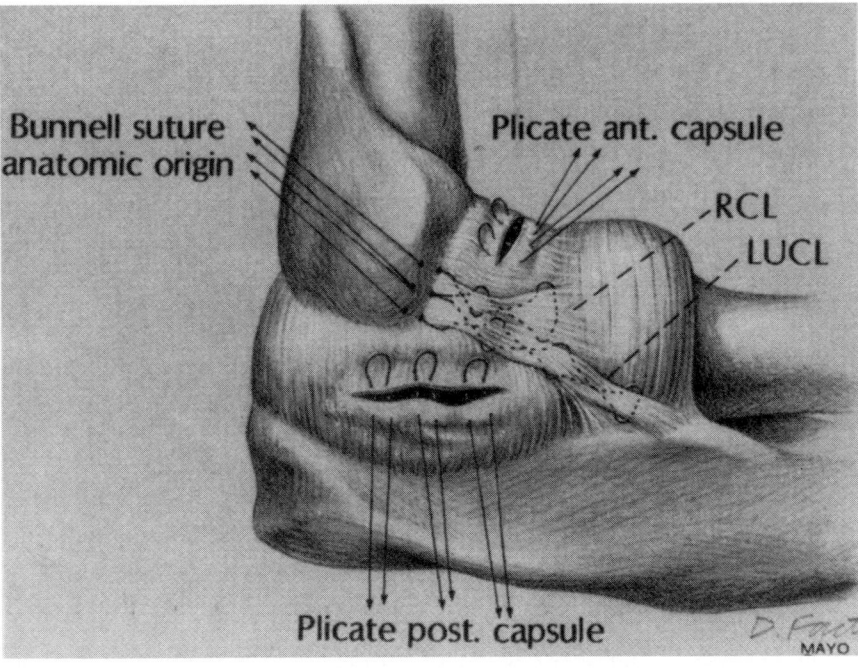

Bunnell suture
anatomic origin

Plicate ant. capsule

RCL

LUCL

Plicate post. capsule

D. Fact
MAYO

B

Figure 56-7 Reconstruction for lateral ligament insufficiency. *A.* Kocher approach with dissection and release of the common extensor tendon reveals lateral ulnar collateral ligament (LUCL). *B.* Imbrication of both the LUCL and the radial part of the radial collateral ligament (RCL) with Bunnell sutures placed through drill holes at the anatomic origin of the ligament. (From Nestor BJ, O'Driscoll SW, Morrey BF: Ligamentous reconstruction for posterolateral instability of the elbow. *J Bone Joint Surg* 74A:1235–1241, 1992. By permission of the Mayo Foundation.)

favorably to excision of the origin of the extensor brevis together with decortication of the origin in the region of the epicondyle.[54–56] Good results have also been reported using Wilhelm's denervation technique. This operation divides several articular nerves to the elbow by section in the region of the extensor origin.[57] A similar division of the extensor carpi radialis longus and brevis muscle origins is also achieved.

Morrey has pointed out the importance of accurate diagnosis for good results. A syndrome of entrapment of the posterior interosseous nerve (PIN) at the arcade of Frohse is important in the differential diagnosis, and there should be a careful examination for any sensory or motor deficiency in branches of the radial nerve. The region of the arcade should be specifically palpated. Tenderness over the arcade, aggravated by resisted supination, and relieved by injection of 2 mL of lidocaine makes a reliable triad for the diagnosis of PIN entrapment.[52] The elbow should be tested for varus instability in slight flexion to unlock the olecranon, and a "pivot shift" test for posterolateral instability should also be performed. In patients with articular disease such as rheumatoid arthritis, care should be taken to exclude a PIN syndrome associated with a synovial cyst.[58] Occasionally a ganglion can also arise in this region and cause impingement of the PIN, with pain in the region of the radial head; this may be mistaken for tennis elbow. Other causes of pain in the region include degenerative arthritis and anconeus or extensor muscle compartment syndrome.[59,60]

MEDIAL EPICONDYLITIS

This condition is sometimes known as golfer's elbow. The tenderness is anterior to the medial epicondyle in the region of the origin of the flexor pronator muscle mass. Such patients represent about 10 percent of all patients with epicondylitis.[61] This overuse syndrome of the common flexor pronator muscle group may occur in golfers who strike the ground or in throwing athletes who have either imperfect technique or an overuse syndrome. If rest and NSAIDs fail, they may be superseded by steroid injections administered into the point of maximal tenderness, which is usually anterior to the medial epicondyle and thus avoids the ulnar nerve. Care must be taken to differentiate this syndrome from attenuation of the MCL. The pain can usually be reproduced by flexion of the wrist of pronation of the forearm against resistance. A careful physical examination with 25° of elbow flexion should identify any accompanying valgus instability. Any attempt to release muscle fibers from the anterior aspect of the medial epicondyle is absolutely contraindicated in the presence of any medial ligament pathology, since the flexor pronator mass is an important secondary stabilizer in these circumstances. Any associated ulnar nerve irritation upon palpation should be carefully noted, as should any ulnar neuropathy. Any accompanying MCL pathology should be dealt with surgically as previously described.

ULNAR NERVE COMPRESSION

The main points of ulnar nerve compression in the cubital tunnel are the arcade of Struthers, the arcuate ligament, and the fascia of the flexor carpi ulnaris.[62] The clinical finding of irritation or neuropathy can be confirmed by electrodiagnostic tests. Several decompressing procedures have been proposed. One may choose to decompress the arcuate ligament and the flexor carpi ulnaris fascia but leave the nerve in its anatomic position. Alternatively, transposition of the nerve anterior to the epicondyle into a submuscular or subcutaneous bed may be preferred. Essential to the success of these operations is the division proximally of the edge of the medial intermuscular septum. Excision of the epicondyle has been proposed as an alternative to anterior transposition. Advocates point out that it removes or releases the compressing structures, including the arcade of Struthers, the arcuate ligament, and the two heads of the flexor carpi ulnaris. At the same time, it preserves the blood supply to the nerve, which can be rendered relatively ischemic after transposition.[63] Removing the epicondyle in effect enlarges the dimensions of the tunnel. Another approach has been to osteotomize the epicondyle and then move the nerve anteriorly to the epicondyle so that it lies in a deep submuscular situation. The epicondyle is then replaced in its normal anatomic situation with two AO screws.[64] Only a few cases are described by the author, and this procedure requires meticulous technique, since the epicondylar fragment is small.

CAUSES AND TREATMENT OF POSTTRAUMATIC ELBOW STIFFNESS

Even with considerable improvements in the management of complex elbow trauma, the stiff elbow remains a troubling sequela of such injuries.

It is important to identify with precision the causes of the restricted motion in the posttraumatic stiff elbow. Lateral tomograms in addition to routine radiographs are most helpful.[65] Capsular contracture, extracapsular scarring, or ectopic bone formation must be carefully assessed. Additionally, in patients who have had intraarticular fractures, it is important that there be a complete assessment of any continuing intraarticular incongruity, malunion, or nonunion. Occasionally, the ankylosis is due to a combination of these extrinsic and intrinsic factors. A rational treatment plan can be constructed only after such a detailed preoperative assessment.

Capsular Contracture

Although arthroscopic capsular release of flexion contractures of the elbow is described,[66] this is an operation in which the risk of neurovascular injury may be unduly high, particularly to the PIN. The problem is made worse when intraarticular capacity and compliance of these capsules in stiff elbows is reduced and adequate distention for elbow arthroscopy is difficult to achieve.[67] The technique of capsular release advocated by O'Driscoll[68] is probably among the safest, but this procedure should not be attempted by the inexperienced arthroscopist (Fig. 56-8). Open anterior capsulotomy was described by Urbaniak and coauthors; they were able to reduce a preoperative flexion deformity averaging 48° to 19° without dividing the brachialis or the biceps.[69] Morrey has described capsulotomy performed through a lateral modified Kocher approach by releasing the extensor carpi radialis longus from the lateral supracondylar ridge of the humerus and then dissecting anteriorly in the extracapsular plane.[70] Good access can be achieved to the posterior capsule through the same incision by reflecting the lateral border of the triceps and the anconeus muscle posteriorly. This gives good access to the posterior compartment of the joint, and exposure is further improved by removing the triceps tendon subperiosteally from the tip of the olecranon. The entire posterior capsule plus the olecranon process is now excised, and the wound is closed if a range of motion from 10 to 140° is achieved; otherwise further procedures are performed (see below).

Ectopic Bone

Myositis ossificans caused by the deposition of new bone in an area of damaged muscle is an uncommon lesion usually seen in the brachialis muscle, and the bone is not contiguous with the humeral cortex (a differentiating point from parosteal sarcoma). More common, in these days of high-speed traffic accidents, is the formation of heterotopic ossification (HO) following head injury and coma. This type of ossification around the elbow can occur following any neurologic illness with prolonged uncon-

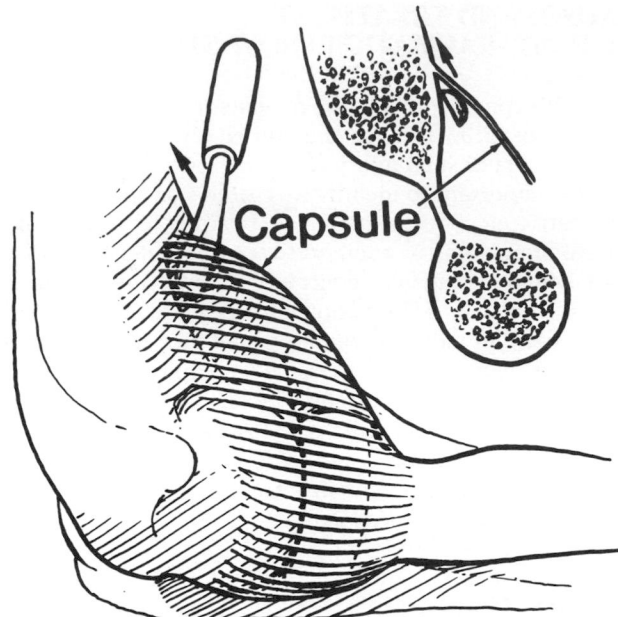

Figure 56-8 Release of contracted capsule utilizing a sweeping motion from distal to proximal with a blunt periosteal elevator under arthroscopic vision. (Reproduced with permission from O'Driscoll SW: Arthroscopic treatment for osteoarthritis of the elbow. *Orthop Clin North Am* 26:691–706, 1995.)

sciousness even in the absence of trauma. The ectopic bone may ossify capsular ligaments and periarticular muscle. It is contiguous with bone and no respecter of anatomic boundaries. It can completely surround the ulnar nerve for several centimeters above and distal to the medial epicondyle, and it can lock up pronation-supination by producing a radial ulnar synostosis. Some form of new bone formation around the elbow can occur in up to 3 percent of cases of elbow trauma.[71] A combination of head and elbow trauma may produce this unwanted complication in as many as 89 percent of cases.[72] Garland has pointed out that a normal alkaline phosphatase level and normal baseline bone scans do not imply that the new bone will not recur after excision.[73] This author recommends three different surgical approaches, depending on the location of the bone—which may be posterolateral, anterolateral, or medial. If ulnar nerve transposition is required, the nerve can be freed from its bony carapace using nerve root decompression techniques and instrumentation.

Garland recommends that the HO not be resected until most of the neurologic motor recovery has occurred in the brain-injured adult. This usually takes 18 months, and he recommended that such a procedure be delayed if significant neurologic recovery is continuing or neurologic recovery has been delayed. Recurrence of the elbow lesions is more common in patients with severe cognitive and physical defects. A poor neurologic recovery and persistent spasticity are associated with recurrence. Prophylactic postoperative radiation is recommended, using 1000 cGy given as 200 cGy/day beginning on the day of surgery.

Indomethacin may be used (25 mg three times a day for 3 months beginning on postoperative day 1).[73]

Interposition Arthroplasty

If preoperative evaluation of the stiff joint indicates associated damage to the articular bearing surface, interposition arthroplasty may be necessary after release of extrinsic contractures or ectopic bone. Failure to achieve a good range of motion (10 to 140°), damage to more than 50 percent of the articular surface, or the need to refashion the articular surface is an indication for interposition.[74,75]

The classic fascial arthroplasty developed by Campbell[76,77] is still popular. After performing the Morrey approach described for extensive capsular release, one can carefully detach the lateral ligament from the humerus (for later accurate reattachment). This step will give good access to the joint for resurfacing with a strip of fascia lata taken from the thigh. The fascia is attached to the lower humerus to clothe the front and back surfaces in the articular region and is then folded back on itself to cover the ulna. The external surfaces of the fascia thus slide upon each other within the new joint.

The technique of cutis arthroplasty was popularized by Vainio, who used it mainly in combination with bone grafting of the deficient olecranon for the treatment of rheumatoid arthritis. Froimsen popularized the procedure in the United States.[78] In the technique of cutis arthroplasty, a thin (0.031- to 0.038-mm) epidermal layer of skin is raised and left attached at the margin of the donor site. The deep dermal layer is then excised from the underlying fat and used as a graft, being sutured snugly over the distal humerus. Froimsen recommends sewing the epidermal layer back into position.[79] Our own preference is to remove it, undermine the margins of the donor area, and obtain a linear scar. The grafted skin is usually removed from the abdomen.

Before application of the interposition membrane, it may be necessary to reconstruct the articular surfaces, securing osteosynthesis of ununited condylar fragments with screws and bone graft if necessary. Where there is complete bony ankylosis, sculpturing of the articular surfaces with a burr may be necessary to give a good articular shape with some intrinsic stability. If the radiocapitellar joint is undamaged, it is unnecessary to involve it in the resurfacing procedure, and the radial head should be preserved if possible. Any bony elements impairing flexion/extension should be dealt with; this includes much of the olecranon process and occasionally the tip of the coronoid. The surgical approach may be modified if there is pathology on both sides of the joint that requires attention; in these cases, a transolecranon approach may be more suitable. Ulnar nerve transposition may also be required. The authors have found that these joints are often quite stable, but careful attention to restoring the integrity of the medial and lateral ligaments is required. If the brachialis tendon is found to be detached, the joint may prove to be unstable in flexion.[46] The authors have found it useful, in these cases, to transpose the biceps tendon into the region of the coronoid (Fig. 56-9).

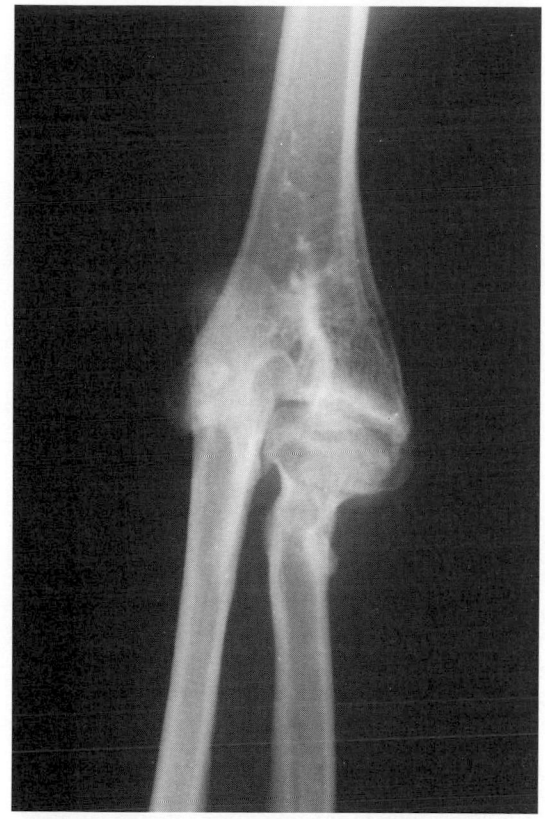

A

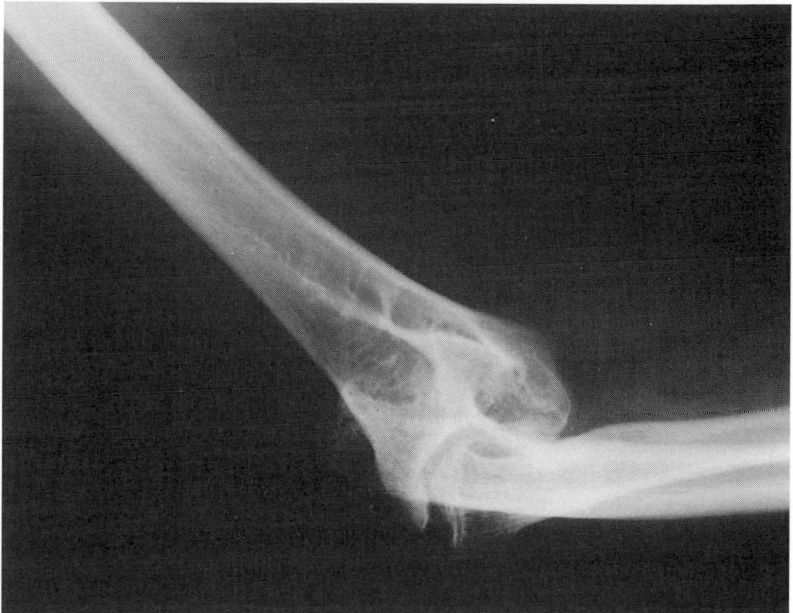

B

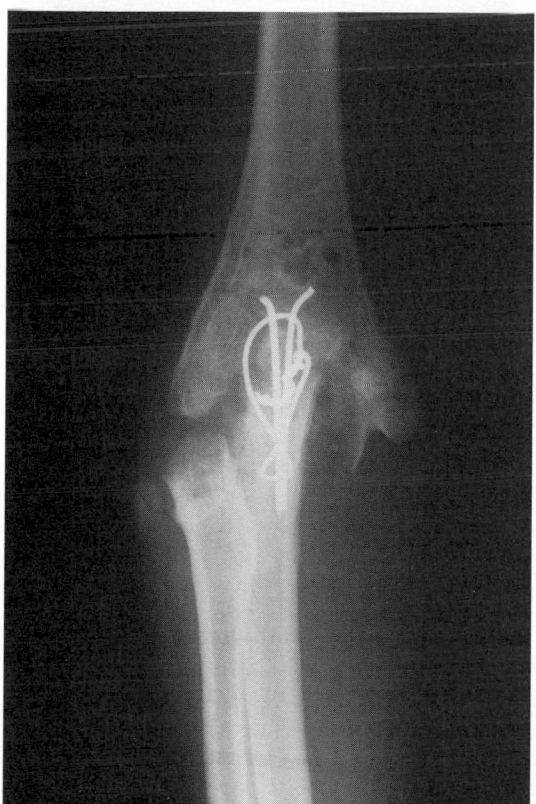

C

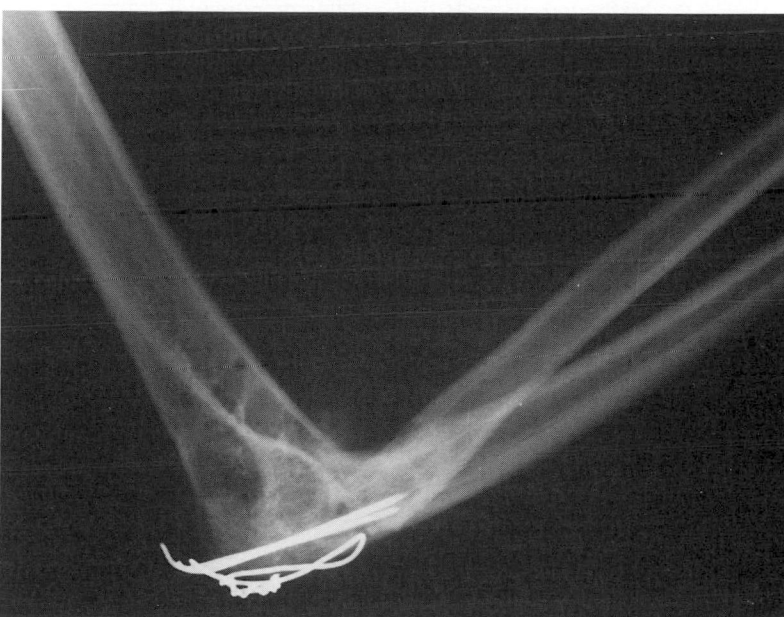

D

Figure 56-9 *A* and *B*. Neglected posterior dislocation of 20 years duration in a 35-year-old female. Elbow ankylosed in extension at 30°. At cutis arthroplasty, the radial head was excised and the ulna relocated. Collateral ligaments were difficult to locate and repair. When the biceps muscle was transferred to the insertion point of the absent brachialis muscle, the elbow stabilized dramatically. *C* and *D*. Good clinical result (30° to 110°) without bracing.

Distraction Arthroplasty

Even after simple capsular release, the fact that a good range of motion is achieved on the operating table does not mean that that motion will be preserved, and a careful postoperative rehabilitation regimen is essential to success. It is sometimes sufficient to splint these elbows in the newly achieved extended position for 48 h, then in 20° of flexion utilizing a continuous passive motion device, and finally early active motion. However, there are additional procedures that should be considered, particularly if the limitation of motion is associated with intraarticular damage. In these cases, a distraction device may be of value, as initially described by Volkov and Oganesian.[80] The biomechanics of the rotation of the elbow are such that the instant center of rotation does not move much more than a couple of millimeters; motion can thus be approximated by a single axis of rotation that passes through the center of the trochlea and the capitellum. A threaded pin can be passed along this single axis and an external device fitted onto the pin and secured to the ulna, so that, as the elbow is moved, the ulna rotates around the axis. Thus the distance between the surfaces of the trochlea and the notch in the ulna remains constant, but the joint can be distracted.[74] A combination of this distraction device plus CPM has been found useful for the first 3 or 4 weeks following soft tissue release and fascial grafting.[75] Adjustable turnbuckle splints are also useful in maintaining motion in the postoperative period and may be necessary for several months.

A sophisticated orthosis that applies incremental static progressive stretch through patient-controlled therapy has recently been described as an alternative to surgery.[81] The biomechanical basis for elbow hinged distraction design has been well described.[82]

The importance of surgical correction of intraarticular nonunions of malunions as a part of reconstruction of the stiff elbow must be emphasized.[83]

ARTHRITIS OF THE ELBOW

Osteoarthritis

Osteoarthritis of the elbow is rare, accounting for only 1 to 2 percent of patients presenting with degenerative arthritis.[84] These patients often suffer problems associated with the impingement of anterior or posterior osteophytes or intraarticular loose bodies. Some of these patients may be victims of osteochondritis dissecans. In some cases, it seems that the development of the disease is linked to an occupation or activity involving repetitive use of the dominant arm.[84] Relief of locking and elbow pain in osteoarthritis has been described using the Outerbridge-Kasiwagi (OK) method.[85] Other authors have confirmed the effectiveness of this procedure, in which a fenestration is made through the olecranon fossa of the distal humerus to give access to the anterior joint space via a posterior approach.[86] This open procedure has been modified and

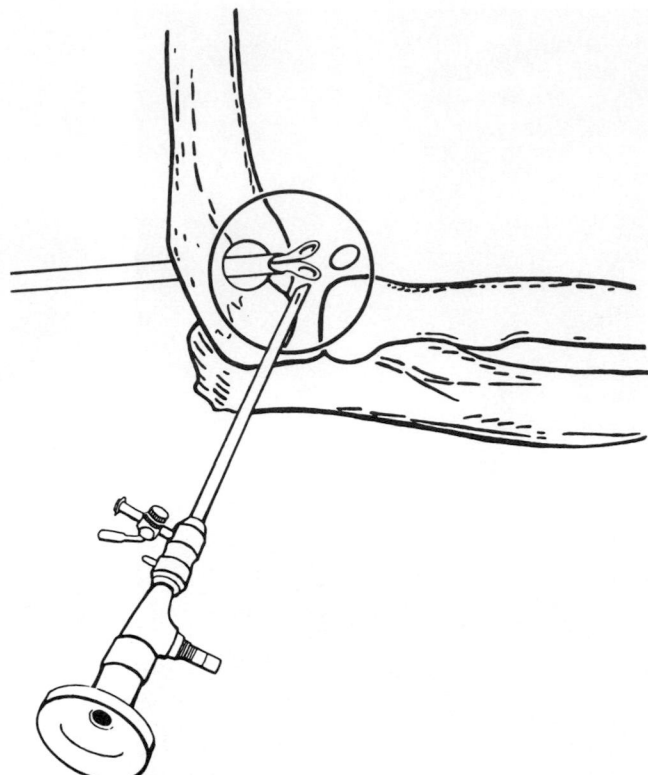

Figure 56-10 A loose body in the anterior joint compartment can be removed arthroscopically utilizing a posterior portal and fenestrating the humerus. (Reproduced with permission from Redden JF, Stanley D: Arthroscopic fenestration of the olecranon fossa in the treatment of osteoarthritis of the elbow. *J Arthroscop Rel Surg* 9:14–16, 1993.

may now be performed arthroscopically (Fig. 56-10). It permits removal of loose bodies and prominent impinging bone spurs of the coronoid.[84,87]

Arthroscopic Surgery of Osteoarthritis

The techniques for establishing arthroscopic portals have been well described by O'Driscoll,[68] and other authors have written useful reviews on the techniques of arthroscopic removal of loose bodies from the elbow.[88,89] The portals most commonly used for this work include the following. (1) The anterolateral portal, 1 cm distal and 1 cm anterior to the lateral epicondyle. Any mistakes in siting this portal will result in damage to the radial nerve or its branches (Fig. 56-11B). This portal is particularly useful for visualizing the medial part of the joint. (2) The anteromedial portal, which is made 1 cm proximal and 1 cm anterior to the medial epicondyle. The anteromedial portal is often established after the anterolateral portal by the use of switching sticks. A rod is inserted into the arthroscopic sheath placed on the lateral side to exit at a previously selected and visualized point on the medial synovium. The portal may then be established safely utilizing a small incision onto the rod from the skin (Fig. 56-11B). The ante-

Figure 56-11 *A.* Portals in common use for arthroscopy. The midlateral portal is made in the soft spot centered in the triangle formed by radial head, capitellum, and olecranon. The posterolateral portal lies more posteriorly. *B.* The anteromedial portal is established by identifying the desired entry point using arthroscopic vision from the anterolateral portal. A switch stick marks the spot and the skin is then cut safely. (From O'Driscoll SW, Morrey BF: Arthroscopy of the elbow. *J Bone Joint Surg* 74A:84–94, 1992. By permission of the Mayo Foundation.)

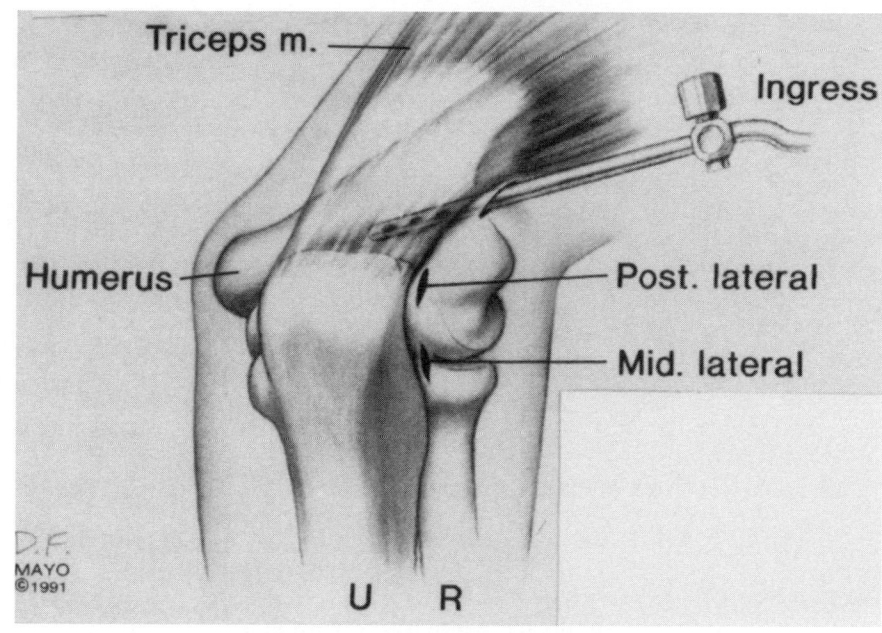

A

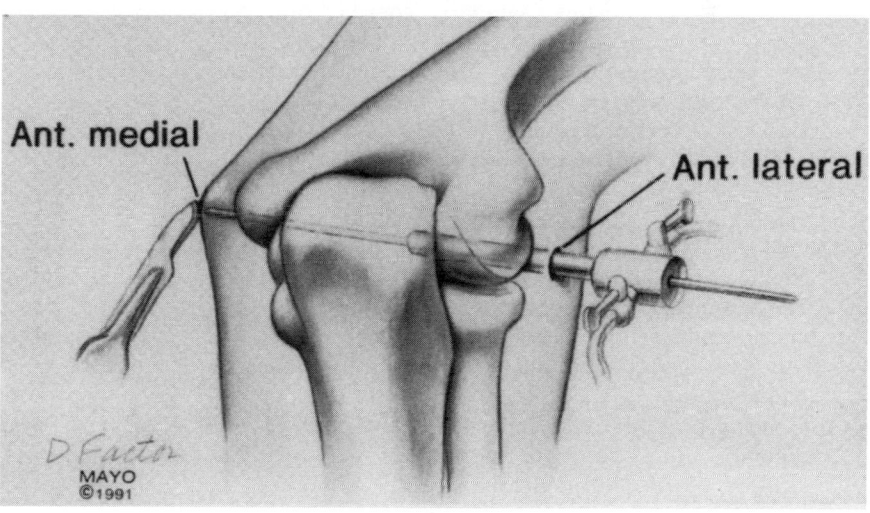

B

rior portals are best made with the elbow flexed at 90° and the capsule fully distended to displace the anterior neurovascular structures away from the anterior portals[68] (Fig. 56-12). (3) The midlateral portal between the capitellum, radial head, and olecranon is the safest portal and is usually established first, and for inspection purposes as well as joint distention (Fig. 56-11*A*). (4) The posterior portal is used for the OK procedure. Most arthroscopic surgery of the elbow is now performed with the patient in the lateral position or prone. Debridement of bone spurs from the olecranon (in throwing athletes) and from the coronoid (in osteoarthritis) as well as the removal of loose bodies can be achieved with safety provided there is meticulous attention to detail.

Osteoarthritis involving the humeroulnar joint is relatively uncommon; however, if pain and limitation of mo-

tion continue after less intrusive surgical procedures or nonoperative treatment, it may be necessary to perform prosthetic arthroplasty or interposition arthroplasty on these patients. One must take care to exclude the following alternative diagnoses:

1. *Spondyloarthropathies.* This is a group of joint diseases characterized by spondylitis. They often present with sacroiliac, ocular, or genital involvement. Included are psoriatic arthropathy, Reiter's disease, and ankylosing spondylitis. The HLA-B27 antigen is detectable in a high proportion of these patients, which, together with the clinical features of the disease, may suggest the appropriate diagnosis.

2. *Gout and pseudogout.* The area of the olecranon is a common site for rheumatoid nodule formation and

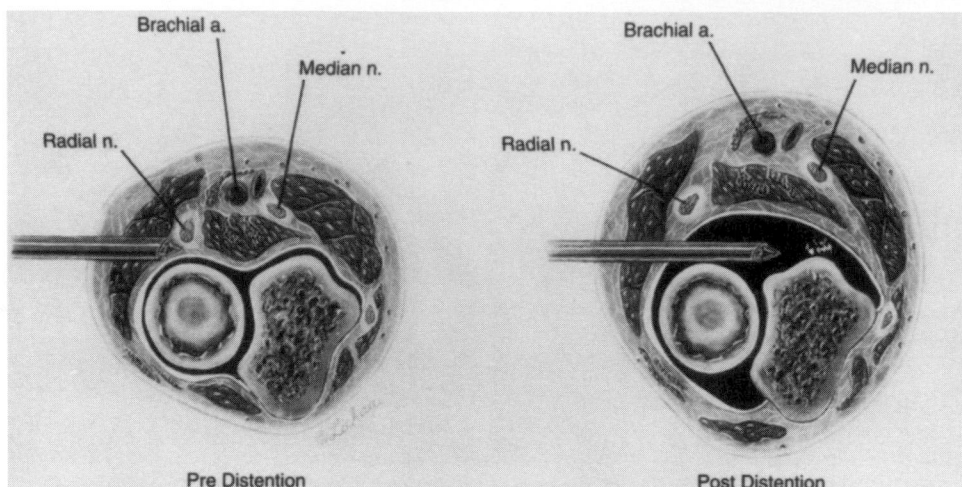

Figure 56-12 In establishing anterior portals, joint distension considerably increases the safety margin with the elbow flexed at 90°. The radial nerve is only a few millimeters away and may be harmed in an undistended joint. (Reproduced with permission from O'Driscoll SW: Arthroscopic treatment for osteoarthritis of the elbow. *Orthop Clin North Am* 26:691–706, 1995.)

also for sodium urate deposition in tophaceous gout. The synovial fluid may show the presence of sodium urate crystals, causing a synovitis. These crystals are often within phagocytes and are identified using a polarizing microscope (with a first-order red compensator), which reveals them as needle-shaped, negatively birefringent crystals.

3. *Calcium pyrophosphate deposition disease* (CPDD). This can present as an acute monoarticular arthritis involving the elbow. Radiologic examination may reveal the typical linear pattern of calcification in the capsule and the normally unseen articular cartilage. The examination of fresh synovial fluid under the polarizing microscope reveals positively birefringent, rhombus-shaped calcium pyrophosphate crystals in this condition.

4. *Septic arthritis.* Septic arthritis of the elbow is uncommon but does occur in patients who are drug abusers because of the proximity of the elbow joint to the common site of injection in the antecubital fossa. Occasionally, sepsis in an olecranon bursa spreads to involve the elbow joint, especially if it is not promptly treated. Rheumatoid patients on steroids are also at risk for septic arthritis, which may involve this joint. One should always be aware that the septic change may have occurred in any joint in this disease. In the young patient, differentiation from acute hematogenous osteomyelitis is important, since the metaphysis of the distal humerus is not intracapsular and involvement of the joint is not therefore inevitable. Careful physical examination and accurate determination of the maximum site of tenderness—together with diagnostic technetium and gallium scans—should help to differentiate a true arthritis from humeral osteomyelitis with a sympathetic effusion. Blood cultures and diagnostic aspiration should support the diagnosis.

Septic arthritis is usually accompanied by severe pain and distress upon the slightest attempt to move the joint. The presentation may be subacute in a patient with rheumatoid arthritis, and the diagnosis can therefore be overlooked. Appropriate antibiotic treatment is based on the identification on the organism involved, which is commonly *Staphylococcus aureus.* A wide variety of other organisms may be identified in patients who are drug abusers.

The use of the arthroscope permits lavage of the joint to reduce the intraarticular bacterial count by dilution. This technique avoids the need for open surgical drainage in some cases. Arthroscopy, early lavage and drainage, and well-managed blood levels of appropriate antibiotics enable controlled assisted active motion to be recommenced as soon as the infection is under control. Early diagnosis and therapeutic motion are necessary for a good result.

Rheumatoid Arthritis of the Elbow

This disabling disease commonly affects the upper limb and causes painful instability on ankylosis of the elbow. Rheumatoid arthritis may be staged radiologically.[90] Stage I shows osteoporosis and soft tissue changes. Stage II demonstrates mild or moderate degrees of bone erosion and a moderately reduced joint space, but not to less than 1 mm. In stage III disease, there is a more advanced situation in which the joint space is markedly narrowed to 1 mm or less, with extensive erosions. In stage IV disease, there is extensive destruction of the articular surfaces with subluxation and ankylosis.[90]

Synovectomy

Synovectomy has long been recognized as a useful procedure for the relief of pain in rheumatoid arthritis.[91–93] However, radiologic deterioration is observed to occur after surgery,[92,93] and at long-term follow-up (beyond 6 years) there is increasing clinical deterioration. Undoubtedly some of this is associated with continued bone erosion and instability.[94–97] Excision of the radial head may accelerate this process.[92,94] The incidence of instability following radial head excision and synovectomy has been reported as between 9.5 and 50 percent.[95–97] Copeland and Taylor[93] confirm that there is radiologic deterioration in patients with stage II and stage III disease after synovectomy, but they state that there is little functional loss for up to 10 years following surgery and therefore no down side to radial head excision, which they have practiced routinely.

The reoperation rate after synovectomy seems to be about 12 percent at a minimum of 5 years follow-up. It seems that synovectomy has no prophylactic effect in arresting what is a progressive disease. There is pain relief as the synovitis is improved. Range of motion seems to be the same or better after the operation. The best indications for the surgery seem to be in stage I and stage II disease. Stage III patients will progress, particularly if instability develops, and stage IV patients will probably progress inexorably and should have a different procedure than synovectomy. The lateral (Kocher) approach is suitable for this. If there are symptoms of ulnar compression, medial and lateral approaches may be used, since ulnar nerve decompression will be required. The midline posterior approach should be avoided, since these patients may have skin problems with large flaps, which are then necessary to access the medial and lateral sides of the joint. A transolecranon approach is not used for this procedure and should be avoided with the eroded olecranon of the severely rheumatoid patient.

In addition to ulnar nerve compromise from rheumatoid synovium, it should be noted that the posterior interosseous nerve (PIN) may be compromised in rheumatoid arthritis. Compression of this nerve can occur when there is a local cystic swelling compressing the nerve against the arcade of Frohse, which should then be decompressed without delay.[58,98]

Arthroscopic techniques for elbow synovectomy have been reported. The hazards are similar to those already described for arthroscopic surgery, and the techniques are still evolving.[99] Synovectomy has been shown to be of little value in juvenile rheumatoid arthritis. There is little relief of pain or improvement in range of motion, and the disease continues to progress.[99a]

PROSTHETIC REPLACEMENT OF THE ELBOW
General Indications

In stages III and IV rheumatoid arthritis, interposition arthroplasty with fascia may be successfully used to tighten up ligamentous instability and relieve pain. In this category, cutis arthroplasty is less favored by the authors because the skin texture is often unsuitable, but favorable results are reported.[100] Prosthetic arthroplasty is an alternative procedure in rheumatoid arthritis provided that bone erosion has not progressed too far. An unconstrained prosthesis will tighten up and stabilize the joint by the spacer effect of the components, bringing lax ligaments back out to length.

However, ligamentous rupture or insufficiency is a contraindication to the use of an unconstrained implant. In such cases and also where bone stock is unsuitable, a semiconstrained stemmed prosthesis should be chosen to stabilize the joint. Ewald et al. do not recommend unconstrained prosthetic arthroplasty for degenerative or posttraumatic arthritis[101]; these patients in any case are usually too young for such consideration. The indications for unconstrained implants in these categories of patients are discussed further on in this chapter.

Contraindications to Prosthetic Arthroplasty

These are similar to those in any other prosthetic joint replacement situation. Ongoing sepsis must be excluded with certainty. It is important that any inadequacies of the soft tissue coverage be carefully evaluated and corrected by plastic surgery prior to prosthetic intervention. Grafted skin must be replaced by appropriate full-thickness flaps. Deficient triceps musculature will mean that the implant may be subcutaneous just above the olecranon and prone to ulcerate through without soft tissue augmentation.

Unconstrained (Surface Replacement) Prostheses

The failure of fully constrained hinge joints in the elbow[102,103] and the success of surface replacement implants in the knee joint led to the development of several surface replacement devices for the elbow. They are utilized primarily in rheumatoid arthritis.

The capitellocondylar prosthesis devised by Ewald has gained popularity in the United States, and there are many reports of results of this implant in the literature.[104–106] This prosthesis consistently provides relief of pain and improvement of function as well as a good range of motion. However, it is not uncommon for these elbows sometimes to lack 30° of extension. The loosening rate at 1.5 percent is exceedingly low.[104] Kaplan-Meier survivorship analysis showed a functional prostheses in 88 percent at 1.4 years (with some early failure) and 83 percent at 5.5 years.[107] Both collateral ligaments of the elbow are essential stabilizers of this implant, and their integrity is a prerequisite for stable function.[108] Ewald and his coauthors describe performing the procedure through a modified Kocher exposure, which preserves the ulnar collateral ligament and the triceps insertion. They also describe cleaning soft tissues from the inside of the ulnar collateral ligament in an effort to restore normal length to that structure and relocate the elbow joint frequently during the operation to avoid prolonged excessive tension on the ulnar nerve. Their account deserves to be read in full.[104] In their expert hands, they experienced only one permanent partial ulnar nerve motor paralysis in 200 cases and 5 permanent partial sensory ulnar nerve injuries. Dislocation occurred in 3.5 percent of patients after implantation. They had a revision rate of only 3 percent; half were for infection and half for continuing dislocation (Fig. 56-13).

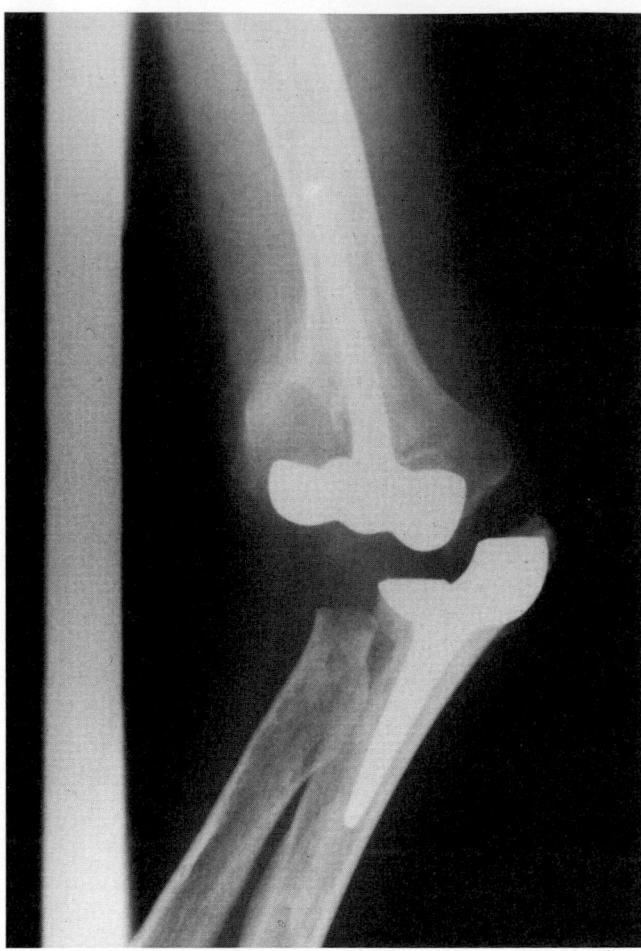

Figure 56-13 The medial collateral ligament is especially important when unconstrained elbow prostheses is being inserted. Here a capitellocondylar prosthesis has dislocated postoperatively, probably because the medial collateral ligament was not preserved during its insertion.

Other authors have confirmed that the important anterior portion of the ulnar collateral ligament is vulnerable to damage during placement of the ulnar component, and such an injury will result in instability.[108] Other authors have reported subluxation or dislocation of the prosthesis in 30 percent of patients, with a 15 percent incidence of ulnar nerve palsy even when the recommended lateral approach to the elbow was adopted.[106]

That ulnar nerve injury and postoperative dislocation are the main problems with resurfacing implants seems to be confirmed by experienced with other prostheses of similar design.[109,110] A high incidence of subsidence of the humeral component was also observed by Kudo and Iwano in their unconstrained prosthesis, leading them to change the design to include an intramedullary stem.[111]

Ewald recommends that the device not be used in patients before the rheumatoid disease has progressed to stage IV and there is excessive bone loss with giant cysts or a deficient trochlear notch. A specific contraindication to using this unconstrained device is joint instability with

a deficient medial collateral ligament. Ewald also stresses the importance of matching the valgus angle of the individual elbow with the appropriate prosthesis (the humeral components have varying angles between the axis of the articulation and the stem). Those rheumatoid patients who have ipsilateral shoulder and elbow disease may have arthroplasties of both joints without compromise. The joint that causes the most pain and disability should be operated on first. If both joints are equally involved, it is recommended that the elbow be operated on first.[112]

Semiconstrained Prostheses

The "sloppy hinge" type of semiconstrained implant is probably not as technically demanding to insert as the unconstrained type. Even if the integrity of the ligaments is compromised, there is sufficient stability in most of these designs (including the Coonrad-Morrey, the Inglis triaxial, and the Pritchard device) to stabilize the elbow. At the same time, there is sufficient laxity built into the articulation that the long-term survival with regard to loosening has been satisfactory.[113–115] The muscles and ligaments absorb some of the forces and moments that will loosen a constrained hinge joint.[116] Since the shape of the lower humerus does not lend itself to stem fixation with intramedullary cement, Morrey and Coonrad have added a titanium plasma–sprayed anterior flange to their device, which lies on the anterior humeral cortex. A bone graft is incorporated between the flange and the cortex to improve resistance to posterior displacement and axial rotation stresses which may be transmitted to the stem (Fig. 56-14). In their hands, semiconstrained designs have given good or excellent results in 90 percent of patients with rheumatoid arthritis at 4 years. The Kaplan-Meier survivorship analysis demonstrates that the prosthesis in 94 percent of these patients will probably survive for at least 7 years. A total of 71 percent of these patients has stage III involvement and 12 percent stage IV involvement with gross instability from the rheumatoid arthritis. Remarkably, no patient had radiographic evidence of loosening with this articulated linked design. Similarly, good survivorship analyses are available for other designs (Fig. 56-15).[117]

The surgical approach at the Mayo Clinic is through a straight posterior incision. The ulnar nerve is mobilized and then transposed anteriorly. The triceps muscle is then separated subperiosteally from the olecranon and displaced laterally in continuity with the forearm fascia and periosteum. As the elbow is flexed, the ulnar nerve lies medially and the triceps lies laterally, exposing the elbow joint (Fig. 56-16).[118] A somewhat similar approach calls for developing a continuous flap consisting of triceps, the posterior tip of the olecranon, and the anconeus; it is described by Wolfe and Ranawat.[119] This flap is also retracted laterally to give access.

The most frequent mode of failure following semiconstrained arthroplasty in patients with inflammatory disease is infection.[117] The routine use of antibiotic-impreg-

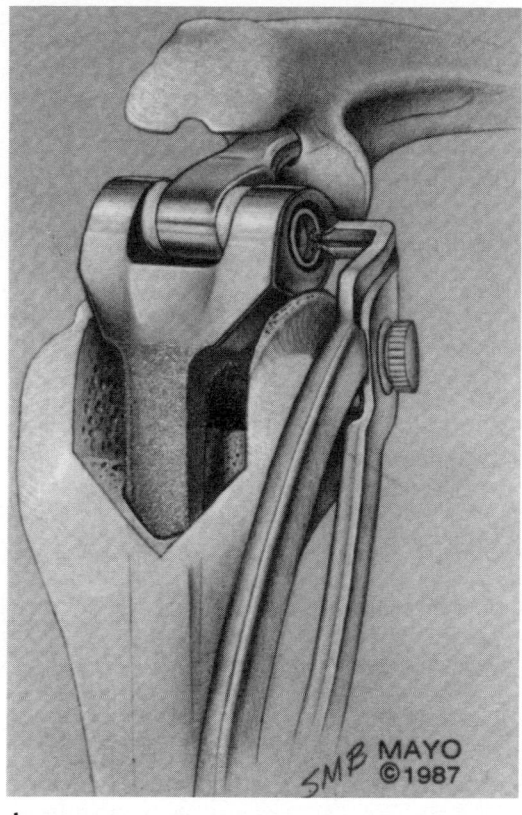

A

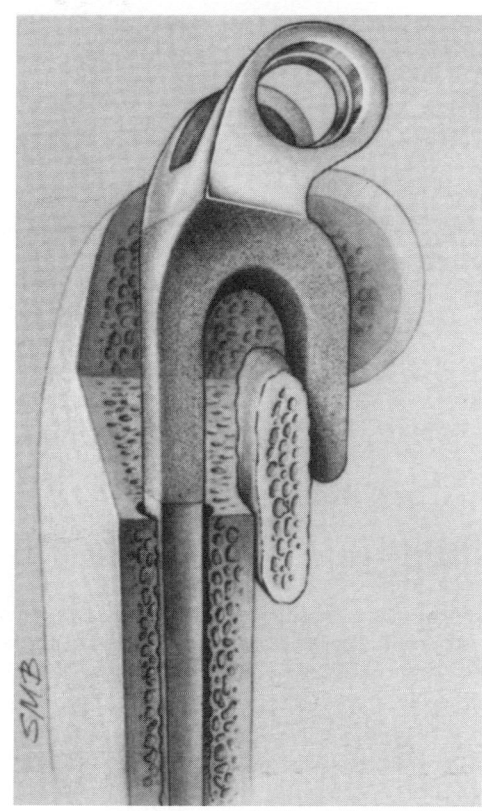

B

Figure 56-14 *A.* The Mayo-Coonrad semiconstrained prosthesis. *B.* Note that bone graft is inserted between the humerus and the anterior flange to further stabilize the component.

(Reproduced with permission from Morrey BF, Adams RA: Semiconstrained arthroplasty for the treatment of rheumatoid arthritis of the elbow. *J Bone Joint Surg* 74A:479–490, 1992.)

nated cement has been shown to reduce the incidence of infection dramatically in these patients and is recommended.[120] Risk factors for infection following primary total elbow arthroplasty have been identified.[120] They are (1) previous operation on the elbow, (2) previous infection in the region of the elbow, (3) psychiatric illness, (4) stage IV rheumatoid arthritis, (5) drainage from the wound after surgery, (6) spontaneous drainage after 10 days, and (7) reoperation for any reason.

In patients with supracondylar nonunion, supracondylar fracture, or traumatic arthritis, implant survival is significantly worse following total elbow arthroplasty than in patients with inflammatory arthritis (Fig. 56-15). These patients have often had several previous surgeries. A prosthesis should be contemplated only in those over age 60.[121] These categories of patients seem to be susceptible to early loosening of the humeral component and also have an increased propensity to become infected.[117] Removal of the metaphyseal/epiphyseal humeral fragment and its replacement with a customized elbow joint for supracondylar nonunions should be avoided. If it fails, the result is an unsalvageable flail elbow. In selected cases, salvage of these cases can be achieved by inserting a stemmed semiconstrained prosthesis, but preserving the epicondyles and their muscle attachments.[120]

Revision of the Failed Total Elbow Prosthesis

Improved joint design and the preservation of bone stock has made the revision problems somewhat less difficult than those following failure of earlier designs. Salvage of a failed unconstrained prosthesis can usually be achieved by the insertion of a semiconstrained prothesis, which will also stabilize an unstable joint. Alternately, conversion to nonprosthetic interposition arthroplasty is possible. Osteolytic damage to the metaphysis and diaphysis seen upon removal of a failed stemmed cemented implant is similar to that experienced in other joints. Occasionally, custom-made long-stemmed implants are required, with accompanying reconstruction of cortical deficiencies by the use of structural allografts.[102,122–124] There are cases in which the cortex is so thin after removal of the cement that it may be impossible to reinsert a total elbow prosthesis.[126] Under these circumstances, if there is instability due to loss of bone stock, the clinical result may be a flail elbow. It is therefore of great importance to be conservative with bone stock at primary surgery for open fractures and when initially inserting a total elbow arthroplasty (TEA).[125] Conservation of the epicondyles and olecranon is critical.

Stabilization of these elbows and also flail elbows following open fractures may be achieved by insertion of seg-

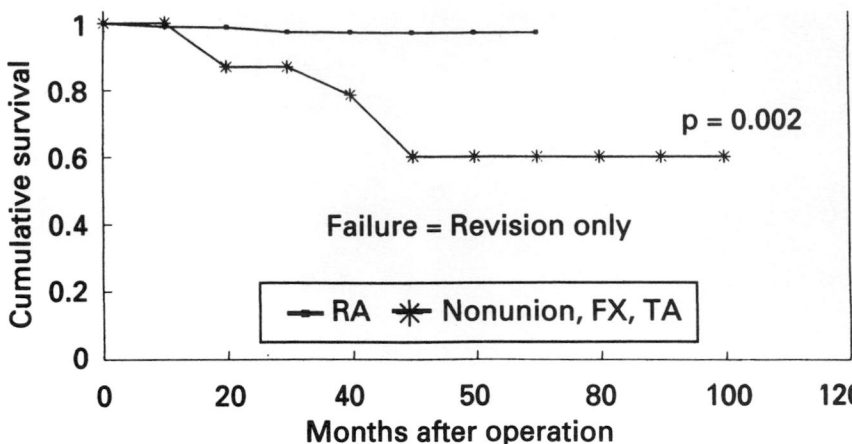

Figure 56-15 Survival of primary total elbow arthroplasty with the Hospital for Special Surgery semiconstrained implant. Note difference between patients with inflammatory arthritis (RA) compared with those with supracondylar nonunions (FX) or traumatic arthritis (TA). Failure in the figure includes all cases revised for loosening of mechanical failure but excludes deep injection. (Reproduced with permission from Kraay MJ, Figgie MP, Inglis AE, et al: Primary semiconstrained total elbow arthroplasty. *J Bone Joint Surg* 74A: 479–490, 1992.)

mental allografts plated to the host humeral diaphysis (Figs. 56-17 and 56-18).[102,123]

Revision for mechanical instability following semiconstrained arthroplasty is usually because the implant has come loose or broken at the articulation. A kit for the triaxial implant can be used to replace a broken bearing with no need to remove a well-fixed prosthesis.[122] A new polyethylene bushing is also included by the manufacturer (Osteonics, USA).

The Infected Prothesis

Any wound problems after surgery can readily result in a deep wound infection in these patients; therefore the smallest area of skin necrosis must be treated aggressively and closely monitored. In the elbow, prosthetic infection often follows a superficial lesion or bursitis. The prosthesis becomes consequently infected. Since the infection often travels from the outside in, early debridement and antibi-

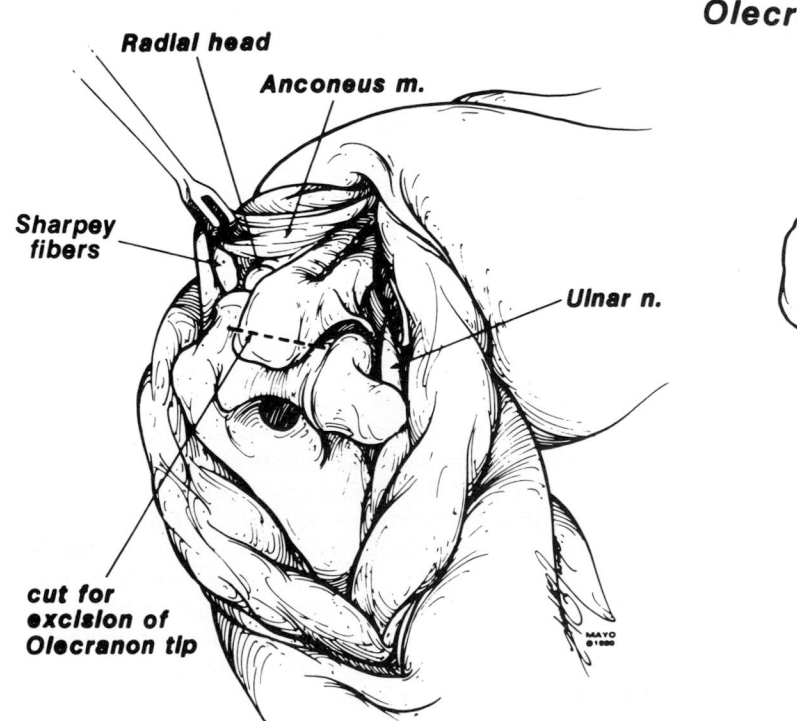

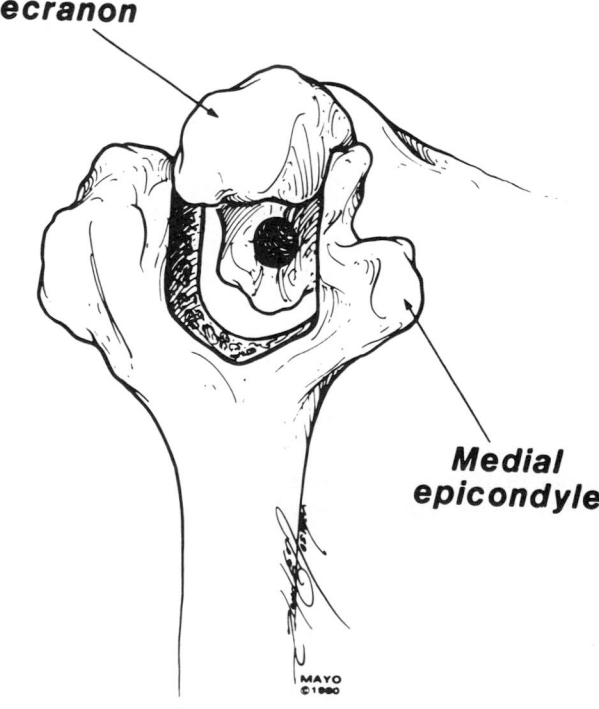

Figure 56-16 *Left:* The Mayo Clinic approach to the elbow for semiconstrained prosthetic arthroplasty. The triceps muscle is reflected laterally in continuity with the ulnar periosteum by separating the Sharpey fibers from their tendinous insertion into the olecranon. The ulnar nerve is transposed and protected. *Right:* Bony section of the tip of the olecranon; the jigged cutout for the humeral component gives good access. Note how relatively insubstantial and prone to fracture is the bone now supporting the medial epicondyle. (Reproduced with permission from Morrey BF, Bryan R, Dobyns JH, Linschied RL: Total elbow arthroplasty. *J Bone Joint Surg* 63A:1054, 1981.)

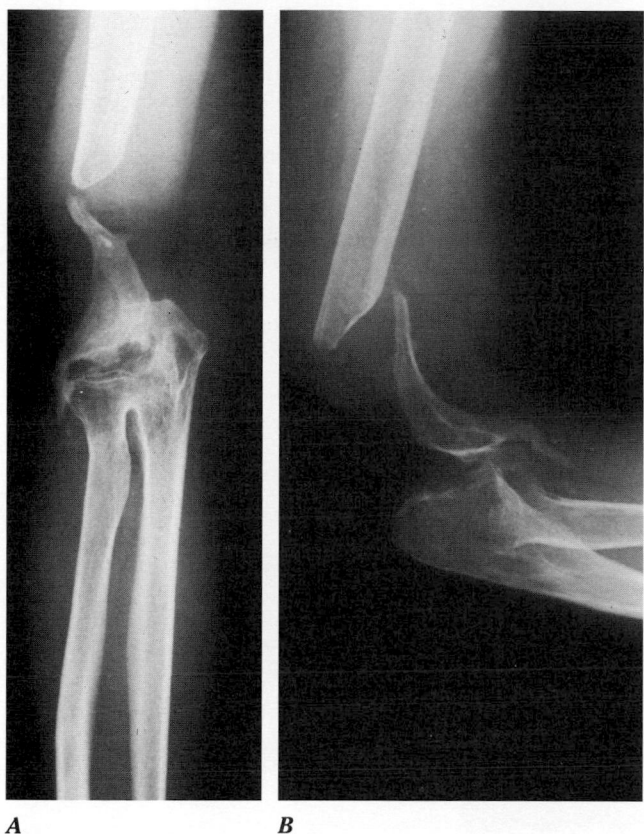

A   *B*

Figure 56-17 Two x-ray views of a flail elbow following a severe open fracture in a young woman. The loss of bone stock was due to a combination of destruction caused by the initial injury and subsequent surgical debridement for infection.

otics can salvage many joints. [120,127] If there are radiographic lucencies and endosteal scalloping or the organism is virulent, the implant must be removed, together with all of the bone cement, and a careful debridement accompany this procedure. Reimplantation strategy—as in the hip and knee—depends on the infecting organism, the quality of the tissues around the elbow, and whether the infection can be eradicated. It may be found that after removal of either a semiconstrained or an unconstrained implant, the elbow is not markedly unstable. If the removal of the implant is not accompanied by a marked increase in pain level, reimplantation may not be necessary or appropriate, particularly in the debilitated patient.

Total Elbow Arthroplasty for Ankylosis

Since taking down an ankylosed on fused elbow usually requires division of the ligaments of the elbow, a semiconstrained type of prosthesis component is necessary. A surprisingly good range of motion can be achieved after taking down an ankylosis that may have existed for many years. Figgie and coauthors recommend a custom-fitted prosthesis[128] inserted via the Bryan-Morrey posteromedial approach to the elbow.[118] The authors have successfully taken down posttraumatic bony fusions in the elbow and

utilized cutis interposition arthroplasty. This should be done only in carefully selected cases, where elbow motion is highly desirable. Prosthetic arthroplasty must be avoided in the younger age group (under 65 years). The authors' preferred approach for cutis arthroplasty in bony ankylosis is transolecranon.

ARTHRODESIS OF THE ELBOW

Arthrodesis of the elbow is rarely performed and has a high failure rate when attempted for the flail elbow with loss of bone stock. It is not indicated in rheumatoid arthritis, since in these patients loss of any mobile joint throws additional stress on proximal and distal joints, which are already diseased. Improved primary treatment and secondary reconstruction of the traumatized elbow has also minimized the requirements for these kinds of procedures.

When arthrodesis is performed, fixation may be achieved by a posterior right-angle plate.[129] The use of autogenous bone may also be required. The position at which the elbow is fused should be decided by the patient's employment.[130] When arthrodesis is indicated for infection, external fixation may be a preferable method of immobilizing the joint.

The unpopularity of elbow arthrodesis seems to be well justified since arthrodesis (whatever the position) of the elbow, unlike that of other joints, causes significant functional impairment. It has been shown that the adjacent shoulder and wrist joints cannot compensate to permit completion of functional activities when this joint is fused.[131]

THE ELBOW AND BLEEDING DIATHESES
Hemophilia

Recognizable arthropathy of the elbow is common in bleeding diatheses and—by contrast with other joints of the upper limb—occurs in 87 percent of hemophiliacs.[132] Interposition arthroplasty has been used to mobilize the virtually ankylosed joints of chronic hemophilic arthropathy.[133,134] However, the silastic membrane utilized in this procedure may fragment[134] and cause long-term problems. Synovectomy has some value in reducing bleeding and pain.[135]

Sickle Cell Disease

The fluid from the uninfected joint may be purulent in sickle cell disease even in the absence of infection, and culture is imperative to confirm an additional septic arthritis. Many polymorphonuclear leukocytes may appear in articular fluid without sepsis.[136,137] Acute gouty arthritis has also been described in this disease, and serum uric acid is often elevated, further complicating

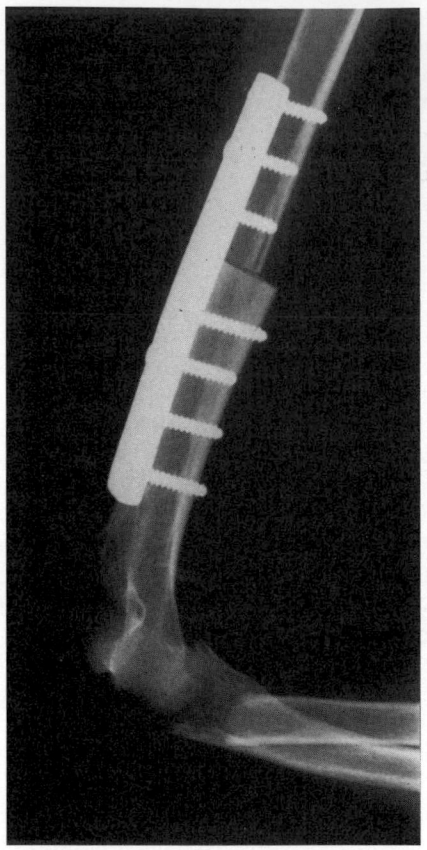

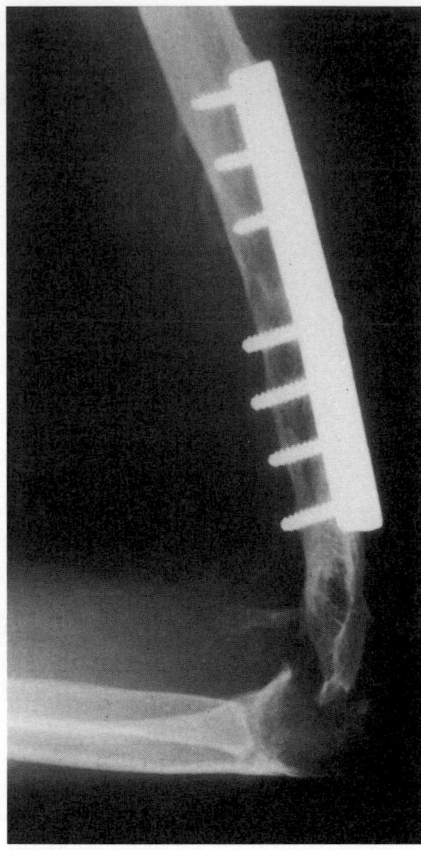

A   *B*

Figure 56-18 *A.* skeletal length and muscle balance have been restored by replacement of the distal humerus with a fresh frozen allograft. Union to the host bone was achieved in 6 months. *B.* Three years later there is considerable erosion in the region of the elbow joint, not only of the allograft but also of the host bone. Sufficient stability persists, however, for useful function without a brace.

the differential diagnosis of acute synovitis from an intraarticular hemorrhage.

SYNOVIAL CHONDROMATOSIS OF THE ELBOW

This disease commonly affects the knee and hip as well as the elbow[138] and is a distinct pathologic entity. Intrasynovial proliferation of microscopic lobules of cartilage, with occasional ossified areas, occurs within the layers of the membrane (Fig. 56-19).[139]

Three phases of the disease are described.[139,140] In stage I, there is active intrasynovial disease but no loose bodies. In stage II, loose bodies are also present, and in stage III, the intrasynovial disease is burned out, with normal or only slightly inflamed synovium; however, there are multiple residual loose bodies. Differentiation should be made from other causes of a few loose bodies, such as osteochondral fracture, osteochondritis dissecans, or osteoarthritis. Treatment consists of removal of loose bodies and as complete a synovectomy as possible. If ossification has occurred, the "loose" bodies may be firmly attached to bone and masses of them may burst through herniations in the capsule, making complete removal hazardous.

OLECRANON BURSITIS

Swelling and erythema over the point of the elbow may indicate bursitis in the olecranon bursa. This can be occupational, due to mechanical irrigation directly in the region of the olecranon tip, or it can arise spontaneously. If unaccompanied by overlying cellulitis or pyrexia, the inflammation may be sterile. A period of rest is then usually enough to cause the fluid-filled cavity to shrink. However, such attacks frequently become chronic, and the patient is left with a permanent fluctuant swelling with some thickening in the bursal tissue. Under these conditions, surgical removal is justified. The surgeon should clearly explain the risk of recurrence, though recurrence can be minimized by careful operative technique. Wound breakdown is a potential complication in this anatomic area and may be avoided by immobilizing the elbow for a week or so with a posterior padded back slab. The proximity of the ulnar nerve makes removal of the bursa without identification and mobilization of the nerve difficult and hazardous. Both an adequate excision and a clear visualization of the nerve can easily be obtained through a midline incision. The floor of the bursa may be removed with a fine sliver of the bone, particularly if there is an associated exostosis.

Aspiration of synovial bursae in unsanitary conditions or with careless technique can lead to infection of the bur-

Figure 56-19 Magnetic resonance image of a 50-year-old recreational weight lifter with elbow now almost completely ankylosed due to joint packed tight with partly ossifying synovial chondromatosis.

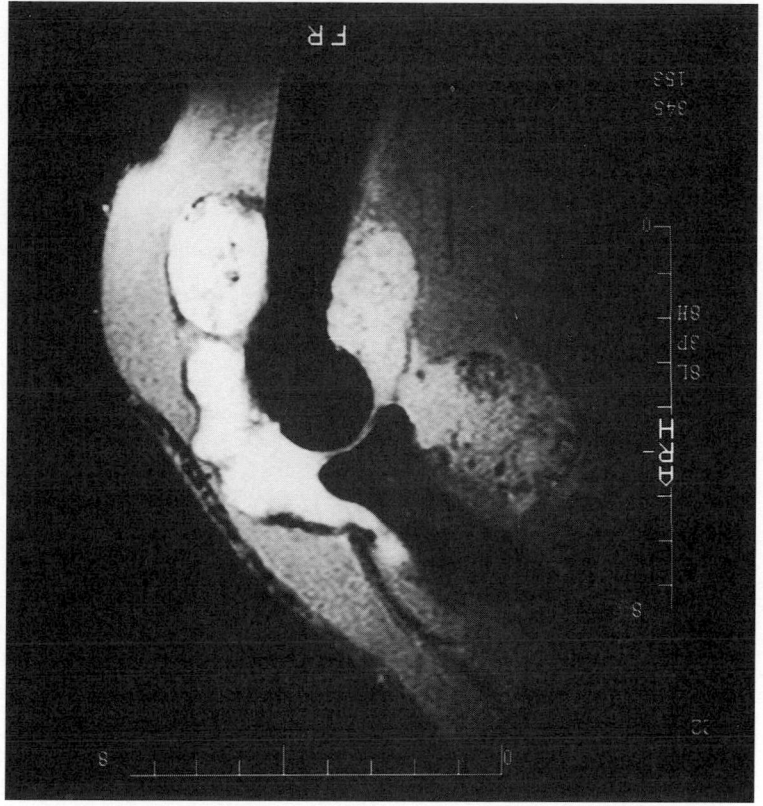

sae, and a bursa can similarly become infected without any obvious predisposing skin abrasion. The patient may be toxic and ill, with a high fever and leukocytosis. In the presence of frank pus, surgical drainage and appropriate immobilization of the elbow are required. Appropriate antibiotic therapy should then resolve the situation. When the acute infection is resolved and the wound is dry, definitive removal of the bursa can be considered.

REFERENCES

1. Boone DC, Azen SP: Normal range of motion of joints in male subjects. *J Bone Joint Surg* 61A:756–759, 1979.
2. Morrey BF, Askew LJ, An KN, Chao EV: A biomechanical study of normal junctional elbow motion. *J Bone Joint Surg* 63A:872–877, 1981.
3. Mall FP: On the angle of the elbow. *Am J Anat* 4:391–404, 1905.
4. Morrey BF, Chao EV: Passive motion of the elbow joint. *J Bone Joint Surg* 58A:501–508, 1976.
5. Youm V, Dryer RF, Thambyrajah K, et al: Biomechanical analysis of forearm pronation supination and elbow flexion-extension. *J Biomech* 12:245–255, 1979.
6. Ewald FF: Total elbow replacement. *Orthop Clin North Am* 6:685–696, 1975.
7. Ishizuki M: Functional anatomy of the elbow joint and three dimensional quantitative motion analysis of the elbow joint. *J Jpn Orthop Assoc* 53:989–996, 1979.
8. London JT: Kinematics of the elbow. *J Bone Joint Surg* 63A:529–535, 1981.

9. Dempster WT: *Space Requirements of the Seated Operator.* Wright Air Development Center Technological Report. 1955, pp 55–159.
10. Burman M: Induced pseudarthrosis of the radius in congenital radioulnar synostosis: Geometric analysis of the consequent mechanical situation. *Bull Hosp Joint Dis* 13:269–321, 1952.
11. Steindler A: *Kinesiology of the Human Body.* Springfield, IL, Charles C. Thomas, 1955, pp 499–507.
12. Ray RD, Johnson RJ, Jameson RM: Rotation of the forearm: An experimental study of pronation and supination. *J Bone Joint Surg* 33A:993–996, 1951.
13. Kapandji IA: *The Physiology of the Joints.* Vol 1. Edinburgh, Churchill Livingstone, 1982.
13a. Potter HP: The obliquity of the arm of the female in extension. The relation of the forearm with the upper arm in flexion. *J Anat Physiol* 29:488–491, 1895.
14. Atkinson WB, Elftman H: The carrying angle of the human arm as a secondary sex character. *Anat Rec* 91:42–49, 1945.
15. Fick R: *Handbuch der Anatomie und Mechanik der Gelenke.* Jena, Gustav Fischer, 1911, pp 304–312.
16. Nagel K: Untersuchungen Uber den Armwinkel des Menschen. *Morphol Anthropol* 10:317–352, 1907.
17. Thompson AR: Some features of the elbow joint. *J Anat* 58:368–373, 1924.
18. Amis AA, Dowson D, Unsworth A, et al: An examination of the elbow articulation with particular reference to variation of the carrying angle. *Eng Med* 6:76–80, 1977.
19. An KN, Morrey BF, Chao EV: Carrying angle of the human elbow joint. *J Orthop Res* 1:369–378, 1984.
20. Wadsworth TG: *The Elbow.* Edinburgh, Churchill Livingstone, 1982.
21. Williams A, Lissner B, in LeVeau B (ed): *Biomechanics of Human Movement.* Philadelphia, Saunders, 1977.

22. Amis AA, Dowson D, Wright V: Elbow joint force predictions for some strenuous isometric actions. *J Biomech* 13:765–775, 1980.

23. Amis AA, Dowson D, Wright V, Miller JH: The derivation of elbow joint forces and their relation to prosthetic design. *J Med Eng Tech* 3:229–234, 1979.

24. Gurtowski J, Stern L, Manley MT, et al: Loosening of semi-constrained elbow prosthesis. *Trans Orthop Res Soc* 8:102, 1983.

25. Regan WD, Korineck SL, Morrey BF, An K: Biomechanical studies of ligaments around the elbow joint. *Clin Orthop* 271:170–179, 1991.

26. Tullos HS, Schwat G, Bennet JB, Woods GW: Factors influencing elbow instability. *AAOS Instr Course Lect* 30:185–199, 1991.

27. Schwab GH, Bennet JB, Woods GW, Tullos HS: Biomechanics of elbow instability: The role of medial collateral ligament. *Clin Orthop* 146:42, 1980.

28. Sojbjerg JO, Wvesen J, Nielsen S: Experimental instability after transection of the medial collateral ligament. *Clin Orthop* 218:186–190, 1987.

29. Morrey BF, An KN: Articular and ligamentous contributions to the stability of the elbow joint. *Am J Sports Med* 11:315–319, 1983.

30. Morrey BF, Tanaka S, An KN: Valgus stability of the elbow. *Clin Orthop* 1265:187–195, 1991.

31. Tullos HS, Erwin W, Woods GW, et al: Unusual lesions of the pitching arm. *Clin Orthop* 88:169–182, 1972.

32. Waris W: Elbow injuries of javelin throwers. *Acta Chir Scand* 93:563–575, 1976.

33. Norwood LA, Schook JA, Andrew JR: Acute medial elbow ruptures. *Am J Sports Med* 9:16–19, 1981.

34. Kuroda S, Sakamaki K: Ulnar collateral ligament tears of the elbow joint. *Clin Orthop* 208:266–271, 1986.

35. Jobe FW, Stark H, Lombardo SJ: Reconstruction of the ulnar collateral ligament in athletes. *J Bone Joint Surg* 68A:1158–1164, 1986.

36. Timmerinon LA, Schwartz ML, Andrews JR: Preoperative evaluation of the ulnar collateral ligament by magnetic resonance imaging and computed tomography arthrography. *Am J Sports Med* 22:26–32, 1994.

37. Osborne G, Cotterill T: Recurrent dislocation of the elbow joint. *J Bone Joint Surg* 48B:340, 1966.

38. Hassman GC, Neer CS II: Recurrent dislocation of the elbow. *J Bone Joint Surg* 57A:1080, 1975.

39. Jacobs RL: Recurrent dislocation of the elbow: A case report and a review of the literature. *Clin Orthop* 74:151, 1971.

40. Linscheid RL: Elbow dislocations. *JAMA* 194:1171, 1965.

41. Osborne GV, Cotterill T: Recurrent dislocation of the elbow joint. *J Bone Joint Surg* 48B:340, 1966.

42. Witvoet J, Tayon B: La luxation recidivante du coude. *Rev Chir Orthop* 60:485, 1974.

43. Durig M, Mueller W, Ruedei TP, Gauer EF: The operative treatment of elbow dislocation in the adult. *J Bone Joint Surg* 61A:239, 1979.

44. Josefsson PO, Gentz CF, Johnelee O, Wendenberg B: Surgical versus non-surgical treatment of ligamentous injuries following dislocation of the elbow joints. *J Bone Joint Surg* 69A:605, 1987.

45. Zeirer FG: Recurrent traumatic elbow dislocation. *Clin Orthop* 169:211, 1982.

46. Dryer RF, Buckwalter JS, Sprague BL: Treatment of chronic elbow instability. *Clin Orthop* 148:254, 1980.

47. King T: Recurrent dislocation of the elbow. *J Bone Joint Surg* 35B:50, 1953.

48. Protzman RR: Dislocation of the elbow joint. *J Bone Joint Surg* 48B:340, 1966.

49. O'Driscoll SW, Morrey BF, Korinek S, An KN: Elbow subluxation and dislocation: A spectrum of instability. *Clin Orthop* 280:186–197, 1992.

50. O'Driscoll SW, Bell DF, Morrey BF: Posterolateral rotary instability of the elbow. *J Bone Joint Surg* 73A:440–446, 1991.

51. Nestor BJ, O'Driscoll SW, Morrey BF: Ligamentous reconstruction for posterolateral instability of the elbow. *J Bone Joint Surg* 74A:1235–1241, 1992.

52. Morrey BF: Reoperation for failed surgical treatment of refractory lateral epicondylitis. *J Shoulder Elbow Surg* 1:47:55, 1992.

53. Coonrad RW, Hooper WR: Tennis elbow: Its causes, natural history, conservative and surgical management. *J Bone Joint Surg* 55A:1177, 1973.

54. Nirschl RP, Petrone FA: Tennis elbow: The surgical treatment of lateral epicondylitis. *J Bone Joint Surg* 61A:832, 1979.

55. Nirschl RP: Tennis elbow. *Orthop Clin North Am* 43:797–800, 1973.

56. Goldberg EJ, Abraham E, Siegel I: The surgical treatment of chronic lateral humeral epicondylitis by common extensor release. *Clin Orthop* 233:208–212, 1988.

57. Wittenberg RH, Schaal S, Muhr G: Surgical treatment of persistent elbow epicondylitis. *Clin Orthop* 278:73–80, 1990.

58. Ishikawa H, Hirohatoa K: Posterior interosseous nerve syndrome associated with rheumatoid synovial cysts of the elbow joint. *Clin Orthop* 254:134–138, 1990.

59. Posch JN, Goldberg BM, Larrey R: Extensor fasciotomy for tennis elbow, a long term follow-up study. *Clin Orthop* 135:179–182, 1978.

60. Abrahamson SO, Sollerman C: Lateral elbow pain caused by anconeus compartment syndrome. *Acta Orthop Scand* 58:589–591, 1987.

61. Bernhang AN: The many causes of tennis elbow. *NY State J Med* 79:1363, 1979.

62. Froimsen AI, Anouchi YS, Seitz WH Jr, Winsberg DD: Ulnar nerve decompression with medial epicondylectomy for neuropathy at the elbow. *Clin Orthop* 265:200–206, 1991.

63. Orgata K, Manske PR, Leske PA: The effect of surgical dissection on the regional blood flow to the upper ulnar nerve in the cubital tunnel. *Clin Orthop* 193:195, 1985.

64. Mass DP, Silverberg B: Cubital tunnel syndrome, anterior transposition with epicondylar osteotomy. *Orthopedics* 9:711–715, 1986.

65. Morrey BF: Past traumatic contracture of the elbow. *J Bone Joint Surg* 72A:601–618, 1990.

66. Scott Jones G, Savoie FH: Arthroscopic capsular release of flexion contractures (arthrofibrosis) of the elbow. *Arthroscopy* 9:277–283, 1993.

67. Gallay SH, Richard RR, O'Driscoll SW: Intraarticular capacity and compliance of stiff and normal elbows. *Arthroscopy* 9:9–13, 1993.

68. O'Driscoll SW: Arthroscopic treatment for osteoarthritis of the elbow. *Orthop Clin North Am* 26:691–706, 1995.

69. Urbaniak JR, Hansen PE, Beissinger SF, Aitken MS: Correction of post-traumatic flexion contracture of the elbow by anterior capsulectomy. *J Bone Joint Surg* 67A:1160–1165, 1985.

70. Morrey BF: Post-traumatic contracture of the elbow. *J Bone Joint Surg* 72A:601–618, 1990.

71. Thompson HC, Garcia A: Myositis ossificans: Aftermath of elbow injuries. *Clin Orthop* 50:129–134, 1967.

72. Garland DE, O'Hollaran RM: Fractures and dislocations about the elbow and the head injured adult. *Clin Orthop* 168:38–41, 1982.

73. Garland DE: Surgical approaches for resection of heterotopic ossification in traumatic brain injured adults. *Clin Orthop* 263:59–70, 1990.

74. Morrey BF: Post-traumatic contracture of the elbow: Operative treatment including distraction arthroplasty. *J Bone Joint Surg* 72A:601–618, 1990.

75. Morrey BF: Post-traumatic stiffness: Distraction arthroplasty. *Orthopedics* 15:863–869, 1992.

76. Campbell WC: Mobilization of joints with bony ankylosis. *JAMA* 83:978, 1924.

77. MacAusland WR: Arthroplasty of the elbow. *N Engl J Med* 236:97, 1947.

78. Vainio K: Arthroplasty of the elbow and hand in rheumatoid arthritis, in Chapchal G (ed): *Synovectomy and Arthroplasty in Rheumatoid Arthritis*. Stuttgart, Thieme Verlag, 1976, 66–70.

79. Froimsen A, Silva JE, Richey WG: Cutis arthroplasty of the elbow joint. *J Bone Joint Surg* 58A:863–865, 1976.

80. Volkov MV, Oganesian OV: Restoration of function in the knee and elbow with a hinged distractor apparatus. *J Bone Surg* 57A:591–600, 1975.

81. Bonnutti PM, Windan JE, Ables BA, Moller BG: Static progressive stretch to reestablish elbow ranged motion. *Clin Orthop* 303:128–134, 1994.

82. Deland JT, Garg A, Walker PS: Biomechanical basis for elbow hinge distractor design. *Clin Orthop* 215:303–315, 1987.

83. McKee MJ, Choon LT, Wilson L, et al: Reconstruction after malunion and non-union of intraarticular fractures of the distal humerus. *J Bone Joint Surg* 76B:614–621, 1994.

84. Morrey BF: Primary degenerative arthritis of the elbow. *J Bone Joint Surg* 74B:409–413, 1992.

85. Kasiwagi D: Osteoarthritis of the elbow joint: Intra-articular changes and the special operative procedure; Outerbridge-Kasiwagi method, in Kasiwagi D (ed): *Elbow Joint*. Amsterdam, Elsevier, 1985, 177–188.

86. Stanley D, Winson IG: A surgical approach to the elbow. *J Bone Joint Surg* 72B:728–729, 1990.

87. Redden JF, Stanley D: Arthroscopic fenestration of the olecranon fossa in the treatment of osteoarthritis of the elbow. *J Arthrop Rel Surg* 9:14–16, 1993.

88. Ogilvie-Harris DJ, Schemitsch E: Arthroscopy of the elbow for removal of loose bodies. *Arthroscopy* 9:5–8, 1993.

89. Greis PE, Halbrecht J, Plancher KD: Arthroscopic removal of loose bodies of the elbow. *Orthop Clin North Am* 26:679–689, 1995.

90. Steinbrocker O, Taegen CH, Batterman RC: Therapeutic criteria in rheumatoid arthritis. *JAMA* 140:659–662, 1979.

91. Inglis AE, Ranawat CS, Straub LR: Synovectomy and debridement of the elbow in rheumatoid arthritis. *J Bone Joint Surg* 53A:622–652, 1971.

92. Porter BB, Richardson C, Vainio K: Rheumatoid arthritis of the elbow: The results of synovectomy. *J Bone Joint Surg* 56B:427–437, 1974.

93. Copeland SA, Taylor JG: Synovectomy of the elbow in rheumatoid arthritis. *J Bone Joint Surg* 61B:69–73, 1979.

94. Rymuszewsky LA, Mackay I, Amis AA, Miller JH: Long term effects of excision of the radial head in rheumatoid arthritis. *J Bone Joint Surg* 66B:109, 1984.

95. Brumfield R, Resnick CT: Synovectomies of the elbow in rheumatoid arthritis. *J Bone Joint Surg* 67A:60, 1985.

96. Rymuszewsky LA, Eichen Blatt M, Hass A, Kessler I: Synovectomy of the elbow in rheumatoid arthritis. *J Bone Joint Surg* 64A:1074, 1982.

97. Vahvanen V, Eskola A, Peltonen J: Results of elbow synovectomy in rheumatoid arthritis: *Arch Orthop Trauma Surg* 110:151–154, 1991.

98. White SH, Goodfellow JW, Mowat A: Posterior interosseous nerve palsy in rheumatoid arthritis. *J Bone Joint Surg* 77B:468–474, 1988.

99. Maradei PE: Arthroscopic elbow synovectomy in rheumatoid arthritis. *J Bone Joint Surg* 77B(suppl 2):143–144, 1995.

99a. Jacobsen ST, Levinson JE, Crawford AH: Late results of synovectomy in juvenile rheumatoid arthritis. *J Bone Joint Surg* 67A:8–15, 1985.

100. Vuspaa V: Anatomical interposition arthroplasty with dermal graft: A study of 51 elbow arthroplasties on 48 rheumatoid patients. *Zeitschr Rheumatol* 46:132–135, 1987.

101. Ewald FC, Scheinberg RD, Thomas WH, et al: Capitellocondylar elbow arthroplasty. *J Bone Joint Surg* 62A:1259–1263, 1980.

102. Dee R: Reconstructive surgery following failed total elbow endoprosthesis. *Clin Orthop* 170:196–203, 1982.

103. Morrey BF, Bryan RS: Complications of total elbow arthroplasty. *Clin Orthop* 170:204–219, 1982.

104. Ewald FC, Simmons ED, Sullivan JA, et al: Capitellocondylar total elbow replacement in rheumatoid arthritis. *J Bone Joint Surg* 75A:498–507, 1993.

105. Trancick T, Wilde AH, Borden LS: Capitellocondylar total elbow arthroplasty. *Clin Orthop* 223:175–180, 1987.

106. Weiland AJ, Weiss APC, Willis RP, Moore JR: Capitellocondylar total elbow replacement: A long term follow-up study. *J Bone Joint Surg* 71A:217–222, 1989.

107. Ruth JT, Wilde AH: Capitellocondylar total elbow replacement: A long term follow-up study. *J Bone Joint Surg* 74A:95–100, 1992.

108. King GJW, Itoi E, Niebur GL, et al: Motion and laxity of the capitellar condylar total elbow prosthesis. *J Bone Joint Surg* 76A:1000–1007, 1994.

109. Burnett R, Rye IS, Souter W: Souter-Strathclyde arthroplasty of the rheumatoid elbow. *Acta Orthop Scand* 62A:52–54, 1991.

110. Lyall HA, Cohen B, Clatworthy M, Constant CR: Results of the Souter-Strathclyde total elbow arthroplasty in patients with rheumatoid arthritis. *J Arthrop* 9:279–284, 1994.

111. Kudo H, Iwano K: Total elbow arthroplasty with a non-constrained surface replacement prosthesis in patients who have rheumatoid arthritis. *J Bone Joint Surg* 72A:355–362, 1990.

112. Friedman RJ, Ewald FC: Arthroplasty of the ipsilateral shoulder and elbow in patients who have rheumatoid arthritis. *J Bone Joint Surg* 69A:661–666, 1987.

113. Inglis AE, Pellici PN: Total elbow replacement. *J Bone Joint Surg* 62A:1252–1258, 1980.

114. Pritchard RW: Long-term follow-up study of semi-constrained elbow prosthesis. *Orthopedics* 4:151–155, 1981.

115. Morrey BF, Adams RA: Semi-constrained arthroplasty for the treatment of rheumatoid arthritis of the elbow. *J Bone Joint Surg* 74A:479–490, 1992.

116. O'Driscoll SW, An KN, Korines S: Kinematics of semi-constrained total elbow arthroplasty. *J Bone Joint Surg* 74B:297–299, 1992.

117. Kraay MJ, Figgie MP, Inglis AE, et al: Primary semi-constrained total elbow arthroplasty. *J Bone Joint Surg* 74A:479–490, 1992.

118. Bryan RS, Morrey BF: Extensive posterior exposure of the elbow: A triceps sparing approach. *Clin Orthop* 166:188–192, 1982.

119. Wolfe SW, Ranawat CS: The osteoanconeus flap. *J Bone Joint Surg* 72A:684–688, 1990.

120. Wolfe SW, Figgie MP, Inglis AE, et al: Management of infection about total elbow prosthesis. *J Bone Joint Surg* 72A:199–212, 1990.

121. Morrey BF, Adams RA, Bryan R: Total replacement for post-traumatic arthritis of the elbow. *J Bone Joint Surg* 73B:607–612, 1991.

122. Figgie HE III, Inglis AE, Ranawat CS, Rosenberg GM: Results of total elbow arthroplasty as a salvage procedure for failed elbow reconstructive operations. *Clin Orthop* 219:185–193, 1985.

123. Fonlkes GD, Mitsunaga MM: Allograft salvage of failed total elbow arthroplasty. *Clin Orthop* 296:113–117, 1993.

124. Kay RM, Eckardt JJ: Total elbow allograft for twice failed total elbow arthroplasty. *Clin Orthop* 303:135–139, 1994.

125. Figgie MP, Inglis AE, Mow C, Figgie HE III: Salvage of nonunion of supracondylar fracture of the humerus by total elbow arthroplasty. *J Bone Joint Surg* 71A:1058–1065, 1989.

126. Figgie MP, Inglis AE, Mow CS, et al: Results of reconstruction for failed total elbow arthroplasty. *Clin Orthop* 253:123–132, 1990.

127. Morrey BF, Bryan RS: Infection after total elbow arthroplasty. *J Bone Joint Surg* 65A:330–338, 1983.

128. Figgie MP, Inglis AP, Mow CS, Figgie HE: Total elbow arthroplasty for complete ankylosis of the elbow. *J Bone Joint Surg* 71A:513–520, 1989.

129. McAuliffe JA, Burkhalter WE, Ouellette EA, Carneiro FS: Compression plate arthrodesis of the elbow. *J Bone Joint Surg* 74B:300–304, 1992.

130. Snider WJ, DeWitt HJ: Functional studies for optimum position for elbow arthrodesis on ankylosis. *J Bone Joint Surg* 55A:1305, 1973.

131. O'Neal OR, Morrey BF, Tanaka S, An KA: Compensatory motion in the upper extremity after elbow arthrodesis. *Clin Orthop* 281:89–96, 1992.

132. Hogh J, Ludlam CA, Macnicol MF: Hemophilic arthropathy of the upper limb. *Clin Orthop* 218:215–231, 1985.

133. Smith MA, Savidge GF: Fountain EJ: Interposition arthroplasty in the management of advanced haemophilic arthropathy of the elbow. *J Bone Joint Surg* 65B:436–440, 1983.

134. Butler-Manuel PA, Smith MA, Savidge GF: Silastic interposition for hemophilic arthropathy of the elbow. *J Bone Joint Surg* 72B:472–474, 1990.

135. Kaye L, Stainsby D, Buzzard B, et al: The role of synovectomy in the management of recurrent hemarthrosis of hemophilia. *Br J Hematol* 49:53, 1981.

136. Gilchrest GS: Hematologic arthritis, in Morrey BF (ed): *The Elbow and Its Disorders.* Philadelphia, Saunders, 1985, pp 674–681.

137. Gilchrest GS, Espinoza IR, Spillburg I, Osterland CK: Joint manifestations of sickle cell disease. *Medicine* 53:295, 1974.

138. Patte GA, Snyder SJ: Synovial chondromatosis of the acromioclavicular joint. *Clin Orthop* 233:205–207, 1988.

139. Milgran JW, Hadesman WM: Synovial chondromatosis in the subacromial bursa. *Clin Orthop* 236:154–159, 1987.

140. Milgram JN: Synovial osteochondromatosis. *J Bone Joint Surg* 59A:792, 1977.

The Hand

CHAPTER 57

Congenital Anomalies of the Hand and Upper Extremity

Melvin P. Rosenwasser and Gina C. Del Savio

In order to study this diverse group of conditions, the International Federation of Hand Societies adopted a classification of limb anomalies based on anatomic and embryologic defects. The classification, outlined by Swanson in the first issue of the *Journal of Hand Surgery,*[1] cites seven major groups: (1) failure of formation of parts, (2) failure of separation of parts, (3) duplication, (4) overgrowth (gigantism), (5) undergrowth (hypoplasia), (6) congenital constriction bands, and (7) generalized skeletal abnormalities.

To develop an appropriate treatment plan for any of these conditions, a thorough understanding of the neuromuscular development of the upper extremity is necessary, such that the proper staging for reconstruction will be integrated into the overall maturation of the child's skills. Most child behaviorists and hand surgeons believe that the hand functions of grasp, release, and pinch are well integrated by the first year and that further refinement, coordination, and control continue into the fourth year. Thumb reconstruction, therefore, is performed at 1 year of age, or when the child is large enough to safely undergo general anesthesia. Earlier surgery may be called for in cases where the deformity is progressive and will alter longitudinal growth if allowed to continue, as with thumb-index syndactyly.

The cause is unknown in more than 50 percent of congenital limb deformities, with the remaining half divided among environmental factors, genetic factors, or a combination of the two. An understanding of the etiology of congenital limb abnormalities is necessary in order to facilitate recognition of possible other organ system abnormalities. It is well established that thalidomide, coumadin, and dilantin are capable of causing limb defects.[2] Genetic factors such as chromosomal errors and inheritance play a major role in determining extremity anomalies. Trisomy 21 (Down's syndrome), trisomy 18, and trisomy 13 are associated with syndactyly, polydactyly, clinodactyly, and camptodactyly. Single gene defects may also cause congenital limb abnormalities such as brachydactly, syndactyly, and camptodactyly through dominant or recessive autosomal inheritance patterns or by sex-linked gene defects.

Acrocephalosyndactyly (Apert's syndrome) is an example of an autosomally dominant transmitted condition, while thrombocytopenia–absent radius syndrome (TAR), which presents with radial clubhand, is an example of an autosomally recessive transmitted condition. When discussing with the parents the risk of sibling deformity, one must emphasize that the risk of recurrence varies with the mode of transmission. A thorough organ system review by the pediatrician to assess corollary systemic anomalies (heart, kidney, hematopoietic) is necessary prior to any reconstructive surgery.

ARM ABNORMALITIES

The shoulder may be involved in congenital defects such as congenital amputation, phocomelia, and arthrogryposis. Upper limb amputations are extremely rare, with a frequency of 1 in 270,000 live births. When amputation is complete, prosthetic rehabilitation is the sole therapeutic option in most cases. Longitudinal deficiencies such as phocomelia yield an extremely short limb. Phocomelia is seen in only 0.8 percent of congenital anomalies but has most often been related to the mother's ingestion of thalidomide. Historically, these deficiencies were treated with prostheses; however, advances in the use of distraction osteogenesis have permitted reconstruction of diminutive extremities.[3–5] The goal of such lengthening varies with the amount and location of the shortening as well as the number and quality of mobile joints. Prosthetic rehabilitation can be performed successfully even in the young child and should not be delayed if this is the treatment of choice. Introduction of such devices past the age of 3 to 5 years will not allow integration for bimanual activities and the child will reject the prosthesis.

The most common congenital anomaly around the elbow is radial head dislocation, with an incidence of 0.16 percent.[6] While most cases are idiopathic, an autosomal recessive familial form has been reported.[7] The dislocation can be anterior, posterior, or lateral. Two-thirds are posterior, with the remainder equally divided between anterior and lateral.

Traditional teaching has been that to be congenital the condition had to be bilateral; however, recent studies report isolated unilateral cases of congenital radial head dislocations.[6,8] The differential diagnosis includes traumatic radial head dislocation, relative shortening of the ulna, and relative lengthening of the radius. Many associated conditions that demonstrate a short ulna may predispose to radial head dislocations.

Ulnar deficiency, multiple exostosis, radioulnar synostoses, and multiple enchondromatosis are only a few conditions that may present with a dislocated radial head. Recognition of a dome-shaped radial head with a long narrow neck, and relative radius lengthening as well as the appropriate history may aid in diagnosis.[6] Capitellar hypoplasia may also be seen but is not a consistent finding. Radial head dislocation leads to a mild to moderate loss of motion at the elbow, with most loss seen in rotation. Surgery is indicated for pain, limited mobility, and cosmesis. While reconstructive procedures are not recommended in childhood, radial head excision may be performed at skeletal maturity for cosmesis, but it will not increase forearm pronosupination.

Congenital radioulnar synostosis of the elbow is a rare but disabling condition when it is complete, especially so when it is bilateral, which it is in 60 percent of the cases.[9] There is no genetic inheritance pattern for this defect, but males have a 2:1 greater incidence, and the anomaly occurs with greater frequency in patients with sex chromosome abnormalities.[9] One-third of synostoses is associated with other congenital anomalies involving all major organ systems as well as generalized skeletal anomalies such as congenital hip dislocation and clubfoot.

Derotational osteotomies have been used to position one forearm (nondominant) into mild supination to aid perineal care and to decrease the pronation deformity in the other forearm (dominant) to neutral or slight pronation.[10]

HAND ABNORMALITIES

The incidence of congenital hand deformities is difficult to ascertain because of the heterogeneity of the population subgroups. Recent figures from the Centers for Disease Control in Atlanta, Georgia,[2] reveal that approximately 1 out of every 1000 live births demonstrates a congenital deformity. Relative incidence as studied by Flatt[11] in a series from Iowa showed syndactyly, polydactyly, camptodactyly, clinodactyly, and radial agenesis to be the five most frequent diagnoses, which accounted for 50 percent of the total. Because the scope of this topic far exceeds the limits of presentation, only these five most common hand deformities are discussed.

Syndactyly

Syndactyly is one of the most common congenital hand deformities, with a frequency of 0.5 to 0.9 in 1000 live births.[2] Of all cases of syndactyly, 20 percent are inherited. If syndactyly is an isolated finding, it is inherited in an au-

tosomally dominant fashion[2] with an incidence of 1 in 200 to 2500 births.[12] It is classified as complex if structures such as nail, bone, tendon, nerve, or blood vessels are conjoined and as simple if only a skin bridge exists. Syndactyly is also classified in terms of its extent: complete if the process extends to the tip of the digit and incomplete if the syndactylization is less.[10]

The most common site is the interspace of the long and ring fingers, followed by the interspace of the ring and little fingers, and then that of the index and long fingers. The thumb-index interspace is rarely involved in isolated cases of syndactyly, but is involved with associated anomalies, such as Apert's syndrome.

Treatment of this condition depends upon its complexity, extension, and location.[12] Division of border digits is done early to prevent progressive angular deformity. Dorsal and volar flaps are raised to resurface the commissures and reestablish the proper web depth and slope. The anatomic constraint to the amount of deepening is the bifurcation of the proper digital arteries. The lateral sides of the separated fingers can only be partially surfaced with the flaps because of the increased surface area of the separate digits, which always require a skin graft. There is an unknown but definite incidence of recurrence of web contracture secondary to longitudinal growth and the contraction of the skin graft. However, in division of simple syndactylies, a normal cosmetic and functional result is to be expected.

Polydactyly

Polydactyly is a very common entity classified by Temtamy and McKusick[13] as follows:

Postaxial
Type A: extra well-formed ulnar digit articulating with a metacarpal
Type B: extra poorly formed ulnar digit, often a skin tag
Preaxial
  Type 1: thumb polydactyly
  Type 2: triphalangeal thumb polydactyly
  Type 3: index polydactyly
  Type 4: polysyndactyly

Genetic transmission of polydactyly differs by its classification: preaxial, sporadic (except for triphalangeal thumbs, which are either autosomal dominant or recessive); central, autosomal dominant; and postaxial, autosomal dominant. The incidence of preaxial polydactyly is 0.08 in 1000 live births, with a predilection for American Indians.[14] The male-to-female ratio is 2.5 to 1. In contrast, one-third of patients with central polydactyly has associated foot anomalies. Postaxial polydactyly differs in that it is less common in Caucasians but more common in blacks, with an incidence of 10.4 per 1000 live births in South Africa. It is also more frequently associated with other organ system anomalies, especially in Caucasians.

Thumb polydactyly has been further classified by Wassel into seven types, according to the level of duplication.[16] Fifty percent of thumb duplications are type IV, which is a duplication of both phalanges and a common metacarpal. In general, it is best to ablate the radial (rudimentary) thumb, but a careful preoperative evaluation will determine which duplicate should be preserved. If the duplication is a triphalangeal thumb, it is most frequently ablated with maximal utilization of bone, skin, and nail matrix to reconstruct the adjacent thumb. It is important to recognize that the remaining thumb must be rebalanced following ablation of the supernumerary digit. The tendon insertions, collateral ligaments, and capsule must be restored or a late collapsing zig-zag deformity will result.[17]

Most fifth-digit duplications (postaxial) are merely skin tags (type B), versus the rare type A (well formed with articulation). Central duplications of the index, middle, or ring fingers are usually complex duplications of the distal and middle phalanges. Postaxial duplication is usually easier to treat, and simple ablation for the skin tag or more formal tissue rearrangement for complete duplication should be performed in the operating suite when the child is around 1 year of age.

CAMPTODACTYLY

Seen in 1 out of 1000 live births with a sporadic inheritance pattern, camptodactyly, or bent finger, is frequently seen involving the proximal interphalangeal joint (PIP) of the fifth finger. The deformity has a bimodal distribution, appearing in either infancy (84 percent) or adolescence (16 percent). It is progressive in 80 percent of the cases and can be functionally limiting when contracture of the PIP joint approaches 90° of flexion. Two-thirds of the cases are bilateral, with a flexion contracture of the PIP joint and compensatory extension of the metacarpophalangeal joint.

The cause is unknown, but a rudimentary or absent intrinsic extensor mechanism has been implicated. At initial evaluation, possible trauma or juvenile aponeurotic fibromatosis as the cause must be ruled out. Trauma can injure the dorsal extensor mechanism, causing a boutonniere deformity, while juvenile aponeurotic fibromatosis involves palmar fascia and skin, creating a flexion deformity.

Conservative treatment of camptodactyly consists of static and dynamic splinting. Patient compliance is critical for success. Surgical treatment of camptodactyly is reserved for severe progressive deformities that have failed conservative treatment because of the loss of joint flexion that occurs after surgical intervention.[18] Releases of the joint capsule, collateral ligaments, volar plate, and flexor digitorum superficialis as well as z-plasty of the skin with skin graft should be followed with static and dynamic splinting and early mobilization. Simultaneous transfers should be avoided so that early mobilization can be achieved. Even in severe cases, no series has proven that soft tissue releases do better than splinting in the long term.[18] In skeletally mature individuals with fixed deformities, a dorsal closing wedge osteotomy is preferred. Excessive straightening may cause nerve or vascular injury and must be avoided.

CLINODACTYLY

Clinodactyly is a bending or curvature in the radioulnar plane usually seen with the fingertip curved toward the midline.[10] Clinodactyly has often been said to be a normal variant with a gentle curvature being present in up to 20 percent of children. Rarely, this curvature is caused by a delta phalanx with progressive angular deformity in an autosomally dominant inheritance pattern with variable penetrance. Clinodactyly rarely requires treatment, but if a delta phalanx is present, an epiphysiodesis and wedge osteotomy will correct and prevent further deformity. Excision of the delta phalanx may be performed but will lead to excessive shortening of the digit.

RADIAL CLUBHAND

Radial clubhand is a manifestation of radial agenesis with a longitudinal deficiency that may be total or partial. It may involve all or part of the extensor muscle mass, radial carpus, or thumb ray. It occurs in 1 in 30,000 births[19] and may be an isolated anomaly, drug-induced (thalidomide), or associated with cardiac and hematologic disorders such as the Holt-Oram[15], TAR (thrombocytopenia absent radius) or VATER (vertebral anomalies imperforate anus tracheoesophageal fistula and/or renal malformation) syndromes.[2] The treatment is based on the child's functional needs. Indeed the European literature advocates no specific treatment for bilateral cases, especially if a rudimentary thumb is present. Most American authors have advocated early splinting of the radial and palmar flexed hand and subsequent centralization of the carpus over the ulna with secondary thumb reconstruction.[19] This reconstruction may be a distraction lengthening and stabilization if adequate thumb components are present or, more likely, will be an index pollicization, which involves a local vascularized transposition with a restoration of thenar intrinsic function. This reconstruction works very well if the index to be pollicized is itself not too hypoplastic. New microsurgical procedures—for example, transplantation of toe to thumb—have provided additional ways of allowing active prehension and longitudinal growth through viable epiphyses.[20,21] Elbow mobility is a prerequisite for centralization procedures for radial clubhand to ensure that hand-to-mouth feeding activities are possible. Centralization or radialization will not always prevent a recurrence. When radial deviation recurs, a wrist arthrodesis may be necessary at skeletal maturity.

LESS COMMON CONGENITAL DEFORMITIES

The above five diagnoses account for one-half of the patients in Flatt's[11] series. The remaining half is represented by less common diagnoses but require the same thoughtful evaluation of functional requirements before any surgical exercise is contemplated. Congenital trigger thumb is easily diagnosed, and treatment can yield a normal hand. Many of the hypoplastic syndromes, including annular congenital bands, may require digital lengthenings via transposition or distraction. It is clear that joint mobility, sensibility, and bilaterality are important determinants of whether the patient will be able to use the reconstructed limb. Each patient is unique, and no algorithm can be fashioned to treat all children with the same diagnosis. Photographs of the end results will often prepare parents and child for what can be realistically expected from reconstruction.

One day, with prenatal screening, in utero imaging, and or manipulation both surgical and genetic, we may be able to intercede and correct these limb anomalies before birth, thus obviating often imperfect reconstruction.

REFERENCES

1. Swanson AB: A classification for congenital limb malformations. *J Hand Surg* 1:8–22, 1976.
2. Goldberg MF, Bartoshesky KE: Congenital hand anomaly: Etiology and associated malformations. *Hand Clin* 1:405–415, 1985.
3. Cattaneo R, Villa A, Catagni MA, Bell D: Lengthening of the humerus using the Ilizarov technique. *Clin Orthop* 250:117–124, 1990.
4. Villa A, Paley D, Catagni MA, et al: Lengthening of the forearm by the Ilizarov technique. *Clin Orthop* 250:125–137, 1990.
5. Matev IB: Thumb reconstruction in children through metacarpal lengthening. *Plast Reconstr Surg* 64:665–669, 1979.
6. Agnew DK, Davis RJ: Congenital unilateral dislocation of the radial head. *J Pediatr Orthop* 13:526–528, 1993.
7. Gunn DR, Pillay ZK: Congenital dislocation of the head of the radius. *Clin Orthop* 34:108–113, 1964.
8. Wiley JJ, Loehr J, McIntyre W: Isolated dislocation of the radial head. *Orthop Rev* 20:973–976, 1991.
9. Simmons BP, Southmayd WW, Riseborough EJ: Congenital radioulnar synostosis. *J Hand Surg* 8A:829–838, 1983.
10. Dobyns JH, Wood VE, Bayne LG: Congenital hand deformities, in Green DP (ed): *Operative Hand Surgery.* New York, Churchill Livingstone, 1993, pp 251–548.
11. Flatt AE: *The Care of Congenital Hand Anomalies.* St. Louis, Mosby, 1977.
12. Eaton CJ, Lister GD: Syndactyly. *Hand Clin* 6:555–575, 1990.
13. Temtamy SA, McKusick V: Polydactyly. *Birth Defects* 3:125–184, 1969.
14. Simmons BP: Polydactyly. *Hand Clin* 1:545–563, 1985.
15. Holt M, Onam S: Familial heart disease with skeletal malformations. *Br Heart J* 22:336–342, 1960.
16. Wassel HD: The results of surgery for polydactyly of the thumb: A review. *Clin Orthop* 64:175–193, 1969.
17. Marks TW, Bayne LG: Polydactyly of the thumb: Abnormal anatomy and treatment. *J Hand Surg* 3:107–116, 1978.
18. Siegert JJ, Cooney WP, Dobyns JH: Management of simple camptodactyly. *J Hand Surg* 15B:181–189, 1990.
19. Lamb DW: Radial clubhand. *J Bone Joint Surg* 59A:1–13, 1977.
20. Buncke HJ: Toe digital transfer. *Clin Plast Surg* 3:49–57, 1976.
21. Buncke HJ, McLean DH, George PT, et al: Thumb replacement: Great toe transplantation by microvascular anastomosis. *Br J Plast Surg* 26:194–201, 1973.

CHAPTER 58

Rheumatoid Disorders of the Hand and Wrist

Jerry L. Ellstein and James W. Strickland

The primary target of rheumatoid arthritis in the hand and wrist is the synovium of tendons and joints. Chronic involvement of peritendinous and periarticular tissues results in the loss of capsular and ligamentous support, joint instability, contractures, and functional impairment. All tissues may be affected, including skin and local blood vessels, the latter leading to secondary vasculitis and Raynaud's phenomenon. Muscle involvement may produce wasting, contracture, and weakness.

Synovial proliferation in the form of tenosynovitis about tendons and pannus formation in the joints of the hand and wrist results in hyperemia, increased fluid production, and thickening of the synovial joint lining. Tendons may be eroded, attenuated, or ruptured by direct synovial invasion, by ischemic changes created by pressure within compartments—such as the flexor tendon sheath in the palm and digit, under the extensor retinaculum, and within the carpal canal—or by erosion from bony spurs created by the invasive disease process. Joint changes ultimately occur in the many diarthrodial joints of the hand and wrist. The earliest changes occur at the joint margins, where synovial reflections are located. Synovial proliferation results in increased fluid production and joint pressure, which reduce cartilage nutrition. Direct invasion of the cartilage by pannus formation also contributes to the loss of the normal smooth joint surface. Capsular and ligamentous support is slowly lost because of chronic distension and direct invasion. Ultimately deformities occur that are characterized by erosions, periarticular osteoporosis, and cyst and spur formation, leading to joint destruction, collapse, subluxation, dislocation, fibrous adhesions, or ankylosis.

Rheumatoid nodules (granulomas), which consist of fibrinoid necrosis, cellular debris, and monocytes, are probably secondary to small vessel vasculitis and are frequently located over the extensor surface of the elbow and the dorsum of the digits. Vasculitis with injury to vessel intima may also be the cause of Raynaud's phenomenon and peripheral neuropathy. Chronic myositis leads to muscular atrophy, weakness, and contracture, with lymphocyte accumulation in the tissues.

No one area of the hand or wrist is immune to the effects of rheumatoid arthritis. A wide variety of dysfunction and deformity may develop, and, although certain recurring patterns are said to be characteristic of the disease, the clinical presentation is highly variable. The particular deformity that develops is dependent on the site, intensity, and duration of the synovitis and may often result in neighboring digits exhibiting different deformities.

CLINICAL DIAGNOSIS AND EXAMINATION

Examination of the hands and wrists reveals increased warmth over affected joints, tenderness, swelling, and palmar erythema. Synovitis presenting as boggy swelling over joints and fullness of the flexor tendon sheaths or dorsum of the wrist is both visible and palpable. Rheumatoid nodules occur in 20 percent of patients. Decreased muscle strength with atrophy frequently accompanies joint involvement and may lead to progressive loss of motion and deformity.

Table 58-1 lists the more common deformities that develop in the hand and wrist in rheumatoid arthritis. Instability or collapse of a single joint may have an untoward effect on the entire balance of the hand. As Landsmeer has shown, the collapse of an intercalated segment of the osseous chain of the hand produces, at contiguous segments, deformity that is often opposite in direction and of equal severity.[41] For example, in the rheumatoid hand, palmar subluxation and ulnar translocation of the carpus result in radial deviation and dorsal displacement of the metacarpals and ulnar deviation and flexion of the digits. Similarly, lateral dislocation of the base of the first metacarpal secondary to basilar joint disease leads to adduction of the first ray hyperextension of the metacarpophalangeal (MCP) joint and reciprocal hyperflexion of the interphalangeal (IP) joint. Correction or stabilization of impending deformity of a joint whose collapse may initiate a multilevel deformity is one of the important considerations for the management of rheumatoid arthritis affecting the wrist and hand.

Sensory and motor neuropathy presenting as carpal tunnel syndrome frequently occurs due to vasculitis of the vasa nervorum or from entrapment resulting from the increased volume produced by flexor tenosynovitis in the carpal canal. Rheumatoid patients should be specifically questioned about symptoms of carpal tunnel syndrome, as this may be an easily overlooked cause of hand discomfort.

Tendon ruptures are not infrequent and may be secondary to attrition over bony spurs or from direct invasion by the diseased synovium (Fig. 58-1). Extensor tendon ruptures (Vaughan-Jackson syndrome) most often involve the common extensors to the fourth and fifth digits and the extensor digiti quinti in association with the caput ulnae syndrome, in which the tendons are eroded over the dorsally prominent distal ulna. The extensor pollicis longus may rupture at Lister's tubercle when it becomes eroded by the rheumatoid process. Involvement of flexor tendons may produce triggering or loss of digital motion; chronic tenosynovial invasion may result in attenuation or rupture of the profundus or superficialis tendons or both. Rupture may also result from attrition over palmar carpal bony irregularities (Mannerfelt syndrome) and most commonly involves the flexor pollicis longus, which ruptures over a prominent trapezial ridge.

Radiographs of the hands and wrists early on may show soft tissue swelling, periarticular osteoporosis, joint space narrowing, and bony erosions. Late findings include progression of the bony erosions from the joint margins to complete joint surface destruction and articular incongruity. Ulnar styloid erosions are characteristic. As the dis-

---

TABLE 58-1 Common Deformities and Tendon Involvement in Rheumatoid Arthritis of the Hand and Wrist

---

Hand deformities

Swan-neck—digits and thumb
Boutonniere—digits and thumb
Joint subluxations
Joint dislocations
Ulnar deviation of digits (ulnar drift)
Radial deviation of the hand
Volar subluxation and supination of the hand and wrist with apparent
  dorsal subluxation of the distal ulna
Digital flexion contractures
Ankylosed joints
Unstable or floppy joints
Stiff joints

Tendon involvement

Vaughan-Jackson syndrome (rupture of extensors to ring and/or small fingers)
Caput ulnae syndrome
Rupture of extensor pollicis longus
Ruptured wrist extensors associated with volar wrist subluxation and dislocation
Subluxation or dislocation of the extensor carpi ulnaris
Extensor tenosynovitis
Triggering digit, palm, wrist
Flexor tenosynovitis
Digital or flexor tendon ruptures (Mannerfelt's syndrome)
Nerve involvement
Carpal tunnel syndrome
Posterior interosseous syndrome
Cubital tunnel syndrome

---

ease progresses, loss of joint space, subluxations, and dislocations can be expected to follow. Partial or complete carpal coalition is seen in advanced cases and in juvenile rheumatoid arthritis. Loss of bone stock with digital short-ening and telescoping may be seen in the advanced stages of arthritis mutilans and in psoriatic arthritis. Bone erosion, often associated with tendon rupture, includes the distal ulna, trapezial ridge, and Lister's tubercle.

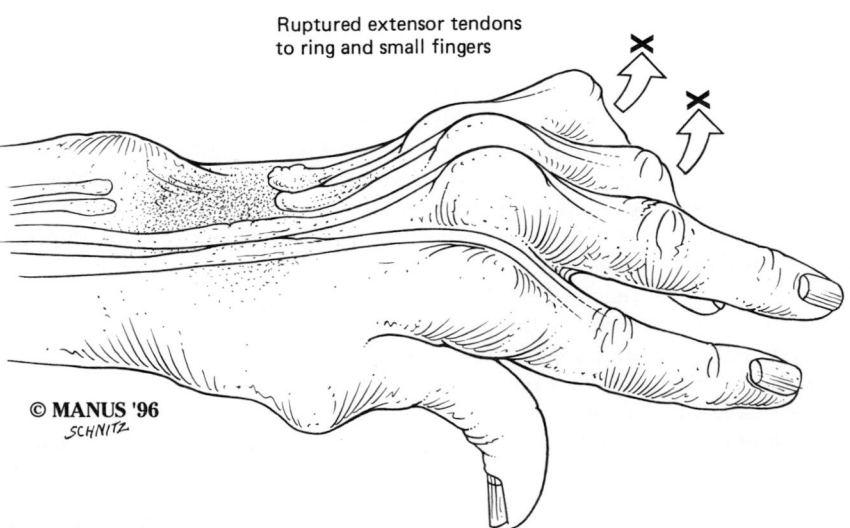

Ruptured extensor tendons
to ring and small fingers

© MANUS '96
SCHNITZ

Figure 58-1 Tendon ruptures are not infrequent occurrences in rheumatoid arthritis. Extensor tendon ruptures (Vaughan-Jackson syndrome[76]) most often involve the common extensors to the fourth and fifth digits and the extensor digiti quinti. This most often occurs in association with the caput ulnae syndrome, in which the tendons are eroded over the dorsally prominent distal ulna. (Reprinted with permission of the Indiana Hand Center.)

TREATMENT

Nonsurgical Treatment

Nonsurgical treatment of rheumatoid arthritis consists of medical management of the disease, including the use of salicylates, steroids, gold injections, antimalarial and immunosuppressant drugs, occasional and judicious use of steroid injections, and an individualized therapy program. The hand therapist can be helpful to patients with rheumatoid arthritis in all stages of disease. Splinting programs may be designed to rest joints, strengthen the hand, provide assistance or modification of the use of the hand in activities of daily living, assist in the evaluation and treatment of individual patient needs, and provide the means to maintain or improve joint motion and strength. It is unlikely, however, that splinting will prevent the development of deformity in patients with chronic and progressive rheumatoid involvement.

Surgical Considerations in the Rheumatoid Patient

The goals of hand surgery in the rheumatoid patient are to help control the medically resistant inflammatory process and to either preserve function prior to the onset of deformity or restore function and correct established deformity. This is accomplished by procedures designed to excise chronic synovial accumulations and reestablish joint alignment, congruity, and stability. The surgeon must carefully evaluate static stability, dynamic stability, and motor balance while recognizing that surgery cannot eliminate the underlying systemic disease and that many procedures may be more palliative than curative. Surgery can be helpful in rheumatoid patients who have severe pain, chronic synovitis unresponsive to medical treatment, tendon ruptures, nerve entrapment, and deformities associated with compromised hand function. Surgical candidates should be well motivated and healthy enough to undergo surgery and the postoperative rehabilitation program. Patients must thoroughly understand the specific goals of surgery and the expected result. Although multiple surgical procedures may be combined at one operation, it is occasionally impossible to complete all indicated procedures at one sitting due to the time constraints or to noncomplementary requirements of postoperative therapy. The patient must be aware of the possible need for additional surgery.

Finally, the timing of hand surgical procedures for the rheumatoid patient must be carefully planned, with consideration of the patient's needs for reconstructive surgery in other anatomic sites. Preference is usually given to lower extremity reconstruction in view of the excessive demands that may be placed on the hands by the need to use crutches and other walking aids. The status of the shoulders and elbows must also be considered. A functionally reconstructed hand will do the patient little good if he or she cannot adequately position it in space.

Operative procedures for the hand and wrist should be individually designed for each patient dependent upon the stage of disease and functional limitations present.

Surgery should not be reserved for the severely deformed hand. Often, better functional preservation or restoration may be provided for a longer period of time if surgical intervention is performed earlier in the course of the disease. Procedures that can help preserve function and relieve pain prior to the onset of deformity include synovectomy, nerve decompression, trigger-finger release, and intrinsic releases. Additional procedures that can be used to help restore function after the onset of deformity include soft tissue reconstruction of joints and tendons, arthroplasty, arthrodesis, and combinations of these techniques.

THE RHEUMATOID WRIST

Initial involvement of the wrist in rheumatoid arthritis is unusual, with the hand affected five times more frequently. However, with time and continuance of the disease, synovitis affects the hand and wrist in most cases. While the characteristic digital deformities that occur in rheumatoid arthritis, including ulnar drift and swan-neck deformities, are not directly the result of rheumatoid wrist collapse, wrist deformity may contribute to their development, worsen preexistent deformity, and compromise surgical correction. Therefore, it is recommended to treat the wrist imbalance prior to or simultaneous with the treatment of finger deformities.

The carpus is suspended in position by ligamentous attachments to both volar radial and dorsal ulnar aspects of the distal radius, including the ulnocarpal complex. Additional wrist stability is provided by the two radial wrist extensors and a single ulnar wrist extensor tendon. The radial ligamentous sling stabilizes the lateral carpal column (scaphoid) and the ulnar sling supports the medial carpal column (triquetrum). Synovitis of the carpus in the closed extensor compartments of the wrist and in the carpal tunnel may locally invade and weaken the ligamentous and tendinous support of the wrist joint.

Development of Deformities

On the radial side of the wrist, attenuation of the deep radioscapholunate of Testut and radioscaphocapitate ligaments causes instability of the scaphoid proximal pole, leading to rotary subluxation of the scaphoid and scapholunate dissociation. This produces radiocarpal shortening and contributes to a radial shift of the metacarpals when accompanied by the changes occurring in the ulnar aspect of the wrist. On the ulnar side of the wrist, synovitis attacks the ligamentous support, including the triangular fibrocartilage that extends from the dorsum of the ulna to the volar wrist capsule. The disease also results in attenuation of the ulnolunate and ulnotriquetral ligaments. Palmar collapse of the ulnar carpus follows, producing a relative supination of the carpus and an increased metacarpal descent. This palmar displacement and supination of the carpus creates a prominent appearance of the distal ulna, which may actually be in its normal anatomic position. Synovitis affecting the distal radioulnar joint may further contribute to the deformity by producing radioulnar dissociation and a true dorsal displacement of the ulna. The distal radioulnar joint becomes painful because of persisting synovitis and crepitus, and the condition has been referred to as the *caput ulnae syndrome.*

With the loss of radiocarpal height and collapse of the carpus, there is a relative excess length of the distal ulna, causing impingement and pain. The clinical manifestations are pain along the ulnar border of the wrist, mostly with forearm rotation.

As the wrist moves in a volar and relatively supinated position, the extensor carpi ulnaris moves with it, becoming volar to the axis of wrist motion and contributing to further carpal displacement encouraged by the unopposed radial wrist tendons.

Tendon Rupture at the Wrist

Impending rupture may often be recognized by pain along the course of the involved tendon. Apparent tendon rupture, with loss of extension of the metacarpophalangeal joints of the index through small fingers, may mimic true tendon rupture. This phenomenon may be caused by two different problems. The first is subluxation of the extensor tendons from their dorsal, biomechanically efficient location atop the metacarpal heads into the valleys or sulcus between the metacarpal heads, where they become volar to the axis of rotation of the metacarpophalangeal joint and become flexors rather than extensors. Careful examination demonstrates subluxation of the extensor tendons to the ulnar side of the metacarpal shafts, ulnar drift of the digits, or even metacarpophalangeal joint dislocation. A complete loss of extension at the metacarpophalangeal joints does not always accompany extensor tendon rupture because of the presence of tendinous interconnections between the finger extensors known as *juncturae tendinum.* Often, when the juncturae alone extend the metacarpophalangeal joint, extension is weak, painful, or incomplete. The second cause of apparent tendon rupture may be a partial or complete posterior interosseous nerve syndrome secondary to rheumatoid synovitis of the elbow and compression of the motor branch of the radial nerve as it passes through the supinator muscle at the arcade of Frohse.[53] Electrodiagnostic tests may be helpful in making the proper diagnosis, although the tenodesis effect that produces digital extension when the wrist is flexed may help demonstrate that the tendons are intact. Fixed joint deformities that limit tendon excursion may also compromise the ability to evaluate tendon integrity clinically.

Rupture of the extensor pollicis longus may easily be overlooked, since the thumb intrinsics may continue to extend the interphalangeal joint. True extensor pollicis longus function may be tested by placing the affected hand flat on a table with the patient extending or lifting the thumb off the table surface while the examiner palpates the extensor pollicis longus distal to Lister's tubercle.

Surgery for the Rheumatoid Wrist

Indications for surgery include chronic flexor or extensor tenosynovitis and joint synovitis when unresponsive to medical management after 3 to 6 months. Either impending or actual tendon rupture is another indication. Because the results of tendon transfer are inversely proportional to the number of tendon ruptures, prompt diagnosis and early treatment should be carried out. While synovial inflammation may recur following synovectomy, it rarely returns to the extent present preoperatively, and tendon rupture seldom occurs. Without surgical intervention, a single tendon rupture is often followed rather rapidly by additional ruptures. When ruptures have occurred, an early surgery is indicated to correct loss of function, prevent additional ruptures, and preserve joint function.

Carpal tunnel syndrome is frequently seen in association with flexor tenosynovitis. Patients should be questioned specifically about symptoms from median nerve compression in an effort to separate that entity from pain associated with arthritic joints. Carpal tunnel release is a simple procedure that may often provide considerable benefit to the rheumatoid patient. Joint subluxation, dislocation, or painful arthritis may be additional surgical indications in the rheumatoid wrist.

The surgical procedures utilized in the management of the rheumatoid wrist may be divided according to whether they are employed early or late in the course of the disease. Prior to the onset of deformity, the following procedures may be appropriate:

1. Synovectomy of the extensor and flexor tendons
2. Synovectomy of the dorsal and volar carpus
3. Carpal tunnel release
4. Restoration of ruptured tendons
   a. Tendon transfer
   b. End-to-side repair and free tendon graft[50]
5. Wrist rebalancing
   a. Tendon transfer[17]
   b. Dorsal stabilization techniques[40]

After the onset of deformity or late in the course of the disease, procedures that may improve function include:

1. Darrach excision of the distal ulna (or its modifications)[16]
2. Hemiresection arthroplasty of the distal radioulnar joint[10]
3. The Sauvé-Kapandji ulnar pseudarthrosis operation[29,54,73]
4. Total wrist arthroplasty[9,25,37,45,68]
   a. Articulated prosthesis[1]
   b. Flexible implant arthroplasty[1]
5. Wrist arthrodesis[40]
   a. Steinmann pins with[14] or without bone graft (Nalebuff)[47,51]
   b. Compression plate fixation with local and/or iliac bone grafting

THE METACARPOPHALANGEAL JOINT IN RHEUMATOID ARTHRITIS

The metacarpophalangeal joints are the keystones of both the longitudinal and the transverse skeletal arches of the hand.[27] They are frequently the site of intense rheumatoid synovitis, which ultimately results in ulnar deviation of the digits and volar subluxation of the proximal phalanx.[32] Dislocation of the metacarpophalangeal joint is the final stage of this deforming progression, and the consequent disruption of the continuity of the longitudinal arch creates an imbalance of forces, which, in turn, leads to a reciprocal distal joint collapse.

Many authors have implicated various factors that contribute to the deformities that occur at the metacarpophalangeal joint in rheumatoid arthritis. These factors have been categorized by Smith and are listed in Table 58-2.

Surgical Treatment of the Rheumatoid Metacarpophalangeal Joint

In the early stages of disease, before deformity has occurred, synovectomy and soft tissue procedures, including intrinsic transfer and extensor tendon realignment, have been recommended.[1,18,22,38,39,43,45,63,68,78]

The indications for surgical synovectomy of the metacarpophalangeal joint include marked synovial proliferation that has not responded well to systemic treatment, has persisted for at least 6 months, is painful, and appears to be progressing to inevitable deformity. Contraindications include joint destruction with articular erosion, instability, irreducible dislocation, or fixed deformity.[13] Synovectomy has not been uniformly successful and is often disappointing because of the rapid return of diseased synovium. It may, however, offer a satisfactory alternative in carefully selected patients who are early in the course of their disease and have no radiographic changes.[23,44,75] Synovectomy may also be combined with extensor tendon relocation and intrinsic release when indicated.

In the late stages of rheumatoid involvement of the metacarpophalangeal joint, resection-interposition arthroplasty utilizing soft tissue or silicone rubber, rebalancing procedures including extensor relocation, intrinsic release, and transfer or arthrodesis may be indicated.[3]

Replacement arthroplasty of the metacarpophalangeal joint using the Swanson or Niebaur design silicone implants (spacers) remains the gold standard because of more predictable pain relief, motion, and stability. Complications of these procedures include infection, implant fracture, and a progressively decreased range of motion. Although synovial infiltration by silicone particles, cyst formation, and local bone resorption have been described, with silicone implants being most frequently implicated, these occur more commonly with silicone wrist or trapezial implants.[39,43,45]

RHEUMATOID ARTHRITIS OF THE PROXIMAL INTERPHALANGEAL JOINT

The proximal interphalangeal joint of the rheumatoid hand may develop either flexion or hyperextension patterns which are commonly referred to as boutonniere and swan-neck deformities, respectively. Swan-neck deformities, which Bunnell has also called the intrinsic plus deformity,[12] are common, occurring in 28 percent of all patients with rheumatoid arthritis, whereas boutonniere deformities occur in 15 percent.[3] Each deformity may also be associated with lateral displacement or subluxation due to either bone erosion or the loss of soft tissue support. Hand function may be greatly compromised as these deformities increase and become fixed.

Swan-Neck Deformity

Swan-neck deformity is a hyperextension deformity of the proximal interphalangeal joint with a concomitant extensor lag of the distal interphalangeal joint, often associated with some degree of metacarpophalangeal joint flexion (Fig. 58-2). Landsmeer defined this deformity as a terminal imbalance of an intercalated segment in a bimuscular biarticular system.[41] Nalebuff and Millender[60] have developed a system that classifies this deformity into four types based on the flexibility of the proximal interphalangeal joint, the amount of intrinsic tightness, and the radiographic changes (Table 58-3).

Multiple factors may contribute to the development of swan-neck deformity of the proximal interphalangeal joint in rheumatoid arthritis. These factors include intrinsic muscle contracture or adhesion, intrinsic muscle shortening secondary to metacarpophalangeal joint synovitis or contracture, intrinsic muscle shortening secondary to mallet deformity of the distal interphalangeal joint, proximal interphalangeal joint synovitis or effusion, flexor tenosynovitis (wrist, palm, or digital sheath), distal profundus entrapment, extensor tendon contracture or adhesion, collateral ligament contracture or adhesion, palmar plate adhesion to bone, capsular contracture, retinacular ligament contracture or adhesion, bony block, joint fibrosis, ankylosis or articular incongruity, dorsal skin contracture,[60,70] and proximal migration of the carpal-hand unit with the "extrinsic minus" phenomenon resulting in muscle imbalance.[70]

The surgical treatment selected for the management of swan-neck deformity is dependent upon the stage of involvement. Early deformities may be amenable to flexor tenosynovectomy and intrinsic release, while later stages are treated by joint arthrodesis or arthroplasty.[1,38,70,77]

Boutonniere Deformity

Boutonniere deformities exhibit flexion at the proximal interphalangeal joint and hyperextension at the distal interphalangeal joint (Fig. 58-3). To some extent, the deformity may also involve some degree of metacarpophalangeal

**TABLE 58-2 Factors Leading to Deformities
at the Metacarpophalangeal Joints in Rheumatoid Arthritis**

1. Forces normally acting on the hand that may promote unlar deviation of the digits in rheumatoid arthritis
   A. Gravity
   B. Lateral pinch pressure
   C. Power grasp[42]

2. Normal anatomy that may contribute to the ulnar deviation of the finger
   A. Asymmetrical shape of metacarpal heads (smaller sloping ulnar condyle)[32]
   B. Unequal collateral ligament length, and their differing orientation[32]
   C. Asymmetry of the intrinsic muscles to the small finger (hypothenars are stronger than third volar interosseous)

3. Rheumatoid involvement that can lead to ulnar deviation and volar subluxations of the metacarpophalangeal joint
   A. Decreased joint stability due to bony erosions of the metacarpal head and base of proximal phalanx
   B. Attrition and stretching of the collateral ligaments by rheumatoid synovitis, allowing the volarly directed flexor tendon force on the proximal phalanx to go unheeded
   C. Stretching of the accessory collateral ligaments by rheumatoid synovitis, allowing ulnar and palmar displacement of the palmar plate and flexor tendons at the base of the finger
   D. Flexor tenosynovitis, with resultant stretching of the flexor tendon sheath pulley system, resulting in ulnar and volar displacement of the flexor tendons
   E. Ulnar dislocation of the extensor digitorum communis due to attenuation and stretching of the radial sagittal band
   F. Rupture of the extensor digitorum communis, creating an unopposed imbalance at the metacarpophalangeal joint
   G. Contracture of the intrinsic muscles, with volar subluxation and ulnar deviation of the digits
   H. Flexion of the fourth and fifth metacarpal bases with grip
   I. Rheumatoid deformities at the wrist, which contribute to radial deviation at the wrist, which contributes to ulnar deviation of the fingers and increases the ulnar-directed extensor and flexor tendon forces at the metacarpophalangeal joint including
      1. Attenuation of the dorsal-radial support system against the strong palmar-ulnar forces
      2. Increased metacarpal descent associated with volar subluxation of the ulnar carpus
      3. Ulnar translocation of the carpus
      4. Radial deviation of the metacarpals

Source: Reproduced with permission from Smith RJ, Kaplan EB: Rheumatoid deformities of the metacarpophalangeal joints of the finger: A correlative study of anatomy and pathology. *J Bone Joint Surg* 49A:31, 1967.

joint hyperextension, and synovitis is again the initiating factor. Chronic dorsal synovitis with capsular swelling results in a gradual attenuation of the central extensor tendon and the more distal triangular ligament. As the extensor tendon lengthens, there is progressive loss of the ability to actively extend the proximal interphalangeal joint. The lateral bands eventually sublux palmward and lose their mobility. They come to lie volar to the axis of the proximal interphalangeal joint, where they act as flexors instead of extensors of the joint. The lateral bands gradually tighten in their subluxed position and produce a secondary hyperextension deformity of the distal interphalangeal joint.

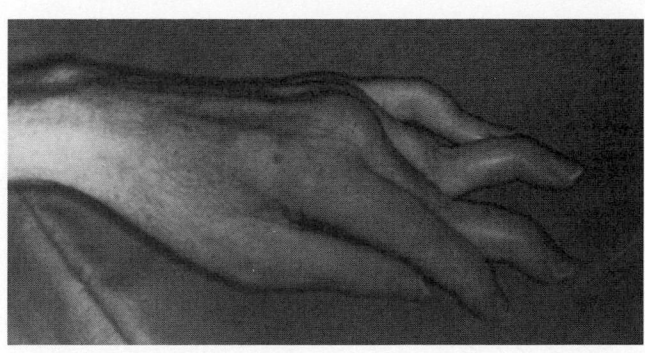

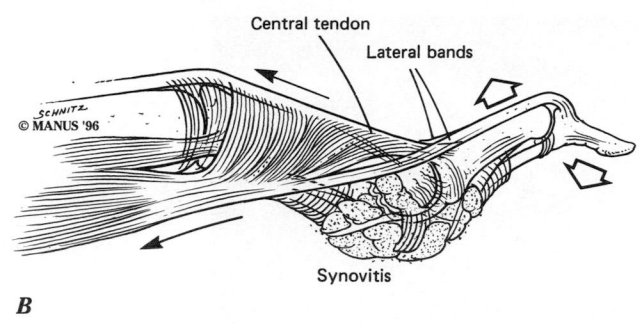

Figure 58.2 Swan-neck deformity in the hand of a patient with rheumatoid arthritis. *A.* Clinical appearance. *B.* Volar synovitis about the proximal interphalangeal joint is one possible cause (see text). (Reprinted with permission of the Indiana Hand Center.)

This terminal hyperextension is further aggravated by shortening of the oblique retinacular ligaments, which further limit active flexion of the distal interphalangeal joint. The retinacular component of the deformity may be demonstrated by extending the proximal interphalangeal joint to its maximum and demonstrating the passive loss of distal joint flexion (intrinsic-intrinsic tightness test). This test may not be entirely reliable in advanced boutonniere deformities, when the shortened and displaced lateral bands produce the same phenomena. As the synovial invasion persists, joint changes ensue, contributing to further stiffness. The metacarpophalangeal joint may become secondarily involved with some degree of compensatory hyperextension, as the extensor tendon, unable to extend the proximal interphalangeal joint, increases its proximal pull at the metacarpophalangeal level. The intrinsic tightness of metacarpophalangeal joint disease, however, may negate this metacarpophalangeal extension influence.

Millender and Nalebuff have developed a classification system, for boutonniere deformities that aids in selecting the proper treatment for each stage of the process (Table 58-4). It should be made clear, however, that the presence of the deformity does not necessarily mean that significantly compromised hand function has occurred.

INVOLVEMENT OF THE DISTAL INTERPHALANGEAL JOINT

Rheumatoid arthritis directly involves the distal interphalangeal joint much less frequently than the proximal two digital joints and must not be confused with coexisting degenerative arthritis involvement. As rheumatoid synovitis erodes the distal finger joint surfaces and atten-

TABLE 58-3 Swan-Neck Deformities

Type	PIP joint flexibility	Treatment
I	Flexible in all positions	Flexor tenosynovectomy
II	Limited with MCP joint extension) (intrinsic tightness)	Flexor tenosynovectomy
III	Limited in all positions of the MCP joint (articular/paraarticular problems)	Arthroplasty, flexible implant, arthrodesis
IV	PIP joint stiff with advanced radiographic changes	Arthroplasty (resection), flexible implant, arthrodesis

Key: PIP, proximal interphalangeal; MCP, metacarpophalangeal.
Source: Reproduced with permission from Nalebuff EA, Millender LH: Surgical treatment of the swan-neck deformity in rheumatoid arthritis. *Orthop Clin North Am* 6:733–752, 1975. And from Kiefhaber TR, Strickland JW: Soft tissue reconstruction for rheumatoid swan-neck and boutonniere deformities: Long-term results. *J Hand Surg* 18A:984–989, 1993.

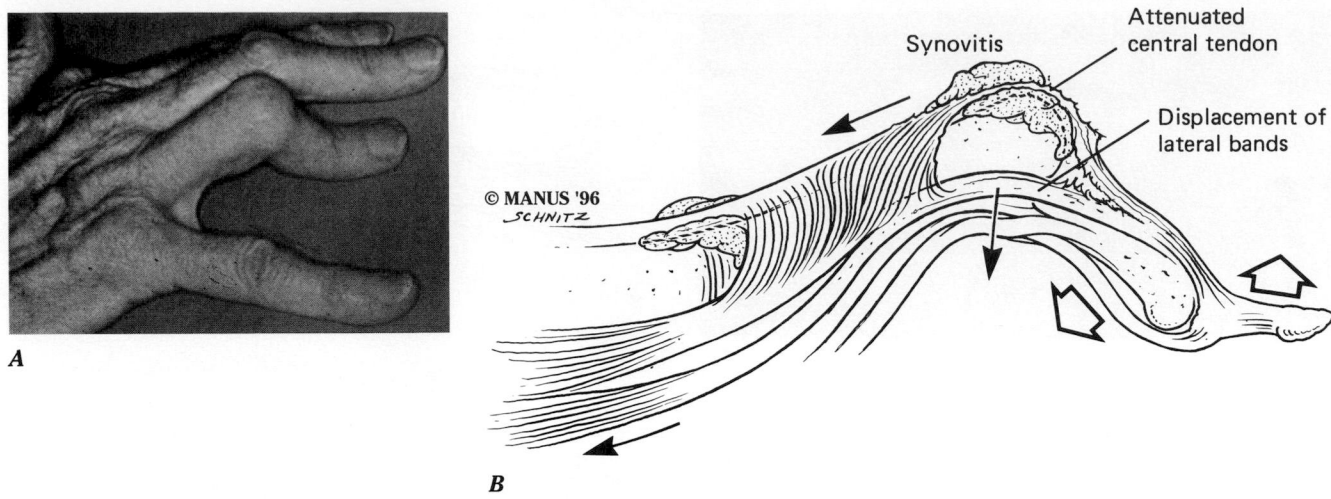

Figure 58.3 Boutonniere deformity in rheumatoid arthritis. *A.* Clinical appearance. *B.* Pathomechanics, showing dorsal synovitis with central slip attenuation and displacement of lateral bands. (Reprinted with permission of the Indiana Hand Center.)

uates the capsule and ligaments about the joint, pain and limited motion result, often associated with joint instability. Mallet deformity occurs with rupture of the terminal extensor tendon, or hyperextension deformity may result from rupture or stretching of the volar plate and long flexor tendon.

In many instances, no treatment is necessary for distal interphalangeal joint involvement in rheumatoid arthritis. Severe deformity, instability, or pain are best managed by arthrodesis. This procedure restores distal joint stability and may improve function at the more proximal finger joints, as strength of the extensor and flexor mechanism is concentrated at those levels.

THE THUMB IN RHEUMATOID ARTHRITIS

In rheumatoid arthritis, as a consequence of joint destruction, instability, or muscle imbalance, the thumb loses its ability to act as a strong opposition post. As grasp-and-pinch function decreases, hand function becomes seriously compromised. The rheumatoid thumb deformities have been classified by Millender et al.[52,55]; Table 58-5 provides a summary of the rheumatoid thumb deformities and their treatment based on this classification system. An additional type of rheumatoid thumb deformity (type V), described by Ratcliff,[64] has been added to the classification in Table 58-5. There can be no question that stabiliza-

TABLE 58-4 Staging and Treatment for the Rheumatoid Boutonniere Deformity

Stage	Deformity	PIP joint	DIP joint	Treatment
I	Mild	10–15° lag	± Hyperextension with positive intrinsic-intrinsic tightness test	Extensor tenotomy over middle phalanx
II	Moderate	30–40° lag	Hyperextended (+) intrinsic-intrinsic tightness test	Central slip shortening, mobilization of lateral bands and tenotomy, or PIP joint fusion
III	Severe	Fixed flexion posture	Hyperextended	PIP joint fusion

Key: PIP, proximal interphalangeal; DIP, distal interphalangeal.
Source: Adapted with permission from Millender LH, Nalebuff EA, Feldon PG: Rheumatoid arthritis, in Green DP (ed): *Operative Hand Surgery.* New York, Churchill Livingstone, 1982. And from Kiefhaber TR, Strickland JW: Soft tissue reconstruction for rheumatoid swan-neck and boutonniere deformities: Long-term results. *J Hand Surg* 18A:984–989, 1993.

TABLE 58-5   Rheumatoid Thumb Deformities and Their Treatment

Type of thumb deformity	Deformity	Joint involved by synovitis	CMC joint	MCP joint	IP joint	Treatment
I	Boutonniere (A + B + C = 57% of rheumatoid thumb deformities)	MCP	—	Flexed	Extended	—
I$_A$ (mild)			—	Flexed passively corrects	Hyperextended, passively corrects	MCP joint synovectomy extensor mechanism reconstruction
I$_B$ (moderate)		MCP		Fixed in flexion with or without joint destruction	Hyperextended, passively corrects	MCP joint arthrodesis or arthroplasty
I$_C$ (severe)		MCP	—	Fixed in flexion	Fixed in hyperextension	Depending on joint status, IP joint: capsulotomy vs. fusion; MCP joint: synovectomy, extensor reconstruction, arthroplasty vs. fusion
III	Swan-neck (a + b + c = 9% of rheumatoid thumb deformities)	CMC	Dorsal and radial subluxation to frank dislocation	Hyperextended 2° metacarpal adduction contracture		
III$_a$ (mild)		CMC	Minimal subluxation and deformity	—	Reciprocal flexion	Conservative management vs. CMC hemiarthroplasty
III$_b$ (moderate)		CMC	Subluxation and deformity	Passively correctable joint hyperextension	Reciprocal flexion	CMC hemiarthroplasty or resection arthroplasty, volar tenodesis of MP joint or MP joint fusion
III$_c$ (severe)		CMC	Dislocation with fixed adduction contracture (of MC)	Fixed hyperextension deformity	Reciprocal flexion	CMC hemiarthroplasty MP joint fusion

(Continued on next page)

TABLE 58-5   Rheumatoid Thumb Deformities and Their Treatment *(Continued)*

Type of thumb deformity	Deformity	Joint involved by synovitis	CMC joint	MCP joint	IP joint	Treatment
IV	Gamekeeper's	CMP	—	Abduction deformity with 2° adduction deformity MC	—	MCP joint synovectomy collateral ligament reconstruction vs. MCP joint fusion and adduction fascia release
II	Combination types I and II (rare)	MP, CMC	Subluxation or dislocation	Flexed	Hyperextended	As types I and II
V[115]	Instability of IP or MP joints due to joint destruction as seen with arthritis mutilans	IP, MCP		Multidirectional instability	Multidirectional instability	Joint fusion using bone graft

Key: CMC, carpal metacarpal; MCP, metacarpophalangeal; IP, interphalangeal;
MC, metacarpal.
Source: Adapted with permission from Millender LH, Nalebuff EA, Feldon PG: Rheumatoid arthritis, in Green DP (ed): *Operative Hand Surgery.* New York, Churchill Livingstone, 1982. And from Kiefhaber TR, Strickland JW: Soft tissue reconstruction for rheumatoid swan-neck and boutonniere deformities: Long-term results. *J Hand Surg* 18A:984–989, 1993.

tion procedures, such as metacarpophalangeal joint or interphalangeal joint arthrodesis, rank at the top of the list of rheumatoid procedures with regard to their ability to restore strong, pain-free thumb function, particularly when good basilar joint motion remains or can be preserved by arthroplasty.

FLEXOR TENOSYNOVITIS AND TENDON RUPTURE

Flexor tenosynovitis has been discussed briefly as a causative factor in many of the deformities of the individual joints of the hand and wrist in rheumatoid arthritis. The significance of this problem cannot be overemphasized; it must be carefully searched for at the level of the wrist, palm, and digits in rheumatoid patients. Because of the depth of the deep transverse carpal ligament, flexor tenosynovitis of the wrist may be less obvious than its extensor counterpart. Symptoms of carpal tunnel syndrome should be carefully sought out in addition to observation of any fullness of the volar wrist or palm, catching (trig-

gering) of the flexor tendons at the wrist level, or digital dysfunction resulting from ruptured or attenuated flexor tendons. As a sign of flexor tenosynovitis, observe for decrease in active range of motion when passive range of motion remains full. Although steroid treatment may occasionally be beneficial, wrist flexor tenosynovectomy and carpal tunnel release are often indicated.

Fullness in the distal palm and digits with evidence of triggering or crepitus is seen in rheumatoid arthritis patients with digital flexor tenosynovitis. When such patients are sufficiently symptomatic, treatment consists of flexor tenosynovectomy. Although incising the A-1 pulley is still the most frequent technique for decompression of the flexor tendon sheath, some authors have advocated decreasing the bulk of the flexor tendon system by excising one slip of the flexor digitorum superficialis.[24] This method may be biomechanically helpful by not increasing the ulnar approach of the flexor tendons and the resultant ulnar drift of the digits. Nalebuff has described four types of rheumatoid trigger-finger problems based on the location of the tendon nodule and whether or not diffuse tenosynovitis is present.[56] For all four types, flexor tenosynovectomy and excision of flexor tendon nodules is the recommended treatment.

Unattended flexor tenosynovitis may contribute to flexor tendon rupture. The most commonly affected tendon is the flexor pollicis longus, with attrition occurring at the level of the trapezial crest or scaphoid.[70] The tendon rupture may be in the wrist, palm, or digit, often requiring surgical exploration to determine the exact site. Care must be taken to distinguish between a flexor tendon rupture and a stenosing tenosynovitis with the digit locked in extension. Flexor tendon ruptures may be treated by tendon graft or tendon transfer.[57,58] On occasion, arthrodesis of the terminal joint for rupture of the profundus or flexor pollicis longus may be a simpler alternative.

MULTIPLE-LEVEL INVOLVEMENT OF THE RHEUMATOID HAND AND WRIST

Some surgeons experienced in the surgical management of the rheumatoid hand favor an aggressive multilevel surgical approach to the complex rheumatoid hand. Complementary reconstructive procedures must be carefully selected and must not present conflicting rehabilitation requirements.[71] General guidelines for the reconstruction of the rheumatoid hand with multiple-level involvement suggest surgical correction of more proximal joints such as the wrist and metacarpophalangeal joints before proceeding further distally. When severe deformities exist, it may be most practical to try to achieve improved motion at one joint level and to stabilize adjacent joints. The benefit of each surgical procedure may be maximized by combining those procedures which are complementary in terms of the postoperative therapy requirements. Above all, the patient's needs, expectations, and motivation must be considered. The mere existence of deformity is not an indication for surgery. The specific reconstructive program must be tailored to the individual rheumatoid patient.

SYSTEMIC LUPUS ERYTHEMATOSUS

Muscular pain and atrophy as well as joint pain are frequent symptoms in this systemic multisystem disease.[11] Although the hallmark of the disease as it affects the hands and wrists are deformities that resemble those of rheumatoid arthritis, the joint changes are nonerosive. Radiographic findings have been reported to include joint effusion, narrowing, juxtaarticular demineralization, subluxation or dislocation, bone infarction, aseptic necrosis, and abnormal calcification. Joint destruction, even in longstanding cases with severe joint disease, is usually scant.[62] Other authors have reported that articular destruction and ankylosis do not occur unless there is coexistent rheumatoid arthritis.[8]

The common hand lesions seen in systemic lupus erythematosus (SLE) include migratory polyarthralgias, flexor tenosynovitis, metacarpophalangeal and proximal inter-

phalangeal arthritis, skin rash, Raynaud's phenomenon, and avascular necrosis of the carpal bones.[5] The pathophysiologic mechanisms producing deformities differ slightly from those of rheumatoid patients in that distention of soft tissue rather than direct destruction and fibrosis of supporting elements appears to be the primary offender. Although both diseases exhibit synovitis, the pannus is not as aggressive in producing deformity in SLE. The synovitis results in stretching of supporting structures, allowing normal muscle-tendon forces to deform the joint.[5]

Surgical treatment of hand involvement with SLE is primarily designed to rebalance the affected soft tissue structures.[8,35] Some authors have reported the inadequacy of soft tissue rebalancing alone and recommend selected joint fusion and implant arthroplasty in combination with soft tissue rebalancing.[11,65]

JUVENILE RHEUMATOID ARTHRITIS

Several distinctions set juvenile rheumatoid arthritis (JRA) apart from rheumatoid arthritis seen in the adult, and these merit consideration. Children affected with JRA in general have a much milder course, resulting in less disability than in adults, with 50 to 70 percent of cases achieving remission.[34] The disease may, however, result in greater joint stiffness and ankylosis than its adult counterpart. Although surgery may play a major role in the early management of the JRA patient, conservative treatment consisting of splinting and exercises is most often recommended.[30] In growing children, reconstructive procedures often used in adults are not appropriate, as epiphyseal arrest may ensue. Even as afflicted children with active disease pass through puberty, their bones are often too narrow and medullary canals too small to make them acceptable candidates for many procedures, such as arthroplasty.[6,70]

In the child with JRA, ulnar deviation of the hand (metacarpals) with radial deviation of the fingers associated with a short ulna may occur.[42] This is opposite to the deformity that occurs most frequently in adults. Boutonniere finger deformities are common, as well as fixed flexion deformities of the interphalangeal joints. Swan-neck deformities are seen infrequently.[15] At the level of the metacarpophalangeal joint, in addition to radial deviation, loss of flexion without loss of extension is seen, as contrasted to adult-onset rheumatoid arthritis, in which ulnar drift and extension deficits are present with the maintenance of reasonable metacarpophalangeal flexion. Intrinsic tightness, so often seen in the adult, was not seen at all in a large reported series of JRA patients.[31] Finally, in the adult with rheumatoid arthritis, dorsal tenosynovitis of the wrist is frequently seen early, while in JRA early clinical signs are a mild loss of complete wrist extension prior to the presence of a palpable synovitis or other clinical findings.[31]

The surgeon's primary function is to follow patients afflicted with JRA closely and detect joint imbalance prior to the development of fixed deformities. The key to the early management is physical therapy with exercise, splinting, and occasional steroid injections.[31] In neglected or unresponsive cases, wedging casts can help bring the subluxed or volarflexed wrist into a functional position, with the hope that this position can then be maintained in an orthosis.[26] Immobilization in this manner may permit spontaneous intercarpal or radiocarpal fusion to take place with the wrist in a functional position.[46] Reconstructive surgery for the wrist can then be reserved for the adult patient.[33]

ARTHRITIS MUTILANS

Arthritis mutilans, main en lorgnette, and *opera-glass hand* are terms used to denote a severe form or variant of rheumatoid arthritis often associated with psoriasis.[19,28,61] It is manifest by extreme resorption of the ends of bones but with sparing of the vessels, nerves, and tendons. In the hand, there is severe shortening, telescoping, and instability of the digits. It has been distinguished from Charcot's neuropathy by the presence of normal nerve conduction.[73] The deformities may be quite severe and are frequently seen about the wrist, elbow, and shoulder joints as well as the ribs, ankles, and toes.[67] In the hand and wrist, significant disability may result and may include unequal shortening of adjacent digits, decreased grasp due to loss of digital length, instability, and angular deformity.[59] The goal of treatment is to preserve or restore length. Early treatment may be more successful than late salvage procedures accomplished with intercalary iliac bone grafts and joint fusions.[59]

PSORIATIC ARTHRITIS

Approximately 5 to 10 percent of patients with rheumatoid disease have psoriasis. According to Flatt, the diagnosis of psoriatic arthritis rather than rheumatoid disease is considered when the seronegative, nodule-free patient has psoriasis and when the disease appears patchy and less symmetrical in distribution.[27] It also may be less progressive in its course. In addition to the usual rheumatoid hand involvement, the distal interphalangeal joint in particular is affected in psoriatic arthritis. Although there may be less synovial proliferation, bone and joint destruction occur. The surgical treatment is much the same as in the rheumatoid patient, although arthrodesis may be more difficult to achieve.

GOUT

Gout may affect the hand and wrist but usually presents earlier and in other locations. Large tophi composed of urate crystals and draining sinuses are occasions for surgical intervention; however, the mainstay of treatment is medical management.[69]

OSTEOARTHRITIS

Osteoarthritis is common in the hands of both men and postmenopausal women. All men and women over the age of 60 years show some physical or radiologic evidence of osteoarthritis, but only 25 percent of the women and 15 percent of the men are symptomatic.[27] The joints most frequently involved are the basilar joints of the thumbs and proximal and distal interphalangeal joints, which exhibit Bouchard's and Heberden's nodes, respectively.

Patients with osteoarthritis can be subdivided into those presenting with Heberden's nodes only, those with generalized osteoarthritis with hand involvement of the thumb basilar joint and distal interphalangeal joints, and those with osteoarthritis affecting the levels of both the proximal and distal interphalangeal joints.[49] Radiographs may show joint space narrowing, subchondral sclerosis, and osteophyte formation. Most patients are best managed medically with aspirin or the nonsteroidal anti-inflammatory drugs.

Painful instability of the thumb carpometacarpal joint is frequently seen in women and may be evaluated with the grind and circumduction tests.[21] Care must be taken to distinguish this condition from more proximal arthritic involvement of the scaphoid, trapezium, and trapezoid articulations. The arthritic process may also be pantrapezial, affecting not only the carpometacarpal joint but also the surrounding trapezial articulations to the trapezoid and scaphoid. Another area of the wrist frequently affected in osteoarthritis is in the scaphoradial joint. The SLAC wrist, or scapholunate advanced collapse pattern, presents with significant degenerative changes at the scaphoradial articulation with sparing of the radiolunate.[78] This may also be seen in calcium pyrophosphate deposition disease.

Surgical treatment for osteoarthritis in the hand and wrist is reserved for cases unresponsive to medical management. Fusions and joint arthroplasties have both been recommended for cases that do not respond satisfactorily to medical management.

REFERENCES

1. Adamson GJ, Gellman H, Brumfield RH Jr, et al: Flexible implant resection arthroplasty of the proximal interphalangeal joint in patients with systemic inflammatory arthritis. *J Hand Surg* 19:378–384, 1064, 1994.
2. Adolfsson L, Nylander G: Arthroscopic synovectomy of the rheumatoid wrist. *J Hand Surg (Br)* 18B:92–96, 1993.
3. American Society for Surgery of the Hand. *Hand Review Course.* New York, ASSH, 1982, p 178.
4. American Society for Surgery of the Hand. *Hand Surgery Update.* New York, ASSH, 1994, pp 173–181.

5. Aptekar RG, Lawless OJ, Decker JL: Deforming non-erosive arthritis of the hand in systemic lupus erythematosus. *Clin Orthop* 100:120–124, 1974.

6. Athreya, BH: The hand in juvenile rheumatoid arthritis, in Proceedings of the First APA Conference on the Rheumatoid Diseases of Childhood. *Arthritis Rheum* 20 (suppl 2):573–574, 1976.

7. Benjamin M, Ralphs JR, Shibu M, Irwin M: Capsular tissues of the proximal interphalangeal joint: Normal composition and effects of Dupuoytren's disease and rheumatoid arthritis. *J Hand Surg (Br)* 18B:371–376, 1993.

8. Bleifeld CJ, Inglis AE: The hand in systemic lupus erythematosus. *J Bone Joint Surg* 56A:1202–1215, 1974.

9. Bosco JA III, Bynum DK, Bowers WH: Long-term outcome of Volz total wrist arthroplasties. *J Arthrop* 9:25–31, 1994.

10. Bowers W: Distal radio-ulnar joint, in Green DP (ed): *Operative Hand Surgery.* New York, Churchill Livingstone, 1982, p 765.

11. Brumfield RH, Patzakis MJ, Conaty P, et al: Surgery of the hand in systemic lupus erythematosus: A preliminary study. *Contemp Orthop* 1:5:42–45, 1979.

12. Bunnell S, Soherty EW, Curtis RM: Ischemic contracture located in the hand. *Plast Reconstr Surg* 3:424, 1948.

13. Burton RI: The rheumatoid hand, in Kilgore, Graham (eds): *The Hand: Surgical and Nonsurgical Management.* Philadelphia, Lea & Feibiger, 1977, p 408.

14. Carroll RE, Dick HM: Arthrodesis of the wrist for rheumatoid arthritis. *J Bone Joint Surg* 53A:1365, 1971.

15. Chaplin D, Pulkki T, Sacrimoa A, Vaninio K: Wrist and finger deformities in juvenile rheumatoid arthritis. *Acta Rheum Scand* 15:206–233, 1969.

16. Clayton ML: The caput ulnae syndrome: Update, in Strickland JW, Steichen JB (eds): *Difficult Problems in Hand Surgery.* St Louis, Mosby, 1982, p 199.

17. Clayton, ML, Ferlic DC: Tendon transfer for radial deviation of the wrist in rheumatoid arthritis. *Clin Orthop* 100:176, 1974.

18. Connor J, Nalebuff EA: Current recommendations for surgery of the rheumatoid hand and wrist. *Curr Opin Rheum* 7:120–124, 1995.

19. Davis J et al: Rehabilitation of the rheumatoid upper limb. *Orthop Clin North Am* 9:559–568, 1978.

20. Duché R, Canovas F, Thaury MN, et al: Flexor tenosynovectomy in rheumatoid arthritis: Short-term and long-term analysis of finger mobility. *Ann Chir Main* 12:85–92, 1993.

21. Eaton RG, Littler W: Ligament reconstruction for the painful thumb carpometacarpal joint. *J Bone Joint Surg* 55A:1655–1666, 1973.

22. El-Gammal TA, Blair WF: Motion after metacarpophalangeal joint reconstruction in rheumatoid disease. *J Hand Surg* 18A:504–511, 1993.

23. Ellison MR, Kelly KJ, Flatt AE: The results of surgical synovectomy of the digital joints in rheumatoid disease. *J Bone Joint Surg* 53A:1041–1060, 1971.

24. Ferlic DC, Clayton ML: Flexor tenosynovectomy in the rheumatoid finger. *J Hand Surg* 3:292, 1978.

25. Ferlic DC, Jolly SN, Clayton ML: Salvage for failed implant arthroplasty of the wrist. *J Hand Surg* 17:917–923, 1992.

26. Findley TW, Halpern D, Easton JKM: Wrist subluxation in juvenile rheumatoid arthritis: Pathophysiology and management. *Arch Phys Med Rehabil* 64:69–74, 1983.

27. Flatt A: *Care of the Arthritic Hand,* 4th ed. St Louis, Mosby, 1983.

28. Froimsen AI: Hand reconstruction in arthritis mutilans. *J Bone Joint Surg* 53A:1377, 1971.

29. Goncalves D: Correction of disorders of the distal radio-ulnar joint by artificial pseudarthrosis of the ulna. *J Bone Joint Surg* 56B:462–463, 1974.

30. Granberry WM, Brewer EJ: Early synovectomy in juvenile rheumatoid arthritis. *Instr Course Lect* 27–32, 1974.

31. Granberry WM, Mangum GL: The hand in the child with juvenile rheumatoid arthritis. *J Hand Surg* 5:105–113, 1980.

32. Hakstan RW, Tubiana R: Ulnar deviation of the fingers, the role of joint structure and function. *J Bone Joint Surg* 49A:299, 1967.

33. Hanff G, Sollerman C, Elborgh R, Pettersson H: Wrist synovectomy in juvenile chronic arthritis (JCA). *Scand J Rheum* 19:280–284, 1990.

34. Hansen V, Konreich H, Berstein B, et al: Prognosis of juvenile rheumatoid arthritis, in Proceedings of the ARA Conference on the Rheumatic Disease of Childhood. *Arthritis Rheum* 20(suppl2): 279–284, 1976.

35. Hastings DE, Evans JA: The lupus hand: A new surgical approach. *J Hand Surg* 3:179–183, 1978.

36. Ishikawa H, Hanyu T, Tajima T: Rheumatoid wrists treated with synovectomy of the extensor tendons and the wrist joint combined with a Darrach procedure. *J Hand Surg* 17A:1109–1117, 1992.

37. Jolly SL, Ferlic DC, Clayton ML, et al: Swanson silicone arthroplasty of the wrist in rheumatoid arthritis: A long-term follow-up. *J Hand Surg* 17A:142–149, 1992.

38. Kiefhaber TR, Strickland JW: Soft tissue reconstruction for rheumatoid swan-neck and boutonniere deformities: Long-term results. *J Hand Surg* 18A:984–989, 1993.

39. Kirschenbaum D, Schneider LH, Adams DC, Cody RP: Arthroplasty of the metacarpophalangeal joints with use of silicone-rubber implants in patients who have rheumatoid arthritis: Long-term results. *J Bone Joint Surg* 75A:3–12, 1993.

40. Kulick RG, DeFiore JC, Straub LR, Ranawat CS: Long term results of dorsal stabilization of the rheumatoid wrist. *J Hand Surg* 6:272, 1981.

41. Landsmeer JMF: Studies in the anatomy of articulation: I. The equilibrium of the "intercalated" bone. *Acta Morphol Neerl Scand* 3:287, 1961.

42. Landsmeer JM: Power grip and precision handling. *Ann Rheum Dis* 21:164–170, 1962.

43. Lanzetta M, Herbert TJ, Conolly WB: Silicone synovitis: A perspective. *J Hand Surg (Br)* 19:479–484, 1994.

44. Lipscomb PR: Is early synovectomy of the small joints of the hand worthwhile? in Camer LM, Chase RA (eds): *Symposium on the Hand,* vol 3. St Louis, Mosby, 1971, pp 29–32.

45. Lundkvist L, Barfred T: Total wrist arthroplasty: Experience with Swanson flexible silicone implants. *Scand J Plast Reconstr Surg Hand Surg* 26:97–100, 1992.

46. Maldonado-Cocco JA, Garcia-Morteo O, Spindler AJ, et al: Carpal ankylosis in juvenile rheumatoid arthritis. *Arthritis Rheum* 23:1251–1255, 1980.

47. Mannerfelt L, Malmsten M: Arthrodesis of the wrist in rheumatoid arthritis: A technique without external fixation. *Scand J Plast Reconstr Surg* 5:124, 1971.

48. Melone CP Jr, Taras JS: Distal ulna resection, extensor carpi ulnaris tenodesis, and dorsal synovectomy for the rheumatoid wrist. *Hand Clin* 7:335–43, 1991.

49. Millender LH: Surgery of the hand in osteoarthritis. *Orthop Rev* 9:73–81, 1980.

50. Millender LH, Nalebuff EA, Albin R, et al: Dorsal tenosynovectomy and tendon transfer in the rheumatoid hand. *J Bone Joint Surg* 56A:601, 1979.

51. Millender LH, Nalebuff EA: Arthrodesis of the rheumatoid wrist: An evaluation of sixty patients and a description of a different surgical technique. *J Bone Joint Surg* 55A:1026, 1973.

52. Millender LH, Nalebuff EA, Felton PG: Rheumatoid arthritis, in Green DP (ed): *Operative Hand Surgery.* New York, Churchill Livingstone, 1982, pp 1161–1262.

53. Millender LH, Nalebuff EA, Holdsworth DE: Posterior interosseous nerve syndrome secondary to rheumatoid synovitis. *J Bone Joint Surg* 55A:753, 1973.

54. Millroy P, Coleman S, Ivers R: The Sauvé-Kapandji operation: Technique and results. *J Hand Surg (Br)* 17B:411–414, 1992.

55. Nalebuff EA: Diagnosis, classification and management of rheumatoid thumb deformities. *Bull Joint Dis* 29:119–137, 1968.

56. Nalebuff EA: Surgical treatment of rheumatoid tenosynovitis in the hand. *Surg Clin North Am* 49:799–809, 1969.

57. Nalebuff EA: Surgical treatment of tendon rupture in the rheumatoid hand. *Surg Clin North Am* 49:811–822, 1969.

58. Nalebuff EA: The recognition and treatment of tendon ruptures in the rheumatoid hand. *AAOS Symposium on Tendon Surgery in the Hand*. St Louis, Mosby, 1975, pp 255–269.

59. Nalebuff EA, Garrett J: Opera-glass hand in rheumatoid arthritis. *J Hand Surg* 1:210–220, 1976.

60. Nalebuff EA, Millender LH: Surgical treatment of the swan-neck deformity in rheumatoid arthritis. *Orthop Clin North Am* 6:733–752, 1975.

61. Nelson LS: The opera-glass hand in chronic arthritis: "La main enlorgnette" of Marie and Leri. *J Bone Joint Surg* 20:1045, 1938.

62. Noon CD, Odone DT, Engleman EP, Splitter SD: Roentgenographic manifestations of joint disease in systemic lupus erythematosus. *Radiology* 80:837–843, 1963.

63. Olsen I, Gebuhr P, Sonne-Holm S: Silastic arthroplasty in rheumatoid MCP joints: 60 joints followed for 7 years. *Acta Orthop Scand* 65:430–431, 1994.

64. Ratcliff AHC: Deformities of the thumb in rheumatoid arthritis. *Hand* 3:138–143, 1971.

65. Shomacker HR, Zweiman B, Bora FW: Corrective surgery for the deforming hand arthropathy of systemic lupus erythematosus. *Clin Orthop* 117:292–295, 1976.

66. Smith RJ, Kaplan EB: Rheumatoid deformities of the metacarpophalangeal joints of the finger: A correlative study of anatomy and pathology. *J Bone Joint Surg* 49A:31, 1967.

67. Soloman WM, Stecher RM: Chronic absorptive arthritis or opera-glass hand: Report of eight cases. *Ann Rheum Dis* 9:209, 1950.

68. Stanley JK, Tolat AR: Long-term results of Swanson silastic arthroplasty in the rheumatoid wrist. *J Hand Surg (Br)* 18B:381–388, 1993.

69. Straub LR, Smith JW, Carpenter GK, Deitz GH: Surgery of gout in the upper extremity. *J Bone Joint Surg* 43A:731–752, 1961.

70. Strickland JW, Ellstein JL: Rheumatoid disorders of the hand and wrist, in Hurst LC, Dee R (eds): *Principles of Orthopaedic Practice*. New York, McGraw-Hill, 1988, pp 646–665.

71. Strickland JW, LaSalle WB: The surgical management of multiple-level deformities of the rheumatoid hand, a practical approach, in Strickland JW, Steicher JB (eds): *Difficult Problems in Hand Surgery*. St Louis, Mosby, 1982, pp 224–240.

72. Swezey RL, Bjarnason H, Austin ES: Nerve conduction studies in resorptive arthropathies: Opera-glass hand. *J Bone Joint Surg* 55A:1680, 1973.

73. Taleisnik J: The Sauvé-Kapandji procedure. *Clin Orthop Rel Res* 275:11023, 1992.

74. Thompson M, Douglas G, Davidson EP: Evaluation of synovectomy in rheumatoid arthritis. *Proc R Soc Med* 66:197–199, 1973.

75. Tonkin MA, Hughes J, Smith KL: Lateral band translocation for swan-neck deformity. *J Hand Surg* 17:260–267, 1992.

76. Vaughan-Jackson OJ: Attrition ruptures of tendons in the rheumatoid hand. *J Bone Joint Surg* 40A:1431, 1958.

77. Watson HK, Ballet FL: The SLAC wrist: Scapholunate advanced collapse pattern of degenerative arthritis. *J Hand Surg* 9A:358–365, 1984.

78. Wilson YG, Sykes PJ, Niranjan NS: Long-term follow up of Swanson's silastic arthroplasty of the metacarpophalangeal joints in rheumatoid arthritis. *J Hand Surg (Br)* 18B:81–91, 1993.

CHAPTER 59

Dupuytren's Contracture

Lawrence C. Hurst
and Marie A. Badalamente

Dupuytren's contracture is a debilitating fibromatosis involving the palmar aponeurosis of the hand. Nodular thickenings form in the palmar fascia and may progress into the longitudinal bands, resulting in fixed flexion contractures of the fingers. The term *Dupuytren's diathesis* refers to the rare predisposition of some patients for multiple areas of involvement. Dupuytren's diathesis is associated with a positive family history and early onset of disease. In patients with Dupuytren's diathesis, involvement may be present in the volar aspects of the hands and the dorsum of the fingers in the form of knuckle pads, in the feet as plantar fibromatosis, and in the penis as Peyronie's disease.[1,2] In 1614, Plater[3] described flexion deformities of the fingers, which were probably Dupuytren's contracture. Sir Ashley Cooper[4] reported the condition in 1822. Despite this, Baron Dupuytren's name appears to be the permanent eponym for this particular fibromatosis because he accurately described the condition in a dissected cadaver hand, correctly identified the palmar fascia as the predominantly involved tissue, and in 1831 presented a clinical case.

Our understanding of the pathobiology of Dupuytren's contracture has progressed slowly. However, the clinical features of the disorder are well defined. As the fibromatosis slowly progresses over a period of years, flexion contractures of the fingers, web space contractures, and distal interphalangeal (DIP) hyperextension contractures all contribute to a significant functional handicap. The normal palmar fascia has been well described.[5–9] The anatomic structures that become involved in Dupuytren's contracture are the longitudinal pretendinous bands, the spiral bands, the natatory ligaments, the lateral digital sheaths, Grayson's ligaments, and Cleland's ligaments[10–13] (Fig. 59-1). The ring and the little fingers are the most frequently involved digits in Dupuytren's disease.[14] However, the radial digits and thumb-index web space may also become involved. In the first web, four separate pathologic cords are possible: a radial longitudinal fibrous cord, a longitudinal cord secondary to the radial distal fibers of the palmaris longus, a distal transverse interdigital cord secondary to involvement of Grapow's ligament, and a transverse proximal web cord secondary to involvement of a proximal transverse commissural ligament. Involvement of these ligaments can result in interference with web width and ultimately with grasp and pinch.[15]

As the fascial ligaments of the hand are progressively changed into pathologic cords by the palmar fibromatosis, the fingers can develop a fixed flexion contracture. Three different pathologic cords can develop in the palm and digits. These are the central cord, the spiral cord, and the lateral cord[11,12,16] (Fig. 59-2). The central cord develops when there is involvement of the pretendinous longitudinal bands and the fibrofatty tissues in the superficial fascia between the neurovascular bundles. Contracture of the middle layer of the pretendinous band is the most common cause of proximal interphalangeal joint contracture. The cord splits just distal to the proximal interphalangeal (PIP) joint and can further split with part going to the bone and part to Grayson's ligaments on the lateral side of the neurovascular bundles. The spiral cord develops when there is involvement of the pretendinous bands, the spiral bands, the lateral digital sheaths, the vertical band, and Grayson's ligament. At surgery, the spiral cord should be approached cautiously, because it can displace the neurovascular bundle medially and superficially, particularly at the level of the first transverse finger crease.[12,17]

The lateral cord results from contracture of the lateral digital sheath. This sheath is formed from the coalescence of the natatory ligament and the spiral band. The ulnar side of the small finger does not have this fascial arrangement; however, another cord can originate from the abductor digiti minimi tendon. The lateral cord generally inserts into the dermis of the finger, and this does not result in severe PIP joint contracture. In the small finger however, it can attach to the middle phalanx via Grayson's ligaments. Here it can cause severe PIP joint contracture. It can also cause DIP joint contracture through a distal extension beyond this joint. It does not cause displacement of the neurovascular bundle.

The retrovascular cord arises from digital fascia dorsal to the neurovascular bundle and appears to be separate from the transverse Cleland's ligaments. The retrovascular cord runs in a longitudinal direction. On its own it does not cause contracture of the PIP joint but, in combination with the lateral cord, it can result in a hyperextension contracture of the DIP joint.

Cord combinations are not uncommon, and they can result in continued contracture after individual cord excision. The most common cord combination is a central cord–lateral cord combination, which results in contracture of the PIP and metacarpophalangeal (MCP) joints. In general, this combination does not result in DIP joint contracture. The neurovascular bundle is drawn centrally. Other common cord combinations include the central cord–spiral cord combination and spiral cord–natatory cord combination. With the central cord–spiral cord combination, the cords, which are initially separate, become a solid sheet encasing the neurovascular bundle.

Finally, the little finger may become contracted because of the cords or because of the involvement of the abductor digiti minimi fascia and tendon.[9,12] Involvement of this intrinsic muscle may partially explain the increased frequency of the severe, persistent, and recurrent contracture in this digit.

The pathohistology of Dupuytren's contracture was first described in the 1940s by Meyerding and also in the now classic work of Gabbiani, Majno, and others.[18,19] These investigators correctly pointed out that the nodules in the affected palmar fascia were composed of smooth, muscle-like cells called *myofibroblasts*. They correctly postulated

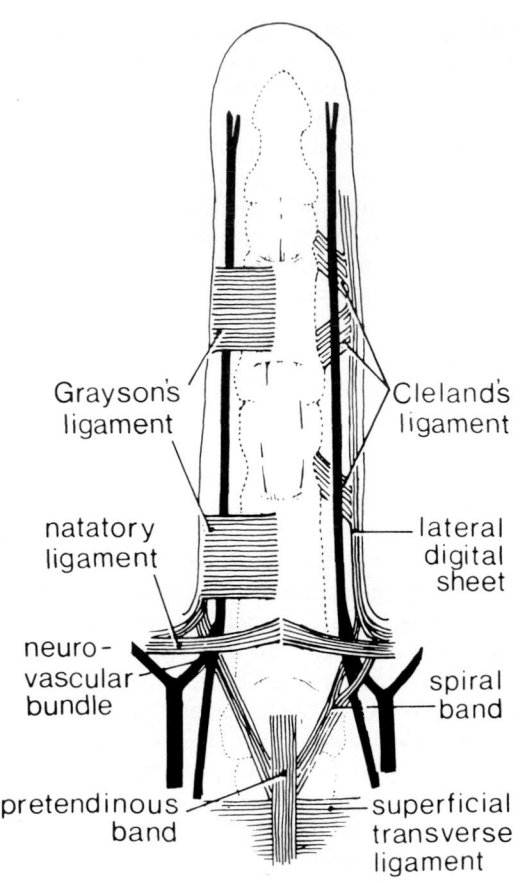

Figure 59-1 The normal structures of the finger that may be involved in Dupuytren's disease are the longitudinal pretendinous bands, spiral bands, natatory ligaments, lateral digital sheaths, and Grayson's and Cleland's ligaments. (Reproduced with permission from McFarlane RM: Patterns of the diseased fascia in the fingers of Dupuytren's contracture. *Plast Reconstr Surg* 54:31, 1974.)

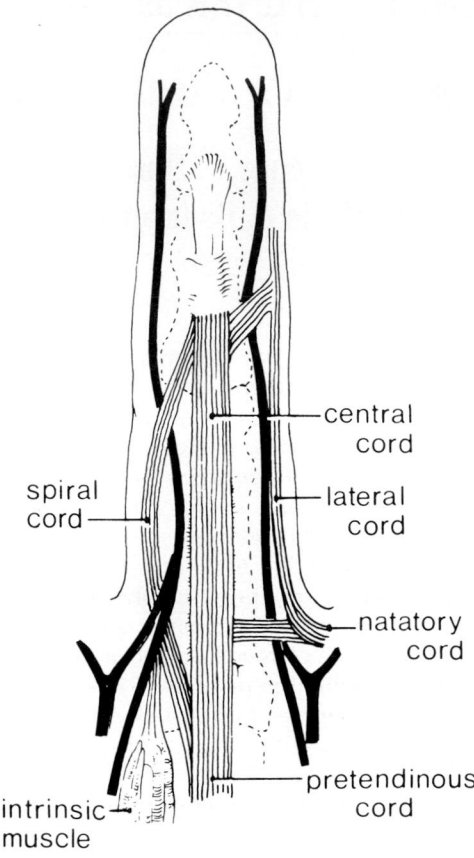

Figure 59-2 Three pathologic cords may develop during the progressive palmar fibromatosis of Dupuytren's disease: the central, the spiral, and the lateral cords. (Reproduced with permission from Chiu HP, McFarlane RM: Pathogenesis of Dupuytren's contracture: A correlative clinical-pathological study. *J Hand Surg* 3:1–10, 1978.)

that myofibroblasts were responsible for contracture of the palmar fascia, overlying skin, and fingers. Myofibroblasts, which are best identified using the electron microscope, have distinct features compatible with contractile ability. These ultrastructural features are bundles of 40- to 80-Å fibrils within the cell cytoplasm oriented parallel to the long axis of the cell, deeply indented nuclei, and the presence of cell-to-cell and cell-to-stroma membrane attachment sites known as *desmosomes* and *hemidesmosomes,* respectively.[18–22] Fibril bundles also contain darkened areas known as *dense bodies* located beneath the cell membrane. The presence of a pH-dependent adenosine triphosphatase (ATPase) has been found to be associated with the fibril bundles in Dupuytren's myofibroblasts.[23] In muscle, this enzyme is associated with cellular contraction.

A mechanism that would explain how myofibroblasts could transmit contractile force from cell to cell and from cell to adjacent collagen was elucidated by Tomasek et al.[24] These authors described fibronectin anchoring strands in a direct collinear and lateral fashion from the intracellular actin/myosin filaments to the extracellular collagen as well as to other myofibroblasts.[24,25] In addition, Tomasek and Rayan have shown in vitro that there is a positive correlation between the expression of alpha smooth muscle actin and the generation of contractile force in myofibroblasts.[26]

Most authors adhere to the concept that the proliferation of myofibroblasts within the nodules of Dupuytren's contracture is a slowly progressive phenomenon. Luck's early report of the stages of cellular progression have since been substantiated.[11] The proliferative stage of the disorder is the first occurrence in which the cellularity in the palmar fascia increases. The second, involutional stage, is characterized by a dense myofibroblast network and less cellular collagen bundles. In the last or residual stage, most myofibroblasts have disappeared and few fibroblasts remain within a dense collagen cord.

The origin of the myofibroblast is unknown. An extrinsic theory has been proposed, which states that the myofibroblasts originate subdermally.[1,27] The puckering of the skin, so commonly seen in the disorder, is purported by this theory to reflect the contracture of the skin toward the underlying fascia because of subdermal involvement.

Recently, the skin has again been implicated by Sugden et al., who suggested that a population of cells termed *dermal dendrocytes* have a role in pathogenesis.[28] Other investigators[19,20,23,29,30] have proposed the intrinsic theory, which states that fascial fibroblasts differentiate into myofibroblasts.

The role that microvascular changes and secondary local hypoxia play in the stimulation of cellular changes in Dupuytren's contracture has also been investigated. It has been suggested that hypoxemia stimulates pericytes and/or vascular fibroblasts to differentiate into myofibroblasts.[27,31,32] This hypoxemia may also explain the presence of high levels of short chain fatty acids and high levels of serum cholesterol and triglycerides[33] in the palmar fascia of patients with Dupuytren's disease.[34] Oxygen free radicals have also been suggested to play a role in the pathobiology of the disease, but a recent report using superoxide dismutase injections for oxygen free radicals showed no clinical benefit.[35]

There is an increased metabolic activity in the diseased tissues from Dupuytren's contracture.[36] Despite the fact that lysosomal enzyme activity and the enzymes involved in glucose catabolism are increased in Dupuytren's fascia,[37] it has not been possible to show conclusively that the increased metabolic rate is secondary to increased enzymatic activity. Rather, it is probable that the increased number of myofibroblasts,[36] which have an increased capacity to synthesize glycosaminoglycans and type III collagen, are responsible for the increased metabolic activity of the diseased tissue.[36,38-40] Myofibroblasts and significantly increased amounts of type III collagen coexist within a matrix of these glycosaminoglycans.[23] Type III collagen undergoes a constant remodeling until the residual stage of the disease, when an inextensible band has been produced.[41,42] Increased amounts of hydroxylysine, increased numbers of reducible cross-links, and the presence of hydroxylysinohydroxynorleucine have all been shown in Dupuytren's contracture.[36,38-43] In addition, collagen abnormalities have recently been shown to be more prevalent in the more grossly diseased fascia.[44] It has been proposed that the enzyme transglutaminase cross-links procollagen, type III peptides to maintain the contracted state of the collagen fibrils.[45] It has also been shown that prostaglandins F_{2a} and E_2 can cause contraction and relaxation of myofibroblasts.[46]

Finally, recent reports by numerous investigators have addressed the issue of exogenous factors that may be responsible for myofibroblast proliferation. In 1992, Lappi et al. reported that basic fibroblast growth factor (b-FGF) as well as b-FGF receptors are present in association with myofibroblasts in vitro. These authors further reported that b-FGF induced myofibroblast proliferation in vitro. That same year, Badalamente and Hurst et al. reported that platelet-derived growth factor (PDGF)[47] was present in association with the proliferative- and involutional-stage myofibroblasts obtained from surgical patients. These authors suggested a role for PDGF as a myofibroblasts mitogen. Badalamente, Sampson, and Hurst et al. have recently demonstrated that transforming growth factor beta$_1$ and beta$_2$ (TGF-β_1 and TGF-β_2) is localized within proliferative and involutional myofibroblasts in situ but not in residual-stage fibroblasts.[48] Their study also showed that exogenous TGF-β could induce myofibroblast proliferation in vitro. In 1994, Burton's group showed b-FGF and PDGF were mitogenic for Dupuytren's tissue and normal palmar fascia. TGF-β stimulated collagen production in normal tissue and tissue from patients with Dupuytren's disease; however, diseased tissue showed more metabolic activity and more sensitivity to growth factors. In 1994, Zamora et al. reported that TGF-β stained cells in "early" nodules.[49] In 1995, Kloen et al.[50] suggested that both TGF and epidermal growth factor (EGF) play a role in Dupuytren's disease.

If the cellular signals for myofibroblast proliferation are defined, then therapeutic inhibitors are a future possibility. At present, it is not known what cellular signal(s) may cause the appearance of nodular myofibroblasts or the endogenous disappearance of the myofibroblasts between the involutional and the residual stages of the disease.

The incidence of Dupuytren's disease is greater in northern European countries and in countries where emigrants are of Celtic origin.[51] The disease is rarely seen in non-Caucasians, but occasional cases have been reported.[52] The incidence of the disease steadily increases with age.[53,54] In one population study in Norway, 36.8 percent of the population between age 70 and 74 showed evidence of Dupuytren's disease. Variable incidences have been reported in the two sexes. Some reports suggest that the incidence is equal, particularly in older men and women,[51] while others report that the incidence is 2 to 10 times greater in men than in women.[55] The most commonly involved digits are the ring and little fingers. The index finger has the lowest incidence of involvement.[15]

The relationship between the incidence of Dupuytren's disease, occupation, and hand trauma remains unclear. Several reports emphatically state that there is no relationship between these three factors.[53,54,56] McFarlane has reported a set of guidelines pertinent to manual work and Dupuytren's disease.[57] Other authors, including Dupuytren himself, stated that injury and/or heavy manual labor do play a role in increasing the incidence of Dupuytren's contracture.[58,59] Probably the best assessment is that trauma aggravates the pathologic process in genetically predisposed individuals.[60]

The highest incidence of Dupuytren's contracture has been reported in patients with associated epilepsy, diabetes mellitus, chronic alcoholism, chronic pulmonary tuberculosis, and chronic lung disease.[53,54,61-63] These associated conditions may simply reflect the rising incidence of Dupuytren's disease in the elderly.

Some 10 percent of the patients with Dupuytren's contracture have a positive family history of this disorder. Dupuytren's disease is probably transmitted as a dominant gene with variable penetrance. This penetrance is almost complete in elderly men but not in women.[64] Myofibroblast karotyping has also shown an abnormal trisomy of chromosome eight.[65] Despite a dominant gene transmission pattern, it was initially reported that patients with Dupuytren's contracture do not show a specific pattern of HLA antigens.[61,66] However, more recently, the presence of HLA-DR3 has been cited in Dupuytren's disease, indicating a higher risk for the formation of connective tissue autoantibodies.[67]

The treatment of Dupuytren's contracture is presently surgical, although nonsurgical methods have been tried. Injections of enzymes, cortisone, superoxide dismutase, massage with vitamin E creams, physical therapy, therapeutic splinting, and radiation have all been ineffective.[1,35,51]

Recently, gamma interferon injections have been investigated with success in a small series of patients, but larger and long-term controlled clinical studies will be necessary to validate this therapy.[68] Also, clostridial collagenase injection has shown safety in vivo in animal models[69] and some merit in vitro as a nonoperative treatment modality.[70]

Presently, the treatment for Dupuytren's contracture remains surgical. The aim of surgical treatment is to relieve the fixed flexion deformities by removal of the pathologic palmar fascia with preservation of the digital arteries and nerves, correction of joint deformities, preservation of uninvolved skin, and maintenance of flexion and grip. Surgery does not cure Dupuytren's disease, but it may modify its progression and improve hand function. It was reported that surgical results could be predicted by the Legge and McFarlane outcome standard formula, which estimates the residual postoperative contracture at the PIP joint.[71] However, this formula is not in widespread clinical use. Surgery is indicated in patients with significant handicap who demonstrate a positive tabletop test. In this test, the patient places the hand on a flat surface. When there are significant contractures of the MCP and/or PIP joints, the fingers and the palm cannot be placed simultaneously on the flat surface, thus demonstrating a positive test. Another indication for surgical treatment is an MCP contracture of greater than 30° or any significant PIP joint contracture.[72] Palmar nodules alone are not an absolute indication for surgical treatment. Pain is also not an indication for surgery. In the proliferative stage, patients without contractures but with painful nodules should be advised that this may resolve as they move into the last, residual stage of the disorder. In patients with severe unrelenting pain, particularly if there is night pain, the possibility of an extremely rare condition—fibrosarcoma of the hand—should be considered.

Patients presenting with mild Dupuytren's disease who have painful associated trigger fingers should have their trigger fingers treated surgically; however, this should include a limited regional fasciectomy at the time of A-1 pulley release. Surgical treatment of the trigger finger without excision of the local fascia may result in an exacerbation of the Dupuytren's disease. In patients with significant Dupuytren's disease and coexisting carpal tunnel syndrome, the Dupuytren's contracture should first be treated surgically while the carpal tunnel syndrome is treated nonoperatively. If, after the Dupuytren's surgery, symptoms of carpal tunnel syndrome continue despite conservative therapy, then carpal tunnel release should be performed as a second procedure.[73] An exception to this may be made when early palmar Dupuytren's disease coexists with carpal tunnel syndrome. In this case, simultaneous carpal tunnel release and limited fasciectomy are usually safe.

Surgical treatment of Dupuytren's contracture is contraindicated when this condition is associated with advanced rheumatoid arthritis,[74] when the hand has trophic changes secondary to vascular insufficiency, and when the patient's general health is such that he or she will not be able to withstand the stress of surgery and anesthesia.[75]

The operative choices for Dupuytren's contracture include fasciotomy, regional fasciectomy, and total (radical) fasciectomy.[51,60] Closed fasciotomy is dangerous, particularly in the digit.[76,77] In the elderly patient, however, fasciotomy may be a useful treatment for a single palmar band or as a preliminary procedure.[51,60] In any case, fasciotomy should be done only by a surgeon who is experienced with this technique. Total fasciectomy has been abandoned because of the significant surgical morbidity associated with it.[78,79] Regional fasciectomy with excision of grossly pathologic fascia is the most popular current procedure.[51,60] However, Tubiana has warned that regional fasciectomy can lead to higher recurrence rate.[75] The extent of the procedure is determined by evaluation of the individual case, with special consideration being given to the patient's age, sex, family history, alcohol history, epileptic history, the presence or absence of knuckle pads, history of previous surgical treatment, and occupation. No matter which operative procedure is employed, the prognosis is particularly poor in young patients with a strong family history—that is, those with Dupuytren's diathesis.[60] Dermatofasciectomy with subsequent placement of full-thickness skin grafts is a useful procedure for recurrent disease, especially in young patients. Hueston has stated that he never saw recurrence beneath a graft, but other authors disagree.[80] More recently, Brotherston et al. studied 46 patients treated by dermatofasciectomy with an 8-year follow-up and found no clinical evidence of recurrence.[81]

Numerous incisions have been used for fasciectomies in Dupuytren's contracture. For example, Skoog and McCash popularized transverse incisions.[59,82] However, others have used midlateral and longitudinal incisions, longitudinal oblique incisions with Z-plasty, V-Y plasty incisions, and zig-zag incisions.[51,60,72,75,83] Whatever incision is employed, it should provide an exposure allowing proper identification of the neurovascular bundles as well as good access to the pathologic tissues in the palm, fingers, and web spaces. Skin flaps should be elevated with as much subcutaneous tissue as possible in order to maintain the subdermal vascular plexuses. Prior to closure, meticulous hemostasis should have been achieved in order to prevent hematoma. If a tourniquet has been used, it is appropriate to lower it and control any vigorous bleeding prior to reapplying the tourniquet and proceeding with surgical closure. Various adjunctive procedures such as volar PIP joint capsulotomy, skin grafts, arthrodeses, arthroplasties, and/or amputations are sometimes needed.[72,75,81,84]

Postoperative care begins in the operating room with the application of a bulky compressive dressing, whether the skin is to be left open or closed. If the wound is closed, then a drain should be left in the wound for 48 h. Bulky dressings are removed at 3 to 5 days and smaller dressings applied and the fingertips are left visible for neurovascular checks. If an open palm technique has been used, frequent early range-of-motion exercises and soaks are mandatory. McCash reports that these open incisions close in 2 to 5 weeks.[82] Our experience shows that this takes closer to 2 months. With the closed-palm technique, the bulky dressings are removed at 3 to 5 days postoperatively, and hand therapy, with static night extension splinting and daytime active range-of-motion exercises, is begun under the supervision of the hand therapist.[85]

The overall postoperative complication rate in Dupuytren's surgery has decreased in recent years from earlier reports.[51,86] Common complications include hand edema, palmar hematoma, skin necrosis, infections, digital nerve laceration, digital artery laceration, joint stiffness, loss of grip strength secondary to loss of finger flexion, reflex sympathetic dystrophy, and digital loss secondary to vascular damage.[86,87] Hematoma often leads to skin necrosis and secondary infection. This sequence is so common that McFarlane has called this a complication triad. McFarlane and McGrouther summarized complications from 1339 operations as follows: infection, 1.3 percent; hematoma, 2.2 percent; skin slough, 4.7 percent; nerve injury, 1.5 percent; arterial injury, 0.8 percent; finger gangrene, 0.1 percent; and other, 2.7 percent.

The results of a 10-year follow-up study show 80 percent good results, with patients demonstrating a normal-appearing palm, full extension, and full flexion.[76,77] However, Hakstian reported recurrence or extension of the disease in 50 percent of McIndoe's patients who were followed from 5 to 25 years, the average follow-up being 11.1 years.[88] His data, and the more recent data of Rebelo et al., reporting a 46 percent recurrence after 10-year follow-up, remind us that surgical treatment does not cure this disorder but only improves hand function temporarily.[89] Since a large percentage of patients with Dupuytren's contracture are elderly, this improvement may last the rest of their lives. In young patients; however, recurrence, further functional loss, and additional surgery should be anticipated in a significant percentage of the operative cases.

REFERENCES

1. Hueston JT: *Dupuytren's Contracture.* Edinburgh, Churchill Livingstone, 1963, pp 54–63.
2. Wheller E, Meals R: Dupuytren's diathesis: A broad-spectrum disease. *Plast Reconstr Surg* 68:781–783, 1981.
3. Elliot D: The early history of contracture of the palmar fascia. Part I. *J Hand Surg (Br)* 13(3):246–253, 1988.
4. Elliot D: The early history of contracture of the palmar fascia. *J Hand Surg (Br)* 14(1):25–29, 1989.
5. Kaplan EB, Milford W: The retinacular system of the hand, in Spinner M (ed): *Kaplan's Functional and Surgical Anatomy of the Hand.* Philadelphia, Lippincott, 1984, pp 245–282.
6. Lamb DW: Dupuytren's disease, in Lamb DW, Kaczynski K (eds): *The Practice of Hand Surgery.* Oxford, England: Blackwell, 1981, pp 476.
7. Milford L: *Retaining Ligaments of the Digits of the Hand.* Philadelphia, Saunders, 1968.
8. Stack H: *The Palmar Fascia.* Edinburgh, Churchill Livingstone, 1973.
9. White S: Anatomy of the palmar fascia on the ulnar border of the hand. *J Hand Surg (Br)* 9B:50–56, 1984.
10. Gosset J: Dupuytren's disease and the anatomy of the palmodigital aponeurosis, in Hueston JT, Tubiana R (eds): *Dupuytren's Disease.* Edinburgh, Churchill Livingstone, 1974, pp 11–23.
11. Luck J: Dupuytren's contracture: A new concept of the pathogenesis correlated with surgical management. *J Bone Joint Surg (Am)* 41A:635–664, 1959.
12. McFarlane R: Patterns of the diseased fascia in the fingers in Dupuytren's contracture. *Plast Reconstr Surg* 54:31–44, 1974.
13. Thomine J: The development and anatomy of the digital fascia, in Hueston JT, Tubiana NR, (eds): *Dupuytren's Disease,* Edinburgh, Churchill Livingstone, 1974, pp 1–9.
14. Brunner J: The dynamics of Dupuytren's disease. *Hand* 2:172–176, 1970.
15. Tubiana NR, Simmons B, DeFrenne H: Location of Dupuytren's disease on the radial aspect of the hand. *Clin Orthop Rel Res* 168:222–229, 1982.
16. McFarlane R: Dupuytren's contracture, in Green D (ed): *Operative Hand Surgery.* London, Churchill Livingstone, 1982, 463–497.
17. Short W, Watson H: Prediction of the spiral nerve in Dupuytren's contracture. *J Hand Surg (Am)* 7:84–86, 1982.
18. Gabbiani G, Majno G: Dupuytren's contracture: Fibroblast contraction? An ultrastructural study. *Am J Pathol* 66:131–138, 1972.
19. Majno G, Gabbiani G, Hirschel H, et al: Contraction of granulation tissue in vitro: Similarity to smooth muscle. *Science* 173:548–550, 1971.
20. Chiu H, McFarlane R: Pathogenesis of Dupuytren's contracture: A correlative clinical-pathological study. *J Hand Surg (Am)* 3:1–10, 1978.
21. Iwasaki H, Muller H, Stutte H, Brennscheidt U: Palmar fibromatosis (Dupuytren's contracture): Ultrastructural and enzyme histochemical studies of 43 cases. *Virchows Arch (Pathol Anat)* 405:41–53, 1984.
22. VandeBerg J, Gelberman R, Rudolph R, et al: Dupuytren's disease: Comparative growth dynamics and morphology between cultured myofibroblasts (nodule) and fibroblasts (cord). *J Orthop Res* 2:247–256, 1984.
23. Badalamente M, Stern L, Hurst L: The pathogenesis of Dupuytren's contracture: Contractile mechanisms of the myofibroblasts. *J Hand Surg (Am)* 8:235–242, 1983.
24. Tomasek J, Schultz R, Haaksma C: Extra cellular matrix–cytoskeletal connections at the surface of the specialized contractile fibroblast (myofibroblast) in Dupuytren's disease. *J Bone Joint Surg* 69A:1400–1407, 1987.
25. Halliday NL, Rayan GM, Zardi L, Tomasek J: Distribution of ED-A and ED-B containing fibronectin isoforms in Dupuytren's disease. *J Hand Surg (Am)* 19:428–434, 1994.
26. Tomasek JJ, Rayan GM: Correlation of alpha smooth muscle actin expression and contraction in Dupuytren's disease fibroblasts. *J Hand Surg (Am)* 20:450–455, 1995.
27. Hueston J, Tubiana R: *Dupuytren's Disease.* GEM monograph I. Edinburgh, Churchill Livingstone, 1974.
28. Sugden P, Andrew J, Andrew S, Freemont A: Dermal dendrocytes in Dupuytren's disease. *J Hand Surg (Br)* 18:662–666, 1993.
29. Millesi H: Neve Gesichtspunkte in der Pathogenese der Dupuytren'schen Kontracturn. *Bruns Beitr Klin Chir* 198:1–25, 1959.
30. Rudolph R, Vandeberg J: The myofibroblast in Dupuytren's contracture. *Hand Clin* 7:683–692, 1991.
31. Davis J: On surgery of Dupuytren's contracture. *Plast Reconstr Surg* 36:277–314, 1965.
32. Kischer C, Speer D: Microvascular changes in Dupuytren's contracture. *J Hand Surg (Am)* 9A:58–62, 1984.

33. Sanderson PL, Morris MA, Stanley JK, Fahmy NR: Lipids and Dupuytren's disease. *J Bone Joint Surg (Br)* 76:923–927, 1992.

34. Rabinowitz J, Osterman A, Bora F, Staeffer J: Lipid composition and de novo biosynthesis of human palmar fat in Dupuytren's disease. *Lipids* 18:371–379, 1983.

35. Weinzierl G, Flugel M, Geldmacher J: Lack of effectiveness of alternative non-surgical treatment procedures of Dupuytren's contracture. *Chirurgie* 64:492–494, 1993.

36. Delbruck A, Reimers E, Schonborn I: A comparative study of the activity of lysosomal and main metabolic pathway enzymes in tissue biopsies and cultured fibroblasts from Dupuytren's disease and palmar fascia. *J Clin Chem Clin Biochem* 19:931–941, 1981.

37. Hooper J, Jabaley M, Chi-Tsung S, et al: Enzymes of glucose metabolism in palmar fascia and Dupuytren's contracture. *J Hand Surg (Am)* 2:62–65, 1977.

38. Bazin S, LeLous M, Duance V, et al: Biochemistry and histology of the connective tissue of Dupuytren's disease lesions. *Eur J Clin Invest* 10:9–16, 1980.

39. Brickley-Parsons D, Glimcher M, Smith R, et al: Biochemical changes in the collagen of the palmar fascia in patients with Dupuytren's disease. *J Bone Joint Surg* 63A:787–797, 1981.

40. Delbruck A, Schroder H: Metabolism and proliferation of cultured fibroblasts from specimens of human palmar fascia and Dupuytren's contracture. *J Clin Chem Clin Biochem* 21:11–17, 1983.

41. Hunter J, Ogdon C, Norris M: Dupuytren's contracture: I. Chemical pathology. *Br J Plast Surg* 28:10–18, 1975.

42. Hunter J, Ogdon C: Dupuytren's contracture: II. Scanning electron microscopic evaluations. *Br J Plast Surg* 28:19–25, 1975.

43. Menzel E, Piza H, Zielinski C, et al: Collagen types and anti-collagen-antibodies in Dupuytren's disease. *Hand* 2:243–248, 1979.

44. Parsons D, Adams S, Smith R, Glimcher M: Collagen polymorphism in Dupuytren's disease. *Trans ORS* 10:116, 1985.

45. Dolynchuk K, Pettigrew N: Transglutaminase levels in Dupuytren's disease. *J Hand Surg* 16A:787–790, 1991.

46. Badalamente M, Hurst L, Sampson S: Prostaglandins influence myofibroblast contractility in Dupuytren's disease. *J Hand Surg* 13A:267, 1988.

47. Badalamente MA, Hurst LC, Grandia S, Sampson SP: Platelet derived growth factor in Dupuytren's disease. *J Hand Surg (Am)* 17A:317–323, 1992.

48. Badalamente MA, Hurst LC, Dowd A, Miyasaka K: The role of TGF-beta in Dupuytren's disease. *J Hand Surg (Am)* 21A:210–215, 1996.

49. Zamora R, Heights R, Kraemer B, et al: Presence of growth factors in palmar and plantar fibromatosis. *J Hand Surg (Am)* 19A:435–441, 1994.

50. Kloen P, Jennings LL, Gebhardt MC, et al: TGF-β: Possible roles in Dupuytren's contracture. *J Hand Surg (Am)* 20:101–108, 1995.

51. McFarlane R: The current status of Dupuytren's disease. *J Hand Surg (Am)* 8A:703–708, 1983.

52. Mennen U, Grabbe R: Dupuytren's contracture in a Negro: A case report. *J Hand Surg (Am)* 4:451, 1979.

53. Early P: Population studies in Dupuytren's contracture. *J Bone Joint Surg* 44B:602–613, 1962.

54. Hueston J: The incidence of Dupuytren's contracture. *Med J Aust* 2:99–1002, 1960.

55. Mikkelsen O: The prevalence of Dupuytren's disease in Norway. *Acta Chir Scand* 138:695–700, 1972.

56. Bell R, Furness J: A study of the effect of recurrent trauma on the development of Dupuytren's contracture. *Br J Plast Surg* 30:149–150, 1977.

57. McFarlane RM: Dupuytren's disease: Relation to work and injury. *J Hand Surg (Am)* 16:775–779, 1991.

58. Larsen R, Takagishi N, Posh J: The pathogenesis of Dupuytren's contracture. *J Bone Joint Surg* 42A:993–1007, 1960.

59. Skoog T: Dupuytren's contracture with special reference to aetiology and improved surgical treatment; Its occurrence in epileptics; Note on knuckle pads. *Acta Chir Scand* 96(suppl 139):11–176, 1948.

60. Hueston J: Current state of treatment of Dupuytren's disease. *Ann Chir Main* 3:81–92, 1984.

61. James J: The genetic pattern of Dupuytren's contracture and idiopathic epilepsy, in Hueston JT (ed): *Dupuytren's Disease*. New York, Grune and Stratton, 1974, pp 37–42.

62. Noble J, Heathcote J, Cohen H: Diabetes mellitus in the aetiology of Dupuytren's disease. *J Bone Joint Surg* 66B:322–325, 1984.

63. Pojer R, Radivojeuie M, Williams F: Dupuytren's disease: Its association with abnormal liver function in alcoholism and epilepsy. *Arch Intern Med* 129:561–566, 1972.

64. Ling R: The genetic factor in Dupuytren's disease. *J Bone Joint Surg* 45B:709–718, 1963.

65. Bonnici AV, Birjandi F, Spencer JD, et al: Chromosomal abnormalities in Dupuytren's contracture and carpal tunnel syndrome. *J Hand Surg (Br)* 17:349–355, 1992.

66. Tait B, Mackay L: HLA phenotypes in Dupuytren's contracture. *Tissue Antigens* 19:240–241, 1982.

67. Neumuller J, Menzel J, Millesi H: Prevalence of HLA-DR3 and autoantibodies to connective tissue components in Dupuytren's contracture. *Clin Imunol Immunopathol* 71:142–148, 1994.

68. Pittet B, Rubbia-Brandt L, Desmouliere A, et al: Effect of gamma interferon on the clinical and biologic evolution of hypertrophic scars and Dupuytren's disease. *Plast Reconstr Surg* 93:1224–1235, 1994.

69. Badalamente MA, Hurst LC: Enzyme injection as a non-operative treatment for Dupuytren's disease. *Drug Delivery* 3(1):35–40, 1996.

70. Starkweather K, Lattuga S, Hurst LC, et al: Collagenase in the treatment of Dupuytren's disease. *J Hand Surg (Am)* 21A:490–495, 1996.

71. Legge L, McFarlane R: Prediction of results of treatment of Dupuytren's disease. *J Hand Surg* 5:608–616, 1980.

72. Hurst LC, Starkweather KD, Badalamente MA: Dupuytren's disease, in Piemer CA (ed): *Surgery of the Hand and Upper Extremity*. Vol 2. New York, McGraw Hill, 1996, pp 1601–1615.

73. Nissenbaum M, Kleinert H: Treatment considerations in CTS with co-existent Dupuytren's disease. *J Hand Surg (Am)* 5:544–547, 1980.

74. McIndoe A, Beare RLB: The surgical management of Dupuytren's contracture. *Am J Surg* 95:197–203, 1958.

75. Tubiana R: The principles of surgical treatment of Dupuytren's contracture, in Hueston JT, Tubiana R (eds): *Dupuytren's Disease*. New York, Grune & Stratton, 1974, pp 71–77.

76. McFarlane R, Jamieson W: Dupuytren's contracture: The management of one hundred patients. *J Bone Joint Surg* 48A:1095–1104, 1966.

77. McFarlane R, Jamieson W: The current status of Dupuytren's disease. *J Hand Surg (Am)* 9A:103–708, 1966.

78. Neckesser EC: Results of wide excision of the palmar fascia for Dupuytren's contracture: Special reference to factors which adversely affect prognosis. *Ann Surg* 160:1007, 1964.

79. Zacharaie L: Extensive vs limited fasciectomy for Dupuytren's contracture. *Scand J Plast Reconstr Surg* 150:150, 1967.

80. Tonkin M, Burke F, Varian JP: Dupuytren's contracture: A comparative study of fasciectomy and dermatofasciectomy in one hundred patients. *J Hand Surg (Am)* 9B:156–162, 1984.

81. Brotherston TM, Balakrishnan C, Milner RH, Brown HG: Long term follow up of dermatofasciectomy for Dupuytren's disease. *Br J Plast Surg* 47:440–443, 1994.

82. McCash C: The open palm technique in Dupuytren's contracture. *Br J Plast Surg* 17:271–280, 1964.

83. Orlando JC, Smith JW, Dorgon D: Dupuytren's contracture: Review of 100 patients. *Br J Plast Surg* 27:211–217, 1974.

84. Moberg E: Three useful ways to avoid amputation in advanced Dupuytren's contracture. *Orthop Clin North Am* 4:1001–1005, 1978.

85. Fietti VG, Mackin EJ: Dupuytren's disease, in Hunter JM, Schneider LH, Mackin EJ, Bell JA (eds): *Rehabilitation of the Hand.* St Louis, Mosby, 1978, pp 147–153.

86. Tubiana R, Fahrer M, McCullough CJ: Recurrence and other complications in surgery of Dupuytren's contracture. *Clin Plast Surg* 8:45–50, 1981.

87. Kleinert HD, Leitch I, Smith DJ, Lubbers LM: Problems in Dupuytren's contracture, in Strickland JW, Steicher JB (eds): *Difficult Problems in Hand Surgery.* St Louis, Mosby, 1982, pp 402–408.

88. Hakstian R: Late results of extensive fasciectomy, in Hueston J, Tubiana R (eds): *Dupuytren's Disease.* New York, Grune & Stratton, 1974, pp 79–83.

89. Rebelo JS, Ferreira JB, Vilao MC, Boleo-Tome J: Dupuytren's disease: Analysis of ten year caseload. *Acta Med Port* 5:463–469, 1992.

================= CHAPTER 60 =================

Tendon Transfers in the Hand and Forearm

Joseph P. Leddy
and Timothy P. Leddy

PRINCIPLES

"A tendon transfer is that procedure in which the tendon of insertion or of origin of the functioning muscle is mobilized, detached or divided, and reinserted into a bony part or into another tendon to supplement or substitute for the action of the recipient tendon."[1] These procedures are utilized in the upper extremity following irreparable nerve damage, loss of function of the musculotendinous unit through trauma or disease, and in certain nonprogressive or slowly progressive neurologic disorders.

Stability of the wrist is essential for good hand function. The synergistic action of wrist flexion accompanies finger extension, whereas wrist extension accompanies finger flexion. However, experience has shown that the use of synergistic transfers is not mandatory and that virtually any muscle in the forearm and hand can be transferred to perform a certain function provided that one adheres to the fundamental principles of transfers. These principles have been outlined by Mayer,[2,3] Steindler,[4] Bunnell,[5,6] Boyes,[1] and others.

Correction of Contractures

The joints must be freely movable, because a transferred muscle tendon unit cannot overcome a fixed joint contracture. Splinting, therapy, and/or surgery may be necessary to release the contracture prior to the transfer.

The skin and soft tissues must be supple and free of scarring. Occasionally, a pedicle or a free flap will have to be constructed prior to the tendon transfer.

Adequate Power in the Transfer

The muscle must be strong enough to perform the desired function. The power of the muscle is determined by its cross-sectional area.[7,8] The transferred muscle will most likely lose some power; therefore, only muscles rated 4+, 5, or better should be considered acceptable donor motors.[9]

Sufficient Amplitude in the Transfer

The amplitude of a muscle is a function of its sarcomere length.[10] The effective amplitude of a muscle can be in-

creased by freeing its fascial attachments (e.g., brachioradialis) or by changing a muscle from a monoarticular to a biarticular one. Since amplitude can be limited by scarring and by adhesions in the area through which the tendon passes, one should choose a donor with more than adequate amplitude for the desired action.

According to Boyes,[1] the following values may be used as a practical guideline for amplitude:

Wrist motors	*33 mm*
Finger extensors	*50 mm*
Finger flexors	*70 mm*

The work capacity of a muscle is determined by the product of its power and amplitude.[1] Table 60-1 lists the forearm muscles and their abbreviations with their work capacities given in kilogram meters (kg·m).

Other abbreviations include the following:

Extensor indicis proprius (EIP)
Extensor digiti quinti proprius (EDQP)
Extensor pollicis brevis (EPB)
Abductor pollicis brevis (APB)

Although the FCU has the greatest work capacity of the wrist motors, its use has been questioned in tendon transfers because of its great importance in wrist function.[1] The wrist works in radial dorsiflexion and ulnar volar flexion (e.g., using a hammer).

Satisfactory Line of Pull Must Be Provided

The best course for a tendon transfer is a straight line of pull through unscarred soft tissues. Each turn or bend in the transferred tendon can set up a point of friction, causing loss of effective power and amplitude. However, it is not always possible for a transferred tendon to pull in a straight line.

Functional Integrity Must Be Preserved

The transferred tendon cannot be expected to perform more than one function or to have separate amplitudes for different motions. If the tendon is split and inserted into different sites, the force of the transfer will be expended on the tighter of the two and only that function will be performed. The transferred muscle tendon unit must be expendable. For instance, if both the FCR and FCU tendons are transferred to the dorsum of the hand and wrist, active wrist flexion will be lost and a permanent dorsiflexion contracture may result.

SURGICAL CONSIDERATIONS

The timing of tendon transfers depends upon the cause of the problem, the prognosis for recovery, and, to some extent, the preference of the patient. If there is no chance for functional recovery, transfers should be performed as soon

TABLE 60-1   Work Capacities of the Forearm Muscles

Muscle	Work capacity, kg·m
Flexor carpi radialis (FCR)	0.8
Extensor carpi radialis longus (ECRL)	1.1
Extensor carpi radialis brevis (ECRB)	0.9
Extensor carpi ulnaris (ECU)	1.1
Abductor pollicis longus (APL)	0.1
Flexor pollicis longus (FPL)	1.2
Flexor digitorum profundus (FDP)	4.5
Flexor digitorum sublimis (superficialis) (FDS)	4.8
Brachioradialis (BR)	1.9
Flexor carpi ulnaris (FCU)	2.0
Pronator teres (PT)	1.2
Palmaris longus (PL)	0.1
Extensor pollicis longus (EPL)	0.1
Extensor digitorum communis (EDC)	1.7

as the patient is ready. If nerve regeneration is expected, then one should wait until the level of functional recovery can be determined.

Early tendon transfers are defined as those performed within 12 weeks of injury. The relative indications for these procedures include (1) proximal nerve lesions, (2) irreparable nerve lesions, and (3) other lesions with a statistically poor chance for acceptable recovery. Prerequisites of early transfer are that the donor tendon be completely expendable and that no imbalance will be created by neural regeneration.[11–13]

Careful planning is essential prior to any surgical procedure, since each patient has different deficits and needs. We recommend the systematic approach. First, a list of the deficient functions should be made. Then, opposite this, a list of available working donor muscles should be compiled. Utilizing these two lists, the surgeon can decide which functions need restoration and which available donors are most appropriate for the tasks. In complex lesions, multiple transfers may be necessary to both sides of the wrist.

Multiple, short transverse incisions are preferable to extended longitudinal incisions for mobilization of donor tendons. The tendons should be handled carefully, and hemostasis should be obtained. There should be good soft tissue coverage over the tendon junctures. Direct end-to-end, end-to-side, side-to-side, or tendon-weave sutures may be utilized.

How does one achieve proper tension in tendon transfers? It is not possible to give one general rule covering all situations; experience is often the best teacher for this particular problem. The surgeon may place the hand in the position that it will assume when the tendon transfer is functioning optimally and then suture the tendon without any tension. It is usually preferable to make the transfer a little tighter rather than a little looser.

RADIAL NERVE PALSY

Problem

There is loss of extension of the wrist and metacarpophalangeal (MCP) joints of the fingers and loss of extension and abduction of the thumb (Fig. 60-1). There is inability to stabilize the wrist in neutral or in extension; therefore, power grasp is severely impaired. The fingers and thumb cannot be widely opened for prehension.

Treatment

Splinting and/or therapy may be necessary to prevent the development of contractures in a patient with radial nerve palsy. Burkhalter is a strong advocate of early tendon transfer because the tendon can serve as an internal splint.[11] He transfers PT to ECRB in an end-to-side fashion as soon as possible after the injury. This stabilizes the wrist, allows some power grasp, and may make external splinting unnecessary. In its transferred state, the PT still functions as a pronator of the forearm. If there is inadequate motor return, further transfers can be done to provide MCP joint extension and thumb extension and abduction. Early tendon transfer is not a universally accepted principle, but it does have some strong advocates.

The patient with a radial nerve palsy needs wrist extension, MCP joint extension, and extension and abduction of the thumb. Many donor motors are available. If there is a posterior interosseous nerve palsy only, extension of the wrist may be intact because of a functioning ECRL, and no transfer will be needed for wrist extension. The sensory deficit is usually not significant in radial nerve palsy.

We prefer the transfers described by Boyes[1]:

PT to ECRL and ECRB
FCR to EPB and APL
FDS long finger to EDC
FDS ring finger to EPL and EIP

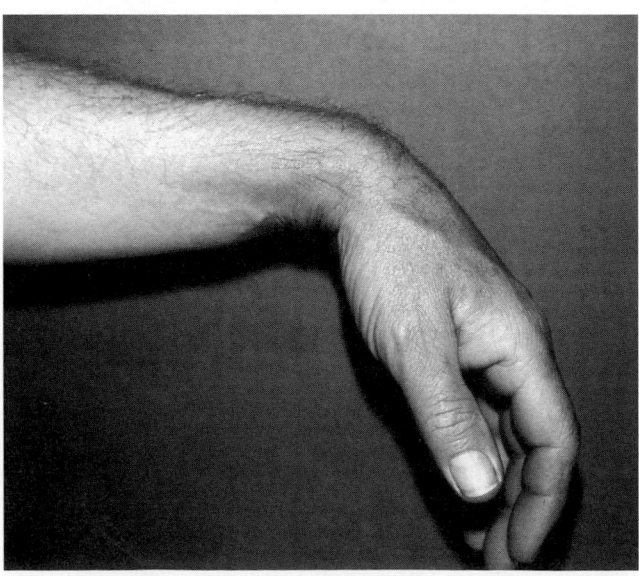

Figure 60-1 Radial nerve palsy.

This set of transfers has several advantages. The FCU, which is the most important muscle in the wrist, is retained.[14] Because of the amplitude of the transferred superficialis tendons, simultaneous wrist and finger extension can be obtained. The FDS muscles of long and ring fingers are passed through a large opening made in the interosseous membrane just proximal to the pronator quadratus muscle. The long finger FDS courses between the profundus mass and the FPL, and that of the ring finger goes along the ulnar side of the FDP. The transferred muscles are well mobilized proximally, so that muscle tissue rather than tendon is in the interosseous opening. This lessens the chance for adherence of the transfer at this site. The FDS of the long finger provides extension of the fingers, and the FDS of the ring finger gives independent extension to the thumb and index finger. The FCR provides strong abduction for the thumb metacarpal.

One of the most common operations for radial nerve palsy is referred to by Green as the *standard (FCU) transfer*[9]:

PT to ECRB
FCU to EDC
PL to rerouted EPL

This operation restores wrist and MCP joint extension and also abduction and extension of the thumb. It is technically easier to perform than the Boyes transfers. However, in the opinion of the authors, its major disadvantage is the use of the FCU as a donor motor. Since the wrist works in radial dorsiflexion and ulnar volar flexion, this important motor should be retained if possible. Other authors,[15] who agree with this concept, have proposed a set of transfers that preserve the FCU:

PT to ECRB
FCR to EDC
PL to rerouted EPL

The reader is referred to the original text for details of operative procedures and postoperative management.

MEDIAN NERVE PALSY

Problems

In median nerve palsy, the sensory deficit is very important. There is loss of sensation over the palmar aspect of the thumb and of the index and long fingers and of the radial half of the ring finger, which are the most important contact areas in the hand. Every attempt at restoring this important function should be made.

The motor deficit in low median nerve injuries at the level of the distal forearm and wrist is loss of the APB, the opponens pollicis, and, to a varying extent, the flexor pollicis brevis. There is great variability in the innervation of the thenar musculature, and approximately one-third of patients with low median nerve palsy will have sufficient power in the remaining flexor pollicis brevis muscle to obviate any type of opposition transfer.

Treatment

If opposition power is insufficient and cannot be returned by neurorrhaphy or nerve grafting, then tendon transfer should be considered. Good skin and supple joints are a prerequisite. If a fixed contracture develops in the first web space, surgery may be necessary to mobilize this prior to opponensplasty.

The history of tendon transfers for opposition of the thumb is long and complex. Much of the early experience was gained from patients with poliomyelitis. There is no simple cookbook formula for opposition transfers in the thumb, and patients must be judged carefully regarding their specific needs and deficits. A strong motor is necessary if the thumb adductor and first dorsal interosseous and the EPL are functioning. If these muscles are paralyzed due to a combined nerve lesion or to some neurologic disorder, then a weaker donor can be utilized. There are many methods of insertion of the tendon transfer; the reader is referred to the classic articles for a description of these.[15]

In isolated low median nerve palsy, the antagonists are functioning and a strong motor is necessary. Bunnell[5] has shown us that the line of pull of the transfer should be from the area of the pisiform. A loop is made in the FCU tendon at the level of the pisiform to act as a fixed pulley. One-half of the FCU tendon is utilized just proximal to the pisiform to fashion this loop, and it is sutured to itself. The ring finger superficialis can be used as a donor tendon unless it was damaged at the time of the injury to the median nerve. This tendon can be divided in the palm just proximal to the A1 metacarpal pulley. Through a separate incision, it is withdrawn into the proximal forearm, placed through the fixed FCU pulley at the level of the pisiform, and then tunneled subcutaneously across the palm to the level of the MCP joint of the thumb, where it can be inserted into the tendon of the APB or into the dorsoulnar aspect of the base of the proximal phalanx. If the FDS of the ring finger is not a suitable donor, other tendons such as the EIP, EDQP, ECU, and the abductor digiti minimi may be utilized.[16,17] If the pulley is made proximal to the pisiform, more abduction will be gained. If it is made distal to the pisiform, there will be more flexion and adduction. This is useful in combined low median and ulnar nerve palsy.

In long-standing cases of median nerve compression at the wrist with loss of thenar function, the Camitz transfer has been advocated.[18] At the time of carpal tunnel release, the palmaris longus tendon, prolonged with a strip of palmar fascia, is inserted into the tendon of the APB to provide palmar abduction of the thumb.

In high median nerve lesions, the entire FDS, the FDP of index and long fingers, and the FPL are also lost (Fig. 60-2). The FCR is not functioning, but the FCU—innervated by the ulnar nerve—is working and provides adequate strength for wrist flexion. Since there is loss of FDS function, the ring finger superficialis cannot be utilized in the opponens transfer. Therefore, one of the alternatives mentioned above is carried out. The FDP of index and long fingers can be attached side to side to the FDP of the ring and little fingers to produce flexion of the index and long fingers, but the power of grasp is not increased. The BR, af-

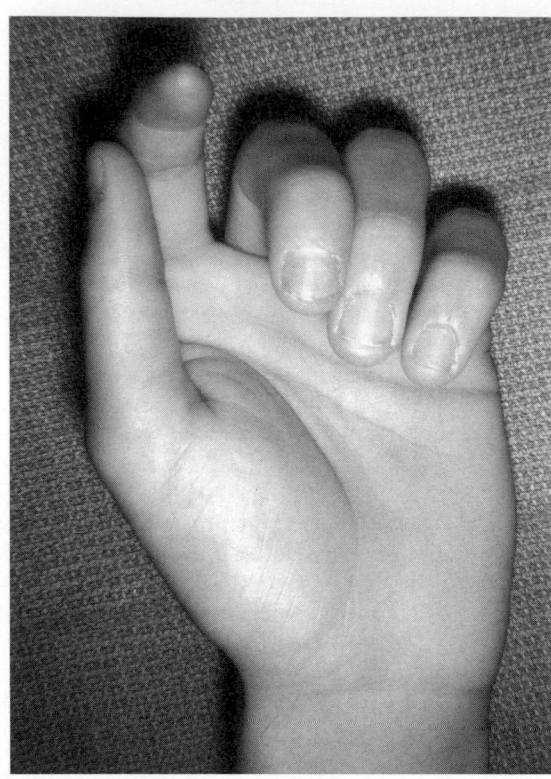

Figure 60-2 High median nerve palsy. There is median sensory loss and weakness or paralysis of APB, opponens pollicis, entire FDS, FDP of index and long, FPL, and FCR.

ter being freed from its fascial attachments in the forearm, can be transferred to the FPL to provide flexion at the interphalangeal (IP) joint of the thumb and power and stability for pinch. If more power is needed for flexion of the index and long fingers, the ECRL can be transferred to the FDP of the index and long fingers.

THE ULNAR NERVE

Problems

There are multiple deficits in ulnar nerve palsy affecting almost all facets of hand function. Proper coordination of finger flexion requires initiation of flexion at the MCP joints. With loss of function of the interossei and the ulnar two lumbricals, there is no independent flexion of the MCP joints. The FDS and FDP act upon the distal interphalangeal (DIP) and proximal interphalangeal (PIP) joints primarily and the MCP joints secondarily. During grasp, therefore, the extrinsic muscles first flex the DIP and PIP joints, curling the fingers into the hand. The MCP joints flex last. Thus, the arc of flexion is shortened, and it is impossible to grasp large objects, which are actually pushed out of the palm during attempted flexion of the fingers. Power grip and stability of pinch are severely impaired. Froment described instability of key pinch with compensatory hy-

perflexion of the IP joint in 1915. The IP joint flexes to increase the mechanical advantage of the EPL as a secondary adductor (Froment's sign). Hyperextension at the MCP joint occurs secondary to loss of the intrinsic musculature of the thumb (Fig. 60-3). Loss of abduction and adduction of the fingers contributes to the impaired dexterity of the hand.

Clawing is most commonly seen in the ring and little fingers, although it may also be seen in the index and long fingers (Fig. 60-4). It is more common in loose-jointed individuals and may not be present in a person with very tight joints that cannot be passively hyperextended. As the MCP joints hyperextend, complete extension of the PIP joints is not possible. If these joints are not properly exercised or splinted, fixed contractures may develop, with the MCP joints in hyperextension and the PIP joints in flexion.

In high ulnar nerve lesions, there is loss of the FCU at the wrist and FDP of the ring and little fingers. Loss of the ulnar two profundi further contributes to the loss of power grip. In low ulnar nerve lesions, there is loss of sensation on the ulnar border of the hand, including the palmar surface of the little finger and the ulnar half of the ring finger.

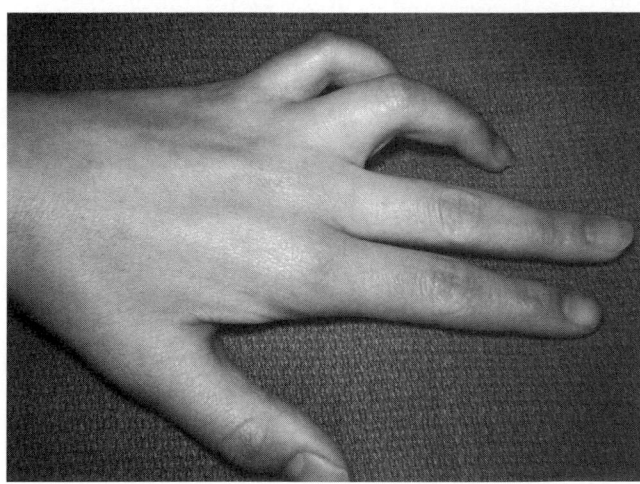

Figure 60-3 Ulnar nerve palsy. There is clawing of ring and little fingers with atrophy of the interossei.

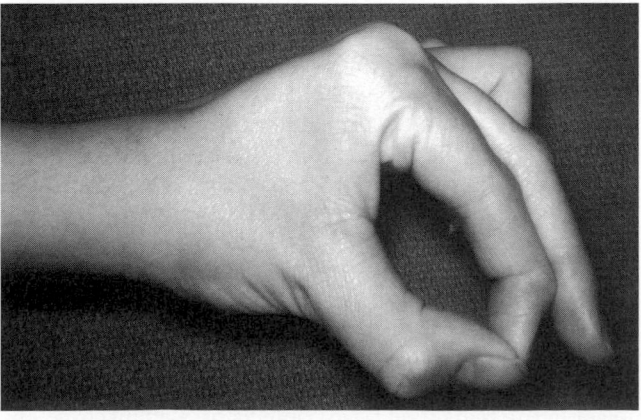

Figure 60-4 Ulnar nerve palsy. Positive Froment sign.

In high ulnar nerve lesions, the same loss if present along with the absence of sensation on the dorsoulnar aspect of the hand. The sensory deficit in an ulnar nerve lesion is significant, but it is not nearly as important as loss of sensation in the median nerve distribution.

Treatment

Once it is obvious that there will be no recovery of motor function after an ulnar nerve lesion, various procedures should be considered. Restoration of pinch function involves bringing the thumb metacarpal toward the index metacarpal with a strong motor. Maintenance of a stable thumb MCP joint as a base upon which to pinch is important. Therefore, tendon transfers for pinch must provide balanced forces to the first metacarpal, the MCP joint, and the index finger. Only a few of the more commonly used transfers are discussed here, but a more complete listing is available in the References.

A BR transfer can restore strong adduction to the thumb.[1] A free tendon graft is required and is attached by a pull-out wire sutured to the base of the proximal phalanx of the thumb on the ulnar volar border. The graft is then passed along the surface of the paralyzed adductor muscle to the ulnar side of the third metacarpal, where it is brought out to the dorsum of the hand between the long and ring finger metacarpals. Here it is attached to the BR muscle, which has been mobilized proximally to increase its excursion. Smith[19] used the ECRB prolonged with a free tendon graft between the bases of the index and long finger metacarpals going across the adductor muscle to be sutured to the base of the proximal phalanx of the thumb on its ulnar side near the adductor tubercle with a pull-out wire and button. Other procedures utilized are the tendon loop operation, the tendon T operation, and transfer of the superficialis. Some authors prefer fusion of either the MCP or IP joint of the thumb[13] with or without an associated transfer to improve abduction of the index finger.[1]

Many different surgical procedures have been devised to compensate for the loss of active MCP joint flexion in the fingers. These procedure fall into two major categories: static and dynamic. If, when MCP joint hyperextension is blocked passively, there is full DIP and PIP joint extension, then static procedures may be helpful in correcting the deformity. These procedures include bone block techniques,[20] arthrodesis of the MCP joints, volar plate capsulorrhaphy,[21,22] capsulodesis and pulley advancement,[6,23,24] and various tenodesis techniques[25] to prevent the hyperextension at the MCP joints. None of the static techniques increase the power of grasp. If fixed contractures are present or if the extensor apparatus has been stretched out over the dorsum of the PIP joints so that full extension here is not possible when MCP joint hyperextension is blocked, then static techniques will not be successful and tendon transfers may be indicated. These transfers are designed to produce primary flexion at the MCP joints,[22] providing synchronous finger flexion and, in some cases, adding to the power of grasp. Stiles advocated using superficialis tendons as transfers to provide MCP joint flexion.[6] However, using a superficialis tendon will not increase

power of grasp. Since then, many other tendons have been utilized including extensor tendons.[1,25]

Normally, the transfer is placed through the lumbrical canal beneath the transverse metacarpal ligament and then inserted into the lateral band of the finger. Because of the development of hyperextension at the PIP joint in some of these patients, many authors prefer to insert the transfer into the A2 pulley or into the proximal phalanx instead of the lateral band. These procedures can increase the power of grasp by adding a new motor unit to the flexor side of the hand.[26] Other procedures have been devised to restore the flattened metacarpal arch[27] and to correct an abduction deformity at the MCP joint of the little finger.[1,28]

In high ulnar nerve palsy, there is loss of flexion at the DIP joints of the ring and little fingers and loss of the FCU. If there is profound weakness in flexion of the ring and little fingers, the FDP of these two fingers can be attached side to side to the functioning FDP of the long finger to provide flexion. Since ulnar deviation is important in wrist flexion, one-half or all of the FCR can be transferred to the FCU to provide ulnar volar flexion at the wrist.[12]

COMBINED NERVE LESIONS

Combined nerve lesions are very difficult problems. They are often associated with injuries such as fractures and tendon or muscle damage (Fig. 60-5). Without proper exercise and splinting, contractures often develop very quickly. There are limited motors available for use in transfer, due to the involvement of more than one nerve. All of the basic principles discussed previously apply to the patient with combined nerve lesions. Goals for rehabilitation must be realistic, since it is usually impossible to replace all of the lost function. Because of the limitation of available motors, static procedures—such as fusion, tenodesis,

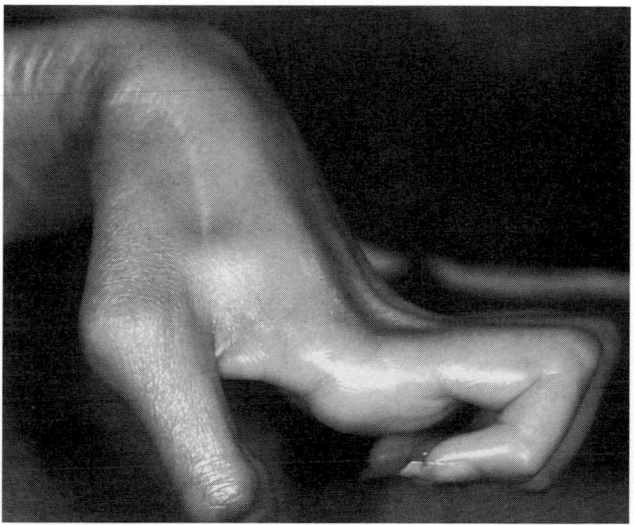

Figure 60-5 Combined nerve lesion following severe injury to the forearm.

and capsulodesis—must often be utilized. Since it is beyond the scope of this chapter to discuss the treatment of the various combined nerve lesions, the reader is referred to other sources for a complete discussion of these intricate problems.[13]

REFERENCES

1. Boyes JH (ed): *Bunnell's Surgery of the Hand,* 5th ed. Philadelphia, Lippincott, 1970.
2. Mayer L: The physiological method of tendon transplantation: Parts I, II, and III. *Surg Gynecol Obstet* 22:182, 298, 422, 1916.
3. Mayer L: The physiological method of tendon transplantation. *Surg Gynecol Obstet* 33:528, 1921.
4. Steindler A: Orthopaedic operations on the hand. *JAMA* 71:288, 1918.
5. Bunnell S: Opposition of the thumb. *J Bone Joint Surg* 20:269, 1938.
6. Bunnell S: Surgery of the intrinsic muscles of the hand other than those producing opposition of the thumb. *J Bone Joint Surg* 24:1, 1942.
7. Lieber RL, Jacobson MD, Fazeli BM, et al. Architecture of the selected muscles of the arm and forearm: Anatomy and implications of tendon transfer. *J Hand Surg* 17A:787, 1992.
8. Zajac FE: How musculotendon architecture and joint geometry affect the capacity of muscles to move and exert force on objects: A review with application to arm and forearm tendon transfer design. *J Hand Surg* 17A:523, 1992.
9. Green DP: Radial nerve palsy, in Green DP (ed): *Operative Hand Surgery.* New York, Churchill Livingstone, 1993, pp 1401–1418.
10. Blix M: Die Lange und die Spannung des Muskels. *Skand Arch Physiol* 3:295, 1891.
11. Burkhalter WE: Early tendon transfer in upper extremity peripheral nerve injury. *Clin Orthop* 104:68, 1974.
12. Omer GE Jr: Ulnar nerve palsy, in Green DP (ed): *Operative Hand Surgery.* New York, Churchill Livingstone, 1993, pp 1449–1466.
13. Omer GE Jr: Combined nerve palsies, in Green DP (ed): *Operative Hand Surgery.* New York, Churchill Livingstone, 1993, pp 1467–1482.
14. Chuinard RG, Boyes JH, Stark HH, Ashworth CR: Tendon transfers for radial nerve palsy: Use of superficialis tendons for digital extension. *J Hand Surg* 6:561, 1978.
15. Brand PW: Tendon transfers in the forearm, in Flynn JF (ed): *Hand Surgery,* 2d ed. Baltimore, Williams & Wilkins, 1975, pp 189–200.
16. Huber E: Hilfsoperation bei medianuslahmung. *Dtsch Z Chir* 162:271, 1921.
17. Litter JW, Cooley SGS: Opposition of the thumb and its restoration by abductor digiti quinti transfer. *J Bone Joint Surg* 45A:1389, 1963.
18. Camitz H: Surgical treatment of paralysis of the opponens muscle of the thumb. *Acta Clin Scand* 65:77, 1929.
19. Smith RJ: Extensor carpi radialis brevis tendon transfer for thumb abduction—A study of power pinch. *J Hand Surg* 8:4, 1983.
20. Mikhail IK: Bone block operation for claw hand. *Surg Gynecol Obstet* 118:1077, 1964.
21. Brown PW: Zancolli capsulorrhaphy for ulnar claw hand. *J Bone Joint Surg* 52A:868, 1970.
22. Zancolli EA: *Structural and Dynamic Basis of Hand Surgery.* Philadelphia, Lippincott, 1966.
23. Leddy JP, Stark HH, Ashworth CR, Boyes JH: Capsulodesis and pulley advancement for the correction of claw finger deformity. *J Bone Joint Surg* 54A:1475, 1972.
24. Leddy JP, Strauss ED: Tendon transfers in Dee R, Mango E, Hurst LC (eds): *Principles of Orthopaedic Practice.* New York, McGraw-Hill, 1988, pp 719–727.
25. Riordan DC: Tendon transfers in hand surgery. *J Hand Surg* 8(suppl):748, 1983.
26. Smith RJ: Surgical treatment of the claw hand, in American Academy of Orthopaedic Surgeons: *Symposium on Tendon Surgery in the Hand.* St. Louis, Mosby, 1975, p 181.
27. Hastings H, McCollam SM: Flexor digitorum superficialis lasso tendon transfer in isolated ulnar nerve palsy: A functional evaluation. *J Hand Surg* 19A:275, 1994.
28. Dellon AL: Extensor digiti minimi tendon transfer to correct abducted small finger in ulnar dysfunction. *J Hand Surg* 16A:819, 1991.

CHAPTER 61

Traumatic Amputations of the Hand and Wrist

John J. Leppard

CARPAL AND METACARPAL LEVEL

Disarticulations at the wrist level allow excellent pronation and supination of the forearm and hand unit. The difficulties of prosthetic fittings have been recently overcome, thus making amputations at this level a more attractive choice than previously thought.

Midpalmar or carpal amputations must be approached carefully. It is a serious mistake for the surgeon to prejudge what is and is not worth saving in an injured or partially amputated palm.[1] An intact radiocarpal joint that allows wrist flexion and extension can be extremely useful to the patient. Replantation may be actively considered (see Chap. 64). A patient who has lost digits can remain extremely functional by utilizing the residual carpus and metacarpals as a broad terminal assist. Frequently, such a patient who is fitted with a terminal prosthesis discards it because the residual function is better without it. The primary reason for this residual function is the intact sensation in the remainder of the carpus hand unit. Thus, preservation of sensate parts is important.

PROXIMAL PHALANX LEVEL

Amputations at the proximal phalanx level lose the flexor power of the superficialis tendon. Intrinsic function allows only weak flexion at the metacarpophalangeal (MCP) joint. Thus, serious consideration should be given in such circumstances to ray resection and reconstruction of the contiguous transverse carpal ligament. This procedure has been a long-time favorite of hand surgeons because it rectifies several predicaments all at once. The obvious deformity of the stubby finger is immediately corrected. Small objects and coins thus no longer slip through the defect that would otherwise exist between the two normal fingers. In addition, the cosmetic influence and cascade of the contiguous digit is closely reapproximated by ray resection. This has significant functional ramifications, because a finger that is left with a short proximal phalanx is frequently bypassed in daily use. The adjacent normal finger assumes most of the functional duties of its amputated neighbor. Exceptions do exist. For example, the problem is not so straightforward when two contiguous digits are amputated at this level. Resection of two contiguous rays would significantly narrow the breadth of such a palm and leave a three-fingered hand. Prosthetic replacement may be preferred.

Ray amputation of the index finger in an otherwise normal hand leads to a satisfactory cosmetic result; nevertheless, a functional residual disability—some weakness of pinch and grip—persists after such an amputation. After ray resection of the long finger, the treating surgeon has two options. The first is reconstruction of the volar intermetacarpal ligament between the index and ring fingers, thus attempting to pull these two digits closer together. The second alternative is the transposition of the index ray to the position of the long finger, as originally described by Carroll.[2] This procedure immediately obliterates the dead space of the middle finger. However, it has been associated with delayed union or nonunion of the osteotomy site in some cases. Similar choices exist for amputations through the ring or small finger. In the case of the ring finger ray resection, transposition of the fifth ray to the ring position can be done. In amputation of the fifth ray, it is important to preserve the hypothenar musculature to serve as adequate padding and cushioning of the ulnar side of the hand. Augmentation of existing interosseous musculature with that of the amputated digit should be discouraged because intrinsic tightness can result.

MIDDLE PHALANX LEVEL

Amputations at the middle phalanx level can remain quite functional if the level is distal to the superficial flexor tendon insertion. In such cases, functional flexion of the proximal interphalangeal (PIP) joint can be maintained. Proximal to this insertion, however, flexion is less likely to be preserved. Consequently, a disarticulation through the PIP joint can be just as functional as a short middle phalangeal amputation.

DISTAL PHALANX LEVEL

In most cases, consideration must be given to the type of fingertip that will result if greater than half of the distal phalanx is amputated. In such cases, very little supportive structure is left for the remaining nail and nail matrix. Often a "hook-nail" deformity or other such unattractive, troublesome situation can result. Thus, it is frequently advisable to remove not only the remainder of the injured nail but also the proximal germinal matrix in order to prevent this deformity. If there is enough distal phalanx to support the nail, the hook-nail deformity will probably be prevented. The rule then is to preserve as much length and distal phalanx as possible, but the patient should be made aware of the continuing possibility of nail deformity. Such a deformity can be surgically corrected later. In distal digital amputations, one should properly identify each terminal digital nerve in carrying out the same careful neurectomy as for more proximal amputations. The bone should be rongeured to form a small contour that will not exert undue pressure on the soft tissues of the terminal portion of the amputation and produce a painful stump. The flexor tendon should never be sutured to the extensor tendon, because it can limit flexor profundus function in the other digits.

After division of the flexor digitorum profundus, a patient may be left with a so-called lumbrical-plus finger.[3] In this situation, flexion of the PIP joint is severely limited secondary to the additional tension exerted through the lumbrical. This muscle has had its origin moved proximally by migration of the flexor profundus tendon, which no longer has an insertion into the distal phalanx. To prevent this, the cut profundus stump can be sutured to the remaining flexor pulley. If a lumbrical-plus finger deformity is noted, it is frequently wise to section the proximal lumbrical as a delayed reconstructive procedure. This problem appears to be especially evident in tip amputations of the index finger.

FINGERTIP LEVEL

Of all amputations sustained traumatically, the one that presents most commonly is the fingertip amputation.

In recent years, hand surgeons have become increasingly aware of the excellent regeneration and self-healing capacity of the finger pulp. This is not surprising, given its rich vascular bed. With thorough and meticulous care, debridement, and regular dressing changes, the finger pulp amputation can shrink, granulate, and epithelialize quite satisfactorily.[4] This "no-surgery technique" is especially indicated in the young child, in whom the ability to heal a distal amputation is most evident. The initial tip discrepancy and cosmetic loss become less and less evident with each year of remaining growth.

This conservative treatment is also applicable to adult partial fingertip amputations. However, in adult patients,

other factors should be considered. Time lost from work can be a very real problem, and the period of such healing is frequently significant. In addition, the hypersensitivity in such an escarified tip that has healed by secondary intention can often be so extreme as to necessitate a more proximal amputation at a later date. This can frequently occur after months of protracted waiting and loss of employment. Thus, the best interest of the patient who is a manual laborer may be to carry out a slightly proximal amputation at the time of primary treatment. Such treatment allows primary closure of the wound and frequently involves the shortest recuperative period.

An alternative to amputation is the resurfacing of the distal pulp via advancement of more proximal undamaged tissue. This is the premise of the Atasoy (triangular volar advancement) and the Kutler (lateral tissue advancement) flap techniques.[5,6]

Sometimes a full-thickness loss that has left the distal phalanx with some degree of soft tissue pulp can be repaired with a split-skin graft. The suggestion has been made that such treatment hastens the actual shrinkage of the defect in the tip by pulling the edges of the wound together. Whether or not this technique hastens the healing any more than treating by secondary intention granulation is conjectural at this point.

When the skin loss extends to the volar surface of the flexor tendon, there is an additional problem. The surgeon is loath to amputate a large portion of the distal phalanx, since the flexor sheath is still intact. However, the techniques so far described will not suffice. In such cases a cross-finger flap is useful (Fig. 61-1).[7] In this procedure, the dorsal untraumatized skin and subcutaneous tissue are carefully dissected and elevated from an adjacent uninjured finger and attached to the traumatized defect in the contiguous injured finger.[8] This procedure replaces the volar surface that has been lost and allows adequate padding and soft tissue coverage of all of the important volar surfaces of the finger. The dorsal aspect of the donor finger is then resurfaced with a free skin graft. This graft

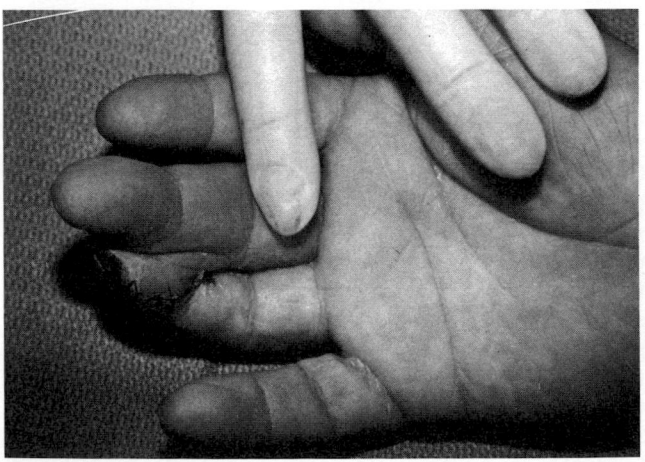

A

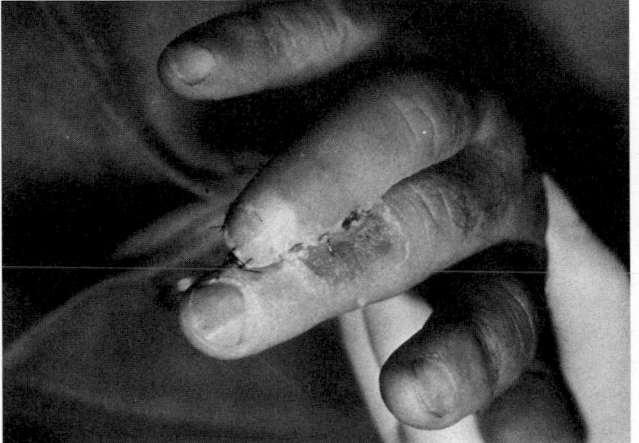

B

Figure 61-1 *A.* The cross-finger flap provides fleshy pulp coverage. *B.* The donor defect is covered with skin graft to the dorsum of the long finger.

can be from the groin or from the flexor surface of the wrist. Detachment of such a pedicle graft is usually safely accomplished at 3 weeks after the attachment. Stiffness of the interphalangeal joints can often be a sequela of such a procedure, but gentle, controlled range-of-motion exercises during the healing phase usually prevent this complication. In addition, the young patient is less likely to experience such joint stiffness. The defect incurred on the dorsum of the donor digit does not result in functional disability, since it is not on the tactile surface of the finger.

An alternative method to the cross-finger flap is the thenar flap (Fig. 61-2). In this procedure, the involved finger is flexed just enough to attach the damaged portion to a pedicle flap raised from the skin and subcutaneous tissues of the thenar area. Some critics of the thenar flap have warned against resultant stiffness of the damaged finger. Therefore this procedure is contraindicated in elderly or arthritic patients or in patients with any condition that might lead to the development of stiffness, including Dupytren's contracture and scleroderma. If the patient is not elderly or arthritic, the degree of flexion contracture can usually be kept to a minimum. The thenar flap technique is useful, particularly in the index and long fingers. In order to minimize PIP joint stiffness, the flap should be disconnected from the thenar area at 12 to 14 days. It

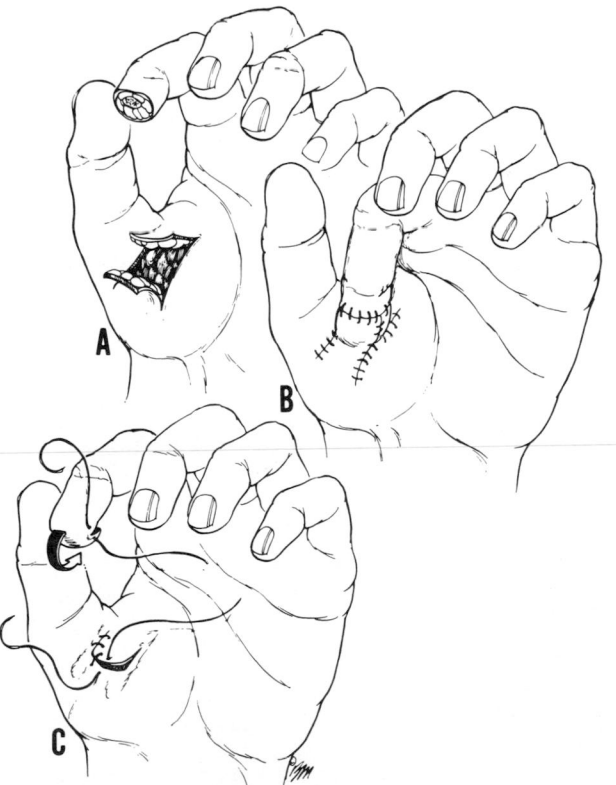

Figure 61-2 *A–C.* The thenar flap works well in the properly selected patient. Residual stiffness is minimized by proper positioning of the digit and aggressive therapy after "release." [Reproduced with permission from Green, DP (ed): *Operative Hand Surgery.* New York, Churchill Livingstone, 1982.]

should not be immediately sutured tightly down at the junction of the proximal end of the flap and the proximal edge of the pulp defect but gently coaxed into place by progressively tightened adhesive strips. Immediate tight suturing of the proximal end of the flap to the finger after disconnecting it from the thenar area causes undue stress on the vascular supply of the flap from the tip of the finger and can result in flap loss.

Reattachment as a composite graft of a fingertip amputation is a valid alternative to complex microsurgical procedures in young children between 1 and 8 years of age, as such tissue will frequently survive.[9]

A reversed digit artery island pedicle flap can also be raised from the dorsum of the proximal phalanx and transposed to cover volar tip amputations.[10]

The Heuston volar flap is raised by an L-shaped incision, with the longitudinal line along the lateral digital border and the transverse line along the proximal interphalangeal joint crease. Dissection must be superficial to the neurovascular bundle. The other bundle is preserved in the base of the flap and provides its blood supply. It must be stressed that horned nail deformities occur when insufficient bone remains beneath the nail matrix. The flap itself can be temporarily transfixed to the underlying bone via a needle until suturing is completed.[11]

The rotational pedicle flaps can also be raised from the dorsal metacarpal region. These flaps have the advantage of being able to close the donor defect primarily.[12]

If revascularization is not feasible, an amputated distal phalanx and its nail matrix can be used as a composite graft to retain length of the digit in the properly selected patient. The palmar skin is removed from the amputated part. The bone with its matrix is held in place via K-wire fixation. Skin coverage over this bone-free tissue graft is achieved via local soft tissue advancement.[13]

The esthetic early results of treatments for dorsal avulsions of the nail bed are superior to those of secondary reconstructions. This defect can be covered via a split-thickness graft of nail matrix harvested from a toe. An alternative method utilizes the advancement of the traditional volar V-Y advancement. If the distalmost portion of the advanced tissue is deepithelialized, it can be attached to the dorsal proximal remnant of the sterile matrix. The tension in the flap is overcome by using a K wire to transfix the soft tissue to the bone. This is left intact for 2 to 3 weeks.[14]

A one-stage dorsal middle phalangeal neurovascular island flap can be used for closure of fingertip partial amputations. The dorsal sensory nerve can be sutured to the recipient proximal digital nerve. Although this procedure is reported to provide excellent two-point discrimination, it requires extensive dissection of the entire finger.[15]

THE THUMB

Amputations of the thumb are managed differently from other digital amputations. The three joints of the thumb axis compose an arc of flexion that compensates for the loss of motion at any one of the individual joints. Such latitude allows the surgeon to consider alternative reconstructive modalities in the thumb, which would not work in the finger. An amputated thumb can be expected to be quite functional as long as the distal portion of the remaining thumb reaches the MCP-joint level of the contiguous index finger. The distal pulp and tip amputation can often be treated in the same manner as fingertip amputations. More proximal levels, however, are matters of concern.

The thumb obviously functions more independently in the hand than the other digits and thus is of greater functional importance, which indicates a need for greater effort in reconstruction and preservation of length than in the digits. Microsurgical replantation and repair probably have no greater use or indication than in all-out attempts at preservation of an amputated thumb. In more distal levels (1 cm or less of thumb lost), where replantation may not be feasible, the volar advancement of Moberg can be utilized (Fig. 61-3). In such a procedure, the volarmost remaining tissue is incised laterally in the midaxial plane, with preservation of both digital neurovascular bundles in the volar flap.[15] This incision must carefully preserve the circulation as well as the sensation to the flap. The flap itself must also be carefully dissected off the flexor sheath of the thumb. Next, the interphalangeal (IP) and MCP joints of the thumb are brought into as much flexion as necessary to gain tip coverage with the flap. Resultant fixed flexion deformities of the thumb joints can occur after this procedure. However, the composite flexion of the joints of the thumb rarely makes this a functional disability. These contractures can also be minimized by aggressive hand therapy. The sutures used to attach the volar advancement flap in the thumb should be left in place for approximately 2 to 3 weeks to prevent proximal migration or wound dehiscence.

More proximal amputations in the thumb (greater than 1 cm of thumb length lost) require other management techniques. Despite the proliferation of more elaborate microsurgical transfers and reconstructions, the surgeon is probably best advised to pursue the most conservative and least risky procedures in thumb reconstruction. The distraction and augmentation techniques can provide a satisfactory thumb. These procedures are most applicable when the amputation level has left the remaining thumb just short of the contiguous index MCP joint. In such case, the thumb amputation should be cleaned and shortened only as much as necessary to allow primary closure after digital neurectomies and contouring of the remaining bone. At a later date, usually months, the technique and risks of distraction and augmentation procedures are explained to the patient in detail. When the tip of the thumb has healed completely with no signs of hyperemia, the first stage, a simple osteotomy in the thumb metacarpal, can be done. A distraction device such as a mini-Hoffman or Jaquet's device is attached via two distally placed and two proximally placed pins. Each pair of pins is separated by the osteotomy site through the thumb metacarpal. To further stabilize the osteotomy and in preparation for its distraction, one or two longitudinally placed Kirschner wires are also used. The wounds are primarily closed over the osteotomy. In the weeks after surgery, the patient is carefully supervised in the twice-daily technique of lengthening the foreshortened thumb. About 1 to 2 mm of distraction per day can be tolerated. If neurologic or vascular compromise at the end of the digit occurs during the distraction schedule, the surgeon should delay or curtail the distraction.

Once an appropriate length of the thumb has been achieved, usually when the distal portion of the thumb reaches the level of the index MCP joint, the distraction of the thumb can be discontinued. At this stage the second phase of the reconstruction is undertaken. The same dorsal incision utilized for the osteotomy is opened. The distracted attenuated periosteum should be incised longitudinally without disrupting these bone-forming tissues. Next, an autogenous iliac graft is obtained, shaped, and cut appropriately to fit neatly into the distraction space of the thumb metacarpal. The graft is usually fixed with percutaneously placed Kirschner wires. These wires can eas-

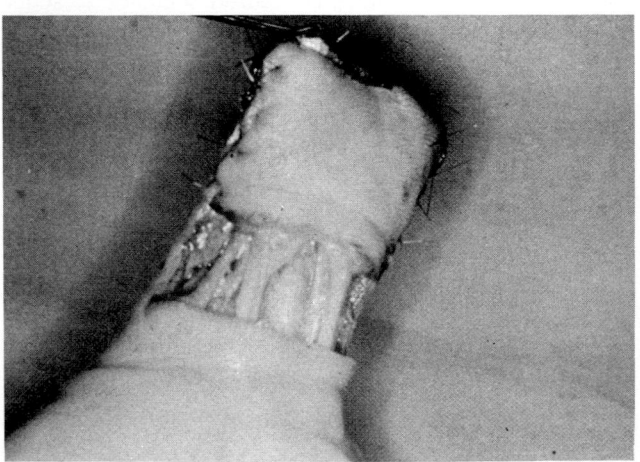
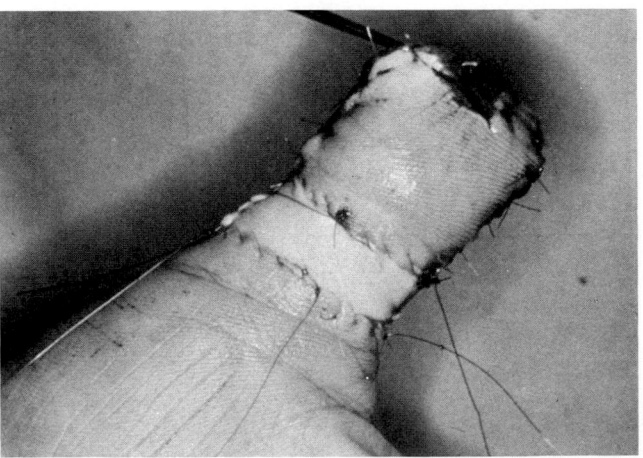

A *B*

Figure 61-3 *A.* Volar advance flap: volar skin proximal to the deficiency is moved distally. *B.* Split skin graft fills the deficiency.

ily be removed in the office once the graft has sufficiently incorporated. Incorporation usually takes 3 to 6 weeks. Once fixation is achieved, the external fixation distraction device can be removed and hand therapy with dynamic and static splinting instituted. Frequently, Z-plasty and first-web-space deepening are necessary as secondary procedures.

Amputations that occur at or proximal to the MCP level are probably best treated at this time with microsurgical composite reconstruction. In one technique (the wraparound), a well-contoured portion of iliac graft is used as a structural extension to the remaining metacarpal of the thumb. This is then covered by donor soft tissues, which are dissected from the great toe. Microsurgical anastomoses of neurovascular structures in the soft tissue graft and the residual portions of the thumb are performed to complete the reconstruction. When this is successfully accomplished, the result is a functional thumb. The residual donor site in the great toe can frequently be treated by skin grafting or by creating a syndactyly to the second toe. A time-honored procedure that is extremely useful for treating patients with thumb amputation is pollicization of the index finger. This still remains the technique of choice in the younger patient. In pollicization after traumatic loss of the thumb, careful assessment of the vasculature of the rat that is to be pollicized should be carried out preoperatively. A dorsal-ulnar pedicle flap can be raised from over the thumb metacarpal to cover distal thumb amputations.[17]

COMPLICATIONS

Painful Stumps, Scars, Neuromas, Cold Intolerance, Phantom Limb Pain

Painful neuromas can usually be avoided by cutting each nerve cleanly while it is placed in maximal traction. This allows the cut nerve to retract into the remaining soft tissue cuff. Painful neuromas that persist months or years after amputation should be treated first with conservative techniques. These include alterations in the prosthesis, aggressive physical or occupational therapy with a specific desensitization program, localized infiltration with cortisone and long-acting local anesthetics, and regular massage by the patients themselves. In this way sensitivity can frequently be minimized.

One of the most resistant conditions is the neuroma of the superficial branch of the radial nerve. The sensitivity caused even by a neuroma-in-continuity can persist despite the fact that no complete laceration of this nerve has occurred during initial injury or surgery.

When a patient shows no improvement, other modalities should be pursued. Some of these are biofeedback, sympathetic blocks, regional Bier's blocks with guanethidine or reserpine, or even sympathectomies. Sometimes the appropriate step at this point is referral to a pain clinic, which has appropriate facilities and staff for administering these techniques.

Contractures, which frequently occur in the amputated portion of the upper extremity, can be minimized by early edema control. Bulky, well-padded, and mild compressive dressings are helpful adjuvants to avoid edema and subsequent contractures. The range of motion of the remaining portions of the upper extremity can be maximized with early active, active-assisted, and passive exercises supervised by a qualified therapist.

Cold intolerance is the same in finger replantations and stump revision after amputation. Thus, the decision between stump revision and replantation after amputations should not be determined on this basis. Cold intolerance is a reflection of the type of injury sustained by the neurovascular bundle.[19]

Phantom limb pain after amputation is presently hypothesized as being the result of plastic changes in the somatosensory cortex.[20] In a recent series of Boswick,[18] phantom pain existed in almost all of 100 patients during the first month postinjury. Continuation of this pain was strongly associated with psychological perception and regressive disability.

Though the long-term prognosis for phantom limb pain and reflex dystrophy is poor, the chance of improvement is maximized when these syndromes are recognized and treated early.[22]

REFERENCES

1. Chase RA: Functional levels of amputation in the hand. *Surg Clin North Am* 40:415–423, 1960.
2. Tubiana R, Roux JP: Phalangization of the first and fifth metacarpals: Indications, operative technique and results. *J Bone Joint Surg* 56A:447–457, 1974.
3. Parkes A: The "limbrical-plus" finger. *Hand* 2:164–167, 1970.
4. Bate JT: Second and third intention healing of finger tip amputations: A salvage procedure. *Clin Orthop* 47:151–155, 1966.
5. Atasoy E, Iokimidis E, Kasdan ML, et al: Reconstruction of the amputated finger tip with a triangular volar flap: A new surgical procedure. *J Bone Joint Surg* 52:921–926, 1970.
6. Freiberg A, Manktelow R: The Kutler repair of finger tip amputations. *Plast Reconstr Surg* 50:371–375, 1972.
7. Brailliar F, Horner RL: Sensory cross-finger pedicle graft. *J Bone Joint Surg* 51A:1264–1268, 1969.
8. Johnson RK, Iverson RE: Cross finger pedicle flaps in the hand. *J Bone Joint Surg* 53A:913–919, 1971.
9. Roszlein R, Simmen B: Fingertip amputations in the child. *Handchiv Mikrochiv Plast Chiv* 23:312–317, 1991.
10. Sapp JW, Allen RJ, Dupin C: A reversed digital artery island flap for the treatment of fingertip injuries. *J Hand Surg* 18A:528–534, 1993.
11. Foucher G, Dellaserra M, Tilquin B, et al: The Hueston flap in reconstruction of fingertip skin loss: Results in a series of 41 patients. *J Hand Surg* 19A:508–515, 1994.
12. Yansit NJ, Ye Z, Sanger JR, et al: The versatile metacarpal and reverse metacarpal artery flap in hand surgery. *Ann Plast Surg* 29:523–531, 1992.
13. Foucher G, Brasa D, Silva J, Boulas J: Reposition-flap technique in fingertip injuries: Review of 21 cases. *Ann Clin Plast Esthet* 37:438–442, 1992.
14. Dumontier C, Tilquin B, Lenoble E, Frucher G: Reconstruction of distal defects of the nail bed by a de-epithelialized palmar advancement flap. *Ann Clin Plast Esthet* 37:553–559, 1992.

15. Hirase V, Kojimat, Matsuuv AS: A versatile one-stage neurovascular flap for fingertip reconstruction: The dorsal middle phalangeal finger flap. *Plast Reconstr Surg* 90:1009–1015, 1992.

16. Keim HA, Grantham SA: Volar flap advancement for thumb and finger tip injuries. *Clin Orthop* 66:109–112, 1969.

17. Brunnell F: Dorso-ulnar thumb flap. *Ann Clin Main Memb Super* 12:105–114, 1993.

18. Boswick JA: Neuroma formation following digital amputations. *J Trauma* 23:136–147, 1983.

19. Nystrom A, Backman C, Bertheim U, et al: Digital amputation, replantation, and cold intolerance. *J Reconstr Microsurg* 7:175–178, 1991.

20. Flor H, Elbert T, Kneckt S, et al: Phantom limb pain as a perceptual correlate of cortical reorganization following amputation. *Nature* 375:482–484, 1995.

21. Elbert T, Flor H, Birbaumer N, et al: Extensive reorganization of the somatosensory cortex in adult humans after nervous system injury. *Neuroreport* 5:2593–2597, 1994.

22. Geertzen J, Eisma W: Amputations and reflex dystrophy. *Prosthet Orthot Int* 18:109–111, 1994.

CHAPTER 62

Tumors of the Hand and Wrist

Harold M. Dick
and Robert J. Strauch

In the hand and upper limb occur the entire range of neoplasms possible in the musculoskeletal system. They are perhaps more dramatic and obvious in the hand because of their constant exposure and potential interference with hand function.

We will first consider the most frequent of these neoplasms, that is, the benign tumors of the hand and wrist.

GANGLIA OF THE HAND AND WRIST

It is estimated that 50 to 70 percent of all soft tissue tumors of the hand and wrist are ganglion cysts (Fig. 62-1A). They appear to be more prevalent in women (3:1), and 70 percent occur between the second and fourth decade of life.[1]

The cause is not known. However, there are various descriptions of etiologic factors including trauma, mucoid degeneration, and synovial herniation of the carpal capsule. Synovial rest cells have been described as well as de novo growths.

There are two common sites of occurrence. Dorsal carpal ganglion cysts, usually arising from the scapholunate ligament, occur in some 60 to 70 percent of series; volar carpal ganglia are most commonly seen at the volar wrist crease between the flexor carpi radialis and the abductor pollicis longus (Fig. 62-1A). Volar carpal ganglia typically stem from the scaphotrapezial joint capsule.[2]

Other variations of the ganglion include the volar ulnar ganglion, originating from the pisotriquetral joint, and the mucous cyst.

The retinacular ganglion cyst (10 to 20 percent) is the third most common ganglion of the hand. It appears only in the pulley areas of the flexor tendon retinacula, usually at the level of the A1 or A2 pulley of the digital flexor tendons. It rarely exceeds 1 cm in diameter.

The mucous cyst is a variant of the ganglion cyst (Fig. 62-1B). It most commonly occurs on the dorsum of the digit at the level of the distal interphalangeal joint and invariably is associated with concurrent osteoarthritis and osteophyte formation.[3]

In certain cases this ganglion may stretch the dorsal skin, groove the nail bed, and, infrequently, break the skin. Following resection, a skin graft and resection of the osteophytes of the distal phalanx may be required. Some authors have reported excellent results and resolution of fingernail deformities with excision of osteophytes only.[4]

Most ganglion cysts are asymptomatic aside from local tenderness. On physical examination, the ganglion cyst is found to be soft to firm; it transilluminates and is 1 to 3 cm in diameter. It is usually relatively immobile. The tuck sign is negative.

Pathologic examination shows a cystic cavity with viscous mucin of glucosamine, albumin, globulin, and a high concentration of hyaluronic acid. This substance is significantly more viscous than joint fluid.

The treatment of the ganglion cyst is usually reassurance for the asymptomatic lesions. Aspiration can be performed for diagnostic purposes, although recurrence is the norm. Aspiration followed by 3 weeks of casting produces resolution of the problem about half the time. When the cysts are surgically excised, they should be traced to their origin, and the joint capsule should not be closed.

When surgical excision is properly performed, recurrence rates of dorsal ganglion cysts should be rare (less than 5 percent),[1] although some centers have reported recurrences in up to 30 percent of cases. Recurrence following surgical excision of volar ganglion cysts is more commonly seen (20 percent).[2] Other complications include sensory neuromas, joint stiffness, and tendon injury.

LIPOMAS OF THE HAND AND UPPER LIMB

Lipomas of the hand and upper limb are among the most common benign tumors. There is an equal incidence in the upper and lower limbs. These lesions are more frequently proximal than distal. Some 10 to 20 percent of upper limb lipomas occur in the hand and wrist area.[5]

There is a greater female incidence of lipomas (2:1), and the tumor is usually seen in the third to sixth decades of life. The most frequent site in the hand is the thenar eminence; the tumors also occur at the level of the proximal phalanx in both the volar and dorsal locations (Fig. 62-2). These growths are usually asymptomatic and are often mistaken for ganglia. They occasionally cause nerve compression symptoms in the proximal volar forearm or the loge de Guyon.

The tumors are soft; they do not transilluminate and are usually nontender and mobile. Lipomas may be radiolucent. This radiolucency on x-ray compared to the surrounding soft tissue and bone is called a Bufolini's sign.

Pathological examination shows an encapsulated soft tissue mass with characteristic yellow fat cells apparent microscopically. The usual treatment is excision for diagnosis and cosmesis. The prognosis is excellent, with a negligible recurrence rate.

BENIGN GIANT CELL TUMORS OF THE TENDON SHEATH

These tumors are also referred to as *xanthofibroma, xanthoma, localized pigmented villonodular tenosynovitis,* and *benign fibrous histiocytomas.*

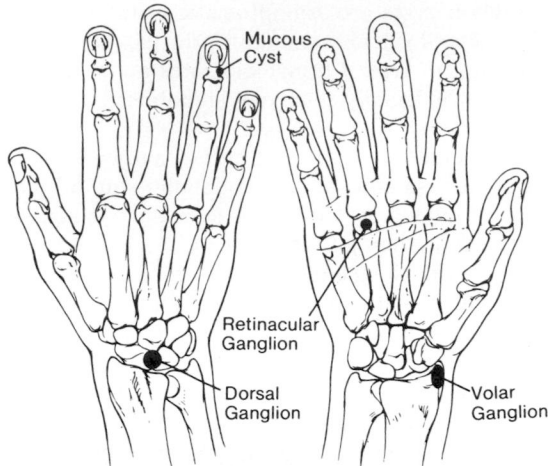

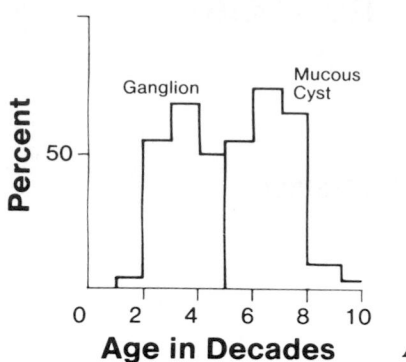

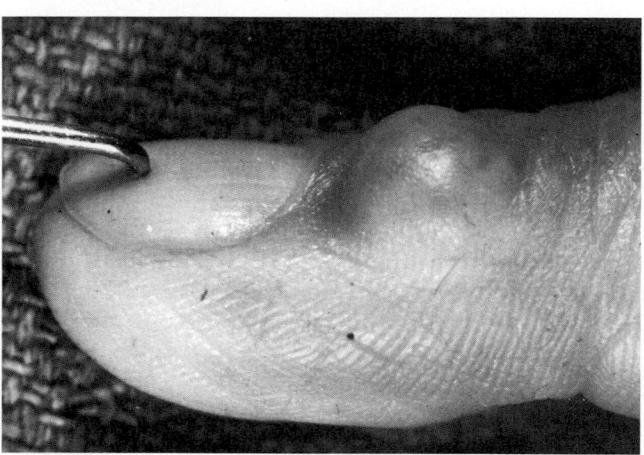

B

Figure 62-1 *A.* Incidence of ganglia in the hand and forearm. *B.* A 65-year-old woman with mucoid cyst at the dorsal distal interphalangeal joint of the right third finger.

Benign giant cell tumor of the tendon sheath is the second most common tumor of the hand after ganglia (Fig. 62-3*A*). It occurs in the mature adult (40 to 60 years old). The tumor is commonly located on the index and middle digits on the volar and dorsal surfaces. It can envelop the neurovascular bundle and present problems in dissection.

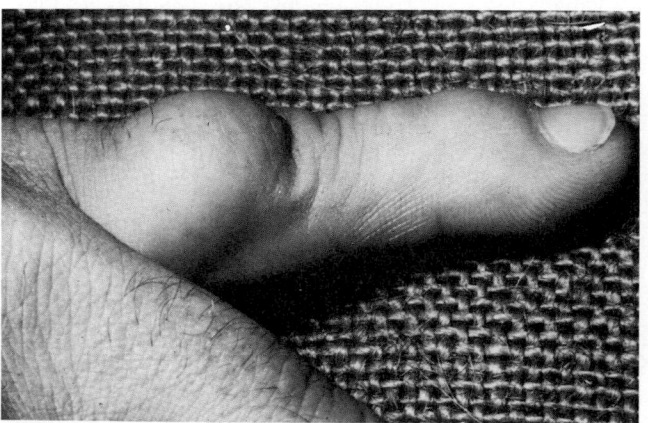

Figure 62-2 A 50-year-old woman with a lipoma of the fifth finger.

The growths are usually painless, but when they encroach upon small joints, they may restrict motion (Fig. 62-3*B*). On physical examination, they are found to be firm and often multilobulated. There are no characteristic x-ray findings, but the tumors can cause bone remodeling and rarely invade the bone.

Pathologic examination shows variable-sized encapsulated yellow tissue with fatty areas. There are classic foam cells, and histologic examination shows histiocytes and small nuclei. The cytoplasm is full of lipoid globules, and characteristic giant cells are found in various new beds.

The treatment of choice is resection, including portions of the tendon sheath or joint capsule if necessary.[6] Recurrence may be a problem if the tumor is not adequately excised. If a joint is severely involved, arthrodesis may be required.

EPIDERMAL CYSTS (INCLUSION CYSTS)

Epidermal inclusion cysts are the most frequent tumors found in the region of the distal phalanx. The cause is thought to be traumatic. There is a 2:1 male predominance, and the mean age is the third decade. The most common site is the volar aspect of the distal phalanx of the index or middle finger.[7]

Epidermal cysts present as painless firm swellings. They do not transilluminate. X-ray examination may reveal a smooth, round or oval radiolucent lesion in the adjacent area of the distal phalanx with thinning of the cortex. On histologic examination, one finds a fibrous capsule with a keratin-filled space. Squamous epithelium may be present and is characteristic of the lesion.

The most effective treatment is surgical excision through a midlateral incision with curettage of the phalanx. Bone grafting may be necessary. There is a low recurrence rate with complete cyst removal.

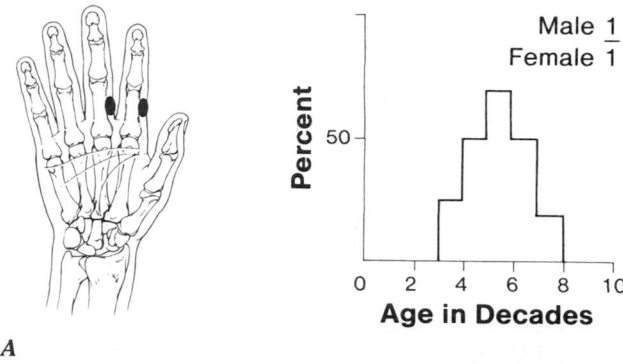

A

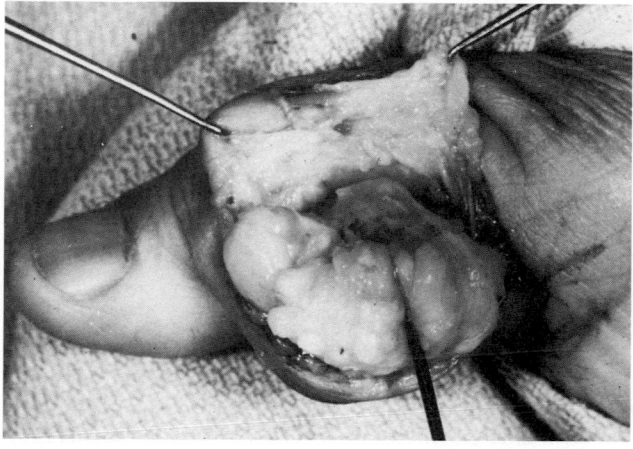

B

Figure 62-3 *A.* Incidence of giant cell tumor of the tendon sheath of the hand and forearm. *B.* Operative specimen of benign giant cell tumor of the flexor aspect of the thumb.

GLOMUS TUMOR

Glomus tumor is among the rarest of hand tumors. Some series estimate that it constitutes 1 to 5 percent of all hand tumors. It occurs in the third to fifth decades of life and is an unusual tumor of childhood and the elderly.

Over 50 percent of glomus tumors occur in the subungual region, although they have been reported in a wide range of sites including all the extremities and the trunk. They usually present with a pathognomonic triad of severe pain, point tenderness, and cold sensitivity.[3]

The physical findings often include ridging of the nail. The area is exquisitely sensitive to touch and temperature testing. A blue spot at the base of the nail is often present. Placing the digit on an ice pack may elicit symptoms. X-rays may show a well-defined, radiolucent, eccentric lesion in the base of the distal phalanx, and MRI may be helpful in locating tumors that are elusive on physical examination.[9]

The lesions are less than 1 cm in diameter. Histologic examination shows polyhedral cells, fibrous stroma, and small blood vessels.

The most effective surgical treatment utilizes loupe magnification and removal of the nail plate. The lesion is usually well encapsulated and exposed via a longitudinal incision in the nail bed followed by careful reapproxima-

tion. The prognosis is excellent and pain relief usually spectacular unless the glomus is not completely removed. Occasionally multicentric glomus tumors are present and should be searched for; all sites require removal for adequate symptom relief.

ENCHONDROMA

Enchondroma is the most common primary bone tumor of the hand (Fig. 62-4). It occurs in the second to fourth decades of life. The most common site is the proximal phalanx of the digits. Enchondroma is usually not symptomatic unless microfracture has occurred. Most of the physical findings of tenderness and swelling are usually due to fracture through the lesion. X-rays reveal a characteristic radiolucent lesion in the diaphyseal or metaphyseal area of the phalanx, with thinned cortex and flecks of calcification. The gross appearance is cartilaginous and ricelike. The histologic examination shows benign cartilage.

The definitive treatment is curettage with bone grafting. An excellent donor source for the bone graft is the distal radius. The prognosis is excellent with a minimal recurrence rate. Surgical treatment is both diagnostic and therapeutic. Left untreated, these lesions have occasionally been reported to develop into chondrosarcomas.[10]

OSTEOCHONDROMA

Osteochondroma occurs rarely as a solitary lesion in the hand (Fig. 62-5*A*). Patients with multiple hereditary osteochondromas will present with multifocal lesions. There is a male preponderance. This lesion is usually diagnosed in the first two decades of life. In the hand, osteochondroma is usually most frequent in the metacarpals and proximal phalanges. It infrequently presents as a subungual lesion. Pain is rarely associated with this tumor. It may, however, produce growth disturbances of shortening, angulation, and flexion/extensions deficits. Multiple osteochondromas typically produce more severe growth disturbances.

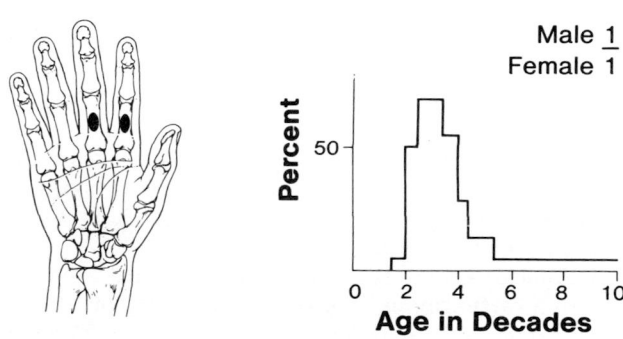

Figure 62-4 Incidence of enchondromas in the hand and forearm.

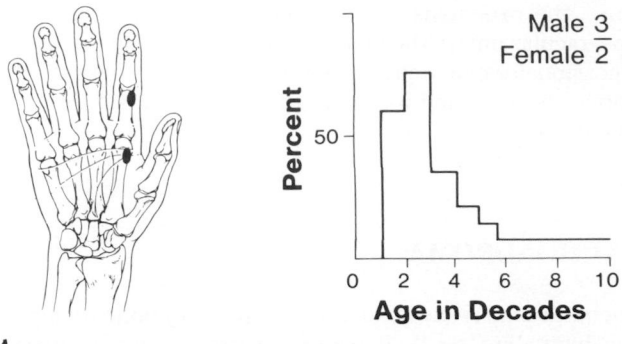

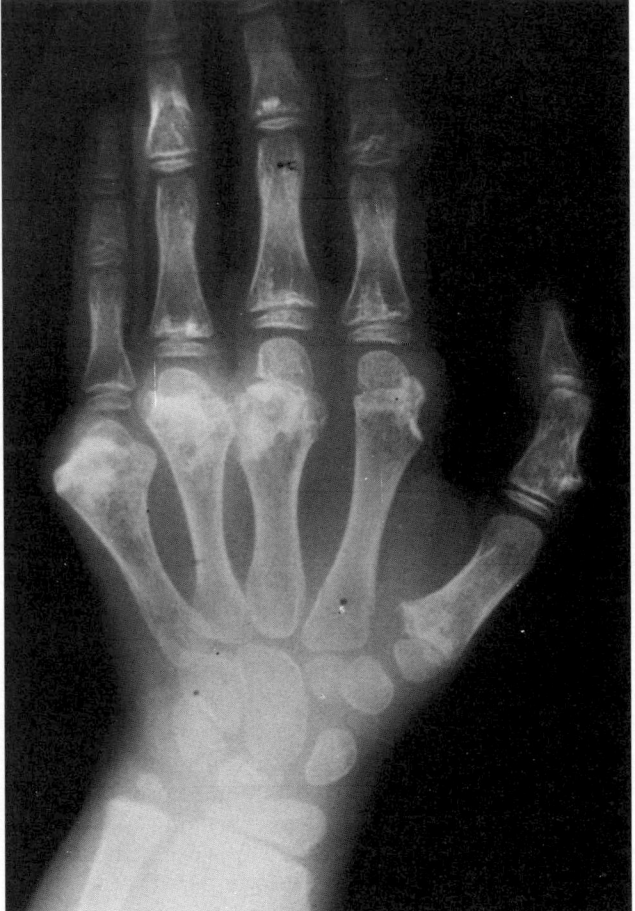

B

Figure 62-5 *A.* Incidence of osteochondroma in the hand and forearm. *B.* A 20-year-old man with multiple osteochondromas of the metacarpals and phalanges.

Physical examination reveals bony prominences at the metaphyseal portions of the small tubular hand bones. X-rays indicate portions of the tumor cortex continuous with normal cortex (Fig. 62-5*B*).

Pathologic examination often reveals normal bone cortex with a cartilaginous cap. Operative treatment may be deferred until skeletal maturity, when osteotomy for angulatory and rotatory correction may be performed concurrent with tumor excision. The prognosis is excellent when the tumor is completely excised. In patients with multiple osteochondromas, malignant degeneration to chondrosarcoma has been reported in 2 to 11 percent of cases.[11]

OSTEOID OSTEOMA

Osteoid osteoma is a rare primary bone tumor.[12,13] There is a 2:1 male predominance. Mean age at presentation is 39 years. Most lesions occur in the proximal phalanges and the carpus. They are virtually never found in the middle phalanges (Fig. 62-6).

The most characteristic finding is the pain relief produced by aspirin, or nonsteroidal anti-inflammatory medications, which are thought to inhibit the increased prostaglandin synthesis of these lesions. There is often localized tenderness when the osteoma is palpable. The classic x-ray appearance reveals eccentric cortical sclerosis with a radiolucent nidus less than 1 cm in diameter. Bone scan and computed tomography (CT) are most helpful in confirming the diagnosis and localizing the nidus. Pathology is diagnostic, showing a soft tissue tumor within a sclerotic cavity. Histology is notable for vascularized osteoid tissue with abundant osteoblasts.

Treatment is curettage of the nidus. A window into the nidus is made by using a dental drill. Localization is frequently facilitated by intraoperative x-rays. Pain relief is dramatic and excellent with nidus removal. Recurrence rates of 13 percent have been reported, usually associated with incomplete removal.

JUVENILE APONEUROTIC FIBROMA

Juvenile aponeurotic fibroma is an uncommon soft tissue tumor, occurring in the first two decades of life; 50 percent occur in the hand and forearm.[14]

This is a painless growth that has spotty calcification on x-ray and the histologic appearance of a cellular tumor, with fat and muscle infiltration. The histologic examination is quite difficult, with many cases being incorrectly diagnosed as a malignancy (fibrosarcoma). Treatment is local surgical resection, which may require skin grafting or local flaps. There is a high recurrence rate even with adequate excision.

MALIGNANT TUMORS OF THE HAND AND FOREARM

Primary malignant tumors of the upper limb below the elbow are fortunately quite rare. All tumors distal to the elbow in patients over 40 years of age should first be viewed as metastatic disease.

If the tumor is thought to be malignant, careful evaluation should be performed prior to biopsy. This includes a complete blood count, determination of sedimentation rate, serum alkaline phosphatase, and serum and urine protein levels when indicated for possible myeloma. Bone scans and chest tomography should be performed to de-

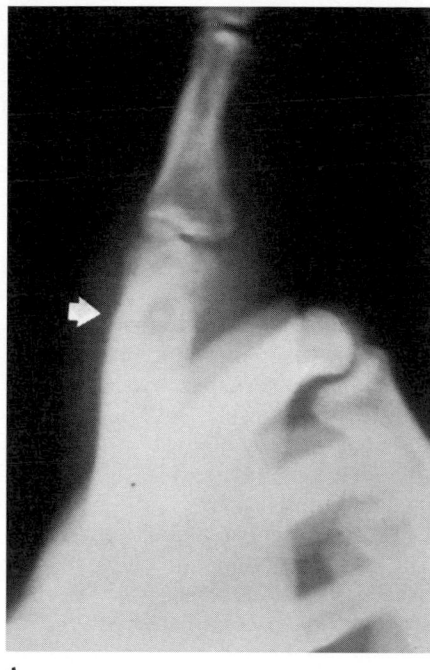

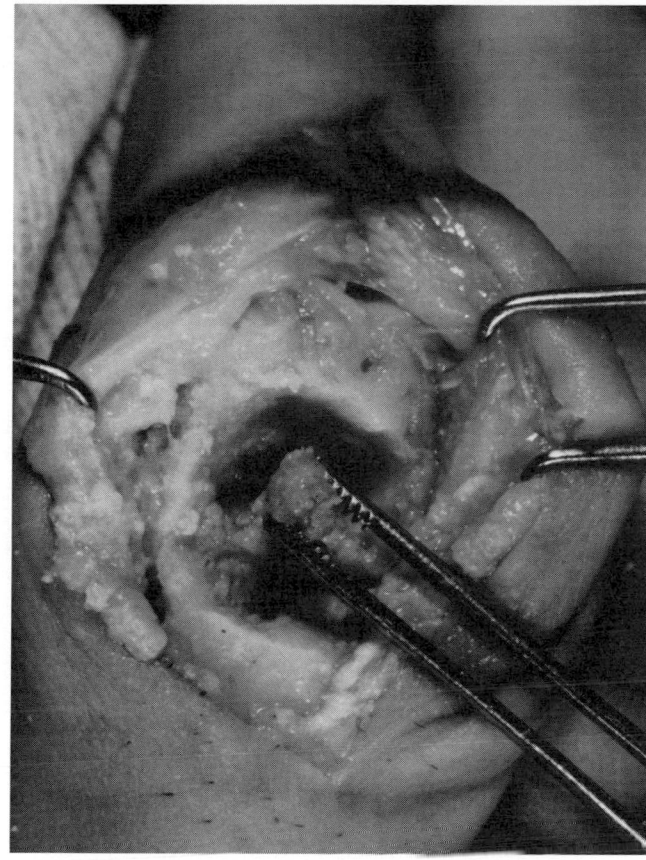

Figure 62-6 *A*. A 19-year-old man with osteoid osteoma (*arrow*) of the proximal phalanx of the right index finger. *B*. Nidus of the osteoid osteoma is exposed with the use of a dental drill.

tect metastases when the tumor biopsy has been identified as malignant. Computed tomography and MRI are invaluable in preoperative assessment and in planning reconstructive alternatives. Smith, in 1977, outlined the objectives of treatment of malignant tumors of the hand: (1) the goal of all malignant-tumor surgery is ablation of the tumor with a satisfactory tumor-free margin; (2) functional reconstruction should rarely be performed at the same time as excision of the tumor; (3) all suspected malignancies should have incisional biopsies; (4) when the diagnosis is agreed upon, the decision for ablation versus preserved hand function requires great experience in oncology and in hand and upper limb reconstruction; and (5) the use of adjuvant chemotherapy and/or radiotherapy may have distinct advantages in the treatment protocol.[15]

The operative planning for reconstruction includes the following: (1) assessment of final skin coverage needs, including possible interim split-thickness grafts or free tissue transfers; (2) the Esmarch bandage should not be used, for fear of "squeezing" tumor cells into the circulation, but pneumatic tourniquet should be used; and (3) any elaborate reconstruction should be deferred until the pathologist has declared the actual specimen "margin-free" of tumor.

We believe that, when possible, the grading and staging of tumors should be done according to the method of Enneking and the Musculoskeletal Tumor Society.[16]

METASTATIC TUMORS OF THE HAND

In all patients over 40 years of age, especially if primary sites are already known (breast, lung, kidney), any painful radiolucent lesion of the upper limb skeleton should be suspected of being metastatic rather than a primary skeletal tumor. The distal phalanx is the most common site. The carpus is the most unlikely site of metastases. Treatment choices are resection or radiation therapy. Prognosis at this stage is poor, with the majority of patients in the end stage of their primary disease.[17]

CHONDROSARCOMA

Benign cartilage tumors of the hand, seen with solitary or multiple enchondromas, may occasionally be precursors of malignant degeneration to chondrosarcoma. Chondrosarcoma is probably one of the most difficult diagnoses to confirm by histology because of the wide variation in mitotic and malignant cells. Much of the diagnosis rests upon the biological behavior of the tumor—i.e., rapid growth, pain, pattern, high recurrence rate, and the x-ray patterns of expansile growth with cortical destruction and extension to the soft tissues.

When the diagnosis is established, ablation by ray resection or amputation is the procedure of choice. The tumor is radioresistant and not sensitive to chemo-therapy.[18]

OSTEOGENIC SARCOMA

Osteogenic sarcoma is a rare primary bone malignancy occurring in the first two decades of life, usually in the distal radius, metacarpals, or phalanges. It is usually a rapidly progressive, painful lesion that is most often lytic, destructive, and intramedullary. Open biopsy and careful diagnosis are mandatory. Differentiation from a benign osteoblastoma may be somewhat difficult.

Treatment is surgical, with ablation of the involved area of bone and often the adjacent joint (Fig. 62-7). Lateral tumor extension in the hand may require adjacent ray resections where indicated to provide adequate margins. Adjuvant chemotherapy is indicated for this tumor and has improved survival.[19]

EWING'S SARCOMA

Ewing's sarcoma is an extremely rare tumor in the hand skeleton. It usually occurs in the first two decades of life, and 20 percent of all Ewing's cases are in the upper extremity. Pain and swelling are the common presenting symptoms. Patients may have an elevated sedimentation rate, leukocytosis, and anemia with a low-grade fever. This may lead to confusion with osteomyelitis. X-rays may reveal a classic "onionskin" appearance due to multiple layers of reactive periosteal new bone formation. This appearance is not, however, pathognomonic for Ewing's.

The treatment of choice is surgical resection with adjuvant chemo- and radiotherapy. Classically, survival rate has been dismal, at 5 to 20 percent by 5 years; however, with improved treatment protocols, results are improving.[20]

SOFT TISSUE MALIGNANT TUMORS

This area comprises a wide range of neoplasms such as synovial sarcomas, epithelioid sarcomas, fibrosarcomas, clear cell sarcomas, malignant fibrous histiocytomas, liposarcomas, leiomyosarcomas, angiosarcomas, neuroectodermal sarcomas, and rhabdomyosarcomas. The mainstay of treatment for these lesions is surgical resection. The role of chemotherapy and radiotherapy for these tumors in adults remains controversial, with some centers reporting benefit while others report no improvement in survival. Once diagnosed, all patients should be evaluated with a whole body bone scan and chest CT scan to detect distant metastases.

The sarcomas seen most commonly in the hand are synovial cell and epithelioid sarcoma in adults and rhabdomyosarcoma in children.

EPITHELIOID SARCOMA

In some series, this is the most common sarcoma involving the hand in adults. It is a highly malignant tumor with a predilection for metastases to regional lymph nodes in addition to systemic metastases. This tumor has a male predominance and typically presents as a single, superficial nodule less than 1 cm in size in patients in their twenties and thirties. It is often ignored until it enlarges, ulcerates, or in-

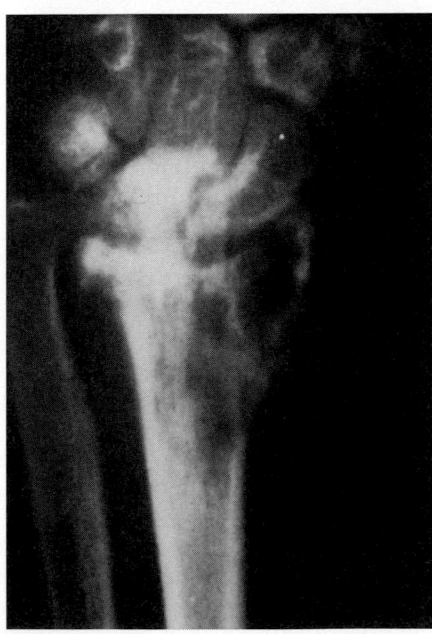

A

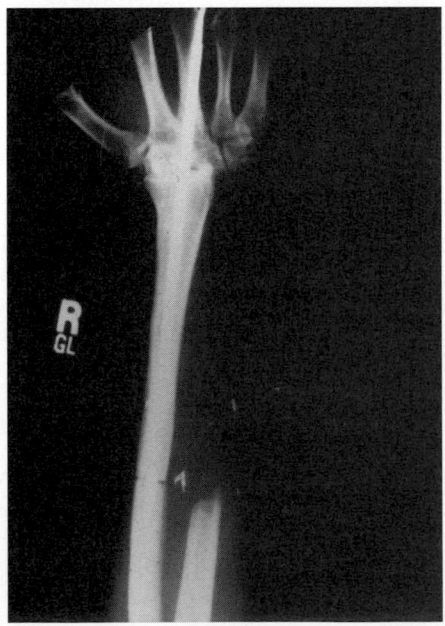

B

Figure 62-7 *A*. A 21-year-old man with an osteosarcoma of the distal radius. *B*. The patient was treated by en bloc re-section and allograft replacement with intramedullary rod fixation.

filtrates. Imaging studies, including MRI, are useful to delineate the extent of the tumor but do not point to a specific diagnosis. Incisional biopsy reveals histologic features of malignant cells with an epithelioid, spindle, or mixed appearance with deeply acidophilic cytoplasm. Immunocytochemical studies are helpful in confirming the diagnosis.[21]

Treatment with marginal surgical resection has led to dismal outcomes with or without adjuvant measures (8 percent survival rate). Disease-free survival at 10 years is significantly improved with wide (margin of normal tissue more than 3 cm) or radical resection (70 percent survival). Adjuvant postoperative radiation therapy does not negate the effect of positive surgical margins. Regional lymph nodes (epitrochlear or axillary) should be sampled at the time of resection if palpable.[22]

SYNOVIAL SARCOMA

Synovial sarcoma has been described as a "great masquerader" and may present with or without pain near a joint; there may be evidence of acute inflammation or a chronic joint contracture. This lesion may lie dormant for months or years or may metastasize within weeks of presentation. It usually afflicts young adults aged 25 to 35, with a slight male predominance. This tumor may also metastasize to regional lymph nodes. X-rays may reveal calcification and bone formation in 20 to 30 percent of cases. In 10 to 20 percent, there may be periosteal reaction, bone erosion, or invasion. Incisional biopsy will often reveal a "biphasic" appearance of the tumor, with epithelial and spindle cell types. Immunocytochemistry can be helpful in confirming the diagnosis.[23]

Treatment involves wide or radical resection, which usually requires a ray or double ray resection when the tumor occurs in the hand. For lesions of the carpus, carpal tunnel, and distal forearm, a below-elbow amputation is preferable. Postoperative radiotherapy is required if a marginal resection is performed but does not negate the effect of positive margins in the hand. Chemotherapy has not been shown to definitively improve survival but is often given on protocol. Overall 5-year survival ranges from 25 to 62 percent; 10 year survival falls to about 30 percent. Lesions involving the hand have a somewhat worse prognosis than synovial cell sarcomas located elsewhere.[23,24]

RHABDOMYOSARCOMA

Rhabdomyosarcoma is the most common soft tissue sarcoma in children. The most common childhood type is embryonal, and the most common type in the extremities is the alveolar subtype of rhabdomyosarcoma. It is seen in children, usually between the ages of 2 to 5 years, with a male predominance. The tumor typically presents as a painless mass that spreads along lymphatic (40 percent) and hematogenous routes. Incisional biopsy will reveal the tumor and histologic diagnosis is aided by the immunoperoxidase antibody technique, which has identified an intermediate protein desmin as a useful marker.

Treatment is often with limb salvage techniques, followed by postoperative radiation and chemotherapy. Prior to adjuvant therapy, the survival rate was under 20 percent. The survival rate has improved with adjuvant therapy to above 70 percent.[23]

REFERENCES

1. Angelides AC, Wallace PF: The dorsal ganglion of the wrist. *J Hand Surg* 1:228–235, 1976.
2. Wright TW, Cooney WP, Ilstrup DM: Anterior wrist ganglion. *J Hand Surg* 19A:954–958, 1994.
3. Newmeyer WL, Kilgore ES, Graham WP: Mucous cysts: The dorsal distal interphalangeal joint ganglion. *Plast Reconstr Surg* 53:313–315, 1974.
4. Gingrass MK, Brown RE, Zook EG: Treatment of fingernail deformities secondary to ganglions of the distal interphalangeal joint. *J Hand Surg* 20A:502–505, 1995.
5. Leffert RD: Lipomas of the upper extremity. *J Bone Joint Surg* 54A:1262–1266, 1972.
6. Moore RJ, Weiland AJ, Curtis RM: Localized nodular tenosynovitis: Experience with 115 cases. *J Hand Surg* 9A:412–417, 1984.
7. Byers P, Salm R: Epidermal cysts of phalanges. *J Bone Joint Surg* 48B:577–581, 1966.
8. Carroll RE, Berman AT: Glomus tumors of the hand. *J Bone Joint Surg* 54A:591–603, 1972.
9. Jablon M, Horowitz A, Bernstein DA: Magnetic resonance imaging of a glomus tumor of the fingertip. *J Hand Surg* 15A:507–509, 1990.
10. Culver JE, Sweet DE, McCue FC: Chondrosarcoma of the hand arising from pre-existent benign solitary enchondroma: Case report and pathological description. *Clin Orthop* 113:128–131, 1975.
11. Wood VE, Molitor C, Mudge MK: Hand involvement in multiple hereditary exostosis. *Hand Clin* 6:685–692, 1990.
12. Bednar MS, McCormack RR, Glasser D, Weiland AJ: Osteoid osteoma of the upper extremity. *J Hand Surg* 18A:1019–1028, 1993.
13. Carroll RE: Osteoid osteoma in the hand. *J Bone Joint Surg* 35A:888–893, 1953.
14. Eisenbaum SL, Eversmann WW: Juvenile aponeurotic fibroma of the hand. *J Hand Surg* 10A:622–625, 1985.
15. Smith RJ: Tumors of the hand: Who is best qualified to treat tumors of the hand? *J Hand Surg* 2:251–252, 1977.
16. Enneking WF: *Musculoskeletal Tumor Surgery.* New York, Churchill Livingstone, 1983.
17. Wu KK, Guise ER: Metastatic tumors of the hand: A report of six cases. *J Hand Surg* 3:271–276, 1978.
18. Dahlin DC, Salvador AH: Chondrosarcomas of bones of the hands and feet: A study of 30 cases. *Cancer* 34:755–760, 1974.
19. Fleegler EJ, Marks KE, Sebek BA, et al: Osteosarcoma of the hand. *Hand* 12:316–322, 1980.
20. Pritchard DJ, Unni KK: Small round cell tumors, in Bogumill GP, Fleegler EJ (eds): *Tumors of the Hand and Upper Limb.* New York, Churchill Livingstone, 1993.
21. Dobyns JH: Epithelioid sarcoma, in Bogumill GP, Fleegler EJ (eds): *Tumors of the Hand and Upper Limb.* New York, Churchill Livingstone, 1993.
22. Steinberg BD, Gelberman RH, Mankin HJ, Rosenberg AE: Epithelioid sarcoma in the upper extremity. *J Bone Joint Surg* 74A:28–35, 1992.
23. Dick HM, Lee DH: Synovial sarcoma and rhabdomyosarcoma, in Bogumill GP, Fleegler EJ (eds): *Tumors of the Hand and Upper Limb.* New York, Churchill Livingstone, 1993.
24. Brien EW, Terek RM, Geer RJ, et al: Treatment of soft tissue sarcomas of the hand. *J Bone Joint Surg* 77A:564–571, 1995.

CHAPTER 63

Tendon Injuries in the Upper Extremity

James W. Strickland

Forearm, wrist, and hand lacerations that divide flexor or extensor tendons will produce a substantial loss of function. In order to manage these injuries most effectively, it is important to fully understand the normal and pathologic anatomy, the mechanics of tendon function, and the biology of tendon nutrition and healing.

This chapter summarizes current concepts of tendon basic science, repair, reconstruction, and rehabilitation. Rapid developments in research and clinical investigation may make some of these concepts outdated; the reader should consult the appropriate journals to update his or her knowledge base.

TENDON STRUCTURE

Tendons are composed of fascicles of long, narrow, spiraling bundles of tendon cells (tenocytes) and primary type I collagen fibers. Both synovial cells and fibroblasts have been identified in the tendon cell population. The surface of individual bundles of collagen is covered by the endotenon, which surrounds the fascicles, blood vessels, and nerves. A fine, fibrous outer layer, the epitenon, is highly cellular and continuous with the endotenon. The epitenon is confluent with the vascular mesenteries of the tendon or mesotendon, which contains arteries destined to provide tendon nutrition.[1]

ANATOMY

Flexor Tendons

In the distal forearm, the extrinsic flexor tendons arise from the flexor muscles. The most superficial group is made up of the flexor carpi radialis, the flexor carpi ulnaris, and the palmaris longus, which act primarily as wrist flexors. The intermediate group consists of the four tendons of the flexor digitorum superficialis, and the deepest group comprises the flexor digitorum profundus and flexor pollicis longus.

At the wrist, the nine long digital flexor tendons enter the carpal tunnel beneath the protective roof of the transverse carpal ligament in company with the median nerve. In this canal, the common profundus tendons to the long, ring, and small fingers divide into the individual tendons that fan out distally and proceed toward the terminal phalanges of these digits. At approximately the level of the distal palmar crease, the paired profundus and superficialis tendons to the index, long, ring, and small fingers and the flexor pollicis longus enter the individual flexor sheaths that house them throughout the remainder of their digital course. These sheaths with their predictable annular pulley arrangement, serve as a protective housing for the flexor tendons, a smooth, gliding synovium-lined surface, and an efficient mechanism to hold the tendons close to the digital bone and joint (Fig. 63-1).[2,3] The A_2 and A_4 annular pulleys arise from the periosteum of the proximal half of the proximal phalanx and the midportion of the middle phalanx, respectively. The A_1, A_3, and A_5 pulleys are joint pulleys that arise successively from the palmar plates of the metacarpophalangeal (MCP), proximal interphalangeal (PIP), and distal interphalangeal (DIP) joints. The palmar aponeurosis pulley is composed of the transverse and vertical fibers of the palmar fascia and is important when other proximal components of the sheath have been lost. The thin, condensable cruciate sections of the sheath—C1 (between A_2 and A_3), C2 (between A_3 and A_4), and C3 (between A_4 and A_5)—collapse to permit the annular pulleys to approximate each other during flexion.

The flexor digitorum superficialis tendons lie on the palmar side of the flexor digitorum profundus tendons until they enter the A_1 entrance of the digital sheath. Within the proximal sheath, the flexor digitorum superficialis tendon divides into two slips that wrap around the flexor digitorum profundus tendon, rejoin dorsally by means of fibers referred to as the chiasma tendinum or Camper's chiasma, and terminate as they insert along the proximal half of the proximal phalanx (Fig. 63-2). The flexor digitorum profundus tendons pass through the flexor digitorum superficialis bifurcation to insert into the proximal aspect of the distal phalanges. A single flexor pollicis longus inserts on the base of the distal phalanx of the thumb.

Extensor Tendons

Extension of the wrist and fingers is produced by the extrinsic extensor muscle tendon system. A superficial layer consists of the abductor pollicis longus, extensor pollicis brevis, brachial radialis, extensor carpi radialis longus, extensor carpi radialis brevis, extensor digitorum communis, and extensor carpi ulnaris. A deeper layer is composed of the extensor indicis proprius, extensor pollicis longus, and extensor digiti quinti. The brachial radialis originates from the epicondylar line proximal to the lateral epicondyle and, because it inserts on the distal radius, does not truly contribute to wrist or digital motion. The extensor carpi radialis longus and brevis insert proximally on the bases of the second and third metacarpals and the extensor carpi ulnaris inserts on the base of the fifth metacarpal. The long digital extensors terminate by insertions on the base of the middle phalanges after receiving and giving fibers to the intrinsic tendons to form the lateral bands that are destined to insert on the bases of the distal phalanx.

At the wrist, the extensor tendons are divided into six dorsal compartments (Fig. 63-3). The first compartment consists of the tendons of the abductor pollicis longus and

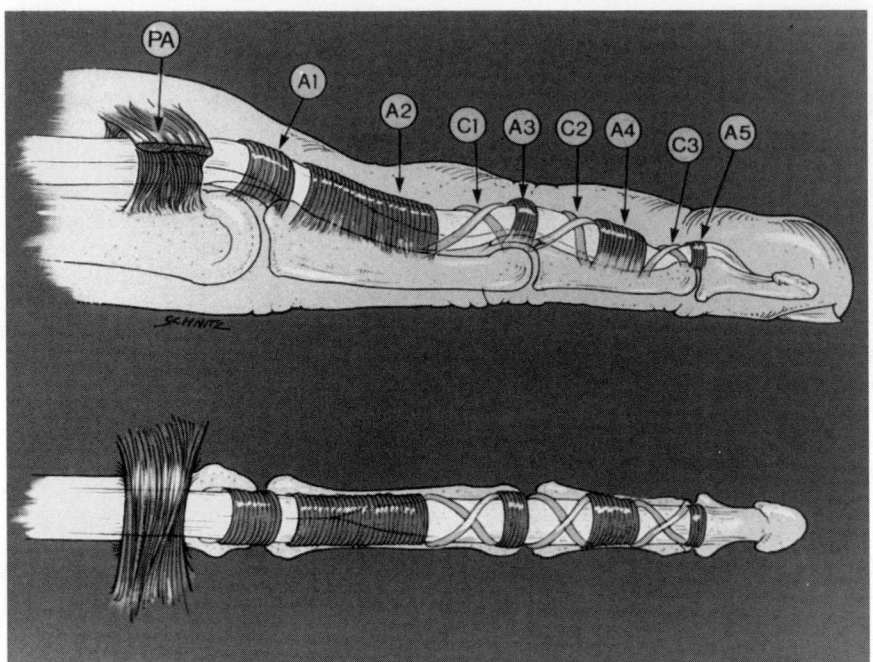

Figure 63-1 The components of the digital flexor sheath are depicted in this drawing. The sturdy annular pulleys (A-1 through A-5) are important biomechanically in keeping the tendons closely applied to the phalanges. The thin, pliable cruciate pulleys collapse to allow full digital flexion. A recent addition has been the palmar aponeurosis pulley, which adds to the biomechanical efficiency of the sheath system. (Modified and reproduced with permission from Idler RS: Anatomy and biomechanics of the digital flexor tendons. *Hand Clin* 1:1:12–13, 1985.)

extensor pollicis brevis and the second compartment houses the two radial wrist extensors, the extensor carpi radialis longus and brevis. The third compartment is composed of the tendon of the extensor pollicis longus, and the fourth compartment allows passage of the four communis extensor tendons and the extensor indicis proprius tendon. The extensor digiti quinti travels through the fifth dorsal compartment, and the sixth compartment houses the extensor carpi ulnaris tendon.

The digital extensor tendons are linked by intratendinous slips called juncturae tendinum. At the level of the metacarpal heads, a complex extensor apparatus forms between the extrinsic extensor tendons and the intrinsic tendons. The long tendon is held in the midline by the sagittal bands, which insert into the transverse metacarpal ligament and palmar plate complex (Fig. 63-4). A circumferential sling is thus created, which helps the extensor digitorum communis to extend the MCP joint. Distally, the interosseous tendons attach to the extensor mechanism and contribute to the extension of the PIP and DIP joints.

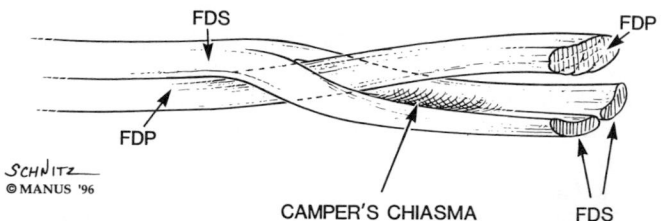

Figure 63-2 Early in the flexor sheath, the flexor digitorum superficialis (FDS) tendon divides and passes around the distal interphalangeal (DIP) tendon. The two portions of the FDS tendon reunite at Camper's chiasma.

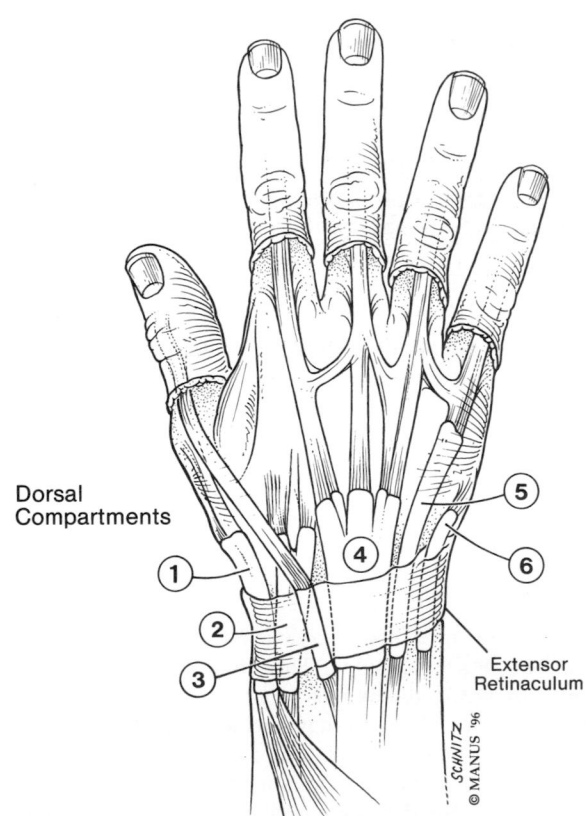

Figure 63-3 Arrangement of the extensor tendons in the compartments of the wrist: (1) abductor pollicis longus and extensor pollicis brevis; (2) extensor carpi radialis longus and brevis; (3) extensor pollicis longus; (4) extensor digitorum communis and extensor indicis proprius; (5) extensor digiti quinti proprius; (6) extensor carpi ulnaris.

Figure 63-4 Extensor mechanism of the digits.

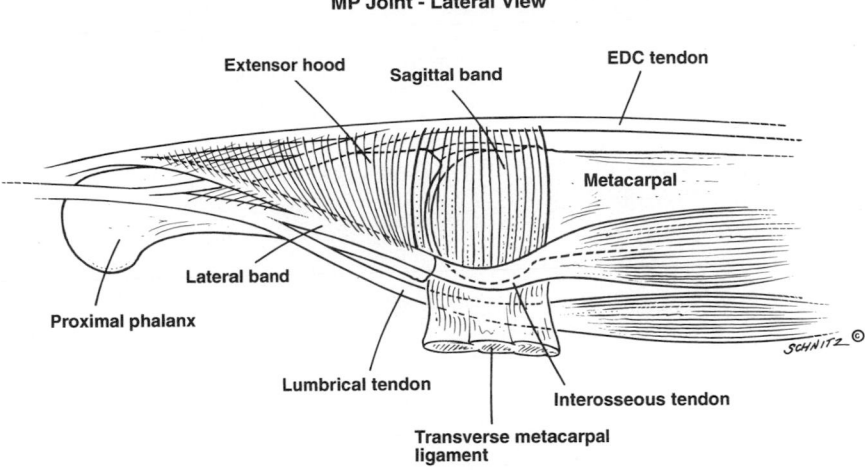

MP Joint - Lateral View

BIOMECHANICAL PROPERTIES

The flexor digitorum profundus acts as the primary digital flexor while the superficialis and the interossei combine for forceful flexion. Digital balance and equilibrium during flexion and extension require a complex integration of extrinsic and intrinsic activity, and strong forces in the neighborhood of 200 N can be achieved during power grip.[4] When there is normal resting tone in the extrinsic and intrinsic muscle groups of the forearm and hand, the wrist and digital joints will be maintained in a balanced position. With the forearm midway between pronation and supination, the wrist dorsiflexed, and the digits in moderate flexion, the hand is in the optimum position from which to function.

Tendons are arranged about joints in pairs so that each musculotendinous unit has at least one antagonistic muscle to balance the involved joint. The wrist is the key joint and has a strong influence on the performance of the long extrinsic muscles at the digital level. Maximal digital flexion strength is facilitated by dorsiflexion of the wrist, which lessens the effective excursion of the antagonistic extensor tendons while maximizing the contractual force of the digital flexors. Conversely, a posture of wrist flexion will markedly weaken grasping power.

At the digital level, MCP joint flexion is a combination of extrinsic flexor power supplemented by the contribution of the intrinsic muscles, whereas PIP joint extension results from a combination of extrinsic extensor and intrinsic muscle action. At the DIP joint, the intrinsic muscles provide a majority of the extensor activity necessary to balance the antagonistic flexor digitorum profundus tendon.

As much as 9 cm of flexor tendon excursion may be required to produce composite wrist and digital flexion, while only about 2.5 cm of excursion is required for full digital flexion with the wrist stabilized in neutral position (Fig. 63-5). The greater the distance the tendon is from the axis of joint rotation, the greater the moment arm and the less motion a given muscle contracture will generate at that joint. Conversely, a shorter moment arm results in

more joint rotation from the same tendon excursion. The moment arm, excursion, and joint rotation produced by the flexor tendons are governed by the constraint of the pulley system. Loss of portions of the digital pulleys may

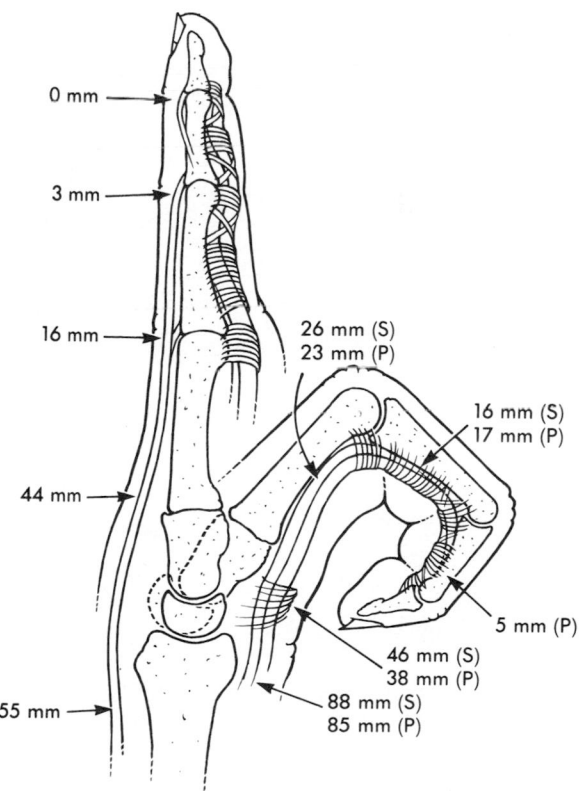

Figure 63-5 The approximate tendon motion necessary to produce full flexion and extension of digital joints at the forearm, wrist, hand, and digital levels are illustrated. P = flexor digitorum profundus; S = flexor digitorum superficialis. (Modified and reproduced with permission from Strickland JW: The management of acute flexor tendon injuries. *Orthop Clin North Am* 14:831–832, 1983.)

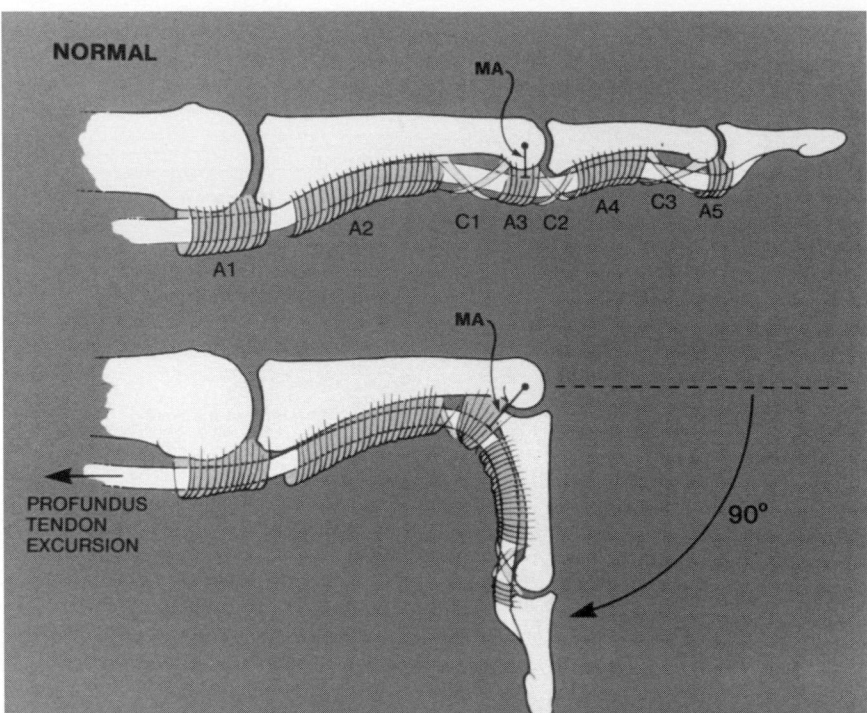

A

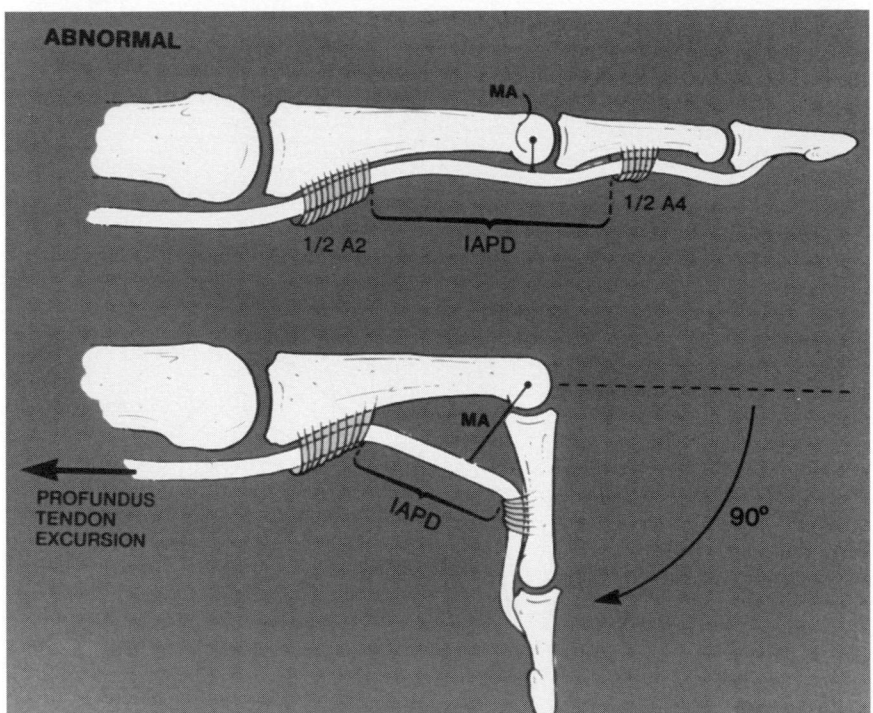

B

Figure 63-6 Function of the finger flexor tendon pulley system. *Top.* The arrangement of the annular (A_1, A_2, A_3, A_4, and A_5) and cruciate (C_1, C_2, and C_3) synovial pulleys of the finger flexor tendon sheath within the intact fibro-osseous canal and the normal moment arm (MA) and flexor digitorum profundus (FDP) tendon excursion as the PIP joint is flexed to 90°. *Bottom.* The biomechanical alteration that results from excision of the distal half of the A_2 pulley; the C_1, A_3, and C_2 pulleys; and the proximal portion of the A_4 pulley. The distance between the distal edge of the A_2 pulley and the proximal edge of the A_4 pulley is the intraannular pulley distance (IAPD). The moment arm is increased and a greater FDP tendon excursion is required to produce 90° of flexion because of the bowstringing that results from the loss of pulley support.

significantly alter the normal integrated balance between the flexor, intrinsic, and extensor tendons. The A_2 and A_4 pulleys are the most important to these mechanical functions: the loss of a substantial portion of either may diminish the digital motion and power or lead to flexion contractures of the interphalangeal joints (Fig. 63-6).[5–7]

TENDON NUTRITION AND HEALING

The nutrition of flexor tendons has several sources: longitudinal vessels enter the tendons in the palm and extend down intratendinous channels; vessels also enter the tendon at the level of the proximal synovial fold or reflection in the distal palm; segmental branches from the paired digital arteries enter the tendons in the flexor tendon sheath through the long and short vinculae; and vessels enter the superficialis and profundus tendons at their osseous insertions. The vascularity of digital flexor tendons is richer dorsally and injection studies have identified consistent areas of avascularity. Both the profundus and superficialis have avascular segments over the proximal phalanx between the synovial reflection and their first vinculum, and the profundus has a second avascular zone over the middle phalanx between its long and short vinculae (Fig. 63-7).[8]

Diffusion of synovial fluid has been shown to be an alternate nutritional pathway for flexor tendons and may actually function more rapidly and completely than vascular perfusion.[9] Tendon sheath fluid contains concentrations of hyaluronic acid and several proteins similar to the composition of normal joint fluid. It may provide a significant contribution to the lubrication and nutrition of gliding flexor tendons. The delivery of nutrients from the synovial fluid is apparently accomplished by a pumping mechanism known as "imbibition," in which the fluid is forced into the interstices of the tendons through small ridges or conduits in the tendon surface, which are oriented at 90° to each other. The pumping process is enhanced by finger flexion as the tendon glides across the fibroosseous pulleys.

The blood supply of the extensor mechanism is not as complex as that of the flexors. Except at the wrist, there is no synovial sheath system and the tendons are well vascularized by adjacent circumferential peritenon.[10] Tendons have both an intrinsic and an extrinsic capability to participate in healing, and the relative contribution of each will depend on the type of injury and the method of repair.[11] While an overview of current concepts of flexor tendon healing is presented here, the cellular events are similar for all tendons. As with other tissues, tendon healing involves three phases: an inflammatory phase, a fibroblastic or collagen-producing phase, and a remodeling phase. The biological events comprised by each of these phases are illustrated in Fig. 63-8.

A healing tendon may be strengthened by the application of tension forces, which may cause a more rapid realignment of the molecules in collagen fibers. Gelberman and coworkers demonstrated that passive mobilization led to a more rapid recovery of tensile strength, fewer adhesions, improved excursion, better nutrition, and minimal repair-site deformation of repaired canine flexor tendons when compared to immobilized repairs.[12–14] They concluded that passive mobilization enhances healing by stimulating maturation of the tendon wounds simultaneously with the remodeling of tendon scar. While may questions remain to be answered, it would appear that the most effective current method of returning strength and excursion to repaired tendons would involve the use of strong gap-reducing suture techniques followed by the application of controlled stress on the repaired tendon.[15,16]

Considerable research is being conducted in an effort to understand the influence that soluble polypeptides, including mitogens (growth factors and hormones), as well as chemotactic and differentiating factors exert on the cellular sequence of tendon healing.[17,18] In various ways, these

Figure 63-7 The blood supply to the flexor tendons within the digital sheath. The segmental vascular supply reaches the flexor tendons by means of long and short vincular connections. The vinculum brevis superficialis (VBS) and the vinculum brevis profundus (VBP) consist of small triangular mesenteries near the insertion of the FDS and FDP tendons. Seen here is the vinculum proximal phalanx. The vinculum longum to the profundus tendon (VLP) arises from the FDS at the level of the PIP joint. The cutaway view depicts the relative avascularity of the palmar side of the flexor tendons in zones I and II compared with the richer blood supply on the dorsal side, which connects with the vincula.

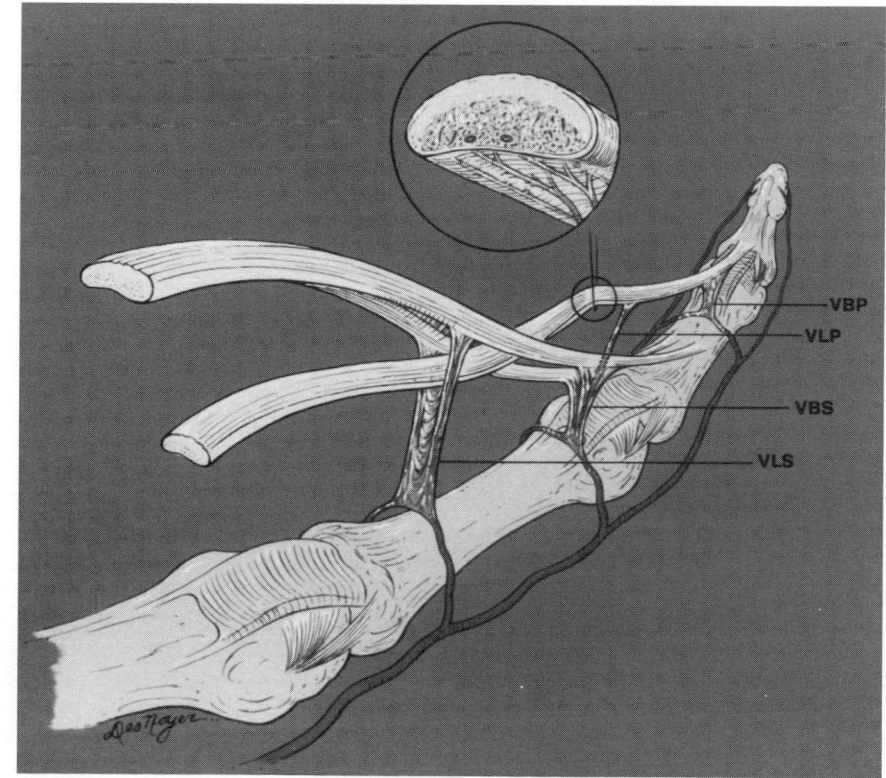

VBP
VLP
VBS
VLS

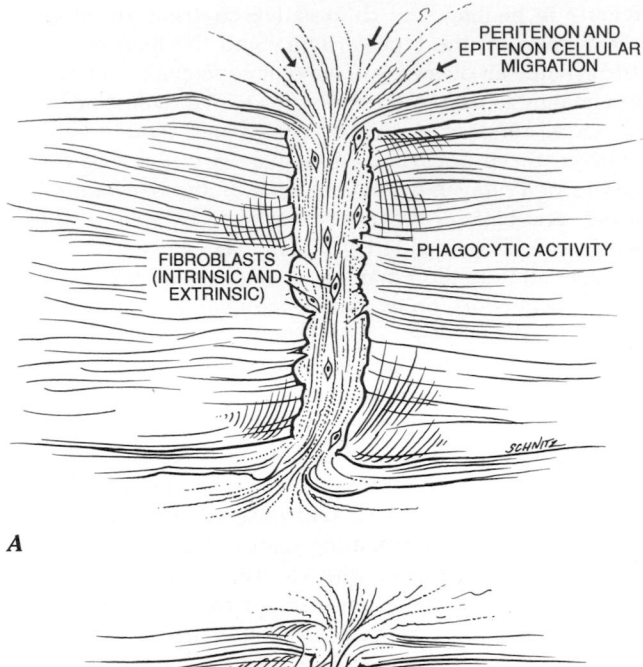

A

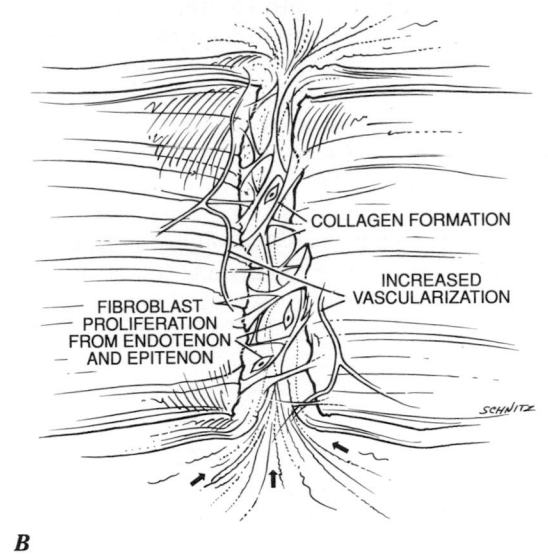

B

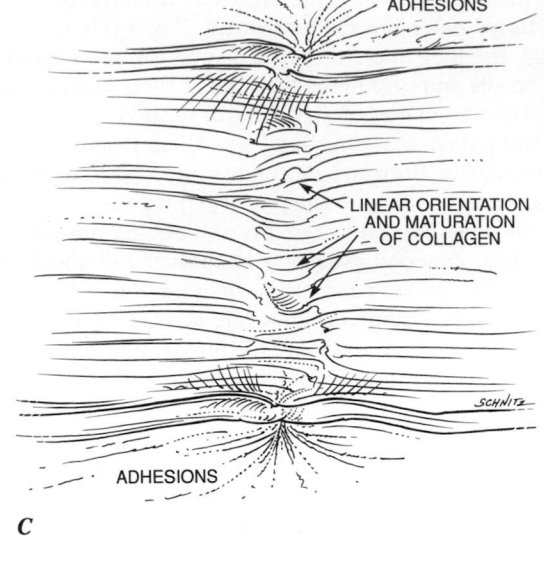

C

Figure 63-8 Tendon healing. Artist's representation of the biological sequence. *A.* At 1 week, an inflammatory response predominates and the laceration site is filled with cells that originate from the extrinsic peritendinous tissues and from the epitenon and endotenon. The cells proliferate; their function is largely phagocysosis and also the synthesis of new collagen. *B.* At 3 weeks, there is marked fibroblastic proliferation from the endotenon and epitenon, and these fibroblasts participate in both the synthesis and resorption of collagen. The fibroblasts and collagen are in a plane perpendicular to the long axis of the tendon and revascularization increases at the repair site, including penetration of the former "avascular zones" by new vessels. *C.* At 8 weeks, the collagen is mature and realigned in linear fashion. Adhesions are stimulated both by the initial trauma to the tendon and sheath and by immobilization.

factors stimulate self-proliferation, matrix synthesis, and cell differentiation. They may act alone or in synergy with other factors and a better understanding of their mechanism of action may lead to improved methods of controlling the biological events associated with tendon healing.

MANAGEMENT OF TENDON INJURIES

Although the continuity of upper extremity tendons is most commonly interrupted by open injuries, both flexor and extensor tendons may experience closed rupture. The diagnosis of tendon disruption is usually fairly obvious to the discerning examiner who carefully observes any alterations in the normal resting posture of the hand and the patient's ability to fully flex and extend the wrist and all thumb and digital joints. When there is doubt as to whether or not a tendon has been completely or nearly completely divided, a

surgical exploration is usually appropriate. Once the tendon injury has been established, repair should be carried out promptly, although not necessarily on an emergency basis.

Flexor Tendon Injuries

Flexor tendon injuries have been divided into several zones on the basis of anatomic characteristics (Fig. 63-9). The most distal zone, zone I, represents the area distal to the insertion of the flexor digitorum superficialis (FDS) where only the profundus tendon can be divided. The area from zone I to the beginning of the flexor tendon sheath at the level of the distal palmar crease is known as zone II and was once referred to as "no man's land" because of the difficulty returning function after one or both flexor tendons had been divided in this area. The zone of lumbrical origin, distal to the distal edge of the transverse carpal ligament, is known as zone III; the carpal tunnel is zone IV; and the distal portion of the forearm is zone V.

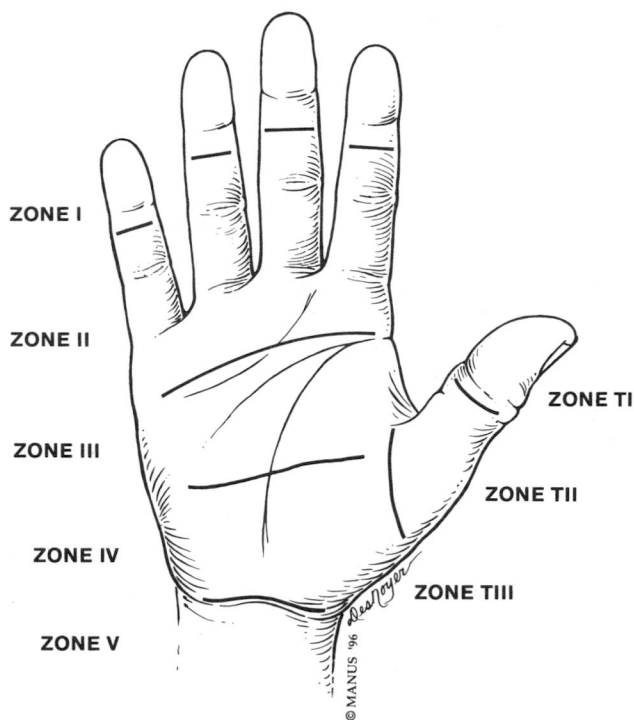

Figure 63-9 The zones of flexor tendon injuries. T = thumb zones.

Surgical Considerations

Numerous methods of tendon suture have been advocated in an effort to satisfy the following characteristics of an ideal repair[15] (Fig. 63-10):

1. Sufficient strength throughout healing to permit the application of early motion stress to the tendon
2. Sutures easily placed in the tendon
3. Secure knot
4. Minimal gapping at the repair site
5. Minimal interference with tendon vascularity
6. Smooth juncture of the tendon ends with minimal bulk

Many current repair methods employ the technique first described by Kirchmayr in 1917 and later popularized by Kessler in 1973, or one of its many variations. Recent evidence supports the conclusion that the number of suture strands crossing the repair strongly influences the strength of the repair.[15,19] Some flexor tendon repair protocols are now adopting four-strand repair methods, which would seem to indicate that those repairs are sufficiently safe to allow the use of controlled active postrepair motion programs with the hope of improving tendon excursion and digital motion.[11,13–15,20–22]

The importance of the use of a peripheral circumferential epitenon suture has been demonstrated by experimental studies to provide a 10 to 50 percent increase in repair strength and a significant reduction in gapping between the tendon ends. These benefits have been further confirmed by experiments that apply both static and cyclic loads to the tendon repair. In addition, strong

epitenon sutures, such as the running lock loop stitch,[23] horizontal mattress,[24] and epitenon/intrafiber methods[25] have been shown to be the strongest of the peripheral suture techniques (Fig. 63-11).

In recent years, many surgeons have advocated repair of the flexor tendon sheath after tendon suture in zone I or II. The stated advantages of sheath repair are that it serves as a barrier to the formation of extrinsic adhesions, provides a quicker return of synovial nutrition, acts as a mold for the remodeling tendon, and results in better tendon sheath biomechanics. Disadvantages include the fact that sheath repair is often technically difficult to accomplish and that the repaired sheath may be narrowed and thus may restrict tendon gliding.

There has also been considerable debate regarding the appropriate management of partial tendon lacerations. Initial investigations created considerable controversy by recommending that partial flexor tendon lacerations should not be repaired. Recent studies have demonstrated that lacerations of less than 60 percent need not be sutured, but that those greater than 60 percent should be repaired, since they may lead to entrapment, rupture, or triggering.[26]

Splints and exercise programs are now routinely implemented during the period following tendon repair in an effort to favorably influence the biological process of collagen synthesis and degradation.[27] Favorable remodeling of the scar around the healing tendon is best accomplished by applying stress to the tendon, which, in turn, transmits the stress to the adjacent scar. Imparting early postrepair motion stress to repaired flexor tendons has been shown to be beneficial for more rapid recovery of tensile strength, fewer adhesions, improved tendon excursion, and minimal repair site deformity. The strength of immediately mobilized tendons has been shown to be twice that of immobilized tendons up to at least 12 weeks following tendon suture.

CONSIDERATIONS BY ZONE

Zone I—Distal Superficialis Insertion

At this level, only the FDP is injured and repair is accomplished by end-to-end suture or by reinsertion of the tendon to the bone of the distal phalanx. The technique of tendon advancement, which involves tendon shortening, is rarely appropriate, particularly if the advancement exceeds 1 cm, because this technique carries the risk of creating a flexion deformity in the finger and influencing the function of adjacent digits.

Zone II—Within the Flexor Tendon Sheath ("No Man's Land")

Injuries in this area may sever the FDP alone or both the FDP and the FDS tendons. In the past, primary tenorrhaphy was not recommended for this difficult area; currently, primary or delayed primary repair is established as the preferred method of treatment of acute flexor tendon divi-

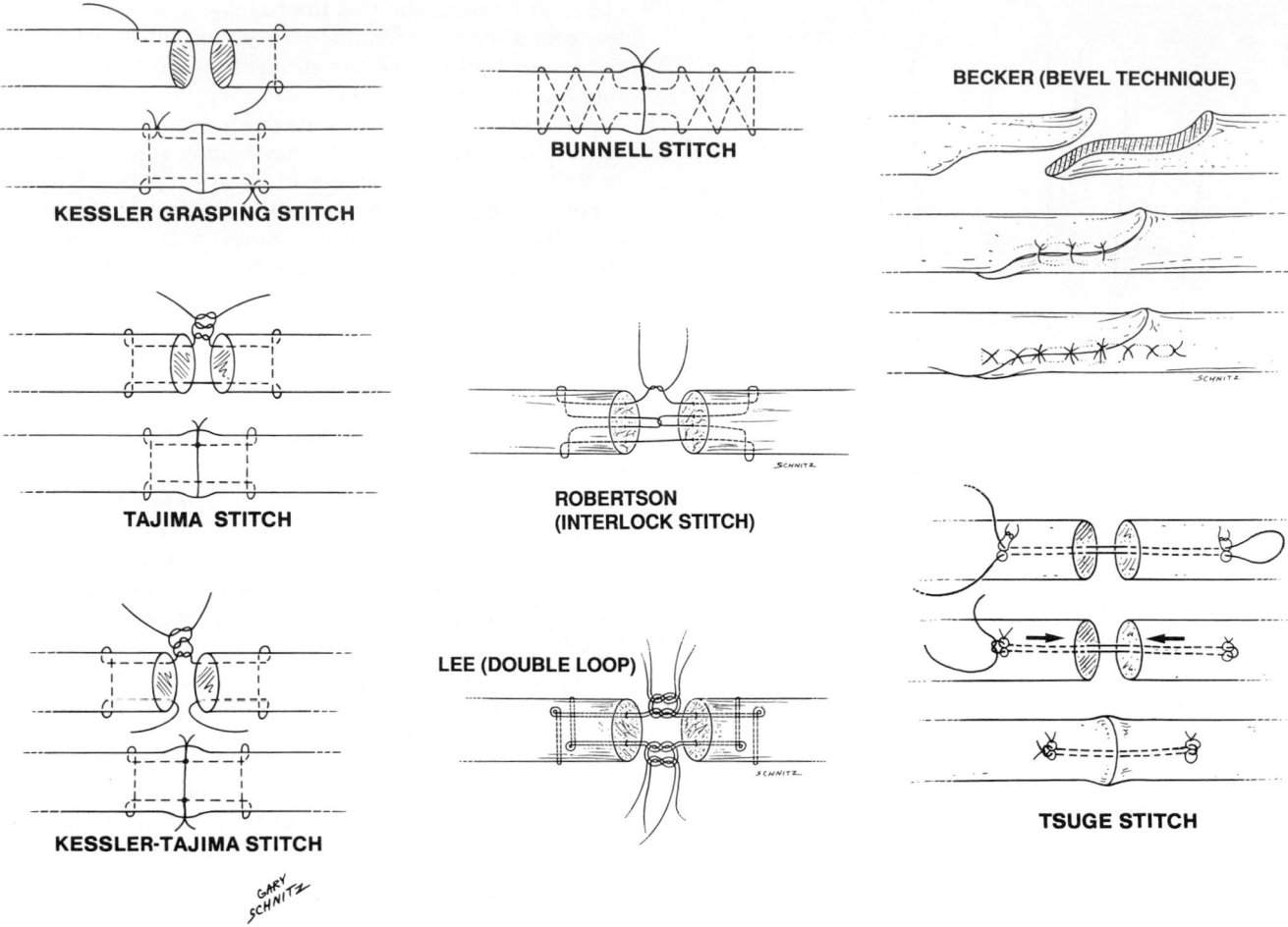

Figure 63-10 End-to-end flexor tendon repair methods. The Robertson and Lee methods are four-strand repairs and approximately twice as strong as the two-strand methods.

sion within the digital sheath. It has also been demonstrated that, in most instances, it is better to repair both the FDP and FDS tendons rather than the profundus alone, as was thought to be the wiser option in the past. Rigorous attention to the principles of atraumatic technique as espoused by Bunnell are of paramount importance in zone II, and early mobilization of repaired zone II tendons has repeatedly been shown to produce superior results.

Zone III—The Palm

In this area, one or both tendons may be injured, and direct repair has a relatively good prognosis because of the absence of the flexor sheath.

Zone IV—The Carpal Tunnel

In this area, the flexor tendons are again enclosed in synovial sheaths and held in a tight compartment, where the recovery of function may be more difficult to achieve after tendon suture. Various combinations of injuries to one or more superficialis or profundus tendons may occur in this

zone, and they are usually accompanied by injury to the median nerve. Primary repair of all severed structures should be carried out before muscle contracture develops. Carefully applied early motion protocols are appropriate in this area.

Zone V—The Wrist and Forearm

Proximal to the transverse carpal ligament, the flexor tendons are less constrained and are surrounded by loose areolar tissue. Flexor tendon repairs in this zone have a more favorable prognosis, although multiple tendon injuries and associated injuries to the major nerves and vessels can compromise the prognosis for good functional recovery.

EXTENSOR TENDON INJURIES

Injuries to the extensor system can occur from the forearm to the distal interphalangeal joint. There are nine zones of injury (Fig. 63-12, Table 63-1).

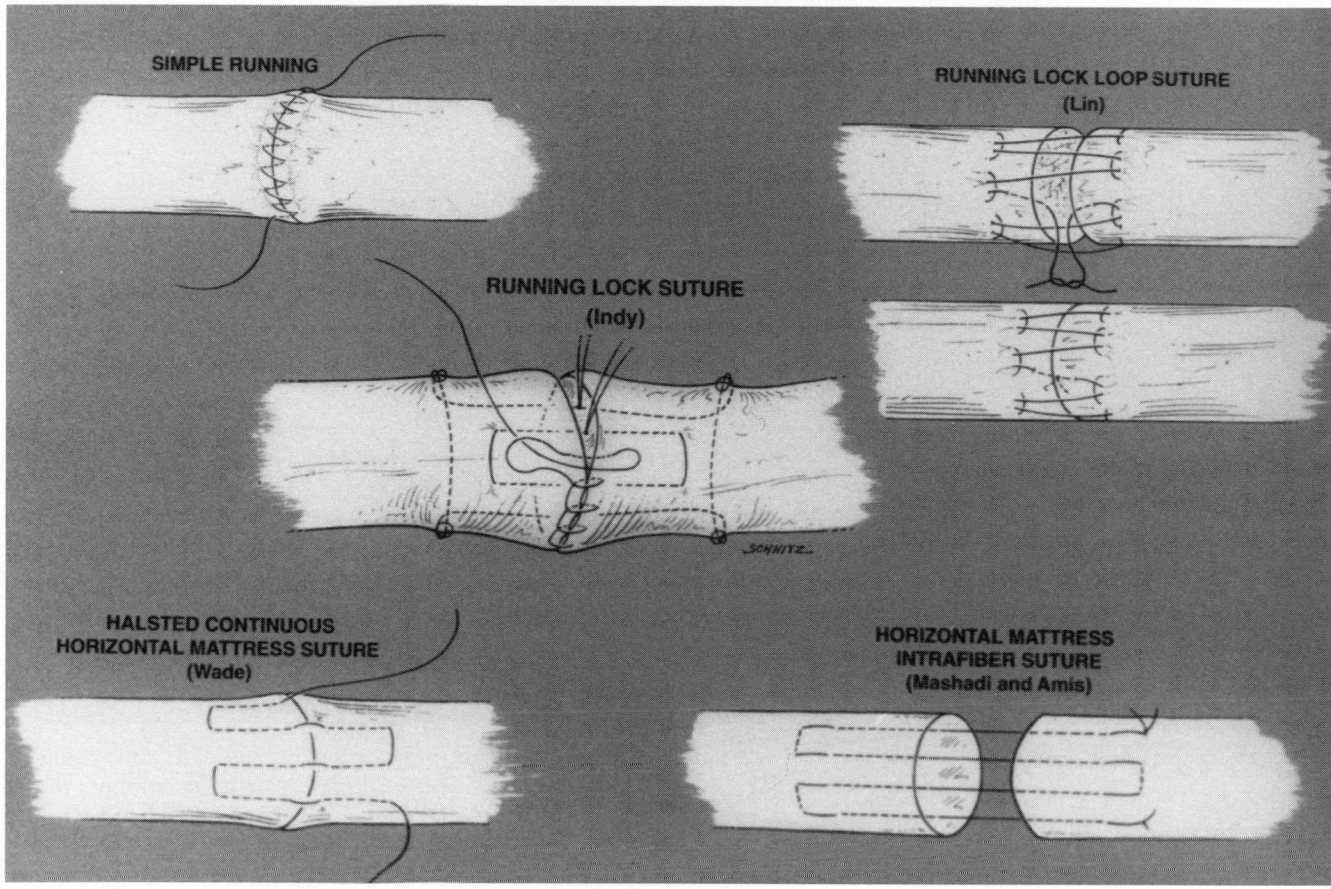

Figure 63-11 Peripheral circumferential suture methods. The "running locking loop"[23] technique and the intrafiber continuous mattress[25] method provide greater strength and resistance to gapping than simple and horizontal mattress running sutures.

Extensor Tendon Injuries at Specific Zones

Zone I—DIP Joint (Mallet Finger)

The loss of continuity of the terminal extensor tendon at or proximal to the level of the DIP joint results in the characteristic flexion deformity known as "mallet finger." In this condition, full passive extension of the involved joint is usually present and there may be some degree of hyperextension of the proximal interphalangeal joint due to unopposed central slip tension and palmar plate laxity. While these injuries may be either closed or open, the usual mechanism of injury is sudden, acute, forceful flexion of the extended digit, which results in avulsion of the extensor tendon with or without a fragment of bone from its dorsal insertion at the base of the distal phalanx.

Mallet finger deformities are classified as follows:[28]

Type I: Closed or open with a loss of tendon continuity with or without a small avulsion fracture (Fig. 63-13)
Type II: Laceration at or just proximal to the DIP joint with loss of tendon continuity
Type III: Deep abrasion with loss of skin, subcutaneous tissue, and tendon substance

Type IV: (a) Transepiphyseal plate fracture in children; (b) hyperflexion injury with fracture of articular surface of 20 to 50 percent; and (c) hyperextension injury with fracture of the articular surface usually greater than 50 percent and with early or late volar subluxation of the distal phalanx.

Type I injuries are the most common and are usually treated by a dorsal or palmar splint. Excellent to good results can be anticipated in the majority of cases in which treatment is provided early. Extension splinting should be continued for 6 to 8 weeks to be effective; several additional weeks of night splinting are recommended. Operative repair of these injuries is contraindicated. A transarticular K wire may be utilized in patients who cannot wear a splint for 6 weeks.

Type II open lacerations of the terminal extensor tendon may be managed by direct repair, whereas type III injuries may not offer the opportunity for extensor tendon repair or reconstruction and may be best managed by arthrodesis of the DIP joint.

The management of type IV injuries is somewhat controversial. Transepiphyseal plate fractures in children

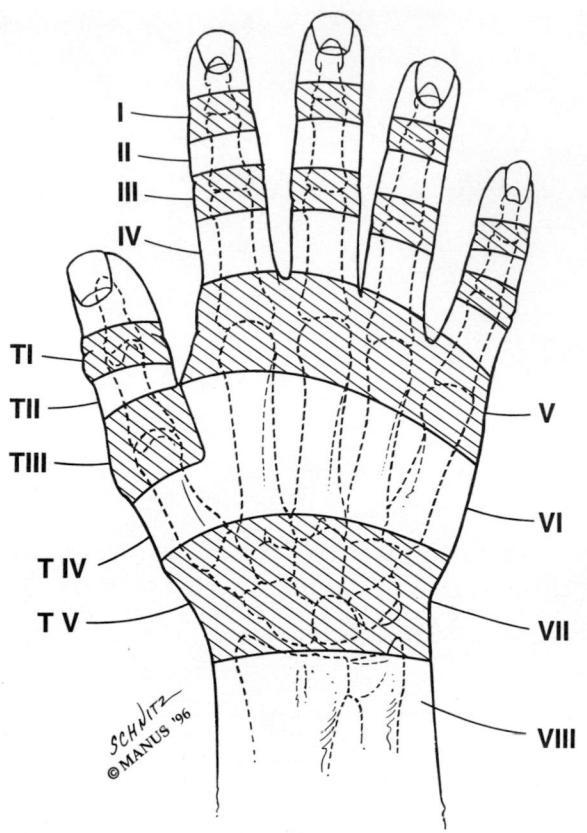

Figure 63-12 The zones of extensor tendon injuries. T = thumb zones.

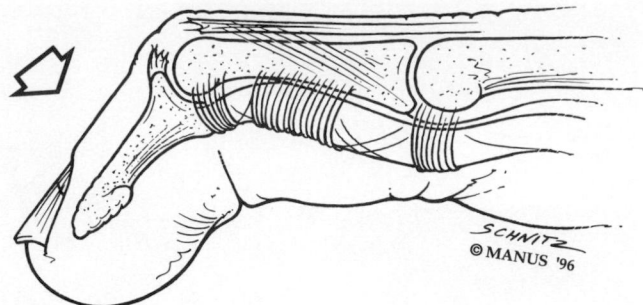

Figure 63-13 Artist's depiction of mallet-finger deformity.

teaching has recommended open reduction and an effort at anatomic repositioning of the fracture. Some have advised nonoperative treatment for all mallet fractures, even with subluxation of the distal phalanx, in the belief that restoration of joint congruity does not influence the end result.

Zone II—Middle Phalanx Finger and Proximal Phalanx Thumb

Extensor tendon injuries in this zone are almost always secondary to direct laceration. Partial lacerations of less than 50 percent of the tendon can be treated by skin wound care alone, followed by immobilization in extension for 2 weeks. Complete lacerations require suture and static splinting of the PIP joint in full extension for 6 weeks.

Zone III—Central Slip Insertion ("Boutonniere")

Interruption of the extensor central slip over the PIP joint will usually be accompanied, over time, by palmar migration of the lateral bands. This results in the loss of extension at the PIP joints and a compensatory hyperextension of the DIP joint, which is referred to as a "boutonniere" deformity (Fig. 63-14). The lesion is often secondary to blunt trauma with acute forceful flexion of the PIP joint, which avulses the central slip from its insertion on the dorsal base of the middle phalanx—with or without an avulsion fracture. The development of the full boutonniere deformity may not occur for as long as 3 weeks after injury, although a tender swollen PIP joint should alert the examiner to the possible underlying pathology. It has been suggested that an early diagnosis of boutonniere deformity might be aided by the findings of weak extension against resistance or a 20° or greater loss of active extension of the PIP joint when the wrist and MCP joints are fully flexed.

The successful management of closed acute boutonniere injuries requires the restoration of the normal tendon balance and precise length relationships of the central slip and lateral bands. This is best achieved by immobilizing the PIP joint in full extension while permitting active and passive exercises at the DIP joint. Extension of the PIP joint may be maintained by static palmar splints or the use of transarticular K wires. Operative intervention is indi-

(a) are usually easily reduced and stable. If they are unstable, small K wires can be used to maintain epiphyseal reduction for several weeks. Articular fractures of less than 50 percent (b) should be reduced as accurately as possible and splinted for 6 weeks provided that there is no subluxation of the distal phalanx. Injuries with articular surface avulsions greater than 50 percent (c) often present with palmar subluxation of the distal phalanx. Historic

TABLE 63-1   Zones of Extensor Tendon Injuries

Zone	Finger	Thumb
I	DIP joint	IP joint
II	Middle phalanx	Proximal phalanx
III	PIP joint	MP joint
IV	Proximal phalanx	Metacarpal
V	MP joint	Carpometacarpal joint/radial styloid
VI	Metacarpal	
VII	Dorsal wrist retinaculum	
VIII	Distal forearm	
IX	Middle and proximal forearm	

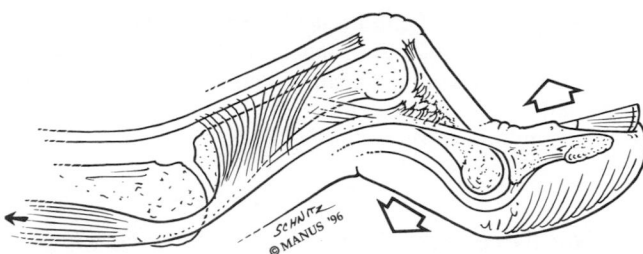

Figure 63-14 Illustration of the pathomechanics of the boutonniere lesion.

cated when the central slip has been avulsed with a bone fragment that is retracted over or proximal to the PIP joint. The bone fragment may be excised or reattached, depending on its size, and the central slip should be reattached to the base of the middle phalanx. Splinting or pinning is usually maintained for 4 to 6 weeks prior to the initiation of general active extension and later passive PIP flexion.

Open lacerations over the PIP joint that sever the extensor insertion are carefully managed in order to prevent infection of the joint. Primary tendon repair should be followed by extension splinting or pinning of the joint for 5 to 6 weeks. The DIP joint may be actively flexed in order to maintain balance between the central slip and the lateral bands.

Zone IV—Proximal Phalanx of the Finger and Metacarpal Thumb

Zone IV lacerations are often partial because the tendon, which is quite intimate with the underlying phalanx, is wide, flat, and curved. Severed lateral bands should be repaired and protected motion begun immediately. Complete lacerations of the central finger tendon must also be sutured to avoid imbalance between the central slip and lateral band, and the PIP joints should then be maintained in full extension for 6 weeks. Lacerations of the thumb extensor pollicis brevis, extensor pollicis longus, or both should be sutured and the thumb MCP joint maintained in full extension for 1 month.

Zone V—Metacarpophalangeal Joint

Injuries to the extensor mechanism over the metacarpophalangeal joint are often secondary to contact with human teeth during fisticuffs. These injuries must be considered as highly contaminated wounds with a potential for septic arthritis. X-rays should be obtained to detect the presence or absence of fracture or foreign bodies, and the wound should be extended to permit inspection of the joint. Following wound care, the wounds are left open and appropriate antibiotics initiated. Because partial or even complete extensor lacerations in this area are rarely associated with significant tendon retraction, they may not re-

quire immediate suture. Splinting with the wrist in extension and the MCP joints in 20 or 30° of flexion is usually adequate.

Simple, uncomplicated lacerations of the extensor mechanism or its expansions may be repaired using simple suture techniques. Failure to repair this type of injury can result in subluxation of the extensor tendon. These injuries are amenable to an earlier mobilization program than more distal extensor tendon injuries, and a gentle dynamic splinting program can be initiated as early as 2 weeks.

Closed rupture of the sagittal bands following a forceful flexion or extension injury of the finger may result in subluxation or dislocation of the extensor tendon at the MCP joint. This injury most commonly occurs on the radial side, leading to ulnar dislocation associated with an inability to fully extend the finger in some degree of ulnar deviation. Because the tendon recentralizes during extension, active digital extension can be maintained once it has been passively achieved. Acute rupture of the sagittal bands can be satisfactorily treated by cast immobilization with the MCP joint in full extension for 4 weeks if the diagnosis is made immediately after the injury. When diagnosis or treatment is delayed, secondary suture is usually possible. If it is not, there are several reconstructive procedures designed to recentralize the extensor tendon and provide stability.

Zone VI—Metacarpal Level

Extensor tendon lacerations in this area have sufficient substance to accept core-type sutures, and the prognosis for gliding is better than in the more distal zones. Postoperative management includes maintaining the wrist in at least 45° of extension and the MCP joints in slight flexion for about 6 weeks.

Zone VII—Wrist Level

Extensor tendon lacerations at the wrist level are almost always associated with injuries to the extensor retinaculum area. The close relationship between the tendons and the retinaculum may increase the likelihood of adhesions and there may, in some cases, be some benefit to excising a component of the retinaculum that overlies an area of tendon repair and the excursion of that repair. It is important to preserve as much retinaculum as possible to prevent bowstringing of the extensor tendons.

Zone VIII—Distal Forearm

These injuries usually occur at the muscle-tendon junction and require the best possible anatomic restoration. Because of the difficulty holding sutures in muscle, it is important to search out stronger fibers within the muscle for proximal suture placement when restoring muscle-tendon relationships. Postoperatively, the wrist is again held in extension and the MCP joints may be allowed to flex 20 or 30° for 4 to 6 weeks.

RECONSTRUCTION FOLLOWING TENDON INJURIES

Secondary Repair

Delayed primary repair of flexor or extensor tendons usually cannot be performed after about 4 weeks, although there are instances when it is possible to effect a repair after an even greater passage of time.

Flexor Tendon Grafting

Free tendon grafting is indicated when both the flexor digitorum profundus and superficialis have been injured (usually in zone II) and for some reason have not been repaired. Prior to tendon grafting, the wound should be well healed and the finger passively supple. The tendon grafting is usually used to reconstruct the profundus tendon only and traverses from the palm to the distal phalanx. It is an important rule never to sacrifice an intact flexor superficialis to perform a tendon graft, and grafting through an intact superficialis requires careful consideration and experience. Loss of DIP flexion alone may not represent a significant functional impairment, and the possibility of the procedure making the finger worse rather than better should be balanced against the patient's age and functional needs.

Staged Tendon Reconstruction

In difficult salvage situations, the placement of a silicone rubber tendon implant in the scarred digit in order to form a pseudosheath favorable for second-stage tendon grafting, has proved to be a very satisfactory procedure.[29] Staged reconstruction should not replace conventional free tendon grafting in digits that have minimal scarring, pliable joints, and an adequate pulley system. When the tendon bed is markedly scarred and there is extensive damage to the sheath system or there are significant joint contractures, the staged tendon reconstruction approach is appropriate. Most of these cases are secondary to failed prior surgical procedures—be they repairs, grafts, or lysis procedures—and it is well known that fingers with severe neurovascular deficiency have a poor prognosis and may be better managed by arthrodesis or amputation.

Stage I of the staged technique consists of preparing a bed in the scarred palm and digit, excising most of the scar tissue, releasing joint contractures, inserting the silicone implant (usually digit to distal forearm), and reconstructing components of the pulley system over the implant. While the implants are usually left to glide with passive digital motion, an active silicone rubber tendon implant is available that allows for distal attachment to the distal phalanx and can be secured to a proximal motor tendon.[30]

Stage II consists of removing the implant and replacing it with a free tendon graft. This stage is usually carried out no sooner than 3 months and must await "tissue equilibrium" with a soft, passively supple digit. The grafting technique is fairly simple and involves attaching the graft to the distal end of the implant through a small incision and pulling it through the channel prepared by the implant into a proximal wound. Proximal and distal graft junctures can then be accomplished with the hope of restoring excellent function to these badly damaged digits.

Pulley Reconstruction

It is often necessary to reconstruct at least the A_2 and A_4 pulleys in order to reestablish the most biomechanically efficient tendon restraint system. Pulleys may be restored utilizing local tissue, one tail of the superficialis tendon (A_3), or autogenous tendon or retinacular material from the dorsal wrist. Synthetic materials have also been advocated and a sufficient width of pulley reconstruction should be carried out to defray the considerable pressure of the tendon/pulley interface during strong digital flexion.

Flexor Tenolysis

Tenolysis should always be considered as a potential final salvage procedure following tendon repair, grafting, or staged reconstruction, and patients should be forewarned that a certain percentage of those procedures result in tendon adherence sufficient to require lysis.[31,32] The procedure must be approached as a major surgical effort with great consideration for patient selection, operative technique, and postoperative management. The procedure is particularly indicated whenever the passive range of digital joint flexion significantly exceeds the patient's ability to actively flex the same joints. The decision to perform a tenolysis should be based on serial joint measurements indicating that there has been no appreciable improvement in active flexion after several months, despite a good therapy program and the conscientious efforts of the patient. All fractures should be healed and wounds should have reached tissue equilibrium with soft, pliable skin and subcutaneous tissues and minimal reaction around scars. In addition, joint contractures must have been overcome or near normal passive range of digital motion achieved. Satisfactory sensation and muscle strength must also be present and the patient must be carefully informed as to the objectives, techniques, postoperative course, and pitfalls of the procedure.

The proper timing for tenolysis following tendon surgery, repair, or graft is somewhat controversial. It is probably best considered for those patients in whom serial examinations have revealed no significant improvement in 3 months or more after repair or graft, provided that the previously mentioned criteria for the procedure had been fulfilled and there has been no improvement in active motion in the previous 4 to 8 months.

In recent years, it has been popular to carry out tenolysis under the use of local anesthesia supplemented by intravenous analgesia or tranquilizing medications. With the patient awake and the forearm musculature functional, the patient is able to actively demonstrate the completeness of the lysis by flexing or extending the involved digits during surgery.

Thorough tenolysis requires wide surgical exposure; the exact incisions employed often depend on the wounds resulting from the original injury and subsequent operative efforts. Flexor or extensor tendons are meticulously extricated from their restricting scar and adhesions. In the case of flexor tendons, the pulley system should be preserved throughout the lysis procedure. When the tendons have been fully freed, the patient can be asked to actively extend and flex the fingers and demonstrate the completeness of the procedure. A rapid and vigorous postoperative therapy program follows, in which every effort is made to preserve the gains achieved in surgery.

CONCLUSION

Restoration of satisfactory wrist and digital function following interruption of flexor or extensor tendons is often a very difficult and frustrating process. Acute surgical repairs and late reconstructive procedures all demand a strong understanding of the normal and pathologic anatomy of the flexor and extensor systems and an appreciation for their biomechanics and biology. The best opportunity for functional recovery also often requires the combined efforts of patient, surgeon, and therapist.

REFERENCES

1. Gelberman R, Goldberg V, An K, Banes A: Tendon, in Woo S, Buckwalter J (eds): *Injury and Repair of the Musculo-skeletal Soft Tissues.* American Academy of Orthopaedic Surgeons Symposium. Park Ridge, IL: AAOS, 1987, pp 5–40.
2. Doyle JR: Anatomy of the finger flexor tendon sheath and pulley system. *J Hand Surg* 13A:4:473–484, 1988.
3. Manske PR, Lesker PA: Palmar aponeurosis pulley. *J Hand Surg* 8:3:259–263, 1983.
4. Schuind F, Garcia-Elias M, Cooney WP, An KN: Flexor tendon forces: In vivo measurements. *J Hand Surg* 17A:291–298, 1992.
5. Strickland JW: Experimental studies of the structure and function of tendon, in *Hand Surgery Update.* Park Ridge, IL: American Academy of Orthopaedic Surgeons, 1996, pp 127–139.
6. Hume EL, Hutchinson DT, Jaeger SA, Hunter JM: Biomechanics of pulley reconstruction. *J Hand Surg* 16A:4:722–730, 1991.
7. Idler RS: Anatomy and biomechanics of the digital flexor tendons. *Hand Clin* 1:1:3–12, 1985.
8. Weber ER: Nutritional pathways for flexor tendons in the digital theca, in Hunter JM, Schneider LH, Mackin EJ (eds): *Tendon Surgery in Hand.* St Louis, Mosby, 1987, pp 91–99.
9. Manske PR, Lesker PA: Nutrient pathways of flexor tendons in primates. *J Hand Surg* 7:436–444, 1982.
10. Manske PR, Lesker PA: Nutrient pathways to extensor tendons within the extensor retinacular compartments: An experimental study in dogs. *Clin Orthop* 181:234–237, 1983.
11. Manske PR, Gelberman RH, Lesker PA: Flexor tendon healing. *Hand Clin* 1:25–34, 1985.
12. Gelberman RH, Khabie V, Cahill CJ: The revascularization on healing flexor tendons in digital sheath: A vascular injection study in dogs. *J Bone Joint Surg* 73A:6:868–881, 1991.
13. Gelberman RH, Botte MJ, Spiegelman JJ, et al: The excursion and deformation of repaired flexor tendons treated with protected early motion. *J Hand Surg* 11:106–110, 1986.
14. Gelberman RH, Woo SLY, Lothringer K, et al: Effects of early intermittent passive mobilization on healing canine flexor tendons. *J Hand Surg* 7:170–175, 1982.
15. Strickland JW: Flexor tendon injuries: I. Foundations of treatment. *J Am Acad Orthop Surg* 3:44–54, 1995.
16. Strickland JW: Flexor tendon injuries: II. Operative technique. *J Am Acad Orthop Surg* 3:55–62, 1995.
17. Gelberman RH, Goldberg V, An KN, et al: Tendon, in Woo SLY, Buckwalter JA (eds): *Injury and Repair of the Musculoskeletal Soft Tissues.* Park Ridge, IL, American Academy of Orthopaedic Surgeons, 1988, pp 5–40.
18. Gelberman RH, Steinberg D, Amiel D, et al: Fibroblast chemotaxis after tendon repair. *J Hand Surg* 16:686–693, 1991.
19. Savage R: In vitro studies of a new method of flexor tendon repair. *J Hand Surg* 10:135–141, 1985.
20. Robertson GA, Al-Quattan MM: A biomechanical analysis of a new interlock suture technique for flexor tendon repair. *J Hand Surg* 17:92–93, 1992.
21. Lee H: Double loop locking suture: A technique of tendon repair for early active mobilization: Part I. Evolution of technique and experimental study. *J Hand Surg* 15:945–952, 1990.
22. Lee H: Double loop locking suture: A technique of tendon repair for early active mobilization: Part II. Clinical experience. *J Hand Surg* 15:953–958, 1990.
23. Lin GT, An KN, Amadio PC, et al: Biomechanical studies of running suture for flexor tendon repair in dogs. *J Hand Surg* 13:553–558, 1988.
24. Wade PJF, Wetherell RG, Amis AA: Flexor tendon repair: Significant gain in strength from the Halsted peripheral suture technique. *J Hand Surg* 14:232–235, 1989.
25. Mashadi ZB, Amis AA: Strength of the suture in the epitenon and within the tendon fibers: Development of stronger peripheral suture technique. *J Hand Surg* 17:172–175, 1992.
26. Bishop AT, Cooney WP III, Wood MB: Treatment of partial flexor tendon lacerations: The effect of tenorrhaphy and early protected mobilization. *J Trauma* 26:301–312, 1986.
27. Strickland JW: Biologic rationale, clinical application, and results of early motion following flexor tendon repair. *J Hand Ther* 2:71–83, 1989.
28. Doyle JR: Extensor tendons—Acute injuries, in Green DP (ed): *Operative Hand Surgery,* 2d ed. New York, Churchill Livingstone, 1988, pp 2055–2060.
29. Hunter JM: Staged flexor tendon reconstruction. *J Hand Surg* 8:789–793, 1983.
30. Hunter JM: Tendon salvage and the active tendon implant: A perspective. *Hand Clin* 1:181–186, 1985.
31. Strickland JW: Flexor tenolysis. *Hand Clin* 1:121–132, 1985.
32. Strickland JW: Tenolysis—A personal experience, in Hunter J, Schneider L, Mackin E (eds): *Tendon Surgery in the Hand.* St Louis, Mosby, 1987, pp 216–233.

CHAPTER 64

Replantation Surgery in the Upper Extremity

Alexander Bee Dagum and M. Ather Mirza

The possibility of reattaching an amputated human part has been the dream of reconstructive surgeons for centuries. The first limb replantation attempts were made in the animal laboratory by Hopfner and Carrel in 1903 and 1906, respectively. However it was not until 1962 that the first arm was replanted by Malt and 1965 that Komatsu and Tamai replanted the first thumb. In the 1970s replantation surgery took off, and by the 1980s many microsurgical centers had been established throughout the world with viability rates on the order of 80 percent.[1]

DEFINITIONS

Microsurgery refers to the field of surgery that uses a microscope to perform all or part of the surgery. In general replantation is facilitated by the use of the microscope to perform the microvascular and neuronal anastomoses. In vessels smaller than 1.5 mm, the magnification of the microscope makes reliably successful anastomoses possible.

Replantation is the reattachment of a completely severed part of the body back to the same body. A complete amputation means that the part has no attachment to the body. This must be distinguished from an incomplete amputation, where a connection between the part and the body exists. An incomplete amputation will usually require arterial anastomosis but not necessarily venous anastomosis. The results are usually better for incomplete amputations, as more structures have been preserved. *Revascularization* refers to reestablishment of vascular flow through an arterial anastomosis in order to prevent tissue necrosis of an incompletely amputated part.

Amputations are classified by the anatomic level of injury and the type of injury.[2,3] The type of injury is important in determining the immediate success and ultimate function of the replantation. There are three types of injuries: guillotine, crush, and avulsion. *Guillotine* refers to a sharp amputation, as seen when a part is severed by a knife or band saw; these injuries have the best success rate and prognosis. *Crush* refers to an amputation that was caused by a large compressive load, with a larger zone of injury, as seen with punch press accidents. *Avulsion amputation* is an injury where the part has been pulled out of the body; this has the poorest success rate and prognosis.

INDICATIONS AND CONTRAINDICATIONS TO REPLANTATION

In general the decision to attempt replantation should be made by a microsurgeon after carefully evaluating the patient and the part. Patients with other serious injuries or illnesses are usually not candidates for replantation. The patient must understand and be committed to a lengthy operation, hospital stay, and course of hand therapy. Except for a thumb and single digit, the average replantation patient may be off work for up to 1 to 2 years and require an average of two further operations such as tenolysis, neurolysis, capsulectomy, or two-stage tendon reconstruction.[2–6]

In the appropriate patient with a guillotine or localized crush amputation, an attempt at replantation should always be tried in a thumb, multiple digits, hand, or distal forearm (Figs. 64-1 and 64-2). Relative indications include a single digit distal to the superficialis insertion or a below- or above-elbow amputation. In a through elbow, very high arm, or single-digit amputation through the proximal phalanx, replantation in general is contraindicated. Children have great capacity for regeneration; thus all amputations in children should be replanted. Avulsed or severely crushed digital amputations should be scrutinized for their salvage and functional potential.

It is the authors' opinion that distal digital amputations, if replantable, do well. Compared to a revision amputation, a distal replant provides better motor and sensory function as well as cosmesis. A distal replant can prevent neuroma formation but may cause a disabling cold intolerance. Average time to return to work is 10 to 12 weeks for a distal replantation as compared to 6 weeks for a revision amputation.

CARE OF THE AMPUTATED PART, AMPUTATION SITE, AND PATIENT

Care of the amputated part is critical to the success and survival of the replant. Cooling to 4°C lowers the metabolic rate of the tissue and doubles its ischemia time. If the warm ischemia time is greater than 12 h or the cool ischemia time is greater than 24 h, replantation is not recommended. The limit of ischemia time for tissue containing a significant amount of muscle is 6 h of warm and 12 h of cool ischemia. Therefore amputations proximal to the carpus should not be replanted if the ischemia time is greater than 6 h of warm or 12 h of cool ischemia.

The amputated part should be gently irrigated with saline or Ringer's lactate and then wrapped in moist saline gauze; it is then placed in a plastic bag in ice water. Alternatively it can be placed in a small container full of saline that is then placed in a container with crushed ice. It is important that the part does not rest on ice or it will sustain a frostbite injury.

A pressure dressing is placed on the amputation stump, which is then elevated and splinted. This will con-

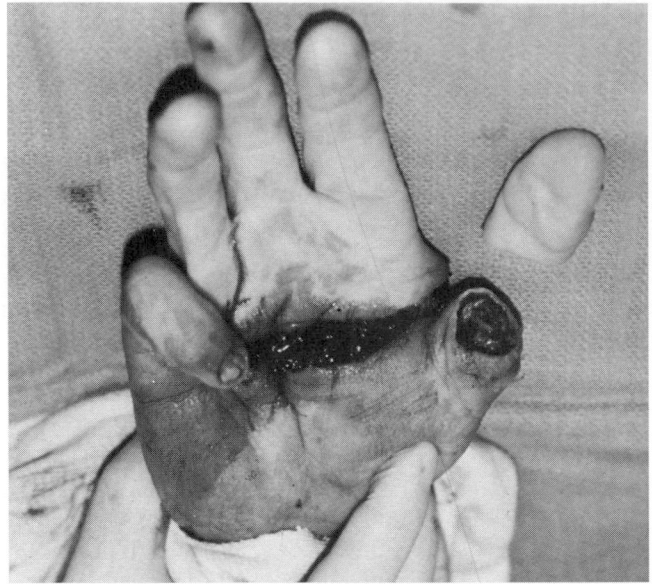

A

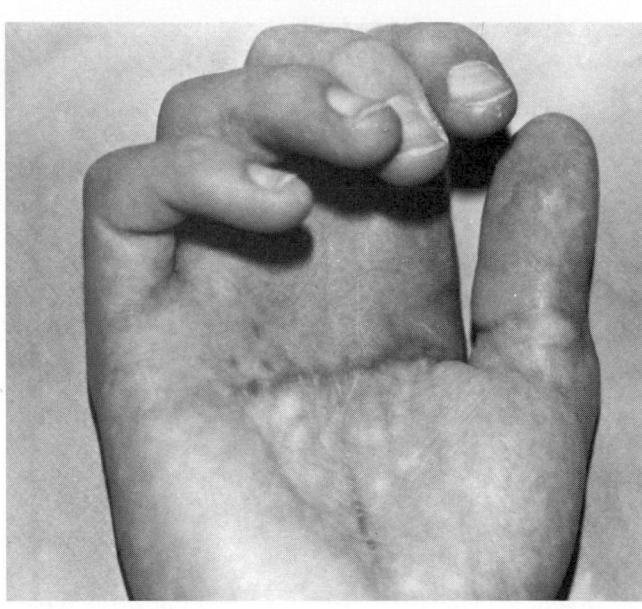

B

Figure 64-1 *A.* Thumb amputation secondary to power saw injury with associated partial amputation involving index and long fingers. All thumb amputations should be considered candidates for replantation if there are no other systemic medical contraindications to the long surgical procedure. *B.* Successful replantation of thumb and revascularizations of digits. Some restriction of finger flexion is noted.

trol bleeding in all cases except where there is a partial vessel laceration. It is important to avoid blind clamping of the vessels with hemostats, as this can seriously injure the neurovascular bundle.

The overall management of the patient always takes precedence. The patient is fully evaluated particularly in more major injuries such as an extremity amputation. In a major injury, the ATLS protocol should be followed. Even experienced emergency room physicians may be overwhelmed by a patient who arrives with an amputated extremity. In the rush to transfer the patient to a replantation center, associated chest or abdominal injuries can be missed.

GENERAL OPERATIVE MANAGEMENT

Replantations are best carried out at a dedicated hand and microsurgical center.[7] Although possible, it is difficult

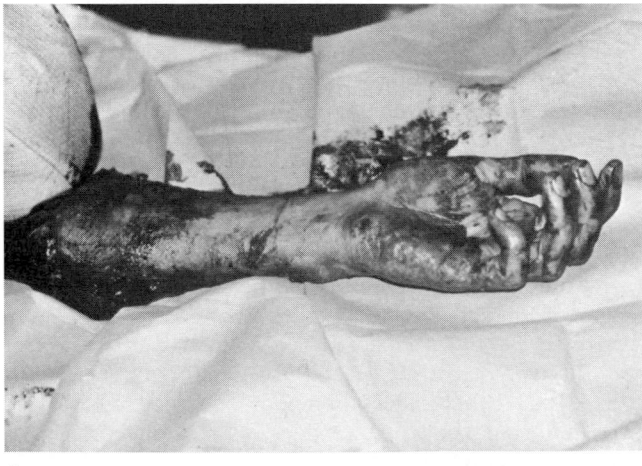

A

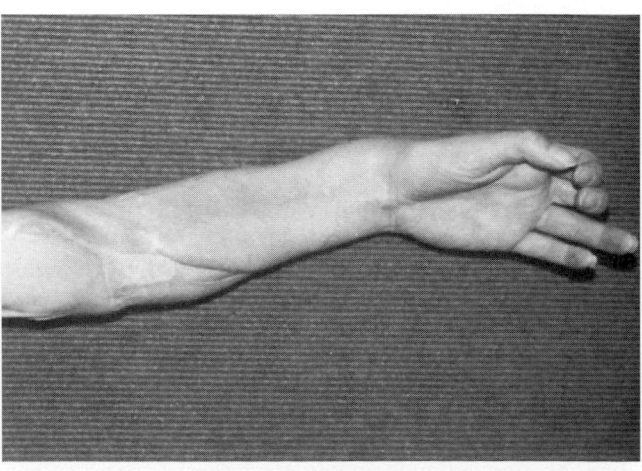

B

Figure 64-2 *A.* Proximal forearm amputation in young male's dominant extremity. *B.* Successful replantation of the upper extremity. Some functional deficits remain because of the deficiencies in nerve regeneration.

for the solo microsurgeon to maintain a high success rate. A dedicated center or group allows for a team approach to these lengthy cases, which may go on for more than 16 h and may require a return to the operating room a day later.

Assessment of the part will reveal a great deal of information about the feasibility of successful replantation. The presence of red streaks on the skin along the course of the digital arteries is called the *Chinese red line sign.* This is caused by severe traction on the neurovascular bundles and thus tearing of the side branches, with hemorrhage on the side of the finger. The *ribbon sign* describes an elongated tortuous and twisted artery with a pigtail appearance. Both these signs are indicative of a severe avulsion injury and usually preclude a successful replantation.

Regional anesthesia in the form of a 0.25 percent bupivacaine brachial plexus block is used for most replantations distal to the carpus. This has the advantage of providing a sympathetic block and increasing proximal blood flow as well as avoiding the complications of prolonged general anesthesia.

The use of two operating teams—one on the part and the other on the amputation stump—constitutes the best approach, in particular when multiple digits are involved. After careful debridement through a slightly curved midlateral incision, each team identifies and tags arteries, veins, nerves, and tendons (Fig. 64-3). The bone is then prepared for osteosynthesis. It is extremely important to get out of the zone of injury; this usually means shortening the bone by 0.5 to 1 cm on the part and the stump, allowing for a tension-free repair of undamaged vessels and nerves. Failure to do this will lead to an unsuccessful replant.

The sequence of repair varies slightly from surgeon to surgeon. The first step is bony fixation, which is carried out either with one or two longitudinal K wires or with interosseous wires. The extensor and flexor tendons are then repaired in the usual manner. If the veins were easily found and of good caliber, they are repaired next under the microscope. The artery is then repaired under the microscope. In cases where good veins are not initially found, it is convenient to repair the artery first, as this will allow for easier identification of useful veins. At least one artery and, if possible, two veins are repaired, as this increases the survival rate. The nerves are then repaired, followed by a loose closure of the skin with only enough sutures to ensure coverage of the vessels. The closure must be tension-free in order to prevent compression of the anastomosis. If this is not possible, a skin graft can be used to cover the vessels. A soft, nonconstricting dressing is then placed on the extremity, which is elevated. It is important that the dressing allow for adequate and easy inspection of the replanted part.

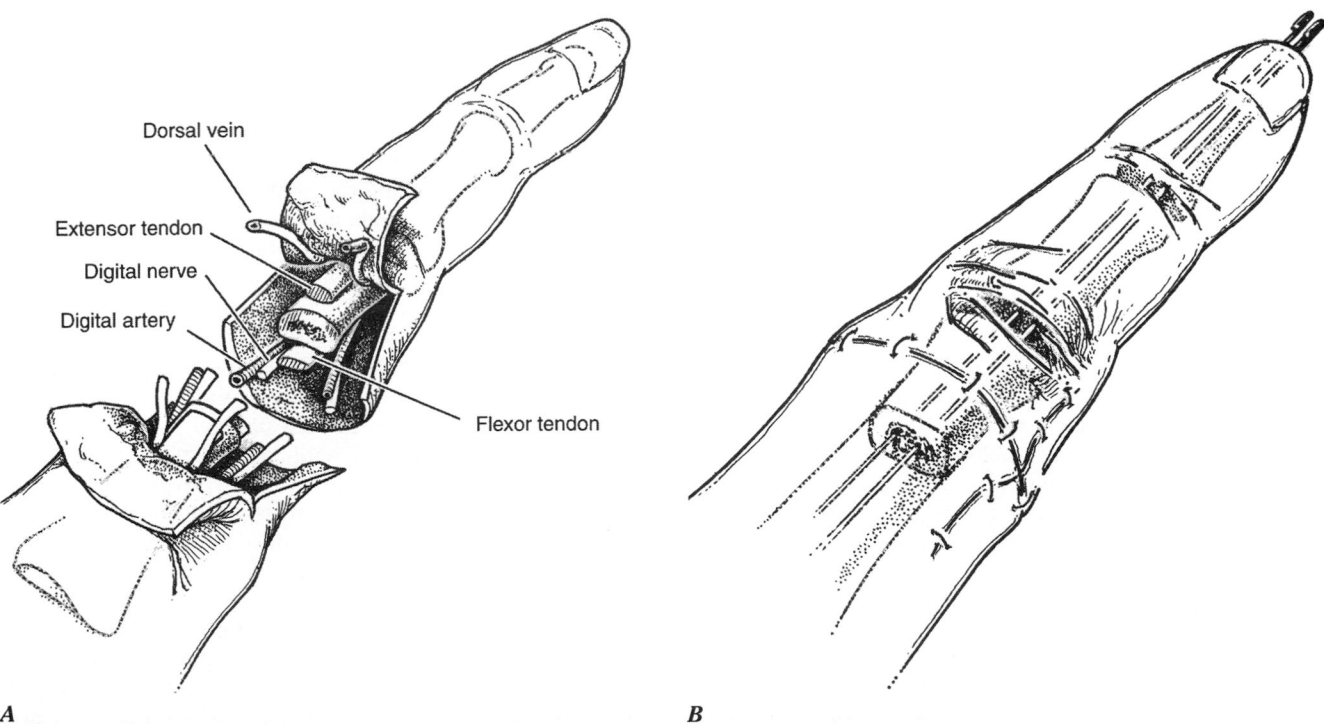

Dorsal vein

Extensor tendon

Digital nerve

Digital artery

Flexor tendon

A

B

Figure 64-3 *A.* A schematic diagram of the surgically prepared amputation part and stump is shown. The bony osteosynthesis will be performed first followed by the flexor and extensor tendons. The dorsal veins will be repaired next followed by the digital arteries and the nerves. *B.* The replanted digit is shown. Note the loose closure to ensure no compression of the repaired dorsal digital veins.

MAJOR LIMB REPLANTATION

Major limb replantation requires expedient management in order to be successful and to prevent major systemic complications.[2–4,6,8] The injuries tend to involve higher energy and therefore require more aggressive shortening of the extremity. The bone is repaired first, followed by the artery. The part is allowed to perfuse and drain prior to venous anastomosis in order to reduce lactate and myoglobinemia, which can lead to life-threatening complications. The muscles are approximated next by sewing the epimysium, followed by repair of the nerves. Last is the repair of the veins. If arrival to the operating room is greater than 6 h postinjury some surgeons recommend the use of a Sundt shunt to quickly establish arterial flow prior to performing bony osteosynthesis, so as to prevent significant muscle necrosis. We find that a Sundt shunt is usually not necessary. Prior to unclamping the venous repair, the patient should be extremely well hydrated; 50 mL of 20 percent mannitol is given to create a urine output greater than 100 mL/h, and the urine should be alkalized by giving 100 mL of $NaHCO_3$ in order to prevent precipitation of the myoglobin and subsequent acute renal failure from acute tubular necrosis. Fasciotomies should routinely be done and the patient brought back to the operating room at 48 h for reassessment.

POSTOPERATIVE MANAGEMENT

Postoperative management is essential to the survival of the replant.[7] The patient is transferred to a microsurgical or intensive care unit step-down bed and kept NPO for 24 h. Intravenous antibiotics are given for 5 days. The room must be kept warm or a warming hood used. The patient is given a caffeine-free diet to prevent vasospasm. Ringer's lactate at 150 mL/h is given for 3 days to maintain a high flow through the repaired vessels. Anticoagulation is used in most replants except for major limb replants or guillotine amputations. The patient is fully heparinized so as to maintain the partial thromboplastin time at 1.5 to 2 times control, or dextran 40 at 25 mL/h is used for 7 days. The dressing is changed at 7 days. Tight dressings can easily interfere with digital vein repairs. The dressing change should be done in an extremely gentle manner to avoid damage to vessels. The patient is then placed in a splint and allowed to ambulate with the extremity elevated. The patient is discharged at 10 days with instructions not to smoke and to continue on a caffeine-free diet for 6 weeks. Aspirin is often recommended for 1 to 3 months after digital replant.

The replanted part is monitored hourly for 72 h and then q 4 h. This involves checking the CTTC: capillary refill, temperature, turgor, and color. Twice a day or if there is cause for concern, the part is pricked with a 21-gauge needle for bleeding; slow, bright red oxygenated blood should be seen. Several monitors are used for continuous assessment of the replanted part. Monitoring includes temperature, laser Doppler, tissue O_2, etc. These are useful in conjunction with good clinical observation. The continuous temperature monitor is the most popular type for replants. A drop of 2°C in an hour is significant of some form of vascular compromise and demands immediate assessment by the surgeon. A rapid temperature drop to less than 28°C signifies an arterial problem, and a gradual temperature drop to less than 30°C signifies a venous problem.[9,10]

COMPLICATIONS

Early complications are mostly vascular and hence directly affect the survival of the part. The nursing team and house staff involved in the care of replants should be competent in the clinical assessment of perfusion to a part and be able to differentiate normal from arterial or venous insufficiency. Arterial compromise is characterized by a pale, cool, prunelike (decrease turgor) part with loss of capillary refill, which, on pinprick, shows no significant bleeding. Venous compromise is characterized by a blue, cool, swollen (increase turgor) part with brisk capillary return, which, on pinprick, has brisk dark-red bleeding. The first step is to take down the dressing and cut one or two stitches if the skin closure appears tight. If this fails to improve vascularity, the patient should immediately be taken back to the operating room. At reexploration, the vessel in question is looked at and the anastomosis redone if need be, with or without vein grafts as the situation dictates. If this restores normal vascular perfusion, there is no need to explore the other vessels (i.e., if a pure arterial thrombosis is encountered and repair of the artery restores normal perfusion, there is no need to look at the veins and vice versa). The success rate in early takebacks that require redoing of an anastomosis is on the order of 50 to 60 percent, certainly making reexploration worthwhile.

Adequate dorsal veins are occasionally not found, in particular in distal digital replantations. An arterial-only replant has only a 20 percent survival rate. Occasionally volar veins may be used or the opposite digital artery anastomosed through a vein graft to a proximal vein, creating an arteriovenous fistula. In general, heparinization of the patient, removal of the nail plate, and rubbing the sterile matrix with a heparin-soaked pledget every half hour for 5 days or application of medicinal leeches (*Hirudo medicinalis*) four times a day for 5 to 7 days will temporarily provide sufficient venous drainage until normal connections are reestablished as the part heals to the stump. Each of these methods will increase the arterial-only replant's survival rate up to 66 to 70 percent. If medicinal leeches are used, the patient should first be started on appropriate antibiotics such as cefotaxime, trimethoprim-sulfamethoxazole, gentamicin, or ciprofloxacin to prevent an *Aeromonas hydrophilia* infection, which can lead not only to loss of the part but also to sepsis.[11] Note that *A. hydrophilia* is not sensitive to cefazolin.

Bleeding can be a major problem postoperatively; it may represent a thrombosed venous anastomosis, arterial or venous anastomotic leak, inadequate hemostasis of the soft tissue, or overanticoagulation. If bleeding persists after correction of overanticoagulation, the patient should be taken back to the operating room, where adequate lighting and equipment facilitates control of hemostasis. Infection is uncommon—less than 2 percent—and is minimized by careful operative debridement, shortening of the bone, and perioperative antibiotics. Localized skin slough is commonly encountered. This is usually not a problem because bone shortening leads to an excess of skin. If vessels become exposed, they can usually be covered with a skin graft. Rarely, a pedicle flap may be necessary.

Late complications are related to functional problems through the one-wound one-scar concept. In other words, all the structures from bone to skin heal as one scar, and thus the important function of differential gliding, which gives our hands their dexterity, is lost. The one guarantee that the surgeon can make to the patient if the digital replant survives is that it will be like cement and require a great deal of therapy and probably secondary surgery in order to improve motion. An early motion protocol to improve tendon gliding and prevent joint contractures is usually not possible because of the increased risk of vessel thrombosis. Late flexor and extensor tendon adhesions are common and usually require tenolysis. Flexor tendon rupture, particularly after tenolysis, is not uncommon and requires two-stage reconstruction. Joint contractures can usually be worked out by the therapist.

Bony nonunion is usually due to inadequate fixation. A 21 percent nonunion has been reported with cross K wire as compared to 8 percent with K wire and interosseous wire and 0 percent with perpendicular interosseous wires. However, with prolonged splinting, one-third of nonunions will go on to unite.[12]

Nerve recovery is dependent on the level and type of injury and comparable to a similar isolated injury. Cold intolerance in the replanted part is common and can be extremely disabling, particularly in colder climates. Although at one time it was felt to improve after 2 years, a recent study showed no improvement in most patients.[13]

RESULTS FOLLOWING REPLANTATION

The survival results of replantation are approximately 80 percent for adults and greater than 70 percent for children less than 10 years old. The lower viability results in children are in part due to the more aggressive approach at attempting replantation as well as smaller vessels with an increased tendency toward spasm.[2–6,8]

The long-term results are variable and dependent on the type and level of injury; the patient's health, age, body habitus, motivation, and compliance with therapy; and the surgeon's expertise. In general, young, healthy, motivated patients with long, supple, skinny fingers do better than their counterparts. The more distal the injury and the sharper the transection, the better the results.

In general, it can be said that for digital replantations, the range of motion postreplant will be approximately 50 percent of normal, with a mean 2-point discrimination of 10 mm and a cosmetic appearance superior to that of a prosthesis. The best results are obtained in thumb, hand, and distal forearm replants.[2–6,6a,8]

RING AVULSION INJURIES

Ring avulsion injuries are common and by definition involve the tearing away of skin plus or minus tendon plus or minus neurovascular bundles plus or minus bone and joint. The pathomechanics is that of a ring caught on a stationary object while the patient continues to move the finger, arm, and body. The mechanical advantage is tremendous, leading to a spectrum of injury from simple laceration to complete amputation of the digit.

The classification of ring avulsion injuries is important with respect to treatment and prognosis. It is based on the circulation of the digit.[13]

Class 1: Circulation is adequate with or without tendon or skeletal injury.

Class 2: Circulation is inadequate (arterial and/or venous) with or without tendon or skeletal injury.

Class 3: There is no circulation with complete degloving or amputation.

Treatment depends on the extent of injury balanced by age, sex, cultural background, and occupation. If circulation is adequate, the injured parts are repaired and a skin graft is usually required for closure to prevent venous constriction. If the circulation is inadequate, arterial and/or venous repairs are performed. This usually requires vein grafts. In general, complete amputations are better served by revision amputation except in a child, a thumb, or possibly if the flexor and extensor tendons are intact.[14,15]

The results of treatment depend on the extent of injuries and patient factors. Return to work in class 1 injuries or revision amputation is approximately 6 to 8 weeks, while for microsurgical salvage it ranges from 9 to 12 weeks. The most common long-term complication is cold intolerance seen in 65 percent of digits. Range of motion for classes 1 and 2 is greater than 75 percent, while for class 3 it is approximately 50 percent.

REFERENCES

1. Buncke HJ: Forty years of microsurgery: What's next? *J Hand Surg* 20A:S34–S45, 1995.
2. Goldner RD: Replantation surgery, in Manske PR (ed): *Hand Surgery Update.* Denver, American Society for Surgery of the Hand, 1994, pp 30-1–30-9.
3. Urbaniak JR: Replantation, in Green DR (ed): *Operative Hand Surgery,* New York, Churchill Livingstone, 1993, pp 1085–1102.
4. Axelrod TS, Buchler U: Severe complex injuries to the upper extremity: Revascularization and replantation. *J Hand Surg* 16A:574–584, 1991.
5. Bowen CVA, Beveridge J, Milliken RG, Johnston GHP: Rotating shaft avulsion amputations of the thumb. *J Hand Surg* 16A:117–121, 1991.

6. Kleinert JM, Graham B: Macroreplantation: An overview. *Microsurgery* 11:229–233, 1990.

6a. Glickman L, Mackinnon S: Sensory recovery following digital replantation. *Microsurgery* 11:236–242, 1990.

7. Mirza MA, Krober KE: Organization and implementation of a community hospital microsurgical service for the management of amputation injuries. *Microsurgery* 5:136–139, 1984.

8. Zucker RM, Stevenson JH: Proximal upper limb replantation in children. *J Trauma* 28:554–547, 1988.

9. Dagum AB, Dowd A: A new technique for monitoring muscle flaps. *Microsurgery* 16:723–726, 1995.

10. Neligan PC: Monitoring techniques for the detection of flow failure in the postoperative period. *Microsurgery* 14:162–164, 1993.

11. Wells MD, Manktelow RT, Boyd JB, Bowen V: The medical leech: An old treatment revisited. *Microsurgery* 14:183–186, 1993.

12. Whitney TM, Lineaweaver WC, Buncke HJ, Nugent K: Clinical results of bony fixation methods in digital replantation. *J Hand Surg* 15A:328–334, 1990.

13. Collins ED Novak CB, Mackinnon SE: Long-term follow-up of cold intolerance following nerve injury (abstr). The American Society for Surgery of the Hand, 50th Annual Meeting. San Francisco, CA, September 1995.

14. Urbaniak JR, Evans JP, Bright DS: Microvascular management of ring avulsion injuries. *J Hand Surg* 6:25–30, 1981.

15. Kay S, Werntz J, Wolff TW: Ring avulsion injuries: Classification and prognosis. *J Hand Surg* 14:204–213, 1989.

CHAPTER 65

Infections of the Upper Extremity

Steven J. Lee, David A. Cutcliffe, and
Lawrence C. Hurst

Infection can turn a highly useful hand and upper extremity into a stiff and painful appendage. Amputation and even loss of life can result from a poorly treated hand infection. Early diagnosis and prompt treatment, including antibiotic therapy and often surgical debridement, are the cornerstones to successful treatment and restoration of hand function.

PATTERNS OF INFECTION IN THE HAND

The fascial spaces of the hand are closed anatomic compartments, which when infected allow abscess formation. Infections enter these spaces by direct puncture or by extension from an adjacent closed-space infection.[1] When abscesses form in these closed compartments, treatment with systemic antibiotics alone is ineffective and surgical drainage is required. A thorough knowledge of the compartmental anatomy of the hand is necessary to approach and surgically drain the abscess.

CELLULITIS

This infection presents as a diffuse swelling, with erythema and ascending lymphangitis. Fluctuation and pus are absent. An attempt may be made to culture the organisms by injecting a small amount of sterile, nonbacteriostatic saline into the area of cellulitis and then withdrawing the fluid for culture. However, the success of obtaining a positive culture is low.[2] *Streptococcus pyogenes* is most often responsible. The treatment involves a combination of elevation, warm soaks, splintage, and antibiotics.

PARONYCHIA AND EPONYCHIA

Paronychia is the most common infection of the hand. This infection can be initiated by foreign material lodging between the nail plate and paronychial tissue or by a hangnail that traumatizes the eponychial tissue. The infection starts as a subcuticular abscess in the paronychial fold. If it involves the eponychium as well as the lateral fold, it is called eponychia. Paronychias are typically polymicrobial

infections that are often caused by both aerobic and anaerobic flora. The most common aerobic organisms are *Staphylococcus aureus,* group A streptococci, and *Eikenella corrodens.* The most common anaerobic organisms include *Bacteroides* species, gram-positive anaerobic cocci, and *Fusobacterium nucleatum.*[3]

Paronychias may be treated initially with warm soaks, splinting, and antibiotics. If this fails to decompress the abscess, incision and drainage are indicated. For more extensive infections including those involving the eponychial fold, a longitudinal incision is made paralleling the proximal nail and extending to its proximal eponychial border. The lateral quarter of the nail is removed to decompress the paronychia and specimens for appropriate cultures, including those for fungi, are taken. Amoxicillin-clavulanic acid (Augmentin) is an effective antibiotic combination against most pathogens isolated.[4]

The surgeon must not overlook a possible concomitant apical abscess, felon, or subungual abscess. A subungual abscess may result from an extension of the paronychia under the nail. This can be distinguished by the presence of a "floating fingernail" or by pain elicited when pressure is applied to the center of the nail. Removal of the devitalized nail is mandatory, and cultures, soaks, splints, and antibiotics are employed, as with eponychia.

In a chronic paronychia, the possibility of tuberculosis, atypical mycobacteria, fungal infection, gout, or even carcinoma should be entertained. Although rare, osteomyelitis of the distal phalanx can also complicate the seemingly trivial paronychia.

FELON

A felon is an abscess of the terminal phalanx pulp. This infection is unique because the pulp consists of closed spaces made up of fatty tissue separated by 15 to 20 fibrous septa running from the periosteum of the distal phalanx to the skin (Fig. 65-1). Although the most common cause is a puncture wound, an overlooked or inadequately treated paronychia or subungual abscess can result in a felon. The most common causative organism is *S. aureus.* On exam, there may initially be a minor wound with some swelling, erythema, and tenderness. Over the next few days, the pulp becomes tense, red, and exquisitely tender. If left untreated, the felon can be complicated by a draining sinus, osteomyelitis of the distal phalanx (seen on x-ray as tuft rarefaction or resorption), obliteration of the digital vessels with subsequent sloughing, flexor tenosynovitis, and pyogenic arthritis of the distal interphalangeal joint. X-rays show soft tissue swelling and possibly bony involvement; it may demonstrate foreign bodies.

If seen early, the felon may be treated with antibiotics and elevation. However, most felons require a combination of incision and drainage and systemic antibiotics. Many different surgical approaches are advocated; however, certain surgical principles should be adhered to.[5] The inci-

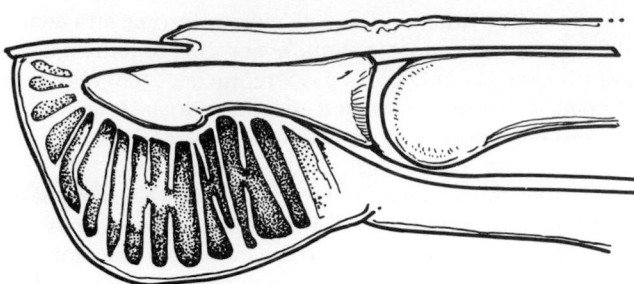

Figure 65-1 Cross-sectional anatomy of a felon. Note fibrous septa and collection of pus in the pulp abscess.

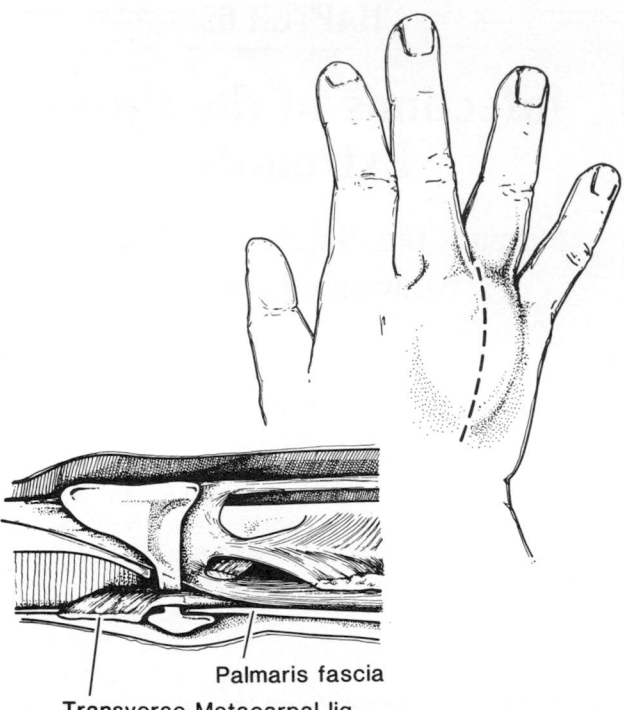

Palmaris fascia
Transverse Metacarpal lig.

Figure 65-2 A web space infection. The hand shows a dorsal swelling and incision. The insert shows the cross-sectional anatomy of a web space infection. Note the dorsal subcutaneous collection of pus communicating with a volar subcutaneous collection to form a dumbbell-shaped abscess. The metacarpophalangeal joint behind the abscess usually does not communicate with the web space infection.

sion should not be too volar, in order to avoid injuring the neurovascular structures. It is placed on the noncontact side of the digit, meaning radially based on the thumb and little finger and ulnarly based in the other digits. The incision should not extend proximally to the flexor tendon sheath or joint, so as to avoid tenosynovitis or pyogenic arthritis respectively. Fish-mouth incisions are notorious for sloughing of the fat pad and thus are discouraged. As such, the two favored incisions are the unilateral longitudinal approach and the classic J or hockey stick incision for more severe felons. The vertical septa are bluntly divided from their periosteal attachments, allowing drainage of all septal compartments. After specimens for culture are obtained, the wound is irrigated and antibiotics are started. The wound is then packed open and allowed to close by secondary intention.[6]

TENDON SHEATH INFECTIONS

Tendon sheath infections are often the result of puncture wounds or lacerations. This closed-space infection can lead to chronic finger stiffness as a result of destruction of the pulley system, adhesions, and liquefaction of the tendon itself. Therefore, prompt recognition with immediate surgical drainage is mandatory. Diagnosis is based on a history of a penetrating injury and Kanavel's four classic signs: tenderness over the involved tendon sheath, pain on passive extension of the finger, flexed attitude of the finger, and fusiform swelling of the involved digit.[1] The ring, middle, and index fingers are the most commonly involved digits.[5] Coagulase-positive *S. aureus* is the most common organism, but gram-negative bacteria may also be responsible for up to 20 percent of the cases.[7] Antibiotic therapy alone (after an attempt to obtain a culture sample by aspiration) may be curative if employed early in the infective process. However, if no improvement occurs within 24 h, incision and drainage should be performed. Postoperative closed irrigation of the tendon sheath may be beneficial.[8] Wounds are left open and closed secondar-

ily except if closed irrigation is used, in which case the wounds are loosely closed. Whirlpool baths, soaks, and active range-of-motion exercises are started approximately 48 h postoperatively.

WEB SPACE INFECTION

A web space ("collar button") abscess is usually caused by a fissure or puncture in the skin between the fingers, from an infected distal palmar callus, or from a septic subcutaneous lesion in the proximal finger. Its boundary is defined dorsally by the webbed skin, volarly by the transverse palmar fascia, radially and ulnarly by the vertical septa. A sagittal section through a web space abscess consists of both dorsal and volar collections of pus with a communicating channel. This dumbbell or "collar-button–shaped" abscess forms as the expanding abscess penetrates the palmar fascia near the superficial transverse metacarpal ligaments (Fig. 65-2). Therefore, on exam, tenderness and swelling are noted on both the dorsal and volar aspects. The adjacent fingers assume an abducted posture. A sinus with purulent drainage may be present. Treatment involves incision and drainage through both dorsal and volar incisions, as drainage of only one side can lead to recurrent infection. Transverse incisions across the web space should be avoided as they can lead to contracture. After culture specimens are obtained, both incisions are irrigated, then packed open or drained, and empiric antibiotics are started. Whirlpool or soaks and active range-of-motion exercises are started immediately.[5]

DEEP SPACE (THENAR AND MIDPALMAR) INFECTIONS

The thenar and midpalmar spaces comprise two more potential closed spaces in the hand (Fig. 65-3). Infection in these spaces occurs through direct puncture wounds; extensions from other adjacent areas, as in the case of flexor tenosynovitis; or abscesses from other closed spaces. The thenar space is bounded radially by the midpalmar oblique septum and long finger profundus tendon and ulnarly and inferiorly by the adductor pollicis muscle. Thenar space infections present as marked swelling, pain, and tenderness over the thenar eminence and first web space, pushing the thumb into abduction.

The midpalmar space is bounded dorsally by the third, fourth, and fifth metacarpals, volarly by the flexor tendons, radially and ulnarly by the midpalmar oblique and hypothenar septum, respectively. Distally, the vertical septa of the palmar fascia serve as its endpoint, while proximally it is limited by a fascial layer at the end of the carpal tunnel. Midpalmar space infections present with swelling not only in the palm, causing it to lose its normal concavity, but also dorsally because the major lymphatic drainage occurs there. Although there is swelling dorsally,

the tenderness, fluctuance, and erythema are localized to the volar aspect overlying the midpalmar space. Because this is adjacent to the flexor tendons of the middle, ring, and little fingers, motion of these fingers is painful and limited. Systemic signs of infection may also be present in both thenar and midpalmar infections.

The treatment for both thenar and midpalmar space infections is incision and drainage. Possible communications and extensions to other closed spaces should be carefully evaluated. After culture specimens are obtained, the wound is irrigated and either packed open or drained, or a continuous irrigation system is employed. Empiric antibiotics are started and later modified. Soaks and active motion exercises are begun the next day.[5]

RADIAL AND ULNAR BURSAL INFECTIONS

The radial and ulnar bursae represent fascial compartments that enclose the flexor tendons (Fig. 65-3). The radial and ulnar bursae are proximal tendon sheath extensions of the flexor pollicis longus and little finger flexor digitorum longus, respectively. Infection occurs through direct puncture of the bursa or through extension of a tendon sheath infection. There is swelling, erythema, and tenderness over the anatomic boundaries of the respective bursa. Treatment is by incision, drainage, and antibiotics. The wounds are left open. Concurrent tendon sheath infections are treated as above. Soaks and active range-of-motion exercises then commence, and the wound is allowed to heal by secondary intention.

HERPETIC WHITLOW

Herpetic whitlow is a viral infection of the fingers caused by contact with the herpes simplex virus. It occurs predominantly in health care workers because of their frequent contact with oral and genital secretions, although it can also be caused by autoinoculation.[9] After an incubation period that ranges between 2 and 20 days, the infection initially manifests itself by intense, throbbing pain and erythema in the involved finger. Vesicles filled with clear and sometimes turbid (not purulent) fluid appear early, then may coalesce to form bullae. Viral shedding averages 12 days, during which time the patient is most infective. The lesions become encrusted and desquamate, and the symptoms subside over 2 to 3 weeks. Although the diagnosis is usually made clinically, laboratory studies can confirm it. Cultures of the fluid from the carefully unroofed vesicles remain the gold standard. Tzanck smears from scraping the base of the vesicle show multinucleated giant cells. Giemsa, Wright, and H&E stains as well as serologic testing can also be utilized but can have significant false-

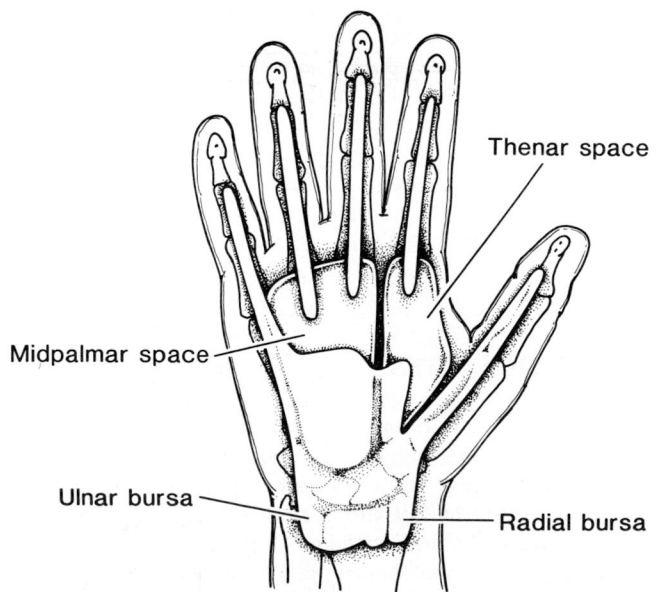

Figure 65-3 Deep spaces, bursae, and digital tendon sheaths of the hand.

negative rates. The treatment for this self-limited disease remains conservative and symptomatic. This infection should not be confused with paronychia or felon, as surgical drainage of herpetic whitlow can lead to disastrous complications such as a secondary bacterial infection, viremia, or encephalitis.[10] Treatment with acyclovir remains controversial in both acute and recurrent cases, although it may have its place in severe or chronic infection or in immunocompromised patients.[11]

HUMAN, DOG, AND CAT BITES

Bite wounds are a major concern for the orthopaedic surgeon. Depending on the inoculum, these wounds may result in stiffness, chronic osteomyelitis, necrotizing fasciitis, amputation, or even death. The incidence of animal bites has been reported from 300 to 700 bites per 100,000 population per year.[12] The majority of bite wounds are caused by dogs (70 percent), cats (10 percent), and humans (15 percent).[13] A far fewer number are caused by venomous creatures (i.e., snakes or spiders), but these can lead to severe morbidity and mortality. The treating physician must also always remember the catastrophic complications of tetanus and rabies.

Dog bites are the most common, but they rarely involve the hand. They usually do not become infected unless there is significant soft tissue injury or joint involvement. Physical examination reveals the marks of a puncture wound with surrounding erythema and cellulitis. Purulent drainage and ascending lymphangitis may or may not be present. Culture often reveals a mixed infection of *Streptococcus, S. aureus,* and *Pasteurella multocida.*[14] A thorough irrigation and debridement with delayed primary closure is indicated. The choice of antibiotics remains controversial, but ampicillin-sulbactam (Unasyn) and amoxicillin-clavulanic acid (Augmentin) provide excellent single-drug therapy.[15]

Although cat bites occur less often than dog bites, they become infected more frequently (30 to 50 percent).[14] The chief pathogen is *P. multocida* in more than 50 percent of cases. Clinically, this infection is characterized by pain, swelling, and a rapid, intense inflammatory response within 24 h. Purulent drainage, lymphangitis, and regional adenopathy may also be present. Given the high infection rate, prophylactic antibiotic treatment seems appropriate for fresh bites. *Pasteurella multocida* soft-tissue infections can be successfully treated with antibiotics and surgical drainage when indicated. Such infections are susceptible to penicillin, the second- and third-generation cephalosporins, tetracyclines, and chloramphenicol, but ampicillin-sulbactam and amoxicillin-clavulanic acid again provide excellent single-drug therapy.[15]

Human bites also deserve special consideration. Although they account for approximately 15 percent of bite wounds, treatment is often delayed because patients either fail to seek immediate medical care or do not state the mechanism of injury (fistfight). Despite this, fistfights probably account for 60 to 80 percent of all human bites.[14]

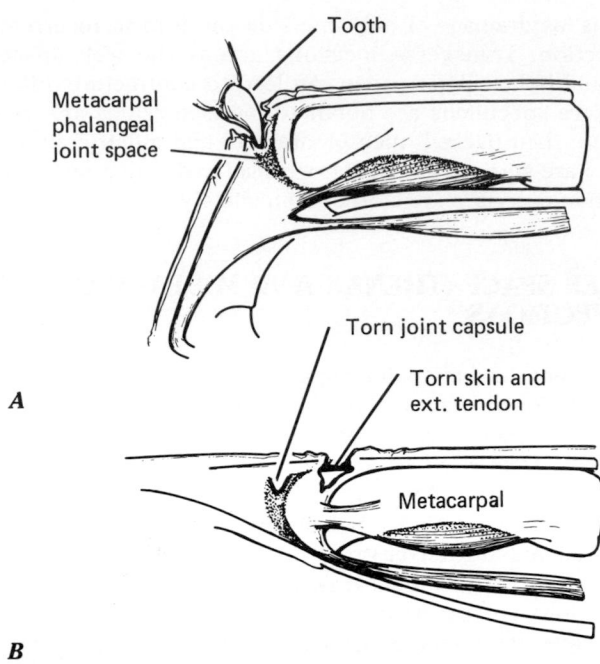

B

Figure 65-4 Mechanism of fistfight injury. *A.* Tooth piercing skin, extensor tendon, and joint capsule as patient strikes opponent in mouth. *B.* Patient releases fist by extending fingers. Hole in joint capsule now covered by intact tendon. Defect in skin and tendon now moves proximally and does not appear to communicate with joint.

The adult human mouth contains many anaerobes that can cause severe infections. Physical examination reveals findings similar to those of other bite wounds. Cultures usually grow an average of three organisms: *S. aureus,* alpha and beta streptococci, and *E. corrodens.* When the fingers are extended, the wound may appear superficial and proximal to the joint; however, thorough irrigation and debridement with exploration for possible metacarpalphalangeal joint involvement is mandatory (Fig. 65-4). Antibiotics are used for even the most superficial wounds. Penicillin for *E. corrodens* and oxacillin or a second- or third-generation cephalosporin for streptococci and *S. aureus* may be used. As with animal bites, ampicillin-sulbactam or amoxicillin-clavulanic acid provide good single-drug coverage.[15]

VENOMOUS BITES

Every year, approximately 10,000 persons sustain venomous snake bites, over 50 percent of which occur in the upper extremity.[16] Some 98 percent of venomous snake bites are inflicted by the Crotalidae snake family (pit viper). These include rattlesnakes, copperheads, cottonmouths (water moccasins), pigmy rattlesnakes, and massasaugas, all of which are characterized by heat-sensitive pits located between the eyes and the nostril. Envenomation, which occurs when a sufficient amount of venom introduced into the body to produce a reaction, causes a wide range of effects. Locally, the venom causes pain, rapid swelling, ecchymosis, and local necrosis, typically within 20 min and no more than 4 h following envenomation. Systemically, the venom causes, among other things, increased capillary permeability and coagulopathy, resulting in a bleeding diathesis, pulmonary edema, hypotension, renal failure, and eventually multiorgan failure.[17]

Immediately following a snake bite, the patient should be kept emotionally and physiologically calm. A tourniquet should be applied but tightened only enough to restrict the superficial lymphatic flow. It should not restrict venous or arterial blood flow. Incision and suction is effective in removing up to 50 percent of the local venom. This is performed by incising each fang mark 1/4 in long and 1/4 in deep and then applying suction. Mechanical suction is preferable to mouth suction, as the venom can be absorbed through oral or gastric disruptions. Once the patient has reached a medical facility, he or she can be reevaluated for signs and symptoms of envenomation. Appropriate resuscitation measures are performed and lab studies—including a complete blood count with platelets, electrolytes, coagulation and bleeding profiles, urinalysis, type and cross match—are obtained. The patient should be treated with antivenin after a skin test for sensitivity is performed. Anaphylaxis and serum sickness are not uncommon even with negative skin tests; therefore resuscitation equipment must be available. Tetanus antitoxin and broad-spectrum antibiotics, including gram-negative coverage, are administered. Because of the rapid swelling, the patient should frequently be checked for signs and symptoms of compartment syndrome. Icing should not be utilized, as its usage has led to increased incidence of thermal injury and increased amputation rates.[18]

NECROTIZING FASCIITIS

Necrotizing fasciitis is a potentially limb- and life-threatening soft tissue infection characterized by rapidly progressing inflammation and necrosis of subcutaneous fascia, fat, skin, and sometimes muscle. The most common causative organism is group A streptococcus, although other aerobic and anaerobic bacteria are frequently isolated. Four factors are important to the pathogenesis of this infection: an anaerobic wound environment, toxic lytic enzymes, bacterial synergy, and thrombosis of nutrient blood vessels.[19]

An early diagnosis is the key to successful treatment and requires a high index of suspicion. Patients who are more susceptible to necrotizing fasciitis include those with impaired host defenses or systemic illness such as chronic renal failure, malignancy, peripheral vascular disease, diabetes, or alcoholism as well as patients on immunosuppressive therapy. Clinically, several classic signs can lead to a diagnosis: skin bullae, edema beyond the area of cellulitis, and absence of lymphangitis can be seen early, while crepitus, fever, and shock are late signs. A leukocytosis of 10,000 to 20,000 is usually found.

The cornerstone of therapy is early adequate surgical debridement with complete removal of all necrotic skin, fascia, fat, and muscle through generous longitudinal incisions. The wound is left open, with subsequent delayed closure or a coverage procedure; a second-look debridement is performed in 24 to 48 h. Antibiotic coverage includes empiric triple therapy with penicillin, an aminoglycoside, and clindamycin until definitive culture results are determined. Adjuvant therapy includes subcutaneous heparin therapy (to reduce the risk of venous thrombosis) as well as nutritional support. The role of hyperbaric oxygen therapy remains controversial. Careful surgical technique, adequate antibiotic regimens, and general medical support have achieved a 91 percent survival rate in these patients.[20]

GAS GANGRENE

Gas gangrene (clostridial myonecrosis) in the upper extremity is an infrequent occurrence but one that can lead to significant morbidity and mortality. It is caused by the gram-positive bacillus *Clostridium, C. perfringens* being the most common species.[21] *Clostridium* grows in tissues with low oxygen tension, the environment often encountered after significant trauma. However, any process that lowers the oxygen tension can result in clostridial infection if contamination with the organism occurs. The toxicity of this infection is due to the production of exotoxins. *Clostridium* produces nine exotoxins, of which the alpha toxin is the most lethal.[22] Intense edema follows infection with little or no inflammatory phase, further reducing the oxygen tension. The infection progresses rapidly and toxemia results.

Early diagnosis is the key to successful treatment. The earliest symptom is pain in the affected area, followed by chills, tachycardia, confusion, and toxemia. In the early stages, the skin is cool and edematous. Later the wound develops a brownish discoloration with foul-smelling drainage.[23] It is at this late stage that crepitance can be present. X-rays will not reveal gas consistently in the early stages, and gas is not pathognomonic for gas gangrene.[24] Nonetheless, x-rays are mandatory and may aid in determining the extent of the infectious process. Gram's stain of the drainage reveals large gram-positive rods.

It cannot be emphasized enough that early diagnosis and treatment of this infection are paramount. Penicillin in dosages of 10 to 24 million U/day in combination with immediate surgical debridement (which may include amputation) and hyperbaric oxygen at 3 atm for 120-min intervals provide optimal care. Tetracycline in dosages of 2 to 4 g/day may be used as an alternative in cases of penicillin allergy. The value of antitoxin is still unproved; but it should be given serious consideration when hyperbaric oxygen is not available.[21] Hyperbaric oxygen not only counteracts the hypoxic environment, thereby haulting progression of the infection, but also neutralizes toxins produced by *Clostridium*. With these regimens, the mortality of this infection has decreased to 25 percent.[21]

ATYPICAL MYCOBACTERIAL INFECTIONS

A majority of chronic hand infections are due to atypical mycobacteria, while most of the remainder are from tuberculosis and fungi. Although these organisms are frequently considered to be opportunistic, they do infect healthy people. By far the most common causative organism is *Mycobacterium marinum,* while *M. kansasii* is the next most common, followed by *M. avium-intracellulare.* Because *M. marinum* can survive only at temperatures of 30 to 32°C, it has been usually described in the hands and feet, and the bursae of the elbow and knees. It is transmitted by direct inoculation, most commonly from exposure to fish tanks, pools, marine bites and injuries, and soil. Typically, the initial trauma is insignificant and often forgotten.

Three characteristic presentations of *M. marinum* have been identified.[25] Type I is a self-limited verrucal lesion. Type II represent single or multiple subcutaneous granulomas, with or without ulceration. Type III are deep infections, involving tenosynovium, bursae, bones, or joints. A presumptive diagnosis should be made with the typical history and compatible exam, noncaseating granulomas seen on biopsy, and negative fungal smears.[26] A definitive diagnosis rests on positive tissue culture, which may take 6 to 8 weeks, and histologic findings of acid-fast bacilli and noncaseating granulomas. Unfortunately, both the culture and visualization of acid-fast bacilli and granulomas may be negative, especially early in the course of the disease. In these cases, a trial of antituberculous medication may be attempted. The differential diagnosis includes tuberculosis, gout, rheumatic synovitis, and fungal infections.

The treatment again relies on a high clinical suspicion. Type I lesions may be treated with observation for 2 to 4 months. If the lesions do not resolve during this period, a biopsy should be performed and minocycline given for 1 month after clinical resolution. Type II (subcutaneous granulomas) lesions should undergo an immediate excision of any well-defined masses; if the cultures prove positive, minocycline should be given for 3 months after the disappearance of any clinical signs or symptoms. Type III (deep) infections require an appropriate surgical procedure such as a tenosynovectomy, synovectomy, arthrodesis, or incision and drainage, followed by minocycline for 3 months after the disappearance of any clinical signs or symptoms. Depending on the sensitivities and resistance, other antituberculous medications typically can involve a combination of tetracycline, rifampin, ethambutol, and isoniazid.[25,26]

TUBERCULOSIS

Tuberculosis of the hand is rare, representing less than 1 percent of extrapulmonary tuberculosis.[27] Nonetheless, it may be a patient's only manifestation of disease. The infection usually begins in the tenosynovium and can then spread to adjacent bones and joints. Signs and symptoms appear insidiously and, early in the course of the disease, are consistent with synovitis. Because of either late patient presentation or misdiagnosis, there is characteristically a significant delay in diagnosis. The differential diagnosis includes rheumatoid arthritis and synovitis, sarcoidosis, nonspecific synovitis, and atypical mycobacterial and fungal infections. A presumptive diagnosis can be made from a biopsy by the presence of acid-fast bacilli

and/or caseating granulomas with giant cells. If untreated, tuberculosis may cause carpal tunnel syndrome, tendon rupture, bony changes, or joint destruction. Also, rice bodies have been noted to occur in tuberculous infections. If they are incidentally found during a carpal tunnel release, synovial biopsies and tuberculosis cultures should be performed. The treatment of tuberculosis lesions in the upper extremity includes open biopsy, surgical debridement, and combination antituberculosis therapy.[27,28]

FUNGAL INFECTIONS

Deep fungal infections in the hand are rare and occur almost exclusively in immunocompromised patients. Several reports have described the isolation of *Candida albicans, Aspergillus flavus, Cryptococcus neoformans,* and *Coccidioides immitis* from deep hand infections. The location of the infection is variable; it may present as a soft tissue abscess, tenosynovitis, or a necrotic ulcer. Draining sinuses may be present. Diagnosis is made by histologic examination and culture from surgically obtained tissue. The mainstays of treatment are systemic antifungal medications with surgical debridement of infected and necrotic tissue.[26]

REFERENCES

1. Kanavel AB: *Infections of the Hand,* 7th ed. Philadelphia, Lea & Febiger, 1943, chap 1.
2. Canoso JJ, Barza M: Soft tissue infections. *Rheum Dis Clin North Am* 19:293–309, 1993.
3. Brook I: Paronychia: A mixed infection. Microbiology and Management. *J Hand Surg* 18B:358–359, 1993.
4. Siegel DB, Gelberman RH: Infections of the hand. *Orthop Clin North Am* 19:779–789, 1988.
5. Nevaiser RJ: Infections, in Green (ed): *Operative Hand Surgery.* New York, Churchill Livingstone, 1993, pp 1021–1038.
6. Stern PJ: Selected acute infections. *AAOS Instr Course Lect* 39:539–546, 1990.
7. Nevaiser RJ: Closed tendon sheath irrigation for pyogenic flexor tenosynovitis. *J Hand Surg* 3:462–466, 1978.
8. Juliano PJ, Eglseder WA: Limited open-tendon-sheath irrigation in the treatment of pyogenic flexor tenosynovitis. *Orthop Rev* 20:1065–1069, 1991.
9. Gill MJ, Denhollander C: DNA restriction analysis of digital and genital isolates of herpes simplex virus from three patients. *J Infect Dis* 158:242, 1988.
10. Hurst LC, Gluck R, Sampson SP, Dowd A: Herpetic whitlow with bacterial abscess. *J Hand Surg* 16:311–314, 1991.
11. Fowler JR: Viral infections. *Hand Clin* 5:613–622, 1989.
12. Weber DJ, Hansen AR: Infections resulting from animal bites. *Infect Dis Clin North Am* 5:663–680, 1991.
13. Callahan M: Dog bite wounds. *JAMA* 244:2327–2328, 1980.
14. Goldstein EJC: Bite wounds and infection. *Clin Infect Dis* 14:633–638, 1992.
15. Levy CS: Treating infections of the hand: Identifying the organism and choosing the antibiotic. *AAOS Instr Course Lect* 39:533–537, 1990.
16. Parrish HM: Incidence of treated snake bites in the United States. *Public Health Rep* 81:269–276, 1966.

17. Seiler JG III, Sagerman SD, Geller RJ, et al: Venomous snake bites: Current concepts of treatment. *Orthopedics* 17:707–714, 1994.

18. Rowland SA: Fasciotomy: The treatment of compartment syndrome, in Green DP (ed): *Operative Hand Surgery.* New York, Churchill Livingstone, 1993, pp 675–694.

19. Lewis R: Necrotizing soft tissue infections. *Surg Infect* 5:693–703, 1992.

20. Schecter W, Meyer A, Schecter G, et al: Necrotizing fasciitis of the upper extremity. *J Hand Surg* 7:15–20, 1982.

21. Present DA, Meislin R, Shaffer B: Gas gangrene: A review. *Orthop Rev* 19:333–341, 1990.

22. Hart GB, Lamb RC, Strauss MB: Gas gangrene: A collective review. *J Trauma* 23:991–995, 1983.

23. Fee NF, Dobranski A, Bisla RA: Gas gangrene complicating open forearm fractures. *J Bone Joint Surg* 59A:135–138, 1977.

24. Nichols RL, Smith JWC: Gas in the wound: What does it mean? *Surg Clin North Am* 55:1289–1296, 1975.

25. Hurst LC, Amadio PC, Badalamente MA, et al: *Mycobacterium marinum* infections of the hand. *J Hand Surg* 12A:428–435, 1987.

26. Gunther SF: Chronic infections. *AAOS Instr Course Lect* 39:547–554, 1990.

27. Gluck R, Riou JP, Margolis IB, Hurst LC: Tuberculosis of the hand and wrist. *NY State J Med* 91:262–264, 1991.

28. Leffert RD, Smith RJ: Tuberculosis of the hand, in Flynn JE (ed): *Hand Surgery,* 3d ed. Baltimore, Williams & Wilkins, 1981, pp 719–730.

CHAPTER 66

Ligamentous Injuries of the Wrist and Hand

Alan J. Schefer, Robert V. Garroway, and Frank C. McCue III

LIGAMENTOUS INJURIES OF THE WRIST

The wrist relies on both ligaments and the contact surfaces of the bones as constraints during normal motion.[1] The ligamentous anatomy of the wrist consists of extrinsic (i.e., radiocarpal) and intrinsic (i.e., intercarpal) ligaments that are completely intracapsular. Table 66-1 reviews the ligamentous anatomy.[2]

The key ligaments of the wrist are volar and intracapsular. The short and long radiolunate and the radioscaphocapitate ligaments are the main radial stabilizers.[3] The radioscapholunate ligament, which was once thought to be important, is now considered most likely to be a neurovascular structure.[3] The ulnocarpal ligaments consist of the ulnolunate and ulnotriquetral ligaments, which make up part of the triangular fibrocartilage complex.[4] The volar ligaments are arranged in a double V configuration with an area of potential weakness at the capitolunate articulation, known as the space of Poirier.[5] The dorsal ligaments play a role as accessory stabilizers of the triquetrolunate and radiocarpal joints.[6]

The interosseous or intrinsic ligaments are much thicker and maintain stability between individual bones within the carpus. These ligaments are much thicker and stronger dorsally and volarly and have a membranous center.[5] The ligaments of the proximal row (scapholunate, lunotriquetral) are the strongest ligaments in the wrist and the most elastic, allowing for the most motion. The distal-row ligaments are quite immobile and rarely rupture.[5] Failure of these ligaments leads to dissociation of individual carpal bones and, in combination with injury to the extrinsic ligament, will lead to radiocarpal dislocation.

Perilunate and Lunate Dislocation

Dislocation of the carpus is usually the result of a high-energy injury with the wrist hyperextended. Dislocation usually occurs at the capitolunate joint at the space of Poirier, with the carpus dislocating dorsally to the lunate. These dislocations can occur with or without a concomitant scaphoid fracture (transscaphoid perilunate dislocation). Mayfield described a progression of injury and progressive perilunar instability (PLI) that provides a logical sequence of this lesion.[7]

The injury begins with instability on the radial side, either rupture of the scapholunate ligament or scaphoid fracture. It should be noted that these injuries are not mutually exclusive and can occur together. The injury progresses ulnarly with capitolunate dislocation and then lunotriquetral disruption. Finally, the dorsal lunocarpal ligaments fail and the lunate dislocates volarly. Lunate dislocation can be considered an end to a continuum of progressive perilunate instability and not as a separate entity. At times both radiographic findings can be seen secondary to the severe instability. Thus the treatment of both is similar.

As with any injury caused by excessive force, concomitant injury at the hand and elbow must be ruled out. Also, a good neurovascular examination must be carried out with particular attention to median nerve function. Acute injuries obviously need to be reduced to restore carpal anatomy.

Acute perilunate and lunate dislocations can usually be reduced closed. Reduction is usually performed under general anesthesia with longitudinal traction, volar stabilization of the lunate, dorsiflexion of the wrist, and then gradual flexion to bring the capitate back into articulation with the lunate.[8] Because of the magnitude of the ligamentous disruption, reduction is usually unstable and cannot be maintained with cast immobilization alone. Stabilization can be accomplished by either closed reduction and percutaneous pinning; if satisfactory reduction is not possible (usually of the scapholunate articulation), open reduction and pinning can be performed. In open reduction, the wrist is approached both dorsally and volarly with repair of the ligaments, direct visualization of reduction, pinning, and release of carpal tunnel. Pins are left in for 8 weeks with an additional 4 weeks of cast immobilization.[8] Associated scaphoid fractures are fixed internally at the time of surgery with wires or screws.

Carpal Instability

Carpal instability can occur secondary to perilunate dislocation if ligaments heal improperly. More commonly, carpal instability is the result of unrecognized isolated ligamentous injury to the wrist.

The bones of the carpus are aligned in two rows (proximal and distal) and are linked by the scaphoid. The biomechanics of the carpus has been investigated by many authors.[8] Normally the bones in each row move in association, secondary to their strong ligamentous attachments. Carpal instability is present when the ligamentous supports are disrupted and the bones move in dissociation (for example, the scaphoid flexes but the lunate extends). This pattern of instability is described as *dissociative carpal instability* in the literature.[9] *Nondissociative carpal instability* has also been described. This pattern exists when the ligaments within each row are functional, providing associative motion, but the ligaments between the two rows of the carpus and the distal forearm are incompetent. This injury will result in abnormal motion between the proximal and distal carpal rows.[9]

For accurate analysis of carpal instability, it is important to evaluate the history, physical examination, and roentgenographic findings systematically. Patients will often complain of weakness, snapping, a click, or a wrist clunk. Pain is usually difficult to localize, but certain provocative maneuvers can guide diagnosis. The Watson

TABLE 66-1   Ligamentous Structures of the Wrist

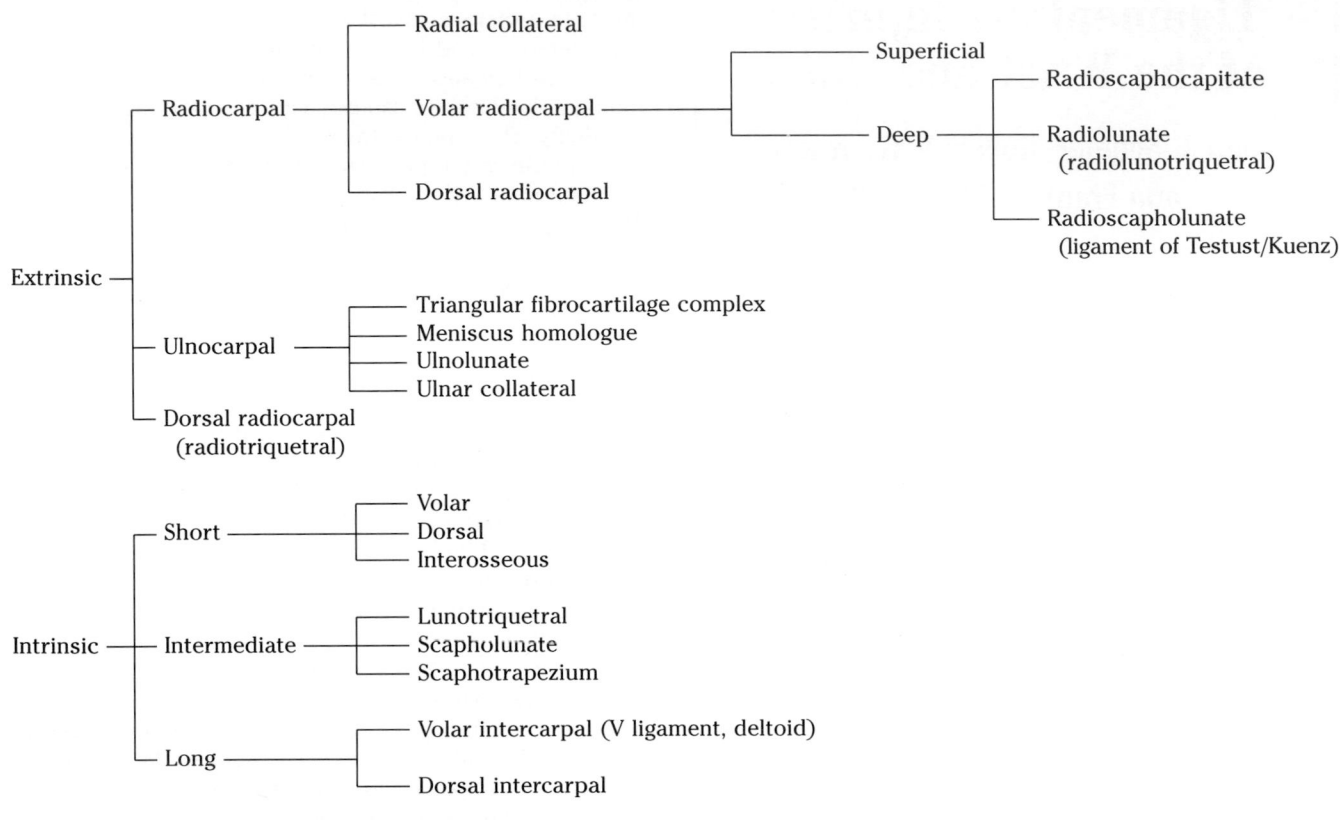

Source: Reproduced with permission from *Regional Review Course in Hand Surgery—Manual.*
New York, American Society for Surgery of the Hand, 1994.

or scaphoid shift test elicits scapholunate dissociation. The examiner causes dorsal subluxation of the proximal pole of the scaphoid on a stabilized radius when the wrist is brought into radial deviation and pressure is kept on the palmar distal pole of the scaphoid.[10] The ballotment test, described by Reagan, helps in diagnosing triquetrolunate dissociation.[11] The test is positive when there is pain on displacement of the triquetrum on a stabilized lunate.

Radiographic analysis can lead to the diagnosis of carpal instability as being either dynamic or static. Dynamic instability requires provocative views of the wrist to demonstrate dissociation that would not be seen on normal anteroposterior (AP), lateral, and oblique radiographs of the wrist. Static instability of the wrist can be seen on a normal wrist series.[9] Gilula and associates recommend that the x-ray evaluation of carpal instability should include a posteroanterior (PA)—in neutral, radial, and ulnar deviation—a clenched-fist AP, a true lateral—in neutral, volar flexion, and dorsiflexion—an oblique view, and a pisotriquetral view.[12] Cine radiographs can be helpful in diagnosing dynamic instability. Arthrography of the wrist by the three-compartment technique can also assist in defining ligamentous disruption, but one must be aware of the high false-positive rates as patients age and the probability of similar defects in the contralateral asymptomatic wrist.[13]

Many normal angles of the carpal bones have been described to help evaluate disruption of the carpus; the reader is referred to Green's textbook for review.[8] Linscheid et al. emphasize the importance of the scapholunate axis as viewed on the neutral lateral. This angle should be between 30 and 60°, average 47°, and is the key to carpal instability (Fig. 66-1).[14]

Dorsal Intercalated Segment Instability (Rotatory Subluxation of the Scaphoid)

Dorsal intercalated segment instability (DISI), or rotatory subluxation of the scaphoid, is the most common form of carpal instability.[8] The term *intercalated segment* refers to the proximal carpal row, which is represented by the lunate x-ray and is intercalated between the distal carpal row and the radius. This injury is most commonly caused by disruption of the scapholunate interosseous ligament, causing rotatory subluxation of the scaphoid, and it can also be present from bony injury, as seen in malunions or nonunions of the scaphoid, malunions of distal radius fractures, or Kienbock's disease. These are known as nondissociative DISI deformities, since there is no ligamentous disruption.[5] The DISI deformity results in the lunate axis pointing dorsally and the scaphoid rotating palmarly.

Radiographically, a DISI deformity will produce a scapholunate angle of 60° or more.[5] On the AP x-ray, a scapholunate gap of 3 mm or greater will be present; this

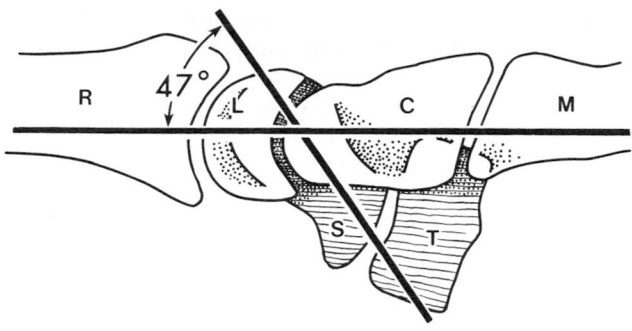

Figure 66-1 Rotary subluxation of the scaphoid is indicated by the gap between scaphoid and lunate.

is commonly known as the Terry Thomas sign, for the British actor who had a large space between his front teeth (Fig. 66-2). The scaphoid appears shorter on the AP film, since it is in a flexed posture and presents a cortical ring sign when it is viewed on end.[9]

Treatment for a DISI deformity will depend on whether it is an acute or chronic injury, a dynamic or static lesion, or if there is any radiocarpal arthritis present. Acute partial injuries of the scapholunate ligament can be treated with closed reduction and pinning.[5] Acute, complete injuries can be treated by open reduction and repair of the ligament through a dorsal approach in combination with a capsulodesis.[15,16] Chronic dissociations that are dynamic can be treated by dorsal capsulodesis, as described by Blatt, to provide a dorsal check rein of scaphoid palmar flexion.[10] Watson would recommend a limited arthrodesis of the scapho-trapezial-trapezoid joint to correct chronic dynamic or static dissociation. He feels that the large multidirectional forces of the wrist cannot be withstood by soft tissue reconstructions and that a more solid construct

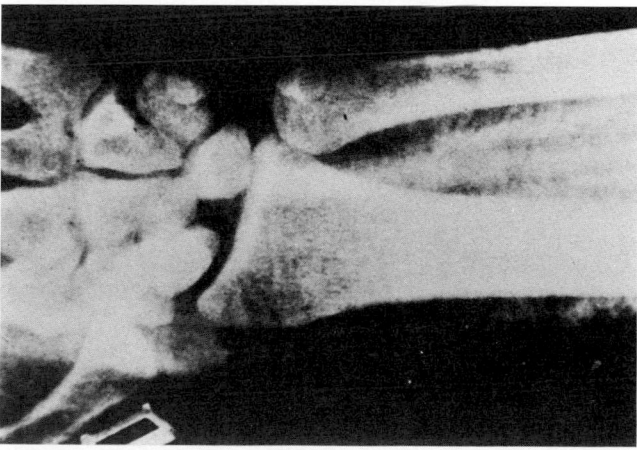

Figure 66-2 Normal carpal alignment in the lateral view is shown. Note that the longitudinal axes of the radius, lunate, capitate, and third metacarpal are in a straight line. The longitudinal axis of the scaphoid makes a 47° angle (average) with this straight line. Up to 60° is considered within normal limits, and 70° or more is clearly pathologic. (Reproduced with permission from Beckenbaugh RD: *Orthop Clin North Am* 15:295, 1984.)

is needed.[10] Finally, if any radiocarpal arthritis exist (scapholunate advanced collapse, or SLAC wrist), a salvage procedure must be used. Radial styloidectomy, four-bone fusion with scaphoid excision, proximal-row carpectomy, or wrist fusion can be selected, depending on the degree of arthritis and the patient's requirements.

Volar Intercalated Segment Instability

Volar intercalated segment instability (VISI) is an uncommon type of carpal instability. It may be recognized on a lateral roentgenogram by a downward tilt of the lunate and a scapholunate axis of 30° or less.[5] It may result from a variety of different injuries causing ulna-sided or dorsal wrist instability. Lunotriquetral instability is the most commonly implicated defect causing VISI.[11] Vegas showed that preservation of the dorsal radiocarpal ligaments was important in preventing a static VISI deformity.[6] Other lesions that have been reported to cause this pattern of instability are triquetrohamate, capitolunate, and scaphotrapezial dissociations.[9]

Treatment for a VISI deformity follows the same approach as that for the DISI deformity. If the injury is acute and partial, treatment can usually be accomplished with closed reduction and casting with or without percutaneous wire fixation.[5] Chronic lesions resulting in dorsal subluxation and volar angulation of the lunate may be treated by various ligamentous reconstructions or capsulodesis if the deformity is dynamic. Intercarpal fusion can be used if a static deformity exists. It should be mentioned that isolated triquetrolunate tears are frequently associated with ulnar impaction and can be treated with an ulna-shortening osteotomy.[5]

Distal Radioulnar Joint Instability

Palmer and Werner introduced the term *triangular fibrocartilage complex* (TFCC).[17] The TFCC (Fig. 66-3) incorporates the dorsal and volar radioulnar ligaments, ulnar collateral ligaments, meniscus homologue, anatomically definable disk, and extensor carpi ulnaris sheath. The complex arises from the ulnar aspect of the lunte fossa of the radius and courses toward the ulnar to insert into the caput ulna. It flows distally and is joined by fibers arising from the ulnar styloid. It then becomes thickened (the meniscus homologue) and inserts distally into the triquetrum, the hamate, and the base of the fifth metacarpal.[17]

A careful physical examination as described by Palmer is essential in diagnosing instability associated with injury to the TFCC.[18] This includes examination of forearm rotation, point tenderness, and clicking on motion or direct pressure. Evidence of instability is noted by manipulations of the distal ulna with attention to wrist symptoms such as clicks and snaps. Posteroanterior and lateral roentgenograms are essential to the exam.

Diagnostic studies include three-compartment wrist arthrograms, MRI, and computed tomography (CT) to assist in evaluating dislocation or subluxation of the distal radioulnar joint. Arthroscopy of this area has become an aid to diagnosis and treatment.[9]

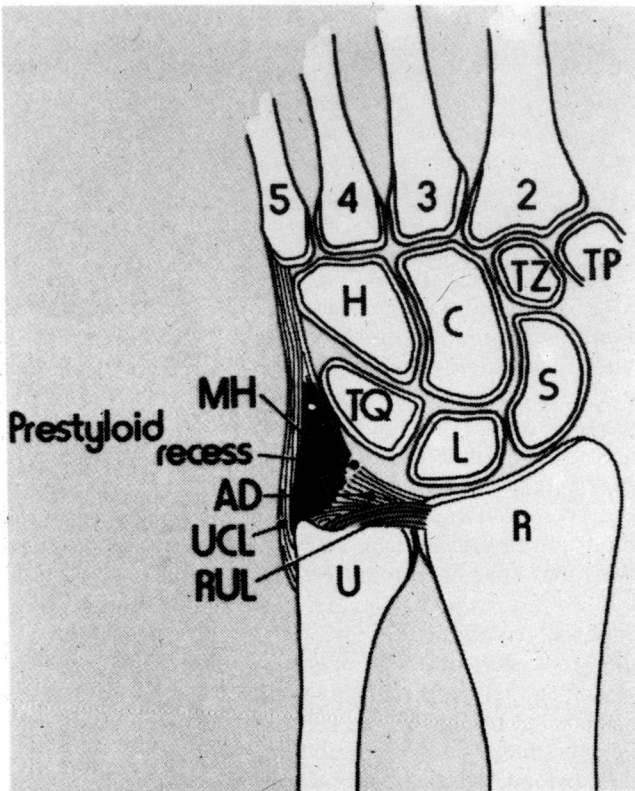

Figure 66-3 TFCC (triangular fibrocartilage complex). Components: RUL = radioulnar ligaments; ULC = ulnar collateral ligament; AD = articular disk; MH = meniscus homologue. Also shown are the radius (R); ulna (U); scaphoid (S); lunate (L); triquetrum (TQ); trapezium (TP); trapezoid (TZ); capitate (C); and hamate (H). (Reproduced with permission from Palmer AK: *Orthop Clin North Am* 15:321–326, 1984.)

Anatomic studies by Palmer have divided TFCC lesions into traumatic and degenerative types.[19] The categories are further subdivided by location of the lesion and degree of degeneration. All traumatic lesions of the TFCC should be treated with immobilization when seen acutely. Central tears may necessitate arthroscopic debridement. Peripheral tears that do not improve with conservative treatment will require arthroscopic or open repair.[20] Late degenerative changes in the area may require ulnar shortening.

Acute subluxation of the distal radioulnar joint (DRUJ) is treated in a long arm cast—in supination for dorsal subluxations and in pronation for volar subluxations. Open reduction is required in late cases or when closed reduction is unsuccessful. Open reduction might need to be combined with direct repair of the TFCC, stabilization with tenodesis, osteotomies of the radius to correct angular deformities, or fusion of the DRUJ and proximal pseudoarthrosis of the ulna (Suave-Kapandji procedure).[10,16]

Carpometacarpal Sprains

Fractures and fracture dislocations of the carpometacarpal joint are covered elsewhere in this volume. Ligamentous

sprains occur in a group of patients whose injury is not severe enough to dislocate or fracture the carpometacarpal joint, who have only minor luxation or pain during stressful maneuvers. Physical findings include point tenderness over the involved joint and reproduction of pain when the joint is stressed by the examiner. Temporary immobilization is the treatment of choice in acute cases, but chronic cases usually require an arthrodesis of the involved joints.[16] In the case of the thumb carpometacarpal (CMC) joint, Lane and Eaton have shown good, reproducible results with ligament reconstruction using a slip of the flexor carpi radialis.[21]

LIGAMENTOUS INJURIES OF THE FINGERS AND THUMB

Ligamentous structures of the hand include the collateral ligaments of the metacarpophalangeal (MCP) and proximal interphalangeal (PIP) joints. Both consist of cordlike collateral ligaments proper and membranous accessory ligaments. The collateral ligaments at the MCP joint are taut in flexion and lax in extension; at the PIP joint, the membranous portion is also tight in extension.

The thumb MCP joint is anatomically unique. On the ulnar aspect of the joint, the adductor pollicis muscle is inserted partly into the ulnar sesamoid bone, partly into the volar plate, and partly through a powerful tendon directly into the proximal phalanx. Additional fibers contribute to the dorsal aponeurosis, which overlies the ulnar collateral ligament of the thumb MCP joint.

The anatomy of the PIP joint is extremely complex. It is a hinged joint that has a range of motion between 0 and 120°. The lateral ligaments and volar plate are thick and strong. The dorsal central slip of the extensor tendon and the volar flexor tendons supplement these capsular ligaments. In addition, the lateral band and its various extensions, the oblique and transverse retinacular ligaments, and both Cleland's and Grayson's ligaments must move and glide freely to allow proper motion. The volar plate has a proximal cul-de-sac that must be free of scar; otherwise, during PIP joint flexion, the base of the middle phalanx cannot glide into the sac.

Ulnar Collateral Ligament Injuries of the Thumb

This injury is often over looked, but it can lead to instability when the thumb is stressed in abduction, thus compromising pinch. It is commonly known as gamekeeper's thumb, describing chronic injury, or skier's thumb, relating to acute lesions.

In acute injuries, the following can occur: local tenderness to pressure over the ulnar collateral ligament, pain in the joint with abduction stress testing, swelling, weakness of pinch, and instability. In tests of stability the affected side should be compared to the uninvolved side, and such tests should be performed with the MCP joint in extension and in flexion.[16] Stress x-ray views comparing

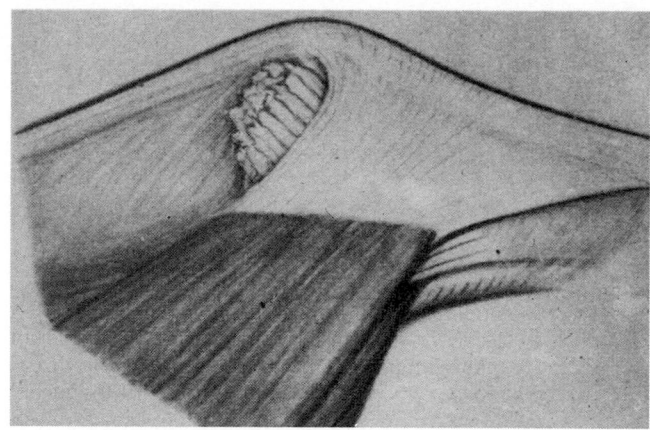

Figure 66-4 Ulnar aspect of the metacarpophalangeal joint of the right thumb. After distal rupture, the ulnar collateral ligament has been folded over. The torn end protrudes proximal to the adductor aponeurosis. (Reproduced with permission from Flynn JD (ed): *Hand Surgery.* Baltimore, Williams & Wilkins, 1966.)

both thumbs or arthrography should be obtained if there is any doubt about the diagnosis.[22,23]

The ulnar collateral ligament usually tears at its distal attachment to the proximal phalanx. Most of these are partial tears and can be treated with immobilization until they heal. Complete tears are more serious because of the clinical instability of the thumb MCP joint. Laxity is measured as at least 20 to 30° greater abduction than that of the opposite thumb.[16] Roentgenograms may show a displaced, rotated avulsion fracture from the proximal phalanx. The ligament can become displaced outside of the adductor aponeurosis (Stener lesion) and cannot heal (Fig. 66-4).[24]

Surgical indications in acute cases include significant involvement of the articular surface, displacement or rotation of the fracture fragment, gross clinical instability, or Stenor lesion.[16,24] The major indications for chronic repair are pain, functional instability, and weakness in pinch.

If the ligament is avulsed with a large articular fragment, open reduction and internal fixation (ORIF) can be performed. If the fracture fragment is small or there is none, the ligament can be attached using a pullout suture technique. If the ligament is torn in its midsubstance, direct repair can be performed with nonabsorbable sutures. A splint or thumb spica cast is worn for 5 weeks. In chronic reconstructions, a slip of the adductor pollicis still attached to the proximal phalanx can be advanced as a dynamic component of the repair.[25] In certain cases in which the ulnar collateral ligament is atrophic or missing, it can be reconstructed with a free tendon graft.

Collateral Ligament Injuries to Metacarpophalangeal Joints

Collateral ligament injuries of the finger MCP joints are less common and usually less disabling than those involving the PIP joint. Since radial and ulnar control are maintained by the intrinsics, lateral instability is usually not a problem.

However, after an avulsion fracture, the distal attachment of the collateral ligament may become interposed in the joint, and this can be disabling. If the collateral ligament becomes interposed or is significantly displaced, open repair becomes necessary.[16] Most other tears can be treated with a short course of splinting and then an 8- to 12-week course of buddy taping to support the healing process.[16]

Injuries to Proximal Interphalangeal Joints Collateral Ligaments

Injuries to the PIP joints are most common on the radial aspect of the digit on which the proximal attachment of the collateral ligament is avulsed. They are usually associated with partial or complete rupture of the volar plate, depending upon the magnitude of the force applied. Injury is caused by a force transmitted to the extended finger. Examination shows generalized tenderness over the collateral ligament. Complete rupture, which creates lateral instability, must be ruled out. This can be demonstrated clinically and radiographically by stress films (Fig. 66-5). Even without obtaining stress films, one may be able to make the diagnosis by routine radiograph if a small bony fragment is associated with an avulsed ligament.

The treatment for a mild sprain of the collateral ligaments is splinting of the finger in a functional position or buddy taping it to the adjacent finger until the pain has subsided and the range of motion can be restored.[26] For injuries in which there is joint laxity and incomplete tearing of the ligament, the finger should be splinted in 30° of flexion.[27] Active motion exercises are begun in 10 to 14 days, with protective splinting for at least 3 weeks.

There is a great deal of controversy concerning treatment of complete tears of the collateral ligaments of the PIP joint. Many believe that conservative treatment is satisfactory. Others feel that the optimal treatment in these cases is open inspection and repair of the torn ligament.[28] In chronic repairs, frequently a free tendon graft is needed to reinforce the repair.

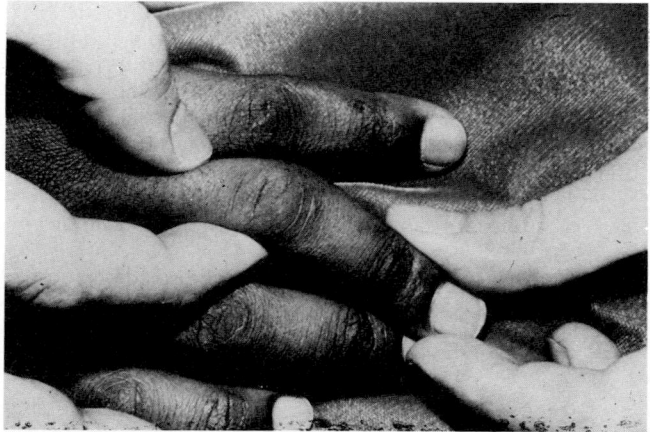

Figure 66-5 Stress roentgenograms confirmed a complete collateral ligament rupture, suspected on physical examination.

Volar Plate Injuries

The volar plate of the PIP joint is composed of a strong, distal fibrocartilaginous tissue that inserts broadly on the base of the middle phalanx. Proximally the plate is thin and membranous as it originates from the proximal phalanx.[16] The volar plate is usually injured by a hyperextension force or a dorsal dislocation. Radiographs may show a small bone chip associated with an avulsion injury.

Volar plate injuries may result in either hyperextension or flexion deformities of the PIP joint. In most cases, the hyperextension deformity is caused by rupture of the volar plate at its distal end. In acute injury, protection by splinting in 25 to 30° of flexion is indicated for 3 weeks, followed by protected motion for 2 to 3 weeks. Disruption of the volar plate distally can result in a swan-neck deformity. Secondary surgical reconstruction is indicated only when the PIP joint locks in hyperextension and subsequently interferes with normal hand function.

Disruption of the volar plate at its proximal membranous portion can result in a pseudoboutonniere deformity.[23,27] This resembles the true boutonniere, but disruption of the central slip is not present. The diagnostic features are as follows: a flexion contracture of the PIP joint, which is more resistant to correction by passive extension than the typical boutonniere; slight hyperextension of the distal interphalangeal (DIP) joint; radiologic evidence of calcification at the distal end of the proximal phalanx (proximal attachment of the volar plate); and a history of hyperextension or twisting injury to the middle joint rather than one of hyperflexion injury.

If the lesion is diagnosed early, extension is more easily obtained by conservative means. The patient must be followed closely, since the deformity may recur. A mild deformity (less than 40° of flexion) will respond to prolonged splinting. For severe injury with a flexion deformity of 45° or more, surgical intervention is usually required for optimal function. Repair consists of release and distal advancement of the scarred proximal volar plate, gouging out the bone spur, and release of the accessory collateral ligament. The PIP joint is maintained in extension for 3 weeks by the use of a K wire along with an external splint.

REFERENCES

1. Weber ER: Concepts governing the rotational shift of the intercalated segment of the carpus. *Orthop Clin North Am* 15:193–208, 1984.
2. *Regional Review Course in hand Surgery: Manual.* New York, American Society for Surgery of the Hand, 1994.
3. Berger RA, Landsmeer JM: The palmar radiocarpal ligaments: A study of adult and fetal human wrist joints. *J Hand Surg* 15A:847–854, 1990.
4. Taleisnik J: The ligaments of the wrist. *J Hand Surg* 1A:110–118, 1976.
5. Ruby LK: Carpal instability. *Instr Course Lect* 45:3–13, 1996.
6. Viegas SF, Patterson RM, Peterson PD, et al: Ulnar sided perilunate instability: An anatomical and biomechanic study. *J Hand Surg* 15A:268–278, 1990.
7. Mayfield JK, Johnson RP, Kilcoyne RK: Carpal dislocations: Pathomechanics and progressive perilunar instability. *J Hand Surg* 5:226–241, 1980.
8. Green DP (ed): *Operative Hand Surgery,* 3d ed. New York, Churchill Livingstone, 1993, pp 861–928.
9. Manske PR (ed): *Hand Surgery Update.* New York, American Society for Surgery of the Hand, 1994.
10. Belberman RH (ed): *The Wrist: Master Techniques in Orthopaedic Surgery.* New York, Raven Press, 1994, pp 135–146, 147–166, 183–194, 195–206.
11. Reagan DS, Linscheid RL, Dobyns JH: Lunotriquetral sprains. *J Hand Surg* 9A:502–514, 1984.
12. Gilula LA, Destouet JM, Weeks PM, et al: Roentgenographic diagnosis of the painful wrist. *Clin Orthop* 187:52–64, 1984.
13. Herbert TJ, Faithfull RG, McCann DJ, Ireland J: Bilateral arthrography of the wrist. *J Hand Surg* 15B:233–235, 1990.
14. Linscheid RL, Dobyns JH, Bequmont JW, Bryan RS: Traumatic instability of the wrist: Diagnosis, classification, and pathomechanics. *J Bone Joint Surg* 54A:1612–1632, 1972.
15. Lavernia CJ, Cohen M, Taleisnik J: Treatment of scapholunate dissociations by ligamentous repair and capsulodesis. *J Hand Surg* 17A:354–359, 1992.
16. Posner MA (ed): Ligament injuries in the wrist and hand. *Hand Clin* 8:603–611, 631–644, 645–653, 653–668, 693–700, 713–732, 733–744, 745–754, 1992.
17. Palmer AK, Werner FW: The triangular fibrocartilage complex of the wrist anatomy and function. *J Hand Surg* 6A:153–162, 1981.
18. Palmer AK: The distal radioulnar joint. *Orthop Clin North Am* 15:321–336, 1984.
19. Palmer AK: Triangular fibrocartilage complex lesion: A classification. *J Hand Surg* 14A:594–606, 1989.
20. Hermansdorfer JD, Kleinman WB: Management of chronic peripheal tears of the triangular fibrocartilage complex. *J Hand Surg* 16A:340–346, 1991.
21. Lane LB, Eaton RG: Ligament reconstruction for the painful "prearthritic" thumb carpometacarpal joint. *Clin Orthop Res* 220:52–57, 1987.
22. Bowers WH, Hurst LC: Gamekeeper's thumb. *J Bone Joint Surg* 59A:519–524, 1977.
23. McCue FC, Hakala MW, Andrews JR, Gieck JH: Ulnar collateral ligament injuries of the thumb in athletes. *Am J Sports Med* 2:70–80, 1974.
24. Stener B: Displacement of the ruptured ulna collateral ligament of the metacarpophalangeal joint of the thumb: A clinical and anatomical study. *J Bone Joint Surg* 44B:869–879, 1962.
25. McCue FC, Baugher WH, Dulund DN, Gleck JH: Hand and wrist injuries in the athlete. *Am J Sports Med* 7:275–286, 1979.
26. McCue FC, Andrews JR, Hakala MW: The coach's finger. *Am J Sports Med* 2:270–275, 1974.
27. McCue FC, Abbot JL: The treatment of mallet finger and boutonniere deformities. *Virginia Med Monthly* 94:623–628, 1967.
28. McCue FC, Honner R, Johnson MC, Gieck JH: Athletic injuries of the proximal interphalangeal joint requiring surgical treatment. *J Bone Joint Surg* 52A:937–956, 1970.

CHAPTER 67

Nerve Injury: Healing, Repair, and Grafting

Alexander Bee Dagum, Lawrence C. Hurst, and Marie A. Badalamente

Peripheral nerve injuries constitute a major source of chronic disability. The published results of nerve repairs in World War II have led clinicians to perceive the outcome of nerve repair as poor.[1] The principles of microsurgery and our improved understanding of nerve biology have greatly advanced our clinical results. Although far from perfect, our results today give patients not only hope but also some degree of function. Now that the technical aspects of nerve repair have been mastered, the next step will be to manipulate the nerve biology in order to improve our outcomes.

This chapter deals with the biological process of nerve regeneration following injury and repair, the technical aspects and results of nerve repair and grafting. A discussion of brachial plexus injuries and of obstetrical brachial plexus palsy is included.

PERIPHERAL NERVE ANATOMY AND PHYSIOLOGY

A nerve consists of axons, Schwann cells, and connective tissue (Fig. 67-1). The outer covering is called the *external epineurium* and consists of collagenous connective tissue. The internal epineurium cushions the fascicles from external pressure and surrounds the perineurium. The perineurium surrounds individual fascicles and consists of flattened cells with prominent basement membranes and tight junctions. The perineurium functions as the blood-nerve barrier. The endoneurium lies inside the perineurium and consists of collagenous tissue surrounding Schwann cells and axons.[2]

A fascicular group consists of two or more fascicles surrounded by internal epineurium. A nerve fascicle consists of multiple nerve fibers surrounded by perineurium. A nerve fiber consists of multiple axons and Schwann cells surrounded by endoneurium. Fascicles are interconnected to form an intraneural plexus known as the *plexus of Sunderland*. This plexus is more marked proximally and absent distally. Its function is to permit nerve stretching without significant fascicular stretching as the extremity is moved. Clinically, this is important, because it allows for group fascicular repair in distal nerve injuries but not in proximal nerve injuries, such as those of the brachial plexus, where only an epineural repair can be carried out. The topography of nerves is therefore constant distally,

with groups of fascicles being either sensory or motor. A good example of this is the median and ulnar nerves at the wrist and distal forearm, where each consists of three fascicles, one of which is motor and the other two sensory. In the median nerve the motor fascicle lies volar and in the ulnar nerve it lies dorsal.[3,4]

The vascular supply of nerves consists of multiple segmental extrinsic nutrient vessels supplying a longitudinally intrinsic oriented vascular plexus in the epineurium, which, in turn, supplies a similar longitudinal intrinsic perineurial vascular plexus. From the perineurial plexus arise longitudinally oriented arterioles, capillaries, and venules that course in the endoneurium and supply the nerve fibers. This extensive longitudinally oriented blood supply allows for mobilization of the uninjured peripheral nerve for up to 50 times its diameter—e.g., approximately 20 cm for the ulnar nerve at the elbow without compromise to its vascularity.

The neuron consists of a soma (cell body) and an axon, which can be several feet long. There exist several axoplasmic transport systems that enable the cell body to communicate with its motor or sensory end organ. These adenosine triphosphate (ATP)–dependent systems maintain the structure and function of the peripheral nerve. There are two antegrade axoplasmic transport systems: fast and slow. The fast system transports neurotransmitters, the slow system transports structural proteins. There is also a retrograde axoplasmic transport system, which recycles neurotransmitters and takes up neurotrophic factors from the end organ.[5]

CLASSIFICATION OF NERVE INJURY

The classification of nerve injuries is important not only for prognosis but also for treatment. There are two major types of classification in use today, that of Seddon (1943) and that of Sunderland (1951).[6,7] Seddon classified nerve injuries into three groups: neuropraxia, axonotmesis, and neurotmesis. Neuropraxia represents a physiologic block of nerve function with anatomic continuity. Axonotmesis corresponds to disruption of the axon and myelin sheath without injury to the endoneurium. Neurotmesis corresponds to complete transection of the nerve. Sunderland expanded Seddon's classification by classifying nerve injuries according to degree of histologic injury, ranging from first-degree to fifth-degree.

A first-degree injury corresponds to a neuropraxia. This represents a localized conduction block with an intact axon with or without segmental demyelination. Electromyographic (EMG) studies will be normal, but nerve conduction studies (NCS) will show some slowing. There will be no advancing Tinel's sign. This is the mildest of injuries, with full recovery occurring within 2 to 6 weeks. The etiology is that of acute nerve compression such as a "Saturday night palsy."

A second-degree injury corresponds to axonotmesis. There is axonal injury with Wallerian degeneration, but the endoneurium remains intact. The axons regenerate along

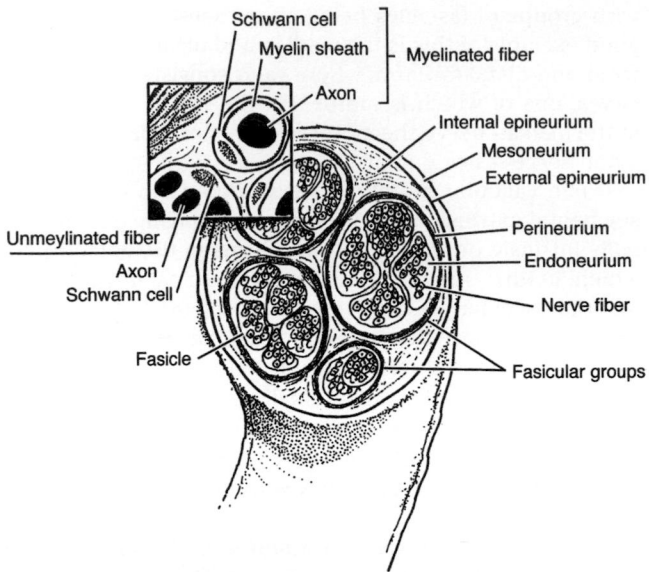

Figure 67-1 A cross section of a peripheral nerve is shown. Note all the structures that make up the nerve and how they relate to Sunderland's classification of progressive nerve injury.

their original endoneurial tubes and show a progressing Tinel's sign and appropriate EMG/NCS changes. Complete recovery is the norm unless the motor targets are more than 12 to 24 in away. The etiology is usually that of a closed stretch injury, such as that sustained by the axillary nerve with a shoulder dislocation.

A third-degree injury corresponds to injury of the axon, myelin, and endoneurium but not perineurium. The fascicle remains intact. Recovery is variable and depends on the axonal injury and hence the amount of fibrosis as well as the type of nerve. Pure motor or sensory nerves do better than mixed nerves, which will lead to increased mismatch. Recovery is incomplete, and it is this type of injury that may benefit from neurolysis. The etiology is usually that of a more severe stretch injury.

In a fourth-degree injury, there is injury to the axon, myelin, endoneurium, and perineurium, with continuity of the nerve maintained by the epineurium. Spontaneous recovery is not expected because the interposed fibrosis and scarring traps sprouting axons. The etiology is usually that of a traction injury from severe stretch or an iatrogenic nerve injection injury. The treatment consists of resection and grafting.

A fifth-degree injury corresponds to neurotmesis. This is a complete nerve transection with gross anatomic separation and therefore injury to the axon, myelin, endoneurium, perineurium, and epineurium. Spontaneous recovery is not possible. The etiology is usually that of a laceration, and treatment consists of surgical repair.

Dellon and Mackinnon expanded on Sunderland's classification by adding a sixth-degree injury. This consists of a combination of injuries from first to fifth degree, as seen in a neuroma-in-continuity.[2]

NERVE REGENERATION

The process by which peripheral nerves regenerate is governed by the inherent ability of the nerve to display neurotropism, neurotrophism, contact guidance, and specificity.[5] *Neurotropism* refers to the influence of axonal growth direction by exerting attraction at a distance by a gradient of diffusible substances produced by the target. This is differentiated from *neurotrophism,* which refers to factors that influence the maturation of peripheral nerve and supports the survival and general growth capabilities of neurons. *Contact guidance* refers to the ability of surrounding tissue to influence the direction of regeneration. *Tissue specificity* refers to the preferential reinnervation of distal nerve tissue by nerve tissue. *End-organ specificity* refers to the preferential reinnervation of motor axons to motor targets rather than sensory targets. Sensory axons do not show this preferential end-organ specificity. *Topographic specificity* refers to preferential reinnervation of analogous distal pathways—i.e., correct muscle with correct motor nerve. Except perhaps at the spinal level, motor nerve topographic specificity is felt to not occur in routine nerve regeneration. Therefore in primary nerve repair, mechanical alignment by the surgeon is the most important determinant of motor and sensory specificity.[8]

The response of peripheral nerve injury depends on the severity of the initial trauma. In first-degree or neuropraxic injuries, the axons respond by demyelination, followed by remyelination by Schwann cells. The damage produces localized slowing or a conduction block over the demyelinated region. Conduction is restored over 2 to 6 weeks as the axons are remyelinated.

In terms of nerve healing and regeneration it is best to discuss the changes as they occur at the different anatomic sites—namely, the nerve cell body, proximal stump, gap site, distal stump, and receptors, understanding, however, that all these changes are taking place simultaneously.

The nerve cell body responds within 12 h after injury with increased RNA synthesis leading to increased protein and lipid synthesis, which are transported along the axonal transport system to the site of injury as a mechanism for the synthesis of membrane proteins necessary for regeneration. The stimulus to axotomy is postulated to be an interruption of neurotrophic substances from the end organ.[5] If the injury is very proximal, death of the cell body occurs and no regeneration takes place.

The proximal axonal stump undergoes Wallerian degeneration to the most proximal node of Ranvier. An outgrowth occurs from the proximal stump, with each axon giving rise to multiple axonal sprouts surrounded by Schwann cells. The tip of such an axonal sprout is known as the *growth cone.* Neurite-promoting factors such as the protein GAP-43 stimulate growth cone membrane formation and advancement of axons. Fingerlike projections known as *filipodia* extend the axonal sprouts and sample the environment.

These growth cones grow through the gap or site of injury. The axonal sprouts that make appropriate contact through the filipodia use the distal Schwann cell basal lamina as a substrate and grow into the now empty endoneurial tubes. Laminin, a potent neurite outgrowth–promoting factor and the major component of basal lamina, acts as the contact guidance to the filipodia. The axonal sprouts that do not make contact undergo degeneration. Axonal sprouting can be blocked by scar tissue, infection, gap size, and tension, leading to necrosis. Clinically, the growth cone region may be localized by eliciting a Tinel's sign. This region is hyperexcitable; thus mechanical tapping produces a pins-and-needles or "electric shock" sensation, known as a *Tinel's sign*.

The distal stump undergoes classic Wallerian degeneration. An influx of Ca^{2+} triggers a sequence of enzymatic degradation by calpains, which begins with proteolysis of axons (axonolysis). Degenerated axons and myelin are phagocytosed by Schwann cells and macrophages over 1 to 3 months, leaving empty neural tubes. These empty tubes, which are composed of Schwann cells and basal lamina, when stuck together give a characteristic appearance under the microscope known as the *bands of Bungner*. Electrophysiologic studies have shown that by 3 to 5 days, motor amplitudes are decreased by 50 percent, and they are absent by 9 days after injury.[9] The clinical significance of this is that the distal motor fascicle can be identified by electrical stimulation up to 1 week after injury.

Regenerating axons grow distally at a rate of 1 to 3 mm per day or just slightly more than an inch a month. The axon must grow from the site of injury all the way to the end-organ receptor. Muscle tissue undergoes progressive, irreversible atrophy and fibrosis if it is not reinnervated by 1 to 2 years. Therefore repair of a very proximal nerve injury such as a brachial plexus is unlikely to result in recovery of intrinsic hand muscles, as they will mostly have undergone atrophy and fibrosis by the time the axons reach the muscle end organ. Sensory receptors such as Meissner's end organs, Ruthni endings, and Merkel cells do not undergo significant degeneration and may be innervated many years later with reasonable results. However, Pacinian corpuscles may fail to be reinnervated as their central axons undergo fibrosis.

The regenerated nerve fiber at completion is smaller in diameter, less well myelinated, and conducts less rapidly than before the injury.

Cortical plasticity plays an important role in the ultimate functional recovery of motor and sensory nerves as some amount of end-organ reinnervation mismatch occurs after nerve regeneration. The cerebral cortex must reprogram itself to compensate for these errors in end-organ reinnervation. The therapeutic modality of sensory reeducation is an excellent example of brain reprogramming that improves sensory recovery after nerve repair and regeneration.[5]

Nerve grafting is the transplantation of peripheral nerve tissue to a new site. In general, healing and nerve regeneration go through similar phases as in primary nerve repair. Survival of nonvascularized autogenous nerve grafts in the first 3 to 5 days is by host bed diffusion, followed by revascularization from direct ingrowth from the periphery and cut ends of the nerve. Failure of revascularization will result in graft fibrosis and therefore blockage of axonal sprout advancement. Neurotization of the graft occurs by the attachment of axonal sprouts by filipodia to

the basal lamina of the nerve graft. The Schwann cell and basal lamina guide axonal growth through the graft to the distal stump. The axon then neurotizes into the distal stump site as described above.

NERVE REPAIR

The goal of nerve repair is to restore preinjury innervation and thus function. Practically, this translates to providing an environment that will maximize axonal regeneration with optimal fascicular orientation.

Timing of Nerve Repair

The timing of nerve repair depends on the type of injury. Open, clean, guillotine-type nerve lacerations are best repaired acutely (primary or delayed primary), as this provides for earlier recovery, better appreciation of the orientation of the nerve, no secondary nerve contraction, and the ability to stimulate the distal motor branches, making them easier to isolate, as in the deep ulnar nerve or the recurrent median nerve. Although this view is controversial, in crush, avulsion, or other untidy wounds, it is better to debride the wound, tag the nerves to the underlying skin with Prolene to prevent secondary contraction, and make it easier to isolate them at secondary surgery. The wound is allowed to heal and, at 3 to 6 weeks, secondary repair is performed in a clean bed.

Although gunshot injuries are open, they are treated as closed injuries. The wound is debrided but no special attempt is made to explore the paralyzed nerves at the time of injury. Because the etiology of the nerve injury is in general a contusion from the blast effect rather than a transection, the type and zone of injury cannot be determined at the time of injury. In fact many will recover on their own, as they will have sustained only a Sunderland first-, second-, or third-degree injury.

The treatment of closed nerve injuries is staged. The following are general guidelines, but timing may vary depending on the type, location, and extent of nerve injury. Stage 1 involves the first 3 months. The nerve injury is treated expectantly. The therapist sees the patient and ensures that he or she maintains full range of motion of all joints and protects anesthetic areas. The patient is followed clinically for proximal-to-distal recovery and a progressing Tinel's sign. At 3 months, an EMG/NCS is performed to assess the extent of injury and evidence of reinnervation. The EMG/NCS precedes clinical findings by about a month.[10]

Stage 2 is from 3 to 6 months. If there is evidence of return of function clinically or electrophysiologically, the patient continues to be followed expectantly. If a plateau occurs or no function has returned, the patient undergoes a nerve exploration.

Stage 3 involves the nerve exploration. At exploration, an external neurolysis is performed through the zone of injury. The nerve is stimulated proximally; if muscle contraction is present or conduction through the zone of injury is detected, the operation is finished. If there is no conduction, the nerve is resected to normal nerve. The nerve is grafted, as primary repair is rarely possible at this stage.

Stage 4 is from the time of nerve exploration and repair to 1 or 2 years later. The patient is followed expectantly with continuation of active hand therapy. Stage 5 is at 2 years, at which time a final assessment is made of the extent of recovery. At this time adjunctive procedures can be carried out in order to improve hand and limb function. These may involve muscle, tendon transfers, free muscle transfers, arthrodesis, or/and amputation.

Technique of Nerve Repair

The nerve is assessed under the microscope for proximal and distal extent of injury. Scarred nerve has a ground-glass appearance and should be sharply resected proximally and distally to normal nerve, as evidenced by sprouting fascicles. A primary repair should be done whenever possible. Transposition of the nerve, as in an ulnar nerve laceration at the elbow, can be helpful in achieving a tension-free end-to-end repair. However, extreme joint positioning or tension at the anastomosis site should be avoided, as this will lead to contractures and necrosis with scarring across the nerve repair. In general, a nerve gap greater than 2.5 cm will require nerve grafts.[2]

The neurorrhaphy is done using standard microsurgical techniques. An epineural repair is performed after careful alignment of the fascicles (Fig. 67-2). An epineural repair involves placement of microsutures through the external epineurium. Fibrin glue has recently been used with apparently equal results to repair with microsutures.

A group fascicular repair or an epineural repair with fascicular group matching can be done when the neural topography is known and no fascicular crossover (plexus of Sunderland) exists, as in the distal ulnar or median nerves or radial nerve at the elbow (Fig. 67-2). The neural maps of Sunderland, Jabaley, and coworkers can be helpful in identifying the neural topography.[3,4,11,12] An epineural repair with fascicular group matching entails aligning the fascicular groups and suturing the external epineurium. A group fascicular repair entails aligning the group of fascicles and suturing the internal epineurium. Theoretically

this is advantageous when there are three or four groups, where each group is either motor or sensory and the groups can be correctly aligned. In the acute injury, alignment of the fascicles under the microscope is relatively straightforward. In secondary reconstruction where a nerve gap exists and nerve grafts are usually required, it is not usually possible to align the fascicular groups visually. It is in these cases that the techniques of awake stimulation or chemical enzyme staining have proved useful in identifying the motor and sensory fascicular groups. Awake stimulation involves stimulating the proximal nerve fascicles. The patients will identify the cutaneous distribution of the sensory group; in the motor group, the stimulation will be localized as a deep dull ache in the middle of the muscle belly. Chemical staining with acetylcholinesterase or cholineacetyltransferase will identify pure motor fascicles, and carbonic anhydrase will locate pure sensory fascicles. The new enzyme stains can be done in less than an hour and therefore intraoperatively; however, they require an experienced neuropathologist for interpretation of the results.[13] The distal groups are identified by dissecting to the level where the nerve branches—Guyon's canal for the ulnar nerve or the carpal tunnel for the median nerve.

Nerve Grafts

Nerve grafts have proved useful in secondary reconstruction where primary repair is not possible or would entail excessive tension or extreme joint positioning. Excessive tension leads to necrosis and fibrosis of the nerve repair with axonolysis and blockage of nerve regeneration.[2,13] Autogenous nonvascularized nerve grafts can be obtained from several sites. The sural nerve is the standard donor and can provide 30 to 40 cm of nerve graft. Other donor nerves that are commonly used are the lateral antebrachial cutaneous, medial antebrachial cutaneous, and sensory branch of the posterior interosseous nerve. In digital nerve gaps of less than 3 cm, autogenous vein conduits and polyglycolic acid tubes have proved useful as alternatives to standard nerve grafts. Vascularized autogenous nerve grafts may be of benefit in severely scarred beds or in the transplantation of large nerve trunks to avoid central necrosis. Allograft nerve grafts have been used but remain experimental and require immunosuppressive therapy for at least 2 years.

RESULTS OF NERVE REPAIR

There have not been many published studies on the results of nerve repair. It is important to note that anatomic motor and sensory reinnervation does not ensure functional recovery. First the axons must regenerate into the distal nerve and establish neural connections to target end organs. The second phase involves return of simple function, such as protective sensation or motor contraction. The third phase entails return of complex movement and discriminative sensation. It is this last phase that is

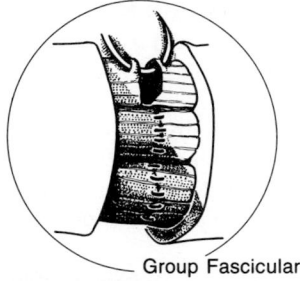
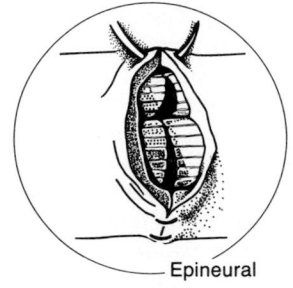

Group Fascicular   Epineural

Figure 67-2 Group fascicular nerve repair and epineural nerve repair are shown.

TABLE 67-1 End-Result Grading System

Motor recovery:

M10	No contraction
M1	Return of perceptible contraction in the proximal muscles
M2	Return of perceptible contraction in both proximal and distal muscles
M3	Return of function in both proximal and distal muscles of such degree that all important muscles are sufficiently powerful to act against resistance
M4	Return of function as in stage M3 with the addition that all synergic and independent movements are possible
M5	Complete recovery

Sensory recovery:

S0	Absence of sensibility in the autonomous area
S1	Recovery of deep cutaneous pain sensibility within the autonomous area of the nerve
S2	Return of some degree of superficial cutaneous pain and tactile sensibility within the autonomous area of the nerve
S3	Return of superficial cutaneous pain and tactile sensibility throughout the autonomous area with disappearance of any previous overreaction
S3+	Return of sensibility as in stage S3 with the addition that there is some recovery of two-point discrimination within the autonomous area
S4	Complete recovery

Source: Introduced by the Nerve Injuries Committee of the (British) Medical Research Council (MRC), 1954.

termed *useful functional recovery.* This takes approximately 2 years to achieve fully, although there may still be improvement for 3 to 5 years. Results of nerve repair may be evaluated using the British Medical Research Council Nerve Injury Committee classification scheme for sensory and motor recovery (Table 67-1). A sensory recovery S3 or better or motor nerve recovery M4 or better is considered useful functional recovery.

The results of nerve repair are variable and depend on surgical and patient factors. Distal nerve injuries do better than proximal ones. Younger patients do better than older patients because of better cortical reorientation, shorter regeneration distance, and improved healing. However, in adults the results can be improved with sensory reeducation. Sensory or pure motor nerve repair does better than mixed nerve repair. A guillotine injury does better than a crush injury, which, in turn, does better than an avulsion injury.

Digital neurorrhaphy produces the best results of any sensory nerve repair, with most series reporting a two-point discrimination of 10 mm, or S3[+] or better in 60 percent of patients and more recently 80 to 90 percent.[2,14,15] Recent reports of digital nerve grafting have reported two-point discrimination in 60 percent of patients.[2,15] The improved results in the past decade can be attributed to the use of microsurgical technique and sensory reeducation.

The results of low median nerve repair show that 50 percent of patients will recover S3 or greater.[2] A recent study using sensory reeducation reported 80 percent of patients recovering S3[+] following median nerve grafting.[16] The reported results of low ulnar nerve repair show 50 percent of patients recovering M4 or M5 motor function.[2] High median and ulnar nerve injuries have a more guarded prognosis.

NEUROMA

Following transection, peripheral nerves form neuromas at their cut ends as the proximal nerve attempts to regenerate.[17] Few neuromas become symptomatic, but when they do, they can be extremely disabling. Common clinical situations that lead to symptomatic neuromas are amputations, inadvertent transection of the radial sensory nerve during DeQuervain's release, or excision of a dorsal ganglion.

In the treatment of neuromas, prevention is the key. In amputations, it is important to transect the nerve well proximal to the amputation site to prevent scarring of the neuroma to the stump, leading to constant irritation and pain. The number of treatment methods for painful neuromas is testament to the lack of a universally successful approach to this difficult clinical problem.[18] In established painful neuromas, an early course of desensitization by the therapist is the first line of treatment and will often alleviate the problem. If nonoperative treatment of the nonoperative nerve fails, the patient should undergo a nerve block with a long-acting local anesthetic. If this fails to alleviate the pain, surgery will usually be unsuccessful. If the neuroma is due to a transected nerve, microsurgical repair with adequate soft tissue coverage is performed. If primary repair is not possible, transposition of the neuroma proximally away from the site of injury and into a minimally mobile vascularized bed has proved to be most effective. Postoperatively, the patient should undergo a course of desensitization.[2,13]

The neuroma-in-continuity is a separate, complicated problem that usually results from an incompletely transected nerve. The goal is to alleviate the pain without downgrading the functioning nerve fascicles. Intraoperative electrophysiologic assessment with a nerve graft bypass procedure of the nonfunctioning fascicular groups and translocation of the neuroma with functioning nerve fascicles deep to the site of the injury has proved useful in treating this condition.[19] Dissection through the neuroma-in-continuity is tedious, usually results in some loss of function, and does not completely alleviate the pain. Covering the nerve with vascularized soft tissue such as a pronator quadratus flap has also been of help.

BRACHIAL PLEXUS INJURIES

Injury to the brachial plexus is a devastating problem resulting in partial to total paralysis of the involved extrem-

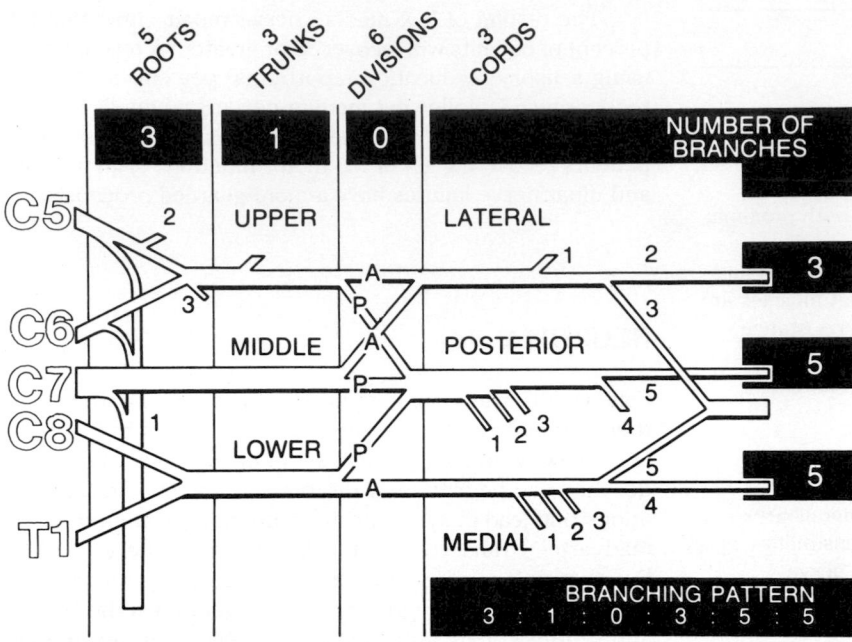

Figure 67-3 *A.* Brachial plexus starting from roots C5, C6, C7, C8, and T1. *B.* The branching pattern of brachial plexus nerves.

A

3	1	0	3	5	5
1 Long thoracic n. 2 Dorsal scapular n. 3 Subclavian n.	1 Suprascapular n.		1 Lateral pectoral n. 2 Musculocutaneous n. 3 Lateral head of Median n.	1 Upper subscapular n. 2 Thoracodorsal n. 3 Lower subscapular n. 4 Axillary n. 5 Radial n.	1 Medial pectoral n. 2 Medial cutaneous nerve of arm 3 Medial cutaneous nerve of forearm 4 Ulnar n. 5 Medial head of Median n.

B

ity. These injuries occur mostly in young patients. Although, with the advent of microsurgery, an improvement in recovery has been obtained, there is still a long way to go for improvement in outcome.[20]

The brachial plexus consists of the anterior rami of the C5, C6, C7, C8, and T1 nerve roots (Fig. 67-3). These lie between the scalenus anterior and medius muscles. In the posterior triangle of the neck, the upper, middle, and lower trunks are formed. At the level of the clavicle, the trunks divide into anterior and posterior divisions. As the divisions enter the axilla, the cords are formed. The anterior divisions of the upper and middle trunks form the lateral cord, which lies lateral to the axillary artery. The anterior division of the lower trunk forms a medial cord, which lies medial to the axillary artery. Posterior to the axillary artery is the posterior cord, which is formed from the union of all three posterior divisions.

Nerve branches from the brachial plexus are arranged according to the 3:1:0:3:5:5 rule (an extension of Last's 3:5:5 rule).[21] There are three branches from the root: the long thoracic nerve, the nerve to subclavius, and the dorsal scapular nerve. There is one branch from the upper trunk: the suprascapular nerve. The divisions have none. The lateral cord has three: the lateral pectoral nerve, the musculocutaneous nerve, and the lateral contribution of the median nerve. The medial cord gives off five branches, including the medial cutaneous nerve of the arm, medial cutaneous nerve of the forearm, medial pectoral nerve, medial contribution of the median nerve, and ulnar nerve. The posterior cord has five branches: the upper and lower subscapular nerves, thoracodorsal nerve, axillary nerve, and radial nerve.

The most common etiology of a brachial plexus injury is direct traction on the plexus. This results in a mixed injury to the plexus, with all the Sunderland degrees of injury coexisting. High-energy injuries such as falling off a motorcycle will lead to more severe trauma, with rupture of the plexal segments and avulsion of the nerve roots. Low-energy injuries, such as a fall from a tree or a "stinger" injury in football, will result in a more reversible injury—i.e., neuropraxia and axonotmesis.

Evaluation of the patient with a brachial plexus injury involves taking a careful history and performing a detailed clinical examination. Every muscle in the shoulder girdle and upper extremity is tested and graded, followed by a sensory examination. A sketch (Fig. 67-3) of the brachial plexus is drawn and the nerves marked as functioning or not. The muscles are listed, a corresponding Medical Research Council (MRC) grade is given, and the sensory distribution is recorded. It is only in this fashion that the patient's progress can be properly evaluated and a surgical plan made.

There are several key points in the evaluation. The presence of a Horner's syndrome (anhydrosis, myosis, ptosis, entropion) suggests avulsion of the C8 and T1 nerve roots. A long thoracic or dorsal scapular nerve palsy suggests corresponding root avulsions. A computed tomography myelogram is useful in evaluating root rupture, with presence of a pseudomeningocele corresponding to an 85 percent probability of root rupture. An elevated hemidiaphragm on chest x-ray is indicative of phrenic nerve injury, which suggests a proximal injury or avulsion and precludes use of intercostal nerves for neurotization. Sensory evoked potentials can be used to evaluate the status of the roots.

There are three types of injury patterns: root avulsion, rupture, and neuroma-in-continuity. In root avulsion, the roots are usually avulsed directly from the spinal cord and are at present not amenable to surgical repair. In a rupture, the nerve is severed; this is a Sunderland fifth-degree injury. A neuroma-in-continuity can have all the Sunderland degrees of injury. A brachial plexus injury will usually contain a mixture of the above injuries. Even in complete brachial plexus palsy, only 11 percent of patients will have all five roots avulsed.[20]

The surgical treatment of brachial plexus palsy (BPP) depends on the type of injury and whether it is open or closed. The treatment management follows the same algorithm as above. Open, clean, sharp lacerations undergo a primary epineural repair. After debridement, gunshot injuries are treated the same as closed injuries in a staged approach. In the brachial plexus, spontaneous recovery of gunshot injury is poor. In the first 3 months, the injury is treated expectantly. If there is no return of function at 3 months or a plateau in functions occurs from 3 to 6 months, the brachial plexus is explored.

At exploration, intraoperative stimulation is carried out. If a normal action potential is present, the nerve just undergoes neurolysis. If no conduction is present, as with a rupture, the nerve is resected under frozen section control until normal nerve is encountered with nerve grafting of the nerve gap. If the root is avulsed, neurotization is considered. Neurotization involves transferring a donor nerve and anastomosing it to the distal nerve that has undergone a root avulsion. The usual donors are the intercostals C3–C6, the accessory nerve past the first branch to the trapezius, and the cervical plexus.[2,22]

In a complete adult BPP that comes to exploration, normal recovery is not possible. Surgical priorities have to be set in the reconstruction of this injury in order to convert a flail, painful upper extremity into a helper arm. The priorities are as follows: a stable, pain-free shoulder with some abduction, restoration of elbow flexion, and restoration of protective sensation to the median or ulnar nerve distribution. If these three priorities are met, one has achieved useful function. Millesi, in a large series of complete BPP treated by microsurgical techniques using the above principles, showed that useful function can be expected in 69 percent of lesions undergoing neurolysis, 72 percent of lesions that are grafted, and 50 percent of lesions that undergo neurotization. Upper BPP, C5–C7, showed 95 percent useful function after neurolysis, 75 percent after nerve graft, and 63 percent after neurotization.[20]

OBSTETRICAL BRACHIAL PLEXUS PALSY

Obstetrical brachial plexus palsy (OBPP) is associated with traumatic deliveries; it has an incidence of 0.4 to 2.5 per 1000 live births. There is usually an element of cephalopelvic disproportion, with large infants. The upper roots of the brachial plexus are usually injured during delivery, when shoulder dystocia necessitates excessive lateral flexion in order to free the shoulder from the pubic arch. The right extremity is affected twice as often as the left, as most babies present left occiput anterior.[23]

A majority of patients show injury to C5 and C6, which is known as *Erb-Duchenne palsy.* Clinically there is loss of shoulder abduction and external rotation, elbow flexion, and forearm supination. The upper extremity assumes a "waiter's tip" position. The next most frequent is a complete palsy. Klumpke's paralysis is an isolated C8 and T1 injury affecting primarily the hand and is quite rare.

The diagnosis is primarily clinical. It is suspected in a newborn when there is absence of upper extremity motion but retention of full passive motion. The differential diagnosis includes fracture of the clavicle or the proximal humeral epiphysis, congenital dislocation, arthrogryposis, cervical spine injury, or cerebral palsy. Frequent examination is necessary to confirm the diagnosis. X-ray views should be taken of the cervical spine, upper extremity, and diaphragm.

The treatment is the same as for all closed nerve injury—expectant at first. It is important to start therapy early to prevent joint contractures. Prospective studies have shown that 50 to 80 percent of patients with OBPP make a complete recovery. Some 40 to 60 percent of OBPP will be neuropraxias and will recover within a month. However, 15 to 20 percent will have a poor outcome.[23] Poor prognostic indicators include complete C8–T1 paralysis, or lack of biceps or deltoid contraction by 3 months. Even with the poor prognostic indicators, there still will be improvement over the ensuing 18 to 24 months. However, these extremities will be markedly smaller and weaker than the opposite extremities. It is these more severe injuries that benefit from surgical exploration and repair.[24,25] The neurolysis of neuroma-in-continuity in the involved nerves in OBPP that require surgical exploration has led to disappointing results, and most surgeons now recommend resection and nerve grafting.[24,25]

REFERENCES

1. Woodall B, Beebe WG: *Peripheral Nerve Regeneration: A Follow-up Study of 3,656 World War II Injuries.* VA Medical Monograph. Washington, D.C., U.S. Government Printing Office, 1956.
2. Mackinnon SE, Dellon AL: *Surgery of the Peripheral Nerve.* New York, Thieme, 1988.
3. Chow JA, Sunderland S, Van Beek AL: Surgical significance of the motor fascicular group of the ulnar nerve in the forearm. *J Hand Surg* 10A:867–872, 1985.

4. Chow JA, Van Beek AL, Bilos ZJ, et al: Anatomic basis for the repair of ulnar and median nerves in the distal part of the forearm by group fascicular suture and nerve grafting. *J Bone Joint Surg* 68A:273–280, 1986.

5. Lundborg G, Dahlin L, Danielsen N, Zhao Q: Trophism, tropism, and specificity in nerve regeneration. *J Reconstr Microsurg* 10:345–353, 1994.

6. Seddon HJ: Three types of nerve injury. *Brain* 66:237, 1943.

7. Sunderland S: A classification of peripheral nerve injuries producing loss of function. *Brain* 74:491, 1951.

8. Brushart TM: Motor axons preferentially reinnervate motor pathways. *J Neurosci* 13:2730–2738, 1993.

9. Chaudhry V, Cornblath DR: Wallerian degeneration in human nerves: Serial electrophysiological studies. *Muscle Nerve* 15:687–693, 1992.

10. Leffert RD: *Brachial Plexus Injuries.* New York, Churchill Livingstone, 1985.

11. Jabaley ME, Wallace WH, Hechler FR: Internal topography of major nerves of the forearm and hand: A current review. *J Hand Surg* 5:1–18, 1980.

12. Sunderland S: *Nerves and Nerve Injuries,* 2d ed. New York, Churchill Livingstone, 1978.

13. Mackinnon SE: Peripheral nerve injuries, in Manske PR (ed): *Hand Surgery Update.* Boulder, Colorado, American Society for Surgery of the Hand, 1994, pp 22-1–22-11.

14. Young L, Wray RC, Weeks PM: A randomized prospective comparison of fascicular and epineural digital nerve repairs. *Plast Reconstr Surg* 68:89–92, 1981.

15. Mailander P, Berger A, Schaller E, Ruhe K: Results of primary nerve repair in the upper extremity. *Microsurgery* 10:147–150, 1989.

16. Novak CB, Kelly L, Mackinnon SE: Sensory recovery after median nerve grafting. *J Hand Surg* 17A:59–68, 1992.

17. Badalamente MA, Hurst LC, Ellstein JE, McDevitt CA: The pathobiology of human neuromas: An electron microscopic and biomechanical study. *J Hand Surg* 10B:49–53, 1985.

18. Williams HB: The painful stump neuroma and its treatment. *Clin Plast Surg* 11:79–84, 1984.

19. Mackinnon SE, Glickman LT, Dagum AB: A technique for the treatment of neuroma incontinuity. *J Reconstr Microsurg* 8:379–383, 1992.

20. Millesi H: Brachial plexus injuries: Management and results, in Terzis JK (ed): *Microreconstruction of Nerve Injuries.* Philadelphia, Saunders, 1987, pp 347–360.

21. Last RJ: *Anatomy, Regional and Applied,* 7th ed. New York, Churchill Livingstone, 1984, pp 25–52.

22. Narakas A: Thoughts on neurotization or nerve transfers in irreparable nerve lesions, in Terzis JK (ed): *Microreconstruction of Nerve Injuries.* Philadelphia, Saunders, 1987, pp 447–451.

23. Brown KLB: Review of obstetrical palsies: Nonoperative treatment, in Terzis JK (ed): *Microreconstruction of Nerve Injuries.* Philadelphia, Saunders, 1987, pp 499–512.

24. Gilbert A, Razaboni R: Indications and results of brachial plexus surgery in obstetrical palsy. *Orthop Clin North Am* 19:91–105, 1988.

25. Clarke HM, Al-Qattan MM, Curtis CG, Zuker RM: Obstetrical brachial plexus palsy: Results following neurolysis of conducting neuromas-in-continuity. *Plast Reconstr Surg* 97:974–982, 1996.

CHAPTER 68

Nerve Entrapment Syndromes in the Upper Extremity

Michael P. Coyle, Jr.

Nerve entrapment lesions are a major cause of peripheral neuropathy. Although they may involve any nerve at any level, these lesions are usually found at predictable locations and share common elements of pathogenesis and neuropathophysiology.

The pathogenesis of peripheral nerve entrapment is multifaceted[1]: (1) anatomic (passage of nerves through or under normal anatomic structures, which thicken, hypertrophy, or fibrose); (2) postural (repetitive motion or positioning of an extremity at extreme ranges of motion); (3) developmental (anomalous, aberrant muscle bellies, fibrous bands); (4) inflammatory (synovitis, tenosynovitis); (5) metabolic and endocrine (pregnancy and the premenstrual phase, diabetes mellitus, hypothyroidism, acromegaly, gout, and pseudogout); (6) tumors (any mass lesion such as a ganglion or lipoma); (7) trauma (acute fracture, dislocation or compartment syndrome, delayed entrapment from healed fracture deformity, or abundant callous formation); and (8) iatrogenic (injections into the nerve, retraction on a nerve during surgery, faulty positioning of an anesthetized patient).

NEUROPATHOPHYSIOLOGIC PROCESSES

Ischemia and mechanical deformation (compression, friction, traction, angulation) are the main causes of nerve pathology in entrapment syndromes.[2] Nerve fibers demonstrate differing susceptibility to these factors. Within a nerve, ischemia and direct pressure affect in sequence larger-diameter fibers before smaller fibers, superficial fibers before deeper fibers, and larger fasciculi surrounded by scanty perineurium before smaller fasciculi with abundant cushioning perineurium. In general, motor fibers are more susceptible to injury than sensory fibers and large myelinated fibers more than fine or unmyelinated ones, with failure occurring in sequential order: motor, proprioceptor, touch, temperature, and pain. Recovery, in general, occurs sequentially in the reverse order.

Ischemia produces a localized segmental conduction block by disrupting the intraneural circulation and possibly causing ischemic necrosis of the myelin sheath.[3] Pressure of 30 mmHg impairs epineural venous flow and axonal transport, 50 mmHg diminishes intrafascicular arterial flow, while 60 to 80 mmHg causes all intraneural blood flow in the compressed nerve segment to cease.

Entrapped nerve fibers are more sensitive to ischemia. In purely ischemic lesions, sensory fibers tend to fail before motor fibers.

Mechanical compression produces structural changes within the nerve secondary to the applied pressure and shear forces.[4] The effects of compression depend upon its magnitude, rate of application, and duration, with the structural deformation greatest at the very edge of the compressed zone. Acute (rapid, severe) compression causes an intussusception of one internodal segment (axon and myelin sheath) into an adjacent internodal segment, producing a pinching-off effect on nerve function. Chronic pressure, however, produces a differential shearing effect on the multiple lamellae of myelin, squeezing the myelin away from the site of compression and forming a bulbous myelin lesion (tadpole configuration) with a segmental tapering of the internodal segments. Varying degrees of segmental demyelination may occur in the area of entrapment.

Friction causes a mechanical irritation of the nerve, producing fibrosis and restricting adhesions that interfere with its physiologic excursion.[2] Stretch elongation is highly dependent upon rate of application. If slowly stretched (months), a nerve can elongate to a remarkable degree without loss of function, whereas very rapid stretch (milliseconds) causes instant conduction loss and even structural rupture. Conduction defects begin to appear at 6 percent elongation and impaired microcirculation at 8 percent. Rapid stretching, however, produces axonal disruption at 6 to 20 percent elongation and microvascular occlusion at 11 to 18 percent elongation. The perineurium provides the main resistance against stretch injury.

The degree of nerve damage is more related to the severity of the compression than to its duration, and permanent nerve damage can occur within a relatively short time. Mild compression may cause only minimal demyelination with widening of the nodal areas. Chronic, severe pressure will produce complete intranodal segmental demyelination with complete nerve conduction block.

Proximal entrapment of a nerve may render it more susceptible to the effects of a more distal entrapment (double-crush phenomenon).[5] This may be due to a diminished axoplasmic flow distally caused by the proximal compression.

Most nerve entrapment lesions represent either a physiologic conduction block (impulse transmission inhibited by local ischemia), neuropraxia (conduction block due to local myelin damage), axonotmesis (loss of axon fiber continuity with intact endoneural tubes and distal Wallerian degeneration), or more likely a combination of these, with different fibers damaged to varying degrees.[3] Consequently, some elements of the lesion will show rapid recovery, with others delayed.

CARPAL TUNNEL SYNDROME

Compression of the median nerve at the wrist—carpal tunnel syndrome (CTS)—is the most common entrapment neuropathy in the upper extremity. The carpal canal is an open-ended, rigid compartment whose floor and walls are the bony carpus and roof the thick transverse carpal ligament. The median nerve lies directly beneath the transverse carpal ligament, with the flexor tendons encased by the synovium of the radial and ulnar bursae deep to it (Fig. 68-1).

Although open-ended, physical forces applied within the rigid confines of the canal mechanically deform the nerve and interfere with its local blood supply. With flexion and extension of the wrist and fingers, there is normal 15-mm excursion of the median nerve and 50-mm excursion of the flexor tendons, causing friction and compression of the nerve against both the tendons and transverse carpal ligament. Reduced cross-sectional area within the carpal canal (carpal stenosis) has been reported, as has increased pressures within the carpal canal in patients with CTS (32 mmHg compared to a normal value of 2.5 mmHg), with a tripling of those values with the wrist in flexion and extension.[6,6a]

Any factor decreasing the space within the carpal canal will cause pressure against the median nerve, the most common such factor being a nonspecific tenosynovitis of the flexor tendons.[7] Trauma may alter the canal or cause posttraumatic scarring and fibrosis, as may inflammatory conditions (rheumatoid arthritis, gout, pseudogout), tumors endocrinopathies (hypothyroidism, acromegaly, diabetes mellitus), or developmental conditions (persistent median artery, abnormal muscle bellies, proximal or hypertrophied lumbrical muscles). Pregnancy or the use of the contraceptive pill can affect the nerve, presumably by increasing retention of extracellular fluid and causing soft tissue swelling within the canal.

Precisely because CTS is so common, with such a broad spectrum of clinical symptoms and findings, the differential diagnosis must include cervical radiculopathy, collagen vascular disorders, thoracic outlet syndrome, Raynaud's phenomenon, reflex sympathetic dystrophy, peripheral neuropathies, and other types of peripheral nerve entrapment (pronator syndrome, anterior interosseous syndrome).[7,8]

CLINICAL DIAGNOSIS

Pain, numbness, and paresthesia are the most frequent complaints.[9] Classic burning pain awakens the patient at night, 2 to 4 h after retiring. Vague complaints (swelling of the fingers and clumsiness) are common. Driving a car, knitting, or vigorous physical activities may precipitate symptoms. Pain may radiate to the forearm.

Most of the nerve fibers of the median nerve within the carpal canal are sensory, explaining the predominance of sensory symptoms and findings.[7] Sensory findings range from a minimal hypesthesia to complete anesthesia of the median nerve–innervated field of the hand (thumb, index, middle and radial half of ring finger, and distal two-thirds of the radial palm). Threshold tests (Semmes-Weinstein monofilament and vibratory tests) measure a single sensory nerve fiber and are more sensitive in evaluating a gradual progressive change in sensory nerve function due to nerve compression than are innervation density tests (two-point discrimination) or pinprick. Sensory comparison should be made with the tip of the ipsilateral little finger as well as with the same digits in the opposite hand. Bilateral CTS is not infrequent.

Provocative tests (Phalen's wrist flexion, Tinel's sign, and direct median nerve compression) give evidence of nerve irritability and local entrapment and are especially helpful in patients with intermittent symptoms or exertional (dynamic) CTS. The direct median nerve compression test is the most sensitive (0.87) and most specific

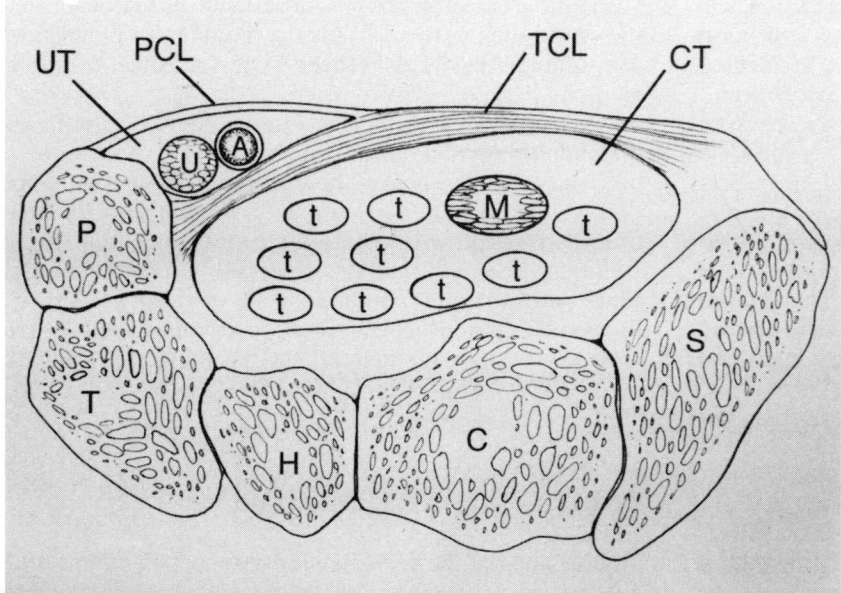

Figure 68-1 Cross section of wrist, illustrating the relationship of the carpal tunnel (CT) and ulnar tunnel (UT) and the location of medial (M) and ulnar nerves. *Key:* TCL, transverse carpal ligament; PCL, palmar carpal ligament; t, tendons; A, ulnar artery; S, scaphoid; C, capitate; H, hammate; T, triquetrum; P, pisiform. (Reproduced with permission from Szabo R, Steinberg D: Nerve entrapment syndromes in the wrist. *J Am Acad Orthop Surg* 2:115–123, 1994.)

(0.90).[10] The time interval required to produce paresthesia or hypesthesia is an indicator of the severity of nerve entrapment. Isolated testing of the abductor pollicis brevis may show thenar muscle weakness, but visible muscle atrophy is a late finding in CTS.

In the majority of cases, a diagnosis can be made with confidence on the basis of a careful clinical history and physical examination.[9] Where the clinical diagnosis is unclear or there is a need to exclude coexisting conditions, electrophysiologic studies should be considered. Prolongation of distal sensory conduction is the most sensitive criterion. In general, prolongation of sensory conduction beyond 3.5 ms and distal motor latency beyond 4.0 ms confirm the clinical diagnosis. Comparison with the ulnar nerve at the wrist gives helpful information. Current electrodiagnostic accuracy in CTS is approximately 85 to 90 percent accurate but false-negative rates have been reported in 8 to 20 percent.[7] Intact conduction in a small percentage of axons will give normal conduction velocities for the whole nerve. A normal study, therefore, does not rule out the clinical diagnosis. These studies are often of greatest value in localizing the site of nerve entrapment.

TREATMENTS OF CARPAL TUNNEL SYNDROME

Patients with mild, intermittent sensory symptoms without neurologic deficit may be treated with conservative measures (neutral wrist splints at night, nonsteroidal anti-inflammatory agents, correction of endocrinopathies, and corticosteroid injections into the carpal canal).[7] Local injection of corticosteroid into the carpal canal has given a high percentage (75 to 81 percent) of short-term symptomatic relief but full relief over 1 year in only 20 percent.[11]

Those with progressing persistent symptoms, with neurologic deficits (marked sensory loss, thenar weakness or atrophy), or significant functional impairment of the hand are candidates for surgical decompression of the carpal tunnel.[9] Release of the transverse carpal ligament enlarges the volume of the carpal canal by 24 percent and changes its shape from oval to circular, with an increase in the palmar dorsal diameter. The standard operation is an open release, directly incising the transverse carpal ligament. More recently, an endoscopic carpal tunnel release has been introduced; quantitative outcomes are nearly identical, but the functional outcomes were achieved more rapidly with endoscopic release.[12] A slightly higher incidence of more serious complications—such as direct injury to nerve and or tendon within the carpal canal—has been noted with the endoscopic release.

Results of surgical release reflect the degree of preoperative neurologic damage.[9] Those with intermittent or mild, persistent symptoms obtain rapid relief. Those with moderate sensory deficits usually regain normal sensation, but over a longer period. Those with long-standing, severe sensory loss or muscle atrophy will obtain relief of pain, but with less than full sensory recovery; the return of thenar muscle function is similar to that of sensation.

Acute CTS associated with trauma is a special problem.[6] This is an acute compartment syndrome involving the median nerve in the carpal tunnel. Increasing pain (particularly if dysesthetic), worsening of CTS symptoms, or progression of neurologic deficits in the presence of trauma are all indications for immediate release of the carpal tunnel. A compartment pressure of more than 45 mmHg is usually found in these circumstances. Delayed surgical release in the presence of significant compression of the median nerve can result in a permanent loss of median nerve function.

Complications of CTS surgery are more common than currently realized (12 percent).[12a] These include reflex sympathetic dystrophy, surgical scar tenderness, and/or hypertrophy, neuromas of the palmar cutaneous branches of both the median and ulnar nerves, postsurgical tenosynovitis, flexor tendon adhesions, and bowstringing of the flexor tendons. Incomplete release of the transverse carpal ligament has frequently been reported,[12b] but this represents inadequate surgery rather than a complication. The use of a volar splint or firm dressing to hold the wrist in slight extension has been advocated to prevent bowstringing as well as to provide constant pressure against the wound to inhibit reflex sympathetic dystrophy. Early active finger range-of-motion exercises encourage nerve and tendon excursion.

PRONATOR TERES SYNDROME

Entrapment of the median nerve in the proximal forearm as it passes between the two heads of the pronator teres is termed *pronator syndrome*.[13,14] The muscle belly or tendinous bands within either head of the pronator teres are the most common cause, although the lacertus fibrosus, ligament of Struthers, and fibrous arch of the flexor digitorum superficialis are also reported as causative factors[15] (Fig. 68-2).

Aching pain, fatigue, and muscle cramping in the proximal forearm are the most frequent subjective complaints.[13,14] Repetitive forearm pronation-supination (using tools or playing tennis) aggravates symptoms. The patient has difficulty in describing and localizing symptoms because the nerve entrapment is often mild and intermittent. Paresthesias may occur with more severe entrapment, but persistent numbness is uncommon. In contrast to CTS, nocturnal paresthesias are rare and wrist position does not exacerbate symptoms.

Local tenderness to deep compression is found over the site of nerve entrapment with reproduction of the patient's symptoms. Tinel's sign may be present over the site of entrapment, but measurable weakness is usually not found in isolated muscle examination. Certain muscle-stressing tests may localize the site of nerve entrapment.[15,16] Pain or paresthesias evoked by resisted pronation of the forearm with the elbow extended implicates the pronator teres; simultaneous resistive flexion of the elbow

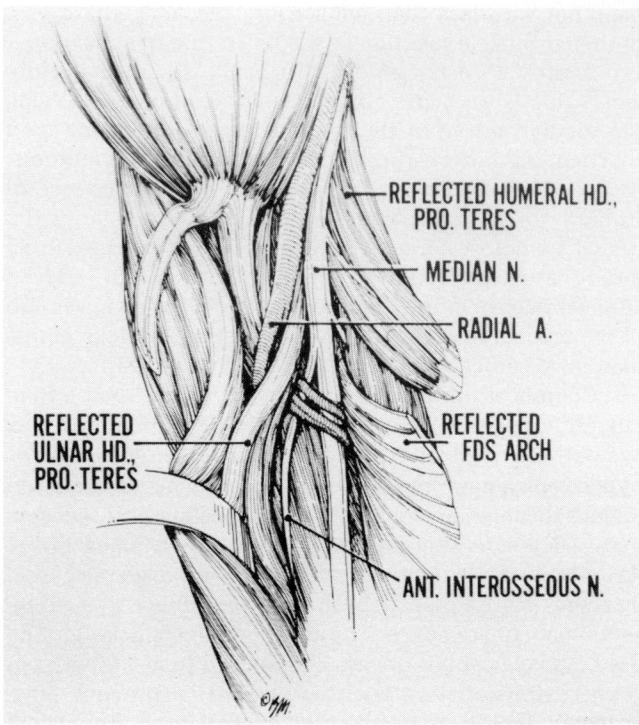

Figure 68-2 Exposure of the median and interosseous nerves by reflection of the humeral (superficial) head of the pronator teres and the radial origin of the flexor digitorum. (Reproduced with permission from Eversman W, in Green DP (ed): *Operative Hand Surgery.* New York, Churchill Livingstone, 1993.)

and supination of the forearm implicates the lacertus fibrosus; while symptoms evoked by the resisted flexion of the proximal interphalangeal joint of the middle finger points to the arch of the flexor digitorum superficialis.

Electrophysiologic studies are frequently of little help, since entrapment is often intermittent.[1,13] Nerve conduction studies have shown delay in only 20 percent; electromyographic studies may occasionally show evidence of denervation. These studies are usually more helpful in excluding other mimicking conditions such as CTS, cervical radiculopathy (C6 or C7 root), thoracic outlet syndrome, muscle strains of the flexor pronator mass, and musculoskeletal overuse syndromes of the forearm and elbow.

Since the majority of pronator syndromes are mild and symptomatically intermittent, conservative treatment should be utilized initially. Avoidance of aggravating activities, modification of sports activities, and changes in work habits as well as the way one uses the extremity may provide lasting relief. Nonsteroidal anti-inflammatory drugs and the use of a resting splint with the elbow and wrist gently flexed and forearm pronated may be of benefit. Conservative treatment and observation for at least 3 months is reasonable.

Persistence or progression of symptoms suggests the need for surgical exploration and neurolysis of the median nerve.[2,13–15] The lacertus fibrosus, any constricting portion of the pronator teres or fibrous bands within that muscle, and the fibrous arch of the flexor digitorum superficialis

are released so that the median nerve has free passage from the elbow through the proximal and middle forearm. The majority of patients show significant improvement in symptoms following surgery, but forearm muscle soreness and tenderness may persist for 6 months. Results of treatment are obviously dependent upon a proper diagnosis and the degree of preexisting nerve damage.

ANTERIOR INTEROSSEOUS SYNDROME

The anterior interosseous nerve arises from the dorsoradial aspect of the median nerve just at or above the superficial head of the pronator teres (Fig. 68-2). Although described as a purely motor nerve innervating the flexor pollicis longus, flexor digitorum profundus to the index and middle fingers, and pronator quadratus, it does carry afferent sensory fibers from the wrist and distal radial ulnar joint. Compression of this nerve produces a distinct entrapment syndrome,[16–18] although an incomplete syndrome of an isolated paresis of the flexor tendon pollicis longus or flexor profundus to the index finger can present.[19]

Spontaneous vague proximal forearm pain is the most common presenting symptom. Often symptoms last for a short interval then resolve, leaving the patient with loss of strength and dexterity in the radial digits and a weakness of pinch.[16] Fine tip-to-tip pinch is impossible due to inability to flex the distal joints of the thumb and index finger. Weak pulp-to-pulp pinch between the thumb and index finger is possible. Weak to absent flexion against resistance is found with flexor pollicis longus and flexor digitorum profundus to the index finger and less commonly to the middle fingers on clinical exam. Pronator quadrator weakness may be elicited by testing pronation with the elbow flexed. Direct pressure over the nerve produces deep pain and tenderness. Tinel's sign is usually negative and no sensory deficit is present. Electrophysiologic studies are most often positive, showing denervation in the affected muscles.[18,19]

In the absence of a direct penetrating wound or an acute compartment syndrome, initial conservative treatment is advocated for a syndrome of recent onset.[1,2,16] Avoiding aggravating forearm motions, nonsteroidal anti-inflammatory medication, and the occasional use of forearm splints have been advocated. A trial of conservative treatment for 12 weeks is advocated by most authors. If there is no improvement or symptoms worsen, surgical exploration is advocated. The most common constricting structure found has been the tendinous origin of the deep head of the pronator teres, which crosses the anterior interosseous nerve at its hilum from the median nerve. Results of surgery, again, are related to the degree of nerve damage present. Most surgical series have reported good recovery of nerve function,[2,16,17,19] but motor recovery may be prolonged (6 to 9 months). Although spontaneous recovery after 18 months of conservative observation has been reported, most series show a more rapid return of nerve function following neurolysis than after prolonged conservative therapy.

ULNAR NERVE ENTRAPMENT

Entrapment of the ulnar nerve occurs at two major sites, with entrapment at the elbow approximately ten times more common than entrapment at the wrist.

Cubital Tunnel Syndrome

Entrapment neuropathy of the ulnar nerve at the elbow is the second most common site of nerve entrapment seen in the upper extremity and has been reported under various titles, including ulnar neuritis, tardy ulnar palsy, and cubital tunnel syndrome.

Anatomic features play a major causative role. At the elbow, the ulnar nerve has a normal excursion of 12 mm; it elongates approximately 4.7 mm during flexion.[20] The medial head of the triceps pushes the nerve 7 mm medially, adding traction. With flexion, the roof of the cubital tunnel (arcuate ligament) becomes taut and the medial collateral ligament bulges inward, compressing the cubital tunnel space. Cubital tunnel compartment pressures rise from 7 mmHg in extension to 24 mmHg at 90° of flexion.[21] Recurrent subluxation or dislocation of the ulnar nerve occurs in 16 percent, exposing it to repetitive minor trauma and soft tissue friction. Other etiologic factors[1,2] include direct trauma to the nerve, late sequelae from previous trauma (cubitus valgus deformity or irregularities in the postcondylar groove), arthritis with compressing proliferative synovitis and osteophytes, loose bodies, or synovial chondromatosis. Tumor masses or anomalous muscles (anconeus epitrochlearis) may rarely encroach upon the nerve.

Dull, aching discomfort about the medial elbow and ulnar aspect of the forearm accompanied by intermittent paresthesias into the ulnar border of the hand are commonly seen. A popping or clicking sensation about the medial epicondyle may be noted, and prolonged flexion of the elbow exacerbates the pain, paresthesias, and numbness. Sensory symptoms predominate early because the sensory fibers lie superficially in the body of the nerve. Awkwardness with fine hand movement, weakness of grip and pinch, and loss of dexterity are later complaints of motor involvement. Patients may be awakened by severe nocturnal dysesthesias involving the ulnar border of the forearm and hand; these are not relieved by shaking the hand but rather by extending the elbow. This complaint may obviously be confused with CTS.

Sensory examination will demonstrate hypesthesia over the ulnar aspect of both palm and dorsum of the hand as well as the entire little finger and ulnar half of ring finger. Because of anomalous innervation, up to 20 percent of patients have ulnar nerve sensation over the entire ring finger and ulnar half of middle finger. The medial forearm has normal sensation, as it is innervated by the medial cutaneous nerve of the forearm derived directly from the brachial plexus. Hypesthesia of the medial forearm implicates a much more proximal nerve lesion.

Tinel's sign is usually present over the ulnar nerve, behind the medial epicondyle, or over the cubital tunnel. Dynamic flexing of the patient's elbow with the examiner's thumb behind the medial epicondyle may sublux or dislo-cate the ulnar nerve and reproduce the patient's symptoms. Likewise, extreme flexion of the elbow maintained for 1 to 2 min may reproduce the pain, paresthesias, or dysesthesia. Motor examination may reveal weakness of pinch and grip strength as well as flexor carpi ulnaris and flexor digitorum profundus to the ring and little fingers. The ulnar intrinsic muscles are more likely to be affected than the ulnar forearm muscles owing to their topographic location within the ulnar nerve. Atrophy of the intrinsic muscles, clawing of the ring and little fingers, and Froment's sign may be present in severe cases. The conduction velocity of the ulnar nerve will usually be reduced across the elbow and electromyographic studies may show denervation potentials in the affected muscles. These studies are of help in localizing the level of the lesion as well as determining the need or urgency of surgical decompression. Although the elbow is the most common site, entrapment may also occur more proximally (arcade of Struthers) as well as more distally within the forearm (anomalous fibrous bands).[1,2,16] Other conditions to be excluded are cervical radiculopathy (C8 to T1), thoracic outlet syndrome, spinal cord pathology (syringomyelia, tumor) cervical spondylosis, superior sulcus tumor (Pancoast tumor), amyotrophic lateral sclerosis, and localized peripheral neuropathy (Dejerine-Sottas disease, neuritis, leprosy).

For patients with intermittent, mild symptoms and no significant neurologic deficits, conservative treatment is advised.[1,2,16] Repetitive flexion-extension motions and prolonged flexion of the elbow should be avoided. A resting splint or a pillow wrapped around the elbow may be used at night to maintain relative elbow extension. Steroidal injections within the cubital tunnel should be avoided. Surgical treatment is indicated for patients with persistent, significant symptoms or neurologic deficit. Anterior transposition of the ulnar nerve has been the most common technique to alleviate the entrapment.[5] Neurolysis of the nerve with placement of the nerve anterior to the elbow joint axis of motion eliminates most of the causative factors (Fig. 68-3). Following anterior transposition, the nerve is left either subcutaneously or placed submuscularly (Learmouth procedure)[22] beneath the flexor pronator muscle mass. Simple surgical decompression of the roof of the cubital tunnel is effective if this is the only site of entrapment.[23] Unfortunately, it does not address any of the other causative factors of this complex syndrome. Medial epicondylectomy decompresses the cubital tunnel by removing its floor.[24,25] The nerve, however, migrates anteriorly and is left in a subcutaneous position next to the bony structures of the medial elbow, subjecting it to repetitive trauma. Despite this, good relief of sensory symptoms and some improvement in motor deficits have been reported with this procedure.

In general, the postoperative relief of paresthesias and dysesthesias is good.[26] Overall, the return of sensation is better than that of motor function. The more severe the pre-existing neurologic deficits and the longer their duration, the less likely it is that a full functional recovery will occur. Functional recovery may slowly continue over a 3- to 5-year period. Higher success rates are found with subcutaneous transpositions and medial epicondylectomy than with sim-

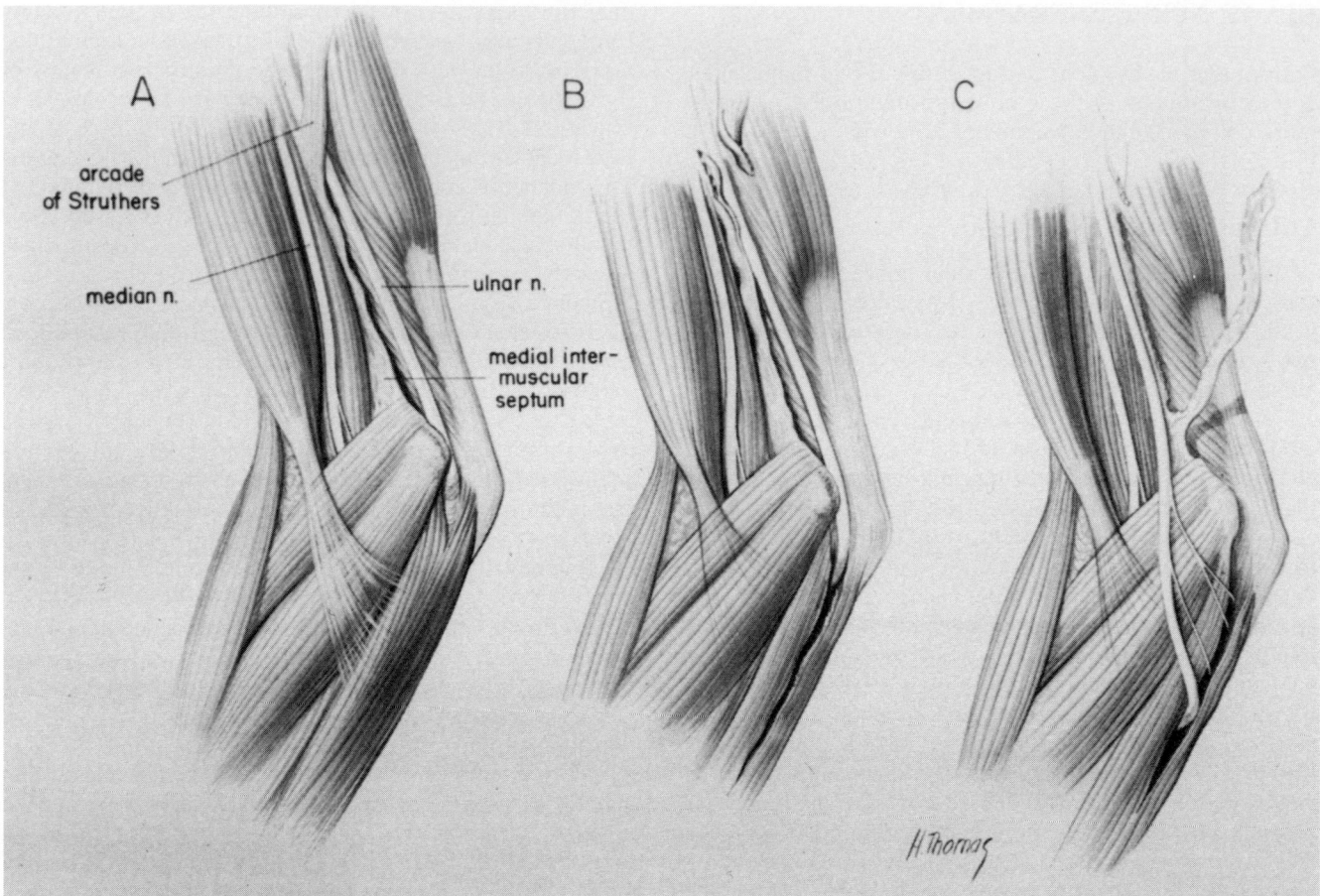

Figure 68-3 *A.* Normal position of the ulnar nerve at the elbow in the postcondylar groove behind the medial epicondyle, with the roof of the cubital tunnel (aponeurosis of humeral and ulnar heads of flexor carpi ulnaris) intact. *B.* Neurolysis of the ulnar nerve with release of the cubital tunnel and arcade of Struthers. *C.* Anterior subcutaneous transposition of the ulnar nerve and motor branches with excision of the medial intermuscular septum. The nerve lies anterior to the elbow joint axis in a straight line. Distal kinking should be prevented. (Reproduced with permission from Spinner M: *Injuries to the Major Branches of the Peripheral Nerves of the Forearm.* Philadelphia, Saunders, 1978.)

ple decompression.[26] The submuscular transposition of Learmouth[22] provides the best relief of symptoms.[26]

Complications from any of the above procedures include a painful hypertrophic scar, neuromas of the medial antebrachial cutaneous nerve, and reflex sympathetic dystrophy. Persistent or recurrent symptoms may be due to kinking of the transposed ulnar nerve, an intact medial intermuscular septum or unreleased arcade of Struthers, or perineural scarring of the nerve back into the postcondylar groove.[27]

Ulnar Tunnel Syndrome

Entrapment neuropathy of the ulnar nerve may occur at the wrist in Guyon's canal,[28] a 4-cm-long ulnar tunnel whose floor comprises the transverse carpal and pisohamate ligaments, its roof is the volar carpal ligament, and its walls are the pisiform and hook of hamate.[27a,28] Only the ulnar artery and nerve course through Guyon's canal (Fig. 68-4). Within the canal, the nerve bifurcates into su-

perficial sensory and deep motor branches separated by the common tendinous origin of the hypothenar muscles. The superficial sensory branch innervates the ulnar palm, little finger, and ulnar half of the ring finger. The deep motor branch loops around the hook of the hamate and innervates all the hypothenar and ulnar innervated intrinsic muscles of the hand except the palmaris brevis, which receives its motor innervation from the sensory branch. The ulnar dorsum of the hand is innervated by the dorsal sensory branch of the ulnar nerve, which leaves the nerve approximately 5 cm proximal to the ulnar styloid.

Guyon's canal is a small closed space; therefore any space-occupying lesion may compromise the ulnar nerve. Ganglia and other soft tissue masses account for 45 percent of reported cases and anomalous muscles another 16 percent.[28] Fractures of the wrist or hook of the hamate, repetitive trauma with thrombosis of the ulnar artery (hypothenar hammer syndrome) edema secondary to burns, inflammatory arthritis, and pseudoaneurysms of the ulnar artery are other causes.

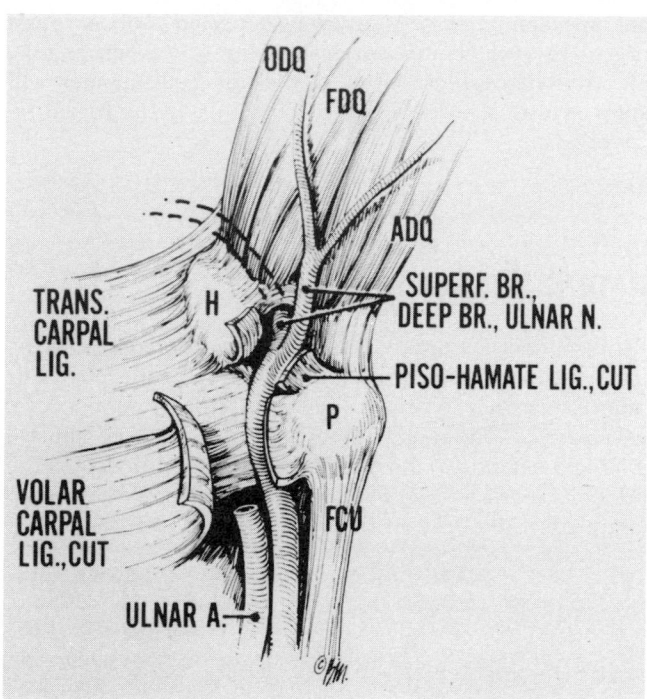

Figure 68-4 Ulnar tunnel (loge of Guyon). The volar carpal and pisohamate ligaments form the roof. The fibrous origin of the hypothenar muscles—opponens digiti quinti (ODQ), flexor digiti quinti (FDQ), and abductor digiti quinti (ADQ)—separates the superficial sensory and deep motor branches and may entrap the deep motor branch. Note the absence of tendons in the ulnar tunnel. (Reproduced with permission from Eversman W, in Green DP (ed): *Operative Hand Surgery.* New York, Churchill Livingstone, 1993.)

Depending upon the level of entrapment within Guyon's canal, the patient may complain of aching discomfort in the ulnar region of the wrist and hand, with varying combinations of weakness, atrophy, paresthesias and hypesthesias.[28,29] Patients may have a pure sensory deficit, pure motor deficit, or combination of both. Careful sensory evaluation is critical in that the abnormal sensation over the ulnar dorsum of the hand implies nerve entrapment proximal to Guyon's canal. A pure motor deficit involving only the ulnar-innervated interosseous and lumbrical muscles implicates entrapment of the deep motor branch at or distal to the hood of the hamate, whereas involvement of both the hypothenar and intrinsic muscles implicates a more proximal canal entrapment. A pure sensory deficit implies a distal lesion within the canal, usually by thrombosis or pseudoaneurysm of the ulnar artery. Allen's test and Doppler studies are helpful diagnostically. The mixed motor and sensory lesion is usually found within the proximal canal, with ganglion and other soft tissue tumors or anomalies the main cause. Magnetic resonance imaging is helpful.

Differential diagnosis must include cubital tunnel syndrome, thoracic outlet syndrome, and cervical root compression. Altered sensation along the medial forearm indicates pathology above the elbow, such as brachial plexus, thoracic outlet, cervical spine, or spinal cord problems.

Examination may reveal local tenderness to deep pressure over the nerve, a positive Tinel's sign, a positive Phalen's (wrist flexion) test, palpable swelling or mass, or calloused skin over the hypothenar eminence. A positive Allen's test (no arterial filling) is present with an ulnar artery thrombosis, and discrete distal fingertip subcutaneous infarcts and subungual splinter hemorrhages can result from distal thrombotic emboli. Cold intolerance and Raynaud's phenomenon may also be noted. Electrophysiologic studies most often show delayed distal motor latency, and denervation fibrillations will often be found in the ulnar intrinsics.

As in all nerve entrapment syndromes, treatment of the ulnar tunnel syndrome depends upon the cause, severity, and duration of the problem.[2,16,28] Mild symptoms and neurologic deficits resulting from a single traumatic episode or from mild repetitive chronic trauma over a short period of time may be treated with rest, splinting, and avoidance of repetitive trauma. Patients who fail to improve or those with more severe neurologic deficits should undergo surgical decompression with complete neurolysis of the nerve and its motor and sensory branches. Coexisting contributory abnormalities should be simultaneously excised (hook of hamate nonunion, ganglion, anomalous muscle, or fibrous band). Vascular abnormalities (thrombosis or pseudoaneurysm) should be resected or undergo vascular reconstruction. Complications include injury to the palmar cutaneous branch of the ulnar nerve and failure to adequately decompress the deep motor branch distal to the hook of the hamate. Resection of the hook of the hamate or pisiform does not result in any functional disability.

RADIAL NERVE ENTRAPMENT

Although injury to the radial and posterior interosseous nerves is far more commonly due to trauma where they lie adjacent to the shafts of the humerus and radius, entrapment neuropathies do occur and are noted at three distinct levels.

As the radial nerve courses posteriorly along the spiral groove of the humerus, it passes through a fibrous arch under the lateral head of the triceps just posterior to the deltoid insertion. Onset of symptoms usually follows vigorous exercise or strenuous physical effort, and patients may present with a partial or complete high radial nerve palsy.[1] These palsies usually resolve spontaneously over several weeks. More distally, the nerve pierces the lateral intermuscular septum, but compression here is usually associated with major trauma, especially fracture of the humerus.

Radial nerve entrapment in the proximal forearm produces a confusing picture of two distinct clinical syndromes—one mainly pain, the other weakness.[30] Although certain compressing structures tend to be associated with one or the other, these syndromes are probably expressions of varying degrees of progressive nerve compression, one mild and intermittent and the other constant.[31]

POSTERIOR INTEROSSEOUS NERVE SYNDROME

This is the syndrome of finger and wrist weakness, often heralded by a deep aching pain in the forearm, that resolves within several days or weeks, only to be followed by weakness and varying degrees of paresis of the wrist and digital extensors. With complete paralysis, there is weak wrist extension in radial deviation, since the extensor carpi radialis longus is innervated by the radial nerve above the elbow. The extensor carpi ulnaris is paralyzed and offers no counterbalance in extension. The metacarpophalangeal joints of all five digits cannot be extended beyond 45°, although the interphalangeal joints can be extended by the intact ulnar intrinsic muscles, giving the appearance of an intrinsic-plus hand. Sensation over the radial dorsum of the hand is normal. More commonly, an incomplete motor paresis is present, with lack of extension either to the long and ring fingers, ring and little fingers, or even isolated to thumb extension. This is associated with weakness of both power grip and wrist extension.

Causative factors of compression[1,30] include mass lesions (ganglia, lipoma, rheumatoid synovitis of the elbow joint, and bicipital tendon bursitis at the radial tubercle), trauma (dislocation at the elbow or Monteggia's fracture with dislocation of the radial head), surgical intervention (resection of the radial head, plating of a proximal radius fracture), and iatrogenic injections in the lateral elbow. The anatomic anomalies found with radial tunnel syndrome are less commonly implicated in posterior interosseous nerve syndrome. Differentiation from a high radial nerve lesion is made by observing the lack of sensory loss and the presence of a functioning brachioradialis and extensor carpi radialis longus. Lead poisoning neuropathy is usually bilateral but may start unilaterally. It produces a full radial motor palsy without any sensory loss, although initially, only the inability to extend the metacarpophalangeal joints of the middle and ring fingers may be seen. Conversion reaction (hysterical wrist drop) may be differentiated by the patient's inability to extend the interphalangeal joints as well as the metacarpophalangeal joints. Polyarteritis may produce a transient isolated posterior interosseous palsy. Last, rupture of the extensor tendons to the thumb or multiple digits, especially in rheumatoid patients, may be differentiated by the tenodesis effect with passive flexion of the wrist. Electrophysiologic nerve studies may show an increased distal motor latency across the arcade of Frohse as well as denervation fibrillations in the affected muscles.

Treatment for posterior interosseous nerve palsy in the presence of a mass lesion should be surgical exploration with removal of the mass. If no mass lesion is present on examination or MR imaging, a period of observation of 8 to 12 weeks before surgical exploration is reasonable. Electromyographic studies of the affected muscles will show electrical evidence of recovery prior to clinical recovery.

RADIAL TUNNEL SYNDROME

Radial tunnel syndrome (resistant tennis elbow) is a dynamic structural compression syndrome of the posterior interosseous nerve causing pain with little or no muscular weakness.[8,30] The radial tunnel begins at the radiohumeral joint and extends to the end of the supinator muscle in the proximal forearm (Fig. 68-5). Four anatomic features may compress the nerve in the radial tunnel: fibrous bands

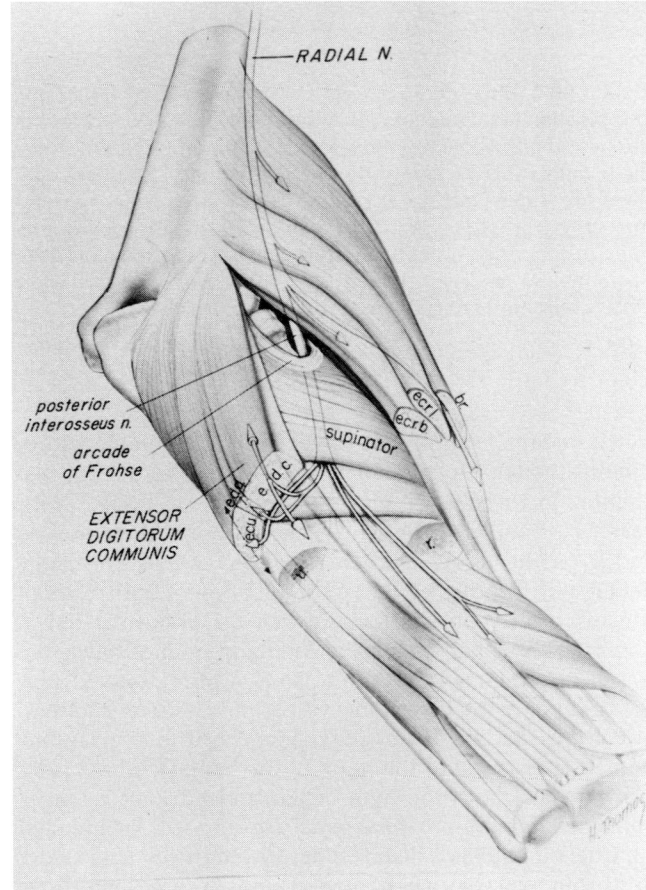

Figure 68-5 The radial tunnel exposed through the internervous plane between the extensor carpi radialis brevis (ECRB) and the extensor digitorum communis (EDC). The fibrous arcade of frohse (superficial head of the supinator muscle) is partially encircling the posterior interosseous nerve. (Reproduced with permission from Spinner M: *Injuries to the Major Branches of the Peripheral Nerves of the Forearm.* Philadelphia, Saunders, 1978.)

that tether the nerve to the radial humeral capsule, a fibrous medial edge along the extensor carpi radialis brevis, a radial recurrent leash of vessels overlying the nerve, and, last, the fibrous arcade of Frohse. This fibrous arcade of the proximal superficial edge of the supinator is normally present in 20 to 30 percent of the population,[16] but it has been found in 80 percent of surgically explored radial tunnel syndromes. Entrapment of the nerve at the distal edge of the supinator has also been reported. No space-occupying mass lesion has been reported in this syndrome.

Dull, aching pain located deep in the extensor muscle mass and often radiating distally to the wrist is the main symptom.[31] Nocturnal pain is frequent. Pain is usually absent upon awakening, but often the patient develops a persistent aching soreness by day's end. Occasional complaint of dysesthesias in the distribution of the superficial radial sensory nerve are noted. Weakness of grip strength is a frequent complaint, particularly with repetitive or prolonged gripping movements. The major differential diagnosis is lateral epicondylitis (tennis elbow), which, however, may occur concomitantly with radial tunnel syndrome (resistant tennis elbow).[32] The most important point of physical diagnosis is the localized tenderness directly over the posterior interosseous nerve 5 cm distal to the lateral epicondyle. Increased pain may be elicited by resisted active supination and passive forced pronation of the forearm, with pain caused by tightening of the proximal edge of the supinator muscle across the nerve. The "middle finger extension test"[8] may aggravate pain symptoms, since the extensor carpi radialis brevis inserts into the base of the third metacarpal, tensing the medial edge of that muscle against the nerve.

The most reliable diagnostic test is a local anesthetic block into the radial tunnel with relief of the pain.[33] A posterior interosseous palsy should accompany the pain relief to indicate accurate placement of the anesthetic block. It may be necessary to inject the lateral epicondyle to rule out the classic tennis elbow tendinitis. Electrophysiologic studies of this condition have been normal. Recently, however, increased motor latencies have been shown in these patients during active forceful supination of the forearm as the study is being performed.

In this pain syndrome, conservative measures are the first form of treatment. Rest of the elbow and wrist from repetitive stressful activity, splinting of the elbow in mild flexion and supination with wrist extension, and a course of nonsteroidal anti-inflammatory medication are indicated. These palsies usually resolve spontaneously over the course of several weeks. Surgical exploration with careful neurolysis of the posterior interosseous nerve throughout its entire course in the radial tunnel is indicated if conservative treatment fails. However, only 70 percent of patients report good to excellent relief of pain following neurolysis.[33]

In the distal forearm, the superficial sensory branch of the radial nerve leaves the cover of the brachioradialis muscle and courses distally on the radial dorsal surface on the distal forearm, wrist, and hand. Traumatic neuritis or compression of this branch produces severe dysesthetic pain over that area, associated with an exquisitely

sensitive Tinel's sign at the site of entrapment and numbness distally.[34] Lacerations, surgery for de Quervain's tendinitis, tight jewelry, watchbands, snug casts, handcuffs, insertion of intravenous needles, and dialysis shunts have all been reported as causes. Complications from this entrapment syndrome or injury can be devastating, leaving the patient with a florid reflex sympathetic dystrophy.

Treatment consists in relieving any physical compression over the nerve. Local steroid injections may be beneficial, but symptoms may take several months to resolve. For persistent, severe symptoms, surgical neurolysis is warranted. If it is entrapped in scarred fibrous tissue, the nerve should be meticulously neurolysed and placed under healthy subcutaneous tissues and skin. If a neuroma is found, the prognosis is much more guarded. A more proximal resection of the nerve underneath the brachioradialis, neurorhaphy of the radial nerve, transposition of the neuroma deeper into the forearm, or capping of the nerve with silicone have all been advocated.

REFERENCES

1. Lister G: *The Hand: Diagnosis and Indications,* 3d ed. Edinburgh, Churchill Livingstone, 1993.
2. Sunderland S: *Nerves and Nerve Injuries,* 2d ed. London, Churchill Livingstone, 1978.
3. Lundborg G, Dahlin LB: Pathophysiology of nerve compression. *Hand Clin* 8:215–227, 1992.
4. Ochoa J: Nerve fiber pathology in acute and chronic compression, in Omer GE, Spinner M (eds): *Management of Peripheral Nerve Problems.* Philadelphia, Saunders, 1980.
5. Osterman AL: Double crush phenomenon: The double crush syndrome. *Orthop Clin North Am* 19:147–155, 1991.
6. Gelberman RH: *Acute Carpal Tunnel Syndrome: Operative Nerve Repair and Reconstruction.* Philadelphia, Lippincott, 1991, pp 939–948.
6a. Gelberman RH, Hergenroeder PT, Hargens AR, Lungborg: Carpal canal pressures. *J Bone Surg* 63A:380–383, 1981.
7. Szabo RM, Steinberg DR: Nerve entrapment syndromes in the wrist. *J Am Acad Orthop Surg* 2:115–123, 1994.
8. Lister GD, Belsole RB, Kleinert HE: The radial tunnel syndrome. *J Hand Surg* 4:52–59, 1979.
9. Phalen GS: The carpal tunnel syndrome: Seventeen years' experience in diagnosis and treatment of 654 hands. *J Bone Joint Surg* 48A:211–228, 1968.
10. Durkan JA: A new diagnostic test for carpal tunnel syndrome. *J Bone Joint Surg* 73A:535–538, 1991.
11. Green DP: Diagnostic and therapeutic value of carpal tunnel injection. *J Hand Surg* 9A:850–854, 1984.
12. Brown RA, Gelberman RH, Seiler JG III: Carpal tunnel release: A prospective, randomized assessment of open and endoscopic methods. *J Bone Joint Surg* 75A:1265–1275, 1993.
12a. MacDonald RI, Lichtman DM, Hanlon JJ, Wilson JN: Complications of surgical release for carpal tunnel syndrome. *J Hand Surg* 3:70–76, 1987.
12b. Langloh ND, Linscheid RL: Recurrent and unrelieved carpal tunnel syndrome. *Clin Orthop* 83:41–47, 1972.
13. Hartz CR, Linscheid RL, Gramse RR, Daube JR: The pronator teres syndrome: Compressive neuropathy of the median nerve. *J Bone Joint Surg* 63A:885–890, 1981.

14. Johnson RK, Spinner M, Shrewsbury MM: Medial nerve entrapment syndrome in the proximal forearm. *J Hand Surg* 4:48–61, 1979.

15. Johnson RK, Spinner M: Median nerve compression in the forearm: The pronator tunnel syndrome, in *Nerve Compression Syndromes—Diagnosis and Treatment*. NJ, Slack, 1989, pp 137–151.

16. Spinner M: Injuries to the major branches of peripheral nerves of the forearm, 2d ed. Philadelphia, Saunders, 1978.

17. Spinner M: The anterior interosseous nerve syndrome. *J Bone Joint Surg* 52A:84–94, 1970.

18. Stern PJ, Fassler PR: *Anterior Interosseous Nerve Compression Syndrome: Operative Nerve Repair and Reconstruction.* Philadelphia, Lippincott, 1991, pp 983–994.

19. Hill NA, Howard FM, Huffer BR: The incomplete anterior interosseous nerve syndrome. *J Hand Surg* 10A:4–16, 1985.

20. Apfelberg DB, Larson SJ: Dynamic anatomy of the ulnar nerve at the elbow. *Plast Reconst Surg* 51:76, 1973.

21. Pechan J, Julis I: The pressure measurement in the ulnar nerve: A contribution to the pathophysiology of the cubital tunnel syndrome. *J Biomech* 8:75–79, 1975.

22. Leffert RD: Anterior submuscular transposition of the ulnar nerve by the Learmouth technique. *J Hand Surg* 7:147–155, 1982.

23. Osborne GV: Compression neuritis of the ulnar nerve at the elbow. *Hand* 2:10, 1970.

24. Craven PR, Green DP: Cubital tunnel syndrome: Treatment by medial epicondylectomy. *J Bone Joint Surg* 62A:986–989, 1980.

25. Froimson A, Zahrawi F: Treatment of compression neuropathy of the ulnar nerve at the elbow by epicondylectomy and neurolysis. *J Hand Surg* 5:391–395, 1980.

26. Dellon AL: Review of treatment results for ulnar nerve entrapment at the elbow. *J Hand Surg* 14A:688–700, 1989.

27. Rogers MR, Bergfield TG, Aulicino PL: The failed ulnar nerve transposition: Etiology and treatment. *Clin Orthop* 269: 193–200, 1991.

27a. Dupont C, Cloutier GE, Pevost Y, Diaon M: Ulnar tunnel syndrome at the wrist. *J Bone Joint Surg* 47A:757–761, 1965.

28. Gelberman RH: *Ulnar Tunnel Syndrome: Operative Nerve Repair and Reconstruction.* Philadelphia, Lippincott, 1991, pp 1131–1143.

29. Shea JD, McClain EJ: Ulnar nerve compression syndrome at and below the wrist. *J Bone Joint Surg* 51A:1095–1103, 1969.

30. Roles NC, Mandsley R: Radial tunnel syndrome; resistant tennis elbow as a nerve entrapment. *J Bone Joint Surg* 54B:499–508, 1972.

31. Moss SH, Switzer HE: Radial tunnel syndrome: A spectrum of clinical presentations. *J Hand Surg* 8:414–420, 1983.

32. Werner CO: Lateral elbow pain and posterior interosseous nerve entrapment. *Acta Orthop Scand* 174(suppl):1–62, 1979.

33. Ritts GD, Wood MB, Linscheid RL: Radial tunnel syndrome: A ten year surgical experience. *Clin Orthop* 219:201–205, 1987.

34. Dellon AL, Mackinnon SE: Radial sensory nerve entrapment in the forearm. *J Hand Surg* 11A:199–205, 1986.

CHAPTER 69

Neuromuscular Disorders in the Upper Extremity

Donald K. Bynum

CEREBRAL PALSY

Surgery of the upper extremity has a definite but limited role in the management of cerebral palsy. The degree of involvement in the upper extremity ranges from essentially none in diplegia to severe in the total-care spastic quadriplegic. The goals of surgery may range from improving function or hygiene to merely enhancing cosmesis. The key to successful surgical treatment is a good matchup of treatment goals, expectations of parents and patient, and surgical procedures. Achieving this matchup may be harder with these patients than in any other field of orthopaedics. This chapter is not intended to go into the details of operative procedures but rather to serve as a general guide to understanding.

General Principles and Preoperative Evaluation

Most of the functional deficits and deformities in patients with cerebral palsy result from excessive spasticity in the flexor muscle groups. Orthopaedic treatment is directed at attempts to rebalance the muscle forces and correct fixed joint contractures and occasional joint instabilities. There are few hard and fast rules to guide the selection process, but the following principles have gained general acceptance. Tendon lengthening gives a more predictable outcome than tendon transfer. Lengthening both weakens the muscle and diminishes the stretch reflex and will not result in a reverse deformity. Muscles that are overactive during opposite functions, i.e., during both grasp and release, may cause a reverse deformity if transferred and should be released or lengthened rather than transferred.[1] Tendon transfers should be performed using muscles that the patient can voluntarily control or muscles that act synergistically.[2,3] Rigid joint or bony deformities cannot be corrected by tendon transfers alone. Joints that cannot be controlled by voluntary muscle actions should be tenodesed or arthrodesed prior to tendon transfer. The surgeon should bear in mind, however, that the tenodesis effect of a movable wrist joint is extremely important and should usually be preserved. Arthrodesis is the last resort in management of the wrist.[1]

Athetosis is a form of cerebral palsy that results in dyskinetic movements or posturing rather than spasticity. In general, surgery should be avoided in athetosis, as the outcome is unpredictable. A possible exception is arthrodesis of a joint in which the arthrodesis has been simulated preoperatively by precise long-term casting, splinting, or pin fixation. However, there is insufficient support of this criterion in the literature to recommend it without reservation.

The factors that correlate best with a successful outcome are intelligence or cognition, sensibility, voluntary muscle control in the hand, motivation, placement of the hand in space, and age of the patient. An IQ of 70 or above is desirable if the patient is to cooperate with a postoperative rehabilitation regimen. The success of hygienic procedures usually does not depend on the patient's IQ.[3]

Most authors agree that good sensibility in the hand is a prerequisite for a good result in which improved function is the goal of surgery. Two-point discrimination, stereognosis, graphesthesia, and texture discrimination are useful tests of sensory impairment. Of these, two-point discrimination is probably the most reliable when the patient is old enough and intelligent enough to cooperate with the test. If two-point discrimination is not better than 10 mm, there is probably insufficient sensory input to control the hand except by visual cues.[3] There is no documentable improvement in sensory function following surgery.

As might be expected, the quality of voluntary muscle control is a good correlate in predicting the success of any operation.[4] Although the need for control in the hand is obvious, the need for control of placement is just as important. The ability to place the involved hand on the head and then to the opposite knee within 5 s is considered a favorable indicator of achieving improved function.[3] Where primitive mass reflexes (tonic neck reflex, etc.) interfere with motor control, there is poor functional potential.[2]

Older patients may have dissociated themselves from the disabled limb and thus would not be good candidates for functional improvement.[5] The pattern of functional deformity can be reliably determined by age 3,[1] so surgery should be performed over the next few years. The patient will not gain more selective muscle control when surgery is performed early but may learn to use the new "pattern" more readily than if the change is delayed.

Candidates for functional improvement should have favorable assessments in at least two and preferably three of the above areas. Cosmetic and hygienic improvements are readily achieved and the decision for surgery rests with those special considerations, not with the other factors mentioned above. Good motivation cannot ensure a good outcome in cerebral palsy surgery; on the other hand, if improved function is the goal, absence of motivation will result in complete failure.

Muscle testing of patients with cerebral palsy is very complicated. Preoperatively, the surgeon must determine not only the strength of a muscle but also the degree of voluntary control of the muscle; the level of activity of the muscle during each separate functional task (phasic activity) such as grasp, release, and pinch; and finally whether the muscle is subject to pathologic reflexes such as the stretch reflex, clonus, or retained infantile reflexes.[1,2,6] This type of examination is difficult, but with experience it can be fairly reliable. A dynamic electromyogram can be used to supplement manual muscle testing.[3]

Another adjunct to the preoperative evaluation is temporary myoneural blockade of the spastic muscles with alcohol, local anesthetic, or botulinum A toxin.[7] Alcohol or botulinum A toxin blockade will last for several weeks. This allows some time for the uninjected muscles to show their true strength.[1] Thus the patient and surgeon will have a better idea of what to expect from tendon lengthening or release.

Treatment of Specific Regions

Shoulder

Surgical correction is seldom required at the shoulder. Typical posturing includes adduction and internal rotation. If this position limits hand placement, lengthening of the pectoralis major and subscapularis is the recommended procedure[6] and should be augmented by aggressive physical therapy postoperatively. Rotational osteotomy of the humerus is rarely indicated.

Elbow

The usual deformity at the elbow is flexion, as either contracture or dynamic "overflow" or a combination of both. When elbow flexion limits hand placement, appropriate correction should be attempted. This will usually occur at 45° or greater contracture.[6] Surgical correction is directed at the primary elbow flexors.[8] Anterior capsulotomy of the elbow may be required in more severe cases or in older children. These procedures result in an average improvement of 40° of extension, retain active elbow flexion sufficient to enable patients to place the hand to the mouth, and provide lasting correction. Loss of supination has not been a problem with these procedures.

Forearm

Pronation contracture of the forearm is common in cerebral palsy.[6] This may be reduced by releasing the pronator teres from its insertion or by rerouting it to act as a supinator.[9] Occasionally the pronator quadratus will require release.[6] Some improvement in supination may follow a flexor-pronator slide or transfer of flexor muscles around the ulnar border of the forearm to the dorsum of the hand or wrist.[10] Neutral rotation is the optimum position and excessive supination should be avoided.[1]

Wrist and Hand

In the wrist and hand, the usual problems are flexed wrists, flexed fingers, and thumb-in-palm deformity. Functionally, the impairments include a poor release of grasp because of the finger flexor spasticity, weak opening of the hand due to weak finger extensors, weak grasp because the wrist is held in flexion during grasp, and inability to open the hand with the thumb retracted out of the palm. Occasional patients will have swan-neck deformity of the fingers. Surgical procedures to improve function are generally aimed at diminishing flexor spasticity, augmenting exten-

sor strength, or creating a more stable joint by arthrodesis, tenodesis, or capsulodesis. Cosmetic and hygienic procedures involve releasing tight contractures and stabilizing joint position by arthrodesis.

A majority of patients who are candidates for functional reconstruction have weak finger extension.[11,12] Surgery may be directed at either weakening the flexor tightness, strengthening finger extension, or both. The flexor-pronator slide has been used successfully in the past as a utilitarian procedure to provide improved function, control, and cosmesis.[13–15] Objections to this procedure are that some patients may lose too much grip strength or may develop a reverse deformity and that the procedure is not selective enough in patients who already have some selective control.[1,2] Another observation is that when the flexor pollicis longus (FPL) origin is released as part of the flexor-pronator slide, the existing balance of the thumb-in-palm deformity is changed. Correction of the thumb deformity must then be delayed until the effects of this rebalancing can be determined.

A more selective approach would combine the clinical classification of Zancolli[16] with the use of preoperative dynamic electromyographic (EMG) evaluation[11] to determine whether lengthening or specific transfers would be appropriate. Patients can be grouped into three categories. In group 1, mild, the patient can fully extend the fingers while the wrist remains flexed 20° or less. Group 2 patients can extend the fingers only while the wrist is flexed more than 20°. This group is also assessed on the basis of whether any degree of active wrist extension is possible while the fingers are held flexed. The group 2A patients have selective wrist extension, whereas the group 2B patients do not. Group 3 patients are severely involved and lack any active extension of either wrist or fingers. Present EMG and clinical data indicate that muscles which are active during a desired activity can be reliably transferred, whereas those that are active during all phases of the grasp-release cycle or when the limb is at rest should be lengthened or released. Muscles with isolated activity in grasp should be transferred preferentially to improve grasp, whereas those with isolated activity in release should be preferentially transferred to improve release.[11] Thus, if the flexor carpi ulnaris (FCU) is overactive during release, it can be tenotomized or lengthened in the mild (group 1) patient or transferred[10] to the extensor digitorum communis (EDC) to augment finger extension in the group 2A patient. If the patient's release is adequate but wrist extension is poor (group 2B), the FCU can be transferred to the extensor carpi radialis brevis (ECRB). This will also enhance grip strength by placing the wrist into a more extended position. The surgeon should confirm preoperatively, however, that the patient has active finger extension when the wrist is passively held in the desired degree of extension (usually neutral). Transfer of the FCU to the EDC is the more reliable procedure.[5,11]

When strengthening of grasp is desired, several alternatives bear consideration. If the FCU is overactive in grasp but not in release, it is logical to transfer it to the ECRB to augment extension. This transfer should not be performed when the FCU is overactive in release and the patient lacks finger extension. Alternatively, a flexor digitorum superficialis (FDS) can be transferred to the ECRB as a synergistic transfer.

In the severely involved hand, the EMGs will show overactivity in all attempted phases of grasp. In that instance, lengthening of all the flexors by proximal muscle slide, Z lengthening of tendons at the wrist, or superficialis to profundus transfer will provide cosmetic and hygienic improvement.[17] Proximal-row carpectomy[18] is an alternative method of effectively weakening tight flexors, which retains wrist motion for its tenodesis effect. This procedure is useful when wrist contracture is so severe that neurovascular structures limit the amount of extension that might be obtained with muscle-tendon lengthenings. Transfers can be combined with proximal-row carpectomy to provide additional balance.

Some patients with spastic cerebral palsy will have swan-neck deformities of the fingers.[19] Tenodesis of the proximal interphalangeal (PIP) joint into flexion using a slip of the FDS[15] provides reliable, durable correction of this problem.

Thumb

The usual deformity of the thumb, the thumb-in-palm deformity, imposes functional problems including small grip span and ineffective grip because the thumb blocks access to the palm. Pinch may be impossible. There are several components of this deformity, any of which can occur in combination with the others. These are adduction contracture of the thumb–index finger web space; malposition of the metacarpophalangeal (MCP) joint, consisting of either flexion contracture or hyperextension; tightness of the flexor pollicis longus (FPL); and weakness of the extrinsic extensors of the thumb. The exact deformity depends on the severity of the imbalance between the intrinsic and extrinsic muscles. Treatment must be individualized, using any of several accepted procedures. Correction of the thumb-in-palm deformity is usually reserved until other upper extremity deformities have been corrected.[20]

In the mildly involved patient, adduction contracture may be the only significant deformity of the thumb. Release of the insertion of the adductor pollicis and the metacarpal origin of the first dorsal interosseous muscle and its fascia has been considered the "classic" release. Myotenotomy of the entire adductor insertion can result in partial loss of adduction and thus loss of any ability to pinch. This complication may be avoided if only the metacarpal origins of the adductor are released[16,21] or, alternatively, if the tendon of insertion of the transverse head alone is released.[3] Electromyograms correlated with clinical follow-up confirm that grip span can be improved, pinch retained, and overcorrection avoided in mildly involved patients if only the transverse fibers of the adductor are released.[3] Z-plasty of the thumb–index finger web space is usually required in all but mild cases. Bone block fusion of the thumb and index metacarpals into an abducted position has not gained wide acceptance because the lack of some residual thumb adduction is felt to impair pinch too severely.[5]

Correction of the flexion deformity requires releasing or recessing the intrinsic insertions or releasing the intrinsic origins. If the intrinsic insertions are released, the MCP joint should be stabilized to prevent hyperextension. Release of the origins of the flexor brevis and part of the abductor brevis as well as the adductor can be performed through a volar–thenar crease incision and may avoid overcorrection of the MCP joint.[21] When stabilization of the MCP joint is necessary, either arthrodesis or capsulodesis[16,22] is effective. Arthrodesis of the MCP joint should place the thumb in position for pulp-to-pulp pinch with the index and long fingers. Frequently, the contribution of the FPL to the deformity is overlooked until correction of wrist flexion increases the tightness of the FPL. The FPL must be released in all but the mildest cases.[1,21] It is important to avoid overlengthening, since instability of the interphalangeal (IP) joint may result.

Weakness of the thumb extensors is variable. Myoneural blockade of the FPL, flexor pollicis brevis (FPB), and adductor pollicis may provide clues as to whether reinforcement of extension will be necessary to correct the thumb-in-palm deformity. Several options are available. A prerequisite to strengthening extrinsic extension is that the MCP joint is stable. Combination extension and abduction is provided when the extensor pollicis brevis (EPL) is rerouted to the radial-volar aspect of the radius[1] and augmented by transferring the brachioradialis, flexor carpi radialis, palmaris longus, or a flexor digitorum superficialis to the FPL. In some instances the surgeon may prefer to augment the extensor pollicis brevis or the abductor pollicis longus,[23] as there may be less tendency for these procedures to destabilize the MCP joint into hyperextension. The procedure chosen will depend on the exact positions of the thumb and wrist and upon the stability of the MCP and trapeziometacarpal joints.

Correction of the thumb-in-palm deformity has been classified and approached systematically[4,24] but remains the most difficult correction of deformity while yet maintaining function of the upper extremity in the patient with cerebral palsy. The least satisfactory results are from attempts to attain opposition by means of opponensplasty.[20] The goals of treatment in the thumb should be to correct the deformity, maintain useful grip, attain pulp-to-pulp pinch (not necessarily tip-to-tip pinch), and, as in all aspects of upper extremity surgery in cerebral palsy, avoid overcorrection.

ARTHROGRYPOSIS

General Comments

Treatment of the upper extremities of patients with arthrogryposis should begin immediately after birth. Splinting and active and passive range-of-motion programs are the initial modes of treatment. Early surgery may occasionally be indicated, but surgery is usually deferred until at least 2 years of age.[25–27] This allows time for the parents, therapists, and physicians to carefully assess the child's functional attributes as well as deficits. In addition, muscle testing becomes more reliable as the child gets older and becomes more cooperative. Patients' adaptations may make surgery unnecessary, and potentially detrimental procedures can then be avoided.[28]

Typical deformities in arthrogryposis include internal rotation and adduction contractures at the shoulders, elbows in either flexion or extension with a limited arc of motion, forearms in pronation, wrists in flexion and ulnar deviation, hands with thumb in palm, and stiff fingers with varying degrees of flexion contracture.[27] Fortunately, the thumb, although adducted, is frequently relatively spared and has some functioning intrinsic muscles. Skin creases are poorly developed, probably reflecting the lack of joint motion.

Associated anomalies in the upper extremities include dislocation of the radial head, radioulnar synostosis, cubital recurvatum, simian hands, syndactyly, constriction bands, and bilateral radial nerve palsy.[27]

Since each patient is unique, treatment should be individualized. Nonetheless, certain goals and principles should guide the therapeutic plan. The two primary functional goals in the upper extremity are self-feeding and independent toilet care. Patients should not be deprived of one of these functions in an effort to provide the other.[25]

Recurrence of corrected deformities is common, especially when muscle balancing alone or osteotomy alone is used.[28] Recurrent deformity "results principally from the rigid and thick capsule and periarticular tissues, which do not stretch as the limb grows. These structures seem to be the key to the successful treatment of arthrogryposis in the growing child."[26] Combinations of soft tissue and bony procedures also seem more durable than either alone. Some specific recommendations are discussed in the paragraphs below and in Table 69-1.

Treatment of Specific Regions

Shoulder

In spite of the frequency of internal rotation contracture of the shoulder, surgical correction is rarely required.[25,26] This is because most activities of personal care, daily living, and hygiene are performed with the shoulder internally rotated to varying degrees. Occasionally, however, internal shoulder rotation is so severe that the hand cannot be brought to the mouth when the elbow is flexed.[3] In such cases, correction of the rotary malalignment should be performed.

Carroll and Hill report performing shoulder fusion prior to triceps transfer for elbow flexion.[29] Most authors recommend derotational osteotomy combined with release or lengthening of the pectoralis major and subscapularis. Soft tissue release alone has failed to provide good lasting correction.[25,26,28] Failure to maintain the de-

---

TABLE 69-1 Summary of Recommended Surgical Treatment in the Arthrogrypotic Upper Extremity

Joint	Problem	Procedure(s)
Shoulder	Internal rotation contracture	Derotational osteotomy, lengthen subscapularis and pectoralis, internal fixation, spica cast
Elbow	Extension contracture, no active flexion	Posterior elbow capsule release, triceps lengthening; pectoralis or triceps flexorplasty
Wrist	Excessive flexion, ulnar deviation	Volar capsule release, transfer FCU to ECRB, also carpectomy, fusion, or osteotomy if severe
Thumb	Thumb in palm	Web deepening plus skin graft or flap, MCP fusion, fractional lengthening of FPL, tendon transfers for abduction and extension when indicated and feasible
Digits	PIP flexion deformity	Volar release plus skin graft if active motion; PIP arthrodesis if severe; no surgery if deformity is mild

Key: PIP, proximal interphalangeal; FCU, flexor carpi ulnaris; ECRB, extensor carpi radialis brevis; MCP, metacarpophalangeal; FPL, flexor pollicis longus.

sired derotation is likely unless a spica cast and/or internal fixation is used to prevent the arm from resting in an internally rotated position during healing.

The staging of shoulder and elbow procedures should be carefully considered in each case. Usually correction of shoulder malrotation is performed prior to tendon transfers for elbow flexion. However, if extension contracture of the elbow makes it difficult to judge the axis of elbow flexion, the surgeon might prefer to perform the elbow release first. If the pectoralis major is to be transferred for elbow flexion, it should not be completely released as part of the shoulder correction. Subsequent myostatic shortening would reduce its effectiveness as an elbow flexion transfer. In such a case a controlled lengthening of the pectoralis might be preferable, or shoulder and elbow correction could be performed simultaneously.

Elbow

The elbow is the critical factor in upper extremity function in the arthrogrypotic patient. Most patients have bilateral fixed extension contractures; only occasional patients have fixed flexion deformity.[25] The goals of treatment at the elbow are to enable patients to actively oppose both hands in a two-handed grip, to get at least one hand to the mouth and one to the perineum, and to push themselves out of a chair.[26,30] In order to achieve these goals, existing elbow motion must be placed into a more functional arc or the motion must be increased; usually, it must be reinforced by a tendon transfer to provide flexion power. The pitfall to avoid is any accidental removal of extension power from both elbows by performing bilateral triceps to biceps transfers.[29]

Probably more benefit is derived from a successful elbow flexorplasty than from any other procedure in an arthrogrypotic patient's upper extremity. The shoulder should be addressed first, if necessary; then the elbow extension contracture released; and then or simultaneously the flexorplasty performed. Posterior elbow release must be performed prior to the development of secondary changes in the bony architecture and is achieved most reliably by posterior capsulotomy combined with triceps tendon lengthening.[27] Extension deformity recurs following flexion osteotomy alone.

Pectoralis Transfer Transfer of the pectoralis major seems to be the best elbow flexorplasty in arthrogrypotic patients.[26] Several variations have been described, but transferring the entire muscle seems superior to transferring only the sternal head.[25,30] Pectoralis transfer can achieve a 90° arc of active motion.[25] This procedure allows preservation of extensor (triceps) function if present and may augment shoulder flexion.[21] The pectoralis transfer can be performed bilaterally, since active elbow extension is not sacrificed; however, tension on the transfers should be adjusted to allow sufficient elbow extension on at least one side for the hand to reach the perineum (Fig. 69-1). The reader is referred to the works of Clark,[31] Carroll and Kleinman,[32] and Brooks and Seddon[33] for details of the pectoralis transfer.

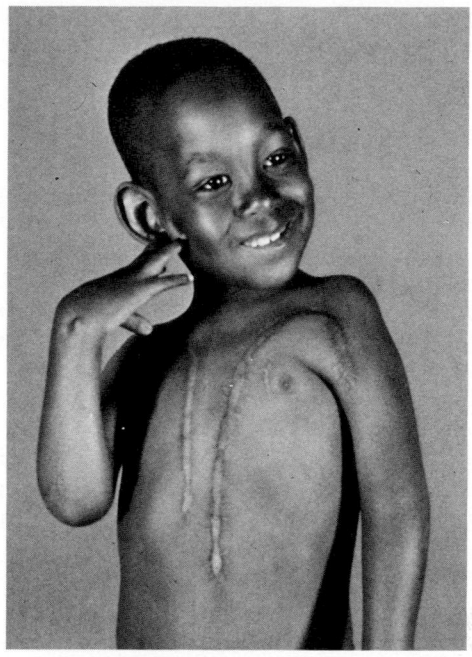

Figure 69-1 This patient has had bilateral pectoralis major transfers for elbow flexion. Active motion is 50 to 105° on the right and 20 to 70° on the left. These arcs allow both hands to function together in bimanual tasks, but they also allow the right hand to reach the mouth and the left hand to reach the perineum. Active elbow extension is preserved although weak.

Triceps Transfer Anterior transfer of the insertion of the triceps is an alternative elbow flexorplasty. Whereas this procedure can provide a good arc of motion in posttraumatic and paralytic cases, the average arc of motion in arthrogrypotics is quite limited, averaging only 43° degrees in one series.[29] Still, some arc of elbow motion is better than none, and any improvement can help the arthrogrypotic patient tremendously. Most patients require release of the elbow extension contracture prior to triceps transfer. The average flexion contracture of the elbow after completion of the triceps transfer is approximately 60°; thus, this procedure should not be performed bilaterally.

Steindler Flexorplasty The Steindler technique of flexorplasty transplants the common flexor-pronator origin proximally and laterally on the humerus.[34] This usually results in a flexion contracture and some active flexion. In the arthrogrypotic patient, this is a weak transfer and in fact tends to aggravate flexion deformity of the wrist and fingers because wrist and finger extension are so weak or absent.[26] Although the Steindler flexorplasty is easier to perform than the pectoralis transfer, it is a less desirable procedure because it provides relatively weak flexion power and aggravates hand deformity.

Wrist

The typical deformity at the wrist is flexion and ulnar deviation. Wrist, finger, and thumb extension are weak or absent. Correction of the deformities may be desirable to improve opposition of the hands and also to improve appearance. Before attempting complete correction, the surgeon should bear in mind that many functions of personal care (perineal hygiene, clothing fastening, etc.) are best performed with the wrist in slight flexion. In general, grip is stronger with the wrist in dorsiflexion, but patients with severe arthrogryposis lack sufficient wrist extensors or muscles for transfer to gain a good arc of wrist motion, and their finger extensor power is too weak to extend the digits against tight finger flexors with the wrist dorsiflexed. In the mildly involved patient, wrist dorsiflexion and power grip can be attained, but this is probably the exception rather than the rule. Those patients with poor elbow motion, especially those with fixed extension, will actually require wrist flexion for optimum function.[25] Finally, neurovascular structures are frequently the limiting factor and may not allow dorsiflexion unless sufficient bone is removed.

There is a high recurrence rate when either soft tissue release or osteotomy is performed alone.[25,28] A key component of correcting these deformities is complete release of the restricting portions of the capsule, but this must be augmented by other measures, such as proximal-row carpectomy or extension osteotomy and transfer of wrist flexors to the dorsum. Long-term night splinting is an integral part of the postoperative regimen and may need to be continued to skeletal maturity.

Although there are problems with recurrent deformity, the benefits to be gained make the effort worthwhile. It has been stated that "correction of the wrist deformity by carpectomy has done more to improve the position of the fingers than any single procedure performed in the hand itself."[26]

Hand

The principal problems in the hand are thumb-in-palm deformity and flexion contractures in the fingers. Despite these problems, arthrogrypotic patients show remarkable adaptability of hand function. A careful, cautious preoperative evaluation is vital, so that as little surgery as necessary is done in the hand. When judiciously selected for surgery, patients can expect some improved function 75 percent of the time.[25]

Thumb function, fortunately, is frequently better spared than that of the other digits. If the thumb-in-palm deformity requires treatment, a variety of procedures are known to be successful. All approaches require web-space deepening. In the vast majority of these cases, the addition of skin (graft or flap) is essential to reduce recurrence. Adductor release, metacarpophalangeal fusion, metacarpal osteotomy, lengthening of the flexor pollicis longus, and tendon transfer for extension-abduction should be performed as necessary to achieve correction.[25,26]

Attempts to improve the total arc of joint motion in the fingers have been unsuccessful, but the functional position of the fingers can be improved. Skin grafting is recommended if contracture release is attempted. If useful grasp is blocked by severely flexed digits, the procedure of choice is probably proximal interphalangeal (PIP) joint arthrodesis in a more functional position.

TETRAPLEGIA

General Comments

The recovery of upper extremity function is the restoration most desired by most patients with tetraplegia. When appropriately selected, 75 percent or more of tetraplegic patients can obtain significant improvement from reconstructive hand surgery.[35–38] Nonetheless, the surgeon must maintain a realistic perspective and not rush, force, or overstate the value of surgery. Suitable criteria include (1) sensibility with two-point discrimination less than 10 mm in at least part of the median nerve distribution, (2) plateau of neurologic recovery—this usually means no sooner than 1 year after injury, (3) grade 4 (Medical Research Council[39]) or better muscles available for transfer, (4) no uncontrolled spasticity, (5) no excessive pain in the hand, and (6) psychological stability and motivation.[39,40] Success depends on proper, detailed preoperative evaluation, selection of procedures, and postoperative rehabilitation.[37,38,41] Advances in microcomputer technology coupled with implantable electrical stimulators may alter treatment and surgical indications in the future.[42]

Historically, tetraplegic injuries have been referred to by the level of injury to the spinal column, i.e., C5 to C6, C7, etc. Neurologic level, however, frequently does not correspond to vertebral level because of asymmetry, incomplete lesions, ascending vascular lesions, and anatomic anomalies. Currently the accepted International Classification[43] is based on (1) presence or absence of useful cutaneous sensibility, (2) lowest-functioning muscle with MRC grade 4 strength, and (3) rating each extremity separately (Table 69-2). Shoulder and elbow function are evaluated independently of the International Classification.

In general terms, realistic goals are to improve the performance of daily activities and to minimize or eliminate the need for splinting. Priority should be to first establish elbow control and then reconstruct the hand.[38,40,41] If the hand is reconstructed first, its rehabilitation or use will be interrupted by the immobilization necessary following triceps reconstruction. Function of the brachioradialis is enhanced by elbow extension; thus triceps reconstruction should be accomplished first so that the tension of a brachioradialis transfer can be set accordingly.

Patients in the lower groups of the International Classification (higher levels of cord injury) are candidates for procedures designed to enhance simple tenodesis grip. Those in the intermediate categories can achieve stronger grasp with some finger intrinsic balance, whereas thumb control can be refined in those in the higher categories. The better hand should be reconstructed first.[38] This would be the dominant hand in the event that both hands are neurologically equal. If they are neurologically unequal, the better hand should be addressed first regardless of previous hand dominance.

TABLE 69-2 International Classification for Surgery of the Hand in Tetraplegia, Edinburgh 1978 (Modified)—Giens 1984[a]

Sensibility, 0 or CU group	Motor characteristics	Description of function
0	No muscle below elbow suitable for transfer	Flexor of the elbow
1	BR	May have weak wrist extension
2	+ ECRL	Extension of the wrist (weak or strong)
3	+ ECRB	Extension of the wrist (weak or strong)
4	+ PT	Extension of the wrist (strong)
5	+ FCR	Flexion of the wrist
6	+ finger extensors	Extrinsic extensors of the fingers
7	+ thumb extensors	Extrinsic extensor of the thumb
8	+ partial digital flexors	Extrinsic flexors of the digits (weak)
9	Lacks only intrinsics	Extrinsic flexors of the digits
x	Exceptions	

[a]Motor grouping assumes that all listed muscles are grade 4 (MRC) or better and a new muscle is added for each group; for example, a group 3 patient will have BR, ECRL, and ECRB rated at least grade 4 (MRC).[39] Assuming 10 mm or less two-point discrimination in the thumb and index finger, the correct classification would be CU 3, where the CU stands for the fact that the patient has adequate cutaneous sensibility. If two-point discrimination was greater than 10 mm (meaning inadequate cutaneous sensibility), the designation 0 would precede the motor group (example, 03).
Key: BR, brachioradialis; ECRL, extensor carpi radialis longus; ECRB, extensor carpi radialis brevis; PT, pronator teres; MRC, Medical Research Council.
Source: McDowell CL, Moberg EA, House JH: Report of the Second International Conference on surgical rehabilitation of the upper limb in tetraplegia (quadriplegia). *J Hand Surg* 11(A):604–608, 1986.

Treatment of Specific Regions

Elbow

When the deltoid and biceps are functioning but the triceps is weak, the patient may be a candidate for reconstruction of elbow control. Patients who have undergone both elbow and hand reconstruction feel that they have benefited the most from reconstruction of triceps function. The best procedure for this seems to be transfer of the posterior one-third of the deltoid to the triceps.[38,41] The posterior one-third of the deltoid is elevated from its insertion, mobilized from the middle third, and elongated using toe extensors,[38,41] tibialis anterior,[44] or fascia lata[37] as graft material. Reinsertion is accomplished through both the distal triceps tendon and the olecranon. Postoperative rehabilitation should rigidly adhere to Moberg's guidelines of graduated increases in motion for 6 weeks, lest the transfer stretch out. This reliable procedure provides the active antagonist for elbow control needed to accurately position the hand in space. Even if the hand cannot be reconstructed, this improves the patient's ability to operate power controls such as those on a wheelchair. Last, if elbow extension is strong enough, the patient's ability to transfer may be improved.

Hand

Prior to Nickel's[45] introduction of the flexor-hinge hand in the 1960s, tenodesis was usually the full extent of treatment offered to patients who fell into groups 1, 2, and 3. The concept of the flexor-hinge hand involved creating tripod pinch and concentrating power at the finger MCP joints by arthrodesing the IP joints. The thumb was shortened and fused into an opposition post. Thus, strong pinch became possible in those patients who had active wrist extension.

Current opinion is based primarily on Moberg's work and favors maintaining a more flexible hand because it is more emotionally acceptable to patients and is also more versatile.[38,41] Key pinch is preferred because it is easier to achieve than tripod pinch, provides a broader surface contact area which enhances stability of pinch, and minimizes the problem of an opposed thumb acting as an obstruction to grasping objects. The tenodesis effect is an integral component of the reconstruction; therefore wrist fusion is rarely indicated.

Review of Groups

Group 0 patients have no active motors below the elbow suitable to function independently as transfers. Brachioradialis function may be sufficiently enhanced by restoration of elbow extension that it can be converted to a wrist extensor to activate a wrist-driven flexor splint.[43]

Groups 1, 2, and 3 patients are candidates for simple hand procedures. These reconstructions depend on strong active wrist extension and the creation of tenodeses to achieve key pinch and simple grasp. The brachioradialis can be transferred to effect wrist extension or to provide limited finger or thumb power.[46] Moberg has developed a widely accepted and reliable procedure that involves pinning the thumb IP joint, releasing the A1 pulley, tenodesing the FPL to the radius, tenodesing the thumb MCP joint to prevent excessive flexion, and releasing the extensor retinaculum to improve the mechanical advantage and strength of wrist extension. Some surgeons[37] prefer to fuse the IP joint rather than to pin it because of a high incidence of pin breakage. Brand[47] describes a rerouting of the FPL, which improves its mechanical advantage without sacrificing the A1 pulley.

When the ECRB is strong enough to act alone for wrist extension (confirmation requires testing under local anesthesia at the time of surgery), more complicated reconstructions can be entertained using the ECRL as a finger flexor transfer. Finger flexor strength introduces an element of clawing to the toneless release action unless an intrinsic toneless or transfer is added. Zancolli's two-stage reconstruction exemplifies this concept. His "lasso"[38,48] procedure is a utilitarian intrinsic transfer that works somewhat in the group 3 patients, even though the FDS is not active.[43]

Reconstruction in groups 4 and 5 patients is similar to that in group 3 patients except that two or more muscles are available for transfer. Digital flexor, extensor, and intrinsic functions must be balanced. This usually requires at least two stages because the flexor and extensor transfers must be immobilized in different positions. Curtis,[49] House and Shannon,[50] and Henderson et al.,[36] among others, have described various combinations of transfers that give good results.

In group 6, the EPL can be attached to the EDC to provide active extension of all the digits. Group 7 patients have all extensors intact. The extensor indicis proprius may be suitable for transfer.

Patients in groups 8 and 9 have flexor digitorum profundus (FDP) and FDS function, respectively. They can be approached as if for low median and ulnar nerve palsies.

House and Shannon[51] have stabilized the thumbs of patients in groups 4 to 7 by means of opponens adductorplasty in one hand and carpometacarpal arthrodesis in the other. The hands with the transfer had stronger lateral pinch, whereas those that were fused had stronger grasp. The patients showed no preference for one over the other but felt that the differences were complementary. Either technique alone is acceptable, thus illustrating both the acceptability and desirability of using different procedures for different goals.

REFERENCES

1. Goldner JL: Upper extremity surgical procedures for patients with cerebral palsy. *Instr Course Lect* 28:36–66, 1979.
2. Hoffer MM: The upper extremity and cerebral palsy, in Fredericks S, Brody G (eds): *Neurological Aspects of Plastic Surgery.* Vol 17. St Louis, Mosby, 1978.
3. Hoffer MM: Cerebral palsy, in Green DP (ed): *Operative Hand Surgery.* New York, Churchill Livingstone, 1993.
4. House JH, Gwathmey FW, Fiddler MO: A dynamic approach to the thumb-in-palm deformity in cerebral palsy: Evaluation and results in 56 patients. *J Bone Joint Surg* 63A:216–225, 1981.
5. Samilson RL, Morris JM: Surgical improvement of the cerebral-palsied upper limb: Electromyographic studies and results in 128 operations. *J Bone Joint Surg* 46A:1203–1216, 1964.
6. Skoff L, Woodbury DF: Current concepts review: Management of the upper extremity in cerebral palsy. *J Bone Joint Surg* 67A:500–503, 1985.
7. Koman LA, Gelberman RH, Toby EB, Poehling GG: Cerebral palsy: Management of the upper extremity. *Clin Orthop* 253:62–74, 1990.
8. Mital MA: Lengthening of the elbow flexors in cerebral palsy. *J Bone Joint Surg* 61A:515–522, 1979.
9. Sakellarides HT, Mital MD, Lenzi WD: Treatment of pronation contractures of the forearm in cerebral palsy by changing the insertion of the pronator radii teres. *J Bone Joint Surg* 63A:645–652, 1981.
10. Green WT, Banks HH: Flexor carpi ulnaris transplant and its use in cerebral palsy. *J Bone Joint Surg* 44A:1343–1352, 1962.
11. Hoffer MM, Perry J, Melkonian GJ: Dynamic electromyography and decision making for surgery in the upper extremity of patients with cerebral palsy. *J Hand Surg* 4:424–431, 1979.
12. Williams P: The management of arthrogryposis. *Orthop Clin North Am* 9:67–88, 1978.
13. Inglis AE, Cooper W: Release of the flexor-pronator origin for flexion deformities of the hand and wrist in spastic paralysis: A study of 18 cases. *J Bone Joint Surg* 48A:847–857, 1966.
14. Page CM: An operation for the relief of flexor contracture in the forearm. *J Bone Joint Surg* 5:233, 1923.
15. Swanson AB: Surgery of the hand in cerebral palsy and muscle origin release procedures. *Surg Clin North Am* 48:1129–1138, 1968.
16. Zancolli EA, Goldner JL, Swanson AB: Surgery of the spastic hand in cerebral palsy: Report of the committee on spastic hand evaluation. *J Hand Surg* 8:766–772, 1983.
17. Braun RM, Vise GT: Sublimus to profundus tendon transfers in the hemiplegic upper extremity. *J Bone Joint Surg* 55A:873, 1973.
18. Omer GE, Capen DA: Proximal row carpectomy with muscle transfers for spastic paralysis. *J Hand Surg* 1:197–204, 1976.
19. Swanson AB: Surgery of the hand in cerebral palsy and the swanneck deformity. *J Bone Joint Surg* 42A:951–964, 1960.
20. Inglis AE, Cooper W, Bruton W: Surgical correction of thumb deformities in spastic paralysis. *J Bone Joint Surg* 52A:253–268, 1970.
21. Matev IB: Surgical treatment of flexion-adduction contracture of the thumb in cerebral palsy. *Acta Orthop Scand* 41:439–445, 1970.
22. Filler BC, Stark HH, Boyes JH: Capsulodesis of the metacarpophalangeal joint of the thumb in children with cerebral palsy. *J Bone Joint Surg* 58A:667–670, 1976.
23. Keats S: Surgical treatment of the hand in cerebral palsy: Correction of thumb-in-palm and other deformities: Report of nineteen cases. *J Bone Joint Surg* 47A:274–284, 1965.
24. Mital MA, Sakellarides HT: Surgery of the upper extremity in retarded individual with spastic cerebral palsy. *Orthop Clin North Am* 12:127–141, 1981.
25. Bennett JB, Hansen PE, Granberry WM, Cain TE: Surgical management of arthrogryposis in the upper extremity. *J Pediatr Orthop* 5:281–286, 1985.
26. Doyle JR, James PM, Larsen LJ, Ashley RK: Restoration of elbow flexion in arthrogryposis multiplex congenita. *J Hand Surg* 5:149–151, 1980.

27. Friedlander HL, Westin GW, Wood WL: Arthrogryposis multiplex congenita. *J Bone Joint Surg* 50A:89–112, 1968.
28. Lloyd-Roberts GC, Lettin AWF: Arthrogryposis multiplex congenita. *J Bone Joint Surg* 52B:494–508, 1970.
29. Carroll RE, Hill NA: Triceps transfer to restore elbow flexion. *J Bone Joint Surg* 52A:239–244, 1970.
30. DeBenedetti M: Restoration of elbow extension power in the tetraplegic patient using the Moberg technique. *J Hand Surg* 4:86–89, 1979.
31. Clark JPM: Reconstruction of biceps brachii by pectoral muscle transplantation. *Br J Surg* 34:180–181, 1946.
32. Carroll RE, Kleinman WB: Pectoralis major transplantation to restore elbow flexion to the paralytic limb. *J Hand Surg* 4:501–507, 1979.
33. Brooks DM, Seddon HJ: Pectoral transplantation for paralysis of flexors of the elbow: A new technique. *J Bone Joint Surg* 41B:35–43, 1958.
34. Steindler A: Reconstruction work on hand and forearm. *NY State Med J* 108:117–119, 1918.
35. Lamb DW, Chan KM: Surgical reconstruction of the upper limb in traumatic tetraplegia. *J Bone Joint Surg* 65B:291–298, 1983.
36. Henderson ED, Lipscomb PR, Elkins EC, et al: Review of the results of surgical treatment of patients with tetraplegia. Proceedings of the American Society for Surgery of the Hand. *J Bone Joint Surg* 52A:1059, 1970.
37. Hente VR, Brown M, Keshian LA: Upper limb reconstruction in quadriplegia: Functional assessment and proposed treatment modifications. *J Hand Surg* 8:119–131, 1983.
38. Moberg E: *The Upper Limb in Tetraplegia.* Stuttgart, Thieme, 1978.
39. Medical Research Council: *Aids to the Investigation of Peripheral Nerve Injuries. War Memorandum No. 7,* 2d rev ed. London, His Majesty's Stationery Office, 1943.
40. McDowell CL, Moberg EA, Graham-Smith A: International conference on surgical rehabilitation of the upper limb in tetraplegia. *J Hand Surg* 4:387–390, 1979.
41. Moberg E: Surgical treatment for absent single hand grip and elbow extension in quadriplegia. *J Bone Joint Surg* 57A:196–206, 1975.
42. Keith MW, Peckham H, Thrope GB, et al: Implantable functional neuromuscular stimulation in the tetraplegic hand. *J Hand Surg* 14A:524–530, 1989.
43. McDowell CL: Tetraplegia, in Green DP (ed): *Operative Hand Surgery.* New York, Churchill Livingstone, 1982, pp 1109–1127.
44. Freehafer AA, Kelly CM, Peckham PH: Tendon transfer for the restoration of upper limb function after a cervical spinal cord injury. *J Hand Surg* 9:887–893, 1984.
45. Nickel VL, Perry J, Garrett AL: Development of useful function in the severely paralyzed hand. *J Bone Joint Surg* 45A:933–952, 1963.
46. Frehafer AA, Mast WA: Transfer of brachioradialis to improve wrist extension in high spinal-cord injury. *J Bone Joint Surg* 49A:648–652, 1967.
47. Brand PF: *Clinical Mechanics of the Hand.* St Louis, Mosby, 1985.
48. Zancolli EA: *Structural and Dynamic Bases of Hand Surgery,* 2d ed. Philadelphia, Lippincott, 1979.
49. Curtis RM: Tendon transfers in the patient with spinal cord injury. *Orthop Clin North Am* 5:415–423, 1974.
50. House JH, Shannon MA: Restoration of strong grasp and lateral pinch in tetraplegia due to cervical spinal cord injury. *J Hand Surg* 1:152–159, 1976.
51. House JH, Shannon MA: Restoration of strong grasp and lateral pinch in tetraplegia: A comparison of two methods of thumb control in each patient. *J Hand Surg* 10:22–29, 1985.

PART VI

The Spine

CHAPTER 70

Fractures and Dislocations of the Spine

Michael F. O'Brien
and Lawrence G. Lenke

Injuries to the axial skeleton occur from the occipitocervical junction to the coccyx. The description of spinal trauma is organized anatomically into upper cervical (C0-C2), subaxial cervical (C3-C7), thoracolumbar, and sacral injuries. The mechanism that results in injury is quite variable. The effect that a specific traumatic event has on the spine depends on the magnitude of the injury as well as the region of the spine involved. Blunt trauma—as experienced in motor vehicle accidents, industrial injuries, falls from heights, and even recreational activities—produces the majority of injuries. Penetrating trauma such as gunshot wounds may also cause significant injuries to the spinal column or neural elements.

When the physician is presented with a spinal injury, there are some key questions to consider: Are there other, perhaps life-threatening injuries? Is there actual or impending neurological damage? What was the mechanism of injury? What are the injured anatomic structures? Can the spine function as a weight-bearing column?

The initial management of the potentially spine-injured patient can be divided into five steps, beginning with immobilization and stabilization in the field and transportation to an appropriate triage facility. Cervical as well as thoracolumbar immobilization should be instituted at the scene to protect the spinal column and neuraxis. Second, medical management is instituted as dictated by the type and extent of the trauma. The third step includes a thorough radiographic documentation of all spinal injuries. This allows proper anatomic alignment of all injured segments, which is the fourth step. Finally, an assessment is made regarding surgical or nonoperative treatment for the injury.

ANATOMY

It is important to understand the regional variations in anatomy and alignment of the spine. These will determine the typical appearances of the uninjured and injured spine. Because of these regional variations in anatomy and biomechanics, each segment maintains a unique position in space with typical loading parameters. Each region is therefore subjected to unique loading forces during trauma, which result in characteristic injuries.

There are two lordotic segments in the spine: the cervical and the lumbar regions. These are separated by a kyphotic segment: the thoracic region. In addition, the sacral-coccygeal area is also kyphotic. There is approximately 25° of cervical lordosis, 35° of thoracic kyphosis, and 50° of lumbar lordosis. This allows the skull to be aligned directly over the pelvis, with the weight-bearing line passing just anterior to S1.

The cross-sectional anatomy of the spine is organized into three columns.[1] The anterior column consists of the anterior longitudinal ligament, the anterior half of the vertebral body, the annulus fibrosus, and the disk. The middle column consists of the posterior half of the vertebral body, annulus, disk, and posterior longitudinal ligament. The posterior column includes the facet joints and neural arches, ligamentum flavum, and interspinous ligaments (Fig. 70-1). Each column contributes to the weight-bearing capacity (Fig. 70-2) of the spine. This three-column concept has been more typically used in the lumbar spine, but it may be usefully extrapolated to both the cervical and thoracic spine.

The three-column theory of spinal stability[1-3] can be applied to the simple classification of spinal injuries, compression fractures, burst fractures, and injuries involving flexion-distraction or fracture-dislocation to assess structural integrity (Table 70-1). Compression fractures are characterized by failure of the anterior column under compression with intact middle and posterior columns; these are stable injuries. When the anterior and middle columns fail under axial loading forces, a burst fracture is produced. Distraction of the middle and posterior columns produces a "seat-belt type" of flexion-distraction injury. These two injury patterns can express varying degrees of instability. Fracture-dislocation injuries are characterized by involvement of all three columns in compression, distraction, rotation, and/or shear. These are typically grossly unstable. A similar classification system based on fracture morphology has recently been suggested by Gaines et al. (Fig. 70-3).[122] The amounts of comminution, fragment apposition, and local kyphosis are assessed to estimate the degree of instability.

Classification systems based on mechanism of injury have been described for both the lumbar[4,5] (Fig. 70-4 and Table 70-2) and cervical spine[6] (Table 70-3). Magerl's classification is based on mechanism, with a description of characteristic injuries for the anterior, middle, posterior, or combined column injuries. Ferguson and Allen's classification[6] for cervical injuries, while complicated, allows accurate identification and understanding of both the injured anatomic structures and the resulting instability.

Because numerous forces may be involved in creating a spinal column injury—including compression, distraction, rotation, torsion, and/or shear—careful attention must be paid to the alterations from normal alignment in the coronal and sagittal planes. These simple concepts will allow at least a provisional estimation of overall spinal stability and lead to the formulation of a treatment plan to reverse effects of the mechanism of injury and stabilize the injured anatomic structures.

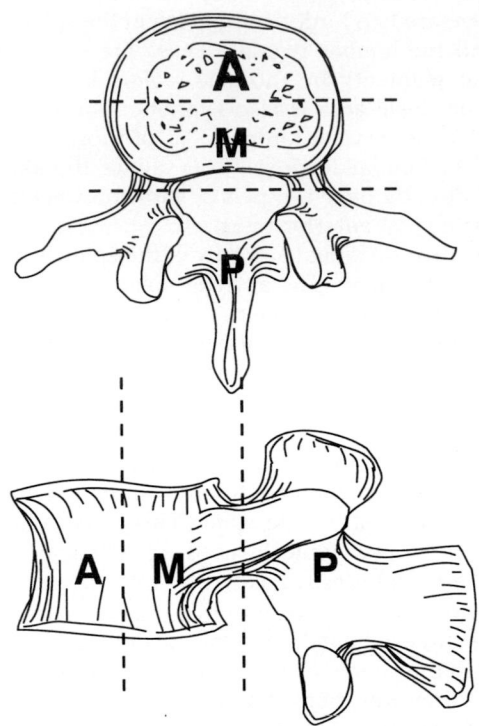

Figure 70-1 Diagrammatic representation of the three columns of the spine: anterior, middle, and posterior.

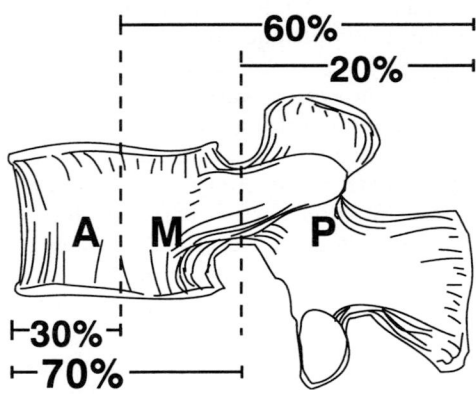

Figure 70-2 Contributions of the three columns of the spine to axial loading.

TABLE 70-1 Fracture Type and Column Involvement

	Anterior	Middle	Posterior
Compression fracture	Yes	No/Yes	No
Burst fractures	Yes	Yes	No/Yes
Flexion-distraction injuries	No/Yes	Yes	Yes
Fracture-dislocations	Yes	Yes	Yes

Reproduced with permission from Haher TR, O'Brien MF, Felmy WT: Thoracic and lumbar fractures: Diagnosis and management, in Bridwell KH, DeWald RL (eds): *Textbook of Spinal Surgery*. Philadelphia, Lippincott, 1991.

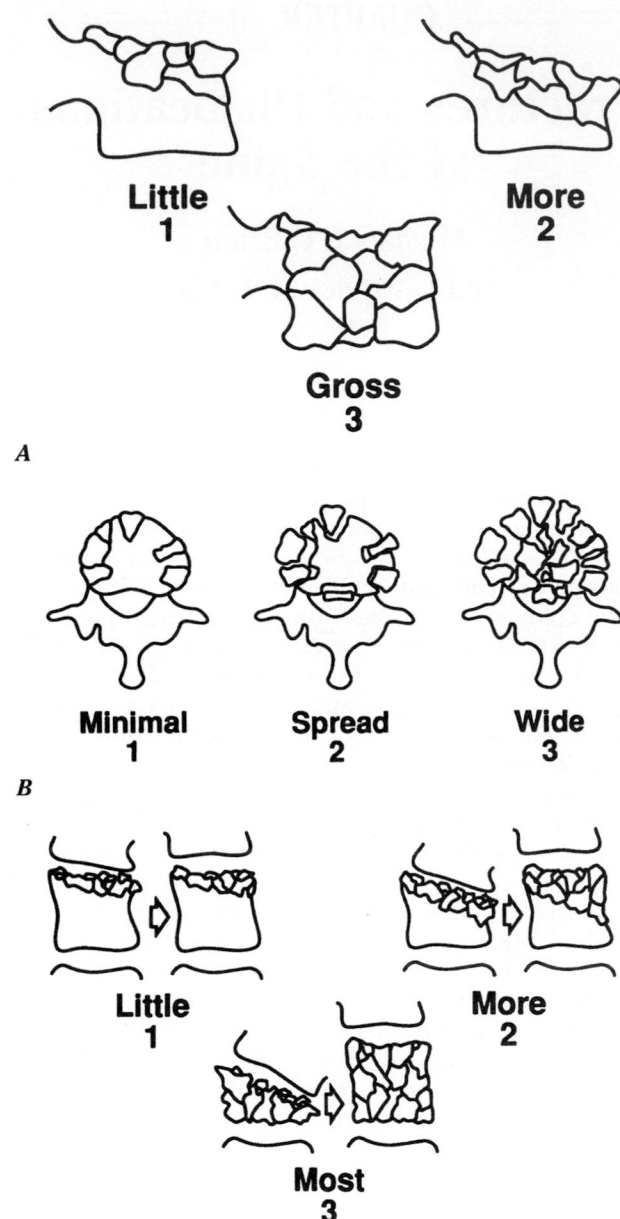

Figure 70-3 *A.* Comminution: *little* (1 point), <30 percent comminution on sagittal reconstruction CT; *more* (2 points), 30 to 60 percent comminution; *gross* (3 points), >60 percent comminution. *B.* Apposition of fragments: *minimal* displacement on axial CT (1 point); *spread* of at least 2 mm of >50 percent of cross section (2 points); *wide* displacement of ≥2 mm of ≥50 percent of cross section (3 points). *C.* Deformity correction: kyphosis correction ≤3° on lateral plain x-rays (1 point); kyphosis correction 4–9° on lateral plain x-rays (2 points); kyphosis correction ≥10° on lateral plain x-rays (3 points). A cumulative score of ≥7 points portends screw failure when these fractures are treated with short-segment posterior pedicle screw constructs without anterior reconstruction. (Reproduced with permission from McCormack T, Karaikovic E, Gaines RW: The load sharing classification of spine fractures. *Spine* 19:1741-1744, 1994.)

Figure 70-4 Mechanistic classification of thoracolumbar fractures by Magerl et al. *A.* Vertebral body compression. *B.* Type B, anterior and posterior element injury with distraction. *C.* Type C anterior and posterior element injury with rotation. (Reproduced with permission from Magerl F, Harms J, Gertzbein SD, et al: A new classification of spinal fractures. Presented at the Societé Internationale Orthopedie et Traumatologie meeting, Montreal, Canada, Sept 9, 1990.)

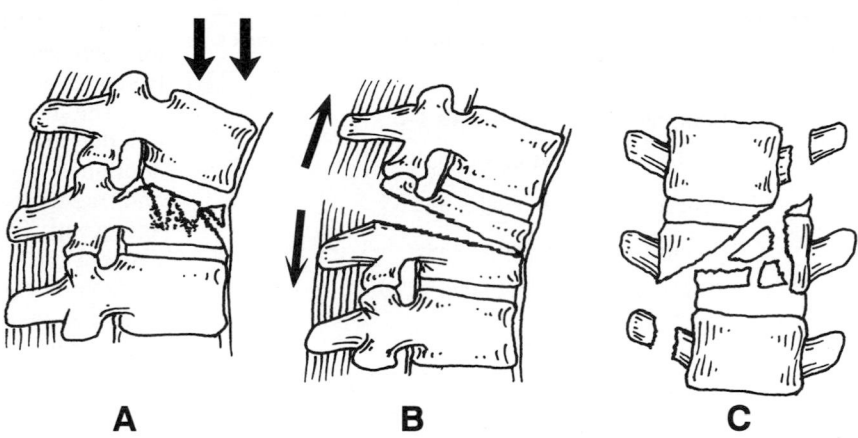

A   **B**   **C**

Osseous Anatomy

There are seven cervical vertebrae between the skull and the thoracic spine. The cervical spine protects the brainstem and spinal cord while supporting the skull and al-

lowing significant flexibility. Approximately 50 to 60 percent of flexion-extension in the cervical spine occurs between the base of the skull and C1. In addition, a significant portion of coronal rotation occurs here. Similarly, 50 to 60 percent of the axial rotation of the cervical spine oc-

TABLE 70-2 Classification of Thoracic and Lumbar Fractures

Type	Group	Subgroup
A. Vertebral body compression	1. Impaction fracture	1. End-plate infarction 2. Vertebral body collapse 3. Wedge impaction
	2. Split fractures	1. Sagittal split 2. Coronal split 3. Pincer fracture
	3. Burst fracture	1. Partial burst 2. Burst split 3. Complete burst
B. Anterior and posterior element injury with distraction	1. Posterior disruption predominantly ligamentous	1. With transverse disruption of the disk 2. With compression of the vertebral body
	2. Posterior disruption including the arch	1. With transverse disruption through the vertebral body 2. With transverse disruption through the disk 3. With compression of the vertebral body
	3. Anterior disruption	1. With hyperextension subluxation of the facet joint 2. Hyperextension spondylosis 3. With posterior facet dislocation
C. Anterior and posterior element injury with rotation	1. Vertebral body compression with rotation	1. Impaction 2. Split 3. Burst
	2. Distraction with rotation	1. Posterior disruption predominantly ligamentous 2. Posterior disruption including the arch 3. Anterior disruption of the disk
	3. Rotational shear	1. Slice fracture of the vertebral body 2. Oblique fracture of the vertebral body

Source: Reproduced with permission from Gertzbein SD: *Fractures of the Thoracic and Lumbar Spine.* Philadelphia, Williams & Wilkins, 1992, p 30.

TABLE 70-3 Mechanistic Classification of Cervical Injuries

Compressive flexion, stages 1–5

Vertical compression, stages 1–3

Distractive flexion, stages 1–4

Compressive extension, stages 1–5

Distractive extension, stages 1 and 2

Lateral flexion, stages 1 and 2

Source: Modified with permission from Allen BL Jr, Ferguson RL, Lehmann TR, et al: A mechanistic classification of closed, indirect fractures and dislocations of the lower cervical spine. *Spine* 7:1–17, 1982.

curs at the C1-C2 articulation. The remaining motion—flexion, extension, rotation, and lateral bending—occurs between C2 and the cervicothoracic junction (Table 70-4).

The anatomy and development of the craniocervical junction are unique (Fig. 70-5). Considerable controversy continues to exist around the question of developmental and traumatic pathology here, particularly in the pediatric age group. The atlas is unique among all vertebrae because it has no vertebral body. During development, its centrum becomes fused to the axis to form the dens. The synchrondoses can be seen into adulthood in some patients. It is often identified on MRI as a disklike structure within the dens. The normal atlas comprises anterior and posterior rings connecting two lateral masses. These lateral masses support the occipital condyles and rest on the lateral masses of C2. The shape of the superior and inferior articulations of C1 to a large degree define the unique movement in the craniocervical junction. The cup-and-ball type of articulation of C0 and C1 allows coronal and sagit-

TABLE 70-4 Range of Motion (Degrees) for the Occipitoatlantoaxial Joint

	Sagittal plane, flexion-extension		Axial plane, rotation		Coronal plane, lateral bending		Sagittal plane, anteroposterior shear, mm	
	C0-C1	C1-C2	C0-C1	C1-C2	C0-C1	C1-C2	C0-C1	C1-C2
Fick[149]	50	0	—	60	30–40	0	—	—
Poirier[150]	50	11	—	30–80	14–40	4	—	—
Jackson[151]	—	—	—	—	—	—	—	2–5
Fielding[152]	35 (+10, −11)	15 (+5, −10)	0	45	—	—	—	—
Werne[153]	13 (4–33)	10 (2–22)	—	47 (22–58)	8 (4–14)	0	—	—
Werne[154]	23 (9–41)		47 (22–58)		8 (4–14)	0	—	—
Hohl[155]	15	15	—	45	—	—	—	—
Penning[156]	30 (25–45)	30 (25–45)	—	—	5	0	—	—
White[157]	13	10	0	47	8	0	—	—
Weisel[158]	—	—	—	—	—	—	1	—
Clark[159]	23 (12–34)	10	5 (3–7)	15 (11–19)	—	—	—	—
Dvorak[160]	—	—	4	42 (38–44)	—	—	—	—
Penning[161]	—	—	1 (2–5)	41 (29–46)	—	—	—	—
Dvorak[162] (active)	—	12 (5–20)	—	—	—	—	—	—
Dvorak[162] (passive)	—	15 (8–22)	—	—	—	—	—	—
Panjabi[163]	25	22	7	39	6	8	—	—
Goel[164]	+7, −17	+5, −5	2.4	28	3.4	4.2	—	—
Grob[165]	—	23 (8–36)	—	36 (29–42)	—	12 (8–19)	—	—
Dickman[166]	—	+13, −10	—	35	—	5	—	—

Source: Reproduced with permission from O'Brien MF, Sutterlin CE: Occipitocervical biomechanics: Clinical and biomechanical implications for posterior occipitocervical stabilization and fusion. *Spine* 10:281–313, 1996.

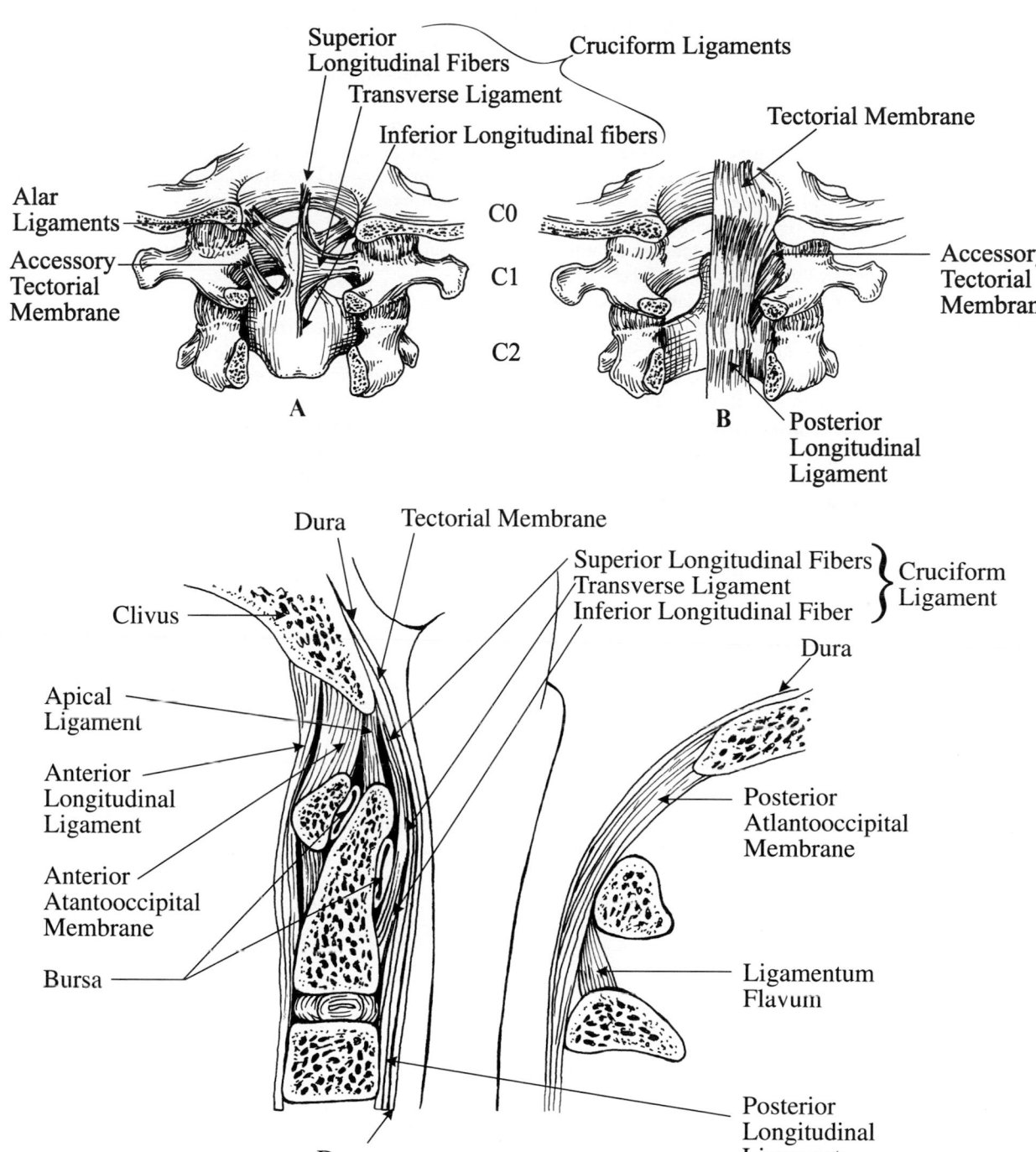

Figure 70-5 Deep (*A*), superficial (*B*), and cross-sectional (*C*) views of the occipitoatlantoaxial ligamentous and osseous anatomy. (Reproduced with permission from O'Brien MF, Sutterlin CE: Occipitocervical biomechanics: Clinical and biomechanical implications for posterior occipitocervical stabilization and fusion. *Spine* 10:281–313, 1996.)

tal rotation. The more horizontal and flattened orientation of the C1-C2 articulation allows predominantly axial rotation. Although the range of motion may be dictated by the osseous anatomy of the articulations from C0 to C1 and C1 to C2, the stability of these joints is almost entirely the result of the ligamentous anatomy.

The remaining cervical vertebrae (C3 through C7) have small vertebral bodies that are concave on the superior surface, each with a rostrally projecting lip (uncus) forming the uncovertebral joint with the vertebral body above. They have corresponding convex inferior surfaces. Arising anterolaterally from the bodies are transverse processes that have both anterior and posterior tubercles. The foramen transversarium is located between the posterior tubercle and the lateral part of the vertebral body. The vertebral artery passes through this foramen, entering at C6 and exiting at C2. The exiting nerve roots pass just posterior to the vertebral arteries at the level of the disk space.

Posterior to the vertebral artery foramen (foramen transversarium) are the lateral masses (articular pillars), which make up that portion of vertebra between the superior and inferior facets. The cervical facet joints are oriented more horizontally than vertically. The superior facet of the caudal vertebra sits anterior to the inferior facet of the rostral vertebra. This allows for a great amount of flexion and extension of the neck but limits lateral bending. Significant lateral bending induces axial rotation as a coupled motion. The rest of the posterior elements of the cervical spine include the laminae and spinous processes, which are posterior and medial to the facet joints and lateral masses.

There are 12 thoracic vertebrae. The differential features are as follows: thin pedicles connect the vertebral bodies to the posterior elements; the transverse processes project posteriorly in a superolateral direction from the posterior parts of the pedicles and are larger in size than the cervical transverse processes. The ventral surface of the transverse process has a costal articulation. The rib cage creates a rigid construct that reduces intersegmental movement in all planes. As in the cervical spine, the facets of the thoracic spine are oriented more in the coronal plane, with the superior facets of the caudal vertebra anterior to the inferior facet of the rostral vertebra. At the thoracolumbar junction, the facet joints change gradually from a coronal to a more sagittal orientation.

The vertebrae of the lumbar spine are larger than the cervical or thoracic vertebrae. The pedicles are wider and broader. The facet joints are oriented sagittally, with the inferior facet of the rostral segment medial to the superior facet of the caudal segment. This allows for significant flexion-extension but less axial rotation. The transverse processes project straight laterally from the superior facets and are quite large. The posterior elements (laminae and spinous processes) are also larger in the lumbar spine. The sacrum and coccyx are normally fused and attach the axial skeleton to the pelvis by the sacrotuberous and sacrospinous ligaments and sacroiliac joint.

Ligamentous Anatomy

The ligamentous anatomy can easily be overlooked when plain x-rays are viewed. However, it is vital to keep these important structures in mind in considering the stability of the spine. This is particularly true at the craniocervical junction and in the cervical spine. Here, significant destabilizing injuries may consist of ligamentous disruption alone. These injuries might easily be overlooked or impossible to see on static plain x-rays. Failure to identify these injuries can result in catastrophic neurologic injury.

The ligamentous anatomy of the upper cervical spine is as unique as its osseous counterpart. To a large degree, the mobility of C0-C1 is dictated by the alar and the apical ligaments. These provide direct connection between the occiput and C2. This direct ligamentous connection allows C1 to act as an intercalated segment between C0 and C2 (Fig. 70-6). Occipital rotation and, to some degree, anteroposterior translation of the occiput on C1 is limited by the alar ligaments. Anteroposterior translation of the occipital–C1 complex on C2 is primarily limited by the transverse ligament[7,8] (see Fig. 70-5).

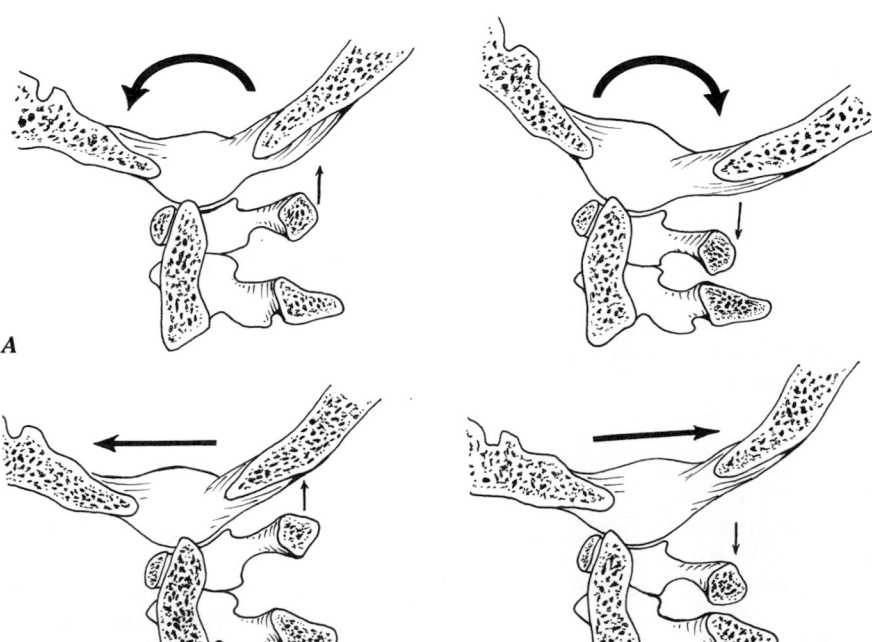

A

B

Figure 70-6 Induced flexion and extension of the atlas relative to C2 occurs as a result of occipital flexion and extension (*A*) and anterior and posterior shear of the occiput (*B*). (Reproduced with permission from O'Brien MF, Sutterlin CE: Occipitocervical biomechanics: Clinical and biomechanical implications for posterior occipitocervical stabilization and fusion. *Spine* 10:281–313, 1996.)

The ligamentous stabilizers of the anterior and middle column are the anterior longitudinal ligament (ALL) and the posterior longitudinal ligament (PLL). These extend the entire length of the spine and insert on the vertebral bodies and disks. The ALL is closely applied and attached to the intervertebral disk and has a ribbon-like structure. The PLL is widest in the upper cervical spine but quite thin, and it narrows as it proceeds caudally. It is typically thin over the vertebral bodies and thickens over the intervertebral disks. The rostral extension of these two ligaments coalesces to insert onto the occiput near the anterior lip of the foramen magnum (basion). The PLL forms the tectorial membrane at the level of C0 and C1.

The supraspinous and the interspinous ligaments, the facet capsules, and the ligamentum flavum are the important stabilizing structures for the posterior column. The ligamentum flavum typically is attached to the ventral caudad surface of the superior lamina and runs to the superior margin of the caudal lamina. Typically, there is a right and a left ligamentum flavum separated by a small fissure, which is where the ligamentum flavum merges with the interspinous and supraspinous ligaments posteriorly and medially. These, in turn, merge with the ligamentum nuchae, which connects all of the cervical spinous processes. The ligamentum flavum is replaced at C0-C1 by the posterior occipitocervical membrane, which is much thinner than the ligamentum flavum. Each facet joint is surrounded by a facet capsule. The posterior ligamentous structures act as a tension band. They are the important stabilizers of the vertebral bodies and disks in flexion.

The intervertebral disks are complex structures made up of an outer annulus fibrosus and an inner nucleus pulposus. The annulus fibrosus is a laminated structure consisting of collagen fibers oriented 30° from the horizontal and 120° to fibers in adjacent layers. The inner layers are attached to the cartilaginous end plates, while the outer fibers are firmly secured to the osseous vertebral bodies. The annulus is responsible for the stability of axial rotation as well as being important in the transmission of compressive stress through the anterior and middle columns. The annulus surrounds and contains the nucleus pulposus, a matrix of protein, glycosaminoglycans, and water. Injury to the intervertebral disk may not be obvious on conventional radiography but must be considered when overall spinal stability and potential neurologic compromise are being evaluated. Magnetic resonance imaging allows direct visualization of the intervertebral disk. This is particularly important in evaluating cervical trauma.[9]

BIOMECHANICS

In the sagittal projection, the spine is made up of four smooth curves: cervical lordosis, thoracic kyphosis, lumbar lordosis, and sacral kyphosis. This complex shape means that flexion-extension and lateral bending will be accompanied by coupled movements. The primary movement will induce flexion, extension, coronal bending, or rotation.[10]

The mobile cervical and lumbar segments are separated by the stiffer thoracic segment. This creates stress risers at the cervicothoracic and thoracolumbar junctions, where the more mobile segments of the spine make a rapid transition into the rigid thoracic spine. Ideally, the center of gravity passes through the cervical vertebral bodies, anterior to the thoracic spine, and just posterior to the mid-lumbar vertebral bodies before intersecting the anterior corner of the sacrum. This implies that most of the spinal column will experience compressive forces anteriorly through the vertebral bodies and that tensile forces will be transmitted through the posterior elements and ligaments. An exception to this simplification occasionally occurs in the lumbar spine, where increased lordosis may allow the center-of-gravity line to pass through the middle or posterior column in the mid- or lower lumbar spine. This may have implications for the treatment of compression and/or burst fractures of the lower lumbar spine. If compression forces can be realigned through the facet joints, the compressed vertebral bodies can be unloaded anteriorly.

The material distribution in the osseous structures matches the load requirements for the spine. The vertebral bodies are well equipped to handle compressive loads, with the majority of the vertebral body being cancellous bone—the primary weight-bearing component in compression.[11-14] The cortical bone is responsible for only about 10 percent of the vertebral body's compressive strength. In addition, the marrow elements, with their viscous properties, create a hydraulic system that provides both strength and a dampening effect, which allows significant energy absorption.[15] The osseous elements in the posterior column are less massive and are designed to be the attachment points for ligamentous and tendinous insertions.

These ligamentous structures are predominantly collagenous and are extremely strong when loaded in tension. Their insertion points on the osseous structures place them at some distance from the instantaneous axis of rotation (IAR), giving them excellent mechanical advantage. These ligaments provide the major stabilizing elements of the posterior column.

The intervertebral disks act as force-transmission and dampening units for the anterior column.[16] The nucleus transmits axial loads from vertebra to vertebra. In addition, they transfer the compressive forces into tension forces within the annulus. The outer layers of the annulus are important rotational stabilizing structures. The annulus is thickest anteriorly and laterally. It thins significantly in the posterior and posterolateral corner. This, in combination with a tight radius of curvature at the posterolateral corner, creates stress risers and probably explains why this is the common site for annular failure, accompanied by disk herniation. Minor focal failures of the annular/nuclear structure, evidenced as high-intensity zones on MRI, or as rents through which dye may leak on diskograms, may result in pain. Catastrophic failure may result in gross instability, which is not easily identified on static plain x-rays.

Instantaneous Axis of Rotation

The instantaneous axis of rotation (IAR) describes the relative motion of an object from one position to another. The IAR is a geometric concept that locates a point in space around which a vertebral body rotates. It is not necessary for the IAR to be contained in a discrete anatomic structure. Regional differences in anatomy will significantly affect the position of the instantaneous axis of rotation. In addition, degenerative changes and loss of anatomic stabilizers will allow the IAR to change its position. Within certain limits, destruction of anatomic structures tends to allow the instantaneous axis of rotation to shift toward the uninjured segments, repositioning it within the intact structures.[17] The shape of the vertebral bodies and their ligamentous attachments to adjacent vertebrae determines the characteristic IAR at each level. A clear understanding of the normal location of the IAR throughout the spine is necessary to understand the normal biomechanics and the effect pathology will have on each spinal segment. Certainly, if an attempt is made to counteract or prevent a deformity with instrumentation or a reduction of deformity is attempted, the location of the IAR must be understood, so that the construct can be placed in the most biomechanically favorable position. This will be at the greatest distance from the IAR, thus maximizing the instrumentation's moment arm and therefore its mechanical advantage.

Based on anatomic studies, the IAR for the occipito-cervical joint in the frontal plane (i.e., lateral bending) has been established to be approximately 2 to 3 mm above the apex of the dens in the midline (Fig. 70-7). Its location is largely dictated by the shape of the articulation between the occipital condyles and the superior articulation of C1. In the sagittal plane (i.e., flexion and extension), the IAR's location is above the dens at approximately the level of the foramen magnum, passing through the spherical mass of the occipital condyles.

For the atlantoaxial joint, the IAR is probably confined to the substance of the dens. This is probably true for both the sagittal and the frontal planes. The IAR for the axial plane is through the dens, which is constrained anteriorly by the anterior arch of the atlas and posteriorly by the transverse ligament; it acts as an eccentrically placed axle about which these two vertebrae move in relation to each other. Because there is little axial rotation between C0 and C1, the IAR for this joint is probably essentially the same as for the atlantoaxial joint, reflecting the IAR of the more mobile C1-C2 articulation.

In the cervical spine, the IAR, for flexion and extension, appears to be in the anterior aspect of the vertebral body. In lateral bending, the IAR is centered in approximately the geographic center of the vertebral body from right to left. In axial rotation, the IAR appears to reside within the vertebral body's cross section.

In the lumbar spine, the IAR for axial rotation is located near the posterior annulus in the vicinity of the facet joints. With destruction of the annulus, the IAR migrates posteriorly. Destruction of the posterior elements causes the IAR to

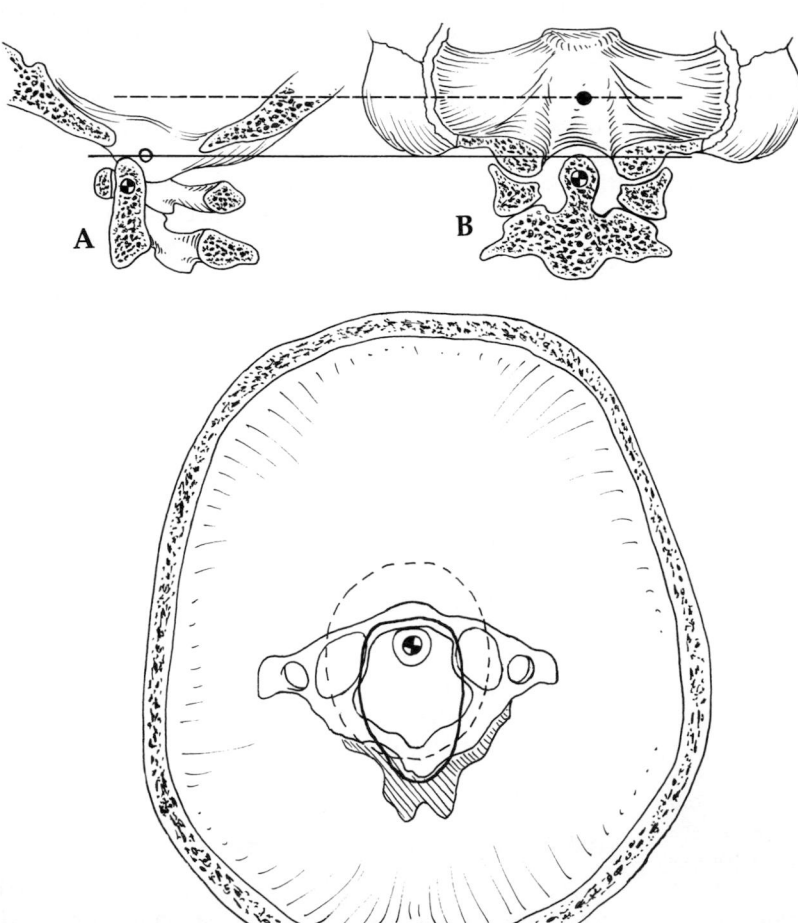

Figure 70-7 The approximate location of the instantaneous axis of rotation (IAR) for the occiput and atlas in the sagittal plane (*A*), coronal plane (*B*), and axial plane (*C*). (Reproduced with permission from O'Brien MF, Sutterlin CE: Occipitocervical biomechanics: Clinical and biomechanical implications for posterior occipitocervical stabilization and fusion. *Spine* 10:281–313, 1996.)

migrate anteriorly. Those structures furthest from the IAR will have the greatest effect on resisting torsion; therefore, the anterior column—consisting of the anterior longitudinal ligament, the anterior aspect of the annulus, and the anterior portion of the vertebral body—is the structure most responsible for controlling rotation in the intact spine.[18,19] Of these structures, the annulus seems to be the most important for resisting rotation. Loss of anterior column integrity renders the lumbar spine incapable of resisting torsion. In the intact lumbar spine, the IAR in flexion is located in the intervertebral disk. Therefore, in flexion and extension, the nucleus pulposus may be considered the center of motion in the sagittal plane. In flexion and with anterior column destruction, the IAR migrates inferiorly and posteriorly. In extension and with posterior column destruction, the IAR migrates inferiorly and anteriorly. This tendency for either anterior or posterior migration is enhanced by additional destruction of the middle column[20] (Fig. 70-8).

Practical biomechanical implications for these findings can be expressed in terms of moment arms and mechanical advantages. For example, in the noninjured erect spine, moments created by the center of gravity and moments created by the paraspinal muscles are in equilibrium. An injury to the anterior column will induce a posterior migration of the IAR, which will give the center of gravity a positive mechanical advantage by increasing its moment arm (i.e., a flexion moment). The spine will remain stable if the paraspinal muscles can increase their force generation across a decreased moment arm sufficiently to offset the force now generated by the center of gravity and its increased moment arm. With anterior and middle column failure, the IAR migrates into the region of the paraspinal musculature (Fig. 70-8B). In this situation, the muscles no longer have an effective moment arm and therefore have no mechanical advantage. They are unable to counteract the forces created by the center of gravity and its longer moment arm, resulting in instability.

Conclusion

Determining the stability of this complex biomechanical structure is sometimes difficult. Injury classifications based on radiographic estimation of anatomic integrity are sometimes useful. The three-column concept of spinal anatomy suggests that a one-column injury is stable, while a three-column injury is grossly unstable. Two-column pathology represents an intermediate or gray zone and these injuries need to be carefully analyzed. The classification popularized by Gaines simplistically but reasonably assumes that the greater the amount of vertebral body destruction and acute deformity, the more instability there will be. However, assessment of static x-rays can be deceiving; dynamic studies are often important in the final determination of biomechanical stability. Thus, in many situations, the question of spinal stability is unclear and rests on the interpretation of pertinent radiographs, a neurologic exam, and a sound clinical and biomechanical judgment.

It is also clear that it is necessary to understand the position of the IAR in the nonpathologic as well as the pathologic spine. Without such understanding, it will be

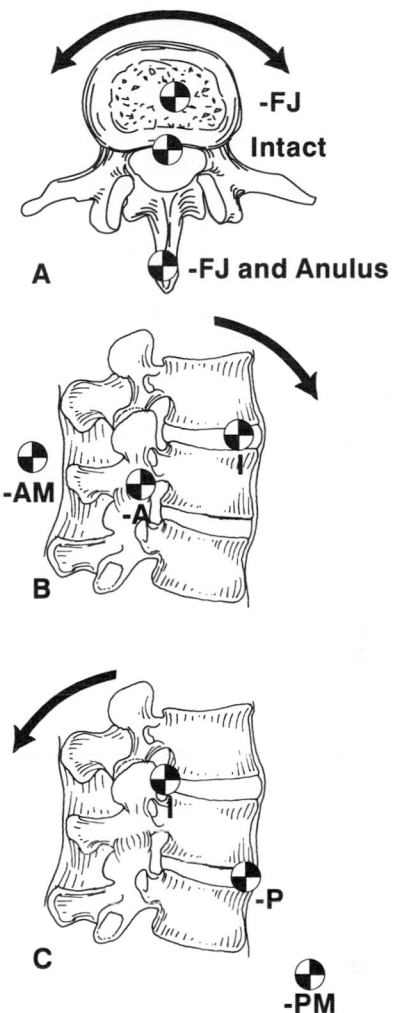

Figure 70-8 The instantaneous axis of rotation (IAR) for the lumbar spine. *A.* The IAR in the intact spine during axial rotation. The IAR is found near the posterior vertebral body wall. With destruction of the facet joints, the IAR moves anteriorly, and with destruction of both the facet joints and the annulus, the IAR moves posteriorly. *B.* The IAR in the intact spine during flexion is identified in the anterior column and near the intervertebral disk. With destruction of the anterior column, the IAR moves posteriorly to the region of the facet joint. With destruction of both the anterior and the middle columns, the IAR moves into the paraspinal muscle area. *C.* The IAR during extension in the intact lumbar spine is located near the posterior vertebral body wall in the region of the disk. With destruction of the posterior elements, the IAR moves toward the anterior column into the region of the next inferior disk. With destruction of both the posterior and middle columns, the IAR moves anterior to the spine.

impossible to appropriately counteract the pathologic biomechanics and reestablish stability to the injured spine.

NEUROLOGIC INJURIES

Neurologic systems fall into two broad categories: upper motor neuron (UMN) and lower motor neuron (LMN) (Fig.

70-9). Based upon the anatomic location of the vertebral column injury, there are three categories of neurologic injury: lesions of the spinal cord (UMN), conus medullaris (UMN), and cauda equina (LMN). Injuries to the cervical and thoracic spine typically affect the spinal cord and nerve roots in the vicinity of the injury.[21] Significant spinal cord injuries are typically accompanied by obvious radiographic evidence of trauma, but this is not always the case. Spinal cord injury without obvious vertebral column injury is a documented phenomenon often seen in children.[22] The distal spinal cord is termed the conus medullaris and usually lies near the thoracolumbar junction at about L1 or L2 (Fig. 70-10). The sacral nuclei that control bowel, bladder, and sexual function are located in the conus.[23,24] Because of the close proximity of the cauda equina, it is often involved with conus injuries[25] (Fig. 70-11). The cauda equina consists of all lumbar and sacral roots below the conus. Neurologic injuries below L2 typically are cauda equina in nature. Injuries to the cauda equina, because they involve peripheral nerves, have a better prognosis for return of function than spinal cord or conus injuries.

Spinal cord injuries typically accompany cervical and thoracic fractures.[26–28] When they occur, they are classified as either complete or incomplete. Complete lesions are characterized by total loss of motor, sensory, and reflex function below the level of injury[29,30] (Table 70-5). These injuries result in varying degrees of quadriplegia in the cervical spine and paraplegia in the thoracic spine. Complete spinal cord injuries of the cervical spine are named by the last functioning cervical root (e.g., C6 quadriplegia). In cervical lesions, one root level may make the difference between the patient's dependence or functional independence. For example, a C3 quadriplegic is ventilator-dependent without any upper or lower extremity function, while patients with a level C6 or below can function independently with mechanical aids (Table 70-6).

When complete spinal cord injuries occur in the thoracic spine, they produce paraplegia. The location of the lesion is irrelevant to the functional outcome for the patient, since the segmental thoracic nerve roots only supply sensation to the thorax and innervation to the intercostal muscles. However, a patient with a proximal thoracic paraplegia may have an increased risk of respiratory problems because of increased intercostal paralysis in comparison with a lower thoracic paraplegic. Patients with complete spinal cord injuries also run a risk of developing spinal deformities and Charcot spinal joints.[31,32]

Incomplete spinal cord injuries are more difficult to classify accurately (Table 70-7). Each injury is unique, involving various regions of the spinal cord and adjacent nerve roots.[33] In practical experience, incomplete lesions rarely fall cleanly into any one category. Classically, these injuries have been categorized into four types: anterior cord, posterior cord, central cord, and Brown-Séquard's syndrome.

Anterior cord syndromes result from injury or destruction to the anterior spinal cord, which contains corticospinal motor tracks and motor horns in the ventral gray matter. This results in motor paralysis with preservation of deep pressure sensation and proprioception due to the intact posterior columns.

The posterior cord syndrome is more rare and results from direct injury to the posterior columns. This causes loss of proprioception and deep pressure sensation. Maintenance of motor function is due to the intact anterior motor columns.

Cervical central cord syndrome results from damage to the central gray matter and the more centrally oriented white matter tracts, which provide motor innervation to the upper extremities. As a result, the upper extremities are more involved than the lower. A similar injury can occur in the thoracic spine. Here, a central cord injury will affect the proximal musculature of the lower extremities more severely than the distal musculature.

In the Brown-Séquard syndrome, half of the spinal cord is damaged in the axial projection. For a right-sided injury, there will be an ipsilateral motor paralysis and loss of position sense due to ipsilateral destruction of the anterior and posterior cell bodies and white matter tracts. In addition, there is a contralateral (left-sided) loss of pain and temperature sensation. The difference in right and left expression of this injury is due to different levels of decussation of the white matter tracts responsible for these functions. The motor tracts and posterior columns decussate in the brainstem, while the sensory tracts decussate one or two levels above where they enter the spinal cord.

Injuries involving the conus medullaris occur with trauma to the thoracolumbar junction and upper lumbar spine. They frequently involve elements of both the lower spinal cord and the cauda equina. Since the conus medullaris usually resides at the level of L1 or L2, vertebral column injuries at this level often result in a combination of sacral upper motor neuron and sacral or lumbar root (LMN) injuries (see Table 70-8). In the acute setting, especially in the face of spinal shock, injuries at this level

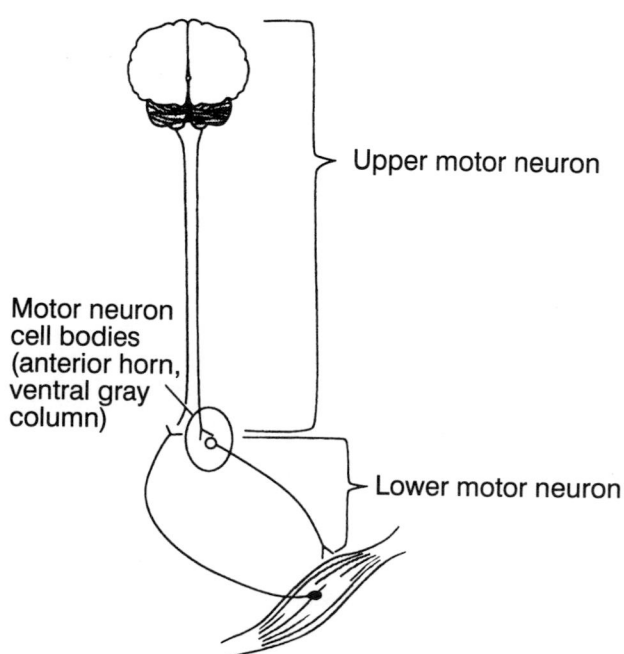

Upper motor neuron

Motor neuron cell bodies (anterior horn, ventral gray column)

Lower motor neuron

Figure 70-9 Schematic anatomy of upper and lower motor neurons. (Reproduced with permission from Haher TR, O'Brien MF, Felmy WT: Thoracic and lumbar fractures: Diagnosis and management, in Bridwell KH, DeWald RL (eds): *Textbook of Spinal Surgery.* Philadelphia, Lippincott, 1991.)

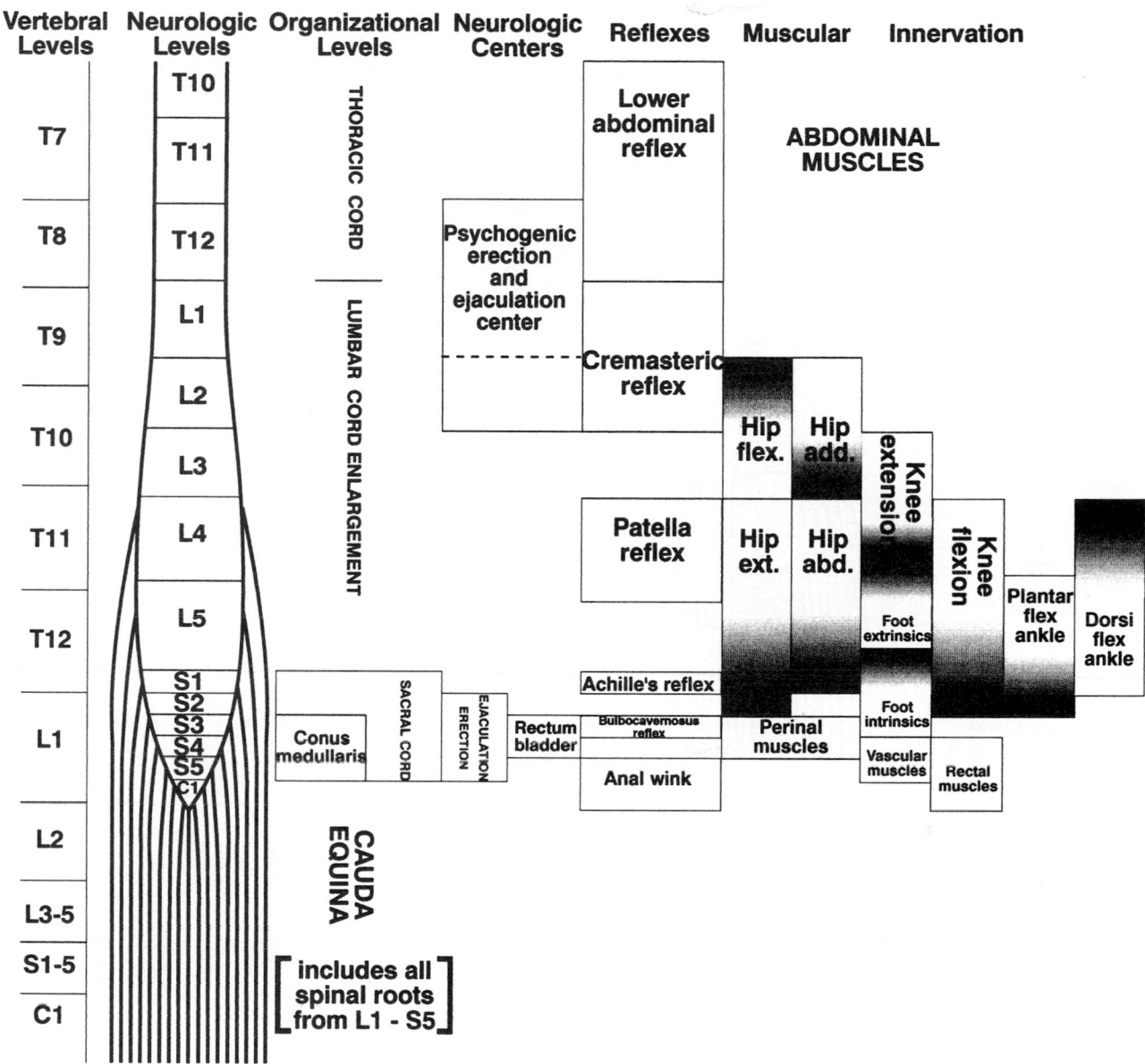

Figure 70-10 Structural and neurologic schema of the vertebral column and spinal cord. The neurologic implications of a vertebral column injury may be traced from left to right across the chart. [Reproduced with permission from Haher TR, O'Brien MF, Felmy WT: Thoracic and lumbar fractures: Diagnosis and management, in Bridwell KH, DeWald RL (eds): *Textbook of Spinal Surgery.* Philadelphia, Lippincott, 1991.]

are difficult to diagnose and describe accurately. Thus, it is possible to regain motor strength in the lower extremities, which are innervated by the involved lumbar nerves (LMN), but to continue to have absent bowel and bladder function due to a conus injury (UMN).

Cauda equina injuries occur with fractures or dislocations involving the L2 vertebral level and below. The neurologic deficit may range from a single nerve root injury to a cauda equina syndrome in which there is marked weakness of both lower extremities and involvement of the nerve roots supplying the bowel and bladder. Though not typically associated with traumatic injuries, an extremely large acute disk herniation may also cause an acute cauda equina syndrome. Emergent decompression is mandatory if neurologic function is to return.

The decrease in the spinal canal's cross-sectional area following fracture or dislocation does not always correlate with the severity of neurologic injury or the prognosis for recovery. This is because the size of the canal and the presence of bone or disk material within it only reflects the final resting place of these fragments. It does not define the magnitude of the energy absorbed, the maximum displacement, or the trajectory of the displaced fragments.[34-36] However, residual spinal canal compromise of greater than 50 percent or an absolute spinal canal AP dimension less than 10 to 13 mm would raise concerns about the possibility of impending neurologic dysfunction, either acutely or chronically. In spite of these concerns—which might prompt decompression—studies have shown that retropulsed bone will of-

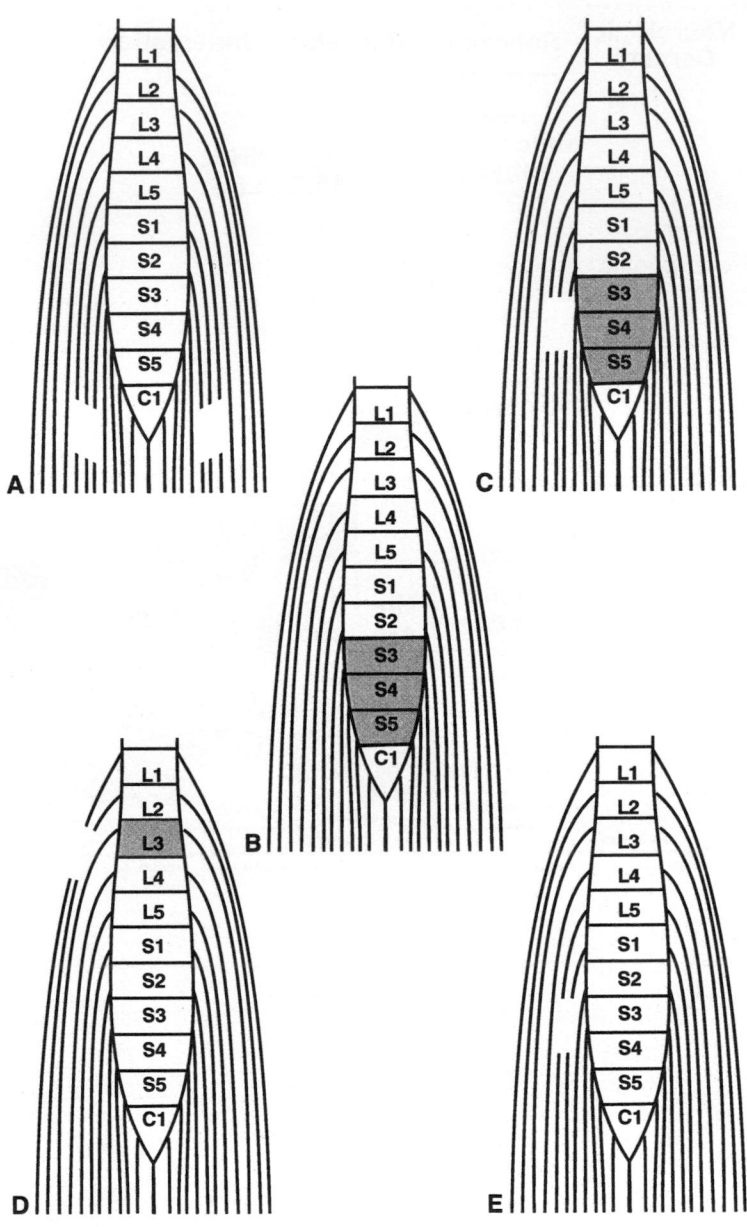

Figure 70-11 Neurologic injuries resulting from thoracolumbar fractures. *A.* Cauda equina injury (LMN) with good chance of recovery. *B.* Conus medullaris injury (LMN) with little chance of recovery. *C.* Conus medullaris with root injuries (LMN) with good chance of root recovery but not for S3-S5 cord segments. *D.* L3 cord injury (LMN), no chance of recovery for L3 segment and below. Conus medullaris symptoms (UMN) with no chance of recovery. Adjacent L2 root lesion (LMN) with good chance of recovery. *E.* Isolated root injury (LMN) with good chance of recovery. [Reproduced with permission from Haher TR, O'Brien MF, Felmy WT: Thoracic and lumbar fractures: Diagnosis and management, in Bridwell KH, DeWald RL (eds): *Textbook of Spinal Surgery.* Philadelphia, Lippincott, 1991.]

ten remodel over time,[37] thus increasing spinal canal dimensions.

Decompression of the spinal canal for complete spinal cord injuries typically does little to improve neurologic outcome. Surgical decompression is recommended for incomplete spinal cord, conus, or cauda equina lesions. These may benefit from rigid immobilization and prompt institution of pharmacologic therapy to counteract the secondary effects of spinal cord injury. Significant improvement in neurologic outcome is possible, especially with cauda equina (LMN) lesions.[38]

Penetrating spinal trauma from gunshot wounds rarely renders the spinal column unstable. However, neurologic injury is frequent. Cervical and thoracic level injuries often produce quadriplegia or paraplegia, respectively. Incomplete injuries are usually Brown-Séquard in nature. Similarly, injury to the cauda equina occurs with lumbar gunshot wounds. Most of the neural damage is secondary

to kinetic energy transference to the neural tissues. Surgical removal of a bullet is rarely indicated except with incomplete spinal cord or cauda equina lesions with a space-occupying fragment of bone or bullet identified. Because of the heat generated, these bullet wounds have a low infection rate unless they have traversed the colon prior to entering the spinal column. This is an indication for elective removal of the bullet if lodged in the spinal column or canal. Shotgun wounds should also be debrided because of the possibility of organic material from the wadding or from foreign material dragged in with the mass of projectile.

Diagnosis

It should be assumed that all multitrauma patients have spinal column injury until proven otherwise. The initial

TABLE 70-5 Functional Goals for Spinal Cord Injuries

Level	Mobility	Transfer	ADL	Bowel Dress	Bladder Care	Attendant Care	Care	Special Equipment
C1-2	Elec. WC	Dependent	Dependent	Dependent	Dependent	Dependent	Full time	Envir. control respirator
C3	Elec. WC	Dependent	Dependent	Dependent	Dependent	Dependent	Full time	Envir. control
C4	Elec. WC	Dependent	Dependent	Dependent	Dependent	Dependent	Full time	Envir. control
C5	Elec. WC	Dependent	Dependent	Dependent	Dependent	Dependent	Full time	Low-effort car controls
C6	Manual WC, van/car	?Independent	Minor assistance	?Independent	Dependent	Dependent	Part time	Adapted utensils tenodesis splints
C7	Manual WC, car	?Independent	Independent	Independent	Dependent	Assist	Part time	
C8	Manual WC, car	Independent	Independent	Independent	Assistance	Minor assist	Minimum time	
T1	Manual WC, car	Independent	Independent	Independent	Assistance	Minor assist	Minimum time	
T2-7	Manual WC, car	Independent	Independent	Independent	Minor assist	Independent	Minimum to none	
T8-9	Manual WC, car, ?exercise ambulation	Independent	Independent	Independent	Independent	Independent	None	?KAFO
T10-11	Manual WC, car, exercise ambulation	Independent	Independent	Independent	Independent	Independent	None	KAFO
T12-L1	Manual WC, car, ?house ambulation	Independent	Independent	Independent	Independent	Independent	None	KAFO
L2-3	Manual WC, car, house ambulation	Independent	Independent	Independent	Independent	Independent	None	KAFO
L4 and below	Community ambulation, ?WC, car	Independent	Independent	Independent	Independent	Independent	None	AFO

Key: ADL, activities of daily living; WC, wheelchair; KAFO, knee-ankle-foot orthosis; AFO, ankle-foot orthosis.

TABLE 70-6   Incomplete Spinal Cord Injuries

Syndrome	Sensory sparing	Motor sparing	Neurologic prognosis	Functional prognosis
Anterior cord	Touch, vibration, joint and pain	None or minimal	Better than complete anterior	Dependent or return
Central cord	All modalities distal > proximal	Distal > proximal	Variable; fair to good	Variable; poor to fair
Brown-Séquard	Contralateral position sense Touch bilateral Pain ipsilateral	Contralateral	Good	Excellent
Posterior cord	Pain, touch	Fair to good; difficult to test	Rare, probably fair to good	Fair
Concussion (Stinger)	Rapid return	Rapid return	Normal within 48 h	Excellent

priorities are for medical management, including securing an airway, ventilation, and hemodynamic stabilization. This should be done as expeditiously as possible and without undue mobilization of the spine. Spinal precautions should be established as soon as the medical condition allows. This includes immobilization of the entire spinal column at the accident site and until a major axial injury is ruled out. As far as possible, multiple evaluations should be performed by the same examiner, so that any evolving neurologic deficits can be detected in a timely fashion. An

TABLE 70-7   Expected Functional Outcome after Spinal Cord Injury

Lowest functioning neurologic level	Lowest functional muscle	Upper extremity function	Trunk control	Lowest extremity function
C1-2	Neck	None	Absent or poor	None
C3	Diaphragm	None	Absent or poor	None
C4	Deltoid	Limited shoulder	Absent or poor	None
C5	Biceps	Elbow flexion, fair shoulder	Absent or poor	None
C6	Wrist extensor	Good shoulder, tenodesis grasp	Absent or poor	None
C7	Triceps	Good shoulder, good elbow, tenodesis grasp	Absent or poor	None
C8	Wrist flexor, finger extrinsics	Good shoulder and elbow, fair hand	Absent or poor	None
T1	Hand extrinsics	Good shoulder, elbow, and hand	Poor to fair	None
T2-7	Intercostals	Normal	Poor to fair	None
T8-9	Upper abdominal	Normal	Fair	None
T10-11	Lower abdominal, quadratus lumborum	Normal	Good	Pelvic control
T12-L2	Hip flexors and adductors	Normal	Normal	Hip flexion
L3-4	Quadriceps	Normal	Normal	Knee extension
L5	Anterior tibial	Normal	Normal	Knee good, ankle fair
S1-S2	Gastrocnemius, gluteals	Normal	Normal	Hip, knee, ankle good

TABLE 70-8 Neurologic Sequelae Resulting from Injuries to the Cauda Equina, Conus Medullaris, and Spinal Cord

Symptoms	Cauda equina root	Conus medullaris	Cord above conus
Sensory deficit	Saddle anesthesia or inappropriate root distribution Loss of bladder sensation	Anesthetic in S3-S5 distribution	Below the level of the lesion
Motor deficit	Possible symmetrical deficits Asymmetrical deficits seen in appropriate root distribution Flaccid paralysis (LMN)	Symmetrical loss of perineal muscles Symmetrical loss of some root intrinsics Flaccid paralysis (LMN)	Below the level of the lesion Flaccid paralysis at the destroyed level (LMN) Possible spastic paralysis below (UMN)
Bowel and bladder changes	No anal sphincter tone Overflow Spastic incontinence Flaccid bladder	No anal sphincter tone Overflow incontinence Flaccid bladder (LMN)	Positive anal sphincter tone incontinent Hyperreflexic bladder (UMN) ⎫ Detrusor-sphincter Spastic urethral sphincter ⎭ Dyssynergia
Sexual function	Loss of reflexogenic erections, positive psychogenic erection Possible emission Possible ejaculation Possible fertility Possible orgasm	Loss of reflexogenic erection, + psychogenic erection Unlikely emission Possible ejaculation Unlikely fertility Unlikely orgasm	All function may be present if lesion is between upper and lower center Positive reflexogenic erection No psychogenic erection *if lesion is above T12* Unlikely emission, fertility, orgasm Possible ejaculation
Reflex changes	No deep tendon or physiologic reflexes below the lesion in the distribution of affected roots	No anal wink No bulbocavernosus reflex Possibly no Achilles reflex	Hyperactive DTR (UMN) + Bulbocavernosus + Anal wink + Achilles
Pathologic reflexes	No pathologic reflexes	No pathologic reflexes	+ Babinski if lesion is above L5
Pain	Low back pain Radicular pain in thigh or leg May be unilateral May be in perineum Symmetrical or asymmetrical	Not significant, usually bilateral when present	

Source: Reproduced with permission from Haher TR, O'Brien MF, Felmy WT: Thoracic and lumbar fractures: Diagnosis and management, in Bridwell KH, DeWald RL (eds): *Textbook of Spinal Surgery.* Philadelphia, Lippincott, 1991.

evolving neurologic deficit may be missed if multiple examiners are responsible for documenting the patient's neurologic status or if a reliable and reproducible notation technique is not used (Fig. 70-12).

Conscious patients with a history of trauma to the head, neck, or back who report any neurologic symptoms, even if only transient, should be immobilized in a cervical collar, maintaining complete head and neck immobilization on a spine board until an appropriate evaluation can be performed. A detailed history—including the mechanism of injury, localization of any neck or back pain, and a

motor and sensory examination of all extremities—is essential. The thorough evaluation of an unconscious patient in the setting of major trauma is more difficult. Nevertheless, suspicion of spinal injury should remain high until thorough examination has ruled out spinal cord or column injury.

A thorough neurologic examination should be performed as soon as possible. This examination should include a complete assessment of motor, sensory, and reflex functions for both the upper and lower extremities. In addition, perineal and perirectal sensation and motor func-

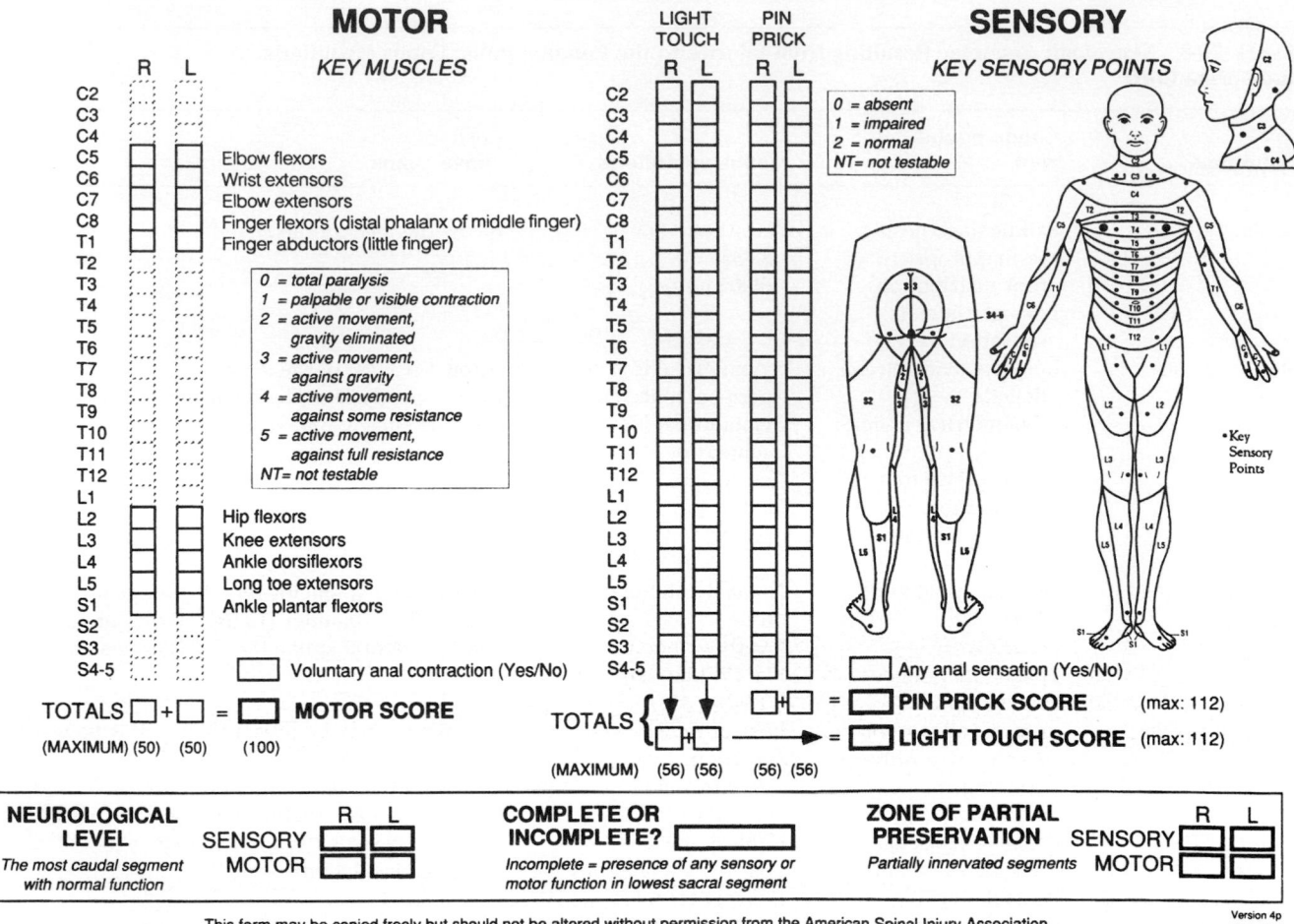

STANDARD NEUROLOGICAL CLASSIFICATION OF SPINAL CORD INJURY

MOTOR

KEY MUSCLES

	R	L	
C2			
C3			
C4			
C5			Elbow flexors
C6			Wrist extensors
C7			Elbow extensors
C8			Finger flexors (distal phalanx of middle finger)
T1			Finger abductors (little finger)

0 = total paralysis
1 = palpable or visible contraction
2 = active movement, gravity eliminated
3 = active movement, against gravity
4 = active movement, against some resistance
5 = active movement, against full resistance
NT= not testable

L2			Hip flexors
L3			Knee extensors
L4			Ankle dorsiflexors
L5			Long toe extensors
S1			Ankle plantar flexors

☐ Voluntary anal contraction (Yes/No)

TOTALS ☐ + ☐ = ☐ **MOTOR SCORE**

(MAXIMUM) (50) (50) (100)

LIGHT TOUCH | **PIN PRICK** | **SENSORY**

KEY SENSORY POINTS

0 = absent
1 = impaired
2 = normal
NT= not testable

☐ Any anal sensation (Yes/No)

TOTALS { ☐ + ☐ = ☐ **PIN PRICK SCORE** (max: 112)

☐ + ☐ → = ☐ **LIGHT TOUCH SCORE** (max: 112)

(MAXIMUM) (56) (56) (56) (56)

• Key Sensory Points

NEUROLOGICAL LEVEL		R	L	COMPLETE OR INCOMPLETE? ☐	ZONE OF PARTIAL PRESERVATION		R	L
The most caudal segment with normal function	SENSORY	☐	☐		Partially innervated segments	SENSORY	☐	☐
	MOTOR	☐	☐	Incomplete = presence of any sensory or motor function in lowest sacral segment		MOTOR	☐	☐

This form may be copied freely but should not be altered without permission from the American Spinal Injury Association

Version 4p
GHC 1992

A

Figure 70-12 *A.* Motor and sensory checklist for posttrauma neurologic examination. *B.* Neurologic impairment scale. (Reproduced with permission from the American Spinal Injury Association.)

ASIA IMPAIRMENT SCALE

☐ **A = Complete:** No motor or sensory function is preserved in the sacral segments S4-S5.

☐ **B = Incomplete:** Sensory but not motor function is preserved below the neurological level and extends through the sacral segments S4-S5.

☐ **C = Incomplete:** Motor function is preserved below the neurological level, and the majority of key muscles below the neurological level have a muscle grade less than 3.

☐ **D = Incomplete:** Motor function is preserved below the neurological level, and the majority of key muscles below the neurological level have a muscle grade greater than or equal to 3.

☐ **E = Normal:** Motor and sensory function is normal.

CLINICAL SYNDROMES

☐ Central Cord
☐ Brown-Sequard
☐ Anterior Cord
☐ Conus Medullaris
☐ Cauda Equina

B

tion need to be assessed to determine the functionality of the sacral roots and sacral cord. Sacral sensory sparing or any trace of distal motor function in the face of spinal cord or cauda equina injury strongly implies the possibility of improved neurologic function. Spinal shock during the first 24 to 72 h can easily give the appearance of, and be misinterpreted as, a complete spinal cord injury in patients who will later be found to have sensory and motor function. Resolution of spinal shock is typically indicated by the return of a bulbocavernosus reflex. This can be tested by performing a digital rectal examination and pulling on either the glans of the penis, the clitoris, or the Foley catheter. This should result in contraction of the anal sphincter when the reflex is present. Presence of a bulbocavernosus reflex in the face of complete loss of distal motor function suggests that the patient has sustained a complete spinal cord injury with little chance for return of neurologic function.

Initial Management

Prior to definitive stabilization, all patients are kept in a supine position on a well-padded mattress and log-rolled every 2 h to decrease cutaneous pressure over bony prominences or over skin desensitized by spinal injury.[39] Because immobilization puts these patients at risk for deep vein thrombosis, mechanical prophylaxis is provided in the form of thigh-high elastic stockings and mechanical compression devices. This is particularly true for the elderly and the severely involved trauma patient.

Careful monitoring of cardiac and pulmonary function is mandatory. In addition, a nasogastric tube is placed for decompression of the gastrointestinal ileus that often accompanies major trauma. Fluid support is maintained with intravenous access. Overall hydration and renal function are accurately measured with the assistance of a Foley catheter. Standard laboratory tests, including complete blood count and blood chemistries, are obtained to verify medical and hemodynamic stability. This is particularly important early in the postinjury period, when internal hemorrhage may be overlooked. Low blood pressure in the setting of acute spinal cord injury may represent internal hemorrhage or spinal shock.[40] Spinal shock results from loss of sympathetic control over the vascular system. This is identified by a low blood pressure without tachycardia. Internal hemorrhage results in low blood pressure combined with tachycardia. Analgesic support is dictated by age, medical status, and the level of pain. Physical therapy for range of motion of uninjured extremities should be started early in the hospital course to prevent contractures.

Patients with injuries of the cervical spine, in addition to this standard regimen, should be treated with cervical traction.[41] They should be placed in traction for reduction of the cervical malalignment regardless of their neurologic status. It is suggested that MRI-compatible occipital fixation devices be used. These can either be Gardner-Wells tongs or, if a halo brace is anticipated to be necessary, either during operative treatment or as part of the postoperative immobilization, a halo ring may be affixed primarily.[42] In using a halo ring as the occipital attachment, care should be taken to ensure that there is no friction between the posterior aspect of the ring and the bed. This can be accomplished either by using a three-quarter ring open in the back or by padding the patient. During placement of Gardner-Wells tongs, the occipital pins are placed one finger's breadth above the superior aspect of the earlobe and in line with the external auditory canal.

The position may be changed so that the pins are either anterior or posterior to the external auditory canal to assist in creating either a flexion or extension vector. Controlling the vector pull is somewhat easier when a halo is used because the multiple fixation points allow rigid fixation to the skull. Gardner-Wells tongs should be equipped with pressure-sensitive "pop-up" pins that indicate when the appropriate tension has been reached. Halo rings are typically fixed to the skull with either predetermined shear-type tightening devices or with slip-clutch–activated torque wrenches. Typically 6 to 8 lb of force is applied through the fixation pins.[43] In applying halo ring devices, care must be taken to avoid the supraorbital and supratrochlear nerve over the middle and medial thirds of the orbits.[44] Posterior pin placement should be below the equator of the skull. The ring must not touch the earlobes. Generally, a finger's breadth is allowed between the ring

and the tip of the earlobes. Anterior pin placement should be approximately 1 to 2 cm above the eyebrows and no further medial than the junction of the middle and lateral thirds of the orbit. Standard fixation with four pins is typically sufficient for older adolescents and adults. In the elderly who are osteoporotic or in children with soft bone, consideration should be given to additional pins; up to six or eight may be used to spread the force of fixation over more surface area. Numerous complications have been reported with the use of halos, including nerve injury, dysphagia from extreme hyperextension to achieve fracture reduction, infection, penetration of the skull with pins, loss of occipital fixation, and loss of reduction.[44,45]

In applying traction for realignment, ligamentous integrity is assumed. This must be verified with lateral x-rays soon after the application of weight. In addition, the neurologic status should be closely watched during the process of realignment with occipital traction. Severe neurologic injuries have been reported with overly aggressive application of traction weight in patients with occult ligamentous injuries.[46] These can result in occipitocervical or cervical dislocations with complete neurologic injuries or death.

When traction is used, 5 lb per cervical level including the skull is a reasonable start. Therefore, a patient with a C4-C5 facet dislocation may require 25 lb for reduction of the malalignment. However, the authors have used up to 85 lb for the reduction of a C5-C6 bilateral facet dislocation in a large, otherwise healthy 20-year-old male with a complete spinal cord injury (Fig. 70-13). The use of weights in excess of 100 lb has been reported. This is not unusual in lower cervical injuries in large adults with significant axial muscle spasm due to acute injury.

When using heavy weights for reduction, care must be taken to assure that the occipital fixation remains good. Gardner-Wells pins may become stressed and bent, losing fixation. In addition, the frame may bend, resulting in loss of occipital fixation. These things are less likely to happen with a halo ring and multiple occipital fixation points.

Once reduction is achieved, minimal weight is required to maintain reduction. As little as 10 to 15 lb is usually sufficient to maintain alignment. Lateral radiographs of the cervical spine should be taken frequently during the realignment process. In addition, after transportation of the patient to and from tests, lateral radiographs should be obtained to ensure that the alignment has not been lost.

Radiographic Examination

Standard screening radiographs for each section of the spine include anteroposterior (AP) and lateral projections. Additionally, in the cervical spine, open-mouth x-rays for visualization of the C1-C2 articulation and the dens are obtained. Right and left oblique radiographs of the cervical spine provide excellent visualization of the neural foramen as well as the facet joints. Oblique x-rays may also be used in the lumbar spine for identification of pars injuries. Lateral flexion-extension x-rays may be useful to document dynamic instabilities, particularly in the cervical and lumbar spine. However, paraspinal muscle spasm accompanying acute injury may prevent adequate voluntary flexion-extension radiographs in the acute setting; these may

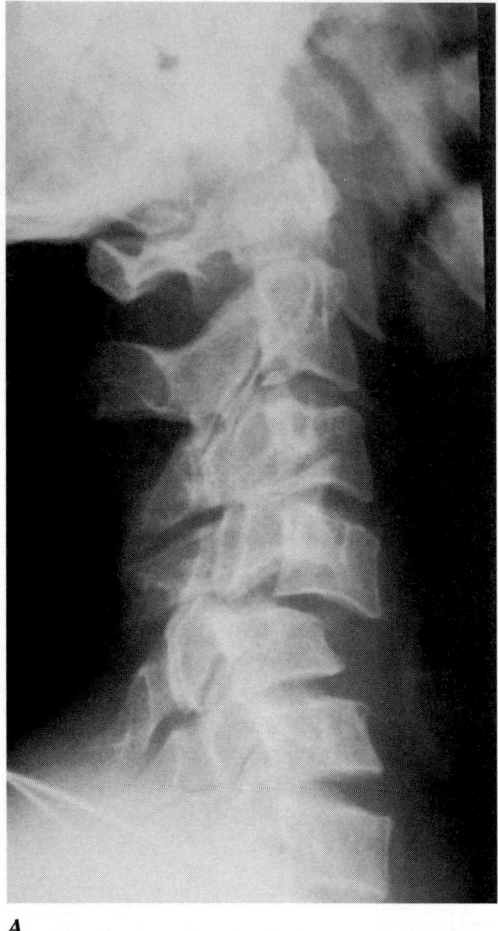

A

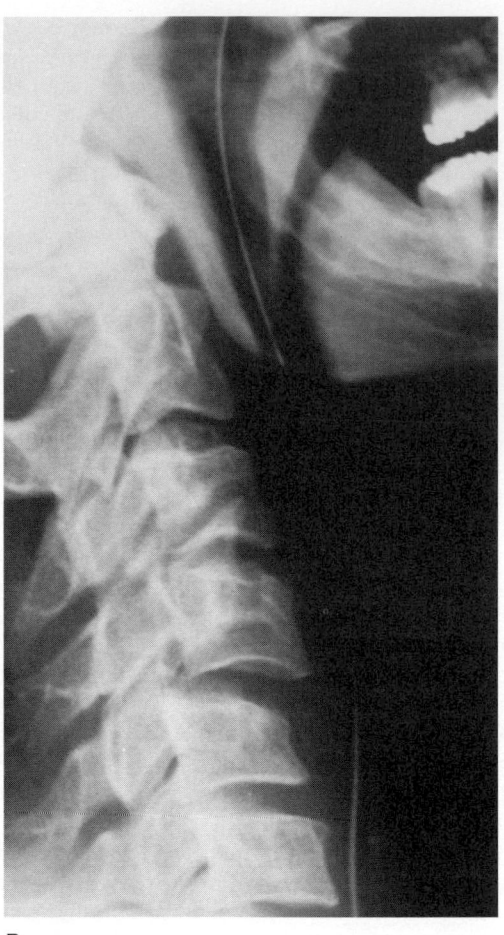

B

Figure 70-13 *A.* Bilateral facet dislocation identified at C4-C5 in a young patient who presented quadriplegic after a diving accident. *B.* Closed reduction in skeletal traction resulted in adequate initial alignment but did not improve the patient's neurologic examination.

need to be done 1 week postinjury to identify subtle instabilities. If an instability is recognized, axial computed tomography (CT) or MRI may help to ascertain if this is a purely ligamentous or an osseous injury. Also, CT scans may be necessary to rule out injuries of the upper cervical spine and cervicothoracic junction.[47]

In the lateral x-rays, the height of all the vertebral bodies should be uniform and symmetrical in comparison with adjacent vertebrae. There should be a smooth transition from segment to segment throughout the vertebral column. When vertebral body height is lost, an anterior angular deformity (i.e., kyphosis) will be evident on lateral radiographs. Compression of the middle column may be accompanied by posterior vertebral body retropulsion into the spinal canal, which may be evident on lateral spinal x-rays. This is more easily identified on transaxial CT scans.

While ligamentous injuries cannot be directly identified on plain radiographs, widened intraspinous distances, opened or subluxed facet joints, or asymmetrical widening of an intradiskal space may be indicative of an injury through ligamentous structures. White and Panjabi's definition of instability as judged on radiographs is helpful to keep in mind in evaluating cervical spine radiographs af-

ter trauma. Instability is indicated if adjacent vertebral bodies show more than 3.5 mm of translation or greater than 11° of intersegmental lordosis or kyphosis in comparison to adjacent segments. While these measurements may not indicate total loss of structural integrity, they probably do reflect significant ligamentous injuries if there is no obvious osseous injury.

In the AP radiographs, each vertebral body should sit directly on top of the one below and have its right- and left-hand borders aligned with those of the vertebral bodies directly adjacent. The pedicles should be placed symmetrically within the outline of the vertebral body. Widening of the distance between the pedicles at one level compared to that at adjacent levels may indicate injury to the middle column.[48] Careful examination should be made of the posterior elements. The posterior elements of a segment are somewhat distal to the corresponding vertebral body. The shadow of the spinous process is usually visible, allowing for comparison of the distances between the interspinous processes at each level. Increased distance between the shadows of the spinous processes may indicate a ligamentous injury involving the posterior column. An offset of the alignment in the spinous processes in the coronal projection (AP) may indicate rotational injury involving a facet fracture or dislocation. In the lumbar spine, minimally displaced but unstable fracture-dislocations can also be identified using this technique. In the lumbar spine, the facet joints should be examined for integrity and alignment. Finally, the transverse processes at each level should be examined for fractures. Transverse process fractures in the cervical spine may be accompanied by neural or vascular injury. Transverse process fractures in the lumbar spine may indicate significant ligamentous injury at the lumbosacral pelvic junction, where the heavy iliolumbar ligaments attach the lower lumbar spine to the pelvis. Fractures or avulsion fractures of the pelvic ring may portend similar instabilities. Similarly, in the thoracic spine, fractures of the transverse process and head/neck of the rib may indicate a severe soft tissue injury.[49] Anteroposterior x-rays are additionally useful for detecting sacral injuries. Asymmetry of the sacroiliac joints may suggest ligamentous disruption. Asymmetry of the sacral foramen and trabeculations may suggest fracture. These may not be obvious and close examination will be required to identify them. Any pelvic or sacral fractures indicate significant trauma and should always make one suspicious of undiagnosed occult spinal fractures.

As many as 10 percent of patients with documented spinal trauma at one level will have another undetected injury at an adjacent or distant site.[50] This is particularly important when these undetected injuries are in the cervical or thoracic spine. In patients who have an identified cervical or thoracic injury with an accompanying spinal cord injury, loss of sensation may make it difficult or impossible to detect vertebral column injuries at more caudal levels. For this reason it is important that in all patients with documented injuries of the spine or vertebral column a screening examination of the entire axial skeleton is done.

SPINAL CORD INJURIES

An in-depth discussion of the physiology and pharmacologic treatment of spinal cord injuries (SCI) is beyond the scope of this chapter.[51] However, it is important to mention some current concepts suggesting that there are two mechanisms—a primary and secondary injury—which contribute to the final neurologic damage in acute spinal cord injuries[52,53] (Fig. 70-14). The primary injury results from the mechanical tissue disruption itself, with its accompanying hemorrhage and cellular destruction (Table 70-9). The secondary injury is the sum of the body's reaction to the local trauma. This involves edema, inflammation, ischemia,[54] and a host of biochemical and cellular responses[55] that expand the zone of injury (Table 70-10). It is important to distinguish between these two cascades, since the primary injury occurs passively over a short interval of time and its immediate consequences are usually irreversible. However, the secondary component of the injury cascade is an actively mediated cellular and molecular process that evolves over many hours and may be manipulated if understood.[56]

A truly effective pharmacologic regimen for the treatment of spinal cord injury has yet to be defined. Numerous agents have been tested experimentally, including excitatory amino acid receptor blockade, gangliosides for stabilization of central nervous system cell membranes, opiate antagonists, calcium ion channel blockers, and steroids (Table 70-11). At this time, the only medication that has been documented to have some beneficial effect in the treatment of spinal cord injuries is methylprednisolone.[57–59] This is administered to the patient as an intravenous bolus of 30 mg/kg over 45 min, followed by continuous intravenous infusion of methylprednisolone at a dose of 5.4 mg/kg per hour for the next 23 h. The exact mechanism of action for its beneficial effect is unknown. It has been postulated that dosing at this level increases spinal cord blood flow, inhibits production of superoxide radicals and deactivates them,[60] decreases edema and inflammation, which improves vascularity and stabilizes cell membranes (Table 70-12). Because these large doses of steroids have been associated with some complications, including poor wound healing and infection, their use needs to be carefully considered. The indication for the use of steroids is cervical spinal injury in all patients with neurologic deficits—also thoracic spinal injuries with incomplete paraplegia and incomplete cauda equina lesions of the lumbar spine with neurologic deterioration. Since it is unlikely that there will be any significant functional improvement after a complete thoracic spinal cord injury, the use of high-dose steroids is probably not warranted. Because the functional outcome in cervical spinal injuries can be highly dependent on regaining even one root level, steroids should be considered even in the face of a complete cervical cord injury.[60]

Significant neurologic deterioration while a patient is on methylprednisolone warrants reconsideration of its use. In addition, because of the high risk of gastrointestinal hemorrhage with large doses of steroids, particularly in the face of the stress of a major spinal cord injury, all patients should be protected with H_2 antagonists such as cimetidine or ranitidine for at least 72 h. It is important to keep in mind that the beneficial effect of the steroids has been quite small, limited to minor improvements in sensation and motor function without significantly changing the grade or the level of serious spinal cord injuries. However, the benefits obtained by regaining even one root level may make their use reasonable.[61]

Injuries of the Upper Cervical Spine (C0-C2)

The unique anatomy and development of the craniocervical junction gives rise to unique biomechanics and injury patterns.[62] The most commonly occurring clinical entities are atlas fractures, atlantoaxial subluxations, odontoid fractures, and C2 traumatic spondylolisthesis (hangman's fractures). Other less common injuries are atlantooccipital dislocations, occipital condyle fractures, and atlantoaxial rotatory subluxation.

Atlas Fractures

Fractures of the atlas typically result from axial impaction of the occipital condyles onto the lateral masses of C1.[63] Atlas fractures represent approximately 10 percent of all

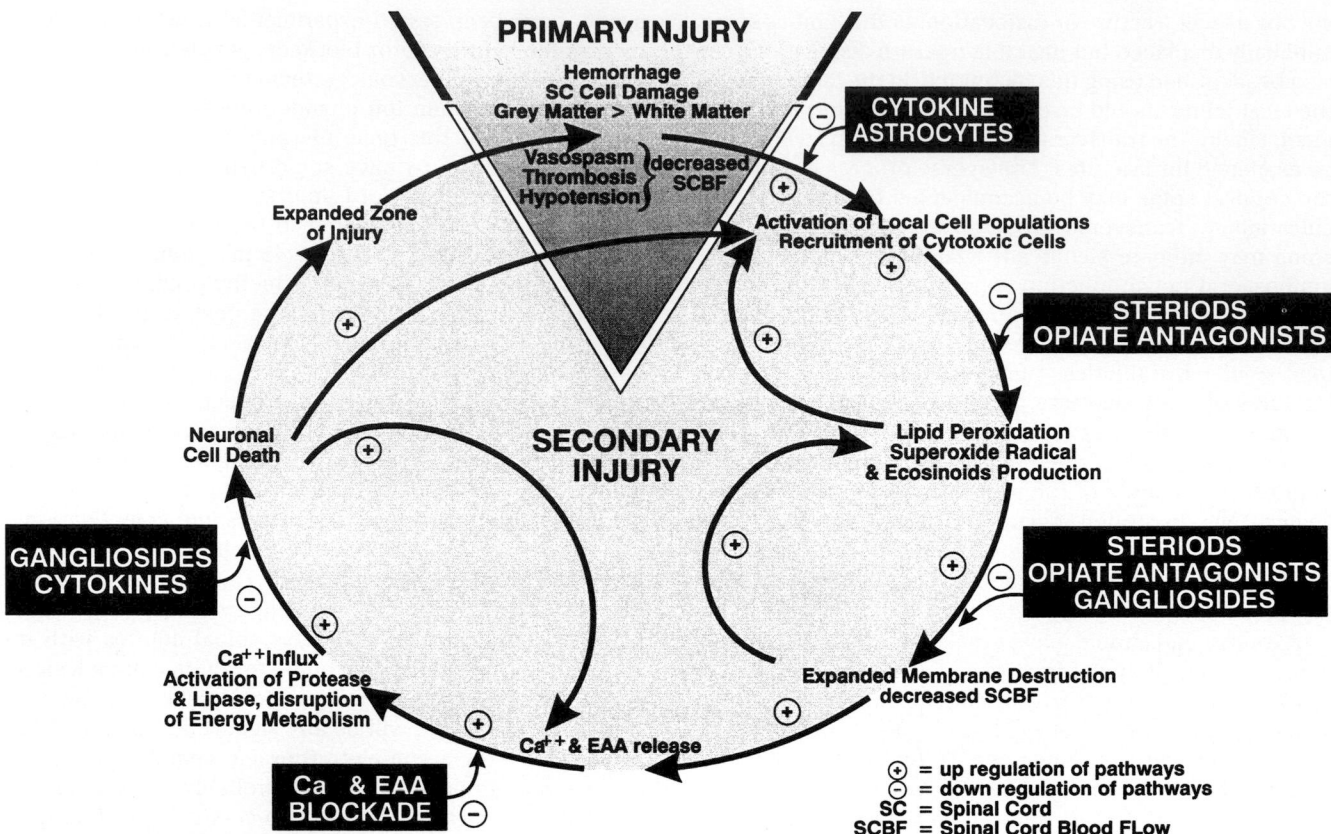

Figure 70-14 Primary and secondary injury cascade in acute spinal cord injury. [Reproduced with permission from O'Brien MF, Lenke LG, Joyce ME: Acute spinal cord injury: Patho- physiology and pharmacologic treatments, in Bridwell KH, DeWald RW (eds): *The Textbook of Spinal Surgery,* 2d ed. Philadelphia, Lippincott-Raven, 1996.]

cervical fractures and 2 percent of all spinal fractures.[64] Because of the mechanism of the injury, nearly 25 percent of atlas fractures are associated with significant craniofacial trauma, including closed head injuries. There is also a high association with noncontiguous spinal fractures. Because of the large space available for the spinal cord at this level, these fractures are not typically associated with neurologic injuries.[65] Fracture patterns can involve the anterior arch, the posterior arch, or both (Fig. 70-15). Isolated fractures of the lateral masses are also possible. Atypical fractures in the horizontal plane have been described. Because of the atlas's ringlike structure, there will typically be at least two fracture lines. Isolated bilateral fractures of

TABLE 70-9   Primary Mediators of Spinal Cord Injury

Mechanical traumatic event
Mechanical tissue disruption
Neural tissue compression/distraction
Hemorrhage
Electrolyte fluxes
Release of metabolites from injured cells

TABLE 70-10   Secondary Mediators of Spinal Cord Injury

Edema
Inflammation
Ischemia
Growth factors
Reperfusion
Calcium flux
Superoxide radicals

TABLE 70-11   Pharmacologic Treatment of Clinical and Experimental Acute Spinal Cord Injury

Antioxidants:
  Methylprednisolone (MP)
  21-Aminosteroids
  Free radical scavengers

Excitatory amino acids (EAA)
Receptor blockers

Gangliosides

Opiate antagonists

Calcium ion channel blockers

TGF-β and astrocytes

TABLE 70-12   Beneficial Effects of Methylprednisolone

Stabilizes cell membranes
Neutralizes superoxide radicals
Limits lipid peroxidation
Decreases accumulation of intracellular calcium
Decreases the release of excitatory amino acids
Decreases tissue edema
May improve spinal cord blood flow

the anterior arch are rare. They may present as comminuted but minimally displaced fracture lines at the junction of the anterior arch and the lateral masses. Bilateral fractures of the posterior arch account for two-thirds of all C1 fractures and are usually the result of hyperextension and axial loading. Failure occurs at the weakest point: the vascular groove for the vertebral artery. The Jefferson fracture is really a burst fracture of the atlas involving bilateral fractures of both the anterior and posterior arches with splaying of the lateral masses. Potential instability with these fractures needs to be assessed.[66] The lateral masses may drift apart if the transverse ligament has been ruptured or avulsed from its attachment to the medial aspect of the C1 lateral mass. If there is more than 6.9 mm of combined C1 lateral mass overhang on C2, this indicates rupture of the transverse ligament. If left unaddressed, this may result in cranial settling as the lateral masses of C1 are forced apart by the occipital condyles. Atlantoaxial instability due to rupture of the transverse ligament or its attachment to C1

may also result. Isolated lateral mass fractures may occur as a result of asymmetrical axial loading of the occiput on C1. If there is no significant comminution and if the ring of C1 has not been compromised, these injuries are stable. Severe comminution may cause asymmetrical settling, resulting in mechanical malalignment of the C0-C1 joint. These injuries are best seen on the open-mouth odontoid views of the C1-C2 complex.

Management of these fractures is still a topic of some debate. Type I and II atlas fractures may be managed in a well-fitting cervical orthosis in a compliant patient; otherwise a halo vest is more appropriate. Type III fractures are managed in a halo vest. In type IV Jefferson fractures, immediate halo vest immobilization is acceptable if the transverse ligament is competent (i.e., less than 6.9 mm of lateral mass displacement and no atlantoaxial subluxation). If there is any evidence of instability, particularly cranial settling as judged by a separation of the lateral masses of more than 6.9 mm,[67] these injuries are unstable and need to be managed with an initial period of 4 to 6 weeks of in-line cervical traction to realign the fragments and allow early consolidation of the fracture. This cannot be accomplished with a halo vest, since axial distraction is not consistently maintained with this device. After this initial period of realignment, a period of halo immobilization is necessary until complete consolidation of the fracture has occurred. While nonsurgical treatment of these fractures is the general rule, there may occasionally be associated fractures of the cervical spine or other contraindications to halo vest immobilization that would prompt surgical intervention for the treatment of these fractures. Nonunion, while rare, may also prompt fusion if it is painful. Provided that the lateral masses can be realigned, C1-C2 transarticular screws would be the

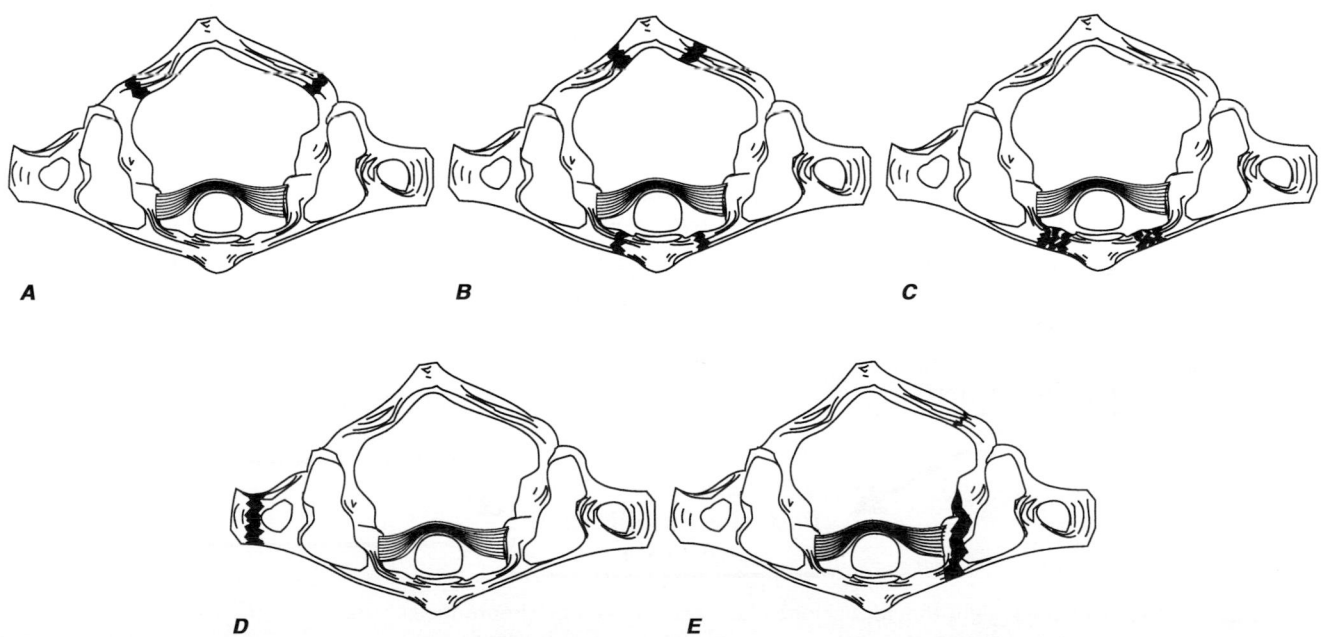

Figure 70-15 Classification of atlas fractures. *A.* Posterior arch fracture. *B.* Burst fracture (Jefferson fracture). *C.* Anterior arch fracture. *D.* Transverse process fracture. *E.* Comminuted, or lateral mass, fracture.

treatment of choice.[68] If this is not possible, either because the technical expertise is not available or there are associated occipital fractures, occipitocervical fusion may be the indicated procedure. Because occipitocervical fusion severely limits the motion of the cervical spine, it should be avoided whenever possible. In the setting of acute trauma, anterior decompression at the craniocervical junction is very unlikely to be required. However, when fractures at the craniocervical junction are irreducible and there is an anterior bony compressive element that puts the neuraxis at risk, a combined anterior and posterior procedure may be necessary (Fig. 70-16). After this fracture is healed, the stability of the C1-C2 complex must be verified. Rupture of the transverse ligament or incompetency due to stretch will result in atlantoaxial instability. Flexion-extension x-rays that reveal more than 5 mm of atlantoaxial subluxation in the adult may prompt fusion of the C1-C2 joint.

Atlantoaxial Subluxation

Atlantoaxial subluxation may be an isolated phenomenon or may accompany fracture of the atlas or dens.[69] Traumatic rupture of the transverse ligament is rare in the absence of an atlas fracture.[70] This injury results from a combination of flexion and anterior translation. Neurologic injury to the spinal cord is unlikely if there is a concomitant fracture of the dens. However, if the dens is intact, it may then become an anterior compressive agent, resulting in upper cervical cord injury. An atlantodens interval (ADI) of more than 3 mm in adults and 4.5 mm in children is pathologic, suggesting anterior translation of C1 on C2. In the awake, cooperative patient, voluntary flexion-extension x-rays can rule out this injury. In those who are unable to cooperate, anterior soft tissue swelling seen on lateral cervical x-rays of the spine should raise suspicion for this injury. In the face of apparently normal radiographs, a subtle avulsion fracture of the medial edge of the lateral mass of C1 at the insertion of the transverse ligament may identify an occult or impending atlantoaxial instability. These avulsion fractures can be clearly identified on CT scans. Halo immobilization is appropriate for documented avulsion fractures of the transverse ligament from the lateral mass of C1. These may heal with osseous union of the avulsed transverse ligament attachment, with only minor residual instability. Magnetic resonance imaging is useful in identifying tears of the transverse ligament itself.

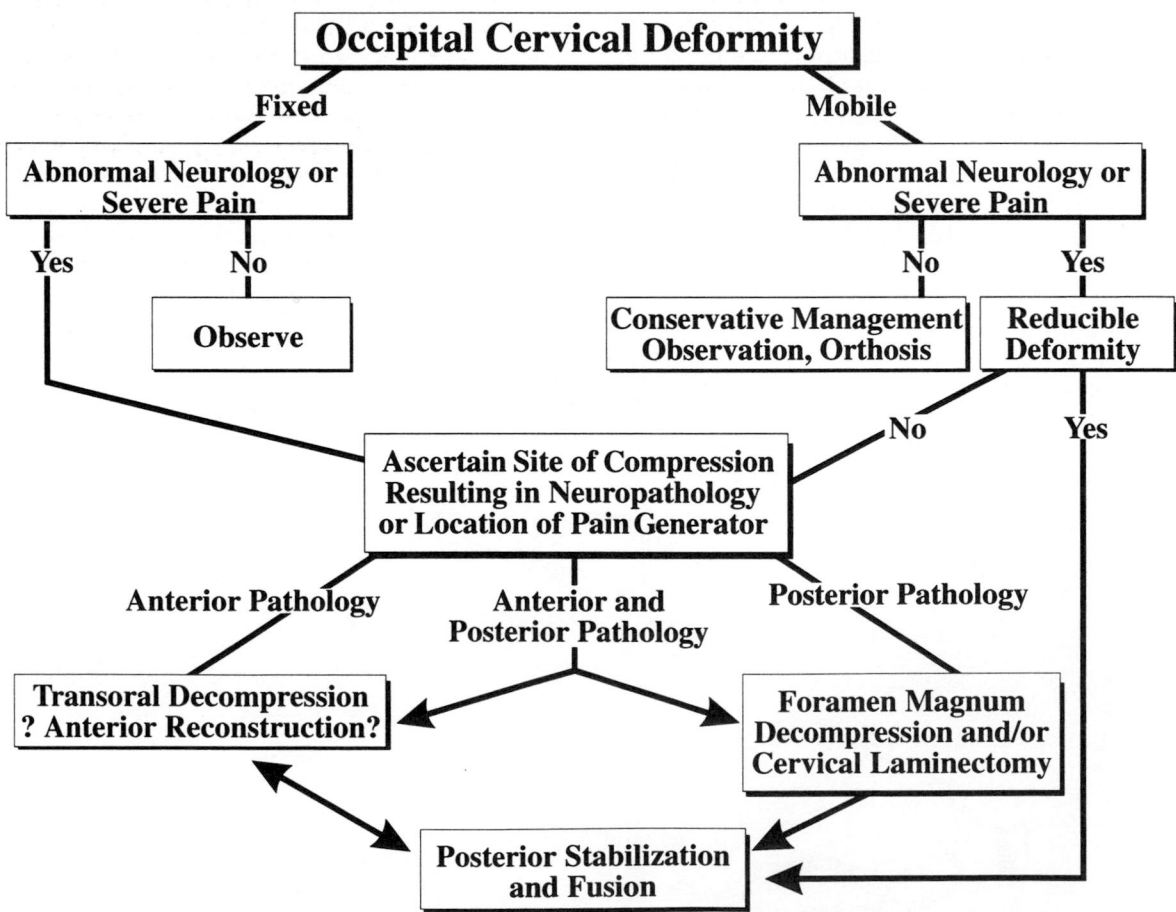

Figure 70-16 Treatment algorithm for occipitoatlantoaxial pathology. (Reproduced with permission from O'Brien MF, Sutterlin CE: Occipitocervical biomechanics: Clinical and biomechanical implications for posterior occipitocervical stabilization and fusion. *Spine* 10:281–313, 1996.)

When this injury is due to ligamentous damage, it is likely that there will be residual instability. Residual ligamentous instability would necessitate fusion of the C1-C2 joint. Posterior wiring techniques for C1-C2 are useful if a solid fusion is obtained. However, from a biomechanical point of view, these fixation techniques are suboptimal in maintaining alignment during the healing process and often result in malreductions and malunions.[71] The placement of transarticular screws fusing C1 to C2, while technically more demanding, represents the state of the art for fusion of this joint[72] (Fig. 70-17). Because of the potential for vertebral artery and neuraxial injury, this procedure should be performed only by those specifically trained in its use. When transarticular screws are supplemented with C1-C2 wiring and bone grafting, a superior biomechanical construct with a high likelihood of fusion is created.[73]

C2 Fractures

Odontoid fractures require a high index of suspicion for identification.[74] These fractures must be ruled out in all patients with neck pain following motor vehicle accidents. Falls in the elderly population with complaints of neck pain warrant careful scrutiny for nondisplaced odontoid fractures.[75] There may be significant translation of C1 either anteriorly or posteriorly as a result of this fracture, and spinal cord injury may occur. Most commonly, the fractured odontoid migrates posteriorly, decreasing the space available for the cord. The incidence of neurologic injury with this fracture is approximately 10 percent.[76] The radiographic views required to identify odontoid fractures are an open-mouth view of the upper cervical spine as well as lateral x-rays of the upper cervical spine. Both sagittal and coronal plane reconstructions will clearly characterize the fracture and the direction of dens displacement. Transaxial CT scans may miss the fracture line if it is in the plane of the axial image.[77] Odontoid fractures have been classified by Anderson and D'Alonzo.[78]

Type I fractures involve fractures of the tip of the dens at the insertion of the alar ligaments (Fig. 70-18). These fractures are relatively rare and are often associated with atlantooccipital dislocations. Rotatory instability may result from loss of alar ligament continuity. When not associated with occipitocervical dislocations, these injuries are typically stable and can be managed with an orthosis for symptomatic relief.

Type II fractures, which are the most common, occur at the base of the odontoid at its junction with the body of the axis. The high incidence of nonunion for this fracture has, in the past, been blamed on a supposedly tenuous blood supply.[79] However, entrapment and interposition of the transverse ligament within the fracture line is probably the more typical reason for ultimate nonunion.[80] In addition, other anatomic reasons for the high incidence of nonunion may be the high ratio of cortical to cancellous bone at the "waisted junction" of the dens and the body of the axis. Other risk factors for nonunion have been identified, namely angulation in the immediate postinjury x-rays, anterior or posterior displacement of more than 4 mm of the fracture fragment, and patient age greater than 40 years.[81] In patients above age 60, treatment is often complicated by delayed diagnosis. This is because the injury often results from minor trauma and is only discovered when the patient complains of persistent neck pain.

Halo immobilization is probably sufficient in most cases for stabilization and successful healing. Halos do not provide rigid fixation, and fusion may be necessary.[78] While fibrous nonunion does not necessarily portend a bad outcome, malunion with kyphotic angulation at the site of the fracture has been shown to result in posttraumatic myelopathy, which develops slowly over years.[80] Posterior fusion of C1 and C2 using either a wiring technique or transarticular screws[82] (Fig. 70-19) may be more appropriate in those patients who are either medically or emotionally unable to tolerate halo immobilization (see Fig. 70-36). Thought should also be given to anterior osteosynthesis with a dens screw in appropriate acute fractures[83] (Fig. 70-20).

This technique provides immediate stabilization without limiting C1-C2 movement.[82] Various techniques have been described for this, using either one or two screws, depending on the available room within the confines of the cortical shell of the dens.[84] Comminution at the site of the fracture, an anterior slope (posterosuperior to anteroinferior) of the fracture line, and fibrous nonunion may be contraindications to this technique. Both C1-C2 transarticular screws and dens screws are technically precise operative procedures that should be attempted only by those specially trained in them.

Type III fractures involve fractures into the body of C2, often involving the articular surfaces of the C1-C2 joint. Because these fractures have a large surface area and a higher ratio of cancellous to cortical bone, they typically unite without operative intervention (Fig. 70-21). Provided that an anatomic reduction can be achieved, the fractures will nearly always go on to uneventful union. Immobilization in a halo vest for 2 to 3 months is usually sufficient. If reduction is difficult to achieve, a short period of halo traction immobilization in bed may realign the fracture fragments.

Hangman's Fractures

Hangman's fractures, or traumatic spondylolisthesis of the axis, are bilateral pars fractures of C2. This fracture is named for the injury identified during judicial hanging with the knot placed in the submental position.[85] Hangman's fractures may result from either hyperextension or flexion[86] (Fig. 70-22).

Type I injuries involve minimally or nondisplaced fractures of the posterior neural arches without angulation of C2 on C3. Type I hangman's fractures are typically stable injuries and are managed with a cervical orthosis for 3 months. This can easily be accomplished in compliant patients. Type II fractures have anterior displacement greater than 3 mm between the fractured elements. There is also increased angulation or translation between C2 and C3 due to disk space injury. These injuries typically result from severe hyperextension and axial loading followed by flexion. This causes posterior annular and disk injury and allows anterior translation and angulation (Fig. 70-23). Type IIa injuries are flexion-distraction variants of type II injuries and result in severe angulation of C2 on C3 with minimal translation of C2 on C3; C2 will appear to hinge anteriorly on the anterior longitudinal ligament. Accurate identification of this injury is important because even min-

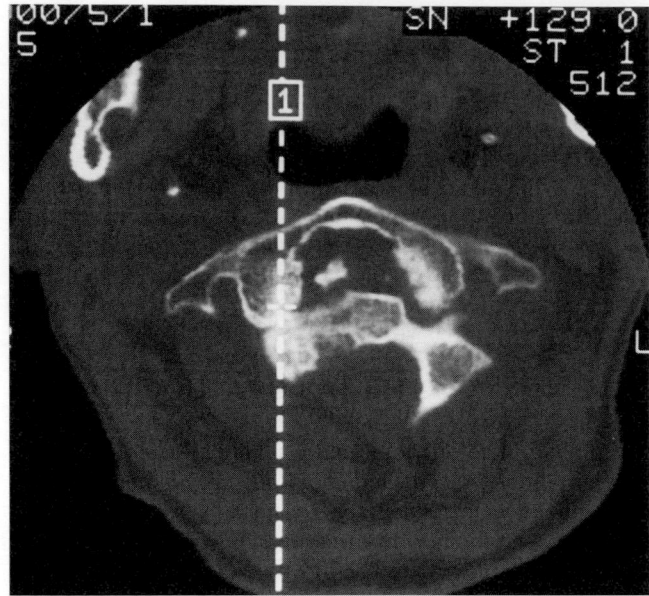

A

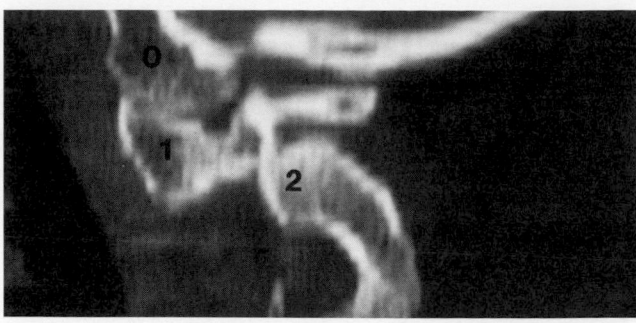

B

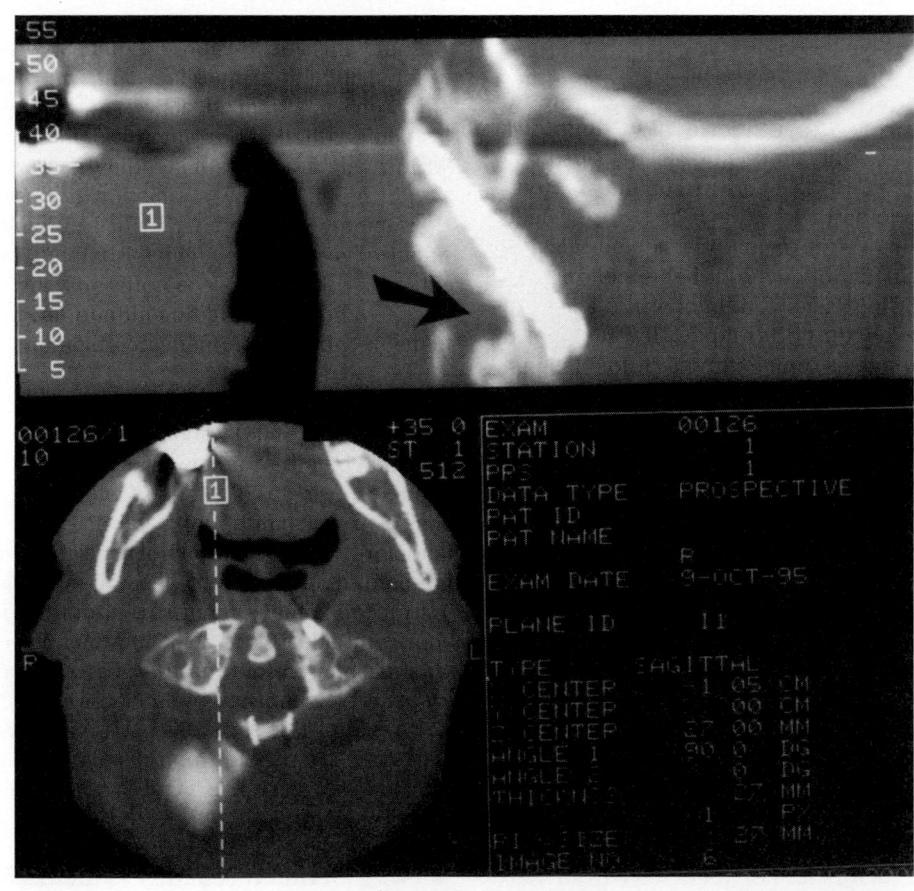

C

Figure 70-17 Preoperative axial (*A*) and sagittal (*B*) CT scans showing a nearly complete C1-C2 dislocation. Postoperative sagittal reconstruction CT scans (*C*) show anatomic reduction of C1 and C2 with correct position of C1-C2 transarticular screws. The vertebral artery foramen in the lateral aspect of C2 (*arrow*) must be avoided when using this technique. Operative (*D*) and postoperative (*E*) sagittal MRIs show decompression by reduction of craniocervical kyphosis.

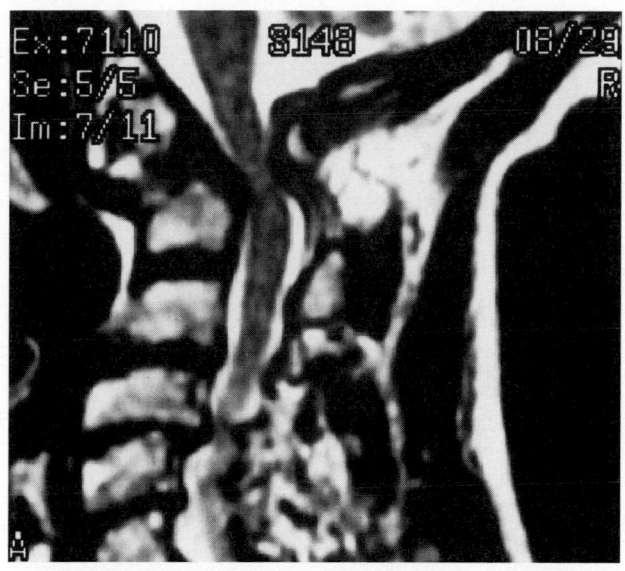

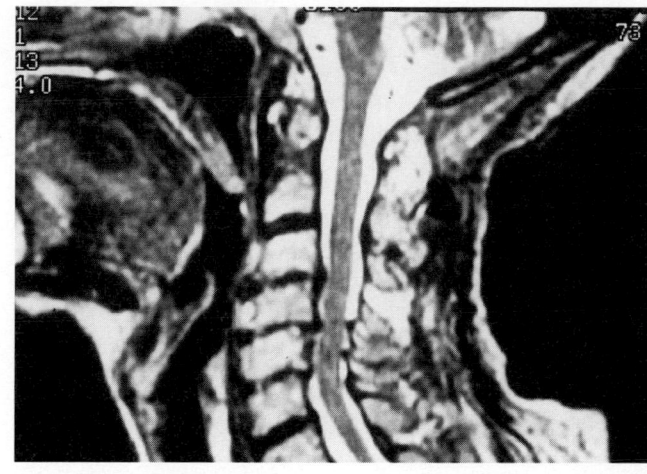

E

D

Figure 70-17 *(Continued)*

imal cervical traction could result in a severe distraction injury between C2 and C3.[87] Type II injuries with less than 5 mm of displacement or minimal angulation can be treated definitively in a halo vest if reduction can be achieved and maintained. Fractures with more than 5 mm of displacement or severe angulation are managed initially in cervical traction with extension for approximately 3 to 6 weeks until initial stability can be documented. Definitive treatment is then in a halo vest. Traction is contraindicated in type IIa fractures. These fractures can be managed with early halo immobilization. Fluoroscopic guidance can help to achieve compression across the fracture site to maintain reduction. Both type I and II fractures can be treated with open reduction and internal fixation if necessary, using C2 pars screws. Care should be taken to investigate the vertebral artery foramen on radiographic studies prior to open reduction. Fractures through the foramen transversarium may indicate a possible vertebral artery laceration, making hemostasis during operative intervention difficult. Type III hangman's fractures are associated with unilateral or bilateral facet dislocations of C2 on C3. These injuries are highly unstable and are associated with a high incidence of neurologic sequelae. This is due in part to the ki-

netic energy required to create this injury. These fractures typically need to be reduced by open techniques when closed reduction is not possible.[87] Posterior stabilization from C2 to C3 after reduction of the C2 facet joints is necessary to establish stability. Typically, traumatic spondylolistheses are not accompanied by neurologic injury because these are "canal-expanding" lesions. However, if there are irregular fractures of the pedicles involving the posterior wall of the vertebral body, a canal-narrowing injury could be created.

Other less commonly identified fractures of C2 involve avulsion fractures of the anteroinferior margin of C2, most probably due to hyperextension injuries with avulsion of the distal tip of C2 by the anterior insertion of the longitudinal ligament. These injuries are usually stable and heal uneventfully. More often, they are identified as incidental findings in a somewhat malreduced but fused position some time after trauma (Fig. 70-24).

Occipitocervical Dislocations

Occipitocervical dislocations are rare injuries resulting from total disruption of all the ligamentous structures con-
(Text continues on page 1265)

Figure 70-18 Dens fracture classification.

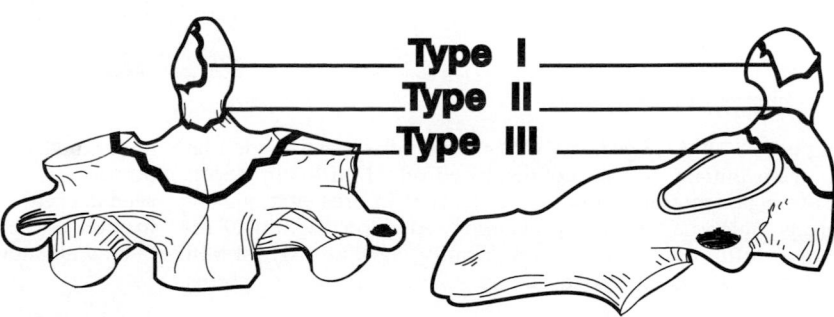

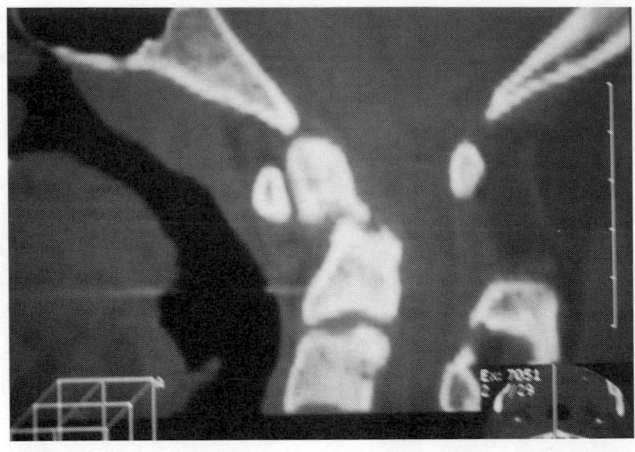

A

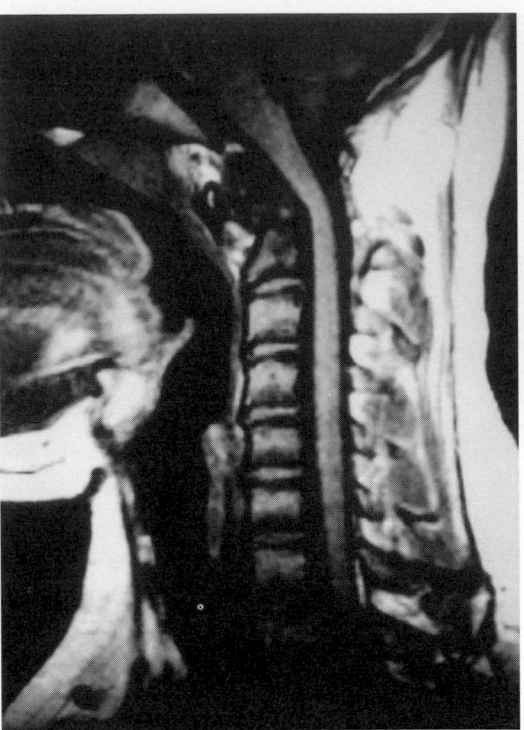

B

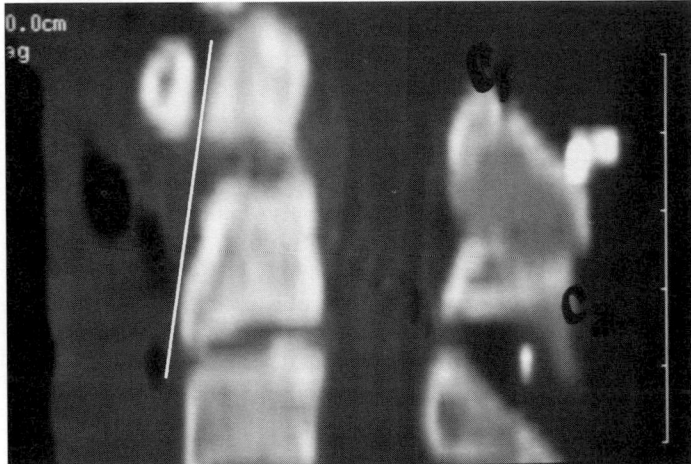

C

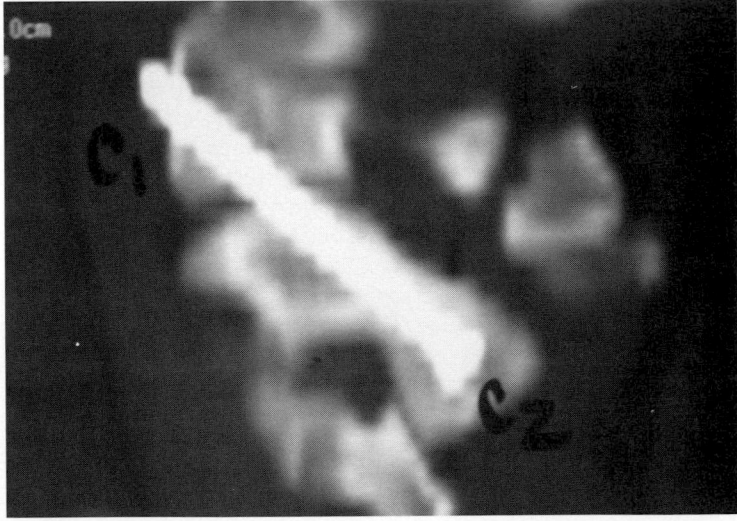

D

Figure 70-19 A 16-year-old patient identified several months after an initially missed nondisplaced odontoid fracture with C1-C2 ligamentous instability. At the time of presentation, a fibrous union had formed, preventing reduction. Sagittal CT reconstruction (*A*) shows the deformity; midline sagittal MRI (*B*) shows the acute kyphosis over which the neural structures are draped, causing mild myelopathic symptoms. Anterior and posterior release (*C*) allowed anatomic alignment. C1-C2 screws seen in sagittal (*D*) and coronal (*E*) reconstructions show good fixation of the joint. Postoperative plain films (*F*) show good overall alignment.

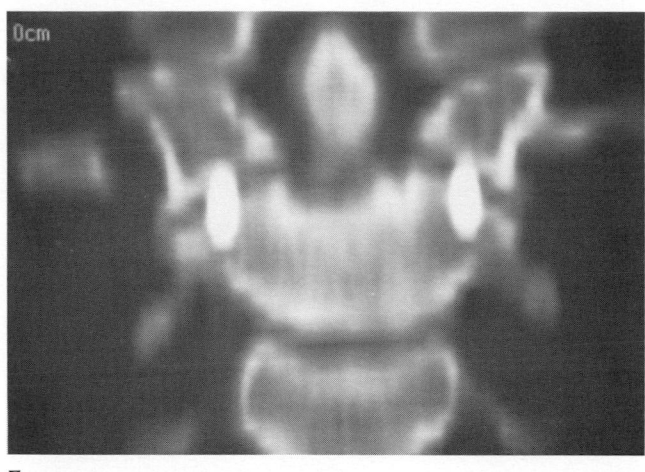

E

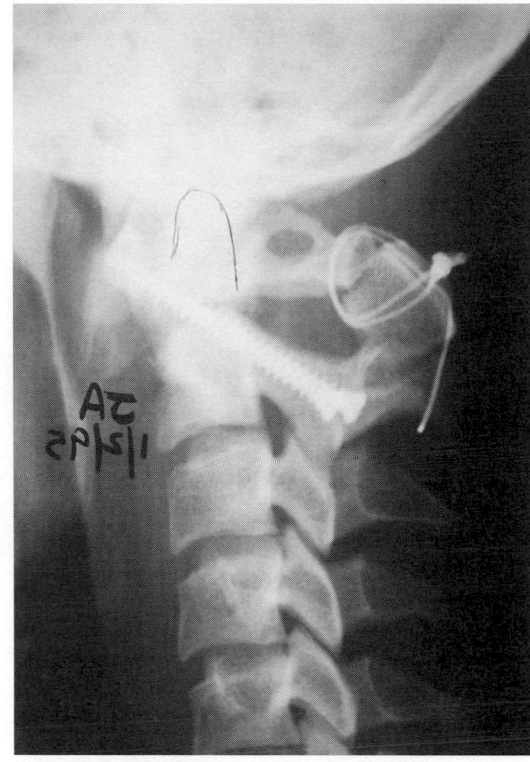

Figure 70-19 *(Continued)*   F

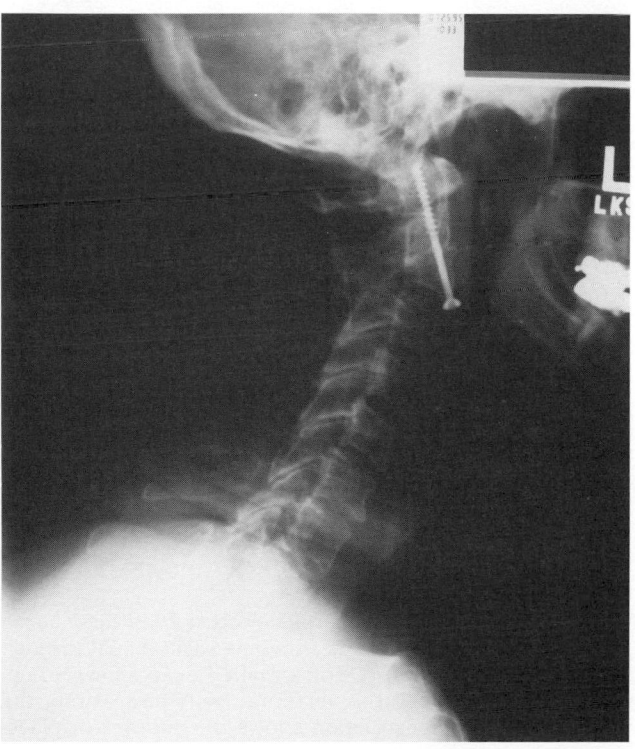

A

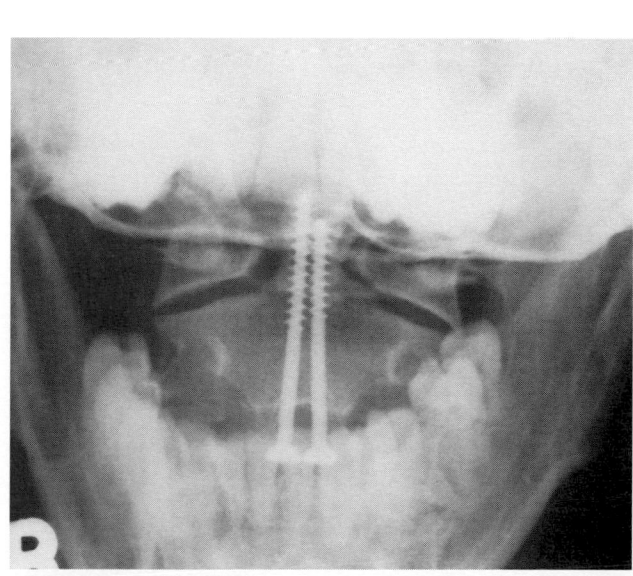

B

Figure 70-20 Type II dens fracture (*A*) fixed with odontoid screws seen in the anterior-posterior (*B*) projection.

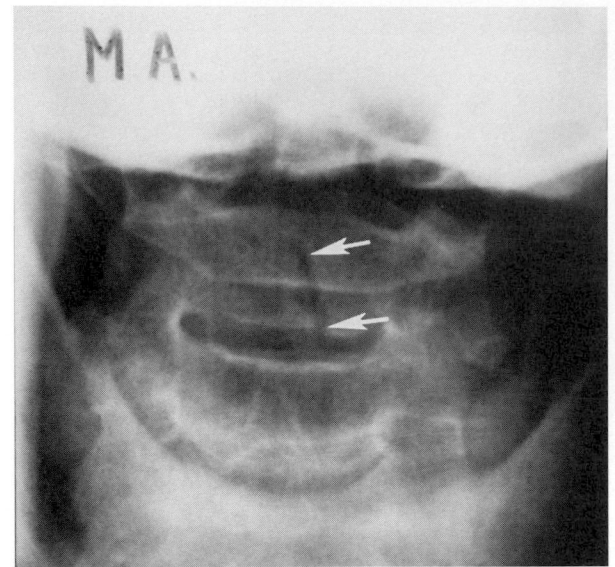

A

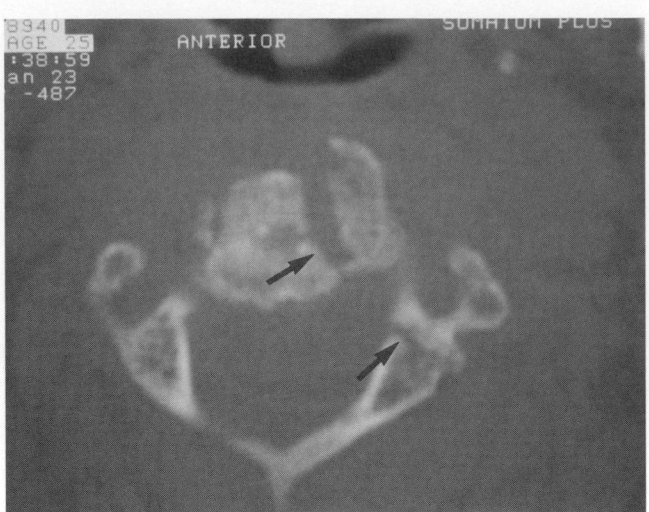

B

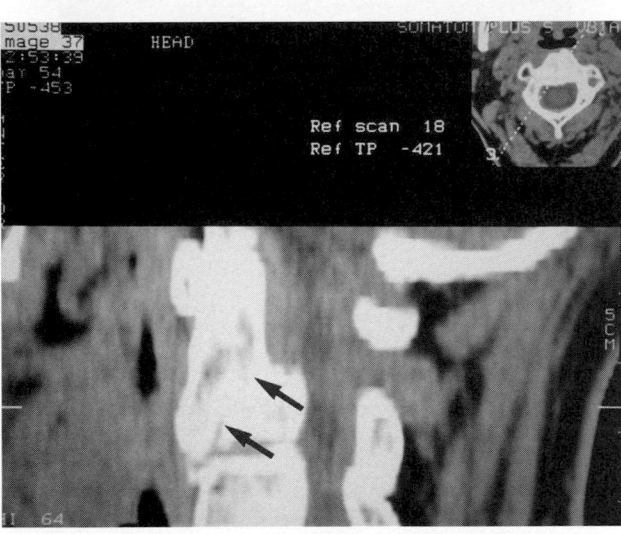

C

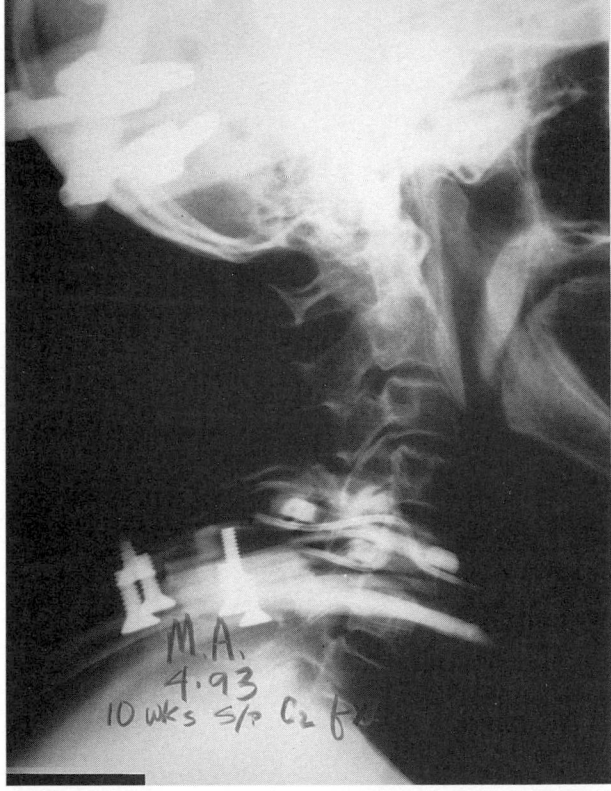

D

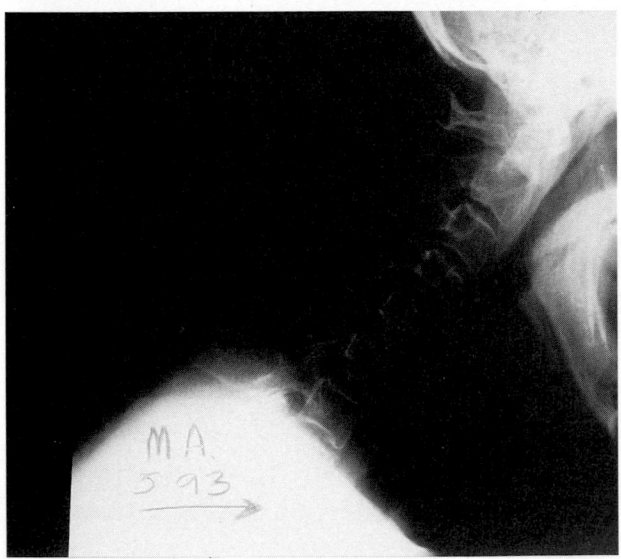

E

Figure 70-21 A type III odontoid fracture identified on an (*A*) open-mouth view. There is a midline sagittal split through the body of C2 (arrows) *B.* Transaxial CT scan shows an unusual fracture through the vertebral body and exiting the pars. *C.* Sagittal reconstruction shows the anterior displacement of the superior aspect of C2. *D.* Anatomic alignment in halo vest. *E.* Fracture consolidated at 4 months with good stability on flexion x-rays.

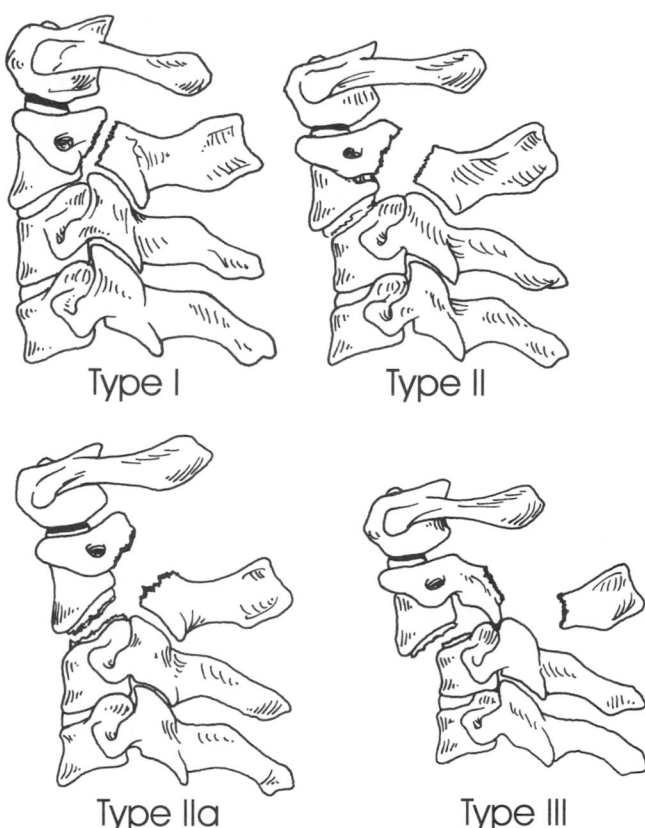

Type I

Type II

Type IIa

Type III

Figure 70-22 Classification of traumatic spondylolisthesis of the axis.

necting the occiput to the cervical spine and may be associated with concomitant C0-C1-C2 fractures.[88] The mechanism of injury is distraction, extension, and/or flexion. These injuries typically result in death due to severe brainstem and spinal cord injury resulting in respiratory arrest. Because of this, these injuries are probably underestimated. They are often reported after forensic examination.[89] Associated noncontiguous spinal fractures and head injuries are typical findings.

Atlantooccipital dislocations are identified on lateral radiographs of the cervical spine or skull. These views profile the atlantooccipital junction quite well. If there is a loss of continuity in the clival-dens line (Fig. 70-25), a gap greater than 5 mm between the basion (anterior margin of the foramen magnum) and the tip of the dens, or significant prevertebral swelling anterior to C1 and C2, there should be a high index suspicion for this injury. The articulation between the occiput and C1 should be carefully examined for symmetry. If plain radiographic evidence is inconclusive and there is suspicion of an atlantooccipital dislocation, fine (1-mm) axial CT slices through the C0-C1 joint supplemented with sagittal and coronal reconstructions may allow more detailed investigation of the atlantooccipital joint. If, on the CT reconstructions or on the plain films, there is more than a 2-mm gap between the occipital condyles and C1, there is

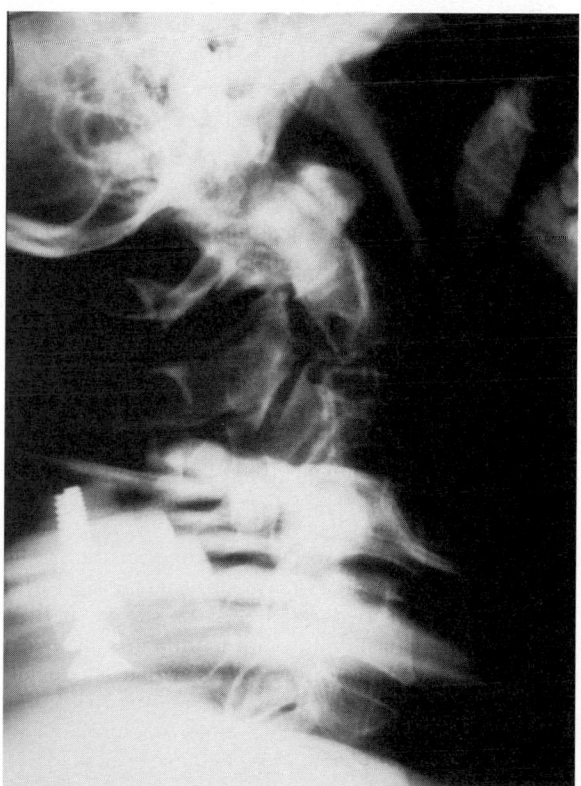

A

B

Figure 70-23 *A.* Apparently stable traumatic spondylolisthesis of the axis with an associated atlas fracture with overall good alignment in a neurologically intact patient. *B.* Prevertebral soft tissue and diskal injury, which was not appreciated at the time and became apparent after a short period of immobilization in a halo vest.

a high likelihood that there has been a rupture of the major ligamentous structures connecting the occiput to the cervical spine.[90]

Examination of plain lateral radiographs with application of the Powers ratio can be used to distinguish between type I and II dislocations. The Powers ratio[91] is defined as the measured distance between the basion and the posterior arch of C1 divided by the measured distance from the opisthion (posterior rim of the foramen magnum) to the anterior arch of C1 (Fig. 70-26). A type I or anterior dislocation is confirmed by a Powers ratio greater than 1. Conversely, type II or posterior dislocation of the occiput is confirmed by a Powers ratio of less than 1, with 1 being normal.

The use of traction in the treatment of atlantooccipital dislocations is risky. Even 5 lb of traction may overdistract the vertebral column and cause spinal cord or brainstem injury. Because of this possible catastrophic complication of using cervical traction, any traction applied during the treatment of a subaxial injury should have initial films taken with light weights to ensure that there is not an occult atlantooccipital instability. The initial treatment for this injury is application of a halo vest to reestablish the stability of the craniocervical junction. Once the patient is stabilized and in no acute cardiorespiratory distress, treatment is with definitive posterior occipitocervical fixation[73,92,93] (Figs. 70-27, 70-28). Continued immobilization in the halo vest may be necessary to augment the internal stabilization until fusion is verified (see Fig. 70-29). Because this injury is ligamentous, nonoperative treatment is unlikely to be successful.

Occipital Condyle Fractures

These fractures occur from combined axial and lateral loading. Mechanistically, two types are identified: avulsion fractures and comminuted compression fractures.[94] These fractures are difficult to visualize on plain radiographs. Supplemental axial CT scans with coronal and sagittal reconstructions may be of use. There must be a high index of suspicion to identify these fractures. Because the lower cranial nerves exit from the base of the skull posterior and medial to the occipital condyles, cranial nerve injuries often accompany these fractures.[95]

Type I fractures (Fig. 70-30) involve comminution of a single occipital condyle, probably due to significant asymmetrical lateral loading. Because the attachment of the alar ligament is in the region of the occipital condyle, rotational instability of the occiput on C2 may result. Type II occipital condyle fractures are essentially basal skull fractures with separation of the occipital condyle from the base of the skull. Type III injuries are avulsion injuries. The medial aspect of the occipital condyle is avulsed by the alar ligament attachment. These may also result in rotatory instability of the occiput on C2.[96]

Immobilization in a cervical orthosis is the treatment for occipital condyle fractures. The type I and type II injuries are stable and can be treated with a hard collar or some other rigid orthosis. Typically, 6 to 12 weeks is sufficient. Type III injuries may be unstable, needing more rigid mobilization in a halo vest for at least 12 weeks. Flexion-extension x-rays should be obtained to document stability prior to discontinuing immobilization. Most fractures heal

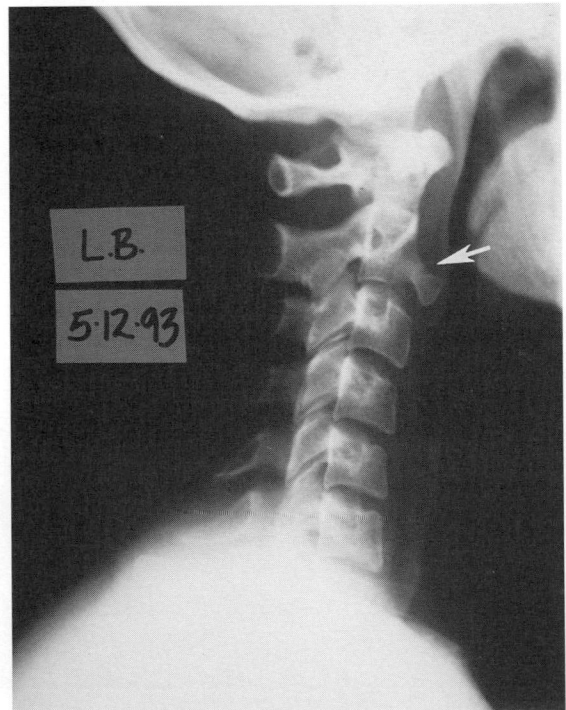

A

B

Figure 70-24 *A.* A minimally displaced anteroinferior avulsion fracture of C2 identified after a motor vehicle accident. *B.* After several months of treatment in a hard collar, x-rays reveal uneventful fusion. The patient remained neurologically intact and had no symptoms following uneventful healing.

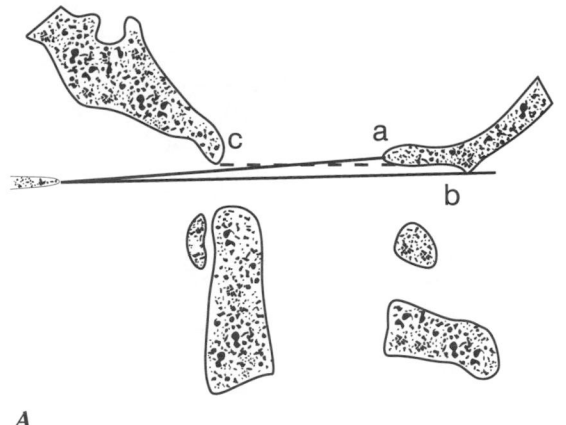

A

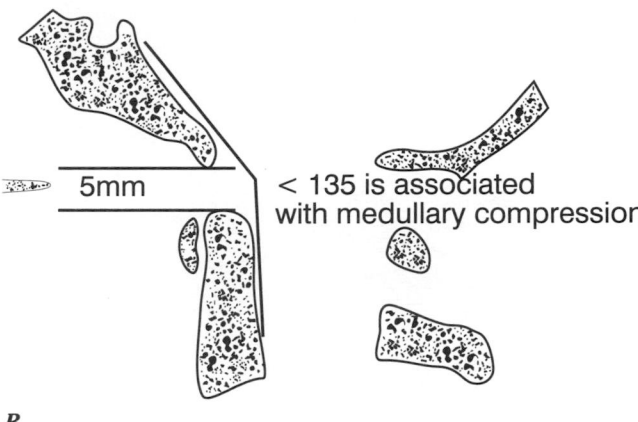

B

Figure 70-25 *A.*Craniometric lines and angles for evaluating the craniocervical junction: a, Chamberlen's line; b, McGregor's line; c, McCrae's line. These represent anatomic alignments for evaluating basilar invagination. *B.* There should be 5 mm of space between the caudal tip of the clivus and the rostral tip of C2. The clivus-canal angle is variable; however, an angle of less than 135° is associated with medullary compression.

uneventfully, although occasionally posttraumatic arthritis may occur. If significant pain results or instability is documented after an appropriate time in immobilization, then posterior occipital cervical fixation and fusion is indicated.

Atlantoaxial Rotatory Subluxation

Another uncommon and often missed injury is the atlantoaxial rotatory subluxation (AARS). These have been classified by Fielding as types I through IV[97] (Fig. 70-31). These injuries are most reliably detected on open-mouth odontoid views. Asymmetry in the anteroposterior projection of the lateral masses of C1 indicates rotation of C1 on C2. In addition, rotatory anteroposterior translation of C1 on C2 can be identified by the "wink sign." This results from the superimposition of the osseous margin of C1 over the superior edge of C2 with asymmetrical obliteration of the C1-C2 joint space on the subluxed side. Axial CT scans are useful to diagnose this injury. The subluxation of the C1-C2 joint can be cleanly identified on the axial CT images. Malalignment can also be seen in coronal reconstructions (Fig. 70-32). This injury is often identified in children who have had minor trauma or recent upper respiratory tract infections, who are found several weeks later to have a "cock robin" position of the head. If these injuries are identified within the first several weeks, reduction can typically be achieved with a short period of cervical traction. Once the injury is reduced, a period of halo immobilization is often successful at maintaining the reduction. If initial attempts at reduction or a trial in the halo vest are unsuccessful, open reduction and internal stabilization may be necessary. If the reduction results in chronic pain or instability, then atlantoaxial arthrodesis is the treatment of choice. These injuries do not typically result in spinal cord injury, since the space available for the cord is usually not significantly reduced. If this injury results from acute rotational trauma, the vertebral artery may be injured or compressed, resulting in vertebrobasilar artery syndrome.[98] Severely decreased flow or loss of flow in one vertebral artery may lead to occlusion of the posterior inferior cerebellar artery on one side. This may result in an ipsilateral lateral medullary infarct, or Wallenberg's syndrome. This is characterized by ipsilateral loss of cranial nerves V, IX, X, and XI, cerebellar ataxia, Horner's syndrome, and contralateral loss of pain and temperature sensation.

Conclusion

The unique anatomy of the craniocervical junction lends itself to unique biomechanics and unique injury patterns. Injuries to this region of the spine run the gamut of neurologic compromise ranging from none to death. Careful attention must be paid to the anatomy of the craniocervical junction in the postinjury period to prevent missed injuries and lay the groundwork for appropriate management. Because injuries to this region of the spine are relatively

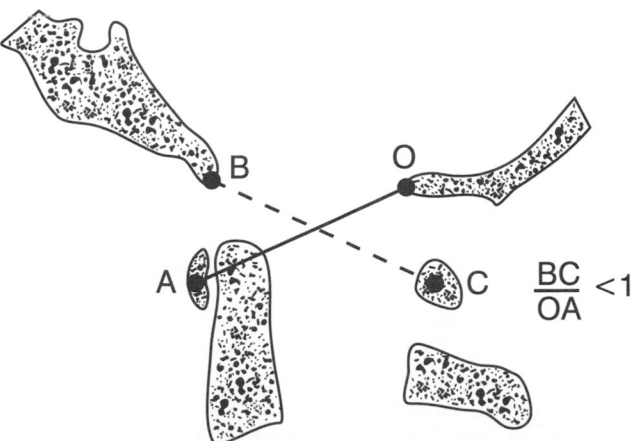

Figure 70-26 The Powers ratio defines the relationship between the occiput and the upper cervical spine. This ratio is normally approximately 0.8. A Powers ratio greater than 1 suggests anterior occipital dislocation; a Powers ratio of less than 0.8 suggests a posterior occipital dislocation.

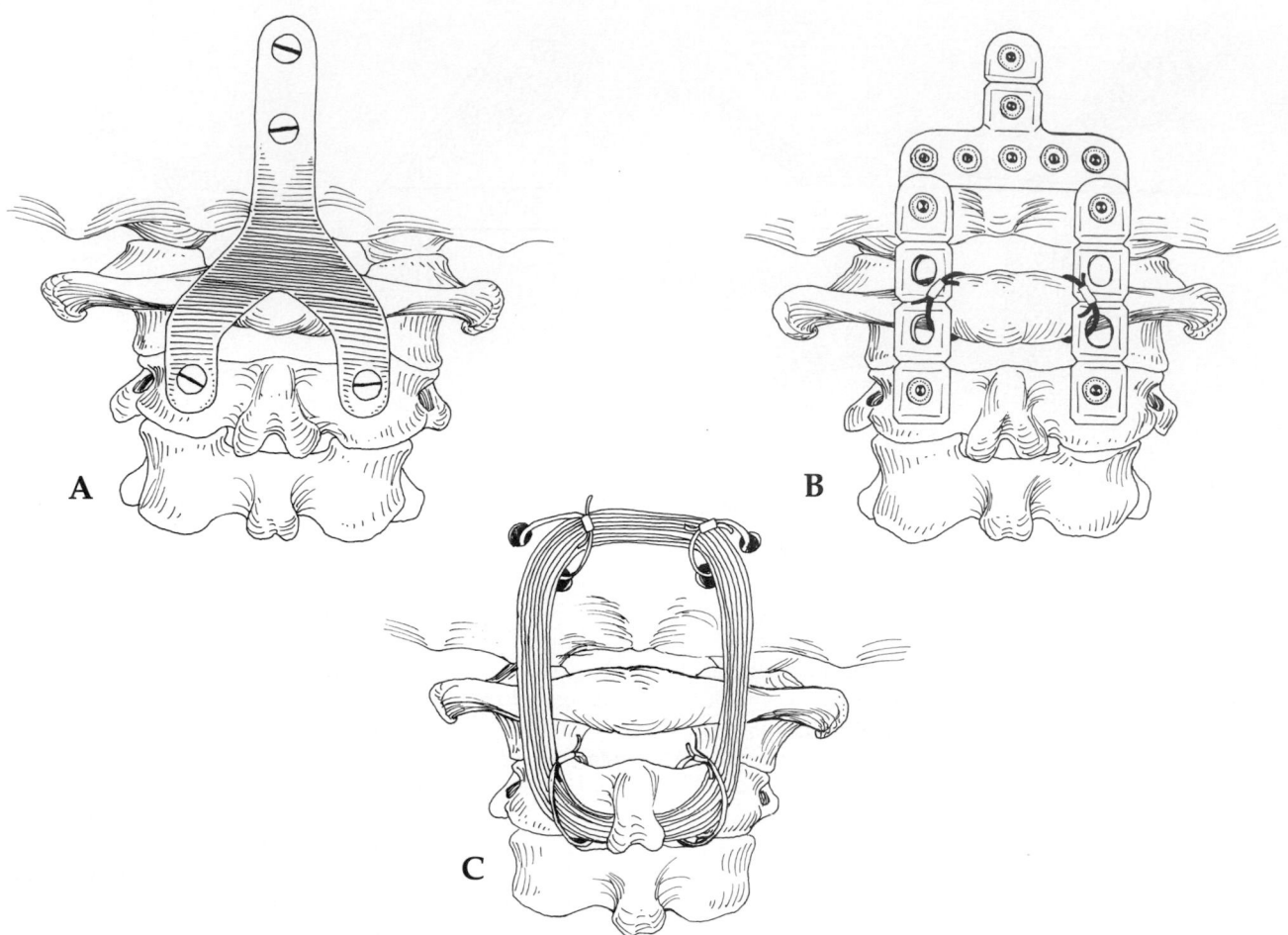

Figure 70-27 Occipitocervical instrumentation techniques. *A.* Y plate. *B.* Axis plate with custom occipital attachment. *C.* Luque rectangle. (Reproduced with permission from O'Brien MF, Sutterlin CE: Occipitocervical biomechanics: Clinical and biomechanical implications for posterior occipitocervical stabilization and fusion. *Spine* 10:281–313, 1996.)

uncommon and treatment techniques are demanding,[99] these injuries can be among the most challenging of all spinal injuries.

INJURIES OF THE SUBAXIAL CERVICAL SPINE

Osseous pathology is often the first and most obvious manifestation of trauma in the subaxial cervical spine. This may not be the case with children, who may have spinal injuries without obvious vertebral deformities.[100] It is essential to accurately identify injuries to the ligamentous structures and distinguish them from normal variants or degenerative changes for complete and accurate assessment. Failure to appreciate these ligamentous injuries may result in vertebral segment translation. In the subaxial spine, there is less tolerance for subtle change in canal dimension because there is less room for the spinal cord. This is in contrast to injuries in the upper cervical spine, which often result in canal-expanding lesions.

For trauma patients with possible injuries of the cervical spine, cross-table lateral and AP x-rays are mandatory. In addition, open-mouth x-rays are often necessary to rule out craniocervical junction injury. Oblique views, while difficult to obtain in the trauma setting, will be useful in cases of potential unilateral and bilateral facet dislocations. It is of critical importance that the C7-T1 junction and preferably the T1 vertebra be clearly visualized on the lateral x-rays of the cervical spine. A swimmer's view or a lateral radiograph with the shoulders being pulled down manually is sometimes necessary to obtain this view. Caution must be exercised in performing these two maneuvers, since even this slight movement may precipitate neurologic deterioration in the unstable spine. When these techniques are felt to be too unsafe or have been unsuccessful, an axial CT scan of the cervicothoracic junction with sagittal reconstructions will also give the same information.[101]

The lateral x-ray is the most useful view for ruling out trauma.[102] Six lines should be evaluated. These should describe smooth, more or less parallel arcs, adjoining similar anatomic regions of the vertebral bodies (Fig. 70-33). Any malalignment could indicate a potential acute vertebral subluxation or dislocation. In addition, lateral and AP x-rays should be inspected for general symmetry of the vertebral body, facet joints, and the spinous processes from vertebra to vertebra.

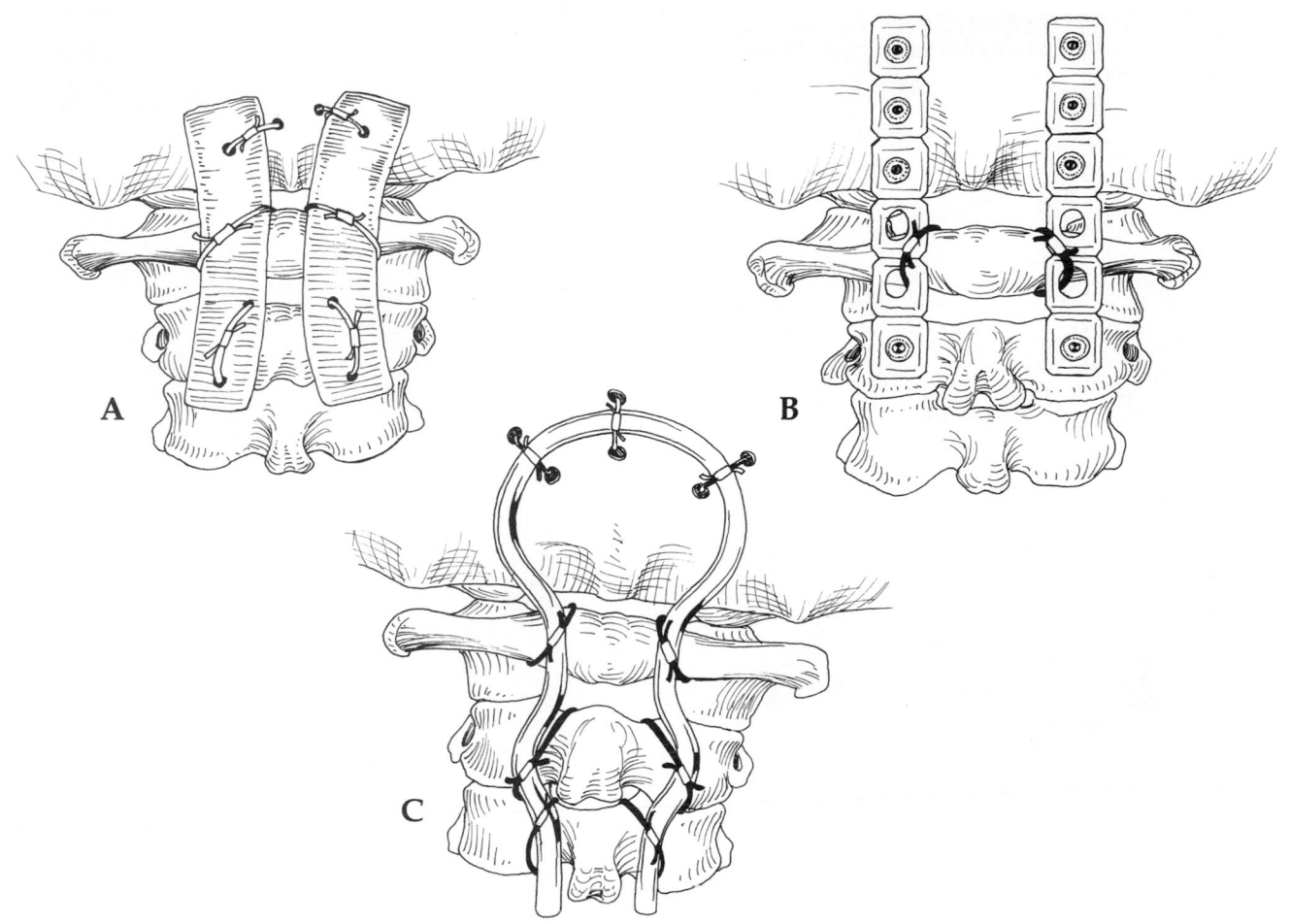

Figure 70-28 Additional methods for fixation of the occipitocervical junction include (*A*) direct wiring of calvarial, iliac crest, or rib strut grafts directly to the osseous structures; (*B*) lateral mass plate fixation without custom occipital attachment; (*C*) Lansford loop with sublaminar and suboccipital cables. (Reproduced with permission from O'Brien MF, Sutterlin CE: Occipitocervical biomechanics: Clinical and biomechanical implications for posterior occipitocervical stabilization and fusion. *Spine* 10:281–313, 1996.)

Additionally, on the lateral x-ray, the retropharyngeal and retrotracheal soft tissue shadows should be inspected for any evidence of soft tissue swelling. This may suggest a regional hematoma at the site of an occult injury. Soft tissue shadows should be no more than 6 mm thick when measured at the level of C2 and less than 2 cm anterior to C6. This is easily remembered as a mnemonic: "six at two and two at six."

Special studies such as MRI, CT, and CT/myelography have specific purposes in the evaluation of spinal trauma. Magnetic resonance imaging allows accurate visualization of soft tissue trauma, including disk, ligament, vascular, and neurologic structures. Computed tomography and CT/myelography allow close inspection of osseous structures as well as accurate identification of neural compression.

Classification

The Ferguson and Allen classification is extremely useful for understanding the mechanism of injury (see Table 70-3). However, it is somewhat cumbersome. The mechanistic classification system of Harris et al. may be somewhat easier to use in the clinical setting[103] (Table 70-13). An understanding of the principles of stability are important if these injuries are to be assessed accurately. Once the mechanism of injury and the injured structures are identified, a treatment plan can be formulated to reverse the mechanism of injury and realign and protect the injured structures.

For simplicity, five morphologic classifications of subaxial injuries are discussed below: isolated posterior element fractures, minor avulsion fractures, compression fractures, vertebral burst fractures, teardrop fractures, and facet injuries.

Isolated Fractures of Posterior Elements of the Cervical Spine

These fractures can include fractures of laminae, articular processes, and spinous processes. Typically due to axial compression with the cervical spine in an extended position, they result from impaction upon adjacent posterior elements. These injuries may include contiguous fractures. In the elderly, hyperextension injuries may be associated with

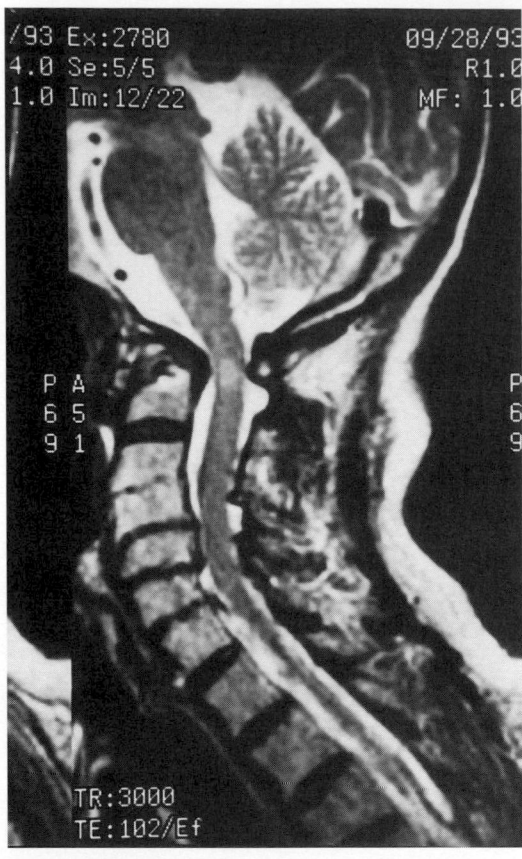

A

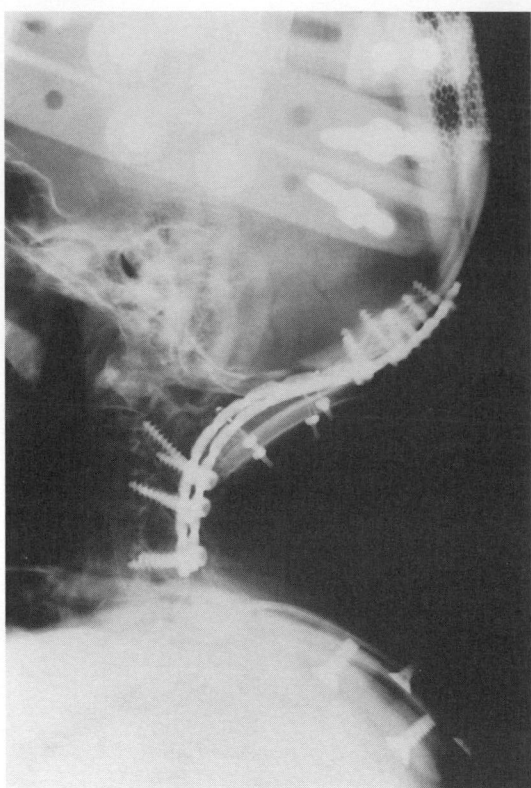

B

Figure 70-29 This elderly rheumatoid patient complained of slowly progressive but mild myelopathic changes in his upper and lower extremities after a minor fall. *A.* The MRI reveals an occipitocervical kyphosis with anterior translation of the occiput on the upper cervical spine. In addition, there is brainstem and spinal cord compression with intramedullary changes. *B.* After spinal cord decompression, fixation and fusion were undertaken with bilateral/lateral mass plates. Distally, lateral mass screws were placed into a previous sub-axial fusion mass, with the most inferior screws crossing the oldest fused facet joint for additional cortical purchase. Superiorly, the plates were bent into the midline to make the screws converge into the thick midline keel of occipital bone. Iliac crest morphinized graft was placed into the craniocervical junction and the occiput to cervical spine was spanned with parietal bone. For the first 2 months postoperatively, the construct and healing fusion were protected further with halo vest immobilization.

a central cord syndrome due to infolding of the ligamentum flavum, which causes a pincer effect against anterior disk bulges or osteophytes. Another manifestation of hyperextension injuries is an anterior avulsion fracture of the inferior lip of a vertebral body (Fig. 70-34). The hyperextension moment causes avulsion of the bony insertion of the anterior longitudinal ligament.

Isolated posterior element fractures due to flexion are less common but do occur. "Clay shoveler's" fracture of the lower cervical spinous processes is an example of such a lesion.

Plain AP and lateral radiographs may not show these injuries if they are nondisplaced. Oblique x-rays are often helpful in identifying them. When facet fractures are nondisplaced, they may be difficult to see, but failure to recognize them may result in gross instability (Fig. 70-35). Radiographic evidence suggesting this type of injury warrants flexion-extension films to prove that there is no instability. When facet fractures are rotated out of their normal coronal orientation, they may have an asymmetric appearance in the frontal plane when compared to adjacent levels. This is often described as a *transverse facet.*

Initial management of these isolated fractures of the posterior elements and minor avulsion fractures is with a cervical orthosis. The majority of these injuries are quite stable and typically are not accompanied by neurologic injuries. Facet fractures may be associated with nerve root irritation. For multiple-level injuries, a halo vest may be a more appropriate way to gain effective control of the cervical spine. In patients who have a complete fracture of the facet joint with a floating lateral mass or when gross malalignment is identified (i.e., a transverse facet), open reduction and internal fixation will be necessary, since these are unstable injuries and cannot be reduced closed.

Compression Fractures

These fractures involve compression of the anterior column with loss of vertebral height of less than 30 percent.

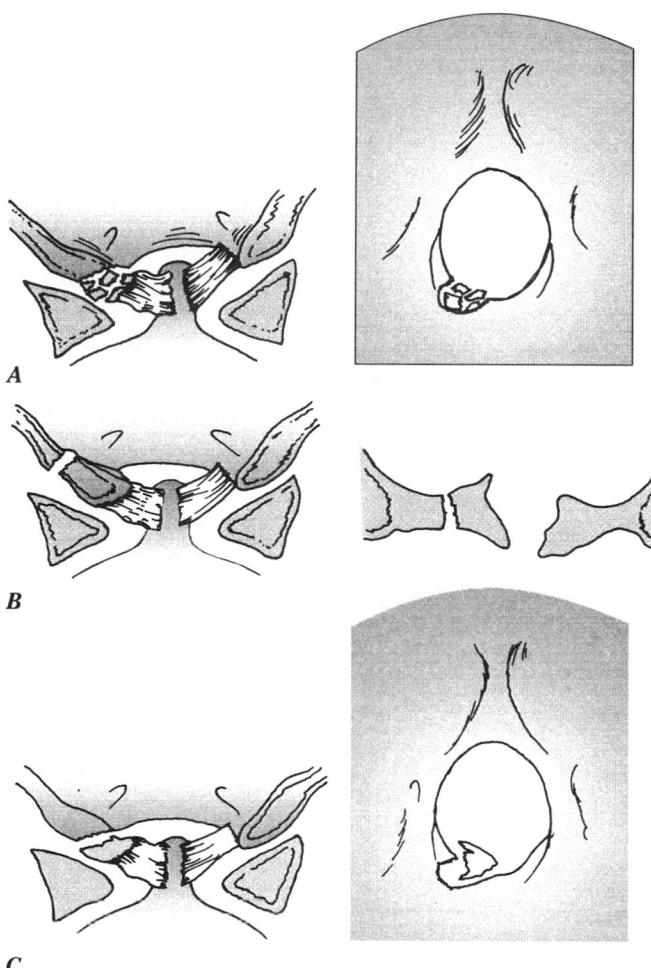

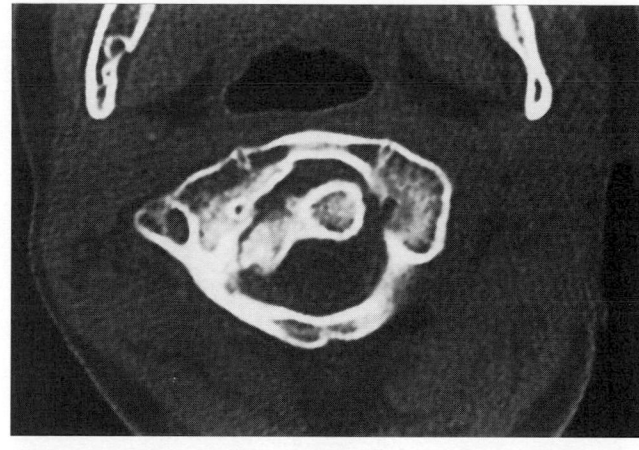

A

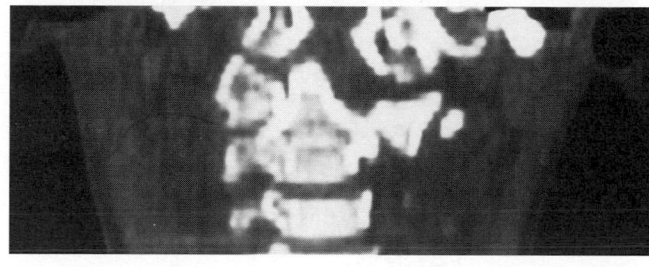

B

Figure 70-32 Transaxial *(A)* and coronal *(B)* CT scan projections of an atlantoaxial rotatory subluxation (AARS) in a child.

Figure 70-30 Occipital condyle fractures. *A.* Type I impaction-type condylar fracture. *B.* Type II basilar skull fracture with inclusion of the occipital condyle. *C.* Type III avulsion-type occipital condyle fracture. (Reproduced with permission from Anderson PA, Montesano PX: Morphology and treatment of occipital condyle fractures. *Spine* 13:731–736, 1988.)

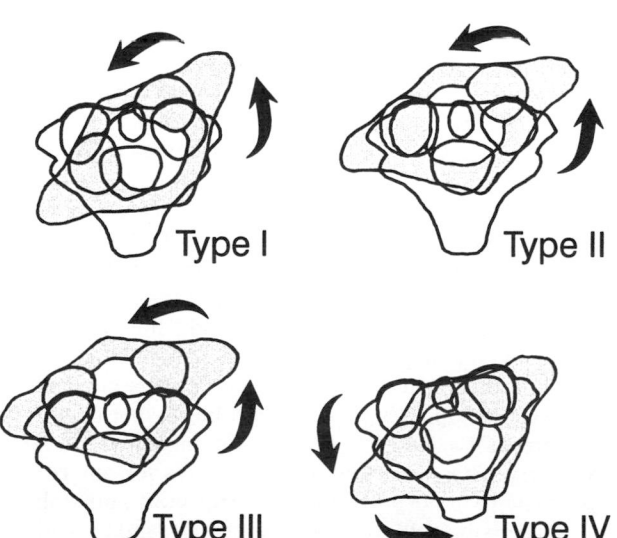

Figure 70-31 Classification of atlantoaxial rotatory subluxations.

In nearly all cases the wall of the posterior vertebral body remains intact. Typically, there is no bony retropulsion into the canal or significant angulation. In compression fractures with more than 50 percent of vertebral body collapse, there is a chance that there may be some segmental instability. This may be made worse if there is posterior column involvement, which would result in kyphosis. Stable injuries can be managed in a cervical orthosis. Any suggestion of acute instability or failure to maintain the reduced position would prompt internal fixation. The presence or development of neurologic deficits should warrant reevaluation of the fracture in an attempt to identify a missed injury either at the site in question or at a remote location.

Burst Fractures

Vertebral burst fractures are usually the result of axial loading and flexion. These injuries are typical of those seen in diving accidents (Fig. 70-36). These are differentiated from simple compression fractures by significant destruction of the vertebral body, often with sagittal or coronal plane fractures much like lumbar burst fractures. Widening between the pedicles is their hallmark.

Burst fractures typically involve posterior retropulsion of the middle column into the spinal canal. For accurate analysis, axial CT scans and/or MRIs are necessary. When collapse of the anterior column is 50 percent or greater, se-

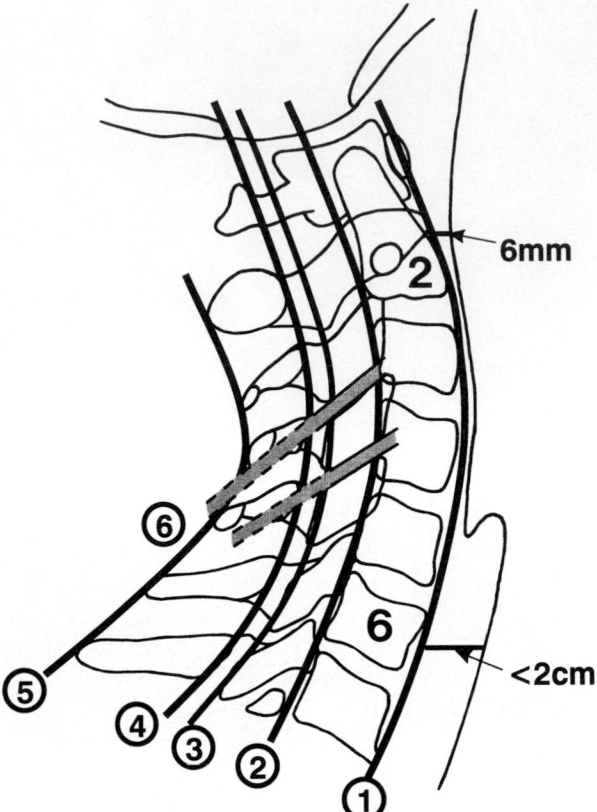

Figure 70-33 Important radiometric lines for evaluation of cervical spine trauma: (1) anterior vertebral body; (2) posterior vertebral body; (3) posterior facet joint; (4) spinolaminar line; and (5) the tips of the spinous processes. These lines should form smooth arcs throughout the cervical spine, as pictured. In addition, adjacent facet joints should be aligned in a parallel fashion. (6) Prevertebral soft tissue should be inspected. There should be approximately 6 mm of prevertebral shadow anterior to C2 and less than 2 cm anterior to C6 ("six at two and two at six").

TABLE 70-13   Mechanistic Classification for Injuries of the Cervical Spine

I. Flexion
   A. Anterior subluxation (hyperflexion sprain)
   B. Bilateral interfacetal dislocation
   C. Simple wedge (compression) fracture
   D. Clay-shoveler (coal-shoveler) fracture
   E. Flexion teardrop fracture

II. Flexion-rotation
   A. Unilateral interfacetal dislocation

III. Extension-rotation
   A. Pillar fracture

IV. Vertical compression
   A. Jefferson bursting fracture of atlas
   B. Burst (bursting, dispersion, axial loading) fracture

V. Hyperextension
   A. Hyperextension dislocation
   B. Avulsion fracture of anterior arch of atlas
   C. Extension teardrop fracture of axis
   D. Fracture of posterior arch of atlas
   E. Laminar fracture
   F. Traumatic spondylolisthesis (hangman's fracture)
   G. Hyperextension fracture-dislocation

VI. Lateral flexion
   A. Uncinate process fracture

VII. Diverse or imprecisely understood mechanisms
   A. Atlantooccipital disassociation
   B. Odontoid fractures

Source: Reproduced with permission from Harris JK Jr, Edeiken-Monroe B, Kapaniky DR: A practical classification of acute cervical spine injuries. *Orthop Clin North Am* 17:15–30, 1986.

vere middle-column and concomitant posterior ligamentous injuries must be considered. Posterior ligamentous injuries may not be readily apparent in this group because collapse of the anterior and middle columns removes the middle-column fulcrum, which would highlight the loss of the posterior tension band. Subtle widening of the interspinous distance, fractures of the posterior elements, asymmetrical alignment, or overriding of adjacent facet joints may suggest posterior-column injury. Because of the potential for neurologic injury, flexion-extension x-rays are contraindicated. Sagittal MRIs may allow visualization of edema and hematoma within the posterior elements, which would raise suspicions for a posterior ligamentous injury.

The initial management of burst fracture with greater than 25 percent loss of vertebral body height, retropulsion of the posterior vertebral body wall, or an accompanying neurologic deficit is cervical tong traction. This is done in an attempt to stabilize the spinal segments and prevent any further injury to the neuraxis. If ligamentotaxis does not realign

the spine and/or decompress the neural canal, consideration should be given to an anterior corpectomy and fusion in the acute setting. A deteriorating neurologic status or an incomplete injury would make surgical decompression the treatment of choice.

Definitive treatment of cervical burst fracture is dependent on the loss of vertebral body height, the amount of retropulsion, neurologic status, kyphotic angulation, and the presence of posterior element injuries. Fractures with less than 25 percent loss of vertebral body height, minimal retropulsion, and kyphosis in a neurologically intact patient can be managed successfully in a halo.[104] This may need to be in place for up to 3 months. With increasing middle-column retropulsion, there is an increased likelihood of spinal cord injury. These patients are candidates for anterior decompression via corpectomy with strut graft and stabilization. This can be achieved by a variety of standard and specialized approaches.[105] If posterior elements are intact and there is no ligamentous instability, the anterior strut graft

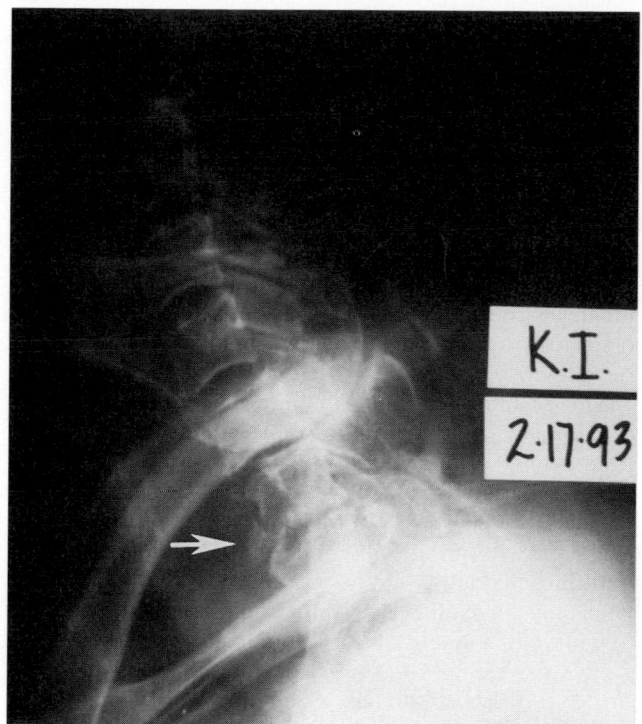

Figure 70-34 An avulsion fracture of the tip of C6 identified in postinjury x-rays.

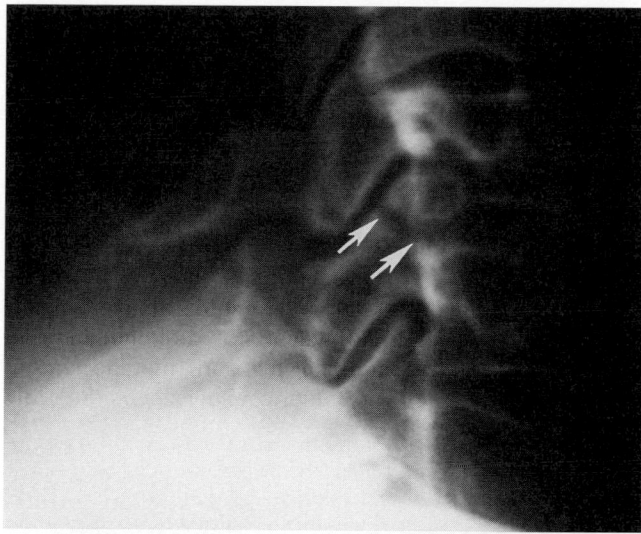

A

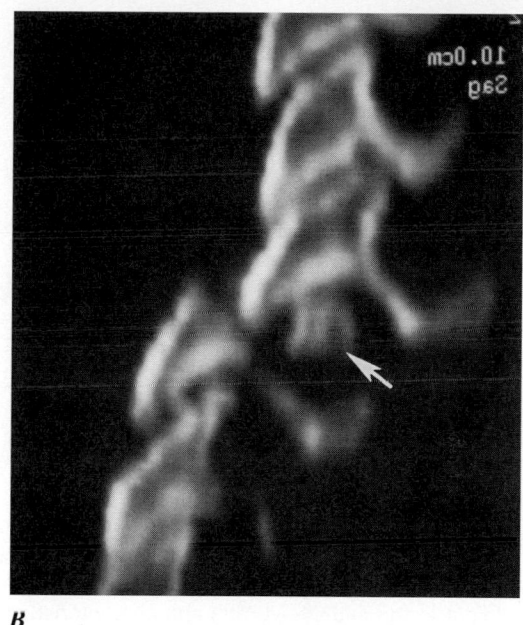

B

Figure 70-35 *A.* Immediate postinjury films revealing nondisplaced facet fracture initially missed in the emergency room after a motor vehicle accident. *B.* Subsequent unilateral dislocation identified 1 month later, when the patient complained of unilateral nerve root irritation and continuing neck pain.

construct can be protected with either a halo vest or an anterior plate.[106] In those patients with significant vertebral body burst fractures and severe ligamentous instability, anterior strut graft with anterior locking plate has been shown clinically to be sufficient. Biomechanical studies, however, suggest that these constructs may be at risk for failure when significant posterior disruption is present or when stressed in flexion. Therefore, in the face of a severe posterior injury, a combined anterior and posterior fusion and stabilization may be prudent.[107] This is also a consideration in the osteoporotic patient who has questionable bone stock for anterior fixation alone. Anterior and posterior reconstruction may also be reasonable in patients who are noncompliant or who have failed prior anterior reconstruction.

Complications in the treatment of burst fractures include lack of appreciation of the posterior ligamentous instability, which results in progressive kyphosis. This may be accompanied by a slowly progressive neurologic deterioration.[108] Patients treated in orthoses for cervical fractures may have undiagnosed ligamentous injuries. Therefore, in patients who are neurologically intact with greater than 50 percent loss of vertebral body height, voluntary flexion-extension radiographs after the compression fracture has healed should be used to rule out any posterior ligamentous injury prior to the development of a chronic fixed kyphotic deformity. Complications in the use of anterior strut grafts and instrumentation include dislodgement with esophageal compression and/or erosion. Posterior dislodgement of strut grafts can cause spinal cord compression. In addition, there is the complication of

strut graft collapse or fracture. Complications related to instrumentation include malpositioning, hardware loosening, and fracture and dislodgement of screws and plates.

Teardrop Fractures

The teardrop fracture-dislocation is a similar injury but with more severe osseous destruction. This is a particular group of fractures associated with severe spinal cord injury and spinal instability. They occur with the neck in a

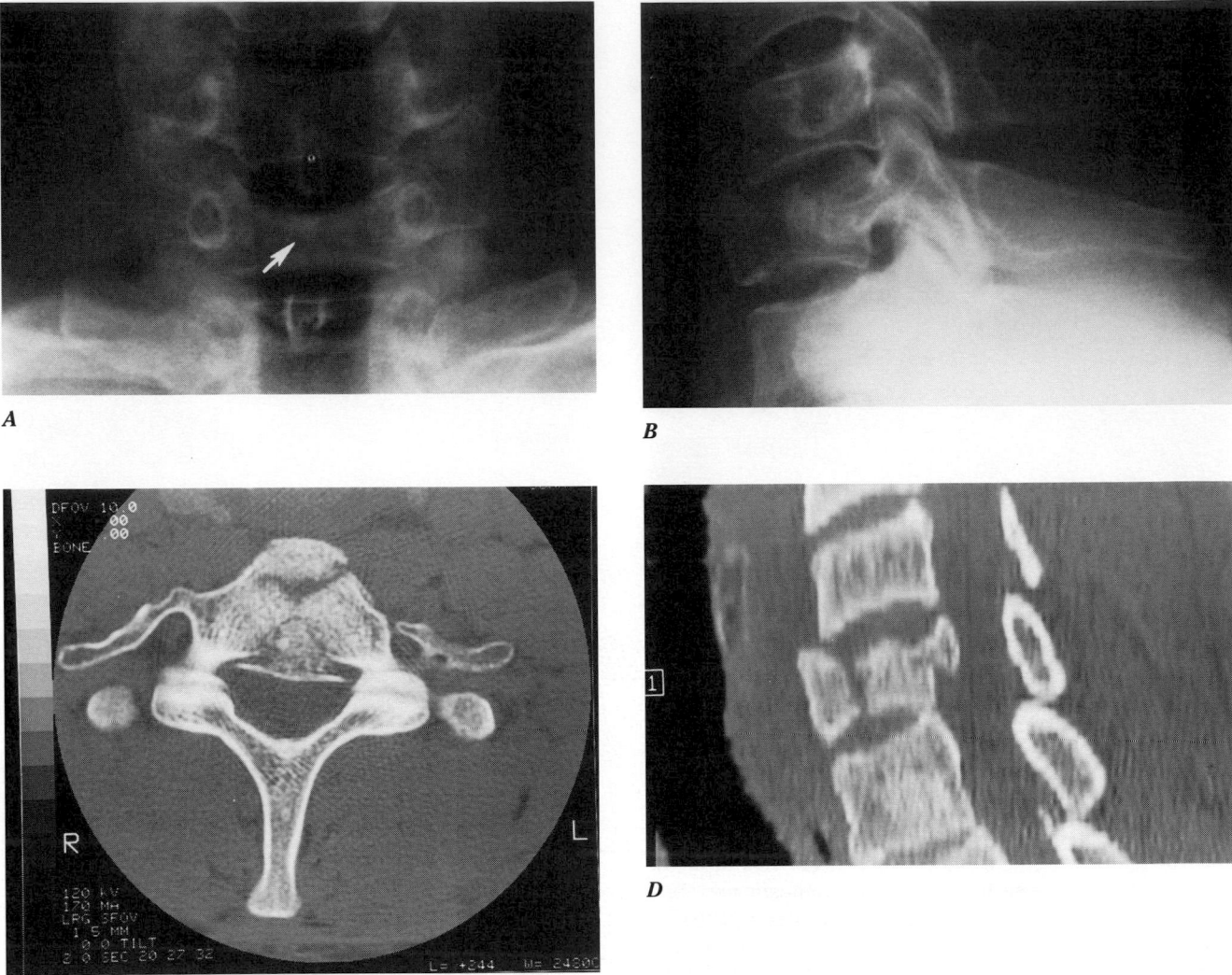

Figure 70-36 Compression fracture of C7 identified several weeks after a climbing accident in a neurologically intact patient complaining of continuing neck pain. *A.* Anteroposterior x-ray shows a sagittal split in the midline (*arrow*) and characteristic pedicle widening. *B.* Lateral x-ray shows anterior fracture fragment, but without posterior body wall retropulsion or vertebral dislocation. *C.* Transaxial CT scan reveals anterior- and middle-column fractures, but without pedicle fractures or posterior element fractures. *D.* Sagittal reconstruction shows the anterior- and middle-column fractures with retropulsion of superoposterior wall. *E.* Postoperative anterioposterior radiograph shows anterior reconstruction after corpectomy. *F.* Lateral x-ray shows tricortical iliac crest graft reconstruction.

flexed position, with the transmission of significant axial compression loads.[109] The mechanism is similar to that of a burst fracture. During impact, the inferior lip of the proximal vertebral body is driven into the superior surface of the caudal vertebral body. This produces a fracture of the distal anterior corner of the superior vertebra, i.e., the teardrop fragment (Fig. 70-37). The true significance of this injury pattern lies in its three-column instability. The teardrop fracture pattern exits through the disk space, causing severe damage to the disk and the annulus. In addition, posterior element injury involving ligamentous and bony structures results in a grossly unstable three-column injury. In addition, the middle column is often retropulsed into the spinal canal, causing either partial or complete

spinal cord injuries. Teardrop fractures are identified on lateral radiographs of the cervical spine, which shows retrodisplacement of the fractured vertebral body. Posterior element fractures or intraspinous widening may also be seen. Transaxial CT scans or MRI scans through the involved segment will demonstrate multiple fracture lines through the vertebral body and diminished spinal canal dimensions, caused by retrolisthesis of the fractured middle column.

Initial management of teardrop fractures is the application of cervical tong traction. This provides immediate stabilization, and usually improves overall alignment. It may also improve the spinal canal dimensions by indirect reduction via ligamentotaxis.

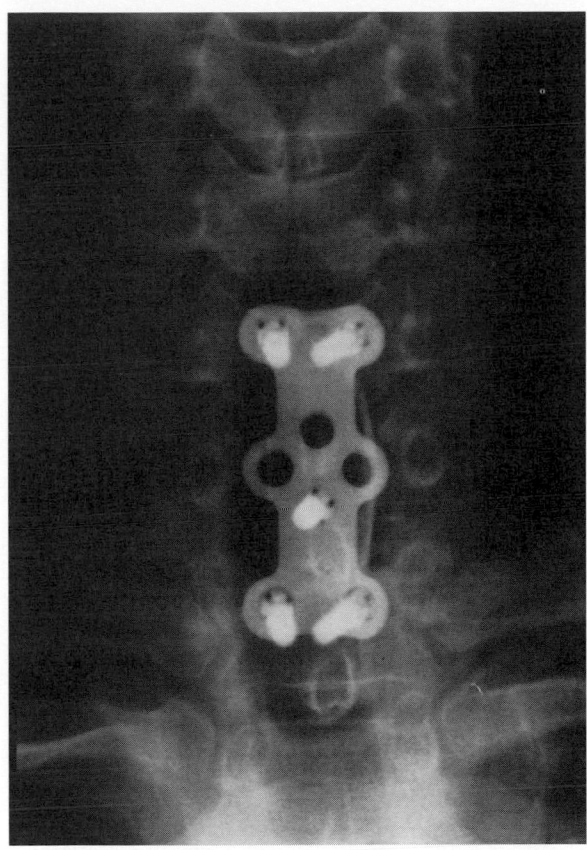

E

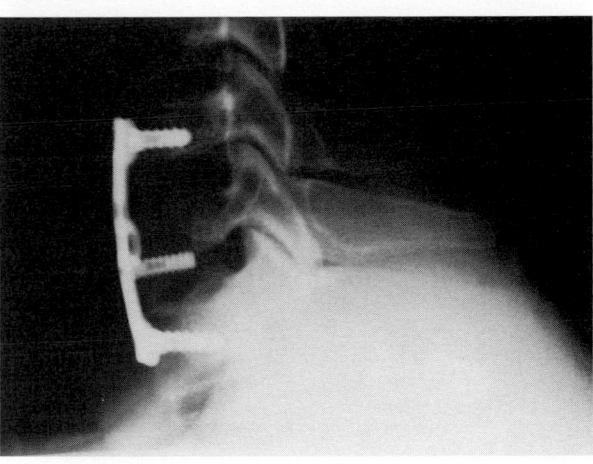

F

Figure 70-36 *(Continued)*

Definitive treatment of teardrop fractures is based on the extent of bony, ligamentous, and neurologic damage. When there is significant spinal canal compression, anterior corpectomy of the retropulsed vertebral body is performed with reduction and reconstruction of the anterior column using autologous iliac crest bone graft. Application of an anterior cervical plate is an option, as previously discussed, to stabilize these segments.[110] Because of the posterior-column instability, if there is any question of the mechanical integrity of the anterior construct, this should be protected with either a halo vest or posterior instrumentation and fusion as necessary.

Complications experienced in the treatment of teardrop fractures typically revolve around unrecognized posterior ligamentous injuries with the subsequent development of postoperative kyphosis. Management of anterior injuries with anterior corpectomy and strut grafting in the face of a significant posterior-column injury has resulted in graft dislodgement and late kyphotic deformity. As previously discussed, this problem can be obviated by both anterior and posterior fusion with internal stabilization.

Facet Subluxations

These injuries are ligamentous in nature and typically allow segmental translation with subluxation or dislocation of adjacent vertebral segments. The primary mechanism of injury is a posterior distraction force applied to an already flexed spine. This produces a spectrum of injuries ranging from a simple intraspinous ligament sprain with mild widening of the intraspinous distance (whiplash injury) to complete ligamentous and facet joint failure producing bilateral facet dislocations. The name *perched facet* has been given to the injury where there is significant anterior subluxation of the superior facet so that its inferior tip is "perched" on the superior tip of the more caudal facet articulation (Fig. 70-38). This arrangement immediately precedes bilateral facet dislocation.

As the facet subluxation proceeds through the spectrum of flexion and distraction to produce a bilateral facet dislocation (see Fig. 70-13), the neurologic sequelae typically increase. The forces involved in bilateral dislocations cause disruption of the posterior ligamentous complex, including the intraspinous ligaments, ligamentum flavum, and both facet capsules, with disruption of intervertebral disks.[111] This allows anterior translation of the superior vertebral body, which decreases the space available for the spinal cord and typically results in complete spinal cord injury.

Unilateral facet fractures (Fig. 70-39) or dislocations may display a variety of neurologic injuries ranging from a completely normal examination to a single nerve root deficit or incomplete spinal cord syndrome.[112] Typically, these do not result in complete spinal cord injuries. Because of the mechanics involved in unilateral facet dislocation, these in-

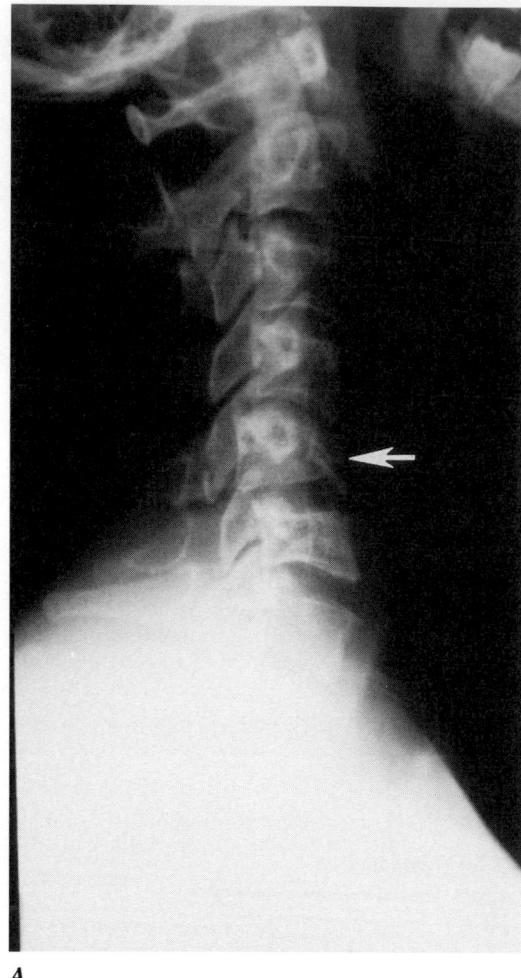

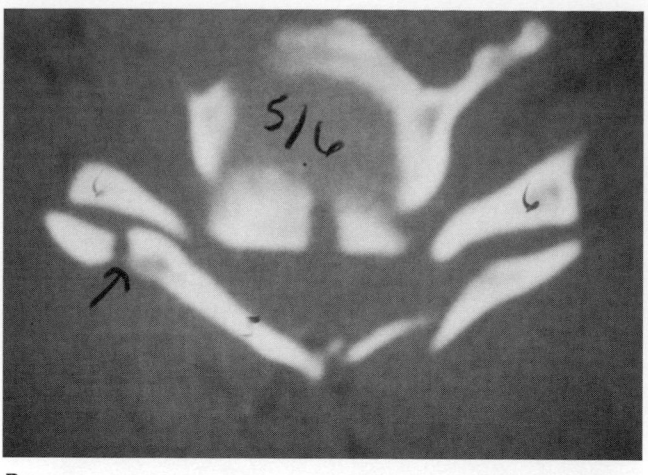

A

B

Figure 70-37 *A.* Lateral radiograph obtained in a young quadriplegic patient after a motor vehicle accident reveals a C5 teardrop fracture (*arrow*) dislocation of the cervical spine. In addition, the retrolisthesis of C5 is clearly identified. *B.* Transaxial CT section through the inferior aspect of C5 reveals the severe comminution and three-column involvement in this injury.

juries are typically associated with significant rotational abnormalities that can be identified on lateral radiographs. They are characterized by approximately 25 percent anterior olisthesis of the cephalad vertebral body on the caudad vertebral body. In contrast, bilateral dislocations typically have more than 50 percent anterior olisthesis. Oblique x-rays nicely document the malalignment of the articular pillars and can easily identify either a bilateral or unilateral dislocation. Anteroposterior radiographs can document a differential shift at the level of injury between the alignment of the spinous processes above and below the injured level. In addition, widening of the intraspinous distance can be seen. Because of the rotational malalignment, the unilateral facet dislocation can be identified by asymmetrical overlap of the articular pillars at the injured level. This has been described as the "bow-tie sign." Bilateral dislocations typically do not show this variable rotation above and below the injury site because both articular pillars have dislocated anteriorly. Axial CT scans are also very helpful in clearly diagnosing these dislocations. Parasagittal CT reconstructions through the articular pillars clearly show the malalignment adjacent to the injured level.

Perched facets are also easily identified on lateral radiographs or sagittal CT reconstructions. These injuries are

characterized by significant kyphosis at the injured level with little anterior translation of the cephalad vertebra.

Initial management of facet subluxations is to place the patient in cervical tong traction for attempted reduction. Because of the documented existence of significant disk herniations with bilateral facet dislocations,[111] extreme care should be taken in attempting to reduce bilateral facet dislocations using closed technique with axial traction. The argument has been made that in patients who have either complete spinal cord injury or significant, progressive neurologic injuries, an attempt at closed reduction without MRI documentation of disk integrity is probably not unreasonable. In a neurologically intact patient with bilateral facet dislocation, which is a rare occurrence when not accompanied by a canal-expanding fracture of the posterior arch, MRI documentation of disk integrity is mandatory.

Because unilateral facet dislocations typically are not complicated by disk herniations, these can be reduced in the emergency room under fluoroscopic guidance using axial cervical traction with gentle manipulation. Facet dislocations accompanied by fractured facets may require open reduction and internal fixation (ORIF).[113] In either unilateral or bilateral dislocations, one should be suspi-

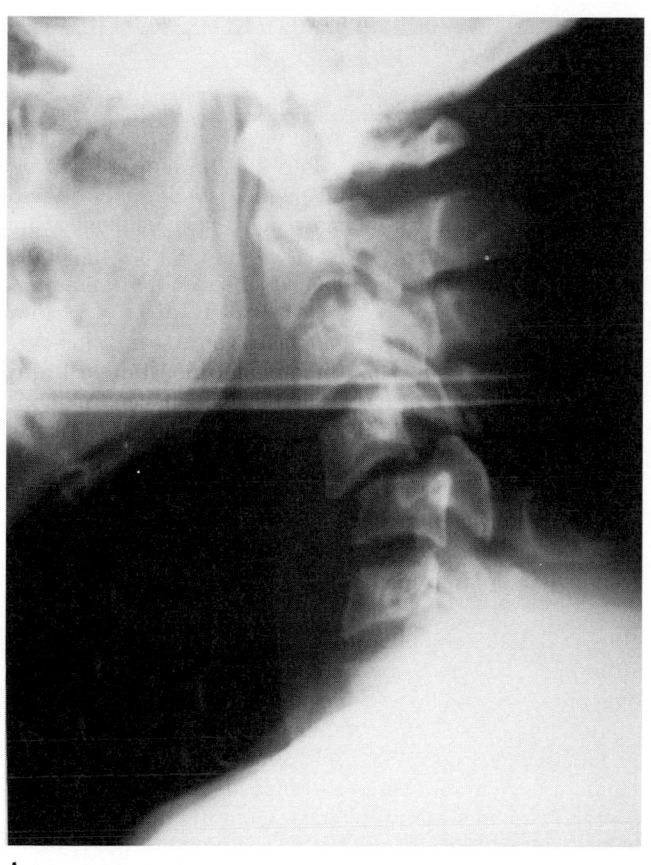 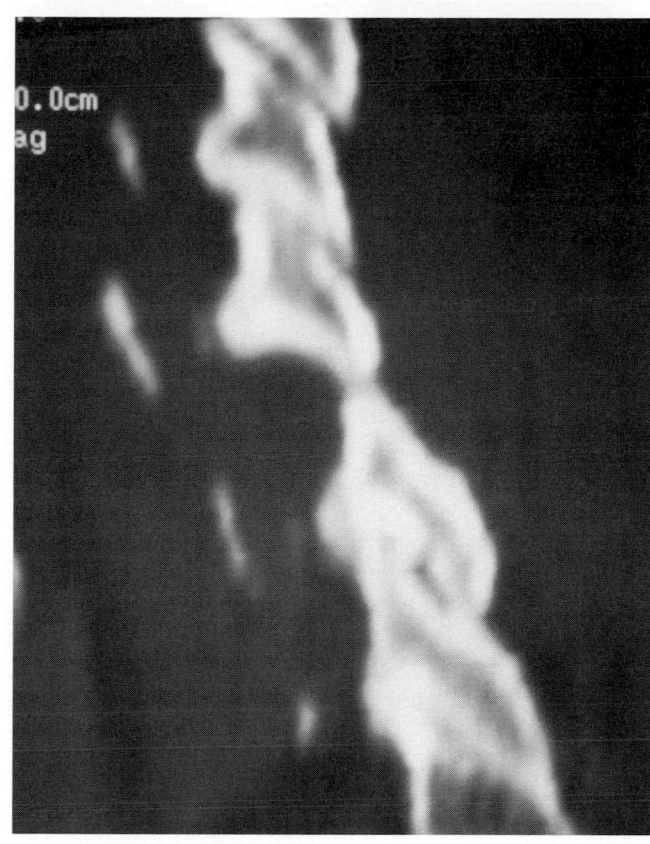

A   *B*

Figure 70-38 *A.* Lateral radiograph shows a perched facet. *B.* Sagittal CT reconstructions clearly show the precarious alignment of the facet joints in this injury.

cious of a disk herniation if there is significant loss of disk height at the injured level on plain lateral radiographs. This should prompt obtaining an MRI prior to attempting closed reduction. In the awake patient, if attempts at closed reduction result in a deterioration of the neurologic status, the reduction maneuver should be halted immediately. Either MRI or a cervical CT myelogram should be performed to identify the cause of the neurologic decline.[114] Open decompression and reconstruction may be necessary.

To attempt closed reduction, occipital tongs are placed as previously described, with the addition of weights in 5-lb increments. Lateral radiographs are taken after the addition of each weight to document that there is no overdistraction and to check for reduction. Once the facet joints have been distracted so that they can be reduced, gentle manipulation of the tongs under fluoroscopic guidance will allow realignment of the facet joint. Then, to effect reduction, the weight is reduced until the facet joints settle down into their anatomic position. Manipulation of the head (upper cervical spine) during the reduction of a unilateral facet dislocation may be necessary to realign the articular pillars on the dislocated side.[115] Once the facet is relocated, 10 to 15 lb may be left on the traction frame to maintain axial alignment and prevent redislocation. Typically, unilateral facet dislocations are more diffi-

cult to reduce, especially those involving fractures of the articular pillar. Because bilateral facet dislocations typically involve more soft tissue injury, they tend to reduce with less traction weight. However, in either unilateral or bilateral subluxations—depending on the degree of soft tissue injury, the patient's body habitus, and paraspinal muscle spasm—traction weights as heavy as 80 to 100 lb may be required to effect reduction.[115] In using traction weights of this magnitude, one must be extremely careful that previously unrecognized or minimally injured segments are not overdistracted. Care must also be taken to ensure that the halo pins are sufficiently tight in the occiput so that they do not tear through the patient's scalp.

After successful reduction, the patient needs to be stabilized in the reduced position until healing occurs. For the treatment of unilateral facet dislocations, halo vests have been advocated by some. However, because this is a ligamentous injury, there is a possibility that this will result in a somewhat hypermobile painful segment. The options of halo immobilization versus internal fixation should be offered to the patient, with the risks and benefits explained. Fusion for unilateral facet dislocations can be accomplished using a variety of posterior techniques. These include intraspinous wiring,[116] facet wiring, hook plates, and lateral mass screws and plates.[117,118] Sublaminar wiring techniques should not be considered in these in-

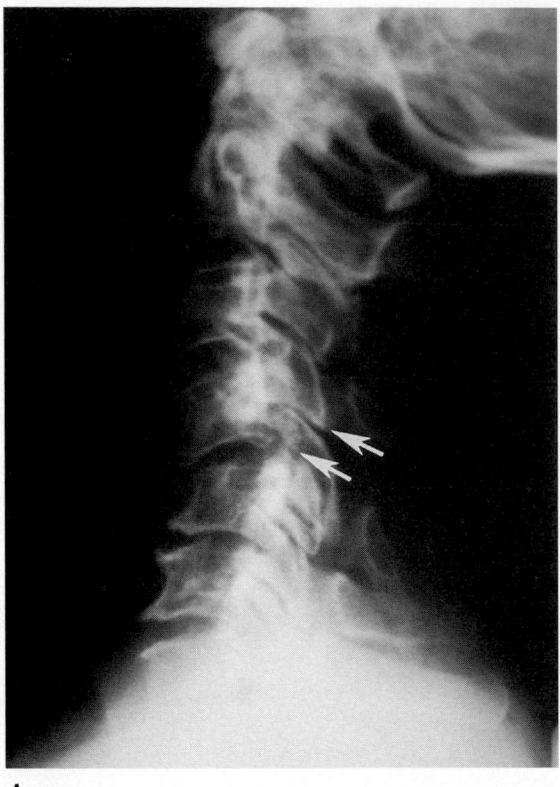

A

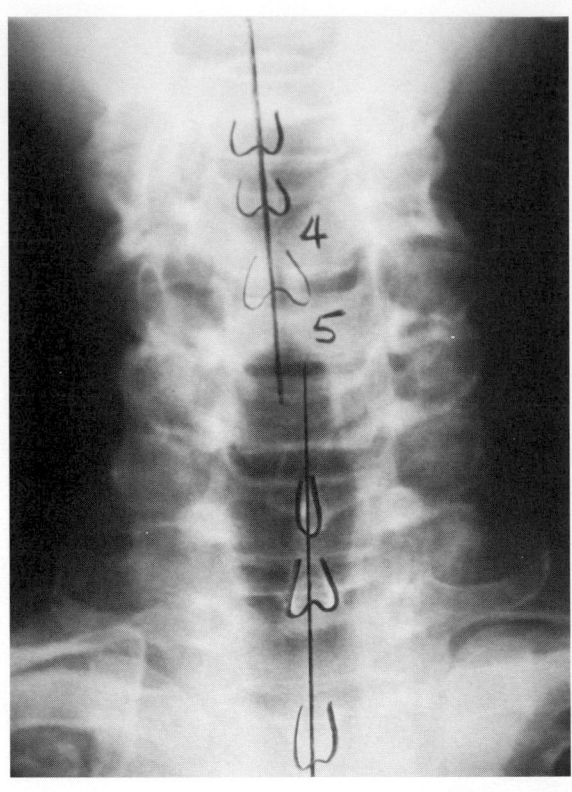

B

Figure 70-39 *A.* A unilateral facet dislocation is clearly identified by the characteristic radiographic findings. There is an acute kyphotic deformity between C4 and C5 with less than 25 percent olisthesis of C4 on C5. The incompletely superimposed trapezoidal shadows of the C4 lateral masses result in the "bow-tie sign." This is clearly seen in the lateral x-rays, also showing the inferior tips of the C4 facet joints (*arrows*). In addition, intraspinous gapping can be identified between the spinous processes. *B.* Anteroposterior x-rays show the coronal deformity with an offset of the spinous processes above and below the injury.

juries since any additional encroachment into the spinal canal may cause significant neurologic injury.

Because bilateral facet dislocations involve a severe soft tissue injury, these in all likelihood will not heal in halo immobilization and will almost certainly require fusion. In patients who have anterior compression due to a herniated disk, the initial treatment would be an anterior diskectomy and fusion at that level to decompress the potentially devastating effects of the disk herniation. After decompression, using a combination of direct manipulation and traction, it is sometimes possible to reduce the bilateral dislocation. This can be followed by anterior reconstruction and fixation. It could be argued that this, while biomechanically not entirely stable, might be sufficient stabilization once the anterior column fuses. If anterior fusion is accompanied by ankylosis of the facet joints, this could easily give adequate support. However, because of the potential instability, serious consideration should be given to additional posterior stabilization to reconstruct the posterior tension band. Following anterior decompression, if reduction cannot be achieved, a posterior approach with open reduction must be performed. This will probably require an anterior-posterior-anterior approach, since an appropriate anterior-column reconstruction is impossible until reduction is achieved.

Complications of cervical facet subluxations encompass both acute and chronic instability. This is frequently due to an unrecognized or undertreated posterior ligamentous injury or failure to reduce an initial kyphotic deformity. Long-term treatment in halo vest immobilization for these soft tissue injuries has been complicated by pin-track infections and an inability to maintain the reduction. This may require either repositioning of the dislocated segment or abandonment of halo immobilization for internal fixation and fusion.[119]

THORACIC AND LUMBAR INJURIES

Fractures of the thoracic, thoracolumbar, and lumbar spine are discussed under four general categories: compression fractures, burst fractures, flexion-distraction injuries (which include both ligamentous and bony Chance-type fractures), and fracture-dislocations.[2,120] Mechanistic classifications—such as those of Ferguson and Allen,[120a]

Magerl,[121a] and Gertzbein[121b]—are necessary for a complete understanding of fracture biomechanics.[4] However, clinical assessment of stability may be more easily understood by considering Denis's classification of the three columns of the spine. This classification suggests that if two columns are intact, the overall structure is stable. If two columns or more are compromised, acute or impending mechanical instability is present.[121] A similar morphologically based assessment of clinical stability has been offered by Gaines et al. in a load-sharing classification for spinal fractures.[122] Suggested as a method to decide if short-segment posterior instrumentation alone is adequate for spinal stabilization after trauma, it attempts to ascertain the structural stability of the anterior and middle columns by making three observations: the amount of vertebral body comminution in the lateral x-rays, the degree of apposition of the fracture fragments in the transaxial plane, and the overall intersegmental deformity present. A score may be obtained from a low of 3 for the most severely comminuted to 9 for the least severely involved fracture.

While compression fractures tend to be stable, fracture-dislocations tend to be grossly unstable. To make the determination regarding the stability of the intervening fracture patterns, such as burst fractures and flexion-distraction injuries, it is important to understand these mechanistic and morphologic classification schemes and have thorough radiographic documentation of the injury.

Compression Fractures

One of the most common and benign of the thoracic and lumbar fractures is the simple compression fracture. The force necessary to produce these injuries varies. In the elderly, minor trauma can be sufficient. In healthy young or middle-aged adults, these fractures require significant axial loading. They typically result in a wedge-shaped appearance of the anterior column with little middle-column involvement. They may be located anywhere throughout the thoracic or lumbar spine but are most commonly found in the midthoracic and midlumbar spine. Since these involve the anterior column only, they are inherently stable fractures. Multiple contiguous compression fractures or compression fractures with more than 50 percent involvement of the anterior column, particularly in the thoracic spine, may be relatively unstable, producing an unacceptable kyphotic deformity.

Diagnosis of compression fractures is normally made on routine lateral radiographs of the affected segment of the spine. If there is some concern about the age of an apparent compression fracture and the clinical examination and/or history is inconclusive, a bone scan may be useful in verifying whether the observed fracture is acute or chronic. If there is concern that a compression fracture is complicated by a middle-column injury, axial CT scans with sagittal reconstructions are an excellent way to document posterior wall and pedicle integrity. In the elderly one must always be aware that compression fractures may stem from an occult neoplastic involvement of the vertebral body.

Management of compression fractures in the thoracic and lumbar spine depends on the age of the patient, location of the injury, amount of kyphotic deformity, and whether there is any evidence of posterior column distraction injury[123] (Fig. 70-40). Elderly patients with multiple osteoporotic compression fractures are often treated symptomatically without any immobilization after a short period of bed rest. Isolated compression fractures of less than 50 percent of the total anterior vertebral body height are stable injuries and can be treated with a spinal orthosis for pain control. In addition, a well-molded orthosis may be able to unload the anterior column by achieving more anatomic alignment during healing. For lesions of the thoracolumbar junction and the lumbar spine, where the maintenance of anatomic alignment is essential for good long-term results, a hyperextension orthosis may be used to try to limit the development of postinjury kyphosis. However, even with a well-molded hyperextension cast or brace, some settling will occur, and in the early period of bracing, frequent lateral x-rays are needed to document maintenance of good alignment. Frequent modification of the brace may be necessary to maintain hyperextension and fracture reduction. For patients with greater than 50 percent compression deformity, it is essential to rule out involvement of the middle column. In addition, it is important to rule out any posterior ligamentous injury prior to attempting treatment in a brace. Sagittal MRIs may document posterior ligamentous injury and suggest a higher degree of instability than suggested by plain x-rays. In patients with significant anterior compression and posterior ligamentous injury, progressive kyphosis, or neurologic deficit, surgical stabilization is necessary. Depending on the degree of anterior compression (see Fig. 70-3), this may necessitate anterior strut grafting with posterior instrumentation or posterior instrumentation alone.

If reduction cannot be maintained in a brace, a period of postural reduction in bed while the fragments begin to coalesce may be necessary. This, however, puts the patient at risk for disseminated intravascular thrombosis, decubiti, pulmonary problems, and other systemic complications. The development of postinjury kyphosis is most often the result of underestimation of anterior column comminution, failure to recognize posterior column ligamentous injuries, and failure to obtain a reduction.

Burst Fractures

Burst fractures represent the next level in the continuum of axial compression injuries. These injuries involve both the anterior and middle columns and may also involve ligamentous or bony injuries of the posterior column. The mechanism is similar to that of compression fractures but with higher-energy axial loading combined with flexion.[11] The name for this injury comes from the bursting effect of the axial compression has on the anterior vertebral body. This injury often results in retropulsion of the posterior vertebral body wall (middle column). These and other high-energy thoracolumbar fractures are often associated with multisystem trauma, such as liver or spleen lacerations, aortic tears, and intraabdominal trauma. Burst frac-

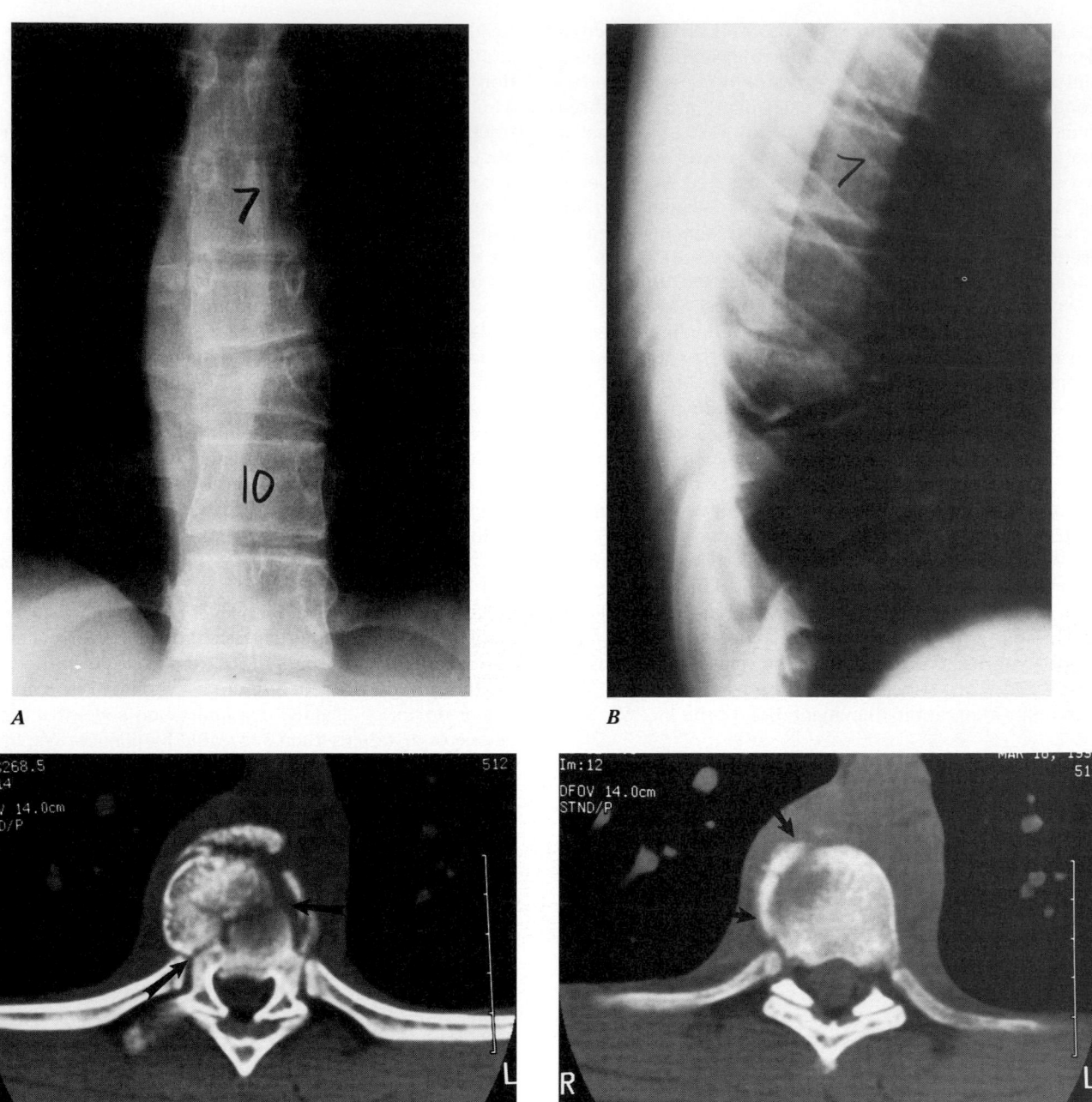

Figure 70-40 Contiguous thoracic fractures identified in a neurologically intact 17-year-old male after a bicycle accident. *A*. Anteroposterior radiographs show a T9 burst fracture with pedicle widening and an asymmetrical compression fracture of T8. *B*. Sagittal projection x-rays show an acute kyphosis be-tween T8 and T10. Transaxial CT scans (*C*) document the burst characteristics of the T9 fracture and transaxial CT scans (*D*) of T8 reveal it to be a compression fracture. This patient was successfully treated in a well-molded hyperextention TLSO orthosis with near anatomic alignment at 4 months.

tures can also occur with minimal apparent trauma in elderly osteoporotic patients.

Initial treatment of patients with thoracic or lumbar fractures includes bed rest with log rolling to decrease the chances of decubitus formation over bony prominences or over desensitized skin. A thorough systems review needs to be performed prior to any definitive treatment of the spinal trauma because of the possibility of coexisting systems injuries. Frequent neurologic examinations are nec-essary to uncover any developing neurologic deficits while definitive treatment is pending. Deterioration in the neurologic examination may prompt emergent surgery.

Definitive treatment of thoracic and lumbar burst fractures depends on neurologic status, patient age, fracture locations, spinal canal compromise, posterior element involvement, coronal or sagittal subluxations, the amount of segmental kyphosis and concomitant multisystem injuries, and body habitus.[122,124,125]

Nonoperative care for these fractures is an accepted method of treatment.[126] Burst fractures can be managed nonoperatively when the patient is neurologically intact, there is minimal segmental kyphosis, or bony retropulsion results in less than 50 percent spinal canal compromise (see Fig. 70-40). It is important to point out that the degree of canal compromise does not always correlate with neurologic injury, and while a very narrow or stenotic postinjury canal may predispose toward the development of neurologic injury in the future, there is no guarantee this will happen even in the face of a severely stenotic canal. Other instances in which nonoperative treatment may be contemplated include those where there is no coronal or sagittal subluxation and no involvement of posterior elements. Treatment can be provided in the form of a hyperextension cast applied to the patient while in the reduced position or with a two-piece hyperextension orthosis padded appropriately to maintain hyperextension and fracture reduction.[127] Patients with thin body habitus, a long torso, and easily palpable bony prominences over the thoracic rib cage and iliac crest are ideal candidates for cast immobilization. In older patients or patients with an obese body habitus, bracing may be ineffective or poorly tolerated, necessitating operative intervention. Low lumbar burst fractures may be ideally suited to cast immobilization because much of the axial load is carried by the posterior elements.[128] However, because of the position of these lesions low in the lumbar spine, these patients may need to have one leg incorporated into a pantaloon-type cast to gain control over the distal segments of the spine through pelvic immobilization.

In patients who are neurologically intact with canal compromise of more than 50 percent, nonoperative treatment is somewhat controversial. The fractures in the majority of these patients will heal uneventfully. If adequate sagittal alignment has been maintained, these patients will probably not experience neurologic sequelae. Typically, the spinal canal will remodel over time to increase the space available for the neural elements. However, with the reduced space available for the neural elements, these patients may be somewhat more sensitive to the development of neurologic sequelae precipitated by axial settling or the development of kyphosis.

Treatment of thoracic burst fractures in an orthosis is somewhat more concerning but is a good option in carefully selected patients. While this region is typically more stable biomechanically than the lumbar spine, the consequences for the development of neurologic injuries (spinal cord) are somewhat more severe than in the lumbar spine (cauda equina). Careful monitoring of both the coronal and lateral x-rays and the patient's neurologic status is mandatory in attempting to treat thoracic burst fractures in this conservative fashion.

The indications for operative management of burst fractures in a neurologically intact or minimally involved patient are three-column injury with subluxation in the coronal or sagittal plane, significant segmental kyphosis at the fracture site, and spinal canal compromise greater than 60 percent.[129] In addition, concomitant injuries or a body habitus not suited to orthotic treatment may lead one to consider surgical options for these fractures. In addition, fractures at the thoracolumbar junction or in the lumbar

spine, where kyphosis is poorly tolerated and apt to develop, may be better treated with ORIF. This can probably be done by a posterior approach with posterior stabilization alone provided that there is no severe anterior column compression.[130] Preservation of the sagittal alignment is important; however, reducing the number of fixed segments above and below the injury is equally important in this mobile region of the spine. At the thoracolumbar junction, instrumentation is typically carried higher up into the thoracic spine, where mobility is less of an issue. This provides a series of good fixation points. Instrumentation below the level of the injury, into the more mobile lumbar spine, is kept to a minimum (see Fig. 70-30). Numerous constructs have been designed to achieve this end. The Edwards rod-and-sleeve system[131] has been used with some success, as have pedicle screws, to create both "multilevel" and "single-level" constructs.[131] Attempting to do limited fixation one level above and one level below the fractured vertebral body with reduction and posterior stabilization alone needs to be carefully contemplated. If this limited fixation is attempted with an unstable anterior column, failure is likely. The load-sharing classification of Gaines et al. is a useful tool to estimate the chances of success with this approach[122] (see Fig. 70-31). Any question of anterior column compromise with this short construct is answered by providing the patient with a well-fitted TLSO orthosis (Fig. 70-41). Long constructs using either Harrington rod or multiple hook rod constructs have been used in the past with good results, with and without sublaminar and spinous process wiring.[133] The problems with these longer constructs are that they immobilize more segments and do little to provide direct reduction forces to the anterior and middle columns. This can only be achieved with longer moment arms on either side of the fracture site. In the neurologically intact patient with significant anterior column destruction, posterior instrumentation is supplemented with an anterior partial corpectomy and strut grafting to reestablish anterior column alignment and continuity. This allows the posterior instrumentation to function as a tension band rather than as a cantilever support for the anterior column, cantilever bending is a mode of loading known to cause pedicle screw failure.

Operative treatment of neurologically involved patients with burst fractures centers around spinal cord, thecal sac, or nerve root decompression[105,134] (Fig. 70-42). This is accomplished via a retroperitoneal or transthoracic approach to the anterior vertebral column.[134] Spinal canal decompression is accomplished via corpectomy or partial corpectomy. It is important to make sure that the spinal canal decompression reaches from pedicle to pedicle. Failure to do so may leave residual middle-column bony elements in the spinal canal. Patients with nerve root lesions and laminar fractures have entrapped nerve roots until proven otherwise. This situation may prompt posterior decompression first.[135] Trauma-induced dural tears are common in this situation.

Fractures from T1 to T10 will typically be approached with a thoracotomy. For fractures at the T11, T12, and L1 levels, a thoracoabdominal approach through the 10th rib will be necessary. This may require incision of the diaphragm to gain access to the thoracolumbar junction. For fractures from L2 to L5, a retroperitoneal flank approach below the diaphragm is usually adequate. Prior to the corpectomy, complete removal of the intervertebral disks above and below the fractured vertebral body is accomplished. This allows clear orientation with respect to the fractured body and the spinal canal and helps define the extent of the surgical dissection. Often a subtotal corpectomy with removal of only the ipsilateral and posterior vertebral body is necessary to gain access to and adequately decompress the thecal sac. This leaves vascularized bone anterior and deep to assist in the healing process. In the thoracic and lumbar spine, extracavitary and pedicular approaches have been advocated by some for limited decompressions.[136] Some of these approaches may allow the placement of structural grafts; however, the working space is limited and the grafts may not be adequate to support force transmission through the anterior column. For simple decompressive procedures, this may be an adequate approach to decompression of the spinal canal.

Following the spinal canal decompression a strut graft is placed between the end plates of the superior and inferior vertebral bodies. Initial success or failure of this surgery rests on the stability and strength of the graft. Ultimately, success depends on the ability of the graft to heal and fuse to the superior and inferior vertebral bodies. Supplemental stabilization can be added in the form of anterior fixation devices such as the Kaneda[137] device (Acromed), Z-plate (Danek),[138] or anterior thoracolumbar locking plate (Synthes). In addition, pedicle-screws/rod constructs can be used. In those patients who do not have an associated posterior ligamentous injury, anterior reconstruction alone with rigid plate fixation may be sufficient. Fractures approached anteriorly as a primary procedure can be followed with posterior fusion and instrumentation for additional stabilization (Fig. 70-43). In patients who do have a concomitant posterior ligamentous injury as evidenced by widened intraspinous distance and high-intensity signal within the posterior ligaments on an MRI or in those who have fractured elements posteriorly, supplemental fixation posteriorly may be needed to provide adequate stabilization. This can be achieved with either a hook-and-rod construct or pedicle fixation, depending on the extent and type of posterior-column injury. Comminuted or fractured posterior elements may not lend themselves to hook-and-rod constructs and may be better suited to pedicle fixation. On the other hand, if it is only necessary to reestablish the posterior-column tension band, a one-level hook-and-rod or a pedicle-screw construct may be entirely sufficient.[139] If the posterior injury consists of a facet capsule disruption without any other obvious bony injury, then the minimally invasive placement of transarticular facet screws or spinous process wiring may be useful in reestablishing continuity through the facet joint or posterior elements. In a highly unstable burst fracture, consideration could be given to posterior alignment and stabilization first in order to maintain the overall alignment and to reduce the spinal deformity. In this way, the screws and rods can be used to reestablish axial and sagittal alignment and achieve decompression by ligamentotaxis[140] (Fig. 70-44). Once the spine is sta-

bilized in this fashion, it is easier to safely approach the anterior aspect of the spinal cord for decompression. Subsequent anterior-column reconstruction is accomplished as previously described.

Complications of nonoperatively treated burst fractures involve residual kyphotic deformity, progressive kyphosis due to unrecognized posterior-column injuries, and vertebral collapse. These complications can exacerbate or create neurologic deficits.[141]

The complications of operative management include failure of instrumentation, failure to adequately reconstruct the anterior column, major vessel injury in the chest or retroperitoneum, and neurologic injuries. In addition, strut grafts may be dislodged, may fracture, or may subside into adjacent vertebral bodies, allowing the development of kyphotic deformity. Anterior dislodgement of strut grafts may cause vascular or intraabdominal injuries. Pseudarthrosis at the fracture site is a rare consequence of either operative or nonoperative treatment.

Fracture-Dislocation

Fracture-dislocation is the result of significant energy applied to the spine. The forces involved may include flexion, distraction, extension, rotation, shear, and axial loading.[1] These injuries by definition involve all three columns of the spine and are extremely unstable. They typically result in profound neurologic deficits.[142] Plain x-rays will show evidence of the grossly malaligned spine in both planes. Occasionally, thoracic subluxations are subtle and may involve only slight lateral translation of one vertebral body upon another or slight olisthesis in the sagittal plane (Fig. 70-45). Because the thoracic region is inherently stable, even slight malalignment portends significant injury. Therefore CT scans are mandatory to assess for unrecognized posterior element fractures that may affect operative management. An axial CT scan may demonstrate two vertebral bodies in the same transaxial slice, indicating dislocation and overriding of vertebral segments. In addition, the "empty-facet sign" identified on axial CT scans is present when there is complete facet dislocation. Unlike burst fractures, the middle column is often intact when the primary mechanism of injury is a shear force. In this instance, the compromise of the vertebral canal is secondary to extreme vertebral malalignment rather than retropulsed bone.

In the unlikely event that this type of injury is not accompanied by complete spinal cord injury, great care must be taken to maintain the alignment of the spine. Spinal precautions are necessary with immobilization on a back board until definitive treatment can be arranged. As with burst fractures, these injuries are often accompanied by numerous multisystem injuries as a result of the large forces involved. Definitive management of dislocations is similar to that of severely unstable burst fractures. Posterior operative reduction and stabilization, preferably with pedicle-screw instrumentation, is accomplished to realign the spine and protect it from further injury dur-

(Text continues on page 1287)

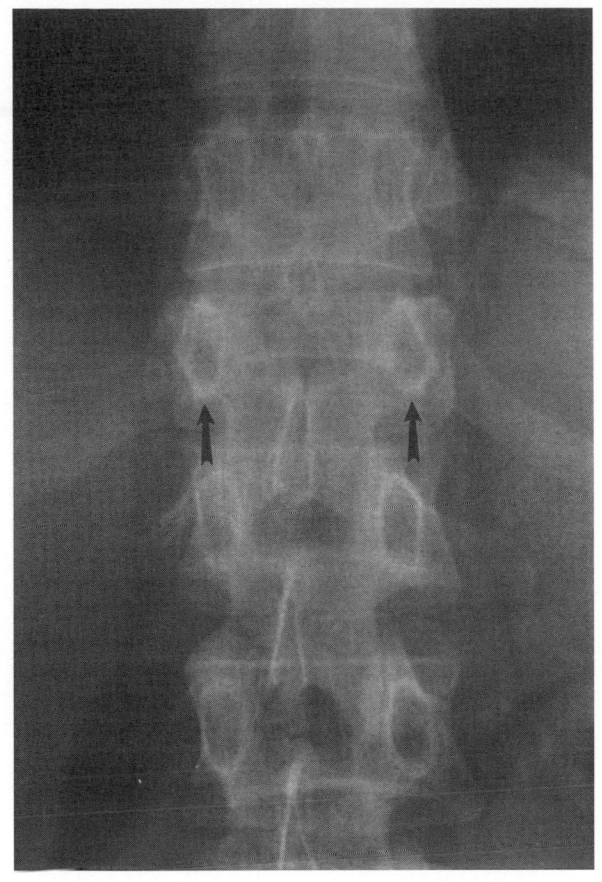

A

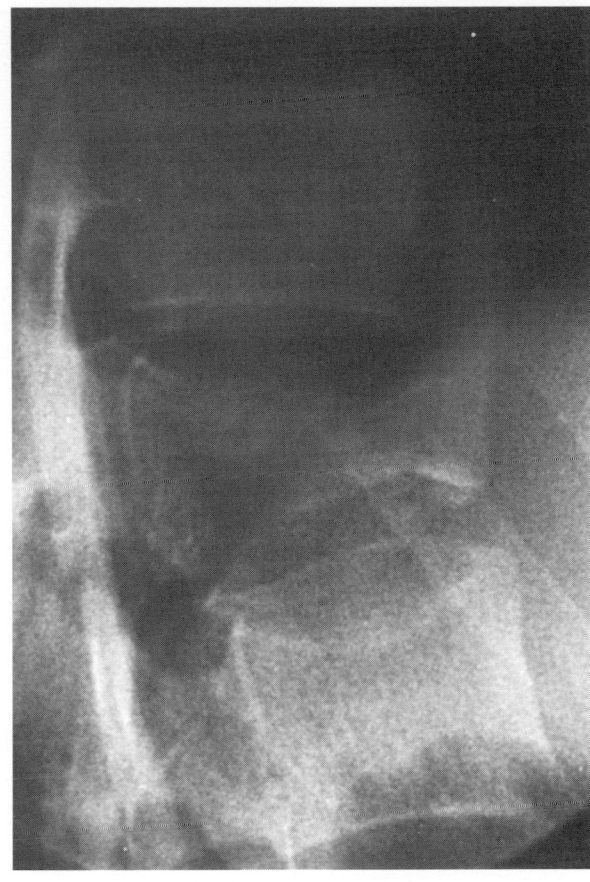

B

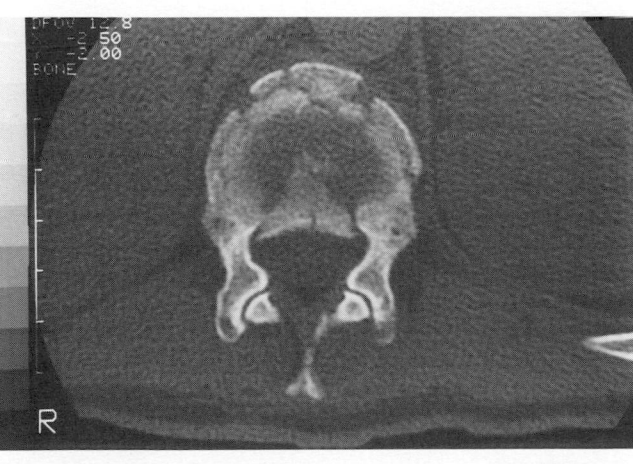

C

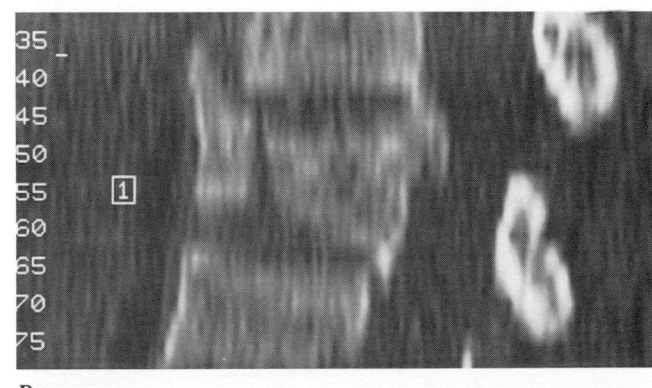

D

Figure 70-41 T12 burst fracture identified after a fall in a neurologically intact patient. *A.* Anteroposterior x-rays show pedicular widening between the pedicles. *B.* Lateral radiograph shows significant anterior and middle-column collapse with retropulsion of middle column into the spinal canal. *C.* Transaxial CT scan reveals the extent of the anterior–middle-column injury. *D.* Sagittal reconstruction shows the anterior and middle-column failure with middle-column retropulsion. *E.* Reestablishment of anterior and middle-column height and overall alignment is documented in lateral postoperative x-ray. *F.* Anteroposterior x-ray postoperatively. This construct was protected in a TLSO brace for 2 months with good results.

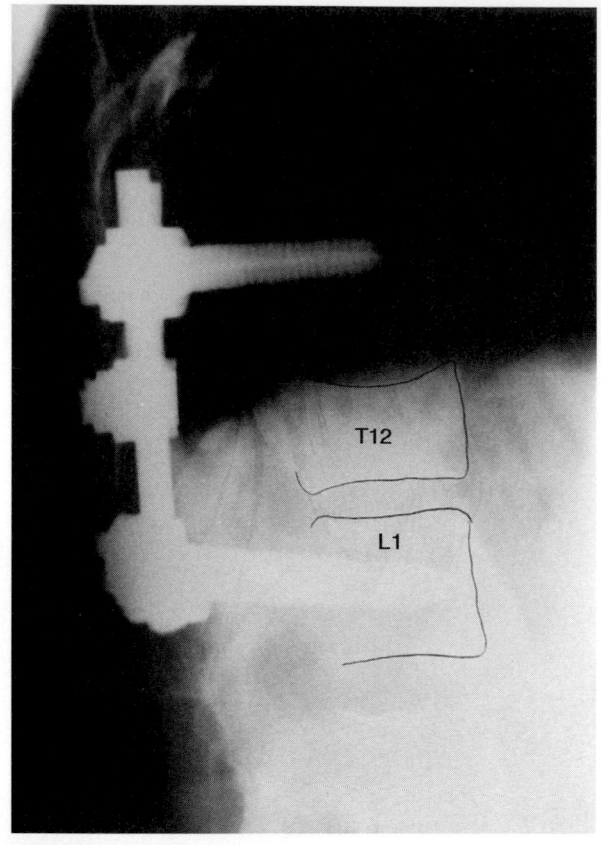

E

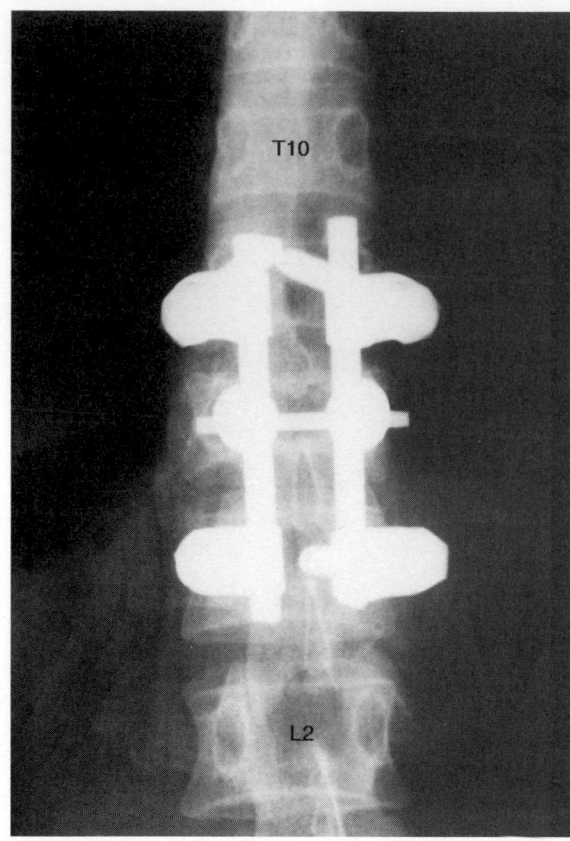

F

Figure 70-41 *(Continued)*

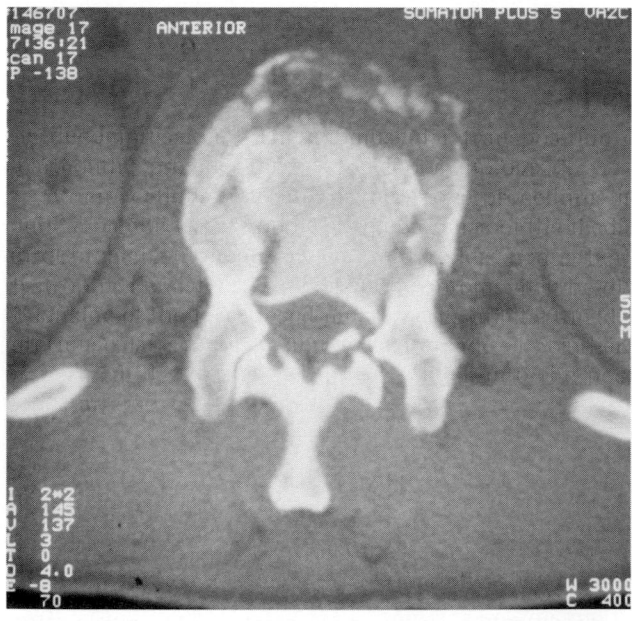

A

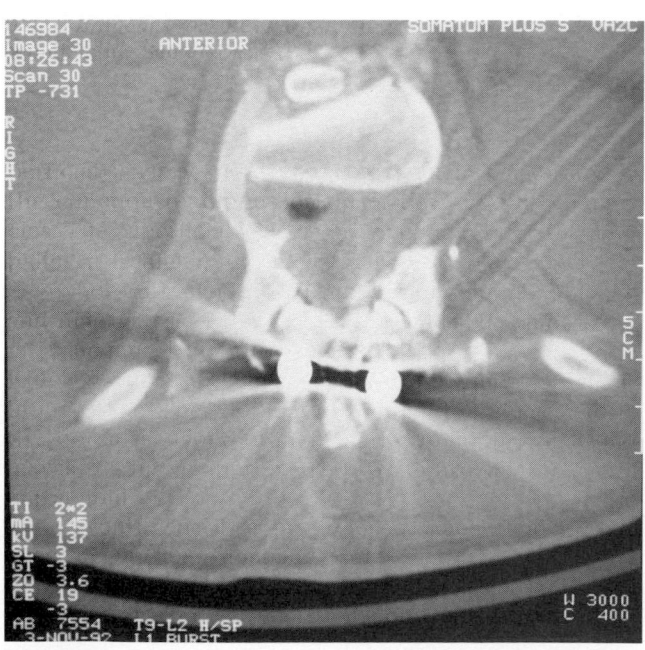

B

Figure 70-42 An L1 burst fracture is identified in a neurologically compromised patient. *A.* Extensive anterior-middle- and posterior-column injury requiring both an anterior decompression and reconstruction supplemented with posterior instrumentation and fusion. *B.* Complete decompression was achieved from pedicle to pedicle.

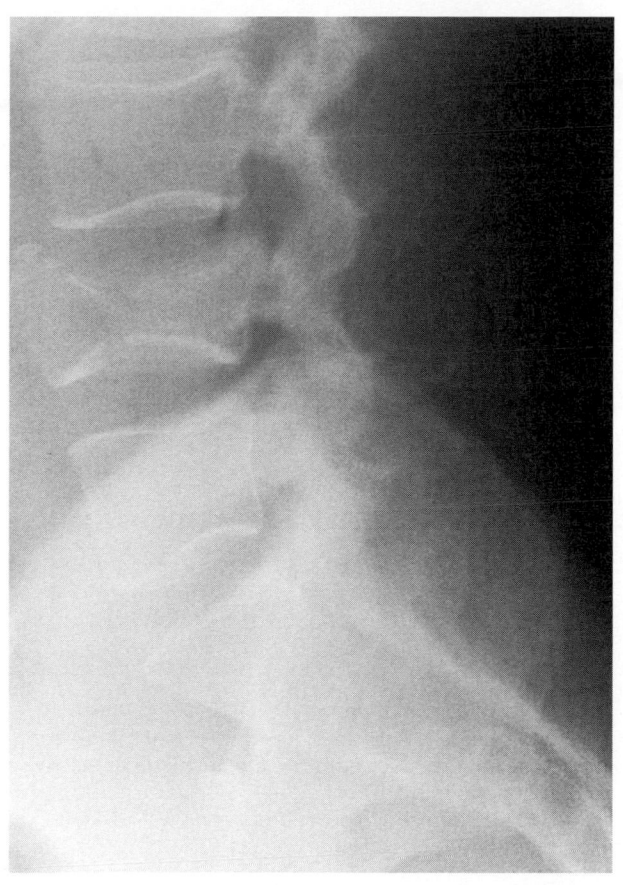

A

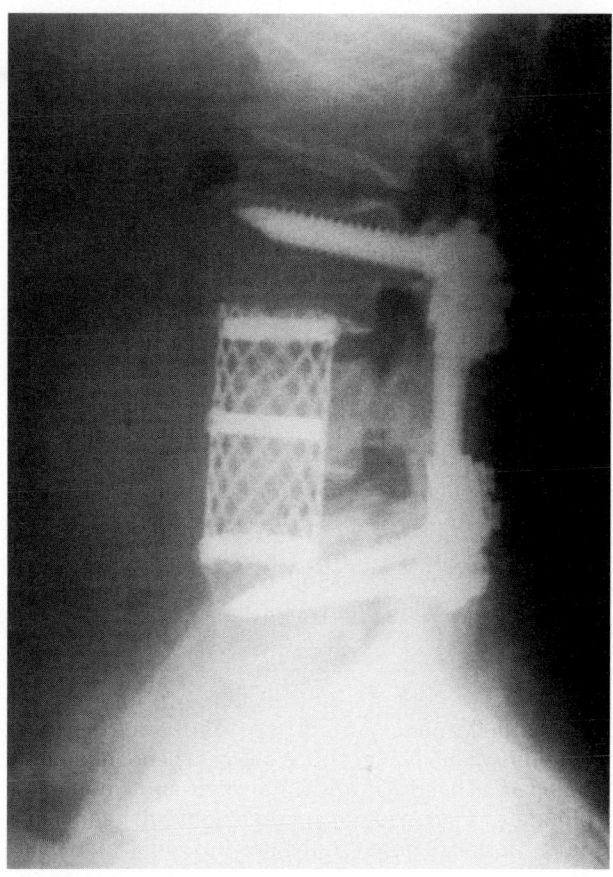

B

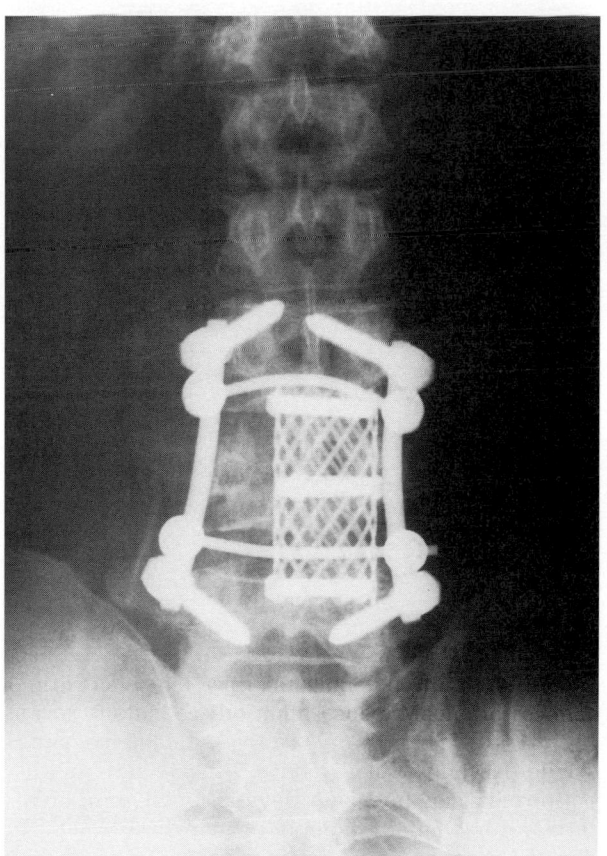

C

Figure 70-43 *A.* This low lumbar burst fracture was identified in a neurologically intact, obese young male after violent tonic-clonic seizures. *B* and *C.* This anteroposterior reconstruction was performed one level above and below the fracture with anterior column reconstruction because the patient was not a good candidate for bracing and there was concern about continued neurologic stability.

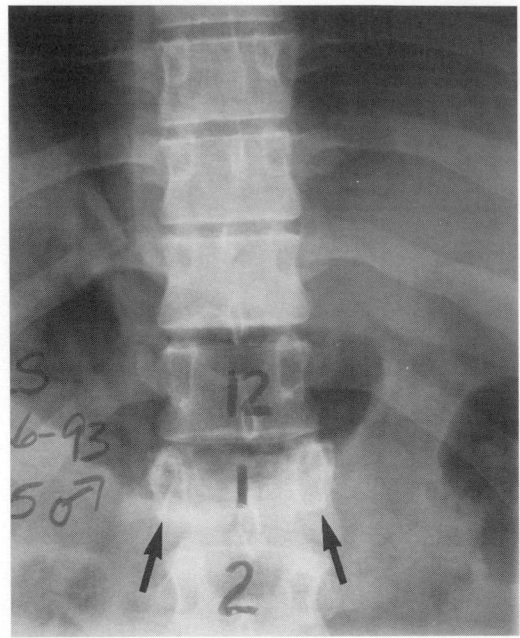

A

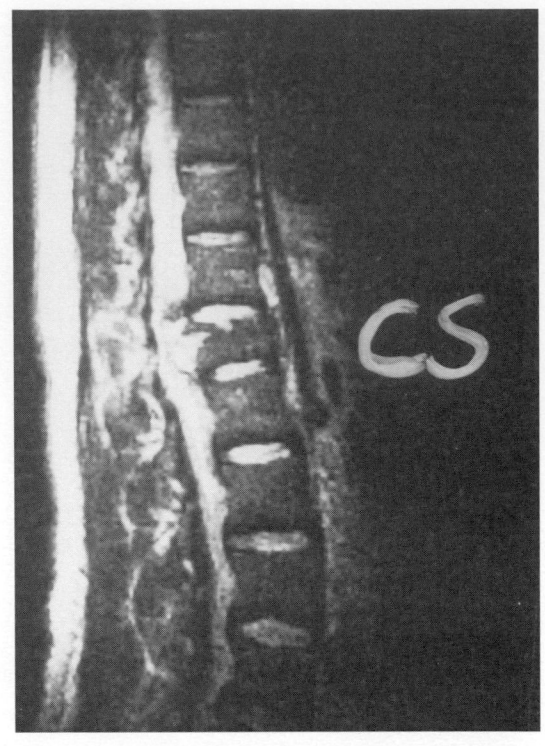

B

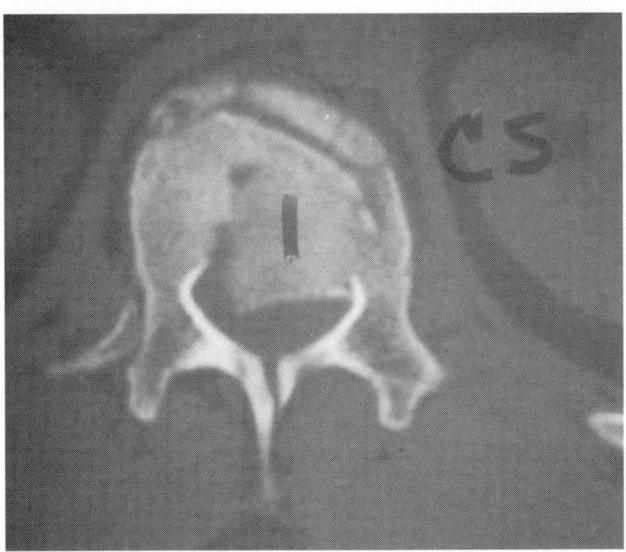

C

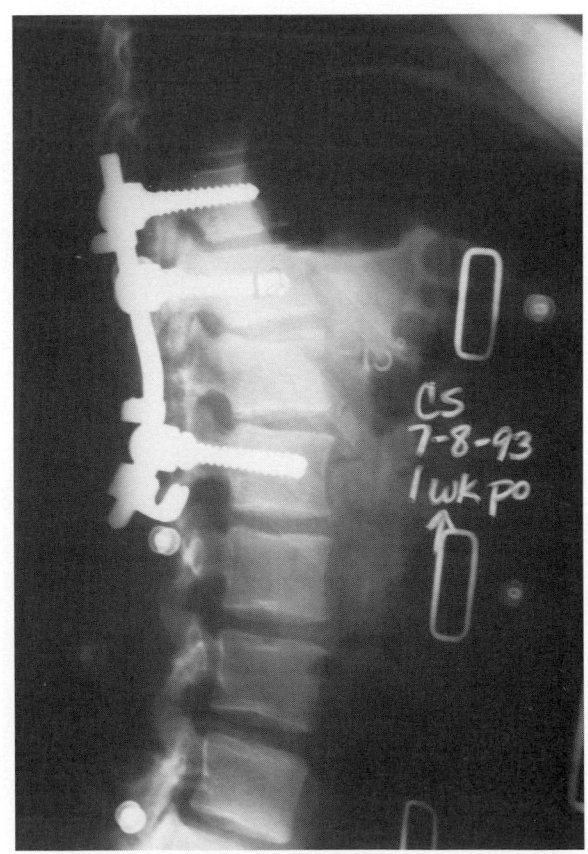

D

Figure 70-44 An L1 burst fracture is clearly identified in the (*A*) anteroposterior x-rays, which show widening between the pedicles. Sagittal MRI (*B*) shows a fractured and retropulsed middle column, which resulted in an incomplete spinal cord injury. Transaxial CT scan (*C*) shows anterior–middle-column involvement with a midline laminar fracture. Significant canal compromise is identified. Lateral radiograph (*D*) after posterior alone instrumentation and fusion from T11 to L2. Significant canal decompression (*E*) has been achieved with ligamentotaxis alone. (Reproduced with permission from Haher TR, O'Brien MF, Felmy WT: Thoracic and lumbar fractures: Diagnosis and management, in Bridwell KH, DeWald RL (eds): *Textbook of Spinal Surgery.* Philadelphia, Lippincott, 1991.)

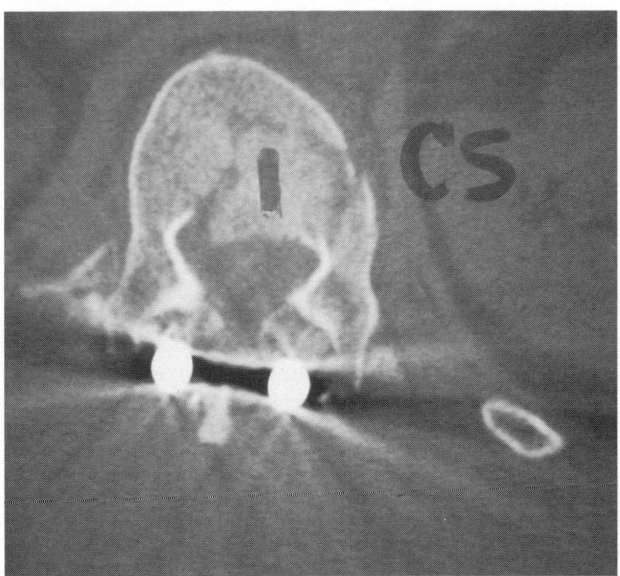

E

Figure 70-44 *(Continued)*

ing the anterior decompressive procedure. Thoracic injuries can be instrumented three to four levels above and below the fracture dislocation using a hook-and-rod construct. In thoracolumbar and lumbar injuries, instrumentation is better suited to a pedicle-screw/rod construct. Limiting the number of distally instrumented and fused segments should be considered in the neurologically involved but potentially ambulatory patient. Maintaining mobile segments may be less of an issue in nonambulatory patients.

The timing for operative reduction and stabilization is determined by the neurologic status and overall medical condition of the patient. The primary indication for emergent operative reduction is an incomplete neurologic injury with a progressive neurologic deficit.[27] Patients with complete spinal cord injuries are stabilized as soon as possible to decrease the duration of enforced bed rest and institute physical therapy as soon as possible. Patients with incomplete neurologic injuries that are improving may be observed until their condition plateaus. If recovery is not deemed satisfactory, decompression may be warranted.[143] Anterior decompression in patients with incomplete spinal cord injury has resulted in neurologic improvement even years after the traumatic event.

Complications of fracture-dislocations of the spine include increased spinal deformity due to inadequate structural realignment and stabilization. Charcot spinal arthropathy below the level of a complete spinal cord injury may be due to accelerated degeneration within a spinal segment lacking protective sensation.

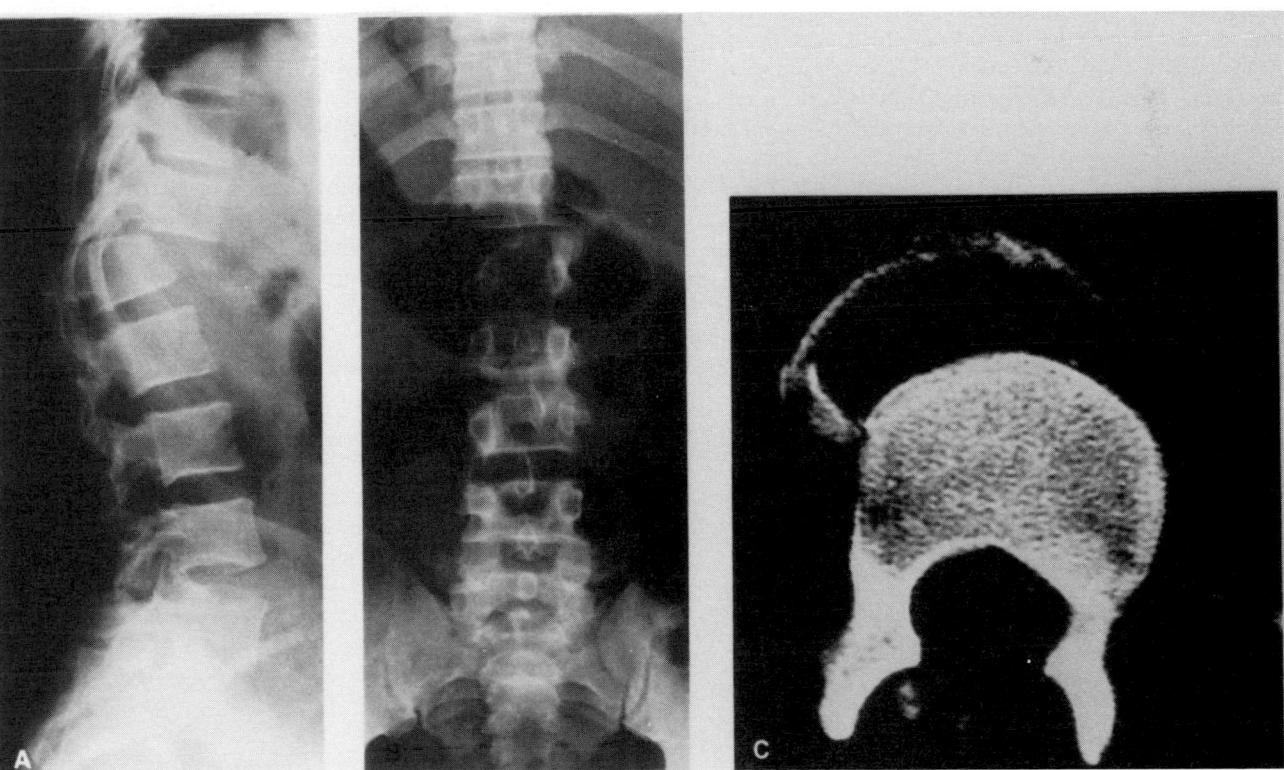

Figure 70-45 T12-L1 fracture dislocation. Lateral (*A*) and AP (*B*) projections show gross malalignment. Axial CT scans (*C*) show both T12 and L1 vertebral bodies in the same image plane, documenting significant displacement of vertebral segments.

Flexion-Distraction Injuries (Chance Injuries)

These injuries often result from flexion and distraction occuring during motor vehicle collisions. Restrained individuals wearing lap belts only are prone to this injury. The mechanism includes acute flexion of the torso over the lap belt with the upper part of the body accelerated forward, causing a distraction moment against the restrained pelvis. The seat belt acts as a fixed fulcrum anterior to the abdomen with distractive forces applied to the spine through the posterior, middle, and anterior columns[144] (Fig. 70-46).

While some flexion-distraction injuries are quite dramatic on presentation, a high index of suspicion must be maintained to discover others. Patients presenting to the emergency room with abrasions or bruises over the lower abdomen must be investigated carefully. A palpable or tender gap over the spinous processes may be the first indication of a flexion-distraction injury. The incidence of neurologic complications in flexion-distraction injuries is low in patients who do not frankly dislocate. These patients may have life-threatening intraabdominal injuries, which need to be addressed prior to spinal stabilization.

Plain lateral radiographs are essential in the diagnosis of these injuries. Lateral radiographs will often document the injury. Chance fractures are typically three-column injuries with the fracture propagating through the bony elements from posterior to anterior. These fractures are easily identified with a gap through the entire osseous structure of the vertebral segment. These injuries may also be entirely ligamentous, with rupture of the intraspinous ligaments, facet capsules, and rupture of the posterior longitudinal ligament, annulus, and disk. There may be a combination of both ligamentous and osseous injuries. If the injury is ligamentous and sustained forces are involved, a bilateral facet dislocation may occur. As in the cervical spine, unilateral dislocations are suspected when there is less than 50 percent anterior olisthesis of the superior vertebral body on the inferior vertebral body. Displacements of 50 percent or more raise the suspicion of a bilateral facet dislocation.

Definitive treatment of flexion-distraction injuries depends upon the anatomic structures involved and the amount of displacement. Lesions occurring entirely through bony elements can be very successfully managed in hyperextension orthoses. When the only osseous injury involves the pars interarticularis, these are best managed with open reduction and internal stabilization, since the pars has little in the way of cancellous bone, making healing less reliable, particularly in the elderly. Chance injuries that result primarily from ligamentous or soft tissue damage need to be addressed with open reduction and internal stabilization, since these ligamentous structures will not heal adequately to provide stability if treated closed. It is usually sufficient to apply a short-segment construct, preferably with pedicle screws in the thoracolumbar and lumbar region to reeestablish the tension band. In addition, fusion is performed. A thoracolumbar orthosis may additionally be worn for several months postoperatively.

As with bilateral facet dislocations in the cervical spine, it is important to identify traumatic disk herniations prior to surgical reduction. Complications of flexion-distraction injuries include inadequate posterior column reduction when closed reduction with external immobilization is the treatment. In addition, failure to recognize the magnitude of ligamentous or soft tissue components of the injury may lead to posttreatment instability. Rarely, traumatic disk herniations may cause neurologic symptoms because of postreduction compression of neural elements by extruded disk fragments.

SACRAL FRACTURES

Sacral fractures occur most frequently in high-energy trauma; however, fractures in the elderly due to osteoporosis, fatigue fractures in children, and sacral insufficiency fractures after radiotherapy have been described.[145]

Physical findings are back and buttock pain with ecchymosis over the sacrum or sacral pain on rectal examination. Specific low lumbar and sacral root neurologic deficit should prompt consideration of this diagnosis.[146]

Sacral fractures typically do not present as isolated injuries and are often accompanied by pelvic fractures. Denis has classified sacral fractures into zone I, zone II, and zone III injuries[147] (Fig. 70-47). Zone I fractures typically are lateral to the neural foramen. Neurologic deficits may result

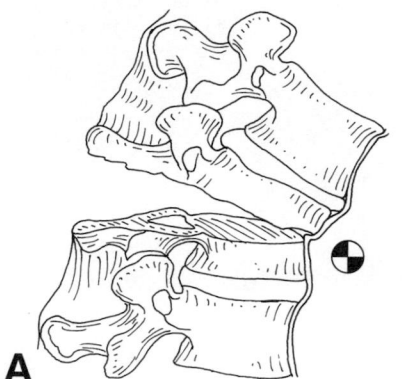

A

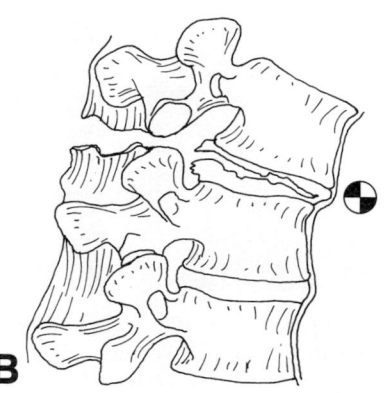

B

Figure 70-46 Diagrammatic representation of an osseous (*A*) and soft tissue (*B*) Chance fracture. The circular symbol defines the axis of rotation for these injuries.

from superior migration of the sacral fracture fragments compressing the L5 nerve root against the distal edge of the L5 transverse process. Zone 1 injuries also include various ligamentous avulsion fractures around the periphery of the sacrum.

Zone II fractures are longitudinal fractures through the sacral foramen. These are associated with a 28 percent incidence of neurologic deficits. Neurologic injury is usually characterized by S1 compression. This is often associated with sciatica. The L5 nerve root may be involved if fracture fragments are displaced superiorly. Other sacral nerve roots may be involved if the fracture extends through their respective foramina causing displacement and reduction in neuroforaminal cross-sectional area. Sacral fractures may result in anesthesia over the sacral dermatomes, impotence, and a flaccid bowel and bladder. Incontinence rarely occurs with unilateral root injuries between S2 and S5. Decreased sensation is a more typical consequence. When there is doubt about the integrity of the structures innervated by the sacral segments, urodynamic studies are helpful in the assessment of bladder motor function. Because these fractures are typically unilateral, involving only the nerve roots on the fractured side, incontinence and sexual dysfunction are typically rare. Evaluation of the Achilles and bulbocavernosus reflex is mandatory in assessing sacral root function.

Zone III fractures involve the central canal and have a higher incidence (57 percent) of neurologic deficits, which may include loss of sphincter tone, saddle anesthesia, and acute cauda equina syndromes (Fig. 70-48). Transverse fractures occur as isolated fractures due to a flexion force imparted to the lower part of the sacrum and the coccyx. This typically results from a fall where the patient lands on his or her buttocks. Below S4 there is little chance of significant neurologic deficit, since the sacral nerve roots exit proximal to this.

Radiographic investigation of suspected sacral fractures is difficult because of the complex shape of the sacrum and the pelvis. Some 50 percent of sacral fractures without neurologic deficits are missed on initial examination. The initial radiographic examination includes lateral and anteroposterior Ferguson projections of the lumbosacral junction. The Ferguson projection centers the proximally directed beam on the sacrum. Radiographic findings associated with sacral fractures are low lumbar transverse process fractures, asymmetrical sacral foramen, and irregular trabeculation of the lateral masses of the proximal sacral segments. Computed tomography scans are the most accurate method of evaluating sacral fractures. The presence of occult sacral fractures is verified on bone scan when the sacral segments are too osteopenic to produce reliable radiographic images.[148]

Isolated sacral fractures without disruption of the anterior pelvic ring or neurologic deficits do not require treatment beyond symptom relief, since they are stable. Patients typically are kept at bed rest and log-rolled until the pain subsides to the point where mobilization may be initiated in approximately 7 to 10 days.

For more severe zone II or III injuries, particularly longitudinal fractures, patients may be mobilized in a non-weight-bearing capacity on the unaffected side. After an

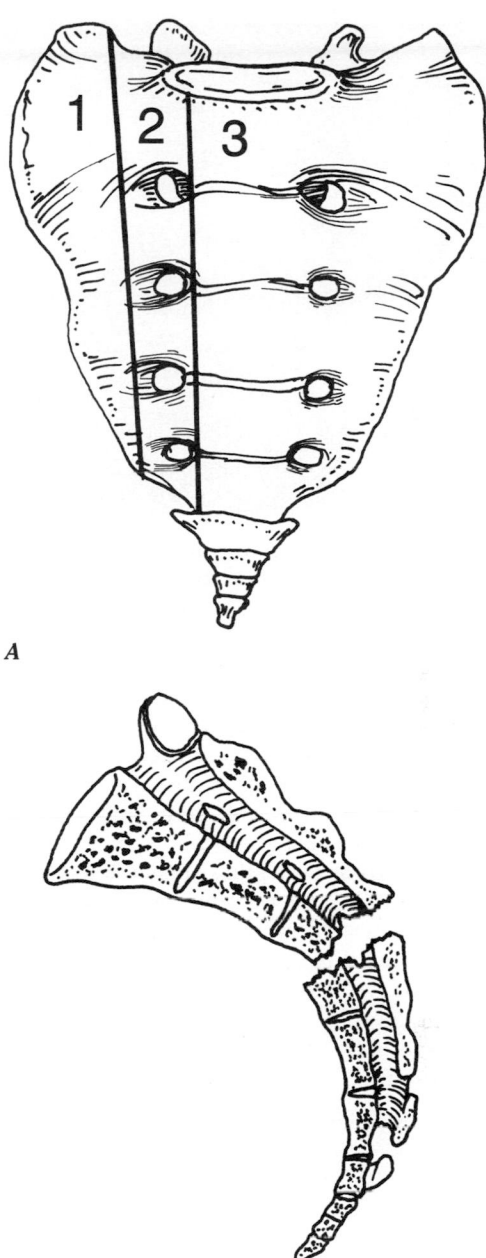

A

B

Figure 70-47 Classification of sacral fractures. *A.* Zone I, zone II, and zone III injuries. *B.* Transverse fractures. (Reproduced with permission from Denis F, Davis S, Comfort T: Sacral fractures: Retrospective analysis of 236 cases. *Clin Orthop* 227:67–81, 1988.)

initial period of bed rest, weight bearing on the fractured side may then be attempted at 4 to 8 weeks. Sacral fractures involving anterior pelvic ring may not be stable and therefore not amenable to this conservative treatment. Management of these fractures is based on the inherent stability within the injured pelvic ring.

Complications of sacral fractures include chronic pain secondary to sacroiliac joint arthritis or changes in the alignment of the sacrum. In addition, loss of voluntary

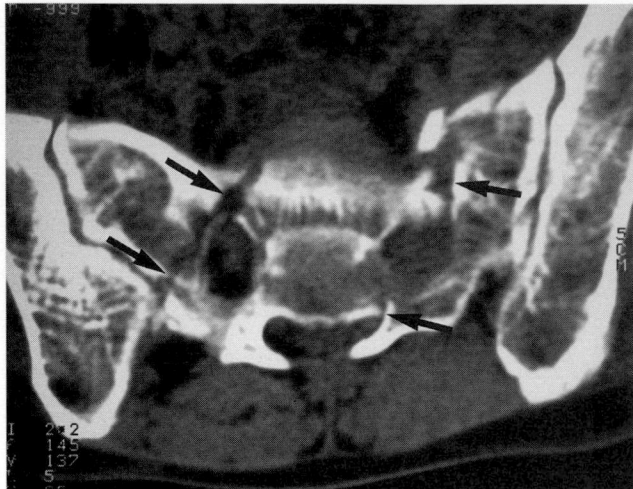

Figure 70-48 Complex sacral fracture with right-sided zone II injury and left-sided comminuted zone II and III injury.

bowel and bladder control may cause functional disability. If sacroiliac arthritis is symptomatic and persistent, arthrodesis may be required for relief of symptoms. Neurologic deficits may be associated with zone II injuries; these are managed with observation, since most such injuries will be neuropraxias that will resolve spontaneously. Neurologic symptoms persisting beyond 6 to 8 weeks may benefit from foraminal decompression. Deficits associated with zone III injuries should undergo aggressive radiologic examination to identify the cause of the neurologic injury. Early posterior decompression may result in return of bowel and bladder control and reversal of foot drop. Late decompression is often complicated by epidural fibrosis and minimal return of function.

REFERENCES

1. Denis F: The three column spine and its significance in the classification of acute thoracolumbar spinal injuries. *Spine* 8:817–831, 1983.
2. Denis F: Spinal instability as defined by the three column spine concept in acute spinal trauma. *Clin Orthop Rel Res* 189:65, 1984.
3. Haher TR, Tozzi JM, Lospinuso MF, et al: The contribution of the three columns of the spine to spinal stability: Biomechanical model. *Paraplegia* 27:432, 1989.
3a. McCormack T, Karaikovic E, Gaines RW: The load sharing classification of spine fractures. *Spine* 19:1741–1744, 1994.
4. Gertzbein SD: Spine update: Classification of thoracic and lumbar fractures. *Spine* 19:626–628, 1994.
5. Ferguson RL, Allen BL: A mechanistic classification of thoracolumbar spine fractures. *Clin Orthop Rel Res* 189:77, 1984.
6. Allen BL Jr, Ferguson RL, Lehmann TR, et al: A mechanistic classification of closed, indirect fractures and dislocations of the lower cervical spine. *Spine* 7:1–27, 1982.
7. Goel VK, Yamanishi TM, Chang H: Development of a computer model to predict strains in the individual fibers of a ligament across the ligamentous occipito-atlanto-axial (C0-C1-C2) complex. *Ann Biomed Eng* 20:667–686, 1992.
8. Goel VK, Clark CR, Galles King Liu Y: Moment rotation relationships of the ligamentous occipito-atlanto-axial complex. *J Biomech* 21:673–680, 1988.
9. Mahale YJ, Silver JR, Henderson NJ: Neurological complications of the reduction of cervical spine dislocations. *J Bone Joint Surg* 75B:403–409, 1993.
10. Mimura M, Moriya H, Watanabe T, et al: Three-dimensional motion analysis of the cervical spine with special reference to the axial rotation. *Spine* 14:1135, 1989.
11. Bozic KJ, Keyak JH, Skinner HB, et al: Three-dimensional finite element modeling of a cervical vertebra: An investigation of burst fracture mechanism. *J Spine Dis* 7:102–110, 1994.
12. Edward WT, Haues WC, Posner I, et al: Variations of lumbar spine stiffness with load. *J Biomech Eng* 109:35, 1987.
13. Fyhrie DP, Schaffler MB: Failure mechanisms in human vertebral cancellous bone. *Bone* 15:105–109, 1994.
14. Snyder BD, Piazza S, Edwards WT, Haynes WC: Role of trabecular morphology in the etiology of age-related vertebral fractures. *Calcif Tissue Int* 53(suppl 1):S14–S22, 1993.
15. Carter DR, Hayes WC: The compressive behavior of bone as a two-phase porous structure. *J Bone Joint Surg* 59A:954, 1977.
16. Broberg KB: On the mechanical behavior of intervertebral discs. *Spine* 8:151, 1983.
17. Haher TR, O'Brien MF, Felmly WT, et al: Instantaneous axis of rotation as a function of the three columns of the spine. *Spine* 17:149, 1992.
18. Haher TR, Felmly WT, Baruch H, et al: The contribution of the three columns of the spine to rotational stability: A biomechanical model. *Spine* 14:663, 1989.
19. Haher TR, Berhman M, O'Brien MF, et al: The effect of the three columns of the spine on the instantaneous axis of rotation in flexion and extension. *Spine* 16:312, 1991.
20. Haher TR, Felmly WT, O'Brien MF, et al: The IAR as a function of the three columns of the spine. Presented at the annual meeting of the Scoliosis Research Society, Amsterdam, the Netherlands, Sept 17, 1989.
21. Bedbrook GM: Spinal injuries with tetraplegia and paraplegia. *J Bone Joint Surg* 61B:267–284, 1979.
22. Babcock JL, Albright J: Spine trauma in children and adolescents. *J Bone Joint Surg [Am]* 58:728, 1976.
23. Bors E, Comarr A: Neurological disturbances of sexual function with special reference to 529 patients with spinal cord injury. *Urol Surv* 10:191, 1960.
24. Comarr AE: Sexual concepts in traumatic cord and cauda equina lesions. *J Urol* 106:375, 1971.
25. Dall BE, Stauffer ES: Neurologic injury and recovery patterns in burst fractures at the T12 or L1 motion segment. *Clin Orthop Rel Res* 233:171–176, 1988.
26. Bohlman HH: Acute fractures and dislocations of the cervical spine: An analysis of 300 hospitalized patients and review of the literature. *J Bone Joint Surg* 61A:1119–1142, 1979.
27. Bohlman HH: Treatment of fractures and dislocations of the thoracic and lumbar spine—Current concepts review. *J Bone Joint Surg* 56A:165, 1985.
28. Bohlman HH: Traumatic fractures of the upper thoracic spine with paralysis: A study of 180 cases. *J Bone Joint Surg* 56A:1299, 1974.
29. Waters RL, Adkins RH, Yakura JS: Definition of complete spinal cord injury. *Paraplegia* 29:573–581, 1991.
30. Waters RL, Yakura JS, Adkins RH, et al: Recovery following complete paraplegia. *Arch Phys Med Rehabil* 73:784–789, 1992.

31. Bradford DS: Deformities of the thoracic and lumbar spine secondary to spinal injury, in Bradford DS, Lonstein JE, Moe JH, et al (eds): *Moe's Textbook of Scoliosis,* 2d ed. Philadelphia, Saunders, 1987, pp 435–463.

32. Brown CW, Jones B, Donaldson DH, et al: Neuropathic (Charcot) arthropathy of the spine after traumatic spinal paraplegia. *Spine* 17:S103–S108, 1992.

33. Waters RL, Adkins RH, Yakura JS, et al: Motor and sensory recovery following incomplete paraplegia. *Arch Phys Med Rehabil* 75:67–72, 1994.

34. Chang DG, Tencer AF, Ching RP, et al: Geometric changes in the cervical spine canal during impact. *Spine* 19:973–980, 1994.

35. Hashimoto T, Kaneda K, Kuniyoshi A: Relationship between traumatic spinal canal stenosis and neurologic deficits in thoracolumbar burst fractures. *Spine* 13:1268, 1988.

36. Panjabi MM, Kifune M, Wen L, et al: Dynamic canal encroachment during thoracolumbar burst fractures. *J Spinal Dis* 8:39–48, 1995.

37. Johnsson R, Herrlin K, Hägglund G, et al: Spinal canal remodeling after thoracolumbar fractures with intraspinal bone fragment: 17 cases followed 1–4 years. *Acta Orthop Scand* 62:125–127, 1991.

38. Gertzbein SD, Court-Brown CM, Marks P, et al: The neurologic outcome following surgery for spinal fractures. *Spine* 13:641, 1988.

39. Garfin SR, Shackford SR, Marshall LF, et al: Care of the multiply injured patient with cervical spine injury. *Clin Orthop Rel Res* 239:19–29, 1989.

40. Levi L, Wolf A, Belzberg H: Hemodynamic parameters in patients with acute cervical cord trauma: Description, intervention, and prediction of outcome. *Neurosurgery* 33:1007–1017, 1993.

41. Breig A: *Skull Traction and Cervical Cord Injury: A New Approach to Improved Rehabilitation.* Berlin, Springer-Verlag, 1989.

42. Lerman JA, Haynes RJ, Koeneman EJ, et al: A biomechanical comparison of Gardner-Wells tongs and halo device uses for cervical spine traction. *Spine* 21:2403–2406, 1994.

43. Botte MJ, Byrne TP, Garfin SR: Application of the halo device for immobilization of the cervical spine utilizing increased torque pressure. *J Bone Joint Surg* 69A:750–752, 1987.

44. Garfin SR, Botte MJ, Waters RL, et al: Complications in the use of the halo fixation device. *J Bone Joint Surg* 68A:320–325, 1986.

45. Botte MJ, Garfin SR, Byrne TP, et al: The halo skeletal fixator. *Clin Orthop Rel Res* 239:12–18, 1989.

46. Fried LC: Cervical spinal cord injury during skeletal traction. *JAMA* 229:181, 1974.

47. Blacksin MF, Lee HJ: Frequency and significance of fractures of the upper cervical spine detected by CT in patients with severe neck trauma. *AJR* 65:1201–1204, 1995.

48. Atlas SW, Regenbogen V, Rogers LF, Kim KS: The radiographic characterization of burst fractures of the spine. *Am J Radiol* 147:575, 1896.

49. el-Khoury GY, Whitten CG: Trauma to the upper thoracic spine: Anatomy, biomechanics, and unique imaging features. *AJR* 160:95–102, 1993.

50. Keenen TL, Antony J, Benson DR: Noncontiguous spinal fractures. *J Trauma* 30:489–491, 1990.

51. O'Brien MF, Lenke LG, Joyce ME: Acute spinal cord injury: Pathophysiology and pharmacologic treatments, in Bridwell KH, DeWald RL (eds): *The Textbook of Spinal Surgery,* 2d ed. Philadelphia, Lippincott-Raven, 1996.

52. Ballentine JD: Pathology of experimental spinal cord trauma. I. Necrotic lesion as a function of vascular injury. *Lab Invest* 39:236, 1978.

53. Finkelstein SD, Gillespie JA, Markowitz RS, et al: Experimental spinal cord injury: Qualitative and quantitative histopathologic evaluation. *J Neurotrauma* 7:29, 1990.

54. Anderson DK, Hall ED: Pathophysiology of spinal cord trauma. *Ann Emerg Med* 22:987–992, 1993.

55. Noble LJ, Cortez SC, Ellison JA: Endogenous peroxidatic activity in astrocytes after spinal cord injury. *J Comp Neurol* 296:674, 1990.

56. O'Brien MF, Lenke LG, Lu J, et al: Astrocyte response and transforming growth factor-beta localization in acute spinal cord injury: An immunohistochemical investigation. *Spine* 19:2321, 1994.

57. Bracken MB, Shepard MJ, Collins WF, et al: A randomized controlled trial of methylprednisolone or naloxone in the treatment of acute spinal cord injury. *N Engl J Med* 322:1405, 1990.

58. Bracken MB, Shepard MJ, Collins WF, et al: Methylprednisolone or naloxone treatment after acute spinal cord injury: A one-year follow-up data. Results of the Second National Acute Spinal Cord Injury Study. *J Neurosurg* 76:23, 1992.

59. Bracken MB: Treatment of acute spinal cord injury with methylprednisolone: Results of a multicenter, randomized clinical trial. *J Neurotrauma* 8(suppl 1):S47–S52, 1991.

60. Hall ED: The neuroprotective pharmacology of methylprednisolone. *J Neurosurg* 76:13, 1992.

61. Benzel EC, Larson SJ: Recovery of nerve root function after complete quadriplegia from cervical spine fractures. *Neurosurgery* 19:809–812, 1986.

62. Fielding JW: Injuries to the upper cervical spine. *Instr Course Lect* 36:483–494, 1987.

63. Shenk MM, Nicholson JT: Fractures of the atlas. *J Bone Joint Surg [Am]* 52:1017–1020, 1970.

64. Fowler JL, Sandhu A, Fraser RD: A review of fractures of the atlas vertebra. *J Spinal Dis* 3:19–24, 1990.

65. Levine AM, Edwards CC: Fractures of the atlas. *J Bone Joint Surg* 73A:680–691, 1991.

66. Hadley MN, Dickman CA, Browner CM, Sonntag VKH: Acute axis fractures: A review of 229 cases. *J Neurosurg* 71:642, 1989.

67. Heller JG, Virsolav S, Hudson T: Jefferson fractures: The role of magnification artifact in assessing transverse ligament integrity. *J Spinal Dis* 6:392–396, 1993.

68. Dickman CA, Sonntag VKH, Marcotte PJ: Techniques of screw fixation of the cervical spine. *Barrow Neurol Inst Q* 8:9–26, 1992.

69. Pedersen AK, Kostuik JP: Complete fracture-dislocation of the atlantoaxial complex: Case report and recommendations for a new classification of dens fractures. *J Spinal Dis* 7:350–355, 1994.

70. Fielding JW, Cochran G, Lawsing JF III, Hohl M: Tears of the transverse ligament of the atlas. *J Bone Joint Surg* 56A:1683, 1974.

71. Hajek PD, Lipka J, Hartline P, et al: Biomechanical study of the C1-C2 posterior arthrodesis techniques. *Spine* 18:173–177, 1993.

72. Grob D, Jeanneret B, Abaebi M, Marlkwalder TM: Atlantoaxial fusion with transarticular screw fixation. *J Bone Joint Surg* 73B:972–976, 1991.

73. Dickman CA, Douglas R, Sonntag WKH: Occipitocervical fusion: Posterior stabilization of the craniovertebral junction and upper cervical spine. *Barrow Neurol Inst Q* 6:2–14, 1990.

74. Ackerson TT, Patzakis MJ, Moore TM, et al: Fractures of the odontoid: A ten-year retrospective study. *Contemp Orthop* 4:54, 1982.

75. Bednar DA, Parikh J, Hummel J: Management of type II odontoid process fractures in geriatric patients: A prospective study of sequential cohorts with attention to survivorship. *J Spinal Dis* 8:166–169, 1995.

76. Dunn ME, Seljeskog EL: Experience in the management of odontoid process injuries: An analysis of 128 cases. *Neurosurgery* 18:306, 1986.

77. Ehara S, el-Khoury GY, Clark CR: Radiologic evaluation of dens fractures: Role of plain radiography and tomography. *Spine* 17:475–479, 1992.

78. Anderson LD, D'Alonzo RT: Fractures of the odontoid process of the axis. *J Bone Joint Surg* 56A:1663, 1974.

79. Althoff B, Goldie IF: The arterial supply of the odontoid process of the axis. *Acta Orthop Scand* 48:622, 1977.

80. Moskovich R, Crockard HA: Myelopathy due to hypertrophic nonunion of the dens: Case report. *J Trauma* 30:222–225, 1990.

81. Clark CR, White AA: Fractures of the dens: A multicenter study. *J Bone Joint Surg* 67A:1340–1348, 1985.

82. Grob D, Jeanneret B, Aebi M, Markwalder IM: Atlanto-axial fusion with transarticular screw fixation. *J Bone Joint Surg* 73:972–976, 1991.

83. Aebi M, Etter C, Coscia M: Fractures of the odontoid process: Treatment with anterior screw fixation. *Spine* 14:1065–1070, 1989.

84. Doherty BJ, Heggeness MH, Esses SI: A biomechanical study of odontoid fractures and fracture fixation. *Spine* 18:178–184, 1993.

85. Benzel EC, Hart BL, Ball PA, et al: Fractures of the C2 vertebral body. *J Neurosurg* 81:206–212, 1994.

86. Effendi B, Roy D, Cornish B, et al: Fractures of the ring and axis: A classification based on the analysis of 131 cases. *J Bone Joint Surg* 63B:319, 1981.

87. Levine AM, Edwards CC: The management of traumatic spondylolistheses of the axis. *J Bone Joint Surg* 67:217, 1985.

88. Eismont FJ, Bohlman HH: Posterior atlanto-occipital dislocation with fractures of the atlas and odontoid process: Report of a case with survival. *J Bone Joint Surg* 60A:397, 1978.

89. Alker GJ, Oh YS, Leslie EV, et al: Post mortem radiology of head and neck injuries in fatal traffic accidents. *Radiology* 114:611, 1975.

90. Lee C, Woodring JH, Goldstein SJ, et al: Evaluation of traumatic atlanto-occipital dislocations. *AJNR* 8:19, 1987.

91. Powers B, Miller MD, Kramer RS, et al: Traumatic anterior atlanto-occipital dislocation. *Neurosurgery* 4:12, 1979.

92. O'Brien MF, Sutterlin CE: Occipitocervical biomechanics: Clinical and biomechanical implications for posterior occipitocervical stabilization and fusion. *Spine* 10:281–283, 1996.

93. Sasso RC, Jeanneret B, Fischer K, Magerl F: Occipitocervical fusion with posterior plate and screw instrumentation. *Spine* 19:2364–2368, 1994.

94. Anderson PA, Montesano PX: Morphology and treatment of occipital condyle fractures. *Spine* 13:731–736, 1988.

95. Harding-Smith J, MacIntosh PK, Sherbon KJ: Fractures of the occipital condyle. *J Bone Joint Surg* 63A:1170, 1981.

96. Dvorak J, Panjabi MM: Functional anatomy of the alar ligaments. *Spine* 12:183–189, 1987.

97. Fielding JW, Hawkins RJ: Atlantoaxial rotatory fixation. *J Bone Joint Surg* 59A:34, 1977.

98. Barton JW, Margolis MT: Rotational obstruction of the vertebral artery at the atlantoaxial joint. *Neuroradiology* 9:117, 1975.

99. Smith MD, Phillips WA, Hensinger RN: Complications of fusion to the upper cervical spine. *Spine* 16:702–705, 1991.

100. Pang D, Wilberger JE: Spinal cord injury without radiographic abnormalities in children. *J Neurosurg* 57:114, 1982.

101. Harris JH, Edeiken-Monroe B: *The Radiology of Acute Cervical Spine Trauma.* Baltimore, Williams & Wilkins, 1987.

102. Daffner RH: Evaluation of cervical vertebral injuries. *Semin Roentgenol* 27:239–253, 1992.

103. Harris JK Jr, Edeiken-Monroe B, Kopaniky DR: A practical classification of acute cervical spine injuries. *Orthop Clin North Am* 17:15–30, 1986.

104. Cooper PR, Maravilla KR, Sklar FH, et al: Halo immobilization of cervical spine fractures. *J Neurosurg* 50:603–610, 1979.

105. Bohlman HH, Eismont FJ: Surgical techniques of anterior decompression and fusion for spinal cord injuries. *Clin Orthop Rel Res* 154:57, 1981.

106. Ripa DR, Kowall MG, Meyer PR Jr, et al: Series of ninety-two traumatic cervical spine injuries stabilized with anterior ASIF plate fusion technique. *Spine* 16:S46–S55, 1991.

107. Cybulski GR, Douglas RA, Meyer PR Jr, et al: Complications in three-column cervical spine injuries requiring anterior-posterior stabilization. *Spine* 17:253–256, 1992.

108. Bohlman HH: Complications of treatment of fractures and dislocations of the cervical spine, in Epps E (ed): *Complications in Orthopaedic Surgery.* Vol 2. Philadelphia, Lippincott, 1978.

109. Kim KS, Chen HH, Russell EJ, Rogers LF: Flexion teardrop fracture of the cervical spine: Radiographic characteristics. *AJR* 152:319–326, 1989.

110. Cabenela ME, Ebersold MJ: Anterior plate stabilization for bursting teardrop fractures of the cervical spine. *Spine* 13:888–891, 1988.

111. Avena MJ, Eismont JF, Green BA: Intervertebral disc extrusion associated with cervical facet subluxation and dislocation. *J Bone Joint Surg* 73A:1555–1560, 1991.

112. Beyer CA, Cabenela ME, Berquist TH: Unilateral facet dislocations and fracture-dislocations of the cervical spine. *J Bone Joint Surg* 73B:977–981, 1991.

113. Hadley MN, Fitzpatrick BC, Sonntag VK, Browner CM: Facet fracture dislocation injuries of the cervical spine. *Neurosurgery* 30:665–666, 1992.

114. Robertson PA, Ryan MD: Neurological deterioration after reduction of cervical subluxation: Mechanical compression by disc tissue. *J Bone Joint Surg* 74B:224–227, 1992.

115. Cotler HB, Miller LS, DeLucia FA, et al: Closed reduction of cervical spine dislocations. *Clin Orthop* 214:185–199, 1987.

116. Neilsen CF, Annertz M, Persson L, et al: Posterior wiring without bony fusion in traumatic distractive flexion injuries of the mid to lower cervical spine: Long-term follow-up in 30 patients. *Spine* 16:467–472, 1991.

117. Anderson PA, Henley MB, Grady MS, et al: Posterior cervical arthrodesis with AO reconstruction plates and bone graft. *Spine* 16(suppl 3):S72–S79, 1991.

118. Heller JG, Carlson GD, Abitbol JJ, Garfin SR: Anatomic comparison of the Roy-Camille and Magerl techniques for screw placement in the lower cervical spine. *Spine* 16(suppl):S552–S557, 1991.

119. Bucci M, Dauser R, Maymond F, et al: Management of post-traumatic cervical spine instability: Operative fusion versus halo vest immobilization. Analysis of 49 cases. *J Trauma* 28:1001, 1988.

120. Bucholz RW, Gill K: Classification of injuries to the thoracolumbar spine. *Orthop Clin North Am* 17:67, 1986.

120a. Ferguson RL, Allen BL: An algorithm for the treatment of unstable thoracolumbar fractures. *Orthop Clin North Am* 17:105–112, 1986.

121. Panjabi MM, Oxland TR, Kifune M, et al: Validity of the three-column theory of thoracolumbar fractures: A biomechanics investigation. *Spine* 20:1122–1127, 1995.

121a. Magerl F, Harms J, Gertzbein SD, et al: A new classification of spinal fractures. Presented at the Societé Internationale Orthopedie et Traumatologie meeting, Montreal, Canada, Sept 9, 1990.

121b. Gertzbein SD, Court-Brown CM: Flexion-distraction injuries of the lumbar spine: Mechanism of injury and classification. *Clin Orthop Rel Res* 227:52, 1988.

122. McCormack T, Karaikovic E, Gaines RW: The load sharing classification of spine fractures. *Spine* 19:1711–1722, 1994.

123. Anderson PA, Henley MB, Rivara FP, et al: Flexion distraction and chance injuries to the thoracolumbar spine. *J Orthop Trauma* 5:153–160, 1991.

124. Denis F, Armstrong GW, Searls K, et al: Acute thoracolumbar burst fractures in the absence of neurologic deficit: A comparison between operative and nonoperative treatment. *Clin Orthop Rel Res* 189:142–149, 1984.

125. James KS, Wenger KH, Schlegel JD, Dunn HK: Biomechanical evaluation of the stability of thoracolumbar burst fractures. *Spine* 19:1731–1740, 1994.

126. Jacobs RR, Asher MA, Snider RK: Thoracolumbar spinal injuries: A comparative study of recumbent and operative treatment in 100 patients. *Spine* 5:463–477, 1980.

127. Knight RQ, Stornelli DP, Chan DP, et al: Comparison of operative versus nonoperative treatment of lumbar burst fractures. *Clin Orthop Rel Res* 293:112–121, 1993.

128. An HS, Vaccaro A, Cotler JM, et al: Low lumbar burst fractures: Comparison among body cast, Harrington rod, Luque rod, and Steffee plate. *Spine* 16:S440–S444, 1991.

129. Esses SI, Botsford DJ, Kostuik JP: Evaluation of surgical treatment for burst fractures. *Spine* 15:667–673, 1990.

130. Abumi K, Panjabi MM, Duranceau J: Biochemical evaluation of spinal fixation devices: Part III. Stability provided by six spinal fixation devices and interbody bone graft. *Spine* 14:1249–1255, 1989.

131. Edwards CC, Levine AM: Early rod-sleeve stabilization of the injured thoracic and lumbar spine. *Orthop Clin North Am* 17:121–145, 1986.

132. Sasso RC, Cotler HB: Posterior instrumentation and fusion for unstable fractures and fracture-dislocations of the thoracic and lumbar spine: A comparative study of three fixation devices in seventy patients. *Spine* 18:450–460, 1993.

133. Bryant CE, Sullivan JA: Management of thoracic and lumbar spine fractures with Harrington distraction rods supplemented with segmental wiring. *Spine* 8:532, 1983.

134. McAfee PC, Bohlman HH, Yuan HA: Anterior decompression of traumatic thoracolumbar fractures with incomplete neurological deficit using a retroperitoneal approach. *J Bone Joint Surg* 67A:89, 1985.

135. Denis F, Burkus JK: Diagnosis and treatment of cauda equina entrapment in the vertical lamina fracture of lumbar burst fractures. *Spine* 16:S433–S439, 1991.

136. Garfin SR, Mowery CA, Guerras J, Marshall LF: Confirmation of the posterolateral technique to decompress and fuse thoracolumbar spine burst fractures. *Spine* 10:218, 1985.

137. Kaneda K, Abumi K, Fijiya M: Burst fractures with neurologic deficits of the thoracolumbar-lumbar spine: Results of anterior decompression and stabilization with anterior instrumentation. *Spine* 9:788, 1984.

138. Zdeblick TA, Warden KE, Zou D, et al: Anterior spinal fixators: A biomechanical in-vitro study. *Spine* 18:513–517, 1993.

139. Benson DR: Unstable thoracolumbar fractures with emphasis on the burst fracture. *Clin Orthop* 220:14, 1988.

140. Vornamen MJ, Bostman OM, Myllynen PJ: Reduction of bone retropulsed into the spinal canal in thoracolumbar vertebral body compression burst fractures: A prospective randomized comparative study between Harrington rods and two transpedicular devices. *Spine* 15:1699–1703, 1995.

141. Bohlman HH: Late progressive paralysis and pain following fractures of the thoracolumbar spine. *J Bone Joint Surg [Am]* 58:728, 1976.

142. Abdel-Fatteh J, Rizk AM: Complete fracture-dislocation of the lower lumbar spine with spontaneous neurologic decompression. *Clin Orthop Rel Res* 251:140–143, 1990.

143. Bohlman HH: Late anterior decompression and fusion for spinal cord injuries: Review of 100 cases with long term results. *Orthop Trans* 4:42, 1980.

144. Gertzbein SD, Court-Brown CM: Flexion-distraction injuries of the lumbar spine: Mechanism of injury and classification. *Clin Orthop Rel Res* 227:52, 1988.

145. Grier D, Wardell S, Sarwark J, Poznaski AK: T1 fatigue fractures of the sacrum in children: Two case reports and a review of the literature. *Skel Radiol* 22:515–518, 1992.

146. Gibbons KJ, Soloniuk DS, Razack N: Neurological injury and patterns of sacral fractures. *J Neurosurg* 72:889–893, 1990.

147. Denis F, Davis S, Comfort T: Sacral fractures: An important problem. Retrospective analysis of 236 cases. *Clin Orthop Rel Res* 227:67–81, 1988.

148. Gotis-Graham I, McGuigan L, Diamond T, et al: Sacral insufficiency fractures in the elderly. *J Bone Joint Surg [Br]* 76:882–886, 1994.

149. Fick R: *Handbuch der Anatomie und Mechanik der Glenke.* Jena, S Fischer Verlag, 1911.

150. Poirier P, Charpy A: Traite d'anatomie humaine. 1:74–89, 1926.

151. Jackson H: Diagnosis of minimal atlantoaxial subluxation. *Br J Radiol* 23:232–245, 1986.

152. Fielding JW: Cinematography of the normal cervical spine. *J Bone Joint Surg* 39A:1280–1285, 1957.

153. Werne S: Studies in spontaneous atlas dislocation. *Acta Orthop Scand Suppl* 23:1–28, 1957.

154. Werne S: The possibilities of movement in craniovertebral joints. *Acta Orthop Scand* 28:165–173, 1959.

155. Hohl M: Normal motion in the upper portion of the cervical spine. *J Bone Joint Surg* 46A:1777–1779, 1964.

156. Penning L: Normal movements of the cervical spine. *AJR* 130:317–326, 1978.

157. White AA, Panjabi MM: The clinical biomechanics of the occipitoatlantoaxial complex. *Orthop Clin North Am* 9:867–878, 1978.

158. Weisel SW, Rothman RH: Occipitoatlanto hypermobility. *Spine* 4:187–191, 1979.

159. Clark CR, Goel VK, Galles K, Liu YK: Kinematics of the occipito-atlanto-axial complex. Cervical Spine Research Society Meeting, West Palm Beach, FL, December 10–13, 1986.

160. Dvorak J, Panjabi MM, Wichmann M, Gerber M: CT functional diagnostics of the rotatory instability of the upper cervical spine: An experimental study in cadavers. *Spine* 12:197–205, 1987.

161. Penning L, Wilmink JP: Rotation of the cervical spine: A CT study in normal subjects. *Spine* 12:732–738, 1987.

162. Dvorak J, Froehlich D, Penning L, et al: Functional radiographic diagnosis of the cervical spine: Flexion/extension. *Spine* 13:748–755, 1988.

163. Panjabi MM, Dvorak J, Duranceau J, et al: Three dimensional movements of the upper cervical spine. *Spine* 13:726–730, 1988.

164. Goel VK, Clark CR, Gallaes King Liu Y: Moment rotation relationships of the ligamentous occipito-atlanto-axial complex. *J Biomech* 21:673–680, 1988.

165. Grob D, Crisco JJ, Panjabi MM, et al: Biomechanical evaluation of four different posterior atlantoaxial fixation techniques. *Spine* 17:480–490, 1992.

166. Dickman CA, Crawford NR, Brantley AG, Sonntag VK: Biomechanical effects of transoral odontoidectomy. *Neurosurgery* 36:1146–1153, 1995.

CHAPTER 71

Spinal Infections and Tumors

Daniel E. Gelb

SPINAL INFECTIONS

Vertebral Osteomyelitis

Vertebral osteomyelitis continues to be a significant clinical problem. The diagnosis is not always obvious; therefore a high index of clinical suspicion must be maintained in order to make an appropriate diagnosis. Osteomyelitis of the spine accounts for approximately 1.5 to 4 percent of all cases of osteomyelitis.[1-3] The most common mechanism of infection is by hematogenous spread. Infection can also be caused by spread from a contiguous focus or direct inoculation. Any invasive procedure, from open surgery to diagnostic and therapeutic injections, can lead to vertebral infection. For example, the rate of infection following cervical discography has been reported to be approximately 0.2 percent.[4]

Hematogenous osteomyelitis occurs most commonly in the distal spine. The lumbar spine accounts for approximately 60 percent of cases.[5-7] The thoracic spine has the next highest rate of infection, with the cervical spine least commonly affected. *Staphylococcus aureus* accounts for nearly 60 percent of cases in most series.[7,8] The next most common organisms are streptococci and Enterobacteriaceae.[6,8] However, more unusual organisms have been reported as well. Patients with sickle cell anemia have a known predisposition toward *Salmonella* osteomyelitis. Several reports have documented an increased rate of *Pseudomonas* infection in intravenous drug abusers.[9,10] Surgery in and around the oropharynx also seems to predispose to infection with unusual organisms.[11-13]

Hematogenous seeding may occur from the genitourinary tract, skin, or respiratory tract.[8] In one series, up to 40 percent of hematogenous osteomyelitis of the spine was associated with urinary tract infection or manipulation.[9] The most common organism in this series was *Escherichia coli*. In most series, the average age of patients with vertebral osteomyelitis is in the sixth decade of life.[1,6-8,14-17] Males are affected twice as often as females.[2,7] Patients with diabetes mellitus appear to be predisposed to vertebral infection[2,6,7,13]; up to 20 percent of patients in some series have diabetes. Bacterial endocarditis can also be a source of infectious emboli.[9,10]

Many patients will have an identifiable source of infection elsewhere. This has been reported in 50 to 78 percent of cases.[6-8] Often, the vertebral column may be seeded after manipulation of the urinary tract. Batson's vertebral plexus provides a valveless series of veins draining the pelvis through the vertebral column. Some have suggested that this is the source of increased vertebral infection following urinary tract manipulation.[6,7] Up to 10 percent of patients with vertebral infections will have a soft tissue focus of infection distal to the site of the spinal infection.[7]

The initial focus of infection is the vertebral end plate. In this area, there is an end-arterial circulation. Septic emboli to these arteries lead to local infarction and necrosis. This allows the infection to become established.[6,8] In adult vertebrae, unlike those of children, there are no intraosseus anastomoses to prevent the establishment of ongoing infection.[18] Commonly, the infection will involve the end plates of two adjacent vertebrae across a disk space. There is a series of intermetaphyseal anastomoses from one vertebra to the next. These anastomoses bypass the segmental arterial circulation. This allows for infectious spread from one vertebra to the next[18] (Fig. 71-1). The disk between two affected end plates is avascular as well; therefore it becomes involved in the infectious process. These peculiarities of vertebral circulation exist in the anterior vertebral column. Therefore the vertebral bodies are much more likely to be affected than the posterior arches. As infection continues, progressive vertebral destruction ensues. In addition, abscess formation may occur. Abscesses may spread to involve the retroperitoneal or retromediastinal spaces. Likewise, abscesses may extend posteriorly into the vertebral canal, leading to epidural abscess formation with neurologic deficit. The infection spreads by direct extension through bone; therefore, when multiple vertebrae are involved, the areas of infection tend to be contiguous. This is in contrast to tuberculosis, which tends to spread more aggressively along fascial planes and may affect noncontiguous areas. In certain cases, infection will progress to involve the meninges and even the spinal cord itself.

Clinical Presentation

The most common clinical finding in hematogenous vertebral osteomyelitis is back pain. This will occur in more than 90 percent of patients.[6,7,19,20] The pain that occurs with osteomyelitis is often characterized by the patient as "deep" or "boring" in nature. Usually, the patient can recall no specific antecedent trauma to account for the pain. In addition, the pain is unrelieved by periods of rest and is also relatively unaffected by changes in position. Patients will often complain of nonspecific constitutional symptoms. Approximately half of them will present with fever.[7] On physical examination, there will often be focal spinal tenderness at the level of vertebral involvement.[19] Neurologic deficit occurs in approximately 30 percent of patients.[6,7,19,20] This may be a sign of either epidural abscess or septic thrombosis of the neurologic structures.[20] Patients with diabetes are somewhat more likely to present with neurologic deficit; this occurs in approximately 50 percent of cases.

Diagnosis

No laboratory abnormalities are 100 percent specific for vertebral infection. The most common characteristic laboratory abnormality seen is an increased erythrocyte sed-

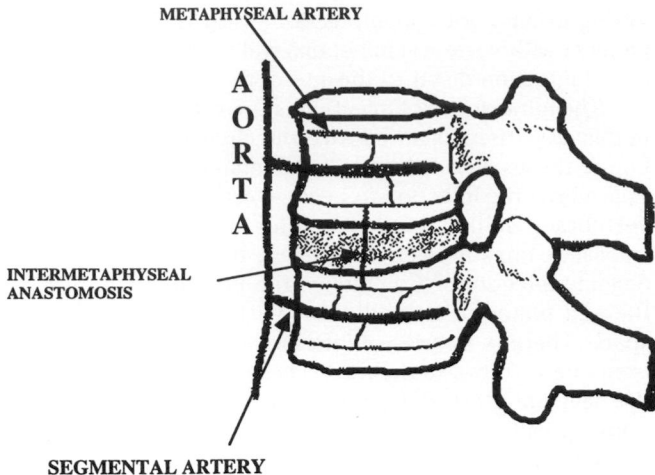

METAPHYSEAL ARTERY

A O R T A

AORTA

INTERMETAPHYSEAL ANASTOMOSIS

SEGMENTAL ARTERY

Figure 71-1 The intermetaphyseal arterial anastomosis allows infection to spread between the end plates of adjacent vertebral bodies, bypassing the segmental arterial circulation.

imentation rate. This occurs in 80 to 100 percent of patients.[4,6,7,24,26] In most patients, the white blood cell count is normal or only sightly elevated. In patients with signs of systemic disease such as fever, blood cultures may be positive. Positive blood culture has been reported in 24 to 56 percent of cases.[6,7]

Since the signs and symptoms of vertebral infection are relatively nonspecific, diagnosis is often delayed. The average time from the onset of symptoms to diagnosis can range from 4 to 6 months in many cases.[14,20]

Diagnostic imaging—along with a high index of suspicion—is crucial to the diagnosis. These earliest x-ray changes may take 2 to 4 weeks to develop.[8,9,14,15] Plain x-rays will show characteristic changes in most cases (Fig. 71-2A and B). Characteristically, pyogenic vertebral osteomyelitis will involve either one or two segments. The initial finding is loss of disk height and of paravertebral soft tissue shadows. Following these early signs, one may see progressive end-plate destruction with loss of end-plate cortical integrity.[14,20] Gas is absent from the disk, and this can be used to differentiate infection from other pathologic entities.[21] (However, rare cases of gas-forming bacterial infections have been reported.) As time goes on, progressive vertebral body destruction is seen in untreated infections. Usually, this leads to fairly symmetrical collapse of both anterior and posterior body height without the development of severe kyphotic deformity, as is seen in tuberculosis. Resolving infection will often go on to spontaneous anterior intervertebral ankylosis (Fig. 71-2C and D). The differential diagnosis of these x-ray changes includes nonpyogenic infection, renal osteodystrophy, ankylosing spondylitis, and rheumatoid arthritis with granuloma formation.[22,23] In contrast, neoplastic vertebral destruction is more likely to be centered in the vertebral body and to spare the disk space.

Computed tomography (CT) has been shown to be more sensitive than plain radiography in the diagnosis of vertebral osteomyelitis.[24,25] Characteristically, one will see

soft tissue swelling in the paravertebral region as well as end-plate fragmentation quite well[8] (Fig. 71-2E). In addition, the affected tissue will have decreased density on CT scan.[16,17] Computed tomography can be used to define the extent of soft tissue involvement. In one series, 16 of 19 patients were found to have unsuspected paravertebral or epidural involvement when they were studied by computed tomography.[17] The combination of contrast myelography followed by computed tomograpy can be used as an excellent modality to define the extent of epidural space involvement[25]; however, this has been supplanted to a large extent by magnetic resonance imaging.

Bone scintigraphy with radiolabeled markers has historically been the imaging study of choice for the diagnosis of vertebral osteomyelitis, but this is changing (see below). Technetium bone scan has been reported to be more than 90 percent sensitive and specific for the diagnosis of osteomyelitis.[8,20] In addition to technetium, other investigators have used indium, gallium, and radiolabeled strontium to increase the accuracy of diagnosis. Indium-labeled white blood cell scanning alone has a reported sensitivity of 25 percent and specificity of 50 percent for the diagnosis of infection. The overall accuracy was reported to be 30 percent. When combined with technetium scans, sensitivity and specificity were increased, for an overall accuracy of 50 percent.[26,27] In another series, 20 of 26 strontium scans were positive, with no false negatives reported.[28] It is important to note that it is possible for the bone scan to show a focal cold spot in the presence of infection.[26] This may be due to an avascular region in the center of the infective focus.

Magnetic resonance imaging, when available, has now emerged as the diagnostic imaging modality of choice in vertebral osteomyelitis. It will show changes sooner than either nuclear bone scintigraphy or plain x-ray.[29] The reported sensitivity and specificity of MRI both exceed 90 percent.[8,30] This is far superior to the results of other imaging modalities. There have been some case reports of active infection that was diagnosed by MRI but not by either CT or bone scan.[31] In addition, the excellent soft tissue resolution obtained with MRI allows one to accurately assess the extent of epidural spread and potential neurologic compromise.

The characteristic findings of early infection on MRI are a decrease in signal from the disk and adjacent end plates on T1-weighted images. This is seen in conjunction with an increase in signal or T2[8,29] (Fig. 71-2F). On the T1-weighted image, there will be a loss of distinction between the end plate and the disk.[32–34] On T2-weighted images, there is loss of the normal intranuclear cleft. These changes are quite specific for infection. Using these criteria, one may differentiate infection from neoplasia, in which one is more likely to see diffuse marrow involvement of a vertebra without involvement of the adjacent disk.[35] Similarly, it has been noted that tuberculous infection will not show increased signal in the disk on T2-weighted images.[8]

The addition of paramagnetic contrast material will increase the information that can be obtained by MRI. Gadolinium has been noted to help distinguish between old degenerative change and active infection.[34] The gadolinium will show increased enhancement on T1-

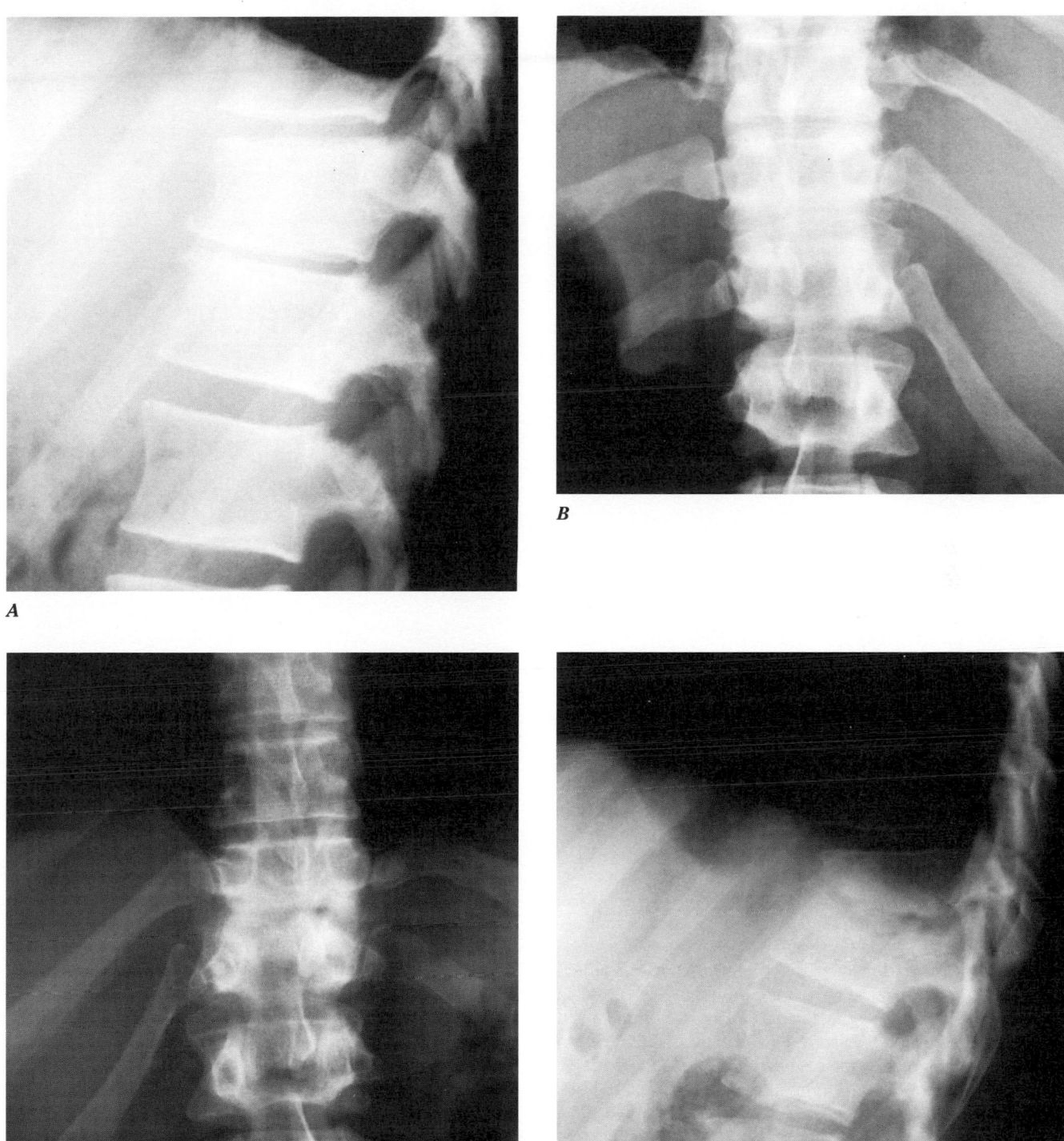

A

B

C

D

Figure 71-2 Radiographic features of pyogenic vertebral osteomyelitis. A 40-year-old man presented with a 4-month history of increasingly severe thoracolumbar back pain following a bout of *Staphylococcus aureus* pneumonia and sepsis. *A* and *B*. Initial plain radiographs showing disk space narrowing and cortical end plate irregularity. *C* and *D*. Plain radiographs following 3 months of treatment with intravenous naficillin and ambulatory bracing in a TLSO, showing attempted spontaneous intervertebral arthrodesis. The patient's symptoms were relieved and he returned to work without restriction. *E*. CT scan, performed for percutaneous biopsy, demonstrating endplate fragmentation. *F*. T2-weighted MRI demonstrating increased signal in bone marrow adjacent to the affected disk space.

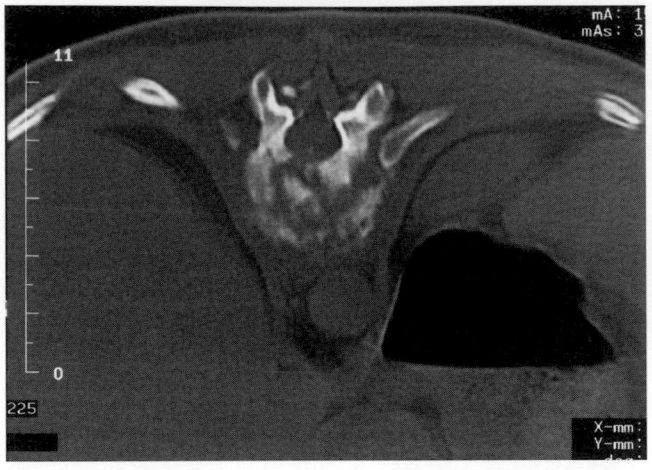

E

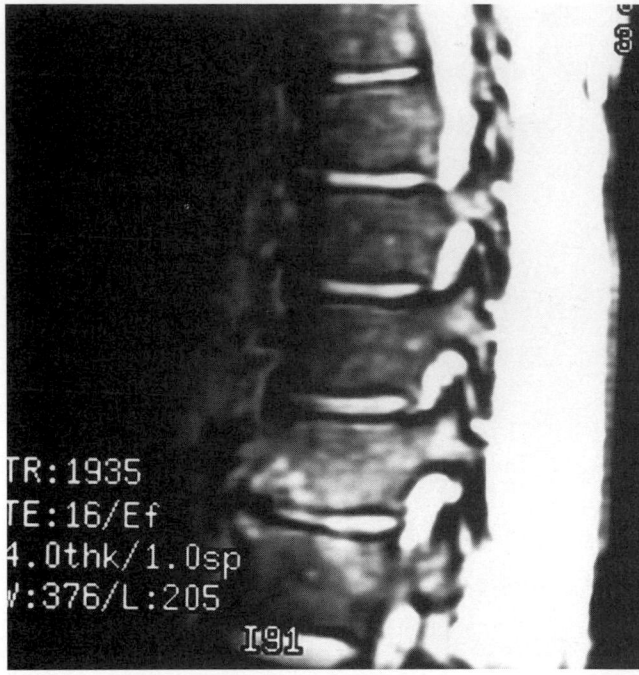

F

Figure 71-2 (*Continued*)

weighted images at the sites of local active infection. This allows one to more accurately differentiate between areas of resolved infection and scar and ongoing abscess.[34,36] Therefore, gadolinium is useful in the evaluation of partially treated infections.

Treatment

Despite the advances in medical imaging in the last decade, tissue sampling remains an important part of the diagnostic/therapeutic algorithm. In cases with classically characteristic radiographic findings and positive blood cultures, treatment can be undertaken based on these results alone. However, in all other cases, tissue should be obtained in order to confirm the diagnosis and isolate the organism to obtain appropriate antibiotic sensitivities. In addition, in any case that is unresponsive to the usual nonoperative methods of treatment and for which tissue has not been obtained, biopsy should be undertaken in order to confirm the diagnosis and rule out the possibility of polymicrobial infection. In most cases, percutaneous biopsy techniques under either fluoroscopic or CT guidance are sufficient to obtain appropriate tissue for diagnosis. The combination of pathologic examination and microbiological cultures is usually sufficient to confirm the diagnosis and isolate the organism. Both should routinely be undertaken in order to avoid misdiagnosis. In one study, an organism was isolated in only about 50 percent of samples, yet 21 of 24 cases were confirmed histologically.[37] The ability to isolate an organism successfully significantly decreases with the institution of antibiotic treatment. Up to 75 percent of pyogenic organisms can be cultured from biopsy specimens if no antibiotic has been previously given. The yield drops to approximately 25 percent in the face of antibiotic coverage.[37] All possible attempts to obtain tissue prior to the institution of antibiotic treatment should be made. If percutaneous techniques are unable to provide sufficient tissue for diagnosis, open biopsy may be undertaken. Tissue from the vertebral body may be obtained through the vertebral pedicle. In the thoracic area, costotransversectomy can also be used to obtain tissue for biopsy. The posterior approach for biopsy is relatively straightforward and has a very low morbidity. However, neither of these approaches allows for adequate decompression of the neural elements. If surgery is to be undertaken for purposes other than biopsy, alternate surgical approaches should be used.

Most pyogenic spinal infections are responsive to nonoperative treatment. The mainstays of treatment are appropriate antibiotics and spinal rest. Selection of an antibiotic should be based on sensitivities obtained from microbiological culture of organisms recovered from biopsy. In order to increase the proportion of positive biopsies for culture, antibiotic treatment should be deferred until after tissue sampling. In cases of overwhelming, life-threatening infection, empiric antibiotics may be started prior to biopsy if necessary. In most cases, a drug active against *Staphylococcus aureus* is appropriate, since this is the most common organism found. Alternative antibiotics may be selected for patients in groups at high risk for infection with other organisms, such as intravenous drug abusers or patients with sickle cell anemia. Some authors have recommended the routine administration of an aminoglycoside in addition to a beta-lactam antibiotic, for synergy, to help clear infection more effectively.[15] The duration of antibiotic treatment must be prolonged in order to ensure its complete resolution. At least 6 to 8 weeks of intravenous therapy is required. The most reliable indicator of resolution of infection is return to the erythrocyte sedimentation rate to the normal range. Intravenous antibiotics should be continued at least until this occurs. Extension of intravenous treatment beyond this point may be indicated to ensure full resolution of the infection. Alternatively, one may consider switching the patient to several weeks of an oral agent following the termination of intravenous treatment. Recommendations for duration of treatment, in total, usually range from 3 to 6 months.[6,7]

Spinal immobilization and rest are important parts of the treatment. Initial treatment should be with both bed rest and spinal immobilization. This can be accomplished either with casting or use of a molded thoracolumbar sacral orthosis (TLSO) brace. The combination of bed rest and spinal immobilization is effective in relieving the patient's pain. Prior to the development of antibiotic therapy, this was the mainstay of treatment. Once symptoms of pain and systemic infection resolve, the patient may be treated with ambulatory casting or bracing. This should be continued at least as long as the antibiotic treatment. The combination of spinal immobilization and antibiotics will lead to a cure in the vast majority of cases.[6] Spontaneous fusion across the affected disk space has been documented to occur in upward of 60 percent of cases.[7] Prior to the introduction of antibiotic treatment, the mortality rate for vertebral osteomyelitis was approximately 30 percent.[7]

Surgery is extremely effective in the treatment of pyogenic spinal osteomyelitis, especially in cases that are unresponsive to nonoperative treatment. As state previously, surgery may be indicated in order to obtain tissue for diagnosis and culture. Other indications for surgery include continued severe systemic symptoms despite appropriate antibiotic therapy, severe, disabling pain, abscess formation, vertebral collapse and progressive kyphosis, as well as the development of neurologic deficits (Table 71-1).[1,7,14,19,38,30] The onset of neurologic deficit or the development of a progressive neurologic deficit are the most urgent indications for operative intervention. In most cases, neurologic deficit is caused by anterior impingement on the neurologic structures. This may occur from epidural abscess formation or vertebral collapse and gibbus formation. Epidural infection occurs in approximately 35 percent of cases of spinal osteomyelitis.[7] Symptomatic

epidural infection is more likely to occur in the thoracic spine as opposed to the lumbar or cervical areas. The organism responsible occurs in the same proportion as those that cause vertebral osteomyelitis in general. Progressive vertebral destruction and collapse leading to gibbus formation may also lead to anterior neurologic compression. Likewise, sequestered vertebral material may be retropulsed into the spinal canal, also causing neurologic deficit.

The mainstay of the surgical treatment of pyogenic vertebral osteomyelitis is debridement of the infected tissue and stabilization of the vertebral column. The focus of infection should be approached directly anteriorly to ensure optimal visualization and adequate debridement. Standard surgical approaches can be utilized, depending on the area of the spinal column affected. In the thoracolumbar and lumbar spine, retroperitoneal approaches are preferred. These can be done with diaphragmatic takedown if necessary. For thoracic lesions, a transthoracic approach by thoracotomy gives the best exposure. In patients absolutely unable to tolerate a thoracotomy, a costotransversectomy approach may be used to drain an abscess and debride vertebral involvement. However, visualization is limited by this exposure and strut grafting after debridement may be difficult. The goal of debridement is to remove all infected tissue completely, down to normal unaffected bone. If there is neurologic compromise, it is essential that the spinal canal be completely cleared of any tissue causing anterior compression of the dura mater. In cases where imaging studies reveal that the focus of infection is primarily posterior, posterior debridement and drainage by wide laminectomy can be employed in order to control infection and attempt to salvage neurologic function.

Following debridement, bone grafting is essential to restore the stability of the spinal column. Structural bone graft of sufficient strength to prevent vertebral collapse is necessary to restore spinal stability. Autogenous graft consisting of tricortical ilium or fibula may be harvested. Structural allograft can also be used. This will prevent the morbidity associated with bone graft harvest, especially when large segments must be spanned. If debridement has been adequate, there appears to be very little risk of infection of the allograft despite the fact that it is avascular and technically a foreign body. Not enough information is available on other types of synthetic vertebral replacements to recommend their use in this setting. With the easy availability of either autogenous or allograft bone, there seems to be very little call for use of other types of materials.

The use of internal fixation in the treatment of osteomyelitis is limited. With adequate anterior bone grafting techniques, sufficient stability can be obtained in most cases that internal fixation is not necessary. Fusion rates following anterior debridement and grafting are reported to be greater than 90 percent.[19] Therefore it seem unnecessary to introduce a metallic foreign body, which could potentially serve as a nidus for further infection. If there is a question of significant instability following anterior debridement and grafting, posterior segmental fixation can be used to maintain spinal alignment and stability in con-

---

TABLE 71-1 Indications for Operative Interventions in Pyogenic Vertebral Osteomyelitis

---

Biopsy for diagnosis and culture

Systemic symptoms despite appropriate antimicrobial therapy

Severe pain

Abscess formation

Vertebral collapse and kyphosis

Neurologic deficit

---

junction with the anterior procedure. In this manner, no metal need be introduced into a potentially contaminated wound site. In cases where posterior debridement has significantly compromised spinal stability because of resection of the facet joints, posterior instrumentation can be used to restore spinal stability. Posterior instrumentation should also be employed in cases where, preoperatively, there is significant kyphotic deformity that is to be corrected surgically. These cases also require anterior strut grafting in order to restore the anterior column and prevent late collapse and hardware failure. Anterior surgery is also useful for the drainage of soft tissue abscesses associated with vertebral osteomyelitis.

Results

Anterior spinal surgery for the treatment of vertebral osteomyelitis carries a mortality rate as high as 25 percent.[40] This is the highest rate for any type of anterior spinal surgery. There have been reports of mycotic aneurysm secondary to vertebral infection.[41] These aneurysms can rupture intraoperatively and lead to catastrophic hemorrhage and death. However, most reports cite cure rates in excess of 90 percent.[1,7,19] Fusion usually occurs within 6 to 8 months following surgery. Correction of kyphotic deformity is quite reliable. Permanent neurologic sequelae occur in approximately 6 percent of patients.[7]

TUBERCULOSIS

Worldwide, *Mycobacterium tuberculosis* is unquestionably the most common source of vertebral infection. Tuberculosis continues to be common in third world countries. Moreover, there has recently been a resurgence of tuberculosis in the United States. This has coincided with the emergence of strains resistant to multiple antibiotics. Although spinal tuberculosis accounts for only 1 percent of all cases of tuberculosis, the spine remains the most common site of skeletal tuberculosis, accounting for approximately 60 percent tuberculous osteomyelitis.[9,42] Spinal tuberculosis is very common among children, with over 50 percent of cases being reported the first decade of life.[43]

The pathophysiology of tuberculous spinal infection is somewhat different from that of pyogenic infection (Table 71-2). The infection may begin either by direct extension from the lung or by hematogenous spread. Like pyogenic infection, tuberculosis usually begins in the vertebral body. The initial site of infection is generally the anterior inferior one-third of the vertebral body. Tuberculosis is unlikely to remain localized to a single vertebral focus and has a propensity to spread along fascial plains. It will spread along the anterior longitudinal ligament to affect multiple contiguous vertebral segments.[9,44] Tuberculosis, therefore, is more likely to involve multiple vertebral bodies and lead to progressive kyphosis as multiple vertebra are destroyed.[45] As the in-

TABLE 71-2 Differences between Pyogenic and Tuberculous Vertebral Osteomyelitis

Pyogenic	Tuberculous
Single vertebral focus	Multisegment involvement
Symmetrical collapse	Kyphosis
Spreads intraosseously	Spreads along fascial planes
Disk destroyed	Disk sequestered
Anterior-column involvement	Three-column involvement
Epidural abscess more common	Paravertebral abscess common
More acute onset	Insidious chronic course

fection spreads, the disk is sequestered rather than being destroyed. As the vertebrae are destroyed, this sequestered disk material may be extruded posteriorly, causing paraplegia.[42] Tuberculosis is well known to cause large paravertebral abscesses. Unlike the case in pyogenic infection, the posterior elements are frequently involved in tuberculous infection. This has been reported in 50 to 70 percent of cases.[8,46] Although the infection may spread along the anterior epidural space, large epidural abscesses are uncommon. However, the infection can progress to involve the meninges and spinal cord directly.[42] Overall, tuberculosis tends to be a more chronic infection with a slow and insidious progression. Symptoms are usually present for a longer time than in pyogenic infection prior to presentation.

It can be very difficult to differentiate infection caused by tuberculosis from pyogenic infection on plain radiographic studies. The patterns of vertebral destruction may be similar. Tuberculosis is more likely to involve multiple vertebrae. At least 50 percent of cases will have involvement of three or more vertebral bodies.[9,44] Since tuberculosis is relatively "disk sparing," it may be mistaken for neoplastic conditions. Other conditions that may appear similar radiographically include actinomycoses, hydatid disease, and brucellosis.[9,44]

Magnetic resonance imaging can be useful to help make the diagnosis. Characteristically, tuberculosis does not show increased signal in the disk space, in contrast to pyogenic vertebral infection.[8] As with other forms of infection, MRI remains the best study to define the extent of the infectious process in soft tissue. Magnetic resonance imaging is also useful to help delineate pus from scar in partially treated or resolving infections, and it can help to assess the degree of direct spinal cord involvement.[46]

Treatment

Several studies have documented that the treatment of spinal tuberculosis using only drug therapy can be effective.[42,47,48] As with other forms of tuberculosis, multiple drug therapy is necessary to combat the infection. The British Medical Research Council, in a controlled trial, found that good results were obtained in 77 percent of patients treated with drug therapy alone.[47] In this study, there were 8 percent poor results. It should be noted that no patient in this series was paraparetic on first presentation. At the end of treatment, only 8 of 265 patients were persistently myelopathic and only 2 were functionally impaired. However, in another study, no patient who presented with neurologic deficit recovered when treated with drug therapy only.[48] Drug treatment should continue for 1 year. Treatment for less than 6 months consistently resulted in failure to control infection. Although drug therapy is effective in eradicating infection and spontaneous anterior arthrodesis can usually be anticipated, it is not effective in reversing significant spinal deformity and the resultant neurologic deficit. In these cases, surgical therapy is necessary.

The surgical treatment of tuberculous spinal infection has been recommended in cases where there is more than 5° of kyphosis segmentally, more than 50 percent of vertebral body destruction, neurologic compromise, or unresponsiveness to medical therapy as well as in cases where a nondiagnostic percutaneous biopsy sample has been obtained.[49] The mainstay of surgical treatment involves complete anterior debridement of the affected tissue in conjunction with anterior strut grafting. This was first described by Hodgson and Stock.[50] Several studies have compared anterior debridement alone with radical debridement and strut grafting[51–53] in both children and adults. In one study involving 80 children, with a 17-year follow up, it was noted that equal rates of fusion and cure were obtained with simple debridement as opposed to radical debridement and grafting. However, simple debridement leads to a significant increase in the residual kyphotic deformity. This was particularly true in the lumbar spine.[51] Likewise in adults, debridement alone produced equal results in terms of fusion, pain, and resolution of neurologic deficit. Once again, better correction of deformity was obtained with anterior strut grafting. These findings were consistent even in the face of prolonged postoperative bed rest. All patients in all studies involving the surgical treatment of tuberculosis received concomitant multidrug therapy. This is certainly necessary to achieve a cure. Following anterior surgery with or without grafting, residual postoperative deformity will usually stabilize between 6 weeks and 6 months postoperatively. After this period, there is usually no progressive deformity. This is true even in children; no disproportionate posterior spinal growth causing increasing kyphosis has been found to occur despite solid anterior arthrodesis.[54] Overall, the rate of neurologic recovery following surgery is very good. In one study, 30 of 32 patients recovered neurologically following anterior decompression, while none deteriorated.[55] Several other studies document similar rates of neurologic recovery.

In certain cases, the use of posterior instrumentation may prove efficacious in the treatment of spinal tuberculosis. Posterior instrumentation can be used to correct deformity and maintain correction during drug treatment.

One study documented an average loss of correction of only 3.4° when patients with short-segment kyphosis, no neurologic deficits, and no large anterior abscess were treated with posterior instrumentation and drug therapy.[56] All patients in this study obtained fusion. In cases where there is significant posterior element or three-column involvement, posterior segmental instrumentation may be used to restore stability to the involved spine.[46,57] In vivo experiments have demonstrated no biofilm production by the *M. tuberculosis,* in contrast to most other pyogenic organisms.[57] In the same study, investigators were able to use posterior hardware effectively without the development of any hardware-related infections. In patients with significant long-segment involvement of the anterior column leading to severe kyphosis, both anterior debridement and strut grafting in combination with posterior segmental instrumentation is the most reliable way of achieving correction of deformity while obtaining a cure.[48,55]

OTHER UNCOMMON INFECTIOUS AGENTS

Aside from the common pyogenic infectious agents and tuberculosis, infection from other, more rare infectious agents may affect the spine. Among these uncommon types of spinal infection are brucellosis, aspergillosis, mucormycosis, coccidiomycosis, candidiasis, and *Kingella kingae* infection.[24,58–66] Some of these organisms such as coccidia or brucella are endemic to the areas in which the infections occur. Often the usual host is in some way immunocompromised. Aspergillosis is seen in renal and cardiac transplant patients.[24,60] Candidiasis may occur in patients with malignant cancer or in neonates.[59,64,65]

Since these organisms are rare causes of spinal infection, there are few large series available to accurately compare different treatment regimens. Most of the literature is composed of case reports or very small series. For most of these rare pathogens, there are no absolutely pathognomonic findings on presentation or radiographs that will make the diagnosis definitively. Aside from a high index of suspicion in patients with predisposing conditions, there is nothing specific to alert the physician that some uncommon agent is responsible for the patient's presentation. Often the radiographic appearance of the infection will mimic that seen typically in pyogenic or tuberculous infections. Most of these infections are rather indolent, and patients characteristically have had a long period of symptoms prior to presentation. Similarly, most of these infections can be treated nonoperatively with appropriate antimicrobial agents. Fungal infections require prolonged treatment with multiple antifungal agents. Successful treatment often takes more than a year.[60,66] In contrast, brucellosis is quite sensitive to quinolone antibiotics, and an 8- to 10-week course of single drug therapy is usually sufficient to eradicate the infection.[67] Indications for operative intervention are the same as for those listed for pyogenic and tuberculous spinal osteomyelitis: infection unresponsive to antibiotic therapy, progressive neurologic deficit, or deformity. Often surgery can speed resolution of infections unresponsive to medical therapy by removing avascular necrotic tissue and allowing better penetration of systemic drug therapy into the affected area. In addition, spinal instability can be corrected and the neurologic structures decompressed to preserve and enhance neurologic function in the face of a developing neurologic deficit.

PENETRATING INJURIES

Penetrating injuries are a fairly common cause of spinal injury. Gunshot wounds rate as the third most common cause of spinal cord injury.[68] However, they account for only a minority of spinal infections. There is little controversy that high-velocity missile injuries require debridement to prevent osteomyelitis. However, low-velocity missile wounds are more common. Infection is most commonly associated with concomitant penetration of the gastrointestinal tract. Low-velocity missile wounds and other low-energy injuries (i.e., knife wounds) that enter dorsally can usually be treated with local wound care and a short course of systemic antibiotics. It is not necessary to remove retained metal fragments. Neurologic injury in the case of gunshot wounds is usually the result of the blast effect. Removal of foreign bodies from within the spinal canal does not generally result in improved neurologic outcome. Operative intervention to remove the fragments only serves to destabilize the spine further. Stab wounds account for the majority of other low-energy penetrating injuries. These most commonly occur in the upper dorsal or cervical area.[69] They may require formal surgical exploration based on general surgical principles for penetrating neck injuries. However, formal debridement of the spine is unnecessary unless there has been pharyngeal contamination.

Recent literature has focused on the appropriate treatment of missile injuries that are complicated by gastrointestinal contamination. Pharyngeal injuries have been associated with a high degree of contamination with oral flora.[70] Infection with *streptococcus* and *Bacteroides* species has been reported. In such cases, formal debridement of the spine is necessary. Some authors have recommended stabilization with a halo brace along with antibiotic therapy consisting of a beta-lactam antibiotic and an aminoglycoside.[70] Transperitoneal injuries have been another area of controversy. Various authors have supported the routine use of formal debridement, while others have recommended antibiotics and observation alone as sufficient treatment.[68,71–74] There have been reports of duodenal injuries resulting in extensive osteomyelitis.[71,72] Other studies have shown a very low rate of spinal osteomyelitis following injuries to the stomach and small bowel only. Most studies do report a significant incidence of spinal infection following gunshot wounds that traverse the colon.[73,74] Based on the data presented in these studies, it seems prudent to recommend the routine formal debridement of the spine in all cases of missile injuries complicated by colonic perforation.

CHILDHOOD DISKITIS

Diskitis is a pediatric affliction presenting with many signs of infection. However, in many cases, it is a self-limited condition that resolves without antibiotic treatment. In addition, many authors have reported inability to consistently culture bacterial organisms from the site of the lesion. For this reason, some authors have questioned whether this entity truly has an infectious etiology.[75]

The pathophysiology of acute disk space infection in children is different from that seen in adults. Prior to maturity, the disk continues to receive blood supply through arteries that penetrate the adjacent vertebral end plates.[76] In this manner, bacteria can spread hematogenously directly into the disk. In the adult, the end-plate arteries do not penetrate the disk; the vertebral end plate rather than the disk becomes the focus of septic infarction. In the adult, the disk is involved secondarily as the infection progresses locally. In the child, the disk may become the primary focus of infection.

The average age at presentation is 2 and 6 years.[43,76–78] Males and females are equally affected.[78] The classic presentation is one of a child complaining of back pain that has gradually increased in intensity for between 2 and 4 weeks.[43,77,79] Usually, the child, who will be irritable and will often refuse to stand or walk, will present with markedly increased spinal rigidity and maintain a posture of fixed hyperlordosis.[80] The child may have a low grade fever as well. Other common complaints include abdominal, pelvic, hip, or leg pain and anorexia. The clinical differential diagnosis includes appendicitis or other intraabdominal processes, psoas abscess, or hip sepsis among others. Up to 90 percent of children will present with an elevated erythrocyte sedimentation rate.[77,79] No other laboratory abnormalities are seen consistently.

The pathognomonic radiographic finding for acute childhood diskitis is disk space narrowing at the level of the involved disk.[43,77,79,80] This will usually appear between 2 and 6 weeks following the onset of symptoms. Disk narrowing is accompanied by loss of cortical distinction of the adjacent vertebral end plates. The most common site of involvement is the distal lumbar spine; L4-5 accounts for 40 percent of cases.[77,78] Involvement never occurs at multiple levels.[81] This can help to distinguish diskitis from other destructive lesions within the spine. Magnetic resonance imaging will show loss of disk height and irregular contour of the vertebral end plates. Increased signal may be seen in the adjacent vertebral bodies on T1-weighted images but not seen on T2-weighted images.[80] Acute diskitis will not show the aggressive, destructive bone changes seen in true osteomyelitis.[35,82,83] Biopsy is rarely required to make the diagnosis. If a biopsy is undertaken, *Staphylococcus* species are the most common organisms isolated.[78] However, cultures of aspirated disk material are positive in only 25 percent of cases.[76,77]

The primary treatment for acute childhood diskitis consists of bed rest and spinal immobilization with a cast.[76] In most cases, this will lead to prompt resolution of symptoms. Initial treatment with antibiotics is not necessary.[43,77,81] Antibiotics can be used for cases that fail to respond to spinal immobilization and rest or in cases with persistent signs of systemic infection, such as fever, increased sedimentation rate, increased white blood cell count, or positive biopsy. In the absence of specific culture results, an antibiotic active against *Staphylococcus* organisms should be selected. Surgery is almost never indicated in the treatment of childhood diskitis.

The results in the treatment of diskitis are usually quite good. In approximately one-quarter of patients, the disk space will undergo spontaneous interbody fusion. In about one-third of cases, the disk height will be restored spontaneously following resolution of symptoms.[77,79] Approximately 50 percent of patients will develop a mild form of scoliosis. The resulting spinal deformity is usually nonprogressive and rarely requires treatment. In one study, 30 percent of patients followed for an average of 7 years reported mild backache.[77]

POSTOPERATIVE WOUND INFECTIONS

Infection following spinal surgery represents a source of significant morbidity. Despite the best efforts of the surgeon, these infections will inevitably occur. Acute postoperative infections may complicate all types of surgery, from simple laminectomies to the most complex reconstructions.

Acute infection can be expected to complicate 1 to 3 percent of all surgical procedures for disk herniation.[84–86] Simple posterior wound infection will usually present with the usual signs and symptoms of wound infection anywhere, including redness, swelling, local pain, and wound drainage. These infections are usually fairly obvious. In most cases, they can be treated successfully with local wound irrigation and drainage measures and suitable antibiotics. Most cases will resolve without permanent sequelae with prompt and appropriate therapy.

An entity that is more difficult to diagnose is an acute postoperative disk space infection. In such cases, there may be no clinical manifestations of difficulties in wound healing. Clinically and radiologically, these infections are similar to vertebral osteomyelitis, which occurs after hematogenous seeding.[85,87] Since there may be no signs of external infection, diagnosis is often delayed; in one study, the average time to diagnosis for this problem was 15 weeks.[85] This complication has been reported to occur after percutaneous lateral diskectomy as well as open diskectomy procedures.[88] *Staphylococcus aureus* is the most common organism isolated.[85] In the clinical setting, continued severe back pain and a persistently elevated erythrocyte sedimentation rate are the two hallmarks of acute postoperative diskitis.[2,85] Characteristic x-ray changes may take several weeks to develop. Boden and colleagues have identified a specific triad of findings on pre- and postcontrast MRI images that are fairly specific for postoperative diskitis (Table 71-3). The combination of changes in the vertebral bone marrow adjacent to the affected disk, the disk space itself, and the posterior annulus fibrosus, when seen together, are highly suggestive of diskitis even before radiographic changes appear.[89]

Treatment of established postoperative diskitis is the same as that for infection occurring after hematogenous

---

TABLE 71-3 MRI Characteristics of Postoperative Diskitis

Decreased signal in bone marrow adjacent to disk space on T1-weighted image

Increased signal in disk space on T2-weighted image

Enhancement of both vertebral bone marrow and disk space on T1-weighted images after administration of intravenous gadopentetate dimeglumine

---

seeding. Bed rest with casting or bracing will lead to spontaneous anterior interbody fusion in approximately 40 percent of cases.[86] However, antibiotics should be used routinely to help ensure that the infection is arrested. The combination of antibiotics and spinal immobilization will lead to cure in almost all cases. Percutaneous disk space biopsy under fluoroscopic or CT guidance should be undertaken to confirm the diagnosis pathologically and isolate the causative organism to identify appropriate antibiotics. Intravenous antibiotics should be employed and should be continued at least until the erythrocyte sedimentation rate returns to normal. The usual duration of antibiotic treatment is between 6 and 12 weeks. Several weeks of oral antibiotics after this can be used to ensure complete eradication of the infection.

The treatment of spinal infection following procedures to fuse the spine presents more challenges and controversies than acute postoperative diskitis. This is especially true when infection occurs following the use of instrumentation to stabilize the spine. These procedures tend to be associated with longer operative times as well as more significant dissection and exposure. More tissue is devitalized and a larger dead space created. The combination of these factors significantly raises the risk for postoperative wound infection. Infection has been reported to occur in approximately 5 percent of cases of spinal instrumentation. The ability of the host to fight infection becomes a significant factor in the prevention of infection. Several studies have documented an increased rate of infection in patients who show laboratory evidence of malnourishment.[90,91] In addition, older patients and those on chronic immunosuppressants such as steroid medications may be at increased risk for the development of infection. Especially in the setting of elective surgery, every effort should be made to optimize the patient's preoperative condition prior to proceeding with surgery. Once infection is established, the presence of a foreign body (i.e., the instrumentation) makes it almost impossible to render the wound free of microorganisms. Most common bacterial organisms secrete a glycocalyx or "slime layer," which inhibits antibiotic penetration and prevents full clearance of organisms despite surgical debridement.

When acute infection occurs following spinal instrumentation, the most common presenting signs is persistent wound drainage. This finding will occur after both anterior and posterior instrumentation procedures.[91,92] The patient may present with other signs of acute infection, such as fever, chills, and localized pain. Rarely will the patient present with a new or progressive neurologic deficit. Overall, these infections are somewhat more virulent than acute postoperative diskitis. In one study, the average time from surgery to diagnosis was 17 days rather than months.[91]

The treatment of spinal wound infections following instrumentation is difficult because in many cases removal of instrumentation may leave the spine dangerously unstable. Instrumentation may be necessary to protect neurologic function or prevent the development of deformity. Its removal would seriously compromise the goals of the original surgery. However, in the presence of retained hardware, it may be impossible to eradicate the infectious organisms completely because of the poor penetration of antibiotics into the glycocalyx secreted by the organisms, which is adherent to the metallic foreign body. Several investigators have reported on various strategies to treat these infections. The common aspect of all these treatment plans is aggressive wound debridement of all devitalized soft tissue along with adequate wound drainage. These interventions combined with appropriate antibiotic therapy will often allow for the control of infection. Wound management can be difficult. In severe, life-threatening sepsis, it is probably best to leave the wound open and packed. After the infection is adequately controlled, delayed wound closure can often be performed. However, it may be difficult to close the wound once the soft tissue has retracted. Allowing the wound to granulate may be successful but can take a long time. Several authors have described local muscle rotation flaps that can be used to obtain wound coverage.[93,94] In order to simplify would management, acute fascial closure can often be performed safely. Wound closure over large drains can also be successful.[95] The author has used continuous irrigation through these drains for several days in conjunction with repeated would debridements to control postoperative infections. Another strategy is to insert antibiotic-containing polymethylmethacrylate beads into the wound to enhance local antibiotic penetration.[96] Whatever the method of wound management chosen, all attempts should be made to maintain the instrumentation *in situ*. Removal of the instrumentation may render the spine unstable and lead to disastrous consequences. Appropriate management of bone graft within the wound is a question that often arises. Certainly any bone graft material that is grossly contaminated by pus should be removed. However, graft material that is covered by healthy-appearing granulation tissue may be left in place as long as the infection is well controlled.

Infection following anterior instrumentation may present with sinus tract formation or groin abscess.[92] This can usually be treated with removal of the instrumentation and administration of antibiotics. Once the infection has been controlled, spinal stability can be restored, if necessary, with posterior instrumentation. Simple bracing may be employed if there is no significant compromise of stability. If bony debridement is necessary to remove frankly infected vertebral body bone, structural bone grafting to restore stability can be employed successfully as long as adequate debridement has been carried out.

At least 6 weeks of intravenous antibiotics should be given to adequately control infection with retained hardware. This duration of therapy is usually more than adequate to control the clinical symptoms of infection. It may be followed by a prolonged course of suppressive oral antibiotics. In most cases, eventual fusion will result.[91] Once this has occurred, antibiotics can be discontinued. If, following the cessation of antibiotic therapy, symptoms such as pain or wound drainage recur, instrumentation can safely be removed with the expectation of cure of infection.

There have been some reports of late infection following seemingly uncomplicated spinal instrumentation procedures.[97] It is unclear whether these infections represent late bacterial seeding of retained instrumentation or whether there is direct contamination at the time of surgery with low-virulence organisms, which only become symptomatic later. It has been theorized that the infections are related to the bulk of the instrumentation inserted and to corrosion at the interconnections of modular components that eventually lose their rigid connection. In one series, the infections presented at an average of 25 months following surgery.[97] These infections presented with either spontaneous drainage or wound fluctuance. The organisms isolated from these infections include *Proprionibacterium, Micrococcus,* and *Staphylococcus epidermidis.* The common characteristic of all these organisms is the need for isolation and extended periods of incubation for growth. Removal of instrumentation resulted in cure in all cases. The authors of this study caution that appropriate surveillance for low-virulence organisms should be undertaken in the scenario of delayed postoperative wound infection.

TUMORS OF THE SPINE

Benign Tumors

According to Dahlin's report on a series of over 6000 tumors, approximately 8 percent of primary benign bone tumors occur in the spine or sacrum.[98] Conversely, among primary spinal tumors, nonmalignant lesions account for 20 to 40 percent of the tumors diagnosed.[98–100] Benign sacral tumors account for 30 percent of the tumors seen in this location.[98,101] As is true with benign bone tumors in other locations, the age distribution of benign spinal tumors is skewed toward the earlier decades (Fig. 71-3). Dahlin reported that 60 percent of benign spinal tumors occurred in the second and third decades of life.[98] Other authors have reported incidences from 37 to 80 percent in the first two decades of life.[99,102] Sacral tumors tend to occur in a slightly older age group. These tumors are usually encountered in the third, fourth, and fifth decades.[101] Tumors in the body of the sacrum in children are more likely to be malignant.[103]

The more common histologic subtypes of benign spine tumors are listed in Table 71-4. Common osseous lesions include osteochondroma, osteoblastoma, and osteoid osteoma. Purely chondrous lesions are more rare. Giant cell tumor, eosinophilic granuloma, hemangioma, and aneurysmal bone cysts all represent significant diagnostic entities. In the sacrum, giant cell tumor and aneurysmal bone cysts are most common.[98,101] Certain tumors have a propensity

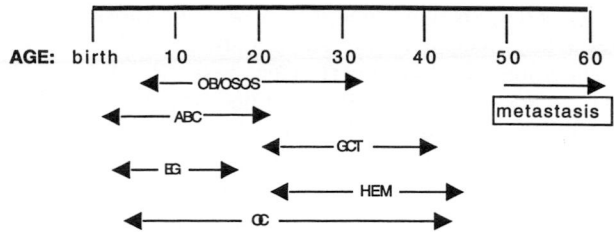

Figure 71-3 The age distribution of some common benign spinal tumors. OB/OSOS, osteoblastoma/osteoid osteoma; ABC, aneurysmal bone cyst; GCT, giant cell tumor; EG, eosinophilic granuloma; HEM, hemangioma; OC, osteochondroma.

to occur either anteriorly in the body or in the posterior elements. Osteoblastoma and osteoid osteomas are known almost always to involve the posterior elements of the particular vertebrae involved. Likewise, eosinophilic granuloma, hemangioma, and giant cell tumor tend to involve the anterior portion of the vertebral body rather than the posterior elements.

Presentation

The most common complaint is pain. This may be either local or radicular in nature. It is important to note that back pain is a very infrequent complaint in the pediatric population unless accompanied by some specific traumatic episode. Ehrlich and Zaleske studied complaints of musculoskeletal pain in a pediatric population. They found that benign neoplasm was the second most common diagnosis following trauma in pain of unclear etiology.[102] Night pain has been known to be associated with certain benign skeletal neoplasms such as osteoid osteoma and osteoblastoma.[103,104] Tumors causing radicular pain may

TABLE 71-4 Common Histologic Subtypes of Benign Spinal Tumors

Tumor[a]	Cervical, thoracic, and/or lumbar	Sacrum
Giant cell tumor	11.4	61.4
Osteoid osteoma	17.7	5.3
Osteoblastoma	14.9	7.0
Hemangioma	14.2	0
Osteochondroma	12.1	5.3
Aneurysmal bone cyst	22.7	14.0
Other[b]	7.0	6.7

[a]Not listed: eosinophilic granuloma.
[b]Includes chondroma, chondroblastoma, chondromyxoid fibroma, neurolemmoma, fibrous histiocytoma.

mimic the presentation of a herniated disk, with unilateral sciatica.[105] Osteoblastoma and osteoid osteomas typically involve the posterior elements in the region of the nerve root, and up to 28 percent of these tumors will present with radicular pain complaints.[103]

Scoliosis has also been reported to be a common finding in patients with benign spinal neoplasms. This may be rapid in progression and is frequently painful.[113] In addition, several authors have noted that patients with benign spinal neoplasms frequently demonstrate extreme rigidity associated with their scoliosis.[103,106] On examination, the prototypical patient will have great difficulty with spinal motion in all planes, including forward flexion. In addition, often these curves show significant coronal decompensation and do not demonstrate the usual compensatory balancing curves above or below the curve involving the lesions. Radiographically as well, the scoliosis will lack the usual structural characteristics associated with idiopathic scoliosis. Commonly, there is absence of both vertebral rotation and wedging. All these factors serve to distinguish this type of scoliosis from idiopathic scoliosis, which may present in a similar age group. Taylor studied adolescents with painful scoliosis and found that fully 50 percent of these patients had osteoid osteomas.[107] Characteristically, the tumor will be found at the concave apex of the curve except for tumors occurring in the lowest lumbar vertebra, in which case the apex of the curve is usually higher.[108]

Myelopathy is more common in tumors involving the cervical and particularly the thoracic spine. The ratio of spinal cord to spinal canal diameter is highest in this area. Focal sensory and motor abnormalities may accompany root involvement. Levine et al. reported a 14 percent incidence of sensory abnormalities and 7 percent focal motor deficits.[109] Incontinence has been reported as a presenting complaint in benign sacral tumors.[110]

Most tumors have a very characteristic radiographic appearance. Osteoid osteoma and osteoblastoma frequently present as sclerotic lesions in the pedicle.[111] Aneurysmal bone cysts and giant cell tumors are most often expansile and lytic.[112,113] Hemangiomas will show coarsened vertical trabeculae. Eosinophilic granuloma is well recognized as a cause of vertebra plana. In a study of 44 benign spinal tumors, from Rome, 43 of 44 x-rays were considered to be abnormal; however only 29 percent showed pathognomonic findings.[99] In osteoblastoma and osteoid osteoma, anywhere from 25 to 50 percent of x-rays will be interpreted falsely as negative.[83,86] Persistent back pain of several weeks' or months' duration that is unresponsive to rest and presents with "normal" x-rays should prompt further investigation with screening studies of occult lesions.[114,115]

Bone scan is a useful screening tool because of its high sensitivity and ability to visualize the entire skeleton. It is the study of choice for painful scoliosis in an adolescent with otherwise normal x-rays.[108,115,116] In one study, bone scan shortened the period prior to diagnosis in osteoid-producing lesions from 35 to 12 months.[104] However, bone scan is nonspecific and its use is limited to screening and localization of suspected lesions. There are no reported cases of false-negative technetium bone scan in osteoblastoma or osteoid osteoma. However, other lesions may be photopenic; hemangioma in particular may present with a cold scan.[117,118]

Once the area of pathology is identified by bone scan or plain x-ray, further imaging with either CT or MRI should be undertaken to fully define the extent and nature of the pathologic lesions. Sagittal and coronal reformatted tomographic images are essential to define the exact anatomic location and extent of lesions. Computed tomography, with its excellent resolution of bony detail, has been recommended as the study of choice to define these lesions.[119] More recently, MRI has been used to study benign spinal neoplasms. This study gives excellent soft tissue resolution, which aids in the assessment of the soft tissue extent of any tumor.[120] In addition, MRI is excellent for determining the level and extent of spinal cord compression in lesions with neurologic deficit.[121] Furthermore, CT myelography is adequate to define areas of neural compression, but it is somewhat more invasive. However, MRI may overestimate the extent of involvement secondary to the inflammatory response surrounding the tumor, which may simulate soft tissue involvement and give the impression of a more aggressive tumor than actually exists.[119,122,123]

Some lesions (osteoid osteoma, hemangioma) may be sufficiently "classic" on preoperative imaging not to require tissue diagnosis prior to definitive surgery. For many lesions, however, the differential diagnosis will include several benign and malignant possibilities—aneurysmal bone cyst (ABC), giant cell tumor, osteoblastoma, eosinophilic granuloma. It is essential to make a definitive diagnosis prior to planning treatment. Frequently, a needle biopsy performed under CT guidance in the radiology suite can obtain sufficient tissue for diagnostic purposes. Open transpedicle biopsy can also be used to obtain tissue for pathologic examination.

Treatment

Benign spinal tumors can be classified according to the stages described by Enneking as either latent (stage 1), active (stage 2), or aggressive (stage 3) lesions.[110] Stage 1 lesions are usually incidental findings that require no treatment (osteochondroma, hemangioma). Tumors that typically present symptomatically as stage 2 are osteoid osteoma, eosinophilic granuloma, hemangioma, osteochondroma, and ABC. Giant cell tumors and osteoblastomas may be stage 2 but are more likely to be stage 3 lesions. Stage 2 lesions in general require en bloc excision or curettage. In stage 3 aggressive lesions, wide excision should be performed. In tumors with neurologic involvement, a marginal or intralesional margin with preservation of neurologic function is preferable to a wide excision. These procedures can then be followed with adjuvant therapy as deemed necessary. Aggressive osteoblastomas and giant cell tumors have a particular propensity to recur after marginal excision and should be resected with wide margins if possible, using a "no touch" technique. In the cervical spine, in addition to the neural structures, margins are often limited by the position of the vertebral

artery. Preoperative angiography with temporary vertebral artery occlusion may show sufficient collateral flow to allow unilateral vertebral artery resection; this can be done to achieve a wide margin, if necessary.[124]

In the thoracic and lumbar spine, wide or marginal margins can be obtained through standard anterior thoracotomy or retroperitoneal approaches. Exposure may be limited in a costotransversectomy approach, which can inadvertently result in undesired contamination of the surgical margins or incomplete excision of the lesions. Posterior lesions can be treated with a standard posterior midline approach and excision of the necessary tissue to achieve the desired margins.

Sacral lesions may be approached either posteriorly or with combined approaches, depending on the extent of the tumor. The large pelvic venous plexus can make the resections very difficult, and heavy blood loss should be anticipated and planned for. Excision of the more proximal portions of the sacrum may interfere with urinary or fecal continence. Some 50 percent of patients will remain continent of urine and stool if both S1 and one S2 root are preserved.[110] If both S1 and S2 roots as well as one S3 root are preserved, 100 percent of patients will maintain adequate sphincter function.[101] The distal sacrum and coccyx can safely be excised without significant compromise. Enneking has recommended cryosurgical techniques for adjuvant therapy in sacral tumors as being superior to polymethylmethacrylate or radiation in stage 3 lesions, when wide resection cannot be performed.[110]

Frequently, with aggressive tumors, the dura mater will be involved, and it may be impossible to dissect the tumor off the dura. In these cases, the dura should be resected with the tumor and the defect patch-grafted.

After removal of the tumor, stabilization and fusion are necessary when resection has compromised spinal stability. Anteriorly, the degree of vertebral body resection will determine the need for stabilization. Except in cases where only limited curettage is performed for small lesions, fusion should be carried out. If a small lesion is amenable to curettage and grafting only, postoperative protection in an orthosis may be advisable until the vertebral body regains its structural integrity. The wearing of an orthosis may also be advisable after anterior or posterior fusions, depending on their length, degree of resection, and the internal stability achieved. However, when in doubt, there is usually little morbidity involved in adding postoperative bracing to the treatment protocol.

Since most patients have a normal life expectancy, constructs that achieve biological stabilization with bony fusions are preferable to other methods, such as polymethylmethacrylate, to ensure long-term stability. Anteriorly, structural bone graft in the form of autograft or allograft may be needed to provide structural support. Autograft tricortical ilium or fibula have sufficient strength to provide structural support, and they incorporate more readily than allograft. However, these advantages must be weighed against the potential donor site morbidity. Other methods of achieving anterior structural support, such as hollow titanium cages, may seem attractive, but there has been insufficient experience with their use for them to be recommended routinely. Internal fixation is recommended to provide immediate stability and promote fusion, especially where allograft is used. However, this may not be feasible in very young patients, where insufficient bone stock may preclude instrumentation.

Complete laminectomy in a skeletally immature patient may lead to progressive kyphosis. In particular, the cervicothoracic junction, midthoracic spine, and thoracolumbar junction are prone to develop kyphotic deformity after laminectomy. In the lumbar spine, where there is preexistent lordosis, progressive kyphosis is less likely to be a problem. Instrumentation and fusion should be included concurrently with resection when complete laminectomy is carried out in high-risk areas. Partial laminar excision need not be followed by fusion, but careful follow-up is mandatory until skeletal maturity is reached, so as to treat any developing deformity. Resection of more than 50 percent of either facet joint should be followed by instrumentation and fusion to prevent instability. Total segmental resection demands posterior stabilization with instrumentation as well as anterior structural grafting.[125]

Postoperative wound complications can ruin an otherwise successful tumor excision. Sacral lesions pose particular problems in this area. In one study, there was an 11 percent incidence of wound infection and an 11 percent incidence of delayed wound healing following excision of benign sacral tumors.[101] This is probably the result of the large dead space created when these tumors are excised. Postoperative closed suction drainage is recommended to help eliminate dead space and prevent hematoma formation. An undrained hematoma may serve as an excellent "culture medium" for the establishment of postoperative infection. Furthermore, prophylactic antibiotics should be used to help prevent infection. Meticulous wound closure technique utilizing multiple layers and nonabsorbable suture will help to prevent wound dehiscence. If postoperative radiation is to be employed, it is probably wise to delay the start of these treatments from a few to several weeks postoperatively until wound healing is well under way. These tenets apply to all spinal levels as well as sacral lesions.

Radiation

Aneurysmal bone cysts and hemangiomas in particular have been reported to respond well to radiation. In ABC, doses less than 30 Gy may be effective,[125,126] but higher doses, from 30 to 40 Gy, are necessary in hemangiomas.[127,128] This should be given as a single course over 6 to 8 weeks for maximal benefit. Doses less than 30 Gy result in a dramatically increased incidence of incomplete resolution.[128] Giant cell tumors may have some radiosensitivity, and this modality can be used to control surgically unresectable lesions.[129,130] However, radiation has been associated with late malignant degeneration in giant cell tumors.[131] Radiation was formerly employed in the treatment of eosinophilic granuloma, but more recently this modality has been shown not to affect the natural history of these lesions.[132–134] Radiation has also been recommended for rapidly increasing neurologic deficits related to tumor compression of neural structures if operative intervention cannot be immediately undertaken.[135] However, radiation does carry with it certain inherent risks. One report noted that 43 percent of children receiving radiation will develop a scoliosis greater than 20°.[136] In addition, the risk of secondary sarcomatous degeneration following radiation is always present. Osteosarcoma and fibrosarcoma are the most common secondary malignancies reported.[136] The reported minimal dose leading to sarcomatous degeneration is 30 Gy, and these sarcomas may not develop for many years following treatment.

Results

Most often, scoliosis will resolve following excision of the tumor; but in certain instances, the curve may become structural and fail to resolve or even progress despite adequate tumor treatment.[107,108,113,137] The duration of symptoms seems to be one factor that affects the ability of the curve to resolve following treatment.[103,104,137] It appears that between 15 and 18 months is a watershed, after which resolution of a curve is less reliable. Also, the age of curve onset seems to affect the ability of the spine to compensate after tumor excision. In one study, patients at or near skeletal maturity or those less than 12 years old were able to resolve their curves, while patients between the ages of 9 and 13½ did not.[137] Furthermore, the magnitude of the scoliosis appeared to effect the chance of progression of this study. Deformity may develop following tumor resection secondary to engendered instability. All patients should be followed for the development of progressive spinal deformity at least until skeletal maturity.

Certain tumors such as osteoblastoma and giant cell tumor tend to be more aggressive and may recur following intralesional excision. From 10 to 20 percent of osteoblastomas will recur; recurrence rate is related to tumor stage and the margins obtained.[138–140] Up to 50 percent of giant cell tumors may recur after intralesional resection.[131] In one study, 8 or 10 patients with continued pain postoperatively following resection of either osteoblastoma or osteoid osteoma had recurrence of tumor.[104] Fairly prompt relief of preoperative symptoms seems to be the best indicator of adequate tumor removal. However, long-term follow-up is necessary to document that lesions do not recur: Computed tomography, with its excellent definition of bony architecture, is the study of choice to screen for recurrence. If instrumentation has been used, once biological fusion has been obtained, it may be advantageous to remove any instrumentation present. In cases of suspected recurrence, this will decrease metal artifact during subsequent imaging studies. In general, recurrent lesions are more problematic than tumors in their primary presentation because of compromised tissues following original treatment. This makes achieving adequate margins more difficult during secondary procedures. Certainly it is best to perform a complete and thorough excision during the first attempt at removal in order to prevent a later recurrence. If documented recurrence occurs, every effort should be made to obtain wide surgical margins during secondary resections. Radiotherapy may be appropriate for unresectable lesions. This is often a reasonable option for recurrent giant cell tumors, which are often radiosensitive, but usually not so for osteoblastoma, which is radioresistant.

Malignant degeneration has been reported to occur most frequently in osteochondroma, osteoblastoma, and giant cell tumor. Up to 10 percent of giant cell tumors will undergo malignant degeneration or metastasize despite benign histologic appearance.[129,131,141] Treatment of malignant degeneration depends on whether or not metastatic spread has occurred and should follow the guidelines for other malignancies.

Malignant Tumors

Malignant neoplastic disease accounts for a significant proportion of the destructive spinal lesions seen. This is especially true in adults where neoplasms are much more likely to be malignant than benign. Likewise, metastatic disease accounts for the majority of malignant lesions seen as opposed to primary tumors arising in the spine itself. Up to 60 percent of patients with metastatic carcinoma will eventually develop metastatic disease prior to their demise; 50 percent of these patients will have metastatic disease to the spine.[142,143] Some 80 to 85 percent of metastatic lesions will occur in the anterior column.[144,145] Posterior element involvement occurs with only about one-seventh the frequency of anterior body involvement.[143] The thoracic spine is the most common site for metastatic tumor involvement, being affected in between 50 and 75 percent of reported cases.[142,146] Of all patients with spinal metastatic disease, approximately 5 to 20 percent will eventually develop neurologic deficits.[142,143] The diagnosis of spinal involvement with metastatic disease is usually a poor prognostic indicator. Most patients will survive less than 1 year following the diagnosis of spinal metastasis.[147–149] The onset of neurologic deficit related to spinal involvement signals an even more dire prognosis.

The metastatic tumors that most commonly affect the spine are the same as those that affect the bony skeleton in general (Table 71-5). Breast, lung, and prostate carcinomas account for the majority of the cases seen.[142,146–148,150]

TABLE 71-5 Common Malignancies Metastatic to the Spine

Breast

Lung

Prostate

Lymphoma

Renal

Thyroid

GI

After these, lymphoma, renal cell carcinoma, thyroid carcinoma, and gastrointestinal malignancies account for the majority of other metastatic lesions. Plasmacytoma/multiple myeloma is the most common primary malignant bone tumor and will commonly present with spinal involvement. Aside from this lesion, other primary malignant tumors are more rarely seen. Chordoma accounts for up to one-half of malignant sacral tumors. A few small series of primary osteosarcoma of the spine have been reported.[151–154] Other primary malignant tumors are rarer still and appear mostly as case reports in the literature.

The pain associated with a malignant spinal neoplasm is classically described as a relentlessly progressive pain that is unresponsive to rest and normal conservative measures. Often, the patient will complain of pain at night, which will awaken him or her from sleep. The most common symptom of malignant neoplasm is local pain, but a patient may present with various neurologic symptoms as well. The new onset of back pain in an adult over the age of 50 without a specific inciting traumatic event should always arouse the suspicion of possible malignancy. Patients may also complain of radicular pain. Occasionally, the first presentation of malignant disease is the rapid onset of significant neurologic deficit in the form of paraparesis or frank paraplegia.

Diagnosis

Diagnostic imaging is important to localize the offending lesion; it is also necessary to define the extent of disease. Often there is scant, plain radiographic evidence even in fairly extensive destructive lesions. Up to 50 percent of the vertebral body must be destroyed prior to being visible on normal radiographs.[143] The most consistent finding to look for is unilateral absence of the cortical pedicle shadow on the anteroposterior radiograph. Once sufficient vertebral destruction has occurred to cause pathologic fracture, it becomes less difficult to localize the lesion. Destructive lesions secondary to malignant disease will usually occur centered in a single vertebral body without compromise of the adjacent disks and end plates. This feature serves to help differentiate tumors from other destructive lesions. Occasionally, in the face of advanced osteoporosis, it can be difficult to determine by plain radiograph whether a true osteolytic lesion is present. Once a tumor is suspected, MRI should be employed to define the anatomic extent of the lesion. This imaging modality gives superior soft tissue detail to define the extent of tumor involvement in the spinal canal as well as in the anterior paravertebral soft tissues. Sagittal reconstructions help to define the extent of bony spinal involvement in segments distant from the main focus of involvement. Up to 9 percent of patients will demonstrate more than one site of spinal canal compromise when appropriate imaging studies are obtained.[143] To a large extent, MRI has supplanted myelography and postmyelographic CT in the investigation of spinal canal compromise. Osteoporotic compression fractures may show diffusely altered marrow signal on MRI as well. Occasionally, acute fracture hematoma can even appear as a paravertebral soft tissue mass. In these cases, CT is often quite helpful because of its superior resolution of bony detail.

Biopsy is usually necessary to confirm the diagnosis. In patients with well-established metastatic disease with a known primary tumor, treatment can be instituted presumptively. In many cases, vertebral metastasis may be the first presentation of a cancer. Biopsy may be the simplest method to establish the diagnosis prior to extensive screening studies to search for a primary tumor. In most cases, CT-guided percutaneous needle biopsy is adequate to obtain sufficient tissue for diagnosis. Occasionally, open biopsy through the vertebral pedicle is necessary when the pathologic diagnosis is uncertain. Appropriate staging studies to assess the extent of tumor spread must also be undertaken prior to any surgical intervention to determine whether the patient is an appropriate surgical candidate and the extent of any planned surgery. These studies should be managed in conjunction with an oncologist who can plan and administer nonsurgical therapies as well.

Treatment

Surgical treatment is not the primary mode of care for individuals suffering from metastatic malignancy. Symptoms of pain related to vertebral structural compromise and neurologic deficit related to extension of tumor within the spinal canal can usually be treated with nonsurgical methods. Radiation, chemotherapy, and, in the appropriate setting, hormonal manipulation all may be used effectively to treat spinal metastases.[145,155–157] Primary malignant tumors arising from within the vertebra will usually require surgical treatment to obtain adequate local control. Prior to undertaking surgical treatment of any spinal tumor, it is important to assess the patient's long-term prognosis. Patients with less than a 2-month survivability are probably not candidates for extensive surgical reconstruction. In addition, the patient who is to undergo surgery should have adequate immunologic function and general nutrition. Malnourished, immunocompromised patients have a much higher rate of postsurgical complications. Since the goal of surgery is to improve the quality of remaining life for these patients and not necessarily to extend it, one must be judicious in selecting appropriate surgical candidates. However, in patients who develop a pathologic fracture with instability, painful kyphosis, or spinal canal impingement with neurologic deficit secondary to a radioresistant tumor or after having received maximal radiation, surgery has a well-defined role in helping to relieve pain and return patients to a functional status for their remaining lives (Table 71-6). Patients who have developed neurologic compromise related to pathologic vertebral fracture with retropulsion of bone and disk fragments into the canal can never be reasonably expected to improve with radiation and chemotherapy alone.

The goal of surgery should be to remove as much tumor as possible, to restore stability to the spinal column immediately, and to provide a construct with reasonable durability to last the rest of the patient's life. In cases of metastatic disease where cure is no longer a possibility, gross debulking of the tumor along with the removal of all retropulsed bone and disk fragments is adequate. In cases of primary malignant tumor confined to one vertebral body, a more radical approach with complete vertebrectomy may be indicated in order to provide a possible cure. Many tumors can be excessively vascular (especially thyroid or renal cell malignancies). Preoperative angiography and embolization is often advisable to avoid large intraoperative blood losses during tumor resection. Decompression can be accomplished through a direct anterior exposure or posterolaterally. Anterior debridement allows for excellent visualization of the pathology and for more thorough decompression. In addition, reconstruction of the anterior column of the spine is facilitated by this approach. The anterior approach is the preferred method in patients who have localized metastatic disease and who are able to tolerate the surgical exposure. In cases of diffuse metastatic spread along the spine, posterior stabilization has the advantage of dealing with the disease at multiple levels. Although spinal canal impingement generally occurs from anterior, this can be dealt with by posterolateral extracavitary or transpedicular decompression techniques. Destruction of the pedicles or the facet joints by tumor mandates posterior stabilization to restore spinal column stability. Often a combined anterior and posterior reconstruction will be necessary to treat certain lesions adequately. Laminectomy alone in the treatment of malignant disease of the spine is generally to be condemned. Only in those rare cases where neural compression arises from a posteriorly situated tumor does laminectomy play a role in the treatment.

Thorough debridement of all tumor back to normal, healthy bone is important to prevent local recurrence. It has been suggested that postoperative local radiation and chemotherapy may be more effective after the removal of most of the gross tumor.[158] Unless local recurrence is prevented, destruction of adjacent segments may lead to failure of anterior constructs.

Anteriorly, the involved vertebra can be approached through standard surgical exposures. Transthoracic, retroperitoneal, thoracolumbar, and lumbar exposures allow access to the spine from T5 to L5. Anterior exposure of the subaxial cervical spine provides excellent access to this area. In the upper thoracic spine, from T1 to T4, standard thoracotomy is usually inadequate. Exposure of these levels may require a sternal splitting procedure.[159] Tumor-

---

TABLE 71-6 Indications for Surgical Treatment of Vertebral Metastases

Greater than 6 weeks survivability
> **and**

Pain unrelieved by maximal conservative therapy
> **or**

Pathologic fracture with instability or painful gibbus deformity

Impending fracture with significant vertebral body destruction

Neurologic deficit
> Canal compromise from radioresistant tumor
> Fracture with bone/disk retropulsion

involved tissue, fractured vertebral fragments, and disk material should be resected back to healthy-appearing, structurally competent vertebral bone above and below. Since most of these patients have a limited life expectancy, it is more important to provide a construct with immediate stability rather than one that is necessarily biological (osseous) for durability. Optimally, patients should be unemcumbered by external immobilization devices postoperatively. Anterior column reconstruction is usually accomplished adequately with a combination of longitudinally placed Steinmann pins and polymethylmethacrylate to fill the anterior column defect. In order to protect the exposed dura from the polymethylmethacrylate, it is important to have some type of substance interposed across the anterior dura during insertion. A large sheet of Gelfoam is usually adequate for this purpose.[155] Errico and Cooper have described a method of using a fenestrated chest tube in order to pressurize the polymethylmethacrylate column to obtain interdigitation in the cancellous bone of the vertebra above and below the defect.[160] Alternatively, a short Harrington rod with hooks at either end can be used to span the defect, and this can be embedded in polymethylmethacrylate. Polymethylmethacrylate is biomechanically sound under compressive forces. This is the major loading mode in anterior column reconstruction. In addition, the material is not weakened by subsequent postoperative irradiation.[158] The use of supplemental instrumentation is especially important in the thoracolumbar and lumbar area. Because of the lordotic curvature in the region, anterior excursion of simple polymethylmethacrylate constructs has been reported.[161] Several reports have documented good long-term survivability of these types of constructs; however, there can be concern that the construct will loosen over time. It has been recommended that, in patients with expected survival of greater than 18 months to 2 years, some sort of biological reconstruction be performed.[143,145] A femoral strut allograft can be used in place of polymethylmethacrylate to provide anterior column support. An alternative is to perform a reconstruction with polymethylmethacrylate and to supplement this with a bone-grafting procedure as well. In this way, both a prosthetic and biological reconstruction is accomplished. If possible, postoperative chemotherapy and irradiation should be delayed up to 6 weeks in these cases to allow for early incorporation of the bone graft, so as to prevent pseudoarthroses.

Complete spondylectomy can be achieved as a staged procedure for cases of malignant primary neoplasm. Following anterior resection and reconstruction, resection of the posterior element and stabilization with instrumentation through a separate exposure can be performed. This type of aggressive surgical resection was found to achieve adequate local control of primary tumors in 6 of 8 cases in one study.[162]

Surgical exposure and resection of sacral lesions can be extremely difficult. Because of the sacrum's position deep within the pelvis, intimately juxtaposed with large vascular structures, bleeding complications are frequent. The sacrum can be resected through a posterior-only approach by developing the retrorectal plane from below after coccygeal resection.

Results

The results of surgery for malignant tumors of the spine have been quite good. With increased understanding of pathomechanics and pathophysiology, improved outcomes have been reported as compared with those of the more distant past. Overall, approximately 90 percent of patients can expect some degree of pain relief and 70 to 80 percent of patients will have some improvement in their neurologic status.[142]

Posterior decompression by laminectomy alone without stabilization is generally to be condemned. Posterior decompression leads to neurologic improvement in only 30 to 40 percent of patients at best.[163] These results are equivalent for patients who have received radiation without surgery.[164,165] Laminectomy is unable to effectively decompress the neural elements, since most compression occurs anteriorly. In order to effectively decompress the spinal canal, some authors recommend posterolateral extracavitary or transpedicle decompression.[144,147] This method may be appropriate for patients who are unable to tolerate thoracotomy or other anterior approaches to the spine because of concurrent medical problems. Surgeons experienced with the technique can effect an adequate decompression. In one study, 8 of 8 patients with less than 6 months to live experienced improvement in their symptoms with posterolateral decompression alone.[144] Posterior decompression techniques may compromise spinal stability through damage to the facets and ligamentous structures. Destabilization may lead to increases in pain, neurologic deficit, or progressive spinal deformity. In order to prevent this complication, posterior decompression procedures should routinely be accompanied by concomitant stabilization with instrumentation. The durability of modern instrumentation systems will exceed the lifespans of most patients. Therefore, instrumentation without simultaneous fusion can be performed to limit surgical time and morbidity.

Posterior stabilization has been shown to be effective in controlling pain secondary to vertebral instability or pathologic fracture. Approximately 90 percent of patients in one study reported pain relief with posterior segmental stabilization using Cotrel-Dubousset instrumentation.[150] In addition, 7 of 15 paraparetic or frankly paraplegic patients in this study regained the ability to walk without a formal spinal decompressive procedure simply through realignment and stabilization of their spinal columns. Likewise, other studies have found that a majority of patients benefit in terms of neurologic function from posterior segmental instrumentation in combination with posterolateral tumor debulking.[166,167] However, the results of these surgeries have been short-lived. Most patients had return of pain within 3 months of surgery. Of six who survived in one study, only three had relief for up to 2 years.[166]

The results of anterior surgery for malignant disease of the spine have proven to be superior to those obtained with posterior procedures. Kevin Harrington is commonly credited with popularizing the anterior reconstruction of the spine for metastatic disease. Several studies have documented pain relief in 80 to 90 percent of patients.[145,163] Up to 70 percent will improve neurologically as well. Some

50 percent of patients can be expected to regain the ability to ambulate, and bowel and bladder recovery can be expected in approximately 30 percent of paraparetic or paraplegic patients.[163] Approximately one-fifth of the patients will not benefit from surgery.[158] Many of these patients will have far advanced disease and will succumb to their malignancy prior to obtaining any real benefit from surgery. Others will have the benefit of surgery compromised by some type of complication. Anterior surgery is limited to disease at a single focus. Metastatic disease at multiple noncontiguous levels is probably better treated with a long posterior segmental instrumentation.

Since many cancer patients are debilitated prior to coming to surgery, complications can be expected to occur. Immunologic compromise and malnutrition are two factors that have been identified as major contributors to postoperative morbidity.[142,167] Likewise, the simultaneous administration of chemotherapy or radiation can interfere with wound healing and be a source of problems.[144] Wound breakdown in areas of previously irradiated skin can be expected. The use of meticulous surgical technique, nonabsorbable suture material for closure, and the retention of staples or skin sutures until the wound is fully healed may help to mitigate some of this difficulty. An acute mortality rate of approximately 5 percent can be expected in this type of surgery.[142,145,149] Most series document a rate of infection of between 3 and 10 percent.[142,163,166] Infection is more common following posterior surgery. New neurologic deficits are exceedingly rare. Likewise, with adequate surgical technique, loss of fixation either anteriorly or posteriorly is uncommon. For posterior constructs, fully segmented instrumentation with multiple hooks, screws, and/or sublaminar wires is recommended because of the anterior column deficiency that is present in most cases.

In most cases, completely clear surgical margins are not obtainable. However, adequate resection remains the most important factor in local control. In primary malignancy, a marginal resection can lead to a recurrence rate of up to 20 percent.[168] As with all oncologic disease, long-term survival depends on the ability of adjuvant chemotherapy and radiation to control and eradicate microscopic disease after surgical resection.

REFERENCES

1. Graziano GP, Sidhu KS: Salvage reconstruction in acute and late sequelae from pyogenic thoracolumbar infection. *J Spinal Dis* 16:199–207, 1993.
2. Stauffer RN: Pyogenic vertebral osteomyelitis. *Orthop Clin North Am* 6:1015–1027, 1975.
3. Rimalovski AB, Aronson SM: Abscess of medulla oblongata associated with osteomyelitis of odontoid process. *J Neurosurg* 29:97–101, 1968.
4. Connor PM, Darden BV: Cervical discography complications and clinical efficacy. *Spine* 18:2035–2038, 1993.
5. Elghazawi AK: Clinical syndromes and differential diagnosis of spinal disorders. *Radiol Clin North Am* 29:651–663, 1991.
6. Perronne C, Saba J, Behloul Z, et al: Pyogenic and tuberculous spondylodiskitis (vertebral osteomyelitis) in 80 adult patients. *Clin Infect Dis* 19:746–750, 1994.
7. Sapico FL, Montgomerie JZ: Pyogenic vertebral osteomyelitis: Report of nine cases and review of the literature. *Rev Infect Dis* 1:754–776, 1979.
8. Smith AS, Blaser SI: Infectious and inflammatory process of the spine. *Radiol Clin North Am* 29:809–827, 1991.
9. Bonakdar-pour A, Gaines VD: The radiology of osteomyelitis. *Orthop Clin North Am* 14:21–37, 1983.
10. Bryan V, Franks L, Torres H: *Pseudomonas aeruginosa* cervical diskitis with chondro-osteomyelitis in an intravenous drug abuser. *Surg Neurol* 1:142–144, 1973.
11. Tucker AL, Hubbard JG: Retropharyngeal infection with disc space involvement and osteomyelitis, following a pharyngeal flap operation. *Plast Reconstr Surg* 53:477–478, 1974.
12. Fein SJ, Torg JS, Mohnac AM, Magsamen BF: Infection of the cervical spine associated with a fracture of the mandible. *J Oral Surg* 27:146–149, 1969.
13. Peereboom D, Poretz DM: *Eikenella corrodens* cervical osteomyelitis: Case report. *Virginia Med* 114:150–153, 1987.
14. Ambrose GB, Alpert M, Neer CS: Vertebral osteomyelitis. *JAMA* 197:619–622, 1966.
15. Hall M, Williams A: Group G streptococcal osteomyelitis of the spine. *Br J Rheum* 32:342–345, 1993.
16. Larde D, Mathieu D, Frija J, et al: Vertebral osteomyelitis: Disk hypodensity on CT. *AJR* 139:963–967, 1982.
17. Burke DR, Brant-Zawadzki: CT of pyogenic spine infection. *Neuroradiology* 27:131–137, 1985.
18. Ratcliffe JF: Anatomic basis for the pathogenesis and radiologic features of vertebral osteomyelitis and its differentiation from childhood discitis. *Acta Radiol Diagn* 26:137–143, 1985.
19. Fang D, Cheung KMC, Dos Remedios IDM, et al: Pyogenic vertebral osteomyelitis: Treatment by anterior spinal debridement and fusion. *J Spinal Dis* 7:173–180, 1994.
20. Kemp HBS, Jackson JW, Jeremiah JD, Hall AJ: Pyogenic infections occurring primarily in intervertebral discs. *J Bone Joint Surg* 55B:698–714, 1973.
21. Resnick D, Niwayama G, Guerra J Jr, et al: Spinal vacuum phenomena: Anatomical study and review. *Radiology* 139:341–348, 1981.
22. Nair S, Vender J, McCormack TM, Black P: Renal osteodystrophy of the cervical spine: Neurosurgical implications. *Neurosurgery* 33:349–355, 1993.
23. Arnold MH, Brooks PM, Ryan M, Francis H: A destructive discovertebral lesion: Septic discitis, ankylosing spondylitis, or rheumatoid arthritis? *Clin Rheum* 8:277–281, 1989.
24. Price AC, Allen JH, Eggers FM, et al: Intervertebral disk-space infection: CT changes. *Radiology* 149:725–729, 1983.
25. McGahan JP, Dublin AB: Evaluation of spinal infections by plain radiographs, computed tomography, intrathecal metrizamide, and CT-guided biopsy. *Diagn Imaging Clin Med* 54:11–20, 1985.
26. Wukich DK, Van Dam BE, Abreu SH: Preoperative indium-labeled white blood cell scintigraphy in suspected ostemyelitis of the axial skeleton. *Spine* 13(10):1168–1170, 1988.
27. Streule K, De Schrijver M, Fridrick R: ^{99}Tcm-labelled HSA-nanocolloid versus ^{111}In oxine-labelled granulocytes in detecting skeletal septic process. *Nucl Med Commun* 9:59–67, 1988.
28. Staheli LT, Nelp WB, Marty R: Strontium 87m scanning. *JAMA* 221:1159–1160, 1972.
29. Kerslake RW, Worthington BS: MRI of the spine. *Clin Radiol* 43:227–233, 1991.
30. Szypryt EP, Hardy JG, Hinton CE, et al: A comparison between magnetic resonance imagining and scintigraphic bone imaging in the diagnosis of disc space infection in an animal model. *Spine* 13:1042–1048, 1988.
31. Lutz JE: Magnetic resonance imaging and the diagnosis of spinal infections. *Ann Intern Med* 15:348, 1988.

32. Modic MT, Masaryk T, Paushter D: Magnetic resonance imaging of the spine. *Radiol Clin North Am* 24:229–245, 1986.

33. Hyman RA, Gorey MT: Imaging strategies for MR of the spine. *Radiol Clin North Am* 26:505–533, 1988.

34. Donovan Post MJ, Bowen BC, Sze G: Magnetic resonance imaging of spinal infection. *Rheum Dis Clin North Am* 17:773–794, 1991.

35. Lamminen HA, Salonen O, Raininko R: MR imaging of the lower spine. *Acta Radiol* 35:532–540, 1994.

36. Donovan Post MJ, Sze G, Quencer M, et al: Gadolinium-enhanced MR in spinal infection. *J Comput Assist Tomogr* 14:721–729, 1990.

37. Cotty PH, Fouquet B, Pleskof L, et al: Vertebral osteomyelitis: Value of percutaneous biopsy. *J Neuroradiol* 15:13–21, 1988.

38. Ducker TB: Continuing controversy of disc space infection. *J Spinal Dis* 1:320–322, 1989.

39. Ducker TB: Disc space infection. *J Spinal Dis* 1:236–242, 1988.

40. Naunheim KS, Barnett MG, Crandall DG, et al: Anterior exposure of the thoracic spine. *Ann Thorac Surg* 57:1436–1439, 1994.

41. Rubery PT, Smith MD, Cammisa FP, Silane M: Mycotic aortic aneurysm in patients who have lumbar vertebral osteomyelitis. *J Bone Joint Surg* 77A:1729–1732, 1995.

42. O'Brien JP: Kyphosis secondary to infectious disease. *Clin Orthop Rel Res* 128:56–64, 1977.

43. Keiser RP, Grimes HA: Intervetevral disk space infections in children. *Clin Orthop Rel Res* 30:163–166, 1963.

44. Smith AS, Weinstein MA, Mizushima A, et al: MR imaging characteristics of tuberculous spondylitis vs vertebral osteomyelitis. *AJNR* 153:399–405, 1989.

45. Buchelt M, Lack W, Kutschera HP, et al: Comparison of tuberculous and pyogenic spondylitis. *Clin Orthop Rel Res* 296:192–199, 1993.

46. Hoffman EB, Crosier JH, Cremin BJ: Imaging in children with spinal tuberculosis. *J Bone Joint Surg* 75B:233–239, 1993.

47. MRC Working Party on Tuberculosis of the Spine: Controlled trial of short-course regimens of chemotherapy in the ambulatory treatment of spinal tuberculosis. *J Bone Joint Surg* 75B:240–248, 1993.

48. Nussbaum ES, Rockwold GL, Bergman TA, et al: Spinal tuberculosis: A diagnostic and management challenge. *J Neurosurg* 83:243–247, 1995.

49. Rezai AR, Lee M, Cooper PR, et al: Modern management in spinal tuberculosis. *Neurosurgery* 36:87–98, 1995.

50. Hodgson AR, Stock FE: Anterior spinal fusion. *Clin Orthop Rel Res* 300:16–23, 1994.

51. Upadhyay SS, See P, Saji MJ, et al: 17-year prospective study of surgical management of spinal tuberculosis in children. *Spine* 18:1704–1711, 1993.

52. Upadhyay SS, Sell P, Saji MJ, et al: Surgical management of spinal tuberculosis in adults. *Clin Orthop Rel Res* 302:173–182, 1994.

53. Upadhyay SS, Saji MJ, Sell P, et al: Longitudinal changes in spinal deformity after anterior spinal surgery for tuberculosis of the spine in adults. *Spine* 19:542–549, 1994.

54. Upadhyay SS, Saju MJ, Sell P, Yau AC: The effect of age on the change in deformity after radical resection and anterior arthrodesis for tuberculosis of the spine. *J Bone Joint Surg* 76A:701–708, 1994.

55. Chen W, Chen C, Shih C: Surgical treatment of tuberculous spondylitis. *Acta Orthop Scand* 66:137–142, 1995.

56. Guven O, Kmano K, Yalcin S, et al: A single stage posterior approach and rigid fixation for preventing kyphosis in the treatment of spinal tuberculosis. *Spine* 19:1039–1043, 1994.

57. Oga M, Arizono T, Takasita M, Suigioka Y: Evaluation of the risk of instrumentation as a foreign body in spinal tuberculosis. *Spine* 18:1890–1894, 1993.

58. Buruma OJS, Craan H, Kunsi MW: Vertebral osteomyelitis and epidural abcess due to mucormycosis. *Clin Neurol Neurosurg* 81:39–44, 1979.

59. Hayes WS, Berg RA, Dorfman HD, Freedman MT: Case report 291. *Skel Radiol* 12:284–287, 1984.

60. Hummel M, Schuler S, Weber U, et al: Aspergillosis with aspergillus osteomyelitis and diskitis after heart transplantation: Surgical and medical management. *J Heart Lung Trans* 12:599–603, 1993.

61. Kashimoto T, Kitagawa H, Kachi H: *Candida tropicalis* vertebral osteomyelitis and discitis. *Spine* 11:57–61, 1986.

62. Dalinka MK, Dinnenberg S, Greendyke WH, Hopkins R: Roentgenographic features of osseous coccidioidomycosis and differential diagnosis. *J Bone Joint Surg* 53A:1157–1164, 1971.

63. Claesson B, Falsen E, Kjellman B: *Kingella kingae* infections: A review and a presentation of data from 10 Swedish cases. *Scand J Infect Dis* 17:233–243, 1985.

64. Shaikh BS, Appelbaum PC, Aber RC: Vertebral disc space infection and osteomyelitis due to *Candida albicans* in a patient with acute myelomonocytic leukemia. *Cancer* 45:1025–1028, 1980.

65. Diament MJ, Weller M, Berstein R: *Candida* infection in a premature infant presenting as discitis. *Pediatr Radiol* 12:96–98, 1982.

66. Sugar AM, Saunders C, Diamond RD: Successful treatment of *Candida* osteomyelitis with fluconazole. *Diagn Microbiol Infect Dis* 13:517–520, 1990.

67. Tekkok IH, Berker M, Ozcan OE, et al: Brucellosis of the spine. *Neurosurgery* 33:838–844, 1993.

68. Kihtir T, Ivatury RR, Simon R, Stahl WM: Management of transperitoneal gunshot wounds of the spine. *J Trauma* 31:1579–1583, 1991.

69. Thakur RC, Khosla VK, Kak VK: Non-missile penetrating injuries of the spine. *Acta Neurochir* 113:144–148, 1991.

70. Jones RE, Bucholz RW, Schaeffer SD, et al: Cervical osteomyelitis complicating transpharyngeal gunshot wounds to the neck. *J Trauma* 19:630–634, 1979.

71. Hales DD, Duffy K, Dawson EG, Delamarter R: Lumbar osteomyelitis and epidural and paraspinous abscesses. *Spine* 15:380–383, 1991.

72. Hales DD, Duffy K, Dawson EG, Delamarter R: Lumbar osteomyelitis and epidural and paraspinous abscesses. *Spine* 16:380–383, 1991.

73. Romanick PC, Smith TK, Kopaniky DR, Oldfield D: Infection about the spine associated with low-velocity-missile injury to the abdomen. *J Bone Joint Surg* 67A:1195–1201, 1985.

74. Miller BR, Schiller WR: Pyogenic vertebral osteomyelitis after transcolonic gunshot wound. *Mil Med* 154:64–66, 1989.

75. Modic MT, Pavlicek W, Weinstein MA, et al: Magnetic resonance imaging of intervertebral disk disease. *Radiology* 152:103–111, 1984.

76. King HA: Back pain in children. *Pediatr Clin North Am* 31:1083–1095, 1984.

77. Spiegel PG, Kengla KW, Isaacson AS, Wilson JC: Intervertebral disc-space inflammation in children. *J Bone Joint Surg* 54A:284–296, 1972.

78. Rocco HD, Eyring EJ: Intervertebral disk infections in children. *Am J Dis Child* 123:448–451, 1972.

79. Peterson HA: Disk-space infection in children. *AAOS Instr Course Lect* 32:50–60, 1983.

80. Heller RM, Szalay EA, Green NE, et al: Disc space infection in children: Magnetic resonance imaging. *Radiol Clin North Am* 26:207–209, 1988.

81. Peterson HA: Disk-space infection in children. *AAOS Instr Course Lect* 28.

82. Eismont FJ, Bohlman HH, Soni PL, et al: Vertebral osteomyelitis in infants. *J Bone Joint Surg* 64B:32–35, 1982.

83. Bonfiglio M, Lange TA, Kim YM: Pyogenic vertebral osteomyelitis. *Clin Orthop Rel Res* 96:234–246, 1973.

84. Miller JH, Wahner HW, Wellman WE: Disk-space infection: Localization with gallium 67. *Minn Med* 60:65–168, 1977.

85. Taylor TKF, Dooley BJ: Antibiotics in the management of postoperative disc space infections. *Aust NZ J Surg* 48:74–77, 1978.

86. Scott M: Surgery of the spinal column and cord. *Prog Neurol Psychiatry* 25:294–304, 1970.

87. Djukic S, Lang P, Morris J, et al: The postoperative spine. *Orthop Clin North Am* 21:603–624, 1990.

88. Blankstein A, Rubinstein E, Ezra E, et al: Disc space infection and vertebral osteomyelitis as a complication of percutaneous lateral discectomy. *Clin Orthop Rel Res* 225:234–237, 1987.

89. Boden DK, Davis DO, Dina TS, et al: Postoperative diskitis: Distinguishing early MR imaging findings from normal postoperative disk space changes. *Radiology* 184:765–771, 1992.

90. Jevsevar KS, Karlin LI: The relationship between preoperative nutritional status and complications after an operation for scoliosis in patients who have cerebral palsy. *J Bone Joint Surg* 75A:880–884, 1993.

91. Stambough JL, Beringer D: Postoperative wound infections complicating adult spine surgery. *J Spinal Dis* 5:277–285, 1992.

92. Robertson PA, Taylor TK: Late presentation of infection as a complication of Dwyer anterior spinal instrumentation. *J Bone Joint Surg* 6:256–259, 1993.

93. Shektman A, Granick MS, Solomon MP, et al: Management of infected laminectomy wounds. *Neurosurgery* 35:307–309, 1994.

94. Seyfer AE: The lower trapezius flap for recalcitrant wounds of the posterior skull and spine. *Ann Plast Surg* 20:414–418, 1988.

95. Dernbach PD, Gomez H, Hahn J: Primary closure of infected spinal wounds. *Neurosurgery* 26:707–709, 1990.

96. Harle A, van Ende R: Management of wound sepsis after spinal fusion surgery. *Acta Orthop Belg* 57:242–246, 1991.

97. Richards BS: Delayed infections following posterior spinal instrumentation for the treatment of idiopathic scoliosis. *J Bone Joint Surg* 77A:524–529, 1995.

98. Dahlin DC, Kirshanan KU (eds): *Bone Tumors: General Aspects and Data on 8,542 Cases.* Springfield IL, Charles C Thomas, 1986.

99. DiLorenzo N, Nardi P, Ciappetta P, Fortuna A: Benign tumors and tumorlike conditions of the spine: Radiological features, treatment, and results. *Surg Neurol* 25:449, 1986.

100. Mirra JM, Picci P: General considerations, in Mirra JM (ed): *Bone Tumors, Clinical, Radiologic, and Pathologic Corrections.* Philadelphia, Lea & Febinger, 1989, p 13.

101. Sung HW, Shu WP, Wang HM, et al: Surgical treatment of primary tumors of the sacrum. *Clin Orthop* 215:91, 1987.

102. Ehrlich MG, Zaleske DJ: Pediatric orthopedic pain of unknown origin. *J Pediatr Orthop* 6:460, 1986.

103. Kirwan EO'G, Hutton PAN, Pozo JL, Ransford AO: Osteoid osteoma and benign osteoblastoma of the spine. *J Bone Joint Surg* 66B:21, 1984.

104. Pettine KA, Klassen RA: Osteoid-osteoma and osteoblastoma of the spine. *J Bone Joint Surg* 68A:354, 1986.

105. Sinar EJ, Marice-Williams RS: Spinal extradural tumour mimicking a lumber disc protrusion. *J R Coll Surg Edinburgh* 32:179, 1987.

106. Richardson RL: A report of 16 tumors of the spinal cord in children: The importance of spinal rigidity as an early sign of disease. *J Pediatr* 57:42, 1960.

107. Taylor LJ: Painful scoliosis: A need for further investigation. *Br Med J* 292:120, 1986.

108. Horsfield D, Macvicar D: A painful adolescent back. *Radiography* 53:1990.

109. Levine AM, Boriani S, Donati D, Campanacci M: Benign tumors of the cervical spine. *Spine* 17:S399, 1992.

110. Enneking WF: Spine, in Enneking WF (ed): *Musculoskeletal Tumor Surgery.* New York, Churchill Livingstone, 1983, p 303.

111. Sweriduk ST, Deluca SA: The sclerotic pedicle. *Am Fam Phys* 35:161, 1987.

112. Kumar R, Guinto FC Jr, Madewell JE et al: Expansile bone lesions of the vertebra. *RadioGraphics* 8:749, 1988.

113. Kozlowski K, Barylak A, Campbell J, et al: Primary sacral bone tumours in children (report of 16 cases with a short literature review). *Australas Radiol* 34:142, 1990.

114. Hayden JW: Back pain in childhood. *Pediatr Clinic North Am* 14:611, 1967.

115. Mohan V, Sabri T, Marklund T, et al: Clinicoradiological diagnosis of benign osteoblastoma of the spine in children. *Arch Orthop Trauma Surg* 110:260, 1991.

116. Villas C, Lopez R, Zubieta JL: Osteoid osteoma in the lumbar and sacral regions: Two cases of difficult diagnosis. *J Spinal Dis* 3:418, 1990.

117. Botsford DJ, Esses SI: Normal radionuclide scan in a giant cell tumor of the spine. *Orthopedics* 14:790, 1991.

118. Makhija M, Bofill ER: Hemangioma: A rare cause of photopenic lesion on skeletal imaging. *Clin Nuclear Med* 13:661, 1988.

119. Crim JR, Mirra JM, Eckardt JJ, Seeger LL: Widespread inflammatory response to osteoblastoma: The flare phenomenon. *Radiology* 177:835, 1990.

120. Davis PC, Hoffman JC Jr, Ball TI, et al: Spinal abnormalities in pediatric patients: MR imaging findings compared with clinical, myelographic, and surgical findings. *Radiology* 166:679, 1988.

121. Masaryk TJ: Neoplastic disease of the spine. *Radiol Clin North Am* 29:829, 1991.

122. Beltran J, Aparisi F, Bonmati LM, et al: Eosinophilic granuloma: MRI manifestations. *Skel Radiol* 22:157, 1993.

123. Woods ER, Martel W, Mandell SH, Crabbe JP: Reactive soft-tissue mass associated with osteoid osteoma: Correlation of MR imaging features with pathologic findings. *Radiology* 186:221, 1993.

124. Shikata J, Yamamuro T, Shimizu Katsuji, et al: Surgical treatment of giant-cell tumors of the spine. *Clin Orthop Rel Res* 278:29, 1992.

125. Bridwell KH, Ogilvie JW: Primary tumors of the spine (benign and malignant), in Bridwell KH, DeWald RL (eds): *The Textbook of Spinal Surgery.* Philadelphia, Lippincott, 1991, p 1143.

126. Ohry A, Lipschitz M, Shemesh Y, et al: Disappearance of quadriparesis due to a huge cervicothoracic aneurysmal bone cyst. *Surg Neurol* 29:307, 1988.

127. Faria SL, Schlupp WR, Chiminazzo H Jr: Radiotherapy in the treatment of vertebral hemangiomas. *Int J Radiat Oncol Biol Phys* 11:387, 1985.

128. Schild SE, Buskirk SJ, Frick LM, Cupps RE: Radiotherapy for large symptomatic hemangiomas. *Int J Radiat Oncol Biol Phys* 21:729, 1991.

129. Turcotte RE, Sim FH, Unni KK: Giant cell tumor of the sacrum. *Clin Orthop Rel Res* 291:215, 1993.

130. Walker DR, Rankin RN, Anderson C, Rock MG: Giant-cell tumour of the sacrum in a child. *Can J Surg* 31:47, 1988.

131. Sanjay BKS, Sim FH, Unni KK, et al: Giant-cell tumours of the spine. *J Bone Joint Surg* 75B:148, 1993.

132. Dickinson LD, Farhat SM: Eosinophilic granuloma of the cervical spine: A case report and review of the literature. *Surg Neurol* 35:57, 1991.

133. Kornberg M: Erythrocyte sedimentation rate following lumbar discectomy. *Spine* 11:766, 1986.

134. Silberstein MJ, Sundaram M, Akbarnia B, et al: Eosinophilic granuloma of the spine: Radiologic case study. *Orthopedics* 8:264, 1985.

135. Martinez-Lage JF, Poza M, Cartagena J, et al: Solitary eosinophilic granuloma of the pediatric skull and spine. *Childs Nerv Syst* 7:448, 1991.

136. Dalinka MK, Mazzeo VP Jr: Complications of radiation therapy. *CRC Crit Rev Diagn Imaging* 23:235, 1985.

137. Ransford AO, Pozo JL, Hutton PAN, Kriwan EOG: The behaviour pattern of the scoliosis associated with osteoid osteoma or osteoblastoma of the spine. *J Bone Joint Surg* 66B:16, 1984.

138. Aulisa L, Tamburrelli F, Galli M: Osteoblastoma of the atlas. *Childs Nerv Syst* 9:115, 1993.

139. Boriani S, Capanna R, Donati D, et al: Osteoblastoma of the spine. *Clin Orthop Rel Res* 278:37, 1992.

140. Dessner DA, Martin DS, Pittman T, Sundaram M: Vertebral osteoblastoma. *Orthopedics* 15:393, 1992.

141. Inci S, Akbay A, Bertan V: Giant-cell tumour of the lumbar spine: Case report. *Paraplegia* 31:412, 1993.

142. Hammerberg KW: Surgical treatment of metastatic spine disease. *Spine* 17:1148–1153, 1992.

143. Harrington KD: Current concepts review metastatic disease of the spine. *J Bone Joint Surg* 68A:1110–1115, 1986.

144. Weller SJ, Rossitch E Jr: Unilateral posterolateral decompression without stabilization for neurological palliation of symptomatic spinal metastasis in debilitated patients. *J Neurosurg* 82:739–744, 1995.

145. Harrington KD: Anterior decompression and stabilization of the spine as a treatment for vertebral collapse and spinal cord compression from metastatic malignancy. *Clin Orthop Rel Res* 233:177–197, 1988.

146. Livingston KE, Perrin RG: The neurosurgical management of spinal metastases causing cord and cauda equina compression. *J Neurosurg* 49:839–843, 1978.

147. Coraddu M, Nurchi GC, Floris F, Meleddu V: Surgical treatment of extradural spinal cord compression due to metastatic tumours. *Acta Neurochir* 111:18–21, 1991.

148. Orcutt FV: Surgical management of spinal metastases. *West J Med* 159:483–484, 1993.

149. Malawski SK: The results of surgical treatment of primary spinal tumors. *Clin Orthop Rel Res* 272:50–57, 1991.

150. Rompe JD, Eysel P Hopf C, Heine J: Decompression/stabilization of the metastatic spine. *Acta Orthop Scand* 64:3–8, 1993.

151. Yoshino MT, Carmody RF: Osteosarcoma of the cervical spine. *AJR* 157:1357, 1991.

152. Shives TC, Dahlin DC, Sim FH, et al: Osteosarcoma of the spine. *J Bone Joint Surg* 68A:660–668, 1986.

153. Bielack SS, Wulff B, Delling G, et al: Osteosarcoma of the trunk treated by multimodal therapy: Experience of the Cooperative Osteosarcoma study group (COSS). *Med Pediatr Oncol* 24:6–12, 1995.

154. Barwick KW, Huvox AG, Smith J: Primary osteogenic sarcoma of the vertebral column: A clinicopathologic correlation of ten patients. *Cancer* 46:595–604, 1980.

155. Harrington KD: The use of methylmethacrylate for vertebral-body replacement and anterior stabilization of pathological fracture-dislocations of the spine due to metastatic malignant disease. *J Bone Joint Surg* 63A:36–46, 1981.

156. Kleinman WB, Kiernan HA, Michelsen WJ: Metastatic cancer of the spinal column. *Clin Orthop Rel Res* 136:166–172, 1978.

157. Raycroft JF, Hockman RP, Southwick WO: Metastatic tumors involving the cervical vertebrae: Surgical palliation. *J Bone Joint Surg* 60A:763–768, 1978.

158. Harrington KD: Anterior cord decompression and spinal stabilization for patients with metastatic lesions of the spine. *J Neurosurg* 61:107–117, 1984.

159. Calliauw L, Dallenga A, Caemaert J: Trans-sternal approach to intraspinal tumours in the upper thoracic region. *Acta Neurochir* 127:227–231, 1994.

160. Errico TJ, Cooper PR: A new method of thoracic and lumbar body replacement for spinal tumors: Technical note. *Neurosurgery* 32:678–681, 1993.

161. Cooper PR, Errico TJ, Martin R, et al: A systematic approach to spinal reconstruction after anterior decompression for neoplastic disease of the thoracic and lumbar spine. *Neurosurgery* 32:1–8, 1993.

162. Sundaresan N, DiGiacinto GV, Krol G, Hughes JE: Spondylectomy for malignant tumors of the spine. *J Clin Oncol* 7:1485–1491, 1989.

163. Kostuik JP, Errico TJ, Gealson TF, Errico CC: Spinal stabilization of vertebral column tumors. *Spine* 13:250–256, 1988.

164. Bednar DA, Brox WT, Viviani GR: Surgical palliation of spinal oncologic disease: A review and analysis of current approaches. *Can J Surg* 34:129–131, 1991.

165. Nicholls PJ, Jarecky TW: The value of posterior decompression by laminectomy for malignant tumors of the spine. *Clin Orthop Rel Res* 201:210–213, 1985.

166. Bridwell KH, Jenny AB, Saul T, et al: Posterior segmental spinal instrumentation (PSSI) with posterolateral decompression and debulking for metastatic thoracic and lumbar spine disease. *Spine* 13:1383–1394, 1988.

167. DeWald RL, Bridwell KH, Prodromas C, Rodts MF: Reconstructive spinal surgery as palliation for metastatic malignancies of the spine. *Spine* 10:21–26, 1985.

168. Gibson JNA, Reid R, McMaster MJ: Fibrocartilaginous mesenchymoma of the fifth lumbar vertebra treated by vertebrectomy. *Spine* 19:1992–1997, 1994.

CHAPTER 72

Degenerative Disorders of the Lumbar and Thoracic Spine

Michael P. Chapman

BACK PAIN: ITS INCIDENCE AND ETIOLOGY

Degenerative changes in the spine are inevitable as we age. However, not everyone with degenerative changes develops symptoms. Regardless of the degree of degenerative change, nearly everyone experiences at least occasional low back pain. The National Health and Nutrition Examination Survey reports that 60 to 80 percent of people have low back pain at some time in their lives, and prevalence rates are around 30 percent—i.e., 3 of 10 adults have low back pain at any given time.[4]

The peak prevalence increases with increasing age. This suggests that the natural degeneration or maturation process of the spine has something to do with the cause of low back pain. However, there is little correlation between the degree of radiographic degeneration and degree of low back pain. In fact, many young people with radiographically "normal" spines have severe low back pain. So what is the cause? This is the subject of considerable debate.

While there are certainly biochemical and histologic changes contributing to the pain, we must first understand what nonphysiologic factors may be contributing.

It is widely accepted that physically demanding work increases the incidence of low back pain and disk herniation. This would include jobs that require frequent bending, lifting, twisting, pushing, and pulling; repetitive work; static work; awkward posture; and vibration. Psychological and psychosocial factors may also play a role. The last two are probably more influential than are the previously mentioned occupational factors contributing to back disability (Table 72-1).

A number of individual factors have been discussed as potential risk factors for low back pain. Advancing age puts a patient at high risk of low back pain, and elderly females have the highest prevalence. The presence of kyphosis and scoliosis and leg-length discrepancy are important risk factors only if these deformities are large. Height, weight, and body build are probably overrated with regard to their importance in low back pain. The very tall and very obese have more low back pain, but otherwise these factors are unimportant. General physical fitness is most important in aiding recovery for a back pain episode, but it is not a predictor of future risk. Smokers have an increased risk of low back pain. Smoking decreases the oxygen tension in spinal tissue such as the disk and therefore increases the risk of disk degeneration. Heredity may also play a role, but most feel the environmental factors are the most important (Table 72-2).

PATHOANATOMIC CONSIDERATIONS

Theoretically, any structure with pain receptors in the lumbar spine may be a cause of back pain (Fig. 72-1). Since pain is a subjective complaint and can occur in the absence of tissue damage, most episodes of back pain are probably due to a local affliction in the supporting structures of the lumbar spine. We can best institute treatment if we have some understanding of the mechanisms of spinal pain.

Diskogenic Pain

The intervertebral disk has long been considered a potential source of low back pain. The fact that disk herniations typically follow one or more episodes of low back pain supports this concept.[107] Also lending support is the provocative pain response following intradiskal injection of hypertonic saline or contrast in the presence of annular tears.[61,64]

TABLE 72-1   Occupational Factors Associated with an Increased Risk of Low Back Pain

Heavy physical work
Frequent bending and twisting
Lifting, pushing, and pulling
Repetitive work
Static work postures
Vibrations
Psychological and psychosocial factors

Source: Reproduced with permission from Andersson GBH: in Weinstein JN, Rydevik BL, Sonntag VKH (eds): *Essentials of the Spine.* New York, Raven Press, 1995, p 6.

TABLE 72-2   Individual Factors Often Discussed as Potential Risk Factors in Low Back Pain

Factor	Importance
Age	Certain
Sex	Probable (age-dependent)
Posture	Low (severe only)
Anthropometry	Low (extremes only)
Muscle strength	Low (work-related)
Physical fitness	Low (work-related)
Spine mobility	Low
Smoking	Probable

Source: Reproduced with permission from Andersson GBH: in Weinstein JN, Rydevik BL, Sonntag VKH (eds): *Essentials of the Spine.* New York, Raven Press, 1995, page 7.

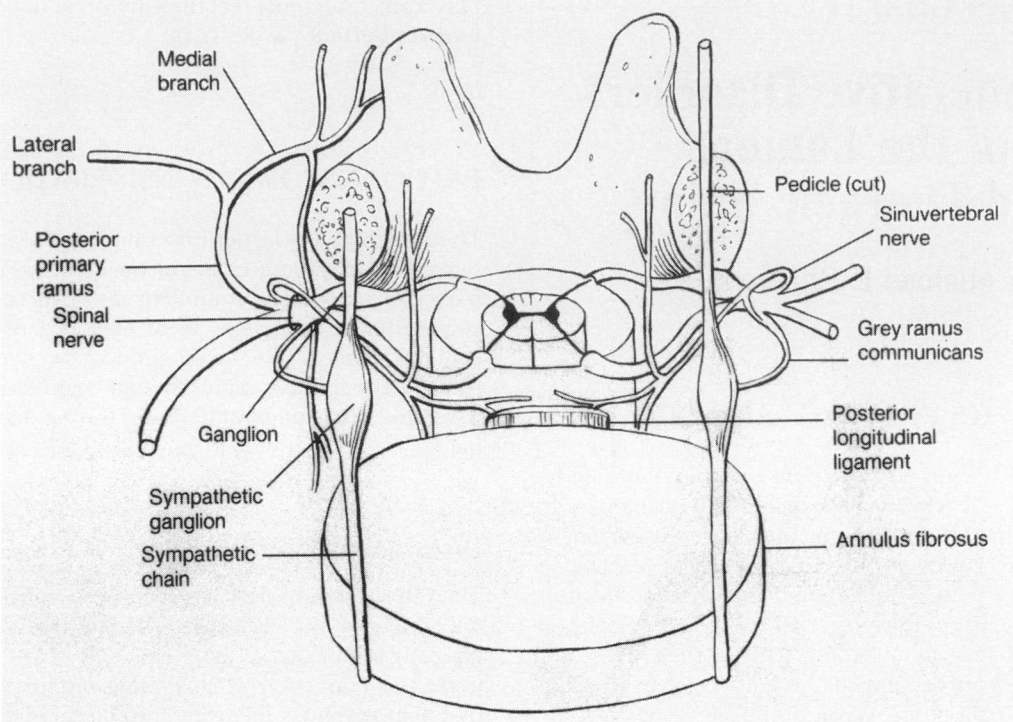

Figure 72-1 Neural innervation of the spine. (Reproduced with permission from Esses SI (ed): *Textbook of Spinal Disorders.* Philadelphia, Lippincott, 1995, page 29.)

Other authors have produced central back pain by stimulating the posterior central annulus and posterior longitudinal ligament.[89,159] Lending further support to the disk as a pain generator is the presence of free nerve endings in the outer layer of the annulus fibrosus and within the anterior and posterior longitudinal ligaments.[14,25,70,95] With the use of immunohistochemical methods, it has been proved that these neural elements are related to spinal pain.[156]

The healthy disk is 90 to 95 percent water, with collagen and proteoglycans making up the rest. The collagen is primarily type 1 in the outermost aspect of the annulus and type 2 in the innermost. The nucleus is type 2 collagen. With aging, this composition changes; the water and proteoglycan content decreases and there is an increase in the keratin sulfate/chondroitin sulfate ratio. This changing composition leads to fragmentation of the disk and fissuring of the annulus.[34,62]

The presence of an annular tear does not necessarily mean that this is a painful disk. In fact, there is very little evidence supporting a mere tear as a pain generator. However, there is some evidence to support the view that asymmetrical radial tears are more likely to be painful than more symmetrical degeneration. Some authors have also demonstrated a decrease in pH within a degenerating disk, which could be irritating to the nerve root.[61,70,106] The pH hypothesis remains controversial.

The intervertebral disk depends exclusively on passive diffusion through the end plates and the peripheral annulus for nutrition. Since this structure is avascular, there is no healing potential for the fissuring and fragmentation that occurs.[101] As such, the process continues

as one ages. Kirkaldy-Willis and Hill have divided the whole process into three distinct phases.[82] The first stage, dysfunction, is generally in the 15- to 45-year age range and is characterized by circumferential and radial tears in the annulus and synovitis of the facets. The next stage, instability, is found in 35- to 70-year-olds and is characterized by internal disk disruption, progressive disk resorption, degeneration of the facets with capsular laxity, subluxation, and joint erosion. The final stage, found in patients over 60, is stabilization, in which the development of hypertrophic bone has led to segmental stiffening or frank ankylosis. Each spinal segment goes through this process at a different rate.

While going through the dysfunction and instability stages, some disks herniate. The explanation of why some do and most do not is probably multifactorial. In a smaller percentage of patients, the disk herniation may be partially due to a familial predisposition.[149] More likely are the previously mentioned occupational factors, which could create a torsional injury damaging the outermost layers of the annulus. Combine this with the loss of compressive stiffness from the degeneration, and an unstable situation develops. This torsional instability may explain the episodic nature of low back pain syndromes.

Facet Joint Pain

The lumbar facet joint has long been considered a potential source of low back pain.[8,41,44] Several studies have reproduced typical low back pain with thigh radiation by injecting hypertonic saline into the facet joint capsule.[61,90,105]

Each facet joint receives innervation from at least two spinal levels.[105] Immunohistochemical techniques and electrophysiologic studies have shown the presence of nociceptors in the facet joints.[6,166]

There are a number of different mechanisms whereby the facets may cause low back pain. One is simply pain from osteoarthritis, similar to arthritis pain from other joints.[83] Another potential mechanism is the compression of the nerve root secondary to the degenerative changes of the facet joint, creating lateral recess stenosis via hypertrophy of the degenerating facet. Last, some feel that pain can be induced by a mechanical blockage of the facet by a synovial fold.[83] This has never been proved.

Facet pain, like other types of pain in the spine, is difficult to localize; there seems to be no specific pain pattern that distinguishes facet pain from other potential types of pain.[98] In an effort to localize the facet joints as the pain source, some authors have utilized facet joint injections as both a diagnostic and therapeutic modality.[33,92,105] Several studies, however, fail to demonstrate significant success with this technique.[71,91] The role of facet injections is, at best, controversial.

Nerve Root Pain

Mixter and Barr[102] were among the first to recognize that compressed nerve roots from a herniated disk resulted in low back pain and sciatica. Verbiest[150] was first to describe spinal stenosis as another cause of radicular pain. In this situation, the nerve roots are compressed by hypertrophied posterior elements and bulging disks. Spondylolysis and spondylolisthesis also have been implicated in nerve root irritation.

Exactly how these conditions cause pain has been the subject of considerable research. Simple compression of a nerve root creates sensory and motor symptoms but no pain.[136] Chronically irritated nerve roots, on the other hand, tend to be painful when compressed.[66,136] Most authors feel that the different reactions of normal and irritated nerve roots are related to one or more of the following factors: (1) alteration in intraneural blood flow; (2) problems with axoplasmic transport; and (3) inflammation, edema, and/or demyelination.[108,123]

Muscle-Induced Pain

The lumbar paraspinal muscles and associated soft tissues have been implicated in spinal pain. Myofascial pain syndrome is a condition in which there are characteristic trigger points that produce the patient's pain when pressure is applied. Trigger point injections can be therapeutic and diagnostically helpful.[137] Another possible muscular source of low back pain is lumbar paraspinal compartment syndrome.[21,117] Deconditioned spinal extensor muscles can also be a source of persistent back pain due to muscle fatigue.

Referred Pain

The wide variation of pain seen clinically for a particular condition (hip pain in an L5-S1 herniated disk, for example) could be explained by referred pain rather than radicular pain.

Referred pain is pain caused by a lesion of a spinal motion segment located in the back and radiating somewhere distal in a nondermatomal pattern, as to the buttocks, thighs, hips, and occasionally the lower leg. Referred pain is often confused with sciatica, but the term *sciatica* should be reserved for nerve root pain in a specific dermatomal distribution. An understanding of the sensory dermatomes and muscle innervations is extremely important in localizing the specific dermatome involved (Fig. 72-2, Table 72-3). Kellgren[81] was the first to label the vague anatomic distributions of referred pain as *sclerotomal,* differentiating it from the more specific dermatomes. The sclerotomes are formed by connective tissue structures such as bone and cartilage. These different parts of the skeleton have innervations that may be related to specific nerve roots, and this is the sclerotomal innervation. The sclerotomal distribution is quite different from the dermatomal distribution. Whereas an L4-5 herniated disk might be expected to cause pain into the dorsum of the foot and to weaken the extensor hallucis longus, problems in the facet joints, ligaments, or disks at this level irritating the same nerve might create a dull pain at the region of the hip and femur rather than radiating into the lower legs.[84]

An understanding of the neuroanatomy of the spinal segments might help to explain how degeneration of the disk or facet or irritation of a ligament can produce referred pain. The sinovertebral nerve is a recurrent branch off the spinal nerve that originates just distal to the dorsal root ganglion and reenters the neural foramen. It divides into superior and inferior branches that supply the periosteum, posterior longitudinal ligament, dura, outer layer of the annulus, and epidural vessels of several adjacent segments. The posterior primary ramus has branches that innervate the facets, paravertebral muscles, fascia, ligaments, and laminae[114] (Fig. 72-1).

The differentiation between referred pain and radiculopathic pain is often difficult. Referred pain is usually poorly localized, dull, and less superficial than root pain.[94] Obviously, an accurate differentiation of referred pain from radiculopathy is important in achieving a good result in the treatment of patients with back and leg pain.

Dorsal Root Ganglion

The dorsal root ganglion (DRG) is considered by many authors a key structure relating to low back and radicular pain.[99,154] Substance P and calcitonin gene–related peptide (CGRP) are the most abundant peptides of the dorsal root ganglion and have been implicated in nociception.[42]

Rydevik et al.[124] feel that mechanical compression of the DRG with resultant intraneural edema and decrease in the cell body's blood supply causes a release of these pain-inducing neural peptides.

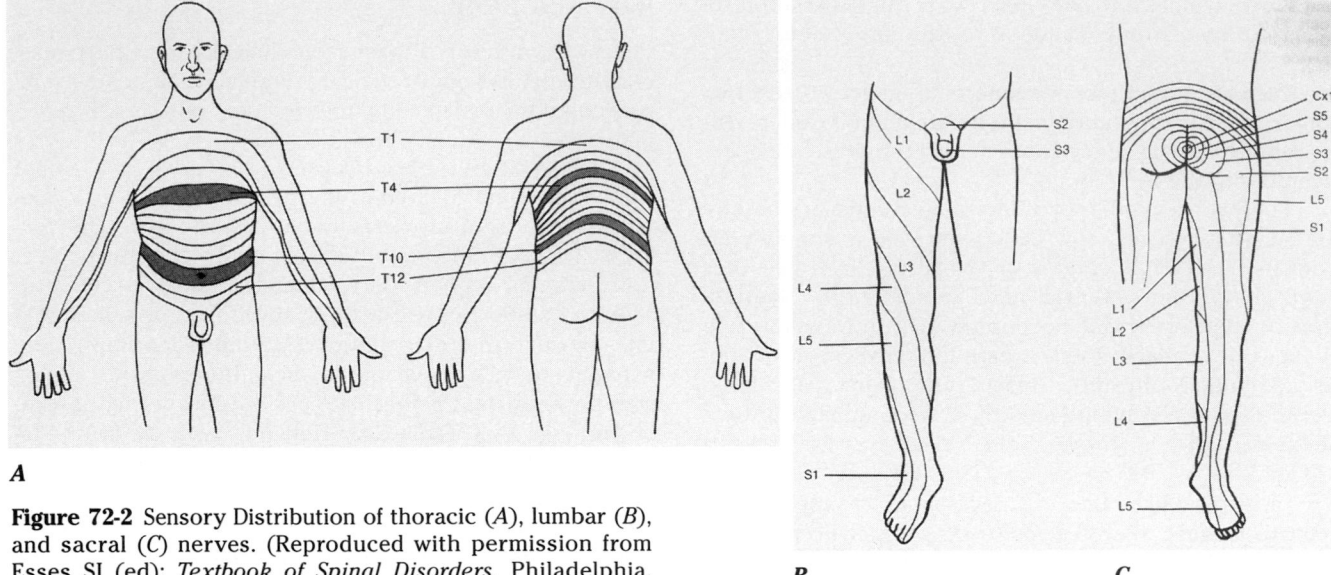

A

Figure 72-2 Sensory Distribution of thoracic (*A*), lumbar (*B*), and sacral (*C*) nerves. (Reproduced with permission from Esses SI (ed): *Textbook of Spinal Disorders*. Philadelphia, Lippincott, 1995, pages 59 and 64.)

B   *C*

Sacroiliac Joint Pain

The sacroiliac (SI) joint has been implicated as another cause of back and buttock pain. There are a number of physical exam maneuvers that can elicit pain in the sacroiliac joint in the hope of differentiating this source from other causes of back pain. The stress test involves applying a medially directed force from each side of the pelvis to stress the sacroiliac joint on each side. This is done with the patient in the supine position. Also, one can stress the sacroiliac joint with the patient prone, pushing inferiorly on the posterior iliac crest and causing a shear force across the ipsilateral joint. Patrick's test, also known as the FABER test (flexion, abduction, and external rotation), can reproduce sacroiliac joint pain. Gaenslen's test also stresses the

sacroiliac joint by extending the hip on one side while the other is maximally flexed. This is done with the patient on his or her side or supine on the side of the examining table. To confirm the SI joint as the primary source of pain, SI joint injections under fluoroscopic control can be diagnostic as well as temporarily therapeutic.[32] Sacroiliac joint arthritis is probably the most common cause of SI joint pain, but there are a number of spondyloarthropathies that can cause pain; these are discussed in Chap. 74.

Piriformis Syndrome

Another proposed etiology of buttock pain and sciatica is piriformis syndrome. The sciatic nerve can be irritated as it passes over the piriformis tendon or there can be an anatomic anomaly of the piriformis that contributes to this syndrome. Reproducing the pain by applying pressure near the piriformis fossa and/or stressing the piriformis muscle can aid in the diagnosis. Again, injections can be both diagnostic and therapeutic. Some authors have reported good results with sectioning of the piriformis tendon to relieve the pain.[87]

Other Sources of Back Pain

The most important factor in determining whether the source of back pain is from one of the various primary disorders of the spine, from a systemic process affecting the spine, or from a process completely unrelated to the spine is the patient's history. The examiner should determine the location of the pain, its quality, and how long it has been present. Constant, unremitting pain, especially at night, is suggestive of a tumor or infection. Constitutional symptoms such as fever, malaise, and weight loss suggest a systemic process. Inflammatory arthritides commonly

TABLE 72-3   Important Muscles and Their Nerve Root Innervation

Muscle	Nerve root innervation[a]
Iliopsoas	L1, L2, L3
Adductors	L2, L3, L4
Quadriceps	L2, L3, L4
Tibialis anterior	L4, L5
Extensor hallucis longus	L5, S1
Hamstrings	L4, L5, S1, S2
Peroneus longus	L5, S1
Gluteus maximus	L5, S1, S2
Gastrocnemius-soleus	S1, S2

[a]Predominant innervation is underlined.
Source: Reproduced with permission from Esses SI (ed): *Textbook of Spinal Disorders*. Philadelphia, Lippincott, 1995, page 63.

involve the spine. Also, numerous visceral sources of back pain must be considered: peptic ulcers, cholecystitis, pancreatitis, retrocecal appendicitis, dissecting abdominal aortic aneurysms, and pyelonephritis. In female patients, pelvic inflammatory diseases and endometriosis can be sources of referred pain to the back, as can prostate disorders in men.[84]

DIAGNOSTICS

Any discussion of spinal imaging should begin with emphasis on the fact that the imaging is simply an aid to diagnosis and by no means foolproof. It is essential that any abnormal findings on the imaging studies be correlated with the history and findings on physical examination. "Abnormal" findings are commonly seen in completely asymptomatic patients. Many imaging techniques are available; all have advantages and disadvantages and none can be used as a general screening exam, since most are overly sensitive and nonspecific. They should be used to confirm information gathered from the history and physical examination.[12]

Before going on to the specifics of the particular imaging modalities, the reader should understand the definitions of *specificity* and *sensitivity*. The sensitivity of a test is its ability to detect disease when present. The specificity is the ability of a test to remain negative in the absence of clinical disease.

Plain Radiographs

In interpreting plain radiographs, one must be aware of the fact that there can be frequent findings of significant degenerative changes in completely asymptomatic patients. There is often no direct relationship between symptoms and the radiographic changes of degenerative disk disease in the lumbar spine.[12] Findings of disk space narrowing, traction osteophytes, end-plate sclerosis, and Schmorl's nodes (lucency in the end plates) are quite prevalent in middle-aged individuals and almost ubiquitous in older individuals. The presence of these radiographic abnormalities does not correlate well with clinical symptoms and has no predictive value in determining who will have back problems in the future. Plain radio-graphs of the lumbar and thoracic spine are useful for detecting infections, tumors, deformities, and the presence of instability. The standard plain radiographic series for the lumbar spine should include anteroposterior (AP), lateral, and spot lateral views of the lumbosacral junction. Flexion/extension views are used when instability is suspected. Oblique radiographs do not need to be obtained routinely, but they are useful in visualizing the pars interarticularis. The AP and lateral views of the spine should be taken with the patient in the upright position and the flexion/extension views should be taken in the supine position.[164] For the evaluation of spinal deformity, standing 36-in x-rays should be obtained.

Computed Tomography

Computed tomography (CT) is a widely available, relatively inexpensive technique for imaging the spine. The CT scan does an excellent job of demonstrating the spine's bony configuration and, to some degree, can also show the soft tissues in graded shadings. The plain CT scan be an extremely valuable diagnostic tool when used appropriately, but, again, a high percentage of asymptomatic people will have abnormal findings. The clinician is again cautioned that it is imperative to be sure that the history and physical examination correlate with the findings on the imaging studies. The primary weakness of plain CT scanning is its relative lack of sensitivity in detecting soft tissue abnormalities. The sensitivity of CT appears to be enhanced by the addition of intradural contrast agents (Fig. 72-3). Computed tomography really should not be a first-line diagnostic radiologic test because of the inherent radiation exposure.

Myelography and Postmyelographic Computed Tomography

The lumbar myelogram has long been considered the "gold standard" for measuring neural compression. Extradural masses show up as filling defects in the contrast, and an intrathecal mass would appear as an outwardly protruding defect. Myelography is quite sensitive in picking up extradural encroachment but not very sensitive in differentiating protrusion coming from bony, malignant, infectious, or disk encroachment on the spinal canal. The primary advantage of myelography is that, as a dynamic test, it measures the ability of the cerebrospinal fluid to flow around extradural lesions.

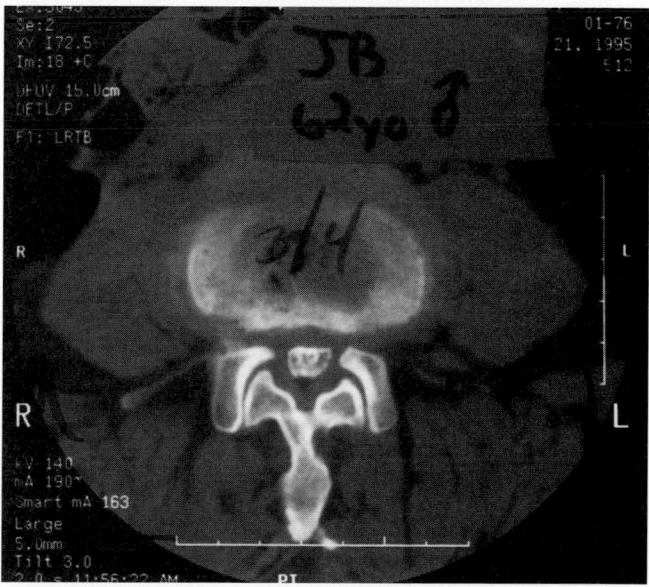

Figure 72-3 Postmyelogram CT scan demonstrating hypertrophic facets with further encroachment on the thecal sac by diffuse bulging of disk and ligamentous hypertrophy.

Disadvantages include the fact that it is an invasive test and often requires an overnight stay in the hospital. Potential complications include leakage of spinal fluid, which can cause severe headache, nausea, vomiting, and dizziness. This usually resolves with bed rest but occasionally requires a blood patch, which involves placement of the patient's own blood in the epidural space at the level of the puncture. The use of water-soluble and nonionic contrast agents has eliminated the problems with the oil-based agents, which included headache, nausea, vomiting, seizures, and arachnoiditis. Myelography, like the other imaging studies, can demonstrate abnormalities in asymptomatic patients.

Myelography is also very useful in dealing with severe deformity. An accurate view of neural encroachment can be obtained in both the coronal and sagittal planes (Fig. 72-4). The spinal deformity tends to pass in and out of the plane of the sagittal cut on the MRI scan. With CT scanning, even with reformatting to create coronal and sagittal images, severe deformities create the same limitations as seen on MRI. A postmyelogram CT scan is very useful in evaluating spinal stenosis. It nicely demonstrates and differentiates between bony and soft tissue encroachment on the dural sac and therefore provides the best "road map" for planning a surgical decompression.

Magnetic Resonance Imaging

Magnetic resonance imaging does not require ionizing radiation or contrast agents. Images are obtained by the detection of extremely small differences in proton density in a magnetic field bombarded with short pulses of radio waves, causing the atoms to vibrate in a specific manner. Variations in proton density, the radiofrequency, and relaxation times to the nonexcited state will modify the MRI image to highlight different tissues. Magnetic resonance imaging affords excellent anatomic resolution and as such is the most sensitive test in picking up early signs of disk degeneration. In T2-weighted images, the intervertebral disk is typically of high signal intensity (white) and degenerated disks appear dark. For the detection of herniated disks, MRI is comparable to CT/myelography. It is superior to all other imaging techniques in the detection of spinal tumors as well as the imaging of spinal infections. The use of gadolinium is helpful in imaging the postoperative spine, as it will enhance scar tissue. The MRI scan has been shown to be overly sensitive in detecting abnormalities in asymptomatic people. Twenty-two percent of asymptomatic subjects under age 60 and 57 percent of those over age 60 had significant abnormalities on their MRI scans. Additionally, the presence of signs of degenerative disk disease were present in 98 percent of subjects

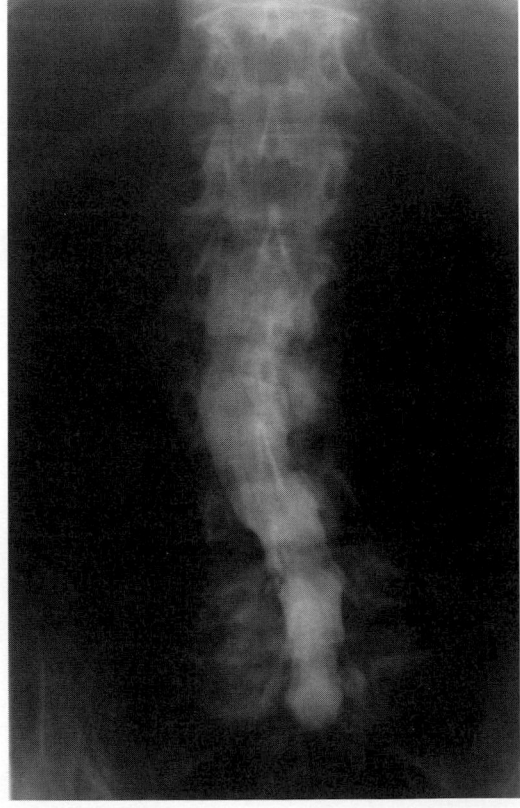

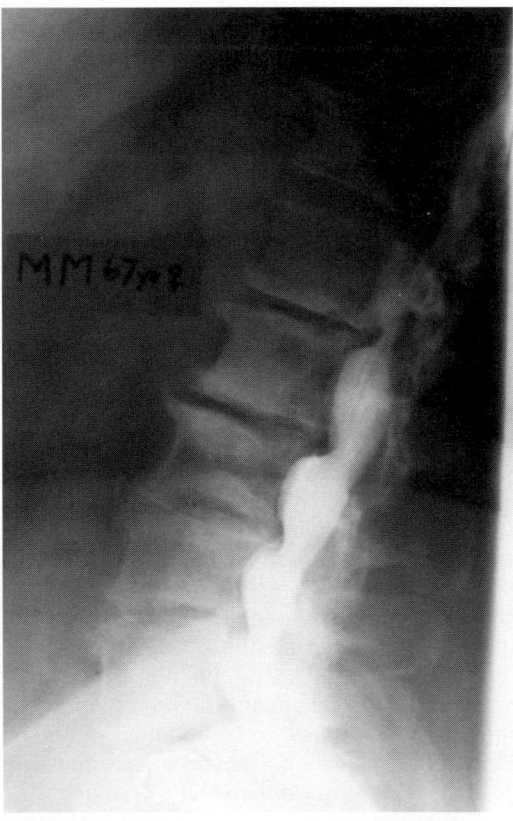

A *B*

Figure 72-4 Anteroposterior and lateral myelograms of patient with degenerative scoliosis.

over the age of 60.[13] The temptation is to ascribe the patient's symptoms to these abnormalities on the MRI scan, but if the imaging studies do not match the history and physical examination, these findings are most likely variations of normal and are not causing any of the patient's symptoms.

Nuclear Imaging

Radionuclide imaging is an excellent modality for studying any process that disturbs the balance of osteoblast and osteoclast activity. Technetium 99m is the most commonly used radiopharmaceutical for bone scanning and tends to concentrate in areas of increased bone production. This would show as a hot spot on a bone scan. Interruption of blood flow to the bone will result in the absence of uptake and present as a cold spot on the bone scan. Bone scans can be used to survey the entire skeleton or to obtain closeup spot views for particular areas of concern. Such scans are also useful in identifying areas of infection, working up tumors, or in diagnosing trauma cases where the plain x-ray is equivocal. Nuclear imaging is commonly used in evaluating the pars interarticularis. Infection, tumors, and trauma tend to increase osteoblastic activity and therefore would be "hot" on bone scans. Some tumors, however, such as multiple myeloma, may not result in increased activity and might present as cold spots on bone scan. Also, bone scanning can be useful in detecting disease in the sacroiliac joints, which can present as low back or buttock pain.

Discography

A diskogram involves injection of contrast material into the intervertebral disk space in an effort to demonstrate some degree of internal disk derangement as well as to see if the injection reproduces the patient's characteristic pain. To be deemed a positive provocative diskogram, the study must reproduce the patient's pain. Reliance on a patient's subjective response instead of specific objective findings makes this a less than perfect test. When it is reserved as a secondary diagnostic tool to be used when less invasive tests are negative or equivocal in the presence of persistent pain that has been refractory to other methods of diagnosis, discography can be a useful modality.[153]

Injection Studies

Some authors recommend a graded spinal anesthesia or differential spinal as a general screening test for chronic, long-standing, and constant lower back and leg pain.[162] Patients who are not relieved of their pain with full spinal anesthesia (nonphysiologic response) are definitely not candidates for surgery. These patients require counseling and aggressive physical therapy. Patients who exhibit the placebo effect should be treated similarly to the nonre-

sponders, and those that are relieved with spinal anesthesia should be studied further to determine the source of their pain.

Nerve root block or selective nerve root infiltration is useful in patients with radicular complaints or inconclusive findings. The test is most useful when the nerve root is entrapped laterally, as in foraminal stenosis.[86,144]

Lumbar facet injection is another relatively simple procedure that may establish a source of back and buttock pain.[41,105] The test is most appropriate for those with primary lower back, buttock, or thigh pain with local tenderness lateral to the midline that is exacerbated by increased lumbar extension. One should keep in mind that the facet joints are rarely the sole cause of back pain, and relief of back pain with this procedure should not be used to predict the success of a spinal fusion.[72]

Electrodiagnostics

Electromyograms (EMGs) can be used for the further evaluation of spinal stenosis. Many patients with symptoms of spinal stenosis can have some degree of stenosis at multiple levels, but some of these levels may be asymptomatic. Electromyograms show changes in approximately 80 percent of patients with stenosis and can therefore be used to help localize appropriate areas for decompression. Electromyography alone should never be used to determine the levels of decompression.[29] Somatosensory evoked potentials (SSEPs) and dermatomal SSEPs are often useful in the preoperative evaluation of patients undergoing surgery for spinal stenosis. These studies tend to be more sensitive than EMGs, but they also have a higher rate of false-positive readings and therefore require close correlation with the clinical symptoms.[45,55]

Psychosocial Testing

The Minnesota Multiphasic Personality Inventory (MMPI) is the most reliable and well-documented test used as a predictor of treatment regardless of the pathologic spinal condition. The test is predictive of preinjury susceptibility to back injury and the potential for failure of treatment.[160] Even when sound objective findings on physical examination and imaging studies might suggest a good surgical outcome, those with abnormal MMPIs were less likely to return to work, less likely to have reduction in their pain, and more likely to have greater disability than similar patients who did not have surgery.[40]

A simple test that is a good screening aid in picking up patients with psychological disturbances is the pain diagram. The pain drawing has been shown to correlate well with clinical results[147] (Fig. 72-5). Last, in examining the patient, one must be sure to check, during the physical examination, for nonorganic findings that can help to identify those patients who have a significant psychological or socioeconomic basis for their pain. These findings include the following:

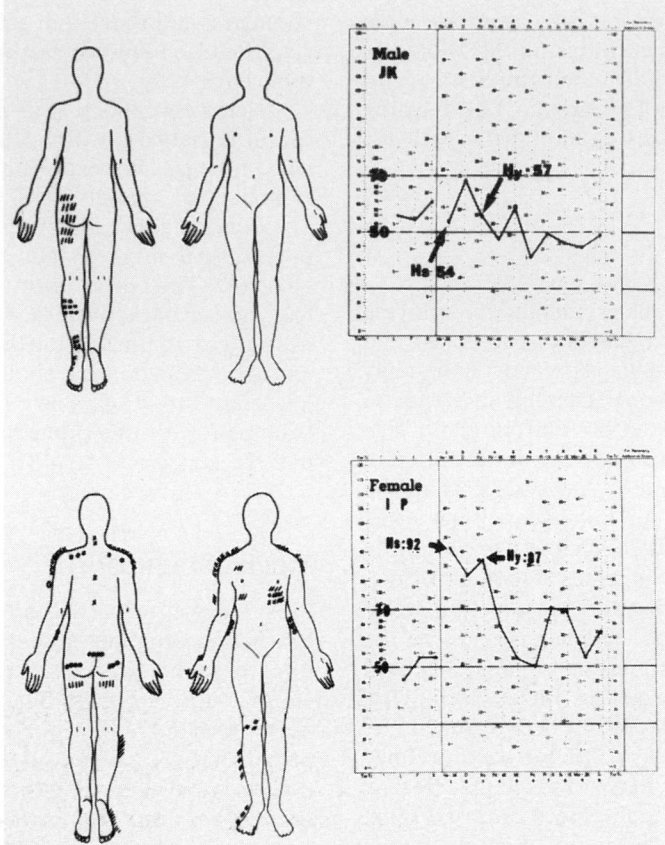

Figure 72-5 *A*. Pain drawing and corresponding MMPI raw score sheet of patient with "conversion V" who was not relieved of pain after disk surgery. *B*. Pain drawing and corresponding MMPI raw score sheet of patient with normal findings who was relieved of pain after disk surgery. (Reproduced with permission from Wood GW II, in Crenshaw AH (ed): *Campbell's Operative Orthopedics,* 8th ed. St Louis, Mosby, 1992, pages 37–39.)

1. Nonorganic tenderness, including either broad superficial tenderness to light touch in the lumbar region and/or widespread deep tenderness in a nonanatomic distribution.
2. Simulation tests whereby one suggests to the patient that a specific exam is being performed, though in fact it is not. For example, low back pain may be produced with either axial loading of the skull or passive rotation of the shoulders and pelvis through the hips.
3. Distraction tests that attempt to reproduce positive physical examination findings while the patient's attention is distracted. One should be suspicious of a positive supine straight-leg-raising test if, in pretending to examine the knee in the sitting position, the examiner is able to get the knee fully extended.
4. Regional disturbances in sensory and motor abnormalities such as give-way weakness and sensory loss in a stocking distribution rather than dermatomal distribution; this probably represents a nonorganic component.
5. Overreaction or pain out of proportion to the examination manifest as inappropriate facial expressions, tremors, collapsing, sweating, or dispropor-

tionate verbalization. These nonorganic findings are termed the *Waddell signs.*[152]

TREATMENT OF LOW BACK PAIN

A vast majority of people experience at least one episode of severe back pain during their lives. The episode is almost always self-limiting, regardless of whether or not the patient seeks treatment. Therefore the treatment for acute episodes of back pain should be symptomatic once one has ruled out the potential nonspinal causes of the pain. The recommendations handed down by the government-sponsored multidisciplinary Committee on the Evaluation and Treatment of Low Back Pain have emphasized the various conservative means of management and cautioned against early surgery in the absence of significant neurologic deficits.[10] No single approach to the treatment of acute back pain was deemed significantly better than any other approach. Generally, short-term bed rest is in order for the initial flareup, but it is rarely indicated for more than 2 days. Extending bed rest beyond this time will result in significant neuromuscular and cardiopulmonary deconditioning. Exercise has become the cornerstone of treatment for back pain.[104]

General Principles of Treatment for Low Back Pain

Various exercise programs have been advocated. Williams introduced flexion exercises consisting of partial sit-ups, pelvic tilts, and stretching of the hip flexors. The theory behind these exercises is that flexing the lumbar spine opens the intervertebral foramina and facet joints, thereby reducing nerve compression. These exercises are therefore theoretically better in more advanced degenerative conditions. The McKenzie system of exercises focuses on finding maneuvers that cause pain to centralize. Stabilization exercises are directed toward maintaining a position of comfort in the spine. Extension exercises, which are less likely to increase the intradiskal pressures and as such are best in patients with possible disk herniations, are aimed at strengthening the back extensor muscles, increasing the range of motion, and shifting the nucleus pulposus of the disk anteriorly. For chronic pain, the goal is generally to strengthen the muscles, especially the spinal extensors.[10]

Aerobic exercises are also important, as there is good evidence that people with increased general fitness and endurance are less vulnerable to back problems.[3,68]

The practitioner should be cautioned that exercise is not a panacea, and the use of standardized exercise regimens that essentially assume all back disorders to be the same should be discouraged. There is no indication that one specific type of exercise program is consistently better than another. Other passive modalities such as heat treatments, ultrasound, chiropractic manipulation, and traction may help relieve the symptoms temporarily but have not been shown to have a significant impact on the natural history of acute back pain.

Lumbosacral braces are among the most common forms of treatment for low back pain, but there is little evidence to document their benefit. While a person may temporarily feel better in an orthosis, one major disadvantage is that there is the potential for deconditioning and laxity of the abdominal and paraspinal musculature with prolonged use.

Analgesics and nonsteroidal anti-inflammatory drugs may help reduce symptoms during an acute flareup of pain, but they must be used judiciously, especially the narcotic analgesics. Muscle relaxants can also play an effective role if used judiciously.

Some authors have advocated "back schools" to educate patients about their condition in hopes of improving their ability to manage their symptoms and bring about an early return to work. The place of these programs in the treatment of spinal disorders remains to be clarified.

Chronic Low Back Pain

The patient with chronic low back pain in the absence of radicular complaints or any neurologic findings is often the most difficult to treat. Again, assuming no evidence of any serious pathologic process, nonoperative management is the cornerstone of treatment for these patients. Nonnarcotic pain medication and exercise programs, including aerobic conditioning and trunk strengthening, as outlined above, should be implemented. Those who have had symptoms for more than 6 months should have a complete psychological assessment. Also, an effort must be made to identify environmental issues that reinforce the pain behaviors, such as ongoing litigation. It is unlikely that a patient would show significant signs of improvement when it is not in his or her financial interest to improve. For the motivated patient who has become deconditioned, work transition programs do appear to offer some benefit.[49,80,96]

Degenerative Disk Disease

For patients who have symptoms of low back pain and have only dark disks on MRI, treatment should initially be the same as for any other patient with idiopathic low back pain, as outlined above. If the pain persists and these patients have been determined not to have any overlying psychological problems or pending litigation undermining their chances for improvement, some authors advocate diskography. This is obviously controversial. In properly selected patients, however, some authors have reported good results when diskography revealed morphologically abnormal disks associated with a significant concordant pain response.[11,24] The workup of degenerative disk disease and the rationale for operative management are discussed later.

THORACIC DISK DEGENERATION

Degenerative disease in the thoracic spine is considerably less common than degenerative conditions of the cervical and lumbar spine. However, it does occur and must be considered in any patient presenting with midback and intrascapular pain as well as radiculopathy in the distribution of the intercostal nerves as well as myelopathy of the lower extremity. Probably the most significant cause for the rare incidence of symptomatic degenerative disk problems in the thoracic spine is the stabilizing effect of the thorax.[2] The facet joints of the lumbar spine are oriented so that flexion is the primary motion, and it is typically the flexion component of motion that injures the annulus acutely. Add torsional loading to an acutely injured annulus and we often see posterior disk herniations in the lumbar spine. At the thoracic segments, we see the splinting effect of the thoracic cage and the decreased height of the thoracic disk compared to the lumbar disks. Finally, the orientation of the facet joints allows torsion as the primary motion. All this accounts for the markedly decreased incidence of thoracic versus lumbar disk degeneration and herniation.[110] In fact, symptomatic displacement of the intervertebral disk in the thoracic spine is such an uncommon event that the incidence has been reported to be 1 per million per year. In other words, approximately one-half of 1 percent of all protruded disks occur in the thoracic spine.[5,7] The first documented report of a thoracic disk herniation was in 1911.[100] Thoracic disk herniations are most common in the fourth decade of life, and three-quarters of them occur below T8.[5] It is very rare for thoracic disk herniations to occur above T4, but it has been reported in the literature.[88]

Symptomatic degeneration of the thoracic disks can occur in any age group, but it is exceedingly rare in adolescents and young adults. Often patients will describe antecedent trauma leading to their current symptoms. A thoracic intervertebral disk can be significantly damaged during a compression fracture, especially when there is evidence of end-plate involvement. The vertebral body can be expected to heal, but the disk can remain symptomatic. In a situation such as this, the physical exam might show local pain with palpation but the neurologic exam would be normal. When the symptoms are more diskogenic, flexion tends to exacerbate the pain; if the condition is more due to facet joint arthritis, extension would be more likely to exacerbate the pain.[32] With symptomatic thoracic disk herniations, there is more likely to be evidence of radiculopathy in the distribution of the intercostal nerve and/or myelopathy.

Diagnostic Evaluation

Ogilvie[110] describes four categories of symptoms in the evaluation of patients with pain possibly emanating from the thoracic spine.

The first category is *mechanical.* Simple disk degeneration may result in axial pain with localized back pain, with typical mechanical features such as improvement with recumbency and exacerbation by activity, especially flexion. Acute herniations in this setting may include pain with a pleuritic character.

The second category is *radicular.* This is pain from a disk herniation impinging on an intercostal nerve and resulting in intercostal girdle pain. Upper thoracic herniations can cause a Horner's syndrome.[39]

Myelopathic symptoms from a thoracic source can present as urge incontinence or lower extremity weakness and can progress to frank paraplegia. This typically occurs from thoracic disk herniations in which the disk material impinges on the spinal cord itself. However, thoracic myelopathy can be caused by other conditions. Congenital spinal stenosis resulting in thoracic myelopathy has been described,[9] as has acquired thoracic stenosis relating to osteophytes or hypertrophy of the posterior elements, including facet hypertrophy and ossification of the ligamentum flavum.[111,134,165]

The last category is *visceral.* This category is important because many visceral conditions can present with symptoms similar to those caused by degenerative disorders of the thoracic spine. The manifestations of thoracic disk disease have been confused with herpes zoster, cardiac disorders, pulmonary problems, or abdominal diseases.[143] More often than not, a complete history and thorough physical examination will minimize the chance of confusion.

The findings on physical examination among these patients can vary widely.[133] A careful sensory exam may disclose a demarcation corresponding to the level of impingement. If muscle weakness is present, it is usually bilateral, and decreased rectal sphincter tone may also be present. Long tract signs such as sustained ankle clonus or a positive Babinski reflex are more often present in herniations of shorter duration. Rarely, patients will present with profound neurologic symptoms, including paraplegia; this might suggest an intradural herniation of a thoracic disk.[142] These patients often present with an anterior cord syndrome (preservation of position and vibratory sense) because the cord impingement is from the anterior.

Imaging studies should probably begin with lateral radiographs of the thoracic spine. These films may show only nonspecific findings of decreased intervertebral disk height and/or hypertrophic changes of the facets, but they may also show calcified disk material in the spinal canal. It has been reported that more than 50 percent of thoracic disk herniations are associated with calcified disk material in the canal.[97] Myelography and postmyelography CT scanning have been used with reasonable success in the past, but myelography is an invasive study. Today, MRI scanning allows us to evaluate the thoracic spine noninvasively. One problem with MRI images is that because they are so sensitive at picking up varying degrees of degeneration, clinical correlation often becomes more difficult. Wood et al.[163] recently reported on thoracic MRI examinations in asymptomatic adults and found evidence of disk degeneration in 55 percent, with actual disk herniations in 37 percent; 40 percent of the latter had more than one level of herniation. With this in mind, the clinician must ensure that a degenerative finding identified on MRI is indeed the source of the patient's pain and not simply a normal variant. This is where some clinicians recommend the provocative diskogram as a diagnostic test. Diskography should not be done only at the index level but also at the disks above and below to achieve an internal control (Fig. 72-6). Whether or not the provocative diskogram is scientifically valid has yet to be shown conclusively.[128] Electromyograms and SSEPs have not proved helpful in the diagnosis of herniated thoracic disks.

Treatment

As in diskogenic conditions of the cervical and lumbar spines, degenerative disk problems of the thoracic spine usually resolve with nonoperative care. Nonsteroidal antiinflammatory drugs, avoiding exacerbating activities, low-impact aerobic exercises, and other active and passive modalities should be tried initially. No scientifically controlled study has demonstrated one of these treatments to be significantly better than any other. Patients can return to activities as tolerated as their symptoms improve.

Patients with an unacceptable level of pain who have not responded to conservative measures and/or patients with significant neurologic deficits related to a specific disk lesion are candidates for surgical intervention. Patients whose pain is the predominant indication for surgery can have a very broad spectrum of findings on their imaging studies.[110] On one end of the spectrum is the

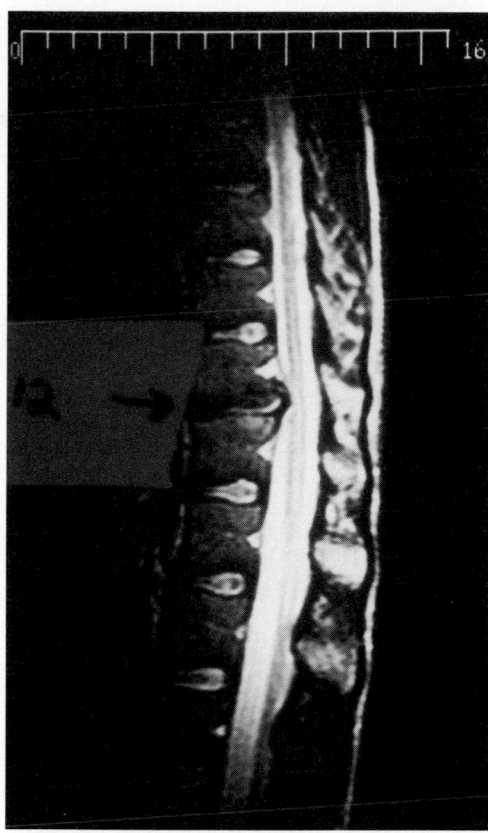

Figure 72-6 Disk herniation (T11–T12) with effacement of the spinal cord. This patient did not have neurologic symptoms but had severe thoracic back pain with a positive provocative diskogram at this level and negative provocation at control levels.

isolated thoracic disk and the presence of normal disks above and below, and with positive pain provocation with thoracic discography. Single-level surgery is indicated in these patients. At the other extreme is the patient with Scheuermann's disease, with evidence of severe disk degeneration at multiple segments. These patients require anterior diskectomy and fusion and posterior instrumentation and fusion of the entire kyphotic deformity when surgery is elected. The most troublesome patients are those in the middle of the spectrum who have unremitting back pain with several levels of disk degeneration on the sagittal MRI. Provocative diskography may help the surgeon to determine which levels, if any, are appropriate for surgery. In these cases, it is extremely important to differentiate the symptoms of thoracic disk disease from other nonspecific musculoskeletal pain syndromes that do not respond to surgery. In general, for symptomatic degenerative disk disease of the thoracic spine in the absence of a deformity such as Scheuermann's kyphosis, surgery is rarely necessary.

In those patients with neurologic findings, a number of approaches have been described for disk excision. Thoracic diskectomy through a laminectomy approach should be condemned. In the lumbar spine, the cauda equina is eas-

ily retractable; therefore diskectomies here are easily done through a laminotomy. In the thoracic spine, however, the spinal cord does not tolerate retraction.[133] Some authors have advocated a transpedicular approach, a costotransversectomy exposure, or an anterolateral decompression for excising herniated thoracic disks.[67,116,125] These approaches are most suitable for laterally oriented disk herniations. A number of authors report high success rates using the transthoracic technique.[15,36] Otani et al. have described an extrapleural anterior exposure for disk excision that requires less dissection than the transthoracic approach and does not require the use of a chest tube.[113] In hopes of lessening the morbidity and the time to recovery of open techniques, the thoracoscopic approach to these conditions is gaining acceptance.[118]

Surgical Technique

Our experience is primarily with the transthoracic approach (Fig. 72-7). The patient is placed in a lateral decubitus position with the "up" side corresponding to the side of the disk herniation and the preoperative imaging studies. If a central disk is the problem, the left side up is chosen, as the aorta is less likely to be injured than the vena cava and, if injured, is more easily repaired. Depending on the slope of the ribs, an incision is made over the rib one or two spaces above the disk in question. Intraoperative x-rays are taken to confirm the level. The parietal pleura is then incised and the segmental artery and vein are ligated anterior to the neural foramen above and below the disk in question. Usually the entire disk is removed back to the posterior longitudinal ligament, and small curets can be used in excising the protruding annulus and marginal osteophytes. Often removal of the base of the rib as well as the pedicle of the adjacent level (eighth rib and pedicle for a T7-T8 herniation) should be performed to help extract the disk material that is lodged in the spinal canal. The indications for performing a fusion at the time of diskectomy are not well established, but usually the harvested rib is used as a strut graft. In patients with a major component of thoracic back pain and in those with segmental degenerative disk disease as seen in Scheuermann's disease, arthrodesis is probably important. Internal fixation or postoperative immobilization is rarely necessary for limited fusions, especially when operating above T10, due to the support provided by the thoracic cage. There may be an indication for rigid internal fixation or postoperative immobilization in an orthosis if surgery is performed at the thoracolumbar junction, because at this level the thoracic cage does not provide intrinsic stability. A chest tube is inserted before wound closure and is removed when the drainage is 30 to 50 mL for an 8-h shift, which usually occurs on the third postoperative day. The patient stands at the bedside on postoperative day 1 and is mobilized as soon as the chest tube is out. In properly selected patients, improvement can be expected, but there is often residual pain or weakness.[119]

Less common than problems related to thoracic disk degeneration is thoracic spinal stenosis defined as nar-

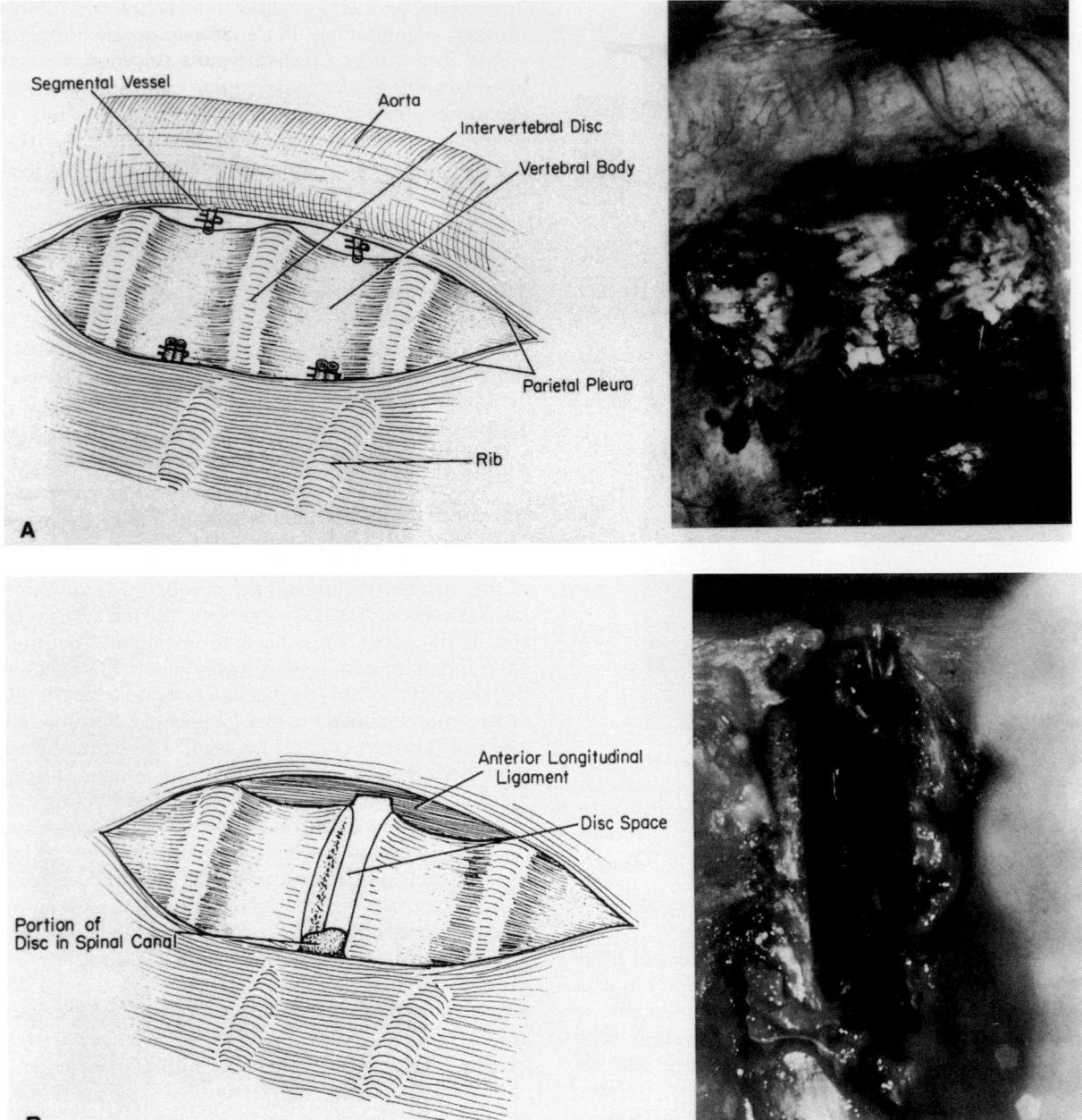

Figure 72-7 Surgery of Thoracic disk herniation. *A.* Exposure of the affected interspace. *B.* Preliminary disk excision. *C.* Completion of diskectomy with removal of compressing fragment. *D.* Trough cut in adjacent vertebral bodies. *E.* Rib graft fusion performed. (Reproduced with permission from Ogilvie JW: Thoracic disk herniation, in Bridwell KH, DeWald RL (eds): *The Textbook of Spinal Surgery.* Philadelphia, Lippincott, 1991, pages 714–716.)

rowing of the AP diameter of the canal to less than 10 mm. Epstein and Schwall describe primary and secondary thoracic spinal stenosis.[31] Primary thoracic stenosis is similar to degenerative spinal stenosis in the cervical and lumbar spine and, in fact, a vast majority of patients with primary thoracic stenosis have accompanying lumbar involvement. The secondary type of stenosis is attributed to endocrinopathies and systemic diseases; it typically involves the entire spinal canal, not just the posterior elements, as with degenerative stenosis. The authors stress the importance of recognizing the presence of primary or secondary thoracic stenosis and the extent of involvement in the adjacent cervical and lumbar regions in order to manage these patients properly.

Complications

The most feared complication in any spinal surgery is direct trauma to the spinal cord; this is avoidable with proper technique. Many surgeons worry about cord in-

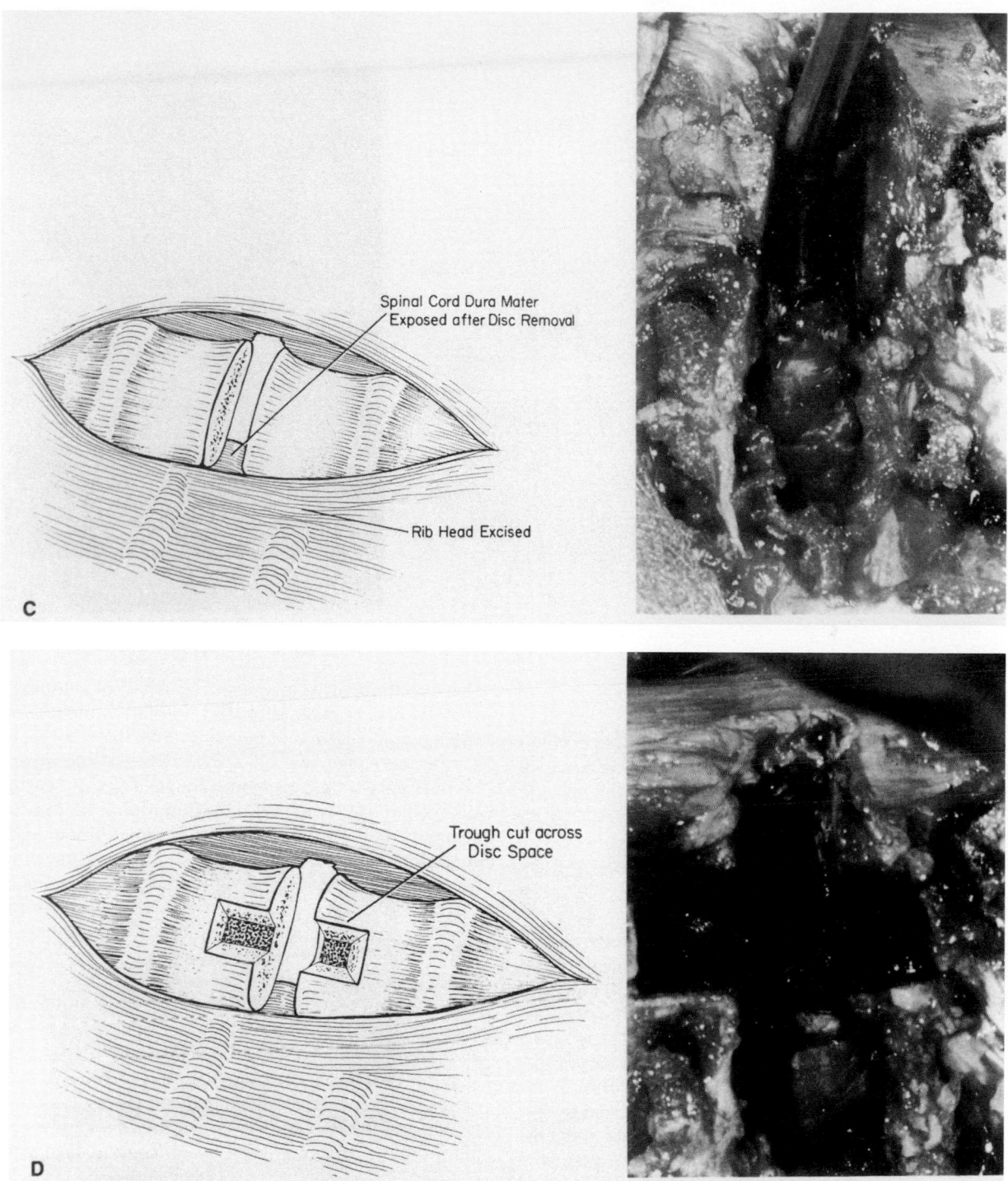

Figure 72-7 (*Continued*)

farct when ligating the segmental vessels, but the experience of Winter et al. suggests that this is exceedingly rare.[161] Other possible complications include persisting neurologic deficit and/or pain and, in those who have had thoracotomy, an intercostal neuritis is occasionally present that may require local nerve blocks. Those cases treated with laminectomy are potentially complicated by iatrogenic neurologic deficits and/or postlaminectomy deformity, including kyphosis and spondylolisthesis.[27,119]

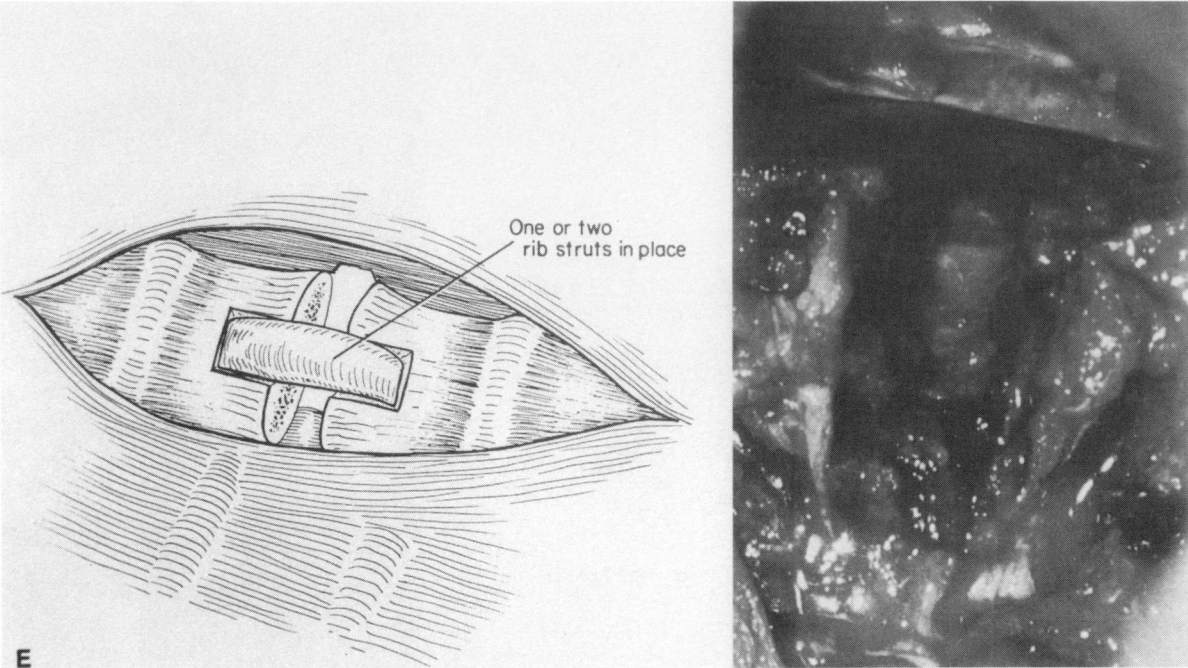

One or two
rib struts in place

E

Figure 72-7 (*Continued*)

LUMBAR DISK DEGENERATION

It is inevitable that degenerative structural changes develop within the spinal motion segments as people age. Some 70 to 80 percent of individuals experience a significant episode of acute low back pain at some point in their lives.[4,63]

Pathophysiology

Being the largest avascular structure in the body, the intervertebral disk depends exclusively on passive diffusion through the central end plates and peripheral annulus for nutrition. Being avascular, it has no potential for healing when structural disruptions occur within it. These structural disruptions then persist indefinitely and can propagate, further compromising the structural integrity of the disk. The aging process of the disk is characterized by histologic and biochemical changes in its cellularity and a decrease in its water content. These universally occurring changes do not usually produce symptoms, but they can lead to progressive rupture of the disk material through the posterior annulus and herniation of disk material into the spinal canal.[19] Adams and Hutton postulate that a herniated nucleus pulposus is the culmination of a series of pathophysiologic events. Asymptomatic intradiskal fissuring and fragmentation occurs, followed by progressive annular disruption progressing from the inner layers to the outer layers. In some patients, this ultimately results in a complete annular rupture with herniation of disk material into the canal.[1] Why some individuals develop symptoms along this continuum and others do not is not entirely known, nor is why certain individuals develop fragmentation and herniation and others do not. Individual factors

that are thought to increase the risk of developing symptomatic disk degeneration and herniation include increasing age and history of smoking. Possible risk factors include decreased overall aerobic fitness and strength of spinal extensor and abdominal muscles, poor posture, and decreased spinal mobility. Occupational factors include heavy physical work; frequent bending, lifting, and twisting; static work postures; vibrations; and psychological and psychosocial factors.[4] While increasing age is considered a risk factor, degenerative changes certainly can take place in younger individuals. Some young patients reporting low back pain demonstrate vertebral end-plate irregularity, anterior Schmorl's nodes, and narrowing of the involved intervertebral disks at the thoracolumbar and lumbar spine; this is termed thoracolumbar Scheuermann's disease.[51] It is felt that in these younger patients the degenerative disease is a manifestation of an intrinsic defect of the disks and/or cartilaginous end plates, resulting in inadequate nutrition and structural weakness or a combination of both, which, in turn, leads to early degeneration.

Signs and Symptoms

Because the interior of the disk is sparsely innervated, the fissuring and fragmentation are usually asymptomatic. The annulus has more nociceptive pain fibers; therefore progressive annular disruption is more likely to produce episodes of back pain that can range from a mild aching to a severe, incapacitating pain.[138] This back pain plus the progressive annular disruption can often cause some associated radiating pain into the pelvis or legs in a nonradicular pattern; this is the referred pain, which is to be distinguished from radicular sciatic pain occurring when a particular nerve root is compressed. The diskogenic pain is typically worse with any flexion or torsional load placed on the disk. Anything requiring the Valsalva maneuver, which will increase intradiskal pressures, also exacerbates the pain, and the pain is typically improved with recumbency or spinal extension, since this decreases the load on the disks.

A disk will not herniate unless there is preexisting degeneration. What we commonly see is a patient with severe back pain that suddenly resolves, only to be replaced by severe leg pain. The pressure on the annulus by the fragment is relieved and may or may not be transferred to the nerve root. In some individuals, the entire process of annular disruption and disk herniation can be asymptomatic and the patient can present with the sciatica. Probably the most common scenario is that the entire process of degeneration and herniation is totally asymptomatic.[13] The pain from progressive annular disruption is termed *diskogenic* and the pain from nerve root compression is termed *radiculopathy.* The variability in symptoms from one individual to the next is tremendous. The pain of some will be primarily diskogenic, while others will have primarily neurologic pain or, often, a combination of the two.

Physical Exam

Patient with primarily diskogenic pain are typically quite stiff, with pain exacerbated by forward flexion, but there are no neurologic findings. Evaluation of the posture of some patients often suggests a herniated disk. An involuntary attempt by the patient to reduce nerve root irritation by leaning to one side in an effort to open up the neural foramen is termed a *sciatic list.* Again, range of motion may be limited due to paravertebral muscle spasm, and forward flexion may increase the symptoms of sciatica. Evaluating for nerve root tension is an important part of the physical exam, and this should be done with both supine straight-leg raising and sitting straight-leg raising. The most specific sign for lumbar disk herniation is a contralaterally positive straight-leg-raising sign. If a disk herniation is suspected at L3-4 or above, a femoral stretch test should be performed.

It is important to understand the muscle innervation of the lower extremity. The level of nerve root irritation can be determined by noting specific muscle group weakness or loss of a particular reflex. Table 72-3 lists the important muscles of the lower extremity and the nerve root innervation. Asymmetrical quadriceps weakness or diminished quadriceps reflex suggests L3 or L4 nerve root compression. Diminished foot dorsiflexion suggests L4 nerve root irritation. Diminished strength of the extensor hallucis longus suggests L5 nerve root compression. Weak plantar flexors and a diminished Achilles reflex suggest S1 problems. The examiner should also make an effort to look for asymmetry in the sensory exam.

Diagnostics

After the physical exam and a thorough history, the examiner should have a good idea as to what the problem is, but other studies are necessary to define it more specifically. Plain radiographs are not particularly useful but should be

obtained to serve as a baseline. Sciatica in a young patient may be associated with an avulsion of the end plate, and this would be seen as an ossified fragment in the canal at the level of the disk. In patients with primarily low back pain, lytic or degenerative spondylolisthesis and/or degenerative disk disease may help explain the patient's symptoms. As mentioned earlier in the chapter, many "abnormalities" seen on imaging studies actually represent variations of normal. A variety of imaging studies plus the history and physical examination help narrow the source of pain.

Magnetic resonance imaging is the optimal study for suspected lumbar disk herniations (Fig. 72-8) but is probably overly sensitive in picking up degenerative disk disease.[103] Degenerated disks appear dark on T2-weighted images. Also, T2-weighted images allow the differentiation of sequestered disk herniations from disk protrusions and extrusions. The use of gadolinium helps in the differentiation between recurrent disk herniations and postoperative scarring as well as in demonstrating intradurally herniated disks.[157] The sensitivity and specificity of MRI compare favorably with those of other imaging modalities. Moreover, MRI is noninvasive and does not require exposure to ionizing radiation. Disadvantages include its cost and difficulty in patients with ferromagnetic implants and those who have claustrophobia.

Myelography in combination with computed tomography (CT) is more useful than either study alone. Magnetic resonance imaging has replaced myelography as the primary imaging modality for the spine, but there are still definite indications. These include the presence of a significant spinal deformity, the presence of metallic implants, and significant claustrophobia.[32]

Crock has popularized the concept of internal disk disruption as a cause of low back pain; diskography can

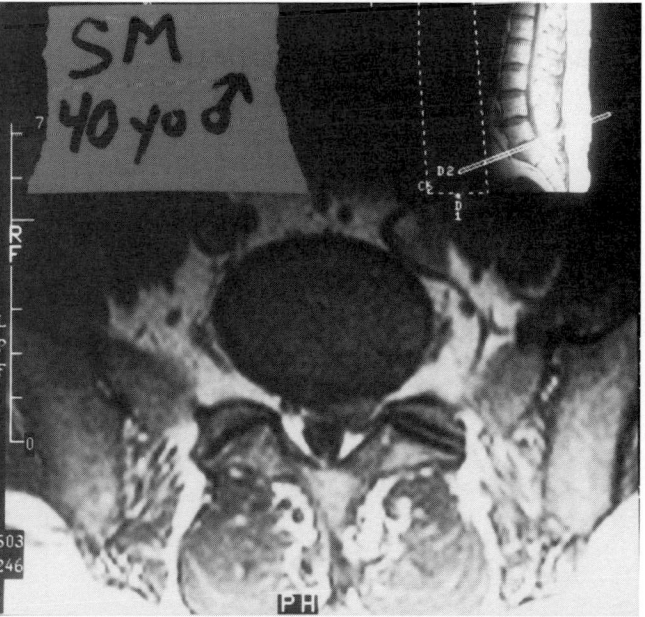

Figure 72-8 T1-weighted image through L5-S1 disk showing large left-sided herniated disk. At surgery, there was a large extruded disk fragment.

help in the evaluation of this syndrome.[26] There are some data to support the use of provocative diskograms as supplemental studies in selected patients.[11,24,153] However, many surgeons feel that there are few objective data to justify accepting this condition as an entity in and of itself. As Spengler states, many patients who have a narrow disk space may, indeed, develop nerve root encroachment syndromes or segmental hypermobility, but the simple presence of disk space narrowing on plain radiographs or a dark disk on T2-weighted MRIs should not justify an operative procedure on a back pain patient.[139] Diskography has not been shown to correlate with these anatomic variations in any scientifically controlled studies.

Electromyography may be useful in objectively documenting motor dysfunction and ascertaining the degree and duration of denervation in selected patients. Somatosensory evoked potentials have been used to measure the sensory integrity of specific nerve roots.

Treatment

Since the vast majority of patients with acute back pain and/or sciatica improve with time, the nonoperative approach remains the cornerstone of treatment. For both acute back pain flareups and sciatica, brief periods of bed rest and specific "back school" programs are efficacious. Nonsteroidal anti-inflammatory drugs can be effective as well. Some report temporary improvement with epidural steroid injections.[10,48]

There are many other treatment modalities that have not been shown to improve the natural history of the problem but may make the patient feel better temporarily and are probably not harmful. Such treatments include the short-term use of braces, heat, ice, biofeedback, traction, manipulation, massage, acupuncture, psychological support, and so on.

The indications for operating on the patient with a herniated disk is a progressive neurologic deficit and/or severe incapacitating pain. A relative indication for proceeding with surgery is failure of conservative therapy. If the patient does not have a progressive neurologic deficit or severe incapacitating pain, the surgeon should try at least 6 weeks of nonoperative management. If there are no signs of improvement at this time, surgery is an option, as is continued conservative therapy. In these patients there is no long-term difference in those with continued conservative therapy versus those who had surgery, and the long-term cost differential is insignificant. Those with prolonged conservative therapy do tend to miss more work than those who have surgery.[128]

The decision to proceed with surgery in patients with degenerative disk disease is considerably more controversial. If the patient demonstrates nonphysiologic pain responses on exam (positive Waddell signs),[151] has litigation pending, is a worker's compensation patient,[37] and/or is a smoker,[46] the patient is likely to do poorly with surgery; therefore the surgeon must proceed cautiously with these patients. When patients have exhausted nonoperative means and do not fall into the above groups and their provocative diskograms are markedly concordant at one or two levels, fusion may be an option. Hanley et al.[49] proposed an algorithm for the treatment of these patients (Fig. 72-9). As stated by these authors, not only is the decision to proceed with surgery controversial, but exactly what surgical procedure to perform is controversial as well (Table 72-4). The reported success rate with spinal fusion in patients with degenerative disk disease varies widely.[37,46,168]

As for lumbar disk herniations, the indications for surgery in the few who do not improve with nonoperative management include severe pain with evidence of nerve root tension, recurrent incapacitating episodes of sciatica, and physical examination findings of impairment of nerve root conduction. As previously emphasized, every patient should be given a chance to improve without surgery, and the vast majority will. It is only the rare patient who requires an urgent or emergent diskectomy due to a seriously progressive neurologic deficit.

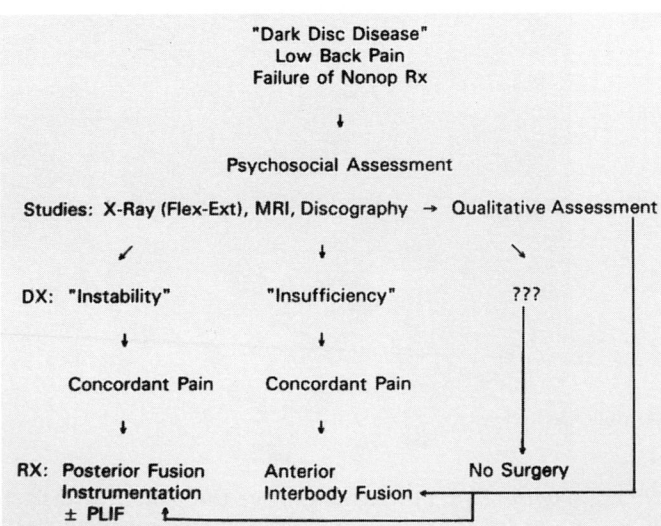

Figure 72-9 Algorithmic approach to "dark disk disease." (Reproduced with permission from Hanley EN Jr, Spengler DM, Wesel S, et al: Controversies in low back pain: The surgical approach. *Instr Course Lect* 43:418, 1994.)

TABLE 72-4 Controversial Treatment Options—Fusion Surgeries[a]

Anterior interbody fusion (ALIF)
  No hardware
  With hardware
Circumferential 360° fusion
Posterior lumbar interbody fusion (PLIF)
  No hardware
  With hardware

[a]Surgical treatment options for patients with degenerative "dark disk disease." These procedures are controversial and not yet scientifically validated.
Source: Reproduced with permission from Hanley EN Jr, Spengler DM, Wesel S, et al: Controversies in low back pain: The surgical approach. *Instr Course Lect* 43:419, 1994.

Spengler et al. proposed an objective evaluation system in selecting possible candidates for surgery. They found that the best predictor of surgical findings is the preoperative imaging study, but the best predictor of outcome was the preoperative psychological assessment[140] (Table 72-5).

Once the patient and the surgeon have decided to proceed with a procedure, there are a number of treatment options. The effort to relieve the symptoms with as little morbidity as possible has been the driving force behind the minimally invasive procedures for herniated disks. Lyman Smith was the first to describe chemonucleolysis for the treatment of sciatica due to a disk herniation.[135] The success rate of chemonucleolysis with chymopapain has been approximately 70 percent.[109] While this is probably the least invasive technique, there are a number of problems with it. The pain relief usually occurs slowly over a period of several weeks; a signifi-

TABLE 72-5 Objective Evaluation System

Category	Maximum points	Assignment of points
Neurologic signs	25	
Weakness consistent with level of lesion		
Associated with positive EMG		25
Associated with negative EMG		10
Atrophy (more than 2 cm)		10
Reflex absent or asymmetrical		
Patient 50 years old or younger[a]		20
Patient older than 50 years[b]		10
No clinical signs; EMG positive		15
Sciatic tension signs	25	
Positive crossed straight-leg-raising test[c]		20
Pelvic list		15
Dysrhythmia of lumbar paraspinal muscles		
during motion of the back		15
Positive ipsilateral straight-leg-raising test[d]		5
Personality factors (score on MMPI)	25	
Normal (includes depression)		25
Abnormal (impulsive or schizophrenic)		10
Elevated hysteria or hypochondriasis scales, or both		
(more than one but less than two standard deviations)		10
Conversion reaction or hysteria		
(more than two standard deviations)		0
Findings on lumbar myelography or computed tomography	25	
Positive and correlates with clinical findings		25
Equivocal nerve root asymmetry		10
Positive but does not correlate with clinical findings		0
Normal		0
	100	

Key: EMG, electromyography; MMPI, Minnesota Multiphasic Personality Inventory.
[a]Add 5 points if the EMG is positive.
[b]Add 15 points if the EMG is positive.
[c]Positive when straight-leg raising on asymptomatic side causes the patient to perceive pain in the asymptomatic buttock, thigh, or leg.
[d]Standard straight-leg-raising test.
Source: Reproduced with permission from Spengler DM, Oullette EA, Battie M, Zeh J: Elective diskectomy for herniation of a lumbar disk. *J Bone Joint Surg* 72A:231, 1990.

cant percentage of patients have severe pain and spasms for up to 3 months following the injection; the enzyme acts on the entire disk, resulting in disk space narrowing and an increase in annular laxity; and a small percentage of patients have had catastrophic complications such as transverse myelitis and anaphylactic reactions.[138] For these reasons, chemonucleolysis is rarely used in this country.

Percutaneous diskectomy is another minimally invasive procedure that again does not address the herniation itself but attempts to decompress the nerve root by removing disk material from the center of the disk space. Using the most objective studies, generally only 50 percent of patients can expect good to excellent results.[43,65]

Laser diskectomy, likewise, does not address the actual pathology, and, as expected, the success rates are dramatically inferior to those of standard diskectomy.[129]

One procedure that may have a role in the future is the endoscopic removal of the herniated disk fragments. This procedure holds more hope than the previously mentioned procedures because it addresses the actual pathology. The instrumentation for this procedure is evolving. Preliminary reports are of 80 percent good results, but final judgment awaits the ability of others to duplicate them.[78]

The gold standard for the treatment of sciatica due to a herniated nucleus pulposus is the hemilaminotomy and diskectomy performed with the use of loupe magnification or operating microscope, in which approximately 85 percent good to excellent results can be expected.[30,140]

Surgical Technique

In planning a diskectomy, the surgeon must carefully review the imaging studies to check the location of the herniation in relation to the nerve root and be sure of the proper level.

Most disk surgeries are performed with the patient under general endotracheal anesthesia, but various regional and local anesthetic techniques have been used. In positioning the patient, it is best to allow the abdomen to hang free, minimizing the congestion of the epidural veins; this, in turn, generally means less bleeding at surgery. The modified kneeling position, using one of the customized tables or frames on the market, are the best at allowing the abdomen to hang free. Loupe magnification with a head lamp or an operating microscope improves the visualization of various structures. Prior to making the incision, a localizing x-ray should be obtained with the use of a paper clip over the spinous process or a spinal needle in the paraspinal muscle away from where the skin incision will be.

After appropriate antibiotic prophylaxis and prepping and draping, a longitudinal incision is made between the spinous processes of the level in question. The paraspinal muscles are elevated subperiosteally out to the level of the facets on the side in question, taking care not to enter the facet capsule. The paraspinal muscles need to be elevated only minimally on the opposite side, and a hemilaminectomy retractor is then placed. Next, the fat pad and the interval between the facet and the ligamentum flavum are debrided. The lateral and inferior

margins of the ligamentum flavum should be clearly delineated; this sometimes requires a partial medial facetectomy. The spinal canal is entered at the inferolateral margin of the ligamentum flavum. This is generally done with a 40° Kerrison rongeur. The ligamentum flavum is then carefully dissected off the lamina. The preoperative imaging study should show whether more of the superior or inferior lamina needs to be removed (Fig. 72-10). At L5-S1, the interspace is occasionally large enough that a hemilaminotomy is not required. Cottonoid patties or bipolar coagulation help control the bleeding of the epidural veins. Once the canal is reached, the nerve root should be identified; it is usually found at the inferolateral margin of the laminotomy. Once identified, it is followed proximally toward the disk space. With the nerve root and dural sac retracted medially, the canal is easily explored to localize the disk herniation. Often a disk fragment will be found already ruptured through the annulus and it is not necessary to use a scalpel to incise the annulus. Following removal of the disk fragment, an effort should be made to find the annular disruption, and this should be entered with a pituitary rongeur. Lose intradiskal fragments must be removed. Following removal of the disk fragments, the nerve root is usually noted to be much more mobile. When one is satisfied that an adequate decompression has been performed, bleeding is controlled with Gelfoam pledgets and cottonoid patties. An interposition graft is usually not necessary with this exposure. The lumbodorsal fascia should be closed with a heavy interrupted suture. The subcutaneous tissues and skin should be closed as separate layers. We generally leave a Hemovac drain in prior to closure and pull it the morning after surgery. Patients are sent home 24 to 36 h after surgery. Some surgeons are performing this procedure on an outpatient basis.[16]

The majority of disk herniations are just lateral to the nerve root as it exits the dural sac. The previously described exposure usually brings the surgeon into the canal just inferior to the disk herniation. Occasionally the disk fragment can be in the axilla of the nerve root, in which case a slightly more medial exposure is warranted. When the disk herniation is not in the traditional location, a slightly different approach is often required. A foraminal disk herniation will compress the cephalad nerve root rather than the more traditional caudal nerve root at that level. In these cases, a partial medial facetectomy is required, and the surgeon generally stands on the opposite side of the table (Fig. 72-11). If the disk herniation is far lateral in an extraforaminal location (Fig. 72-12), it should be approached through a paramedian incision made two finger breadths lateral of the midline on the involved side (Fig. 72-13). The muscles are split down to the intertransverse ligament, which is sharply dissected off the inferior medial border of the transverse process and reflected caudally and laterally. The nerve root is identified just caudal to the transverse process. It should be retracted laterally to allow extraction of the disk fragments.[138] The standard posterolateral disk herniation tends to entrap the nerve root exiting under the pedicle of the lower vertebra (L4-5 posterolateral disk herniation entraps L5 nerve root) and a standard far lateral disk herniation will entrap the nerve root that has already exited under the pedicle of the above

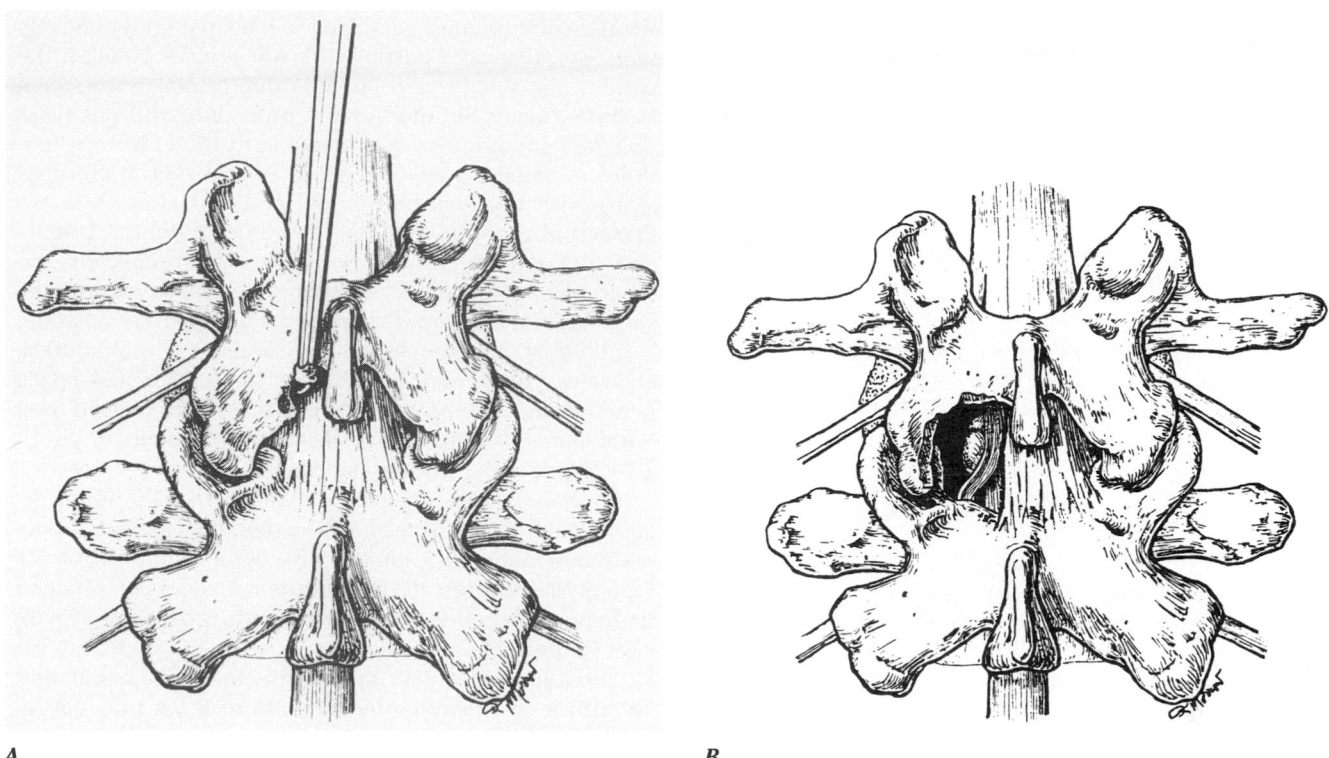

A   *B*

Figure 72-10 *A.* Partial medial facetectomy performed with 3-mm 40° Kerrison. *B.* Appropriately positioned hemilaminotomy centered over nerve root. (Reproduced with permission from Spencer DL: Lumbar intervertebral disk surgery, in Bridwell KH, DeWald RL (eds): *The Textbook of Spinal Surgery.* Philadelphia, Lippincott, 1991, pages 681 and 682.)

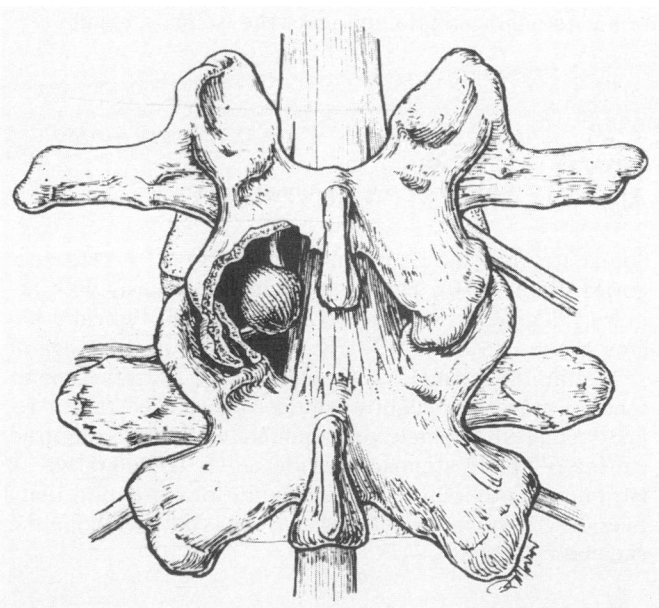

Figure 72-11 Lumbar intervertebral disk surgery. (Reproduced with permission from Spencer DL, Lumbar intervertebral disk surgery, in Bridwell KH, DeWald RL (eds): *The Textbook of Spinal Surgery.* Philadelphia, Lippincott, 1991.)

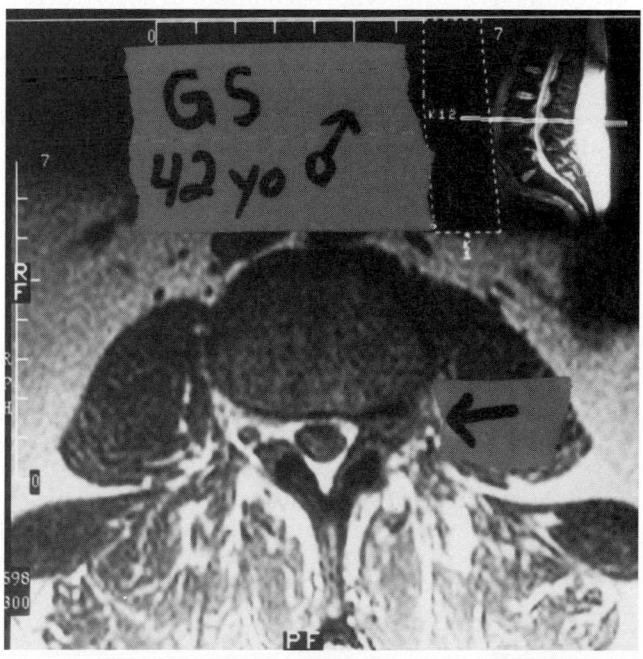

Figure 72-12 T2-weighted image demonstrating far lateral disk herniation at L3-L4. At surgery, the L3 nerve root was tented over the disk fragment.

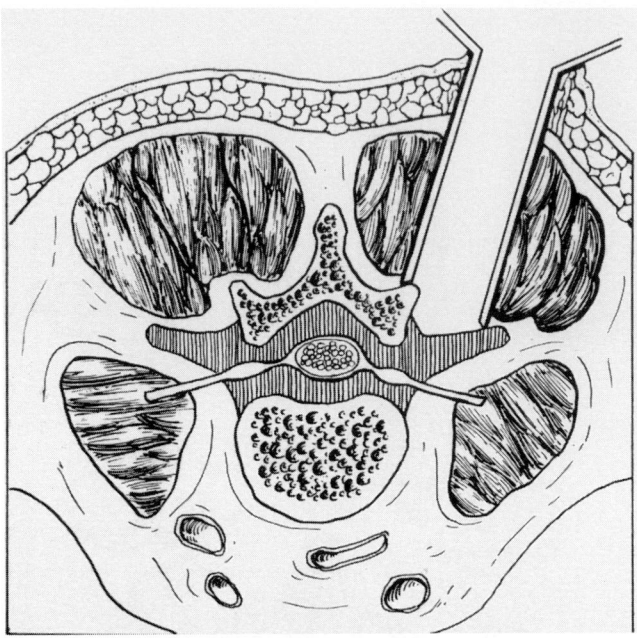

Figure 72-13 Lumbar intervertebral disk surgery. (Reproduced with permission from Spencer DL, Lumbar intervertebral disk surgery, in Bridwell KH, DeWald RL (eds): *The Textbook of Spinal Surgery.* Philadelphia, Lippincott, 1991, page 685.)

vertebra (L4-5 far lateral disk herniation entrapping the L4 nerve root).

Postoperative Care

Postoperatively, patients are encouraged to do a great deal of walking and to avoid prolonged sitting as well as bending, twisting, and lifting. Most patients with sedentary jobs can return to work within 1 to 2 weeks, but more physically demanding jobs require 6 to 8 weeks to recover not only from the surgery but from the overall deconditioning.

Recurrent disk herniations can occur in 5 to 10 percent of patients.[48] When performing surgery on a recurrent disk herniation, the surgeon must perform an additional laminotomy inferolateral and superior to the original hemilaminotomy. This makes it possible to avoid reentering through scar tissue. If the recurrent pain is truly due to a recurrent herniated disk, the results are quite good.[53] If the pain is primarily due to nerve root injury or scar formation, the results are much less rewarding. Most surgeons would recommend a concomitant arthrodesis for a third herniation at one level. Some recommend an arthrodesis for a second herniation at L4-5 because it is adjacent to the relatively immobile L5-S1 segment and thus is theoretically subject to more stresses than the other disks.[49]

Complications

The most common complication is incomplete relief of symptoms. This is usually due to diagnostic inaccuracy. If the patient's primary complaint is back pain, it is unlikely that operating on a bulging disk will provide relief. If the patient has sciatic pain but it is due primarily to spinal stenosis, again the diskectomy procedure will not help. This last situation is most common in the elderly, where there is usually some degree of lateral recess stenosis along with the disk herniation, and this should be addressed at the time of surgery. Another potential complication is operating on the wrong level. Intraoperative radiographs are mandatory and should be repeated until the surgeon is absolutely certain of the appropriate location.

Complications such as dural tears, nerve root injuries, and injury to the iliac vessels due to anterior disk space penetration are rare if meticulous technique is used. Any dural tear with spinal fluid leakage should be repaired with a 6-0 stitch and a tapered needle.

If there is a suspicion of a retained fragment following surgery, an MRI is usually not helpful, due to the postoperative hematoma. A lumbar myelogram followed by CT scan is the best test in this situation. If there is a retained fragment, it should be removed with repeat surgery as soon as possible.

Postoperative disk space infection can occur and should be suspected whenever there is an unusual increase in low back pain weeks or months following the surgery. Patients generally have an elevated sedimentation rate. Imaging studies show changes in the vertebral end plates and often disk space narrowing. An MRI in this situation is often helpful. Treatment generally involves a needle aspiration for culture and antibiotic therapy. Rarely is surgery required. Superficial infections and persistent wound drainage should be treated with surgical debridement and closure over drains.

The overall complication rates are approximately 8 percent for intraoperative problems, and 4 percent for postoperative problems.[141] Fortunately, most complications are minor and do not affect the ultimate result.

SPINAL STENOSIS AND DEGENERATIVE INSTABILITY

Spinal stenosis can be classified into one of several categories (Table 72-6). This section deals primarily with acquired degenerative spinal stenosis, which typically begins in the late fifties or early sixties. The average age of presentation for females is the early to mid-seventies; males tend to present at slightly younger ages. Most recent reports suggest a female predominance.[93] Other acquired causes of spinal stenosis include either degenerative or isthmic spondylolisthesis and conditions creating bony overgrowth, such as Paget's disease and diffuse idiopathic skeletal hyperostosis (DISH).

Pathophysiology

A useful guideline for spinal canal diameter is a midsagittal diameter of more than 11.5 mm and an overall area of

TABLE 72-6   Classification of Spinal Canal Stenosis

Congenital/developmental
   Idiopathic
   Achondroplastic
   Osteopetrosis

Acquired
   Degenerative
      Central
      Lateral recess and foraminal
      Degenerative spondylolisthesis
   Iatrogenic
      Postlaminectomy
      Postfusion
      Postdiskectomy
   Miscellaneous disorders
      Acromegaly
      Paget's
      Fluorosis
      Ankylosing spondylitis
   Traumatic

Combined
   Any combination of congenital, developmental, or acquired
   stenosis

Source: Reproduced with permission from Merkovic S, Garfin SR: Spinal stenosis: History and physical examination. *Instr Course Lect* 43:435, 1994.

more than 1.45 cm^2.[148] Most authors would agree that a midsagittal diameter of the canal of less than 10 mm or overall area of less than 100 mm^2 represents absolute stenosis, and that relative stenosis is a midsagittal diameter between 10 and 13 mm.[156] However, symptoms do not always correspond to canal size.

To understand the pathogenesis of spinal stenosis, the reader must understand the three-joint complex. This complex is made up of the intervertebral disk and the two facet joints. Degeneration can start in any one of these segments, but generally all three joints are involved. Typically, synovitis in the facet joints causes the joint cartilage to thin and the facet capsule to loosen. This loosening subsequently allows for greater spinal motion and the degeneration of the disk is accelerated. In an effort to stabilize itself, the spine forms osteophytes. Often the spine does fuse and the process is arrested, but these osteophytes can narrow the spinal canal. Osteophytes in the superior articular facet narrow the lateral recess, osteophytes in the inferior facet can narrow the spinal canal, and the degenerative narrowing of the disk can create foraminal stenosis. Disk narrowing also creates bulging of the annulus and redundancy of the ligamentum flavum, and this can contribute to the narrowing of the spinal canal.[156] The epidural fat pad has also been implicated in the narrowing of the canal.[60]

Many patients with spinal stenosis also have spondylolisthesis. This condition, which occurs five to six times more frequently in women, is felt to be due to generalized ligamentous laxity related to hormonal factors before the onset of menopause.[58] The arthritis of the facet joints and the subsequent loss of structural support is also implicated. One study recently noted an increased incidence of sagittal facet joint orientation in patients with degenerative spondylolisthesis, and this predisposes to forward slippage. The reason most slippages occur at L4-5 is because of the preponderance of coronal facet joint orientation at L5-S1.[47] When slips are present, they rarely exceed 25 to 30 percent of the width of the subjacent vertebrae, and progression of the slippage occurs in approximately 30 percent of the patients.[58]

If the spine is unable to stabilize itself, the instability of the facets and disk degeneration progresses, leading to more and more stenosis and/or instability. The size of the spinal canal and lateral recess and neural foramen continue to decrease, and this subsequently puts pressure on the neural elements, compromising their vascular supply. The resulting ischemic neuritis is felt to be a primary cause of the leg pain of spinal stenosis.[115,122] Degenerative disk disease, facet arthritis, and degenerative instability account for the back pain in these patients.

Adults with isthmic spondylolisthesis can develop back and leg pain later in life due to progressive disk degeneration at the olisthetic segment; this slippage can progress and cause radiculopathies as well.[38]

Clinical Presentation

Patients will typically present with a history of an insidious onset of back and leg pain. The distribution of the pain in the legs is dependent upon the level of the stenosis. Usually the symptoms are bilateral. The leg pain is usually worse with standing and walking. Sitting or lying and flexing the spine forward usually relieves the pain. A classic history is one of leg pain upon walking distances, but the patient is able to walk when leaning forward on a shopping cart or walking uphill. This is because the forward-flexed position increases the area in the spinal canal. Another common history is symptoms that are worse at night; this occurs because the sleeping posture decreases the area in the spinal canal. In very severe cases, the symptoms can be less reliably relieved by sitting or flexing forward; a neurogenic bladder may develop in the most severe cases.

Differential Diagnosis

Since the majority of these patients are elderly and many of them smoke, the surgeon must be aware of the possibility of a vascular etiology for the leg pain. Table 72-7 summarizes the difference between neurogenic claudication, vascular claudication, and the back pain of lumbar spondylosis without spinal stenosis. Peripheral neuropathy must also be considered in making the differentiation from neurogenic claudication. Such neuropathy can be due to diabetes, a history of exposure to toxins, and/or alcoholism. The symptoms will generally be in a glove-and-stocking distribution. Vibratory sensation is often dimin-

TABLE 72-7 Differential Diagnosis of Signs and Symptoms

Findings	Neurogenic claudication	Vascular claudication	Lumbar spondylosis
Signs			
Neurologic examination	Occasional findings, usually asymmetrical	Rare findings, symmetrical if present	No findings, negative
Straight-leg raise	Negative, rarely positive	Negative	Negative
Femoral stretch test	Negative, rarely positive	Negative	Negative
Pulses	Present or symmetrically diminished	Diminished or absent, often asymmetrical	Symmetrical
Skin	Normal	Hair loss	Normal
Bicycle test	Negative/positive with lumbar hyperextension	Positive	Negative
Symptoms			
Pain			
Type	Vague cramping, aches, sharp, burning in legs	Tightness, cramping (usually in calf)	Dull, ache (in the low back)
Location	Back, buttocks, legs	Leg muscles	Back
Radiation	Common proximal to distal	Localized in legs	Localized back
Exacerbation	Standing (particularly with trunk extended) Walking—less Bicycling—none, unless trunk extended	Walking, bicycling (lower extremity activities)	General activities, bending, standing, twisting, lifting
Improvement	Sitting, flexing, squatting	Standing, cessation of muscular activity	Decreased activity, rest
Time to relief	Slow	Quick	Slow
Walking uphill	No pain	Pain	±Pain
Walking downhill	Pain (lumbar hyperextension)	Pain	±Pain
Back pain	Common	Uncommon	Common
Limitation of spinal movement	Common	Uncommon	Common

Source: Reproduced with permission from Merkovic S, Garfin SR: Spinal stenosis: History and physical examination. *Instr Course Lect* 43:436, 437, 1994.

ished, and the symptoms are often unrelated to activity. Other problems that can mimic spinal stenosis include epidural neoplasms and synovial cysts.[130,145]

Physical Examination

The neurologic exam in these people is often normal if the symptoms have not been present for a long time. The patients may complain of leg weakness, but in most cases this is not dramatic on exam. When motor deficits are present, they usually affect the L5 nerve root distribution, because L4-5 is the most frequently involved level. If sensory changes are present, the examiner must consider a peripheral neuropathy as the cause. Reflexes are commonly diminished in a symmetrical distribution in the elderly, so this finding is probably not significant, but asymmetrical reflexes are. The straight-leg-raising test is usually negative unless a concurrent disk herniation is present. The presence of long tract signs should make the examiner look for coexisting cervical stenosis. Diminished pedal pulses and absence of shin hair raise the suspicion of a vascular etiology for the leg pain.

Most patients are able to bend forward with little difficulty but have difficulty with extension, and this often exacerbates the pain. Upon inspection of the back, the lumbar spine is often flattened.

Diagnostics

One provocative test that we commonly employ is the exercise bike/treadmill test. Theoretically a patient with claudication secondary to spinal stenosis should be better able to ride a bicycle with the spine in a flexed position than to walk on a treadmill, and someone with vascular claudication or a combination of both conditions will have difficulty with both these exercises. This helps differentiate between neurogenic claudication and vascular claudication and also gives a good baseline, objective, functional assessment. Often arterial Doppler studies are needed to rule out a vascular etiology definitively. Patients in whom peripheral neuropathy is being ruled out often need EMG, nerve conduction studies, and consultation with a neurologist.

Workup with imaging studies should also begin with plain radiographs. These will show if there is any preexisting congenital stenosis as well as signs of disk degeneration, facet degeneration, and the presence of degenerative spondylolisthesis and degenerative scoliosis, which suggests segmental instability. The plain AP and lateral x-rays should be done with the patient standing, and supine flexion/extension films should be used to determine the degree of instability[164] (Fig. 72-14).

In the absence of deformity, MRI is an excellent screening modality. It is noninvasive and has the ability to differentiate tissues and assess the status of intervertebral disks. Disadvantages include its relatively high cost, the inability to use it in the presence of ferromagnetic implants, and the fact that many patients experience claustrophobia during imaging. Also, MRI is still inferior to CT scanning in evaluating bony detail. In patients with isthmic spondylolisthesis and clinical evidence of radiculopathy, MRI has been shown to effectively demonstrate the lateral recess and foraminal stenosis, which are the likely sources of the leg pain.[73]

Myelography, with a water-soluble contrast agent followed by CT scanning remains the gold standard. The myelogram makes possible visualization of multiple levels in the presence of deformity and allows for a more dynamic study in which images can be obtained with the patient flexing, extending, and so on. Also, the combined study gives an excellent view of the central and lateral canal and will define any extradural cause of compression (Fig. 72-15). The disadvantage is that it is an invasive study and often requires an overnight stay in the hospital.

Electromyograms commonly show changes in these patients, and they can help localize the appropriate areas for decompression. Similarly, SSEPs can also be useful in a complicated differential.[85]

Treatment

Nonoperative Management

Most patients should initially be tried on a vigorous outpatient physical therapy program. Flexion exercises as well as stretching exercises and strengthening for the back extensors and hip flexors can help increase the range of motion and reduce the anterior pelvic tilt. The patient should be encouraged to try to stay as aerobically fit as possible. Passive modalities such as traction, ultrasound, transcutaneous electrical nerve stimulators, and so on often provide relief, albeit usually temporary.

Nonsteroidal anti-inflammatory medications often help. Since the majority of these patients are elderly, the clinician must watch for the frequent gastrointestinal side

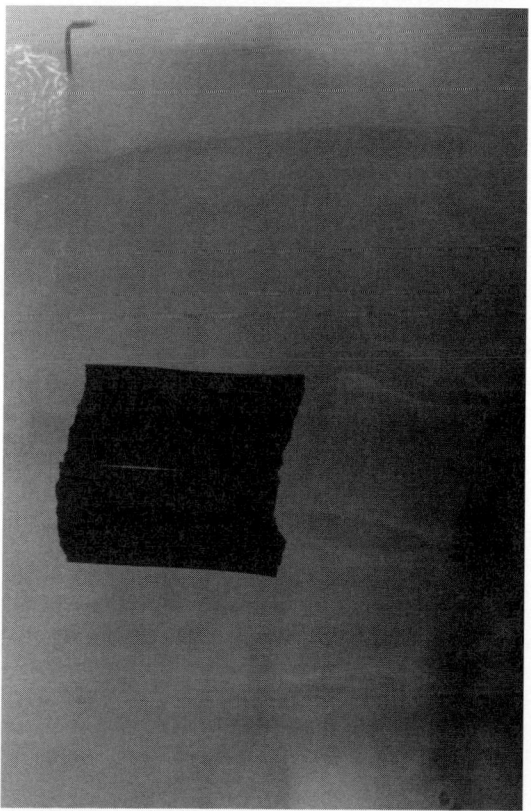

A   *B*

Figure 72-14 Patient with L4-5 degenerative spondylolisthesis with approximately 5 mm of motion noted on the flexion/extension films.

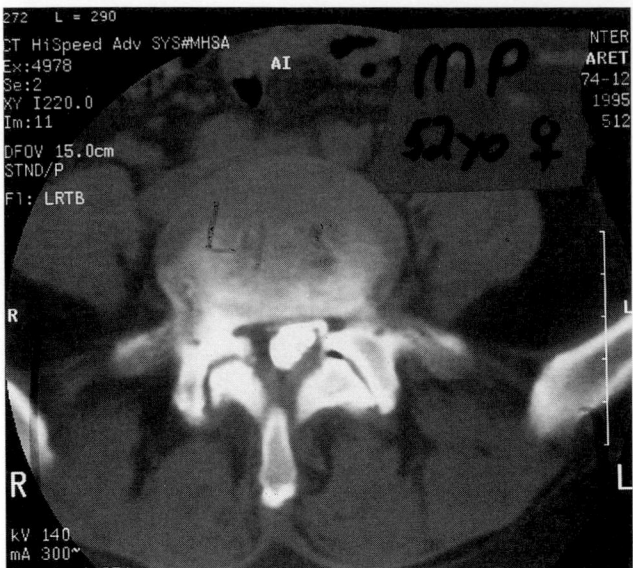

Figure 72-15 Postmyelogram CT scan demonstrating the contrast-enhanced nerve root on the left and no such finding on the right.

effects. Low-dose tricyclic antidepressants often help with the night pain. The majority of patients can expect some improvement with this aggressive nonoperative approach.[112]

Many clinicians prescribe epidural steroids for these patients. These drugs rarely provide long-term relief but are probably beneficial in the treatment of patients who are not good surgical candidates. These injections can also be helpful in predicting which patients are likely to benefit from surgery. If epidural steroids give 50 percent or better relief for 1 week to patients who have had symptoms for less than 1 year, 95 percent of such patients will have a good result 1 year after surgery. If the symptoms have been present for more than 1 year and the epidural steroid does not provide 50 percent improvement, then only 5 percent will be improved with surgery.[28]

As the symptoms become more severe, there is less likelihood that these methods will be successful in providing significant relief. In contemplating surgery, it should be stressed to the patient that this is purely an elective procedure except in the presence of bowel or bladder dysfunction. The decision to proceed should be entirely up to the patient, and it should be stressed that a delay in surgery of months or years will typically not be a problem.[75]

Surgical Techniques for Decompression of Lumbar Stenosis

Once a patient has exhausted an appropriate nonoperative course of treatment and other causes of pain have been ruled out, he or she is considered for surgical intervention. These patients require a thorough medical evaluation by their internists preoperatively. Once a patient is deemed an appropriate candidate for surgery, the surgeon

must, as accurately as possible, determine the source of pain so as to focus the decompression just at those symptomatic levels. Also, many of these patients require a concomitant spinal fusion, and every effort must be made to rule out the presence of instability. Usually the need for spinal fusion can be predicted preoperatively, but there is the occasional case where the extent of the decompression necessitates a fusion. Therefore the possibility of fusion should be discussed with every patient preoperatively (Fig. 72-16).

The patient should be given a general anesthesia and positioned such that the abdomen is allowed to hang free, reducing the venous distention and thusly keeping intraoperative bleeding at a minimum. Some surgeons prefer the modified kneeling position with a flattened lumbar lordosis, while others prefer to keep the hips more extended to preserve the patient's natural lordosis and thus make it possible to observe the stenotic conditions in a more natural position. Also, if a fusion is being planned, keeping the spine lordotic will minimize the chance of fusing the spine into hypolordosis. Loupe magnification with fiberoptic headlights optimizes the visualization.

The specific technique of decompression depends on where the preoperative imaging studies show the pathology to be. Patients can have simply a central canal stenosis, a lateral recess stenosis, a foraminal stenosis, or a combination of all three. Central canal stenosis requires exposure of the spinous processes and the lamina by elevating the paraspinal muscles subperiosteally from the midline to the facets. The facet joint capsules are not disturbed. The spinous processes and interspinous ligament of the level involved are removed. With care to protect the dura, the lamina is subsequently removed with a Kerrison rongeur. The decompression should always begin from the area of least stenosis. The lamina is removed out to the most medial portion of the facets and the pars must be preserved if a fusion is not being done. The ligamentum flavum must be removed in its entirety. If, after removal of the ligamentum flavum, compression on the dura persists, it is usually due to facet hypertrophy. In fact, only a minority of patients will be adequately decompressed with only a central decompression. In these cases there is usually congenital stenosis with short pedicles. The majority require a lateral decompression.

A partial medial facetectomy can usually be done with a 45° Kerrison rongeur. Up to 50 percent of each facet joint or up to 100 percent of one facet joint can be removed without significantly compromising stability. Passing a probe out the neural foramen and retracting the nerve root medially will show if the decompression is adequate (Fig. 72-17). If the patient does not have much in the way of midline stenosis but has significant lateral recess stenosis, the spinous processes and interspinous ligaments can be preserved and the decompression consists of a laminotomy and partial facetectomy.

The lateral recess is commonly divided into three zones: an entrance zone, a middle zone, and an exit zone.[23] If only the entrance zone is stenotic, a partial medial facetectomy will provide adequate decompression. The middle zone is the area underneath the pars interarticularis. Its boundaries are the vertebral body anteriorly, the pars

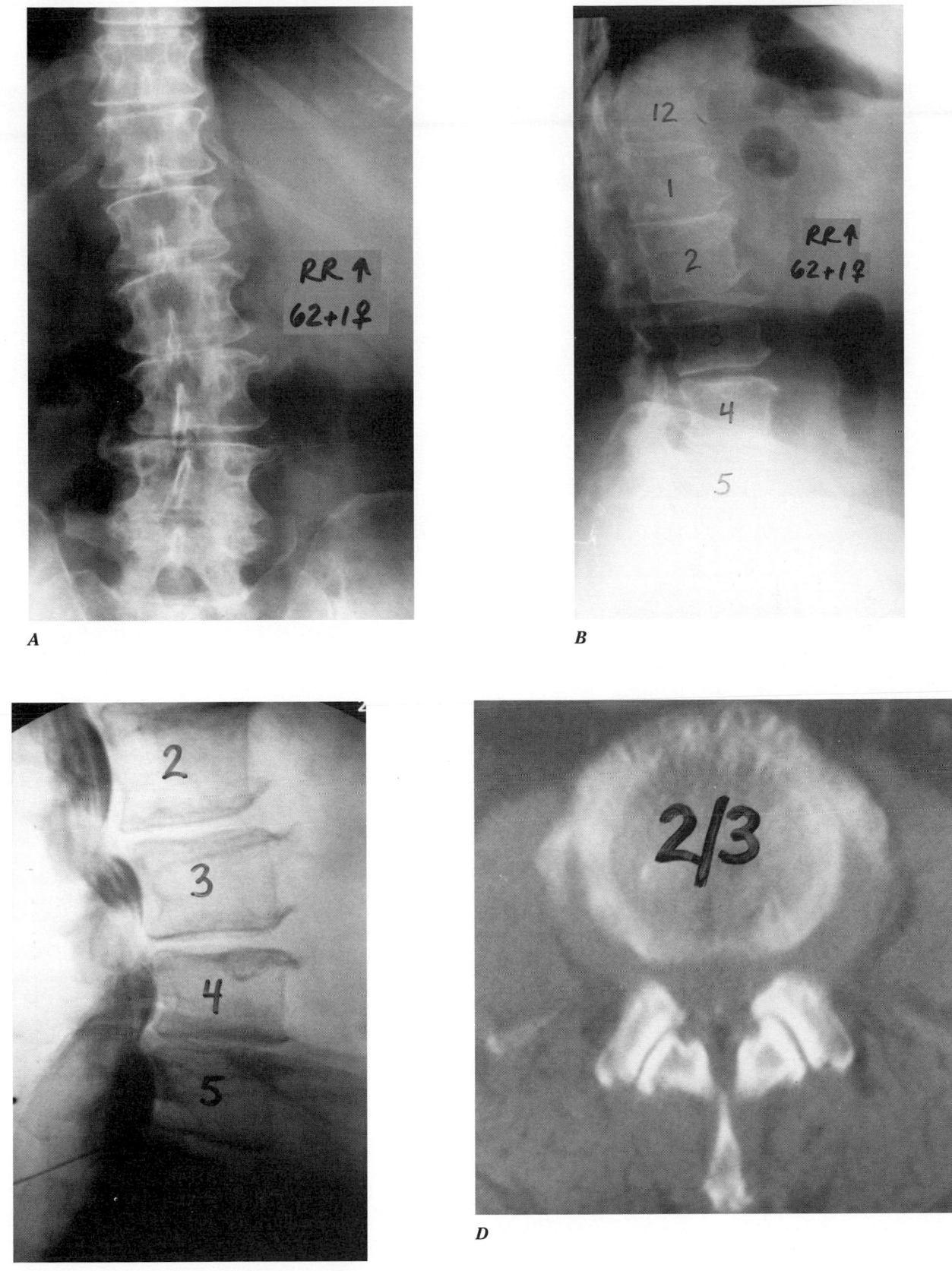

Figure 72-16 R.R. is a 62 + 1-year old male with neurogenic claudication. His (*A*) coronal and (*B*) lateral lumbar radiographs show bilevel degenerative disk disease and a small degenerative scoliosis with many stabilizing osteophytes. A CT lateral myelogram (*C*) showed spinal stenosis in the lumbar spine and a postmyelographic CT scan showed spinal stenosis that was severe at L2-L3, (*D*) moderate at L3-L4, (*E*) and mild at L4-L5 (*F*). He underwent a decompressive laminectomy from L2-3 to L5-S1 with good relief of his symptomatology and no change in the position of his spine (*G*).

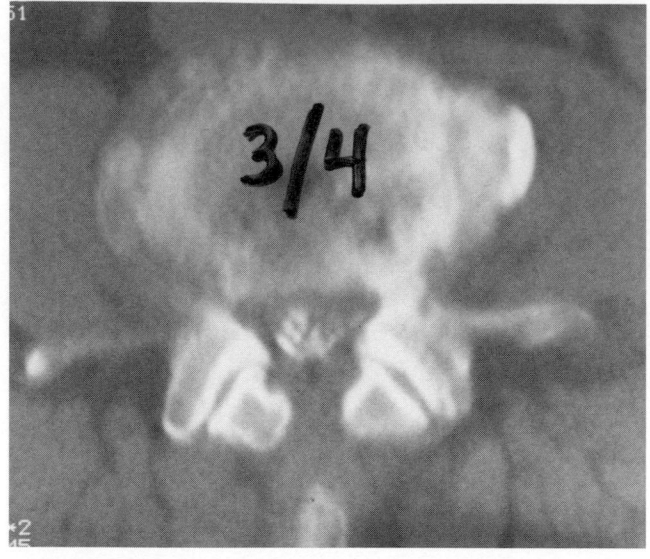

E

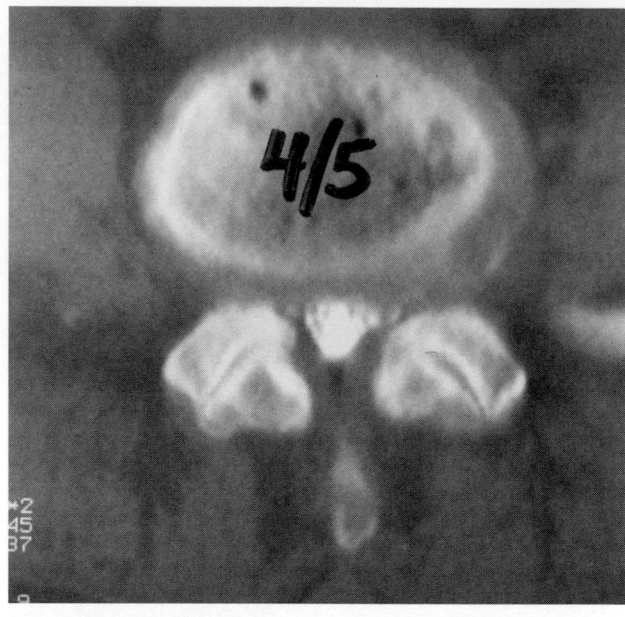

F

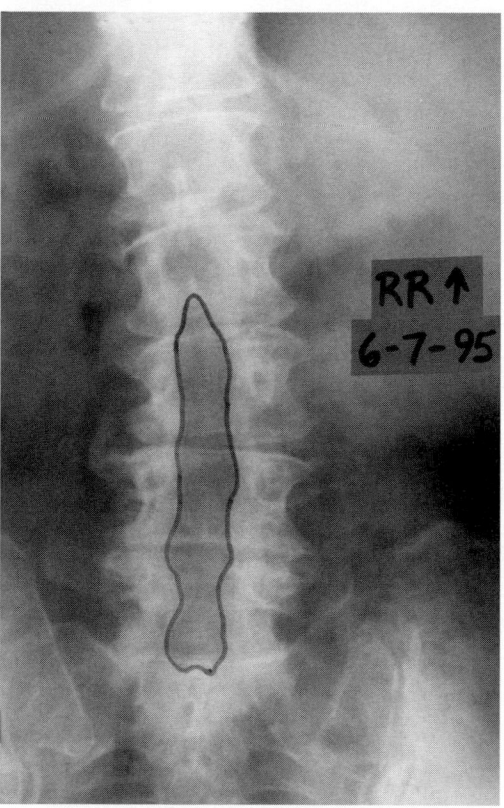

G

Figure 72-16 (*Continued*)

interarticularis posteriorly, and the pedicle and foramen laterally. Often the dorsal root ganglion, which is the widest portion of the nerve root, lies in this area and thus can be easily compressed. Total facetectomy is the surest way of decompressing this, but it can lead to instability. If the disks are very degenerated with collapsing and bridg-

ing osteophytes, even with total unilateral facetectomy, fusion may not be required.[156] The exit zone boundaries are made up by the disk anteriorly and the facet joint of the caudal segment posteriorly. Again, total facetectomy provides the surest decompression, but increases the risk of instability.

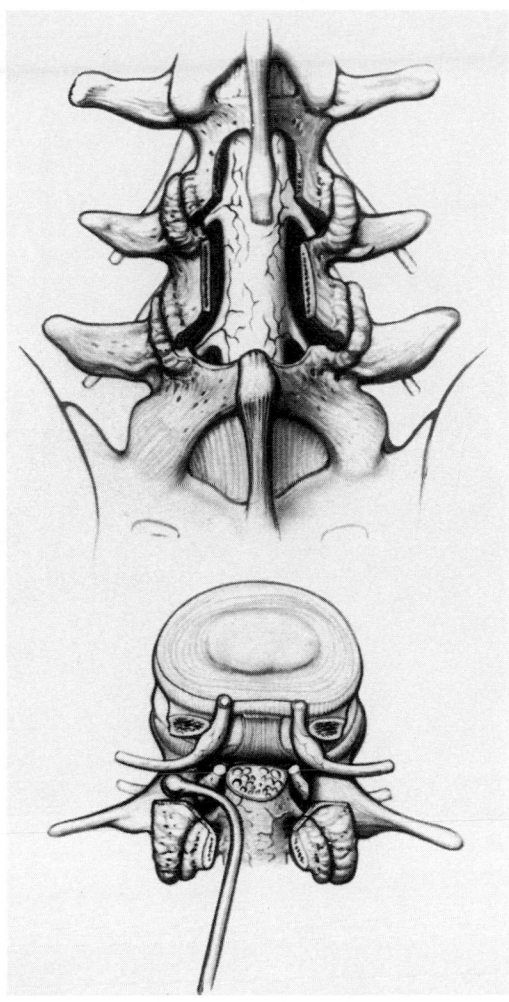

Figure 72-17 Spinal stenosis decompression. A probe is passed out the neuroforamen to check adequacy of decompression. (Reproduced with permission from Whiffen JR, Neuwirth MG: Spinal stenosis, in Bridwell KH, DeWald RL (eds): *The Textbook of Spinal Surgery.* Philadelphia, Lippincott, 1991, page 644.)

Results

Decompressive surgery does not stop the degenerative process in the lumbar spine; for this reason, stenosis can recur due to bone regrowth in the surgical defect.[23] In spite of this, most properly selected patients undergoing a decompressive laminectomy do quite well. In a metaanalysis of the literature, Turner et al. found that 64 percent of the patients had good to excellent outcomes after surgery.[146] Other studies have shown similar success rates.[20,52,131] Katz et al. reported good results in those patients whose preoperative pain was primarily leg pain, but those bothered predominantly by back pain and those with greater medical comorbidity did less well following their surgery for degenerative lumbar spinal stenosis.[79] Other studies have reported factors that predict a poor outcome; these include significant comorbidities including diabetes mellitus, the presence of compensation or litigation factors, no relief of symptoms from prior surgical procedures, objective postoperative sensory deficit, and female sex.[54,132]

Johnsson et al. compared two similar groups of patients, one that had decompressive surgery and one that did not. They used a visual analog-scale estimation to determine degree of improvement, finding that 60 percent of those treated surgically and 33 percent of the untreated patients reported feeling better. However, neurophysiologic changes progressed in all the patients, and this was more pronounced in the treated group. This certainly lends support to a trial of nonoperative treatment for such patients.[76]

DEGENERATIVE SPONDYLOLISTHESIS

Patients with spinal stenosis and degenerative spondylolisthesis must be approached a little differently than a patient with straightforward stable spinal stenosis. In spondylolisthesis, in addition to the stenosis caused by the hypertrophic facets and ligamentum flavum and the bulging of the disk, the inferior margin of the lamina of the cephalad vertebra and the posterior margin of the caudad vertebra often compress the thecal sac. Also, the nerve root is usually trapped between the superior border of the caudad vertebral body and the hypertrophic anterior listhetic inferior facet of the cephalad vertebra. All this usually means that a fairly extensive central and lateral decompression is called for, requiring at least the removal of the spinous processes and lamina and a partial medial facetectomy. A number of authors have evaluated decompression alone in the presence of a spondylolisthesis versus decompression and fusion. Most reports suggest that those who received the fusion clearly do better.[18,35,56,59] The study by Herkowitz and Kurz[60] is the only prospective study in this group, but it very clearly shows the advantages of fusion in decompressing spinal stenosis in the presence of degenerative spondylolisthesis (Fig. 72-18).

While almost every patient with spinal stenosis and degenerative spondylolisthesis should have a fusion along with decompression, Whiffen and Neuwirth propose specific criteria for those that may not need a fusion.[156] These criteria include (1) no evidence of instability on the supine preoperative flexion/extension radiographs defined as translation of greater than 3.5 mm; (2) no associated degenerative scoliosis of greater than 10°; (3) minimal osteoporosis; (4) no compression fractures at the level of the planned decompression; and (5) no symptoms or history of prolonged mechanical back pain. They add that if a fusion is not planned preoperatively, it may become necessary at the time of surgery by either (1) taking more than one-third of the medial facet, (2) fracture or weakening of the pars interarticularis, and/or (3) removal of the intervertebral disk. If there is a question of whether or not the patient needs a fusion, it is probably best to err on the side of fusion, since results with secondary surgery, if it becomes necessary, tend to be less rewarding.

Other indications for concomitant arthrodesis along with decompression include some cases of scoliosis and/or kyphosis. There are also patients who require a second decompressive laminectomy at the same segment with or

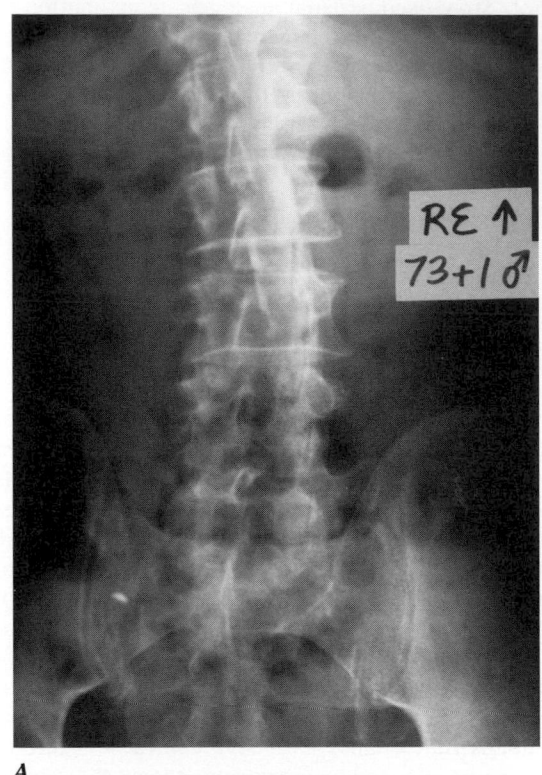

A

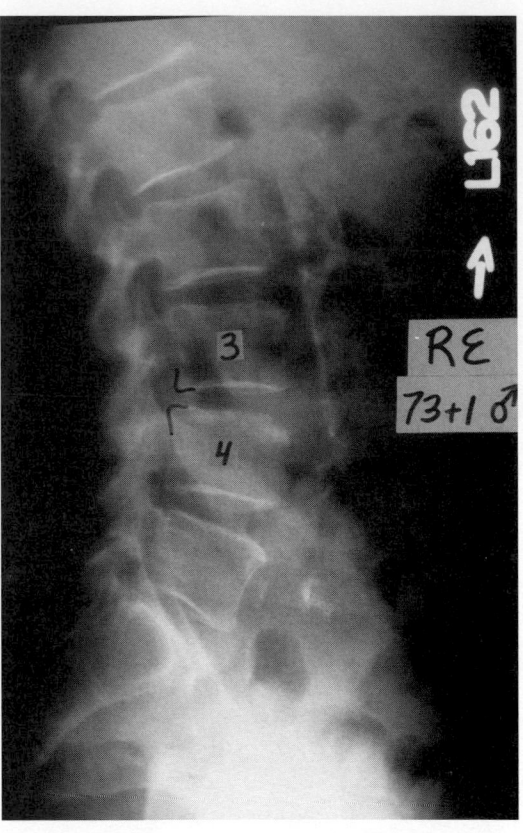

B

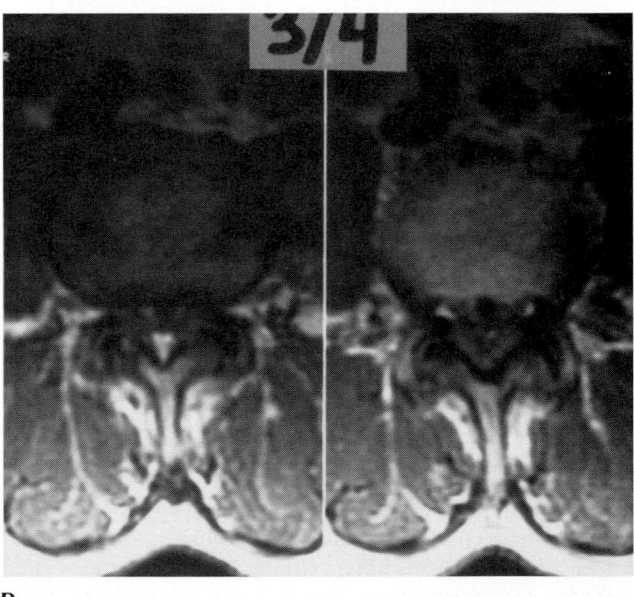

D

C

Figure 72-18 R.E. is a 73 + 1-year-old male with his (*A*) coronal and (*B*) lateral lumbar radiographs showing a small degenerative spondylolisthesis at L3-L4. His (*C*) lateral MRI showed potential spinal stenosis at L3-L4, also seen on his (*D*) axial MRI images. He underwent a single-level decompressive laminectomy pedicle instrumentation and fusion from L3-L4. His 2½ year postoperative (*E*) coronal and (*F*) lateral radiograph show a solid fusion.

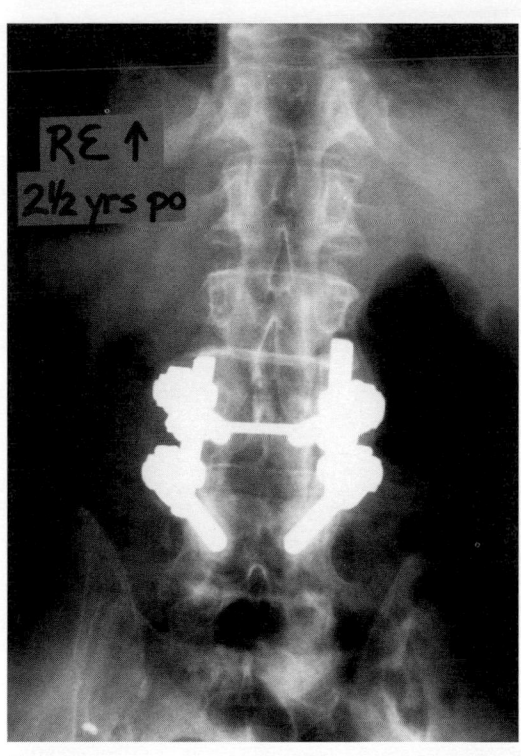

E

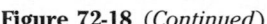

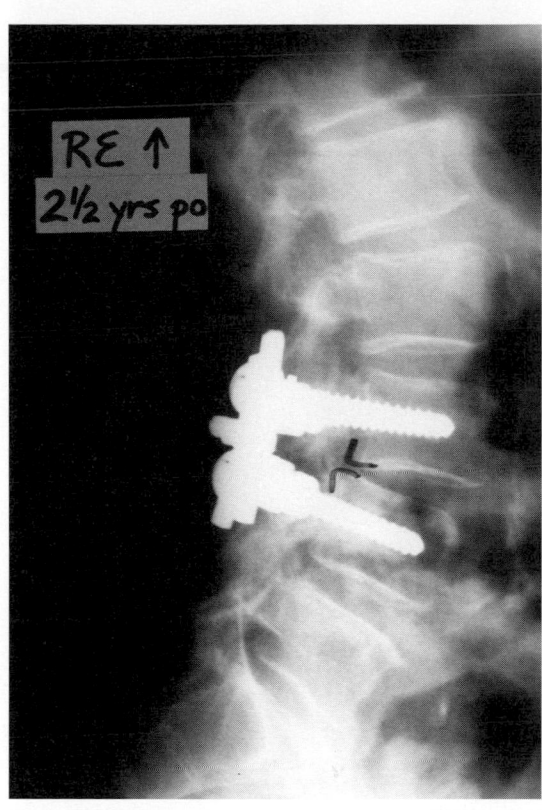

F

Figure 72-18 (*Continued*)

without iatrogenic spondylolisthesis. In the former group, fusion might not be necessary if the deformity is stable; in this latter group, revision decompression further compromises the facet joints, putting the patient at risk for segmental instability.[57]

When the decision has been made to add a fusion to the procedure, the options are fusion with or without instrumentation. There is a preponderance of data suggesting that an intertransverse process fusion in the presence of pedicle instrumentation provides the best environment for obtaining a solid arthrodesis.[18,57,156,167]

Obviously, each patient must be evaluated individually in determining exactly what procedure to perform. We can, however, make some general recommendations regarding when to fuse. Patients with preoperative spondylolisthesis and preoperative evidence of instability manifest as greater than 3.5 mm of motion on flexion/extension films or documented progression of degenerative scoliosis should be fused, as should radical decompressions involving total or subtotal facetectomies (Fig. 72-19). The fusion should be done with instrumentation systems via the pedicles, utilizing the patient's autogenous bone. Every effort should be made to maintain a normal lumbar lordosis when performing a fusion, so as to minimize the risk of developing a transition syndrome above or below the fusion.[22]

Bridwell and DeWald have offered specific treatment recommendations for patients with degenerative scoliosis.

They divide patients into one of four groups (Table 72-8), depending on amount of coronal deformity, sagittal deformity, degree of stenosis, and amount of subluxation. Patients in group I receive conservative management involving muscle-strengthening exercises. Group II patients receive decompression alone. Group III patients receive decompression with posterior instrumentation and fusion. Group IV patients, due to the increased coronal and sagittal imbalance, along with the decompression and posterior instrumentation and fusion, also require anterior surgery using structural grafts to help restore the sagittal alignment and increase the foraminal cross-sectional area.[17] Hanley et al.[49] offer treatment algorithms in working up these difficult patients with stenosis and instability (Fig. 72-20).

Most authors agree that isthmic spondylolisthesis arises before adulthood and is often asymptomatic in adolescence. In fact, it has been estimated that 4 to 6 percent of adults have defects in the pars interarticularis.[38,121,151] Many of these previously asymptomatic or mildly symptomatic patients end up with low back pain and radiculopathy later in adult life.[38] The olisthetic disk may undergo degeneration, leading to an increase in slippage and/or low back pain with or without radiculopathy.

In these adult patients who fail conservative management, surgery can provide relief. A Gill procedure is done posteriorly to fully decompress the nerve roots, and the L5 nerve root should be traced out far laterally. Then seg-

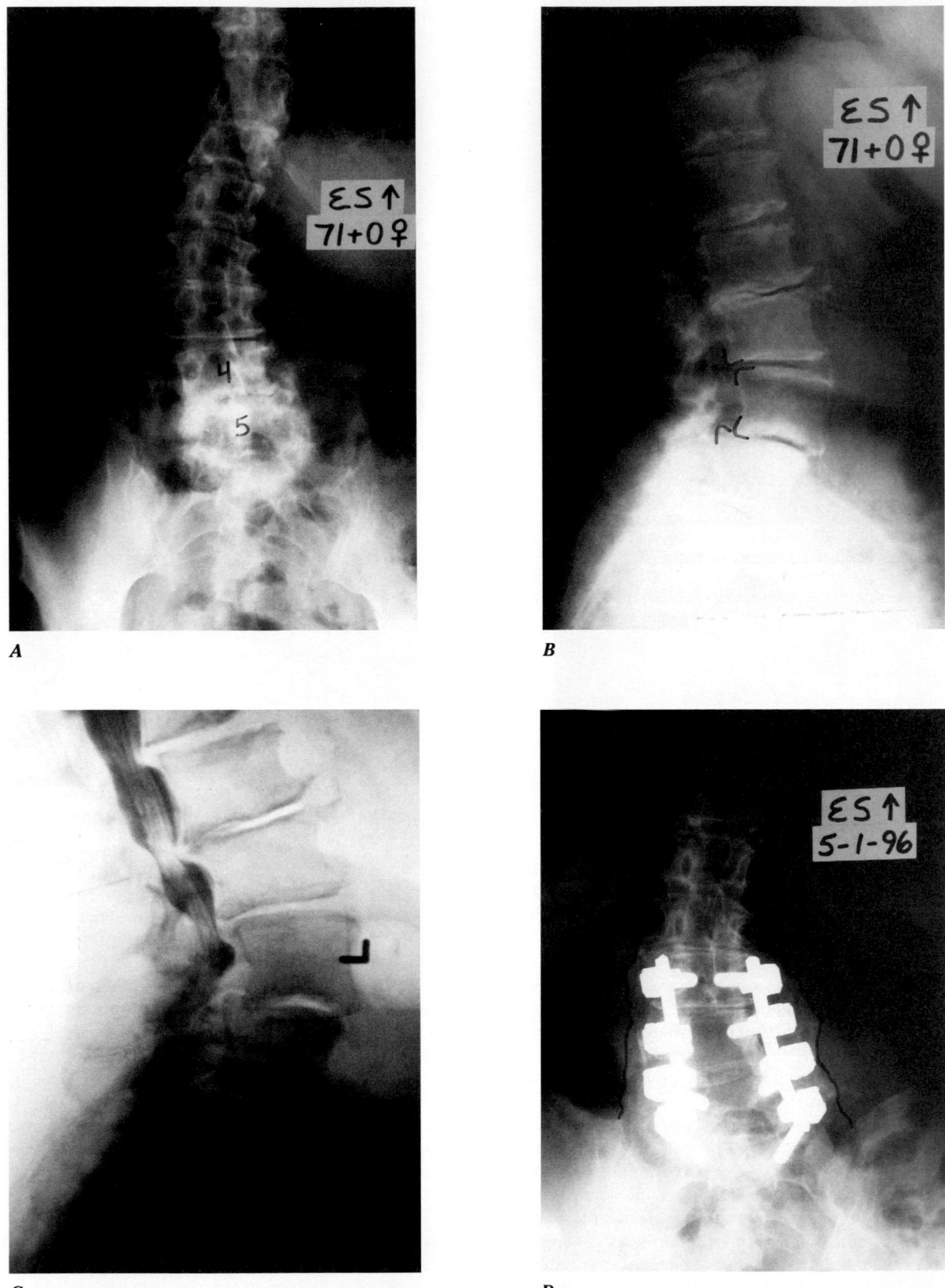

A

B

C

D

Figure 72-19 E.S. is a 71-year-old female with severe neurogenic claudication. Her (*A*) coronal and (*B*) lateral radiographs show a degenerative scoliosis with multilevel degenerative disk disease as well as a retrolisthesis at L3 on L4 and a degenerative spondylolisthesis at L4 on L5. *C.* Lumbar myelography showed a complete block of contrast on the lateral myelogram at L4-L5, with moderate stenosis at L3-L4 as well. She underwent a decompressive laminectomy from L3-S1 along with instrumentation and fusion to stabilize those segments, which was required because of her preoperative instability and the wide decompression necessary to free her lateral recesses. Her postoperative coronal (*D*) and (*E*) lateral radiographs show instrumented fusion with no change at the degenerated transition level above.

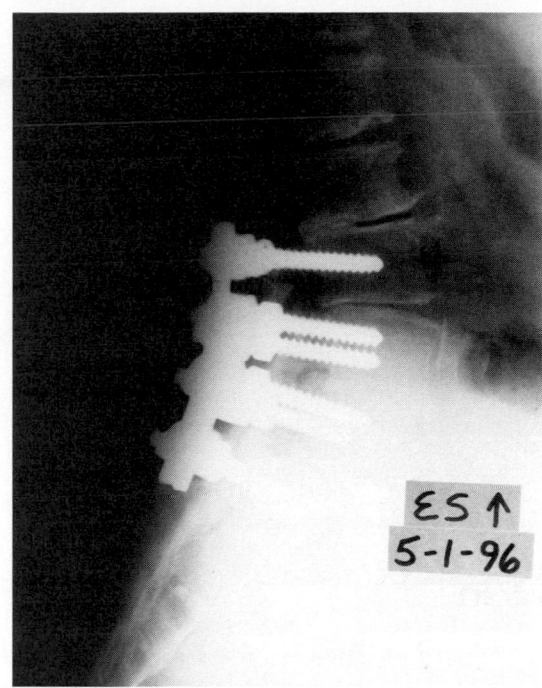

E

Figure 72-19 (*Continued*)

mental instrumentation is placed from L5 to the sacrum; if the slip is of high grade, instrumentation should be extended to the pelvis. If the proximal segment is degenerated as well, the fusion can be carried up one level. In low-grade slips, an anterior arthrodesis can be performed using a posterior lumbar inner-body fusion technique. In higher

grades, we place a strut graft from L5 to the sacrum through a separate anterior approach. We generally do not attempt to reduce high-grade slips in adults, but this has been done successfully.[69]

Postoperative Care

Patients receiving decompression without fusion are generally ambulated the evening of surgery or the next morning. Most are able to leave the hospital within a week of surgery and are encouraged to walk as much as possible. In the short term, the patient should avoid excessive bending, lifting, and twisting, but by 4 to 6 weeks postoperatively, they are able to take part in a more vigorous rehabilitation program. If there is a concern with instability, such a patient can be fitted with a lumbosacral corset postopertively. Those with sedentary jobs can usually return to work within 2 to 4 weeks. Those with more physically demanding jobs may require more thorough work hardening and more aggressive therapy, but most should be able to return to work by 6 to 8 weeks.

In patients who have had spinal fusion, we again ambulate them the morning after surgery. Most of these patients are fitted with a low-profile thoracolumbar sacral orthosis (TLSO) to wear when they are standing or sitting. They are encouraged to do a great deal of walking in the short term but to avoid bending, lifting, and twisting. The brace is usually discontinued by about 4 months postoperatively. At that point the patient can begin activities such as gentle swimming and riding an exercise bike. By 7 or 8 months, these patients can often start light jogging or a noncompetitive game of tennis. By a year postop, they are usually able to go back to their preoperative activities.

TABLE 72-8 Classification of Spinal Lesions

Coronal	Sagittal (L1 to sacrum)	Stenosis	Subluxation, mm
I (10° to 25°)	A. −40° to −60°	+	1. < 2
II (26° to 35°)	B. −20° to −39°	+ +	2. 2–5
III (36° to 45°)	C. 0° to −19°	+ + +	3. 5–10
IV > 45° or > 3 cm deviation from CVA	D. Frank kyphosis	+ + + +	4. >10
I (10° to 25°)	A. −40° to −60°	+	1. <2
II (26° to 35°)	B. −20° to −39°	+ +	2. 2–5
I (10° to 25°)	A. −40° to −60°	+ + +	1. <2
II (26° to 35°)	B. −20° to −39°	+ + + +	
	C. 0° to −19°		
II (26° to 35°)	A. −40° to −60°	+ + +	1. <2
III (36° to 45°)	B. −20° to −39°	+ + + +	2. 2–5

Source: Reproduced with permission from Spencer DL: Lumbar intervertebral disk surgery, in Bridwell DH, DeWald RL (eds): *The Textbook of Spinal Surgery.* Philadelphia, Lippincott, 1991, page 685.)

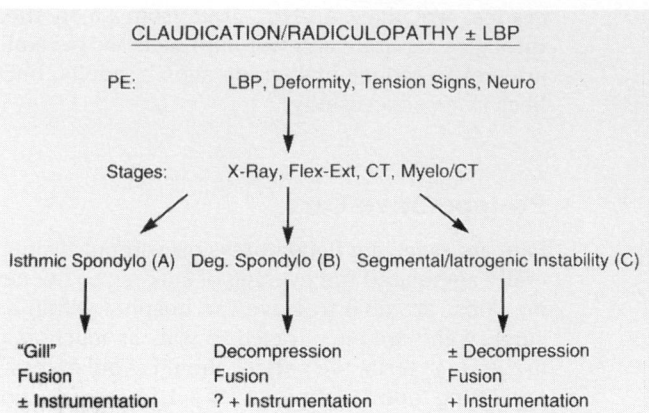

Figure 72-20 Stenosis and instability. (Reproduced with permission from Hanley EN Jr, Spengler DM, Wesel S, et al: Controversies in low back pain: The surgical approach. *Instr Course Lect* 43:418, 1994.)

Complications

Potential complications of this surgery include iatrogenic instability (in those that have received decompression alone) as well as dural tears, arachnoiditis, infection, nerve injury, and epidural fibrosis.

The risk of postoperative instability when there is no preexisting evidence of instability is low, but when it does occur it compromises the ultimate result.[50,74,120]

Dural tears occur in approximately 5 percent of decompression cases and the incidence is slightly higher in revision cases. When there is a significant leakage of cerebrospinal fluid, it should be repaired with a 5 or 6-0 suture. Large tears may require a fascial graft, and hard-to-reach areas may require the use of fibrin glue. In severe tears, occasionally a subarachnoid catheter is required to reduce the cerebrospinal fluid pressure. The dural tears do not affect the ultimate long-term result.[77]

Arachnoiditis or intrathecal fibrosis can best be minimized by careful handling of the neural tissues, but once present, it responds poorly to treatment.

Infections occur in 1 to 2 percent of previously unoperated patients; the risk increases to 5 percent in those who have had prior surgery. All wound infections should be treated with irrigation and debridement and closure over drains with appropriate antibiotic therapy.

Typically the most common patient concern is the risk of nerve injury, but this is exceedingly rare with good surgical technique, especially if magnification is used with surgery. When pedicle instrumentation is used, stimulating the pedicle screws and measuring potentials distally can suggest whether a pedicle screw is too close to a nerve root, thus minimizing the risk of nerve root injury from instrumentation.

If surgery has failed to relieve the symptoms, one must consider an inadequate decompression or bony regrowth. Also postoperative instability or, in a case that was fused, the development of a pseudoarthrosis can lead to persistent pain. Flat-back syndrome, neural injury, and/or arachnoiditis can lead to chronic pain as well; psychoneurosis can also lead to persistent pain.[159]

SUMMARY

Surgery for degenerative disorders of the spine can be very rewarding for both patient and the physician in the properly selected cases. In patients whose quality of life is dramatically impaired, even elderly patients, surgery can be offered as an elective procedure.[126]

REFERENCES

1. Adams MA, Hutton WC: Gradual disc prolapse. *Spine* 10:524–531, 1985.
2. Agostini E, Mognoni G, Tori G, Miserocki G: Forces deforming rib cage. *Respir Physiol* 2:105–108, 1956.
3. Alaranta H, Tallroth K, Soukka A, Heliovaara M: Fat content of lumbar extensor muscles and low back disability: A radiographic and clinical comparison. *J Spinal Dis* 6:137–140, 1993.
4. Andersson GB: in Weinstein JN, Rydevik BL, Sonntag VKH (eds): *Essentials of the Spine.* New York, Raven Press, 1994, chap 1.
5. Arce CA, Dohrmann GH: Herniated thoracic disks. *Neurol Clin* 3:383–392, 1985.
6. Ashton IK, Ashton SJ, Gibson JM, et al: Morphological basis for back pain: The demonstration of nerve fibers and neuropeptides in the lumbar facet joint capsule, but not in ligamentum flavum. *J Orthop Res* 10:72–78, 1992.
7. Awwad EE, Martin DS, Smith KR Jr, Baker BK: Asymptomatic versus symptomatic herniated thoracic disk: Their frequency and characteristics as detected by computed tomography after myelography. *Neurosurgery* 28:180–186, 1991.
8. Badgley CE: The articular facet in relation to low back pain and sciatic radiation. *J Bone Joint Surg* 23:481–496, 1941.
9. Barnett GH, Hardy RW Jr, Little JR, et al: Thoracic spinal canal stenosis. *J Neurosurg* 66:338–344, 1987.
10. Bijos S, Bowyer O, Braen G, et al: *Acute Low Back Problems in Adults: Clinical Practice Guidelines.* AHCPR Publication #95-0642. Rockville, MD, Agency For Health Care Policy and Research, Public Health Service, U.S. Department of Health and Human Services, December 1994.
11. Blumenthal SL, Baker J, Dossett A, Selby DK: The role of anterior lumbar fusion for internal disc disruption. *Spine* 13:566–569, 1988.

12. Boden SD: in Weinstein JN, Rydevik BL, Sonntag VKH (eds): *Essentials of the Spine.* New York, Raven Press, 1994, chap 1.

13. Boden SD, Davis DO, Dina TS: Abnormal lumbar spine MRI scans in asymptomatic subjects: A prospective investigation. *J Bone Joint Surg* 72A:403–408, 1990.

14. Bogduk N, Tynan W, Wilson AS: The nerve supply to the human lumbar intervertebral discs. *J Anat* 132:39–56, 1981.

15. Bohlman HH, Zdeblick TA: Anterior excision of herniated thoracic discs. *J Bone Joint Surg* 70A:1038–1047, 1988.

16. Bookwalter JW III, Busch SW, Nicely D: Ambulatory surgery is safe and effective in radicular disk disease. *Spine* 19:526–530, 1994.

17. Bridwell KH, Dewald RL: Spinal Surgery Symposium. Decompression: Cervical, thoracic and lumbar—Who should be decompressed and how. St Louis, Missouri, May 10–13, 1995.

18. Bridwell KH, Sedgewick TA, O'Brien MF, et al: The role of fusion and instrumentation in the treatment of degenerative spondylolisthesis with spinal stenosis. *J Spinal Dis* 6:461–472, 1993.

19. Brinckmann P, Porter RW: A laboratory model of lumbar disc protrusion: Fissure and fragment. *Spine* 19:228–235, 1994.

20. Caputy AJ, Luessenhop AJ: Long-term evaluation of decompressive surgery for degenerative lumbar stenosis. *J Neurosurg* 77:669–676, 1992.

21. Carr D, Gilbertson L Frymoyer J, et al: Lumbar paraspinal compartment syndrome: A case report with physiologic and anatomical studies. *Spine* 10:816–820, 1985.

22. Chapman MP, Bridwell KH, Lenke LG, et al: Assignment of risk factors for transition syndrome: An analysis of patients who have broken down above or below a solid fusion. Presentation at the 30th Annual Meeting of the Scoliosis Research Society, Asheville, NC, September 13–16, 1995.

23. Chen Q, Baba H, Kamitani K, et al: Postoperative bone regrowth and lumbar spinal stenosis. *Spine* 19:2144–2149, 1994.

24. Colhoun E, McCall IW, Williams L, Pullicino VNC: Provocation discography as a guide to planning operations on the spine. *J Bone Joint Surg* 70B:267–271, 1988.

25. Coppes MH, Marani E, Thomer RT, et al: Innervation of annulus fibrosus in low back pain (letter). *Lancet* 336:189–190, 1990.

26. Crock HV: Internal disk disruption. *Spine* 11:650–653, 1986.

27. Curcin A, Lucas PR: Spondylolisthesis after posterolateral thoracic discectomy: Case report and literature review. *Spine* 17:1254–1256, 1992.

28. Derby R, Kine G, Saal J, et al: Response to steroid and duration of radicular pain as predictors of surgical outcome. *Spine* 17:S176–S183, 1992.

29. Eisen A, Hoirch M: The electrodiagnostic evaluation of spinal lesions. *Spine* 8:98–106, 1983.

30. Eismont FJ, Currier B: Current concepts review: Surgical management of lumbar intervertebral disk disease. *J Bone Joint Surg* 71A:1266–1271, 1989.

31. Epstein NE, Schwall G: Thoracic spinal stenosis: Diagnostic and treatment challenges. *J Spinal Dis* 7:259–269, 1994.

32. Esses SI (ed): *Textbook of Spinal Disorders.* Philadelphia, Lippincott, 1994.

33. Fairbank JCT, Park WM, McCall IW, O'Brien JP: Apophyseal injection of local anesthetic as a diagnostic aid in primary low back syndrome. *Spine* 6:598–605, 1981.

34. Farfan HF, Huberdeau RM, Dubow HI: Lumbar intervertebral disc degeneration. *J Bone Joint Surg* 54A:492–510, 1972.

35. Feffer HL, Wiesel SW, Cuckler JM, Rothman RH: Degenerative spondylolisthesis: To fuse or not to fuse. *Spine* 10:287–293, 1985.

36. Fidler MW, Goedhart ZD: Excision of prolapse of thoracic invertebral disk: A transthoracic technique. *J Bone Joint Surg* 66B:518–522, 1984.

37. Franklin GM, Haug J, Heyer NJ, et al: Outcome of lumbar fusion in Washington State Worker's Compensation. *Spine* 19:1897–1903, 1994.

38. Fredrickson B, Baker D, McHolick W, Lubicky J: The natural history of spondylolysis and spondylolisthesis. *J Bone Joint Surg* 66A:699–707, 1984.

39. Gelch MM: Herniated thoracic disk at T1-2 level associated with Horner's syndrome: Case report. *J Neurosurg* 48:128–130, 1978.

40. Gentry WD: Chronic back pain: Does elective surgery benefit patients with evidence of psychologic disturbance? *South Med J* 75:1169–1170, 1982.

41. Ghormley RK: Low back pain with special reference to the articular facet with presentation of an operative procedure. *JAMA* 101:1773–1777, 1933.

42. Gibson SJ, Polak JM, Bloom SR, Wall PD: The distribution of nine peptides in rat spinal cord with special emphasis on the substantia gelatinosa and on the area around the central canal. *J Comp Neurol* 201:65–79, 1981.

43. Gill K: Percutaneous lumbar diskectomy. *J Am Acad Orthop Surg* 1:33–40, 1993.

44. Goldthwait JE: The lumbosacral articulation: An explanation of many cases of lumbago, sciatica, and paraplegia. *Boston Med Surg J* 164:365–372, 1911.

45. Gonzalez EG, Hajdu M, Bruno R, et al: Lumbar spinal stenosis: Analysis of pre- and post-operative somatosensory evoked potentials. *Arch Phys Med Rehabil* 66:11–15, 1985.

46. Gribb SA, Lipscomb HJ: Results of lumbosacral fusion for degenerative disk disease with and without instrumentation: Two- to five-year follow-up. *Spine* 17:349–355, 1992.

47. Grobler L, Robertson P, Novotny J, et al: Etiology of spondylolisthesis: Assessment of the role played by lumbar facet morphology. *Spine* 18:80–92, 1993.

48. Hanley EN: Management of syndromes related to herniated discs: Essentials of the spine. *J Spinal Dis* 6:137–140, 1993.

49. Hanley EN, Spengler DM, Wesel S, et al: Controversies in low back pain: The surgical approach. *Instr Course Lect* 43:415–423, 1994.

50. Hazlett JW, Kinnard P: Lumbar apophyseal process excision and spinal instability. *Spine* 7:171–176, 1982.

51. Heithoff KB, Gundry CR, Burton CV, Winter RB: Juvenile diskogenic disease. *Spine* 19:335–340, 1994.

52. Herno A, Airaksenen O, Saari T: Long-term results of surgical treatment of lumbar spinal stenosis. *Spine* 18:1471–1474, 1993.

53. Herron LD: Recurrent lumbar disk herniation: Results of repeat laminectomy and discectomy. *J Spinal Dis* 7:161–166, 1994.

54. Herron LD, Mangelsdorf C: Lumbar spinal stenosis: Results of surgical treatment. *J Spinal Dis* 4:26–33, 1991.

55. Herron LD, Trippi AC, Gonyeau M: Intraoperative use of dermatomal somatosensory evoked potentials in lumbar stenosis surgery. *Spine* 12:379–383, 1987.

56. Herron LD, Trippi AC: L4-5 Degenerative spondylolisthesis: The results of treatment by decompressive laminectomy without fusion. *Spine* 14:534–538, 1989.

57. Herkowitz HN: Lumbar spinal stenosis: Indications for arthrodesis and spinal instrumentation. *Instr Course Lect* 43:425–433, 1994.

58. Herkowitz HN: Spine update: Degenerative lumbar spondylolisthesis. *Spine* 20:1084–1090, 1995.

59. Herkowitz HN, Kurz LT: Degenerative spondylolisthesis with spinal stenosis: A prospective study comparing decompression with decompression and intertransverse process arthrodesis. *J Bone Joint Surg* 73A:802–808, 1991.

60. Herzog RJ, Kaiser JA, Saal JS: The importance of posterior epidural fat pad in lumbar central canal stenosis. *Spine* 16:S227–S232, 1991.

61. Hirsch C, Ingelmark BE, Miller M: The anatomical basis for low back pain. *Acta Orthop Scand* 33:1–17, 1963.

62. Hirsch C, Schajowicz F: Studies on the structural changes in the lumbar annulus fibrosis. *Acta Orthop Scand* 22:184–231, 1952.

63. Holbrook TL, Grazier K, Kelsey JL, Stauffer RN: *The Socioeconomic Impact of Selected Musculoskeletal Disorders.* Chicago, American Academy Orthopedic Surgery, 1994.

64. Holt EP: The questions of lumbar discography. *J Bone Joint Surg* 50A:720–726, 1968.

65. Hoppenfeld S: Percutaneous removal of herniated lumbar discs: Fifty cases with ten-year follow-up. *Clin Orthop Rel Res* 238:92–97, 1989.

66. Howe JF, Laser JD, Calvin WH: Mechanosensitivity of dorsal root ganglion and chronically injured axons: A physiologic basis for the radicular pain of nerve root compression. *Pain* 3:25–41, 1977.

67. Hulme A: The surgical approach to thoracic intervertebral disc protrusions. *J Neurol Neurosurg Psychiatry* 23:133–137, 1960.

68. Hultman G, Nordin M, Saraste H, Ohlsen H: Body composition, endurance strength, cross-sectional area, and density of erector spinae muscles in men with and without low back pain. *J Spinal Dis* 6:114–123, 1993.

69. Hu SS, Bradford DS, Transfeldt EE, Cohen M: Reduction of high-grade spondylolisthesis using Edwards instrumentation. *Spine* 21:367–371, 1996.

70. Jackson HC, Winkelmann RK, Bickel WH: Nerve endings in the human spinal column and related structures. *J Bone Joint Surg* 48A:1272–1281, 1966.

71. Jackson RP: The facet syndrome: Myth or reality? *Clin Orthop Rel Res* 279:110–121, 1992.

72. Jackson RP, Jacobs RR, Montesano PX: Facet joint injections in low back pain: A prospective statistical study. *Spine* 13:966–971, 1988.

73. Jinkins JR, Rauch A: Magnetic resonance imaging of entrapment of lumbar nerve roots in spondylolytic spondylolisthesis. *J Bone Joint Surg* 76A:1643–1648, 1994.

74. Johnsson KE, Redlund, Johnell I, et al: Preoperative and postoperative instability in lumbar spinal stenosis. *Acta Orthop Scand Suppl* 251:67–68, 1993.

75. Johnsson KE, Rosen I, Uden A: The natural course of lumbar spinal stenosis. *Clin Orthop Rel Res* 218:82–86, 1992.

76. Johnsson KE, Uden A, Rosen I: The effect of decompression on the natural course of spinal stenosis: A comparison of surgically treated and untreated patients. *Spine* 16:615–619, 1991.

77. Jones AAM, Stambough JL, Balderston RA, et al: Long-term results of lumbar spine surgery complicated by incidental durotomy. *Spine* 14:443–446, 1989.

78. Kambin P: Arthroscopic microdiskectomy. *Arthroscopy* 8:287–295, 1992.

79. Katz JN, Lipson SJ, Brick GW, et al: Clinical correlates of patient satisfaction after laminectomy for degenerative lumbar spinal stenosis. *Spine* 20:1155–1160, 1995.

80. Kellett KM, Kellett DA, Nordholm LA: Effects of an exercise program on sick leave due to back pain. *J Phys Ther* 71:283–293, 1991.

81. Kellgren JH: Sciatica. *Lancet* 1:561–564, 1941.

82. Kirkaldi-Willis WH, Hill RJ: More precise diagnosis for low back pain. *Spine* 4:102–109, 1979.

83. Kirkaldi-Willis WH: Managing low back pain, 2d ed. New York, Churchill Livingstone, 1983.

84. Klein JD, Garfin SR: in Weinstein JN, Rydevik BL, Sonntag VKH (eds): *Essentials of the Spine.* New York, Raven Press, 1994, chap 1.

85. Kondo M, Matsuda H, Kureya S, Shimazu A: Electrophysiological studies of intermittent claudication in lumbar stenosis. *Spine* 14:862–866, 1989.

86. Krempen JF, Smith BS: Nerve-root injection: A method for evaluation of the etiology of sciatica. *J Bone Joint Surg* 56A:1435–1444, 1974.

87. Kuehle JW, Simmons EH, Hard R, Mendel FC: Variations of sciatic nerve in relation to piriformis syndrome and nerve compression as a cause of sciatica. Presented at 30th Annual Meeting of Scoliosis Research Society, Asheville, NC, September 13–16, 1995.

88. Kumar R, Buckley TF: Briefly noted: First thoracic disc protrusion. *Spine* 11:499, 1986.

89. Kuslich SD, Ulstrom CL, Michael CJ: The tissue origin of low back pain and sciatica: A report of pain response to tissue stimulation during operation on the lumbar spine using local anesthesia. *Orthop Clin North Am* 22:181–187, 1991.

90. Lewis T, Kellgren JH: Observations relating to referred pain viscerometed reflexes and other associated phenomena. *Clin Sci* 4:47–71, 1939.

91. Lilius G, Laasonen EM, Myllynen PT, et al: The facet joint syndrome. *J Bone Joint Surg* 71B:681–684, 1989.

92. Lippitt AB: The facet joint and its role in spinal pain: Management with facet joint injections. *Spine* 9:746–750, 1984.

93. Lipson S: Clinical diagnosis of spinal stenosis. *J Semin Spine Surg* 1:143–144, 1989.

94. Ljunggren AE: Descriptions of pain and other sensory modalities in patients with lumbago, sciatica, and herniated intervertebral discs. *Pain* 16:265–276, 1983.

95. Malinsky J: The ontogenetic development of nerve terminations in the intervertebral discs of man. *Acta Anat* 38:96–113, 1959.

96. Mayer TG, Gatchel RJ, Kishino N, et al: Objective assessment of spine function following industrial injury: A prospective study with comparison group and one-year follow-up. *Spine* 10:482–493, 1985.

97. McAllister VL, Sage MR: The radiology of thoracic disc protrusion. *J Clin Radiol* 27:291–299, 1976.

98. McCall WE, Park WM, O'Brien JP: Induced pain referral from posterior lumbar elements in normal subjects. *Spine* 4:441–446, 1979.

99. Melzack R, Wall PD: Pain mechanism: A new theory. *Science* 150:971–979, 1965.

100. Middleton FG, Teacher H: Injury of the spinal cord due to rupture of an intervertebral disk during muscular effort. *Glasgow Med J* 76:1–6, 1911.

101. Miller JAA, Schmatz C, Schultz AB: Lumbar disk degeneration: Correlation with age, sex, and spine level in 600 autopsy specimens. *Spine* 13:173–178, 1988.

102. Mixter WJ, Barr JS: Rupture of the intervertebral disk with involvement of the spinal canal. *N Engl J Med* 211:210–215, 1934.

103. Modic MT, Ross JS: Magnetic resonance imaging in the evaluation of low back pain. *Orthop Clin North Am* 22:283–301, 1991.

104. Mooney V: Treating low back pain with exercise. *J Musculoskel Med* 12:2436–2442, 1995.

105. Mooney V, Robertson J: The facet syndrome. *Clin Orthop Rel Res* 115:149–156, 1976.

106. Nachemson A: Intradiskal measurement of pH in patients with lumbar rhizopathies. *Acta Orthop Scand* 40:23–42, 1969.

107. Nachemson A: The lumbar spine: An orthopedic challenge. *Spine* 1:59–71, 1976.

108. Nobuhiro H, Hwan-Mo L, Weinstein JN: The source of pain in the lumbar spine, in Bridwell KH, Dewald RL (eds): *The Textbook of Spinal Disorders,* 2d ed. Philadelphia, Lippincott, 1996.

109. Nordly EJ, Wright PH: Efficacy of chymopapain in chemonucleolysis: A review. *Spine* 19:2578–2583, 1994.

110. Ogilvie JW: Thoracic disk herniations, in Bridwell KH, DeWald RL (eds): *The Textbook of Spinal Surgery,* 2d ed. Philadelphia, Lippincott, 1996.

111. Okada K, Oka S, Tohge K, et al: Thoracic myelopathy caused by ossification of the ligamentum flavum: Clinical pathologic study and surgical treatment. *Spine* 16:280–287, 1991.

112. Onel D, Sari H, Donmez C: Lumbar spinal stenosis: Clinical/radiologic therapeutic evaluation in 145 patients: Conservative treatment or surgical intervention? *Spine* 18:291–298, 1993.

113. Otani K, Yoshida M, Fuji E, et al: Thoracic disk herniation: Surgical treatment in 23 patients. *Spine* 13:1262–1267, 1988.

114. Oudenhoven RC: The role of laminectomy, facet rhizotomy and epidural steroids. *Spine* 4:145–147, 1979.

115. Parke WW: The significance of venous return impairment in ischemic radiculopathy and myelopathy. *Orthop Clin North Am* 22:213–221, 1991.

116. Patterson RH Jr, Arbit E: A surgical approach through the pedicle to protruded thoracic disks. *J Neurosurg* 48:768–772, 1978.

117. Peck D: Evidence for the existence of compartment syndromes of the axial muscles. *Anat Rec* 199:198A, 1981.

118. Regan JJ, Mack MJ: Endoscopic anterior thoracic diskectomy: A prospective evaluation of the first 36 cases. Presentation at the 10th Annual Meeting of the North American Spine Society, Washington, DC, October 18–21, 1995.

119. Ridenour TR, Haddad SF, Hitchon PW, et al: Herniated thoracic disks: Treatment and outcome. *J Spinal Dis* 6:218–224, 1993.

120. Robertson PA, Grobler LJ, Novotny JE, Katz JN: Postoperative spondylolisthesis at L4-5: The role of facet joint morphology. *Spine* 18:1483–1490, 1993.

121. Roche MB, Rowe GG: Incidence of separate neural arch and coincident bone variations: A survey of 4,200 skeletons. *Anat Rec* 109:233–252, 1951.

122. Rydevik B: Neurophysiology of cauda equina compression. *Acta Orthop Scand Suppl* 251:52–55, 1993.

123. Rydevik BL, Brown MD, Lundberg G: Pathoanatomy and pathophysiology of nerve root compression. *Spine* 9:7–15, 1984.

124. Rydevik BL, Myers RR, Powell HC: Pressure increases in the dorsal root ganglion following mechanical compression. *Spine* 14:574–576, 1989.

125. Safdari H, Baker RL II: Microsurgical anatomy and related techniques to an intervertebral transthoracic approach to thoracic disk herniations. *Surg Neurol* 23:589–593, 1985.

126. Sanderson PL, Wood PLR: Surgery for lumbar spinal stenosis in old people. *J Bone Joint Surg* 75B:393–397, 1993.

127. Schellhas KP, Pollei SR, Dorwart RH: Thoracic diskography: A safe and reliable technique. *Spine* 19:2103–2109, 1994.

128. Schvartzman L, Weingarten E, Sherry H, et al: Cost-effectiveness analysis of extended conservative therapy vs surgical intervention in the management of herniated lumbar intervertebral disks. *Spine* 17:176–182, 1992.

129. Sherk HH, Black JD, Prodoehl JH, Cummings RS: Laser diskectomy. *Orthopedics* 16:573–576, 1993.

130. Shimazaki K, Nishida H, Harada Y, Hirohata K: Late recurrence of spinal stenosis and claudication after laminectomy due to an ossified extradural pseudocyst. *Spine* 16:221–223, 1991.

131. Silvers HR, Lewis PJ, Asch HL: Decompressive lumbar laminectomy for spinal stenosis. *J Neurosurg* 78:695–701, 1993.

132. Simpson JM, Silveri CP, Balderston RA, et al: The results of operations on the lumbar spine in patients who have diabetes mellitus. *J Bone Joint Surg* 75A:1823–1829, 1993.

133. Singounas EG, Kypriades EM, Kellerman AJ, Garvan N: Thoracic disk herniation. Analysis of 14 cases and review of the literature. *Acta Neurochir* 116:49–52, 1992.

134. Smith DE, Godersky JC: Thoracic spondylosis: An unusual cause of myelopathy. *Neurosurgery* 20:569–573, 1987.

135. Smith L: Enzyme dissolution of the nucleus pulposus in humans. *JAMA* 187:137–140, 1964.

136. Smyth MJ, Wright V: Sciatica and the intervertebral disk—An experimental study. *J Bone Joint Surg* 40A:1401–1418, 1958.

137. Sola AE, Williams RL: Myofascial pain syndrome. *Neurology* 6:91–95, 1956.

138. Spencer DL, Bernstein AJ: Lumbar and intervertebral disk surgery, in Bridwell KH, DeWald RL (eds): *Textbook of Spinal Surgery,* 2d ed. Philadelphia, Lippincott, 1996.

139. Spengler DM: Perspectives on the indications and surgical management of patients with selected degenerative disorders of the lumbar spine, in Bridwell KH, DeWald RL (eds): *Textbook of Spinal Surgery,* 2d ed. Philadelphia, Lippincott, 1996.

140. Spengler DM, Ouellette EA, Battie M, Zeh J: Elective diskectomy for herniation of a lumbar disk. *J Bone Joint Surg* 72A:230–237, 1990.

141. Stolke D, Sollmann WP, Seifert V: Intra- and postoperative complications in lumbar disk surgery. *Spine* 14:56–59, 1989.

142. Stone JL, Lichtor T, Banerjie S: Intradural thoracic disk herniation. *Spine* 19:1281–1284, 1994.

143. Tahmouresie A: Herniated thoracic intervertebral disk—An unusual presentation: Case report. *Neurosurgery* 7:623–625, 1980.

144. Tajima T, Furukawa K, Kuramochi E: Selective lumbosacral radiculopathy and block. *Spine* 5:68–77, 1980.

145. Travlos J, DuToit G: Primary spinal epidural lymphoma mimicking lumbar spinal stenosis. *Spine* 16:377–379, 1991.

146. Turner JA, Ersek M, Herron L, Deyo R: Surgery for lumbar spinal stenosis: Attempted meta-analysis of the literature. *Spine* 17:1–8, 1992.

147. Uden A, Landin LA: Pain drawing and myelography in sciatic pain. *Clin Orthop Rel Res* 216:124–130, 1987.

148. Ullrich CG, Binet EF, Sanecki MG, Kieffer SA: Quantitative assessment of the lumbar spinal canal by computed tomography. *J Radiol* 134:137–143, 1980.

149. Varlotta GP, Brown MD, Kelsey JL, Golden AL: Familial predisposition for herniation of a lumbar disk in patients who are less than 21 years old. *J Bone Joint Surg* 73A:124–128, 1991.

150. Verbiest H: A radicular syndrome from developmental narrowing of the lumbar vertebral canal. *J Bone Joint Surg Br* 36:230–237, 1954.

151. Virta L, Ronnemaa T, Osterman K, et al: Prevalence of isthmic lumbar spondylolisthesis in middle-aged subjects from eastern and western Finland. *J Clin Epidemiol* 45:917–922, 1992.

152. Waddell G, McCulloch JA, Kummel E, Venner RM: Nonorganic physical signs in low back pain. *Spine* 5:117–125, 1980.

153. Walsh TR, Weinstein JN, Spratt RF, et al: Lumbar diskography: A controlled prospective study. *J Bone Joint Surg* 72A:1081–1088, 1990.

154. Weinstein JN: Mechanism of spinal pain: The dorsal root ganglion and its role as a mediator of low back pain. *Spine* 11:999–1001, 1986.

155. Weinstein JN, Claverie W, Gibson S: The pain of diskography. *Spine* 13:1344–1348, 1988.

156. Whiffen JR, Neuwirth MG: Spinal stenosis, in Bridwell KH, DeWald RL (eds): *Textbook of Spinal Surgery,* 2d ed. Philadelphia, Lippincott, 1996.

157. Whittaker CK, Bernhardt M: Magnetic resonance imaging shows gadolinium enhancement of intradural herniated disks. *Spine* 19:1505–1507, 1994.

158. Wiberg G: Back pain in relation to nerve supply of the intervertebral disk. *Acta Orthop Scand* 19:211–218, 1949.

159. Wiltse L: Salvage of failed lumbar spinal stenosis surgery, in Hopp E (ed): *Spine: State of the Art Reviews.* Vol 1. Philadelphia, Hanley and Belfus, 1987, pp 421–456.

160. Wiltse LL, Rocchio P: Preoperative psychological tests as predictors of success of chemonucleolysis in the treatment of the low back pain syndrome. *J Bone Joint Surg* 57A:478–483, 1975.

161. Winter RB, Lonstein JE, Denis F, et al: The risk of paraplegia secondary to segmental vessel ligation: An analysis of 1197 consecutive anterior operations. Presentation at the 30th Annual Meeting of the Scoliosis Research Society, Asheville, NC, September 13–16, 1995.

162. Wood GW III: Lower Back Pain and Disorders of Intervertebral Disks, in Crenshaw AH (ed): *Campbell's Operative Orthopedics,* 8th ed., St Louis, Mosby, 1992.

163. Wood KB, Garvey TA, Gundry C, Heithoff KB: Magnetic resonance imaging of the thoracic spine: Evaluation of asymptomatic individuals. *J Bone Joint Surg* 77A:1631–1638, 1995.

164. Wood KB, Popp CA, Transfeldt EE, Geissele AE: Radiographic evaluation of instability in spondylolisthesis. *Spine* 19:1697–1703, 1994.

165. Yamamoto I, Matsumae M, Ikeda A, et al: Thoracic spinal stenosis: Experience with seven cases. *J Neurosurg* 68:37–40, 1988.

166. Yamashita T, Cavanaugh JM, El-Bohy AA, et al: Mechanosensitive afferent units in the lumbar facet joint. *J Bone Joint Surg* 72A:865–870, 1990.

167. Yuan HA, Garfin SR, Dickman CA, Mardjetko SM: A historical cohort study of pedicle screw fixation in thoracic, lumbar and sacral spinal fusions. *Spine* 19:S2279–S2296, 1994.

168. Zdeblick TA: A prospective randomized study of lumbar fusions: Preliminary results. *Spine* 18:983–991, 1993.

CHAPTER 73

Degenerative Diseases and Disk Disorders of the Cervical Spine

Christopher L. Hamill

ANATOMY OF THE CERVICAL SPINE

The osseous component of the cervical spine consists of seven cervical vertebrae, the third through the seventh having a similar type of configuration. These cervical vertebrae bear the least weight; therefore, their bodies are relatively small with respect to the size of the vertebral arch and vertebral foramen. The diameter is greater transversely than it is in the anteroposterior (AP) direction. The lateral edges of the superior surface of these lower vertebrae are sharply turned upward to form the uncinate process (joint of Luschka). However, the most distinguishing feature of the cervical vertebrae is the transverse foramen. This acts as a protective column for the transmission of the vertebral arteries up into the foramen magnum. The third through the seventh cervical vertebrae have equally divided amounts of motion in the flexion-extension planes. The C5-6 interspace is generally considered to have the largest range.[165] The lateral bending and axial rotation predominantly seen at the occipital atlantoaxial joints are somewhat limited in the caudal segments. This has been well shown by Lysell.[95] The amount of rotation between the occiput and C1 remains controversial. The range of motion for one-sided axial rotation is from 3 to 8°.[24,40,110,173] Major axial rotation in the cervical spine is located between C1 and C2.[115] The articular surface of the C1-2 lateral masses has a convex orientation in the sagittal plane. This allows for considerable mobility in all planes. Approximately 60 percent of the rotation in the cervical spine is postulated to occur between the occiput, C1, and C2. The remaining 40 percent occurs in the lower region of the cervical spine. The presence of pathologic motion at the C1-2 interface can lead to kinking of the contralateral vertebral artery when there is greater than 30° of rotation.[142] When the rotation is greater than 45°, kinking of the ipsilateral vertebral artery has also been found to occur.[173]

Translatory movements at the occipitoatlantal joint complex are small. The amount of translation between the C1-2 articulation is also minimal because of the fit of the ring of C1 about the dens. During the translation in the midsagittal plane, the distance between the anterior portion of the dens and posterior portion of the anterior aspect of C1 is clinically significant. The normal translation is thought to be between 2 and 3 mm and is used as a guide for the integrity of the transverse ligament. Jackson found the normal range of motion at the atlantodens interval in children to be as great as 4.5 mm.[85] The ligamentous complex of the C1-C2 articulation has important implications for the stability of this joint. The transverse ligament provides the main stabilizer ligament for the C1-C2 complex. The symmetrically placed alar ligament connects the occiput and atlas to the dens and acts as a secondary restraint for the translation around C1-2.

The range of motion in the middle and lower cervical spine has been found to be the most evenly distributed throughout the motion segments. There is a slight increase in the amount of flexion/extension that occurs at the C5-6 level. This increased motion has also been found to have a causal relationship between the incidence of cervical spondylosis at this interspace.[165] Maximum sagittal plane translation occurring in the lower cervical spine under physiologic loads has been suggested by White and Panjabi to be 3.5 mm. This measurement is used for the upper limits of normal.[164]

The ligamentous structures play an important role in the maintenance of stability and the smooth arc of rotation occurring both in the upper and lower cervical spine. Key ligamentous structures for C1-2 articulation include the atlantodens ligament, which runs between the anterior portion of the dens and the caudal portion of the anterior ring of C1; the atlantooccipital ligament between the cephalad portion of the anterior ring of C1 and the tubercle of C0, which has also been postulated to be a continuation of the anterior longitudinal ligament; and the posterior atlantooccipital ligament connecting the posterior ring of C1 to the occiput. The dentate ligament consists of the alar and apical ligaments. The alar ligaments are important in the limitation of actual rotation and side bending of the C0/C1-C2 complex and have been postulated to be injured in the whiplash-type mechanism.[39] The cruciate ligament, the major portion of the transverse ligament, is considered by most to be the most important ligament of the C0/C1-C2 complex. It is the largest and strongest ligament and must be torn to have anterior dislocation of C1-2. An intact ligament will prevent more than 3 mm of anterior displacement of C1 on C2.[57] Instability detected in the C0/C1-C2 complex has been well described. It has been found by Fielding and colleagues[57] to be dependent upon the integrity of the transverse ligament. Bilateral overhang of the lateral masses totaling 7 mm or more is indicative of a rupture of the transverse ligament. C1-C2 fusion for the prevention of neurologic injury is recommended. The tectorial membrane is a continuation of the posterior longitudinal ligament. Its exact function has yet to be described, but it is postulated to limit flexion and extension of the C1-C2 joint.[161]

Instability of the lower cervical spine has received considerable attention in the literature. The anatomic structures important in the maintenance of the stability of the cervical spine are shown in Fig. 73-1, illustrating both the lateral and coronal views. The main structures responsible for stability have been postulated by Holdsworth to be the supraspinous and intraspinous ligaments as well as the ligamentum flavum. However, other investigators have not considered ligamentous structures as crucial.[80] In the lower cervical spine, at the level of the intervertebral disk, the annulus is a stabilizing structure.[4] Munro's experimental studies on cadaver spines have shown not only the intervertebral disk but also the anterior and pos-

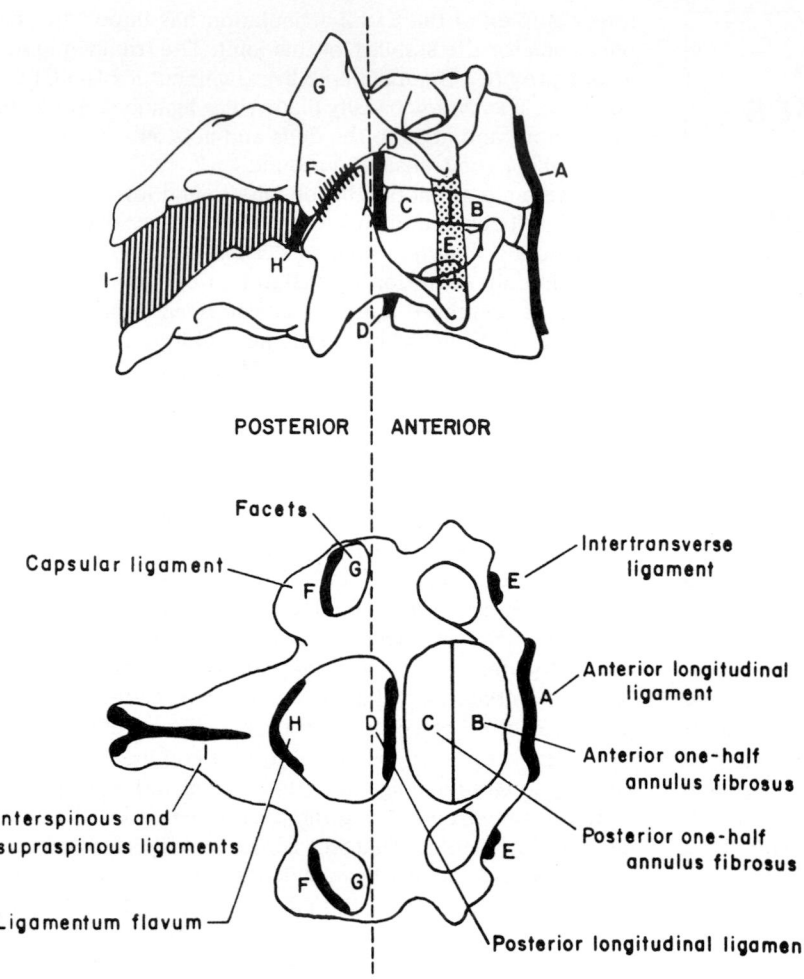

POSTERIOR | ANTERIOR

Facets

Capsular ligament

Intertransverse ligament

Anterior longitudinal ligament

Anterior one-half annulus fibrosus

Posterior one-half annulus fibrosus

Interspinous and supraspinous ligaments

Ligamentum flavum

Posterior longitudinal ligament

Figure 73-1 Schematic illustration of the ligamentous structures that participate in the stabilization of the middle and lower cervical spine. The components are divided into anterior and posterior elements. Anatomic components posterior to the posterior longitudinal ligaments are defined as the posterior elements. The posterior longitudinal ligament and all the anatomic components anterior to it are defined as the anterior elements. In the experiments on clinical stability, ligaments were cut in the alphabetical order indicated in the diagram from anterior to posterior and in reverse alphabetical order from posterior to anterior.

terior longitudinal ligaments to be the important stabilizing structures.[105] The radiographic criterion for cervical spinal instability in the sagittal plane is displacement or translation greater than 3.5 mm on either standard or dynamic flexion-extension lateral radiographs; this should be considered pathologic.[162] White and Panjabi have shown that greater than 11° of relative sagittal plane angulation should be considered potentially unstable. This 11° is relative to the angulation above or below the level of consideration.[164]

SPONDYLOSIS

Spondylosis is the presence of degenerative changes throughout the spine. In the cervical region, most of these changes occur around the two facet joints, the intervertebral disks, and the two uncovertebral joints. Presenting symptoms usually include a generalized degenerative type of neck pain. Severe forms of spondylosis can lead to myelopathy or a myeloradicular type of symptomatology secondary to compromise of the canal from hypertrophic changes of the uncinate process anteriorly as well as the

facet joint posteriorly.[45,49,50] The relative significance of degenerative disk disease with the concomitant production of osteophytes and spurs depends upon location and size. The radiographic classification of stenosis of the cervical spine has been well documented. The true diameter of the cervical spine canal in the sagittal plane is shown in Fig. 73-2. The sagittal plane diameter has also been described by using two different types of classification: (1) developmental anterior posterior diameter and (2) spondylotic anterior-posterior diameter (Fig. 73-3). While these two radiographic assessments are technique-dependent, the development of Pavlov's ratio[113] has become the standard to detect the presence or absence of cervical spine stenosis. This ratio is calculated by the size of the canal divided by the AP diameter of the vertebral body. A value of greater than 1 mm is normal; between 1 mm and 0.8 mm indicates relative stenosis; and less than 0.8 means absolute stenosis. Relative numbers to describe cervical AP diameter include averages of 17 mm at the midvertebral level, with absolute stenosis being less than 10 mm.

The sagittal diameter of the cord measures between 0.8 and 1.3 cm, with the soft tissues occupying another 2 to 3 mm. The presence of a congenitally stenotic canal renders the patient more susceptible to myelopathy and neurologic injuries secondary to insignificant trauma. The most

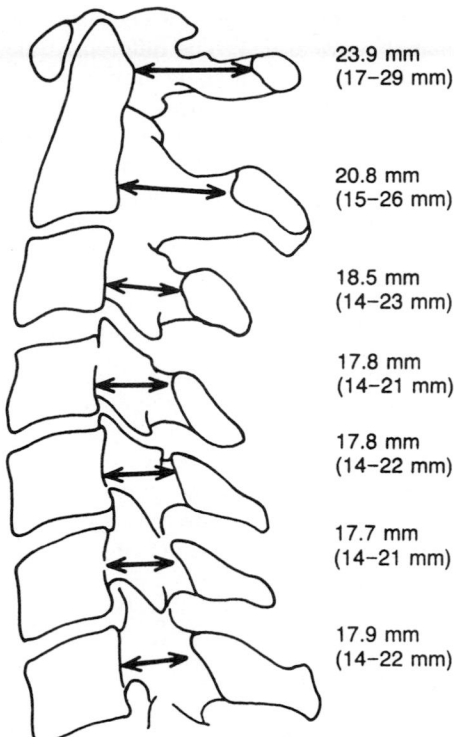

23.9 mm
(17–29 mm)

20.8 mm
(15–26 mm)

18.5 mm
(14–23 mm)

17.8 mm
(14–21 mm)

17.8 mm
(14–22 mm)

17.7 mm
(14–21 mm)

17.9 mm
(14–22 mm)

Figure 73-2 The true sagittal plane diameter of the cervical spinal canal. The upper portion has relatively more space for the spinal cord, even though the cord is larger there. The means are presented for each level, with the range presented in parentheses. We must always keep in mind that clinical x-ray measurements represent a 20 to 30 percent magnification of the real linear distances.

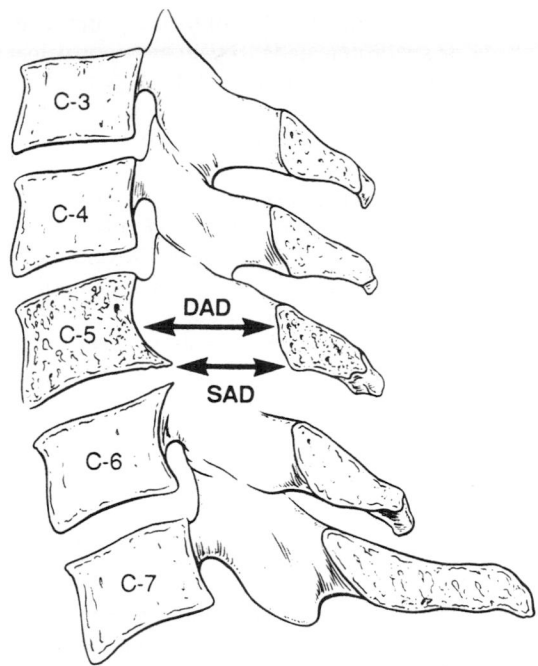

Figure 73-3 This is an illustration of two important concepts—development anteroposterior diameter (DAD) and the spondylotic anteroposterior diameter (SAD). These are generally measured as simple linear diameters. Because of differences in source-to-object-to film distances, there is potential for variation. In general, 14 mm can be chosen as a representative for the lowest limits of normal. The SAD is an important measurement. The developmental diameter may not be the important functional diameter if there is an osteophyte (spur) that significantly reduces the canal space.

common of these are a central cord syndrome as well as more significant quadriparesis or quadriplegic events. The underlying stenotic changes also makes patients more symptomatic in earlier years.[43,44,46,48,53–55,109,158,159,172] The cervical spinal cord's maximum sagittal diameter is 10 mm in the adult.[3] Edwards and LaRocca looked at 63 patients with symptomatic cervical spondylosis and found that 40 patients were in the narrow canal group and 23 patients were noted to have an average or above average midcervical spinal canal measurement. They computed a spondylosis index, which is the difference between the developmental segmental sagittal diameter and the spondylotic segmental sagittal diameter. This represents the amount of narrowing due to disease.[59] The spondylosis index was an average of 2.084 mm per segment in the symptomatic group versus 3.45 mm per segment for the asymptomatic group. Of the 214 patients they reviewed for clinical spondylosis, 63 patients exhibited symptoms referable to the cervical spine alone.[41] Symptoms are exacerbated during hyperextension or hyperflexion, and this can result in acute or chronic neural injury.[18,21,38,43,114] Hyperextension causes cervical cord and root compression between the anterior disks, the degenerative spurs, and the posterior hypertrophied facets and ligamentum flavum. With continuous compression, there is also an accompanying thickening of the cord and nerve roots. Hyperflexion leads the neural struc-

tures to become lengthened and tethered across the anterior spurs and disks. The presence of foraminal spondylotic changes causes additional cord insult because of decreased cord mobility.

Differential Diagnosis

Cervical spondylosis, radiculopathy, and myelopathy must be differentiated from other local and systemic diseases causing similar symptomatology. The most common differential in cervical radiculopathy includes both intra- and extraspinal tumors; entrapment syndromes involving median, ulnar, and radial nerves; and diseases or disorders of the thoracic outlet, brachial plexus, and shoulder. Tumors associated with a large soft tissue mass can cause unilateral radiculopathy. These patients usually present with pain in the neck, shoulder, and arm. The pain is frequently constant and typically worse at night. Many extraspinal tumors may also cause cervical radiculopathy. Tumors of the thyroid, upper esophagus, and pharynx and apical carcinomas of the lung (Pancoast's tumor) may encroach on the brachial plexus or subclavian vessels. These patients can present with Horner's syndrome, shoulder girdle pain, and profound unilateral upper extremity weakness. Many upper extremity entrapment syndromes can also present with upper extremity numbness, paresthesias, or sensory and motor loss. The pronator syndrome leads to pain in the proximal lower forearm and sensory loss in the radial $3\frac{1}{2}$ digits of the hand, with weakness in all median nerve innervating muscles. The symptomatology can be elicited depending on the location of compression by certain specific resisted forearm movements. These include flexion of the elbow against resistance between 90° and 135°, where compression is from the ligament of Struthers or lacertus fibrosus. Symptoms increasing by resistance to forced voluntary pronation of the forearm may suggest compression by the pronator teres muscle. Exacerbation of symptoms by resisted flexion of the long finger flexor digitorum superficialis can cause compression at the aponeurotic arch of the pronator muscle. The anterior interosseous syndrome may mimic a C8 radiculopathy with motor weakness of the flexor pollicis longus, pronator quadratus, and flexor digitorum profundus of the index finger. Carpal tunnel syndrome presents with night pain, paresthesias, and numbness of the radial $3\frac{1}{2}$ digits. The symptoms can usually be elicited with Phelan's or Tinnel's test. These sensory symptoms may mimic C6 or C7 radiculopathy, but no motor weakness is found. Compression of the ulnar nerve can occur at the cubital tunnel or Guyon's canal. Cubital tunnel syndrome typically can present as a C8 or T1 nerve root radiculopathy. These conditions can be especially difficult to differentiate. Electrodiagnostic studies that show significant conduction delay across the elbow are useful in this regard. Compression of the ulnar nerve at Guyon's canal can also mimic a C8 or T1 radiculopathy. Compression of the radial nerve, most commonly at the elbow, is generally called radial tunnel syndrome. This can occur at the arcade of Frohse, tendinous bands from the extensor carpi radialis brevis, or the leash of vessels that supply the brachioradialis and extensor carpi radialis longus muscles. A C7 radiculopathy may mimic radial nerve compression. However, a C7 radiculopathy involves the triceps muscle, which is normally spared in a radial nerve compression syndrome at the elbow. The thoracic outlet syndrome is related to pathology of the subclavian axillary artery vein complex, where the two lower brachial plexus nerve roots pass from the base of the neck through the axilla. These structures may be compressed by bony elements, cervical ribs, an enlarged first thoracic rib, the clavicle, and/or muscle (scalenus anticus and pectoralis minor or both). Brachial plexus disorders including brachial plexopathy and idiopathic brachial neuritis may also present as a difficult differential from a cervical radiculopathy. Electromyography (EMG) and nerve conduction studies are extremely useful in the differential diagnosis of these two disorders.

Cervical myelopathy must be differentiated from other neurologic degenerative syndromes, particularly in amyotrophic lateral sclerosis and multiple sclerosis.

CERVICAL DISK DISEASE WITH ASSOCIATED RADICULOPATHY

The presence of cervical radiculopathy should be defined by pain radiating down a dermatomal distribution into the arm. The most common cause for cervical radiculopathy is a herniated cervical disk. The differential diagnosis alluded to earlier involves ruling out any radiating arm pain secondary to compressive neuropathy in the arm. Which herniated disk is causing the radiculopathy can usually be determined by a thorough history and physical examination. There are occasional radiculopathies involving the C2 nerve root; however, these are extremely rare.

C3 Radiculopathy

The C3 nerve root can be compressed by a herniation involving the C2-3 disk. This is a very uncommon interspace for disk herniation to occur. The sensory distribution of the C3 nerve root includes the posterior aspect of the neck, the posterior suboccipital region, and the ear. The pain can be extremely difficult to differentiate from muscle tension headaches. There is no detectable motor involvement in a C3 nerve root lesion.

C4 Radiculopathy

C4 radiculopathy can present with neck and shoulder pain. There is no significant motor deficit. The radiating pain can be present at the base of the neck, extending to the midshoulder and posteriorly to the scapula. There are no reflex changes secondary to a C4 radiculopathy.

C5 Radiculopathy

The C5 nerve root deficit secondary to compressive radiculopathy is found in the deltoid muscle. Patients will usually complain of difficulty with elevation of the arm. There might also be a weakness of the supraspinatus-infraspinatus and a decrease in the biceps reflex on the affected side.

C6 Radiculopathy

Herniations between the C5 and C6 disks most commonly compress the C6 nerve root. The pain will radiate across the top of the neck along the biceps muscle into the lateral aspect of the forearm and onto the dorsal surface of the hand between the thumb and index finger. Accompanying muscle weakness will be seen in the biceps as well as the wrist extensor. The biceps reflex and the brachioradialis reflex will be diminished in C6 radiculopathy. This is usually the second most common radiculopathy present.

C7 Radiculopathy

The most common area of disk herniation in the cervical spine is the C6-7 level. C7 radiculopathy presents with pain radiating across the back of the shoulder down the triceps posterolateral aspect of the forearm and into the middle finger. The triceps reflex is usually involved. Weakness of a C7 radiculopathy is seen in the triceps muscle and finger extensors.

C8 Radiculopathy

C7-T1 disk herniation will cause C8 radiculopathy. The patient will complain of numbness in the small finger and the medial half of the ring finger. The C8 root supplies most of the small intrinsic muscles of the hand. The patient will lose fine fingertip movement and grip strength. Electromyography nerve conduction studies are especially useful in distinguishing ulnar nerve compression from a C8 radiculopathy.

Generally, patients will give a history of some chronic type of neck pain. These symptoms are usually consistent with degenerative disk disease. They will complain of intermittent exacerbation of their neck pain. However, when the disk herniation occurs, they will have partial or even complete relief of their neck pain with new onset arm pain. Patients will often complain that the pain wakes them up from sleep. They can present with a characteristic pose, with the forearm on top of the head for relief of the arm pain. This is the body's attempt to open the neuroforamen on the involved side. They also will tilt the head to try to relieve the pain from the disk herniation. Cervical extension can exacerbate the pain. When the neck is immobilized, they may feel more comfortable. A collar should not extend the neck, as this can exacerbate the patient's pain. As previously stated, cervical radiculopathy can be confused with intraarticular pathology of the shoulder. On the physical examination, it is important to elucidate the syndromes secondary to radiculopathy. This can be done with cervical compression or cervical traction to alleviate or exacerbate the pain syndrome.

PAIN MECHANISMS

The rich innervation by the sinuvertebral nerve has been postulated to be responsible for various pain syndromes observed in approximately 50 percent of the patients with acute cervical disk disease.[106,140,158] The nerves that arise in a postganglionic fashion from the dorsal root ganglion and then reenter the spinal canal through the superior neuroforamen carry both pain and sympathetic fibers. They innervate multiple contiguous intraspinal structures: dura, posterior longitudinal ligaments, anterior longitudinal ligament, external annular fibers, facet joints, joint capsules, cancellous bone, and the nerve roots themselves.[101,106] The disk space and cartilage end plates have no neural elements.[101,106,140,158] Most studies on acute disk herniation will give a range of 50 to 90 percent of the patients having severe arm pain accompanied by paresthesias.[101,106,107,118,137,139–141] The dermatomal distribution can help determine the site of pathologic involvement; however, the sinuvertebral anastomatosis can make these findings nonanatomic.[118,120] With accompanying cord com-

promise, dysesthesias and hyperesthesias may accompany radicular symptoms. Patients with C2 to C4 disk disease can present with referred pain to the head or retroocular, occipital, or paraspinal discomfort.[101] C5 root disease can be difficult to differentiate from bursitis, tendinitis, or rotator cuff tears. Chest pain may also arise from C5 to T1 nerve root irritation, although C8 is the most frequently involved root.[106]

PHYSICAL EXAMINATION
Motor Evaluation

Ninety percent of patients with cervical radiculopathy also exhibit some form of motor dysfunction.[101,107] However, the severity of neurologic dysfunction does not always correlate with the size of the disk herniation.

Sensory Examination

Compression from the cervical disk on the lateral spinothalamic track is responsible for contralateral loss of pain and temperature sensation. The posterior columns, which are located dorsally and function in position and vibratory sense, may also be directly or indirectly compressed. There may be a direct compression of the posterior column due to a loss of disk space height and infolding of the hypertrophied ligamentum flavum in stenosis, disk disease, or spondylosis. Indirectly, there may be a mass type of effect, whereby the cord is directly compressed anteriorly and indirectly compressed posteriorly. These effects are usually seen in the patients who have cervical myelopathy and loss of position sense, causing an unsteady and wide-base gait.

Reflex Examination

A C4-5 disk herniation will involve the C5 nerve, which would cause a diminished biceps reflex. As previously stated, a C5-6 disk herniation will involve the C6 nerve root. The biceps reflex will be diminished, as well as the brachoradialis reflex. A C6-7 disk herniation will involve the C7 nerve root and the triceps reflex would be diminished with nerve root compression.

DIAGNOSTIC TESTS
Plain X-ray Studies

A wide range of radiographic changes can be seen in patients who have cervical disk disease. Scoville found that 50 percent of cervical x-rays were normal in patients with overt disease.[140,141] He found only 20 percent of the x-ray tests were helpful but not specific, showing only diffuse multilevel degenerative changes. In his study, he found that calcified lateral disks and osteophytes on plain radiographs were the most diagnostic of symptomatic cervical disease.[90,141] The typical cervical spinal changes seen would be loss of disk space, anterior listhesis, or retrolisthesis. The more severe cases have loss of cervical lordosis. Uncovertebral joint changes include hypertrophy, particularly in the lower cervical spine, with involvement of the neuroforamen. Osteophyte formation typically occurs posteriorly, posterolaterally, laterally, and anteriorly. These changes can be diffusely found throughout the cervical spine or limited to a specific level. Increased motion secondary to degenerative disk disease causes facet hypertrophy. The uncovertebral joints can also undergo degenerative changes and spurring, with resultant narrowing of the neuroforamen at that level.

Computed Tomography of the Cervical Spine

Plain computed tomography (CT) of the cervical spine has been supplanted by the MRI scan. The CT scan is still, however, valuable for looking at the bony anatomy of the cervical spine. The amount of cervical stenosis can be accurately depicted on the CT scan. The presence of a disk herniation can be visualized; however, CT does not do this as well as the MRI scan. Computed tomography after myelography is the gold standard for the determination of cervical spinal stenosis. The addition of contrast material will improve the quantitative analysis of cord compression and add specificity in correlating structural changes with symptomatology. The CT/myelogram can also be used postoperatively for the determination of surgical decompression. This is not advocated for routine use; however, it is an excellent test in the postoperative setting. The disadvantage of myelography stems from its invasive nature.

Magnetic Resonance Imaging of the Cervical Spine

Routine MRI of the cervical spine consists of T1- and T2-weighted images in different gradient echo or spin echo sequences. These are obtained in the sagittal and axial planes. The noninvasive nature of MRI makes it an ideal test for screening the cervical spine. Its ability to display anatomic structures in multiple planes and its power to characterize different types of tissue make it an invaluable diagnostic technique. Image quality is subject to technical factors and the size of the scanner magnet. There are several studies attesting to the accuracy of the MRI, with a correlation as high as 90 percent of surgically confirmed cervical disk herniations. The resolution of MRI can also allow examination of the neuroforamen in the cervical spine. Although MRI is not routinely used with contrast, MRI with gadolinium can be used postoperatively to differentiate scarring from recurrent disk herniations.

Diskography

The use of cervical diskography in the evaluation of patients with diskogenic pain has remained controversial since its introduction in 1955. Numerous surgeons have used diskography as a diagnostic tool to decide whether or not to perform surgery on a given patient.[88,136,146,147,166] There are others who do not feel that cervical diskography has merit.[28,81,89] Some authors even believe that MRI reflects degenerative changes in the intervertebral disk more accurately and could eventually replace invasive diskography.[61,104,108]

The technique of diskography varies among practitioners. The basic technique to obtain a diskogram is to place a small-gauge needle anteriorly under fluoroscopic control into the disk space and then injecting the disk space with a water-soluble contrast. At this point, a lateral radiograph is obtained for documentation of needle placement. If the patient does have reproduction of the presenting symptomatology upon injection, the diskogram would be considered positive. The amount of dye accepted as well as the amount of resistance encountered during injection helps to determine if the disk in question is degenerated. In 1976, Roth[136] further refined the technique of diskography by using local anesthetic after a positive pain response is obtained. The positive diskogram now meant loss of the pain response with the injection of a small amount of local anesthetic after a positive diskogram had been obtained. Roth reported 93 percent good to excellent surgical results after anterior cervical disk excision and fusion in those who had positive diskograms and 76 percent good to excellent results when only saline contrast diskography was done. Whitecloud and Seago[166] reviewed their operative fusion results in patients who have positive cervical diskograms and found 70 percent good to excellent results at follow-up. In 1975, Simmons published a study on 456 diskograms in the cervical spine on 114 patients, 91 percent of which were diagnostic.[146] Recent studies have tried to correlate cervical diskography and MRI patterns with diskogenic disease. Parfenchuck and Janssen[112] attempted this correlation with cervical diskogenic pain and predictable MRI patterns. They looked at 52 patients with cervical diskogenic pain who had both cervical MRI and cervical diskography with postdiskography CT scan. Their conclusions were that several MRI patterns did correlate well with positive or negative cervical diskography but others were equivocal. In their study, MRI did not detect approximately 27 percent of the painful disks and had a false-positive rate of 33 percent. They therefore felt that the high false-positive and false-negative rates of MRI prevented it from replacing provocative diskography as the definitive test of choice in cervical diskogenic pain. They concluded that the postdiskography morphology of cervical disks is of little diagnostic value as compared to that of disks in the lumbar spine where the morphologic pattern is important.

TREATMENT

Conservative Therapy

Conservative management of cervical disk disease has been found to be successful by some authors in 80 to 90 percent of cases.[83] Some have found that neck pain resolves in 85 percent of patients, with fewer than 12 percent remaining disabled for more than 3 months.[101] The treatment for these patients involves a 4- to 6-week course of nonsteroidal anti-inflammatory drugs (NSAIDs), limited use of a cervical collar, and "tincture of time." Use of cervical traction can alleviate pain due to cervical disease; however, the pathophysiology for which traction works remains controversial.[137,158] Use of isometric neck-strengthening exercises in conservative care may be beneficial; however, it must be used after the acute pain resolves. Pain without any radicular component should be treated with long, aggressive isometric neck-strengthening exercises and general aerobic conditioning. Most patients with mechanical neck pain will have resolution of their symptomatology with time and strengthening exercises. The limited use of a cervical collar may be beneficial. Some authors even feel that adequate emotional and physiotherapeutic support is necessary.[137,158] Multimodality pain centers staffed with therapists and psychologists have been beneficial in treatment of the whole patient.[158] Trigger-point injections have also been used to try to break the inflammatory cycle of the myofascial type of pain. The use of NSAIDs has been beneficial and is a mainstay in the conservative treatment of patients with cervical pathology. Those patients with herniated cervical disks can have a large inflammatory component to the radiculopathy. The use of NSAIDs can be effective in the treatment of these patients. Narcotic medication for acute pain has also been part of the initial treatment of patients with disk herniations. Muscle relaxants can be helpful in acute exacerbations of cervical disk herniation, which may be accompanied by painful muscle spasms. Many short-acting muscle relaxants are now on the market; however, it should be noted that most of these medications are habit-forming.

All patients with cervical neck pain from spondylosis or disk herniation should initially be treated conservatively. This involves the selective use of a soft cervical collar for immobilization, NSAIDs, and possibly physical therapy. The use of traction remains controversial. Some studies have found it to be potentially harmful in the acutely injured cervical spine.[19,64,70,178] Traction should never be prescribed without x-ray demonstration of a stable cervical spine. Cervical traction is contraindicated in situations including malignancy, cord compression, infection, and rheumatoid arthritis. The use of traction can be either mechanical or manual, continuous or intermittent, and sitting or supine. There are many types of home traction therapy where the minimal weight is approximately 5 lb, with a maximum of 10 lb pulling in slight flexion. Other physical therapy modalities include moist heat, transcutaneous electrical nerve stimulation (TENS), and even ultrasound. However, there are no scientific data to support the use of these modalities. Any patient undergoing this type of conservative management should also be placed on NSAIDs. It has been found that most patients will respond to this approach of immobilization and pharmacotherapy in the first few weeks. Those who begin to improve can then start on a well-supervised physical therapy regime, including isometric neck-strengthening and range-of-motion exercises. Conservative management should be aggressive in its approach to treating patients.

The optimal duration of conservative care remains controversial. Patients with radiculopathy secondary to disk herniations may be candidates for operative intervention between 6 weeks and 6 months. Those who complain predominantly of cervical neck pain should continue to be managed conservatively for longer periods of time.

Surgical Management

Cervical spinal pathology and symptomatology dictate the type of operative procedure that would be best suited for these patients. The factors that need to be addressed are (1) the type of disk herniation—soft versus hard (spondylotic spurs), (2) the location of the disk herniation—central versus posterolateral, and (3) the preoperative cervical alignment. The approaches include anterior with and without fusion, laminotomy/foraminotomy, laminoplasty, and laminectomy. Indications for surgery in cervical radiculopathy include the following:

1. Significant arm pain that has not responded to a trial of conservative treatment
2. A neurological deficit associated with radicular pain, including muscle weakness
3. The proper corresponding imaging study, including a myelogram with postmyelogram CT or MRI

A decision as to the type of approach, as stated previously, remains controversial.

Anterior Surgical Approaches

The anterior approach to the cervical spine has been demonstrated to be safe and effective for the treatment of cervical spondylosis, cervical disk herniation, and cervical myelopathy. There are many different techniques of anterior cervical fusion. These include the horseshoe-shaped graft of Smith and Robinson,[148,149] the dowel graft of Cloward,[26] the iliac strut graft of Bailey and Badgley,[5] and the keystone graft of Simmons and Bhalla.[147] The approach to the anterior cervical spine can be from the right or the left. Advantages of the left-sided approach are comfort of a right-handed surgeon and less risk of injury to the recurrent laryngeal nerve. On the left side, the recurrent laryngeal nerve enters the thoracic cavity within the carotid sheath, loops under the aortic arch, and then ascends into the neck besides the trachea and esophagus. The right side is more variable; there, the recurrent laryngeal nerve can cross anteriorly behind the thyroid, thus leaving itself more susceptible to injury on approach to the right side of the cervical spine. The left side does have disadvantages, especially in the lower cervical spine at the cervicothoracic junction, with the risk of injury to the thoracic duct. The incision on the cervical spine can be either transverse or longitudinal, following the border of the sternocleidomastoid muscle. Landmarks used for skin incision include the hyoid bone at the level of C3, the thyroid cartilage at the level of C4-5, and the cricoid cartilage at C6. The skin and platysmal incisions are in the same direction. The carotid sheath is retracted laterally, with the esophagus and trachea being retracted medially. The paravertebral fascia and longus colli muscles are then dissected away from the vertebral bodies. At this point, a spinal needle should be inserted into the disk and a lateral radiograph obtained. This will determine the level of the cervical spine with the most accuracy. The disk in question is then removed and cervical fusion is performed.

The Smith-Robinson technique involves the removal of the disk in question to the posterior longitudinal ligament. Most surgeons feel that the posterior longitudinal ligament should be preserved to maintain stability; however, if there are extruded fragments, partial removal of the posterior longitudinal ligament can be performed.[135,149,150] When the disk has been adequately removed, a horseshoe-shaped iliac graft is obtained from the iliac crest. Cortical bone is carefully preserved to maintain the graft strength. Cervical traction is applied and the graft is countersunk approximately 1 to 2 mm below the surface of the anterior vertebral body. To avoid graft resorption, the graft should measure 5 mm in height.[11]

The question of whether posterior osteophytes need to be removed or whether they will be reabsorbed with cervical fusion remains somewhat unanswered. Most authors feel that removal of posterior osteophytes is not routinely necessary, since resorption will occur with solid bony fusion.[29,117,119,120,133] The resection of these osteophytes can carry a high risk of iatrogenic cord injury, especially in patients with small spinal canals. Most surgeons feel that when compression by an osteophyte is thought to cause a significant neurologic problem, removal of the entire vertebral body should be performed. This would allow for adequate decompression and reduce the risk to the spinal cord. Use of the Smith-Robinson graft technique has been highly successful in fusion of the cervical spine. A factor that has contributed to graft failure is improper size. A graft that is too short in the longitudinal or transverse direction leads to inadequate distraction and decompression of the neuroforamen. When the graft is too large, there will be too much compression, which can lead to collapse of the graft and subsequent kyphosis above the operative level. Surgical failure can also occur when grafts are retropulsed posteriorly into the cord or extruded anteriorly into the esophagus and trachea.

The Cloward technique also involves the anterior approach to the cervical spine. After adequate exposure has been obtained, a circular drill, centered over the involved disk space, is used to remove a dowel type of segment. The resection includes the disk material along with portions of the superior and inferior vertebral bodies. Resection of disk and end plates to the posterior longitudinal ligament is performed. A slightly larger dowel is then harvested from the iliac crest. Cervical traction is applied and the graft is then placed. This technique is not as popular as the Smith-Robinson approach.

The Simmons-Bhalla technique is also known as the keystone graft. It involves complete removal of the disk back to the posterior longitudinal ligament. After disk removal, end-plate resection with beveling upward into the vertebral body above and downward into the vertebral body below is performed. The resection, which is carried posteriorly to the level of the posterior cortex, maintains part of the posterior cortex to prevent posterior retropul-

sion of the graft, and the defect is then measured. A rectangular graft is obtained from the iliac crest and shaped to fit the trough. The ends are beveled to allow for locking in of the graft. Care should be taken to countersink the graft (Fig. 73-4). Cancellous bone can then be placed around any areas that do not have good contact. In their original study, Simmons and Bhalla looked at 84 patients; they treated 68 with the keystone technique and 17 with the dowel technique. They found that 80 percent of the patients having keystone techniques had an excellent or good result, as opposed to only 64.8 percent with the dowel type of procedure. The patients who had a poor result all had multiple-level fusions. There was no incidence of nonunion using the keystone technique. Critics of this technique base their argument on the removal of the superior and inferior end plates, causing collapse of the levels fused. This apparent collapse will then lead to kyphosis and possible neuroforaminal narrowing.

Emery et al.[42] used the standard Robinson anterior cervical interbody fusion technique with modification. They compared 31 patients having a standard technique and 29 patients having a modified technique with respect to settling of bone graft, kyphotic angulation, and pseudarthrosis as well as pain outcome. They found that their modified technique of burring of the end plates for cervical interbody arthrodesis resulted in a detectable but not clinically important amount of graft settling but a higher success rate for arthrodesis. They found a pseudarthrosis rate of 4.4 percent versus 12 percent in an earlier group they had studied, comprising 122 patients with 195 surgical levels. A statistically significant loss of height occurred. This was approximately 1.3 mm and was not deemed clinically significant enough to cause foraminal encroachment from settling. Their conclusion was that the modified Robinson technique improved the pseudarthrosis rate with a small but measurable amount of height loss due to graft settling; however, this was not deemed to be clinically significant. Bohlman et al.[13] in 1993 used cervical anterior diskectomy and arthrodesis for cervical radiculopathy with the Robinson technique. They treated 122 patients with an average follow-up of 6 years and a range of 2 to 15 years. Preoperatively, 118 patients had pain in the arm and 55 had weakness in one or more roots. A one-level procedure was done in 62 of the 122 patients; a two-level procedure in 48; a three-level procedure in 11, and a four-level procedure in 1. The investigators found a pseudarthrosis in 24 of the 195 operatively treated segments. Of these, 16 were symptomatic, with 4 warranting revision. Bohlman et al. found that at the most recent follow-up, 53 of the 55 patients had resolution of their motor deficit. Their technique involves a tricortical iliac crest graft, which provides an excellent fit, and at least a 5 mm disk space height distraction for foraminal opening and to relieve pressure on the nerve root. Postoperatively, 108 of the 122 patients returned to work, with 81 having no pain in the neck or arm at the time of the latest follow-up. Of the 91 patients who had been employed preoperatively, 79 returned to their preoperative employment and 11 did not return to work. No patients had neurologic injury or graft dislodgement, but graft collapse did occur in one patient.

The complications of anterior cervical diskectomy and fusion can be broken down into those occurring at the graft site and those in the neck. The most common postoperative complications are transient sore throat, hoarseness, or difficult in swallowing.[22,73,167] More serious complications include vascular injuries to the carotid vessels and vertebral arteries as well as esophageal and tracheal perforations. Injury to the recurrent laryngeal nerve was the single largest neurologic complication in more than 36,000 cases reviewed in 1982.[58] The most serious complications of spinal cord injury have been reported in the literature. Flynn et al., reporting on the experience of a large group of neurosurgeons, found significant permanent radiculomyelopathy in 100 out of 36,657 patients.[58] Other surgical complications included graft extrusion, resorption, and retropulsion. These complications have been described with all types of grafting techniques.[127,128,171] Pseudarthrosis rates have been found to be inversely proportional to the number of levels fused.[29,132] However, the presence of a pseudarthrosis does not always suggest a poor surgical outcome. Some authors could not find a significantly different result between solid fusion and pseudarthrosis.[35,128] The results for anterior cervical fusions have been satisfactory in over 90 percent of the patients studied.[11,26,29,35,36,63,72,131,132,147,165,168,171] These studies, however, have shown that single-level fusions do better than multiple-level fusions in terms of postoperative surgical outcome and fusion rates.

Complications at the donor site include hematoma, infection, injury to the lateral femoral cutaneous nerve, and persistent pain over the iliac crest. These problems do not usually lead to long-term disabilities. To prevent these complications careful placement of the iliac crest incision is recommended. Most authors suggest staying at least 1 cm behind the anterosuperior iliac crest to prevent laceration of the nerve.

Anterior Cervical Disk Excision without Fusion

In the early 1960s, Hirsch published his results of simple diskectomy without fusion in the treatment of cervical radiculopathy.[129,133] He had small numbers but excellent results, and over the years many authors[7,8,66,94,99,129,134,152,174] have corroborated these findings on anterior cervical diskectomy without fusion. These articles are mostly in the neurosurgical literature. Many authors have reported success rates similar to those of cervical diskectomy and fusion. They have reported spontaneous fusion in up to 75 percent of patients having simple diskectomy. The procedure was most successful in patients with minimal spondylosis. However, only two reports of prospective anterior cervical diskectomy with and without fusion exist in the literature. Martin studied 51 patients nonrandomly assigned to anterior cervical diskectomy (ACD) or anterior cervical diskectomy with fusion (ACF) by the Cloward technique.[99] The results between the two groups were comparable, with 92 percent having good or excellent results. Most of the patients were operated on for radicular pain. However, 20 percent appeared to be operated upon for neck pain alone. There was no clear explanation of complications associated with either procedure, and the follow-up was less than

1 year. Rosenorn et al.[134] randomly assigned 63 patients with cervical radiculopathy to ACD or ACF by the Cloward technique, using allograft in 19 patients. These authors found that ACD patients returned to work more quickly than ACF patients and had more excellent or good results at 1-year follow-up. This study is less than optimal from the cervical fusion standpoint of the Cloward technique and using allograft. Watters and Levinthal[160] retrospectively reviewed the outcome of 126 patients treated with ACD or ACF. They found that patients having ACD alone had significantly reduced mean operative time, blood loss, and hospital stay. There were 16 complications for ACF patients, 15 of which were graft-related. There were 4 complications for ACD patients. The investigators found no difference in return to work between the two groups. Their long-term follow-up demonstrated an equal amount of neck and arm pain in both groups. The report did not describe how the patients were selected for the type of procedure performed or indicate whether the presence of cervical spondylosis contraindicated the ACD procedure alone. The authors did not recommend routine removal of the posterior longitudinal ligament and felt that not doing so is an excellent way to prevent the serious complications and instability reported with ACD in other studies. The remarkable uniformity of results between the two groups led them to believe that neither ACD nor ACF was a superior surgical procedure for the symptomatic cervical disk.

Posterior Surgical Approaches

Posterior surgical approaches have been used predominantly by neurosurgical spinal surgeons to treat disk disease and spondylosis irrespective of the location of the disk herniation.[16,46,48,50,53–55,67,71,121,139–141,170] The posterior approach is felt by some to improve visualization of nerve root decompression and to have increased versatility for multilevel exploration as compared with the anterior approach. The posterior approach can be used to treat posterior, posterolateral, lateral, anterolateral, or even, some feel, anterior disk herniations. Controversy still surrounds the best operation for a lesion that is midline anterior to the cord.[54,139–141,169] Epstein, Farter, and Scoville have outlined modifications in posterior techniques that can be used to expose these anterior lesions from the back.[48,53–55,141] The removal of posterolateral herniations through a keyhole foraminotomy or hemilaminectomy with appropriate unilateral or bilateral facetectomy has been well established.[21,54] These studies found that approximately 91 percent of such patients improved with this procedure.[139–141] Some authors feel that only a posterior approach will directly relieve posterolateral compression from an infolded ligamentum flavum, shingled laminae, or posterior spurs from the hypertrophied facet joint. The problem with the posterior approach for anterolateral or central disk herniations is that in order to approach these pathologies, a full laminectomy—including two levels above and below the level of major disease—is necessary. This multilevel laminectomy can include medial facetectomy, either unilateral or bilateral, to untether the nerve root sleeves enough to allow the cord and root to migrate away from the single or multiple central defects.[15] There

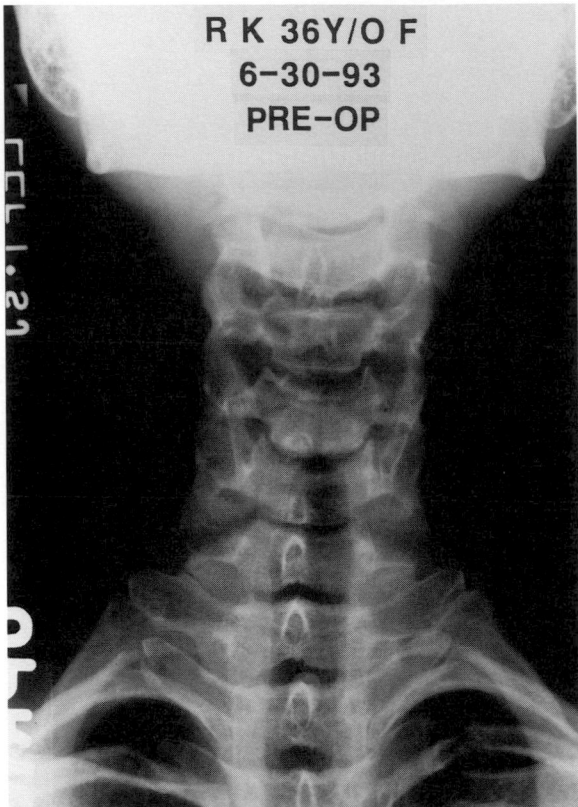

A

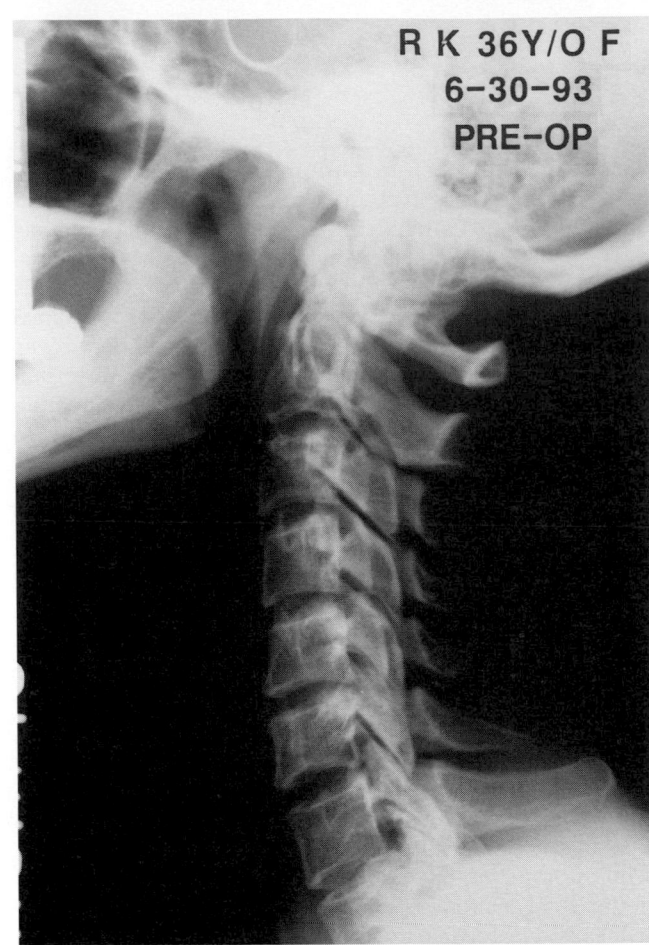

B

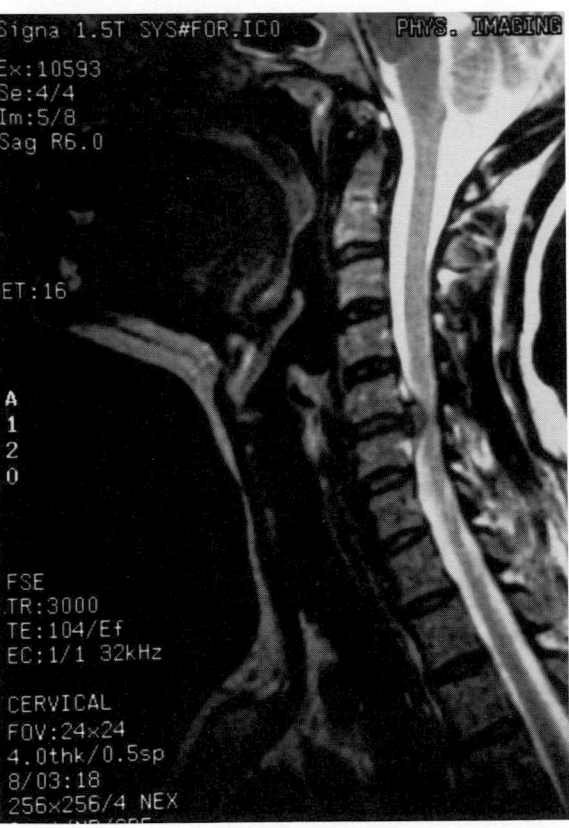

C

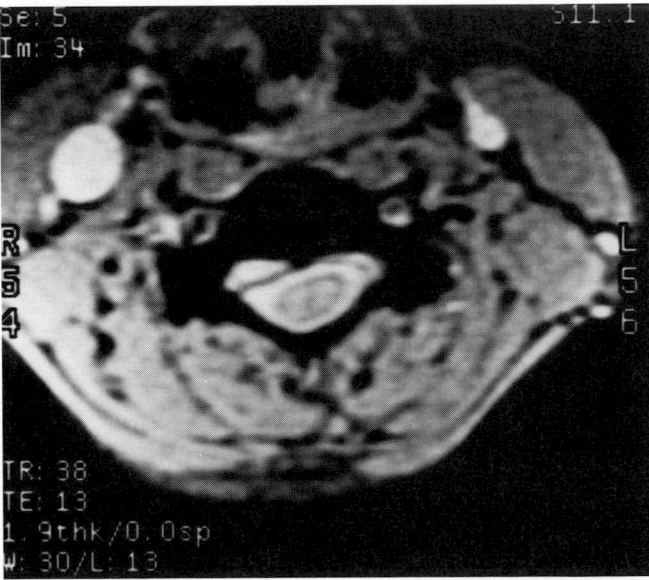

D

Figure 73-4 R.K. is a 36-year-old female with a 6-month history of right arm pain and a C6 radiculopathy. The (*A*) coronal and (*B*) lateral cervical spine films were unremarkable except for a slight loss of disk height seen on the lateral x-ray at C5-6. A (*C*) lateral and (*D*) axial MRI scan at C5-6 shows the large right-sided disk herniation. The patient underwent an anterior cervical diskectomy and keystone fusion. At 2 years postoperatively, the (*E*) coronal and (*F*) lateral extension x-rays demonstrate a well-healed fusion (*Continued*).

1360

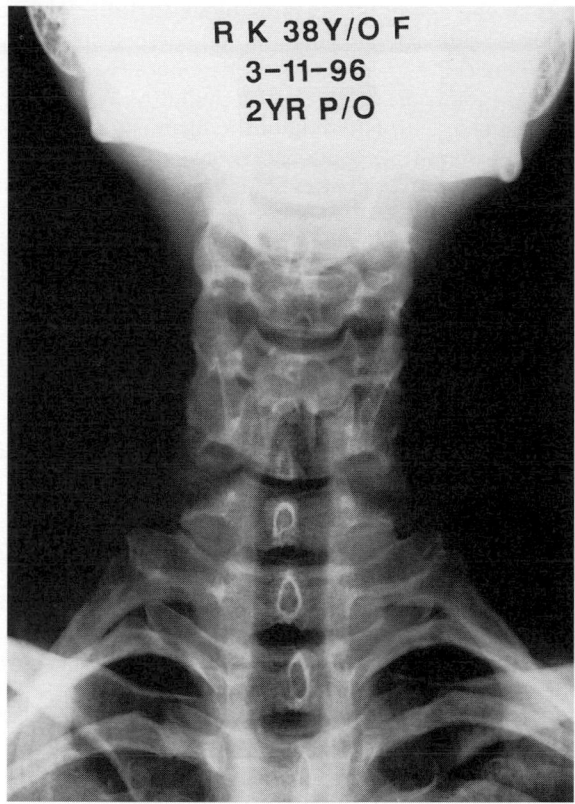

E

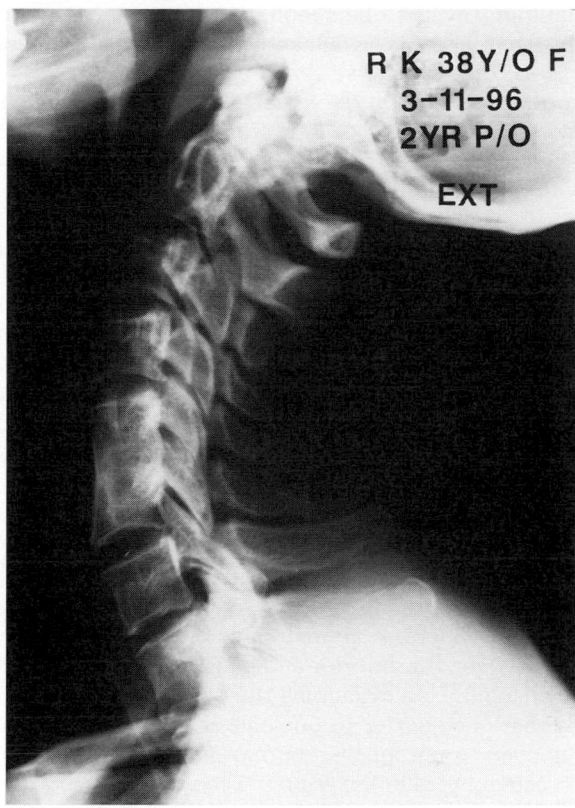

F

Figure 73-4 *(Continued)*

are reports in the literature suggesting that if this surgical approach does not allow sufficient exposure, the dura should be opened and a transdural approach adopted. These authors do not advocate this type of radical procedure for something that could be performed through an anterior procedure alone. There are numerous complications from dural procedures, including pseudomeningocele formation, arachnoiditis, and dural leak.

An anterior procedure has been deemed the treatment of choice for midline soft disk herniations, symptomatic myelopathy from midline hard disk protrusions at one or two levels, and disk herniations with bilateral radiculopathy. The posterior approach can be used for unilateral radiculopathy at one or more levels, cervical myelopathy with spinal cord compression at three or more levels without the presence of preoperative kyphosis, and spinal cord compression secondary to congenital spinal stenosis or acquired stenosis from posterior compression.[145]

Keyhole Foraminotomy

Keyhole foraminotomy to treat lateral soft and hard disk herniations was originally proposed in the 1940s.[140] It was originally planned with the patient in the sitting position but is now more commonly performed with the patient prone and the cervical spine parallel to the floor. This allows for partial collapse of the epidural veins and reduces the risk of air embolism. An incision approximately 3 cm

long is made over the appropriate spinous processes and a subperiosteal dissection is then performed. The laterally placed laminotomy forms a circular or keyhole type of exposure. Under magnification, the nerve root is then exposed by unroofing the foramen. The nerve root is usually found tight against the inferior surface of the facet joint. The lateral extent of the foraminotomy is determined by passing an angled instrument out of the foramen. If the instrument can slip comfortably between the tissues around the nerve root and bony foramen, the foraminotomy is complete. The operation is complete if the patient has hard disk pathology. If the patient does need removal of a disk fragment, the cuff of veins around the nerve root must be taken down. The root is then retracted to allow for disk removal. With this technique, stability is preserved, with both exposure and mobilization of the nerve root being performed.

The complications associated with posterior nerve root decompression are low. They include failure to operate at the correct level of root injury and inadequate foraminotomy.

Hemilaminectomy

The hemilaminectomy procedure has been described by Faiger[55] to be the procedure of choice for patients with mono- or polyradicular syndromes due to lateral disk herniations or spondylosis. The hemilaminectomy and accompanying medial facetectomies and foraminotomies allow multiple levels to be simultaneously explored and decompressed. There is significantly more removal of bone in this procedure to expose the root; therefore, the risk of postoperative instability is real. Some authors feel that careful attention to the preservation of the lateral aspects of the facet joints during laminectomy should maintain stability of the cervical spine. However, if the facets are sacrificed, subluxation and swan-neck deformity may occur. The denervation of the posterior cervical spinal muscles can also lead to a prolonged recovery time. The cervical muscles attached to the large spinous process of C2 should be preserved. Sim et al. found that only 3 percent of patients will develop cervical kyphosis or swan-neck deformity following cervical laminectomy.[144a] It has been well established that children are much more at risk for the development of kyphosis after cervical laminectomy. The procedure should be avoided or intraoperative stability should be performed on children having cervical laminectomy performed.

A decision to use an anterior approach instead of a posterior approach depends on the site of pathology and the operating surgeon's familiarity with the technique. Raynor in 1983 looked at anatomic and radiographic evaluation between the anterior and posterior approach of the cervical spine.[124] In evaluating the posterior approach, he found that one-quarter to one-half of the facet joint must be removed to unroof the neuroforamen and that the anterior osteophytes in the region of the uncovertebral joint are difficult to reach. He also found that with the anterior approach, the amount of root decompression is usually overestimated. He found that the lateral limits of decompression anteriorly must be beyond direct visualization to equal that obtained posteriorly. Plain x-rays of the cervical spine reflected few if any anatomic alterations accomplished by an operation. Oblique x-ray films do not visualize the entrance of the anatomic foramen, and osteophytes seen on this view may be well anterior to the neural canal. Raynor found that greater exposure of a root can be performed posteriorly under direct vision. For an equal amount of decompression to be performed with the anterior exposure, the work is done beyond the limit of direct visualization. The osteophytes arising from or near the uncovertebral joints can cause root compression and spondylosis, and it can be relatively easy to reach them from an anterior exposure. By the posterior approach, it is difficult to decompress this area of the uncovertebral joint. This study does not address the importance of disk space distraction through the use of anterior cervical graft for fusion. It has been shown that this distraction will decompress the nerve root by restoring the foraminal height and removing the infolding of the ligamentum flavum.

CERVICAL SPINAL STENOSIS

The cervical spine and the effect of stenosis on the area has been well studied from the 1950s through the 1980s. Clark and Robinson in 1956[25] published a review of 120 patients with cervical spondylotic myelopathy (CSM). The authors described the clinical manifestation of myelopathy as spasticity and weakness that most often is gradual in onset and occurs at the age of 50 years or older. In 1967, Brain and Wilkinson[16] published a monograft on cervical spondylosis. They defined it as a progressive degenerative disease involving the joints of Luschka and including osseous spurring and thickening with infolding of the ligamentum flavum. In 1977, Robinson et al.[130] published an important article on the etiology and treatment of CSM, in which they suggested that the basic pathology of spondylosis was a production of chondroosseous spurs. More recently and with the arrival of refined technology, the pathophysiology of cervical myelopathy has been proposed to be multifactorial, the most important conditions being congenital cervical spinal stenosis with progressive cervical spondylosis, direct cord compression, and impairment of the blood supply to the cord. Mechanical factors are also felt to play a significant role.[17] The normal sagittal diameter of the spinal canal and the diameter of the spinal cord and their association has been well documented.[2,3] There is a general agreement that the average sagittal diameter of the canal from C3 to C7 ranges from 15 to 25 mm, with an average of 17 mm.[77,79,141] These determinations were based on a standard lateral x-ray with the tube 6 ft from the actual film. If the diameter of the canal is less than 13 mm, the canal is stenotic by definition. The average diameter of the cervical spinal cord from C1 to C7 has been documented to be an average of 10 mm, with a range from 8.5 to 11.5 mm.[2,32,52,111,116,126] Pavlov et al., in 1987,[113] looked at 23 patient athletes with cervical spine neuropraxia. Two methods of measurements were performed, the conventional sagittal diameter being measured from the posterior surface of the vertebral body to the nearest point of the corresponding laminar line, and the ratio method with the sagittal diameter of the spinal canal being divided by the sagittal diameter of the corresponding vertebral body. The investigators found the ratio method to be a reliable determination for cervical spinal stenosis, and it is independent of technical variables. Their determination was that a ratio of greater than 1 meant no significant stenosis. A ratio of spinal canal to vertebral body of 0.8 or less indicated significant cervical spinal stenosis, with a range of 0.8 to 1 as relative stenosis in the cervical spine. Edwards and LaRocca[41] retrospectively reviewed 63 patients with symptomatic cervical spondylosis. They performed measurements of segmental sagittal diameter at the level of the pedicle and measurements of spondylotic segmental sagittal diameter at the level of the disk. They determined a spondylosis index that was computed as a difference between the two measurements, with 2.08 mm per segment for patients with narrow canals and 3.29 per segment for patients with wider canals. They felt that canal dimensions were determinants of symptom production and neurologic compromise (Fig. 73-5). The importance of an improved blood supply to the spinal cord has been well established in CSM.[37,62,78,82,143] The mechanism has been proposed to occur through interruption in the sucal and terminal vessels of the anterior spinal artery. A large chondroosseous spur in conjunction with a congenitally narrow canal may produce this direct neural compression.[154,157] The second mechanism of vascular ischemia has been postulated to be due to tethering and compression of the foraminal and radicular feeder arteries to the cord. This vascular ischemia can be attributed to osteophytes in the foramen as well as thickening of the ligamentum flavum.

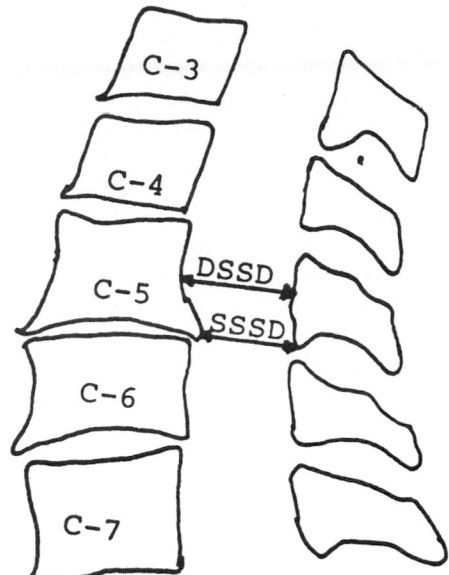

Figure 73-5 Measurement of the cervical developmental segmental sagittal diameter (DSSD) and the spondylotic segmental sagittal diameter (SSSD). Using a standard 72-in lateral radiograph, the pedicle–vertebral body junction is identified. A perpendicular line is drawn to the posterior margin of the spinal canal as determined by the most anterior bony landmark for the segment. A second perpendicular line is drawn at the level of the disk to the segmental connecting line posteriorly. The difference between the two measurements is the spondylosis index and represents the amount of narrowing due to the disease process. DSSD = 16 mm; SSSD = 13 mm. The spondylosis index is 3 mm for the C5-6 level. (Reproduced with permission from Burrows EH: *J Bone Joint Surg* 45A:1171, 1963.)

In 1977, Hoff et al.[78] proposed that cervical myelopathy involves compression and ischemia of the cord. Bohlman and Emery in 1988[12] postulated that CSM is a multifactorial disease. They have found that most patients with the disease present with a variation of the anterior cord syndrome, with eventual loss of posterior column modalities of position and vibratory sense. Their hypothesis is that the disease in its early stages is secondary to anterior cord compression and ischemia in association with congenital cervical stenosis. The electrophysiologic changes that occur—leading to alteration in evoked potentials—increase as the disease becomes more severe.[32,92,144,175,177] The authors postulated that many intrinsic changes occur within the spinal cord, including blockage of axoplasmic flow, distortion of the cord tissue, stretching of the intrinsic transverse terminations of the anterior spinal artery, and, in more severe cases, demyelination of the white matter. The end stage is cystic degeneration and destruction of the spinal cord. Most authors agree that patients with CSM have congenital cervical stenosis. The addition of other factors can then lead to symptoms consistent with myelopathy. Cervical spondylotic myelopathy can be produced by a herniated nucleus pulposus in a narrow spinal canal, which usually leads to an acute onset of myelopathic signs. A more common etiology of CSM is a slow degenerative process that usually occurs over multiple levels of the cervical spine. The combination of a hard disk

and posterior osteophyte formation anterior to the spinal cord in conjunction with infolding of the ligamentum flavum posteriorly can lead to myelopathy. The condition is usually gradual in onset, with disk degeneration occurring first, leading to osteoarthritic changes and subluxation of the vertebral bodies. The autostabilizing effect of facet joint hypertrophy and thickening of the ligamentum flavum leads to spinal canal compromise, with the sagittal diameter less than 13 mm. These patients are not only suffering from symptomatology of their disease but are also at significant risk for cord injury with minimal trauma.

Another cause of CSM, more frequently found in Japan, is ossification of the posterior longitudinal ligament (OPLL). This condition may be isolated or segmental and can present with radiculopathy or myelopathy.[96] It has become more prevalent in the United States mainly because of improved recognition of the disease entity and improved radiographic diagnosis.

The Natural History of Cervical Spondylotic Myelopathy

In 1956, Clark and Robinson[25] separated patients with myelopathy due to cervical spondylosis from those with cord changes induced by acute disk herniation. They observed that once the disorder is recognized, complete remission never occurs and spontaneous regression of neurologic deficits is unusual. Seventy-five percent of their cases had progressive myelopathy. This progression was episodic in that two-thirds had ongoing deterioration and in one-third the condition had stabilized. Lees and Turner in 1963[93] reviewed 44 patients who had myelopathy on presentation and compared them to 51 patients who had cervical spondylosis. They found that the behavior of the disease was the same, whether it was present for more or less than 10 years, and that there was an initial development of symptoms followed by a static period or one of improvement. They found that this was "a condition in which there are long periods without new or worsening symptoms. Exacerbations can occur at long or shorter intervals for many years." The authors established that CSM was a disease marked by long periods of nonprogressive disability. However, Symon and Lavender[155] in 1967 reviewed the results of treatment given by Lees and Turner. Their findings were not as positive as those noted by the latter authors. They found that only 18 percent of the patients changed category for the better. Symon and Lavender therefore challenged the benefits of conservative care and noted that over 60 percent of the patients had a steady, progressive course of deterioration.

The literature regarding the natural history of CSM does not include a clear prognostic indicator as to which patients are at risk for progression of their disease. Some patients will maintain a given minor level of dysfunction indefinitely, while others will deteriorate relentlessly. Ideally the patient who presents with minor deficits without recent progression should be closely observed and treated conservatively. Those who are moderately or severely disabled when first seen may not be candidates for conservative care and might improve with early surgical intervention.[91]

History and Physical Findings

Patients with CSM can present with four different types of syndromes.[56] The patient may present with (1) primary root- or radicular-type symptoms or (2) long tract signs only. The most common presentation is (3) a combination of the two syndromes and the least common type is (4) that of primary vascular involvement. Typically, the patients will have compression of one or more nerve roots, showing lower motor neuron findings from this compression as well as upper motor neuron findings at the levels below the lesion. Patients will also often complain of difficulty with walking and maintaining balance. They do not usually complain of significant weakness but can have difficulty with fine finger movements. Some patient might present with Lhermitte's sign, in which flexion or extension of the neck produces "electric shocks" in their arms and legs. The sensory disturbance in patients with CSM can be confusing. Compression may occur at the spinothalamic tract, affecting contralateral pain and temperature sensation. Patients who have posterior column involvement can have ipsilateral loss of position and vibratory sense. This is the predominant tract involved in loss of gait. The third area of sensory involvement can be the dorsal root ganglion, with subsequent decrease in dermatomal sensation. The sensory changes usually occur at the level below the area of compression.

Reflex changes occurring in CSM are consistent with lower motor neuron involvement at the level of the lesion and upper motor neuron findings below the level of the lesion. Therefore, reflexes are diminished at the level of the lesion and hyperactive below it. The Hoffman reflex or sign occurs when the ipsilateral interphalangeal joint of the thumb and index finger flex when the volar surface of the terminal phalanx of the long finger is flicked. Extension of the patient's neck by the patient or the examiner during testing increases the sensitivity of Hoffman's sign.[34] The inverted radial reflex is spontaneous flexion of the digits when the brachioradialis reflex is elicited. This sign is felt to be pathognomonic of CSM because it indicates spondylotic compression of the cord at the fifth and sixth cervical levels. The physiology behind this mechanism stems from interference with the reflex arc of the brachioradialis at the sixth cervical level with cord compression. This causes an upper motor neuron lesion with spontaneous contraction of the finger flexors. The patients with severely involved CSM might have abnormal plantar responses.

Nurick classified cervical spondylotic myelopathy based on the gait patterns of these patients.[109] Nurick grade 0 patients have only root symptoms. Nurick grade I patients have signs of cord involvement—i.e., hyperreflexia—but have normal gait. Nurick grade II patients have gait abnormalities, but these are not severe enough to alter activities of daily living. Nurick grade III patients have cord involvement and increased gait abnormalities that prevent them from seeking gainful employment and affect activities of daily living. Nurick grade IV patients walk only with assistance, and patients with grade V spondylotic myelopathy are chair- or bedridden (Table 73-1). The Japanese Orthopaedic Association (JOA) has devised a scale to further quantitate neurologic involvement. This scale looks at motor function, arm and leg sensations, and bladder function. The maximum number of points obtainable is 17 (Table 73-2).

Diagnostic Studies

The differential diagnosis of patients with CSM must include metabolic, congenital, rheumatologic, and neural degenerative disease entities.[102] The metabolic considerations include acromegaly and gigantism, while the list of congenital syndromes includes Arnold-Chiari malformation, achondroplasia, Morquio's syndrome, Down's syndrome, and Klippel-Feil anomaly.[9,27,68,98,123,138,153] Patients with atlantoaxial instability from ligamentous laxity may also have cord compression. These patients usually have rheumatoid arthritis, Still's disease, ankylosing spondylosis, or Paget's disease.[1,23,31,33,52,68,97,100] Patients must also be differentiated from those with neurodegenerative syndromes such as amyotrophic lateral sclerosis—multiple sclerosis being the most common—as well as combined systems diseases.

The initial workup of patients with CSM should include AP, lateral, flexion, and extension lateral and oblique radiographs of the cervical spine. The plain films help to identify many different pathologic processes such as degenerative subluxation, congenital stenosis, spondylotic stenosis, and

---

TABLE 73-1   Nurick's Classification of Disability in Spondylotic Myelopathy

Grade	Description
I	Signs of cord involvement, normal gait
II	Mild gait impairment, ADL[a] normal, able to be employed
III	Gait abnormality that prevents employment and normal ADL
IV	Able to ambulate only with assistance
V	Chairbound or bedridden

[a]ADL, activities of daily living.
Source: Reproduced with permission from Nurick S: The pathogenesis of the spinal cord disorder associated with cervical spondylosis. *Brain* 95:87–100, 1972.

TABLE 73-2   The Assessment Scale Proposed by the Japanese Orthopaedic Association

---

I.   Motor dysfunction of the upper extremity
              Score
                        0 = Unable to feed oneself
                        1 = Unable to handle chopsticks, able to eat with a spoon
                        2 = Chopsticks handled with much difficulty
                        3 = Chopsticks handled with slight difficulty
                        4 = None

II.   Motor dysfunction of the lower extremity
              Score
                        0 = Unable to walk
                        1 = Able to walk on flat floor with walking aid
                        2 = Able to walk up and/or down stairs with handrail
                        3 = Lack of stability and smooth reciprocation
                        4 = None

III.   Sensory deficit
        A. The upper extremity
              Score
                        0 = Severe sensory loss or pain
                        1 = Mild sensory loss
                        2 = None
        B. The lower extremity, same as A
        C. The trunk, same as A

IV.   Sphincter dysfunction
              Score
                        0 = Unable to void
                        1 = Marked difficulty in micturition (retention, strangury)
                        2 = Difficulty in micturition (pollakiuria, hesitation)
                        3 = None

---

foraminal narrowing. Pavlov's ratio, as stated previously, remains the best indicator of cervical spinal stenosis. Those patients with a Pavlov's ratio of 0.8 or less are considered to be stenotic. The next test for the workup of CSM should be an MRI. This study will give excellent anatomic detail to determine the severity of spinal cord compression and canal compromise.[103] Monitoring of somatosensory evoked potentials and cortical evoked potentials does have a role in the workup of patients with CSM. Electromyographic studies can be useful in differentiating peripheral nerve compression and neuropathies from CSM. The gold standard for the diagnosis of CSM is the myelogram with a postmyelogram CT. A myelogram can give the more exact degree of nerve root compression as well as the bony architecture in relation to spinal cord compression, but it is invasive. The MRI is beneficial in its ability to differentiate intramedullary disease (cysts, syrinxes, hydromyelias, tumors, and neurodegenerative syndromes) from extramedullary disease.

Conservative Treatment

Conservative management of CSM revolves around immobilization of the neck with a semirigid orthosis. Immobilization diminishes the irritation and compression on the spinal cord. Isometric exercises can be used in conjunction with cervical immobilization. Bohlman believes that if the patients are having difficulty walking and their MRIs or other radiographs indicate severe spinal cord compression, a more aggressive approach should be carried out that includes surgical decompression and stabilization.[10]

Surgical Treatment

The most common treatment for CSM historically has been the laminectomy at one or more levels.[47,48,84] On follow-up, these patients have shown significant immediate improvement but, on long-term follow-up, eventual deterioration.[30,65] The poor long-term results of laminectomy are related to the loss of spinal stability. The laminectomy procedure should not be performed in the face of loss of normal cervical lordosis or kyphosis. Decompressive laminectomies of the involved levels should be performed with appropriate foraminotomies when radicular pain is present. The lamina is removed completely in a laminectomy and up to 50 percent of the medial aspect of the facet can be removed without fear of destabilization.[125] The postoperative rehabilitation program in these patients includes physical therapy with range-of-motion and isometric neck-strengthening exercises to maintain paravertebral muscle strength and prevent possible swan-neck deformity.

A variation of the laminectomy first reported by Hirabayashi and coworkers in 1977 to replace ordinary laminectomy[74-77] was termed *expansive open-door laminoplasty*. This technique was devised to prevent post-laminectomy complications, including increased risk of the long-term postoperative malalignment syndromes. The operative procedure involves the midline approach and subperiosteal dissection of the laminae in question. Two bony gutters are made on the medial margins of the facets. This can be done with a high-speed drill. The medial side of the gutter is thinned enough to cut the wall of the ligamentum flavum between the laminae at both upper and lower ends of the laminoplasty. The medial wall is resected using a Kerrison rongeur. The bony gutter on the hinge side is made slightly more lateral to prevent instability in the laminar hinge. Stay sutures are then placed on the deep musculature and facet capsule on the hinge side. The laminae are spread and the stay sutures are tied around the bases of the spinous process to prevent the collapse of the laminae back down. The patient is kept in a brace for approximately 3 to 6 months postoperatively.

Indications for expansive open-door laminoplasty include the treatment of spinal canal stenosis, extensive OPLL, and spondylosis over four spinal segments. Hirabayashi and coworkers reported on 90 cases with a follow-up of 9.5 years maximum and 3 years on average. They used the Japanese Orthopaedic Association's scoring criteria, as described previously. In most of the 90 cases, the results from this procedure were good. There were no cases where the patient's clinical symptoms worsened; however, the investigators did find weakness of the muscles innervated by C5 and C6 on the open side. They found that the postoperative canal diameter increased 3 to 5 mm on average as compared with the preoperative films. Fujiwara et al.[60] examined 50 patients treated for CSM. They computed the compression ratio—which is equal to the sagittal diameter divided by the transverse diameter times 100—and found this to be the best predictor of recovery after surgery. They found that the compression ratio at the level of maximum compression did not correlate with the preoperative JOA score or with postoperative neurologic recovery. The transverse area at maximum compression did show a positive correlation with the postoperative JOA score and the recovery rate. Fujiwara et al. found that patients with a transverse area less than 30 mm^2 had a poor prognosis. They found that the ability to predict the postoperative JOA score depended on the postoperative transverse area at the maximum compression level followed by age at surgery and the preoperative JOA score. Herkowitz in 1988[72] surveyed 45 patients with a minimum 2-year follow-up who had undergone anterior fusion, cervical laminectomy, or cervical laminoplasty for management of multiple-level cervical radiculopathy due to cervical spondylosis. He found that the overall success rate for those using anterior fusion and decompression was 92 percent—66 percent for cervical laminectomy and 86 percent for cervical laminoplasty. When the success rate was evaluated for unilateral versus bilateral radiculopathy, anterior fusion provided the best results. Herkowitz found pseudarthrosis in 22 of the 58 levels, for a 37 percent rate of pseudarthrosis; however, this did not correlate with the presence or absence of a good result. This is shown by 92 percent of the patients undergoing anterior fusion having satisfactory results. Herkowitz's conclusions were that anterior cervical diskectomy and fusion is the procedure of choice for multiple-level spondylotic radiculopathy. The laminoplasty procedure is indicated in patients with developmental cervical canal stenosis, failed anterior fusion, or prior anterior neck surgery. Cervical laminectomy should be performed in those patients who have failed cervical laminoplasty or those with anterior bony ankylosis. Anterior decompression and fusion at one or more levels for cervical myelopathy and radiculopathy have been found to be safe and effective methods of treatment.[6,14,29,42,69,147,148,163,165] These procedures were especially effective for those patients who presented with ataxia, hyperreflexia, and varying degrees of weakness with an anterior or central cord syndrome. Such patients will have preoperative studies that include myelography and MRI showing that the majority of the pathology is anterior, causing cord compression. These patients do extremely well with anterior decompression and autogenous fusion (Fig. 73-6). The extent of the compression should be based on the preoperative studies. Typically speaking, if a two-level corpectomy is performed, an iliac bone graft can be used; however, with longer decompressions, Zdeblick and Bohlman recommend the use of autogenous fibular grafts.[179] There is a significant donor-site morbidity with use of autofibula. Some authors feel that allograft fibula might be indicated for the treatment of multiple-level cervical decompression in the face of CSM. Fernyhough et al. examined 126 consecutive multilevel diskectomy and vertebrectomy cases for spondylosis using autograft and allograft fibular struts for reconstruction. They found that the nonunion rate was markedly increased with an increasing number of motion segments included in the fusion.[20,29,35,63,128,133,165,171,176] They found that it takes approximately 24 months for the fibular strut graft to become incorporated and recommended supplemental posterior wiring of the spinous process to enhance the likelihood of fusion. In 1989, Zdeblick and Bohlman considered the problem of cervical kyphosis and myelopathy. They looked at 14 patients over 18 years who were treated with anterior decompression and arthrodesis. An average of 2.25 vertebral bodies were removed and a subsequent fusion over 3.25 levels on average was executed. Eight patients were treated with a fibular graft that spanned an average of 4.1 levels. Three grafts dislodged, but two of these patients had posterior instability that caused the graft dislodgement. With the technique of corpectomy and anterior decompression, 13 out of 14 patients had excellent return of neurofunction, with 9 patients having complete recovery of function.

Complications

This technically difficult surgical procedure can be fraught with complications related to the bone graft, soft tissues of the neck, or the neurologic system. Graft complications include graft collapse, graft extrusion, and pseudarthrosis.

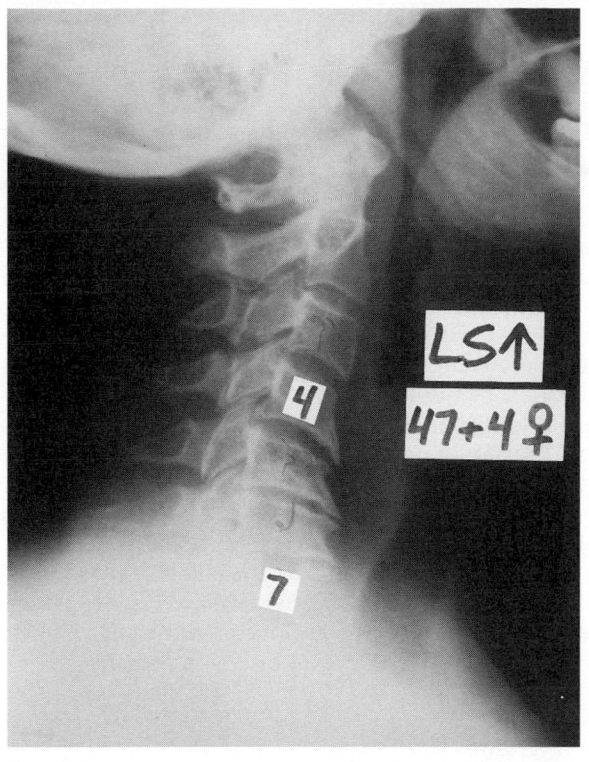

A

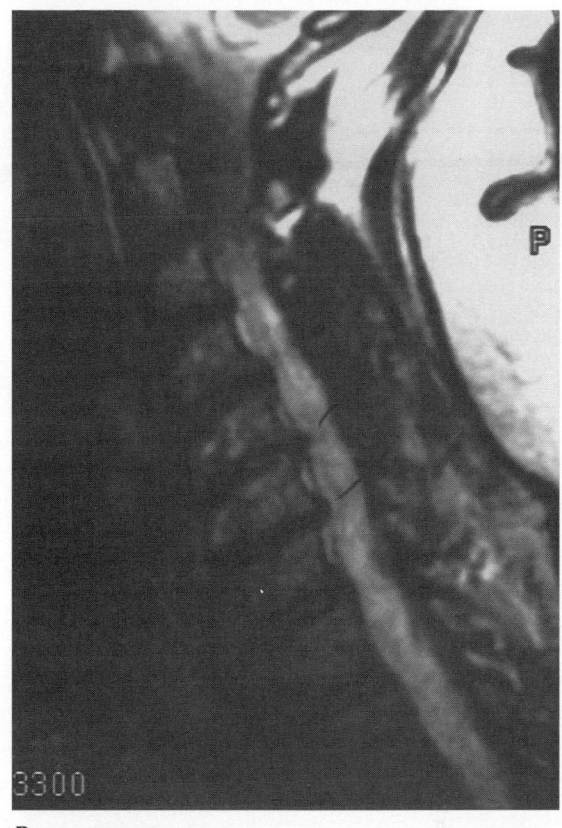

B

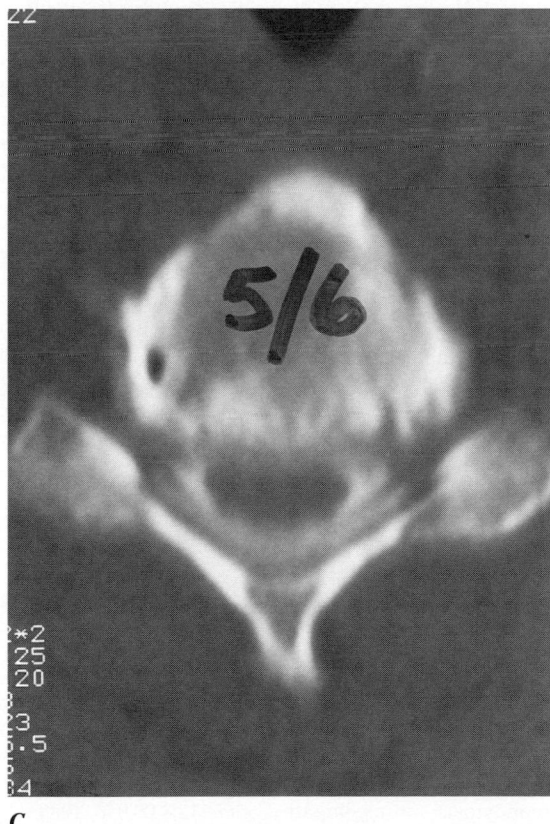

C

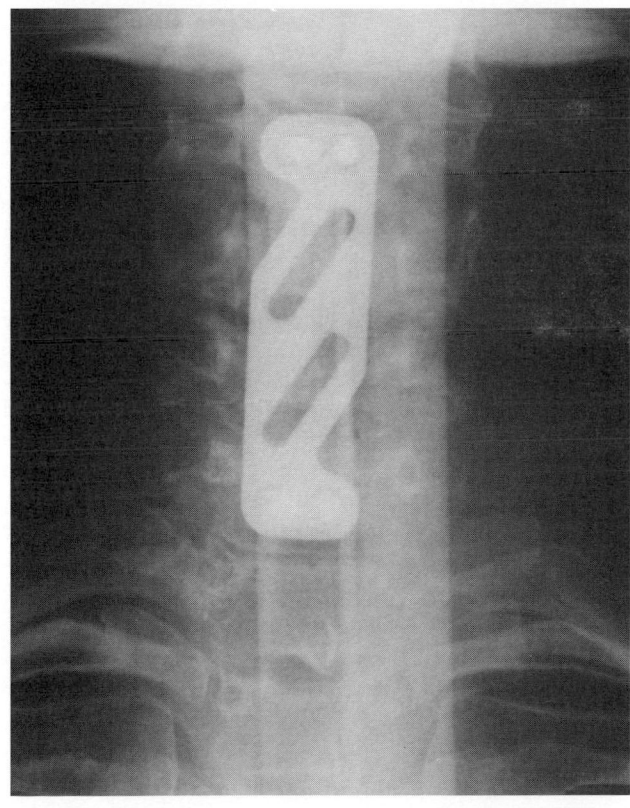

D

Figure 73-6 L.S., a 47-year-old female, presented with cervical spondylotic myelopathy. Her (*A*) lateral cervical spine radiograph demonstrates marked degenerative changes from C4 to C7. Her (*B*) lateral MRI scan shows cervical stenosis at C4-5, C5-6, and C6-7. Her postmyelographic axial CT scan (*C*) at C5-6 shows central and lateral recess stenosis. She underwent an anterior C5 and C6 cervical corpectomy, anterior spinal fusion from C4 to C7, autogenous iliac crest strut grafting, and an anterior cervical plate spanning C4 to C7 for stabilization. Her postoperative AP (*D*) and lateral (*E*) x-rays show her instrumentation and fusion. (*Courtesy of Lawrence G. Lenke, M.D.*)

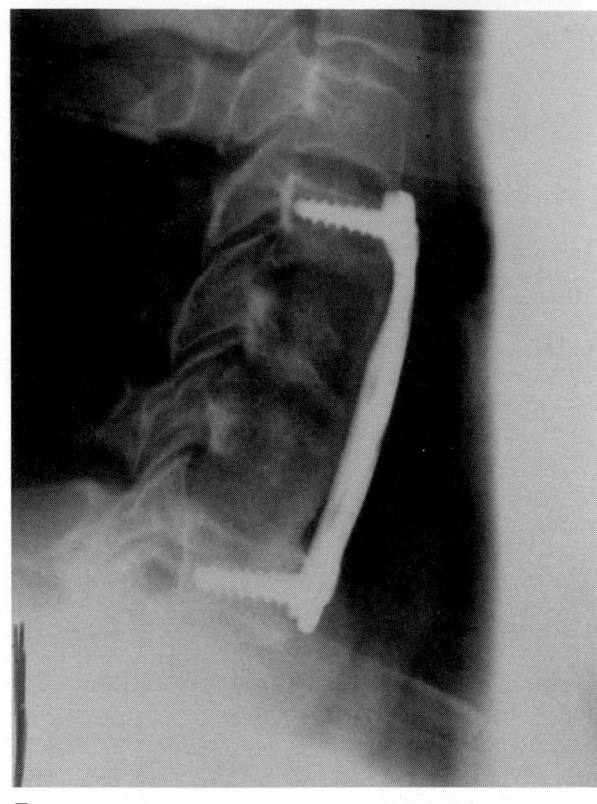

E

Figure 73-6 *(Continued)*

of OPPL causing anterior compression on the spinal cord, and it can present in isolation or over multiple segments.[51,86]

The treatment recommendations for OPLL include posterior decompression. However, some authors do advocate anterior decompression. The disease entity of OPLL has historically been treated with laminectomy or, more recently, laminoplasty. Use of anterior decompression can be fraught with potentially fatal complications.[96,151,163] These are centered around the absence of dura or the ossification of the PLL to the dura and the inability to remove the ligament without major disruption of dural tissue. The anterior decompression, however, is indicated for OPLL in the case where there is an associated kyphosis of the cervical spine. This is treated with the anterior floating method in which the disk and a portion of the vertebrae are removed to allow the ossified PLL to be pulled forward without actually being removed.[87,156] Those patients in whom kyphosis is associated with OPLL have not done well with only a posterior decompression.

The problem of graft extrusion is more common in the elderly osteoporotic patient. Once this occurs, revision surgery is indicated, because these grafts can lead to significant soft tissue damage in the anterior aspect of the neck. Those patients who are at higher risk for neurologic injury secondary to severe cord compression might be candidates for perioperative steroid administration. This is usually continued for approximately 24 h after surgery and tapered gradually. There is no scientific evidence supporting this conclusion; however, it does make sense empirically. It is not recommended to produce hypotension in these patients during their surgical procedure because the blood supply to the cord secondary to the compression is already tentative.

OSSIFICATION OF THE POSTERIOR LONGITUDINAL LIGAMENT

Ossification of the posterior longitudinal ligament (OPLL) has been well described in Asian patients.[76,96] There has been increased identification of this clinical entity through improved radiologic and histologic features in non-Asian patients.[96] It has been discovered that approximately half of patients with OPLL have diffuse idiopathic skeletal hyperostosis (Forestier's disease).[96,122] The best diagnostic test has been found to be the CT scan. The pathophysiology is that

REFERENCES

1. Afshani E, Girdani BR: Atlanto-axial dislocation in chondrodysplasia punctate. *Radiology* 102:399, 1972.
2. Alker G: Neuroradiology of cervical spondylotic myelopathy. *Spine* 13:850–853, 1988.
3. Arnold JG, Jr: The clinical manifestations of spondylochondrosis (spondylosis) of the cervical spine. *Ann Surg* 141:872–889, 1955.
4. Bailey RW: Observations of cervical intervertebral disc lesions in fractures and dislocations. *J Bone Joint Surg* 45A:461, 1963. (A very good presentation of some of the logical and practical aspects of this topic.)
5. Bailey RW, Badgley CE: Stabilization of the cervical spine by anterior fusion. *J Bone Joint Surg* 42A:565–594, 1960.
6. Bernard TN Jr, Whitecloud TS III: Cervical spondylotic myelopathy and myeloradiculopathy: Anterior decompression and stabilization with autogenous fibula strut graft. *Clin Orthop* 221:149–160, 1987.
7. Bertalanffy H, Eggert H-R: Clinical long-term results of anterior discectomy without fusion for treatment of cervical radiculopathy and myelopathy: A follow-up of 164 cases. *Acta Neurochir* 90:127–135, 1988.
8. Bertalanffy H, Eggert H-R: Complications of anterior cervical discectomy without fusion in 450 consecutive patients. *Acta Neurochir* 99:41–50, 1989.
9. Blaw ME, Langer LO: Spinal cord compression in Morguio-Brailsford's disease. *J Pediatr* 74:593–600, 1969.
10. Bohlman HH: Cervical spondylosis and myelopathy. *AAOS Instr Course Lect* 44:81–97, 1995.
11. Bohlman H: Degenerative arthrosis of the lower cervical spine, in Evarts CM (ed): *Surgery of the Musculoskeletal System.* Vol 2. New York, Churchill Livingstone, 1983, pp 25–35.
12. Bohlman HH, Emery SE: The pathophysiology of cervical spondylosis and myelopathy. *Spine* 13:843–846, 1988.
13. Bohlman HH, Emery SE, Goodfellow DB, Jones PK: Robinson anterior cervical discectomy and arthrodesis for cervical radiculopathy: Long-term follow-up of one hundred and twenty-two patients. *J Bone Joint Surg* 75A:1298–1307, 1993.
14. Bopni M, Cherubino P, Denar V, et al: Multiple subtotal somatectomy: Technique and evaluation of a series of 39 cases. *Spine* 9:358–362, 1984.

15. Brackett CE: The posterior midline approach to a cervical disc. *J Neurosurg* 38:668–671, 1973.

16. Brain L, Wilkinson M (eds): *Cervical Spondylosis and Other Disorders of the Cervical Spine.* Philadelphia, Saunders, 1967.

17. Brieg A, Turnbull I, Hassler O: Effects of mechanical stresses on the spinal cord in cervical spondylosis. *Brain* 75:187–225, 1952.

18. Brieg A, Turnbull I, Hassler O: Effects of mechanical stresses on the spinal cord in cervical spondylosis: A study of fresh cadaver material. *J Neurosurg* 25:45–56, 1966.

19. British Association of Physical Medicine: Pain in the neck and arm: A multicentre trial of the effects of physiotherapy. *Br Med J* 1:253, 1966.

20. Brown MD, Malinin TI, Davis PB: A roentgenographic evaluation of frozen allografts versus autografts in anterior cervical spine fusion. *Clin Orthop* 119:231–236, 1976.

21. Brunton FJ, Wilkinson JA, Wise KSH, Simonis RB: Cineradiography in cervical spondylosis as a means of determining the level for anterior fusion. *J Bone Joint Surg* 44B:399–404, 1982.

22. Bulgar R, Rejowski J, Beatty R: Vocal cord paralysis associated with anterior cervical fusion: Considerations for prevention and treatment. *J Neurosurg* 62:657–661, 1985.

23. Bull JW, Nixon W, Pratt RC: The radiological criteria and familial occurrence of primary basilar impression. *Brain* 78:229–247, 1955.

24. Clark CR, Goel VK, Galles K, Liu YK: Kinematics of the occipito-katlanto-axial complex. *Trans Cerv Spine Res Soc* 1986.

25. Clark E, Robinson PK: Cervical myelopathy: A complication of cervical spondylosis. *Brain* 79:483, 1956.

26. Cloward RB: The anterior approach for ruptured cervical discs. *J Neurosurg* 15:602, 1958.

27. Cohen ME, Rosenthal AD, Matson DD: Neurological abnormalities in achondroplastic dwarfs. *J Pediatr* 71:367–376, 1967.

28. Collins HR: An evaluation of cervical and lumbar discography. *Clin Orthop* 107:133–138, 1975.

29. Connolly ES, Seymour RJ, Adams JE: Clinical evaluation of anterior cervical fusion for degenerative cervical disc disease. *J Neurosurg* 23:431–437, 1965.

30. Crandall PH, Gregorius FK: Long-term follow-up of surgical treatment of cervical spondylotic myelopathy. *Spine* 2:139–146, 1977.

31. Cruishank B: Pathology of ankylosing spondylosis. *Clin Orthop* 74:43–58, 1971.

32. Cusick JF: Monitoring of cervical spondylotic myelopathy. *Spine* 13:877–880, 1988.

33. DeAndrade JR, Macnab I: Anterior occipitocervical fusion in rheumatoid arthritis. *Arthritis Rheum* 12:423–426, 1969.

34. Denno JJ, Meadows GR: Early diagnosis of cervical spondylotic myelopathy: A useful clinical sign. *Spine* 16:1353–1355, 1991.

35. DePalma A, Rothman R, Lewinnek G, Canale ST: Anterior interbody fusion for severe cervical disc degeneration. *Surg Gynecol Obstet* 134:755–758, 1972.

36. Dillin W, Booth R, Cuckler J et al: Cervical radiculopathy: A review. *Spine* 11:988–991, 1986.

37. Doppman JL: The mechanism of ischemia in anteroposterior compression of the spinal cord. *Invest Radiol* 10:543–551, 1975.

38. Dunsker SB, Colley DP, Mayfield FH: Kinematics of the cervical spine. *Clin Neurosurg* 25:174–183, 1978.

39. Dvorak J, Panjabi MM: Functional anatomy of the alar ligaments. *Spine* 12:183, 1987. (Highly recommended to anyone with detailed interest in the normal and abnormal function of this region.)

40. Dvorak J, Panjabi MM, Gerber M: CT-functional diagnostics of the rotatory instability of the upper cervical spine: An experimental study in cadavers. *Spine* 12:197, 1987.

41. Edwards WC, LaRocca H: The developmental segmental sagittal diameter of the cervical spinal canal in patients with cervical spondylosis. *Spine* 8:20–27, 1983.

42. Emery SE, Bolesta MJ, Banks MA, Jones PK: Robinson anterior cervical fusion: Comparison of the standard and modified techniques. *Spine* 19:660–663, 1994.

43. Epstein BS, Epstein JA, Jones MD: Anatomicoradiological correlations in cervical spine discal disease and stenosis. *Clin Neurosurg* 25:148–173, 1978.

44. Epstein JA, Carras R, Hyman RA, Costa S: Cervical myelopathy caused by developmental stenosis of the spinal canal. *J Neurosurg* 51:362–367, 1979.

45. Epstein JA, Carras R, Lavine LS, Epstein BS: The importance of removing osteophytes as part of the surgical treatment of myeloradiculopathy in cervical spondylosis. *J Neurosurg* 30:219–226, 1969.

46. Epstein JA, Epstein BS, Lavine LS: Cervical spondylotic myelopathy: The syndrome of the narrowed canal teated by laminectomy, foraminotomy, and the removal of osteophytes. *Arch Neurol* 8:307–317, 1963.

47. Epstein JA, Epstein NE: The surgical management of cervical spinal stenosis, spondylosis, and myeloradiculopathy by means of the posterior approach, in The Cervical Spine Research Society Editorial Committee (Ed): *The Cervical Spine,* 2d ed. Philadelphia, Lippincott, 1989, pp 625–643.

48. Epstein JA, Janin Y, Carras R, Lavine LS: A comparative study of the treatment of cervical spondylotic myeloradiculopathy: Experience with 50 cases treated by means of extensive laminectomy, foraminotomy, and excision of osteophytes during the past 10 years. *Acta Neurochir (Wien)* 61:89–104, 1982.

49. Epstein JA, Davidoff IM: Chronic hypertrophic spondylosis of the cervical spine with compression of the spinal cord and nerve roots. *Surg Gynecol Obstet* 35:27–38, 1951.

50. Epstein JA, Lavine LS, Aaronson HA, Epstein BS: Cervical spondylotic radiculopathy: The syndrome of foraminal constriction treated by foraminotomy and the removal of osteophytes. *Clin Orthop* 41:113–122, 1965.

51. Epstein NE: Ossification of the posterior longitudinal ligament in evolution in 12 patients. *Spine* 19:673–681, 1994.

52. Epstein NE, Epstein JA, Carras R, et al: Coexisting cervical and lumbar spinal stenosis: Diagnosis and management. *Neurosurgery* 15:489–496, 1984.

53. Fager CA: Results of adequate posterior decompression in the relief of spondylotic cervical myelopathy. *J Neurosurg* 38:684–692, 1973.

54. Fager CA: Management of cervical disc lesions and spondylosis by posterior approaches. *Clin Neurosurg* 24:488–505, 1977.

55. Fager CA: Posterior surgical tactics for the neurological syndromes of cervical disc and spondylotic lesions. *Clin Neurosurg* 25:118–144, 1978.

56. Ferguson RJC, Caplan LR: Cervical spondylitis myelopathy. *Neurol Clin North Am* 3:373–382, 1985.

57. Fielding JW, Cochran GVB, Lansing JF, Hohl M: Tears of the transverse ligament of the atlas: A clinical biomechanical study. *J Bone Joint Surg* 56A:1683, 1974.

58. Flynn TB: Neurologic complications of anterior fusion. *Spine* 7:536–539, 1982.

59. Friedenberg ZB, Miller WT: Degenerative disc disease of the cervical spine: A comparative study of asymptomatic and symptomatic patients. *J Bone Joint Surg* 45A:6 1171-1178, 1963.

60. Fujiwara K, Yonenobu K, Ebara S, et al. The prognosis of surgery for cervical compression myelopathy. *J Bone Joint Surg* 71B:393–398, 1989.

61. Gibson MJ, Buckley J, Mawhinney R, et al: Magnetic resonance imaging and discography in the diagnosis of disc degeneration: A comparative study of 50 discs. *J Bone Joint Surg [Br]* 68:369–373, 1986.

62. Gooding MR, Wilson CB, Hoff JT: Experimental cervical myelopathy: Effects of ischemia and compression of the canine cervical spinal cord. *J Neurosurg* 43:9–17, 1975.

63. Gore D, Sepic S: Anterior cervical fusion for degenerated or protruded discs. *Spine* 9:667–671, 1984.

64. Greenfield J, Ilfeld FW: Acute cervical strain. *Clin Orthop* 122:196–200, 1977.

65. Gregorius FK, Estrin T, Crandall PH: Cervical spondylotic radiculopathy and myelopathy: A long-term follow-up study. *Arch Neurol* 33:618–625, 1976.

66. Grisoli F, Graziani N, Fabrizi AP, et al: Anterior discectomy without fusion for treatment of cervical lateral soft disc extrusion: A follow-up of 120 cases. *Neurosurgery* 24:853–859, 1989.

67. Guidetti B, Fortuna A: Long-term results of surgical treatment of myelopathy due to cervical spondylosis. *J Neurosurg* 30:714–721, 1969.

68. Gulati DR, Rout D: Atlantoaxial dislocation with quadriparesis in achondroplasia. *J Neurosurg* 40:394–396, 1974.

69. Hanai K, Fujiyoshi F, Kiamei K: Subtotal vertebrectomy and spinal fusion for cervical spondylotic myelopathy. *Spine* 11:310–315, 1986.

70. Harris W: Cervical traction: review of the literature and treatment guidelines. *Phys Ther* 57:8, 1977.

71. Henderson CM, Hennessey RG, Shuey HM, Shackelford EG: Posterior lateral foraminotomy as an exclusive operative technique for cervical radiculopathy: A review of 846 consecutively operated cases. *Neurosurgery* 15:504–512, 1983.

72. Herkowitz HN: A comparison of anterior cervical fusion, cervical laminectomy and cervical laminoplasty for the surgical management of multiple level spondylotic radiculopathy. *Spine* 13:774–780, 1988.

73. Herkowitz HN: The surgical management of cervical spondylotic radiculopathy and myelopathy. *Clin Orthop* 239:94–108, 1989.

74. Hirabayashi K: Expansive open-door laminoplasty for cervical spondylotic myelopathy. *Shujutsu* 32:1159–1163, 1978.

75. Hirabayashi K, Miyakawa J, Uzawa M: Canal-expansive laminoplasty as a new method of cervical posterior decompression. *Chubu Seisai-shi* 22:417–419, 1979.

76. Hirabayashi K, Miyakawa J, Satomi K, et al: Operative results and postoperative progression of ossification among patients with ossification cervical posterior longitudinal ligament. *Spine* 6:354–364, 1981.

77. Hirabayashi K, Wantanabe K, Wakano K, et al: Expansive open-door laminoplasty for cervical spinal stenotic myelopathy. *Spine* 8:693–699, 1983.

78. Hoff J, Nishimura M, Pitts L, et al: The role of ischemia in the pathogenesis of cervical spondylotic myelopathy: A review and new microangiographic evidence. *Spine* 2:100–108, 1977.

79. Hoff JT, Wilson CB: Microsurgical approach to the anterior cervical spine and spinal cord. *Clin Neurosurg* 26:513–528, 1979.

80. Holdsworth FW: Fractures, dislocations and fracture dislocations of the spine. *J Bone Joint Surg* 45B:6, 1963. (A classic article so frequently referred to that it could be considered required reading for anyone interested in the question of clinical stability of the spine.)

81. Holt EP: Fallacy of cervical discography: Report of 50 cases in normal subjects. *JAMA* 188:799–801, 1964.

82. Hukuda S, Wilson CB: Experimental cervical myelopathy: Effects of compression and ischemia on the canine cervical cord. *J Neurosurg* 37:631–652, 1972.

83. Hunt WE: Cervical spondylosis natural history and care indications for surgical decompression. *Clin Neurosurg* 27:466–480, 1980.

84. Ishida Y, Suzuki K, Ohmori K, et al: Critical analysis of extensive cervical laminectomy. *Neurosurgery* 24:215–222, 1989.

85. Jackson H: The diagnosis of minimal atlanto-axial subluxation. *Br J Radiol* 23:672, 1950.

86. Jamjoom A, Williams C, Cummins B: The treatment of spondylotic cervical myelopathy by multiple subtotal vertebrectomy and fusion. *Br J Neurosurg* 6:249–255, 1991.

87. Kamikozuru M: Significance of the anterior floating method for cervical myelopathy due to the ossification of the posterior longitudinal ligament. *Nippon Seikeigeka Gakkai Zasshi* 65:431–440, 1991.

88. Kikuchi S, Macnab I, Moreau P: Localisation of the level of symptomatic cervical disc degeneration. *J Bone Joint Surg [Br]* 63:272–277, 1981.

89. Klafta LA: The diagnostic inaccuracy of the pain response in cervical discography. *Cleve Clin Q* 36:35–39, 1969.

90. Kosary IZ, Braham J, Schaked I, Schaked R: Microsurgery in anterior approach to cervical discs. *Surg Neurol* 6:275–277, 1976.

91. LaRocca H: Cervical spondylotic myelopathy: Natural history. *Spine* 13:854–855, 1988.

92. Leblhuber F, Reisecker F, Boehm-Jurkovic H, et al: Diagnostic value of different electrophysiologic tests in cervical disk prolapse. *Neurology* 3:1879–1881, 1988.

93. Lees F, Turner JWA: Natural history and prognosis of cervical spondylosis. *Br Med J* 2:1607–1610, 1963.

94. Lunsford LD, Bissonette DJ, Jannetta PJ, et al: Anterior surgery for cervical disc diseases: Part 1. Treatment of lateral cervical disc herniation in 253 cases. *J Neurosurg* 53:1–10, 1980.

95. Lysell E: Motion in the cervical spine. *Acta Orthop Scand* 123 (suppl): 1969. (The most exhaustive and carefully done study of the kinematics of the lower cervical spine.)

96. McAfee PC, Regan JJ, Bohlman HH: Cervical cord compression from ossification of the posterior longitudinal ligament in non-Orientals. *J Bone Joint Surg* 69B:569–575, 1987.

97. Martel W: The occipito atlanto axial joints in rheumatoid arthritis and ankylosing spondylitis. *Am J Roentgenol* 86:223–240, 1961.

98. Martel W, Uyham R, Stimson CW: Subluxation of the atlas causing spinal cord compression in a case of Down's syndrome with a "manifestation of an occipital vertebra." *Radiology* 93:839–240, 1961.

99. Martins AN: Anterior cervical discectomy with and without interbody bone graft. *J Neurosurg* 44:290–295, 1976.

100. Mathews JA: Atlanto-axial subluxation in rheumatoid arthritis. *Ann Rheum Dis* 28:260–266, 1969.

101. Mayfield FH: Cervical spondylosis: Observations based on surgical treatment of 400 patients: Neurosurgical aspects of the spinal cord and column. *Postgrad Med* 38:345–357, 1965.

102. Michie RH, Clark M: Neurological syndrome associated with cervical and craniocervical anomalies. *Arch Neurol* 18:241–247, 1968.

103. Modic MT, Ross JS, Masaryk TJ: Imaging of degenerative disease of the cervical spine. *Clin Orthop* 239:109–120, 1989.

104. Modic MT, Weinstein MA, Pavlicek W: Magnetic resonance imaging of the cervical spine. *AJR* 141:1129–1136, 1983.

105. Munro D: Treatment of fractures and dislocations of the cervical spine complicated by cervical cord and root injuries: A comparative study of fusion vs nonfusion therapy. *N Engl J Med* 264:573, 1961.

106. Murphy F: Sources and patterns of pain in disc disease. *Clin Neurosurg* 15:343–351, 1968.

107. Murphy F, Simmons JCH, Brunson B: Surgical treatment of laterally ruptured cervical disc: Review of 648 cases, 1939–1972. *Clin Neurosurg* 20:9–16, 1972.

108. Nachemson A: Editorial comment: Lumbar discography—where are we today? *Spine* 14:555–557, 1989.

109. Nurick S: The pathogenesis of the spinal cord disorder associated with cervical spondylosis. *Brain* 95:87–100, 1972.

110. Panjabi M, Dvorak J, Duranceau J, et al: Three-dimensional movements of the upper cervical spine. *Spine* 13:726, 1988.

111. Panjabi M, White A III: Biomechanics of nonacute cervical spinal cord trauma. *Spine* 13:838–842, 1988.

112. Parfenchuck TA, Janssen ME: A correlation of cervical magnetic resonance imaging and discography/computed tomographic discograms. *Spine* 19:2819–2825, 1994.

113. Pavlov H, Torg JS, Robie B, Jahre C: Cervical spinal stenosis: Determination with vertebral body ratio method. *Radiology* 164:771, 1987. (This is an excellent and important article which contains comprehensive and useful review of the literature on normal and abnormal cervical spinal canal diameters.)

114. Penning L: *Function and Pathology of the Cervical Spine.* Baltimore, Williams & Wilkins, 1968.

115. Penning L: Normal movements of the cervical spine. *Am J Roentgenol* 130:317, 1979.

116. Penning L: Some aspects of plain radiography of the cervical spine in chronic myelopathy. *Neurology* 12:513–519, 1962.

117. Penning L, VaDer Zwaag P: Biomechanical aspects of spondylotic myelopathy. *Acta Radiol* 5:1090, 1966.

118. Perneczky A, Sunder-Plassman M: Intradural variant of cervical nerve root fibers potential cause of misinterpreting the segmental location of cervical disc prolapse from clinical evidence. *Acta Neurochir (Wien)* 62:79–83, 1980.

119. Perry S, Nickel VL: Total cervical spine fusion for neck paralysis. *J Bone Joint Surg* 41A:37–60, 1959.

120. Phillips DG: Surgical treatment of myelopathy with cervical spondylosis. *Neurol Neurosurg Psychiatry* 36:879–884, 1973.

121. Piepgras DG: Posterior decompression for myelopathy due to cervical spondylosis: Laminectomy alone versus laminectomy with dentate ligament section. *Clin Neurosurg* 24:509–515, 1977.

122. Pouchot J, Watts CS, Esdaile JM, et al: Sudden quadriplegia complicating ossification of the posterior longitudinal ligament and diffuse idiopathic skeletal hyperostosis. *Arthritis Rheum* 30:1069–1072, 1987.

123. Ramsey J, Bliznack J: Klippel-Feil syndrome with renal agenesis and other anomalies. *Am J Roentgenol* 113:460–463, 1971.

124. Raynor RB: Anterior or posterior approach to the cervical spine: An anatomical and radiographic evaluation and comparison. *Neurosurgery* 12:7–13, 1983.

125. Raynor RB, Pugh J, Shapiro I: Cervical facetectomy and its effect on spine strength. *J Neurosurg* 63:278–282, 1985.

126. Reid JD: Effects of flexion-extension movements of the head and spine upon the spinal cord and nerve roots. *J Neurol Neurosurg Psychiatry* 23:214–221, 1960.

127. Riley L: Anterior cervical spine surgery. *Instr Course Lect* 27:154–158, 1978.

128. Riley L, Robinson R, Johnson K, Walker A: The results of anterior interbody fusion of the cervical spine. *J Neurosurg* 30:127–133, 1969.

129. Robertson JT, Johnson SD: Anterior cervical discectomy without fusion: Long-term results. *Clin Neurosurg* 27:440–449, 1980.

130. Robinson RA, Afeiche N, Dunn EJ, et al: Cervical spondylotic myelopathy: Etiology and treatment concepts. *Spine* 2:89–99, 1977.

131. Robinson RA, Smith GW: Anterolateral cervical disc removal and interbody fusion for cervical disc syndrome. *Bull Johns Hopkins Hosp* 96:223–224, 1955.

132. Robinson RA, Smith GW: The treatment of certain spine disorders by anterior removal of the intervertebral disc and interbody fusion. *J Bone Joint Surg* 40A:607, 1958.

133. Robinson R, Walker A, Ferlic D, Wieckling DK: The results of anterior interbody fusion of the cervical spine. *J Bone Joint Surg* 44A:1569–1587, 1962.

134. Rosenorn J, Hansen EB, Rosenorn M-A: Anterior cervical discectomy with and without fusion: A prospective study. *J Neurosurg* 59:252–255, 1983.

135. Rosomoff HL, Rossman F: Treatment of cervical spondylosis by anterior cervical discectomy and fusion. *Arch Neurol* 14:392–398, 1966.

136. Roth DA: Cervical analgesic discography: A new test for the definitive diagnosis of the painful-disk syndrome. *JAMA* 235:1713–1714, 1976.

137. Rothman HL, Rossman F: The acute cervical disc. *Clin Orthop* 109:59–68, 1975.

138. Sarpyener MD: Congenital stricture of the spinal canal. *J Bone Joint Surg* 27:70–79, 1945.

139. Scoville WB: Cervical spondylosis treated by bilateral facetectomy and laminectomy. *J Neurosurg* 18:423–428, 1961.

140. Scoville WB, Whitcomb BB: Lateral rupture of cervical intervertebral disks. *Postgrad Med* 39:174–180, 1966. (Neurosurgical aspects of the spinal cord and column—chap 5).

141. Scoville WB, Dohrmann GH, Corkill G: Late results of cervical disc surgery. *J Neurosurg* 45:203–210, 1976.

142. Selecki BR: The effects of rotation of the atlas on the axis: Experimental work. *Med J Aust* 1:1012, 1969.

143. Shimomura Y, Hukuda S, Mizuno S: Experimental study of ischemic damage to the cervical spinal cord. *J Neurosurg* 28:565–581, 1968.

144. Shinomiya K, Komori H, Matsuoka T, et al: Neuroradiologic and electrophysiologic assessment of cervical spondylotic amyotrophy. *Spine* 19:21–25, 1994.

144a. Sim FH, Svien HJ, Bickel WH, James JM: Swan-neck deformity following extensive cervical laminectomy *J Bone Joint Surg* 36A:564–570, 1974.

145. Simeone FA: Surgical management of cervical radiculopathy: Posterior approach, in Rothman HL, Simeone FA (eds): *The Spine,* 3d ed. Philadelphia, Saunders, 1992.

146. Simmons EH: An evaluation of discography in the localization of symptomatic levels in discogenic diseases of the spine. *Clin Orthop* 108:57–59, 1975.

147. Simmons EH, Bhalla SK: Anterior cervical discectomy and fusion: A clinical and biomechanical study with eight-year follow-up. *J Bone Joint Surg [Br]* 51:226–237, 1969.

148. Smith GW, Robinson RA: The treatment of certain cervical-spine disorders by anterior removal of the intervertebral disc and interbody fusion. *J Bone Joint Surg* 40A:607–624, 1958.

149. Smith GW, Robinson RA: Anterior lateral cervical disc removal and interbody fusion for cervical disc syndrome. *Bull Johns Hopkins Hosp* 96:223–224, 1955.

150. Smith GW, Robinson RA: The treatment of cervical spine disorders by anterior removal of the intervertebral discs and interbody fusion. *J Neurosurg* 46:223–238, 1977.

151. Smith MD, Bolesta MH, Leventhal M, et al. Postsurgical cerebrospinal-fluid fistula associated with erosion of the dura: Findings after anterior resection of ossification of the posterior longitudinal ligament in the cervical spine. *J Bone Joint Surg* 74A:270–277, 1992.

152. Synder GM, Bernhardt M: Anterior cervical fractional interspace decompression for treatment of cervical radiculopathy: A review of the first 66 cases. *Clin Orthop* 246:92–99, 1989.

153. Spillane JD: Three cases of achondroplasia with neurological complications. *J Neurol Neurosurg Psychiatry* 15:246–252, 1952.

154. Suh TH, Alexander L: Vascular system of the human spinal cord. *Arch Neurol Psychiatry* 41:659–677, 1939.

155. Symon L, Lavender P: The surgical treatment of cervical spondylotic myelopathy. *Neurology* 17:117–127, 1967.

156. Tsuyama N: Ossification of the posterior longitudinal ligament of the spine. *Clin Orthop* 184:71–84, 1984.

157. Turnbull IM: Microvasculature of the human spinal cord. *J Neurosurg* 35:141–147, 1971.

158. Verbiest H: The management of cervical spondylosis. *Clin Neurosurg* 20:262–294, 1972.

159. Verbiest H: The lateral approach to the cervical spine. *Clin Neurosurg* 20:295–305, 1972.

160. Watters WC III, Levinthal R: Anterior cervical discectomy with and without fusion: Results, complications, and long-term follow-up. *Spine* 19:2343–2347, 1994.

161. Werne S: Studies in spontaneous atlas dislocation. *Acta Orthop Scand* 23(suppl):1957. (One of the most complete and thorough presentations of the biomechanical and clinical aspects of C1-C2.)

162. White AA, Johnson RM, Panjabi MM, Southwick WO: Biomechanical analysis of clinical stability in the cervical spine. *Clin Orthop* 109:85, 1975.

163. White AA, Panjabi MM: Biomechanical considerations in the surgical management of cervical spondylotic myelopathy. *Spine* 13:856–860, 1988.

164. White AA, Panjabi MM: *Clinical Biomechanics of the Spine,* 2d ed. Philadelphia, Lippincott, 1990.

165. White AA, Southwick WO, DePonte RJ, et al. Relief of pain by anterior cervical spine fusion for spondylosis: A report of 65 patients. *J Bone Joint Surg* 55A:525, 1973.

166. Whitecloud RS, Seago RA: Cervical discogenic syndrome. Results of operative intervention in patients with positive discography. *Spine* 12:313–316, 1987.

167. Whitecloud T: Complications of anterior cervical fusion. *Instr Course Lect* 27:222–227, 1978.

168. Whitecloud T: Management of radiculopathy and myelopathy by the anterior approach, in Cervical Spine Research Society (eds): *The Cervical Spine.* Philadelphia, Lippincott, 1983, pp 441–424.

169. Whitecloud T III, LaRocca H: Fibular strut graft in reconstructive surgery of the cervical spine. *Spine* 1:33–43, 1976.

170. Williams RW: Microcervical foraminotomy: A surgical alternative for intractable radicular pain. *Spine* 8:708–716, 1983.

171. Williams J, Allen M, Harkess J: Late results of cervical discectomy and interbody fusion: Some factors influencing the results. *J Bone Joint Surg* 50A:277–286, 1968.

172. Wolf BS, Khilnani M, Malis LI: The sagittal diameter of the bony cervical spinal canal and its significance in cervical spondylosis. *J Mount Sinai Hosp* 23:283–292, 1956.

173. Worth DR: Cervical spine kinematics (thesis). School of Medicine, Flinders University of South Australia, 1985. (A comprehensive review of methodologies for the study of cervical spine kinematics.)

174. Yamamoto I, Ikeda A, Shibuya N, et al: Clinical long-term results of anterior discectomy without interbody fusion for cervical disc disease. *Spine* 16:272–279, 1991.

175. Yiannikas C, Shahani BT, Young RR: Short-latency somatosensory-evoked potentials from radial, median, ulnar, and peroneal nerve stimulation in the assessment of cervical spondylosis: Comparison with conventional electromyography. *Arch Neurol* 43:1264–1271, 1986.

176. Yonenobu K, Fuji T, Ono K, et al: Choice of surgical treatment for multisegmental cervical spondylotic myelopathy. *Spine* 10:710–716, 1985.

177. Yu TL, Jones SJ: Somatosensory evoked potentials in cervical spondylosis: Correlation of median, ulnar and posterior tibial nerve responses with clinical and radiological findings. *Brain* 108(pt 2):273–300, 1985.

178. Zhongda L: A study of the effect of manipulative treatment on 158 cases of cervical syndrome. *J Trad Chin Med* 7:205–208, 1987.

179. Zdeblick TA, Bohlman HH: Cervical kyphosis and myelopathy: Treatment by anterior corpectomy and strut-grafting. *J Bone Joint Surg* 71A:170–182, 1989.

CHAPTER 74

Spinal and Pelvic Manifestations of Rheumatoid Arthritis and the Spondyloarthropathies

Christopher L. Hamill

ANKYLOSING SPONDYLITIS

Ankylosing spondylitis was previously described as rheumatoid spondylitis but recently has become a disease entity in its own right. Ankylosing spondylitis is more common in males, with a predilection to affect the spine and major joints, whereas rheumatoid arthritis is more common in females and affects the major and small joints more commonly than the spine. The incidence of ankylosing spondylitis varies from 2 to 3 per thousand.[1] The first change that occurs in the skeleton of a patient with ankylosing spondylitis is in the sacroiliac joints. These changes usually occur on the iliac side, with patchy periarticular osteopenia. This is followed by loss of definition with superficial erosions and then subchondral sclerosis with an apparent widening of the joint.[2] Areas of increased density are noted, with eventual bridging of the joint and loss of the joint space. The next skeletal change that occurs in the spine usually appears at the thoracolumbar and lumbosacral areas. This is followed by midlumbar upper thoracic and cervical vertebral body changes. However, the rapidity, order, and extent of the involved changes are variable.[3] The earliest changes in the spine include osseous erosion of the anterior corners of the vertebral bodies, which leads to a squaring of the anterior aspects of the vertebral bodies (Fig. 74-1). A subsequent reparative process leads to prominence of the vertebral body corners and a relatively osteopenic midsection. Reconstitution of the anterior concavity of the body is a sign of a fully evolved disease process (Fig. 74-2). The spine progresses on to lose its normal lumbar lordosis in early disease evolution. The annulus and the adjacent anterior longitudinal ligament ossify, which produces vertically oriented marginal syndesmophytes that are classic for the inflammatory seronegative spondyloarthropathies.[4] These are different from the horizontally oriented osteophytes, commonly known as *traction spurs,* seen in degenerative disk disease (Fig. 74-3). The end-stage symmetrical syndesmophyte formation leads to the pathognomonic "bamboo spine" of ankylosing spondylitis. Ossification of the spine, loss of cervical and lumbar lordosis, and increasing thoracic kyphosis may result in a severe kyphotic deformity of the spine. A clinical awareness of this disease entity can help prevent the severe, disabling deformity that these patients can develop. Physicians should be alert to the insidious onset of low back pain in young male patients that is worse in the morning and better as the day progresses. On physical examination, these patients will show decreased lengthening of the spine on forward bending, decreased lateral bending, and decreased chest expansion with possibly sacroiliac or costochondral tenderness. The early radiographic changes, as stated, occur at the sacroiliac joints and then progress to the axial skeleton to squaring of the lumbar vertebrae, as discussed previously. Laboratory tests including an HLA-B27 antigen test and a bone scan showing increased uptake at the sacroiliac joint are imperative to complete the diagnosis.

The common pathologies of the cervical spine in patients with ankylosing spondylitis, from most prevalent to least prevalent, are (1) atlantoaxial subluxation, (2) subaxial fracture deformity with instability, (3) occipitoatlantal destruction with painful deformity, and (4) fixed kyphotic deformity due to loss of normal cervical lordosis and normal cervicothoracic extension angle.[5] The development of clinical instability at the atlantoaxial joint is a multifactorial process. Patients with a solid cervical spine might have increased stress at the C1-C2 area. The inflammatory component of the disease entity also might lead to loss of transverse and alar ligament integrity. This then may lead to atlantoaxial subluxation and neurologic compromise secondary to cord compression. These patients can also go on to autostabilize in a subluxed position. It is recommended that all patients undergoing general anesthesia with the diagnosis of ankylosing spondylitis have preoperative flexion-extension radiographs taken. If there is gross instability, especially when associated with spinal cord compression, operative stabilization is required. There are many different techniques to obtain the stabilization.

KYPHOTIC DEFORMITY OF THE CERVICAL SPINE

Those patients who present with a severe kyphotic deformity occurring primarily in the cervical spine are plagued by this severely disabling condition. They might have severely marked restriction in their field of vision, interference with skin care, and eventual difficulty with everyday activities such as opening the mouth (from a chin-on-chest deformity). Once the disease has progressed to a chin-on-chest deformity, there are not many useful conservative measures in the treatment of these patients. The indications for surgical correction depend largely on the extent of the deformity, the age and condition of the patient, the feasibility of correction, and the willingness of the patient to accept the risk of surgical correction.[5] Once surgical intervention has been decided upon, it is important to assess the actual site of deformity in the patient. It is important to remember that these patients commonly have ankylosis of their hip joints and their lumbar, thoracic, and cervical spines. The angle from chin-brow to vertical is the

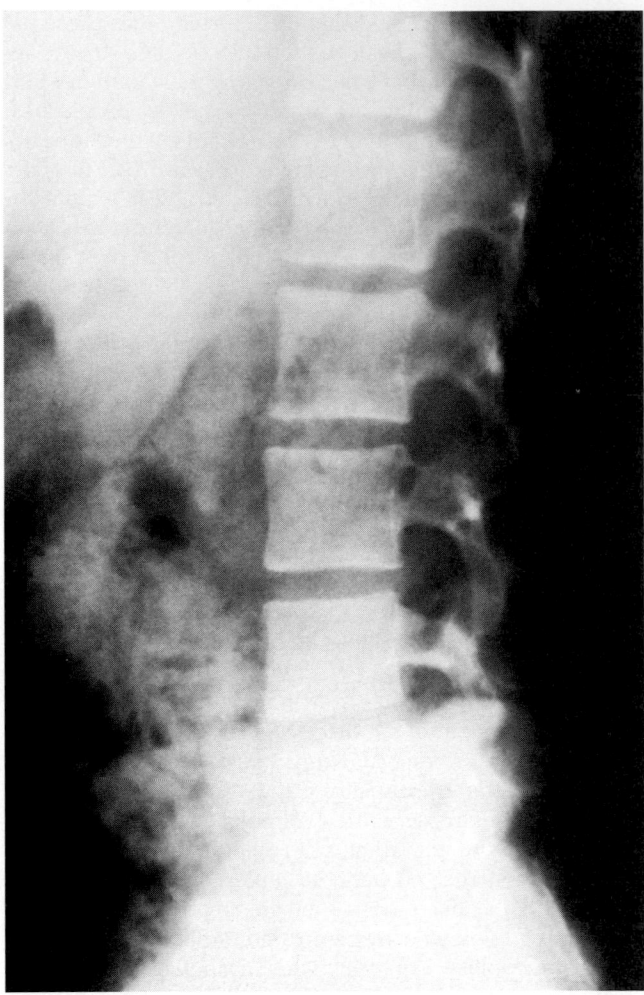

Figure 74-1 A lateral radiograph of the lumbar spine with early changes of ankylosing spondylitis. Note the squaring off of the anterior aspects of the lumbar vertebrae.

most reliable measure of trunk deformity. This is measured between the line from the brow to the chin to the vertical when the patient stands with hips and knees extended (Fig. 74-4). Two types of patients will present with a significant kyphotic deformity of the cervical spine: (1) patients with long-standing disease or (2) those with acute onset of flexion deformity. Those patients with ankylosing spondylitis who have increasing flexion deformity and pain should be presumed to have a fracture until proven otherwise. The fractures that occur in these patients are of a shear pattern that usually occurs at the base of the neck.[6] These patients will give a history of gradual loss of position of their head throughout the day, with return to normal alignment after an evening of rest. Visualization of C6-T2 is extremely difficult in these patients because of the severe osteopenia. Therefore, lateral computed tomography (CT) or sagittal reconstruction of CT scans is important to visualize this area of injury. Those patients with an acute injury do not need a cervical osteotomy but do need cranial halo traction along the line of the current neck position with a slow correction into the preinjury status. These patients are then placed into a well-molded halo

cast for approximately 12 months. It should be noted that this is a gradual process and care must be taken to avoid causing a neurologic deficit with an overly hasty correction of the cervical spinal deformity.

Patients who have a fixed painless kyphotic deformity of the cervical spine may require a resection-extension osteotomy for correction of the deformity. The level between the C7 and T1 vertebrae is selected for correction. Mason et al. and Urist[7,8] have pointed out the certain benefits of performing an osteotomy at this level. They found that the canal is relatively wide at this level of the cervical cord and that the eighth cervical nerve root has reasonable flexibility. It is the least important of any of the cervical nerve roots. Also, at this level the vertebral artery and veins usually pass in front of the transverse process of the seventh cervical nerve root. They enter the transverse foramen at the sixth cervical vertebra. This anatomic position of the vertebral artery places it at less risk for injury during the extension osteotomy. The closing based wedge osteotomy is performed under local anesthetic with the patient in the sitting position. The exact details of the osteotomy extend beyond the scope of this chapter. Generally, the patient is fitted preoperatively with a well-molded halo cast. In the sitting position under local anesthetic, the spine is dissected subperiosteally, allowing identification of the C7 lamina, which is then removed entirely along with the spinous process and lower lamina of C6 as well as the upper portion, spinous process, and lamina of T1. The remaining arches of C6 and T1 are undercut to avoid impingement following correction. The pedicles of C7 and T1 are noted and the eighth nerve root is identified. The amount of bone to be removed is indicated by the amount of correction required. This is determined by the preoperative angle from chin-brow to vertical. It is important to remove the inferior margins of the base of the pedicles at C7 and T1 to avoid impingement on the eighth cervical nerve root when the extension osteotomy is performed. When the decompression has been adequately performed, the patient is given a small dose of a short-acting general anesthetic, and when this has taken its full effect, the closed osteoclasis is performed. This may be followed by an audible crack. The patient is then awakened and asked to move all his or her extremities. Once this has been done, the bone removed from the decompression is used for fusion. Sutures placed in the fascia before the osteotomy was performed are then closed. The subcutaneous layers are closed in the standard fashion and the skin is closed with a subcuticular stitch. The patient is then reattached to the halo cast and walked to the hospital bed. Results from this type of surgery can be extremely gratifying for the patient as well as the surgeon (Fig. 74-5).

LUMBAR OSTEOTOMY

The second most common spot for corrective osteotomy is the lumbar spine. This osteotomy can be performed at one of multiple levels. In order to prevent potential neurologic complications of this procedure in the upper lum-

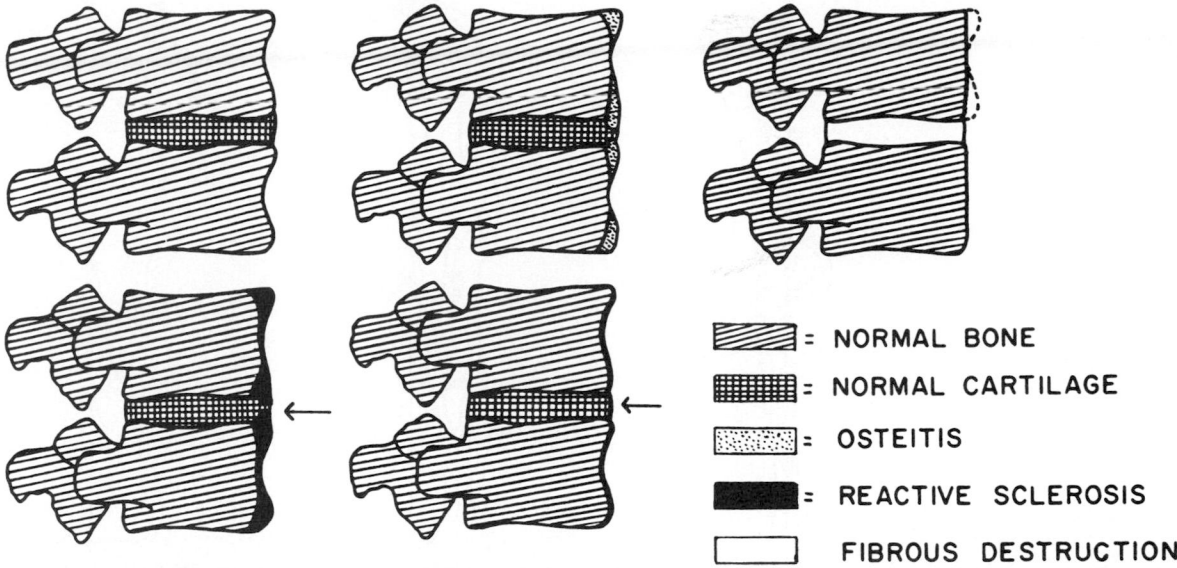

= NORMAL BONE

= NORMAL CARTILAGE

= OSTEITIS

= REACTIVE SCLEROSIS

= FIBROUS DESTRUCTION

Figure 74-2 Schematic representation of stages in the developing pathology of ankylosing spondylitis of the lumbar vertebrae as seen radiologically. *Upper left*: Normal. *Upper center*: Osteitis (x-ray osteopenia). *Upper right*: Osteoclastic destruction of bone (x-ray will show bone destruction and squaring of vertebra). *Lower left*: Reossification. X-ray will show restoration of normal contour of vertebra, sclerosis, and syndesmophyte formation (*arrow*). *Lower right*: Partial resorption of new bone. X-ray will show minimal sclerosis and syndesmophyte (*arrow*). (Reproduced with permission from Smuckler N: Arthritis of the spine, in Rothman R, Simeone FA (eds): *The Spine,* 2d ed. Vol II. Philadelphia, Saunders, 1982.)

bar spine, the level of the conus must be determined. Other types of injuries include aortic disruption and superior mesenteric artery syndrome. The Smith-Peterson technique entails osteoclasis following removal of a posterior wedge. The technique described by Thomassen involves removal of a wedge of bone from the posterior aspect of the fused vertebral bodies and intervening disk space[9] (Fig. 74-6). Postsurgically, these patients usually remain in a brace or some form of protection for approximately 1 year. Most recently a technique described by Thiranont and Netrawichien described a transpedicular decancellation closing wedge vertebral osteotomy. These authors reported on a technique involving six patients, with an average of 36° correction for each osteotomy performed. They had no neurologic injury. Their technique involves a standard approach to the posterior aspect of the spine. The osteotomy site is L2. They remove the entire posterior elements and the pedicles bilaterally of L2; a decancellation of the body of L2 is then performed.[10] Their correction is gradually obtained by elevating the two ends of the operating table that were previously flexed. They use 18-gauge sublaminar wires and Luque shaped rods for their fixation. This procedure to shorten the posterior column theoretically will decrease the risk for vascular injury, superior mesenteric artery syndrome, and paraplegia.

THE DIFFERENTIAL DIAGNOSIS

The differential diagnosis for ankylosing spondylitis includes sacroiliitis associated with osteitis condensans ilii. This disease most commonly occurs in pregnant females.

(Text continues on page 1379)

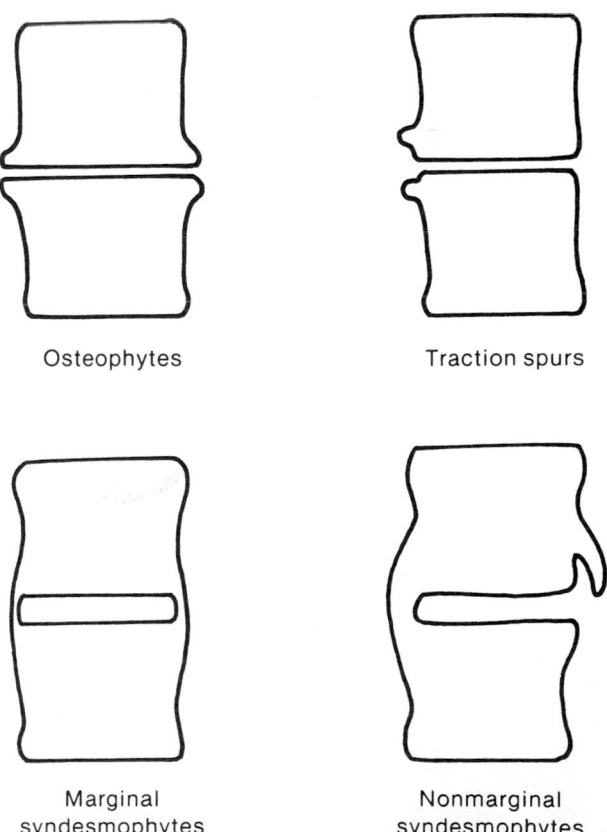

Osteophytes

Traction spurs

Marginal syndesmophytes

Nonmarginal syndesmophytes

Figure 74-3 Osteophytes and syndesmophytes, representative of diskogenic and inflammatory spondylitis. (Reproduced with permission from Booth RE Jr: Pathogenesis of signs and symptoms in spinal disorders. *Instr Course Lect* 34: 1985.)

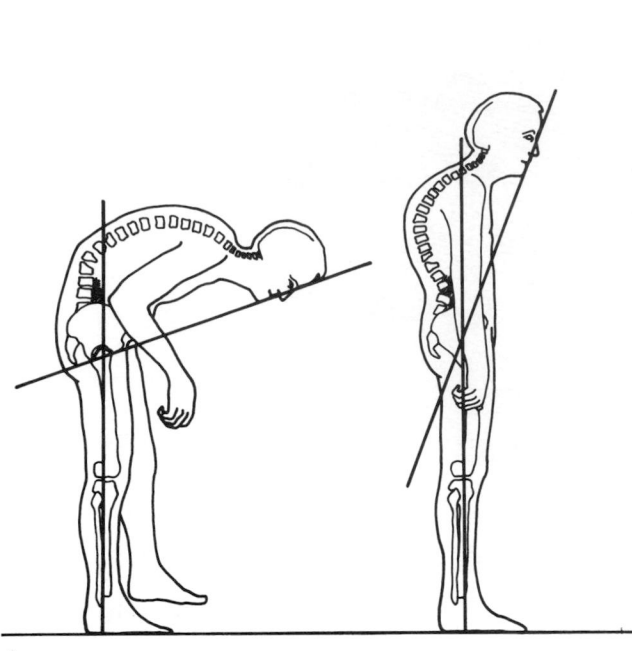

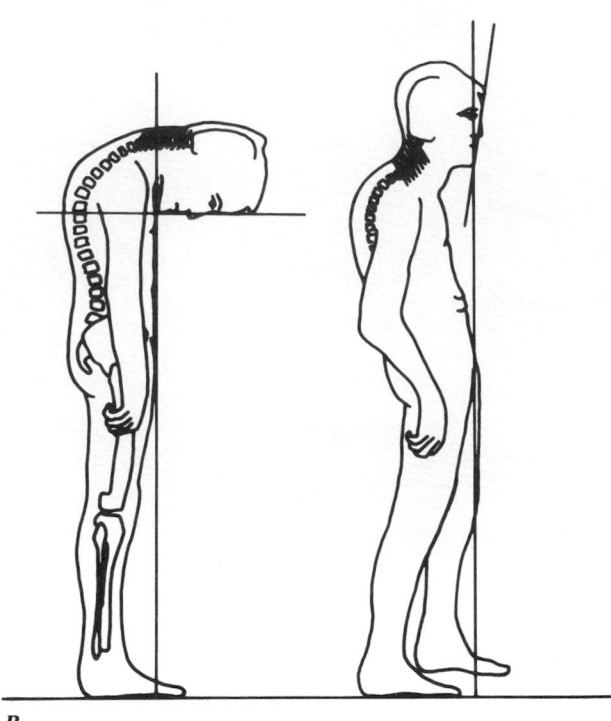

A

B

Figure 74-4 Technique for measuring the degree of kyphotic or flexion deformity of the spine in ankylosing spondylitis. The angle formed by a line from the brow to the chin to the vertical is measured with the patient standing with the hips and knees extended and the neck in either its fixed or neutral position. *A.* Chin-brow to vertical angle measuring thoracolumbar deformity. *B.* Chin-brow to vertical angle measuring cervical deformity. (Reproduced with permission from Simmons EH: Ankylosing spondylitis: Surgical considerations, in Rothman R, Simeone FA (eds): *The Spine,* 3d ed. Philadelphia, Saunders, 1992, pp. 1447–1511.)

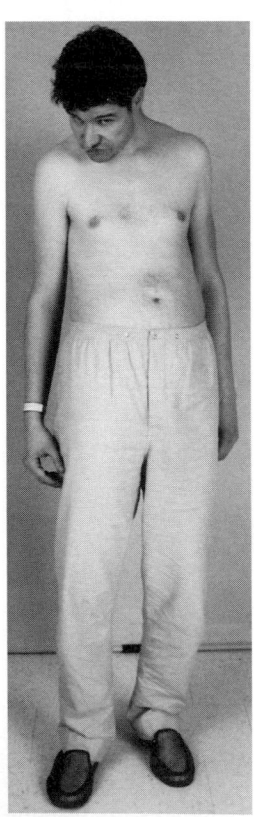

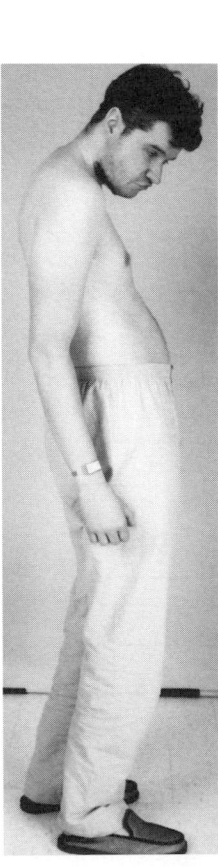

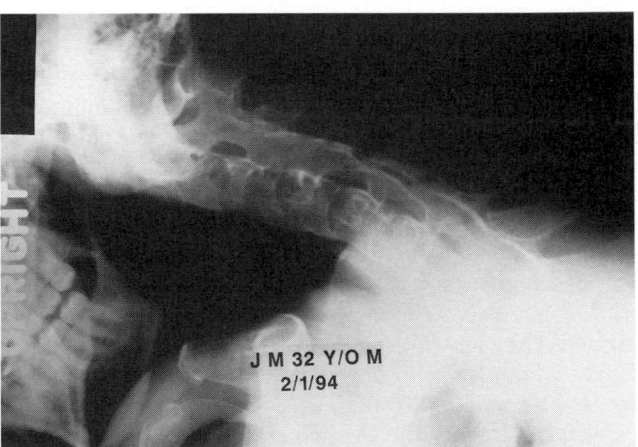

A

B

C

Figure 74-5 J.M. is a 32-year old male with ankylosing spondylitis who presented with this markedly rotated chin-on-chest deformity as seen on his clinical (*A*) frontal and (*B*) lateral photos. His (*C*) lateral cervical spine film demonstrates his autofused cervical spine with a marked cervical thoracic flexion deformity. His planning x-ray (*D*) demonstrates the amount of bone required to be removed posteriorly, beginning at the base of the posterior disk at C7-T1. He underwent a posterior closing wedge osteotomy with postoperative halo vest placement and a posterior autogenous fusion from C6-T1. His 2-year postoperative (*E*) frontal and (*F*) lateral x-rays demonstrate his solid fusion in the extended position. His postoperative clinical photos demonstrate his improved head and neck posture in (*G*) frontal and (*H*) lateral views.

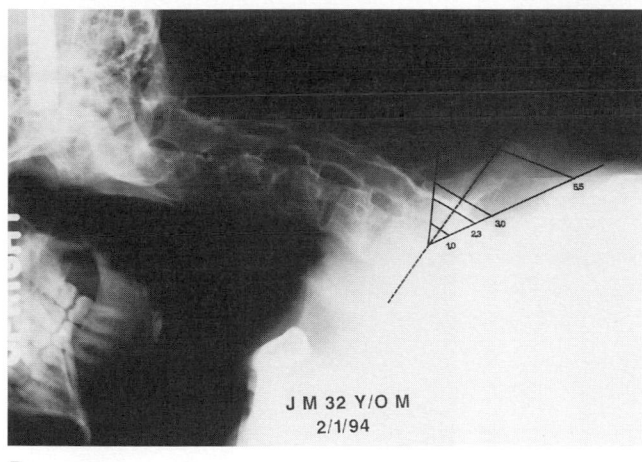

D

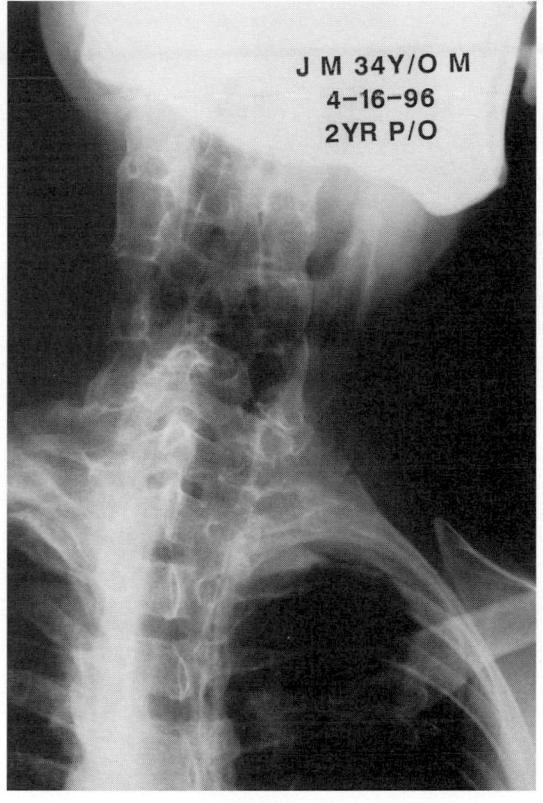

E

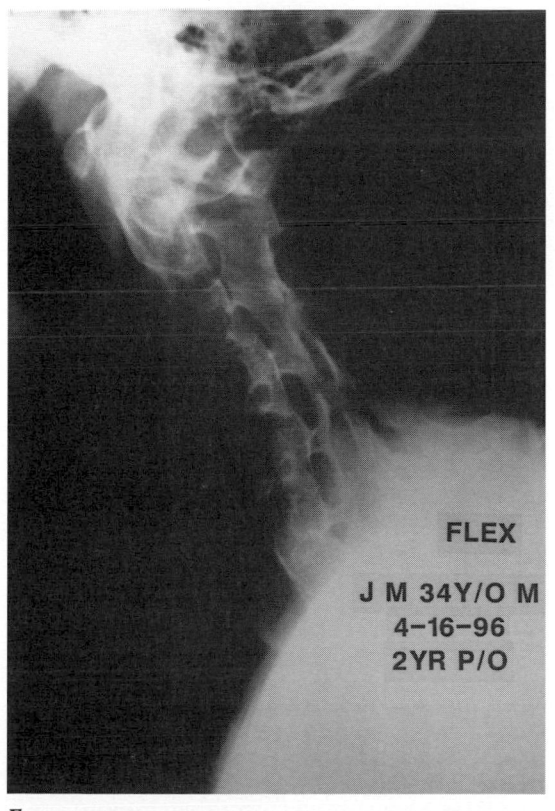

F

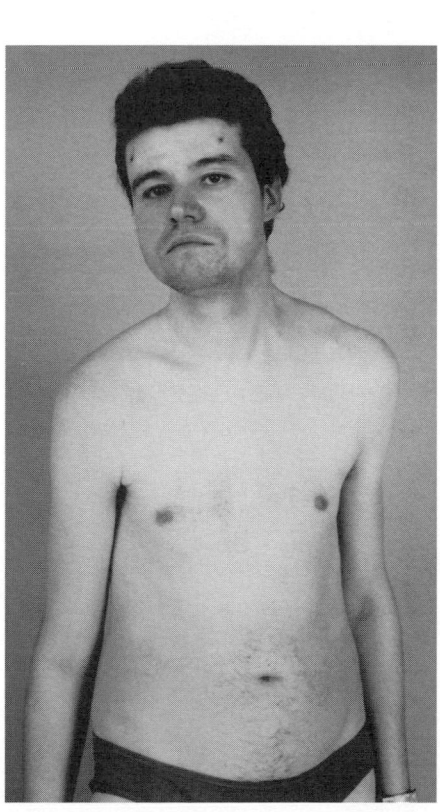

G

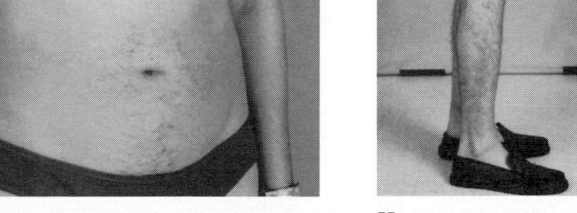

H

Figure 74-5 *(Continued)*

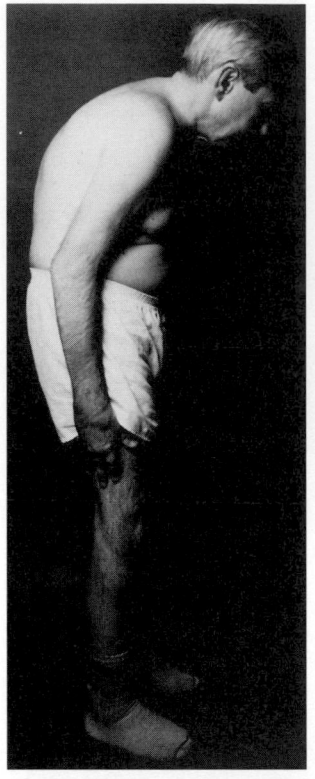

A

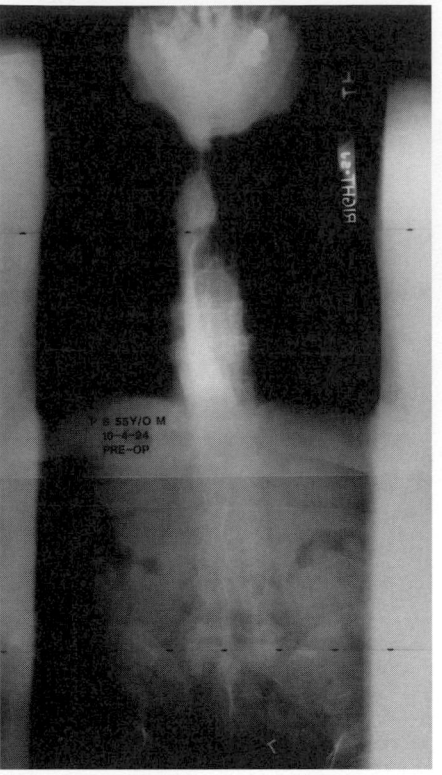

B

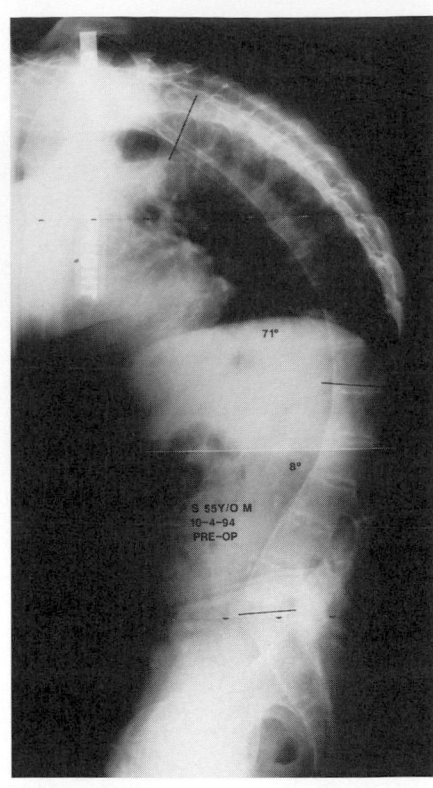

C

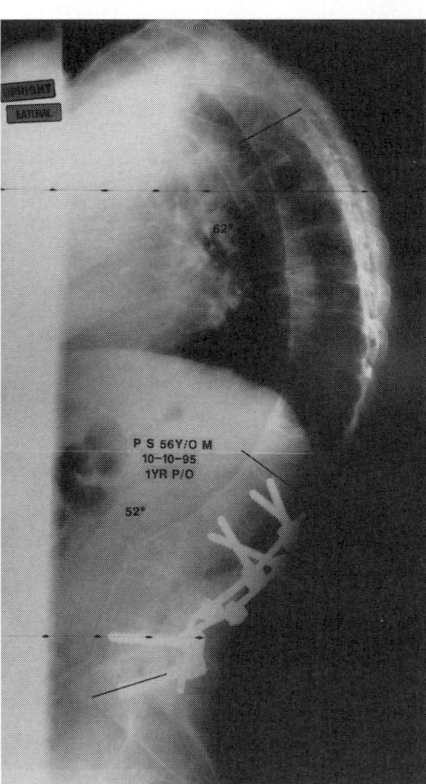

D

E

Figure 74-6 T.S. is a 55-year old male with ankylosing spondylitis who presented with this marked forward flexion posture as seen on his (*A*) lateral preoperative photo. His (*B*) coronal and (*C*) lateral radiographs of the entire spine demonstrate his autofused spine in a position of marked thoracic and lumbar kyphosis. His lateral lumbar planning radiograph (*D*) demonstrates the posterior osteotomy bone removal for correction of his deformity through the L3-L4 disk. He underwent a corrective osteotomy of the lumbar spine centered at L3-L4. His 1-year postoperative (*E*) coronal and (*F*) lateral radiographs demonstrate his healed extension osteotomy. His (*G*) postoperative clinical photo demonstrates his improved posture and forward site of view.

Figure 74-6 *(Continued)*

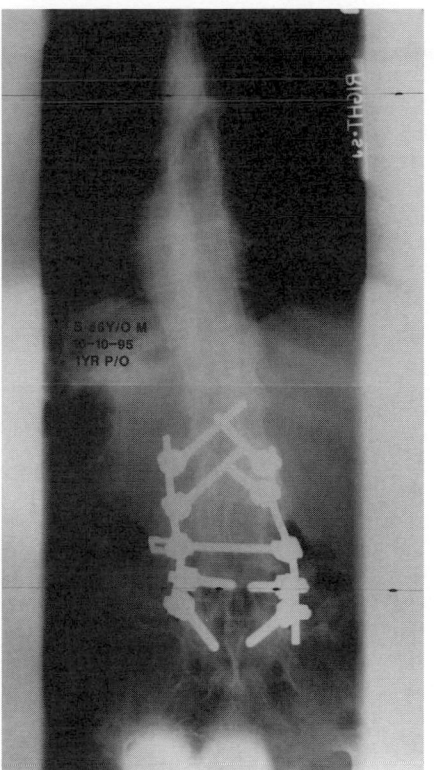

F

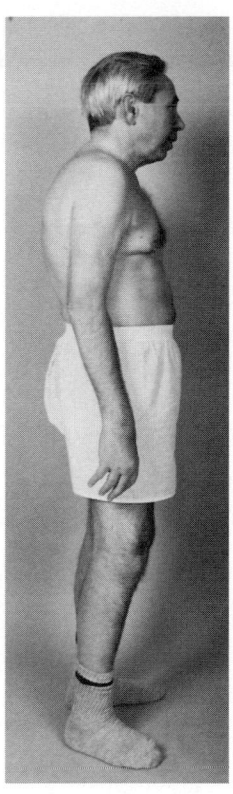

G

The radiographic picture involves sclerotic changes in the medial portion of the ilium next to the sacroiliac joint. The triangle-shaped sclerotic area may be either unilateral or bilateral. The laboratory test of HLA-B27 antigen is negative. This helps the differential. Fibrodysplasia ossificans progressiva, a rare hereditary disorder, can lead to fusion of both the sacroiliac joint and the spine. These patients are also plagued by a diffuse heterotrophic bone formation that differentiates it from ankylosing spondylitis. Juvenile rheumatoid arthritis must also be differentiated from ankylosing spondylitis. Patients with juvenile rheumatoid arthritis are less than 6 years of age, with diffuse pain, usually in the upper spine. Ankylosing spondylitis is in the sacroiliac or lumbar regions. Juvenile rheumatoid arthritis is not associated with an increased incidence of HLA-B27.

lantoaxial, atlantodental, and neurocentral joints.[11] The upper cervical spine is the most frequently involved with atlantoaxial subluxation, this being the most common manifestation of rheumatoid arthritis of the cervical spine. The second most commonly involved areas are the occipitoatlantal and atlantoaxial joints, with resultant cranial settling. The third type of involvement is subaxial subluxation. These involvements are not mutually exclusive and all three processes can occur simultaneously in a given patient. Ranawat[12a] has developed a very useful classification for the evaluation of patients with rheumatoid arthritis (Table 74-1). Class I is normal. Patients with subjective weakness and hyperreflexia and paraesthesias belong to class II. The presence of objective weakness with long tract signs is categorized as class III. Class III is further subdivided into IIIA

RHEUMATOID SPONDYLITIS

The synovium-lined articulations of the cervical spine are frequently involved in the disease process of rheumatoid arthritis. In fact, the majority of rheumatoid patients have cervical spinal involvement.[11,12] This may be difficult to differentiate from generalized rheumatoid arthritis, especially in the patients with chronic debilitating disease and multiple joint involvement. The pathophysiology involved in rheumatoid arthritis of the cervical spine resembles that of peripheral joint involvement. Synovitis and the development of pannus will lead to ligamentous, cartilaginous, and bony destruction with resultant instability in the cervical spine. The primary joints include the atlantooccipital, at-

TABLE 74-1 Ranawat Classification of Neurologic Deficit

Class I	Pain, no neurologic deficit
Class II	Subjective weakness, hyperreflexia, dysethesias
Class III	Objective weakness, long-tract signs
Class III A	Ambulatory
Class III B	Nonambulatory

Source: Reproduced with permission from Boden SD: Rheumatoid arthritis of the cervical spine: Surgical decision making based on predictors of paralysis and recovery. *Spine* 19:2275–2290, 1994.

and IIIB. The IIIA patients are ambulatory and the IIIB patients are nonambulatory. Some authors feel that the Ranawat grading system is too broad to be useful. Other grading scales include the Frankel[12b] spinal cord injury scale (Table 74-2) or the American Spinal Injury Association (ASIA) grading scale (Table 74-3). These, however, are more useful for the assessment of traumatic lesions and are inadequate for describing lesions at the craniovertebral junction. Zeidman and Ducker[12c] have proposed a modification of the Nurick rating scale that incorporates upper extremity function (Table 74-4). All the grading scales fail to completely describe the function of patients with rheumatoid arthritis. The ideal scale would evaluate the upper and lower extremities separately and provide a score for each.

NATURAL HISTORY

Our understanding of the natural history of rheumatoid arthritis of the cervical spine remains incomplete. Rana[13] reported a series of 41 patients who had atlantoaxial subluxation and were followed for 10 years. They found that 61 percent of the patients were unchanged; however, 27 percent had progressive subluxation. In a long-term study Weismann et al.[14] found that patients with 9 mm or more of anteroposterior subluxation and associated cranial settling were more likely to have cord compression. Boden et al.[15] reviewed 73 patients all for an average of 7.1 years to determine the predictors of paralysis and recovery. They found that 42 of these patients developed paralysis and 35 underwent surgery. They recommended surgical intervention when the posterior atlantodens interval was equal to or less than 14 mm, when atlantoaxial subluxation was present with more than 5 mm of cranial settling, or when subaxial subluxation was present, leading to a spinal cord diameter of less than or equal to 14 mm.

CLINICAL PRESENTATION

These patients may be difficult to evaluate because they have multifocal involvement secondary to their rheumatoid arthritis. They might have silent involvement of the

TABLE 74-2   Frankel Grading Scale

Frankel grade	Lesion
A	Complete neurologic injury
B	Preserved sensation only
C	Preserved motor— nonfunctional
D	Preserved motor—functional
E	Normal motor function

Source: Reproduced with permission of Zeidman SM, Ducker TB: Rheumatoid arthritis: Neuroanatomy, compression, and grading deficits. *Spine* 19:2259–2266, 1994.

TABLE 74-3   American Spinal Injury Association (ASIA) Grading Scale

Range	10–100
Upper extremity	Biceps, wrist extensors, triceps, flexor profundus, hand intrinsics
Lower extremity	Iliopsoas, quadriceps, tibialis anterior, extensor hallucis longus, gastrocnemius

Ratings: 0, absent; 1, trace; 2, poor; 3, fair; 4, good; 5, normal.
Source: Reproduced with permission of Zeidman SM, Ducker TB: Rheumatoid arthritis: Neuroanatomy, compression, and grading deficits. *Spine* 19:2259–2266, 1994.

cervical spine associated with their severe peripheral joint involvement. Review of a large series of rheumatoid patients by Menezes and associates[16] found that the patients with cranial settling have clinical symptoms including occipital pain, myelopathy, blackout spells, and brainstem signs. Rana and coworkers[17] concluded that these patients also have subtle involvement of the fifth cranial nerve. These patients may present with signs of myelopathy including pyramidal tract involvement, such as hyperreflexia, positive Babinski's sign, and loss of proprioception, all indicative of spinal cord compromise secondary to compression of the cervical spine. Because, on the basis of the neurologic examination, this may be difficult to differentiate from severe peripheral joint involvement, objective assessment of the cervical spine by somatosensory evoked potentials (SSEPs) has gained significant interest.[18,19] Indeed, most of the signs and symptoms of cervical involvement are subtle. A sudden increase in neck pain accompanied by loss of ambulatory status and the development of bowel or bladder incontinence must be considered as potential signals of cervical spine pathology.

RADIOGRAPHIC WORKUP

Initial radiographic evaluation should comprise plain radiographs including anteroposterior, open-mouth odontoid, and lateral flexion-extension dynamic views. Instability of the cervical spine is determined by the criteria of White and associates (Fig. 74-7). By these criteria, an anteroposterior displacement from the subaxial spine greater than 3.5 mm is defined as constituting instability. Atlantoaxial subluxation exists when the anterior atlantoodontoid interval (the distance between the posterior edge of the anterior ring of the atlas and the anterior surface of the odontoid process as measured along the transverse axis of the ring of the atlas) is more than 3.5 to 4 mm.[20] The posterior atlantoodontoid interval (the distance between the posterior surface of the odontoid process and the anterior edge of the posterior ring of the atlas as measured along the posterior of the ring of the atlas) has also been shown to have important ramifications for the evaluation of patients with rheumatoid arthritis. There are many measurements for the assessment of basilar invagination (cranial settling), which include McRae's line (Fig. 74-8). McRae's line

TABLE 74-4 Zeidman and Ducker Modification of Nurick Grading Scale

Grade	Root signs	Cord involvement	Gait	Hand function
0	Yes	No	Normal gait	Normal
I	Yes	Yes	Normal gait	Slight
II	Yes	Yes	Mild abnormality	Functional
III	Yes	Yes	Severe abnormality	Cannot button
IV	Yes	Yes	Only with assistance	Severe
V	Yes	Yes	Chair-bound or bedridden	Useless

Source: Reproduced with permission of Zeidman SM, Ducker TB: Rheumatoid arthritis: Neuroanatomy, compression, and grading deficits. *Spine* 19:2259–2266, 1994.

is drawn from the anterior aspect of the foramen magnum to its posterior aspect. Protrusion of the tip of the dens above the transversely drawn McRae's line is indicative of cranial settling. McGregor's line, drawn from the hard palate to the caudal surface of the basiocciput, is indicative of basilar invagination when migration of the odontoid tip is more than 4.5 mm cephalad to the line.

The arrival of MRI evaluation has further enhanced our ability to determine spinal cord compression in pa-tients with rheumatoid arthritis. This modality provides more detailed information about the soft tissue lesions causing spinal cord compression, especially at the cra-niovertebral junction, and MRI has also been established as the best method for evaluating the craniocervical re-gion. The diameter of the spinal canal is significantly de-creased in the flexed position.[22,23] The difference between the diameter of the neutral and flexed positions is highly significant. Recommendations are for surgical intervention in patients who have a spinal cord diameter of less than 6 mm in flexion. Severe pain and cranial migration of the axis were also justifications for surgical intervention.

UPPER CERVICAL SPINE

Atlantoaxial subluxation (AAS) is the most common afflic-tion of patients with rheumatoid arthritis and is secondary to a combination of etiologies in the joints involving the occiput, C1, and C2. Factors that have been shown to be correlative with AAS include the use of steroids, seroposi-tivity, subcutaneous nodules and mutilating rheumatoid disease.[24] An atlanto-dens interval over 3.5 mm is found in 20 to 25 percent of patients with rheumatoid arthritis.[13,14,25] Increased subluxation at this joint indicates loss of in-tegrity of the transverse ligament. When the subluxation is

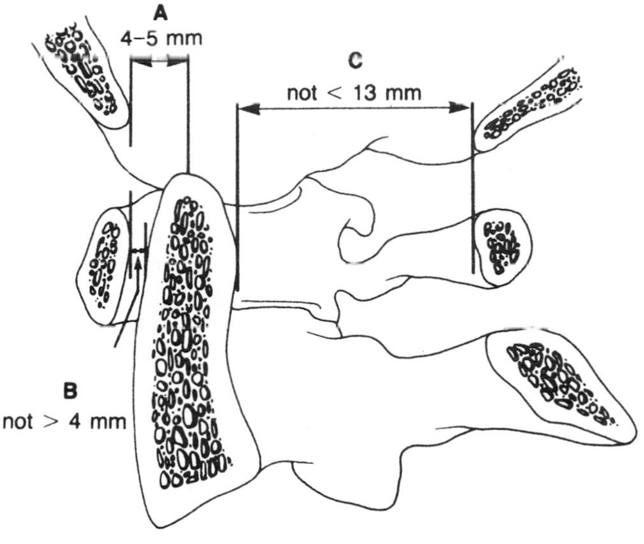

Figure 74-7 C0-C1-C2 lateral view: **A,** The distance between the basion of the occiput and the top of the dens is 4 to 5 mm. An increase of more than 1 mm in this distance with flex-ion/extension views is believed to indicate instability of C0-C1 if one assumes that the transverse ligament of the atlas is in-tact. **B,** The distance between the anterior border of the dens and the posterior border of the right of C1 should not be greater than 4 mm. **C,** There is another important measure-ment that we must consider. We refer to the distance between the posterior margin of the dens and the anterior cortex of the posterior ring of C1. This distance is of concern should it be less than 13 mm. (Modified with permission from White AA, Panjabi MM, Posner I, et al: Spinal stability: Evaluation and treatment. *Instr Course Lect* 30:1982).

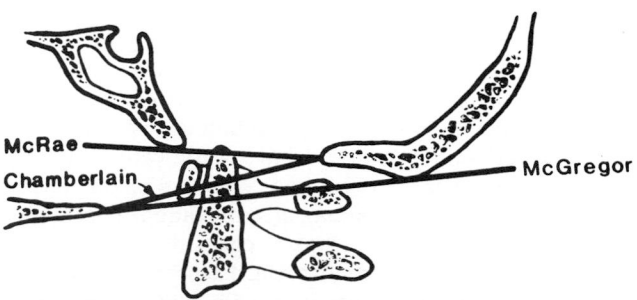

Figure 74-8 Diagrammatic representation for measurement of basilar invagination. (Reproduced with permission from Kricun ME: *Imaging Modalities in Spinal Disorders*. Philadelphia, Saunders, 1988.)

greater than 7 mm, it is thought to indicate disruption of the alar ligaments.[26] Posterior and lateral atlantoaxial subluxation has also been described; however, it is much less common than anterior subluxation.[27] For posterior displacement to occur, the odontoid and the anterior arch of C2 must be destroyed. Basilar invagination occurs when destruction occurs at both C1 and C2 as well as the occiput and C1. The odontoid process actually migrates cephalad through the arch of C1 to cause compression of the spinal cord. The MRI is a useful adjunct to visualize this area. Recently there have been developments to improve the predictors of paralysis and potential for neurologic recovery in patients with rheumatoid arthritis.

This involves a measurement of the posterior atlantodental interval (PADI), which is measured from the posterior wall of the dens to the anterior aspect of the C1 lamina. The use of the PADI with a cutoff less than or equal to 14 mm yields a sensitivity (ability) to detect those with paralysis of 97 percent. The most important predictive value using posterior atlantodental intervals is 94 percent, meaning that if the PADI is greater than 14 mm, there is a 94 percent chance that the patient will not have paralysis.[27] Boden recommends that plain x-rays be taken; if the PADI is less than 14 mm, then further diagnostic screening tools are recommended. If the PADI is less than 14 mm, an MRI to evaluate the space available for the cord is indicated. If the MRI demonstrates the cervical medullary angle of less than 135°, a cord diameter cross-section of less than 6 mm, or space available for the cord of less than 13 mm, then posterior atlantoaxial fusion should be considered.[27] If the PADI is greater than 14 mm on plain radiographs and the patient is asymptomatic, observation is warranted. Those patients with less atlantoaxial subluxation and any significant degree of basilar invagination need an MRI scan to evaluate the space available for the cord. These patients warrant an aggressive approach, especially if there is any evidence of cord compression. Cervical traction for reduction of the invagination followed by occipitocervical fusion should be performed.

THE PREDICTORS OF NEUROLOGIC RECOVERY

Recent data have suggested that the preoperative PADI and the postoperative diameter of the subaxial canal are the best predictors of potential for neurologic recovery.[27] These studies have shown that patients whose PADI is less than 10 mm before surgery had a poor prognosis for return of motor function. Those who had a posterior interval of greater than 14 mm did have significant motor recovery after surgical intervention. This was also found to be true for patients with subaxial subluxation. Those with a residual postoperative subaxial canal diameter of less than 14 mm showed a trend toward less recovery. Also several factors have appeared not to be strongly correlated with recovery from surgery. These include age, gender, duration of paralysis, PADI, and the preoperative percentage slippage of the vertebral body.

ATLANTOAXIAL SUBLUXATION WITH BASILAR INVAGINATION

Patients exhibiting basilar invagination with atlantoaxial subluxation warrant aggressive treatment. An MRI scan in flexion is advisable to quantitate the amount of actual cord compression. If there is evidence of cord compression on MRI scan from basilar invagination, cervical traction is appropriate. After the basilar invagination is reduced, these patients warrant an occipitocervical fusion. If cord compression cannot be relieved with traction, then fusion should be extended to a normal level. Either a C1 laminectomy or odontoid resection then must be performed in addition to the occipitocervical fusion. Those patients with isolated fixed basilar invagination and no symptoms may warrant observation.

SUBAXIAL SUBLUXATION

The presence of subaxial subluxation and no neurologic deficit does not warrant surgical intervention, especially if the canal diameter is greater than 14 mm. If, however, the diameter of the subaxial canal is less than 14 mm, further diagnostic testing including MRI is warranted. The MRI will allow evaluation of the true space available for the cord. If this space is less than 13 mm, surgical arthrodesis is indicated. This usually can be performed posteriorly. However, if the subluxation cannot be readily reduced, anterior decompression might be warranted in addition to posterior stabilization.

Complications

Some studies will report a clinical success rate of cervical fusion in rheumatoid patients of from 60 to 90 percent. The most common complications include death (5 to 10 percent), infection, wound dehiscence, wire breakage and loss of reduction, nonunion (5 to 20 percent), and late subaxial subluxation.[24]

DIFFUSE IDIOPATHIC SKELETAL HYPEROSTOSIS

Diffuse idiopathic hyperostosis (DISH), also known as Forestier's disease, is distinguished from ankylosing spondylitis by both its clinical and radiologic presentation. It occurs due to ossification of Sharpee's fibers and of the anterior longitudinal ligament from the anterior cortex of the vertebral body (Fig. 74-9). The new bone forms at the waist of the vertebral body and extends across to the neighboring vertebral body. New bone formation does not cause narrowing of the intervertebral disk space or osteopenia of the involved vertebral body.[28] New bone does not incorporate the horizontal

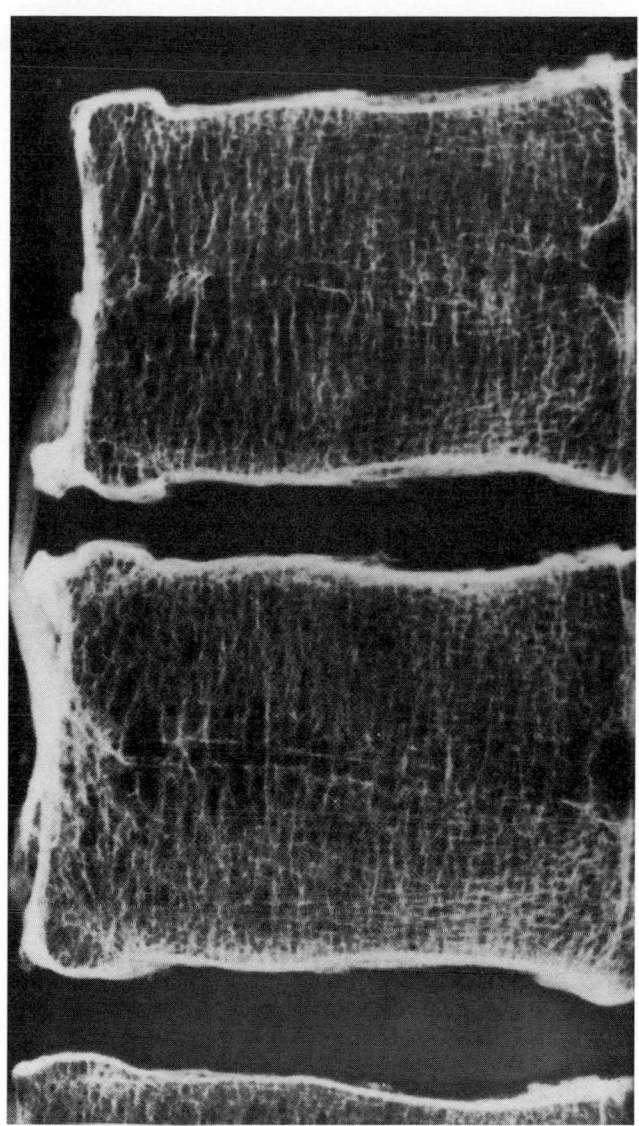

Figure 74-9 Radiography of an autopsy specimen of a patient with early DISH. The ossification of the anterior longitudinal ligament originating in Sharpey's fibers at the point of attachment of the ligament to the waist of each vertebra now extends across the intervertebral space at several levels. It is distinct from the cortex and the small marginal osteophytes, which are associated with some degenerative disk disease. (Reproduced with permission from Fornaster VL, et al: Spinal entheseal new bone formation: The early changes of spinal diffuse idiopathic skeletal hyperostosis. *J Rheumatol* 10:939–947, 1983.)

marginal osteophytes that are associated with degenerative disk disease. If four continuous vertebrae are affected, the diagnosis of DISH is confirmed. Patients with DISH will also exhibit absence of apophyseal joint ankylosis as well as changes in the sacroiliac joint. These patients will not show flattening of the anterior aspect of the vertebral body, as do patients with ankylosing spondylitis.

Clinical Features

This disease entity most commonly affects males near middle age or elderly patients. They will present with mild to moderate pain; however, they do not usually complain of stiffness. Some patients may even experience dysphagia because anterior osteophytes in the cervical spine are impinging on the esophagus. They will rarely have spinal stenosis when ossification of the posterior longitudinal ligament occurs. The disease is associated with a normal incidence of HLA-B27 antigen.[1] Some 10 percent of the DISH patients will have diabetes and 22 percent will have hypertension.[30] The treatment of these patients is symptomatic with anti-inflammatory drugs and physiotherapy to maintain motion. Surgery is rarely required to remove the osteophytes.[31]

CRYSTAL-INDUCED ARTHROPATHIES

There is no pathognomonic sign attributed to spinal symptomatology with crystal-induced arthropathy. In those patients who are suspected of the diagnosis of gout and who present with spinal pain, a trial of indomethacin may be warranted for the acute attack. These patients will have a history of gouty arthropathy secondary to their prolonged uricemia. Their hyperuricemia may be due to increased production of uric acid, diminished secretion of uric acid, or a combination of both. The most common radiologic finding of patients with spondylitis secondary to gout is typically punched out areas of bone lysis 5 mm or more in diameter.[32] The definitive diagnosis of gouty arthritis is made on the identification of monosodium urate crystals. These crystals may be distinguished from the calcium pyrophosphate crystals of pseudogout by a polarizing light microscope. The uric acid crystals are negatively birefringent needle-shaped structures.

SPONDYLITIS ASSOCIATED WITH INFLAMMATORY BOWEL DISEASE

Both Crohn's disease and ulcerative colitis have been shown to be associated with sacroiliitis and spondylitis. These disease entities and their spinal manifestations are clinically and radiographically similar to ankylosing spondylitis. The spinal manifestations similar to ankylosing spondylitis have been found in 15 to 60 percent of patients with Crohn's disease and ulcerative colitis.[33] There appear to be two different forms of spondylitis in patients with inflammatory bowel disease. The first is relatively mild and asymptomatic. In the second, the patient is HLA-B27 positive and has a much more progressive and aggressive form of spondylitis. It has been found that the progressive spondylitis, very classically similar to ankylosing spondylitis, will not be affected by colectomy in these patients.

THE PROGRESSIVE SPONDYLITIS IN PSORIATIC ARTHRITIS

Approximately one-fifth of the patients with psoriatic arthritis develop spondylitis during the course of their disease.[34] The cause and pathogenesis of psoriatic arthritis remain unknown, but are probably multifactorial. There is experimental and parental evidence suggesting an immunologic basis.[11] The clinical presentation of these patients is similar to that seen in Reiter's syndrome. Typically, psoriatic skin lesions present in the third decade. The lesions are primarily papules or micropapules. Patients will usually have involvement of the small joints in the hands and feet in an asymmetrical fashion. In a study by Lambert and Wright,[20] spondylitis was noted in 40 percent of the 130 patients with psoriatic arthritis. However, spondylitis was a predominant clinical feature in only 5 percent of these patients. The spinal involvement is consistent with findings described in Reiter's syndrome, with an asymmetrical, patchy type involvement. In the more severe form, this can resemble ankylosing spondylitis. Treatment is conservative with the use of rest, physical therapy, and anti-inflammatory agents.

REITER'S SPONDYLITIS

Reiter's syndrome is the presence of peripheral arthritis with urethritis, conjunctivitis, and frequently mucocutaneous lesions. The most sensitive and specific variable for the recognition of Reiter's syndrome is an episode of arthritis lasting at least 1 month after an episode of urethritis or cervicitis.[35] Men are more commonly affected and it is usually most prevalent in the third decade. Most investigators feel that this is a postinfectious, reactive form of arthritis. The clinical presentation is polyarthritis with urethritis or cervicitis. Again, the arthritis is asymptomatic, with a predilection for large and small joints of the lower extremities. Heel pain ranks second to synovitis of the knee as the main musculoskeletal manifestation. The ocular involvement consists primarily of a mild conjunctivitis. Symptoms of back pain may occasionally be seen, as well as sacroiliitis, in especially long-standing cases, in approximately 20 to 30 percent of patients.[36] However, in contrast, ankylosing spondylitis sacroiliac involvement is frequently unilateral in this disease. Late consequences in Reiter's syndrome are becoming better known. These include cardiac complications, atrioventricular block, and pulmonary fibrosis. Radiographically, juxtaarticular osteoporosis, joint space narrowing, and erosive changes may be seen.[37] Spinal involvement in Reiter's syndrome is less severe and extensive than in ankylosing spondylitis. The treatment of this entity remains controversial. Reiter's syndrome is a chronic condition with no cure.

BEHÇET'S SYNDROME

This is a rare seronegative disease that involves multiple systems. Its main characteristics are oral and genital ulcers, uveitis, and central nervous system involvement. Other manifestations include arthritis, thrombophlebitis, and skin lesions.[38–40] Males are affected more frequently than females. The disease is endemic to eastern Mediterranean areas as well as Japan. It more commonly involves the appendicular skeleton and is usually asymmetrical. Sacroiliitis and spondylitis have been reported in patients with Behçets syndrome. It is also associated with vasculitis involving the aorta, vena cava, and gastrointestinal tract. The etiology of the disease is unknown, but theories have included both viral and aberrant immune systems hypotheses. Large joints, especially the knee, are commonly involved. Sacroiliitis is associated with the syndrome.[41] Treatment again is symptomatic, which usually involves aspirin or other nonsteroidal anti-inflammatory drugs. More recently, use of immunosuppressive agents has been reported to have some positive results.[42]

ALKAPTONURIA AND OCHRONOSIS

Alkaptonuria is an inborn error of metabolism in which homogentisic acid cannot be oxidized. This autosomal recessive inherited condition is secondary to a lack of the enzyme homogentisic acid oxidase, causing large quantities of homogentisic acid to appear in the urine. This produces a brownish-black discoloration in the urine. A form of this acid can be deposited in tissues, leading to the term *ochronosis* as a description of the dark-yellow appearance of the pigment under a microscope. The pigment is usually deposited in connective tissue, involving fibrocartilage and hyaline cartilage. The most common manifestation of alkaptonuria/ochronosis is spondylosis. It presents as a waferlike calcification, with subsequent ossification of the intervertebral disk. Marginal syndesmophytes may form and thereby bridge the intervertebral disk space. However, unlike those with ankylosing spondylitis, these patients do not usually have fusion of the sacroiliac joint. Ochronosis can be detected by homogentisic acid in the urine. These patients will usually present with stiffness as their primary complaint. They can have marked limitation of motion or even ankylosis of the lumbar and thoracic spines. The earliest radiographic changes in these patients include calcification of the intervertebral disk and narrowing of the disk space. The treatment is symptomatic.

NEUROPATHIC SPONDYLOARTHROPATHY

Neuropathic arthropathy occurs secondary to alteration in the pain sensation of the affected joint. The absence of the protective sensory motor reflexes causes excessive loads or range of motion, leading to joint destruction. In the vertebral column, this is most often associated with tabes dorsalis, but it has also been associated with syringomyelia and diabetes mellitus.[43,44] Syphilis has been found to affect primarily the posterior column of the spinal cord, resulting in impaired proprioception. Loss of the protective mechanism can lead to spinal deformity and cord impingement. The proposed mechanism involves injury to the ligamentous and capsular structures with subsequent lack of protective sensation. However, a normal inflammatory response will occur. These patients will present with deformity, instability, crepitation, and hypermobility of the spine. The lumbar spine is most commonly involved in tabes dorsalis; however, syringomyelia more commonly affects the cervical spine. Radiographically, changes consistent with advanced spondylosis are seen, including osteophyte formation, facet hypertrophy, and vertebral body sclerosis.[45] The differential diagnosis includes severe osteoarthritis, DISH, infection, tumor, and Paget's disease. Treatment is centered around spinal stabilization. Conservative bracing to allow for adequate healing of the fracture and damaged soft tissue does not usually play a role in treatment. Intractable pain or progressive weakness can serve as indicators for surgery. This surgical undertaking must be aggressive and usually involves both anterior and posterior fusion with instrumentation.

REFERENCES

1. Simmons EH: Ankylosing spondylitis: Surgical considerations, in Rothman R, Simeone FA (eds): *The Spine,* 3d ed. Philadelphia, Saunders 1992.
2. Cruickshank B: Pathology of ankylosing spondylitis. *Clin Orthop* 74:43–58, 1971.
3. Berens DS: Roentgen features of ankylosing spondylitis. *Clin Orthop* 74:2–33, 1971.
4. Romanus R, Yden S: *Pelvo-spondylitis Ossificans.* Chicago, YearBook, 1955.
5. Simmons EH: The cervical spine in ankylosing spondylitis, in Bridwell KH, DeWald RL (eds): *Textbook of Spinal Surgery,* 2d ed. Philadelphia, Lippincott-Raven. In press.
6. Rosenthal M, Bahns I, Muller W: Increased frequency of HLA-B8 in hyperostatic spondylosis. *J Rheum* 4(suppl 3):94–96, 1977.
7. Mason C, Cozen L, Adelstein L: Surgical correction of flexion deformity of the cervical spine. *Calif Med* 79:244, 1953.
8. Urist MR: Osteotomy of the cervical spine: Report of a case of ankylosing rheumatoid spondylitis. *J Bone Joint Surg* 40A:833, 1958.
9. Thomassen E: Vertebral osteotomy for correction of kyphosis in ankylosing spondylitis. *Clin Orthop* 194:142–152, 1985.
10. Thiranont N, Netrawichien P: Transpedicular decancellation closed wedge vertebral osteotomy for treatment of fixed flexion deformity of spine in ankylosing spondylitis. *Spine* 18:2517–2522, 1993.
11. Brewerton DA, Nichols A, Laffrey M, et al: HLA-B27 and arthropathies associated with ulcerative colitis and psoriasis. *Lancet* 1:956–958, 1974.
12. Dilsen N, Ergenbi T, Konice M, et al: Virus-like particles in the glomerular basement membrane in a case of Behçet's disease with amyloidosis, in Duffy JD (ed): Summary of internal symposium on Behçet's disease. *J Rheumatol* 5:229–233, 1978.
12a. Ranawat CS, O'Leary P, Pellicci P, et al: Cervical fusion in rheumatoid arthritis. *J Bone Joint Surg* 61(A):1003–1010, 1979.
12b. Frankel HL: The value of postural reduction in the initial management of closed injuries of the spine. *Paraplegia* 7:179–192, 1969.
12c. Zeidman SM, Ducker TB: Rheumatoid arthritis: Neuroanatomy, compression, and grading deficits. *Spine* 19:2259–2266, 1994.
13. Rana NA: Natural history of atlantoaxial subluxation in rheumatoid arthritis. *Spine* 14:1054–1056, 1989.
14. Weissman BNW, Aliabadi P, et al: Prognostic features of atlantoaxial subluxation in rheumatoid arthritis patients. *Radiology* 144:745–751, 1982.
15. Boden SD, Dodge LD, Rechtine GR, Bohlman HH: Rheumatoid arthritis of the cervical spine: A twenty year analysis with predictors of paralysis and recovery. *J Bone Joint Surg* 75A:1282–1297, 1993.
16. Menezes AH, VanGilder JC, Clark CR, El-Khoury GY: Odontoid upward migration in rheumatoid arthritis. *J Neurosurg* 63:500–509, 1985.
17. Rana NA, Taylor AR: Upward migration of the odontoid peg in rheumatoid arthritis. *Proc R Soc Med* 64:717–718, 1971.
18. Toolanen G, Knibestol M, Larsson SE, Landman K: Somatosensory evoked potentials (SSEPs) in rheumatoid cervical subluxation. *Scand J Rheumatol* 16:17–25, 1987.
19. Toolanen G, Larsson SE, Fagerlund M: Medullary compression in rheumatoid atlantoaxial subluxation evaluated by computerized tomography. *Spine* 11:191–194, 1986.
20. Lambert JR, Wright V: Psoriatic spondylitis: A clinical and radiological description of the spine in psoriatic arthritis. *Q J Med* 46:411, 1977.
21. White AA, Panjabi MM: *Clinical Biomechanics of the Spine.* 2d ed. Philadelphia, Lippincott, 1990.
22. Dvorak J, Grob D, Baumgartner H, et al: Functional evaluation of the spinal cord by magnetic resonance imaging in patients with rheumatoid arthritis and instability of upper cervical spine. *Spine* 14:1057–1064, 1989.
23. Kawaida H, Sakou T, Morizono Y, Yoshikuni N: Magnetic resonance imaging of upper cervical disorders in rheumatoid arthritis. *Spine* 14:1144–1148, 1989.
24. Boden SD, Dodge LD, Bohlman HA, et al: Rheumatoid arthritis of the cervical spine: Predictors of paralysis and recovery. Presented at the Annual Meeting of the Cervical Spine Research Society, Palm Desert, CA, December 1992.
25. Clark CR, Goetz DD, Meanness AH: Arthrodesis of the cervical spine in rheumatoid arthritis. *J Bone Joint Surg* 71A:381–392, 1989.
26. Fielding JW, Hensinger RN, Hawkins RJ: Os odontoideum. *J Bone Joint Surg* 62A:376, 1980.
27. Boden SD: Rheumatoid arthritis of the cervical spine: Surgical decision making based on predictors of paralysis and recovery. *Spine* 19:2275–2280, 1994.
28. Conlon PW, Isdale IC, Rose BS: Rheumatoid arthritis of the cervical spine. *Ann Rheum Dis* 25:120–126, 1966.
29. Utsinger PD: Diffuse idiopathic skeletal hyperostosis, in Sokoloff L (ed): *Clinics in Rheumatic Diseases.* Vol 11. Philadelphia, Saunders, 1985, pp 325–351.
30. Harris J, Carter A, Glick E, Storey G: Ankylosing hyperostosis: Clinical and radiological features. *Ann Rheum Dis* 33:210–215, 1974.

31. Lambert JR, Tepperman PS, Kimerez J, Newman A: Cervical spine diseases and dysphagia. *Am J Gastroenterol* 76:35–40, 1981.

32. Simpson JM, Booth RE Jr: Arthritis of the spine, in Rothman R, Simeone FA (eds): *The Spine,* 3d ed. Philadelphia, Saunders, 1992.

33. McEwen C, Ditata D, Lingg C, et al: Ankylosing spondylitis and spondylitis accompanying ulcerative colitis, regional enteritis, psoriasis and Reiter's disease: A comparative study. *Arthritis Rheum* 14:291, 318, 1971.

34. Wright VA, Chamberlin MA: Behçet's syndrome. *Bull Rheum Dis* 29:972–977, 1979.

35. Wilkens RF, Arnett FC, Bitter T, et al: Reiter's syndrome: Evaluation of preliminary criteria for definite disease. *Arthritis Rheum* 24:844, 1981.

36. Oates JK, Young AC: Sacroiliitis in Reiter's disease. *Br Med J* 1:1013–1015, 1959.

37. Reynolds DF, Gonka GW: Radiological aspects of Reiter's syndrome (venereal arthritis). *J Fac Radiol (Lond)* 9:44, 1958.

38. Behçet H: Uber rezidivierende Apthose, durch ein virus verusachte Geschwure am Mund, am Auge und an den Genitalien. *Dermatol Wochenschr* 105:1152, 1937.

39. Oshima Y, Shimizu T, Yokohari R, et al: Clinical studies on Behçet's syndrome. *Ann Rheum Dis* 22:36, 1963.

40. Simmons EH: The surgical correction of flexion deformity of the cervical spine in ankylosing spondylitis, in Cervical Spine Research Society (eds): *The Cervical Spine.* Philadelphia, Lippincott, 1989, p 573.

41. Mignucci LA, Bell GR: Differential diagnosis of sciatica, in Rothman R, Simeone FA (eds): *The Spine,* 3d ed. Philadelphia, Saunders, 1992.

42. Buckley CE, Gillis JP: Cyclophosphamide therapy of Behçet's disease. *J Allerg* 43:273–283, 1969.

43. Campbell DJ, Doyle JO: Tabetic Charcot's spine: Report of eight cases. *Br Med J* 1:1018, 1954.

44. Culling J: Charcot's disease of the spine. *Proc R Soc Med* 67:1026, 1974.

45. Resnick D, Shaul SR, Robins JM: Diffuse idiopathic skeletal hyperostosis (DISH): Forestier's disease with extraspinal manifestations. *Radiology* 122:1, 1977.

CHAPTER 75

The Pediatric Spine

Lawrence G. Lenke

The pediatric spine is a growing and dynamic structure of axial support, allowing varying degrees of flexibility while protecting the neural elements. The pediatric spine may be involved in pathology encompassing the spinal column, neural elements within the spinal canal, or a combination of both. This chapter covers the common disease states encountered in the pediatric spine from an orthopedic perspective.

PATIENT EVALUATION

In the pediatric age range, patients typically present for evaluation of the spine for three different reasons: pain somewhere along the spinal axis; deformity of the spinal column in either the coronal or sagittal planes; or because of distal neurologic abnormalities that seem to be emanating from the spine. Often patients present in only one of these categories, but occasionally they might fall into two or even all three. Thus, the history obtained and the physical examination performed must always be extremely thorough and inclusive of multiple diagnostic possibilities.

The history obtained from a pediatric patient with a spinal abnormality should be thorough. Responses from parents or caretakers are an essential part of an adequate history. Birth and developmental milestones should be recorded, along with any other relevant aspects of the birth history. Developmental milestones should be briefly discussed and elaborated upon if they have been significantly delayed. The primary reason for evaluation is then discussed in detail. For a patient presenting with spinal pain, its onset, relationship to activities, and any prior accidents, injuries, or similar episodes should be noted. Factors that have relieved or exacerbated the pain and treatments rendered thus far are also important to identify. Activity-related pain, especially with extension, may indicate a stress fracture of the pars interarticularis of the lumbar spine; constant, boring pain that increases at night, awakening the patient, may indicate a spinal column tumor. Important questions to determine the severity of the problem and how it has affected the child include whether school has been missed because of the pain and also whether the pain has interfered with the child's recreational and play activities. One should always be more suspicious of a serious spinal problem when a pediatric patient's recreational or play activity has been severely compromised because of the pain. It is important to note any medications that have been taken for the pain and the response to the medications. It is also important to know whether the pain is increasing in frequency and severity or improving over time.

For patients presenting for evaluation of a spinal deformity, the history should begin with documenting the first time the deformity was noted and by whom. Often the first to note a spinal deformity are the patient's parents, grandparents, pediatrician, or school nurse if the child is part of a school screening program. Any history of significant pain in a patient presenting with a deformity should also be investigated. Almost all spinal deformities in young patients are asymptomatic. Patients with very large deformities may have fatigue-type pain in the lower back following prolonged sitting or standing. However, by and large, significant axial pain in a patient with a spinal deformity should warrant further detailed investigation.

It is always important to assess the relative skeletal maturity of the patient being evaluated for a spinal abnormality, especially a deformity that may be progressive during the growing years. Thus, recent growth trends in both males and females should be obtained, as well as the menarcheal status of females. In patients who have older siblings, inquiry into the relative height difference between the older siblings and the patient will provide information on the patient's remaining growth. A family history of any significant spinal deformities will also help to determine the genetic implications of spinal deformity.

In all pediatric patients presenting for spinal evaluation, a neurologic history must also be obtained. Any weakness, sensory abnormalities (paresthesias, tingling, numbness), or complaints of radicular pain should be documented. Recent changes in bowel and bladder habits must also be detailed. Any overt clumsiness, difficulty climbing steps or stairs, or early fatigue with activities should alert the physician to potential neurologic changes.

A past medical history including medical illnesses, previous hospitalizations, and prior surgical procedures should be obtained. Current medications and allergies are also documented. Normally, the patient's pediatrician or family physician can provide additional information in these areas if required.

PHYSICAL EXAMINATION

The physical examination of a pediatric spinal patient should be performed in a consistent and reproducible manner. Males should have only shorts on so the entire trunk and torso can be visualized. Modesty is important for females; however, a back-opening gown is essential to allow observation of the posterior torso and trunk. Observation of overall coronal and sagittal alignment is performed first. Skin lesions such as café-au-lait spots indicating neurofibromatosis or hairy patches indicative of spinal canal abnormalities are searched for. The overall balance of the patient's head, trunk, and torso over the pelvis is noted (Fig. 75-1). Any waistline asymmetry or trunk shift suggests a scoliosis deformity. In a relaxed position, the shoulders should be level, with the head directly centered on the pelvis. Leg lengths are assessed

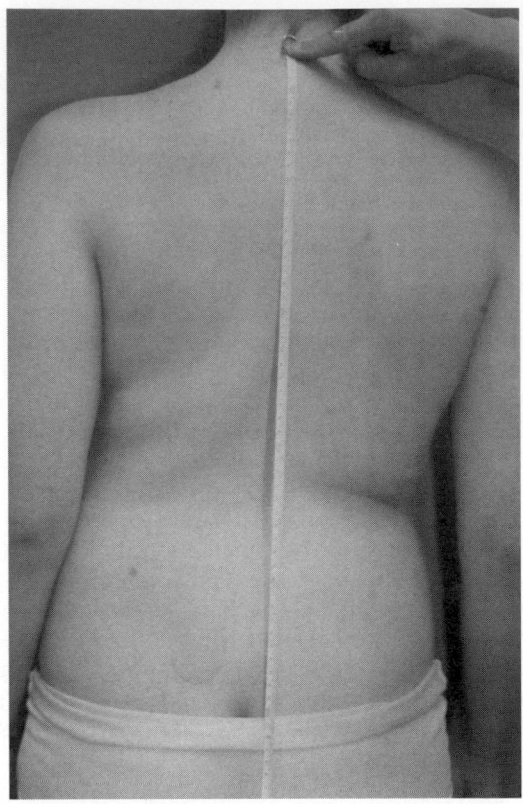

Figure 75-1 Physical examination of the posterior torso and back region. A ruler dropped from the base of the neck should bisect the midgluteal crease if the plumbline is balanced. Any visible trunk shift or waistline asymmetry indicates a structural scoliosis deformity.

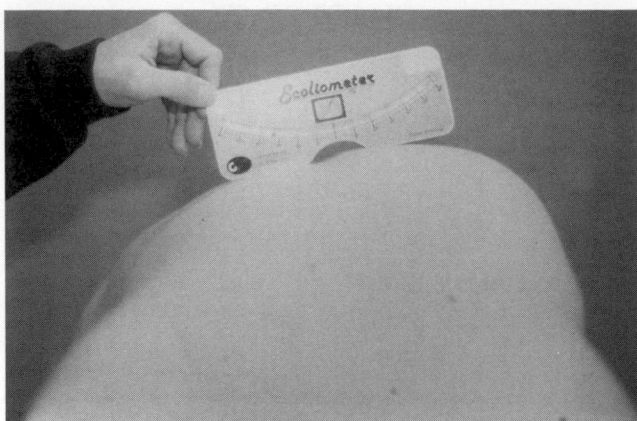

Figure 75-2 On forward bending, asymmetry in the thoracic or lumbar region is detected on a scoliometer. This measures the angle of trunk rotation in both the thoracic and lumbar spine. Measurements are made in degrees, and normally any increment greater than 5° indicates a scoliosis deformity that requires further investigation.

quickly by palpating the tops of the iliac crests and noting any side-to-side difference. A forward bending test is then performed to assess the flexibility of the spine by seeing how far the fingertips can reach with the knees fully extended. Most pediatric patients should be able to touch their toes or the floor with this maneuver without too much difficulty. Severely limited back flexion may be indicative of more serious spinal pathology, such as spondylolisthesis. While the patient is bending forward, any asymmetry in the thoracic or lumbar region is noted as a potential clinical manifestation of spinal deformity. A scoliometer measures the angle of trunk rotation in the thoracic and lumbar spine, and this measurement should be made on any patient with any type of asymmetry (Fig. 75-2). Next, spinal movements of extension, rotation, and side bending are performed and quantitated. Also, range of motion of the neck through all movements is performed and documented.

A dynamic neurologic exam is then performed with the patient standing. This includes normal gait, tandem gait, toe and heel gait, single-leg stance, jogging in place, squatting, and jumping. If the patient can readily perform all of these activities in an efficient manner, a significant motor abnormality to the lower extremities is very unlikely.

The static exam, during which the patient sits and lies down, is then performed. While sitting, the patient is asked to straighten out each leg. This simultaneously performs a neurologic stretch test of the distal lumbar nerve roots (as the straight-leg-raise procedure), checks quadriceps strength with the leg straight, and also assesses any hamstring tightness. Specific motor testing of the lower and upper extremities may then be performed in each major motor group bilaterally. Sensory testing is performed in a similar fashion to evaluate specific dermatomes. Upper and lower extremity reflexes, including clonus and Babinski testing, logically follows. Range of motion of the knees and hips is assessed in those patients with atypical lower extremity complaints.

Following a complete history and thorough physical exam, the patient's condition should be placed into one of the three categories (allowing that there may be some overlap): spinal pain syndrome, spinal deformity, or a primary neurologic abnormality of the spinal cord or nerve roots. Diagnostic imaging modalities then serve to confirm the diagnostic suspicion.

RADIOGRAPHIC EVALUATION

Radiographic evaluation of a child who presents with spinal pain or deformity should start with anteroposterior and lateral radiographs of the affected part of the spine. In patients who have pain, the x-ray should center on the specific painful region of the spine, whether it be cervical, thoracic, and/or lumbar. In a patient who presents with a spinal deformity, long cassette radiographs showing the entire spinal column and pelvis should be obtained. In evaluating spondylolysis with or without a spondylolisthesis, oblique views as well as a Ferguson anteroposterior (30° cephalocaudal) view are helpful in defining pathology of the pars interarticularis region at L5 and profiling the L5 transverse processes and sacral alar region (Fig. 75-3). In spinal deformity patients who are to undergo surgery, flexibility x-rays consisting of right and left supine side-bending films as well as push-prone dynamic correction films are extremely helpful in assessing curve correctability. In patients being evaluated for a kyphotic deformity, hyperextension lateral x-rays also demonstrate the flexibility of the deformity. It is important to obtain the initial spinal radiographs in an upright position to appreciate the position of the spine with weight bearing (Fig. 75-4).

Bone Scan

In a child or adolescent with significant back or neck pain and nondiagnostic radiographs, a technetium-99 bone scan should be performed. This is very sensitive for finding stress reactions or fractures, diskitis, and bony tumors, but it is nonspecific. It should study the entire spine and pelvis.

Single photon emission computed tomography (SPECT), a newer technique, combines bone scan with CT technology. Recent reports have shown that SPECT imaging is more sensitive than plain scanning for diagnosing stress fractures and is more precise in pinpointing the spe-

cific anatomic location. Such scans have become very helpful in properly identifying pars interarticularis stress reactions and fractures (Fig. 75-5).

Computed Tomography

Computed tomography is not of much help as a screening study in the pediatric population. However, it is still useful in evaluating suspicious bony lesions seen on radiographs or bone scans. Also, CT scans are useful to evaluate neural compression in the spinal canal following myelography. However, MRI has recently eliminated the need for myelograms in most pediatric clinical situations.

Magnetic Resonance Imaging

Current MRI scanning techniques have revolutionized evaluation of the pediatric spine. An MRI scan will evaluate neural elements, the intervertebral disks, the vertebral body marrow, and the soft tissues supporting and surrounding the spine. The MRI is a powerful diagnostic tool that must be utilized appropriately in patients whose clinical symptoms and signs warrant the exam. It is certainly

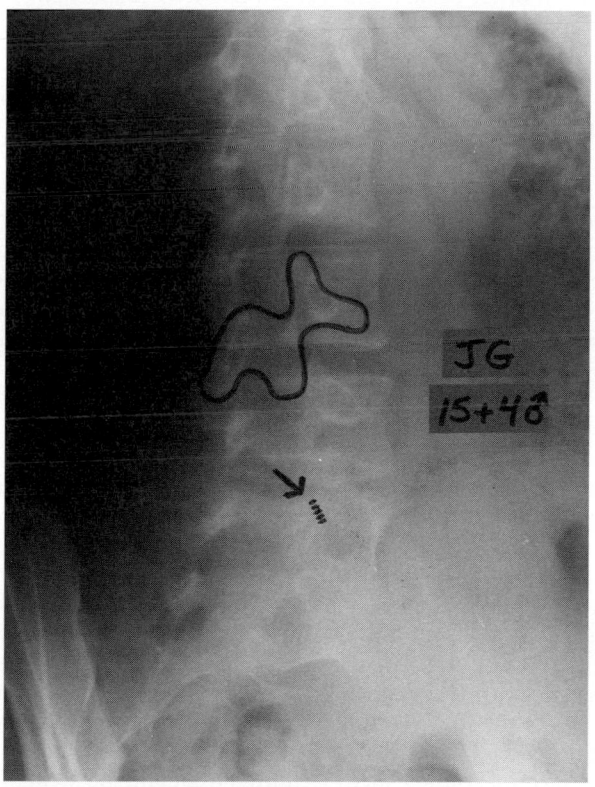

A

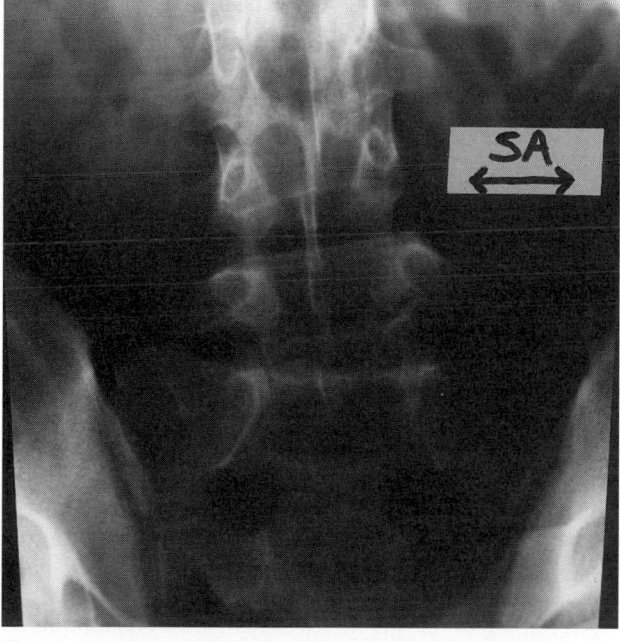

B

Figure 75-3 *A.* An oblique view of the lumbar spine profiles the "Scottie dog." The ear of the dog is the superior facet, the nose is the transverse process, the eye is the pedicle, the neck is the pars interarticularis region, the body is the lamina, and the forefoot is the inferior articular facet. The arrow points to a crack in the neck of the Scottie dog, indicating a pars interarticularis defect. *B.* A Ferguson AP view of the lumbosacral spine profiles this region best because it is a true AP of the lumbosacral junction, paralleling the L5-S1 disk. Note that the L5 pedicles, transverse processes, and sacral alae are visible.

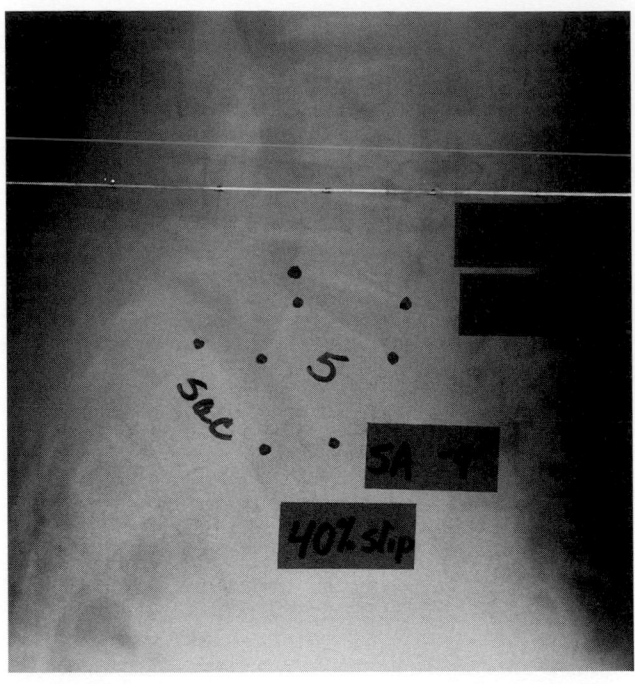

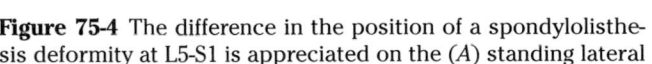

A

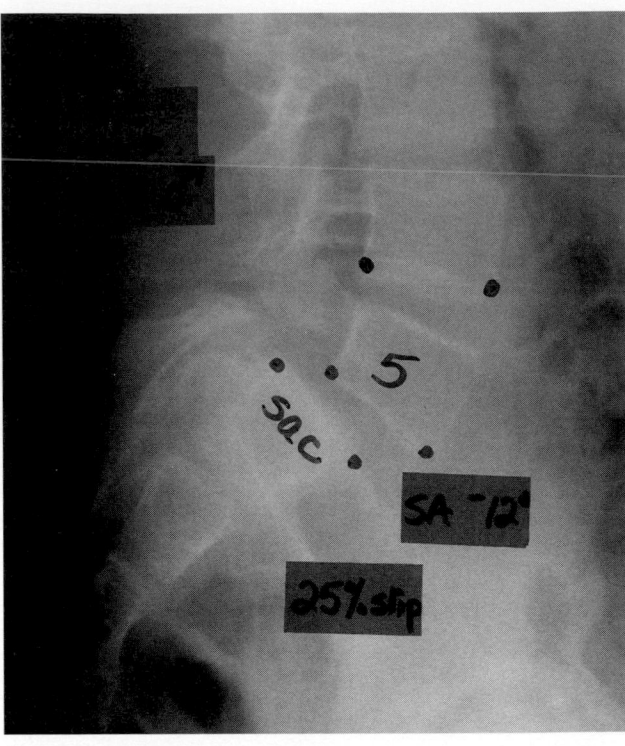

B

Figure 75-4 The difference in the position of a spondylolisthesis deformity at L5-S1 is appreciated on the (*A*) standing lateral view, which shows a 40 percent slip, versus the (*B*) supine lateral view of the same patient, showing a 25 percent slip.

the procedure of choice for spinal neurologic deficits, spinal cord tumors and syringomyelia, diskitis, spinal column tumors, and other conditions.[165] An MRI can also be used as a screening tool to evaluate the spinal canal for abnormalities in patients with atypical spinal deformities. Certainly, any patient with an atypical curve pattern (such as a left thoracic scoliosis) or a congenital scoliosis or abnormal history or physical exam should have a total spinal MRI prior to operative correction of the deformity (Fig. 75-6). As a screening tool in these circumstances, the MRI should include sagittal sections of the cervical, thoracic, and lumbar spine, with axial views of the occipitocervical, cervicothoracic, thoracolumbar, and lumbosacral spine. This protocol should detect nearly all types of spinal canal abnormalities causing a specific spinal deformity.

Laboratory Evaluation

A laboratory evaluation may be indicated in patients presenting with various complaints and associated clinical findings of the spine. The diagnosis of conditions such as suspected infection, rheumatologic disease, lymphoma, or leukemia benefits from appropriate laboratory studies. These include a complete blood count, sedimentation rate, electrolytes, liver and blood enzymes, and urinalysis. Occasionally, studies such as HLA-B27, rheumatoid factor, and antinuclear antibody will be obtained if a rheumatologic condition is being considered.

DIFFERENTIAL DIAGNOSIS OF PEDIATRIC SPINAL PAIN

A differential diagnosis should be established following a careful history and physical examination of a pediatric patient who presents with spinal pain. Radiographic evaluation and laboratory tests will often elucidate or confirm a specific diagnosis. As a general guide, lumbar spinal pain in children can be divided into five categories: mechanical, developmental, inflammatory, neoplastic, and psychiatric disorders (conversion reaction).

Specific entities of the various categories include postural, muscular, and overuse syndromes along with herniated disks among the mechanical disorders; spondylolysis with or without spondylolisthesis and Scheuermann's disease in the developmental category; diskitis, osteomyelitis, and juvenile rheumatoid arthritis among the inflammatory disorders; tumors of the vertebral column, spinal cord or canal, as well as metastatic tumors in the category of neoplastic disorders; and finally psychosomatic back pain, which is the most common conversion reaction seen as a cause of back pain.

Several studies have attempted to define the incidence of back pain in children. It appears that somewhere between 10 and 25 percent of children have definite back pain; however, it is unknown exactly how many of them will have a specific diagnosis.[25] Several studies have shown that spondylolysis and spondylolisthesis are the most common causes of back pain in children.[78,79,91] Somewhat sur-

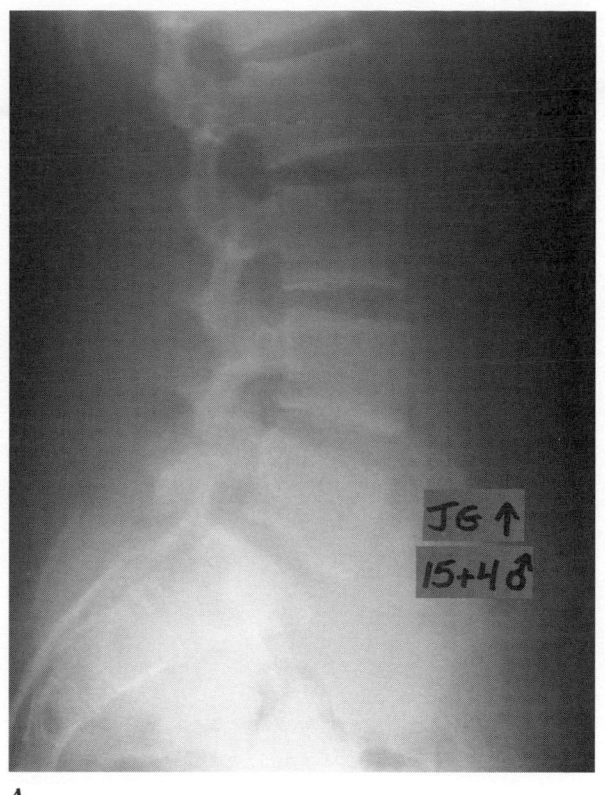

A

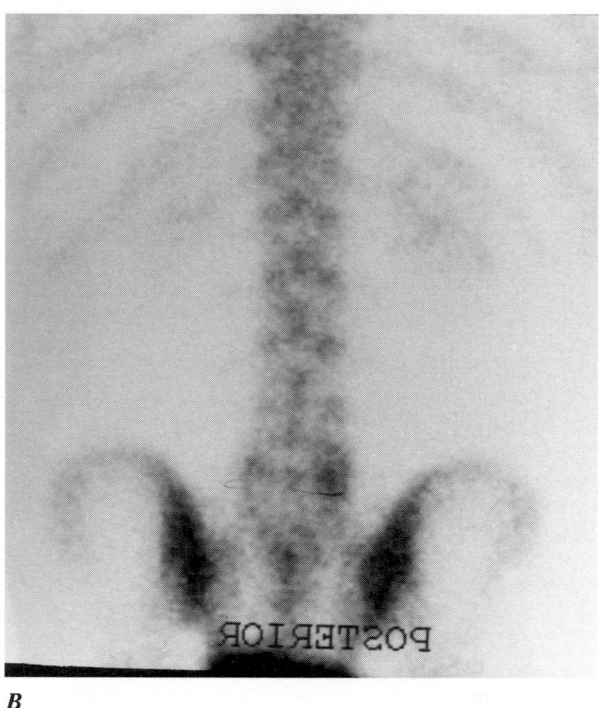

B

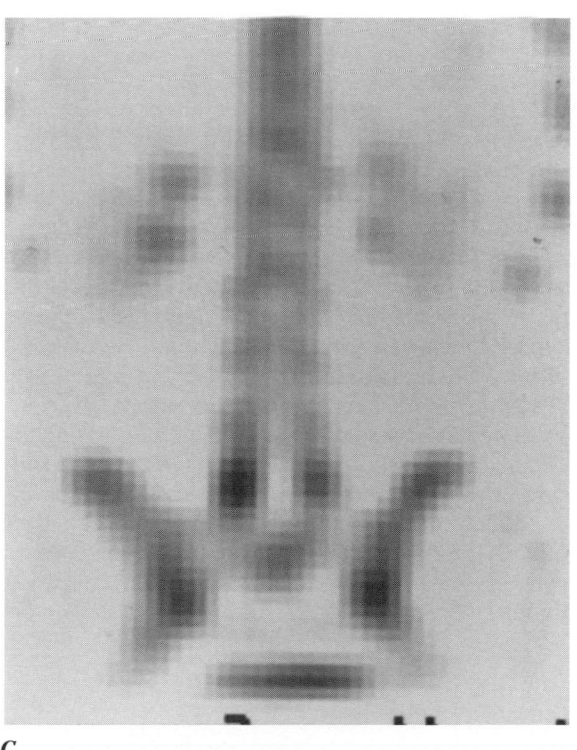

C

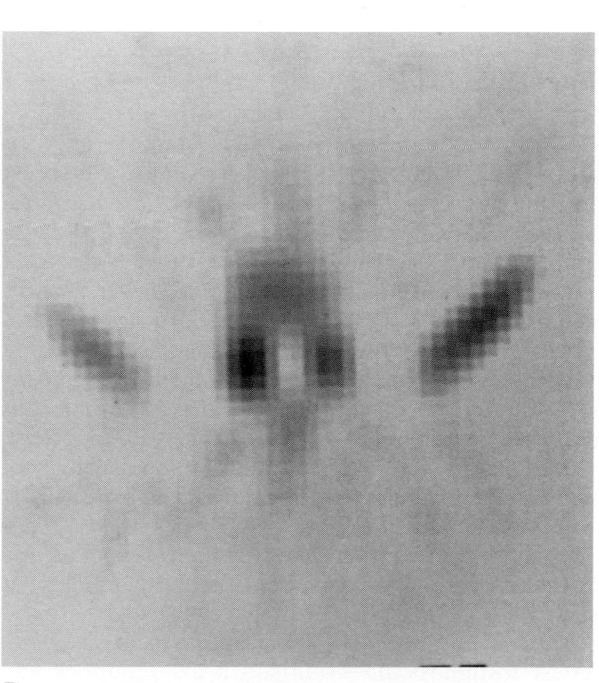

D

Figure 75-5 This 15 + 4-year-old male complained of lumbosacral pain with activity. *A.* His lateral lumbar spine x-ray suggested a possible pars defect at L5. *B.* A technetium bone scan showed a vague increase of uptake in the right L5 region. *C.* A coronal SPECT scan demonstrates the abnormality, with (*D*) further definition on the axial image.

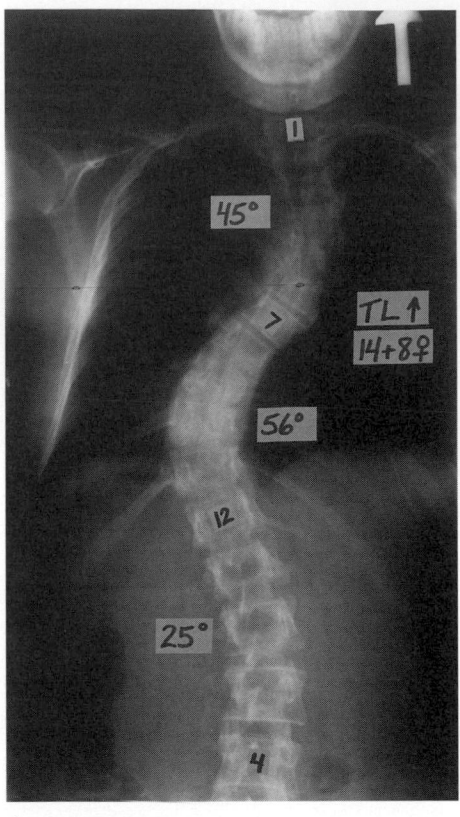

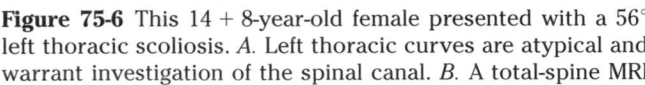

A

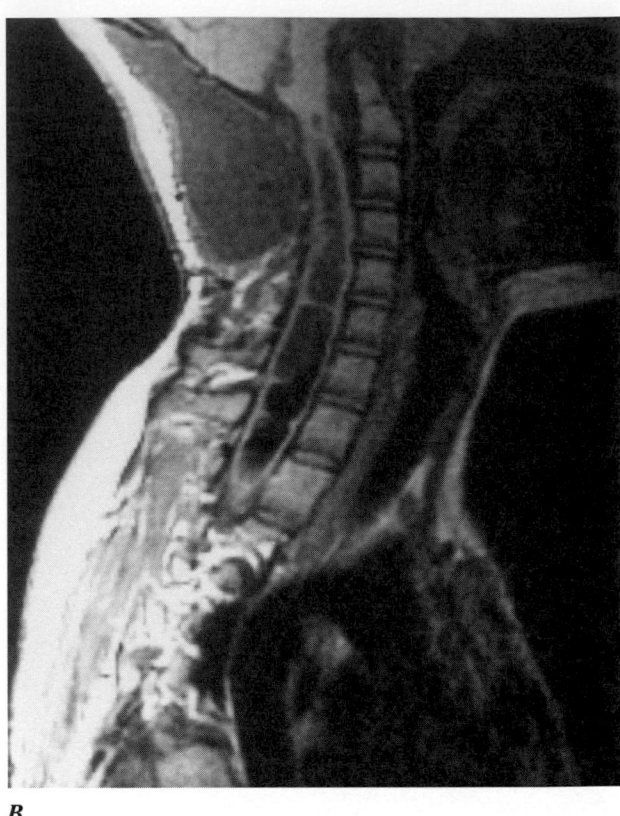

B

Figure 75-6 This 14 + 8-year-old female presented with a 56° left thoracic scoliosis. *A.* Left thoracic curves are atypical and warrant investigation of the spinal canal. *B.* A total-spine MRI revealed an extensive syrinx extending throughout the entire cervical spine.

prisingly, there is a high incidence of tumors along the spinal column and cord in patients presenting with back pain: 6 percent in one series and 11 percent in another.[150] Thus, overall, in children under the age of 10 who present with back pain, diskitis and spinal tumors are occasionally the cause (Fig. 75-7). In patients over the age of 10, spondylolysis, spondylolisthesis, and Scheuermann's disease are much more likely to be the etiology.[82] However, it must be remembered that tumors can occur at any age and should always be considered in the differential diagnosis of a child with significant axial pain. Overuse syndrome and back strains should be diagnosed only after all other causes have been excluded.

Disk protrusions and herniations, although much rarer than in adults, may develop in children and especially adolescents.[88,95] Males are more commonly affected than females, and three factors have been implicated for being significant in the etiology: trauma, congenital spinal anomalies, and a familial predisposition to herniated disks.[186,190] The history is usually one of lumbar spinal pain with varying degrees of stiffness that eventually leads to buttock and/or leg pain specifically. There may be a normal neurologic exam; however, there is almost invariably a positive straight-leg-raising test because of the neural irritation. The diagnosis is confirmed via CT or more commonly MRI.

As in adults, the two most common levels for adolescent disk herniation will be L4-L5 and L5-S1. One must always include in the differential diagnosis for this age group a slipped ring apophysis, which may simulate a herniated disk[54] (Fig. 75-8). As in adults, conservative treatment is indicated initially; but if symptoms persist, surgical diskectomy produces good to excellent results in the majority of patients.[32,115] However, one must remind the patient that the degenerative processes continue in the affected disc.

Psychosomatic back pain is occasionally seen, but other organic causes of pain must be eliminated. Often, these children or adolescents will have experienced significant psychosocial events in the past that initiated and have tended to exacerbate their complaints of pain. Careful psychological support for both the patient and caregivers is essential to the diagnosis and appropriate treatment.

PEDIATRIC DISKITIS AND OSTEOMYELITIS

Like other areas of the immature skeleton, the spine in young children is prone to bacterial infections.[27,62]

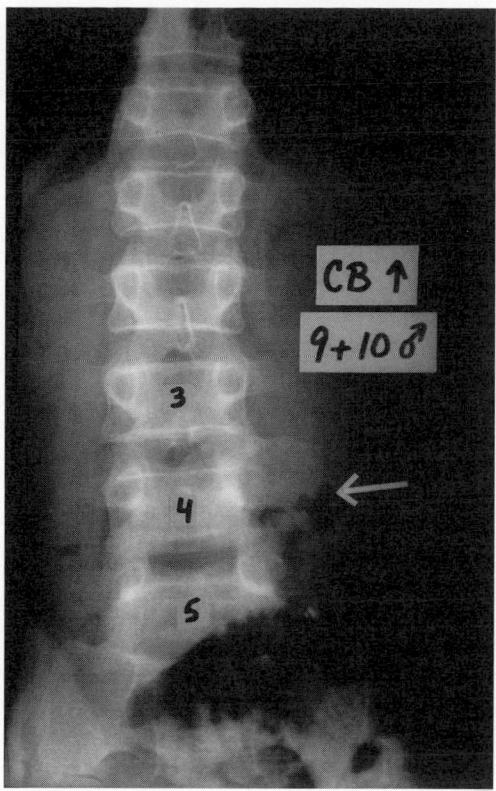

A

B

Figure 75-7 C.B., a 9 + 10-year-old male, presented with significant back and right thigh pain that prevented him from going to school and playing sports. *A.* His AP x-ray of the lumbar spine demonstrated an expansile lesion of the right transverse process and pedicle of L4, with further definition seen on the axial CT scan (*B*). This required surgical excision, which documented an aneurysmal bone cyst.

Although traditionally vertebral osteomyelitis was thought to be caused by a bacterial organism, the etiology of diskitis is more speculative. Recently, with the advent of newer imaging modalities, especially MRI, it has become evident that both diskitis and vertebral osteomyelitis are variations of a similar theme, depending on the area and chronicity of involvement, bacterial involvement, and host reactivity.[74] The pathoanatomy surrounding the onset of bacterial infection of the spine stems from the perforating vascular channels seen in the vertebral end plate, which make the adjacent vertebrae and avascular disks susceptible to bacterial infection.[72] In recent years, a change has been noted in the amount of diskitis (versus osteomyelitis) that is seen. This may be due to the availability of both bone scans and MRIs, which result in earlier diagnosis and thus appropriate antibiotic treatment of suspected spinal infections. Thus, currently, vertebral osteomyelitis with significant vertebral body destruction is rarely seen in young children.[195]

The diagnosis of spinal infection should be entertained in any child or teenager with back pain and limited spinal range of motion of unexplained etiology.[27] A screening bone scan or MRI will confirm the suspicion prior to any radiographic changes, such as end-plate erosions, sclerosis, or disk space narrowing, which are all rather late findings of diskitis (Fig. 75-9).

Following confirmatory radiologic studies, biopsy of the suspected lesion should be performed. Normally, the patient undergoes a closed needle biopsy of the region under CT guidance. Blood cultures are also taken. The white blood cell count is usually normal; however, the erythrocyte sedimentation rate (ESR) will be mildly or highly elevated.

The hallmark of treatment of pediatric spinal infections is immobilization and antibiotics. A spinal orthosis is fabricated to decrease motion in the affected part of the spine. Appropriate antibiotics are chosen following the biopsy results. If the biopsy is inconclusive, broader-spectrum coverage to include at least *Staphylococcus aureus* and *Streptococcus* is indicated. Consultation with the infectious disease service is helpful in these circumstances, due to the prolonged (4 to 6 weeks) antibiotic treatment necessary.

Clearly, the goal in managing pediatric spinal infection is early diagnosis and prompt institution of the above-mentioned nonoperative treatment regimens. In some chronic cases, vertebral osteomyelitis with abscess formation may require surgical drainage and more extensive antibiotic therapy; however, this is rarely encountered.

PEDIATRIC SPINAL DEFORMITY —THE CORONAL PLANE

Idiopathic Scoliosis

Traditionally, idiopathic scoliosis has been divided into three categories according to the age of onset of the deformity: infantile, 0 to 3 years; juvenile, 4 to 10 years; adolescent, above age 10 years to adulthood. Thus, the date when the child is first diagnosed radiographically with

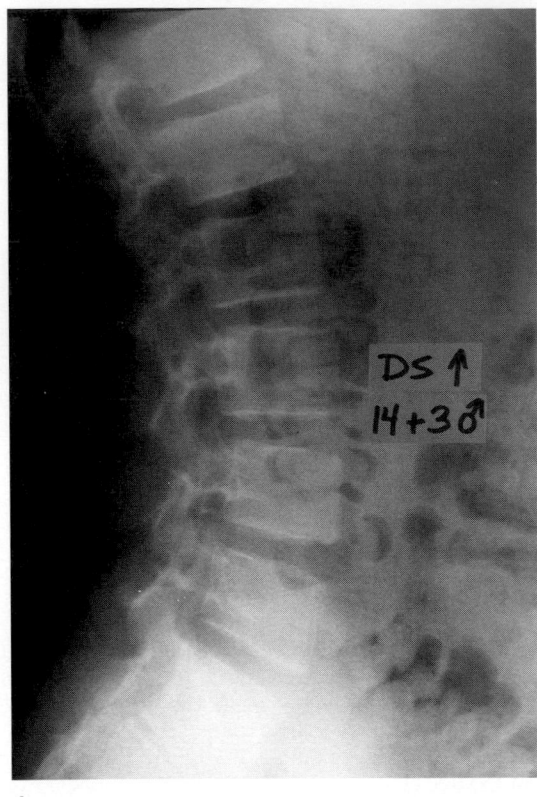

A

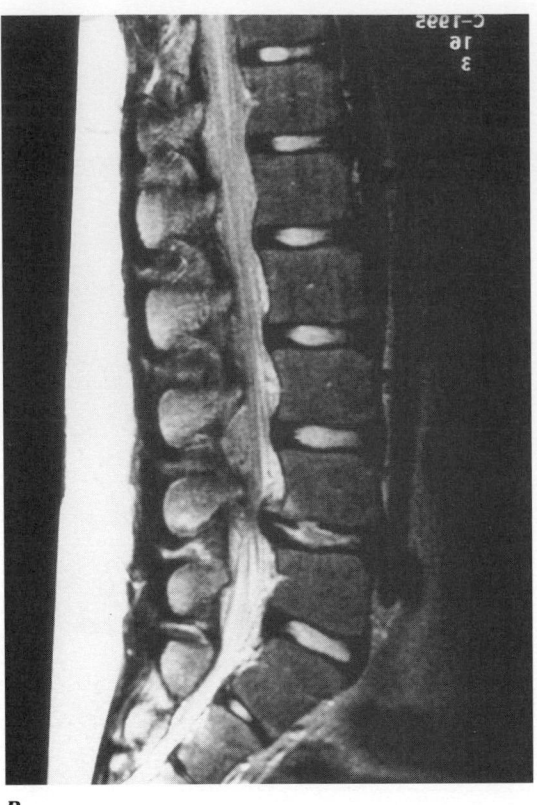

B

Figure 75-8 D.S., a 14-year-old male, presented with minimal pain in the low back but severe pain bilaterally in the lower extremities. He had a positive bilateral straight-leg-raising test at approximately 45° and L5 symptomatology on his physical exam. His lumbar spine lateral x-ray (*A*) was unremarkable. A lumbar spine MRI (*B*) documented a slipped ring apophysis with neural compression. He underwent surgical excision with complete relief of his symptomatology.

scoliosis is the recorded date of onset. Obviously, young children may have a significant scoliosis that does not present for treatment until much later, but the classification will proceed with the age at which the diagnosis was made. The prognosis and treatment are different for these three categories of idiopathic scoliosis and thus are discussed separately. Adolescent idiopathic scoliosis is encountered much more frequently than the other two categories because of the tendency for idiopathic curves to develop and progress during the adolescent growth spurt. As in all ages of presentation, idiopathic scoliosis is a diagnosis of exclusion, and it is essential to rule out other causes on the basis of a thorough history, physical examination, and radiologic studies.

Infantile Idiopathic Scoliosis

The infant or child with more than 10° of scoliosis presenting between birth and 3 years of age is classified as having infantile idiopathic scoliosis if all other etiologies are excluded. Scoliosis presenting in an infant or very young child may be secondary to a congenital spinal anomaly, a myopathy, a neuromuscular disorder, or other non-idiopathic diagnoses. Thus, a complete birth history, developmental record, and review of systems is an essential part of the evaluation. If the history, examination, and radiographs exclude other diagnoses in a child up to age 3, then the diagnosis of infantile idiopathic scoliosis is made.[58,112] It is unclear whether spinal cord imaging with MRI is necessary in these young patients. There certainly does appear to be a subgroup of "idiopathic" patients who may have significant pathology referable to the central nervous system, which may be seen on a screening MRI; however, the true incidence of these spinal canal anomalies in the infantile age group is unknown (Fig. 75-10).

It is important to document whether a significant thoracic deformity is present at a very young age, for, if progressive, these may carry a high risk of subsequent cardiopulmonary compromise. These patients not only have the stigma of a spinal deformity but may also have associated serious health problems.[66] At birth, although all of the conductive pulmonary airways are complete, only a small number of the respiratory bronchioles and alveoli have been formed.[78] Formation of these terminal branches continues until the age of 8, when a full complement of alveoli is seen as in the adult. Restriction of the thoracic cage has a variable effect upon future lung development, depending upon the age of onset of significant restriction.

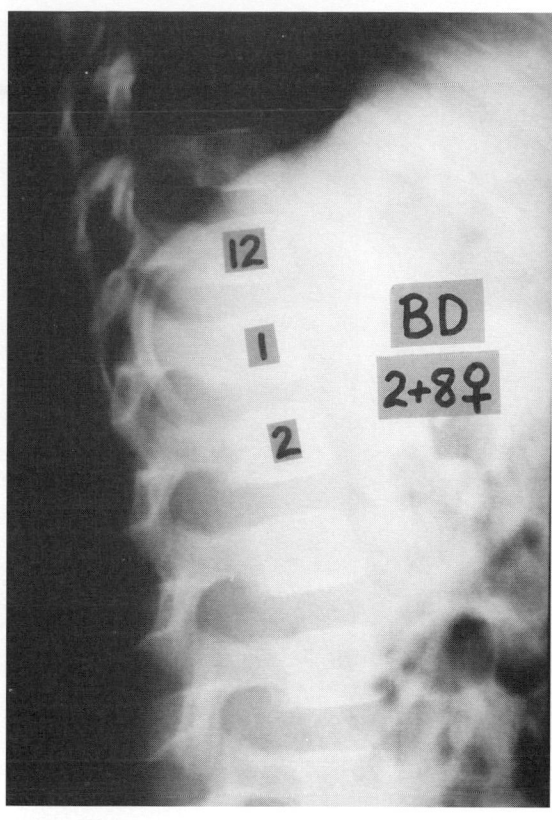

A

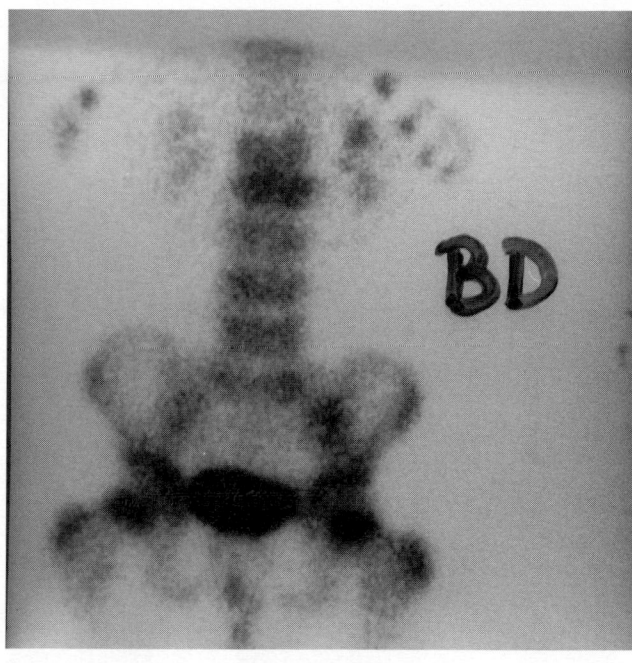

B

Figure 75-9 This 2 + 8-year-old patient presented with lumbar back pain and limited spinal range of motion. A lateral spinal x-ray (*A*) suggested decreased disk height at L1-L2. A bone scan (*B*) demonstrated increased uptake at this level as well.

Patients with infantile scoliosis and a progressive deformity tend to form far less than the normal number of alveoli, which may be an irreversible condition. The secondary consequence of reduced alveoli is the development of an inadequate pulmonary vascular system. This vascular system appears to develop and remodel in response to the developing alveoli. Thus, it responds to the amount of lung tissue present rather than to any systemic signal of chronologic or physiologic age. This may be a cause of pulmonary arterial hypertension and associated cor pulmonale that are inevitable complications of significant pulmonary hypertension.[66,185] Thus, it is imperative to avoid the relentless progression of infantile idiopathic curves, for this may pose a major health risk to the child in later years.

Fortunately, significant infantile curves are infrequently encountered, and some of these will resolve spontaneously. In 1951, James[111] noted that only 4 of 33 cases of early-onset idiopathic scoliosis resolved. A follow-up series that included 212 patients demonstrated that 64 percent progressed and 36 percent resolved.[112] In the 1960s, several published series of early-onset scoliosis showed that a convincing majority of the curves were resolving spontaneously.[130] Currently, it is believed that a significant portion of these curves will resolve, and that there is a declining overall incidence of infantile curves.[187] A decline in incidence may be due to postnatal positioning of the infant in the crib. Traditionally, European countries have favored the supine position versus the prone position favored in North America. This has been suggested as a potential rea-

son why European countries have had a higher incidence of infantile spinal deformity than North American countries. Mehta[149] felt that a floppy and hypotonic baby was less able to resist thoracic deformation than a normal baby with normal muscular tone. Wynne-Davies[217] noted a higher prevalence of congenital heart disease, developmental dysplasia of the hip, breech delivery, older mother, and inguinal hernia among infantile idiopathic scoliotics. However, there were no significant genetic differences between early- and late-onset patients.

In contrast to later-onset idiopathic scoliosis, males are much more commonly affected by infantile scoliosis than are females, and thoracic curves tend to be convex to the left in 75 percent of infantile cases. As in later-onset scoliosis, though, initial curve size and the amount of associated rotation are strong prognostic factors for progression. Mehta[149] found that inclination of the ribs on each side of the apical vertebrae could provide information as to which curves would progress and which would resolve. In this method, the apical rib-vertebra angles are drawn on each side of the apical body, with the convex angle being more acute and the concave angle being more obtuse. If the difference between the angles, noted as the rib-vertebra angle difference (RVAD), exceeds 20°, the curve is much more likely to be progressive. Calculation of the RVAD on an infant's serial spinal x-rays is important in assessing the risk of progression[149] (Fig. 75-11).

On physical examination, it is critical to assess the entire body for other growth abnormalities, including de-

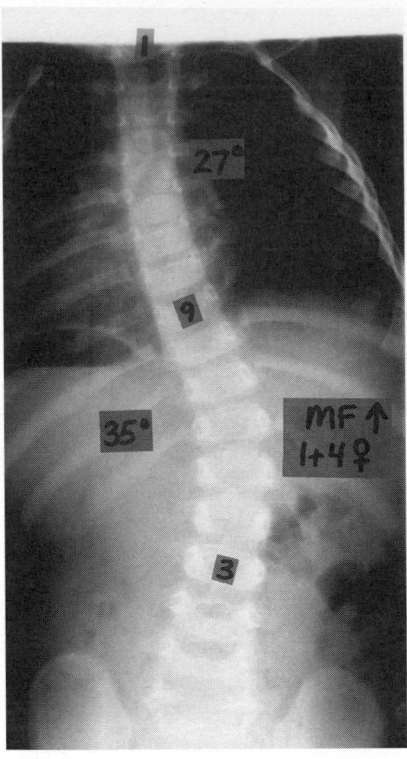

A

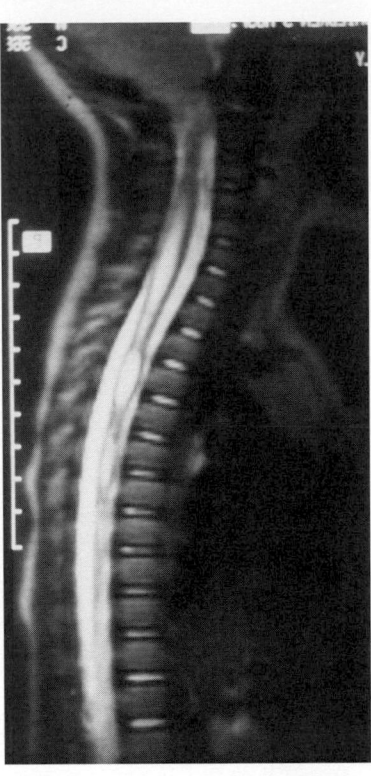

B

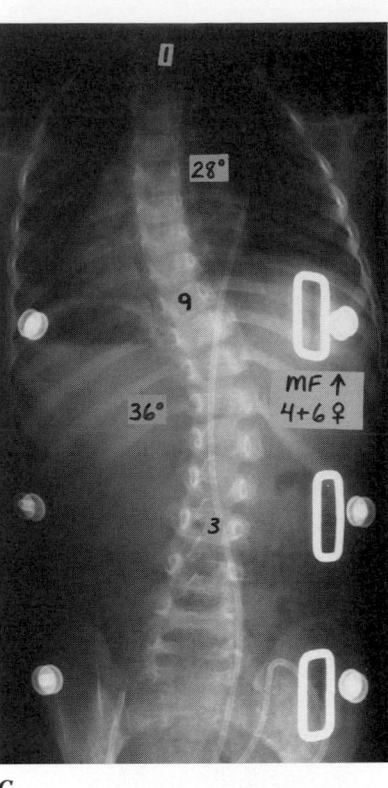

C

Figure 75-10 M.F. was 1 + 4 years old when she was diagnosed with infantile idiopathic scoliosis. Her coronal x-ray (*A*) showed a 35° right thoracolumbar curve. Because of her young age, a screening MRI (*B*) was performed, which showed an extensive syrinx of her cervical-thoracic spine. She was treated with a syringoperitoneal shunt and a clamshell brace. At age 4 + 6, her coronal x-ray (*C*) demonstrates that her scoliosis has been maintained at 36°.

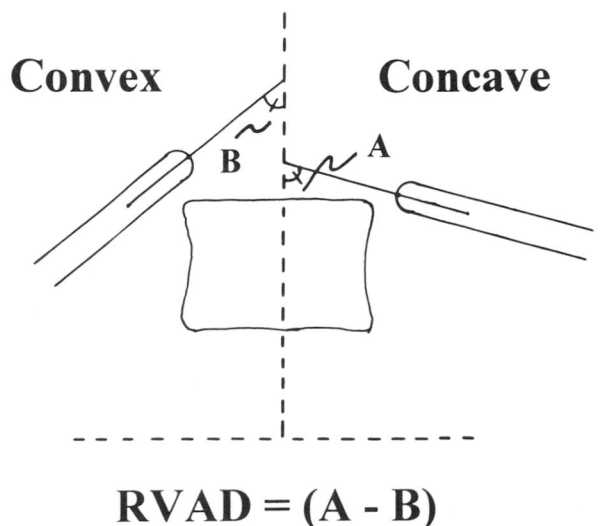

$$RVAD = (A - B)$$

Figure 75-11 Schematic drawing showing calculation of the rib–vertebral angle difference (RVAD). A line paralleling the medial aspect of the convex rib creates angle B, while the line paralleling the medial aspect of the concave rib to the midline forms angle A. The RVAD equals angle A minus angle B.

creased joint motion, asymmetrical extremities, neurologic abnormalities, facial asymmetries, skin lesions, and general muscular tone. The amount of rib deformity and the flexibility of the curvature should be assessed by suspending the child and pushing in on the convexity. If there is any suspicious component to the historical or physical examination, MRI scanning of the spinal canal should be performed. Currently, there is no complete study showing the incidence of an abnormal neural axis on MRI imaging in infantile idiopathic scoliosis.

The treatment of infantile idiopathic scoliosis ranges from observation, bracing, serial casting, to various surgical procedures. Observation is in order for small curves that have an RVAD below 20°. For curves that have shown progression and are over 30°, a trial of a body jacket or Milwaukee-type orthosis may be indicated. It is unclear whether bracing affects the natural history of infantile idiopathic curves at risk for progression.[147] In this manner, serial casting with an elongation-derotation-flexion (EDF) cast may be indicated. This is usually placed on a standard Cotrel EDF casting frame with the patient (as an outpatient) under a light general anesthetic. Normally the cast can be tolerated for 3 to 4 months, and casting is repeated until the deformity has improved or resolved completely. Normally there is little point in continuing cast treatment after the age of 4 or 5, where the infantile growth spurt has plateaued. One must be sure that the thoracic rib cage is not being molded adversely from pressure effects of either casting or bracing.

In curves that are progressive past 40° and have an RVAD greater than 20°, surgery may be indicated. If the sagittal plane is not excessively kyphotic, "growing" rod instrumentation may act as an internal splint to allow further axial growth prior to surgical fusion (Fig. 75-12). For curves not amenable to a growing rod, anterior convex apical fusion over four or five segments and posterior fusion (acting as a convex growth arrest procedure) may be indicated.[6] If circumferential fusion is planned and the infant's posterior elements are large enough, pediatric-type instrumentation can be inserted; this affords some correction and secures the spine during the healing phase, along with supplementary casting or bracing. If the spine is too small to instrument, then it is mandatory to place the patient in a body cast postoperatively. It is true that axial growth will cease over the fused levels. However, allowing a progressive deformity to continue unabated will produce a far worse deformity than fusing the spine at an earlier age in appropriate cases. It is essential to perform a circumferential fusion on these patients to avoid the "crankshaft phenomenon" due to continued anterior spinal growth in the presence of a solid posterior fusion.

Juvenile Idiopathic Scoliosis

Juvenile idiopathic scoliosis occurs between the ages of 4 and 10 years. Scoliosis in this age range may present as a small curve that spontaneously regresses, a slowly progressive curve that responds to nonoperative treatment, or a progressive curve that requires surgery. Juvenile idiopathic curves are reported in anywhere from 12 to 21 percent of patients with idiopathic scoliosis.[114] Juvenile curves occur more frequently in females than males in a 2:1 to 4:1 ratio.[81,142,189] As one proceeds from younger to older juveniles, the female-to-male ratio increases to similar levels as seen for adolescent idiopathic scoliosis. Thoracic curves are most common, with both left thoracic and more commonly right thoracic curves noted. Lumbar curves are quite rare, occurring in only 1 percent of cases.[81] Approximately 70 percent of juvenile idiopathic curves progress and require some form of treatment, and approximately 50 percent of these will require surgery.[189]

Appropriate x-rays of the entire spine in the coronal and sagittal planes are needed to follow progression. Because of the reportedly high incidence of intraspinal pathology occurring in juvenile-onset scoliosis, these patients should be considered to have their spinal canals evaluated with MRI scans[126] (Fig. 75-13). Anomalies such

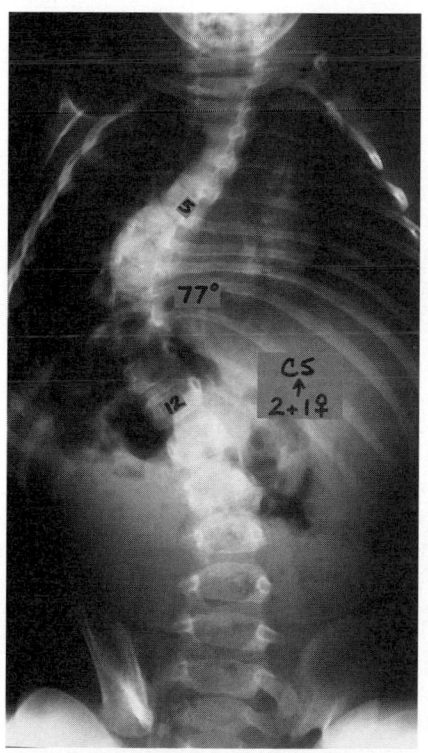
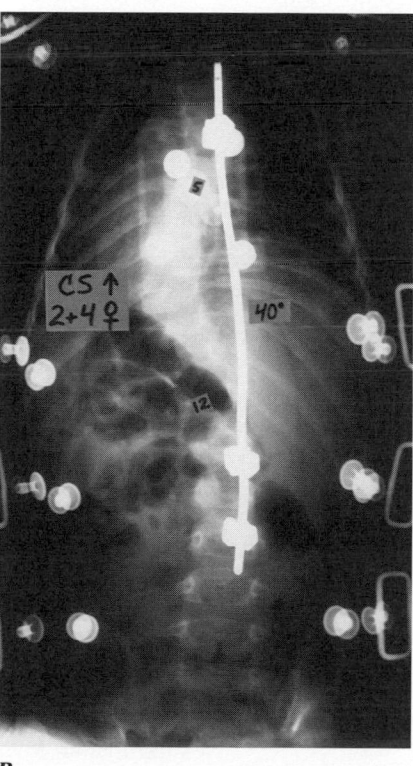
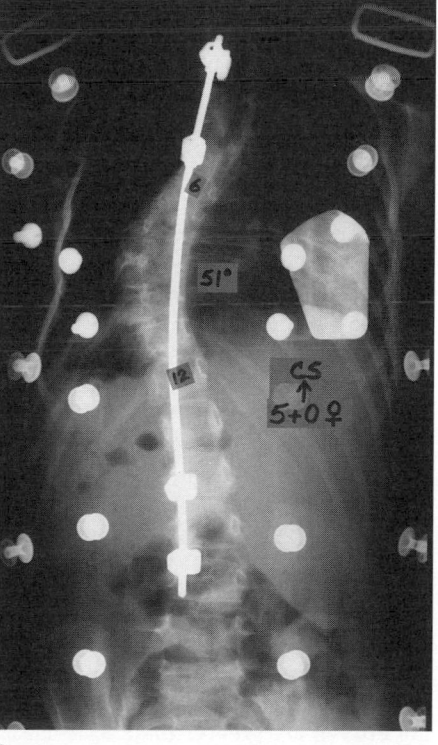

A   *B*   *C*

Figure 75-12 C.S., a 2 + 1-year-old female, presented with a 77° left thoracic infantile idiopathic scoliosis (*A*). Left thoracic curves are actually more common in the infantile population. Because of the size and stiffness of the curve, it was treated initially with a subcutaneous infantile "growing rod" (*B*). This was maintained for approximately 2 1/2 years, when she underwent a definitive anterior apical fusion from T6 to T12 and posterior fusion from T2 to L3 (*C*).

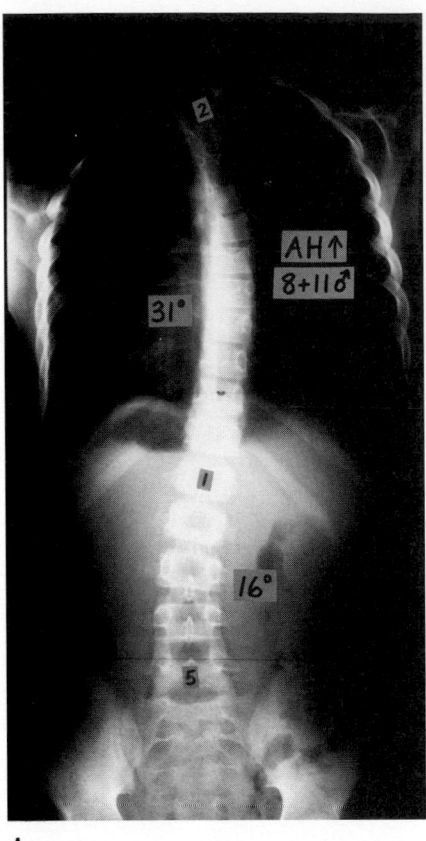
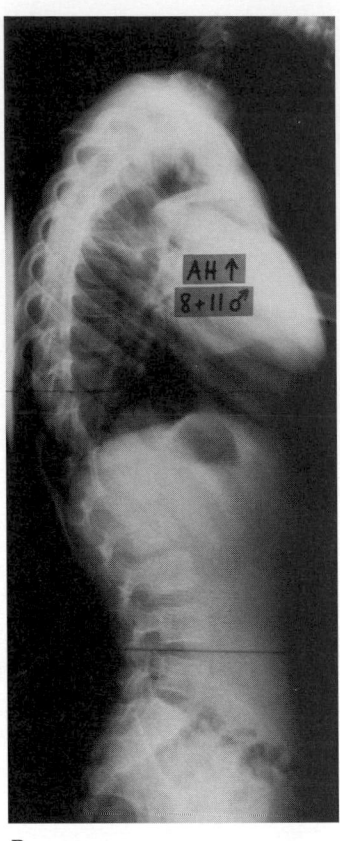
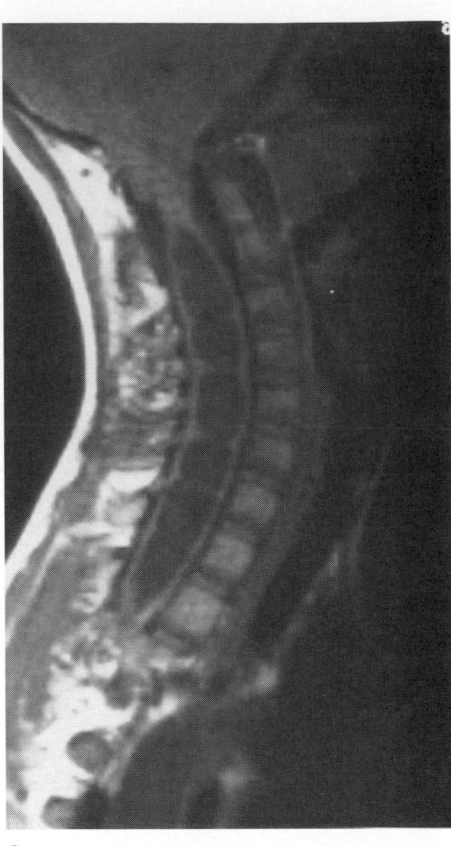

A   *B*   *C*

Figure 75-13 A.H, an 8 + 11-year-old male, presented with (*A*) a 31° right thoracic juvenile idiopathic scoliosis. His physical examination, including a detailed neurologic examination, was unremarkable. Imaging of his sagittal plane (*B*) showed normal thoracic kyphosis and lumbar lordosis. Because of his diagnosis of juvenile idiopathic scoliosis, he underwent a total-spine screening MRI exam, which revealed (*C*) a large cervical syrinx that required neurosurgical intervention.

as syringomyelia, tethered cords, and Arnold-Chiari malformations, among others, have been noted in these patients, with an incidence of 20 to 25 percent of cases evaluated by MRI.[126] As in infantile idiopathic scoliosis, measuring the RVAD as suggested by Mehta is useful in helping predict which curves will respond positively to bracing[149] (see Fig. 75-11).

Brace treatment is indicated for those curves greater than 25° with documented progression.[189] Traditionally, the Milwaukee brace was prescribed and worn initially 20 to 23 h a day. If stabilization of the curve occurred, bracing time was then decreased or the brace might often be worn only during sleep, because of relatively slow growth during the juvenile years. An underarm Boston-type orthosis may also be effective in curves suitable to this type of brace (Fig. 75-14). In curves that have progressed past 40 to 45°, bracing may be indicated to attempt to delay surgical correction until a more skeletally mature spine is achieved. However, suboptimal results occur when bracing curves are greater than 40° (Fig. 75-15).

Indications for surgical treatment of juvenile idiopathic scoliosis are fairly similar to those for adolescent scoliosis. However, bracing may be indicated for a slightly longer time if longitudinal growth is still occurring. Occasionally, as in infantile scoliosis, a "growing" rod type of instrumentation may further delay a definitive fusion procedure in these patients. This rod should be placed within the stable zone at the most proximal and distal aspects and often requires serial lengthening every 6 months or so. Usually an orthosis is mandatory anytime the child is out of bed, so as to further secure the instrumentation. Excessive thoracic kyphosis (greater than 45°) is a relative contraindication to this procedure, for it is hard to stabilize the instrumentation on a kyphotic spine without dislodging the hooks from the posterior elements.

For curves reaching 50°, definitive fusion surgery may be indicated, especially if "growing" instrumentation is not an option.[189] Because of the risk of continued anterior growth following a posterior fusion—termed the "crankshaft phenomenon"—these children usually require combined anterior and posterior fusions.[73] This is certainly true for those much younger than age 10 both chronologically and skeletally. Posterior instrumentation is very helpful for improving curve correction as well as promoting a solid fusion. Many "pediatric" systems are available that are appropriate for juvenile-sized spines. However, because the bony purchase is often less than optimal, bracing is often required in juvenile patients postoperatively.

Winter[204] devised a formula for determining potential lost axial growth after spinal fusion in these skeletally im-

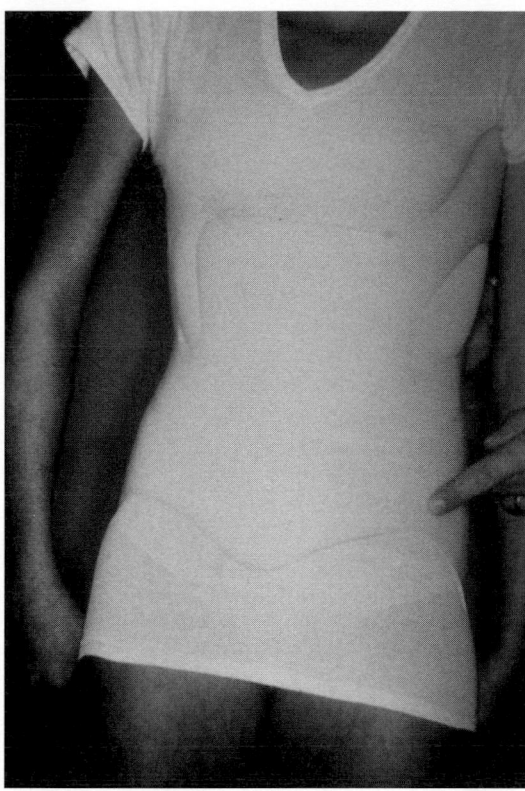

Figure 75-14 Picture of a patient wearing a Boston-type thoracolumbar sacral orthosis (TLSO).

mature patients. One can multiply 0.07 by the number of segments fused and then multiply that by the number of years of growth remaining. This will be the amount in centimeters of axial growth lost by spinal fusion in the juvenile patient. However, the parents and child must be informed that allowing a progressive curve to proceed untreated may often mean surgical correction at a later date and may provide less correction and an even shorter trunk and torso in the long run. If surgical fusion of the skeletally immature spine is deemed necessary, clinical judgment must be utilized to ascertain whether both anterior and posterior fusions are necessary to prevent loss of correction and deterioration of cosmesis secondary to the crankshaft phenomenon.

Adolescent Idiopathic Scoliosis

Adolescent idiopathic curves are those detected after the age of 10 and extending up to the age of 21. Adolescent idiopathic curves are the most common deformities presenting to a pediatric spinal specialist. If 10° is the minimal level of curvature required to diagnose scoliosis, the prevalence of adolescent idiopathic curves is approximately 2 to 3 percent (ages 14 to 16). As curve magnitude increases, the overall prevalence decreases. Although the overall female predominance of 3.6:1 for all curve magnitudes is seen, there is an overwhelming female predominance of approximately 10:1 in curves greater than 30°. Typical curve patterns seen include right thoracic (90 percent), double major (right thoracic, left lumbar), left and right

thoracolumbar and lumbar, and double thoracic (left upper thoracic, right main thoracic) curves. Of note, a primary left thoracic curve pattern is known to be associated with a fairly high incidence of intraspinal anomalies such as syringomyelia and warrants investigation of the spinal canal with an MRI exam prior to any treatment[43,160,172] (see Fig. 75-6).

The main concern in the skeletally immature patient with idiopathic scoliosis relates to the risk of curve progression.[56,163,192] In the immature patient, the risk of progression is related primarily to the amount of growth potential remaining as well as specific factors relating to the curve.[46,193] Overall, five factors have been determined to influence the probability of curve progression in the skeletally immature patient, such that a greater risk of progression occurs: (1) the younger the patient at the time of diagnosis; (2) in premenarcheal females; (3) patients with lower Risser grade at curve detection (Fig. 75-16); (4) patients with larger curve magnitude at detection; and (5) in association with thoracic hypokyphosis.[133] These factors should be taken into account when counseling patients regarding the risk of progression. Using the aforementioned criteria, the scenario of the patient who is at high risk of progression includes a 34° right thoracic scoliosis in a 12-year-old premenarcheal Risser 0 female. Lonstein and Carlson have developed nomograms and tables to help predict the risk of curve progression.[133] This information is useful in counseling families and patients in order to help determine appropriate treatment.[70]

Bracing is the only nonoperative treatment to have a role in the treatment of adolescent idiopathic scoliosis. Electrical stimulation of the convex aspect of the scoliosis has not proven to change the natural history of this condition and is thus currently not widely utilized.[11] Bracing of adolescent idiopathic scoliosis is indicated only in those patients who have significant spinal growth remaining. The immediate goal is to improve the short-term natural history of curve progression. The long-term goal is to keep curves below 40° once skeletal maturity is achieved. Currently, bracing is recommended for skeletally immature patients with 30 to 45° curves at presentation and those with 25 to 30° curves that have documented 5° of progression already.[134,153] A Boston-type orthosis (underarm) is the most common brace utilized for adolescent thoracic idiopathic scoliosis[17,18,77,210] (see Fig. 75-14). A recent prospective, multicenter study documented the effectiveness of underarm Boston-type bracing in the skeletally immature patient with thoracic adolescent idiopathic scoliosis.[156] Occasionally, a Milwaukee brace, or cervical-thoracic-lumbar-sacral orthosis (CTLSO), may be required for thoracic curves with a high apex (T7 and above) and also to control double thoracic curves (Fig. 75-17). For thoracic scoliosis, one must be aware that bracing may often accentuate both thoracic hypokyphosis and lordosis and may be contraindicated, due to adverse consequences for pulmonary function, in cases where progressive loss of thoracic kyphosis is documented radiographically.[211] One must also recognize that compliance with brace wear may be less than optimal in these patients.[71]

Indications for surgical correction of adolescent idiopathic scoliosis are based on our knowledge of its natural

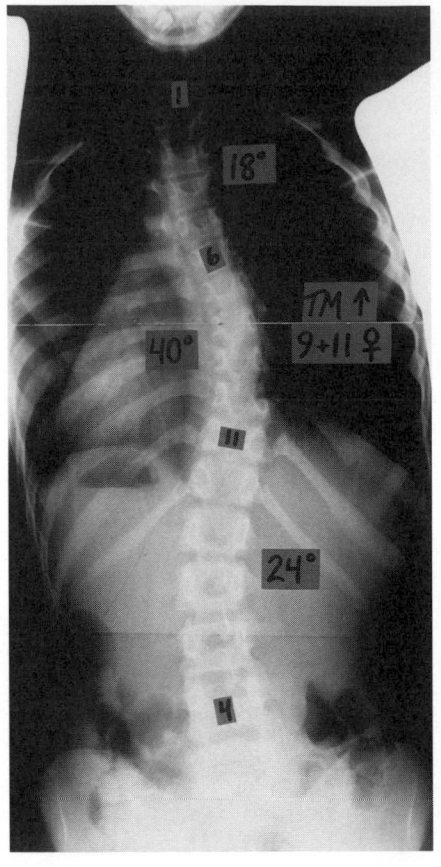

A

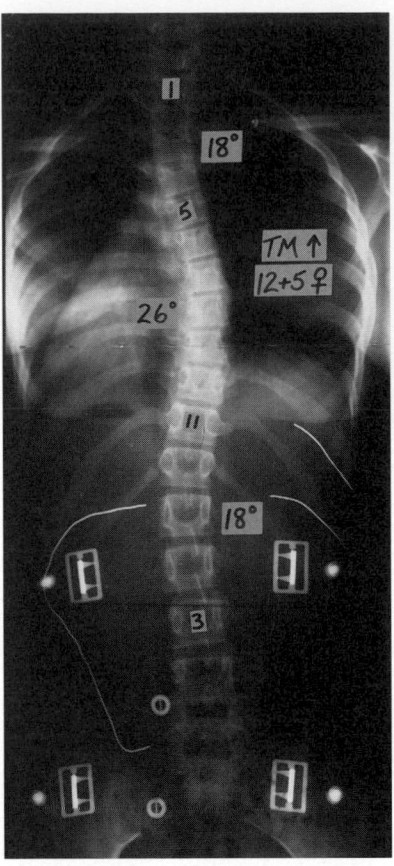

B

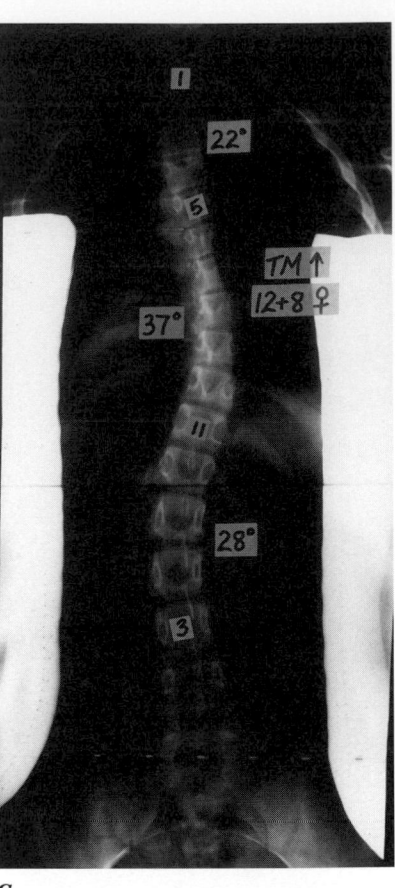

C

Figure 75-15 T.M., a 9 + 11-year-old female, presented with (*A*) a 40° juvenile right thoracic idiopathic scoliosis. Risser 0 at that time, she was placed into a Boston underarm orthosis, which she wore for nearly 3 years. Her in brace x-ray (*B*) at age 12 + 5 years shows her deformity to be well corrected in the brace at 26° in the right thoracic region and 18° in the left lumbar region. At this point she was nearing skeletal maturity and had reached menarche 1 1/2 years earlier. Therefore she was told to wear her brace only at night. When she was 12 + 8 years of age, her x-ray (*C*) without the brace showed maintenance of her spinal curves at 37° in the thoracic region and 28° in the lumbar region, her thoracic curve being less than the initial 40° at presentation.

history when it is untreated.[10,76,194] Basically, curves greater than 40° most commonly progress at 1 to 2° per year following skeletal maturity. However, skeletally immature patients are at risk for a more rapid increase in curve magnitude during the adolescent growth spurt.

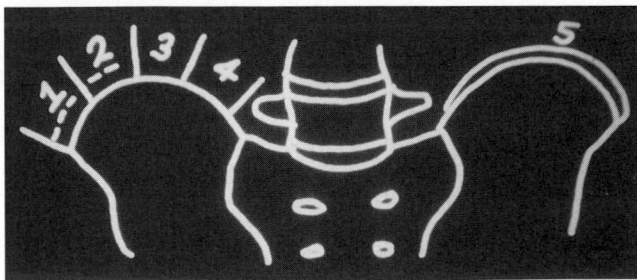

Figure 75-16 Schematic for the evaluation of skeletal maturity via the Risser sign. Risser 0 indicates skeletal immaturity, while Risser 5 indicates full skeletal maturation.

Currently, surgical recommendations vary somewhat depending upon the degree of skeletal maturity, curve magnitude, sagittal plane alignment, and the patient's clinical appearance. In simple terms, curves over 50° are treated surgically; curves under 40° are either braced in the immature patient or observed in the more mature patient; and curves between 40 and 50° are in a gray zone and are analyzed individually. Certainly in those patients who are skeletally immature and have curves greater than 40 to 50°, surgery is recommended because of the high risk of curve progression in these patients.

There are both radiographic and clinical criteria for optimal surgical success in these patients. The radiographic criteria include having a well centered fusion mass with the appropriate fusion levels included in the surgery. Ideally, when fusing to L2 and below, the lowest instrumented vertebra (LIV) should be bisected by the center sacral line, horizontal to the top of the iliac crest, and neutral in rotation.[158] The center sacral line bisects the sacrum and is perpendicular to a line drawn horizontally to the top of the iliac crest[113] (Fig. 75-18). The center

Figure 75-17 A Milwaukee brace is rarely required in adolescent idiopathic scoliosis but is occasionally used when the apex is above T7 or a double thoracic curve pattern is present; and it is also used for some kyphotic deformities. It includes a chin piece that aids in stabilizing the upper thoracic region, along with the appropriate pads and a pelvic girdle. Here is the (*A*) frontal and (*B*) lateral view of the brace.

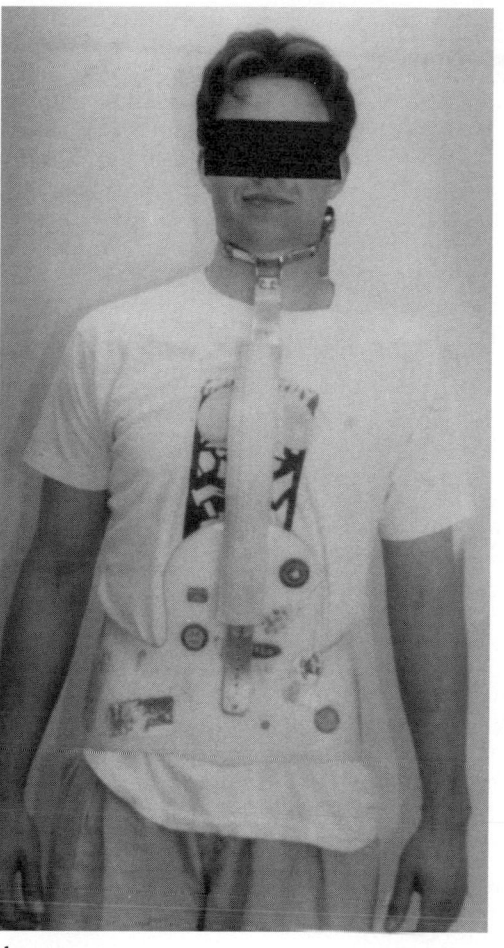

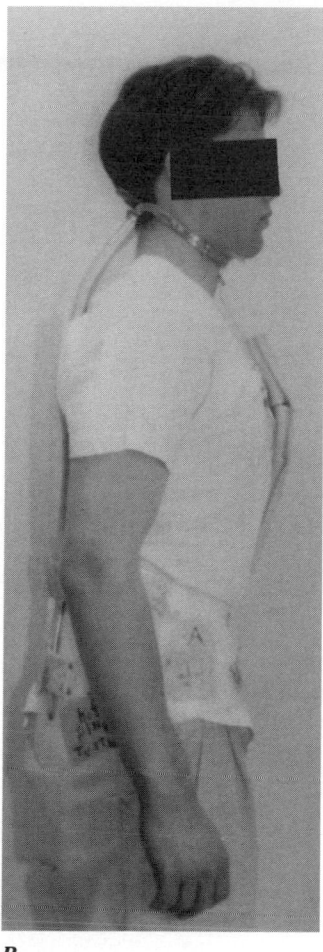

A   *B*

sacral line is important in choosing the stable vertebra, which is the most proximal lumbar vertebra bisected by this line, as the LIV for most scoliosis fusions.[113]

In the sagittal plane, a smooth and harmonious sagittal contour of thoracic kyphosis, a neutral to slightly lordotic thoracolumbar junction, and appropriate instrumented and noninstrumented lumbar lordosis are important.[20] It has become increasingly apparent that sagittal alignment, especially of the thoracolumbar and lumbar spine, may prove extremely important for the long-term surgical success of scoliosis fusions.[38] In this regard, fusing the lumbar spine flat promotes hyperextension of the lower lumbar disks, with resultant premature degeneration and production of the flat-back syndrome.[55]

The clinical goals of surgery for idiopathic scoliosis include having the base of the neck centered over the pelvis, thus producing a balanced plumbline. The shoulders should be level to the horizontal pelvis. The thoracic rib hump deformity should ideally also be improved both for cosmetic reasons and to limit the potential development of late scapulothoracic pain. It is becoming increasingly apparent that scoliosis patients are truly concerned about their overall physical appearance and specifically the degree of their deformity. In this regard, postoperative patients report increased satisfaction following curve cor-

rection that allows the torso and trunk to appear more normal (Fig. 75-19). Following a scoliosis fusion, most postoperative patients prefer to have their bodies appear as normal as possible.

In patients being prepared for surgery, the minimal preoperative studies include long-cassette AP and lateral standing radiographs along with the supine right- and left-side bending films assessing the flexibility of all curves of the thoracic and lumbar spine. A traction or push-prone film provides a dynamic assessment of the effect that correction of the main structural curve has upon adjacent curves (Fig. 75-20). Simplistically, the proximal fusion level is the neutral vertebra at the upper end of the most structural curve. The distal fusion level is normally the stable vertebra, which is the most proximal lumbar vertebra bisected by the center sacral line.

The routine use of preoperative MRI scans in adolescent idiopathic scoliosis is still somewhat controversial. Certainly, any patient with an atypical curve pattern such as the left thoracic curve, an unusual sagittal plane, an abnormal neurologic exam, more rapid curve progression than can be accounted for by skeletal growth alone, or any unusual pain or limitation of back flexibility should undergo preoperative MRI scanning[107] (Fig. 75-21). A large curve magnitude in and of itself does not appear to be an

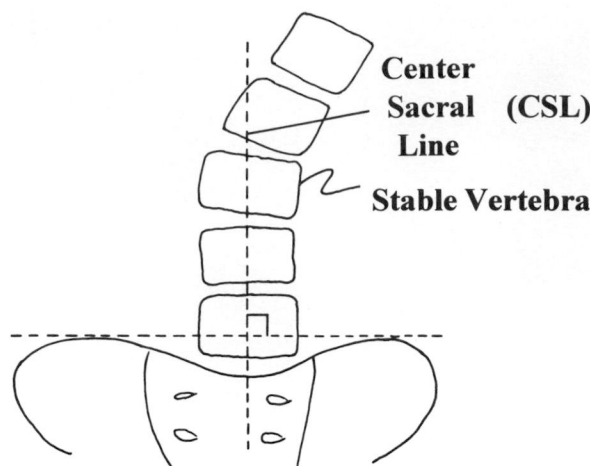

Figure 75-18 The center sacral line (CSL) bisects the proximal sacrum and is perpendicular to a horizontal line at the top of the iliac crest. The most proximal lumbar vertebra bisected by this line is known as the stable vertebra.

indication for a preoperative scan.[160] Pulmonary function testing is probably indicated only for patients being considered for thoracotomies or thoracoplasties, those who have any type of significant pulmonary history, or those

with a severely lordotic thoracic sagittal contour.[1]

Adolescent idiopathic scoliosis is classified anatomically into thoracic (apex T2-T11), thoracolumbar (apex T12-L1), and lumbar (apex L2-L4) curves. Thoracic curves are most commonly classified into five types via the King classification[113] (Fig. 75-22). When two or three structural curves are identified, these are noted as double and triple major scoliosis, respectively.

The modern era of segmental spinal fixation began with the introduction of Cotrel-Dubousset instrumentation in the 1980s.[24] Prior to this, Harrington instrumentation was the gold standard of spinal instrumentation.[55] Although many different forms of segmental fixation are currently available, the benefits derived from these systems are quite similar. These include the stable fixation provided, which obviates external immobilization; ability to perform selective compression and distraction forces on the same rod at different locations; and better control of the sagittal plane, especially in the lumbar spine.[122] Most adolescent idiopathic curves are approached posteriorly alone for instrumentation and fusion. Indications for anterior releases and fusion followed by posterior instrumentation and fusion include patients with large curve magnitudes (greater than 75 to 80°), patients who are extremely skeletally immature (Risser 0, premenarcheal), and those with a significant kyphotic sagittal alignment over the scoliotic segments. Many or most thoracolumbar

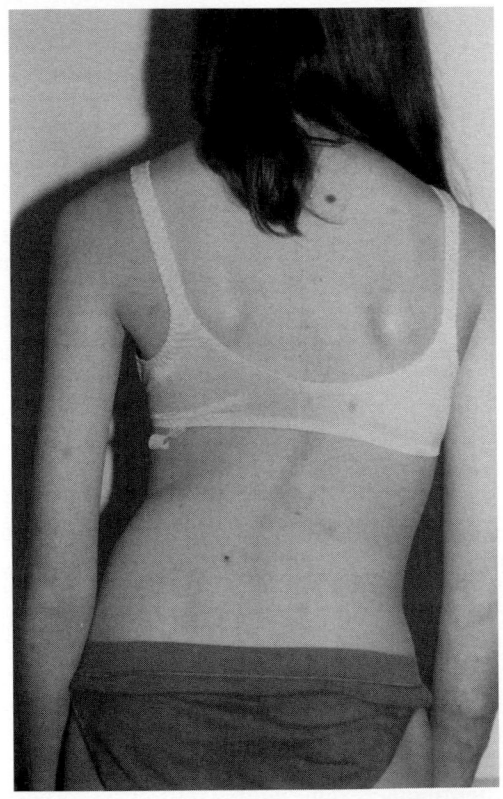

A

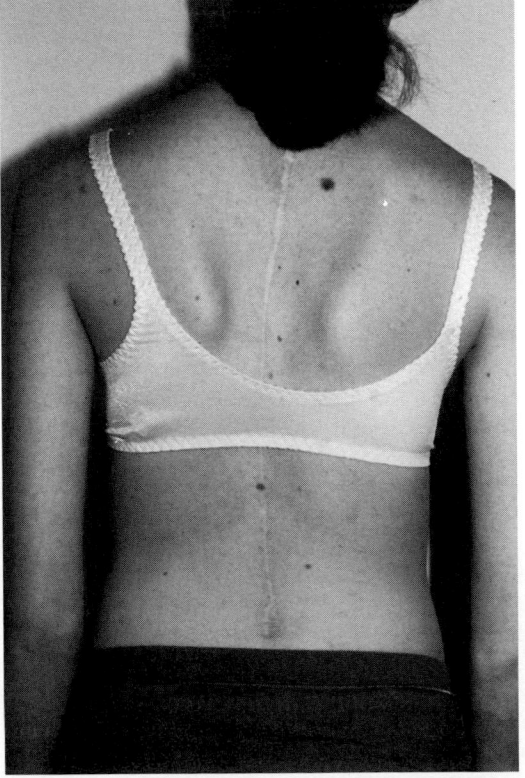

B

Figure 75-19 Preoperative coronal photo (*A*) of an adolescent idiopathic scoliosis patient demonstrating a right trunk shift as well as coronal decompensation to the right. Two-year post-operative photo (*B*) showing normalized trunk and plumbline alignment following a posterior spinal fusion with thoracoplasty.

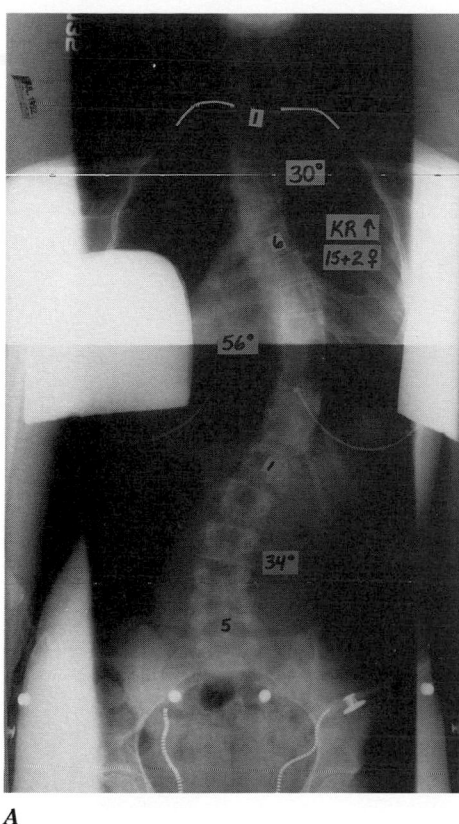
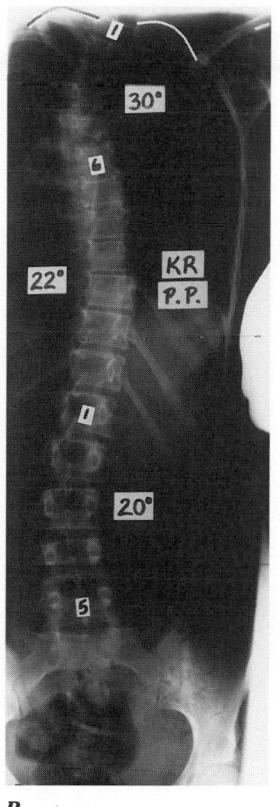
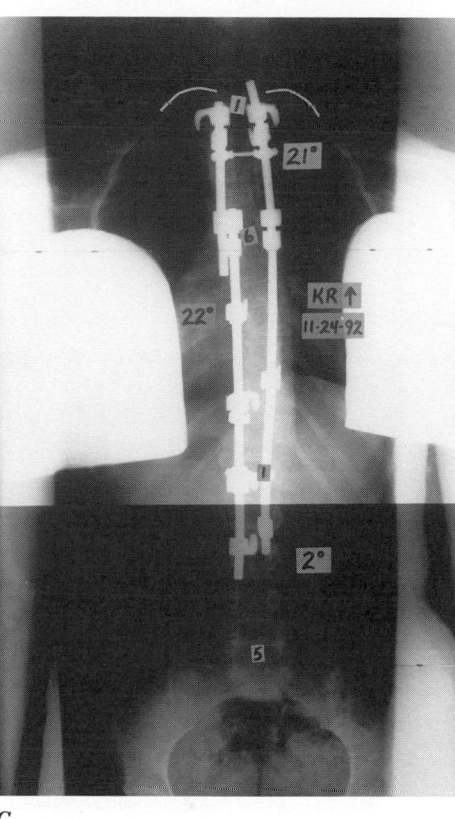

A   *B*   *C*

Figure 75-20 K.R., a 15 + 2-year-old female, has a 56° right thoracic idiopathic scoliosis. Her coronal x-ray (*A*) also demonstrates a 30° left thoracic scoliosis with slightly positive T1 tilt in that her first rib is slightly higher than the right. A push-prone coronal x-ray (*B*) demonstrates active correction of the main thoracic curve down to 22°. The left upper thoracic curve is maintained at 30°, with marked elevation of the left first rib versus the right. Thus, this curve pattern must be treated as a double thoracic curve, and both thoracic curves must be instrumented and fused. Postoperative x-ray (*C*) following a T2-L2 posterior spinal fusion with instrumentation shows good correction of the scoliosis with level first rib heights and well-balanced shoulders.

and lumbar curves are more appropriately treated with anterior instrumentation and fusion. This usually allows a shorter fusion level and the ability in selected cases to perform isolated correction of just the thoracolumbar and lumbar components while leaving the compensatory thoracic curve alone. Additionally, anterior instrumentation and fusion of thoracic curves is an available technique for improving thoracic kyphosis in those patients who are hypokyphotic or frankly lordotic in the sagittal plane. This may also be useful to save distal fusion levels where posterior instrumentation and fusion would be required for thoracic scoliosis.

King et al. classified thoracic scoliosis into five types[113] (see Fig. 75-22). A King I curve is a thoracic and lumbar curve where the lumbar curve is larger and less flexible than the thoracic curve, though both curves are usually structural and require fusion. Occasionally, only the lumbar curve requires fusion in a King type I curve as long as shoulder balance will be maintained postoperatively. If both curves are treated, normally posterior instrumentation and fusion are performed to L3 or L4, depending upon the lumbar curve magnitude, flexibility, rotation, and apical distance from the center sacral line (Fig. 75-23).

A King II curve is a primary thoracic curve with a compensatory lumbar curve that crosses the midline but is less structural and more flexible than the thoracic curve. Ideally, a King II curve can undergo selective thoracic fusion, thus leaving the mobile lumbar spine below unfused. This curve has been somewhat troublesome for scoliosis surgeons since the advent of segmental spinal fixation because of the problem of early postoperative coronal decompensation[39,120] (Fig. 75-24). While many theories have been popularized for both the production and treatment of these decompensations, our experience has been that the problem occurs with both improper identification of which King II curves can successfully undergo selective thoracic fusion as well as the difficulty in performing specific instrumentation sequences that will allow a balanced lumbar spine below the instrumented thoracic spine.[120] We prefer analyzing the relative ratios between thoracic and lumbar curve magnitude, rotation, and deviation from the midline at the apex of both curves to help classify them. When the aforementioned thoracic to lumbar ratios are 1.2:1 or greater, these curves may be classified as true type II curves. These curves may then be treated with selective thoracic instrumentation and fusion provided that a thoracolumbar junctional

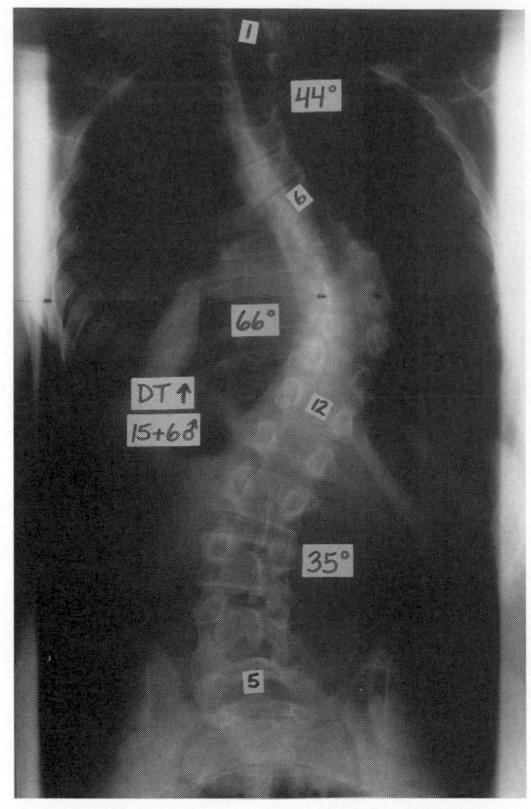

A

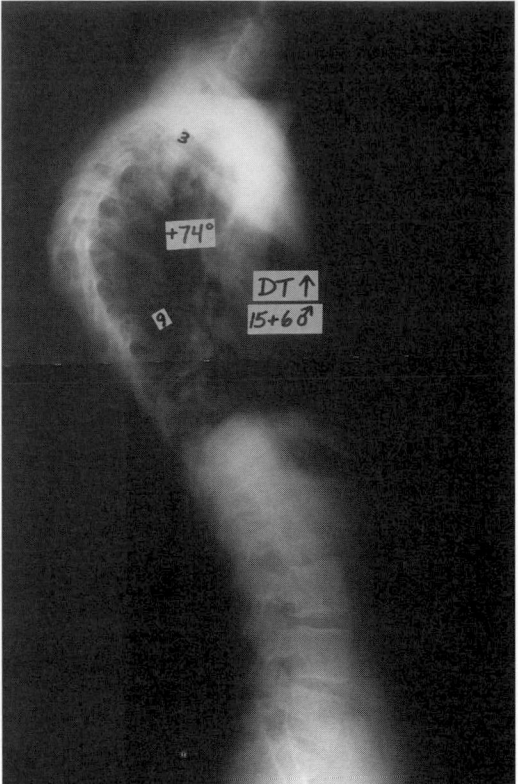

B

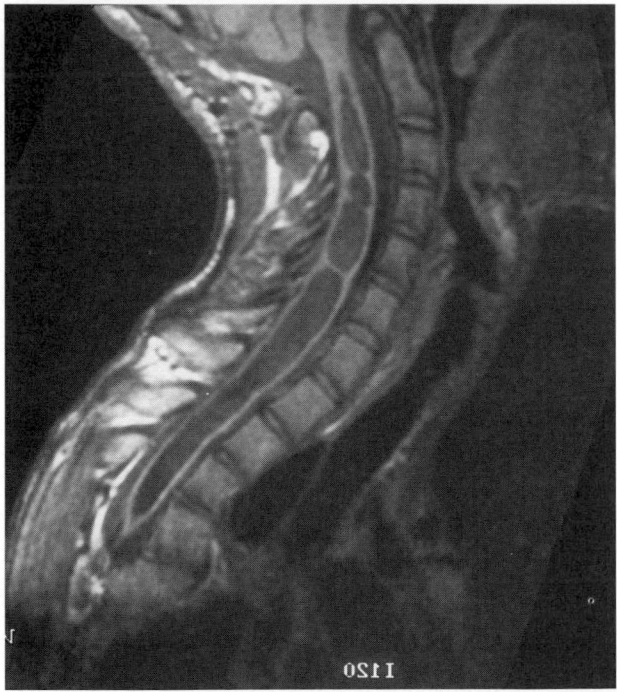

C

Figure 75-21 D.T., a 15 + 6-year-old male, presented with this (*A*) 44° proximal left thoracic, 66° main right thoracic idiopathic-appearing scoliosis. His history and exam were otherwise unremarkable except for excessive thoracic kyphosis. His sagittal x-ray (*B*) showed 74° of kyphosis from T3 to T9. Because of the increased thoracic kyphosis prior to his planned scoliosis fusion, he underwent a total-spine MRI scan, which showed (*C*) a large cervicothoracic syrinx and an Arnold-Chiari type II malformation requiring neurosurgical intervention. This reinforces the importance of considering adolescent idiopathic scoliosis to be a diagnosis of exclusion. Although the coronal x-ray was that of a "typical" adolescent idiopathic deformity, the sagittal x-ray demonstrating marked thoracic hyperkyphosis was atypical and warranted the MRI scan prior to correction of the spinal deformity.

kyphosis is not present and the magnitude of the lumbar curve is less than 65°.

Once an appropriate King II curve is identified for selective thoracic fusion, it is important to limit thoracic curve correction by avoiding a full 90° rod rotation ma-

neuver and relying more on selective compression and distraction forces. As a guideline, one should not correct the thoracic curve beyond the side-bending correction of the lumbar curve. It is also important to leave tilt to the lowest instrumented vertebra at the thoracolumbar junction,

(*Text continues on page 1407.*)

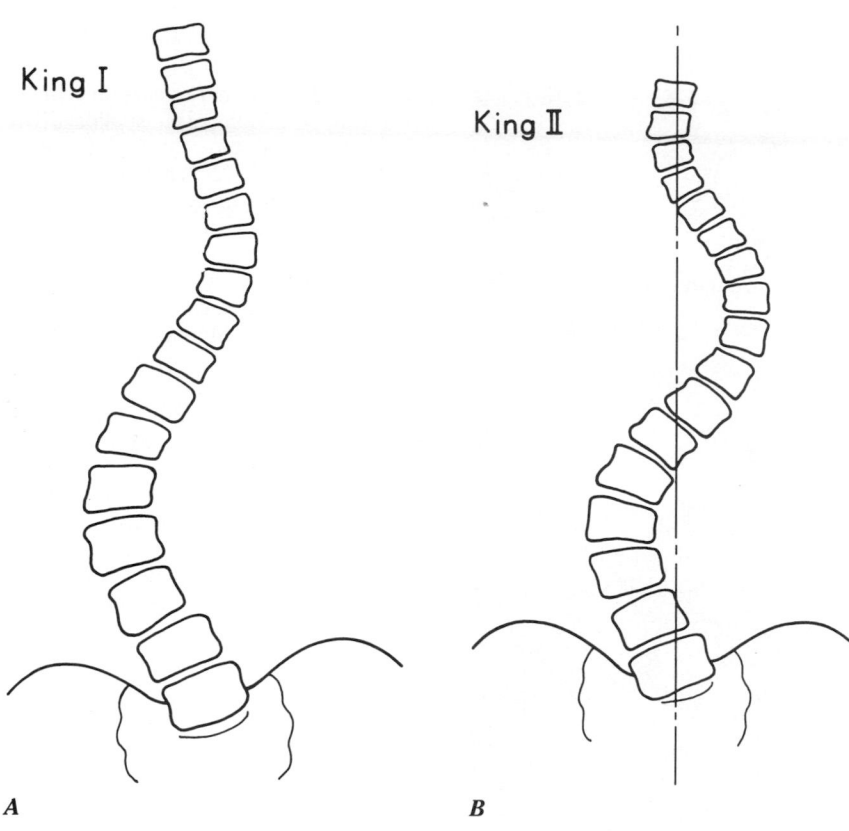

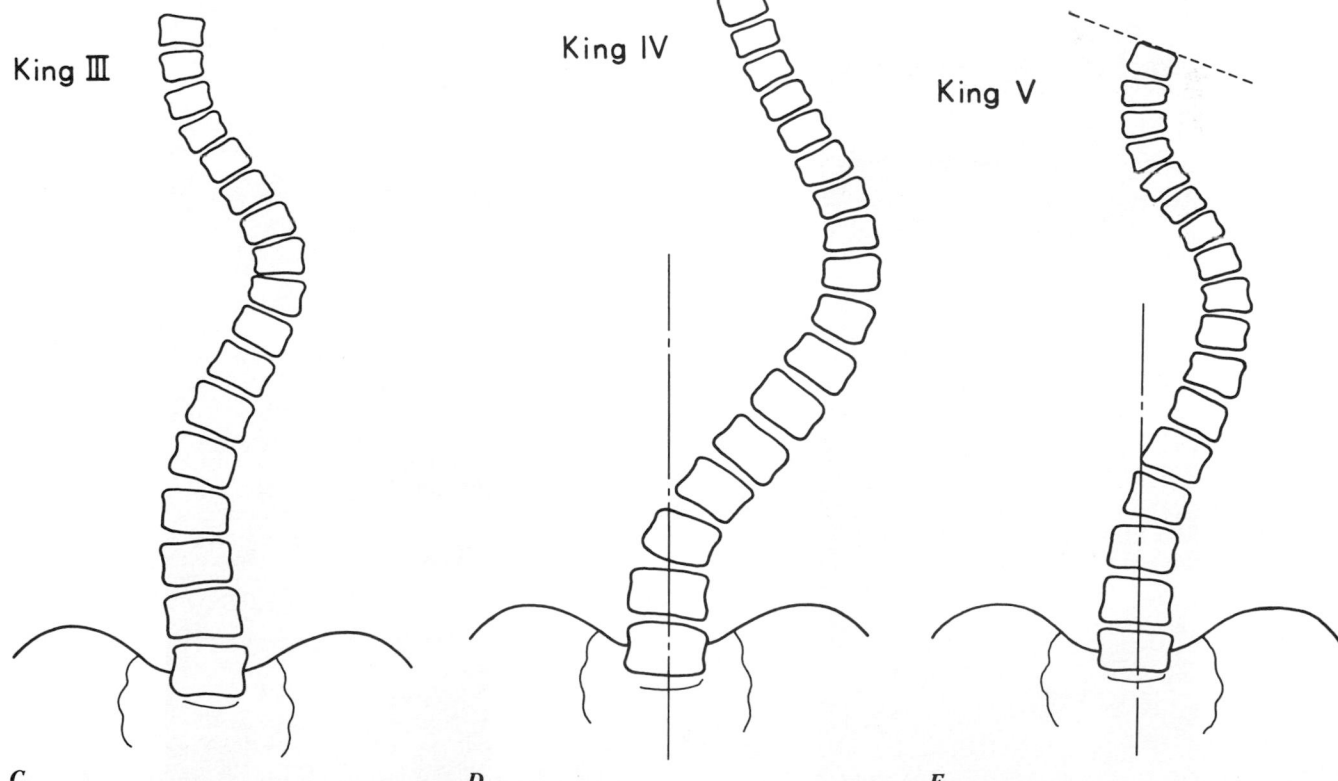

Figure 75-22 The King classification, I through V. *A.* A type I curve is a right thoracic–left lumbar curve where the lumbar curve is more structural and less flexible than the thoracic curve. *B.* A type II curve is a right thoracic–left lumbar curve where the thoracic curve is more structural and less flexible than the lumbar curve. Certain type II curves may undergo selective thoracic instrumentation and fusion. *C.* A type III curve is a right thoracic curve with the lumbar curve not crossing the midline and not structural. *D.* A type IV curve is a long right thoracic curve with a lower apex (T8-T10), where L4 is tilted into the curve but is the stable vertebra. *E.* A type V curve is a double thoracic curve with a proximal left thoracic–main right thoracic curve. It is noted by a positive T1 tilt where the left side of T1 is high and the right side of T1 is low, thus elevating the left first rib above the right first rib.

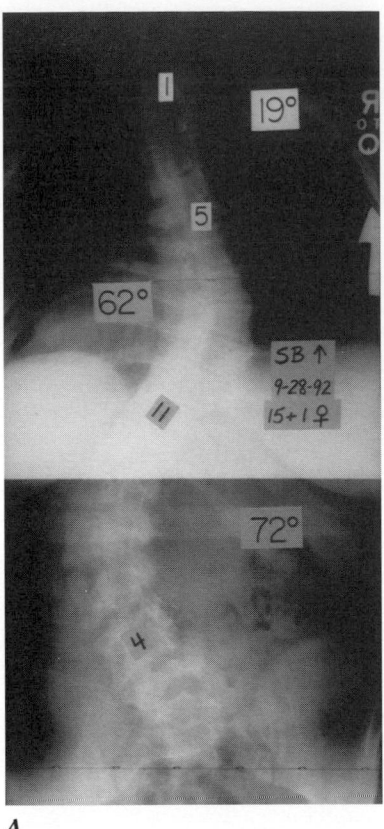

A

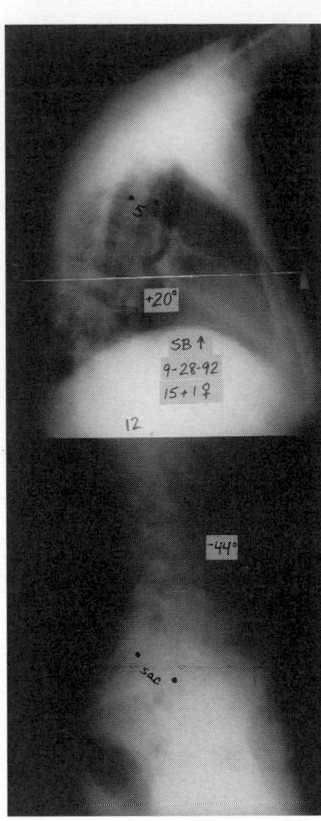

B

Figure 75-23 S.B., a 15-year-old female, has a King type I idiopathic scoliosis. The preoperative coronal x-ray (*A*) showed a 62° right thoracic, 72° left lumbar curve. The lumbar curve had more rotation and deviation from the midline; it was stiffer than the thoracic curve, thus satisfying the criteria for a King type I deformity. *B.* The sagittal plane showed mild thoracic hypokyphosis and lumbar hypolordosis. The patient was treated with a posterior instrumentation and fusion from T4 to L4, with iliac crest bone graft. Her 2 + 2-year postoperative coronal x-ray (*C*) shows correction of her scoliosis to 35° in the thoracic region and 40° in the lumbar region, with a well-balanced spine. *D.* The patient's sagittal x-ray shows mild improvement in thoracic kyphosis and lumbar lordosis with a harmonious and balanced sagittal plane.

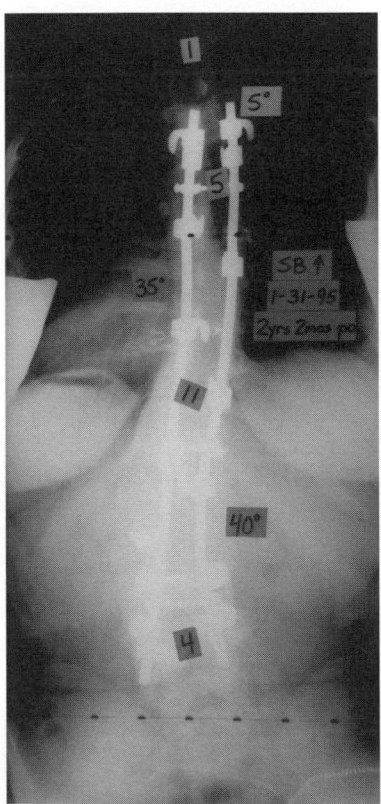

C

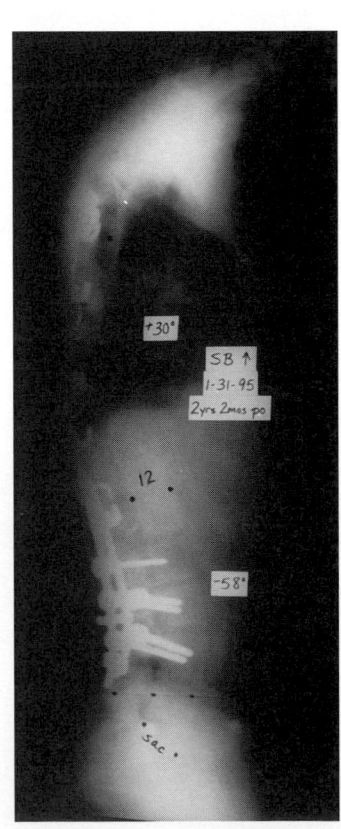

D

Figure 75-24 A.B., a 10 + 6-year-old female, has a 42° right thoracic, 37° left lumbar curve (in a brace); she had been treated elsewhere. Her 7-month postoperative x-ray following a T6-T12 posterior instrumentation and fusion shows marked progression of her left lumbar curve with coronal decompensation to the left.

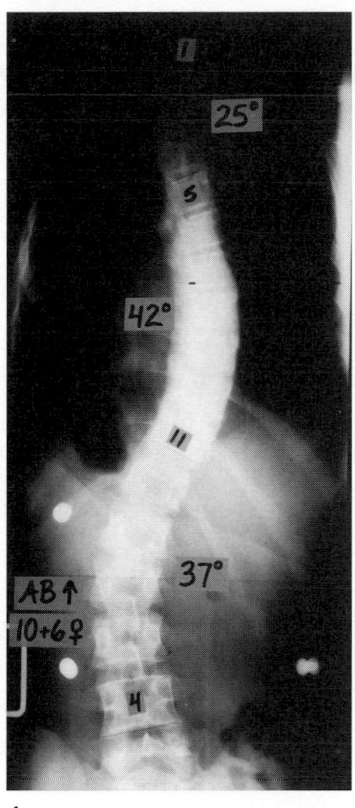

A

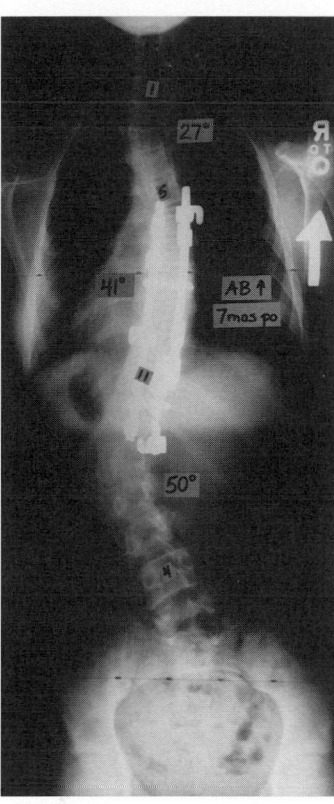

B

as most of these curves have their fusion ending at either T12 or L1, whichever is the most stable (Fig. 75-25). Anterior thoracic instrumentation and fusion may also allow selective thoracic fusion of more flexible thoracic type II curves. Whether these curves are treated posteriorly or anteriorly, the goal is modest correction of the thoracic deformity to accommodate the lumbar spine below and produce a well-balanced spine. Some surgeons advocate instrumentation and fusion down to L2 or L3 in King type II curves. By using bilateral pedicle screw fixation at L1, L2, and L3, the lumbar curve may be derotated and the fusion stopped at L3 or even occasionally L2.[121]

King type III curves are standard right thoracic curves without structural components either above in the upper thoracic region or below in the lumbar spine. These curves are treated with segmental instrumentation and fusion to the stable vertebra, which is usually L1, L2, or L3. The specific types of correction maneuvers depend upon many factors, including curve flexibility, location of the apex, preoperative shoulder balance, and the alignment of the thoracic sagittal plane (Fig. 75-26).

The King IV curve is also a right thoracic curve but extends into the lower lumbar spine such that L4 is tilted into the curve but is the stable vertebra. These curves usually require instrumentation and fusion that extends into the lower lumbar spine, usually L3 or L4 if treated posteriorly (Fig. 75-27). In select cases of flexible curves, instrumentation and fusion may end one level proximal to the stable vertebra, with a well-balanced spine produced.[121]

King V curves are double structural thoracic curves where the left upper thoracic curve as well as the main right thoracic curve must be instrumented and fused. Radiographically, a structural upper thoracic curve is noted by a positive T1 tilt, elevation of the left versus right first rib, and a curve that is greater than 35° upright and bends out to no less than 20° on side bending.[124] It is important always to assess the structural characteristics of the left upper thoracic curve even when the shoulders are level or the right shoulder is slightly higher preoperatively in the treatment of a main right thoracic scoliosis. Greater correction of the main thoracic curve will potentially elevate the left shoulder if the aforementioned structural characteristics are present (see Fig. 75-20). Postoperative shoulder imbalance is poorly tolerated by scoliosis patients; thus every attempt should be made to obtain optimal shoulder alignment during scoliosis correction.

Double Major Curves

Double major curve patterns have thoracic and lumbar curves of equal structural characteristics. Typically, a right thoracic–left lumbar curve pattern will be present, with a variable sagittal plane alignment. Many of these curves are optimally treated by a rod rotation maneuver of the left-sided rod. This 90° counterclockwise rod rotation transforms the coronal plane deformity into thoracic kyphosis above and lumbar lordosis below (Fig. 75-28). Although hooks are commonly utilized in the thoracic and lumbar spine, the placement of convex lumbar pedicle screws ap-

(Text continues on page 1411.)

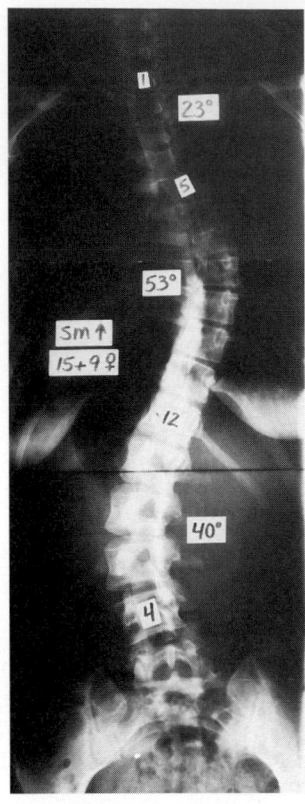

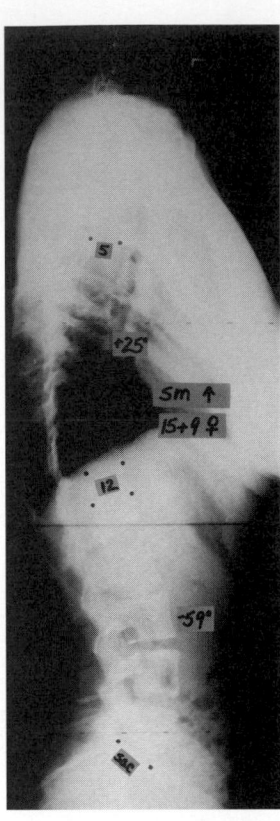

A

B

Figure 75-25 S.M., a 15 + 9-year-old female, has a King type II adolescent idiopathic scoliosis. Her coronal preoperative radiograph (*A*) shows a 53° right thoracic, 40° left lumbar curve. The right thoracic curve has a larger magnitude, is stiffer on side bending than the lumbar curve, has about equal rotation at the apex, but shows more deviation from the midline than the lumbar curve. Thus, this curve does satisfy criteria for selective thoracic instrumentation and fusion. The sagittal x-ray (*B*) demonstrates the absence of a significant thoracolumbar kyphosis. The patient underwent a selective thoracic instrumentation and fusion from T4 to T12, which was her stable vertebra, with selective compression and distraction forces and avoidance of overcorrection of the thoracic curve. She had a thoracoplasty rib resection procedure for correction of her rib hump and as a source of autogenous bone graft. A postoperative x-ray (*C*) in the coronal plane shows a well-balanced spine and correction of the thoracic curve to 30° and spontaneous correction of the lumbar curve to 31°. *D.* The patient's sagittal alignment postoperatively has remained unchanged.

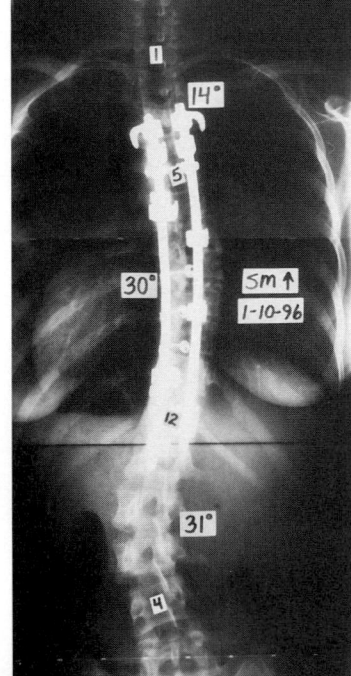

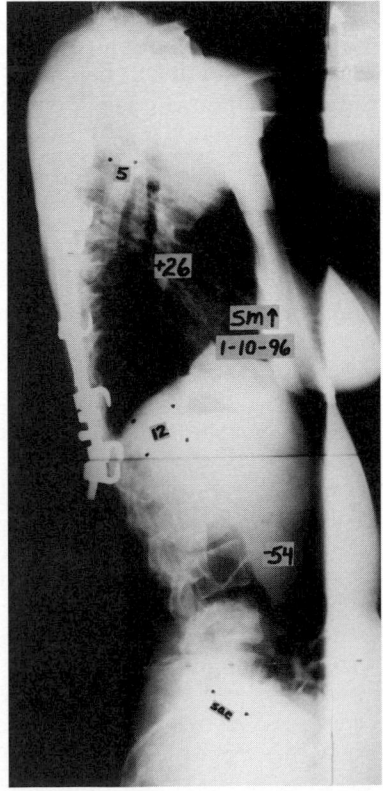

C

D

Figure 75-26 J.C., a 15 + 10-year-old female, has (*A*) a 48° right thoracic King type III idiopathic scoliosis. Her stable vertebra is L3. *B.* Imaging of the sagittal plane shows thoracic hypokyphosis of +10°. The patient underwent a posterior spinal fusion with CD instrumentation from T5 to L2, with a 90° rod rotation maneuver of her left-sided rod for both correction of her scoliosis and production of more normal thoracic kyphosis. Her 2-year postoperative coronal x-ray (*C*) shows a well-balanced spine with 18° of scoliosis and the lowest instrumented vertebra (L2) stable and horizontal to the pelvis. *D.* The patient's postoperative lateral x-ray shows a normalized sagittal plane with improvement of thoracic kyphosis to 23°. This improved thoracic kyphosis was secondary to the 90° rod rotation maneuver, which placed the coronal deformity into increased thoracic kyphosis in the sagittal plane.

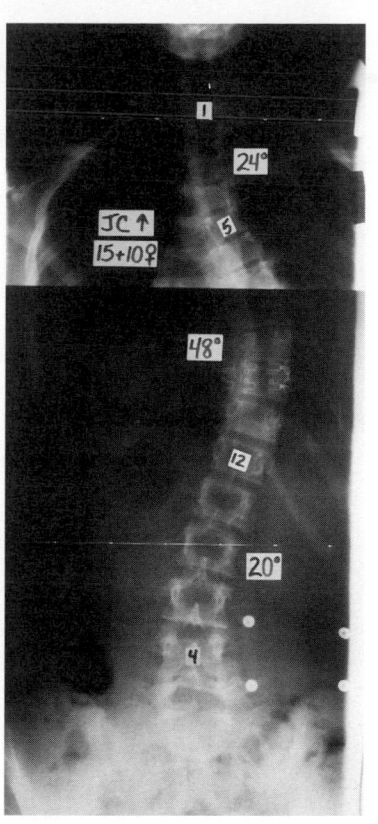

A

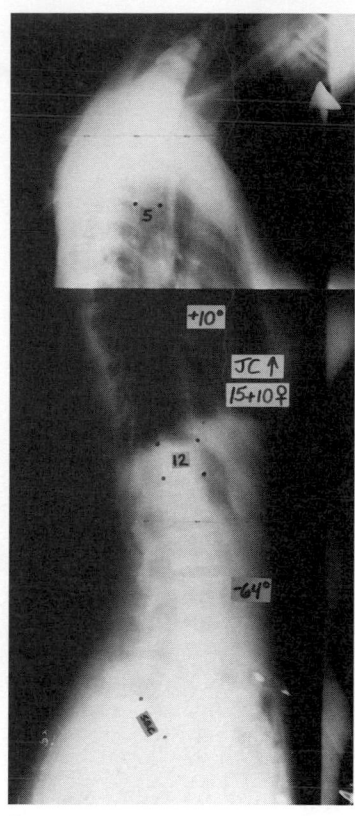

B

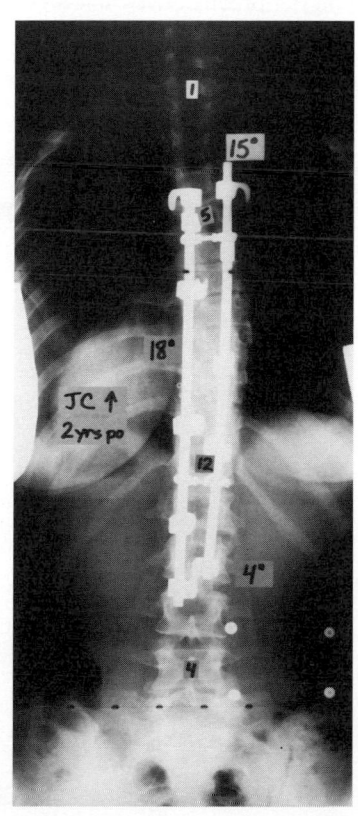

C

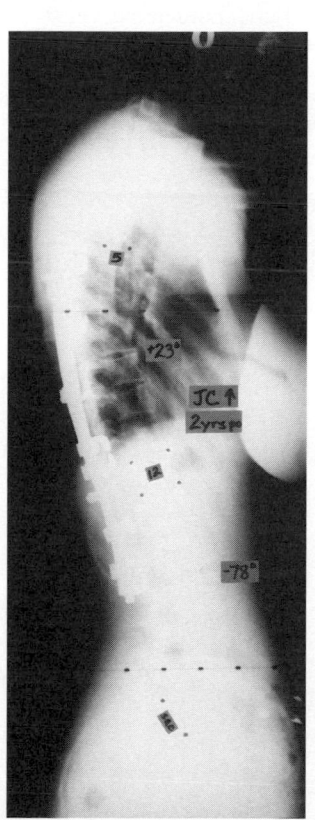

D

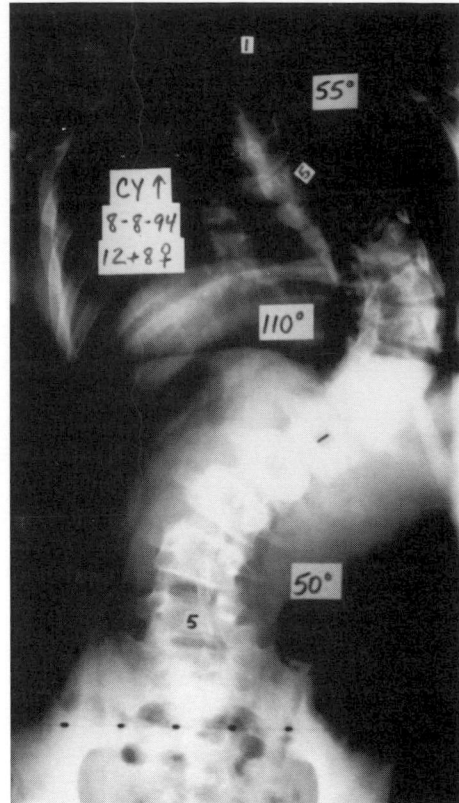

A

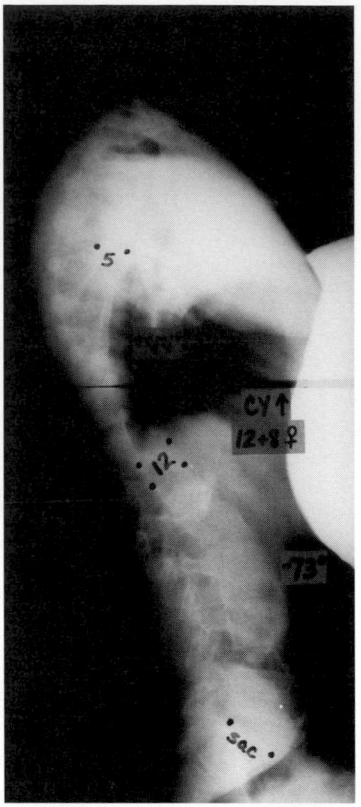

B

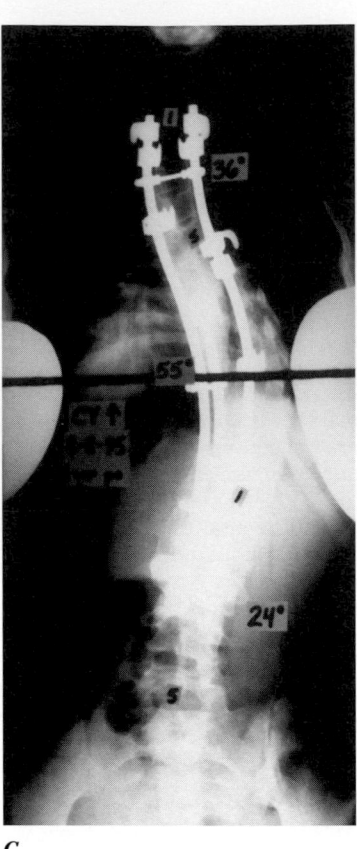

C

Figure 75-27 C.Y., a 12 + 8-year-old skeletally immature female, presented with a 110° thoracic scoliosis. It is important in the case of these large curves to rule out any associated causes such as connective tissue disorders, genetic syndromes, and so on. *A.* Her presenting x-ray showed a 110° right thoracic King type IV deformity where L4 is stable but still tilted into the concavity of the main right thoracic curve. *B.* The sagittal plane was fairly unremarkable. Because of the magnitude of the deformity and the patient's skeletal immaturity, she underwent a same-day anterior and posterior fusion. The first stage anterior included diskectomies and autogenous rib fusion from T5 to L1.

She was then prepared for her posterior instrumentation and fusion, which extended from T2 to L3 with iliac crest bone graft. Her 1-year postoperative coronal x-ray (*C*) shows a balanced spine with approximately 50 percent correction of the main thoracic deformity to 55° and a well-healed spinal fusion. The patient's lateral postoperative x-ray (*D*) shows maintenance of a normal alignment. Her preoperative clinical photo (*E*) demonstrates her marked truncal deformity. Her postoperative clinical photo (*F*) demonstrate restoration of more normal truncal alignment with level shoulders and a balanced plumbline.

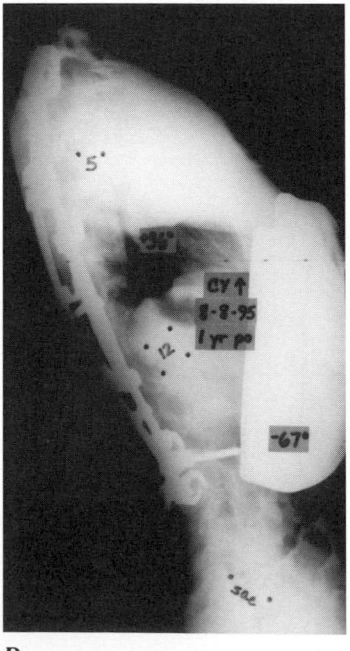

D

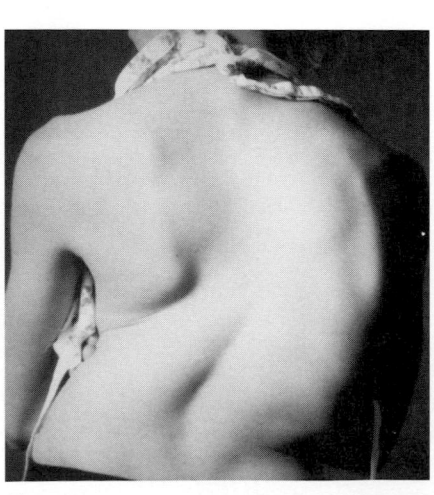

E

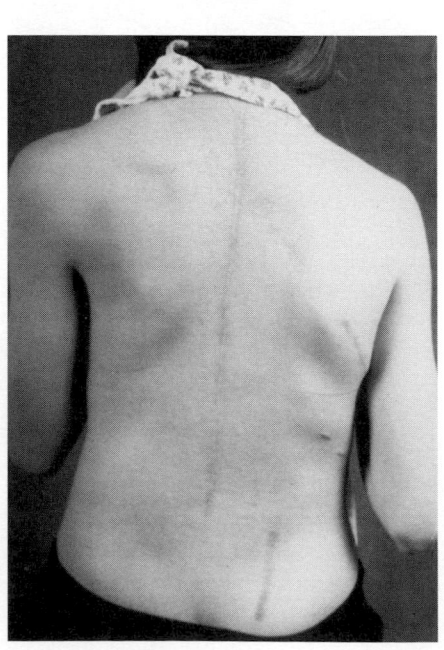

F

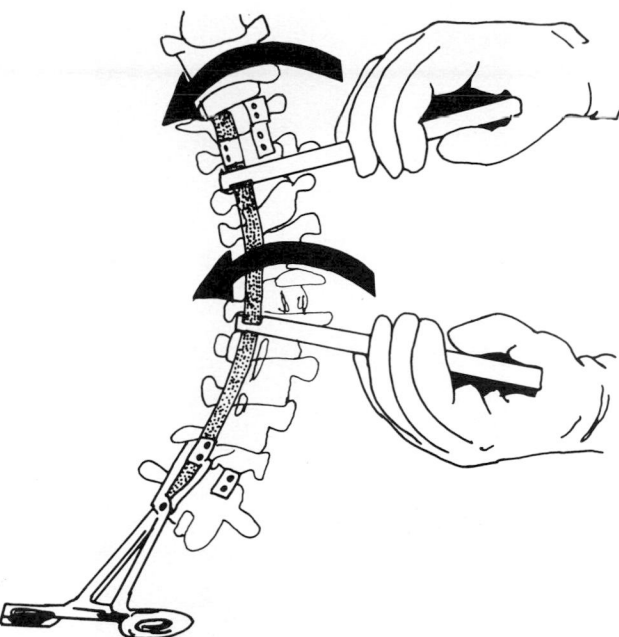

Figure 75-28 Schematic drawing of a 90° rod rotation maneuver for a right thoracic scoliosis whereby the coronal deformity is placed into sagittal thoracic kyphosis with 90° counterclockwise rotation of the rod.

pears to provide superior three-column attachment to the spine to maximize both coronal and sagittal correction[91] (Fig. 75-29). It is important to maintain instrumented lumbar lordosis in the sagittal plane, for this may optimize the long-term function and health of the unfused lumbar spine below.

Thoracolumbar and Lumbar Curves

In thoracolumbar curves, the apex of the deformity is centered between T12 and L1, while in lumbar curves, the apex is between L2 and L4. These curves are much more commonly associated with coronal imbalance to the same side as the convexity of the scoliosis. These curves may produce waistline asymmetry and trunk shifts, which are cosmetically objectionable to adolescent patients. These curves are most commonly treated with anterior instrumentation and fusion as the primary corrective technique. This usually allows fusing less distal lumbar levels, which is an important goal for curves such as these, based in the thoracolumbar and lumbar spine. Following thorough diskectomies, structural bone graft or cages packed with morcellized bone are placed in the anterior half of the disk space prior to the application of segmental compression forces on the convexity of the curve. These structural grafts or cages in the anterior half of the disk spaces allow for improved sagittal plane correction and avoidance of instrumentation kyphosis, which is a known consequence of anterior convex compression. Thus the goal for sagittal plane correction is to have the thoracolumbar spine in a neutral to slightly lordotic position, with increasing lumbar lordosis as one proceeds distally along

the lumbar spine. Using the aforementioned techniques, we have been able to maintain adequate coronal correction while maintaining or even enhancing instrumented lumbar lordosis in treating thoracolumbar and lumbar curves with anterior compression instrumentation. Currently, the use of solid anterior rods with screw and staple fixation of the vertebral bodies instrumented is the preferred technique (Fig. 75-30).

The short-term results after segmental spinal fixation of adolescent idiopathic scoliosis have been quite good. Postoperative coronal decompensation in King type II curves is less commonly encountered due to better definition and more appropriate treatment of these curve types. Results 5 to 10 years after segmental spinal fixation for adolescent idiopathic scoliosis are now becoming available, with favorable radiographic and clinical results thus far. Certainly, though, long-term (more than 10 to 20 years) follow-up will be needed to confirm the short- and midterm results. Thus far, the main advantages of segmental spinal fixation appear to be improved control of the sagittal plane with less reliance on external immobilization postoperatively. Although they are well accepted in the thoracolumbar and lumbar spine, the future of anterior instrumentation and fusion for thoracic scoliosis is uncertain. Regardless of the operative approach or the type of instrumentation, the goal still remains to obtain a solid fusion of the spine in a well-balanced position.

Complications of Scoliosis Surgery

Although one of the most feared complications of scoliosis surgery is postoperative spinal cord injury with subsequent paralysis, this is a fairly rare event. The use of spinal cord monitoring with or without a wake-up test to document lower extremity neurologic function following correction of scoliosis and other spinal deformities should be routine. The rate of deep wound infection is less than 1 percent, and cardiac and pulmonary problems are also infrequently encountered in healthy patients with spinal deformities. Certainly these risks increase in patients who have concomitant disease processes, such as neuromuscular disorders. The pseudarthrosis rate in idiopathic patients utilizing autogenous bone graft should be at most 1 to 2 percent. However, it is possible for rigid segmental spinal fixation to hide asymptomatic pseudarthroses; thus long-term follow-up is warranted.

Congenital Scoliosis

Congenital scoliosis is a lateral curvature of the spine secondary to development of vertebral anomalies producing imbalance of longitudinal growth. Although the vertebral anomalies are present at birth, the clinical deformity may not become evident until later in childhood, when a scoliosis develops and the diagnosis is made with radiographs. The hallmark of congenital scoliosis is a radiograph showing vertebral anomalies in part of the curvature.[174]

McMaster reported on the natural history of 251 congenital scoliosis patients and found that all degrees of curve severity were seen at all different ages.[148] He found that severe curves were extremely rigid and that their sur-

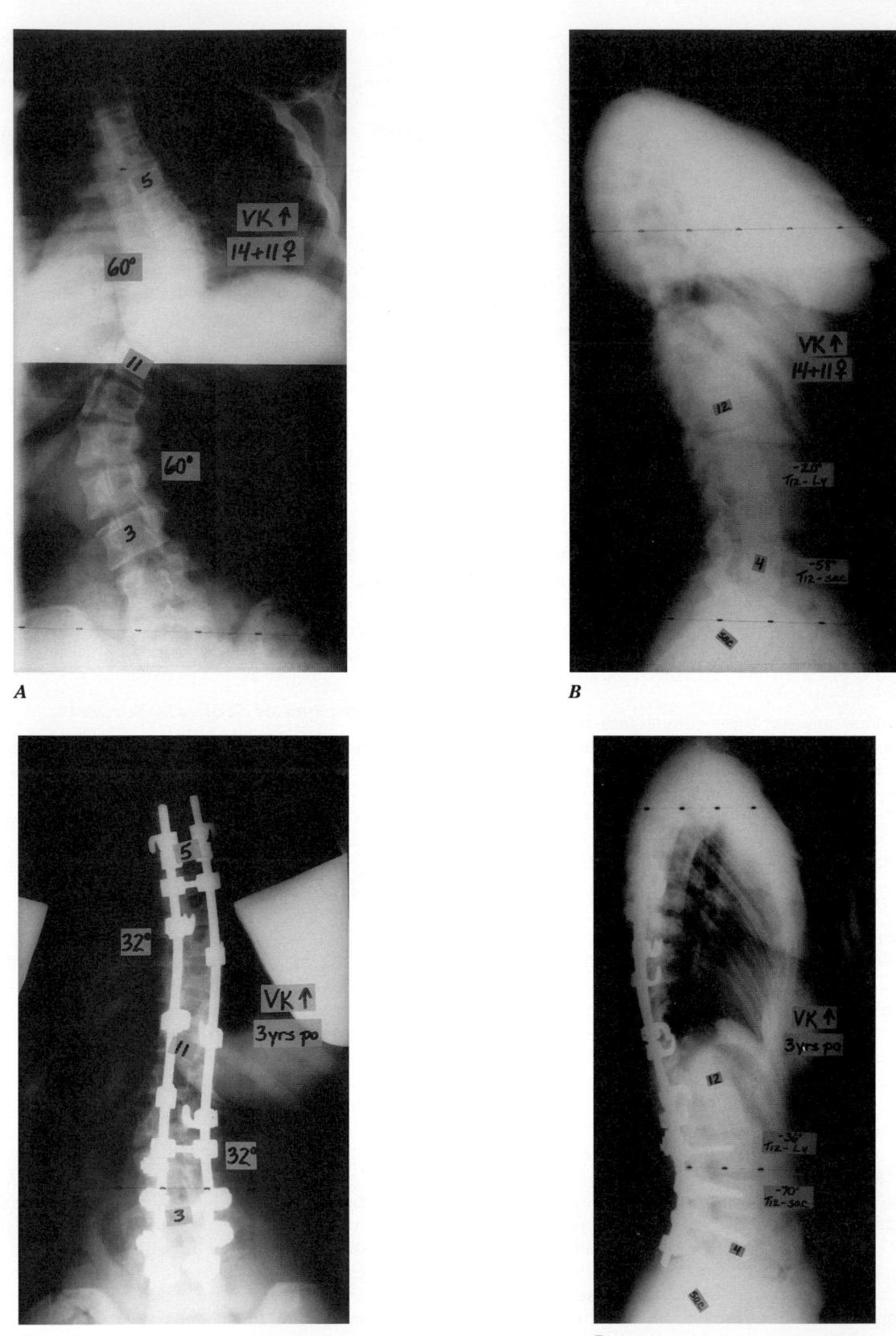

A

B

C

D

Figure 75-29 V.K., a 14 + 11-year-old female, has (*A*) a 60° right thoracic, 60° left lumbar double major idiopathic scoliosis. Both the thoracic and lumbar curves have nearly equal Cobb measurements, apical rotation, apical deviation from the midline, and side-bending flexibility. Thus both curves need to be instrumented and fused. Her sagittal plane (*B*) was unremarkable. She underwent a posterior instrumentation and fusion from T4 to L4, including a 90° rod rotation maneuver of the left-sided rod. This allowed correction of the scoliosis (*C*) and production of a normal sagittal plane (*D*).

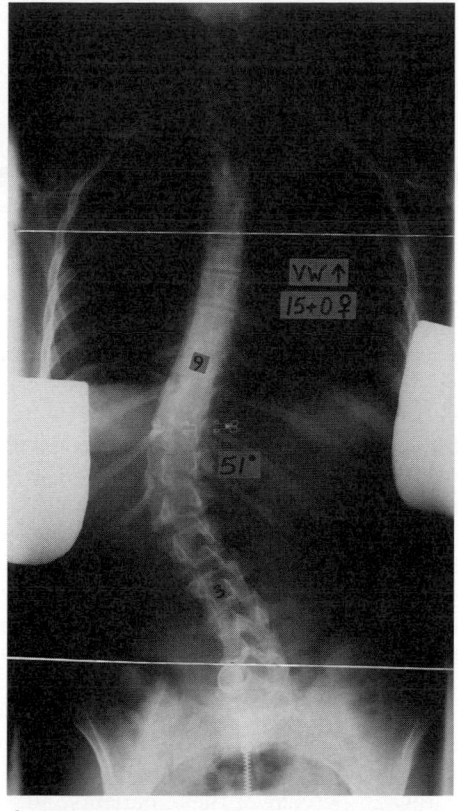

A

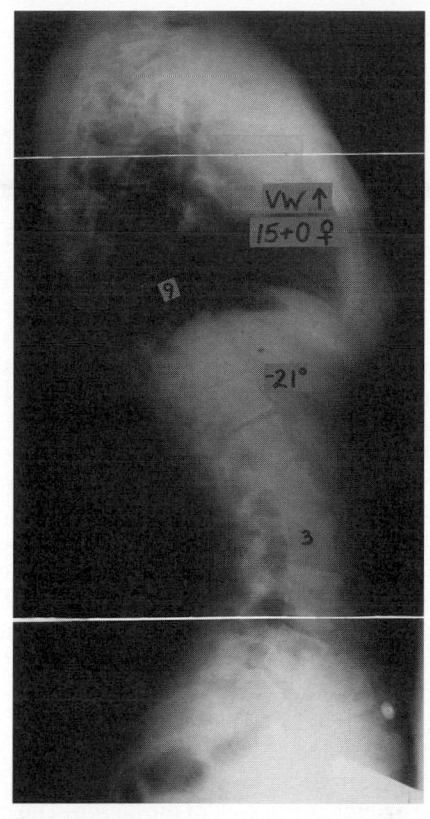

B

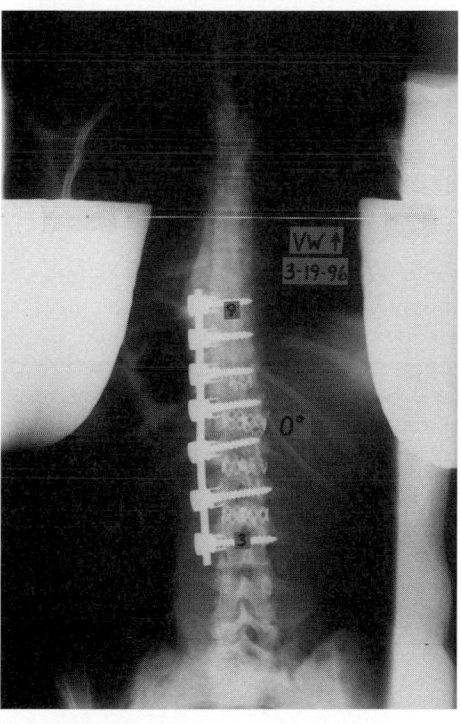

C

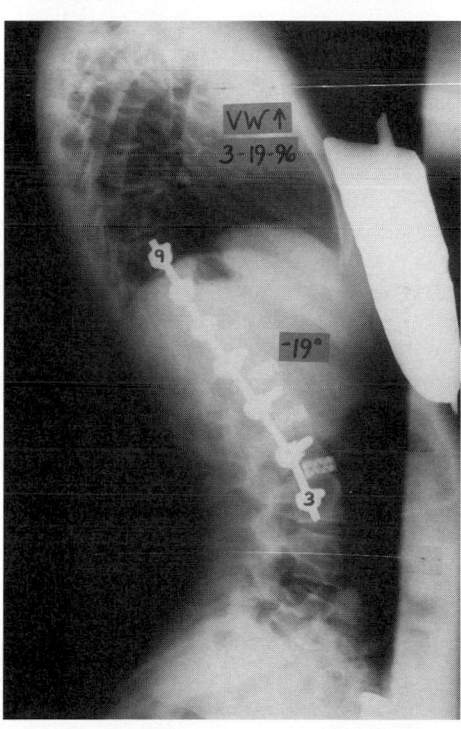

D

Figure 75-30 V.W., a 15-year-old female, presented with this (*A*) 51° left thoracolumbar idiopathic scoliosis. The apex of the curve is T12 and thus dictates the thoracolumbar classification. The spine was inherently flexible both above and below this deformity, as noted on side-bending x-rays. The preoperative sagittal plane (*B*) is unremarkable, with 21° of lordosis between T9 and L3, the intended anterior instrumentation and fusion levels. By a left thoracoabdominal approach, she underwent diskectomies and fusions at each level from T9 to L3. She had autogenous rib graft placed in the disk spaces, with structural cages placed in the anterior half of the lower four disks to help maintain appropriate sagittal alignment during correction of the anterior convex compression of her coronal plane deformity. Postoperative x-ray (*C*) shows complete correction of the scoliosis with the anterior solid rod–screw stable construct. Her radiographic and clinical alignments are perfect. Her postoperative sagittal x-ray (*D*) shows maintenance of appropriate thoracolumbar and lumbar sagittal alignment with the cages noted in the anterior half of the lower four instrumented disks.

gical correction was often difficult and dangerous. Therefore, it is important to anticipate which congenital curves are at risk of rapid deterioration so that prophylactic treatment may be initiated when the curve is smaller and more controllable.

Winter et al.,[213] in a landmark study involving 234 children, established a radiographic classification based on the types of vertebral anomalies present. They also discussed the potentially serious prognosis for certain types of congenital scoliosis. Congenital scoliosis is classified into defects of segmentation, defects of formation, and mixed or unclassifiable anomalies (Fig. 75-31). Approximately 80 percent of cases are classified, with the remaining 20 percent unclassifiable for a variety of reasons. Occasionally, there are massive anomalies where the scoliosis is so severe that it obscures the individual radiographic characteristics. Defects of segmentation may be either unilateral, as in an unsegmented bar, or bilateral, as in a block vertebra. The unilateral unsegmented bar is among the most common causes of congenital scoliosis, consisting of bony fusion of the facet joints and disk spaces unilaterally with contralateral growth continuing.

Defects of formation are divided into complete unilateral and partial unilateral lack of formation. The most common complete unilateral defect of formation is a hemivertebra, which is another common cause of congenital scoliosis. There are four different types of hemivertebra, depending upon the pathologic anatomy and relationship to adjacent vertebrae. These types include (1) the segmented (nonincarcerated) with a viable disk above and below the hemivertebra—this is the most common; (2) the semisegmented, with a disk above or below the deformity but not both; (3) the nonsegmented, or without a growth plate above and below; and (4) the incarcerated, which has a growth plate above and below but is accommodated by the vertebral bodies above and below, thus minimizing the deformity (see Fig. 75-31A). It is most important to recognize a unilateral unsegmented bar along with a contralateral hemivertebra at an early stage, because this combination produces the most severe and rapidly progressive type of congenital scoliosis.[213]

It is important to examine other organ systems for associated anomalies with congenital scoliosis. Because of the close association of the spinal cord and the spinal column, it is not unexpected for neural and vertebral malformations to coexist. Scanning with MRI is a noninvasive and sensitive way of looking for intraspinal lesions. Using MRI, Bradford et al.[33] noted a 38 percent incidence of intraspinal anomalies in 42 patients with congenital spinal deformities. Lesions encountered included diastematomyelia, diplomyelia, tethered spinal cords, syringomyelia, and low-lying conus (Fig. 75-32). Although an intraspinal anomaly may not be immediately obvious on clinical examination, clues such as skin abnormalities (e.g., hairy patch, dimple), neurologic abnormalities, extremity shortening, or a cavus foot may provide physical clues. Even though MRI is not mandatory for all patients with congenital scoliosis, it should be done in any patient with suspicious clinical or radiographic findings and certainly as a preoperative study in those patients who undergo spinal deformity correction.[33]

Other organ systems having anomalies associated with congenital scoliosis include the genitourinary system, affected in up to 25 percent of patients. Thus, a screening renal ultrasound should be obtained routinely on these patients. Klippel-Feil syndrome may also be found in approximately 25 percent of these patients, and congenital heart disease in 10 percent.[99]

The prognosis for congenital scoliosis with respect to curve progression and severity depends on three factors: the type of vertebral anomaly present and the degree of growth imbalance, the location of the anomaly, and the age of the patient at the time of diagnosis.[213] Unfavorable characteristics include a unilateral unsegmented bar with a contralateral hemivertebra at the same level[157]; a lesion in the thoracic or thoracolumbar spine; and an obvious clinical deformity presenting in the first few years of life. Depending on the various factors, curve progression may be much more malignant than curve magnitudes of similar size in idiopathic scoliosis during skeletal growth.

In planning the treatment of congenital scoliosis, the goal is to produce a balanced spine with as little deformity as possible at the end of growth. The key factors that combine to produce this goal are early diagnosis, anticipation, and prevention of rapid deterioration. Once the congenital scoliosis is diagnosed, a referral to a scoliosis specialist is

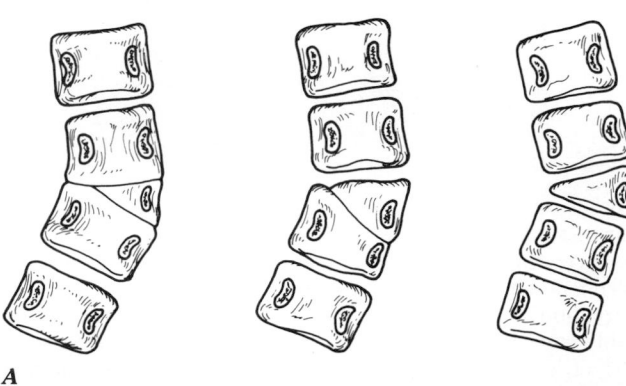

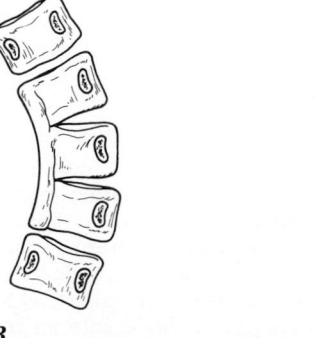

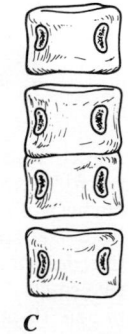

A   *B*   *C*

Figure 75-31 Classification of congenital scoliosis. *A.* Failure of formation (hemivertebra) of a vertebra, which is either fully segmented, partially segmented, or nonsegmented. *B.* Unilateral lack of segmentation (unilateral bar). *C.* Block vertebra.

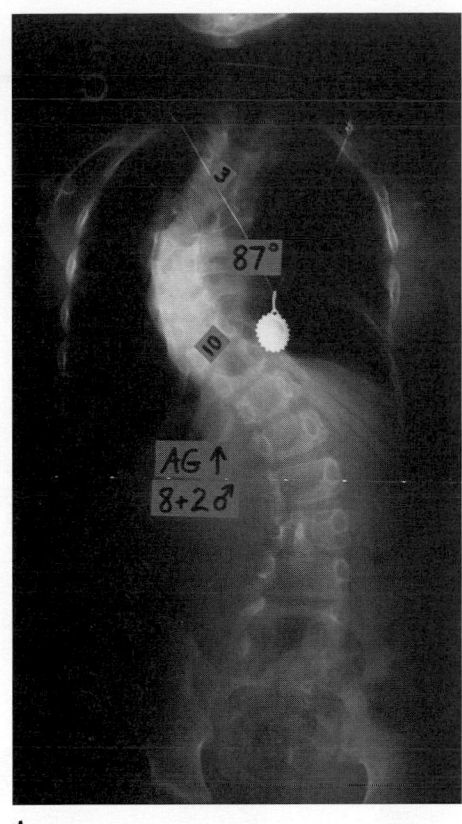

A

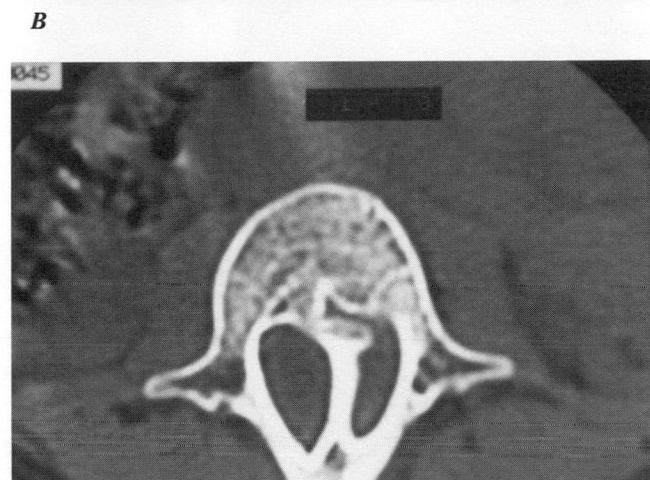

B

C

Figure 75-32 *A*. An 87° left thoracic congenital scoliosis. A screening MRI scan (*B*) demonstrated a diastematomyelia with two hemicords noted. An axial CT scan (*C*) shows the bony spike separating the spinal canal in half.

indicated. Often the best view of the anomaly will be noted on early radiographs of the baby's spine, prior to the formation of the major sagittal curves that will obscure some of the coronal profile. Patients should be followed carefully every 4 or 6 months to document any progression and obtain a better appreciation of the natural history of the evolving deformity. Some types of congenital scoliosis have such a bad prognosis that surgical treatment is required no matter how young the patient. Other types may be observed and lead to a well-balanced spine with an ultimate mild and acceptable deformity. Once significant progression occurs, early operative treatment is necessary to prevent further deterioration (Fig. 75-33).

Bracing has a minimal role in the treatment of congenital scoliosis.[215] In fact, for young children with congenital scoliosis, the application of a plaster jacket or brace can actually constrict the chest and have an adverse effect on the developing respiratory system. The Milwaukee brace is sometimes advantageous, helping to improve spinal alignment by controlling secondary compensatory

curves above or below the congenital curve.[215] An under-arm orthosis may be sufficient for patients with a secondary thoracolumbar and lumbar curve. If the brace is not controlling overall spinal alignment and the congenital curve continues to progress, the patient normally requires surgery at that juncture. Following surgery, however, a spinal orthosis may often help to control overall spinal alignment and the development of compensatory curves that were not included in the fusion.

Surgical Treatment

Surgical treatment is indicated in congenital scoliosis when nonoperative treatment has been unsuccessful in preventing progression and also in severe curves. Numerous factors determine the type of surgery for each particular deformity. Successful surgical treatment requires selecting the correct procedure and performing it at the optimal age. Occasionally, prophylactic surgical procedures are applied to young patients with small curves to prevent fur-

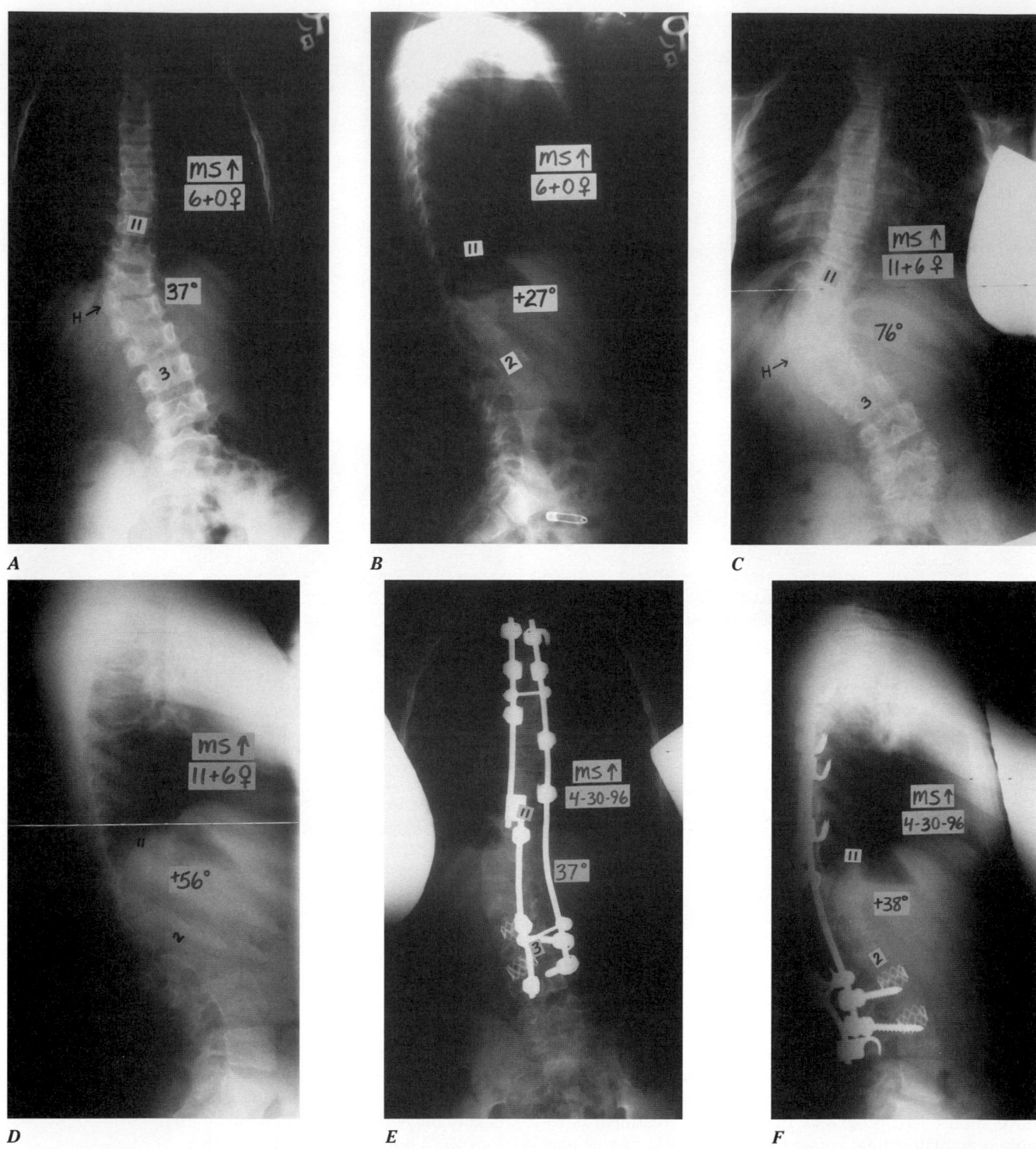

Figure 75-33 M.S., a 6-year-old female, presented with (*A*) a left thoracolumbar congenital scoliosis due to a hemivertebra. Her sagittal x-ray (*B*) at that point showed 27° of kyphosis from T11 to T12. Surgical fusion was discussed; however, the patient's family refused to consider this and did not return until the patient was 11 + 6. *C.* At that time, her scoliosis had increased to 76° and was associated with a significant clinical deformity as well (see *G*). *D.* Her sagittal kyphosis had also increased to 56°. The patient's family agreed to surgical correction, which consisted of a same-day anteroposterior hemivertebra excision, fusion, and instrumentation. Because of the great magnitude of the curve, the posterior instrumen-

tation and fusion extended from T4 to L4. The patient's postoperative x-rays (*E*) show correction of her main deformity to 37°, with improved truncal alignment. Her postoperative sagittal x-ray (*F*) shows decreased thoracolumbar kyphosis to 38°. Her preoperative clinical photo (*G*) demonstrates significant truncal deformity. The postoperative photo (*H*) demonstrates improved clinical alignment. This case addresses the importance of careful follow-up in patients with congenital scoliosis. Ideally, a shorter fusion done at the time of initial presentation would have corrected the deformity while leaving more motion segments free above and below the congenital anomaly.

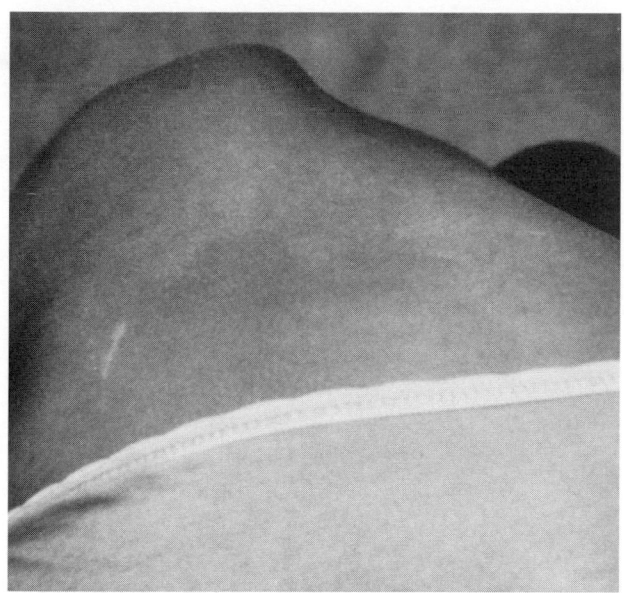

G

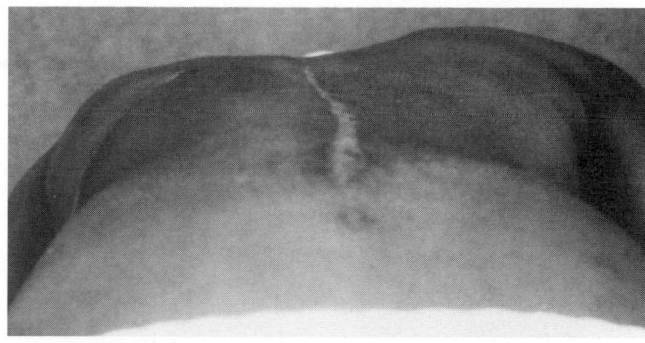

H

Figure 75-33 *(Continued)*

ther deterioration by optimizing growth and balance of the spine. Patients with congenital scoliosis who have undergone surgery must be followed closely to ensure that the goals of the procedure have been maintained long-term.

Combined convex anterior hemiepiphysiodesis and posterior hemiarthrodesis is a method of prophylactic arrest of convex growth.[213] The ideal candidate is a child under the age of 5 years with a small but progressive congenital scoliosis, a curve less than 40°, and concave growth potential at the site of the anomaly. The objective of the surgery is to balance growth of the spine by preventing convex growth and permitting concave growth. Bone graft is placed in the convex half of the disk spaces as well as in the convex aspect of the posterior elements of the spine. A postoperative cast or brace is maintained for approximately 6 months until the convex growth arrest has healed.

Excision of a fully segmented hemivertebra is an attractive procedure, for it entirely removes the primary cause of the scoliosis and provides an opportunity to close the resultant open wedge, thus fully correcting and fusing only a single level of spine.[31] This is especially attractive in the lumbar spine and at the lumbosacral junction with hemivertebra that often produce marked coronal imbalance (Fig. 75-34). To excise the hemivertebra, the spine should be approached both anteriorly and posteriorly. Anteriorly, the hemivertebral body and pedicle are excised as far back as possible, as are the adjacent disks and vertebral end plates. Posteriorly, the posterior elements of the hemivertebra are removed along with the transverse process and posterior aspect of the pedicle. If possible, the wedge defect created is then closed down with instrumentation over one level of the spine and fusion is performed. This is performed much more easily and safely in the lumbar versus the thoracic spine. The use of a postoperative spica cast is normally required following surgery until the single-level osteotomy is thoroughly healed. The best results following hemivertebra resection occur if the

scoliosis can be nearly completely corrected. When curves are quite large and structural or have fixed compensatory curves associated with the congenital component, results tend to be less than optimal and may deteriorate with time.

Prophylactic fusion in situ is the optimal surgical treatment for patients with a small congenital scoliosis caused by a unilateral unsegmented bar with or without a contralateral hemivertebra.[214] These anomalies produce very rigid deformities with a high potential for progression. Usually a concomitant anterior spinal fusion is required to prevent further progression. Normally just one or two levels above and below the anomalous vertebra are included in the fusion, and a postoperative spinal orthosis is required for approximately 6 months during the healing phase.

Posterior spinal fusion with moderate correction of congenital scoliosis is the treatment of choice in the case of moderately severe but flexible curves in older children and adolescents.[214] The fusion procedure is normally performed from the upper neutral vertebra to the lower stable vertebra of the scoliosis. A preoperative MRI or myelographic study of the spinal canal is essential prior to intraoperative correction of the deformity. It is always safer to attempt to correct the deformity by shortening the spinal column (convex compression) than by lengthening it (concave distraction). Because of the inherently high risk of associated intraoperative correction, it is important to perform spinal cord monitoring with or without a wake-up test during correction of the deformity. In treating congenital spinal deformities, it is important to remember that the main objective is to achieve overall trunk and spinal balance rather than excessive correction of the scoliotic deformity.

A spinal osteotomy to correct a fixed congenital scoliosis is rarely needed; however, it is a method of obtaining a balanced spine, which would be impossible with other

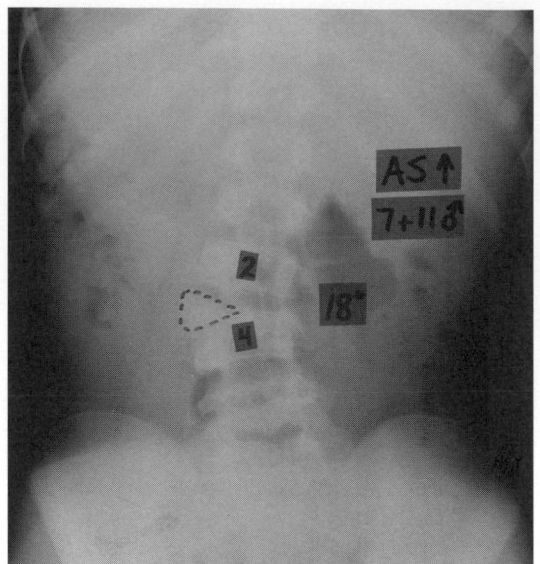

A

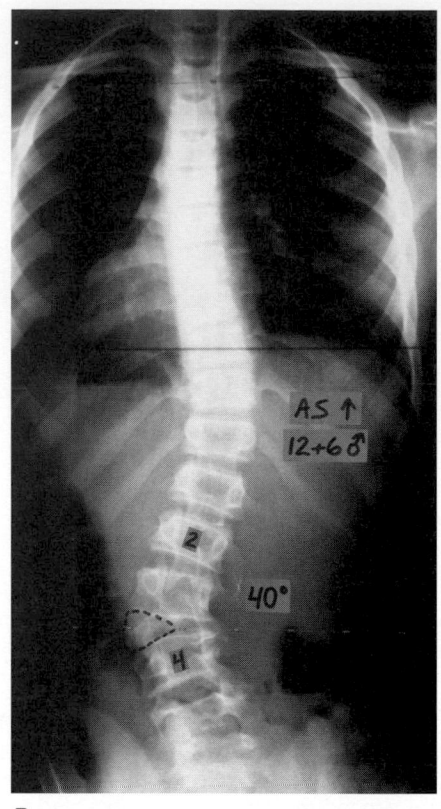

B

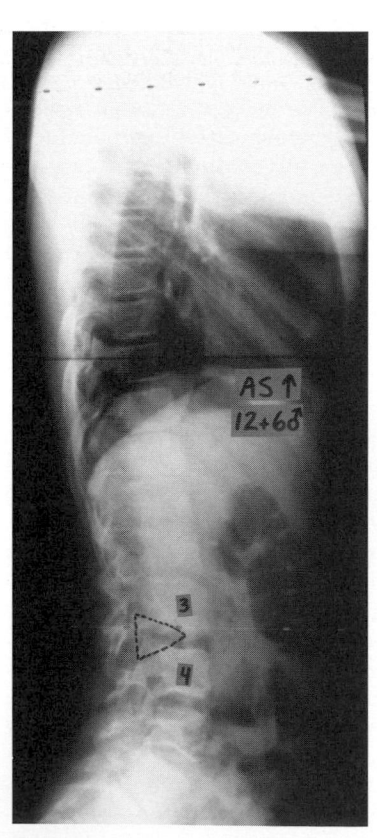

C

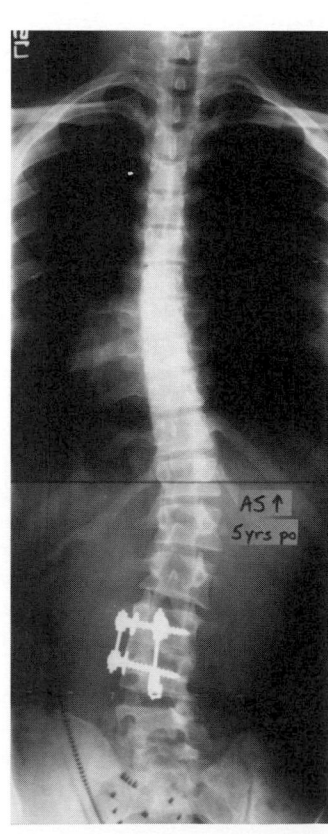

D

Figure 75-34 A.S., a 7 + 11-year-old male, presented with a fully segmented L3 hemivertebra that produced (*A*) an 18° congenital left lumbar scoliosis. He was followed closely, and by age 12 + 6 his congenital scoliosis (*B*) had increased to 40°. His curves above continued to be compensatory. *C.* His sagittal plane was unremarkable. The patient thus underwent a same-day anteroposterior hemivertebra excision and single-level fusion. Anteriorly, the hemivertebral segment was removed back to the base of the pedicle. Also, the disk between the L3 and L4 segments was completely excised. Posteriorly, the elements at that level were excised and then both anterior and posterior compression instrumentation was utilized to close the defect. A single-level fusion was also performed. The 5-year long-cassette coronal x-ray (*D*) shows the single-level fusion and a well-balanced spine with minimal scoliosis. The lateral x-ray (*E*) demonstrates the well-healed anterior spine fusion and good clinical balance of the spine. (Courtesy of Keith H. Bridwell, MD.)

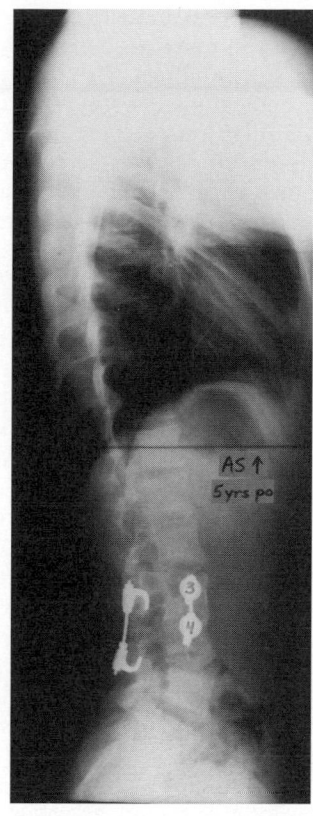

E

Figure 75-34 *(Continued)*

Society into either neuropathic or myopathic conditions (Table 75-1). Neuropathic conditions have been divided into upper and lower motor neuron lesions based on the primary location of neural abnormality. Thus, upper motor

---

TABLE 75-1   Classification of Structural Scoliosis

I. Idiopathic
  A. Infantile: 0–3 years
    1. Resolving
    2. Progressive
  B. Juvenile: 4 years to puberty onset
  C. Adolescent: puberty onset to epiphyseal closure

II. Neuromuscular
  A. Neuropathic
    1. Upper motor neuron lesion
      a. Cerebral palsy
      b. Spinocerebellar degeneration
        i. Friedreich's ataxia
        ii. Charcot-Marie-Tooth disease
        iii. Roussy-Levy syndrome
      c. Syringomyelia
      d. Spinal cord tumor
      e. Spinal cord trauma
      f. Other
    2. Lower motor neuron lesion
      a. Poliomyelitis
      b. Other viral myelitides
      c. Traumatic
      d. Spinal muscular atrophy
      e. Myelomeningocele (paralytic)
    3. Dysautonomia (Riley-Day)
    4. Other
  B. Myopathic
    1. Arthrogryposis
    2. Muscular dystrophy
      a. Duchenne (pseudohypertrophic)
      b. Limb-girdle
      c. Facioscapulohumeral
    3. Fiber-type disproportion
    4. Congenital hypotonia
    5. Myotonia dystrophica
    6. Other

III. Congenital
  A. Failure of formation
    1. Wedge vertebra
    2. Hemivertebra
  B. Failure of segmentation
    1. Unilateral bar
    2. Bilateral ("fusion")
  C. Mixed

IV. Neurofibromatosis

V. Mesenchymal
  A. Marfan's syndrome
  B. Homocystinuria
  C. Ehlers-Danlos syndrome
  D. Other

(Continued on next page)

---

methods. This requires both anterior and posterior procedures. The anterior procedure entails disk excision and osteotomy through unsegmented bars. Posteriorly, posterior osteotomies are performed at the same sites as anterior osteotomies with division of the unsegmented bar on the concavity posteriorly. Following both anterior and posterior osteotomies, the spine can be corrected posteriorly by applying posterior compression instrumentation to close the convexity of the wedge osteotomy. This effectively shortens the spinal column and relaxes the neural structures and thus is the safest method of correcting these deformities. Posterior fusion is performed over the entire length of the scoliosis. It is evident that congenital scoliosis is much more amenable to treatment if the curves are small and require less extensive surgical correction. Thus, it is probably wiser to correct a smaller deformity at a younger age rather than to allow the deformity to progress and perform an extensive procedure on an older child.[213] Congenital scoliosis is still a potentially serious condition that can result in severe deformity and cardiopulmonary compromise. Thus, close attention to these patients by the pediatric spinal surgeon is certainly warranted.

Neuromuscular Scoliosis

Neuromuscular spinal deformities include abnormalities of the neuromuscular system. Patients with these deformities have been classified by the Scoliosis Research

TABLE 75-1 *(Continued)* **Classification of Structural Scoliosis**

VI. Traumatic
   A. Fracture or dislocation (nonparalytic)
   B. Surgical
      1. Postlaminectomy
      2. Postthoracoplasty
   C. Irradiation

VII. Extraspinal contractures
   A. Postempyema
   B. Burns
   C. Other

VIII. Osteochondrodystrophies
   A. Achondroplasia
   B. Spondyloepiphyseal dysplasia
   C. Diastrophic dwarfism
   D. Mucopolysaccharidoses
   E. Other

IX. Tumor
   A. Vertebral column
      1. Benign
      2. Malignant
   B. Spinal cord

X. Rheumatoid disease

XI. Metabolic disease
   A. Rickets
   B. Juvenile osteoporosis
   C. Osteogenesis imperfecta

XII. Related to lumbosacral area
   A. Spondylolysis and spondylolisthesis
   B. Congenital anomalies of lumbosacral region

XIII. Infection of bone
   A. Acute
   B. Chronic

neuron abnormalities include diseases such as cerebral palsy, syringomyelia, and spinal cord tumors. The lower motor neuron diseases include entities such as spinal muscular atrophy and poliomyelitis. Certain entities such as myelodysplasia and trauma to the spinal cord may have both upper and lower motor neuron involvement. Myopathic conditions include diseases such as muscular dystrophy, arthrogryposis, and other myopathies.

The prevalence of spinal deformity in neuromuscular conditions is much higher than that of idiopathic scoliosis—between 25 and 100 percent. In general, the greater the neuromuscular involvement, the greater the incidence and severity of scoliosis. Additional components of neuromuscular disorders include problems such as limb contractures, hip dislocations, seizures, mental retardation, and insensate skin, among others. Patients may be classified by their ambulatory status as either being community, household, or minimal ambulators or nonambulatory, confined to a wheelchair. Patients with neuromuscular disor-

ders may be of fairly normal intelligence or severely mentally deficient, with minimal to no communication with others and their surroundings. These patients may also have significant medical histories of respiratory illnesses, malnutrition, and other joint and extremity conditions.[141]

The scoliotic curve patterns seen in neuromuscular disorders are quite varied. Certainly thoracic scoliosis with hypokyphosis or lordosis in the sagittal plane, typical of "idiopathic scoliosis," is occasionally seen. However, many of these patients present with long "C"-type sweeping curves that involve almost the entire thoracic and lumbar spine, extending from the neck into the pelvis, with the sacrum and pelvis being a part of the curve (Fig. 75-35). In the sagittal plane, kyphosis is also frequently seen in neuromuscular curves. It can either be the result of actual collapse of the spine, as seen in myelodysplasia, or a "kyphosing scoliosis" due to excessive vertebral rotation at the apex of the curve, which appears as a posterior spinal angulation (kyphosis) rather than as a lateral deformity (scoliosis). Kyphosis presents a greater clinical challenge to the spinal surgeon and usually warrants more aggressive treatment.

The evaluation of patients with neuromuscular scoliosis must begin with an accurate diagnosis as well as consultation with appropriate subspecialists, including a neurologist, a pulmonologist, a geneticist, and occasionally a cardiologist, among others. The radiographic evaluation includes radiographs obtained in an upright position, standing in those patients who are ambulatory and sitting

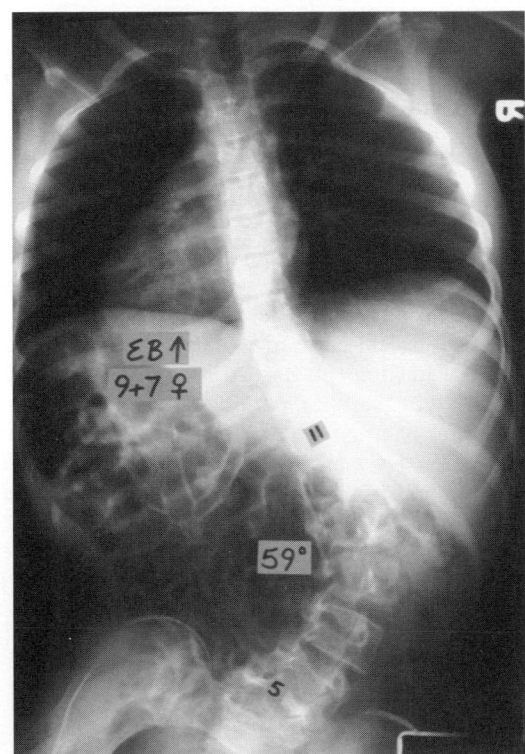

Figure 75-35 E.B., a 9 + 7-year-old female, has cerebral palsy and a 59° right thoracolumbar scoliosis extending to the pelvis with the formation of pelvic obliquity.

in nonambulators. A true appreciation of the magnitude of the spinal deformity, pelvic obliquity, and spinal imbalance will be obtained when minimal to no support is provided to the patient when the radiographs are obtained.

The treatment of neuromuscular scoliosis is either nonoperative with observation, bracing, or wheelchair modifications or operative with spinal fusion. Orthotic treatment of neuromuscular scoliosis is more demanding than that of idiopathic scoliosis.[45] It usually produces more skin problems and is required for a longer period of time. Surgical fusion entails posterior fusion either with or without an anterior fusion.[80] Most deformities require fusion of the majority of both the thoracic and lumbar spine. Often, the pelvis must be included in the fusion, especially in nonambulators with pelvic obliquity.[5] Because of the multitude of medical problems associated with neuromuscular disorders, the complication rate following spinal reconstructive surgery for these patients is much higher than for patients with idiopathic scoliosis, especially regarding respiratory insufficiency, intraoperative blood losses, and pseudarthrosis rates.[132]

Cerebral Palsy

Cerebral palsy, which designates the most common neuromuscular condition, is an all-inclusive term for static encephalopathy. Thus, it includes all nonprogressive brain disorders occurring before, at the time of, or directly after birth. Because of the generalized brain involvement, all aspects of cerebral function may be affected, producing mental retardation, seizures, and delayed motor development. The motor involvement of patients with cerebral palsy is divided into four types: spastic, flaccid, athetoid, or mixed. The most common form is spastic quadriplegia with or without good head control; if head control is lacking, the condition is noted as total body involvement or spastic pentaplegia.

Curve patterns seen in cerebral palsy include scoliosis, kyphosis, lordosis, or a combination. Scoliosis is present in approximately 25 percent of all cerebral palsy patients but is much higher (65 to 75 percent) in spastic quadriplegics. Kyphosis is commonly seen in patients with generalized torso imbalance and is often treated nonoperatively. Lordosis commonly occurs in two situations: in those nonambulatory patients with hip flexion contractures and in severely involved spastic patients with extensor muscle overactivity.

The evaluation of a cerebral palsy patient includes an overall assessment of the medical history, concentrating on the pulmonary history, nutritional status, seizures, and communication skills. The ambulatory status is important to define, and also whether there has been any change or progressive loss of ambulatory ability with continued skeletal growth. In nonambulators, it is important to assess sitting balance and whether it is slowly deteriorating due to pelvic obliquity (Fig. 75-36). Hip and knee flexion contractures and dislocated, adducted hips are also commonly seen in these patients.

Observation of spinal deformities is undertaken in those patients with small deformities of less than 30° or in those with minimal deformity that are relatively skeletally

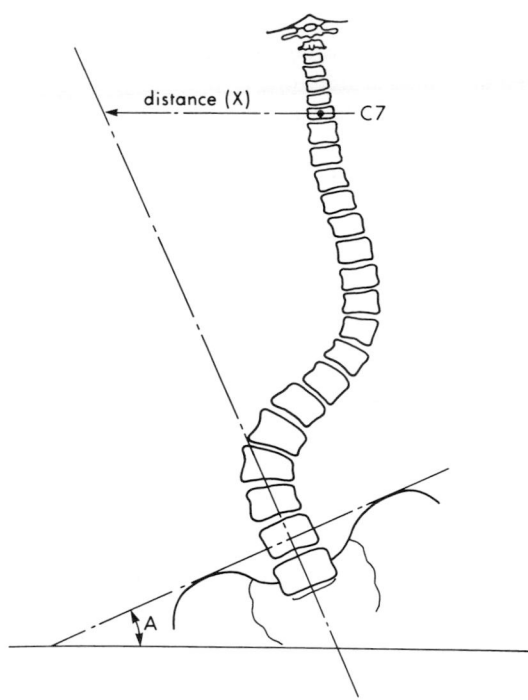

Figure 75-36 Assessment of pelvic obliquity in the neuromuscular patient. The pelvic obliquity angle (*A*) is noted as the angle from the top of the iliac crests to the horizontal. The distance from the C7 vertebra to the center sacral line drawn from the pelvis below to the neck above (X) notes the distance from the base of the neck and the relative decompensation of the top of the spine to the pelvis.

mature. Far and away, these are the minority of cerebral palsy patients that present to spine specialists. Many patients require nonoperative treatment consisting of either curve control with an orthosis or, in nonambulatory patients, seating support. It is important to work closely with a skilled orthotist to determine the best type of orthosis. These patients are often quite difficult to brace successfully and thus must be followed very closely during periods of skeletal growth.[45]

Surgical correction is indicated once the scoliosis progresses over 50° in a growing child, but it involves a true assessment of the functional aspects occurring with the spinal deformity.

This requires input from all caregivers—including parents, attendants, therapists, and teachers—to gain a full appreciation of the change in the patient's functional level. Often cases such as deteriorating sitting ability or greater difficulty in swallowing and eating are clinical responses to progressive spinal deformity.

Once surgical correction is decided upon, the length of fusion and whether posterior or circumferential anterior and posterior fusion is required must be determined.[42] The length of fusion is decided upon by the ambulatory status. In patients who are good ambulators and apparently will stay ambulatory, fusion levels similar to those of idiopathic scoliosis can be chosen. Normally these patients are fused posteriorly unless a significantly rigid or kyphotic curve is present, which would require an anterior release and fusion preceding the posterior fusion.

This situation is different in nonambulators who are wheelchair-bound. Even if these patients have minimal pelvic obliquity, we usually recommend instrumentation and fusion from high up in the thoracic spine (T2 or T3) into the pelvis. Because of the risk of developing pelvic obliquity following fusion to L4 or L5 in a nonambulator, we recommend fusing all nonambulators to the pelvis, irrespective of the curve pattern (Fig. 75-37). The decision whether to do an anterior fusion along with a posterior fusion in this circumstance is based upon three factors: the degree of curvature, the degree of spasticity, and the potential for harvesting autogenous bone graft.[42,68] In patients with large, stiff curves (greater than 75°) or those with a significant kyphosis, we recommend a preliminary anterior release and fusion prior to the posterior fusion (Fig. 75-38). We also tend to perform an anterior fusion if minimal autogenous bone graft is available for the posterior fusion, as in severely spastic patients with small iliac crests in whom it will be difficult to harvest an iliac crest graft along with performing Galveston fixation into the pelvis,[4] and who also are too frail to allow harvesting of posterior rib cage bone. However, in more flaccid patients, often the use of fresh-frozen allograft bone for a posterior fusion will provide adequate bone for a solid posterior fusion to form.[40]

We still prefer Luque-type instrumentation with segmental sublaminar 16- or 18-gauge wires bilaterally, linked to a 3/16- or 1/4-in Luque rod, depending on the size of the patient and the size of the pelvis.[26,41,139] Proximal and distal cross links provide a rectangular construct to increase support and also allow the Galveston component of the rods to lock into the iliac crests. Postoperative bracing is used for most patients as additional support for these osteoporotic spines. The operative goals include obtaining a balanced spine with the head centered over a level pelvis and with a fairly normalized sagittal plane for either ambulating or sitting.[183]

Myelomeningocele Spinal Deformity

Patients with myelomeningocele are prone to develop spinal deformities, most commonly scoliosis. Myelo-

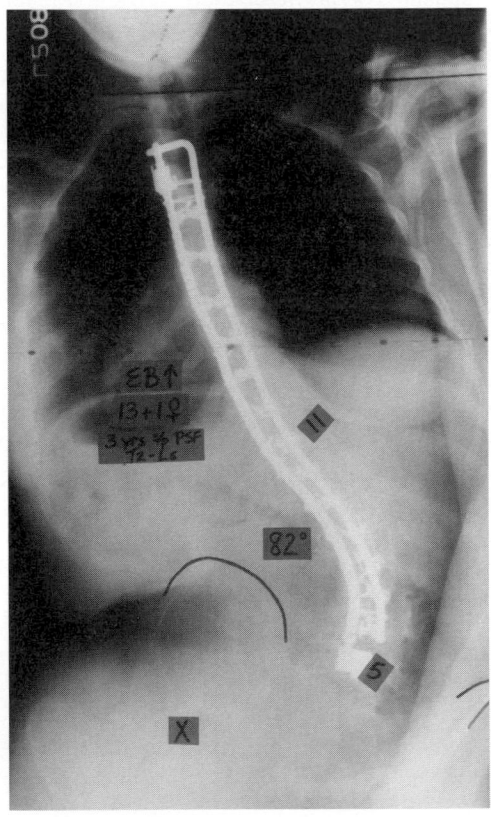

A

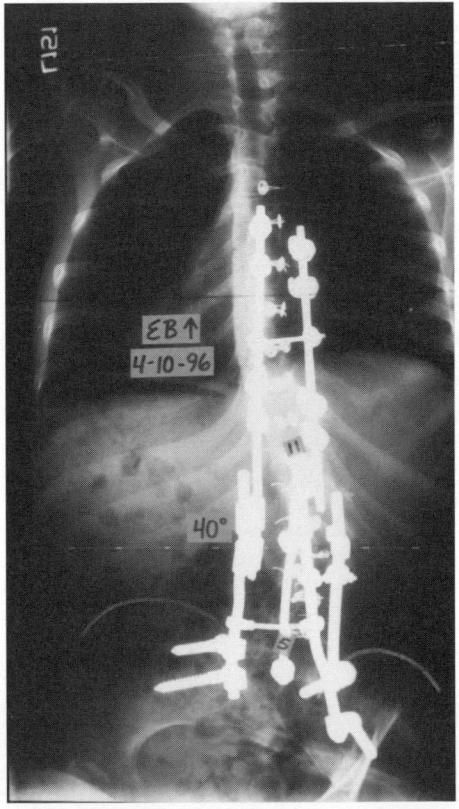

B

Figure 75-37 E.B., a 9 + 7-year-old female, has spastic quadriplegic cerebral palsy and is a nonambulator. She developed a 59° right lumbar neuromuscular scoliosis with pelvic obliquity (see Fig. 75-35). Shortly thereafter, she underwent posterior spinal fusion from T3 to L5. By the time of presentation to us, her pelvic obliquity and truncal malalignment (*A*) had increased. This stresses the importance of fusing nonambulatory cerebral palsy patients with pelvic obliquity to the pelvis during the initial surgery to correct sitting imbalance. She required a complex anterior and posterior corrective osteotomy with instrumentation and fusion extending into the pelvis. The postoperative coronal x-ray (*B*) demonstrates her improved truncal alignment and position of her pelvis in relation to her spine.

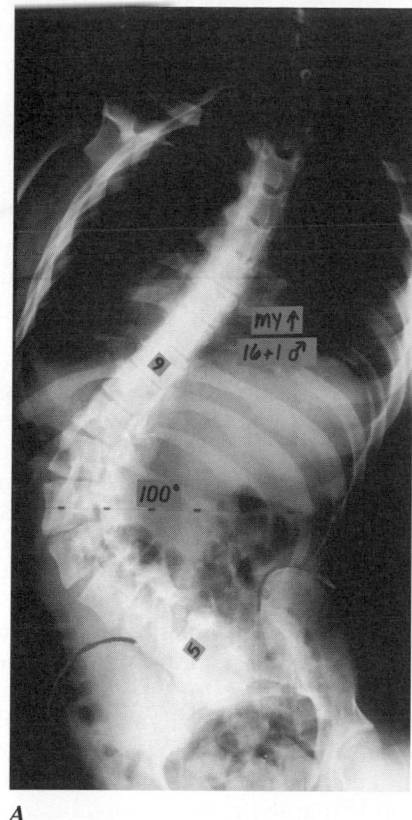

A

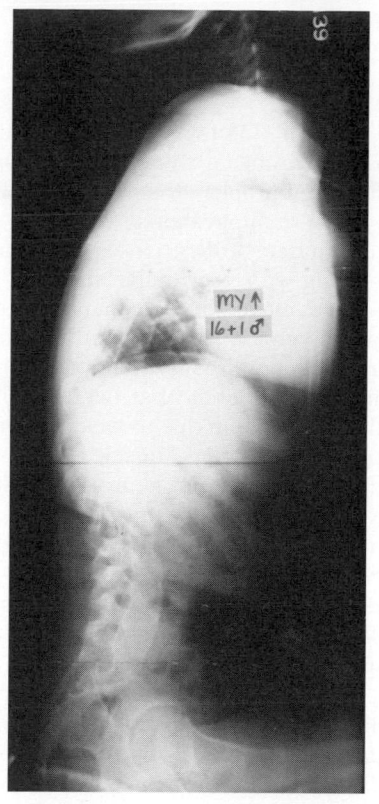

B

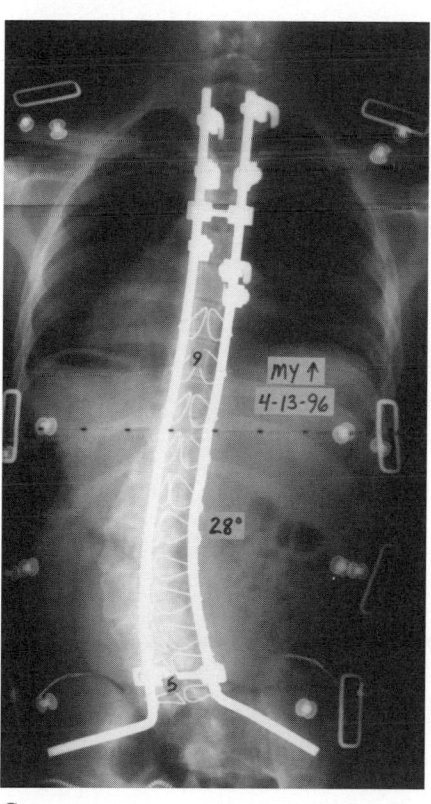

C

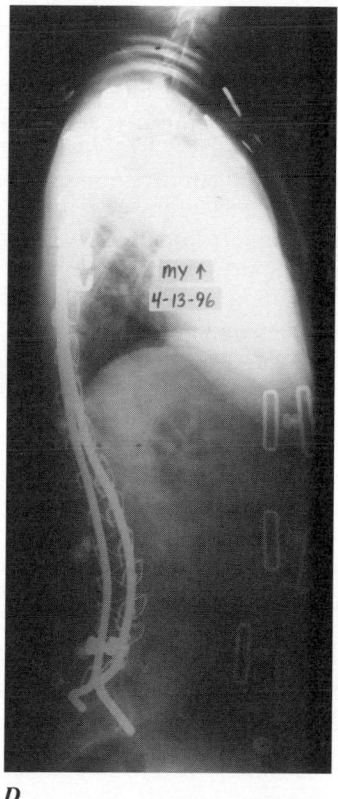

D

Figure 75-38 M.Y., a 16-year-old male, is a spastic quadriplegic with cerebral palsy and (*A*) a 100° left thoracolumbar neuromuscular scoliosis with pelvic obliquity. *B.* His sagittal plane is fairly unremarkable. He underwent a same-day anterior release and fusion from T10 to the sacrum with a combination of structural allograft iliac wedges as well as autogenous rib graft for anterior fusion along with a posterior instrumentation and fusion using allograft fresh-frozen femoral head and iliac crest autograft. The patient's postoperative coronal x-ray (*C*) shows improvement in the scoliosis to 28°, with a well-balanced spine over a level pelvis. *D.* His fusion maintained normal sagittal contours, which are important for sitting as well.

meningocele, or spina bifida, is an acquired defect in the posterior vertebral arches with or without dysplasia of the spinal cord and membranes. It is a complex disorder that affects many other organ systems. At birth, neurosurgical closure of the skin defect of either exposed dura or actual neural tissue along with ventricular shunting prevents infection and brain damage. Urologic management often consists of urinary diversion for the control of urinary tract infections and hydronephrosis. Orthopaedic management tries to minimize deformities that occur in the lower extremities and spinal column due to lack of appropriate nervous innervation to the trunk muscles and lower extremity, depending on the extent of neurologic deficit.

These patients are graded based on the most distal functioning neurologic segment of the spinal column. Thus, low-level myelomeningocele includes patients with a functional L5 level who are ambulatory and occasionally have bowel and bladder control. In contrast, patients with high-level myelomeningocele, at the T10 or T11 level, are almost always paraplegic and lack bowel and bladder control. The incidence of paralytic scoliosis in myelomeningocele correlates with the level of paralysis. According to Hall et al., there is a 100 percent incidence of spinal deformity and paralysis in patients having a T12 level or higher, 90 percent at L1, 80 percent at L2, 70 percent at L3, 60 percent at L4, 25 percent at L5, and 5 percent at S1.[109] Three basic types of spinal deformity occur in patients with myelomeningocele: developmental (paralytic), congenital, and mixed, with both developmental and congenital abnormalities.[67]

Developmental or paralytic deformities are the most common type of spinal deformity, seen in approximately 50 to 80 percent of patients.[109,127,128] These deformities are usually not present at birth but gradually develop during growth; most are present by the age of 10. These deformities generally continue to progress, especially during the adolescent growth spurt and beyond.[15]

The most common type of developmental paralytic curve is a long sweeping C-shaped scoliosis from the middle or lower thoracic spine extending to the sacrum, frequently producing pelvic obliquity (Fig. 75-39). This pelvic obliquity may interfere with ambulation and proper sitting balance and cause skin problems as well. Most commonly, thoracic lordoscoliosis is present; however, developmental kyphosis can be seen, especially with increasingly high levels of involvement.[13]

Patients with myelomeningocele may have congenital anomalies of the spine in addition to the paralytic component producing a scoliotic deformity. Frequently, these patients have a mixed developmental and congenital component, with either one or both contributing to the deformity. Perhaps the most difficult problem seen is congenital lumbar kyphosis. This usually occurs in high-level patients and can progress rapidly to produce deformities greater than 100° by the age of 3 or 4.[13,15] Severe kyphosis can result in skin ulceration as well as loss of sitting balance, with an excessively short abdominal wall. Often, a compensatory lordosis of the thoracic spine results, which may impair respiratory function.

The diagnosis of myelomeningocele is usually obvious at birth, due to the open skin defect posteriorly. Following satisfactory skin closure and possible shunting for any associated hydrocephalus, these children ideally should be followed in specialized centers offering a comprehensive team approach to management, including pediatricians, orthopedists, neurosurgeons, urologists, orthotists, social workers, and physical and occupational therapists.[128] Because of the frequent occurrence of spinal deformity, these patients should be monitored closely and radiographed at frequent intervals during their growth to document the onset and follow the progression of these deformities. In low-level ambulatory patients, spinal deformities may produce trunk imbalance and difficulty with gait, warranting treatment. The goal in managing nonambulatory myelomeningocele patients is the maintenance of appropriate sitting ability with a level pelvis and maximal torso length. This provides freedom to use the upper extremities for activities other than trunk support.

Treatment of spinal deformities involves various nonoperative and operative methods. Nonoperative treatment entails bracing with either a spinal orthosis with or without wheelchair modifications for nonambulators. The purpose of bracing is to control curve progression and maintain optimal trunk balance until the optimal age of spinal fusion.[127] Paralytic deformities have a better response rate than congenital deformities; however, orthoses rarely correct a deformity or prevent progression leading to an inevitable spinal fusion. Nevertheless, they can improve standing and/or sitting balance in these patients until a more appropriate age (10 to 11 in girls and 12 to 13 in boys) for spinal fusion. Possible contraindications to orthotic management include obesity, skin irritation, and noncompliance.[138] Problems with skin breakdown must be carefully monitored in these patients, who are often insensate over a good portion of the braced trunk and torso.

Surgical management of spinal deformity is common due to the progressive nature of these deformities.[3,128] Although the degree of deformity is an important surgical indication, paramount is functional ability—such as maintenance of ambulation or optimization of sitting balance and avoidance of skin problems in wheelchair-bound patients.[138] In the majority of these patients, a combined anterior and posterior procedure is required.[138,146,162] The missing bone stock posteriorly makes attainment of a spinal fusion by the posterior route alone difficult. Thus, the anterior route is quite attractive in these patients due to a large surface area for fusion.[182] Only those low-level patients treated for a deformity above the bifid region are considered for a posterior only procedure (Fig. 75-40).

The majority of patients treated for high-level myelomeningocele spinal scoliosis will require a combined anterior and posterior spinal fusion to the pelvis. This normally entails a staged anterior multilevel diskectomy, fusion, and possibly anterior spinal instrumentation in an attempt to correct the lumbar deformity and pelvic obliquity. About 1 to 2 weeks later, a posterior spinal fusion is performed from the high thoracic region (T2 or T3) to the sacrum, using Galveston technique into the iliac wings[5] (Fig. 75-41). Proximal thoracic and thoracolumbar fixation is performed with either hooks or wires, with button wires wrapped around the pars region of the bifid lumbar seg-

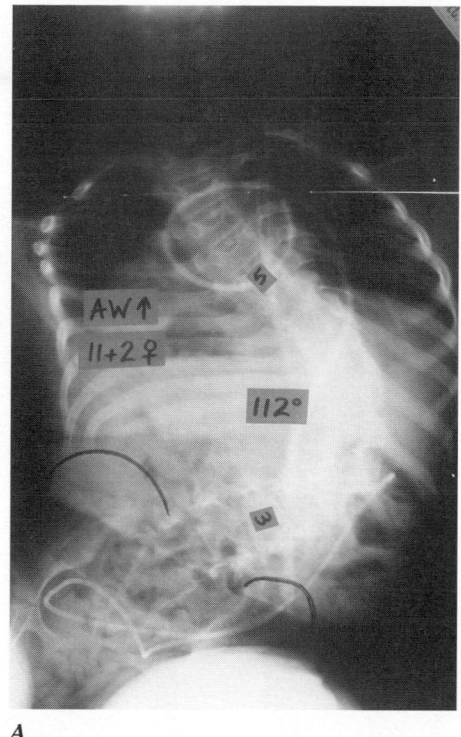

A

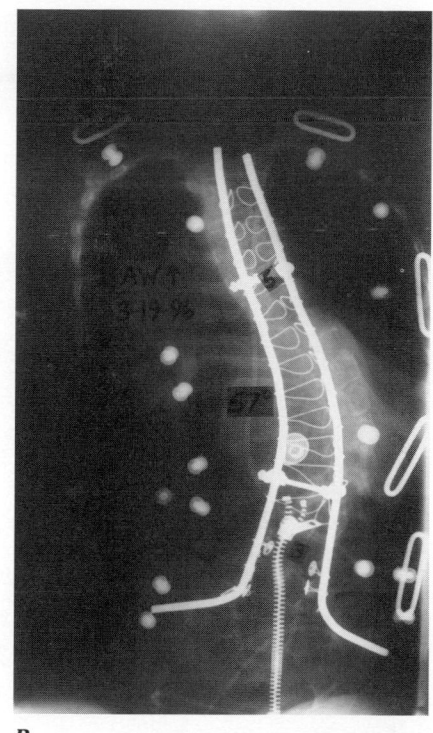

B

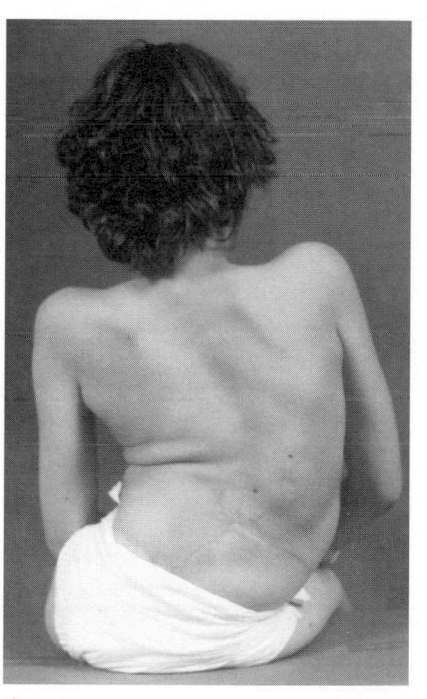

C

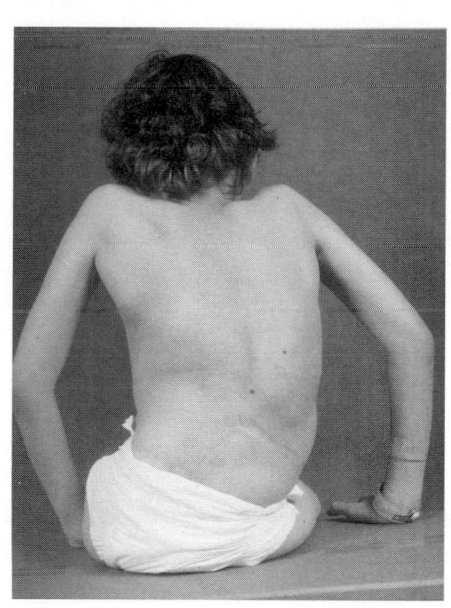

D

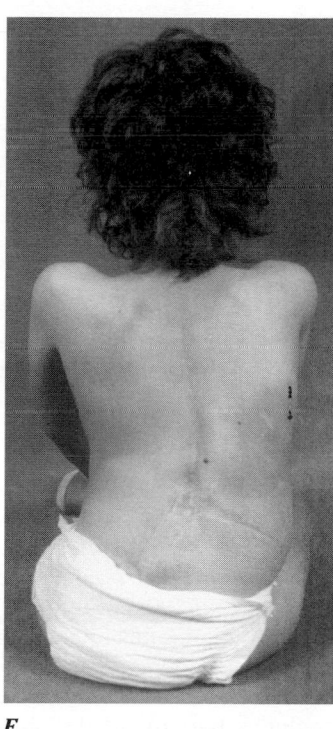

E

Figure 75-39 A.W., an 11 + 2-year-old female, has a high-level myelomeningocele as well as progressive scoliosis, pelvic obliquity, and difficulty with sitting balance. Her unsupported upright sitting x-ray (*A*) shows a 112° neuromuscular type of scoliosis with pelvic obliquity. She underwent staged anterior and posterior spinal fusion. Her anterior fusion was performed from T6 to the sacrum. A second-stage posterior instrumentation and fusion extended from T2 to the pelvis, using sublaminar and pars wires in the bifid areas of her middle and lower lumbar spine. The patient's postoperative coronal x-ray (*B*) demonstrates correction of her scoliosis to 57°, with improved clinical alignment and pelvic obliquity. Her preoperative sitting clinical photo (*C*) demonstrates her truncal shift and pelvic obliquity, with the necessity to use her arms (*D*) to control her position when sitting for any length of time. The patient's postoperative clinical photo (*E*) demonstrates improved truncal alignment and pelvic obliquity, so that she could sit for a long time without relying on her upper extremities for support.

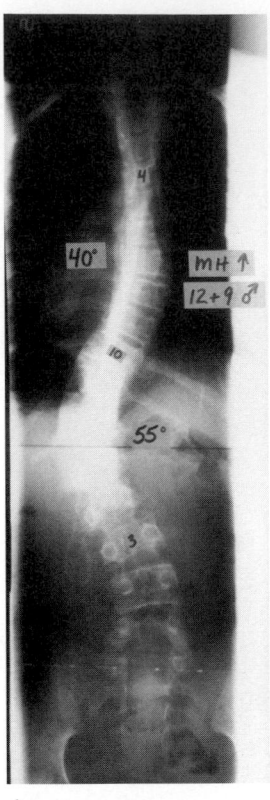
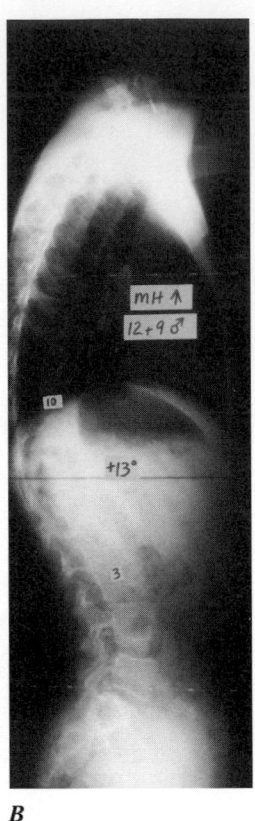
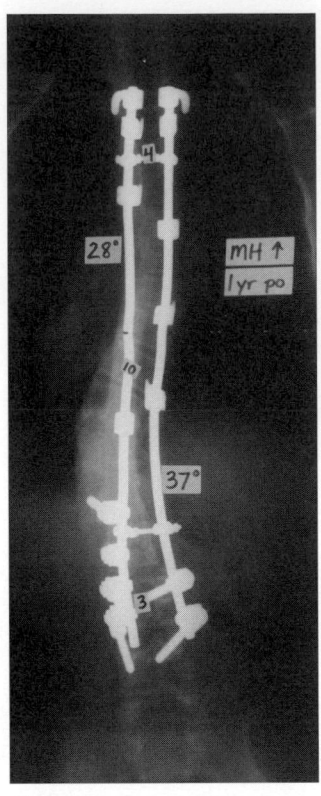
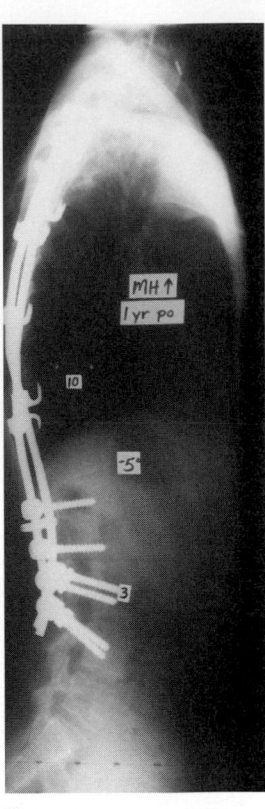

A   *B*   *C*   *D*

Figure 75-40 M.H., a 12 + 9-year-old male, has a low-level myelomeningocele with an L5 functional level. He has posterior elements present all the way down to L5. His coronal x-ray (*A*) showed a 30° right thoracic, 55° left thoracolumbar scoliosis. The sagittal plane (*B*) showed a very mild thoracolumbar junctional kyphosis. He underwent a posterior instrumenta-tion and fusion from T3 to L4 using segmental spinal fixation and lumbar pedicle screws. Autogenous iliac crest graft was used for the fusion. The patient's 1-year postoperative coronal x-ray shows good balance of the spine in the coronal (*C*) and sagittal (*D*) planes.

ments performed as well.[138] Spinal instrumentation in these patients is quite difficult to place due to the soft osteoporotic bone as well as the frequent occurrence of multiple congenital anomalies. Postoperative bracing is usually required for 6 months to a year, until fusion is complete.

Surgical management of complex myelomeningocele deformities is a challenging endeavor. Complications are many and often unavoidable.[108] The most common complications include wound problems, pseudarthrosis, spinal fluid leak, and respiratory problems due to poor nutrition. Neurologic complications related to proximal abnormalities of the neural axis, such as syringomyelia or Arnold-Chiari malformation, are possible.[89] Our current protocol includes hyperalimentation before, during, and after the staged spinal fusions. An inverted "Y" incision is made posteriorly, with the apex above the bifid region.[138] This avoids the midline open segments of the spinal column and thus lessens the risk of obtaining a spinal fluid leak during the procedure. Although not without significant risks, it is possible to obtain a solid spine fusion and improved sitting balance in these patients, which is helpful to both the patients and their caregivers.

A special problem in myelomeningocele patients is congenital lumbar kyphosis.[13,129,168] These curves are usu-ally rapidly progressive and result in a severe deformity. Although some patients can do reasonably well with these types of deformity, they often cause skin ulceration at the apex of the deformity, a shortened trunk, and proximal thoracic lordosis, which can severely limit pulmonary function. Thus, in these patients, surgical resection of the kyphosis is often advantageous. Currently, the best results are obtained by wide resection of the kyphosis posteriorly with osteotomies and instrumentation from the high thoracic region into the sacrum[103,129] (Fig. 75-42). Sacral fixation is performed with a specially bent rod that loops the distal ends of the rods anterior to the sacral ala, as recommended by Dunn and McCarthy.[138] Covering the area of instrumentation with healthy skin and subcutaneous tissue is important in preventing postoperative wound breakdowns. Lubicky has recommended a myocutaneous flap as a durable soft tissue cover.[138] However, resection of the bony kyphosis usually increases the amount of posterior tissue available for soft tissue reconstruction.

Muscular Dystrophy

The two most common types of muscular dystrophy include Duchenne and Becker.[49,64] These are believed now to represent two ends of this spectrum of diseases. They

Figure 75-41 S.V., a 12 + 8-year-old female, has (*A*) a 50° left lumbar myelomeningocele scoliosis and associated pelvic obliquity. She is a nonambulator and has an approximately L2 functional level. She underwent a staged anterior instrumentation and fusion from T11 to L5 and posterior instrumentation and fusion from T2 to the pelvis. Her 2-year postoperative coronal x-ray (*B*) shows improvement of her scoliosis and pelvic obliquity as well as overall spinal alignment with a solid fusion.

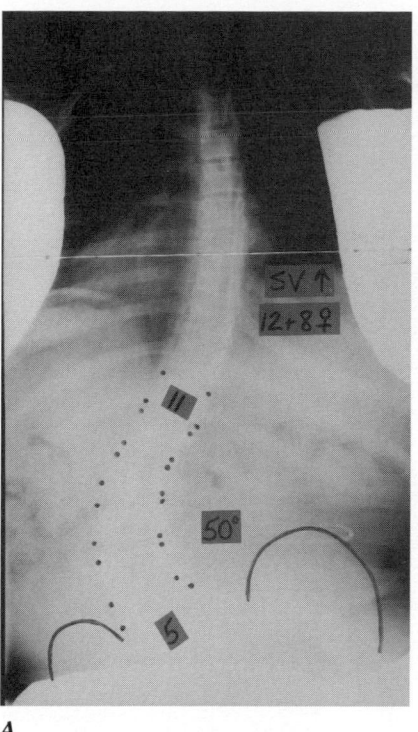

A

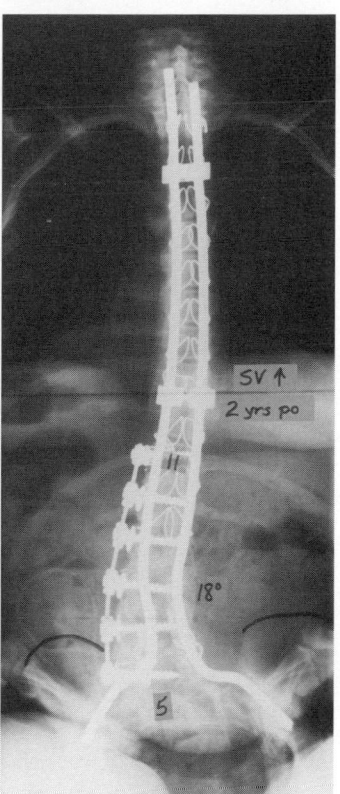

B

occur mainly in boys and are characterized by proximal muscle weakness with a sex-linked recessive inheritance pattern. Children with Duchenne muscular dystrophy are more severely affected than those with Becker muscular dystropy.[49] The diagnosis of muscular dystrophy is usually made in the young child, due to delayed motor milestones. Often, these children are noted to be clumsy and to have difficulty running, although that may be noted only retrospectively. Other clinical findings include enlarged calf muscles, mild Achilles contractures, quadriceps weakness, and gluteus maximus weakness, as indicated by a positive Gower's sign. Later on, a wide-based lordotic stance and waddling Trendelenburg gait becomes manifest. The diagnosis is confirmed by laboratory findings of highly elevated levels of creatinine phosphokinase, 50 to 100 times normal, and a muscle biopsy characterized by split fibers, degenerating fibers, and deposition of fibrous tissue.[49] The gene defect has been isolated to the Xp21 locus of the chromosome. In normal children, this gene produces the protein dystrophin, which is a structural component of normal muscle fibers. Patients can be classified into the Duchenne versus the Becker type of dystrophy by the dystrophic level in the muscle biopsy: less than 3 percent of normal, Duchenne; 3 to 10 percent of normal, severe Becker dystrophy; and 20 percent or more of normal, mild Becker dystrophy.

The clinical course of patients with Duchenne muscular dystrophy is one of progressive deterioration in muscle function and thus overall function.[105] These patients usually become wheelchair-bound by 11 to 13 years of age and subsequently develop a progressive thoracolumbar scoliosis.[105] The progressive spinal deformity produces a decline in pulmonary function, which directly contributes to an earlier death due to cardiopulmonary failure and/or respiratory infections. The disease course is less aggressive in the Becker type of muscular dystrophy, with the patients often still able to walk into their twenties and beyond.

The incidence of progressive scoliosis in Duchenne muscular dystrophy is approximately 95 percent or higher.[105,151] This almost always occurs within several years after the patient becomes wheelchair-bound and greatly interferes with sitting balance and upper extremity function. Concomitant with an increased spinal deformity is a decline in respiratory function.[93,110,116,151] Unfortunately, the combination of both of these can lead to an earlier demise. The forced vital capacity is the best pulmonary function value to monitor in these patients. This begins to decline rapidly once the patients become wheelchair-bound, usually deteriorating to approximately 25 percent of normal until death.[116] Studies have shown that early surgical treatment of these patients, due in part to the stabilization of pulmonary function, can extend survival for several years.[184]

Bracing has little or no role in the treatment of these patients because only curve progression is slowed while the systemic manifestations of the disease continue. Eventually, the braced spinal deformity begins to progress rapidly, and by this time the patient may be too debilitated with decreased pulmonary function to withstand surgery. Certainly, all patients should be fitted with a well-contoured wheelchair seat.

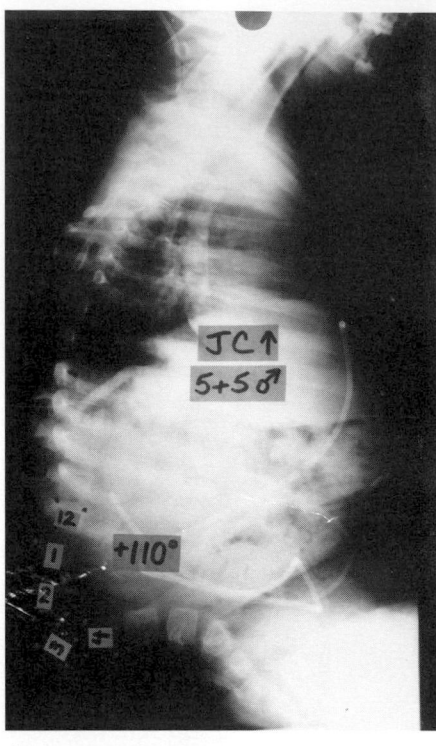

A

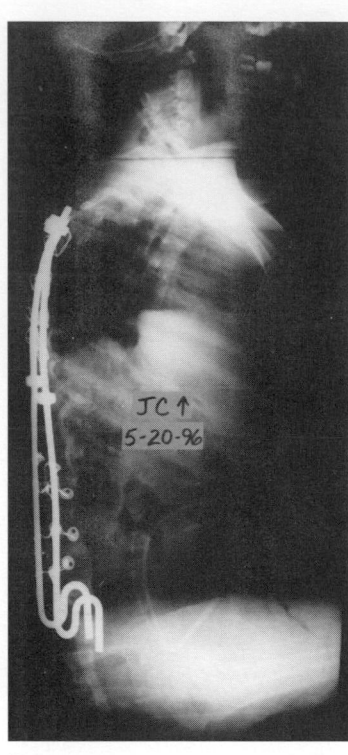

B

Figure 75-42 J.C., a 5 + 5-year-old male, has a high-level myelomeningocele with a 110° low lumbar fixed kyphosis. He underwent a posterior apical kyphectomy with reconstruction of the proximal and distal ends of his spinal column with bilateral Luque rods bent with a Dunn-McCarthy bend to sit over the anterior aspect of the sacrum. Postoperative lateral x-ray (*B*) demonstrates complete correction of the lumbar kyphosis. (Courtesy of Keith H. Bridwell, MD.)

Posterior spinal instrumentation and fusion is the treatment of choice for this type of scoliosis[64,184] (Fig. 75-43). Ideally, it should be performed once the patients are unable to ambulate and are wheelchair-bound. The instrumentation and fusion should extend from the upper thoracic spine to the sacrum so as to prevent or correct pelvic obliquity. However, some authors suggest that these patients will usually succumb to their progressive disease before the development of a severe pelvic obliquity deformity.[86] Commonly, Luque instrumentation with segmental sublaminar and/or Wisconsin wiring is performed.[5] This allows prompt postoperative mobilization without the use of an external orthosis. Postoperative respiratory complications are occasionally unavoidable. Basically, patients with preoperative pulmonary function better than 30 percent of normal usually tolerate the procedure well, with minimal time spent on a ventilator postoperatively. Patients with respiratory function between 20 and 30 percent of normal may require prolonged ventilatory support. Patients with less than 20 percent of normal function probably will not get off the ventilator and thus may be inoperable. The ultimate goal in the treatment of this deformity is the maintenance of an upright sitting posture, which slows the inevitable respiratory decline and thus maximizes quality of life for these patients.

Spinal Muscular Atrophy

Spinal muscular atrophy (SMA) encompasses a group of inherited conditions characterized by degeneration of the anterior horn cells of the spinal cord. Clinical elements common to all patients include symmetrical limb and trunk weakness and muscular atrophy affecting the lower extremities and proximal muscles more than the upper extremities and distal muscles. Intelligence and sensation are usually normal. The incidence is 1 in 15,000 live births. Scoliosis, joint contractures, and hip dislocations are the most common orthopaedic conditions associated with the disease.

The reported incidence of scoliosis in SMA varies but is probably between 50 and 60 percent.[19,79,176] If one follows patients to skeletal maturity, it is apparent that most of them will develop scoliosis.[176] As in many neuromuscular diseases, a spinal deformity that occurs in patients with SMA develops because of muscle weakness. This leads to a progressive collapsing spinal deformity that is often independent of the patient's growth pattern.

Three types of SMA have been characterized: type I or Werdnig-Hoffmann disease, which is an acute type; type II, or intermediate/severe chronic childhood SMA; and type III, or mild childhood SMA, known as Kugelberg-Welander disease. Most patients with the acute or type I form are severely involved and succumb to the disease at a young age. The prognosis is brighter for those with the chronic childhood forms, including type II and especially type III. Often these patients will ambulate up to age 20 or so, and occasionally patients show minimal deterioration with aging.

The occurrence of a spinal deformity should generally be anticipated in patients with SMA. Most patients are diagnosed in childhood with their deformity, and the strongest factor relating to the occurrence and progression of scoliosis seems to be the level of motor function.[79,176]

Common characteristics of all types of SMA are symmetrical muscular atrophy, fasciculations—especially of the tongue, and trembling of the hands. Diagnosis is based

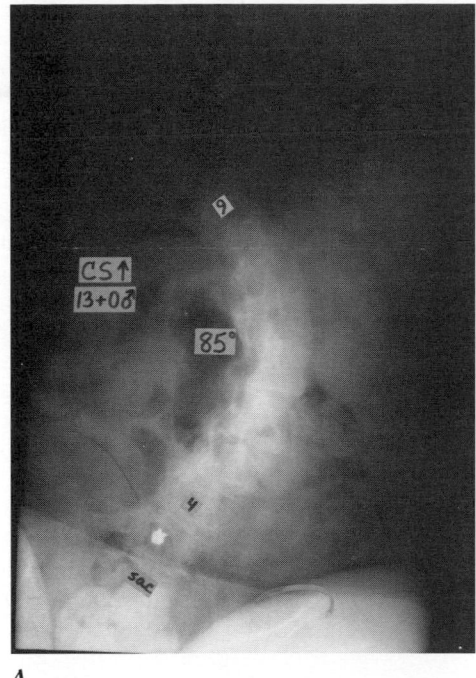

A

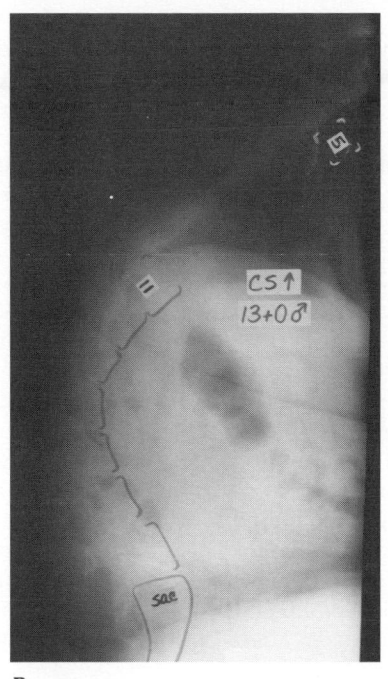

B

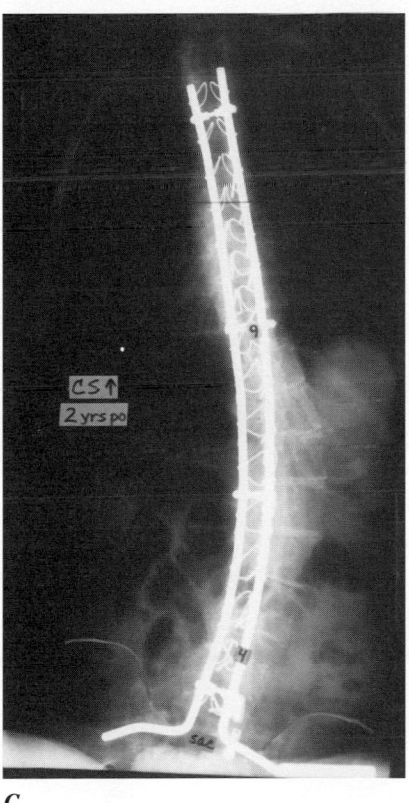

C

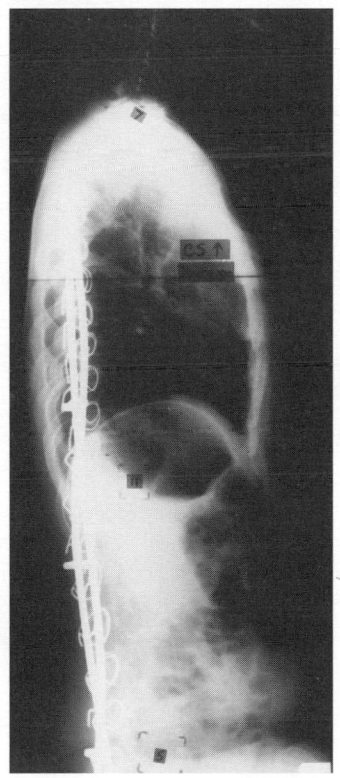

D

Figure 75-43 C.S., a 13-year-old male, has Duchenne muscular dystrophy. He was nonambulatory for approximately 2 years prior to seeking treatment for his spinal deformity. His sitting unsupported coronal x-ray (*A*) demonstrates an 85° neuromuscular scoliosis with associated pelvic obliquity. The sagittal plane (*B*) shows global kyphosis of the entire thoracic and lumbar spine due to muscle weakness. His pulmonary function was still greater than 30 percent of the predicted; thus he was a candidate for posterior instrumentation and fusion to correct his deformity, improve his sitting posture, and slow his inevitable pulmonary decline. His 2-year postoperative coronal (*C*) and sagittal (*D*) x-rays show correction in both planes. (Courtesy of Keith H. Bridwell, MD.)

on the clinical features and genetic evidence of the affected family. The pyramidal long tracts are not involved.

The treatment of spinal deformity in SMA patients is primarily operative.[65,164,171] Certainly, orthoses may be used, with the objective of reducing the rate of progression while helping to maintain a proper sitting posture. However, as in other neuromuscular disorders, orthoses will not avoid development or ultimate progression of the deformity. Certainly, patients who function at a higher level can benefit from a brace more than those with severe weakness, who often tolerate a brace poorly. Generally, orthoses are indicated in children with deformities between 20 and 40°. Once the deformity progresses to more than 50°, regardless of the age of the child, spinal fusion must be considered.

Surgical treatment of these patients involves segmental spinal instrumentation from the upper thoracic spine to the pelvis using Luque rods and sublaminar wires and a Galveston technique for pelvic fixation[8] (Fig. 75-44). It is recommended that these curves be operated once they reach 50 to 60°, avoiding those curves that have progressed to 100° or more.[166] The anterior procedure on these pa-

tients adds considerable pulmonary risk and should be avoided if possible. Thus, the smaller, more manageable deformity can be treated by posterior instrumentation and fusion alone. Fusion is performed with local autogenous bone graft procured during the procedure and supplemented judiciously with allograft bone. We prefer fresh-frozen femoral head allograft cut into small pieces. Our results have been quite acceptable when this type of allograft is placed in flaccid SMA patients approached posteriorly alone.[40] It is best to avoid use of a postoperative orthosis in these frail patients. Anterior releases and fusions combined with posterior instrumentation and fusion must be performed if there is a severe fixed lumbar curve with pelvic obliquity. However, the surgeon must consider the added risk in these procedures, which must often be staged because of potential pulmonary complications. Certainly, the complication rate is higher in patients who are older and have more severe curves; it approaches 40 percent in patients who undergo surgery.[164] It is important to thoroughly evaluate pulmonary function preoperatively, often with the assistance of a pulmonologist, in order to assess the relative risks of undergoing a spinal fusion.

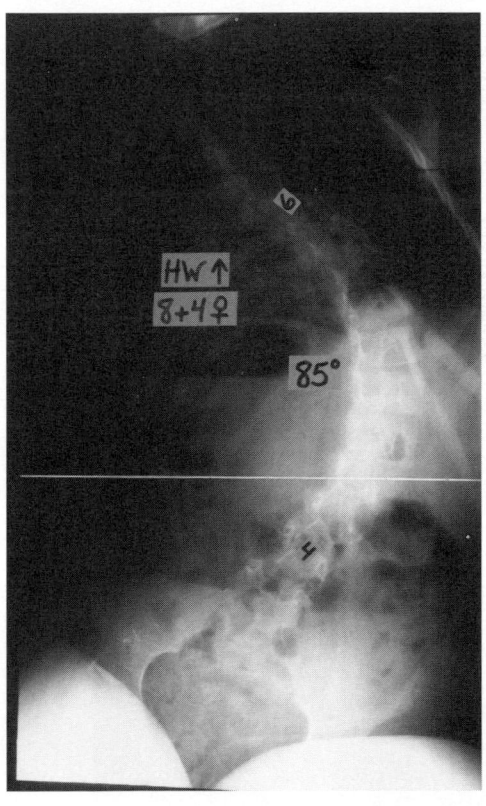

A

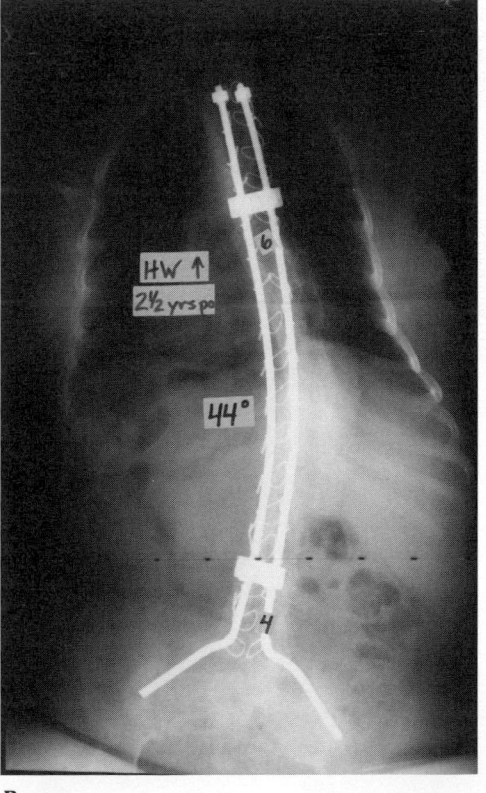

B

Figure 75-44 H.W., an 8 + 4-year-old female, has type II childhood spinal muscular atrophy and is a nonambulator. Upon presentation, her coronal x-ray (*A*) shows an 85° neuromuscular scoliosis with pelvic obliquity. Her poor pulmonary function did not allow consideration of anterior fusion. She was thus treated with single-stage posterior instrumentation and fusion from T2 to the pelvis with Luque rods, sublaminar wires, and Galveston fixation into her pelvis. Her 2 ½-year postoperative coronal x-ray (*B*) demonstrates maintenance of the correction at 44° and a suspected solid spinal fusion. It is often difficult, in these osteoporotic patients, to document a solid fusion. However, when the correction is maintained and instrumentation is intact at 2 years postoperative, the spine is considered fused. Fusion was performed with allograft fresh-frozen femoral head and local bone harvested during the laminotomies performed for the passage of sublaminar wires.

Friedreich's Ataxia

Friedreich's ataxia is the most common hereditary progressive spinocerebellar degenerative disease. However, over 57 hereditary ataxic syndromes have been identified thus far. Barbeau et al.[16] have proposed a clinical classification based on five factors: inheritance pattern, progression pattern, age at first onset of symptoms, state of deep tendon reflexes, and the type of ataxia. According to this classification, Friedreich's ataxia is defined as a progressive autosomal recessive syndrome of early onset with decreased or absent reflexes and a predominant spinocerebellar incoordination.[16]

The prevalence of Friedreich's ataxia is approximately 1 per 100,000 population.[47] Males and females are equally affected, and the geographic distribution is worldwide. Chamberlain et al.[53] have mapped the gene responsible for Friedreich's ataxia to chromosome 9. Unfortunately, the biochemical disorder has not yet been identified.

Because of the large number of ataxic syndromes, it is important to establish a clear diagnosis for patients suspected of having Friedreich's ataxia. Harding[94] modified a classification system initially developed by Geoffroy et al.; this is now universally accepted: group I, typical Friedreich's ataxia; group Ia, complete picture; group Ib, incomplete picture; group IIa, atypical Friedreich's ataxia; group IIb, not Friedreich's ataxia.

The primary signs and symptoms used for diagnosing group I Friedreich's ataxia include onset prior to age 25, progressive ataxia of limbs and gait, absent knee and ankle jerks, extensor plantar responses, decreased motor and nerve conduction velocities with smaller or absent sensory action potentials, and dysarthria. Secondary symptoms and signs present in most cases but not essential for diagnosis include scoliosis, weak lower limbs, distal loss of joint position and vibration sense, abnormal electrocardiograms, and difficulty with ambulation, among others.[117] Other less common symptoms and signs include optic atrophy, nystagmus, distal weakness, partial deafness, and pes cavus, among others.

The prevalence of scoliosis in Friedreich's ataxia has been found to be close to 100 percent.[47] Males and females are equally affected, and left- and right-sided curves are seen with equal frequency. Approximately 80 percent of cases have typical idiopathic types of deformities, while 20 percent will have typical neuromuscular deformities with long sweeping curves, including pelvic obliquity.[100]

The natural history of scoliosis in these patients is somewhat variable.[47] Approximately one-third will have minimally progressive deformities not requiring treatment. Also on average, patients with Friedreich's ataxia survive only until the third decade of life, so that many do not live long enough to experience the detrimental effects of progressive scoliosis. However, curve progression can occur to a significant degree during the adolescent growth spurt; and these high-risk curves must be closely monitored and appropriately treated.

Nonoperative treatment in these patients has generally been unsuccessful and is not recommended.[47,118] Bracing is often poorly tolerated and impairs walking ability in these patients, who are often struggling to continue walking in the first place. Thus, surgery is the only treatment that can clearly alter their prognosis by providing curve correction and stabilization of progressive curves.[47,63,118] Indications for surgery are quite similar to those for adolescent idiopathic scoliosis and include all progressive deformities of more than 50° in the frontal plane. Most surgeons dealing with the surgical treatment of Friedreich's ataxia have utilized Harrington or Luque instrumentation.[47,63,118] Although newer segmental spinal instrumentation systems currently appear to be a logical choice, no published reports are available to document their success. Most ambulatory patients can be treated short of the sacrum using the fusion levels established for idiopathic scoliosis. An anterior fusion is required only for large and rigid curves prior to posterior instrumentation and fusion (Fig. 75-45). The results of surgery among these patients are quite good as long as the curves treated are of moderate severity. It is important to recognize that neurophysiologic monitoring of these patients intraoperatively may be difficult or impossible. Thus, plans to perform a wake-up test following correction of the deformity should be discussed and carried out.

Poliomyelitis

The orthopaedic manifestations of poliomyelitis are due to destruction of the anterior horn cells of the spinal cord, which causes a flaccid paralysis. Due to widespread immunization in North America, reports of new cases are extremely rare.[57] Accordingly, patients presenting with spinal deformities due to polio are usually adults with significant curves (Fig. 75-46). Associated problems include respiratory insufficiency due to both thoracic respiratory muscle paralysis and truncal deformity. There is also pain secondary to the pelvic obliquity and spinal deformity as well as a progressive decline in endurance secondary to cardiopulmonary problems. Brace treatment is usually not helpful for these patients.[57]

It was specifically for these patients that Luque developed his method of segmental spinal instrumentation in the mid-1970s.[139] Its advantages were (1) the ability to contour rods to achieve physiologic sagittal alignment; (2) distribution of the corrective forces over multiple segments, thus decreasing the pull-out force on each individual segment; (3) the ability to fix the spinal pelvic unit as one using Galveston fixation; and (4) rapid postoperative immobilization without the use of external support. Many of these patients require a first-stage anterior release and fusion, especially patients with kyphosis, which is very common.[68,144,159]

Neurofibromatosis

Classic neurofibromatosis as described by von Recklinghausen in 1982 is inherited as an autosomal dominant trait with variable expressivity. Some 10 to 40 percent of patients with neurofibromatosis will develop a spinal deformity.

To help establish a diagnosis, Riccardi in 1981 differentiated two types of neurofibromatosis on the basis of their clinical manifestations.[170] Primary features include multiple

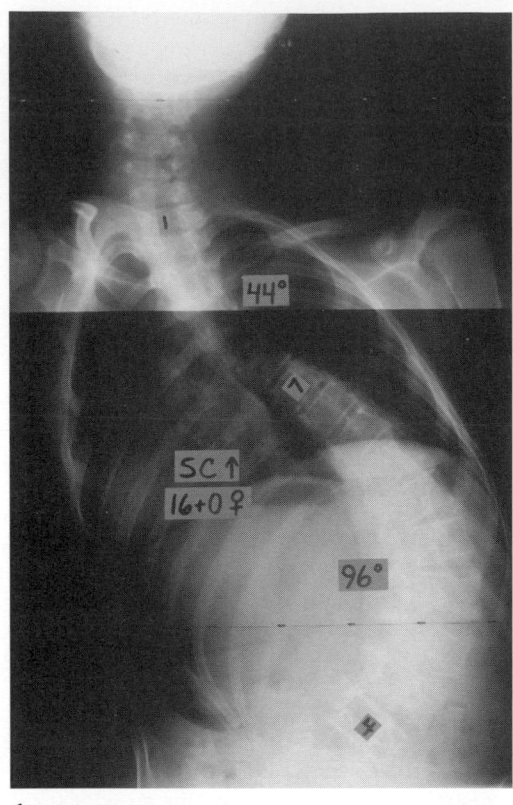

A

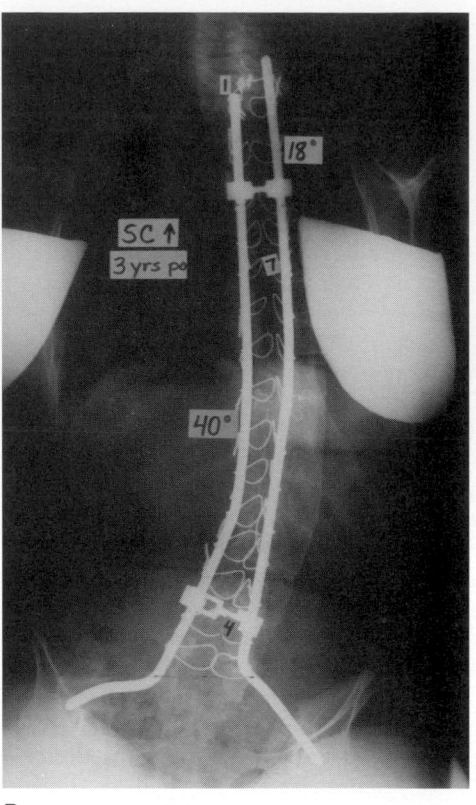

B

Figure 75-45 S.C., a 16-year-old female, has severe Friedreich's ataxia, which has left her wheelchair-bound. *A.* She presented with a 96° neuromuscular-type scoliosis with pelvic obliquity. Because of the magnitude of the curve and its stiffness, she underwent a staged anterior and posterior spinal fusion. Her an-terior fusion extended from T10 to the sacrum and her posterior fusion from T2 to the pelvis. Her 3-year postoperative coronal x-ray (*B*) demonstrates that her scoliosis has improved to 40°, with a concomitant improvement in her spinal balance and pelvic obliquity.

café au lait spots, multiple neurofibromas, and Lich nodules (pigmented iris hamartomas). Café-au-lait spots are not considered diagnostic unless more than six are found with a diameter greater than 1.5 cm.[170] In children, 5 or more café-au-lait spots each 0.5 cm or more in diameter is considered pathognomonic for neurofibromatosis.[59]

Two types of scoliosis are found in neurofibromatosis patients: dystrophic and nondystrophic.[60] Dystrophic scoliosis occurs along with dystrophic changes, including vertebral body wedging, marked apical vertebral rotation, scalloping of the vertebral body, foraminal enlargement, transverse process spindling, and rib penciling[50] (Fig. 75-47). Dystrophic curves are usually located in the thoracic area; they tend to be very short, involving only four to six vertebrae, and are inherently progressive. In many cases, they are associated with kyphosis in the sagittal plane; however, lordosis may occasionally be seen. Dystrophic curves tend to progress rapidly and are also associated with abnormalities of the cervical spine, which should be examined prior to surgical treatment.[61]

Nondystrophic curves resemble and behave just like idiopathic curves; thus treatment is similar to that of patients with idiopathic scoliosis. However, prior to any sur-gical intervention in these patients, imaging of the spinal canal as with MRI is indicated to check for intraspinal neurofibroma or other abnormalities.[82] Certainly dystrophic curves will involve a higher incidence of intraspinal abnormalities than nondystrophic curves.[140]

Orthotic treatment may be helpful with the nondystrophic curves but has not been found effective with progressive dystrophic ones.[52] For progressive dystrophic curves with concomitant severe and rigid kyphosis, anterior releases followed by skeletal traction may be helpful prior to posterior instrumentation and fusion so as to obtain correction more safely.[52,106] Overcorrection of the stiff short deformity must be avoided. Even progressive rigid curves should undergo spinal fusion, for paraplegia may result in untreated cases.[60,191] Segmental spinal fixation along with postoperative external immobilization is helpful to improve the fusion rate in these curves, which are prone to be associated with pseudarthrosis, especially those with a significant kyphotic deformity.[180,212] Occasionally, anterior strut grafts are necessary to control the kyphotic progression of the deformity.[209] Rarely, a lordotic thoracic sagittal alignment will be encountered in these patients; this can severely compromise pulmonary function.[207]

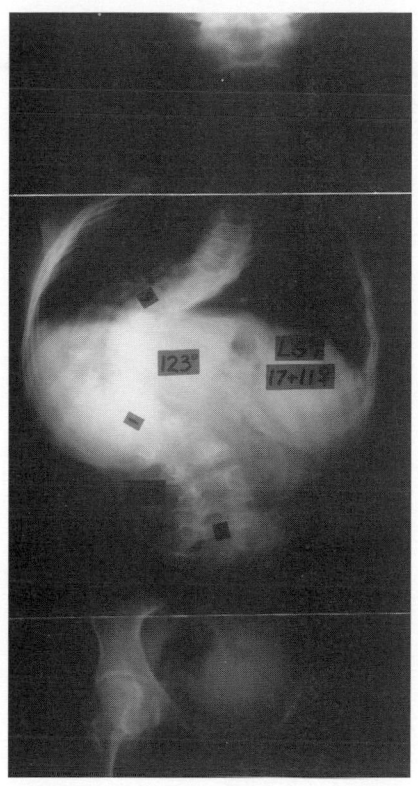

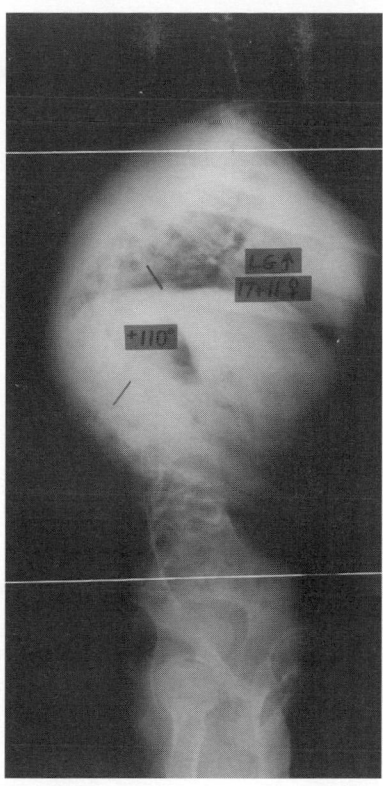

A   *B*

Figure 75-46 L.G, a female of almost 18, has a known history of polio. She presented for treatment for her severe kyphoscoliosis deformity. Her coronal x-ray (*A*) demonstrated a 123° left thoracolumbar scoliosis. *B*. Her sagittal plane showed 110° kyphosis centered over the same levels as her coronal plane deformity. She underwent a staged anterior release and fusion followed by posterior instrumentation and fusion for correction and stabilization of her deformity.

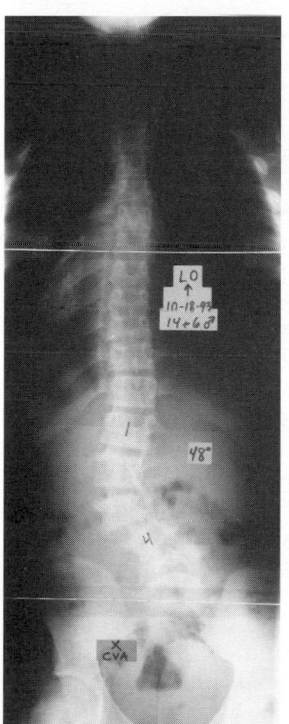

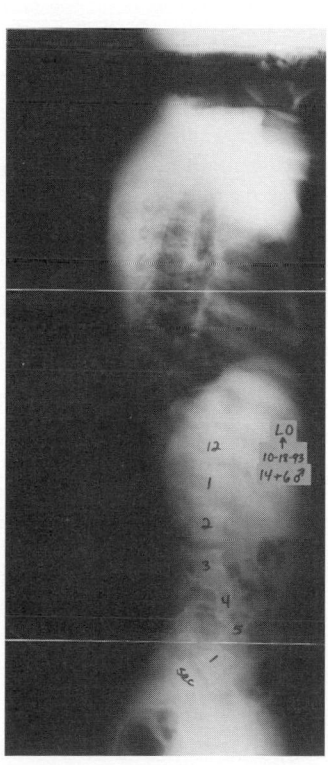

A   *B*

Figure 75-47 Coronal (*A*) and sagittal (*B*) x-rays of a lumbar curve in a case of dystrophic neurofibromatosis, with associated severe vertebral rotation, scalloping of the vertebral bodies, and rather sharp angulation to the curve.

Marfan's Syndrome

Marfan's syndrome is a prototypical hereditary connective tissue disorder. Recently, abnormalities of the fibrillin gene have been confirmed as its phenotypic manifestation.[119] It is inherited as an autosomal dominant trait and has cardiovascular, ocular, and skeletal manifestations. Scoliosis occurs in 40 to 75 percent of patients with Marfan's syndrome; it is often progressive and can become severe[23] (Fig. 75-48). Males are affected as often as females, and the deformity frequently presents in the infantile and juvenile age groups. Scoliosis is the primary deformity; however, kyphoscoliosis or more commonly lordoscoliosis may occur in the thoracic spine. Lumbar curves are often hypokyphotic and may result in disabling back pain. The natural history of scoliosis in Marfan's syndrome is one of steady progression, usually leading to severe and rigid deformities.[23,161]

Orthotic treatment for Marfan's scoliosis has a fairly poor prognosis. Correction that may be obtained is lost after the brace is discontinued.[161] The Milwaukee brace is used in young patients with mild to moderate flexible curves under 40 to 50°. Larger rigid curves are unresponsive to orthotic treatment and should be considered for fusion. If a patient is braced, it is imperative to make sure that the brace is not accentuating thoracic lordosis, which will cause pulmonary deterioration. Lumbosacral spondylolisthesis may also be encountered and should be assessed during the evaluation.[205]

Infantile and juvenile patients with flexible curves and fairly normal sagittal alignment may be considered for sub-

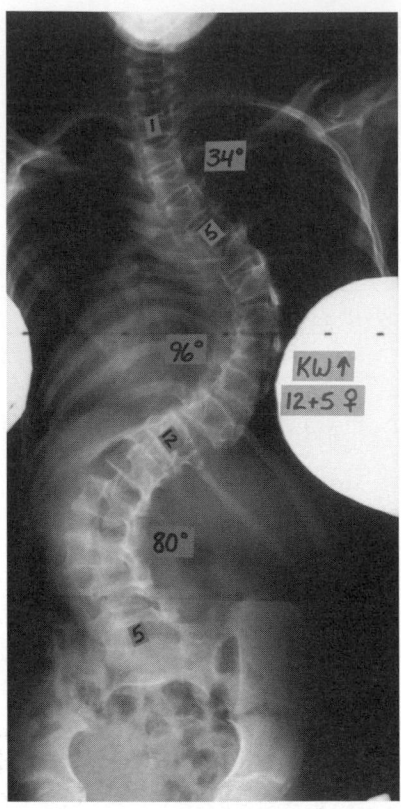

A

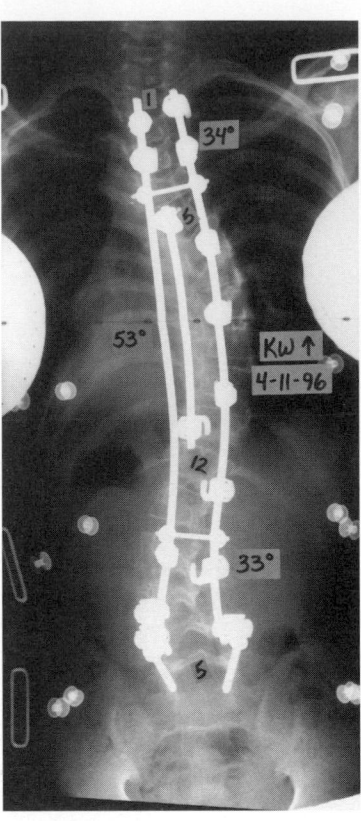

B

Figure 75-48 K.W., a 12 + 5-year-old female with Marfan's syndrome, presented with this large spinal deformity. The coronal long-cassette x-ray (*A*) showed a 96° right thoracic, 80° left lumbar scoliosis. *B.* This necessitated a posterior instrumentation and fusion from T2 to L5 to control the deformity in this skeletally immature patient.

cutaneous rod procedures with intermittent lengthenings. Because these young patients often have flexible curves, this may allow axial growth to occur prior to definitive spinal fusion (Fig. 75-49).

Spinal fusion for Marfan's scoliosis is treated similarly to idiopathic scoliosis.[175] However, prior to surgery, a thorough cardiovascular evaluation is needed to exclude aortic aneurysms and cardiac valvular lesions with potential for cardiac failure. Occasionally, patients will need cardiothoracic surgery prior to spinal fusion.

Large curves (greater than 90 to 100°) often need perioperative halo gravity traction to ensure safe correction. Anterior procedures are done with indications similar to those of idiopathic scoliosis. Patients who are severely lordotic through the thoracic spine may need an anterior closing wedge osteotomy procedure prior to posterior instrumentation and fusion with posterior translation of the spinal column.[175,206] Overall, the pseudarthrosis rates in Marfan's patients and those with idiopathic scoliosis are quite similar and the results of surgical fusion should also be about the same.

Neuropathic Causes of Spinal Deformity

Since idiopathic scoliosis is a diagnosis of exclusion, all efforts should be made to confirm that diagnosis via a complete history and thorough physical examination. Any history of abnormal neurologic symptoms—such as numbness or weakness in a particular extremity, difficulty with bowel or bladder control, or persistent, unexplained spinal or extremity pain—should suggest a potential neuropathic cause of scoliosis. Similarly, any abnormality in the physical examination—including asymmetrical upper extremity, lower extremity, or abdominal reflexes; peripheral weakness or sensory changes; as well as any gait abnormalities—should raise suspicion for some type of neural axis abnormality. Any patient with a suspicious history or physical examination should undergo prompt MRI examination, certainly prior to any corrective spinal surgical procedure.

Certain radiographic characteristics warrant increased suspicion for a nonidiopathic diagnosis. Probably one of the most common radiographic abnormalities associated with an abnormal neural axis is a primary left thoracic curve. It has been shown in several studies that there is somewhere between a 25 and 40 percent incidence of syringomyelia in primary left thoracic scoliosis. Also, any unusual curve progression not accounted for by skeletal growth alone, curve rigidity, or otherwise atypical curve patterns—such as sharply angular curves, cervicothoracic curves, or left thoracic–right lumbar double major curves—should undergo MRI investigation prior to surgical fusion. Recently, juvenile scoliosis with an otherwise idiopathic appearance has been shown to coincide in approximately 20 to 25 percent of cases with abnormalities of the neural axis.[125] Thus, patients age 10 and under who are undergoing a scoliosis fusion should have preoperative MRI scanning even with an otherwise normal history, examination, and radiographs.

Figure 75-49 A.T., a 6 + 7-year-old female with known Marfan's syndrome, had developed an 82° right thoracic scoliosis (*A*) at this very young age. To help control her significant deformity while allowing continued axial growth, she underwent a posterior subcutaneous rod placement with subsequent lengthenings over time. X-ray (*B*) following her first lengthening showed improvement of her curve to 37°. Note that she has continued to wear a brace for improved control of her deformity along with the subcutaneous rod.

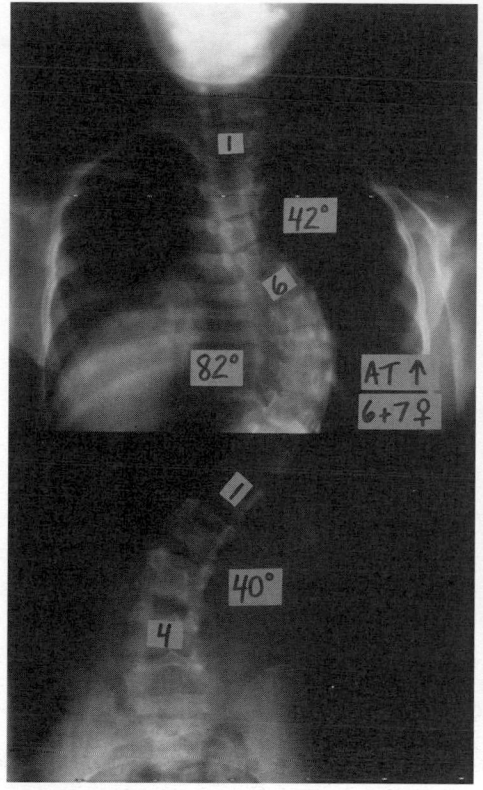

A

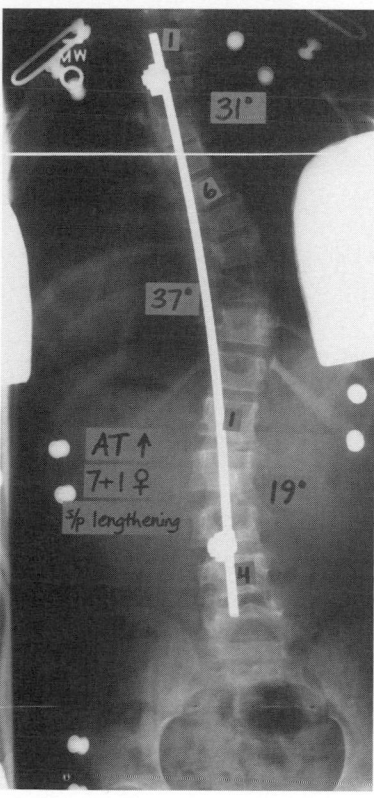

B

Certainly any patient with unexplained spinal pain, with or without radiographic progression of the deformity, should raise suspicion for a spinal canal or spinal column abnormality. Neural axis abnormalities such as syringomyelia, tethered cord, Arnold-Chiari malformations, and spinal tumors such as osteoid osteoma or osteoblastoma may occur in association with or as the principal cause of spinal deformity[2,90,96,104,145] (Fig. 75-50). Often, only subtle radiographic signs such as increased thoracic kyphosis may indicate these abnormalities. Thus, it is imperative that the physician caring for patients with spinal deformities always have nonidiopathic diagnoses in mind. The curve magnitude in and of itself may not be a justification for preoperative MRI scanning, since a study by O'Brien et al. showed no increased evidence of spinal canal abnormalities associated with curve magnitudes greater than or equal to 70° in otherwise "idiopathic" patients.[160] Certainly in our cost-conscious health care environment, screening examinations such as a total spine MRI should be used prudently, but not at the risk of misdiagnosis. This exam must include sagittal images of the cervical, thoracic, and lumbar spine, with axial images of the occipitocervical, cervicothoracic, thoracolumbar, and lumbosacral junctions for completeness. These studies should be reviewed by a neuroradiologist as well as the attending spine surgeon. The goal is to truly exclude all nonidiopathic patients that have neural axis abnormalities presenting with a spinal deformity.

Spinal Deformity and Skeletal Dysplasia

Although fairly rare for most orthopedists to evaluate, patients with skeletal dysplasia may present with spinal deformity.[83] Although well over 120 different short-stature syndromes have been described, with this number increasing annually, there are many commonalities to these syndromes of which pediatric spine specialists should be aware.[22,102,188] Some of these syndromes may be apparent at birth; however, many are discovered later, following growth, when shortening of the trunk versus the extremities becomes more noticeable. Syndrome identification is aided by noting the location of the limb shortening. The term *rhizomelia* refers to shortening of the proximal limb (e.g., achondroplasia); *mesomelia* describes midlimb shortening; and *acromelia* describes shortening of the distal limb, such as short hands and feet. Early on, the most common spinal change is platyspondylia (flattened vertebral bodies), which may or may not progress to a spinal deformity such as scoliosis or kyphosis. Consultation with a geneticist is useful both to confirm the diagnosis and to counsel the family regarding the risks of having future children with similar skeletal dysplasias.

Achondroplasia is the most common skeletal dysplasia requiring treatment for spinal abnormalities.[188] These are rhizomelic patients in whom the upper arm and thigh segments are the shortest components. These patients usually present with muscle hypotonia and developmental

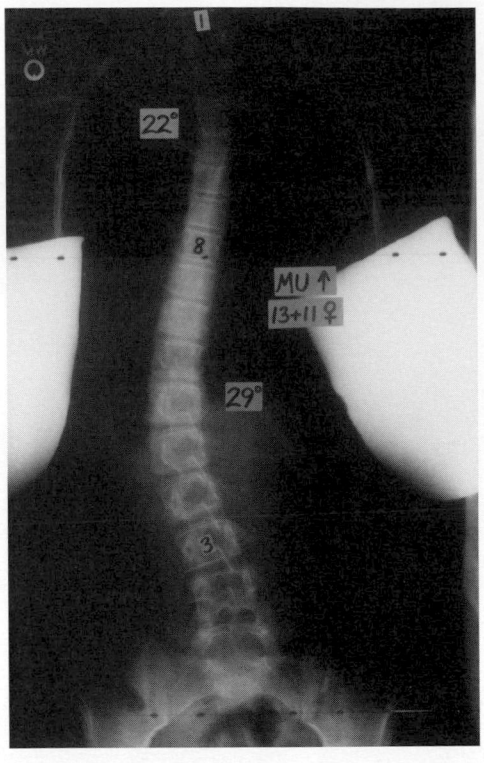

A

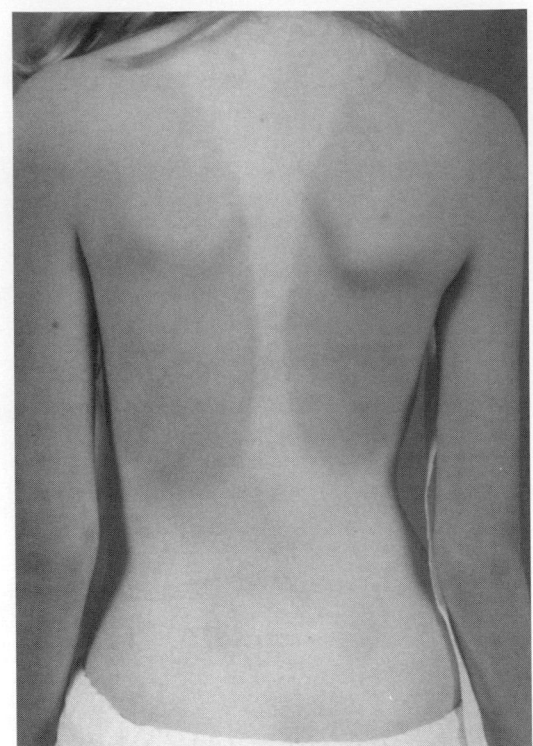

B

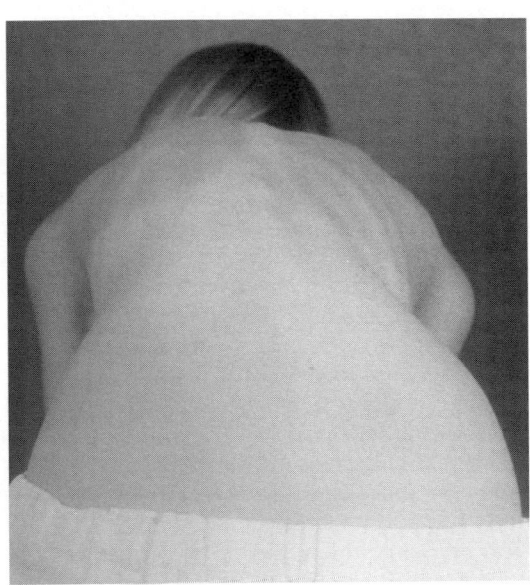

C

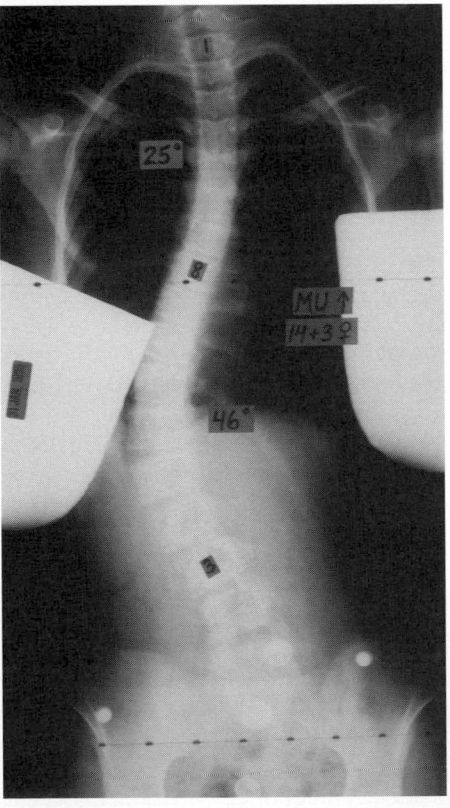

D

Figure 75-50 M.V., a 13 + 11-year-old female, presented for evaluation of a mild spinal deformity. Her presenting x-ray (*A*) showed a 29° left thoracolumbar scoliosis. Her upright clinical photo (*B*) demonstrated her minimal deformity, while her forward bending test (*C*) demonstrated the rotational component of her scoliosis. Her deformity was observed at this point, and she returned 4 months later complaining of increased lower lumbar pain. Her physical exam—except for her deformity—was unremarkable. *D.* At this point her curve had increased to 46°. She was placed in a brace and had a total-spine MRI, which demonstrated a tethered spinal cord. She then underwent surgery to release her spinal cord. This, however, did not control her spinal deformity.

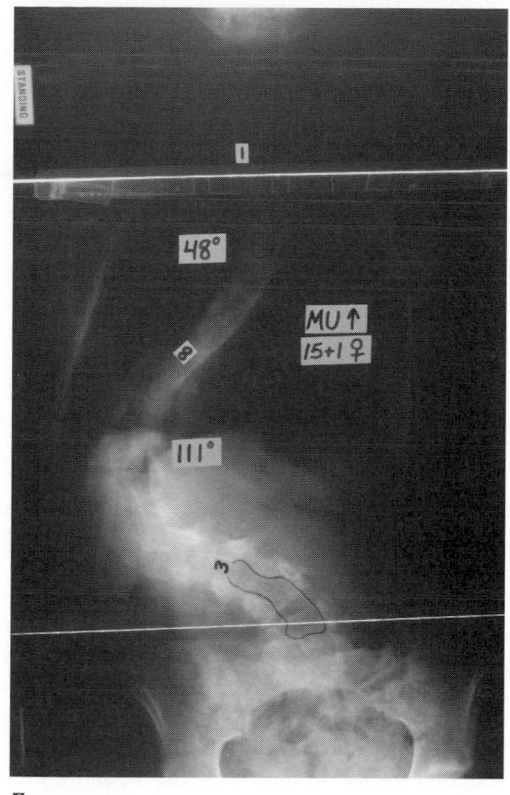

E

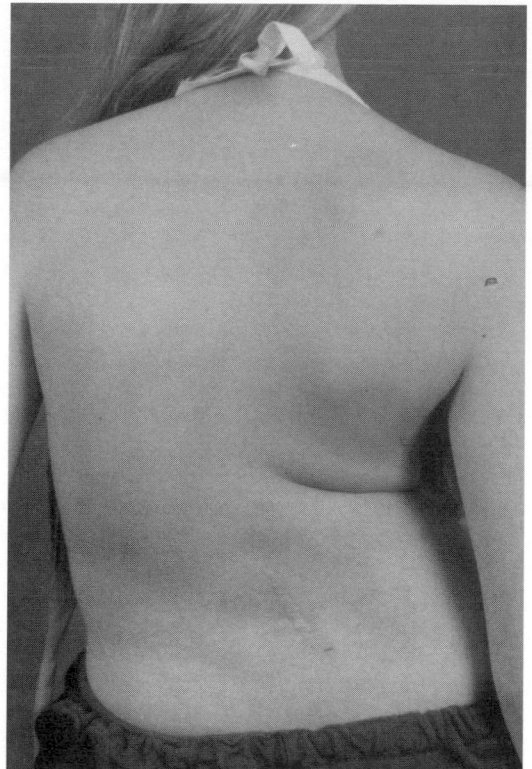

F

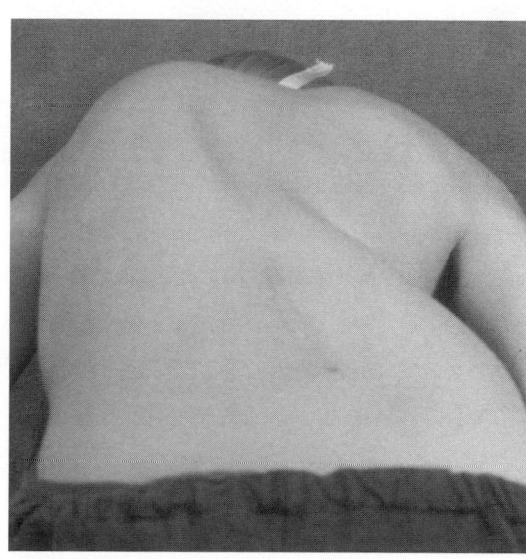

G

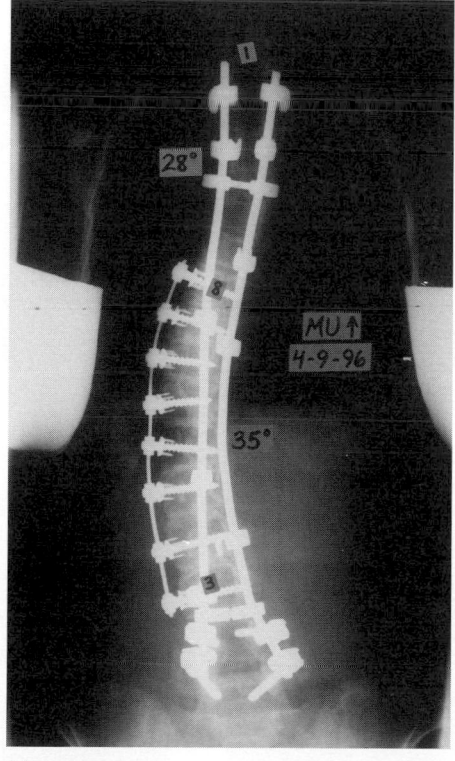

H

Figure 75-50 *(Continued)* Her long-cassette x-ray (*E*) 8 months later showed a marked increase in her scoliosis to 111°. Her laminectomy defect was also noted from L3 to the sacrum. *F* and *G.* The patient's clinical upright and bending photos also demonstrated a marked clinical deterioration in her deformity. She underwent a staged anterior and posterior spinal fusion to correct her deformity and stop the progression. Her anterior instrumentation and fusion were performed from T8 to L3. The second-stage posterior instrumentation and fusion went from T2 to L5. This patient's postoperative coronal x-ray (*H*) demonstrates correction of her scoliosis to 35°, with improved clinical alignment.

delay. Spinal radiographs show progressive narrowing of the interpedicular distance from the upper lumbar spine to the sacrum on coronal views and often thoracolumbar kyphosis on the lateral views. These patients tend to develop spinal stenosis either at the occipitocervical junction or in the thoracolumbar and lumbar spine, which may lead to neurologic sequelae (Fig. 75-51).

The treatment of achondroplastic spinal abnormalities is based upon the degree of abnormality and the natural history of the specific problem. Some 90 percent of patients with thoracolumbar kyphosis improve without specific treatment.[208] Thus, observation is the most appropriate early course of management. After age 5 or 6, kyphosis with vertebral body wedging greater than 40° normally does not spontaneously correct and anterior and posterior surgical fusion may be indicated. Care must be taken to avoid placing implants in the spinal canal, for these patients' spinal canals are narrowed, and such placement may increase the risk of neurologic sequelae.

Achondroplastic patients are at risk for insidious neurologic compression of either nerve roots or spinal cord. Often, the progressive decrease in the patient's ability to walk long distances is due to spinal claudication. The symptoms are improved by flexion of the spine, which optimizes the space in the spinal canal. Bladder abnormalities from sacral root compression may also occur

and be part of the presentation. Treatment of achondroplastic spinal stenosis is somewhat controversial, since these patients are often kyphotic over the stenotic levels. Following evaluation with MRI with or without a CT/myelogram, spinal decompression is indicated. Whether a fusion should be performed is debatable. For multilevel disease, we recommend midline decompression, sparing the facet joints bilaterally. Fusion should be entertained for patients with kyphosis of more than 40 to 50° over the apex of the decompressed levels. This increases the neurologic risk of the procedure; often in situ fusion with instrumentation must be performed to avoid neurologic sequelae.

Pseudoachondroplasia is an autosomal dominant condition characterized by rhizomelia and normal trunk size. These patients have normal facies, abnormal joint laxity, and no narrowed distances between the pedicles, which helps distinguish this condition from achondroplasia.[21] These patients may develop atlantoaxial instability with subsequent myelopathy, platyspondyly, scoliosis, or excessive thoracic kyphosis or lumbar lordosis. If these patients' spinal deformities do require surgical treatment, segmental spinal fixation may be utilized, since the spinal canal is not as stenotic as those in achondroplasia. Thus, the intraoperative neurologic risk for these patients is much lower.

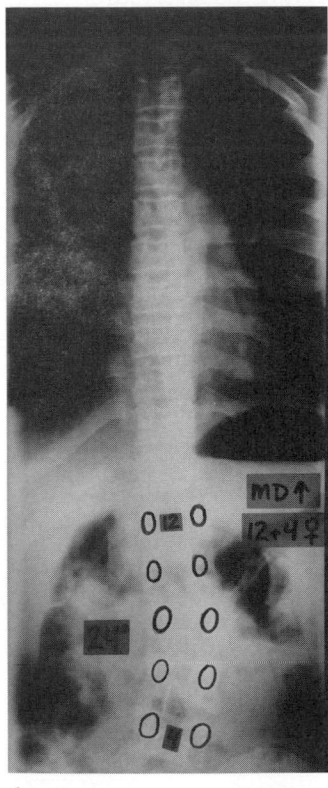

A

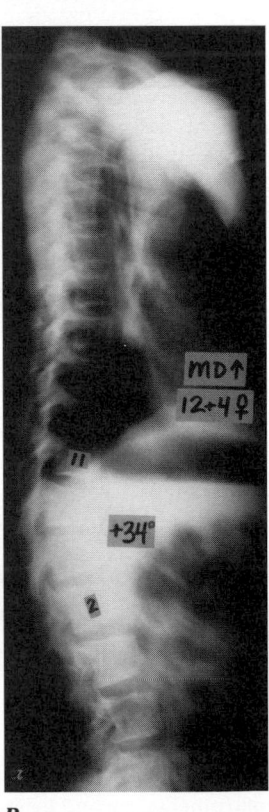

B

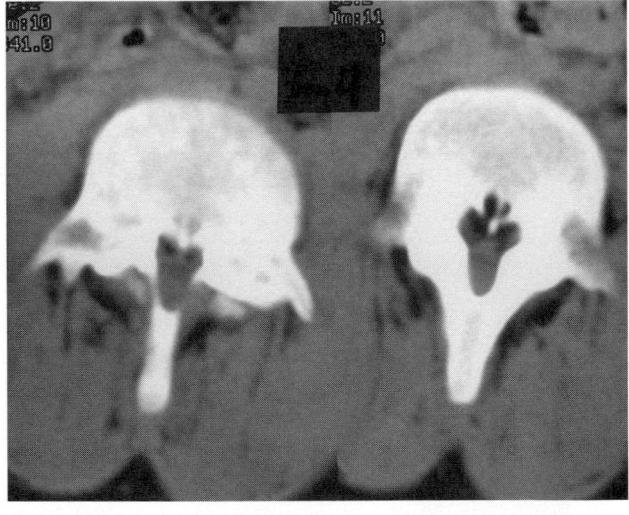

C

Figure 75-51 M.D., a 12 + 4-year-old male, has achondroplasia. His lumbar coronal x-ray (*A*) shows narrowed distances between the pedicles and his lateral x-ray (*B*) shows a moderate thoracolumbar junctional kyphosis of 34°. An axial CT scan (*C*) at the L4 level demonstrates the extremely stenotic spinal canal.

PEDIATRIC SPINAL DEFORMITY —THE SAGITTAL PLANE

The last decade has seen a tremendous increase in the appreciation of sagittal spinal alignment. Our knowledge of "normal" cervical, thoracic, and lumbar sagittal alignment in the pediatric patient has improved. Thus, norms for global, regional, and segmental sagittal alignment at every level of the thoracic and lumbar spine are known, and alignments that deviate significantly from these norms produce sagittal plane pathologies.

Normative regional alignments of cervical lordosis ($-30°$), thoracic kyphosis (T1–T12, $+45°$), and lumbar lordosis (T12-sacrum, $-60°$), are fairly well accepted.[20] In addition, the sagittal vertical axis (SVA) or sagittal plumbline described as a vertical line from the midpoint of the C7 vertebral body should fall posterior to the lumbosacral disk (Fig. 75-52). Thus, most asymptomatic children stand in negative sagittal balance. Segmental thoracic kyphosis is found throughout the thoracic spine; it is maximal at the apex and minimal at the cervicothoracic and thoracolumbar junctions. Thoracolumbar alignment (T10-L2) should be neutral to slightly lordotic (0, $-10°$), with lumbar lordosis increasing segmentally from the upper to lower lumbar spine such that the majority of lumbar lordosis occurs from the L4-5 and L5-S1 disk spaces.[20] Thus, the surgeon engaged in reconstructive procedures of the spine in the pediatric population must keep these sagittal alignments in mind so as to optimize the health of the unfused spine both above and below the fusion.

Pathologies involving the sagittal plane are most commonly due to increased kyphosis, primarily in the thoracic spine but also at the thoracolumbar junction and lumbar spine (Table 75-2). Rarely, lordosis of the thoracic spine or hyperlordosis of the thoracic or lumbar spine may occur and require treatment.

Postural kyphosis, defined as an increase in flexible thoracic kyphosis between 45 and 70°, is also described as a postural round-back deformity (Fig. 75-53). These patients present mainly for their poor cosmetic appearance and occasionally because of increased thoracic back pain

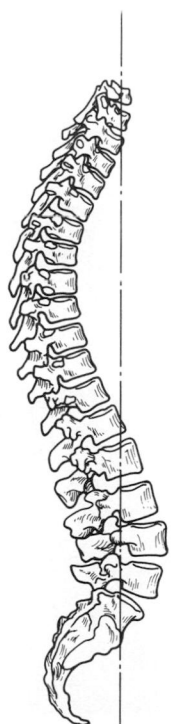

Figure 75-52 Schematic of a sagittal plumbline or sagittal vertical axis (SVA) as a vertical line drawn from the midportion of the body of C7. This line should fall at the posterior edge of the lumbosacral disk or slightly behind it.

TABLE 75-2   Classification of Kyphosis

I. Postural

II. Scheuermann's disease

III. Congenital
    A. Defect of segmentation
    B. Defect of formation
    C. Mixed

IV. Neuromuscular

V. Myelomeningocele
    A. Development
    B. Congenital

VI. Posttraumatic
    A. Acute
    B. Congenital

VII. Postsurgical
    A. Postlaminectomy
    B. Following excision of vertebral body

VIII. Postirradiation

IX. Metabolic
    A. Osteoporosis
        1. Senile
        2. Juvenile
    B. Osteogenesis imperfecta
    C. Other

X. Skeletal dysplasias
    A. Achondroplasia
    B. Mucopolysaccharidoses
    C. Other

XI. Collagen disease
    A. Ankylosing spondylitis
    B. Other

XII. Tumor
    A. Benign
    B. Malignant
        1. Primary
        2. Metastatic

XIII. Inflammatory

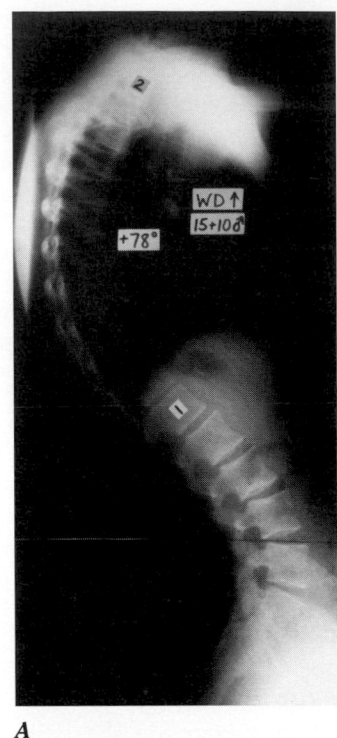

A

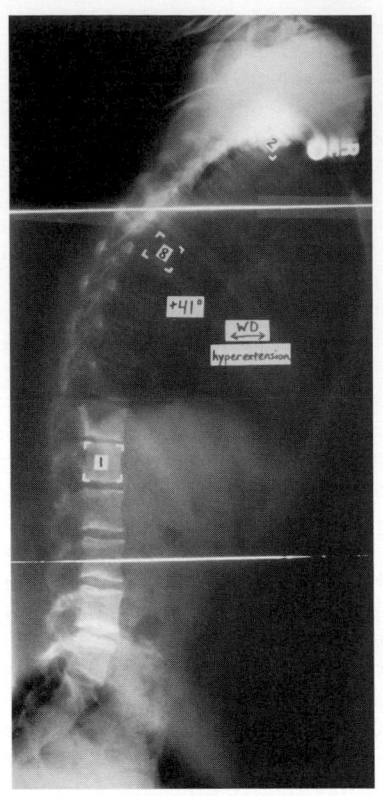

B

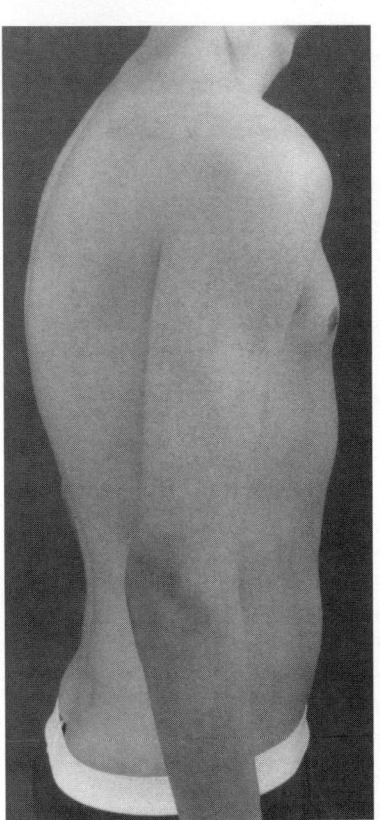

C

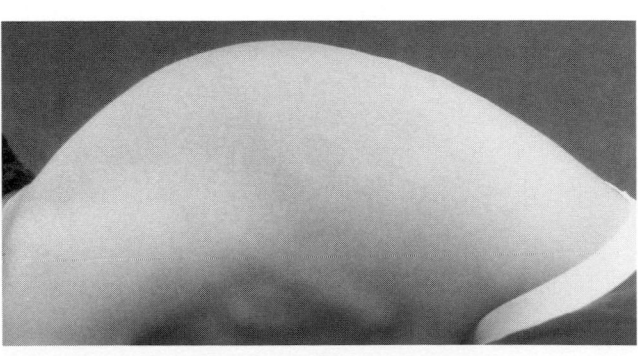

D

Figure 75-53 W.D., a 15 + 10-year-old male, presented for "poor posture." His long-cassette lateral x-ray (*A*) showed 78° of global kyphosis from T2 to L1 with no wedging of his disk spaces or vertebral bodies. A hyperextension lateral x-ray (*B*) shows his improved kyphosis to 41° from T2 to L1. His clinical photo (*C*) with active correction of his posture demonstrates the flexibility. A forward bend photo (*D*) demonstrates the global kyphosis present.

due to poor posture and spinal extensor muscle tone. The key element in postural round back is flexibility of the kyphosis and the absence of skeletal dysplasias and metabolic diseases.[97] Having the patient arch the back with the shoulders retracted should significantly improve the deformity.

Scheuermann's Kyphosis

Scheuermann's kyphosis was described in 1921 as a thoracic kyphotic deformity characterized by vertebral wedging and a subsequent growth disturbance of the vertebral end plate.[137] Scheuermann's kyphosis affects between 0.5 and 8 percent of healthy subjects, with a preponderance of males being affected.[155] The cause of Scheuermann's kyphosis is still controversial, with theories including aseptic necrosis of the ring apophysis, abnormal endochondral ossification due to a weakened cartilaginous end plate, a mechanical growth deficiency due to deleterious anterior compressive forces on the growth centers,[87] and genetic transmission, which has been shown via autosomal dominant inheritance with a high degree of penetrance and variable expressivity.[137]

The onset of Scheuermann's kyphosis is usually prior to puberty, around age 10. Early forms are probably neglected and often labeled postural kyphosis. The main clinical difference between postural and Scheuermann's kyphosis is the rigidity of the kyphotic curve, especially at the apex.[87] There are two main forms of Scheuermann's kyphosis, the more common thoracic type with the apex between T7 and T9 and the less common thoracolumbar type with the apex between T10 and L1.[137]

Over the past decade, there have been increasing reports of lumbar abnormalities describing a third type of Scheuermann's disease. This form seems to occur primarily in male patients who are athletically active or perform hard labor. Radiographically, lumbar Scheuermann's is characterized by irregular vertebral end plates, Schmorl's nodules, and a reduction in disk space height that is not associated with wedging. Usually, these lesions appear to be localized to the anterior rim of the vertebral body and are coined "anterior marginal detachments." Lumbar hypolordosis or frank kyphosis are the resultant radiographic abnormalities and typically produce lumbar back pain.

Patients normally present for either cosmetic deformity or pain. Both the thoracic and thoracolumbar types of Scheuermann's kyphosis may produce pain, which is often most severe during the period of rapid growth. The pain usually tends to decline following skeletal maturity. Often, areas above or below the kyphosis are subjected to excessive load, causing painful symptoms. Scheuermann's kyphosis by itself should not produce neurologic symptoms. However, there are reports of paraparesis due to thoracic disk herniations or compression fractures.

Radiographic criteria for the diagnosis of Scheuermann's kyphosis include hyperkyphosis greater than 40°; irregular upper and lower vertebral end plates with loss of disk space height; and wedging of 5° or more in three consecutive vertebrae (Sorenson criteria).[137]

The natural history of Scheuermann's kyphosis during the growth spurt is variable. Lowe[137] suggested that if residual kyphosis remained at less than 60° at skeletal maturity, the patient had an excellent prognosis for minimal problems in adult life. Murray et al.[155] followed 61 patients with Scheuermann's kyphosis for an average of 31.7 years and compared them with 34 normal controls. The overall conclusion was that the clinical and functional natural history of Scheuermann's kyphosis tended to be benign. However, excessive kyphosis (greater than 65 to 70°) may cause morphologic and structural biomechanical imbalances that can lead to curve progression and future difficulties. One other aspect not easily quantified is the altered cosmetic appearance and self-esteem of these patients.

Treatment for Scheuermann's kyphosis is usually conservative.[37] Adolescents with a moderate thoracic kyphosis (40 to 60°) without evidence of progression require only postural exercises and infrequent follow-up. Their prognosis is quite good. For curves between 50 and 75° in skeletally immature patients, bracing may prove beneficial.[177] Flexibility is an important variable in choosing between an active correction system (Milwaukee brace) and a passive one (antigravity cast). The goal is reconstitution of the vertebral end plate, and this is possible only if the thoracic vertebrae maintain optimal growth potential over a sufficiently long period of time.[35,177] For patients with less flexible deformities, placement of serial hyperextension casts with intervening bracing may be advantageous. It takes a motivated patient and dedicated staff to optimize this treatment regimen.

Orthotic management of Scheuermann's kyphosis usually requires between 12 and 24 months of treatment. Kyphosis will recur if significant anterior vertebral body growth has not been achieved. It appears that a spinal orthosis or casting is not indicated in most patients nearing or already having achieved skeletal maturity.

Surgery may be considered for skeletally mature patients with greater than 75° of kyphosis. Since the recent report showing a potentially benign natural history for many of these patients,[155] the surgeon should be selective in determining which patients should undergo operative treatment. Probably the two most common indications for surgery are spinal pain and unacceptable cosmetic appearance. However, these are both subjective; thus it is wise to be cautious in counseling these patients. We tend to recommend surgical correction only for large curves greater than 80 to 90° associated with significant axial pain[30,36] (Fig. 75-54). Surgical treatment consists of an anterior release and fusion as well as a posterior instrumentation and fusion performed under the same anesthesia on the same day.[30,101] This includes thorough anterior diskectomies and releases, leaving the posterior longitudinal ligament intact, with packing of the disk spaces with autogenous rib graft harvested from the thoracotomy approach. The patient is then placed prone with segmental spinal instrumentation extending from the upper thoracic spine (T2 or T3) to the upper or midlumbar spine. The goal is posterior column shortening and minimal anterior column lengthening.

It is important not to fuse these patients too short, for instrumentation failure or sagittal malalignment will oc-

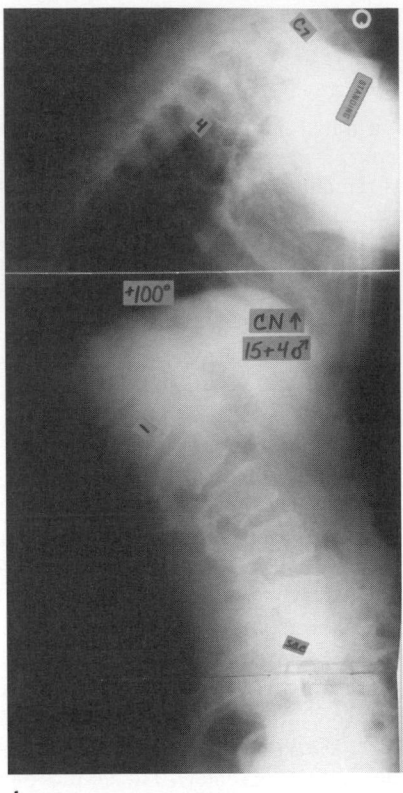

A

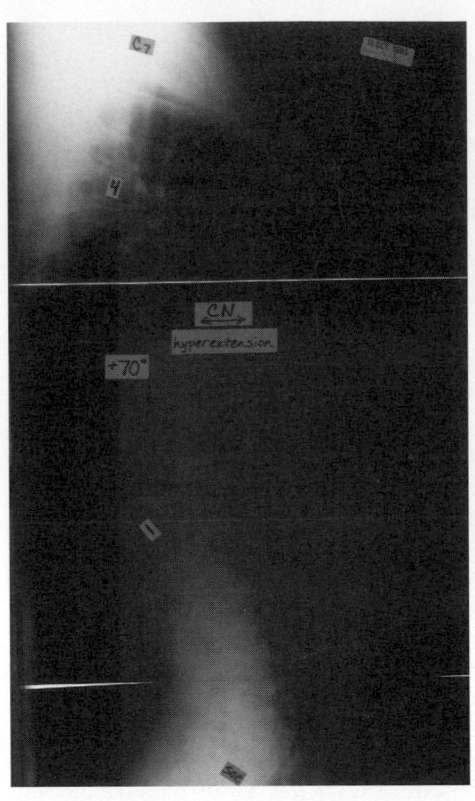

B

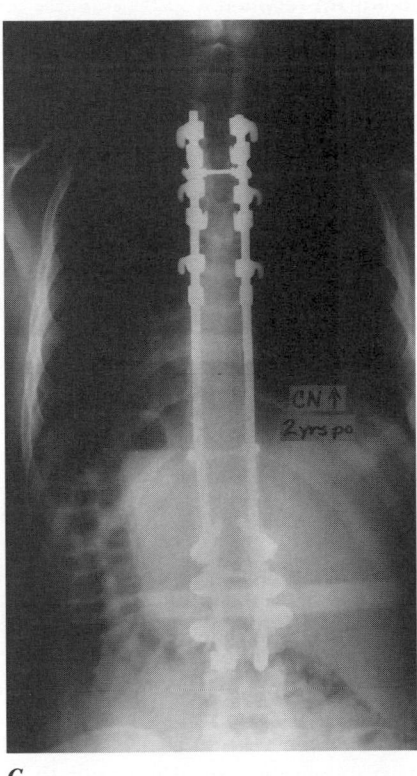

C

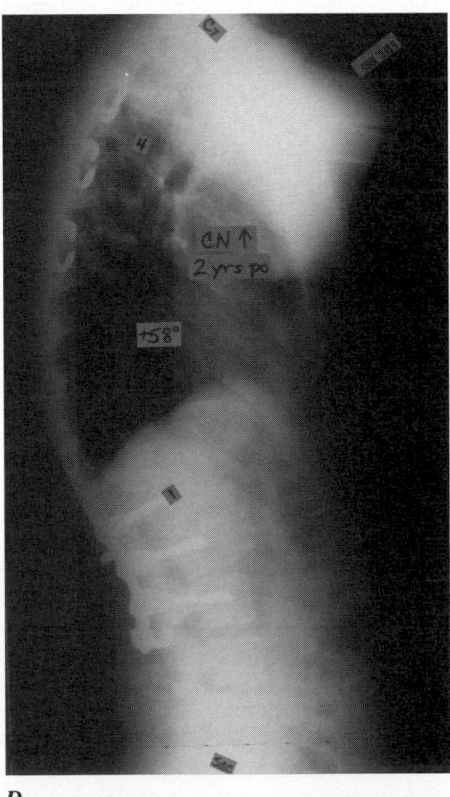

D

Figure 75-54 C.N., a 15 + 4-year-old male, presented with lower thoracic and lumbar back pain as well as poor posture. His lateral long-cassette x-ray (*A*) showed a 100° Scheuermann's kyphosis within an apex of approximately T9. A hyperextension lateral x-ray (*B*) over the bump centered at the apex of his thoracic deformity improved the kyphosis to 70°. Because of his significant deformity, he underwent same-day anterior and posterior spinal fusion. Anteriorly, through a right fifth rib thoracotomy, he had T5-L1 anterior release and fusion and was then placed prone to undergo a T2-L3 instrumentation and fu-

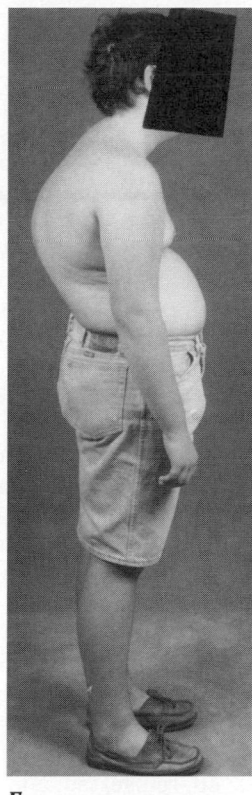

E

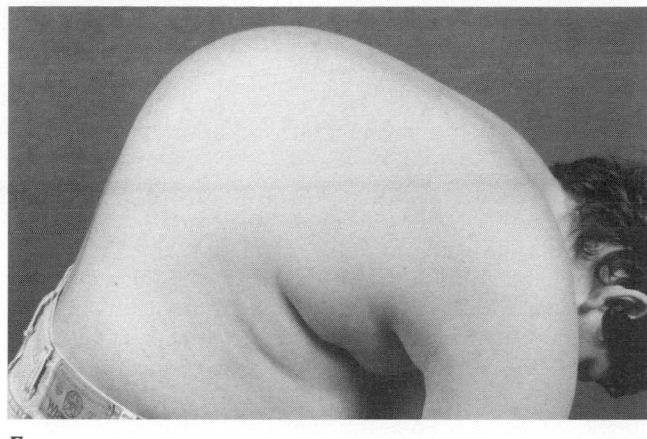

F

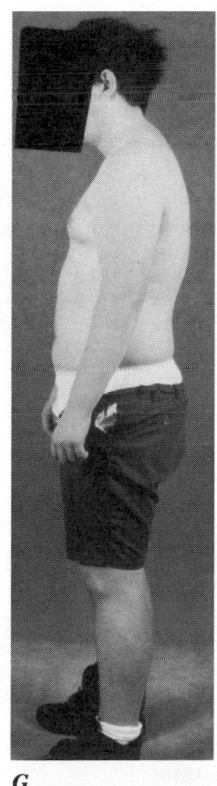

G

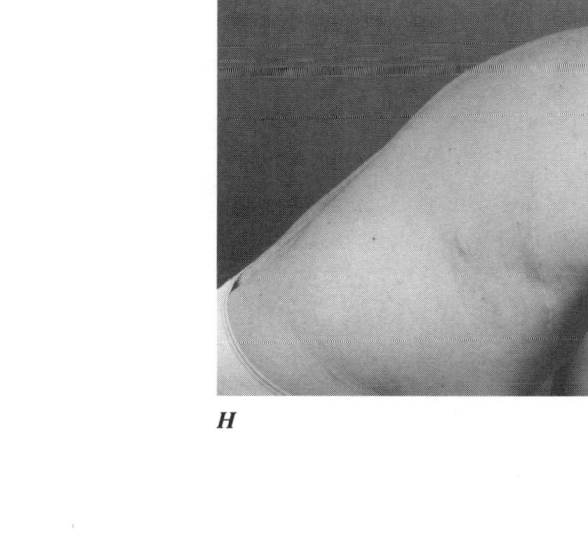

H

Figure 75-54 (*Continued*) sion with correction of his deformity by posterior compression and cantilever forces. His 2-year postoperative coronal (*C*) and lateral (*D*) x-rays show solid spinal fusion with a thoracic kyphosis measuring 58°. The patient's preoperative upright clinical photo (*E*) demonstrates his increased thoracic kyphosis and overall poor posture. On bending forward (*F*), his large thoracic gibbus deformity becomes manifest. His postoperative upright posture (*G*) shows marked improvement. On bending forward (*H*), he is seen to have a more normal thoracic posterior contour.

cur.[137] The lowest instrumented vertebra (LIV) is chosen from both the standing and supine hyperextension x-ray. On the standing x-ray, the fusion must proceed so that the LIV is distal to the first lordotic disk. A sagittal vertical line drawn from the posterior edge of the sacrum should intersect the intended LIV. On a hyperextension long-cassette lateral x-ray, the intended LIV should be close to a horizontal position. Normally, all of these parameters will indicate that the LIV will be L1 in those patients with a high thoracic apex (approximately T6), L2 when the thoracic apex is T8, and L3 when the apex is approximately T10.

The results of surgical treatment are variable, primarily depending on whether concomitant anterior and posterior fusions are performed as well as on the type of instrumentation utilized to correct the deformity.[30,36] Bradford et al. observed improvement in the results of Harrington compression instrumentation for the treatment of Scheuermann's kyphosis when a concomitant anterior arthrodesis was performed.[30] The use of segmental spinal instrumentation systems such as the Cotrel-Dubousset system has recently been shown to provide good postoperative results; however, follow-up thus far is rather short.[137] We prefer a segmental spinal system with four to six pairs of claw hooks above the apex and three pairs of pedicle screws below the apex in the thoracolumbar and lumbar spine down to the LIV. Cantilever bending forces are utilized to shorten the posterior column of the spine when seating the rods into the distal screws. Postoperative bracing is recommended for approximately 7 months, until anterior arthrodesis is confirmed on radiographs.

Complications related to the surgery for Scheuermann's kyphosis are similar to those observed in any type of major spinal surgery. The most frequently occurring complication is pseudarthrosis, followed by instrumentation failure and secondary loss of correction. These complications are minimized by concomitant anterior release and arthrodesis, secure posterior internal fixation, and choice of the correct proximal and distal fusion levels. Neurologic sequelae are rare; they may be due to vascular etiologies from circumferential spinal exposures during same-day anterior and posterior reconstructions, direct mechanical insults if the spinal canal is lengthened, or improper instrumentation. The use of spinal cord monitoring along with a wake-up test as indicated is mandatory in these procedures.[135]

Postlaminectomy Kyphosis

When a multilevel cervical or thoracic laminectomy is performed in children due to intraspinal pathology, a progressive kyphosis may ensue. Two factors govern the occurrence of spinal deformity in such instances: the age of the patient and the anatomic level of the laminectomy.[154,203,218] It is apparent that younger patients have a much higher risk of a progressive deformity than older adolescents or adults.[131] Also, laminectomies occurring in the upper thoracic and cervical region are more likely to produce kyphotic deformities than those in the lower thoracic or lumbar region.[181] In one study,[219] spinal deformity occurred in 100 percent of patients with cervical laminectomy, 36 percent of patients with thoracic laminectomy, and no patients with lumbar laminectomy. Although kypho-

sis, lordosis, or scoliosis, or combinations are all possible, kyphosis following multilevel laminectomy is the most common deformity (Fig. 75-55). Besides the obvious lack of posterior column support, production of a kyphotic deformity occurs due to wedging of the vertebral bodies from the abnormal anterior compression forces on the immature growing structures as well as hypermobility between vertebral bodies. Since the lumbar spine normally has a lordotic curvature, posterior laminectomy does not increase anterior compressive loads; thus kyphosis is much less likely to occur.[219]

The best way to manage postlaminectomy spinal deformity is prevention. Facetectomy should be avoided if at all possible. Surgical fusion of the remaining structures (facet joints and transverse processes) with autogenous bone graft concomitant with the laminectomy may suffice to prevent subsequent deformity and should be considered in every case of multilevel laminectomy in children.[48] Another procedure that may be useful during intraspinal pediatric neurosurgery is laminaplasty. In this procedure, both laminae are divided as close to the pedicle as possible, with the laminae and spinous processes removed as one piece, preserved, reinserted, and sutured in place at the conclusion of the intraspinal procedure. Postoperative bracing is required to prevent deformity and instability.

Once a kyphotic spinal deformity occurs, bracing will not correct it.[203] Surgical fusion is required to correct and stabilize the deformity. In the cervical spine, anterior fusion with bone grafts between the vertebral bodies is necessary.[51] In the thoracic spine, an anterior release and fusion followed by a posterior fusion with instrumentation is needed. Postoperative bracing or casting will be required, depending upon the type and amount of instrumentation placed. For large structural deformities, the use of halo gravity traction separating the anterior and posterior fusions is helpful to correct the kyphotic deformity slowly and safely over time with the patient awake (Fig. 75-56). A definitive posterior instrumentation and fusion well proximal and distal to the laminectomy may then be performed with the patient prone in cervical traction to safely optimize correction of the deformity.

A spinal deformity may also occur following either rib or chest wall resection or after irradiation.[9,67,75,173] In young patients with prior thoracotomy, the incidence of scoliosis increases convex to the site of removal.[75] Young children receiving radiation to the immature spine may develop a spinal deformity because of the adverse effects on normal endochondral maturation.[173] Patients must be followed in both of these areas during their growth to watch for the occurrence of any spinal deformity.

Congenital Kyphosis

Congenital kyphosis can be divided into three types, according to the basic defects: failure of formation, failure of segmentation, and rotatory dislocation of the spine[216] (Fig. 75-57). Failure of formation occurs due to total or partial absence of one or more vertebral bodies. Failure of formation often produces more angular gibbus deformities,

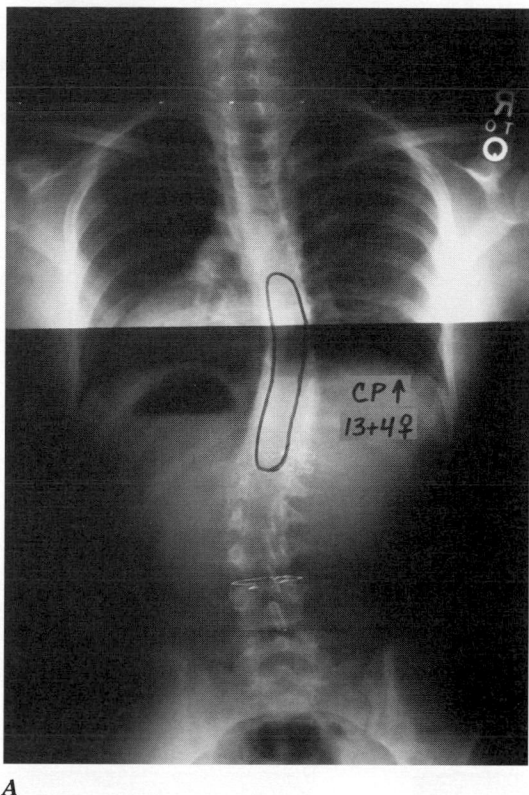

A

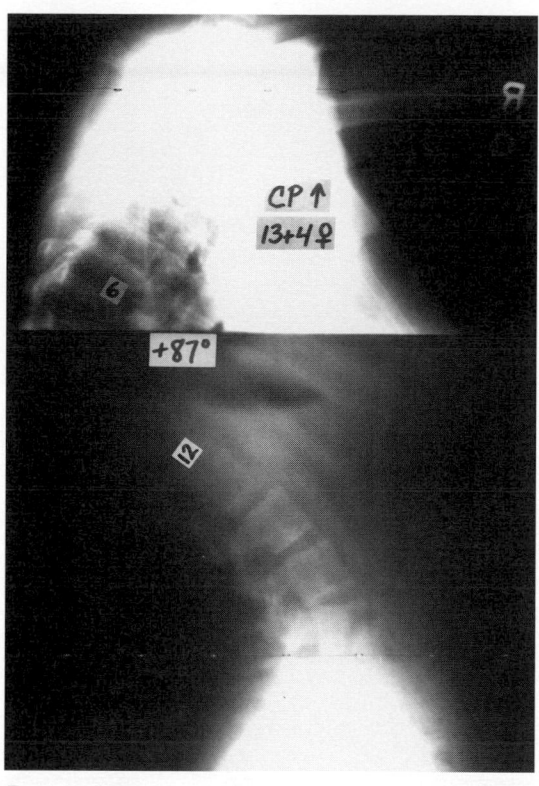

B

Figure 75-55 C.P., a 13 + 4-year-old female, had an astrocytoma that was excised 3 years prior to presentation. Her coronal x-ray (*A*) shows her thoracic laminectomy (outlined in black) involving the middle and lower thoracic spine. Her sagittal x-ray (*B*) shows that 87° of middle and lower thoracic postlaminectomy kyphosis has developed.

which increases the neurologic risk for the spinal cord spanning the apex of the deformity. Failure of segmentation produces a congenital kyphosis involving one or multiple levels. When the failure is strictly anterior, a pure kyphosis results. However if the failure is anterolateral, a kyphoscoliosis will result. The resulting kyphosis generally has a more rounded shape; thus there is less neurologic risk to the spinal cord. The third type of congenital kyphosis, a mixed variety, involves failures of formation and segmentation simultaneously. This may lead to a variety of kyphotic conditions, depending upon the contributions of each as well as the location of the aberrant vertebral bodies and segmentation defects.

Evaluation and treatment of congenital kyphosis begins with assessment of the degree of deformity, flexibility, state of the spine above and below the kyphosis, and the growth potential at the site of the deformity, which may lead to progression. Evaluation with MRI for any intraspinal anomalies is mandatory prior to surgical intervention. Bracing has no role in the treatment of a congenital kyphotic deformity but may be useful in stabilizing compensatory curves above and below the deformity following surgical stabilization of the apex.[216]

The hallmark of treatment of congenital kyphosis is anterior and posterior spinal fusion spanning the kyphotic segments.[216] For most patients who are neurologically intact, excessive correction and/or anterior spinal decompression is potentially dangerous and should be avoided.

Most patients are treated with in situ anterior and posterior spinal fusion, with posterior instrumentation placed following postural reduction (Fig. 75-58). Active correction of kyphosis with instrumentation is dangerous and should be avoided. For those rare patients who have neurologic compromise secondary to an angular kyphosis, anterior decompression with subsequent anterior spinal cord transposition may be necessary. This carries with it a high risk of further neurologic sequelae and thus must be discussed thoroughly with both the patient and his or her family. Preoperative halo gravity traction of an angular kyphosis without prior decompression is dangerous, as the spinal cord may become tented over the fixed anterior structures, producing neurologic compromise.[216] Following successful anterior and posterior fusion, the risk of neurologic sequelae is nil. In summary, early treatment should be provided, not necessarily to correct the deformity but primarily to prevent any worsening of the deformity or onset of progressive neurologic sequelae.

Spondylolysis and Spondylolisthesis

Spondylolysis, a defect in the pars interarticularis in the posterior column of the lumbar spine, is the most common cause of low back pain in childhood and adolescence.[29,150] The defect is rare in children under 5 years of age. The incidence increases to 6 percent by age 7; how-

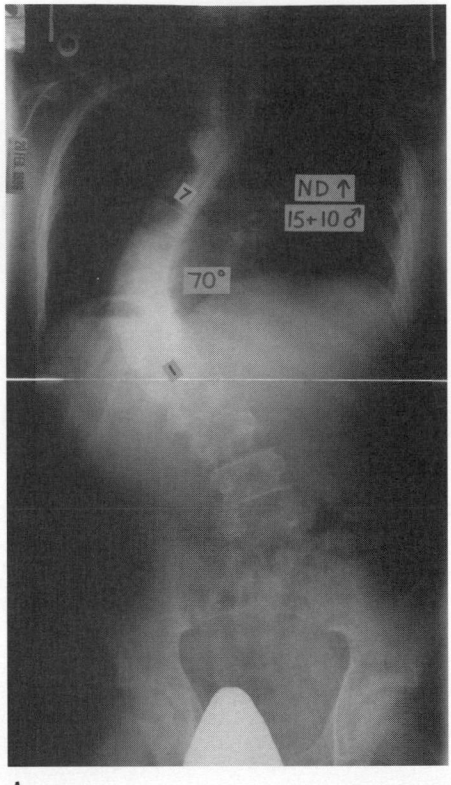

A

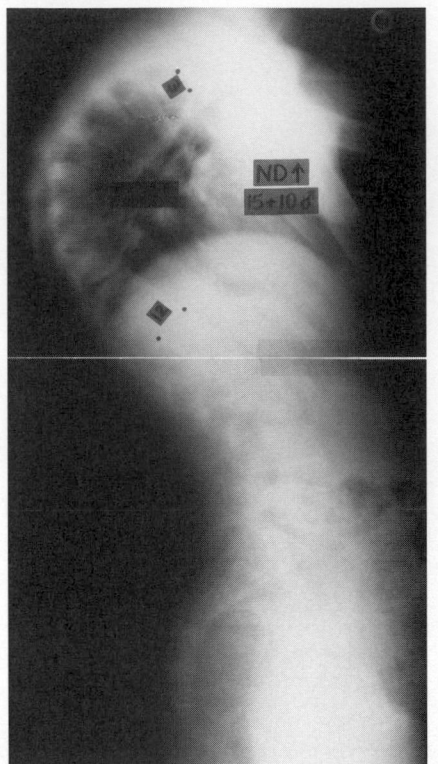

B

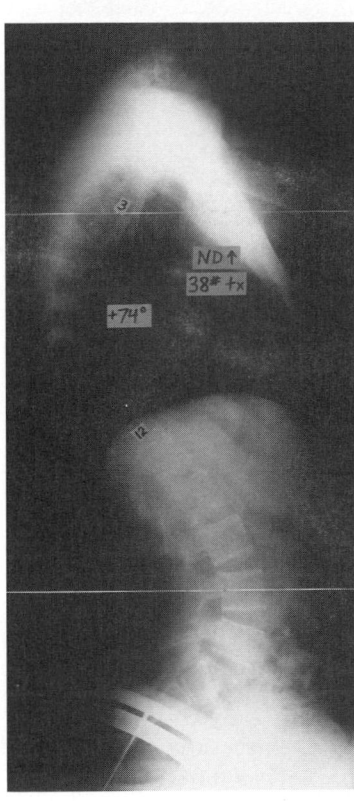

C

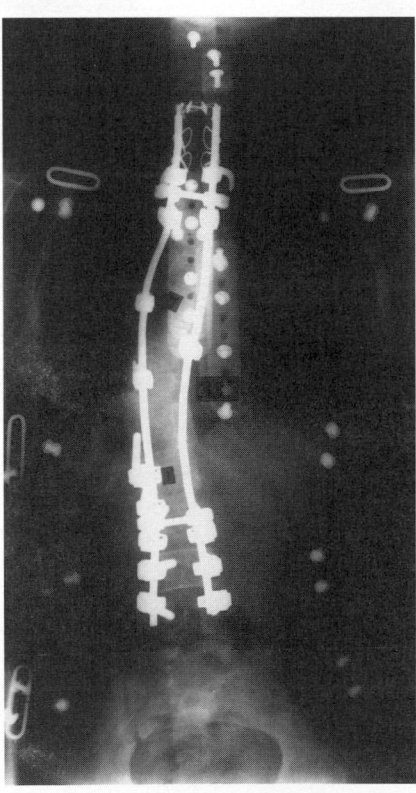

D

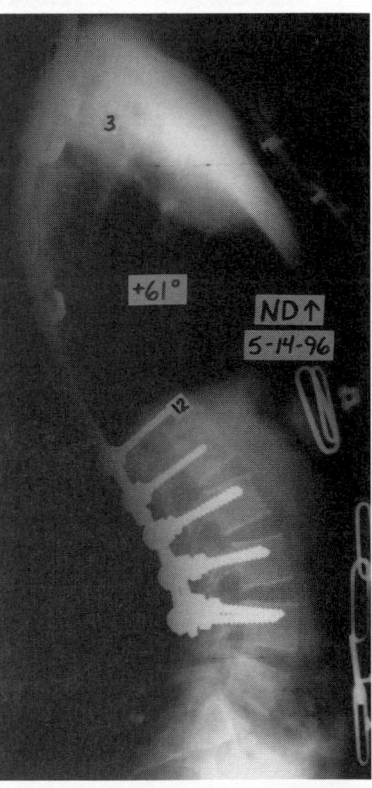

E

Figure 75-56 N.D., a 15 + 10-year-old male, was found to have a thoracic oligodendroglioma that required neurosurgical resection via a posterior laminectomy. When he presented to us, N.D. had a 70° left thoracic scoliosis deformity (*A*) as well as a 109° thoracic kyphosis (*B*). He underwent staged anterior and posterior spinal fusion. His anterior fusion was performed between T4 and T12. He was then placed in halo-wheelchair gravity traction for 6 weeks to slowly improve his deformity. His lateral x-ray (*C*) with 38 lb of traction sitting shows improvement of his thoracic kyphosis to 74°. *D*. He then underwent a posterior instrumentation and fusion from C7 to L4 with segmental fixation including thoracolumbar and lumbar pedicular instrumentation. N.D.'s postoperative coronal x-ray shows improvement of his scoliosis to 33°. *E*. His postoperative upright lateral x-ray shows decreased kyphosis to 61°.

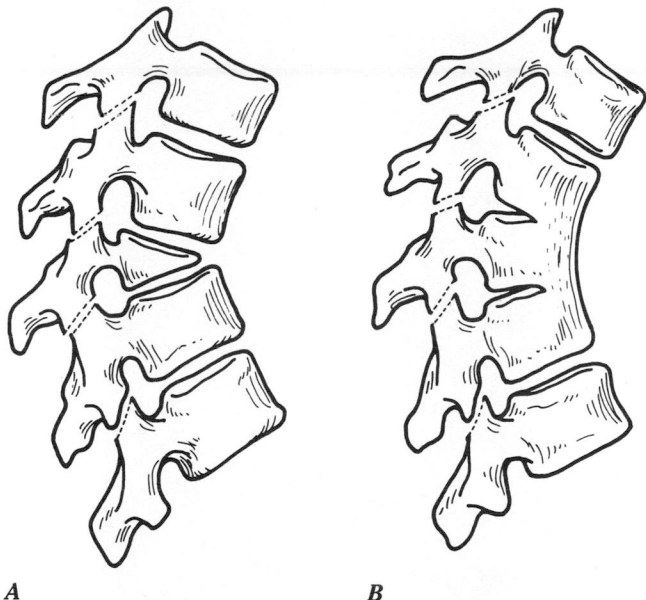

A   *B*

Figure 75-57 Schematic diagram of congenital kyphosis. *A.* Anterior failure of formation. *B.* Anterior failure of segmentation.

ever, older children and adolescents may develop the lesion as well.[8] If there are bilateral defects in the pars, spondylolisthesis may result. Spondylolisthesis, or forward slippage of one vertebra on another, is classified into five major types according to Wiltse et al.[196,197] We will discuss primarily the type I or the dysplastic condition as well as the type II or isthmic spondylolisthesis due to defects in the pars interarticularis. More recently, Marchetti and Bartolozzi[143] have classified spondylolisthesis into developmental versus acquired types. The developmental types included all the previously described dysplastic types, which are further subdivided into high dysplastic and low dysplastic, depending on the degree of slippage and abnormality seen. The acquired types include acute traumatic pars defects that occur in adolescents undergoing specific trauma and are differentiated because these do not produce significant lumbosacral deformities, as can the developmental types.

Anatomically, the primary defect producing spondylolisthesis in childhood is located at the pars interarticularis.[200] However, it is important to differentiate whether a defect has a developmental or an acquired etiology. Developmental defects tend to be associated with dysplastic lumbosacral facet joints, spina bifida occulta of the sacrum, dysplastic L5 posterior elements, and rounded sacrums. All of these tend to produce a more unstable slip that is prone to progression, with resultant sagittal imbalance (Fig. 75-59). In contrast, acquired pars defects are known to occur following increased, repeated stress on the pars region.[85,125] Thus, it is known that sports such as gymnastics and football, which impose high axial loads and extension forces on the lumbar spine, pose a higher risk of producing acute pars fatigue fractures.[98] Genetic inheritance studies have shown a predisposition to pars le-

sions in certain families. However, environmental stresses are probably equally if not more important.

The most common presentation for children and adolescents with spondylolysis with or without olisthesis is back pain. This may or may not be accompanied by leg pain, which may rarely be the primary complaint. Also, occasionally the patient presents with an atypical gait or a spinal deformity, which may occur in high-grade developmental spondylolisthesis. In acquired lesions, pain associated with certain sporting activities is common, occasionally with a history of a specific event associated with the onset of the symptoms.[125] Physical examination will vary, depending upon the degree of spondylolisthesis. In patients with spondylolysis, the typical exam will show fairly localized lumbar back pain, minimal tenderness, and paraspinal muscle spasm. There may be decreased forward flexion of the spine secondary to tight hamstrings; pain is usually aggravated with forced hyperextension.[98] Straight-leg raising may produce some limitations secondary to tight hamstrings without true nerve root tension signs. In patients with low-grade developmental spondylolisthesis, the picture is similar to that described above. However, those with high-grade developmental spondylolisthesis may present with an antalgic forward gait with knee flexion, a foreshortened trunk and resultant prominent buttocks, and overall forward sagittal imbalance. The most extreme form of this is seen in patients who present with a "spondylo crisis." These patients have severe back and lower extremity limitations as well as possible bowel and bladder abnormalities due not only to their excessive lumbosacral deformity but also to tight L5 and sacral nerve roots from the excessive slippage of L5 on the sacrum. Prompt workup and treatment is necessary for these challenging patients.

It must be remembered that patients with bilateral pars defects occurring early in the developmental stage may often tolerate a fair amount of more anterior olisthesis before the cauda equina becomes compressed. In contrast, patients with a developmental pars elongation that effectively impinges on the posterior elements on the lumbosacral cauda equina, with resultant forward slippage, do tend to have more severe neurologic compression with a lesser degree of olisthesis (Fig. 75-60). The degree of spinal canal occlusion is noted on either an MRI or a CT/myelogram. Patients with severe cauda equina compression may present with lower extremity weakness, sacral sensory abnormalities, and subtle functional bladder problems. Urodynamic evaluation may be indicated to detect any urinary abnormality.

Radiologic evaluation of pediatric patients with spondylolysis or spondylolisthesis initially involves plain radiographs. Standing AP and lateral lumbar spine films are the initial studies performed. It is important to obtain a standing lateral x-ray, as a subtle olisthesis may not be evident on a supine view.[136] Some 80 percent of isthmic spondylolisthesis occurs at L5-S1, with L4-5 the next most common level. Oblique lumbar films are occasionally necessary to further delineate the pars defect. The posterior elements are thus rotated into a projection such that a defect at the pars level corresponds to the neck region of a "Scottie dog," which portrays the posterior elements diagrammatically

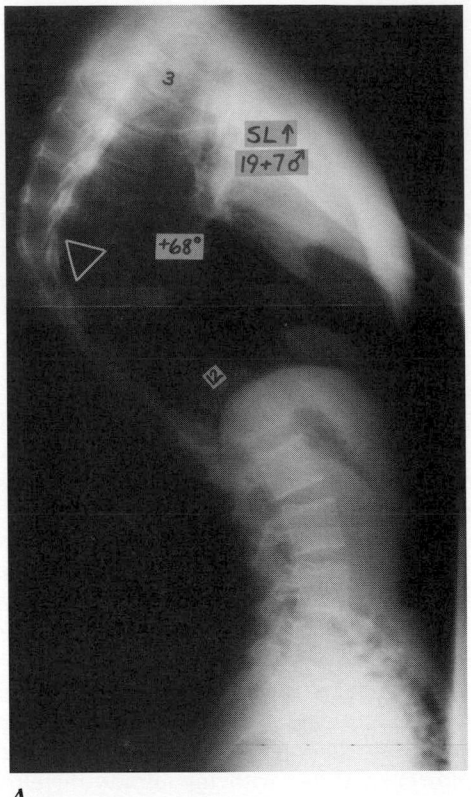

A

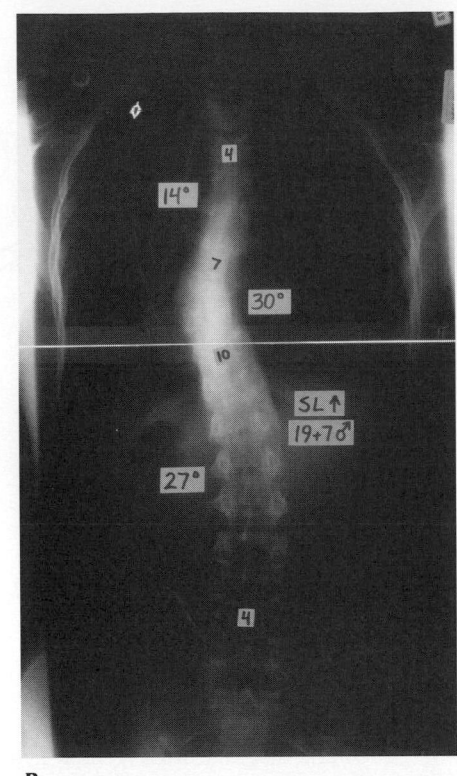

B

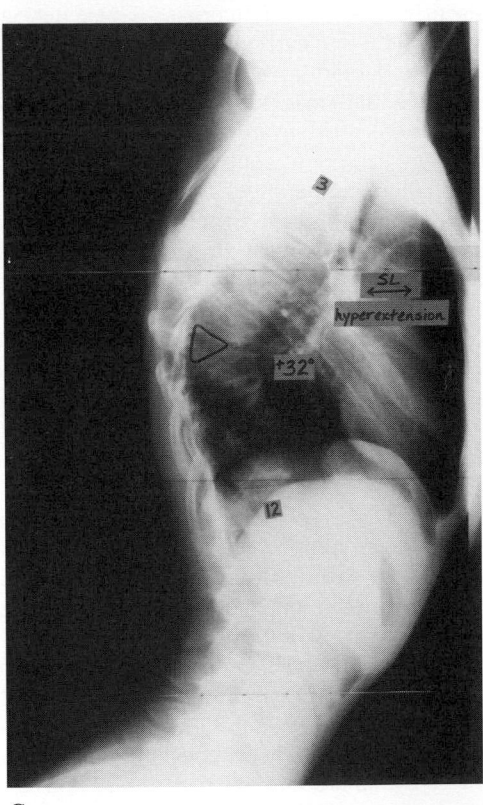

C

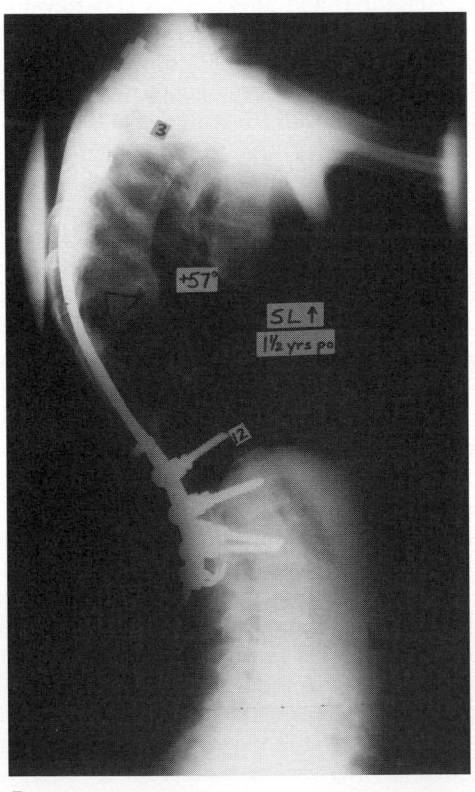

D

Figure 75-58 S.L., a 19 + 7-year-old male, presented with a 68° thoracic congenital kyphosis (*A*) due to anterior failure of formation. His coronal x-ray (*B*) demonstrated a small 30° left thoracic scoliosis due to uneven failure of formation in the coronal plane. A hyperextension x-ray (*C*) on a bump demonstrated correction above and below the deformity with no real change at the apex. S.L. thus underwent a same-day anterior release and fusion from T4 to T12 and a same-day posterior instrumentation and fusion from T2 to L2. The patient's postoperative lateral x-ray (*D*) shows modest correction of his deformity with overall good sagittal balance. His coronal x-ray (*E*) shows his overall alignment and instrumentation.

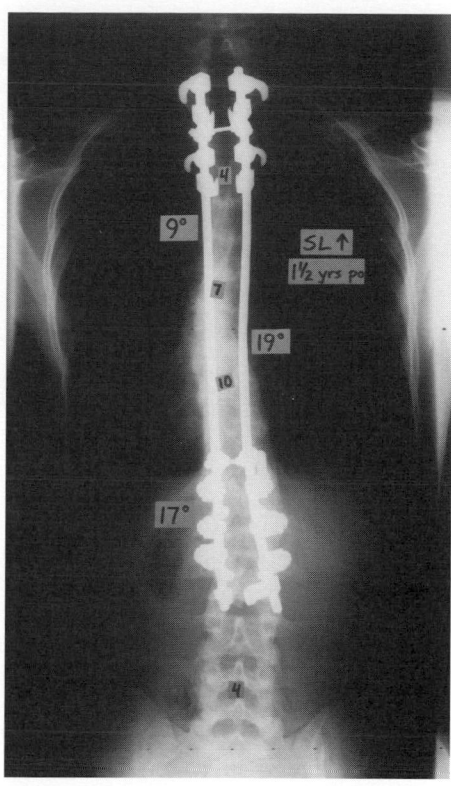

E

Figure 75-58 *(Continued)*

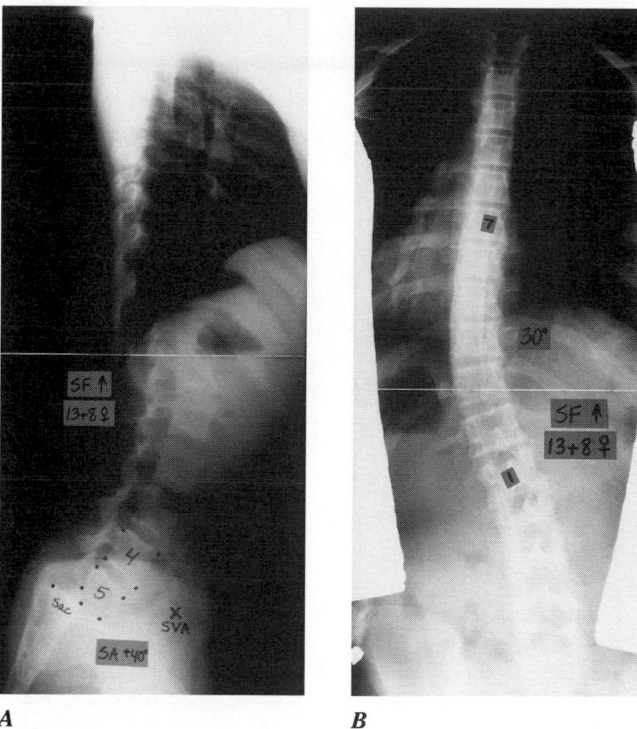

A   *B*

Figure 75-59 S.F., a 13 + 8-year-old female, has a high dysplastic developmental spondylolisthesis. Her long-cassette lateral x-ray (*A*) demonstrates her severe spondylolisthesis, a kyphotic slip angle, and marked forward sagittal imbalance of her entire spine on her pelvis. Her coronal x-ray (*B*) demonstrates "sciatic scoliosis" due to her tight lower lumbar and sacral nerve roots.

(see Fig. 75-3). For many patients with spondylolisthesis, a Ferguson AP or 30° caudal-cephalic view profiles the lumbosacral region more clearly[123] (see Fig. 75-3).

Many measurements can be obtained from the lateral lumbosacral radiographs (Fig. 75-61). The amount of slippage is graded either by the Meyerding classification (grades I through IV) or by the percentage of slip. The Meyerding classification breaks the proximal aspect of the sacrum into quartiles, with the slippage at L5 on the sacrum categorized by its degree: grade I, 25 percent or less; grade II, 25 to 50 percent; grade III, 50 to 75 percent; and grade IV, 75 to 100 percent. Grade V or spondyloptosis is where the L5 vertebral segment is entirely below a horizontal line drawn from the top edge of the sacrum. Similarly, the percentage of slip is calculated from the degree of displacement of L5 on the sacrum from the total anteroposterior length of the proximal sacrum. In this respect, it is a more precise determination. The second most important measurement is the slip angle, or angle of lumbosacral sagittal alignment. Normally, the L5-S1 disk is in 25 to 30° of lordosis, and thus the slip angle is negative. As L5 slips forward on the sacrum due to disk degeneration, a more kyphotic lumbosacral alignment ensues. Thus, kyphotic slip angles represent a more advanced degree of deformity and must be analyzed in context with the degree of forward translation as well. In high-grade developmental slips, the sacrum becomes more vertical as well, which aggravates the lumbosacral kyphosis.

Bone scans are indicated in patients with back pain and no obvious spondylolisthesis but possible acute pars fractures or stress reactions. Recently, SPECT scanning has enabled us to delineate the stress fracture region more precisely.

On CT scans through the affected region, it is occasionally difficult to distinguish the pars defect from the facet joint. The pars defect will be seen on an axial CT scan slice immediately distal to the level of the pedicle and will be more horizontal in alignment. The L5-S1 facet joint will be more distal to the level of the pars lesion, with approximately 45° obliquity and the smooth contour of the facet joints.

On MRI, spondylolisthesis will invariably demonstrate a degenerated lumbosacral disk with any significant amount of slippage. In evaluating an L5-S1 slip, it is important to note the degree of hydration and thus the possible degeneration occurring at the L4-5 segment. This may directly influence surgical planning as to whether the L4-5 joint should be included in a surgical fusion. A good-quality MRI exam will show the lumbosacral spinal canal as well as the exiting L5 nerve root regions, confirming any suspected neural compression. However, often a CT/myelogram is still the optimal study to profile the exiting L5 nerve roots, lumbosacral cauda equina, and bony anatomy prior to operative intervention.

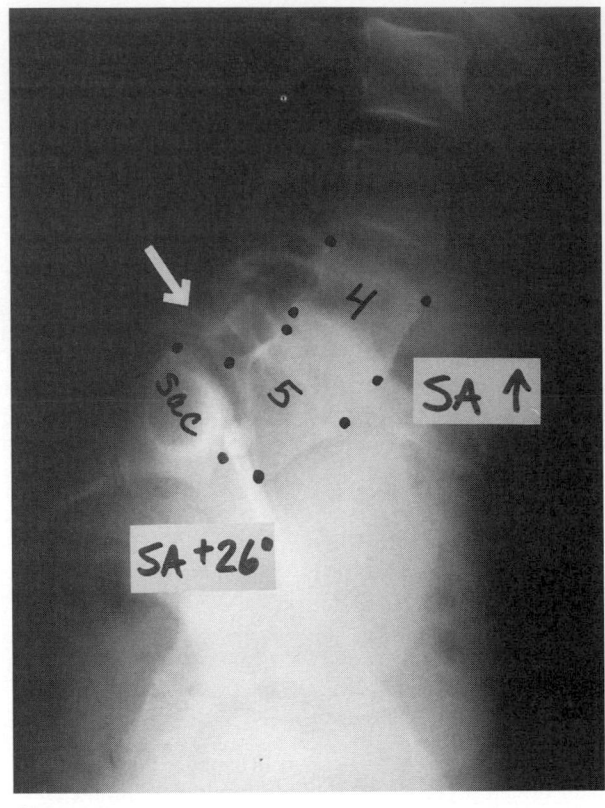

A

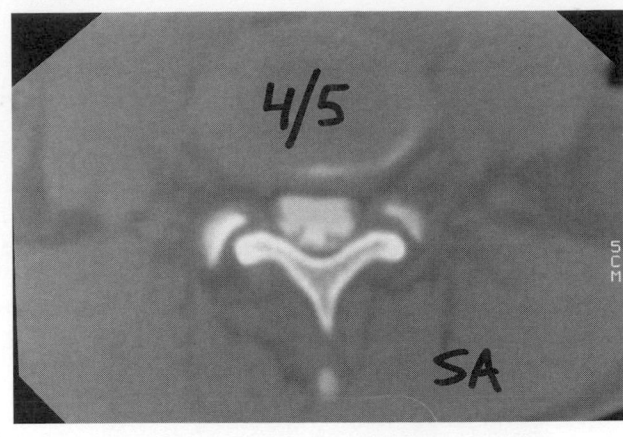

B

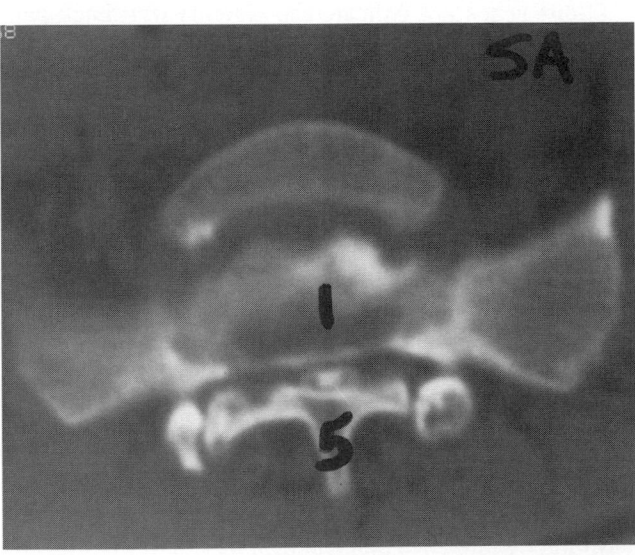

C

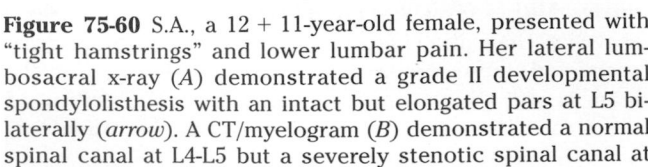

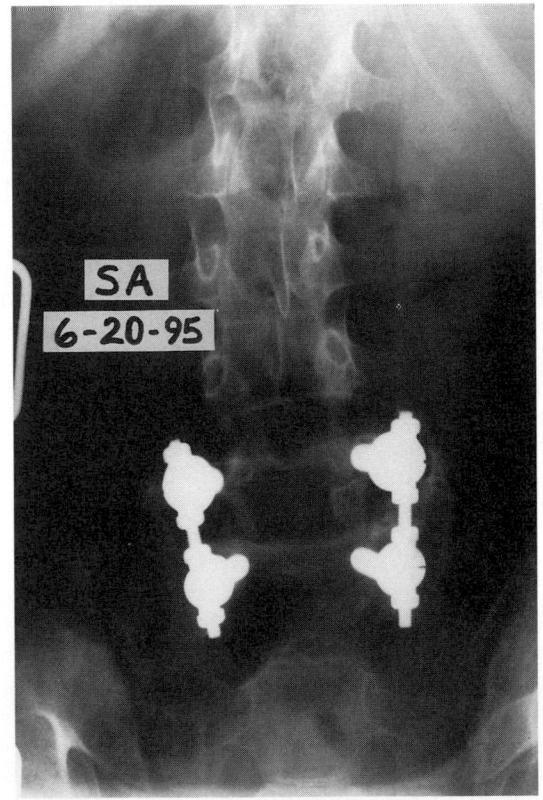

D

Figure 75-60 S.A., a 12 + 11-year-old female, presented with "tight hamstrings" and lower lumbar pain. Her lateral lumbosacral x-ray (*A*) demonstrated a grade II developmental spondylolisthesis with an intact but elongated pars at L5 bilaterally (*arrow*). A CT/myelogram (*B*) demonstrated a normal spinal canal at L4-L5 but a severely stenotic spinal canal at L5-S1, with subluxed facets. *C.* The patient underwent a wide L5 and S1 decompression with instrumentation and fusion from L5 to the sacrum. Her Ferguson AP x-ray (*D*) confirms a solid arthrodesis bilaterally. Her lateral x-ray (*E*) shows mild correction of her fused deformity.

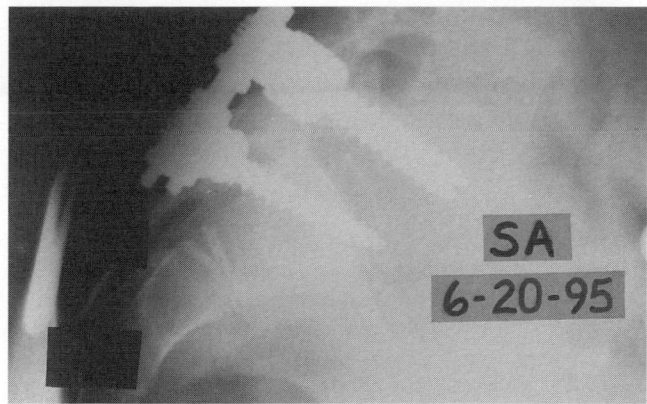

E

Figure 75-60 *(Continued)*

Surgical treatment is recommended for slips greater than 50 percent in both symptomatic and asymptomatic patients.[98] In patients with less than a 50 percent slip, surgery may be indicated following failure of a conservative treatment program. In skeletally mature young adults, surgery is based upon symptoms alone, since further slip is unlikely in the third decade and beyond.[28,98] Where the pars defects in spondylolysis have no or minimal (less than 3 or 4 mm) slips, it is an attractive alternative to try to fuse them operatively, as initially popularized by Buck[44] and then by Bradford and Iza.[34] If successful, this should create a more normal biomechanical posterior column to resist the increased forces that occur at the disk space when bilateral pars defects are present in the posterior column. Our results of surgical pars fusions evaluated critically by CT scans have been less successful than those diagnosed by radiographs alone. However, this may be a pertinent treatment option in select cases, especially of those defects occurring above L5 in the lumbar spine (Fig. 75-62).

The standard operative management of spondylolisthesis in children is bilateral intertransverse process fusion in situ.[98] If the slip is less than 50 percent, an L5-S1 fusion may be sufficient; but for slips greater than 50 percent, fusion should extend from the transverse processes at L4 down to the sacral ala (Fig. 75-63). A Gill laminectomy and bilateral L5 nerve root decompressions are normally not required for patients with small to moderate slips and neutral slip angles. The operative approach may be either via the direct midline or more commonly via a paraspinal muscle splitting approach, as popularized by Wiltse, which avoids the midline structures and allows direct access to the lateral elements, where fusion will be performed.[198] Following the in situ fusion, patients are immobilized in either a cast or single pantaloon brace that includes one thigh. Whether the patient is kept supine or is allowed to ambulate is decided on an individual basis.

It is important to critically assess the fusion status on postoperative spot lateral and Ferguson AP radiographs.[123] Although most studies have shown excellent results following in situ fusion for low-grade spondylolisthesis,[92,199] the true bilateral solid fusion rate for these patients may be less than anticipated when strict radiographic criteria

The majority of children with spondylolysis and low-grade (I and less) spondylolisthesis are treated conservatively, with activity restriction.[98] If the onset is recent, a bone scan may confirm a recent pars fracture that may be amenable to a period of brace or cast immobilization to achieve fracture healing. However, sometimes patients have had symptoms for some time and the radiographic and bone scan appearance is that of a more chronic lesion. In these circumstances, conservative treatment consists of activity limitation, abdominal strengthening, hamstring stretching, and anti-inflammatory drugs. If the patient's symptoms do not subside, brace immobilization is a form of more aggressive activity modification and may improve the patient's symptoms. In skeletally immature patients with developmental spondylolisthesis, continued radiographic follow-up is important to assess for possible slip progression. The risk factors that increase the likelihood of slip progression in these patients include younger age, female sex, presence of spina bifida, wedging of the L5 vertebral body, rounding of the anterior sacral dome, and hyperlordosis.[98,178,199] It is unusual for further slippage to occur following skeletal maturation.

Figure 75-61 Various radiographic parameters measured off the lateral lumbosacral radiograph.

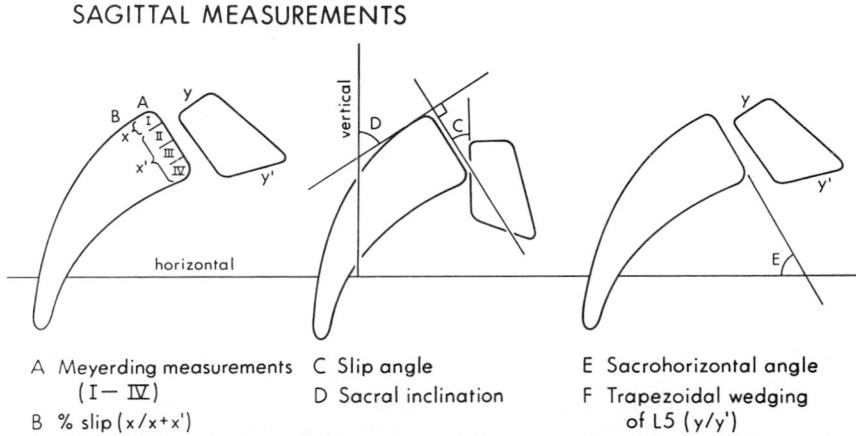

SAGITTAL MEASUREMENTS

A Meyerding measurements (I – IV)
B % slip (x/x+x')
C Slip angle
D Sacral inclination
E Sacrohorizontal angle
F Trapezoidal wedging of L5 (y/y')

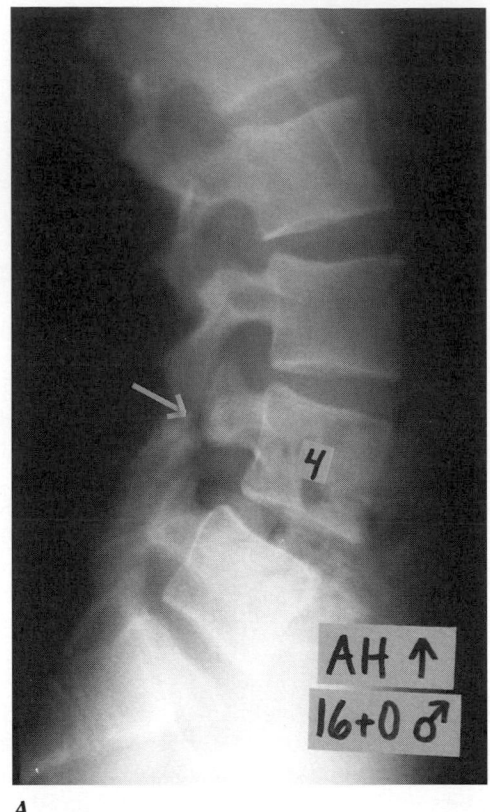

A

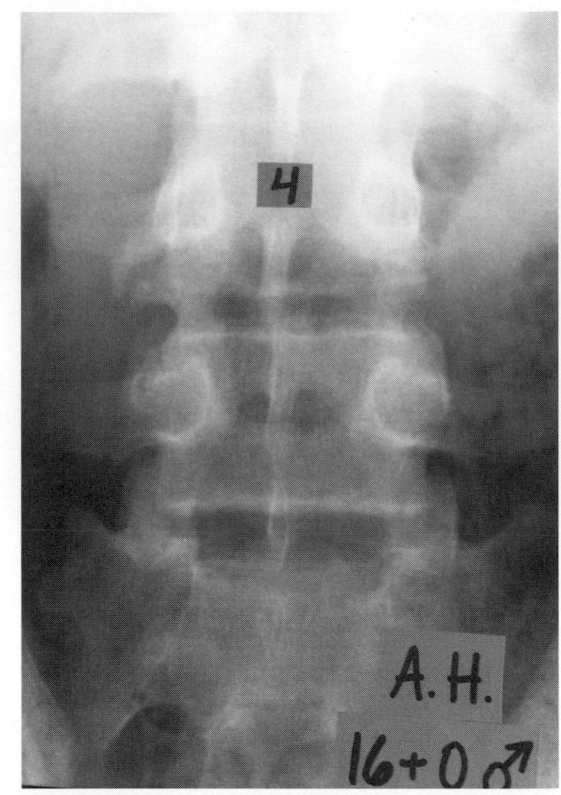

B

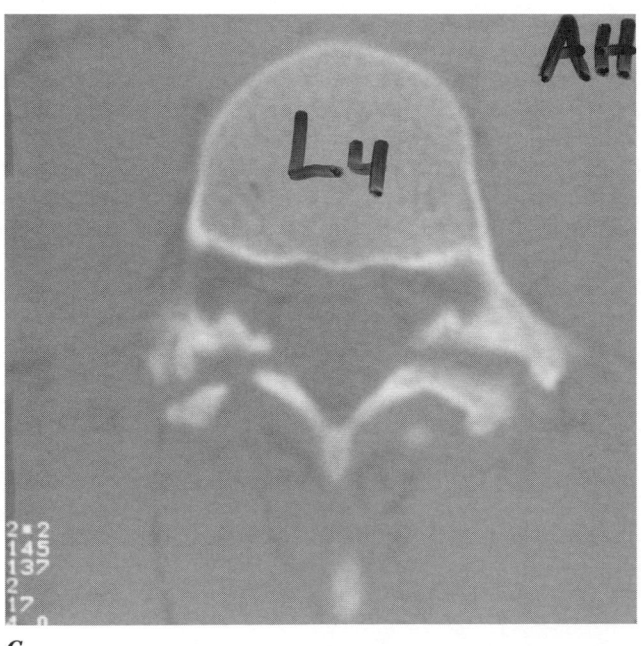

C

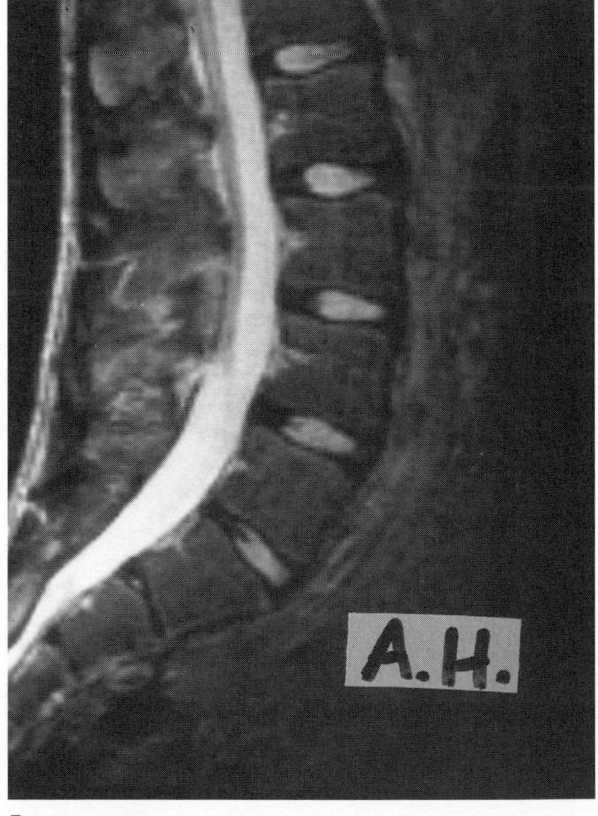

D

Figure 75-62 A.H., a 16-year-old male, presented with a 2-year history of intermittent back pain that prevented him from participating in high school sporting activities. His lumbar lateral x-ray (*A*) confirmed bilateral spondylolysis at L4 (*arrow*), with a minimal olisthesis. His Ferguson AP x-ray (*B*) profiles his L4, L5, and S1 regions. The irregular area directly underneath the pedicles of L4 are visualized and indicative of the bilateral pars defects present. The patient's chronic pars defects are visible on the axial CT scan (*C*) directly beneath the pedicles bilaterally at L4. He underwent an MRI scan (*D*), which showed normal hydration to the L4-5 disk. Following failure of conservative treatment, A.H. underwent a surgical attempt at bilateral L4 instrumented pars fusions. Through a posterior approach, bilateral pedicle screws were placed at L4 and wired to the

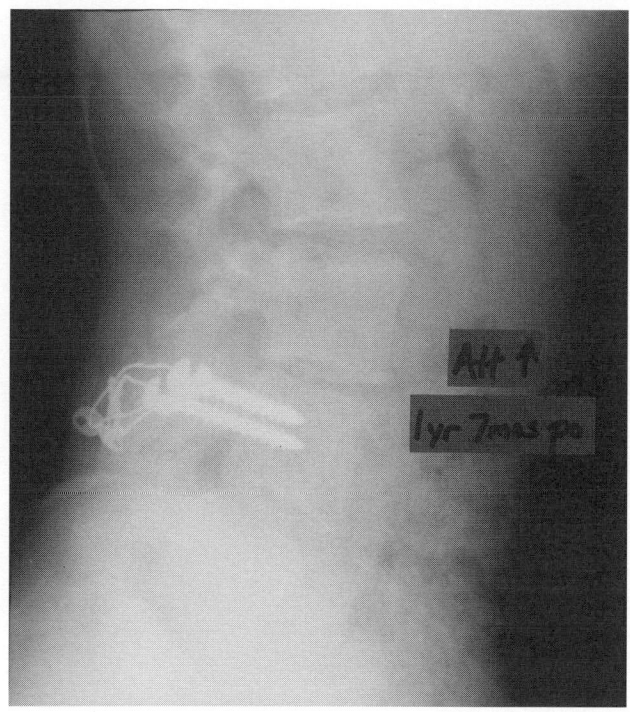

E

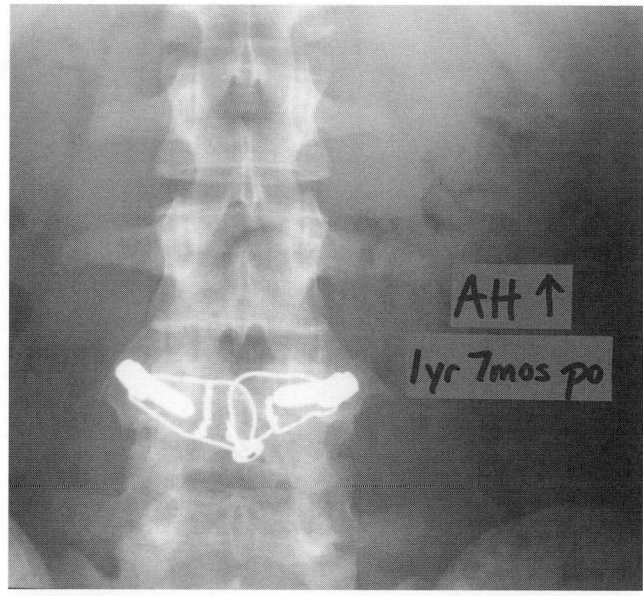

F

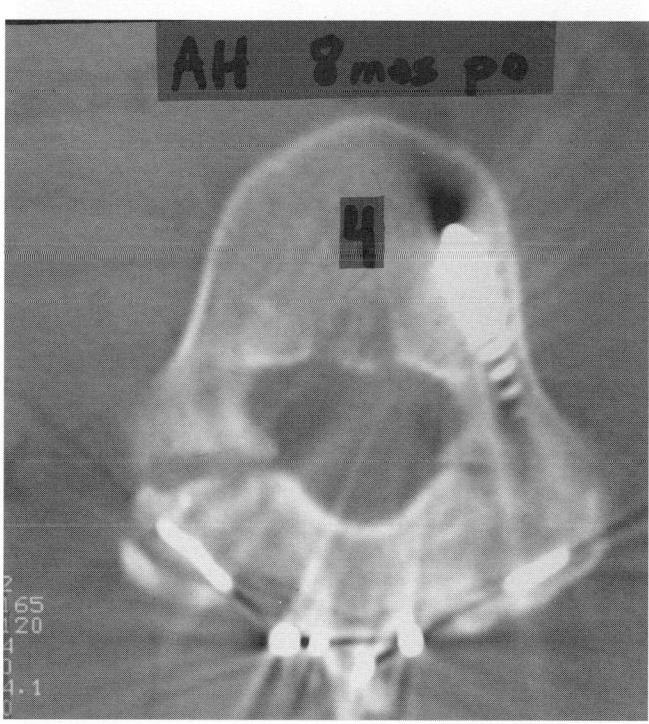

G

Figure 75-62 *(Continued)* loose posterior elements at L4 bilaterally with 16-gauge button wires. The patient's 1-year lateral x-ray (*E*) shows no change in his sagittal alignment. His postoperative AP x-ray (*F*) shows apparent solid fusion of the bilateral pars defects. A postoperative CT scan (*G*) documents fusion of the left pars region with a persistent defect in the right pars region.

are utilized.[123] However, even without definitive evidence of fusion, the early functional results for these patients are quite good, probably due in part to the activity restriction following surgery.

In patients with high-grade developmental slips with marked cosmetic deformity and neurologic sequelae, there has been recent interest in reduction with primary correction of the lumbosacral kyphosis via a reduction maneuver[28,69,179] (Fig. 75-64). These procedures involve de-

compression of the lumbosacral cauda equina and L5 and sacral nerve roots as well as instrumented reduction in an attempt to improve the kyphotic slip angle and obtain a solid bilateral intertransverse process arthrodesis. Usually, an anterior spinal fusion in the form of either intradiskal lumbosacral bone grafts or a dowel graft from the L5 vertebral body into the sacrum is also performed as a second-stage procedure. These types of reduction procedures are a major undertaking, with a high complication risk, in-

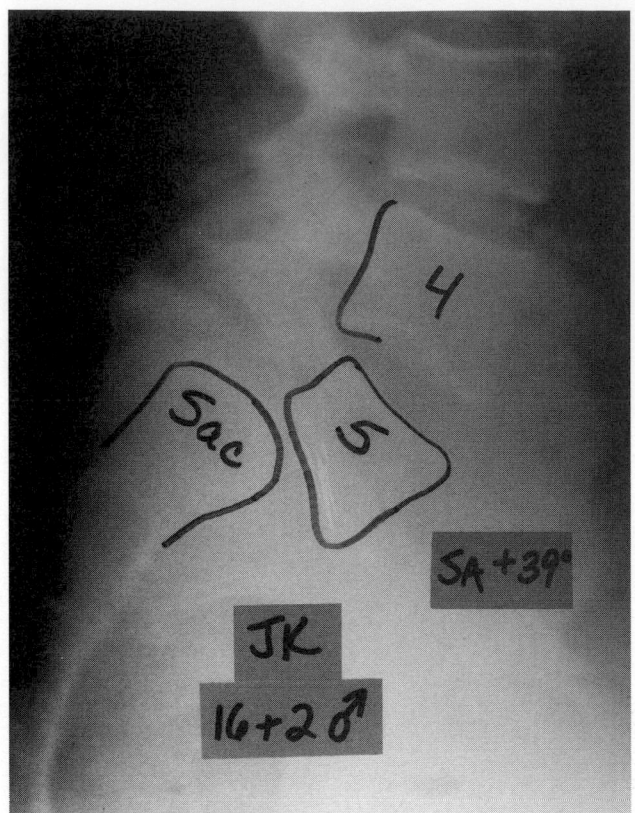

A

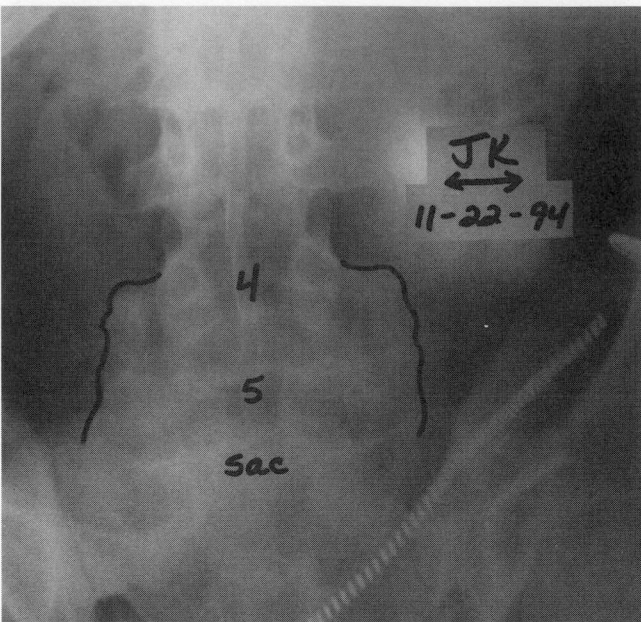

B

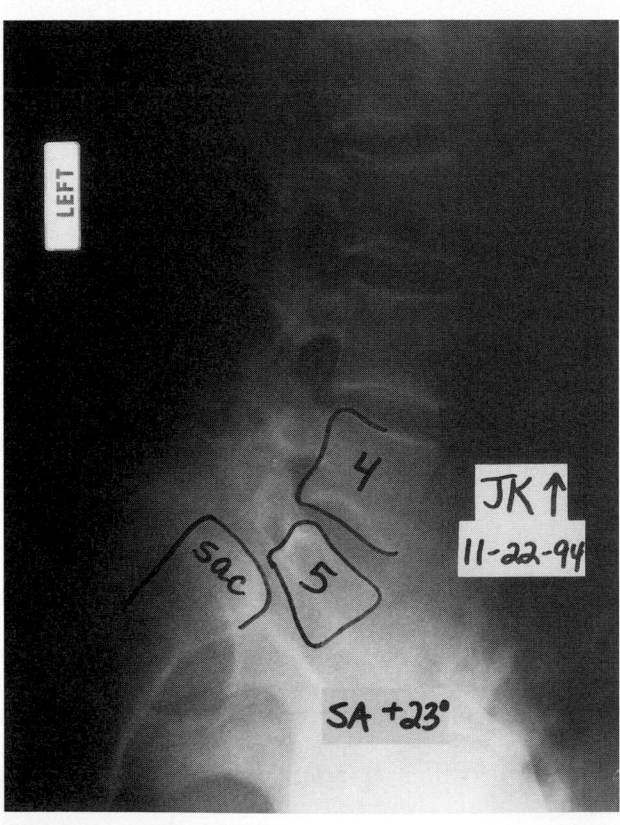

C

Figure 75-63 J.K., a 16 + 2-year-old male, has grade III isthmic spondylolisthesis of L5 on S1 (*A*). He underwent posterolateral spinal fusion from L4 to the sacrum through a paramedian approach with autogenous iliac crest bone graft and postoperative extension casing. His 9-month postoperative Ferguson AP x-rays show a solid spinal fusion (*B*). His postoperative lateral x-ray (*C*) shows no change in position of his spine with a well-healed L4-to-sacrum fusion.

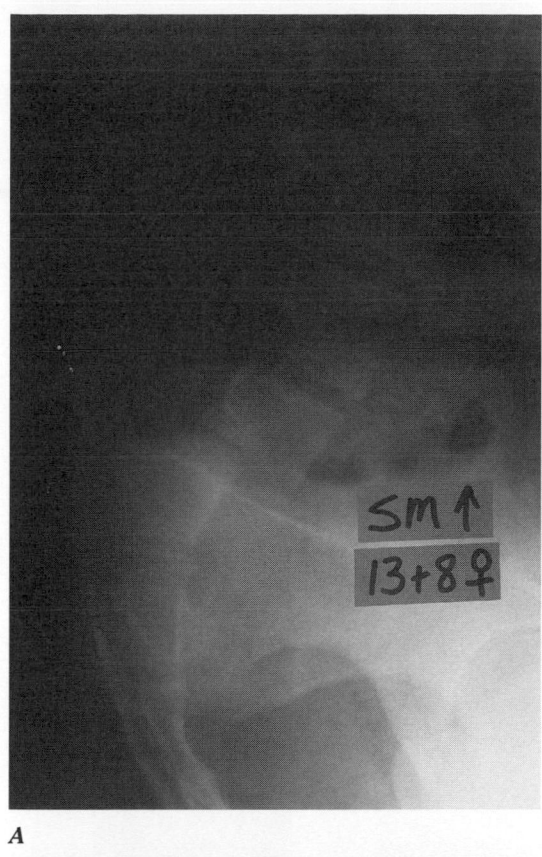

A

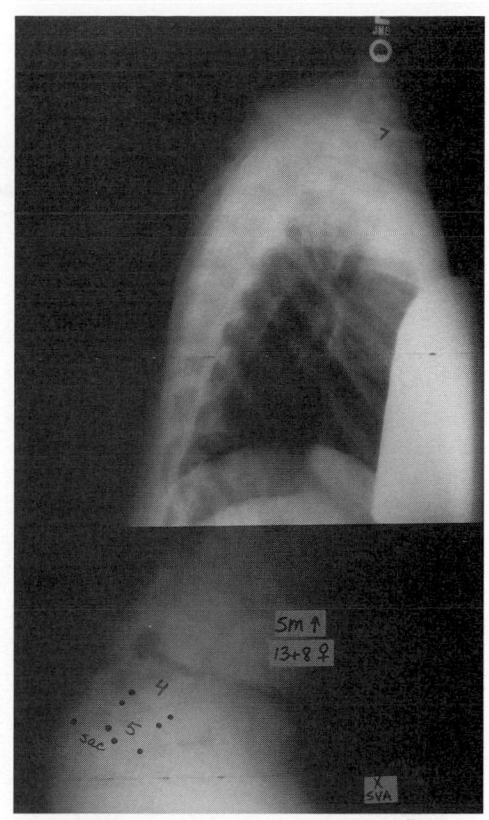

B

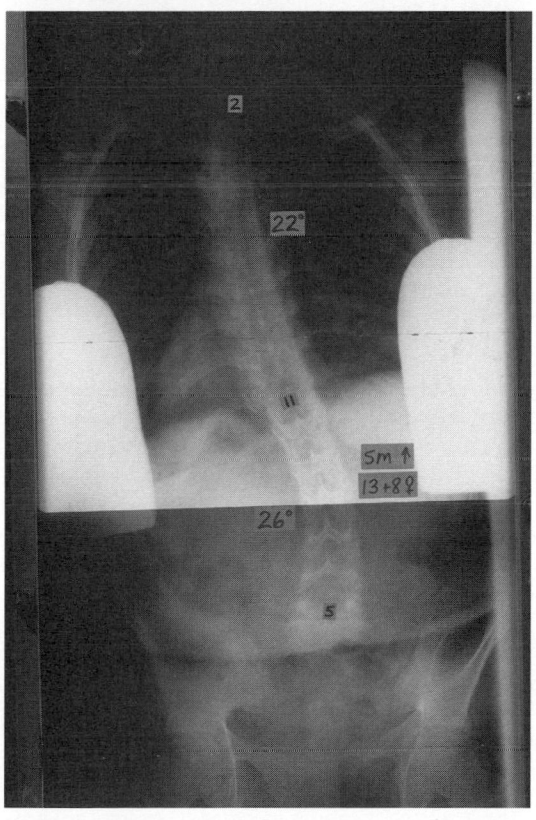

C

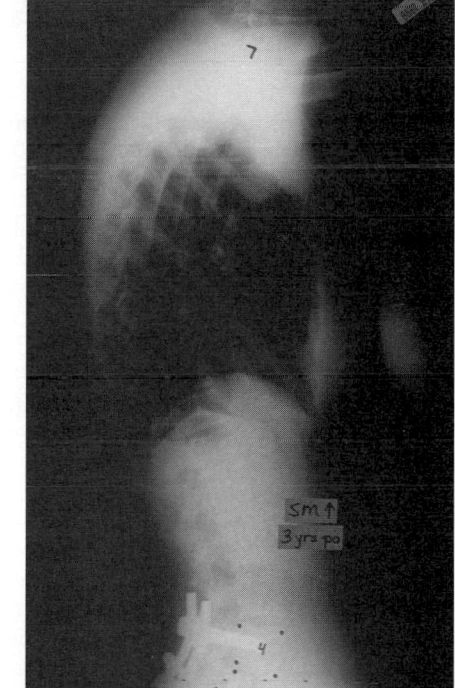

D

Figure 75-64 S.M., a 13 + 8-year-old female, presented with a severe spondylolisthesis deformity. Her lateral upright lumbosacral radiograph (*A*) demonstrates a grade IV high dysplastic developmental spondylolisthesis with a severely kyphotic slip angle and a vertical sacrum. S.M.'s long-cassette x-ray (*B*) demonstrates the marked sagittal imbalance of her entire spine anterior to the sacrum and her sagittal vertical axis (SVA) 15 cm anterior to her L5-S1 disk. Her long-cassette coronal x-ray (*C*) demonstrates "sciatic scoliosis" due to tight lower lumbar and sacral nerve roots. The patient's physical exam was consistent with her high-grade spondylolisthesis. She underwent a posterior instrumented reduction consisting of bilateral L5 and S1 nerve root decompressions and a reduction procedure with posterior instrumentation and fusion from

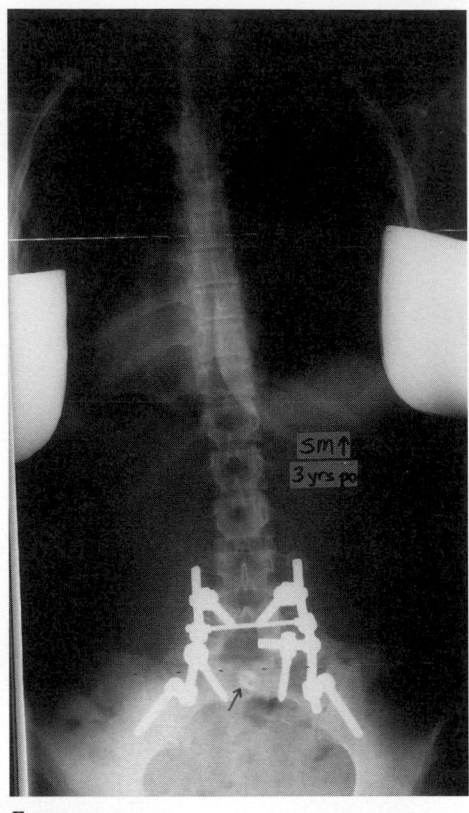

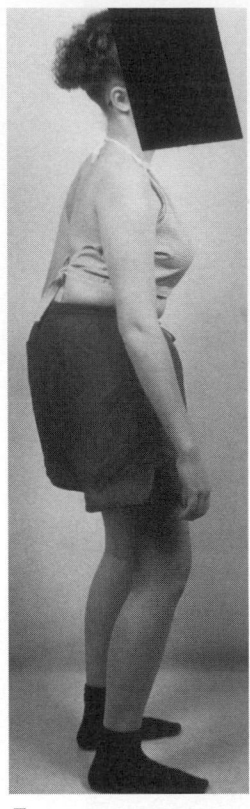

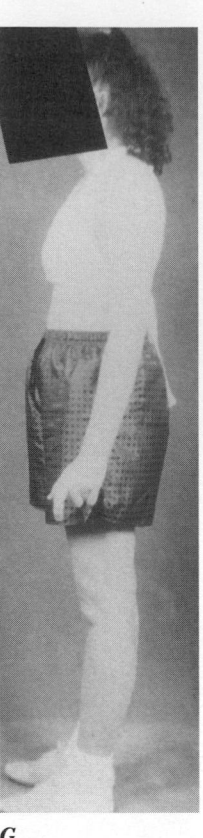

E   *F*   *G*

Figure 75-64 *(Continued)* L4 to the sacrum. Her 3-year post-operative long-cassette x-ray (*D*) demonstrates improved lumbosacral as well as overall spinal alignment, with the sagittal vertical axis falling at the level of the lumbosacral disk. S.M.'s 3-year postoperative long-cassette coronal x-ray (*E*) demonstrates solid spinal fusion as well as the anterior fibular graft that was placed as a second procedure from the L5 body into the S1 body via an anterior approach. The patient's preoperative clinical photo (*F*) demonstrates her shortened trunk, prominent buttocks, flexed knees, and overall forward pitch of sagittal alignment. Her postoperative clinical alignment (*G*) shows normalization of the appearance of her overall trunk and lower extremities. (Courtesy of Keith H. Bridwell, MD.)

cluding neurologic sequelae. Reduction may also be achieved by a variety of other methods, including hyperextension casting and skeletal traction. No one technique has yet shown itself to be completely satisfactory and thus universally accepted.

In order to help ascertain whether a reduction procedure is indicated, we utilize a standing long-cassette lateral x-ray as well as a supine hyperextension lumbosacral x-ray on a bolster. Patients with a forward sagittal imbalance, where a vertical line drawn from the body of the C7 segment falls several centimeters in front of the lumbosacral disk, have a greater tension force on their lumbosacral area and a higher nonunion rate with uninstrumented, unreduced posterior fusions in situ. In contrast, patients with an appreciably reducible slip angle on supine hyperextension x-rays may undergo treatment with an in situ instrumented fusion from either L4 or L5 to the sacrum with pedicle screw fixation in order to stabilize the slip during fusion. It is also important to assess the size of the L5 transverse processes and their relation to the sacral ala. Large L5 transverse processes that are closely approximated to the sacral ala have a much higher fusion rate than small, wispy transverse processes that are positioned anterior to the sacral ala because of the high degree of spondylolisthesis and a kyphotic slip angle. It is important to assess all these factors so as to optimize surgical treatment.

Patients with spondylolysis and spondylolisthesis frequently have coexisting scoliosis (Fig. 75-65). The majority of the curvatures are mild, with curves rarely greater than 20°. However, there is a sciatic type scoliosis of nerve root tension in high-grade developmental spondylolisthesis that may produce a larger scoliosis. These curves normally have minimal rotation and respond to appropriate fusion treatment of the spondylolisthesis. In contrast, patients with idiopathic scoliosis have an incidence of lumbosacral spondylolisthesis similar to that of the general population (approximately 6 percent). If both idiopathic scoliosis and spondylolisthesis coexist, each should be treated independently while both conditions are followed. If the scoliosis requires treatment, then every attempt should be made to avoid fusing into the lower lumbar spine, so as to avoid increased stress on the spondylolisthetic segment. Occasionally, it is necessary to fuse both the scoliosis and the spondylolisthesis simultaneously in patients who must have their spinal deformity fused to the sacrum. Adequate fixation and autogenous bone grafting must be obtained in

Figure 75-65 A.S., a 16 + 7-year-old male, presented with a thoracic deformity and lumbar spinal pain. His long-cassette coronal x-ray (*A*) demonstrates a 52° right thoracic scoliosis. His long-cassette lateral x-ray (*B*) demonstrates a grade II isthmic spondylolisthesis at L5-S1.

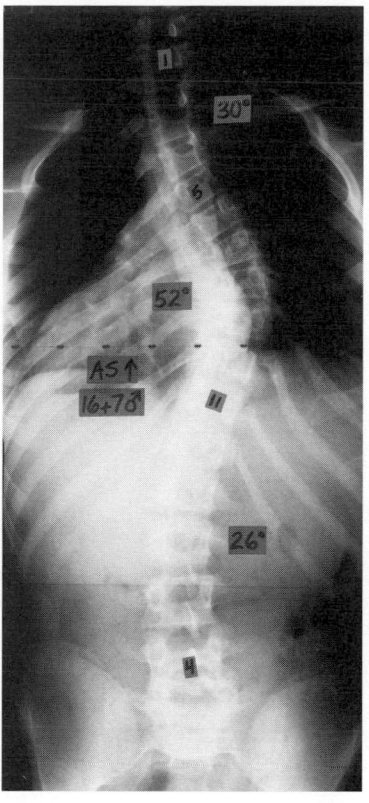

A

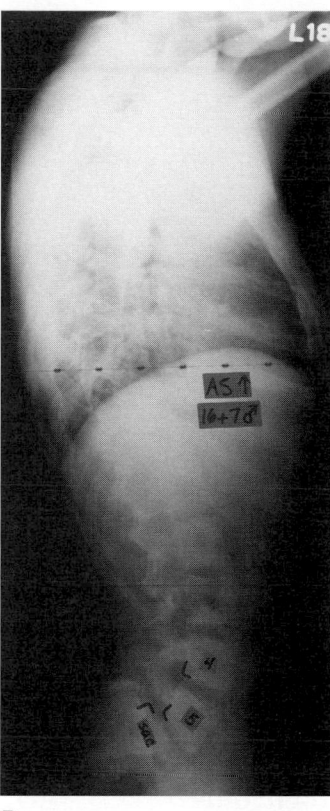

B

the L5 and sacral segments to produce an adequate arthrodesis.

Sagittal Plane Lordosis

Pathologic lordosis of the spine is manifest as any degree of lordosis in the thoracic spine and hyperlordosis of the thoracolumbar and lumbar spine (Table 75-3). In the thoracic spine, the most common cause of a lordotic sagittal alignment is idiopathic scoliosis. Normally the spine is hypokyphotic over the apex of the scoliosis, but it may also be frankly lordotic, even when total thoracic sagittal alignment from T1 to T12 is slightly kyphotic. However, there are certainly some patients with idiopathic scoliosis who have a generalized lordotic alignment to the entire thoracic region. This usually has a detrimental effect on pulmonary function and thus the patient's ultimate functional as well as cosmetic outcome.[141,211] It is important to follow sagittal alignment when contemplating bracing an idiopathic scoliosis patient, for it is known that spinal orthoses aggravate thoracic lordosis. Thus bracing should be stopped if progression of lordosis is noted radiographically. In addition, the surgical treatment of a patient with idiopathic scoliosis and a lordotic thoracic sagittal alignment should strive to improve overall thoracic kyphosis, not only to optimize the cosmetic appearance but also to improve long-term pulmonary function. Marked thoracic hyperlordosis found in a patient with an apparently idiopathic scoliosis should raise concern for possible entities

such as neuromuscular disease, Marfan's syndrome, or congenital posterior element bars that would produce a greater degree of lordosis.[206,207]

Congenital lordosis occurs because of posterior failure of segmentation or, less likely, formation with resultant excessive anterior growth. In the thoracic spine, severe rigid lordotic deformities may occur at a young age, and these may cause severe pulmonary restriction. Once this condition is recognized, prompt anterior spinal fusion is required to reverse the lordotic growth potential. Congenital lordosis may also occur in the lumbar spine; however, this must produce a hyperlordosis to become clinically and radiographically apparent.

Neuromuscular disorders may cause thoracic lordosis or lumbar hyperlordosis. Patients with myelomeningocele lumbar kyphosis may develop a hyperlordotic deformity of the thoracic spine to compensate for the kyphotic lumbar deformity. Wheelchair-bound patients often develop hip flexion contractures that predispose to lumbar hyperlordosis in the sitting position. Spastic cerebral palsy patients may also develop severe thoracolumbar and lumbar hyperlordotic deformities that interfere with sitting, proper use of the upper extremities, pulmonary function, and proper nutrition (Fig. 75-66).

The treatment of neuromuscular lumbar hyperlordotic deformities is challenging. Bracing does not have a role in these patients, who are almost exclusively nonambulatory. If surgery for a concomitant scoliotic deformity is performed, anterior lumbar compression instrumentation will decrease the lumbar hyperlordosis. In patients without a coronal plane deformity, a thorough anterior release and fusion, followed by skeletal traction and then posterior Luque instrumentation and fusion to pull the individual segments of the lumbar spine posteriorly, and thus out of hyperlordosis, may be indicated. However, if these patients have adequate ability to sit, observation alone is indicated.

THE PEDIATRIC CERVICAL SPINE

Torticollis

Torticollis is defined as a head tilt and rotatory deformity that may present at birth or soon thereafter. The differential diagnosis of torticollis is quite large, including both congenital and acquired diagnoses. Congenital spinal anomalies such as unilateral absence of the C1 facet, Klippel-Feil syndrome (Fig. 75-67), and odontoid anomalies such as odontoid hypoplasia may present with torticollis. Acquired conditions such as atlantoaxial rotary subluxation, Arnold-Chiari malformation, and inflammatory syndromes such as retropharyngeal abscesses may also produce tilting and/or rotary deformity of the head and neck in children. However, congenital muscular torticollis is by far the most common cause in the infant and young child.

Congenital muscular torticollis appears in a high proportion of breech or otherwise difficult births. Although the exact cause is unknown, it is believed to be the result of local compression to the soft tissues of the neck, which somehow leads to pathologic fibrosis of the sternocleidomastoid muscle. The deformity is caused by sternocleidomastoid contracture with the head tilted toward the involved side and the chin rotated toward the opposite side. The involved sternocleidomastoid is often nontender but palpable as a taut structure in the anterior lateral neck region. There are varying degrees of tightness to the muscle, producing variable motion to the neck. Radiographs of the cervical spine should always be obtained to ensure that the deformity is truly a muscular torticollis and not associated with congenital vertebral lesions of the cervical spine (Fig. 75-68). Plain x-rays of the cervical spine in these children should be normal. Since up to 20 percent of children with congenital muscular torticollis have developmental dysplasia of the hip, careful examination of the

hips and an appropriate radiographic study and/or ultrasound should be performed if any suspicion exists regarding the status of the hips.

Treatment of congenital muscular torticollis consists of conservative measures of stretching exercises performed by the caregivers and guided by a physical therapist. Often, modifying the child's toys and crib so that the neck will be stretched in the optimal position is indicated. Surgery is recommended only if the deformity persists past 1 year of age and progress is not being made with stretching exercises. Although many surgical procedures have been described, a Z-plasty release of the sternal attachment of the muscle has produced many satisfactory results in one series. A postoperative brace maintaining alignment of the head and neck is desirable, along with stretching exercises when the muscle is healed.

Atlantooccipital Anomalies

Occipitocervical synostosis, basilar impression, and odontoid anomalies are the most common developmental malformations of the occipitovertebral junction. These lesions arise from faulty development of the skull and adjacent vertebral skeleton during the embryonic stage. The bony vertebral anomalies produce not only abnormal motion of the upper cervical spine but also neurologic abnormalities of a potentially altered spinal canal. Clinically, the appearance of these anomalies is similar to those seen in patients with Klippel-Feil syndrome, who have short, broad necks, restricted movement, low hairlines, and torticollis. Although neurologic symptoms can occur during childhood, they often present much later in life, in the fifth or sixth decade. Most commonly, children present with neck and occipital pain, vertigo, torticollis, ataxia, and even dysphagia.

Standard x-rays may be difficult to obtain because of the fixed bony deformities and the overlying shadows of the mandible, occiput, and foramen magnum. The best way to detail the upper cervical spine is to take a lateral x-ray of the skull rather than the midcervical spine. Although there are many commonly used lines to determine basilar impression—such as McRae, Chamberlain, and McGregor—the basic issue is whether the tip of the odontoid process is protruding into the foramen magnum and thus potentially narrowing the area for the proximal spinal cord and distal brainstem.

Flexion/extension x-rays should always be taken in these patients and others who have suspected C1-C2 instability. Pediatric C1-C2 instability due to transverse ligament abnormalities is diagnosed when the distance is greater than 4 mm between the anterior aspect of the odontoid and the posterior aspect of the anterior ring of C1 (Fig. 75-69). In patients with an atlantodental interval (ADI) greater than 4 mm, this narrows the space available for the cord and may require operative attention to correct the instability. Thus when symptoms and/or signs of an unstable C1-C2 complex are present, a posterior C1-C2 fusion is indicated. Preliminary traction to attempt reduction is helpful and makes the surgery safer. Rarely, a posterior decompression of the occiput and/or proximal cervical spine is necessary, depending on the amount and correctability of neural compression.

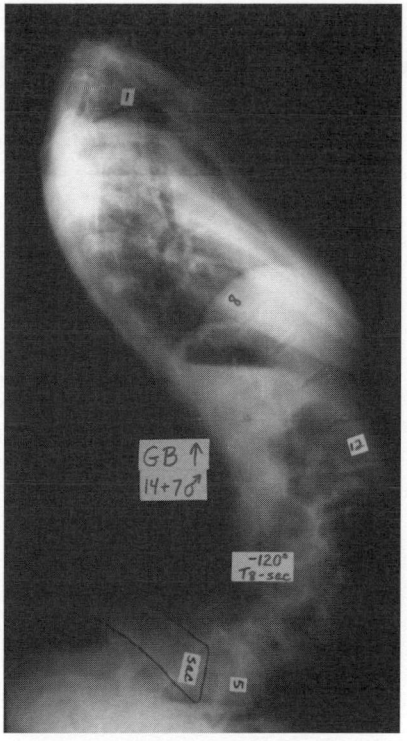

A

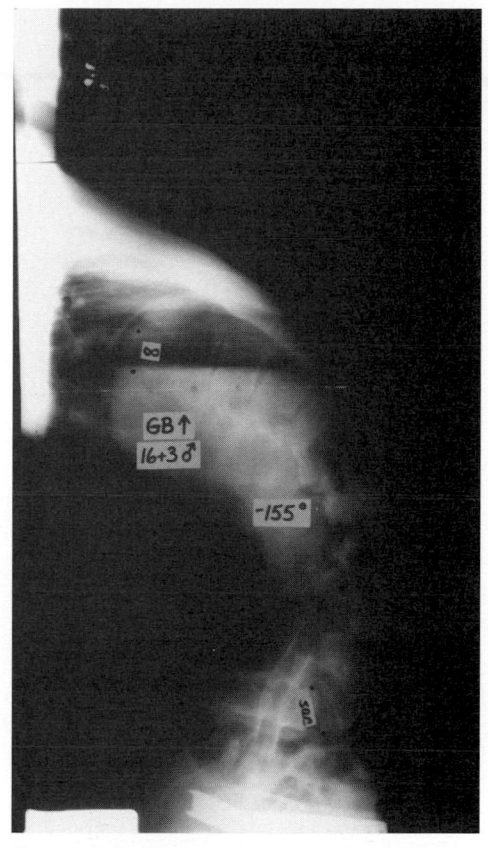

B

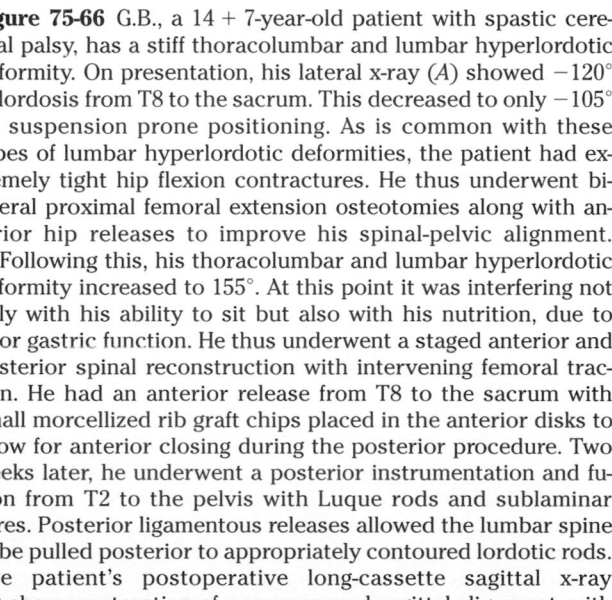

Figure 75-66 G.B., a 14 + 7-year-old patient with spastic cerebral palsy, has a stiff thoracolumbar and lumbar hyperlordotic deformity. On presentation, his lateral x-ray (*A*) showed −120° of lordosis from T8 to the sacrum. This decreased to only −105° on suspension prone positioning. As is common with these types of lumbar hyperlordotic deformities, the patient had extremely tight hip flexion contractures. He thus underwent bilateral proximal femoral extension osteotomies along with anterior hip releases to improve his spinal-pelvic alignment. *B.* Following this, his thoracolumbar and lumbar hyperlordotic deformity increased to 155°. At this point it was interfering not only with his ability to sit but also with his nutrition, due to poor gastric function. He thus underwent a staged anterior and posterior spinal reconstruction with intervening femoral traction. He had an anterior release from T8 to the sacrum with small morcellized rib graft chips placed in the anterior disks to allow for anterior closing during the posterior procedure. Two weeks later, he underwent a posterior instrumentation and fusion from T2 to the pelvis with Luque rods and sublaminar wires. Posterior ligamentous releases allowed the lumbar spine to be pulled posterior to appropriately contoured lordotic rods. The patient's postoperative long-cassette sagittal x-ray (*C*) shows restoration of a more normal sagittal alignment, with the T8-to-sacrum lordosis decreased to −73°. His coronal x-ray

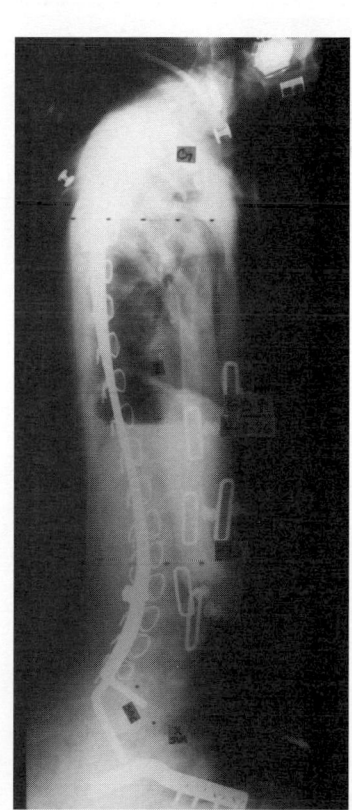

C

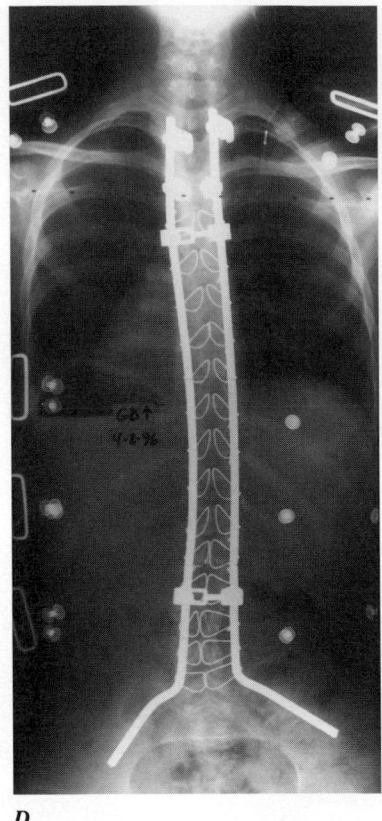

D

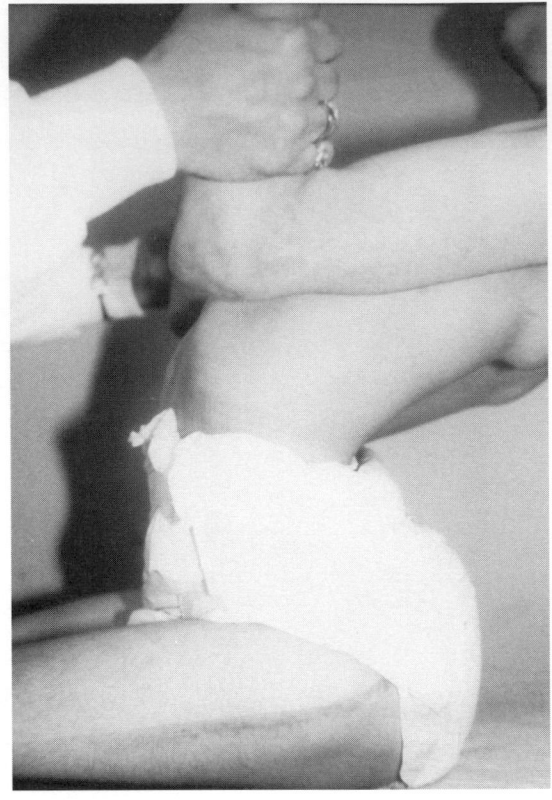

E

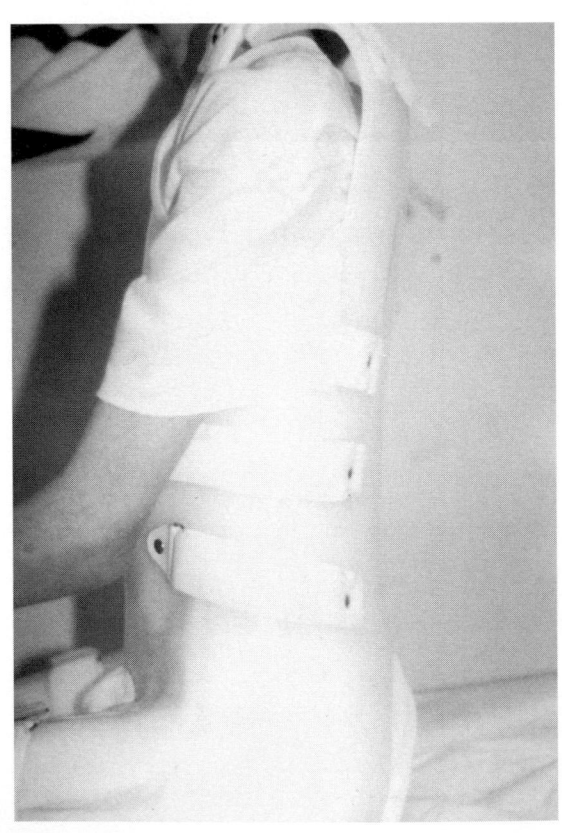

F

Figure 75-66 *(Continued)* (*D*) shows fixation and Galveston rod placement into the iliac wings bilaterally. The patient's preoperative sitting photo (*E*) demonstrates his severe deformity. His postoperative sitting photo (*F*) demonstrates a more normal sitting posture and overall alignment of the trunk and pelvis.

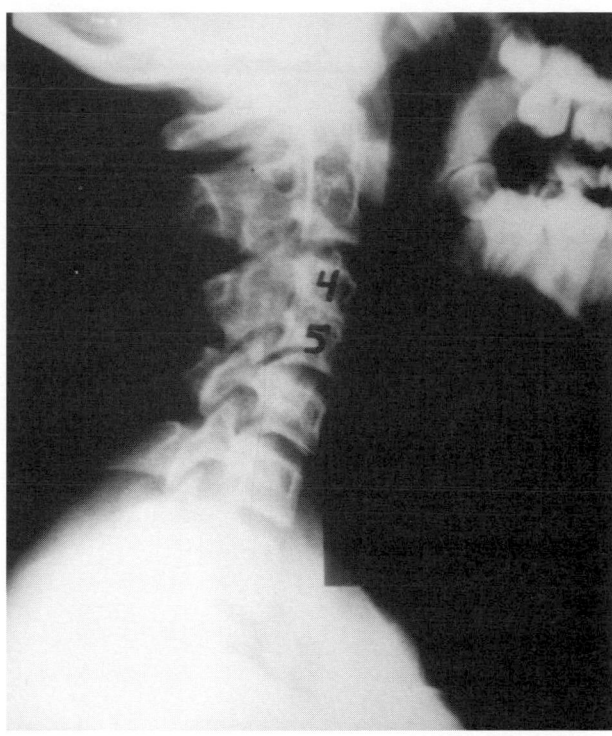

Figure 75-67 A patient with Klippel-Feil syndrome with anterior fusion of C2-C3 and C4-C5 as well as posterior fusion of those levels.

The incidence of C1-C2 instability in children with Down's syndrome is extremely high, estimated from 9 to 22 percent. It is often a gradual and progressive lesion that may produce neurologic sequelae. Most Down's syndrome patients are asymptomatic, but some may present with myelopathy due to spinal cord compression. Radiographically, an atlantodental interval on flexion/extension lateral radiographs of more than 4 or 5 mm indicates the instability. Normal ranges of motion at the atlantooccipital intervals have not been as well defined. In normal patients, however, there should be no translation between the occiput and C1. When the plain x-rays indicate instability, MRI scanning in neutral, flexion, and extension, if needed, can be utilized to determine the extent of encroachment on the spinal cord. If this is substantial, prophylactic proximal cervical spinal stabilization is indicated. Also, for those patients who do show symptoms and signs of myelopathy, posterior C1-C2 fusion is indicated. Preoperative traction is useful to reduce the deformity and thus make surgical correction safer. It is known that Down's syndrome patients seem to be at much higher risk for postoperative neurologic and other complications following these types of surgeries. They also have a higher pseudarthrosis rate even when immobilized in a halo postoperatively. Even if their surgeries are successful, Down's patients may develop instability at levels above or below the fusion later on. Thus, these patients should be approached with caution and followed carefully.

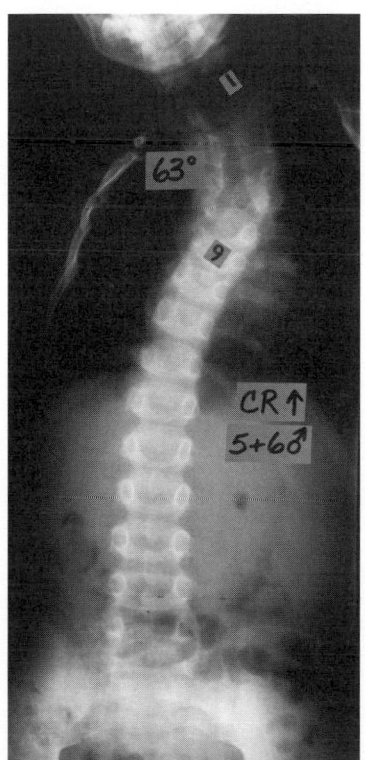

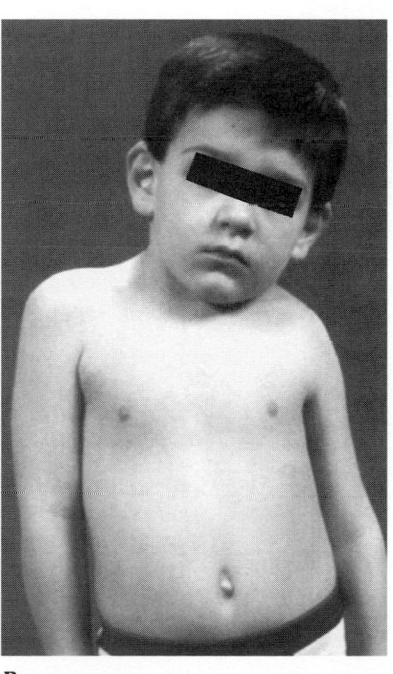

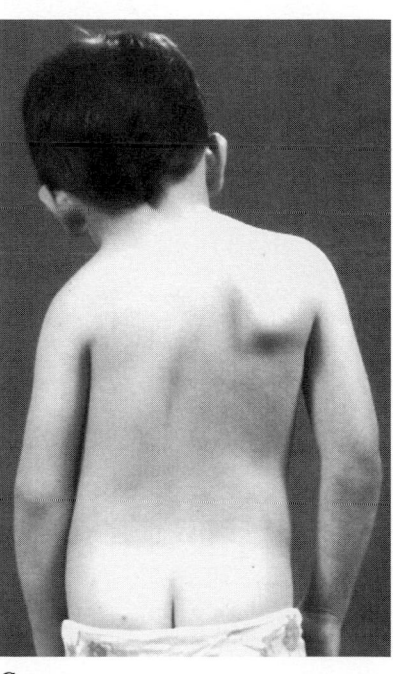

Figure 75-68 C.R., a 7-year-old patient, has congenital upper thoracic scoliosis and resultant torticollis. His upright coronal x-ray (A) at age 5 + 6 shows 63° upper thoracic scoliosis. Frontal (B) and posterior (C) clinical photos document his torticollis.

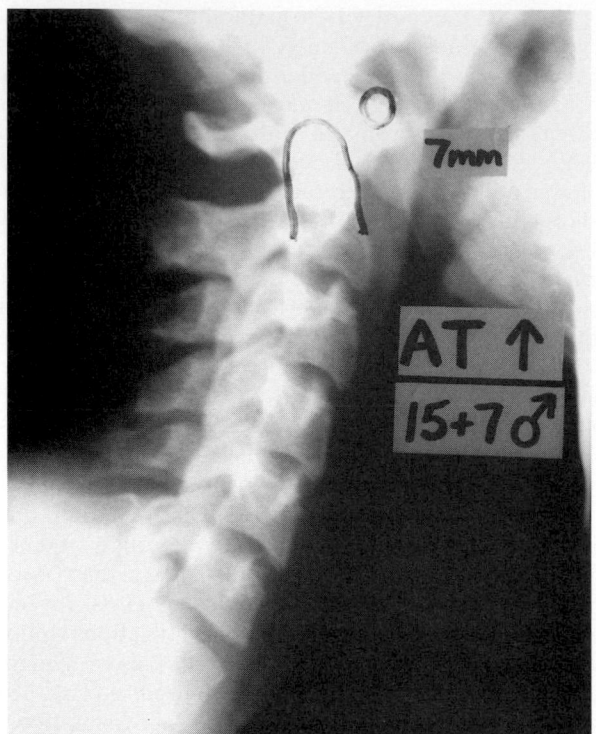

A

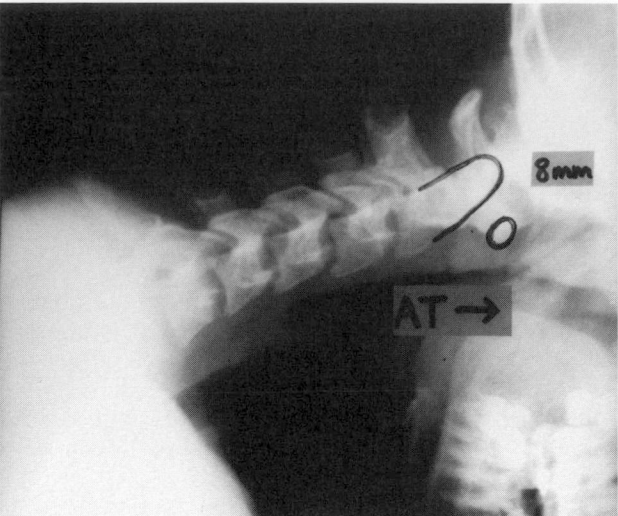

B

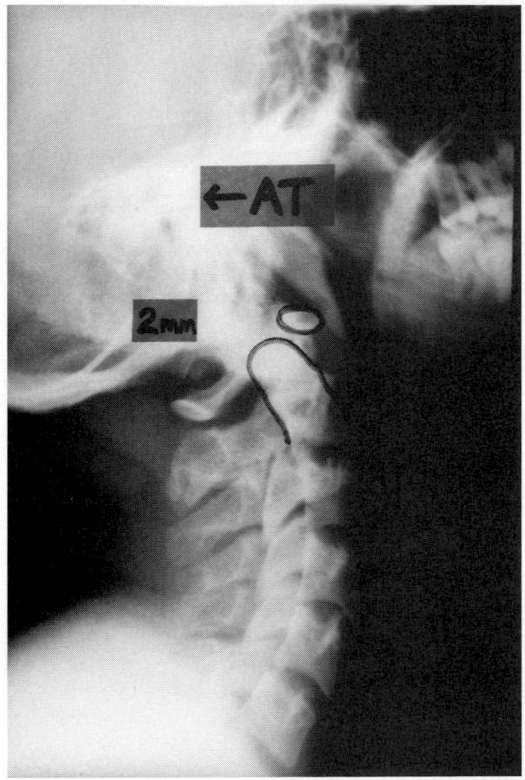

C

Figure 75-69 A.T., a 15 + 7-year-old male, presented with a long history of upper neck pain. His upright neutral lateral x-ray (*A*) shows a 7-mm atlantodental interval. On forward flexion (*B*), this increased to 8 mm. On extension (*C*), it was reduced to 2 mm.

Atlantoaxial Rotary Displacement

Atlantoaxial rotary displacement is one of the more common causes of childhood torticollis. The vast majority of these cases recover spontaneously without treatment; however, some of them may present with a fixed torticollis often termed fixed atlantoaxial displacement. The onset usually is spontaneous following minor or major trauma, upper respiratory infection, or head and neck surgery. Muscular torticollis of the sternocleidomastoid muscle follows the bony rotary displacement. Radiographs are often difficult to interpret because of the difficulty in positioning the patient as well as the pain associated with the condition. The diagnosis is made with an axial CT scan, which shows the rotation of C1 on C2.

Patients with rotary subluxation of less than 1 week's duration can be treated with immobilization in a soft tissue collar and rest. Close follow-up is indicated. If the reduction fails to occur spontaneously, hospitalization and the use of halter traction with muscle relaxants and analgesics is the next step. If no reduction is obtained or a patient presents in a chronic (greater than 6 weeks) and fixed position, a posterior C1-C2 fusion is performed in the fixed position. A forceful or manipulative reduction is to be avoided. Positioning in a halo cast or vest is done after the fusion. This can be expected to provide satisfactory alignment.

REFERENCES

1. Aaro S, Ohlund C: Scoliosis and pulmonary function. *Spine* 9:220–222, 1984.
2. Albright AL, Gartner JC, Wiener ES: Lumbar cutaneous hemangiomas as indicators of tethered spinal cords. *Pediatrics* 83:977–980, 1989.
3. Allen BL Jr, Ferguson RL: The operative treatment of myelomeningocele spinal deformity. *Orthop Clin North Am* 10:845–862, 1979.
4. Allen BL, Ferguson RL: L-rod instrumentation for scoliosis in cerebral palsy. *J Pediatr Orthop* 2:87–96, 1982.
5. Allen BL, Ferguson RL: The Galveston technique of pelvic fixation with L-rod instrumentation of the spine. *Spine* 9:388–394, 1984.
6. Andrew T, Piggott H: Growth arrest for progressive scoliosis: Combined anterior and posterior fusion of the convexity. *J Bone Joint Surg [Br]* 67:193–197, 1985.
7. Andrish J, Kalamchi A, MacEwen GD: Sacral agenesis: A clinical evaluation of its management, heredity, and associated anomalies. *Clin Orthop* 139:52–57, 1979.
8. Aprin H, Bowen JR, MacEwen GD, Hall JE: Spine fusion in patients with spinal muscular atrophy. *J Bone Joint Surg [Am]* 64:1179–1187, 1982.
9. Arkin AM, Pack GT, Ransohoff NS, Simon N: Radiation induced scoliosis: A case report. *J Bone Joint Surg [Am]* 32:401–404, 1950.
10. Ascani E, Bartolozzi P, Logroscino CA, et al: Natural history of untreated idiopathic scoliosis after skeletal maturity. *Spine* 11:784–789, 1986.
11. Axelgaard J, Brown JC: Lateral electrical surface stimulation for the treatment of progressive idiopathic scoliosis. *Spine* 8:242–260, 1983.
12. Banerian KG, Wang AM, Samberg LC, et al: Association of vertebral endplate fracture with pediatric lumbar intervertebral disc herniation: Value of CT and MR imaging. *Radiology* 177:763–765, 1990.
13. Banta JV, Hamanda JS: Natural history of the kyphotic deformity in myelomeningocele. *J Bone Joint Surg [Am]* 58:279, 1976.
14. Banta JV, Nichols O: Sacral agenesis. *J Bone Joint Surg [Am]* 51:693–703, 1969.
15. Banta JV, Whiteman S, Dyck PM, et al: Fifteen year review of myelodysplasia. *J Bone Joint Surg [Am]* 58:726, 1976.
16. Barbeau A, Sadibelouiz M, Sadibelouiz A, Roy M: A clinical classification of hereditary ataxias. *Can J Neurol Sci* 11:501–505, 1984.
17. Bassett GS, Bunnell WP: Effect of a thoracolumbosacral orthosis on lateral trunk shift in idiopathic scoliosis. *J Pediatr Orthop* 6:182–185, 1986.
18. Bassett GS, Bunnell WP, MacEwen GD: Treatment of idiopathic scoliosis with the Wilmington brace: Results in patients with a twenty to thirty-nine-degree curve. *J Bone Joint Surg [Am]* 68:602–605, 1986.
19. Benady SG: Spinal muscular atrophy in childhood: Review of 50 cases. *Dev Med Child Neurol* 20:746–757, 1978.
20. Bernhardt M, Bridwell KH: Segmental analysis of the sagittal plane alignment of the normal thoracic and lumbar spines and thoracolumbar junction. *Spine* 14:717–721, 1989.
21. Bethem D, Winter RB, Lutter L: Disorders of the spine in diastrophic dwarfism: A discussion of nine patients and review of the literature. *J Bone Joint Surg [Am]* 62:529–536, 1980.
22. Bethem D, Winter RB, Lutter L, et al: Spinal disorders or dwarfism: Review of the literature and report of eighty cases. *J Bone Joint Surg [Am]* 63:1412–1425, 1981.
23. Birch JG, Herring JA: Spinal deformity in Marfan syndrome. *J Pediatr Orthop* 7:546–552, 1987.
24. Birch JG, Herring JA, Roach JW, et al: Cotrel-Dubousset instrumentation in idiopathic scoliosis: A preliminary report. *Clin Orthop* 227:24–29, 1988.
25. Blumel J, Evans EB, Eggers GWN: Partial and complete agenesis or malformation of the sacrum with associated anomalies. *J Bone Joint Surg [Am]* 41:497–518, 1959.
26. Boachie-Adjei O, Lonstein JE, Winter RB, et al: Management of neuromuscular spinal deformities with Luque segmental instrumentation. *J Bone Joint Surg [Am]* 71:548–562, 1989.
27. Boston HC Jr, Bianco AJ Jr, Rhodes KH: Disk space infections in children. *Orthop Clin North Am* 6:953–964, 1975.
28. Boxall D, Bradford DS, Winter RB, Moe JH: Management of severe spondylolisthesis in children and adolescents. *J Bone Joint Surg [Am]* 61:479–495, 1979.
29. Bradford DS: Management of spondylolysis and spondylolisthesis. *AAOS Instr Course Lect* 32:151–162, 1983.
30. Bradford DS, Ahmed KB, Moe JH, et al: The surgical management of patients with Scheuermann's disease: A review of twenty-four cases managed by combined anterior and posterior spine fusion. *J Bone Joint Surg [Am]* 62:705–712, 1980.
31. Bradford DS, Boachie-Adjei O: One-stage anterior and posterior hemivertebral resection and arthrodesis. *J Bone Joint Surg [Am]* 72:536–540, 1990.
32. Bradford DS, Garcia A: Herniations of the lumbar intervertebral disk in children and adolescents: A review of 30 surgically treated cases. *JAMA* 210:2045–2051, 1969.
33. Bradford DS, Heithoff KB, Cohen M: Intraspinal abnormalities and congenital spine deformities: A radiographic and MRI study. *J Pediatr Orthop* 11:36–41, 1991.
34. Bradford DS, Iza J: Repair of the defect in spondylolysis or minimal degrees of spondylolisthesis by segmental wire fixation and bone grafting. *Spine* 10:673–679, 1985.
35. Bradford DS, Moe JH, Montalvo FJ, Winter RB: Scheuermann's kyphosis and roundback deformity: Results of Milwaukee brace treatment. *J Bone Joint Surg [Am]* 56:740–758, 1974.
36. Bradford DS, Moe JH, Montalvo FJ, Winter RB: Scheuermann's kyphosis: Results of surgical treatment by posterior spine arthrodesis in twenty-two patients. *J Bone Joint Surg [Am]* 57:439–448, 1975.
37. Bradford DS, Moe JH, Winter RB: Scheuermann's juvenile kyphosis and postural roundback deformity, in Rothman RH, Simeone FA (eds): *The Spine*. Vol I. Philadelphia, Saunders, 1975, pp 361–385.

38. Bridwell KH, Betz RR, Capelli AM, et al: Sagittal plane analysis in idiopathic scoliosis patients treated with Cotrel-Dubousset instrumentation. *Spine* 15:921–926, 1990.

39. Bridwell KH, McAllister JW, Betz RR, et al: Coronal decompensation produced by Cotrel-Dubousset "derotation" maneuver for idiopathic right thoracic scoliosis *Spine* 16:769–777, 1991.

40. Bridwell KH, O'Brien MF, Lenke LG, et al: Posterior spinal fusion supplemented with only allograft bone in paralytic scoliosis: Does it work? *Spine* 19:2658–2666, 1994.

41. Broom MJ, Banta JV, Renshaw TS: Spinal fusion augmented by Luque rod segmental instrumentation for neuromuscular scoliosis. *J Bone Joint Surg [Am]* 71:32–44, 1989.

42. Brown JC, Swank S, Specht L: Combined anterior and posterior spine fusion in cerebral palsy. *Spine* 7:570–573, 1982.

43. Brumberg JA, Latchaw RE, Kanal E, et al: Magnetic resonance imaging of spinal dysraphism. *Radiol Clin North Am* 26:181–205, 1988.

44. Buck JE: Direct repair of the defect in spondylolisthesis. *J Bone Joint Surg [Br]* 52:432–437, 1970.

45. Bunch WH: The Milwaukee brace in paralytic scoliosis. *Clin Orthop* 110:63–68, 1975.

46. Bunnell WP: The natural history of idiopathic scoliosis before skeletal maturity. *Spine* 11:773–776, 1986.

47. Cady RB, Bobechko WP: Incidence, natural history, and treatment of scoliosis in Friedreich's ataxia. *J Pediatr Orthop* 4:673–676, 1984.

48. Callahan RA, Johnson RM, Margolis RN, et al: Cervical facet fusion for control of instability following laminectomy. *J Bone Joint Surg [Am]* 59:991–1002, 1977.

49. Cambridge W, Drennan JC: Scoliosis associated with Duchenne muscular dystrophy. *J Pediatr Orthop* 7:436–440, 1987.

50. Casselman ES, Mandell GA: Vertebral scalloping in neurofibromatosis. *Radiology* 131:89–94, 1979.

51. Cattell HS, Clark GL Jr: Cervical kyphosis and instability following multiple laminectomies in children. *J Bone Joint Surg [Am]* 49:713–720, 1967.

52. Chaglassian JH, Riseborough EJ, Hall JE: Neurofibromatous scoliosis: Natural history and results of treatment in thirty-seven cases. *J Bone Joint Surg [Am]* 58:695–702, 1976.

53. Chamberlain S, Shaw J, Rowland A, et al: Mapping of mutation causing Friedreich's ataxia to human chromosome 9. *Nature* 334:248–250, 1988.

54. Clark JE: Apophyseal fracture of the lumbar spine in adolescence. *Orthop Rev* 20:512–516, 1991.

55. Cochran T, Irstam L, Nachemson A: Long-term anatomic and functional changes in patients with adolescent idiopathic scoliosis treated by Harrington rod fusion. *Spine* 8:576–584, 1983.

56. Collis DK, Ponseti IV: Long-term follow-up of patients with idiopathic scoliosis not treated surgically. *J Bone Joint Surg [Am]* 51:425–445, 1969.

57. Colonna PC, Von Saal F: A study of paralytic scoliosis based on 500 cases of poliomyelitis. *J Bone Joint Surg [Am]* 23:335–353, 1941.

58. Conner AN: Developmental anomalies and prognosis in infantile idiopathic scoliosis. *J Bone Joint Surg [Br]* 51:711–713, 1969.

59. Crawford AH: Neurofibromatosis in childhood. *AAOS Instr Course Lect* 30:56–74, 1981.

60. Crawford AH: Pitfalls of spinal deformities associated with neurofibromatosis in children. *Clin Orthop* 245:29–42, 1989.

61. Crawford AH, Bagamery N: Osseous manifestations of neurofibromatosis in childhood. *J Pediatr Orthop* 6:72–88, 1986.

62. Crawford AH, Kucharzyk DW, Ruda R, Smitherman HC: Diskitis in children. *Clin Orthop* 266:70–79, 1991.

63. Daher YH, Lonstein JE, Winter RB, Bradford DS: Spinal deformities in patients with Friedreich's ataxia: A review of 19 patients. *J Pediatr Orthop* 5:553–557, 1985.

64. Daher YH, Lonstein JE, Winter RB, Bradford DS: Spinal deformities in patients with muscular dystrophy other than Duchenne: A review of 11 patients having surgical treatment. *Spine* 10:614–617, 1985.

65. Daher YH, Lonstein JE, Winter RB, Bradford DS: Spinal surgery in spinal muscular atrophy. *J Pediatr Orthop* 5:391–395, 1985.

66. Davies G, Reid L: Effect of scoliosis on growth of alveoli and pulmonary arteries and on right ventricle. *Arch Dis Child* 46:623–632, 1971.

67. DeRosa GP: Progressive scoliosis following chest wall resection in children. *Spine* 10:618–622, 1985.

68. DeWald RL, Faut MM: Anterior and posterior spinal surgery for paralytic scoliosis. *Spine* 4:401–409, 1979.

69. DeWald RL, Faut MM, Taddonio RF, Neuwirth MG: Severe lumbosacral spondylolisthesis in adolescents and children: Reduction and staged circumferential fusion. *J Bone Joint Surg [Am]* 63:619–626, 1981.

70. Dickson RA: Conservative treatment for idiopathic scoliosis. *J Bone Joint Surg [Br]* 67:176–181, 1985.

71. DiRaimondo CV, Green NE: Brace-wear compliance in patients with adolescent idiopathic scoliosis. *J Pediatr Orthop* 8:143–146, 1988.

72. Doyle JR: Narrowing of the intervertebral-disc space in children: Presumably an infectious lesion of the disc. *J Bone Joint Surg [Am]* 41:1191–1200, 1960.

73. Dubousset J, Herring JA, Shufflebarger H: The crankshaft phenomenon. *J Pediatr Orthop* 9:541–550, 1989.

74. du Lac P, Panuel M, Devred P, et al: MRI of disc space infection in infants and children: Report of twelve cases. *Pediatr Radiol* 20:175–178, 1990.

75. Durning RP, Scoles PV, Fox OD: Scoliosis after thoracotomy in tracheoesophageal fistula patients: A follow-up study. *J Bone Joint Surg [Am]* 62:1156–1159, 1980.

76. Edgar MA, Mehta M: Long term follow-up of fused and unfused idiopathic scoliosis. *J Bone Joint Surg [Br]* 70:712–716, 1988.

77. Emans JB, Kaelin A, Bancel P, et al: The Boston bracing system for idiopathic scoliosis: Follow-up results in 295 patients. *Spine* 11:792–801, 1986.

78. Emery JL, Mithal A: The number of alveoli in the terminal respiratory unit of man during late intrauterine life and childhood. *Arch Dis Child* 35:544–547, 1960.

79. Evans GA, Drennan JC, Russman BS: Functional classification and orthopaedic management of spinal muscular atrophy. *J Bone Joint Surg [Br]* 63:516–522, 1981.

80. Ferguson RL, Allen BL: Staged correction of neuromuscular scoliosis. *J Pediatr Orthop* 3:555–562, 1983.

81. Figueiredo UM, James JI: Juvenile idiopathic scoliosis. *J Bone Joint Surg [Br]* 63:61–66, 1981.

82. Flood BM, Butt WP, Dickson RA: Rib penetration of the intervertebral foraminae in neurofibromatosis. *Spine* 11:172–174, 1986.

83. Ford M, Silverman FN, Kozlowski K: Spondyloepiphyseal dysplasia (pseudoachondroplastic type). *J Roentgenol Radium Ther Nucl Med* 86:462–472, 1961.

84. Fredrickson BE, Baker D, McHolick WJ, et al: The natural history of spondylolysis and spondylolisthesis. *J Bone Joint Surg [Am]* 66:699–707, 1984.

85. Frennered AK, Danielson BI, Nachemson AL: Natural history of asymptomatic isthmic low-grade spondylolisthesis in children and adolescents: A seven-year follow-up study. *J Pediatr Orthop* 11:209–213, 1991.

86. Galasko CS, Delaney C, Morris P: Spinal stabilization in Duchenne muscular dystrophy. *J Bone Joint Surg [Br]* 74:210–214, 1992.

87. Greene TL, Hensinger RN, Hunter LY: Back pain and vertebral changes simulating Scheuermann's disease. *J Pediatr Orthop* 5:1–7, 1985.

88. Grobler LJ, Simmons EH, Barrington TW: Intervertebral disc herniation in the adolescent. *Spine* 4:267–278, 1979.

89. Hall PV, Lindseth RE, Campbell RL, Kalsbeck JE: Myelodysplasia and developmental scoliosis: A manifestation of syringomyelia. *Spine* 1:48–56, 1976.

90. Hall WA, Albright AL, Brunberg JA: Diagnosis of tethered cords by magnetic resonance imaging. *Surg Neurol* 30:60–64, 1988.

91. Hamill CL, Lenke LG, Bridwell KH, et al: The use of pedicle screw fixation to improve correction in the lumbar spine of patients with idiopathic scoliosis. Is it warranted? *Spine* 21:1241–1249, 1996.

92. Hanley EN Jr, Levy JA: Surgical treatment of isthmic lumbosacral spondylolisthesis: Analysis of variables influencing results. *Spine* 14:48–50, 1989.

93. Hapke EJ, Meek JC, Jacobs J: Pulmonary function in progressive muscular dystrophy. *Chest* 61:41–47, 1972.

94. Harding AE: Friedreich's ataxia: A clinical and genetic study of 90 families with an analysis of early diagnostic criteria and intrafamilial clustering of clinical features. *Brain* 104:589–620, 1981.

95. Hashimoto K, Fujita K, Kojimoto H, Shimomura Y: Lumbar disc herniation in children. *J Pediatr Orthop* 10:394–396, 1990.

96. Hendrick EB, Hoffman HJ, Humphreys RP: The tethered spinal cord. *Clin Neurosurg* 30:457–463, 1983.

97. Hensinger RN: Kyphosis secondary to skeletal dysplasias and metabolic disease. *Clin Orthop* 128:113–128, 1977.

98. Hensinger RN: Spondylolysis and spondylolisthesis in children and adolescents. *J Bone Joint Surg [Am]* 71:1098–1107, 1989.

99. Hensinger RN, Lang JE, MacEwen GD: Klippel-Feil syndrome: A constellation of associated anomalies. *J Bone Joint Surg [Am]* 56:1246–1253, 1974.

100. Hensinger RN, MacEwen GD: Spinal deformity associated with heritable neurological conditions: Spinal muscular atrophy, Friedreich's ataxia, familial dysautonomia, and Charcot-Marie-Tooth disease. *J Bone Joint Surg [Am]* 58:13–23, 1976.

101. Herndon WA, Emans JB, Micheli LJ, Hall JE: Combined anterior and posterior fusion for Scheuermann's kyphosis. *Spine* 6:125–130, 1981.

102. Herring JA: The spinal disorders in diastrophic dwarfism. *J Bone Joint Surg [Am]* 60:177–182, 1978.

103. Heydemann JS, Gillespie R: Management of myelomeningocele kyphosis in the older child by kyphectomy and segmental spinal instrumentation. *Spine* 12:37–41, 1987.

104. Hood RW, Riseborough EJ, Nehme AM, et al: Diastematomyelia and structural spinal deformities. *J Bone Joint Surg [Am]* 62:520–528, 1980.

105. Hsu JD: The natural history of spine curvature progression in the nonambulatory Duchenne muscular dystrophy patient. *Spine* 8:771–775, 1983.

106. Hsu LC, Lee PC, Leong JC: Dystrophic spinal deformities in neurofibromatosis: Treatment by anterior and posterior fusion. *J Bone Joint Surg [Br]* 66:495–499, 1984.

107. Huebert HT, MacKinnon WB: Syringomyelia and scoliosis. *J Bone Joint Surg [Br]* 51:338–343, 1969.

108. Hull WJ, Moe JN, Lai C, Winter RB: The surgical treatment of spinal deformities in myelomeningocele. *J Bone Joint Surg [Am]* 57:1767, 1974.

109. Hull WJ, Moe JN, Winter RB: Spinal deformity in myelomeningocele: Natural history, evaluation, and treatment. *J Bone Joint Surg [Am]* 56:1767, 1974.

110. Inkley SR, Oldenburg FC, Vignos PJ Jr: Pulmonary function in Duchenne muscular dystrophy related to stage of disease. *Am J Med* 56:297–306, 1974.

111. James JIP: Two curve patterns in idiopathic structural scoliosis. *J Bone Joint Surg [Br]* 33:399–406, 1951.

112. James JIP, Lloyd-Roberts GC, Pilcher MF: Infantile structural scoliosis. *J Bone Joint Surg [Br]* 41:719–735, 1959.

113. King HA, Moe JH, Bradford DS, et al: The selection of fusion levels in thoracic idiopathic scoliosis. *J Bone Joint Surg [Am]* 65:1302–1313, 1983.

114. Koop SE: Infantile and juvenile idiopathic scoliosis. *Orthop Clin North Am* 19:331–337, 1988.

115. Kurihara A, Kataoka O: Lumbar disc herniation in children and adolescents: A review of 70 operated cases and their minimum 5-year follow-up studies. *Spine* 5:443–451, 1980.

116. Kurz LT, Mubarak SJ, Schultz P, et al: Correlation of scoliosis and pulmonary function in Duchenne muscular dystrophy. *J Pediatr Orthop* 3:347–353, 1983.

117. Labelle H, Beauchamp M, Lapierre L, et al: Pattern of muscle weakness and its relation to loss of ambulatory function in Friedreich's ataxia. *J Bone Joint Surg* 7:496–497, 1987.

118. Labelle H, Tohme S, Duhaime M, Allard P: Natural history of scoliosis in Friedreich's ataxia. *J Bone Joint Surg [Am]* 68:564–572, 1986.

119. Lee B, Godfrey M, Vitale E, et al: Linkage of Marfan syndrome and a phenotypically related disorder to two different fibrillin genes. *Nature* 253:279–281, 1991.

120. Lenke LG, Bridwell KH, Baldus C, Blanke K: Preventing decompensation in King type II curves treated with Cotrel-Dubousset instrumentation: Strict guidelines for selective thoracic fusion. *Spine* 17:274–281, 1992.

121. Lenke LG, Bridwell KH, Baldus C, et al: Ability of Cotrel-Dubousset instrumentation to preserve distal lumbar motion segments in adolescent idiopathic scoliosis. *J Spinal Dis* 6:339–350, 1993.

122. Lenke LG, Bridwell KH, Baldus C, et al: Cotrel-Dubousset instrumentation for adolescent idiopathic scoliosis. *J Bone Joint Surg [Am]* 74:1056–1067, 1992.

123. Lenke LB, Bridwell KH, Bulles D, et al: Results of in-situ fusion for isthmic spondylolisthesis. *J Spinal Dis* 5:433–442, 1992.

124. Lenke LG, Bridwell KH, O'Brien MF, et al: Recognition and treatment of the proximal thoracic curve in adolescent idiopathic scoliosis treated with Cotrel-Dubousset instrumentation. *Spine* 19:1589–1597, 1994.

125. Letts M, Smallman T, Afanasiev R, Gouw G: Fracture of the pars interarticularis in adolescent athletes: A clinical-biomechanical analysis. *J Pediatr Orthop* 6:40–46, 1986.

126. Lewonowski K, King JD, Nelson MD: Routine use of magnetic resonance imaging in idiopathic scoliosis patients less than eleven years of age. *Spine* 17(6 suppl):S109–S116, 1992.

127. Lindseth RE: Myelomeningocele, in Morrissy RT (ed): *Lovell and Winters' Pediatric Orthopaedics,* 3d ed. Philadelphia, Lippincott, 1990, pp 507–538.

128. Lindseth RE: Myelomeningocele. *AAOS Instr Course Lect* 40:271–291, 1991.

129. Lindseth RE, Stelzer L Jr: Vertebral excision for kyphosis in children with myelomeningocele. *J Bone Joint Surg [Am]* 61:699–704, 1979.

130. Lloyd-Roberts GC, Pilcher MF: Structural idiopathic scoliosis in infancy. *J Bone Joint Surg [Br]* 47:520–523, 1965.

131. Lonstein JE: Post-laminectomy kyphosis. *Clin Orthop* 128:93–100, 1977.

132. Lonstein JE, Akbarnia A: Operative treatment of spinal deformities in patients with cerebral palsy or mental retardation: An analysis of one hundred and seven cases. *J Bone Joint Surg [Am]* 65:43–55, 1983.

133. Lonstein JE, Carlson JM: The prediction of curve progression in untreated idiopathic scoliosis during growth. *J Bone Joint Surg [Am]* 66:1061–1071, 1984.

134. Lonstein JE, Winter RB: The Milwaukee brace for the treatment of adolescent idiopathic scoliosis: A review of one thousand and twenty patients. *J Bone Joint Surg [Am]* 76:1207–1221, 1994.

135. Lonstein JE, Winter RB, Moe JH, et al: Neurologic deficits secondary to spinal deformity: A review of the literature and report of 43 cases. *Spine* 5:331–355, 1980.

136. Lowe RW, Hayes TD, Kaye J, et al: Standing roentgenograms in spondylolisthesis. *Clin Orthop* 117:80–84, 1976.

137. Lowe TG: Current concept review: Scheuermann disease: *J Bone Joint Surg [Am]* 72:940–945, 1990.

138. Lubicky J: Myelomeningocele spinal deformity, in Bridwell KH, DeWald RH (eds): *Textbook of Spinal Surgery,* 2d ed. Philadelphia, Lippincott-Raven. In press.

139. Luque ER: Segmental spinal instrumentation for correction of scoliosis. *Clin Orthop* 163:192–198, 1982.

140. Major MR, Huizenga BA: Spinal cord compression by displaced ribs in neurofibromatosis: A report of three cases. *J Bone Joint Surg [Am]* 70:1100–1102, 1988.

141. Makley JT, Herndon CH, Inkley S, et al: Pulmonary function in paralytic and nonparalytic scoliosis before and after treatment: A study of sixty-three cases. *J Bone Joint Surg [Am]* 50:1379–1390, 1968.

142. Mannherz RE, Betz RR, Clancy M, Steel HH: Juvenile idiopathic scoliosis followed to skeletal maturity. *Spine* 13:1087–1090, 1988.

143. Marchetti PG, Bartolozzi P, Binavzi R, Briccoli A: New classification of spondylolisthesis. *Orthop Transactions* 12:241, 1988.

144. Mayer PJ, Dove J, Ditmanson M, Shen YS: Post-poliomyelitis paralytic scoliosis: A review of curve patterns and results of surgical treatment in 118 consecutive patients. *Spine* 6:573–582, 1981.

145. McLone DG, Herman JM, Gabrieli AP, Dias L: Tethered cord as a cause of scoliosis in children with a myelomeningocele. *Pediatr Neurosurg* 16:8–13, 1990–91.

146. McMaster MJ: Anterior and posterior instrumentation and fusion of thoracolumbar scoliosis due to myelomeningocele. *J Bone Joint Surg [Br]* 69:20–25, 1987.

147. McMaster MJ, MacNicol MF: The management of progressive infantile idiopathic scoliosis. *J Bone Joint Surg [Br]* 61:36–42, 1979.

148. McMaster MJ, Ohtsuka K: The natural history of congenital scoliosis: A study of two hundred and fifty patients. *J Bone Joint Surg [Am]* 64:1128–1147, 1982.

149. Mehta MH: The rib-vertebral angle in the early diagnosis between resolving and progressive infantile scoliosis. *J Bone Joint Surg [Br]* 54:230–243, 1972.

150. Micheli LJ: Low back pain in the adolescent: Differential diagnosis. *Am J Sports Med* 7:362–364, 1979.

151. Miller F, Moseley CF, Koreska J, Levison H: Pulmonary function and scoliosis in Duchenne dystrophy. *J Pediatr Orthop* 8:133–137, 1988.

152. Millner PA, Helm RH, Dickson RA: Early onset idiopathic scoliosis: Natural history and outcome. *J Bone Joint Surg [Br suppl II]* 74:303–304, 1992.

153. Moe JH, Kettleson DN: Idiopathic scoliosis: Analysis of curve patterns and the preliminary results of Milwaukee-brace treatment in one hundred sixty-nine patients. *J Bone Joint Surg [Am]* 52:1509–1533, 1970.

154. Moe JH, Winter RB, Bradford DS, Lonstein JE: Post laminectomy spine deformity, in *Scoliosis and Other Spinal Deformities.* Philadelphia, Saunders, 1978, pp 595–600.

155. Murray PM, Weinstein SL, Spratt KF: The natural history and long-term follow-up of Scheuermann's kyphosis. *J Bone Joint Surg [Am]* 75:236–248, 1993.

156. Nachemson AL, Peterson LE: Effectiveness of treatment with a brace in girls who have adolescent idiopathic scoliosis. *J Bone Joint Surg [Am]* 77:815–822, 1995.

157. Nasca RJ, Stilling FH, Stell HH: Progression of congenital scoliosis due to hemivertebrae and hemivertebrae with bars. *J Bone Joint Surg [Am]* 57:456–466, 1975.

158. Nash CL Jr, Moe JH: A study of vertebral rotation. *J Bone Joint Surg [Am]* 51:223–229, 1969.

159. O'Brien JP, Yau ACMC, Gertzbein S, Hodgson AR: Combined staged anterior and posterior correction and fusion of the spine in scoliosis following poliomyelitis. *Clin Orthop* 110:81–89, 1975.

160. O'Brien MF, Lenke LG, Bridwell KH, Blanke K: Preoperative spinal canal investigation in "large" adolescent idiopathic scoliosis curves (70 degrees–140 degrees). *Spine* 9:1606–1610, 1994.

161. Orcutt FV, DeWald RL: The special problems which the Marfan syndrome introduces to scoliosis. *J Bone Joint Surg [Am]* 56:1763, 1974.

162. Osebold WR, Mayfield JK, Winter RB, Moe JH: Surgical treatment of the paralytic scoliosis associated with myelomeningocele. *J Bone Joint Surg [Am]* 64:841–856, 1982.

163. Perdriolle R, Vidal J: Thoracic idiopathic scoliosis curve evolution and prognosis. *Spine* 10:785–791, 1985.

164. Phillips DP, Roye DP, Jr, Farcy JP, et al: Surgical treatment of scoliosis in a spinal muscular atrophy population. *Spine* 15:942–945, 1990.

165. Phillips WA, Hensinger RN, Kling TF Jr: Management of scoliosis due to syringomyelia in childhood and adolescence. *J Pediatr Orthop* 10:351–354, 1990.

166. Piasecki JO, Mahinpour S, Levine DB: Long-term follow-up of spinal fusion in spinal muscular atrophy. *Clin Orthop* 207:44–54, 1986.

167. Piggott H: The natural history of scoliosis in myelodysplasia. *J Bone Joint Surg [Br]* 62:54–58, 1980.

168. Reigel DH: Kyphectomy and myelomeningocele repair, in Ransohoff J (ed): *Modern Techniques in Surgery.* Vol. 13: *Neurosurgery.* Mt Kisco, NY, Futura, 1979, pp 1–9.

169. Renshaw TS: Sacral agenesis: A classification and review of twenty-three cases. *J Bone Joint Surg [Am]* 60:373–383, 1978.

170. Riccardi VM: Von Recklinghausen neurofibromatosis. *N Engl J Med* 305:1617–1627, 1981.

171. Riddick MF, Winter RB, Lutter LD: Spinal deformities in patients with spinal muscle atrophy: A review of 36 patients. *Spine* 7:476–483, 1982.

172. Rindahl MA, Colletti PM, Zee CS, Taber P: Magnetic resonance imaging of pediatric spinal dysraphism. *MRI* 7:217–224, 1989.

173. Riseborough EJ, Grabias SL, Burton RI, Jaffe N: Skeletal alterations following irradiation for Wilms' tumor: With particular reference to scoliosis and kyphosis. *J Bone Joint Surg [Am]* 58:526–536, 1976.

174. Rivard C, Nairbait Z, Vithoff HK: Congenital vertebral malformation. *Orthop Rev* 8:135–139, 1979.

175. Robins PR, Moe JH, Winter RB: Scoliosis in Marfan's syndrome: Its characteristics and results of treatment in thirty-five patients. *J Bone Joint Surg [Am]* 57:358–368, 1975.

176. Russman BS, Melchreit R, Drennan JC: Spinal muscular atrophy: The natural course of disease. *Muscle Nerve* 6:179–181, 1983.

177. Sachs B, Bradford D, Winter R, et al: Scheuermann kyphosis: Follow-up of Milwaukee brace treatment. *J Bone Joint Surg [Am]* 69:50–57, 1987.

178. Saraste H: Long-term clinical and radiological follow-up of spondylolysis and spondylolisthesis. *J Pediatr Orthop* 7:631–638, 1987.
179. Scaglietti O, Frontino G, Bartolozzi P: Technique of anatomical reduction of lumbar spondylolisthesis and its surgical stabilization. *Clin Orthop* 117:165–175, 1976.
180. Shufflebarger HL: Cotrel-Dubousset instrumentation in neurofibromatosis spinal problems. *Clin Orthop* 245:24–28, 1989.
181. Sim FH, Svien HJ, Bickel WH, Janes JM: Swan-neck deformity following extensive cervical laminectomy: A review of twenty-one cases. *J Bone Joint Surg [Am]* 56:564–580, 1974.
182. Sriram K, Bobechko WP, Hall JE: Surgical management of spinal deformities in spina bifida. *J Bone Joint Surg [Br]* 54:666–676, 1972.
183. Stanitski CL, Micheli LJ, Hall JE, Rosenthal RK: Surgical correction of spinal deformity in cerebral palsy. *Spine* 7:563–569, 1982.
184. Sussman MD: Advantage of early spinal stabilization and fusion in patients with Duchenne muscular dystrophy. *J Pediatr Orthop* 4:532–537, 1984.
185. Swank SM, Winter RB, Moe JH: Scoliosis and cor pulmonale. *Spine* 7:343–354, 1982.
186. Taylor TKF: Lumbar intervertebral disc prolapse in children and adolescents. *J Bone Joint Surg [Br]* 64:135–136, 1982.
187. Thompson SK, Bentley G: Prognosis in infantile idiopathic scoliosis. *J Bone Joint Surg [Br]* 62:151–154, 1980.
188. Tolo VT: Spinal deformity in short-stature syndromes. *AAOS Instr Course Lect* 39:399–405, 1990.
189. Tolo VT, Gillespie R: The characteristics of juvenile idiopathic scoliosis and results of its treatment. *J Bone Joint Surg [Br]* 60:181–188, 1978.
190. Varlotta GP, Brown MD, Kelsey JL, Golden AL: Familial predisposition for herniation of a lumbar disc in patients who are less than twenty-one years old. *J Bone Joint Surg [Am]* 73:124–128, 1991.
191. Veliskakis KP: Neurofibromatosis and scoliosis: Significance of the short angular spine curvature. *J Bone Joint Surg [Am]* 52:883, 1970.
192. Weinstein SL: Idiopathic scoliosis: Natural history. *Spine* 11:780–783, 1986.
193. Weinstein SL, Ponseti IV: Curve progression in idiopathic scoliosis: Long-term follow-up. *J Bone Joint Surg [Am]* 65:447–455, 1983.
194. Weinstein SL, Zavala DC, Ponseti IV: Idiopathic scoliosis: Long-term follow-up and prognosis in untreated patients. *J Bone Joint Surg [Am]* 63:702–712, 1981.
195. Wenger DR, Bobechko WP, Gilday DL: The spectrum of intervertebral disc-space infection in children. *J Bone Joint Surg [Am]* 60:100–108, 1978.
196. Wiltse LL: Etiology of spondylolisthesis. *Clin Orthop* 10:48–60, 1957.
197. Wiltse LL: Spondylolisthesis in children. *Clin Orthop* 21:156–163, 1961.
198. Wiltse LL: The paraspinal sacrospinalis-splitting approach to the lumbar spine. *Clin Orthop* 91:48–57, 1973.
199. Wiltse LL, Hutchinson RH: Surgical treatment of spondylolisthesis. *Clin Orthop* 35:116–135, 1964.
200. Wiltse LL, Widell EH Jr, Jackson DW: Fatigue fracture: The basic lesion in isthmic spondylolisthesis. *J Bone Joint Surg [Am]* 57:17–22, 1975.
201. Winter RB: Congenital absence of the lumbar spine and sacrum: One-stage reconstruction with subsequent two-stage spine lengthening. *J Pediatr Orthop* 11:666–670, 1991.
202. Winter RB: Convex anterior and posterior hemiarthrodesis and hemiepiphyseodesis in young children with progressive congenital scoliosis. *J Pediatr Orthop* 1:361–366, 1981.
203. Winter RB: Postlaminectomy kyphosis, in Lovell WW, Winter RB (eds): *Pediatric Orthopaedics.* Vol 2. Philadelphia, Lippincott, 1978, pp 645–646.
204. Winter RB: Scoliosis in spinal growth. *Orthop Rev* 6:617–620, 1977.
205. Winter RB: Severe spondylolisthesis in Marfan syndrome: Report of two cases. *J Pediatr Orthop* 2:51–55, 1982.
206. Winter RB: Thoracic lordoscoliosis in Marfan syndrome: Report of two patients with surgical correction using rods and sublaminar wires. *Spine* 15:233–235, 1990.
207. Winter RB: Thoracic lordoscoliosis in neurofibromatosis: Treatment by a Harrington rod with sublaminar wiring. *J Bone Joint Surg [Am]* 66:1102–1106, 1984.
208. Winter RB, Herring JA: Kyphosis in an achondroplastic dwarf. *J Pediatr Orthop* 3:250–252, 1983.
209. Winter RB, Lonstein JE, Anderson M: Neurofibromatosis hyperkyphosis: A review of 33 patients with hyperkyphosis of 80 degrees or greater. *J Spinal Dis* 1:39–49, 1988.
210. Winter RB, Lonstein JE, Drogt J, Noren CA: The effectiveness of bracing in the nonoperative treatment of idiopathic scoliosis. *Spine* 11:790–791, 1986.
211. Winter RB, Lovell WW, Moe JH: Excessive thoracic lordosis and loss of pulmonary function in patients with idiopathic scoliosis. *J Bone Joint Surg [Am]* 57:972–977, 1975.
212. Winter RB, Moe JH, Bradford DS, et al: Spine deformity in neurofibromatosis: A review of one hundred and two patients. *J Bone Joint Surg [Am]* 61:677–694, 1979.
213. Winter RB, Moe JH, Eilers VE: Congenital scoliosis: A study of 234 patients treated and untreated. *J Bone Joint Surg [Am]* 50:1–47, 1968.
214. Winter RB, Moe JH, Lonstein JE: Posterior spinal arthrodesis for congenital scoliosis: An analysis of two hundred and ninety patients five-nineteen years old. *J Bone Joint Surg [Am]* 66:1188–1197, 1984.
215. Winter RB, Moe JH, MacEwen GD: The Milwaukee brace in the nonoperative treatment of congenital scoliosis. *Spine* 1:85–96, 1976.
216. Winter RB, Moe JH, Wang JF: Congenital kyphosis: Its natural history and treatment as observed in a study of 130 patients. *J Bone Joint Surg [Am]* 55:223–256, 1973.
217. Wynne-Davies R: Infantile idiopathic scoliosis: Causative factors, particularly in the first six months of life. *J Bone Joint Surg [Br]* 57:138–141, 1975.
218. Yasuoka S, Peterson HA, Laws ER Jr, MacCarty CS: Pathogenesis and prophylaxis of postlaminectomy deformity of the spine after multiple level laminectomy: Difference between children and adults. *Neurosurgery* 9:145–152, 1981.
219. Yasuoka S, Peterson HA, MacCarty CS: Incidence of spinal column deformity after multilevel laminectomy in children and adults. *J Neurosurg* 57:441–445, 1982.
220. Zamani MH, MacEwen GD: Herniation of the lumbar disc in children and adolescents. *J Pediatr Orthop* 2:528–533, 1982.

CHAPTER 76

Rehabilitation after Spinal Cord Injury

Oksana Volshteyn

Rehabilitation of a patient with spinal cord injury (SCI) begins as soon as the patient becomes medically and surgically stable and there is no longer an immediate threat to survival. There is a growing body of scientific evidence showing improved neurologic and functional outcome when early stabilization and decompressive procedures of the spine are done.[1,2] Early surgical intervention also allows early mobilization of the patient and initiation of an aggressive rehabilitation program, which reduces morbidity and mortality by reducing the period of prolonged bed rest. The latter poses a high risk of secondary medical complications and delays the initiation of functional restoration.[1,3]

There are currently 18 model spinal cord injury centers in the United States. All of them have been funded and supported by the National Institute on Disability and Rehabilitation Research (NIDRR). There are well-documented benefits when SCI patients are rehabilitated in such centers. Model systems provide high-quality care in a more efficient and cost-effective way.[6,7]

Model spinal cord injury systems integrate and coordinate emergency treatment and transport services with level 1 trauma centers. Utilization of standardized protocols at all levels of emergency and acute care is an integral part of their function, which allows a consistent, timely, and organized approach to SCI management and provides the highest quality of care.[8] Acute services should closely collaborate with comprehensive medical rehabilitation services so that coordinated treatment programs can be delivered as a continuum of care.

SPINAL CORD INJURY SYNDROMES

Injuries to the spinal cord may result in commonly recognized syndromes based on the neuroanatomic area of involvement. Each syndrome carries characteristic features and prognosis for functional and neurologic recovery.

Central cord syndrome (CCS) is quite common and most frequently the result of hyperextension injury to the cervical spine, especially in older patients with preexisting degenerative spine changes. In CCS, the central gray matter and middle portion of long tracts carrying motor and sensory fibers to the upper extremities and thorax are more involved than those to lower extremities. Sacral segments are usually spared, with intact bowel and bladder function.

Prognosis is good for regaining mobility and ambulatory function; however, hand function might remain quite impaired, necessitating assistance for self-care activities.[38] Age of CCS patient was shown to be a critical predictor of recovery of ambulation. Some 97 percent of CCS patients who are under 50 years old become ambulatory, as compared with 41 percent of patients over 50 years of age.[39]

Anterior cord syndrome involves injury to the anterior two-thirds of the cord, which is in the territory of the anterior spinal artery with sparing of the posterior columns. In incomplete injuries, there are various degrees of motor paralysis of both upper and lower extremities and impairment of pain and temperature sensation below the level of the injury. Neurologic and functional recovery depends on the degree and extent of injury.

Brown-Séquard syndrome is a hemisection of the spinal cord with the impairment of motor function and proprioception (touch, position, vibration) on the ipsilateral side to the injury and loss of pain and temperature sensation on the contralateral side. This dissociation of sensory and motor presentation is based on the fact that corticospinal tracts and posterior column tracts (gracilis and cuneatus) deccusate at the level of the lower brain stem as compared to the spinothalamic tract, which crosses over to the opposite side at the segmental levels within the spinal cord itself. Of all motor syndromes due to incomplete spinal cord injury, the Brown-Séquard type has the best prognosis for ambulatory recovery, approximating 90 percent.[40]

Posterior cord syndrome is quite rare and produces loss or impairment of vibration and proprioception with sparing of motor pain, and temperature sensation. There is difficulty in identifying the movement and position of the parts of the body below the level of the injury. There is also a problem with sensory discrimination and ability to recognize objects and their qualities by touch, even though touch pressure sensation is relatively intact. Tasks that require simultaneous analysis of spatial and temporal characteristics of the stimulus are usually difficult to perform.[41] Prognosis for functional improvement is usually fair, especially as related to fine motor coordination and the function of distal upper extremities.

Conus medullaris syndrome generally results from injury to the sacral cord and produces areflexic bowel and bladder, impotence, impaired or absent sensation in the sacral dermatomes, and sometimes weakness of leg muscles. Prognosis for the restoration of bowel and bladder function is usually poor.

Cauda equina syndrome involves injury to the lumbosacral nerve roots within the neural canal and presents as asymmetrical paralysis of lower extremities, radicular sensory loss, and areflexic bowel and bladder. Neuropathic pain might be quite prominent. Prognosis for ambulatory function is very good; however, recovery of bladder, bowel, and sexual function is poor.

Mixed spinal cord injury syndromes are probably the most common presentation of spinal cord injury and require accurate neurologic evaluation. Prognosis in this group depends on the localization and extent of injury as well as associated trauma and pre-existing conditions.[41]

THE AMERICAN SPINE INJURY ASSOCIATION: STANDARDS OF NEUROLOGIC CLASSIFICATION OF SPINAL CORD INJURY

It is important to have a uniform classification of spinal cord injury in order to be able to use the same terminology in accurate communication between clinicians and researchers. The American Spine Injury Association (ASIA) developed such standards of classification, which are now being widely used in clinical practice and investigative work.[29,30]

The Neurologic Level

All injuries are being classified by the neurologic level and the degree of injury. Injuries to the cervical cord result in tetraplegia. Injuries to the thoracic, lumbar, and sacral spine that include the conus medullaris and cauda equina result in paraplegia. The numerical level of injury is defined as the most caudal normal motor and sensory segment on both sides of the body. As a result of overlap of innervation of muscles from more than one spinal segment, three-fifths strength is considered adequate to define muscle as normal if the immediately rostral muscle is four-fifths or better.

Motor neurologic level is determined by the key muscle groups (Fig. 76-1). Sensory level is determined by the last normal dermatome by testing for pain and light touch sensation. There are 28 dermatomes on each side of the body. The key point within each dermatome is shown in Fig. 76-1. If the patient is unable to discriminate sharp and dull sensation, the score is 0 for pain.

Motor and Sensory Index Scores

To document changes in motor and sensory function after the injury, whether this change takes place as a natural course of illness or is affected by therapeutic intervention, motor and sensory index scores are calculated during the initial assessment and subsequent reevaluations. The motor score is based on 10 key muscles on each side of the body, graded from 0 to 5, 0 being total paralysis and 5 being normal for the maximal total score of 100 points (Fig. 76-1). Sensory score for both pinprick and light touch is graded from 0 (absent) to 2 (normal) for each side of the body, with a total maximal score of 112 for each (Fig. 76-1). Injury is considered complete if no motor or sensory function is preserved below the zone of partial preservation, including the lowest sacral segment. Sacral sensation includes sensation at the anal mucocutaneous junction and deep anal sensation. Motor function is determined by the presence of voluntary contraction of the external anal sphincter. If injury remains complete within the first 72 hours, it is unlikely that there will be any further recovery regardless of treatment.[9] Thorough neurological evaluation during this period is extremely important for the estimation of prognosis and development of comprehensive rehabilitation plan.

American Spine Injury Association Impairment Scale

The ASIA Impairment Scale,[36] which replaced the Frankel Classification,[37] is based on the definition of complete and incomplete injury and further classifies incomplete injuries by the extent of preservation of motor and sensory function below the neurological level. The scale has five classes: A, B, C, D, and E, as shown in Table 76-1.

TABLE 76-1   ASIA Impairment Scale

A = Complete: No motor or sensory function is preserved in the sacral segments S4-S5.

B = Incomplete: Sensory but not motor function is preserved below the neurological level and extends through the sacral segments S4-S5.

C = Incomplete: Motor function is preserved below the neurological level, and the majority of key muscles below the neurological level have a muscle grade less than 3.

D = Incomplete: Motor function is preserved below the neurological level, and the majority of key muscles below the neurological level have a muscle grade greater than or equal to 3.

E = Normal: Motor and sensory function is normal.

Source: Reproduced with permission from *International Standards for Neurological and Functional Classification of Spinal Cord Injury—Revised.* Chicago, American Spinal Association, 1992.

PREDICTION OF NEUROLOGIC AND FUNCTIONAL OUTCOME

Neurologic Outcome

The prognosis of neurologic recovery depends on the level of spinal cord injury as well as its type and severity. It can be best predicted based on accurate neurologic examination. The timing of the neurologic examination as related to the onset of injury is very important. It has been shown that neurologic examination at 72 h postinjury gives a quite reliable estimate of the extent of the injury, which allows for more accurate prognosis.[9] Seventy-two hours was considered a better time mark. Immediately after the injury, examination might not be accurate because of the presence of other associated injuries. The level of consciousness might be too impaired to allow appropriate examination, and the patient might be undergoing surgical procedures for other injuries and trauma.

The spinal cord injury itself may be evolving, either to reflect further deterioration secondary to hemorrhage or edema and ongoing autodestructive processes.[10] Alterna-

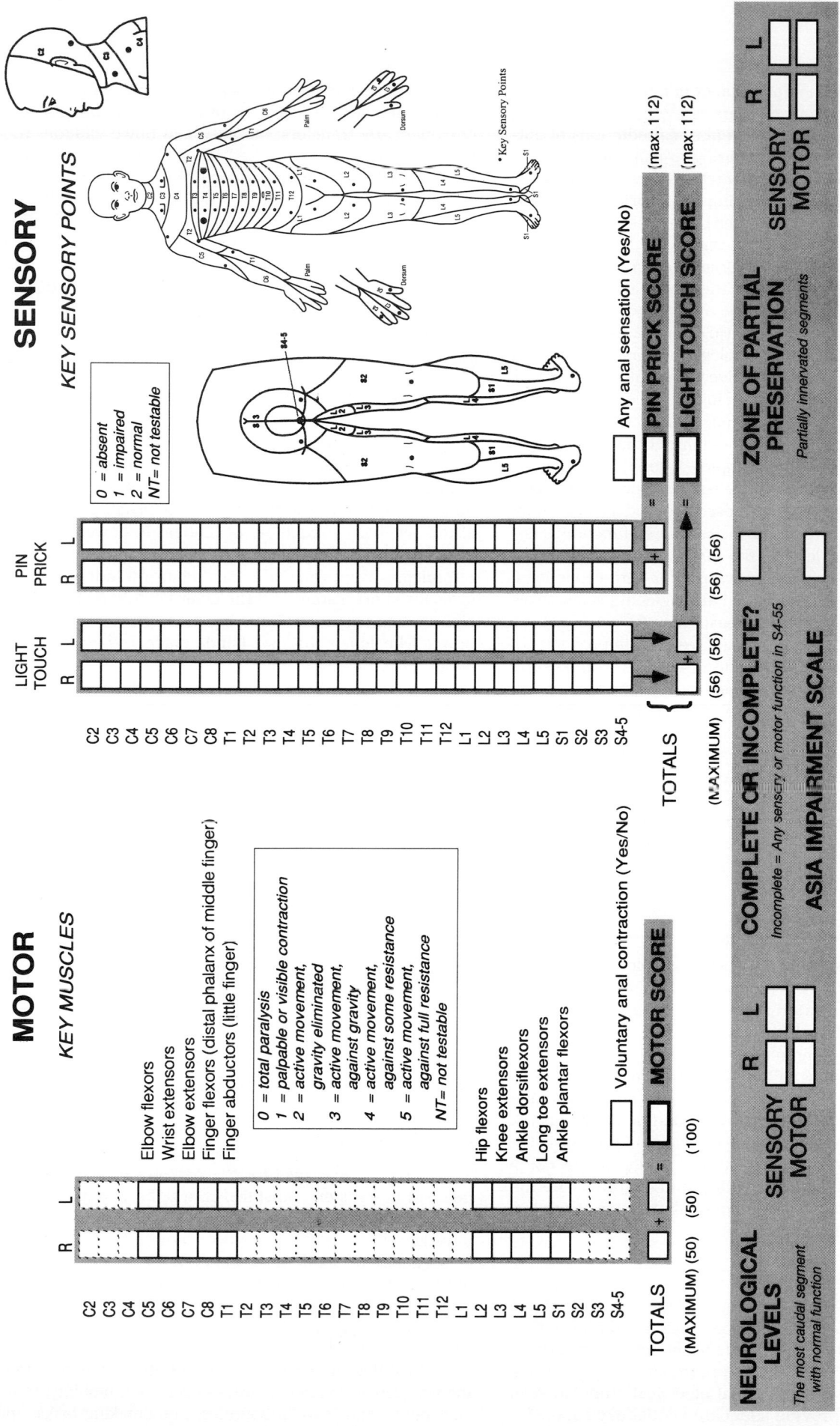

Copyright, American Spinal Injury Association, from "International Standards for Neurological and Functional Classification of Spinal Cord Injury", Revised 1996.

Figure 76-1 Standard neurologic classification of spinal cord injury.

tively, there may be an improvement in function as a result of resolution of transient neuropraxia.[11,12]

Motor testing has produced better predictions of outcome than sensory testing.[1] Sparing of pain and temperature sensation (spinothalamic tract) carries a more favorable prognosis than does sparing of proprioception and vibration sense (posterior column) due to the proximity of the former to the cortocospinal tract.[13,14]

When long-term prognosis for motor recovery and functional potential is being assessed, the examination at 1 month postinjury has been shown to be a very good predictor of individual muscle or groups of muscles function at 1 year.[18–20] Of patients with complete tetraplegia and paraplegia at 30 days, 90 and 96 percent respectively, remain complete at 1 year.[18,19] Recovery in the zone of injury can continue for an extended period of time and as long as 2 years postinjury.[21] The rate of recovery in the zone of injury is faster in incomplete lesions as opposed to complete ones.[22] Recovery below the zone of injury in complete lesions is poor and ranges between 0 to 9 percent.[23] In those who undergo late conversion to incomplete lesions, the recovered function is not useful. In incomplete lesions, the early appearance of motor function carries a favorable prognosis for better functional outcome. Most of the neurologic improvement usually takes place within the first 9 months postinjury.[18–20]

Over the past 20 years there have been improvements in care at the scene of injury and in transportation of the patient. Prompt surgical intervention when appropriate[2] and such protocols as the use of methylprednisolone[17] have contributed to the reduction observed in the severity of these injuries. Complete injuries have declined by 11.6 percent while the number of incomplete injuries has increased by 10.4 percent.[15] There has also been a decline in complete tetraplegia by 10 percent and an increase in incomplete paraplegia by 6 percent.[15]

Functional Outcome

Functional outcome in patients with complete injuries can be estimated based on the neurologic level of injury. However, the anticipated function may differ from what the patient actually achieves, whether in the home environment or in the community.

Many factors play an important role in determining a patient's true functional capacity. These factors include the presence of associated medical conditions, the degree of spasticity or sensory loss, age, availability of assistive devices, environmental modifications, family and peer support, and the patient's motivation and attitude. The following represents expected functional outcome at various levels of spinal cord injury.

C3-4 Tetraplegia

Patients at the C3 level and above are ventilator-dependent. If the phrenic nerve is intact, an implanted phrenic nerve pacemaker, whether simultaneous or alternating, may be of benefit for functional electrical stimulation of the diaphragm to provide adequate ventilatory support.

Patients at the C4 level are usually ventilator-free. Tetraplegics at C3-4 levels require complete assistance in personal care, transfers, mobility, and bowel/bladder routine. They require motorized wheelchairs and are independent with wheelchair locomotion using either head, chin, or sip-and-puff control. They can interact with the environment through environmental control units (sophisticated computerized equipment) to operate phone, TV/radio, computer, lights, doors, emergency systems, etc. For community transportation, they need lift-equipped vans with tie-down systems.

C5 Tetraplegia

Patients with C5 tetraplegia can feed themselves and perform limited self-care activities such as grooming, dressing, and bathing with appropriate setup and the use of assistive devices such as a balanced forearm orthosis (BFO), stabilizing wrist-hand orthosis, or universal cuffs with built-in adaptations for utensils, pencil, brush, etc. Patients at this level are completely dependent in bowel and bladder care and require full-time attendant care. C5 tetraplegics can propel a manual chair on indoor flat surfaces for short distances if the chair is equipped with special rim coating and oblique hand-rim projections. With a power wheelchair that has hand controls, they can move about independently.

C6 Tetraplegia

At this level, patients become independent in basic activities of daily living (ADLs) with the help of adaptive equipment and assistive devices related to feeding, upper-body hygiene, and dressing. Patients are also independent with bed mobility and manual wheelchair propulsion indoors as well as for short distances on flat outdoors. For community locomotion, they require a power wheelchair with hand controls. Wheelchair, bed, and toilet transfers continue to require assistance for the majority of patients; however, for those who are motivated and acquire an appropriate skill, there is a potential for independence with the transfer boards. Bladder care remains dependent. However, some patients can achieve independence with their bowel routine by using assistive equipment. For community transportation, these patients can drive independently in vans with hand controls.

C7 Tetraplegia

This is the critical level for the patients to become independent in transfers, most self-care skills, and ADLs. Many patients, though, continue to require the use of assistive devices.

Manual wheelchair propulsion becomes functional outdoors to include rough terrain and slopes.

C8-T1 Tetraplegia

Patients at this level are essentially totally independent from the wheelchair level in all areas of self-care, mobility, transfers, bowel and bladder routines, homemaking tasks, and wheelchair locomotion on all surfaces. They are independent with community transportation and can drive regular cars with hand controls. They are also independent in placing the manual wheelchair into the car. At this level patients can live independently in wheelchair-accessible housing.

T2-T10 Thoracic Paraplegia

Patients in this category are independent from the wheelchair level in all mobility skills and ADLs. A frequently raised question in this group is the potential for ambulation. In spite of the development of several sophisticated orthotic systems, ambulation is not a functional activity for these patients[26,27] and the orthotic rejection rate is as high as 75 percent for community ambulation.[27,28] The major limiting factor is the high energy requirement which prevents the patient from sustaining ambulation for long enough distances.[24,25] However, this approach might still be useful for short household distances, especially in non-wheelchair-accessible areas or as a form of exercise that might have some positive effect on the cardiovascular system and bowel function.

For those patients who are persistent in their request for gait training, it is preferable to have them use training orthoses so that they can decide on their own whether ambulation is a realistic goal.

T11-L2 Paraplegia

These patients have some potential for independent community ambulation with knee-ankle-foot orthoses (KAFOs) and crutches. They can only achieve short distances, however, and realistically ambulate functionally mainly indoors. For the most part, for outdoor community ambulation, such patients will continue to use a wheelchair.

Criteria for functional community ambulation include normal trunk control, good pelvic control, good hip flexors, functional quadriceps strength at least on one side, and preservation of proprioception in hips and knees.[25]

L3-S2 Paraplegia

These patients are independent in ambulation on all surfaces indoors and outdoors with an ankle-foot orthosis (AFO), crutches, canes, or a walker. A wheelchair is not required.

MEASUREMENT OF FUNCTIONAL OUTCOME

It is important to have objective and valid documentation of patient's progress within a rehabilitation program in order to demonstrate the effectiveness and efficiency of rehabilitation treatment and justify the need and high cost of rehabilitation services.

A number of assessment tools are available to measure functional outcome. The Functional Independence Measure (FIM) has been endorsed by the American Spinal Injury Association as the main instrument to measure functional progress and outcome in patients with spinal cord

injury (SCI).[29,30] The FIM has come into wide use in the United States and is gaining acceptance internationally; it was adopted by the Spinal Cord Injury Data Base for clinical and research purposes (Table 76-2).

The FIM focuses on six domains of function: self-care, sphincter control, mobility, locomotion, communication, and

---

TABLE 76-2 Elements of the Functional Independence Measure (FIM)[a]

L E V E L S	7 Complete Independence (Timely, Safely) 6 Modified Independence (Device)	No Helper
	Modified Dependence 5 Supervision 4 Minimal Assist (Subject = 75%+) 3 Moderate Assist (Subject = 50%+) **Complete Dependence** 2 Maximal Assist (Subject = 25%+) 1 Total Assist (Subject = 0%+)	Helper

	ADMIT	DISCH
Self Care A. Eating B. Grooming C. Bathing D. Dressing-Upper Body E. Dressing-Lower Body F. Toileting	☐	☐
Sphincter Control G. Bladder Management H. Bowel Management	☐	☐
Mobility Transfer: I. Bed, Chair, Wheelchair J. Toilet K. Tub, Shower	☐	☐
Locomotion L. Walk/wheelchair M. Stairs	W ☐ C ☐	W ☐ C ☐
Communication N. Comprehension O. Expression	A ☐ V ☐ V ☐ N ☐	A ☐ V ☐ V ☐ N ☐
Social Cognition P. Social Interaction Q. Problem Solving R. Memory	☐	☐
Total **FIM**	☐	☐

NOTE: Leave no blanks; enter 1 if patient not testable due to risk.

[a]For explanation, see text.

Source: Reproduced with permission from *Guide for the Use of the Uniform Data Set for Medical Rehabilitation.* Buffalo, NY, Center for Functional Assessment Research, State University of New York at Buffalo, 1990.

social cognition. Each domain is further divided into specific activities, so that there is a total of 18 items. Each of those items is evaluated on a seven-point scale, with 1 being total assist and 7 being complete independence.[31] It should be kept in mind that the FIM was developed for the disabled population in general and is not always sensitive to small functional changes in the spinal cord injury SCI population.

The Quadriplegia Index of Function (QIF) was developed specifically for tetraplegics, and has been shown to be more sensitive and highly specific for small functional gains in SCI patients.[32,33] This scale was found to have good interrater reliability but needs further testing on a large number of patients.

The patient's ability to function within the social environment is being defined by six dimensions based on the World Health Organization (WHO) definition: physical independence, mobility, occupation, social integration, orientation, and economic self-sufficiency.[34] At this time the best measure of handicap in the SCI population is considered to be the Craig Handicap Assessment and Reporting Technique (CHART).[35] This scale makes it possible not only to measure individual limitations in the community but can also play a significant role in the development of appropriate strategies to reduce handicap in the SCI population.

TABLE 76-3 Multidisciplinary Rehabilitation Team

Physician (physiatrist, consultants)

Rehabilitation nursing, clinical nurse specialists

Physical therapist

Occupational therapist

Therapeutic recreational specialist

Psychologist

Social worker

Vocational counselor

Nutritionists

Rehabilitation engineer

Orthotist-prosthetist

Equipment vendors

Program coordinator/case managers

Patient and family

Chaplain

THE MULTIDISCIPLINARY REHABILITATION TEAM

A multidisciplinary team approach has become an integral part of the rehabilitation process and is an essential component in achieving successful outcomes. The team is composed of health care professionals who have a high level of expertise in spinal cord management. Each team member has a well-defined role in the SCI rehabilitation program and brings to the team the skills of his or her respective discipline (Table 76-3). However, within the team, the concept of remaining discipline-specific becomes less important. It is not an individual discipline that determines the success of the program but genuine teamwork.[4]

CONTINUUM OF REHABILITATION CARE FOR SPINAL CORD INJURY PATIENTS

Rehabilitation during the Acute Phase of Spinal Cord Injury

Rehabilitation during the acute phase after SCI emphasizes the prevention of secondary complications and initiation of rehabilitation process.

The rehabilitation consultation team develops an initial rehabilitation plan of treatment within 48 to 96 h after injury. This plan emphasizes prevention of skin breakdown and pressure sores through an appropriate schedule of turning and the utilization of specialty beds and mattresses, prevention of joint contractures by proper positioning and splinting of extremities, and maintenance of

muscle length and tendon extensibility through range-of-motion and stretching exercises. A program of strengthening exercises for weakened muscles as well as supportive respiratory care for high tetraplegics is initiated. Also, training for basic self-care activities such as grooming, feeding, and dressing is initiated. Bowel and bladder retraining programs can be started during this phase, in consultation with rehabilitation nurses.

Bladder drainage is initially maintained by an indwelling catheter. If there is an injury to the lower genitourinary system, cystostomy with a suprapubic catheter is indicated. Once the patient becomes medically and surgically stable and there is no need for ongoing intravenous fluids, a bladder retraining program with intermittent catheterizations is initiated.

A bowel program is initiated when bowel sounds are restored and the patient starts oral feeding. Common practice is to follow a scheduled bowel routine with suppositories along with a combination of stool softeners, stimulants, and bulk-forming preparations. This program should be adjusted to the patient's individual bowel habits as they existed prior to the injury. During this phase, patient and family are introduced to the concept of multidisciplinary SCI rehabilitation and given initial education regarding the physical and functional sequelae of SCI.

Once acute issues related to the injury are resolved and the spine is appropriately stabilized, whether surgically or through the application of appropriate orthotic devices, the patient is ready for transfer to the comprehensive inpatient rehabilitation service. The SCI rehabilitation team works closely with the staff of the acute medical and surgical services to ensure the transfer of all appropriate medical information and to prepare the patient and family for the next phase of rehabilitation management.

Comprehensive Inpatient Medical Rehabilitation Program

An inpatient rehabilitation program for SCI patients is best delivered either in the specialized rehabilitation unit of an acute care hospital or in a free-standing rehabilitation facility.

Team members develop the rehabilitation plan within 24 h of admission to include short- and long-term goals and to identify the treatment strategies and resources necessary to achieve those goals. The emphasis of the inpatient program is on reducing disability through enhancing residual function in the areas of ADLs, self-care, mobility, locomotion, assistance in adaptation to disability, and facilitation of appropriate community reintegration.

Ongoing education becomes an integral part of the rehabilitation program and covers a wide range of topics, including basic knowledge about SCI, potential medical complications and their recognition and prevention, bowel and bladder management, sexuality, knowledge about specialty adaptive and assistive equipment, and community resources. Family members or designated caregivers are taught the essentials of multisystem care and assistive mobility skills.

The patient begins high-intensity therapy programs usually for 4 to 6 h daily. These include progressive strengthening exercises for both affected and normal muscles. Stretching exercises are done to maintain functional range of motion and as a basic therapeutic approach for spasticity treatment. The patient works on balance and coordination activities as well as mobility tasks including bed mobility and wheelchair, toilet, and bathtub transfers. He or she also masters wheelchair locomotion and initiates ambulation training when and if appropriate.

The patient is provided with appropriate adaptive equipment and assistive devices such as a balanced forearm orthosis (BFO) to assist with feeding and grooming, a static and dynamic wrist-hand orthosis (WHO) to augment hand function and facilitate grasp for various ADLs, assistive devices for dressing and hygiene, and specialty tools for homemaking activities and cooking. A decision is made regarding the appropriate transfer equipment, hospital bed, wheelchair and cushion, toilet and bathing equipment, and environmental control unit (ECU). All team members contribute to the decision making on equipment needs, along with the input from patient and family. If necessary, the occupational therapist makes a home visit to evaluate for accessibility and provide recommendations for modifications and adaptations.

Throughout the inpatient rehabilitation period and at discharge, the patient's functional status is measured and documented by using functional outcome measurement instruments such as the FIM and QIF, etc., described elsewhere in this section.

Long-Term Rehabilitation Care for Spinal Cord Injury Patients

Over the past decade there has been almost a 50 percent decrease in length of stay in the initial rehabilitation hospital,[7] much of which is attributed to more effective and efficient delivery of rehabilitation care, and a further decrease in length of stay is anticipated.[42] Now, there is not enough time within the inpatient stay to accomplish necessary psychosocial goals. It becomes critical, therefore, to continue to maintain these patients in a structured multidisciplinary setting after hospital discharge, so that the rehabilitation process can be continued until the patient achieves a satisfactory level of functioning in the community.

Many patients continue with outpatient physical and occupational therapies to further increase muscle strength, improve level of physical fitness, work on high-level wheelchair mobility skills, continue with ambulation training, further work on hand dexterity and function, and enhance abilities in self-care and ADLs. They also require regular psychological counseling. Patients are encouraged to attend support groups where they have an opportunity to share their feelings and experiences with peers with the same disability, develop new social relationships, and learn about new advances in the SCI field.

Lifelong Rehabilitation Care

Patients with SCI require lifelong follow-up. This can best be accomplished through the organized system of SCI rehabilitation clinics, which have a structure in place to coordinate medical care throughout the network of multidisciplinary specialists and consultants.

The most common long-term medical problems in the SCI population include chronic urinary tract dysfunction, pressure sores, nutritional problems, deconditioning, degenerative arthritis and focal entrapment neuropathies of the upper extremities, issues of chronic pain, musculoskeletal pathologic conditions such as postural abnormalities, contractures, and spasticity, and depression.

Frequently medical and social problems are interrelated, and unless a thorough evaluation is done and the complexity of the situation established and seen to, care might become fragmented, sporadic, uncoordinated, and doomed to failure. That again proves the need for multidisciplinary involvement as an essential part of long-term follow-up.

The life span of SCI patients has improved significantly over the past two decades. Individuals with SCI over the age of 60 now make up about 8.5 percent, as compared with 4.5 percent two decades ago.[7] With significantly improved care overall for SCI patients, there has been a shift in morbidity and mortality. Previously, renal failure and other urinary tract complications were the leading cause of death.[4] As a result, these problems have received substantial clinical and research attention, and significant progress has been made toward reducing urinary tract complications. Most recent studies have shown that respiratory disease, particularly pneumonia, has become a leading cause of death in tetraplegic patients, followed by heart disease, suicide, and septicemia.[43] In paraplegia, suicide, septicemia, and heart disease are now the leading causes of death.[43] In SCI patients over the age of 60, heart disease has become the leading cause of death. This shift indicates that the aging SCI population incurs the same medical problems as the able-bodied geriatic population. Health care professionals involved in SCI care need to develop appropriate plans and have resources available to be able to meet the health care needs of SCI patients throughout their lives.

SPECIAL EQUIPMENT FOR SPINAL CORD INJURY PATIENTS

Wheelchairs

Since the wheelchair becomes the primary means of locomotion for most SCI patients, appropriate prescription of a wheelchair is very important.[45] Decision making regarding wheelchair selection should take into consideration the patient's neurologic level of injury, functional abilities, age, weight, level and type of activity; the chair's durability, portability, appearance, access to the environment, and cost should also be considered.

Each patient must be individually measured for precise fitting, which is critical in preventing postural abnormalities and skin breakdown as well as assuring maximal performance. Measurements are taken with the patient sitting in the wheelchair—including wheelchair depth and width; the height of the back, seat, armrests, and footrests; and the length of the armrests. Wheelchairs can be manual or power-operated; the decision regarding either one or both is based predominantly on neurologic level, the patient's functional ability, and the type of activity involved.

Power wheelchairs allow patients with C6 levels and above to achieve independence in mobility. For those with injuries below C6, a power wheelchair might be indicated if they are involved in high-level activities on the job, at school, or generally in the community; if they are required to travel long distances for extended periods of time on various surfaces; or if they are older and have associated medical conditions that will make the use of a manual wheelchair very strenuous.

When a power wheelchair is prescribed for a high-level tetraplegic patient, it should have either a reclining or tilt-in-space system to provide independence in pressure relief for prevention of pressure sores, allow quick response to orthostatic hypotension episodes, provide improved ventilation and a position of comfort for rest, and accommodate easier transfers. The mobility of power chairs is controlled through the microprocessor, which allows the information to be programmed and saved as it would be in a computer. The type of control module is selected based on patient's functional abilities. A C4 tetraplegic requires either chin, head, or sip-and-puff controls. C5-6 tetraplegics use a manual control in the form of a joystick.

It is important to remember that a power wheelchair requires a van for transportation equipped with a wheelchair tie-down system and lift. If such a van is not available, the high tetraplegic patient should have the option of using a manual wheelchair to travel long distances.

Patients with injuries below the C6 level are independent with manual wheelchair propulsion. Manual wheelchairs are manufactured in a great variety of models to accommodate the wide range of functional needs of a wheelchair user.

When a manual wheelchair is prescribed, the first consideration should be given to the frame design, which is either folding or rigid. Folding chairs are easier to lift into the car. They are more compact and ride better on rough terrains. Rigid-frame wheelchairs are more durable and have greater push efficiency. However, they require disassembly for transportation. Based on their weight and size, wheelchairs are divided into standard, ultralight, lightweight, heavy-duty, extra heavy duty, and high-strength lightweight. High strength and light weight are essential to allow higher levels of performance independence. Other wheelchair components that need to be specified when the prescription is made include the following:

1. Rear wheels can be either spoked or made of molded plastic. The latter are heavy but essentially maintenance-free and more durable.
2. Tires can be pneumatic, solid, or pneumatic with solid inserts. Pneumatic tires give a smoother ride and are appropriate for soft surfaces such as grass, sand, and thick carpet. Solid tires provide little shock absorption on hard surfaces; however, they far outlast pneumatic tires and require no maintenance.
3. Casters come in different sizes and can be pneumatic or solid. Larger-size casters allow easier push over obstacles.
4. Leg rests can be rigid, which makes them stronger and more durable and provides an advantage for sports wheelchairs. Elevating leg rests are helpful in decreasing dependent edema and minimizing orthostatic hypotension. Swing-way removable leg rests allow for better transfer and fit in tighter spaces.
5. Arm-rest selection includes removable flip-back or tubular swing-way. Rests can be full or desk length to fit under most tables or desks.
6. The back of the wheelchair can be firm or sling upholstery. A firm back is important to maintain good posture, decrease deformity, and improve respiration. High tetraplegics require a high back with head support. Active paraplegics with good truncal musculature can use a lower back.

To improve wheelchair stability, the rear axle is moved more posteriorly. The height of the seat is lowered and camber is added to the rear wheels. Every SCI patient must have an individually selected seating cushion to best meet the needs of appropriate pressure distribution. This lowers the risk of pressure sores and allows the patient to sit for extended periods of time in various environmental conditions.

Environmental Control Units

Environmental control units (ECUs) allow patients with high-level tetraplegia to achieve independence in many environmental interactive functions and greatly increase effectiveness and efficiency of function. These units vary from very simple systems to control a single device such as a phone or TV set to complex centralized systems with computer control and multiple connections to include electrical appliances, household items, radio/TV/entertainment center, air conditioning, computer, page turner, etc. They are especially helpful for the patients who stay home alone, providing easy access to emergency communication and door locks. An ECU can be operated by a voice-recognition device, joystick, or breath-control switch.

Robotic Devices

The notion that robots can replace the need for attendant care is very attractive. Currently available industrial stationary and mobile devices are quite complex, very costly, and require extensive training. There are no devices specifically designed to assist disabled patients, although many laboratories around the world are engaged in experimental work to create such systems.

Functional Electrical Stimulation

The use of electrical current to evoke functional movement in paralyzed muscles is called *functional electrical stimulation* (FES). Muscle must have intact peripheral nerve to be appropriate for FES. Electrical stimulation can be applied either directly to the nerve or to the muscle at the motor point.[46,47]

Currently available systems can be classified as follows:

1. Surface electrical stimulation systems, which require daily application of surface electrodes to a number of specific muscles. They have the disadvantage of providing only limited function and poor repeatability. There is only one FDA-approved system currently available for clinical use. It is called Parastep and is manufactured by Sigmetics Inc.
2. Hybrid systems, which use braces in combination with surface electrical stimulation. These systems are simple and safe, and they reduce energy load. However, they have the disadvantage of being difficult to don, have poor cosmesis, and provide limited function.
3. Implanted electrical stimulation systems, which require extensive surgery for the implantation of electrodes. There are problems with system reliability, the possibility of infection, and the high cost of the procedure as well as the cost of maintenance. However, these systems provide improved function and cosmesis.

The FES control modes can be either open- or closed-loop systems. Open-loop control is more frequently used. The patient triggers stimulation externally and has the option of choosing a particular computer-stored program with a preset sequence of muscle stimulation and parameters for intensity, frequency, and duration. Closed-loop systems use sensors from the muscles, skin, and joints, providing constant feedback to the computer, which modulates the appropriate force, frequency, and duration of muscle contraction.

These systems have been successfully used to improve hand function in tetraplegic patients and enable them to perform most simple ADLs. Frequently though, additional corrective and restorative hand surgery is required to augment the effectiveness of FES.

For locomotion, FES can be used by both complete and incomplete SCI patients. The protocol usually consists of muscle restrengthening, standing, and gait training.

The major exclusion factors for FES include the presence of a lower motor neuron lesion, joint contractures, poorly controlled spasticity, skin problems, urinary tract infection, autonomic dysreflexia, poor truncal balance, history of substance abuse, and cognitive problems. The psychological impact on the patient involved in FES must also be considered. Those who have unrealistic goals and high expectations are usually at risk for developing depression secondary to their failure to achieve the desired level of function.

Currently FES is not being widely used for routine clinical rehabilitation practice. Those who are accepted in FES programs are trained in specialized and centralized centers because the necessary procedures are quite lengthy and expensive, requiring highly trained personnel.

Future of FES systems will belong to implanted closed-loop systems. Questions of muscle physiology—especially as related to muscle fatigue, sensory feedback, and safety—must be solved before FES systems can become truly functional and user-friendly.

PSYCHOSOCIAL ISSUES IN SPINAL INJURY PATIENTS

Spinal cord injury has a devastating impact on a person's life. It destroys the patient's lifestyle and future plans. Adjustment to disability due to SCI poses a major challenge even to emotionally stable and mature individuals. Acceptance of disability and the belief that one can have a productive life after the injury becomes the main point in the development of coping mechanisms and adjustment strategies for SCI patients.

The main goal of psychological rehabilitation is to reach the point where disability is no longer the main focus of a patient's life. There is a temporal sequence of phases of psychosocial adjustments to SCI.[48,49] These usually occur in the following order: shock, anxiety, denial, depression, anger, and adjustment. Not all of these phases appear in each individual patient, and reactions may overlap. Fluctuation back and forth can also be observed. A number of factors influence this process, the most significant including preinjury personality, especially such attributes as independence, motivation, self-esteem, optimism, power control, problem-solving ability, and situational conditions such as financial resources, social support network, access to medical care, and overall socioeconomic status.

Depression has been the most frequent psychological symptom in the SCI population. It becomes a part of the mourning process associated with the loss of body functions. However, depression is not a universal phenomenon among persons who have sustained SCI; its incidence ranges from 12 to 50 percent. These figures are much higher than the rates of 5 to 10 percent reported for the general population.[51] It has been shown that an SCI patient's self-perceived handicap is a significant predictor of depression and distress.[50] Those who believe that they have control over their lives and health are generally less likely to be depressed.

SPECIAL MEDICAL ISSUES IN SPINAL CORD INJURY CARE

Neurogenic Bladder

During the acute phase after SCI, the bladder is best managed by indwelling catheter to provide continuous drainage and close control of intake, output, and electrolyte balance. Once the patient becomes medically stable and no longer requires a continuous large volume of intravenous fluids, a bladder retraining program can be initiated.

The goal of bladder retraining after SCI is to achieve effective bladder emptying at regular intervals to less than 100 mL of residual urine and to maintain an infection-free low-pressure areflexic bladder system in order to prevent upper genitourinary tract deterioration and renal failure.

Intermittent catheterizations have become a standard of neurogenic bladder management, whether it is an upper motor neuron hyperreflexic bladder or a lower motor neuron or hyporeflexic bladder. Intermittent catheterizations are performed initially every 4 to 6 h based on the estimated need for a fluid intake requirement of about 2000 mL/24 h and urinary output of 60 to 100 mL/h. Fluid is closely monitored and distributed in such a way that most of it is taken between the early morning and late afternoon hours. It is generally recommended that the bladder should not hold more than 500 mL so as to prevent complications. During the hospital stay, intermittent catheterizations are performed using sterile technique. In the home environment, however, the patient can use clean technique.

If there is a problem with incontinence between catheterizations in the case of upper motor neuron hyperreflexic bladder, anticholinergic drugs such as oxybutynin and propanthelene may be prescribed to inhibit detrusor activity. If patient is not able to tolerate the side effects of those drugs, then an external collecting system should be used in addition to intermittent catheterizations.

Many patients are able to achieve catheter-free emptying of the bladder with low postvoiding residuals. Since bladder function remains involuntary, continence is maintained through the use of an external collecting system. To facilitate the initiation of the voiding reflex, stimulation of the upper motor neuron bladder contraction can be done by tapping of the lower abdomen, scratching the inner thigh, or pulling on the pubic hair. In case of the lower neuron bladder, the Valsalva or Crede maneuver facilitates bladder emptying through the production of increased intraabdominal pressure.

In female patients, if bladder continence cannot be maintained by intermittent catheterizations and use of anticholinergic medication, long-term use of an indwelling catheter might become a choice, since there is no currently available external collecting system for females.

Urodynamic studies provide objective and very useful information regarding the bladder's functional activity and help to select appropriate management strategy. Urodynamic studies permit more accurate classification of the bladder type, provide information regarding detrusor and sphincter activity, assess bladder compliance, measure intravesicular pressure, and provide a urethral pressure profile. They also establish the presence or absence of detrusor sphincter dyssynergia (DSD). This is a phenomenon that occurs when the detrusor muscle and sphincter contract at the same time, thus obstructing urinary flow. Treatment options may include pharmacologic intervention to change the dynamics of the bladder, usually a combination of an anticholinergic, adrenergic blocker, and antispasticity drug, or surgical management, such as sphincterotomy, if conservative measures have failed.

Urinary tract infection (UTI) is the most frequent medical complication of neurogenic bladder. It has been reported that UTI is present in 80.4 percent of individuals with spinal cord injury overall, ranging from 73.8 percent in persons with incomplete paraplegia to 87.4 percent in those with complete tetraplegia.[52] Uncomplicated urinary tract infection can be successfully treated with oral antibiotics based on the urinary culture and sensitivity, usually for 10 to 14 days. In cases of asymptomatic bacteriuria, the presence of pyuria may be used as an indication for treatment, even though pyuria in SCI patient is usually a poor indicator of tissue invasion. The general consensus is that asymptomatic bacteriuria need not be treated routinely with antibiotics in otherwise healthy persons with SCI. However, the presence of urea-producing organisms associated with stone formation may warrant antibiotic treatment.[53] The use of prophylactic antibiotics has not been shown to be statistically significant and efficacious in preventing recurrent UTI.[53]

Long-term care of the neurogenic bladder should include regular reevaluations of the urinary system, to including urinalysis, culture, kidney ultrasound, renal scan, cystoscopy, intravenous pyelography, and urodynamic studies.

The rehabilitation physician needs to work closely with the urologist to provide a comprehensive assessment of the genitourinary system so that timely and appropriate management can be instituted.

Neurogenic Bowel

In the acute stage after SCI, paralytic ileus is common; during this time, patient should take nothing by mouth. Over a period of several days, ileus usually resolves spontaneously. Once bowel sounds reappear, oral food intake can be resumed. A bowel retraining program usually starts with enema cleansing, with subsequent institution of routine bowel care including the use of bisacodyl suppositories every other day in combination with oral stool softeners, stimulants, and bulking agents. Suppositories are usually given at the same time of the day and emphasis is placed on utilizing the natural gastrocolic reflex to facilitate bowel emptying. Frequently, additional digital stimulation and evacuation are necessary to achieve more complete evacuation and prevent bowel accidents.

Autonomic Dysreflexia in Spinal Cord Injury

Autonomic dysreflexia (AD) is a clinical syndrome that affects patients with SCI above the major sympathetic outflow; it is most commonly seen with injuries at or above the T6 level. The initial episode most commonly occurs within the first 6 months after the injury. Autonomic dysreflexia affects 30 to 85 percent of patients with high SCI.[54]

The most frequent trigger of AD is a noxious stimulus below the level of the injury, which induces generalized sympathetic activity resulting in vasoconstriction and hypertension. This activity is unopposed because of the lack of parasympathetic feedback resulting from SCI. Hypertension is the primary cause of morbidity and mortality associated with AD, which may lead to seizures, status epilepticus, intracerebral and subarachnoid hemorrhage, coma, and death. Effect on cardiovascular system may cause hemodynamic changes leading to heart failure.

The most common presenting symptoms include bilateral pounding headache in the back of the head or between the eyes, sweating and flushing above the lesion and pallor and piloerection below the lesion, visual disturbances, nasal congestion, and chest pain. In addition, centrally activated vagal activity causes bradycardia. Patients with AD are usually restless and anxious.[55]

The most common provoking stimuli for initiation of AD originate within lower urinary tract and include bladder and urethral distention or spasm, obstructed indwelling catheter, catheterization procedure, urinary tract infection, epididymitis, testicular torsion, and stones. The second most common trigger for AD arises from anorectal stimulation, especially from bowel distention due to fecal impaction or irritation from rectal suppositories. Other provoking stimuli include such diverse factors as cutaneous irritations, pressure sores, ingrowing toenail, or tight clothing. Acute abdominal conditions, bone injuries, passive stretch of joints and muscles, and sexual intercourse may trigger AD as well. Even the use of nasal decongestants by SCI patients may induce AD. It is important to be aware of the possibility of AD during pregnancy in SCI patients, especially during labor and delivery.

When an episode of AD presents as a medical emergency, speedy determination of causative factors is imperative. Blood pressure needs to be closely monitored. The patient is usually sat up at 90° and all tight clothing removed. Since the lower urinary tract is the most common cause, the bladder needs to be checked for distention and catheterized.[9] If an obstruction is present in the indwelling catheter, the catheter needs to be changed.

If bowel distension is found to be a causative factor, the anal sphincter and rectum need to be anesthetized first by the instillation of dibucaine ointment, with subsequent manual evacuation in 15 to 20 min.

If the above measures do not relieve symptoms and decrease blood pressure, pharmacologic treatment is indicated, along with further evaluation to determine the cause of AD. For oral medication, currently the drug of choice is a calcium channel blocker such as nifedipine, which is given sublingually in the dose of 10 mg and may be repeated in 30 min. Other useful drugs include ganglion blocking agents (mecamylamine, trimethaphan), alpha adrenergic blockers (phenoxybenzamine, terazosine), sympatholytic agents (guanethidine), and direct arteriodilators (hydralazine, diazoxide). In the case of severe uncontrollable blood pressure direct arterial infusion of vasodilators such as sodium nitroprusside is indicated.

In SCI patients who are at a high risk for development of autonomic dysreflexia, prevention becomes no less important than appropriate management. Patients, families, and health care personnel, especially in the emergency rooms, need to be educated about AD. Pharmacologic prophylaxis is indicated prior to diagnostic and treatment procedures in susceptible patients.

Heterotopic Ossification

Heterotopic ossification (HO) may occur in the periarticular soft tissues following SCI, traumatic brain injury, or burns. It has been reported to occur in 16 to 53 percent of SCI patients,[56] developing below the level of the injury, and it is most commonly seen in the hip—a little less commonly in the knee. It can also be seen in the shoulder, elbow, and paravertebral areas. The joint space is generally preserved. Heterotopic ossification usually develops within the first year after the injury with the highest incidence between the first and the fourth months. However, there are reports of late HO formation at 5 to 7 years after the injury. Those SCI patients with complete lesions, spasticity, and pressure sores have a much higher risk of developing HO. The incidence of HO in cervical and thoracic lesions is higher than in lumbar lesions.

The most common initial symptom of HO is a decreased range of motion in the joint, followed by localized swelling associated with redness and warmth.

The differential diagnosis of HO includes thrombophlebitis, cellulitis, joint infection, hematoma, local trauma, and fracture. A venogram may be necessary to rule out deep vein thrombosis, since HO may lead to false-positive Doppler or ultrasonography studies. Triple-phase bone scan is considered to be the test of choice, with high sensitivity and specificity, when clinical signs are already present; it usually precedes findings on plain x-rays by 2 to 4 weeks.

Alkaline phosphatase may be elevated up to 7 weeks prior to clinical symptoms; however, it is not specific, since SCI patients may have significant associated bone trauma. Initially, HO presents as a hypervascular inflammatory mass. As it matures, the amorphous calcium phosphate composing HO is replaced by hydroxyapatite crystals.[57] Maturation of HO might take 12 months. It may be up to 2 years before the bone scan reverts to normal.

Prevention of HO in SCI patients remains controversial. Radiation therapy and non-steroidal anti-inflammatory drugs such as indomethacin have not been shown to be effective in SCI patients. Didronel (etidronate disodium) is the drug of choice in SCI patients. It inhibits calcium phosphate precipitation and slows conversion of amorphous calcium into crystalline form. However, even though the extent of HO formation is less in those who received Didronel, the final incidence remains about the same.

The most detrimental complications of HO are severe contractures, compromise of venous and lymphatic flow, and nerve entrapment. Patients with HO also have a much higher incidence of pressure sores and urinary tract infections.

Surgical removal of HO becomes necessary when it severely compromises the patient's functional abilities (especially sitting posture) or when secondary complications develop. Serial bone scans are necessary to determine the maturity of HO. Patients who need surgery usually require Didronel treatment 2 weeks prior to the surgery and up to 1 year afterwards. No less important is an ongoing physical therapy program to maintain range of motion in the involved joints.

Spasticity

Spasticity is a hallmark of upper motor neuron disorder and is present in spinal cord injuries above conus medullaris. The definition of spasticity includes muscle hypertonia with increased resistance to passive movements of the joint, which is velocity-dependent and has associated features such as hyperreflexia, muscle spasms, and clonus. In SCI, spasticity results from the loss of descending inhibition as well as structural reorganization of the segmental circuits. Spasticity is not present immediately after spinal cord injury and appears only after resolution of the spinal shock phase. The incidence of spasticity was found to be lower in persons with paraplegia below T7 as compared with those with levels of T7 and above.[58] The highest incidence of spasticity was also reported to be in persons classified as Frankel class B (complete motor, incomplete sensory below the level of the injury), 67.9 percent; and C (incomplete motor and sensory with motor nonfunctional), 64.6 percent; followed by Frankel class A (complete motor and sensory), 59.5 percent.[58]

As a negative phenomenon, spasticity predisposes to contracture development and skin breakdown. It interferes with the performance of ADLs such as transfers, bed mobility, sitting posture, driving, self-care activities. It may present a problem to the maintenance of hygiene and sexual function. It can also interfere with sleep. In SCI patients spasticity can be exacerbated by associated medical conditions such as urinary tract infection, pressure sores, intraabdominal pathology, or virtually any noxious stimuli below the level of the injury. A decision to treat spasticity is based on how much it interferes with the patient's ability to perform functional activities, how much discomfort it produces, and whether there are associated medical complications.

Treatment includes the avoidance of noxious stimuli, a regular stretching program, and proper positioning in bed and wheelchair. Use of local applications of heat and cold and appropriate splinting and casting are also important components of the initial management. When pharmacologic intervention is required, baclofen (Lioresal) has become the drug of choice in spasticity after SCI.[59] Baclofen is a gamma-aminobutyric acid (GABA) agonist, which produces a presynaptic inhibition of motor neurons. Baclofen inhibits both monosynaptic and polysynaptic reflexes through binding to GABA B receptors at the presynaptic terminals, inhibiting calcium influx and thus suppressing the release of excitatory neurotransmitters. The usual initial dose is 5 mg orally three times a day, which may be titrated up over several weeks to a total dose of up to 200 mg. The most common side effect is sedation; however, the most dangerous side effect is seizure, which may occur when the medication is suddenly discontinued.

Diazepam (Valium) facilitates the postsynaptic effect of GABA, resulting in an increase in presynaptic inhibition. The usual initial dose is 2 mg twice or three times a day, which is slowly increased up to 40 to 60 mg per day in divided doses. The most common side effect is, again, sedation. It can, however, precipitate depression and may cause an increasing weakness of useful muscles in SCI patients. Dantrolene sodium (Dantrium) has a direct effect on the muscle by inhibiting calcium reuptake into the sarcoplasmic reticulum, thus reducing muscle action potential. It is metabolized predominantly by the liver and causes gastrointestinal side effects such as nausea, vomiting, and diarrhea. Hepatotoxicity, however, is considered to be the most serious side effect of dantrolene and may occur in about 1 percent of patients. Abnormal liver function tests are dose-dependent and reversible. The initial dose of dantrolene is 25 mg per day, which is slowly increased up to 400 mg per day. Other drugs that have been shown to reduce spasticity in SCI patients include alpha$_2$ adrenergic agonist such as clonidine at a dose of 0.1 mg twice a day; however, tolerance of this drug is poor secondary to hypotension and syncope.

For severe spasticity with a poor response to oral medication, intrathecal baclofen might be an option.[60] With this method, baclofen is infused into the subarachnoid space through an implantable pump, which permits a steady delivery of medication at high concentrations into the cerebrospinal fluid. Most patients can be maintained on 300 to 800 μg per day. The pump reservoir is usually implanted subcutaneously in the abdominal wall and must be refilled every 6 to 12 weeks. Possible side effects include overdose, infection, and system malfunction.

Local procedures such as phenol or alcohol nerve blocks are usually not indicated in SCI unless there is a severe superimposed local increase in muscle tone. Musculocutaneous nerve block may be employed to decrease elbow flexion tone or obturator nerve block to decrease lower extremity adductor spasticity, improve peroneal hygiene, and decrease scissoring during gait. Spinal blocks using intrathecal phenol or alcohol may be of benefit in severe intractable generalized spasticity. Patients need to be carefully evaluated prior to such procedures, since complications include parasthesias as well as urinary and fecal incontinence. Neurosurgical procedures such as rhizotomy and myelotomy are performed infrequently and are usually reserved for severe cases only. Orthopedic procedures such as tenotomies and tendon transfers may be useful in association with other therapeutic interventions.

CONCLUSION

Rehabilitation of the SCI patient continues throughout the patient's lifespan. It requires a competent, dedicated, and committed rehabilitation team that provides a continuum of services beginning from the point of injury until the patient is successfully functioning in the community.

REFERENCES

1. Maynard FM, Reynolds GG, Fountain S, et al: Neurological prognosis after traumatic quadriplegia: Three-year experience of California Regional Spinal Cord Injury Care System. *J Neurosurg* 50:611–616, 1979.
2. Murphy KP, Opitz JL, Cabanela M, Ebersold MJ: Cervical fracture and spinal cord injury: Outcome of surgical and nonsurgical management. *Mayo Clin Proc* 65:949–959, 1990.
3. Garfin SR, Botte MJ, Waters RL, et al: Complications in the use of the halo fixation device. *J Bone Joint Surg [Am]* 68:320–325, 1986.
4. Melvin JL: Interdisciplinary and multidisciplinary activities and ACRM. *Arch Phys Med Rehabil* 61:379–380, 1980.
5. Lundberg LB: What is leadership? *Gen Nurs* 12:32–33, 1982.
6. Stover SL, Fine PR: *Spinal Cord Injury: The Facts and Figures.* Birmingham, University of Alabama at Birmingham, 1986.
7. Stover SL, DeLisa JA, Whiteneck GG: *Spinal Cord Injury, Clinical Outcomes from the Model Systems.* Aspen, CO, Aspen Publications, 1995.
8. Meyer PR: The integral relationship between emergency medical systems and acute spinal cord injury care: Spinal cord injury: The model. Proceedings of the National Consensus Conference on Catastrophic Illness and Injury. Atlanta, Shepard Center for Treatment of Spinal Injuries, 1990.
9. Brown PJ, Marino RJ, Herbison GJ, et al: The 72 hour examination as a predictor of recovery in motor complete quadriplegia. *Arch Phys Med Rehabil* 72:546, 1991.
10. Nuftchi NE, Demeny M, Demopoulos H, et al: Spinal cord regeneration. *Prog Clin Biol Res* 39:63, 1980.
11. Blight AR, Young W: Central axons in injured cat spinal cord recover electrophysiological function following remyelination by Schwann cells. *J Neurol Sci* 91:15–34, 1989.
12. Young W: The post-injury responses in trauma and ischemia: Secondary injury or protective mechanisms. *Cent Nerv Syst Trauma* 4:27–52, 1987.
13. Crozier K, Graziani V, Ditunno JF: Prognosis for ambulation based on sensory examination in patients who are initially motor complete. *Arch Phys Med Rehabil* 72:119, 1991.
14. Folman Y, Masri WE: Spinal cord injury: Prognostic indicators. *Injury* 20:92, 1989.
15. Stover SL, Benefits of the model spinal cord injury system of care, in Apple DF, Hudson LM (eds): *Spinal Cord Injury: The Model.* Proceedings of the National Consensus Conference on Catastrophic Illness and Injury, Atlanta, 1990, Georgia Regional Spinal Cord Injury Care Systems.
16. Ditunno JF, Cohen ME, Formal C, Whiteneck G: Functional outcomes, in Stover SL, DeLisa JA, Whiteneck G (eds): *Spinal Cord Injury: Clinical Outcomes from the Model Systems.* Aspen Publishers, Inc. Gaithersburg, Maryland, 1995.
17. Bracken MB, Shepard MJ, Collins WF, et al: A randomized controlled trial of methylprednisolone or naloxone in the treatment of acute spinal cord injury: Results of the Second National Acute Spinal Cord Injury Study. *N Engl J Med* 322:1405–1411, 1990.
18. Waters RL, Adkins RH, Yakura JS, Sie I: Motor and sensory recovery following complete tetraplegia. *Arch Phys Med Rehabil* 74:242–247, 1993.
19. Waters RL, Adkins RH, Yakura JS, Sie I: Recovery following complete paraplegia. *Arch Phys Med Rehabil* 73:784–789, 1991.
20. Waters RL, Adkins RH, Yakura JS, Sie I: Motor and sensory recovery following incomplete paraplegia. *Arch Phys Med Rehabil* 75:67–73, 1994.
20a. Waters RL, Adkins RH, Yakura JS, Sie I: Motor and sensory recovery following incomplete tetraplegia. *Arch Phys Med Rehabil* 75:306–311, 1994.
21. Ditunno JF, Stover SL, Freed MM, et al: Motor recovery of the upper extremities in traumatic quadriplegia: A multicenter study. *Arch Phys Med Rehabil* 73:431, 1992.
22. Mange KC, Ditunno JF, Herbison GJ, et al: Recovery of strength at the zone of injury in motor complete and motor incomplete cervical spine cord injured patients. *Arch Phys Med Rehabil* 71:562, 1990.
23. Young JS, Dexter WR: Neurological recovery distal to the zone of injury in 172 cases of closed, traumatic spinal cord injury. *Paraplegia* 16:39, 1978.
24. Gordon EE, Vandenwalde H: Energy requirement in paraplegic ambulation. *Arch Phys Med Rehabil* 37:276–285, 1956.
25. Hussey RW, Stauffer ES: Spinal cord injury: Requirements for ambulation. *Arch Phys Med Rehabil* 54:544–547, 1973.
26. Mikelberg R, Reid S: Spinal cord lesions and lower extremity bracing: An overview and follow up study. *Paraplegia* 19:379–385, 1981.
27. Heinemann AW, et al: Mobility for persons with spinal cord injury: An evaluation of two systems. *Arch Phys Med Rehabil* 68:90–93, 1987.
28. Merkel KD, et al: Energy expenditure of paraplegic patients standing and walking with two knee-ankle-foot orthoses. *Arch Phys Med Rehabil* 65:121–124, 1984.
29. Ditunno JF: Functional assessment in central nervous system trauma. *J Neurotrauma* 9:301–305, 1992.
30. *International Standards for Neurological and Functional Classification of Spinal Cord Injury—Revised.* Chicago, American Spinal Injury Association, 1992.
31. *Guide for the Use of the Uniform Data Set for Medical Rehabilitation.* Buffalo, NY, Center for Functional Assessment Research, State University of New York at Buffalo, 1990.
32. Gresham GE, Labi ML, Dittman CC, et al: The quadriplegia index of function (QIF): Sensitivity and reliability demonstrated in a study of thirty quadriplegic patients. *Paraplegia* 24:38, 1986.
33. Knight P, Huang M, Marino RJ, et al: Evaluating self-care in quadriplegia: Superiority of the quadriplegia index of function over the functional independence measure. *J Am Paraplegia Soc* 15:144, 1992.
34. World Health Organization: *International Classification of Impairments, Disabilities and Handicaps: A Manual of Classification Relating to the Consequences of Disease.* Geneva, World Health Organization, 1980.

35. Whiteneck GG, Charlifue SW, Gerhart KA, et al: Quantifying handicap: A new measure of long term rehabilitation outcomes. *Arch Phys Med Rehabil* 73:519, 1992.

36. Ditunno JF: New spinal cord injury standards—1992. *Paraplegia* 30:90, 1992.

37. Frankel HL, Hancock DO, Hyslop G, et al: The value of postural reduction in initial management of closed injuries of the spine with paraplegia and tetraplegia: 1. *Paraplegia* 7:179, 1969.

38. Stauffer ES: Neurologic recovery following injuries to the cervical spinal cord and nerve roots. *Spine* 9:532, 1984.

39. Penrod LE, Hedge SK, Ditunno JF: The effect of age on prognosis for ambulation in acute traumatic central cord syndrome (CCS). Abstracts Digest, ASIA 14th Annual Scientific Meeting, 1988, p 75.

40. Bosch A, Stauffer ES, Nickel VL: Incomplete traumatic quadriplegia: A ten-year review. *JAMA* 216:473, 1979.

41. Ozer MN, Gibson L: Neurological consultation for persons with spinal cord injury. *Arch Phys Med Rehabil* 1:340, 1987.

42. Stover SL: Review of forty years of rehabilitation issues in spinal cord injury. *J Spinal Cord Med* 18:3–175, 1995.

43. DeVito MJ, Kartus PL, Stover SL, et al: Cause of death for patients with spinal cord injuries. *Arch Intern Med* 149:1761, 1989.

44. Whiteneck GG, Charlifue SW, Frankel HL, et al: Mortality, morbidity, and psychosocial outcomes of persons spinal cord injured more than 20 years ago. *Paraplegia* 30:617–630, 1992.

45. Tracker J, Sprigle S, Morris B: *Understanding the Technology When Prescribing Wheelchairs.* Washington, DC, RESNA Press, 1994.

46. Marsolais EB, Kobetic R: Functional walking in paralyzed patients by means of electrical stimulation. *Clin Orthop* 175:3036, 1983.

47. Petrofsky JS, Phillips CA: Computer controlled walking in the neurologically paralysed individual. *J Neurol Orthop Surg* 4:153, 1983.

48. Weller DJ, Miller PM: Emotional reactions of patients, family and staff in acute care period of spinal cord injury. *Soc Work Health Care* 2:369, 1977.

49. Hohmann GW: Psychological aspects of treatment and rehabilitation of spinal cord injured persons. *Clin Orthop* 112:81, 1975.

50. Tate D, Forchheimer M, Maynard F, et al: Predicting depression and psychological distress in persons with spinal cord injury based on indicators of handicap. *Am J Phys Med Rehabil* 73:3–175, 1994.

51. Craig AR, Hancock KM, Dickson M, et al: Psychological consequences of spinal injury: A review of the literature. *Aust NZ J Psychiatry* 24:418, 1990.

52. Cardenas DD, Farrell-Roberts L, Sijski ML, et al: Management of gastrointestinal, genitourinal, and sexual function, in Stover SL (ed): *Spinal Cord Injury: Clinical Outcomes from the Model Systems.* Aspen Publishers, Inc. Gaithersburg, Maryland, 1995.

53. National Institute on Disability and Rehabilitation Research Consensus Statement: The prevention and management of urinary tract infection among people with spinal cord injuries. *J Am Paraplegia Soc* 15:194–207, 1992.

54. Colachis SC: Autonomic hyperreflexia with spinal cord injury. *J Am Paraplegia Soc* 15:171–186, 1992.

55. Lee BY, Karmakar MG, Herz BL, et al: Autonomic dysreflexia revisited. *J Spinal Cord Med* 18:2–75, 1994.

56. Finerman GA, Stover SL. Heterotopic ossification following hip replacement or spinal cord injury: Two clinical studies with EHDP. *Metab Bone Dis Relat Res* 3:337–342, 1981.

57. Jensen LL, Halar E, Little J, Brook MM: Neurogenic heterotopic ossification: Special review. *Am J Phys Med* 66:351–363, 1988.

58. Maynard FM, Karunas RS, Warming WP: Epidemiology of spasticity after spinal cord injury. *Arch Phys Med Rehabil* 71:566–569, 1990.

59. Whyte J, Robinson K: *The Practical Management of Spasticity in Children and Adults.* Philadelphia, Lea & Febiger, 1990, 10:1–25.

60. Abel NA, Smith RA: Intrathecal baclofen for treatment of intractable spinal spasticity. *Arch Phys Med Rehabil* 75:54–57, 1994.

INDEX

Note: Page numbers followed by t and f indicate table and figures, respectively.